ROBBINS PATHOLOGIC BASIS OF DISEASE

RAMZI S. COTRAN, M.D.

Frank Burr Mallory Professor of Pathology
Harvard Medical School
Chairman, Department of Pathology
Brigham and Women's Hospital
Boston, Massachusetts

VINAY KUMAR, M.D.

Charles T. Ashworth Professor of Pathology
Southwestern Medical School
The University of Texas
Southwestern Medical Center at Dallas
Dallas, Texas

STANLEY L. ROBBINS, M.D.

Visiting Professor of Pathology
Harvard Medical School
Senior Pathologist
Brigham and Women's Hospital
Boston, Massachusetts

4th Edition

W.B. SAUNDERS COMPANY
HARCOURT BRACE JOVANOVICH, INC.
Philadelphia ■ London ■ Toronto ■ Montreal ■ Sydney ■ Tokyo

W. B. SAUNDERS COMPANY
Harcourt Brace Jovanovich, Inc.

The Curtis Center
Independence Square West
Philadelphia, PA 19106

Library of Congress Cataloging-in-Publication Data
Robbins, Stanley L. (Stanley Leonard), 1915–
    [Pathologic basis of disease]
    Robbins' pathologic basis of disease.— 4th ed./Ramzi S.
Cotran, Vinay Kumar, Stanley L. Robbins.
      p.   cm.
    Rev. ed. of: Pathologic basis of disease. 3rd ed./Stanley L.
Robbins, Ramzi S. Cotran, Vinay Kumar. 1984.
    Includes bibliographies and index.
    ISBN 0-7216-2302-6
    1. Pathology.   I. Cotran, Ramzi S., 1932–   .   II. Kumar, Vinay.
III. Title.   IV. Title: Pathologic basis of disease.
    [DNLM: 1. Pathology.   QZ 4 R634p]
RB111.R62   1989
616.07—dc20
DNLM/DLC
for Library of Congress   89-6261
                                            CIP

Listed here are the latest translated editions of this book together with the language of the translation and the publisher.

Portuguese *(4th edition)*—Editora Guanabara Koogan S.A., Rio de Janeiro, Brazil

Spanish *(4th edition)*—2 volumes, McGraw-Hill Interamericana de Espana, Madrid, Spain

Yugoslavian *(1st edition)*—Serbo-Croat, Skolska Knjiga, Zagreb, Yugoslavia

Italian *(3rd edition)*—Piccin Nuova Libraria S.p.A., Padova, Italy

French *(2nd edition)*—Piccin Nuova Libraria S.p.A., Padova, Italy

Persian *(3rd edition)*—Sherkat Sahami TCHEHR, Tehran, Iran

Editor: W. B. Saunders Staff
Developmental Editor: Linda Mills
Designer: W. B. Saunders Staff
Production Manager: Carolyn Naylor
Manuscript Editor: Constance Burton
Staff Illustrators: Karen Giacomucci, Risa Clow, Glenn Edelmayer, Sharon Iwanczuk
Illustration Coordinator: Brett MacNaughton
Indexer: Ann Cassar

Robbins Pathologic Basis of Disease   ISBN 0-7216-2302-6

Last digit is the print number: 9   8   7   6   5

*To
Kerstin
To
Raminder
and to
Elly
with love*

Preface

THE DATABASE OF biomedical knowledge, as all interested observers know, is expanding at an astonishing rate. Witness the growth of molecular genetics and its rapid application to the understanding and diagnosis of disease; the growing awareness of the complexity of regulatory circuits governing the immune response and inflammation; and the penetrations that have been made into the roles of oncogenes and antioncogenes in the origins of cancer. Any textbook of pathology, then, requires revision periodically if it is to keep abreast of this deluge of new information.

Our major goals for this edition are:

- To bring to the bedside the remarkable advances that have been made in the understanding of the biomolecular origins of disease, drawing on the most recent reports (as the abundant references will attest) as well as the standard classics.
- To present accurately and clearly the dynamics and development of clinical diseases from their very beginnings (i.e., etiology and pathogenesis), through the dysfunctions caused by lesions, to the clinical implications.
- To devote space to subjects in proportion to their clinical importance or biologic relevance to fundamental processes, providing complete discussions of the significant conditions without permitting the book to become unwieldy.
- To maintain the essential morphologic descriptions that represent the backbone of pathology, incorporating the current molecular, immunologic, and other techniques that enhance accurate interpretation of the pathogenesis and diagnosis of lesions.
- Above all, to be meticulous about the organization and clarity of the writing, recognizing that readability illuminates a text and enhances understanding and learning.

Only the users of this book can tell to what extent these goals have been met, but such shortfalls as may exist surely cannot stem from lack of trying.

This book is written primarily as a teaching text. With recognition of the constraints on a student's time, rigorous efforts have been made to achieve as much brevity as is compatible with thoroughness and sufficient discussion to permit easy understanding. We reasoned that it is better to unfold a rounded, full story rather than attempt to achieve brevity by short, more difficult to comprehend telegraphic condensations. Topics, be they cell injury, inflammation, or systemic disorders such as amyloidosis, systemic lupus erythematosus, and **AIDS**, are discussed as a piece rather than dispersed into parts based on particular tissue or organ involvements. Detailed outlines are given at the beginning of each chapter, offering the student an immediate overview of the content and organization and facilitating a teacher's selection of specific segments for course instruction.

Effort has been made to maintain an organization of the subject matter compatible with most teaching programs. Thus, about the first third of the book is devoted to general pathology, i.e., cell injury, inflammation, hemodynamic derangements including thrombosis and infarction, the role of immunity in producing disease, and a general discussion of neoplasia. The remainder of the text is a systematic presentation of disorders divided into rational categories, e.g., environmental disease, pediatric diseases, vascular disease, heart disease, and pulmonary disease. Because this is designed as a teaching text, the coverage is not intended to be encyclopedic, but it is sufficiently broad and detailed, we believe, to be helpful to pathologists, residents in training, and biomedical and basic scientists and to clinicians who wish to review and refresh their understanding of the origins of clinical dysfunctions.

It may fairly be asked, "How does this edition differ from its predecessor?" The simple and, we believe, valid answer is— greatly. Aside from the extensive rewriting, which involves in many instances complete chapters and careful reconsideration of previous text, the changes are wide ranging. New chapters and sections have been added on aging, the head and neck, the eye, and soft tissue tumors. Many lesions and disorders that were poorly understood at the time of the previous edition have now been detailed in much greater depth—for example, the basic defects in diabetes mellitus, the origins of neoplasia, and the etiology and immunopathogenesis of **AIDS**. The improved diagnostic accuracy provided by immunocytochemical and molecular techniques has been amply detailed. Encouraged by the positive response to the use of schematic illustrations in our "smaller" book, *Basic Pathology*, colored diagrams, drawings, and flow charts have been introduced to the extent that they enhance the understanding of the text matter. Numerous illustrations have been replaced and many added to better document the nature of anatomic changes. The writing is liberally referenced to provide guidance to those who wish to pursue subjects of particular interest. The same three authors of previous editions prepared most of this text to ensure uniformity and continuity of writing. But however seasoned in teaching and however broad their interests, the advice of specialist consultants was sought to bring expertise to particular fields, thus enhancing accuracy and authenticity.

We only hope that we have succeeded in transmitting to the reader the excitement of our greatly increased understanding of the pathologic basis of disease.

Acknowledgments

THE COMPLETION OF this edition brings us to the time to express our thanks to all those who helped along the way. Our only regret is our inability, because of limitations of space or lapses of memory, to mention by name each and every one of our "samaritans," because all made contributions to the progress and are deserving of our gratitude. To those wittingly or unwittingly unsung, our apologies and thanks.

Foremost among those to whom we are deeply indebted are our editorial assistants and secretaries—Ms. Cathleen Curtin (RC), Ms. Beverly Shackelford and Ms. Mary Helen Solano (VK), and Ms. Robin Lee (SLR). Without their expert help in library research, preparation of reams of manuscript, patient proofing of immeasurable "miles" of writing, and unobtrusive organization of their "bosses," there would be no text.

Special thanks are owed to our contributors of individual chapters; some participated in the previous edition, and a few joined us afresh. They are cited in the following pages as well as with their specific chapters. The depth of their knowledge and clarity of their writing are documented in their contributions.

New to this edition is a Board of Consultants, experts in particular fields, whose knowledge, perspectives, and suggestions we sought to enhance the clarity and accuracy of the writing. Their names are listed below, but here we wish to express our gratitude for their help because, however broadly experienced writers may be, they cannot be expert in all areas.

Consultants

Dr. Max Goodman, Massachusetts Eye and Ear Infirmary, Harvard Medical School.

Dr. Jose Hernandez, University of Texas Southwestern Medical School.

Dr. Lester Kobzik, Brigham and Women's Hospital – Harvard Medical School.

Dr. Janice Lage, Brigham and Women's Hospital – Harvard Medical School.

Dr. Robert W. McKenna, University of Texas Southwestern Medical School.

Dr. Joseph Rutledge, Children's Hospital and Medical Center, University of Washington School of Medicine.

Dr. Frederick Schoen, Brigham and Women's Hospital – Harvard Medical School.

Dr. Arlene Sharpe, Brigham and Women's Hospital – Harvard Medical School.

Dr. Ricardo Uauy, University of Texas Southwestern Medical School.

Dr. Noel Weidner, Brigham and Women's Hospital – Harvard Medical School.

Many colleagues, senior and relatively junior, have been extremely helpful in many ways, including enlightening us with their thoughts about controversial or emerging areas, offering critiques of the writing, or providing us with choice illustrative material. In alphabetical order, from Brigham and Women's Hospital – Harvard Medical School they are: Drs. Jon Aster, Gilbert Brodsky, Joseph Corson, James Crawford, Mark Flomenbaum, John Godleski, Nabila Haikal, Morris Karnovsky, Lester Kobzik, Richard Mitchell, Helmut Rennke, Marcel Seiler, Joseph Semple, Charles Serhan, Sandor Szabo, and William Welch; from the University of Texas Southwestern Medical School: Drs. Maximilian Buja, Dennis Burns, Edwin Eigenbrodt, Pam Jensen, Mary Lipscomb, Julie Sandstad, Nancy Schneider, Fred Silva, and Patrick Stout; as well as Drs. Jag Bhawan (Boston University School of Medicine), Loren Borud (Harvard Medical School), Robert Jennings (Duke University School of Medicine), Manjeri Venkatachalam (University of Texas School of Medicine at San Antonio), and Patrick Ward (University of Minnesota School of Medicine at Duluth). VK also wishes to thank Dr. Michael Bennett and his other colleagues for their support in the research laboratory during his absence.

Our publisher, W.B. Saunders, also deserves recognition and thanks. They were most generous in their commitment of resources and efforts to produce the best book possible. Ms. Linda Mills, our developmental editor, must be singled out in particular. Throughout the sometimes arduous and hectic "gestation" of this text, she was an unflappable tower of strength and unfailing source of good humor. Her dedication to this edition went far beyond duty. Many other individuals contributed unstintingly, among them Ms. Carolyn Naylor, Ms. Constance Burton, and Mr. Lewis Reines, President of W.B. Saunders, who graciously and gracefully acceded to virtually all our requests and consistently offered encouragement and support.

Similarly, we wish the W. B. Saunders Illustration Department, Ms. Lynn Waltman, and Ms. Amy Boches, to know how grateful we are for their skill and help. Their artistry has undoubtedly embellished these pages. Special thanks go to Mr. Anthony Merola and Ms. Linda Bolding for their invaluable help with the photography.

Not to be forgotten are our wives, Kerstin Cotran, Raminder Kumar, and Elly Robbins, to whom it must have appeared that we would never be done with the writing. Their reading of these words is proof that "we have indeed finished," and we thank them for their unending tolerance of our "compulsion."

Finally, each of us wishes to express to his two coauthors gratitude for their patience and good humor, respect for their dedication to the common effort, and appreciation for their collegiality. Although we did not always agree on every point, we always listened carefully, and we finished the writing still good friends.

R.C.
V.K.
S.R.

Contents

1

Cellular Injury and Adaptation

Translated literally, pathology is the study (logos) of suffering (pathos). As a science, pathology focuses on the structural and functional consequences of injurious stimuli on cells, tissues, and organs and ultimately the consequences on the entire organism.

Traditionally the study of pathology is divided into *general pathology*, and *special* or *systemic pathology*. The former is concerned with the basic reactions of cells and tissues to abnormal stimuli that underlie *all diseases*. The latter examines the specific responses of specialized organs and tissues to more or less well-defined stimuli. In this book we will first cover the principles of general pathology and then proceed to specific disease processes as they affect particular organs or systems.

The four aspects of a disease process that form the core of pathology are (1) its cause (etiology), (2) the mechanisms of its development (pathogenesis), (3) the structural alterations induced in the cells and organs of the body (morphologic changes), and (4) the functional consequences of the morphologic changes (clinical significance).

1. **Etiology or Cause.** The concept that certain abnormal symptoms or diseases are "caused" is as ancient as recorded history. For the Acadians (2500 BC), if someone became ill, it was either his own fault (for having sinned) or the makings of outside agents, such as bad smells, cold, evil spirits, or gods.[1] In more modern terms, there are the two major classes of etiologic factors: *genetic* and *acquired* (infectious, nutritional, chemical, physical, etc.). Knowledge or discovery of the primary cause remains the backbone on which a diagnosis can be made, a disease understood, or a

treatment developed. But the concept of *one cause* leading to *one disease*—developed largely from the discovery of specific infectious agents as the causes of specific diseases—is no longer sufficient. Although it is true that there would be no malaria without malarial parasites, no tuberculosis without tubercle bacilli, and no gout without a derangement in urate metabolism, not all individuals infected with these organisms or born with the metabolic abnormality develop the disease, or develop it at the same rate and with the same severity. Genetic factors clearly affect environmentally induced maladies, and the environment may have profound influences on genetic diseases.

2. **Pathogenesis.** Pathogenesis refers to the sequence of events in the response of the cells or tissues, or the whole organism, to the cause—from the initial stimulus to the ultimate expression of the manifestations of the disease. *The study of pathogenesis remains one of the main domains of the science of pathology.* Even when the initial infectious or molecular cause is known, it is many steps removed from the expression of the disease. For example, to understand gout is to know not only the molecular pathways of uric acid metabolism, but also the biochemical and morphologic events leading to a painful toe or a kidney stone. Although from the late nineteenth century up to the 1950s, pathology was largely limited to the study of the morphologic consequences of disease, chemical, immunologic, and molecular mechanisms clearly underlie the morphologic changes and these, fortunately, have become the domain of modern pathology.

3. **Morphologic Changes.** The morphologic changes refer to the structural and associated functional alter-

1

ations in cells or tissues that are either characteristic of the disease or diagnostic of the etiologic process.
4. **Functional Derangements and Clinical Significance.** The nature of the morphologic changes and their distribution in different organs or tissues influence normal function and determine the clinical features (symptoms and signs), course, and prognosis of the disease.

Virtually all forms of tissue injury start with molecular or structural alterations in *cells*, a concept first put forth in the 19th century by Rudolf Virchow, known as the "father" of modern pathology. We will therefore begin our consideration of pathology by the study of the origins, molecular mechanisms, and structural changes of cell injury.

DEFINITION AND CAUSES OF CELLULAR INJURY AND ADAPTATION

The normal cell is confined to a fairly narrow range of function and structure by its genetic programs of differentiation and specialization, constraints of neighboring cells, the availability of metabolic substrates, and the finite capacities of its primary and alternative metabolic pathways. It is said to be in a homeostatic *"steady state,"* able to handle normal physiologic demands. Somewhat more excessive physiologic stresses or some pathologic stimuli may bring about a number of *cellular adaptations* in which a new but altered steady state is achieved, preserving the viability of the cell. For example, the bulging muscles of the "muscle men" and women engaged in "pumping iron" are cellular adaptations. The increase in muscle mass reflects the increase in size of the individual muscle fibers. The workload is thus shared by a greater mass of cellular components, and each muscle fiber is spared excess work and so escapes injury. The enlarged muscle cell achieves a new equilibrium, permitting it to survive at a higher level of metabolic activity. This adaptive response is called *hypertrophy*. Conversely, *atrophy* is an adaptive response in which there is a decrease in the size and function of cells. Other cell adaptations occur and these are considered later in this chapter.

If the limits of adaptive capability are exceeded, or when no adaptive response is possible, a sequence of events follows, loosely termed *cell injury*. Cell injury is *reversible* up to a certain point, but if the stimulus persists or is severe enough from the beginning, the cell reaches the point of no return, and suffers *irreversible cell injury* and cell death. For example, if the blood supply to a segment of the heart is cut off for 10 to 15 minutes and is then restored, the myocardial cells experience injury but can recover and function normally. However, if blood flow is not restored until one hour later, the myocardial fiber dies. *Adaptation, reversible injury*, and *cell death*, then, should be con-

sidered states along a continuum of progressive encroachment on the cell's normal function and structure (Fig. 1–1). Whether specific types of stress induce an adaptive response, reversible injury, or cell death depends on the nature and severity of the stress and on many other variables relating to the intrinsic state of the cell itself.

The causes of reversible cell injury and cell death range from the external gross physical violence of an automobile accident to internal endogenous causes, such as a subtle genetic lack of a vital enzyme that impairs normal metabolic function. Most adverse influences can be grouped into the following broad categories.

HYPOXIA. Hypoxia, an extremely important and common cause of cell injury and cell death, impinges on aerobic oxidative respiration. Loss of blood supply (ischemia), which occurs when arterial flow is impeded by arteriosclerosis or by thrombi, is the most common cause of hypoxia. Another cause is inadequate oxygenation of the blood due to cardiorespiratory failure. Loss of the oxygen-carrying *capacity* of the blood, as in anemia or carbon monoxide poisoning (producing a stable carbon monoxyhemoglobin that blocks oxygen carriage), is a third, less frequent basis for oxygen deprivation. Depending on the severity of the hypoxic state, cells may adapt, undergo injury, or die. For example, if the femoral artery is narrowed, the skeletal muscle cells of the leg may shrink in size (atrophy). This reduction in cell mass achieves a balance between metabolic needs and the available oxygen supply. More severe hypoxia will induce injury and cell death.

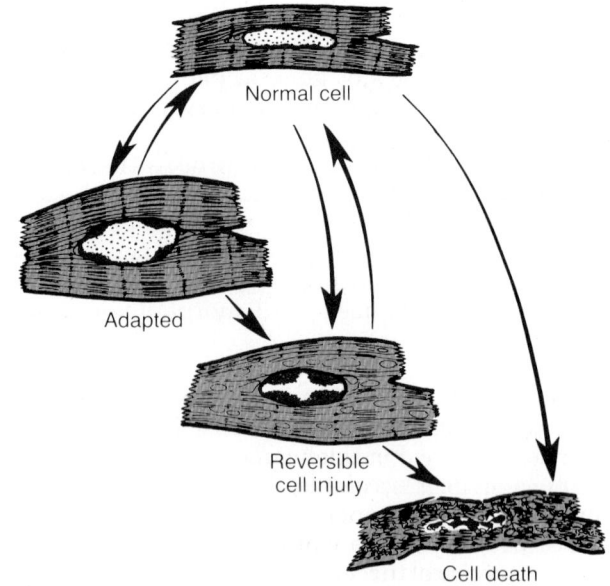

Figure 1–1. The relationships among normal, adapted, reversibly injured, and dead myocardial cells. The cellular adaptation depicted here is hypertrophy, and the type of cellular injury is ischemic necrosis.

PHYSICAL AGENTS. Physical agents include mechanical trauma, extremes of temperature (burns and deep cold), sudden changes in atmospheric pressure, radiation, and electric shock (see Chapter 9, Environmental Pathology).

CHEMICAL AGENTS AND DRUGS. The list of chemicals that may produce cell injury defies compilation. Simple chemicals such as glucose or salt in hypertonic concentrations may cause cell injury by deranging the fluid and electrolyte homeostasis of cells. Even oxygen, in high concentrations, is severely toxic. Trace amounts of agents known as *poisons,* such as arsenic, cyanide, or mercuric salts, may destroy sufficient numbers of cells within minutes to hours to cause death. Other substances, however, are our daily companions: environmental and air pollutants, insecticides, and herbicides; industrial and occupational hazards, such as carbon monoxide and asbestos; social stimuli, such as alcohol and narcotic drugs; and the ever-increasing variety of therapeutic drugs.

INFECTIOUS AGENTS. These agents range from the submicroscopic viruses to the large tapeworms. In between are the rickettsiae, bacteria, fungi, and higher forms of parasites. The ways by which this heterogeneous group of biologic agents causes injury are diverse and are discussed in greater detail in Chapter 7 (Infectious Diseases).

IMMUNOLOGIC REACTIONS. These may be life-saving or lethal. Although the immune system serves in the defense against biologic agents, immune reactions may, in fact, cause cell injury. The anaphylactic reaction to a foreign protein or a drug is a prime example, and reactions to endogenous self-antigens are thought to be responsible for a number of so-called autoimmune diseases (see Chapter 5).

GENETIC DERANGEMENTS. Genetic defects as causes of cellular injury are of major interest to biologists today (see Chapter 4). The genetic injury may result in as gross a defect as the congenital malformations associated with Down's syndrome or in subtle alterations in the coding of hemoglobin responsible for the production of hemoglobin S in sickle cell anemia. The many inborn errors of metabolism arising from enzymic abnormalities, usually an enzyme lack, are excellent examples of cell damage due to subtle alterations at the level of DNA.

NUTRITIONAL IMBALANCES. Even today nutritional imbalances continue to be major causes of cell injury. Protein-calorie deficiencies cause an appalling number of deaths, chiefly among underprivileged populations. Deficiencies in specific vitamins are found throughout the world (see Chapter 8). Ironically, nutritional excesses have become important causes of cell injury among the overprivileged. Excesses of lipids predispose to atherosclerosis, and obesity is an extraordinary manifestation of the overloading of some cells in the body with fats. Atherosclerosis

is virtually endemic in the United States, and as any look down the street reveals, obesity is rampant.

MECHANISMS OF CELL INJURY

The molecular mechanisms responsible for cell injury are complex. As we have seen, injury to cells may have many causes, and probably there is no common final pathway of cell death. There are, however, a number of considerations that are useful to remember.

1. Although it is not always possible to determine the precise biochemical site of action of an injurious agent, four intracellular systems are particularly vulnerable: (a) *maintenance of the integrity of cell membranes,* upon which the ionic and osmotic homeostasis of the cell and its organelles is dependent, (b) *aerobic respiration* involving oxidative phosphorylation and production of ATP, (c) *synthesis of enzymic and structural proteins,* and (d) *preservation of the integrity of the genetic apparatus* of the cell.

2. *The structural and biochemical elements of the cell are so closely related that whatever the precise point of initial attack by the damaging agent, injury at one locus leads to wide-ranging secondary effects.* For example, impairment of aerobic respiration disrupts the energy-dependent sodium pump that maintains the ionic and fluid balance of the cell, resulting in alterations in the intracellular content of ions and water.

3. *The morphologic changes of cell injury become apparent only after some critical biochemical system within the cell has been deranged.* As would be expected, the morphologic manifestations of lethal damage take more time to develop than those of reversible damage. For example, cell swelling is a reversible morphologic change, and this may occur in a matter of minutes; however, unmistakable light microscopic changes characteristic of cell death do not occur in the myocardium until 10 to 12 hr after total ischemia, yet we know that irreversible injury occurs within 20 to 60 min. Obviously, ultrastructural alterations occur earlier than light microscopic changes.

4. *Reactions of the cell to injurious stimuli depend on the type of injury, its duration, and its severity;* thus, small doses of a chemical toxin or ischemia of short duration may induce reversible injury, whereas large doses of the same toxin or more prolonged ischemia might lead either to instantaneous cell death or to slow, irreversible injury leading in time to cell death.

5. *The consequences of cell injury depend not only on the type, duration, and severity of the stimulus but also on the type, state, and adaptability of the cell.* The cell's nutritional and hormonal status and its metabolic needs are important in its response to injury. How vulnerable is a cell, for example, to loss of blood supply and hypoxia? The striated muscle cell in the leg can be placed entirely at rest when deprived of its blood supply; not so, the striated muscle of the heart (Table 1–1). Exposure of two individuals to identical concentrations of a toxin, such as tetrachloride, may

Table 1-1. Susceptibility of Cells to Ischemic Necrosis

High	Neurons (3-5 min)
Intermediate	Myocardium, hepatocytes, renal epithelium (30 min-2 hr)
Low	Fibroblasts, epidermis, skeletal muscle (many hours)

be without effect in one and may produce cell death in the other. This may be due, as we shall see, to the amounts of hepatic enzymes that convert carbon tetrachloride to toxic by-products. Differences in the nutritional state or in potentiating factors, such as alcohol consumption, influence the ability of the two individuals and their cells to withstand injury.

With certain injurious agents, the mechanisms and loci of attack are well defined. Cyanide represents an intracellular asphyxiant in that it inactivates cytochrome oxidase. Certain anaerobic bacteria, such as *Clostridium perfringens*, elaborate phospholipases, which attack phospholipids in cell membranes. Other isolated examples exist, but the modes of action of many injurious agents are more complex. Recent work, however, suggests a central role for *oxygen* in cell injury (Fig. 1-2). Lack of oxygen clearly underlies the pathogenesis of cell injury in ischemia, but it also is clear that *partially reduced activated oxygen species* are important mediators of cell death in many pathologic conditions. As we shall see, these free radical species cause lipid peroxidation and other deleterious effects on cell structure. In the following discussions, we shall concentrate on four of the common causes and mechanisms of cell injury: (1) *hypoxic injury*, (2) *injury induced by free radicals, including activated oxygen species*, (3) some forms of *chemical injury*, and (4) injury induced by *viruses*.

ISCHEMIC AND HYPOXIC INJURY

Sequence of Events and Ultrastructural Changes

The sequence of morphologic and biochemical changes following acute hypoxic injury has been studied extensively in humans, in experimental animals, and in culture systems,[2-5] and reasonable schemes concerning the mechanisms underlying these changes have emerged (Fig. 1-3). A useful model for hypoxic injury has been occlusion of one of the main coronary arteries and examination of the cardiac muscle in the areas supplied by the artery. Besides the relevance of this model to human myocardial infarction, the cellular changes in the heart can also be correlated with physiologic and electrophysiologic alterations.

REVERSIBLE CELL INJURY. *The first point of attack of hypoxia is the cell's aerobic respiration, i.e., oxidative phosphorylation by mitochondria.*[2] As the oxygen tension within the cell decreases, there is loss of oxidative phosphorylation, and the generation of adenosine triphosphate (ATP) slows down or stops.

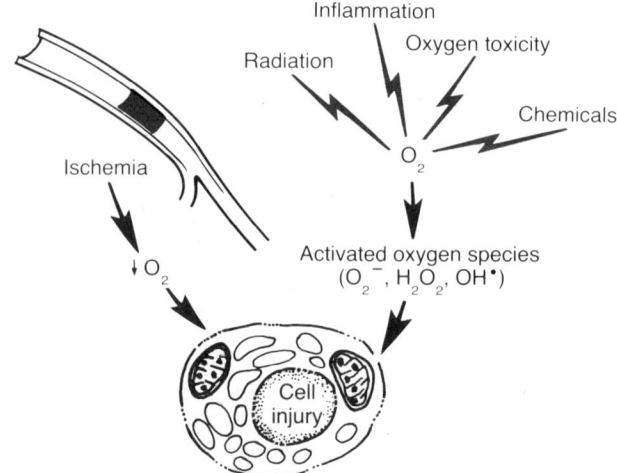

Figure 1-2. The critical role of oxygen in cell injury. Ischemia causes cell injury by reducing cellular oxygen supplies, whereas other stimuli, such as radiation, induce damage via toxic activated oxygen species.

This loss of ATP—the energy source—has widespread effects on many systems within the cell. Heart muscle, for example, ceases to contract within 60 sec of coronary occlusion. (Note, however, that noncontractility does not mean cell death.) The decrease in cellular ATP and associated increase in adenosine monophosphate (AMP) stimulate phosphofructokinase and phosphorylase activities. This results in an increased rate of *anaerobic glycolysis* designed to maintain the cell's energy sources by generating ATP from glycogen. Glycogen is thus rapidly depleted, a phenomenon that can be appreciated histologically if tissues are stained for glycogen (such as with the periodic acid–Schiff [PAS] stain). ATP is also generated anaerobically from creatine phosphate, through the action of the enzyme *creatine kinase*. Glycosis results in the accumulation of lactic acid and inorganic phosphates from the hydrolysis of phosphate esters. *This reduces the intracellular pH.* At this early period there is also *early clumping of nuclear chromatin*, apparently caused by the reduced pH.[5]

One of the earliest and most common manifestations of ischemic injury (and for that matter, other types of injury) is *acute cellular swelling* (cellular edema) (Figs. 1-4 and 1-5), caused by an impairment of cell volume regulation by the plasma membrane. You will recall that mammalian cells possess a high intracellular osmotic colloidal pressure, exerted by a greater intracellular than extracellular concentration of protein. To balance this, sodium is maintained at a lower intracellular than extracellular concentration by an energy-dependent sodium pump (ouabain sensitive Na^+, K^+-ATPase), which also keeps the concentration of potassium significantly higher intracellularly than extracellularly. *Failure of this active transport, owing to diminished ATP and ATPase, causes sodium to accumulate intracellularly with diffusion of potassium out of the cell.* The net gain of

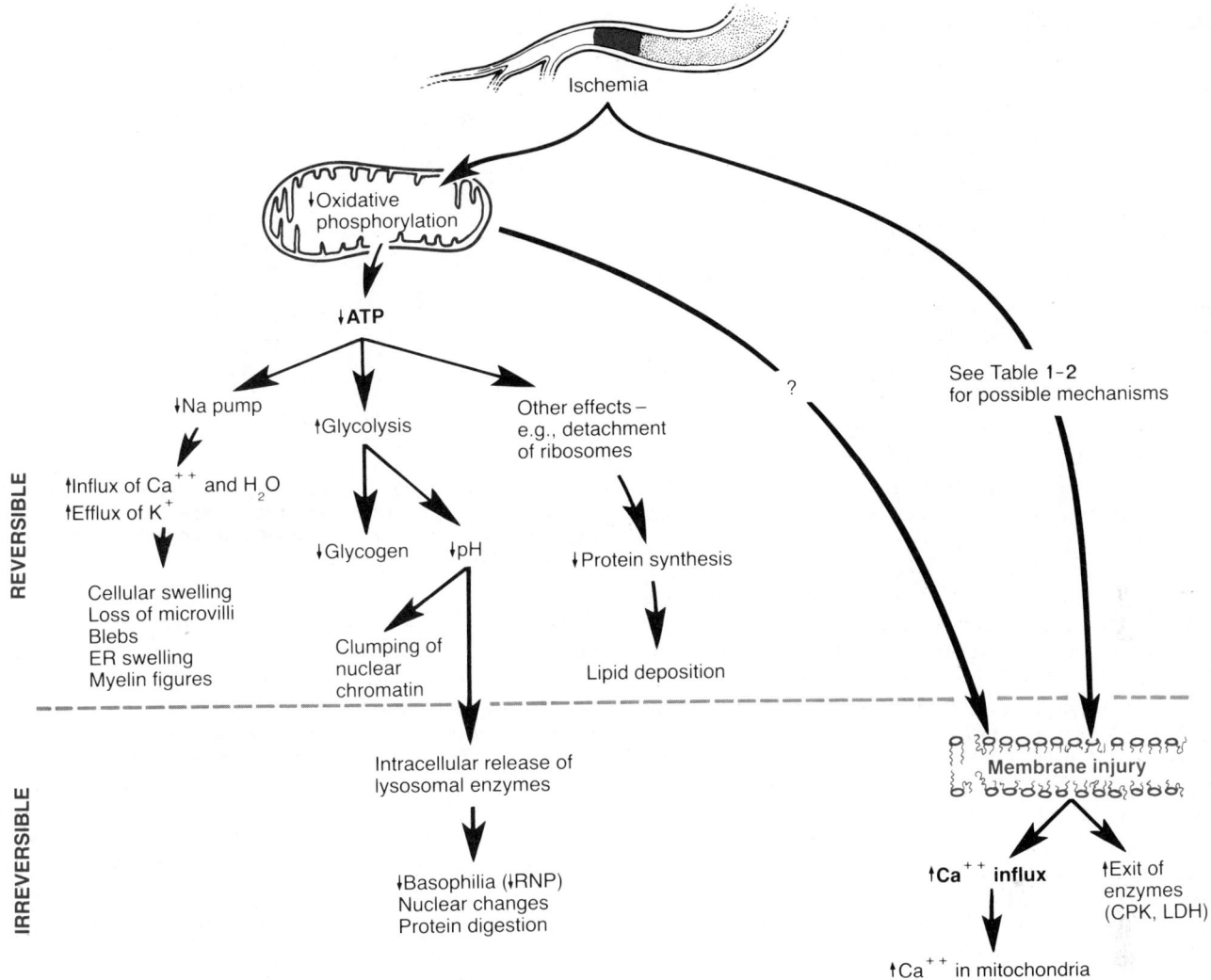

Figure 1–3. Postulated sequence of events in ischemic injury. Note that although reduced oxidative phosphorylation and ATP levels have a central role, ischemia causes direct membrane damage by mechanisms outlined in Table 1–2.

solute is accompanied by an isosmotic gain of water and consequent cell swelling. The movement of fluid and ions into the cell is associated with *early dilation of the endoplasmic reticulum.* A second mechanism for cell swelling in ischemia is the increased intracellular osmotic load, engendered by the accumulation of catabolites such as inorganic phosphates, lactate, and purine nucleosides.[5]

The next phenomenon to occur is *detachment of ribosomes from the granular endoplasmic reticulum* and *dissociation of polysomes into monosomes,* probably due to disruption of the energy-dependent interactions between the membranes of the endoplasmic reticulum and its ribosomes. If hypoxia continues, other alterations take place and, again, are reflections of increased membrane permeability and diminished mitochondrial function. *Blebs* may form at the cell surface (Figs. 1–5 and 1–6), and cells that possess microvilli (such as proximal tubular epithelial cells) begin to lose their normal microvillous structure.

"Myelin figures," derived from plasma as well as organellar membranes, may be seen within the cytoplasm or extracellularly. They are thought to result from dissociation of lipoproteins with unmasking of phosphatide groups, promoting the uptake and intercalation of water between the lamellar stacks of membranes. At this time the mitochondria are usually swollen, owing to loss of volume control by these organelles; the endoplasmic reticulum remains dilated; and the entire cell is markedly swollen, with increased concentrations of water, sodium, and chloride and a decreased concentration of potassium. Up to a certain time, *all the above disturbances are reversible if oxygenation is restored.*

IRREVERSIBLE INJURY. If ischemia persists, irreversible injury ensues. As will be detailed later, *there is no universally accepted biochemical explanation for the transition from reversible injury to cell death.* However, irreversible injury is associated morpho-

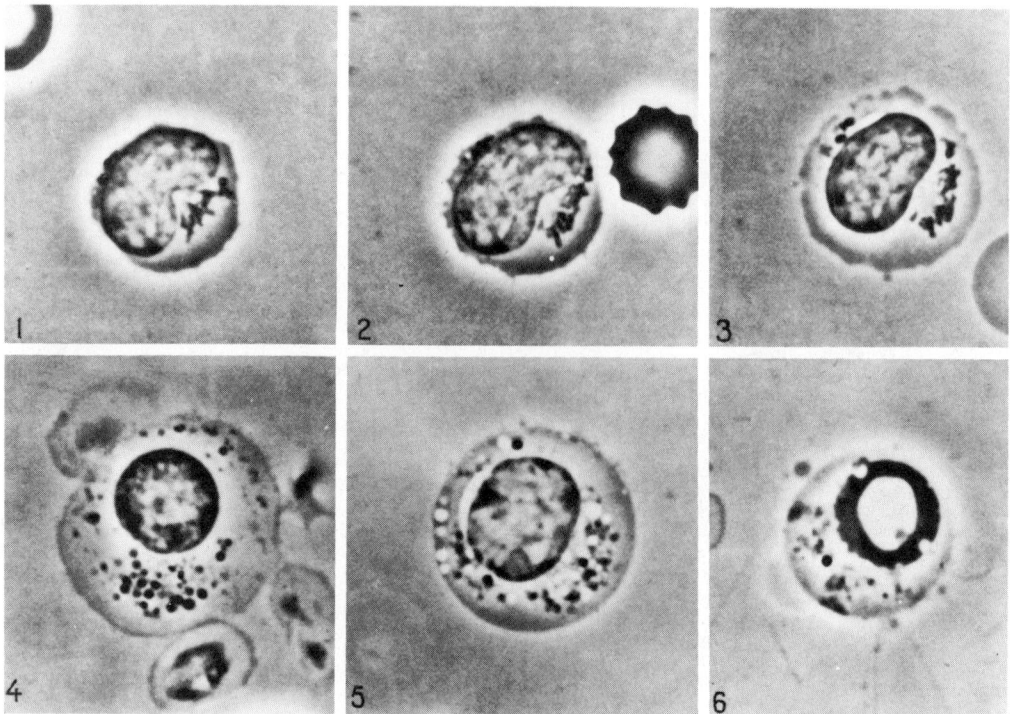

Figure 1–4. Phase micrographs depicting stages of cell death in blood lymphocyte. *1,* Normal lymphocyte; *2,* slight cytoplasmic edema; *3,* increasing cytoplasmic edema; *4* and *5,* disappearance of the nuclear depression; *6,* nuclear pyknosis. (From Bessis, M.: Living Blood Cells and Their Ultrastructure. New York, Springer-Verlag, 1972.)

logically with severe vacuolization of the mitochondria (Figs. 1–5 and 1–7), including their cristae; extensive damage to plasma membranes; swelling of lysosomes; and—particularly if the ischemic zone is reperfused—massive calcium influx into the cell.

Large flocculent amorphous densities develop in the mitochondrial matrix (Fig. 1–7). In the myocardium, these are indications of irreversible injury and can be seen as early as 30 to 40 min after ischemia. There is continued loss of proteins, essential coenzymes, and

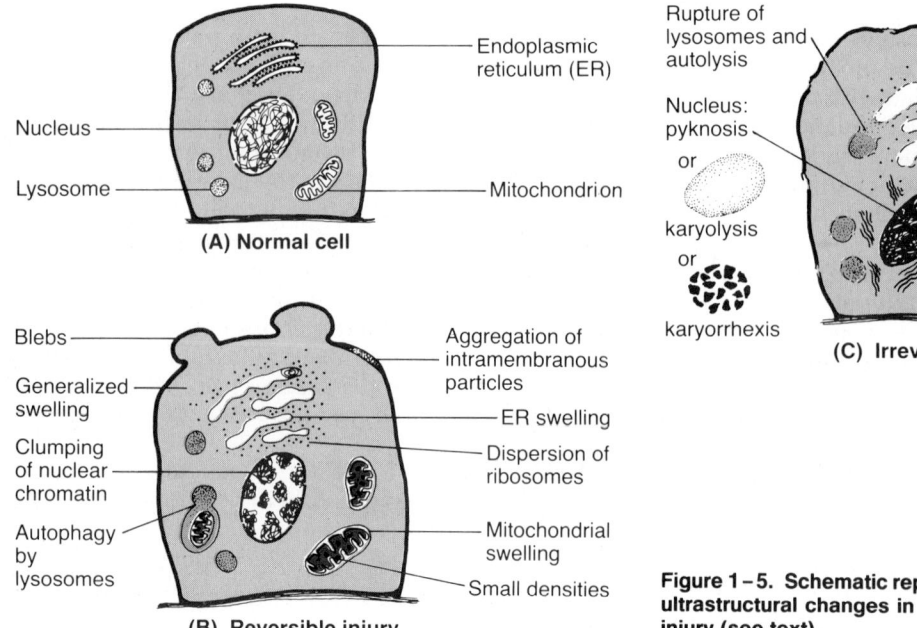

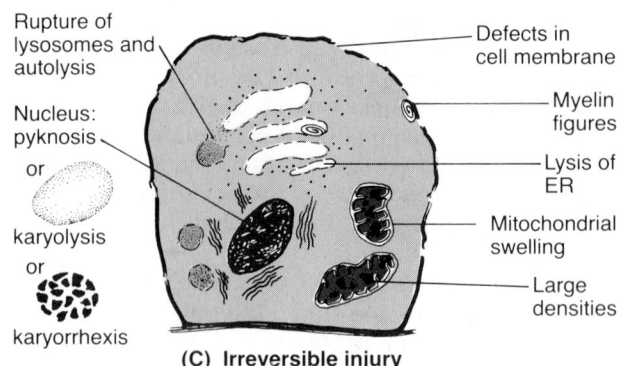

Figure 1–5. Schematic representation of a normal cell (A) and the ultrastructural changes in reversible (B) and irreversible (C) cell injury (see text).

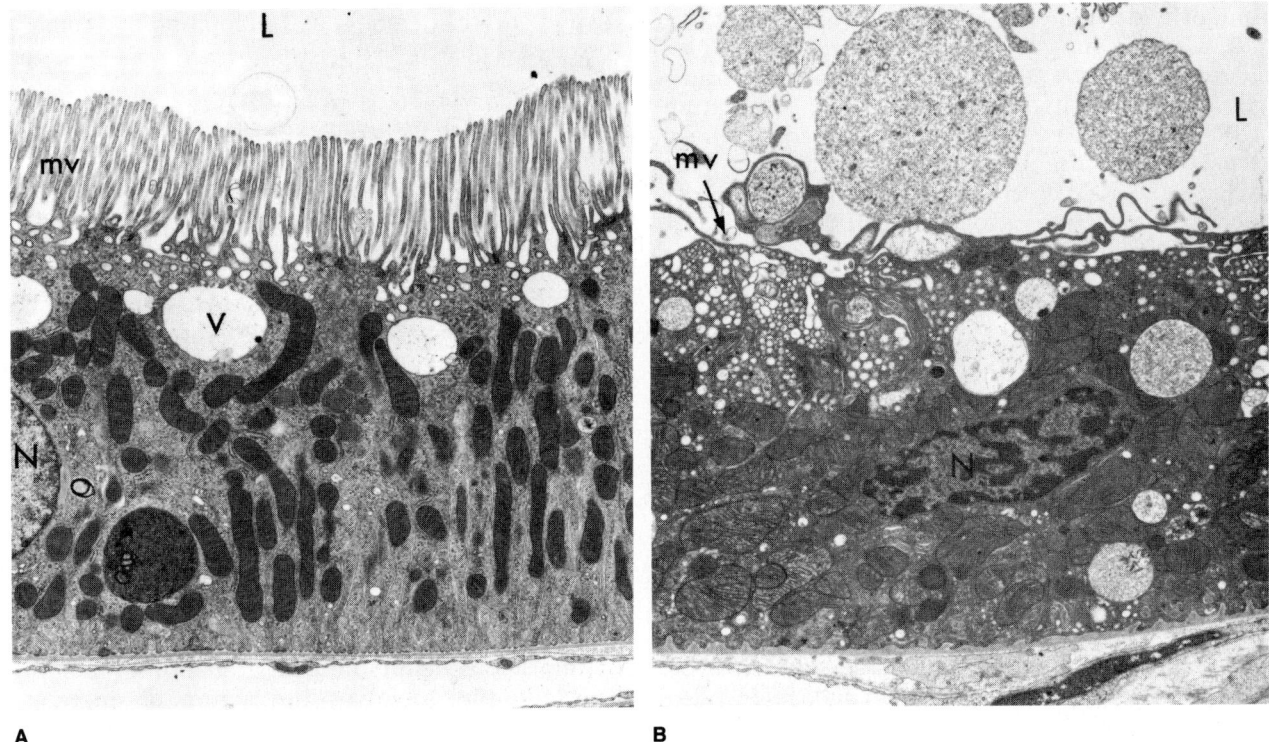

A   **B**

Figure 1–6. *A,* Electron micrograph of normal epithelial cell of proximal kidney tubule. Note abundant microvilli (mv) lining the lumen (L). N = nucleus; V = apical vacuoles (which are normal structures in this cell type). *B,* Epithelial cell of the proximal tubule showing reversible ischemic changes. The microvilli (mv) are lost and have been incorporated in apical cytoplasm; blebs have formed and are extruded in the lumen (L). Mitochondria are slightly dilated. (Compare with *A.*)

ribonucleic acids from the hyperpermeable membranes. The cells may also leak metabolites, which are vital for the reconstitution of ATP, thus further depleting net intracellular high-energy phosphates.

The falling pH (due to glycolysis, lactate accumulation, and breakdown of phosphate esters) together with changes in the ionic composition of the cell leads to *injury to the lysosomal membranes, followed by leakage of their enzymes into the cytoplasm and activation of their acid hydrolyses.* Lysosomes contain RNAases, DNAases, proteases, phosphatases, glucosidases, and cathepsins. Activation of these enzymes leads to enzymatic digestion of cell components evidenced by loss of ribonucleoprotein, deoxyribonucleoprotein, and glycogen, and the various *nuclear changes* described later (p. 17).

Following cell death, cell components are progressively degraded, and there is widespread leakage of cellular enzymes into the extracellular space and, conversely, entry of extracellular macromolecules from the interstitial space into the dead cells. Finally, the dead cell may become replaced by large masses composed of phospholipids in the form of myelin figures. These are then either phagocytosed by other cells or degraded further into fatty acids. *Calcification* of such fatty acid residues may occur with the formation of calcium soaps.

At this point in the story, we should note that leakage of intracellular enzymes across the abnormally permeable plasma membrane, and into the

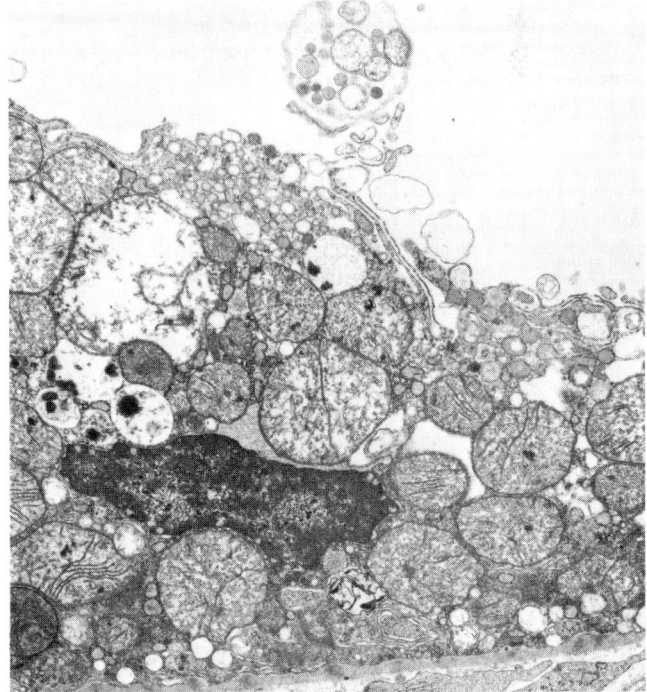

Figure 1–7. Proximal tubular cell showing irreversible ischemic injury. Note the markedly swollen mitochondria containing amorphous densities, disrupted cell membranes, and dense pyknotic nucleus.

serum, provides important clinical parameters of cell death. Cardiac muscle, for example, contains glutamic-oxaloacetic transaminase (GOT), pyruvic transaminases, lactic dehydrogenase (LDH), and creatine kinase (CK). Elevated serum levels of such enzymes, and particularly the isoenzymes specific for heart muscle (e.g., CK-MB), are valuable clinical criteria of myocardial infarction, a locus of cell death in heart muscle discussed in some detail on page 608.

Mechanisms of Irreversible Injury

The sequence of events for hypoxia was described as a continuum from its initiation to the ultimate digestion of the lethally injured cell by lysosomal enzymes. But at what stage did the cell actually die? And what is the critical biochemical event responsible for the "point of no return"? The duration of hypoxia necessary to induce irreversible cell injury varies considerably according to the cell type and the nutritional and hormonal status of the animal (Table 1–1). In the liver, between one and two hours of ischemia are required to produce irreversible damage to liver cells. In the brain, neurons suffer irreversible damage after three to five minutes. The state of nutrition of the cell is also important. Liver cells of rats fed a normal diet contain abundant glycogen and have a higher potential for survival after ischemia than do the liver cells of starved rats.

What then are the critical events for lethal hypoxic injury? Two phenomena consistently characterize irreversibility after ischemia and these point the finger to the two most likely contributing events. The first is the *inability to reverse mitochondrial dysfunction* (lack of oxidative phosphorylation and ATP generation) upon reperfusion or reoxygenation, and the second is the development of *profound disturbances in membrane function.*[7]

ATP Depletion

ATP depletion clearly contributes to the functional and structural consequences of ischemia, as described earlier (Fig. 1–3). It would be reasonable to consider that progressive depletion of ATP in itself at some critical juncture constitutes the lethal event. In favor of a primary role for ATP depletion are the following observations. High-energy phosphate in the form of ATP is required for many synthetic and degradative processes within the cell, and cells that show resistance hypoxic cell injury are those that are able to generate ATP anaerobically or conserve ATP by reducing its consumption.[2] Infusion of ATP-rich solutions protects against ischemic injury in some experimental models.[8] In the myocardium, the marked depletion of ATP is closely related to the development of lethal injury.[5] However, although numerous alterations in mitochondrial structure and function are found in ischemic tissues, it has been possible experimentally to dissociate these changes as well as ATP depletion from the inevitability of cell death.[9] It is now thought that the role of ATP depletion in irreversibility is its contribution to the second critical event in ischemia—cell membrane damage—discussed next.

Cell Membrane Damage

A great deal of evidence indicates that cell membrane damage is a central factor in the pathogenesis of irreversible cell injury.[7] As should be well known, the cell membrane consists of a lipid-protein mosaic made up of a bimolecular layer of phospholipids and globular proteins embedded within the lipid bilayer.[10] An intact plasma membrane is essential to the maintenance of normal cell permeability and volume. Loss of volume regulation, increased permeability to extracellular molecules such as inulin, and demonstrable plasma membrane ultrastructural defects occur in the earliest stages of irreversible injury.

Several biochemical mechanisms have been identified as contributors to such membrane damage (Table 1–2).

1. *Progressive loss of phospholipids.* Normally, the turnover of membrane phospholipids is coupled to their resynthesis so that the integrity of the cell membrane is maintained. Degradation of membrane phospholipids involves the action of endogenous *phospholipases,* whose activation is strongly calcium dependent. In some ischemic tissues (e.g., liver) irreversible ischemic injury is associated with a marked (50%) decrease in the content of membrane phospholipids.[11] One postulated explanation for phospholipid loss is increased phospholipid degradation owing to activation of endogenous phospholipases (Fig. 1–8).[11] This activation of phospholipases may in turn be the result of increased cytosolic calcium concentration induced by ischemia. It should be remembered that the normal intracellular calcium concentration is extremely low ($\pm 10^{-7}$ M), and that such calcium is sequestered in mitochondria and endoplasmic reticulum. Oxygen deprivation releases sequestered calcium and raises cytosolic calcium, and most recent studies suggest that increased cytosolic calcium *precedes* the onset of irreversible injury in models of ischemia or hypoxia.[13–16] Whether calcium is the primary mediator of irreversibility is unsettled.[17] Progressive phospholipid loss can also presumably occur owing to *decreased reacylation or de novo synthesis* of phospholipids, which involves ATP-dependent steps as well as appropriate substrate availability (Fig. 1–8).[18,19]

Table 1–2. Possible Mechanisms of Membrane Damage in Irreversible Cell Injury

Progressive loss of phospholipids
   Increased degradation
   Decreased synthesis
Cytoskeletal alterations
   Activation of proteases
   Damage to cytoskeletal-membrane connections
   Physical effects of cell swelling
Free radical–induced injury
Lipid breakdown products

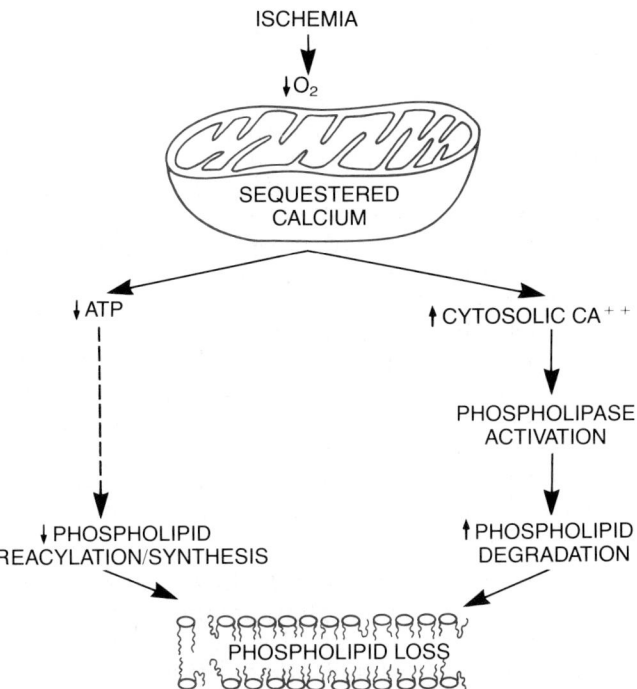

ISCHEMIA

↓O₂

SEQUESTERED
CALCIUM

↓ATP

↑CYTOSOLIC CA⁺⁺

PHOSPHOLIPASE
ACTIVATION

↓ PHOSPHOLIPID
REACYLATION/SYNTHESIS

↑ PHOSPHOLIPID
DEGRADATION

PHOSPHOLIPID LOSS

Figure 1-8. **Possible mechanisms of phospholipid loss induced by ischemia. On the right, increased phospholipid degradation due to calcium-induced activation of phospholipase. On the left, decreased phospholipid reacylation or de novo synthesis, possibly related to ATP depletion.**

2. *Cytoskeletal abnormalities.* It has recently been proposed that cell membrane damage, at least in the myocardium, is due to hypoxia-induced injury to intermediate cytoskeletal filaments, which anchor the myocardial myofibrils to each other and to the sarcolemma (the cell membrane of myocardium).[20] In the presence of cell swelling, which occurs in ischemia, this cytoskeletal damage results in detachment of the cell membrane from the cytoskeleton, rendering the membrane susceptible to stretching and rupture.[21] In support of this hypothesis, there is evidence of increased degradation of the cytoskeletal protein vinculin in ischemia.[22] A potential mechanism for such increased degradation is activation of intracellular *proteases*, induced by increased cytosolic calcium.

3. *Toxic oxygen radicals.* As will be discussed in detail later, partially reduced oxygen free radicals are highly toxic molecules, which cause injury to cell membranes and other cell constituents. There is now evidence that such free radicals are produced at very low levels in ischemic myocardium during ischemia, but that there is an increase in free radical production *on restoration of blood flow.*[23] Reperfusion results in a paradoxical effect — an increase in damage called *reperfusion injury.* This injury can be reduced by antioxidants in some,[24] but not all,[25] models of ischemia. *The toxic oxygen species are thought to be produced largely by polymorphonuclear leukocytes that infiltrate the site of ischemia during reperfusion.*[25] It must be emphasized that if reperfusion does not occur, lethal ischemic cell injury will still eventually ensue, but toxic oxygen species are not involved under these conditions.

4. *Lipid breakdown products.* These include unesterified free fatty acids, acyl carnitine, and lysophospholipids, catabolic products that are known to accumulate in ischemic cells as a result of phospholipid degradation.[26] They have a detergent effect on membranes. They also either insert into the lipid bilayer of the membrane or exchange with membrane phospholipids, potentially causing changes in permeability and electrophysiologic alterations. Indeed, there is a high degree of correlation between the intracellular level of unesterified free fatty acid and irreversible cell injury in cells with marked reductions of ATP.[27]

Whatever the mechanism(s) of membrane injury, the resultant loss of membrane integrity causes further influx of calcium from the extracellular space, where it is present in high concentrations ($> 10^{-3}$ M), into the cells.[28] When, in addition, the ischemic tissue is reperfused to some extent, as may occur in vivo, the scene is set for massive influx of calcium. This calcium influx may be the "coup de grace" that determines irreversible injury, not only after ischemia but also in toxic injury.[7] Calcium is taken up avidly by mitochondria after reoxygenation and permanently poisons them, inhibits cellular enzymes, denatures proteins, and causes the cytologic alterations characteristic of coagulative necrosis.

It is evident that the precise molecular events that initiate irreversible cell damage are still incompletely understood. Indeed, it is likely that several mechanisms, acting at more than one locus, underlie cell death. *For now it must suffice to say that hypoxia affects oxidative phosphorylation and hence the synthesis of vital ATP supplies, that membrane damage is critical to the development of lethal cell injury, and that calcium is an important mediator of the biochemical alterations leading to cell death.*

FREE RADICALS AND CELL INJURY

It can be deduced from our discussion of hypoxic cell injury that any agent that can cause damage to the cell membrane, or to the membranes of critical cell organelles, can trigger a sequence of events that, in the end, may mimic those occurring in hypoxia. Indeed, a large number of chemical, physical, and infectious agents as well as the process of immune lysis cause irreversible injury by damage to cell membranes. One important mechanism of membrane damage, already alluded to in the discussion of reperfusion injury, is injury induced by free radicals, particularly by activated oxygen species.[29-31] It is emerging as a final common pathway of cell injury in such varied processes as chemical and radiation injury, oxygen and other gaseous toxicity, cellular aging, microbial killing by phagocytic cells, inflammatory damage, tumor destruction by macrophages, and others (Fig. 1-2).

Free radicals are chemical species that have a

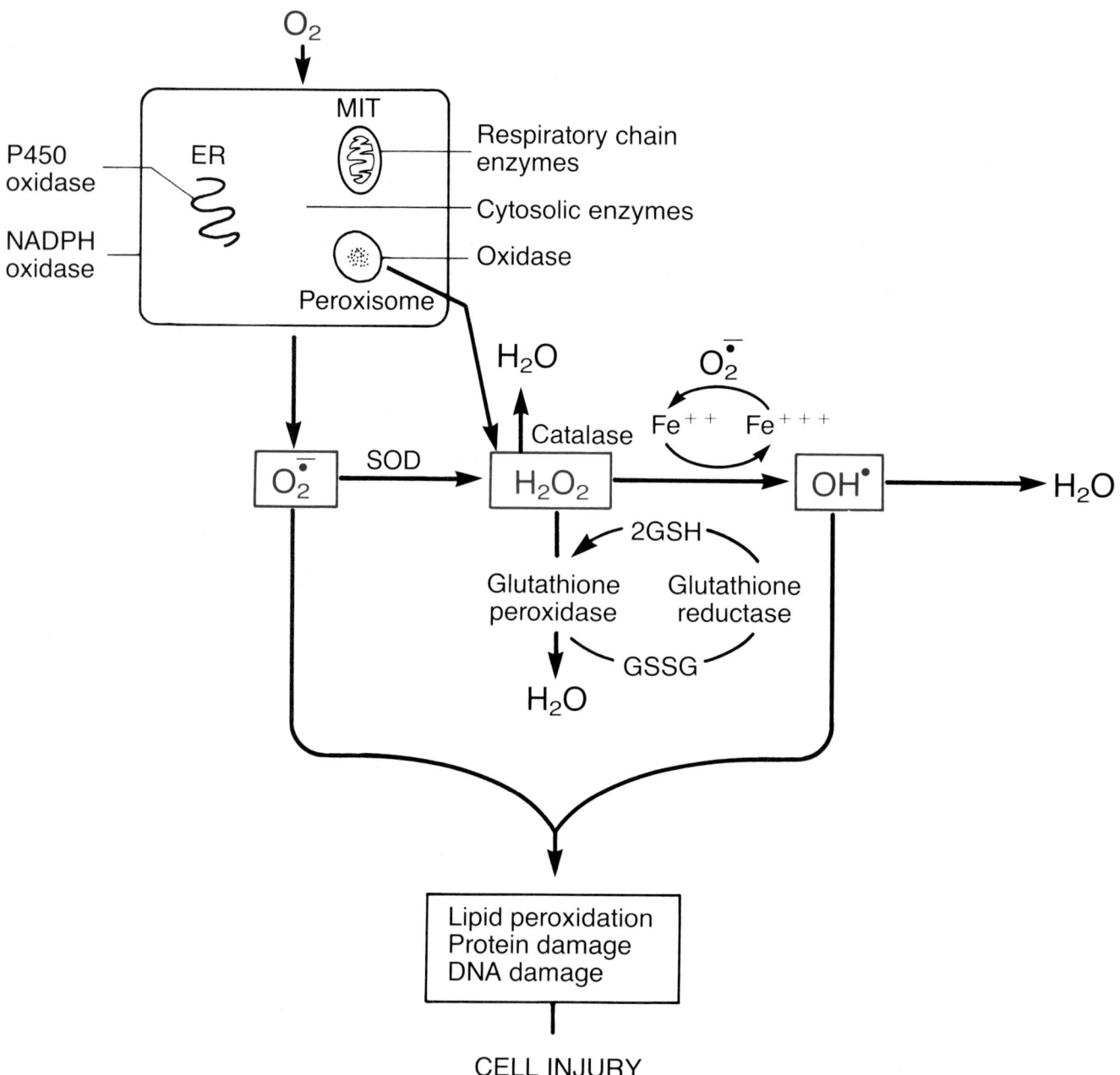

Figure 1–9. Formation of reactive oxygen species and anti-oxidant mechanisms in biologic systems. O_2 is converted to superoxide ($O_2^{\cdot-}$) by oxidative enzymes in the ER, mitochondria, plasma membrane, peroxisomes, and cytosol. $O_2^{\cdot-}$ is converted to H_2O_2 by dismutation and thence to OH· by the Cu^{++}/Fe^{++} catalyzed Fenton reaction. H_2O is also derived directly from oxidases in peroxisomes. Not shown is another potentially injurious radical, singlet oxygen. Resultant free radical damage to lipid (peroxidation), proteins, and DNA leads to various forms of cell injury. Note that superoxide catalyzes the reduction of Fe^{+++} to Fe^{++}, thus enhancing OH· generation by the Fenton reaction. The major antioxidant enzymes are SOD, catalase, and glutathione peroxidase.

single unpaired electron in an outer orbital. In such a state the radical is extremely reactive and unstable and enters into reactions with inorganic or organic chemicals — proteins, lipids, carbohydrates — particularly with key molecules in membranes and nucleic acids. Moreover, free radicals initiate autocatalytic reactions whereby molecules with which they react are themselves converted into free radicals to thus propagate the chain of damage.

Free radicals may be *initiated* within cells (1) by the absorption of radiant energy (e.g., ultraviolet light, x-rays), (2) by endogenous, usually oxidative, reactions that occur during normal metabolic processes, or (3) by enzymic metabolism of exogenous chemicals or drugs (e.g., $CCl_3^{\cdot}$, a product of CCl_4). An unpaired electron can be associated with almost any atom, but oxygen- and carbon-centered free radicals are of greatest biologic relevance.

Oxygen-derived radicals. As should be well known, oxygen normally undergoes a four-electron reduction to H_2O, catalyzed by cytochrome oxidase. However, the presence of intracellular oxygen also allows the inadvertent production of partially reduced toxic intermediate oxygen species. The three most important such species are superoxide (O_2^-), hydrogen peroxide (H_2O_2), and hydroxyl ions ($OH \cdot$). These can be produced by the activity of a variety of oxidative enzymes, in different sites of the cells — cytosol, mitochondria, lysosomes, peroxisomes, and plasma membrane (Fig. 1–9).

Superoxide is generated either directly during auto-oxidation in mitochondria, or enzymatically by cytoplasmic enzymes such as xanthine oxidase, cytochrome P450, and other oxidases.

$$O_2 \xrightarrow{\text{oxidase}} O_2^-$$

Once produced, O_2^- can be inactivated either spontaneously or, more rapidly, by the enzyme superoxide dismutase (SOD), forming H_2O_2.

$$O_2^- + O_2^- + 2H^+ \xrightarrow{\text{SOD}} H_2O_2 + O_2$$

Hydrogen peroxide is produced either by the dis-

mutation of O_2^- as just explained, or directly by oxidases present in peroxisomes — the catalase-containing organelles present in many organs (Fig. 1–9).

Hydroxyl radicals are generated (1) by the hydrolysis of water caused by *ionizing radiation*

$$H_2O \longrightarrow H \cdot + OH \cdot$$

or (2) by interaction with transitional metals (e.g., iron, copper) in the Fenton reaction

$$Fe^{++} + H_2O_2 \longrightarrow Fe^{+++} + OH \cdot + OH^-$$

or (3) through the Haber-Weiss reaction:

$$H_2O_2 + O_2^- \longrightarrow OH \cdot + OH^- + O_2$$

Iron is particularly important in toxic oxygen injury. Most of free iron is in the ferric (Fe^{+++}) form and has to be reduced to the ferrous (Fe^{++}) form to be active in the Fenton reaction. This reduction can be enhanced by superoxide, and thus superoxide ion is important in $OH \cdot$ generation.

The main effects of these reactive species are on *membrane, lipid*, sulfydryl bonds of *proteins*, and nucleotides of *DNA* (Fig. 1–9).[32–35] In the presence of oxygen they may cause peroxidation of lipids

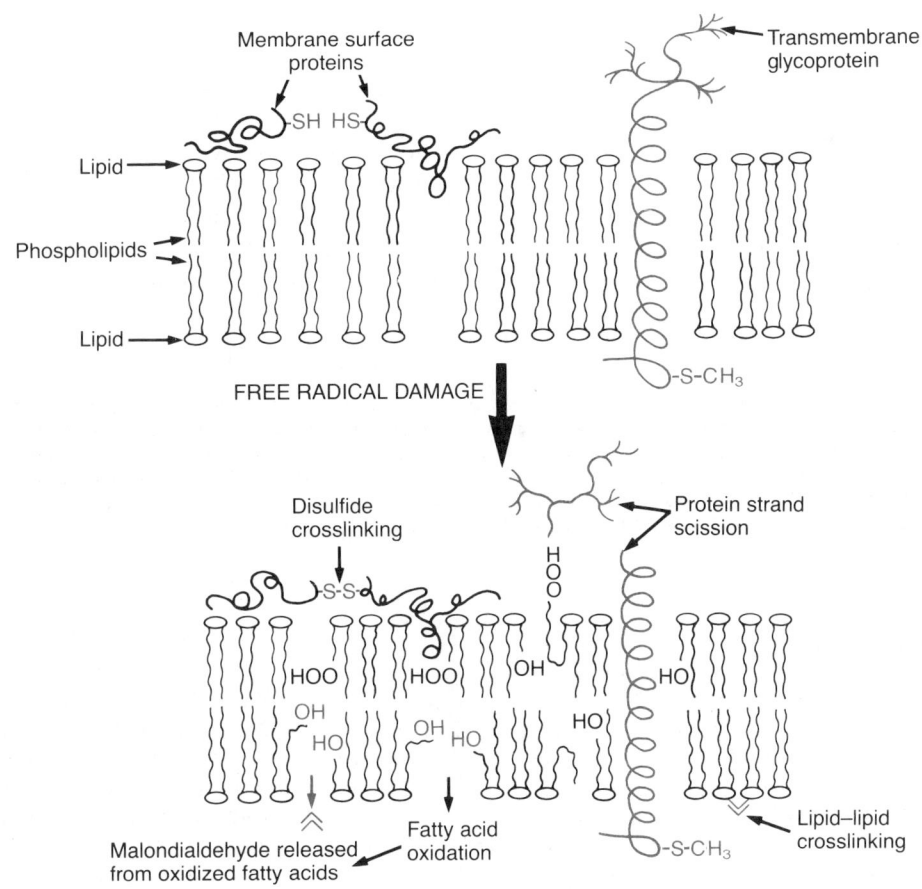

Figure 1–10. Certain mechanisms of free radical damage to membranes (in lower panel) including disulfide crosslinking of membrane surface proteins, protein strand scission, lipid-lipid crosslinking, and fatty acid peroxidation (lipid peroxidation). The latter leads to release of derivatives such as malondialdehyde. (Modified from Freeman B.A., and Crapo V.D.: Biology of disease: Free radicals and tissue injury. Lab Invest. 47:412, 1982.)

within cellular and organellar membranes and cause damage to endoplasmic reticulum, mitochondria, and other microsomal components. Cross linking of proteins by the formation of disulfide bonds (the most labile amino acids are methionine, histidine, cystine, and lysine) may also occur and raise havoc through the cell, in particular inactivating enzymes, especially sulfhydryl enzymes (Fig. 1–10). Interactions with DNA induce mutations in the genetic code, which, if not repaired, induce cellular derangements as well as inhibition of DNA replication. All three oxygen-derived radicals are involved in such DNA damage.[36]

Lipid peroxidation is one well-studied (but not always the primary) mechanism of free radical injury.[29,37] It is initiated by hydroxyl radicals, which react with unsaturated fatty acids of membrane phospholipids to generate organic acid free radicals, which in turn react quickly with oxygen to form *peroxides.* *Peroxides* themselves then act as free radicals, initiating an autocatalytic chain reaction, resulting in further loss of unsaturated fatty acids and in extensive membrane damage.

Once free radicals are formed, how does the body get rid of them? They may spontaneously decay. Superoxide, for example, is unstable and decays spontaneously into oxygen and hydrogen peroxide. There are, however, several systems that contribute to *termination* or inactivation of free radical reactions. These include:

1. Endogenous or exogenous *antioxidants* (e.g., vitamin E; sulfhydryl-containing compounds such as cysteine, glutathione, and D-penicillamine; serum proteins such as ceruloplasmin and transferrin), which either block the initiation of free radical formation or inactivate (e.g., scavenge) free radicals. Transferrin is thought to act as an antioxidant by binding free iron, which, as we have seen, can catalyze free radical formation.

2. *Enzymes.* These include:

a. *Superoxide dismutase,* which converts superoxide to H_2O_2.

b. *Catalase,* present in peroxisomes, which decomposes H_2O_2

$$2 H_2O_2 \longrightarrow O_2 + 2 H_2O$$

c. *Glutathione peroxidase,* which catalyzes the ability of reduced glutathione (GSH) to release hydrogen from $-SH$ to a hydroxyl radical or to H_2O_2.

$$2 OH\cdot + 2GSH \longrightarrow 2 H_2O + GSSG$$

or

$$H_2O_2 + 2GSH \longrightarrow 2 H_2O + GSSG$$

In many pathologic processes the final effects of stimulus-inducing free radicals depend on the net balance between free radical formation and termination.

Examples of Free Radical Injury

As stated earlier, free radicals are now thought to be involved in many pathologic and physiologic processes,[29,30] to be discussed throughout this book. Here we shall introduce only some examples of free radical injury.

CHEMICAL INJURY. The toxicity of many chemicals and drugs can be attributed either to conversion of these chemicals to free radicals or to formation of oxygen-derived toxic metabolites. Later in this chapter we will discuss carbon tetrachloride poisoning as one example of chemical free radical damage.

INFLAMMATION. Toxic oxygen metabolites produced by leukocytes and other cells in the course of inflammation play an important role in inducing tissue damage and in elaborating chemotactic agents (p. 57).[34]

MICROBIAL KILLING. Bacteria ingested by leukocytes are killed within the phagolysosomes. The lethal damage to bacteria is largely dependent on the oxidative burst that occurs in leukocytes during phagocytosis, resulting in release of oxygen radicals (p. 50).

IRRADIATION INJURY. The role of free radicals in tissue damage induced by *irradiation* is well documented. $-OH\cdot$ and $H\cdot$ produced by radiolysis are known to add to the bases of nucleic acids and to abstract hydrogen from pentose to release organic free radicals (p. 50).

OXYGEN AND OTHER GAS TOXICITY. Exposure to high concentrations of oxygen, ozone, and other gases results in lung damage, and this action also appears to be mediated by free radical formation. Because superoxide dismutase and catalase inactivate some of the toxic radicals of oxygen, administration of these enzymes will diminish the severity of lung damage.

AGING. In its simplest form, the so-called *"free radical" theory of aging* supposes that the formation of free radicals is more frequent in aging organisms, resulting in lipid peroxidation and membrane damage. Theoretically, increased lipid peroxidation with aging might occur as a result of (1) continuous increased formation of free radicals caused by environmental agents; (2) diminished availability of antioxidants for unknown reasons; or (3) a loss of diminution of activity of some of the compounds or enzymes that catalyze the inactivation of toxic free radicals, e.g., superoxide dismutase (see also Chapter 11).

There is also increasing evidence that oxidation products play a role in the development of *atherosclerosis* (p. 567) and in *carcinogenesis.*

CHEMICAL INJURY

Chemicals induce cell injury by one of two general mechanisms: (1) Some chemicals can act *directly* by combining with some critical molecular component or cellular organelle. For example, in *mercuric chlo-*

ride poisoning, mercury binds to the sulfhydryl groups of the cell membrane and other proteins, causing increased membrane permeability and inhibition of ATPase-dependent transport. In such instances the greatest damage is usually to the cells that utilize, absorb, excrete, or concentrate the chemicals — in the case of mercuric chloride, the gastrointestinal tract and kidney. Many antineoplastic chemotherapeutic agents and antibiotic drugs also induce cell damage by direct cytotoxic effects. (2) Most other toxic chemicals are not biologically active but must be converted to reactive toxic metabolites, which then act on target cells. Although these metabolites might cause membrane damage and cell injury by *direct covalent binding* to membrane protein and lipids, by far the most important mechanism of membrane injury involves the formation of *reactive free radicals* and subsequent lipid peroxidation,[38] as detailed earlier.

CCl$_4$-Induced Cell Injury

One of the best characterized models of free radical injury is the chemical injury produced in the liver by *carbon tetrachloride (CCl$_4$) poisoning.*[29,38] This halogenated hydrocarbon is used widely in the drycleaning industry and represents a prototype for chemical injury by many similar compounds. The toxic effect of carbon tetrachloride is due to conversion of CCl$_4$ to the *highly reactive toxic free radical* CCl$_3\cdot$ (CCl$_4$ + e $\rightarrow$ CCl$_3\cdot$ + Cl$^-$) in the smooth endoplasmic reticulum (SER) by the mixed-function oxidase system of enzymes involved in the metabolism of lipid-soluble drugs and other compounds (cytochrome P-450).[38] The CCl$_3\cdot$ initiates lipid peroxidation, as has been described for hydroxyl radicals (p. 12); there is initially autoxidation of the unsaturated (polyenoic) fatty acids present within the membrane phospholipids, and formation of organic peroxides after reaction with oxygen. *This reaction is autocatalytic* in that new radicals are formed from the peroxide radicals themselves. There is thus rapid breakdown of the structure and function of the endoplasmic reticulum. *It is no surprise, therefore, that CCl$_4$-induced liver cell injury is both severe and extremely rapid in onset.* Within less than 30 min of CCl$_4$ administration, there is a decline in hepatic protein synthesis. Swelling of the cisternae of the endoplasmic reticulum can be seen early with the electron microscope, and within less than two hours there is dissociation of the ribosomes from the membranes of the endoplasmic reticulum (Fig. 1–11), followed by disaggregation of the free polysomes.

The next event that occurs is an accumulation of lipid within the cytoplasm, beginning in the endoplasmic reticulum. This lipid accumulation is attributable to the inability of cells to synthesize lipoprotein from triglycerides and "lipid acceptor protein." As will be detailed in the section on fatty change (p. 21), triglycerides can leave the hepatic cell only after they have been incorporated into lipoprotein. Thus, failure of lipid acceptor protein synthesis leads to marked

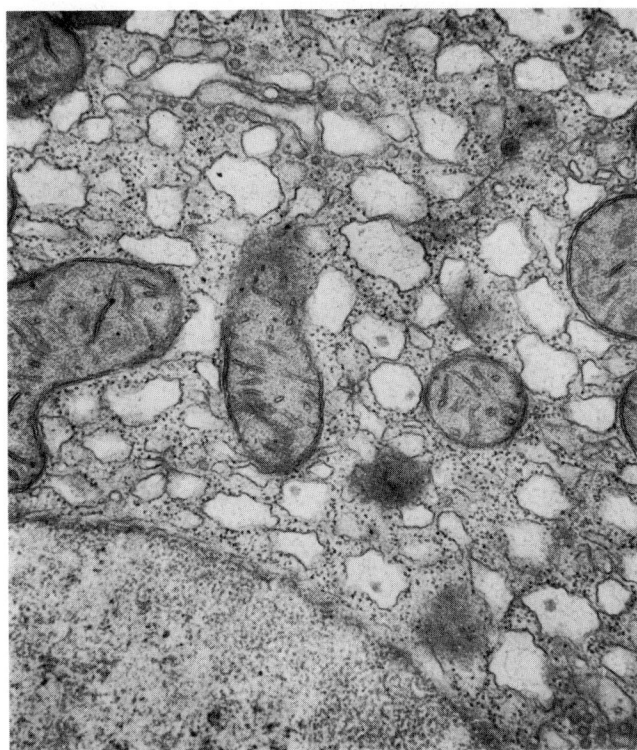

Figure 1–11. Rat liver cell four hours after carbon tetrachloride intoxication; with swelling of endoplasmic reticulum and shedding of ribosomes. Mitochondria at this stage are unaltered. (Courtesy of Dr. O. Iseri.)

increases in intracellular triglycerides and the characteristic fatty liver of CCl$_4$ poisoning.

This is followed by progressive swelling of the cells due to increased permeability of the plasma membrane. Plasma membrane damage is thought to be caused by relatively stable fatty aldehydes, which are produced by lipid peroxidation in the SER but are able to diffuse to the cell membrane.[39] Plasma membrane damage also results in a massive influx of calcium, which accumulates in the mitochondria. The progressive damage to the cell after these events is similar to that which occurs in hypoxic injury (Fig. 1–12).

VIRUS-INDUCED CELL INJURY

Viruses that induce cellular changes are of two types: (1) *cytolytic/cytopathic* viruses, which cause various degrees of cell injury and cell death, and (2) *oncogenic* viruses, which stimulate host cell replication and may produce tumors. The detailed mechanisms of viral infection are reviewed in Chapter 7. Here we are concerned with the cytopathic effects of viruses and some of the mechanisms by which cell injury occurs.[39]

Viruses are thought to cause cell injury by one of two general mechanisms. The first is the direct cytopathic effect, in which rapidly replicating virus particles interfere with some aspect of cell metabolism and thus cause cellular damage. The second mechanism involves the induction of an immunologic response

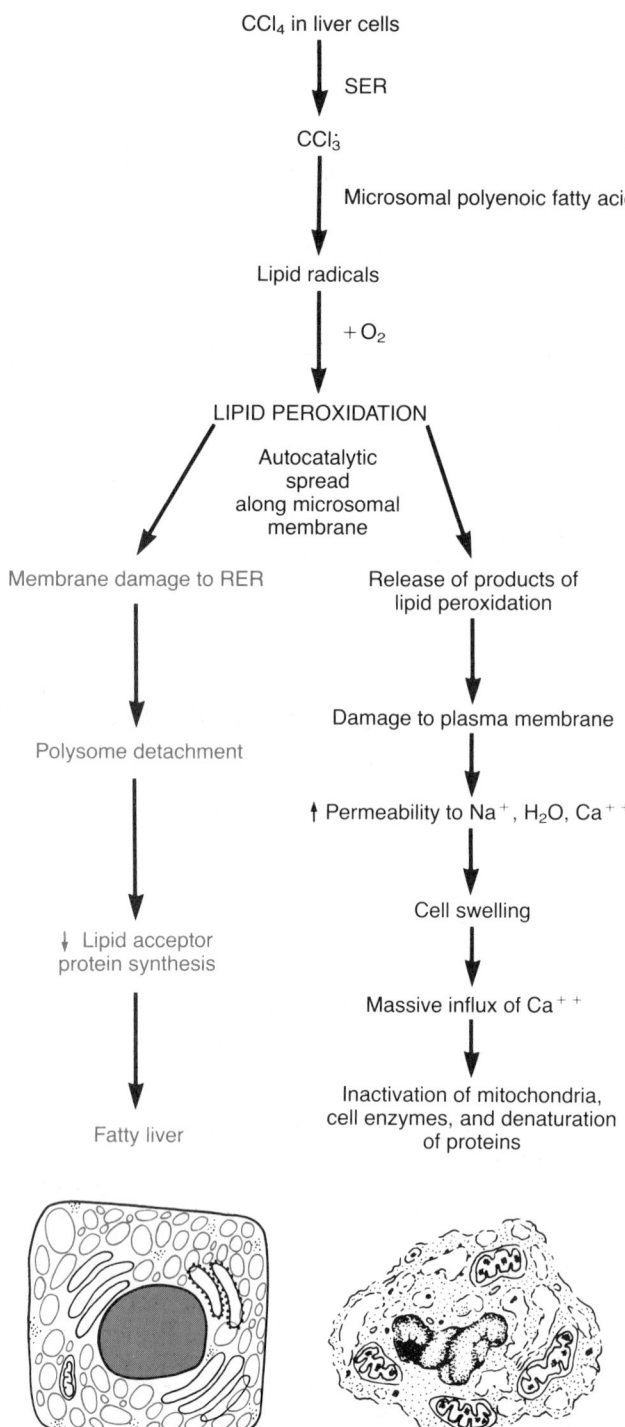

Figure 1–12. Sequence of events leading to fatty change and cell necrosis in CCl₄ toxicity. SER: smooth endoplasmic reticulum.

against viral or virus-altered cell antigens and the destruction of the cell by either antibody or cell-mediated reactions. The damage to hepatocytes caused by hepatitis B virus, for example, is mediated by cytolysis induced by T lymphocytes.

Most directly cytopathic viruses have a high degree of specificity for certain cell types (viral tropism), caused in part by the presence of membrane receptors on host cells, which interact with specific viral structures (Fig. 1–13). The interactions between viruses and receptors allow the virus to attach to, and then enter and injure, the host cell. In such viral infections as poliomyelitis, adenovirus infection, and influenza, specific viral polypeptides are responsible for these interactions; in the case of reovirus a single surface protein, the sigma 1 polypeptide, accounts for the specificity of this agent for certain cells of the central nervous system. Following attachment, viruses enter the cells by different pathways, including phagocytosis, endocytosis in coated vesicles, and direct fusion of enveloped virus with the cell membrane. Following entry into the cell, active replication of the viruses ensues (Fig. 1–13A).

The nature of the cell response to viral replication depends on the specific viral agent and the species of the host cells (Fig. 1–13B), and may take several forms: (1) *Cell lysis,* apparently due to major subversion of cellular metabolism caused by explosive viral replication, is at one end of the spectrum. Some viral proteins may insert into the plasma membrane, increasing its permeability. Many viruses *alter synthesis of proteins and macromolecules* by host cells. For example, the poliovirus is known to inhibit the formation of regulatory gene sequences that initiate protein synthesis. The ultimate effect is *cell membrane injury* with loss of volume regulation and eventual cell death. (2) Some viruses, including the poxvirus and reoviruses, cause *cytoskeletal alterations,* such as disruption of vimentin intermediate filaments and organizational changes in microtubules. Several common respiratory viruses cause additions or deletions in the number of microtubules in cilia of epithelial cells, thus interfering with ciliary motion and with clearance of particles from respiratory passages. (3) Cells sometimes respond to infection with the measles or herpes virus by the *formation of syncytial or multinucleate giant cells,* caused by cell-to-cell fusion. This fusion appears to require the insertion of viral glycoproteins into host surface membranes and a viral effect on the cytoskeleton. (4) Certain virus infected cells develop *inclusion bodies* containing virions or viral proteins in nuclei or cytoplasm (p 314). But recall that cell death is at one end of the spectrum of viral interactions with cells; at the other end is transformation caused by oncogenic viruses (p. 275).

In concluding this discussion of the pathogenesis of cellular injury induced by hypoxia, chemicals, and viruses, several points should be made. Cells sustain biochemical injuries long before they undergo alteration in their structure. Alterations in one intracellular locus have ramifications affecting a host of additional systems. The tiny pebble cast into the pool causes only a minute splash, but the ripples propagate and ultimately affect the entire pool. Irreversible injury may well be not the result of damage to a single locus or system, but the summation of many disruptions that eventually overcome the cell's capacity to adapt. Whatever the Achilles' heels of the cell may be, they are undoubtedly biochemical processes that,

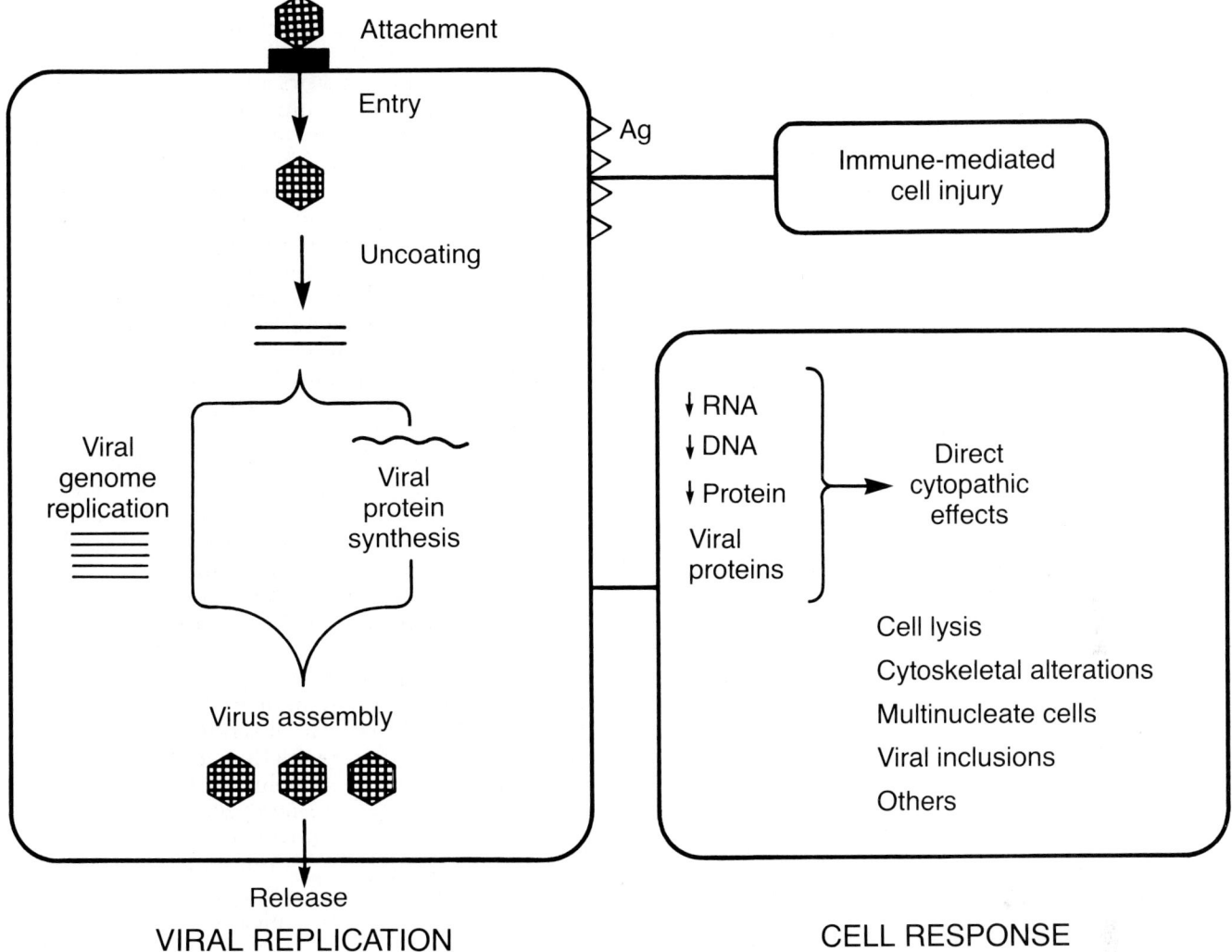

Figure 1–13. Simplified scheme of viral replication and the two mechanisms of cell injury: immune mediated and direct cytopathic (see text). Ag: antigen.

when dislocated, lead in time to observable morphologic change.

MORPHOLOGY OF INJURED CELLS

ULTRASTRUCTURAL CHANGES

We can now examine the morphologic changes in reversibly and lethally injured cells, and we shall begin with the ultrastructural changes. These have been alluded to in the discussion of the pathogenesis of cell injury.

Changes ascribable to alterations in the plasma membrane are seen early in cell injury, reflecting the disturbances in ion and volume regulation induced by loss of ATP. These include cell swelling, formation of cytoplasmic blebs, blunting and distortion of microvilli, creation of myelin figures, and deterioration and loosening of intercellular attachments. These changes can occur rapidly and are readily reversible. In later stages, breaks are seen in both the membranes enclos-

ing the cell and those of the organelles (Figs. 1–5 and 1–6), which denote irreversible injury.

Mitochondrial changes occur extremely rapidly after ischemic injury but are delayed in some forms of chemical injury. Early after ischemia, the mitochondria appear condensed. However, this is quickly followed by *swelling of mitochondria* due to the ionic shifts that occur in the mitochondrial inner compartment. Characteristic *amorphous densities* appear as early as 30 min after ischemia in the myocardium, where they correlate with the onset of irreversibility. These densities consist of lipids or lipid-protein complexes, but with reperfusion, dense granules appear that are very rich in *calcium*. The latter also occur in chemical injury. With irreversible injury also comes increased swelling of mitochondria, which may assume large, bizarre forms. Finally, there is outright rupture of the mitochondrial membranes, followed by progressively increased calcification.

Dilation of the *endoplasmic reticulum* occurs early after injury, probably due to changes in ion and water movement. This is followed by detachment of ribosomes and disaggregation of polysomes, with a decrease of protein synthesis (Fig. 1–11). These responses are also reversible, but with further injury (or early on, as in the case of CCl_4, due to lipid peroxidation) there is progressive fragmentation of the endoplasmic reticulum and formation of intracellular aggregates of myelin figures.

Changes in the *lysosomes* generally appear late. In the stages of reversible injury, lysosomes may be swollen, but there is no evidence of leakage of lysosomal enzymes at this stage. However, after the onset of lethal injury, lysosomes rupture and eventually may disappear as recognizable structures from the disfigured carcass of the dead cell.

LIGHT MICROSCOPIC PATTERNS

Reversible Injury

In classic pathology, the morphologic changes resulting from nonlethal injury to cells were termed degenerations, but today they are more simply designated *reversible injuries.* Two patterns can be recognized under the light microscope: *cellular swelling* and *fatty change.* Cellular swelling appears whenever cells are incapable of maintaining ionic and fluid homeostasis. *Fatty change,* under some circumstances, may be another indicator of reversible cell injury. It is a less universal reaction, principally encountered in cells involved in and dependent on fat metabolism, such as the hepatocyte and myocardial cell. As it is a form of intracellular accumulation, it is described later in this chapter.

> **Cellular swelling** is the first manifestation of almost all forms of injury to cells, resulting from a shift of extracellular water into the cell caused by mechanisms described earlier. It is a difficult morphologic change to appreciate with the light microscope; it may be more apparent at the level of the whole organ. When it affects all cells in an organ, it causes some pallor, increased turgor, and increase in weight of the organ. Microscopically, enlargement of cells is most often discernible by compression of the microvasculature of the organ as, for example, the hepatic sinusoids and the capillary network within the renal cortex.
>
> If water continues to accumulate within cells, small clear vacuoles appear within the cytoplasm. These vacuoles represent distended and pinched-off or sequestered segments of the endoplasmic reticulum. This pattern of nonlethal injury is sometimes called **"hydropic change"** or **"vacuolar degeneration"** (Fig. 1–14). Swelling of cells is reversible.

Cell Death — Necrosis

Cells can be recognized as dead with the light microscope only after they have undergone the sequence of changes referred to as necrosis. *Necrosis may be defined as the morphologic changes that follow cell death in a living tissue or organ, resulting from the progressive degradative action of enzymes on the lethally injured cell.*

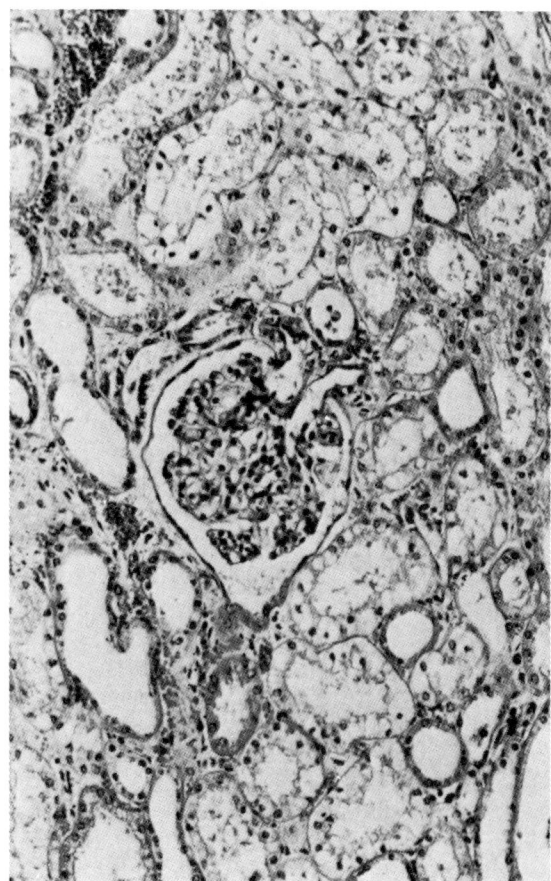

Figure 1–14. Marked cellular swelling (hydropic degeneration) of renal tubular epithelial cells seen in the center field above and below the glomerulus. The cleared, vacuolated cells contain dark displaced nuclei.

THE NECROTIC CELL. *Necrosis is the sum of the morphologic changes that follow cell death in a living tissue or organ.*[40] Except for the typical findings in "normal" tissues placed immediately in fixatives (which are dead but not necrotic), necrosis is the major morphologic manifestation of irreversible cell injury. It has already been made clear that cells die some time before such lethal injury can be identified with the light microscope.

Two essentially concurrent processes bring about the changes of necrosis: (1) enzymic digestion of the cell and (2) denaturation of proteins. The catalytic enzymes are derived either from the lysosomes of the dead cells, in which case the enzymic digestion is referred to as *autolysis,* or from the lysosomes of immigrant leukocytes, termed *heterolysis.*

> The dead cell usually shows increased eosinophilia, attributable in part to the loss of normal basophilia imparted by the RNA in the cytoplasm and in part to increased binding of eosin to denatured intracytoplasmic proteins. The cell may have a more glassy homogeneous appearance than normal cells, due mainly to the loss of glycogen particles.

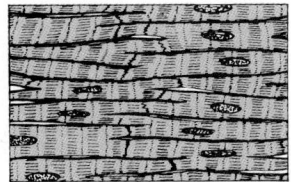
Normal cells

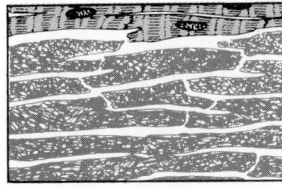
Coagulative necrosis

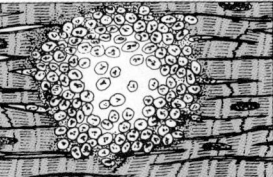
Liquefactive necrosis

Figure 1–16. Schematic representation of coagulative and liquefactive necrosis in myocardium.

When lysosomal enzymes have digested the cytoplasmic organelles, the cytoplasm becomes vacuolated and appears moth-eaten. Finally, calcification of the dead cells may occur in some instances.

Nuclear changes also occur in sublethally and lethally injured cells (Fig. 1–5). The earliest observed ultrastructural change is a reversible clumping of the chromatin to create large aggregates attached to the nuclear membrane and to the nucleolus. As the degradative changes in the cell progress, however, nuclear degeneration may follow along one of two pathways. In some cells, the nucleus progressively shrinks and becomes transformed to a small, dense wrinkled mass of tightly packed chromatin, an alteration called nuclear **pyknosis.** With time, this chromatin undergoes progressive dissolution **(karyolysis),** apparently as a result of the hydrolytic action of the DNases of lysosomal origin. In other cells, after undergoing pyknosis, the nucleus may break up into many clumps, a process called **karyorrhexis.** Eventually the nucleus disappears.

A somewhat distinctive morphologic pattern of cell death has been renamed *apoptosis*[41] (derived from Greek for "dropping off"). It usually involves single cells, or clusters of cells, which appear on sections stained with hematoxylin and eosin (H and E) as round or oval masses of intensely eosinophilic cytoplasm often with dense chromatin fragments (Fig. 1–15). The fragments are taken up and degraded by adjacent phagocytic cells. Apoptosis is thought to be responsible for the programmed destruction of cells during embryogenesis and for hormone-dependent involution, as occurs, for example, in the endome-

trium. It also occurs in certain pathologic conditions. Examples are the acidophil or *Councilman body* seen in the liver in toxic or viral hepatitis, and cell injury to target cells induced by cytotoxic T lymphocytes (p. 183). In the latter example the nuclear changes precede and are required for the eventual cell lysis that occurs in the target cell.[42] It is thought that the alterations initially involve rapid DNA damage and condensation of nuclear chromatin, probably through activation of an endogenous endonuclease,[43] but it is not clear how the nuclear changes lead to cell injury.

Types of Necrosis

The death of cells is not always followed by immediate dissolution of the cellular carcass. Different pathways may be followed depending on the balance between progressive proteolysis, coagulation of protein, and calcification, resulting in the emergence of distinctive morphologic types of necrosis (Fig. 1–16). Although in all instances these types of necrosis clearly signify previous cell death, the characteristic histologic types sometimes give a clue to the cause of cell injury and will therefore be described in some detail.

COAGULATION NECROSIS. Coagulation necrosis is the most common pattern of necrosis and is characterized by conversion of the cell to an acidophilic, opaque "tombstone" (Fig. 1–16). This usually occurs with loss of the nucleus but with preservation of the basic cellular shape, permitting recognition of the cell outlines and tissue architecture (Fig. 1–17). This pattern of necrosis results most commonly from sudden severe ischemia in such organs as the kidney, heart, and adrenal gland. Presumably the pattern results from denaturation, not only of structural proteins but also of enzymic proteins, which blocks the proteolysis of the cell. Ultimately, the necrotic myocardial cells are removed by fragmentation and phagocytosis of the cellular debris by leukocytes or by the action of proteolytic enzymes brought in by such cells.

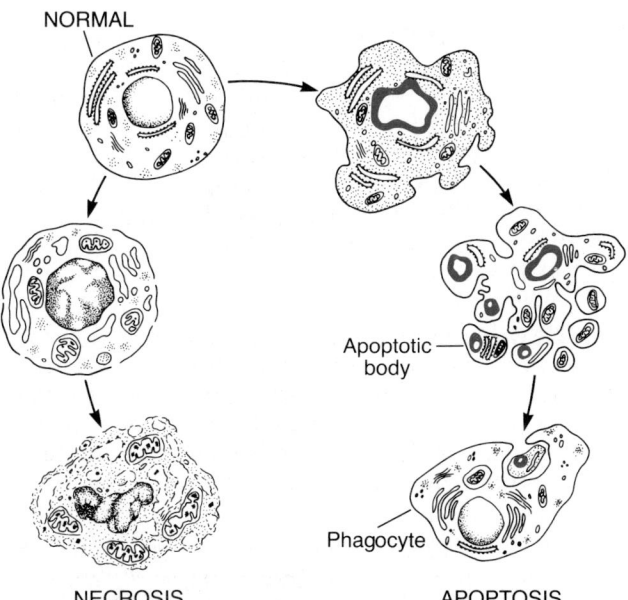

NORMAL

Apoptotic body

Phagocyte

NECROSIS   APOPTOSIS

Figure 1–15. Cell necrosis and apoptosis. In apoptosis the initial changes consist of nuclear chromatin condensation and fragmentation, followed by phagocytosis of apoptotic bodies. (Adapted from Walker et al.[41]).

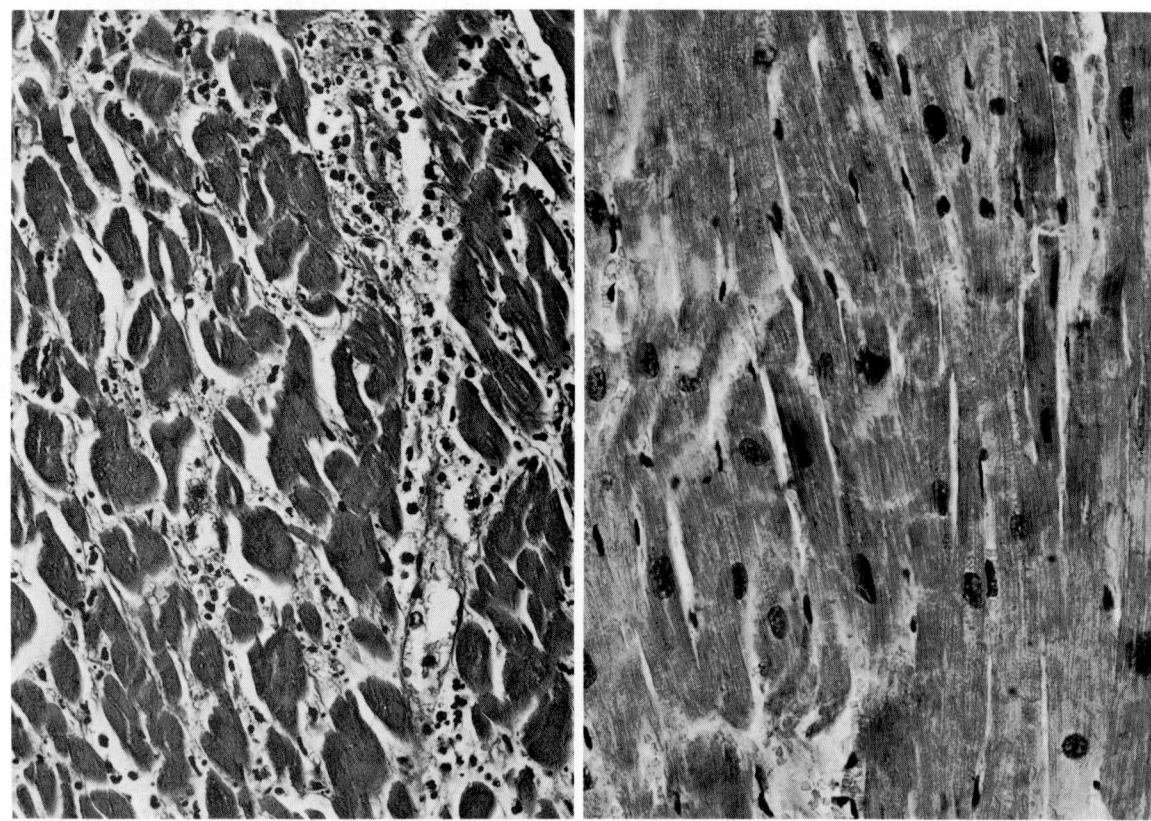

Figure 1–17. *Left,* necrotic cardiac muscle cells with well-preserved outlines. The nuclei have disappeared, and the cytoplasm is coagulated and granular. *Right,* preserved normal muscle for comparison.

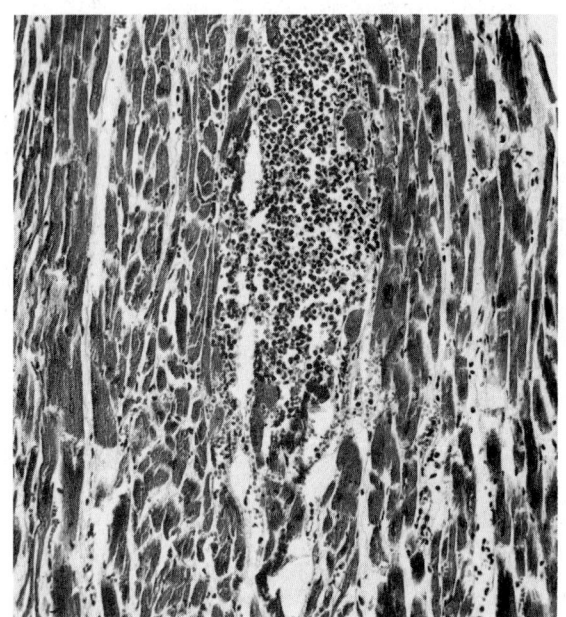

Figure 1–18. Liquefaction necrosis of a focus in the myocardium caused by bacterial seeding. The focus is filled with white cells, creating a myocardial abscess.

LIQUEFACTION NECROSIS. Liquefaction necrosis results from the action of powerful hydrolytic enzymes and occurs when autolysis and heterolysis prevail over conditions that favor denaturation of proteins. This pattern is characteristic of ischemic destruction of brain tissue. It is also commonly encountered in bacterial lesions, presumably because enzymes of bacterial and leukocytic origin contribute to the digestion of dead cells (Fig. 1–18). Brain tissue undergoing liquefaction necrosis is eventually converted to a cystic structure filled with debris and fluid. These cysts are the hallmarks of areas of past brain infections.

FAT NECROSIS. This is the specific morphologic pattern of cell death encountered in adipose tissue due to the action of lipases. It is most commonly seen in *acute pancreatic necrosis,* in which pancreatic enzymes cause patchy necrosis of the pancreas and of fatty depots throughout the abdomen. Powerful lipases are activated and released, and these destroy not only the pancreatic substance itself, but also fat cells in and about the pancreas and throughout the peritoneal cavity. These lipases catalyze the decomposition of triglycerides that leak from adjacent damaged adipose cells to produce free fatty acids. Histologically, the necrosis takes the form of foci of shadowy outlines of necrotic fat cells, the lipid content of which has been lipolyzed, surrounded by an inflammatory reaction (Fig. 1–19). The released fatty acids then complex with calcium to create calcium soaps, which appear in tissue sections as amorphous, granular, basophilic deposits. To the naked eye, the necrotic foci appear opaque and chalky white. Fat necrosis can also be induced by trauma, particularly in breast adipose tissue.

CASEOUS NECROSIS. This is another distinctive type of necrosis that is a combination of coagulative and liquefactive necrosis encountered principally in the center of tuberculous infections (Fig. 1–20). The characteristic appearance of this type of necrosis is that of soft, friable, whitish-gray debris resembling clumped cheesy material, hence the term caseous necrosis. This appearance has been attributed to the capsule of the tubercle bacillus *Mycobacterium tuberculosis*, which contains lipopolysaccharides, but the exact interaction of this material with dead cells is not well understood. Microscopically the cells are not totally liquefied nor are their outlines preserved, creating a distinctive amorphous granular debris (Fig. 1–21). The caseous necrosis is enclosed within a granulomatous inflammatory wall.

GANGRENOUS NECROSIS. Although gangrenous necrosis in reality does not represent a distinctive pattern of cell death, the term is still commonly used in surgical clinical practice. It is usually applied to a limb, generally the lower leg, which has lost its blood supply and has subsequently been attacked by bacterial agents. The tissues in this case have undergone

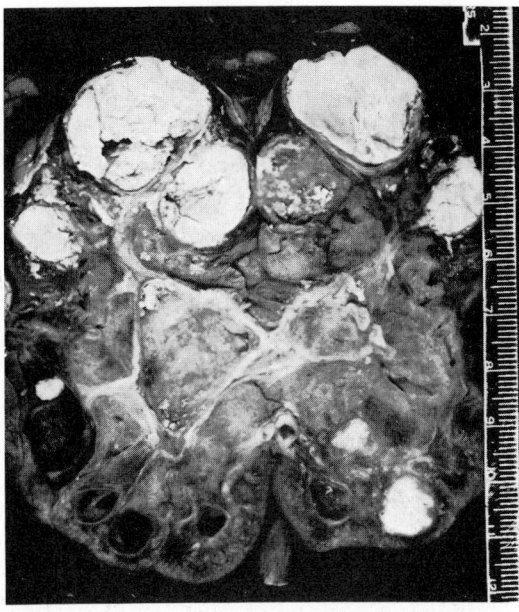

Figure 1–20. A tuberculous kidney with multiple discrete large foci of caseous necrosis. The caseous debris is yellow-white and cheesy.

ischemic cell death and coagulative necrosis modified by the liquefactive action of the bacteria and the attracted leukocytes. When the coagulative pattern is dominant, the process may be termed *dry gangrene*. Alternatively, when the liquefactive action is more pronounced, it may be designated *wet gangrene*.

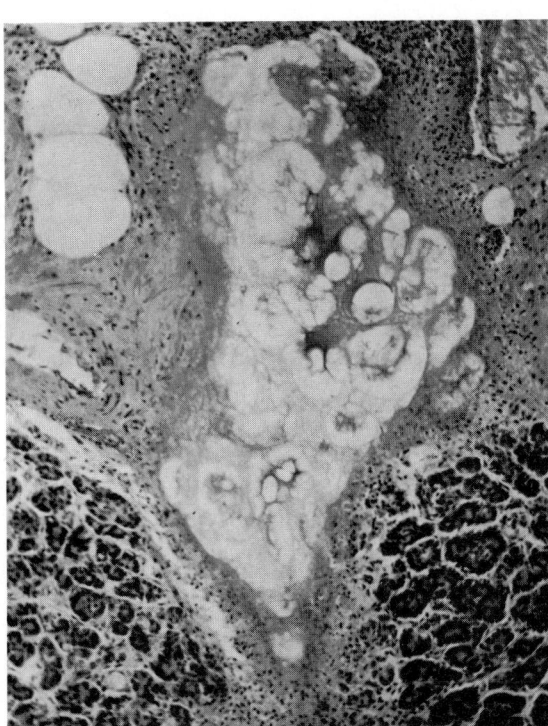

Figure 1–19. A sharply circumscribed focus of enzymatic necrosis of fat. Shadowy outlines of fat cells persist, surrounded by a zone of inflammation. The focus is surrounded by normal pancreatic substance.

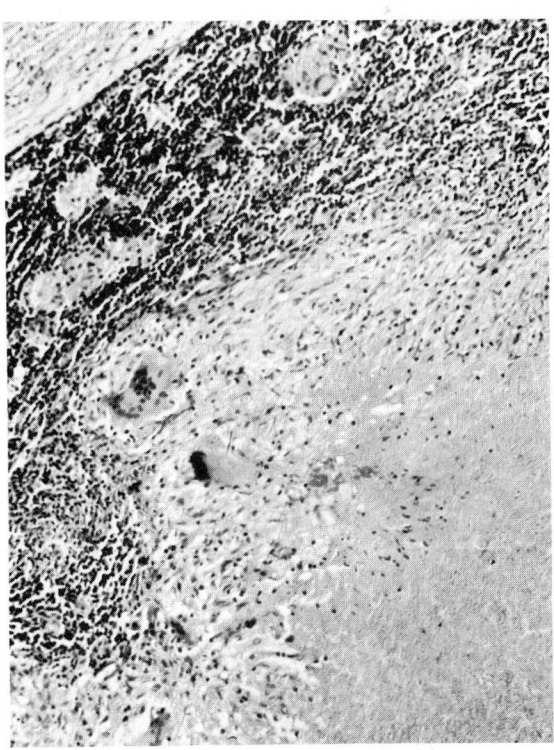

Figure 1–21. A tubercle. A large area of caseous tuberculosis is seen in lower right.

INTRACELLULAR ACCUMULATIONS

Under some circumstances, normal cells may accumulate abnormal amounts of various substances. The stockpiled substances fall into three categories: (1) *a normal cellular constituent* accumulated in excess, such as lipid, protein, and carbohydrates; (2) *an abnormal substance*, which may be a product of abnormal metabolism; and (3) *a pigment*, i.e., a colored substance. These substances may accumulate either transiently or permanently, and they may be harmless to the cells, but on occasion may also be severely toxic. The location of the substance may be in either the cytoplasm or the nucleus; in the former location *it is most frequently within lysosomes*. In some instances the cell may be producing the abnormal substance, and in others it may be merely storing products of pathologic processes occurring elsewhere in the body.

The processes that result in abnormal intracellular accumulations in non-neoplastic cells are many, but most can be divided into three general types (Fig. 1–22).

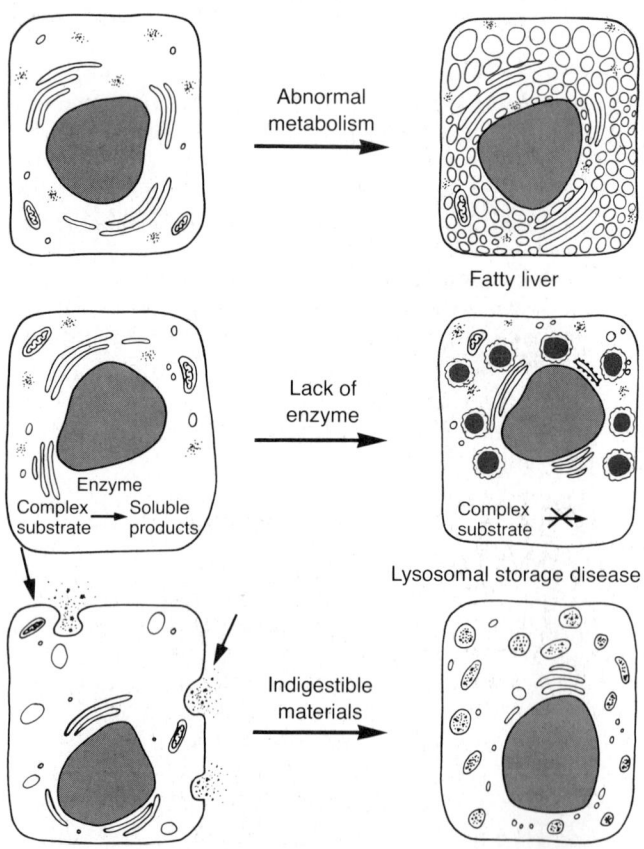

Figure 1–22. The major general mechanisms of intracellular accumulation: (1) abnormal metabolism, as in fatty change in the liver; (2) deficiency of critical enzymes that prevent breakdown of substrates—which accumulate in lysosomes, as in lysosomal storage diseases; and (3) inability to degrade phagocytosed particles, as in hemosiderosis and carbon pigment accumulation.

1. *A normal endogenous substance is produced at a normal or increased rate, but the rate of metabolism is inadequate to remove it.* An example of this type of process is *fatty change* in the liver, due to intracellular accumulation of lipids, mostly triglycerides.
2. *A normal or abnormal endogenous substance accumulates because it cannot be metabolized.* The most common cause of such failure of metabolism is *lack of an enzyme* that blocks a specific metabolic pathway, so that some particular metabolite cannot be used. Enzyme lack is due to a genetically determined inborn error of metabolism, and resulting diseases are referred to as *storage diseases*. Clinical entities result from the abnormal accumulations and are discussed more fully later (p. 144).
3. *An abnormal exogenous substance is deposited* and accumulates because the cell has neither the enzymic machinery to degrade the substance nor the ability to transport it to other sites. Accumulations of carbon particles, and such nonmetabolizable chemicals as silica particles, are examples of this type of alteration.

Whatever the nature and origin of the intracellular accumulation, it implies the storage of some product by individual cells. If overload is due to a systemic derangement and can be brought under control, the accumulation is reversible. On the other hand, in genetic storage diseases, because the metabolic error is not correctable, accumulation is progressive, and the cells may become so overloaded as to cause secondary injury, leading in some instances to death of the tissue and the patient.

LIPIDS

Fatty Change

Fatty change refers to any abnormal accumulation of fat within parenchymal cells. The term embraces the older terms *fatty degeneration* and *fatty infiltration*, which are misleading because neither a degenerative nor an infiltrative process is necessarily involved in the pathogenesis of the lipid accumulation. The more noncommittal term *fatty change* embraces the different pathogenetic mechanisms that may lead to accumulation of neutral fat within cells.

The appearance of fat vacuoles within cells, whether small or large, represents an absolute increase in intracellular lipids. It does not represent so-called unmasking of the normal fat content of cells. Although itself an indicator of nonlethal injury, fatty change is sometimes the harbinger of cell death and, in many situations, is encountered in cells adjacent to those that have died and undergone necrosis. Fatty change is often seen in the liver, since it is the major organ involved in fat metabolism, but it may also occur in heart, muscle, kidney, and other organs.

Pathogenesis of Fatty Liver

Under normal conditions, lipids are transported to the liver from adipose tissue and from the diet. From adipose tissue, lipids are released and transported in only one form—free fatty acids. Dietary lipids, on the other hand, are transported either as chylomicra (lipid particles consisting of triglyceride, phospholipid, and protein) or as free fatty acids (the latter being derived mainly from medium-chain triglycerides containing C_8 and C_{10} fatty acids). Free fatty acids enter the liver cell, and most are esterified to triglycerides. Some are converted to cholesterol, incorporated into phospholipids, or oxidized in mitochondria into ketone bodies. Some fatty acids are synthesized from acetate within the liver proper. *In order to be secreted by the liver, intracellular triglyceride must be complexed with specific apoprotein molecules called "lipid acceptor proteins" to form lipoproteins.*

Excess accumulation of triglycerides within the liver may result from defects in any one of the events in the sequence from fatty acid entry to lipoprotein exit (Fig. 1–23).[44] (1) *Excessive entry of free fatty acids into the liver.* In starvation, for example, adipose tissue fats are mobilized, and more fatty acids are brought to the liver, where they are synthesized into triglycerides. Corticosteroids also produce lipid mobilization from adipose tissue. (2) *Enhanced fatty acid synthesis.* (3) *Decreased fatty acid oxidation.* Both (2) and (3) result in increased esterification of fatty acids to triglycerides. (4) *Increased esterification of fatty acids to triglycerides, due to an increase in alpha-glycerophosphate,* the carbohydrate backbone involved in such esterification. This is thought to be one effect of alcohol poisoning. (5) *Decreased apoprotein synthesis.* As stressed earlier, this protein is necessary for the conversion of triglycerides to lipoproteins for excretion. This mechanism is the cause of lipid accumulation produced by carbon tetrachloride, phosphorus, and protein malnutrition. (6) *Impaired lipoprotein secretion from the liver.* This seems to be involved in an experimental model of fatty liver induced by the administration of orotic acid.

It should be apparent that different types of disturbances may affect the control of fat transport and metabolism, and that an individual etiologic agent may act at more than one locus within the complex process of fat metabolism. Alcohol, at least in industrialized countries, is perhaps the most common cause of fatty liver. Alcohol is a hepatotoxin that alters mitochondrial and microsomal functions. Increased free fatty acid synthesis, diminished triglyceride utilization, decreased fatty acid oxidation, a block in lipoprotein excretion, and enhanced lipolysis—thus increasing delivery and uptake of free fatty acids—have all been implicated in alcohol-induced fatty liver.[45] Other causes of fatty liver include protein malnutrition, diabetes mellitus, obesity, hepatotoxins, and certain chronic illnesses. Acute fatty liver of pregnancy[46] is an often fatal but fortunately rare condition in which the pathogenesis is unknown.

The significance of fatty change depends on the cause and severity of accumulation. It may have no effect on cellular function when mild. More severe fatty change may impair cellular function, but unless

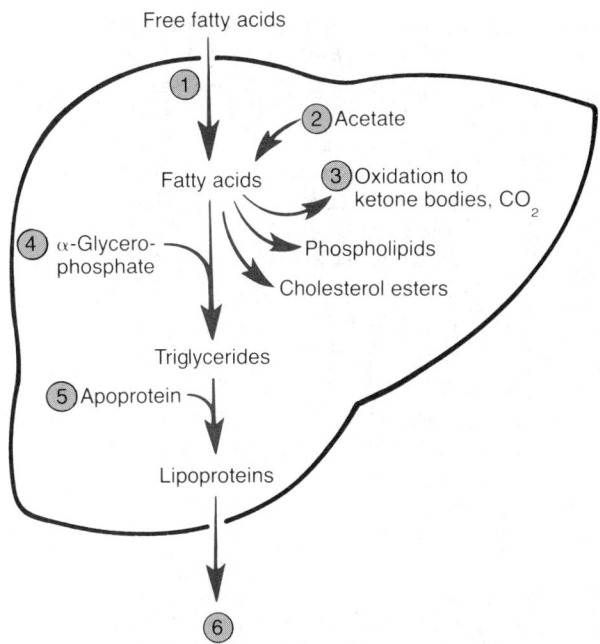

Figure 1–23. Possible mechanisms in the pathogenesis of fatty liver. The illustration depicts the uptake and metabolism of fatty acids by the liver, formation of triglycerides, and secretion of lipoproteins. Defects in any of the six numbered steps can lead to accumulation of triglycerides and fatty liver (see text).

some vital intracellular process is irreversibly impaired (such as in carbon tetrachloride poisoning), fatty change per se is reversible. The liver in the alcoholic, for example, may become enormously enlarged, leading to a progressive form of fibrosis of the liver termed *cirrhosis* (p. 941). However, in the alcoholic who has not yet developed fibrosis and who wisely adopts an alcohol-free balanced diet, it is quite remarkable to observe the return of the enlarged fatty liver to normal. As a severe form of injury, therefore, fatty change may be a harbinger of cell death, *but it should be emphasized that cells may die without undergoing fatty change.*

Fatty change is most often seen in the liver and heart, but it may occur in other organs.

LIVER. In the liver, mild fatty change may not affect the gross appearance. With progressive accumulation, the organ enlarges and becomes increasingly yellow until, in extreme instances, the liver may weigh 3 to 6 kg and be transformed into a bright yellow, soft, greasy organ.

Fatty change begins with the development of minute, membrane-bound inclusions (liposomes) closely applied to the endoplasmic reticulum. It is first manifested light microscopically by the appearance of small fat vacuoles in the cytoplasm around the nucleus. As the process progresses, the vacuoles coalesce to create cleared spaces that displace the nucleus to the periphery of the cell (Fig. 1–24). Occasionally, contiguous cells rupture, and the enclosed fat globules coalesce to produce so-called fatty cysts.

HEART. Lipid, as neutral fat, is quite frequently found in heart muscle in the form of small droplets. It occurs in two patterns. In one, prolonged moderate hypoxia, such as that produced by profound anemia, induces a "thrush breast" or "tigered" effect. Here the intracellular deposits of fat create grossly apparent bands of yellowed myocardium, alternating with bands of darker, red-brown, uninvolved myocardium. In the other pattern of fatty change, such as that produced by more profound hypoxia or some forms of myocarditis (e.g., diphtheritic), the myocardial cells are uniformly affected and the entire myocardium becomes flabby. Histologically, the fat in the myocardial cell tends to be distributed in minute cytoplasmic vacuoles. Diphtheria bacillus causes a fatty heart through the production of an exotoxin that interferes with the metabolism of carnitine, a cofactor for the oxidation of long-chain fatty acids.

In all organs, fatty change appears as clear vacuoles within parenchymal cells. Intracellular accumulations of water or polysaccharides (such as glycogen) may also produce clear vacuoles, and it becomes necessary to resort to special techniques to distinguish these three types of clear vacuoles. The identification of lipids requires the avoidance of fat solvents commonly employed in paraffin embedding for routine hematoxylin and eosin stains. To identify the fat, it is necessary to prepare frozen tissue sections of either fresh or aqueous formalin-fixed tissues. The sections may then be stained with Sudan IV or Oil Red-O, both of which impart an orange-red color to the contained lipids. The periodic acid–Schiff (PAS) reaction is commonly employed to identify glycogen, although it is by no means specific. When neither fat nor polysaccharide can be demonstrated within a clear vacuole, it is presumed to contain water or fluid with low protein content.

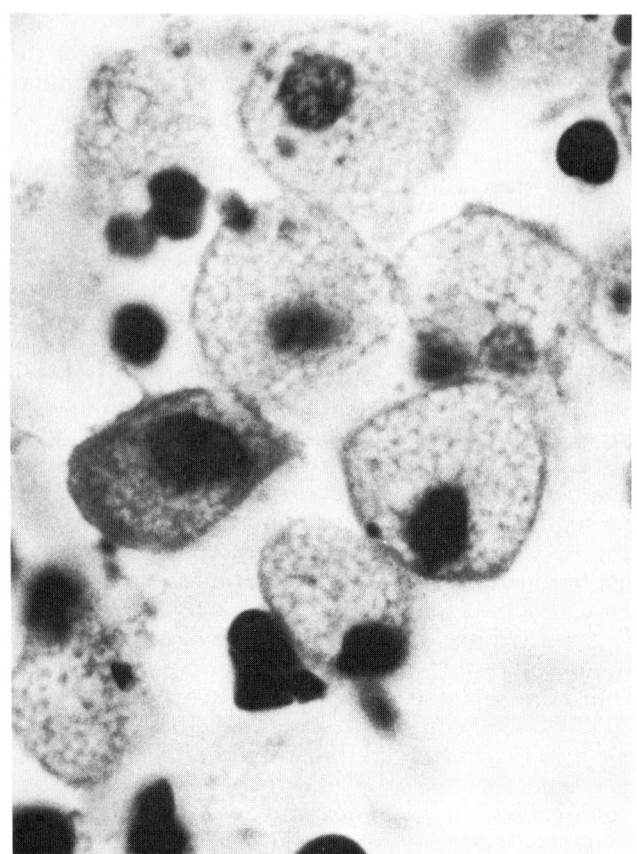

Figure 1–25. Lipid-laden macrophage (foam cell) from a focus of necrosis and inflammation, due to phagocytosis of lipids derived from injured cells.

Other Lipid Accumulations

As detailed in the previous section, the overload of parenchymal liver cells by triglycerides is termed "fatty change." By quite different mechanisms, intracellular accumulations of cholesterol and cholesterol esters are encountered in a variety of diseases. The most important disorder is atherosclerosis, in which smooth muscle cells and macrophages within the intimal layer of the aorta and large arteries are filled with lipid. Such cells appear foamy, and aggregates of them in the intima produce the cholesterol-laden atheromas characteristic of this serious disorder. Many of these fat-laden cells rupture, releasing the lipids into the ground substance of the intima. The mechanisms of lipid accumulation in these cells in atherosclerosis are discussed in Chapter 12. The extracellular cholesterol esters may crystallize in the shape of long needles, producing quite distinctive clefts in tissue sections.

Intracellular accumulations of cholesterol and cholesterol esters within macrophages are also characteristic of acquired and hereditary hyperlipidemic states (p. 140). Usually, these lesions are found in the subepithelial connective tissue of the skin and in tendons, producing tumorous masses known as *xanthomas.*

Foamy macrophages can also occur in foci of cell injury and inflammation, owing to phagocytosis of lipid derived from injured cells (Fig. 1–25).

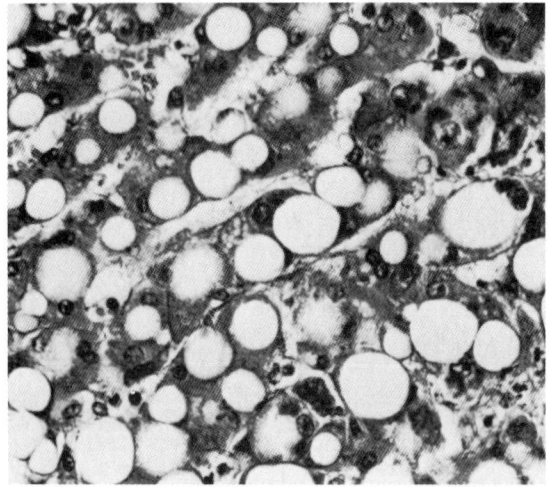

Figure 1–24. High-power detail of marked fatty change of liver. The variability in size of vacuoles is evident. In some cells, the well-preserved nucleus is squeezed into the displaced rim of cytoplasm about the fat vacuole.

Stromal Infiltration of Fat or Fatty Ingrowth

This is a form of *accumulation of lipids that has a mechanism and connotation completely different from those of intracellular fatty accumulation*. It is discussed at this time merely to differentiate it from the condition described as fatty change. Fatty ingrowth refers to the accumulation of lipids *within stromal connective tissue cells*.

Fatty ingrowth is most commonly encountered in the heart and pancreas, where adult adipose cells appear within the connective tissue stroma. In the heart, the right ventricle is generally more severely affected than the left. Usually, there is an increase of subepicardial fat that extends in continuity as finger-like projections between the muscle bundles (Fig. 1–26A). These insinuations may extend throughout the thickness of the myocardium to appear beneath the endocardium as small yellow deposits. The adult fat cells separate but do not damage the adjacent myocardial cells (Fig. 1–26B). In the pancreas, the fat is found in the connective tissue septa of the pancreatic lobules.

As far as is known, stromal infiltration of fat rarely affects cardiac or pancreatic function.

OTHER INTRACELLULAR ACCUMULATIONS

Proteins

Excesses of proteins within the cells sufficient to cause morphologically visible droplets occur principally in the renal epithelial cells of the proximal convoluted tubules and in plasma cells. The former example is seen in renal diseases associated with protein loss in the urine (proteinuria). If a protein leaks across the glomerular filter, it passes into the proximal tubule where it is reabsorbed by the epithelial cell through pinocytosis. Pinocytotic vesicles fuse with lysosomes to produce phagolysosomes, which appear as pink hyaline droplets within the cytoplasm of the tubular cell (Fig. 1–27). These aggregations do not impair cellular function. If the underlying cause for the proteinuria can be controlled, the protein excess is metabolized and the droplets disappear.

Plasma cells engaged in active synthesis of immunoglobulins may become overloaded with their synthetic product to produce large, homogeneous eosinophilic inclusions called *Russell bodies*. With an electron microscope, such Russell bodies are found to be localized within hugely distended cisternae of the endoplasmic reticulum, where protein synthesis occurs.

Glycogen

Excessive intracellular deposits of glycogen are seen in patients with an abnormality in either glucose or

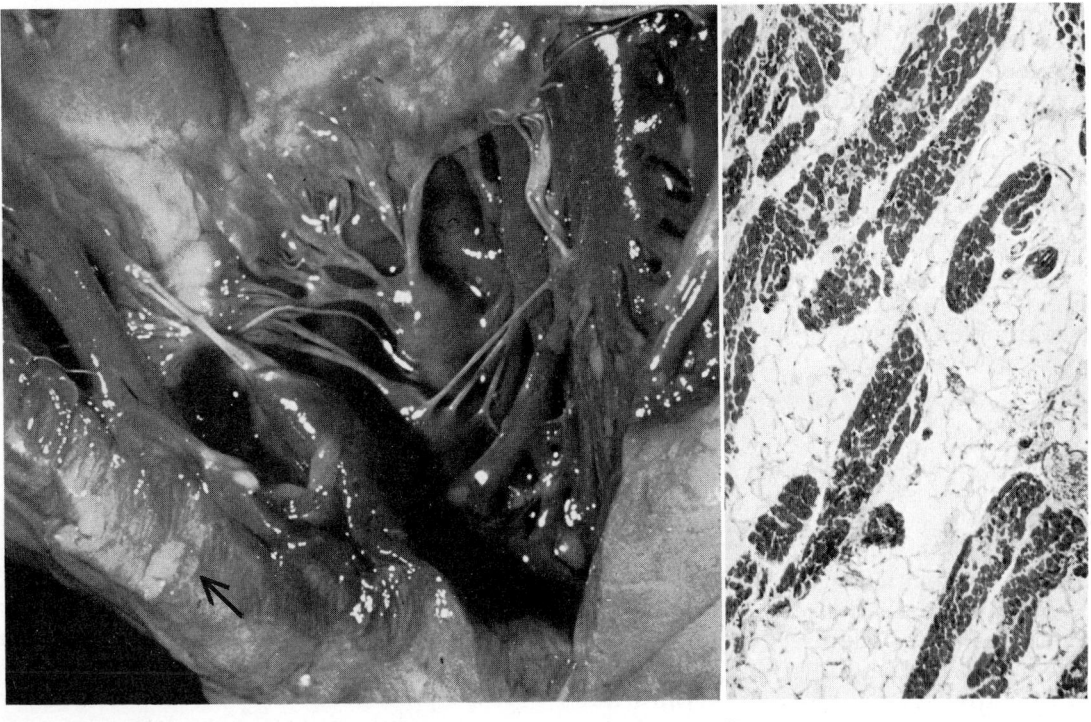

A   B

Figure 1–26. *A,* Stromal fatty infiltration (fatty ingrowth) of the heart. Streaks of yellow fat extending through the myocardium are visible on cross section of the ventricular wall *(arrow).* Small, pale yellow deposits are also present subendocardially in the columnae carneae. *B,* Stromal fatty infiltration (fatty ingrowth) of the heart. A microscopic detail to demonstrate normal myocardial fibers separated by adult fat tissue.

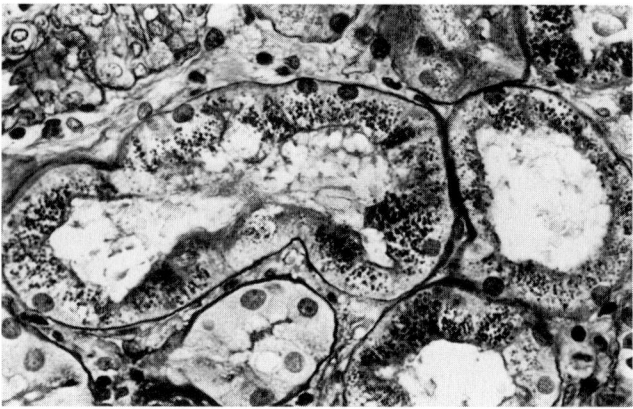

Figure 1–27. Hyaline droplets in the renal tubular epithelium.

glycogen metabolism. Whatever the clinical setting, the glycogen masses appear as clear vacuoles within the cytoplasm. Glycogen is best preserved in nonaqueous fixatives; for its localization, tissues are best fixed in absolute alcohol. Staining with Best's carmine or the PAS reaction imparts a rose-to-violet color to the glycogen, and diastase digestion prior to staining will serve as a further control by hydrolyzing the glycogen.

Diabetes mellitus is the prime example of a disorder of glucose metabolism. In this disease, glycogen is found in the epithelial cells of the distal portions of the proximal convoluted tubules and sometimes in the descending loop of Henle, as well as within liver cells, beta cells of the islets of Langerhans, and heart muscle cells. The intracellular glycogen produces marked vacuolization of the cytoplasm of renal tubular cells so that they appear to be entirely cleared (Fig. 1–28).

Glycogen also accumulates within the cells in a group of closely related disorders, all genetic, collectively referred to as the *glycogen storage diseases*, or *glycogenoses* (p. 144). In these diseases, some abnormal or normal form of glycogen cannot be metabolized. These diseases represent instances in which massive stockpiling of substances within cells causes secondary injury and cell death.

Complex Lipids and Carbohydrates
In certain forms of storage diseases resulting from inborn errors of metabolism, abnormal complexes of carbohydrates and lipids accumulate that cannot be metabolized normally (p. 144). These substances collect within cells throughout the body, principally those in the reticuloendothelial system. Examples include the mucopolysaccharidoses and Gaucher's, Tay-Sachs, and Niemann-Pick diseases, in which the abnormal products are complex lipids. The abnormal metabolites in all the storage diseases overflow into the blood and are phagocytized by reticuloendothelial cells, which thus become enlarged and develop an apparent foaminess to their cytoplasm, often producing massive splenomegaly and hepatomegaly. These intracellular deposits may become extreme and cause death not only of the cell but also of the patient.

Pigments
Pigments are colored substances, some of which are normal constituents of cells (e.g., melanin), whereas others are abnormal and collect in cells only under special circumstances.[47] The various pigments differ greatly in origin, chemical constitution, and biologic significance. Pigments can be either exogenous, coming from outside the body, or endogenous, synthesized within the body itself.

The most common *exogenous pigment* is *carbon* or coal dust, which is a virtually ubiquitous air pollutant of urban life. When inhaled, it is picked up by macrophages within the alveoli and is then transported through lymphatic channels to the regional lymph nodes in the tracheobronchial region. Accumulations of this pigment blacken the tissues of the lungs (*anthracosis*) and the involved lymph nodes. In coal miners and those living in heavily polluted environments, the aggregates of carbon dust may induce a fibroblastic reaction or even emphysema, and thus cause a serious lung disease known as *coal worker's pneumoconiosis. Tattooing* is a form of localized, exogenous pigmentation of the skin. The pigments inoculated are phagocytized by dermal macrophages in which they reside for the remainder of the life of the embellished. Although the pigments do not evoke any inflammatory response, they have a distressing habit of persisting as a reminder of bygone follies.

Endogenous pigments include lipofuscin, melanin, and certain derivatives of hemoglobin.

LIPOFUSCIN. Lipofuscin is an insoluble pigment, also known as lipochrome, and "wear-and-tear" or aging pigment. Its importance lies in its being the telltale sign of free radical injury and lipid peroxidation. The term is derived from the Latin (fuscus =

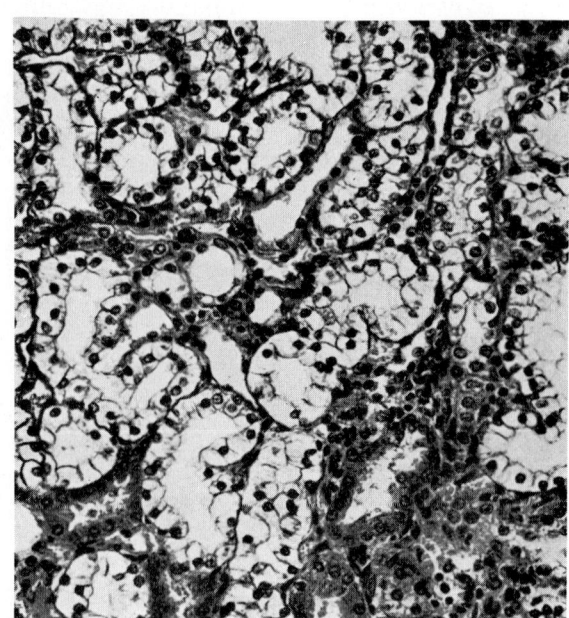

Figure 1–28. Glycogen vacuolation of the kidney. The epithelial cells of the affected tubules have distinct, well-preserved nuclei and sharp cell membranes.

brown), thus brown lipid. In tissue sections it appears as a yellow-brown, finely granular intracytoplasmic pigment. It is seen in cells undergoing slow, regressive changes and is particularly prominent in the liver and heart of aging patients, or patients with severe malnutrition and cancer cachexia. It is usually accompanied by organ shrinkage *(brown atrophy)*. On electron microscopy, the granules are highly electron dense, often have membranous structures in their midst, and are usually in a perinuclear location (Fig. 1–29).

Lipofuscin represents the indigestible residues of autophagic vacuoles (p. 28) formed during aging or atrophy. It appears to be composed of polymers of lipids and phospholipids complexed with protein,[48] *suggesting that it is derived through lipid peroxidation of polyunsaturated lipids of subcellular membranes.* With progressive polymerization, the lipofuscin loses its lipid characteristics, including its solubility in organic solvents and its staining with Sudan dyes. Lipofuscin is not injurious to the cell or its functions.

MELANIN. Melanin (derived from the Greek word *melas,* meaning black) is an endogenous, non–hemoglobin-derived, brown-black pigment formed when the enzyme tyrosinase catalyzes the oxidation of tyrosine to dihydroxyphenylalanine in melanocytes. It is the skin pigment, and its disorders are discussed in detail in Chapter 27. For all practical purposes, melanin is the only endogenous *brown-black* pigment. The only other that could be considered in this category is homogentisic acid, a black pigment that occurs in patients with alkaptonuria, a rare metabolic disease. Here the pigment is deposited in the skin, connective tissue, and cartilage, and the pigmentation is known as ochronosis.

HEMOSIDERIN. Hemosiderin is a hemoglobin-derived, golden-yellow to brown granular or crystalline pigment in which form iron is stored in cells. Iron metabolism and the synthesis of ferritin and hemosiderin are considered in detail on page 686. Suffice it to say here that iron is normally carried by transport proteins, transferrins. In cells it is normally stored in association with a protein, apoferritin, to form ferritin micelles, which can be identified with the electron microscope as characteristic, closely packed dense particles (6 nm in radius) arranged in tetrads.[49] Ferritin is a constituent of many cell types under normal conditions. *When there is a local or systemic excess of iron, ferritin forms hemosiderin granules,* which are easily seen with the light microscope. Thus, hemosiderin pigment represents aggregates of ferritin micelles (Fig. 1–30). Under normal conditions small amounts of hemosiderin can be seen in the mononuclear phagocytes of the bone marrow, spleen, and liver, all actively engaged in red cell breakdown.

In many pathologic states, excesses of iron cause hemosiderin to accumulate within cells, either as a localized process or as a systemic derangement. Under all circumstances the hemosiderin (having ferric ions in the ferritin micelles) can be visualized by such histochemical procedures as the Prussian blue reaction. In this reaction, which can be applied to both gross and histologic sections of tissue, colorless potassium ferrocyanide reacts with the ferric ions to create an insoluble blue ferric ferrocyanide. This reaction helps to differentiate the golden pigmentation of hemosiderin from that produced by lipofuscin, and can exclude non–iron-containing melanin.

Local excesses of iron and hemosiderin result from gross hemorrhages or the myriad minute hemorrhages that accompany severe vascular congestion. The best example of localized hemosiderosis is the common bruise. Following local hemorrhage, the area is at first red-blue. With lysis of the erythrocytes, the hemoglobin eventually undergoes transformation

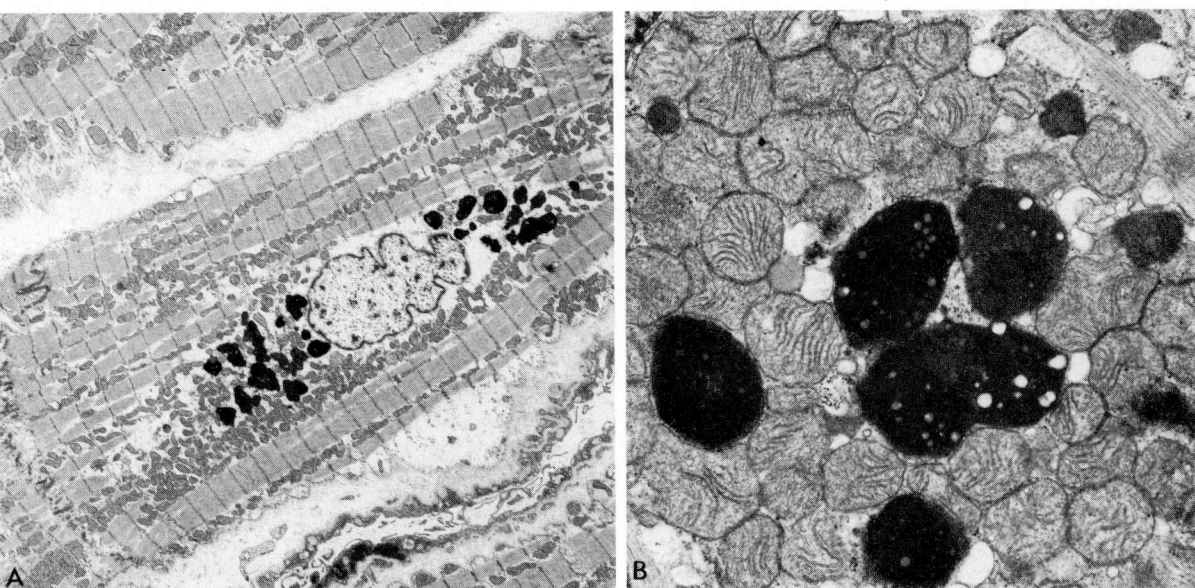

Figure 1–29. Lipofuscin. Lipofuscin granules in myocardial fiber. *A,* Low magnification, showing perinuclear localization. *B,* Electron-dense bodies are composed of lipid-protein complexes.

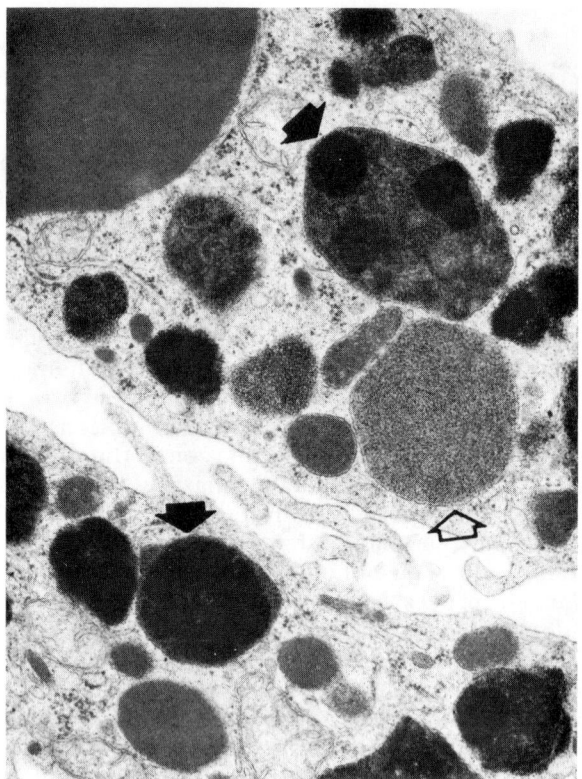

Figure 1–30. Hemosiderin granules in human splenic sinusoidal lining cells. Ferritin micelles *(open arrow)* are concentrated within phagosomes. The osmiophilic material *(arrows)* is probably lipid. A recently engulfed (undigested) red blood cell is present in the upper left hand corner.

to hemosiderin. Macrophages take part in this process by phagocytizing the red cell debris, and then lysosomal enzymes eventually convert the hemoglobin, through a sequence of pigments, into hemosiderin. The play of colors through which the bruise passes reflects these transformations. The original red-blue color of hemoglobin is transformed to varying shades of green-blue, comprising the local formation of biliverdin (green bile), then bilirubin (red bile), and thereafter the iron moiety of hemoglobin is deposited as golden-yellow hemosiderin.

Whenever there are causes for *systemic overload of iron*, hemosiderin is deposited in many organs and tissues, a condition called *hemosiderosis*. It is seen with (1) increased absorption of dietary iron, (2) impaired utilization of iron, (3) hemolytic anemias, and (4) transfusions, as the transfused red cells constitute an exogenous load of iron. These conditions are discussed in Chapter 14.

The morphologic appearance of the pigment and its staining reactions are identical whatever the mechanism of its accumulation. It appears as a coarse, golden, granular pigment lying within the cell's cytoplasm. When the basic cause is the localized breakdown of red cells, the pigmentation is found at first in the reticuloendothelial cells in the area. In systemic hemosideroses, it is found at first in the mononuclear phagocytes of the liver, bone marrow, spleen, and lymph nodes and in scattered macrophages throughout other organs such as the skin, pancreas, and kidneys. With progressive accumulation, parenchymal cells throughout the body (principally in the liver, pancreas, heart, and endocrine organs) become pigmented.

In most instances of systemic hemosiderosis, the intracellular accumulations of pigment do not damage the parenchymal cells and so do not impair organ function. However, the more extreme accumulations of iron in a disease called *hemochromatosis* (p. 950) are associated with liver and pancreatic damage, resulting in liver fibrosis and diabetes mellitus.

BILIRUBIN. Bilirubin is the normal major pigment found in bile. It is derived from hemoglobin but contains no iron. Its normal formation and excretion are vital to health, and jaundice is a common clinical disorder due to excesses of this pigment within cells and tissues. Bilirubin metabolism and jaundice are discussed in detail on page 913.

Bilirubin pigment within cells and tissues is visible morphologically only when the patient is rather severely jaundiced for some period of time. Even though this pigment is distributed throughout all tissues and fluids of the body, the *accumulations are most evident in the liver and kidneys.* In the liver, particularly with diseases caused by obstruction of the outflow of bile (such as cancers of the common bile duct or head of the pancreas), bilirubin is encountered within bile sinusoids, Kupffer cells, and hepatocytes. *In all these sites, it appears as a mucoid, green-brown to black, amorphous, globular deposit.* In advanced cases of such obstructive jaundice, the aggregates of pigment may be quite large, creating so-called bile lakes. These may cause necrosis of hepatocytes in the focal area. Bilirubin pigment is encountered in the renal tubular epithelial cells in various forms of jaundice.

SUBCELLULAR ALTERATIONS

Certain conditions are associated with rather distinctive alterations in cell organelles or cytoskeleton. Some of these alterations coexist with those described for acute lethal injury; others represent more chronic forms of cell injury, and others still are adaptive responses that involve specific cellular organelles. Here we shall touch on only some of the more common or interesting of these reactions.

LYSOSOMES: HETEROPHAGY AND AUTOPHAGY

As should be well known, lysosomes contain a variety of hydrolytic enzymes including acid phosphatase, glucuronidase, sulfatase, ribonuclease, collagenase, and so on. These enzymes are synthesized in the rough endoplasmic reticulum and then packaged into vesicles in the Golgi apparatus (Fig. 1–31). At this stage they are called *primary lysosomes*. Primary lysosomes fuse with membrane-bound vacuoles that contain material to be digested (the latter called *phagosomes*), forming *secondary lysosomes* or *phagolysosomes*.

Phagolysosomes originate in one of two ways: *Heterophagocytosis* refers to the uptake of materials from the external environment through the process of *endocytosis*. Uptake of particulate matter is known as *phagocytosis*, and that of soluble smaller macromolecules as *pinocytosis*. Heterophagy is most common in the "professional" phagocytes, such as

AUTOPHAGY   HETEROPHAGY

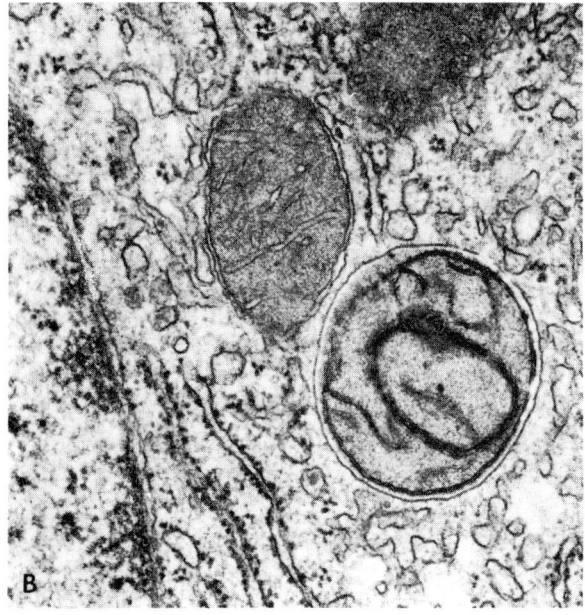

Figure 1–31. *A*, Schematic representation of autophagy *(left)* and heterophagy *(right)*. (Redrawn from Fawcett, D.W.: A Textbook of Histology. 11th ed. Philadelphia, W.B. Saunders Co., 1986, p. 17.) *B*, Electron micrograph of an autolysosome containing a degenerating mitochondrion and amorphous material.

neutrophils and macrophages, but it also occurs to a certain extent in many other cell types. Examples of heterophagocytosis include the uptake and digestion of bacteria by neutrophilic leukocytes, the removal of necrotic cells by macrophages, and the reabsorption of protein that may filter across the renal glomerulus by the pinocytotic vesicles of the proximal convoluted tubules (heteropinocytosis).

Autophagocytosis is the second process by which phagolysosomes are formed. In many instances, individual cell organelles, such as mitochondria or endoplasmic reticulum, suffer focal injury and must then be digested if the cell's normal function is to be preserved. The lysosomes involved in such autodigestion are called *autolysosomes* and the process is called *autophagy*. Autophagy is particularly pronounced in cells undergoing atrophy.

Both heterophagy and autophagy are very common intracellular processes and will be alluded to repeatedly in subsequent discussions of specific pathologic conditions such as inflammation, atrophy, and others. The enzymes in the lysosomes are capable of breaking down most proteins and carbohydrates, but some lipids remain undigested. Lysosomes with undigested debris may persist within cells as *residual bodies* or may be extruded. Certain indigestible pigments, such as carbon particles inhaled from the atmosphere, or pigment inoculated in tattoos, can persist in phagolysosomes of macrophages for decades.

Lysosomes are also wastebaskets in which cells sequester abnormal substances, particularly those of macromolecular nature, when these cannot be adequately metabolized. For example, in some hereditary diseases known as *lysosomal storage* disorders, deficiencies of certain enzymes that degrade mucopolysaccharides cause abnormal amounts of these compounds to be sequestered in the lysosomes. Such diseases are characterized by lysosomal deposits in cells all over the body, particularly in neurons, with often severe neurologic abnormalities.

HYPERTROPHY OF SMOOTH ENDOPLASMIC RETICULUM

Hypertrophy of smooth endoplasmic reticulum is an interesting adaptive response, first described in hamster liver cells[50] following administration of phenobarbital to these animals (Fig. 1–32). It is known that protracted human use of this hypnotic agent leads to a state of increased tolerance, so that repeated identical doses lead to progressively shorter time spans of sleep. The patients have thus "adapted" to the medication. The basis of this adaptation is induction of increased volume (hypertrophy) of the smooth endoplasmic reticulum (SER) of hepatocytes. Phenobarbital and other drugs are detoxified in the SER by the mixed-function oxidase electron transport pathway, the cytochrome P-450–multienzyme complex. P-450 catalyzes the metabolism of many other exogenous compounds, including CCl_4, potentially carcinogenic hydrocarbons, steroids, and insecticides. It is noteworthy that cells adapted to one drug have increased capacity to detoxify other drugs handled by the system, or endogenous metabolic products, such as bilirubin and bile acids.

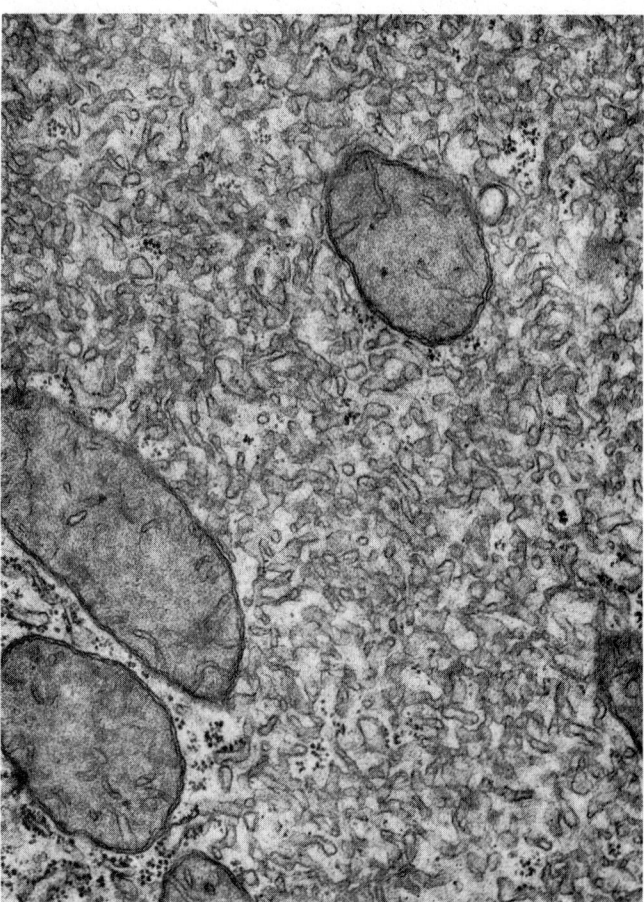

Figure 1–32. Electron micrograph of liver from phenobarbital-treated rat showing marked increase in smooth ER. (From Jones, A.L., and Fawcett, D.W.: Hypertrophy of the agranular endoplasmic reticulum in hamster liver induced by phenobarbital. J. Histochem. Cytochem., *14*:215, 1966. Courtesy of Dr. Fawcett.)

MITOCHONDRIAL ALTERATIONS

We have seen that mitochondrial dysfunction plays an important role in acute cell injury. In addition, however, various alterations in the number, size, and shape of mitochondria occur in some pathologic conditions. For example, in hypertrophy and atrophy there is an increase and decrease, respectively, in the number of mitochondria in cells. Mitochondria may assume an extremely large and abnormal shape (megamitochondria) (Fig. 1–33). These can be seen in the liver in alcoholic liver disease and in certain nutritional deficiencies, in skeletal muscle fibers in some myopathies, and in other cells in which there is alteration in mitochondrial growth and replication. In addition, large and highly pleomorphic mitochondria are seen commonly in tumor cells.

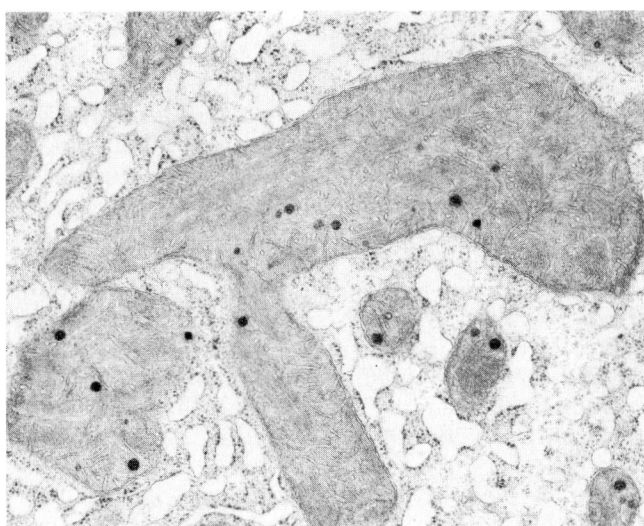

Figure 1–33. Enlarged, abnormally shaped mitochondria from liver of patient with alcoholic cirrhosis. Note also crystalline formations in mitochondria.

ABNORMALITIES OF CYTOSKELETON, CONTRACTILE PROTEINS, AND MEMBRANE SKELETON

Abnormalities of these components are emerging as important determinants of certain disease states, and these will be alluded to repeatedly throughout the book. The *cytoskeleton* consists of microtubules (20 to 25 nm in diameter), thin actin filaments (6 to 8 nm), thick myosin filaments (15 nm), and various classes of intermediate filaments (10 nm).[51,52] Several other nonpolymerized and nonfilamentous forms of contractile proteins also exist. Cytoskeletal abnormalities may be reflected by defects in cell function, such as cell locomotion and intracellular organelle movements, or in some instances by intracellular accumulations of fibrillar material. Only a few examples will be cited.

Functioning myofilaments and microtubules are essential for various stages of leukocyte migration and phagocytosis, and functional deficiencies of the cytoskeleton appear to underlie certain defects in leukocyte movement toward an injurious stimulus (chemotaxis, p. 46), or the ability of such cells to perform phagocytosis adequately. For example, a defect of microtubule polymerization in the *Chédiak-Higashi syndrome* causes delayed or decreased fusion of lysosomes with phagosomes in leukocytes, and thus impairs phagocytosis (p. 51). Cytochalasin B, a drug that inhibits microfilament function, also affects phagocytosis. Other drugs, such as colchicine, cause disruption of microtubules, thus blocking mitosis in the metaphase; morphologically, colchicine causes aggregations of crystalline tubulin within the cytoplasm. Defects in the organization of microtubules in spermatozoa inhibit sperm motility and cause male sterility, and a microtubule defect in the cilia of respi-ratory epithelium interferes with the ability of such epithelium to clear inhaled bacteria and predisposes to lung infections (the immotile cilia syndrome) (p. 777).

Intermediate filaments are constituents of a variety of cell types. The principal intermediate filaments are *keratin* filaments, *neurofilaments, glial* filaments, *vimentin,* and *desmin.* Intermediate filaments are thought to mechanically integrate the organelles within the cytoplasm. Two common histologic entities have been traced to accumulations of intermediate filaments. One is the *Mallory body,* or "alcoholic hyalin," an eosinophilic intracytoplasmic inclusion in liver cells (Fig. 1–34A), which is highly characteristic of alcoholic liver disease but whose nature until recently has been obscure. Such inclusions are now known to be composed largely of intermediate filaments (Fig. 1–34B) of predominantly *prekeratin* composition,[53] suggesting that a cytoskeletal defect with loss of intracellular organization may be one mechanism of cell injury in alcoholic liver disease. Another is the *neurofibrillary tangle* found in the brains of patients with Alzheimer's disease, an important cause of presenile dementia. These tangles contain microtubule-associated proteins and neurofilaments, and are thought to represent the end stage of a disrupted neuronal cytoskeleton.[54]

Finally, mention should be made of the *"mem-*

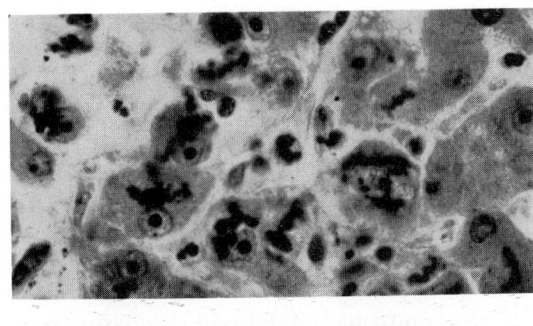

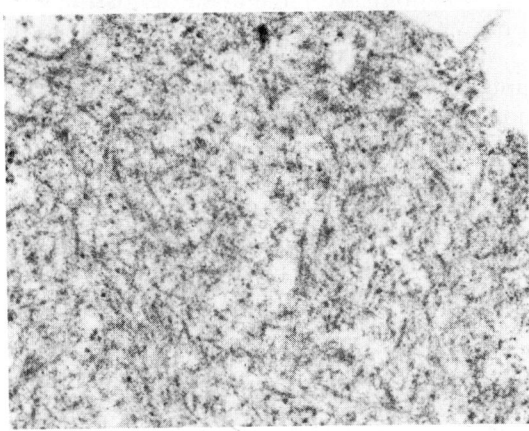

Figure 1–34. *A,* The liver of alcohol abuse (chronic alcoholism). Hyaline inclusions in hepatic parenchymal cells appear as dark, irregular networks disposed about the nuclei. *B,* Electron micrograph of alcoholic hyalin. The material is composed of intermediate (prekeratin) filaments and an amorphous matrix.

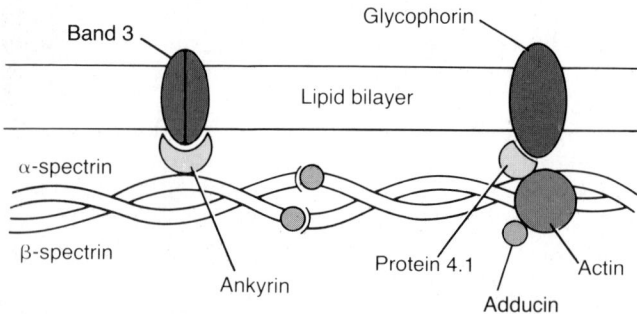

Figure 1–35. Schematic view of the proteins that form the cyto-skeleton of the red cell membrane. Spectrin consists of alpha- and beta-chains that lie on the inner surface of the cell membrane and are connected to membrane glycoproteins (band 3, glycophorin) through ankyrin and protein 4.1.

brane skeleton," the filamentous meshwork of proteins lining the inner membrane surface of most cells. In the erythrocyte, the major proteins consist of *spectrin, actin, protein 4.1,* and *ankyrin* (Fig. 1–35), and their interactions determine the structural stability of the cell membrane.[55] Membrane skeletal flaws may account for some important red cell disorders (p. 663). For example, in some patients with *hereditary spherocytosis,* in which the red cells are spheroid rather than discoid (and more prone to fragmentation), the defect in red cell shape may be caused by abnormal or deficient spectrin that is incapable of binding protein 4.1 and thus unable to maintain the stability of the red cell membrane.[56] Since spectrin and protein 4.1–like molecules are also present in other cell types (e.g., platelets, endothelium),[57] defects in membrane skeletal proteins may play a role in other forms of cell injury.

CELLULAR ADAPTATIONS OF GROWTH AND DIFFERENTIATION

Up to this point we have been discussing regressive alterations induced in cells by potentially lethal stimuli. As we explained earlier, cells must constantly adapt, even under normal conditions, to changes in their environment. These physiologic adaptations usually represent responses of cells to normal stimulation by hormones or endogenous chemical substances, for example, as in the enlargement of the breast and induction of lactation by pregnancy. Pathologic adaptations may have similar mechanisms, but they provide the cells with the ability to modulate their environment and perhaps escape injury. Cellular adaptation, then, is a state that lies intermediate between the normal, unstressed cell and the injured, overstressed cell.

There are numerous types of cellular adaptations. Some involve up- or down-*regulation of specific cellular receptors* involved in metabolism of certain components—for example, in the regulation of cell-surface receptors involved in the uptake and degrada-

tion of low-density lipoproteins (LDL) (p. 140). Others are associated with the *induction of new proteins* by the cells. Such proteins may protect cells from certain forms of injury (e.g., heat shock proteins[58]) or may make cells more adhesive for other cells (as, for example, in the induction of adhesive molecules on endothelial cells in inflammation (p. 46). Other adaptations involve a switch by cells from producing one type of a family of proteins to another, or to markedly overproduce one protein; such is the case in cells producing various types of collagens and extracellular matrix proteins in chronic inflammation and fibrosis (p. 78). Recent molecular techniques have increased our understanding of how such cellular responses occur—at levels of *receptor binding,* or *signal transduction,* or *transcription,* or *translation,* or *regulation of protein packaging and release*—as will be alluded to in other chapters in this book.

In this section we will consider the adaptive changes in cell growth and differentiation that are particularly important in pathologic conditions. These include atrophy (decrease in cell size), hypertrophy (increase in cell size), hyperplasia (increase in cell number), metaplasia (change in cell type), and dysplasia. Some of the intracellular accumulations, discussed earlier, such as fatty change, can be considered forms of cell adaptation.

ATROPHY

Shrinkage in the size of the cell by loss of cell substance is known as atrophy. It represents a form of adaptive response. When a sufficient number of cells are involved, the entire tissue or organ diminishes in size, or becomes atrophic.

The causes of atrophy are the following:

1. decreased workload
2. loss of innervation
3. diminished blood supply
4. inadequate nutrition
5. loss of endocrine stimulation
6. aging

When a limb is immobilized in a plaster cast, or when muscles become paralyzed from loss of innervation as in poliomyelitis, atrophy of muscle ensues. In late adult life, the brain undergoes progressive atrophy, presumably as arteriosclerosis narrows its blood supply (Fig. 1–36) and the gonads shrink with depletion of endocrine stimulation. Some of these stimuli are physiologic (e.g., the loss of endocrine stimulation following the menopause), whereas others are clearly pathologic (e.g., loss of nerves). However, the fundamental cellular change is identical in all, representing a retreat by the cell to a smaller size at which survival is still possible. By bringing into balance cell volume and lower levels of blood supply, nutrition, or trophic stimulation, a new equilibrium is achieved. Although *atrophic cells may have diminished function, they are not dead.*

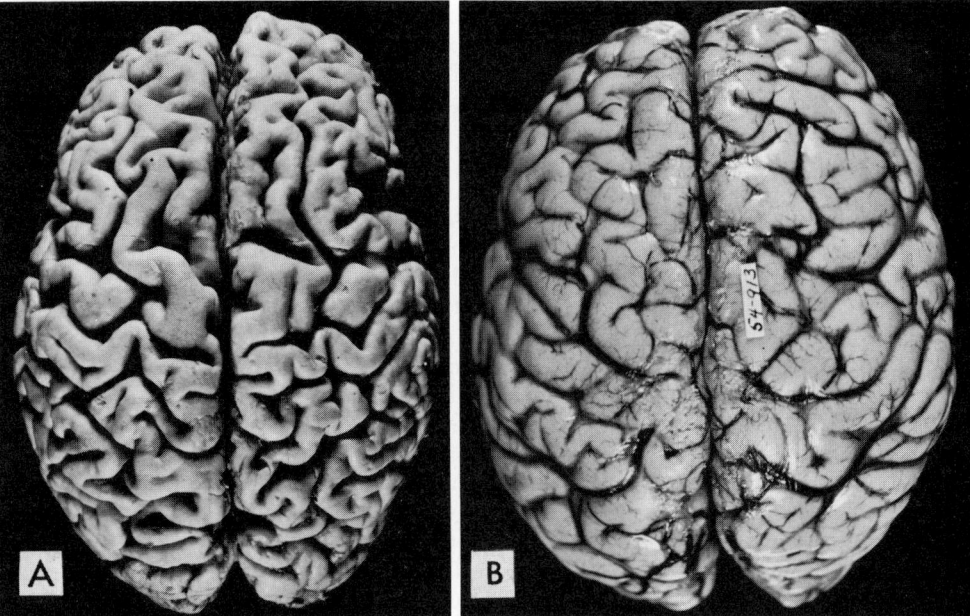

Figure 1-36. *A*, Physiologic atrophy of the brain in an 82-year-old male. The meninges have been stripped. *B*, Normal brain of 36-year-old male.

Atrophy represents a reduction in the structural components of the cell. The cell contains fewer mitochondria and myofilaments and a lesser amount of endoplasmic reticulum. The biochemical mechanisms responsible for atrophy are incompletely understood, but it must be stressed that there is a finely regulated balance between protein synthesis and degradation in normal cells, and either decreased synthesis, increased catabolism, or both may cause atrophy. Hormones, particularly insulin, thyroid hormones, glucocorticoids, and prostaglandins, influence such protein turnover. Thus, only slight increases of degradation over a long period of time may result in atrophy, as seems to occur in some muscle dystrophies.

In many situations atrophy is also accompanied by marked increases in the number of *autophagic vacuoles*. As stated earlier, these are membrane-bound vacuoles within the cell that contain fragments of cell components (e.g., mitochondria, ER), which are destined for destruction, and into which the lysosomes discharge their hydrolytic contents. The cellular components are then digested. The formation of autophagic vacuoles can be surprisingly rapid. For example, in experimental occlusion of the portal venous blood supply to the liver lobe, large numbers of autophagic vacuoles are formed within 5 to 10 min after the blood supply is occluded.

Some of the cell debris within the autophagic vacuole may resist digestion and persist as membrane-bound *residual bodies* that may remain as a sarcophagus in the cytoplasm. An example of such residual bodies is the *lipofuscin granules*, discussed earlier (p. 24). When present in sufficient amounts, they impart a *brown discoloration* to the tissue (brown atrophy).

Obviously, atrophy may progress to the point at which cells are injured and die. If the blood supply is inadequate even to maintain the life of shrunken cells, injury and cell death may supervene. The atrophic cells are then replaced by connective and adipose tissue.

HYPERTROPHY

Hypertrophy refers to an increase in the size of cells and, with such change, an increase in the size of the organ. Thus, the hypertrophied organ has no new cells, just larger cells. The increased size of cells is due not to an increased intake of fluid, called cellular swelling or edema, but to the synthesis of more structural components.

Hypertrophy can be *physiologic* or *pathologic* and is caused by increased functional demand or by specific hormonal stimulation. The physiologic growth of the uterus during pregnancy involves both hypertrophy and hyperplasia. The cellular hypertrophy is stimulated by estrogenic hormones through smooth muscle estrogen receptors, which allow for interactions of the hormones with nuclear DNA, eventually resulting in increased synthesis of smooth muscle proteins and increase in cell size. This is then physiologic hypertrophy effected by hormonal stimulation. Hypertrophy as an adaptive response was cited earlier in the discussion of muscular enlargement. The striated muscle cells in both the heart and skeletal muscle are most capable of hypertrophy, perhaps because they cannot adapt to increased metabolic demands by mitotic division and the formation of more cells to share the work.

The change that produces hypertrophy of striated muscle appears to be principally increased workload, implying an increase in metabolic activity. There is synthesis of more membranes, more enzymes, more ATP, and more filaments capable of achieving an equilibrium between the demand and the cell's functional capacity. The greater number of myofilaments means an increased workload but with a level of metabolic activity per unit volume of cell not different from that borne by the normal myofilament. Thus, the draft horse readily pulls the load that would break the back of a pony.

Perhaps the best example of adaptive hypertrophy occurs in the heart in a variety of cardiovascular diseases that place increased burdens on the myocardium (Fig. 1–37). In patients with hypertension (high blood pressure), the heart, which must contract against increased pressures in the aorta, hypertrophies and may achieve weights of 700 to 800 gm instead of the normal weight of 350 gm. Cardiac hypertrophy also occurs secondary to diseased cardiac valves. When valves are damaged, there is incomplete emptying of the cardiac chambers and stretching of the cardiac muscle fibers. The precise signal for hypertrophy under these conditions is unknown. ATP depletion, stretching of muscle fibers, activation by cell degradation products, and hormonal factors (e.g., thyroid hormones) have all been implicated.[59] Whatever the mechanism, there follows increased RNA synthesis, increased protein synthesis, and the formation of a greater number of all organelles, including mitochondria, sarcoplasmic reticulum, and especially myofibrils.

Whatever the exact mechanism of hypertrophy, it eventually reaches a limit beyond which enlargement of muscle mass is no longer able to compensate

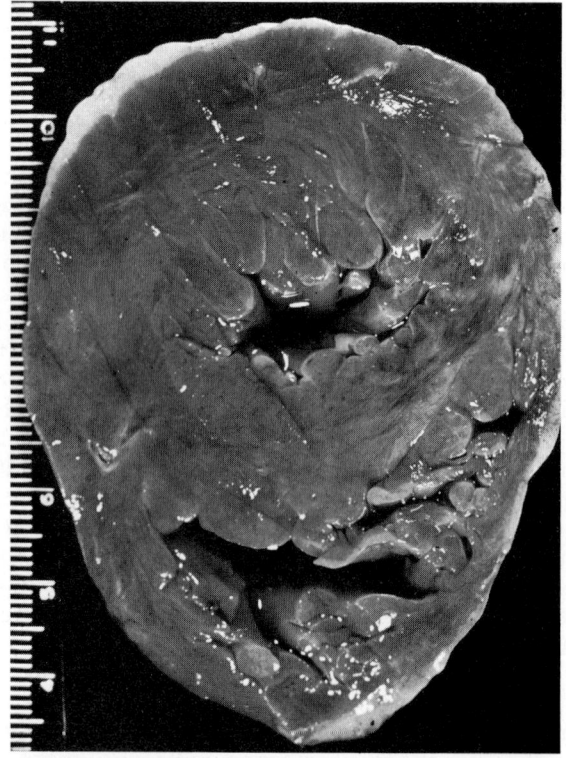

Figure 1–37. Cross section of a heart with marked left ventricular hypertrophy. The left ventricular wall (top) is over 2 cm in thickness (normal = 1 to 1.5 cm). In the interventricular septum, the mottled, dark area is a focus of fresh ischemic necrosis (myocardial infarct).

for the increased burden, and cardiac failure ensues. At this stage, a number of "degenerative" changes occur in the myocardial fibers, of which the most important are lysis and loss of myofibrillar contractile elements. The limiting factors for continued hypertrophy and the causes of the regressive changes are poorly understood; they may be due to limitation of the vascular supply to the enlarged fibers, diminished oxidative capabilities of mitochondria, or alterations in protein synthesis and degradation.

Hypertrophy can also occur at the level of individual organelles, as in the example of hypertrophy of the smooth endoplasmic reticulum described earlier (p. 28).

HYPERPLASIA

Just as enlargement of cells, hypertrophy, represents a response to increased functional demand, cells capable of mitotic division may divide when stressed or stimulated to increased activity. *Hyperplasia therefore constitutes an increase in the number of cells in an organ or tissue, which may then have increased volume.* Hypertrophy and hyperplasia are closely related and often develop concurrently. Both hypertrophy and hyperplasia take place if the cellular population is capable of synthesizing DNA, thus permitting mitotic division.

Not all adult cell types have the same capacity for hyperplastic growth. Although epidermis, intestinal epithelium, hepatocytes, fibroblasts, and bone marrow cells can undergo profound hyperplasia, nerve cells and, for all practical purposes, cardiac and skeletal muscle cells have no capacity for hyperplastic growth. Intermediate among these are such tissues as bone, cartilage, and smooth muscle. The determinants of cell growth control are discussed more fully on page 76.

Hyperplasia traditionally has been divided into *physiologic* and *pathologic* hyperplasia.

PHYSIOLOGIC HYPERPLASIA. The two most common types of physiologic hyperplasia are (1) *hormonal hyperplasia*, best exemplified by the proliferation of the glandular epithelium of the female breast at puberty and during pregnancy, and the physiologic hyperplasia that occurs in the pregnant uterus; and (2) *compensatory hyperplasia*, e.g., the hyperplasia that occurs when a portion of the liver is removed (partial hepatectomy). The ancient Greeks knew of the capacity of the liver to regenerate. According to the myth, Prometheus was chained to a mountain, and his liver was daily devoured by a vulture, only to regenerate anew every night.[60] In fact, the mitotic activity of hepatocytes increases after partial hepatectomy, eventually restoring the liver to normal weight. At this time (usually 12 days after partial hepatectomy in the rat), further growth stops. This is therefore a regulated form of hyperplasia that results in *regeneration* of the liver without appreciable increase in size or abnormal function. A similar sequence occurs in the epidermis following skin abrasion. If the superficial skin layers are removed, cells of the basal layer undergo increased mitotic activity that results in regeneration of the superficial layers and restoration of the original skin.

The model of partial hepatectomy has been especially useful in following the sequence of events and mechanisms involved in compensatory hyperplasia. In the normal mature liver, only 0.5 to 1.0% of cells are dividing at any one time, as can be shown autoradiographically by injecting tritiated thymidine into the experimental animal. An increase in the number of DNA-synthesizing cells begins as early as 12 hr after hepatectomy and peaks between one and two days, when about 10% of all cells may be involved in DNA synthesis (Fig. 1–38). Subsequently, DNA synthesis declines, and by the time the liver mass is restored (at one to two weeks), the liver cells become quiescent again.

There is substantial evidence that cell proliferation in this setting is initiated and subsequently potentiated by polypeptide growth factors and hormones (e.g., glucagon).[61] Current studies implicate *transforming growth factor α* (p. 77), produced by the remnant liver cells, as an important stimulator of hepatic cell regeneration.[62] Initiation of cell growth is associated with specific and sequential increases in the expression of proto-oncogenes (e.g., *c-fos, c-myc,*

and *c-ras,* p. 282) involved in cell proliferation.[62] Conversely, cessation of cell growth, after the liver mass has been restored, appears to be caused by growth *inhibitors* produced in the liver itself. One of these growth inhibitors is transforming growth factor *β* (TGF *β*, p. 77), a polypeptide produced by nonparenchymal cells of the liver after the major wave of cell division.[63]

PATHOLOGIC HYPERPLASIA. Most forms of *pathologic hyperplasia are instances of excessive hormonal stimulation or are the effects of growth factors on target cells. An example of hormonally induced hyperplasia is hyperplasia of the endometrium.* After a normal menstrual period, there is a rapid burst of proliferative activity, which might be viewed as reparative proliferation or physiologic hyperplasia in the endometrium. As is well known, this proliferation is potentiated by pituitary hormones and ovarian estrogen. It is brought to a halt by the rising levels of progesterone, usually about 10 to 14 days before the anticipated menstrual period. In some instances, however, the balance between estrogen and progesterone is disturbed. This results in absolute or relative increases in the amount of estrogen, or both, with consequent hyperplasia of the endometrial glands. Although this form of hyperplasia is a common cause of abnormal menstrual bleeding, the hyperplastic process remains controlled nonetheless: if the estrogenic stimulation abates, the hyperplasia disappears. Thus, it responds to regular growth control of cells. As will be discussed in the chapter on neoplasia (p. 250), it is this response to normal regulatory control mechanisms that differentiates benign pathologic hyperplasias from cancer. However, it should be stressed here that *pathologic hyperplasia constitutes a fertile soil in which cancerous proliferation may eventually arise.* Thus, patients with hyperplasia of the endometrium are at increased risk of developing endometrial cancer (see p. 73).

Hyperplasia is also an important response of connective tissue cells in wound healing, in which proliferating fibroblasts and blood vessels (granulation tissue, p. 73) aid in repair. Under these circumstances mitogenic growth factors are responsible for the hyperplasia; for example, a factor derived from platelets (platelet-derived growth factor) is released when blood clots, binds to receptors on the surface of fibroblasts, and stimulates fibroblast proliferation (p. 75). Stimulation by growth factors is also involved in the hyperplasia that is associated with certain *virus infections,* such as papilloma viruses, causing skin warts. These warts are composed largely of masses of hyperplastic epithelium.

Although hypertrophy and hyperplasia are, by definition, two distinct processes, it is clear that in many instances both occur together and, further, are triggered by the same mechanism. Estrogen-induced growth in the uterus is the classic example. Uterine epithelium and smooth muscle undergo both increased DNA synthesis and enlargement of cells. In

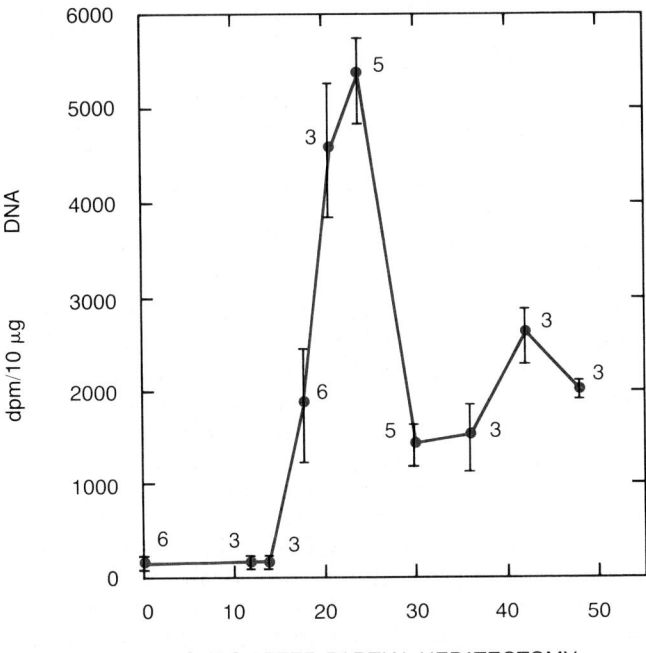

Figure 1–38. One-hour incorporation of ³H-thymidine into hepatic DNA in 200-gm male Sprague Dawley rats at intervals after partial hepatectomy. Vertical lines indicate the standard error of the mean, numbers the number of rats per point. (From Bucher, N.L.R., and McGowan, J.A.: Regulatory mechanisms. *In* Wright, R., Albert, K.G.M.M., Karran, S., and Millward-Sadler, G.H. [eds.]: Liver and Biliary Disease. Philadelphia, W.B. Saunders Co., 1979, pp. 210–227.)

fact, there is probably more hypertrophy than hyperplasia in this condition. Both processes are initiated by binding of estrogen to a receptor complex in the cytoplasm of target cells. Even in nondividing cells that undergo only hypertrophy (such as myocardial fibers), events occur that result in an increase in or derepression of DNA synthesis; the nuclei thus have a much higher DNA content than normal myocardial cells. In fact, a large percentage of cells from severely hypertrophied hearts are polyploid, and large, bizarre nuclei are seen in hypertrophied myocardial fibers. A likely explanation for such polyploidy is that the cells arrest in the G_2 phase of the cell cycle without undergoing mitosis.

METAPLASIA

Metaplasia is a reversible change in which one adult cell type (epithelial or mesenchymal) is replaced by another adult cell type. It, too, may represent an adaptive substitution of cells more sensitive to stress by other cell types better able to withstand the adverse environment. Such adaptive metaplasia is best seen in the squamous metaplasia that occurs in the respiratory tract in response to chronic irritation. In the habitual cigarette smoker, the normal columnar ciliated epithelial cells of the trachea and bronchi are often replaced focally or widely by stratified squamous epithelial cells. Similar changes may be encountered in chronic infections of the bronchi and bronchioles. Stones in the excretory ducts of the salivary glands, pancreas, or bile ducts may cause replacement of the normal secretory columnar epithelium by nonfunctioning stratified squamous epithelium (Fig. 1–39). A

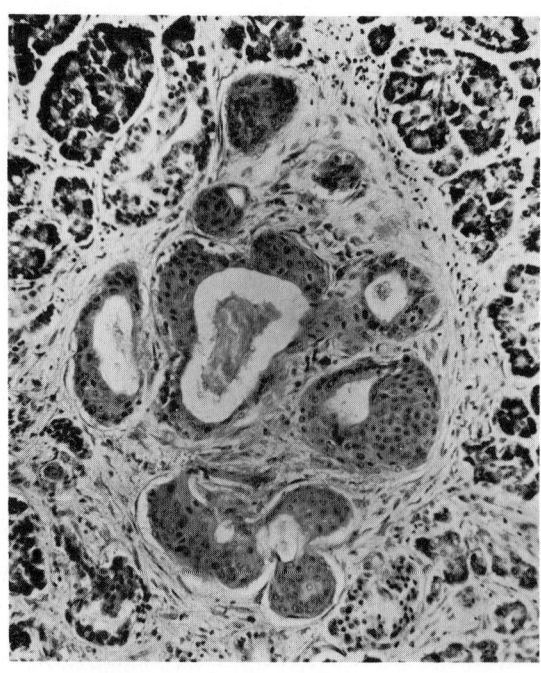

Figure 1–39. Metaplastic transformation of adult columnar epithelial cells to adult stratified squamous cells in pancreatic ducts.

deficiency of vitamin A induces squamous metaplasia in the respiratory epithelium. In all these instances, the more rugged stratified squamous epithelium is able to survive under circumstances in which the more fragile specialized epithelium most likely would have succumbed.

Although the squamous metaplastic cells in the respiratory tract, for example, are capable of surviving, an important protective mechanism—mucus secretion—is lost. Thus, epithelial metaplasia is a two-edged sword and, in most circumstances, represents an undesirable change. *Moreover, the influences that predispose to such metaplasia, if persistent, may induce cancer transformation in metaplastic epithelium.* Thus, the common form of cancer in the respiratory tract is composed of squamous cells.

Metaplasia may also occur in mesenchymal cells but less clearly as an adaptive response. Fibroblasts may become transformed to osteoblasts or chondroblasts to produce bone or cartilage where it is normally not encountered. For example, bone is occasionally formed in soft tissues, particularly in foci of injury. This process represents a form of "divergent differentiation."

DYSPLASIA

Dysplasia is a controversial term in pathology, used both loosely and commonly. Strictly speaking, *dysplasia means deranged development; however, in common usage it is applied to either epithelial or mesenchymal cells, principally the former, that have undergone proliferation and atypical cytologic alterations involving cell size, shape, and organization.* It is not an adaptive process but is considered here because it is closely related to hyperplasia; indeed, it is sometimes called *atypical hyperplasia.*

Epithelial dysplasia presents as a loss of normal orientation of one epithelial cell to the other, accompanied by alterations in cellular size and shape, nuclear size and shape, and staining characteristics. It is most commonly encountered in lining epithelia, mostly squamous epithelia—for example, in the uterine cervix. The dysplastic stratified squamous epithelium is thickened by hyperplasia of basal cells, accompanied by disordered maturation of the cells as they proceed to the surface layers. Mitotic figures are found only in the basal layer in normal cervical mucosa but, in dysplastic cervical epithelium, they may be found in the middle levels or even toward the surface. The increased proliferative activity produces greater amounts of DNA and more intense basophilia of the nuclei (Fig. 1–40). Although mitoses are increased in number, they are usually not abnormal, as is characteristic of cancer.

Dysplastic changes also are frequently encountered in the metaplastic squamous epithelium of the respiratory tract in habitual cigarette smokers. *In both the cervix and the respiratory tract, such dysplasia is strongly implicated as a precursor of cancer.* Dysplastic changes are often found adjacent to foci of cancer-

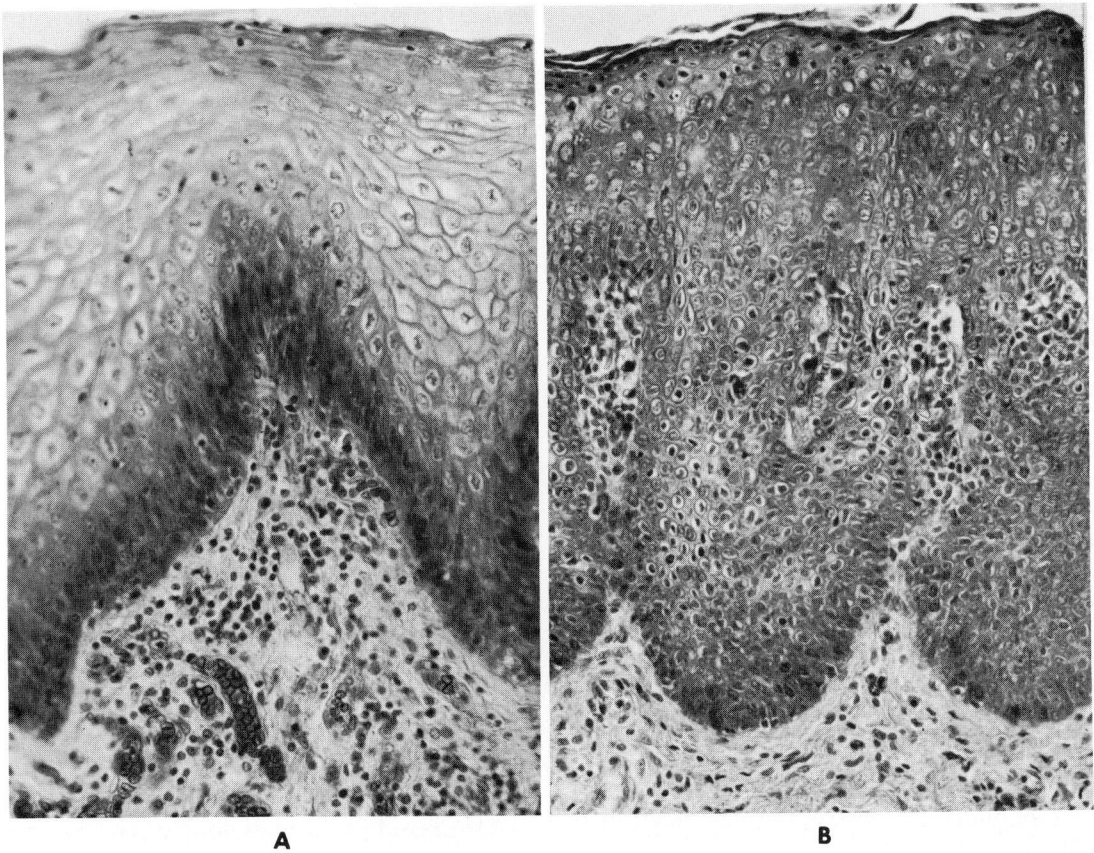

A   **B**

Figure 1–40. *A,* Normal stratified squamous epithelium. *B,* Dysplastic stratified squamous epithelium. The basal cells are hyperplastic and form a zone many cells thick. The dysplastic cells are deeply chromatic and disorganized.

ous transformation and, in long-term studies of cigarette smokers, epithelial dysplasia almost invariably precedes in time the appearance of cancer. However, from many clinical studies, it is known that dysplasia does not necessarily progress to cancer. The changes may be reversible and, with removal of the putative inciting causes, the epithelium may revert to normal.

SUNDRY ALTERATIONS

CALCIFICATION

Pathologic calcification implies the abnormal deposition of calcium salts, together with smaller amounts of iron, magnesium, and other mineral salts. It is a common process occurring in a variety of pathologic conditions. When the deposition occurs in nonviable or dying tissues, it is known as *dystrophic calcification;* it may occur despite normal serum levels of calcium and in the absence of derangements in calcium metabolism. In contrast, the deposition of calcium salts in vital tissues is known as *metastatic calcification,* and it almost always reflects some derangement in calcium metabolism, leading to hypercalcemia.

DYSTROPHIC CALCIFICATION. This alteration is encountered in areas of necrosis, whether they are of coagulative, caseous or liquefactive type, and also in foci of enzymic necrosis of fat. Calcification is almost inevitable in the atheromas of advanced atherosclerosis, which, as will be seen, are focal intimal injuries in the aorta and larger arteries characterized by the accumulation of lipids (p. 564). It also commonly develops in aging or damaged heart valves, further hampering their function (Fig. 1–41). Whatever the site of deposition, the calcium salts appear macroscopically as fine, white granules or clumps, often felt as gritty deposits. Sometimes, a tuberculous lymph node is virtually converted to stone.

Histologically, with the usual H and E stain, the calcium salts have a basophilic, amorphous granular, sometimes clumped appearance. They can be *intracellular, extracellular,* or *in both locations.* In the course of time, *heterotopic bone* may be formed in the focus of calcification. On occasion, single necrotic cells may constitute seed crystals that become encrusted by the mineral deposits. The progressive acquisition of outer layers may create lamellated configurations called *psammoma bodies* because of their resemblance to grains of sand. Some types of papillary cancers (e.g., thyroid) are apt to develop psammoma bodies. Strange concretions emerge when calcium iron salts gather about long slender spicules of asbestos in the lung, creating exotic, beaded dumbbell forms.

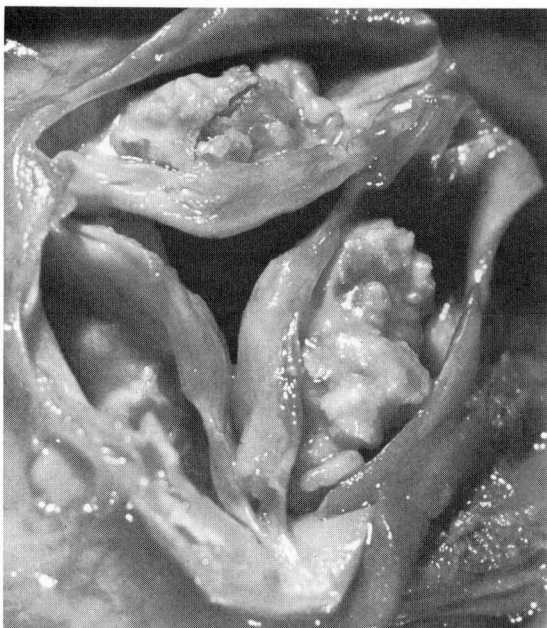

Figure 1–41. A view looking down onto the unopened aortic valve in a heart with calcific aortic stenosis. The semilunar cusps are thickened and fibrotic. Behind each leaflet are seen irregular masses of piled-up dystrophic calcification.

The pathogenesis of dystrophic calcification is beginning to be unraveled.[64,65] The final common pathway is the formation of crystalline calcium phosphate mineral in the form of an apatite similar to the hydroxyapatite of bone. The process has two major phases: *initiation* (or nucleation) and *propagation*, which can occur within cells and extracellularly. Initiation in *extracellular* sites occurs in membrane-bound *vesicles*, about 200 nm in diameter; in cartilage and bone they are known as *matrix vesicles*, and in pathologic calcification they are derived from degenerating or aging cells. It is thought that calcium is concentrated in these vesicles by its affinity for acidic phospholipids, and phosphates accumulate possibly as a result of the action of membrane-bound phosphatases. Initiation of *intracellular* calcification occurs in the *mitochondria* of dead or dying cells that accumulate calcium, as described earlier. After mineral initiation in either location, propagation of crystal formation occurs, dependent on the concentration of Ca^{++} and PO_4 in the extracellular spaces, the presence of mineral inhibitors, and the presence of collagen. Collagen itself appears to enhance the rate of crystal growth, but whether there is mineralization of collagen independent of cellular calcification is controversial.[67]

Although dystrophic calcification may be simply a telltale sign of previous cell injury, it is often a cause of organ dysfunction. Such is the case in calcific valvular disease and arteriosclerosis, as will become clear in further discussion of these diseases.

METASTATIC CALCIFICATION. This alteration may occur in normal tissues whenever there is hypercalcemia. Hypercalcemia also accentuates dystrophic calcification. The causes of hypercalcemia include hyperparathyroidism, vitamin D intoxication, systemic sarcoidosis, milk-alkali syndrome, hyperthyroidism, idiopathic hypercalcemia of infancy, Addison's disease (adrenocortical insufficiency), increased bone catabolism associated with disseminated bone tumors (such as multiple myeloma and metastatic cancer) and leukemia, and decreased bone formation as occurs in immobilization. Hypercalcemia also arises in some instances of advanced renal failure with phosphate retention, leading to secondary hyperparathyroidism.

Metastatic calcification may occur widely throughout the body but principally affects the interstitial tissues of the blood vessels, kidneys, lungs, and gastric mucosa. In all these sites, the calcium salts morphologically resemble those described in dystrophic calcification. Thus, they may occur as noncrystalline amorphous deposits or, at other times, as hydroxyapatite crystals. Metastatic calcification appears to begin also in mitochondria, except in kidney tubules where it develops in the basement membranes, probably in relation to extracellular vesicles budding from the epithelial cells.

In general, the mineral salts cause no clinical dysfunction but, on occasion, massive involvement of the lungs produces remarkable x-ray films and respiratory deficits. Massive deposits in the kidney (nephrocalcinosis) may in time cause renal damage.

HYALINE CHANGE

The term hyalin is a widely used descriptive histologic term rather than a specific marker for cell injury. *Hyalin refers to any alteration within cells or in the extracellular space, which gives a homogeneous, glassy, pink appearance in routine histologic sections stained with H and E.* It may then represent an intracellular accumulation or be the consequence of extracellular deposits. This tinctorial change is produced by a variety of alterations and does not represent a specific pattern of accumulation. Thus, it is important, when describing hyaline change, to be cognizant of the possible mechanisms of its formation. In some instances the mechanism is clearly known; in others it is obscure.

Some examples of *intracellular hyaline* change are the following: (1) The hyaline droplets seen in the proximal tubular epithelial cells of the kidney have already been referred to (p. 24). In most instances they represent reabsorption of excessive amounts of protein that have leaked across the glomerular filter. (2) In plasma cells, spherical hyaline deposits represent aggregates of immunoglobulin synthesized in the rough endoplasmic reticulum of the cell, so called Russell bodies. (3) Many viral infections are associated with the appearance of hyaline inclusions within either the cytoplasm or the nucleus. In some instances these are accumulations of viral nucleoproteins. (4) As described earlier, the characteristic hyaline inclusions in the liver cells of alcoholics, "alcoholic hyalin," consist of aggregates of prekeratin intermediate filaments.

Extracellular hyalin has been somewhat more difficult to analyze. Collagenous fibrous tissue in old scars may appear hyalinized, but the physicochemical mechanism underlying this change is not clear. In longstanding hypertension and diabetes mellitus the walls of arterioles, especially in the kidney, become hyalinized. As we shall see (p. 1066), such *hyaline arteriolosclerosis* in renal vessels has important diagnostic and pathogenetic implications. It appears that much of the hyalin is composed of precipitated plasma proteins that have leaked across injured endothelium into the arteriolar wall. There is also some reduplication of the basement membrane of the arterioles. Another example of extracellular hyalin is the hyalinization of glomeruli of the kidney when these undergo chronic damage. Here the hyalin appears to be a conglomeration of plasma proteins, basement membrane material, and mesangial matrix (p. 1024). With H and E stains, the protein *amyloid* (p. 211) also has a hyaline appearance. But this is a very specific fibrillar protein, with characteristic biochemical composition. Amyloid can be clearly identified by its special staining characteristics with the Congo red stain, with which it appears red and shows bipolar refringence.

Thus, although one continues to use the convenient term hyaline, it is important to recognize the multitude of mechanisms that produce this change and the implications of the alteration when it is seen in different pathologic conditions. It is apparent that the various forms of cellular derangement cover a wide spectrum, ranging from the reversible and irreversible forms of cell injury to the less ominous forms of intracellular accumulations, including pigmentations. Reference will be made to all these alterations throughout this book because all organ injury and, ultimately, all clinical disease arise from derangements in cell structure and function.

1. Majno, G.: The Healing Hand: Man and Wound in the Ancient World. Boston, Harvard University Press, 1975, p. 43.

2. Hochachka, P.W.: Defense strategies against hypoxia and hypothermia. Science 231:234, 1986

3. Jennings, R.B., and Steenbergen, C., Jr.: Nucleotide metabolism and cellular damage in myocardial ischemia. Ann. Rev. Physiol. 47:727, 1985

4. Borgens, M., et al.: Changes in ultrastructure and calcium distribution in the isolated working heart after ischemia. Am. J. Pathol. 126:92, 1986.

5. Reimer, K.A., and Ideker, R.E.: Myocardial ischemia and infarction. Hum. Pathol. 18:462, 1987.

6. Trump, B., and Arstila, A.: Pathobiology of Cell Membranes, Vol. 3. New York, Academic Press, 1983.

7. Farber, J.: Membrane injury and calcium homostasis in the pathogenesis of coagulative necrosis. Lab. Invest. 47:114, 1982.

8. Venkatachalam, M.A., et al.: Salvage of ischemic cells by impermeant solute and ATP. Lab. Invest. 49:1, 1983.

9. Mittnacht, S., Jr., and Farber, J.L.: Reversal of ischemic mitochondrial dysfunction. J. Biol. Chem. 256:3199, 1982.

10. Katz, A.M., and Messineo, F.C.: Lipid-membrane interactions and the pathogenesis of ischemic damage in the myocardium. Circ. Res. 48:1, 1981.

11. Chien, K.R., et al.: Phospholipid alterations in canine ischemic myocardium. Temporal and topographical correlations with Tc-99-m-PPi accumulation and an *in vitro* sarcolemmal calcium permeability defect. Circ. Res. 48:711, 1981.

12. Nayler, W.G.: The role of calcium in the ischemic myocardium. Am. J. Pathol. 102:262, 1981.

13. Marban, E., et al.: Intracellular free calcium concentration measured with 19F NMR spectroscopy in intact ferret hearts. Proc. Natl. Acad. Sci. U.S.A. 84:6005, 1987.

14. Steenbergen, C., et al.: Elevation in cystolic free calcium concentration early in myocardial ischemia in perfused rat heart. Circ. Res. 60:700, 1987.

15. Nicotera, P., et al.: Cytosolic-free calcium and cell killing in hepatoma cell exposed to chemical anoxia. FASEB J. 3:59, 1989.

16. Buja, L.M., et al.: Altered calcium homeostasis in the pathogenesis of myocardial ischemic and hypoxic injury. Cell Calcium 9:205, 1988.

17. Bonventre, J.: Mediators of ischemic renal injury. Ann. Rev. Med. 39:531, 1988.

18. Chien, K.R., et al.: Accumulation of unesterified arachidonic acid in ischemic canine myocardium: Relationship to a phosphatidylcholine deacylation-reacylation cycle and depletion of membrane phospholipids. Circ. Res. 54:313, 1984.

19. Das, D.K., et al.: Role of membrane phospholipids in myocardial injury induced by ischemia and reperfusion. Am. J. Physiol. 251:H71, 1986.

20. Ganote, C.E., and VanderHeide, R.S.: Cytoskeletal lesions in anoxic myocardial injury: A conventional and high-voltage electron microscopic and immunofluorescence study. Am. J. Pathol. 129:327, 1987.

21. Steenbergen, C., et al.: Volume regulation and plasma membrane injury in aerobic, anaerobic, and ischemic myocardium *in vitro*: Effects of osmotic cell swelling on plasma membrane integrity. Circ. Res. 57:864, 1985

22. Steenbergen, C., et al.: Cytoskeletal damage during myocardial ischemia: Changes in vinculin immunofluorescence staining during total *in vitro* ischemia in canine heart. Circ. Res. 60:478, 1987.

23. Bolli, R., et al.: Demonstration of free radical generation in (stunned) myocardium of intact dogs. J. Clin. Invest. 82:476, 1988.

24. Burton, K.P., and Massey, K.D.: Alterations in membrane phospholipids, mechanisms of free radical damage and antioxidant protection during myocardial ischemia and reperfusion. *In* Signal, P.K. (ed.): Free Radicals in the Pathophysiology of Heart Disease. Boston, Martinus Nijhoff, 1987.

25. Richard, V.J., et al.: Therapy to reduce free radicals during early reperfusion does not limit the size of myocardial infarcts caused by 90 minutes of ischemia in dogs. Circulation 78:473, 1988.

26. Corr, P.B., et al.: Amphipathic metabolites and membrane dysfunction in ischemic myocardium. Circ. Res. 55:135, 1984.

27. Venkatachalam, M.A., et al.: Energy thresholds that determine membrane integrity and injury in a renal epithelial cell line (LLC-PK₁). J. Clin. Invest. 81:745, 1988.

28. Cheung, J.Y., et al.: Calcium and ischemic injury. N. Engl. J. Med. 314:1670, 1986.

29. Halliwell, B.: Oxidants and human disease: some new concepts. FASEB J. 1:358, 1987.

30. Halliwell, B., and Gutteridge, J.M.C.: Free Radicals in Biology and Medicine. New York, Oxford University Press, 1985.

31. Freeman, B.A., and Crapo, J.D.: Biology of disease: Free radicals and tissue injury. Lab. Invest. 47:412, 1982.

32. Klebanoff, S.J.: Phagocytic cells: Products of oxygen metabolism. *In* Gallin, J., et al. (eds.): Inflammation: Basic Principles and Chemical Correlates. New York, Raven Press, 1988, pp. 391–444.

33. Slater, T.F.: Free radical mechanisms in tissue injury. Biochem. J. 222:1, 1984.

34. Henson, P.M., and Johnson, R.B., Jr.: Tissue injury in inflammation: Oxidants, proteases and cationic proteins. J. Clin. Invest. 79:669, 1987.

35. Taylor, A., et al. (eds.): Physiology of Oxygen Radicals. Baltimore, Williams & Wilkins, 1986.

36. Imlay, J.A., and Linn, S.: DNA damage and oxygen radical toxicity. Science 240:1302, 1988.

37. Dormandy, T.L.: In praise of peroxidation. Lancet 2:1126, 1988.

38. Farber, J.C.: Xenobiotics, drug metabolism and liver injury. *In*

Farber, E., et al. (eds.): Pathogenesis of Liver Diseases. Baltimore, Williams & Wilkins, 1987.

39. Sharpe, A., and Fields, B.: Pathogenesis of viral infections: Basic concepts derived from the neovirus model. N. Engl. J. Med. *312:*486, 1985.

40. Majno, G., et al.: Cellular death and necrosis: Chemical, physical, and morphologic changes in rat liver. Virchows Arch. *333:*421, 1960.

41. Walker, N.I., et al.: Patterns of cell death. *In* Jasmin, G. (ed.): Methods and Achievements in Experimental Pathology. Basel, S. Kargen, 1988, pp. 18–54.

42. Duke, R.C., and Cohen, J.J.: The role of nuclear damage in the lysis of target cells by cytotoxic T-lymphocytes. *In* Podack, E.R. (ed.): Cytologic Lymphocytes and Complement, Vol. 2. Boca Raton, CRC Press, 1988, pp. 35–48.

43. Duke, R.C., et al.: Endogenous endonuclear induced DNA fragmentation: an early event in cell mediated cytolysis. Proc. Natl. Acad. Sci. U.S.A. *80:*6361, 1983.

44. Podolsky, K., and Isselbacher, K.J.: Derangements of hepatic metabolism. *In* Harrison's Principles of Internal Medicine. New York, McGraw-Hill Book Co., 1987, p. 1309.

45. Geokas, M.C., et al.: Ethanol, the liver and the gastrointestinal tract. Ann. Intern. Med. *95:*198,1981.

46. Riely, C.A.: Acute fatty liver of pregnancy. Semin. Liver Dis. *7:*47, 1987.

47. Wolman, M.: Pigments in Pathology. New York, Academic Press, 1969.

48. Toubald, R.D., et al.: Studies on the chemical nature of lipofuscin (age pigment) isolated from normal human brain. Lipids *10:*383, 1975.

49. Richter, G.W.: A review. The iron-loaded cell — the cytopathology of iron storage. Am. J. Pathol. *91:*361, 1978.

50. Jones, A.L., and Fawcett, D.W.: Hypertrophy of the agranular endoplasmic reticulum in hamster liver induced by phenobarbital. J. Histochem. Cytochem. *14:*215, 1966.

51. Nagle, R.: Intermediate filaments: A review of basic biology. Am. J. Surg. Pathol. *12*(S1):4, 1988.

52. Brandle, E.R., and Gabbiani, G.: The role of cytoskeletal and cyto-contractile elements in pathologic processes. Am. J. Pathol. *110:*361, 1983.

53. Katsuma, Y., et al.: Changes in cytokeratin intermediate filament cytoskeleton associated with Mallory body formation in mouse and human liver. Hepatology, *7:*1215, 1987.

54. Perry, G. (ed.): Alteration of the Neuronal Cytoskeleton in Alzheimer Disease. New York, Plenum Press, 1987.

55. Marchesi, V.T.: The cytoskeletal system of red cell membrane. Hosp. Pract. *20:*113, 1985.

56. Becker, P.S., and Lux, S.E.: Hereditary spherocytosis and related disorders. Clin. Hematol. *14:*15, 1985.

57. Fox, J.E., and Boyles, J.K.: The membrane skeleton — a distinct structure that regulates the function of cells. Bioessay *8:*14, 1988.

58. Lindquist, S.: The heat shock response. Annu. Rev. Biochem. *55:*1151, 1986.

59. Zak, R.: Cardiac hypertrophy: Biochemical and cellular relationships. Hosp. Pract. *18:*23, 1983.

60. Baserga, R.: The Biology of Cell Reproduction. Cambridge, Harvard University Press, 1985.

61. Alison, M.R.: Regulation of hepatic growth. Physiol. Rev. *66:*49, 1986.

62. Fausto, N., and Mead, J.E.: Regulation of liver growth: Proto-oncogenes and transforming growth factors. Lab. Invest. *60:*4, 1989.

63. Braun, L., et al.: Transforming growth factor mRNA increases during liver regeneration: A possible paracrine factor in growth regulation. Proc. Natl. Acad. Sci. U.S.A. *85:*1539, 1988.

64. Anderson, H.C.: Calcific disease. A concept. Arch. Pathol. Lab. Med. *107:*341, 1983.

65. Schoen, F.J., et al.: Calcification: pathology, mechanisms and strategies of prevention. J. Biomed. Material Res. *22:*A1, 1988.

Inflammation and Repair

INFLAMMATION

Inflammation is best defined as *the reaction of vascularized living tissue to local injury.* Invertebrates with no vascular system, single-celled organisms, and multicellular parasites all have their own responses to local injury. These include phagocytosis of the injurious agent; entrapment of the irritant by specialized cells (hemocytes), which then ingest it; and neutralization of noxious stimuli by hypertrophy of the cell or one of its organelles.[1] All these reactions have been retained in other forms of life, but what characterizes the inflammatory process in higher forms is *the reaction of blood vessels,* leading to the accumulation of fluid and blood cells. This makes the reaction more complex but also more fascinating to unravel.

The inflammatory response is closely intertwined with the process of *repair.* Inflammation serves to destroy, dilute, or wall off the injurious agent, but in turn it sets into motion a series of events that, as far as possible, heal and reconstitute the damaged tissue. Repair begins during the early phases of inflammation but reaches completion usually after the injurious influence has been neutralized. During repair, the injured tissue is replaced by *regeneration* of native parenchymal cells, by filling of the defect with fibroblastic scar tissue *(scarring),* or most commonly by a combination of these two processes.

Humans owe to inflammation and repair their ability to contain injuries and heal defects. Without inflammation, infections would go unchecked, wounds would never heal, and injured organs might remain permanent festering sores. *However, inflammation and repair may be potentially harmful.* Inflammatory reactions underlie the genesis of rheumatoid arthritis, life-threatening hypersensitivity reactions, and some forms of fatal renal disease. Reparative efforts may lead to disfiguring scars or fibrous bands that cause intestinal obstruction or limit the mobility of joints. For this reason our pharmacies abound with "anti-inflammatory drugs," which supposedly limit the normal inflammatory reaction. The ideal drug would be one that enhances the salutary effects of inflammation yet controls its harmful sequelae. As our understanding of the mechanisms of inflammation increases, so will our ability to foster its beneficial effects.

HISTORICAL HIGHLIGHTS

Inflammation has a rich and ancient history, intimately linked to the history of wars, wounds, and infections.[1-3] Space here does not allow for any but the briefest of historical perspectives.

Cornelius Celsus, a Roman writer of the first century AD, described the four cardinal signs of inflammation: *rubor, tumor, calor,* and *dolor* (redness, swelling, heat, and pain). In 1793, the Scottish surgeon *John Hunter* noted what is now considered an obvious fact: that inflammation is not a disease but a nonspecific response that has a "salutary" effect on its host.[4] *Julius Cohnheim* (1839–1884) provided one of the first microscopic descriptions of inflammation. He observed **39** injured blood vessels in thin, transparent membranes, such as the mesentery and tongue of the frog. Noting the initial vasodilation and changes in blood flow, the subsequent edema due to increased vascular permeability, and the characteristic leukocyte emigration, he wrote descriptions that can hardly be improved upon.[5]

The Russian biologist *Elie Metchnikoff* discovered the process of *phagocytosis* by observing the ingestion of rose thorns by amebocytes of starfish larvae (1882) and of bacteria by mammalian leukocytes (1884).[6] He concluded that the purpose of inflammation was to bring phagocytic cells to the injured area to engulf invading bacteria. At that time, Metchnikoff contradicted the prevailing theory that the purpose of inflammation was to bring in factors from the serum to neutralize the infectious agents. It soon became clear that both cellular (phagocytosis) and serum factors (antibodies) were critical to the defense against microorganisms, and in recognition of this both Metchnikoff and Paul Ehrlich (who developed the humoral theory) shared the Nobel Prize in 1908.

To these names must be added that of *Sir Thomas Lewis* who, on the basis of simple experiments involving the inflammatory response in skin, established the *concept that chemical substances, locally induced by injury, mediate the vascular changes of inflammation.* This fundamental concept underlies the important discoveries of *chemical mediators* of inflammation and of potent anti-inflammatory agents.

ACUTE INFLAMMATION

It is common to think of bacteria or other microbes as the cause of inflammation, but almost all causes of cell injury cited earlier (Chapter 1) may also provoke inflammation. These causative factors include microbial infections, physical agents (such as burns, radiation, and trauma), chemicals (toxins and caustic substances), necrotic tissue, and all types of immunologic reactions.

Inflammation is divided into acute and chronic patterns — useful terms, provided that certain qualifications of their meaning are appreciated.[7] *Acute inflammation* is of relatively short duration, lasting for a few minutes, several hours, or one to two days, and its main characteristics are the exudation of fluid and plasma proteins (edema) and the emigration of leukocytes, predominantly neutrophils. Regardless of the nature of the injurious agent, acute inflammation is more or less stereotypic. *Chronic inflammation,* on the other hand, is less uniform. Of longer duration, chronic inflammation is associated histologically with the presence of lymphocytes and macrophages and with the proliferation of blood vessels and connective tissue. But many factors modify the course and histologic appearance of chronic inflammation, and these will become apparent later in this chapter.

Many of the vascular and cellular responses of inflammation are mediated by chemical factors derived from the action of the inflammatory stimulus on plasma or cells. A series of such chemical mediators, acting together or in sequence, then influence the evolution of the inflammatory response. But it is important to remember that certain stimuli, such as toxins, bacteria, and ischemia, *cause cell necrosis directly,* and that the necrotic tissue, in turn, can trigger the elaboration of inflammatory mediators. Such is the case with the acute inflammation following myocardial infarction.

The arena of the inflammatory response is the vascularized connective tissue, including plasma, circulating cells, blood vessels, and cellular and extracellular constituents of connective tissue (Fig. 2–1). The student should be familiar with the structure, biology, and biochemistry of these components. The circulating cells that are important in inflammation include *neutrophils, monocytes, eosinophils, lymphocytes, basophils,* and *platelets.* The connective tissue cells are the *mast cells,* which intimately surround *blood vessels;* the connective tissue *fibroblasts;* and occasional resident macrophages and lymphocytes. The extracellular connective tissue consists of *basement membrane,* and the various types of *collagen, elastin,* and *proteoglycans* (heparan sulfate, chondroitin sulfate, hyaluronic acid). *Fibronectin* and *laminin* are glycoproteins that, together with some types of collagen (IV and V), are present in basement membranes.

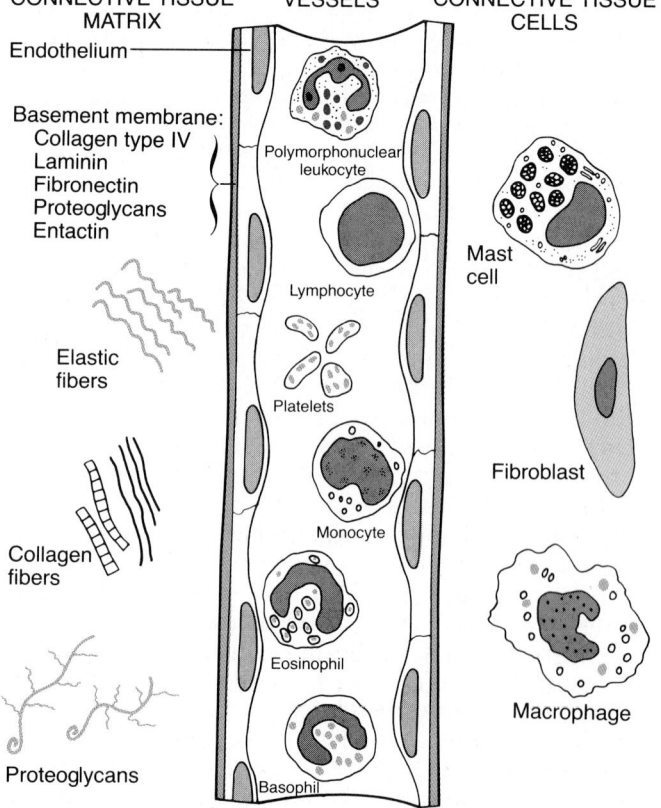

Figure 2–1. Intravascular cells and connective tissue matrix and cells involved in the inflammatory response.

Certain terms must be defined before we describe specific features of inflammation. The escape of fluid, proteins, and blood cells from the vascular system into the interstitial tissue or body cavities is known as *exudation.* An *exudate* is an inflammatory extravascular fluid that has a high protein concentration, much cellular debris, and a specific gravity above 1.020. It implies significant alteration in the normal permeability of small blood vessels in the area of injury. In contrast, a *transudate* is a fluid with low protein content (most of which is albumin) and a specific gravity of less than 1.012. It is essentially an ultrafiltrate of blood plasma and results from hydrostatic imbalance across the vascular endothelium. In this situation, the permeability of the endothelium is normal. *Edema* denotes an excess of fluid in the interstitial tissue or serous cavities; it can be either an exudate or a transudate. *Pus,* a *purulent exudate,* is an inflammatory exudate rich in leukocytes (mostly neutrophils) and parenchymal cell debris. Lysosomal enzymes are present in pus, and the extent of proteolysis that they produce determines the viscosity of the material.

The local clinical signs of acute inflammation are the heat, redness, swelling, and pain immortalized by Celsus. A fifth clinical sign, loss of function *(functio laesa),* was later added by Virchow. These signs of the inflammatory response are induced by (1) *changes in vascular flow and caliber* (also referred to as hemodynamic changes), (2) *changes in vascular permeability,* and (3) *leukocytic exudation.* These three reactions may overlap and some share common mediator mechanisms. In general, however, the structural and biochemical basis of each of these responses is sufficiently different to require separate consideration.

CHANGES IN VASCULAR FLOW AND CALIBER

Changes in vascular flow and caliber are best observed in thin, transparent injured tissues by time-lapse cinematography. Beginning very early after injury, they develop at varying rates, depending on the severity of the injury. The changes occur in the following order.

1. First, there is *transient vasoconstriction of arterioles.* This is an inconstant finding, and with mild forms of injury it disappears within three to five seconds. With more severe injury, such as a burn, vasoconstriction may last several minutes.

2. The next and fundamental event is *vasodilation,* which first involves the arterioles and then results in opening of new microvascular beds in the area. *Thus comes about the increased blood flow — the hallmark of the early hemodynamic changes in acute inflammation* and the cause of the heat and the redness. At this stage, the increased blood volume in the vasodilated vessels may result in sufficient increases in local hydrostatic pressure to cause fleeting transudation of protein-poor fluid into the extravascular space.

3. *Slowing of the circulation* follows, brought about by *increased permeability of the microvasculature,* with the outpouring of protein-rich fluid into the extravascular tissues. This results in concentration of the red cells in small vessels and increased viscosity of the blood. In histologic sections, this phenomenon is reflected by the presence of dilated small vessels packed with red cells — termed *stasis.*

4. As stasis develops, one begins to see peripheral orientation of leukocytes, principally neutrophils, along the vascular endothelium, a process termed *leukocytic margination.* Leukocytes stick to the endothelium at first transiently, then more avidly; soon afterward they migrate through the vascular wall into the interstitial tissue, the latter process being called *emigration.*

The time scale of these events is variable. With mild stimuli the stages of stasis may not become apparent until 15 to 30 minutes have elapsed, whereas, with severe injury, stasis may occur in but a few minutes. Furthermore, if the injurious agent is diffusible or if there is a gradient of injury, the vessels closest to the stimulus show evidence of severe and rapid hemodynamic changes, whereas those at the periphery have mild alterations. Thus, if a local burn is inflicted on the skin, the area immediately adjacent to the burn may show complete stasis, whereas more peripheral areas may still be vasodilated.

CHANGES IN VASCULAR PERMEABILITY

Normal Permeability and Structure of Microcirculation

We have seen that, in the early stages, vasodilation and increased hydrostatic pressure may result in some degree of *transudation.* However, this is soon overshadowed by *increased vascular permeability and exudation of plasma proteins, the mark of acute inflammatory edema.* Increased permeability in inflammation occurs in the microcirculation, which includes the small arterioles, capillaries, and venules. In these segments the exchange of substances occurs between the blood and tissues.

According to Starling's hypothesis, the normal fluid balance is maintained by two opposing sets of forces (Fig. 2–2A). Those that cause fluid to move out of circulation are the osmotic pressure of interstitial fluid and the intravascular hydrostatic pressure; those that cause fluid to move in are the osmotic pressure of plasma proteins and the tissue hydrostatic pressure. The balance of these forces is such that, in peripheral muscle capillaries, there is a net small movement of fluid outward, but this fluid normally drains into the lymphatics, and no edema occurs. Factors that tend either to increase intravascular hydrostatic pressure or to decrease intravascular osmotic pressure will result in increased movement of fluid out of the capillary and consequent edema. In these instances, however, the edema is a transudate. *In inflammatory*

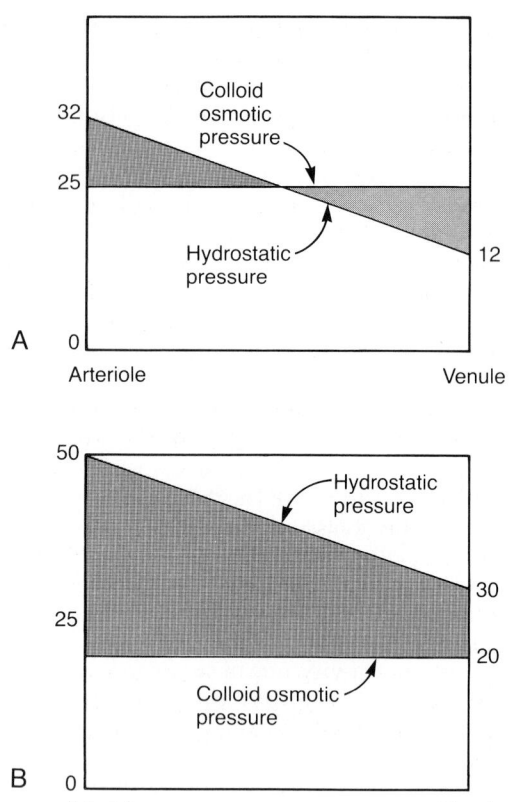

Figure 2–2. Blood pressure and plasma colloid osmotic forces in normal and inflamed microcirculation. A, Normal hydrostatic pressure of about 32 mm Hg at arterial end of capillary and 12 mm Hg at venous end. Mean capillary pressure equals colloid osmotic pressure (horizontal line). B, Acute inflammation. Mean capillary pressure is increased because of arteriolar dilatation, while osmotic pressure is reduced because of protein leakage across venule. Result is net excess of extravasated fluid. (Redrawn from Wright, G.P.: An Introduction to Pathology. 3rd ed. London, Longmans, Green and Co., 1958.)

edema there is loss of high-protein fluid owing to a leaky endothelium and therefore a reduction of the intravascular osmotic pressure, accompanied by increased osmotic pressure of the interstitial fluid, both leading to impairment of the return of fluid to the blood on the venous end of the capillary (Fig. 2–2*B*). There is thus a marked *outflow* of fluid.

Normal fluid exchange is critically dependent on an intact endothelium. Normal endothelium is a thin, simple, squamous epithelium adapted to permit free, rapid exchange of water and small molecules between plasma and interstitium, but to limit the passage of plasma proteins with increased restriction as the size of the protein increases. The endothelial lining of all arterioles and venules and of most capillaries in the body is of the *continuous* type, having an unbroken cytoplasmic layer with closely apposed intercellular junctions. *Fenestrated* endothelium is characteristic of endocrine organs, intestines, and the renal glomerulus, and *discontinuous* or *open* endothelium occurs in the liver, spleen, and bone marrow. Physiologic studies[8,9] explain normal capillary permeability for small lipid-insoluble molecules by the existence of water-

filled "small pores" 6 nm in radius, or slits about 8 nm wide. There is also a postulated system of large pores (25-nm radius) to account for the small quantities of protein and other large solutes that normally cross the capillary wall.

Electron microscopists generally agree that *micropinocytotic vesicles* represent the large pores, but the morphologic equivalent of the small-pore system is still uncertain. There are two views. One is that the small-pore system is represented by continuous trans-endothelial channels formed by fusing pinocytotic vesicles (transcytosis),[10,11] and the other view holds that open *intercellular junctions* transfer the small lipid-insoluble molecules across the capillary wall.[12] Whichever the route in capillaries, it is clear that intercellular junctions are less structurally complex and more permeable in *small venules*.[12] Furthermore, junctions are labile structures and are susceptible to being widened by a variety of physical and chemical factors. As we shall see, most chemical mediators of inflammation cause increased vascular permeability by opening gaps in *intercellular* junctions.

Various polyanionic molecules, such as sialoglycoproteins and heparan sulfate, are localized in specific domains on the luminal surface of endothelium (e.g., vesicles, fenestrae, intercellular junctions).[14] These anionic sites may well play a role in normal and increased vascular permeability by repelling anionic molecules and facilitating the transport of cationic proteins. Such a role for anionic sites has been shown in the case of the renal glomerulus (p. 1014).

It must be emphasized that, despite its relatively simple structure, the vascular endothelial cell is a functionally and metabolically active cell capable of secretion of a variety of biologically important molecules. These include hormones (prostaglandins), procoagulant (factor VIII) and anticoagulant (plasminogen activator) factors, and connective tissue proteins (e.g., collagens).[15,16] (See Table 12–1, p. 556.)

Patterns and Morphologic Basis of Increased Vascular Permeability

Increased vascular permeability is seen clinically as *edema*. It can be demonstrated or quantitated experimentally by measurement of the escape of intravenously injected dyes or radiolabeled protein into injured areas. Some dyes such as colloidal carbon (particles 25 to 30 nm in diameter), are normally taken up by the reticuloendothelial (mononuclear phagocyte) system but not by endothelial cells. However, carbon particles leak across injured endothelium but are too large to cross the basement membrane. They are thus trapped between the basement membrane and the endothelium. Leaky vessels are therefore "labeled" with carbon and can thus be visualized on light and electron microscopy.

With such techniques, three general types of response in the rise and ebb of vascular leakage can be demonstrated in the skin of animals exposed to various types of injury (Fig. 2–3): (1) *the immediate-*

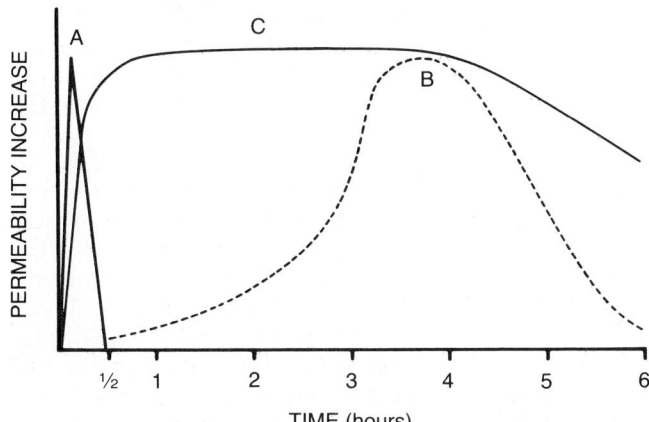

Figure 2–3. Patterns of increased vascular permeability in inflammation. A shows the immediate transient response; B shows the delayed response; and C shows the immediate sustained response.

transient response, (2) *the immediate-sustained response* and (3) *the delayed-prolonged response.*[17]

The immediate-transient response usually begins directly after injury, reaches a peak by five to ten minutes, and phases out within 15 to 30 minutes. *The*

response is elicited by histamine and most other chemical mediators and by mild injury (such as heating the skin at 54°C for five seconds). Majno and co-workers[18,19] used the carbon-labeling technique and found that immediate-transient leakage induced by histamine and most other chemical mediators[20] occurred *exclusively* (1) *from small- and medium-sized venules* less than 100 μm in diameter, leaving the capillaries unaffected (Fig. 2–4), and (2) through gaps (0.5 to 1.0 μm in width) *between the endothelial cells* (Fig. 2–5B). The mechanism by which gaps form turns out to be quite simple: they are caused by actual *contraction* of endothelial cells and widening of the junction. Similar changes are seen in the immediate-transient responses induced by mild thermal injury,[20] and these can be inhibited by antagonists of histamine. Why do histamine-type mediators act exclusively on venules? We do not know for sure, but some evidence suggests that venular endothelium has a higher concentration of high-affinity binding sites (receptors) for histamine than does arteriolar or capillary endothelium.[21]

Immediate-sustained reactions are encountered in severe injuries, usually associated with necrosis of endothelial cells. Leakage starts immediately after in-

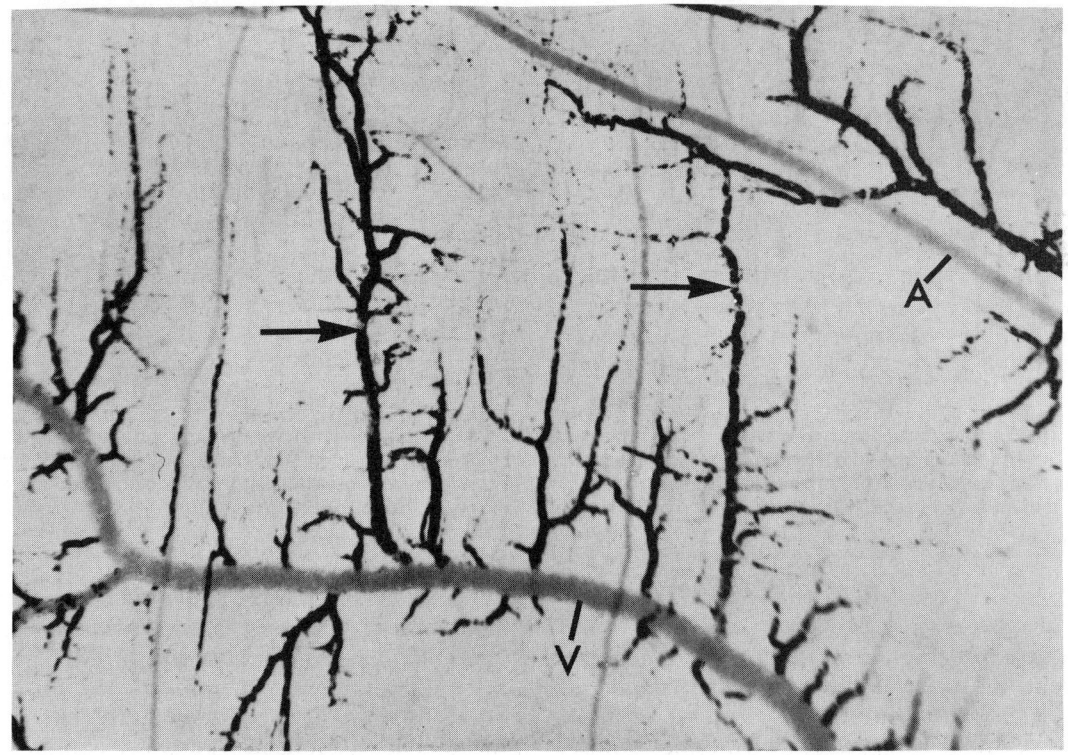

Figure 2–4. Vascular leakage as induced by most chemical mediators. This is a laminar muscle of the rat (cremaster), fixed, cleared in glycerin, and examined unstained by transillumination. One hour prior to sacrifice, bradykinin was injected over this muscle, and colloidal carbon was given intravenously; bradykinin caused small gaps to appear between endothelial cells in some vessels. Plasma, loaded with carbon, escaped, but most of the carbon particles were retained by the basement membrane of the leaking vessels, with the result that these became "labeled" in black. *Note that not all the vessels leak* — only the venules, and then only within a certain caliber range. A = arteriole; V = small vein; arrows point to blackened, leaking venules. The capillary network is very faintly visible in the background. (Courtesy of Dr. Guido Majno.)

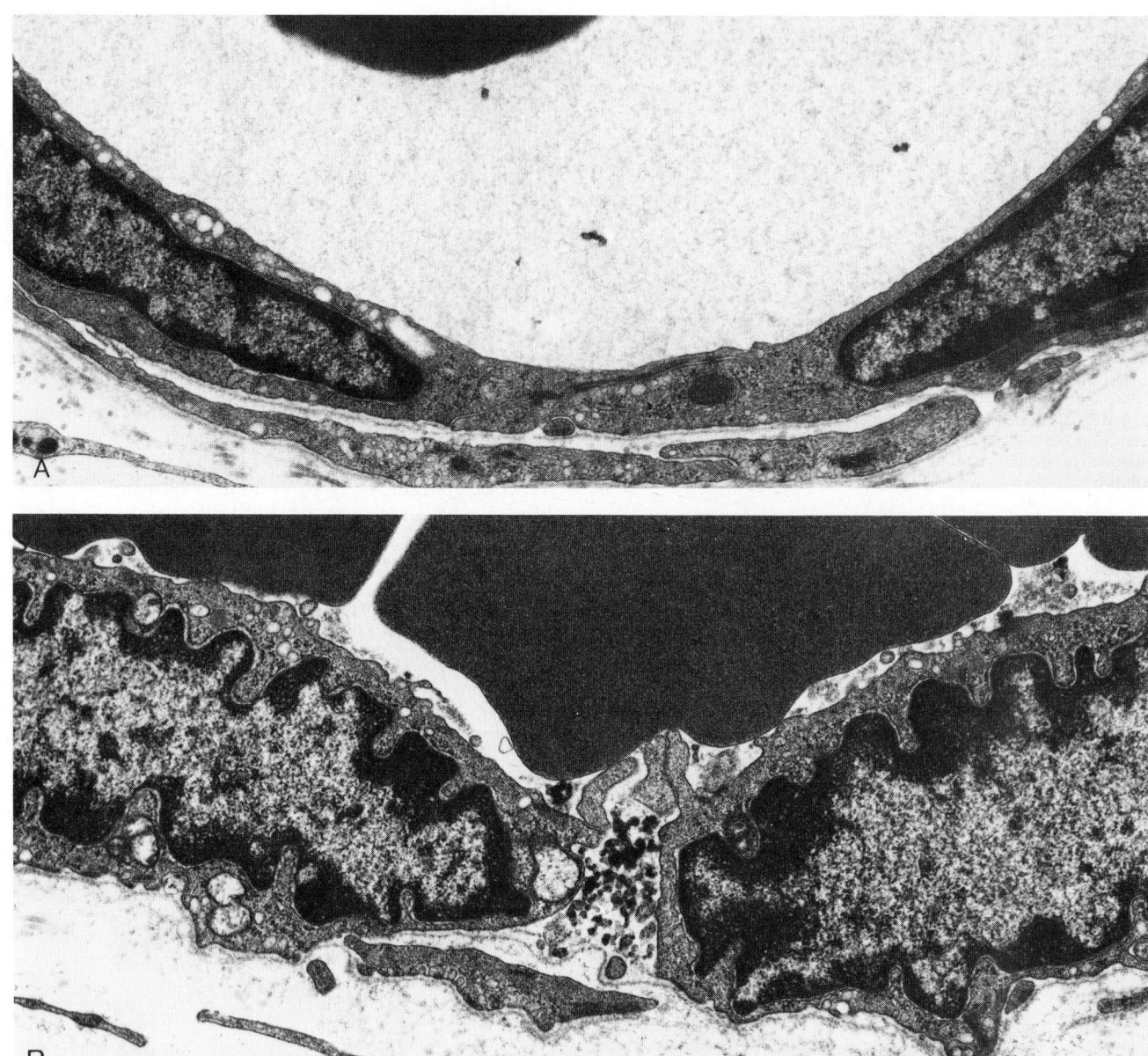

Figure 2–5. *A,* Electron micrograph of wall of normal venule, showing closed intercellular junction and flattened endothelial cells. *B,* Venule after injection of a histamine-type mediator, showing an intercellular gap through which injected black carbon particles have leaked. Note that the cells have bulged into the lumen and their nuclei show many indentations, suggesting contraction. (From Joris, I.J., et al.: The mechanism of vascular leakage induced by leukotriene E4. Am. J. Pathol. *126*:19, 1987.).

jury, is sustained at a high level for several hours, and continues for one to several days until the damaged vessels are either thrombosed or repaired. *All levels of the microcirculation are affected, including venules, capillaries, and arterioles.* Severe endothelial cell damage, with frequent sloughing of endothelial cells and platelet adhesion to endothelium are present. *Here the mechanism for increased permeability appears to be direct damage by the injurious stimulus.* The classic example is the increased permeability that occurs after a severe burn.[23]

Delayed-prolonged leakage is a curious type of response that *begins after a delay, lasts for several hours or even days, and involves venules and capillaries.* This response is relatively common, occurring after mild-to-moderate thermal injury, after x-ray or ultraviolet irradiation, with certain bacterial toxins, and in delayed (type IV) hypersensitivity reactions (p. 182). One common example of a delayed response is seen in sunburn, which is appreciated only several hours after a person has left the beach! In the delayed phase, leakage occurs in both venules and capillaries.[17] In the capillaries, the leakage is largely due to direct injury to the endothelium by the initial stimulus. Electron microscopy shows the leakage to be predominantly intercellular, but curiously there is no endothelial cell contraction.[24] Why gaps form in capillaries with this type of direct injury and why the leakage is delayed are not known.

Before we leave this discussion, it should be noted that although it is possible to separate the three patterns in the experimental model, the patterns in most inflammatory reactions of man overlap because there is a graded severity of injury from the center to the periphery of injured sites. In addition, different chemical mediators may be activated at consecutive phases of the inflammatory response and account for sustained and prolonged responses.

CELLULAR EVENTS: LEUKOCYTIC EXUDATION AND PHAGOCYTOSIS

The accumulation of leukocytes—principally neutrophils and monocytes—is the most important feature of the inflammatory reaction. Leukocytes engulf and degrade bacteria, immune complexes, and the debris of necrotic cells, and their lysosomal enzymes contribute in other ways to the defensive response. But, as we shall see, leukocytes during these defensive reactions may themselves prolong inflammation and increase tissue damage by the release of enzymes, chemical mediators, and toxic radicals.

The sequence of these "leukocyte events" can be divided into (1) margination, (2) adhesion, (3) emigration toward a chemotactic stimulus, (4) phagocyto- *sis and intracellular degradation, and (5) extracellular release of leukocyte products (Fig. 2–6).*

Margination

In normally flowing blood, the red and white cells within microvessels are confined to the axial central column, leaving a relatively cell-free layer of plasma in contact with the vessel wall. As slowing and stagnation of the flow occur, the white cells appear to fall out of the central column to assume positions in contact with the endothelium. The cells first tumble slowly along the walls of the capillaries and venules, coming to rest finally at some point. In time, the endothelium appears to be virtually lined by such cells, a phenomenon called *pavementing.*

Adhesion

Following margination, white cells adhere in great numbers to the endothelial surface, resembling "pebbles or marbles over which a stream runs without disturbing them." Since this process of leukocyte-endothelial adhesion is a prelude to all the subsequent cellular events, its mechanism is of prime importance.

Although a number of factors may influence adhesion (e.g., Ca^{++}, surface charge) recent evidence[25] suggests that *increased leukocytic adhesion in inflammation involves specific interactions between complementary "adhesion molecules" present on the leukocyte and endothelial surfaces.*[26] The surface expression of these adhesion molecules is either induced, or enhanced, or altered by inflammatory agents and chemical mediators (Table 2–1), resulting in increased adhesivity. *Some agents act on leukocytes,*

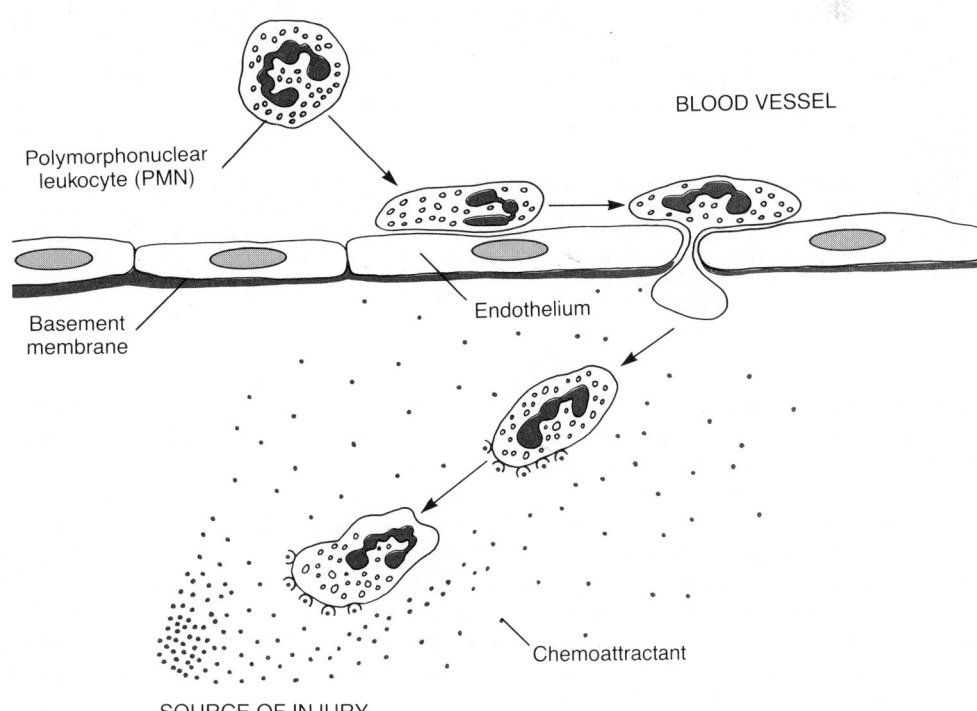

Figure 2–6. Sequence of leukocytic events in inflammation. The leukocytes adhere to endothelium, crawl toward an endothelial junction, and emigrate through it and toward chemoattractants emanating from the source of injury.

Polymorphonuclear leukocyte (PMN)

BLOOD VESSEL

Basement membrane

Endothelium

Chemoattractant

SOURCE OF INJURY

Table 2–1. Endothelial-Leukocyte Adhesion

MEDIATORS
Bacterial products (Endotoxin)
Complement fragments (C5a)
Chemotactic peptides
Leukotriene B4 (LTB$_4$)
Platelet activating factor
Transferrin
Cytokines (IL-1 and TNF)
MECHANISMS
Stimulation of leukocyte adhesion molecules (C5a, LTB$_4$)
Stimulation of endothelial adhesion molecules (IL-1, endotoxin)
Both effects (TNF)

others on endothelial cells, and still others on both cell types.

One group of adhesion molecules on leukocytes consist of a family of three glycoproteins (LFA-1; MO-1; and p 150,95), which are heterodimers with identical β subunits (molecular weight, 95,000) but different α subunits of molecular weight 150,000 to 180,000[27] (Fig. 2–7, *left*). In normal unstimulated leukocytes, they are present in an intracellular vesicular compartment, as well as on the cell surface. Certain inflammatory mediators, including chemotactic complement fragments, stimulate a rapid increase in these proteins on the leukocyte surface as well as increased leukocyte adhesion to endothelium.[26]

The most telling proof of the importance of adhesion molecules is the existence of a genetic deficiency in the leukocyte adhesion proteins (leukocyte adhesion deficiency), characterized by recurrent bacterial infections and impaired leukocyte adhesion.[27] Patients with this disorder have a deficiency in the biosynthesis of the β chain shared by these proteins. In contrast to the leukocyte-dependent effect on adhesion induced by complement fragments, inflammatory mediators such as interleukin-1 (IL-1) (p. 58) stimulate leukocyte adhesion by inducing synthesis of adhesive surface proteins *on endothelial cells*—an endothe-lium-dependent effect.[28] Two such proteins are ELAM-1 (endothelial leukocyte adhesion molecule-1), which is involved in IL-1–stimulated neutrophil adhesion to endothelium[28] and ICAM-1 (intracellular adhesion molecule-1), which mediates adhesion of lymphocytes, neutrophils, and monocytes.[29,29a] ICAM-1 serves as a receptor for the LFA-1 molecule of leukocyte adhesion protein. Certain mediators increase adhesion by both leukocyte and endothelial-dependent effects.[29] Just as certain mediators increase leukocyte adhesion to endothelium, others inhibit adhesion and may serve to terminate the adhesive events in inflammation.[30]

Emigration and Chemotaxis

Emigration refers to the process by which motile white cells escape from the blood vessels to the perivascular tissues. Neutrophils, eosinophils, basophils, monocytes, and lymphocytes all use the same pathway. Following adhesion, the leukocytes move slightly along the endothelial surface and insert large pseudopods into the junctions between the endothelial cells[31] (Fig. 2–6). They crawl through widened interendothelial junctions, eventually to assume a position between endothelial cell and basement membrane (Fig. 2–8). They may stay at that site for short periods, but they eventually traverse the basement membrane and escape into the extravascular space. Red cells may also leave blood vessels, particularly in severe injuries. Unlike the white cell, the red cell seems to be passively and unwillingly shoved out of the leaky, injured vessel by the intraluminal pressure in the wake of emigrating leukocytes.

The cell type present in the inflammatory response varies with the age of the inflammatory lesion and with the type of stimulus. In most types of acute inflammation, *neutrophils predominate in the first six to 24 hours, being replaced by monocytes in 24 to 48 hours.* Although this sequence can be explained in different ways, three factors account for it best: (1)

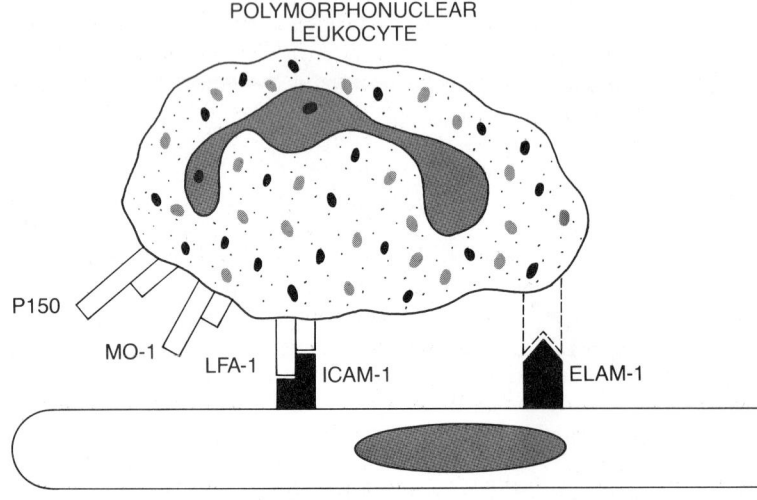

POLYMORPHONUCLEAR
LEUKOCYTE

P150
MO-1
LFA-1
ICAM-1
ELAM-1

STIMULATED ENDOTHELIAL CELL

Figure 2–7. Examples of adhesion molecules on leukocytes (LFA1, MO1, P150) and inflamed endothelium (ELAM-1, ICAM-1). ICAM-1 is a ligand for LFA-1. The ligand for ELAM-1 on the leukocyte is currently unknown.

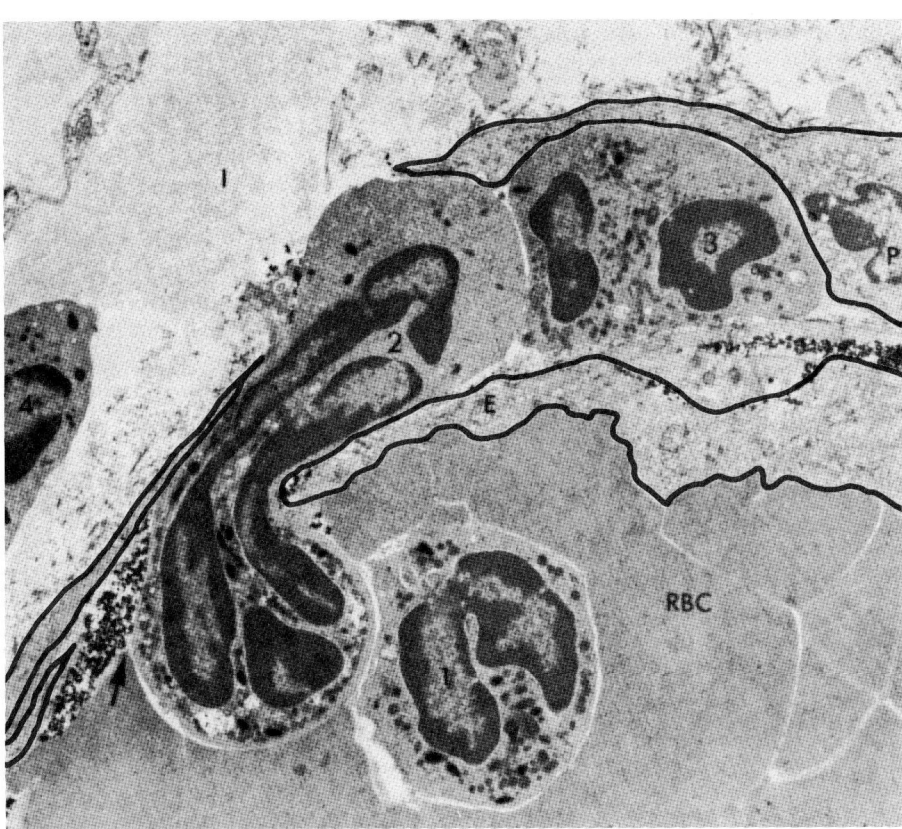

Figure 2–8. Venule ten hours after injection of an inflammation-provoking toxin. Four polymorphonuclear leukocytes are seen: 1 is in the lumen; 2 is squeezing through (emigrating from) the lumen into the perivascular space; 3 is trapped between the endothelium (E) and pericyte (P); and 4 is already in the interstitium (I). The endothelial cells and pericytes are outlined in red.

short-lived neutrophils disintegrate and disappear after 24 to 48 hours, whereas monocytes survive much longer in tissues; (2) monocyte emigration is sustained long after neutrophil emigration ceases[32]; and (3) chemotactic factors for neutrophils and monocytes are activated at different periods of the response. There are many exceptions to this pattern of cellular exudation: in infection produced by Pseudomonas organisms, neutrophils predominate over two to four days; in viral infections, lymphocytes may be the first cells to arrive; in some hypersensitivity reactions, eosinophilic granulocytes may be the main cell type.

Chemotaxis is defined as the unidirectional migration of cells toward an attractant or, more simply, locomotion oriented along a chemical gradient (Fig. 2–6). The term should be differentiated from *chemokinesis*, which is the accelerated *random* locomotion of cells. All granulocytes, monocytes, and, to a lesser extent, lymphocytes respond to chemotactic stimuli with various rates of speed.

Many early workers studied chemotaxis, but the development of Boyden's micropore filter technique[33] turned the early expeditions to "fish" for chemoattractants into an international sport. With Boyden's technique, leukocytes are placed in one compartment of a chamber, separated by a porous filter membrane from a second compartment into which the chemotactic substance is placed. If a chemotactic influence is present, the leukocytes crawl across the pores of the filter. Quantitation of chemo-

taxis can be done by counting the cells either on the stained filter membrane or in the second chamber. Some chemotactic factors operate only on the polymorphonuclear leukocytes, others only on monocytes, and some affect both types of white cells.

Both exogenous and endogenous substances can act as attractants.[34] The most significant chemotactic agents for neutrophils are (1) *bacterial products;* (2) *components of the complement system,* particularly C5a (p. 54); and (3) *products of the lipoxygenase pathway of arachidonic acid metabolism,* particularly leukotriene B_4 (discussed in detail in the section on chemical mediators). *Soluble bacterial factors* with chemotactic activity can be isolated from filtrates of a variety of organisms, including *Staphylococcus albus, S. aureus,* and *Escherichia coli.* Some of these are peptides that possess an N-formyl-methionine terminal amino acid, an observation that led to the synthesis of simple oligopeptides that are highly chemotactic for leukocytes.[35] Others are lipid in nature and resemble the endogenously produced lipoxygenation products of arachidonic acid metabolism. Chemotactic substances for monocytes are discussed on page 64.

But how does the headless leukocyte "see" (or "smell") the chemotactic agents, and how do these diverse substances actually induce directed cell movement? Although not all the answers are known, several important steps and second messengers are recognized (Fig. 2–9).[36,37] *First and foremost is the presence of specific receptors for chemotactic agents on the cell membranes of leukocytes.* The binding of the

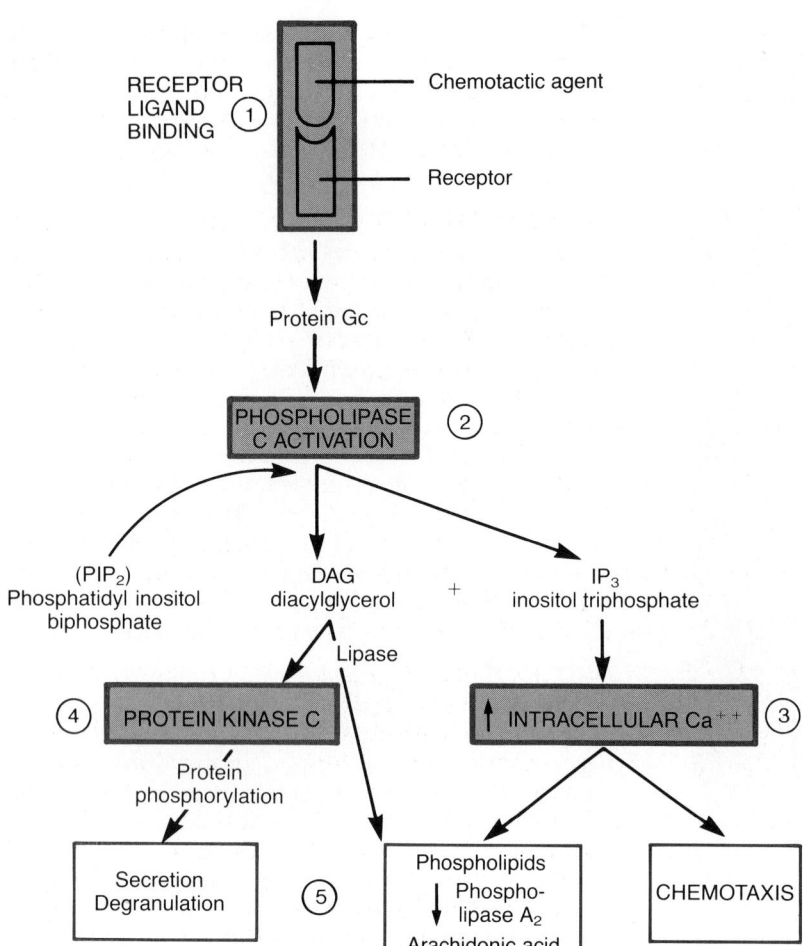

Figure 2–9. Biochemical events in leukocyte activation. The key events are (1) receptor-ligand binding (2) phospholipase-C activation, (3) increased intracellular calcium, and (4) activation of protein kinase C. The biologic activities (5) resulting from leukocyte activation include chemotaxis, elaboration of arachidonic acid metabolites, secretion, and degranulation.

ligand to the receptor is rapid, and if about 20% of the receptors are occupied there is increased random locomotion as well as chemotaxis. Chemotactic agents at higher concentrations also cause leukocyte "activation" (i.e., degranulation of storage vesicles and production of toxic oxygen products) (p. 57). Occupancy of receptors activates phospholipase C, mediated by a unique G-protein termed Gc. Phospholipase C activation results in the hydrolysis of a membrane phospholipid, phosphatidylinositol-4,5-biphosphate (PIP_2), to inositol-1,4,5-triphosphate (IP_3) and diacylglycerol (DAG). IP_3 causes the release of calcium from intracellular stores, *and it is the increased ionic calcium within the cytosol* that triggers the assembly of contractile elements responsible for cell movement. Increased intracellular Ca^{++} also activates phospholipase A_2, which, as we shall see (p. 56), converts membrane phospholipids to arachidonic acid and triggers the formation of arachidonic acid metabolites. Subsequently, sustained PIP_2 hydrolysis results in a stimulation of Ca^{++} *influx* across the leukocyte plasma membrane, and such Ca^{++} influx appears important in the consequent leukocyte activation. In addition, DAG, through its activation of protein kinase C, is involved in various phases of leukocyte degranulation and secretion,[37] which occur when there is a very strong chemotactic stimulus or during phagocytosis (p. 49).

The mechanisms of actual locomotion in leukocytes are beginning to be unraveled. The phagocyte moves by extending a pseudopod (lamellipod) that pulls the remainder of the cell in the direction of extension, just as an automobile with front-wheel drive is pulled by the motor in front (Fig. 2–10). The interior of the pseudopod consists of a branching network of filaments composed of *actin* as well as the contractile protein *myosin*. The phagocyte uses rapid association and dissociation of actin from monomer to fibrillar form to expand and contract the pseudopod when it is required to move. This phenomenon is controlled by calcium ions and a number of regulatory proteins, such as *actin binding protein, gelsolin, profilin,* and *calmodulin.* The last is a calcium-binding protein that controls the assembly of myosin molecules. Precisely how myosin interacts with actin in the pseudopod to produce contraction is unknown. However, movement is very dependent on intracytoplasmic calcium gradients that affect the action of the actin regulatory proteins.[38,39]

Phagocytosis and Degranulation

Phagocytosis and the release of enzymes by neutrophils and macrophages constitute two of the major benefits derived from the accumulation of leukocytes at the inflammatory focus.[40,41] Phagocytosis involves three distinct but interrelated steps (Fig. 2–11).

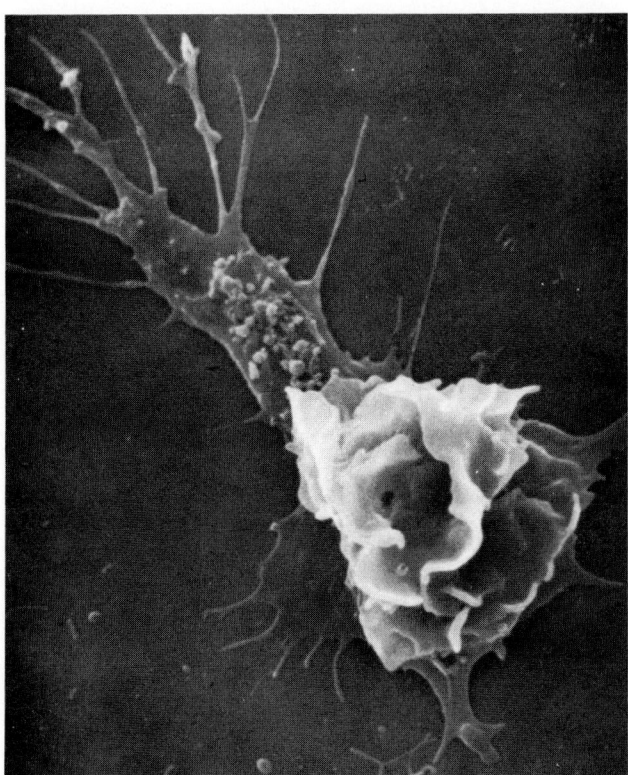

Figure 2–10. Scanning electron micrograph of a moving leukocyte in culture showing a pseudopod (upper left) and a trailing tail. (Courtesy of Dr. Morris J. Karnovsky, Harvard Medical School.)

First, the particle to be ingested becomes attached to the surface of the leukocyte, a phenomenon that requires some kind of *recognition* by the leukocyte. The second step is *engulfment*, with subsequent formation of a phagocytic vacuole. The third is *killing* or *degradation* of the ingested material.

RECOGNITION AND ATTACHMENT. Neutrophils and macrophages on occasion recognize and engulf bacteria or extraneous matter (e.g., latex beads) in the absence of serum, *but most microorganisms are not recognized until they are coated by naturally occurring serum factors called opsonins.* The two major opsonins are: (1) IgG (subtypes 1 and 3), presumably naturally occurring antibody against the ingested particle; and (2) C3b, the so-called "opsonic fragment of C3," generated by activation of complement by immune or nonimmune mechanisms[42] (p. 53). Opsonized particles attach to groups of corresponding *receptors* on the surface of neutrophils and macrophages: one group for the Fc fragment of the IgG molecules (called FcγR) and the other group for C3b.

ENGULFMENT. Engulfment occurs once the phagocyte recognizes a particle's foreignness. Binding of the opsonized particle to the FCγR is sufficient to trigger engulfment, but binding to the C3b receptors requires an activation of such receptors before engulfment occurs. Such activation is accomplished by simultaneous binding to extracellular fibronectin and laminin or by soluble products of stimulated T-lymphocytes. During engulfment, extensions of the cytoplasm (pseudopods) flow around the object to be engulfed, eventually resulting in complete enclosure of the particle within a phagosome created by the cytoplasmic membrane of the cell (Figs. 2–11 and 2–12). The limiting membrane of this phagocytic vacuole

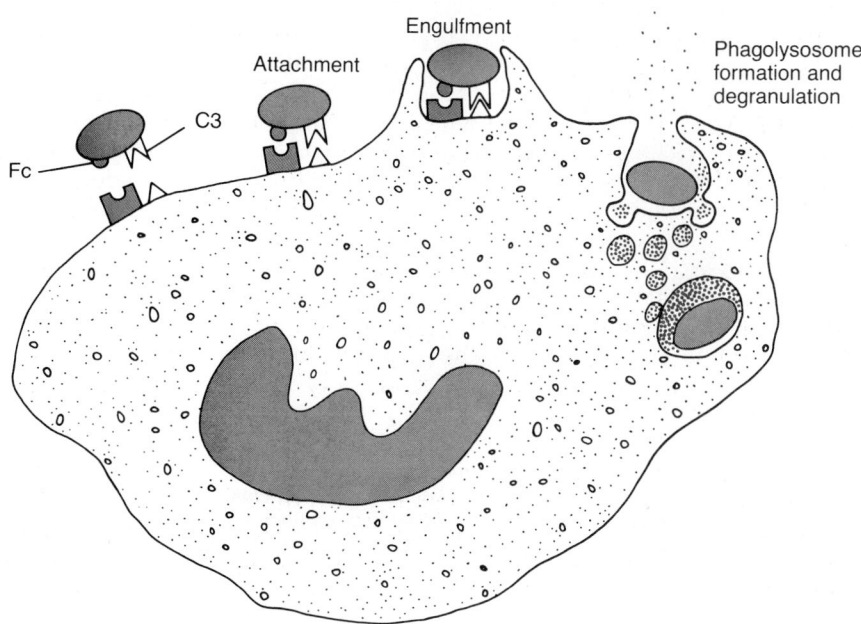

Figure 2–11. Phagocytosis of a particle (e.g., bacterium) involves attachment and binding of Fc and C3b to receptors on the leukocyte membrane, engulfment, and fusion of granules (in red) with phagocytic vacuoles, followed by degranulation. Note that during phagocytosis, granule contents may be released extracellularly.

then fuses with the limiting membrane of a lysosomal granule, resulting in discharge of the granule's contents into the phagolysosome. In the course of this action, the neutrophil and the monocyte become progressively degranulated. *During this process of degranulation there is some leakage of hydrolytic enzymes as well as metabolic products (e.g., hydrogen peroxide) from the phagocytizing leukocyte into the external medium,* probably through unclosed channels from the phagolysosome to the exterior. This process is aptly termed "regurgitation during feeding"; it is important because some of the leaked enzymes have proteolytic activity and may cause tissue damage.

Many of the biochemical events involved in phagocytosis and degranulation are similar to those described for chemotaxis (Fig. 2–9). The process is associated with receptor-ligand binding, phospholipase C activation, diacylglycerol and IP_3 production, protein kinase C activation, and increased concentration of cytosolic calcium, the latter two acting as second messengers to initiate cellular events that involve contractile proteins, microfilaments, and microtubules.[1,43]

KILLING OR DEGRADATION. The ultimate step in phagocytosis of bacteria is killing and degradation.

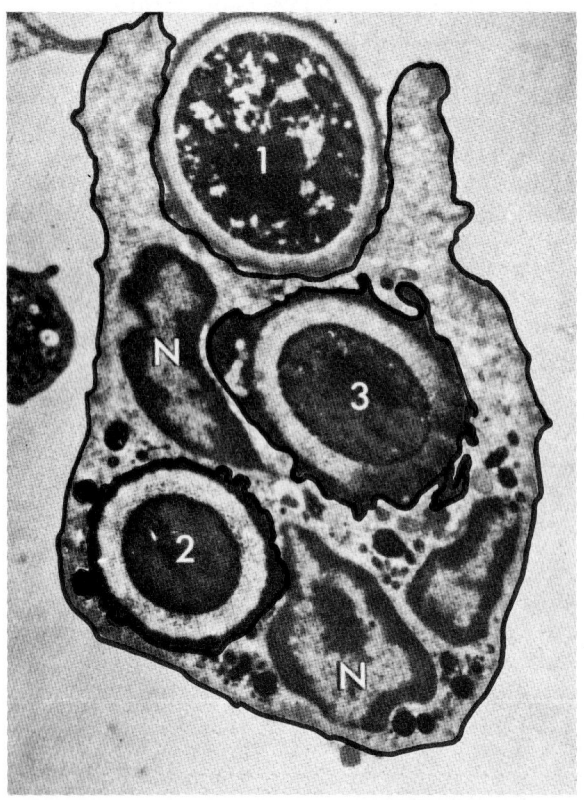

Figure 2–12. Neutrophil, stained for myeloperoxidase (black reaction product), showing phagocytosis of three yeast particles. Particle 1 is being engulfed and particle 2 shows fusion with granules; the granules have emptied their contents around particle 3. N = nucleus. (Courtesy of Dr. M. J. Karnovsky, Department of Pathology, Harvard Medical School.)

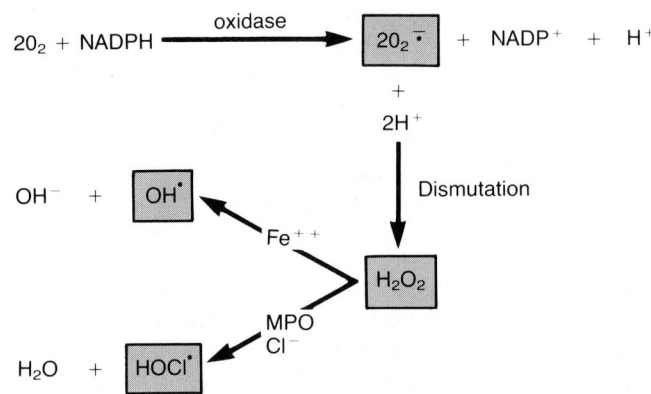

Figure 2–13. Summary of oxygen-dependent bactericidal mechanisms.

Two categories of bactericidal mechanisms are recognized: oxygen-dependent and oxygen-independent.

OXYGEN-DEPENDENT BACTERICIDAL MECHANISMS (FIG. 2–13). Phagocytosis is an energy-dependent phenomenon that stimulates numerous intracellular events, including *a burst in oxygen consumption, glycogenolysis, increased glucose oxidation via the hexose-monophosphate shunt, and production of reactive oxygen metabolites.*[41,45,46] The generation of oxygen metabolites is attributable to the rapid activation of an oxidase (NADPH oxidase), which oxidizes NADPH (reduced nicotinamide adenine dinucleotide) and in the process reduces oxygen to superoxide ion (O_2^-).

$$2O_2 + NADPH \xrightarrow{\text{oxidase}} 2O_2^- + NADP^+ + H^+$$

Superoxide is then converted into H_2O_2, mostly by spontaneous dismutation. The NADPH oxidase is present on the membrane or, when the membrane is invaginated, in the phagolysosome. Thus, the hydrogen peroxide is produced within the lysosome. These oxygen metabolites are the principal killers of bacteria, acting in one of two ways:

The H_2O_2-Myeloperoxidase-Halide System (Myeloperoxidase-Dependent Killing). The quantities of H_2O_2 produced in the phagolysosome are insufficient to induce effective killing of bacteria. However, the azurophilic granules of neutrophils contain the enzyme *myeloperoxidase* (MPO), which, in the presence of a halide such as Cl^-, converts H_2O_2 to $HOCl\cdot$, a powerful oxidant and antimicrobial agent.[46] A similar mechanism is also effective against fungi, viruses, protozoa, and helminths. Most of the H_2O_2 is eventually broken down by catalase into H_2O and O_2 (p. 12), and some is destroyed by the action of glutathione oxidase. Blood monocytes also contain MPO granules and use the H_2O_2-MPO-halide system for bacterial killing.

The most cogent argument for the relevance of the H_2O_2-myeloperoxidase system is the existence of a disease — *chronic granulomatous disease of child-*

hood (CGD) — characterized by an inherited enzymic defect that results in the failure of production of H_2O_2 during phagocytosis. Abrogation of the H_2O_2-myeloperoxidase-halide killing system makes these patients unusually susceptible to recurrent infections.

Myeloperoxidase-Independent Killing. Though the H_2O_2 myeloperoxidase-halide system is by far the most efficient bactericidal system in neutrophils, myeloperoxidase-deficient leukocytes are capable of killing bacteria (albeit more slowly than control cells). This MPO-independent system also requires oxygen. Superoxide, and hydroxyl radicals, extremely reactive radicals also formed during oxidative metabolism (Fig. 2–13), have been implicated in such killing. Mature activated *macrophages* under various conditions also produce H_2O_2 but do not contain MPO. They may thus kill bacteria by producing sufficient quantities of H_2O_2 or other toxic radicals, such as hydroxyl ions.

OXYGEN-INDEPENDENT MECHANISMS. Bacterial killing can also occur in the absence of an oxidative burst, by substances in the leukocyte granules. These include: *bactericidal permeability increasing protein (BPI)*, a highly cationic granule-associated protein that causes permeability changes in the outer membrane of the microorganisms[47]; *lysozyme*, which hydrolyzes the muramic acid-N-acetyl-glucosamine bond, found in the glycopeptide coat of all bacteria; *lactoferrin*, an iron-binding protein present in specific granules; and *major basic protein (MBP)*, a cationic protein of eosinophils, which has limited bactericidal activity but is cytotoxic to many parasites.[48]

Following killing, acid hydrolases found in azurophil granules degrade the bacteria within phagolysosomes. The pH of the phagolysosome drops to between 4 and 5 after phagocytosis, this being the optimal pH for the action of such enzymes.

Although most organisms are readily killed by the scavenger cells, some are sufficiently virulent to destroy their captor. Others, such as the tubercle bacillus, appear to survive happily within the phagocyte. Indeed, the persistence of organisms within phagocytes poses a problem in the eradication of such infections as tuberculosis. Thus enclosed, the microorganism is protected against the action of antibacterial drugs and other defense mechanisms. When these phagocytic cells migrate through lymphatic pathways, infections such as tuberculosis may be spread.

Extracellular Release of Leukocyte Products

The membrane perturbations that occur in neutrophils and monocytes after receptor-ligand binding during chemotaxis and phagocytosis result in the release of products not only within the phagolysosome, but also potentially into the extracellular space. The most important of these substances are (1) *lysosomal enzymes*; (2) *oxygen-derived active metabolites*, de-

tailed earlier; and (3) *products of arachidonic acid metabolism*, including prostaglandins and leukotrienes. These products are powerful mediators of vascular and cellular effects of inflammation and of tissue damage, and they serve to amplify the effects of the initial inflammatory stimulus.[49]

The actual release of lysosomal enzymes during phagocytosis occurs in at least three ways[50,51]:

1. *Regurgitation during feeding* may occur when the phagocytic vacuole remains transiently open to the outside before complete closure of the phagolysosome, permitting escape of lysosomal hydrolases, as explained earlier (see Fig. 2–11).
2. *Reverse endocytosis* (or frustrated phagocytosis) occurs when white cells are exposed to potentially ingestible materials (such as immune complexes) on flat surfaces, such as capillary endothelium. Attachment of the immune complexes to the leukocyte triggers membrane movement, but, because of the flat surface, phagocytosis does not occur, and lysosomal enzymes are released into the medium. This interesting phenomenon occurs in certain forms of immune complex–induced glomerular injury (p. 1024).
3. *Cytotoxic release* occurs when the neutrophil dies and is disrupted, its lysosomal enzymes rupturing into the extracellular space. Some particles (urate crystals and silica) are toxic to lysosomal membranes, allowing intracellular release of lysosomal enzymes.

Defects in Leukocyte Function

The significance of leukocyte adhesion, emigration, chemotaxis, and phagocytosis in the body's defense against bacterial infections cannot be underestimated. The best evidence for an in vivo role for these phenomena is the vulnerability to infection of patients suffering from acquired or genetic deficiencies in any of the factors that may affect the white cell — *from the moment it sticks to the endothelium, through its journey across the venular wall, to the ultimate battle within its phagolysosomes.* Although the diseases associated with these deficiencies are discussed in later chapters, it is useful here to list the *basic defects* that underlie the specific disorders of leukocytic function.[52,53]

1. *Defects in numbers of circulating cells* (e.g., neutropenia, toxic depression of bone marrow resulting from radiotherapy or chemotherapy).
2. *Defects in adherence* have been reported in diabetics, after acute alcohol intoxication, and after intake of certain drugs such as corticosteroids. *Leukocyte adhesion deficiency* is an autosomal recessive disorder, localized to chromosome 21, caused by a deficiency of the biosynthesis of the β chain of the leukocyte adhesion proteins described earlier (p. 46).[27]
3. *Defects in migration and chemotaxis* may be caused by (a) *an intrinsic abnormality of leukocytes*, such as occurs in diabetes, and the *Chédiak-Higashi syndrome* (a genetic disease in which there are several defects in

leukocytes, including impaired chemotaxis); (b) *a defect in chemotactic factor generation,* such as genetic or acquired C5 deficiency or immunoglobulin deficiency; (c) *serum chemotactic inhibitors* (for example, C5 inactivators), which are present in small amounts in normal serum but are markedly increased in patients with cirrhosis, sarcoidosis, and other diseases; and (d) *inhibitors of leukocyte locomotion,* which include some drugs (chloroquine) and poorly defined serum factors present in patients with malignancy, rheumatoid arthritis, and other isolated diseases.

4. *Defects in phagocytosis* may also be caused by an intrinsic cellular defect (e.g., diabetes, neutrophil "actin dysfunction"), or a deficiency of immunoglobulin or complement, resulting in decreased opsonization of particles.

5. *Defects in microbicidal activity* may be caused by the following:

a. *Impaired H_2O_2 production,* such as *chronic granulomatous disease* (CGD). CGD is an inherited, most commonly X-linked disease of male children and infants, characterized by recurrent infections and death at an early age. The neutrophils do not develop the typical "respiratory burst" upon phagocytosis. H_2O_2 production is deficient, leading to failure of the important MPO-H_2O_2-halide killing system. Catalase-positive organisms (e.g., *Staphylococcus aureus*), which destroy the little H_2O_2 that is produced, most frequently cause infections, whereas catalase-negative bacteria or bacteria that form their own H_2O_2 are killed normally by CGD leukocytes.[54]

b. *Myeloperoxidase deficiency* is a rare autosomal recessive disorder. Because H_2O_2 and O_2^- themselves may be sufficiently bactericidal, most patients are in good health, although some have recurrent infections.

c. *Severe deficiency of leukocyte glucose-6-phosphate dehydrogenase (G6PD);* because this enzyme is required to produce NADPH in the hexose monophosphate (HMP) shunt, its absence results in H_2O_2 deficiency and a defect similar to that seen in CGD.

6. *Mixed defects.* In some diseases (e.g., diabetes, Chédiak-Higashi syndrome), more than one defect is involved. In the latter disease, for example, there is neutropenia, impaired chemotactic response, delayed or decreased fusion of lysosomes with phagosomes, and deficient degranulation. The disease is a rare autosomal recessive disorder characterized by the presence of giant lysosome-like granules in the leukocytes and other granule-containing cells. The basic defect may be in microtubule polymerization. Leukocyte defects increase the susceptibility of these patients to infection. As described later (p. 82), corticosteroids also interfere with a variety of leukocyte functions.

CHEMICAL MEDIATORS OF INFLAMMATION

Injury precipitates the inflammatory response, but released chemicals mediate it. Their existence was long suspected for two reasons: (1) Whatever the nature of the injury, the ensuing inflammatory changes constituted a fairly uniform, almost stereotyped reaction, and (2) inflammation developed in tissues deprived of their nervous connections. Since Lewis's discovery of histamine, the active search for other mediators has uncovered a perplexing multitude of candidates. The list of possible mediators (almost all discovered from studies in vitro) increases with every edition of this book. We must now determine which are significant in man and what roles each plays.

Mediators can originate from *plasma,* from *cells,* or conceivably from *damaged tissue* (Fig. 2–14). They can be divided into the following groups:

• Vasoactive amines: histamines and serotonin
• Plasma proteases:
  (1) the kinin system (bradykinin and kallikrein);
  (2) the complement system (C3a; C5a; C5b–C9);
  (3) the coagulation-fibrinolytic system (fibrinopeptides, fibrin degradation products)
• Arachidonic acid (AA) metabolites:
  (1) via cyclooxygenase (endoperoxides, prostaglandins, thromboxane);
  (2) via lipoxygenase (leukotriene; HPETE; HETE)
• Lysosomal constituents (proteases)

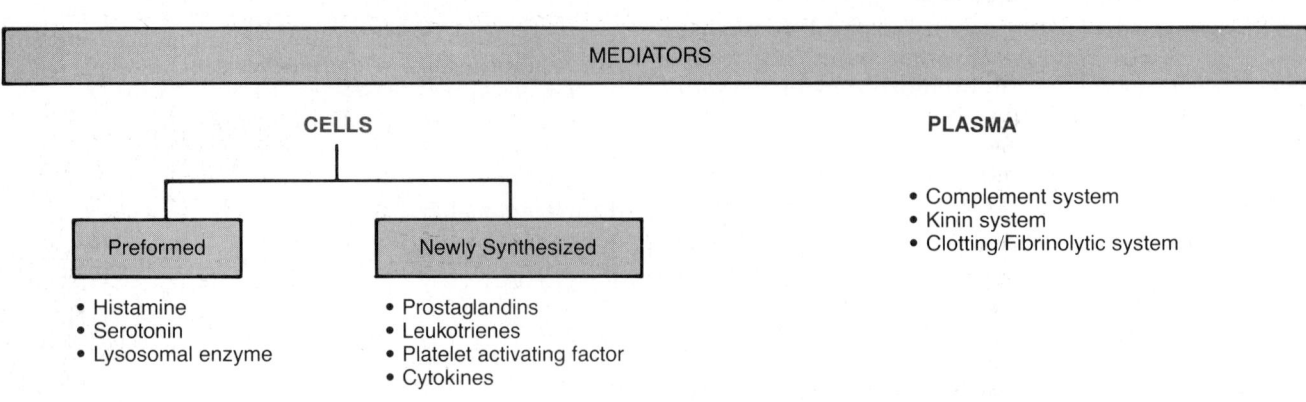

Figure 2–14. Chemical mediators of inflammation.

- Oxygen-derived free radicals
- Platelet activating factors (**PAF**)
- Cytokines
- Growth factors

Vasoactive Amines

Histamine and serotonin (5-hydroxytryptamine) are believed to be mediators in the immediate active phase of increased permeability. In humans, histamine is stored and is immediately available largely in the granules of the mast cells in tissues and basophils in the blood. Serotonin likewise is present in the mast cells of such rodents as rat and mouse and in platelets. These amines cause vasodilation and increased vascular permeability, the latter being restricted to venules. Histamine acts on the microcirculation mainly through H1-type receptors.[55]

Many agents release amines from mast cells. Principal among these are (1) *physical agents,* such as trauma or cold; (2) *immunologic reactions,* through a well-known mechanism involving receptors on the mast cell surface that bind with IgE (p. 174); (c) *C3a and C5a,* fragments of complement that induce increased vascular permeability (for which reason they are called *anaphylatoxins);* (d) *histamine-releasing factors* from neutrophils, monocytes, and platelets; and (e) *interleukin-1.*

Histamine can be isolated from inflammatory sites in early inflammation, and H1 histamine antagonists suppress the immediate-transient response induced by mild injury. However, the content of histamine dwindles within the first 60 minutes, and antihistaminics have no effect on the delayed permeability responses. *Thus, histamine is important mainly in early inflammatory responses* and in immediate IgE-mediated hypersensitivity reactions.

Release of histamine and serotonin from *platelets* (the platelet release reaction) is stimulated when platelets aggregate after contact with collagen, thrombin, ADP, and antigen-antibody complexes. Platelet aggregation and release are also stimulated by platelet activating factor (PAF) derived from mast cells during IgE-mediated reactions. In this way the platelet release reaction results in increased permeability during immunologic reactions. As will be discussed later, PAF itself has many inflammatory properties.

Plasma Proteases

Three interrelated systems—the complement, kinin, and clotting systems—are active within this category. The kinins are highly vasoactive; complement components are both vasoactive and chemotactic.

THE COMPLEMENT SYSTEM. The complement system consists of 20 component proteins (together with their cleavage products), which are found in greatest concentration in plasma.[57] This system functions in the immune system by mediating a series of biologic reactions, all of which serve in the defense against microbial agents. These biologic reactions include increased vascular permeability, chemotaxis, opsonization prior to phagocytosis, and lysis of target organisms.

The complement system consists of *activating* and *effector* sequences. Activation occurs rapidly and efficiently via the *classic* pathway, initiated by antigen-antibody complexes, or more slowly by the *alternate* pathway, initiated by a variety of largely nonimmunologic stimuli. As a result of activation, proteolytic cleavage products are elaborated, with profound inflammatory effects. Both pathways converge into the common pathway of a membrane attack complex (Fig. 2–15).[58]

The *classic pathway* is initiated by binding of an antigen-antibody complex to the C1q subunit of C1, which self-activates and cleaves C4 and C2; the resulting cleavage fragments form a complex C4b2a, also called *C3 convertase.* C3 convertase is an important enzyme, because it splits C3 into two critical fragments: C3a and C3b. C3a is released, but C3b forms a trimolecular complex with C4b2a, (C5 convertase). C5 convertase interacts with C5 to break off C5a; C5b combines with C6 and C7 into a C5b67 complex. Further binding of C5b67 with C8 and C9 produces C5b–9, the membrane attack complex.

In the alternate complement pathway, C3 is activated directly (thus bypassing C1, C4, and C2) by such stimuli as bacterial endotoxins, complex polysaccharides, cobra venom, and aggregated globulins, particularly IgA. The C3 convertase of this system is

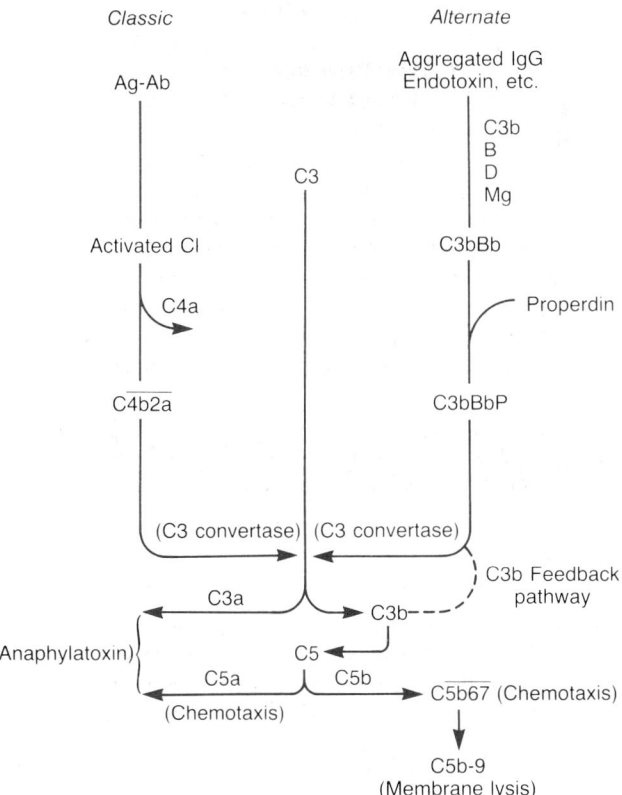

Figure 2–15. Complement system (see text).

formed by interactions of factors B, D, and C3b in the presence of magnesium (see also p. 1041).

The principal components of the complement system that have biologic activity in inflammation are as follows:

1. *C3a* increases vascular permeability. In addition to being produced by the classic and alternate pathways, *C3 can be directly cleaved* (at least in vitro) by plasmin, bacterial proteases, and other C3-cleaving enzymes found in various tissues.

2. *C5a* induces increased vascular permeability and is highly chemotactic to neutrophils, eosinophils, basophils, and monocytes. It is released by complement activation or by direct cleavage by trypsin, bacterial proteases, and enzymes found in neutrophil lysosomes and macrophages. C5a is rapidly converted in human serum to *C5a des Arg*, which is also chemotactic in the presence of a serum polypeptide called *cochemotoxin*. C5a also increases the adhesion of leukocytes to endothelium by increasing the surface expression of the leukocyte adhesion molecules (p. 46).

The permeability-increasing components of C3a and C5a are called *anaphylatoxins*. They act mainly by liberating histamine from mast cells and platelets. C5a also activates the lipoxygenase pathway of arachidonic acid metabolism in neutrophils and macrophages, leading to the formation of additional mediators of increased permeability and chemotaxis from these cells. Concomitant release of oxygen-derived radicals may also cause tissue damage and production of other chemotactic lipids, as we shall see (p. 57). Thus, C5a in vivo is a powerful inflammatory agent.

3. *C3b and C3bi* are important opsonins, recognizing receptors on neutrophils, macrophages, and eosinophils.

4. *C5b-9*, the membrane attack complex (MAC), is the final lytic component of complement and is involved in injury to parenchymal cells.[58] The complex inserts into lipid bilayers and forms transmembrane channels that increase cell permeability, causing cell lysis. MAC also stimulates arachidonic acid metabolism and production of reactive oxygen metabolites by macrophages and other cells.

THE KININ SYSTEM. The kinin system is one of three mediator systems directly triggered by surface activation of Hageman factor (Fig. 2–16). This system results in the ultimate release of the vasoactive nonapeptide *bradykinin*, a potent agent that increases vascular permeability. *Bradykinin also causes contraction of smooth muscle, dilation of blood vessels, and pain when injected into the skin. It is not chemotactic.* The cascade that eventually produces kinin is shown in Figure 2–16.[59] It begins with the activation of factor XII of the intrinsic clotting system (Hageman factor) by contact with surface-active agents, such as collagen, basement membrane, and endotoxin. A fragment of factor XII (prekallikrein activator, or factor XIIA) is produced, and this converts plasma prekallikrein into an active proteolytic form, the enzyme *kallikrein*. The latter cleaves a plasma-glycoprotein precursor, *high-molecular-weight kininogen* (HMWK), to produce *bradykinin* (HMWK also acts as a cofactor or catalyst in the activation of Hageman factor). The action of bradykinin is short-lived because it is quickly inactivated by an enzyme called *kininase. Of importance is that kallikrein itself is a potent activator of Hageman factor*, allowing for autocatalytic amplification of the initial stimulus. Kallikrein has chemotactic activity, and it causes aggregation of neutrophils in vitro.

THE CLOTTING SYSTEM. The clotting system (p. 57) is a series of plasma proteins that can be activated by Hageman factor (Fig. 2–16). The final step of the cascade is the conversion of fibrinogen to fibrin by the action of thrombin. During this conversion, *fibrinopeptides* are formed, which induce increased vascular permeability and chemotactic activity for leukocytes.

The *fibrinolytic system* contributes to the vascular phenomena of inflammation in several ways, but mainly by means of the kinin system (Fig. 2–16). Plasminogen activator (released from endothelium, leukocytes, and other tissues) or kallikrein cleaves plasminogen, a plasma protein that binds to the evolving fibrin clot to generate *plasmin*, a multifunctional protease. Plasmin is important in lysing fibrin clots, but in the context of inflammation it has the following actions: (1) it activates Hageman factor (XII), releasing factor XIIA, which initiates the cascade to generate bradykinin; (2) it cleaves C3, the third component of complement, to produce C3 fragments; and (3) it degrades fibrin to form "fibrin split products," which may have permeability-inducing properties.

SUMMARY OF PLASMA PROTEASES. From this discussion of the complex mediators generated by the kinin, complement, and clotting systems, a few general conclusions can be drawn:

1. *Bradykinin, C3a, and C5a (as mediators of increased vascular permeability), and C5a (as the mediator of chemotaxis), are the most likely to be important in vivo.*

2. *C3 and C5* are central because they can be generated (at least in vitro) by three different groups of influences: (a) classic immunologic reactions; (b) alternate complement pathway activation; and (c) agents with little immunologic specificity, such as bacterial products, plasmin, and some serine proteases found in normal tissue.

3. *Activated Hageman factor (factor XIIA)* initiates the clotting, fibrinolytic, and kinin systems. The products of this initiation—kallikrein, factor XIIA, and plasmin, but particularly kallikrein—can, by feedback, activate Hageman factor, resulting in profound amplification of the effects of the initial stimulus.

Arachidonic Acid Metabolites: The Prostaglandins and Leukotrienes

Oxygenated arachidonic acid derivatives have roles in a variety of biologic and pathologic processes, only

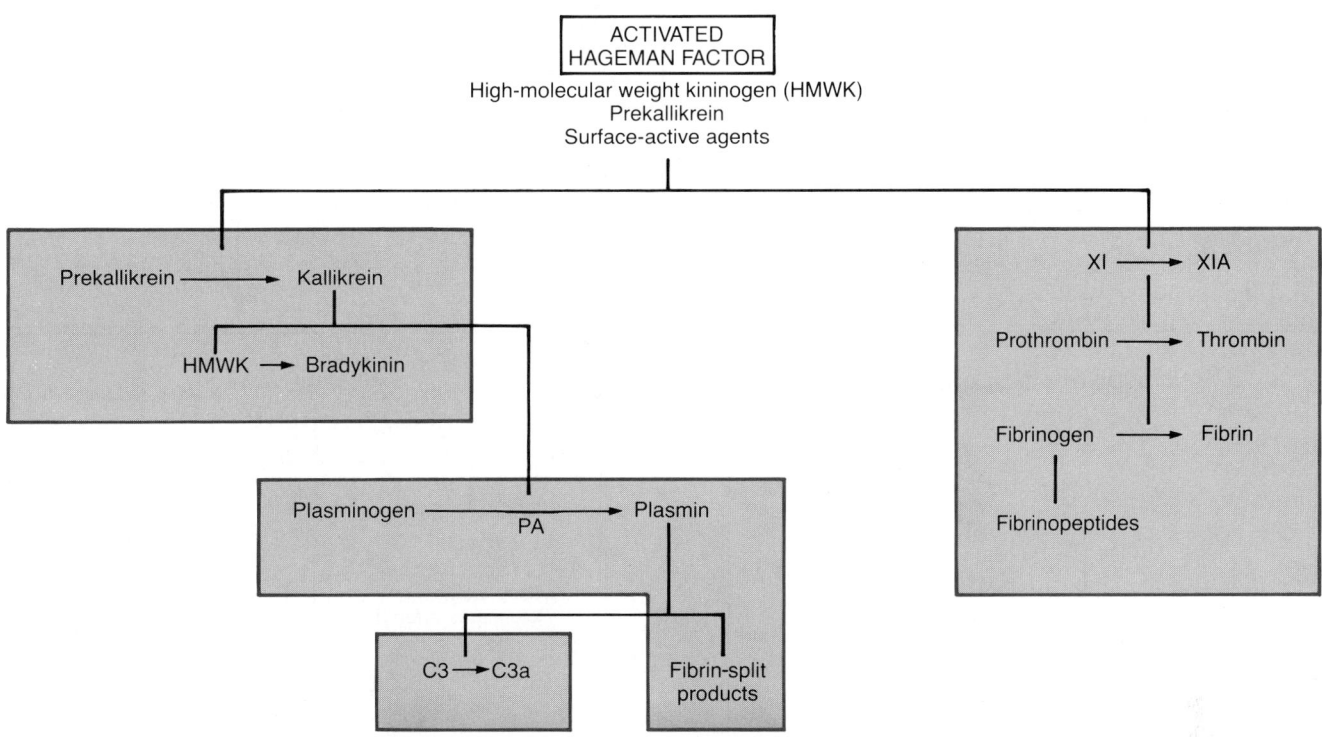

Figure 2–16. Plasma mediator systems triggered by activation of Hageman factor. PA = plasminogen activator.

one of which is inflammation. These compounds are involved in the processes of hemostasis and thrombosis and in cardiovascular, pulmonary, renal, and endocrine pathophysiology. Here we review briefly the arachidonic acid cascade and its major products and highlight those that appear to be important mediators of various aspects of the inflammatory response[62] (Fig. 2–17).

Prostaglandins and related compounds are best thought of as *autocoids*, or local short-range hormones, which are formed rapidly, exert their effects locally, and then decay spontaneously or are destroyed enzymatically.

Arachidonic acid (AA) is a 20-carbon polyunsaturated fatty acid (5,8,11,14-eicosatetraenoic acid) that is derived directly from dietary sources or by conversion from the essential fatty acid *linoleic acid*. It does not occur free in the cell but is normally esterified in membrane phospholipids, particularly in the carbon 2 position of phosphatidylcholine and phosphatidylinositol. In order for arachidonic acid to be utilized by the cell to make eicosanoids, it must first be released from phospholipids. This is accomplished through the activation of cellular phospholipases by mechanical, chemical, and physical stimuli or by other mediators (e.g., C5a). Following activation, biosynthesis of the metabolites of arachidonic acid occurs by one of two major pathways (Fig. 2–17).

THE CYCLOOXYGENASE PATHWAY. A fatty acid cyclooxygenase transforms arachidonic acid rapidly into the prostaglandin endoperoxide PGG_2, which in turn is converted enzymatically into PGH_2. In the conversion of PGG_2 to PGH_2, a free radical of oxygen is generated. PGH_2 is then converted enzymatically into three products: (1) *thromboxane A_2* (TXA_2), found in platelets and other cells, a short-lived (half-life of seconds), potent platelet aggregator and blood vessel constrictor; (2) *prostacyclin* (PGI_2), found predominantly in the vessel wall, a potent inhibitor of platelet aggregation and vasodilator; and (3) in many sites the more stable prostaglandins PGE_2, $PGF_2\alpha$, *and PGD_2*, which have a variety of actions on vascular tone and permeability. Each of these steps is carried out by specific enzymes (e.g., thromboxane synthetase, prostacyclin synthetase) present within the target cell. Aspirin, indomethacin, and other nonsteroidal anti-inflammatory drugs inhibit cyclooxygenase.

THE LIPOXYGENASE PATHWAY. The lipoxygenase pathway involves the conversion of AA by fatty acid lipoxygenases into hydroperoxy derivatives (hydroperoxyeicosatetraenoic acid [HPETE]; 12-HPETE in platelets and 5-HPETE and 15-HPETE in leukocytes).[60,61] 5-HPETE may undergo peroxidation to hydroxyeicosatetraenoic acid (HETE), the latter being a potent chemotactic stimulus for neutrophils. 5-HPETE also gives rise to the *leukotrienes*, so designated because of their conjugated triene chain and their initial isolation from leukocytes. An unstable 5,6-epoxy derivative, *leukotriene A_4* (LTA_4), is then enzymatically converted to *leukotriene B_4*, or by addition of a glutathione residue to *leukotriene C_4* (LTC_4) LTC_4 is then converted to *leukotriene D_4* (LTD_4) and subsequently to *leukotriene E_4*. Leukotriene B_4 is a potent chemotactic agent that causes

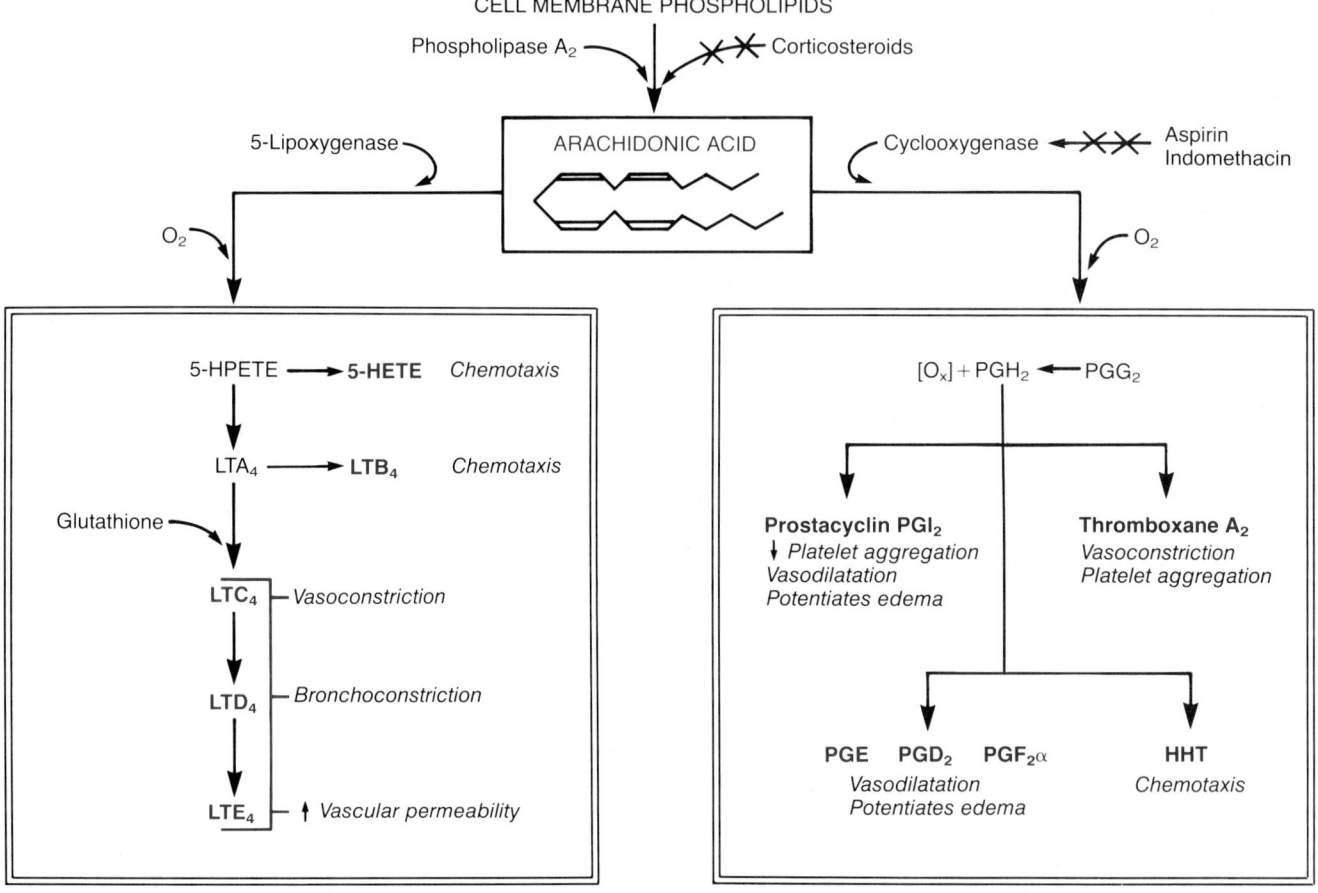

Figure 2–17. Arachidonic acid metabolites in inflammation.

aggregation of leukocytes; LTC_4, LTD_4, and LTE_4 all cause vasoconstriction, bronchospasm, and increased vascular permeability.

Neutrophils also produce trihydroxymetabolites of arachidonic acid called *lipoxins.*[61] These metabolites have powerful proinflammatory effects in vitro, but their role in vivo is only currently being investigated.

Table 2–2 summarizes the principal actions of arachidonic acid metabolites. The evidence for their involvement in inflammation can be summarized as follows:

Table 2–2. Inflammatory Actions of Arachidonic Acid Metabolites

ACTION	METABOLITE
Vasoconstriction	Thromboxane A_2, HPETE, endoperoxides, leukotrienes C_4, D_4, E_4
Vasodilatation	PGI_2, PGE_1, PGE_2, PGD_2
Increased Vascular Permeability	Leukotrienes C_4, D_4, E_4
Chemotaxis	Leukotriene B_4, HHT, HPETE, HETE

• *Prostaglandins and leukotrienes* can be detected in the fluids and exudates of inflammatory reactions and in anaphylactic reactions in the lungs.

• *Drugs such as corticosteroids, aspirin, and indomethacin* have anti-inflammatory properties because they inhibit the biosynthesis of prostaglandins (Fig. 2–17).

• *Prostaglandin E and prostacyclin* are probably the most important mediators of inflammatory vasodilation. They also markedly potentiate the permeability-increasing and chemotactic effects of other mediators.

• *The cysteinyl-containing leukotrienes C_4, D_4, and E_4* cause intense vasoconstriction and increase vascular permeability. The vascular leakage, as with histamine, is restricted to venules. They are also potent bronchoconstrictors.[63]

• *Leukotriene B_4* causes aggregation and adhesion of leukocytes to venular endothelium and is a powerful chemotactic agent.[64] Some of the other products of lipoxygenase metabolism, such as HETE, are also chemotactic.

• *The prostaglandins* are also involved in the pathogenesis of pain and fever in inflammation. PGE_2 causes a marked increase in pain produced by intradermal injection of suboptimal concentrations of histamine and bradykinin, and prostaglandin production is involved in the causation of fever during severe infections (p. 70).

• *Diets rich in fish oil* contain essential fatty acids of the *omega 3* (ω3) variety (e.g., *linolenic acid*) rather than ω2 linoleic acid found in most animal or vegetable fat. The ω3 fatty acids serve as poor substrates for conversion to active metabolites of the cyclooxygenase, and particularly the lipoxygenase, series. In experimental animals and in vitro there is considerable evidence that such diets inhibit platelet aggregation and prevent certain inflammatory processes (see also p. 559).[65]

Lysosomal Constituents

Neutrophils and monocytes contain lysosomal granules, which when released may contribute to the inflammatory response. *Neutrophils* exhibit two main types of granules (Fig. 2–18). The smaller *specific* (or secondary) granules contain lactoferrin, lysozyme, alkaline phosphatase, leukocyte adhesion molecules (p. 45), and (in human neutrophils) collagenase. The large *azurophil* (or primary) granules contain myeloperoxidase, lysozyme, bactericidal factors, cationic proteins, acid hydrolases, and some neutral proteases (elastase). The three last-mentioned products are the lysosomal constituents that have potential inflammatory activities.[66]

The *cationic proteins* are a heterogeneous group of proteins that (1) increase vascular permeability either directly or by releasing histamine from mast cells; (2) cause chemotaxis of monocytes (neutrophil chemotactic factor, NCF); and (3) inhibit the movement of other neutrophils and eosinophils. *Acid proteases* degrade proteins at an acid pH. Their most likely action is to degrade bacteria and debris *within* the phagolysosomes, where an acid pH is readily reached. *Neutral proteases,* on the other hand, are capable of degrading various extracellular components. These enzymes (collagenase, elastase, cathepsins, and so forth) can attack collagen, basement membrane, fibrin, elastin, and cartilage, resulting in the tissue destruction characteristic of purulent and deforming inflammatory processes. Neutral proteases can also release a kinin-like peptide from kininogen.

The *monocytes* and *macrophages* also contain acid hydrolases, collagenase, elastase, and plasminogen activator. These may be particularly active in chronic inflammatory reactions (p. 63).

Lysosomal constituents thus have numerous effects. The initial leukocytic infiltration, if unchecked, can potentiate further increases in vascular permeability, chemotaxis, and tissue damage. These harmful proteases, however, are held in check by a system of *antiproteases* in the serum and tissue fluids.[67] Foremost among these is *alpha-1-antitrypsin*, which is the major inhibitor of neutrophilic elastase. It follows, therefore, that a deficiency of these inhibitors may lead to sustained action of leukocyte proteases, as is the case in patients with alpha-1-antitrypsin deficiency (p. 769). *Alpha-2-macroglobulin* is another antiprotease found in serum and various secretions.

Oxygen-Derived Free Radicals

As we have seen, reactive oxygen metabolites, elaborated in neutrophils and macrophages, may be released extracellularly after exposure to chemotactic agents, immune complexes, or a phagocytic challenge. These metabolites have been implicated in the following responses.

1. *Endothelial cell damage with resultant increased vascular permeability.* For example, activation of C5a in vivo causes neutrophilic aggregation, endothelial cell damage, and increased permeability of lung capillaries; the latter can be prevented by previous treatment of the animals with H_2O_2 and OH· scavengers, which suggests that these species mediate the endothelial damage.[68]

2. *Inactivation of antiproteases*, such as alpha-1-antitrypsin, discussed earlier. Potentially this may lead to unopposed protease activity with increased destruction of structural components of tissue, such as elastin. Inactivation appears to result from oxidation of methionyl residues on the antiprotease molecule *to the sulfoxide* with loss of biologic activity.

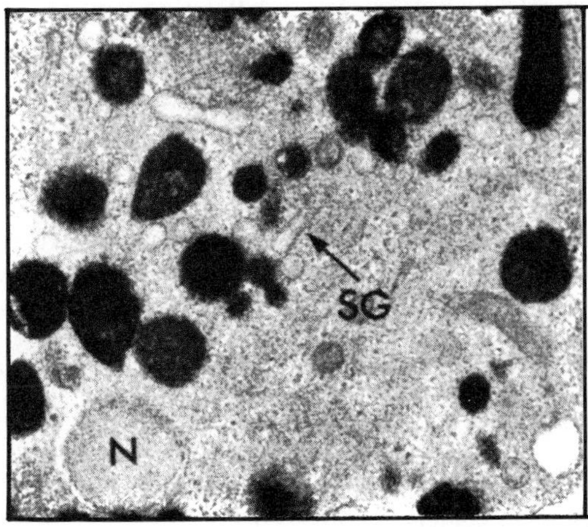

Figure 2–18. Ultrastructure of neutrophil granules stained for peroxidase activity and their constituents. The large peroxidase-containing granules are the azurophil granules; the smaller peroxidase-negative ones are the specific granules (SG). N: portion of nucleus.

SPECIFIC GRANULES
Lactoferrin
Lysozyme
Alkaline phosphatase
Collagenase
Leukocyte adhesion molecules

AZUROPHIL GRANULES
Myeloperoxidase
Lysozyme ← Bactericidal factors
Cationic proteins
Acid hydrolases
Neutral proteases (elastase)

3. *Injury to other cell types* (tumor cells, red cells, parenchymal cells), ascribed to a variety of oxygen metabolites.

Serum, tissue fluids, and target cells possess antioxidant protective mechanisms that detoxify these potentially harmful oxygen-derived radicals. These antioxidants have been discussed in Chapter 1, but to repeat, they include (1) the copper-containing serum protein *ceruloplasmin;* (2) the iron-free fraction of serum *transferrin;* (3) the enzyme *superoxide dismutase,* which is found or can be activated in a variety of cell types; (4) the enzyme *catalase,* which detoxifies H_2O_2; and (5) *glutathione peroxidase,* another powerful H_2O_2 detoxifier. *Thus, the influence of oxygen-derived free radicals in any given inflammatory reaction depends on the balance between the production and inactivation of these metabolites by cells and tissues.*

Platelet Activating Factor (PAF)

PAF has been known for years as a factor, derived from antigen-stimulated IgE-sensitized basophils, which causes aggregation of platelets and release of their active constituents (such as histamine and serotonin).[70-72] The chemical structure of PAF has been documented as a lipid—acetyl glycerol ether phosphocholine (AGEPC) (Fig. 2–19). PAFs are not stored as preformed mediators but are rapidly generated after cell stimulation.

In addition to platelet stimulation, PAF causes vasoconstriction and bronchoconstriction, and at extremely low concentrations it induces vasodilation and increased venular permeability with a potency 100 to 10,000 times greater than that of histamine. PAF also causes increased leukocyte adhesion to endothelium and chemotaxis in vitro and early leukocytic infiltration when injected into the skin. Thus, PAF can elicit most of the cardinal signs of inflammation. A variety of cells types, including basophils, neutrophils, monocytes, and endothelium, can elaborate PAF.[72]

PAF appears to act directly on target cells, but it also stimulates the synthesis of other mediators, particularly prostaglandins and leukotrienes, by leukocytes and other cells. In addition, there is synergism of its actions with those of other autocoids. The recent availability of synthetic PAF antagonists may soon clarify its role in mediating inflammatory responses in vivo.

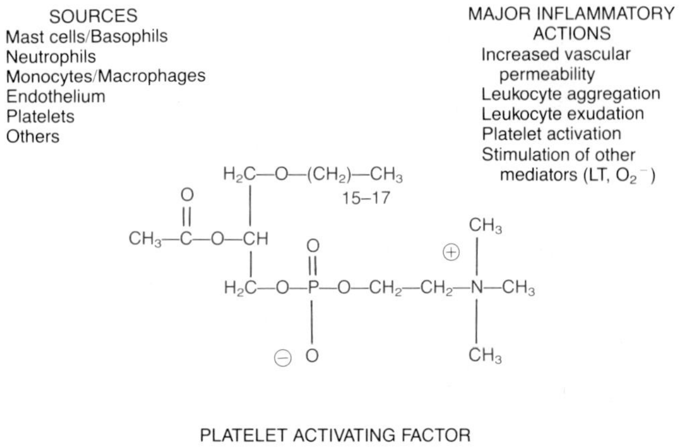

Cytokines

Certain *polypeptide* products of activated lymphocytes and monocytes—called *lymphokines* and *monokines,* respectively—have long been known to be involved in cellular responses in immunology, such as lymphocyte recruitment and lymphocyte proliferation (p. 168). Recently it has become clear that some of these products have additional effects that play an important role in the inflammatory response.[74] Similar polypeptides *(cytokines)* are produced by many nonlymphoid cell types. Two of the cytokines that appear to be important mediators of inflammation are *interleukin-1* (IL-1) and *tumor necrosis factor* (TNF).[73,74] Although different gene products, they share many biologic properties.[75]

IL-1 was originally isolated from activated macrophages but is produced by virtually all cell types, including lymphocytes and vascular endothelium. Production of IL-1 in vitro can be stimulated by endotoxin, immune complexes, toxins, physical injury, and a variety of inflammatory processes. *TNF* (also called *cachectin,* because it is thought to be involved in the cachexia of chronic infection and tumors, p. 294)[76] was originally described as a product of stimulated macrophages that caused lysis of certain tumor cell lines in vitro and hemorrhagic tumor necrosis in vivo. IL-1 and TNF induce the same spectrum of biologic effects, particularly in acute phases of inflammation, and also act synergistically.

In general, IL-1 and TNF (and most other cytokines) induce their effects in three ways: they can act on the same cell that produces them (an *autocrine* effect); on cells in the immediate vicinity (as in lymph nodes and joint spaces; a *paracrine* effect); or systemically, as with any other hormone (endocrine effect). Their most important actions in inflammation are the local effects on endothelium, the systemic "acute phase" reactions, and the effect on fibroblasts (Fig. 2–20). The latter is relevant to the process of repair and is discussed later (p. 77). The effects of IL-1 and TNF on endothelium include the following:

1. Induction and synthesis of surface adhesion molecules, which stimulate increased adhesion of neutrophils, monocytes, and lymphocytes to the endothelium.
2. Induction of synthesis and release of PGI_2, a potent vasodilator and inhibitor of platelet aggregation.
3. Stimulation of synthesis of platelet activating factor (PAF).
4. Increase in procoagulant and decrease in anticoagulant properties of endothelial cells, rendering the endothelial surface potentially thrombogenic (p. 94).

SOURCES
Mast cells/Basophils
Neutrophils
Monocytes/Macrophages
Endothelium
Platelets
Others

MAJOR INFLAMMATORY ACTIONS
Increased vascular permeability
Leukocyte aggregation
Leukocyte exudation
Platelet activation
Stimulation of other mediators (LT, O_2^-)

PLATELET ACTIVATING FACTOR

Figure 2–19. Structure, sources, and main inflammatory actions of PAF. LT = leukotrienes.

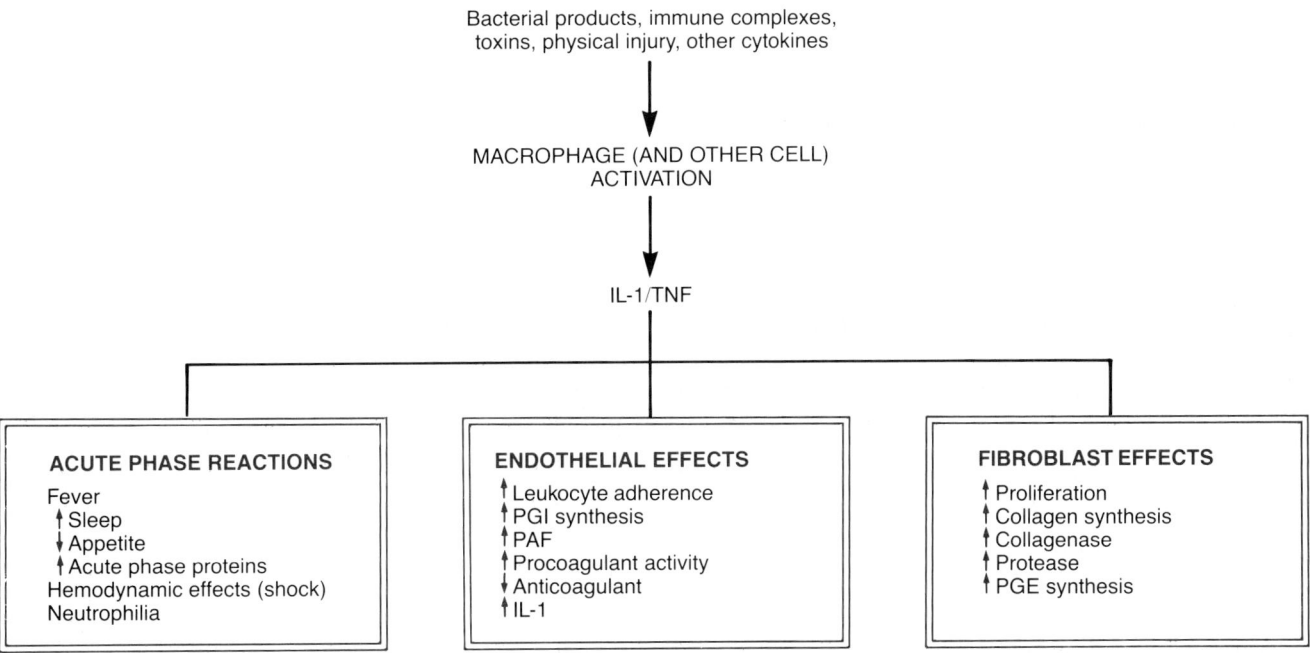

Bacterial products, immune complexes,
toxins, physical injury, other cytokines

↓

MACROPHAGE (AND OTHER CELL)
ACTIVATION

↓

IL-1/TNF

ACUTE PHASE REACTIONS	ENDOTHELIAL EFFECTS	FIBROBLAST EFFECTS
Fever	↑ Leukocyte adherence	↑ Proliferation
↑ Sleep	↑ PGI synthesis	↑ Collagen synthesis
↓ Appetite	↑ PAF	↑ Collagenase
↑ Acute phase proteins	↑ Procoagulant activity	↑ Protease
Hemodynamic effects (shock)	↑ Anticoagulant	↑ PGE synthesis
Neutrophilia	↑ IL-1	

Figure 2–20. Major effects of interleukin-1 (IL-1) and tumor necrosis factor (TNF) in inflammation.

Both IL-1 and TNF also induce the systemic *acute phase responses* (p. 70) associated with infection or injury, including fever, the production of slow-wave sleep, the release of neutrophils into the circulation, the release of ACTH and corticosteroids, and, particularly for TNF, the hemodynamic effects of septic shock—hypotension, decreased vascular resistance, increased heart rate, and decreased blood pH (p. 70).

Growth Factors and Other Mediators

Other mediators that have chemotactic activity for leukocytes are fragments derived from the breakdown of collagen or fibronectin and certain growth factors. These factors have additional roles in chronic inflammation and wound healing and are discussed on page 76.

Summary of Chemical Mediators of Acute Inflammation

Table 2–3 summarizes the major actions of the principal mediators. The multiplicity of proposed mediators is eloquent testimony not only to the current excitement about the biochemical basis of inflammation, but also to the fact that we are still unsure of the precise events involved in mediation of the inflammatory response. When Lewis suggested the existence of histamine, one mediator was clearly not enough. Now we are wallowing in them! Yet from this morass we can tentatively extract a few mediators that may be relevant in vivo (Table 2–4). *For increased vascular permeability, histamine, the anaphylatoxins (C3a and C5a), the kinins; leukotrienes C,D, and E; and PAF are almost certainly involved, at least early in the course of inflammation. For chemotaxis, complement fragments C5a, AA lipoxygenase products (leukotriene B$_4$), and other chemotactic lipids are the most likely protagonists. Also, the important role of prostaglandins in vasodilation, pain, and fever and in potentiating edema cannot be denied. IL-1 and TNF are involved with vascular events and with acute phase reactions. Lysosomal products and oxygen-derived radicals are the most likely candidates as causes of the ensuing tissue destruction.*

Two points must be re-emphasized before the discussion of mediators is closed. The first is that the *different mediator systems, although discussed separately, are intimately intertwined.* One example, cited earlier, is the role of activated Hageman factor in the kinin, clotting, and fibrinolytic cascades. Another is the influence of chemotactic agents or phagocytic stimuli themselves on leukocytes; these result in activating the arachidonic acid cascade and releasing proteases and oxygen-derived free radicals from leukocytes. These interactions may explain prolonged inflammatory responses, in which mediators may be activated in sequence.

The second point is that *with all these mediators there seems to be an intelligent system of checks and balances.* If not, inflammation would take over the world or would run riot! But these chemicals are either tightly sequestered within cells or are present in plasma or tissue as precursor forms that must go through many steps before becoming activated, or must by synthesized de novo. Thus, the molecular mechanisms responsible for the rate-limiting steps involved are of primary importance in understanding inflammation. Conversely, once activated or re-

Table 2–3. Summary of Mediators of Acute Inflammation

		ACTION		
MEDIATOR	SOURCE	Vascular Leakage	Chemotaxis	Other
Histamine and serotonin	Mast cells, basophils, and platelets	+	–	
α Bradykinin	Plasma substrate	+	–	Pain
α C3a C5a	Plasma protein via liver; macrophages	+ +	– +	Opsonic fragment (C3b) Leukocyte adhesion
Prostaglandins	Most cells, from membrane phospholipids	Potentiate other mediators	–	Vasodilation, pain, fever
α Leukotriene B_4	Leukocytes	–	+	Leukocyte adhesion
Leukotriene C_4, D_4, E_4	Leukocytes, mast cells	+	–	Bronchoconstriction, vasoconstriction
Lysosomal components Cationic proteins	Leukocytes	+	+	Immobilization of neutrophils
Neutral proteases	Leukocytes	+	–	Tissue damage
Oxygen metabolites	Leukocytes	+		Endothelial damage, tissue damage
PAF	Leukocytes; other	+	+	Bronchoconstriction
IL-1 and TNF	Macrophages; other	–	+	Acute phase reactions Leukocyte adhesion

leased, these mediators are quickly inactivated or destroyed. Some of the inactivators are known, such as kininase, which destroys bradykinin; chemotactic factor inactivators, which neutralize C5a; antioxidants, which scavenge oxygen-derived free radicals; and antiproteases, which neutralize elastase and collagenase. Others are more obscure. However, the more we know about these checks and balances, the better we can modify the inflammatory response.

The discussion of mediators completes the basic description of the relatively uniform pattern of the inflammatory reaction encountered in most injuries. Recall that, although hemodynamic, permeability, and

Table 2–4. Most Likely Mediators in Inflammation

Vasodilation
  Prostaglandins
Increased Vascular Permeability
  Vasoactive amines
  C3a and C5a (through liberating amines)
  Bradykinin
  Leukotriene C_4, D_4, E_4, PAF
Chemotaxis
  C5a
  Leukotriene B_4
  Other chemotactic lipids
  Bacterial products
Fever
  IL-1; TNF
  Prostaglandins
Pain
  Prostaglandins
  Bradykinin
Tissue Damage
  Neutrophil and macrophage lysosomal enzymes
  Oxygen metabolites

white cell changes have been described sequentially and may be initiated in this order, all these phenomena in the fully evolved reaction to injury are concurrent in a seemingly chaotic but remarkably organized multiring circus. As might be expected, many variables may modify this basic process. Particularly important are (1) the nature and intensity of the injury, (2) the site and tissue affected, and (3) the responsiveness of the host—nutrition, adequacy of the cardiovascular system, drug therapy, existence of predisposing disorders such as diabetes mellitus and cancer, and the presence of previously acquired immunity to the offender.

LYMPHATICS IN ACUTE INFLAMMATION

The system of lymphatics and lymph nodes filters and "polices" the extravascular fluids. Together with the *mononuclear phagocyte system* (p. 61) it represents a secondary line of defense that is called into play whenever a local inflammatory reaction fails to contain and neutralize injury.

Lymphatics are extremely delicate channels that are difficult to visualize in ordinary tissue sections because they readily collapse. They are lined by continuous thin endothelium with loose, overlapping cell junctions; scant basement membrane; and no muscular support, except in the larger ducts. Lymph flow in inflammation is increased and helps drain the edema fluid from the extravascular space. Because the junctions of lymphatics are loose, lymphatic fluid eventually equilibrates with extravascular fluid. Not only fluid but also leukocytes and cell debris may find their way into lymph. Valves are present in collecting lymphatics, allowing lymph content to flow only proximally. Delicate fibrils, attached at right angles to the walls of the lymphatic vessel, extend into the adjacent tissues and serve to maintain patency of the lymphatic channels.

In severe injuries the drainage may transport the offending agent, be it chemical or bacterial. The lymphatics may become secondarily inflamed *(lymphangitis)*, as may the draining lymph nodes *(lymphadenitis)*. Therefore, it is not uncommon in infections of the hand, for example, to observe red streaks along the entire arm up to the axilla following the course of the lymphatic channels, accompanied by painful enlargement of the axillary lymph nodes. The nodal enlargement is usually caused by hyperplasia of the lymphoid follicles and also by hyperplasia of the phagocytic cells lining the sinuses of the lymph nodes. This constellation of nodal histologic changes is termed *reactive* or *inflammatory lymphadenitis*.

Fortunately, the secondary barriers sometimes contain the spread of the infection, but in some instances they are overwhelmed, and the organisms drain through progressively larger channels and gain access to the vascular circulation, thus inducing a *bacteremia*. The phagocytic cells of the liver, spleen, and bone marrow constitute the next line of defense, but in massive infections, bacteria seed distant tissues of the body. The heart valves, meninges, kidneys, and joints are favored sites of implantation for blood-borne organisms, and in such a fashion endocarditis, meningitis, renal abscesses, and septic arthritis may develop.

MONONUCLEAR PHAGOCYTES

Before we proceed to a discussion of the subsequent course of acute inflammation, we shall review some aspects of the biology of mononuclear phagocytes — ubiquitous cells that are involved in all phases of the healing or progression of the inflammatory response.[77]

Mononuclear phagocytes have always been known as the scavenger cells of the body. This traditional role, known since the time of Metchnikoff, remains one of their most important functions. In inflammation, they are abundant after the very early stages, when they avidly engulf and digest foreign particles, debris from injured cells, red cells, proteins that have leaked out, and even their predecessors, the neutrophils, after the latter have finished their own job of ingestion. Macrophages, however, have much wider functions in biology and pathology.[77,78] They have a fundamental role in specific immunity through a relationship with the lymphocyte,[78a] as will be further developed in the chapter on immunity (Chapter 5). Here we describe the normal physiology of macrophages and their established or postulated roles in inflammation.

Monocytes and macrophages belong to the mononuclear phagocyte system (MPS) (also known as the reticuloendothelial system **RES**). The **MPS** consists of cells in the bone marrow, peripheral blood, and tissues that are highly specialized for the function of endocytosis (pinocytosis and phagocytosis) and intracellular digestion. In connective tissue of organs, they are termed *histocytes* or *resident macrophages*. They originate from a committed stem cell in the bone marrow through a *monoblast* stage to form the *promonocytes*. Promonocytes are capable of rapid division, giving rise to the peripheral blood *monocyte*. The blood monocyte is a smaller cell, is more functionally active, does not divide, and forms 4 to 8% of the total white count. Its average transit time in the blood is about 32 hours, appreciably longer than that of the neutrophil or eosinophil. The monocyte is characterized by large numbers of pinocytotic vesicles, ruffling of the surface membrane, a variable number of lysosomes, and an active Golgi apparatus (Fig. 2–21).

There is little question now that the origin of the vast majority of macrophages in an inflammatory focus is the blood monocyte[78] (see also p. 64). Although there is substantial evidence that the resident macrophages listed in Table 2–5 are bone marrow–derived, such macrophages frequently acquire differing biochemical and structural characteristics, depending on their microenvironment. Nevertheless, macrophages from various sites share some general properties that make them unique. The cells are mobile (although slower than neutrophils). They are capable not only of *phagocytosis* of relatively large particles but also of *pinocytosis* of soluble molecules. The uptake of particles is carried out in part as a result of the presence on the macrophage of cell surface receptors for the Fc fragment of immunoglobulin and the third component of complement (C3b). Macrophages possess a large repertoire of hydrolytic enzymes, which explains their capacity to degrade various materials rapidly. Most importantly, mononuclear phagocytes are pluripotential cells, having the property of becoming "activated" by external stimuli. The term "activated macrophage" refers to cells that are larger and have a more ruffled cyto-

Table 2–5. The Mononuclear Phagocyte (Reticuloendothelial) System

Stem Cells (Committed) *Monoblasts* *Promonocytes* }	BONE MARROW
Monocytes	BLOOD
Macrophages	TISSUES Inflammatory macrophages Liver (Kupffer cells) Lung (alveolar macrophages) Connective tissue (histiocytes) Bone marrow (macrophages) Spleen and lymph nodes (fixed and free macrophages) Serous cavities (pleural and peritoneal macrophages) Nervous system (microglial cells) Bone (osteoclasts) Skin (?Langerhans' cells) Lymphoid tissue (?dendritic cells)

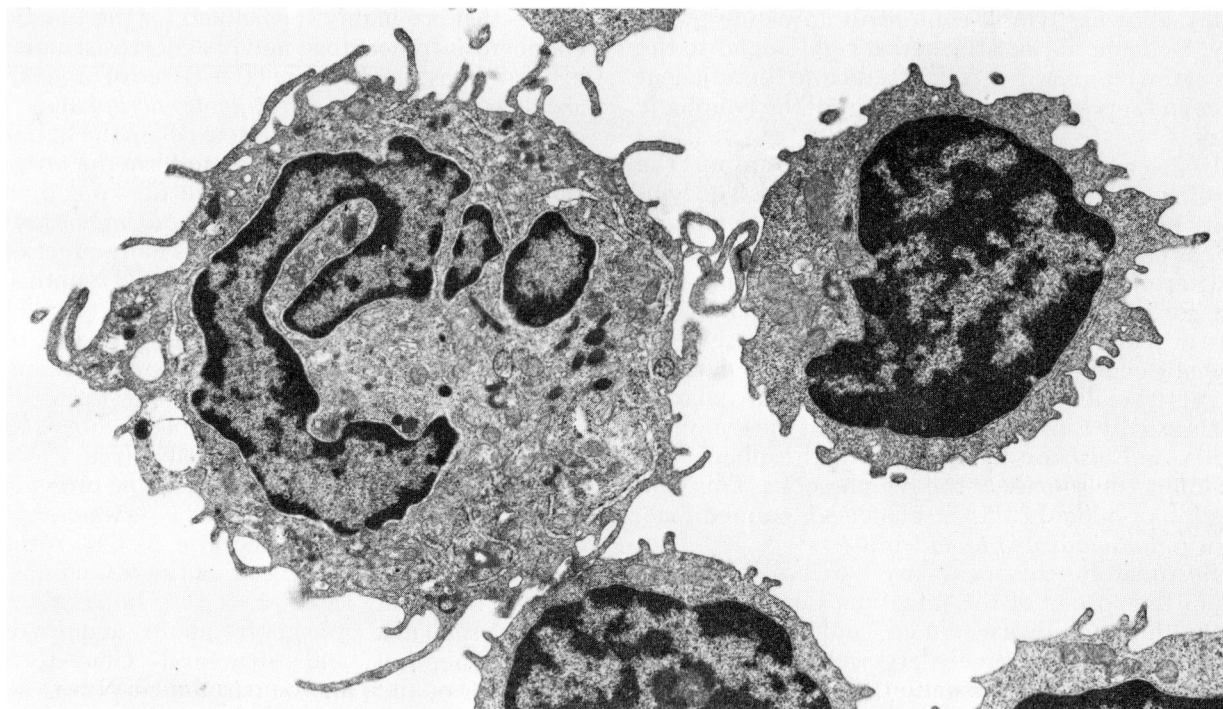

Figure 2–21. Electron micrograph of peripheral blood monocyte *(left)* and lymphocyte. Note the abundant cytoplasm, indented nucleus, ruffled surface membrane, and lysosomes of the monocyte.

plasm, increased numbers of mitochondria, increased levels of hydrolytic enzymes and lysosomes, greater membrane activity with increased endocytosis, more active metabolism, and a greater ability to kill both intracellular bacteria and malignant tumor cells. This state of activation can be triggered by (1) *lymphokines (principally γ interferon)* produced by *immune-sensitized* activated T lymphocytes (p. 182); or (2) *nonimmunologic interactions* that "perturb" the cell membrane (e.g., contact with certain bacterial products, such as endotoxin, or other chemicals, or phagocytosis) (Fig. 2–22).

Activated macrophages have the potential to secrete a wide variety of products, many of which are active in inflammation. The spectrum of biologic activities induced is phenomenal — and all from one cell type.[79,80] *Furthermore, the versatility of the macrophage is such that secretion of these products can be regulated* (increased or decreased) by interactions between the cell and its environment — other cells, extracellular matrix components (e.g., fibronectin), and serum (complement), as well as exogenous agents. Thus macrophages may become "deactivated," favoring resolution of the inflammatory response. One of the known deactivators is transforming growth factor *β*, a product of several cell types present in inflammation, including endothelium, platelets, and T cells.[81] In addition, the macrophages are long-lived and can readily migrate to all tissues; thus their secretory properties may affect many pathophysiologic responses.

Among the important classes of macrophage products are the following:

1. *Neutral proteases* such as collagenase and elastase, which degrade connective tissue components, and plasminogen activator, which activates the elaboration of the fibrinolytic agent plasmin.
2. *Chemotactic factors* for other leukocytes.
3. *Arachidonic acid metabolites,* both cyclooxygenase and lipoxygenase products, which cause vasodilation, increased vascular permeability, and chemotaxis.
4. *Reactive oxygen metabolites.*
5. *Complement components* of both the classic and alternate pathways.
6. *Coagulation factors* (e.g., factor V, thromboplastin), which may be important in converting fibrinogen to fibrin locally.
7. *Growth-promoting factors* for fibroblasts, blood vessels, and myeloid progenitor cells.
8. *Cytokines,* such as IL-1 and TNF.
9. Other biologically active agents that cause inflammation (PAF) or have antiviral activity (interferon).

Although many of these factors and properties are beneficial in responding to injurious agents, unregulated macrophage activation may have a deleterious effect, and indeed — as we shall see — macrophages play a role in the pathogenesis of certain chronic diseases, such as atherosclerosis and rheumatoid arthritis.

Besides its importance in inflammation and immunity, the MPS (particularly the Kupffer cells of the liver and splenic macrophages) is the main line of defense against bacteria in the bloodstream and serves to control the hematogenous dissemination of organisms. The system is also involved in the removal

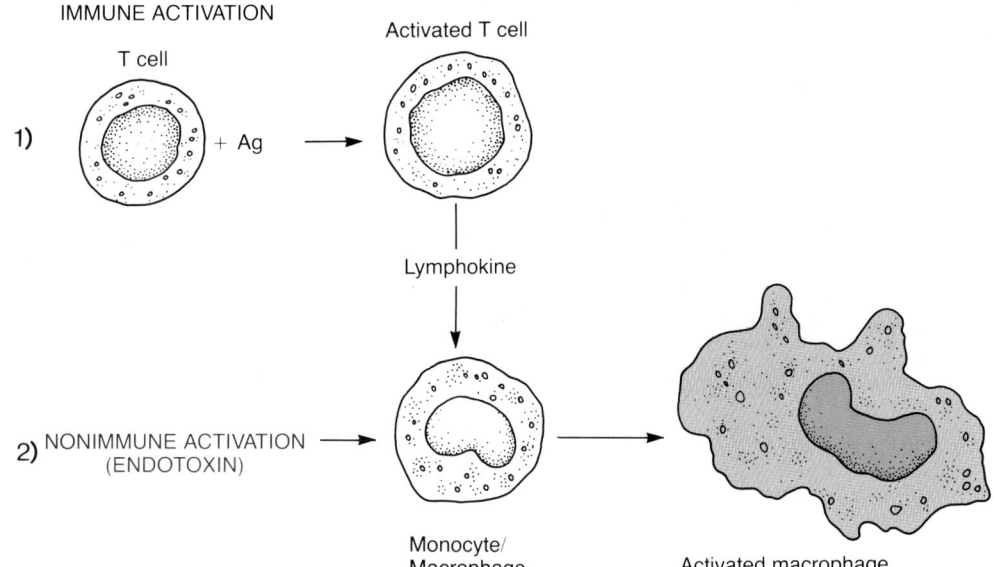

IMMUNE ACTIVATION

Figure 2–22. Two stimuli for macrophage activation: lymphokines (γ interferon) from immune activated T cells and nonimmunologic stimuli such as endotoxin. Ag: antigen.

and phagocytosis of unwanted materials floating about in the blood or sequestered in organs. The capacity of the MPS to recognize such products is remarkable. Included are obsolescent or injured red cells, white cells, and platelets; coagulation products; antigen-antibody complexes; and foreign macromolecules such as complex lipids and carbohydrates synthesized by the body in some of the inborn errors of metabolism (the basis for so-called storage diseases) (p. 144).

CHRONIC INFLAMMATION

DEFINITION AND CAUSES

Acute inflammation may have one of four outcomes:
• complete *resolution,* with restoration of the site of acute inflammation to normal; this is the usual outcome when the injury is mild, such as from a superficial burn or limited trauma, or when there has been little tissue destruction;
• *healing by scarring* (p. 73), which occurs after substantial tissue destruction, or when the inflammation occurs in tissues that do not regenerate, or when there is abundant fibrin exudation;
• *abscess formation,* which occurs particularly in infections with pyogenic organisms; and
• progression to *chronic inflammation.*
 Although the transition from acute to chronic inflammation is often difficult to pinpoint, chronic inflammatory responses have some features sufficiently unique to warrant a separate description.
 Clinically, chronic inflammation in various organs arises in one of three ways:

1. *It may follow acute inflammation,* either because of the persistence of the inciting stimulus, or because of some interference in the normal process of healing. For example, infection of the lung by some species of bacteria may begin as an acute inflammation (pneumonia), but persistence of these organisms or their products leads to tissue destruction, a smoldering inflammation, and a chronic lung abscess.
2. *Repeated bouts of acute inflammation* may also be responsible, with the patient showing successive attacks of fever, pain, and swelling. In this case, histologic examination will show evidence of acute inflammation, healing (between attacks), and chronic inflammation, as seen in recurrent infections of the gallbladder (cholecystitis) and kidney (pyelonephritis).
3. *More curiously, chronic inflammation may begin insidiously* as a low-grade smoldering response that does not follow classic symptomatic acute inflammation. This last form includes some of the most common and disabling diseases of humans, such as rheumatoid arthritis, tuberculosis, and chronic lung disease. Such diseases occur in one of the following settings:
a. persistent infection by *intracellular* microorganisms (e.g., tubercle bacilli, viral infection), which are of low toxicity but evoke an immunologic reaction.
b. prolonged exposure to nondegradable but potentially toxic substances (e.g., silicosis and asbestosis in the lung).
c. immune reactions, particularly those perpetuated against the individual's own tissues (autoimmune diseases, such as rheumatoid arthritis).

CELLS AND MEDIATORS

The histologic hallmarks of chronic inflammation are (1) *infiltration by mononuclear cells,* principally macrophages, lymphocytes, and plasma cells; (2) *proliferation of fibroblasts* and, in many instances, *small blood vessels* (Fig. 2–23); (3) increased connective tissue (fibrosis); and (4) tissue destruction.
 Infiltration by monocytes or macrophages is a

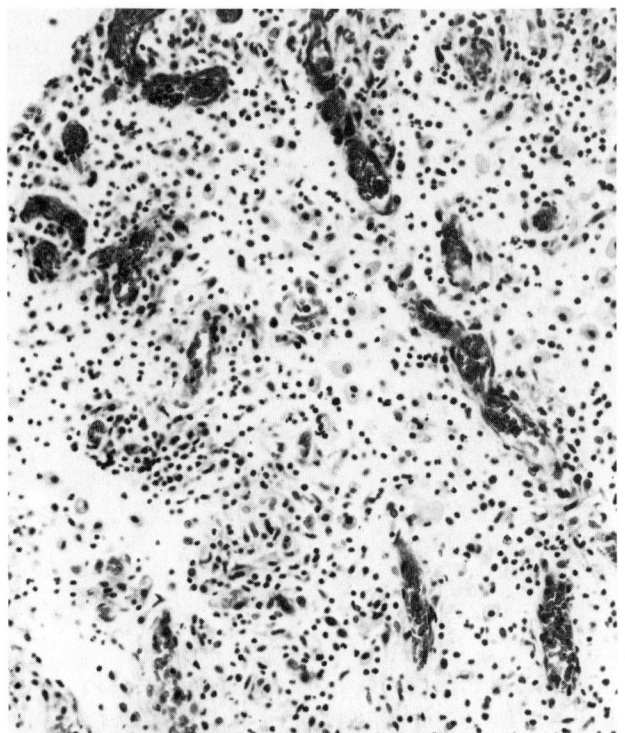

Figure 2–23. Focus of chronic inflammation showing infiltration by macrophages (pale large cells) and lymphocytes, and proliferation of small vessels.

particularly important component of chronic inflammation. As discussed previously, monocytes begin to emigrate relatively early in acute inflammation, and within 48 hours they constitute the predominant cell type. When the monocyte reaches the extravascular tissue it undergoes transformation into a much larger cell, the macrophage, which may become "activated." In short-lived acute inflammation, if the irritant is eliminated, these macrophages eventually disappear (either dying off or making their way into the lymphatics and lymph nodes). If the injurious agent is not eliminated, as for example in a tuberculous infection, with some immunologic reactions, or in the presence of a stubborn irritant, macrophage accumulation may persist for prolonged periods of time.

Accumulation of macrophages occurs in three ways, each predominating in different types of infection (Fig. 2–24):

1. *Continued recruitment of monocytes from the circulation,* which results from the steady release of chemotactic factors. This is numerically the most important source for macrophages. Chemotactic stimuli for monocytes include C5a; fibrinopeptides; neutrophilic cationic proteins; lymphokines; certain growth factors, such as platelet-derived growth factor (PDGF) and transforming growth factor β (TGFβ); and fragments from the breakdown of collagen and fibronectin. Each of these may play a role under given circumstances; for example, lymphokines are almost certainly involved during delayed-hypersensitivity immune reactions.

2. *Local proliferation* (by mitotic division) *of macro-*

phages after their emigration from the bloodstream. This is an unusual event, but it has been documented in some experimental models.

3. *Prolonged survival and immobilization of macrophages* within the site of inflammation. This is especially evident when the irritants such as inert lipids and carbon particles are of low virulence.

The macrophage is a central figure in chronic inflammation because of the great number of biologically active products it can produce (p. 62). Some of these products are toxic to tissues (e.g., oxygen metabolites, proteases), others cause influx of other cell types (e.g., lymphocytes, neutrophils), and still others cause fibroblast proliferation and collagen deposition (e.g., IL-1). *All of these effects contribute to progressive tissue damage and to the consequent functional impairment.*

The mechanisms that lead to the recruitment and proliferation of fibroblasts, to vascular proliferation, and to collagen accumulation and fibrosis in chronic inflammation are similar to those that contribute to wound healing and are described on page 76.

Other types of cells present in chronic inflammation are lymphocytes, plasma cells, eosinophils, and mast cells. *Plasma cells* produce antibody, directed

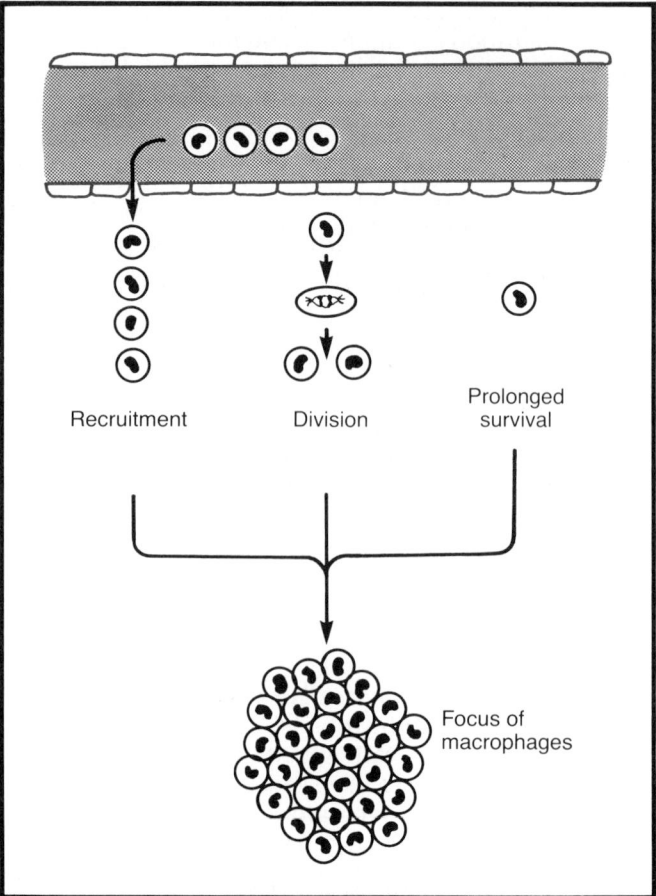

Figure 2–24. Three mechanisms for macrophage accumulation. By far the most important is recruitment from the microcirculation. (Adapted from Ryan, G., and Majno, G.: Inflammation. A Scope Publication. Upjohn Co.)

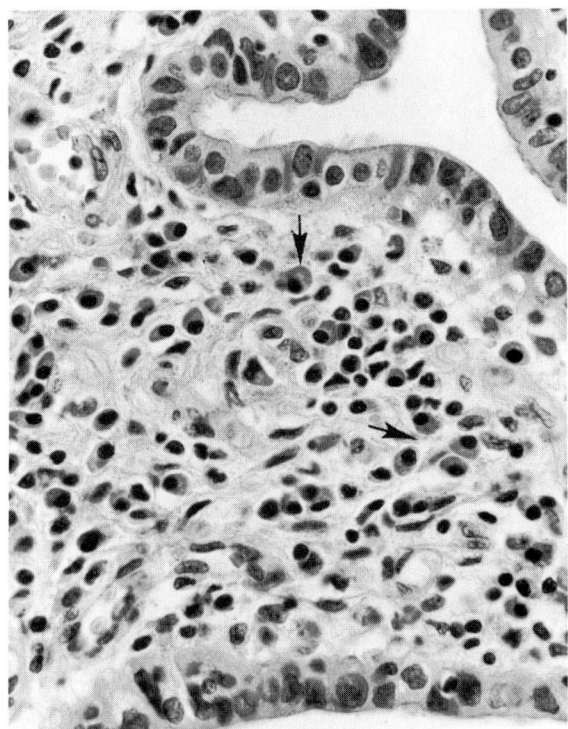

Figure 2–25. Chronic inflammation of the fallopian tube. The subepithelial connective tissue is infiltrated with mononuclear white cells, principally plasma cells marked by eccentric nuclei *(arrows).*

cytes is discussed in detail in Chapter 5. *Eosinophils* are characteristic of immunologic reactions mediated by IgE and of parasitic infections. Eosinophils respond to chemotactic agents derived largely from mast cells (p. 176). Although their precise functions are still speculative, their granules contain *major basic protein* (MBP), a highly cationic 14,000 MW protein, which is toxic to parasites but also causes lysis of mammalian epithelial cells. They may thus be of benefit in parasitic infections but contribute to tissue damage in hypersensitivity states.[81a]

Although polymorphonuclear leukocytes are usually considered the hallmarks of acute inflammation, many forms of chronic inflammation, lasting for months, continue to show large numbers of neutrophils and to form *pus.* In chronic inflammation of bone (osteomyelitis), a neutrophilic exudate can persist for many months. In actinomycosis, a disease induced by organisms with a particular ability to attract neutrophils, the center of the lesion abounds with neutrophils months or years after the initial infection. Here, then, chronic and acute responses coexist. Conversely, the presence of lymphocytes does not always mean that inflammation has been present for long periods. This is especially true of viral infections. In acute hepatitis or viral myocarditis, for example, lymphocytes predominate even in the first few days of the acute disease.

either against persistent antigen in the inflammatory site or against altered tissue components (Fig. 2–25). *Lymphocytes* are mobilized in both antibody- and cell-mediated immunologic reactions, but also, for unknown reasons, in nonimmunologic inflammation. They have a unique reciprocal relationship to macrophages in chronic immune-mediated inflammation (Fig. 2–26). Lymphocytes can be activated by contact with antigen. Activated lymphocytes produce *lymphokines*, and these, as we have seen, are major stimulators of monocytes and macrophages; they cause monocyte chemotaxis as well as macrophage activation and differentiation (γ interferon). Products of activated macrophages (monokines) in turn influence both T- and B-cell functions. The role of lympho-

CHRONIC GRANULOMATOUS INFLAMMATION

Some agents evoke a distinctive pattern of chronic inflammation, referred to as granulomatous inflammation.[80] Granulomatous diseases, such as tuberculosis, leprosy, and schistosomiasis, are of major worldwide public health importance. *Granulomas are small, 0.5- to 2-mm collections of modified macrophages called "epithelioid cells," usually surrounded by a rim of lymphocytes* (Fig. 2–27). The modified macrophages have abundant, pale-pink, plump cytoplasm, resembling an epithelial cell. Like all macrophages, epithelioid cells are derived from blood monocytes. They are less phagocytic than macro-

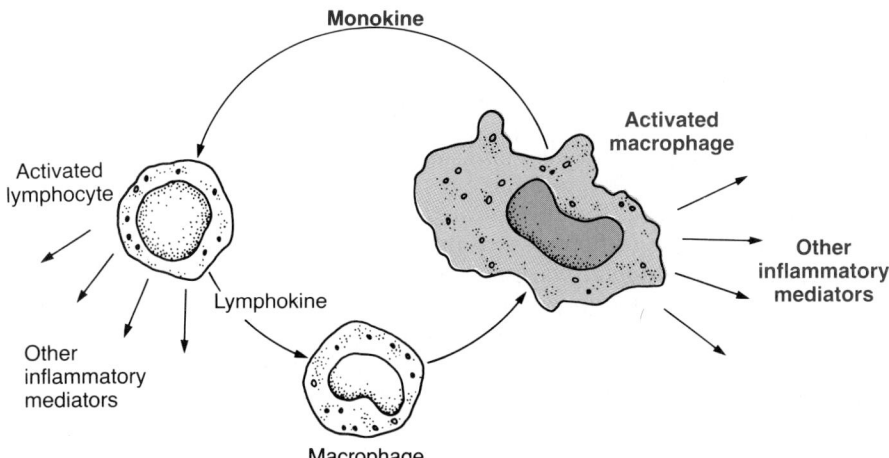

Figure 2–26. Macrophage-lymphocyte interactions in chronic inflammation. Activated lymphocytes and macrophages influence each other and also release inflammatory mediators that affect other cells.

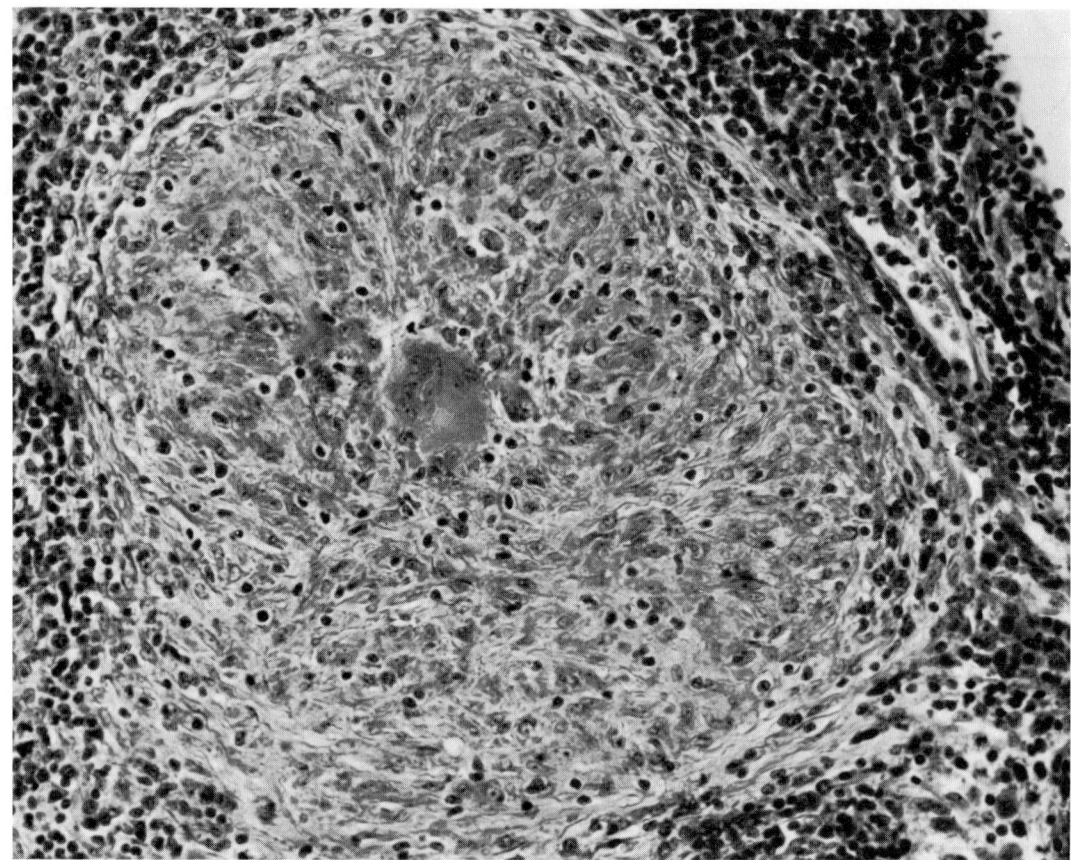

Figure 2–27. A granuloma with a central Langhans'-type giant cell surrounded by epithelioid cells (large pale cells) and lymphocytes.

phages but are rich in endoplasmic reticulum, Golgi apparatus, vesicles, and vacuoles. Their appearance suggests that the cells may be adapted for extracellular secretion rather than phagocytosis.

Another feature of the granuloma is the presence of *Langhans' or foreign body – type giant cells.* These are formed by the coalescence and fusion of epithelioid cells, with only rare internal nuclear division. They may achieve diameters of 40 to 50 μm and may contain as many as 50 nuclei. The nuclei are sometimes arranged around the periphery (creating a horseshoe pattern), giving rise to the traditional Langhans'-type giant cell (Fig. 2 – 28). Giant cells also are formed in the presence of large amounts of indigestible material, and indeed they often conglomerate around a foreign body and have scattered nuclei (hence the term foreign body – type giant cell) (Fig. 2 – 29).

Fibroblasts, plasma cells, and, at times, neutrophils can be seen in a granuloma, but the presence of the characteristic cell (the epithelioid cell) is required for the diagnosis of granulomatous inflammation. *The diagnosis of granulomatous inflammation based on lymph node biopsy significantly limits the number of possible causes.* The classic example of granulomatous disease is tuberculosis, but sarcoidosis, deep fungal infections, reactions to a foreign body, brucellosis, schistosomiasis, cat-scratch disease, syphilis, and leprosy all evoke this pattern. In clinical practice, the most common causes are reaction to a foreign body, tuberculosis, and sarcoidosis.

In tuberculosis, the granuloma is referred to as a *tubercle* and is *classically characterized by the presence of central caseous necrosis.* In contrast, caseating necrosis is rare in other granulomatous diseases. The morphologic patterns in the various granulomatous diseases may be sufficiently different to allow reasonably accurate diagnosis by an experienced pathologist (Table 2 – 6); however, there are so many atypical presentations that it is always necessary to identify the specific etiologic agent. The agent can be identified histologically (as in the case of a refractile foreign body that can be detected by polarization microscopy), by special stains for organisms (e.g., acid-fast stains for tubercle bacilli), by culture methods (in tuberculosis, fungal disease), and by serologic studies (e.g., in syphilis). In sarcoidosis, the etiologic agent is unknown (p. 427).

Two factors appear to determine the formation of granulomas. One factor is evident — the presence of indigestible organisms (such as the tubercle bacillus) or particles (such as mineral oil, complex polysaccharides, and polymers). In addition, experimental studies indicate that *granulomatous inflammation is potentiated by,*[82] *or sometimes requires, the presence of cell-mediated immunity to the inciting agent. Indeed,*

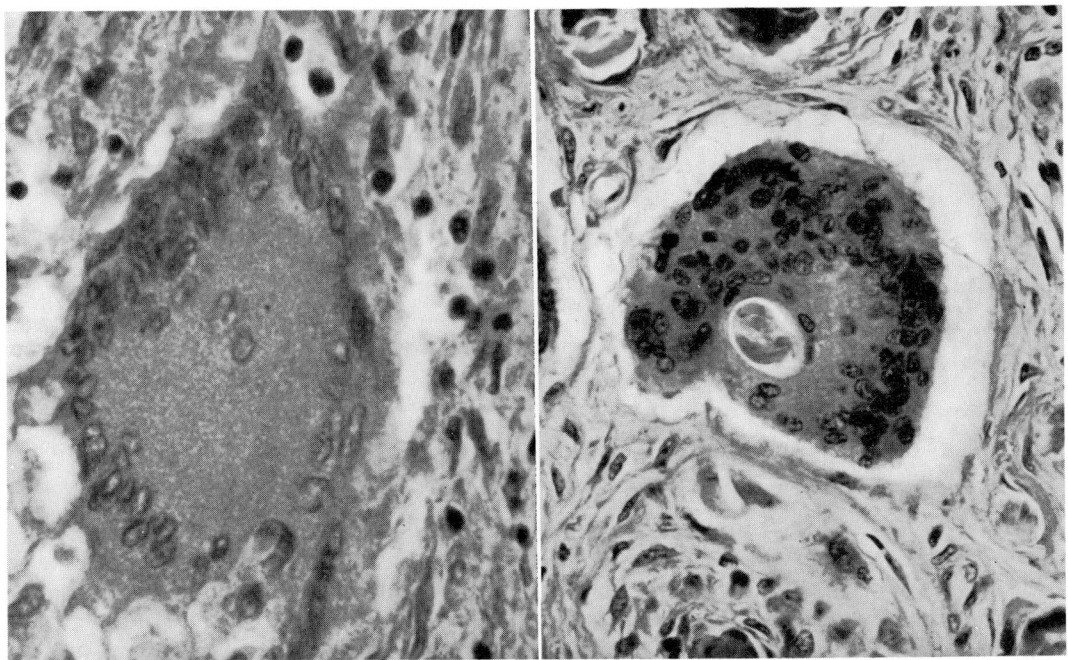

Figure 2–28   Figure 2–29

Figure 2–28. Detail of a Langhans'-type giant cell in the margin of a tubercle.

Figure 2–29. Detail of a foreign body–type giant cell containing a foreign body.

Table 2–6. Examples of Granulomatous Inflammations

DISEASE	CAUSE	TISSUE REACTION
Bacterial Tuberculosis	*Mycobacterium tuberculosis*	*Noncaseating tubercle (granuloma prototype):* a focus of epithelioid cells, rimmed by fibroblasts, lymphocytes, histiocytes, occasional Langhans' giant cell; *caseating tubercle:* central amorphous granular debris, loss of all cellular detail; acid-fast bacilli
Leprosy	*Mycobacterium leprae*	Acid-fast bacilli in macrophages; granulomas and epithelioid types
Syphilis	*Treponema pallidum*	*Gumma:* Microscopic to grossly visible lesion, enclosing wall of histiocytes; plasma cell infiltrate; center cells are necrotic without loss of cellular outline
Cat-scratch disease	*Gram-negative bacillus*	Rounded or stellate granuloma containing central granular debris and recognizable neutrophils; giant cells uncommon
Parasitic Schistosomiasis *Fungal*	*Schistosoma mansoni, S. haematobium, S. japonicum*	Egg emboli; eosinophils
	Cryptococcus neoformans	Organism is yeast-like, sometimes budding; 5 to 10 μm; large, clear capsule
	Coccidioides immitis	Organism appears as spherical (30–80 μm) cyst containing endospores of 3 to 5 μm each
Inorganic Metals and Dusts Silicosis, berylliosis		Lung involvement; fibrosis
Unknown Sarcoidosis		*Noncaseating granuloma:* giant cells (Langhans' and foreign-body types); asteroids in giant cells; occasional Schaumann's body (concentric calcific concretion); no organisms

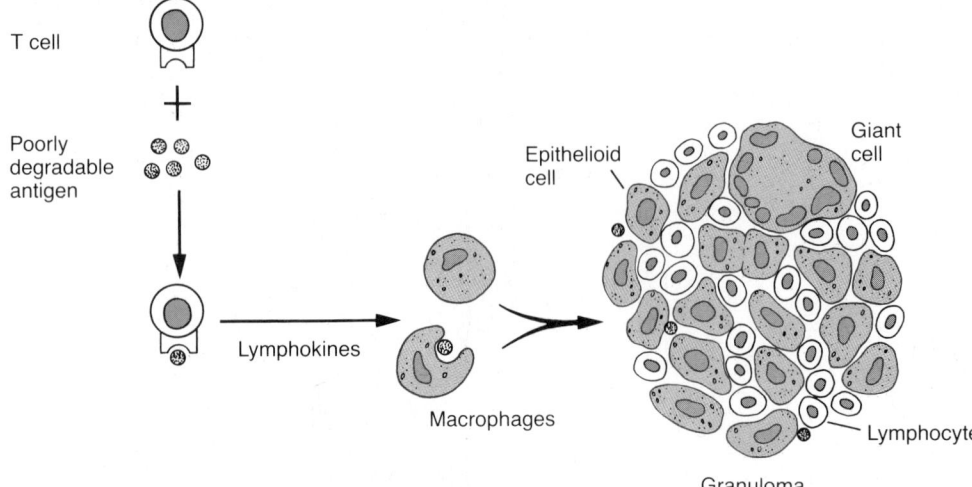

Figure 2–30. Mechanisms of granuloma formation—lymphokines (γ interferon, IL-4) play a role in activating macrophages and forming giant cells. (Modified from Sell, S.: Immunology, Immunopathology, and Immunity. 4th ed. Amsterdam, Elsevier, 1987.)

products of activated T cells (γ-interferon and possibly interleukin 4) enhance the transformation of monocytes to epithelioid cells and multinucleate giant cells in culture[83,84] (Fig. 2–30).

To summarize, granulomatous inflammation is a specific type of chronic inflammation characterized by accumulations of modified macrophages (epithelioid cells) and initiated by a variety of infectious and noninfectious agents. The presence of *poorly digestible irritants or T cell–mediated immunity (with production of γ-interferon) to the irritant, or both*, appears to be necessary for granuloma formation.

MORPHOLOGIC PATTERNS IN ACUTE AND CHRONIC INFLAMMATION

The severity of the reaction, its specific causation, and the particular tissue and site involved all introduce morphologic variations in the basic patterns of acute and chronic inflammation. For example, the fluid, protein, and cell content of an exudate depend on the specific causative agent and its intensity. Thus, major characteristic patterns of acute and chronic inflammation can be differentiated on the basis of the nature of the exudate and on the morphologic variables introduced by location.

SEROUS INFLAMMATION

Serous inflammation is marked by the outpouring of a thin fluid that, depending on the site of injury, is derived from either the blood serum or the secretions of mesothelial cells lining the peritoneal, pleural, and pericardial cavities. The skin blister resulting from a burn (Fig. 2–31) represents a large accumulation of fluid, either within or immediately beneath the epidermis of the skin. This type of exudate, seen early in the development of most acute inflammatory reactions, is the dominant pattern in mild injuries and is characteristic of certain causative agents, such as tuberculous pleuritis, often referred to as pleurisy with effusion.

FIBRINOUS INFLAMMATION

The exudation of large amounts of plasma proteins, including fibrinogen, and the precipitation of masses

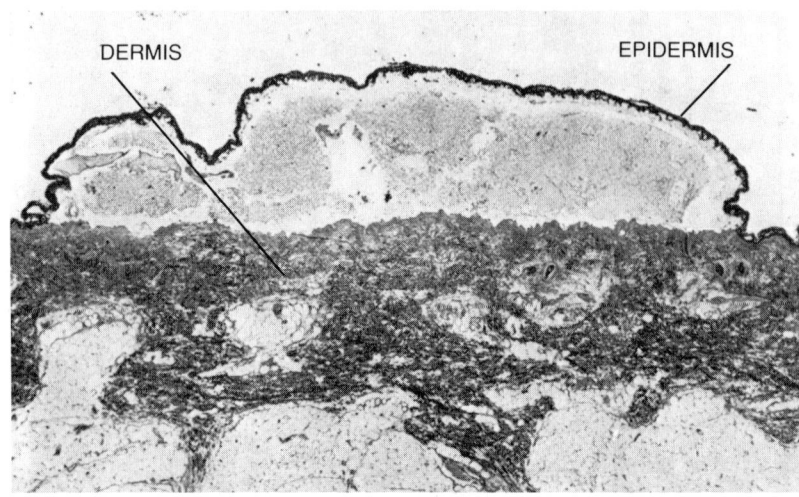

Figure 2–31. A low-power view of a cross section of a skin blister. The epidermis has been lifted off the dermis by the focal collection of fluid.

of fibrin are characteristic of certain inflammatory responses involving the body cavities, such as the pleural cavity and pericardial sac. In fibrinous pericarditis, the space may become virtually filled with large masses of rubbery fibrin loosely gluing the parietal and visceral pericardium *("bread and butter" pericarditis)*. Histologically, fibrin is identified by its tangled, threadlike eosinophilic meshwork, although it occasionally presents as large masses of solid amorphous eosinophilic coagulum (Fig. 2–32).

A fibrinous exudate may often be reabsorbed (resolution of the exudate) but invites ingrowth of fibroblasts and capillary buds, which transform the proteinaceous precipitate into a vascularized connective tissue, a process referred to as *organization* of the exudate. Organization of a fibrinous pleuritis or pericarditis may obliterate these serosal cavities and hamper the function of the organs now tied down to surrounding structures.

SUPPURATIVE OR PURULENT INFLAMMATION

This form of inflammation is characterized by the production of large amounts of pus or purulent exudate. Certain organisms (e.g., staphylococci) produce this localized suppuration and are therefore referred to as pyogenic (pus-producing) bacteria. A common example of an acute suppurative inflammation is acute appendicitis (Fig. 2–33). In this situation, masses of polymorphonuclear leukocytes are found diffusely or in local aggregates throughout the mucosa, and coagulated pus may layer the surface and fill the lumen (Fig. 2–33).

An *abscess* is an example of a localized suppurative inflammation. *Abscesses are localized collections of pus* caused by suppuration buried in a tissue, organ, or confined space. They are produced by the deep seeding of pyogenic bacteria into a tissue. An abscess starts as a focal accumulation of neutrophils in a space created by liquefactive necrosis of the native cells of

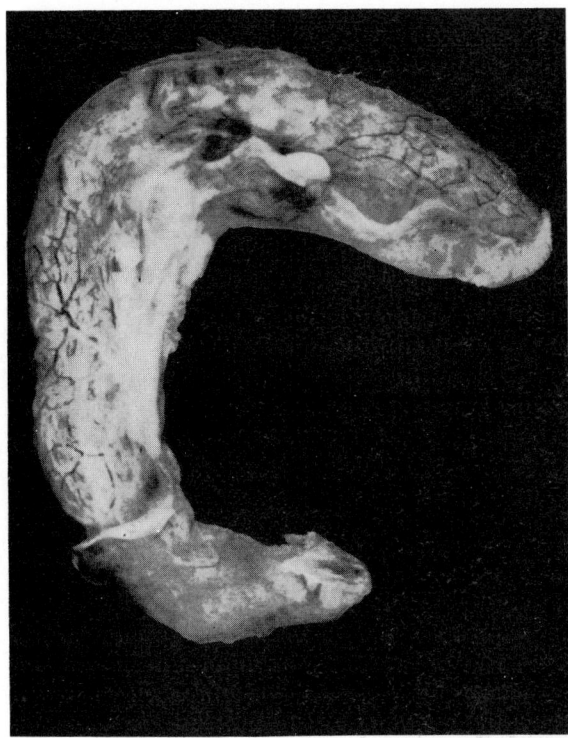

Figure 2–33. A gross view of acute appendicitis. The covering serosa is heavily layered with a pale fibrinosuppurative exudate.

the tissue. As it develops, it may expand as a result of the progressive necrosis of surrounding cells. The central region appears as a mass of necrotic white cells and tissue cells. There is usually a zone of preserved neutrophils about this necrotic focus, and outside this region vascular dilation and parenchymal and fibroblastic proliferation occur, indicating the beginning of repair. In time, the abscess may become walled off by connective tissue that serves as a limiting barrier to further spread.

ULCERS

An ulcer is a local defect, or excavation, of the surface of an organ or tissue, which is produced by the sloughing (shedding) of inflammatory necrotic tissue. Ulceration can occur only when an inflammatory necrotic area exists on or near a surface. It is most commonly encountered in (1) inflammatory necrosis of the mucosa of the mouth, stomach, intestines, or genitourinary tract, and (2) subcutaneous inflammations of the lower extremities in older persons who have circulatory disturbances that predispose to extensive necrosis. Such lesions are best exemplified by the peptic ulcer of the stomach or duodenum (Fig. 2–34). In the acute stage, there is intense polymorphonuclear infiltration and vascular dilation in the margins of the defect. With chronicity, the margins and base of the ulcer develop fibroblastic proliferation, scarring, and the accumulation of lymphocytes, macrophages, and plasma cells.

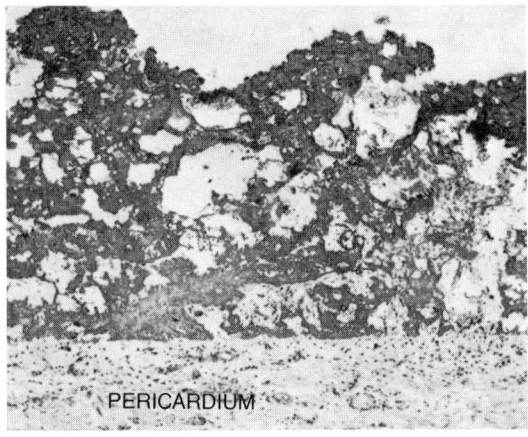

PERICARDIUM

Figure 2–32. The microscopic appearance of the shaggy, amorphous fibrinous exudate on the pericardial surface.

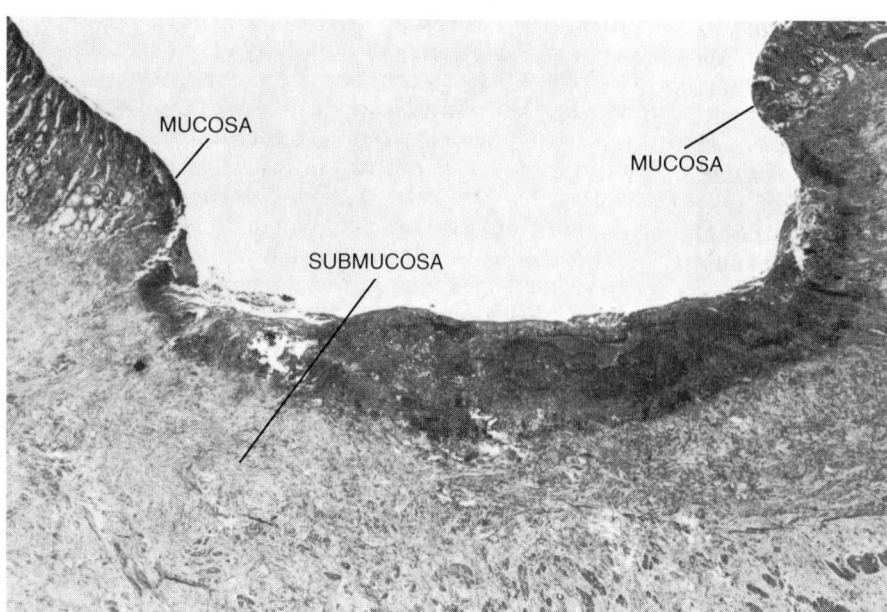

Figure 2–34. A low-power cross section of duodenal ulcer crater with a dark inflammatory exudate in the base.

SYSTEMIC EFFECTS OF INFLAMMATION

Anyone who has suffered a severe sore throat or a respiratory infection has experienced the systemic manifestations of acute inflammation. Fever is one of the most prominent systemic manifestations, especially when the inflammation is associated with infection. Bacteremia usually induces fever with dramatic swings in temperature, producing so-called spikes on the temperature chart. Violent shaking chills are known to all those who have had the flu. In addition to fever, the systemic manifestations of inflammation, known collectively as *acute phase reactions*, include: increase in slow-wave sleep; decreased appetite; increased degradation of proteins; hypotension and other hemodynamic changes; the synthesis of acute phase proteins by the liver, including C-reactive protein, serum amyloid A (p. 210), complement, and coagulation proteins; and a variety of changes in peripheral blood leukocytes.

IL-1 and TNF are important mediators of these reactions.[85] The following sequence of events is thought to account for *fever* (Fig. 2–35). IL-1 or TNF, or both, produced by leukocytes (and perhaps other cell types) in response to infectious agents or to immunologic and toxic reactions are released into the circulation. They reach the brain and interact with *vascular* receptors in the thermoregulatory center of the hypothalamus. *Either by the direct action of the cytokines or, more likely, through the induction of local prostaglandin (PGE) production*, information is transmitted from the anterior through the posterior hypothalamus to the vasomotor center, resulting in sympathetic nerve stimulation, vasoconstriction of skin vessels, decrease in heat dissipation, and fever.

Leukocytosis is a common feature of inflammatory reactions, especially those induced by bacterial infection. The leukocyte count usually climbs to 15,000 or 20,000 cells/ml, but sometimes it may reach extraordinarily high levels of 40,000 to 100,000 cells/ml. These extreme elevations are referred to as *leukemoid reactions*, because they are similar to the white cell counts obtained in leukemia. The leukocytosis occurs initially because of *accelerated release* of cells from the bone marrow postmitotic reserve pool (caused by IL-1 and TNF) and is associated with a rise in the number of more immature neutrophils in the blood ("shift to the left"). However, pro-

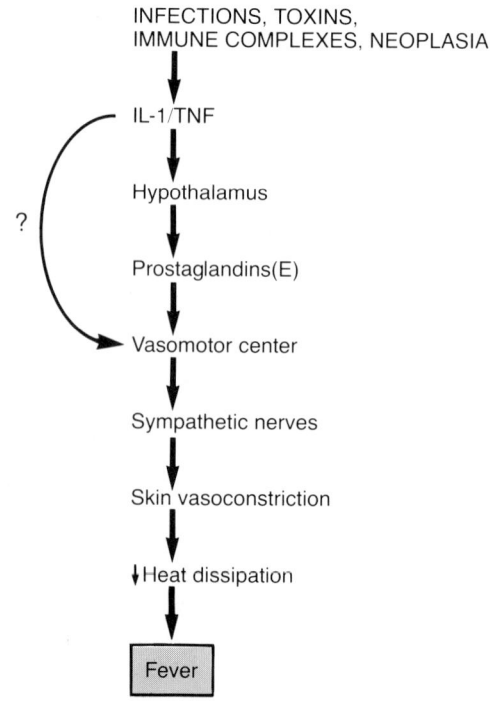

Figure 2–35. Mechanism of fever (see text).

longed infection also induces proliferation of precursors in the bone marrow, caused by increased production of *colony-stimulating factors* (CSFs) (p. 658). This stimulation of CSF production is also mediated by IL-1 and TNF.[86]

Most bacterial infections induce *neutrophilia,* but infectious mononucleosis, mumps, and German measles are exceptions and produce a leukocytosis by virtue of an absolute increase in the number of lymphocytes *(lymphocytosis).* In an additional group of disorders, which includes bronchial asthma, hay fever, and parasitic infestations, there is an absolute increase in the number of eosinophils, creating an *eosinophilia.*

Certain systemic inflammatory states, such as typhoid fever, infections caused by viruses, rickettsiae, and certain protozoal infections, are associated with decreases in the number of circulating white cells *(leukopenia).* Leukopenia is also encountered in infections that overwhelm patients debilitated by disseminated cancer or rampant tuberculosis.

Although the early reaction pattern of the inflammatory response is quite stereotyped, it is soon modified by a number of variables pertaining to both intruder and host that introduce striking departures from the basic theme. Perhaps the most important is the duration of the inflammatory process, but the causative agent, the location of the injury, and the nature of the exudate all contribute heavily to the ultimate character of the reaction. Even these modifiers do not tell the whole story because an important component has, to this point, been omitted—the changes induced by the reparative response. The repair of injury begins almost as soon as the inflammatory changes have begun, and so it constitutes a sequence of events as important as that of inflammation.

HEALING AND REPAIR

REGENERATION
Labile Cells
Stable Cells
Permanent Cells
REPAIR BY CONNECTIVE TISSUE — GRANULATION TISSUE
WOUND HEALING

Primary Union (Healing by First Intention)
Secondary Union (Healing by Second Intention)
MECHANISMS INVOLVED IN REPAIR
Growth Factors
Cell-Cell and Cell-Matrix

Interactions
Collagenization and Wound Strength
  Collagen
  Other extracellular matrix components
  Wound strength

FACTORS MODIFYING THE QUALITY OF THE INFLAMMATORY-REPARATIVE RESPONSE
Systemic influences
Local influences
PERSPECTIVE ON INFLAMMATORY-REPARATIVE RESPONSE

The body's attempts to heal damage induced by local injury begin very early in the process of inflammation and, in the end, result in *repair and the replacement of dead or damaged cells by healthy cells.* Repair usually involves two distinct processes: (1) *regeneration,* which is the replacement of injured tissue by parenchymal cells of the same type, sometimes leaving no residual trace of the previous injury; and (2) *replacement by connective tissue,* which in its permanent state constitutes a scar. In most instances, both processes contribute to repair. This chapter describes the healing of *skin wounds* as a prototype of the repair process in inflammation, but first let us review some of the general features of regeneration and connective tissue repair.

REGENERATION

The cells of the body are divided into three groups on the basis of their regenerative capacity: labile, stable, and permanent cells. Labile cells continue to proliferate throughout life; stable cells retain this capacity, although they do not normally replicate; and permanent cells cannot reproduce themselves after birth.

LABILE CELLS

Labile cells continue to proliferate throughout life, replacing cells that are continually being destroyed. Labile cells include surface epithelia, such as stratified squamous surfaces of the skin, oral cavity, vagina, and cervix; the lining mucosa of all the excretory ducts of the glands of the body (e.g., salivary glands, pancreas, and biliary tract); the columnar epithelium of the gastrointestinal tract, uterus, and fallopian tubes; and the transitional epithelium of the urinary tract.

The cells of the *splenic, lymphoid, and hematopoietic tissues* are also labile cells. Bone marrow is in a state of active hematopoiesis throughout life. Destruction of hematopoietic cells is rapidly compensated for by proliferation of persisting elements. The embryonic precursors of splenic and lymphoid cells (primitive mesenchymal stem cells) survive postnatally, proliferating and differentiating to replace lost elements.

STABLE CELLS

Stable cells usually demonstrate a low normal level of replication. However, these cells can undergo rapid

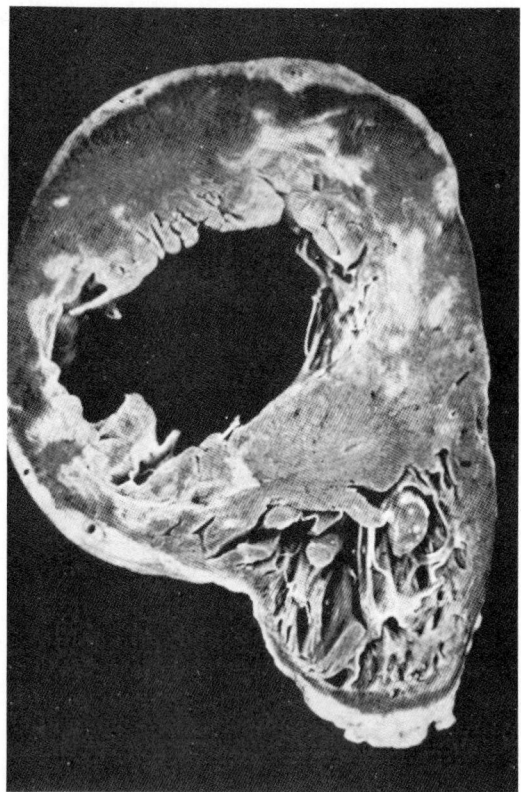

Figure 2–36. Myocardial fibrosis. The cross section of the ventricular myocardium shows pale scars of fibrous tissue that have been caused by ischemic necrosis of foci within the myocardium.

stitute the liver lobule. By contrast, a large liver abscess that destroys hepatocytes and connective tissue framework is followed by scarring.

The *connective tissue and mesenchymal cells* (fibroblasts, endothelium, smooth muscle, chondrocytes, and osteocytes) are quiescent in adult mammals. However, all proliferate in response to injury, and fibroblasts in particular proliferate widely, constituting the connective tissue response to inflammation (see section on "Repair by Connective Tissue").

PERMANENT CELLS

To the group of permanent cells belong the nerve cells, which cannot undergo mitotic division in postnatal life, and the skeletal and cardiac muscles cells, the regenerative attempts of which (at least in mammals) are of no practical importance. Neurons destroyed in the central nervous system (CNS) are permanently lost. They are replaced by the proliferation of the CNS supportive elements, the glial cells. The situation is somewhat more complicated with respect to the neurons of the peripheral nerves, as detailed in Chapter 29. When the cell body is destroyed, the entire structure (i.e., the cell body and extended axon) degenerates totally. If the cell body is spared and only the peripheral axon is injured, regeneration of a new process may proceed from the cell body or from the remaining proximal axonal segment.

The precise mode of regeneration of *skeletal muscle* is still somewhat uncertain. It may occur (1)

division in response to a variety of stimuli and are thus capable of reconstitution of the tissue of origin. In this category are the parenchymal cells of virtually all the glandular organs of the body, such as liver, kidney, and pancreas; mesenchymal cells such as fibroblasts, smooth muscle cells, osteoblasts, and chondroblasts; and vascular endothelial cells. The regenerative capacity of stable cells is best exemplified by the ability of the liver to regenerate after hepatectomy and following toxic, viral, or chemical injury.

Although labile and stable cells are capable of regeneration, it does not necessarily follow that there will be restitution of normal structure. *The underlying framework or supporting stroma of the parenchymal cells must be present to permit orderly replacement. The basement membrane appears to be the main structural component necessary for organized regeneration, forming a "scaffold" for the replicating parenchymal cells.* When basement membranes are disrupted, cells may proliferate in a haphazard fashion and produce disorganized masses of cells bearing no resemblance to the original arrangement. Alternatively, scarring may ensue. To use the liver as an example, hepatitis virus necessarily destroys parenchymal cells without injuring the more resistant connective tissue cells or framework of the liver lobule. Thus, after viral hepatitis, regeneration of liver cells may completely recon-

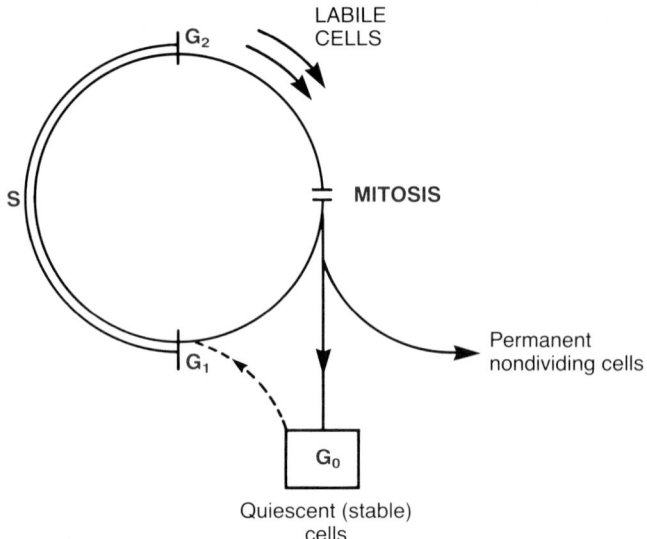

Figure 2–37. Cell populations and the phases of the cell cycle. Continuously dividing cells (labile cells) go around the cell cycle from one mitosis to the next. Nondividing cells have left the cycle and are destined to die without dividing again. Quiescent G_0 cells are neither cycling nor dying and can be induced to reenter the cycle by an appropriate stimulus. (Modified from Baserga, R.: The cell cycle. N. Engl. J. Med. 304:453, 1981.)

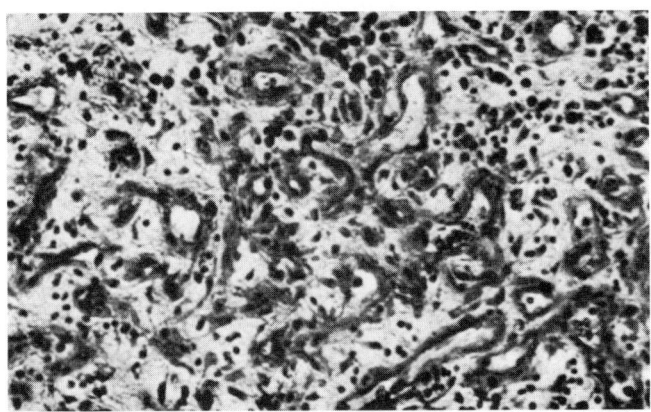

Figure 2–38. Active granulation tissue containing numerous vascular channels and inflammatory white cell exudate in a loose fibrous tissue stroma.

from the budding of old fibers, (2) by the fusion of myoblasts, or (3) by transformation of the satellite cells found attached to the endomysial sheaths of all multinucleated skeletal cells. If the ends of severed muscle fibers are closely juxtaposed, muscle regeneration in mammals can be excellent, but this is a condition that can rarely be attained under practical conditions. As to *cardiac muscle,* it is fair to state that if cardiac muscle has regenerative capacity, it is limited, and most large injuries to the heart are followed by connective tissue scarring (Fig. 2–36). Certainly, scarring follows the all too common myocardial infarction in man.

Another way of looking at these cell types is to consider their relationship to the cell growth cycle, which should be familiar to you (Fig. 2–37). *Continuously dividing (labile) cells* follow the cell cycle from one mitosis to the next. *Nondividing (permanent) cells* have left the cell cycle and are destined to senesce and die. *Quiescent (stable) cells* can be considered to be in G_0 but can be stimulated into G_1 by an appropriate stimulus. Arrest at G_2 before entering mitosis results in the appearance of polyploid cells — characteristic

of cells that have undergone hypertrophy but cannot undergo division. Except for nondividing tissues, *tissues of adults consist of a mixture of cells that includes continuously dividing cells, quiescent cells that occasionally go back to the cell cycle, and nondividing cells.*

REPAIR BY CONNECTIVE TISSUE — GRANULATION TISSUE

As mentioned earlier, healing starts very early in inflammation when the macrophages begin digesting whatever invading organisms have survived the neutrophilic attack, as well as necrotic debris from dead parenchymal cells and neutrophils. Sometimes as early as 24 hours after injury, fibroblasts and vascular endothelial cells begin proliferating to form (by three to five days) the specialized type of tissue (granulation tissue) that is the hallmark of healing inflammation. The term "granulation tissue" derives from its pink, soft granular appearance on the surface of wounds, but it is the histologic features that are characteristic: the *proliferation of new small blood vessels and of fibroblasts* (Fig. 2–38).

New vessels originate by budding or sprouting of pre-existing vessels, a process called *angiogenesis or neovascularization. Angiogenesis* is an important biologic process, which, as we shall see (p. 254), is also involved in the progressive growth of tumors.[87] At least four steps are needed in the development of a new capillary[88] (Fig. 2–39): (1) enzymatic degradation of the basement membrane of the parent vessel, to allow formation of a capillary sprout; (2) migration of endothelial cells toward the angiogenic stimulus; (3) proliferation of endothelial cells, just behind the leading front of migrating cells; and (4) maturation of endothelial cells and organization into capillary tubes. These new vessels have leaky interendothelial junctions, allowing the passage of proteins and red cells into the extravascular space.[89] Thus, *new granulation tissue is often edematous.* Indeed, this leakiness accounts for much of the edema that persists in heal-

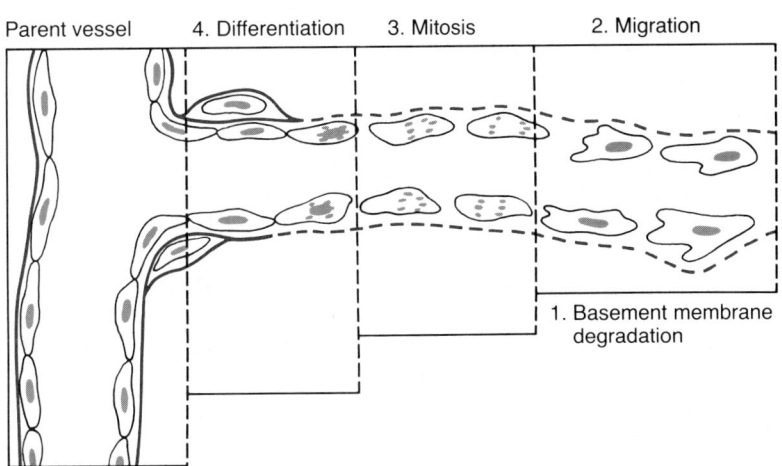

Figure 2–39. Four steps in angiogenesis. Parent mature vessel is on the left. 1. Basement membrane and ECM matrix degradation. 2. Endothelial migration. 3. Endothelial proliferation (mitoses). 4. Organization and maturation. (Adapted from Ausprunk, D.H.: *In* Houck, J.C. (ed.): Chemical Messengers of the Inflammatory Process. Amsterdam, Elsevier/North Holland, 1979.)

ing wounds, long after the acute inflammatory response has subsided.

In newly developing granulation tissue, fibroblasts proliferate, acquire increased amounts of rough endoplasmic reticulum, and appear in histologic sections as large, plump ("juicy") cells. Fibroblasts are active in synthesizing proteoglycans and collagen. In early stages, more glycoproteins are formed; later on, collagen predominates. *Some of the large fibroblasts in granulation tissue acquire features of smooth muscle cells* (thus the term *myofibroblast*): They develop large indented nuclei, prominent bundles of cytoplasmic fibrils with peripheral condensations, and large amounts of contractile proteins in their cytoplasm.[90]

Macrophages are almost always present in granulation tissue, busily ridding the area of extracellular debris, fibrin, and other foreign matter; and, if the appropriate chemotactic stimuli persist, neutrophils, eosinophils, and lymphocytes will also be seen. Mast cells are also present in great numbers. With further healing, there is an increase in extracellular constituents, mostly collagen, with a decrease in the number of active fibroblasts and new vessels. Many of the blood vessels characteristic of early stages undergo thrombosis and degeneration, and their various cells are resorbed and digested by macrophages. The end result of granulation tissue is a scar composed of inactive-looking, spindle-shaped fibroblasts, dense collagen, fragments of elastic tissue, extracellular matrix, and relatively few vessels (Fig. 2–40).

With this background on parenchymal regeneration and the formation of granulation tissue, we can now turn to a discussion of the healing of skin wounds.

WOUND HEALING

PRIMARY UNION (HEALING BY FIRST INTENTION)

The least complicated example of wound repair is the healing of a clean surgical incision (Fig. 2–41). The wound edges are approximated by surgical sutures,

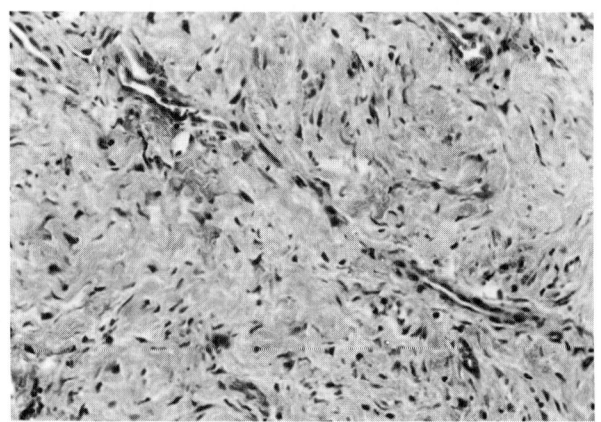

Figure 2–40. Healed scar composed of packed fibroblasts and dense collagen with only scattered compressed vascular channels.

and healing occurs without significant bacterial contamination and with a minimal loss of tissue. Such healing is referred to surgically as "primary union" or "healing by first intention." The incision causes the death of a limited number of epithelial cells as well as of dermal adnexa and connective tissue cells; the incisional space is narrow and immediately fills with clotted blood, containing fibrin and blood cells; dehydration of the surface clot forms the well-known scab that covers the wound and seals it from the environment almost at once.

Within 24 hours, neutrophils appear at the margins of the incision, moving toward the fibrin clot. The epidermis at its cut edges thickens as a result of mitotic activity of basal cells and, within 24 to 48 hours, spurs of epithelial cells from the edges both migrate and grow along the cut margins of the dermis and beneath the surface scab to fuse in the midline, thus producing a continuous but thin epithelial layer.

By day 3, the neutrophils have been largely replaced by macrophages. *Granulation tissue* progressively invades the incisional space. Collagen fibers are now present in the margins of the incision, but at first these are vertically oriented and do not bridge the incision. Epithelial cell proliferation continues, thickening the epidermal covering layer.

By day 5, the incisional space is filled with granulation tissue. Neovascularization is maximal. Collagen fibrils become more abundant and begin to bridge the incision. The epidermis recovers its normal thickness, and differentiation of surface cells yields a mature epidermal architecture with surface keratinization.

During the second week, there is continued accumulation of collagen and proliferation of fibroblasts. Leukocytic infiltrate, edema, and increased vascularity have largely disappeared. At this time, the long process of blanching begins, accomplished by the increased accumulation of collagen within the incisional scar, accompanied by regression of vascular channels.

By the end of the first month, the scar comprises a cellular connective tissue devoid of inflammatory infiltrate, covered now by an intact epidermis. The dermal appendages that have been destroyed in the line of the incision are permanently lost. Tensile strength of the wound increases thereafter, but it may take months for the wounded area to obtain its maximal strength.

SECONDARY UNION (HEALING BY SECOND INTENTION)

When there is more extensive loss of cells and tissue, such as occurs in infarction, inflammatory ulceration, abscess formation, and surface wounds that create large defects, the reparative process is more complicated. *The common denominator in all these situations is a large tissue defect that must be filled.* Regeneration of parenchymal cells cannot completely reconstitute the original architecture. Abundant granulation tissue grows in from the margin to complete the repair.

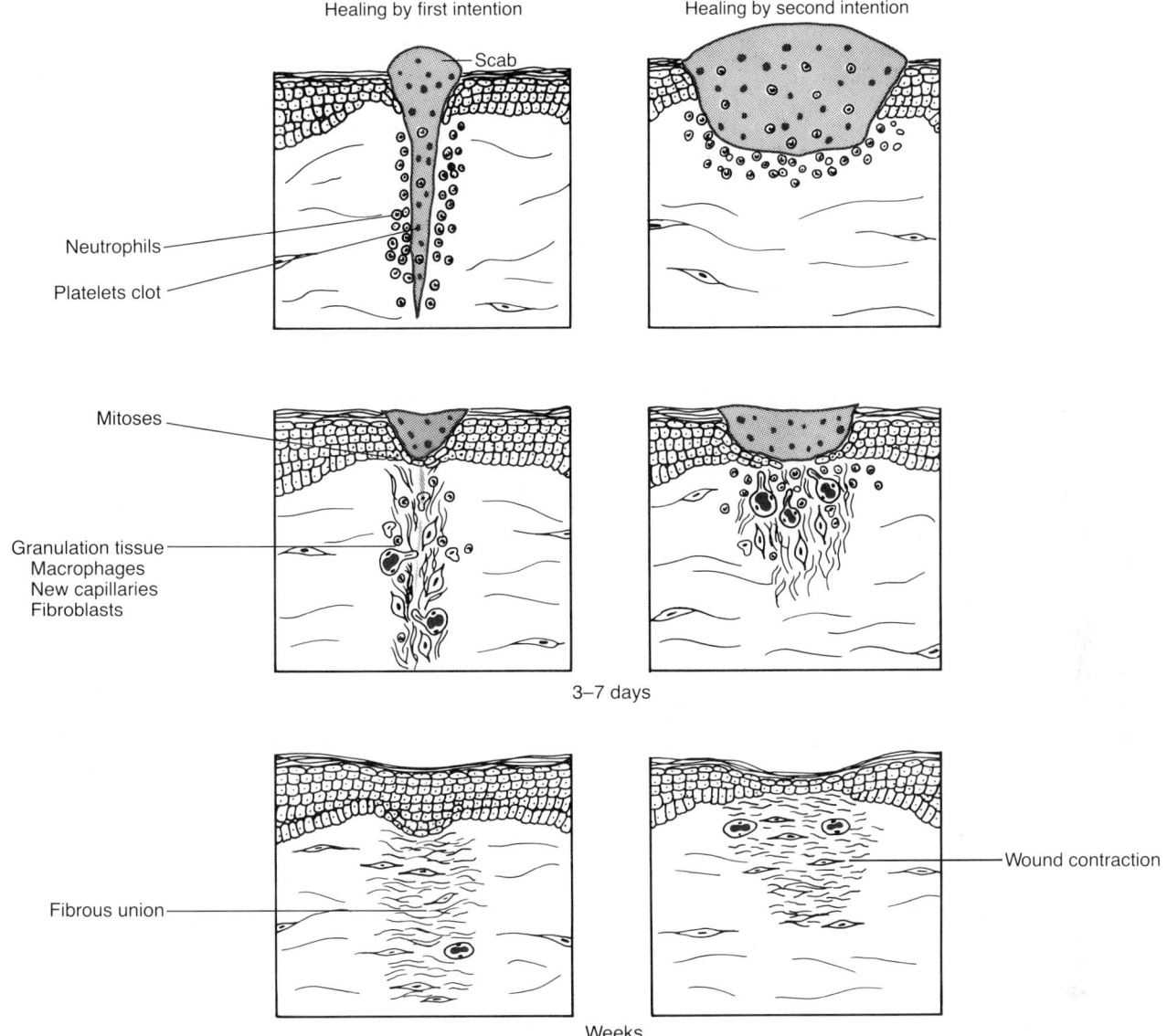

Healing by first intention   Healing by second intention

Scab

Neutrophils

Platelets clot

Mitoses

Granulation tissue
Macrophages
New capillaries
Fibroblasts

3–7 days

Fibrous union

Wound contraction

Weeks

Figure 2–41. Steps in wound healing by first intention (left) and second intention (right). In the latter, the resultant scar is much smaller than the original wound, owing to wound contraction.

This form of healing is referred to as "secondary union" or "healing by second intention" (Fig. 2–41, right).

Secondary healing differs from primary healing in several respects:

1. Inevitably, large tissue defects initially have more fibrin and more necrotic debris and exudate that must be removed. Consequently, the *inflammatory reaction is more intense.*

2. *Much larger amounts of granulation tissue are formed.* When a large defect occurs in deeper tissues, such as in a viscus, granulation tissue bears the full responsibility for its closure, because drainage to the surface cannot occur.

3. Perhaps the feature that most clearly differentiates primary from secondary healing is the phenomenon of *wound contraction,* which occurs in large surface

wounds.[91] A defect of about 40 cm² in the area in the skin of a rabbit is reduced in approximately six weeks to 5 to 10% of its original size, largely by contraction. The myofibroblasts have been implicated, by some,[92] but not others,[93] in this wound contraction.[92] Wound contraction contributes heavily to the repair of large surface defects, making it clear that whatever the dimension of a scar, the initial area of necrosis or tissue loss must have been greater.

As may be expected, events sometimes go awry in wound healing. Many aberrations relate to the management of the wound and the state of health of the wounded person. However, two deviations in particular may occur in the completely normal individual who has received optimal care. The first is the formation of excessive amounts of granulation tissue. The excess, referred to as *exuberant granulations,* or more

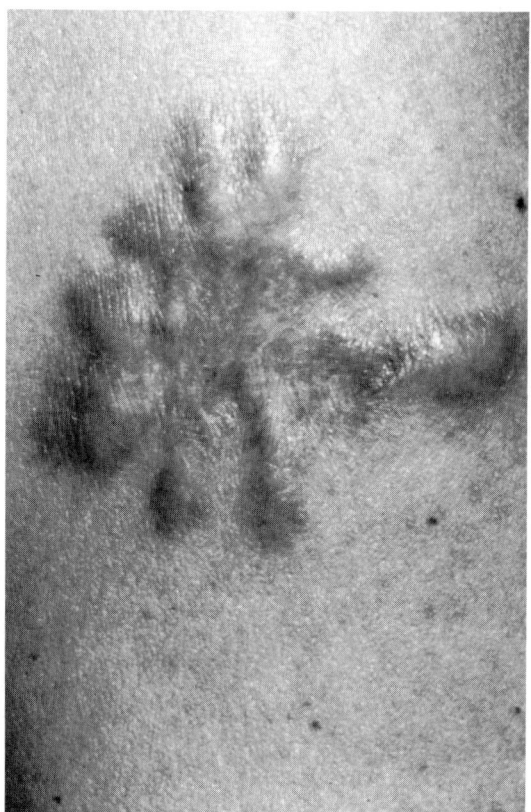

Figure 2–42. Close-up gross photograph of a *keloid* on the skin of the forearm. The irregular tumor-like lesion is firm and consists of abundant amounts of dense collagen.

grandiloquently as *proud flesh*, may protrude above the margins of the closing defect and block re-epithelialization. Happily, the problem is readily managed by either surgical excision or cauterization of the excess. The second abnormality, for mysterious reasons encountered most often in blacks, is *keloid* formation. In this situation, an abnormal amount of collagen is present in the connective tissue, producing a large, bulging, tumorous scar (Fig. 2–42). The tendency to form keloids appears to be an individual genetic characteristic. Keloid formation can be a troublesome problem, particularly on exposed skin areas, because it is disfiguring and exceedingly difficult to manage clinically; excision may be followed only by recurrence.

MECHANISMS INVOLVED IN REPAIR

Having described the sequence of events in repair, we can now turn to the mechanisms underlying these events. Wound healing is an extremely complex phenomenon involving a number of well-orchestrated processes, including *regeneration of parenchymal cells, migration and proliferation of both parenchymal and connective tissue cells, synthesis of extracellular* matrix proteins, remodeling of connective tissue and parenchymal components, and collagenization and acquisition of wound strength.[94] The mechanisms underlying these events are beginning to be understood and here we address three of the more important features: (1) *the role of growth factors*, which are central to the growth of fibroblasts and blood vessels and the regeneration of epithelial cells; (2) *cell-cell and cell-matrix interactions;* and (3) *extracellular matrix synthesis and collagenization.*

GROWTH FACTORS

It is now thought that normal growth in populations of cells is controlled by the opposing effects of growth stimulators and growth inhibitors. An excess of growth stimulators or a deficiency of growth inhibitors will lead to net proliferation, and in the case of cancer, uncontrolled proliferation, as we shall see (p. 252). Although growth can be accomplished by shortening the cell cycle or decreasing the rate of cell loss (as occurs in tumors), *the most important factors are those that recruit G_0 cells into the cell cycle.*[95]

Although many growth factors (including nutrients) have been described, current interest is focused on a number of *polypeptide growth factors* present in serum or produced by cells, which stimulate proliferation of a variety of cell types.[96] Some of these substances are *competence factors*, which do not stimulate DNA synthesis but render cells in G_0 or G_1 competent to do so; others are *progression factors*, which stimulate DNA synthesis in competent cells. Certain growth factors also initiate cell migration, differentiation, and tissue remodeling and may be involved in various stages of wound healing.[97] The principal polypeptide growth factors are the following (Table 2–7):

1. *Epidermal growth factor (EGF)*, a 6045-dalton polypeptide, purified from submaxillary glands of mice or from human urine (urogastrone).[98] First discovered by its ability to cause precocious separation of the eyelids of newborn mice (a true eye-opener!), EGF is mitogenic for a variety of epithelial cells and fibroblasts in vitro. EGF is a progression factor, and it stimulates cell division by binding to specific tyrosine kinase EGF receptors on the cell membrane, clustering of cell-bound EGF, phosphorylation of EGF receptor protein, internalization and lysosomal degradation of bound EGF with its receptor, followed eventually by onset of RNA synthesis and a commitment to DNA synthesis. Precisely how the second message—from EGF binding to RNA and DNA synthesis—is transmitted is now under active study.
2. *Platelet-derived growth factor (PDGF)*. This is a highly cationic protein composed of two chains (A and B) of approximately 30,000 daltons.[99] PDGF is stored in the platelet α granules and released upon platelet activation. It can also be produced by activated macrophages, endothelium, smooth muscle cells, and a

Table 2-7. Activities of Major Growth Factors Involved in Chronic Inflammation

	PDGF	FGF	TGF-β	TGF-α/EGF	IL-1 or TNF
Angiogenesis in vivo	o	+	+*	+*	+*
Chemotaxis					
Monocytes	+	?	+	?	+
Fibroblasts	+	+	+	o	?
Endothelium	o	+	?	+	?
Mitogenesis					
Fibroblasts	+	+	±	+	+
Endothelium	o	+	−	+	o or −
Collagen synthesis	+	?	+	?	+
Collagenase secretion	+	+	+	+	+

+ = Stimulates; − = inhibits; o = no effect; * = effect may be indirect.

PDGF = platelet-derived growth factor; FGF = fibroblast growth factor; TGF-α = transforming growth factor α; TGF-β = transforming growth factor β; IL-1 = interleukin-1; TNF = tumor necrosis factor; EGF = epidermal growth factor.

Modified from Sprugel et al.: Effects of growth factor in vivo. Am. J. Pathol. *129*:601, 1987.

variety of tumor cells. PDGF causes both migration and proliferation of fibroblasts, smooth muscles, and monocytes, but it has many other proinflammatory properties as well. Like EGF, PDGF binds to specific receptors that have protein kinase activity, but unlike EGF, it triggers the cell cycle by acting as a competence factor and thus it requires a progression factor for mitogenesis. Plasma, EGF, and insulin—like growth factors—can serve as progression factors in this process. PDGF has recently been shown to be active in vivo: when applied directly to surgical incisions in rats, there is enhancement of monocyte influx, collagen synthesis, and tensile strength in the wounds.[100]

3. *Fibroblast growth factor(s) (FGFs)*. First described as fibroblast mitogens extracted from bovine brain and pituitary, FGFs represent a family of polypeptide growth factors that have many other activities, including, in particular, *the ability to induce all the steps necessary for new blood vessel formation (angiogenesis)*, both in vivo and in vitro.[101] As you recall, these steps include basement membrane degradation, endothelial cell migration, proliferation, and capillary tube formation. FGFs have a strong affinity for heparin (heparin-binding growth factors), and consist of basic groups and acidic groups. Basic FGF is present in the extracts of many organs and is elaborated by activated macrophages, whereas acidic FGF is confined to neural tissue.

4. *Transforming growth factors (TGFα and TFGβ)*.[96] These factors were initially extracted from sarcoma virus–transformed cells and were thought to be involved in transformation of normal cells to cancer. TGFα has homology to EGF, binds to the EGF receptor, and produces most of the biologic activities of EGF. TGFβ, on the other hand, has more varied and often conflicting effects. TGFβ is a *growth inhibitor* to most cell types in culture, and is implicated in cessation of cell growth after partial hepatectomy (p. 33).

TGF-β stimulates fibroblast chemotaxis and the production of collagen and fibronectin by cells, at the same time inhibiting collagen degradation—all these effects favoring fibrogenesis. It "deactivates" macrophages (p. 62). TGF-β can be produced by different cell types, including platelets, endothelium, T cells, and macrophages.

5. *IL-1 and TNF*, discussed earlier, are mitogenic mediators that are chemotactic for fibroblasts, and they increase the synthesis of both collagen and collagenase by fibroblasts. They are thought to play a role in the fibroplasia and remodeling of connective tissue in inflammation. TNF is also angiogenic in vivo.

Before leaving the topic of growth factors, several points should be made. First, in addition to the growth stimulators described, *a number of growth inhibitors are known to be produced in inflammation.* One of these, TGFβ, was already considered. Others include α-interferon, prostaglandin E$_2$, and heparin; all three inhibit fibroblast and smooth muscle proliferation in vitro.

Second, as we have described, growth factors have effects on cell locomotion, contractility, and differentiation—effects that may be as important to wound healing as the growth effects.

Third, *macrophages*, which may be abundant in healing wounds, may play a central role in these processes, because they can be induced to secrete growth factors (PDGF, FGF, IL-1, or TNF), growth inhibitors (TGFβ, prostaglandins), and a variety of enzymes that may be involved in tissue degradation and organization.[79]

Finally, as we shall see later in Chapter 6, the genes encoding for some of these growth factors show extensive sequence homology with *oncogenes* (for example, PDGF with *c-sis* and the EGF receptor with *c-erb b*), suggesting involvement of these growth factors in cancer formation.

CELL-CELL AND CELL-MATRIX INTERACTIONS

When certain normal cell lines are placed in culture, they proliferate, eventually to form a confluent monolayer of cells, *after which proliferation ceases.* Malignant cells do not display this phenomenon but continue growing; thus, a clear understanding of the mechanisms may shed light on the initiation of neoplastic growth. The cessation of division may in part be ascribed to "contact inhibition," analogous to the contact inhibition of cell movement. However, many lines of evidence indicate that contact inhibition is also dependent on cell density within the culture dish.[102] This *density-dependent regulation of cell growth* may be caused by (1) limitation of any one of the various materials in the microenvironment that surrounds the crowded cells, (2) the number of receptor sites for the growth factors, or (3) accumulation of growth inhibitors in the culture medium. Whatever the signals, *the density-dependent regulation of cell growth is as important in vivo as it is in culture. As stated earlier, most cells capable of regenerating in response to injury usually cease proliferating after the defect caused by the injury has healed.* In the case of liver regeneration after hepatectomy, this cessation of growth is now being ascribed to production of TGF-β by nonparenchymal cells in the liver, as we have seen (p. 33).

Of current interest is the influence of *interactions with extracellular matrix on cell migration, proliferation, and differentiation.*[103] The type of collagen in the matrix, the presence of fibronectin or of laminin, and the nature of the proteoglycans in the pericellular areas all seem to affect these processes. For example, endothelial cells grown on laminin or type I collagen–coated culture dishes have a higher rate of replication when exposed to growth factors than cells grown on type IV (basement membrane) collagen. If grown on type IV collagen, these cells organize into tube-like structures.[103] Fibronectin or fibronectin fragments promote migration of endothelial cells and fibroblasts into an area of injury, a process that is critical to wound healing.

But how do these extracellular matrices induce their intracellular signals? Although the precise answer is unknown, it is now clear that cells possess *surface receptors that recognize extracellular matrix proteins* (Fig. 2–43).[104,105] These receptors are *transmembrane glycoproteins*, and their intracellular domains interact with elements of the cytoskeleton to signal cell locomotion or differentiation. One particular group of such receptors is the *integrins*, which belong to a supergene family including (1) the fibronectin receptors, (2) receptor glycoproteins on the platelet surface (p. 95), and (3) the leukocyte adhesion molecules described earlier (p. 46). Interestingly, many integrins bind the matrix proteins by recognizing the specific amino acid sequence of the tripeptide *arginine-glycine-aspartic acid* (RGD), a sequence that is thought to play a key role in cell adhesion (see also Fig. 2–45).

As stated earlier, the presence of *fibrin* is associated with the influx of inflammatory cells, fibroblasts, and new vessels and the formation of granulation tissue in wound healing. Pure fibrin-containing gels induce fibroplasia and angiogenesis in experimental animals.[106] Whether fibrin itself (or some degradation product of fibrin) or secondary factors derived from infiltrating leukocytes are the proximate mediators in these fibrin-induced reactions is unclear.

The nature of the factors that regulate cell growth, and of the stimuli for cell migration, proliferation, and differentiation in inflammatory repair in vivo is now under intensive investigation, and our understanding of the mechanisms will undoubtedly expand rapidly. Table 2–7 is a current summary of the factors that seem to be most important in mediating angiogenesis, fibroblast migration and proliferation, and collagen deposition in wound healing; Figure 2–43 is a postulated model of the interactions between growth factors, extracellular matrix, and cell responses in wound healing.[108]

COLLAGENIZATION AND WOUND STRENGTH

The development of wound strength is undoubtedly related to the proliferation of fibroblasts and the laying down of collagen and other extracellular elements in healing wounds. In this section we will briefly review a few details of the biology of connective tissue extracellular matrices and then discuss the development of wound strength.

Collagen

Collagen is the most common protein in the animal world, providing the extracellular framework for all multicellular organisms. Without collagen, man would be reduced to a clump of cells, interconnected by a few neurons! Consisting of a family of molecules, each a genetically distinct type, collagen is a major component of fibrous tissue, basement membranes, bone, cartilage, and other specialized tissues, such as cornea and heart valves. The essential product of the fibroblast, collagen ultimately provides the tensile strength of healing wounds.[109]

The metabolism of collagen in normal tissues involves a balance between biosynthesis and degradation.[110] The fundamental unit of collagen is the collagen molecule *(tropocollagen)* — a long rod, 300 × 1.5 nm, with a molecular weight of 285,000. Each collagen molecule is made up of three separate polypeptide chains (α chains) wrapped tightly together into a triple left-handed helix. Each α chain has a triple repetitive amino acid sequence, with every third amino acid being *glycine*. On the basis of the biochemical composition of the chains, 11 types of collagen are recognized, each characteristic of the tissue from which it is derived (Table 2–8). Types I, II, and III,

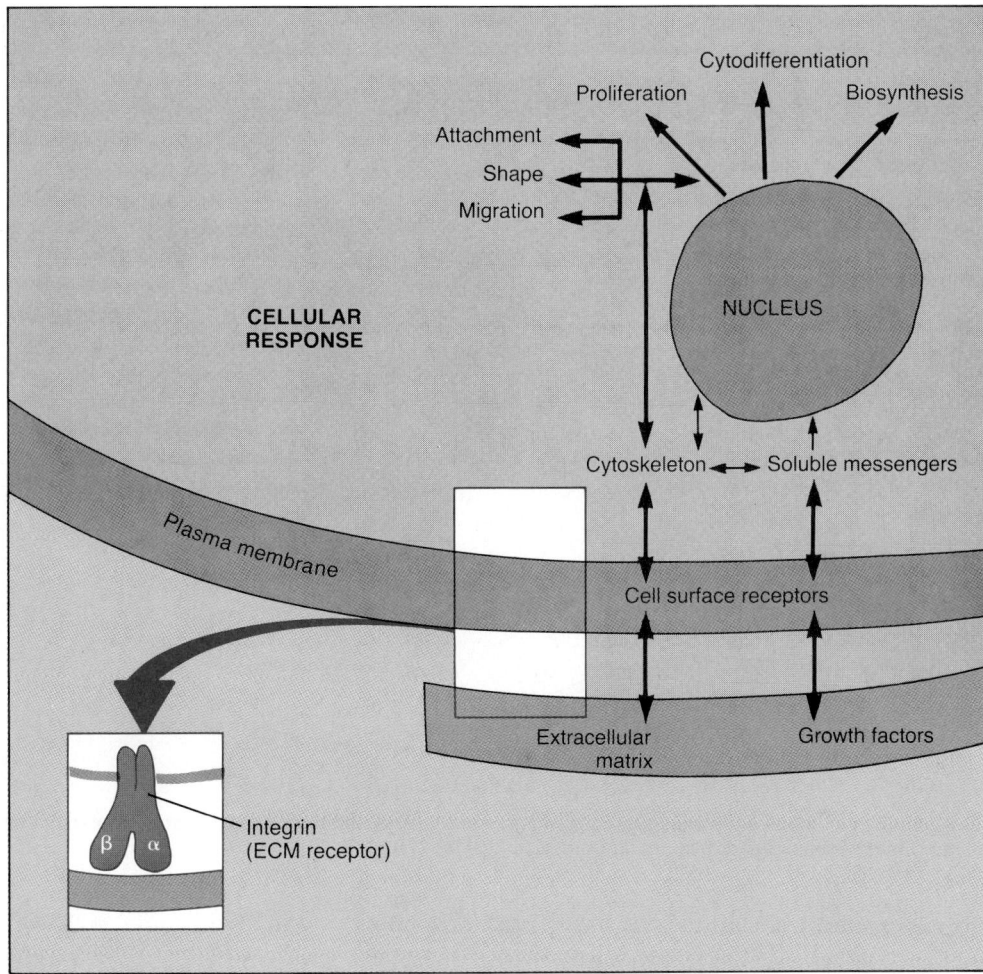

Figure 2–43. Scheme of possible mechanisms by which extracellular matrix (ECM) and growth factors influence cell shape, motility, and growth. Receptors for ECM, such as the integrins — which recognize the RGD sequence (p. 78) — interact with the cytoskeleton and initiate the production of diffusible second messengers, which act on both nucleus and cytoplasm to cause the cell responses, as illustrated. Cell surface receptors to growth factors also initiate second messengers, which modulate cell growth, locomotion, and differentiation. (Adapted from Madri, J., et al.: *In* Simionescu, N., and Simionescu, M. (eds.): Endothelial Cell Biology. New York, Plenum Publishing, 1988.)

are the interstitial or fibrillar collagens. In Type I collagen each molecule packs with one-fourth stagger with respect to adjacent molecules. The overlap produces the 67-nm banding of the collagen fibril. Types IV to XI do not form fibrils but appear as amorphous materials in interstitial tissue or basement membranes.

Synthesis of collagen (Fig. 2–44) is initiated by DNA transcription from specific genes coding for the polypeptide chains, followed by processing of mRNA

Table 2–8. Types of Collagen

TYPE	CHAINS	CHARACTERISTICS	DISTRIBUTION
I	α 1(I), α 2(I)	Bundles of banded fibers with high tensile strength	Skin (80%), bone (90%), tendons, most other organs
II	α 1(II)	Thin fibrils; structural protein	Cartilage (50%), vitreous humor
III	α 1(III)	Thin fibrils; pliable	Blood vessels, uterus, skin (10%)
IV	α 1(IV), α 2(IV)	Amorphous	All basement membranes
V	α 1(V, α2(V)), α 3(V)	Amorphous/fine fibrils	2–5% of interstitial tissues, blood vessels Interstitial tissues
VI	α 1(VI), α 2(VI)	Function unknown	
VII	α 1(VII)	Function unknown	
VIII	α 1(VIII)	Probably amorphous	Endothelium-specific
IX	α 1(IX), α 2(IX), α 3(IX)	Possible role in maturation of cartilage	Cartilage
X	α 1(X)		

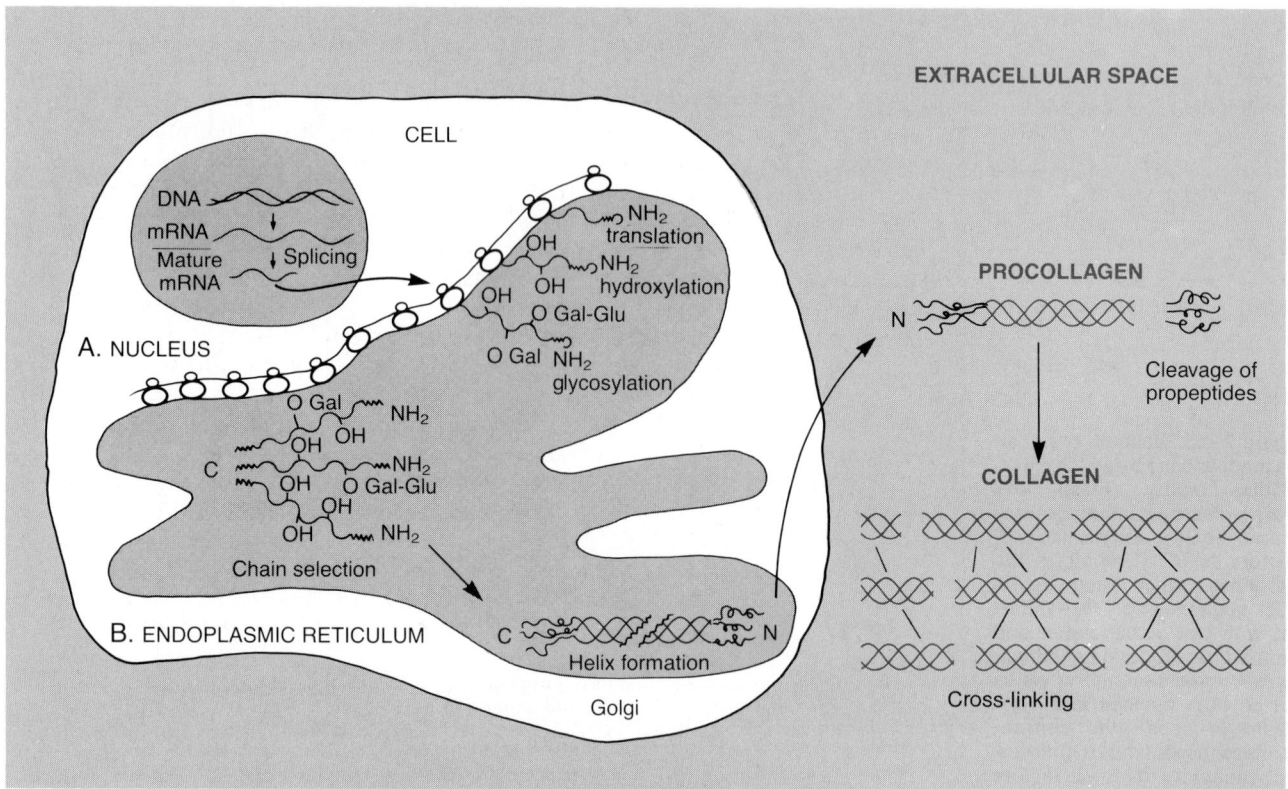

Figure 2–44. Steps in synthesis of collagen (see text). (Adapted from Krieg, T., et al.: Molecular defects of collagen metabolism in the Ehlers-Danlos syndrome. Int. J. Dermatol. *20*:415, 1981.)

precursor and translation (synthesis) of the α chains on ribosomes.[110] The α chains subsequently come off the ribosomes into the cisternae of the rough endoplasmic reticulum (RER), where they undergo a series of biochemical modifications of the chains, activated by specific enzymes. One of these modifications is the hydroxylation of proline in the α position, providing collagen with its characteristic high content of hydroxyproline (about 10%). This hydroxylation, which is dependent on the availability of ascorbic acid (vitamin C), is important because it is necessary to hold the three α chains in the cisternae of the RER.

As mentioned, the triple helix is assembled in the cisternae of the RER. At this stage the procollagen molecule is still soluble and contains an extra length of polypeptide and C terminal at the ends of the chain. It is transported through the Golgi apparatus and larger vacuoles to the cell surface. During or shortly after excretion from the cell, procollagen peptidases clip the terminal peptide chains, promoting formation of fibrils. *True fibrils form in the extracellular space,* and these collagen fibrils give strength to connective tissue.

Another critical extracellular modification is *lysine oxidation,* because this results in *cross linkages* between α chains of adjacent molecules and is *the basis of the structural stability of collagen.* Indeed, inhibition of lysine oxidation results in malformation of the skeleton, skin, and blood vessels, as occurs in some forms of human disorders of collagen (i.e., Mar-

fan's syndrome, p. 138). *Thus, cross linking is a major contributor to the tensile strength of collagen.*

Collagen fibers are very hardy and in the native state are resistant to digestion. However, *collagenase,* which is present in a variety of cell types (fibroblasts, macrophages, polymorphonuclear leukocytes, synovial cells, and some epithelial cells), can cleave collagen under physiologic conditions, cutting the triple helix into two unequal fragments, which are then susceptible to digestion by other proteases.[111] Fortunately, however, collagenase is present in these cells in the inactive form, *procollagenase.* The conditions regulating activation of the precursor molecule are obviously of great importance but are not well understood. However, it is thought that the collagenase of neutrophils, macrophages, and fibroblasts plays a role in degrading collagen in inflammation and wound healing. Degradation might aid in the débridement of injured sites and also in the remodeling of connective tissue necessary for healing of the defect. However, it may have a harmful effect because collagenase contributes to continuing tissue damage in rheumatoid arthritis and other inflammatory disorders.

Collagens of types IV and V, together with laminin, fibronectin, and heparan sulfate proteoglycan, are components of the basement membranes. Types IV and V exhibit no fibrils, and although they are readily degraded by selected neutral proteases derived from leukocytes, they are resistant to the collagenases found in skin.

Other Extracellular Matrix Components

Fibroblasts also synthesize *elastic fibers* and secrete the various glycosaminoglycans (GAG) and other components of the extracellular matrix.

Elastic fibers consist of two protein components: the more abundant *elastin*, which is amorphous on electron microscopy, and the *elastic microfibril*, composed of a specialized glycoprotein.[112] Mature elastin fibers are made of individual polypeptide chains, called tropoelastin, of about 70,000 daltons, which are covalently connected by cross linkages (desmosine and isodesmosine). Elastin has an extremely long half-life, exceeding the life of the individual, but a number of elastases produced by certain bacteria, neutrophils, and macrophages may play a role in local degradation of elastic tissue in inflammation. Indeed, as discussed in Chapter 16, unchecked activity of elastase may be a major factor in the pathogenesis of *emphysema*, a common and debilitating disease in which the lung loses its normal elasticity.

Laminin is the most abundant glycoprotein in the basement membranes (see Fig. 6–21, p. 258). *A large (800,000- to 1,000,000-dalton) cross-shaped structure, laminin spans the basement membrane* and binds on the one hand with specific receptors on the surface of cells and on the other hand with matrix components such as collagen type IV and heparan sulfate. Laminin is believed to mediate cell attachment to connective tissue substrates and, in culture, to alter the growth, survival, morphology, differentiation, and motility of various cell types. For example, it stimulates endothelial cell migration and replication and causes formation of neurite processes in cultured neural cells.

Proteoglycans consist of glycosaminoglycans (hyaluronic acid, heparin, chondroitin, dermatan, keratan, and heparan sulfate) linked covalently to a protein core.[109] They have diverse roles in regulating connective tissue structure and permeability and in modulating cell differentiation (see also p. 149).

Fibronectin is a large (440,000 dalton) multifunctional glycoprotein consisting of two chains held together by disulfide bonds. Associated with cell surfaces, basement membranes, and pericellular matrices, fibronectin is produced by fibroblasts, monocytes, endothelial cells, and other cells. An important characteristic of fibronectins is their ability to bind on the one hand with a number of other macromolecules (including collagen, fibrin, heparin, and proteoglycans) and on the other to cells via the previously described integrin receptors (p. 78, Fig. 2–45). For these reasons, it is thought that fibronectin is involved in interactions (e.g., attachment and spreading) of cells with the extracellular matrix. In healing skin wounds, a large quantity of fibronectin, mostly plasma-derived, appears in the extracellular matrix in the first two days after wounding. Thereafter, fibronectin is actively synthesized by proliferating endothelial cells.[114] Fibronectin in healing wounds may induce cell migration and possibly tissue organization. As alluded to earlier, fibronectin fragments are chemotactic for fibroblasts and also promote organization of endothelial cells into capillary tubes in vitro.

Fibroblasts and myofibroblasts are the cells that secrete collagens, elastin, and proteoglycans in healing wounds, but the mechanisms that stimulate or terminate such secretion at different phases are still poorly understood. Growth factors and other factors derived from macrophages, platelets, and lymphocytes have been shown to stimulate collagen accumulation in cultures; other agents, such as corticosteroids and parathyroid hormone, depress collagen synthesis. IL-1 and TNF stimulate collagenase formation by fibroblasts. The point to emphasize is that the healing wound is a dynamic and changing environment. Different mechanisms, occurring at different times and involving interaction between cells and local factors (e.g., oxygen tension, pH, immune reactions), most likely trigger the release of chemical signals that modulate the synthesis or degradation of extracellular matrix proteins, as well as migration and proliferation of cells. The details of these mechanisms are unknown, but it is remarkable that despite the many seemingly disjointed activities, the pattern of wound healing is so well orchestrated.

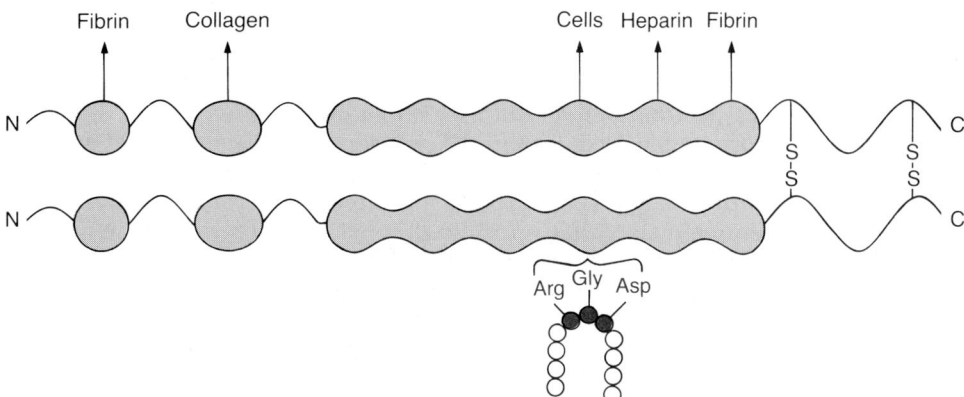

Figure 2–45. The fibronectin molecule consists of a dimer held by S—S bonds. Note the various domains that bind to extracellular matrices, and the cell-binding domain containing an ARG/GLY/ASP sequence.

Wound Strength

We now turn to the crucial questions of how long it takes for a skin wound to achieve its maximal strength and which substances contribute to this strength. There are variations that depend on the site of the wound, the species, and the depth of the incision.[115] From the welter of facts, however, a general impression emerges. Carefully sutured wounds have approximately 70% of the strength of unwounded skin immediately after surgery, largely due to the placement of the sutures. When sutures are removed, usually at the end of the first week, wound strength is approximately 10%. A rapid increase in wound strength takes place over the next four weeks. This rate of increase then slows and virtually plateaus at approximately the third month after the original incision. This plateau is reached at about 70 to 80% of the tensile strength of unwounded skin, and indeed may persist for life.

The recovery of tensile strength can therefore be represented by a sigmoid curve terminating in a plateau below the original level of the unwounded skin. The structural or biochemical explanation of this curve still eludes us. It is not merely a function of collagen synthesis, because the curve of tensile strength does not parallel that of collagen increase in the wound, but it may be related to the type of collagen produced. Thus, although adult skin collagen is type I, collagen deposited early in granulation tissue is type III, that characteristic of embryonic skin. During maturation of the scar, type III is again replaced by adult type I collagen.

FACTORS MODIFYING THE QUALITY OF THE INFLAMMATORY-REPARATIVE RESPONSE

Many systemic and local host factors influence the adequacy of the inflammatory-reparative response. Only a few of the most important are discussed here.

SYSTEMIC INFLUENCES

Age is probably not a major influence on the inflammatory-reparative response. There is a prevailing "general wisdom" that the elderly heal more slowly than the young, but very little controlled data in the experimental animal exist to support this notion.

Nutrition has a profound effect on the healing of wounds. Many workers have confirmed the deleterious effects of prolonged protein starvation on wound healing. Synthesis of collagen appears to be inhibited in protein-deficient animals. A high-protein diet hastens the rate of tensile strength gain. It has not been possible to isolate specific critical amino acids, but methionine and cystine supplementations have been reported to have a beneficial effect on the healing process in the protein-depleted animal. Of the many influences, the best documented is the need for adequate levels of vitamin C for the synthesis of normal collagen. As mentioned earlier, vitamin C enhances the conversion of proline to hydroproline and of lysine to hydroxylysine. Thus, deficiencies of this nutrient (scurvy) result in impaired synthesis of normal collagen. Absence of hydroxyproline will result in failure to achieve fibrillogenesis. Many enzymes, such as the metalloenzymes and DNA and RNA polymerases, are *zinc dependent*. Wound healing is delayed in patients with zinc deficiency and is restored to normal by zinc administration.

Hematologic derangements, such as deficiency of neutrophils in the circulating blood (granulocytopenia) or defects in leukocyte chemotaxis and phagocytosis, are well-documented bases for increased susceptibility to bacterial infection. Wound infection greatly slows the entire reparative process. In bleeding disorders there is excessive extravasation of blood into the wounded areas, serving as a substrate for bacterial growth and significantly slowing repair.

Diabetics have an increased susceptibility to serious infections, owing to a variety of factors, including diminished neutrophil chemotaxis and decreased phagocytic capacity. These patients are more vulnerable to bacterial invasion and consequent delays in wound healing.

Glucocorticosteroids have a well-documented anti-inflammatory effect, affecting numerous components of the inflammatory response.[116] One common mechanism for these anti-inflammatory effects may be the ability of glucocorticoids to enhance the production of a specific family of proteins called *lipocortins*.[117] Lipocortins inhibit phospholipase A_2, which, as may be recalled (see Fig. 2–17), is the enzyme necessary for the release of arachidonic acid from membrane phospholipids. Reduced synthesis of active metabolites of arachidonic acid follows.

The action of steroids in vivo on the healing phase is less clear. Although there are several effects on fibroblasts in vitro, if cortisone is administered to animals two days after injury, healing is not impaired, suggesting that it acts early in the response and probably does not primarily affect the healing phase. We may conclude by noting that steroids unquestionably block or retard the inflammatory-reparative response. *Clinically a wound in any patient receiving appreciable amounts of corticosteroids during or following surgery should be watched carefully.*

LOCAL INFLUENCES

Infection is the single most important local cause for delayed healing. Indeed, if the generalized and local factors that adversely influence repair are examined, infection is the final common pathway by which most retard the process of healing.

Adequacy of blood supply in an area of injury is an obvious important influence. From all that has been said before, it must be apparent that vascularization of the focus is a key factor in both inflammation and repair. Arterial disease that limits blood flow and venous abnormalities that retard drainage are well-documented impairments to the healing of wounds.

Foreign bodies and, of course, sutures constitute impediments to healing. The surgeon is faced with a dilemma in closing an incision: the wound will have almost no intrinsic strength during the immediate postoperative period save that conferred by sutures, which are themselves an obstacle to healing. The puncture wounds in the epidermis invite bacterial contamination, and the suture material excites an inflammatory and foreign-body reaction. One old but interesting study contends that a single suture enhances the invasiveness of staphylococci by a factor of 10,000. Fragments of wood, steel, glass, and even bone are equally undesirable. The surgeon must ply between Scylla and Charybdis by using sutures judiciously and removing all extraneous foreign bodies.

The tissue in which the injury has occurred is also a factor to be considered. Perfect repair can occur only in tissues made up of stable and labile cells, whereas all injuries to tissues composed of permanent cells must inevitably give rise to scarring and, at the most, very slight restoration of specialized elements. The location of the injury, or the character of the tissue in which the injury occurs, likewise is of considerable importance from yet another standpoint. There are many situations in the body in which inflammations arising within tissue spaces develop extensive exudates that fill these spaces, but in which there is no associated necrosis of fixed tissue cells. Under these circumstances, repair may occur by digestion of the exudate, initiated by the proteolytic enzymes of leukocytes, and resorption of the dissolved exudate. This mechanism of dealing with an exudative inflammation

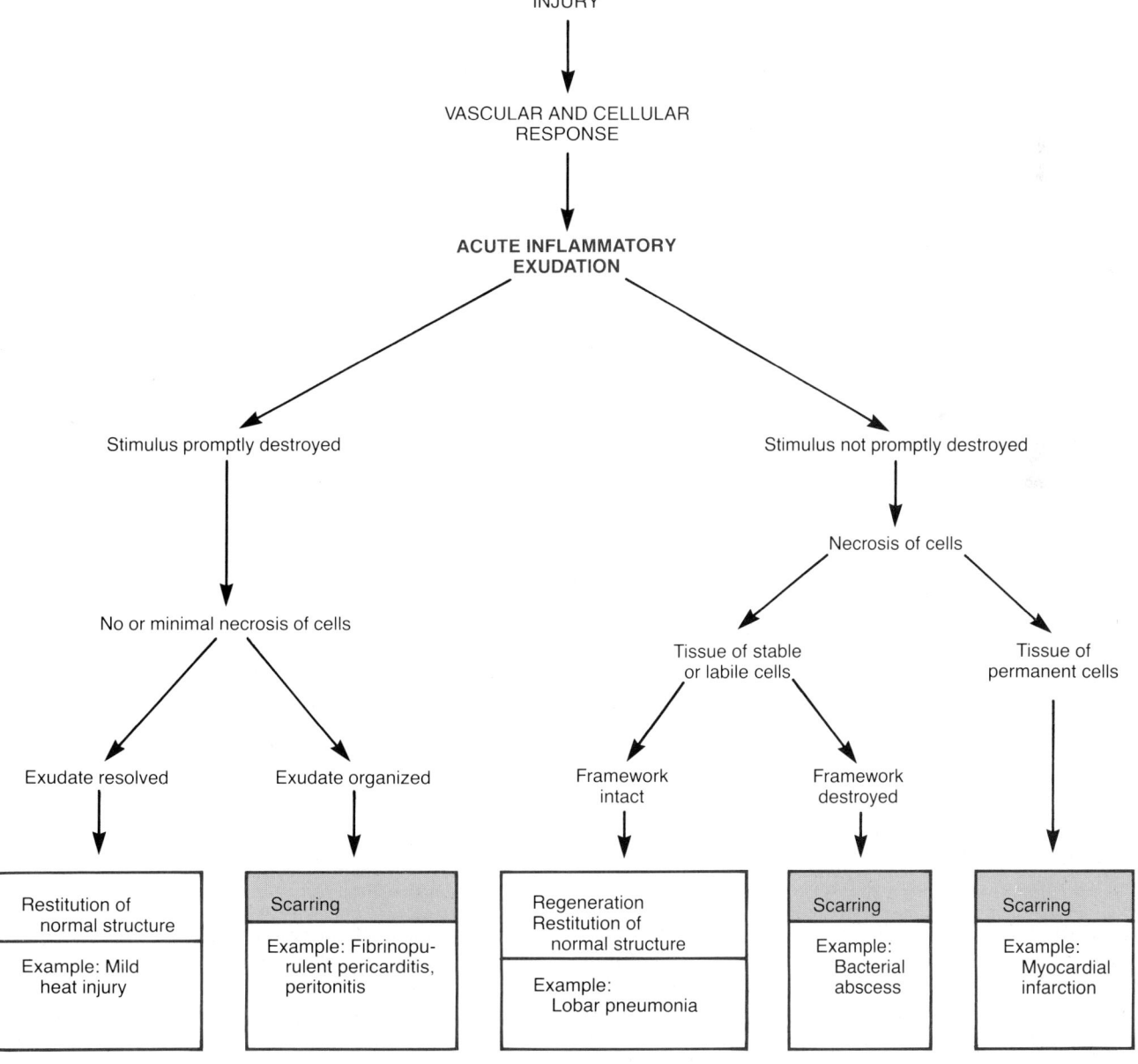

Figure 2–46. Pathways of reparative response.

is called *resolution*. No necrosis of fixed tissue cells has occurred, so perfect restitution of the pre-existing architecture is attained. Conversely, in the presence of substantial necrosis, granulation tissue grows into the exudate and converts it into masses of fibrous tissue, referred to as *organization*.

These processes of resolution or organization of inflammatory exudates are also observed in inflammations within other tissue spaces of the body (i.e., peritoneal, pericardial, and pleural cavities and joint spaces). Overall, most injuries of the body do not resolve without tissue necrosis and result in some connective tissue proliferation and therefore some degree of scarring. Finally, even when scarring is complete, another hazard occurs consequent upon a lag in the return of tensile strength of the collagen fibers. A rise in tension may bring about undue stretching of the scar, with hernia formation when the abdominal wall is affected.

In concluding this discussion of host factors, suffice it to say that many involve issues of considerable clinical importance. The correction of nutritional deficiencies, avoidance of steroid therapy, wise use of sutures, careful débridement and removal of foreign bodies, and, in general, scrupulous attention to all the influences that may hamper the inflammatory response are all responsibilities of the clinician.

PERSPECTIVE ON INFLAMMATORY-REPARATIVE RESPONSE

The full spectrum of events, from the initial reaction to injury to the ultimate tissue repair, has been presented. An injury may have little consequence and may be dealt with readily, or it may culminate in severe destruction and damage. A perspective of the various pathways is offered in Figure 2–46. This overview makes clear that not all injuries result in permanent damage; some are resolved with perfect reconstitution of the native tissue. Most often, however, some residual scarring persists.

1. Majno, G.: The Healing Hand: Man and Wound in the Ancient World. Cambridge, Harvard University Press, 1975.
2. Weissman, G.: Inflammation: Historical perspectives. *In* Gallin, J.I., et al. (eds.): Inflammation: Basic Principles and Clinical Correlates. New York, Raven Press, 1988, p. 5.
3. Majno, G.: Inflammation and infection. Historical highlights. *In* Majno, G., and Cotran, R. S. (eds.): Current Topics in Inflammation and Infection. Baltimore, Williams & Wilkins Co., 1982, p. 1.
4. Hunter, J.: A Treatise of the Blood, Inflammation, and Gunshot Wounds. Vol. I. London, J. Nicoli, 1794.
5. Cohnheim, J.: Lectures in General Pathology. (Translated by McKee, A.D., from the second German edition, Vol. I.) London, New Sydenham Society, 1889.
6. Heifets, L.: Centennial of Metchnikoff's discovery. J. Reticuloendothel. Soc. 31:381, 1982.
7. Ryan, G., and Majno, G.: Acute inflammation, a review. Am. J. Pathol. 86:185, 1977.

8. Landis, E.M., and Pappenheimer, J.R.: Exchange of substances through the capillary wall. *In* Hamilton, W.F., and Dow, P. (eds.): Handbook of Physiology. Section 2, Vol. II. Washington, D.C. American Physiological Society, 1963, p. 961.
9. Renkin, E.M.: Capillary transport of macromolecules: Pores and other endothelial pathways. J. Appl. Physiol. 58:315, 1985.
10. Milici, A.J., et al.: Transcytosis of albumin in capillary endothelium. J. Cell Biol. 105:2603, 1987.
11. Simionescu, M.: Receptor-mediated transcytosis of plasma molecules by vascular endothelium. *In* Simionescu, N., and Simionescu, M. (eds.): Endothelial Cell Biology in Health and Disease. New York, Plenum Press, 1988, p. 69.
12. Karnovsky, M.J.: The ultrastructural basis of transcapillary exchange. J. Gen. Physiol. 52:645, 1970.
13. Simionescu, N., et al.: Structural basis of permeability in sequential segments of the microvasculature of the diagram. II. Pathways followed by microperoxidase across the endothelium. Microvasc. Res. 15:17, 1978.
14. Simionescu, M., et al.: Differentiated microdomains on the luminal surface of capillary endothelium. II. Partial characterization of their anionic sites. J. Cell Biol. 90:614, 1981.
15. Jaffe, E.: Cell biology of endothelial cells. Hum. Pathol. 18:236, 1988.
16. Cotran, R.S.: Cellular components of inflammation: Endothelial cells. *In* Kelley, W.N., et al. (eds): Textbook of Rheumatology, 3rd ed. Philadelphia, W.B. Saunders Co., 1989.
17. Cotran, R.S., and Majno, G.: A light and electron microscopic analysis of vascular injury. Ann. N.Y. Acad. Sci. 116:750, 1964.
18. Majno, G., et al.: Studies on inflammation. II. Effects of histamine and serotonin along the vascular tree: A topographic study. J. Biophys. Biochem. Cytol. 11:607, 1961.
19. Majno, G., and Palade, G.E.: Studies on inflammation. I. The effect of histamine and serotonin on vascular permeability: An electron microscopic study. J. Biophys. Biochem. Cytol. 11:571, 1961.
20. Joris, I., et al.: The mechanism of vascular leakage induced by leukotriene E4: Endothelial contraction. Am. J. Pathol. 126:19, 1987.
21. Cotran, R.S.: Delayed and prolonged vascular leakage in inflammation. III. Immediate and delayed vascular reactions in skeletal muscle. Exp. Molec. Pathol. 6:143, 1967.
22. Heltianu, C., et al.: Histamine receptors of the microvascular endothelium revealed *in situ* with a histamine-ferritin conjugate: Characteristic high-affinity binding sites in venules. J. Cell Biol. 93:357, 1982.
23. Cotran, R.S., and Remensynder, J.P.: The structural basis of increased vascular permeability after graded thermal injury: Light and electron microscopic studies. Ann. N.Y. Acad. Sci. 150:495, 1968.
24. Gabbiani, G., and Badonnel, M.C.: Early changes of endothelial cells after thermal injury. Microvasc, Res. 10:65, 1975.
25. Hoover, R.L., and Karnovsky, M.J.: Leucocyte-endothelial interactions. *In* Nossel, H., and Vogel, H. (eds.): Pathobiology of the Endothelial Cell. New York, Academic Press, 1982, p. 357.
26. Harlan, J.M.: Leukocyte-endothelial interactions. Blood 65:513, 1985.
27. Anderson, D.C., and Springer, T.A.: Leukocyte adhesion deficiency. An inherited defect in the Mac-1, LFA-1, p150,95 glycoproteins. Ann. Rev. Med. 38:175, 1987.
28. Bevilacqua, M.P., et al.: Identification of an inducible endothelial-leukocyte adhesion molecule, ELAM-1. Proc. Natl. Acad. Sci. U.S.A. 84:9238, 1987.
29. Dustin, M.L. and Springer, T.A.: Lymphocyte function associated antigen-1 (LFA-1) interaction with intercellular adhesion molecule-1 (ICAM-1) is one of the least 3 mechanisms for T-lymphocyte adhesion to cultured endothelial cells. J. Cell Biol. 107:321, 1988.
29a. Smith, C.W., et al.: Recognition of an endothelial determinant for CD18–dependent human neutrophil adherence and transendothelial migration. J. Clin. Invest. 82:746, 1988.
30. Wheeler, E., et al.: Cultured human endothelial cells produce an inhibitor of leukocyte adhesion. J. Clin. Invest. 82:1211, 1988.
31. Marchesi, V.T.: The site of leucocyte emigration during inflammation. Q. J. Exp. Physiol. 46:115, 1961.
32. Issekutz, T.B., et al.: The in-vivo quantitation and kinetics of monocyte migration into acute inflammatory tissue. Am. J. Pathol. 103:47, 1981.
33. Boyden, S.: The chemotactic effect of mixtures of antibody and

antigen on polymorphonuclear leukocytes. J. Exp. Med. *115*:453, 1962.

34. Becker, E.L., and Ward, P.: Chemotaxis. *In* Parker, C.W. (ed.): Clinical Immunology. Philadelphia, W.B. Saunders Co., 1980, p. 272.

35. Schiffman, E., et al.: N-Formylmethionyl peptides as chemoattractants for leukocytes. Proc. Natl. Acad. Sci. U.S.A. *72*:1059, 1975.

36. Sandborg, R., and Smolen, J.: Early biochemical events in leukocyte activation. Lab Invest. *59*:300, 1988.

37. Snyderman, R., and Uhing, R.J.: Phagocytic cells: Stimulus-response coupling mechanisms. *In* Gallin, J.I., et al. (eds.): Inflammation: Basic Principles and Clinical Correlates. New York, Raven Press, 1988, p. 309.

38. Stossel, T.P., et al.: Non-muscle actin binding proteins. Ann. Rev. Cell Biol. *1*:353, 1985.

39. Stossel, T.: The mechanical responses of white blood cells. *In* Gallin, J.I., et al. (eds.): Inflammation: Basic Principles and Clinical Correlates. New York, Raven Press, 1988, p. 325.

40. Becker, E.: The formylpeptide receptor of the neutrophil. A search and conserve operation. Am. J. Pathol. *129*:16, 1987.

41. Silverstein, S.C., et al.: Endocytosis. Annu. Rev. Biochem. *46*:669, 1977.

42. Unkeless, J.C., and Wright, S.D.: Phagocytic cells: FC and complement receptors. *In* Gallin, J.I., et al. (eds.): Inflammation: Basic Principles and Clinical Correlates. New York, Raven Press, 1988, p. 343.

43. Hokin, L.E.: Receptors and phosphoinositide-generated second messengers. Ann. Rev. Biochem. *54*:189, 1985.

44. Boxer, G.J., et al.: Polymorphonuclear leukocyte function. Hosp. Pract. *20*:69, 1985.

45. Babior, B.M.: The respiratory burst of leukocytes. J. Clin. Invest. *73*:599, 1984.

46. Klebanoff, S.J.: Phagocytes — products of oxygen metabolism. *In* Gallin, J.I., et al. (eds.): Inflammation: Basic Principles and Clinical Correlates. New York, Raven Press, 1988, p. 391.

47. Weiss, J., et al.: Oxygen independent intracellular mechanisms. J. Clin. Invest. *69*:959, 1985.

48. Young, J.D., et al.: Mechanism of membrane damage mediated by human eosinophil cationic protein. Nature *321*:613, 1986.

49. Harlan, J.M.: Consequences of leukocyte vessel wall interactions in inflammatory and immune reactions. Semin. Thromb. Hemost. *13*:434, 1987.

50. Weissman, G., et al.: Release of inflammatory mediators from stimulated neutrophils. N. Engl. J. Med. *303*:27, 1980.

51. Henson, P.M., et al.: Phagocytic cells. Degranulation and secretion. *In* Gallin, J.I., et al. (eds.): Inflammation: Basic Principles and Clinical Correlates. New York, Raven Press, 1988, p. 363.

52. Rotrosen, D., and Gallin, J.I.: Disorders of phagocyte function. Annu. Rev. Immunol. *5*:127, 1987.

53. Curnutte, J.T., and Boxer, L.A.: Clinically significant phagocytic cell defects. *In* Swartz, M., and Remington, J. (eds.): Current Clinical Topics in Infectious Disease. New York, McGraw-Hill Book Co. (in press).

54. Babior, B.M., and Crowley, C.A.: Chronic granulomatous disease and other disorders of oxidative killing by phagocytes. *In* Stanbury, J.C., et al. (eds.): The Metabolic Basis of inherited Disease. New York, McGraw-Hill Book Co., 1983, p. 1956.

55. Busse, W.W.: Histamine: Mediator and modulator in inflammation. *In* Houck, J.C. (ed.): Chemical Messengers of the inflammatory Process. Amsterdam, Elsevier/North-Holland, 1979, p. 1.

56. Galli, S.J., et al.: Basophils and mast cells: Morphologic insights into their biology, secretory patterns and function. Prog. Allergy *34*:1, 1984.

57. Ross, G.D. (ed.): Immunobiology of the complement system. New York, Academic Press, 1986.

58. Muller-Eberhard, H.J.: The membrane attack complex of complement. Annu. Rev. Immunol. *4*:503, 1986.

59. Kozin, F., and Cochrane, C.G.: The contact activation system of plasma: Biochemistry and pathophysiology. *In* Gallin, J.I., et al. (eds.): Inflammation: Basic Principles and Clinical Correlates. New York, Raven Press, 1988, p. 101.

60. Samuelsson, B., et al.: Leukotrienes and lipotoxins: Structures, biosynthesis and biological effects. Science *237*:1171, 1987.

61. Parker, C.W.: Lipid mediators produced through the lipooxygenase pathway. Annu. Rev. Immunol., *5*:65, 1987.

62. Serhan, CN.: Lipooxygenase products of human leukocytes: formation and actions of lipoxins. Int. J. Immunopathol. Pharmacol. *1*:73, 1988.

63. Feuerstein, G., and Hallenback, J.M.: Leukotrienes in health and disease. FASEB J. *1*:186, 1987.

64. Palmblad, J., et al.: Leukotriene B_4 is a potent and stereospecific stimulator of neutrophil chemotaxis and adherence. Blood *58*:658, 1981.

65. Leaf, A., and Weber, P.C.: Cardiovascular effects of omega 3 fatty acids. N. Engl. J. Med. *318*:549, 1988.

66. Van Ver Alk, P., and Herman, C.J.: Leukocyte functions. Lab. Invest. *55*:127, 1987.

67. Janoff, A., and Carp, H.: Proteases, antiproteases, and oxidants: Pathways of tissue injury during inflammation. *In* Majno, G., and Cotran, R. S. (eds.): Current Topics in Inflammation and Infection. Baltimore, Williams & Wilkins Co., 1982, p. 62.

68. Fantone, J.C., and Ward, P.A.: Role of oxygen-derived free radicals and metabolites in leukocyte-dependent inflammatory reactions. Am. J. Pathol. *107*:397, 1982.

69. Perez, H.D., et al.: Generation of chemotactic lipid from arachidonic acid by exposure to a superoxide generating system. Inflammation *4*:313, 1980.

70. McManus, L.M.: Pathobiology of platelet activating factor. Pathol. Immunopathol. Res. *5*:104, 1986.

71. Winslow, C.M., and Lee, M.L. (eds.): New Horizons in Platelet Activating Factor Research. New York, John Wiley & Sons, 1987.

72. Pinckard, R.N., et al.: Platelet activating factors. *In* Gallin, J.I., et al. (eds.): Inflammation: Basic Principles and Clinical Correlates. New York, Raven Press, 1988, p. 139.

73. Dinarello, C.A., and Mier, J.W.: Lymphokines. N. Engl. J. Med. *317*:940, 1987.

74. Dinarello, C.A.: Biology of interleukin-1. FASEB J. *2*:108, 1988.

75. Le, J., and Vilček, J.: Tumor necrosis factor and interleukin 1: Cytokines with multiple overlapping biological activities. Lab. Invest. *56*:234, 1987.

76. Sherry, B., and Cerami, A.: Cachectin/tumor necrosis factor. J. Cell Biol. *107*:269, 1988.

77. Roska, A.K., and Lipsky, P.: Monocyte and macrophages. *In* Kelley, W.N., et al. (eds.): Textbook of Rheumatology, 3rd ed. Vol. I. Philadelphia, W.B. Saunders Co., 1989.

78. Johnston, R.B., Jr.: Monocytes and macrophages. N. Engl. J. Med. *318*:747, 1988.

78a. Unanue, E.R., and Allen, P.M.: The basis for the immunoregulatory role of macrophages and other accessory cells. Science *236*:551, 1987.

79. Nathan, C.F.: Secretory products of macrophages. J. Clin. Invest. *79*:319, 1987.

80. Adams, D.O., and Hamilton, T.A.: Phagocytic cells. Cytotoxic activities of macrophages. *In* Gallin, J.I., et al. (eds.): Inflammation: Basic Principles and Clinical Correlates. New York, Raven Press, 1988, p. 471.

81. Tsunawaki, S., et al.: Deactivation of macrophages by transforming growth factor. Nature *334*:260, 1988.

81a. Gelich, G.J.: Current understanding of eosinophil function. Hosp. Pract. *23*:137, 1988.

82. Unanue, E.R., and Benacerraf, B.: Immunological events in experimentally induced granulomas. Am. J. Pathol. *71*:349, 1973.

83. Weinberg, J.B., et al.: Recombinant human gamma interferon induces human monocyte polykaryon formation. Proc. Natl. Acad. Sci. U.S.A. *81*:4554, 1984.

84. McInnes, A., and Rennick, D.M.: Interleukin-4 induces cultured monocytes/macrophages to form giant multinucleated cells. J. Exp. Med. *167*:598, 1988.

85. Dinarello, C.A., et al.: Tumor necrosis factor (cachectin) is a endogenous pyrogen and induces IL-1. J. Clin. Invest. *77*:1734, 1986.

86. Broudy, V.C., et al.: Tumor necrosis factor stimulates human endothelial cells to produce granulocyte/macrophage colony stimulating factor. Proc. Natl. Acad. Sci. U.S.A. *83*:7467, 1987.

87. Folkman, J., and Klagsburn, M.: Angiogenic factors. Science *235*:442, 1987.

88. Ausprunk, D.H.: Tumor angiogenesis, *In* Houck, J.C. (ed.): Chemical Messengers of the Inflammatory Process. Amsterdam, Elsevier/North Holland, 1979, p. 317.

89. Schoefl, G.I. Studies of inflammation. III. Growing capillaries: Their structure and permeability. Virchows Arch. Pathol. Anat. *337*:97, 1963.

90. Ryan, G. B., et al.: Myofibroblasts in human granulation tissue. Hum. Pathol. 5:55, 1974.

91. Billingham, R.E., and Russell, P.S.: Studies on wound healing, with special reference to the phenomenon of contracture in experimental wounds in rabbit skin. Ann. Surg. *144*:961, 1956.

92. Skalli, O., and Gabbiani, G.: The biology of the myofibroblast relationship to wound contraction and fibrocontractive diseases. *In* Clark, R.A.F., and Henson, P. M. (eds.): The Molecular and Cellular Biology of Wound Repair. New York, Plenum Publishing, 1988, p. 373.

93. Eddy, R.J., et al.: Evidence for non-muscle nature of the myofibroblast of granulation tissue. Am. J. Pathol. *130*:252, 1988.

94. Colvin, R.B.: Roles of fibronectin in wound healing. *In* Mosher, D. F. (ed.): Fibronectin. New York, Academic Press. In press.

95. Baserga, R.: The Biology of Cell Reproduction. Cambridge, Harvard University Press, 1985.

96. Deuel, T.F.: Polypeptide growth factors: Roles in normal and abnormal cell growth. Annu. Rev. Cell Biol. *3:*443, 1987.

97. Sporin, M.B., and Roberts, A.B.: Peptide growth factors are multifunctional. Nature *332*:217, 1988.

98. Carpenter, G., and Cohen, S.: Epidermal growth factor. Annu. Rev. Biochem. *48*:193, 1979.

99. Ross, R., et al.: The biology of the platelet-derived growth factor. Cell *46*:155, 1986.

100. Pierce, G.F., et al.: In vivo incisional wound healing augmented by platelet-derived growth factor and recombinant c-*sis* gene homodimeric proteins. J. Exp. Med. *167*:974, 1988.

101. Joseph-Silverstein, J., and Rifkin, D.B.: Endothelial cell growth factors and the vessel wall. Semin. Thromb. Hemost. *13*:304, 1987.

102. Holley, R.W.: Control of growth of mammalian cells in cell culture. Nature *258*:487, 1975.

103. Furcht, L.T.: Critical factors controlling angiogenesis: Cell products, cell matrix and growth factors. Lab. Invest. *55*:505, 1986.

104. Buck, C.A., and Horwitz, A.F.: Cell surface receptors for extracellular matrix proteins. Ann. Rev. Cell Biol. *3*:179, 1987.

105. Hynes, R.O.: Integrins — a family of cell surface receptors. Cell *48*:549, 1987.

106. Dvorak, H.F., et al.: Fibrin-containing gels induce angiogenesis: Implications for tumor stroma generation and wound healing. Lab. Invest. *57*:673, 1987.

107. Sprugel, K.H., et al.: Effects of growth factors *in vivo*. Am. J. Pathol. *129*:601, 1987.

108. Madri, J., et al.: Endothelial cell – extracellular matrix interactions: matrix as a modulator of cell function. *In* Simionescu, N., and Simionescu, M. (eds.): Endothelial Cell Biology. New York, Plenum Publishing, 1988, p. 167.

109. Postlethwaite, A.E. and Kang, A.H.: Fibroblasts in inflammation. *In* Gallin, J.I., et al. (eds.): Inflammation: Basic Principles and Clinical Correlates. New York, Raven Press, 1988, p. 577.

110. Fleischmajer, R., et al.: Biology, chemistry and pathology of collagen. Ann. N.Y. Acad. Sci. *460*:1, 1985.

111. Prockop, D.J.: How does a skin fibroblast make type I collagen fibers? J. Invest. Dermatol. *79*:35, 1982.

112. Krane, S.M.: Collagenases and collagen degradation. J. Invest. Dermatol. *79*:83s, 1982.

113. Sandberg, L.B., et al.: Elastin structure, biosynthesis, and relation to disease states. N. Engl. J. Med. *304*:566, 1981.

114. Colvin, R.B.: Wound healing processes in thrombosis and hemostasis. *In* Gimbrone, M.A., Jr. (ed.): Vascular Endothelium in Hemostasis and Thrombosis. New York, Churchill Livingstone, 1986, pp. 220 – 241.

115. Peacock, E.E., and Van Winkle, W.: Wound Repair, 3rd ed. Philadelphia, W.B. Saunders Co., 1985.

116. Bowen, D.L., and Fauci, A.L.: Adrenal corticosteroids. *In* Gallin, J.I., et al. (eds.): Inflammation: Basic Principles and Clinical Correlates. New York, Raven Press, 1988, p. 877.

117. DiRosa, M., et al.: Multiple control of inflammation by glucocorticoids. Agents Actions *17*:284, 1986.

Fluid and Hemodynamic Derangements

EDEMA
HYPEREMIA AND CONGESTION
HEMORRHAGE
THROMBOSIS
Normal Hemostasis
    Endothelium and subendo-
        thelium

    Platelets
    Coagulation system
Thrombogenesis
Disseminated Intravascular
  Coagulation
EMBOLISM
Pulmonary Embolism

Systemic Embolism
Amniotic Fluid Embolism
Air or Gas Embolism (Caisson
  Disease or Decompression
  Sickness)
Fat Embolism
INFARCTION
SHOCK

All cells and tissues of the body are critically dependent on a normal fluid environment and on adequate blood supply. Either or both of these supporting systems may be deranged in a wide variety of clinical settings, and therefore fluid imbalances (edema or dehydration) and hemodynamic disturbances (hemorrhage, thrombosis, embolism, and infarction) are not only commonplace but also life-threatening. Myocardial infarction is the predominant cause of death in industrialized nations (p. 605). Edema of the brain or lungs and pulmonary embolism also are major causes of death. Severe hemorrhage is a frequent cause of morbidity and mortality, especially in this day of automobile and industrial accidents.

EDEMA

Edema is the term generally used for the accumulation of excess fluid in the intercellular (interstitial) tissue spaces or body cavities. Cells, too, may accumulate an abnormal amount of fluid, but this phenomenon is referred to as a cell swelling or cellular edema, described on page 16. Edema may occur as a localized process (e.g., with inflammation or with swelling of the leg when the venous outflow is obstructed), or it may be systemic with heart failure or the nephrotic syndrome (p. 1033) characterized by heavy proteinuria due to abnormal glomerular permeability. When edema is severe and generalized and causes diffuse swelling of all tissues and organs in the body, particularly noticeable in the subcutaneous tissues, it is called *anasarca.* Collection of edema fluid in the peritoneal cavity is known as *ascites;* in the pleural cavity as *hydrothorax;* and in the pericardial sac as *pericardial effusion,* or *hydropericardium.* Noninflammatory edema fluid such as accumulates in heart failure and renal disease is protein-poor and is referred to as a *transudate.* In contrast, inflammatory edema related to increased endothelial permeability is protein-rich and is caused by the escape of plasma proteins (principally albumin), and possibly leukocytes, to form an *exudate.* The differentiation of a transudate from an exudate was presented on page 41. *Here we are principally concerned with the noninflammatory transudation of fluid related to hemodynamic derangements.*

PATHOGENESIS. Water constitutes roughly 60% of the body weight of a lean adult. One third of it is extracellular fluid; the remainder is intracellular. Thus in a 70 kg adult there are about 42 liters of total body water, 28 of which are within cells. Of the 14 liters of extracellular fluid, about one third, say 4 liters, is intravascular and the remaining 10 liters interstitial. The volume of each compartment is maintained within remarkably narrow limits in health, but as you know, there is constant interchange among them. Each compartment has one solute whose osmotic activity largely determines its volume: serum proteins, principally albumin, for the intravascular compartment; sodium for the extracellular compartment; and potassium for the intracellular compartment. When the total body sodium increases, there is expansion of the interstitial and vascular volumes. The exchange between the intravascular and interstitial compartments is governed by Starling's forces (see p. 41). Fluid moves from the intravascular to the interstitial compartment at the arteriolar end of the microcirculation largely under the influence of the hydrostatic pressure of the blood. It returns to the intravascular compartment at the venular end mainly because of the osmotic pressure of the blood. Critical to this active interchange is a normal endothelial semipermeable barrier. There is a small net loss of fluid into the interstitial tissue spaces; this fluid is drained off through lymphatics, ultimately to be returned to the bloodstream. Thus the volume of interstitial fluid depends on the hydrostatic pressure of the blood in the microcirculation, the level of plasma proteins, the sodium content of the body, and the adequacy of the lymphatic drainage.

Edema constitutes in essence an abnormal expansion of the interstitial fluid or the accumulation of fluid in some "third extracellular space" such as the peritoneal or pleural cavity. Any perturbation of the delicate balance between the production of interstitial fluid and its return to the blood through either reabsorption or lymphatic drainage will result in edema. The major noninflammatory perturbations causing edema are divided into pathophysiologic categories in Table 3–1.

PATHOPHYSIOLOGIC CATEGORIES OF EDEMA.

INCREASED HYDROSTATIC PRESSURE. An increase in hydrostatic pressure in the venular end of the microcirculation raises the filtration pressure and at the same time opposes the oncotic pressure of the plasma proteins, and so flow from the vascular to the interstitial compartment is increased, resulting in edema. The prime example of this form of edema is seen in congestive heart failure. When it affects primarily right ventricular function, the edema is systemic in distribution and involves all tissues and

Table 3–1. Pathophysiologic Categories of Edema

I. Increased hydrostatic pressure
  A. Impaired venous return
    1. Congestive heart failure
    2. Constrictive pericarditis
    3. Cirrhosis of liver (ascites)
    4. Obstruction or narrowing of veins
      a. Thrombosis
      b. External pressure
      c. Inactivity of the lower extremities with long periods of dependency
  B. Arteriolar dilatation
    1. Heat
    2. Neurohumoral excess or deficit
II. Reduced oncotic pressure of plasma—hypoproteinemia
  A. Protein-losing glomerulopathies—nephrotic syndrome
  B. Cirrhosis of liver (ascites)
  C. Malnutrition
  D. Protein-losing gastroenteropathy
III. Sodium retention
  A. Excessive salt intake with reduced renal function
  B. Increased tubular reabsorption of sodium
    1. Reduced renal perfusion
    2. Increased renin-angiotensin-aldosterone secretion
IV. Lymphatic obstruction
  A. Inflammatory
  B. Neoplastic
  C. Postsurgical
  D. Postirradiation

Modified from Leaf, A., and Cotran, R.S.: Renal Pathophysiology, 3rd ed. New York, Oxford University Press, 1985, p. 146.

organs. Constrictive pericarditis acts in a similar manner. When the cardiac failure affects the left ventricle, the lungs are primarily affected.

However, the pathogenesis of cardiac edema is far more complex. Congestive heart failure also reduces cardiac output and therefore the so-called effective arterial blood volume. Reduction in renal blood flow triggers the renin-angiotensin-aldosterone axis, resulting in renal retention of sodium and water (secondary aldosteronism). At the same time there is renal vasoconstriction with a reduced glomerular filtration rate (GFR) and increased tubular reabsorption of salt and water. However, the resultant expansion of the intravascular volume constitutes a further burden on the failing heart, with consequent increase in venous pressure and edema formation. Thus a vicious cycle sets in that can be broken only by improvement in cardiac function with restoration of the balance of Starling's forces. Increased hydrostatic pressure may also produce localized edema, as occurs most commonly in one or both legs owing to thrombosis of major outflow veins, narrowing of the veins by external pressure (a large gravid uterus), or incompetence of the venous valves secondary to varicosities. Cirrhosis of the liver commonly produces an abnormal accumulation of fluid in the peritoneal cavity (ascites), discussed in more detail on page 942. Here it suffices that although the basis for this edema is complex, the two principal influences are portal hypertension (increased hydrostatic pressure) and decreased synthesis of plasma proteins. Arteriolar dilatation, such as occurs in the skin as a compensatory mechanism to increase blood flow and dissipate heat, is an uncommon cause of increased hydrostatic pressure and edema.

REDUCED ONCOTIC PRESSURE OF PLASMA. Lowering of the protein content of the plasma (hypoproteinemia) reduces the osmotic force responsible for reabsorption of interstitial fluid. In most circumstances, the critical level of plasma protein is about 2.5 gm/dl. Although a less common clinical basis for edema than increased hydrostatic pressure, *hypoproteinemia tends to produce the most severe form of generalized edema (anasarca).* The nephrotic syndrome is associated with the most extreme examples of hypoproteinemia (p. 1033). In this syndrome, damage to the normal glomerular filtration barrier leads to massive proteinuria. Less severe proteinuria and hypoproteinemia may be encountered with other forms of glomerulopathy, e.g., acute glomerulonephritis. Hypoproteinemia also may arise because of reduced synthesis of plasma proteins as is most commonly associated with diffuse liver disease, particularly cirrhosis. As noted above, cirrhosis also causes portal hypertension, contributing to the development of ascites. Severe protein malnutrition as occurs in kwashiorkor (p. 436) and protein-losing gastroenteropathy may also result in hypoproteinemia and edema. Whatever the basis for the reduced oncotic pressure of the plasma, the edema reduces the intravascular volume

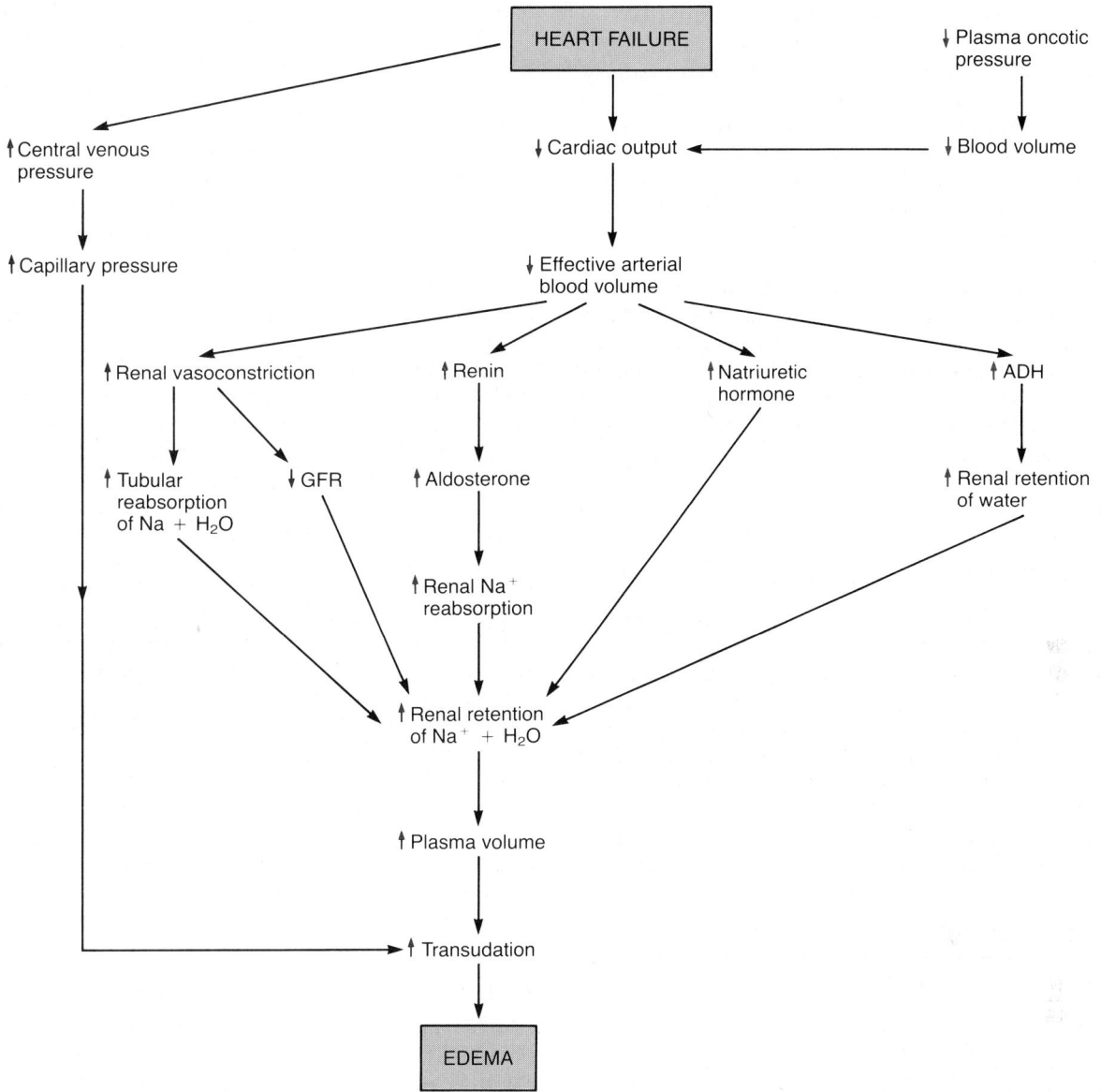

Figure 3-1. Projected sequence of events leading to systemic edema in heart failure and with reduced plasma oncotic pressure.

and effective arterial blood flow, setting in motion the train of events encountered in congestive heart failure and the vicious cycle detailed in Figure 3-1.

SODIUM RETENTION. With normal cardiac and renal function, excessive intake of sodium is soon corrected by renal excretion, although it may transiently increase intravascular volume, blood pressure, and interstitial fluid volume. When there is reduction in renal function as may occur with poststreptococcal glomerulonephritis (p. 1029) or acute renal failure (p. 1048), sodium retention causes expansion of the intravascular fluid volume and, secondarily, the interstitial fluid volume. Retention of sodium may also occur as a secondary phenomenon in any setting of reduced intravascular volume, e.g., congestive heart failure. *Ultimately it is the sodium content of the body that determines the volume of the interstitial fluid compartment,* and for this reason salt intake is restricted in the presence of systemic edema.

LYMPHATIC OBSTRUCTION. Interference with lymphatic drainage is an obvious cause for expansion of the interstitial fluid volume. Almost always, this form of edema is localized to a restricted lymphatic field, e.g., an axillary or inguinal region. Although the normal endothelial lining is relatively impermeable to the passage of proteins, a small amount of albumin leaks into the interstitial space along with the normal interchange of fluid between vascular and interstitial compartments. Thus, with lymphatic obstruction, neither the small amount of fluid lost from the intravascular compartment nor the protein within the interstitial fluid can be drained off, thus reducing the net effective osmotic pressure of the blood. In this manner edema, sometimes called *lymphedema,* appears. It is typically seen in the upper extremity following radical mastectomy with removal of the axillary nodes. It is also encountered with axillary radiation. Chronic infection with the filarial worm *Wuchereria bancrofti* induces lymphatic blockage, most often in the inguinal regions, producing epidermal thickening and massive edema of the external genitalia and legs sufficient to justify the designation *elephantiasis*.

MORPHOLOGY. The anatomic changes produced by edema depend on its severity, the rapidity with which it occurs, and the underlying cause. Indeed, the interstitial fluid compartment may expand as much as several liters before peripheral edema becomes manifest clinically or morphologically. Finger pressure over edematous subcutaneous tissue will displace the interstitial fluid from the dermal and subcutaneous connective tissues to leave pitted depressions, often referred to clinically as pitting edema (Fig. 3–2). The two most common systemic causes—cardiac failure and renal disease—produce slightly different patterns of edema. In **cardiac failure,** the accumulation of fluid is most severe in the dependent portions of the body and hence is referred to as **dependent edema.** When the patient is ambulatory, fluid collects first in the lower extremities, particularly over the dorsal aspects of the feet and ankles. If the patient is confined to bed, fluid may accumulate over the sacral region.

Edema of renal origin, such as is encountered in the nephrotic syndrome, is generally of greater severity than is cardiac edema. All regions of the body are affected equally, but the edema is most manifest in those tissues that have a loose connective tissue matrix. **Renal edema is therefore classically identified by edema of the face, particularly of the eyelids.**

Although considerable emphasis has been placed on subcutaneous edema, the visceral tissues likewise participate in generalized edema. Edematous viscera are slightly enlarged, pale, and heavier than normal; show somewhat tense capsules; and, on section, have a glistening appearance.

When well defined, edema is apparent microscopically as a thin, serous precipitate that separates the cellular and fibrillar elements of the tissue. This pink deposit represents the protein and solutes of the edema fluid. As the parenchymal cells swell, gland lumina and small vessels are compressed.

Edema of the brain and edema of the lungs are the most life-threatening forms of abnormal fluid retention.

Edema of the brain is described in some detail on page 1389. It suffices here that it may be localized to the region about focal lesions (e.g., neoplasms, abscesses) or generalized involving the entire brain, as for example in encephalitis, hypertensive crises, and obstruction to the venous outflow of the brain. Trauma may cause localized or generalized edema depending on its nature and distribution (p. 1413). When the entire brain is involved it is heavier than normal; the sulci are narrowed, and the swollen gyri are flattened where they press against the skull. On section, the white matter may appear unusually soft and gelatinous, and the peripheral layer of gray matter is widened. The ventricles are usually compressed. Histologically, the edema, whether localized or generalized, is marked by widening of the interfibrillar spaces of the brain substance; this gives a loose appearance to the white and gray matter. Swelling of the neuronal and glial cells may also be present. The perivascular (Virchow-Robin) spaces become unusually widened and form clear halos about the small vessels.

Pulmonary edema is a very common clinical problem, discussed in some detail on page 759. Here it is necessary to indicate only that it is a major manifestation of left ventricular failure and is also encountered in renal disease, shock, diffuse alveolar damage (p. 760), infections within the lungs, and hypersensitivity states when the lungs are target organs. The edema is usually confined to, or most marked in, the lower lobes. In far-advanced edema, however, all lobes may be involved and assume a rubbery gelatinous consistency. Sectioning of the lobes permits the free escape of frothy, sanguineous fluid representing a mixture of air and edema fluid (Fig. 3–3). On histologic examination, the edematous fluid first accumulates about the septal capillaries with widening of the septa. As the process evolves, a proteinaceous fluid escapes into the alveolar spaces, which is not retained in the histologic section. Its presence is often marked by a granular, pink coagulate within the alveolar spaces. When present for any period of time, intra-alveolar edema fluid is prone to secondary infection, producing so-called **hypostatic pneumonia.**

CLINICAL SIGNIFICANCE. In the brain and the lungs, edema may be fatal, but subcutaneous edema and edema of other viscera are usually of little functional significance. Swelling of the brain, when generalized, leads to increased intracranial pressure with resultant headaches, projectile vomiting, and convulsive seizures. Herniation of the brain stem or cerebellar tonsils into the foramen magnum may precipitate death. Cerebral edema may develop within hours of brain injury, requiring immediate corrective steps to save the patient's life. Pulmonary edema is important because it impedes the normal ventilatory function of the lungs. Characteristically, as the respired air bubbles through the proteinaceous fluid within the alveolar spaces, a variety of abnormal breath sounds called rales are produced. In severe pulmonary edema, the collection of fluid in the respiratory passages gives rise to extremely loud rales, popularly and appropriately termed the death rattle. Edema of the lungs (with the attendant hazards of hypostatic pneumonia) is one of the most serious complications of cardiac and renal insufficiency and frequently triggers the demise of these vulnerable patients.

HYPEREMIA AND CONGESTION

The terms hyperemia and congestion are elegant medical expressions for an increased volume of blood in an affected tissue or part. *Hyperemia, also called active hyperemia to differentiate it from congestion or*

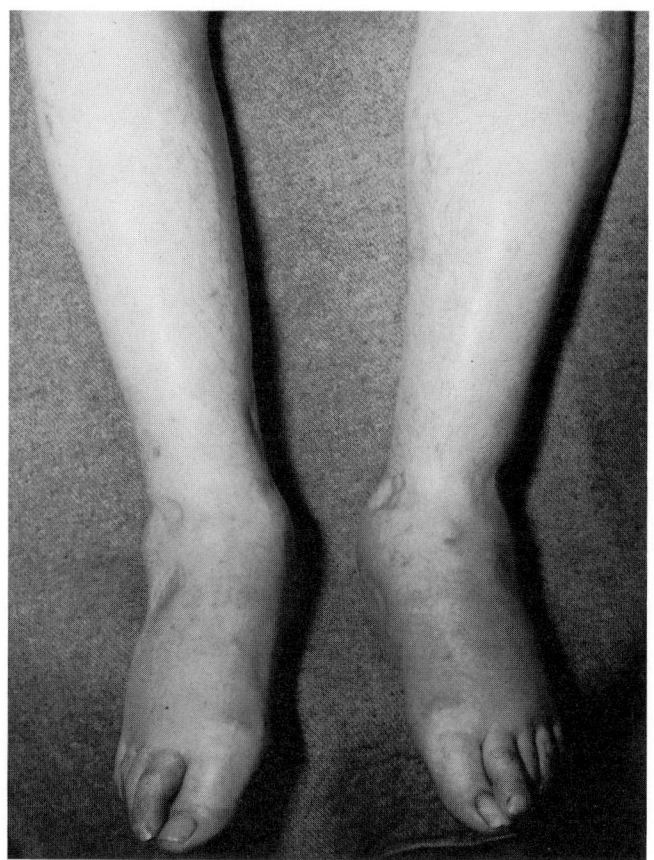

Figure 3–2. Dependent edema of the lower legs illustrating "pitting" about the ankles.

passive hyperemia, occurs when arterial and arteriolar dilatation produces an increased flow of blood into capillary beds, with opening of inactive capillaries. Congestion or passive hyperemia, on the other hand, results from impaired venous drainage.

Active hyperemia causes increased redness in the affected part. The arterial and arteriolar dilatation is brought about by sympathetic neurogenic mechanisms or the release of "vasoactive" substances (as discussed in Chapter 2). Active hyperemia of the skin is encountered whenever excess body heat must be dissipated, such as in muscular exercise and febrile states. Blushing is another example of hyperemia induced by neurogenic mechanisms.

Congestion, or *passive hyperemia,* causes an intensified blue-red coloration in affected parts as venous blood is dammed back. The blue tint is accentuated when the congestion leads to an increase of deoxygenated hemoglobin in the blood—*cyanosis.* Congestion may occur as a systemic phenomenon in congestive heart failure when both left and right ventricles are decompensated; may affect only the pulmonary circuit in left ventricular failure; or may affect the entire body, sparing the lungs, in right ventricular decompensation. Congestion can, of course, occur as a localized process when, for example, the venous return of blood to an extremity is obstructed or involves only the portal circulation when there is portal

hypertension secondary to cirrhosis of the liver. *Congestion of capillary beds is closely related to the development of edema, and so congestion and edema commonly occur together.*

MORPHOLOGY. Cut surfaces of acutely hyperemic and/or congested organs are excessively bloody and wet. With long-standing congestion, called **chronic passive congestion,** the stasis of poorly oxygenated blood causes chronic hypoxia, which may lead to degeneration or even death of parenchymal cells. Minute hemorrhages from capillary rupture may be converted in time to hemosiderin-laden scars. The lungs, liver, and spleen develop the most obvious manifestations of chronic passive congestion.

Acute and chronic passive congestion of the lungs and consequent pulmonary edema are encountered whenever there is elevated left atrial pressure and consequent elevated pulmonary venous pressure. Acute congestive changes are typically seen after a significant left ventricular myocardial infarct. The congestion promptly leads to edema, which leaks into the airspaces and so accounts for the often used clinical term "wet lungs." The most extreme form of chronic lung congestion is associated with rheumatic mitral stenosis, but it may also appear with any

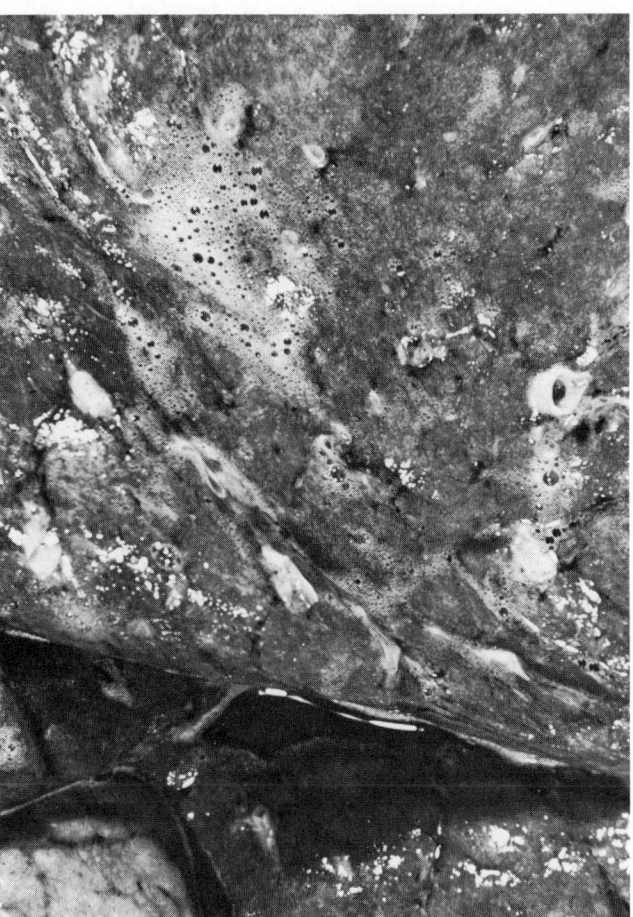

Figure 3–3. Pulmonary edema. The "wet" lungs of left ventricular failure. A frothy fluid oozes out of the transected surface.

condition causing reduced left ventricular output. Microscopically, the alveolar capillaries are engorged with blood and often become tortuous, with small aneurysmal dilatations (Fig. 3–4). Rupture of distended capillaries may cause minute intra-alveolar hemorrhages and the breakdown and phagocytosis of the red cell debris eventually lead to the appearance of hemosiderin-laden macrophages ("heart failure" cells) in the alveolar spaces. In severe forms of chronic passive congestion, the alveolar septa are widened both by the dilatation of alveolar capillaries and by edema fluid that collects within the interstitium of the alveolar septa (congestion and edema). In time, the edematous septa become fibrotic and, together with the hemosiderin pigmentation, constitute the basis for the designation **brown induration.** The long-standing congestion and consequent pulmonary hypertension may cause progressive thickening of the walls of the pulmonary arteries and arterioles (p. 764).

Acute and chronic passive congestion of the liver results from right-sided heart failure or, more rarely, from obstruction of the inferior vena cava or hepatic vein. The first changes include a dusky red cyanosis and increase in liver size and weight. On liver section, there is an excessive ooze of blood, and the central veins may appear prominent. With chronic congestion, the central regions of the lobule

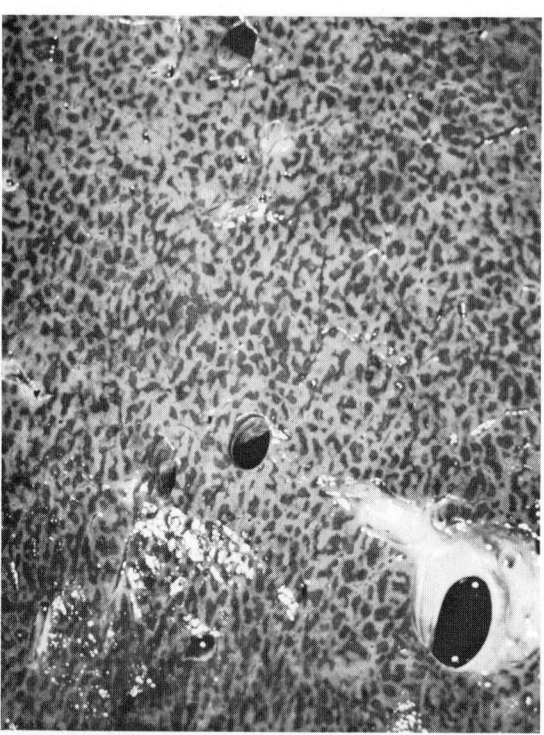

Figure 3–5. Chronic passive congestion of the liver. On the cut surface, the central congested areas appear darker than the pale peripheral portions of the lobules and thus compose the so-called nutmeg pattern.

become red-blue, surrounded by a zone of uncongested liver substance, descriptively referred to as the **nutmeg liver** (Fig. 3–5). Microscopically, the central vein and the vascular sinusoids of the centrilobular regions are distended with blood. The central hepatocytes frequently become atrophic secondary to chronic hypoxia, whereas the peripheral hepatocytes, suffering from less severe hypoxia, develop fatty change.

With severe cardiac failure the central hepatocytes may become necrotic and the centrilobular zone hemorrhagic, producing so-called **central hemorrhagic necrosis.** Arcidi and colleagues have suggested that, whereas chronic passive congestion of the liver is related to elevation of the systemic venous pressure, the subsequent development of central hemorrhagic necrosis reflects hypoxia due to reduction in the circulating blood volume and hepatic blood flow.[1] Thus, **centrilobular necrosis** may appear in shock from any cause without preceding chronic passive congestion. With long-standing chronic passive congestion, particularly when associated with death of central hepatocytes, fibrous thickening of the walls of the central veins eventually appears. Extension of this fibrous tissue into the surrounding lobule creates the distinctive anatomic pattern called cardiac sclerosis or sometimes "cardiac cirrhosis" (p. 921).

Chronic passive congestion of the spleen produces at first a slightly enlarged, tense, cyanotic organ that on section freely exudes blood and collapses slightly, so that the capsule becomes wrinkled. With time, the pulp becomes progressively more firm. In the early stages, the

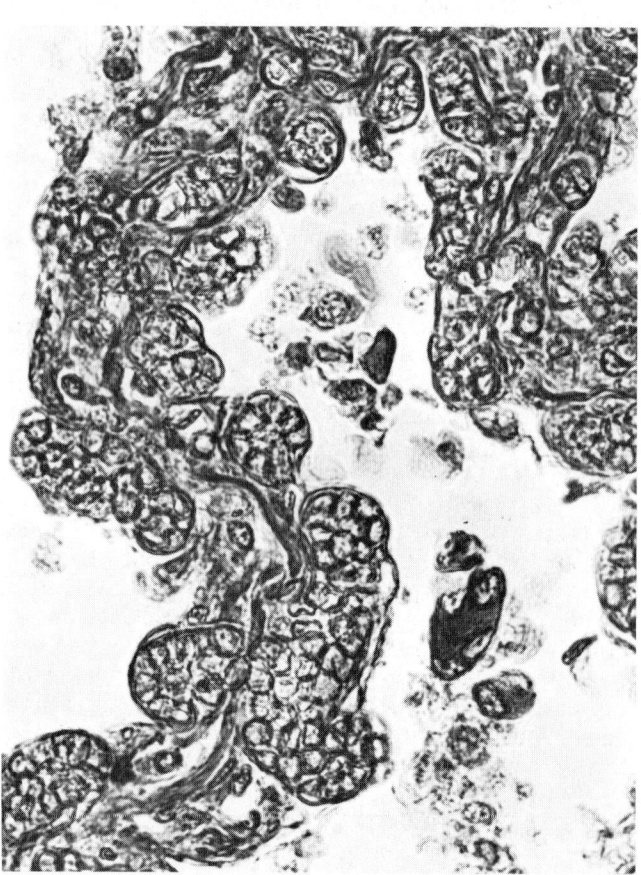

Figure 3–4. Marked congestion of pulmonary alveolar capillaries; a microscopic detail showing the widened and tortuous capillaries. Their lumina now permit the passage of two to three red cells abreast of each other.

spleen usually does not exceed 250 to 300 gm in weight (normal = 150 gm). Microscopically, marked sinusoidal dilatation is present, accompanied by foci of recent hemorrhage and possible hemosiderin deposits. In long-standing chronic congestion, the organ progressively enlarges and may weigh up to 500 to 700 gm. Fibrous thickening and hemosiderin deposits within the edematous, congested, sinusoidal walls produce the characteristic anatomic pattern of **congestive splenomegaly** (p. 750). Sometimes focal hemorrhages, followed by repair, yield **siderofibrotic** nodules of scar tissue laden with hemosiderin.

HEMORRHAGE

Rupture or laceration of a blood vessel is the obvious cause of hemorrhage. If a significant amount of released blood accumulates within a tissue, it is referred to as a *hematoma.* For example, with rupture of the aorta, usually due to some underlying aortic disease, large mediastinal or retroperitoneal hematomas may be produced. If the blood escapes into a serous cavity, it is referred to appropriately as *hemothorax, hemopericardium,* or *hemoperitoneum.* Smaller hemorrhages, usually encountered in the skin, mucous membranes, and serosal surfaces, are known as *petechiae* (minute), *purpura* (up to approximately 1 cm), or *ecchymoses* (when large and blotchy). Microscopic hemorrhages may be produced in loose tissues, such as the lung, merely by marked congestion followed by escape of erythrocytes—a phenomenon referred to as *red cell diapedesis.*

The causes of hemorrhage are too numerous to be detailed and include trauma as well as diseases that primarily (e.g., atherosclerosis) or secondarily (e.g., an extending erosive cancer) attack vessel walls. Worthy of special mention in this context are hypertension and the hemorrhagic diatheses. Retinal and, more ominously, cerebral hemorrhages are encountered in hypertensive patients. The latter is a frequent cause of death in patients having marked (malignant) hypertension. The hemorrhagic diatheses constitute a group of clinical disorders having in common an increased bleeding tendency. Scurvy, platelet deficiencies, and a lack of any one of the clotting factors are the principal causes of hemorrhagic diatheses (p. 691).

CLINICAL SIGNIFICANCE. The significance of hemorrhage depends on the amount of blood loss, its rate of escape, and the site of the hemorrhage. Acute losses of up to 10 to 15% of blood volume and slow losses of even greater amounts have little clinical significance. Larger or more rapid losses may cause hemorrhagic (hypovolemic) shock. But even relatively small amounts of hemorrhage in the brain or pericardial sac may produce sufficient increases of pressure to cause death. It is obvious that external bleeding or hemorrhage into the gastrointestinal tract represents a permanent loss of vital iron. However, if bleeding occurs in a body tissue or cavity (peritoneal, pleural), progressive breakdown of the hemoglobin permits resorption of the iron and its reutilization. In the course of this resorption of hemoglobin, increased amounts of bilirubin are formed and may cause transient jaundice. This sequence is associated particularly with massive gastrointestinal bleeding because even though much of the red cell mass is excreted, some is rapidly digested, with rapid resorption of large amounts of the hemoglobin precursor of bilirubin.

THROMBOSIS

The formation of a clotted mass of blood within the noninterrupted cardiovascular system is termed *thrombosis,* and the mass itself a *thrombus. A thrombus must be differentiated from a blood clot.* The thrombus is formed by a complex process involving the interaction of blood vessel walls, the formed elements of the blood, notably the platelets, and the plasma coagulants that constitute the blood clotting system. In contrast, a blood clot involves only the coagulation sequence, and thus clotting occurs, as you know, when blood is drawn into a test tube or when a blood vessel is severed. Clotting also occurs in extravascular accumulations of blood (hematomas), and after death there is post-mortem clotting of the blood in the cardiovascular system. The composition of thrombi may also differ from that of blood clots. Thrombi that arise in the rapidly moving arterial or cardiac circulation are composed largely of fibrin and platelets and thus bear little resemblance to a blood clot. However, with very sluggish venous flow thrombi may closely resemble blood clots, as will be explained shortly.

Clearly the development of a blood clot is lifesaving when a large vessel ruptures or is severed. However, when a thrombus develops in the unruptured cardiovascular system, it may be life-threatening. Thrombi may (1) diminish or obstruct vascular flow, causing ischemic injury to tissues and organs, or (2) become dislodged or fragment to create emboli. An *embolus* is an intravascular solid, liquid, or gaseous mass carried in the bloodstream to some site removed from its origin or from its point of entrance into the cardiovascular system. Most emboli are derived from thrombi. Indeed, thrombosis and embolism are so closely interrelated as to give rise to the term *thromboembolism. Infarcts* are localized areas of ischemic necrosis of tissues caused most commonly by sudden reduction of the arterial supply or sometimes by reduced venous drainage of the area. They are usually caused by thromboembolic occlusion of a vessel. Infarctions of the heart, lungs, and brain collectively account for more deaths than all forms of cancer and infectious disease together and are the dominating clinical problems today in all industrialized nations.

Before turning to the pathophysiology of thrombosis, it is desirable to first review normal hemostasis.

NORMAL HEMOSTASIS

Nature has designed complex but ingenious systems to maintain the fluidity of the blood in the vascular system yet allow the rapid formation of a solid plug of blood to close holes made by ruptures or other forms of injury to blood vessels. *Thrombosis is, to a considerable extent, a pathologic extension of the normal hemostatic mechanism*; it is dependent on three important components: (1) the *vascular wall*, with its lining endothelium and underlying subendothelial connective tissues; (2) *platelets*, essential for thrombus formation; and (3) *soluble coagulation proteins* present in the plasma and in certain cells in inactive forms, but poised to be triggered along a cascade that ends in the deposition of the ultimate insoluble product *fibrin*. Before each of the components is considered separately, the events in hemostasis will be briefly described.

1. *With vascular injury there is a brief period of vasoconstriction, which in small vessels (principally arterioles) serves to reduce blood loss.*
2. *Much more important, the injury to endothelial cells exposes highly thrombogenic subendothelial connective tissue, to which the platelets adhere and undergo so-called contact activation, i.e., a shape change, a release reaction, and further aggregation of more platelets. This platelet reaction occurs within minutes of injury and is called primary hemostasis.*
3. *Virtually simultaneously, release of tissue factors at the site of injury in combination with platelet factors activates the plasma coagulation sequence, forming fibrin. This requires a longer time for completion and is referred to as secondary hemostasis.*
4. *Ultimately a permanent hemostatic plug is pro-*duced by the combined activities of (a) endothelial cells, (b) platelets, and (c) the coagulation sequence as follows.*

Endothelium and Subendothelium

Normal endothelium has a completely thromboresistant surface, but when injured it can profoundly promote thrombosis. These effects are accounted for by two general mechanisms. The *passive mechanisms* have long been known. Not only is the endothelium thromboresistant, but also it insulates the circulating blood elements from the highly thrombogenic subendothelium; endothelial injury and denudation exposes the subendothelial connective tissue. The *active mechanisms* involve a number of both antithrombotic and prothrombotic factors that endothelial cells possess on their surface or can actively elaborate (Fig. 3–6). Under normal conditions, these opposing properties are in balance and a nonthrombogenic surface is maintained, but perturbations by a variety of stimuli can tip the balance either toward the prothrombotic side, causing clotting/thrombosis, or toward the antithrombotic side, predisposing to ineffective hemostasis and excessive bleeding.[2]

There are several *antithrombotic factors* on endothelial cells (Fig. 3–6). Two of these protect against the unchecked action of thrombin, which, as we shall see, is the terminal enzyme of the coagulation cascade that converts fibrinogen to fibrin. (1) *Thrombomodulin*, a surface protein, binds thrombin and in so doing converts thrombin into an activator of *protein C*, a plasma protein that is a potent anticoagulant in its activated form. Protein S, synthesized by endothelial cells, serves as a cofactor for the anticoagulant activity of activated protein C.[3] (2) *Heparin-like molecules* on

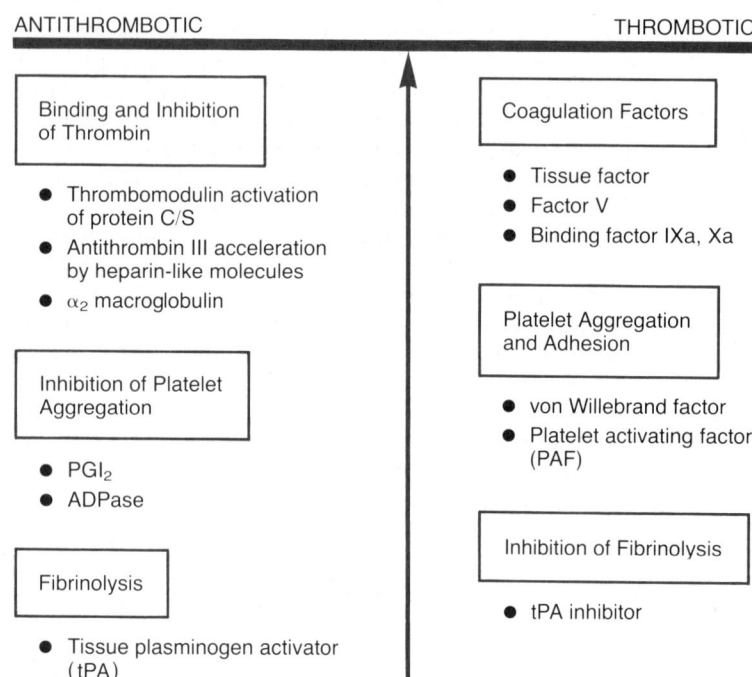

ANTITHROMBOTIC   THROMBOTIC

Binding and Inhibition of Thrombin

- Thrombomodulin activation of protein C/S
- Antithrombin III acceleration by heparin-like molecules
- α_2 macroglobulin

Inhibition of Platelet Aggregation

- PGI$_2$
- ADPase

Fibrinolysis

- Tissue plasminogen activator (tPA)

Coagulation Factors

- Tissue factor
- Factor V
- Binding factor IXa, Xa

Platelet Aggregation and Adhesion

- von Willebrand factor
- Platelet activating factor (PAF)

Inhibition of Fibrinolysis

- tPA inhibitor

Figure 3–6. The endothelial thrombotic/antithrombotic balance. The major factors favoring and inhibiting thrombosis are shown.

the endothelium also markedly accentuate the effects of antithrombin III, a plasma protein that efficiently inactivates thrombin, and several other clotting factors such as XIIa, XIa, Xa, and IXa.[4] *Endothelial cells also inhibit platelet aggregation by several mechanisms.* They have the capacity to convert the strongly proaggregating adenosine diphosphate (ADP) released from platelets to adenine nucleotide platelet inhibitors. *Much more important is their elaboration of prostacyclin (PGI$_2$), a potent inhibitor of platelet aggregation and a strong vasodilator.*[5] Indeed, with endothelial cell injury and activation of the coagulation sequence, the formation of thrombin at the site of injury stimulates the surrounding endothelial cells into more active synthesis of PGI$_2$. In addition, endothelial cells react against blood clots and thrombi by synthesizing tissue plasminogen *activators*, which promote fibrinolytic activity in the blood (p. 54), clear fibrin deposits from the endothelial surface, and also participate in the resolution of intravascular thrombi.[6]

The schizophrenic endothelial cell, on the other hand, can promote thrombosis by virtue of its procoagulant activities (Fig. 3–6). For example, the extrinsic clotting pathway can be activated by tissue factor (thromboplastin) present in minute amounts of normal endothelium, but stimulated by endotoxin and by cytokines, such as interleukin-1 (IL-1) and tumor necrosis factor (TNF).[7] Endothelial cells synthesize and secrete von Willebrand factor (vWF), which is a necessary cofactor for the adherence of platelets to subendothelial components, and they can be stimulated to secrete platelet-activating factor (PAF), a platelet activator and aggregator. Endothelial cells also secrete an inhibitor of plasminogen activator, which depresses fibrinolysis and therefore favors persistence of thrombi (see p. 54).[6]

The *subendothelial connective tissues* not only support the endothelial monolayer but also are thrombogenic. They consist of various types of collagen, elastin, glycosaminoglycans, fibronectin, laminin, and thrombospondin. Although several components such as basement membrane and elastin promote platelet adherence, the most potent stimulus for platelet adhesion and activation is fibrillar collagen, which also provides contact activation of clotting factors in the so-called intrinsic pathway of blood coagulation.[8] Fibronectin serves to stabilize cell-to-cell and cell-to-substrate attachments in the normal endothelial lining. It also becomes cross-linked to fibrin and facilitates anchorage of hemostatic plugs. Thus, damage to the endothelial cell barrier exposes the highly thrombogenic subendothelium, initiating hemostasis and thrombosis.

Platelets

It is already evident that *platelets* play a central role in normal hemostasis and therefore also in thrombosis. Despite their lack of a nucleus, head, and heart, these tiny structures (about 2 μm in diameter) are amazingly versatile. At sites of endothelial cell injury they are capable of (1) *adhesion and shape change*, (2) *secretion (release reaction)*, and (3) *aggregation, collectively referred to as platelet activation*. In addition, as you remember, platelets are capable of synthesizing prostaglandin derivatives, notably thromboxane (TxA$_2$). They also maintain the integrity of the normal endothelial layer, since patients who suffer a platelet deficiency (thrombocytopenia) are prone to purpuric bleeding. With vascular and endothelial cell injury, the following sequence of platelet events unfolds.

1. *Adhesion refers to attachment of platelets to sites of endothelial cell injury, where subendothelial elements, particularly fibrillar collagen, are exposed* (Fig. 3–7). Whether platelets possess specific collagen receptors is uncertain, but as already mentioned, vWF is necessary for such adhesion and serves as a molecular bridge between platelets and collagen, acting through glycoprotein receptors (mostly GpIb) (Fig. 3–8; also see p. 696). Genetic deficiencies of vWF or of the glycoprotein receptors result in defects in platelet adhesion. The platelets at first attach themselves by long pseudopods but then spread broadly to become tightly adherent. The shape transformations are mediated by intraplatelet actomyosin microfilaments and by microtubules.

2. *Secretion — the release reaction —* of the contents of platelet granules follows soon after adhesion. Platelets contain two major types of granules — *alpha granules* and *dense bodies*.[9] *Alpha granules* contain fibrinogen, fibronectin, platelet-derived growth factor, an antiheparin (platelet factor 4), and platelet-specific proteins, i.e., cationic proteins and beta-thromboglobulin. Beta-thromboglobulin has no known function, but when found in the plasma it serves as an indicator of platelet activation. *Dense bodies* are rich in ADP and ionized calcium and also contain histamine, epinephrine, and serotonin (5-HT). Calcium is necessary in the coagulation sequence, and the ADP is a potent mediator of platelet aggregation, as will shortly be discussed. With platelet activation and the release reaction, a phospholipid complex called platelet factor 3 becomes activated or in some manner exposed on the platelet surface. This phenomenon is of some importance since it provides a site on the platelet surface where coagulation factors such as IXa and VIIIa and Ca^{++} bind to activate factor X. In this manner, platelet activation contributes to the intrinsic pathway of blood clotting and the formation of thrombin.

3. *Platelet aggregation (implying platelet-platelet interadherence) closely follows adhesion and secretion.* A major contributor to aggregation is the formation of thromboxane A$_2$ (TxA$_2$) by activated platelets. TxA$_2$ is also a vasoconstrictor.

In addition, the adherent and activated platelets release ADP to thus set into motion an autocatalytic reaction with the build-up of an enlarging platelet aggregation known as the *temporary or primary hemostatic plug*. This primary aggregation is reversible, but with the activation of the coagulation sequence

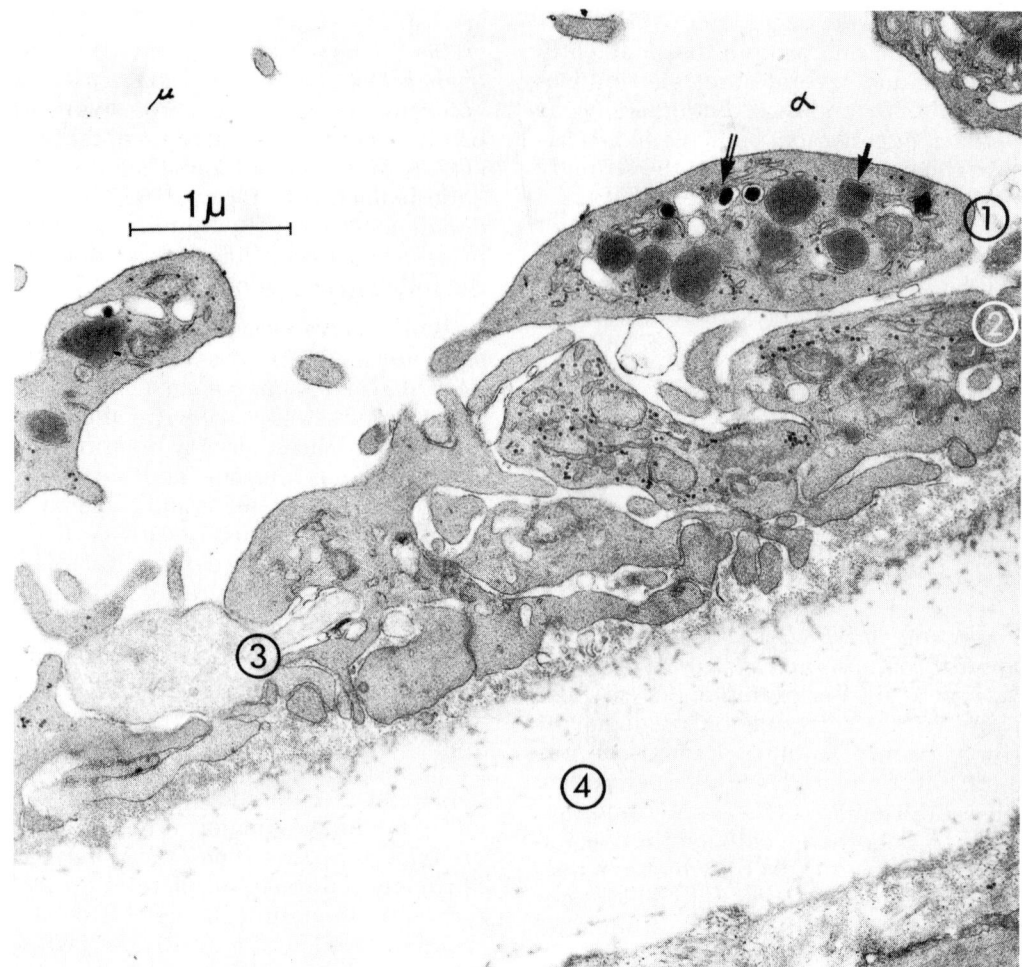

Figure 3–7. Platelet adherence to subendothelial connective tissue at focus of endothelial loss. 1, Intact platelet with pseudopod (thin arrow is alpha granule, thick arrow is dense body); 2, partially degranulated platelet; 3, degranulated platelet "ghost"; 4, internal elastic lamina. (From Haudenschild, C., and Studer, A.: Early interactions between blood cells and severely damaged rabbit aorta. Eur. J. Clin. Invest. 2:1, 1971.)

through the mediation of platelet factor 3, thrombin is generated. *Thrombin is a powerful platelet agonist.* The combination of thrombin, ADP released from platelets, and TxA₂ synthesized by the platelets induces platelet contraction (mediated by the intraplatelet actomyosin) to create a fused mass of platelets—*"viscous metamorphosis"*—constituting a definitive or "secondary hemostatic plug." Most significantly, thrombin causes the conversion of fibrinogen within and about the platelet aggregate to fibrin, producing in essence a mortar for the "platelet bricks," further stabilizing the plug and anchoring it via fibronectin to its site of origin.

In vitro, a variety of agents—ADP, thrombin, collagen, serotonin, catecholamines, and TxA₂—are platelet activators. Among these, ADP, thrombin, epinephrine, and TxA₂ are probably most important in vivo. These platelet agonists bind to membrane receptors and inhibit adenyl cyclase (thus decreasing intraplatelet levels of cAMP. The decreased cAMP induces platelet aggregation, which involves an interaction between platelet membrane glycoprotein re-

ceptors (GPIIb, IIIa) and plasma- or platelet-derived fibrinogen (Fig. 3–8).[10] Conversely, increased cAMP levels inhibit aggregation. Prostacyclin, the potent antiaggregating agent, acts by binding to specific platelet receptors and activating adenyl cyclase to raise the levels of intraplatelet cAMP, thereby inhibiting the function of fibrinogen-binding receptors.

The complex sequence of platelet events can be summarized as follows (Fig. 3–9): (1) Platelets recognize sites of endothelial injury and adhere to exposed subendothelial collagen, thus becoming activated. (2) With activation they secrete a variety of products stored in granules (among them ADP and fibrinogen) and synthesize thromboxane A₂. (3) Platelet factor 3 is unmasked and helps activate several coagulation factors in the intrinsic coagulation sequence. (4) Concomitantly, the release of tissue factor from injured cells and endothelial cells participates in activation of the extrinsic coagulation sequence. (5) The ADP released from platelets initiates the formation of a temporary hemostatic plug of aggregated platelets, soon converted into a larger "secondary plug" under the influ-

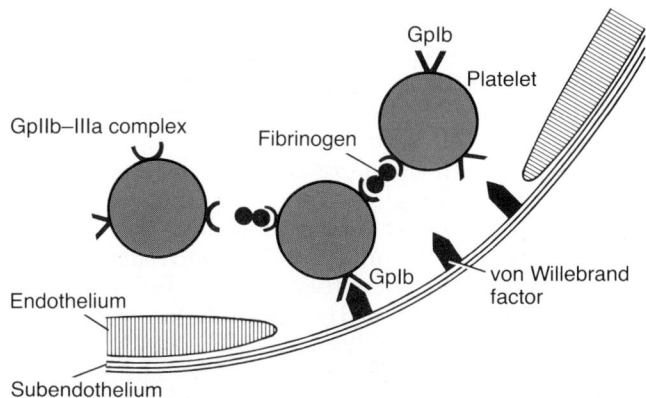

Figure 3-8. Platelet adhesion and aggregation. Von Willebrand factor serves as a bridge between subendothelial collagen and platelet receptors (GpIb). Aggregation involves fibrinogen, which serves as a link between receptors (GpIIb-IIIa) on adjacent platelets.

ence of ADP, thrombin and thromboxane (platelet agonists). (6) The deposition of fibrin (derived from platelets and plasma fibrinogen) into and about the platelet aggregate stabilizes and anchors it.

Thus, a platelet deficiency, in either number or function, will lead to potentially serious bleeding disorders, as discussed on page 692.

Coagulation System

The *coagulation system* is the third component of the hemostatic process and a major contributor to thrombosis. It is not necessary to describe the details of the coagulation system because it is well presented in Figure 3-10.[11] Only general principles and newer concepts will be highlighted.

• The coagulation sequence comprises, in essence, a series of transformations of proenzymes to activated enzymes culminating in the formation of thrombin, which converts soluble fibrinogen into the insoluble fibrous protein fibrin.

• Each reaction in the coagulation pathway results from the assembly of a reaction complex composed of an *enzyme* (activated coagulation factor), a *substrate* (proenzyme form of coagulation factor), and a *cofactor* (reaction accelerator). These components are assembled on a *phospholipid surface* and held together by *calcium ions.* Thus clotting tends to remain localized to sites where such an assembly can occur, e.g., on the surface of activated platelets. One of the key reactions in blood clotting, conversion of factor X to Xa, is illustrated in Figure 3-11.

It has been customary to divide the blood coagulation scheme into an *extrinsic* and an *intrinsic* pathway, both of which converge at the point where factor X is activated (see Fig. 3-10). However, it is now clear that such a division is probably an artifact of in vitro testing methods and that there are several interconnections between the so-called intrinsic and extrinsic pathways. An important example of such

"crosstalk" between pathways is that the conversion of factor IX to IXa occurs not only by the "contact-activated" factors of the intrinsic pathway but also by factor VII of the extrinsic pathway (Fig. 3-10).[11a] The fact that patients with congenital deficiencies of the contact-activated factors (such as factor XII, prekallikrein, and high molecular weight kininogen) do not have any bleeding disorders has cast serious doubts on the in vivo significance of these factors in hemostasis.

ANTICOAGULANT MECHANISMS. An intricate system of checks and balances maintains the fluidity of the blood and localizes a clot to the site of injury, thus preventing a chain reaction leading to the coagulation of the entire cardiovascular system. It is noteworthy

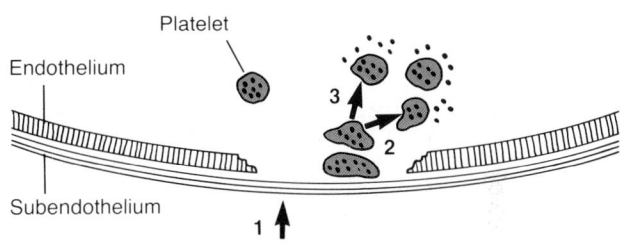

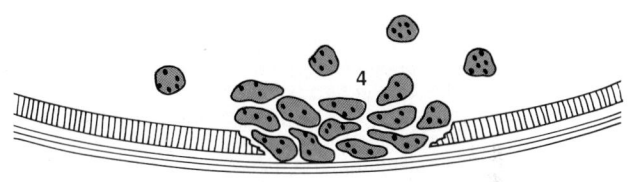

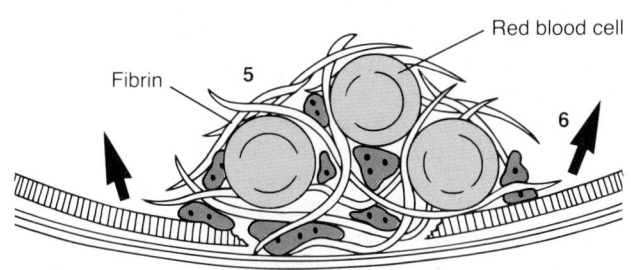

Figure 3-9. Summary of thrombogenesis. 1, Endothelial injury releases tissue factor and exposes subendothelial connective tissues. 2, Platelet adherence and plasma clotting system are triggered. 3, Granule release and prostaglandin generation begin. 4, Platelet aggregation induced by released ADP and vasoconstriction (5HT, thromboxanes) result in primary (temporary) hemostatic plug. 5, Thrombin, thromboxanes, and endoperoxides promote release reaction and irreversible aggregation; amorphous platelet mass and trapped red cells are enmeshed in fibrin to form definitive (permanent) hemostatic plug. 6, Endothelial plasminogen activator and plasma antithrombin check rapid clotting. (Time scale: steps 1-4, seconds to minutes; steps 5-6, several minutes.) (Courtesy of Dr. Michael Gimbrone, Department of Pathology, Brigham and Women's Hospital.)

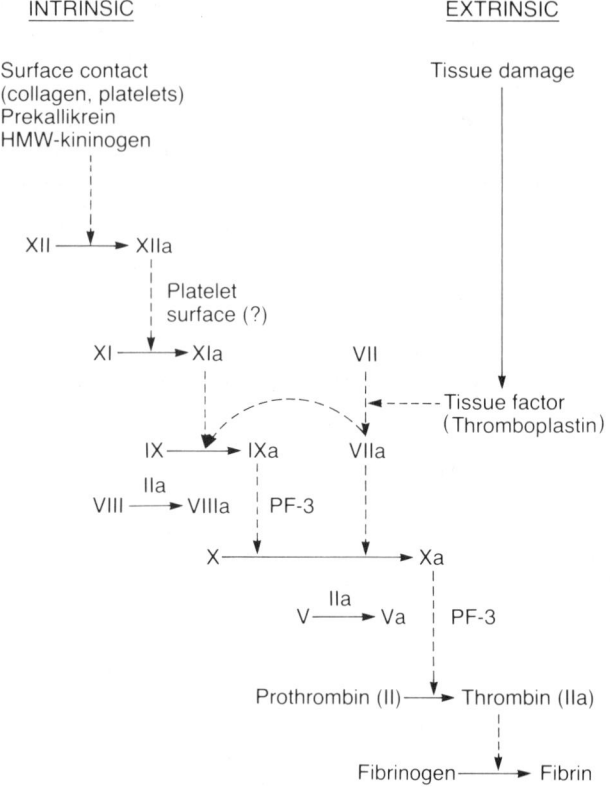

INTRINSIC

EXTRINSIC

Surface contact
(collagen, platelets)
Prekallikrein
HMW-kininogen

Tissue damage

XII ——→ XIIa

Platelet
surface (?)

XI ——→ XIa   VII

IX ——→ IXa   VIIa

Tissue factor
(Thromboplastin)

IIa
VIII ——→ VIIIa   PF-3

X ——————→ Xa

IIa
V ——→ Va   PF-3

Prothrombin (II) ——→ Thrombin (IIa)

Fibrinogen ——→ Fibrin

Figure 3–10. The intrinsic pathway is initiated when blood comes in contact with the negatively charged de-endothelialized vascular surface. Factor XII is activated, and, in a sequential reaction, factors XI and IX are activated. On the platelet surface, factors IXa and VIII interact with calcium and activate factor Xa. In the extrinsic pathway, tissue thromboplastin is released after vessel wall injury activates factor VII, which in turn activates factor X. Then, on the platelet surface, factors Xa and Va interact with calcium and catalyze the conversion of prothrombin to thrombin. Thrombin converts fibrinogen to fibrin monomers and activates factor XIII, which in turn is converted to fibrin polymers in the developing clot. Note that factor VII from the extrinsic pathway may activate factor IX in the intrinsic pathway. (See text.) (Illustration by Ilil Arbel.)

that sufficient thrombin is generated by the clotting of only 1 ml of blood to coagulate all the fibrinogen in 3 liters of blood. These control mechanisms can be characterized as (a) depletion of clotting factors, (b) clearance of activated factors, (c) inhibition by activated proteases, and (d) fibrinolysis.

Depletion of clotting factors by dilution when there is active blood flow past the local site or by utilization-exhaustion when flow is blocked serves to slow or check the clotting process.

Clearance of activated clotting factors is accomplished by the liver and mononuclear phagocyte system. This mechanism is effective only when there is flow of blood from the site of injury. With sufficient stasis the activated factors cannot be cleared.

Normal human blood contains a variety of *protease inhibitors*, which may act on one or more coagulation factors. *Antithrombin III* in the presence of hep-

arin is the principal inhibitor of thrombin, but it also inactivates clotting factors XIIa, XIa, Xa, and IXa. *Protein C* is a vitamin K–dependent plasma protein. In the presence of thrombomodulin on the endothelial cell surface it is activated by thrombin to a protease capable of inactivation of factors Va and VIIIa. It might be noted here that an acquired or hereditary deficiency of or defect in antithrombin III or protein C predisposes to thrombosis. *C′1 inactivator* blocks the classic pathway of activation of complement but also neutralizes XIa, XIIa, and plasma kallikrein. Other protease inhibitors active on coagulation factors include alpha-2-macroglobulin, alpha-1-antitrypsin, alpha-2-plasmin inhibitor, and heparin cofactor II.

The *fibrinolytic system* (Fig. 3–12) provides a critically important mechanism for the dissolution of fibrin clots.[6] The major enzymes capable of digesting fibrin are leukocyte-derived proteases and *plasmin*. The proteolytic conversion of plasminogen, a normal plasma protein, to plasmin is accomplished either by a factor XII–dependent pathway (involving HMWK and prekallikrein) or by well-characterized *plasminogen activators (PA)*. There are two distinct groups of PAs: (1) *Urokinase-like PA (uPA)* is present in plasma and various tissues and activates plasminogen *in the fluid phase*; (2) *tissue-type PA (tPA)*, whose principal site of synthesis is the endothelial cell, is active *when attached to fibrin*. This last property makes tPA a potentially much more useful therapeutic agent. The fibrin split products, once released, serve as potent

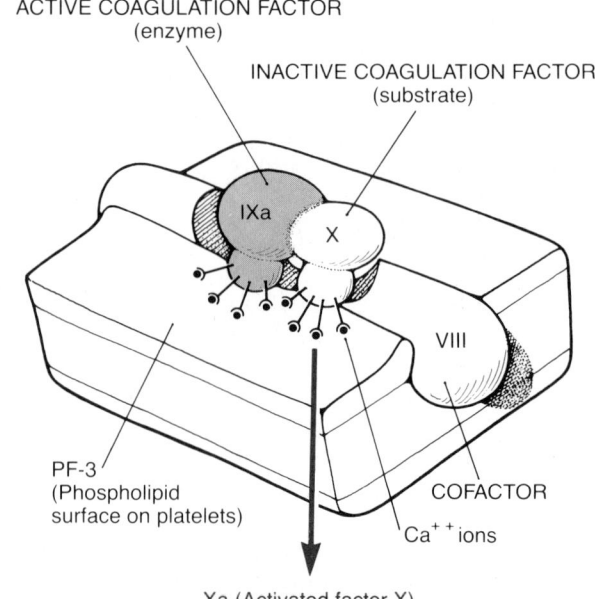

ACTIVE COAGULATION FACTOR
(enzyme)

INACTIVE COAGULATION FACTOR
(substrate)

IXa   X

VIII

PF-3
(Phospholipid
surface on platelets)

COFACTOR

Ca⁺⁺ ions

Xa (Activated factor X)

Figure 3–11. A schematic illustration of the conversion of factor X to factor Xa. The reaction complex, consisting of an enzyme (factor IXa), a substrate (factor X), and a reaction accelerator (factor VIII), is assembled on the surface of platelets. Ca⁺⁺ ions hold the assembled components together and are essential for the reaction. (Modified from Mann, K.G.: Clin. Lab. Med. 4:217, 1984.)

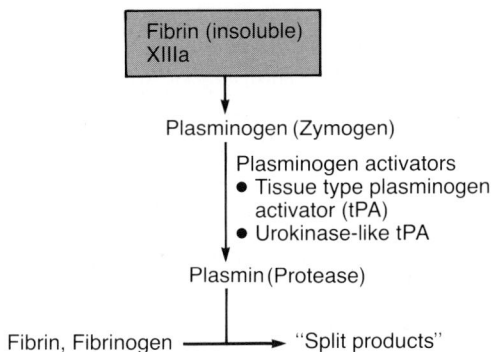

Figure 3–12. The fibrinolytic system illustrating the activation of plasminogen by either a factor XII–dependent pathway or administered plasminogen activators.

anticoagulants. Endothelial cells also elaborate an inhibitor of tPA (tPA-1). Thus the fibrinolytic activity on the surface of endothelium presents a balance between activator and inhibitor properties, which can be perturbed by certain stimuli. For example, the cytokines IL-1 and TNF (which, as you recall, augment tissue factor activity) stimulate tPA inhibitor synthesis. Both these activities of the cytokines favor thrombus formation, and indeed these mediators have been implicated in the intravascular thrombosis that sometimes accompanies severe infections.[2,7] Conversely, certain tumor-promoting agents and tumor extracts increase tPA synthesis by endothelium, thus potentiating fibrinolysis.

Against this background of normal hemostasis we can now consider thrombogenesis.

THROMBOGENESIS

Three major influences predispose to thrombosis: (1) injury to endothelium, (2) alterations in normal blood flow, and (3) alterations in the blood (hypercoagulability). Endothelial injury is the major and most frequent influence and the only one that, by and of itself, may lead to thrombosis. However, it is probably not requisite when the other two influences are operative.

Endothelial injury is particularly important in the formation of thrombi in the heart and arteries. This is amply documented in man by the frequency with which thrombi develop in the left ventricle at sites of myocardial infarction and on ulcerated plaques in advanced atherosclerosis of the aorta and arteries and particularly the coronary arteries (p. 557). Diabetics with their predisposition to severe atherosclerosis are extremely vulnerable to arterial thrombi. Thrombi also develop within the cardiac chambers when there has been injury to the endocardium, as may occur with cardiac surgery, infections of the myocardium, or immunologic myocardial reactions. Inflammatory valve disease (and prosthetic valves) are favored sites for thrombus formation. In addition to such overt causes, covert damage (not visible even by electron microscopy) may be produced by a variety of influ-

ences. The hemodynamic stress in hypertension or the turbulent flow in arterial disorders is thought to be injurious to endothelial cells. Other potential bases for damage to endothelial cells are: radiation injury; chemical agents of exogenous origin (derivatives of cigarette smoke, for example) or of endogenous origin (hypercholesterolemia, homocystine); bacterial toxins or endotoxins; and immunologic injuries (in transplant rejection, immune complex deposition). Whatever the cause of injury to endothelium, it is a potent thrombogenic influence, as has already been made clear.[12,13]

Alterations in normal blood flow, as encountered with turbulence, contribute to the development of arterial and cardiac thrombi, while stasis (sluggish blood flow) contributes to venous thrombosis.[14] In normal flow the larger particles, such as white cells and red cells, occupy the central, most rapidly moving axial stream. The smaller platelets are carried in the more slowly moving laminar stream outside the central column. The periphery of the bloodstream adjacent to the endothelial layer moves most slowly and is free of all formed blood elements. Stasis and turbulence (causing countercurrents and local pockets of stasis) provide four important dimensions: (1) They disrupt laminar flow and bring platelets into contact with the endothelium; (2) they prevent the dilution by the fresh flow of blood and hepatic clearance of the activated coagulation factors; (3) they retard the inflow of inhibitors of clotting factors and permit the build-up of thrombi; and (4) turbulence may damage the endothelium, favoring platelet and fibrin deposition while at the same time reducing the local release of prostacyclin and tissue plasminogen activator.

The roles of turbulence or stasis are clearly documented in many clinical situations involving both the arterial and the venous sides of the circulation. Thrombi often form, as mentioned earlier, overlying ulcerated atherosclerotic plaques. Here the ulceration not only exposes subendothelial elements but also causes local turbulence. Thrombi are also prone to occur in the aorta and arteries within abnormal dilatations referred to as aneurysms. Frequently the thrombus completely fills the abnormal dilatation up to the pre-existent normal level of the vessel wall, when laminar flow is presumably re-established. In the heart, not only do myocardial infarctions provide sites of endothelial injury, but the necrotic muscle does not contract, and so some element of stasis is added. In healed rheumatic heart disease, for example, mitral stenosis causes the left atrium to expand and fail to empty. When arrhythmias such as atrial fibrillation (common in rheumatic heart disease) supervene, the stage is set for atrial and auricular thrombosis.

Stasis is undoubtedly the prime factor in the more slowly moving venous circulation. Most thrombi that develop in abnormally dilated varicose veins arise within the pockets created by venous valves, where presumably there is increased stasis or turbulence.[15] Certainly there is no discernible evidence of endothelial injury, and the basis for thrombogenesis within veins lacking obvious endothelial damage is unclear.

Stasis may have more subtle origins. Hyperviscosity syndromes such as polycythemia, cryoglobulinemia, and macroglobulinemia increase resistance to flow and induce stasis in small vessels. In sickle cell anemia the deformed red cells tend to log-jam, and the stasis predisposes to thrombosis. Similarly there is a thrombotic diathesis in the rare condition known as giant cavernous hemangioma (Kasabach-Merritt syndrome). Here the neoplastic large vascular spaces result in stasis and turbulence, and also provide poorly endothelialized surfaces that may lead to thromboses both within the tumor and elsewhere. Stasis and turbulence, then, are potent thrombogenic influences, particularly when combined with endothelial injury.

Hypercoagulability of the blood has been invoked to explain an increased incidence of thrombosis in individuals lacking other known or potential mechanisms to explain reasonably their thrombotic diathesis. Although hypercoagulability undoubtedly exists as a clinical phenomenon, it has not yet been possible to establish a battery of laboratory tests to reliably identify it.[16] *Nonetheless, an increased tendency to thrombosis is indisputably associated with a variety of conditions, to name only a few now: deficiency of antithrombin III or protein C; the nephrotic syndrome; following severe trauma (including fractures) or burns; disseminated cancer; and during late pregnancy and following delivery.* The basis for the hypercoagulability is certainly not the same in all these settings and indeed is not always understood.[17] *Ultimately it must involve increased levels of activated procoagulants such as fibrinogen, prothrombin, and factors VIIa, VIIIa, and Xa; or increased numbers (or stickiness) of platelets and/or decreased levels of inhibitors such as antithrombin III, protein C, and fibrinolysins.* But, it should be cautioned, often other factors such as immobilization with vascular stasis and injury to vessels provide plausible mechanisms for the thrombotic diathesis without invoking hypercoagulability. The best understood and prototypic hypercoagulable condition is a hereditary deficiency of antithrombin III; here there can be no dispute about cause and effect. The thrombotic diathesis in these individuals is manifested in adolescence or early adult life and frequently leads to premature death.[18] When we turn to the other hypercoagulable states mentioned, the pathogenesis is less certain. With the nephrotic syndrome, urinary excretion of antithrombin III and increased plasma levels of procoagulants have been observed, but most weight is accorded the depressed plasma levels of antithrombin III. With extensive injuries, as for example fractures or burns, release of tissue factor has been incriminated, and with disseminated cancer, secretion by tumor cells of thrombogenic factors or absorption of procoagulant products from necrotic tumor cells has been proposed. Further comments will be made later about some of the other hypercoagulable conditions.

The hazard of thrombosis attributable to hypercoagulability is influenced by race, age, smoking, obesity, and synergism (concurrent thrombogenic influences). The contribution of *race* is a complete mystery, but nonetheless, the death rate from pulmonary embolism secondary to venous thrombosis is about 100 times higher in Israel than in Japan, and analogously, postoperative thrombosis was found to be significantly higher in English women than in Thai women undergoing the same operations by the very same surgeons.[19] With *advancing age*, a number of influences, as will be pointed out later, predispose to thrombus formation, but of particular relevance with respect to hypercoagulability is an increased aggregability of platelets, reduced release of PGI_2, and reduced fibrinolytic response. *Smoking*, possibly because of absorption of some endotheliotoxin from smoke, increases the hazard of thrombosis. This is best borne out by the data to be presented later documenting that users of oral contraceptives who are smokers have a substantially greater risk of developing thrombi than those who do not smoke. *Obesity*, in some ill-defined manner, increases the predisposition. Impaired fibrinolysis and reduced physical activity are suspected but not proved. Relative to *synergism*, the risk of concurrent smoking and oral contraceptives is many-fold greater than the combined risks. Many factors must be considered then in the predisposition to thrombosis.

MORPHOLOGY. Thrombi may occur anywhere in the cardiovascular system: within the cardiac chambers, arteries, veins, or capillaries. They are of variable size and shape, dictated by their site of origin and the circumstances leading to their development. When formed within a cardiac chamber or the aorta they may have apparent laminations called the lines of Zahn. These are produced by alternating layers of paler platelets admixed with some fibrin, separated by darker layers containing more red cells. However, the laminations may not be evident in thrombi formed within smaller arteries or veins. Moreover, thrombi formed in the slower-moving flow in veins sometimes closely resemble coagulated blood, but close inspection will reveal traversing or tangled pale strands of aggregated platelets and fibrin, but well-defined lines of Zahn are rarely evident.

Mural thrombi generally occur in the more capacious lumina of the heart chambers and aorta. Myocardial infarcts or cardiac arrhythmias are common antecedents to the thrombi that form in the heart, while atherosclerosis or aneurysmal dilatations are almost invariable precursors of aortic thrombus formation. The mural thrombi, which are generally formed in these sites, do not fill the entire lumen, in part because of the rapid flow of blood past them, and in part because occlusion would be incompatible with survival except in extraordinarily rare instances (Fig. 3–13).

In addition to arising within the cardiac chambers, thrombotic masses under special circumstances may build up on the heart valves, particularly the mitral and aortic

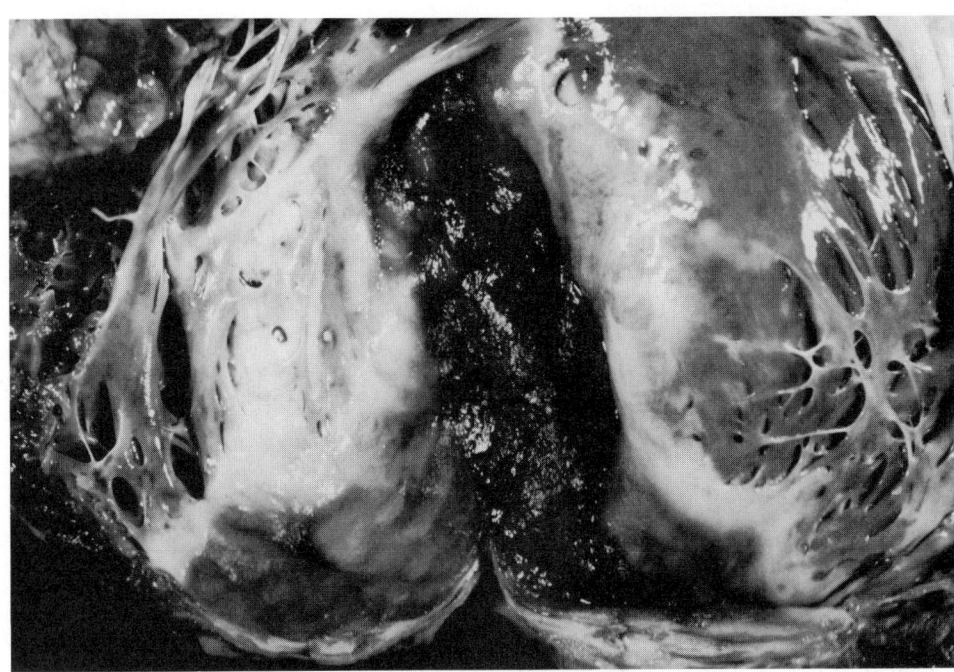

Figure 3–13. A mural thrombus in the left ventricle overlying a large area of pale white fibrosis representing a healed myocardial infarct.

valves. In this setting, the thrombi are referred to as **vegetations.** The most common antecedent is a blood-borne bacterial infection that seeds the heart valves, and thus provides a site of injury on which a thrombotic mass of fibrin and platelets builds up to produce so-called **infective vegetative endocarditis** (p. 633). Less commonly, **nonbacterial bland thrombotic vegetations** (verrucous endocarditis) appear, particularly in patients having systemic lupus erythematosus (p. 201) and in those already debilitated by some fatal illness such as disseminated cancer, or some lymphomatous-leukemic disorder (although they sometimes appear in young individuals not having a fatal illness). In these settings, hypercoagulability of the blood is predicated but without substantial proof.

Arterial thrombi are usually **occlusive,** although they may be mural in such large vessels as the iliacs and common carotids. Occlusive thrombi are most frequently encountered in descending order in the coronary, cerebral, and femoral arteries. Almost always the thrombus is superimposed on an atherosclerotic lesion, but uncommonly, other forms of vascular disease such as acute vasculitis and traumatic injury are involved. They are usually gray-white and friable, made up of tangled strands and layers of fibrin and platelets creating lines of Zahn. Moreover, they are usually firmly attached to the damaged arterial wall. Contraction of the freshly formed thrombus may provide a slitlike lumen, restoring some flow; under this circumstance, the original thrombotic mass may enlarge (propagate) at both the upstream and the downstream ends.

Venous thrombi are also known as phlebothromboses and sometimes inappropriately as **thrombophlebitis** in the mistaken impression that inflammation of the veins induced the thrombi. Venous thrombi are almost invariably occlusive and, in fact, often form quite accurate casts of the vessel in which they arise, even revealing the markings of the venous valves. Thrombi are frequently found in superficial varicose veins, but these rarely embolize and so are more bothersome locally than serious. More significant, phlebothrombosis is encountered preponderantly in the veins of the lower extremity (90% occur in deep leg veins) in approximately the following descending order of frequency: calf, femoral, popliteal, and iliac veins (Fig. 3–14). Less commonly, venous thrombi may develop in the periprostatic plexus and the ovarian and periuterine veins. **Those in the larger outflow veins of the legs, e.g., the popliteal, femoral, and iliac veins, are the most serious because they may embolize.** Thrombi in smaller veins, such as those in the calf muscles, less frequently embolize. All venous emboli are red-blue, perfect casts of the vessels in which they are located, and only ill-defined, pale gray, tangled strands of fibrin permit differentiation from post-mortem clots. They are often attached to the underlying vessel wall, further evidence favoring thrombosis over post-mortem clotting. In the sluggish venous circulation, worsened by the thrombotic occlusion, propagation may occur both in the direction of the venous flow and distally. Presumably stasis is the major causal influence.

The *differentiation of post-mortem clots from venous thrombi* may be important, as for example when searching for the origin of pulmonary emboli, and may be difficult, as noted before. The post-mortem clot is usually a rubbery, gelatinous coagulum and lacks the fibrin strands and attachment to the underlying wall. Large post-mortem clots may show sedimenting of red cells, creating a "chicken fat" clear yellow coagulated plasma overlying a "currant jelly" cyanotic dark red base, with pardon for the penchant

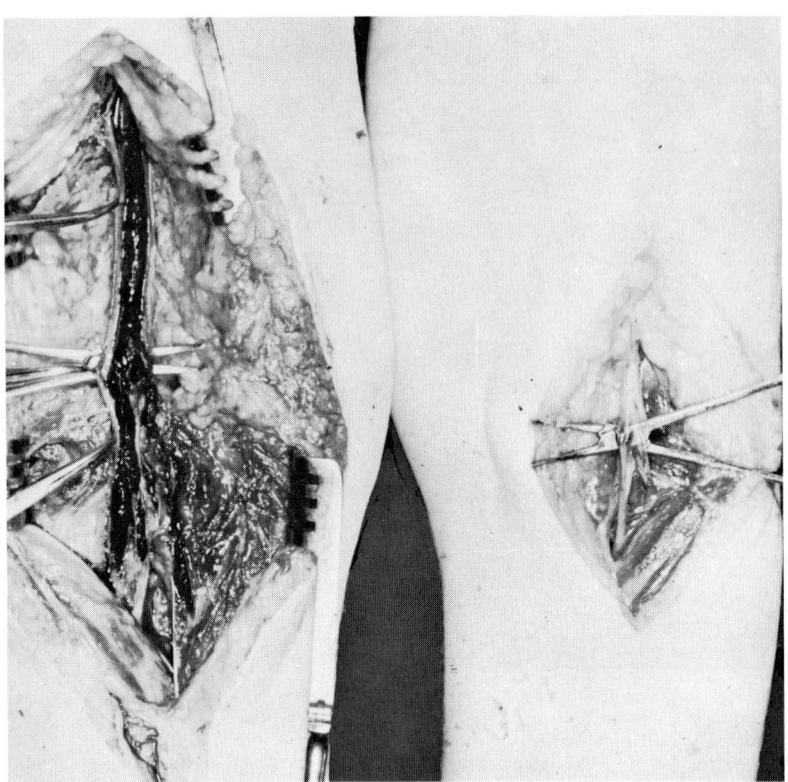

Figure 3-14. The popliteal veins exposed to demonstrate a large thrombus on the left and the normal vein for comparison on the right.

pathologists have for likening distasteful lesions to sometimes tasty foods.

FATE OF THE THROMBUS. If a patient survives the immediate ischemic effects of a newly developed thrombus, what happens thereafter? One of a number of pathways may be followed. *The thrombus may (1) propagate and, by its enlargement, eventually cause obstruction of some critical vessel; (2) give rise to an embolus (discussed in the next section) and thus be carried away in part or in whole from its site of origin; (3) be removed by fibrinolytic action; or (4) become organized and possibly recanalized* (Fig. 3-15). The last two potentials require further consideration here. A thrombus provokes prompt activation of the plasminogen-plasmin system. The efficacy of such fibrinolysis depends mainly on the size of the thrombus and its age. Many (perhaps most) small calf vein thrombi undergo complete dissolution *(resolution)*; in contrast, complete lysis of large venous thrombi in the major outflow veins of the legs is uncommon.[20] The endogenous fibrinolytic response can be augmented by the administration of thrombolytics. Such therapy is most effective within the first few hours of development of the thrombus, probably because freshly formed fibrin is more susceptible to lysis than is older fibrin, after undergoing polymerization.

Almost from the beginning of its formation, the trapped white cells and platelets begin to modify the thrombus to initiate the process of *organization*. The neutrophils, and especially the macrophages, phagocytize fragments of fibrin and cell debris; in addition, proteolytic enzymes, derived both from the white cells and from endothelial cells, begin to digest the coagulum. When a thrombus is quite large, the central region is protected from the diluting effect of the blood flow about the margins, and here the build-up of lytic enzymes may be sufficient to produce *central softening*. Such a sequence is particularly likely to occur in large thrombi within the cardiac chambers or aneurysmal sacs. In passing, bacteremic seeding of such a digestate may convert the softened thrombus to a mass of pus. Concurrently fibroblasts and capillaries proliferate and invade the base of the thrombus where it is attached to the underlying vessel wall. In time, the entire intravascular mass is organized and converted essentially into a vascularized connective tissue. The capillary channels may anastomose to produce thoroughfares that traverse the thrombus and, indeed, provide new channels through which blood flow may at least in part be re-established, a process known as *canalization of the thrombus* (Fig. 3-16). The regrowth of the endothelial cells over the surface of the thrombus covers it, thereby excluding it from the flow of blood. Since fibrous tissue contracts in the course of weeks to months, the thrombus is virtually incorporated within the vessel wall or cardiac chamber as a fibrous lump or thickening.

CLINICAL CORRELATION. Some of the disorders and clinical settings frequently associated with thromboses have already been mentioned in the discussion of thrombogenesis. Many more are cited in Table 3-2. As noted there, the risk of thrombus is significantly higher in some conditions than in others, and whether "high risk" or "lower risk," the underly-

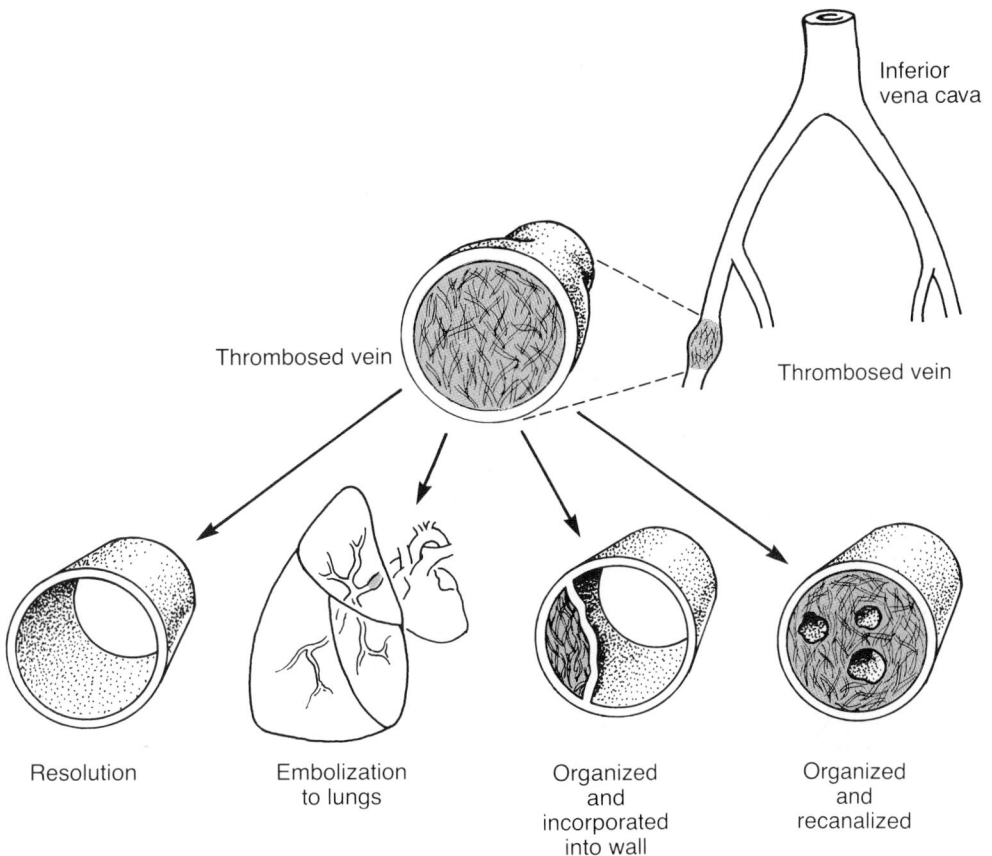

Figure 3-15. The potential outcomes following venous thrombosis.

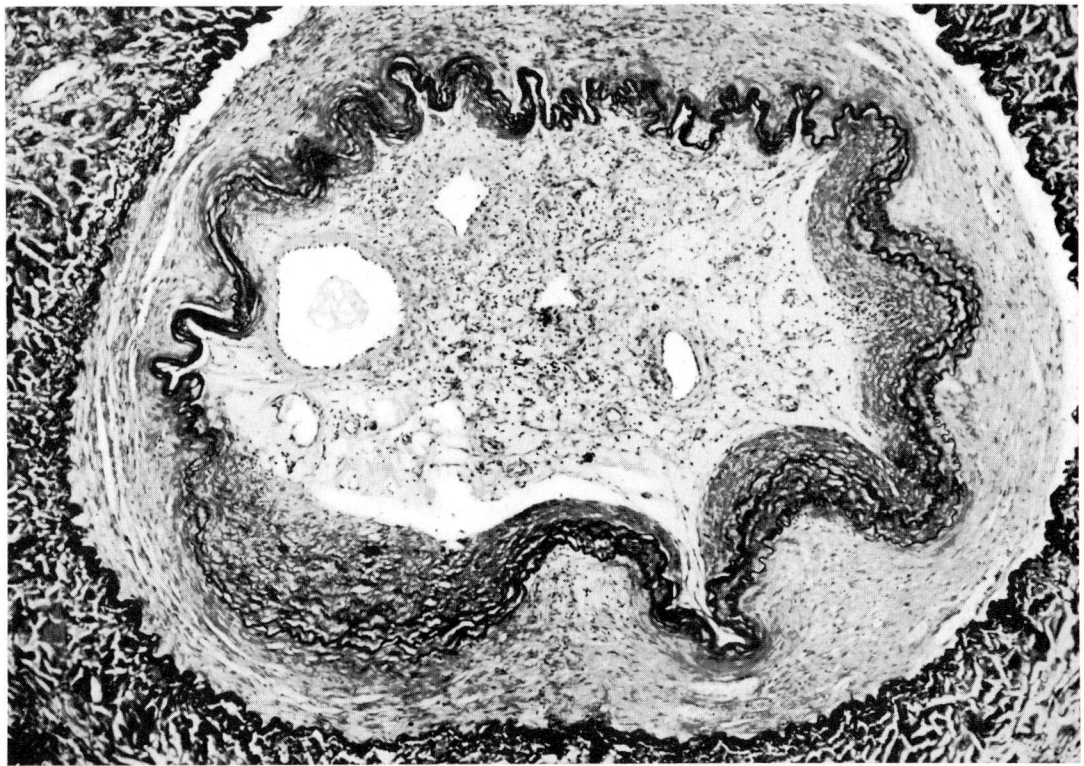

Figure 3-16. A low-power view of a thrombosed artery stained for elastic tissue. The lumen is delineated by the partially degenerated internal elastic membrane and is totally filled with organized clot, now traversed by many newly formed recanalized channels.

Table 3-2. Major Clinical Disorders or Situations Associated With an Increased Risk of Thrombosis

DEFINED MECHANISMS	THEORETICAL MECHANISMS
High Risk	
Antithrombin III deficiency	Cardiac failure
Protein C deficiency	Cancer
Prolonged bed rest or immobilization	Acute leukemia
	Myeloproliferative disorders
Myocardial infarction	Prosthetic cardiac valves
Tissue damage (including surgery, fractures, burns)	Disseminated intravenous coagulation
	Thrombotic thrombocytopenia
	Homocystinuria
Lower Risk	
Atrial fibrillation	Late pregnancy/post delivery
Cardiomyopathy	Oral contraceptives
Nephrotic syndrome	Hyperlipidemia
	Lupus anticoagulant
	Sickle cell anemia
	Prostacyclin deficiency
	Smoking
	Thrombocytosis

ing mechanism may be reasonably well defined or only theoretical. In clinical practice, the most frequently encountered settings with thrombosis are as follows.

Advanced age, bed rest, and immobilization, when they occur together, create a high risk for thrombosis. As pointed out, with advancing years there may well be hypercoagulability; reduced physical activity with poor venous drainage from the legs; underlying atherosclerosis with endothelial injury; and possibly some element of cardiac failure with sluggish circulation. Bed rest further reduces the milking action of the muscles in the lower legs. Thus the elderly are particularly vulnerable when some additional event such as a fracture or cancer (discussed later) adds yet another thrombogenic influence.

Decompensated cardiac disease in general imposes an increased risk of thrombosis. Among the cardiac diseases, myocardial infarction invokes the greatest risk; approximately 20 to 25% of individuals sustaining a myocardial infarct develop a mural thrombus in the left ventricle. Involved are endothelial injury, poor ventricular contraction with turbulence and stasis, and possibly hypercoagulability. Atrial fibrillation, particularly when associated with rheumatic mitral stenosis, predisposes to mural thrombosis within the left auricle (sometimes both auricles) presumably as a result of marked stasis. Cardiomyopathy carries the implications of endothelial injury, cardiac dilatation with poor contractility, and possibly hypercoagulability.

Tissue damage, whether related to soft tissue trauma, fractures, burns, or the postoperative state, constitutes a "high-risk" predisposition to thrombosis. The incidence of thrombi in the veins of the lower legs in patients sustaining hip fracture is about 50%.[21] Operative in all these settings are release of tissue factor, reduced fibrinolytic activity, vascular injury, physical inactivity, and, in those with hip fractures, immobilization and usually advanced age.

The relationship between *cancer* (usually disseminated) and thrombosis was first noted by Trousseau who, indeed, correctly deduced the existence of his own internal (pancreatic) cancer from the appearance of multiple superficial disparate venous thrombi. This thrombotic diathesis, which appears asynchronously in multiple veins, often termed *migratory thrombophlebitis* or *Trousseau's syndrome,* has now been associated with all forms of visceral cancer. Release of thrombogenic factors or absorption of procoagulant products from necrotic tumor cells and impaired fibrinolysis have been implicated.[22]

Late pregnancy and the postdelivery period are associated with about a sixfold increase in the development of thrombi, usually in the leg veins, giving rise to the older designation "milk leg" or "phlegmasia alba dolens" (painful white leg). In the last trimester of pregnancy, compression of the inferior vena cava by the gravid uterus, increased distensibility of the veins with slowing of the circulation, reduced fibrinolytic activity, and hypercoagulability may be involved. Following delivery, there is trauma to vessels and the potential for the entrance of amniotic fluid bearing platelet-aggregating and procoagulant factors into the pelvic veins. However, all these proposed mechanisms are more theoretical than established.

The use of *oral contraceptives* as formulated in the past has been implicated in a fivefold increased death rate from circulatory diseases owing mainly to (1) myocardial infarction following coronary artery thrombosis, (2) stroke associated with thromboembolism within the cerebral circulation, and (3) pulmonary embolism from thrombi within the veins of the lower legs. The estrogen content of the oral contraceptives used in the past was held to be responsible for an increase in concentrations of plasma fibrinogen, prothrombin, and factors VII, VIII, and X as well as decreased antithrombin III and fibrinolytic activity. However, these changes may be epiphenomena rather than causal. Whatever the basis, concomitant cigarette smoking substantially increases the risk. More details on this important problem are found on page 488.

Whatever the clinical circumstances, the significance of a thrombus depends, as would be expected, on its size and particularly on its site, i.e., arterial or venous.

Arterial thrombi in small vessels are occlusive and usually cause infarction of the dependent tissues (although there are exceptions, as discussed more fully on page 113). Two of the major killers in affluent societies, myocardial infarction and cerebral infarction (encephalomalacia), are related to thrombi in atherosclerotic vessels. In general, arterial thrombi come to attention promptly because of the distal organ injury (infarction) that they induce. Occlusive arterial thrombi rarely embolize, since they are firmly wedged into the vessel at their sites of origin. However, thrombi in the cardiac chambers or aorta are prime origins for emboli because they are almost always mural lesions and are vulnerable to fragmentation by the rapid and turbulent flow of passing blood. The favored sites of lodgment of such emboli are discussed later (p. 108).

Venous thrombosis (phlebothrombosis) rarely causes infarction of the dependent tissues because collateral bypass channels soon enlarge sufficiently to maintain the venous drainage of the affected part. There are, however, exceptions where bypasses do not exist, as in the ovarian blood supply, and venous infarction may result. Venous thrombi nonetheless may cause local problems (to be discussed later). Far more important, *venous thrombi such as those arising in the large veins of the leg are of greatest concern because they are prone to break loose or fragment, and embolize almost always to the lungs as is discussed in the next section. In contrast, those of the calf veins or other sites are rare sources of pulmonary emboli.*[23]

In addition, *occlusive venous thrombi in the major outflow vessels of the leg may cause local signs and symptoms.* Edema of the lower leg is one of the more common manifestations. Analogously, thrombosis of the superficial veins of the leg, when varicosities are present, may cause some localized edema and predispose the skin in the affected area to infections following trivial trauma, with the development of indolent varicose ulcers that are most difficult to control. Thrombosed veins may be painful and tender to palpation. Thus, with thrombi in the veins of the calf muscles, dorsiflexion of the foot may elicit pain known as *Homans' sign.* Similarly, simply squeezing the calf muscles will also elicit pain. The painfulness of some thrombosed veins has led to the mistaken belief that the veins were inflamed—hence the term "thrombophlebitis" mentioned earlier.

Over half of thrombi in the large veins of the legs, i.e., popliteal, femoral, and iliac veins, are asymptomatic and recognized only when they have embolized, sometimes to cause death. Thus the prevention or early detection of venous thrombi, particularly in hospitalized patients, is an issue of grave clinical concern.

In closing this discussion of thrombosis it is important to point out that, although many settings are known to significantly increase the risk, thrombogenesis is ultimately a puzzling and unpredictable phenomenon. It may occur at any time, under any conditions, and indeed appears surprisingly often in healthy ambulant individuals without apparent provocation or known predisposition.[24]

DISSEMINATED INTRAVASCULAR COAGULATION (DIC)

A variety of disorders ranging from obstetric difficulties to advanced cancer may be complicated by the sudden or insidious development of myriad fibrin thrombi in the microcirculation—DIC—followed in some cases by active fibrinolysis and a bleeding diathesis. With the development of the multiple thrombi, there is rapid consumption of platelets, prothrombin, fibrinogen, and factors V, VIII, and X (hence the synonyms *consumption coagulopathy* and *defibrination syndrome*); at the same time, the plasminogen-plasmin system is activated and fibrin(ogen) degradation products are formed, having an anticoagulation effect. In this manner a thrombotic disorder ends up as a bleeding disorder. It should be emphasized that DIC is not a primary disease; rather it complicates the course of any condition associated with activation of thrombin through either the intrinsic or the extrinsic pathway. Because it is closely related to thrombotic thrombocytopenic purpura (and several other conditions), it is discussed later along with the bleeding diatheses (p. 698).

EMBOLISM

An embolus is a detached intravascular solid, liquid, or gaseous mass that is carried by the blood to a site distant from its point of origin. Virtually 99% of all emboli arise in thrombi (thromboembolism). Rare forms of emboli include fragments of bone or bone marrow, atheromatous debris from ruptured atherosclerotic plaques, droplets of fat, bits of tumor, foreign bodies such as bullets, and bubbles of air or nitrogen. *Unless otherwise qualified, the term embolus implies thromboembolism.* Inevitably, emboli lodge in vessels too small to permit their further passage, resulting in partial or complete occlusion of the vessel. Depending on their site of origin, emboli may come to rest anywhere within the cardiovascular system and are best discussed from the standpoint of whether they lodge in the pulmonary or systemic circulations, thus producing differing clinical effects.

PULMONARY EMBOLISM

Pulmonary embolism is the most common preventable cause of death in hospitalized patients. This important complication of thrombosis is discussed more fully on page 762; only an overview is presented here.

Occlusion of a large or medium-sized pulmonary artery is embolic in origin until proved otherwise. Thrombotic occlusion of these vessels is very uncommon, and is encountered virtually only when pulmonary hypertension has led to atherosclerotic or other hypertensive changes in the pulmonary arterial tree or with chest trauma. The true incidence of pulmonary embolism, particularly fatal pulmonary embolism, is not known for many reasons. Some occur in ambulant patients; these are usually small and clinically silent and so pass unrecognized. Even among hospitalized patients, not more than a third are diagnosed ante mortem. Moreover, when the diagnosis of a fatal pulmonary embolism is made clinically, it is proved to be incorrect by post-mortem examination in approximately 50% of cases.[25] Unfortunately, autopsy data vary widely. Some hospital analyses report pulmonary emboli in from less than 1% of a series of unselected cases to the extreme of 64%.[26] If only fatal pulmonary emboli are considered, autopsies reveal an incidence of about 0.3% in hospitalized medical patients, approaching 1% in surgical patients, and rising to about 5 to 8% in patients with a hip fracture.[21] Whatever the precise incidence, pulmonary embolism is a major clinical problem, especially among hospitalized patients; annually it causes about 50,000 deaths in the United States.

Over 95% of all pulmonary emboli arise in thrombi within the large veins of the lower legs — popliteal, femoral, and iliac veins. It is of clinical significance that even when a patient has a well-documented pulmonary embolus, venous thrombosis can be found in only 20 to 70% of instances, depending on the use of such invasive procedures as venography. Thrombi within the superficial veins of the legs (usually associated with varicosities), veins of the calf muscles, or such other sites as the veins in the pelvis — the periprostatic, broad ligament, periovarian, and uterine veins — are uncommon sources of emboli.

Depending on the size and length of the embolic mass it may occlude the main pulmonary artery (usually when coiled upon itself) (Fig. 3–17), impact astride the bifurcation (a *saddle embolus*), or pass out into the progressively smaller branching pulmonary arteries (Fig. 3–18). Often there are multiple emboli, perhaps sequentially, or a large mass fragments to produce a shower of smaller emboli impacting in a number of vessels. Indeed the patient who survives a pulmonary embolism has about a 30% chance of developing a second one, and the probabilities keep rising with each subsequent event. Rarely, an embolus may pass through an interatrial or interventricular

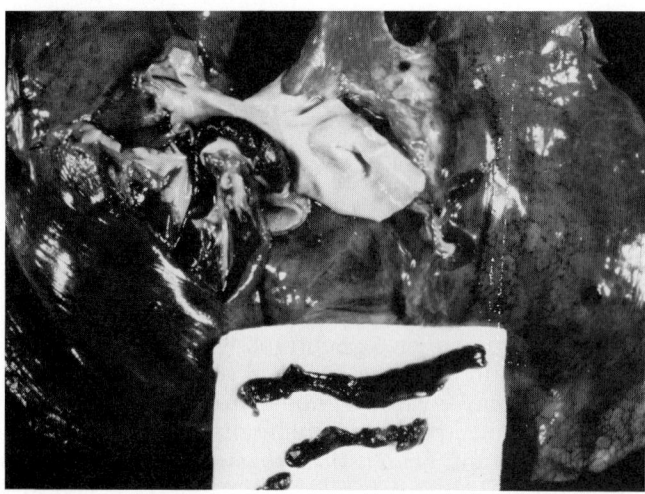

Figure 3–18. Pulmonary embolism. Large emboli fill the main pulmonary arterial vessels on the left. Several extricated fragments are shown below.

defect, when the pressure in the right heart exceeds that in the left heart, to gain access to the systemic circulation (*paradoxical embolism*).

Since the clinical consequences of a pulmonary embolus are discussed more fully on page 762, only summary comments will be offered here.

— The significance of a pulmonary embolus depends on the size and location of the occluded artery, the number of emboli, the proportion of the entire arterial tree obstructed, and the underlying cardiorespiratory status of the patient.

— *Most pulmonary emboli (60 to 80%) are clinically silent* because they are small; the embolic mass is often promptly (within hours) removed by fibrinolytic activity; and the collateral bronchial circulation, in the absence of cardiac failure, is sufficient to sustain the viability of the affected lung parenchyma.

— *Sudden death, acute right heart failure (acute cor pulmonale), or cardiovascular collapse may occur (5% of cases)* when more than 60% of the total pulmonary vasculature is obstructed by a large embolus or multiple, simultaneous, small emboli. Massive pulmonary embolism is one of the few causes of literally instantaneous death, even before the patient has experienced chest pain or dyspnea. As you know, infarction could not occur under such circumstances.

— *Obstruction of relatively small-sized pulmonary branches (10 to 15% of cases) that behave as end-arteries usually causes pulmonary infarction* (described on p. 111). Sometimes a more proximal, larger embolus fragments to obstruct smaller vessels and thus produces infarcts hours or even days after the acute embolic event. Typically, patients sustaining an infarct manifest dyspnea owing in some part to reduction of functioning lung volume, but in greater part related to reflex, humoral, or neural vasoconstriction and bronchoconstriction. Chest pain usually appears due to sterile inflammation of the overlying pleura and sometimes hemoptysis. Syncope may also de-

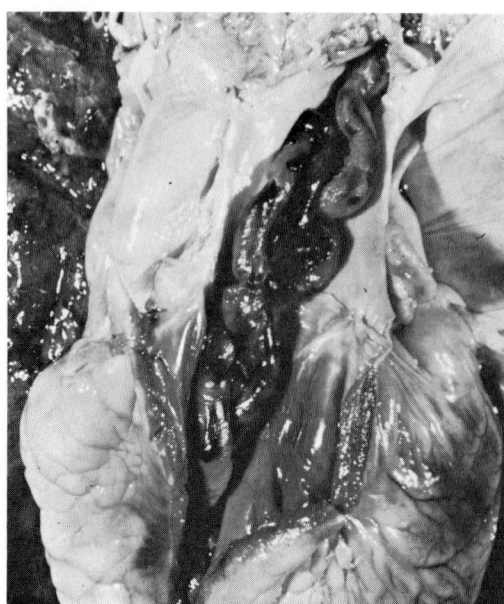

Figure 3–17. A large coiled embolus from the veins of the lower leg lies in the right ventricle and pulmonary artery, almost completely covering the pulmonary valve.

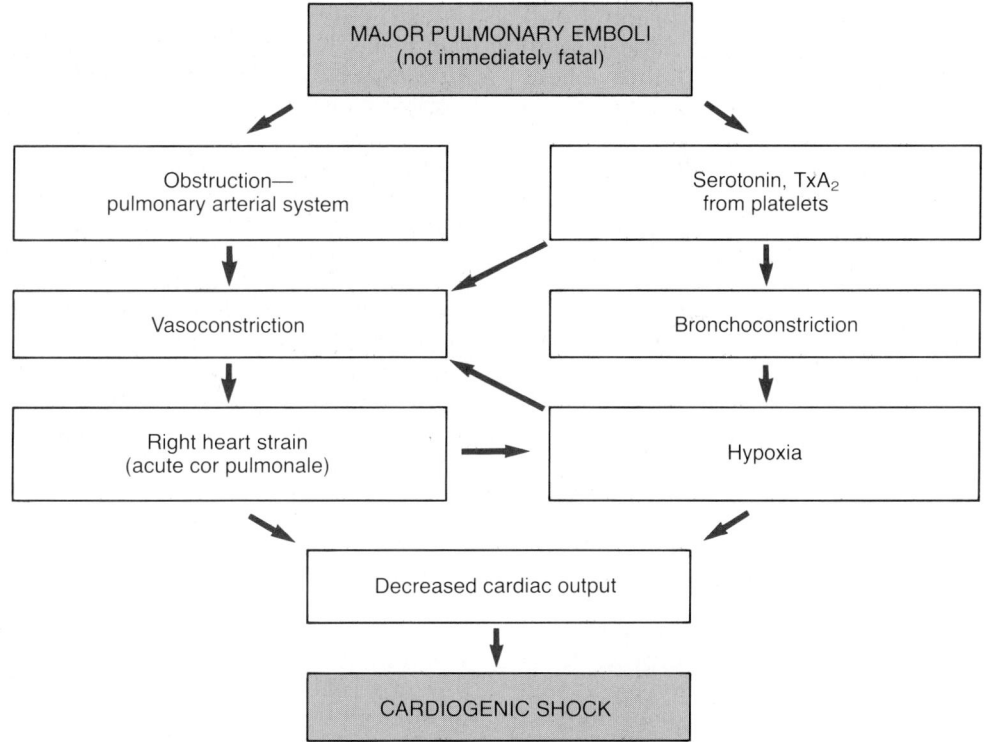

Figure 3–19. Pathophysiology of shock with pulmonary embolism.

velop depending on the size and number of emboli and extent of the pulmonary vascular obstruction.

—*Embolic obstruction of middle-sized arteries (10 to 15% of cases) that are not end-arteries is usually not associated with pulmonary infarction, but instead results in more centrally located pulmonary hemorrhage.* In these more proximal locations, the bronchial circulation and anastomoses within the pulmonary arterial vasculature are sufficient to maintain the viability of the subtended parenchyma if the patient's cardiorespiratory status is normal. However, should there be cardiac failure or underlying pulmonary disease, such proximal emboli may cause large infarcts. Patients with hemorrhage usually manifest dyspnea and/or hemoptysis, but rarely pleuritic chest pain because the central hemorrhage does not involve the pleura. Radiologically an area of hemorrhage clears in a few days because there is no tissue necrosis and subsequent scarring as occurs with an infarct. Depending on the size and number of vessels obstructed, patients with these significant emboli may go into shock (Fig. 3–19).

—Uncommonly, multiple emboli lead to pulmonary hypertension, chronic right heart strain (chronic cor pulmonale), and in time pulmonary vascular sclerosis (p. 764) with progressively worsening dyspnea. An overview of the variable consequences of a pulmonary embolus is offered in Figure 3–20.

Prompt recognition and early effective treatment significantly modify the outcome of a pulmonary embolus in those who survive the initial insult. Even without treatment, angiographic and scan studies reveal about a 10 to 20% improvement in perfusion

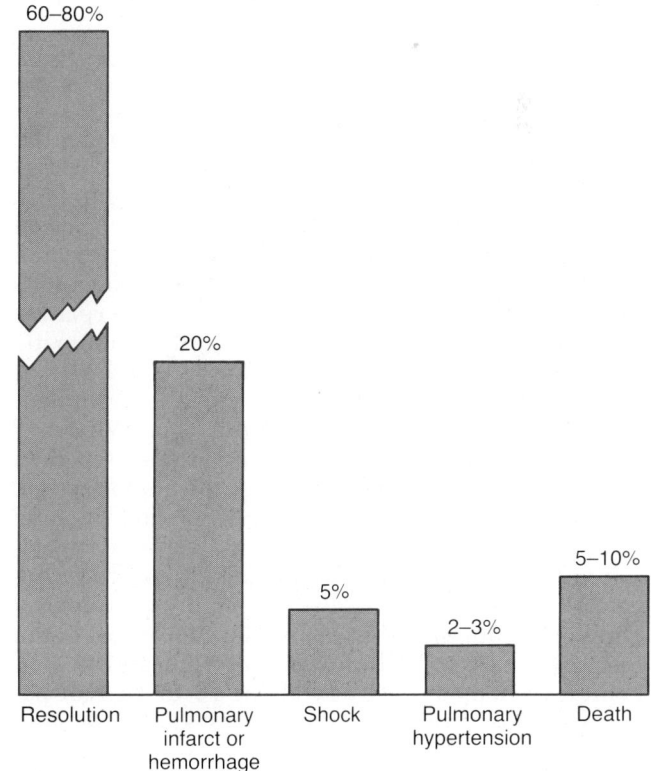

Figure 3–20. Consequences of pulmonary thromboembolism.

within the first 24 hours (following an obstructive pulmonary embolus) and often complete resolution within weeks or months.[27] The rate of improvement and its completeness depend largely on the size and age of the embolus. While some of the restoration of blood flow may result from contraction of the thrombotic mass or fragmentation, spontaneous fibrinolysis plays a major role. If this endogenous response is augmented promptly by fibrinolytic agents such as urokinase or tissue-plasminogen activator, the rate and completeness of the resolution is substantially increased. Thus the mortality rate of diagnosed pulmonary embolism before fibrinolytic agents was 30 to 40%, but with current methods of treatment is now reduced to 5 to 10%.[28] Unfortunately, even with a high index of suspicion and state-of-the-art methods of diagnosis, only one out of three fatal pulmonary emboli is discovered ante mortem.

What is the fate of an embolus if it does not resolve? As with a thrombus, the thromboembolus may undergo organization and essentially be incorporated within the wall of the pulmonary artery as an endothelium-covered fibrous mass. Such mural projections contribute to the development of pulmonary hypertension and subsequent pulmonary vascular sclerosis, including pulmonary atherosclerosis (p. 764). Occasionally and inexplicably, organization of a thromboembolus creates delicate, insignificant, bridging fibrous webs. The clinical consequences then of a pulmonary embolus are indeed diverse; at one end of the spectrum they represent catastrophic "bolts out of the blue," but at the other end they are furtive "nothings," leaving only mere wispy tell-tales of past events.

SYSTEMIC EMBOLISM

This term refers to emboli that travel through the arterial circulation. *Most arterial emboli (80 to 85%) arise from thrombi within the heart.* About 60 to 65% arise within the left ventricle secondary to myocardial infarction and only about 5 to 10% from atrial thrombi in rheumatic heart disease. Cardiomyopathy accounts for an additional 5%.[29] Of interest is that the relative contributions of myocardial infarction and rheumatic heart disease represent a complete reversal of that which obtained about 30 to 40 years ago, a testament to the drop in incidence of rheumatic fever. Whatever the underlying heart disease, arrhythmias such as atrial fibrillation increase the risk of embolization. Less common sources of arterial emboli include thrombi developing in relation to ulcerated atherosclerotic plaques, aortic aneurysms, infective endocarditis, valvular or aortic prostheses, and paradoxical embolism from venous thrombi that gain access to the left side of the circulation through a right-to-left congenital cardiac anomaly. In about 10 to 15% of patients the source of the embolus is unknown. In general there is a 30% recurrence rate of systemic emboli.

In contrast to venous emboli, *arterial emboli follow a much more varied pathway, but they almost always cause infarction.* Emboli from infective endocarditis caused by virulent organisms produce septic infarcts that may be rapidly converted to large abscesses. The major sites of lodgment of all systemic emboli are the lower extremities (70 to 75%), the brain (10%), visceral (10%—includes mesenteric, renal, and splenic), and the upper limbs (7 to 8%).[30] The site of lodgment and the size of the embolus within the systemic vessels are obvious critical determinants of its significance. Embolic occlusion of the femoral artery is disastrous inasmuch as it causes infarction (gangrene) of the lower extremity, but it is not necessarily life-threatening. In contrast, a much smaller embolus that occludes the middle cerebral artery may lead to death in days, or even hours. On the other hand, impaction in the circle of Willis, depending on the state of the cerebral vessels, may be entirely compensated for by collateral flow. As with pulmonary emboli, prompt diagnosis and effective treatment—general supportive measures, anticoagulation, embolectomy—have greatly improved the prognosis of both life and limb. However, a significant mortality rate persists, largely related to the serious cardiovascular diseases that occasioned the thromboembolism.

AMNIOTIC FLUID EMBOLISM (INFUSION)

This extremely grave complication usually of labor and the immediate post-partum period has become a major cause of maternal mortality as the other fatal complications, e.g., hemorrhage, toxemia, pulmonary embolism, have been better controlled. Fortunately, amniotic fluid embolism, or as some would prefer *amniotic fluid infusion*, is uncommon, with an incidence of about 1 per 50,000 deliveries, but it incurs a mortality rate of 86%.[31] The clinical presentation is striking—suddenly and without warning, profound respiratory difficulty with deep cynanosis and cardiovascular shock appear, followed rapidly in some cases by clonic-tonic convulsions and profound coma. If the patient survives the initial crisis, within a few hours marked pulmonary edema usually becomes evident and in about half the cases excessive bleeding from the uterus and any injuries to the birth canal (attributed to the development of DIC). Sometimes nonspecific premonitory manifestations such as chills, nausea and vomiting, apprehension, and agitation usher in the acute crisis. Although an advanced age for pregnancy, multiparity, and tumultuous labor are thought to predispose, amniotic fluid embolism may appear in any obstetric setting including abortion and cesarean delivery.

The underlying cause is the infusion of amniotic fluid with all of its contents into the maternal circulation following a tear in the placental membranes and rupture of uterine and/or cervical veins. As a consequence, *epithelial squames from fetal skin, lanugo hair, fat from vernix caseosa, mucin from the fetal respiratory or gastrointestinal tract, and occasionally bile from meconium contamination of the amniotic fluid can be found in the victim's pulmonary microcirculation at post-mortem examination* (Fig. 3–21).[32] Often there is also marked pulmonary edema and changes typical of ARDS (p. 760), and in occasional cases fibrin thrombi within the pulmonary microcirculation; their relative rarity may merely reflect active fibrinolysis.

Although, clearly, the infusion of amniotic fluid into the maternal circulation triggers the onset of this disorder, the precise basis for the clinical manifestations is still poorly understood. At one time the straightforward understanding was obstruction of the pulmonary circulation by the particulate material within the amniotic fluid, e.g., squames, fat globules, possibly augmented by fibrin thrombi. Although such a mechanism undoubtedly is an important contributor, both clinical and experimental studies suggest that more than mechanical blockage is involved.[33]

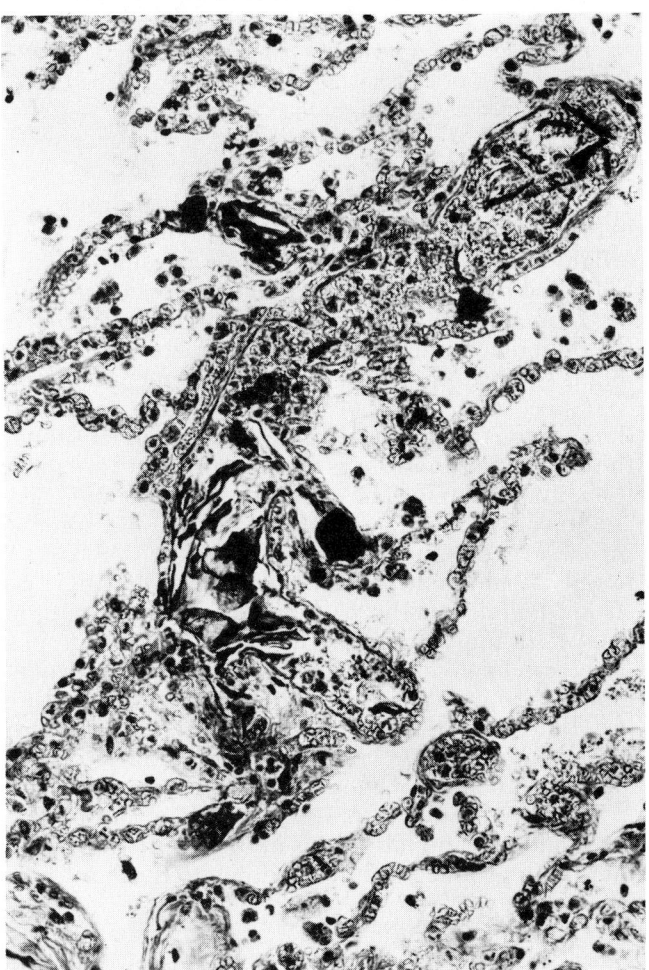

Figure 3–21. Amniotic embolism. Masses of dark mucous debris and desquamated squames are present in the pulmonary vessels and alveolar capillaries.

There is a poor correlation at post-mortem examination between the amount of amniotic fluid debris found in the vessels and the rapidity of the fatal course. Moreover, instillation of the supernatant of amniotic fluid into the arterial side of the circulation in animals has produced a similar syndrome. Thus, it is suspected that some humoral factor in amniotic fluid causing pulmonary vasoconstriction and impaired cardiac contractility is responsible for the respiratory and cardiac decompensation. Prostaglandin F_{2a}, the levels of which increase in amniotic fluid during labor, has been incriminated but without proof.[34] Further investigation is required to unravel the cause of this rare but disastrous disorder to spare the infant from being born into a motherless world. To date, "this cause of maternal death remains unpredictable and largely unpreventable."[35,36]

AIR OR GAS EMBOLISM (CAISSON DISEASE OR DECOMPRESSION SICKNESS)

Bubbles of air or gas within the circulation obstruct vascular flow and damage tissues just as certainly as thrombotic masses. The injury is now referred to as barotrauma. Air or gas may gain access to the circulation during delivery or abortion when it is forced into ruptured uterine venous sinuses by the powerful contractions of the uterus. Air embolization may also occur during the performance of a pneumothorax when a large artery or vein is ruptured or entered accidentally. It may also be observed when injury to the lung or the chest wall opens a large vein and permits the entrance of air during the negative pressure phase of inspiration. These bubbles of air act as physical masses. Many small bubbles may coalesce to produce frothy, gaseous masses, sufficiently large to occlude a major vessel, usually in the lungs or brain. Aggregates of larger size may become trapped in the chambers of the right heart and block the orifice of the pulmonary artery. Sudden death may result. Large quantities of air, probably somewhere in the neighborhood of 100 cc, are required to produce problems; the small amounts commonly introduced during intravenous therapy are of no significance, since they rapidly dissolve in the plasma.

When air or gas embolism is suspected, it is necessary at autopsy to open the heart and major pulmonary trunks under water to detect the escaping gas. At times the frothy appearance of the blood calls attention to the presence of the gaseous bubbles.

A specialized form of gas embolism known as *caisson disease* or *decompression sickness* occurs in persons exposed to sudden changes in atmospheric pressure. Those at particular risk are scuba and deep sea divers and workers engaged in underwater tunneling and the construction of foundations for offshore drilling platforms. With shallow dives, compressed air may be used, but with the deeper levels involved in tunnel and caisson work, compressed mixtures of oxygen and helium are used (to avoid nitrogen narcosis). Whatever the gas, when it is breathed under high pressure, increased amounts dissolve in the blood, tissue fluids, and fat. If the individual decompresses too rapidly, the gases come out of solution as minute bubbles. Oxygen is readily soluble, but nitrogen and helium tend to persist to form gaseous emboli within the blood vessels and tissues.[37]

There are two types of decompression sickness, acute and chronic. The *acute form* is commonly known as "the bends" or "the chokes." The acute obstruction of small blood vessels in and around the joints and skeletal muscles causes the patient to double up in pain; a similar process may produce acute respiratory distress, while involvement of the cerebral vessels may lead to obtundation, coma, and sometimes death. *The chronic form of decompression sickness is more properly referred to as caisson disease.* Here, the presumed persistence of gaseous emboli leads to multiple foci of ischemic necrosis throughout the skeletal system, favored sites being the heads of the femurs, tibia, and humeri. The precise pathogenesis of this ischemic necrosis of bone is not well understood, and there is a suspicion that platelet activation, intravascular coagulation, and hypoxic damage to marrow fat cells, causing their swelling and thus narrowing of the marrow vasculature, may contribute to the avascular necrosis.[38] Once bone necroses have appeared there is no effective treatment save time and possibly reconstructive surgery, but during the acute stages of gas embolism, recompression of the individual followed by slow decompression permits the slow resolubilization of the gaseous emboli.

FAT EMBOLISM

Microglobules of intravascular fat can be identified at post-mortem examination in almost all patients dying soon after fractures of large bones such as the femur and pelvis or after significant soft tissue trauma or burns. Much less often they are seen with a variety of nontraumatic diseases such as diabetes mellitus, sickle cell anemia, and pancreatitis. However, in only 0.5 to 5% of traumatic cases are they associated with the appearance of the so-called fat embolism syndrome about 24 to 72 hours following the injury — marked by progressive pulmonary insufficiency and mental deterioration often accompanied by thrombocytopenia, petechiae in the conjunctivae and upper portions of the body, and sometimes globules of fat in the urine. *It is important therefore to differentiate the mere presence of fat globules in the circulation (often within the microvessels of the lungs) from the fat embolism syndrome with its 10 to 15% mortality rate.* In the classic syndrome, large numbers of fat globules can be visualized, usually in the microcirculation of the lungs and often in the brain and kidneys. The morphology is best considered before turning to the pathogenesis.

MORPHOLOGY. The diagnosis of this condition when suspected can sometimes be confirmed during the autopsy by gentle pressure on fresh slices of lung tissue immersed in saline, which releases the fat globules and permits them to float to the surface. Microscopic demonstration of the fat emboli within the microvessels, principally of the lungs, brain, and kidneys is difficult and often rests on sharply demarcated, cleared spaces where the blood has been displaced (Fig. 3–22). Often it is necessary to use frozen sections and fat stains, thereby avoiding the usual solvents employed in paraffin embedding of tissues. In addition, there are a variety of pulmonary changes comprising essentially pulmonary edema, congestive atelectasis, and the escape of protein-rich fluid into the alveolar spaces with the formation of hyaline membranes — namely the adult respiratory distress syndrome (ARDS) (p. 760). The central nervous system changes are extremely variable and depend on the severity of brain involvement and the duration of survival. At an early stage the brain may appear entirely normal on gross inspection, but it may contain microemboli of fat, demonstrable by the methods just described. Over the course of a few days, cerebral edema may appear, accompanied by microfoci of hemorrhage, most visible in the white matter. Well-developed microinfarcts are sometimes present but are uncommon. Characteristically there are petechiae of the skin (most prominent over the upper body), conjunctivae, and serosal membranes.

Traditionally, the fat embolism syndrome has been attributed to the release and embolism of microglobules of fat from fatty marrow or adipose tissue, following rupture of sinusoids or venules. Most would be trapped in the lungs, causing embolic occlusion of the pulmonary microvessels, but some of the globules might squeeze through into the systemic circulation to impact in the brain. Although most are trapped in the pulmonary circulation, the quantity of fat seen in the lungs post mortem is rarely sufficient to explain the clinical course. The syndrome is occasionally encountered in nontraumatic conditions, and some of the observed pulmonary changes, i.e., ARDS, are not readily attributable to the fat globules. Thus there is a strong belief that the pathogenesis of the symptom complex is multifactorial. The many mechanisms proposed can be divided basically into (1) embolism of fat globules from fat depots as mentioned, (2) emulsion instability with the intravascular formation of microglobules of fat, (3) chemical injury to microvessels, and (4) activation of the coagulation system.

The *emulsion instability theory* proposes that chylomicrons and fatty acids in the circulation agglomerate to produce droplets, adding to those released from fat depots.[39]

The *chemical injury theory* suggests that the elevated plasma levels of free fatty acids induce toxic injury to the microvessels, principally in the lungs, resulting in diffuse capillary leakage and the production of ARDS (p. 760). Toxic injury to the capillaries could also account for the significant pulmonary

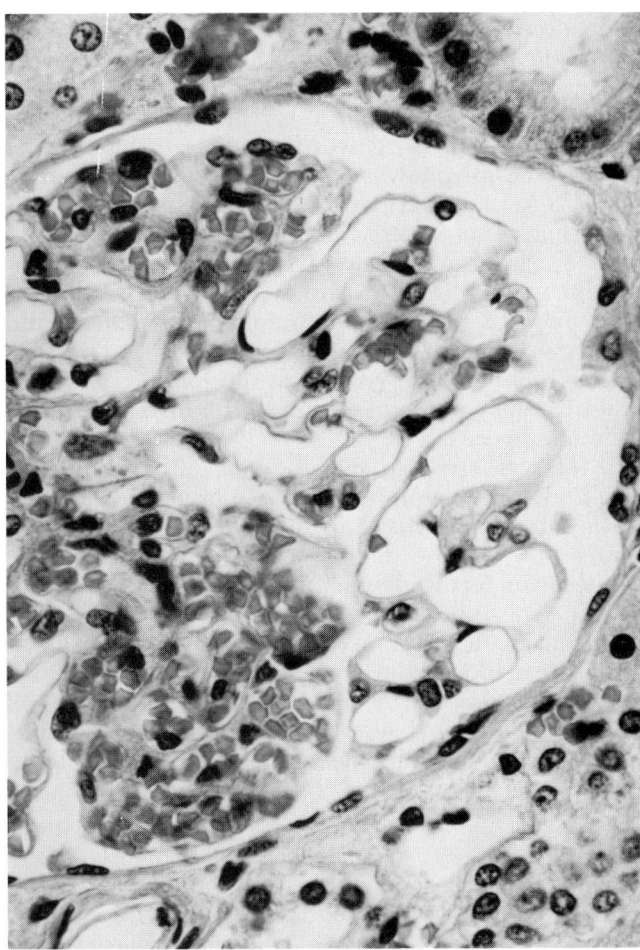

Figure 3–22. Fat embolism in the kidney. The seemingly empty glomerular capillaries are plugged with lipid vacuoles. Contrast with unoccluded congested capillaries on the left.

edema that is sometimes encountered. The cerebral component could then relate to the hypoxia produced by the pulmonary changes.

Activation of coagulation, with the production essentially of DIC, might well contribute to fibrin thrombi in the lungs and elsewhere. Although such thrombi are rarely observed anatomically, active fibrinolysis could explain their disappearance by the time of death. Furthermore, the release from platelets of vasoactive amines and peptides with their vasocontrictive effects could further contribute to the hypoxemia and cerebral hypoxia.

Any one or several of these mechanisms in concert may in one or another setting contribute to the development of the fat embolism syndrome.

INFARCTION

An infarct is a localized area of ischemic necrosis in an organ or tissue, resulting most often from sudden reduction of its arterial supply or occasionally its venous drainage. However, vascular occlusion does not necessarily produce an area of ischemic necrosis, as will

soon be seen. It may cause only atrophy or focal cell death or may even be without effect. *Interruption of the arterial blood supply to a tissue produces ischemic necrosis more certainly than does venous obstruction.* Thrombosis of veins may lead to pulmonary arterial embolism, but if the thrombus remains in situ it may cause only stasis for a brief period until the increased venous pressure distal to the obstruction leads to dilatation of bypasses, which at least partially restores the vascular flow in the affected tissue. However, in organs having a single venous outflow channel devoid of bypass channels, occlusion of this outflow may induce infarction. Examples of this are seen when the venous drainage of the testis or ovary is blocked. Arterial flow must soon come to a standstill, since it has no escape through venous bypasses, and infarction often develops.

The vascular obstruction is usually caused by thrombosis and/or embolism. More rarely, narrowing of a vessel and infarction may be caused by other forms of vascular disease, such as a large atherosclerotic plaque, or by compression of vessels by expansile tumors or inflammatory fibrous adhesions. Spasm of coronary arteries is another possible mechanism that may contribute to myocardial infarction. Vascular narrowing or occlusion may also result from the twisting of the pedicle of a mobile viscus, such as a loop of bowel or the ovary. The venous drainage or arterial supply of loops of bowel, which become trapped in narrow-mouthed hernia sacs, may also become severely reduced or totally compromised. External pressures and torsions usually lead to embarrassment of venous flow, since the veins are more readily compressed than the arteries.

TYPES OF INFARCTS. Infarcts are classified on the basis of their color and the presence or absence of bacterial contamination. Infarcts are either *anemic (white)* or *hemorrhagic (red)*.

White infarcts are encountered (1) with arterial occlusion and (2) in solid tissues. When a solid tissue is deprived of its arterial circulation, the infarct may be transiently hemorrhagic, but most become pale in a very short time. At the moment of vascular occlusion, blood from anastomotic peripheral vessels flows into the focus of injury, producing the initial hemorrhagic appearance. If the tissue affected is solid, the seepage of blood is minimal. Soon after the initial extravasation, the red cells are lysed, and the released hemoglobin pigment either diffuses out or is converted to hemosiderin. In solid organs, therefore, the arterial infarct will soon (24 to 48 hours) become pale. The heart, spleen, and kidneys are representative of solid, compact organs that tend to have pale infarcts (Fig. 3–23).

Red infarcts are encountered usually (1) with venous occlusions, (2) in loose tissues, (3) in tissues with a double circulation, and (4) in tissues previously congested. The loose, honeycombed tissue of the lung provides an example of hemorrhagic infarction secondary to arterial obstruction. At the moment of in-

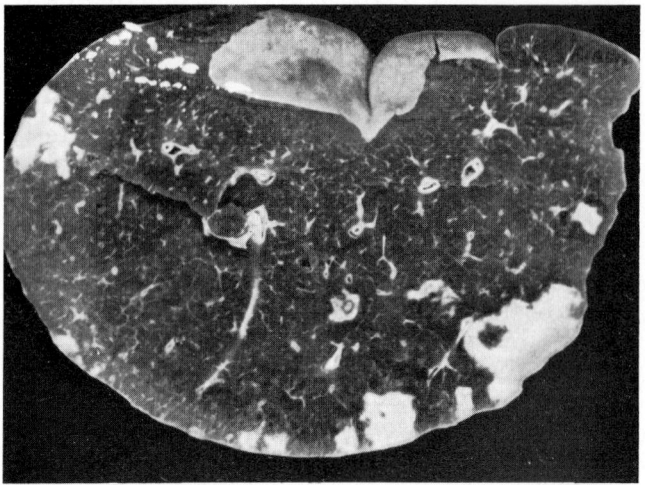

Figure 3-23. Multiple small, peripheral, pale infarcts in a spleen viewed in cross section.

farction, large amounts of hemorrhage collect in the spongy pulmonary parenchyma, so the arterial infarction remains red (Fig. 3-24). Venous occlusion leads to hemorrhagic infarction as occurs, for example, with twisting of the pedicle of the ovary. The thin-walled ovarian veins are occluded first, causing intense congestion and infarction with or without occlusion of the artery. The small intestine is another site where hemorrhagic infarcts typically occur. Venous occlusions or even arterial occlusions may cause hemorrhagic

infarction of long segments of the intestine. The explanation lies in the rich arterial anastomoses between the many branches of the superior mesenteric artery, which permit arterial flow to the injured segment through anastomosing arcades. Indeed, this type of vascular supply may well protect against ischemic damage (p. 113). Hemorrhagic arterial infarction is sometimes encountered in the brain as well. An embolus to a large artery such as the middle cerebral may produce a nonhemorrhagic area of cerebral infarction. Soon thereafter, the embolus may shatter, and the fragments may move into smaller, more peripheral branches. Reflow through the major trunk may yield extensive hemorrhage into the primary area of ischemic necrosis.

Infarcts are also classified as either *septic* or *bland*, depending on the presence or absence of bacterial infection in the area of necrosis. Bacterial contamination may be due to organisms present in the tissue prior to the development of the ischemic necrosis, as in infarction of a lung already affected by bacterial pneumonia; may be brought to the area by an infected blood clot, as occurs with embolization of a fragment of bacterial vegetation from a heart valve; or may result from bacteremic seeding of the margins of the area of ischemic necrosis.

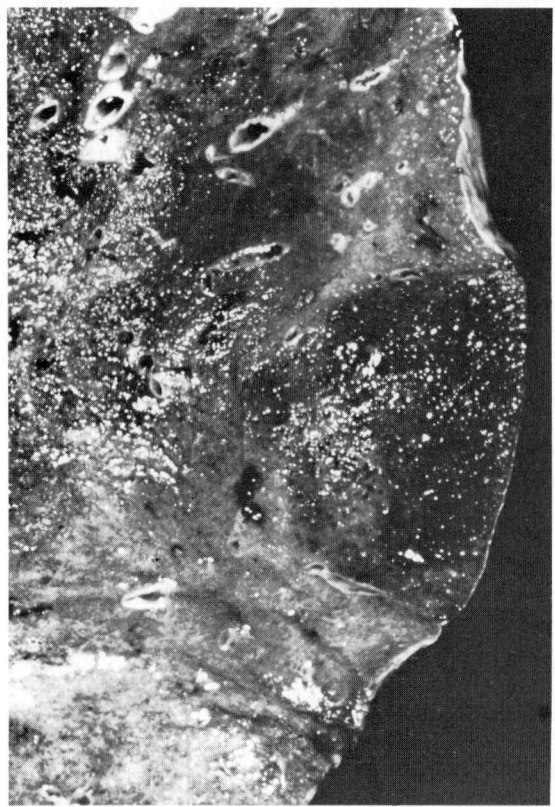

Figure 3-24. A sharply circumscribed hemorrhagic infarct in the lung.

MORPHOLOGY. Whether hemorrhagic or pale, all infarcts tend to be wedge-shaped, with the apex of the wedge pointing toward the focus of vascular occlusion. Since all the dependent tissue out to the periphery of the organ is affected, the external aspect of the organ forms the base of the wedge. The exact outline of the infarct may be quite variable, and sometimes maplike patterns result from the preservation of small marginal areas of tissue that have different and unaffected sources of blood supply.

A few hours after onset, all infarcts are somewhat poorly defined, are slightly darker in color than normal, and have a firmer consistency than surrounding normal tissue. During the next 24 hours, the demarcation becomes better defined, and the color change is more intense. In solid organs, the infarct may then appear paler than normal as the small amounts of red cells are lysed, whereas in the spongy tissues the massive hemorrhage makes the lesion red-blue. The firmer consistency of the infarct is due to the suffusion of blood or inflammatory exudation.

In the course of several days, pale infarcts become yellow-white and sharply demarcated, while the appearance of the pulmonary hemorrhagic infarcts remains relatively unchanged. The margins of both types of infarcts tend to become better defined by a narrow rim of hyperemia due to the marginal inflammatory response. The involved surface of the organ is usually covered by an inflammatory exudation, which is commonly fibrinous. In venous thrombosis and infarction as, for example, in the small intestine, the areas of hemorrhagic necrosis may be somewhat poorly delimited.

The characteristic cytologic change of all infarcts, save those in the brain, is ischemic coagulative necrosis of the affected cells (p. 17) (Fig. 3-25). If the vascular occlusion has occurred only a few hours prior to the death of the patient, there may be no demonstrable cellular change, since there may have been insufficient time for enzymic alteration of the dead cells. If the patient survives for about 12 to 18 hours, only hemorrhagic suffusion may be present.

Inflammatory exudation begins after the first few hours and becomes better defined over the next few days. The inflammatory reaction is followed by a fibroblastic, reparative response beginning in the preserved margins. Some parenchymal regeneration may occur at the periphery where the underlying framework of the organ has been spared. However, in most cases the necrotic focus is eventually replaced by scar tissue, sometimes taking many months (Fig. 3–26).

The brain is an exception to these generalizations. When it suffers ischemic necrosis the affected area promptly and rapidly undergoes **liquefaction** (p. 18).

With septic infarction the lesion is converted to an abscess and, if seen at a very late stage, may be unrecognizable as an infarct. The inflammatory reaction is correspondingly greater, but the eventual sequence of organization follows the pattern already described.

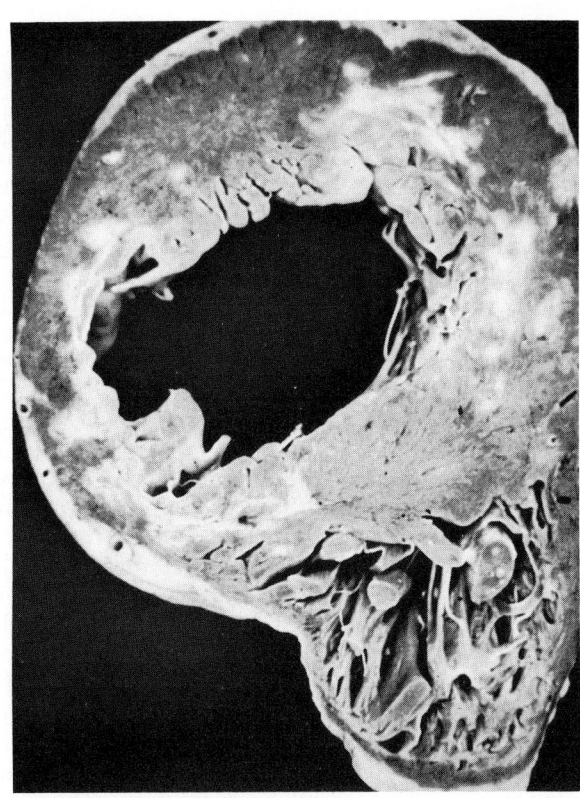

Figure 3–26. Numerous old myocardial infarcts have resulted in scattered pale fibrous scars throughout the myocardium.

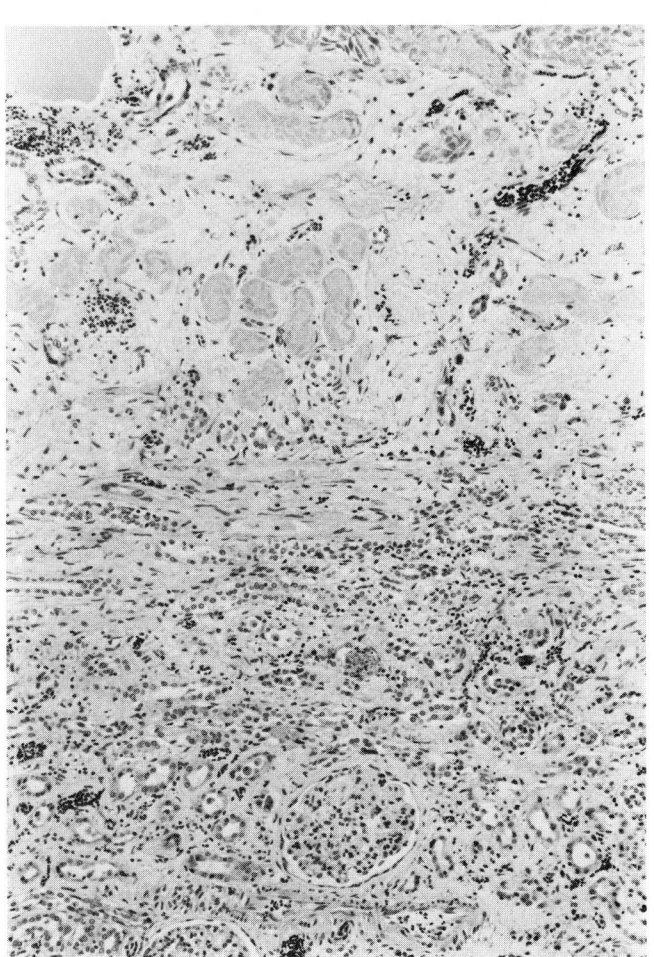

Figure 3–25. The margin of a renal infarct in detail. Outlines of coagulated tubules remain (above), and the unaffected renal parenchyma is below.

FACTORS CONDITIONING SEVERITY OF INJURY RESULTING FROM VASCULAR OCCLUSION.

Both arterial and venous vascular obstructions may be without effect or may cause only atrophy or single cell necroses. The extent to which a tissue is disturbed by occlusion of its venous or arterial connections depends on a number of factors: (1) the general status of the blood and the cardiovascular system, (2) the anatomic pattern of the vascular supply, (3) the rate of development of the occlusion, and (4) the vulnerability of the tissue to ischemia.

GENERAL STATUS OF BLOOD AND CARDIOVASCULAR SYSTEM. Any systemic alteration, such as anemia or hypoxemia, that reduces the oxygen-carrying capacity of the blood, or the velocity and volume of blood flow through the tissue, predisposes to infarction. Sickle cell anemia is a special case; it is characterized by logjamming of the misshapen erythrocytes adding stasis to the hypoxemia. Infarctions are common in these patients. In the very aged patient with marked coronary atherosclerosis, myocardial infarction may occur subsequent to the development of severe anemia or sudden drops in blood pressure, even in the absence of total occlusion of a vessel. Cardiac failure, blood loss, and shock impair the oxygenation of all tissues and thereby render tissues vulnerable to further diminution of their vascular supply.

ANATOMIC PATTERNS OF ARTERIAL SUPPLY. The various tissues and organs of the body receive their arterial supply through one of four patterns: (1) a double blood supply; (2) parallel arterial systems; (3) a "single" arterial supply with rich interarterial anastomoses; and (4) a "single" arterial supply with few anastomoses, insufficient to provide adequate bypass channels, so-called end-arteries. Obviously there are many gradations between the last two patterns. The lungs and the liver are examples of organs fortunately provided with dual blood supplies. In individuals having a normal hematologic and cardiovascular status, the bronchial circulation is capable of preventing ischemic necrosis when a radicle of the pulmonary artery is obstructed. Similarly, infarction is extremely uncommon in the liver because the portal supply of blood may be adequate even when the hepatic arterial flow is compromised. However, in the presence of cardiac failure, severe anemia, or reduced oxygenation of the blood, occlusion of one system may precipitate ischemic necrosis.

Parallel arterial systems are encountered in the forearm and brain. Either the radial or the ulnar artery is sufficient to sustain the vitality of the tissues of the forearm when the other is occluded. The brain with its circle of Willis is protected from ischemic injury resulting from an occlusion at any point *in* the circle of Willis or in one of the major arteries *supplying* the circle. Such a proposition, of course, implies the absence of pre-existing vascular disease within the circle of Willis. These comments should not be construed to apply to the arterial supply to the brain *derived from* the circle of Willis. Occlusion of one of the cerebral or cerebellar arteries will, of course, cause infarction of the dependent region of the brain.

The small intestine is the prototype of a tissue enjoying an arterial supply with rich interarterial anastomoses. The branches of the superior mesenteric artery are interconnected by looping arcades, enabling blood to bypass focal occlusion. If, however, one of the primary divisions of the superior mesenteric artery or the main artery itself is obstructed, the arcades cannot provide compensation.

The kidney is the unfortunate victim of an arterial supply composed of end-arteries. The major branches of the renal artery supply well-defined segments of the kidneys, and occlusion of one of the major branches or, of course, the main renal artery is almost invariably followed by ischemic necrosis.

The heart is an example of an organ having an intermediate pattern of fairly rich interarterial anastomoses that may compensate for narrowing or occlusion of one of the three main trunks of the coronary arterial system. Perfusion techniques have confirmed the presence of fine interarterial anastomoses joining each of the major coronary trunks to the others.[40] When one major trunk is compromised, the collateral supply from an unaffected trunk may suffice to prevent ischemic injury.

Thus, the anatomic pattern of the vascular supply of a tissue materially modifies the consequence of a vascular occlusion.

RATE OF DEVELOPMENT OF OCCLUSION. Slowly developing occlusions are far better tolerated than those occurring suddenly, since they provide an opportunity for alternative pathways and collaterals to become activated.

VULNERABILITY OF TISSUE TO ISCHEMIA. Tissues of the body vary widely in their susceptibility to ischemic hypoxia. The neurons of the central nervous system are undoubtedly the most sensitive, and complete anoxia for a period of only a few minutes may produce irreversible changes. Indeed, a hierarchy of vulnerability to ischemia has been described for the varying cell types within the brain.[41] Cerebral cortical neurons are most sensitive to hypoxia, followed in order by those in the cerebellum and by those in the basal ganglia. The glial cells are more resistant than neurons but also have differing sensitivities. The epithelial cells of the proximal convoluted renal tubules (more so than the other tubular segments) and the myocardial cells are likewise exquisitely sensitive to hypoxia. By contrast, the mesenchymal tissues of the body are in general quite resistant. The robustness of the fibroblast may permit the framework and stroma of a tissue to remain vital despite ischemic necrosis of its more sensitive parenchymal cells.

CLINICAL SIGNIFICANCE OF INFARCTION. In the United States, over half of all deaths are caused by cardiovascular disease. Most of these cardiovascular deaths result from myocardial and cerebral infarctions. Coronary heart disease alone accounts for about 30% of all the mortality, and myocardial infarction is by far the predominant cause of fatal coronary heart disease. Cerebral infarction (encephalomalacia) is also the most frequent type of central nervous system disease. Pulmonary infarction is an extremely common complication in a variety of clinical settings, as has been indicated in previous considerations. Renal infarction does not have the paramount importance of these other forms mentioned. It is, nonetheless, an occasional cause of renal failure and death and is a not uncommon cause of clinical signs and symptoms. Ischemic necrosis (gangrene) of the lower extremities is a relatively unusual clinical problem in the population at large but is a major concern in diabetics. Infarction of tissues, therefore, is a common cause of clinical illness.

Thrombosis, embolism, and infarction may strike without notice, but even worse, they are proverbial vultures, stalking every ill, bedridden, and aged patient who regrettably is least able to cope with them.

SHOCK

Shock, commonly called circulatory collapse, may develop following any serious assault on the body's homeostasis, such as profuse hemorrhage, severe trauma or burns, extensive myocardial infarction, massive pulmonary embolism, or uncontrolled bacterial sepsis. *Whatever the clinical provocation, at the most fundamental level shock constitutes widespread hypoperfusion of cells and tissues due to reduction in the blood volume or cardiac output, or redistribution of blood resulting in an inadequate effective circulating volume.* Incident to the perfusion deficit, there is insufficient delivery of oxygen and nutrients to the cells and tissues (some more than others) and inadequate clearance of metabolites. The cellular hypoxia induces a shift from aerobic to anaerobic metabolism, resulting in increased lactate production and sometimes lactic acidosis. While at the outset the hemodynamic and metabolic derangements are correctable and induce reversible injury to cells, persistence or worsening of the shock state leads to irreversible injury and death of cells and sometimes, unhappily, the patient.

The hemodynamic derangements in the many clinical states sometimes complicated by shock can be divided into four pathophysiologic categories (Table 3–3). In considering these pathophysiologic derangements, it should be recalled that at the level of the cell, blood flow is more important than blood pressure, but obviously the driving force for the flow is the pressure head. Arterial blood pressure, in turn, depends on the cardiac output and the peripheral resistance.[42] The basis then of the reduced perfusion of cells in hypovolemic and cardiogenic shock is evident and most simply stated is — inadequate cardiac output. In an otherwise healthy individual, an acute loss of 10 to 15% of the blood volume is without effect because compensatory mechanisms, such as vasoconstriction, increased heart rate, and myocardial contractility, maintain the pressure and flow. However, compensatory mechanisms cannot compensate for a greater loss of blood volume. Analogously, excessive exudation from extensive skin burns or combined hemorrhage and exudation from large traumatic wounds may also cause hypovolemic shock, sometimes called, respectively, burn shock and traumatic shock. Cardiogenic shock is best viewed as "pump failure." As is evident from Table 3–3, this may occur for a number of reasons, but most important is a large myocardial infarct with loss of effective function of about 45% of the left ventricular myocardium.[43]

When we come to septic shock, the pathogenesis is complex and not well understood. Most commonly it is related to gram-negative sepsis, e.g., *E. coli,* Klebsiella-Enterobacter, Pseudomonas, Serratia, and Bacteroides, with release into the circulation of their endotoxic lipopolysaccharides (particularly the lipid-A moiety), hence the common term "endotoxic shock." However, a similar syndrome can be produced by infections with gram-positive organisms, e.g., streptococci or pneumococci, or more specifically the peptidoglycans in their cell walls. In contrast to the normal to reduced cardiac output and pale, cool, sweaty skin (due to sympathetic vasoconstriction of the microcirculation of the skin vessels) seen in hypovolemic or cardiogenic shock, patients with early septic shock often have a normal or increased cardiac output and a warm, dry skin.[44] Underlying this hyperdynamic phase of septic shock is arteriolar dilatation with a dramatic reduction in systemic vascular resistance. There follows dilatation of the peripheral microcirculation affecting principally the capillary and venular beds and the veins (the so-called capacitance vessels). *The net consequence is peripheral pooling of blood with reduction in the effective circulating blood volume, lowered cardiac output, hypotension, and inadequate perfusion of cells and tissues.*

The pathogenesis of the distributive defect is somewhat controversial. Bacterial products — lipid-A or peptidogylcans — induce a cascade of events. It begins with toxic injury to cell membranes, including endothelial cells, leukocytes, and platelets, activating both the intrinsic and the extrinsic pathways of coagulation (sometimes leading to DIC). Toxic free radicals and vasoactive agents (cited later) are released from these injured cells. Complement is activated through the alternate pathway with the formation of the vasoactive fractions C_{5a} and C_{3a}; they induce the synthesis and release from leukocytes and endothelial cells of toxic free radicals and vasoactive agents (cited later). Damaged platelets release vasoactive substances, e.g., histamine, serotonin, epinephrine, and thromboxane, and the kallikrein-kinin system is activated (to cite only some of the tangle). *Thus comes about arteriolar dilatation, peripheral pooling, and diffuse toxic cell injury, the major hallmarks of early septic shock.* But soon thereafter the diffuse endothelial damage and vasoactive mediators lead to wide-ranging membrane damage, with electrolyte imbalances and increased transudation and exudation of fluid out of the cellular and vascular compartments adding hypovolemia to the complex of events (Fig. 3–27). It might be mentioned in passing that anaphylactic shock (not included in Table 3–3) is also the consequence of peripheral pooling of blood.

SECONDARY MEDIATORS OF SHOCK. Although we speak of loss of blood volume or cardiac output or peripheral pooling of blood as the proximate mecha-

Table 3–3. Classification of Shock

TYPE OF SHOCK	CLINICAL EXAMPLES	PRINCIPAL MECHANISMS
Cardiogenic	Myocardial infarction Rupture of heart Arrhythmias Cardiac tamponade Pulmonary embolism	Failure of myocardial pump due to intrinsic myocardial damage or extrinsic pressure or obstruction to outflow
Hypovolemic	Hemorrhage Fluid loss — e.g., vomiting, diarrhea, burns	Inadequate blood or plasma volume
Septic	Overwhelming bacterial infections: gram-negative septicemia ("endotoxic shock") or gram-positive septicemia	Peripheral vasodilatation and pooling of blood; cell membrane injury, endothelial cell injury with disseminated intravascular coagulation
Neurogenic	Anesthesia, spinal cord injury	Peripheral vasodilatation with pooling of blood

Drawn from Robbins, S.L., and Kumar, V.: Basic Pathology, 4th ed. Philadelphia, W.B. Saunders Company, 1987, p. 79.

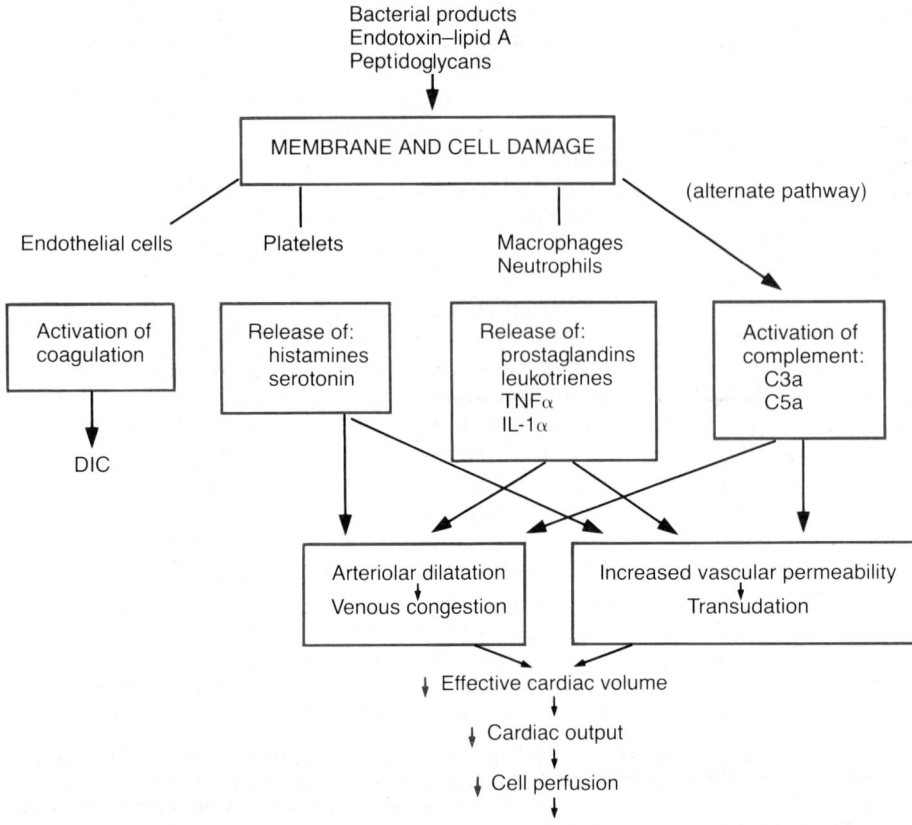

Figure 3–27. A potential schema of the development of septic shock.

nisms of shock, a large number of chemical factors, some mentioned earlier, others listed below, have been invoked as secondary mediators in most forms of shock.[44a]

> Catecholamines
> Histamine
> The kinin system
> Complement activation (C_{5a} and C_{3a})
> Prostaglandins
> Leukotrienes
> Interleukin-1
> Interferon (alpha and gamma)
> Endorphins
> Platelet activating factor
> Tumor necrosis factor-α (TNF-α)
> Myocardial depressant factor

The evidence implicating these mediators is more substantial for some than for others and in many instances is derived from animal studies whose relevance to humans remains uncertain. Only limited comments are indicated, therefore. Reduced venous return and decreased cardiac output with fall in blood pressure seen ultimately in all forms of established shock activates baroreceptors, triggering sympathetic discharge, release of catecholamines, activation of the renin-angiotensin axis, and secretion of

antidiuretic hormone.[45] The net effect of these changes is in part protective, with arteriolar vasoconstriction (following the initial vasodilatation in septic shock), increased cardiac rate, augmented myocardial contractility, and conservation of fluid by the kidney. But the vasoconstrictive reaction is a two-edged sword. On the one hand, the constriction of vessels in the skin, muscles, and splanchnic bed is more pronounced than in the heart and brain, shunting blood to these vital organs. On the other hand, the vasoconstriction further reduces the perfusion of cells and so worsens the ischemic injury, particularly to the gut mucosa, potentiating bacterial invasion and the release of toxic products.

Simultaneously, the sympathetic homeostatic response leads to the hypothalamic release of ACTH and beta-endorphins and to increased synthesis and release of glucocorticoids. In laboratory animals including nonhuman primates, there is evidence that endorphins by and of themselves worsen the hemodynamic deterioration and that the opiate antagonist—naloxone—produces marked hemodynamic improvement in hypovolemic and endotoxic shock.[46] To date no similar benefits have been recorded for humans. Elevated plasma levels of prostaglandins and metabolites of thromboxane A_2 (TxA_2) have been observed in experimental shock models and of TxA_2 in humans suffering from severe septic shock.[47] PGE_2 and PGI_2 (prostacyclin) are vasodilators and may contribute to the reduced vascular resistance in early septic shock; PGF_2 and TxA_2 are potent vasoconstrictors and may participate along with sympathetic mechanisms in supporting the cardiac output. However, most of the relevant evidence is animal-derived with as yet few well-established correlations in humans. In addition, leukotrienes (particularly LTE_4) and platelet activating factor (PAF), presumably derived from neutrophils and endothelial cells, have been observed in experimental models, but their contribution to the clinical state remains unresolved.

To add to the complexity, several lines of experimental evidence suggest that the production of prostaglandins, leukotrienes, platelet activating factor, and interleukin-1 is signaled by the release of tumor necrosis factor-α (TNF-α) from monocytes/macrophages activated in septic shock by bacterial products.[48] Extending these observations to humans, increased serum levels of TNF-α have been demonstrated in patients with endotoxic shock related to meningococcal septicemia.[48a] TNF-α and IL-1 may well be the ultimate and essential mediators of septic shock and possibly other forms as well.[49] One additional putative player in the ever-expanding cast of characters in shock needs mention — myocardial depressant factor (MDF). Produced in the ischemic pancreas, MDF induces splanchnic vasoconstriction, depresses myocardial contractility, and enhances membrane leakiness.[50] Although such actions could contribute to the progressive hemodynamic deterioration in uncontrolled shock, the evidence that it does is tenuous.

STAGES OF SHOCK. Shock is a progressive disorder that, if unhalted, spirals downward into ever deeper levels of hemodynamic and metabolic deterioration. The progression may be tumultuous and the patient may go into profound shock within minutes, say, of a massive hemorrhage. More often it evolves over a span of hours. This progression has been arbitrarily divided into three stages: (1) "early," "compensated" shock; (2) "progressive," "decompensated" shock; and (3) "irreversible" shock. Admittedly there are no hallmarks delimiting one stage from the next, but nonetheless a consideration of each stage permits an overview of the full spectrum of the shock state (Fig. 3–28).

"Early," "compensated" shock implies a relatively minor deficiency in the circulating blood volume such that compensatory mechanisms, e.g., constriction of the arteriolar bed, augmentation of heart rate, increased secretion of ADH, and activation of the renin-angiotensin-aldosterone axis are sufficient to maintain the blood pressure and cardiac output at near-normal levels. It is important to note that the blood pressure can be normal in the early stage of shock and indeed usually is normal in the previously hypertensive patient.[51] The precariousness of this stage when all compensatory reserves have been fully activated may be difficult to discern.

The *"progressive," "decompensated" stage of shock* appears with persistence of the shock, especially when an additional stress is imposed on an individual in "compensated" shock. In this stage, despite intense arteriolar constriction and increased heart rate, there is a decline in blood pressure and cardiac output. Tachypnea is common because of the reduced

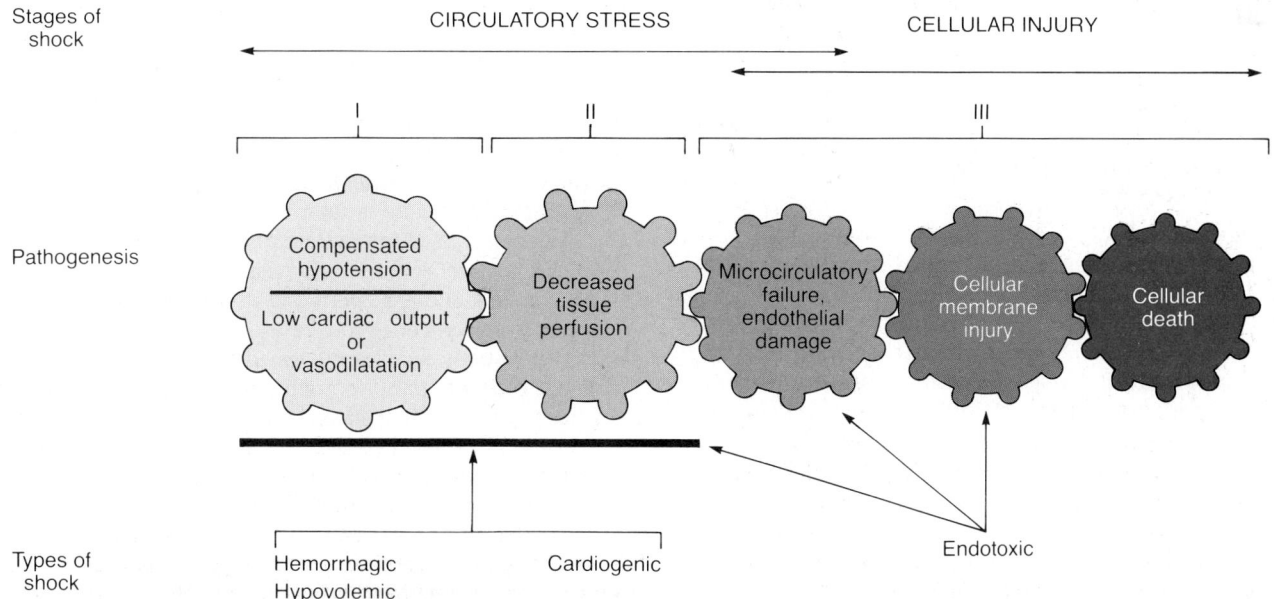

Figure 3–28. Pathogenesis and stages of shock. Stage I is nonprogressive, stage II is progressive, and stage III is irreversible. Note that endotoxic shock is multifactorial; it is associated with vasodilatation, decreased tissue perfusion, endothelial damage, and direct cellular injury. (Modified from Wyngaarden, J.B., and Smith, L.H., Jr.: Cecil Textbook of Medicine, 17th ed. Philadelphia, W.B. Saunders Co., 1985, p. 212.)

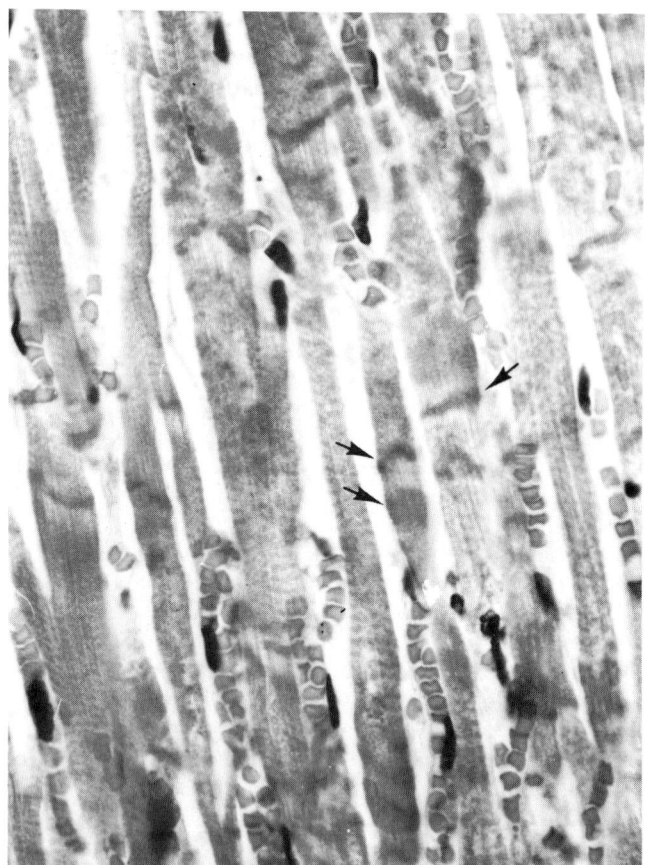

Figure 3 – 29. Contraction bands *(arrows)* in a heart suffering from hypoperfusion. The heavy bands should not be confused with the more delicate cross striations of cardiac myocytes.

pulmonary perfusion and, as will be seen, the development of changes leading to the adult respiratory distress syndrome (ARDS). A marked reduction in urinary output *(oliguria)* may appear owing to reduced renal blood flow. The oxygen deficit forces the cells to revert to anaerobic glycolysis, leading to a metabolic lactic acidosis. Reduced hepatic clearance of lactate contributes to *the acidosis that constitutes one of the characteristic metabolic features of all forms of fully developed shock.* Individuals with pre-existing coronary atherosclerosis are at risk of developing angina or, even worse, a myocardial infarct. It is evident at this point that matters have gone from bad to worse!

"Irreversible" shock is a term that is applied to the clinical situation in which even correction of the hemodynamic derangement does not halt the downward spiral. This stage is marked by progressive reduction in the cardiac output attributed by some to the release of myocardial depressant factor, progressive fall in the blood pressure, and worsening of the metabolic acidosis. The reduced blood flow to the brain, heart, and kidneys leads to ischemic cell death in these organs with progressively deepening obtundation and coma, progressive renal failure, and uremia. The respiratory difficulties become more marked with the worsening pulmonary edema and ARDS. Ultimately,

the perfusion deficit disrupts the integrity of all membranes with unrestrained shifts in fluid and electrolytes between cells and interstitial tissue, accounting for the oft-repeated statement, Shock not only stops the machine, but also wrecks the machinery. Nonetheless, the designation "irreversible" should be used guardedly because, as everyone knows, "It's not over until it's all over."

MORPHOLOGY. As expected, the changes induced by shock take the form of hypoxic injury. The cellular and subcellular alterations have been meticulously detailed by Trump[52,53] and were described on page 4. While such cellular injury is bodywide, certain organs are more severely affected than others because of shunting of blood to the heart and brain and away from other organs, and because of differing cellular vulnerabilities to hypoxic and metabolic injury.

The principal threats to life stem from injury to the brain, heart, lungs, and kidneys, but morphologic changes are frequent in the gastrointestinal tract, adrenals, and liver.

The **brain** suffers so-called hypoxic encephalopathy, described in detail on page 1402.

The **heart** is affected in all forms of shock, whether cardiogenic in origin or some other form. Obviously in cardiogenic shock there is the primary cardiac or extracardiac disease that initiated the shock syndrome.

Two types of distinctive **cardiac** change appear in all forms of shock: (1) subepicardial and subendocardial hemorrhages and necroses and (2) zonal lesions, also called banding.[54,55] The necroses range from isolated fiber ischemic lesions to larger areas of involvement comprising micro- or macroinfarcts. The zonal lesions constitute opaque transverse "contraction bands" (p. 610) within a myocyte usually close to an intercalated disc, accompanied by shortening and scalloping of the sarcomere, fragmentation of the Z bands, distortion of the myofilaments, and displacement of the mitochondria away from the intercalated disc (Fig. 3 – 29). These lesions are not distinctive of shock and may appear following the use of catecholamines, with the use of the heart-lung bypass pump in cardiac surgery, and with reperfusion of the myocardium after an interval of ischemia.

The **lung** is quite resistant to ischemia and so may not be affected in pure hypovolemic shock. But anatomic alterations are prominent in shock incited by bacterial sepsis and trauma, and are referred to as "shock lung." The pulmonary changes are generically referred to as "adult respiratory distress syndrome" or "diffuse alveolar damage" and are encountered in many other clinical settings (discussed on page 760). In essence they include severe intraseptal edema, followed later by the collection of edema fluid and exuded plasma proteins within the alveolar spaces.

The **kidneys** are major targets in severe shock, principally affecting the tubules at all levels of the nephron. The tubular lesions are referred to as acute tubular necrosis (ATN). Once again, ATN is not limited to the shock state and so is described in detail on page 1048.

The **adrenal** changes encountered in shock constitute the reaction of this gland to all forms of stress, and hence might be designated as the "stress response." They take the forms of lipid depletion and scattered necrosis of isolated cells in the cortex beginning in the zona reticularis and spreading outward.

The **gastrointestinal tract** may develop patchy, mucosal hemorrhages and necroses designated as "hemorrhagic gastroenteropathy," described on page 864.

The **liver** sometimes accumulates fat within the hepatocytes. In severe shock states, central necrosis may appear within the lobule.

With certain exceptions, the cellular and organ changes encountered in shock are reversible if the patient survives. Thus, regeneration of renal tubular cells, adrenocortical cells, hepatocytes, and gastrointestinal mucosa may restore the normal architecture of these organs. Loss of neurons from the brain and of myocytes within the heart and development of pulmonary septal fibrosis may constitute irreversible damage, but cellular injury severe enough to lead to such changes is encountered only in the patient with extreme, usually lethal forms of shock. In those who survive, therefore, the function of these organs is usually not detectably altered.

CLINICAL CORRELATIONS. The *initial threats* to the life of the patient in shock arise from the medical, surgical, or obstetric catastrophe that initiated the shock state. However, the cerebral and cardiac changes described worsen the early crisis. If these hazards are survived, metabolic acidosis, shifts in electrolyte levels, and respiratory difficulties occur. The pulmonary changes in particular markedly increase the amount of work required for a given level of alveolar ventilation, giving rise to the clinical term "lung stiffness."

The "fortunate" patient survives to enter a *second phase* of clinical problems, dominated by renal dysfunction. This may appear any time from the second to the sixth day and is characterized in 50 to 75% of patients by oliguria, reflecting the reduction of renal blood flow and glomerular filtration and the impaired tubular function. The oliguria may persist for days to a few weeks, with urine levels of only a few milliliters a day. Typically the urine sodium level remains high. The clinical dilemma is now dominated by the signs and symptoms of fluid overload, hyperkalemia, acidosis, and sometimes uremia. Fortunately, ATN is reversible, and with appropriate therapy most patients can be maintained during this period of renal shutdown to recover fully from this phase.

The *third* or *diuretic phase* begins with a steady increase in urine volume, reaching possibly 3 liters per day. This urinary flood heralds a regeneration of the tubular epithelium, but tubular malfunction persists, and various electrolyte imbalances may now occur. For somewhat obscure reasons, in this stage of the course, vulnerability to infections is increased, perhaps because of reduced immunologic competence, and about 20% of deaths occur during the diuretic phase, mostly from ATN.

Despite all these therapeutic nightmares, most patients survive when the inciting cause of the shock can be controlled. Thus, patients with hypovolemic and neurogenic shock have the best prognosis, with a mortality below 10%. Present-day methods of supportive therapy have reduced the mortality of cardiogenic shock to 30 to 60%. With septic shock, the mortality depends, of course, on control of the primary infection, but on average is 40 to 50%. Disturbing as these data may be, they represent significant improvements over those that prevailed in the past.

1. Arcidi, J.M., Jr., et al.: Hepatic morphology in cardiac dysfunction: A clinicopathologic study of 1000 subjects at autopsy. Am. J. Pathol. *104*:159, 1981.
2. Gimbrone, M.A., Jr.: Vascular endothelium: Nature's blood container. In Gimbrone, M.A., Jr. (ed): Vascular Endothelium in Hemostasis and Thrombosis. New York, Churchill Livingstone, 1986, p. 1.
3. Esmon, N.L.: Thrombomodulin. Semin. Thromb. Hemost. *13*:454, 1987.
4. Marcum, J.A., and Rosenberg, R.D.: Anticoagulantly active heparin sulfate proteoglycan and the vascular endothelium. Semin. Thromb. Hemost. *13*:464, 1987.
5. Weksler, B., and Jaffe, E.A.: Prostacyclin and the endothelium. In Gimbrone, M.A., Jr. (ed.): Vascular Endothelium in Hemostasis and Thrombosis. New York, Churchill Livingstone, 1986, p. 40.
6. Hekman, C.A., and Loskutoff, D.J.: Fibrinolytic pathways and the endothelium. Semin. Thromb. Hemost. *13*:514, 1987.
7. Bevilacqua, M.P., et al.: Recombinant tumor necrosis factor induces procoagulant activity in cultured human vascular endothelium: Characterization and comparison with the actions of interleukin 1. Proc. Natl. Acad. Sci. U.S.A. *83*:4533, 1986.
8. Hawiger, J.: Adhesive interactions of blood cells and the vessel wall. In Coleman, R.W., Hirsh, J., Marder, V.J., and Salzman, E.W. (eds.): Hemostasis and Thrombosis: Basic Principles and Clinical Practice. Philadelphia, J.B. Lippincott Company, 1987, p. 182.
9. Shattil, S.J., and Bennett, J.S.: Platelets and their membranes in hemostasis: Physiology and pathophysiology. Ann. Intern. Med. *94*:108, 1980.
10. Coleman, R.W., et al.: Overview of hemostasis. In Coleman, R.W., Marder, V.J., Salzman, E.W., and Hirsh, J. (eds.): Hemostasis and Thrombosis: Basic Principles and Clinical Practice. Philadelphia, J.B. Lippincott Company, 1987, p. 3.
11. Baugh, R.F., and Houghie, C.: The chemistry of blood coagulation. Clin. Haematol. *8*:3, 1979.
11a. Furie, B., and Furie, B.C.: The molecular basis of blood coagulation. Cell *53*:505, 1988.
12. Wall, R.T., and Harker, L.A.: The endothelium and thrombosis. Annu. Rev. Med. *31*:361, 1980.
13. Spaet, T.H., and Gaynor, E.: Vascular endothelial damage and thrombosis. Adv. Cardiol. *4*:47, 1970.
14. Wessler, S., and Yiu, E.T.: On the mechanism of thrombosis. Prog. Hematol. *6*:201, 1969.
15. Hume, M., et al.: Venous Thrombosis and Pulmonary Embolism. Cambridge, Harvard University Press, 1970, p. 25.
16. Kitchens, C.S.: Concept of hypercoagulability. A review of its development, clinical application, and recent progress. Semin. Thromb. Hemost. *11*:293, 1985.
17. Brozovic, M.: Physiologic mechanisms in coagulation and fibrinolysis. Br. Med. Bull. *33*:231, 1977.
18. Bic, R.L.: Clinical relevance of antithrombin III. Semin. Thromb. Hemost. *8*:276, 1983.
19. Chumnijaraki, T., and Poshyachinda, V.: Postoperative thrombosis in Thai women. Lancet *1*:1357, 1975.
20. Gallus, A.S., and Hirsch, J.: Treatment of venous thromboembolic disease. Semin. Thromb. Hemost. *2*:291, 1976.
21. Becker, D.M.: Venous thromboembolism. Epidemiology, diagnosis, prevention. J. Gen. Intern. Med. *1*:402, 1986.
22. Al-Mondhiry, H.: Tumor interaction with hemostasis. The rationale

for use of platelet inhibitors and anticoagulants in treatment of cancer. Am. J. Hematol. *16*:193, 1984.

23. Hirsch, J., et al.: Epidemiology and pathogenesis of venous thrombosis. J. Am. Coll. Cardiol. *8*:104B, 1986.

24. Hull, R., et al.: Diagnostic efficacy of impedance plethysmography for clinically suspected deep vein thrombosis: A randomized trial. Ann. Intern. Med. *102*:21, 1985.

25. Hull, R.D., et al.: Pulmonary angiography, ventilation lung scanning, and venography for clinically suspected pulmonary embolism with abnormal perfusion scan. Ann. Intern. Med. *98*:891, 1983.

26. Freiman, D.C., et al.: Frequency of pulmonary embolism in man. N. Engl. J. Med. *27*:1278, 1965.

27. Fred, H.L., et al.: Rapid resolution of pulmonary thromboemboli in man. J.A.M.A. *196*:1137, 1966.

28. Kakkar, V.V., and Adams, P.C.: Preventive and therapeutic approach to venous thromboembolic disease and pulmonary embolism — Can death from pulmonary embolism be prevented? J. Am. Coll. Cardiol. *8*:146B, 1986.

29. England, R., and Magee, H.R.: Peripheral arterial embolism 1961–1985. Aust. N.Z. J. Surg. *57*:27, 1987.

30. Elliot, J.J., Jr., et al.: Arterial embolization. Problems of source, multiplicity, recurrence, and delayed treatment. Surgery *88*:833, 1980.

31. Morgan, M.: Amniotic fluid embolism. Anaesthesia *34:*20, 1979.

32. Roche, W.D., Jr., and Norris, H.J.: Detection and significance of maternal pulmonary amniotic fluid embolism. Obstet. Gynecol. *43*:729, 1974.

33. Price, T.M., et al.: Amniotic fluid embolism. Three case reports with a review of the literature. Obstet. Gynecol. Surv. *40*:462, 1985.

34. Rodgers, B.M., et al.: Effects of amniotic fluid on cardiac contractility and vascular resistance. Am. J. Physiol. *220*:1979, 1971.

35. Dolyniuk, M., et al.: Rapid diagnosis of amniotic fluid embolism. Obstet. Gynecol. *61*:288, 1983.

36. Editorial: Amniotic fluid embolism. Lancet *2*:398, 1979.

37. Thomas, I.H.: Caisson disease of bone: The seed and the soil. J.R. Coll. Surg. Edinb. *28*:347, 1983.

38. Gregg, P.J., and Walder, D.N.: Caisson disease of bone. Clin. Orthop. *210*:43, 1986.

39. Gossling, H.R., and Donohue, T.A.: The fat embolism syndrome. J.A.M.A. *241*:2740, 1979.

40. Robbins, S.L., et al.: Demonstration of intercoronary anastomoses in human hearts with a low viscosity perfusion mass. Circulation *33*:733, 1966.

41. Krainer, L.: Pathological effects of cerebral anoxia. Am. J. Med. *25*:258, 1958.

42. Seeley, H.F.: The pathophysiology of haemorrhagic shock. Br. J. Hosp. Med. *37*:14, 1987.

43. Resnekov, L.: Cardiogenic shock. Chest *83*:893, 1983.

44. Wilson, R.F.: The pathophysiology of shock. Intensive Care Med. *6*:89, 1980.

44a. Zimmerman, J.J., and Dietrick, K.A.: Current perspectives on septic shock. Pediatr. Clin. North Am. *34*:131, 1987.

45. Bond, R.F., and Johnson, G.: Vascular adrenergic interactions during hemorrhagic shock. Fed. Proc. *44*:281, 1985.

46. McIntosh, T.K., et al.: Endorphins in primate hemorrhagic shock: Beneficial action of opiate antagonists. J. Surg. Res. *40*:265, 1986.

47. Feuerrstein, G., and Hallenbeck, J.M.: Prostaglandins, leukotrienes, and platelet-activating factor in shock. Annu. Rev. Pharmacol. Toxicol. *27*:301, 1987.

48. Beutler, B., and Cerami, A.: Cachectin: More than a tumor necrosis factor. N. Engl. J. Med. *316*:379, 1987.

48a. Girardin, E., et al.: Tumor necrosis factor and interleukin-1 in the serum of children with severe infectious purpura. N. Engl. J. Med. *319*:397, 1988.

49. Ziegler, E.J.: Tumor necrosis factor in humans. N. Engl. J. Med. *318*:1533, 1988.

50. Lefer, A.M.: Interaction between myocardial depressant factor and vasoactive mediators with ischemia and shock. Am. J. Physiol. *252*:R193, 1987.

51. Billhardt, R.A., and Rosenbush, S.W.: Cardiogenic and hypovolemic shock. Med. Clin. North Am. *70*:853, 1986.

52. Trump, B.F., et al.: The application of electron microscopy and cellular biochemistry to the autopsy. Observations on cellular changes in human shock. Hum. Pathol. *6*:499, 1975.

53. Trump, B.F.: The role of cellular membrane systems in shock. *In* The Cell in Shock. The Proceedings of a Symposium on Recent Research Developments and Current Clinical Practice in Shock. Kalamazoo, Michigan, Upjohn Symposium, 1974, p. 16.

54. Hackel, D.B., et al.: The heart in shock. Circ. Res. *35*:805, 1974.

55. McGovern, V.J.: Hypovolemic shock with particular reference to the myocardial and pulmonary lesions. Pathology *12*:63, 1980.

Genetic Disorders

The study of genetics truly has reached the promised land. The technology is now at hand to manipulate— "engineer"—the genetic code, carrying with it the hope of alleviating or curing mutations.

Much of the recent progress in medical genetics has resulted from the spectacular advances in molecular biology, involving recombinant DNA technology. It is possible, for example, to excise human DNA by using restriction enzymes and to clone the excised fragments in appropriate cloning vectors. When a known DNA fragment is used to detect whether an unknown DNA fragment or m-RNA carries complementary nucleotide sequences, it is termed a **DNA probe.** The underlying principle in the applications of DNA probe analysis is *molecular hybridization.* Hybridization can take place between complementary strands of either DNA or RNA to form DNA:DNA and RNA:RNA hybrids, or between a DNA and an RNA strand to form a DNA:RNA hybrid. A variety of techniques utilizing DNA probes are now routinely used for research and diagnosis.[1] The details of these techniques are available in standard texts of molecular biology.[2] Here we will summarize the basic principles underlying some of the commonly employed methods.

• *Southern blotting* (or Southern blot analysis) involves DNA:DNA hybridization. In this procedure DNA extracted from the cells to be analyzed is digested by one or more restriction enzymes. These bacterial enzymes recognize a specific sequence of base pairs and cut the DNA wherever this sequence occurs. The multitude of DNA fragments so produced are separated on the basis of size by gel electrophoresis. The fragments are then denatured into single strands and transferred onto nitrocellulose membranes. A radiolabeled DNA probe is then applied to the nitrocellulose paper. If any DNA fragment on the paper contains a sequence complementary to that of the probe, hybridization occurs. Because the probe is radioactive, the hybridizing band can be revealed by autoradiography.

• *Northern blotting* (or Northern blot analysis) involves m-RNA:DNA hybridization. This procedure is utilized to detect whether a given gene is being transcribed. Total cellular m-RNA is extracted and subjected to agarose gel electrophoresis that separates m-RNA species on the basis of size. As in Southern blotting, the subsequent steps involve transfer (blotting) to nitrocellulose paper, hybridization with a labeled probe, and autoradiography. By this procedure the presence or absence of a given m-RNA as well as the size of the transcript can be determined.

• *Dot blotting* differs from Southern and Northern blotting in that it does not involve restriction digestion or size fractionation. RNA or DNA to be tested is applied or "dotted" onto a nitrocellulose membrane and probed with a radiolabeled DNA probe.

• *In situ hybridization* allows detection of specific DNA or m-RNA sequences in situ—i.e., within the cells. Unlike Northern and Southern blotting, the nucleic acids are not extracted from the cells, but, rather, probes are applied directly to appropriately preserved and treated tissue sections. This technique not only allows detection of genes or their products (or both) but also permits their localization within specific cells within the tissue.

The advances in molecular genetics have had a major impact in several areas of clinical medicine. At a practical level, molecular probes are proving increasingly useful in the diagnosis of genetic as well as nongenetic (e.g., infectious) diseases. The diagnostic applications of recombinant DNA technology will be detailed at the end of this chapter (p. 157). Here we will briefly mention some *therapeutic applications* of this technology, followed by a brief discussion of the strategies that can now be applied to unravel the molecular basis of human diseases.

In the last few years several cloned human genes have been induced to synthesize their products in unsuspecting bacteria. This ability to engineer large quantities of scarce biologically active products promises to revolutionize the treatment of certain diseases. Witness, for example, the recent availability of ultrapure recombinant growth hormone. As recently as 1985 growth hormone–deficient children had to be treated with hormone extracted from cadaver pituitaries. Not only was the availability of the human hormone limited, but in addition some pituitary extracts transmitted a virus that caused fatal Creutzfeldt-Jakob disease (p. 1401) in the recipients. Besides hormones, a variety of other biologic products such as factor VIII, thrombolytic agents, and immunomodulators (interleukin-2, interferons) are either already in clinical use or will shortly be available. Another exciting application on the horizon is the production of vaccines. Recombinant hepatitis B vaccine is now in use, and work is in progress to produce vaccines for influenza, malaria, and possibly AIDS.

At a more basic level, recombinant DNA technology has made a major impact on the understanding of the molecular basis of human disease. Two general strategies have been employed (Fig. 4–1).

• *Classic genetics:* This is the traditional approach that has been successfully utilized to study a variety of inborn errors of metabolism, such as phenylketonuria and disorders of hemoglobin synthesis. Common to these genetic diseases is a knowledge of the abnormal gene product and the corresponding protein. When the affected protein is known, a variety of methods can be employed to isolate the normal gene, clone it, and ultimately determine the molecular changes that affect the gene in patients with the disorder.

• *Reverse genetics:* Because in many common single-gene disorders, such as cystic fibrosis, there is no clue to the nature of the gene product that is defective, an alternative strategy called new genetics or "reverse genetics" has been employed. This approach initially ignores the biochemical clues from the phenotype and relies instead on the chromosomal localization of the mutant gene. Approximate location of the gene is accomplished by linkage to known "marker genes" that are in close proximity to the disease locus. Once the region in which the mutant gene lies has been localized within reasonably narrow limits, the next step is to clone several pieces of DNA from the relevant segment of the genome. Expression of the cloned DNA in vitro, followed by identification of the protein products, can then be used to identify the aberrant protein encoded by the mutant genes. This approach has been used successfully in several diseases, such as chronic granulomatous disease (a disorder of leukocyte microbicidal function) and, more recently, Duchenne's muscular dystrophy (a hereditary disorder characterized by progressive muscle weakness).[3]

With this background of "new genetics" we can turn next to the time-honored classification of human diseases into three categories: (1) those environmentally determined, (2) those genetically determined, and (3) those in which both environmental and genetic factors play a role. Microbiologic infections at

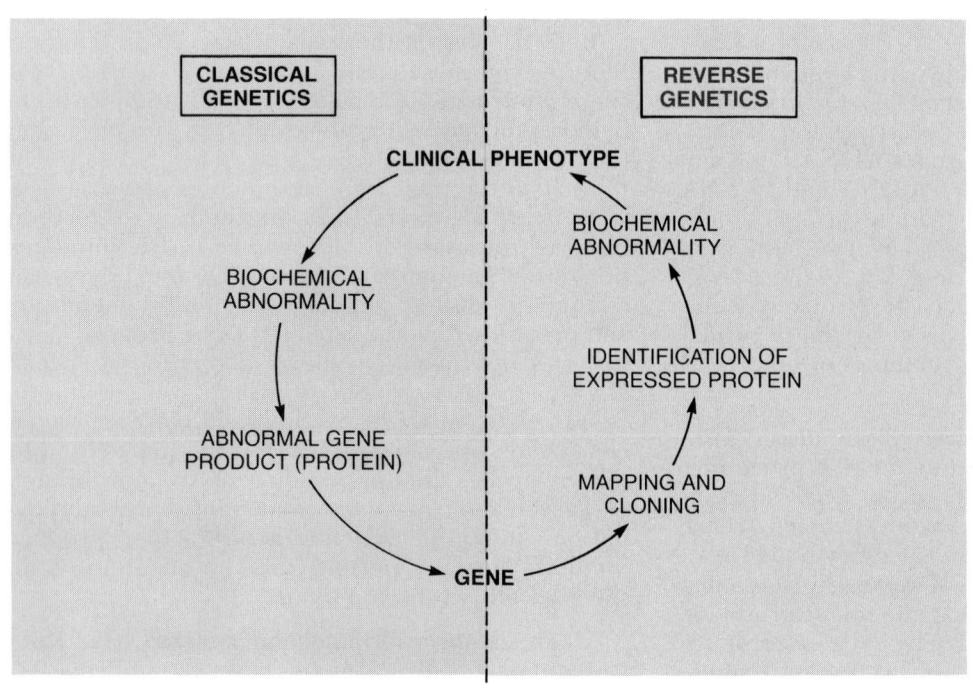

Figure 4–1. A schematic illustration of the strategies employed in classic and reverse genetics. The classic approach begins with relating the clinical phenotype to biochemical-protein abnormalities, followed by isolating the mutant gene. The reverse genetic strategy begins by mapping and cloning the disease gene without any knowledge of the gene product. Identification of the gene product and the mechanism by which it produces the disease follows the isolation of the mutant gene.

first sight might appear to be representative of the first category; however, even here, with the expansion of knowledge about the role of immune response genes in the control of immunocompetence, it is evident that microbiologic infections — and all disorders to a greater or lesser degree — are conditioned by the genotype. Perhaps automobile accidents are examples in which the environment totally determines the nature of the disease. Into the third category just mentioned fall many of the important diseases of man such as peptic ulcer, diabetes mellitus, atherosclerosis, schizophrenia, and probably most cancers, in which clearly both nature and nurture play significant roles.

Recognizing the complexity of this nature-nurture interplay, our interest here is with those diseases in which nature (i.e., the genetic component) plays a major if not determinant role. The genetic diseases encountered in medical practice represent only the tip of the iceberg, that is, those with less extreme genotypic errors permitting full embryonic development and live birth. It is estimated that 50% of spontaneous abortuses during the early months of gestation have a demonstrable chromosomal abnormality; there are in addition numerous smaller detectable errors and many others still beyond our range of identification. About 1% of all newborn infants possess a gross chromosomal abnormality.[4] How many more mutations remain hidden? For years we have marveled at the biologic precision in the processes of mitosis and meiosis, but it is now unmistakably evident that there is far more slippage in these processes than has been appreciated. Fortunately, among the many with mutations, only the "fittest" survive. Nonetheless, in the United States alone these "fittest" add up to 12 million with some genetic disease, imposing in the aggregate an enormous health problem.

It is beyond the scope of this book to review normal human genetics. It is necessary, however, to clarify several commonly used terms — *hereditary*, *familial*, and *congenital*. Hereditary disorders, by definition, are derived from one's parents and are transmitted in the gametes through the generations and therefore are familial. The term *congenital* simply implies "born with." It should be noted that some congenital diseases are not genetic, as for example congenital syphilis. On the other hand, not all genetic diseases are congenital; patients with hereditary Huntington's disease, for example, begin to manifest their condition only after the third or fourth decade of life.

Genetic disorders fall into three major categories: (1) those arising in chromosomal aberrations; (2) those related to mutant genes of large effect; and (3) diseases with multifactorial (polygenic) inheritance. The first category includes disorders that have been shown to be the consequence of numerical or structural abnormalities in the chromosomes. The second category, sometimes referred to as mendelian disorders, includes many relatively rare conditions such as the storage diseases and inborn errors of metabolism, all

resulting from single gene mutations of large effect. Most of these conditions are hereditary and familial. The third category includes some of the most common disorders of humans, such as hypertension and diabetes mellitus. Multifactorial or polygenic inheritance implies that usually both genetic and environmental influences condition the expression of a phenotypic characteristic or disease. The genetic component involves the additive result of multiple genes of small effect; the environmental contribution may be small or large, and in some cases it is required for expression of the phenotypic attribute.

Before we turn to a consideration of specific entities, the normal karyotype will be reviewed, as well as the nature and causes of mutations.

THE NORMAL KARYOTYPE — CYTOGENETICS

As is well-known, human somatic cells contain 46 chromosomes; these comprise 22 homologous pairs of autosomes and two sex chromosomes, XX in the female and XY in the male. The study of chromosomes — karyotyping — is the basic tool of the cytogeneticist. The usual procedure of producing a chromosome spread is to arrest mitosis in cultured cells in metaphase by the use of colchicine, and then to stain the chromosomes. In a metaphase spread, the individual chromosomes take the form of two chromatids connected at the centromere to create the familiar "X" and wishbone conformations. *If the centromere connects the chromatids in their center, the chromosome is said to be metacentric; if the centromere is eccentrically placed, the chromosome is said to be submetacentric. In some chromosomes, the centromere is almost, but not quite, at the end of the chromatids. These are acrocentric chromosomes,* all of which can bear small projections on their short arms. The projections are known as *satellites* and are involved in the formation of nucleoli. Prior to 1970 the techniques utilized in karyotyping resulted in solid, dark staining of the chromosomes, and hence only limited distinction of chromosomes was possible; they were classified into seven groups (A through G) on the basis of their size and the position of the centromere.

In 1970, Caspersson and colleagues described the identification of each individual chromosome on the basis of a distinctive and reliable pattern of alternating light and dark bands along the length of the chromosome.[5] Although a number of *banding techniques* have since been developed, G (Giemsa) banding is the most widely utilized. A normal male karyotype with G banding is illustrated in Figure 4–2. In recent years, the resolution obtained by banding techniques has been dramatically improved by obtaining the cells in prophase. The individual chromosomes appear markedly elongated, and up to 1500 bands per karyotype may be recognized.[6] The use of these banding techniques permits certain identifica-

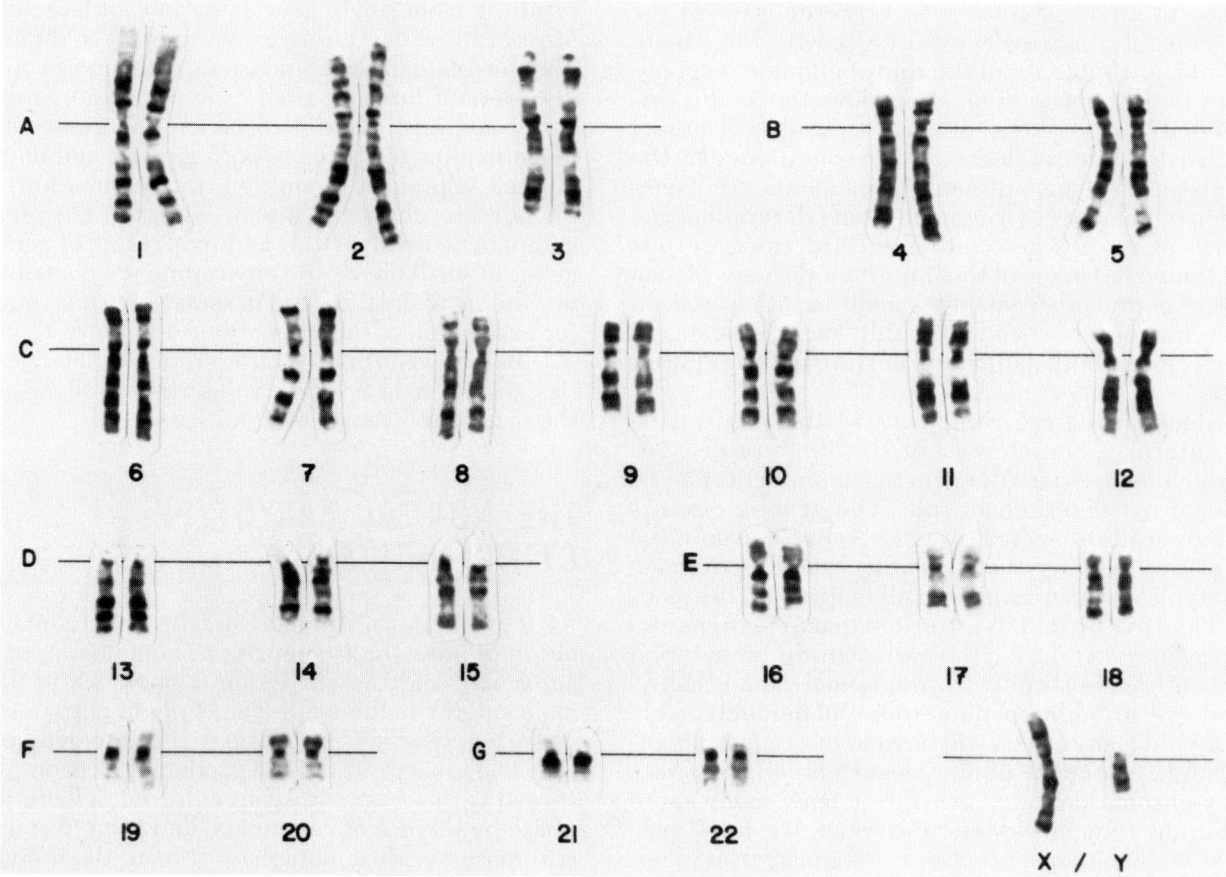

Figure 4–2. A normal male karyotype with G banding. (Courtesy of Dr. Nancy R. Schneider, Department of Pathology, Southwestern Medical Center, Dallas, Texas.)

tion of each chromosome, as well as delineation of precise breakpoints and other subtle alterations, to be described later.

Before this discussion of the normal karyotype is concluded, reference must be made to commonly used cytogenetic terminology. Karyotypes are usually described using a shorthand system of symbols. In general, the following order is utilized: total number of chromosomes is given first, followed by the sex chromosome complement, and finally the description of any abnormality. For example, a male with trisomy 21 is designated 47,XY,+21. The symbols denoting structural alterations of chromosomes are described along with the abnormalities in a later section. Here we should mention that the short arm of a chromosome is designated "p" (for petit) and the long arm is referred to as "q" (the next letter of alphabet). In a banded karyotype, each arm of the chromosome is divided into two or more regions by prominent bands. The regions are numbered (1, 2, 3, etc.) from the centromere outward. Each region is further subdivided into bands and sub-bands, and these are ordered numerically as well (Fig. 4–3). Thus, the symbol Xp21.2 refers to a chromosomal segment located on the short arm of the X chromosome, in region 2, band 1 and sub-band 2.

MUTATIONS

The term mutation refers to a heritable alteration in the genome. Some mutations involve large segments of the genome and therefore produce visible alterations in the structure of a chromosome. Such chromosomal aberrations and their consequences are described later (p. 127). Many mutations, however, are submicroscopic. They may result in partial or complete deletion of a gene, or more often affect a single base. For example, a single nucleotide base may be *substituted* by a different base, resulting in a *point mutation* (Fig. 4–4). Less commonly, one or two base pairs may be *inserted* or *deleted* from the DNA, leading to alterations in the reading frame of the DNA strand; hence these are referred to as *frame shift* mutations (Fig. 4–5). The consequences of mutations are varied, depending on several factors, including the type of mutation and the genomic site affected by it. Details of specific mutations and their effects are discussed along with the relevant disorders throughout this text. Here we will briefly review some general principles relating to the effects of mutations.

• *Mutations within coding sequences.* A point mutation (single base substitution) may alter the code in a trip-

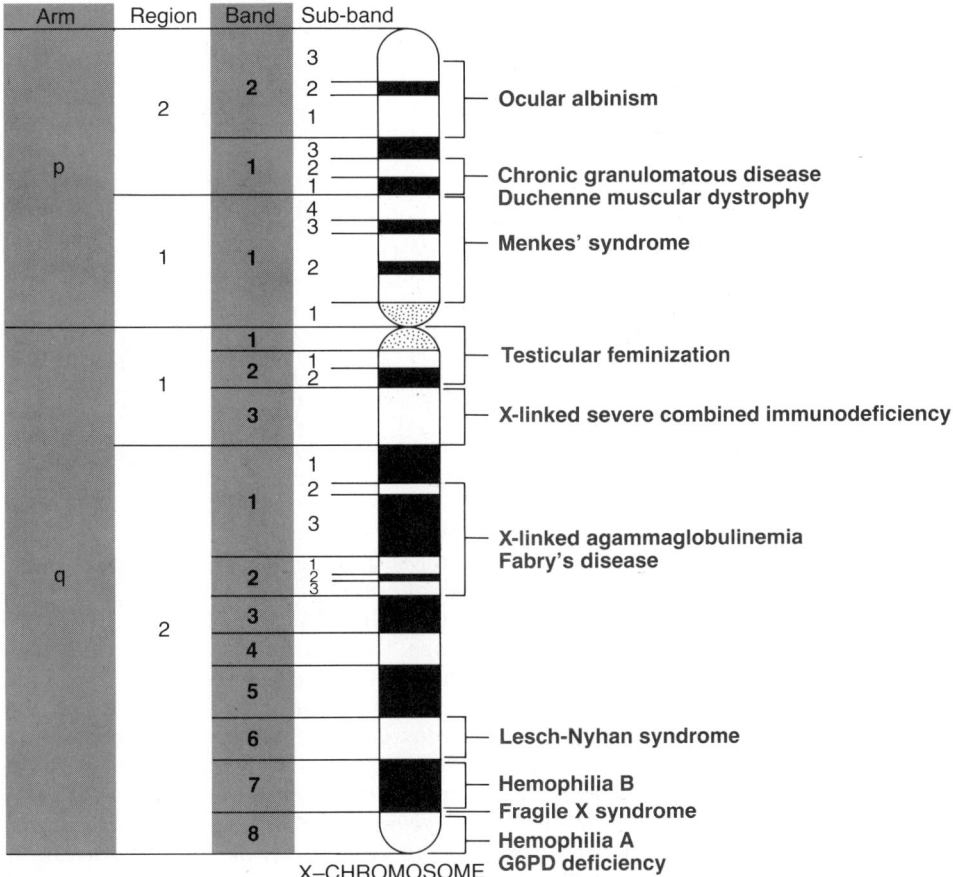

Figure 4–3. Details of a banded karyotype of the X chromosome (also called idiogram). Note the nomenclature of arms, regions, bands, and sub-bands. On the right side, the approximate locations of some genes that cause disease are indicated.

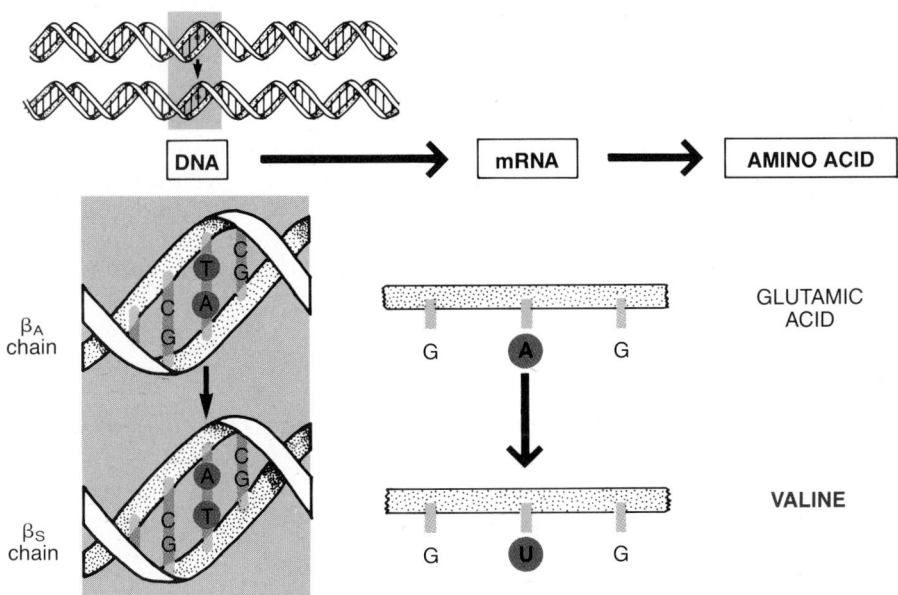

Figure 4–4. Schematic illustration of a point mutation resulting from a single base pair change in the DNA. In the example shown, a CTC to CAC change alters the meaning of the genetic code (GAG to GTG in the opposite strand), leading to replacement of glutamic acid by valine in the polypeptide chain. This change, affecting the sixth amino acid of the normal β-globin (β_A) chain, converts it to sickle β-globin (β_S).

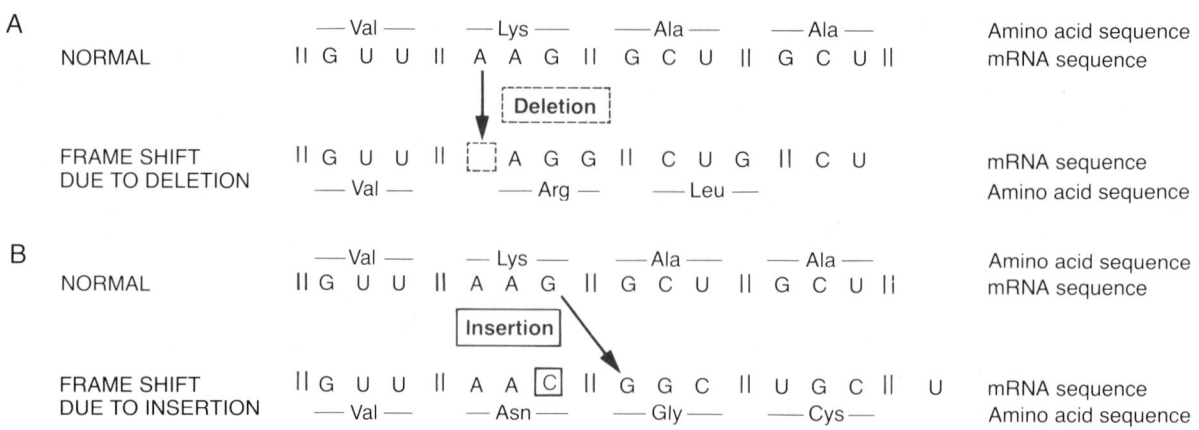

Figure 4–5. Schematic illustration of mutations that alter the reading frame by *(A)* deletion of a base or *(B)* insertion of a base.

let of bases and lead to the replacement of one amino acid by another in the gene product. Because these mutations alter the meaning of the genetic code, they are often termed "missense mutations." An excellent example of this type is the sickle mutation affecting the β-globin chain of hemoglobin (p. 666). Here the nucleotide triplet CTC (or GAG in mRNA), which codes for glutamic acid, is changed to CAC (or GUG in mRNA), which codes for valine (Fig. 4–4). This single amino acid substitution alters the physicochemical properties of hemoglobin, giving rise to sickle cell anemia. Besides producing an amino acid substitution, a point mutation may change an amino acid codon to a chain terminator or *stop codon* ("nonsense mutation"). Taking again the example of β-globin, a point mutation affecting the codon for glutamine (CAG) creates a stop codon (UAG) if U is substituted for C (Fig. 4–6). This change leads to premature termination of β-globin gene translation, and the resulting short peptide is rapidly degraded. The affected individuals lack β-globin chains and develop a severe form of anemia called β⁰ thalassemia (p. 671).

• *Mutations within noncoding sequences.* Deleterious effects may also result from mutations that do not involve the exons. As is well-known, transcription of DNA is initiated and regulated by promoter and enhancer sequences that are found downstream or upstream of the gene. Point mutations or deletions involving these regulatory sequences can lead to a marked reduction in or total lack of transcription. Such is the case in certain forms of hereditary hemolytic anemias (p. 672). In addition, point mutations

within introns lead to defective splicing of intervening sequences. This, in turn, interferes with normal processing of the initial m-RNA transcripts and results in a failure to form mature m-RNA transcripts. Therefore, translation cannot take place and the gene product is not synthesized (p. 672).

To summarize, mutations can interfere with protein synthesis at various levels. Transcription may be suppressed with gene deletions and point mutations involving promoter sequences. Abnormal mRNA processing may result from mutations affecting introns or splice junctions, or both. Translation is affected if a stop codon (chain termination mutation) is created within an exon. And, finally, some point mutations may lead to the formation of an abnormal protein without impairing any step in protein synthesis. As will be discussed later, the phenotypic effects of mutant genes are determined at least in part by the nature of proteins involved (e.g., enzymes, structural proteins, or regulatory proteins).

The cause or causes of most mutations are largely unknown. However, certain environmental influences such as radiation, chemicals, and viruses increase the rate of so-called "spontaneous" mutations. Because the mutagenic potential of environmental agents is linked to their role in carcinogenesis, they are discussed later in Chapter 6 (p. 268).

Against this background we can now turn our attention to the three categories of previously mentioned genetic disorders (p. 123): *(1) chromosomal (cytogenetic) disorders with visible chromosomal abnormalities, (2) mendelian disorders having origin in a*

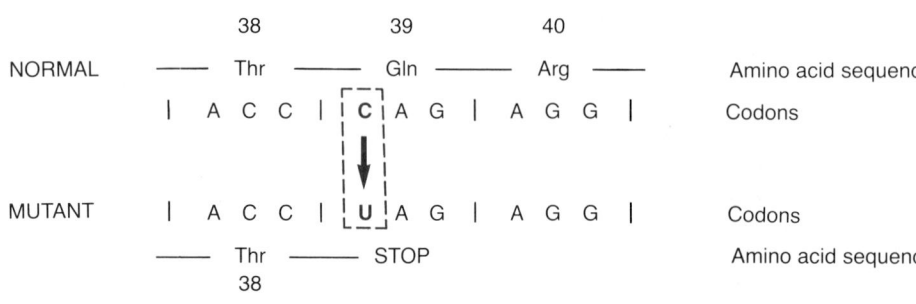

Figure 4–6. Point mutation leading to premature chain termination. Partial mRNA sequence of the β-globin chain of hemoglobin showing codons for amino acids 38 to 40. A point mutation (C → U) in codon 39 changes glutamine (Gln) codon to a stop codon, and hence protein synthesis stops at the 38th amino acid.

mutation of a single gene of large effect, (3) disorders having origin in multifactorial inheritance. To these three we can add another group to include the few entities having variable modes of transmission. The number of disorders assigned to each of these categories grows apace with each passing year. Undoubtedly we have no more than scratched the surface in investigating these categories. Although individually rare, in the aggregate genetic disorders are not uncommon. It is estimated that they account for approximately 15% of the pediatric admissions in teaching hospitals. Some will be dealt with in subsequent chapters; here, we will confine our discussion to some of those which are more important and common.

CYTOGENETIC DISORDERS

The aberrations underlying cytogenetic disorders may take the form of an abnormal number of chromosomes or alterations in the structure of one or more chromosomes. The normal 46 count is known as the *2n* or *diploid number*. The first meiotic reduction division in the formation of gametes halves the number to the *n* or *haploid count of 23*. The normal count would be expressed as 46,XX for the female and 46,XY for the male. Any exact multiple of the haploid number is called *euploid*. However, if an error occurs in meiosis or mitosis and a cell acquires a chromosome complement that is not an exact multiple of 23, it is referred to as *aneuploidy*. The usual causes for aneuploidy are *nondisjunction* and *anaphase lag*. The former occurs when a homologous pair of chromosomes fails to disjoin at the first meiotic division, or the two chromatids fail to separate either at the second meiotic division or in somatic cell divisions, resulting in two aneuploid cells. When nondisjunction occurs during gametogenesis, the gametes formed have either an extra chromosome $(n + 1)$ or one less chromosome $(n - 1)$. Fertilization of such gametes by normal gametes would result in two types of zygotes — trisomic $(2n + 1)$, or monosomic $(2n - 1)$. In anaphase lag, one homologous chromosome in meiosis or one chromatid in mitosis lags behind and is left out of the cell nucleus. The result is one normal cell and one cell with monosomy. As will be seen, monosomy or trisomy involving the sex chromosomes, or even more bizarre aberrations, are compatible with life and are usually associated with variable degrees of phenotypic abnormalities. On the other hand, *monosomy involving an autosome generally represents loss of too much genetic information to permit live birth or even embryogenesis, but a number of autosomal trisomies do permit survival.* With the exception of trisomy 21, all yield severely handicapped infants who almost invariably die at an early age.[7]

Occasionally, *mitotic errors in early development give rise to two or more populations of cells in the same individual, a condition referred to as mosaicism.* This can result from mitotic errors during the cleavage of the fertilized ovum or in somatic cells. Mosaicism affecting the sex chromosomes is relatively common. In the division of the fertilized ovum an error may lead to one of the daughter cells receiving three sex chromosomes, while the other receives only one, yielding, for example, a 45,X/47,XXX mosaic. All descendent cells derived from each of these precursors will thus have either a 47,XXX count or a 45,X count. Such a patient would be a mosaic variant of Turner's syndrome, with the extent of phenotypic expression dependent on the number and distribution of the 45,X cells. If the error occurs at a later cleavage, the mosaic will have three populations of cells, with some possessing the normal 46,XX complement, i.e., 45,X/46,XX/47,XXX. Repeated mitotic errors may lead to many populations of cells. Elderly males show a propensity for loss of the Y chromosome in varying proportions of cells.

Autosomal mosaicism appears to be much less common than that involving the sex chromosomes. An error in an early mitotic division affecting the autosomes usually leads to a nonviable mosaic with autosomal monosomy. Rarely, the loss of a nonviable cell in embryogenesis is tolerated, yielding a mosaic, e.g., 46,XY/47,XY,+21. Such a patient would be a trisomy 21 mosaic with partial expression of the Down's syndrome depending on the proportion of cells expressing the trisomy.

A second category of chromosomal aberrations is associated with changes in the structure of chromosomes. To be visible by currently available banding techniques, a fairly large amount of DNA (approximately 4 million base pairs), containing several thousand genes, must be involved. Structural changes in chromosomes usually result from chromosome breakage followed by loss or rearrangement of material. Such alterations occur spontaneously at a low rate that is increased by exposure to environmental mutagens such as chemicals and ionizing radiations. In addition, several rare autosomal recessive genetic disorders — Fanconi's anemia, Bloom's syndrome, and ataxia-telangiectasia — are associated with such a high level of chromosomal instability that they are known as "chromosome-breakage syndromes." As discussed later (p. 266) there is a significantly increased risk of cancers in all these conditions. In the following section we will briefly review the more common forms of alterations in chromosome structure and the symbols used to signify them.

In *translocation*, a segment of one chromosome is transferred to another (Fig. 4–7). In one form, called *balanced reciprocal translocation*, there are single breaks in each of the two chromosomes, with exchange of genetic material. Such a translocation might not be disclosed without banding techniques. A balanced reciprocal translocation between the long arm of chromosome 2, which has been shortened, and the short arm of chromosome 5, which has been lengthened, would be written 46,XX,t(2q–;5p+). This individual has 46 chromosomes with altered morphology of one of the chromosomes 2 and one of the chromosomes 5. Because there has been no loss of genetic material, the individual

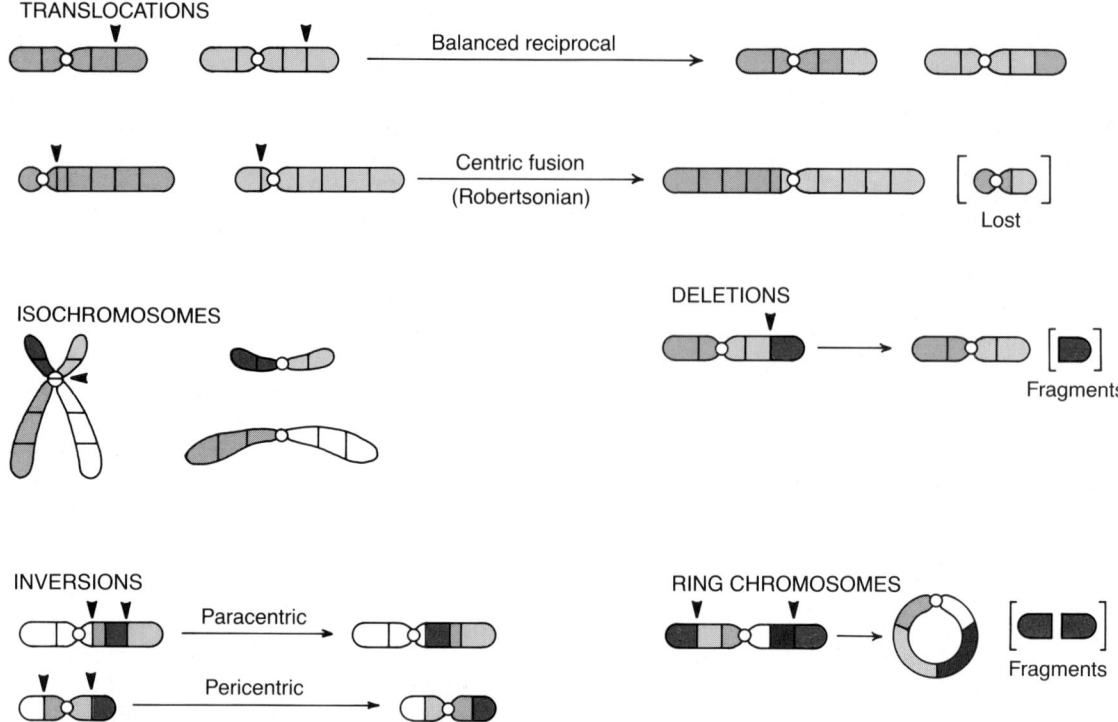

Figure 4–7. Types of chromosomal rearrangements.

will be phenotypically normal. However, a balanced translocation carrier is at increased risk of producing abnormal gametes. For example, in the case cited above a gamete containing one normal chromosome 2 and a translocated chromosome 5 may be formed. Such a gamete would be unbalanced since it would not contain the normal complement of genetic material. Subsequent fertilization by a normal gamete would lead to the formation of an abnormal (unbalanced) zygote, resulting in spontaneous abortion or birth of a malformed child. The other important pattern of translocation is called a *Robertsonian translocation* (or centric fusion), a reciprocal translocation between two acrocentric chromosomes. Typically the breaks occur close to the centromeres of each chromosome, affecting the long arm in one and the short arm in the other. Transfer of the segments then leads to one very large chromosome and one extremely small one. Often, the small product is lost (Fig. 4–7); however, it carries so little genetic information that this loss is compatible with a normal phenotype, and Robertsonian translocation between two chromosomes is encountered in apparently normal individuals. The significance of this form of translocation also lies in the production of abnormal progeny, as discussed later with Down's syndrome.

Isochromosome formation results when the centromere divides in a transverse plane rather than in the normal long axis of the chromosome. Thus, the misdivision gives rise to two chromosomes, one consisting of, for example, two short arms only and the other consisting of two long arms (Fig. 4–7). Both these chromosomes now have genetic information that is morphologically identical in both arms. The most common isochromosome present in live births involves the long arm of the X and is designated i(Xq). Because isochromosomes of the short arm of X do not occur, i(Xq) is associated with monosomy for genes on the short arm of X.

Deletion refers to loss of a portion of chromosome. It may be terminal or interstitial. Terminal deletions result from a single break in the arm of a chromosome, producing a fragment with no centromere, which is then lost at the next cell division. This might be designated as 46,XY,16p− to indicate loss of some part of the short arm of chromosome 16 (Fig. 4–7). One can specify in which region and at what band the break and deletion has occurred, as, for example, 46,XY,del(16)(p14), meaning a break point in region 1 band 4 of the short arm of chromosome 16. Interstitial deletions occur when there are two breaks in the chromosome followed by loss of the region between the breaks.

Inversion refers to a rearrangement that involves two breaks within a single chromosome with reincorporation of the inverted segment (Fig. 4–7). Such an inversion involving only one arm of the chromosome is known as paracentric. If the breaks are on opposite sides of the centromere, it is known as pericentric. Inversions are perfectly compatible with normal development.

A *ring chromosome* is a special form of deletion. It is produced when a deletion occurs at both ends of a chromosome with fusion of the damaged ends

(Fig. 4–7). If significant genetic material is lost, phenotypic abnormalities result. This might be expressed as 46,XY,r(14). Ring chromosomes do not behave normally in meiosis or mitosis and usually result in serious consequences.

All these structural anomalies at one time or another have been described for both autosomes and sex chromosomes. The use of banding techniques has begun to disclose an additional great variety of minor structural abnormalities in chromosomes involving differences in the size of certain bands, largely composed of heterochromatin. Because the heterochromatin contains little genetic information that is transcribed into messenger RNA, it would not be expected to have much effect on the phenotype. However, even minor structural changes may have importance. In the process of repair of a break, one or more genes may be lost. It has been observed that even in balanced translocations that are acquired rather than inherited, mental retardation and other abnormalities may result. Moreover, phenotypically normal parents who have a balanced structural abnormality such as inversion or a balanced translocation are more prone to suffer meiotic errors in gametogenesis, and therefore they are at increased risk of having miscarriages or chromosomally unbalanced and abnormal children, or both.

Many more numerical and structural aberrations are described in specialized texts, and the number of abnormal karyotypes encountered in genetic diseases increases with each passing month. As pointed out earlier, the clinically important chromosome disorders represent only the "tip of the iceberg." It is estimated that approximately 7.5% of all conceptions have a chromosomal abnormality, most of which are not compatible with survival or live birth. Thus, chromosome abnormalities are identified in 50% of early spontaneous abortuses and in 5% of stillbirths and infants who die in the immediate postnatal period. Even in live-born infants the frequency is approximately 0.5 to 1.0%. Many of the early deaths are attributable to gross structural malformations or severe developmental defects in the brain. It is beyond the scope of this book to discuss most of the clinically recognizable chromosomal disorders. Hence we will focus our attention on those few that are most common.

CYTOGENETIC DISORDERS INVOLVING AUTOSOMES

Several of the major autosomal disorders are presented in Table 4–1.

Trisomy 21 (Down's Syndrome)

Down's syndrome is the commonest of the chromosomal disorders and a major cause of mental retardation. In the United States the incidence in newborns is about 1 in 700. Approximately 95% of affected individuals have trisomy 21, so their chromosome count is 47 (Fig. 4–8); most others have normal chromosome numbers, but the extra chromosomal material is present as a translocation. As mentioned earlier, the most common cause of trisomy and therefore of Down's syndrome is meiotic nondisjunction. The parents of such children have a normal karyotype and are normal in all respects.

Maternal age has a strong influence on the incidence of Down's syndrome. It occurs once in 1550 live births in women under the age of 20 years, in contrast to 1 in 25 live births for mothers over 45 years of age.[8] The correlation with maternal age suggests that in most cases the meiotic nondisjunction of chromosome 21 occurs in the ovum. Indeed, recent studies have confirmed that in 80% of cases, the extra chromosome 21 is of maternal origin.[7] Although many hypotheses have been advanced, the reason for the increased susceptibility of the ovum to nondisjunction remains unknown.[7] In 20% of cases the extra chromosome 21 is of paternal origin. No effect of paternal age has been found in these cases.[9]

In about 4% of all cases of Down's syndrome, the extra chromosomal material derives from the inheritance of a parental chromosome bearing a translocation of the long arm of chromosome 21 to another acrocentric chromosome, e.g., 22 or 14. Because the fertilized ovum already possesses two normal autosomes 21, the translocated material provides the same triple gene dosage as trisomy 21. Such cases are frequently familial and the translocated chromosome is inherited from one of the parents, who is most frequently a carrier of a Robertsonian translocation, e.g., mother with karyotype 45,XX, −14, −21, +t (14q 21q). Theoretically the carrier parent has a one in three chance of bearing a live child with Down's syndrome; however, the observed frequency of affected children in such cases is much lower. The reasons for this discrepancy are not well understood.

Approximately 1% of Down's syndrome patients are mosaics, usually having a mixture of cells with 46 and 47 chromosomes. This results from mitotic nondisjunction of chromosome 21 during an early stage of embryogenesis. Symptoms in such cases are variable and milder, depending on the proportion of abnormal cells. Clearly, in cases of translocation or mosaic Down's syndrome, maternal age is of no importance.

The diagnostic clinical features of this condition, listed in Table 4–1, are usually readily evident, even at birth. The flat facial profile, oblique palpebral fissures, and epicanthic folds account for the older, unfortunate designations "mongolism" and "mongolian idiocy." Down's syndrome is a leading cause of mental retardation. The mental retardation is severe; approximately 80% of those afflicted have an intelligence quotient (IQ) of 25 to 50. Ironically, these severely disadvantaged children usually have a gentle, shy manner and are far more easily directed than their more fortunate siblings, less burdened with chromosomes. It should be pointed out that some mosaics with Down's syndrome have very mild pheno-

Table 4–1. Disorders Associated with the Autosomes

DISORDER	EXAMPLES OF KARYOTYPE	APPROXIMATE PERCENTAGE OF CASES	MATERNAL AGE	CLINICAL FEATURES
Down's Syndrome *(1 in 700 births)*				
Trisomy 21 type	47,XX,+21 47,XY,+21	95%	Increased	1. Mental retardation
				2. Flat facial profile
				3. Oblique palpebral fissures
Translocation type	46,XX,−14,+t(14q21q) 46,XY,−22,+t(21q22q)	4%	Normal	4. Epicanthic folds
				5. Muscle hypotonia
				6. Cardiac defects
Mosaic type	46,XX/47,XX,+21	1%	Normal	7. Susceptibility to infection
				8. Susceptibility to acute leukemia
				9. Hyperflexibility
				10. Lack of Moro reflex
				11. Abundant neck skin
				12. Broad and/or short trunk
				13. Dysplastic ears
				14. Horizontal palmar crease
				15. Dysplastic pelvis (on radiographs)
				16. Dysplastic middle phalanx (on radiographs)
Trisomy 18 (Edwards' Syndrome) *(1 in 8000 births)*				
Trisomy 18 type	47,XX,+18 47,XY,+18	90%	Increased	1. Mental retardation and failure to thrive
				2. Prominent occiput
				3. Micrognathia and low-set ears
				4. Hypertonicity
Mosaic type	46,XX/47,XX,+18	10%	Normal	5. Flexion of fingers (second and fifth digits overlapping third and fourth)
				6. Rocker bottom feet
				7. Cardiac, renal, and intestinal defects
				8. Short sternum and small pelvis
Trisomy 13 (Patau's Syndrome) *(1 in 6000 births)*				
Trisomy 13 type	47,XX,+13 47,XY,+13	Over 80%	Increased	1. Microcephaly and mental retardation
				2. Arrhinencephaly
Translocation type	46,XX,−14,+t(14q13q)	10%	Normal	3. Scalp defect
				4. Microphthalmia
Mosaic type	46,XX/47,XX,+13	10%	Normal	5. Cleft lip and cleft palate
				6. Polydactyly
				7. Abnormal ears
				8. Cardiac dextroposition and interventricular septal defect
				9. Extensive visceral defects
Cri du Chat (Cat-cry) Syndrome *(1 in 50,000 births)*				
	46,XX,5p− 46,XY,5p−		Normal	1. Mental retardation
				2. Microcephaly and round facies
				3. Mewing cry
				4. Epicanthic folds

typic changes and may even have normal or near-normal intelligence.

In addition to the phenotypic abnormalities and the mental retardation already noted some other clinical features are worthy of note.

• Approximately 40% of the patients have congenital heart disease, most commonly septal defects, which are responsible for the majority of the deaths in infancy and early childhood.
• Children with trisomy 21 have an 18- to 20-fold increased risk of developing acute leukemia,[10] chiefly lymphoblastic, but other types have also been noted. Curiously the increased frequency of leukemia is confined to the pediatric age group.
• Serious infections, particularly of the respiratory tract, are an important cause of morbidity and mortality in Down's syndrome. Quite mysteriously, however, consistent laboratory evidence for significant immune dysfunction is lacking.

Despite all these problems, improved medical care has increased the longevity of patients with trisomy 21. Currently the average estimated life expectancy is around 30 years and about 25% of individuals live up to the age of 50. With increased survival, another aspect of this disease has come to light. Virtually all patients with Down's syndrome over the age of 35 develop pathologic changes in the brain that are identical to those seen in Alzheimer's disease, a form of dementia (p. 1427).[11] A significant proportion (25 to 40%) of these patients also demonstrate cognitive changes characteristic of Alzheimer's dementia.

Although the karyotype and clinical features of trisomy 21 have been known for well over two decades, little is known about the molecular basis of Down's syndrome. Recent advances in gene mapping, however, have begun to penetrate the mystery. As mentioned earlier, Down's syndrome occurs not only in association with a complete extra copy of chromosome 21, but also when there is a triple dose of the genetic material carried by the long arm of chromosome 21 (translocation variant). By a careful study of

patients exhibiting partial trisomy 21, it has been determined that the region of chromosome 21 that is required for the full expression of Down's syndrome is limited to the 21q22 band.[12] Genes located within this "obligate Down's syndrome region" must be critical to the pathogenesis of the Down's syndrome phenotype (Fig. 4–9). Although this region of chromosome 21 is large enough to accommodate several hundred genes, only a handful have been assigned to this band. These include the genes encoding for GART (an enzyme involved in purine biosynthesis), cell surface receptor for interferon α/β, ets-2 (an oncogene), and possibly the amyloid β-protein that is deposited in the cerebral lesions of Alzheimer's disease. Is one or more of these genes related to the causation of Down's syndrome? It has been argued that excessive purine biosynthesis due to an extra copy of the GART gene may be responsible for mental retardation; the dysregulated expression of the onco-

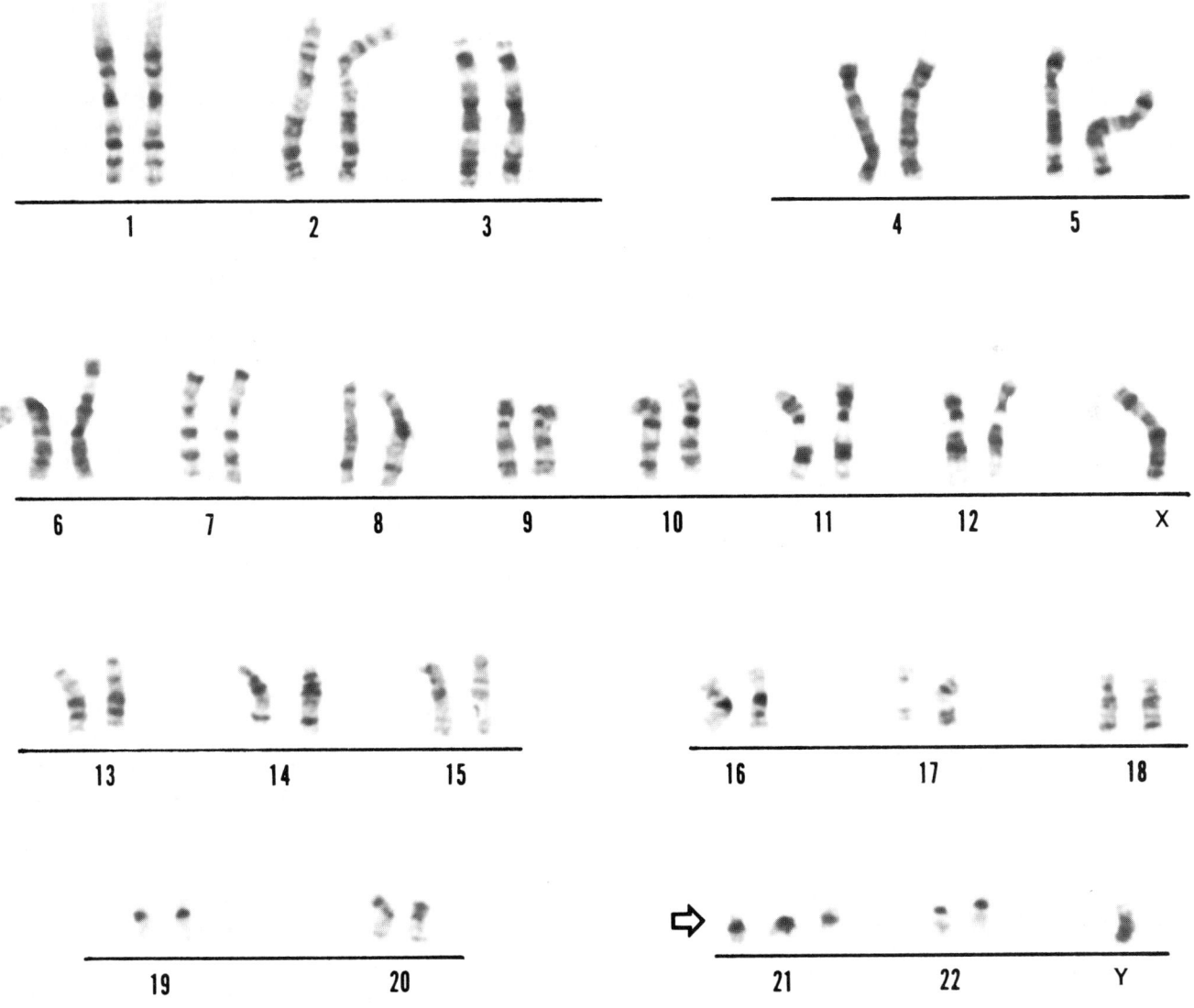

Figure 4–8. G-banded karyotype of a male with trisomy 21. (Courtesy of Dr. Patricia Howard-Peebles, Southwestern Medical School, Dallas, Texas.)

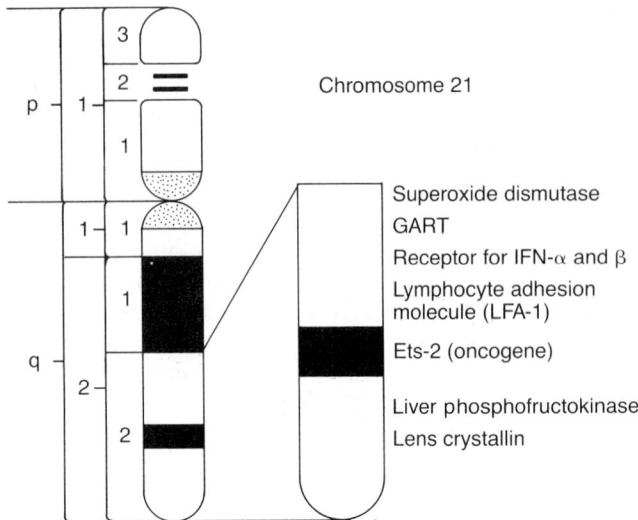

Figure 4–9. Idiogram of chromosome 21. The obligate Down's syndrome region 21q22 is enlarged, and genes mapped to this region are indicated. The orientation of these genes with respect to each other is not known.

gene ets-2 could be linked to the increased risk for leukemia; and the possible overproduction of amyloid β-protein could predispose to the premature Alzheimer's disease.[13] Although these scenarios seem plausible, they must be considered speculations at present.

Other Trisomies

A variety of other trisomies involving chromosomes 8, 9, 22, 18, and 13 have been described. Only trisomy 18 (Edward's syndrome) and trisomy 13 (Patau's syndrome) are common enough to merit brief description. As noted in Table 4–1, they share several karyotypic and clinical features with trisomy 21. Thus, most cases of Edward's and Patau's syndromes result from meiotic nondisjunction and therefore carry a complete extra copy of chromosomes 18 and 13, respectively. As in Down's syndrome, an association with increased maternal age is also noted. However, in contrast to trisomy 21, the malformations are much more severe and wide ranging. As a result, only rarely do these infants survive beyond the first year of life. Most succumb within a few weeks to months.

Cri du Chat Syndrome (5p−)

Deletion of the short arm of chromosome 5 (5p−) was so named because affected infants up to the age of one year have the characteristic cry of a cat. The major clinical features are given in Table 4–1. The mental retardation is quite severe, and congenital heart anomalies (usually ventricular septal defects) are present in about 25%. In general, these children thrive better than those with the trisomies, and some survive into adult life. As the infant grows older, the kitten cry and high vocal register improve, rendering diagnosis more difficult.

Other deletion syndromes involving virtually every chromosome have been identified with the new banding techniques. A variety of congenital malformations are encountered in association with the deletions, including abnormalities of the brain, mental retardation, microcephaly, hypertelorism, congenital heart disease, and malformations of the face, hands, and ears.

CYTOGENETIC DISORDERS INVOLVING SEX CHROMOSOMES

The genetic diseases associated with karyotypic changes involving the sex chromosomes are far more common than those related to autosomal aberrations. Furthermore, imbalances (excess or loss) of sex chromosomes are much better tolerated than similar imbalances of autosomes. In large part this latitude relates to two factors that are peculiar to the sex chromosomes: (1) lyonization or inactivation of all but one X chromosome, and (2) the small amount of genetic material carried by the Y chromosome. We will discuss these features briefly to aid our understanding of sex-chromosomal disorders.

In 1961, Mary Lyon outlined the X-inactivation, or what is commonly known as the Lyon hypothesis. It states that *(1) only one of the X chromosomes is genetically active, (2) the other X of either maternal or paternal origin undergoes heteropyknosis and is rendered inactive, (3) inactivation of either the maternal or paternal X occurs at random among all the cells of the blastocyst on or about the 16th day of embryonic life, and (4) inactivation of the same X chromosome persists in all the cells derived from each precursor cell.* Thus, the great preponderance of normal females are in reality mosaics and have two populations of cells, one with an inactivated maternal X and the other with an inactivated paternal X. Herein lies the explanation of why females have the same dosage of X-linked active genes as the male. The inactive X can be seen in the interphase nucleus as a darkly staining small mass in contact with the nuclear membrane known as the Barr body or X chromatin. Barr bodies are present in all somatic cells of normal females, but they are most readily demonstrated in smears of buccal squamous epithelial cells. Although the Lyon hypothesis provides a satisfactory explanation for the observation that females do not have double dosage of X-linked genes, it fails to account for the somatic and gonadal abnormalities that are invariably associated with imbalances of X chromosome number. For example, if only one X chromosome is active, why should patients with the 45,X (Turner's syndrome) or 47,XXY (Klinefelter's syndrome) have any abnormalities? These questions, along with some other recent observations, have led to the following modifications of the Lyon hypothesis:

• First, it is now accepted that, although one X chromosome is inactivated in all cells during embryogenesis, it is selectively reactivated in germ cells prior to the first meiotic division.[14] Thus it seems that both X chromosomes are required for normal gametogenesis.

• Second, it seems that X-inactivation does not involve the entire chromosome. For example, there is definite molecular and cytogenetic evidence that certain genes located in the Xq26-27 region remain active on both X chromosomes in normal females.[15]

With respect to the Y chromosome, it is well-known that it is both necessary and sufficient for male development. Indeed *irrespective of the number of X chromosomes, the presence of a single Y determines the male sex*. The gene that dictates testicular development (testis-determining factor) has been located on its distal short arm.[16]

With this background we can review some features that are common to all sex chromosome disorders.

• *In general, they induce subtle, chronic complaints relating to sexual development and fertility.*
• *They are often difficult to diagnose at birth, and many are first recognized at the time of puberty.*
• *In general, the higher the number of X chromosomes, in both male and female, the greater the likelihood of mental retardation.* The most important disorders arising in aberrations of sex chromosomes are cited in Table 4–2 and will be described briefly here.

Klinefelter's Syndrome

Klinefelter's syndrome is best defined as male hypogonadism that occurs when there are two or more X chromosomes and one or more Y chromosomes. It is one of the most frequent forms of genetic disease involving the sex chromosomes, as well as one of the most common causes of hypogonadism in the male. The incidence of this condition is approximately 1 in 850 live male births. It can rarely be diagnosed before puberty, particularly because the testicular abnormality does not develop before early puberty. The major clinical features are presented in Table 4–2. Particularly characteristic are the eunuchoid body habitus with abnormally long legs, the small atrophic testes often associated with a small penis, and the lack of such secondary male characteristics as deep voice, beard, and male distribution of pubic hair. The mean IQ is somewhat lower than normal, but mental retardation is uncommon. It should be noted, however, that this typical pattern is not seen in all cases, the only consistent finding being hypogonadism. Plasma gonadotropin levels, particularly FSH, are consistently elevated, whereas testosterone levels are variably reduced. Mean plasma estradiol levels are elevated by an as yet unknown mechanism. The ratio of estrogens and testosterone determines the degree of feminization in individual cases.

Klinefelter's syndrome is the principal cause of male infertility. The reduced spermatogenesis is re-

Table 4–2. Disorders Associated with the Sex Chromosomes

DISORDER	EXAMPLES OF KARYOTYPE	APPROXIMATE INCIDENCE	MATERNAL AGE	CLINICAL FEATURES
Klinefelter's Syndrome	47,XXY 46,XY/47,XXY	1 in 850 male births	Slightly increased	1. Testicular atrophy and azoospermia 2. Eunuchoid body habitus 3. Increase in sole-to–os pubis length 4. Gynecomastia 5. Female distribution of hair
Variants of Klinefelter's Syndrome	48,XXXY 49,XXXXY 48,XXYY	Rare	Increased	1. More severe mental retardation 2. Cryptochidism 3. Hypospadias 4. Radioulnar synostosis
Double Y Males	47,XYY	1 in 1000 male births	Normal	1. Phenotypically normal 2. Most over 6 feet tall 3. (?) Increased aggressive behavior
Turner's Syndrome (Gonadal Dysgenesis)	45,X	1 in 3000 female births	Normal	1. Short stature 2. Primary amenorrhea
Defective second X chromosome	46,XXp– 46,XXq–		Normal Normal	3. Infertility 4. Webbing of neck 5. Cubitus valgus
	46,X,i(Xq)		Normal	6. Peripheral lymphedema 7. Broad chest and wide-spaced nipples
Mosaicism	45,X/46,XX		Normal	8. Low posterior hairline 9. Pigmented nevi 10. Coarctation of aorta
Multiple X Females	47,XXX 48,XXXX	1 in 1200 female births	Increased	1. Mental retardation 2. Menstrual irregularities 3. Many affected persons normal and fertile
True Hermaphrodites				1. Testicular and ovarian tissue 2. Varying genital abnormalities
Most cases	46,XX			
Some mosaics	46,XX/47,XXY	Rare	Normal	

lated to several patterns of morphologic change in the testis. In some patients, the testicular tubules are totally atrophied and replaced by pink, hyaline, collagenous ghosts. In others, the dysgenesis is manifested by apparently normal tubules interspersed with atrophic tubules. In some patients, all tubules are primitive and appear embryonic, consisting of cords of cells that never developed a lumen or progressed to mature spermatogenesis. Hyperplasia of the Leydig cells has been reported in all these variants. According to some authors, however, there is no true Leydig cell hyperplasia but the Leydig cells appear prominent owing to atrophy and crowding of the tubules.[17]

The classic pattern of Klinefelter's syndrome is associated with a 47,XXY karyotype (82% of cases). This complement has been explained by nondisjunction during the meiotic divisions in one of the parents. The extra X chromosome is of maternal origin in 60% and of paternal origin in 40% of the cases. Advanced maternal age and irradiation of either parent have been suggested as relevant in the causation of this condition. In addition to this classic karyotype, some patients with Klinefelter's syndrome have been found to have a variety of mosaic patterns, most of them being 46,XY/47,XXY. Others are 47,XXY/48,XXXY and variations on this theme. Rare individuals have also been found to possess 48,XXXY or 49,XXXXY karyotypes. Such polysomic X individuals have further physical abnormalities, including cryptorchidism, hypospadias, more severe hypoplasia of the testes, and skeletal changes, such as prognathism and radioulnar synostosis.

XYY Syndrome

Supernumerary Y chromosomes may be found in the male, giving rise to 47,XYY, or even greater Y polysomy. Approximately 1 in 1000 live-born males has one of these karyotypes. Nearly all are phenotypically normal, but the individuals frequently are excessively tall and may be susceptible to severe acne. From present data it appears that the intelligence of these individuals is in the normal range.

Most controversial is the impact of extra Y chromosomes upon behavior. These karyotypes have been identified with increased frequency among inmates of penal institutions. The behavioral difficulties take the form of antisocial (not violent), delinquent, impulsive acting-out disorders.[18] From recent studies it appears that only about 1 to 2% of individuals with XYY phenotypes exhibit such deviant behavior; the overwhelming preponderance are no more antisocial than their peers who have fewer Y chromosomes.

Turner's Syndrome

This syndrome results from complete or partial monosomy of the X chromosome and is characterized primarily by hypogonadism in phenotypic females. In approximately 57% of the patients an entire X chromosome is missing, resulting in the 45,X karyotype. The remaining 43% have other abnormalities as described later. It should be emphasized that only about 3% of fetuses with the 45,X karyotype survive to birth. The surviving infants are severely affected, and unlike several other sex-chromosomal aneuploidies, the diagnosis of the 45,X variant of Turner's syndrome can often be made at birth or in early childhood.

Approximately 43% of the patients with Turner's syndrome do not carry the 45,X karyotype. Of these, (1) 40% have a complete deletion of the small arm of the X chromosome resulting in the formation of an isochromosome of the long arm X[46,X,i(Xq)], (2) 23% have a partial deletion of the small arm (Xp−), and (3) the remaining 37% are mosaics. It is important to appreciate the karyotypic heterogeneity associated with Turner's syndrome because it is responsible for significant variations in phenotype. In contrast to the patients with monosomy X, those who are mosaics or who have deletions (e.g., 46,XXq−) may have an almost normal appearance and may present only with primary amenorrhea.

The most severely affected infants generally present during infancy with edema (owing to lymph stasis) of the dorsum of the hand and foot, and sometimes swelling of the nape of the neck. The latter is related to markedly distended lymphatic channels, producing a so-called cystic hygroma (p. 593). As these infants develop, the swellings subside but often leave bilateral neck webbing and persistent looseness of skin on the back of the neck. Congenital heart disease is also common, particularly preductal coarctation of the aorta and aortic stenosis with endocardial fibroelastosis, anomalies that may account for some of the early deaths.

The principal clinical features in the adolescent and adult are cited in Table 4–2. At puberty there is failure to develop normal secondary sex characteristics. The genitalia remain infantile, breast development is inadequate, and there is little pubic hair. The mental status of these patients is usually normal, but a few may exhibit some retardation. Of particular importance in establishing the diagnosis in the adult is the shortness of stature (rarely exceeding 150 cm in height) and the amenorrhea. To be noted, *Turner's syndrome is the single most important cause of primary amenorrhea,* accounting for approximately one third of the cases.

As mentioned earlier, both X chromosomes are essential for normal development of the ovaries. To understand the pathogenesis of Turner's syndrome it is essential to review normal ovarian development. It has been said that "ovary is the most precisely doomed structure in the human body: it carries in its makeup the destruction of its own seeds."[19] During fetal development, ovaries contain as many as 7 million oocytes. However, the oocytes begin to disappear *in utero,* so that by birth there are about 3 million left, and by menarche their numbers have already dwindled to a mere 400,000. Further loss continues after puberty, and when menopause occurs fewer than 10,000 remain. In Turner's syndrome fetal ovaries develop normally early in embryogenesis, but the absence of the second X chromosome leads to an accelerated loss of oocytes, which is complete by the age of 2 years. In a sense, therefore, "menopause occurs before menarche,"[19] and the ovaries are reduced to atrophic fibrous strands, devoid of ova and follicles *("streak ovaries")*. The reduced estrogen output by the ovaries leads to elevated pituitary gonadotropin secretion.

Multi-X Females

Karyotypes with one to three extra X chromosomes have been described and are not uncommon, being found in about 1 in 1200 newborn females. Most of these women, according to current thought, are entirely normal. However, a variety of random findings may be present. As mentioned, there is an increased tendency to mental retardation in proportion to the number of extra X chromosomes. Thus, mental retardation is seen in all with the 49,XXXXX karyotype, whereas most with 47,XXX are unaffected. Some women have amenorrhea or occasionally other menstrual irregularities.

Hermaphroditism and Pseudohermaphroditism

The problem of sexual ambiguity is exceedingly complex, and only limited observations are possible here. For more details, reference should be made to specialized texts.[20] It will be no surprise to medical students that the sex of an individual can be defined on several levels. *Genetic sex* is determined by the presence or absence of a Y chromosome. No matter how many X chromosomes are present, a single Y chromosome dictates testicular development and the genetic male gender. The initially indifferent gonads of both the male and the female embryos have an inherent tendency to feminize, unless influenced by Y chromosome–dependent masculinizing factors. The testis determining factor (TDF) has been located on the distal short arm of Y. Another gene that has been mapped to the long arm of Y codes for a cell surface antigen (H-Y antigen) that is present on all male cells. *Gonadal sex* is based on the histologic characteristics of the gonads. *Ductal sex* depends on the presence of derivatives of the müllerian or wolffian ducts. *Phenotypic* or *genital sex* is based on the appearance of the external genitalia. Sexual ambiguity is present whenever there is disagreement among these various criteria for determining sex.

The term true hermaphrodite implies the presence of both ovarian and testicular tissue. In contrast, a pseudohermaphrodite represents a disagreement between the phenotypic and gonadal sex, i.e., a female pseudohermaphrodite has ovaries but male external genitalia; a male pseudohermaphrodite has testicular tissue but female-type genitalia. Disappointingly, karyotypic analyses have not shed much light on these difficult problems of intersex. Indeed, as will be seen, hormonal influences may induce sexual ambiguity completely apart from the genotype of the individual.

True hermaphroditism, implying the presence of both ovarian and testicular tissue, is an extremely rare condition. In some cases there is a testis on one side and an ovary on the other, whereas in other cases there may be combined ovarian and testicular tissue, referred to as ovotestes. Most of these individuals have a uterus and other ductal structures reminiscent of those found in both male and female. The external genitalia are usually ambiguous and could be interpreted either as a bifid scrotum or enlarged labia with a small penis or enlarged clitoris. The karyotype is 46,XX in two thirds of patients; most of the remaining are mosaics (e.g., XX/XXY) in which a Y-bearing cell line is present. The mechanism of aberrant gonadal differentiation is not clear. In those with the 46,XX karyotype there seems to be a translocation of the Y chromosome to the X chromosome or an autosome. Mosaics, obviously, have both X and Y chromosomes. Thus, true hermaphrodites are a heterogeneous group, having in common the presence of two X chromosomes as well as a complete or partial Y chromosome, in at least some of the cells.

Female pseudohermaphroditism is much less complex. The genetic sex in all cases is XX and the development of the gonads (ovaries) and internal genitalia is normal. Only the external genitalia are ambiguous or virilized. The basis of female pseudohermaphroditism is excessive and inappropriate exposure to androgenic steroids during the early part of gestation. Such steroids are most commonly derived from the fetal adrenal affected by congenital adrenal hyperplasia, which is transmitted as an autosomal recessive trait. Biosynthetic defects in the pathway of cortisol synthesis are present in these cases that lead secondarily to excessive synthesis of androgenic steroids by the fetal adrenal cortex (p. 1260). Less commonly, the virilizing steroids are maternal in origin. Androgen-secreting maternal tumors (e.g., the Sertoli-Leydig cell tumor), or more commonly administration of androgens or progestins to the mother during pregnancy, underlie such cases.

Male pseudohermaphroditism represents the most complex of all disorders of sexual differentiation. These individuals possess a Y chromosome and thus their gonads are exclusively testes, but the genital ducts or the external genitalia are incompletely differentiated along the male phenotype. Their external genitalia are either ambiguous or completely female. Male pseudohermaphroditism is extremely heterogeneous, with a multiplicity of causes. Common to all is defective virilization of the male embryo, which usually results from genetically determined defects in androgen synthesis or action, or both. In the vast majority androgen synthesis is normal but androgen action is impaired. The most common form, called *complete testicular feminization*, results from a mutation in the structural gene for the androgen receptor. This gene is located on the X chromosome, and hence complete testicular feminization is inherited as an X-linked recessive disorder.

MENDELIAN DISORDERS

All mendelian disorders are the result of expressed mutations in single genes of large effect transmitted by autosomal dominant, autosomal recessive, or X-linked modes of inheritance. It is not necessary to detail Mendel's laws here, as every student in biology, and possibly every garden pea, has learned about them at an early age. Only some comments of medical relevance will be made.

The number of mendelian disorders known has grown to monumental proportions. In a recent edition of his book, McKusick has listed over 4000 disorders.[21] It is estimated that every individual is a carrier of five to eight deleterious genes. Fortunately, most of these are recessive and therefore do not cause serious phenotypic effects. About 80 to 85% of these mutations are familial. The remainder represent new mutations acquired de novo by an affected individual. Obviously, such a proband (index patient) will have a normal family pedigree but, on the other hand, could be the forebear of affected generations to come. The extent to which mutations are expressed varies widely. Two variants associated with autosomal dominant inheritance are recognized: (1) *Penetrance* is expressed in mathematical terms: thus, 50% penetrance indicates that 50% of those who carry the gene express the trait. The factors that affect penetrance are not clearly understood, but this possibility is of obvious importance in genetic counseling. (2) In contrast to penetrance, if a trait is seen in all the individuals carrying the mutant gene but is expressed differently among individuals, the phenomenon is called *variable expressivity*. For example, polydactyly may be expressed in the toes or in the fingers as one or more extra digits.

Some autosomal mutations produce partial expression in the heterozygote and full expression in the homozygote. Sickle cell anemia is caused by substitution of normal hemoglobin (HbA) by hemoglobin S (HbS). When an individual is homozygous for the mutant gene, all the hemoglobin is of the abnormal HbS type, and even under normal atmospheric pressures of oxygen the disorder is fully expressed, i.e., sickling deformity of all red cells and hemolytic anemia. In the heterozygote only a proportion of the hemoglobin is HbS (the remainder being HbA), and therefore red cell sickling and possibly hemolysis occur only when there is exposure to lowered oxygen tension. This is referred to as the sickle cell trait to differentiate it from full-blown sickle cell anemia.

Although gene expression is usually described as dominant or recessive, it should be remembered that in some cases both alleles of a gene pair may be fully expressed in the heterozygote—a condition called *codominance*. Histocompatibility and blood group an-tigens are good examples of codominant inheritance as well as *polymorphism*. The latter implies the existence of multiple allelic forms of a single gene.

A single mutant gene may lead to many end effects, termed *pleiotropism*, and conversely mutations at several genetic loci may produce the same trait (*genetic heterogeneity*). Sickle cell anemia may serve as an example of pleiotropism. In this hereditary disorder, not only does the point mutation in the gene give rise to HbS, which predisposes the red cells to hemolysis, but in addition the abnormal sickled red cells tend to cause a logjam in small vessels, inducing, for example, splenic fibrosis, organ infarcts, and bone changes. The numerous differing end-organ derangements are all related to the primary defect in hemoglobin synthesis. On the other hand, profound childhood deafness, an apparently homogeneous clinical entity, results from 16 different types of autosomal recessive mutations. Recognition of genetic heterogeneity is not only important in genetic counseling, but is also relevant in the understanding of the pathogenesis of some common disorders, such as diabetes mellitus (p. 994).

BIOCHEMICAL BASIS OF MENDELIAN DISORDERS

Mendelian disorders result from alterations involving single genes, implying that these diseases result from a primary abnormality in a *single protein molecule*. Broadly speaking, three kinds of proteins may be affected by mutation—enzymes, structural proteins, and regulatory proteins. To some extent the pattern of inheritance of the disease is related to the kind of protein affected by the mutation, as will be described later.

The mechanisms involved in single-gene mendelian disorders can be classified into four categories: *(1) enzyme defects and their consequences; (2) defects in membrane receptors and transport systems; (3) alterations in the structure, function, or quantity of non-enzyme proteins; and (4) mutations resulting in unusual reactions to drugs.*

ENZYME DEFECTS AND THEIR CONSEQUENCES.

Mutations may result in the synthesis of a defective enzyme with reduced activity or in a reduced amount of a normal enzyme. In either case, the consequence is a metabolic block. Figure 4–10 provides an example of an enzyme reaction in which the substrate S is converted by intracellular enzymes E_1, E_2, and E_3 into an end product P through intermediates I_1 and I_2. In this model the final product P exerts feedback control on enzyme E_1. A minor pathway producing small quantities of M_1 and M_2 also exists. The biochemical consequences of an enzyme defect in such a reaction may lead to three major consequences: *(1) Accumulation of the substrate*, which, depending on the site of block, may be accompanied by accumulation of one or both intermediates. Moreover, an increased concentration of I_2 may stimulate the minor pathway and thus lead to

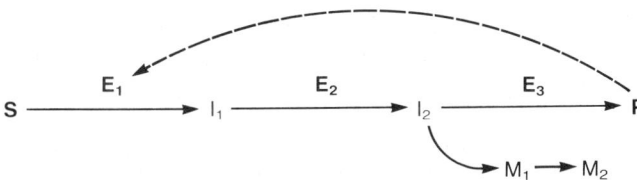

Figure 4–10. A schema illustrating the conversion of a substrate (S) to the end product (P), through several intermediates (I), brought about by enzymes (E). P exerts feedback inhibition of E_1. M denotes products of minor pathways.

an excess of M_1 and $\tilde{M_2}$. Under these conditions tissue injury may result if the precursor, the intermediates, or the products of alternate minor pathways are toxic in high concentrations. For example, in galactosemia, the deficiency of galactose-1-phosphate uridyltransferase (p. 532) leads to the accumulation of galactose and consequent tissue damage. A deficiency of phenylalanine hydroxylase (p. 530) results in the accumulation of phenylalanine. Excessive accumulation of complex substrates within the lysosomes due to deficiency of degradative enzymes is responsible for a group of diseases generally referred to as *lysosomal storage diseases* (p. 144). *(2) An enzyme defect can lead to a metabolic block and a decreased amount of end product* that may be necessary for normal function. For example, a deficiency of melanin may result from lack of tyrosinase, which is necessary for the biosynthesis of melanin from its precursor tyrosine. This results in the clinical condition called albinism, to be discussed later (p. 143). If the end product is a feedback inhibitor of the enzymes involved in the early reactions (in Figure 4–10 it is shown that P inhibits E_1), the deficiency of the end product may permit overproduction of intermediates and their catabolic products, some of which may be injurious at high concentrations. A prime example of a disease with such an underlying mechanism is the Lesch-Nyhan syndrome (p. 1356). *(3) Failure to inactivate a tissue-damaging substrate.* This is best exemplified by alpha-1-antitrypsin ($\alpha1$-AT) deficiency. Patients who have an inherited deficiency of serum $\alpha1$-AT are unable to inactivate neutrophil elastase in their lungs. Unchecked activity of this protease leads to destruction of elastin in the walls of lung alveoli, leading eventually to pulmonary emphysema (p. 769).

DEFECTS IN RECEPTORS AND TRANSPORT SYSTEMS. Many biologically active substances have to be actively transported across the cell membrane. This is generally achieved by one of two mechanisms —through initial binding to a specific receptor site followed by internalization, or via a carrier protein. A genetic defect in a receptor-mediated transport system is exemplified by familial hypercholesterolemia, in which inadequate synthesis of receptors leads to defective transport of low-density lipoproteins (LDL) into the cells and secondarily to excessive cholesterol synthesis by complex intermediary mechanisms (p. 140). In Hartnup's disease, on the other hand, the transport system for tryptophan (and certain other amino acids) across the intestinal cells is defective. Because tryptophan is a precursor of the vitamin nicotinamide, symptoms of pellagra (p. 453) develop.

ALTERATIONS IN STRUCTURE, FUNCTION, OR QUANTITY OF NONENZYME PROTEINS. Genetic defects resulting in alterations of structural proteins often have widespread secondary effects, as exemplified by sickle cell disease (p. 666). Indeed, the hemoglobinopathies, sickle cell disease being one, all of which are characterized by defects in the structure of the globin molecule, best exemplify this category. In contrast to the hemoglobinopathies, the group of thalassemias results from mutations in genes that affect the amount of globin chains synthesized. Thalassemias are associated with reduced amounts of structurally normal α- or β-globin chains (p. 670). Other examples of genetically defective structural proteins that we shall discuss in this chapter involve collagen and are exemplified by Marfan's and Ehlers-Danlos syndromes.

GENETICALLY DETERMINED ADVERSE REACTIONS TO DRUGS. Certain genetically determined enzyme deficiencies are unmasked only after exposure of the affected individual to certain drugs. This special area of genetics, called pharmacogenetics, is of considerable clinical importance.[22] The classic example of drug-induced injury in the genetically susceptible individual is associated with a deficiency of the enzyme glucose-6-phosphate dehydrogenase (G6PD). Under normal conditions, G6PD deficiency does not result in disease, but on administration, for example, of the antimalarial drug primaquine, a severe hemolytic anemia results (p. 665).

Despite the usefulness of a pathogenetic classification, based on the nature of the underlying biochemical defect, mendelian disorders are generally classified according to their mode of inheritance, a tradition followed in the succeeding sections.

AUTOSOMAL DOMINANT DISORDERS

The general rules that govern the transmission of autosomal dominant disorders are well-known and will not be repeated here.[8] Only a few salient features are summarized here.

• Mutations usually involve complex structural proteins, such as collagen, or those that function as regulatory proteins, such as low-density lipoprotein receptors.
• Clinical features can be modified by reduced penetrance and variable expressivity, discussed earlier.
• There may be delayed age of onset of clinical features, as occurs in Huntington's disease.
• In every autosomal dominant disorder a proportion of the affected individuals owe their disorder to de novo mutations affecting the gametes of their parents. These patients do not have affected parents and their siblings are not affected, neither do they incur an increased risk of developing the disease. The propor-

Table 4-3. Autosomal Dominant Disorders

DISORDER	CHAPTER, PAGE
Familial hypercholesterolemia	Chapter 4, p. 140
Adult polycystic kidney disease	Chapter 21, p. 1020
Huntington's disease	Chapter 29, p. 1430
Hereditary spherocytosis	Chapter 14, p. 663
Marfan's syndrome	Chapter 4, p. 138
von Willebrand's disease	Chapter 14, p. 696
Neurofibromatosis	Chapter 4, p. 139
Tuberous sclerosis	Chapter 29, p. 1441
Hereditary hemorrhagic telangiectasia	Chapter 12, p. 590
Familial colonic polyposis	Chapter 18 p. 896
Ehlers-Danlos syndromes (some variants)	Chapter 4, p. 155
Osteogenesis imperfecta	Chapter 28, p. 1318
Acute intermittent porphyria	Chapter 27, p. 1306
von Hippel–Lindau disease	Chapter 4, p. 140

tion of individuals who develop the disease due to new mutations is related to the effect of the disease on reproductive fitness. A marked reduction in the reproductive ability is associated with a high frequency of cases arising from new mutations.

Table 4–3 provides a listing of the more common autosomal dominant disorders. Many are discussed more logically in other chapters, as indicated in the table. A few autosomal dominant conditions not considered elsewhere are discussed here, either because of their frequency or because they illustrate significant genetic principles.

Marfan's Syndrome

Marfan's syndrome is an uncommon but interesting *disorder of the connective tissues of the body, manifested principally by changes in the skeleton, eyes, and cardiovascular system.*[23] Because affected individuals have unusually long, slender extremities, particularly elongation of the fingers, this entity has also been termed *arachnodactyly* (spider fingers). Approximately 70 to 85% of the cases are familial and transmitted by autosomal dominant inheritance. The remainder are sporadic and arise from new mutations. In contrast to Down's syndrome, in which the risk for the offspring rises with maternal age, it is the paternal age that is important in the sporadic cases of Marfan's syndrome; fathers of affected children are about seven years older than the average.

Skeletal abnormalities are the most striking feature of Marfan's syndrome. Typically, the patient is unusually tall with exceptionally long extremities and long, tapering fingers and toes. Because the tall stature is contributed largely by the lower segment of the body, the ratio of the upper segment (top of the head to the pubis) to the lower segment (top of pubic ramus to the floor) is significantly lower than the norm for the age, race, and sex. The joint ligaments in the hands and feet are lax, suggesting that the patient is double-jointed; typically, the thumb can be hyperextended back to the wrist. The head is commonly dolichocephalic (long-headed) with bossing of the frontal eminences and prominent supraorbital ridges. Because President Abraham Lincoln possessed many of these physical characteristics it is strongly suspected that he had Marfan's syndrome. A variety of spinal deformities may appear, including kyphosis, scoliosis, or rotation or slipping of the dorsal or lumbar vertebrae. The chest is classically deformed, presenting either pectus excavatum (deeply depressed sternum) or a pigeon-breast deformity. Subcutaneous fat is usually scant, and muscular development is poor; thus, these patients have a long, gaunt appearance, sometimes marked by the many distortions of the body habitus mentioned.

The **ocular changes** take many forms. Most characteristic is bilateral subluxation or dislocation (usually outward and upward) of the lens, referred to as ectopia lentis. This abnormality is so uncommon in persons who do not have this genetic disease that the finding of bilateral ectopia lentis should raise the suspicion of Marfan's syndrome. The axial length of the globe is markedly increased, predisposing to severe myopia and retinal detachment. The cornea is relatively flat, further exaggerating the visual problems. All these ocular changes relate to a basic defect in connective tissue and impaired support of the ocular structures.

Cardiovascular lesions are the most life-threatening features of this disorder. The two most common lesions are mitral valve prolapse and, of greatest importance, dilatation of the ascending aorta owing to cystic medionecrosis. Histologically, the changes in the media are virtually identical to those found in cystic medionecrosis not related to Marfan's syndrome (p. 582). **Loss of medial support results in progressive dilatation of the aortic valve ring and the root of the aorta, giving rise to severe aortic incompetence.** Weakening of the media also predisposes to an intimal tear, which may initiate an intramural hematoma that cleaves the layers of the media to produce a dissecting aneurysm (p. 582). After cleaving the aortic layers for considerable distances, sometimes back to the root of the aorta or down to the iliac arteries, the hemorrhage often ruptures through the aortic wall. Such a calamity is the cause of death in 30 to 45% of these individuals.

Although mitral valve lesions are more frequent, they are clinically less important than aortic lesions. Loss of connective tissue support in the mitral valve leaflets makes them soft and billowy, creating the so-called "floppy valve" (p. 628). Valvular lesions, along with lengthening of the chordae tendineae, frequently give rise to mitral regurgitation. Similar changes may affect the tricuspid, and rarely the aortic, valves. Echocardiography greatly enhances the ability to detect the cardiovascular abnormalities and is therefore extremely valuable in the diagnosis of Marfan's syndrome.

Although the lesions just described typify Marfan's syndrome, it must be emphasized that there is great variation in the clinical expression of this genetic disorder. Patients with prominent eye or cardiovascular changes may have few skeletal abnormalities, whereas others with striking changes in body habitus have no eye changes. Although variability in clinical expression may be seen within a family, interfamilial variability is much more common and extensive. The most likely explanation for the varied expression of Marfan's syndrome is genetic heterogeneity, i.e., different mutations produce similar phenotypes.

It is disappointing to report that, despite all the striking clinical findings, the basic nature of the underlying connective tissue defect is still obscure. It is logical to suspect some defect in collagen or elastin — the two structural proteins of connective tissue. Indeed, a variety of changes in collagen and elastin have been reported by several workers, but so far no consistent pattern has emerged.[24] Based on recent advances in the understanding of molecular defects in other hereditary connective tissue disorders (e.g., Ehlers-Danlos syndromes, p. 155, and osteogenesis imperfecta, p. 1318) it can be safely assumed that Marfan's syndrome is caused by a variety of mutations, either in one particular gene or in several genes.[25]

Although the precise nature of the connective tissue defect is not clear (and may well differ in different families), much interest has centered on the concept that the basic defect in Marfan's syndrome is decreased formation of cross-linkages in collagen or elastin fibers, or both, which impairs their tensile strength. Indeed, in rats fed sweet pea meal derived from the seeds of *Lathyrus odoratus*, marfanoid manifestations develop owing to defects in collagen cross-linkages. The active ingredient responsible for the production of *lathyrism* is β-aminopropionitrile, which blocks cross-linkages in collagen and elastin fibers by inhibiting the enzyme lysyl-oxidase (p. 80). Because lysyl-oxidase is a copper-dependent enzyme, the search for possible genetic metabolic derangements led to the study of *Menke's syndrome*, an X-linked recessive disorder of man marked by a block in the intestinal absorption of copper. In this rare metabolic disorder, changes in aortic collagen and elastin are present that are attributable to the deficiency of the cross-linking enzyme lysyl-oxidase. However, there is no evidence of any impairment of copper metabolism or lysyl-oxidase activity in Marfan's syndrome. Defective cross-link formation could also be brought about by mutations that affect critical lysine or histidine residues in the collagen chains, but preliminary studies have failed to reveal mutations within or close to the structural genes for collagen types I, II, or III.[26] Alternatively some workers have postulated that the primary defect in Marfan's syndrome involves elastin fibers and that the defects in collagen are secondary.[27] This may well be the case, at least in some situations, as Marfan's syndrome is in all probability a genetically heterogeneous disorder.

As an autosomal dominant syndrome to be anticipated in 50% of the offspring of an affected parent, Marfan's syndrome is of tragic significance. The average age at death is between 30 and 40 years.[28] The great majority of these deaths are caused by rupture of dissecting aneurysms, followed in importance by cardiac failure. Unhappily, there are no satisfactory means of consistently preventing these calamitous consequences, even when the diagnosis is established at an early age.

Neurofibromatosis

Neurofibromatosis is a relatively common disorder with a frequency of almost 1 in 3000.[29] Although approximately 50% of the patients have a definite family history consistent with autosomal dominant transmission, the remainder appear to represent new mutations, perhaps affecting the same gene or genes. In familial cases, the expressivity of the disorder is variable but the penetrance is 100%. *There is more than one form of neurofibromatosis, pointing to genetic heterogeneity.*[30] Most common is the *von Recklinghausen's disease*, or classic neurofibromatosis, which has three major features: (1) multiple neural tumors dispersed anywhere on or in the body; (2) numerous pigmented skin lesions, some of which are "café au lait" spots; and (3) pigmented iris hamartomas, also called Lisch nodules. A bewildering assortment of other abnormalities (cited later) may accompany these cardinal manifestations.

The neurofibromas arise within or are attached to nerve trunks anywhere in the skin, including the palms and soles, as well as in every conceivable internal site, including the cranial nerves (particularly the acoustic nerve). Acoustic neuromas when they occur in classic neurofibromatosis are unilateral, in contrast to the bilateral tumors in the central or acoustic form of neurofibromatosis, to be described later. On the surface of the body, neurofibromas generally occur in profusion and range from discrete, soft, yielding, subcutaneous nodules less than 1 cm in diameter, to moderate-sized pedunculated lesions, to huge, multilobar pendulous masses, 20 cm or more in greatest diameter. The latter, referred to as plexiform neurofibromas, diffusely involve subcutaneous tissue and contain numerous tortuous, thickened nerves; the overlying skin is frequently hyperpigmented. These may grow to massive proportions, causing striking enlargement of a limb or some other body part (vividly depicted in the movie *Elephant Man*). Similar tumors may occur internally, and in general the deeply situated lesions tend to be large. Microscopically neurofibromas are composed of a proliferation of all the elements in the peripheral nerve, including neurites, Schwann cells, and fibroblasts. Typically, these components are dispersed in a loose, disorderly pattern, often in a loose, myxoid stroma. Elongated, serpentine Schwann cells predominate, with their slender, spindle-shaped nuclei. The loose disorderliness of the microscopic architecture helps to differentiate these neural tumors from related neurilemmomas (schwannomas) (p. 1445). Neurilemmomas composed entirely of Schwann cells virtually never undergo malignant transformation, whereas the neurofibromas of von Recklinghausen's disease become malignant in about 3% of patients.[31] Malignant transformation is most common in the very large plexiform tumors attached to large nerve trunks of the neck or extremities. The superficial lesions, despite their size, rarely become malignant.

The cutaneous pigmentations, the second major component of this syndrome, are present in over 90% of patients. Most commonly they appear as light brown **café au lait** macules, with generally smooth borders, often located over nerve trunks. They are usually round to ovoid, with their long axes parallel to the underlying cutaneous nerve. Although normal individuals may have a few café au lait spots, it is a clinical maxim that when six or more spots over 1.5 cm in diameter are present, the patient is likely to have neurofibromatosis.

Lisch nodules are present in over 94% of patients who are six years or older. They do not produce any symptoms but are helpful in establishing the diagnosis.

A wide range of associated abnormalities has been reported in these patients. Perhaps most common (30 to 50% of patients) are skeletal lesions, which take a variety of forms, including (1) erosive defects due to contiguity of neurofibromas to bone, (2) scoliosis, (3) intraosseous cystic lesions, (4) subperiosteal bone cysts, and (5) pseudarthrosis of the tibia. Patients with von Recklinghausen's disease have a two- to four-fold greater risk of developing other tumors, especially meningiomas, optic gliomas, and pheochromocytomas.[31] However, a slight increase in the frequency of some non-neurogenic tumors including Wilms' tumor, rhabdomyosarcoma, and acute nonlymphocytic leukemias has also been reported.

Although some patients with this condition have normal mentality, there is an unmistakable tendency for reduced intelligence. When neurofibromas arise within the gastrointestinal tract, intestinal obstruction or gastrointestinal bleeding may occur. Narrowing of a renal artery by a tumor may induce hypertension. The range of clinical presentations is almost limitless, but ultimately the diagnosis rests on the concurrence of multiple café au lait spots and multiple skin tumors. However, these cardinal features may not be well developed at birth, and in many patients the disease is not discovered until adult life. The skin pigmentations become more evident with age as giant melanosomes in epidermal cells accumulate melanin, and the neural tumors, though small at first, slowly enlarge.

There are three other genetic variants of neurofibromatosis,[29] of which only the *central or acoustic form* is common enough to merit discussion. In these patients, bilateral acoustic nerve tumors are invariably present with or without skin tumors. Café au lait spots are present but Lisch nodules in the iris are not found.

As with most mendelian disorders, the genetic basis of von Recklinghausen's disease is unknown. Although the neurofibromatosis gene had not been identified at the time of this writing, its location on chromosome 17 in the region 17q12-17q22 has been established.[32] It is interesting to note that the gene encoding the nerve growth factor receptor has also been mapped to the same region of chromosome 17, raising the intriguing possibility that proliferation of neural elements, a hallmark of neurofibromatoses, may result from an abnormal response of nerve cells to nerve growth factor. In contrast to the classic form of neurofibromatosis, the gene for the central or acoustic form has been mapped to chromosome 22q11, confirming that this variant is genetically distinct.[33]

von Hippel–Lindau Disease

von Hippel–Lindau disease is a rare autosomal dominant disorder characterized by *a variety of benign and malignant neoplasms widely dispersed throughout the body.*[34] The most common and characteristic neoplasms are retinal hemangioblastoma (retinal angiomatosis), sometimes referred to as von Hippel's tumor, and hemangioblastoma of the cerebellum, sometimes called Lindau's tumor. The other common tumors are hemangioblastoma of the medulla oblongata or spinal cord; angiomas of the liver and kidney; adenomas of the kidney and epididymis; renal cell carcinoma; adrenal pheochromocytoma; and cysts of the pancreas, kidney, and epididymis. Less frequently present are angiomas and cysts in a number of other organs, including lungs, spleen, omentum, adrenal gland, and ovary. In this roster the most important are the hemangioblastomas of the central nervous system, because these are the immediate cause of death in over half of all patients. Retinal angiomatosis is also of significance because it causes visual disturbances that are the presenting symptoms in many patients. Attention should also be directed to the renal cell carcinoma, as this is found in up to 50% of the patients, is usually bilateral, and presents at an earlier age than sporadic, nonfamilial cases of this tumor cell type. It is a major cause of death when present. Interestingly, the gene for von Hippel–Lindau disease has been mapped to the chromosome 3p25, a region that is often deleted in sporadic cases of renal cell carcinoma.[35] This observation supports the idea of "recessive cancer genes" discussed later in Chapter 6, p. 289.

Familial Hypercholesterolemia

This "receptor disease" is the consequence of a *mutation in the gene encoding the receptor for low-density lipoprotein (LDL) that is involved in the transport and metabolism of cholesterol.* As a consequence of receptor abnormalities there is loss of feedback control and elevated levels of cholesterol that induce premature atherosclerosis, leading to a greatly increased risk of myocardial infarction.[36]

Familial hypercholesterolemia (FH) is possibly the most frequent mendelian disorder. Heterozygotes with one mutant gene, representing about 1 in 500 individuals, have from birth a two- to threefold elevation of plasma cholesterol level, leading to tendinous xanthomas and premature atherosclerosis in adult life (p. 557). Homozygotes, having a double dose of the mutant gene, are much more severely affected and may have five- to sixfold elevations in plasma cholesterol levels. These individuals develop skin xanthomas and coronary, cerebral, and peripheral vascular atherosclerosis at an early age. Myocardial infarction may develop before the age of 20 years (p. 605). Large-scale studies have found that familial hypercholesterolemia is present in 3 to 6% of survivors of myocardial infarction.

An understanding of this disorder requires that we briefly review the normal process of cholesterol metabolism and transport. About 93% of the body's total cholesterol is located within cells, whereas 7% circulates in the plasma. Low-density lipoproteins (LDL) constitute the major transport form of cholesterol in the plasma. As might be expected, the level of plasma cholesterol is influenced by its synthesis and catabolism. Figure 4–11 illustrates that liver plays a crucial role in both these processes.[37] The first step in this complex sequence is the secretion of very low–density lipoproteins (VLDL) by the liver into the bloodstream. VLDL particles are rich in triglycerides, although they do contain lesser amounts of cholesteryl esters. The principal function of VLDL particles is to transport triglycerides from the liver to the peripheral tissues. When a VLDL particle reaches the capillaries of adipose tissue or muscle, it is cleaved by lipoprotein lipase, a process that extracts most of the triglycerides. The resulting molecule, called intermediate-density lipoprotein (IDL), is reduced in triglyceride content and enriched in cholesteryl esters, but it

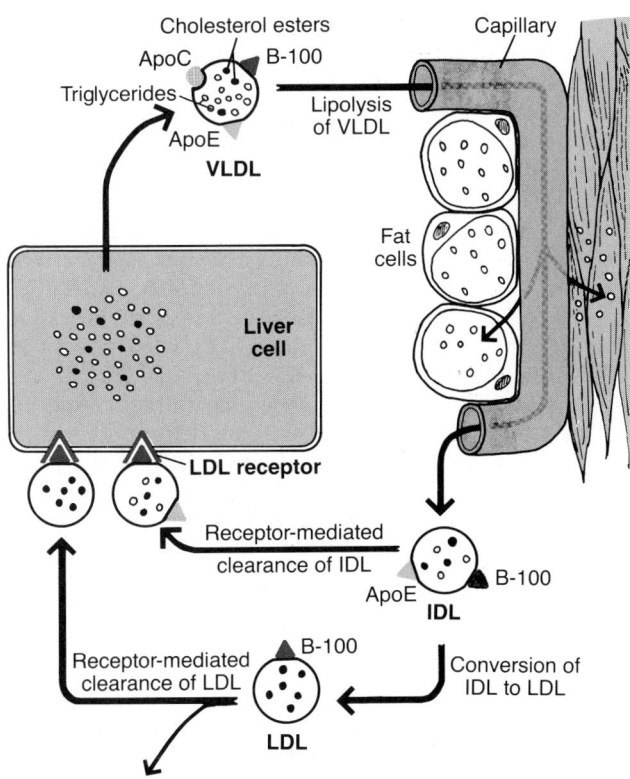

Figure 4–11. Schematic illustration of LDL metabolism and the role of liver in its synthesis and clearance. Lipolysis of VLDL by lipoprotein lipase in the capillaries releases triglycerides that are then stored in fat cells and used as a source of energy in skeletal muscles.

retains two of the three apoproteins (B-100 and E) present in the parent VLDL particle (Fig. 4–11). After release from the capillary endothelium, the IDL particles have one of two fates. Approximately 50% of newly formed IDL is rapidly taken up by the liver through a receptor-mediated transport. The receptor responsible for the binding of IDL to liver cell membrane recognizes both apoprotein B-100 and apoprotein E. However, it is called the LDL receptor because it is also involved in the hepatic clearance of LDL, as described later. In the liver cells IDL is recycled to generate VLDL. The IDL particles not taken up by the liver are subjected to further metabolic processing that removes most of the remaining triglycerides and apoprotein E, yielding the cholesterol-rich LDL. *It should be emphasized that IDL is the immediate and major source of plasma LDL.* There appear to be two mechanisms for removal of LDL from plasma, one mediated by a receptor-dependent process and the other by a receptor-independent pathway. Although many cell types, including fibroblasts, lymphocytes, smooth muscle cells, hepatocytes, and adrenocortical cells, possess high-affinity receptors that recognize apoprotein B-100 of the LDL molecule, approximately 70% of the plasma LDL appears to be cleared by the liver, utilizing a relatively sophisticated transport process (Fig. 4–12). The first step involves binding of LDL to cell surface receptors, which are clustered in specialized regions of the plasma membrane called *coated pits.* Following binding, the coated pits containing the receptor-bound LDL are internalized by invagination to form coated vesicles, after which they migrate within the cell to fuse with the lysosomes. Here the LDL dissociates from the receptor, which is recycled to the surface. In the lysosomes the LDL molecule is enzymically degraded, the apoprotein part being hydrolyzed to amino acids, whereas the cholesteryl esters are broken down to free cholesterol. This in turn crosses the lysosomal membrane to enter the cytoplasm, where it is utilized for membrane synthesis and as a regulator of cholesterol homeostasis. Three separate processes are affected by the released intracellular cholesterol: (1) Cholesterol *suppresses* cholesterol synthesis within the cell by inhibiting the activity of the enzyme 3-hydroxy-3-methylglutaryl (3HMG) CoA reductase, which is the rate-limiting enzyme in the synthetic pathway; (2) the cholesterol *activates* the enzyme acyl-coenzyme A:cholesterol acyltransferase, favoring esterification and storage of excess cholesterol; (3) cholesterol *suppresses* the synthesis of LDL receptors, thus protecting the cells from excessive accumulation of cholesterol.

The transport of LDL not involving LDL receptors alluded to earlier appears to take place in the cells of the mononuclear phagocytic system, but may also occur in other cells (p. 559). The amount catabolized by this pathway is directly related to the plasma cholesterol level.

As mentioned earlier, FH results from mutations in the gene specifying the receptor for LDL. Hetero-

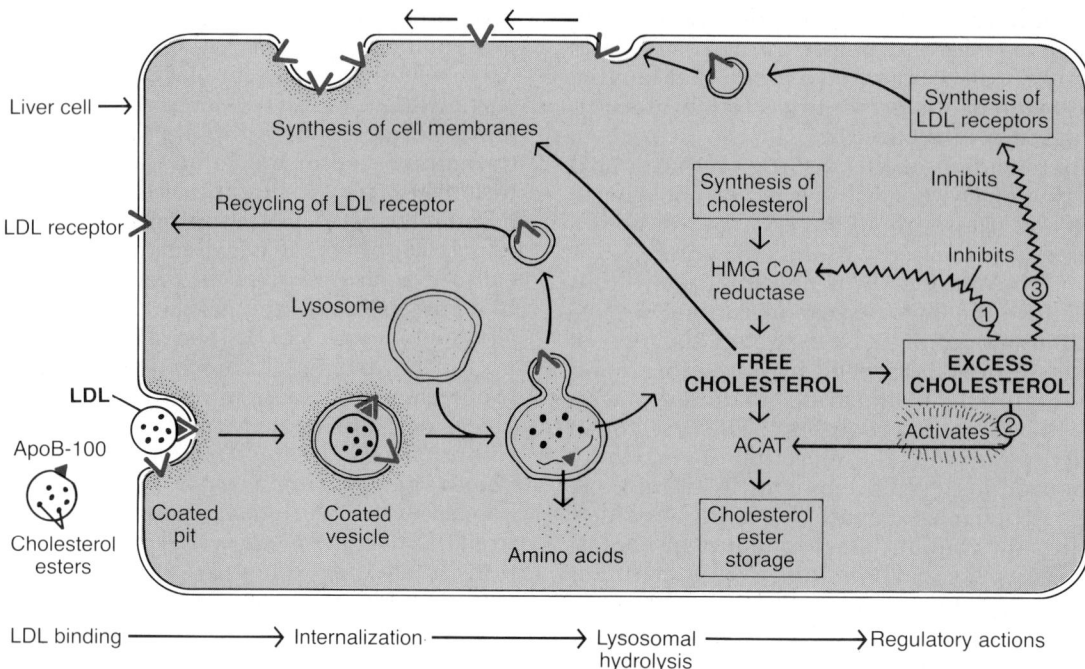

Figure 4–12. Sequential steps in LDL receptor pathway in cultured mammalian cells. LDL = low-density lipoprotein; HMG CoA reductase = 3-hydroxy-3-methyl-glutaryl CoA reductase; ACAT = acyl CoA:cholesterol acyltransferase.

zygotes with FH possess only 50% of the normal number of high-affinity LDL receptors, as they have only one normal gene. As a result of this defect in transport, the catabolism of LDL by the receptor-dependent pathway is impaired and the plasma level of LDL increases approximately twofold. Homozygotes have virtually no normal LDL receptors in their cells and have much higher levels of circulating LDL. In addition to defective LDL clearance, both the homozygotes and heterozygotes have increased synthesis of LDL. In homozygotes production of LDL is estimated to be two- to threefold above normal, whereas in heterozygotes there is a 30% increase. The mechanism of increased synthesis that contributes to hypercholesterolemia also results from a lack of LDL receptors (Fig. 4–11). Recall that IDL, the immediate precursor of plasma LDL, also utilizes hepatic LDL receptors (apoprotein B-100 and E receptors) for its transport into the liver. In FH, impaired IDL transport into the liver secondarily diverts a greater proportion of plasma IDL into the precursor pool for plasma LDL.

We mentioned earlier the LDL receptor–independent transport of LDL into the phagocytic cells. Normally, the amount of LDL transported along this pathway is less than that mediated by the receptor-dependent mechanisms. However, in the face of hypercholesterolemia there is a marked increase in the LDL receptor–independent traffic of LDL cholesterol into the cells of the mononuclear phagocyte system and possibly the vascular walls. This is responsible for the appearance of xanthomas and may also contribute to the pathogenesis of premature atherosclerosis.

The molecular genetics of FH has proved to be extremely complex. The human LDL receptor gene located on chromosome 19 is extremely large, spanning a distance of about 45 kilobases. At least 12 different point mutations and one partial deletion of the LDL receptor gene have been identified.[38] Depending on the mutation the receptor may not be synthesized, or the m-RNA is transcribed but the resultant receptor protein is defective. The mutant protein may fail to be transported to the cell surface, fail to bind to LDL, or fail to cluster in coated pits. Despite this marked genetic heterogeneity, the FH phenotypes can be grouped into three major classes: *(1) Receptor-negative disease,* the most common form, characterized by the absence of functional receptors. The LDL binding by cells from homozygotes with receptor-negative disease is less than 2% of normal. *(2) Receptor-defective disease,* in which the mutant allele specifies a receptor protein with reduced binding activity. Cells from homozygotes bind from 1 to 10% of normal LDL particles. *(3) Internalization defect,* which is extremely rare and is characterized by the presence of a receptor protein that can bind LDL normally but cannot internalize the bound LDL.

For their discoveries of the critical role of LDL receptors in cholesterol homeostasis Michael Brown and Joseph Goldstein were awarded the Nobel Prize in 1985. Their research has stimulated several studies designed to lower plasma cholesterol by increasing the number of LDL receptors.[39] One strategy that has proved to be successful is based on the ability of certain drugs (e.g., lovastatin) to suppress intracellular cholesterol synthesis by inhibiting the enzyme HMG CoA reductase. This in turn allows greater synthesis of LDL receptors (Fig. 4–12). Recent studies indicate that such a therapeutic approach lowers plasma cholesterol levels not only in patients with FH but also

in patients with the more common nongenetic forms of hypercholesterolemia.[40,41] The impact of such interventions may well have far-reaching effects on the management of hypercholesterolemia, which, as we shall see, is a major risk factor in the pathogenesis of atherosclerosis (p. 558).

AUTOSOMAL RECESSIVE DISORDERS

Autosomal recessive inheritance is the single largest category of mendelian disorders. Nonetheless, these mutant genes are relatively rare in the population. In contrast to autosomal dominant diseases, the following features generally apply to most autosomal recessive disorders.

• In affected (homozygous) individuals, the clinical manifestations tend to be more uniform.
• Complete penetrance is common.
• Age of onset is frequently early in life.
• In many cases enzyme proteins (rather than structural proteins) are affected by the mutation.

The category of autosomal recessive disease includes almost all the inborn errors of metabolism. As mentioned previously, these are syndromes in which the mutation leads to deficient functional activity of a specific enzyme. The various consequences of enzyme deficiencies were discussed on page 136. Mechanisms other than enzyme deficiency may also be involved. Increasingly we have become aware that there is another category of genetic metabolic diseases characterized by inborn errors of transport. These are essentially "membrane disorders." The Fanconi syndrome, characterized by glycosuria, aminoaciduria, chronic acidosis, vitamin D–resistant rickets, and osteomalacia, represents such a transport disorder. Thus, autosomal recessive errors in metabolism involve a wide range of mechanisms. The more common of these conditions are listed in Table 4–4. Most are presented elsewhere in the text; a few that involve multiple organs will be described here.

Albinism

Among the genetic metabolic disorders, albinism is, happily, one of the less serious. It constitutes the hereditary inability to synthesize melanin. There are two clinical variants: *ocular albinism* and *oculocutaneous albinism*. In the former, which in the vast majority of cases is inherited as an X-linked recessive trait, the lack of pigmentation is limited to the eye; in the latter, hair, skin, and eye pigmentation is affected.[42]

Almost a dozen genetic variants of oculocutaneous albinism have been identified, all transmitted as autosomal recessive traits. In some forms, there are associated defects in other organ systems, notably the hematopoietic cells. Biochemically albinism can be classified into two categories: "tyrosinase negative" and "tyrosinase positive." As you recall, tyrosine is the substrate from which melanin is produced. Tyrosinase catalyzes the formation of dihydroxyphenylalanine (dopa) from tyrosine. Dopa is one of the intermediaries in the formation of the dark brown-black

Table 4–4. Autosomal Recessive Disorders

DISORDER	CHAPTER, PAGE
Sickle cell anemia	Chapter 14, p. 666
β-thalassemia	Chapter 14, p. 670
Cystic fibrosis	Chapter 10, p. 533
Phenylketonuria	Chapter 10, p. 530
Galactosemia	Chapter 10, p. 532
Wilson's disease	Chapter 19, p. 956
Hemochromatosis	Chapter 19, p. 950
Severe combined immunodeficiency	Chapter 5, p. 222
Alpha-1-antitrypsin deficiency	Chapter 16, p. 769
Albinism	Chapter 4, p. 143
Alkaptonuria	Chapter 4, p. 143
Lysosomal storage diseases	Chapter 4, p. 144
Ehlers-Danlos syndromes (some variants)	Chapter 4, p. 155

pigment melanin. The basis of hypopigmentation in the tyrosinase positive variants is not understood. In both types of metabolic defect, individuals have a dermatosensitivity to solar exposure, greater in the tyrosinase-negative type. When exposed to sunlight, the skin is prone to develop wrinkles, but, more important, there is an increased frequency of solar keratosis and of basal cell and squamous cell carcinomas.

In the eye, the lack of pigment in the iris and retina leads to exquisite sensitivity to bright light and impaired visual acuity. Astigmatism, myopia, and other visual disturbances may also be present. The lack of the "sun shield" in the skin and eye predisposes to actinic-induced melanocarcinomas at these sites.

Alkaptonuria (Ochronosis)

In this autosomal recessive disorder, *the lack of homogentisic oxidase blocks the metabolism of phenylalanine-tyrosine at the level of homogentisic acid.* Thus, homogentisic acid accumulates in the body. A large amount is excreted, imparting a black color to the urine if allowed to stand and undergo oxidation.

The retained homogentisic acid selectively binds to collagen in connective tissues, tendons, and cartilage, imparting to these tissues a blue-black pigmentation **(ochronosis)** most evident in the ears, nose, and cheeks. **The most serious consequences of ochronosis, however, stem from deposits of the pigment in the articular cartilages of the joints.** In some obscure manner, the pigmentation causes the cartilage to lose its normal resiliency and become brittle and fibrillated.[43] Wear-and-tear erosion of this abnormal cartilage leads to denudation of the subchondral bone, and often tiny fragments of the fibrillated cartilage are driven into the underlying bone, worsening the damage. The vertebral column, particularly the intervertebral disc, is the prime site of attack, but later the knees, shoulders, and hips may be affected. The small joints of the hands and feet are usually spared.

Although the metabolic defect is present from birth, the degenerative arthropathy develops slowly and usually does not become clinically evident until the fourth decade of life. Although it is not life threatening, it may be severely crippling. The disability may be as extreme as that encountered in the severe forms of osteoarthritis (p. 1346) of the elderly, but unfortunately in alkaptonuria the arthropathy occurs at a much earlier age.

Lysosomal Storage Diseases

Lysosomes are key components of the "intracellular digestive tract." They contain a battery of hydrolytic enzymes, which have two special properties. First, they can function in the acid milieu of the lysosomes. Second, these enzymes constitute a special category of secretory proteins that, unlike most others, are destined for secretion not into the extracellular fluids but into an intracellular organelle. This latter characteristic requires special processing within the Golgi apparatus that will be reviewed briefly. Like all other secretory proteins, lysosomal enzymes (or acid hydrolases as they are sometimes called) are synthesized in the endoplasmic reticulum and transported to the Golgi apparatus. Within the Golgi complex they undergo a variety of post-translational modifications, of which one is worthy of special note. This involves the attachment of terminal mannose-6-phosphate groupings to some of the oligosaccharide side chains. The phosphorylated mannose residues may be viewed as an "address label" that is recognized by specific receptors found on the inner surface of the Golgi membrane. Lysosomal enzymes bind to these receptors and are thereby segregated from the numerous other secretory proteins within the Golgi. Subsequently, small transport vesicles containing the receptor-bound enzymes are pinched off from the Golgi and proceed to fuse with the lysosomes. Thus the enzymes are targeted to their intracellular abode, and, as indicated in Figure 4–13, the vesicles are shuttled back to the Golgi. As will be discussed later, genetically determined errors in this remarkable sorting mechanism may give rise to one form of lysosomal storage disease.

The lysosomal acid hydrolases catalyze the breakdown of a variety of complex macromolecules.[44] These large molecules may be derived from the metabolic turnover of intracellular organelles (autophagy), or they may be acquired from outside the cells by phagocytosis (heterophagy). With an inherited deficiency of a functional lysosomal enzyme, catabolism of its substrate remains incomplete, leading to the accumulation of the partially degraded insoluble metabolite within the lysosomes. Stuffed with incompletely digested macromolecules, these organelles become large and numerous enough to interfere in normal cell functions, giving rise to the so-called *lysosomal storage disorders* (Fig. 4–14). When first discovered in 1963 it was thought that this category of diseases resulted exclusively from mutations that lead to reduced synthesis of lysosomal enzymes ("missing enzyme syndromes"). However, in the last two decades research focusing on the molecular pathology of

lysosomal storage diseases has led to the discovery of several other defects.[45] Some of these are as follows:

• Synthesis of catalytically inactive protein that cross reacts immunologically with the normal enzyme. Thus by immunoassays the enzyme levels appear to be normal.
• Defects in post-translational processing of the enzyme protein. Included in this category is a failure to attach the mannose-6-phosphate "marker," the absence of which prevents the enzyme from following its correct path to the lysosome. Instead, the enzyme is secreted outside the cell.
• Lack of an enzyme activator or protector protein.
• Lack of a substrate activator protein: In some instances proteins that react with the substrate to facilitate its hydrolysis may be missing or defective.
• Lack of a transport protein required for egress of the digested material from the lysosomes.

It should be evident, therefore, that the concept of lysosomal storage disorders has to be expanded to in-

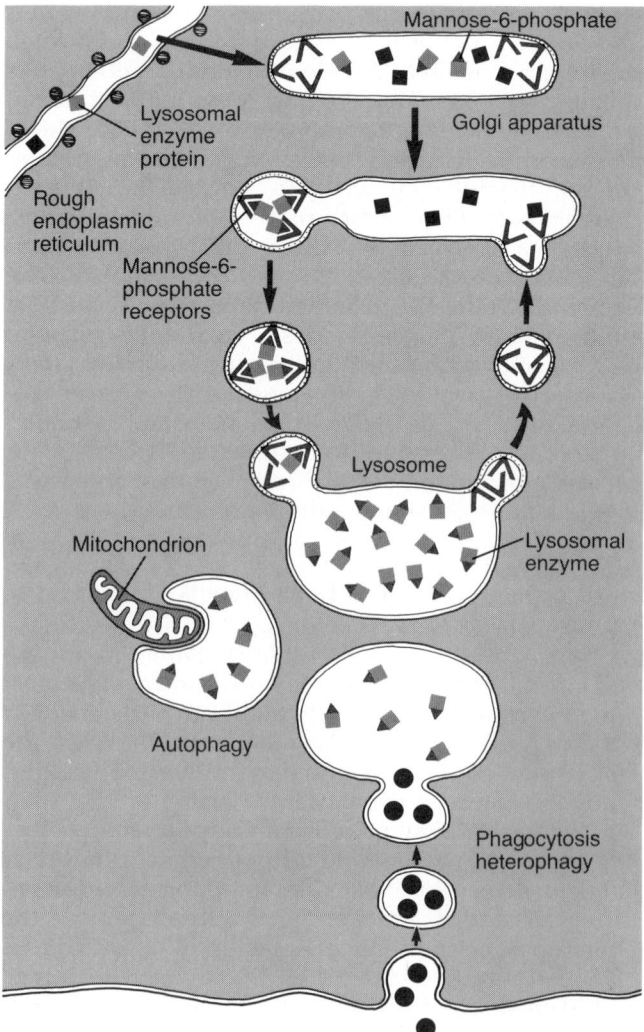

Figure 4–13. Synthesis and intracellular transport of lysosomal enzymes.

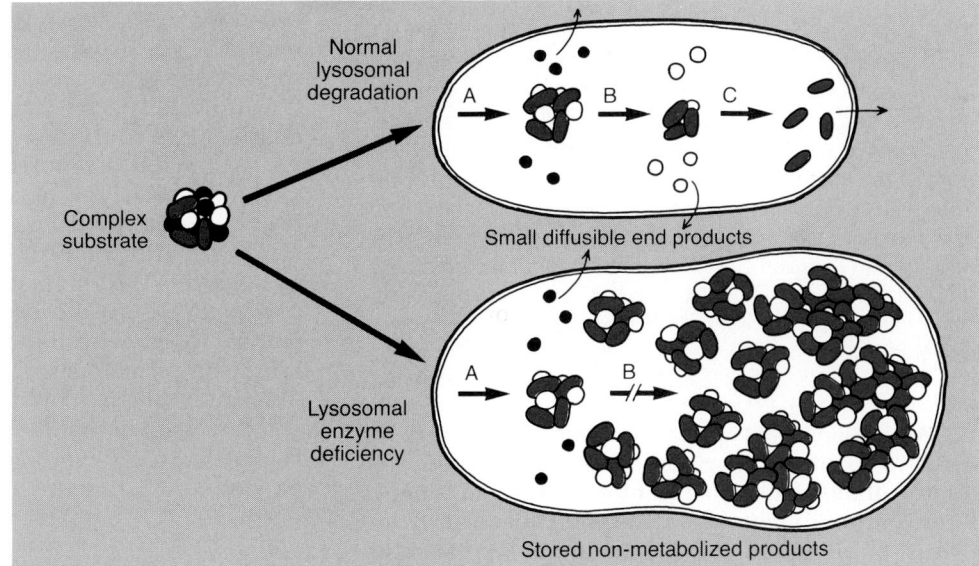

Figure 4-14. A schematic diagram illustrating the pathogenesis of lysosomal storage diseases. In the example illustrated, a complex substrate is normally degraded by a series of lysosomal enzymes (A, B, and C) into soluble end products. If there is a deficiency or malfunction of one of the enzymes (e.g., B), catabolism is incomplete and insoluble intermediates accumulate in the lysosomes.

clude the lack of any protein essential for the normal function of lysosomes.

Several distinctive and separable conditions are included among the lysosomal storage diseases (Table 4–5). In general the distribution of the stored material, and hence the organs affected, is determined by two interrelated factors: (1) the site where most of the material to be degraded is found, and (2) the location where most of the degradation normally occurs. *For example, brain is rich in gangliosides and hence defective hydrolysis of gangliosides as occurs in G_{M1}- and G_{M2}-gangliosidoses results primarily in storage within neurons and neurologic symptoms.* On the other hand defects in degradation of mucopolysaccharides affect virtually every organ because mucopolysaccharides are widely distributed in the body. Because cells of the mononuclear phagocyte system are especially rich in lysosomes and are involved in the degradation of a variety of substrates, organs rich in phagocytic cells such as the spleen and liver are frequently enlarged in several forms of lysosomal storage disorders. The ever-expanding number of lysosomal storage diseases can be divided into rational categories on the basis of the biochemical nature of the accumulated metabolite, thus creating such subgroups as *the glycogenoses, sphingolipidoses (lipidoses), mucopolysaccharidoses, and mucolipidoses.* Within a category, individual entities may closely resemble one another, not only clinically but also biochemically. It therefore is often necessary, and always desirable, to confirm clinical impressions by biochemical identification of the accumulated metabolite or the enzyme deficiency, or both. Only one among the many glycogenoses results from a lysosomal enzyme deficiency, and so this family of storage diseases will be considered later (p. 151). Only the most common disorders among the remaining groups will be considered here; the others must be left to specialized texts and reviews.[46]

TAY-SACHS DISEASE (G_{M2}-GANGLIOSIDOSIS TYPE 1). The autosomal recessive Tay-Sachs disease is the prototype and the most important of the gangliosidoses. As can be seen from Table 4–5, there are other gangliosidoses separated into G_{M1} and G_{M2} categories, each further subdivided into distinctive entities. Tay-Sachs disease, a G_{M2}-gangliosidosis, is particularly prevalent among Jews, in particular among those of Eastern European (Ashkenazic) origin in whom a carrier rate of 1 in 30 has been reported. The specific enzyme dysfunction in Tay-Sachs disease is a deficiency of hexosaminidase A, while the activity of the other isoenzyme, hexosaminidase B, is increased. Hexosaminidase A catalyzes the degradation of G_{M2}-ganglioside, and so in this condition it accumulates.

The hexosaminidase A is absent from virtually all the tissues that have been examined, including leukocytes and plasma, and so G_{M2}-ganglioside accumulates in many tissues (e.g., heart, liver, spleen), but it is the involvement of neurons in the central and autonomic nervous systems and retina that dominates the clinical picture. Depending on the duration of survival, the weight of the brain may be normal or decreased, but in patients surviving one or more years it is usually increased, sometimes more than 50%, owing to the accumulation of ganglioside in cells. On histologic examination, the neurons are ballooned with cytoplasmic vacuoles, each of which comprises a markedly distended lysosome filled with gangliosides (Fig. 4–15). Stains for fat such as oil red O and Sudan black are positive. With the electron microscope, several types of cytoplasmic inclusions can be visualized, the most prominent being whorled configurations within lysosomes composed of onionskin layers of membranes.[47] In time there is progressive destruction of neurons, proliferation of microglia, and accumulation of complex lipids in phagocytes within the brain substance. A similar process occurs in the cerebellum as well as in neurons throughout the basal ganglia, brain stem, spinal cord, and dorsal root ganglia, and the neurons of the autonomic nervous system.[48] The ganglion cells in the retina are similarly swollen with G_{M2}-ganglioside, particularly at the margins of the macula. A **cherry-red spot** thus appears in the macula, representing accentuation of the normal color of the macular choroid contrasted with the pallor produced by the swollen ganglion cells in the remainder of the retina. As the retinal ganglion cells die from the accumulation of lipid, the cherry-red spot may disappear in patients with protracted disease.

Affected infants appear quite normal at birth but begin to manifest signs and symptoms at about six months of age. There is relentless motor and mental deterioration, beginning with motor incoordination, mental obtundation leading to muscular flaccidity, blindness, and increasing dementia. The blindness and progressive mental deterioration account for the older designation of this condition as *amaurotic (having blindness) familial idiocy.* Sometime during the early course of the disease the characteristic, but not pathognomonic, cherry-red spot appears in the macula of the eye grounds in almost all patients. Over the span of one or two years a complete, pathetic vegetative state is reached, followed, usually too late, by death at two to three years of age.

Antenatal diagnosis is possible by identification of the deficiency of hexosaminidase A in cultured fibroblasts derived from amniotic fluid. It is also possible to identify heterozygote carriers who have enzyme levels intermediate between those of controls and homozygous affected infants. In 1978 the AB variant of G_{M2}-gangliosidoses was described. Clinically it is indistinguishable from Tay-Sachs disease, but levels of hexosaminidase A and B are paradoxically elevated! It is now known that the basic defect in this condition is lack of an *activator protein*, which must bind to the G_{M2} substrate to allow its hydrolysis by hexosaminidases.

NIEMANN-PICK DISEASE. This autosomal recessive disorder is characterized by an accumulation of sphingomyelin as well as cholesterol in reticuloendothelial and parenchymal cells in many organs throughout the body. *Niemann-Pick disease is clini-*

Table 4–5. Lysosomal Storage Diseases

DISEASE	ENZYME DEFICIENCY	MAJOR ACCUMULATING METABOLITES
Glycogenosis		
Type 2 — Pompe's disease	α-1,4-glucosidase (lysosomal glucosidase)	Glycogen
Sphingolipidoses		
G_{M1}-gangliosidosis	G_{M1}-ganglioside β-galactosidase	G_{M1}-ganglioside, galactose-containing oligosaccharides
Type 1 — infantile, generalized		
Type 2 — juvenile		
G_{M2}-gangliosidosis		
Tay-Sachs disease	Hexosaminidase A	G_{M2}-ganglioside
Sandhoff disease	Hexosaminidases A and B	G_{M2}-ganglioside, globoside
G_{M2}-gangliosidosis, A B variant	Ganglioside activator protein	G_{M2}-ganglioside
Sulfatidoses		
Metachromatic leukodystrophy	Arylsulfatase A	Sulfatide
Multiple sulfatase deficiency	Arylsulfatases A, B, C; steroid sulfatase; iduronate sulfatase, heparan N-sulfatase	Sulfatide, steroid sulfate, heparan sulfate, dermatan sulfate
Krabbe's disease	Galactosylceramidase	Galactocerebroside
Fabry's disease	α-Galactosidase A	Ceramide trihexoside
Gaucher's disease	Glucocerebrosidase	Glucocerebroside
Niemann-Pick disease	Sphingomyelinase	Sphingomyelin
Mucopolysaccharidoses		
Several types (see p. 150)	Several types (see p. 150)	Dermatan sulfate, heparan sulfate, keratan sulfate, chondroitin sulfate
Mucolipidoses (ML)		
I-cell disease (MLII) and pseudo–Hurler polydystrophy	Deficiency of phosphorylating enzymes essential for the formation of mannose-6-phosphate recognition marker (see p. 144); acid hydrolases lacking the recognition marker cannot be targeted to the lysosomes but are secreted extracellularly	Mucopolysaccharide, glycolipid
Other Diseases of Complex Carbohydrates		
Fucosidosis	α-Fucosidase	Fucose-containing sphingolipids and glycoprotein fragments
Mannosidosis	α-Mannosidase	Mannose-containing oligosaccharides
Aspartylglycosaminuria	Aspartylglycosamine amide hydrolase	Aspartyl-2-deoxy-2-acetamido-glycosylamine
Other Lysosomal Storage Diseases		
Wolman's disease	Acid lipase	Cholesterol esters, triglycerides
Acid phosphate deficiency	Lysosomal acid phosphatase	Phosphate esters

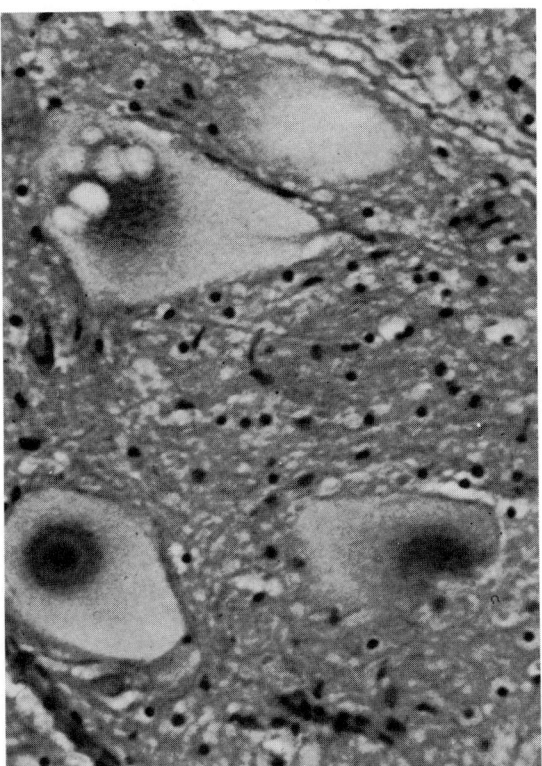
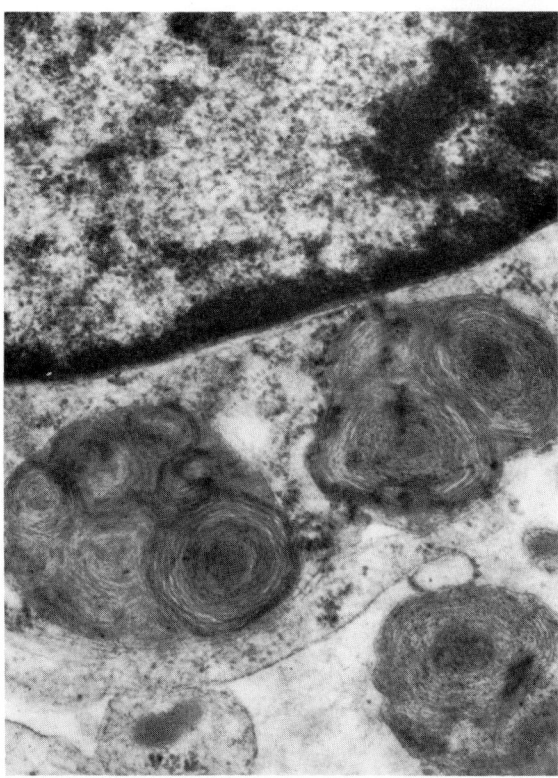

Figure 4–15. Ganglion cells in Tay-Sachs disease. *A,* Under the light microscope, a large neuron at the top has obvious lipid vacuolation with karyolysis and granularity of nucleus. *B,* Portion of a neuron under the electron microscope shows prominent lysosomes with whorled configurations. Part of the nucleus is shown above. (Electron micrograph courtesy of Dr. Joe Rutledge, Southwestern Medical School, Dallas, Texas.)

cally, biochemically, and genetically heterogeneous. By biochemical criteria two major groups can be distinguished: those patients with a deficiency of the sphingomyelin cleavage enzyme, sphingomyelinase, and others in which this enzyme activity is normal.[49] In each of these two categories several subgroups have been recognized. Remarks here will be confined largely to sphingomyelinase deficient, type A variant, representing 75 to 80% of all cases. *This is the severe infantile form with extensive neurologic involvement, marked visceral accumulations of sphingomyelin, and progressive wasting and early death within the first three years of life.* To provide a perspective on the differences between the variants of Niemann-Pick disease we need only point out that in type B, for example, patients have organomegaly but generally no central nervous system involvement. The basis of lipid accumulation in variants with normal sphingomyelinase activity is unknown. The possibility exists that there may be deficiency of an activator protein.

In the classic infantile type A variant, the deficiency of sphingomyelinase is almost complete. Sphingomyelin is a ubiquitous component of cellular (including organellar) membranes, and so the enzyme deficiency blocks degradation of the lipid, resulting in its progressive accumulation within lysosomes, particularly within cells of the mononuclear phagocyte system (Fig. 4–16). Affected cells become

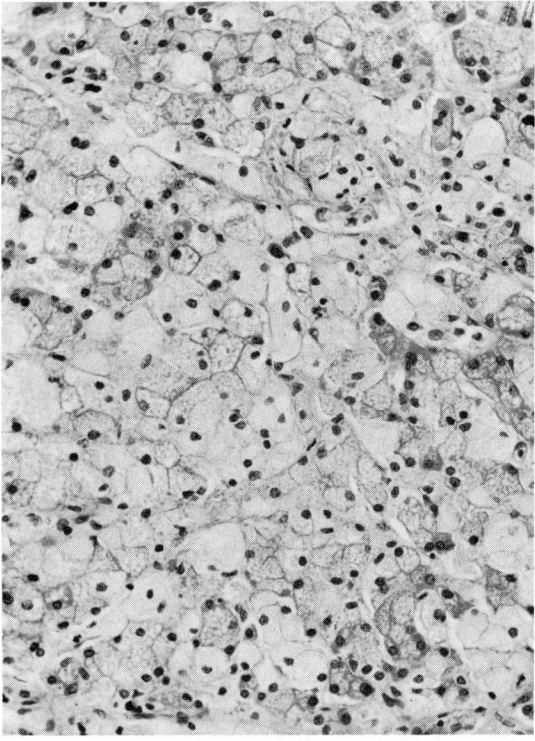

Figure 4–16. Niemann-Pick disease in bone marrow. The marrow space is virtually filled with fairly regular lipid-filled macrophages.

enlarged, sometimes to 90 μm in diameter, secondary to the distention of lysosomes with sphingomyelin and cholesterol. Innumerable small vacuoles of relatively uniform size are created, imparting a foaminess to the cytoplasm. In frozen sections of fresh tissue, the vacuoles stain for fat with Sudan black B and oil red O. Electron microscopy confirms that the vacuoles are engorged secondary lysosomes that often contain membranous cytoplasmic bodies (MCB) resembling concentric lamellated myelin figures. Sometimes the lysosomal configurations take the form of parallel palisaded lamellae, creating so-called zebra bodies.[50]

The lipid-laden phagocytic foam cells are widely distributed in the spleen, liver, lymph nodes, bone marrow, tonsils, gastrointestinal tract, and lungs. The involvement of the spleen generally produces massive enlargement, sometimes to ten times its normal weight, but the hepatomegaly is usually not quite so striking. The lymph nodes are generally moderately to markedly enlarged throughout the body. Often the color of these organs is paler than usual owing to the massive accumulations of sphingomyelin.

Involvement of the brain and eye deserves special mention. In brain the gyri are shrunken and the sulci widened. The cortex is somewhat softer than usual, while the underlying white matter is abnormally firm. The neuronal involvement is diffuse, affecting all parts of the nervous system. Vacuolation and ballooning of neurons is the dominant histologic change, which in time leads to cell death and loss of brain substance.[48] A retinal cherry-red spot similar to that seen in Tay-Sachs disease (p. 146) is present in about one third to one half of affected individuals. Its origin is similar to that described in Tay-Sachs disease, except that the accumulated metabolite is sphingomyelin.

Clinical manifestations may be present even at birth but almost certainly become evident by six months of life. The infants typically have a protuberant abdomen because of the hepatosplenomegaly. Accumulation of sphingomyelin and cholesterol in subcutaneous phagocytic cells may produce small skin xanthomas. Once the manifestations appear, they are followed by progressive failure to thrive, vomiting, fever, and generalized lymphadenopathy as well as progressive deterioration of psychomotor function. Death comes as a release, usually within the first or second year of life.

The diagnosis is established by biochemical assays for sphingomyelinase activity in liver or bone marrow biopsy. Affected individuals as well as heterozygous carriers can be recognized antenatally by enzyme assays in cultured fibroblasts obtained by amniocentesis.

GAUCHER'S DISEASE. This autosomal recessive disorder is characterized by a deficiency of glucocerebrosidase that normally cleaves the glucose residue from ceramide. As a result, glucocerebroside accumulates, principally in the phagocytic cells of the body but sometimes also in central nervous system neurons. In the normal individual, glucocerebrosides are continually formed from the catabolism of glycolipids derived mainly from the cell membranes of senescent leukocytes and erythrocytes. This pathway is the predominant source of glucocerebrosides that accumulate within the mononuclear phagocytic cells; the accumulations in the neurons may in part be derived from the turnover of gangliosides in the nervous system, which is quite rapid in the neonatal period. Three clinical subtypes of Gaucher's disease have been distinguished. *The classic form, called type I, is the adult type of Gaucher's disease, sometimes called the noncerebral form, in which the storage of glucocerebrosides is limited to the mononuclear phagocytes throughout the body without involving the brain. Splenic and skeletal involvements dominate this pattern of the disease.* It is found principally in Jews of European stock and accounts for at least 80% of all cases of Gaucher's disease. Patients with this disorder have reduced but detectable levels of glucocerebrosidase activity. Longevity is shortened but not markedly. *The type II form of Gaucher's disease is the infantile acute cerebral pattern. This infantile disease has no predilection for Jews. In these patients there is virtually no detectable glucocerebrosidase activity in the tissues.* Hepatosplenomegaly is also seen in this form of Gaucher's disease, but the clinical picture is dominated by progressive central nervous system involvement, leading to death at an early age. A third pattern, type III, is sometimes distinguished, intermediate between types I and II. These patients are usually juveniles and have the systemic involvement characteristic of type I, but have progressive central nervous system disease that usually begins in the second or third decade of life. The levels of glucocerebrosidase activity in this variant are intermediate between those found in types I and II. These specific patterns run within families, resulting from different allelic mutations in the structural gene for the enzyme. Recently the normal glucocerebrosidase gene has been cloned, and the molecular analysis of the normal and mutant genes has revealed that a single base substitution (proline for leucine) in exon 10 is highly correlated with the development of neurologic symptoms.[51]

The glucocerebrosides accumulate in massive amounts within phagocytic cells throughout the body in all forms of Gaucher's disease. In addition neuronal storage occurs in types II and III. The distended phagocytic cells, known as **Gaucher cells,** are found in the spleen, liver, bone marrow, lymph nodes, tonsils, thymus, and Peyer's patches. Similar cells may be in both the alveolar septa and the air spaces in the lung. In contrast to the lipid storage diseases already discussed, Gaucher cells rarely appear vacuolated but instead have a fibrillary type of cytoplasm likened to crumpled tissue paper (Fig. 4–17). Gaucher cells are often enlarged, sometimes up to 100 μm in diameter, and have one or more dark, eccentrically placed nuclei.[48] PAS staining is usually intensely positive. With the electron microscope, the fibrillary cytoplasm can be resolved as elongated, distended lysosomes, containing the stored lipid in stacks of bilayers.[52]

The accumulation of Gaucher cells produces a variety of gross anatomic changes. The spleen is enlarged in the adult form of the disease, sometimes up to 10 kg. It too may appear uniformly pale or have a mottled surface owing to focal accumulations of Gaucher cells. The lymphadenopathy is mild to moderate and is bodywide. The accumulations of Gaucher cells in the bone marrow may produce small focal areas of bone erosion or large, soft, gray tumorous masses that cause skeletal deformities or destroy sufficient bone to give rise to fractures. Occasionally, aggregates of distended phagocytes are found in the lungs and other organs, particularly the endocrine glands. In patients with cerebral involvement, Gaucher cells are seen in the Virchow-Robin spaces, and arterioles are surrounded by swollen adventitial cells. Neurons appear shriveled and are progressively destroyed.

The clinical course of Gaucher's disease depends on the clinical subtype. In the type I pattern, symptoms and signs first appear in adult life and are related to splenomegaly or bone involvement. Most commonly, there is pancytopenia or thrombocytopenia secondary to hypersplenism. Pathologic fractures and bone pain occur if there has been extensive expansion of the marrow space. Although the disease is progressive in the adult, it is compatible with long life. In types II and III, central nervous system dysfunction, convulsions, and progressive mental deterioration dominate, although organs such as the liver, spleen, and lymph nodes are also affected.

The diagnosis of homozygotes and the detection of heterozygous carriers can be made through measurement of glucocerebrosidase activity in peripheral blood leukocytes or in extracts of cultured skin fibroblasts. Prenatal diagnosis is also possible using cultured fetal fibroblasts.

As with all lysosomal storage diseases, the prospects for treatment remain bleak, but some advances are being made. Because the fundamental defect resides in mononuclear phagocytic cells originating from marrow stem cells, bone marrow transplantation has been attempted, but with limited success. More recent attempts are directed toward correction of the enzyme defect by transfer of the normal glucocerebrosidase gene into the patient's cells.[53]

MUCOPOLYSACCHARIDOSES (MPS). The mucopolysaccharidoses are another form of lysosomal storage disease. They make up a group of closely related syndromes that result from genetically determined deficiencies of specific lysosomal enzymes involved in the degradation of mucopolysaccharides (glycosaminoglycans). The mucopolysaccharides that accumulate in the MPS are dermatan sulfate, heparan sulfate, keratan sulfate, and chondroitin sulfate.[54] The enzymes involved in each of the MPS cleave terminal sugars from the polysaccharide chains disposed along a polypeptide or "core protein." When there is a block in the removal of a terminal sugar, the remainder of the polysaccharide chain is not further

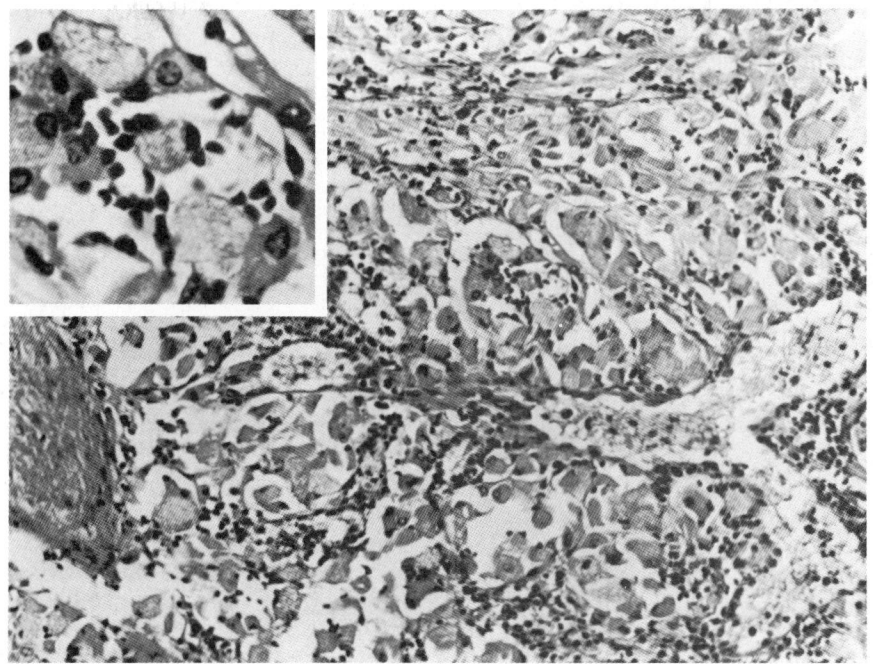

Figure 4-17. Gaucher's disease involving the spleen. The entire field is made up of lipid-laden cells of varying size with sharp cell boundaries, abundant granular cytoplasm, and small eccentric nuclei. Inset shows Gaucher cells at higher magnification. (Courtesy of Dr. Joe Rutledge, Southwestern Medical School, Dallas, Texas.)

degraded, and thus these chains accumulate within lysosomes in various tissues and organs of the body. Severe somatic and neurologic changes result.

Several clinical variants of MPS, classified numerically from MPS I to MPS VII, have been described, each resulting from the deficiency of one specific enzyme. All the MPS except one are inherited as autosomal recessive traits; one variant, called Hunter's syndrome, is an X-linked recessive (Table 4–6). Within a given group (e.g., MPS I, characterized by a deficiency of α-L-iduronidase) subgroups exist that result from different mutant alleles at the same genetic locus. Thus, the severity of enzyme deficiency and the clinical picture even within subgroups is often different.

In general, the MPS are progressive disorders, characterized by involvement of multiple organs, including liver, spleen, heart, and blood vessels. Most are associated with coarse facial features, clouding of the cornea, joint stiffness, and mental retardation. Urinary excretion of the accumulated mucopolysaccharides is often increased.

The accumulated mucopolysaccharides are generally found in mononuclear phagocytic cells, endothelial cells, intimal smooth muscle cells, and fibroblasts throughout the body. Common sites of involvement are thus the spleen, liver, bone marrow, lymph nodes, blood vessels, and also the heart.

Microscopically, affected cells are distended and have apparent clearing of the cytoplasm to create so-called balloon cells. The cleared cytoplasm can be resolved as numerous minute vacuoles, which, with the electron microscope, can be visualized as swollen lysosomes filled with a finely granular PAS-positive material that can be identified biochemically as mucopolysaccharide. Similar lysosomal changes are found in the neurons of those syndromes characterized by central nervous system involvement. In addition, however, some of the lysosomes in neurons are replaced by lamellated zebra bodies like those seen in Niemann-Pick disease. Hepatosplenomegaly, skeletal deformities, valvular lesions, and subendothelial arterial deposits, particularly in the coronary arteries and lesions in the brain, are common threads that run through all the MPS. In many of the more protracted syndromes, coronary subendothelial lesions lead to myocardial ischemia. Thus, myocardial infarction and cardiac decompensation are important causes of death.

Some data relating to clinical manifestations of the better characterized variants are provided in Table 4–6. Further details can be found in recent reviews.[46,54] With these syndromes, biochemical identification of the accumulated metabolite or spe-

Table 4–6. Some Selected Mucopolysaccharidoses (MPS)

NAME	GENETICS	ACCUMULATED PRODUCT	ENZYME DEFICIENCY	LIFE EXPECTANCY	CLINICAL FEATURES
MPS I H (Hurler)	AR	Heparan sulfate Dermatan sulfate	α-L-Iduronidase	6 to 10 years	1. Onset 6 to 8 months 2. Dwarfism 3. Corneal clouding 4. Hepatosplenomegaly 5. Valvular lesions 6. Coronary artery lesions 7. Skeletal deformities 8. Joint stiffness 9. Progressive mental retardation
MPS I S (Scheie)	AR	Heparan sulfate Dermatan sulfate	α-L-Iduronidase	Normal	1. Onset after 5 years 2. Near-normal height 3. Corneal clouding 4. Aortic valvular lesions 5. Finger stiffness 6. Normal intelligence
MPS II (Hunter) (Wide range of severity)	X-R	Heparan sulfate Dermatan sulfate	L-Iduronosulfate sulfatase	Second decade to normal	1. Severe cases similar to Hurler's syndrome, but no corneal clouding 2. Deafness 3. Retinal degeneration common 4. Intelligence normal in mild cases; mildly retarded in severe cases
MPS III (Sanfilippo) Subtypes A, B, C, & D	AR	Heparan sulfate	Heparan N-sulfatase (in type A)	Second to third decade	1. Onset after 3 years 2. Mild somatic features with severe mental retardation are characteristic
MPS IV (Morquio) (Wide range of severity, possibly several forms with different enzyme deficiencies)	AR	Keratan sulfate Chondroitin sulfate	N-Acetylgalacto-samine-6-sulfatase	Third to sixth decade	1. Severe skeletal deformities such as dwarfism, thoracolumbar gibbus, kyphoscoliosis 2. Normal intelligence 3. Aortic vavular lesions

AR = Autosomal recessive; X-R = X-linked recessive.

cific enzyme deficiency, or both, is necessary to differentiate unmistakably one from the others. Prenatal diagnosis is now possible.

Glycogen Storage Diseases (Glycogenoses)

A number of genetic syndromes have been identified that result from some metabolic defect in the synthesis or catabolism of glycogen. The best understood and most important category includes the *glycogen storage diseases* resulting from a hereditary defi-ciency of one of the enzymes involved in the synthesis or sequential degradation of glycogen. Depending on the tissue or organ distribution of the specific enzyme in the normal state, *glycogen storage in these disorders may be limited to a few tissues, be more widespread while not affecting all tissues, or be systemic in distribution.*

The significance of a specific enzyme deficiency is best understood from the perspective of the normal metabolism of glycogen (Fig. 4–18). As is well known, glycogen is a storage form of glucose. Glyco-

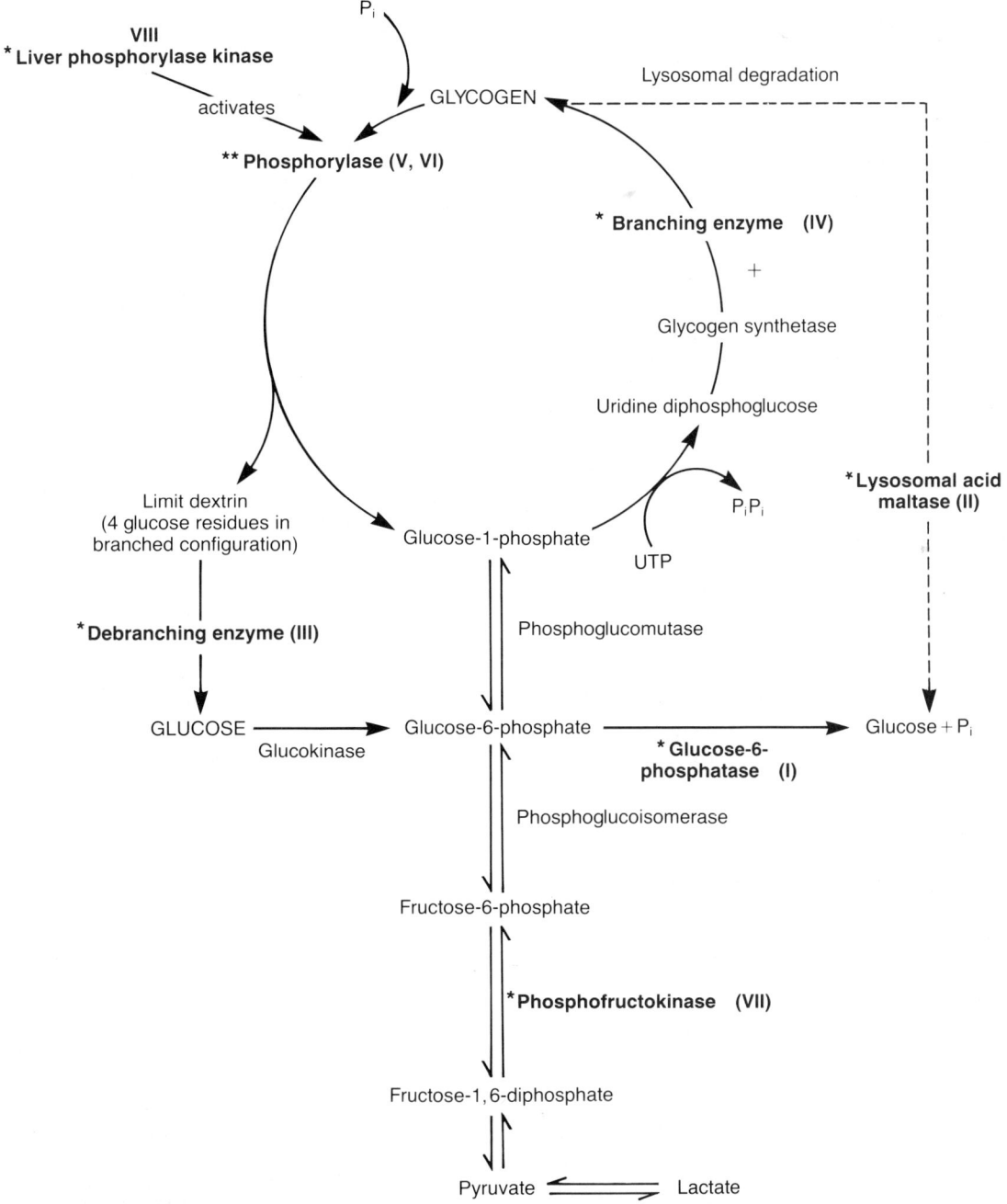

Figure 4–18. Pathways of glycogen metabolism. Asterisks mark the enzyme deficiencies associated with glycogen storage diseases. Roman numerals indicate the type of glycogen storage disease associated with the given enzyme deficiency. Types V and VI result from deficiencies of muscle and liver phosphorylases, respectively. (After Howell, R. R., and Williams, J. C.: The glycogen storage disease. *In* **Stanbury, J. B., et al. [eds.]: Metabolic Basis of Inherited Diseases. 5th Ed. New York, McGraw-Hill Book Co., 1983, p. 144.)**

gen synthesis begins with the conversion of glucose to glucose-6-phosphate by the action of a hexokinase (glucokinase). A phosphoglucomutase then transforms the glucose-6-phosphate to glucose-1-phosphate, which in turn is converted to uridine diphosphoglucose. A highly branched, very large polymer is then built up (molecular weight up to 100,000,000), containing up to 10,000 glucose molecules linked together by α-1,4-glucoside bonds. The glycogen chain and branches continue to be elongated by the addition of glucose molecules mediated by glycogen synthetases. During degradation distinct phosphorylases in the liver and muscle split glucose-1-phosphate from the glycogen until about four glucose residues remain on each branch, leaving a branched oligosaccharide called limit dextrin. This can be further degraded only by the debranching enzyme. In addition to these major pathways, glycogen is also degraded in the lysosomes by acid maltase. If the lysosomes are deficient in this enzyme, the glycogen contained within them is not accessible to degradation by cytoplasmic enzymes such as phosphorylases.

On the basis of specific enzyme deficiencies and the resultant clinical pictures, glycogenoses have traditionally been divided into a dozen or so syndromes designated by roman numerals, and the list continues to grow. Rather than describing each syndrome, we will offer a more manageable classification that is based on the pathophysiology of these disorders.[55] According to this approach, glycogenoses can be divided into three major subgroups.

• *Hepatic forms.* As is well-known, liver is a key player in glycogen metabolism. It contains enzymes that synthesize glycogen for storage and ultimately break it down into free glucose, which is then released into the blood. An inherited deficiency of hepatic enzymes that are involved in glycogen metabolism therefore leads not only to the storage of glycogen in the liver but also to a reduction in blood glucose level (hypoglycemia) (Fig. 4–19). Deficiency of the enzyme glucose-6-phosphatase (von Gierke's disease or type I glycogenosis) is a prime example of the hepatic-hypoglycemic form of glycogen storage disease (Table 4–7). Other examples include lack of liver phosphorylase and debranching enzyme, both involved in the breakdown of glycogen (Fig. 4–19). In all these cases glycogen is stored in many organs, but it is the *hepatic enlargement and hypoglycemia that dominate the clinical picture.*

• *Myopathic forms.* In the striated muscles, as opposed to the liver, glycogen is used predominantly as a source of energy. This is derived by glycolysis, which leads ultimately to the formation of lactate (Fig. 4–19). If the enzymes that fuel the glycolytic pathway are deficient, glycogen storage occurs in the muscles and is associated with muscular weakness owing to impaired energy production. Examples in this category include deficiencies of muscle phosphorylase (McArdle's disease, type V glycogenosis), muscle phosphofructokinase (type VII glycogen storage dis-

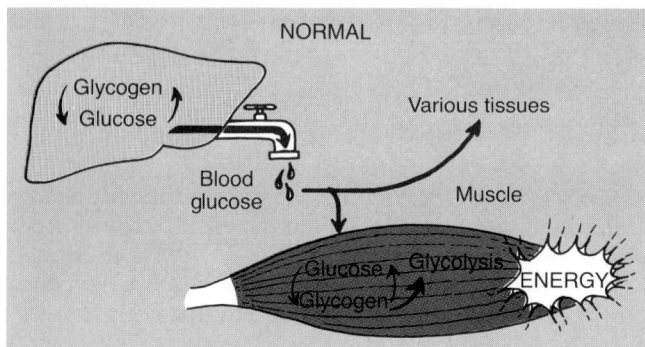

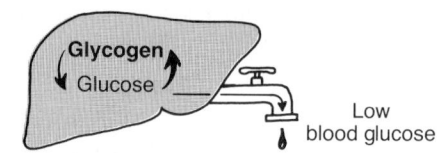

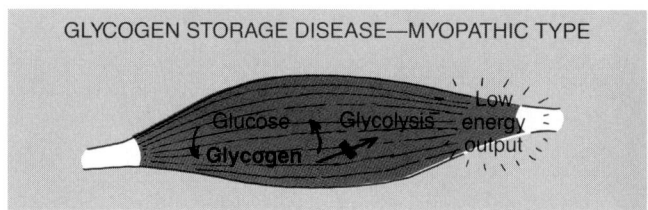

Figure 4–19. A simplified scheme of normal glycogen metabolism in the liver and skeletal muscles *(top).* The middle panel illustrates the effects of an inherited deficiency of hepatic enzymes involved in glycogen metabolism. The lower panel shows the consequences of a genetic deficiency in the enzymes that metabolize glycogen in skeletal muscles.

ease), and several others.[56] *Typically the myopathic forms present with muscle cramps following exercise and a failure of exercise-induced rise in blood lactate levels owing to a block in glycolysis.*

• Glycogen storage diseases associated with (1) deficiency of α-glucosidase (acid maltase) and (2) lack of branching enzyme do not fit into the hepatic or myopathic categories just described. They are associated with glycogen storage in many organs and death early in life. Acid maltase is a lysosomal enzyme, and hence its deficiency leads to lysosomal storage of glycogen (type II glycogenosis, Pompe's disease) in all organs, but cardiomegaly is most prominent. Brancher glycogenosis (type IV) is associated with widespread deposition of an abnormal form of glycogen with detrimental effects on the brain, heart, skeletal muscles, and liver.

The principal features of some important examples from each of the aforementioned three categories are summarized in Table 4–7. Details of other forms may be found in specialized texts.[57]

SEX-LINKED (X-LINKED) DISORDERS

All sex-linked disorders are X-linked, almost all X-linked recessive. The only gene assigned with cer-

Table 4–7. Principal Subgroups of Glycogenoses

CLINICOPATHOLOGIC CATEGORY	SPECIFIC TYPE	ENZYME DEFICIENCY	MORPHOLOGIC CHANGES	CLINICAL FEATURES
Hepatic Type	Hepatorenal—von Gierke's disease (type I)	Glucose-6-phosphatase	Hepatomegaly—intracytoplasmic accumulations of glycogen and small amounts of lipid; intranuclear glycogen. Renomegaly—intracytoplasmic accumulations of glycogen in cortical tubular epithelial cells	Failure to thrive, stunted growth, hepatomegaly, and renomegaly. Hypoglycemia due to failure of glucose mobilization, often leading to convulsions. Hyperlipidemia and hyperuricemia resulting from deranged glucose metabolism; many patients develop gout and skin xanthomas. Bleeding tendency due to platelet dysfunction. Mortality approximately 50%
Myopathic Type	McArdle's syndrome (type V)	Muscle phosphorylase	Skeletal muscle only—accumulations of glycogen predominant in subsarcolemmal location	Painful cramps associated with strenuous exercise. Myoglobinuria occurs in 50% of cases. Onset in adulthood (> 20 years). Muscular exercise fails to raise lactate level in venous blood. Compatible with normal longevity
Miscellaneous Types	Generalized glycogenosis—Pompe's disease (type II)	Lysosomal glucosidase (acid maltase)	Mild hepatomegaly—ballooning of lysosomes with glycogen creating lacy cytoplasmic pattern. Cardiomegaly—glycogen within sarcoplasm as well as membrane-bound. Skeletal muscle—similar to heart (see Cardiomegaly)	Massive cardiomegaly, muscle hypotonia, and cardiorespiratory failure within two years. A milder adult form with only skeletal muscle involvement presenting with chronic myopathy

tainty to the Y chromosome is the determinant for testes; although a few additional phenotypic characteristics have tentatively been assigned to the Y chromosome, none has been proved to be Y chromosome-related.

X-linked recessive inheritance accounts for a small number of well-defined clinical conditions. The Y chromosome, for the most part, is not homologous to the X, and so mutant genes on the X are not paired with alleles on the Y. Thus, the male is said to be *hemizygous* for X-linked mutant genes, so these disorders are expressed in the male. The heterozygous female will usually not express the full phenotypic change because of the paired normal allele. However, because of inactivation of one of the X chromosomes in the female, it is remotely possible for the normal allele to be inactivated in most cells, permitting full expression of heterozygous X-linked conditions in the female. Much more commonly, the normal allele is inactivated in only some of the cells, and thus the heterozygous female expresses the disorder partially. An illustrative condition is *glucose-6-phosphate dehydrogenase (G6PD) deficiency*. Transmitted on the X chromosome, this enzyme deficiency, which predisposes to red cell hemolysis in patients receiving certain types of drugs (p. 665), is expressed principally in males. In the female a proportion of the red cells may be derived from marrow cells with inactivation of the normal allele. Such red cells are at the same risk of undergoing hemolysis as the red cells in the hemizygous male. Thus, the female is not simply a carrier of this trait but also is susceptible to drug-induced hemolytic reactions. However, because the proportion of defective red cells in heterozygous females depends on the random inactivation of one of the X chromosomes, the severity of the hemolytic reaction is almost always less in heterozygous women than in hemizygous men.

There are only a few *X-linked dominant* conditions. These disorders are transmitted by an affected heterozygous female to half her sons and half her daughters, and by an affected male parent to all his daughters but none of his sons, if the female parent is unaffected. Most of the X-linked conditions will be covered elsewhere in the text (Table 4–8). Only two remain to be discussed here.

Table 4–8. X-Linked Recessive Disorders

Fabry's Disease

Fabry's disease is also known by the imposing appellation angiokeratoma corporis diffusum universale. The angiokeratoma consists of a dermal cavernous hemangioma with overlying hyperkeratotic thickening of the epidermis. These lesions present clinically as red-blue, slightly elevated nodules, rarely over 1 cm in diameter. Fabry's disease belongs to the category of lysosomal storage diseases already discussed. Unlike the other variants, Fabry's disease is transmitted on the X chromosome. Underlying this disorder is a genetic error in the metabolism of the glycosphingolipid ceramide trihexoside, resulting in its systemic accumulation in endothelial, pericytic, and smooth muscle cells of blood vessels; in ganglion cells; in perineural cells of the autonomic nervous system; in reticuloendothelial, myocardial, and connective tissue cells; in epithelial cells of the cornea; and most dramatically in the kidney glomeruli and tubules. The deficient lysosomal enzyme has been identified as trihexosylceramide α-galactosidase. The storage product imparts a foaminess to the affected cells, which, on higher resolution, can be resolved as lamellated whorls reminiscent of myelin figures. In adolescence and young adult life, skin lesions (angiokeratomas) and central nervous system symptoms dominate the presentation of this disease, but most patients die in middle life of progressive renal failure owing to the kidney involvement.

Fragile X Syndrome

An X-linked pattern of mental retardation has been seen in many kindreds with familial mental retardation.[58] Approximately 30 to 50% of such cases are associated with a cytogenetically detectable alteration in the X chromosome, thus setting them apart from other X-linked mendelian disorders. The cytogenetic abnormality is usually seen as a discontinuity

of staining or secondary constriction (Fig. 4–20) in an unbanded karyotype. It is referred to as a fragile site because it is particularly liable to chromatid breaks when cells are cultured under appropriate conditions. It should be noted that fragile sites are not peculiar to the X chromosome; many such sites have been found on several autosomes, but without any obvious associated clinical disorders.

Over the last several years it has been recognized that the fragile X syndrome is an extremely common hereditary form of mental retardation. Among genetic causes of mental retardation it is second only to Down's syndrome.[59,60] As with all X-linked diseases, the fragile X syndrome affects males. However, analyses of several pedigrees reveal some patterns of transmission not typically associated with other X-linked recessive disorders. For example, there are well-documented cases in which apparently normal males transmitted the faulty X chromosome to their daughters (who subsequently gave birth to retarded sons). Another peculiar feature is the relatively high (30%) incidence of affected females. Although banding studies have localized the fragile site to band Xq27.3, the mutant gene has yet to be identified; hence the unusual patterns of transmission remain unexplained. Clinically the affected males are moderately to severely retarded (IQ 35 to 50). Although a variety of physical abnormalities have been reported, they are often mild and not readily detected. *The only distinctive physical feature is enlarged testes (macroorchidism).* Diagnosis depends upon clinical features, family history, and, most importantly, the demonstration of fragile X chromosome by karyotypic studies.

DISORDERS WITH MULTIFACTORIAL INHERITANCE

As pointed out earlier, the multifactorial disorders are believed to result from the combined actions of environmental influences and two or more mutant genes having additive effects. The genetic component, then, exerts a dosage effect—the greater the number of inherited deleterious genes, the more severe the expression of the disease. Because environmental factors significantly influence the expression of these genetic disorders, the term *polygenic inheritance* is misleading.

A number of normal phenotypic characteristics are governed by multifactorial inheritance, such as hair color, eye color, skin color, height, and intelligence. These characteristics exhibit a continuous variation in population groups, producing the standard bell-shaped curve of distribution. However, environmental influences significantly modify the phenotypic expression of multifactorial traits. For example, certain subsets of diabetes mellitus have many of the features of a multifactorial disorder. It is well recognized clinically that individuals often first manifest this disease following weight gain. Thus,

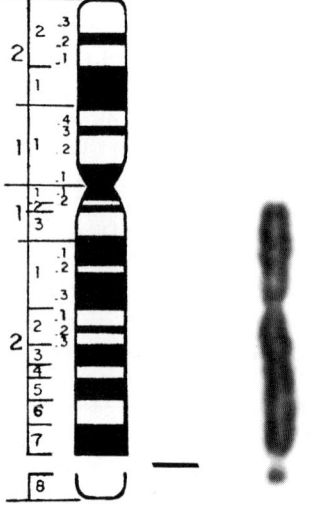

Figure 4–20. Fragile X, seen as discontinuity of staining. (Courtesy of Dr. Patricia Howard-Peebles, Southwestern Medical School, Dallas, Texas.)

obesity as well as other environmental influences unmasks the diabetic genetic trait. Nutritional influences may cause even monozygous twins to achieve different heights. The culturally deprived child cannot achieve his or her full intellectual capacity.

The following features characterize multifactorial inheritance. These have been established for the multifactorial inheritance of congenital malformations and, in all likelihood, obtain for other multifactorial diseases.[61]

1. The risk of expressing a multifactorial disorder is conditioned by the number of mutant genes inherited. Thus, the risk is greater in sibs of patients having severe expressions of the disorder.

2. Environmental influences significantly modify the risk of expressing the disease.

3. The rate of recurrence of the disorder (in the range of 2 to 7%) is the same for all first-degree relatives, i.e., parents, sibs, and offspring, of the affected individual. Thus, if parents have had one affected child, the risk that the next child will be affected is between 2 and 7%. Similarly, there is the same chance that one of the parents will be affected.

4. The likelihood that both identical twins will be affected is significantly less than 100%, but is much greater than the chance that both nonidentical twins will be affected. Experience has proved, for example, that the frequency of concordance for identical twins is in the range of 20 to 40%.

5. The risk of recurrence of the phenotypic abnormality in subsequent pregnancies depends on the outcome in previous pregnancies. When one child is affected there is up to a 7% chance that the next child will be affected, but after two affected sibs the risk rises to about 9%.

6. Severity of expression of the disease may range along a bell-shaped curve or may be discontinuous. Despite the polygenic mode of inheritance, a threshold may exist beyond which individuals are at risk. Thus, for some multifactorial disorders it appears that inheritance of a certain number of mutant genes is required before the disorder is expressed. As stated before, however, environmental influences still play a role.

Assigning a disease to this mode of inheritance must be done with caution. It depends on many factors, but first of all on familial clustering and the exclusion of mendelian and chromosomal modes of transmission. A range of levels of severity of a disease is suggestive of multifactorial inheritance but, as pointed out earlier, variable expressivity and reduced penetrance of mendelian mutant genes may also account for this phenomenon. Because of these difficulties there is often disagreement as to whether the pedigree conforms to a mendelian or multifactorial pattern, as is the case, for example, with diabetes mellitus and epilepsy. The problem is well put in the statement: "multifactorial inheritance is a geneticist's nightmare."

In contrast to the mendelian disorders, which must be considered uncommon, the multifactorial

Table 4–9. Multifactorial Disorders

DISORDER	CHAPTER, PAGE
Cleft lip or cleft palate (or both)	Chapter 17, p. 817
Congenital heart disease	Chapter 13, p. 618
Coronary heart disease	Chapter 13, p. 601
Hypertension	Chapter 21, p. 1062
Gout	Chapter 28, p. 1355
Diabetes mellitus	Chapter 20, p. 994
Pyloric stenosis	Chapter 18, p. 841

group includes some of the most common ailments to which humans are heir (Table 4–9). Most of these disorders are described in appropriate chapters elsewhere in this book.

DISORDERS WITH VARIABLE GENETIC BACKGROUNDS

To this category belong those conditions associated with a variety of genotypic aberrations.

CONGENITAL MALFORMATIONS

Congenital malformations are structural abnormalities that are extremely common causes of spontaneous abortion, stillbirth, and pediatric disease. About 2% of infants have such malformations.[61] Because they have greatest clinical impact in postnatal life and infancy, they are considered in greater detail on page 519. You should note that the term congenital means "born with." *Only some of the congenital anomalies are genetic in origin and have variable modes of transmission,* including (1) cytogenetic aberrations, (2) mendelian inheritance, and (3) multifactorial inheritance. *Some are due to environmental influences,* such as fetal exposure to teratogenic drugs or viral infections during pregnancy.

It is important to identify the genotypic aberrations underlying those malformations of genetic origin. Those involving cytogenetic aberrations (e.g., Turner's syndrome, p. 134) are not familial, so the risk of recurrence in subsequent pregnancies is considerably less than in the case with the mendelian and multifactorial modes of inheritance.

EHLERS-DANLOS SYNDROMES (EDS)

Ehlers-Danlos syndromes are a clinically and genetically heterogeneous group of disorders that result from some defect in collagen synthesis or structure. As such they belong to the same category of diseases as Marfan's syndrome (p. 138) and osteogenesis imperfecta (p. 1318). EDS are discussed here because the mode of inheritance encompasses all three mendelian patterns. This should not be surprising as biosynthesis of collagen is a complex process that can be disturbed by genetic errors that may affect any one of the 20 structural collagen genes or by mutations involving the genes encoding enzymes necessary for post-transcriptional modifications of collagen. Because abnormalities of collagen are fundamental in the pathogenesis of EDS it would be advisable to review collagen structure and synthesis, discussed in Chapter 2. We should recall that there are at least 10 genetically distinct collagen types, having somewhat characteristic tissue distribution. As we shall see, to some extent the clinical heterogeneity and variable modes of transmission of EDS can be explained on the basis of the specific collagen type involved and the nature of the molecular defects.

Traditionally EDS have been subdivided into ten variants according to predominant clinical manifestations and the pattern of inheritance. It is beyond the scope of this book to discuss each variant individually, and the interested reader is referred to several excellent reviews for such details.[62,63] Instead we will first summarize the important clinical features that are common to most variants, and then correlate some of the clinical manifestations with the underlying molecular defects in collagen synthesis or structure.

As might be expected, tissues rich in collagen such as skin, ligaments, and joints are frequently involved in most variants of EDS. Because the abnormal collagen fibers lack adequate tensile strength, *skin is hyperextensible, and the joints are hypermobile.* These features permit grotesque contortions, such as bending the thumb backward to touch the forearm and bending the knee forward to create almost a right angle. Indeed it is believed that most contortionists have one of the EDS. However, a predisposition to joint dislocation is one of the prices paid for this virtuosity. *The skin is extraordinarily stretchable, extremely fragile, and vulnerable to trauma.* Minor injuries produce gaping defects, and surgical repair or any surgical intervention is accomplished with great difficulty because of the lack of normal tensile strength. *The basic defect in connective tissue may lead to serious internal complications.* These include rupture of the colon and large arteries (EDS type IV), ocular fragility with rupture of cornea and retinal detachment (EDS type VI), and diaphragmatic herniae (EDS type I).

The biochemical and molecular bases of these abnormalities are known in only a few forms of EDS. These will be described briefly as they offer some insights into the perplexing clinical heterogeneity of EDS. Perhaps the best characterized is *type VI, the most common autosomal recessive form of EDS.* It results from reduced activity of lysyl hydroxylase, an enzyme necessary for hydroxylation of lysine residues during collagen synthesis. Because hydroxylysine is essential for the cross linking of collagen fibers, a deficiency of lysyl hydroxylase results in the synthesis of collagen that lacks normal structural stability. It is interesting to note that only collagens types I and III are affected in this disorder; the hydroxylation of collagens types II, IV, and V is normal. This observation has raised several questions about the molecular basis of lysyl hydroxylation. Are there different isoenzymes of lysyl hydroxylase with different substrate specifici-

ties? Alternatively, it could be that different domains of the lysyl hydroxylase molecule are utilized for binding to various collagen types, and only the region essential for interaction with types I and III collagen is affected by the mutation that produces EDS type VI. Resolution of these questions awaits cloning of the lysyl hydroxylase gene.

Type IV EDS results from abnormalities of type III collagen. This form is genetically heterogeneous because at least three distinct mutations affecting the structural gene for collagen type III can give rise to this variant. Some mutations affect the rate of synthesis of pro $\alpha 1$ (III) chains; others affect the secretion of type III procollagen; and still others lead to the synthesis of structurally abnormal type III collagen. These molecular studies provide a rational basis for the pattern of transmission and clinical features that are characteristic of this variant. First, because EDS IV results from mutations involving a structural protein (rather than an enzyme protein), an autosomal dominant pattern of inheritance would be expected (p. 137). Second, because blood vessels and intestines are known to be rich in collagen type III, an abnormality of this collagen is consistent with severe defects (e.g., spontaneous rupture) in these organs.

In EDS type VII, the fundamental defect is in the conversion of type I procollagen to collagen. It will be recalled (p. 80) that this step in collagen synthesis involves cleavage of noncollagen peptides at the N- and C-terminals of the procollagen molecule. This is accomplished by N- and C-terminal specific peptidases. *The defect in the conversion of procollagen to collagen in type VII EDS has been traced to two distinct mutations.* In one form there is a deficiency of the enzyme procollagen-N-peptidase. In the other, a mutation in the type I collagen gene results in the synthesis of structurally abnormal pro $\alpha 2$(I) chains that resist cleavage of N-terminal peptides. These two distinct mutations have the same ultimate effect — impaired formation of collagen type I — but because the mutations affect different kinds of proteins (enzyme vs. structural protein) the patterns of inheritance are different. Thus type VII EDS resulting from deficiency of the enzyme N-terminal peptidase is transmitted as an autosomal recessive (as are most other missing enzyme syndromes), whereas in patients who owe their disease to mutation of type I collagen gene, the transmission follows an autosomal dominant pattern. This serves as an excellent example of how an understanding of the molecular pathology has helped resolve apparently divergent patterns of inheritance in a disease that appears to be clinically homogeneous.

Finally, EDS type IX is worthy of brief mention because it illustrates how trace metals can affect connective tissues. The primary defect in this variant involves copper metabolism. These patients have very high levels of copper within the cells but serum copper and ceruloplasmin levels are low. The molecular basis of abnormal copper distribution is not yet known, but its effect is to reduce the activity of the copper-dependent enzyme lysyl oxidase, which is essential for cross-linking of collagen and elastin fibers. Because the genes that regulate copper metabolism map on the X chromosome, this variant of EDS (unlike most others) is inherited as an X-linked recessive trait.

To summarize, the common thread in EDS is some abnormality of collagen. However, these disorders are extremely heterogeneous. At the molecular level a variety of defects, varying from mutations involving structural genes for collagen to those involving enzymes that are responsible for post-transcriptional modifications of m-RNA have been detected. Such molecular heterogeneity results in the expression of EDS as a clinically heterogeneous disorder with several patterns of inheritance.

NEOPLASIA

Cancer and genotype are intimately related on a variety of levels. There is a strong possibility that some alteration of the genetic code—namely, one or more mutations—initiates the formation of malignant neoplasms, as discussed on page 291. Well documented is the fact that certain inherited genotypes predispose to the development of cancers (p. 266). For example, inheritance of a specific autosomal dominant mutation clearly predisposes to the development of retinoblastomas. At yet another level are the cytogenetic abnormalities observed in cancer cells. Both numerical and structural alterations in chromosomes have been observed in cancer cells in vitro as well as in the cells of malignant neoplasms of both animals and man. These and the questions raised about their pathogenetic significance are discussed on pages 260 and 733. There is still another level at which the genome and cancer interrelate, namely, the chromosomal breakage syndromes predisposing to both mutations and cancers. Four autosomal recessive diseases—Fanconi's anemia, Bloom's syndrome, ataxia-telangiectasia, and xeroderma pigmentosum—are characterized by an increased susceptibility to various forms of neoplasia. The fundamental defect in all four of these conditions may be an inability to repair DNA mutations acquired during life, thus increasing the risk of developing cancer (p. 266).

DISEASE DIAGNOSIS BY RECOMBINANT DNA METHODS

Less than a decade ago recombinant DNA technology was considered an arcane tool utilized primarily in basic science research. However, with the rapid transfer of technology from "the bench to the bed" it is now clear that DNA fragments or "probes" can be powerful tools for the diagnosis of human disease, both genetic and acquired.[64-66] In the following section we will briefly review the diagnostic applications of molecular techniques, as they relate to genetic disorders and infectious diseases.

GENETIC DISEASES

Historically, the diagnosis of mendelian or "simple" genetic diseases has depended on the identification of abnormal gene products (e.g., mutant hemoglobin or enzymes) or their clinical effects such as anemia or mental retardation (e.g., phenylketonuria). However, it is now possible to identify gene mutations and offer gene diagnosis for several mendelian disorders, and the list continues to grow. Nucleic acid hybridization for the diagnosis of inherited diseases has several distinct advantages over other techniques.

• First, it is remarkably sensitive. The amount of DNA required for diagnosis can be readily obtained from approximately 10^5 cells. Furthermore, recent improvements allow greater than 200,000-fold amplification of the target DNA by the polymerase chain reaction and hence as few as 100 cells may suffice![67]

• Second, all cells of the body contain the same DNA, and therefore all are affected in inherited genetic disorders. In other words, the test is not dependent on a gene product that may be produced only in certain cells (e.g., erythroid cells) or expression of a gene which may occur late in life. These two features have profound implications for in utero (prenatal) diagnosis because sufficient numbers of cells can be obtained either by removing 10 to 20 ml of amniotic fluid or from biopsy of 1 mg of chorionic villus that can be performed as early as the first trimester.

There are two fundamentally different approaches to the identification of genetic diseases related to an aberrant gene: *(1) direct gene diagnosis involving detection of the mutation, and (2) gene tracking, an indirect method based on detecting linkage of the disease gene with a harmless "marker gene." Each of these will be discussed briefly.*

Direct Gene Diagnosis

This may well be considered the "diagnostic biopsy of the human genome."[66] The principle of detecting the mutant gene is the same as for a traditional diagnostic test, i.e., to detect some important qualitative difference from normal in the DNA sequence of the gene in question. There are two variations of direct gene diagnosis that depend upon the nature of the mutation.

• One technique relies on the fact that some mutations alter or destroy certain restriction sites on the normal DNA. For example, in the normal β-globin gene (HbA) there are three sites that are specifically recognized by the restriction enzyme Mst II (Fig. 4–21). The sickle mutation responsible for sickle cell anemia (p. 666) involves a single base pair change from *CCTGAGG* to *CCTGTGG*, in the sixth codon of the β-globin chain. The enzyme Mst II recognizes and cleaves the normal *CCTGAGG* sequence but not the altered sequence, hence the mutant (hemoglobin S) gene loses one of the three Mst II cutting sites. When DNA from a normal individual is digested with Mst II

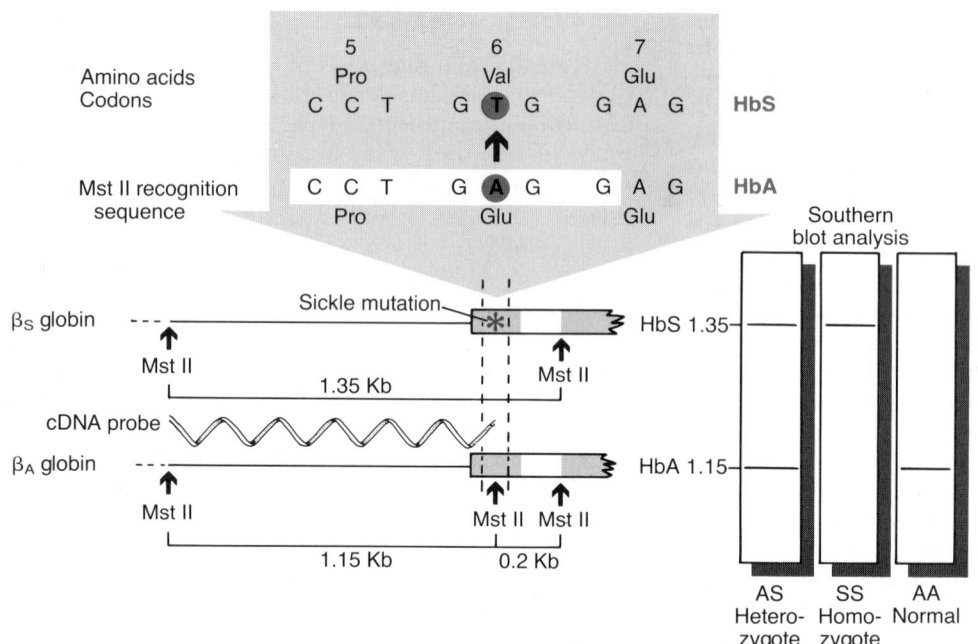

Figure 4–21. Direct gene diagnosis: detection of the sickle mutation by Southern blot analysis. An A → T substitution in the sixth codon of the β_A globin gene yields the β_S allele. This substitution eliminates an Mst II recognition site in the β globin DNA. Thus, when digested with Mst II and probed with an appropriate cDNA, the β_S allele generates a 1.35 Kb fragment, rather than the normal 1.15 Kb fragment.

and hybridized with the radioactive 1.15 kilobase (Kb) cDNA probe specific for the 5′ end of β-globin gene, a single 1.15 Kb band that reacts with the probe is detected on Southern blot analysis (such a band results from the formation of identical 1.15 Kb fragments from each of the two normal chromosomes). On the other hand, a similar analysis of DNA from the cells of a patient homozygous for the HbS gene leads to the formation of a single 1.35 Kb band, owing to the loss of the Mst II sites from both chromosomes. In individuals heterozygous for the sickle mutation, the normal chromosome yields a 1.15 Kb band, whereas the chromosome carrying the mutation gives rise to the 1.35 Kb band. Thus Southern blot analysis reveals two different-sized bands, allowing the detection of a heterozygote carrier.

• Although the methodology just described has proved to be very useful in the diagnosis of sickle cell anemia, its general applicability is limited because most point mutations that cause disease do not alter the cutting sites of any known restriction enzyme. An illustrative example is that of α-1-antitrypsin (α1-AT) deficiency, which in many cases is associated with single G → A change in the α1-AT gene, producing the so-called Z allele (p. 769). In such cases an alternative strategy for the detection of mutant genes can be used (Fig. 4–22). This approach utilizes synthesis of two short (18 to 20 bases long) oligonucleotides that have at their center the single base by which the normal and mutant genes differ. The two oligonucleotides, which differ by only one base, can be radiolabeled and utilized in a Southern blot analysis. The oligonucleotide containing the sequence of the normal gene hybridizes with both the normal and the mutant DNA, but hybridization to the mutant DNA is unstable owing to the single base pair mismatch. Thus, under stringent conditions of hybridization, the

labeled normal probe produces a strong autoradiographic signal with DNA from a normal individual, no signal in the DNA extracted from a patient homozygous for the mutant gene, and a faint signal with DNA from a heterozygote. With the probe containing the mutant sequence the pattern of hybridization is reversed. Of course heterozygotes will react with both probes because they carry one normal and one mutant gene.

Indirect DNA Diagnosis: Gene Tracking

It must be evident from the preceding discussion that direct gene diagnosis is possible only if the mutant gene and its normal counterpart have been identified and cloned, and if their nucleotide sequences are known. In a large number of genetic diseases, including some that are relatively common, such as cystic fibrosis, information about the gene sequence or sometimes even the chromosomal location of the gene is lacking. Obviously, direct gene diagnosis is not possible in these situations. Therefore, alternate strategies, such as "gene tracking," have to be employed. *Stated simply, gene tracking asks the question "has this family member or fetus inherited the same relevant chromosome region(s) as a previously affected family member?"*[68] This principle can be illustrated by considering cystic fibrosis (CF), a relatively common autosomal recessive disease (p. 533). A child who has CF must have received two chromosomes carrying the CF gene, one from each of the two unaffected heterozygous parents. In a subsequent pregnancy such a couple could be expected to give birth to an affected, carrier, or normal child. In a situation like this an antenatal determination of the fetal genotype can be made by detecting whether the conceptus had inherited both, one, or neither of the parental chromosomes that carry the CF gene. It follows, therefore, that the success of such a strategy depends upon the ability to distinguish the chromosome that carries the mutation from its normal homologous counterpart. This is accomplished by exploiting naturally occurring variations in DNA sequences that give rise to the so-called restriction fragment length polymorphisms (RFLPs). Because RFLPs form the backbone of indirect DNA diagnosis, these will be discussed briefly.

Examination of DNA from any two persons will reveal variations in the DNA sequences involving approximately one nucleotide in every 200 to 500 base pair stretch. Most of these variations occur in noncoding regions of the DNA and are hence phenotypically silent. However, these single base pair changes may abolish or create recognition sites for restriction enzymes, thereby altering the length of DNA fragments produced after digestion with certain restriction enzymes. Using appropriate DNA probes that hybridize with sequences in the vicinity of the polymorphic sites, it is possible to detect the DNA fragments of different lengths by Southern blot analysis. *To summarize, the term restriction fragment length polymorphism (RFLP) refers to variation in fragment length between individuals that results from DNA sequence polymorphisms.*

With this background we can discuss how RFLPs can be used in gene tracking. As illustrated in Figure 4–23, if an individual is heterozygous for an RFLP, it is often possible to distinguish the bands produced by each of the two chromosomes in a Southern blot analysis. In the illustrated example, chromosome A has two restriction sites (7.6 Kb apart) whereas chromosome B has a DNA sequence polymorphism that results in the creation of an additional (third) restriction site for the same enzyme. When DNA from such an individual is digested with the appropriate restriction enzyme and probed with a cloned DNA fragment that hybridizes with a stretch of sequences between the restriction sites, chromosome A will yield a 7.6 Kb band whereas chromosome B will produce a smaller 6.8 Kb band. Thus, on Southern blot analysis two bands will be noted. We can now discuss how this technique can be extended to perform indirect gene diagnosis of an autosomal recessive disease such as CF. Let us assume that chromosomes A and B represent two number 7 chromosomes of an individual who is heterozygous for the CF gene, and that the CF gene

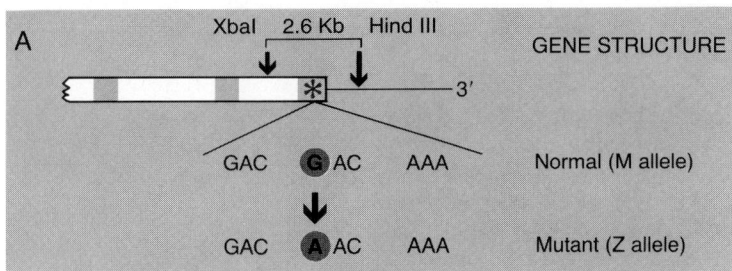

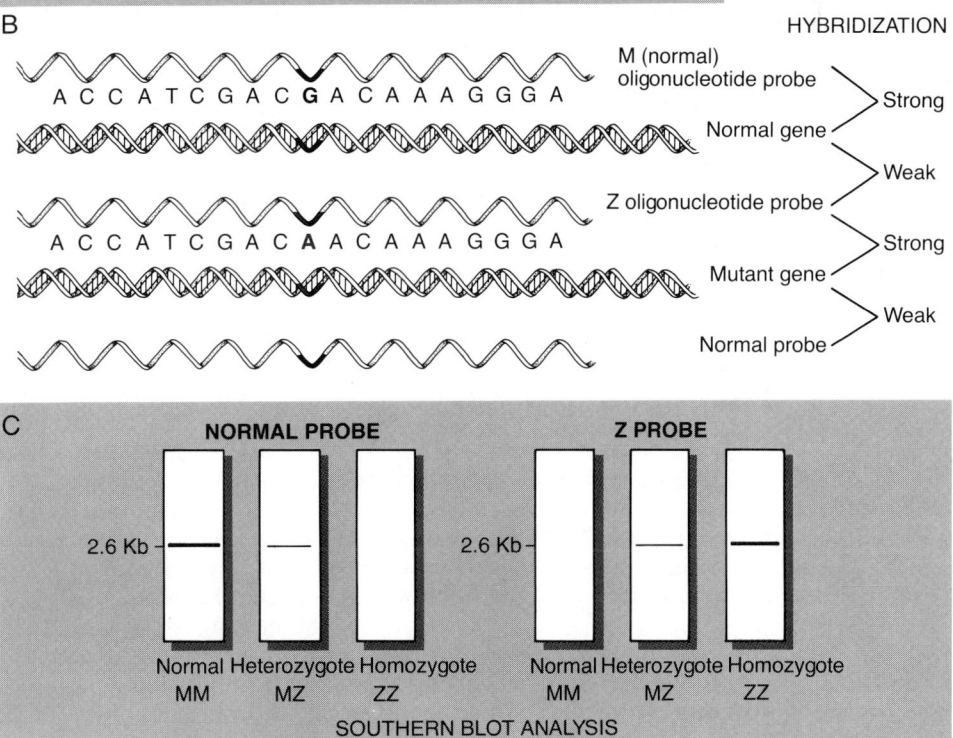

Figure 4–22. Direct gene diagnosis by using an oligonucleotide probe, and Southern blot analysis. Panel A shows that a G → A change converts a normal α-1-antitrypsin allele (allele M) to a mutant Z allele. This change involves exon V of the α-1-antitrypsin gene, which lies between restriction sites for the enzymes Xba I and Hind III. Panel B illustrates the principle of oligonucleotide probe analysis. Two synthetic oligonucleotide probes, one corresponding in sequence to the normal allele (M allele probe) and the other corresponding to the mutant allele (Z allele probe), are lined up against normal and mutant genes, and the expected pattern of hybridization with different combinations is indicated on the right. Panel C diagrams the results of Southern blot analysis when DNA from normal individuals or those heterozygous or homozygous for the mutant Z allele is digested (with Xba I and Hind III) and probed with the normal (M) or Z oligonucleotide probe.

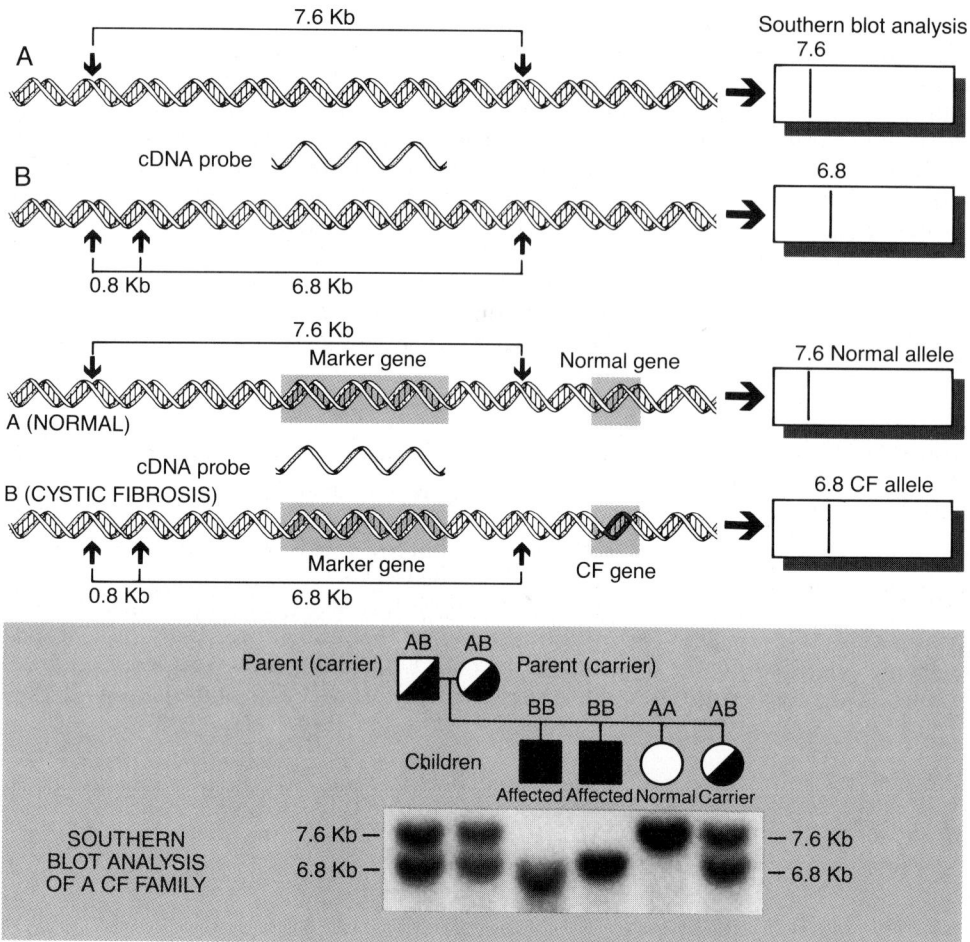

Figure 4–23. Schematic illustration of the principles underlying RFLP analysis in the diagnosis of genetic diseases. Details are described in the text. Note that the distance between the marker gene (p *met* D) and the CF gene is approximately 600 Kb. They are shown closer for simplicity and to emphasize linkage. The Southern blot analysis shown in the lower panel was performed on Ban 1 digest of DNA probed with the p *met* D probe. (Southern blot courtesy of Dr. Arthur L. Beaudet, Howard Hughes Medical Institute and Baylor College of Medicine, Houston, Texas.)

and its normal counterpart are in close proximity to the polymorphic DNA site. Also present in this region is a "marker" gene that is distinct from the CF gene, but whose presence can be detected by available cDNA probes. Under these conditions, Southern blot analysis of DNA extracted from the parents and siblings of a CF patient could be expected to produce an RFLP pattern like that indicated in Figure 4–23. Such an analysis makes it possible to track the transmission of a single chromosome region through a family and to see if a particular single gene disease is co-inherited with a polymorphic site. It is therefore possible to utilize this method for antenatal diagnosis by examining fetal DNA. However, because the probe does not identify the disease gene itself, certain limitations become apparent:

• First, for prenatal diagnosis several relevant family members must be available for testing. In the case of cystic fibrosis, for example, a DNA sample from a previously affected child is necessary to determine the RFLP pattern that is associated with the homozygous CF genotype.
• Second, key family members must be heterozygous for an RFLP, i.e., the two homologous chromosomes must be distinguishable. This may require the use of

multiple restriction enzymes and several different probes for closely linked genes.
• Third, normal exchange of chromosomal material between homologous chromosomes (recombination) during gametogenesis may lead to "separation" of the mutant gene from the polymorphism pattern with which it had been previously co-inherited. This may lead to an erroneous genetic prediction in a subsequent pregnancy. Obviously, the closer the linkage, the lower the degree of recombination and thus a false test. The likelihood of such an error is also minimized by probing for two closely linked marker genes that flank the disease gene.

The probes utilized in RFLP studies may be complementary to functional genes that are linked to the disease gene or to DNA sequences of no known function ("anonymous probes"). An additional advantage of this technique is that if the chromosomal location of the marker gene is known, the chromosomal location of the polymorphic site (and thus the linked mutant gene) can be determined. As an example, Gusella and colleagues screened for RFLP linkage in Huntington's disease with a series of anonymous probes derived from normal genomic DNA. One of the probes, a 12 Kb piece of cloned DNA located on chromosome 4, showed close linkage to Huntington's disease, thereby mapping the gene for Huntington's disease to chromosome number 4.[69] In addition to the two examples already cited (cystic fibrosis and Huntington's disease), RFLPs have been useful in the antenatal or presymptomatic diagnosis of Duchenne muscular dystrophy (p. 1368), polycystic kidney disease (p. 1020), and Lesch-Nyhan syndrome, and the list continues to grow.

RECOMBINANT DNA TECHNIQUES IN THE DIAGNOSIS OF INFECTIOUS DISEASES

As every organism has a DNA sequence that is unique to that microbe, DNA probes can be used not only to detect infectious agents but also to distinguish closely related organisms. This technique can be applied to virtually all classes of pathogens—i.e., bacteria, viruses, and parasites. It is particularly advantageous if the organisms are impossible or difficult to grow. Because the most common objective in the diagnosis of infectious diseases is to detect the presence or absence of microbe-specific DNA or RNA sequences, dot blot hybridization is employed (p. 121). This requires neither cleavage with enzymes nor size fractionation and can be performed rapidly. Under optimal conditions of hybridization the test can detect as few as 10^2 or 10^3 organisms within one to two days. Another form of DNA hybridization that has diagnostic utility in the detection of infectious agents is in situ hybridization performed on tissue sections or cytology specimens. This allows not only detection but also cellular localization of the infecting organism. Nucleic acid hybridization tests are currently available for a variety of microorganisms, including Chlamydia, Salmonella, Mycoplasma, hepatitis B virus, cytomegalovirus, herpes simplex virus, human immunodeficiency virus, and human papilloma viruses.

OTHER DIAGNOSTIC APPLICATIONS OF RECOMBINANT DNA TECHNIQUES

Two other areas in which DNA probe analysis is proving to be of value are (1) the diagnosis of cancer and (2) forensic pathology. As alluded to earlier in this chapter, there is little doubt that neoplastic transformation is associated with some alteration of the genotype. The nature of the genetic alterations that are related to carcinogenesis is discussed in Chapter 6. Suffice it to say here that recombinant DNA techniques can be readily applied to detect the subtlest of alterations in gene structure or expressions that may accompany malignant transformation.

DNA probe analysis has obvious implications for forensic pathology as each human has a unique set of expressed genes and silent DNA polymorphisms. Thus definite identification of individuals or their tissues can be accomplished by utilizing appropriate, usually multiple, gene probes. Such techniques have already proved to be extremely useful in cases of rape and disputed paternity. In closing, it should be mentioned that progress in recombinant DNA technology is occurring at a dizzying, awe-inspiring pace. Witness the recent description of a technique whereby a single hair follicle has been utilized for genetic analysis.[70] It is safe to assume that DNA probes will soon find applications in many more areas of medicine.

So we come to the end of this chapter, but by no means the end of the role of genetics in the diseases of man. Additional instances appear throughout this book.

1. Craig, R.K.: Methods in molecular medicine. Br. Med. J. *295*:646, 1987.
2. Darnell, J., et al. (eds.): Molecular Cell Biology. Washington, D.C., Scientific American Books, 1986.
3. Rowland, L.P.: Dystrophin: A triumph of reverse genetics and the end of the beginning. N. Engl. J. Med. *318*:1392, 1988.
4. Baldwin, V.J., et al.: Diagnostic pathologic investigation of the malformed conceptus. *In* Rosenberg, H.S., and Bernstein, J. (eds.): Perspectives in Pediatric Pathology. Vol. 7. New York, Masson Publishing USA, Inc., 1982, p. 65.
5. Caspersson, T., et al.: Analysis of human metaphase chromosome set by aid of DNA-binding fluorescent agents. Exp. Cell Res. *62*:490, 1970.
6. Francke, U., and Oliver, N.: Quantitative analysis of high-resolution trypsin–Giemsa bands of human prometaphase chromosomes. Hum. Genet. *45*:137, 1978.
7. Hassold, T.J., and Jacobs, P.A.: Trisomy in man. Annu. Rev. Genet. *18*:69, 1984.
8. Thompson, M.W.: Genetics in Medicine. Second edition. Philadelphia, W.B. Saunders Co., 1986, p. 121.
9. Juberg, R.C., and Mowrey, P.N.: Origin of non-disjunction in trisomy 21 syndrome: All studies compiled, parental age analysis, and international comparisons. Am. J. Med. Genet. *16*:111, 1983
10. Ganick, D.J.: Hematologic changes in Down's syndrome. CRC Crit. Rev. Oncol. Hematol. *6*:55, 1986.
11. Karlinsky, H.: Alzheimer's disease in Down's syndrome. A review. J. Am. Geriatr. Soc. *34*:728, 1986.
12. Watkins, P.C., et al.: Molecular genetics of human chromosome 21. J. Med. Genet. *24*:257, 1987.
13. Patterson, D.: The causes of Down's syndrome. Sci. Am. *257*:52, 1987.
14. Gartler, S.M., and Riggs, A.D.: Mammalian X-chromosome inactivation. Annu. Rev. Genet. *17*:155, 1983.
15. Krauss, C.M., et al.: Familial premature ovarian failure due to interstitial deletion of the long arm of the X-chromosome. N. Engl. J. Med. *317*:125, 1987.
16. Simpson, E., et al.: Separation of the genetic loci for the H-Y antigen and for testis determination on human Y chromosome. Nature *326*:876, 1987.
17. Ahmad, K.M., et al.: Leydig cell volume in chromatin-positive Klinefelter's syndrome. J. Clin. Endocrinol. Metab. *33*:517, 1971.
18. Money, J., et al.: Cytogenetics, hormones and behavior disability: Comparison of XXY and XYY syndromes. Clin. Genet. *6*:370, 1974.
19. Federman, D.D.: Mapping the X-chromosome. Minding its p's and q's. N. Engl. J. Med. *317*:161, 1987.
20. Grumbach, M.M., and Conte, F.A.: Disorders of sexual differentiation. *In* Wilson, J.D., and Foster, D.W. (eds.). Williams' Textbook of Endocrinology. Seventh edition. Philadelphia, W.B. Saunders Co., 1985, p. 312.
21. McKusick, V.A.: Mendelian Inheritance in Man. Seventh edition. Baltimore, Johns Hopkins University Press, 1986.
22. Agarwal, D.P., and Goedde, H.W.: Pharmacogenetics and ecogenetics. Experientia *42*:1148, 1986.

23. Pyeritz, R.E.: The Marfan syndrome. Am. Fam. Physician *34*:83, 1986.

24. Pope, F.M., et al.: Clinical and genetic heterogeneity of the Marfan syndrome. Curr. Probl. Dermatol. *17*:95, 1987.

25. Pope, F.M., and Nichols, A.C.: Molecular abnormalities of collagen in human disease. Arch. Dis. Child. *62*:523, 1987.

26. Ogilvie, D.J., et al.: Segregation of all four major fibrillar collagen genes in the Marfan syndrome. Am. J. Hum. Genet. *41*:1071, 1987.

27. Perejda, A., et al.: Marfan's syndrome: Structural, biochemical, and mechanical studies of aortic media. J. Lab. Clin. Med. *106*:376, 1985.

28. Pyeritz, R.E.: Marfan syndrome. *In* Emery, A.E.H., and Rimoin, D.L. (eds.): Principles and Practice of Medical Genetics. New York, Churchill Livingstone, 1983, p. 829.

29. Riccardi, V.M., and Eichner, J.E.: Neurofibromatosis: Phenotype, natural history and pathogenesis. Baltimore, Johns Hopkins University Press, 1986.

30. Marutza, R.L., and Eldridge, R.: Neurofibromatosis 2 (bilateral acoustic neurofibromatosis). N. Engl. J. Med. *318*:684, 1988.

31. Bader, J.L.: Neurofibromatosis and cancer. Ann. N. Y. Acad. Sci. *486*:57, 1986.

32. Seizinger, B.R., et al.: Genetic linkage of von Recklinghausen neurofibromatosis to nerve growth factor receptor gene. Cell *49*:589, 1987.

33. Seizinger, B.R., et al.: Common pathogenetic mechanism for three tumor types in bilateral acoustic neurofibromatosis. Science *236*:317, 1987.

34. Huson, S.M., et al.: Cerebellar hemangioblastoma and von Hippel–Lindau disease. Brain *109*:1297, 1986.

35. Seizinger, B.R., et al.: von Hippel–Lindau disease maps to the region of chromosome 3 associated with renal cell carcinoma. Nature *332*:268, 1988.

36. Brown, M.S., and Goldstein, J.L.: How LDL receptors influence cholesterol and atherosclerosis. Sci. Am. *212*:58, 1984.

37. Vega, G.L., and Grundy, S.M.: Mechanisms of primary hypercholesterolemia in humans. Am. Heart J. *113*:493, 1987.

38. Russell, D.W., et al.: The LDL receptor in familial hypercholesterolemia: Use of human mutations to dissect a membrane protein. Cold Spring Harbor Symp. Quant. Biol. *51*:811, 1987.

39. Illingworth, D.R., and Sexton, G.J.: Hypocholesterolemic effects of mevinolin in patients with heterozygous familial hypercholesterolemia. J. Clin. Invest. *74*:1972, 1984.

40. Garg, A., and Grundy, S.M.: Lovastatin for lowering cholesterol levels in non-insulin-dependent diabetes mellitus. N. Engl. J. Med. *318*:81, 1988.

41. Grundy, S.M.: Drug therapy: HMG-CoA reductase inhibitors for treatment of hypercholesterolemia. N. Engl. J. Med. *319*:24, 1988.

42. Kinnear, P.E., et al.: Albinism. Surv. Ophthalmol. *30*:75, 1985.

43. O'Brien, W.M., et al.: Biochemical, pathologic and clinical aspects of alcaptonuria, ochronosis and ochronotic arthropathy. Review of world literature (1584–1962). Am. J. Med. *34*:813, 1963.

44. Editorial. Lysosomal storage diseases. Lancet *2*:898, 1986.

45. Tager, J.M.: Inborn errors of cellular organelles: An overview. J. Inherited Metab. Dis. *10*(Suppl. 1):3, 1987.

46. Glew, R.H., et al.: Lysosomal storage diseases. Lab. Invest. *53*:250, 1985.

47. Volk, B.W., et al.: The gangliosidoses. Hum. Pathol. *6*:555, 1975.

48. Arey, J.B.: The lipidoses: Morphologic changes in the nervous system in Gaucher's disease, G_{M2}-gangliosidoses and Neimann-Pick disease. J. Clin. Lab. Sci. *5*:475, 1975.

49. Levade, T., et al.: Sphingomyelinases and Neimann-Pick disease. J. Clin. Chem. Clin. Biochem. *24*:205, 1986.

50. daSilva, V., et al.: Niemann-Pick's disease. Clinical, biochemical and ultrastructural findings in a case of infantile form. J. Neurol. *211*:61, 1975.

51. Tsuji, S., et al.: A mutation in the human glucocerebrosidase gene in neuropathic Gaucher's disease. N. Engl. J. Med. *316*:570, 1987.

52. Lee, R.E., et al.: Gaucher's disease: Clinical, morphologic and pathogenetic considerations. Pathol. Annu. *12*:309, 1977.

53. Sorge, J., et al.: Complete correction of the enzymatic defect of type I Gaucher disease fibroblasts by retroviral-mediated gene transfer. Proc. Natl. Acad. Sci. U.S.A. *84*:906, 1987.

54. Muenzer, J.: Mucopolysaccharidoses. Adv. Pediatr. *33*:269, 1986.

55. Beaudet, A.L.: The glycogen storage diseases. *In* Braunward, E., et al. (eds.).: Harrison's Principles of Internal Medicine. Eleventh edition. New York, McGraw Hill Book Co., 1986, p. 1643.

56. DiManro, S., et al.: Metabolic myopathies. Am. J. Med. Genet. *25*:635, 1986.

57. Emery, A.E.H., and Rimoin, D.L.: Principles and Practice of Medical Genetics. New York, Churchill Livingstone, 1983, p. 1272.

58. Turner, G., and Jacobs, P.: Marker (X)-linked mental retardation. Adv. Hum. Genet. *13*:83, 1983.

59. Pembrey, M., and Baraitser, M.: Recently recognized chromosomal defects of clinical importance. Postgrad. Med. J. *62*:131, 1986.

60. Brown, T.W., et al.: The fragile X syndrome. Ann. N.Y. Acad. Sci. *477*:129, 1986.

61. Nelson, K., and Holmes, L.B.: Malformations due to presumed spontaneous mutations in newborn infants. N. Engl. J. Med. *320*: 19, 1989.

62. Uitto, J., and Shamban, A.: Heritable skin diseases with molecular defects in collagen and elastin. Dermatol. Clin. *5*:63, 1987.

63. Byers, P.H., and Holbrook, K.A.: Molecular basis of clinical heterogeneity in the Ehlers-Danlos syndrome. Ann. N. Y. Acad. Sci. *460*:298, 1986.

64. Antonarkis, S.E.: Diagnosis of genetic disorders at the DNA level. N. Engl. J. Med. *320*:153, 1989.

65. Caskey, C.T.: Disease diagnosis by recombinant DNA methods. Science *23*:1223, 1987.

66. McKusick, V.A. The morbid anatomy of the human genome: A review of gene mapping in clinical medicine. Medicine *67*:1, 1988.

67. Orkin, S.H.: Genetic diagnosis by DNA analysis. Progress through amplifications. N. Engl. J. Med. *317*:1023, 1987.

68. Pembrey, M.: Impact of molecular biology on clinical genetics. Br. Med. J. *295*:711, 1987.

69. Gusella, J., et al.: A polymorphic DNA marker genetically linked to Huntington's disease. Nature *306*:234, 1983.

70. Higuchi, R., et al.: DNA typing from single hairs. Nature *332*:43, 1988.

BASIC IMMUNOLOGY

Man lives in a hostile environment, literally immersed in a sea of pathogens ranging from viruses to worms seeking to invade and to destroy tissues and cells. Yet most humans manage not only to survive but indeed thrive in this potentially hostile milieu, without seeming effort. This *immunitas* (Latin, freedom from disease) is dependent on the existence of a complex and highly sophisticated defense system that is often subdivided into two major categories, *innate* and *adaptive*, each endowed with a *humoral* and *cellular* arm (Fig. 5–1). The innate resistance system may be viewed as the first line of defense. Its cellular components, depicted in Figure 5–1, are ideally suited for this role because their actions do not depend on prior sensitization or "priming" by the antigens present on their target cells (e.g., microbes, tumor cells) and furthermore they do not possess the fine antigen specificity that is characteristic of the adaptive (or specific) immune responses. Thus, for example, a given macrophage can whet its appetite by ingesting a wide variety of antigenically distinct bacteria or viruses at its very first encounter. Complement, the major humoral component of innate immunity, was described in Chapter 2. The principal cellular components of the adaptive immune responses are T and B lympho-cytes. As will be detailed later, each T and B lymphocyte is genetically programmed to recognize only one antigenic determinant, by means of an antigen-specific receptor on its surface, and hence these cells display exquisite antigen specificity. During evolution, humans have developed the ability to recognize myriads of foreign antigens and hence a normal individual must possess antigen-specific cells that can react with a staggering number of antigens. Because the human body is not merely a bag of lymphocytes (as many immunologists believe!), it follows that in unprimed individuals the number of lymphocytes that can react to any given specific antigen must be extremely small. However, when challenged with an antigen, say in the form of a microbial infection, antigen-specific lymphocytes divide and expand to effectively handle the offending organism. Such clonal expansion of T and B lymphocytes is a complex multistep process involving both differentiation and cell division; therefore, it takes at least a few days, sometimes weeks, before the process is completed. Because of this requirement, specific immune responses are better suited as the second line of defense, which eventually becomes the major protective mechanism.

Although the distinctions between innate and induced immunity and the cellular and humoral effector systems are helpful in resolving the complexity of the host defense systems, *it is extremely important to remember that there are multiple interconnections and "cross talk" among the various components* (Fig. 5–1).

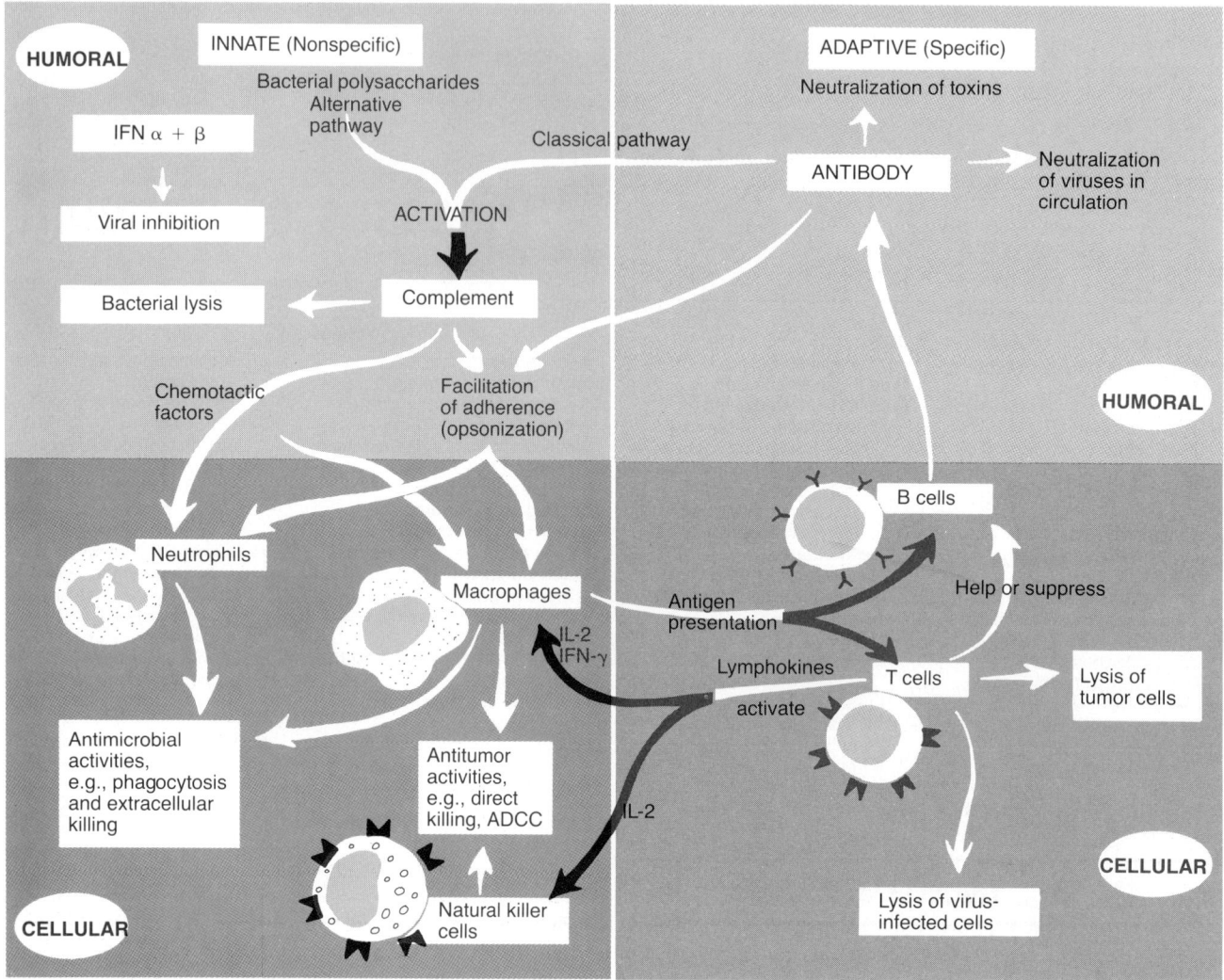

Figure 5–1. Adaptive and innate immunity. A schematic illustration of their humoral and cellular components, and interactions among them.

Recall that the complement cascade, an important nonspecific humoral component, can be triggered directly by an invading organism (the alternate pathway) or by antibodies formed in the course of a specific immune response. Complement, in turn, plays an important role in modulating the function of neutrophils and macrophages, as detailed earlier (p. 54). Macrophages are not only important effector cells in the expression of innate immunity, but also, as antigen-presenting cells, they play an important role in triggering specific immune responses mediated by B and T lymphocytes. The latter, as is well known, mediate cellular immunity and in addition they regulate the function of antibody-producing B cells, as well as that of macrophages and natural killer (NK) cells. The physiologic significance of these interactions is often evident when a genetic or acquired disease selectively destroys just one component of this finely tuned "orchestra," as is exemplified by the acquired immunodeficiency syndrome (AIDS). In this dis-

order, the destruction of a subset of T cells by the human immunodeficiency virus (HIV) produces a cascade of effects that eventually cripple almost the entire host defense apparatus (p. 224).

Although vital to survival, the immune system is like the proverbial two-edged sword. On the one hand, immunodeficiency states render humans easy prey to infections and possibly tumors; on the other hand, a hyperactive immune system may cause fatal disease, as in the case of an overwhelming allergic reaction to the sting of a bee. In yet another series of derangements, the immune system may lose its normal capacity to distinguish self from non-self, resulting in the emergence of immunity against one's own tissues and cells (autoimmunity). In this chapter, we consider diseases caused by too little immunity as well as those resulting from too much immunologic reactivity. But first, we review some recent advances in the understanding of lymphocyte biology, to be followed by a brief description of the histocompatibility genes, because their products are relevant to several immunologically mediated diseases and to the rejection of transplants.

GENERAL FEATURES OF THE IMMUNE SYSTEM

T Lymphocytes

T lymphocytes arise from stem cells in the bone marrow that migrate to the thymus, where they undergo differentiation into mature T cells and then leave the thymus. Mature T cells circulate in the blood and also seed peripheral lymphoid tissues, such as the *paracortical areas of lymph nodes and periarteriolar sheaths of the spleen*. With the use of monoclonal antibodies it has been possible to define several cell-surface markers on developing and mature T cells (Table 5–1). Some, such as CD3 and CD2, are present on all peripheral T cells, whereas others define functionally distinct subsets. For example, CD4 and CD8 molecules are expressed on two nonoverlapping subsets of peripheral T cells. CD4 constitutes the marker on approximately 60% of mature T cells, whereas CD8 is expressed on about 30% of T lymphocytes. Thus, in normal healthy individuals, the CD4 to CD8 ratio is approximately 2. This may be altered in various diseases. Although initially discovered as markers for T cells, most of these molecules have now been shown to be associated with particular T-cell functions, of which there are two broad categories:

1. *Cellular immune reactions.* These include several phenomena in which T cells play a pivotal role. Examples are cytotoxic (killer) T cells reactive against virally infected cells and foreign histocompatibility antigens. Killer T cells are CD3+ (like all mature T cells), but in addition, most of them express CD8. Another expression of cellular immunity is the delayed hypersensitivity reaction (mediated by CD4+ cells) to be described later.
2. *Regulatory functions:* T cells also regulate the function of other T cells, B cells, and hematopoietic stem cells, as well as several nonhematopoietic cells. Their immunoregulatory functions are expressed either as facilitation or as suppression of the response. Thus CD4+ *helper-inducer cells* provide "help" in the generation of cytotoxic T cells and antibody-secreting B cells. On the other hand, a subset of CD8+ cells serves to damp the immune responses. These regulatory functions are mediated for the most part by the secretion of soluble factors called lymphokines, to be described later.

As mentioned earlier, T and B lymphocytes are genetically programmed to recognize specific antigens by means of antigen-specific cell-surface receptors. Until recently, the nature of T-cell antigen receptor (TCR) was an enigma. However, recent advances in molecular biology have provided tools

Table 5–1. Some Immune Cell Antigens Detected by Monoclonal Antibodies

ANTIGEN DESIGNATION*	COMMENTS
Primary T Cell–Associated	
CD2	Receptor for sheep erythrocytes; present on all T cells (peripheral and intrathymic) and NK cells
CD3	Present on all peripheral T cells; associated with the T-cell antigen receptor
CD4	Present on 60% of peripheral T cells and some monocytes; a marker for T helper-inducer cells
CD5	Present on all T lymphocytes, peripheral and intrathymic
CD7	Present on all T lymphocytes
CD8	Present on 30% of peripheral T cells; marker for cytotoxic cells
CD25	Receptor for interleukin-2; present on activated T cells, B cells, and monocytes
Primary B Cell–Associated	
CD19	Present on B cells, from pre-B stage to mature B cells; absent from plasma cells
CD20	Appears on pre-B cells after CD19; otherwise similar to CD19 in distribution
CD10	Common acute lymphoblastic leukemia (CALLA) antigen; present on pre-B cells
Primary Monocyte- or Macrophage-Associated	
CD13	Present on blood monocytes and granulocytes
CD33	Present on myeloid stem cells and mature monocytes
CD11b	Present on monocytes, granulocytes, and some NK cells; receptor for complement (C3b)
Primarily NK Cell–Associated	
CD16	Present on all NK cells and granulocytes; low-affinity receptor for Fc portion of IgG
Present on All Leukocytes	
CD45	
CD11a	

* The antigens are designated by the prefix CD (cluster designation) (based on Third International Workshop on Human Leukocyte Differentiation Antigens as reported by Shaw, S.: Immunol. Today 8:1, 1987.)

that have allowed the discovery and detailed descriptions of the TCR.[1,2] It is now apparent that in approximately 95% of the T cells, *the TCR consists of a disulfide-linked heterodimer made up of an α- and a β-polypeptide chain*, each having a variable (antigen binding) and a constant region, somewhat analogous to immunoglobulin molecules. In a minority of T cells, another type of TCR, constituted of two distinct polypeptide chains termed γ and δ, has been recognized (TCR γ/δ). *Unlike TCR α/β+ cells, these cells do not express either CD4 or CD8 on the cell surface.* Both TCR α/β and TCR γ/δ are noncovalently linked to the CD3 molecular complex, which itself is composed of at least three invariant proteins (Fig. 5–2). Although

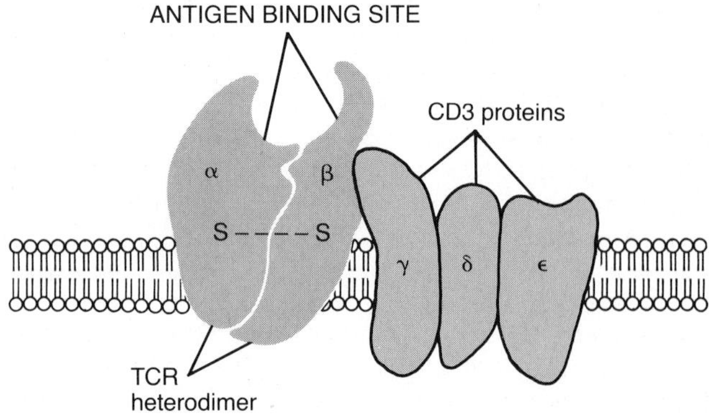

ANTIGEN BINDING SITE

CD3 proteins

α   β

S – – – S

γ   δ   ε

TCR
heterodimer

Figure 5–2. The T-cell receptor (TCR) complex. A schematic illustration of the TCR α and β polypeptide chains linked to the CD3 molecular complex.

antigen recognition is mediated by the variable segments of the α and β polypeptide chains of the TCR, the postrecognition steps involving transduction of activating signals are believed to be the property of CD3 protein complex.[3]

Although the TCR is distinct from immunoglobulins that are known to function as the antigen receptors utilized by B cells, recent studies indicate that the genetic organization of the TCR is remarkably similar to that of immunoglobulins. Figure 5–3 depicts a portion of human chromosome 7, on which the genes

for the β-chain of the T-cell receptor are located. It may be noted that the β-chain of the TCR is assembled from four separate genes, each belonging to a group of genes segregated into four regions. These are designated V, D, J, and C (to indicate *variable*, *diversity*, *joining*, and *constant* segments). As might be expected, every somatic cell contains the T-cell receptor genes (in the so-called germ-line configuration shown in Fig. 5–3), but they are expressed only in T lymphocytes. Transcription of the TCR genes is preceded by a remarkable phenomenon called gene rearrangement, whereby genes—one gene each from the V, D, and J regions—come to lie next to each other by elimination of the intervening DNA. The rearranged DNA is then transcribed to form mRNA. During processing of the mRNA, the intervening sequences between the VDJ and the C regions are spliced off, so that the products of the VDJ and C regions come together. The other chains (α, γ, and δ) are synthesized in an analogous manner. *The phenomenon of the TCR gene rearrangement, which occurs only in T cells during their maturation in the thymus, has enormous theoretical and practical significance.*

• It provides a mechanism by which it is possible to have numerous antigen-specific T cells. Because a complete α- and β-chain of the T-cell receptor is produced by a combination of one of the several genes in each of the V, D, J, and C regions, it is possible to

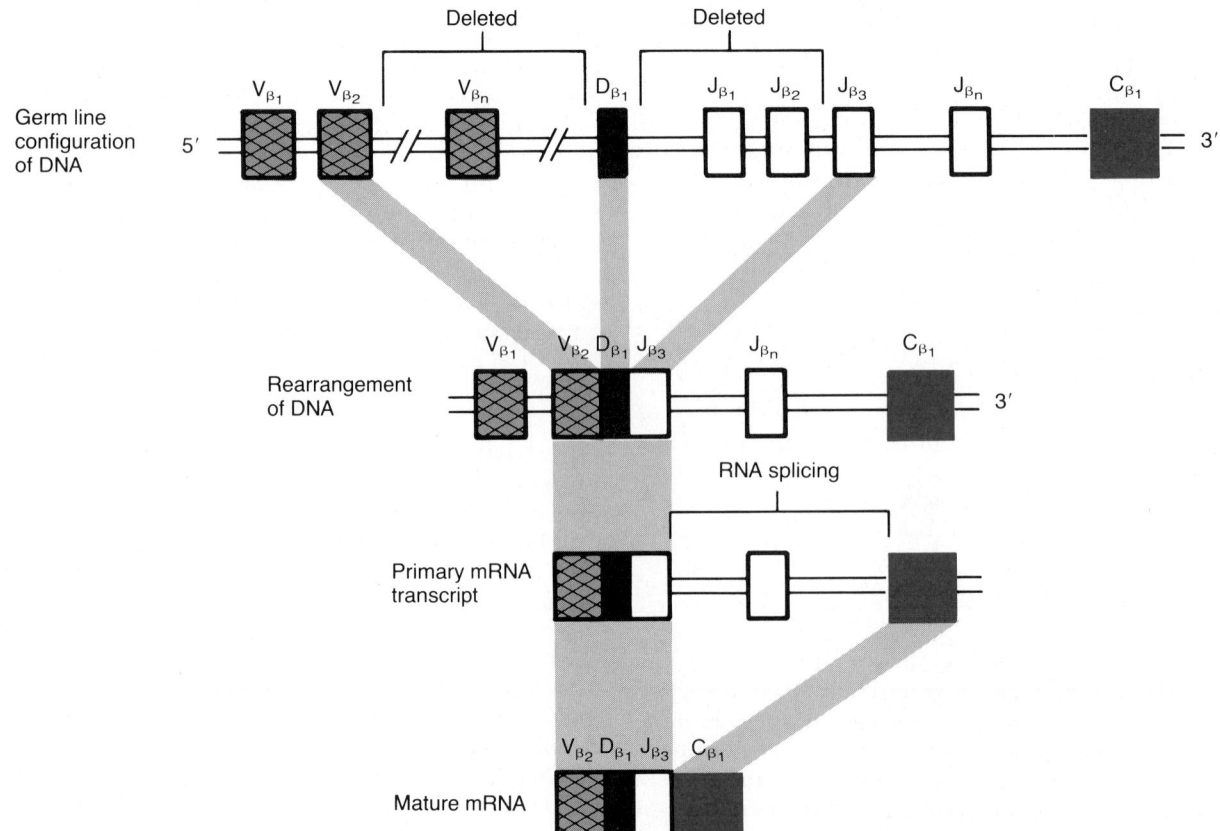

Figure 5–3. Rearrangement and transcription of the β-chain genes of the T-cell antigen receptor.

generate enormous diversity in the TCR. Each TCR, resulting from a specific combinatorial rearrangement of the α- and β-chain genes, has a unique genetically determined structure that is specific for only one of a myriad of antigens.

• At a practical level, the knowledge that each T cell has a unique DNA rearrangement makes it possible to distinguish polyclonal (non-neoplastic) proliferations of T lymphocytes from monoclonal (neoplastic) proliferations. The technique of Southern blot analysis (described on p. 121) is utilized for such studies.

As alluded to earlier, several of the T-cell surface markers are function-associated molecules. CD4 and CD8, although not linked to TCR, are believed to facilitate interactions between T cells and other cells by increasing the avidity of cell-to-cell contact. CD4 molecules bind to class II molecules of the major histocompatibility complex (MHC), whereas CD8 molecules interact with class I molecules. As will be discussed later, corecognition of class I or class II MHC molecules and antigen is a fundamental property of T cells.

B Lymphocytes

B lymphocytes are present in the blood and lymphoid tissue, including bone marrow. In human blood they constitute 10 to 20% of the lymphocyte population. *In lymph nodes they are found in the superficial cortex, forming lymphoid follicles. In the spleen they are found in the white pulp organized as lymphoid follicles, usually having pale-staining central areas called germinal centers.* As is well known, B cells express surface immunoglobulin, which can be identified by fluorescence microscopy or flow cytometry after the cells have been incubated with anti-immunoglobulin antibodies labeled with fluorescein isothiocyanate. This procedure is utilized clinically to identify and quantitate B cells. In addition, as with T cells, several monoclonal antibodies directed against B cell-surface molecules have been described (Table 5–1).[4] Some of the B cell-specific surface markers, such as CD19 (formerly termed B4), appear early in B-cell differentiation, prior to the expression of surface immunoglobulin, and are therefore useful in determining the histogenesis of certain leukemias of childhood (p. 724).

It has been known for quite some time that monomeric IgM, present on the surface of all B cells, constitutes the antigen receptor of B cells. The specificity of the surface immunoglobulin is identical to that of the immunoglobulin that is secreted when the B cell becomes a plasma cell. The genetic basis of the diversity of the B-cell repertoire (i.e., the existence of numerous B cells programmed to recognize only one antigen) has been clarified by the studies that were initiated by Susuma Tonegawa (recipient of the 1987 Nobel Prize). There are remarkable similarities in the organization of immunoglobulin genes and genes of the T-cell receptor. Thus, in mice the immunoglobulin heavy chain is assembled from a pool of approximately 200 V, 12 D, and 4 J segments. In addition, there are eight constant region genes (Cμ, Cγ, Cδ, and so on) corresponding to the immunoglobulin isotypes and their subclasses. Genes in the immunoglobulin light chain have a similar organization, except that they lack the D-region genes. During B-cell maturation there is somatic rearrangement of the DNA, as was described for T cells. Given the numbers of genes in the V, D, and J regions for heavy chains and light chains, it is not difficult to estimate that antibodies with greater than 10^7 specificities can arise by unique combinatorial rearrangements of the immunoglobulin genes. As mentioned earlier with respect to T cells, it is important to note the practical application of this knowledge. *Because in a given B cell and its progeny only one of the several million possible DNA rearrangements occurs, it is feasible to distinguish between clonal (neoplastic, p. 250) and polyclonal (reactive) proliferations of B cells by extracting the DNA and subjecting it to Southern blot analysis.*

Macrophages

Macrophages are a part of the mononuclear phagocyte system and as such their origin, differentiation, and role in inflammation were discussed in Chapter 2. Here we need only to emphasize that macrophages play several roles in the immune response.[5] Some surface antigens present on monocytes and macrophages are listed in Table 5–1.

• First, they are required to process and present antigen to immunocompetent T cells. Because T cells (unlike B cells) cannot be activated by soluble antigens, presentation of processed, membrane-bound antigens by macrophages or other antigen-presenting cells (e.g., Langerhans' cells, discussed later) is obligatory for induction of cell-mediated immunity. The processed antigen is presented in conjunction with class II histocompatibility antigens to CD4 + T cells.
• They produce a variety of soluble factors,[6] including interleukin-1 (IL-1), which promotes the differentiation of both T and B lymphocytes. It should be noted that IL-1 has multiple targets and numerous other effects, some of which are described elsewhere in this text and also summarized in Table 5–2 (Chapter 2, p. 58; Chapter 3, p. 117).
• Macrophages lyse tumor cells by secreting toxic metabolites and proteolytic enzymes and as such may play a role in immunosurveillance.
• Macrophages are important effector cells in certain forms of cell-mediated immunity, such as the delayed hypersensitivity reaction.

NK Cells

In recent years much interest has focused on a novel cell type, called the natural killer (NK) cells.[7] These cells are capable of lysing a variety of tumor cells, virus-infected cells, and some normal cells, *without previous sensitization.* NK cells are found in the peripheral blood and the lymphoid tissues of man as well as a variety of animal species. Although NK cells share

Table 5-2. Cytokines

NAME	SOURCE	TARGET CELLS AND BIOLOGIC PROPERTIES
Interleukin-1	Virtually any cell, including monocytes, macrophages, endothelium, keratinocytes, and glial cells	Activates resting T cells; is a cofactor for other hematopoietic growth factors; induces sleep, fever, ACTH release, and other systemic acute-phase responses; stimulates synthesis of other lymphokines (IL-2, IFN-γ); stimulates production of collagenases; increases bone resorption by osteoclasts; activates macrophages; renders endothelial cells more adhesive for leukocytes
Tumor necrosis factor-α (TNF-α)	Macrophages, activated T cells, NK cells	Mimics many actions of IL-1 on T cells, B cells, macrophages, and endothelial cells; induces acute-phase reactions; inhibits lipoprotein lipase in fat cells; inhibits hematopoietic stem cells; cytotoxic to some tumor cells
Interleukin-2 (IL-2)	Activated T cells	Stimulates growth of activated T and B cells; activates and promotes growth of NK cells; activates monocytes
Interleukin-3 (IL-3)	Activated T cells	Supports growth of pluripotential hematopoietic stem cells; growth factor for mast cells
Interleukin-4 (IL-4)	Activated T cells	Growth and differentiation factor for activated B and T cells; growth factor for mast cells; increases expression of HLA class II antigens on B cells
Interleukin-5 (IL-5)	Activated T cells	Induces differentiation of activated B cells into antibody-producing plasma cells
Interleukin-6 (IL-6)	Activated T cells, fibroblasts, monocytes	Enhances maturation of activated T and B cells; stimulates growth of hematopoietic progenitor cells; inhibits growth of fibroblasts
Interferon-γ (IFN-γ)	Activated T cells, NK cells	Activates macrophages and induces expression of HLA class II molecules on macrophages and many other cells; suppresses hematopoietic progenitor cells; activates endothelial cells; antiviral activity

some cell-surface antigens with T cells and macrophages, they are believed to be distinct from mature T cells, B cells, or macrophages. They are CD3$^-$ but express two markers, CD16 and Leu 19, that are useful for their identification. Morphologically they are somewhat larger than small lymphocytes and possess granules in their cytoplasm; they have therefore been described as *large granular lymphocytes.* NK cells utilize two distinct mechanisms to lyse their target cells. One, termed antibody-dependent cellular cytotoxicity, utilizes NK cell surface Fc-receptors and antibodies directed against the target-cell antigens and will be described later (p. 177). The other involves direct interaction between NK cells and their target cells and utilizes NK cell receptors that have not yet been fully characterized (Fig. 5-4). Because of their ability to lyse tumor cells and virus-infected cells in vitro, without previous immunization, they are considered to be important as the first line of defense against tumors and virus infections. Furthermore, it is possible to rapidly activate and expand their numbers by

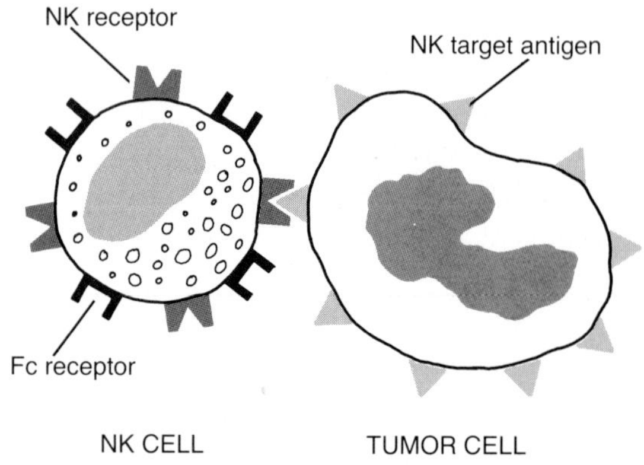

culturing with interleukin-2 in vitro. The resulting population, often referred to as lymphokine-activated killer (LAK) cells, is currently being evaluated as an immunotherapeutic tool in the treatment of certain forms of cancer.[8]

Dendritic and Langerhans' Cells

Dendritic cells and Langerhans' cells include a population of cells that are all characterized by dendritic cytoplasmic processes and the presence of large amounts of cell-surface class II molecules. Dendritic cells are found in the lymphoid tissues, and somewhat similar cells within the epidermis have been called Langerhans' cells. By virtue of cell-surface class II molecules, dendritic cells and Langerhans' cells are extremely efficient in antigen presentation, and some investigators believe that they are the most important antigen-presenting cells in the body. It should be noted that although they share antigen-presenting capacity with macrophages, unlike the latter cell type they are weakly or not at all phagocytic.

Cytokines: Messenger Molecules of the Immune System

It is well known that the induction and regulation of immune responses involves multiple interactions among cells of the immune system, many of which result from the release of polypeptide mediators. Depending on the source of the mediators they have been called *lymphokines* (lymphocyte-derived) or *monokines* (monocyte-derived). However, in recent years it has become apparent that the target spectrum of these soluble mediators extends beyond cells of the immune system, and conversely, some mediators originally thought to be produced only by lymphocytes or monocytes can be generated by many nonlymphoid cells. Hence, the term *cytokines* is now preferred. It is impossible to list all the cytokines and their sources and actions because new factors, and

Figure 5-4. A schematic representation of the direct tumor cell killing by NK cells. Note that the Fc receptor of NK cells is not involved.

previously unknown actions of the better characterized factors, are being discovered with each passing day. Many cytokines are still defined by their activities, but by the end of 1988, genes encoding at least 17 cytokines had been cloned and their products purified. Of these, some that are produced primarily by the cells of the immune system are listed in Table 5–2. Details about these and other cytokines may be found in several recent reviews.[9–13] Here we will summarize some salient features that are associated with the actions of many cytokines:

• Cytokines induce their effects in three ways: (1) they act on the same cell that produces them (*autocrine* effect), such as occurs when IL-2 produced by activated T cells promotes T-cell growth, (2) they affect other cells in their vicinity (*paracrine* effect), as occurs when IL-1 produced by antigen-presenting cells affects T cells during the induction of an immune response (p. 184), and (3) they affect many cells systemically (*endocrine* effect), the best examples in this category being IL-1 and TNF-α that produce the acute-phase response during inflammation.

• Cytokines mediate their effects by binding to specific high-affinity receptors on their target cells. For example, IL-2 activates T cells by binding to high-affinity IL-2 receptors (IL-2R). Blockade of the IL-2R by monoclonal antibodies directed against the receptor prevents T-cell activation. This observation provides a means by which T-cell activation, when undesirable (as in transplant rejection), may be controlled.

• Production of cytokines and responsiveness to cytokines are tightly regulated by environmental stimuli and other cytokines. For example, resting T cells produce little if any IFN-γ; however, during cell-mediated immune response against tubercle bacilli, they produce IFN-γ and many other lymphokines that activate and immobilize macrophages, an action that is necessary for containing the infection. Environmental influences on cytokine production may well be mediated by cytokines themselves; for example, TNF-α regulates the synthesis or release (or both) of IL-1 and hematopoietic growth factor by endothelial cells.

The knowledge gained about cytokines is not merely of academic interest; it has practical therapeutic ramifications as well. First, by regulating cytokine production or action it may be possible to control the harmful effects of inflammation or tissue-damaging immune reactions. Second, cytokines produced by recombinant DNA technology can be administered to enhance immunity against cancer or microbial infections (immunotherapy). Both these avenues are currently being pursued on an experimental basis in humans.

HISTOCOMPATIBILITY ANTIGENS

Although originally identified as antigens that evoke rejection of transplanted organs, histocompatibility antigens are now considered important in the regulation of the immune response as well as in resistance or susceptibility to a growing list of diseases. The histocompatibility antigens and the corresponding genes are complex in structure and organization and are still incompletely understood. Here we summarize only the salient features of human histocompatibility antigens, primarily to facilitate understanding of their role in rejection of organ transplants and in disease susceptibility. A detailed description may be found in specialized texts.[14]

It is well known that when an individual receives an organ transplant obtained from a genetically dissimilar donor, the transplanted organ is rejected by immunologic mechanisms. In this process of rejection, the recipient's immune system recognizes the histocompatibility antigens displayed on the cell surfaces of the donor organ. Several genes code for histocompatibility antigens, but those that code for the most important transplantation antigens are clustered on a small segment of chromosome 6. This cluster of genes constitutes the human major histocompatibility complex (MHC) and is also known as the HLA complex (Fig. 5–5). It is equivalent to the murine H-2 complex.

The initials HLA stand for human leukocyte antigens, as MHC-encoded antigens were initially de-

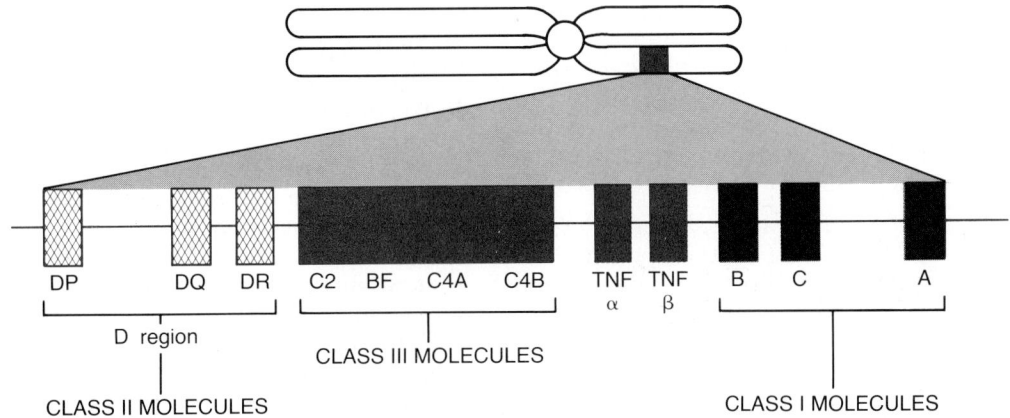

Figure 5–5. A schematic representation of the HLA complex and its subregions on human chromosome 6. The class III genes are not shown individually; they map within the region shown as a solid red rectangle. The relative distances between various genes and regions are not drawn to scale, and in some cases are unknown.

tected on the white cells. The HLA system is highly polymorphic—that is, there are several alternative forms (alleles) of a gene at each locus. This, as we shall see, constitutes a formidable barrier in organ transplantation.

Based on their chemical structure, tissue distribution, and function, the MHC gene products are classified into three categories.[15]

1. *Class I antigens* are coded by three closely linked loci designated HLA-A, HLA-B, and HLA-C (Fig. 5–5). Each of these molecules is a heterodimer, consisting of a polymorphic glycoprotein of 45,000 daltons (heavy chain) linked noncovalently to a smaller nonpolymorphic peptide called $\beta2$-microglobulin. The latter is encoded by a gene on chromosome 15. Class I antigens are present on virtually all nucleated cells and platelets.

2. *Class II antigens* are coded for in a region known as HLA-D. These antigens were initially defined by a phenomenon called the *mixed lymphocyte reaction*, which occurs when lymphocytes from two individuals who have differing HLA-D regions are cultured together in vitro. T lymphocytes from one individual recognize ("see") foreign class II antigens on the cells of the other individual and respond by proliferation. If there is genetic identity at the HLA-D region, proliferation does not occur. Recent studies have identified three subregions, DP, DQ, and DR, within the originally defined HLA-D region. *Class II antigens* differ from class I antigens in several respects. Chemically, they exist as bimolecular complexes, but both of their constituent polypeptide chains are polymorphic. These, labeled α and β, have molecular weights of 34,000 daltons and 29,000 daltons, respectively. Unlike class I antigens, their tissue distribution is quite restricted; they are found mainly on antigen-presenting cells (monocytes and macrophages, dendritic cells), B cells, and some activated T cells. However, several other cell types, such as vascular endothelium, fibroblasts, and renal tubular epithelial cells, can be induced to express class II antigens by γ-interferon, a lymphokine produced by activated T cells.

3. *Class III proteins* are those components of the complement system (C2, C4, and Bf) that are coded for within the MHC. Recent studies indicate that genes for the cytokines TNF-α and TNF-β are also encoded within the MHC.[16] Although genetically linked to class I and II antigens, class III molecules and the cytokine genes do not act as histocompatibility (transplantation) antigens and will not be discussed further.

As already mentioned, a feature shared by class I and class II genes is the high degree of polymorphism. Each of the several alleles at these loci is designated by a number, such as HLA-A1, HLA-B5, and so forth. (Those alleles that have not been fully characterized are identified by a W—e.g., HLA-BW4.) *All class I determinants and most (but not all) of the class II determinants evoke the formation of humoral antibodies in genetically nonidentical individuals.* This makes it possible to type these antigens by conventional serologic techniques such as antibody- and complement-mediated lysis. Sera of multiparous women (who are immunized by the paternal antigens of the fetus) have traditionally served as a useful source of such anti-HLA antibodies. However, it is now possible to raise monoclonal anti-HLA antibodies by immunizing rodents with human cells.

As mentioned above, certain class II antigens cannot be detected by serologic techniques. They are detected by the mixed lymphocyte reaction described earlier and are designated HLA-D antigens, to distinguish them from the serologically defined D-region antigens, such as HLA-DR and HLA-DQ. However, unlike the case with DP, DQ, and DR loci, there is no single definable HLA-D locus within the HLA-D region. It is believed that the responding T cells in the mixed lymphocyte reaction are detecting an array of HLA-DP, HLA-DQ, and/or HLA-DR antigens, some of which are not serologically detectable. Because HLA antigens form an allelic series, an individual inherits only one determinant from each parent and can have no more than two different antigens for every locus. Thus, cells of a heterozygous individual will express six different class I HLA antigens, three of maternal origin and three of paternal origin. Owing to the polymorphism at the major HLA loci, innumerable combinations of antigens can exist, and therefore each individual in a noninbred population is likely to have a more or less unique antigenic profile, like a fingerprint on the cell surface.

Significance of HLA Complex

ORGAN TRANSPLANTATION.
As stated earlier, HLA antigens were discovered in the course of transplantation studies, and they continue to present formidable barriers to the success of clinical organ transplantation. HLA antigens of the graft evoke both humoral and cell-mediated responses, which lead eventually to graft destruction, as discussed on page 183. Because the severity of the rejection reaction is related to the degree of HLA disparity between the donor and recipient, HLA typing is of immense clinical significance in the selection of the donor-recipient combinations.

REGULATION OF IMMUNE RESPONSE.
Class I and II HLA antigens play important but distinct roles in the induction and expression of cellular as well as humoral immunity.

Class I antigens are involved primarily in regulating the function of CD8+ cytotoxic T cells, which are believed to be important in resistance against virus infections. It can be demonstrated experimentally that *cytotoxic T cells specifically sensitized against a virus can recognize and lyse only those virus-infected cells that bear self class I molecules* (Fig. 5–6). The basis of this phenomenon of HLA restriction seems to be that class I HLA antigens provide specific sites that are modified by virus infection and constitute the target antigen for the T cell receptors of cytotoxic (CD8+) T cells. Because virus-infected cells can be

HLA-CLASS I RESTRICTED KILLING

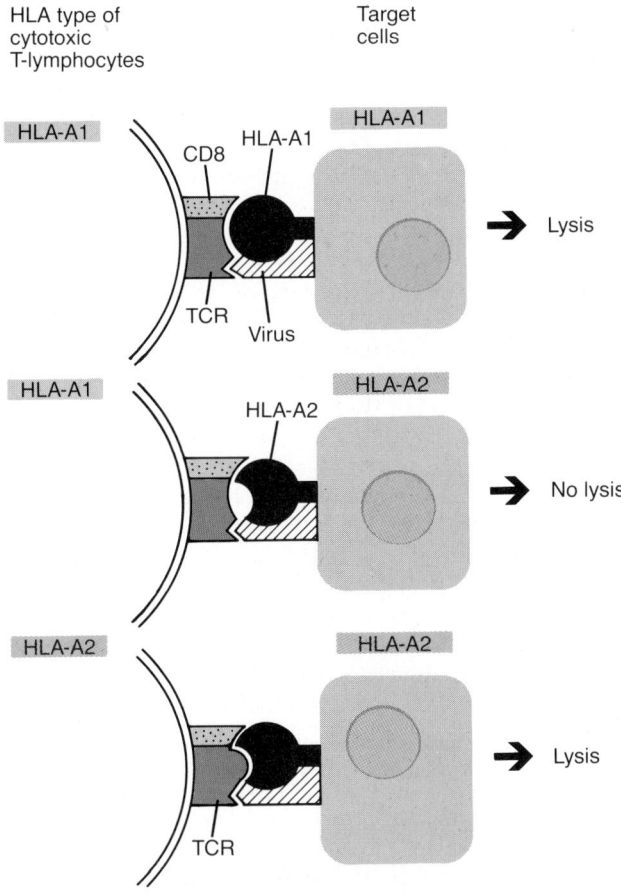

Figure 5–6. A schematic illustration of the role of HLA antigens in the lysis of virus-infected cells by CD8 positive cytotoxic T lymphocytes. Note that cytotoxic T cells from HLA-A1 or HLA-2 positive donors can lyse only those virus-infected cells that carry self-HLA antigens. The CD8 molecule, unlike the T-cell receptor, is invariant and plays an accessory role in T cell–mediated killing.

recognized only in the context of class I MHC antigens, it makes "good sense" to have widespread expression of class I HLA antigens.

Class II antigens are particularly important in cell-to-cell interactions, especially in the activation of CD4+ T cells. In contrast to CD8+ killer T cells that recognize antigens in association with class I MHC antigens, CD4+ helper T cells recognize antigens only in the context of class II antigens on the surface of macrophages or other antigen-presenting cells. The role of class II antigens in the induction of T helper cells may also have an important bearing on the genetic regulation of the immune response. It is well known that the magnitude of immune responses is controlled by immune response (Ir) genes that map within the HLA-D region. Indeed, it is now believed that class II genes function as Ir genes. How class II antigens influence the magnitude of the immune response is not fully understood. It is conceivable that certain class II alleles may code for cell-surface (class II) molecules that form highly immunogenic complexes with a given antigen (Fig. 5–7). This in turn

would translate into a vigorous activation of T-helper cells and a strong immune response. The consequence of inheriting such a class II gene would depend upon the nature of the antigen and the type of immune response generated. For example, if the antigen were ragweed pollen and the response were production of IgE antibody, the individual would be genetically prone to attacks of sneezing (p. 176). On the other hand, good responsiveness to influenza virus may well mean a sniffle-free winter.

HLA AND DISEASE ASSOCIATION. A variety of diseases have been found in association with certain HLA types (Table 5–3). The best known is the association between ankylosing spondylitis and HLA-B27; individuals who possess HLA-B27 antigen have a 90-fold greater chance (relative risk) of developing this disease than those who are negative for HLA-B27. The diseases that show association with HLA can be broadly grouped into the following categories: (1) *inflammatory diseases*, including ankylosing spondylitis and several postinfectious arthropathies, all associated with HLA-B27; (2) *inherited errors of metabolism*, such as hemochromatosis (HLA-A3) and 21-hydroxylase deficiency (HLA-BW47); (3) *autoimmune diseases*, including autoimmune endocrinopathies, associated with alleles at the DR locus; and (4) *complement deficiency* syndromes. The mechanisms underlying these associations are not understood at present. Clearly, with diseases as diverse as enzyme deficiency syndromes and autoimmune disorders, no single mechanism of association is likely. In view of the physiologic role of the HLA complex in regulation of the immune response, it is somewhat easier to speculate on the possible mechanisms that may underlie the associations with immunologically mediated diseases. The following two mechanisms have been proposed.[17]

• *Involvement of immune response genes.* It was mentioned previously that HLA class II genes can regulate immune responsiveness. Accordingly, an association between certain autoimmune diseases and HLA-DR antigens may result from an exaggerated immune response to autoantigens.

• *Direct participation of HLA macromolecules in disease.* There are two possible mechanisms by which

Table 5-3. Association of HLA with Disease

DISEASE	HLA ALLELE	RELATIVE RISK
Ankylosing spondylitis	B27	87.4
Postgonococcal arthritis	B27	14.0
Acute anterior uveitis	B27	14.6
Rheumatoid arthritis	DR4	5.8
Chronic active hepatitis	DR3	13.9
Primary Sjögren's syndrome	DR3	9.7
Insulin-dependent diabetes	DR3	5.0
	DR4	6.8
	DR3/DR4	14.3
Hemochromatosis	A3	8.2
21-Hydroxylase deficiency	BW47	15.0

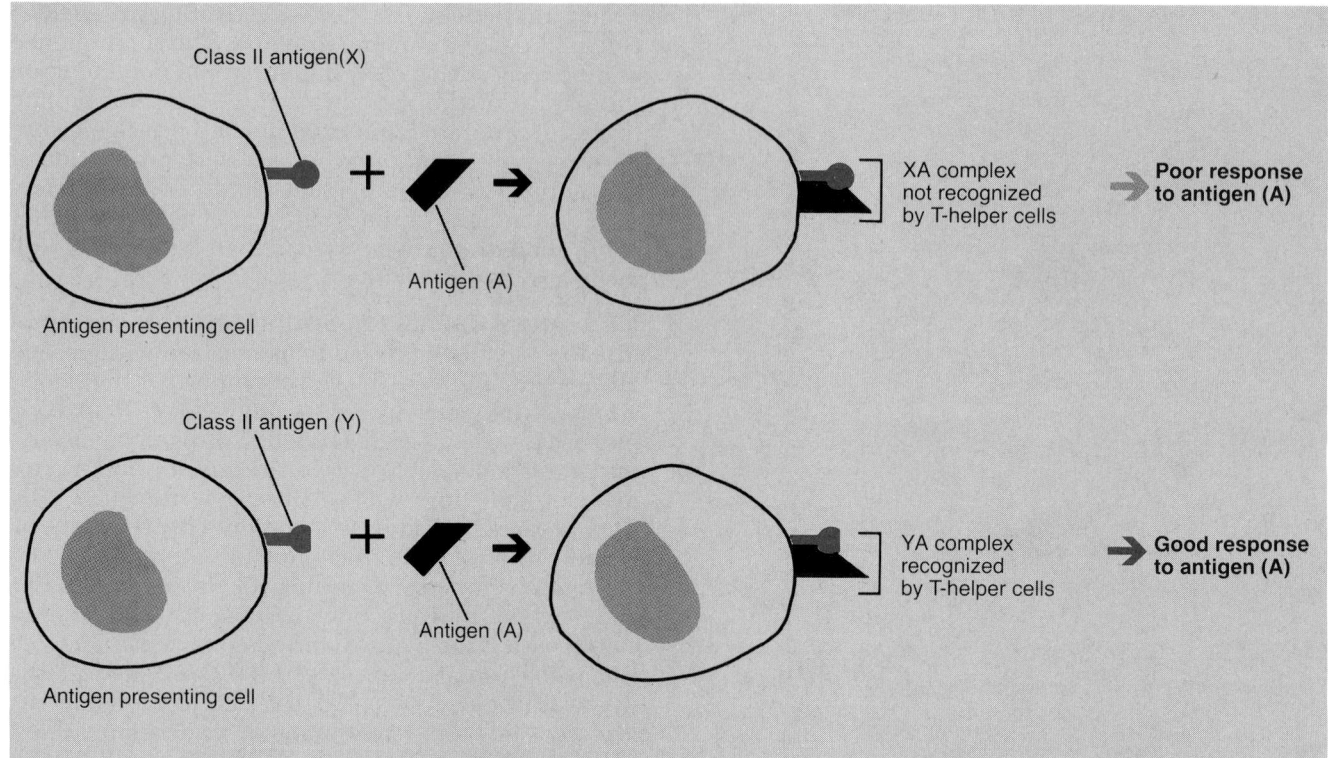

Figure 5–7. Schematic illustration of the proposed role of class II antigens in the genetically determined regulation of the immune response. As explained in the text, the magnitude of the immune response against a given antigen (A) may be determined by the nature of class II gene products expressed on the antigen presenting cell.

HLA molecules may participate directly in disease. First, pathogens may share a cross-reacting antigen with HLA and be protected from an immune response by the host's tolerance for self-HLA antigens ("molecular mimicry"). This in effect would provide the pathogen an "immunologic permit" to invade and destroy tissues at will. Alternatively, a strong immune response may be mounted against the invading pathogen, but because of the sharing of determinants between the microbe and the HLA antigen, immunologically mediated damage may be inflicted on normal tissues.[18] Second, certain HLA molecules may provide receptors for viruses, and this may either facilitate virus-cell interaction or provide a target for host immune cells to destroy virus-infected cells. In the former case, the presence of a given HLA type would favor virus-induced disease, whereas in the latter case it would favor removal of virus-infected cells.

DISORDERS OF THE IMMUNE SYSTEM

Having reviewed some recent advances in basic immunology, we can now turn to general disorders of the immune system and some specific immunologic

diseases. These will be discussed under four broad headings: (1) *hypersensitivity reactions*, which form the mechanisms of immunologic injury in a variety of diseases discussed throughout this book; (2) *autoimmune diseases*, which are caused by immune reactions against self; (3) *amyloidosis*, a poorly understood disorder having immunologic association; and (4) *immunologic deficiency syndromes*, which result from relatively distinct, often genetically determined defects in some components of the normal immune response.

MECHANISMS OF IMMUNOLOGIC TISSUE INJURY (HYPERSENSITIVITY REACTIONS)

Humans live in an environment teeming with substances capable of producing immunologic responses. Contact with antigen leads not only to induction of a protective immune response, but also to reactions that can be damaging to tissues. Exogenous antigens occur in dust, pollens, foods, drugs, microbiologic agents, chemicals, and many blood products used in clinical practice. The immune responses that may result from such exogenous antigens take a variety of forms, ranging from annoying but trivial discomforts such as itching of the skin to potentially fatal disease such as bronchial asthma. The various reactions produced are called *hypersensitivity reactions*, and these can be initiated either by the interaction of antigen with humoral antibody or by cell-mediated immune mechanisms.

Tissue-damaging immune reactions may be evoked not only by exogenous antigens but also by those that are intrinsic to the body (endogenous). This distinction is of value because it indicates that some disorders—those due to exogenous antigens—are essentially environmental and as such are theoretically preventable. Poison ivy contact dermatitis could be eradicated as a disease by mere avoidance of contact with the plant, as could hay fever resulting from inhalation of plant pollens. On the other hand, many of the most important immune diseases are caused by homologous and autologous antigens intrinsic to humans. The disorders triggered by homologous antigens result from the genetic and antigenic dissimilarities among individuals. Transfusion reactions and graft rejection are examples of immunologic disorders evoked by homologous antigens. Appropriate cross matching of donor and recipient could preclude such reactions. The third category of disorders, those incited by autologous antigens, constitutes the important group of autoimmune diseases, to be discussed later in this chapter. These diseases appear to arise because of the emergence of immune responses against self antigens.

Hypersensitivity diseases can be classified on the basis of the immunologic mechanism that mediates the disease (Table 5–4). This approach is of value in clarifying the manner in which the immune response ultimately causes tissue injury and disease.

- In *type I disease*, the immune response releases vasoactive and spasmogenic substances that act on vessels and smooth muscle, thus altering their function.
- In *type II disorders*, humoral antibodies participate directly in injuring cells by predisposing them to phagocytosis or lysis.
- *Type III disorders* are best remembered as "immune complex diseases," in which humoral antibodies bind antigens and activate complement. The fractions of complement then attract neutrophils, which, partly through the release of neutrophilic lysosomal enzymes, produce tissue damage.

- *Type IV disorders* involve tissue injury in which cell-mediated immune responses with sensitized lymphocytes are the cause of the cellular and tissue injury.

Prototypes of each of these immune mechanisms are presented in the following sections.

TYPE I HYPERSENSITIVITY (ANAPHYLACTIC TYPE)

Anaphylaxis may be defined as a rapidly developing immunologic reaction occurring within minutes after the combination of an antigen with antibody bound to mast cells or basophils in individuals or animals previously sensitized to the antigen. It may occur as a systemic disorder or as a local reaction. The systemic reaction usually follows an intravenous injection of an antigen to which the host has already become sensitized. Often within minutes a state of shock is produced, which is sometimes fatal. Local reactions depend on the portal of entry of the allergen and take the form of localized cutaneous swellings (skin allergy, hives), nasal and conjunctival discharge (allergic rhinitis and conjunctivitis), hay fever, bronchial asthma, or allergic gastroenteritis (food allergy).

In humans, type I reactions are mediated by IgE antibodies.[19] An allergen stimulates B lymphocyte production of IgE, principally at the mucosal site of entry of the antigen and in the draining lymph nodes. This process requires the assistance of T-helper cells and is under the regulatory influence of T-suppressor cells. IgE antibodies formed in response to an allergen have a strong tendency to attach to mast cells and basophils through cell surface receptors for the Fc portion of IgE heavy chain (Fig. 5–8). *When a mast cell or basophil, armed with cytophilic IgE antibodies, is reexposed to the specific allergen, a series of reactions takes place, leading eventually to the release of a variety of powerful mediators responsible for the clinical expression of type I hypersensitivity reactions.* In the first step in this sequence, antigen (allergen) is bound to the IgE antibodies previously attached to the mast cells. In this process, multivalent antigens bind to more than one IgE molecule and cause cross

Table 5-4. Mechanisms of Immunologically Mediated Disorders

TYPE	PROTOTYPE DISORDER	IMMUNE MECHANISM
I Anaphylactic type	Anaphylaxis, some forms of bronchial asthma	Formation of IgE (cytotropic) antibody → release of vasoactive amines and other mediators from basophils and mast cells
II Cytotoxic type	Autoimmune hemolytic anemia, erythroblastosis fetalis, Goodpasture's syndrome	Formation of IgG, IgM → binds to antigen on target cell surface → phagocytosis of target cell or lysis of target cell by C8,9 fraction of activated complement or antibody-dependent cellular cytotoxicity (ADCC)
III Immune complex disease	Arthus reaction, serum sickness, systemic lupus erythematosus, certain forms of acute glomerulonephritis	Antigen-antibody complexes → activated complement → attracted neutrophils → release of lysosomal enzymes and other toxic moieties
IV Cell-mediated (delayed) hypersensitivity	Tuberculosis, contact dermatitis, transplant rejection	Sensitized thymus-derived T lymphocytes → release of lymphokines and T cell-mediated cytotoxicity

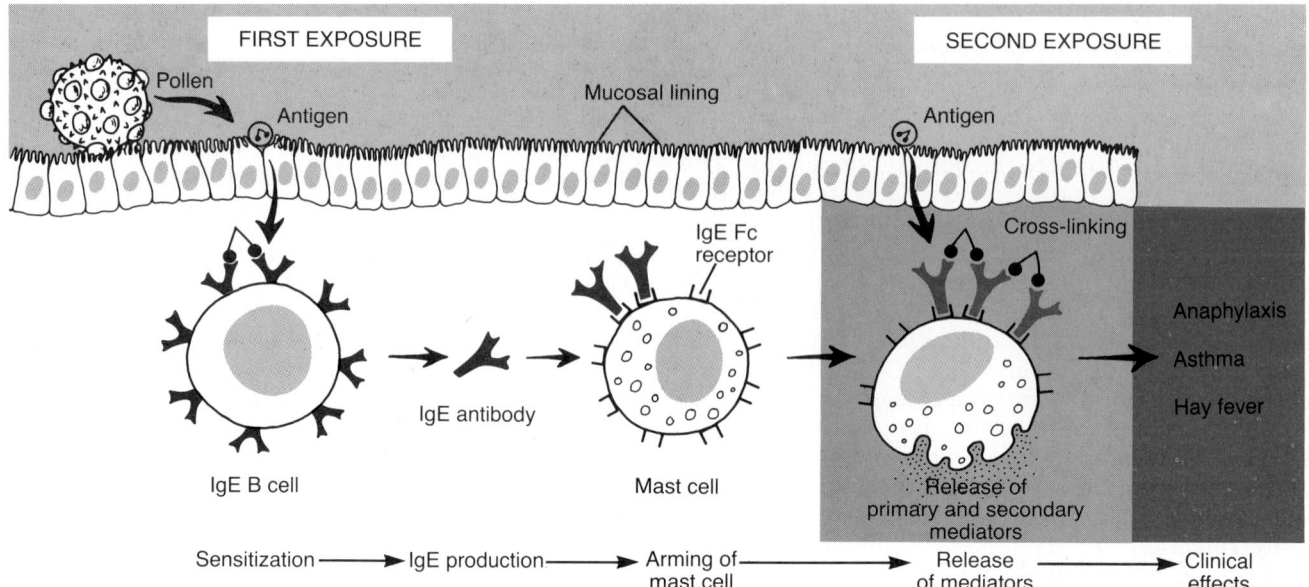

Figure 5–8. Sequence of events leading to type I hypersensitivity. (Modified from Roitt, I., et al.: Immunology. New York, Gower Medical Publishing, 1985, p. 19.2.)

linkage of adjacent IgE antibodies. The bridging of IgE molecules leads to perturbations of the IgE-Fc receptors and initiates two parallel and interdependent processes — one leading to *mast cell degranulation with discharge of preformed (primary) mediators* and the other involving *de novo synthesis and release of secondary mediators, such as leukotrienes.*

Degranulation of mast cells is an active process that requires influx of calcium and depends on an intact glycolytic pathway.[20] Involved in the complex sequence is an initial rapid increase in cAMP, followed by a fall to baseline levels within five minutes (Fig. 5–9). The transient elevation of cAMP activates cAMP-dependent protein kinases. These in turn are responsible for phosphorylation of the membrane around mast cell granules. Phosphorylation and other alterations of the perigranular membranes render them permeable to water and calcium, resulting in marked swelling of the granules (visible with the electron microscope). Simultaneously, calcium-activated enzymes release energy required for the assembly of microtubules and microfilaments. These contractile elements of the cytoskeleton cause the movement of swollen granules toward the cell surface, where they fuse with the cell membrane and spill their contents. In addition to IgE-mediated triggering, mast cell degranulation can also be brought about by a variety of other physical and chemical stimuli. Among the mast cell secretagogues are breakdown products of complement (C3a and C5a, anaphylatoxins), some drugs such as codeine and morphine, mellitin (present in bee venom), and such physical stimuli as sunlight, trauma, heat, and cold.[21] Regardless of the stimulus, degranulation of mast cells is a very finely regulated process, an understanding of which can be used to therapeutic advantage. For example, it was men-

tioned earlier that one of the early events in mast cell triggering is a transient increase in the levels of cAMP. If cAMP levels are *persistently* elevated, as can be achieved by β-adrenergic agents such as epinephrine, mast cell degranulation is prevented, and the symptoms of type I hypersensitivity are relieved.

As indicated earlier, triggering of mast cells leads to the release of preformed (primary) and newly synthesized (secondary) mediators that are described in the following paragraphs.

PRIMARY MEDIATORS. Primary mediators are contained within the mast cell granules and include (1) *histamine,* which causes intense bronchial smooth muscle contraction, increased vascular permeability, and increased secretion by nasal, bronchial, and gastric glands; (2) several *eosinophil chemotactic factors of anaphylaxis* (ECF-A), which account for the presence of these cells in allergic reactions; (3) *neutrophil chemotactic factors;* and (4) *granule-matrix–derived mediators,* such as heparin, neutral proteases (e.g., trypsin), and some less well defined factors (e.g., inflammatory factors of anaphylaxis).[22] The last mentioned are tightly bound to the proteoglycan matrix of the granule and participate in the so called "late-phase reactions" of type I hypersensitivity, described later.

SECONDARY MEDIATORS. Secondary mediators are generated by a complex series of reactions in the mast cell membranes, leading to the generation of *arachidonic acid* from membrane phospholipids by activated phospholipase A_2, phospholipase C, and diacylglycerol lipase.[23] Arachidonic acid, you may recall, is the parent compound from which leukotrienes and prostaglandins are derived by the 5-lipoxygenase and cyclooxygenase pathways, respectively (p. 55). Each of these is considered separately.

• Leukotrienes are extremely important in the pathogenesis of type I hypersensitivity. *Leukotrienes C_4, D_4, and E_4* are the most potent vasoactive and spasmogenic agents known. On a molar basis, leukotrienes C_4 and D_4 are several thousand times more active than histamine in increasing vascular permeability and causing bronchial smooth muscle contraction. They are also remarkably potent stimulators of mucus secretion in the airways. Because leukotriene release is slower than that of histamine, in the past leukotrienes were designated a slow-reactive substance of anaphylaxis (SRS-A). *Leukotriene B_4* is highly chemotactic for neutrophils, eosinophils, and monocytes.

• Among the arachidonic acid metabolites generated by the cyclooxygenase pathway, *prostaglandin D_2* is the most abundant mediator produced by the human lung mast cells. It causes intense bronchospasm and vasodilatation, as well as increased mucus secretion.

• *Platelet activating factor* (PAF, p. 58) is another secondary mediator that causes platelet aggregation and release of histamine. In addition, it also has other potent biologic effects, such as bronchoconstriction, vasodilatation, and increased vascular permeability, all of which are independent of histamine release. Although PAF production is also initiated by the activation of phospholipase A_2, it is not a product of arachidonic acid metabolism.

In summary, a variety of chemotactic, vasoactive, and spasmogenic compounds listed in Table 5–5 mediate type I hypersensitivity reactions. Some are released rapidly from sensitized mast cells and are believed to be responsible for the intense immediate reactions associated with conditions such as bronchial asthma. The initial tissue response usually becomes manifest within five to 30 minutes after exposure to an allergen and tends to subside within 60 minutes. In many individuals, however, the so-called allergic reaction recurs within two to eight hours, without additional exposure to antigen, and can last for two to three days. This "late phase reaction" is characterized by a more intense infiltration of the tissues, with eosinophils, neutrophils, monocytes, and basophils,[24] as well as tissue destruction in the form of mucosal epithelial cell damage. *It is believed that the late phase inflammatory response is mediated largely by factors that are bound to the proteoglycan matrix of mast cells and are released slowly from the granule matrix.* These factors include low- and high-molecular-weight "inflammatory factors of anaphylaxis" (IF-A), which are strongly chemotactic for neutrophils and eosinophils, and neutral proteases such as trypsin and chymotrypsin, which can cleave complement components to gener-

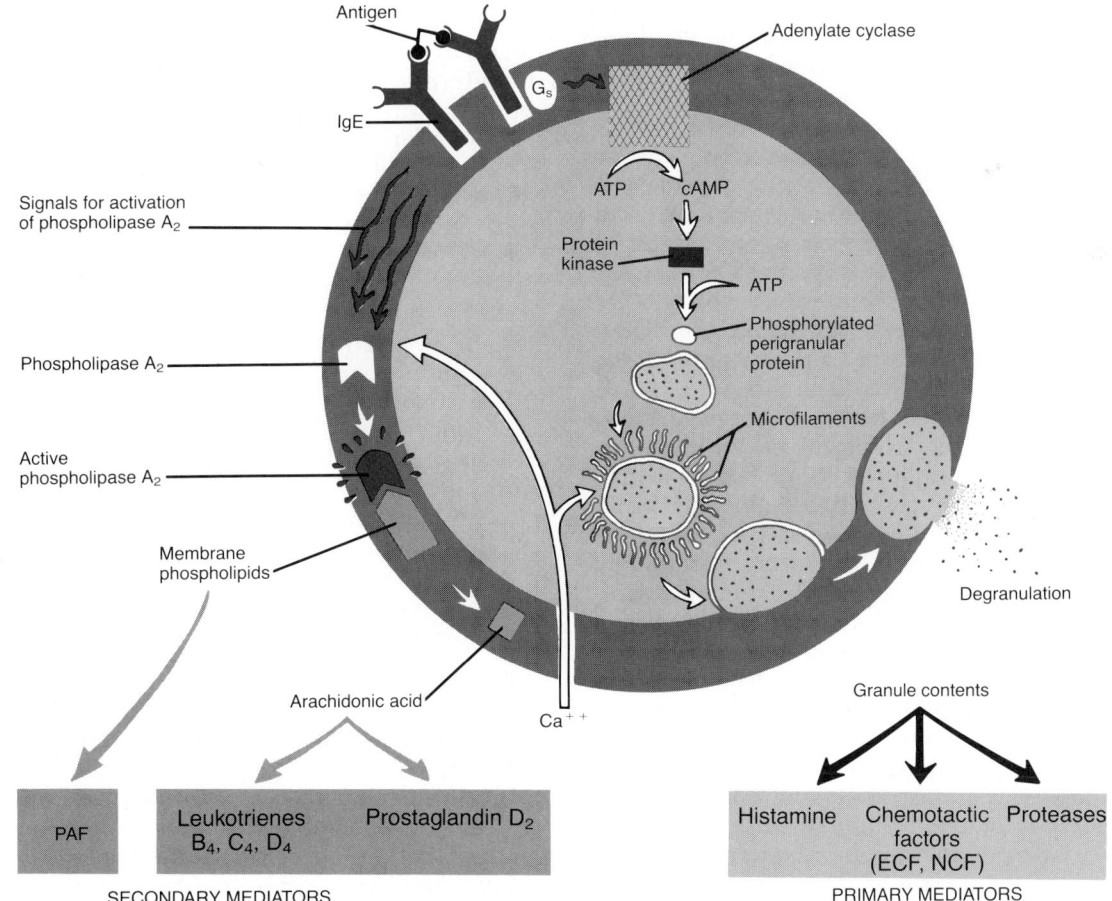

Figure 5–9. Activation of mast cells in type I hypersensitivity and release of their mediators.

Table 5-5. Summary of the Action of Mast Cell Mediators in Type I Hypersensitivity

ACTION	MEDIATOR	SOURCE
Chemotaxis	Leukotriene B$_4$	Membrane phospholipids
	Eosinophil chemotactic factor of anaphylaxis	Intragranular
	Neutrophil chemotactic factor of anaphylaxis	Intragranular
	Inflammatory factors of anaphylaxis	Intragranular (granule matrix)
Vasoactive (vasodilatation, increased vascular permeability)	Histamine	Intragranular
	PAF (platelet activating factor)	Membrane lipids
	Leukotrienes C$_4$, D$_4$, E$_4$	Membrane lipids
	Neutral proteases that activate complement	Intragranular (granule matrix)
	Prostaglandin D$_2$	Membrane lipids
Smooth muscle spasm	Leukotrienes C$_4$, D$_4$, E$_4$	Membrane lipids
	Histamine	Intragranular
	Prostaglandins	Membrane lipids
	PAF	Membrane lipids

ate additional inflammatory and chemotactic factors. The accumulated neutrophils and monocytes also produce distinct "basophil degranulating factors" and the lipid-derived mediators listed earlier, thereby setting up a vicious circle of congestion, edema, inflammation, and mucus production. It should be evident that, unlike the early reactions, the late phase responses are not inhibited by antihistaminic drugs, but glucocorticoids are effective because of their broad-spectrum anti-inflammatory effect.[25]

With this background of the mechanisms involved in type I hypersensitivity, we can turn to its systemic and local manifestations.

Systemic Anaphylaxis

In humans, systemic anaphylaxis may occur after administration of heterologous proteins (e.g., antisera), hormones, enzymes, polysaccharides, and drugs (such as the antibiotic penicillin). The severity of the disorder varies with the level of sensitization. However, the shock dose of antigen may be exceedingly small, as, for example, the tiny amounts used in ordinary skin testing for various forms of allergies. Within minutes after exposure, itching, hives, and skin erythema appear, followed shortly thereafter by a striking contraction of respiratory bronchioles and the appearance of respiratory distress. Laryngeal edema will result in hoarseness. Vomiting, abdominal cramps, diarrhea, and laryngeal obstruction follow, and the patient may go into shock and even die within the hour. At autopsy, some patients may be found to have pulmonary edema and hemorrhage, whereas others show hyperdistention of the lungs along with right-sided cardiac dilatation, a reflection of the constricted pulmonary vasculature. It is obvious that the effect of anaphylaxis must always be borne in mind when a therapeutic agent is administered. Although patients at risk can generally be identified by a previous history of some form of allergy, the absence of such a history does not preclude the possibility of an anaphylactic reaction.

Local Anaphylaxis

These reactions are exemplified by so-called atopic allergy. The term "atopy" implies a genetically controlled predisposition to develop localized anaphylactic reactions to inhaled or ingested allergens. About 10% of the population suffers from allergies involving localized anaphylactic reactions to extrinsic allergens, such as pollen, animal dander, house dust, fish, and the like. Specific diseases include urticaria, angioedema, allergic rhinitis (hay fever), and some forms of asthma, all discussed elsewhere in this book. Of interest is the familial predisposition to the development of this type of allergy. A positive family history of allergy is found in 50% of atopic individuals. The mode of inheritance is unclear, but it is most likely multifactorial. Although there are no significant associations between HLA antigens and atopic diseases as a group, significant association between some HLA loci and immune responses against certain allergens has been noted (e.g., HLA-D2 and ragweed allergen 5). Furthermore, IgE antibody production to some pollen extracts has been correlated with specific HLA haplotypes in certain families.

Before we close the discussion of type I hypersensitivity, it should be noted that the IgE antibodies may also play a protective role in several parasitic infections.[26] Large amounts of IgE antibodies are regularly produced in response to many helminthic infections. Figure 5–10 provides a schematic illustration of the process by which they serve to inflict damage on the schistosome larvae. It should be noted that:

- IgE-sensitized mast cells degranulate on contact with worm antigens and thereby attract other leukocytes, such as eosinophils, by release of chemotactic factors.
- In addition to mast cells, Fc receptors for IgE may be present on eosinophils, platelets, and some macrophages that are attracted to the worms.
- IgE-armed leukocytes attach to the surface of parasites and inflict damage by a variety of mechanisms. For example, eosinophils are capable of mediating

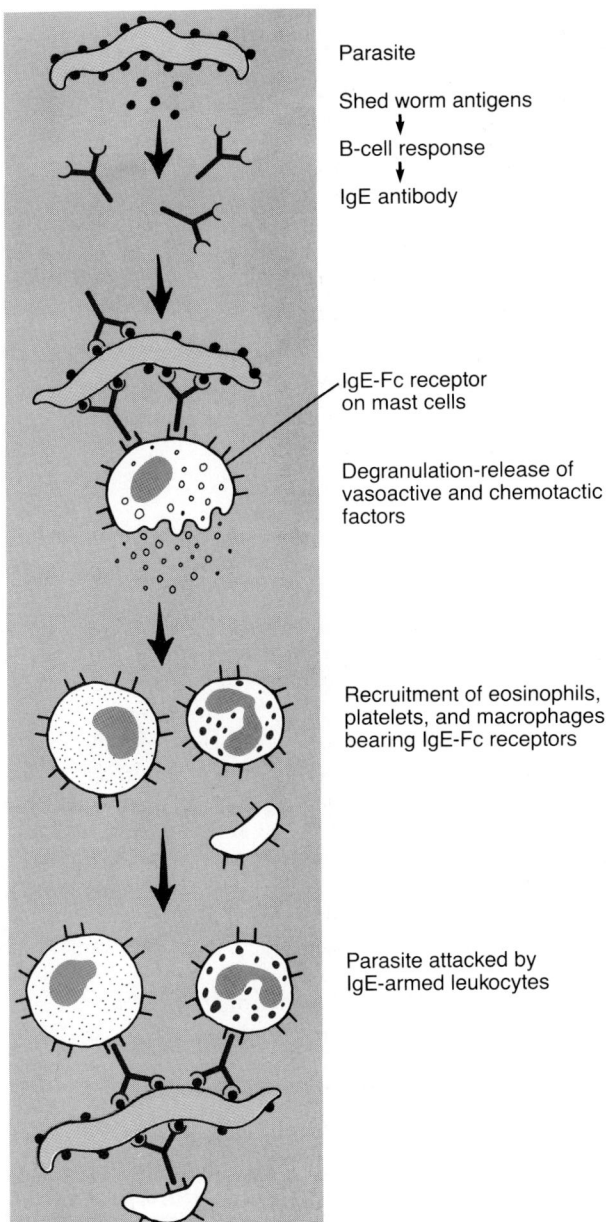

Parasite

Shed worm antigens

↓

B-cell response

↓

IgE antibody

IgE-Fc receptor
on mast cells

Degranulation-release of
vasoactive and chemotactic
factors

Recruitment of eosinophils,
platelets, and macrophages
bearing IgE-Fc receptors

Parasite attacked by
IgE-armed leukocytes

Figure 5–10. IgE-mediated destruction of parasites.

antibody-dependent cellular cytotoxicity (described later); macrophages, on the other hand, release toxic oxygen metabolites and lysosomal enzymes.

TYPE II HYPERSENSITIVITY

Type II hypersensitivity is mediated by antibodies directed toward antigens present on the surface of cells or other tissue components. The antigenic determinants may be intrinsic to the cell membrane, or they may take the form of an exogenous antigen adsorbed on the cell surface. In either case the hypersensitivity reaction results from the binding of antibodies to normal or altered cell-surface antigens. Three different antibody-dependent mechanisms involved in this type of reaction are depicted in Figure 5–11 and described below.

COMPLEMENT-DEPENDENT REACTIONS. There are two mechanisms by which antibody and complement may mediate type II hypersensitivity: direct lysis and opsonization. In the first pattern, antibody (IgM or IgG) reacts with an antigen present on the surface of the cell, causing activation of the complement system and resulting in the assembly of the membrane attack complex that disrupts membrane integrity by "drilling holes" through the lipid bilayer. In the second pattern, the cells become susceptible to phagocytosis (opsonization) by fixation of antibody or C3b fragment to the cell surface (p. 54). This form of type II hypersensitivity most commonly involves blood cells—red blood cells, white blood cells, and platelets—but the antibodies can also be directed against extracellular tissue (e.g., glomerular basement membrane in anti-GBM nephritis, p. 1024). Clinically, such reactions occur in the following situations: (1) *transfusion reactions,* in which cells from an incompatible donor react with autochthonous antibody of the host; (2) *erythroblastosis fetalis,* in which there is an antigenic difference between the mother and the fetus, and antibodies from the mother (of the IgG class) cross the placenta and cause destruction of fetal red cells; (3) *autoimmune hemolytic anemia, agranulocytosis, or thrombocytopenia,* in which individuals produce antibodies to their own blood cells, which are then destroyed; (4) *certain drug reactions,* in which antibodies are produced that react with the drug, which may be complexed to red cell antigen (p. 678).

ANTIBODY-DEPENDENT CELL-MEDIATED CYTO-TOXICITY (ADCC). This form of antibody-mediated cell injury does not involve fixation of complement but instead requires the cooperation of leukocytes. The target cells, coated with low concentrations of IgG antibody, are killed by a variety of *nonsensitized* cells that have Fc receptors. The latter bind to the target by their receptors for the Fc fragment of IgG, and *cell lysis proceeds without phagocytosis.* ADCC may be mediated by monocytes, neutrophils, eosinophils, and NK cells. Thus it would seem that NK cells can kill their targets by two independent mechanisms: (1) spontaneous cytotoxicity mediated by an as yet unidentified NK cell receptor (Fig. 5–4), and (2) lysis of antibody-coated targets via Fc receptors (Fig. 5–11). Although in most instances IgG antibodies are involved in ADCC, in certain cases (for example eosinophil-mediated cytotoxicity against parasites described earlier) IgE antibodies are utilized. ADCC may be relevant to the destruction of targets too large to be phagocytosed, such as parasites or tumor cells (p. 297), and it may also play some role in graft rejection.

EFFECTS OF ANTIRECEPTOR ANTIBODIES. Although cytotoxicity is the most common consequence of the interaction between antibody and cell-bound

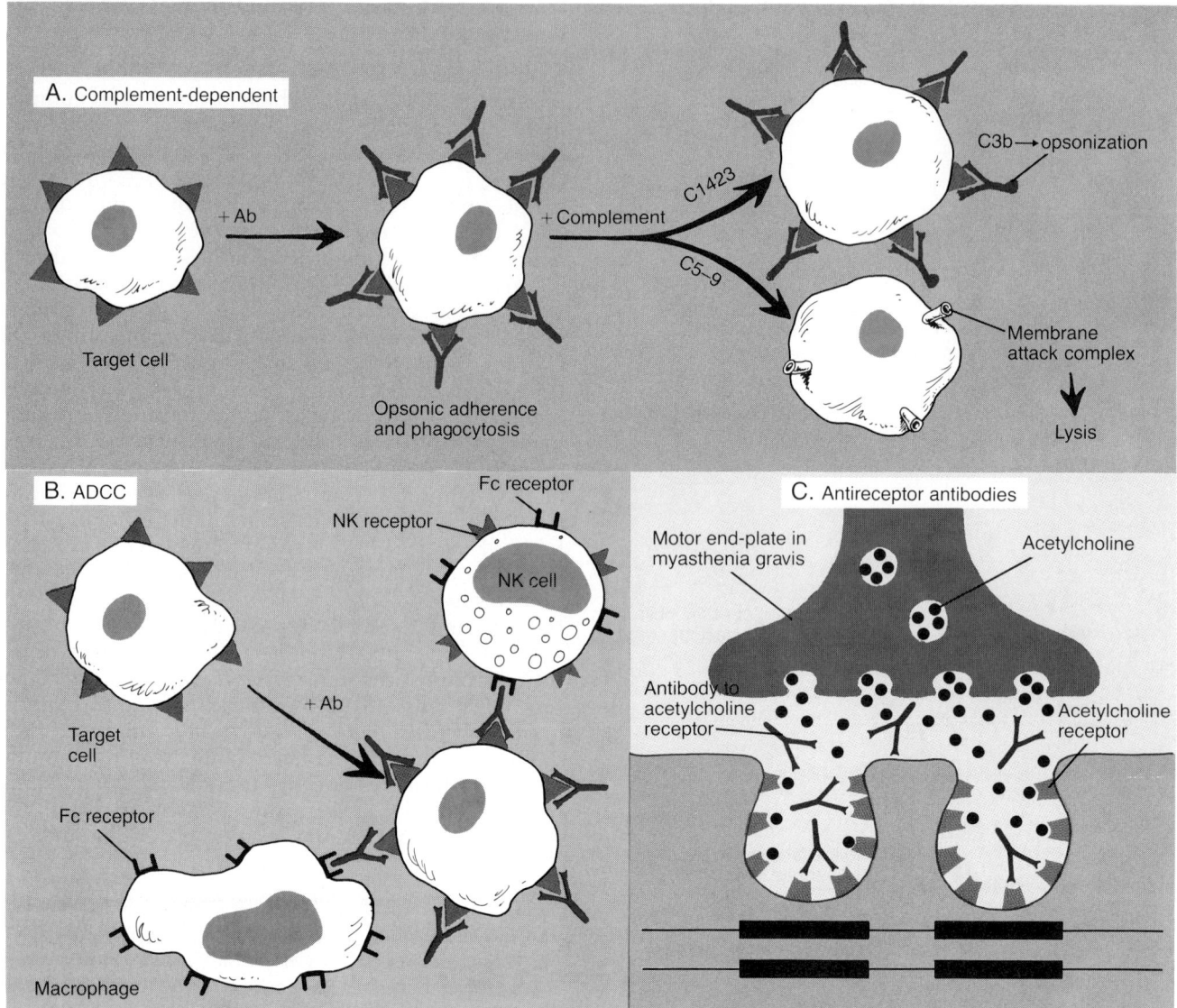

Figure 5–11. A schematic illustration of three different mechanisms of antibody-mediated injury in type II hypersensitivity. *A,* Complement-dependent reactions that lead to lysis of cells or render them susceptible to phagocytosis. *B,* Antibody-dependent cellular cytotoxicity. IgG-coated target cells are killed by cells that bear Fc receptors for IgG (e.g., NK cells, macrophages). *C,* Antireceptor antibodies disturb the normal function of receptors. In this example, acetylcholine receptor antibodies impair neuromuscular transmission in myasthenia gravis.

antigen, this may not always be the case. A variety of diseases result from noncytotoxic interactions between cell surface receptors and antireceptor antibodies. For example, in myasthenia gravis, muscle weakness results from impaired neuromuscular transmission brought about by anti-acetylcholine receptor antibodies (Fig. 5–11) (p. 1366).

TYPE III HYPERSENSITIVITY (IMMUNE COMPLEX–MEDIATED)

Type III hypersensitivity reaction is induced by antigen-antibody complexes that produce tissue damage as a result of their capacity to activate a variety of serum mediators, principally the complement system. The toxic reaction is initiated when antigen combines with antibody, whether within the circulation (circulating immune complexes) or at extravascular sites where antigen may have been deposited (in situ immune complexes). Some forms of glomerulonephritis in which immune complexes are formed in situ following initial implantation of the antigen on the glomerular basement membrane are discussed later on page 1027. Complexes formed in the circulation produce damage, particularly as they localize within blood vessel walls or when they are trapped in filtering structures, such as the renal glomerulus. *It should be pointed out at the outset that the mere formation of antigen-antibody complexes in the circulation does not imply the presence of disease;* indeed, immune complexes are

Table 5-6. Some Antigens Associated with Immune Complex Disorders

ANTIGENS		CLINICAL MANIFESTATIONS
Exogenous		
1. Infectious agents		
Bacteria:	Streptococci	Glomerulonephritis, infective endocarditis
	Yersinia enterocolitica	Arthritis
	Treponema pallidum	Glomerulonephritis
Viruses:	Hepatitis B	Polyarteritis nodosa
	Cytomegalovirus	
Parasites:	Plasmodium sp.	Glomerulonephritis
	Schistosoma sp.	
Fungi:	Actinomycetes	Farmer's lung
2. Drugs or Chemicals		
Foreign serum (antithymocyte globulin)		Serum sickness
Quinidine		Hemolytic anemia
Heroin		Glomerulonephritis
Endogenous		
Nuclear antigens		Systemic lupus erythematosus
Immunoglobulins		Rheumatoid arthritis
Tumor antigens		Glomerulonephritis

formed during many immune responses, and may perhaps represent a normal mechanism of antigen removal. The factors that determine whether the immune complexes formed in circulation will be pathogenic are not fully understood, but some possible influences are discussed later.

Two general types of antigens cause immune complex–mediated injury: (1) the antigen may be *exogenous*, such as a foreign protein, a bacterium, or a virus, but (2) under some circumstances the individual can produce antibody against self components — *endogenous antigens* (Table 5–6). The latter can be trace components present in the blood or, more commonly, antigenic components in cells and tissues. Immune complex–mediated diseases can be *generalized*, if immune complexes are formed in the circulation and are deposited in many organs, or *localized* to particular organs such as the kidney (glomerulonephritis), joints (arthritis), or the small blood vessels of the skin if the complexes are formed and deposited locally (the local Arthus reaction). These two patterns are considered separately.

Systemic Immune Complex Disease

Acute serum sickness is the prototype of a systemic immune complex disease; it was at one time a frequent sequel to the administration of large amounts of foreign serum (e.g., horse antitetanus serum) used for passive immunization. It is now seen infrequently and in different clinical settings. For example, in one report 11 of 12 patients who were injected with horse antithymocyte globulin for treatment of aplastic anemia developed serum sickness.[27]

For the sake of simplicity, the pathogenesis of systemic immune complex disease can be resolved into three phases: *(1) formation of antigen-antibody complexes in the circulation, and (2) deposition of the immune complexes in various tissues, thus initiating (3) an inflammatory reaction in dispersed sites throughout the body* (Fig. 5–12). The *first phase* is initiated by the introduction of antigen into the circulation and its interaction with immunocompetent cells, resulting in the formation of antibodies. Approximately five days after serum injection, antibodies directed against the serum components are produced; these react with the antigen still present in the circulation to form anti-

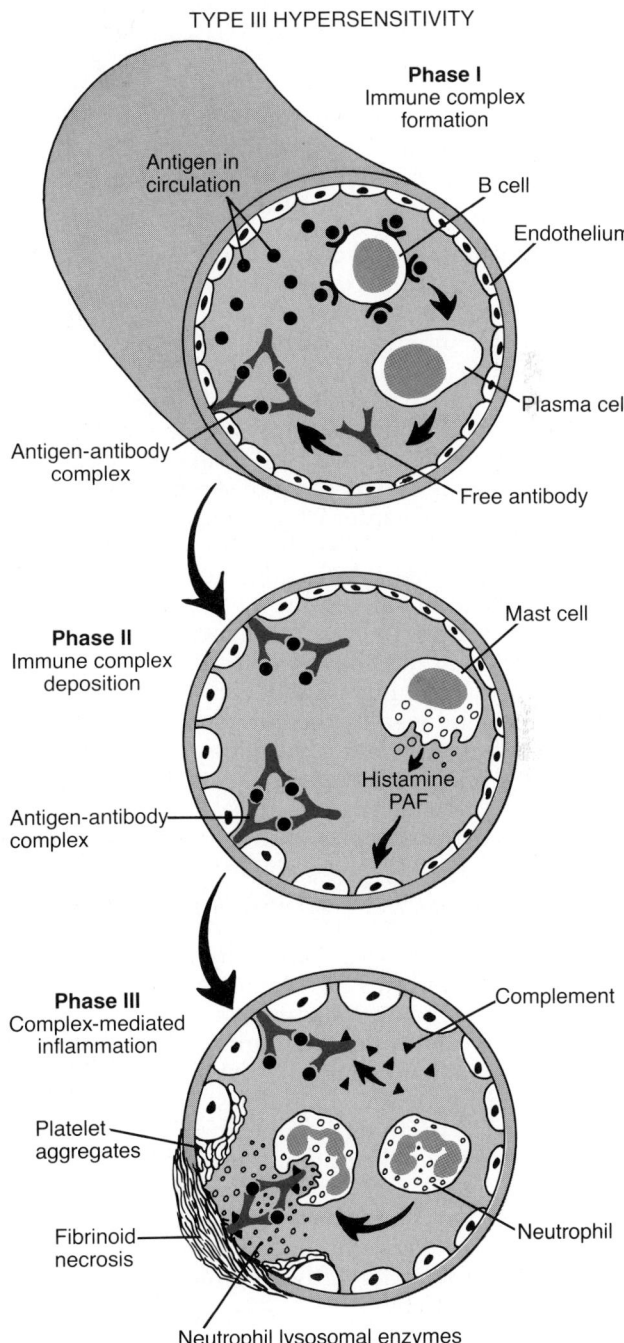

TYPE III HYPERSENSITIVITY

Phase I Immune complex formation

Antigen in circulation
B cell
Endothelium
Antigen-antibody complex
Plasma cell
Free antibody

Phase II Immune complex deposition

Mast cell
Antigen-antibody complex
Histamine PAF

Phase III Complex-mediated inflammation

Complement
Platelet aggregates
Fibrinoid necrosis
Neutrophil
Neutrophil lysosomal enzymes

Figure 5–12. Schematic illustration of the three sequential phases in the induction of systemic type III (immune complex) hypersensitivity.

gen-antibody complexes. In the *second phase*, antigen-antibody complexes formed in the circulation are deposited in various tissues. The factors that determine whether immune complex formation will lead to tissue deposition and disease are not fully understood, but two possible influences are:

• Size of the complexes seems to be important. Very large complexes formed in great antibody excess are rapidly removed from the circulation by the MPS cells and are therefore relatively harmless. The most pathogenic complexes are of small or intermediate size (formed in slight antigen excess), circulate longer, and bind less avidly to phagocytic cells.
• Because the mononuclear phagocyte system normally filters out the circulating immune complexes, its overload or intrinsic dysfunction increases the probability of persistence of immune complexes in circulation and tissue deposition.

In addition, several other factors, such as charge of the immune complexes (anionic versus cationic), valency of the antigen, avidity of the antibody, the affinity of the antigen to various tissue components, the three-dimensional (lattice) structure of the complexes, and hemodynamic factors, influence their tissue deposition.[28] Because most of these influences have been investigated with reference to deposition of immune complexes in the glomeruli, they are discussed further in Chapter 21 (p. 1027). In addition to the renal glomeruli, the favored sites of immune complex deposition are joints, skin, heart, serosal surfaces, and small blood vessels.

For complexes to leave the microcirculation and deposit within or outside the vessel wall, an increase in vascular permeability must occur. It is thought that IgE antibody induced by the antigen shortly after injection binds to circulating basophils and releases histamine and platelet activating factor. The latter induces platelets to aggregate and release their amines (serotonin and histamine) through the platelet-release reaction (p. 95). These amines then separate the endothelial cells and allow the complexes to enter the vessel wall. *This is then a "miniature" type I anaphylactic reaction, occurring transiently in type III reactions.* Once complexes are deposited in the tissues they initiate an acute inflammatory reaction (*phase three*). It is during this phase (approximately ten days after antigen administration) that clinical features such as fever, urticaria, arthralgias, lymph node enlargement, and proteinuria appear.

Wherever complexes deposit, the tissue damage is similar (Fig. 5–13). *Central to this mechanism is activation of the complement cascade (p. 53) and the elaboration of biologically active fragments.* As will be recalled, complement activation has several proinflammatory effects:

• release of C3b, the opsonin that promotes phagocytosis of particles and organisms;
• production of chemotactic factors, which direct the migration of polymorphonuclear leukocytes and monocytes (C5 fragments, C5b67);

• release of anaphylatoxins (C3a and C5a), which increase vascular permeability and cause contraction of smooth muscle; and
• formation of membrane attack complex (C5–9), causing cell membrane damage or even cytolysis.

Phagocytosis of antigen-antibody complexes by leukocytes drawn in by the chemotactic factors results in the release or generation of a variety of additional proinflammatory substances, including prostaglandins, vasodilator peptides, and chemotactic substances, as well as several lysosomal enzymes, including proteases capable of digesting basement membrane, collagen, elastin, and cartilage. Tissue damage may also be mediated by free oxygen radicals produced by activated neutrophils. Immune complexes have several other effects: they cause aggregation of platelets and activate Hageman factor; both of these reactions augment the inflammatory process and initiate the formation of microthrombi (Fig. 5–13). The resultant pathologic lesion is termed vasculitis if it occurs in blood vessels, glomerulonephritis if it occurs in renal glomeruli, arthritis if it occurs in the joints, and so on.

It is clear from the foregoing that complement-fixing antibodies (i.e., IgG and IgM) will induce these lesions. Because IgA can activate complement by the alternate pathway, IgA-containing complexes may also induce tissue injury. The important role of complement in the pathogenesis of the tissue injury is supported by the observation that experimental manipulations that deplete serum complement levels greatly reduce the severity of the lesions, as does depletion of neutrophils. *During the active phase of the disease, consumption of complement decreases the serum levels.*

The morphologic consequences of immune complex injury are dominated by acute necrotizing vasculitis, with deposits of fibrinoid and intense neutrophilic exudation permeating the entire arterial wall, much like the changes that we shall describe for polyarteritis nodosa (Fig. 5–14). Affected glomeruli are hypercellular because of swelling and proliferation of endothelial and mesangial cells, accompanied by neutrophilic and monocytic infiltration. *The complexes can be seen on immunofluorescence microscopy as granular lumpy deposits of immunoglobulin and complement,* and on electron microscopy as electron-dense deposits along the glomerular basement membrane (Figs. 21–9 and 21–11, pp. 1026 and 1027). Endocarditis takes the form of edema and increased vascularity of the heart valves, and the vegetations that develop over the inflamed valves have more than a passing resemblance to acute rheumatic lesions. In due course all lesions tend to resolve, owing to catabolism of the immune complexes. This is particularly true if the disease results from a single large exposure to antigen (e.g., acute poststreptococcal glomerulonephritis and acute serum sickness).

A chronic form of serum sickness results from repeated or prolonged exposure to an antigen. Continuous antigenemia is necessary for the development of

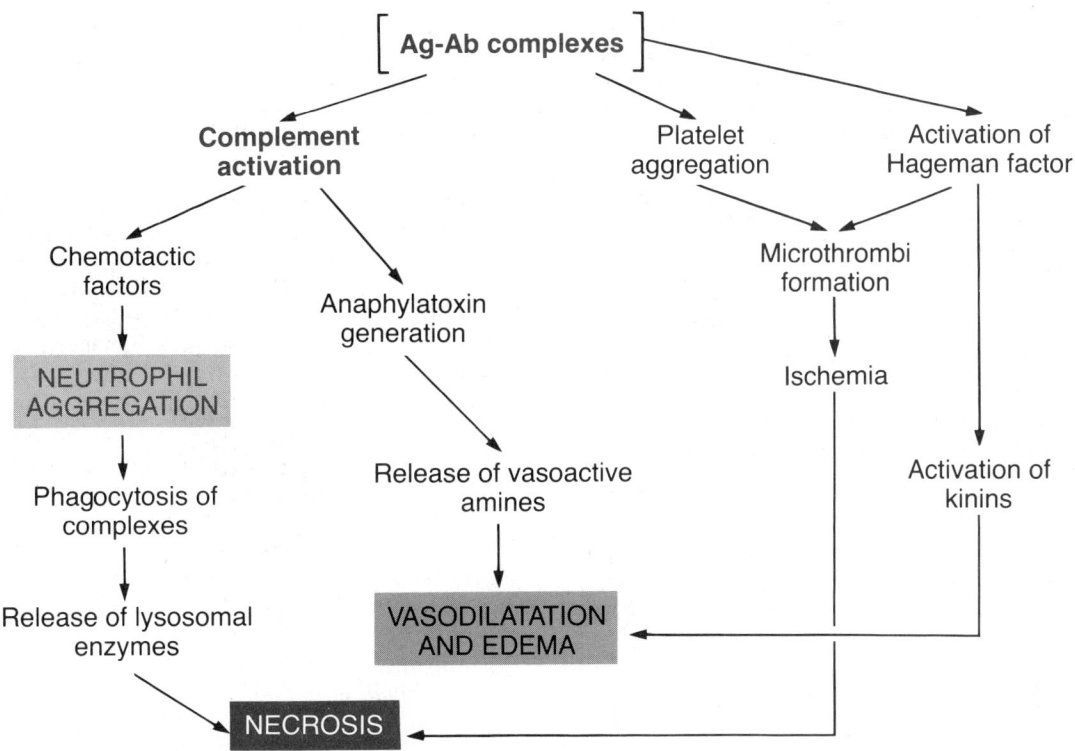

Figure 5–13. Schematic representation of the pathogenesis of immune-complex–mediated tissue injury. The morphologic consequences are depicted as boxed areas.

chronic immune complex disease, because, as stated earlier, complexes in antigen excess are the ones most likely to be deposited in vascular beds. This occurs in several human diseases, such as systemic lupus erythematosus, which is associated with persistent exposure to autoantigens. Often, however, despite the fact that the morphologic changes and other findings suggest immune complex disease, the inciting antigens are unknown. Included in this category are rheumatoid arthritis, polyarteritis nodosa, membranous glomerulonephritis, and several vasculitides.

Local Immune Complex Disease (Arthus Reaction)

The Arthus reaction may be defined as a localized area of tissue necrosis resulting from acute immune complex vasculitis, usually elicited in the skin. The reaction can be produced experimentally by intracutaneous injection of antigen in *an immune animal having circulating antibodies against the antigen.* Because of the excess of antibodies, as the antigen diffuses into the vascular wall, large immune complexes are formed, which precipitate locally and trigger the inflammatory reaction already discussed. Unlike IgE-mediated type I reactions, which appear immediately, the Arthus lesion develops over a few hours and reaches a peak four to ten hours after injection, when it can be seen as an area of visible edema with severe hemorrhage followed occasionally by ulceration. Immunofluorescent stains will disclose complement, immunoglobulins, and fibrinogen precipitated within the vessel walls, usually the venules. On light microscopy,

these produce a smudgy eosinophilic deposit that obscures the underlying cellular detail, an appearance termed *"fibrinoid"* necrosis of the vessels (Fig. 5–14). Rupture of these vessels may produce local hemorrhages, but more often the vascular lumina undergo

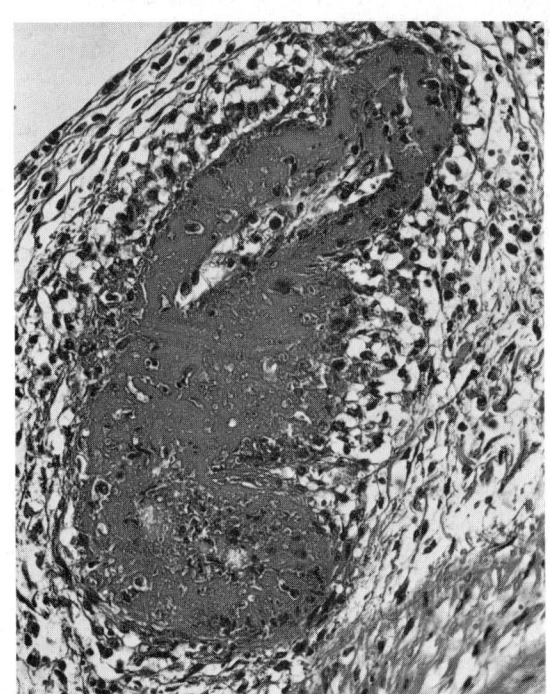

Figure 5–14. Immune complex vasculitis. Acute fibrinoid necrosis of walls of small vessels.

thrombosis, adding an element of local ischemic injury.

TYPE IV HYPERSENSITIVITY (CELL-MEDIATED)

The cell-mediated type of hypersensitivity is initiated by specifically sensitized T lymphocytes. It includes the classic *delayed-type hypersensitivity reactions* and *T-cell–mediated cytotoxic reactions.* It is the principal pattern of immunologic response to a variety of intracellular microbiologic agents, particularly *Mycobacterium tuberculosis,* but also to many viruses, fungi, protozoa, and parasites. So-called contact skin sensitivity to chemical agents and graft rejection are other instances of cell-mediated reactions. The two forms of type IV hypersensitivity are described next.

Delayed-Type Hypersensitivity

The best known example of delayed hypersensitivity is the *tuberculin reaction,* which is produced by the intracutaneous injection of tuberculin, a protein-lipopolysaccharide component of the tubercle bacillus. In a previously sensitized individual, reddening and induration of the site appears in eight to 12 hours, reaches a peak in 24 to 72 hours, and thereafter slowly subsides. An extremely sensitive patient may indeed develop necrosis at the site of injection. Morphologi-

cally the lesion is characterized by the accumulation of mononuclear cells in the subcutaneous tissue and deep and superficial dermis (Fig. 5–15). There is predominant accumulation around small veins and venules, producing a characteristic perivascular "cuffing." Varying numbers of polymorphonuclear leukocytes may also be present, depending on the intensity of the reaction and the amount of necrosis. A small number of basophils is usually present at the site of cutaneous delayed hypersensitivity reaction in man, but in certain species they may form a prominent part of the cellular reaction.[29] Increased vascular permeability associated with widening of interendothelial gaps is a constant feature beginning four to six hours after injection of antigen and reaching a peak by 12 to 24 hours. Fibrin deposition in the interstitium appears to be the main cause of the *induration,* which is characteristic of delayed hypersensitivity skin lesions. Such induration can be prevented by anticoagulants in experimental animals and in man. With certain persistent or nondegradable antigens, the initial perivascular mononuclear cell infiltrate is replaced by granulomas over a period of two to three weeks.

Delayed hypersensitivity reactions are initiated by specifically sensitized T lymphocytes, generated during the initial contact with the antigen. Sensitization involves CD4+ T cells that recognize processed antigens on the surface of antigen-presenting cells in association with class II molecules. Memory T cells gen-

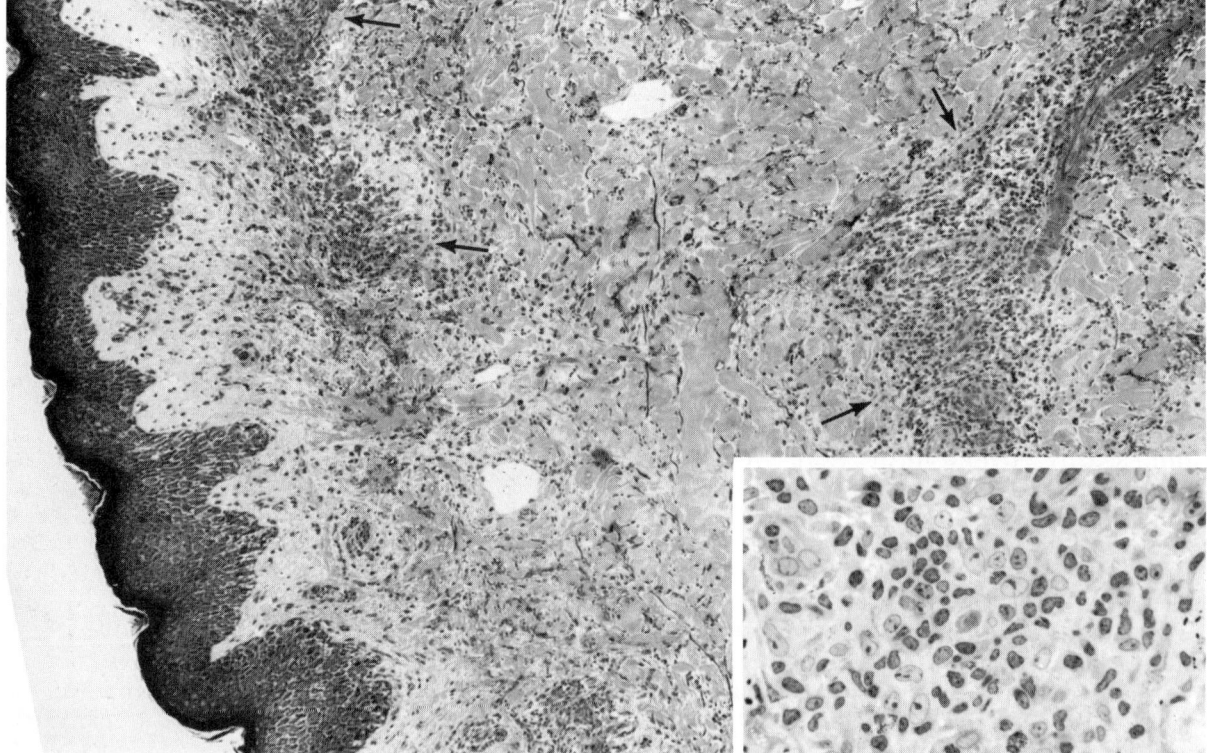

Figure 5–15. A 48-hour delayed hypersensitivity skin reaction in man elicited with tuberculin. There are superficial and deep perivascular infiltrates of mononuclear cells *(arrows).* Note edema *(pale areas)* of superficial dermis. *Inset:* Higher-power view of mononuclear perivascular infiltrate. (From Dvorak, H.: Delayed hypersensitivity. *In* Zweifach, B.W., et al. (eds.): The Inflammatory Process. Vol. III. New York, Academic Press, 1974.)

erated during the initial sensitization remain in circulation for a long time, often several years. When the individual is reexposed to the specific antigen (e.g., tuberculin), memory T lymphocytes are stimulated to divide and release a variety of *lymphokines*. The function of lymphokines is to amplify the response by recruiting inflammatory cells, activating them, and keeping them at the site. In a fully developed delayed hypersensitivity reaction, therefore, only a very small percentage of the mononuclear cell infiltrate is made up of the antigen-specific T cells that initiated the reaction. Among the lymphokines *the most important appear to be the ones that result in the accumulation and activation of macrophages within the lesion*. These include macrophage chemotactic factors, macrophage inhibitory factors, IL-1, TNF-α, and IFN-γ. Macrophages are required for the development of the prominent inflammatory reaction and tissue damage in delayed hypersensitivity reactions. The various ways by which activated macrophages induce tissue injury and continued inflammation were discussed in detail in the chapter on the inflammatory response (Chapter 2).

T Cell–Mediated Cytotoxicity

In response to certain antigens including virus-infected cells, tumor cells, and incompatible (allogeneic) tissue cells, the immune system responds by the generation of cytotoxic T cells (CTLs). The process of CTL generation is complex and still incompletely understood. Some aspects of this process are considered later in relation to rejection of organ transplant. We do know, however, that the vast majority of cytotoxic T cells and their precursors belong to the CD8+ subset of T cells. The process of T cell–mediated lysis is initiated by the recognition of a cell-surface antigen by the T-cell receptor. In this process, the CTL binds avidly and specifically to its target cell and then delivers a lytic signal. The biochemical basis of the "lethal hit" delivered by T cells is under intense scrutiny, as an understanding of this process may allow the development of therapeutic agents that prevent T cell–mediated tissue damage in conditions such as graft rejection. Currently three mechanisms of T-cell cytotoxicity (acting singly or in concert) are being investigated:[30] (1) Pore formation in target cell membrane followed by permeability changes that lead to osmotic death; according to this schema, granules within the cytoplasm of cytotoxic T cells contain pore-forming proteins (perforins, cytolysins) that bind to the target cell membrane and assemble into pores or channels, similar to those produced by the membrane attack complex of complement; (2) release of molecules such as TNF-β (lymphotoxin) that may injure the cell membrane directly; and (3) release of proteolytic enzymes, especially serine esterases that may damage the cell membrane directly or activate precursors of other cytotoxic molecules.

It should be remembered that CTL-mediated cytolysis is highly specific and that adjacent ("innocent bystander") cells are not damaged. Critical to such specificity is the ability of CTLs to recognize the cells bearing the appropriate target antigens. It is now abundantly clear that class I HLA antigens play an extremely important role in the process by which CD8+ CTLs recognize their target cells. For example, CTL generated during a virus infection can recognize the virus-infected cell only in association with self cell-surface HLA antigens, as discussed previously (see Fig. 5–6). The lysis of virus-infected cells by CTL prior to the synthesis of new virions can lead in due course to elimination of the viral infection. Tumor antigens expressed on the cancer cells may also be viewed as modified class I antigens, thus evoking a CTL response that may contribute to immunosurveillance (p. 297).

TRANSPLANT REJECTION

Transplant rejection is discussed here because it appears to involve several of the hypersensitivity reactions discussed earlier. One of the goals of present-day immunologic research is successful transplantation of tissues in humans without immunologic rejection. Although the surgical expertise for the transplantation of skin, kidneys, heart, lungs, livers, spleen, bone marrow, and endocrine organs is now well in hand, it regrettably outpaces thus far our ability to confer on the recipient permanent acceptance of foreign grafts. Histocompatibility, a concept necessary for an understanding of transplant rejection, was reviewed earlier (p. 169). Here we cover the mechanisms involved in rejection and the anatomic changes and patterns of rejection injury.[15,31,32]

Mechanisms Involved in Rejection

Graft rejection depends on recognition by the host of the grafted tissue as foreign. The antigens responsible for such rejection in humans are those of the major histocompatibility antigen (HLA) system. *Rejection is a very complex process in which both cell-mediated immunity and circulating antibodies play a role;* moreover, the relative contributions of these two mechanisms to rejection vary among grafts and are often reflected in the histologic features of the rejected organs.

T CELL–MEDIATED REACTIONS. The critical role of T cells in transplant rejection has been documented both in humans and in experimental animals. But how do T lymphocytes cause graft destruction? Both activation of CD8+ cytotoxic T cells (CTLs) and delayed hypersensitivity reactions triggered by activated CD4+ helper cells seem to be involved (p. 182). The generation of CTLs and antibodies in response to allogeneic HLA antigens is depicted schematically in Figure 5–16. The T cell–mediated reaction is initiated when the recipient's lymphocytes encounter the donor's HLA antigens. The presentation of the foreign HLA antigens may take place within the grafted organ (as depicted) or after the shed donor antigens are carried to the regional lymph nodes. It is believed

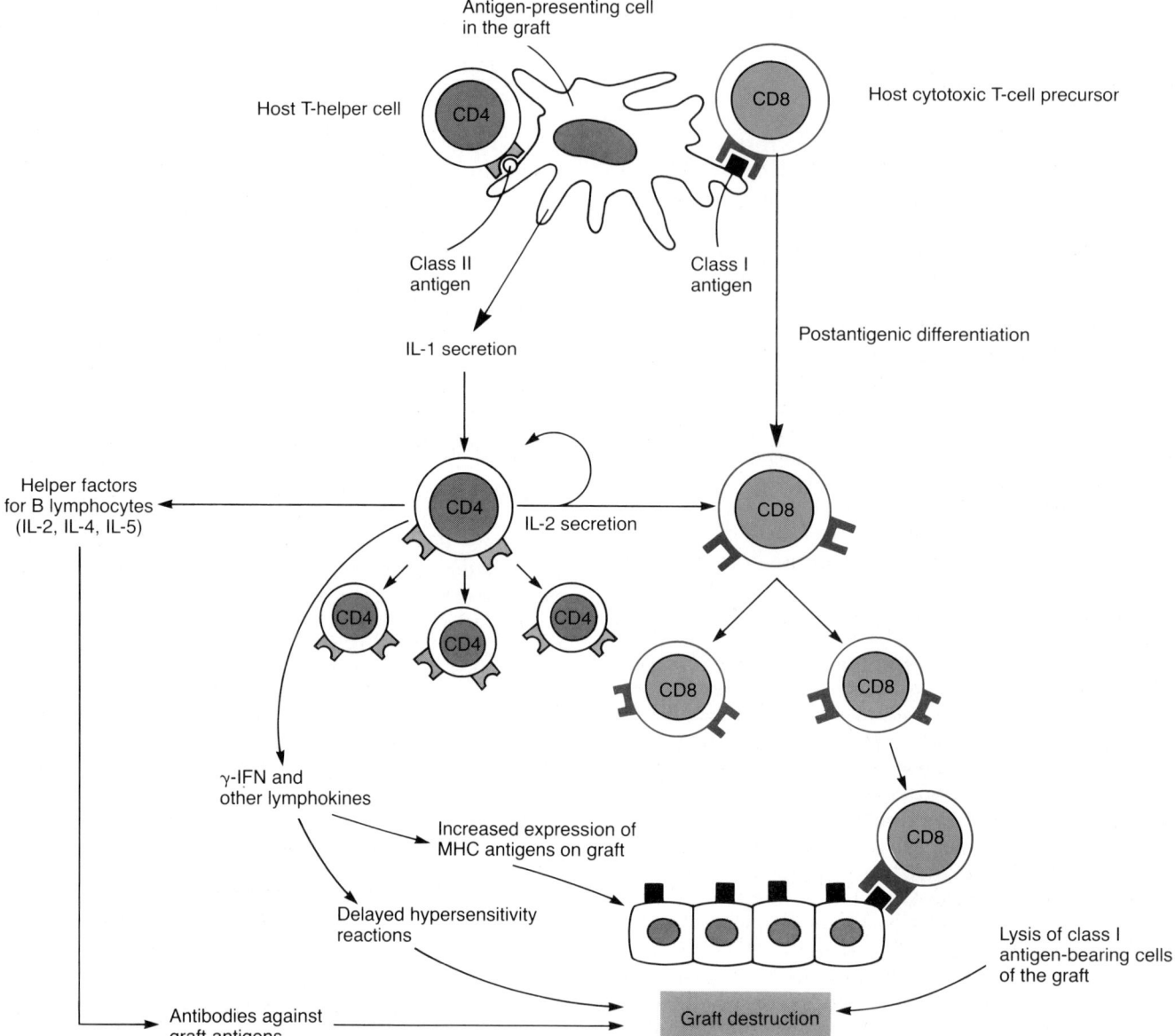

Figure 5–16. Schematic representation of events that lead to the destruction of histoincompatible grafts. Class I and class II antigens of the graft donor are recognized by CD8+ cytotoxic T cells and CD4+ helper cells, respectively, of the host. The interaction of the CD4+ cells with class II antigens leads to the release of interleukin 1 (IL-1) from the antigen presenting cells. IL-1 promotes the proliferation of CD4+ cells and the release of interleukin 2 (IL-2) from the cells. IL-2 further augments the proliferation of CD4+ cells and also provides helper signals for the differentiation of class I–specific CD8+ cytotoxic cells. In addition to IL-2, a variety of other soluble mediators (lymphokines) that promote B-cell differentiation and participate in the induction of a local delayed hypersensitivity reaction are produced by CD4+ helper cells. Eventually, several mechanisms converge to destroy the graft: (1) lysis of cells that bear class I antigens by CD8+ cytotoxic T cells, (2) antigraft antibodies produced by sensitized B cells, and (3) nonspecific damage inflicted by macrophages and other cells that accumulate as a result of the delayed hypersensitivity reaction.

that the donor lymphoid cells ("passenger lympho-cytes"), especially dendritic cells contained within the grafts, are the most important immunogens, as they are rich in both class I and class II antigens. The CD4+ helper T-cell subset is triggered into prolifera-tion by recognition of the class II specificities; this is similar to the mixed lymphocyte reaction that occurs in vitro (p. 170). At the same time, precursors of CD8+ CTL (pre-killer T cells), which bear receptors for class I HLA antigens, differentiate into mature CTLs. This process of differentiation is complex and incompletely understood. Involved are interactions

of antigen-presenting cells, T-cell subsets, and release of cytokines such as IL-1 and IL-2 (Fig. 5–16). Once mature CTLs are generated, they lyse the grafted tis-sue. In addition to the specific cytotoxic T cells, lym-phokine-secreting CD4+ T cells are also generated by sensitization, as in the delayed hypersensitivity reac-tion. This leads to increased vascular permeability and local accumulation of mononuclear cells (lympho-cytes and macrophages), as described previously. Ac-cording to some investigators, the delayed hypersen-sitivity with its attendant microvascular injury, tissue ischemia, and destruction mediated by accumulated macrophages is an important mechanism of graft destruction.[29]

ANTIBODY-MEDIATED REACTIONS.

Earlier studies suggested no role for humoral antibody, as transplantation immunity could not be transferred by serum. It is now thought, however, that humoral responses are important in at least two types of rejection in human kidney transplant recipients:

1. *Preformed circulating antibodies* occur in transplant recipients who have encountered the foreign antigen *before transplantation*. This may occur as a result of presensitization of a recipient by blood transfusions, previous pregnancies, or infections with HLA cross-reacting bacterial or viral surface antigens. In this circumstance, rejection occurs almost immediately after transplantation, owing to the fixation of circulating antidonor antibody to the vascular bed of the graft. The antigenic components of endothelial cells are the initial points of contact of the host immune recognition and effector mechanisms. The resulting reaction is termed "hyperacute rejection." The antidonor antibodies responsible for hyperacute rejection may be directed against HLA or blood-group antigens.

2. In recipients not previously sensitized to transplantation antigens, exposure to the class I and class II HLA antigens of the donor may evoke antibodies, as depicted in Figure 5–16. The antibodies formed by the recipient may cause injury by several mechanisms, including complement-dependent cytotoxicity, antibody-dependent cell-mediated cytolysis, and the deposition of antigen-antibody complexes. The initial target of these antibodies in *rejection appears to be the graft vasculature*. Thus, antibody-dependent rejection phenomena in the kidney are reflected histologically by a vasculitis, sometimes referred to as "rejection vasculitis." The interaction of specific antibody with antigen initiates complement-dependent tissue injury and triggers other mediators of inflammation, namely, platelet aggregation and release, and neutrophil lysosomal leakage as well as coagulation, fibrinolysis, and activation of the kinin cascade (p. 54).

MORPHOLOGY OF REJECTION REACTIONS.

On the basis of the timing, the morphology, and the underlying mechanism, rejection reactions are classified as hyperacute, acute, and chronic. **The morphologic changes in these patterns are described as they relate to renal transplants.** Similar changes are encountered in any other vascularized organ transplant.

HYPERACUTE REJECTION. This form of rejection is attributable to the presence in the recipient of **preformed** circulating antibodies directed against donor-specific antigens. It usually occurs within minutes after transplantation and can be recognized by the surgeon just after the graft vasculature is anastomosed to the recipient's. In contrast to the nonrejecting kidney graft, which rapidly regains a normal pink coloration and normal tissue turgor and

promptly excretes urine, a hyperacutely rejecting kidney rapidly becomes cyanotic, mottled, and flaccid and may excrete a mere few drops of bloody urine. In some cases, the process occurs more slowly over a period of hours or one to two days. This variation in onset appears to relate directly to the recipient's titer of circulating cytotoxic complement-dependent antibody. The histologic lesions are characteristic of the classic Arthus reaction. In the first hour, increased numbers of neutrophils are present on the arteriolar endothelium and within the glomerular and peritubular capillaries. Immunoglobulin and complement are deposited in the vessel wall, and electron microscopy will disclose early endothelial injury together with fibrin-platelet thrombi. **These early lesions point to an antigen-antibody reaction at the level of vascular endothelium.** Subsequently these changes become diffuse and intense, the glomeruli undergo thrombotic occlusion of the capillaries, and fibrinoid necrosis occurs in arterial walls (Fig. 5–17). The kidney cortex then undergoes outright infarction (necrosis) and such nonfunctioning kidneys are eventually removed. Fortunately, cross-matching of the donor's lymphocytes with the recipient's serum prior to transplantation has diminished the frequency of this dramatic complication.

ACUTE REJECTION. This may occur within days of transplantation in the untreated recipient or may appear suddenly months or even years later, when immunosuppression has been employed and terminated. As suggested earlier, acute graft rejection is a combined process in which both cellular and humoral tissue injuries play parts. In any one patient, one or the other mechanism may predominate. Histologically, humoral rejection is associated with vasculitis, whereas cellular rejection is marked by an interstitial mononuclear cell infiltrate.

Acute cellular rejection is most commonly seen within the initial months after transplantation and is often accom-

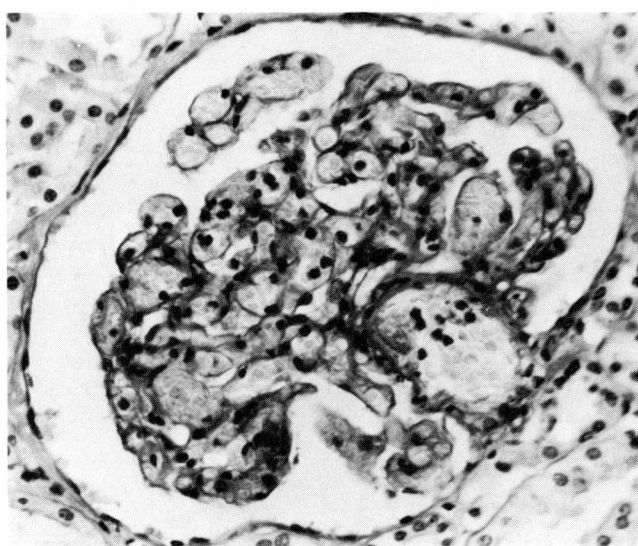

Figure 5–17. Hyperacute rejection. Glomerulus shows marked dilation of hilar arteriole and glomerular capillaries, which are filled with red cells, platelets, and occasional neutrophils. Vascular endothelium is focally absent. (Courtesy of Dr. G. J. Busch.)

panied by the abrupt onset of clinical signs of renal failure. Histologically, there may be extensive interstitial mononuclear cell infiltration and edema, as well as mild interstitial hemorrhage (Fig. 5–18). In humans, the mononuclear cell infiltrate consists primarily of medium-sized and small lymphocytes, along with some large "transformed" lymphocytes, which have abundant basophilic cytoplasm and a vesicular nucleus. As might be expected, immunoperoxidase staining reveals both CD4+ and CD8+ lymphocytes. In many cases interleukin-2 receptors, which appear on activated T cells, can be demonstrated.[33] Some plasma cells can also be identified, especially in long-standing cases. Glomerular and peritubular capillaries contain large numbers of mononuclear cells that may also invade the tubules, causing focal tubular necrosis. The recognition of cellular rejection is important because, in the absence of an accompanying arteritis, patients promptly respond to immunosuppressive therapy.

Acute rejection vasculitis (humoral rejection) is seen most commonly in the first few months after transplantation or when immunosuppressive therapy is discontinued. Such patients show immediate and persistent poor function of the graft and do not respond to high-dose immunosuppressive therapy. The histologic lesions consist of necrotizing vasculitis with endothelial necrosis; neutrophilic infiltration; deposition of immunoglobulins, complement, and fibrin; and thrombosis. The process may evolve to extensive glomerular necrosis and cortical arteriolar thrombosis, with resulting cortical infarction. Almost all these patients will also

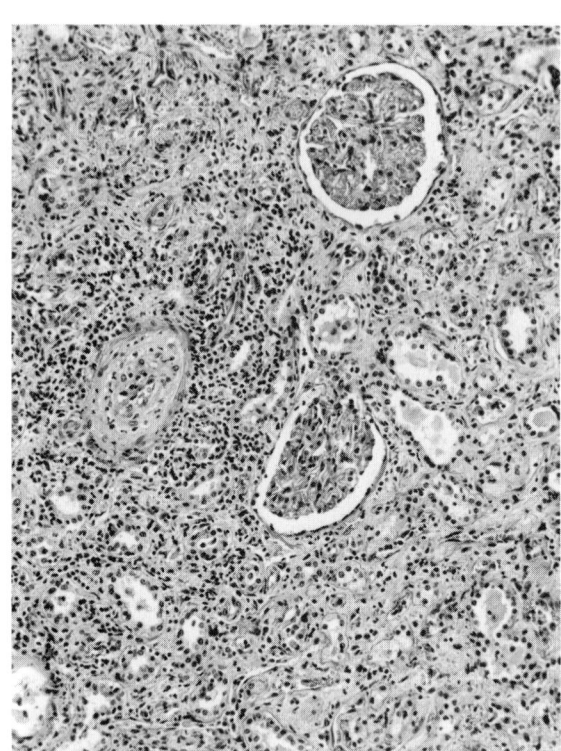

Figure 5–19. Chronic transplant rejection of kidney. There is marked tubular atrophy, increased interstitial fibrosis, and mononuclear cell infiltration. The vessel at left center has a markedly thickened wall with virtual obliteration of the lumen. The glomeruli show some ischemic axial thickening.

have evidence of acute cellular rejection. More common than this acute type of vasculitis is so-called **subacute vasculitis,** which is also seen in greatest intensity during the first months after transplantation. Clinically, patients with subacute vasculitis have a course punctuated by repeated episodes of clinical rejection with altered renal function. The arterial lesions are rather characteristic. **The major alterations are in the intima,** which is markedly thickened by a cushion of proliferating fibroblasts, myocytes, and foamy macrophages, often leading to luminal narrowing or obliteration. The thickened intima may be infiltrated by scattered neutrophils and mononuclear cells, and the walls of most of these arteries show deposits of immunoglobulin and complement.

CHRONIC REJECTION. Because most instances of acute graft rejection are more or less controlled by immunosuppressive therapy, chronic changes are commonly seen in the renal allograft (Fig. 5–19). Patients with chronic rejection present clinically with a progressive rise in serum creatinine level (an index of renal dysfunction) over a period of four to six months. **The vascular changes** consist of dense intimal fibrosis, principally in the cortical arteries, the lesion probably being the end stage of the proliferative arteritis described in acute and subacute stages. These vascular lesions result in renal ischemia manifested by glomerular ischemic simplification and obsolescence, interstitial fibrosis and tubular atrophy, and shrinkage of the renal parenchyma. The decline in renal function is proportional to

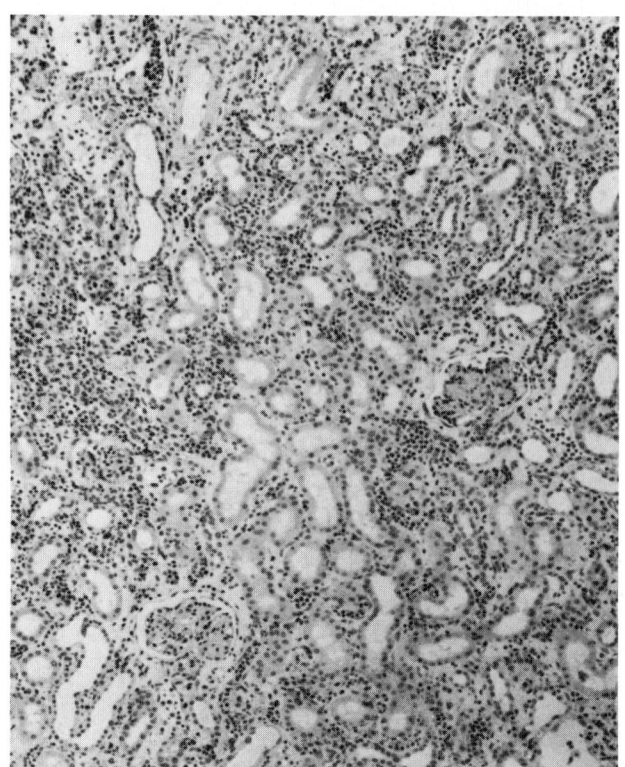

Figure 5–18. Acute cellular rejection of a renal allograft manifested by a diffuse interstitial mononuclear cell infiltrate and interstitial edema with separation of tubules. (Courtesy of Dr. G. J. Busch.)

the degree of interstitial fibrosis and tubular atrophy. An acute arteritis may sometimes be superimposed on the chronic lesions, and in these instances immunoglobulin and complement are present, suggesting a humoral rejection crisis. Together with the vascular lesions, chronically rejecting kidneys usually have interstitial mononuclear cell infiltrates containing large numbers of plasma cells and numerous eosinophils. This is taken as an indication of chronic cell-mediated rejection, but in truth it must be said that delineation of the pathogenetic mechanisms in chronic graft rejection is much more difficult than it is in the acute forms and is further complicated by the contribution of ischemic damage to progressive renal dysfunction.

The glomeruli in chronic graft rejection show no consistent pattern of injury. They may be entirely normal in appearance or may show ischemic changes that may be difficult to distinguish from recurrent glomerular disease.[34-36]

Methods of Increasing Graft Survival

1. Because HLA antigens are the major targets in transplant rejection, minimization of the HLA disparity between the donor and recipient would be expected to influence graft survival. Indeed, in the case of intrafamilial (related donor) kidney transplants, a markedly beneficial effect of matching for class I antigens has been observed. For example, HLA-identical sibling transplants have survival rates of about 90% at three years, whereas the graft survival is reduced to 75% if the donor and recipient share only one haplotype. In cadaver renal transplants, matching for HLA class I antigens has at best a modest effect on graft acceptance. Additional matching for class II antigens results in a definite improvement in graft survival. In all likelihood, this benefit is derived because class II antigen reactive CD4+ helper cells that play an important role in the induction of both cellular and humoral immunity are not triggered. It should be noted, however, that effective immunosuppression, particularly with cyclosporine, may mask the beneficial effects of HLA matching.

2. Except in the case of identical twins, who are obviously matched for all possible histocompatibility antigens, *immunosuppressive therapy* is a practical necessity in all other donor-recipient combinations. Even HLA-identical siblings may differ at several minor histocompatibility loci, which can evoke slow rejection. At present, drugs such as azathioprine, steroids, cyclosporine, and antilymphocyte antibodies (such as monoclonal anti-CD3) are employed.[37,38] As mentioned earlier, introduction of cyclosporine as an immunosuppressive agent has had a major impact on clinical organ transplantation. Cyclosporine seems to suppress the activation of CD4+ helper T cells, once again pointing to the pivotal role these cells play in allograft rejection. Although immunosuppression has produced significant gains in terms of graft survival, it should be remembered that immunosuppressive therapy is like the proverbial double-edged sword. The price paid in the form of increased susceptibility to opportunistic fungal, viral, and other infec-

tions is not small. Furthermore, cyclosporine is itself a nephrotoxic drug.

3. Paradoxical as it may seem, *previous blood transfusions* have been definitely proved to be of benefit in allowing greater survival of the transplanted kidneys, especially in cadaver renal transplants. Although blood transfusions do carry the definite risk of presensitization, such risk is small, contrary to earlier expectations. The exact mechanisms underlying this peculiar observation are unknown.

Transplantation of Liver

The success of kidney transplantation has spurred the efforts to transplant a variety of other organs, such as liver, heart, lungs, and pancreas. Indeed, in the last eight years over 1000 liver transplantations have been performed in the United States, and liver transplantation has become a viable treatment modality for a variety of conditions.[39] *The leading indications for liver transplantation in children include extrahepatic biliary atresia and metabolic disorders such as α-1-antitrypsin deficiency and Wilson's disease; in adults, nonalcoholic cirrhosis, primary biliary cirrhosis, sclerosing cholangitis, and certain resectable neoplasms have been the most common indications.* Unlike the case with renal transplantation, HLA matching is not a prime consideration in liver transplants. There are several reasons for this difference in donor selection: (1) unlike kidney, liver seems to be a "privileged" organ that is much less susceptible to transplant rejection; this peculiar property may be related to the fact that HLA antigens are expressed poorly on hepatocytes; (2) because the transplanted liver has to be snugly "fitted" in the space previously occupied by the host liver, the size of the donor organ is of major importance, especially in children; thus size takes precedence over HLA match; and (3) experience with the use of cyclosporine and other immunosuppressive drugs in renal transplants suggests that with effective immunosuppression the detrimental effects of an HLA mismatch can be overcome to a great extent.

Despite the favorable factors mentioned previously, transplanted livers do undergo rejection reactions. Two patterns of rejection are recognized. **Acute rejection** (within the first two months) is characterized by a triad of histologic features: (1) mixed portal inflammatory infiltrate consisting of lymphocytes, neutrophils, and eosinophils, (2) mononuclear or polymorphonuclear cholangitis, and (3) portal or central vein inflammation, characterized by swelling of the endothelial cells and collection of inflammatory cells under the subendothelial space.[40] **Chronic rejection** is associated with continued portal tract inflammation, with evidence of fibrosis and severe destruction of bile ductules to the point that many portal tracts may be completely devoid of bile ducts. In addition, there is marked arteriolar thickening and hyalinization. With current surgical techniques and immunosuppressive therapy the one-year survival of grafts is approximately 70%, falling to 62% by the end of the second year.

Transplantation of Hematopoietic Cells

Mention should be made of the special features of transplantation of bone marrow. Use of this form of therapy for hematologic malignancies, aplastic anemias, and certain immunodeficiency states is increasing. In most of the conditions in which bone marrow transplantation is indicated, the recipient is irradiated with lethal doses either to destroy the malignant cells (e.g., leukemias) or to create a graft bed (aplastic anemias). Two major problems arise in bone marrow transplantation: graft-versus-host disease (GVH) and transplant rejection.

Graft-versus-host disease occurs in any situation in which immunologically competent cells or their precursors are transplanted into immunologically crippled recipients. Recipients of bone marrow transplants are immunodeficient because of either primary disease or prior treatment of the disease with drugs or irradiation. When such recipients receive normal bone marrow cells from allogeneic donors, the immunocompetent T cells derived from the donor marrow recognize the recipient's tissue as "foreign" and react against them. The relevant antigens, as might be expected, belong to the HLA complex. Antirecipient CTL (p. 183) as well as lymphokine-producing T cells are generated. Although any organ may be affected, the predominant clinical manifestations of GVH relate to the involvement of skin, liver, and intestinal mucosa. GVH disease and its attending complications, mainly infections, are often lethal; better matching of the donor and recipients at the HLA locus reduces the possibility of a GVH reaction. Another approach, which has been quite successful, is to remove all the mature T cells from the donor bone marrow prior to transplantation. This can be achieved by pretreating the bone marrow cells with anti–T-cell antibodies and complement.

Even if GVH can be ameliorated, there remains the problem of *rejection* of the grafted marrow. Indeed, recent studies indicate that while T-cell depletion of the marrow reduces the severity and frequency of GVH, it leads to a significant reduction in stem cell engraftment. Two factors may be responsible for graft failure under these circumstances:[41] (1) some T cells and their soluble products, such as hematopoietic growth factors, may be essential for the optimal growth of the transplanted stem cells; and (2) T-cell–depleted marrow is at a greater risk for rejection by the host (host anti-graft rejection). What cells may be responsible for the rejection of bone marrow in those receiving lethal doses of irradiation? Most evidence points to natural killer (NK) cells as being responsible for the recognition and rejection of allogeneic stem cells, but radiation-resistant T cells may also be involved.[42]

AUTOIMMUNE DISEASES

The evidence is now compelling that an immune reaction against "self-antigens"—autoimmunity—is the cause of certain diseases in humans.[43] In recent years a growing number of diseases have been attributed to autoimmunity (Table 5–7), but it must be confessed that in many the evidence is not firm. This is because autoantibodies can be found in the serum or tissues of a remarkably large number of apparently normal individuals, particularly in older age groups. Apparently innocuous autoantibodies are also formed following damage to tissue and may serve a physiologic role in the removal of tissue breakdown products. Furthermore, recent investigations of cellular interactions involved in the normal immune response indicate that recognition of self-histocompatibility antigens is required for normal cell-to-cell interactions (p. 170). These observations indicate that some forms of autorecognition are normal and physiologic. How, then, does one define "pathologic" autoimmunity?

Ideally, at least three requirements should be met before a disorder can be categorized as truly due to autoimmunity: (1) the presence of an autoimmune reaction, (2) clinical or experimental evidence that such a reaction is *not secondary* to tissue damage but is of primary pathogenetic significance, and (3) the absence of another well-defined cause of the disease. Unfortunately, these requirements are met in only a few diseases, such as systemic lupus erythematosus (SLE) and autoimmune blood dyscrasias.

The autoimmune disorders form a spectrum on one end of which are conditions in which autoantibodies are directed against a single organ or tissue, therefore resulting in localized tissue damage. A classic example is Hashimoto's thyroiditis, in which the antibodies have absolute specificity for thyroid constituents. At the other end of the spectrum is SLE, in which a diversity of antibodies results in widespread lesions throughout the body. In SLE, autoantibodies

Table 5-7. Autoimmune Diseases

SINGLE ORGAN OR CELL TYPE	SYSTEMIC
Probable	*Probable*
Hashimoto's thyroiditis	Systemic lupus erythematosus
Autoimmune hemolytic anemia	Rheumatoid arthritis
	Sjögren's syndrome
Autoimmune atrophic gastritis of pernicious anemia	Reiter's syndrome
Autoimmune encephalomyelitis	*Possible*
Autoimmune orchitis	Polymyositis-dermatomyositis
Goodpasture's syndrome*	Systemic sclerosis (scleroderma)
Autoimmune thrombocytopenia	Polyarteritis nodosa
Insulin-dependent diabetes mellitus	
Myasthenia gravis	
Graves' disease	
Possible	
Primary biliary cirrhosis	
Chronic active hepatitis	
Ulcerative colitis	
Membranous glomerulonephritis	

*Target is basement membrane of glomeruli and alveolar walls.

react with nuclear constituents of virtually every cell within the organism. In the middle of the spectrum falls Goodpasture's syndrome, in which antibodies to basement membranes of lung and kidney induce lesions and symptoms in these organs. It is obvious that autoimmunity implies loss of self-tolerance, and the question arises as to how this happens. Before we look for answers to this question, we should review the mechanisms of immunologic tolerance and self-tolerance.

IMMUNOLOGIC TOLERANCE

Immunologic tolerance is a state in which the individual is incapable of developing an immune response to a specific antigen. Self-tolerance refers to lack of responsiveness to an individual's antigens, and obviously it underlies our ability to live in harmony with our own cells and tissues. Several mechanisms, albeit not well understood, have been postulated to explain the tolerant state. Two of these are worth consideration: clonal deletion and suppression of autoreactive lymphocytes.

CLONAL DELETION. According to this concept, initially developed by Burnet, immature clones of lymphocytes that bear receptors for self-antigens are eliminated (deleted) from the lymphoid system during development. This seemed to be a reasonable explanation for the observations made by the Nobel prize–winning experiments of Medawar, in which mice exposed to foreign histocompatibility antigens in utero became tolerant to them in adult life. According to this hypothesis autoimmune diseases are thought to result from the emergence of "forbidden clones" of lymphocytes reactive against self-antigens, probably owing to somatic mutations. Although plausible and supported by some experimental evidence, the *clonal deletion hypotheses cannot readily explain the well-documented presence of lymphocytes that bear receptors for self-antigens, such as DNA, myelin, collagen, and thyroglobulin, in normal humans.* To resolve this dilemma, it has been proposed that during development the *immature B cells go through a phase during which contact with an antigen leads to functional paralysis without physical deletion.*[44] According to this concept, described as "clonal anergy," lymphoid cells that express receptors for self-antigens continue to exist in adult life but cannot be triggered to form antibody.

SUPPRESSION OF AUTOREACTIVE LYMPHOCYTES. Although some form of clonal deletion or anergy may indeed contribute to maintenance of self-tolerance, several lines of evidence suggest that additional failsafe mechanisms must also be involved. The presence of self-reactive lymphocytes in normal humans, and the ease with which autoimmune diseases can be produced in experimental animals, suggests that *self-tolerance is maintained by mechanisms that actively suppress immune responses against self.* Notice that this concept differs from clonal anergy in

that the autoreactive cells are believed to be intrinsically capable of responding unless restrained by some form of regulatory or suppressor mechanisms. Several such controlling mechanisms have been recently reviewed.[45] Only a brief summary is presented here:

SUPPRESSOR CELLS. Immune response to a variety of heterologous antigens generates T cells capable of suppressing B cell and T-helper cell responses. It is believed that T-suppressor cells are part of the normal regulatory circuits that control the magnitude and the duration of an immune response.[46] It has also been suggested that one of the physiologic functions of T-suppressor cells may be to prevent autoimmune reactions.[47] Loss of suppressor cells might then lead to immune reactions against self.

IDIOTYPE–ANTI-IDIOTYPE NETWORKS. To understand the relevance of idiotype–anti-idiotype networks, we must recall that the antigen-combining sites of antibody molecules as well as T-cell receptors are composed of variable regions (or V domains) whose three-dimensional structure has a lock-and-key complementarity to the antigenic determinants that they recognize. It is now well established that the variable regions of the T and B cell receptors themselves are "antigenic" and can therefore evoke the formation of antibodies directed against themselves.[48,49] *The antigenic determinants on the V domains are called idiotypes, and the antibodies elicited against them are termed anti-idiotypic antibodies* (Fig. 5–20). A subsequent antibody response against the anti-idiotype may result in the production of anti-anti-idiotypes, and so on; indeed such a network of anti-idiotypic antibodies that was predicted to exist by the Nobel Laureate Niels Jerne has been found. The nature of anti-idiotypic antibodies and their ef-

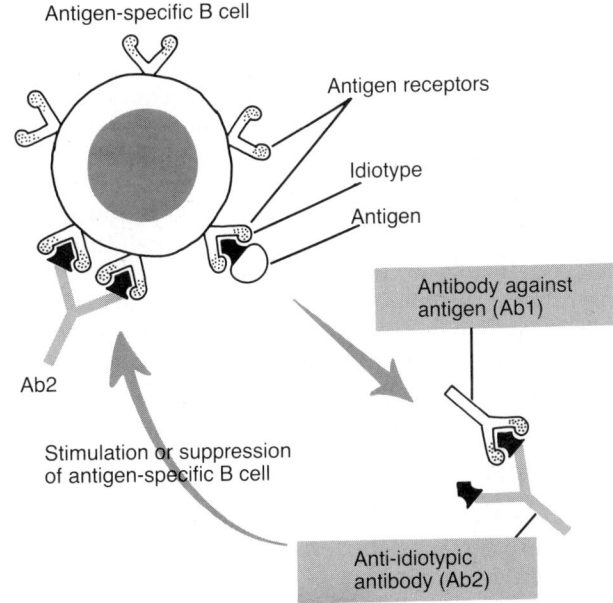

Figure 5–20. Anti-idiotypic antibodies that are internal images of the antigen. These may regulate the antigen-specific B cells.

fects is an extremely complex subject, which will not be considered here. For the present discussion, it suffices to note that *if the anti-idiotypic antibody is directed against the antigen-combining site of the original antibody (Fig. 5–20), the configuration of its own V-region will resemble the antigen itself.* Such an anti-idiotypic antibody (Ab2) (being an internal image of the antigen) could interact with the antigen-specific B cell or T cell and deliver a stimulatory or a suppressive signal. Thus, anti-idiotypic antibodies have the potential to regulate immune responses and are believed to perform such a function in vivo. Perturbations of the idiotype–anti-idiotype network can result in autoimmune diseases, as is discussed later.

In closing this discussion it should be pointed out that the concepts of clonal deletion and peripheral suppression should not be viewed as mutually exclusive. Prevention of autoreactivity is so important for the body that it is likely to involve a series of mechanisms.

CELLULAR BASIS OF TOLERANCE. Before discussing the mechanisms underlying autoimmune disease it is necessary to review the cellular interactions involved in the immune response and see how tolerance may be achieved at the cellular level. Recall that the antibody response against several antigens requires the cooperation of T-helper cells with antibody-secreting B cells. The T-helper cells recognize carrier determinants presented to them by antigen-presenting cells in association with class II MHC antigens. The activated T-helper cells then deliver helper signals to B cells that recognize the haptenic determinants (Fig. 5–21). It follows then that, regardless of the mechanism (i.e., clonal anergy or suppressor influences), tolerance can be maintained if either the T-helper cells or the B cells (or both) are rendered inactive. Indeed, in experimental systems both T- and B-cell tolerance can be demonstrated, but T and B cells differ with respect to the dosage of antigen required to induce tolerance. In general, T-helper cells are rendered tolerant with small doses of the antigen (low-zone tolerance) and the tolerance is long-lasting. On the other hand, B-cell tolerance requires exposure to larger amounts of antigen and is relatively short-lived. In the case of self-tolerance it is proposed that the inability to respond results from T-cell tolerance, whereas B cells are fully competent. *It follows, therefore, that if the nontolerant B cells could be activated, autoimmunity might result.* This and other mechanisms of autoimmune diseases are discussed next.

MECHANISMS OF AUTOIMMUNE DISEASES

Although it would be attractive to explain all autoimmune diseases by a single mechanism, it is now clear that there are a number of ways by which tolerance can be bypassed, thus terminating a previously unresponsive state to autoantigens. More than one defect might be present in each disease, and the defects vary from one disorder to the other. Furthermore, the pathogenesis of autoimmunity appears to involve immunologic, genetic, and viral factors interacting through complicated mechanisms that are poorly understood. Here we can only scratch the surface of the rapidly evolving area of investigation into the mechanisms of autoimmunity. First we discuss the initiating immunologic mechanisms and then the role of genetic and viral factors is reviewed briefly.

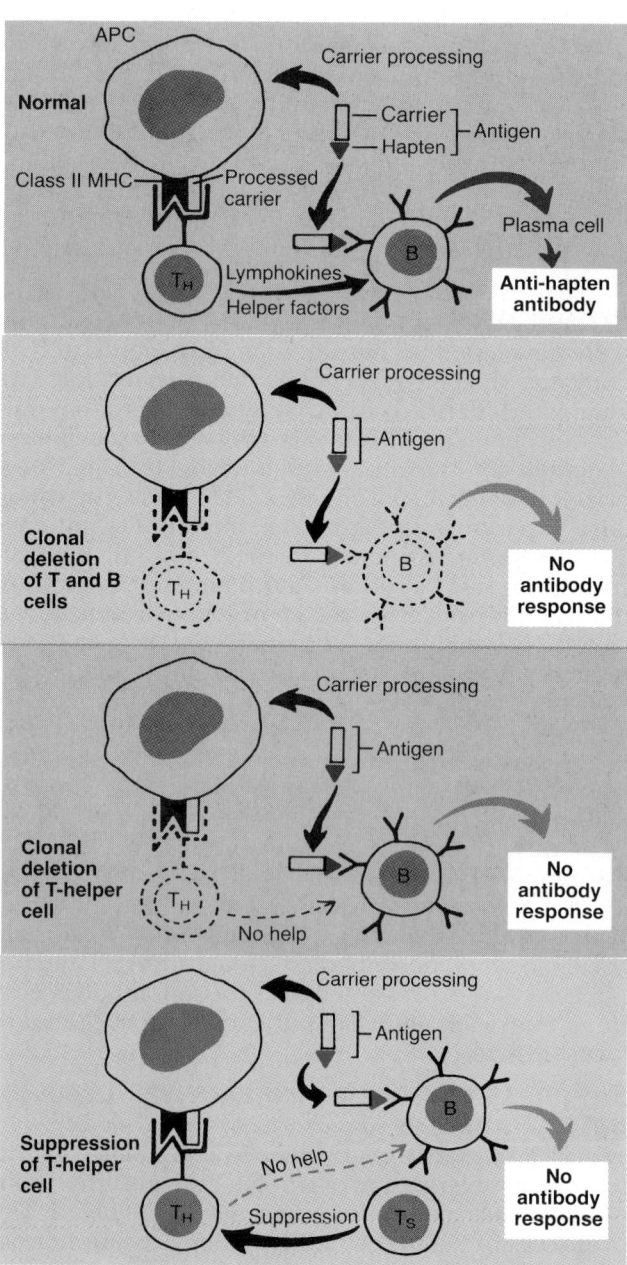

Figure 5–21. Schematic illustration of the cell interactions involved in normal antibody response and the proposed mechanisms of self tolerance: clonal deletion of T and B cells, and clonal deletion or suppression of T-helper cells. APC = antigen-presenting cell; T_H = T-helper cell; T_s = T-suppressor cell.

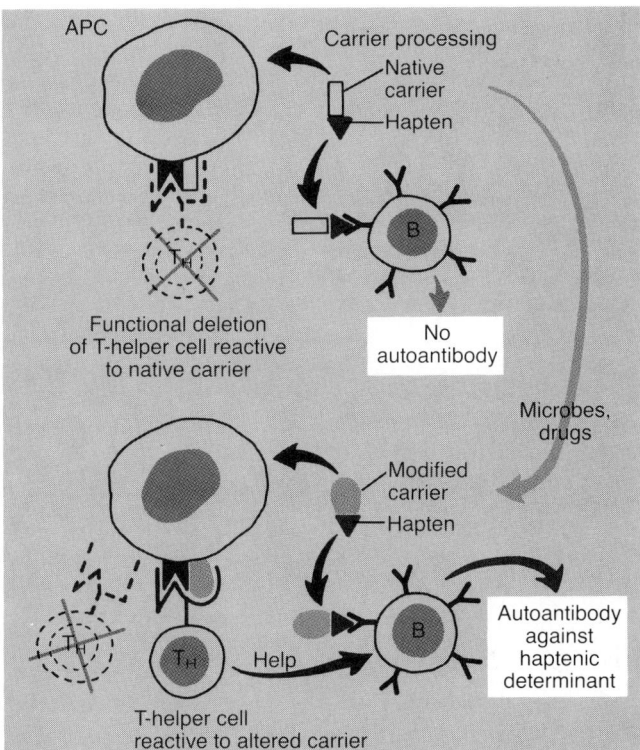

Figure 5–22. Tolerance of self-antigen (native carrier–hapten complex) due to lack of T-cell help, and the loss of self-tolerance by T-helper cell bypass.

The initiating mechanisms in autoimmunity can best be understood in terms of those discussed for tolerance. Four general mechanisms for loss of self-tolerance have been postulated:

BYPASS OF T-HELPER CELL TOLERANCE. It can be deduced from our earlier discussion that tolerance may be broken if T-cell tolerance for the carrier is lost or bypassed (Fig. 5–22). This can be accomplished experimentally in several ways, some of which may have relevance to human autoimmunity.

MODIFICATION OF THE MOLECULE. If a potentially autoantigenic determinant (hapten) is complexed to a new carrier, the carrier part of the complex may be recognized by nontolerant T cells as foreign. The latter would then cooperate with the hapten-specific B cells, leading to the production of autoantibodies. This modification of the molecule could arise in several ways:

• *Complexing of self-antigens with drugs or microorganisms.* Autoimmune hemolytic anemia associated with drugs (e.g., antihypertensive agent alpha-methyldopa) may be due to an alteration of the red cell surface, thus providing a new carrier for an Rh antigen-hapten that stimulates B cells.
• *Partial degradation of autoantigen.* This could expose new antigenic determinants. Thus, partially degraded collagen and enzymatically altered thyroglobulin or gamma globulin are more immunogenic than

the native species. The autoantibodies to gamma globulin (rheumatoid factor) induced during some bacterial, viral, and parasitic infections may well be due to alterations of gamma globulin by either the microorganisms or lysosomal hydrolases.

CROSS REACTIONS. Several infectious agents cross react with human tissues through their haptenic determinants. The infecting microorganisms may trigger an antibody response by presenting the cross-reacting haptenic determinant in association with their own carrier, to which the T-helper cells are not tolerant. The antibody so formed may then damage the tissue that shares the cross-reacting determinants. There is evidence that rheumatic heart disease sometimes follows streptococcal infection because an antibody to streptococcal M protein cross reacts with the M protein in the sarcolemma of cardiac muscle.

POLYCLONAL B-CELL ACTIVATION. Another mechanism by which the T-cell tolerance may be bypassed is through the direct activation of autoreactive B cells. Several microorganisms and their products are capable of causing polyclonal (i.e., antigen nonspecific) activation of B cells.[50] The best investigated among these is bacterial lipopolysaccharide (endotoxin), which can induce mouse lymphocytes to form anti-DNA, antithymocyte, and anti–red cell antibodies in vitro. Infection of B cells with Epstein-Barr virus (EBV) could also achieve the same effect because human B cells bear receptors for EBV. It should be pointed out that the *B-cell activation observed in human and animal models of autoimmune diseases could also result from genetically determined, intrinsic B-cell abnormalities* or loss of T-suppressor cell influence. These are discussed later.

IDIOTYPE BYPASS MECHANISMS. Anti-idiotypic responses may induce autoimmunity by at least two pathways.

LIGAND MIMICRY BY ANTI-IDIOTYPIC ANTIBODIES. This mechanism applies principally to those conditions that are mediated by antireceptor antibodies (Fig. 5–23). Anti-idiotypic antibodies (Ab2) formed against the idiotype of antihormone antibody (Ab1) would be expected to resemble the hormone (internal image). Hence such anti-idiotypic antibodies react with the hormone receptor and can mimic hormone action, as is noted in Graves' disease where antibodies "simulate" TSH and so activate thyroid cells.

PERTURBATION BY MICROBIAL INFECTIONS. *The anti-idiotypic network may be perturbed by microbial infections.* If the microbial antigens (Fig. 5–23B) or idiotypic determinants of antibodies against them (Fig. 5–23C) cross react with the immunoglobulin idiotype on autoreactive B lymphocytes, production of autoantibodies may be triggered. In either case, a T-helper cell that bears anti-idiotypic receptors is initially stimulated, which in turn provides helper signals to the self-reactive B cells.

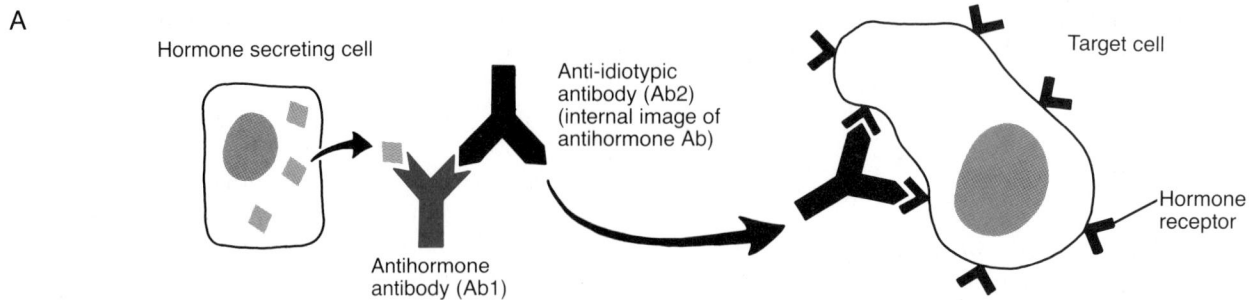

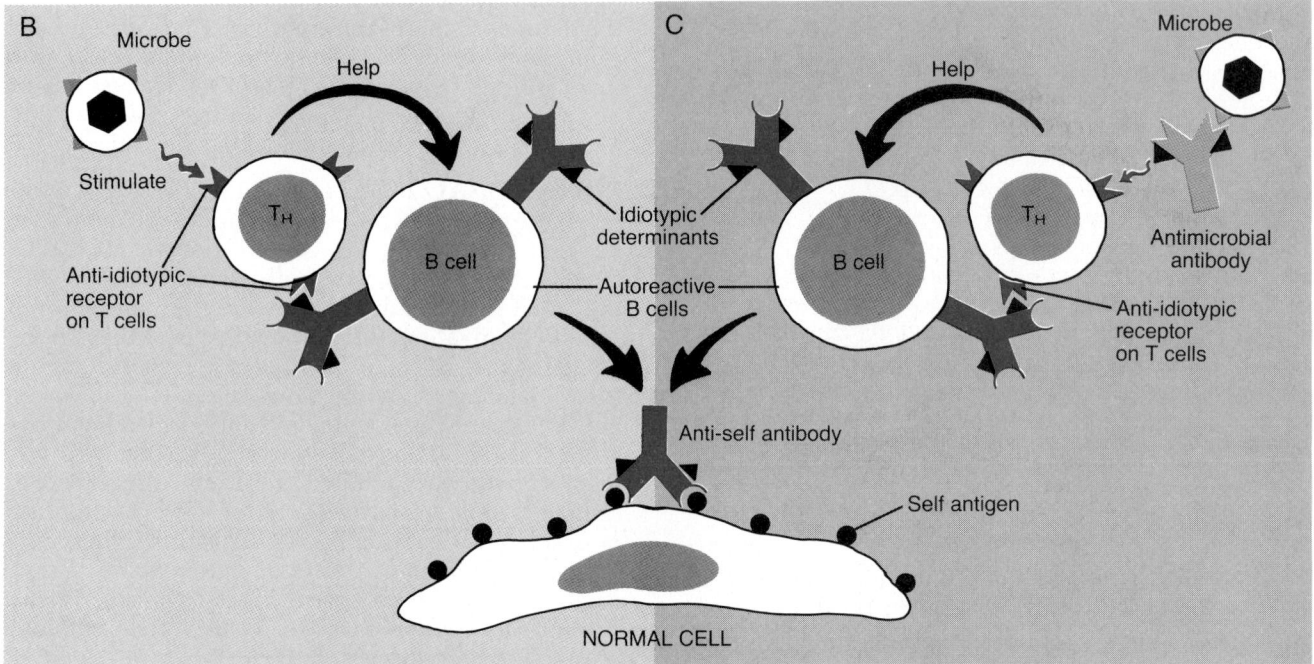

Figure 5–23. Idiotype bypass mechanisms. *A,* Ligand mimicry by anti-idiotypic antibody (Ab2) directed against the antigen (hormone) binding site of antihormone antibody (Ab1) mimics the action of the hormone by binding to the hormone receptors on appropriate target cells. Note that Ab2 is an internal image of the hormone. *B* and *C,* Autoreactive B cells are triggered by T cells that bear receptors for the idiotype of autoantibodies. The T-helper cells are stimulated because the microbial antigen *(B)* or idiotype of antibody against microbial antigen *(C)* cross reacts with the idiotype on autoreactive antibodies.

IMBALANCE OF T-SUPPRESSOR-HELPER FUNCTION. It may be expected from our discussion of T-suppressor cells that any loss of suppressor T-cell function will contribute to autoimmunity and, conversely, excessive T cell help may drive B cells to extremely high levels of autoantibody production. Experimental evidence indeed suggests that this is true. There is an age-associated loss of T-suppressor cells in the NZB × NZW (F1) mice, which develop an autoimmune disease similar to SLE as they age. Defects in T-suppressor cell function or numbers (or both) have also been reported in human SLE, but this subject remains controversial.[51] Enhanced T-helper cell function manifested in the form of chronic hypersecretion of T-helper factors is seen in the lupus erythematosus–prone MRL-1pr/1pr mice, and a somewhat similar increase in helper cell activity is also noted in certain patients with SLE.

EMERGENCE OF A SEQUESTERED ANTIGEN. Regardless of the exact mechanism by which self-tolerance is achieved (clonal deletion or suppressive influences), it is clear that induction of tolerance requires interaction between the antigen and the immune system. It follows, then, that any self-antigen that is completely sequestered is likely to be viewed as foreign if introduced into the circulation, and an immune response will develop. Spermatozoa, myelin basic protein, and lens crystalin may fall into this category of sequestered antigens. Indeed, trauma to the testes involving the release of sperm into the tissues is followed by the appearance of antibodies to spermatozoa.[52] Seductive as this theory may be, it is probably not a major mechanism of autoimmune reactions in humans and is applicable only to the special situations cited.

Several other immunologic abnormalities, including thymic defects and defects in macrophages, have also been implicated in loss of self-tolerance. For a discussion of these, the reader is referred to a recent review.[45]

GENETIC FACTORS IN AUTOIMMUNITY.

There is little doubt that, both in laboratory animals and in humans, genetic factors determine the frequency and the nature of autoimmune diseases.[53] This conclusion is based on the following two lines of evidence: (1) familial clustering of several human autoimmune diseases, such as systemic lupus erythematosus, autoimmune hemolytic anemia, and autoimmune thyroiditis; and (2) linkage of several autoimmune diseases with HLA, especially class II, antigens. It should be recalled that class II antigens are intimately involved in the regulation of immune cell interactions and therefore in the magnitude of the immune response. Thus, it is conceivable that certain class II alleles may facilitate immune responses against autoantigens. Individuals who possess such genes would therefore be at greater risk of developing autoimmune disease when appropriately stimulated with self-antigens. Recent molecular analyses of class II antigens have provided compelling evidence for this hypothesis. For example, the presence or absence of a single amino acid (aspartic acid) at position 57 in the β-chain of the DQ molecule is strongly correlated with resistance or susceptibility to insulin-dependent diabetes mellitus.[54]

Certain genotypes may also constitute fertile soils for the initiation of abnormal immune responses by environmental agents. Included among such agents are microorganisms, particularly viruses, which are the perennial scapegoats in most diseases of obscure causation.

MICROBIAL AGENTS IN AUTOIMMUNITY.

A variety of microbes, including bacteria, mycoplasmas, and viruses, have been implicated in triggering autoimmunity at one time or another. Viruses have received the greatest notoriety because of their involvement in the autoimmune diseases afflicting NZB and NZB $\times$ NZW (F1) mice.

Viruses theoretically may trigger autoimmune reactions in several ways. First, viral antigens and autoantigens may become associated to form immunogenic units and bypass T-cell tolerance, as described earlier (p. 191). Second, some viruses (such as EBV) are nonspecific, polyclonal B-cell mitogens and may thus induce formation of autoantibodies. Third, viral infection may result in loss of suppressor T-cell function by mechanisms that at present are not entirely clear. Viruses and other microbes, particularly certain bacteria such as streptococci and Klebsiella, may share cross-reacting epitopes with self-antigens or self-idiotypes, as discussed earlier. It must be obvious that there is no dearth of possible and some plausible mechanisms by which infectious agents may participate in the pathogenesis of autoimmunity. However, at present there is no clear evidence to implicate any microbe in the causation of human autoimmune diseases. Yet, the search must go on, for if we will not look, we shall not find!

MECHANISMS OF TISSUE DAMAGE IN AUTOIMMUNE DISEASES.

Autoimmune tissue injury could be mediated by antibodies or by T-cell–mediated reactions. Both types II and III hypersensitivity mechanisms have been implicated. For example, opsonization and phagocytosis of red blood cells seems to be the principal mechanism of red cell destruction in autoimmune hemolytic anemia (p. 677). On the other hand, fixation of anti–basement membrane antibody and complement to the glomerular basement membrane seems to be the trigger for glomerular injury in Goodpasture's syndrome (p. 1031). Antibodies directed against β-cells of the pancreatic islets may be responsible for type I (insulin-dependent) diabetes mellitus (p. 995). Both of these are examples of type II hypersensitivity. Type III reactions, initiated by deposition of circulating immune complexes, are the major mechanisms of tissue injury in SLE. In addition to their cytotoxic effects, antibodies may also induce diseases by other mechanisms. In one group of autoimmune disorders, formation of antireceptor antibodies leads to a variety of disease manifestations. Included in this group are: (1) myasthenia gravis, in which anti-acetylcholine receptor antibodies impair myoneural transmission by accelerating the degradation or by blocking of muscle acetylcholine receptors (p. 1366); (2) Graves' disease, in which antibodies to the TSH receptor on thyroid cells mimic the action of TSH, leading to hyperthyroidism (p. 1224); and (3) certain forms of diabetes mellitus, in which anti–insulin receptor antibodies render the cells resistant to the action of insulin (p. 995). In pernicious anemia, on the other hand, the autoantibodies are formed against a biologically active molecule, the intrinsic factor, which is blocked or neutralized, leading to impaired absorption of vitamin B_{12} (p. 683).

As stated earlier, the autoimmune diseases of man range from those in which the target is a single tissue, such as the autoimmune hemolytic anemias and thyroiditis, to those in which a host of self-antigens evoke a constellation of reactions against many organs and systems. In this chapter we deal principally with those presumed autoimmune diseases that are primarily of a systemic nature, and we leave most single-tissue diseases to specific chapters throughout the book. For reference, however, Table 5–7 (p. 188) lists both systemic and organ-specific autoimmune disorders.

SYSTEMIC LUPUS ERYTHEMATOSUS (SLE)

Systemic lupus erythematosus is the classic prototype of the multisystem disease of autoimmune origin, characterized by a bewildering array of autoantibodies, particularly antinuclear antibodies. *Acute or in-*

Table 5-8. The 1982 Revised Criteria for Classification of Systemic Lupus Erythematosus*

CRITERION	DEFINITION
1. Malar rash	Fixed erythema, flat or raised, over the malar eminences, tending to spare the nasolabial folds
2. Discoid rash	Erythematous raised patches with adherent keratotic scaling and follicular plugging; atrophic scarring may occur in older lesions
3. Photosensitivity	Skin rash as a result of unusual reaction to sunlight, by patient history or physician observation
4. Oral ulcers	Oral or nasopharyngeal ulceration, usually painless, observed by a physician
5. Arthritis	Nonerosive arthritis involving two or more peripheral joints, characterized by tenderness, swelling, or effusion
6. Serositis	(a) Pleuritis—convincing history of pleuritic pain or rub heard by a physician or evidence of pleural effusion, or (b) Pericarditis—documented by electrocardiogram or rub or evidence of pericardial effusion
7. Renal disorder	(a) Persistent proteinuria greater than 0.5 g/dl or greater than 3+ if quantitation not performed, or (b) Cellular casts—may be red blood cell, hemoglobin, granular, tubular, or mixed
8. Neurologic disorder	(a) Seizures—in the absence of offending drugs or known metabolic derangements, e.g., uremia, ketoacidosis, or electrolyte imbalance, or (b) Psychosis—in the absence of offending drugs or known metabolic derangements, e.g., uremia, ketoacidosis, or electrolyte imbalance
9. Hematologic disorder	(a) Hemolytic anemia—with reticulocytosis, or (b) Leukopenia—less than 4.0×10^9/L (4000/mm^3) total on two or more occasions, or (c) Lymphopenia—less than 1.5×10^9/L (1500/mm^3) on two or more occasions, or (d) Thrombocytopenia—less than 100×10^9/L (100×10^3/mm^3) in the absence of offending drugs
10. Immunologic disorder	(a) Positive lupus erythematosus cell preparation, or (b) Anti-DNA antibody to native DNA in abnormal titer, or (c) Anti-Sm—presence of antibody to Sm nuclear antigen, or (d) False-positive serologic test for syphilis known to be positive for at least six months and confirmed by negative *Treponema pallidum* immobilization or fluorescent treponemal antibody absorption test
11. Antinuclear antibody	An abnormal titer of antinuclear antibody by immunofluorescence or an equivalent assay at any point in time and in the absence of drugs known to be associated with drug-induced lupus syndrome

*The proposed classification is based on 11 criteria. For the purpose of identifying patients in clinical studies, a person shall be said to have systemic lupus erythematosus if any four or more of the 11 criteria are present, serially or simultaneously, during any interval of observation. From Tan, E. M., et al: The revised criteria for the classification of systemic lupus erythematosus. Arthritis Rheum. 25:1271, 1982.

sidious in its onset, it is a chronic, remitting and relapsing, often febrile illness characterized principally by injury to the skin, joints, kidney, and serosal membranes. Virtually every other organ in the body, however, may also be affected. Indeed, the clinical presentation of SLE is so variable that the American Rheumatism Association has developed criteria for diagnosis of this disorder (Table 5–8). At one time SLE was thought to be a fairly rare disease, but improved methods for diagnosis and an increased awareness that it may be mild and insidious have revealed that its prevalence may be as high as one in 2500 in certain populations[55]. Like most autoimmune diseases, SLE is predominantly a disease of women, with a frequency of 1 in 700 among women between the ages of 20 and 64 and a female-to-male ratio of 9:1. The frequency is even higher in American black women (1 in 245). Although lupus erythematosus usually arises in the second and third decades, it may become manifest at any age, even in early childhood.

ETIOLOGY AND PATHOGENESIS. The cause of SLE remains unknown, but the existence of a limitless number of antibodies in these patients against self-constituents indicates that the *fundamental defect in SLE is a failure of the regulatory mechanisms that sustain self-tolerance.* Antibodies have been identified against an array of nuclear and cytoplasmic components of the cell that are neither organ- nor species-specific. Apart from their value in the diagnosis and management of patients with SLE, these antibodies are of major pathogenetic significance, as, for example, in the immune complex–mediated glomerulonephritis so typical of this disease.

Antinuclear antibodies (ANAs) are directed against several nuclear antigens and can be grouped into four categories:[56] *(1) antibodies to DNA, (2) antibodies to histones, (3) antibodies to nonhistone proteins bound to RNA, and (4) antibodies to nucleolar antigens.* Table 5–9 lists several ANAs and their association with SLE, as well as with other autoimmune diseases to be discussed later. Several techniques are employed to detect ANAs. Clinically, the most commonly utilized method is indirect immunofluorescence, which detects a variety of nuclear antigens, including DNA, RNA, and proteins (collectively called generic ANA). The pattern of nuclear fluorescence suggests the type of antibody present in the patient's serum. Four basic patterns are recognized:

- *Homogeneous or diffuse staining* usually reflects antibodies to deoxyribonucleoprotein, histone, and, occasionally, double-stranded DNA.
- *Rim or peripheral staining* patterns are most commonly indicative of antibodies to double-stranded DNA.
- *Speckled pattern* refers to the presence of uniform or variable-sized speckles. This is one of the most commonly observed patterns of fluorescence and therefore the least specific. It reflects the presence of antibodies to non-DNA nuclear constituents, such as histones and ribonucleoproteins. These components of the nucleus are easily extractable with buffered salt solutions and hence they are also called *extractable nuclear antigens* (ENAs). Examples of ENAs include Sm antigen and SS-A and SS-B reactive antigens (Table 5–9).
- *Nucleolar pattern* refers to the presence of a few discrete spots of fluorescence within the nucleus and represents antibodies to nucleolar RNA. This pattern is reported most often in patients with systemic sclerosis.

It must be emphasized, however, that the patterns are not absolutely specific for the type of antibody. The immunofluorescence test for ANA is positive in virtually every patient with SLE, but it is not specific because patients with other autoimmune diseases also frequently score positive with this "generic" ANA test (Table 5–9). *Furthermore, approximately 10% of normal individuals have low titers of these antibodies.*

Detection of antibodies to specific nuclear antigens requires specialized techniques. Of the approximately 30 nuclear antigen-antibody systems,[57] some that are clinically useful are listed in Table 5–9. It will be noted that *antibodies to double-stranded DNA and the so-called Smith (Sm) antigen are strongly suggestive of SLE.*

Although antibodies to double-stranded DNA are highly specific for SLE, some studies have challenged the conventional wisdom that native DNA is the immunogen that triggers the formation of anti-DNA antibodies.[58] Doubts arose when it was found that monoclonal anti-DNA autoantibodies derived from lupus erythematosus patients could react not only with DNA but also with RNA, certain polynucleotides, and even phospholipids. This unexpected "polyspecificity" of the monoclonal anti-DNA antibodies[59,60] can be readily explained by assuming that they react to an antigenic determinant that recurs in different molecules. One such epitope is believed to reside in the sugar-phosphate backbone that is com-

Table 5-9. Antinuclear Antibodies in Various Autoimmune Diseases*

NATURE OF ANTIGEN	ANTIBODY SYSTEM	DISEASE, % POSITIVE					
		SLE	Drug-Induced LE	Systemic Sclerosis —Diffuse	Systemic Sclerosis —CREST	Sjögren's Syndrome	Polymyositis
Many nuclear antigens (DNA, RNA, proteins)	Generic ANA (indirect IF)	>95	>95	70–90	70–90	50–80	40–60
Native DNA	Anti-double stranded DNA	40–60	<5	<5	<5	<5	<5
Histones	Anti-histone	70	>95	<5	<5	<5	<5
Ribonucleoprotein (Smith antigen)	Anti-Sm	20–30	<5	<5	<5	<5	<5
Ribonucleoprotein	Nuclear RNP	40	<5	15	10	<5	<5
Ribonucleoprotein	SS-A(Ro)	30–40	<5	<5	<5	70–95	10
Ribonucleoprotein	SS-B(La)	15	<5	<5	<5	60–90	<5
DNA topoisomerase I	Scl-70	<5	<5	40–70	10	<5	<5
Centromeric proteins	Anticentromere	<5	<5	<10	90	<5	<5
Histidyl-tRNA synthetase	Jo-1	<5	<5	<5	<5	<5	25

Boxed entries indicate high correlation. ANA = antinuclear antibodies; RNP = ribonucleoprotein.

*Modified from Tan, E. M., et al.: Antinuclear antibodies (ANAs): Diagnostically specific immune markers and clues towards understanding systemic autoimmunity. Clin. Immunol. Immunopathol. *47*:121, 1988; McCarty, G. A.: Autoantibodies and their relation to rheumatic diseases. Med. Clin. North Am. *70*:237, 1986; and Bernstein, R. M., and Mathews, M. B.: Autoantibodies to intracellular antigens, with particular reference to t-RNA and related proteins in myositis. J. Rheumatol. *14*(Suppl. 13):83, 1987.

mon to several polynucleotides and certain phospholipids. Indeed, it has been possible to produce monoclonal antibodies that bind to DNA by immunizing mice with certain phospholipids. By contrast, it has been difficult to induce anti-DNA antibodies when native DNA was used as an immunogen.[53] With respect to the pathogenesis of autoimmunity in SLE, these results imply that (1) anti-DNA antibodies in SLE may not arise in response to DNA (which is poorly immunogenic) but by autoimmunization against other immunogens (phospholipids?) that share determinants with DNA; and (2) the array of autoantibodies produced in SLE may not be as broad as is suggested by their different biologic activities. Thus, a single autoantibody may register as an ANA, as an anticoagulant (owing to reactivity with phospholipids essential for clotting, p. 97), or as a false-positive result in the VDRL test for syphilis (p. 369).

Given the presence of all these autoantibodies, we still know little about the mechanism of their emergence. Three converging lines of investigation hold center stage today: genetic predisposition, a fundamental abnormality in the immune system, and some nongenetic (environmental) factors.

GENETIC FACTORS. The evidence that supports a genetic predisposition takes many forms.

• There is a high rate of concordance (50 to 60%) in monozygotic twins.[53]
• Family members have an increased risk of developing SLE.
• Up to 20% of clinically unaffected first-degree relatives reveal autoantibodies and other immunoregulatory abnormalities, discussed later.
• Approximately 6% of patients with SLE have inherited deficiencies of complement components, especially C2. It seems unlikely that reduced levels of complement per se are involved in disease susceptibility. Because complement genes map within HLA, the association of complement deficiencies with SLE suggests that genetic influences, possibly certain HLA-linked immune response genes, play a role in the appearance of the disease.
• In North American white populations there is a positive association between SLE and the DR-2 and DR-3 genes of the HLA complex.

The role of class II HLA genes in the pathogenesis of SLE is most likely related to their immunoregulatory functions. It should be noted, however, that many immune disorders other than SLE are associated with HLA-DR3, and many individuals with this genotype are clinically unaffected. It follows therefore that the genes in the *D region confer only a general predisposition to autoimmunity, and genes in addition to HLA must also be involved.* More importantly, other (nongenetic) factors must act to convert genetic susceptibility to clinical disease.

NONGENETIC FACTORS. There are many indications that, in addition to genetic factors, several *environmental* or nongenetic factors must be involved in the pathogenesis of SLE. The most clear example comes from the observation that drugs such as hydralazine, procainamide, and D-penicillamine can induce an SLE-like response in humans.[61] Exposure to ultraviolet light is another environmental factor that exacerbates the disease in many individuals. How ultraviolet light acts is not entirely clear, but it is strongly suspected to modulate the immune response. For example, it induces keratinocytes to produce IL-1, a factor known to activate T and B cells. *Viruses* have also been suspected to be the cause of SLE. Although viruses could well initiate autoimmune reactions by a variety of mechanisms that were discussed earlier (p. 193), there is no hard evidence to support any role for viruses or other infectious agents in human SLE. *Sex hormones* seem to exert an important influence on the occurrence and manifestations of SLE. During the reproductive years the frequency of SLE is ten times greater in women than in men, and exacerbation has been noted during normal menses and pregnancy. Some recent data suggest that lupus erythematosus patients have an alteration in estrogen metabolism that results in hyperestrogenic effects, and estrogens may enhance antibody synthesis.[62,63]

IMMUNOLOGIC FACTORS. With all the immunologic findings in SLE patients, there can be little doubt that some fundamental derangement of the immune system is involved in the pathogenesis of SLE. Although a variety of immunologic abnormalities affecting both T cells and B cells have been detected in patients with SLE,[64,65] there is overwhelming evidence that B-cell hyperactivity is fundamental to the pathogenesis of SLE.[66] The activation of B cells is polyclonal, and as such *there is increased production of antibodies to both self and nonself antigens.* It not only is reflected by hypergammaglobulinemia and production of autoantibodies in vivo, but it can also be readily demonstrated in vitro. B cells isolated from the blood of lupus erythematosus patients show eight to ten times higher proliferative capacity and secrete excessive amounts of immunoglobulins per cell. What is the basis of this B cell hyperactivity? As discussed earlier (p. 191) it could result from one or more of the following mechanisms: (1) an inherited intrinsic defect in B cells, rendering them refractory to regulation; (2) polyclonal activation by infectious or other environmental agents; (3) excessive stimulation of intrinsically normal B cells by T-helper cell hyperactivity; and (4) a primary defect in T-suppressor cell circuits. Thus we are faced with the question of which of these mechanisms is "truly" responsible for B cell hyperactivity. Mercifully, the answer seems to be "all of the above!" Thus, it seems that SLE is a syndrome that can result from several different forms of immunologic derangements. As with different animal models of the disease,[67,68] a genetically determined defect in T-helper cells may be paramount in some patients, whereas in others, a combination of intrinsic B cell hyperactivity and decreased activity of T-suppressor cells may be critical to autoantibody formation.[45,69] It should also be remembered that in a patient with full-blown lupus erythematosus it is often difficult to distinguish between primary and secondary immunoregulatory abnormalities. For example, in a given patient excessive T-cell help may be primary, but formation of autoantibodies against T-suppressor cells may lead to a secondary loss of T-cell suppression.

Regardless of the exact sequence by which autoantibodies are formed, they are clearly the mediators of tissue injury. *Most of the visceral lesions are mediated by immune complexes (type III hypersensitivity).* DNA–anti-DNA complexes can be detected in the glomeruli and small blood vessels. Low levels of serum complement and granular deposits of complement and immunoglobulins in the glomeruli further support the immune complex nature of the disease. On the other hand, *autoantibodies against red cells, white cells, and platelets mediate their effects via type II hypersensitivity.* There is no evidence that ANAs, which are involved in immune complex formation, can penetrate intact cells. However, if cell nuclei are exposed, the ANAs can bind to them. In tissues, nuclei of damaged cells react with ANAs, lose their chromatin pattern, and become homogeneous, to produce so-called *LE bodies or hematoxylin bodies. Related to this phenomenon is the LE cell, which is seen only in vitro. Basically, the LE cell is any phagocytic leukocyte (neutrophil or macrophage) that has engulfed the denatured nucleus of an injured cell* (Fig. 5–24). The demonstration of LE cells involves the microscopic examination of white cells in vitro. If the withdrawn

Table 5-10. Clinical Manifestations of Systemic Lupus Erythematosus

CLINICAL MANIFESTATION	PREVALENCE IN PATIENTS, %
Hematologic	100
Arthritis	90
Skin	85
Fever	83
Fatigue	81
Weight loss	63
Renal	50
Pleurisy	46
Myalgia	33
Pericarditis	25
Gastrointestinal	21
Raynaud's phenomenon	20
Central nervous system	20
Ocular	15
Peripheral neuropathy	14
Pneumonitis	11
Parotid gland enlargement	8
Liver disease	2

From Condemi, J.J.: The autoimmune diseases. J.A.M.A. *258*:2920,1987.

blood is agitated, a sufficient number of leukocytes can be damaged to thus expose their nuclei to ANAs. The binding of ANAs to nuclei denatures them, and subsequent fixation of complement renders antibody-coated nuclei strongly chemotactic for phagocytic cells. The LE cell test is positive in up to 70% of the patients with SLE. However, with new techniques for detection of ANA, this test is now largely of historical interest.

To summarize, SLE appears to be a heterogeneous disorder of multifactorial origin resulting from complex interactions among genetic, hormonal, and environmental factors acting in concert to produce pronounced B-cell activation, and resulting in the secretion of several polyspecific antibodies. In this complex web, each factor may be necessary but not enough for the clinical expression of the disease; the relative importance of various factors may vary from individual to individual.

MORPHOLOGY. The morphologic changes in SLE are extremely variable, reflecting the variability of the clinical manifestations and the course of the disease in individual patients. It can also be said that none of these morphologic changes is pathognomonic. It is the constellation of clinical, serologic, and morphologic changes that is essential for diagnosis (Table 5–8). The frequency of individual organ involvement is shown in Table 5–10. The most characteristic lesions are found in the blood vessels, kidneys, connective tissue, and skin.

An acute necrotizing **vasculitis involving small arteries and arterioles** may be present in any tissue, although skin and muscles are most commonly affected. The arteritis is characterized by fibrinoid deposits in the vessel walls. In chronic stages, vessels undergo fibrous thickening with luminal narrowing. Frequently a perivascular lymphocytic infiltrate is present, sometimes accompanied by signif-

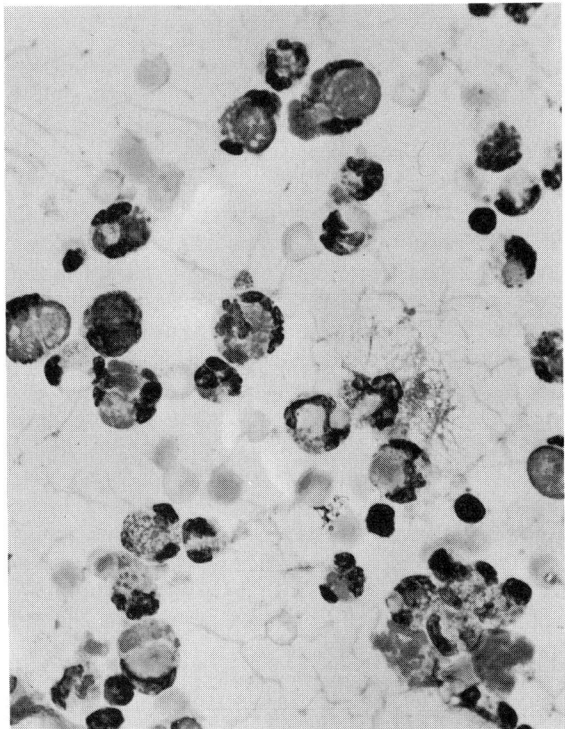

Figure 5–24. A cluster of LE cells (in vitro reaction) demonstrating homogeneous inclusions that have distorted the enclosing polymorphonuclear leukocytes.

icant edema and an increase in ground substance. In the spleen, these vascular lesions involve the central penicilliary arteries and are characterized by marked perivascular fibrosis, producing so-called **onionskin** lesions (Fig. 5–25). Immunoglobulins, DNA, and C3 have been found in these vessel walls, supporting the theory that they may be DNA–anti-DNA complexes.

KIDNEY. On light microscopic examination, the kidney appears to be involved in 60 to 70% of cases, but if **immunofluorescence and electron microscopy are included in the examination of biopsy material, almost all cases of SLE will show some renal abnormality.**[70,71] According to the World Health Organization (WHO) morphologic classification of lupus nephritis, five patterns are recognized: (1) normal by light, electron, and immunofluorescent microscopy (class I), which is quite rare; (2) mesangial lupus glomerulonephritis (class II); (3) focal proliferative glomerulonephritis (class III); (4) diffuse proliferative glomerulonephritis (class IV); and (5) membranous glomerulonephritis (class V). It should be noted, however, that none of these patterns is specific for lupus (p. 1022).

Mesangial lupus glomerulonephritis is the mildest of the lesions and is seen in those patients who have minimal clinical manifestations, such as mild hematuria or proteinuria. It occurs in approximately 10% of the patients. There is a slight-to-moderate increase in the intercapillary mesangial matrix as well as in the number of mesangial cells. Despite the very mild histologic changes, **granular mesangial deposits of immunoglobulin and complement are**

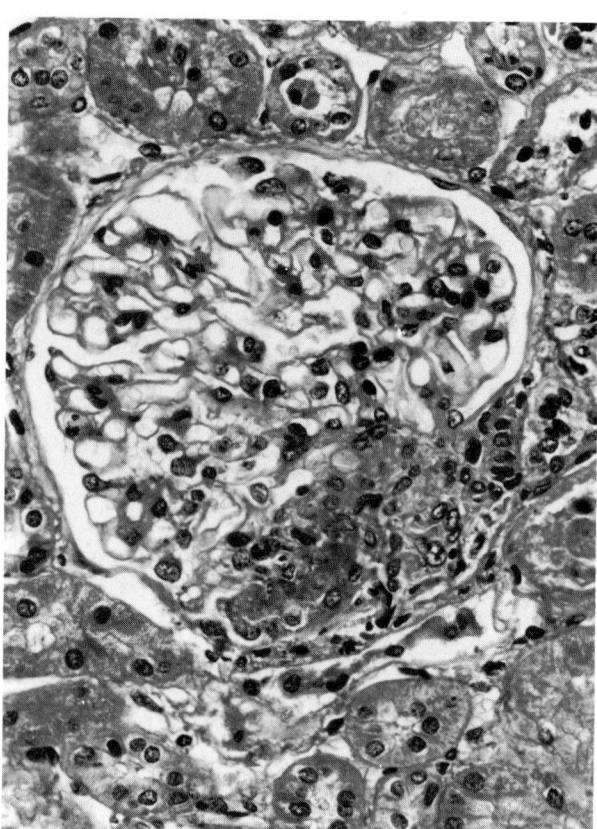

Figure 5–26. Segmental proliferation and necrosis of a glomerular lobule from a case of focal proliferative lupus nephritis. (Courtesy of Dr. Fred Silva, Department of Pathology, Southwestern Medical School, Dallas, Texas.)

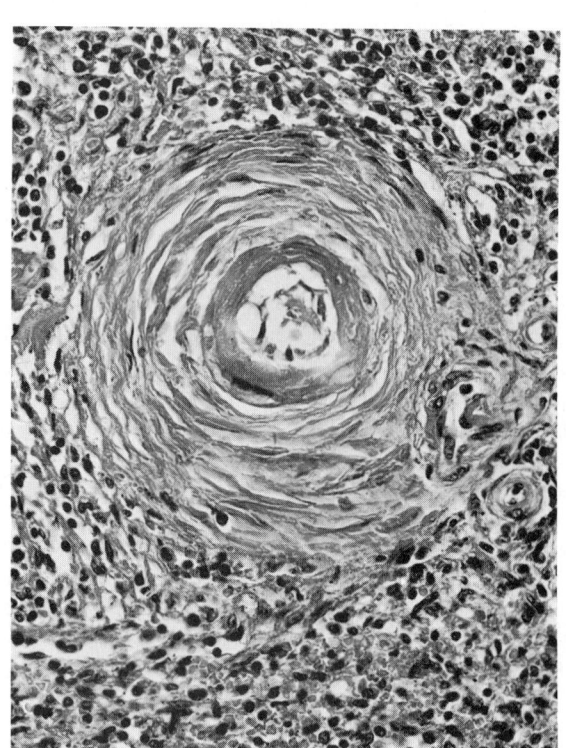

Figure 5–25. Lupus erythematosus—concentric periarterial fibrosis in the spleen.

always present. Such deposits presumably reflect the earliest change, because filtered immune complexes accumulate primarily in the mesangium. The other changes to be described are usually superimposed on the mesangial changes.

Focal proliferative glomerulonephritis is seen in about one third of initial biopsies of these patients. As the name implies, this is a focal lesion, affecting usually fewer than 50% of the glomeruli and generally only portions of each glomerulus. Typically, one or two tufts in an otherwise normal glomerulus exhibit swelling and proliferation of endothelial and mesangial cells, infiltration with neutrophils, and sometimes fibrinoid deposits and intracapillary thrombi (Fig. 5–26). Hematoxylin bodies may be present, and fragmentation and breakdown of nuclei produce an appearance described as "nuclear dust." Focal lesions may be associated with relatively mild clinical manifestations: recurrent hematuria and moderate proteinuria with only occasional mild renal insufficiency. However, some patients with focal lesions may have more severe clinical disease progressing to renal failure.[72]

Diffuse proliferative glomerulonephritis is the most serious of the renal lesions in SLE, occurring in 45 to 50% of patients who are biopsied. Anatomic changes are dominated by proliferation of endothelial, mesangial, and sometimes epithelial cells (Fig. 5–27). Most or all glomeruli are

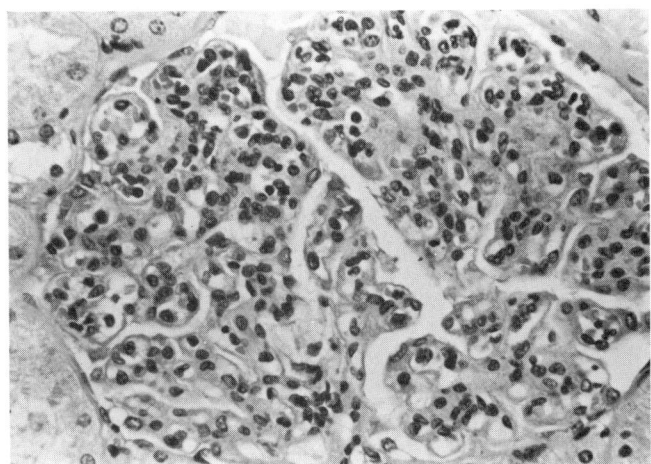

Figure 5–27. Diffuse proliferative lupus nephritis. Note hypercellularity throughout glomerular tuft.

involved in both kidneys, and the entire glomerulus is almost always affected. Patients with diffuse lesions are usually overtly symptomatic, showing microscopic or gross hematuria, proteinuria (including the nephrotic syndrome), hypertension, and frequently a diminution of glomerular filtration rate.

Membranous glomerulonephritis occurs in 10% of patients and is a designation given to glomerular disease in which the principal histologic change consists of widespread thickening of the capillary walls. The lesions are very similar to those encountered in idiopathic membranous glomerulonephritis, described more fully on page 1034. Patients with this histologic change almost always have severe proteinuria or the overt nephrotic syndrome.

All four types are thought to have the same general pathogenetic mechanism, that is, the deposition of DNA–anti-DNA complexes within the glomeruli. Thus, deposits of immunoglobulin and complement are regularly present in the mesangium, either alone or along the entire basement membrane, and sometimes massively throughout the entire glomerulus (Fig. 5–28). Why this same pathogenetic mechanism produces such different histologic lesions (and clinical manifestations) in different patients is not entirely clear. It is likely, as we shall see (p. 1027), that the physical and chemical characteristics of the complexes and the state of the glomerular capillary wall both play a role in the pattern of deposition of complexes and also in the histologic change.

Electron microscopy demonstrates electron-dense immune complexes in three locations within the glomerulus: (1) all histologic types show large amounts of deposits in the mesangium; (2) in membranous glomerulonephritis (class V), the deposits are predominantly between the basement membrane and the visceral epithelial cell (subepithelial), a location similar to that of deposits in other types of membranous nephropathy; (3) subendothelial deposits (between the endothelium and the basement membrane) are particularly characteristic of SLE, because they are noted in few other types of glomerulonephritis (Fig. 5–29). When extensive, subendothelial deposits create a peculiar thickening of the capillary wall, which can be seen by means of

light microscopy as a "wire loop" lesion (Fig. 5–30). Such "wire loops" are often found in the diffuse proliferative type of glomerulonephritis (class IV) but can also be present in the focal (class III) and membranous types (class V). They usually reflect active disease and generally indicate a poor prognosis.

Although the specific types of lesions may persist in individual patients throughout the course of the disease, cases of mesangial or focal glomerulonephritis can progress to diffuse proliferative glomerulonephritis, with a more serious clinical course.[72]

In addition to these glomerular lesions, vasculitis similar to that seen in other affected tissues and organs is sometimes found in cortical arterioles.

Changes in **the interstitium and tubules are also frequently present in patients with SLE,** especially in association with diffuse proliferative glomerulonephritis. In a few cases, tubulointerstitial lesions may be the dominant abnormality.[73] As we shall see in the chapter on kidney diseases (p. 1061), granular deposits composed of immunoglobulin and complement similar to those seen in glomeruli are present in the tubular basement membranes in about 50% of patients with SLE, a pattern indicative of so-called tubular immune complex disease.

SKIN. The skin is often involved. Characteristic erythema affects the facial "butterfly" area (bridge of the nose and cheeks) but also the extremities and trunk. Urticaria, bullae, maculopapular lesions, and ulcerations also occur. Exposure to sunlight incites or accentuates the erythema. Histologically, the involved areas show liquefactive degeneration of the basal layer of the epidermis together with edema at the dermal junction. In the dermis there are variable degrees

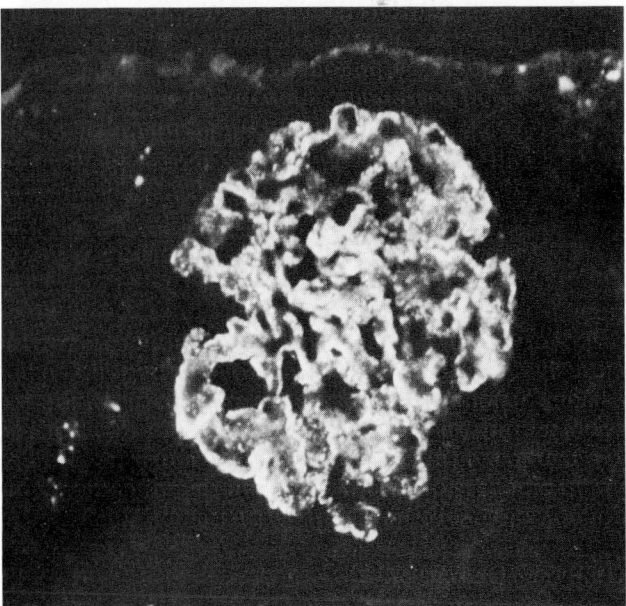

Figure 5–28. Immunofluorescence micrograph stained for IgG from glomerulus with diffuse proliferative lupus nephritis showing abundant deposition of immunoglobulin. (Courtesy of Dr. Fred Silva, Department of Pathology, Southwestern Medical School, Dallas, Texas.)

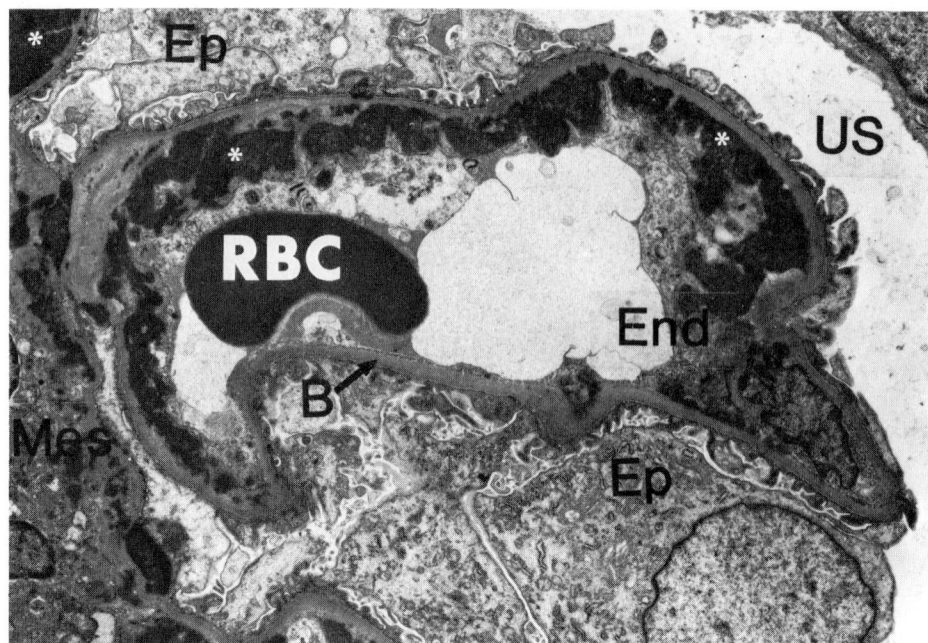

Figure 5–29. Electron micrograph of renal glomerular capillary loop from patient with systemic lupus erythematosus nephritis. Subendothelial dense deposits correspond to "wire loops" seen by light microscopy. End = endothelium; Mes = mesangium; Ep = epithelial cell with foot processes; RBC = red blood cell in capillary lumen; B = basement membrane; US = urinary space; * = electron-dense deposits in subendothelial location. (Courtesy of Dr. Edwin Eigenbrodt, Department of Pathology, Southwestern Medical School, Dallas, Texas.)

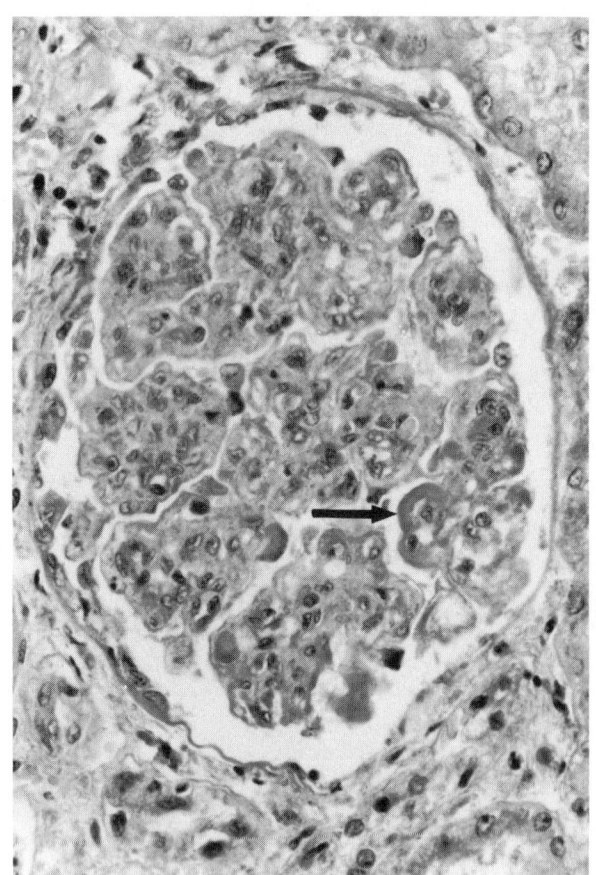

Figure 5–30. Lupus nephritis. A glomerulus with "wire loop" thickening of the basement membrane. (Courtesy of Dr. Fred Silva, Department of Pathology, Southwestern Medical School, Dallas, Texas.)

of fibrosis, perivascular mononuclear infiltrate, and occasionally fibrinoid change in the vessel wall. **Immunofluorescence microscopy shows deposition of immunoglobulin and complement along the dermoepidermal junction.** The presence of immunoglobulin in both involved and non-involved skin in SLE distinguishes the skin lesions from those seen in other connective tissue disorders, such as dermatomyositis and scleroderma, as well as from chronic discoid lupus erythematosus. In the latter disorders, only involved areas of the skin are positive.

JOINTS. Joint involvement is frequent, the typical lesion being a nonerosive synovitis with little deformity. The latter fact distinguishes this arthritis from that seen in rheumatoid disease. In the acute phases of arthritis in SLE there is exudation of neutrophils and fibrin into the synovium and a perivascular mononuclear cell infiltrate in the subsynovial tissue; however, the severe mononuclear infiltration of the subsynovium and the intense synovial hyperplasia characteristic of rheumatoid arthritis are unusual.

CENTRAL NERVOUS SYSTEM. The pathologic basis of CNS symptoms is not entirely clear. It has often been ascribed to acute vasculitis with resultant focal neurologic symptoms. However, histologic studies of the nervous system in patients with neuropsychiatric manifestations of SLE fail to reveal significant vasculitis. Instead, noninflammatory occlusion of small vessels by intimal proliferation is often noticed. These changes are believed to result from damage to the endothelium by antibodies to phospholipids. In addition, recent studies suggest that neuron-reactive antibodies may cause functional impairment without inflicting cell damage.[74]

PERICARDITIS AND OTHER SEROSAL CAVITY INVOLVEMENT. Inflammation of the serosal lining membranes may be acute, subacute, or chronic. During the acute phases, the mesothelial surfaces are sometimes covered with fibrinous exudate. Later they become thickened, opaque, and coated with a shaggy fibrous tissue that may lead to partial or total obliteration of the serosal cavity. In areas of acute involvement, even when the pericardial sac appears normal on gross inspection, there is microscopic evidence of edema; focal vasculitis with a perivascular, mononuclear, inflammatory infiltrate; and fibrinoid necrosis, sometimes containing hematoxylin bodies. These acute changes are replaced in time by fibroblastic proliferation, together with diffuse or focal lymphocytic and plasma cell infiltration.

HEART. In addition to pericarditis, cardiac valves or the myocardium are affected in about half of the cases. The endocardial alterations **(nonbacterial verrucous endocarditis or Libman-Sacks endocarditis),** when present, constitute one of the most striking anatomic findings of lupus erythematosus. Vegetations occur on the mitral and tricuspid valves. These may be small, warty excrescences or, in some cases, friable, berry-like masses of amorphous material that vary in size from less than 1 mm to 3 or 4 mm in diameter (Fig. 5–31). They may occur singly, but more often they occur multiply in random fashion anywhere on the valvular leaflets, usually on the surfaces exposed to the forward flow of blood but sometimes behind the cusps. Infrequently, the vegetations extend onto the mural endocardium of the cardiac chambers or onto the chordae tendineae.

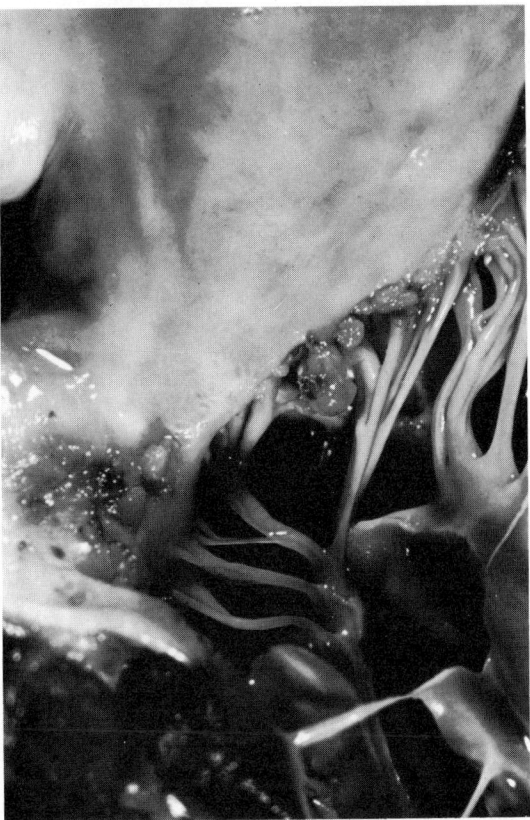

Figure 5–31. Libman-Sacks endocarditis of the mitral valve in lupus erythematosus. The small vegetations attached to the margin of the valve leaflet are easily seen.

The vegetations in SLE must be differentiated principally from those formed in bacterial endocarditis and acute rheumatic endocarditis. In infective endocarditis, the vegetations tend to be considerably larger (0.5 to 2.0 cm) than those in lupus erythematosus, and only rarely are they as widely dispersed. More often, infective vegetations occur singly or in two or three discrete foci, and only very infrequently are they positioned behind the cusps. In rheumatic endocarditis, the vegetations are small, are confined to the lines of closure of the leaflets on the surface exposed to the forward flow of blood, and almost never extend behind the cusps.

Characteristic histologic alterations in Libman-Sacks endocarditis are found underlying the vegetations. Increased ground substance, "fibrinoid necrosis," and, in the later stages, increased vascularization, fibroblastic proliferation, and neutrophilic and mononuclear cell infiltration constitute the inflammatory changes. The vegetation itself may be composed in part of fibrin, but more characteristically is made up of necrotic debris, fibrinoid material, and trapped disintegrating fibroblasts and inflammatory cells. Hematoxylin bodies are sometimes found within the fibrinoid. Organization may, in time, convert the vegetation into a nodule of organized connective tissue. Focal areas of acute-to-chronic inflammation containing fibrinoid may be found throughout the heart in the connective tissue of the endocardium and myocardium, about blood vessels, and in the interfascicular connective tissue planes. Myocardial arterioles and small arteries may suffer acute necrotizing injury with mural deposition of fibrinoid, but myocardial fibers are injured by the resultant ischemia only in the florid, acute cases when the vascular damage is severe and causes thrombosis in lumina.

SPLEEN. The spleen may be moderately enlarged. Capsular thickening is common, as is follicular hyperplasia. Plasma cells are usually numerous in the pulp and can be shown to contain immunoglobulins of the IgG and IgM variety by fluorescence microscopy. As mentioned earlier, the central penicilliary arteries show thickening and perivascular fibrosis, producing the so-called onionskin lesions.

LUNGS. In addition to pleuritis and pleural effusions, interstitial pneumonitis and diffuse fibrosing alveolitis can occur in SLE. As its name indicates, fibrosing alveolitis consists of filling of the alveolar spaces with fibrous tissue, often containing many inflammatory cells. There is evidence that DNA–anti-DNA complexes may contribute to the pathogenesis of this alveolitis.

OTHER ORGANS AND TISSUES. Acute vasculitis may be seen in the portal tracts of the liver accompanied by lymphocytic infiltrates, creating nonspecific portal triaditis. LE cells in the bone marrow may be strongly indicative of lupus erythematosus. Lymph nodes may be enlarged and contain hyperactive follicles as well as plasma cells, changes that are indicative of B-cell activation.

CLINICAL COURSE. It should be evident from Tables 5–8 and 5–10 that SLE is a multisystem disease and as such it is highly variable in its clinical presentation. Typically the patient is a young woman with a butterfly rash over the face, fever, pain but no deformity in one or more peripheral joints (feet, ankles, knees, hips, fingers, wrists, elbows, shoulders), pleuritic chest pain, and photosensitivity. However, in many patients the presentation of SLE is subtle and puzzling, taking forms such as a febrile illness of unknown origin, abnormal urinary findings, or joint disease masquerading as rheumatoid arthritis or rheumatic fever. Antinuclear antibodies can be found in virtually 100% of patients. However, ANAs can also be found in patients with other autoimmune disorders (Table 5–9). *As mentioned earlier, antibodies against double-stranded DNA and Sm antigen are considered strongly suggestive of SLE.* A variety of clinical findings may point toward renal involvement, including hematuria, red cell casts, proteinuria, and, in some cases, the classic nephrotic syndrome (p. 1033). Laboratory evidence of some hematologic derangement is seen in virtually every case, but in some patients they may be the presenting manifestation as well as the dominant clinical problem. In still others, mental aberrations, including psychosis or convulsions, may constitute prominent clinical problems.

The course of the disease is variable and almost unpredictable. Rare acute cases result in death within weeks to months. More often, with appropriate therapy, the disease is characterized by flareups and remissions spanning a period of years or even decades. During acute flareups, increased formation of immune complexes and the accompanying complement activation often results in hypocomplementemia. Disease exacerbations are usually treated by corticosteroids or immunosuppressant drugs such as cyclophosphamide and azathioprine.[75] Even without therapy, in some patients the disease may run a benign course with skin manifestations and mild hematuria for years. The outcome has improved significantly in the recent past. In one recent large multicenter study the survival was 90% at one year, 86% at five years, and 76% at ten years.[76] The most common causes of death are renal failure and intercurrent infections, followed by cardiac failure, pulmonary disease, and CNS disease.

As mentioned earlier, involvement of skin along with multisystem disease is fairly common in SLE. In addition, two syndromes have been recognized in which the cutaneous involvement is the most prominent or exclusive feature.

CHRONIC DISCOID LUPUS ERYTHEMATOSUS. Chronic discoid lupus erythematosus is a disease in which the skin manifestations may mimic SLE but systemic manifestations are rare. It is characterized by the presence of skin plaques showing varying degrees of edema, erythema, scaliness, follicular plugging, and skin atrophy surrounded by an elevated erythematous border. The face and scalp are usually affected, but widely disseminated lesions occasionally occur. The disease is usually confined to the skin, but 5 to 10% of patients with discoid lupus erythematosus

develop multisystem manifestations after many years.[77] The LE cell test is rarely positive, but about 35% of patients show a positive ANA test. Antibodies to double-stranded DNA are rarely present, and immunofluorescence studies of skin biopsies show the same deposition of immunoglobulin and C3 at the dermoepidermal junction that is seen in SLE. *However, in contrast to SLE, normal uninvolved skin does not show such fluorescence.*

SUBACUTE CUTANEOUS LUPUS ERYTHEMATOSUS. This condition also presents with predominant skin involvement and can be distinguished from chronic discoid LE by several criteria. It is characterized by widespread but superficial and nonscarring lesions and mild systemic disease. Furthermore there is a very strong association with antibodies to the SS-A antigen and with the HLA-DR3 genotype. Thus, the term subacute LE seems to define a group intermediate between SLE and lupus erythematosus localized only to skin.[78]

DRUG-INDUCED LUPUS ERYTHEMATOSUS. An interesting lupus erythematosus–like syndrome develops in patients receiving a variety of drugs, including hydralazine (given for hypertension), procainamide, isoniazid, and D-penicillamine, to name only a few of the approximately 46 therapeutic agents that have been implicated.[61] Many are associated with the development of ANAs, but most do not have symptoms of lupus erythematosus. For example 80% of the patients receiving procainamide are positive for ANAs, and one third of these manifest clinical symptoms such as arthralgias, fever, and serositis. *Although multiple organs are affected, renal and CNS involvement is distinctly uncommon.* As compared to idiopathic SLE, there are serologic and genetic differences as well. Anti–double-stranded DNA antibodies are rare, but there is an extremely high frequency of antihistone antibodies. Persons with the HLA-DR4 antigen are at a greater risk of developing lupus erythematosus following administration of hydralazine. These patients seem to have a genetically determined inability to acetylate the amine or hydralazine moiety of these compounds adequately through the hepatic N-acetyl-transferase system.[79] Presumably these "slow acetylators" develop accumulations of nonacetylated metabolites of these drugs, which covalently bind to a nucleoprotein or to cellular macromolecules, producing antigenic complexes. Antihistone antibodies and eventually lupus erythematosus disease are thus induced.[80] Drug-induced LE represents an interesting example of how a genetic *metabolic* defect may lead to autoimmunity. Fortunately, the disease remits after withdrawal of the offending drug.

SJÖGREN'S SYNDROME

Sjögren's syndrome is a clinicopathologic entity characterized by dry eyes (keratoconjunctivitis sicca) and dry mouth (xerostomia) resulting from immunologically mediated destruction of the lacrimal and salivary glands. It occurs as an isolated disorder (primary form), also known as the *sicca syndrome,* or more often in association with another autoimmune disease (secondary form). Among the associated disorders, rheumatoid arthritis is the most common, but some patients have SLE, polymyositis, scleroderma, vasculitis, mixed connective tissue disease, or thyroiditis.

ETIOLOGY AND PATHOGENESIS. As we shall see in the description of morphology, the decrease in tears and saliva (sicca syndrome) is the result of *lymphocytic infiltration* and fibrosis of the lacrimal and salivary glands. The infiltrate contains predominantly T cells and some B cells, including plasma cells that secrete antibody locally.[81] Most of the infiltrating T cells are CD4+ and may serve as helper cells for antibody synthesis. It is not clear, however, whether the tissue damage is mediated by the few cytotoxic T cells that infiltrate the gland or by autoantibodies, several of which can be found in the serum. About 75% of patients have rheumatoid factor (p. 1351) irrespective of whether coexisting rheumatoid arthritis is present or not. ANAs are detected in 50 to 80% of patients, and a positive LE test is present in 25%. A whole host of antibodies have also been identified, including autoantibodies to salivary duct cells, smooth muscle mitochondria, gastric parietal cells, and thyroid antigens. Most important, however, are antibodies directed against ribonucleoprotein antigens, which have been designated SS-A(Ro) and SS-B (La) (Table 5–9, p. 195). The frequency of these autoantibodies varies widely, but it is generally accepted that with highly sensitive techniques both can be detected in up to 90% of the patients. Of the two antibodies, anti-SS-B is considered more specific for Sjögren's syndrome, because anti-SS-A antibodies are also detected in a fair number of patients with other diseases, particularly SLE. Furthermore, it appears that patients with Sjögren's syndrome who have high titers of antibodies to SS-A are more likely to have extraglandular manifestations, such as cutaneous vasculitis and central nervous system disease.[82] In Sjögren's syndrome associated with rheumatoid arthritis there is a high frequency of antibodies to yet another nuclear antigen, called rheumatoid-associated nuclear antigen (RANA). Both serologic and immunogenetic studies suggest that patients with secondary Sjögren's syndrome (associated most often with rheumatoid arthritis) make up a subset that is distinct from those with primary Sjögren's syndrome. The latter seem to show higher frequency of HLA-DR3, whereas patients with associated rheumatoid arthritis show a positive correlation with HLA-DR4. *To summarize, Sjögren's syndrome is associated with several autoantibodies, although the spectrum is not as broad as in SLE. Anti-SS-A and anti-SS-B are the two most common antibodies, hence they are considered to be important serologic markers of this disorder.*

As might be expected from the presence of autoantibodies, a variety of functional abnormalities have been detected in the T cells, B cells, and macrophages, many of which are similar to those described in SLE and need not be repeated (p. 196).[83] Although it seems logical to assume that autoimmunity is involved in the pathogenesis of Sjögren's syndrome, the triggering mechanisms are not clear. As in SLE, genetic predisposition, viruses, and deranged immunoregulation are believed to be involved, but their precise roles and interactions remain to be elucidated.[84]

MORPHOLOGY. As mentioned earlier, lacrimal and salivary glands are the major targets of the disease, although other exocrine glands, including those lining the respiratory and gastrointestinal tracts and the vagina, may also be involved.

The earliest histologic finding in both the major and minor salivary glands is **periductal lymphocytic infiltration.** The cells are predominantly small lymphocytes, but large lymphocytes and plasma cells may also be present, as may lymphoid follicles with germinal centers (Fig. 5–32). The ductal lining epithelial cells may show hyperplasia, thus obstructing the ducts. Later there is atrophy of the acini, fibrosis, and hyalinization, and still later in the course, atrophy and fatty replacement of parenchyma. In some cases the lymphoid infiltrate may be so intense as to give the appearance of a lymphoma; however, the benign appearance of the lymphocytes, the heterogeneous population of cells, and the preservation of lobular architecture of the gland differentiate the lesions from those of lymphoma.

The lack of tears leads to drying of the corneal epithelium, which becomes inflamed, eroded, and ulcerated; the oral mucosa may atrophy, with inflammatory fissuring and ulceration; and dryness and crusting of the nose may lead to ulcerations and even perforation of the nasal septum. When the respiratory passages are involved, secondary laryngitis, bronchitis, and pneumonitis may appear. Atrophic gastritis may also occur. In approximately 25% of cases, extraglandular tissues such as kidneys, lungs, skin, CNS, and muscles are also involved. **In contrast with SLE, glomerular lesions are extremely rare in Sjögren's syndrome.** However, defects of tubular function, including renal tubular acidosis, uricosuria, and phosphaturia, are often seen and are associated histologically with a **tubulointerstitial nephritis** (p. 1061). There is infiltration of the renal interstitium by monocytes, plasma cells, and macrophages and often a pronounced degree of fibrosis. Tubules are atrophied and may be invaded by lymphoid and plasma cells.

CLINICAL MANIFESTATIONS. Approximately 90% of the patients with Sjögren's syndrome are women between the ages of 40 and 60 years. As might be expected, symptoms result from inflammatory destruction of the exocrine glands. The keratoconjunctivitis produces symptoms of blurring of vision, burning and itching, and thick secretions accumulate in the conjunctival sac. The xerostomia results in difficulty in swallowing solid foods, a decrease in the ability to taste, cracks and fissures in the mouth, and dryness of

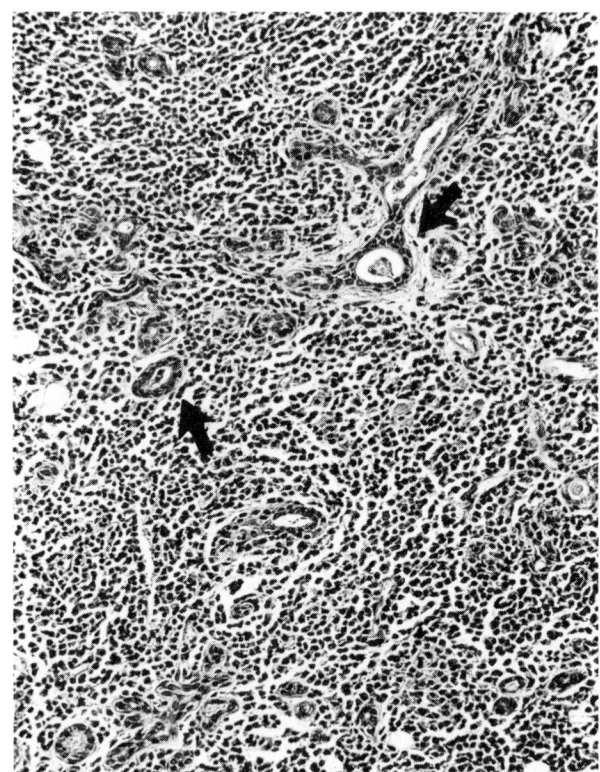

Figure 5–32. Sjögren's syndrome—submandibular gland. The intense lymphocytic and plasma cell infiltration virtually obscures the native architecture. Only a few residual ducts *(arrows)* can be identified.

the buccal mucosa. Parotid gland enlargement is present in half the patients; dryness of the nasal mucosa, epistaxis, recurrent bronchitis, and pneumonitis are other symptoms. The 60% of patients who have an accompanying autoimmune disorder such as rheumatoid arthritis also have the symptoms and signs of that disorder.

The combination of lacrimal and salivary gland inflammatory involvement was once called *Mikulicz's disease.* However, the name has now been replaced by *Mikulicz's syndrome,* broadened to include lacrimal and salivary gland enlargement of whatever cause. Sarcoidosis, leukemia, lymphoma, and other tumors likewise produce Mikulicz's syndrome. Thus, *biopsy of the lip (to examine minor salivary glands) is essential for the diagnosis of Sjögren's syndrome.*

The lymph nodes of patients with Sjögren's syndrome show not only enlargement but also a pleomorphic infiltrate of cells with frequent mitoses. The appearance has been described as "pseudolymphoma" because not all the criteria of malignant lymphoma are satisfied. However, clear-cut malignant lymphomas mostly of the B-cell type have developed in the salivary glands and lymph nodes in some patients, and it is believed that patients with Sjögren's syndrome have an approximately 40-fold higher risk of developing lymphoid malignancies. This has led to the statement that the disorder lies "somewhere between hyperplasia and neoplasia."

SCLERODERMA (PROGRESSIVE SYSTEMIC SCLEROSIS)

Although the term "scleroderma" is ingrained in the literature through common usage, this disease is better named progressive systemic sclerosis (PSS), as it is characterized by excessive fibrosis *throughout the body.* The skin is most commonly affected, but the gastrointestinal tract, kidneys, heart, muscles, and lungs also are frequently involved. In some patients the disease appears to remain confined to the skin for many years, but in the majority it progresses to visceral involvement and death from renal failure, cardiac failure, pulmonary insufficiency, or intestinal malabsorption. In recent years, the clinical heterogeneity of systemic sclerosis has been recognized by classifying the disease into two major categories:[85] (1) *diffuse scleroderma,* characterized by widespread skin involvement at onset, with rapid progression and early visceral involvement, and (2) *CREST syndrome* (an acronym for calcinosis, Raynaud's phenomenon, esophageal dysmotility, sclerodactyly, and telangiectasia), associated with relatively limited skin involvement often confined to fingers and face. Visceral involvement occurs late, hence the clinical course is relatively benign.

Several other variants and related conditions, such as eosinophilic fasciitis, are far less frequent and are not described here.[85]

ETIOLOGY AND PATHOGENESIS. Progressive systemic sclerosis is a disease of unknown cause. Three main lines of investigation have been pursued to explain the excessive deposition of collagen. One is concerned with the factors leading to altered collagen synthesis, another with possible immunologic derangements, and still another with microvascular abnormalities.[86]

Regardless of the initiating event, it is obvious that activation of fibroblasts must be a part of the final common pathway in the pathogenesis of this disease. Indeed, fibroblasts from patients with PSS when cultured in vitro synthesize twice as much collagen as normal fibroblasts, but the collagen itself is not abnormal. Thus, increased biosynthesis of normal collagen is established, but what triggers the fibroblasts to choke the tissues with collagen remains unknown.

Early skin lesions of PSS show infiltration of the dermis with T lymphocytes before fibrosis occurs, and some patients manifest T-cell sensitization to collagen.[87] Conceivably, a delayed hypersensitivity to collagen or some other connective tissue component might cause the release of cytokines such as TNF-α and IL-1, which can attract fibroblasts and promote collagen synthesis. The newly deposited collagen may well perpetuate a vicious circle of cytokine release and more collagen production. The presence of nonspecific serologic abnormalities, such as hypergammaglobulinemia (50% of cases), ANAs (70 to 90% of cases), and rheumatoid factor (25% of cases), points to a possible role for disordered humoral immunity as

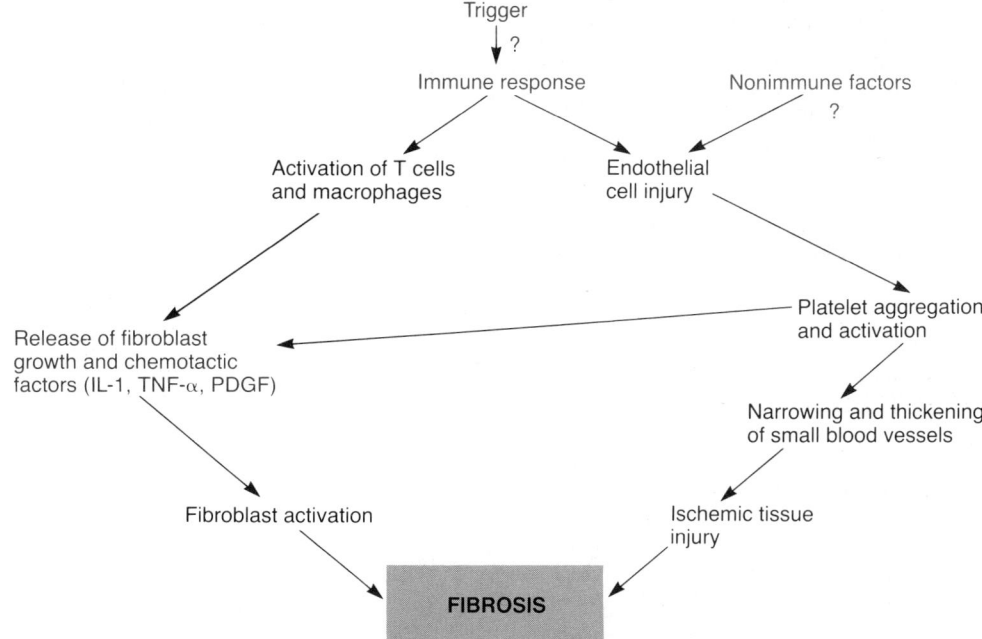

Figure 5–33. A schematic illustration of the possible mechanisms leading to progressive systemic sclerosis.

well. Recently two ANAs more or less limited to systemic sclerosis have been described. One of these, called Scl-70 (Table 5–9, p. 195), is present in up to 70% of patients with the diffuse variant of PSS,[57,88] whereas the other, an anticentromere antibody, is found in 80 to 90% of the patients with the CREST syndrome. It is of interest to note that the frequency of anticentromere antibody is quite low in diffuse scleroderma (Table 5–9). In addition to antibodies against nuclear targets, antibodies directed against collagen types I and IV and against laminin have also been found in the serum of some patients with PSS. Whether these represent primary sensitization against connective tissue components or result from tissue injury is not clear.

Finally, it has been suggested that PSS is a disease of the microvasculature[89] that results from recurrent injury to the endothelium. A serum factor cytotoxic to endothelial cells has been described in some but not all cases. It is also conceivable that vasculature is damaged by autoantibodies or antigen-antibody complexes. Telltale signs of endothelial injury (increased levels of factor VIII—von Willebrand's factor) and increased platelet activation (e.g., increased levels of circulating platelet aggregates) have been noted. According to this view, repeated cycles of endothelial injury followed by platelet aggregation lead to release of platelet factors that increase vascular permeability and stimulate fibroblasts. Thus, initially there is perivascular edema that is followed by periadventitial fibrosis and eventual ischemic injury caused by widespread narrowing of the microvasculature.

To summarize, PSS is associated with a variety of immunologic abnormalities, changes in the microvasculature, and excessive fibrosis. Although the antigens that trigger the (auto-) immune response have not been *identified, it seems reasonable to postulate that immunologic mechanisms lead to fibrosis either by elaboration of cytokines that activate fibroblasts or by inflicting damage on the small blood vessels (Fig. 5–33), or by both.*

MORPHOLOGY. Virtually all organs may be involved in PSS. The prominent changes occur in the skin, alimentary tract, musculoskeletal system, and kidney, but lesions also are often present in the blood vessels, heart, lungs, and peripheral nerves.

SKIN. A great majority of patients have diffuse, sclerotic atrophy of the skin, which usually begins in the fingers and distal regions of the upper extremities and extends proximally to involve the upper arms, shoulders, neck, and face. In the early stages, affected skin areas are somewhat edematous and have a doughy consistency. Histologically there is edema and perivascular lymphocytic infiltrates, together with swelling and degeneration of collagen fibers, which become eosinophilic. Capillaries and small arteries (150 to 500 μm in diameter) may show thickening of the basal lamina, endothelial cell damage, and partial occlusion. With progression, the edematous phase is replaced by progressive fibrosis of the dermis, which becomes tightly bound to the subcutaneous structures. There is marked increase of compact collagen in the dermis along with thinning of the epidermis, loss of rete pegs, atrophy of the dermal appendages, and hyaline thickening of the walls of dermal arterioles and capillaries (Fig. 5–34). Focal and sometimes diffuse subcutaneous calcifications may develop, especially in patients with the CREST syndrome. In advanced stages, the fingers take on a tapered, claw-like appearance with limitation of motion in the joints (Fig. 5–35), and the face becomes a drawn mask. Loss of blood

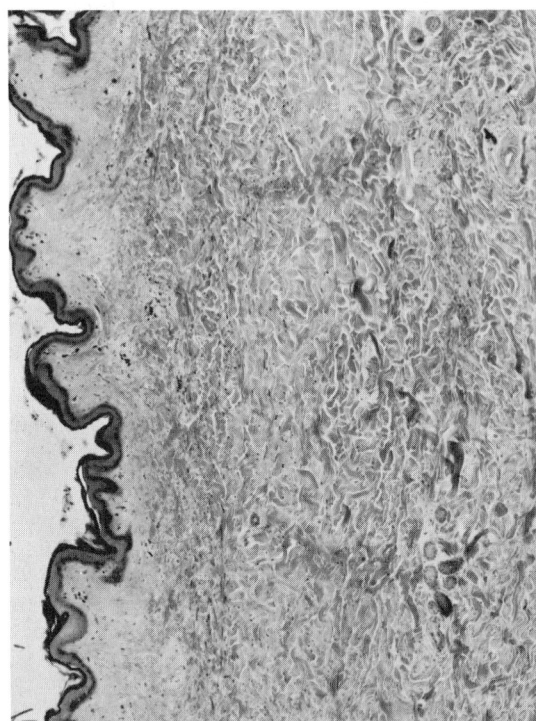

Figure 5–34. Systemic sclerosis. Atrophy of skin with dense sclerosis of dermal tissue and atrophy of skin adnexa.

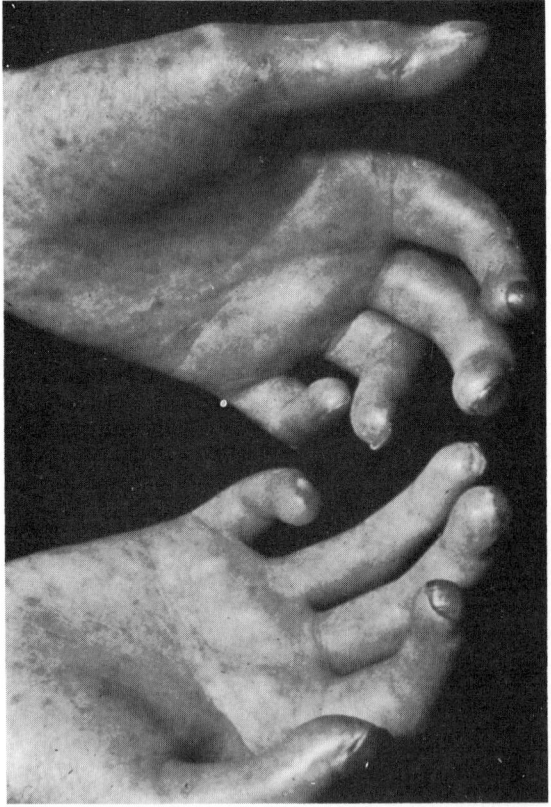

Figure 5–35. Advanced systemic sclerosis. The extensive subcutaneous fibrosis has virtually immobilized the fingers, creating a clawlike flexion deformity.

supply may lead to cutaneous ulcerations and to atrophic changes in the terminal phalanges. Sometimes the tips of the fingers undergo autoamputation.

ALIMENTARY TRACT. The alimentary tract is affected in over half the patients. Progressive atrophy and collagenous fibrous replacement of the muscularis may develop at any level of the gut but is most severe in the esophagus. The lower two thirds of the esophagus often develops a rubber-hose inflexibility. The mucosa may be thinned and ulcerated, and there is excessive collagenization of the lamina propria and submucosa. Milder changes occur in the walls of the small intestine and colon. Loss of villi and microvilli is the anatomic basis for the malabsorption syndrome sometimes encountered. Vessel walls contain perivascular mononuclear cell infiltrates and show hyaline collagenous thickening.

MUSCULOSKELETAL SYSTEM. Inflammatory synovitis is common in PSS. The changes consist of infiltrates of lymphocytes and plasma cells, sometimes gathered into focal aggregates, associated with hypertrophy and hyperplasia of the synovial soft tissues. Fibrosis later ensues. It is evident that these changes are closely reminiscent of rheumatoid arthritis, but joint destruction is not common in PSS. As in polymyositis (p. 208), the muscles may be affected, beginning usually with the proximal groups. Interfiber edema and perivascular infiltrates of lymphocytes and plasma cells make up the early changes, followed by progressive interstitial fibrosis and sometimes regressive alterations in the fibers themselves. However, in systemic sclerosis, the primary change involves the interstitium, whereas in polymyositis, fiber damage is a prominent early lesion. Thickening of the basement membrane of the microcirculation and microvascular sclerosis accompany the interstitial fibrosis.

KIDNEYS. Renal abnormalities occur in two thirds of patients with PSS.[90] The most prominent are those in the vessel walls. Interlobular arteries (150 to 500 μm in diameter) show intimal thickening as a result of deposition of mucinous or finely collagenous material, which stains histochemically for glycoprotein and acid mucopolysaccharides (Fig. 5–36). There is also concentric proliferation of intimal cells. These changes may resemble those seen in malignant hypertension, but it has been stressed that in scleroderma the alterations are restricted to vessels 150 to 500 μm in diameter and are not always associated with hypertension. Hypertension, however, occurs in 30% of patients with scleroderma, and in 7 to 10% it takes an ominously malignant course (malignant hypertension). In hypertensive patients, vascular alterations are more pronounced and are often associated with fibrinoid necrosis involving the arterioles together with thrombosis and infarction. When this occurs it becomes difficult to differentiate the lesions of scleroderma from those of other types of malignant hypertension (p. 1066). Such patients often die of renal failure, which accounts for about 50% of deaths in patients with PSS. Glomerular changes are nonspecific and consist mainly of slightly increased cellularity of the mesangium and

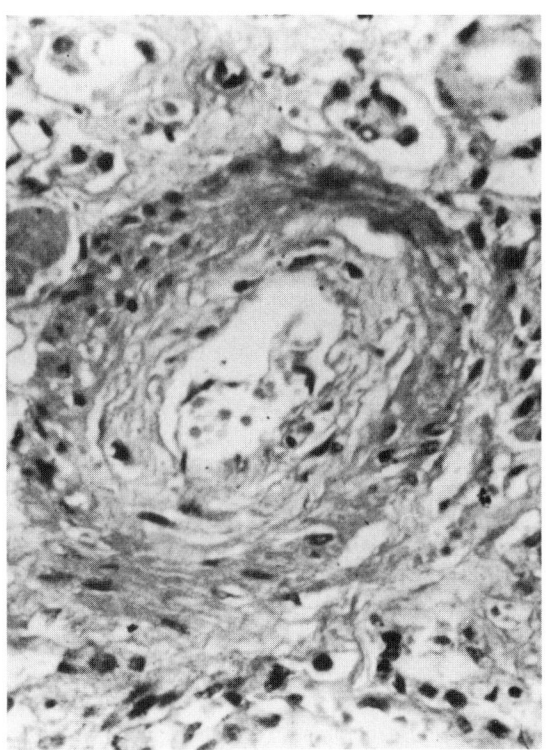

Figure 5–36. Systemic sclerosis. Small renal artery showing intimal thickening.

localized irregular thickening of the basement membrane. Some of these changes may be related to the hypertension.

LUNGS. A diffuse interstitial and alveolar fibrosis may appear in the lungs, with variable fibrous thickening of small pulmonary vessels.[91] In some instances the alveolar walls thicken, and in others there is an apparent distention of alveolar spaces and rupture of septa, leading to cystlike cavities. In later stages, honeycomb changes and severe interstitial fibrosis may ensue. Thus, patients with PSS have a pulmonary picture very much like that of idiopathic pulmonary fibrosis (p. 791), and indeed PSS must be considered in the differential diagnosis of diffuse pulmonary interstitial disease.

OTHER ORGANS. Small arterial lesions similar to those seen in the kidneys are present in many organs, including the skin, muscle, gastrointestinal tract, pancreas, synovium, vasa vasorum, and CNS. In the heart, interstitial fibrosis with perivascular infiltrates can occur; the fibrosis may involve the conduction system, leading to atrioventricular conduction defects and arrhythmias, or it may result in progressive cardiac failure. Sometimes a peripheral neuropathy occurs owing to loss of blood supply to the axis cylinders, resulting from perineural and vascular sclerosis.

CLINICAL COURSE. PSS is primarily a disease of women (female-to-male ratio, 3 : 1) with a mean age of onset around 40 years. In most cases, the disease presents with symmetric edema and thickening of the hands and fingers or with Raynaud's phenomenon (p. 579). Often Raynaud's phenomenon manifested as episodic vasoconstriction of the arteries and arterioles of the extremities precedes all other symptoms. Articular manifestations in the form of pain and stiffness of the finger and knee joints may mimic rheumatoid arthritis. Dysphagia attributable to esophageal fibrosis and its resultant hypomotility is present in more than 50% of patients. Eventually, destruction of the esophageal wall leads to atony and dilatation, especially at its lower end. Abdominal pain, intestinal obstruction, or malabsorption syndrome with weight loss and anemia reflect involvement of the small intestine. Respiratory difficulties due to the pulmonary fibrosis may result in right-sided cardiac dysfunction, and myocardial fibrosis may cause either arrhythmias or cardiac failure. Mild proteinuria occurs in up to 70% of patients, but rarely is the proteinuria so severe as to cause a nephrotic syndrome. The most ominous manifestation is malignant hypertension, with the subsequent development of fatal renal failure, but in its absence progression of the disease may be slow. The disease tends to be more severe in blacks, especially black women.

As mentioned earlier, the so-called CREST syndrome is characterized by calcinosis (C), Raynaud's phenomenon (R), esophageal dysfunction (E), sclerodactyly (S), telangiectasia (T), and the presence of anticentromere antibodies. Patients with the CREST syndrome have relatively limited involvement of skin, often confined to fingers and face, and calcification of the subcutaneous tissues. Raynaud's phenomenon and involvement of skin are the initial manifestations and often the only manifestations for several years. Involvement of the viscera, including esophageal lesions, pulmonary hypertension, and biliary cirrhosis, occurs late, and in general the patients live longer than those with PSS with its diffuse visceral involvement at the outset.

Localized scleroderma, to be distinguished from PSS, is characterized by skin manifestations only. *Morphea* (one of the localized forms) refers to the presence of localized patches of violaceous or lilac, sometimes itchy skin lesions that may appear on any part of the body. Morphea may be widespread and chronic and may involve the fingers with contractures. Because the localized forms do not involve the internal organs, it is unlikely that they have any relationship to PSS.

POLYMYOSITIS-DERMATOMYOSITIS

Polymyositis refers to a chronic inflammatory myopathy of uncertain cause.[92] Clinically it is characterized by symmetric muscle weakness, often accompanied by a skin rash (dermatomyositis). Although a rare disease, it is one of the more frequent myopathies. The disease is most common in the 40- to 60-year-old age group, but a variant affecting children between the ages of 5 and 15 years is also recognized. Overall, females are affected about twice as often as males. The clinical expressions of polymyositis are extremely varied and so have been subclassified as follows:

• Group I: Adult polymyositis (without skin involvement)
• Group II: Adult dermatomyositis
• Group III: Polymyositis or dermatomyositis with malignancy
• Group IV: Childhood dermatomyositis
• Group V: Polymyositis or dermatomyositis associated with other immunologic disorders such as SLE, systemic sclerosis, or Sjögren's syndrome.

The detailed description of these groups is beyond the scope of this book and may be found in recent reviews.[92,93]

ETIOLOGY AND PATHOGENESIS. Although the cause of the disease is unknown, its close association with other diseases of presumed autoimmune causation points to an immunologic origin. Several patients have ANAs (p. 195), but the specificities of the ANAs detected in this disease have not been fully defined. *Recent studies suggest that patients with polymyositis have a predilection to form antibodies against transfer RNA (tRNA) synthetases.*[57] The best characterized among these antibodies is directed against histidyl tRNA synthetase, the so called Jo-1 antigen. This antibody is found in 25% of adults with myositis (group I) and is considered highly specific for this condition. Quite interestingly, virtually all patients who have the Jo-1 antibody develop interstitial lung disease, and they also demonstrate a significant association with HLA-DR3. Thus, *it seems that the presence of Jo-1 antibody defines a subset of patients with a somewhat distinct serologic, genetic, and clinical profile.*

Whether anti-Jo-1 or any other antibodies play a role in the pathogenesis of these disorders is unknown, except possibly in childhood dermatomyositis (group IV). In these patients there is widespread vasculitis involving the skin and gastrointestinal tract. Deposits of IgG, IgM, and complement can be identified in the blood vessels, suggesting immune complex–mediated tissue injury. The nature of the inciting antigen remains unknown.

There is increasing suspicion that muscle injury is mediated by sensitized T cells. This view is supported by the demonstration of activated CD4+ and CD8+ lymphocytes within the inflamed muscle. Some of these lymphocytes seem to be specifically sensitized to muscle antigens, as they proliferate and release cytotoxic lymphokines when cultured with skeletal muscle homogenates. What initiates autosensitization is as obscure as in other autoimmune diseases. As usual, microbial agents are the prime suspects, especially viruses of the Coxsackie B group. These viruses have been isolated from a few cases with polymyositis, and serologic findings suggest that the occurrence of polymyositis in children (group IV) may well be linked to previous infection with Coxsackie virus.[94]

Further support for a viral association comes from the observed similarities between the amino acid sequence of some viral proteins and histidyl tRNA synthetase, the antigenic protein for the Jo-1 antibody. Thus molecular mimicry (p. 172) may be in play.[95]

MORPHOLOGY

STRIATED MUSCLE. Symmetric involvement of striated muscles is present in all cases of polymyositis and dermatomyositis. The first groups to be affected are almost always the proximal muscles of the lower and upper extremities (i.e., muscles of the pelvic and shoulder girdles). Thereafter, muscles of the neck and posterior pharynx, intercostals, and diaphragm may be affected. Although in severe cases the involvement may be more generalized, in contrast to myasthenia gravis, ocular muscles are almost always spared, and distal muscle involvement is seen in only 20 to 25% of patients.

At the onset, the muscles are normal in gross appearance, possibly slightly enlarged owing to diffuse edema. With advance of the disease, they become atrophic and yellowish-gray as the muscle fibers are replaced by fibrous tissue and fat. Histologically, there is focal or extensive muscle fiber death manifested by vacuolation and fragmentation of the sarcoplasm. Usually readily evident is invasion of necrotic fibers by scavenger phagocytic cells engulfing the cellular debris. A prominent mononuclear interstitial inflammatory infiltrate is apparent. Immunocytochemical studies reveal that most of the infiltrating lymphocytes are T lymphocytes that also bear class II antigens and IL-2 receptors, indicating that they are activated. Regeneration of injured but surviving muscle cells may become apparent in the later stages, producing large vesicular sarcolemmal nuclei accompanied by sarcoplasmic basophilia (Fig. 5–37).

SKIN. The skin rash seen in approximately 50% of patients may be quite variable, or it may be virtually diagnostic. **The classic rash takes the form of a lilac or heliotrope discoloration of the upper eyelids,** with periorbital edema, accompanied by a scaling erythematous eruption or dusky red patches over the knuckles, elbows, knees, medial malleoli, forehead, face, neck and upper chest, and back. Histologically, dermal edema is seen in the early stages, with mononuclear infiltrates surrounding the dermal vessels. The changes are followed in the later stages by fibrosis and sometimes calcification.

OTHER SYSTEMS. In children, and in some acute involvements in adults, widespread necrotizing vasculitis may be present, involving the lungs, kidneys, heart, and other organs. This vasculitis is reminiscent of that encountered in polyarteritis. These acute lesions may lead to vascular fibrosis. Transitory arthritis may appear during the acute phases of the disease, but chronic synovitis is rare. Diffuse interstitial fibrosis of the lung is frequently present in patients who have anti-Jo-1 antibodies.

CLINICAL FEATURES. Although polymyositis-dermatomyositis is a multisystem disorder, muscle weakness and eventual motor disability are the most im-

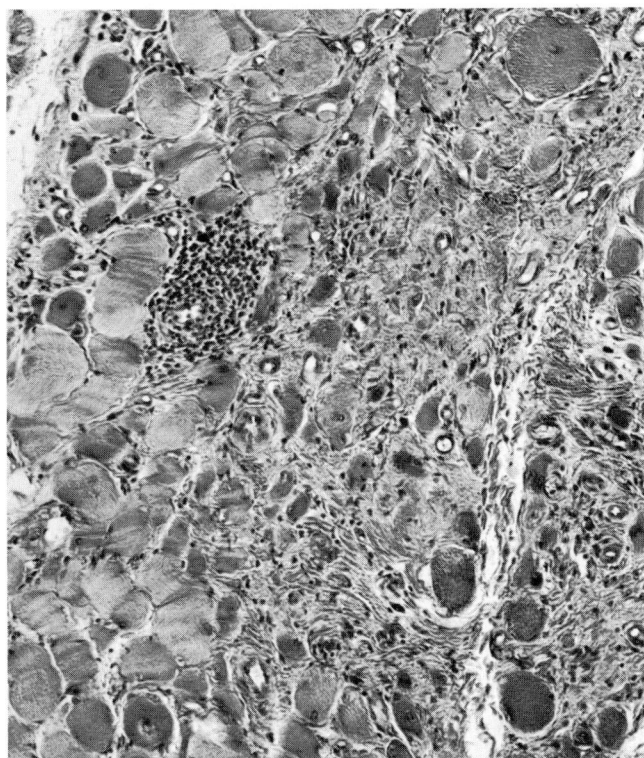

Figure 5–37. A section of striated muscle with interstitial fibrosis, leukocytic infiltration, muscle cell atrophy, and variability in muscle fiber size due to regenerative activity.

portant clinical findings. The proximal nature of the muscular involvement helps to differentiate this disease from some of the dystrophies (p. 1368). In chronic cases, the patients may be confined to a wheelchair or bed. In patients with dermatomyositis, the skin rash may or may not be distinctive. Involvement of skin may be followed by sufficient dermal fibrosis and skin atrophy to cause stiffness of the fingers. Raynaud's phenomenon occurs in about one third of the patients. The involvement of joints is usually mild and rarely causes joint destruction. Dysphagia, due to involvement of the pharyngeal muscles, can be a disabling and serious clinical problem. Patients with diffuse interstitial pulmonary fibrosis develop significant pulmonary impairment (p. 789).

The association of malignancy with polymyositis-dermatomyositis in adults was mentioned earlier, but the exact frequency of tumors and the pathogenetic basis of the increased tumor risk remain uncertain.[96] For our present discussion it is sufficient to note that (1) there is a general agreement that a higher than normal frequency of visceral cancers is seen in patients with polymyositis-dermatomyositis; (2) males and females are affected equally, but adults with dermatomyositis seem to be at greater risk than those with myositis alone; (3) visceral cancers (involving mainly breast, ovary, lungs, and stomach) are present in 15 to 20% of the cases; and (4) in patients who have cancer, the other manifestations of the disease are indistinguishable from those occurring in patients without malignancy.

The diagnosis of polymyositis-dermatomyositis is made by excluding other well-defined diseases of muscles, such as myasthenia gravis, and by the following criteria: (1) proximal muscle weakness, (2) elevations of muscle-derived enzymes in the serum (creatine kinase, aldolase, transaminases, and lactic dehydrogenase), (3) characteristic changes on electromyography, (4) abnormal biopsy findings that are consistent with myositis, and (5) the presence of cutaneous lesions compatible with dermatomyositis.

It is difficult to provide a prognosis for a disease as heterogeneous as polymyositis-dermatomyositis. With immunosuppressive therapy the overall five-year survival is about 75%. Children have a better prognosis than adults.

MIXED CONNECTIVE TISSUE DISEASE (MCTD)

This term was coined in 1972 to describe the disease seen in a group of patients who were identified clinically by the coexistence of features suggestive of SLE, polymyositis, and scleroderma, and serologically by high titers of antibodies to nuclear ribonucleoprotein. Two other factors have been considered important in lending distinctiveness to MCTD—the paucity of renal disease and an extremely good response to corticosteroids, both of which could be considered as indicative of a good long-term prognosis.

MCTD may present with arthritis, swelling of the hands, Raynaud's phenomenon, abnormal esophageal motility, myositis, leukopenia and anemia, fever, lymphadenopathy, and hypergammaglobulinemia. These manifestations suggest SLE, polymyositis, and scleroderma. Approximately 80% of the patients are female, presenting between the ages of 30 and 60 years. Although serologic overlap with SLE occurs, the unifying feature of MCTD is the speckled pattern of nuclei on immunofluorescence (p. 195) and the presence of antibodies against ribonucleoproteins in extremely high titers. Over the last 15 years, as more patients with clinical and serologic features consistent with the diagnosis of MCTD have been identified, a controversy has developed over whether MCTD constitutes a distinct disease or is a heterogeneous mixture of subsets of SLE, scleroderma, and polymyositis.[97] According to this view, because overlapping of clinical features is not uncommon among autoimmune diseases, MCTD cannot be considered a distinct clinicopathologic entity; furthermore, many patients with an initial diagnosis of MCTD develop features most consistent with systemic sclerosis.

However, others[57] who continue to support the notion of MCTD as a distinct disorder argue that, whereas the presence of anti-RNP antibody by itself is not diagnostic, the absence of antibodies to native DNA and Sm antigen (which characterize SLE) is important in defining MCTD. Furthermore, the frequency of severe nephritis, arthritis, or severe CNS involvement is distinctly less than that in classic SLE. We can leave the resolution of this semantic issue to experts, but take note that although in general the various "rheumatic diseases" present with distinctive clinical and serologic features, several patients manifest overlapping features that defy simple categorization.

POLYARTERITIS NODOSA (PN) AND OTHER VASCULITIDES

Polyarteritis nodosa belongs to a group of diseases characterized by necrotizing inflammation of the walls of blood vessels and showing strong evidence of an immunologic pathogenetic mechanism. The general term *noninfectious necrotizing vasculitis* differentiates these conditions from those due to direct infection of the blood vessel wall (such as occurs in the wall of an abscess) and serves to emphasize that any type of vessel may be involved—arteries, arterioles, veins, or capillaries.

Noninfectious necrotizing vasculitis is encountered in many clinical settings. Many classifications are available, and these depend on the size of the involved blood vessels, the anatomic site, the histologic character of the lesion, or the clinical manifestations.[98] A detailed classification and description of vasculitides is presented in the chapter on the diseases of blood vessels, in which the immunologic mechanisms are also discussed (p. 570).

POSSIBLE IMMUNE DISORDERS

Immunologic mechanisms are suspected of contributing to a large number of diseases in addition to those already described in this chapter. Some of the entities are discussed in the chapters dealing with individual organs and systems. One disease—amyloidosis—requires description at this point. New observations provide strong evidence that in most patients some derangement in the immune apparatus underlies this disease, and as a systemic disease it cannot be assigned to any single organ or system.

AMYLOIDOSIS

Amyloid is a pathologic proteinaceous substance, deposited between cells in various tissues and organs of the body in a wide variety of clinical settings. Because amyloid deposition appears so insidiously and sometimes mysteriously, its clinical recognition ultimately depends on morphologic identification of this distinctive substance in appropriate biopsy specimens. Macroscopically, painting the cut surface of affected organs with an iodine solution imparts a yellow-red color to sufficiently large deposits of amyloid that is transformed into blue or violet after the application of dilute sulfuric acid. This technique was first employed over a century ago by Virchow, who interpreted the results to be starchlike, hence the designation "amyloid." *With the light microscope and standard tissue stains, amyloid appears as an amorphous, eosinophilic, hyaline, extracellular substance that, with progressive accumulation, encroaches on and produces pressure atrophy of adjacent cells.* To differentiate amyloid from other hyaline deposits (e.g., collagen, fibrin) a variety of histochemical techniques (p. 216) are employed. Perhaps most widely used is the Congo red stain, which under ordinary light imparts a pink or red color to tissue deposits, but far more dramatic and specific is the green birefringence of the stained amyloid when observed by polarizing microscopy (Fig. 5–38).

The clinical circumstances under which amyloidosis appears, and the distribution of the deposits throughout the body, are extremely varied. In the past the term *primary amyloidosis* was used to describe amyloid deposition in patients who did not have any detectable underlying disease, whereas patients with some chronic inflammatory disease were classified as having *secondary amyloidosis*. More recently, attention has been directed to the chemical composition and origins of amyloid as possible bases for classification. Despite the fact that all deposits have a uniform appearance and tinctorial characteristics, *it is quite clear that amyloid is not a chemically distinct entity.* There are two major and several minor biochemical forms. These are deposited by several different pathogenetic mechanisms, and therefore *amyloidosis should not be considered a single disease; rather, it is a group of diseases sharing in common the deposition of similar-appearing proteins.*[99] At the heart of the morphologic uniformity is the remarkably uniform physical organization of amyloid protein, which we consider first. This is followed by a discussion of the chemical nature of amyloid.

PHYSICAL NATURE OF AMYLOID. Although amyloid has a bland, uninteresting appearance with the light microscope, high resolution has disclosed a remarkably complex substructure. *The amorphous deposits are in fact largely made up of nonbranching fibrils of indefinite length and a diameter of approximately 7.5 to 10 nm* (Fig. 5–39). This electron microscopic structure is identical in all types of amyloidosis. The fibrils may appear singly, in laterally aggregated bundles, or in an interlocking meshwork. In addition to these nonbranching slender fibrils, a minor second component is always present in amyloid, known as the P component. With the electron microscope it appears as a pentagonal, doughnut-shaped structure having an external diameter of approximately 9 nm and an internal diameter of 4 nm. Each pentagon is composed in turn of five globular subunits.

It now appears to be well established that *the major factor responsible for the optical features by which amyloid deposits are classically identified in histologic section is the physicochemical aggregation of amyloid fibrils, yielding a "cross-β" pleated sheet on*

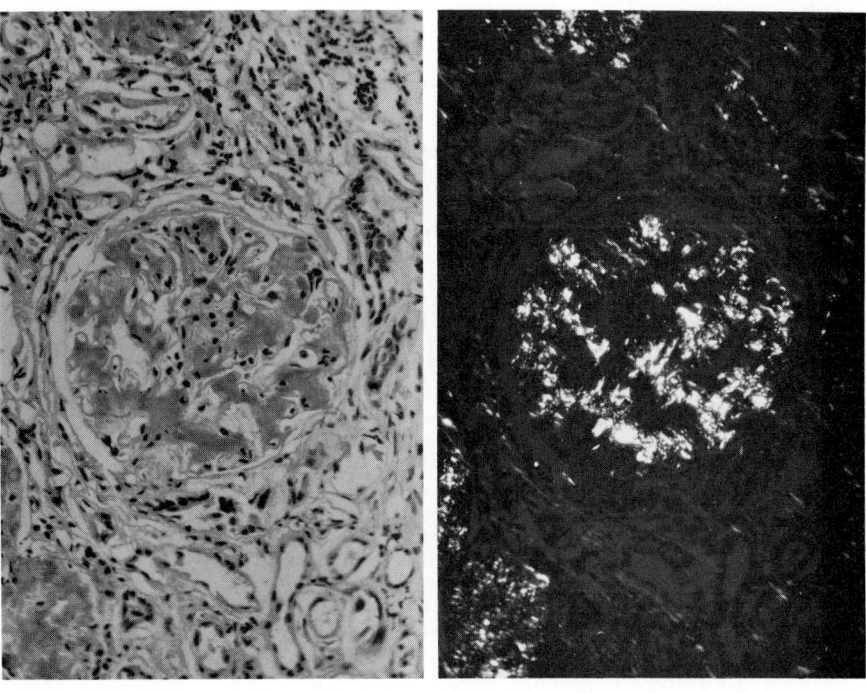

Figure 5–38. *A,* Amyloidosis of the glomerulus. *B,* Note birefringence of the deposits after Congo red staining. (From Cohen, A.S.: The constitution and genesis of amyloid. Int. Rev. Exp. Pathol. *4*:172, 1965.)

A   B

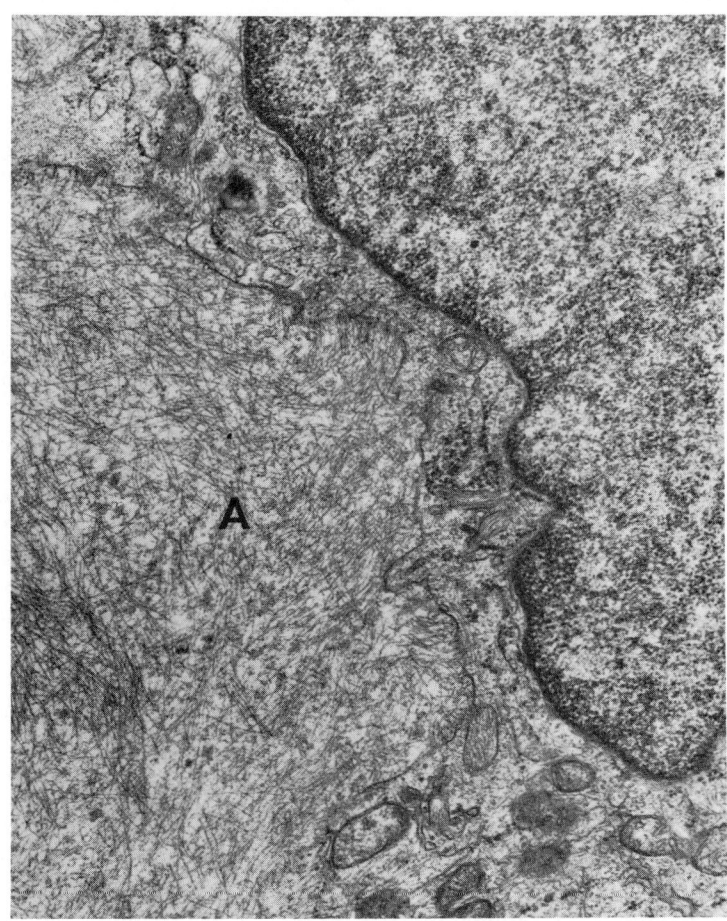

Figure 5–39. Amyloidosis of the spleen under the electron microscope. The amyloid deposit *(A)* adjacent to a reticular cell contains a feltwork of delicate fibrils (×22,500). (From Cohen, A.S.: The constitution and genesis of amyloid. Int. Rev. Exp. Pathol. *4*:178, 1965.)

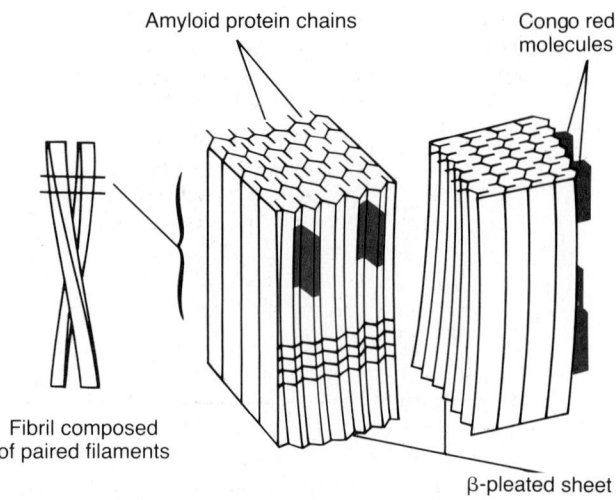

Amyloid protein chains

Congo red molecules

Fibril composed of paired filaments

β-pleated sheet

Figure 5–40. Structure of an amyloid fibril, depicting the β-pleated sheet structure and binding sites for the Congo red dye, which is used for diagnosis of amyloidosis. (After Glenner, G.G.: Amyloid deposit and amyloidosis. The β-fibrilloses. N. Engl. J. Med. 52:148, 1980, by permission of The New England Journal of Medicine.)

x-ray crystallographic analysis[100] (Fig. 5–40). Stated in another way, any fibrillar protein deposition that yields a β-pleated sheet will give rise to what is recognized as amyloid. This physicochemical aggregation gives to amyloid its polariscopic characteristics. The increased intensity of the birefringence of Congo red–stained amyloid is related to the high order of regularity and parallelism of the dye molecules bound to the aggregated fibrils.

CHEMICAL NATURE OF AMYLOID. Major advances in our understanding of amyloidosis have emerged from elucidation of the chemical structure of amyloid. Approximately 90% of the amyloid material consists of fibril proteins, the remaining 10% being the P component, which is a glycoprotein.[100] *Two chemically distinct major classes of amyloid fibril proteins have been identified; one, called AL (amyloid light chain) is derived from plasma cells (immunocytes) and contains immunoglobulin light chains; the other, designated AA (amyloid-associated), is a unique nonimmunoglobulin protein synthesized by the liver.*

These two amyloid proteins are deposited in distinct clinicopathologic settings. The AL protein is made up of complete immunoglobulin light chains, the NH_2-terminal fragments of light chains, or both. Most of the AL proteins analyzed are composed of λ light chains (particularly λ VI type) or their fragments, but in some cases κ chains have been identified. As might be expected, the amyloid fibril protein of the AL type is produced by immunoglobulin-secreting cells, and their deposition is associated with some form of B-cell dyscrasia. The archetype is multiple myeloma, a tumor of plasma cells that may be associated with the deposition of amyloid of the AL type. In multiple myeloma it can be demonstrated that the amyloid fibril protein is derived from the circulating light chains (i.e., Bence Jones protein, p. 739). In fact,

Glenner has been able to create a fibrillar precipitate that has the typical ultrastructure of amyloid fibrils by proteolytic digestion of λ Bence Jones proteins in vitro.[100]

The second major class of amyloid fibril protein (AA) does not have structural homology to immunoglobulins or any known protein. It has a molecular weight of 8500 and consists of 76 amino acid residues. The AA protein is found in those clinical settings described later as "secondary amyloidosis." AA fibrils are derived from a larger (12,000 daltons) precursor in the serum called SAA (serum amyloid–associated) protein that is synthesized in the liver and circulates in association with the HDL3 subclass of lipoproteins.

Several other biochemically distinct proteins have been found in amyloid deposits[101] in a variety of clinical settings:

• *Transthyretin* is a normal serum protein that binds and transports thyroxine and retinol, hence the name *trans-thy-retin*. It was previously called prealbumin, because it precedes serum albumin on serum electrophoresis. Because it has no relationship to serum albumin, however, the term prealbumin is misleading. *A mutant form of transthyretin (and its fragments) is deposited in a group of genetically determined disorders referred to as familial amyloid polyneuropathies.* In each of these conditions the transthyretin deposited in the tissues differs from its normal counterpart by a single amino acid, involving most commonly the substitution of methionine for valine at position 30.[102] Another variant form of transthyretin is deposited in *amyloidosis associated with aging.*[101]

• *β_2-Microglobulin*, a component of the MHC class I molecules (p. 170) and a normal serum protein, has recently been identified as the amyloid fibril subunit in the amyloidosis that complicates the course of patients on *long-term hemodialysis.*

• *β_2-Amyloid protein*, a 4000-dalton peptide (also called A_4) constitutes the core of cerebral plaques found in Alzheimer's disease, as well as the amyloid deposited in walls of cerebral blood vessels in patients with Alzheimer's disease. The A_4 protein is believed to be derived from a much larger 79,000 dalton precursor that has the characteristics of a transmembrane glycoprotein.[103]

• In addition to the foregoing, amyloid deposits derived from diverse precursors such as hormones (procalcitonin, proinsulin) and keratin have also been reported.

The P component is distinct from the amyloid fibrils but is closely associated with them in all forms of amyloidosis. It constitutes approximately 10% of the amyloid substance and has been found to be identical to a normal α_1-serum glycoprotein. It has a molecular weight of 180,000 to 220,000 daltons and a striking structural homology with C-reactive protein, which is an acute-phase reactant. In addition to the amyloid fibril proteins and the P component, some investigators have reported the presence of sulfated glycosaminoglycans in several forms of amyloid deposits.[104]

CLASSIFICATION OF AMYLOIDOSIS.

Amyloidosis has been classified in a variety of ways, none of which is quite satisfactory. This is not entirely surprising, because amyloidosis as defined by morphologic criteria appears to be a single disease, yet chemical analyses reveal that amyloid is quite heterogeneous. The clinical classification of amyloidosis is based on tissue distribution and the presence or absence of a readily identifiable predisposing condition. Thus, amyloid may be *systemic* (generalized), involving several organ systems, or *localized*, when deposits are limited to a single organ, such as the heart.

SYSTEMIC AMYLOIDOSIS.

The systemic, or generalized, pattern is subclassified into *primary amyloidosis* when associated with some immunocyte dyscrasia or *secondary amyloidosis* when it occurs as a complication of an underlying chronic inflammatory or tissue destructive process. *Hereditary* or familial amyloidosis constitutes a separate albeit heterogeneous group, with several distinctive patterns of organ involvement. In contrast to the clinical classification, the chemical classification is based entirely on the chemical nature of the amyloid fibril and its precursor protein. In the classification presented here (Table 5–11) we have attempted to take into account clinical settings, anatomic distribution, and chemical composition of amyloid.

IMMUNOCYTE DYSCRASIAS WITH AMYLOIDOSIS.

Amyloidosis in this category is usually systemic in distribution and is of the AL type. In the United States this is the most common form of amyloidosis.[105] In many of these cases, the patients have some form of plasma cell dyscrasia. Best defined is the occurrence of systemic amyloidosis in 5 to 15% of patients with multiple myeloma, a form of plasma cell neoplasia characterized by multiple osteolytic lesions throughout the skeletal system (p. 740). The cancerous plasma cells in multiple myeloma characteristically synthesize abnormal amounts of a single specific immunoglobulin (monoclonal gammopathy), producing an M (myeloma) protein spike on serum electrophoresis. In addition to the synthesis of whole immunoglobulin molecules, only the light chains (referred to as Bence Jones protein) of either the κ or the λ variety may be elaborated and found in the serum. By virtue of the small molecular size of the Bence Jones protein, it is frequently excreted in the urine. Almost all the patients with myeloma who develop amyloidosis have Bence Jones proteins in the serum or urine, or both, but it should be remembered that a great majority of myeloma patients who have free light chains do not develop amyloidosis. Clearly, therefore, *the presence of Bence Jones proteins, although necessary, is by itself not enough to produce amyloidosis.* We shall discuss later the other factors such as the type of light chain produced ("amyloidogenic potential") and the subsequent handling (degradation?) that may have a bearing on whether Bence Jones proteins will be deposited as amyloid (p. 215). Amyloidosis may also be encountered in a variety of other B-cell neoplasms that are much less common. These include Waldenström's macroglobulinemia, heavy-chain disease, solitary plasmacytomas, and nodular malignant lymphoma.[100] All these conditions are examples of a monoclonal gammopathy.

Table 5–11. Classification of Amyloidosis

CLINICOPATHOLOGIC CATEGORY	ASSOCIATED DISEASES	MAJOR FIBRIL PROTEIN	CHEMICALLY RELATED PRECURSOR PROTEIN
Systemic (Generalized) Amyloidosis			
Immunocyte dyscrasias with amyloidosis (primary amyloidosis)	Multiple myeloma and other monoclonal B-cell proliferations	AL	Immunoglobulin light chains, chiefly λ type
Reactive systemic amyloidosis (secondary amyloidosis)	Chronic inflammatory conditions	AA	SAA
Hemodialysis-associated amyloidosis	Chronic renal failure	β_2-microglobulin	β_2-microglobulin
Hereditary amyloidosis			
(1) Familial Mediterranean fever	—	AA	SAA
(2) Familial amyloidotic neuropathies (several types)	—	Transthyretin*	Transthyretin
Localized Amyloidosis			
Senile cardiac	—	Transthyretin	Transthyretin
Senile cerebral	Alzheimer's disease	A4 (β-protein)	?
Endocrine, e.g., medullary carcinoma of thyroid	—	Procalcitonin	Calcitonin

* Transthyretin is also known as prealbumin. The transthyretins deposited as amyloid are mutant forms of normal transthyretin.

AL = amyloid light chain; AA = amyloid associated (protein); SAA = serum amyloid associated (protein).

The great majority of patients with AL amyloid do not have classic multiple myeloma or any other overt B-cell neoplasm; such cases have been traditionally classified as primary amyloidosis because their clinical features derive from the effects of amyloid deposition without any other associated disease. However, in virtually all such cases, monoclonal immunoglobulins or free light chains, or both, can be found in the serum or urine.[105] Most of these patients also have a modest increase in the number of plasma cells in the bone marrow, which presumably secrete the precursors of AL protein. Clearly, these patients have an underlying B-cell dyscrasia ("covert myeloma") in which production of an abnormal protein, rather than production of tumor masses, is the predominant manifestation. Whether the condition of most of these patients would evolve into multiple myeloma if they lived long enough can only be a matter for speculation.

REACTIVE SYSTEMIC AMYLOIDOSIS. The amyloid deposits in this pattern are systemic in distribution and are composed of AA protein. This category is commonly referred to as secondary amyloidosis because it is secondary to the associated inflammatory condition. The feature common to most of the conditions associated with reactive systemic amyloidosis is protracted breakdown of cells resulting from a wide variety of infectious and noninfectious chronic inflammatory conditions. At one time tuberculosis, bronchiectasis, and chronic osteomyelitis were the most important underlying conditions, but with the advent of effective antimicrobial chemotherapy the importance of these conditions has diminished. More commonly now, reactive systemic amyloidosis complicates rheumatoid arthritis, other connective tissue disorders such as dermatomyositis and scleroderma, and inflammatory bowel disease, particularly regional enteritis and ulcerative colitis. Among these, the most frequent associated condition is rheumatoid arthritis. Amyloidosis is reported to occur in 14 to 26% of patients with rheumatoid arthritis. These figures, obtained from autopsy studies, may be somewhat higher than the true frequency of amyloidosis in an unselected group of rheumatoid arthritis patients. Recent studies indicate that heroin abusers who inject the drug subcutaneously have a very high occurrence rate of generalized AA amyloidosis.[106] The chronic skin infections associated with "skin-popping" of narcotics seem to be responsible for amyloidosis in this group of patients.

Reactive systemic amyloidosis may also occur in association with nonimmunocyte-derived tumors, the two most common being renal cell carcinoma and Hodgkin's disease.

HEMODIALYSIS-ASSOCIATED AMYLOIDOSIS. Patients on long-term hemodialysis for renal failure develop amyloidosis due to deposition of β_2-microglobulin. This protein is present in high concentrations in the serum of patients with renal disease and is retained in circulation because it cannot be filtered through the usual dialysis membranes. In some series as many as 70% of the patients on long-term dialysis developed amyloid deposits in the synovium, joints, and tendon sheaths.[107]

HEREDOFAMILIAL AMYLOIDOSIS. A variety of familial forms of amyloidosis have been described. Most of them are rare and occur in limited geographic areas. The most common and best studied is an autosomal recessive condition called *familial Mediterranean fever*. This is a febrile disorder of unknown cause characterized by attacks of fever accompanied by inflammation of serosal surfaces, including peritoneum, pleura, and synovial membrane. This disorder is encountered largely in individuals of Armenian, Sephardic Jewish, and Arabic origins. It is associated with widespread tissue involvement indistinguishable from reactive systemic amyloidosis. The amyloid fibril proteins are identical to AA proteins, suggesting that this form of amyloidosis is related to the recurrent bouts of inflammation that characterize this disease.

In contrast to familial Mediterranean fever, a group of autosomal dominant familial disorders is characterized by deposition of amyloid predominantly in the nerves—peripheral and autonomic.[102] These familial amyloidotic polyneuropathies have been described in different parts of the world. For example, neuropathic amyloidosis has been identified in individuals in Portugal, Japan, Sweden, and the United States. As mentioned previously, in all of these genetic disorders variant forms of transthyretin are deposited as amyloid fibrils.

LOCALIZED AMYLOIDOSIS. Sometimes amyloid deposits are limited to a single organ or tissue without involvement of any other site in the body. The deposits may produce grossly detectable nodular masses or be evident only on microscopic examination. Nodular (tumor-forming) deposits of amyloid are most often encountered in the lung, larynx, skin, urinary bladder, tongue, and the region about the eye.[108] Frequently there are infiltrates of lymphocytes and plasma cells in the periphery of these amyloid masses, raising the question of whether the mononuclear infiltrate is a response to the deposition of amyloid or instead is responsible for it. At least in some cases the amyloid consists of AL protein[100] and may therefore represent a localized form of immunocyte-derived amyloid.

ENDOCRINE AMYLOID. Microscopic deposits of localized amyloid may be found in certain endocrine tumors, such as medullary carcinoma of the thyroid gland, islet tumors of the pancreas, pheochromocytomas, and undifferentiated carcinomas of the stomach, and in the islets of Langerhans in patients with diabetes mellitus. In all these settings the amyloidogenic proteins seem to be derived by enzymic conversion of the polypeptide hormones or prohormones.

AMYLOID OF AGING. Two well-documented forms of amyloid deposition occur with aging.

Senile cardiac amyloidosis refers to the deposition of amyloid in the heart of elderly patients (usually in the eighth and ninth decades of life). Such deposition is usually asymptomatic but can cause serious cardiac dysfunction. In some, but not all, cases the amyloid protein appears to be a mutant form of transthyretin, suggesting that, as with other conditions associated with deposition of this protein, senile cardiac amyloidosis may also have a genetic basis.[101,109] In addition to cardiac involvement there may also be deposition of amyloid in the lungs, pancreas, or spleen, suggesting that senile cardiac amyloidosis may well be a systemic disorder.

Senile cerebral amyloidosis refers to the deposi-

tion of A_4 (or β-amyloid) protein in the cerebral blood vessels and plaques of patients with Alzheimer's disease (p. 1427).

PATHOGENESIS OF AMYLOID FORMATION. Although our knowledge of amyloidogenesis is far from complete, certain basic principles seem to apply (Fig. 5–41):

• All forms of amyloid are derived from soluble precursors that can be found in circulation.
• In some cases, there is an increase in the level of serum precursors (e.g., immunoglobulin light chains, SAA, β_2-microglobulin) that appear to be structurally normal; in others (e.g., transthyretin) a genetic defect results in the production of a structurally abnormal precursor protein.

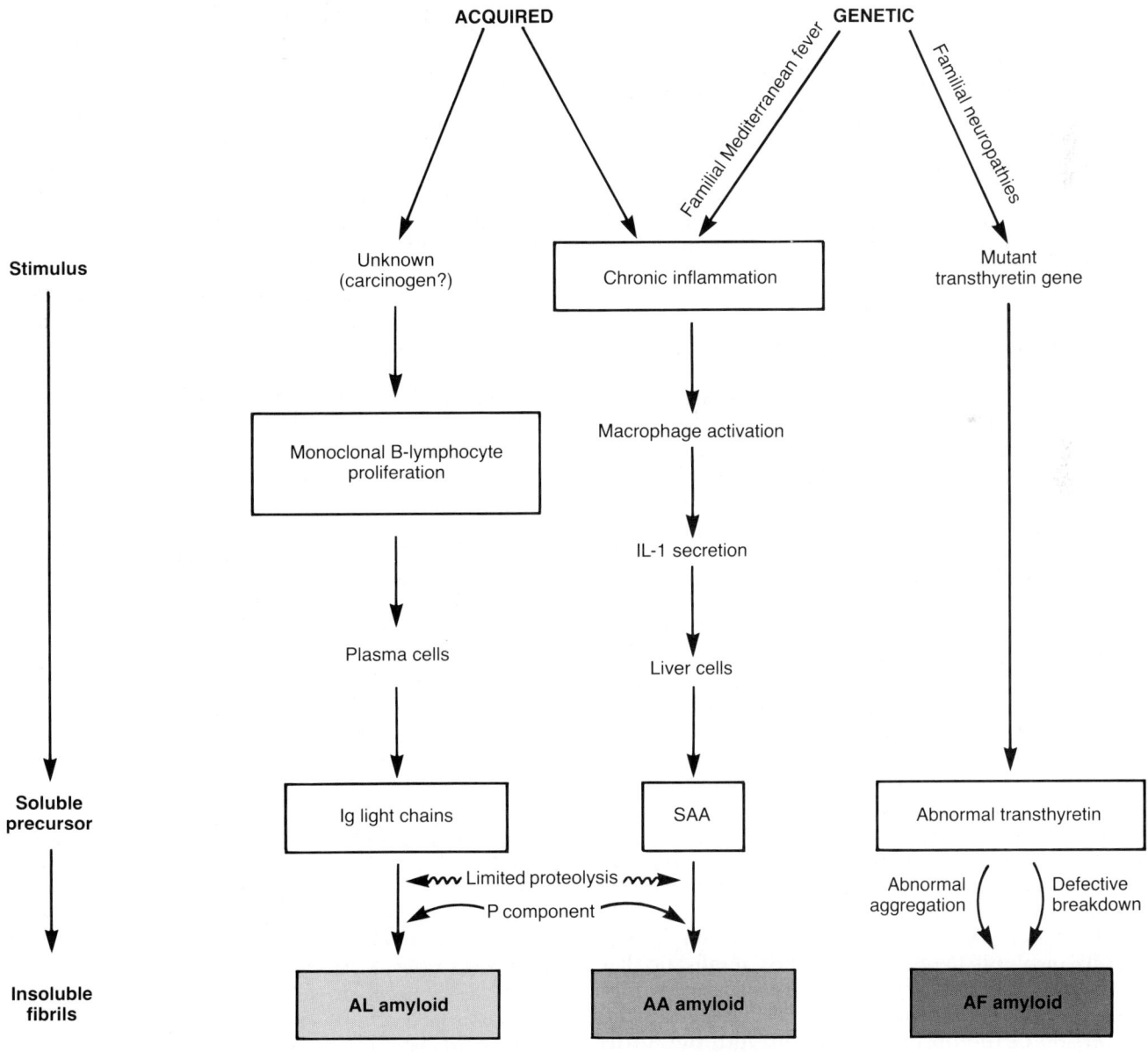

Figure 5–41. Pathogenesis of amyloidosis.

• The conversion of soluble precursors to their insoluble form (i.e., amyloid) involves some form of processing or proteolytic degradation.

However, several critical questions remain unanswered. Taking first the case of reactive systemic amyloidosis, we know that SAA is an acute phase reactant whose levels increase several hundred fold within 24 hours of acute inflammation in normal healthy individuals. This increase is brought about by the release of IL-1 from macrophages, which in turn enhances the synthesis of SAA by liver cells. With chronic tissue destruction and inflammation there is a sustained increase in SAA levels, presumably due to continued activation of macrophages. However, *increased production of SAA by itself cannot be sufficient for the deposition of amyloid because amyloidosis is an uncommon consequence of chronic inflammation.* It is believed that SAA is normally degraded to soluble end products by the action of monocyte-associated serine esterases and that in individuals who develop amyloidosis the inability to metabolize SAA properly leads to the generation of insoluble AA molecules. What is the nature of the processing defect? Does it involve a single enzyme or several factors? The questions remain unanswered.

The case of *immunocyte-derived* amyloid (AL) is somewhat less complex. We know that some stimulus, possibly carcinogenic, induces uncontrolled B-cell proliferation and hence excessive synthesis of the soluble precursor proteins (immunoglobulin light chains). As already discussed, the derivation of amyloid-like fibrils from light chains by limited proteolysis has been demonstrated. Unknown, however, is why only a small fraction of individuals with circulating free light chains develop amyloidosis. Are some light chains more amyloidogenic than others? This would seem to be supported by the observation that AL amyloid is derived largely from the λ VI light chain family. In addition to their amyloidogenic potential, the subsequent cleavage of light chains by the mononuclear phagocyte system may also be important, as discussed earlier.

In contrast to the two examples already cited, in familial amyloidosis the deposition of transthyretins as amyloid fibrils does not result from overproduction of transthyretins. Because the amyloid deposits contain both intact transthyretins and their fragments, it has been proposed that genetically determined alterations of structure render the transthyretins prone to abnormal aggregation and proteolysis.

In summary, several factors must act in concert to produce amyloidosis. These include quantitative or qualitative changes in the precursor proteins, coupled with defective or deficient proteolysis as well as some as yet undefined influences.[99] Because the amyloid fibrils are insoluble in physiologic fluids, it must be that the process of fibrillogenesis takes place in proximity to the sites of deposition. The cells involved in the conversion of the precursor proteins into the fibrils are not fully characterized, but macrophages seem to be the most likely candidates. Whether the conversion of the soluble precursors into amyloid occurs intracellularly within phagocytes or close to the plasma membrane in the ground substance is not yet resolved.

MORPHOLOGY. There are no consistent or distinctive patterns of organ or tissue distribution of amyloid deposits in any of the categories cited. Nonetheless, a few generalizations can be made. Amyloidosis secondary to chronic inflammatory disorders tends to yield the most severe systemic involvements. Kidneys, liver, spleen, lymph nodes, adrenals, and thyroid, as well as many other tissues, are classically involved. Although immunocyte-associated amyloidosis cannot reliably be distinguished from the secondary form by its organ distribution, more often it involves the heart, gastrointestinal tract, peripheral nerves, skin, and tongue. In addition, bizarre distributions, such as amyloidosis of the eye and respiratory tract, are encountered more often in patients with immunocyte-associated amyloidosis. However, the same organs affected by reactive systemic amyloidosis (secondary amyloidosis), including kidneys, liver, and spleen, may also contain deposits in the immunocyte-associated form of the disease.

As noted earlier, the histologic diagnosis of amyloid is based almost entirely on its staining characteristics. The most commonly used staining technique utilizes the dye Congo red, which under ordinary light imparts a pink or red color to amyloid deposits. Under polarized light the Congo red–stained amyloid shows a green birefringence (Fig. 5–38). This reaction is shared by all forms of amyloid and is due to the cross-β-pleated configuration of amyloid fibrils. Other methods of differentiating amyloid from hyaline deposits include somewhat less specific histochemical techniques. For example, amyloid stains metachromatically (violet to pink) with crystal violet or methyl violet. It yields secondary fluorescence in ultraviolet light with the dyes thioflavine T and S. For routine diagnosis, birefringence after Congo red staining is the most widely practiced and reliable tool. Confirmation can be obtained by electron microscopy. AA, AL, and transthyretin amyloid can be distinguished in histologic sections. AA protein loses affinity for Congo red after pretreatment with potassium permanganate, whereas other forms of amyloid do not. Immunoperoxidase staining with specific antisera reactive with various chemical forms of amyloid is also useful in the identification of amyloid fibril proteins.[110]

Because the pattern of organ involvement in different clinical forms of amyloidosis is variable, each of the major organ involvements is described separately.

KIDNEY. Amyloidosis of the kidney is the most common and potentially the most serious form of organ involvement. In most reported series of patients with amyloidosis, renal amyloidosis is the major cause of death. On gross inspection, the kidney may appear normal in size and color or it may be enlarged, pale gray, waxy, and firm. In advanced cases it may be shrunken and contracted due to vascular narrowing induced by the deposition of amyloid within arterial and arteriolar walls.

Histologically, the selective sites of amyloid involvement are primarily the glomeruli, but the interstitial peritubular tissue, arteries, and arterioles are also affected. The glomerular deposits first appear as subtle thickenings of the mesangial matrix, accompanied usually by barely discernible, uneven widening of the basement membranes of the glomerular capillaries. In time, the mesangial depositions and the deposits along the basement membranes cause capillary narrowing and distortion of the glomerular vascular tuft. With the electron microscope, the fibrillar accumulations are observed to begin on the endothelial side of the basement membrane and then appear to flood over the basement membrane to abut on the contiguous podocytes (Fig. 5–42). In many instances, the epithelial cells lose their foot processes. With progression of the glomerular amyloidosis, the endothelial cells are enveloped, the capillary lumina are obliterated, and the obsolescent glomerulus is flooded by confluent masses or interlacing broad ribbons of amyloid (Fig. 5–43). Often the enlarged damaged vascular tufts obliterate the urinary space, and with time all normal architecture is wiped out.

The peritubular deposits also begin in apposition to the tubular basement membranes and extend progressively into the intertubular connective tissue as well as encroach on the tubular lumina. The overlying tubular epithelium may be unaffected or may undergo regressive changes. Often, proteinaceous casts fill these tubular lumina. In cases of myeloma-associated amyloidosis, the casts sometimes exhibit birefringence with Congo red stain, suggesting that they are composed of amyloid proteins. The vascular involvement takes the form of pink, hyaline thickening of arterial and arteriolar walls, often with narrowing of the lumina. With such ischemia, widespread tubular atrophy and interstitial fibrosis superimpose themselves upon the basic deformity produced by the amyloidosis.

SPLEEN. Amyloidosis of the spleen may be inapparent grossly or may cause moderate-to-marked splenomegaly

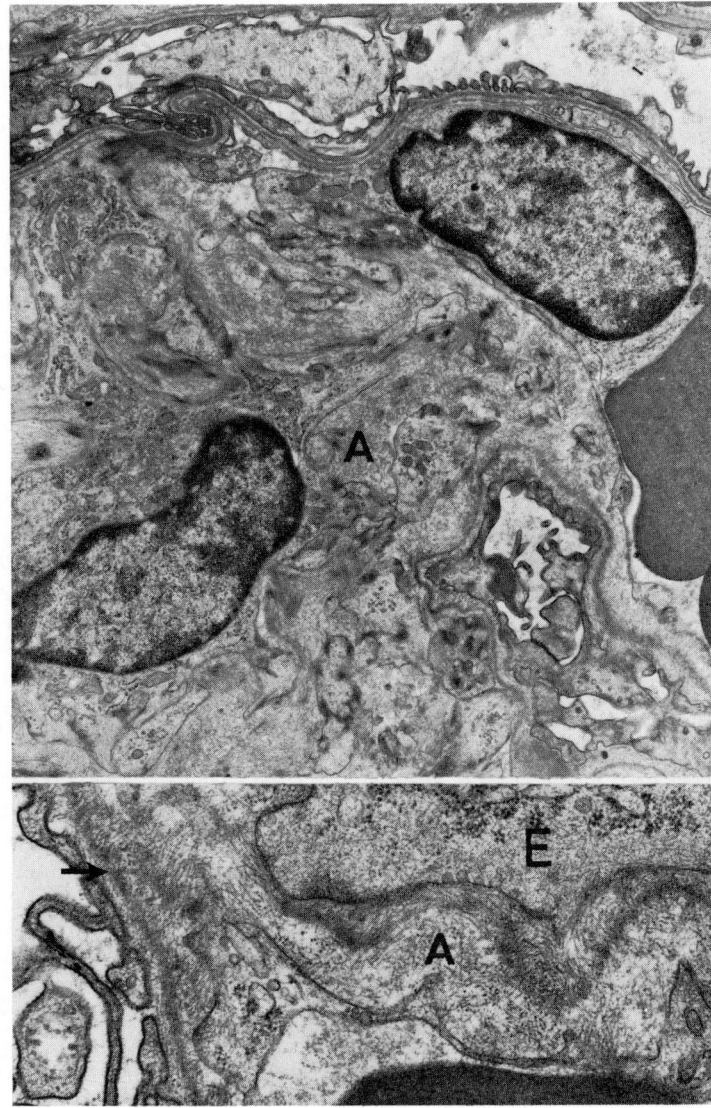

Figure 5–42. Amyloidosis in the kidney under the electron microscope to illustrate the subendothelial location of the amyloid deposit (A). In the lower figure ($\times$23,000), the location between the basement membrane *(arrow)* and the endothelial cell (E) is clearly shown. (From Cohen, A.S.: The constitution and genesis of amyloid. Int. Rev. Exp. Pathol. 4:176, 1965.)

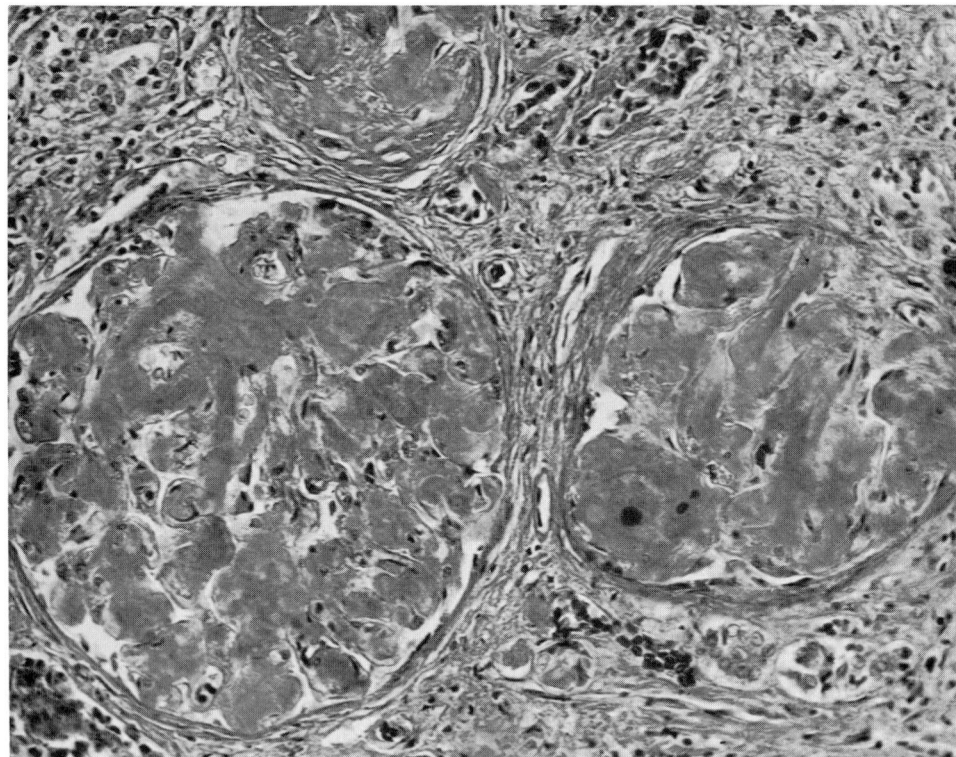

Figure 5–43. Amyloidosis of the kidney. The glomerular architecture is almost totally obliterated by the massive accumulation of amyloid.

(up to 800 gm). It is believed that the amyloid deposits begin in the perifollicular regions, but almost always, by the time they are observed in postmortem studies, the deposits are far more widespread. For completely mysterious reasons, one of two patterns emerges. In one the deposit is largely limited to the splenic follicles, producing tapioca-like granules on gross inspection, designated "sago spleen." Histologically, the entire follicle may be replaced in advanced cases. In the other pattern, the amyloid appears to spare the follicles and instead involves the walls of the splenic sinuses and connective tissues framework in the red pulp (Fig. 5–44). Fusion of the early deposits gives rise to large, maplike areas of amyloidosis, creating what has been designated the "lardaceous" spleen (Fig. 5–45). Ultrastructural studies indicate that the early deposits always occur between cells or in immediate apposition to the basement

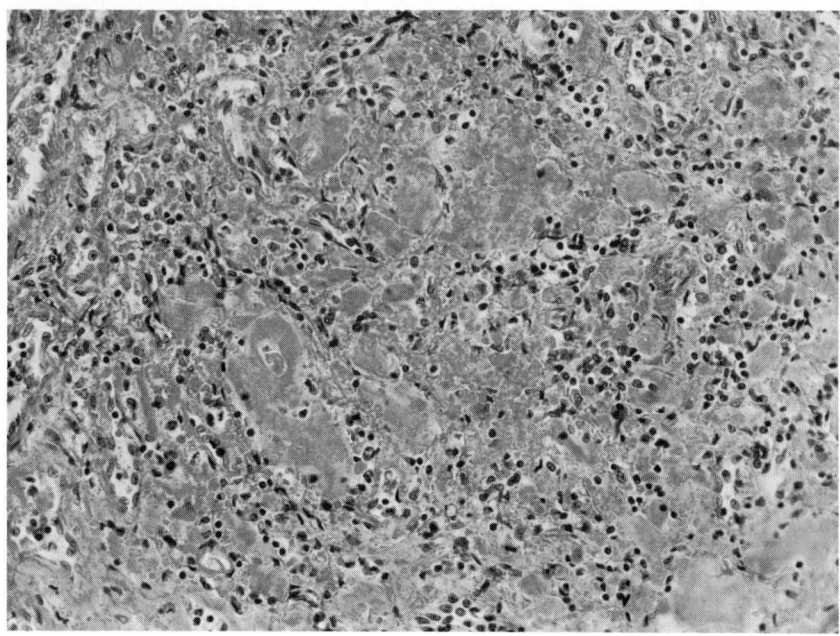

Figure 5–44. Amyloidosis of the spleen. The coalescent masses of amyloid surround the spleen cells.

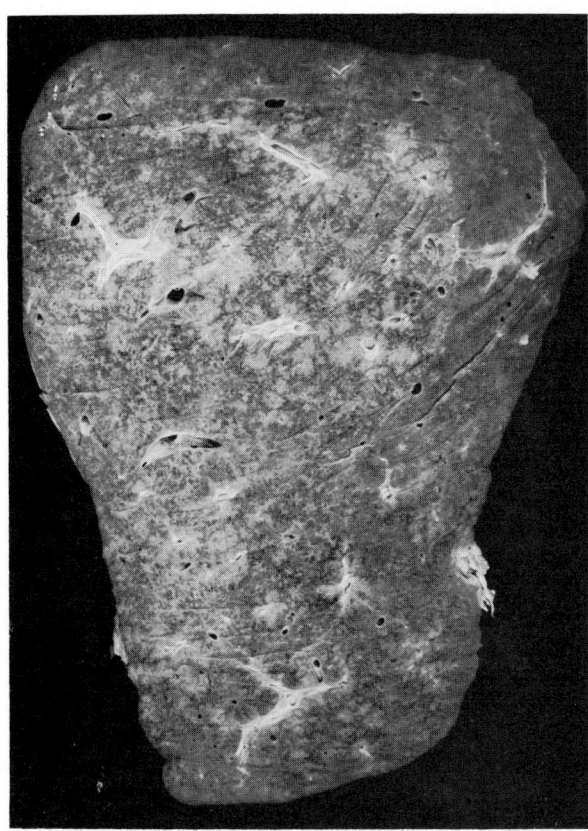

Figure 5–45. Amyloidosis of spleen. The focal deposits appear paler than the surrounding substance and in some areas are confluent. The pattern is that known as "lardaceous."

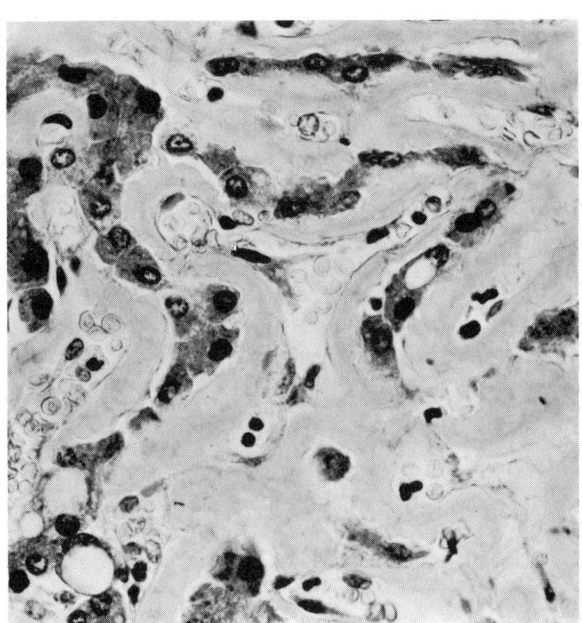

Figure 5–46. Amyloidosis of the liver. Pressure atrophy of hepatic cords by amyloid. Some cells are compressed and distorted, while others have been replaced by the amyloid deposit.

membranes of the mononuclear phagocytic (reticuloendothelial) cells of the splenic sinuses, as well as within the walls of small blood vessels.

LIVER. Here again, the deposits may be grossly inapparent or may cause moderate-to-marked hepatomegaly. With enlargement, the liver assumes a pale, waxy-gray, firm appearance. The amyloid appears first in the space of Disse and then progressively encroaches on adjacent hepatic parenchymal cells and sinusoids. In time, deformity, pressure atrophy, and disappearance of hepatocytes occur, causing total replacement of large areas of liver parenchyma (Fig. 5–46). Vascular involvement and Kupffer cell depositions are frequent. Normal liver function is usually preserved despite sometimes quite severe involvement of the liver.

HEART. Amyloidosis of the heart may occur in any form of systemic amyloidosis, much more commonly in persons with immunocyte-derived disease. In some patients it represents an isolated organ involvement, and almost invariably the patient is over 70 years of age **(amyloid of aging).** The heart may be enlarged and firm but more often it shows no significant changes on cross section of the myocardium. Somewhat distinctive findings, when present, are pink-to-gray pinpoint or nodular elevations of the endocardium, having a dewdrop appearance. Histologically, the deposits begin in focal subendocardial accumulations and within the

myocardium between the muscle fibers. Expansion of these myocardial deposits eventually causes pressure atrophy of myocardial fibers (Fig. 5–47). Vascular and subepicardial accumulations may also occur. In most cases the deposits are separated and widely distributed, but when

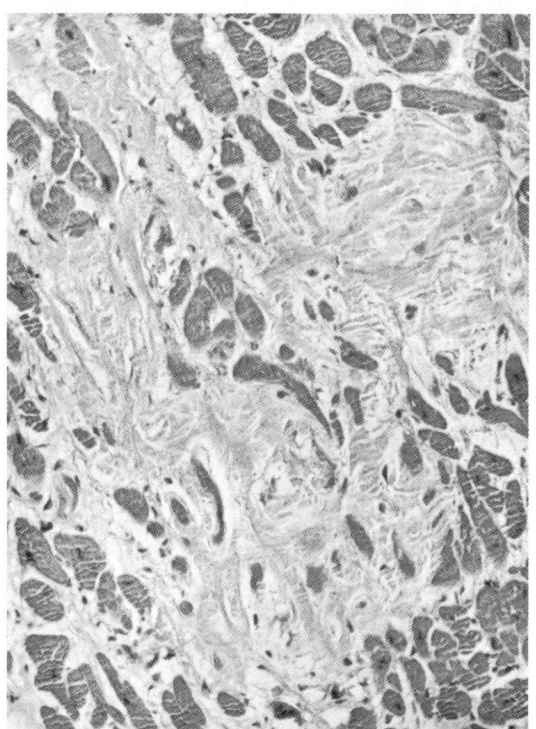

Figure 5–47. Amyloidosis of aging in the heart. The amyloid surrounds isolated myocardial fibers and has caused atrophy of others.

they are subendocardial the conduction system may be damaged, accounting for the electrocardiographic abnormalities noted in some patients.

OTHER ORGANS. Amyloidosis of other organs is generally encountered in systemic disease. The adrenals, thyroid, and pituitary are common sites of involvement. In the adrenals, the intercellular deposits begin adjacent to the basement membranes of the cortical cells, usually first in the zona glomerulosa. With progression, the deposits encroach on cortical cells and advance into the deeper layers of the cortex. Large sheets of amyloid may replace considerable amounts of the cortical parenchyma. Similar patterns are seen in the thyroid and pituitary. The gastrointestinal tract may be involved at any level, from the oral cavity (gingiva, tongue) to the anus. The early lesions are largely vascular in origin but eventually extend to involve the adjacent areas of the submucosa, muscularis, and subserosa. Coalescence of these small deposits may produce plaques or bands of firm gray substance. Nodular depositions in the tongue may cause macroglossia, giving rise to the designation **tumor-forming amyloid of the tongue.** The respiratory tract may be involved focally or diffusely from the larynx down to the smallest bronchioles. As mentioned earlier, a distinct chemical form of amyloid has been found in the brain of patients with Alzheimer's disease. It involves so-called plaques as well as blood vessels (p. 1427). Amyloidosis of peripheral and autonomic nerves is a feature of several familial amyloidotic neuropathies. Curiously, depositions of amyloid in patients on long-term hemodialysis are most prominent in the carpal ligament of the wrist, resulting in compression of the median nerve (carpal tunnel syndrome). These patients may also have extensive amyloid deposition in the joints.

CLINICAL CORRELATION. Amyloidosis may be found as an unsuspected anatomic change, having produced no clinical manifestations, or it may cause death. The symptoms depend, as you might expect, on the magnitude of the deposits and on the particular sites or organs affected. Clinical manifestations at first are often entirely nonspecific, such as weakness, weight loss, lightheadedness, or syncope. Somewhat more specific findings appear later and most often relate to renal, cardiac, and gastrointestinal involvement, but hepatomegaly and splenomegaly and alterations in serum protein levels may also be present.

Renal involvement is the dominating and most life-threatening feature of most cases of reactive systemic (secondary) amyloidosis, including those patients with familial Mediterranean fever. It may also be present (although less consistently) in patients with amyloidosis associated with immunocyte dyscrasias. Proteinuria and casts, both protein and occasionally cellular, are the principal urinary findings in renal amyloidosis. The proteinuria of renal amyloidosis is an important cause of the nephrotic syndrome (p. 1033), as it may be sufficiently severe to induce hypoalbuminemia. Progressive obliteration of glomeruli in advanced cases ultimately leads to renal failure and uremia. It is worth noting that, unlike most causes of renal failure, amyloidosis is not usually associated with hypertension.

Cardiac amyloidosis is extremely common in patients with immunocyte-derived amyloidosis, but it is less frequently present in those with reactive systemic amyloidosis. It is also encountered as an isolated involvement in patients of advanced age. Whether clinical manifestations will appear depends on the severity and extent of the amyloid deposits. When symptomatic, the typical presentation is the insidious onset of congestive heart failure. The most serious aspects of cardiac amyloidosis are the conduction disturbances and arrhythmias that may prove fatal. Occasionally, cardiac amyloidosis produces a restrictive pattern of cardiomyopathy and masquerades as chronic constrictive pericarditis (p. 646).

Gastrointestinal amyloidosis may be entirely asymptomatic, or it may present in a variety of ways. Nodular (tumor-forming) amyloidosis of the tongue may cause sufficient enlargement and inelasticity to hamper speech and swallowing. Depositions in the stomach and intestine may lead to malabsorption, diarrhea, and disturbances in digestion.

Even when amyloidosis is suspected on the basis of the clinical findings, resort must be made to biopsy followed by Congo red staining to demonstrate deposition of amyloid. The most common sites biopsied are the kidney, when renal manifestations are present, or rectal or gingival tissues in patients suspected of having systemic amyloidosis. In two recent studies, examination of abdominal fat aspirates stained with Congo red was found to be an extremely sensitive and specific technique for the diagnosis of systemic amyloidosis. Because this technique is extremely simple and safe, it is likely to find widespread use in the future.[111,112]

In suspected cases of immunocyte-associated amyloidosis, serum and urine protein electrophoresis and immunoelectrophoresis should be performed. Bone marrow aspirates in such cases often show plasmacytosis even in the absence of overt multiple myeloma.

The prognosis for patients with generalized amyloidosis is poor. Those with immunocyte-derived amyloidosis (not including multiple myeloma) have a median survival of 14 months after diagnosis. Patients with myeloma-associated amyloidosis have a poorer prognosis. The outlook for patients with reactive systemic amyloidosis is somewhat better and depends to some extent on the control of the underlying condition. Resorption of amyloid after treatment of the associated condition has been reported, but this is a rare occurrence.

IMMUNOLOGIC DEFICIENCY SYNDROMES

The immunologic deficiency syndromes are experiments of nature that beautifully document the complexities inherent in man's immune system. Nowhere has the relevance of the individual components of immunologic function been more distinctly shown than when deficiencies of single components have given rise to distinctive disorders. Indeed, many of the important concepts of immunology either arose from or were confirmed by the study of clinical examples of specific immunodeficiencies. Traditionally, immunodeficiency disorders are considered according to the primary component or components involved (i.e., the B cell, the T cell, the undifferentiated stem cell, or complement)[113]; however, in view of the major cell interactions between T and B lymphocytes and macrophages, these distinctions are not always clear-cut.

Immunodeficiencies can also be divided into the primary immunodeficiency disorders, which are almost always genetically determined, and secondary immunodeficiency states, arising as complications of infections, malnutrition, aging, or side effects of immunosuppression, irradiation, or chemotherapy for cancer and other autoimmune diseases. Both primary and secondary immunodeficiency disorders are being discovered with increasing frequency because of new laboratory methods that can detect various cellular and humoral components of the immunologic reaction. Here we briefly discuss some of the more important primary immunodeficiencies, to be followed by a more detailed description of the acquired immunodeficiency syndrome (AIDS), the most devastating example of secondary immunodeficiency.

PRIMARY IMMUNODEFICIENCIES

The primary immunodeficiency diseases are genetically determined and may affect specific immunity (i.e., humoral and cellular) or nonspecific host defense mechanisms mediated by complement proteins and cells such as phagocytes or NK cells. Most primary immunodeficiencies manifest themselves in infancy, between six months and two years of life, and they are noted because of the susceptibility of infants to recurrent infections. Detailed classification of the primary immunodeficiencies according to the suggested cellular defect may be found in the WHO report on immunodeficiency and in other specialized sources.[113,114] Only a few examples are presented here.

X-linked Agammaglobulinemia of Bruton

This is one of the most common forms of primary immunodeficiency and is characterized by the virtual absence from the serum of immunoglobulins, although small amounts of IgG may sometimes be present. It is an X-linked disease restricted to males. Severe recurrent infections usually begin at eight to nine months of age, when the infant becomes depleted of maternal immunoglobulins.[115] The most common offending organisms are pyogenic (e.g., staphylococcus, *Haemophilus influenzae*), and patients have recurrent conjunctivitis, pharyngitis, otitis media, bronchitis, pneumonia, and skin infections. Most viral and fungal infections are handled normally, because cell-mediated immunity is the pre-

dominant mode of defense against these pathogens. However, there are some curious and important exceptions to this generalization; affected individuals are at particular risk for development of vaccine-associated paralytic poliomyelitis as well as fatal echovirus encephalitis. Susceptibility to hepatitis and to enterovirus infections is also increased.

The classic characteristics, first described by Bruton, are those that would be expected from a primary B-cell deficiency. B cells are virtually absent in the blood except in very rare cases. Pre-B cells, which are large lymphoid cells with intracytoplasmic IgM but no surface immunoglobulins, are found in normal numbers in the bone marrow. The lymph nodes and spleen lack germinal centers, and plasma cells are absent from the lymph nodes, spleen, bone marrow, and connective tissue. Tonsils in particular are poorly developed or rudimentary. There are, however, normal numbers of circulating and tissue T cells, and T-cell function as measured by delayed hypersensitivity tests and allograft rejection is normal. For reasons that remain mysterious, there is a remarkably high frequency of various autoimmune connective tissue diseases in these patients, and about 20% of them may develop an indolent form of rheumatoid-like arthritis, which responds to gamma globulin therapy. Dermatomyositis, lupus erythematosus, and diffuse vasculitis are also relatively common in these patients.

Common Variable Immunodeficiency

This relatively common but poorly defined derangement probably represents a heterogeneous group of disorders. It may be congenital or acquired, sporadic or familial (with an inconstant mode of inheritance). *The feature common to all patients is hypogammaglobulinemia, generally affecting all the antibody classes but sometimes only IgG.* According to the WHO classification there are three different forms of common variable immunodeficiencies: (1) with predominant (intrinsic) B cell defect; (2) with predominant immunoregulatory T-cell disorder marked by (a) deficiency of T-helper cells or (b) presence of activated T-suppressor cells; and (3) with autoantibodies to T and B cells. Most patients belong to the first category. They have *normal levels of circulating B cells,* which can recognize antigens and proliferate but fail to differentiate into plasma cells. Histologically the B-cell areas (i.e., the lymphoid follicles in the lymph nodes, spleen, and the gut) are markedly hyperplastic. These histologic findings support the notion that B cells can proliferate in response to antigen recognition, but terminal differentiation of B cells is abnormal. The symptoms are those of antibody deficiency—that is, recurrent bacterial infections. Infestation with the intestinal parasite *Giardia lamblia* is also quite common and may lead to a sprue-like syndrome. Another peculiar feature is the occurrence in multiple organs of noncaseating granulomas without any known microbial cause.

These patients also have a high frequency of autoimmune diseases, including rheumatoid arthritis, pernicious anemia, and hemolytic anemia. Lymphoid malignancy sometimes develops several years after the immunologic deficiency is diagnosed.

Isolated IgA Deficiency

Isolated IgA deficiency is a very common immunodeficiency that occurs in about one in 600 individuals and consists of the virtual absence of *both serum and secretory IgA*. It may be familial or acquired in association with toxoplasmosis, measles, or some other virus infection. It is generally believed that most individuals with this disease are completely asymptomatic, but according to some authorities IgA deficiency is commonly associated with some form of illness.[116] Because IgA is the major immunoglobulin in external secretions, mucosal defenses are weakened and infections occur in the respiratory, gastrointestinal, and urogenital tracts. Symptomatic patients commonly present with recurrent sinopulmonary infections and diarrhea. Recent reports suggest that some individuals previously classified as having selective IgA deficiency are also deficient in IgG_2 and IgG_4 subclasses of immunoglobulin G. This group of patients is particularly prone to develop infections.[117] In addition, IgA-deficient patients have a high frequency of respiratory tract allergy and a variety of autoimmune diseases, particularly SLE and rheumatoid arthritis. The basis of the increased frequency of autoimmune and allergic diseases is not known. Because secretory IgA normally acts as a mucosal barrier against foreign proteins and antigens, it could be speculated that unregulated absorption of foreign protein antigens triggers abnormal immune responses in vivo.

The basic defect is in the differentiation of IgA B lymphocytes. Normally, the first IgA B cells are detected in the 12-week-old fetus. These immature cells have surface IgM and IgD in addition to IgA. Transition to mature IgA B cells starts at birth, and in adults only 10% of the IgA B cells express surface IgM and IgD; the majority express only IgA. In most patients with selective IgA deficiency the number of IgA-positive B cells is normal, but most of them express the immature phenotype and very few of these cells can be induced to transform into IgA plasma cells in vitro. Serum antibodies to IgA are found in approximately 40% of the patients. Whether this finding is of any etiologic significance is unknown, but it has important clinical implications. When transfused with blood containing normal IgA, some of these patients develop severe, even fatal anaphylactic reactions.

DiGeorge's Syndrome (Thymic Hypoplasia)

This is an example of selective T-cell deficiency that derives from failure of development of the third and fourth pharyngeal pouches. The latter give rise to the thymus, the parathyroids, some of the clear cells of the thyroid, and the ultimobranchial body. Thus, these patients have total absence of cell-mediated immune responses (owing to hypoplasia or lack of the thymus), tetany (owing to lack of the parathyroids),

and congenital defects of the heart and great vessels. In addition, the appearance of the mouth, ears, and facies may be abnormal. Absence of cell-mediated immunity is reflected in low levels of circulating lymphocytes and a poor defense against certain fungal and viral infections. Sometimes the lymphocyte counts may be normal, in which case virtually all are **B** cells. Plasma cells are present in normal numbers in lymphoid tissues, but the thymic-dependent paracortical areas of the lymph nodes and the periarteriolar sheaths of the spleen are depleted. Immunoglobulin levels tend to be normal.

Support for the idea that this syndrome is directly attributable to maldevelopment of the thymus also comes from the successful treatment of some patients with this disease by transplantation of fetal thymus or thymic epithelium. The syndrome is not genetically determined but appears to be the result of intrauterine fetal damage before the eighth week of gestation. Patients with "partial" DiGeorge's syndrome, who have an extremely small but histologically normal thymus, have also been recorded. T-cell function improves with age in these children, so that by 5 years of age many have no T-cell deficit.

Some children present with severe defects in cell-mediated immunity without associated malformations or parathyroid dysfunction. The immunoglobulin levels are normal or increased, or there is selective deficiency of some isotypes. This condition is not very well defined, but is sometimes referred to as *Nezelof's syndrome.*

Severe Combined Immunodeficiency Disease (SCID)

This is an extremely serious form of inherited immunodeficiency syndrome characterized by defects in both T cell–mediated and humoral immunity. This disorder is heterogeneous with respect to both pattern of inheritance and underlying defects in T and B cells. Two modes of transmission are recognized— autosomal recessive and X-linked recessive. Many patients with the autosomal recessive form of SCID lack the enzyme adenosine deaminase (ADA) in their cells. The implications of enzyme deficiency in the pathogenesis of the immunologic abnormalities are discussed later.

Although all patients show impairment of both T- and B-cell functions, in general there is greater loss of T-cell immunity. Most patients are severely lymphopenic and lack mature T lymphocytes in the blood. When bone marrow cells from some SCID patients are incubated with normal thymic epithelial cells or thymic hormones they fail to differentiate normally, suggesting a defect in the stem cells. However, other patients have shown improvement in T-cell functions after transplantation of thymus, which suggests that the defect may lie in the ability of the thymus to provide signals for differentiation of stem cells.[118] It seems, therefore, that there are two mechanisms of impaired T-cell immunity in SCID: a defect in stem cells, or abnormal differentiation of normal stem cells due to thymic abnormalities.

Investigations into the basis of impaired humoral immunity also indicate heterogeneity. Some patients have a stem cell defect, leading to an extreme paucity of mature B cells in the peripheral blood, whereas others have normal or even increased numbers of B cells that are unable to function. In the latter group of patients, lack of adequate T-helper cells or excessive T-suppressor cell function, or both, have been implicated.[119] Recent studies reveal another level of heterogeneity: in some patients, virtually all of the circulating lymphocytes have the phenotypic and functional characteristics of NK cells.[116] The significance of this finding will be discussed later.

In summary, SCID in most cases results from defects of lymphoid stem cells involving both T-cell and B-cell precursors. As might be expected, lymph nodes, spleen, tonsils, and appendix show virtual absence of any lymphoid tissue, but the pathognomonic histologic finding is in the thymus gland, which fails to descend from the neck into the anterior mediastinum and is devoid of lymphoid cells or Hassall's corpuscles. The blood vessels are very small, indicating that the thymus is fetal rather than involuted. The gland seems to be arrested at the stage at which it resembles the thymus of a six- to eight-week-old fetus. Infants are incapable of any of the immunologic functions—they do not produce antibodies, exhibit very small amounts of IgG and no IgM or IgA in the serum, and fail to reject skin allografts or to develop delayed hypersensitivity reactions. They succumb during the first year of life, usually to such opportunistic organisms as *Pseudomonas*, *Candida*, or *Pneumocystis carinii*, or infections with viruses such as cytomegalovirus and varicella and herpes-simplex viruses. Some patients develop graft-versus-host disease mediated by transplacental transfer of maternal T lymphocytes. Because SCID is usually caused by defects in stem cells, grafting of normal bone marrow stem cells is the treatment of choice. In many patients, full immunologic reconstitution can be achieved by transplantation of sibling bone marrow. The donor marrow has to be depleted of mature T cells to prevent fatal graft-versus-host disease (p. 188). However, as mentioned earlier, NK cells that are present in some of these patients can recognize transplanted allogeneic marrow stem cells, thereby preventing successful engraftment.

Approximately 50% of patients with the autosomal recessive form of SCID lack the enzyme ADA in their red cells and leukocytes. This enzyme is involved in the metabolism of adenosine and deoxyadenosine to inosine and 2′-deoxyinosine, respectively. Deficiency of ADA leads to the accumulation of deoxyadenosine and its derivatives, such as deoxyATP, which are toxic to lymphocytes.[120] In addition to bone marrow transplantation, treatment of this variant of SCID has been attempted by infusion of normal ADA-containing erythrocytes. This has resulted in immunologic improvement in some, but not all, patients. More exciting, however, is the prospect of gene therapy because the gene for human ADA has been cloned and successfully introduced and expressed in primate cells in culture. Thus, it would seem that the insertion of the ADA gene into the patient's own marrow stem cells, followed by reinfusion of the transfected marrow, may offer the possibility of cure without the attendant problems of graft-versus-host disease. This is currently an area of intense investigation.

Immunodeficiency with Thrombocytopenia and Eczema (Wiskott-Aldrich Syndrome)

This remarkable syndrome has been deemed "curious," "enigmatic," or "confusing" because its immunologic defects are so difficult to explain. *It is an X-linked recessive disease characterized by thrombocytopenia, eczema, and a marked vulnerability to recurrent infection, ending in early death.* The thymus is morphologically normal, at least early in the course of the disease, but there is progressive secondary depletion of lymphocytes in the peripheral blood and in the paracortical (thymus-dependent) areas of the lymph nodes, with variable loss of cellular immunity. Patients may exhibit normal responses to such protein antigens as tetanus and diphtheria toxoid, but classically they show a poor antibody response to polysaccharide antigens. IgM levels in the serum are low, but levels of IgG are usually normal. Paradoxically, the levels of IgA and IgE are often elevated. Patients are also prone to develop malignant lymphomas. Whether the failure to respond to polysaccharides results from a defect in antigen recognition and processing or a qualitative deficiency of lymphocyte B-cell function is unclear. There is at present no unifying hypothesis to explain all these defects. Stem cell replacement by T cell–depleted haplo-identical bone marrow has resulted in complete correction of immunologic and platelet abnormalities in some patients.

Immunodeficiency Associated with Deficiency of Cell Membrane Molecules

A large number of membrane-associated proteins have been found to be essential for leukocyte and lymphocyte functions that involve cell-to-cell interactions, such as phagocytosis, interactions between T and B cells, and T-cell activation. Many of these functions involve HLA molecules (already discussed) as well as a family of glycoproteins collectively referred to as *leukocyte adhesion proteins.*[121] There are three leukocyte adhesion proteins: (1) *LFA-1 (lymphocyte-function–associated antigen)*, present on lymphocytes, monocytes, and neutrophils, (2) *Mac-1* (which is identical to complement receptor 3 that binds fixed iC3b fragments), present on neutrophils, monocytes, eosinophils, and NK cells, and (3) *p150,95*, present on all leukocytes. Each of these glycoproteins is a dimer with a distinct α subunit and a common 95,000-dalton β subunit. Two immunodeficiency syndromes associated with a lack of these cell surface proteins are worthy of brief consideration:

• *Bare lymphocyte syndrome.* Patients with this syndrome lack either class I HLA antigens or both class I and class II antigens on their cell surfaces. Because these HLA antigens are necessary for normal functioning of lymphocytes (p. 170), their absence from the cell surface results in varying degrees of immunodeficiency. Typically there is impairment of both cellular and humoral responses with bacterial, viral, and fungal infections. The lymphoid organs are hypoplastic, but lymphopenia is not significant.

• *Leukocyte-adhesion protein deficiency.* This condition results from an inherited defect in the biosynthesis of the β subunit of leukocyte-adhesion proteins.[122] Because the β subunit is common to LFA-1, Mac-1, and p150,95, these glycoproteins are not expressed on the surface of lymphocytes, neutrophils, monocytes, and other leukocytes. Affected patients have recurrent bacterial infections and impaired wound healing. Lymphocyte (T cell, NK cell)-mediated cytotoxicity is impaired, as are T- and B- lymphocyte interactions in antibody synthesis. Although patients with deficiency of leukocyte adhesion proteins are not common, they provide the most telling proof of the *in vivo* relevance of these glycoproteins.

Genetic Deficiencies of the Complement System

Inherited deficiencies of complement proteins represent primary immunodeficiency states but, unlike the other forms described previously, do not involve primary defects in the lymphocytes. However, the various components of the complement system play a critical role in inflammatory and immunologic responses (p. 53). Deficiency of specific complement components may predispose to certain diseases, much like the predisposition that occurs with selective deficiencies of the immune system, discussed earlier. The end result of defects in complement, particularly C3, is an increased susceptibility to bacterial infection and, with C2 deficiency, a greater risk of connective tissue diseases similar to those that occur in the primary immunodeficiencies. The deficiencies of the later-acting components of the classic pathway (C5-8) result in recurrent neisserial (gonococcal, meningococcal) infections. Thus far, hereditary deficiencies have been described for almost all the classic components of the complement system and two of the inhibitors.[123,124] Some of these deficiencies occur relatively often: for example, the C2 deficiency state occurs with a frequency of about 1% in the general population.

ACQUIRED IMMUNODEFICIENCY SYNDROME (AIDS)

In June 1981, the Centers for Disease Control (CDC) of the United States reported that five young male homosexuals in the Los Angeles area had contracted *Pneumocystis carinii* pneumonia. Two of the patients died. This report signaled the beginning of an epidemic of a disease characterized by profound immunosuppression associated with opportunistic infections, the development of certain tumors (especially multifocal Kaposi's sarcoma), and frequent involvement of the CNS, which has come to be known as acquired immunodeficiency syndrome (AIDS). By mid-1988, more than 55,000 patients with AIDS had been reported in the United States, and on the basis of serologic data, it is estimated that approximately 1,500,000 individuals have been infected with the virus likely to cause AIDS.[125] With a problem of this magnitude, it might be expected that there is a rapidly growing body of literature devoted to AIDS. Here we summarize only the salient epidemiologic, etiologic, immunologic, and clinical features of this new scourge, realizing fully that many of the statements will have to be modified before the ink is dry on the printed page.[126,127,128]

EPIDEMIOLOGY. Initially, the CDC defined AIDS as a "disease at least moderately predictive of a defect in cell-mediated immunity, occurring in a person with no known cause for diminished resistance to that disease." Although this definition is still of some value for epidemiologic and surveillance studies, it does not take into account the established role of human immunodeficiency virus (HIV) in the pathogenesis of AIDS, nor that HIV infection may present with a variety of other manifestations not included in the original definition. In recognition of these new developments and in an effort to provide uniformity to the diagnosis of AIDS and other HIV-related syndromes, the CDC has proposed a revised classification (effective January 1, 1988) that divides the spectrum of HIV infections into three categories.[129]

• *Group I:* HIV infection with specified secondary infections or malignant neoplasms. The secondary conditions affecting patients in this group are given in Table 5–12 (this group includes patients with full-blown AIDS, as originally recognized).
• *Group II:* HIV infection with other specified manifestations in the absence of the secondary infections and neoplasms included in the first category (this includes patients previously referred to as having pre-AIDS and AIDS-related complex, or ARC).
• *Group III:* HIV infections not classifiable in the above two categories (this includes certain manifestations of acute HIV infection such as acute lymphadenitis, aseptic meningitis, and a syndrome resembling infectious mononucleosis).

Because the full spectrum of HIV infections is not yet known, it is likely that with additional clinical experience and research further modifications of this classification will be forthcoming.

Although the AIDS epidemic was first described in the United States, and this country has approximately 70% of the reported cases, AIDS has now

Table 5–12. Selected Secondary Infections and Neoplasms Found in Patients with HIV Infection—Group I

Protozoal and Helminthic Infections
    Cryptosporidiosis or isosporidiosis (enteritis)
    Pneumocystosis (pneumonia or disseminated infection)
    Toxoplasmosis (pneumonia or CNS infection)
    Strongyloidosis (pneumonia, CNS infection, or disseminated infection)
Fungal Infections
    Candidiasis (mouth, lung, skin or nails, disseminated)
    Cryptococcosis (CNS infection)
    Coccidioidomycosis (disseminated)
    Histoplasmosis (disseminated)
    Other opportunistic mycoses
Bacterial Infections
    Mycobacteriosis ("atypical," e.g., *M. avium-intracellulare* and *M. tuberculosis* infection, disseminated)
    Nocardiosis (pneumonia, meningitis, disseminated)
    Salmonella infections
Viral Infections
    Cytomegalovirus (pulmonary, intestinal, or CNS infections)
    Herpes simplex virus (localized or disseminated)
    Varicella zoster virus (localized or disseminated)
    Progressive multifocal leukoencephalopathy
Malignant Neoplasms
    Burkitt's lymphoma
    Kaposi's sarcoma
    Immunoblastic lymphoma (B cells)
    Primary CNS lymphomas

been reported from over 100 countries around the world.[130] Epidemiologic studies in the United States have identified five groups at risk for developing AIDS. In late-1988, the case distribution in these groups was as follows:

1. *Homosexual or bisexual males* constituted by far the largest group, accounting for 71.4% of the reported cases.[125] This included 7% who were intravenous drug abusers as well.
2. *Intravenous drug abusers* with no previous history of homosexuality composed the next largest group, representing about 18.4% of all patients.
3. *Hemophiliacs*, especially those who received large amounts of factor VIII concentrates prior to 1985, made up 1% of all cases.
4. *Blood and blood component recipients* who are not hemophiliacs, but who received transfusions of whole blood or components (e.g., platelets, plasma), composed 2.5% of the patients.
5. *Heterosexual contacts* of members of other high-risk groups constituted 3.9% of the patient population.

Approximately 2.8% of the patients did not belong to any of the high-risk groups mentioned, and the mode of transmission in these cases remains unidentified. The epidemiology of AIDS in Africa is quite different from the patterns seen in the United States. This may relate to the pattern of transmission of HIV, especially through heterosexual contact, as is discussed later.[130]

AIDS VIRUS. There is now overwhelming evidence that AIDS is caused by a virus known previously as HTLV-III, LAV, or ARV, but now called the human immunodeficiency virus (HIV). Before we discuss the role of HIV in the causation of AIDS, it is essential that we review the structure of this virus so as to gain a better understanding of its pathogenicity.[127,131,132]

HIV belongs to the family of human retroviruses, which includes human T-cell leukemia virus-I (HTLV-I). Both share tropism for the CD4 molecule, and hence CD4+ T cells are important targets of viral infection. Despite this similarity, there are important biologic and molecular differences among human retroviruses, which form the basis of their subdivision into two categories: (1) *Transforming retroviruses* include human T-cell leukemia virus type I (HTLV-I) and HTLV-II; HTLV-I, the prototype of this group, like many other transforming animal retroviruses (e.g., murine, feline, and bovine leukemia viruses), is noncytolytic and causes neoplastic transformation of its target cells, giving rise to a T-cell leukemia; and (2) *cytopathic retroviruses* include HIV-1 and the more recently described HIV-2. Unlike transforming retroviruses, these two are cytolytic for T cells and hence they produce profound immunodeficiency rather than primary neoplasms. Based on comparisons of morphology, genomic structure, antigenic cross reactivity, and biologic behavior, they are more closely related to the lentivirus family of animal retroviruses than to the transforming human retroviruses. Examples of lentiviruses in animals include visna virus of sheep, equine infectious anemia virus, feline immunodeficiency virus, and simian T-cell leukemia virus-III (STLV-III or SIV). All the viruses in this group, like HIV, are characterized by cytopathic effects in vitro and slow progressive fatal disease in vivo.[133]

Like most C-type retroviruses, the HIV-1 virion is spherical in shape and contains an electron-dense core surrounded by a lipid envelope derived from the host cell membrane during budding of the virus from the infected cell. The virus core contains several core proteins, two strands of genomic RNA, and the enzyme reverse transcriptase that is characteristic of all retroviruses (Fig. 5–48). Studding the viral envelope are two viral glycoproteins, gp120 and gp41. The former projects outward and, as we shall see, is important for the attachment of the virus to its target cells. The structure of HIV-1 proviral genome has been investigated extensively.[131,132,134] It is approximately 10 kilobases in length, and it contains the *gag*, *pol*, and *env* genes that code for the core proteins, reverse transcriptase, and envelope proteins, respectively (Fig. 5–49). *In addition to these three standard retroviral genes, HIV contains at least five other genes*, some of which exert regulatory functions that may well affect its pathogenicity. Figure 5–49 indicates the relative position and possible functions of four of these genes (i.e., *vif, tat III, rev* and *nef*). The fifth gene, called *vpr*, has been mapped, but its function is not yet clear.[135,136] It is beyond the scope of this book to detail the functional significance of these HIV-specific genes, but it is worth noting that both *tat III* and *rev* are potent positive regulatory elements essential

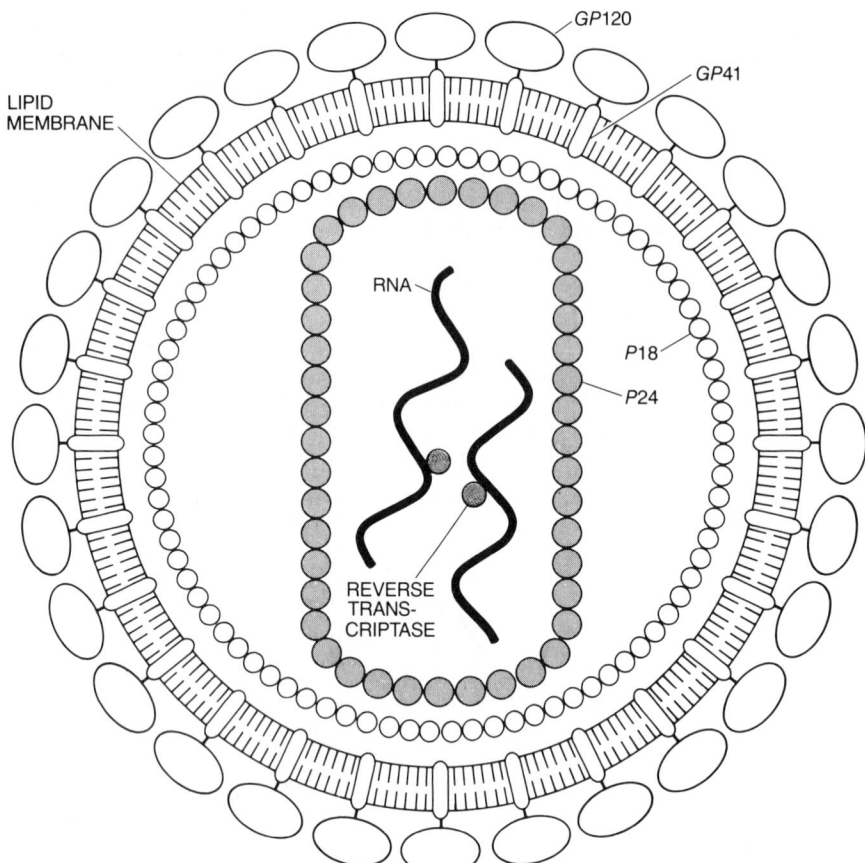

Figure 5–48. HIV virion, or virus particle, is a sphere that is roughly 1000 Angstrom units (one ten-thousandth of a millimeter) across. The particle is covered by a membrane, made up of two layers of lipid material, that is derived from the outer membrane of the host cell. Studding the membrane are glycoproteins. Each glycoprotein has two components: *gp*41 spans the membrane and *gp*120 extends beyond it. The membrane-and-protein envelope covers a core made up of proteins designated *p*24 and *p*18. The viral RNA is carried in the core, along with several copies of the enzyme reverse transcriptase. (From Gallo, R.C.: The AIDS virus. Sci. Am: *256:*46, 1987.)

for the optimal transcription and translation of viral structural genes.[137] Thus, it would seem that the products of these genes may be suitable targets for potential anti-HIV drugs. With this background of HIV structure we can discuss the etiology and pathogenesis of AIDS.

ETIOLOGY AND PATHOGENESIS. As mentioned earlier the *evidence linking HIV-1 in the causation of AIDS is strong.*[131,138] The virus has been isolated repeatedly from the lymphoid cells, semen, vaginal secretions, saliva, breast milk, tears, urine, serum, and cerebrospinal fluid of patients with AIDS and those at

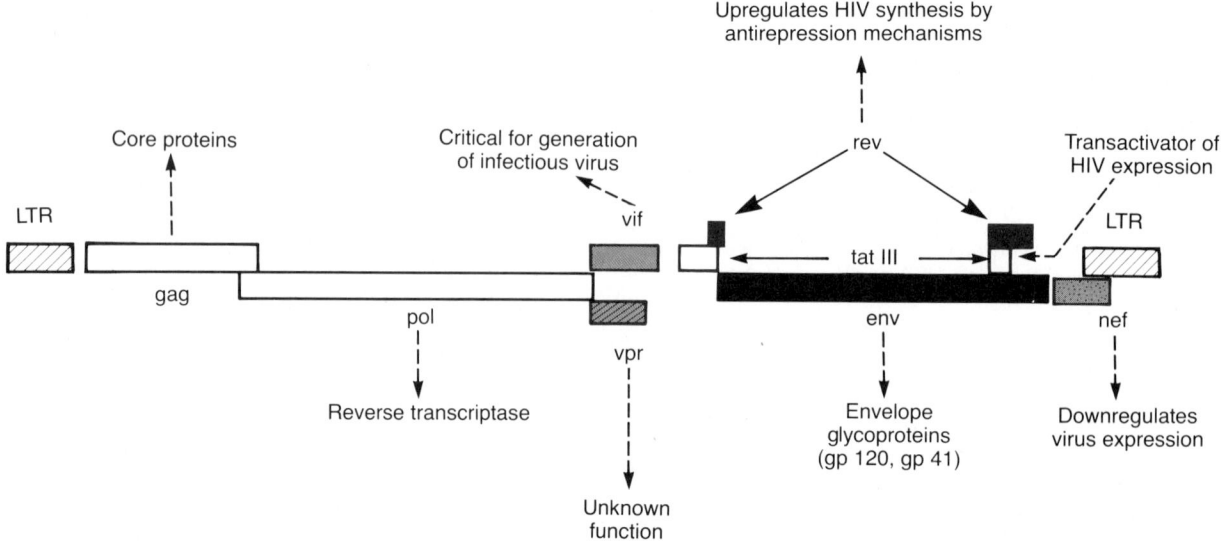

Figure 5–49. HIV proviral genome. The eight identified genes of HIV and their recognized functions are illustrated. The genes outlined in red are unique to HIV; others are shared by all retroviruses. (Modified from Fauci, A.S.: The human immunodeficiency virus: infectivity and mechanism of pathogenesis. Science *239:*617, 1988.)

risk of developing AIDS. In no instance has HIV-1 been recovered from a normal donor. Antibodies to HIV-1 envelope and core proteins have been found in more than 90% of patients with AIDS; by contrast, antibodies are almost never detected in healthy populations outside the defined risk groups. Several methods have been used to detect anti-HIV antibodies; these include the enzyme-linked immunosorbent (ELISA) technique, which is generally used for screening, and if the results are positive they are confirmed by the more specific Western blot analysis. Furthermore, the simian immunodeficiency virus (SIV) has similar genetic organization as HIV-1 and cross reacts with it serologically, causing an AIDS-like illness in captive macaques.

Based on accumulating evidence summarized in several recent publications,[126,127,133] the following discussion covers the mode of HIV infection and subsequent development of AIDS. This will be presented under five broad headings:

- Transmission of HIV-1
- HIV infection of lymphocytes and monocytes
- Central nervous system involvement by HIV
- HIV-associated changes in immune functions
- Natural history of HIV infection

Most of the information presented has been derived from studies with HIV-1, the causative agent of AIDS in the United States and Central Africa. HIV-2 causes a similar disease primarily in West Africa.[130,139] It is interesting to note that HIV-2 has greater (70%) sequence homology with SIV than with HIV-1 (40%), pointing to a possible common ancestry.

TRANSMISSION OF HIV-1. Transmission of HIV-1 occurs through one or more of three routes: *sexual contact, parenteral inoculation,* and *passage of the virus from infected mothers to their newborns.*

Venereal transmission is clearly the predominant mode of infection in the United States. Because the vast majority of patients in the United States are homosexual or bisexual males, most sexual transmission has occurred among homosexual men. The risk of infection increases with the number of sexual partners and with the frequency of anal receptive intercourse, which predisposes to rectal trauma in the receptive partner. It is believed that the virus is carried in lymphocytes present in the semen and enters the recipient's body through abrasions in rectal mucosa.[140] Heterosexual transmission, although currently of less quantitative importance in the United States, is probably the most common mode by which HIV is spread outside the U.S.A. (including Haiti).[141] Even in the United States, the rate of increase of heterosexual transmission is beginning to outpace transmission by other means. For example, whereas all newly reported cases of AIDS increased by 46% between August 1986 and August 1987, heterosexually transmitted cases (excluding those in persons born outside the United States) increased by 85% in the same period. Heterosexual spread has been documented in female sexual partners of intravenous drug abusers, hemophiliacs, and bisexual males with AIDS or at risk for AIDS. Although there is some evidence for increased risk with anal intercourse, most heterosexual transmission of HIV occurs with vaginal intercourse. In the United States heterosexual transmission is being largely perpetuated by intravenous drug abusers, and therefore the incidence of AIDS acquired by this route is highest in those areas with high prevalence of intravenous drug abuse (e.g., New York metropolitan area and Florida).

In contrast to the United States experience, heterosexual transmission seems to be the dominant mode of HIV infection in Africa. There are compelling epidemologic data that support this idea:

- The male-to-female ratio of cases of AIDS is approximately 1:1 in Africa, compared with 12:1 in the United States.
- The risk of seropositivity in Central and East Africa is associated with number of heterosexual partners each year, contact with prostitutes, and a history of sexually transmitted disease. Prostitutes in these areas have an extremely high prevalence of HIV-1 infection (25 to 88%).
- The highest rates of HIV-1 infection are seen in the sexually active age groups.
- Most importantly, 90% of AIDS patients in Africa have no identifiable risk factors, such as homosexuality and intravenous drug abuse.

Although male-to-female transmission is firmly established in both the United States and Africa, the frequency and risk of female-to-male spread is not as clear. HIV-1 has been found in vaginal and cervical secretions and more recently in monocytes and endothelial cells within the submucosa of the uterine cervix[142]; therefore, female-to-male transmission may well occur. For reasons not entirely clear, it seems that this mode of HIV-1 transmission is not particularly common in the United States,[143,144] but it may well be important in the spread of AIDS in Africa.[145]

Parenteral transmission of HIV occurs in three groups of individuals: intravenous drug abusers, hemophiliacs who receive factor VIII concentrates, and random recipients of blood transfusion. Of these three, intravenous drug abusers constitute by far the largest group and the one in which spread is the most difficult to control. Transmission occurs by sharing of needles, syringes, and other paraphernalia contaminated with HIV-containing blood. This group occupies a pivotal position in the AIDS epidemic because it represents the principal link in the transmission of HIV-1 to other adult populations through heterosexual activity.

Transfusion-associated AIDS has been caused by as little as one unit of whole blood, but it is more often related to transfusion of pooled blood components from multiple donors, as in the case of hemophiliacs, who receive lyophilized factor VIII concentrates. As might be expected, blood transfusion is an extremely efficient mechanism of transmission, with approximately 90% of those who receive infected blood developing HIV infection.[126] Fortunately, the screening of donated blood for anti-HIV antibodies, inactivation of the virus by heat treatment of clotting factor concentrates, and more rigid exclusion of donors at risk for AIDS since 1985 have substantially reduced the risk of transfusion-associated AIDS. Nevertheless, a very small but definite risk of acquiring HIV-1 by blood transfusions persists. The reasons for this are two fold; first, the antibody test for HIV-1 is not foolproof. False-negative tests, although very infrequent (four to five per million donors screened) do occur. Second, as is discussed later, antibodies may take three to 17 weeks to develop ("window period") following HIV-1 infection. During this period, seronegative blood may well be infectious.[146]

Finally, *perinatal transmission* could occur during pregnancy or in the immediate postpartum period. Infection *in utero* by the transplacental route has been documented.[147] Other possible routes of transmission include exposure to maternal blood and other infected fluids during birth, and transmission through breast milk. Precise estimates of the rate of perinatal transmission are lacking because the serum of infants born to HIV-infected mothers contains maternally derived antibodies, and therefore diagnosis based on serologic findings alone is difficult. Regardless of the precise route or rate of perinatal transmission, it is clear that in the United States approximately 80% of children with AIDS are known to have an HIV-infected parent.

Because of the uniformly fatal outcome of AIDS, there has been much concern in the lay public and among health care workers regarding the spread of HIV-1 outside the high-risk groups. However, results obtained from several studies (summarized in references 126 and 127) indicate that AIDS cannot be transmitted by casual (nonsexual) contact, even within a family unit (where family members shared household facilities, including beds, toilets, kitchens, and eating utensils). Furthermore, the risk of acquiring AIDS by occupational exposure to patients infected with HIV-1 or to HIV-1–containing fluids is extremely small. By mid-1988, the CDC had data on 15 health care workers worldwide who had acquired HIV-1 infection with no reported nonoccupational risk factors. In almost every case the infection was acquired parenterally by needlestick injury or contact of nonintact skin with infected blood in laboratory accidents. The current estimates suggest that the risk of seroconversion after accidental needlestick exposure is approximately 0.5%, and lower with other forms of exposure.[125] Although it is comforting to note that the risk of occupation-related HIV-1 infection is extremely small, it is imperative that all health care workers abide by the safety guidelines issued by the CDC.[148]

HIV INFECTION OF LYMPHOCYTES AND MONOCYTES. Critical to the pathogenesis of AIDS is the depletion of the CD4+ helper T cells; therefore attention is focused first on the events that lead to the infection and destruction of CD4+ T cells, after which HIV infection of monocytes and its consequences are discussed (Fig. 5–50).

There is abundant evidence that *the CD4 molecule is in fact the high-affinity receptor for HIV-1, HIV-2, and the related SIV (STLV-III)*. Infection with HIV involves binding of the envelope glycoprotein gp120 with the CD4 molecule, followed by internalization of the virus. This explains the selective tropism of HIV for the CD4+ T cells and its ability to infect other CD4+ cells, particularly macrophages. The molecular mechanisms that underlie this initial step in the HIV life cycle are not entirely clear but are the subject of intense investigation. The search is on to precisely map the HIV-binding domains on the CD4 protein[149] and attempts are also under way to localize the CD4 binding region of HIV gp120.[150] Insights derived from such investigations may allow the development of therapeutic tools that limit or prevent HIV infection by preventing CD4-gp120 interactions.

Once internalized, the viral genome undergoes reverse transcription leading to the formation of proviral DNA that is integrated into the host genome. The proviral DNA is then transcribed to form genomic RNA and mRNA. Translation of viral mRNA results in the formation of the HIV proteins. Some of these, such as *tat III, rev,* and *vif,* have regulatory functions mentioned earlier; others, such as the products of *env, pol* and *gag* genes, are assembled with the genomic mRNA; and finally the complete virion particles bud from the cell surface. *It is important to note that the steps following integration of proviral DNA into the host genome occur only when the infected cell is activated, as may occur with antigenic stimulation of helper T cells.* In an inactive cell, the viral life cycle is restricted at the stage of integration and the infection enters a *latent phase,* which may have a bearing on the natural history of HIV infection, to be discussed later.

As mentioned earlier, depletion of CD4+ T cells is a key event in the causation of AIDS. But how T cells are destroyed is far from clear. Several possibilities, each supported by at least some experimental data, have been suggested.[151]

• A feature peculiar to HIV, not shared by many other retroviruses, is the accumulation of large amounts of unintegrated proviral DNA in the host cell. Evidence from some other virus systems suggests that such accumulation may cause cell death, but the precise mechanism remains mysterious.

• CD4–viral glycoprotein interactions seem to be intimately involved in inducing cell death. The major support for this notion comes from the observation that whereas some monocytes and macrophages express CD4 and can be infected with HIV, these cells are quite refractory to cytopathic effects. Because the density of the CD4 molecule on monocytes is significantly lower than on helper T cells, it is possible that the level of CD4 on the target cell surface may be a determinant of the cytopathic effect.

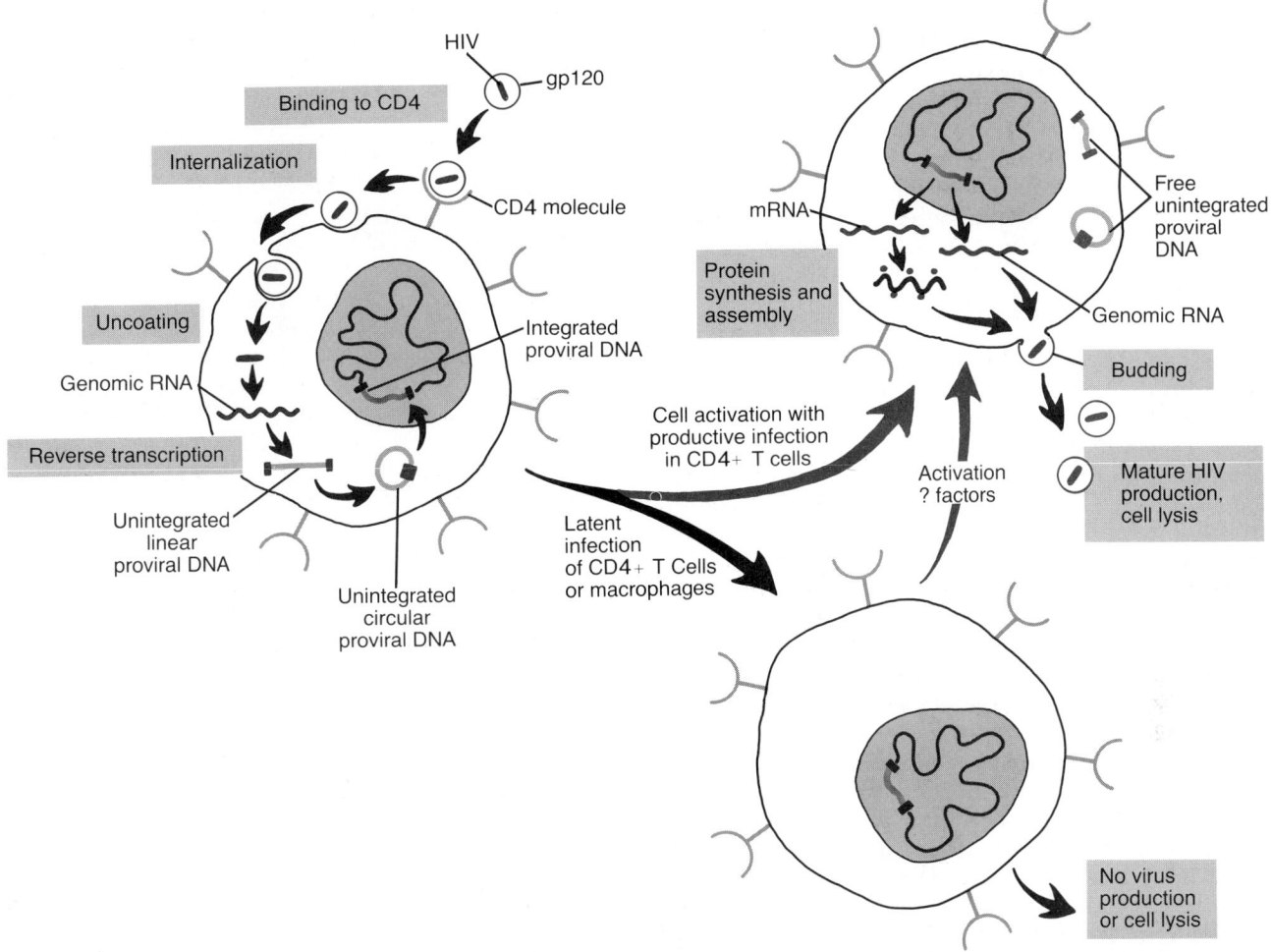

Figure 5–50. The life cycle of HIV. CD4+ target cells (T cells, macrophages) are infected. Productive infection (top right) leads to cytopathic effects, whereas cells with latent infection (bottom right) survive and may persist for prolonged periods. (Modified from Fauci, A.S.: The human immunodeficiency virus: infectivity and mechanism of pathogenesis. Science 239:617, 1988.)

• Fusion of infected cells with formation of syncytia (giant cells) may be a mechanism of cell death. In tissue culture, the gp120 expressed on productively infected cells binds to the CD4 molecules on uninfected T cells, followed by cell fusion. Fused cells develop "ballooning" and usually die within 48 hours.
• Autoimmune reactions may occur against lymphocytes that express *env* glycoproteins (gp120). Surface expression of gp120 may occur in cells that are infected with HIV or in uninfected CD4+ cells that are coated with circulating gp 120.

Because only a very small fraction of circulating cells (approximately 1 in 10^5) of AIDS patients express viral mRNA or surface proteins at any given time, mechanisms other than direct cytolysis have also been suggested to explain the profound T-cell deficiency. For example, it is possible that a CD4 T cell precursor (expected to occur in a low frequency) may be infected with HIV, resulting in impaired production of mature CD4+ cells. Speculations abound,

but definitive data are scarce, and this continues to be one of the many peculiarities of HIV infection that currently defy explanation.

In addition to quantitative defects in CD4+ cells, there are qualitative defects as well. Best characterized is the inability of CD4+ cells to respond to antigens even when the antigen is presented by normal HLA-compatible antigen-presenting cells. This defect can be detected early in the course of HIV infection, prior to severe depletion of CD4+ cells. The functional impairment of CD4+ T cells may be explained in a variety of ways. Following HIV infection, the CD4-HIV complex is internalized and the T cell no longer expresses CD4 molecules. Even if the infection remains latent (i.e., the T cell survives), such a cell would not be able to respond to antigen, because CD4 molecules must interact with class II MHC antigens during antigen recognition (p. 171).

Although depletion of CD4+ cells is the most dramatic outcome of HIV infection, *it is now apparent that monocytes and macrophages express CD4 and are infected by HIV. However, unlike CD4+ T cells, mon-*

ocytes are relatively refractory to the cytopathic effects of HIV. This has two important implications: first, monocytes and macrophages may well be the major reservoir for HIV in the body, and second, they provide a safe vehicle for HIV to be transported to various parts of the body, particularly the central nervous system. Another subtle but perhaps equally important consequence of monocyte infection may be direct transfer of HIV from the monocytes to CD4+ T cells when the two cells come in close contact in the process of antigen presentation.

Low-level chronic or latent infection of T cells and monocytes is probably an important feature of HIV infection. It is widely believed that integrated provirus, without virus expression (latent infection) could remain in the cells from months to years, thus accounting for the long, often variable incubation period of AIDS. Completion of the viral life cycle in latently infected cells occurs only following cell activation, which in the case of CD4+ T cells results in cell lysis. Such activation in vivo may result from antigenic stimulation especially by other infecting microorganisms, such as CMV, EBV, hepatitis B virus, or herpes simplex virus. The life style of most AIDS patients in the United States places them at increased risk of recurrent exposure to other sexually transmitted diseases, and in Africa, socioeconomic conditions probably impose a higher burden of chronic microbial infections. There may be other, as yet unidentified, noninfectious cofactors that may affect the duration of latent infection and hence the incubation period. Much needs to be learned about the influences that awaken HIV from its slumber within the host cell DNA because once aroused the "submicroscopic giant" is virtually unstoppable.

CENTRAL NERVOUS SYSTEM INVOLVEMENT BY HIV. The pathogenesis of neurologic manifestations deserves special mention because, in addition to the lymphoid system, the nervous system is a major target of HIV infection. Three potential mechanisms capable of causing neuronal injury have been suggested (Fig. 5–51).

• *Monocyte-macrophage mediated effects.* According to this view, infected monocytes act as a vehicle ("the Trojan horse") for entry of HIV into the brain. Once in the brain, the monocytes are somehow activated to release cytokines and enzymes that either are directly toxic to neurons or recruit other tissue-damaging inflammatory cells. The pivotal role of monocytes in the pathogenesis of neurologic manifestations is supported by the detection of HIV footprints (mRNA, envelope glycoprotein antigens) in monocytes and multinucleated giant cells, derived by their fusion in cerebral lesions.

• *Direct infection of neuronal tissue or endothelial cells* may be involved as some reports point to the presence of HIV virions within neurons, oligodendrocytes, and astrocytes (reviewed in references 127 and 152) and CD4 on the surface of some of these cells. Infection of endothelial cells by HIV has also been reported,[153]

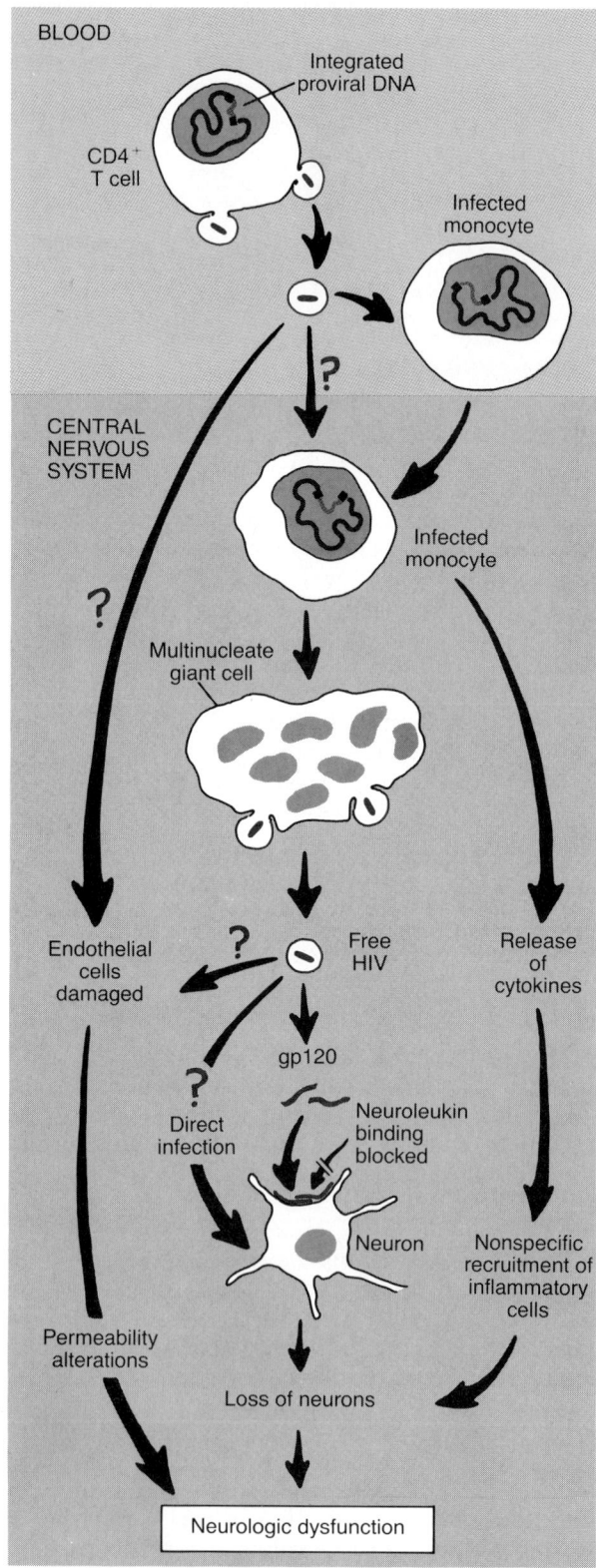

Figure 5–51. Possible mechanisms of HIV-induced central nervous system injury and dysfunction. (Adapted from Ho, D.D., et al.: Pathogenesis of infection with human immunodeficiency virus. New Engl. J. Med. 317:278, 1987.)

leading to the suggestion that permeability abnormalities in small vessels may disrupt the blood-brain barrier and cause neurologic dysfunction.

• *Involvement of neuroleukin.* A novel explanation of neurologic impairment is offered by some investigators who noted that neuroleukin, a growth factor for neurons, shares partial (30%) sequence homology with HIV-gp120.[154] In preliminary experiments, gp120 inhibited neuroleukin-induced growth of neurons, presumably by competing with neuroleukin for binding to the neurons (Fig. 5–51).

HIV-ASSOCIATED ALTERATIONS IN IMMUNE FUNCTIONS. As might be surmised from the discussion of pathogenesis and virology, there is a profound suppression of cell-mediated immunity. Loss of CD4+ cells leads to an inversion of CD4-to-CD8 ratio in the peripheral blood (Table 5–13). It may be recalled that the normal CD4-to-CD8 ratio is close to 2, whereas in patients with AIDS a ratio of 0.5 is not uncommon. Although inversion of CD4-to-CD8 ratio is a particularly consistent finding in AIDS, it should be noted that it is not diagnostic.

The loss of CD4+ cells has ripple effects on the function of other cells of the immune system (Fig. 5–52), because CD4+ helper-inducer cells are the source of lymphokines such as IL-2, IFN-γ, macrophage chemotactic factors, hematopoietic growth factors, and growth and differentiation factors (IL-4, IL-5) for B cells. Paradoxically, patients with AIDS typically have hypergammaglobulinemia and circulating immune complexes owing to polyclonal B-cell

Table 5–13. Major Abnormalities of Immune Function in AIDS

Lymphopenia
Predominantly due to selective loss of the CD4 + helper-inducer T cell subset; inversion of CD4-to-CD8 ratio
Decreased in vivo T-cell Function
Susceptibility to opportunistic infections
Susceptibility to neoplasms
Decreased delayed-type hypersensitivity
Altered in vitro T-cell Function
Decreased proliferative response to mitogens, alloantigens, and soluble antigens
Decreased specific cytotoxicity
Decreased helper function for pokeweed mitogen–induced B-cell immunoglobulin production
Decreased IL-2 and IFN-γ production
Polyclonal B-cell Activation
Hypergammaglobulinemia and circulating immune complexes
Inability to mount a de novo antibody response to a new antigen
Refractoriness to the normal signals for B-cell activation in vitro
Altered Monocyte or Macrophage Functions
Decreased chemotaxis
Decreased HLA class II antigen expression

activation. This may result from the influence of many factors, such as infection with CMV and EBV, both of which are polyclonal B cell activators; HIV glycoprotein may itself activate B cells. As mentioned earlier, gp120 shows sequence homology with neuroleukin, known to activate B cells. *Despite the presence of spontaneously activated B cells, patients with AIDS are unable to mount an antibody response to a new antigen.* This could in part be due to lack of T cell help, but

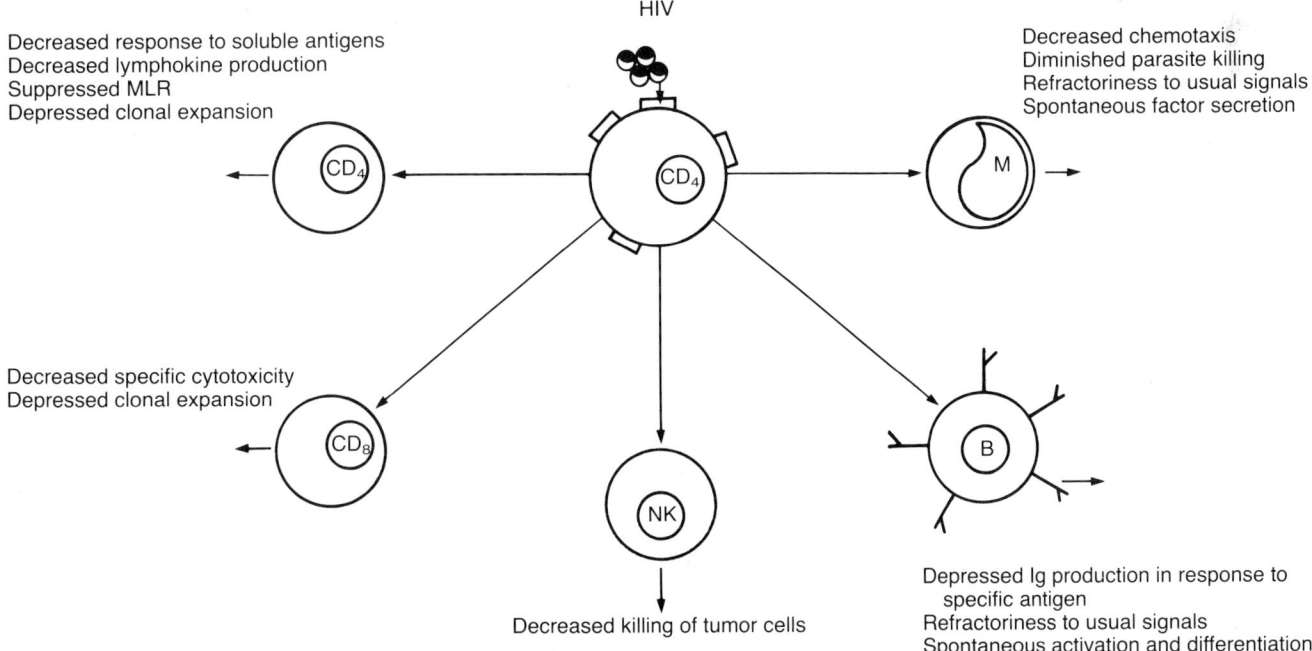

HIV

Decreased response to soluble antigens
Decreased lymphokine production
Suppressed MLR
Depressed clonal expansion

Decreased chemotaxis
Diminished parasite killing
Refractoriness to usual signals
Spontaneous factor secretion

Decreased specific cytotoxicity
Depressed clonal expansion

Depressed Ig production in response to specific antigen
Refractoriness to usual signals
Spontaneous activation and differentiation

Decreased killing of tumor cells

Figure 5–52. Modulation of the human immune system by direct infection by human immunodeficiency virus of the CD4 helper/inducer lymphocyte subset. Infection with HIV results in diverse functional defects due to the central role of the helper/inducer cell on other immune functions. These defects result in a lack of inductive function for other T cells, cytotoxic cells (natural killer [*NK*] and CD8), and monocytes *(M)* and a lack of helper function for the B cell *(B)*. MLR = mixed lymphocyte response. (Modified from Bowen, D.L., et al.: Immunopathogenesis of the acquired immunodeficiency syndrome. Ann. Intern. Med. *103*:704, 1985.)

there seem to be intrinsic defects in B cells as well. Impaired humoral immunity renders these patients prey to certain pyogenic infections, and it renders serologic diagnosis of certain infections such as syphilis unreliable.[155]

NATURAL HISTORY OF HIV INFECTION. We still do not have enough clinical, serologic, and virologic information to trace the entire course of events from the time of HIV infection to the development of AIDS. The initial response to virus infection seems to be the formation of antibodies that may be detected in the serum between three and 17 weeks following presumed exposure. What happens after seroconversion is an area of much uncertainty, and the outcome may depend on the existence of host (genetic) factors, viral strain, and the presence or absence of poorly defined cofactors (e.g., infections with other organisms that may activate T-helper cells). One possible sequence of events, ending in full-blown **AIDS**, is illustrated in Fig. 5–53 and outlined here.[127,156]

• *Acute illness* resembling influenza or infectious mononucleosis may develop in 30 to 50% of the pa-

tients. The symptoms include sore throat, myalgias, fever, rash, and sometimes aseptic meningitis. The peripheral blood may show changes resembling infectious mononucleosis.[157]

• *Persistent generalized lymphadenopathy* develops in some patients following the acute illness and in others without any previous signs or symptoms. Constitutional symptoms may be associated with lymphadenopathy; they are usually mild and at least in some cases reversible. Immunologic abnormalities (depletion of CD4+ cells) are generally modest.

• *AIDS-related complex* (ARC) is characterized by long-lasting fever (3 months or longer) that may be intermittent or continuous, weight loss, and diarrhea. The immunologic tests in patients with ARC are clearly abnormal; CD4+ cell count is usually reduced to a level two standard deviations or greater below normal and the CD4-to-CD8 ratio is reversed. In addition, anemia, thrombocytopenia, and hypergammaglobulinemia are also frequently present.

Several qualifying statements must be made regarding the sequence just outlined. *First,* there is a long and variable latent period between seroconver-

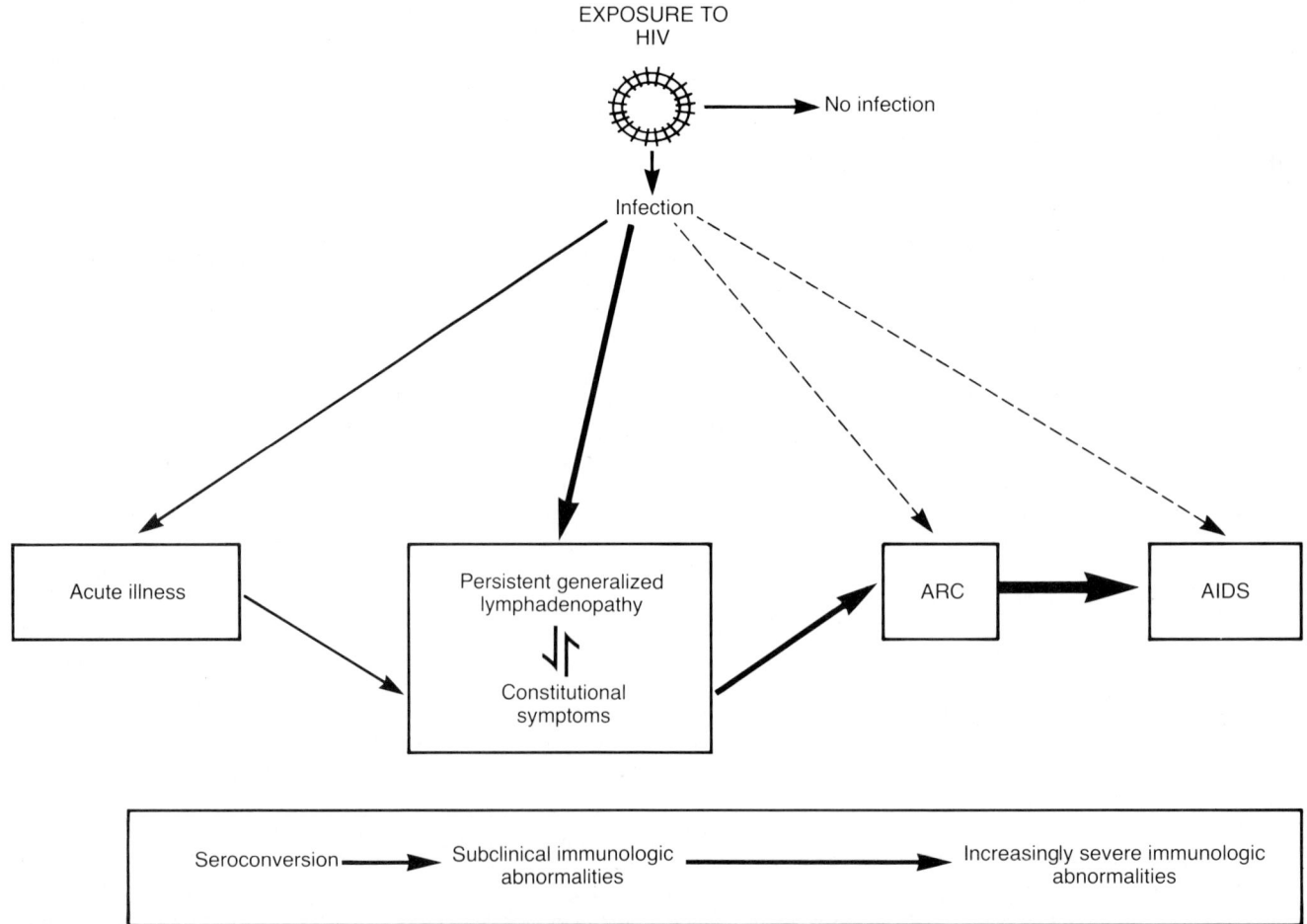

Figure 5–53. **Natural history of HIV infection, leading to the development of AIDS. The heavier arrows represent the most likely sequence of events. It is not clear whether the intermediate outcomes of HIV infection (e.g., persistent generalized lymphadenopathy) represent stages in the development of AIDS or, in some cases, stable end-points.**

sion and clinical expression of AIDS. The current estimates vary between two and eight years.[126] The duration of the incubation period depends on the mode of transmission (e.g., parenteral versus sexually acquired) as well as on the previously discussed factors that may convert latent infection to productive cytopathic infection. *Second,* it is still not proved that all individuals who have been infected (as indicated by seroconversion) will develop AIDS. Current estimates suggest that 25 to 35% of those who are infected develop AIDS in five to seven years. Because of the long and variable incubation period, much longer follow-up of large cohorts, currently in progress, will be required to ascertain the precise percentage of seropositive individuals who develop AIDS. *Third,* the intermediate outcomes of HIV-1 infection (e.g., seropositive asymptomatic carriers, persistent generalized lymphadenopathy without constitutional symptoms) could well be stages in the progression of AIDS,[156] but in some they may be stable endpoints of uncertain duration and clinical relevance.[158] In general it seems that the CD4+ counts are of predictive value; patients with the most extensive or rapid fall of CD4+ cells are the most likely to develop AIDS. Hence, it is reasonable to assume that patients with ARC are at the greatest risk of developing AIDS.

CLINICAL FEATURES. Most of the clinical manifestations of HIV infection can be surmised from the foregoing discussion, and therefore we offer only a brief summary here. In the United States the typical patient with fully developed AIDS is a young homosexual male or an intravenous drug abuser, presenting with fever, weight loss, and persistent generalized lymphadenopathy. Pneumonia caused by the opportunistic protozoan *Pneumocystis carinii,* which rarely affects healthy individuals, is seen in approximately 50% of cases. A variety of other (often multiple) opportunistic infections, including CMV, candidiasis, toxoplasmosis, herpes virus infections, and infections caused by typical and atypical mycobacteria have also been found in these patients (Table 5–12). Recent studies have begun to identify a wide spectrum of pyogenic bacterial infections as well, related presumably to defects in humoral immunity.[159] About 25% of patients present with Kaposi's sarcoma, a multicentric neoplasm that is extremely rare in the United States (p. 591). Unlike the course of sporadic cases, Kaposi's sarcoma in patients with AIDS follows an aggressive clinical course. It should be noted that Kaposi's sarcoma is unevenly distributed among the various risk groups for AIDS. It is far more common among homosexual men than among IV drug abusers or patients belonging to other risk groups. In addition to Kaposi's sarcoma, several other tumors, mostly lymphoid, have been reported in patients with AIDS. These include non-Hodgkin's lymphomas, Burkitt's lymphoma, and Hodgkin's disease. The last-mentioned has an atypical, particularly aggressive course in AIDS patients.[160]

As discussed earlier, involvement of the CNS has emerged as a significant problem in the AIDS population. Seventy-five to 90% of patients demonstrate some form of neurologic involvement at autopsy, and in many there are clinical manifestations as well. Sometimes neurologic manifestations may be the sole or the earliest presenting feature of AIDS.[161] At least four syndromes—an acute aseptic meningitis, a subacute encephalitis, a vacuolar myelopathy, and a peripheral neuropathy—have been described (p. 1398).[152]

MORPHOLOGY. The anatomic changes in the tissues (with the exception of lesions in the brain) are neither specific nor diagnostic.[162,163] In general the pathologic features of AIDS are those characteristic of widespread opportunistic infections, Kaposi's sarcoma, and lymphoid tumors. Most of these lesions have been discussed elsewhere, because they also occur in non-AIDS patients. To appreciate the distinctive nature of lesions in the CNS, they are discussed in the context of other disorders affecting the brain (p. 1398). Some recent studies point to the existence of an AIDS-associated nephropathy[164] that is also described later (p. 1037). Here we concentrate on changes in the lymphoid organs.

Biopsy specimens from enlarged lymph nodes in the early stages of AIDS or ARC reveal nonspecific follicular hyperplasia with mild or minimal paracortical hyperplasia. Hyperplastic follicles are often devoid of mantle zone lymphocytes, but they are usually well demarcated and can be distinguished from follicular lymphoma (a neoplasm) (p. 712). The medulla shows intense plasmacytosis. These changes, affecting primarily the B-cell areas of the node, are the morphologic counterparts of the polyclonal B-cell activation and hypergammaglobulinemia that is seen in patients with AIDS (p. 231). In addition to changes in the follicles, the sinuses show increased cellularity due primarily to an increase in histiocytes, but contributed to also by immunoblasts (B cells) and plasma cells.

With the onset of full-blown AIDS, the frenzy of B-cell proliferation subsides and gives way to a pattern of severe follicular involution and generalized lymphocyte depletion. These "burned-out" lymph nodes are usually seen at autopsy and may harbor numerous opportunistic pathogens. **Because of profound immunosuppression, the inflammatory response to infections both in the lymph nodes and at extranodal sites may be sparse or atypical.** For example, mycobacteria do not evoke granuloma formation because CD4+ cells are deficient. In the empty appearing lymph nodes and in other organs the presence of infectious agents may not be readily apparent without the application of special stains. As might be expected, lymphoid depletion is not confined to the nodes; in later stages of AIDS, spleen and thymus also appear to be "wastelands."

Many tumors prey upon patients with AIDS (Table 5–12). Non-Hodgkin's lymphomas, involving the nodes as well as extranodal sites such as liver, gastrointestinal tract, and bone marrow, are second only to Kaposi's sarcoma in frequency. They are primarily high-grade diffuse B-cell neoplasms (p. 714). It may well be that the origin of these tumors is related to long-term polyclonal B-cell proliferation in the face of deteriorating T cell immunity, as has been postulated for the evolution of Burkitt's lymphoma (p. 734). Indeed, cytogenetic changes similar to those noted in Burkitt's tumor have also been found in the AIDS lymphomas.

AIDS: THE FUTURE.

Since the discovery of AIDS in 1981, and its causative agent in 1983–1984, there have been significant advances in our understanding of this disorder. That the AIDS epidemic was recognized quite early in its course, and the etiologic agent discovered rapidly thereafter, is a tribute to the concerted efforts of epidemiologists, immunologists, and molecular virologists. Despite the rapid, rather hectic pace of progress in AIDS research, the prognosis of patients with AIDS remains dismal. A recent study estimated an 85% five-year mortality.[165] With time, true mortality is likely to approach 100%. Although the causative virus has been identified, it has proved to be extremely complex and hence many hurdles will have to be crossed before a vaccine can be developed.[166] Among these hurdles are the following.

- Recent molecular analyses have revealed an alarming degree of variability (polymorphism) in the extracellular envelope glycoprotein (gp120) of HIV isolates[167] obtained from different, and sometimes the same, patients. However this variation is not randomly distributed throughout the *env* gene. Several constant and variable domains have been identified. In constant domains the sequence homology is greater than 80% among different isolates, but in the most variable domains, sequence conservation is 20 to 30%. This degree of variability has profound clinical implications. If the variable regions are important antigenic targets for an immune response, the task of vaccine development may be extremely difficult. However, the presence of conserved regions within gp120 offers some hope. It is likely that they contain amino acid sequences that are critical for those properties of HIV that are shared by all strains. These would include binding to CD4, internalization, and infectivity. There is some suggestion that conserved sequences may evoke neutralizing antibody responses.[168]
- We still know little about the nature of protective immunity against HIV. Patients with AIDS have antibodies against HIV, but they do not seem to be protective. Is resistance predominantly cell-mediated? If so, the antigens that can induce protective cellular immunity have to be identified. Because several strains of HIV may infect a person, a recurrent selection for a weakly immunogenic variant may occur in vivo, frustrating the induction of protective immunity.
- Even if protective antibodies or cells could be generated, only cells expressing the viral antigens would be eliminated. HIV that exists in a latent form in vivo may well escape immune destruction. We still do not know enough about latency and the mechanisms that convert latent to active infection.

Despite all its wiles, the HIV cannot be long on the loose, surrounded as it is by an army of investigators in hot pursuit.

Currently, the only antiviral drug that is of some value to the treatment of AIDS is 3'-azido-3'-deoxythymidine (AZT). As an inhibitor of reverse transcriptase, it is a logical choice.[169] The ongoing research into the function of genes unique to the HIV family (e.g, *tat III, rev*) may well yield novel therapeutic agents that inhibit viral replication or activation by affecting the function of these gene products.

We must close this discussion on the somber note that despite the frantic, almost dizzying pace at which AIDS research is proceeding, it is unlikely that a vaccine suitable for mass prophylaxis or a magic drug will appear on the horizon in the immediate future. Hence efforts to stem the tide of the AIDS epidemic must continue to be focused on preventive measures.

---

1. Royer, H.D., and Reinherz, E.L.: T lymphocytes: Ontogeny, function and relevance to clinical disorders. N. Engl. J. Med. *317*:1136, 1987.

2. Davis, M.M.: Molecular genetics of T-cell antigen receptors. Hosp. Pract. *23*:157, 1988.

3. Clevers, H., et al.: The T cell receptor/CD3 complex: A dynamic protein ensemble. Ann. Rev. Immunol. *6*:629, 1988.

4. Zola, H.: The surface antigens of human B lymphocytes. Immunol. Today *8*:308, 1987.

5. Johnston, R.G., Jr.: Monocytes and macrophages. N. Engl. J. Med. *318*:747, 1988.

6. Nathan, C.F.: Secretory products of macrophages. J. Clin. Invest. *79*:319, 1987.

7. Ortaldo, J.R., and Longo, D.L.: Human natural lymphocyte effector cells: Definition, analysis of activity, and clinical effectiveness. J. Natl. Cancer Inst. *80*:999, 1988.

8. Rosenberg, S.A. (moderator): New approaches to the immunotherapy of cancer using interleukin-2. Ann. Intern. Med. *108*:853, 1988.

9. Smith, K.A.: Interleukin-2: Inception, impact, and implication. Science *240*:1169, 1988.

10. Dinarello, C.A., and Mier, J.W.: Lymphokines. N. Engl. J. Med. *317*:940, 1987.

11. Cerami A., and Beutler, B.: The role of cachetin/TNF in endotoxic shock and cachexia. Immunol. Today *8*:280, 1988.

12. Miyajima, A., et al.: Co-ordinate regulation of immune and inflammatory responses by T-cell derived lymphokines. FASEB J. *2*:2462, 1988.

13. Billian, A.: Gamma-interferon: The match that lights the fire. Immunol. Today *9*:37, 1988.

14. Male, D., et al.: Advanced Immunology. Philadelphia, J. B. Lippincott Co., 1987, p. 51.

15. Bach, F., and Sachs, D.H.: Transplantation immunology. N. Engl. J. Med. *317*:489, 1987.

16. Spies, T., et al.: Genes for the tumor necrosis factor α and β are linked to the human major histocompatibility complex. Proc. Natl. Acad. Sci. U.S.A. *83*:8699, 1986.

17. Zabriskie, J.B., and Gibofsky A.: Genetic control of susceptibility to infection with pathogenic bacteria. Curr. Top. Microbiol. Immunol. *124*:1, 1986.

18. Shoenfeld, Y., and Isenberg, D.A.: Mycobacteria and autoimmunity. Immunol. Today *9*:178, 1988.

19. Serafin, W.E., and Austen, K.F.: Mediators of immediate hypersensitivity reactions. N. Engl. J. Med. *317*:30, 1987.

20. Ishizaka, T., et al.: IgE-mediated triggering signals for mediator release from human mast cells and basophils. Fed. Proc. *43*:2840, 1984.

21. Friedman, M.M., and Kaliner, M.A.: Human mast cells and asthma. Am. Rev. Resp. Dis. *135*:1157, 1987.

22. Kaliner, M.A.: The late phase reaction and its clinical implications. Hosp. Pract. *22*:73, 1987.

23. Ishizaka, T., et al.: Activation of mast cells and basophils for mediator release. Int. Arch. Allergy Appl. Immunol. *82*:327, 1987.

24. Lichtenstein, L.M.: The nasal late-phase response — an in vivo model. Hosp. Pract. *23*:119, 1988.

25. Pipkorn, U., et al.: Inhibition of mediator release in allergic rhinitis by pretreatment with topical glucocorticoids. N. Engl. J. Med. *317*:1506, 1987.

26. Capon, A., et al.: From parasites to allergy: A second receptor for IgE. Immunol. Today 7:15, 1986.

27. Lawley, J.J., et al.: A prospective clinical and immunologic analysis of patients with serum sickness. N. Engl. J. Med. *311*:1407, 1984.

28. Mannik, M.: Mechanisms of tissue deposition of immune complexes. J. Rheumatol. *13*(Suppl. 14):35, 1987.

29. Dvorak, H.F., et al.: Cellular and vascular manifestations of cell-mediated immunity. Hum. Pathol. *17*:122, 1986.

30. Young, J.D., and Liu, C.: Multiple mechanisms of lymphocyte-mediated killing. Immunol. Today 9:140, 1988.

31. Kirkpatrick, C.H.: Transplantation immunology. JAMA *258*: 2993, 1987.

32. Mason, D.W., and Morris, P.J.: Effector mechanisms in allograft rejection. Ann. Rev. Immunol. *4*:119, 1986.

33. Helderman, J.H., et al.: The interleukin 2 receptor detected by fine-needle aspiration specimens. Transplant. Proc. *20*:675, 1988.

34. Busch, G., et al.: Human renal allografts: Analysis of lesions in long-term survivals. Hum. Pathol. *2*:253, 1971.

35. Porter, K.A.: Renal transplantation. In Heptinstall, R.H.: Pathology of the Kidney. Boston, Little, Brown & Co., 1983, p. 1455.

36. McPhaul, J.J., et al.: Renal transplantation: Some contemporary problems. In Wilson, C.B., et al. (eds.): Immunologic Mechanisms of Renal Disease. New York, Churchill Livingstone, 1979, p. 323.

37. Mandel, T.E.: Transplantation: 1988 Immunol. Today *10*:1, 1989.

38. The Canadian Multicenter Transplant Study Group: A randomized clinical trial of cyclosporine in cadaveric renal transplantation. N. Engl. J. Med. *314*:1219, 1986.

39. Sabesin, S.M., and Williams, J. W.: Current status of liver transplantation. Hosp. Pract. *22*:75, 1987.

40. Snover, D.C., et al.: Liver allograft rejection. An analysis of the use of biopsy in determining outcome of rejection. Am. J. Surg. Pathol. *11*:1,1987.

41. Storb, R.: Critical issues in bone marrow transplantation. Transpl. Proc. *19*:2774, 1987.

42. Murphy, W.J., et al.: Acute rejection of murine bone marrow allografts by NK cells and T cells: Differences in kinetics and target cells recognized. J. Exp. Med. *166*:1499, 1987.

43. Rose, N.R., and Mackey, I.R. (eds.): The Autoimmune Diseases. Orlando, Fl, Academic Press, Inc., 1985.

44. Nossal, G.J.V.: Cellular mechanism of immunologic tolerance. Am. Rev. Immunol. *1*:33, 1983.

45. Theofilopoulos, A.N.: Autoimmunity. In Stites, D.P., et al. (eds.): Basic and Clinical Immunology, 6th edition. Los Altos, CA, Appleton and Lange, 1987, p. 29.

46. Asherson, G.L., et al.: An overview of T-suppressor cell circuits. Ann. Rev. Immunol. *4*:37, 1986.

47. Gibson, J., et al.: A role of suppressor T cells in induction of self-tolerance. Proc. Natl. Acad. Sci. U.S.A. *82*:5150, 1985.

48. Burdette, S., and Schwartz, R.S.: Idiotypes and idiotypic networks. N. Engl. J. Med. *317*:219, 1987.

49. Kantor, F.S.: Autoimmunities: Diseases of dysregulation. Hosp. Pract. *23*:75, 1988.

50. Goodman, M.G., and Weigle, W.O.: Role of polyclonal B cell activation in self/non-self discrimination. Immunol. Today 2:54, 1981.

51. Horowitz, D.A.: Functional properties of CD8 positive lymphocyte subjects in systemic lupus erythematosus. J. Rheumatol. *14*(Suppl. 13):49, 1987.

52. Rose, N.R., et al.: Genetic control of autoimmune disease. In Rose, N.R., et al. (eds.): Developments in Immunology, Vol. 1. New York, Elsevier/North Holland, 1978.

53. Shoenfeld, Y., and Schwartz, R.S.: Immunologic and genetic factors in autoimmune disease. N. Engl. J. Med. *311*:1019, 1984.

54. Todd, J.A., et al.: A molecular basis for MHC Class II – associated autoimmunity. Science *240*:1003, 1988.

55. Michet, C.J., Jr., et al.: Epidemiology of systemic lupus erythematosus and other connective tissue diseases in Rochester, Minnesota, 1950 through 1979. Mayo Clin. Proc. *60*:105, 1985.

56. Christian, C.L., and Elkon, K.B.: Auto-antibodies to intra-cellular antigens. Am. J. Med. *80*:53, 1986.

57. Tan, E.M., et al.: Antinuclear antibodies (ANAs): Diagnostically specific immune markers and clues towards understanding systemic autoimmunity. Clin. Immunol. Immunopathol. *47*:121, 1988.

58. Schwartz, R.S.: Monoclonal lupus autoantibodies. Immunol. Today *4*:68, 1983.

59. Jacob, L., et al.: Human systemic lupus erythematosus sera contain antibodies against cell-surface proteins that share epitopes with DNA. Proc. Natl. Acad. Sci. U.S.A. *83*:6970, 1986.

60. Rauch, J., et al.: Polyfunctional properties of hybridoma lupus anticoagulant antibodies. J. Rheumatol. *14*(Suppl. 13):132, 1987.

61. Hess, E.: Drug-related lupus. N. Engl. J. Med. *318*:1460, 1988.

62. Sthoeger, Z.M., et al.: Regulation of the immune response by sex-hormones. I. In vitro effects of estradiol and testosterone on pokeweed mitogen-induced human B cell differentiation. J. Immunol. *141*:91, 1988.

63. Lahita, R.G.: The influence of sex hormones on the disease systemic lupus erythematosus. Springer Seminar Immunopathol. *9*:305, 1986.

64. Graninger, W., et al.: Etiologic and pathogenetic aspects of systemic lupus erythematosus: A critical approach. In Smolen, J.S., and Zielinski, C.C. (eds.): Systemic Lupus Erythematosus: Clinical and Experimental Aspects. New York, Springer-Verlag, 1987, p. 6.

65. Horowitz D.A.: Lymphocytes and immunoregulation in SLE. In Wallace, D.J., and Dubois, E.L. (eds.): Dubois' Lupus Erythematosus. 3rd ed. Philadelphia, Lea & Febiger, 1987, p. 194.

66. Pisetsky, D.S.: Systemic lupus erythematosus. Med. Clin. North Am. *70*:337, 1986.

67. Laskin, C.A., and Smith, H.R.: Relevance of murine models of systemic lupus erythematosus to human disease. In Smolen, J.S., and Zielinski, C.C. (eds.): Systemic Lupus Erythematosus: Clinical and Experimental Aspects. New York, Springer-Verlag, 1987, p. 73.

68. Mihara, M., et al.: Immunologic abnormality in NZB/NZW F1 mice: Thymus-independent occurrence of B cell abnormality and requirement for T cells in the development of autoimmune disease as evidenced by analysis of the athymic nude individuals. J. Immunol. *141*:85, 1988.

69. Morimoto, C., et al.: A defect of immunoregulatory T cell subsets in systemic lupus erythematosus patients demonstrated by anti 2H4 antibody. J. Clin. Invest. *79*:762, 1987.

70. Silva, F.G.: The nephropathies of systemic lupus erythematosus. In Rosen, S. (ed.): Contemporary Issues in Surgical Pathology, Vol. I. Pathology of Glomerular Diseases. New York, Churchill Livingstone, 1983, p. 79.

71. Ulrich, W., and Syré, G.: Pathology. In Smolen, J.S., and Zielinski, C.C. (eds.): Systemic Lupus Erythematosus: Clinical and Experimental Aspects. New York, Springer-Verlag, 1987, p. 204.

72. Balow, J.E. (moderator): Lupus nephritis (NIH Conference). Ann. Intern. Med. *106*:79, 1987.

73. Gur, H., et al.: Chronic predominant interstitial nephritis in a patient with systemic lupus erythematosus: A follow up of three years and review of literature. Ann. Rheum. Dis. *46*:617, 1987.

74. Blaustein, H.G.: Neuropsychiatric manifestations of systemic lupus erythematosus. N. Engl. J. Med. *317*:309, 1987.

75. McCune, W.J., et al.: Clinical and immunologic effects of monthly administration of intravenous cyclophosphamide in severe systemic lupus erythematosus. N. Engl. J. Med. *318*:1423, 1988.

76. Ginzler, E., and Berg, A.: Mortality in systemic lupus erythematosus. J. Rheumatol. *14*(Suppl. 13):218, 1987.

77. Luger, T.A., and Bensch, D.: Cutaneous manifestations. In Smolen, J.S., and Zielinski, C.C. (eds.): Systemic Lupus Erythematosus: Clinical and Experimental Aspects. New York, Springer-Verlag, 1987, p. 227.

78. Sontheimer, R: Subacute cutaneous lupus erythematosus. Clin. Dermatol. *3*:58, 1985.

79. Woosley, R.L., et al.: Effect of acetylator phenotype on the rate at which procainamide induces antinuclear antibodies. N. Engl. J. Med. *298*:1157, 1987.

80. Totoritis, M.C., and Rubin, R.L.: Drug-induced lupus: Genetic, clinical and laboratory features. Postgrad. Med. *78*:149, 1985.

81. Fox, R.I., et al.: Primary Sjögren's syndrome: Clinical and immunopathologic features. Semin. Arthritis Rheum. *14*:77, 1984.

82. Provost, T., et al.: Sjögren's syndrome. Cutaneous, immunologic, and nervous system manifestations. Neurol. Clin. *5*:405, 1987.

83. Moutsopoulos, H.M.: Immunologic similarities and differences between systemic lupus erythematosus and Sjögren's syndrome. *In* Smolen, J.S., and Zielinski, C.C. (eds.): Systemic Lupus Erythematosus: Clinical and Experimental Aspects. New York, Springer-Verlag, 1987, p. 196.

84. Fox, R.I., et al.: Potential role of Epstein-Barr virus in Sjögren's syndrome. Rheum. Dis. Clin. North Am. *13*:275, 1987.

85. Rocco, V.K., and Hurd, E.R.: Scleroderma and scleroderma-like disorders. Semin. Arthritis Rheum. *16*:22, 1986.

86. Haustein, U.F., et al.: Pathogenisis of progressive systemic sclerosis. Int. J. Dermatol. *25*:286, 1986.

87. Padula, S.J., et al.: Cell-mediated immunity in rheumatic disease. Hum. Pathol. *17*:254, 1986.

88. Jorzabek-Chorzelska, M., et al.: Scl-70 antibody — a specific marker of systemic sclerosis. Br. J. Dermatol. *115*:393, 1986.

89. Leroy, E.C.: The vascular defect in scleroderma (systemic sclerosis). Acta Med. Scand. Suppl. *715*:165, 1987.

90. Oliver, J.A., and Cannon, P.J.: The kidney in scleroderma. Nephron *18*:141, 1977.

91. Owens, G.R., and Follansbee, W.P.: Cardiopulmonary manifestations of systemic sclerosis. Chest *91*:118, 1987.

92. Callen, J.P.: Dermatomyositis. DM *33*:237, 1987.

93. Hochberg, M.C., et al.: Adult onset polymyositis-dermatomyositis: An analysis of clinical and laboratory features and survival in 76 patients with a review of literature. Semin. Arthritis Rheum. *15*:168, 1986.

94. Christensen, M.L., et al.: Prevalence of Coxsackie B virus antibodies in patients with juvenile dermatomyositis. Arthritis Rheum. *11*:1365, 1986.

95. Walker, E.J., and Jeffrey, P.D.: Polymyositis and molecular mimicry, a mechanism of autoimmunity. Lancet *1*:605, 1986.

96. Callen, J.P.: Dermatomyositis. Neurol. Clin. *5*:379, 1987.

97. Leroy, E.C.: Systemic Sclerosis (Scleroderma). *In* Wyngaarden, J.B. and Smith, L.H. (eds.): Cecil Textbook of Medicine. 18th edition. Philadelphia, W.B. Saunders Co., 1988, p. 2021.

98. Cupps, T.R., and Fauci, A.S.: The Vasculitides. Philadelphia, W.B. Saunders Co., 1981.

99. Cohen, A.S., and Connors, L.E.: The pathogenesis and biochemistry of amyloidosis. J. Pathol. *151*:1, 1987.

100. Glenner, G.G.: Amyloid deposits and amyloidosis. The β-fibrilloses. N. Engl. J. Med. *302*:1333, 1980.

101. Caston, E.M., and Frangione, B.: Human amyloidosis, Alzheimer disease and related disorders. Lab. Invest. *58*:122, 1988.

102. Benson, M.D.: Hereditary amyloidosis — disease entity and clinical model. Hosp. Pract. *23*:125, 1988.

103. Anderton, B.H.: Alzheimer's disease. Progress in molecular pathology. Nature *325*:658, 1987.

104. Snow, A.D., et al.: Sulfated glycosaminoglycans: A common constituent of all amyloids? Lab. Invest. *56*:120, 1987.

105. Kyle, R.A., and Greipp, P.R.: Amyloidosis (AL): Clinical and laboratory features of 229 cases. Mayo Clin. Proc. *58*:665, 1983.

106. Neugarten J., et al.: Amyloidosis in subcutaneous heroin abusers. Am. J. Med. *81*:635, 1986.

107. Bardin, T., et al.: Synovial amyloidosis in patients undergoing long-term hemodialysis. Arthritis Rheum. *28*:1052, 1985.

108. Kyle, R.A.: Amyloidosis. Clin. Haematol. *11*:151, 1982.

109. Cornwell, G.G., et al.: Evidence that the amyloid fibril protein in senile systemic amyloidosis is derived from normal prealbumin. Biochem. Biophys. Res. Commun. *29*:648, 1988.

110. Chastonay, P., and Hurlimann, J.: Characterization of different amyloids with immunologic techniques. Pathol. Res. Pract. *181*:657, 1986.

111. Duston, M.A., et al.: Diagnosis of amyloidosis by abdominal fat aspiration. Analysis of four years' experience. Am. J. Med. *82*:412, 1987.

112. Gertz, M.A., et al.: Utility of subcutaneous fat aspiration for the diagnosis of systemic amyloidosis (immunoglobulin light chain). Arch. Intern. Med. *148*:929, 1988.

113. Primary immunodeficiency disease: Report of a World Health Organization study group. Clin. Immunol. Immunopathol. *40*:166, 1986.

114. Rosen, F.S., et al.: The primary immunodeficiencies. N. Engl. J. Med. *311*:235, 300, 1984.

115. Buckley, R.H.: Humoral immunodeficiency. Clin. Immunol. Immunopathol. *40*:13, 1986.

116. Buckley, R.H.: Immunodeficiency diseases. J.A.M.A. *258*:2841, 1987.

117. Ugazio, A.G., et al.: Recurrent infections in children with selective IgA deficiency. Birth Defects *19*:169, 1983.

118. Hong, R.M., et al.: Reconstitution of B- and T-lymphocyte function in severe combined immunodeficiency disease after transplantation with thymic epithelium. Lancet *2*:1270, 1976.

119. Pahwa, S.G., et al.: Heterogeneity of B-lymphocyte differentiation in severe combined immunodeficiency disease. J. Clin. Invest. *66*:543, 1980.

120. Hirschhorn, R.: Adenosine deaminase deficiency. Hosp. Pract. *22*:149, 1987.

121. Bierer, B.E., and Burakoff, S.J.: T-cell adhesion molecules. FASEB J. *2*:2584, 1988.

122. Anderson, D.C., and Springer, T.A.: Leukocyte adhesion deficiency. An inherited defect in the Mac-1, LFA-1 and P150,95 glycoproteins. Ann. Rev. Med. *38*:175, 1987.

123. Fries, L.S., et al.: Inherited deficiencies of complement and complement-related proteins. Clin. Immunol. Immunopathol. *40*:37, 1986.

124. Stoppa-Lyonet, D., et al.: Altered C1 inhibitor genes in type I hereditary angioedema. N. Engl. J. Med. *317*:1, 1987.

125. Update: Acquired immunodeficiency syndrome and human immunodeficiency virus infection among health care workers. MMWR *37*:229, 1988.

126. Curran, J.W., et al.: Epidemiology of HIV infection and AIDS in the United States. Science *239*:610, 1988.

127. Fauci, A.S.: The human immunodeficiency virus: Infectivity and mechanisms of pathogenesis. Science *239*:617, 1988.

128. Harawi, S.J., and O'Hara, C.J. (eds.): Pathology and Pathophysiology of AIDS and HIV-Related Diseases. London, Chapman and Hall Medical, 1989.

129. Human immunodeficiency virus (HIV) infection classification. MMWR *36*(Suppl. 7):1, 1987.

130. Piot, P., et al.: AIDS: An international perspective. Science *239*:573, 1988.

131. Gallo, R.C., and Montagnier, L.: AIDS in 1988. Sci. Am. *259*:41, 1988.

132. Haseltine, W.A., and Wong-Staal, F.: The molecular biology of the AIDS virus. Sci. Am. *259*:52, 1988.

133. Ho, D.D., et al.: Pathogenesis of infection with human immunodeficiency virus. N. Engl. J. Med. *317*:278, 1987.

134. Gallo, R.C., and Streicher, H.Z.: Human T-lymphotropic retroviruses (HTLV-I, II, and III): The biologic basis of adult T-cell leukemia-lymphoma and AIDS. *In* Broder, S. (ed.): AIDS. Modern Concepts and Therapeutic Challenges. New York, Marcel Dekker, 1987, p. 1.

135. Rosen, C.A., et al.: Intragenic cis-acting *art* gene-responsive sequences of human immunodeficiency virus. Proc. Natl. Acad. Sci. U.S.A. *85*:2071, 1988.

136. Hoxie, J.: Editorial: Current concepts in the virology of infection with human immunodeficiency virus. Ann. Intern. Med. *107*:406, 1987.

137. Sadie, M.R., et al.: Site-directed mutagenesis of two trans-regulatory genes (tat-III, trs) of HIV-1. Science *239*:910, 1988.

138. Gallo, R.C., et al.: The etiology of AIDS. In De Vita, V.T., Jr., et al. (eds.): AIDS: Etiology, Diagnosis, Treatment and Prevention. Philadelphia, J.B. Lippincott Co., 1985, p. 31.

139. Clavel, F., et al.: Human immunodeficiency virus type 2 infection associated with AIDS in West Africa. N. Engl. J. Med. *317*:1110, 1987.

140. Friedland, G., and Klein, R.S.: Transmission of the human immunodeficiency virus. N. Engl. J. Med. *317*:1125, 1987.

141. Johnson, A.M.: Heterosexual transmission of human immunodeficiency virus. Br. Med. J. *296*:1017, 1988.

142. Pomerantz, R.J., et al.: Human immunodeficiency virus infection of the uterine cervix. Ann. Intern. Med. *108*:321, 1988.

143. Des Jarlais, D.C., et al.: Intravenous drug use and the heterosexual transmission of the human immunodeficiency virus. N.Y. State Med. J. *87*:283, 1987.

144. May, R.M.: HIV infection in heterosexuals. Nature *331*:655, 1988.

145. Quinn, T.C., et al.: AIDS in Africa: An epidemiologic paradigm. Science *234*:955, 1986.

146. Ward, J.A., et al.: Transmission of human immunodeficiency virus (HIV) by blood transfusions screened as negative for HIV-antibody. N. Engl. J. Med. *318*:473, 1988.

147. Lapointe, N., et al.: Transplacental transmission of HTLV-III virus. N. Engl. J. Med. *312*:1325, 1985.

148. Agent summary statement of human immunodeficiency viruses (HIVs) including HTLV-III, LAV, HIV-1, and HIV-2. MMWR *37*(Suppl. 4): 1988.

149. Jameson, B.A., et al.: Location and chemical synthesis of a binding site for HIV-1 on the CD4 protein. Science *240*:1335, 1988.

150. Kowalaski, M., et al.: Functional regions of the envelope glycoprotein of the human immunodeficiency virus type I. Science *237*:1351, 1987.

151. Edelman, A.S., and Zolla-Pazner, S.: AIDS: a syndrome of immune dysregulation, dysfunction, and deficiency. FASEB J. *3*:22, 1989.

152. Price, R.W., et al.: The brain in AIDS: Central nervous system HIV-1 infection and AIDS-dementia complex. Science *239*:586, 1988.

153. Wiley, C.A., et al.: Cellular virus infection within brains of acquired immunodeficiency syndrome patients. Proc. Natl. Acad. Sci. U.S.A. *83*:7089, 1986.

154. Lee, M.R., et al.: Functional interaction and partial homology between human immunodeficiency virus and neuroleukin. Science *237*:1047, 1987.

155. Tramont, E.C.: Syphilis in the AIDS era. N. Engl. J. Med. *316*:1600, 1987.

156. Seligmann, M., et al.: Immunology of human immunodeficiency virus infection and the acquired immunodeficiency syndrome. An update. Ann. Intern. Med. *107*:234, 1987.

157. Tindall, B., et al.: Characterization of the acute clinical illness associated with human immunodeficiency virus infection. Arch. Intern. Med. *148*:945, 1988.

158. Daul, C.B., et al.: Human immunodeficiency virus infection in hemophiliac patients. A three year prospective evaluation. Am. J. Med. *84*:801, 1988.

159. Witt, D.J., et al.: Bacterial infections in adult patients with the acquired immune deficiency syndrome (AIDS) and AIDS-related complex. Am. J. Med. *82*:900, 1987.

160. Knowles, D.M., et al.: Lymphoid neoplasia associated with the acquired immunodeficiency syndrome (AIDS). Ann. Intern. Med. *108*:744, 1988.

161. Navio, B.A., and Price, R.W.: The acquired immunodeficiency syndrome dementia complex as the presenting or sole manifestation of the human immunodeficiency virus infection. Arch. Neurol. *44*:65, 1987.

162. Waisman, J., et al.: AIDS: An overview of the pathology. Pathol. Res. Pract. *182*:729, 1987.

163. Jaffe, E., et al.: Pathology of AIDS. In Broder, S. (ed.): AIDS, Modern Concepts and Therapeutic Challenges. New York, Marcel Dekker, 1987, p. 143.

164. Rao, T.K.S., et al.: The types of renal disease in the acquired immunodeficiency syndrome. N. Engl. J. Med. *316*:1062, 1987.

165. Rothenberg, R., et al.: Survival with the acquired immunodeficiency syndrome: Experience with 5833 cases in New York City. N. Engl. J. Med. *317*:1279, 1987.

166. Barnes, D.M.: Obstacles to an AIDS vaccine. Science *240*:719, 1988.

167. Nizon, M., and Montagnier, L.: Genetic variability in human immunodeficiency virus. Ann. N.Y. Acad. Sci. *511*:376, 1987.

168. Ho, D.D., et al.: Second conserved domain of gp 120 is important for HIV infectivity and antibody neutralization. Science *239*:1021, 1988.

169. Fischl, M.A., et al.: The efficacy of azidothymidine (AZT) in the treatment of patients with AIDS and AIDS-related complex. N. Engl. J. Med. *317*:185, 1987.

6

Neoplasia

In the United States each year, well over 1 million individuals learn for the first time that they have some type of cancer. Fortunately, many of these tumors can be cured. Nonetheless, according to American Cancer Society estimates, cancer caused approximately 500,000 deaths in 1989, accounting for about 22% of all deaths.[1] Only cardiovascular diseases cause more deaths. The discussion that follows deals with both benign tumors and cancers; understandably, the latter receive more attention. The focus is on the basic morphologic and behavioral characteristics and our present understanding of the origins of tumors. We will also discuss the interactions of the tumor with the host, and the host response to tumor. Although the discussion of therapy is beyond our scope, with many forms of malignancy, notably the leukemias and lymphomas, there are now dramatic improvements in five-year survival rates. A greater proportion of cancers are being cured or arrested today than ever before.

DEFINITIONS

Neoplasia literally means "new growth," and the new growth is a "neoplasm." The term "tumor" was originally applied to the swelling caused by inflammation. Neoplasms also may induce swellings, and by long precedent the non-neoplastic usage of "tumor" has passed into limbo; thus, the term is now equated with neoplasm. Oncology (Greek "oncos" = tumor) is the study of tumors or neoplasms. *Cancer is the common term for all malignant tumors.* Although the ancient origins of this term are somewhat uncertain, it probably derives from the Latin for crab, "cancer"— presumably because a cancer "adheres to any part that it seizes upon in an obstinate manner like the crab." A major focus of the practicing pathologist is the anatomic differentiation of benign and malignant tumors, carrying with it the implication of their probable clinical behavior. It will become evident, however, that all benign tumors are not completely innocent, just as all malignant tumors are not completely evil. Moreover, some neoplasms fall in the gray area both clinically and anatomically between benign and malignant.

Although all physicians know what they mean when they use the term "neoplasm," it has been surprisingly difficult to develop an accurate definition. The eminent British oncologist Sir Rupert Willis has come closest—"A neoplasm is an abnormal mass of tissue, the growth of which exceeds and is uncoordinated with that of the normal tissues and persists in the same excessive manner after cessation of the stimuli which evoked the change."[2] To this characterization we might add that the abnormal mass is purposeless, preys on the host, and is virtually autonomous. It preys on the host insofar as the growth of the neoplastic tissue competes with normal cells and tissues for energy supplies and nutritional substrate. Inasmuch as these masses may flourish in a patient who is wasting away, they are to a degree autonomous. Later it will become evident that such autonomy is not complete. All neoplasms ultimately depend on the host for their nutrition and vascular supply; many forms of neoplasia require endocrine support.

NOMENCLATURE

All tumors, benign and malignant, have two basic components: (1) proliferating neoplastic cells that constitute their *parenchyma* and (2) *supportive stroma* made up of connective tissue and blood vessels. Although parenchymal cells represent the proliferating "cutting edge" of neoplasms and so determine their nature, the growth and evolution of neoplasms are critically dependent on their stroma. An adequate stromal blood supply is requisite, and the stromal connective tissue provides the framework for the parenchyma. In some tumors the stromal support is scant, and so the neoplasm is soft and fleshy. Sometimes the parenchymal cells stimulate the formation of an abundant collagenous stroma — referred to as *desmoplasia*. Such tumors as, for example, some cancers of the female breast are stony hard or scirrhous. The nomenclature of tumors is, however, based on the parenchymal component. *The suffix "oma" denotes a benign neoplasm.* Benign mesenchymal tumors (those arising in muscle, bones, tendon, cartilage, fat, vessels, and lymphoid and fibrous tissue) are classified histogenetically according to parenchymal cell type, e.g., lipoma, fibroma, angioma. Benign epithelial neoplasms are variously classified, some on the basis of their cells of origin, others on microscopic architecture, and still others on their macroscopic patterns.

Adenoma is the term applied to the benign epithelial neoplasm that forms glandular patterns, as well as to the tumors derived from glands but not necessarily reproducing glandular patterns. On this basis a benign epithelial neoplasm that arises from renal tubular cells growing in the form of numerous tightly clustered small glands would be termed an adenoma, as would a heterogeneous mass of adrenal cortical cells growing in no distinctive pattern. Benign epithelial neoplasms producing microscopically or macroscopically visible finger-like or warty projections from epithelial surfaces are referred to as *papillomas*. Those that form large cystic masses as in the ovary are referred to as *cystadenomas*. Some tumors produce papillary patterns that protrude into cystic spaces and are called *papillary cystadenomas* (Fig. 6–1). When a neoplasm, benign or malignant, produces a macroscopically visible projection above a *mucosal* surface and projects, for example, into the gastric or colonic lumen, it is termed a *polyp*. The term polyp preferably is restricted to benign tumors. Malignant polyps are better designated polypoid cancers.

Malignant tumor nomenclature essentially follows the same schema used for benign neoplasms with

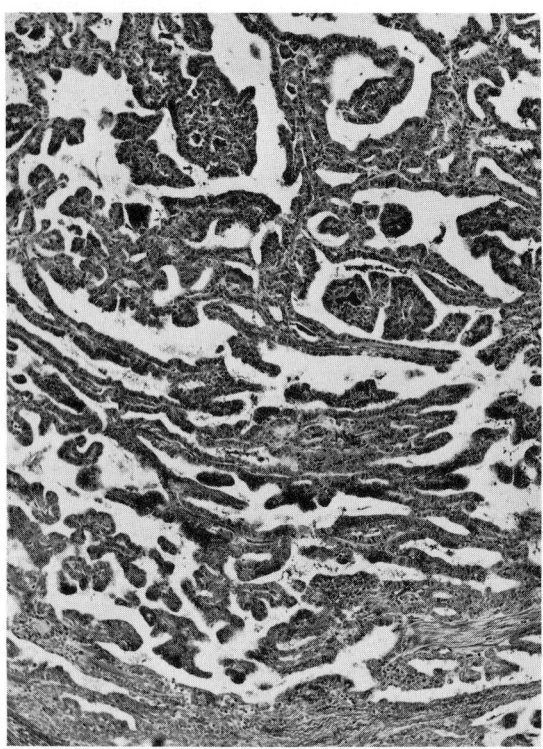

Figure 6–1. Papillary cystadenoma. The papillary tumor fills a small cystic space.

certain additions. *Cancers arising in mesenchymal tissue are called sarcomas* (Greek "sar" = fleshy) because they usually have very little connective tissue stroma and so are fleshy, e.g., fibrosarcoma, liposarcoma, and leiomyosarcoma for smooth muscle cancer, and rhabdomyosarcoma for a cancer arising in striated muscle. *Malignant neoplasms of epithelial cell origin, derived from any of the three germ layers, are called carcinomas.* Thus, cancer arising in the epidermis of ectodermal origin is a carcinoma, as is a cancer arising in the mesodermally derived cells of the renal tubules and the endodermally derived cells of the lining of the gastrointestinal tract. Carcinomas may be further qualified. One with a glandular growth pattern microscopically is termed an *adenocarcinoma*, and one producing recognizable squamous cells arising in any of the stratified squamous epithelia of the body would be termed a *squamous cell carcinoma*. It is further common practice to specify, when possible, the organ of origin, e.g., a renal cell adenocarcinoma or bronchogenic squamous cell carcinoma. Not infrequently, however, a cancer is composed of very primitive undifferentiated cells and must be designated merely as a poorly differentiated or undifferentiated malignant tumor or, when possible, undifferentiated carcinoma or undifferentiated sarcoma.

In most neoplasms, benign and malignant, the parenchymal cells bear a close resemblance to each other, as though all were derived from a single cell, as indeed we know to be the case with many cancers. Infrequently, divergent differentiation of a single line of parenchymal cells creates what are called *mixed tumors*. The best example is the *mixed tumor of salivary gland origin*. These tumors contain epithelial components scattered within a myxoid stroma that sometimes contains islands of apparent cartilage or even bone (Fig. 6–2). All these elements, it is believed, arise from epithelial and myoepithelial cells of salivary gland origin; thus, the preferred designation of these neoplasms is *pleomorphic adenoma*. This schizophrenic morphology presumably reflects variable expression of several programs of differentiation that are repressed and hidden in the genome of all cells in a multicellular organism. The great majority of neoplasms, even mixed tumors, are composed of cells representative of a single germ layer. The *teratoma*, in contrast, is made up of a variety of parenchymal cell types representative of more than one germ layer, usually all three. They arise from totipotential cells and so are principally encountered in the gonads, but rarely in sequestered primitive cell rests elsewhere. These totipotential cells differentiate along various germ lines, producing, for example, tissues that can be identified as skin, muscle, fat, gut epithelium, tooth structures, and, indeed, any tissue of the body (Fig. 6–3). A particularly common pattern is seen in the ovarian *cystic dermoid teratoma*, which differentiates

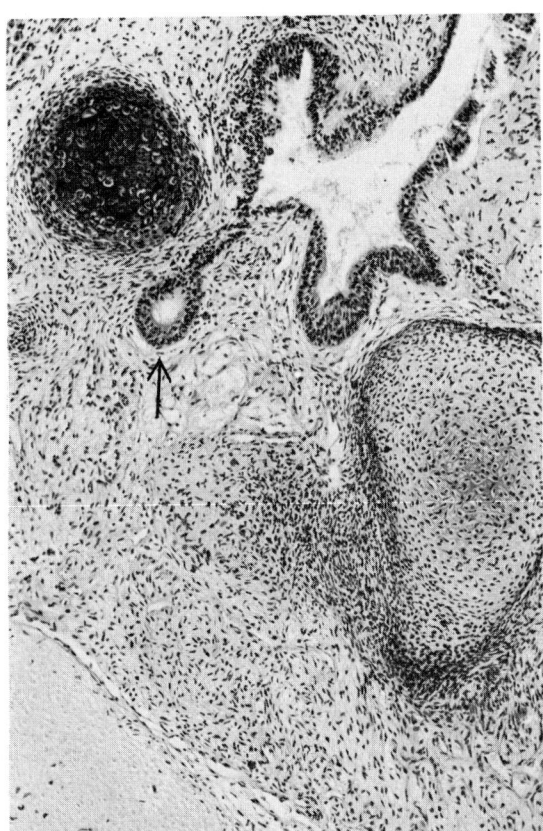

Figure 6–3. A teratoma. Three distinct types of adult tissues are seen: a circular island of darkly stained cartilage (mesodermal) in the upper left, a large nest of stratified squamous epithelial cells (ectodermal) on the right, and in the center a gland space lined by columnar cells resembling intestinal tract mucosa (endodermal) (*arrow*).

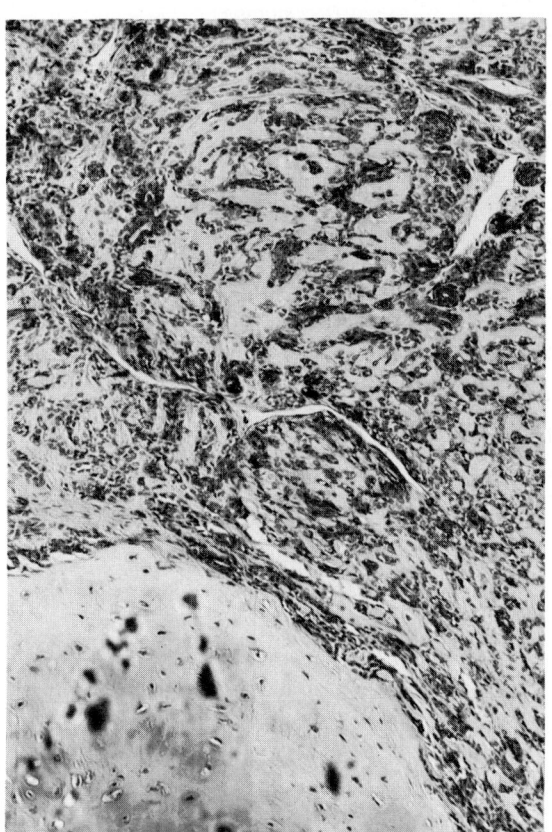

Figure 6–2. A mixed tumor of salivary gland origin (pleomorphic adenoma). There is a large plate of pseudocartilage in the lower field. The remainder of the tumor is composed of small cords and nests of epithelial cells separated by pale areas of loose connective tissue.

principally along ectodermal lines to create a cystic tumor lined by skin replete with hair, sebaceous glands, and tooth structures.

The nomenclature of the more common forms of neoplasia is presented in Table 6–1. It is evident from this compilation that there are some inappropriate but deeply entrenched usages. For generations, carcinomas of hepatocytic origin have been called "hepatomas," although correctly they should be referred to as hepatocellular carcinomas, or liver cell carcinomas. Analogously, carcinomas of melanocytes, e.g., melanocarcinomas, are stubbornly called "melanomas," just as certain carcinomas of testicular origin are referred to as seminomas. Other instances will be encountered in which innocent designations belie ugly behavior. Irrational as such usage may be, it is probably more irrational to expect man to be rational. The converse is also true when ominous terms are applied to usually trivial lesions. An ectopic rest of normal tissue is sometimes called a *choristoma*—as, for example, a rest of adrenal cells under the kidney capsule (p. 537). Occasionally a pancreatic nodular rest in the mucosa of the small intestine may mimic a neoplasm, providing some partial justification for the use of a term that implies a tumor. Analogously, aberrant dif-

Table 6–1. Nomenclature of Tumors

TISSUE OF ORIGIN	BENIGN	MALIGNANT
I. Composed of one parenchymal cell type		
A. Tumors of mesenchymal origin		***Sarcomas***
(1) Connective tissue and derivatives	Fibroma	Fibrosarcoma
	Myxoma	Myxosarcoma
	Lipoma	Liposarcoma
	Chondroma	Chondrosarcoma
	Osteoma	Osteogenic sarcoma
(2) Endothelial and related tissues		
Blood vessels	Hemangioma	Angiosarcoma
	Capillary	
	Cavernous	
Lymph vessels	Lymphangioma	Lymphangiosarcoma
Synovia		Synovioma (synoviosarcoma)
Mesothelium (lining cells of body cavities)		Mesothelioma
Brain coverings	Meningioma	Invasive meningioma
Glomus	Glomus tumor	
(3) Blood cells and related cells		
Hematopoietic cells		Myelogenous leukemia
		Monocytic leukemia
Lymphoid tissue		Malignant lymphomas
		Lymphocytic leukemia
		Plasmacytoma (multiple myeloma)
Langerhans' cells		Histiocytosis X
Monocyte-macrophage		? Histiocytic lymphoma
		? Hodgkin's disease
(4) Muscle		
Smooth muscle	Leiomyoma	Leiomyosarcoma
Striated	Rhabdomyoma	Rhabdomyosarcoma
B. Tumors of epithelial origin		***Carcinomas***
(1) Stratified squamous	Squamous cell papilloma	Squamous cell or epidermoid carcinoma
(2) Basal cells of skin or adnexa		Basal cell carcinoma
(3) Skin adnexal glands		
Sweat glands	Sweat gland adenoma	Sweat gland carcinoma
Sebaceous glands	Sebaceous gland adenoma	Sebaceous gland carcinoma
(4) Epithelial lining		
Glands or ducts—well-differentiated group	Adenoma	Adenocarcinoma
	Papilloma	Papillary carcinoma
	Papillary adenoma	Papillary adenocarcinoma
	Cystadenoma	Cystadenocarcinoma
Poorly differentiated group		Medullary carcinoma
		Undifferentiated carcinoma (simplex)
(5) Respiratory passages		Bronchogenic carcinoma
		Bronchial "adenoma"
(6) Neuroectoderm	Nevus	Melanoma (melanocarcinoma)
(7) Renal epithelium	Renal tubular adenoma	Renal cell carcinoma (hypernephroma)
(8) Liver cells	Liver cell adenoma	Hepatoma (hepatocellular carcinoma)
(9) Bile duct	Bile duct adenoma	Bile duct carcinoma (cholangiocarcinoma)
(10) Urinary tract epithelium (transitional)	Transitional cell papilloma	Papillary carcinoma
		Transitional cell carcinoma
		Squamous cell carcinoma
(11) Placental epithelium	Hydatidiform mole	Choriocarcinoma
(12) Testicular epithelium (germ cells)		Seminoma
		Embryonal carcinoma
II. More than one neoplastic cell type— mixed tumors—usually derived from one germ layer		
(1) Salivary glands	Pleomorphic adenoma (mixed tumor of salivary gland origin)	Malignant mixed tumor of salivary gland origin
(2) Renal anlage		Wilms' tumor
III. More than one neoplastic cell type derived from more than one germ layer— teratogenous		
(1) Totipotential cells in gonads or in embryonic rests	Mature teratoma, dermoid cyst	Immature teratoma

ferentiation may produce a mass of disorganized but mature specialized cells or tissue indigenous to the particular site, referred to as a *hamartoma* (p. 537). Thus, a hamartoma in the lung may contain islands of cartilage, blood vessels, bronchial-type structures, and lymphoid tissue. Indeed, sometimes the lesion is purely cartilaginous, or purely angiomatous. Although these might be construed as benign neoplasms, the complete resemblance of the tissue to normal cartilage or blood vessels and the occasional admixture of other elements favor a hamartomatous origin. In any event, the hamartoma is totally benign.

The nomenclature of tumors is important, because specific designations have specific clinical implications. The historically sanctified term "seminoma" connotes a form of carcinoma that tends to spread to lymph nodes along the iliac arteries and aorta. These cancers in their sites of origin in the testes tend to be resectable in almost all cases. Further, the spread into the abdominal lymph nodes, should it be present, can usually be eradicated by radiotherapy; thus, very few patients with seminomas die of their neoplasm. By contrast, the embryonal carcinoma of the testis is not radiosensitive, tending to invade locally beyond the confines of the testis and to spread throughout the body. There also are other varieties of testicular neoplasms, and so the designation "cancer of the testis" tells little of its clinical significance.

CHARACTERISTICS OF BENIGN AND MALIGNANT NEOPLASMS

In the great majority of instances, the differentiation of a benign from a malignant tumor can be made morphologically with considerable certainty; sometimes, however, a neoplasm defies categorization. It has been said, "All tumors need not of necessity be either benign or malignant." Certain anatomic features may suggest innocence while others point toward cancerous potential. Ultimately, all morphologic diagnosis is subjective and constitutes prediction of the future course of a neoplasm. Occasionally this prediction is confounded by a marked discrepancy between the morphologic appearance of a tumor and its biologic behavior: An innocent face may mask an ugly nature. However, such deception or ambiguity is not the rule; in general, there are criteria by which benign and malignant tumors can be differentiated, and they behave accordingly. These differences can conveniently be discussed under the following headings: (1) differentiation and anaplasia; (2) rate of growth; (3) local invasion; and (4) metastasis.

A concluding chart on page 250 summarizes the differential points.

DIFFERENTIATION AND ANAPLASIA

The terms *differentiation* and *anaplasia* apply to the parenchymal cells of neoplasms. *Differentiation refers* *to the extent to which parenchymal cells resemble comparable normal cells, both morphologically and functionally.* Well-differentiated tumors are thus composed of cells resembling the mature normal cells of the tissue of origin of the neoplasm. Poorly differentiated or undifferentiated tumors have primitive-appearing, unspecialized cells (Figs. 6–4 and 6–5). *In general, all benign tumors are well differentiated.* The neoplastic cell in a benign smooth muscle tumor—a leiomyoma—so closely resembles the normal cell as to make it impossible to recognize it as a tumor cell on high-power examination. Only the massing of these cells into a nodule discloses the tumorous nature of the lesion. One may get so close to the tree that one loses sight of the forest. In such benign tumors, mitoses are extremely scant in number, and the few present are normal in appearance.

Malignant neoplasms, in contrast, range from well differentiated to undifferentiated. Malignant neoplasms composed of undifferentiated cells are said to be anaplastic. Indeed, lack of differentiation, or *anaplasia*, is considered a hallmark of malignant transformation. Literally, anaplasia means "to form backward," implying a reversion from a high level of differentiation to a lower level. However, there is substantial evidence that cancers arise from reserve or stem cells present in all specialized tissues. The well-differentiated cancer evolves from maturation or specialization of undifferentiated cells as they proliferate, whereas the undifferentiated malignant tumor derives from proliferation without maturation of the transformed cells. Lack of differentiation, then, is not the consequence of dedifferentiation.

Lack of differentiation, or anaplasia, is marked by a number of morphologic and functional changes. Both the cells and their nuclei characteristically display pleomorphism—variation in size and shape. Cells may be found that are many times larger than their neighbors, and other cells may be extremely small and primitive-appearing. Characteristically, the nuclei contain an abundance of DNA and are extremely dark-staining (hyperchromatic). The nuclei are disproportionately large for the cell, and the nuclear-cytoplasmic ratio may approach 1:1 instead of the normal 1:4 or 1:6. The nuclear shape usually is extremely variable, and the chromatin often is coarsely clumped and distributed along the nuclear membrane. Large nucleoli are usually present in these nuclei, reflecting the synthetic activity of these cells.

As compared with benign tumors and some well-differentiated malignant neoplasms, undifferentiated tumors usually possess large numbers of mitoses, reflecting the higher proliferative activity of the parenchymal cells. It should be noted, however, that the presence of mitoses does not necessarily indicate that a tumor is malignant, or that the tissue is neoplastic. Many normal tissues exhibiting rapid turnover, such as bone marrow, have numerous mitoses, and non-neoplastic proliferations such as hyperplasias contain many cells in mitosis. More important as a morpho-

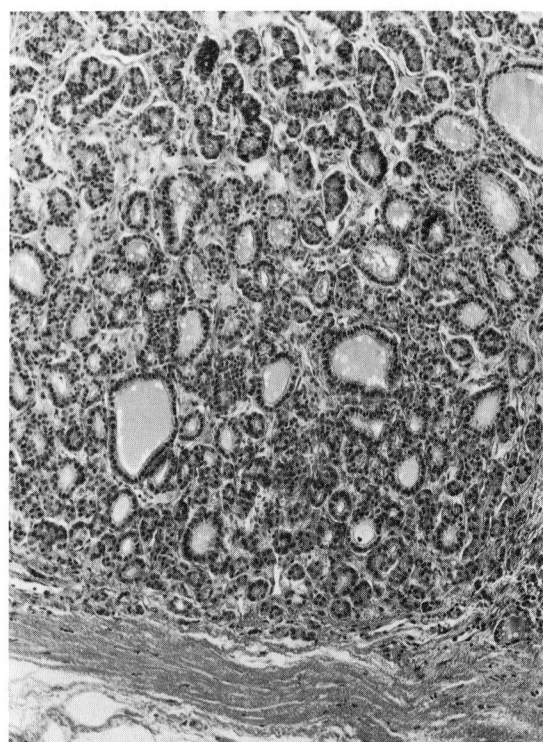

Figure 6–4. A well-differentiated benign thyroid adenoma. The fibrous capsule is in the lower field. The tumor faithfully reproduces thyroid follicles filled with colloid.

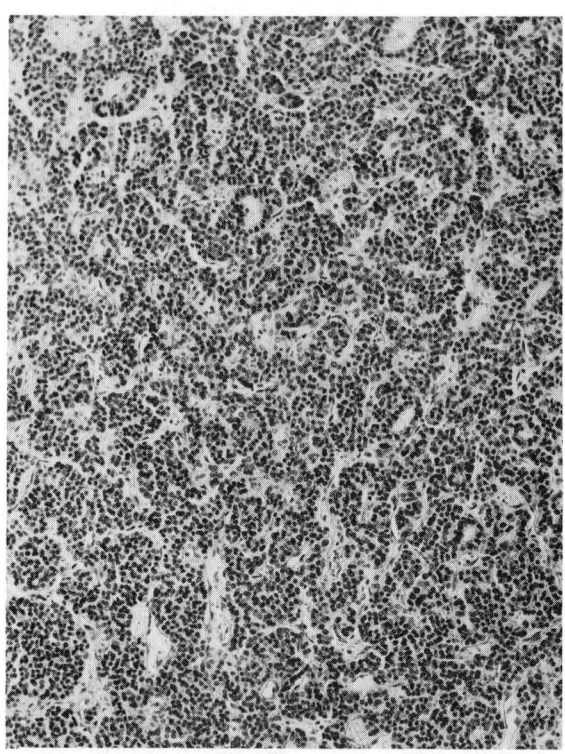

Figure 6–5. A moderately differentiated thyroid carcinoma. The tumor cells comprise disorganized cords of cells, and only occasional follicular spaces suggest a thyroid origin.

logic feature of malignant neoplasia are atypical and bizarre mitotic figures sometimes producing tripolar, quadripolar, or multipolar spindles (Fig. 6–6). Often, the mitotic jumble possesses abnormally large spindles in one area and shrunken, puny spindles in other regions.

Another important feature of anaplasia is the formation of *tumor giant cells*, some possessing only a single huge polymorphic nucleus, while others have two or more nuclei. These giant cells are not to be confused with inflammatory Langhans or foreign body giant cells, which possess many small, normal-appearing nuclei. In the cancer giant cell, the nucleus is hyperchromatic and is too large in relation to the cell (Fig. 6–7). In addition to the cytologic abnormalities described above, the orientation of anaplastic cells is markedly disturbed. Sheets or large masses of tumor cells grow in an anarchic, disorganized fashion. Although these growing cells obviously require a blood supply, often the connective tissue–vascular stroma is scant, and indeed in many anaplastic tumors, large central areas undergo ischemic necrosis. As mentioned at the outset, malignant tumors differ widely in the extent to which their morphologic appearance deviates from the norm. On one end of the spectrum are the extremely undifferentiated, anaplastic tumors, and at the other end are cancers that bear striking resemblance to their tissues of origin. Certain well-differentiated adenocarcinomas of the thyroid, for example, may form normal-appearing fol-

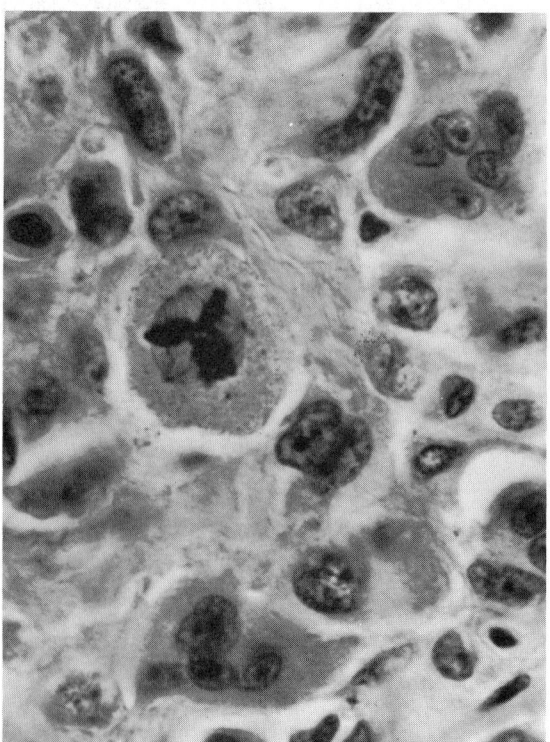

Figure 6–6. High-power detail of anaplastic tumor cells to show cellular and nuclear variation in size and shape. The prominent cell in the center field has an abnormal tripolar spindle.

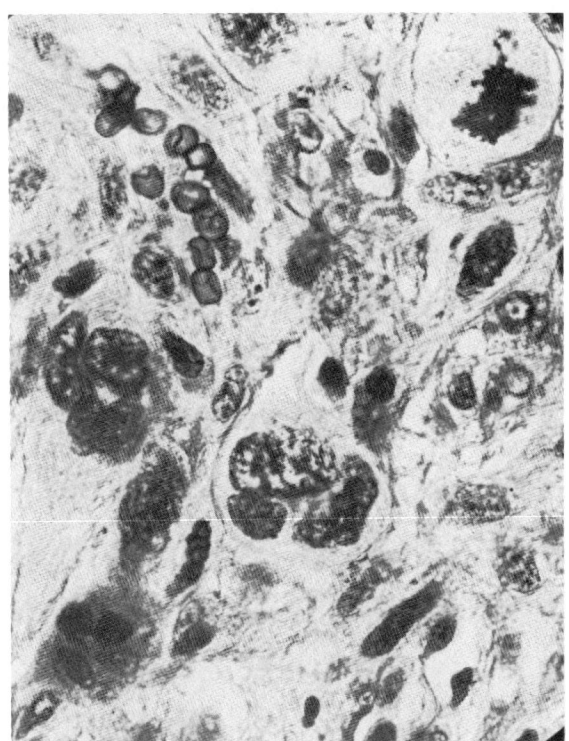

Figure 6-7. Anaplastic tumor cells with prominent multinucleate tumor giant cells and an abnormal mitotic figure in the upper right field.

licles, and some squamous cell carcinomas contain cells that do not differ cytologically from normal squamous epithelial cells. Thus, the morphologic diagnosis of malignancy in well-differentiated tumors may sometimes be quite difficult. In between the two extremes lie tumors that are loosely referred to as "moderately well differentiated."

Electron microscopic studies of neoplastic cells have yielded no great surprises. Well-differentiated cells, whether from benign or malignant neoplasms, deviate little from their normal forebears. With loss of differentiation in cancer cells, there is progressively marked accentuation of the nuclear chromatin in clumps along the membrane, simplification of the rough endoplasmic reticulum, increase of free ribosomes, and greater pleomorphism of the mitochondria. Various organelles may be reduced in size or number or distributed throughout the cell in abnormal patterns.

Turning to the functional differentiation of neoplastic cells, as you might presume, the better the differentiation of the cell, the more completely it retains the functional capabilities found in its normal counterparts. Thus, benign neoplasms and well-differentiated cancers of endocrine glands frequently elaborate the hormones characteristic of their origin. Well-differentiated squamous cell carcinomas of the epidermis elaborate keratin just as well-differentiated hepatocellular carcinomas elaborate bile. Indeed, there are few differences in the enzyme profiles of well-differentiated tumor cells from those of their normal counterparts. As one descends the scale of differentiation, enzymes and specialized pathways of metabolism are lost and the cells undergo functional simplification. Highly anaplastic undifferentiated cells then, whatever their tissue of origin, come to resemble each other more than the normal cells from which they have arisen, a phenomenon referred to as *biochemical convergence.* However, in some instances, unanticipated functions emerge. Some cancers may elaborate fetal proteins (antigens) not produced by the comparable cells in the adult (p. 302). Analogously, cancers of nonendocrine origin may assume hormone synthesis to produce so-called ectopic hormones. For example, bronchogenic carcinomas may produce adrenocorticotropic hormone, parathyroid-like hormone, insulin, and glucagon, as well as others. More will be said about these phenomena later (p. 294), but for now it suffices to state that in the process of cancerous transformation, either repressed genes are derepressed or new DNA sequences are formed. *Despite exceptions, the more rapidly growing and the more anaplastic a tumor, the less likely there will be specialized functional activity.*

In summary, *the cells in benign tumors are almost always well differentiated and resemble their normal cells of origin; the cells in cancer are more or less differentiated, but some loss of differentiation is always present.*

RATE OF GROWTH

The generalization can be made that *most benign tumors grow slowly over a period of years, whereas most cancers grow rapidly, sometimes at an erratic pace,* and eventually spread and kill their hosts. However, such an oversimplification must be extensively qualified. Some benign tumors have a higher growth rate than malignant tumors. Moreover, the rate of growth of benign neoplasms may not be constant over time. Factors such as hormone dependence, adequacy of blood supply, and very likely unknown influences may affect their growth. For example, leiomyomas (benign smooth muscle tumors) of the uterus are very common. Not infrequently, repeated clinical examination of women bearing such neoplasms over the span of decades discloses no significant increase in size. After the menopause, the neoplasms may atrophy and later be found to be replaced largely by collagenous, sometimes calcified, tissue. On the other hand, leiomyomas frequently enter a growth spurt during pregnancy. Presumably these neoplasms are to some extent dependent on the circulating levels of steroid hormones, particularly estrogens.

In general, *the growth rate of tumors correlates with their level of differentiation, and thus most malignant tumors grow more rapidly than do benign lesions.* There is, however, a very wide range of behavior. At one extreme are some highly aggressive cancers that seem to appear suddenly, increase in size virtually under observation, and explosively disseminate to cause death within a few months of discovery. At the other extreme are those that grow more slowly than benign tumors and may even enter periods of dormancy lasting for years. Indeed, on occasion, cancers have been observed to decrease in size and even spontaneously disappear, but the handful of "miracles" fills only a small volume.[3] To examine this variable behavior more closely, we will consider what is known about the life history of cancer, involving the cell kinetics of cancer growth and the influences that modify the growth of malignant tumors, in a later section (p. 251).

LOCAL INVASION

Nearly all benign tumors grow as cohesive expansile masses that remain localized to their site of origin and do not have the capacity to infiltrate, invade, or metastasize to distant sites, as do cancers. Because they grow and expand slowly, they usually develop a rim of compressed connective tissue, sometimes called a fibrous *capsule*, that separates them from the host tissue. This capsule is derived largely from the stroma of the native tissue as the parenchymal cells atrophy under the pressure of expanding tumor. Such encapsulation tends to contain the benign neoplasm as a discrete, readily palpable, and easily movable mass that can be surgically enucleated (Figs. 6–8 and 6–9). Although a well-defined cleavage plane exists around most benign tumors, in some it is lacking. Thus, hemangiomas (neoplasms composed of tangled blood vessels) are often "unencapsulated," and in-

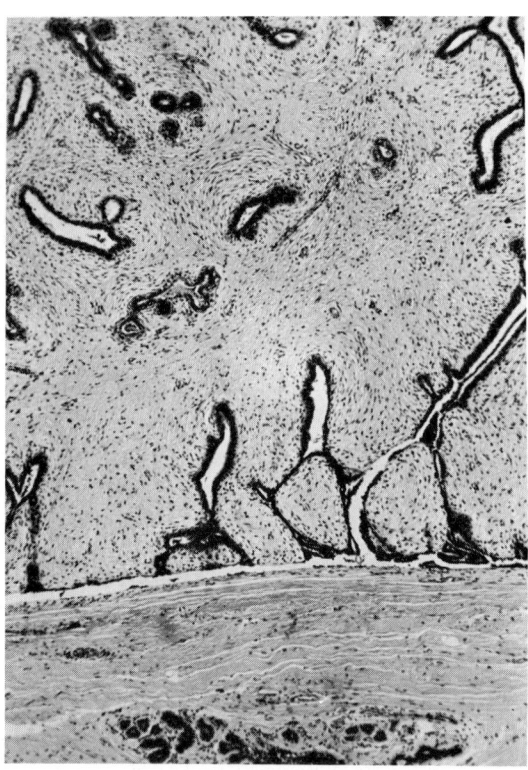

Figure 6–9. Microscopic view of fibroadenoma of breast seen in Figure 6–8. The fibrous capsule (*below*) separates the sharply delimited tumor mass from the surrounding breast substance.

deed may appear to permeate the site in which they arise (commonly the dermis of the skin).

Cancers grow by progressive infiltration, invasion, and destruction of the surrounding tissue. In general, they are poorly demarcated from the surrounding normal tissue and a well-defined cleavage plane is lacking (Fig. 6–10). However, slowly expanding malignant tumors may develop an apparently enclosing fibrous capsule and may push along a broad front into adjacent normal structures (Fig. 6–11). Histologic examination of such apparently encapsulated masses will almost always disclose tiny crablike feet penetrating the margin and infiltrating the adjacent structures.

Most cancers are obviously invasive and can be expected to penetrate the wall of the colon or uterus, for example, or fungate through the surface of the skin. They recognize no normal anatomic boundaries and often permeate lymphatics, blood vessels, and perineural spaces. Such invasiveness makes their surgical resection exceedingly difficult and even if the tumor appears well circumscribed, it is necessary to remove a considerable margin of apparently normal tissues about the infiltrative neoplasm; this is referred to as "radical surgery." *Next to the development of metastases, invasiveness is the most reliable feature that differentiates malignant from benign tumors.* We should note here that some cancers seem to evolve from a preinvasive stage referred to as *carcinoma in situ.* This is best illustrated by carcinoma of the uter-

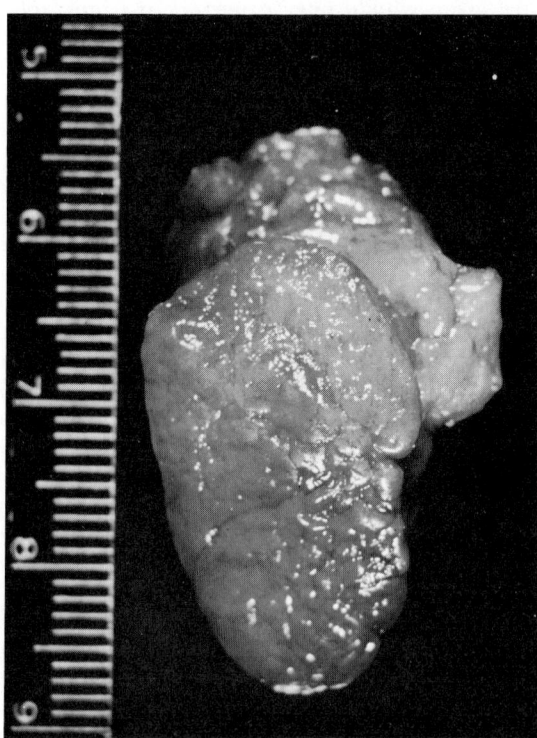

Figure 6–8. Gross view of fibroadenoma of breast. The discrete tumor bulges above the level of the surrounding breast substance as it extrudes from its tight encapsulation.

ine cervix (p. 1142). In situ cancers display the cytologic features of malignancy (p. 244) without invasion of the basement membrane (Fig. 6–12). They may be considered one step removed from frank cancer, and indeed with time almost all penetrate the basement membrane and invade the subepithelial stroma.

Although all tissues in the body can be invaded by cancers, there are differences in their vulnerability. The connective tissue stroma of organized tissues is the favored invasive path of most malignant tumors. Within the connective tissue, elastin fibers are much more resistant to the destructive effects of cancers than are collagen fibers. This difference may relate to a high ratio of collagenase relative to elastase in malignant invading tumors. Nonetheless, densely compacted collagen such as is encountered in membranes, tendons, joint capsules, and so forth resists invasion for long periods. Cartilage is probably the most resistant of all tissues to invasion, but it is not absolute. Several factors have been invoked: (1) the physiochemical characteristics of the matrix, (2) the biologic stability and slow turnover of cartilage, and (3) the elaboration of inhibitory substances such as antiangiogenesis factor or inhibitors of enzymes involved in the growth and invasiveness of cancer cells. Arteries are much more resistant to invasion than are veins and

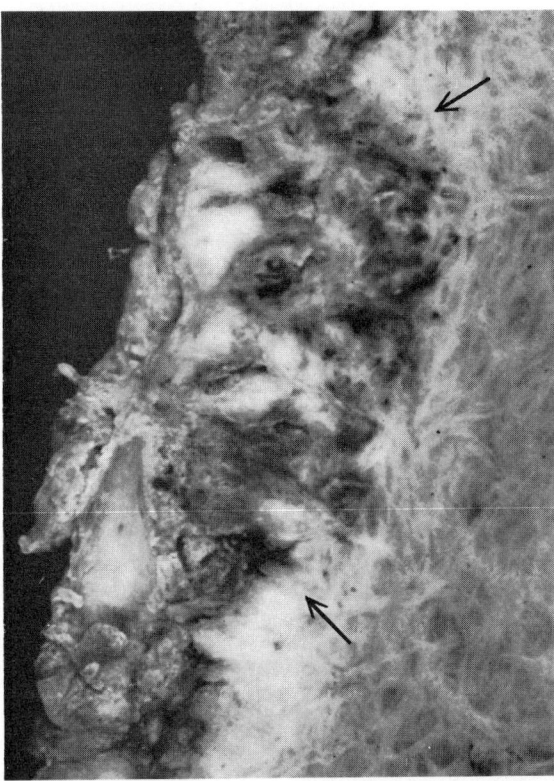

Figure 6–10. Close-up view of adenocarcinoma of endometrium. The malignant tumor (*arrows*) extends into the underlying muscular wall of the uterus. There is no sharp line of delimitation from the surrounding normal tissue.

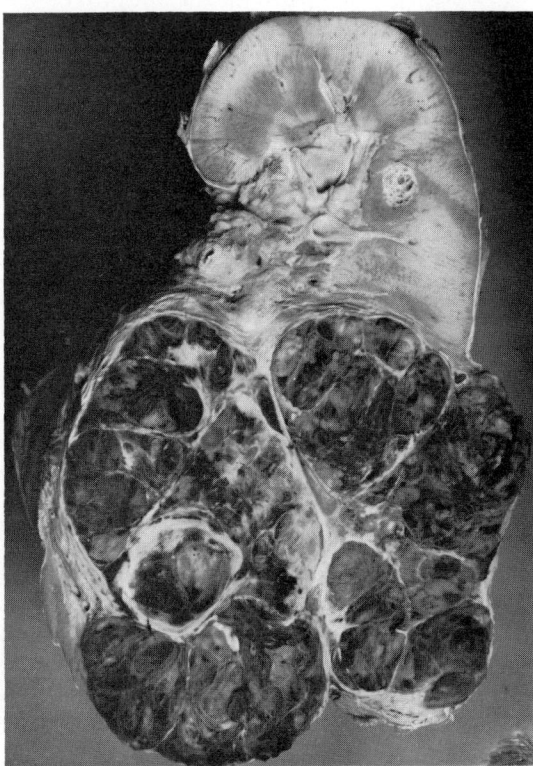

Figure 6–11. Renal cell carcinoma. The malignancy deceptively appears to be well encapsulated.

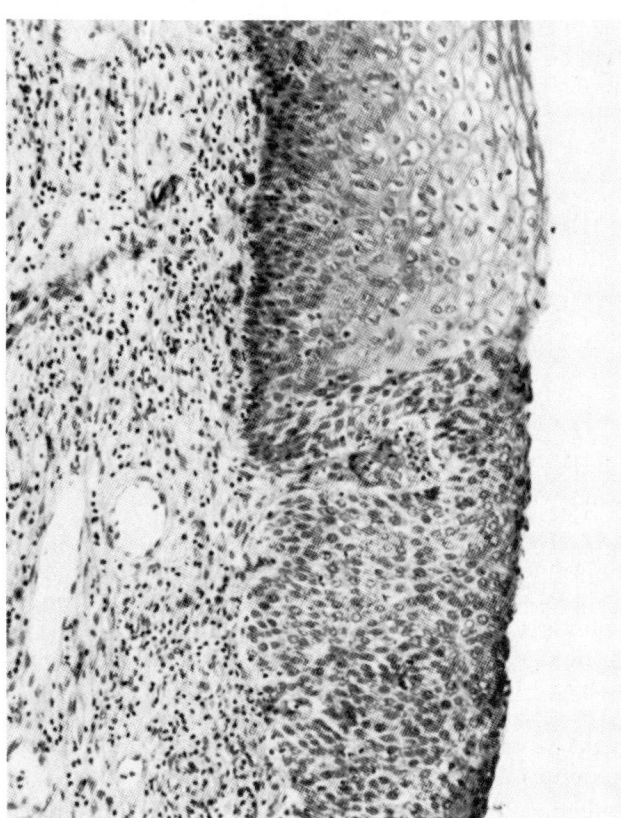

Figure 6–12. Carcinoma in situ of cervix. The normal cervical mucosa is above. There is a sharp transition to the hyperchromatic disorderly cancer cells below, showing no evidence of normal maturation from basal layer to surface. There is no extension of cancer beyond the confines of the mucosa.

lymphatic channels. The resistance to invasion is conventionally ascribed to the thickness of the arterial walls, but it may also be attributable to the elastin content of arterial walls and their elaboration of protease inhibitors.

METASTASIS

Metastases are tumor implants discontinuous with the primary tumor. *Metastasis unequivocally marks a tumor as malignant because benign neoplasms do not metastasize.* The invasiveness of cancers permits them to penetrate into blood vessels, lymphatics, and body cavities, providing the opportunity for spread. *With few exceptions, all cancers can metastasize.* The major exceptions are most malignant neoplasms of the glial cells in the central nervous system, called gliomas, and basal cell carcinomas of the skin. Both are highly invasive forms of neoplasia (the latter being known in the older literature as rodent ulcers because of their invasive destructiveness), but they rarely metastasize.

In general, the more aggressive, the more rapidly growing, and the larger the primary neoplasm, the greater the likelihood that it will metastasize or already has metastasized. However, there are innumerable exceptions. Small, well-differentiated, slowly growing lesions sometimes metastasize widely, and conversely, some rapidly growing lesions remain localized for years. No judgment can be made, then, about the probability of metastasis from pathologic examination of the primary tumor. Many factors relating to both invader and host are involved, as will be pointed out later.

Pathways of Spread

Dissemination of cancers may occur through one of three pathways: (1) direct seeding of body cavities or surfaces, (2) lymphatic spread, and (3) hematogenous spread. Although direct transplantation of tumor cells, as for example on surgical instruments, may theoretically occur, it is exceedingly rare and, in any event, an artificial mode of dissemination that will not be discussed further. Each of the three major pathways will be described separately.

SEEDING OF BODY CAVITIES AND SURFACES.
This may occur whenever a malignant neoplasm penetrates into a natural "open field." Most often involved is the peritoneal cavity, but any other cavity —pleural, pericardial, subarachnoid, and joint spaces—may be affected. Such seeding is particularly characteristic of carcinomas arising in the ovaries, when not infrequently all peritoneal surfaces become coated with a heavy layer of cancerous glaze. Remarkably, the tumor cells may remain confined to the surface of the coated abdominal viscera without penetrating into the substance. Superficial seedings have as much impact on the host as deep seedings. Sometimes, mucus-secreting ovarian and appendiceal carcinomas fill the peritoneal cavity with a gelatinous neoplastic mass referred to as *"pseudomyxoma peritonei."*

LYMPHATIC SPREAD.
Transport through lymphatics is the most common pathway for the initial dissemination of carcinomas (Fig. 6–13), but it should be remembered that sarcomas may also use this route. The emphasis on lymphatic spread for carcinomas and hematogenous spread for sarcomas is misleading, since ultimately there are numerous interconnections between the vascular and lymphatic systems. *The pattern of lymph node involvement follows the natural routes of drainage.* Since carcinomas of the breast usually arise in the upper outer quadrants, they generally disseminate first to the axillary lymph nodes. Cancers of the inner quadrant may drain through lymphatics to the nodes within the chest along the internal mammary arteries. Thereafter, the infraclavicular and supraclavicular nodes may become involved. Bronchogenic carcinomas arising in the major respiratory passages metastasize first to the perihilar tracheobronchial and mediastinal nodes. However, local lymph nodes may be bypassed— "skip metastasis"—because of venous-lymphatic anastomoses, or because inflammation or radiation has obliterated channels.

In many cases the regional nodes serve as effective barriers to further dissemination of the tumor, at least for a time. Conceivably the cells, after arrest within the node, may be destroyed. A tumor-specific immune response may participate in this cell destruction. Drainage of tumor cell debris or tumor antigens, or both, will also induce reactive changes within nodes. Thus, enlargement of nodes may be caused by (1) the spread and growth of cancer cells, (2) follicular hyperplasia, or (3) proliferation of paracortical T cells and sinus histiocytosis (proliferation of sinus endothelial cells and histiocytes) initiated by the products released from the primary lesion. It should be noted,

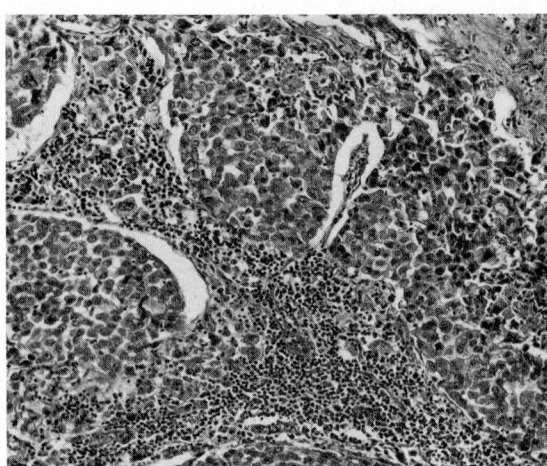

Figure 6–13. Portion of a lymph node with sinuses distended by metastatic tumor.

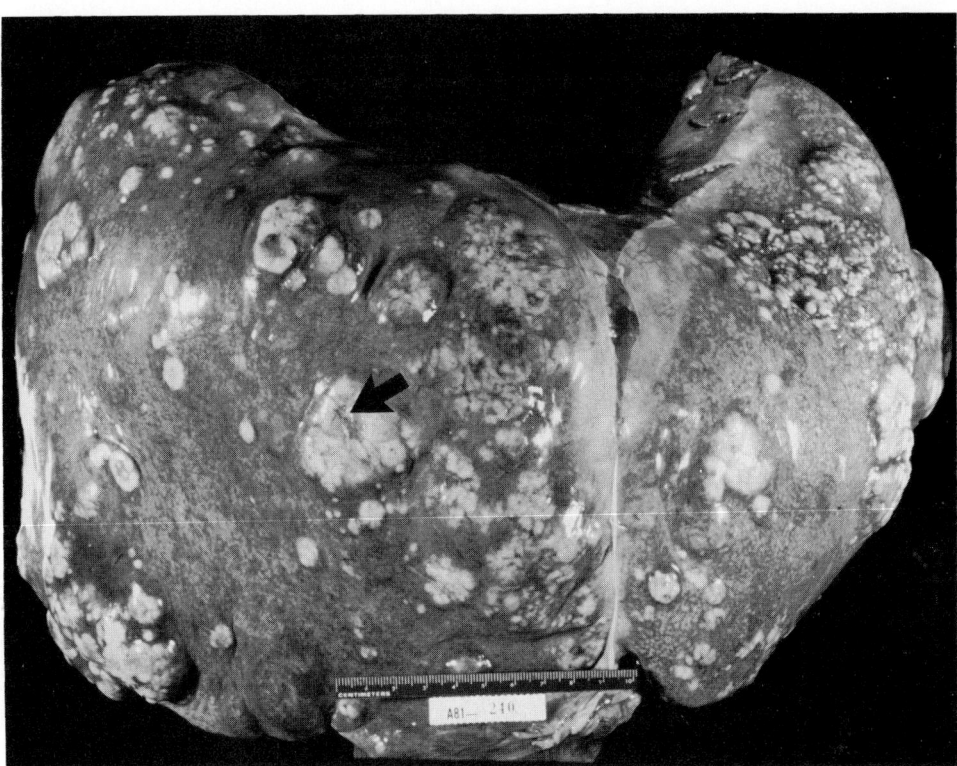

Figure 6–14. Carcinoma metastatic to liver. Note umbilication (*arrow*) of large implant caused by central necrosis of tumor. (Courtesy of Dr. Lawrence Weiss, Brigham and Women's Hospital.)

therefore, that *nodal enlargement in proximity to a cancer does not necessarily mean dissemination of the primary lesion.*

HEMATOGENOUS SPREAD. This pathway is typical of sarcomas but is also utilized by carcinomas. Arteries, as mentioned, are less readily penetrated than are veins. However, arterial spread may occur when tumor cells pass through the pulmonary capillary beds or pulmonary arteriovenous shunts, or when pulmonary metastases themselves give rise to additional tumor emboli. In such arterial spread, a number of factors (to be discussed) condition the patterns of distribution of the metastases. With venous invasion, the blood-borne cells follow the venous flow draining the site of the neoplasm. Understandably, the liver and lungs are most frequently involved secondarily in such hematogenous dissemination (Fig. 6–14). All portal area drainage flows to the liver, and all caval blood flows to the lungs. Cancers arising in close proximity to the vertebral column often embolize through the paravertebral plexus, and this pathway is probably involved in the frequent vertebral metastases of carcinomas of the thyroid and prostate.

Certain cancers have a propensity for invasion of veins. The renal cell carcinoma often invades the branches of the renal vein and then the renal vein itself to grow in a snakelike fashion up the inferior vena cava, sometimes reaching the right side of the heart. Hepatocarcinomas often penetrate portal and hepatic radicles to grow within them into the main venous channels. Remarkably, such intravenous growth may not be accompanied by widespread dissemination. Histologic evidence of penetration of small vessels at the site of the primary neoplasm is obviously an ominous feature. However, such changes must be viewed guardedly because, for reasons discussed later, they do not indicate the inevitable development of metastases.

The differential features discussed in this overview of the specific characteristics of benign and malignant tumors are summarized in Table 6–2.

GRADING AND STAGING OF CANCER

Comparison of end results of various forms of cancer treatment, particularly between clinics, requires some degree of comparability of the neoplasms being assayed. To this end, systems have been derived to express, at least in semiquantitative terms, the level of differentiation, or *grade,* and extent of spread of a cancer within the patient, or *stage,* as parameters of the clinical gravity of the disease.

Grading of a cancer is based on the degree of differentiation of the tumor cells and the number of mitoses within the tumor as presumed correlates of the neoplasm's aggressiveness. Thus, cancers are classified as grades I to IV with increasing anaplasia. Criteria for the individual grades vary with each form of neoplasia and so will not be detailed here, but all attempt, in essence, to judge the extent to which the tumor cells resemble or fail to resemble their normal

Table 6–2. Comparisons Between Benign and Malignant Tumors

CHARACTERISTICS	BENIGN	MALIGNANT
Differentiation/anaplasia	Well-differentiated; structure may be typical of tissue of origin	Some lack of differentiation with anaplasia; structure is often atypical
Rate of growth	Usually progressive and slow; may come to a standstill or regress; mitotic figures are rare and normal	Erratic and may be slow to rapid; mitotic figures may be numerous and abnormal
Local invasion	Usually cohesive and expansile well-demarcated masses that do not invade or infiltrate the surrounding normal tissues	Locally invasive, infiltrating the surrounding normal tissues; sometimes may be seemingly cohesive and expansile
Metastasis	Absent	Frequently present; the larger and more undifferentiated the primary, the more likely are metastases

counterparts. Unfortunately, the grading of cancers is replete with shortcomings. The level of differentiation may differ somewhat from one area to the next in large tumors, creating sampling errors, and it may change as the tumor evolves. Most often, cancers become progressively undifferentiated as more vigorous, less specialized clones outgrow the better differentiated ones. Moreover, the correlation between histologic appearance and biologic behavior is less than perfect. In recognition of these problems and in order to avoid spurious quantification, it is common practice to characterize a particular neoplasm in descriptive terms, e.g., well-differentiated, mucin-secreting adenocarcinoma of the stomach, or highly undifferentiated, retroperitoneal malignant tumor — probably sarcoma. In general, with few exceptions such as soft tissue sarcomas, grading of cancers has proved of less clinical value than has staging.

The staging of cancers is based on the size of the primary lesion, its extent of spread to regional lymph nodes, and the presence or absence of blood-borne metastases. Two major staging systems are currently in use, one developed by the Union Internationale Contre Cancer (UICC), and the other by the American Joint Committee (AJC) on Cancer Staging. The UICC employs a so-called *TNM system — T* for primary tumor, *N* for regional lymph node involvement, and *M* for metastases. The TNM staging varies for each specific form of cancer, but there are general principles. With increasing size the primary lesion is characterized as T1 to T4. Occasionally a T0 is added to indicate an in situ lesion. N0 would mean no nodal involvement, whereas N1–N3 would denote involvement of an increasing number and range of nodes. M0 signifies no distant metastases, while M1 or sometimes M2 indicates the presence of blood-borne metastases and some judgment as to their number.

The AJC employs a somewhat different nomenclature and divides all cancers into stages 0 to IV, incorporating within each of these stages the size of the primary lesion as well as the presence of nodal spread and distant metastases. The use of these systems of staging and more details will emerge later in the consideration of specific tumors. However, it merits emphasis here that staging of neoplastic disease has assumed great importance in the selection of the best form of therapy for the patient, as is most clearly exemplified in the treatment of Hodgkin's disease (p. 719).

BIOLOGY OF TUMOR GROWTH

The natural history of most malignant tumors can be divided into four phases: (1) malignant change in the target cell, referred to as *transformation*, (2) *growth* of the transformed cells, (3) local *invasion*, and (4) distant *metastases*. At the risk of disturbing those with orderly minds, we will first consider altered growth properties of malignant cells in vivo and in vitro, followed by the mechanisms involved in local and distant spread; carcinogenic agents and the mechanisms involved in neoplastic transformation will be discussed in a later section (p. 267).

TUMOR CELL GROWTH

Growth that exceeds and is uncoordinated with that of the normal tissues is a fundamental feature of neoplasms. Before we consider how tumors grow, we should discuss whether tumors are monoclonal (arising from a single cell that has undergone neoplastic transformation) or multiclonal (arising by proliferation of several cells transformed independently).

Clonality of Tumors

A variety of approaches have been used to address this issue, the most common of which is the study of tumors in women, who are heterozygous for X-linked marker enzymes.[4] It may be recalled that glucose-6-phosphate dehydrogenase (G6PD), of which there are many isoenzymes, is encoded by a gene on the X chromosome. As explained on page 132, there is random inactivation of one X chromosome in all cells of the female embryo at the blastocyst stage. Thus, all organs in females are a complex of two populations of cells, one population having an active X chromosome of maternal origin and the other of paternal origin. In some women, most often black women, the two X chromosomes each encode a different G6PD isoenzyme. *Most neoplasms in these women (heterozygous for G6PD isoenzymes) express only a single isoenzyme,*

strongly suggesting that they are monoclonal in origin.
If the tumors were polyclonal, chance alone would dictate expression of both variants (Fig. 6–15). With the development of molecular tools that allow distinction between the maternal and paternal chromosomes by restriction fragment length polymorphism (p. 159), it is possible to examine the pattern of X chromosome inactivation at the level of the genome. In recent studies employing this technique, all 50 of the colonic tumors examined (20 carcinomas and 30 adenomas) and the majority of parathyroid adenomas displayed monoclonal patterns of X inactivation,[5,6] whereas the normal cells adjacent to the tumors revealed polyclonal patterns of X inactivation, as expected. Additional evidence of monoclonality of tumors comes from the following observations:

• In chronic myelogenous leukemia, a malignant tumor of myeloid stem cells, all cells possess a distinctive (nonrandom) translocation referred to as Philadelphia chromosome (p. 728).
• In tumors of T and B lymphocytes, monoclonality is indicated by the presence of identical and unique rearrangements of T and B cell receptor genes, detected by Southern blot analysis (p. 167).

Nonetheless, in a minority of instances, cancers appear to be polyclonal and sometimes multifocal in origin, as for example multiple colonic polyposis. Furthermore, some investigators have cautioned that the presence of a clonal marker (e.g., X chromosome inactivation) in a clinically detectable tumor does not prove that the tumor started with the transformation of a single cell, but only that one clone of the several that may have been present has overgrown the others during progressive growth of the tumor.[7]

Kinetics of Tumor Cell Growth

In any event, if a cancer is monoclonal, and the original transformed cell is about 10 μm in diameter, one can ask the question, "How long does it take to produce a clinically overt mass?" It can be readily calculated that the original transformed cell must undergo at least 30 population doublings to produce 10^9 cells (weighing approximately 1 gm), which is the smallest clinically detectable mass. In contrast, only 10 further doubling cycles are required to produce a tumor containing 10^{12} cells (weighing approximately 1 kg), which is usually the maximum size compatible with life (Fig. 6–16). These are minimal estimates, based on the assumption that all descendants of the transformed cell retain the ability to divide, and that there is no loss of cells from the replicative pool. This concept of tumor as a "pathologic dynamo" is not entirely correct, as we shall soon discuss.[8] Nevertheless, this calculation highlights an extremely important concept about tumor growth, i.e., *by the time a solid tumor is clinically detected, it has already completed a major portion of its life cycle.* This, as we shall see, is a major impediment in the treatment of cancer. But first let us examine the veracity of the assumption that a malignant tumor is a pathologic dynamo — a mass of rapidly and relentlessly dividing cells! To resolve this issue it is necessary to address the following questions that relate to tumor cell kinetics:

• What is the doubling time of tumor cells?
• What is the fraction of accumulating cells that remains in the replicating pool?
• What is the rate at which cells are shed and lost in the growing lesion?

The cell cycle of tumors, like that of all other cells, can be divided into phases, as illustrated in Figure 6–17. Although intuitively one may be inclined to think that tumor cells divide more rapidly than do normal cells, actual measurements speak to the contrary. The mean values of the DNA synthetic phase and total cell cycle time for several acute leukemias and solid tumors are in the range of 20 hours and 60 hours, respectively. These values are somewhat longer than the corresponding figures for normal hemopoietic precursor cells and proliferating epithelial cells in the intestinal crypts. *Thus it can be safely concluded that growth of tumors is not commonly associated with a shortening of cell cycle time.*[8]

The proportion of cells within the tumor population that are in the proliferative pool is referred to as the *growth fraction* (GF). A crude estimate of the frac-

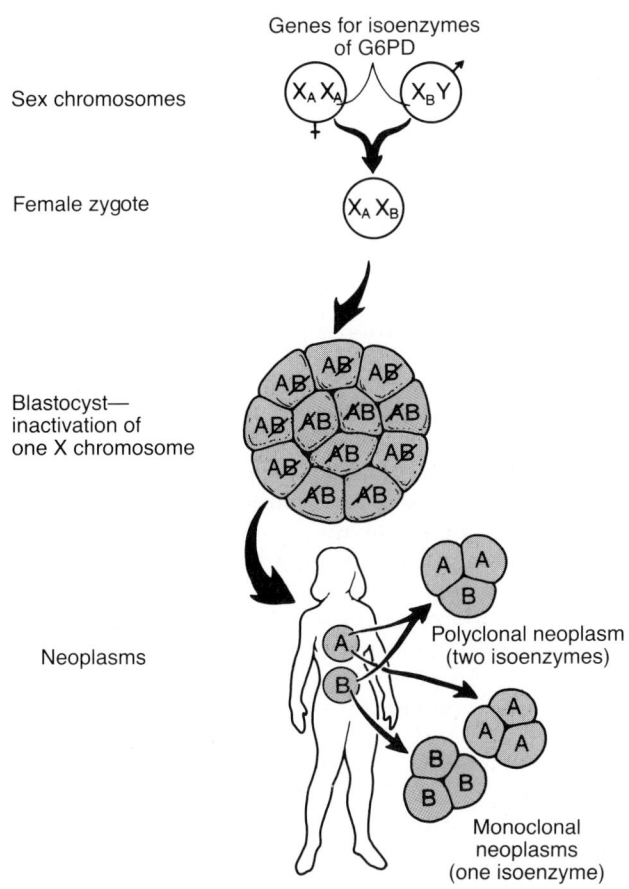

Figure 6–15. Diagram depicting the use of isoenzyme cell markers as evidence of the monoclonality of neoplasms.

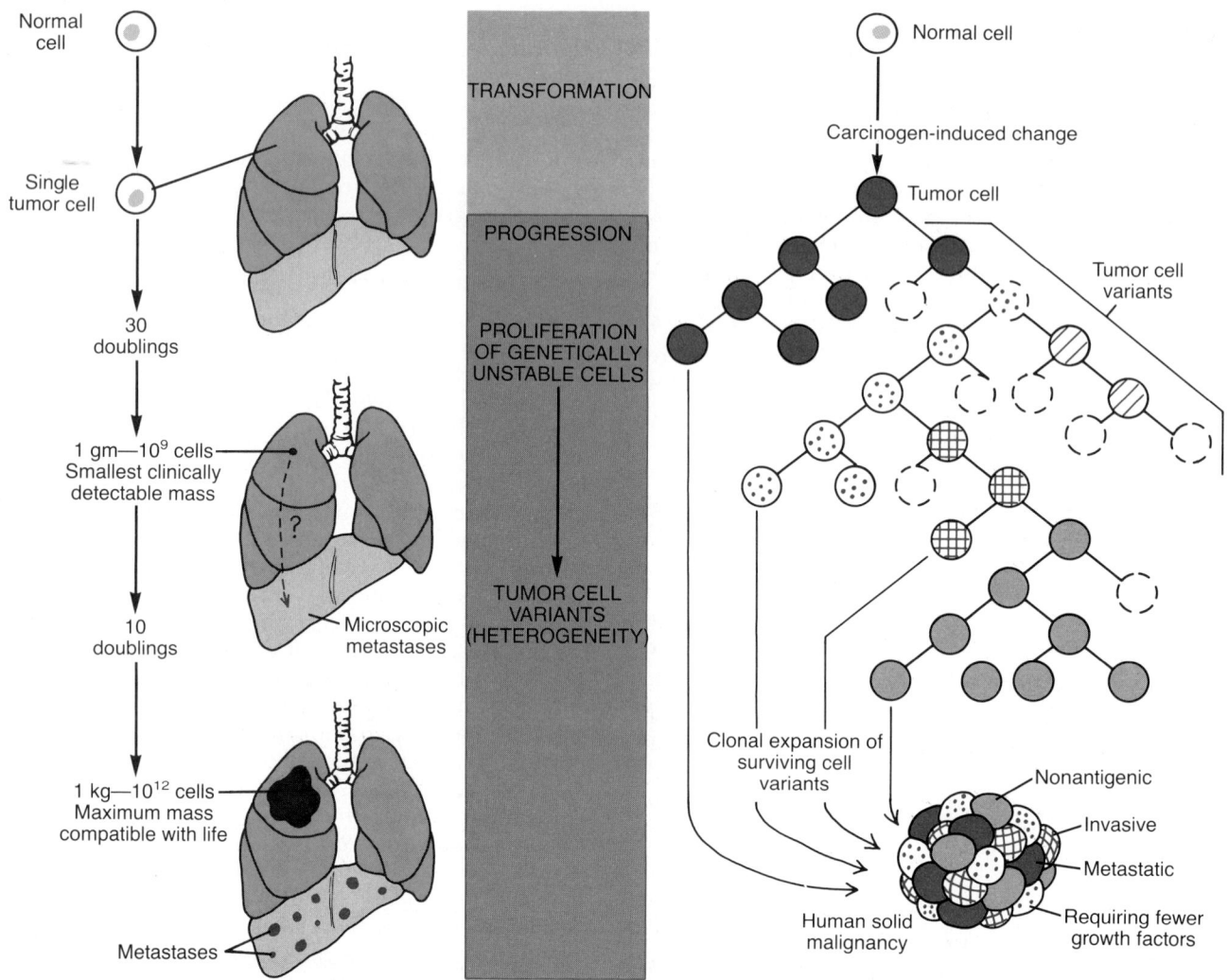

Figure 6–16. Biology of tumor growth. The left panel depicts minimal estimates of tumor cell doublings that precede the formation of a clinically detectable tumor mass. It is evident that by the time a solid tumor is detected, it has already completed a major portion of its life cycle as measured by cell doublings. The right panel illustrates clonal evolution of tumors and generation of tumor cell heterogeneity. New subclones arise from the descendants of the original transformed cell, and with progressive growth the tumor mass becomes enriched for those variants that are more adept at evading host defenses and are likely to be more aggressive. (Adapted from Tannock, I.F.: Biology of tumor growth. Hosp. Pract. 18:81, 1983.)

tion of proliferating cells in a given population can be obtained by calculating the *labeling index*. This is performed quite simply by incubating a sample of the tumor with ^{3}H-thymidine, a procedure that labels cell nuclei that are in the S-phase. It is then possible to calculate the ratio of labeled cells to total cells by autoradiography. It is interesting to note that the typical values of labeling index in many solid tumors vary between 2 and 8%.[8] This rate of proliferation is slower than that in a normal renewing epithelium such as the intestine (labeling index around 16%). Only in very aggressive and rapidly growing tumors (such as high-grade lymphomas), and possibly in the preclinical phase of other tumors, do the labeling indices approach about 30%. By modifications of autoradiographic labeling technique, and more recently by flow cytometry, it is possible to get a fairly accurate estimate of the GF of tumors. Such studies have re-

vealed that the *majority of cells within a clinically detectable tumor are not in the replicative pool.* Even in certain rapidly growing tumors, the GF is approximately 20%. In a growing tumor the daughter cells may leave the proliferative pool by one of three mechanisms: (1) Cancer cells are less cohesive than normal cells and are therefore continuously lost by shedding; (2) some cells differentiate—a process associated with loss of self-renewing capacity; and (3) cells may enter into G_0 (from which they can be potentially recruited back). It has been calculated that approximately 75 to 90% of tumor cells are lost from the replicating pool by one or more of these mechanisms. Given all these observations, how then do tumors increase in size? *Tumors grow, and grow progressively, not because they are pathologic dynamos but because there is an imbalance between cell production and cell loss. The fine homeostasis between cell growth and cell loss that is the hallmark of normal cell proliferation is disrupted in tumors.*

There are several important conceptual and practical lessons to be learned from the study of tumor cell kinetics.

• The rate of tumor growth depends upon the growth fraction and the degree of imbalance between cell production and cell loss. Some leukemias and lymphomas, and certain lung cell cancers (small cell carcinoma), have a relatively high growth fraction; their clinical course is rapid. By comparison, many common tumors such as cancer of the colon and breast have low growth fractions, and cell production exceeds cell loss by only about 10%; they tend to grow at a much slower pace.

• The growth fraction of tumor cells has a profound effect on their susceptibility to cancer chemotherapy. Since most anticancer agents act on cells that are actively synthesizing DNA, it is not difficult to imagine that a tumor which contains 5% of all cells in the replicating pool will be slowly growing but relatively refractory to treatment with drugs that kill dividing cells. Paradoxically, otherwise aggressive tumors (such as certain lymphomas) that contain a large pool of dividing cells literally melt away with chemotherapy, and even cures may be effected.

• Frequency of mitoses in a neoplasm is at best a crude reflection of rate of growth. If the cell cycle time is prolonged, as occurs in some tumors, many more mitoses will be visible at any given time, but whether the tumor grows rapidly or not will depend on other factors such as growth fraction and rate of cell loss.

We can now return to the question posed earlier: "How long does it take for one transformed cell to produce a clinically detectable tumor containing 10^9 cells?" If every one of the daughter cells remained in cell cycle and no cells were shed or lost, we could anticipate the answer to be 90 days (30 population doublings, with a cell cycle time of three days; see Fig. 6–16). In reality, *the latent period before which a tumor becomes clinically detectable is quite unpredictably long, probably years, emphasizing once again that human cancers are diagnosed only after they are fairly advanced in their life cycle.* After they become clinically detectable, the average volume-doubling time for such common killers as cancer of the lung and colon is about two to three months. However, as might be anticipated from the discussion of the variables that affect growth rate, the range of doubling time values is extremely broad, varying from less than one month for some childhood cancers to more than one year for certain salivary gland tumors. Cancer is indeed an unpredictable disorder.

Host Factors Affecting Tumor Growth

Factors other than cell kinetics modify the rate of growth. Most important among these is blood supply. Folkman has demonstrated that tumor cells in culture can grow in the absence of vascularization only up to nodules in the range of 1 to 2 mm in diameter.[9] However, when these nodules are implanted in tissue and develop a blood supply from the surrounding host tissues, further growth ensues. Support for the idea that tumor growth is absolutely dependent upon vascularization also comes from observations of human tumors in vivo. Necrosis commonly occurs in solid tumors. A careful examination often reveals that the necrotic region is parallel to a tumor blood vessel and separated from it by a 1 to 2 mm zone of viable tumor cells. Presumably, the 1 to 2 mm zone around blood vessels represents the maximal distance across which

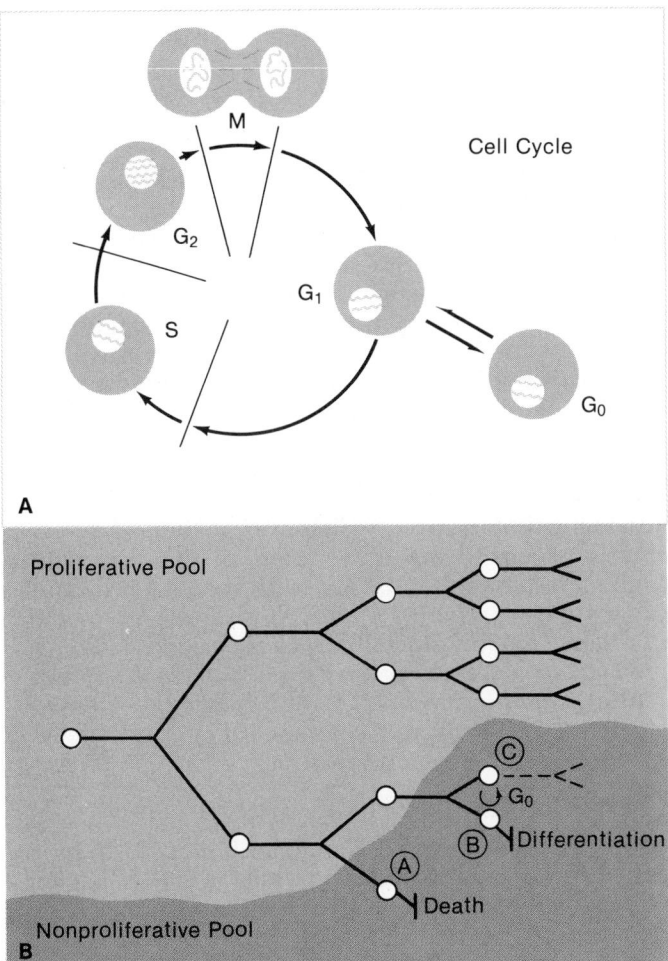

Figure 6–17. *A,* A diagrammatic representation of the events during the cell cycle. M is the period of mitosis—approximately one hour from prophase to cell division. G_1 reflects normal cell metabolism prior to DNA synthesis and usually constitutes more than half the total cell generation time. Cells not actively undergoing replication are described as being G_0; here they may remain indefinitely or be recruited back into the cycle. The DNA synthetic (S) phase is generally 6 to 24 hours. *B,* A schematic representation of tumor growth. As the cell population expands, a progressively higher percentage of cells leaves the proliferative pool by death (A), by differentiation (B), or by entering resting phase G_0 (C) from which they may be recruited back into the proliferative pool if the population size is reduced. (From Wyngaarden, J.B., and Smith, L.H. (eds.): Cecil Textbook of Medicine. 18th ed. Philadelphia, W.B. Saunders Co., 1988.)

oxygen and other nutrients in blood can readily diffuse.

How do growing tumor masses become vascularized? Studies by Folkman and colleagues suggest that tumor cells themselves secrete an angiogenesis factor. The tumor angiogenesis factor seems capable of effecting the entire series of events involved in the formation of capillaries[10] (p. 73). It was thought initially that tumor angiogenesis factor was uniquely tumor derived. Recent studies indicate, however, that this factor belongs to the family of heparin-binding growth factors that are ubiquitous in tissues. All factors of this family, including angiogenesis factor extracted from tumors, are structurally related to each other and, because of their ability to stimulate the growth of fibroblasts as well, have been called fibroblast growth factors.[11] These recent observations raise two interesting issues: (1) Can agents that antagonize angiogenesis factors be developed to prevent tumor neovascularization and hence control the growth of tumors? (2) How is the release of such ubiquitous angiogenic factors controlled in vivo, and what turns on their production by tumor cells?

In addition to blood supply, hormones influence the growth rate, particularly of cancers arising in hormonally responsive tissues (e.g., breast, uterus, endometrium, ovary, and prostate). The normal cells in such locations have steroid receptors, as do many of the cancers, and so carcinomas of the breast may sometimes become explosive in their growth during pregnancy; conversely, the use of antiestrogenic agents or surgical removal of the ovaries and sometimes adrenals and pituitary gland may markedly slow the growth of breast carcinomas. Unfortunately, however, such hormonal manipulations are rarely more than palliative measures. Suffice it to say that *host factors influence growth rate.*

Tumor Progression and Heterogeneity

Given the fact that most human tumors are clonal, i.e., derived from the proliferation of a single transformed cell, one can ask whether all cells within a tumor mass are phenotypically and genotypically identical to the cell of origin. There is mounting evidence that by the time cancers (even those in which proof of clonal origin still exists) become clinically detectable, their constituent cells are extremely heterogeneous. *Subsets that differ in their karyotype, invasiveness, growth rate, hormonal responsiveness, metastatic abilities, and susceptibility to antineoplastic drugs can be readily identified in the descendants of a single transformed cell.* Foulds, who first recognized that tumor growth was associated with heterogeneity, referred to this as *tumor progression* and defined it as "acquisition of permanent, irreversible qualitative changes in one or more characteristics of a neoplasm."[12] Although the mechanisms involved in tumor progression are not fully understood, most investigators believe that neoplastic transformation is associated with the acquisition of genetic instability. This renders the cells sus-

ceptible to a high rate of random mutation during clonal expansion (see Fig. 6–16). The fate of the subclones generated within the tumor is strongly influenced by host selection pressures that are both immune and nonimmune. Thus, cells that are highly immunogenic may be destroyed by host lymphoid cells, whereas those that have reduced oxygen or nutrient requirements would have a growth advantage. An emerging tumor, therefore, tends to be enriched for those subclones that are more adept at survival, growth, invasion, and metastasis.[13,14]

Tumor progression and the resultant tumor cell heterogeneity have important biologic and clinical consequences.[14,15]

• As discussed earlier (p. 251), when clinically detected, most tumors are in a late stage of their natural history, having already undergone at least 30 (and possibly many more) population doublings. If tumor cell heterogeneity is generated by spontaneous mutations, it seems likely that the greater the interval between transformation and clinical detection, the greater will be the number of divisions the cells have undergone, and therefore the greater will be the likelihood that the tumor will contain mutant subclones that have a higher growth rate, greater metastatic potential, and resistance to drugs. Conversely, small lesions have the least probability of containing subsets that are very invasive and therefore have the best prognosis. Indeed, the importance of treating a small tumor burden with chemotherapy has been clearly established.[15]

• In many tumors, progression prior to clinical detection is associated with generation of subclones with high metastatic potential and with seeding of distant organs. *Recognition of this likelihood has led to the development of treatment protocols designed to eliminate metastases even if they are not detectable by currently available means.* This approach has yielded gratifying results in the treatment of certain cancers of the breast, bone, and testis.

Growth of Tumor Cells in Vitro

Much has been learned about the biology of tumor cells by studying the phenotype and growth behavior of cancer cells in vitro. In tissue culture, tumor cells demonstrate several differences from normal cells. These changes have been noted in a large variety of tumor cells and are summarized below:

• *Apparent escape from regulatory controls.* Normal cells grown in culture containing serum continue to divide until they form a confluent monolayer, at which time further replication ceases because of "contact inhibition" or "density-dependent inhibition." Transformed cells are not "contact inhibited" and are less subject to "density-dependent inhibition of growth" (possibly reflecting lowered requirements for supportive growth factors such as are present in serum). Thus, when transformed cells are grown in

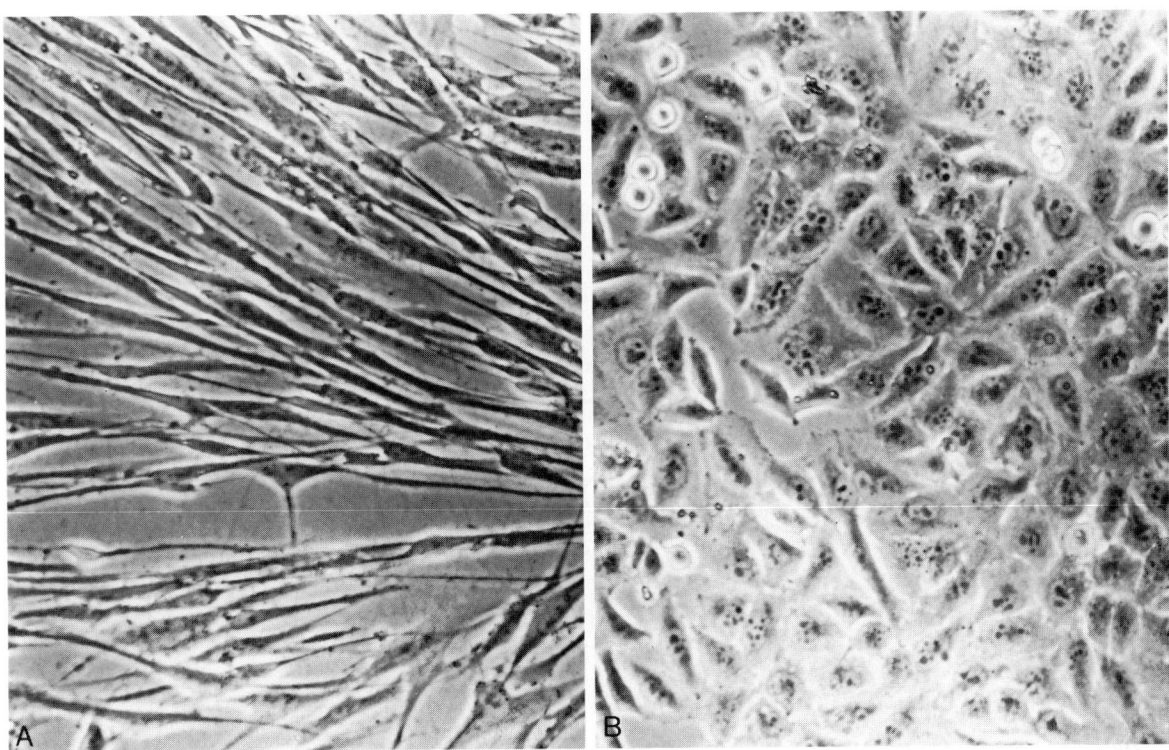

Figure 6–18. *A,* Orderly, oriented growth in culture of normal fibroblasts. Compare with disoriented, random growth of transformed fibroblasts in *B.* (Courtesy of Dr. Tom Wright, Brigham and Women's Hospital and Harvard Medical School, Boston, Massachusetts.)

culture, they pile up in multilayered, disorderly masses (Fig. 6–18).

• *Reduced serum requirement for growth.* Transformed cells generally grow well in media containing less serum than that needed by nontransformed cells. This property reflects reduced requirement for growth factors contained in serum. Many transformed cells synthesize and secrete polypeptide growth factors (p. 285) that stimulate their own growth.

• *Anchorage-independence.* Most normal cells will grow only when they are anchored to a solid surface. Tumor cells, however, are anchorage independent and will therefore grow in soft agar.

• *Failure to maturate.* By not undergoing terminal differentiation and cell death, transformed cells retain for longer periods their viability and capacity to replicate and accumulate.

• *Transformed cells are "immortal."* Normal cells capable of being maintained in subculture undergo a finite number of cell divisions before they perish; transformed cells can be subcultured indefinitely (some have been maintained for decades).

• *Transplantability.* In contrast to normal differentiated cells, fully transformed cells grown in vitro can form tumors when injected into syngeneic hosts.

• *Reduced cohesiveness.* Because of changes in the glycosylation of cell surface proteins, and alterations in the amount of certain glycoproteins (such as fibronectin), tumor cells tend to be less cohesive. This may facilitate invasiveness.

MECHANISMS OF INVASION AND METASTASIS

Invasion and metastasis are biologic hallmarks of malignant tumors. They are the major cause of cancer-related morbidity and mortality, and hence the subjects of intense scrutiny. In order for tumor cells to break loose from a primary mass, enter blood vessels or lymphatics, and produce a secondary growth at a distant site, they must go through a series of steps[14] that are summarized in Figure 6–19. Each step in this sequence is subject to a multitude of influences, and hence at any point in the sequence the breakaway cell may not survive. Studies in experimental animals indicate that despite the fact that millions of cells are released into the circulation each day from a 1 cm³ primary tumor, only a few metastases are produced. What then is the basis of the apparent inefficiency of this process? Do metastases develop from a few randomly surviving tumor cells that all have similar metastatic potential, or does a subpopulation of cells exist within the parent tumor that has unique abilities to negotiate the metastatic cascade? A series of experiments performed by Fidler and colleagues strongly supports the latter possibility.[16] One such experiment is illustrated in Figure 6–20. It is apparent from this and other experimental models of tumor metastases that each tumor contains several subclones with variable degrees of metastatic potential. Only a select population that can detach from the primary tumor, invade the host tissues, enter the circulation and survive in it, extravasate from the blood vessels, and grow at the new site will be successful at forming metastases.

Thus it appears that, as with several other attributes, fully evolved cancers are heterogeneous with respect to metastatic potential. As previously discussed, such heterogeneity may result from new mutations in genetically unstable replicating cells of

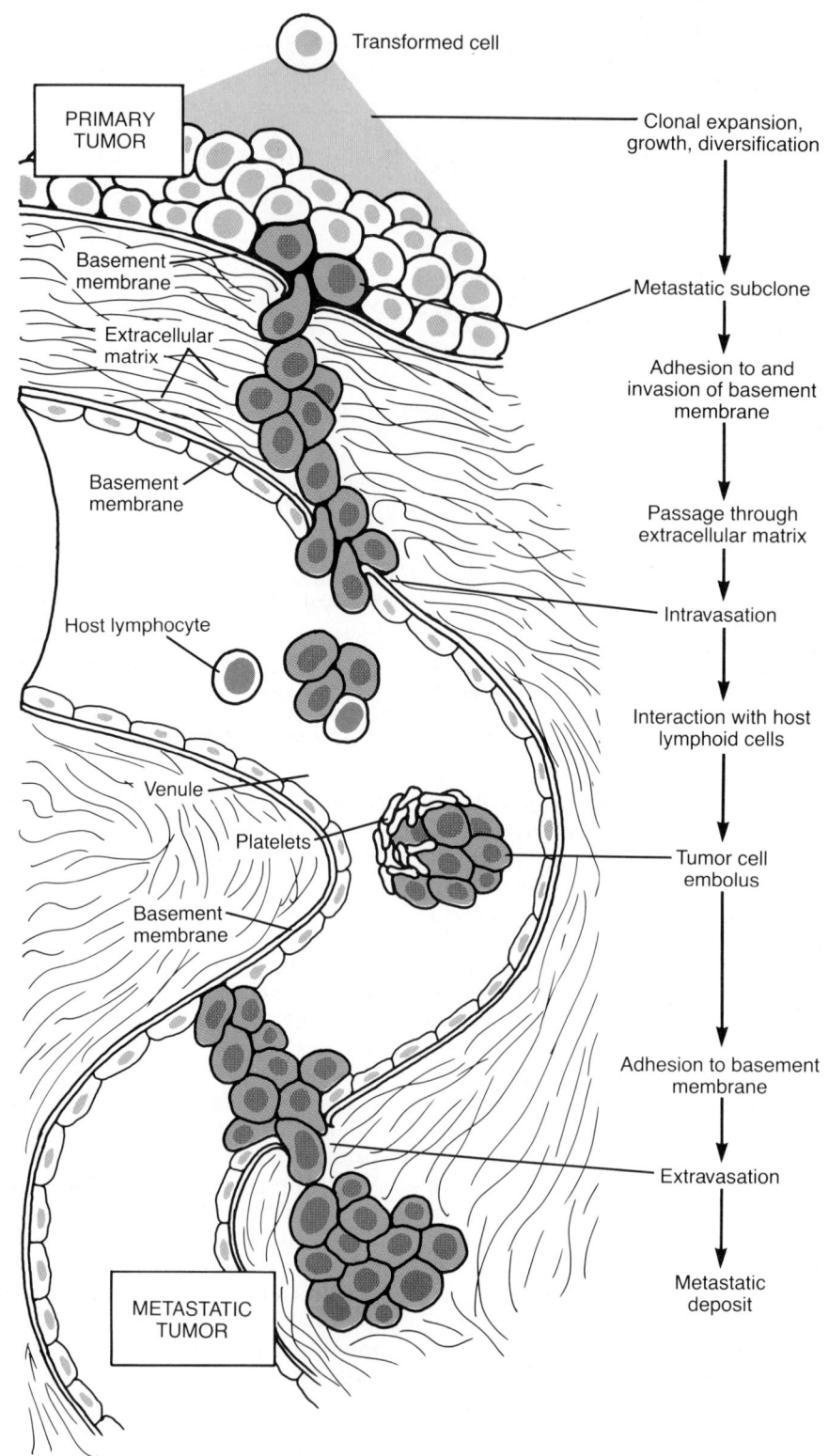

Figure 6–19. The metastatic cascade. A schematic illustration of the sequential steps involved in the hematogenous spread of a tumor.

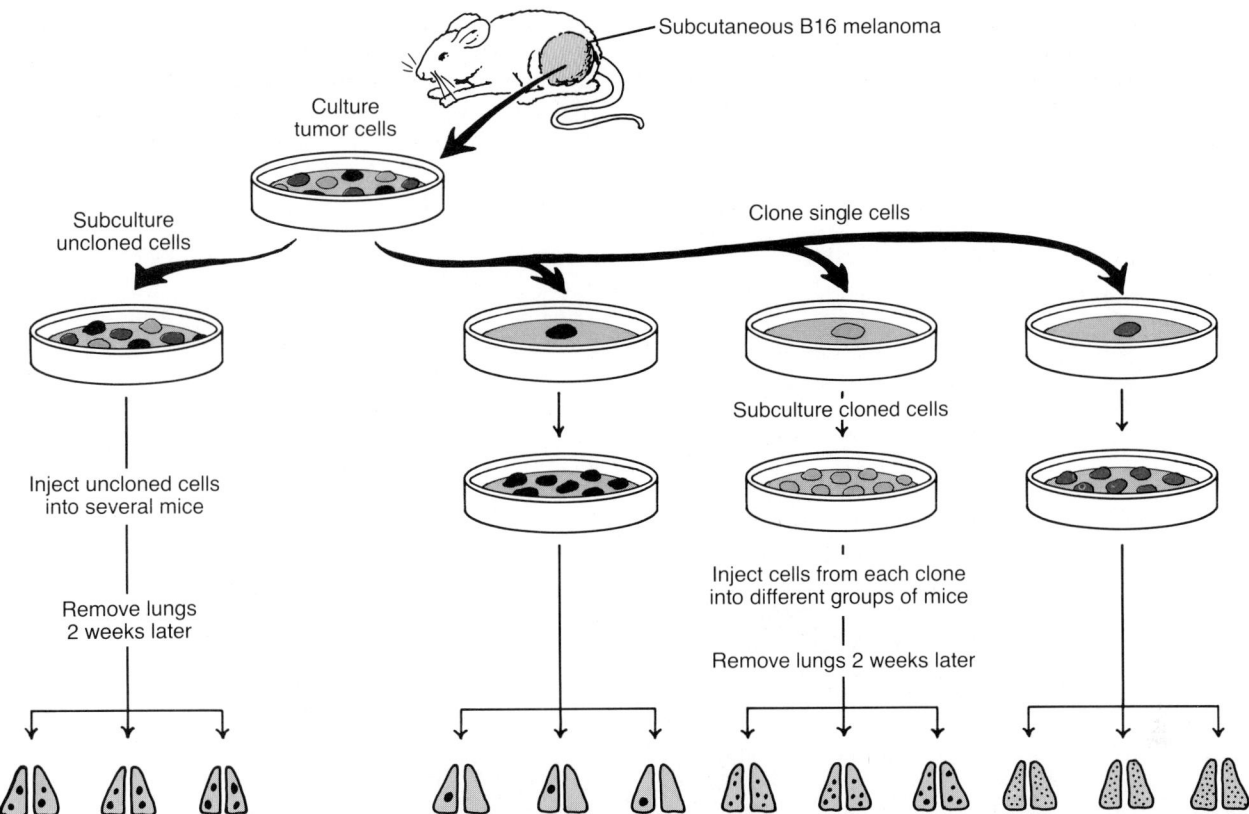

Figure 6–20. Schematic illustration of tumor cell heterogeneity with respect to metastatic ability. A primary tumor contains subclones that differ in their ability to form metastases. When such a heterogeneous population is injected intravenously into mice, each animal receives a mixture of cells with varying levels of metastatic potential, and hence the lungs of each animal reveal approximately equal numbers of metastases. However, if cells from the primary tumor are cloned prior to the experiment, populations with differing metastatic abilities are separated. This experimental design is based on studies of Fidler and colleagues.[16]

evolving neoplasms. Alternatively, it may result from variable expression of genes in different subsets of tumor cells.[17] Whatever the mechanism, it bears repetition (p. 251) that by the time a primary tumor is detected, most of its natural history within the patient has already elapsed, and therefore it may well contain subclones with metastatic potential (see Fig. 6–16). For reasons not entirely clear, the rate at which metastatic variants are generated within primary tumors varies considerably. In some, such as osteogenic sarcoma, micrometastases are almost always present at the time of diagnosis, whereas in others, typified by certain salivary gland cancers, metastases occur late and infrequently.

INTERACTIONS OF TUMOR CELLS WITH EXTRACELLULAR MATRIX

A review of Figure 6–19 will reveal that tumor cells must penetrate the extracellular matrix at several stages in the metastatic cascade. The first barrier carcinomas must cross is the basement membrane, which is a highly specialized sheet of extracellular matrix. Next the tumor cells must penetrate the interstitial matrix and gain access to the circulation by traversing the vascular basement membrane. Eventually this cycle is repeated when the tumor cells leave the vas-

culature and set up shop in the extracellular matrix (ECM) of the distant organ. Thus *an important attribute of metastatic cells is the ability to attach to, degrade, and penetrate the ECM.*

Since tumor cells must interact with the ECM at several steps in the metastatic cascade, we will briefly review the composition and organization of ECM before we discuss the biochemical basis of these interactions. *ECM can be divided into two major categories: basement membranes and interstitial connective tissue.*[18] Basement membranes are condensed sheetlike structures that separate epithelial and endothelial cells from the interstitial connective tissue. They consist of a highly cross-linked meshwork of type IV collagen, specific glycoproteins such as laminin, and heparan sulfate proteoglycan. Type IV collagen accounts for as much as 60% of the total matrix protein, whereas laminin is the major noncollagenous component. Much interest is focused on the laminin molecule, since it seems to be the glue that keeps the basement membrane together. Laminin has high affinity for type IV collagen and proteoglycans, and it also binds to epithelial cell membrane via high-affinity laminin receptors that are found on the epithelium. The multiple functions of laminin are mediated by distinct domains within this large cross-shaped molecule (Fig. 6–21A). The globular ends of the three short arms

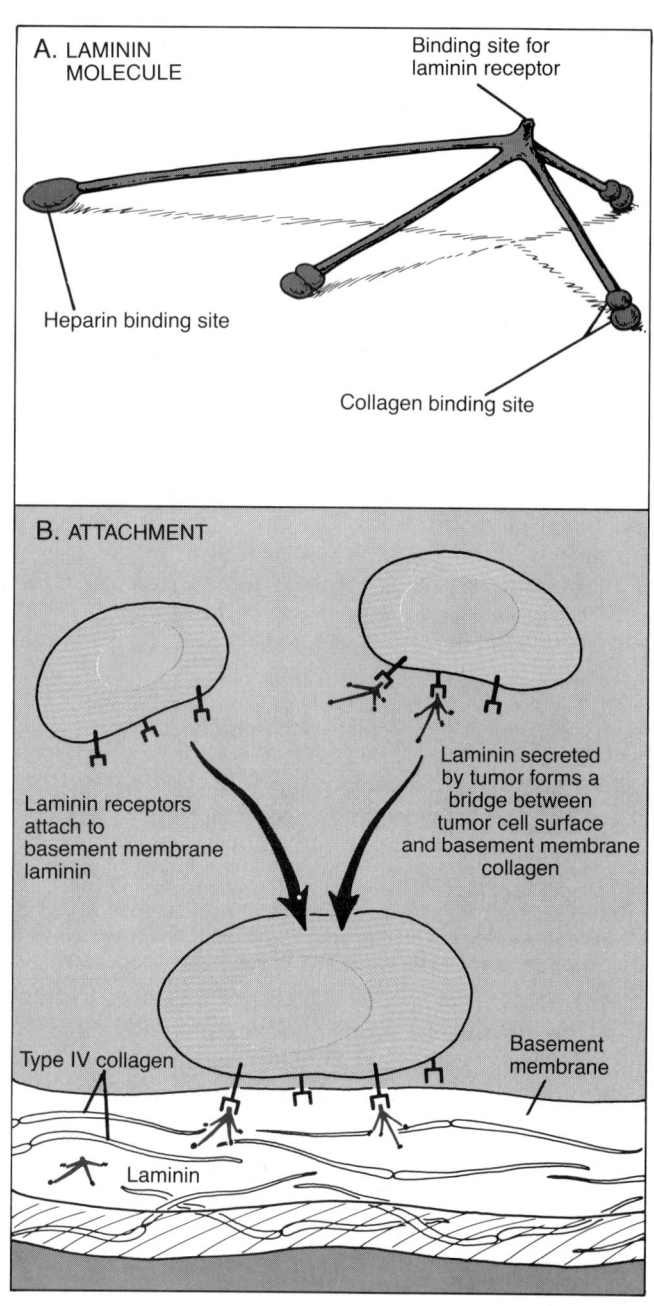

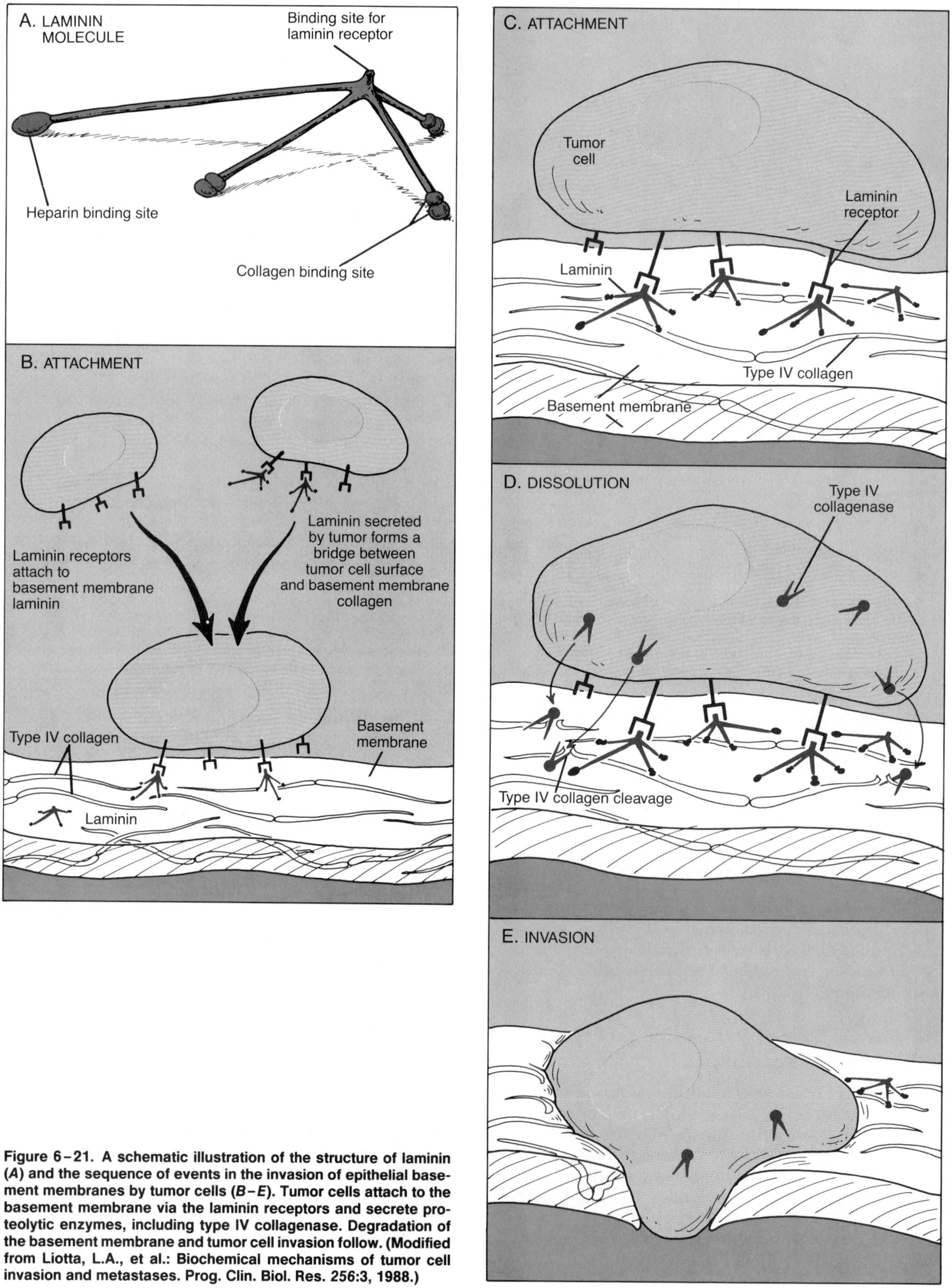

A. LAMININ MOLECULE

Binding site for laminin receptor

Heparin binding site

Collagen binding site

B. ATTACHMENT

Laminin receptors attach to basement membrane laminin

Laminin secreted by tumor forms a bridge between tumor cell surface and basement membrane collagen

Type IV collagen

Basement membrane

Laminin

C. ATTACHMENT

Tumor cell

Laminin receptor

Laminin

Type IV collagen

Basement membrane

D. DISSOLUTION

Type IV collagenase

Type IV collagen cleavage

E. INVASION

Figure 6-21. A schematic illustration of the structure of laminin (*A*) and the sequence of events in the invasion of epithelial basement membranes by tumor cells (*B-E*). Tumor cells attach to the basement membrane via the laminin receptors and secrete proteolytic enzymes, including type IV collagenase. Degradation of the basement membrane and tumor cell invasion follow. (Modified from Liotta, L.A., et al.: Biochemical mechanisms of tumor cell invasion and metastases. Prog. Clin. Biol. Res. 256:3, 1988.)

bind to type IV collagen, whereas the long arm contains the heparin-binding site. The laminin receptor on epithelial cells binds to the central cross-shaped region. As we shall see, these different regions play distinct roles in the adhesion of tumor cells to basement membranes.

As with basement membranes, collagen is the most abundant protein of the interstitial extracellular matrix. However, the type of collagen varies; type I collagen is the predominant type (and is usually codistributed with type III collagen) in all interstitial connective tissues except in cartilage, where type II collagen is specifically found. Interspersed in the collagen meshwork are proteoglycans, and glycoproteins such as fibronectin. Proteoglycans retain fluid in the tissues, and their major function is to maintain the normal shape and volume of the connective tissue. Fibronectin, on the other hand, is the major adhesion-promoting protein of the interstitial tissues. Although laminin and fibronectin are biochemically distinct, they share several properties. Like laminin, fibronectin is a multifunctional-multidomain molecule that can bind to collagen, fibrin, proteoglycans, and hyaluronic acid, among others. Cells adhere to fibronectin via a cell surface receptor that recognizes a short tripeptide sequence Arg-Gly-Asp (RGD).[19] The elucidation of this sequence has enabled detailed investigations of the role of tumor cell adhesion to fibronectin during invasion and metastasis.

With this review of the structure of ECM we can return to the mechanisms by which tumor cells invade and disseminate. According to Liotta and colleagues, invasion can be resolved into three steps:[20]

• Attachment of tumor cells to matrix components such as laminin and fibronectin.
• Secretion of proteolytic enzymes that locally degrade the matrix components.
• Migration of the tumor into the degraded zone of ECM.

Cyclic repetition of these three steps would lead to progressive invasion by the advancing tumor cells. Each of these steps will now be examined in some detail (Fig. 6–21).

Adhesion of Tumor Cells to Extracellular Matrix

There is substantial experimental evidence that receptor-mediated attachment of tumor cells to laminin and fibronectin is important for invasion and metastasis.[21,22] This hypothesis is supported by the observation that the density of laminin receptors on breast cancer cells is positively correlated with invasiveness and number of lymph node metastases. Two mechanisms may be involved:

• Tumor cells bind to the basement membrane laminin via unoccupied cell surface laminin receptors.
• Several tumor cells secrete high amounts of laminin, which occupy their laminin receptors. These cells display increased (rather than decreased) metastatic

potential. This apparent paradox has been resolved by experiments in which the role of various fragments of cell-bound laminin on metastatic behavior was investigated. It seems that laminin receptors on tumor cells bind to the secreted laminin at the cross-shaped intersection of the laminin arms. This leaves the globular collagen-binding domains at the ends of the short arms free to bind type IV collagen in the basement membranes.[20] Thus laminin forms *a bridge between the laminin receptor on the cell and type IV collagen in the basement membranes* (Fig. 6–21B).

The ability to bind fibronectin is also believed to be important in invasion and metastasis. To understand the experimental basis of this conclusion it should be recalled that cell adhesion to fibronectin is mediated by a receptor that recognizes the amino acid sequence RGD (Fig. 2–45, p. 81). Short synthetic peptides that contain the RGD sequence will occupy the fibronectin receptor on cells and block their adhesion to fibronectin. Blockade of the fibronectin receptor on tumor cells by RGD-containing peptides markedly inhibits the formation of lung metastases, presumably by preventing the adhesion of tumor cells to fibronectin in the extracellular matrix.[21]

Degradation of Extracellular Matrix

After attachment to the components of the basement membrane or interstitial extracellular matrix, tumor cells must create passageways for migration. Invasion of the matrix is not due merely to passive growth pressure but requires active enzymatic degradation of the ECM components.[23] In some experimental studies, tumor cells collected from venules draining the tumor demonstrated greater ECM-degrading activity than did the general population of cells within the tumor. Thus it seems that tumor cells entering the circulation represent a subpopulation selected for the ability to secrete enzymes capable of degrading vascular basement membranes. Since the composition of the basement membranes and interstitial connective tissue is different, we will discuss the degradation of these two forms of ECM separately.

Different components of the basement membrane are degraded by distinct mechanisms. Type IV collagen is specifically cleaved by a metalloproteinase referred to as type IV collagenase. This enzyme can be isolated from murine sarcomas and melanomas and human fibrosarcoma cell lines. Liotta and colleagues[20,24] have provided compelling evidence supporting a role for type IV collagenase in tumor cell invasion that can be summarized as follows:

• There is a correlation between metastatic potential of several sublines of a mouse melanoma and the amount of enzyme synthesized by the cell lines in vitro.
• When fibroblasts were transformed by certain oncogenes in vitro, all transformants that had high metastatic propensity secreted large amounts of collagenase IV, whereas those that were transformed (i.e., tumorigenic) but nonmetastatic had lower levels.

• Tumor cells that were able to degrade (and traverse) a matrix containing type IV collagen in vitro were found to be metastatic in vivo. Cells that failed to traverse this barrier were nonmetastatic.

Several other enzymes secreted by tumor cells, including glycosidases and nonspecific proteinases (elastase, cathepsins, and plasmin), have also been implicated in the degradation of basement membranes.[18,23] Of these, plasmin is of particular interest. It can break down several noncollagenous matrix molecules such as laminin and protein cores of proteoglycans. Furthermore, plasmin activates type IV collagenase, which is secreted in a latent form by tumor cells. As is well known, plasmin itself has to be generated from its inactive precursor plasminogen by plasminogen activator (PA). Increased levels of PA are frequently found in malignant cells. Because of its ability to regulate the activation of plasmin and plasmin-dependent type IV collagenase, PA may play an important role in invasion.

Degradation of interstitial collagens (types I and III) presumably occurs by interstitial collagenases. Many tumor cells are known to secrete collagenases, and a positive correlation between tumor invasiveness and the level of interstitial collagenases has been reported. In addition to secreting proteolytic enzymes themselves, it is very likely that cancer cells interact with host fibroblasts and other mesenchymal cells and stimulate them to secrete collagenases.

The most obvious effect of matrix destruction is to create a passage for invasion by tumor cells. In addition, *cleavage products of matrix components, derived from collagen and proteoglycans, have growth-promoting, angiogenic, and chemotactic activities.* The latter may promote the migration of tumor cells into the loosened ECM.

Migration of Tumor Cells

Malignant cells are far less cohesive than normal cells. In histologic sections of invasive tumors, it is not uncommon to find small groups of tumor cells separated from the main mass at the leading edge of the tumor. These observations suggest that invading tumor cells are motile, but little is known about the locomotion of tumor cells.[25] It may result in part from chemotactic fragments of ECM, as described above. In addition, some tumors may secrete factors that stimulate their own motility by autocrine mechanisms.[20]

VASCULAR DISSEMINATION AND HOMING OF TUMOR CELLS

Once in circulation, tumor cells are particularly vulnerable to destruction by natural and adaptive immune defenses. The details of tumor immunity will be considered later (p. 296). Suffice it to say that natural killer (NK) cells seem to be particularly important in controlling hematogenous spread of tumors.

Within the circulation, tumor cells tend to aggregate in clumps. This is favored by homotypic adhesions among tumor cells as well as heterotypic adhesion between tumor cells and blood cells, particularly platelets (see Fig. 6–19). Formation of platelet-tumor aggregates seems to enhance tumor cell survival and implantability. In experimental tumor models, thrombocytopenia (reduction in platelets) reduces the number of lung metastases produced by tumor cells introduced into the circulation. Tumor cells aggregated with platelets may be protected from attack by lymphoid cells.[26]

The site at which circulating tumor cells leave the capillaries to form secondary deposits is related in part to the anatomic localization of the primary tumor (p. 249). However, many observations suggest that natural pathways of drainage do not wholly explain the distributions of metastases. For example, prostatic carcinoma preferentially spreads to bone, bronchogenic carcinomas tend to involve the adrenals and the brain, and neuroblastomas spread to the liver and bones. Cell surface properties, most likely receptors, on the cancer cell and on the endothelial cells appear to underlie such distributions.[27] In the laboratory it has been possible to select sublines from a variety of cancers — notably the B-16 mouse melanoma — that will selectively "home" to specific organs such as the lung, liver, brain, or ovary. In the case of a "lung subline" it can be shown that irrespective of where the cancer cells are introduced into the vascular system, they selectively "home" to the lung. When normal lung tissue is implanted into the thigh of the animal, the cancer cells unerringly colonize it and the native lungs. The fact that this "homing" attribute relates to the cell surface is documented by the ability to transfer "lung preference" to other cancer cell lines by fusing onto them vesicles of plasma membrane shed by pulmonary homing subline. Conversely, it has long been observed that malignant neoplasms rarely metastasize to skeletal muscles and seldom to the spleen. Although this could be attributable to the presence of protease inhibitors in these tissues ("unfavorable soil"), conceivably it may relate to the lack of receptor interactions between tumor cells and endothelial cells in these tissues. However, despite all the foregoing considerations, the localization of metastases cannot be predicted with any form of cancer. Evidently many tumors have not read all of the experimental literature.

KARYOTYPIC CHANGES IN TUMORS

With each passing year it becomes more certain that the malignant cells of most types of human cancer have chromosomal abnormalities and that in many types of cancer the defects are consistent. With high-resolution banding techniques, karyotypic alterations have now been identified in a great many transformed and cancerous cells, and there is a strong possibility that gene changes are present in all.[28,29]

In certain types of neoplasms in humans the karyotypic abnormality is nonrandom and common, which strongly suggests that it is a primary event in the development of the malignant state. Such observations and others underlie the current widely held proposition that the origins of cancers lie within particular genes — "oncogenes" (discussed later, p. 282). However, it should be cautioned that cytogenetic abnormalities may merely reflect fragile sites within chromosomes vulnerable to breaks and rearrangements in a rapidly replicating population.[30] Moreover, even when a nonrandom, potentially "primary" alteration has appeared, tumor progression is often accompanied by ever greater karyotypic deviation. Thus the karyotype may vary somewhat among the many clones making up a fully evolved cancer. Nonetheless, it is usually possible to identify a modal pattern and nonrandom abnormalities and to differentiate them from secondary changes.

Specific abnormalities have been identified in most leukemias and lymphomas and an increasing number of nonhematopoietic tumors, with the promise of many more to come. *The most common types of nonrandom structural abnormalities in tumor cells are (1) balanced translocations, (2) chromosome deletions, and (3) cytogenetic manifestations of gene amplification.*[31] In addition, there may be gains and losses of whole chromosomes. In general, numerical changes are less specific. Some examples of karyotypic changes in tumors are presented in Table 6–3. Many of these will be described with later consideration of specific forms of neoplasia. Only a few examples from each category of structural changes are presented here.

BALANCED TRANSLOCATIONS. *Most notable and first described is the Philadelphia (Ph1) chromosome in chronic myelogenous leukemia (CML), comprising a reciprocal and balanced translocation between chromosomes 22 and, usually, 9 (and in a small percentage, a translocation to other chromosomes).* As a consequence, chromosome 22 appears somewhat abbreviated. This change is present in over 90% of cases of CML and indeed constitutes a reliable marker of the disease. The Ph1 chromosome can be identified in the myeloblastic, erythroblastic, and megakaryocytic lines of cells. Indeed, the few cases of CML lacking the Ph1 chromosome tend to be more resistant to therapy and to have a worse prognosis. As we shall see later (p. 289), a putative oncogene is present at, or close to, the breakpoint in chromosome 9, suggesting that a shift in the location of the oncogene is fundamental to the development of CML. As another example, in *over 90% of the instances of Burkitt's lymphoma, the cells have a translocation, usually between chromosomes 8 and 14,* and less often between 8 and 2 or 22. Once again, an apparent oncogene has been assigned to the breakpoint on chromosome 8 (see Fig. 6–32). Analogous karyotypic abnormalities have been associated with many other varieties of leukemia and lymphoma.

DELETIONS. Chromosomal deletions are the second most prevalent structural chromosome abnormality in

Table 6–3. Some Neoplasms with a Specific Associated Chromosomal Abnormality

DISEASE	CHROMOSOME DEFECT
Leukemias	
Chronic myelogenous leukemia	t(9;22)
Acute nonlymphocytic leukemia	
M1	t(9;22)
M2	t(8;21)
M3	t(15;17)
M4	inv (16)
M4, M5	t(11;*)
M1, M2, M4, M5, M6	del 5q
	del 7q
	+8
Chronic lymphocytic leukemia	+12
Acute lymphocytic leukemia	
L1–L2	t(9;22), t(1;19), t(4;11)
L3	t(8;14)
Lymphomas, Non-Hodgkin's	
Burkitt's, small noncleaved cell (non-Burkitt), diffuse large cell	t(8;14)
Follicular small cleaved, follicular mixed	t(14;18)
Small cell lymphocytic	+12
Small cell lymphocytic, follicular small cleaved, diffuse large cell	t(11;14)
Diffuse large cell, follicular small cleaved cell, immunoblastic	del 6q
Carcinomas and Sarcomas	
Neuroblastoma, disseminated	del 1p
Small cell lung carcinoma	del 3p
Papillary cystadenocarcinoma of ovary	t(6;14)
Retinoblastoma	del 13q
Wilms' tumor	del 11p
Colorectal adenocarcinoma	del 17p, t(17;*)
Renal cell carcinoma	del 3p, t(3;*)
Testicular tumors	i(12p)
Ewing sarcoma	t(11;22)
Liposarcoma, myxoid	t(12;16)
Benign Solid Tumors	
Mixed parotid gland tumor	t(3;8)
Meningioma	−22
Lipoma	t(3;12)
Leiomyoma	t(12;14)

* Various chromosomes.

Drawn and modified from Yunis, J.J.: The chromosomal basis of human neoplasia. Science *221*:227, 1983. (Courtesy of Dr. Nancy Schneider, Department of Pathology, University of Texas, Southwestern Medical School, Dallas, Texas.)

tumor cells. Although they have been found in several leukemias, they are more common in solid tumors of nonhematopoietic origin. The study of deletions in two embryonal tumors of childhood, retinoblastoma and Wilms' tumor, have provided important insights into the origin of cancer. Deletion of chromosome 13, band q14, is associated with retinoblastoma, and deletion of chromosome 11, band p13, is associated with Wilms' tumor. In some individuals these deletions occur as inherited chromosomal abnormalities (affecting all cells), increasing greatly their risk of developing these tumors (p. 266). Detailed molecular studies of tumor DNA derived from both sporadic and familial cases of retinoblastoma and Wilms' tumor have revealed subtle genetic alterations at the breakpoints on chromosomes 13 and 11, respectively, in almost all cases. From these cytogenetic and molecular studies arose the concept that loss of some normal "cancer suppressor genes" located on chromosomes 13 and 11 is related to the development of these tumors. This important concept of tumorigenesis is discussed in detail later in this chapter (p. 289).

CYTOGENETIC CHANGES ASSOCIATED WITH GENE AMPLIFICATION. There are two karyotypic manifestations of gene amplification: homogeneously staining regions (HSRs) on single chromosomes and double minutes (DMs) (see Fig. 6–33). The latter are seen as very small paired fragments of chromatin (not attached to any chromosome). Although initially observed in tumor cells that had become drug resistant by amplification of genes encoding for the enzymes affected by the drug, DMs and HSRs have been observed de novo in some spontaneously arising tumors. Neuroblastomas represent the best studied example in which gene amplification is associated with HSRs. The amplified gene is an oncogene called N-*myc*, and as we shall discuss later (p. 289), amplification of oncogenes may have a bearing on their role in causation of tumors.

Quite intriguing are the observations relating to the existence of nonrandom karyotypic changes in benign neoplasms such as lipomas, meningiomas, and colonic adenomas. Traditionally, the presence of clonal karyotypic abnormalities has been associated with malignant transformation.[32] The challenge now is to determine the significance of karyotypic abnormalities in benign neoplasms. Do they represent one of the several steps involved in malignant transformation, or are they secondary abnormalities in cells that are genetically unstable?

PREDISPOSITION TO CANCER

Because cancer is a disorder of cell growth and behavior, its ultimate cause has to be defined at the cellular and subcellular levels. However, study of cancer patterns in populations can contribute substantially to knowledge about the origins of cancer. For example,

the concept that chemicals can cause cancer arose from the astute observations of Sir Percival Pott, who related the increased incidence of scrotal cancer in chimney sweeps to chronic exposure to soot. Thus, major insights into the etiology of cancer can be obtained by epidemiologic studies that relate particular environmental, racial (hereditary?), and cultural influences to the occurrence of malignant neoplasms. In addition, certain diseases associated with an increased risk of developing cancer can provide insights into the pathogenesis of malignancy. Therefore, the following discussion will review a number of factors relating to both the patient and the environment that influence predisposition to cancer.

GEOGRAPHIC AND RACIAL FACTORS

In some measure, an individual's likelihood of developing a cancer is expressed by national incidence and mortality rates. For example, it is sobering to realize that residents of the United States have about a one in five chance of dying of cancer. There were, it is estimated, about 502,000 deaths from cancer in 1989, representing 22% of all mortality and 1,010,000 new cases of life-threatening cancer diagnoses.[1] These data do not include an additional 500,000, for the most part readily curable, nonmelanoma cancers of the skin and 40,000 to 50,000 cases of carcinoma in situ, largely of the uterine cervix. The major organ sites affected and overall frequency are cited in Table 6–4. The rank order of these forms of malignant neoplasia has not materially changed over the past few decades save for a progressive decline in death rates from carcinoma of the stomach in both males and females. Lung and prostate cancer have led the grim parade in males since the 1950s, as has carcinoma of the breast in females. However, the death rates for many forms of cancer have significantly changed over the years (Table 6–5).[33] Many of the temporal comparisons are noteworthy. In males the overall cancer death rate has significantly increased, whereas in females it has fallen slightly. The increase in males can be laid largely at the doorstep of lung cancer. The improvement in females is mainly attributable to a significant decline in death rates from cancers of the

Table 6–4. Estimated Cancer Incidence for 1989 by Site and Sex

	MALE (505,000)			FEMALE (505,000)	
Rank	*Site*	*No. Cases (%)*	*Rank*	*Site*	*No. Cases (%)*
1.	Prostate	103,000 (20.3)	1.	Breast (invasive)	142,000 (28.1)
2.	Lung	101,100 (20.0)	2.	Colorectum	78,000 (15.4)
3.	Colorectum	73,000 (14.4)	3.	Lung	54,000 (10.6)
4.	Bladder	34,500 (6.8)	4.	Endometrium	34,000 (6.7)
5.	Hodgkin's disease and lymphomas	21,000 (4.1)	5.	Hodgkin's disease and lymphomas	19,200 (3.8)
6.	Leukemia	15,200 (3.0)	6.	Pancreas	14,000 (2.7)
7.	Stomach	11,900 (2.3)	7.	Cervix (invasive)	13,000 (2.5)
8.	Pancreas	13,000 (2.5)	8.	Leukemia	12,100 (2.3)

From Cancer statistics 1989. CA *39*:12, 1989.

Table 6–5. 30-Year Trends in Age-Adjusted Cancer Death Rates Per 100,000 Population 1950–52 to 1980–82

SITES	SEX	1950–52	1980–82	PERCENT CHANGES	COMMENTS
All sites	Male	169.8	216.0	+ 27	Steady increase mainly due to lung cancer.
	Female	146.7	135.4	− 8	Slight decrease.
Bladder	Male	7.2	6.5	*	Slight fluctuations; overall no change.
	Female	3.1	1.9	− 39	Some fluctuations; noticeable decrease.
Brain	Male	3.5	4.7	+ 34	Steady slight increase in both sexes;
	Female	2.3	3.2	+ 39	reasons unknown.
Breast	Male	0.3	0.2	*	Constant rate.
	Female	25.9	26.6	+ 3	Slight fluctuations; overall no change.
Colon and rectum	Male	25.8	25.3	*	Slight fluctuations; overall no change.
	Female	24.9	18.0	− 28	Slight fluctuations; noticeable decrease.
Esophagus	Male	4.7	5.5	+ 17	Some fluctuations; slight increase.
	Female	1.2	1.5	*	Slight fluctuations; overall no change in female.
Kidney	Male	3.3	4.8	+ 45	Steady slight increase.
	Female	2.0	2.2	*	Slight fluctuations; overall no change.
Leukemia	Male	7.7	8.7	+ 13	Early increase, later leveling off and decrease.
	Female	5.3	5.1	*	Slight early increase, later leveling off.
Liver	Male	6.7	4.7	− 30	Some fluctuations. Steady decrease in both
	Female	7.7	3.5	− 55	sexes.
Lung	Male	23.7	72.1	+204	Steady increase in both sexes due to
	Female	4.9	29.9	+510	cigarette smoking.
Oral	Male	6.1	5.5	*	Slight fluctuations; overall no change in both
	Female	1.5	2.3	*	sexes.
Ovary	Female	8.1	7.9	− 2	Steady increase, later leveling off and decrease.
Pancreas	Male	8.4	10.5	+ 25	Steady increase in both sexes, then leveling off;
	Female	5.5	7.0	+ 27	reasons unknown.
Prostate	Male	20.7	22.8	+ 10	Fluctuations throughout; overall slight increase.
Skin	Male	3.2	2.7	*	Slight fluctuations; overall no change in
	Female	2.0	1.4	*	both sexes.
Stomach	Male	23.6	8.1	− 66	Steady decrease in both sexes; reasons
	Female	12.8	3.8	− 70	unknown.
Uterus	Female	20.7	7.6	− 63	Steady decrease.

* Percent changes not listed because they are not meaningful.

From American Cancer Society: Cancer Facts and Figures, 1986, p. 23.

uterus, stomach, and liver, notably carcinoma of the cervix, one of the most frequent forms of malignant neoplasia in females. Striking is the alarming increase in deaths from carcinoma of the lung in both sexes. Although the percentage change is greater for females than for males, this is merely the spurious consequence of the relative rarity of cancer of the lung in females years ago. The rising slope of the curve is about the same in both sexes, and neither current-day efforts to control smoking nor "low tar" cigarettes have yet shown signs of reducing the awesome mortality rate. In females carcinomas of the breast are about three times more frequent than those of the lung. However, because of a striking difference in the cure rates of these two cancers, bronchogenic carcinoma became the leading cause of cancer deaths in women by 1989. The decline in the number of deaths caused by uterine cancer probably relates largely to the earlier diagnosis and better cure rate made possible by the Papanicolaou smear. Much more mysterious is the downward trend in deaths from stomach and liver carcinomas. Could this be due to a decrease in some dietary carcinogens?

Remarkable differences can be found in the inci-

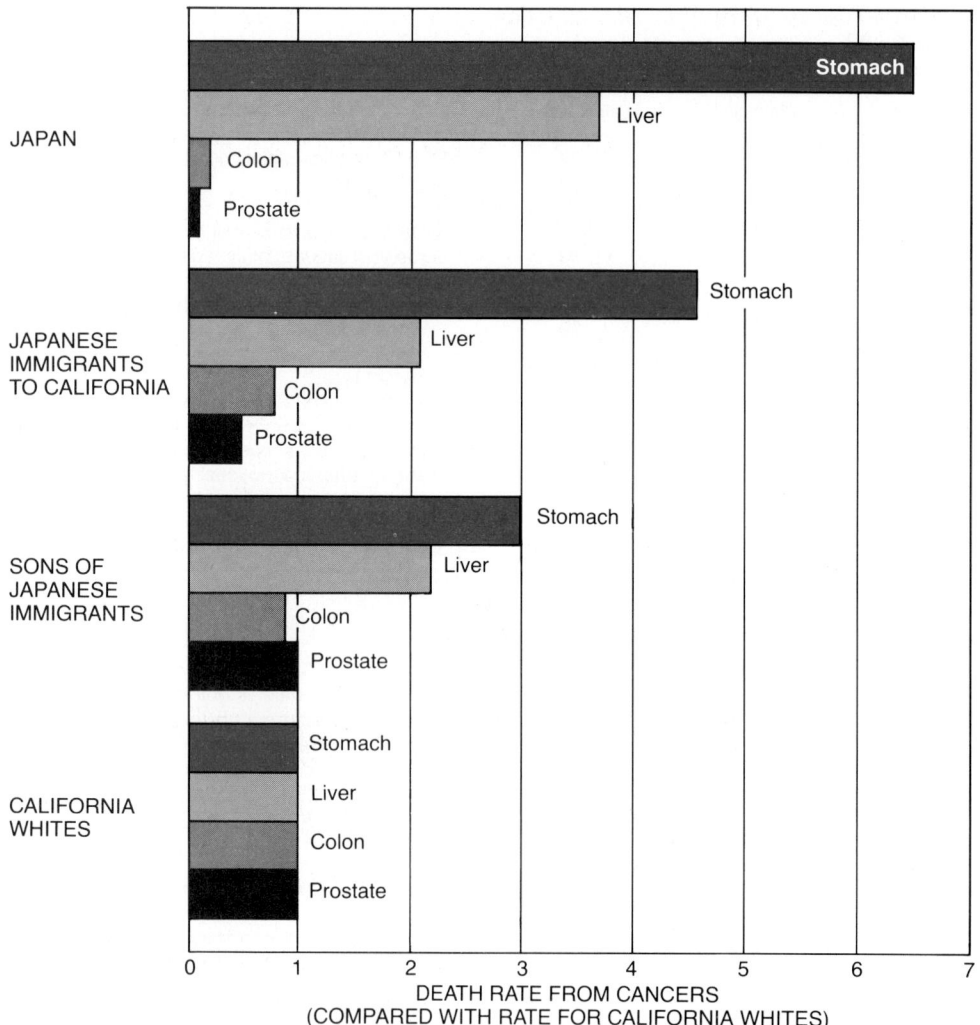

Figure 6–22. Change in incidence of various cancers with migration from Japan to the United States provides evidence that the cancers are caused by components of the environment that differ in the two countries. The incidence of each kind of cancer is expressed as the ratio of the death rate in the population being considered to that in a hypothetical population of California whites with the same age distribution; the death rates for whites are thus defined as 1. The death rates among immigrants and immigrants' sons tend consistently toward California norms. (From Cairns, J.: The cancer problem. *In* Readings from Scientific American—Cancer Biology. New York, W.H. Freeman and Co., 1986, p. 13. © 1975 by Scientific American, Inc. All rights reserved.)

dence and death rates of specific forms of cancer around the world. For example, the death rate for stomach carcinoma in both males and females is seven times higher in Japan than in the United States. In contrast, the death rate from carcinoma of the lung is slightly more than twice as great in the United States as in Japan and, indeed, in Scotland is almost twice as high as in the United States. Skin cancer deaths, largely caused by melanocarcinomas, are six times more frequent in New Zealand than in Iceland, which is probably attributable to differences in sun exposure. While racial predispositions cannot be ruled out, it is generally believed that most of these geographic differences are the consequence of environmental influences. This is best brought out by comparing mortality rates for Japanese immigrants to the United States, and Japanese born in the United States of immigrant parents (Nisei) with those of long-term residents of both countries. Figure 6–22 indicates that cancer mortality rates for first-generation Japanese immigrants are intermediate between those of natives of Japan and of California, and the two rates come closer with each passing generation. This points strongly to environmental and cultural rather than

genetic predisposition. Yet enigmas remain—the death rate for breast cancer in females is higher in Denmark than in Sweden, yet environmental differences between these two countries are not immediately apparent. Many hypotheses have been offered. For example, differences in number of pregnancies, age of the mother at first birth, and breast-feeding practices may be involved because they tend to reduce the uninterrupted cyclic estrogenic stimulation of the breast, particularly in the early decades. Thus, cultural differences may influence the geographic distribution of certain cancers, but in some cases it seems difficult to rule out racial genetic predisposition. In this connection, the age-standardized mortality rate for prostate cancer in United States blacks is more than twice the rate of whites.

ENVIRONMENTAL AND CULTURAL INFLUENCES

Cancer risks lurk behind virtually every door. They can be found in the environment and particularly within certain occupations. The carcinogenicity of ultraviolet rays and many drugs will be discussed in a later section. Asbestos, vinyl chloride, and 2-naphthylamine can serve as examples of occupational hazards, and many others are discussed on page 495. The risks may be incurred in lifestyle and personal exposures, for example, the role of nutrition, considered on page 464. Overall, mortality data indicate that persons more than 25% overweight have a higher death rate from cancer than do their "trim" neighbors. Alcohol abuse alone increases the risk of carcinomas of the oropharynx (excluding lip), larynx, and esophagus, and through the intermediation of alcoholic cirrhosis, carcinoma of the liver. Smoking, particularly of cigarettes, has been implicated in cancer of the mouth, pharynx, larynx, esophagus, pancreas, and bladder but most significantly is responsible for about 77% of lung cancer among males and 43% among females (p. 797). Indeed, cigarette smoking has been called the single most important environmental factor contributing to premature death in the United States. Alcohol and tobacco together multiply the danger of incurring cancers in the upper aerodigestive tract. The risk of cervical cancer is linked to age at first intercourse and the number of sex partners. These associations point to a possible causal role for venereal transmission of cervical viral infections. It begins to appear that everything one does to gain a livelihood or for pleasure is fattening, immoral, illegal, or, even worse, oncogenic.

AGE AND CHILDHOOD CANCER

Age is an important influence on the likelihood of being afflicted with cancer. As everyone knows, most carcinomas occur in the later years of life (55 years and over). Each age group has its own predilection to certain forms of cancer, as is evident in Table 6–6. Here the striking increase in mortality from cancer in the age group 55 to 74 years should be noted. The decline in deaths in the 75-year-and-over group merely reflects the dwindling population reaching this venerable age. Also to be noted is that children under the age of 15 are not spared. Indeed, cancer accounts for slightly more than 10% of all deaths in this group in the United States and is second only to accidents. Acute leukemia and neoplasms of the central nervous system are responsible for approximately 60 to 75% of these deaths. The common neoplasms of infancy and childhood include neuroblastoma, Wilms' tumor, retinoblastoma, acute leukemias, and rhabdomyosarcomas. These are discussed in Chapter 10 and elsewhere in the text.

Table 6–6. Mortality for the Five Leading Cancer Sites for Males by Age Group, United States — 1985

ALL AGES *All Cancer* *246,914*	UNDER 15 *All Cancer* *1,042*	15–34 *All Cancer* *4,029*	35–54 *All Cancer* *25,733*	55–74 *All Cancer* *136,869*	75+ *All Cancer* *79,220*
Lung 83,854	Leukemia 418	Leukemia 679	Lung 8,926	Lung 53,756	Lung 20,996
Colon & Rectum 27,612	Brain & CNS 230	Skin 469	Colon & Rectum 2,247	Colon & Rectum 14,749	Prostate 15,132
Prostate 25,943	Non-Hodgkin's Lymphomas 66	Brain & CNS 444	Brain & CNS 1,272	Prostate 10,488	Colon & Rectum 10,422
Pancreas 11,542	Connective Tissue 50	Non-Hodgkin's Lymphomas 438	Non-Hodgkin's Lymphomas 1,214	Pancreas 6,652	Pancreas 3,672
Leukemia 9,442	Bone 33	Hodgkin's Disease 301	Skin 1,208	Stomach 4,485	Bladder 3,380

Mortality for the Five Leading Cancer Sites for Females by Age Group, United States — 1985

ALL AGES *All Cancer* *214,649*	UNDER 15 *All Cancer* *798*	15–34 *All Cancer* *3,608*	35–54 *All Cancer* *27,001*	55–74 *All Cancer* *106,299*	75+ *All Cancer* *76,921*
Breast* 40,383	Leukemia 296	Breast 649	Breast 8,297	Lung 24,322	Colon & Rectum 14,542
Lung* 38,839	Brain & CNS 192	Leukemia 347	Lung 4,960	Breast 20,301	Breast 11,131
Colon & Rectum 28,839	Bone 41	Uterus 347	Colon & Rectum 1,911	Colon & Rectum 12,200	Lung 9,279
Pancreas 11,560	Bladder 36	Brain & CNS 321	Uterus 1,778	Ovary 6,380	Pancreas 5,211
Ovary 11,531	Non-Hodgkin's Lymphomas 36	Non-Hodgkin's Lymphomas 202	Ovary 1,666	Pancreas 5,542	Ovary 3,346

Source: Vital Statistics of the United States, 1985. From CA — A cancer journal for Clinicians *39*:7, 1989.

* In 1989, lung cancer overtook breast cancer as the leading cause of cancer deaths in females (p. 263).

HEREDITY

One frequently asked question is: "My mother and father both died of cancer. Does that mean I am doomed to get it?" On the basis of current knowledge, the answer must be carefully qualified.[34,35] The evidence now indicates that for a large number of types of cancer, including the most common forms, there exist not only environmental influences but also hereditary predispositions. For example, lung cancer is in most instances clearly related to cigarette smoking, yet mortality from lung cancer has been shown to be four times greater among nonsmoking relatives (parents and siblings) of lung cancer patients than among nonsmoking relatives of controls. Similar data (a twofold increase) were obtained with smoking relatives. So it appears that genetic influences may contribute to the development of cancer even when there are clearly defined environmental factors. A genetic predisposition to breast cancer in females can also be shown. What role heredity plays in the predisposition to particular breast cancers cannot be quantified. Clearly, women who have no family history of this cancer may develop the disease, but presumably those from families with a history of breast cancer are at some increased risk.

In general, the risk of the same neoplasm developing in close relatives of a cancer patient is about three times greater than in control populations. There is an even greater familial risk with particular forms of cancer, notably certain tumors of childhood and carcinomas of the breast and colon. Childhood retinoblastoma offers the most striking example of the role of heredity. Approximately 40% of the retinoblastomas are familial. The predisposition to this tumor shows an autosomal dominant pattern of inheritance.[36] Carriers of this gene have a 10,000-fold increased risk of developing retinoblastoma, usually bilateral. They also have a greatly increased risk of developing a second cancer, particularly osteogenic sarcoma. As will be discussed later, a "cancer suppressor" gene has been mapped to chromosome 13. Loss of both normal alleles (acquired homozygosity) at this locus is associated with the development of retinoblastoma and osteosarcoma. In familial cases, one mutant retinoblastoma gene is inherited through germ cells, and the patient is therefore heterozygous, having one normal and one mutant gene. Homozygosity at the retinoblastoma locus is acquired by a (second) somatic mutation that affects only the retinal cells (p. 290). Multiple polyposis coli is another hereditary disorder marked by an extraordinarily high risk of cancer. Individuals who inherit the autosomal dominant mutation have at birth, or soon thereafter, innumerable polypoid adenomas of the colon, and in virtually 100% of cases are fated to develop a carcinoma of the colon by age 50. Besides the dominantly inherited cancerous or precancerous disorders, there is a small group of autosomal recessive conditions collectively referred to as "chromosomal or DNA instability syndromes" and characterized by some defect in DNA repair

mechanisms, which increases the predisposition to cancer.[37] Homozygotes with xeroderma pigmentosum, for example, have the fully expressed condition, which includes a strong predisposition to sunlight-induced melanocarcinomas and basal cell and squamous cell carcinomas of the skin, in addition to other non-neoplastic cutaneous and ocular abnormalities. Heterozygotes, who of course are much more common, do not express the complete clinical condition but nonetheless have a predisposition (albeit less marked) to sunlight-induced malignancies of the skin. A list of some of the more common cancerous and precancerous disorders in which heredity plays a major role is presented in Table 6–7.

It is impossible to estimate the contribution of heredity to the total human burden of cancer. However, the best "guesstimates" suggest that about 5% of all cancers are genetic.[38] The remainder, then, must be largely environmental in origin or so-called "spontaneous"; it is highly likely, however, that genetic predisposition contributes to some proportion of so-called "environmental" and "spontaneous" cancers. For example, individuals with xeroderma pigmentosum develop cancers of the skin only with exposure to the mutational effects of radiant energy. The converse is equally true: Environmental factors must contribute to the initiation of many hereditary neoplasms. *It is best then to consider heredity and environment as the two ends of a spectrum of predisposing influences.* At the extremes are those neoplasms fated to appear because of heredity or because of environment, but in between are the great majority of cancers that have varying proportions of both influences, depending on where they fall within the spectrum.

ACQUIRED PRENEOPLASTIC DISORDERS

The only certain way to avoid cancer is not to be born; to live is to incur the risk. However, the risk is greater than average under many circumstances, as is evident from the predisposing influences discussed earlier. Certain clinical conditions are also of importance. Because cell replication is involved in cancerous transformation (p. 270), regenerative, hyperplastic, and dysplastic proliferations are fertile soil for the origin of a malignant neoplasm. There is a well-defined association between certain forms of endometrial hyperplasia and endometrial carcinoma (p. 1150), and between cervical dysplasia and cervical carcinoma. The bronchial mucosal metaplasia and dysplasia of habitual cigarette smokers are ominous antecedents of bronchogenic carcinoma. About 80% of hepatocellular carcinomas arise in cirrhotic livers, which are characterized by active parenchymal regeneration. Other examples could be offered, but although these settings constitute important predispositions, it must be appreciated that in the great majority of instances they are not complicated by neoplasia.

Certain non-neoplastic disorders—*the chronic*

Table 6-7. Hereditary Neoplasms and Preneoplastic Conditions

DISORDER	INHERITANCE	FEATURES
Hereditary Neoplasms		
Retinoblastoma	AD	Often bilateral; susceptibility to second tumors, especially osteosarcoma; retinoblastoma locus mapped to 13q14
Familial polyposis coli	AD	Multiple adenomatous polyps and adenocarcinomas of the colon; some families have osteomas, lipomas, and fibromas (Gardner's syndrome)
Multiple endocrine neoplasia I	AD	Adenomas of the pituitary, parathyroid, and pancreatic islet cells
Multiple endocrine neoplasia II	AD	Medullary carcinoma of the thyroid, pheochromocytoma, and parathyroid tumors
Hereditary Preneoplastic ***Conditions***		
Phakomatoses		
Neurofibromatosis (von Recklinghausen's disease)	AD	Gliomas of the brain and optic nerve, acoustic neuroma, meningioma, and pheochromocytoma
Tuberous sclerosis	AD	Glial tumors; hamartomatous growths in several organs
von Hippel–Lindau syndrome	AD	Hemangioblastomas of cerebellum and retina; renal cell carcinoma and pheochromocytoma; gene mapped to 3p25
DNA-chromosomal instability		
Xeroderma pigmentosum	AR	Basal and squamous cell carcinoma of skin; malignant melanomas in patients exposed to UV light
Bloom's syndrome	AR	Acute leukemias, various carcinomas
Fanconi's anemia	AR	Acute leukemias, squamous cell carcinomas, and hepatomas
Ataxia-telangiectasia	AR	Acute leukemia, lymphoma, breast cancer in females
Immune deficiency syndromes		
X-linked agammaglobulinemia	XR	Lymphomas and leukemias
Wiskott-Aldrich syndrome	XR	Acute leukemias and lymphomas
X-linked lymphoproliferative syndrome	XR	Abnormal response to EB virus; EBV-induced B cell immunoblastic lymphomas
Cancer family syndrome	AD	Cancers of multiple organs: colon, endometrium, breast, and lung

AD = autosomal dominant; AR = autosomal recessive; XR = X-linked recessive.

atrophic gastritis of pernicious anemia, solar keratosis of the skin, the chromosomal breakage syndromes, chronic ulcerative colitis, and leukoplakia of the oral cavity, vulva, and penis—have such a well-defined association with cancer that they have been termed "precancerous conditions." This designation is somewhat unfortunate, since in the great majority of instances no malignant neoplasm emerges. Nonetheless, the term persists because it calls attention to the increased risk. Analogously, certain forms of benign neoplasia constitute "precancerous conditions." The villous adenoma of the colon, as it increases in size, develops cancerous change in up to 50% of cases. The myriad adenomatous colonic polyps characteristic of familial multiple polyposis coli are almost always followed eventually by carcinoma of the colon. The multiple neurofibromas of hereditary neurofibromatosis often give rise to neurogenic sarcomas. It might be asked: Is there not a risk with all benign neoplasms? Although some risk may be inherent, a large cumulative experience indicates that *most benign neoplasms do not become cancerous.* Nonetheless, numerous examples could be offered of cancers arising, albeit rarely, in benign tumors: for example, a leiomyosarcoma beginning in a leiomyoma, and carcinoma appearing in long-standing pleomorphic adenomas. Generalization is impossible because each type of benign neoplasm is associated with a particular level of risk ranging from virtually never to frequently. Only follow-up studies of large series of each neoplasm can establish the level of risk, and always the question remains: Was the tumor an indolent form of cancer from the outset or was there a malignant focus in the benign tumor?

CARCINOGENIC AGENTS AND THEIR CELLULAR INTERACTIONS

A large number of agents induce neoplastic transformation of cells in vitro and cancers in experimental animals. These agents fall into the following categories: (1) chemical carcinogens, (2) radiant energy, and (3) oncogenic viruses. Radiant energy and certain chemical carcinogens are documented causes of cancer in humans, and the evidence linking viruses to certain types of clinical neoplasia grows ever stronger. Indeed, epidemiologic studies hint strongly that 80 or even 90% of human cancers are related to lifestyle and other environmental influences.[39] The following discussion will deal largely with observations of particular pertinence to humans and relevant experimental data. Agents will be considered separately, but it is important to note that several may act in concert or synergize the effects of others. *There is strong experimental and clinical evidence that neoplastic transformation is a progressive process involv-*

ing multiple steps and "multiple hits."[40] Furthermore, there is growing belief that all etiologic factors ultimately affect the function of two sets of genes: (1) *proto-oncogenes*, so named because they are considered to be precursors of cancer genes or *oncogenes*, and (2) cancer suppressor genes, or anti-oncogenes. As will be discussed later, proto-oncogenes and cancer suppressor genes are normal components of the human genome, whose products are involved in the physiologic regulation of cell growth.

CHEMICAL CARCINOGENESIS

Although John Hill earlier called attention to the association of "immoderate use of snuff" and the development of "polypusses" (polyps), we owe largely to Sir Percival Pott our awareness of the potential carcinogenicity of chemical agents. Pott astutely related the increased incidence of scrotal skin cancer in chimney sweeps to chronic exposure to soot. A few years later, on the basis of this observation, the Danish Chimney Sweeps Guild ruled that its members must bathe daily. No public health measure since that time has so successfully controlled a form of cancer! Over the succeeding two centuries, hundreds of chemicals have been shown to transform cells in vitro and to be carcinogenic in animals. Some of the most potent (e.g., the polycyclic aromatic hydrocarbons) have been extracted from fossil fuels or are products of incomplete combustions. Some are synthetic products created by industry or for the study of chemical carcinogenesis. Some are naturally occurring components of plants and microbial organisms. Most important, a significant number (including, ironically, some medical drugs) have been strongly implicated in the causation of cancers in humans.[41]

Steps Involved in Chemical Carcinogenesis

Neoplastic transformation of cells in culture and the induction of cancers in vivo by chemical carcinogens is a dynamic process. It involves sequential generations of cells that go through multiple steps (Fig. 6–23) that can be broadly divided into two stages: *initiation and promotion.*[42] The classic experiments that allowed the distinction between initiation and promotion were performed on mouse skin and are outlined in Figure 6–24. The following concepts relating to the initiation-promotion sequence have emerged from these experiments:

• Initiation results from exposure of cells to an appropriate dose of a carcinogenic agent (initiator); an initiated cell is in some manner altered, rendering it likely to give rise to a tumor (groups 2 and 3). However, initiation alone is not sufficient for tumor formation (group 1).

• Initiation is rapid and irreversible, and has "memory." This is illustrated by group 3, in which tumors were produced even if the application of the promoting agent was delayed for several months after a single

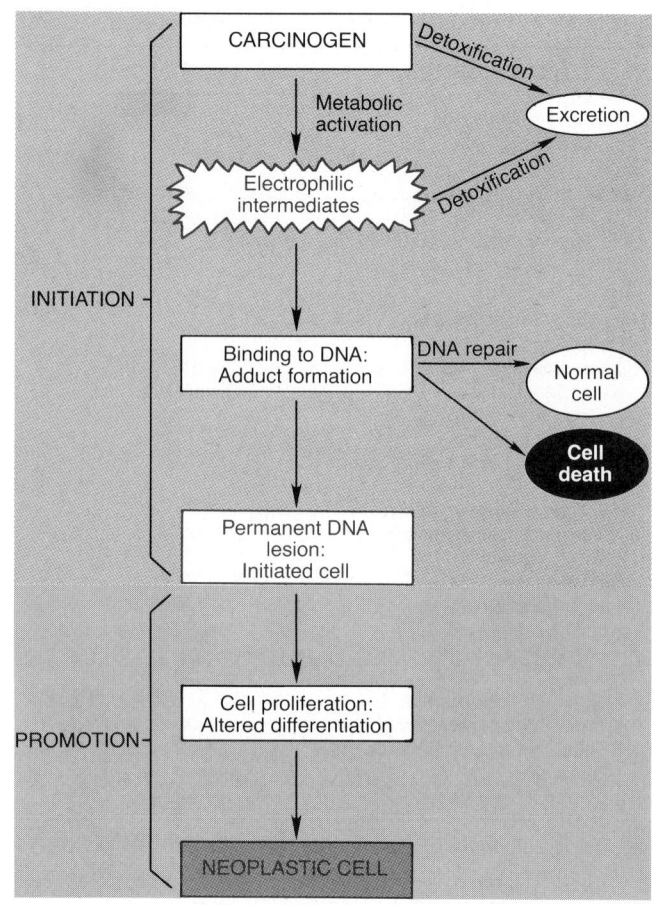

Figure 6–23. The general scheme of events in chemical carcinogenesis. (Modified from Tannock, I.F., and Hill, R.P. (eds.): The Basic Science of Oncology. New York, Pergamon Press, 1987, p. 92.)

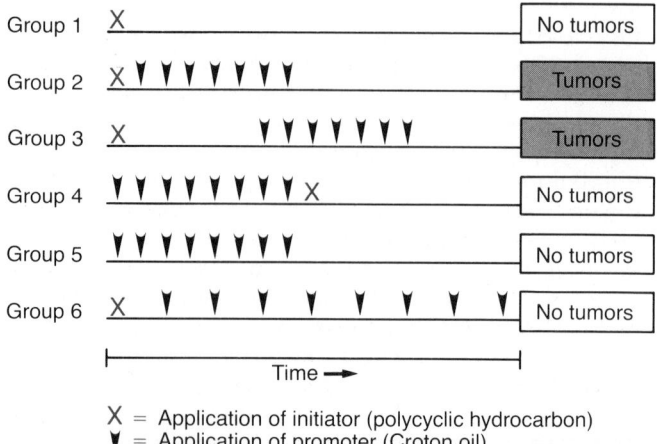

X = Application of initiator (polycyclic hydrocarbon)
⅄ = Application of promoter (Croton oil)

Figure 6–24. Experiments demonstrating the initiation and promotion phases of carcinogenesis in mice. Group 2 — application of promoter repeated at twice-weekly intervals for several months; Group 3 — application of promoter delayed for several months and then applied twice weekly; Group 6 — promoter applied at monthly intervals.

application of the initiator. *Because initiation is irreversible, it is believed that initiating carcinogens produce permanent changes in the DNA of target cells.*

• *Promoters can induce tumors in initiated cells, but they are nontumorigenic by themselves* (group 5). Furthermore, tumors do not result when the promoting agent is applied before, rather than after, the initiating agent (group 4). This indicates that, *in contrast to the effects of initiators, the cellular changes resulting from the application of promoters are reversible.* It is unlikely, therefore, that promoters affect the DNA directly.

• That the effects of promoters are reversible is further documented in group 6, in which tumors failed to develop in initiated cells if the time between multiple applications of the promoter was sufficiently extended.

• Because the effects of initiators are irreversible, multiple divided doses achieve the same result as a comparable dose administered at one time. In contrast, there is a threshold level for promoters; thus, subthreshold or widely spaced doses are without effect.

Although the concepts of initiation and promotion have been derived largely from experiments involving induction of skin cancer in mice, more recent studies indicate that these stages are also discernible in the development of cancers of the liver, urinary bladder, breast, colon, and respiratory tract.[43,44]

It should be noted that some chemicals possess the capability of both initiation and promotion, as evidenced by their ability to induce tumors without any added factors. They are called "complete carcinogens" to distinguish them from "incomplete carcinogens," which are defined as agents capable only of initiation. With this brief overview of the two major steps in carcinogenesis, we can examine initiation and promotion in more detail, following the outline in Figure 6–23.[45,46]

Initiation of Carcinogenesis

Chemicals that initiate carcinogenesis are extremely diverse in structure and include both natural and synthetic products (Table 6–8). They fall into one of two categories: (1) *direct-acting* compounds, which do not require chemical transformation for their carcinogenicity; or (2) *indirect-acting* or *procarcinogens*, which require metabolic conversion in vivo to produce *ultimate carcinogens* capable of transforming cells. All direct-acting and ultimate carcinogens have one property in common: They *are highly reactive electrophiles* (have electron-deficient atoms) *that can react with nucleophilic (electron-rich) sites in the cell.* These reactions are nonenzymatic and result in the formation of covalent adducts (addition products). The electrophilic reactants may attack several electron-rich sites in the target cells, including DNA, RNA, and proteins, thus sometimes producing lethal damage. In initiated cells the interaction is obviously nonlethal, and as we shall discuss later, DNA is the primary target.

Table 6–8. Major Chemical Carcinogens

DIRECT-ACTING CARCINOGENS
Alkylating Agents
Beta-propiolactone
Dimethyl sulfate
Diepoxybutane
Anticancer drugs (cyclophosphamide, chlorambucil, nitrosoureas, and others)

Acylating Agents
1-Acetyl-imidazole
Dimethylcarbamyl chloride

PROCARCINOGENS THAT REQUIRE METABOLIC ACTIVATION
Polycyclic and Heterocyclic Aromatic Hydrocarbons
Benz(a)anthracene
Benzo(a)pyrene
Dibenz(a,h)anthracene
3-Methylcholanthrene
7,12-Dimethylbenz(a)anthracene

Aromatic Amines, Amides, Azo Dyes
2-Naphthylamine (beta-naphthylamine)
Benzidine
2-Acetylaminofluorene
Dimethylaminoazobenzene (butter yellow)

Natural Plant and Microbial Products
Aflatoxin B_1
Griseofulvin
Cycasin
Safrole
Betel nuts

Others
Nitrosamine and amides
Vinyl chloride, nickel, chromium
Insecticides, fungicides
Polychlorinated biphenyls (PCBs)

METABOLIC ACTIVATION OF CARCINOGENS. Save for the few direct-acting alkylating and acylating agents that are intrinsically electrophilic, most chemical carcinogens require metabolic activation for conversion into ultimate carcinogens.[47] The metabolic activation of the procarcinogen to an electrophile may be a single-step reaction or may involve multiple steps in which one or more less reactive intermediates (proximate carcinogens) may be formed. Other metabolic pathways may lead to the inactivation (detoxification) of the procarcinogen or its derivatives. Thus the carcinogenic potency of a chemical is determined not only by the inherent reactivity of its electrophilic derivative but also by the balance between metabolic activation and inactivation reactions. To understand how metabolic activation may be modulated, we will briefly review the mechanisms involved in the formation of ultimate carcinogens.

Most of the known carcinogens are metabolized by cytochrome P-450–dependent mono-oxygenases. This enzyme system is located mainly in the microsomal fraction of the endoplasmic reticulum, but is also present in nuclei. Several factors, both environmental and genetic, are known to affect the activity of these oxidative enzymes, and hence the potency of the procarcinogen. In mice, for example, it has been possible to correlate the carcinogenic potency of polycyclic hydrocarbons with genetically determined levels of the enzyme (aryl hydrocarbon hydroxylase) involved in the formation of reactive metabolites. In humans, a similar correlation between genetically determined levels of aryl hydrocarbon hydroxylase and occurrence of lung cancer in smokers has been noted in some (but not all) studies. The well-known susceptibility of young animals to chemical carcinogenesis may also relate, in part, to immaturity of enzyme systems that can detoxify the chemical. Drugs, such as phenobarbital, that are known to induce microsomal enzymes may enhance tumorigenesis in experimental animals by increasing the levels of the cytochrome P-450 oxygenase system. Suffice it to say that numerous factors, including age, sex, species, and hormonal and nutritional status of the individual, may modify the carcinogenic effect of a chemical by affecting its metabolism.

In addition to the cytochrome P-450 system-dependent activation, several other metabolic pathways, including peroxidative oxidation, reduction reactions, and glutathione conjugation, have been implicated in the generation of reactive carcinogenic metabolites. Details relating to these may be found in specialized reviews and texts.[45,48]

MOLECULAR TARGETS OF CHEMICAL CARCINOGENS. As mentioned earlier, both direct-acting carcinogens and electrophilic derivatives of procarcinogens are capable of forming covalent adducts with several cellular targets. There is convincing evidence, however, that initiation results primarily from interaction with DNA. The irreversible nature of initiation and the persistence of initiated cells both point to a heritable change involving DNA. *Indeed, it is almost an axiom in the field of chemical carcinogenesis that initiating agents are mutagens.* The mutagenic potential of chemical carcinogens has been investigated, most commonly using the *Ames test.* This test utilizes the ability of a chemical to induce mutations in the bacterium *Salmonella typhimurium.* The test organisms are selected for their *inability* to synthesize histidine and are incubated with the potential carcinogen along with liver homogenate (to provide the necessary enzymes for metabolic activation). *If the metabolites are mutagenic, they cause some organisms to mutate and acquire a functional histidine gene,* which in turn allows the mutants to grow on histidine-free culture medium. The number of bacterial colonies that grow under these conditions provides a rough measure of mutagenicity. Chemical carcinogens have also been shown to be mutagenic in mammalian cell cultures. The vast majority (70 to 90%) of known chemical carcinogens score positive in the Ames test. Conversely, most but not all chemicals that are mutagenic in vitro are carcinogenic in vivo. Because of the high correlation between mutagenicity and carcinogenicity, the Ames test is frequently used to screen chemicals for their carcinogenic potential.

That DNA is the primary target for chemical carcinogens seems fairly well established, but there is no single or unique alteration that can be associated with initiation of chemical carcinogenesis. Depending on the carcinogen, the bases, phosphate groups, or the three-dimensional structure of the DNA may be altered.[49] However, carcinogen-induced changes in DNA do not necessarily lead to initiation, since several forms of DNA damage can be repaired by cellular enzymes. Indeed, it is very likely that environmentally induced insults to DNA are far more common than is the occurrence of cancer. This is best exemplified by the rare hereditary disorder xeroderma pigmentosum (XP), which is associated with a defect in DNA repair and a greatly increased vulnerability to skin cancers caused by UV light and some chemicals (p. 274).

ONCOGENES AS GENETIC TARGETS OF CHEMICAL CARCINOGENS. Although it seems reasonably certain that changes in DNA are crucial to the initiation of chemical carcinogenesis, the critical genetic targets remain to be identified. Much recent attention has been focused on the activation of proto-oncogenes by chemical carcinogens.[50] Since the role of proto-oncogenes in the origin of cancer will be discussed in detail later, only brief comments relevant to chemical carcinogenesis will be presented. Proto-oncogenes are a set of cellular genes that play an integral role in controlling normal growth and differentiation (p. 282). It has been suggested that initiating carcinogens, in some cases, induce mutations in proto-oncogenes to produce oncogenes, which in turn give rise to the abnormalities in growth and differentiation. This view is supported by the observation that several chemically induced tumors in rodents, and certain human tumors, are associated with point mutations in the *ras* oncogenes (see also p. 287).[51] As will be pointed out later, recessive cancer genes and other regulatory sequences may also be targeted by carcinogenic chemicals.

THE INITIATED CELL. In the preceding sections we noted that unrepaired alterations in the DNA are essential first steps in the process of initiation. However, changes in DNA are not enough to produce an initiated cell. *For the change to be heritable, the damaged DNA template must be replicated. Thus, for initiation to occur, carcinogen-altered cells must undergo at least one cycle of proliferation, so that the change in DNA becomes "fixed" or permanent.* The dependence of initiation on cell division has been established most clearly in experimentally induced liver tumors[43] but is probably a general feature of chemical carcinogenesis. In the liver, many chemicals are activated to reactive electrophiles, yet most of them do not produce cancers unless the liver cells proliferate within 72 to 96 hours of the formation of DNA adducts. In tissues that are normally quiescent, the mitogenic stimulus may be provided by the carcinogen itself, because many cells die owing to toxic effects of the carcinogenic chemical, thereby stimulating regeneration in the surviving cells. Alternatively, cell proliferation may be induced by concurrent exposure to biologic agents such as viruses and parasites, dietary factors, or hormonal influences.

It must be remembered *that initiated cells are not tumor cells; they do not have growth autonomy, and they do not have readily identifiable unique genotypic or phenotypic markers.* Unlike normal cells, however, they are susceptible to the action of promoters, and give rise to tumors when appropriately stimulated by promoting agents.

Promotion of Carcinogenesis

The significant features of promotion, for instance reversibility and dose-threshold, have already been discussed. Here we will concentrate on the possible mechanisms involved in tumor promotion. Promoters include several substances such as phorbol esters, phenols, hormones, and drugs (e.g., phenobarbital). There is no unifying principle to explain the activity of this diverse group of chemicals. In contrast to initiators, however, *promoting agents are not electrophilic compounds and they do not damage the DNA. Their actions seem to be epigenetic, involving altered expression of genetic information in the cells.*

12-O-Tetradecanoyl phorbol-13-acetate (TPA) is the most widely used tumor promoter, and therefore its effects on cells have been extensively investigated. It binds to cell membranes and induces a number of phenotypic changes in a wide variety of biologic systems. The cellular effects of TPA can be grouped into the following categories:

• Partial mimicry in normal cells of the transformed phenotype in vitro.
• Induction or inhibition of differentiation.
• Stimulation of secretory responses in a variety of cell types such as platelets, neutrophils, and T lymphocytes.
• Modulations of many membrane activities.

The pleotropic effects of TPA strongly suggest that its actions are mediated through some central regulatory pathway within the cells. Indeed, recent studies have demonstrated that TPA specifically binds to and activates protein kinase C (PKC), a ubiquitous enzyme that catalyzes the phosphorylation of numerous protein substrates at seryl and threonine residues. As will be detailed later (see p. 282 and Fig. 6–29), PKC is an integral part of signal transduction mechanisms in cells.[52] The ability of the tumor promoter TPA to activate protein kinase C rests on its structural similarity to diacylglycerol, the physiologic activator of protein kinase C (see Fig. 6–29). It is now established that protein kinase C is the cellular receptor for TPA. Thus when a cell is exposed to TPA, it is tricked into believing that it has received a physiologic signal for activation of protein kinase C.

The protein targets that get phosphorylated by protein kinase C are too numerous to list.[53] Of particular interest in the context of neoplastic transformation are receptors for growth factors, such as epidermal growth factor, interleukin-2, and insulin, and membrane proteins that regulate ion channels. For example, activated protein kinase C increases intracellular pH by phosphorylating the N^+/H^+ exchanger. Cytoplasmic alkalization seems to be causally related to cellular activation and growth in response to several physiologic growth factors. Many other examples of TPA-induced alterations in cellular functions could be cited. Suffice it to say that TPA leads to a cascade of protein phosphorylations that alter the function of membrane-associated receptors, ion channels, and cytoplasmic proteins. These changes, in turn, induce cell proliferation and modulate cell differentiation and the numerous other effects of TPA mentioned earlier.

Induction of mitogenesis, resulting in clonal expansion of initiated cells, seems to be an important attribute of TPA and other promoters. However, a number of agents that induce cellular proliferation in the target tissues are not active as promoters.[54] We must conclude, therefore, that much remains to be learned about the biochemical mechanisms of promotion.

Carcinogenic Chemicals

Before closing this discussion of chemical carcinogenesis, we will briefly describe some initiators (Table 6–8) and promoters of chemical carcinogenesis, with special emphasis on those that have been linked to cancer development in humans.

DIRECT-ACTING ALKYLATING AGENTS. These agents are activation independent, and in general, they are weak carcinogens. Nonetheless, they have importance because many therapeutic agents (e.g., cyclophosphamide, chlorambucil, busulfan, melphalan, and others) fall into this category. These are used as anticancer drugs but regrettably have been documented to induce lymphoid neoplasms, leukemia, and other forms of cancer.[55] Some alkylating agents, such as cyclophosphamide, are also powerful immunosuppressive agents and are therefore used in treatment of immunologic disorders including rheumatoid arthritis and Wegener's granulomatosis. Although the risk of induced cancer with these agents is low, judicious use of them is indicated. Alkylating agents appear to exert their therapeutic effects by interacting with and damaging DNA, but it is precisely these actions that render them also carcinogenic.

POLYCYCLIC AROMATIC HYDROCARBONS. These agents represent some of the most potent carcinogens known. They require metabolic activation and can induce tumors in a wide variety of tissues and species. Painted on the skin, they cause skin cancers; injected subcutaneously, they evoke sarcomas; introduced into a specific organ, they cause cancers locally. The formation of the final reactive products—the "ultimate carcinogens"—has been elegantly detailed for many of the aromatic hydrocarbons.[56] Involved are the microsomal endoplasmic reticulum–associated mono-oxygenases already discussed. The "ultimate carcinogens" for many of the polycyclic hydrocarbons are now known to be dihydrodiol epoxides. These epoxides are strong electrophilic reactants and combine with nucleophilic sites in the target cells, including DNA, RNA, and proteins. The polycyclic hydrocarbons are of particular interest as carcinogens because they are produced in the combustion of tobacco, particularly with cigarette smoking, and may well contribute to the causation of lung cancer. They are also produced from animal fats in the process of broiling meats and are present in smoked meats and fish.

AROMATIC AMINES AND AZO DYES. Agents in this category were the first to reveal the requirement of metabolic activation of most carcinogens. The carcinogenicity of most aromatic amines and azo dyes is exerted mainly in the liver, where the "ultimate carcinogen" is formed by the intermediation of the cytochrome P-450 oxygenase systems. Thus, fed to rats, acetylaminofluorene and the azo dyes induce hepatocellular carcinomas but not cancers of the gastrointestinal tract. An agent implicated in human cancers, beta-naphthylamine, is an exception. In the past it has been responsible for a 50-fold increased incidence of bladder cancer in heavily exposed workers in aniline dye and rubber industries.[57] After absorption it is hydroxylated into an N—OH derivative and then detoxified by conjugation with glucuronic acid. Other products are also formed but are less strong electrophiles. When excreted in the urine, the nontoxic conjugate is split by the urinary enzyme glucuronidase to again release the electrophilic reactant, thus inducing bladder cancer. Regrettably, humans are one of the few species to possess the urinary glucuronidase. Some of the azo dyes were developed to color food, e.g., butter yellow to give margarine the appearance of butter, and scarlet red to impart the seductive coloration of certain foods such as maraschino cherries. These dyes are now federally regulated in the United States because of the fear that they may be dangerous to humans.

NATURALLY OCCURRING CARCINOGENS. Among the approximately 30 known chemical carcinogens produced by plants and microorganisms, the potent hepatic carcinogen aflatoxin B1 is most important. It is produced by some strains of *Aspergillus flavus* that thrive on improperly stored grains and peanuts. A strong correlation has been found between the dietary level of this hepatocarcinogen and the incidence of hepatocellular carcinoma in some parts of Africa and the Far East. The aflatoxin requires metabolic activation by hepatic microsomal oxygenases to yield a dihydrodiol epoxide as the "ultimate carcinogen." It may be noted that infection with hepatitis B virus has also been strongly correlated with these cancers, raising the possibility that the aflatoxin and the virus collaborate in the production of this form of neoplasia, as discussed on page 959.

NITROSAMINES AND AMIDES. These carcinogens are of interest because of the possibility that they are formed in the gastrointestinal tract of humans (p. 465) and so may contribute to the induction of some forms of cancer, particularly gastric carcinoma. Like most other carcinogens, the nitroso-compounds require activation, which again involves the microsomal P-450 system. The ultimate carcinogenic derivatives are alkyl diazonium ions that are strongly electrophilic.

MISCELLANEOUS AGENTS. *Scores of other chemicals* have been indicted as carcinogens. Only a few that represent important industrial hazards will be mentioned.[58] Occupational exposure to *asbestos* has been associated with an increased incidence of bronchogenic carcinomas, mesotheliomas, and gastrointestinal cancers, as discussed in detail on page 479. Concomitant cigarette smoking heightens the risk of bronchogenic carcinoma manyfold.[59] It is somewhat sobering to realize that a number of cases of mesothelioma have been reported among individuals whose only exposure to asbestos was household contact with asbestos workers. *Vinyl chloride* is the monomer from which the polymer polyvinyl chloride is fabricated. It was first identified as a carcinogen in animals, but investigations soon disclosed a scattered incidence of the extremely rare hemangiosarcoma of the liver among workers exposed to this chemical. *Chromium, nickel,* and other metals, when volatilized and inhaled in industrial environments, have caused cancer of the lung. Skin cancer associated with arsenic is also well established. Similarly, there is reasonable evidence that many insecticides, such as aldrin, dieldrin, and chlordane and the polychlorinated biphenyls, are carcinogenic in animals, and the unpleasant citations could be continued.

PROMOTERS OF CHEMICAL CARCINOGENESIS. Certain promoters may contribute to cancers in humans.[60] Saccharin and cyclamates have been shown to promote the induction of bladder cancer in rats previously given marginal doses of carcinogens. Whether these artificial sweeteners are also initiators or promoters in humans is a hotly debated issue, addressed on page 465. Suffice it here to note that epidemiologic studies, while yielding conflicting results, disclose no solid evidence of carcinogenicity in the dosages customarily used by humans. Hormones such as the estrogens serve in animals as promoters of liver tumors. The prolonged use of diethylstilbestrol is implicated in the production of postmenopausal endometrial carcinoma and in the causation of vaginal cancer in offspring exposed in utero, as discussed on page 1138.[61] The action of many promoters is limited to specific cells and tissues. With such specificity, surface receptors on target cells are postulated and, as discussed earlier, this seems to be the case for phorbol esters.

Chemical Carcinogenesis: Summary

The study of chemical carcinogens has provided many insights into the fundamental nature of carcinogenesis. These can be summarized as follows:

• The great majority of chemical carcinogens are mutagens. Either directly or following enzymatic activation, the carcinogens bind directly to DNA, inducing miscoding errors during transcription and replication.

• The critical genes whose structure and function are altered by chemical carcinogens may be dominantly acting oncogenes or recessive cancer suppressor genes (pp. 282 and 289).

• The carcinogenicity of chemical agents is dose dependent, and multiple fractional doses over time have the same oncogenicity as a single comparable dose. The interval between fractional doses can be considerably extended, and thus the critical carcinogenic effect, termed initiation, is virtually irreversible.

• The expression of the initial mutagenic event requires the subsequent exposure to so-called *promoters*, such as phorbol ester, which by themselves are nonmutagenic and nontumorigenic. Promoters induce clonal proliferation of initiated cells and alter their differentiation programs by activating enzymes that are part of the physiologic signal transduction pathways.

• The two-stage initiation-promotion sequence is followed by tumor progression involving the generation of multiple phenotypically diverse subclones that arise by the imposition of new mutations on already aberrant cells. Thus it appears that carcinogenesis involves multiple stages, multiple genes, and probably multiple mechanisms.

• Diverse oncogenic influences may act in concert to induce cell transformation. Cells previously exposed to radiant energy are more vulnerable to chemical carcinogens, and the latter synergize with the transforming action of oncogenic viruses. Thus has arisen the concept of cocarcinogenesis. Tobacco smoke residue, with its polycyclic aromatic hydrocarbons, also contains nitrosamines and other chemicals that may serve as cocarcinogens. In addition, it contains phenolic promoters, making it a dangerous witches' brew. The increasing frequency of cancer with advancing age in humans might well be due to cumulative exposure over the years to a variety of carcinogenic influences, although other explanations may exist.

RADIATION CARCINOGENESIS

Radiant energy, whether in the form of the ultraviolet (UV) rays of sunlight or as ionizing electromagnetic and particulate radiation, can transform virtually all cell types in vitro and induce neoplasms in vivo in both humans and experimental animals.[62,63] UV light is clearly implicated in the causation of skin cancers, and ionizing radiations of medical, occupational, and, lamentably, atomic bomb origins have produced a variety of forms of malignant neoplasia. Although the contribution of radiation to the total human burden of cancer is probably small, the well-known latency of radiant energy and its cumulative effect require extremely long periods of observation and make it difficult to ascertain its total significance. Only now, almost four decades later, is an increased incidence of breast cancer becoming apparent among females exposed during childhood to the A-bomb.[63] Moreover, its possible additive or synergistic effects on other potential carcinogenic influences add yet another dimension. Although the mode of action of radiant energy on target cells is still imperfectly understood, the weight of evidence implicates the production of damage to DNA. The effects of UV light on DNA differ somewhat from those of ionizing radiations, requiring separate consideration of these two forms of radiant energy.

Ultraviolet Rays

There is ample evidence from epidemiologic studies that *UV rays* derived from the sun induce an increased incidence of squamous cell carcinoma, basal cell carcinoma, and melanocarcinoma of the skin.[64] The degree of risk depends on the intensity of exposure and the quantity of light-absorbing "protective mantle" of melanin in the skin. Thus, persons of European origin who have fair skin that repeatedly gets sunburned but stalwartly refuses to tan, and who live in locales receiving a great deal of sunlight (e.g., Queensland, Australia, close to the equator), have the highest incidence of melanocarcinoma. UV rays have a number of effects on cells, including inhibition of cell division, inactivation of enzymes, induction of mutations, and in sufficient dosage, killing of cells. These biologic effects are discussed in greater detail in the general consideration of radiant energy (p. 504). *The carcinogenicity of UV light is attributed to its formation of pyrimidine dimers in DNA. When unrepaired, these dimers lead to larger transcriptional errors and, in some instances, cancer.* Studies in mice suggest that more is involved than UV-induced mutations alone.[65] The UV light simultaneously activates T-suppressor cells and so inhibits cell-mediated immunity, which permits the emergence of highly antigenic skin tumors.[66] Whether these findings apply to humans is still under study, but in any event the UV-induced mutations apparently serve as the initiating mechanism and the immune changes as either potentiators or promoters.

Supportive evidence for the mutagenic effects of UV radiant energy comes from a small group of autosomal recessive hereditary diseases, all characterized by some anomaly in DNA metabolism, particularly repair mechanisms. Several methods of DNA repair have been identified,[67] the one most pertinent to our discussion being referred to as *excision-repair*. In this process, segments of DNA containing an altered base (owing to the effects of radiation) are recognized by a series of enzymes that remove the damaged base and replace it with a normal nucleotide, using the intact complementary strand as a template. At least four enzymes are required for this process: (1) an endonuclease to cut the DNA close to the lesion, (2) an exonuclease to remove the damaged segment, (3) a DNA polymerase to synthesize new DNA for filling the gap, and (4) a ligase to patch the new DNA.

Much of our present awareness of the probable role of mutation in the induction of cancer comes from investigations of the increased vulnerability of individuals with xeroderma pigmentosum (XP) to cancer.[68] Those with this condition can be divided into several distinct groups, each having some defect in excision-repair of DNA, the major subset lacking endonucleases for excision of the dimer. With such impairments these individuals have a markedly increased predisposition to skin cancers, predominantly in the sun-exposed areas of the body. In vitro skin fibroblasts from these patients are also abnormally sensitive to UV light as well as to some chemical carcinogens. However, it is of interest that there is *no* increased incidence of the common forms of lethal cancer, e.g., carcinomas of the lung, breast, and colon, in XP. Possibly the exposure of skin to UV light far exceeds that of internal organs to ingested mutagens that may cause damage to DNA. Three other hereditary "chromosome instability syndromes"—ataxia-telangiectasia, Fanconi's anemia, and Bloom's syndrome—are also characterized by predisposition to cancer. In ataxia-telangiectasia there is a predisposition to leukemia, thought to relate to the lack of a full complement of endonucleases and thus an inability to excise and repair gamma ray–induced DNA damage. However, other factors such as an immune deficiency, characteristic of this condition, may also be involved. The molecular defect in DNA repair in Fanconi's anemia and Bloom's syndrome has not been clearly defined, but there are observations suggesting defects in DNA repair and/or DNA replication.[69] Individuals with Bloom's syndrome have a markedly increased incidence of all forms of cancer, including the most common types. *These syndromes offer strong evidence that defective DNA metabolism and, more specifically, repair mechanisms predispose to cancer, and therefore that alterations in DNA represent at least one pathway to neoplastic transformation.*

Ionizing Radiation

Electromagnetic (x-rays, gamma rays) and particulate (alpha particles, beta particles, protons, neutrons) radiations are all carcinogenic.[70] The evidence is so voluminous that only a few examples will suffice. Many of the pioneers in the development of roentgen rays developed skin cancers. Miners of radioactive elements in central Europe and the Rocky Mountain region of the United States have suffered a tenfold increased incidence of lung cancers. The follow-up of survivors of the atomic bombs dropped on Hiroshima and Nagasaki has disclosed a markedly increased incidence of leukemia—principally acute and chronic myelocytic leukemia—after an average latent period of about seven years. Decades later, the leukemia risk in those heavily exposed is still above the level for control populations, as is the mortality rate from thyroid, breast, colon, and pulmonary carcinoma as well as others.[62] Even therapeutic irradiation has been documented to be carcinogenic. Thyroid cancers have developed in approximately 9% of those exposed during infancy and childhood to head and neck radiation. The previous practice of treating a form of arthritis of the spine known as ankylosing spondylitis with therapeutic irradiation has yielded a 10- to 12-fold increase in the incidence of leukemia years later.

To conclude this doleful litany, mention should be made of the residents of the Marshall Islands who were exposed on one occasion to accidental fallout from a hydrogen bomb test that contained thyroid-seeking radioactive iodines. As many as 90% of the children under the age of ten years on Rongelap Island developed thyroid nodules within 15 years, and it is significant that about 5% of these nodules proved to be thyroid carcinomas. It is evident that radiant energy—whether absorbed in the pleasant form of sunlight, through the best intentions of a physician, or by tragic exposure to an atomic bomb blast—has awesome carcinogenic potential.

Mechanisms of Radiation Carcinogenesis

Although radiant energy is clearly oncogenic, the precise event responsible for neoplastic transformation is obscure. Radiant energy causes chromosomal breakage, translocations, and point mutations; alters proteins; and inactivates enzymes. It also injures membranes. How it exerts all these effects is still debated (see the general discussion of radiant energy on p. 505). Two theories dominate current thinking: (1) The radiation directly ionizes critical cellular macromolecules; or (2) according to the "indirect theory," it first interacts with water or molecular oxygen to produce free radicals that mediate the damage. Through either pathway the DNA sustains injury, thus in effect inducing a somatic mutation. Indeed, *the carcinogenicity of ionizing radiation appears to correlate best with its mutagenicity.* In turn, the mutagenicity depends on a number of factors including (1) radiation quality, (2) dose, (3) dose rate, (4) DNA repair, and (5) host factors. On a dose-for-dose basis, particulate radiations having high LET (linear energy transfer) values (p. 505), such as neutrons and alpha particles, are more dangerous than low LET radiations, such as x-ray and gamma rays. As with chemical carcinogenesis, the critical genetic targets have not been identified with certainty. Activation of proto-oncogenes resulting from radiation-induced mutation is an attractive hypothesis that is supported by some experimental evidence.[71]

Ill-defined host factors also play a role. Clearly, fetuses, infants, and children are more vulnerable than adults. Thyroid cancer following radiation to the head and neck in adults is rare compared with its frequency in persons irradiated in childhood. Immune competence, hormonal influences, and cell type influence the carcinogenicity of radiation. The lack of clear understanding of these modifying factors and widely variable individual susceptibility make it impossible to establish "safe" tolerable levels of radiation exposure. This is a principal concern of regulatory agencies and of those who live in proximity to sources of radiant energy (e.g., nuclear energy installations and waste dumps), adding to the inevitable background exposure of sunlight and cosmic radiation.

In humans there is a hierarchy of vulnerability to radiation-induced cancers. Most frequent are the leukemias, save for chronic lymphocytic leukemia, which, for unknown reasons, almost never follows radiation injury. Cancer of the thyroid follows closely but only in the young. In the intermediate category are cancers of the breast, lungs, and salivary glands. In contrast, skin, bone, and the gastrointestinal tract are relatively resistant to radiation-induced neoplasia, even though the gastrointestinal mucosal cells are vulnerable to the cell-killing effects of radiation and the skin is in the pathway of all external radiation. Nonetheless, the physician dare not forget: *Any* cell can be transformed into a cancer cell by sufficient exposure to radiant energy.

VIRAL ONCOGENESIS

A large number of viruses have proved to be oncogenic in a wide variety of animals, ranging from amphibia to our first cousins, the primates, and the evidence grows ever stronger that certain forms of human cancer are of viral origin. Oncogenic viruses fall into two classes: DNA and RNA viruses. The major agents documented to cause cancer in animals and suspected of being involved in human neoplasia are presented in Table 6 – 9. In the following discussion, the better characterized and most intensively studied agents will be presented, followed by the mechanisms of carcinogenesis as it relates to each of the two categories of tumor viruses.

DNA Oncogenic Viruses

As indicated in Table 6 – 9, several DNA viruses have been associated with the causation of cancer in animals. Some, such as adenoviruses, cause tumors only in laboratory animals, whereas others, such as the bovine papilloma viruses, cause benign as well as malignant neoplasms in their natural hosts. Demonstrated viral oncogenicity in animals has led to great interest in the possible role of viruses in human cancers and the mechanisms involved in neoplastic transformation.

Of the various DNA viruses, three (papilloma viruses, Epstein-Barr virus, and hepatitis B virus) are of particular interest because they have been implicated in the causation of human cancer. Whether they are directly oncogenic or act indirectly by facilitating the action of other carcinogens is the object of much scrutiny. We will first discuss the evidence linking DNA viruses to human cancers, followed by the possible mechanisms of oncogenesis derived largely from studies with laboratory animals.

HUMAN PAPILLOMA VIRUSES (HPV). Papilloma viruses were among the first to be associated with human neoplasia. As early as 1907 Ciuffo demonstrated that human warts (benign epithelial tumors, papillomas of the skin) were caused by a cell-free transmissible agent. In 1933 Shope discovered that papilloma viruses were the etiologic agent of papillomas in rabbits. Since then, the role of human papilloma viruses in the causation of benign epithelial warts has been firmly established, and there is accumulating evidence that they may cause certain human cancers as well.[72-74]

Although it is still not possible to propagate HPV in tissue culture (a major impediment to their study), molecular cloning of their genomes has revealed approximately 50 genetically distinct types of HPV. Each of the HPV types is usually associated with a particular set of clinical and pathologic entities (Table 6 – 10). The initial evidence suggesting that HPV may cause cancer came from the study of epidermodysplasia verruciformis (EV), a rare disease characterized by multiple skin warts and defective cell-mediated immunity. In approximately 30% of these patients, some of the warts that are present on sun-exposed areas of the skin undergo cancerous transformation. Although several HPV types have been identified in individual benign warts in EV (Table 6 – 10), associated cancers have been shown to contain DNA of only a few HPV types, usually HPV-5, 8, or 14. These data suggest that certain papilloma viruses can act in concert with immune deficiency and exposure to UV light to produce malignant change. This hypothesis is supported by the observation that skin cancers arising in the sun-exposed areas of some immunosuppressed renal allograft recipients also contain HPV-5 DNA. In addition to these rare cancers, evidence has now begun to emerge that papilloma viruses may play a role in the genesis of anogenital cancers, particularly carcinoma of the uterine cervix.[73-75] The relationship between tumors of the female genital tract and HPV is discussed in Chapter 24 (p. 1142). Suffice it to say that:

• Squamous cell carcinomas of the cervix contain HPV in 90 to 95% of the cases.[76] HPV-16 is found most commonly (50%), followed by HPV-18 (20%).
• Presumed precursors of squamous cell carcinoma (including carcinoma in situ) consistently contain HPV-16 or 18.
• Benign genital warts are associated with distinct HPV types, predominantly HPV-6 and 11. Lesions containing these viruses may develop into verrucous carcinomas that are locally invasive but not metastatic.
• Molecularly cloned fragments of certain HPV types and the related bovine papilloma viruses can cause transformation of mouse cell lines in vitro, indicating that these viruses contain oncogenic sequences.

To summarize, HPV have clearly proved to be etiologic agents of benign squamous papillomas. In some instances (such as epidermodysplasia verruciformis), HPV-induced benign lesions progress to squamous cell carcinomas. Thus the oncogenic potential of certain HPV types is clearly established. An etiologic role for HPV in anogenital cancers is suggested by the more or less regular presence of viral footprints in the cancer cells. HPV may act alone, or, more likely, in concert with other risk factors (p. 1142).

EPSTEIN-BARR VIRUS (EBV).

This virus, a member of the herpes family, has been implicated in the pathogenesis of two types of human tumors, Burkitt's lymphoma and undifferentiated nasopharyngeal carcinomas.[77,78] Both these neoplasms are reviewed in detail on pages 715 and 814, respectively, and therefore only their association with EBV will be discussed here. Burkitt's lymphoma is a neoplasm of B lympho-

cytes that is the most common childhood tumor in Central Africa and New Guinea. A morphologically identical lymphoma occurs sporadically throughout the world. The association between African Burkitt's lymphoma and EBV is quite strong.

• Approximately 98% of African tumors carry the EBV genome and the EBV-determined nuclear antigen (EBNA).
• One hundred percent of the patients have elevated antibody titers against viral capsid antigens.
• Serum antibody titers against viral capsid antigens are correlated with the risk of developing the tumor.

Table 6–9. Oncogenic Viruses

Family	Virus	Host of Origin	Associated Tumors	Other Risk Factors
		DNA VIRUSES		
Hepadenovirus	Hepatitis B group (HBV)	Man, woodchuck, ducks	Liver cancer	In man: alcohol, smoking, fungal toxins, other viruses
Papovavirus	Polyoma	Mouse	Various carcinomas and sarcomas	
	SV 40	Monkey	Sarcomas in rodents	
	Human papilloma viruses (HPV)	Man	Genital, laryngeal, and skin warts (papillomas)	
			Skin cancer in patients with epidermodysplasia verruciformis	Sunlight, genetic disorders possibly affecting immunity
			In situ and invasive cancers of the vulva and uterine cervix	
			Laryngeal cancer	X-irradiation, smoking
	Bovine papilloma viruses (BPV)	Cattle	Genital, alimentary, and skin warts	
			Esophageal cancer	Possibly carcinogens and immune suppressants in ingested bracken fern
		Other mammals (rabbits, dogs)	Papillomas may progress to carcinomas	Experimentally, carcinogens such as methylcholanthrene
Adenovirus	Types 2, 5, 12	Man	None in man; sarcomas in hamsters	
Herpesvirus	Marek's disease	Fowl	Neurolymphomatosis	Genetic predisposition of unknown basis
	H. ateles and *H. samiri*	Monkey	Lymphoma, leukemia	
	Epstein-Barr virus	Man	Burkitt's lymphoma	Malaria (polyclonal B-cell activation)
			Immunoblastic lymphoma	Immune deficiency (renal transplant recipients, AIDS)
			Nasopharyngeal carcinoma	Histocompatibility antigen genotype
	Herpes simplex type 2	Man	Cancer of uterine cervix?	
	Cytomegalovirus	Man	Kaposi's sarcoma?	Immune deficiency, histocompatibility antigen genotype

Table 6 – 9. Oncogenic Viruses *Continued*

Family	Virus	Host of Origin	Associated Tumors	Other Risk Factors
		RNA VIRUSES (RETROVIRUSES)		
Type B	Mammary tumor virus	Mouse	Mammary adenocarcinoma	Pregnancy (hormone levels)
Type C	Avian leukemia-sarcoma complex	Chicken	Various sarcomas, some carcinomas, lymphomas, and leukemia	Genetic susceptibility affecting virus penetration, replication, and spread
	Mouse leukemia and sarcoma viruses		Various sarcomas, leukemias, and lymphomas	Genetic susceptibility affecting virus penetration, replication, and spread
	Feline leukemia virus		Leukemias and lymphomas	
	Bovine leukemia virus		Leukemias and lymphomas	
	Primate leukemia-sarcoma viruses		Leukemias in apes; sarcomas in monkeys	
Type D	Human T-cell leukemia virus-1		Adult T-cell leukemia/ lymphoma	

Boxed entries highlight human tumors that show strong associations with the corresponding virus.

? indicates association is doubtful in man.

Modified from Wyke, J.A.: Viruses and cancer. *In* Franks, L.M., and Teich, N. (eds): Introduction to the Cellular and Molecular Biology of Cancer. New York, Oxford University Press, 1986, p. 176.

• EBV exhibits strong tropisms for human B cells. It infects B cells by binding to the B cell – specific receptor for the third component of complement. The infected B cells are immortalized and can be propagated indefinitely in vitro.

Although these data strongly support the idea that EBV is intimately involved in the causation of Burkitt's lymphoma, several other observations suggest that additional factors must be involved. *First,* EBV infection is not limited to the geographic locales where Burkitt's lymphoma is found. Indeed, EBV is a ubiquitous virus that asymptomatically infects almost all adults worldwide. *Second,* EBV is known to cause infectious mononucleosis, a self-limited disorder (p. 323) in which B cells are infected. *Third,* the EBV genome can be found in only 15 to 20% of cases of Burkitt's lymphoma outside Africa, but both the endemic (African) and the sporadic cases of Burkitt's lymphoma have a t(8;14) translocation (p. 715), which influences the activation of the c-*myc* oncogene (p. 288). *Finally,* although EBV infection immortalizes B cells in vitro, these cells do not acquire the transformed phenotype (p. 254) or form tumors when

Table 6 – 10. Some HPV Types and Associated Lesions

HPV TYPE	TYPE OF WART	HPV TYPE	TYPE OF CANCER
1	Deep, painful plantar wart		None
2,4,7	Common skin warts		None
5,8,9,12,14,15, 17,19 – 25,28,29	Benign lesions seen in epidermodysplasia verruciformis (EV)	5,8,14	Skin cancer associated with EV
6,11	Anogenital and laryngeal papillomas (condyloma acuminatum)	6,11	Verrucous carcinoma (genital)*
		16,18,33	Carcinoma of cervix, oral cancer
		30,40	Laryngeal cancer
42	Vulvar papilloma		

* Locally invasive but not metastatic.

Data compiled from Ostrow, R.S., and Faras, A.J.: The molecular biology of human papillomaviruses and pathogenesis of genital papillomas and neoplasms. Cancer Metas. Rev. 6:383, 1987; and Lutzner, M.A.: Papillomaviruses and neoplasia in man. *In* Fenoglio-Preiser, C.M., et al.: (eds): New Concepts in Neoplasia as Applied to Diagnostic Pathology. Baltimore, Williams & Wilkins, 1986, p. 133.

injected into appropriately conditioned mice in vivo. It appears, therefore, that EBV serves as one factor in the multistep development of Burkitt's lymphoma (p. 734). In normal individuals, EBV infection is readily controlled by effective immune responses, and hence the vast majority of infected individuals remain asymptomatic or develop self-limited infectious mononucleosis. In regions of Africa where Burkitt's lymphoma is endemic, concomitant malaria (also endemic in those regions) impairs immune competence, allowing uncontrolled EBV-driven B cell proliferation. The actively dividing B cell population is at increased risk of developing mutations such as the t(8;14) translocation that seems to be a consistent feature of this tumor. The fact that in nonendemic areas 80% of the tumors do not harbor the EBV genome but do possess the specific translocation suggests that more than one pathway may exist for the development of Burkitt's lymphoma.

Nasopharyngeal carcinoma is the other tumor associated with EBV infection. This tumor is endemic in Southern China, in some parts of Africa, and in Arctic Eskimos. Unlike Burkitt's lymphoma, 100% of nasopharyngeal carcinomas obtained from all parts of the world contain EBV DNA. In addition, antibody titers to viral capsid antigens are greatly elevated, and in endemic areas patients develop IgA antibodies prior to the appearance of the tumor.

The 100% correlation between EBV and nasopharyngeal carcinoma suggests that EBV plays a role in the genesis of this tumor, but (as with Burkitt's tumor) the restricted geographic distribution indicates that genetic or environmental cofactors, or both, also contribute to its etiology.

HEPATITIS B VIRUS. Epidemiologic studies, discussed in greater detail on page 959, strongly suggest a close association between hepatitis B virus (HBV) infection and the occurrence of liver cancer (hepatocellular carcinoma). HBV is endemic in countries of the Far East and Africa, and correspondingly these areas have the highest incidence of hepatocellular carcinoma. Studies in Taiwan indicate that those who are infected with HBV have a greater than 200-fold increased risk of developing liver cancer as compared with uninfected individuals in the same area. HBV DNA has been found in several cell lines derived from human hepatic cancers. However, as with EBV, the evidence is not sufficient to ascribe a direct causative role to HBV. It is likely that HBV infection acts in concert with the regenerative activity of liver cirrhosis, or other environmental (e.g., dietary) factors or possibly predisposes to other carcinogenic influences (p. 959).

Mechanism of Action of DNA Viruses

The mechanisms by which DNA viruses cause neoplastic transformation are as varied as the viruses themselves. Some DNA viruses, such as HPV, contain transforming sequences (oncogenes) and can transform cells in vitro; others, exemplified by hepatitis B virus, do not encode any known transforming genes and hence must act indirectly. Regardless of the precise mechanism, certain features are shared by many oncogenic DNA viruses.

• To be transformed by a virus, the cell must survive the infection in good health. Cells in which viral replication can be completed are called permissive; such cells cannot be transformed because they die with the release of newly formed virus. In contrast, nonpermissive cells, which do not allow the virus to complete its life cycle, can be transformed into neoplastic cells.
• With most oncogenic DNA viruses, only those portions of the genome that are transcribed early in the viral life cycle (prior to viral DNA replication and synthesis of viral capsid proteins) are essential for transformation. Cloned fragments of the viral DNA, which include only the early region of the genome, can induce transformation when transfected into suitable cells in vitro.
• In nonpermissive cells, oncogenic DNA viruses usually form stable associations with the host cell genome. This usually occurs by integration of viral DNA into chromosomes. However, only those integration events that interrupt late viral genes can produce transformed cells. One such example is illustrated in Figure 6–25, in which integration of SV40 DNA allows transcription of early genes (essential for transformation) but prevents viral multiplication by interfering with replication of late viral genes.

The protein products of several transforming "early genes" have been identified, and recent studies have begun to unravel the molecular basis of their action. Much of the work has been performed with papovaviruses (SV40 and polyoma virus) and adenoviruses that are not associated with tumors in humans. However, since these studies provide important insights into the mechanisms of carcinogenesis, they will be briefly described.[79]

The early regions of polyoma and SV40 viruses code for several proteins referred to as T proteins (or T antigens). There are three polyoma T proteins (large, middle, and small), and two SV40 T proteins (large and small). When primary cultures of rodent cells are transfected with a cDNA encoding the polyoma large T protein, they become immortal and their requirements for growth factor in the medium are reduced, but they do not assume the fully transformed phenotype, nor do they form tumors in vivo. Introduction of polyoma middle T into these cells induces the malignant phenotype (e.g., loss of density-dependent inhibition, p. 254). *These studies provide firm evidence that cancer, even when caused by highly oncogenic viruses, is a multistep process.*

Although the function of the polyoma large T protein is not fully understood, it localizes in the nucleus and is believed to regulate DNA synthesis. Quite interestingly, polyoma middle T protein associates with a normal cell membrane protein referred to as cellular *src* (pronounced sarc). The *src* protein is a tyrosine kinase, whose activity is increased 50-fold

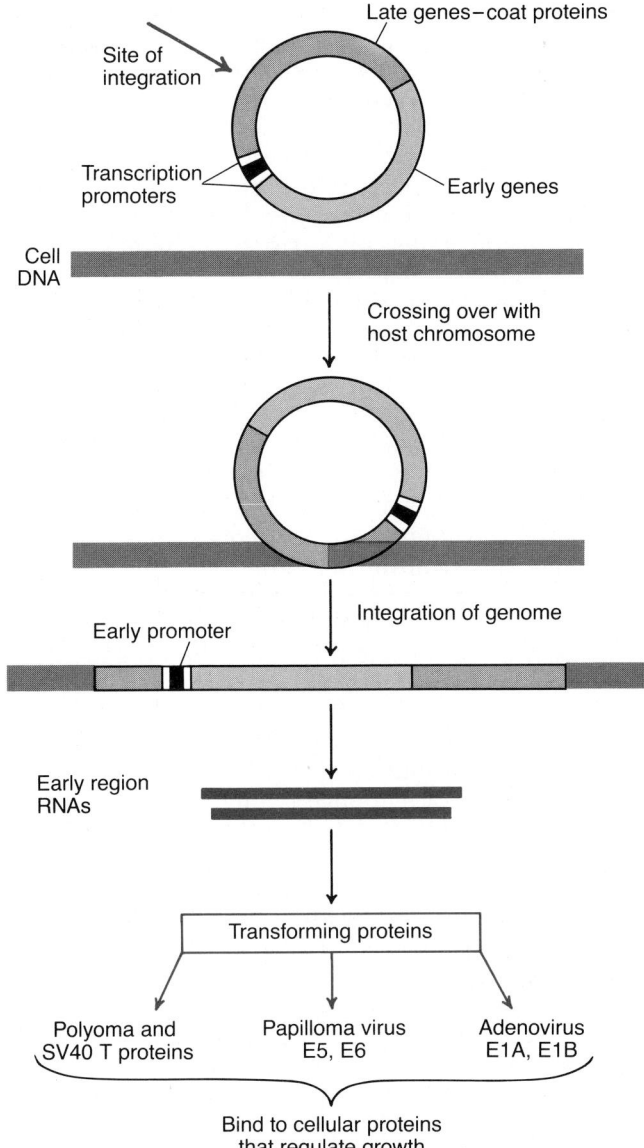

Site of integration

Late genes–coat proteins

Transcription promoters

Early genes

Cell DNA

Crossing over with host chromosome

Early promoter

Integration of genome

Early region RNAs

Transforming proteins

Polyoma and SV40 T proteins

Papilloma virus E5, E6

Adenovirus E1A, E1B

Bind to cellular proteins that regulate growth

Figure 6–25. Schematic illustration of how a DNA virus (such as SV40) may integrate into a host chromosome and lead to neoplastic transformation. Integration within the late region prevents viral replication, but allows transcription of early genes that encode for transforming proteins. (Modified from Watson, J.D., et al.: Molecular Biology of the Gene. 4th ed. Menlo Park, California, Benjamin/Cummings Publishing Co., 1987, p. 1016.)

by association with polyoma middle T. As will be discussed later, transformation induced by Rous sarcoma virus (a retrovirus) is also associated with a large increase in the enzymatic activities of a mutant *src* protein. This observation illustrates another fundamental aspect of carcinogenesis. *Diverse carcinogenic influences may affect common regulatory pathways by different mechanisms.*

Another example that illustrates this point is provided by investigations relating to the transforming proteins of SV40 and adenoviruses. These two viruses belong to different families and transform different cell types in vitro (see Table 6–9). However, trans-

forming proteins of both these viruses (SV40 large T, and adenovirus E1B) bind to a common nuclear protein (p53) in the nucleus. In normal cells, p53 levels are extremely low owing to its short half-life, but in SV40 and adenovirus-transformed cells, p53 levels are markedly increased, possibly as a result of binding with SV40 large T and adenovirus E1B proteins. Thus, it would seem that these two viral proteins effect transformation by subverting the physiologic mechanisms that regulate the levels of a normal nuclear protein. The normal functions of p53 protein are not fully understood, but several pieces of experimental evidence suggest that it upregulates DNA synthesis.[80]

Recent studies indicate that in addition to stimulating the functions of growth-promoting proteins such as p53, DNA oncogenic viruses may act by "neutralizing" the action of growth-inhibitory molecules produced by cancer suppressor genes.[81,82] The nature of these genes and their interaction with DNA viral proteins will be described later (p. 289).

In the preceding discussion we focused on those DNA viruses that encode transforming genes. To this group belong the human papilloma viruses, which have been implicated in human cancer. Although detailed studies are not yet available, it is likely that early proteins of HPV transform cells by mechanisms similar to those implicated in carcinogenesis by SV40, polyoma, and adenoviruses. EBV, the other potential human oncogenic virus, seems to contain genes that can immortalize B cells but cannot fully transform them without additional mutations, induced, for example, by chromosomal translocation. The transforming potential of the human hepatitis B virus is the least understood and is discussed later (p. 959) along with hepatocellular carcinomas.

RNA Oncogenic Viruses

All oncogenic RNA viruses are retroviruses; i.e., they contain the enzyme reverse transcriptase, which allows reverse transcription of viral RNA into virus-specific DNA. Although only one member of this virus family (HTLV-1) is known to be associated with a human tumor, the study of oncogenic animal retroviruses has provided spectacular insights into the genetic basis of cancer. To understand this unfolding drama we will briefly review the life cycle, structure, and oncogenicity of animal retroviruses.

The essential steps in the life cycle of replication-competent retroviruses are illustrated in Figure 6–26. Their genomes contain three sets of genes: *gag*, *pol*, and *env*, bounded on either side by untranslated repeated sequences referred to as long terminal repeats (LTRs) (Fig. 6–27). The LTRs contain promoter and enhancer sequences for the synthesis of adjacent viral RNA. The *gag* coding region carries sequences of the virion core proteins; the *pol* region encodes for *reverse transcriptase*; and the *env* gene products are envelope glycoproteins.

Oncogenic retroviruses can be broadly grouped into three classes on the basis of their transforming activity and genomic structure: (1) acute transform-

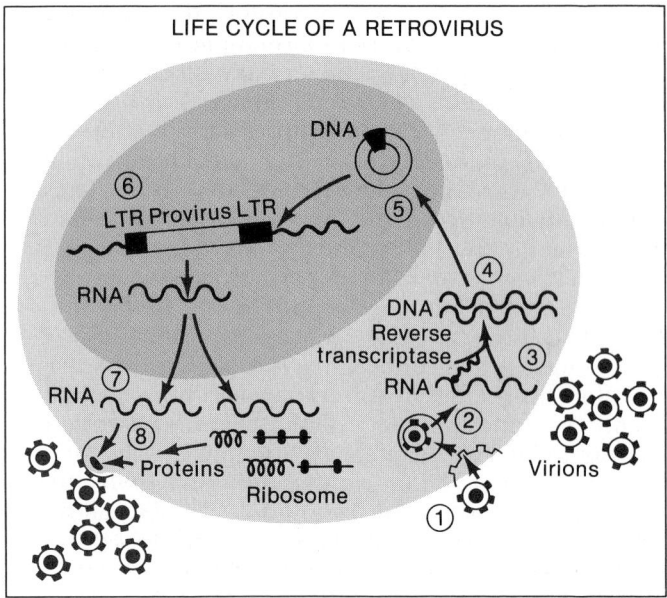

Figure 6–26. Retroviral life cycle: (1) Retrovirus enters the cell by a specific receptor; (2) virus is uncoated in an endosome; and (3) viral RNA is transcribed to double-stranded viral DNA (4) and is transported to the nucleus (5) and integrates into the cellular genome (6). Viral DNA is transcribed as genomic RNA and viral messenger RNA (7), which is translated into new viral protein and assembled at the cell membrane to complete the viral life cycle by budding (8). (From Wyngaarden, J.B., and Smith, L.H. (eds.): Cecil Textbook of Medicine. 18th ed. Philadelphia, W.B. Saunders Co., 1988, p. 1794.)

ing viruses; (2) slow transforming viruses; and (3) human T-cell leukemia virus.

ACUTE TRANSFORMING VIRUSES. These include many transforming type C viruses of animals that are characterized by rapid induction of tumors in infected animals. Many of these viruses are also capable of transforming cells in vitro. Molecular dissection of

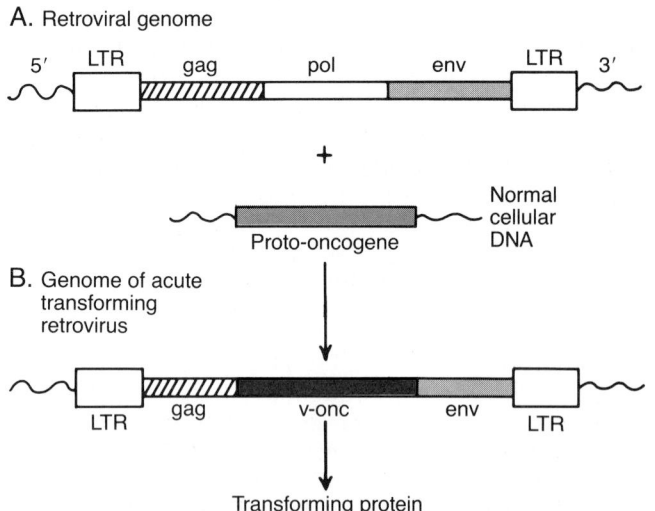

Figure 6–27. Genomic structure of a replication-competent retrovirus (A) and transduction of a proto-oncogene into the retrovirus genome, producing an acute transforming virus (B).

their genomes has revealed that all except one member (Rous sarcoma virus) of this group have lost genetic information coding for their replicative genes (i.e., they are replication defective). New genetic information is inserted in place of the deleted material (Fig. 6–27). By a variety of molecular techniques it is possible to show that the new set of sequences is responsible for their transforming ability; because these cancer-causing genes are a part of the viral genome, they are called *viral oncogenes* or v-*oncs*.[83] Within the past decade, approximately 20 v-*oncs* have been identified. Each of these is given a separate name, a three-letter word that relates the oncogene to the virus from which it was isolated. For example, the v-*onc* contained in *feline* sarcoma virus is designated *fes*, whereas the oncogene in *simian* sarcoma virus is referred to as *sis*. Soon after the first discovery of v-*oncs*, two important questions were raised: (1) Where did the v-*onc* sequences come from? (2) How do v-*oncs* cause transformation?

Answers to the first question came from DNA-hybridization studies, which indicated that the v-*onc* sequences are almost identical to sequences found in the normal cellular DNA of nearly all species in the biologic kingdom (including yeast, slime mold, and humans). These normal genes are referred to as *proto-oncogenes*, in recognition of their transforming potential. Many lines of evidence strongly suggest that v-*oncs* are not viral genes at all; instead they represent wayward copies of proto-oncogenes that became incorporated (transduced) into the viral genome during the process of viral replication within a normal cell. Thus v-*oncs* may be viewed as mere passengers in the viral genome, endowing the virus with the ability to transform cells, at the expense of the ability to replicate. (Such replication-defective acutely transforming viruses often occur in association with a replication-competent "helper virus" that provides the genes for completing the viral life cycle.) *The conservation of proto-oncogenes throughout evolution in species as diverse as yeasts and humans suggests that they play essential roles, probably in cell differentiation and regulation of cell proliferation* (p. 282). We shall return to this subject later, but first we must clarify the distinction between the terms proto-oncogene and *cellular oncogene* (c-*onc*). Often these two are used interchangeably. However, it should be understood that the term proto-oncogene refers to those cellular sequences that are not oncogenic in the physiologic state but may give rise to or behave as cancer-causing genes. This may occur when proto-oncogenes are transduced into acutely transforming retroviruses, giving rise to v-*oncs*, or when the normal structure or expression of proto-oncogenes is altered in situ so that they acquire transforming properties and are converted into cellular oncogenes (c-*oncs*).

We come next to the question of how v-*oncs*, derived as they are from otherwise harmless normal DNA sequences (proto-oncogenes), cause malignant transformation. Two possibilities, both supported by experimental evidence, exist:

• During transduction (proto-oncogene → v-*onc*), mutations occur that render v-*oncs* structurally different from their normal cellular forebears. Although there are significant homologies between several v-*oncs* and the corresponding proto-oncogenes, in most cases the genes are not identical. Such genetic damage may alter the gene products sufficiently to induce unregulated growth.

• Because transduction brings proto-oncogenes into the proximity of potent retroviral promoters, they are expressed at a high level. Sustained and abundant expression of an otherwise normal gene may cause uncontrolled growth.

Thus it seems that both qualitative and quantitative changes may explain why the transduced oncogenes of retroviruses cause cancer despite the fact that they are derived from normal cellular genes.

SLOW TRANSFORMING RETROVIRUSES. These viruses do not have oncogenes, are replication competent, and display the typical retroviral genomic organization already discussed (Fig. 6–27). Because many viruses in this category cause leukemias in rodents, they have also been called chronic leukemia viruses. The mechanism by which they cause neoplastic transformation has been referred to as *insertional mutagenesis*, since the proviral DNA is always found to be inserted (integrated) near a proto-oncogene (Fig. 6–28). The presence of strong retroviral promoters in the vicinity (usually upstream) of the proto-

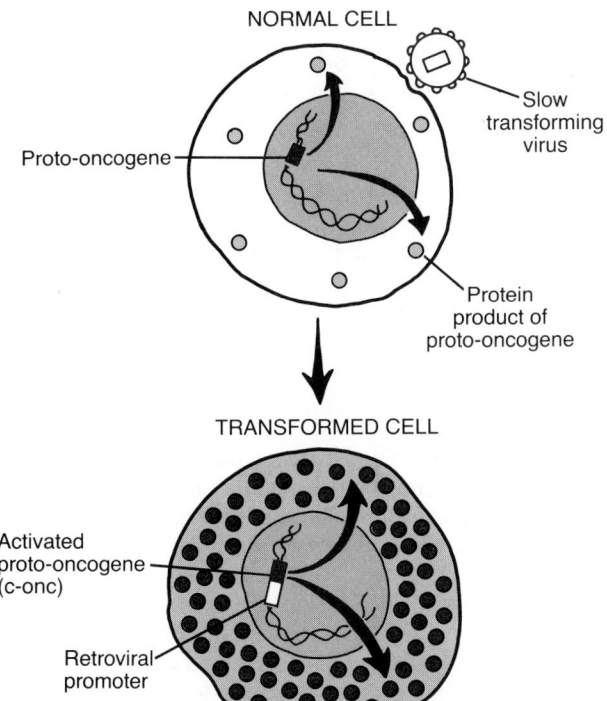

Figure 6–28. Retrovirus-induced neoplastic transformation by insertional mutagenesis. A slow transforming virus infects a normal cell and integrates next to a proto-oncogene. Viral promoters cause increased transcription of the proto-oncogene product.

oncogene leads to increased transcription and conversion to a c-*onc*. Another consequence of proviral insertion near a proto-oncogene may be to induce a structural change in the cellular gene. Thus both genetic damage and enhanced expression of proto-oncogenes may underlie neoplastic transformation by this group of viruses. Several proto-oncogenes (e.g., c-*mos*, c-*myc*, c-*myb*, c-*H-ras*) encountered as v-*oncs* in acutely transforming viruses are also involved in tumorigenesis by insertional mutagenesis. However, some proto-oncogenes have never been found in viruses and were discovered only by exploring the integration site of tumor viruses. For example, mouse mammary tumor virus (MMTV) is a replication-competent retrovirus whose life cycle and genome resemble those of slow transforming leukemia viruses. Analysis of MMTV-induced tumors has shown that the proviral DNA is integrated into one of two regions referred to as *int*-1 or *int*-2. These regions are believed to contain two previously unidentified proto-oncogenes.

HUMAN T-CELL LEUKEMIA VIRUS. This represents the third group of oncogenic retroviruses and the only one that is implicated in the causation of human cancer.[84] It is associated with a form of T-cell leukemia/lymphoma that is endemic in certain parts of Japan and the West Indies but is found sporadically elsewhere. Like HIV, HTLV-1 has strong tropism for CD4 cells (p. 225), and hence this subset of T cells seems to be the sole target for neoplastic transformation. The evidence linking HTLV-1 in the causation of adult T-cell leukemia/lymphoma (ATL) can be summarized as follows.[85]

• HTLV-1 has been repeatedly isolated from neoplastic cells of patients with ATL.

• HTLV-1 proviral sequences can be detected in DNA of leukemic T cells but not in DNA of other lymphoid cells of the same patient, indicating that the virus is acquired by infection and not transmitted in germline.

• The tumor cells contain one to two copies of HTLV-1 provirus in the same chromosomal location in each cell (i.e., the integration shows a clonal pattern). This means that the tumor was derived from the clonal expansion of a single transformed cell that must have been infected prior to transformation, ruling out the possibility that HTLV-1 is a passenger virus.

• Cultured neoplastic T cells release HTLV-1 that can immortalize T cells in vitro.

• Antibodies against HTLV-1 are found in over 90% of patients with ATL.

Despite impressive evidence linking HTLV-1 with ATL, the molecular mechanisms of transformation are obscure. Unlike acute transforming viruses, HTLV-1 does not contain a v-*onc*, and because analysis of leukemic T cells from different patients does not reveal any consistent site of integration, the insertional-mutational activation of a c-*onc* can be ruled out. The genomic structure of HTLV-1 reveals *gag*, *pol, env*, and *LTR* regions typical of other retroviruses, but unlike other retroviruses, it contains a fourth region (between the *env* gene and 3' LTR) called *tat* (a similar region is also noted in HIV-1, p. 225). It is believed that the secrets of its transforming activity are locked within the *tat* region. This conclusion seems to be supported by recent data using transgenic mice. In these animals, cloned *tat* gene was introduced into the germline by microinjection of fertilized eggs. High levels of *tat* gene were expressed in skeletal muscles of such transgenic mice, all of which developed multiple tumors by 17 weeks of age.[86] The *tat* region encodes at least three proteins, one of which causes enhanced transcription of HTLV-1 by acting on the 5' LTR. More important, for transformation, is the observation that *tat* gene product induces activation of IL-2 and IL-2R genes in infected T cells. Thus HTLV-1 infected T cells seem to have turned on the production of a T-cell growth factor (IL-2) and its receptor (IL-2R), thus setting up an autocrine system for growth and proliferation. This causes polyclonal T-cell proliferation (because the virus infects several T cells), and must therefore be an early event in transformation. Some additional genetic changes, as yet unidentified, must occur because fully developed leukemic cells continue to express IL-2R but do not require IL-2 for proliferation. We return once again to the familiar refrain of multiple steps in the development of tumors.

ONCOGENES AND CANCER

As discussed above, the study of transforming retroviruses provided cancer researchers with the first glimpse of proto-oncogenes. However, at the same time it became obvious that most human tumors are not caused by retroviral infection. These observations raised several important questions about proto-oncogenes. Do they don their malignant mask only when captured by retroviruses, or can they metamorphose into cancer genes without leaving the cell? Could mutagenic chemicals alter these genes so as to unleash their oncogenic potential? These questions can be distilled into one central issue: Do nonviral tumors contain sequences that have the potential to cause cancer? Help came in the early 1980s, when progress in recombinant DNA technology and DNA-mediated gene transfer (DNA-transfection) made it possible to tackle this problem head on.[87]

In their quest to find oncogenes, Robert Weinberg and his colleagues extracted DNA from a human bladder carcinoma cell line and transfected it into NIH/3T3 mouse fibroblast cell line. The 3T3 cells grow continuously in culture but, like normal cells, are contact inhibited and do not form tumors when injected into immunosuppressed mice. Following transfection with tumor DNA, however, the 3T3 cells formed foci of transformed cells that showed anchorage-independent growth in soft agar and formed tumors in athymic nude mice. In contrast, transfec-

tion with DNA from normal human cells failed to transform 3T3 cells. The conclusion from these experiments was unescapable: DNA of the bladder carcinoma cells contained sequences (oncogenes) that caused transformation of 3T3 fibroblasts in vitro. During the years following these pioneering studies a large number of human and animal tumors have been tested for the presence of oncogenic DNA by transfection assay, of which 20 to 25% have scored positive. Many of these transforming DNA sequences have turned out to be homologous to *ras* proto-oncogenes that are the forebears of the v-*oncs* contained in Harvey (H) and Kirsten (K) sarcoma viruses. Others, such as c-*neu*, represent novel c-*oncs* that have never been found in retroviruses (Table 6–11). *To summarize, normal cellular genes (proto-oncogenes) may become oncogenic (v-oncs) by retroviral transduction or by influences that alter their behavior in the natural host, thereby converting them into cellular oncogenes.* Two questions follow: (1) What are the physiologic functions of proto-oncogenes? and (2) How do the normally "civilized" proto-oncogenes acquire the pernicious role of cellular oncogenes? These two issues will be discussed separately in the ensuing sections, but it will soon become evident that it is difficult to dissociate them completely.

PRODUCTS OF PROTO-ONCOGENES AND THEIR FUNCTIONS

It was mentioned earlier that proto-oncogenes are likely to play essential roles in the differentiation and proliferation of normal cells. To explore the mechanisms by which the products of proto-oncogenes affect cell proliferation, we will briefly review the sequence of events that take place during normal cell growth. These can be resolved into three steps:

- The interaction of an external factor ("first messenger") with the cell membrane, leading to signal transduction through the cell membrane.
- Transmission of the transduced signal from the inner leaflet of the plasma membrane across to the nucleus via so-called second messengers.
- Initiation of DNA transcription and replication, leading ultimately to cell division.

Figure 6–29 illustrates a simplified scheme of two forms of signal transduction that are relevant to the present discussion. One prototypic pathway is initiated when a growth factor binds to its receptor on the cell surface and transmits activating signals through a guanine-binding (G) protein to the enzyme phospholipase C (PLC). Activated PLC cleaves the membrane phospholipid phosphatidylinositol-4,5 biphosphate (PIP_2) into two second messengers, inositol triphosphate (IP_3) and diacylglycerol (DG). The IP_3 diffuses into the cytoplasm, where it causes Ca^{2+} to be released from intracellular stores in the endoplasmic reticulum. In turn, Ca^{2+} stimulates calmodulin-dependent protein kinases. The DG remains in the

Table 6-11. Selected Oncogenes: Retroviral and Nonretroviral

ONCOGENE	ASSOCIATION *Retrovirus*	*Human Tumor* (Method of Identification)	SUBCELLULAR LOCATION OF ONCOGENE PROTEIN	PROPERTY OR FUNCTION OF PROTEIN
Class I: protein kinases				
src	Rous sarcoma virus	—	Plasma membrane	Tyrosine-specific kinase
yes	Avian sarcoma virus	—	Plasma membrane	Tyrosine-specific kinase
abl	Abelson murine leukemia virus	Chronic myeloid leukemia (translocation)	Plasma membrane	Tyrosine-specific kinase
fes	Feline sarcoma virus	Acute myeloid leukemias (translocation)	Plasma membrane	Tyrosine-specific kinase
erb-B	Avian erythroblastosis virus	Squamous cell carcinoma cell lines (amplification)	Transmembrane	EGF receptor/tyrosine kinase
neu(erb-B2)	—	Breast cancer (amplification)	Transmembrane	Tyrosine kinase resembles EGF receptor
fms	Feline sarcoma virus	—	Transmembrane	CSF-1 receptor/tyrosine kinase
ros	Avian sarcoma virus	—	Transmembrane	Tyrosine kinase, related to growth factor receptors
mos	Moloney murine sarcoma virus virus	—	Cytoplasm	Serine/threonine kinase
Class II: GTP-binding proteins				
H-ras	Harvey murine sarcoma virus	A large variety of human cancers, e.g., bladder, lung, colon, leukemias, neuroblastomas (transfection)	Plasma membrane	GTP-binding proteins with GTPase activity
K-ras	Kirsten murine sarcoma virus			
N-ras	—			
Class III: growth factors				
sis	Simian sarcoma virus	—	Secreted	Related to platelet-derived growth factor
int-2	Mouse mammary tumor* virus	—	Secreted	Related to fibroblast growth factor
Class IV: nuclear proteins				
myc	Avian myelocytomatosis virus	Burkitt's lymphoma (translocation) Small cell lung cancer (amplification)	Nucleus	Nuclear binding protein
L-myc	—	Small cell lung cancer (amplification)	Nucleus	?
N-myc	—	Neuroblastoma (amplification)	Nucleus	?
myb	Avian myeloblastosis virus	Colon carcinoma lines (amplification)	Nucleus	?
fos	Murine osteosarcoma virus	—	Nucleus	?
Class V: unclassified				
bcl-2	—	Follicular lymphomas (translocation)	?	?
met	—	Osteosarcoma	?	?

* *Int-2* is not a v-*onc* of mouse mammary tumor virus. It was detected by insertional mutagenesis caused by the virus. GTP = guanine triphosphate.

membrane, where it activates protein kinase C. This sequence of events is often referred to as the PIP$_2$ pathway.

The other pathway, exemplified by the response of cells to epidermal growth factor (EGF), utilizes the EGF receptor. This receptor spans the plasma membrane and has an external EGF-binding domain and an internal tyrosine-specific protein kinase domain. Binding of an EGF molecule to the receptor presumably changes the receptor conformation and activates tyrosine kinase activity of the intracellular domain. Some growth factor receptors, such as the PDGF receptor, can trigger both pathways because they possess intrinsic tyrosine kinase activity and can also initiate phosphoinositol turnover via G proteins. It will be noted (Fig. 6–29) that all these pathways lead to activation of protein kinases — enzymes that phosphoryl-

ate proteins. Phosphorylation of proteins alters their functional state, and it is generally believed that such changes play an important role in regulating cell proliferation. Possibly certain cytoplasmic proteins convey mitogenic signals to the nucleus after they are phosphorylated near the cell membrane. *To summarize, stimulation of normal cell proliferation often depends upon external signals provided by growth factors (p. 76). The signal is received by a receptor on the cell membrane, which transfers the message through the membrane into the cytoplasm and ultimately to the nucleus. Proto-oncogenes have been found to function at each step of the mitotic cascade, as indicated in Figure 6–29.*

In the following discussion the products of proto-oncogenes are grouped according to their subcellular localization and their role in signal transduction.

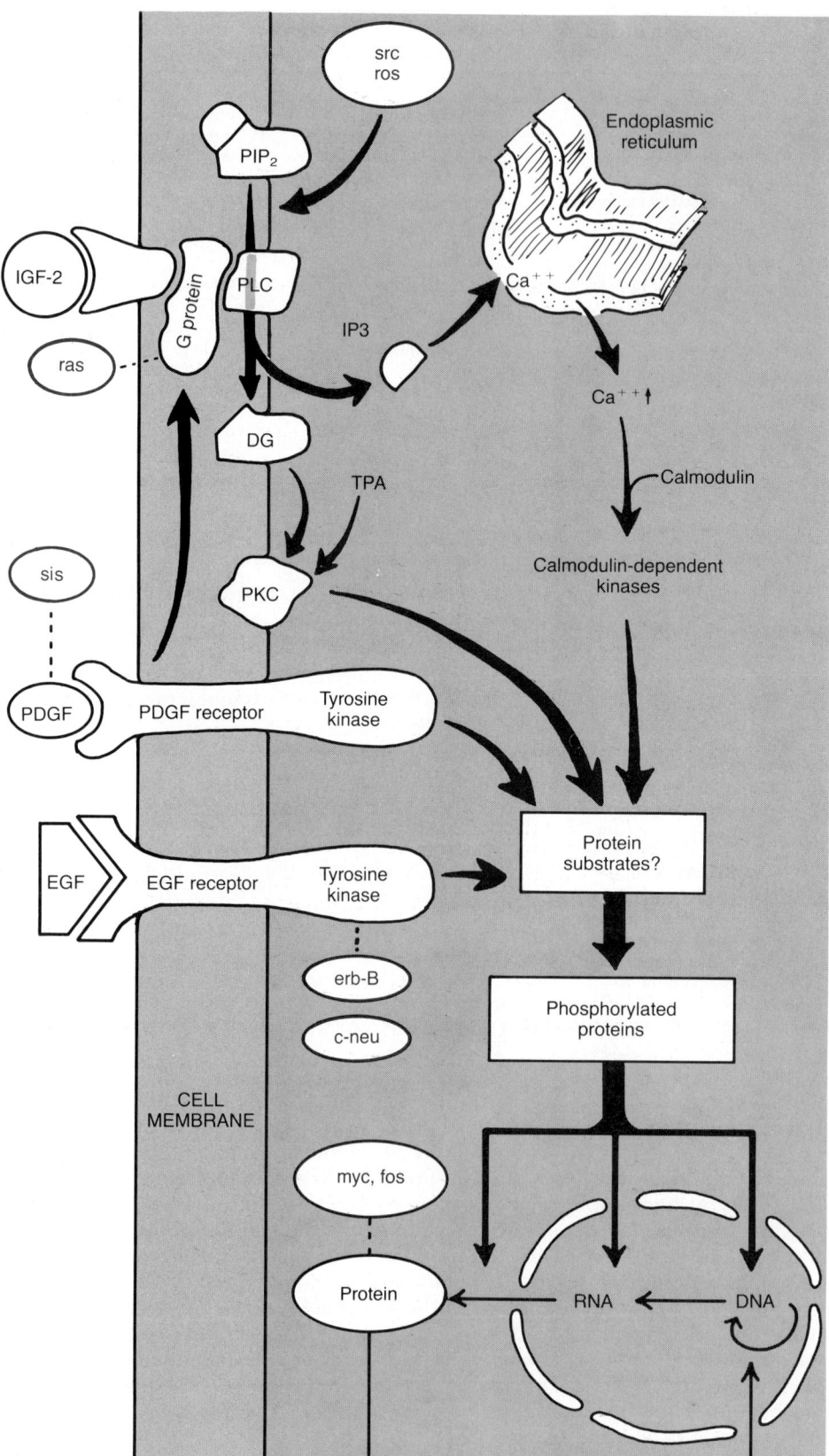

Figure 6–29. Normal signal transduction pathways and the possible sites at which oncogenes may act to distort signal transmission. The activated oncogenes are enclosed in red circles. One pathway, triggered, for example, by insulin-like growth factor-2 (IGF-2), leads to cleavage of phospholipid phosphatidylinositol biphosphate (PIP$_2$), resulting in the generation of diacylglycerol (DG) and inositol triphosphate (IP$_3$). The other prototypic pathway is triggered by the binding of epidermal growth factor (EGF) to its receptor, leading to activation of the receptor-associated tyrosine kinase. Platelet-derived growth factor (PDGF) activates both these pathways. All forms of signal transduction lead ultimately to phosphorylation of certain cytoplasmic proteins, which in turn trigger mitosis. Note that the tumor promoter TPA directly activates protein kinase C (PKC).

GROWTH FACTORS. A number of polypeptide growth factors that stimulate proliferation of normal cells have been described[88] and are discussed in Chapter 2 (p. 76). Three growth factors, PDGF, EGF, and colony stimulating factor-1 (CSF-1) appear to be related to oncogene activity, although others such as IL-2, and transforming growth factors α and β (TGF-α, TGF-β) may also be associated with the pathogenesis of cancer.

PDGF is produced by platelets, macrophages, endothelium, smooth muscle cells, and, as we shall see, several tumor cells. It is referred to as a *competence factor*; i.e., it does not stimulate DNA synthesis directly but renders cells in G_0 or G_1 competent to respond to progression factors, such as EGF, that trigger DNA synthesis. Several observations point to a role for PDGF in cell transformation:

• The v-*sis* oncogene of the simian sarcoma virus (SSV) encodes a transforming protein that shares extensive sequence homology with the B chain of PDGF.
• As with other transforming genes of retroviruses, v-*sis* is derived from the normal gene (proto-oncogene) that encodes PDGF, i.e., the c-*sis* gene.
• SSV-transformed cells secrete a PDGF-like molecule that can act as a mitogen for fibroblasts.
• Several human osteosarcoma, fibrosarcoma, and glioma cells lines transcribe c-*sis* and secrete a series of polypeptides that are structurally and immunologically related to PDGF. Since these tumor cells also bear PDGF receptors, they are continuously activated by the secreted PDGF-like mitogen.

Thus it seems that activation of c-*sis* can lead to constitutive production of PDGF, which in turn may stimulate growth of tumor cells by an autocrine mechanism. However, it should be noted that antisera to PDGF are only partially effective or sometimes ineffective in arresting the growth of the PDGF-producing tumor cells in vitro. These results suggest that factors other than PDGF must also be involved in the autocrine growth of these tumor cells. In this connection it is interesting to note that PDGF by itself cannot transform normal cells. However, the synergistic action of PDGF, TGFs, and insulin-like growth factors can cause anchorage-independent growth of fibroblasts.

PROTEIN TYROSINE KINASES. Approximately 20 of the known proto-oncogenes code for protein kinases, enzymes that catalyze the transfer of a phosphate group to a number of target proteins. Phosphate groups may be added to proteins at the threonine, serine, or tyrosine residues by specific kinases. The majority of the proto-oncogenes (e.g., c-*src*, c-*erb* B) phosphorylate tyrosine residues exclusively (Table 6–11), but a few are serine/threonine–specific kinases (e.g., c-*mos*). The protein kinase family of oncogenes can be further divided into two groups based on their subcellular locations and possible functions: (1) protein kinases that are associated with membrane (cell surface) receptors, and (2) kinases that are cytoplasmic proteins.

MEMBRANE RECEPTORS WITH PROTEIN KINASE ACTIVITY. Receptors for EGF, PDGF, IGF-1, and CSF-1 fall into this category. They are transmembrane proteins with tyrosine kinase activity associated with their cytoplasmic domain (Fig. 6–29). Three oncogenes that encode for members of this receptor family have been found: (1) the proto-oncogene c-*erb* B and its viral counterpart v-*erb* B, the transforming gene of the avian erythroblastosis virus code for the EGF receptor; (2) the c-*neu* gene, which has no viral counterpart, encodes for a protein that is very similar to but distinct from EGF receptor; and (3) the proto-oncogene c-*fms* and its viral counterpart v-*fms*, the transforming gene of feline sarcoma virus, code for the receptor for the myeloid cell growth factor CSF-1. The protein products of these genes are present in normal cells and yet do not result in malignant transformation. The reason for this may be that their oncogenic forms, although homologous, have important differences from their normal precursors. This seems to be true at least for v-*erb* B. The protein product of this v-*onc* is a truncated form of EGF receptor that is missing most of the external EGF-binding domain. Normally when EGF binds to EGF receptor, two events occur: (1) The EGF-EGF receptor complex is internalized, and (2) the tyrosine kinase activity of the cytoplasmic domain is activated. Internalization of the receptor presumably protects the cells from persistent stimulation with EGF. The protein product of v-*erb* B cannot bind EGF, and hence it remains in the cell membrane. Furthermore, it seems that the tyrosine kinase activity of v-*erb* B protein is always being expressed. Thus the simplest hypothesis to explain the transforming ability of v-*erb* B protein is that it mimics an occupied EGF receptor and thus continuously stimulates cell growth. Unlike v-*erb* B, the v-*fms* codes for the entire CSF-1 receptor (including the extracellular portion), but there seem to be mutations in the intracellular domain that may cause the receptor to remain turned on. In contrast to the EGF and CSF-1 receptors, the protein product of the c-*neu* gene is structurally normal, but its expression is markedly increased on human breast cancer cells owing to gene amplification (p. 289).

CYTOPLASMIC PROTEINS WITH TYROSINE KINASE ACTIVITY. Another type of tyrosine protein kinase activity is associated with oncogene products that are associated with the inside of cell membranes. The best studied examples in this category are v-*src* and its cellular homolog c-*src*. They encode for a phosphoprotein with a molecular weight of 60 kd that is sometimes referred to as pp60^{src}. In cells transformed by v-*src*, a number of proteins with phosphorylated tyrosine have been identified. These include enzymes such as lactic dehydrogenase, phosphoglycerate mutase, and vinculin, a cytoskeletal protein. Although it is still not clear which of the several substrates that are phosphorylated by v-*src* are critical for transformation, much interest has focused on *vinculin*. This component of the cytoskeletal network of mesenchymal cells is situated at areas of contact between cells known as focal adhesion plaques (Fig. 6–30). It has been suggested that change in the phosphorylation pattern of vinculin could be responsible for some of the phenotypic changes associated with transformation (decreased cohesiveness, rounding up), but how these are related to uncontrolled growth is not clear. There is some evidence that the *src* protein can also act as a phospholipid kinase (i.e., can phosphorylate lipids) and therefore trigger mitosis via the phosphatidylinositol pathway of signal transduction (p. 282). However, all these scenarios are speculative, and the truth is that we still do not know how v-*src* transforms cells. We do know, however, that although both v-*src* and c-*src* have tyrosine kinase activity and extensive sequence homology, point mutations and genetic substitutions differentiate the two.

GTP BINDING PROTEINS (*ras* Proteins).

The *ras* family of oncogenes has been studied most intensely because *ras* oncogenes are the transforming genes most frequently found in human cancer.[89,90] Their salient features can be summarized as follows:

• There are three members in the *ras* gene family, referred to as H-*ras*, K-*ras*, and N-*ras*. The first two were detected initially as the v-*oncs* of *Harvey rat* sarcoma and *Kirsten rat* sarcoma viruses, and hence their nomenclature. N-*ras* has no viral homolog and was discovered by transfection of DNA obtained from human neuroblastomas.

• All *ras* genes code for highly related 21 kd proteins (p21) that have been found in almost every living organism.

• Located on the inner side of plasma membrane, *ras* proteins bind guanine nucleotides (GTP and GDP) with high affinity and possess intrinsic GTPase activity.

The location and functional activities of *ras* proteins closely resemble those of G proteins. These proteins are known to play a role in the transduction of external (cell surface) signals, initiated by growth factors, hormones, or neurotransmitters, to cellular effectors such as adenylate cyclase and phospholipase C (the enzyme that triggers the PIP_2 pathway) (see Fig. 6–29). Because of their similarity to G proteins, it has been suggested that *ras* proteins are also involved in signal transduction, as is illustrated in Figure 6–31. In the inactive state *ras* proteins (p21) bind GDP; when cells are stimulated by certain ligand-receptor interactions, p21 becomes activated by exchanging GDP for GTP. The activated *ras* protein in turn activates (or inactivates) adenylate cyclase. This alters the intracellular cAMP levels and has pleotropic effects on a variety of kinases that regulate, among other activities, cell division. However, the activation of p21 is transient because its intrinsic GTPase activity hydrolyzes GTP to GDP and concomitantly returns the protein to its inactive form.

Conversion of *ras* proto-oncogene into oncogenes usually involves a point mutation that reduces the ability of mutant *ras* protein to hydrolyze GTP. This leads to sustained activation of the *ras* protein and the adenylate cyclase system. The cell then behaves as if it is under continual stimulation by the external signal.

NUCLEAR PROTEINS.

The products of several oncogenes such as *myc*, *fos*, and *myb* are found only in the nucleus. The *myc* (myelocytomatosis) oncogene was isolated from four separate avian retroviruses that

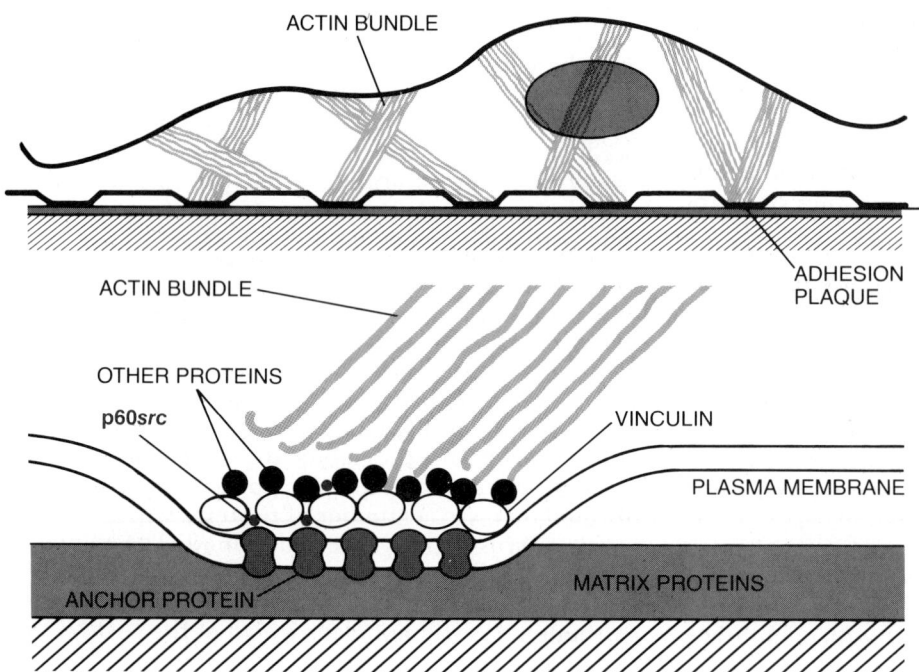

Figure 6–30. Adhesion plaques anchor cells to surfaces and serve as internal anchors for bundles of actin filaments (*top*). The protein vinculin is localized in adhesion plaques, where it may link actin bundles to an anchor protein (*bottom*). In cells transformed by the Rous sarcoma virus, p60*src* (*color*) is also detected primarily in adhesion plaques and the vinculin is found to be phosphorylated on tyrosine. Phosphorylation by p60*src* may disrupt the vinculin link (*left*) and so contribute to the characteristic disorganization of actin bundles in transformed cells. (From Hunter, T.: The proteins of oncogenes. Sci. Am. *251*:75, 1984. Used by permission. © 1984 by Scientific American, Inc. All rights reserved.)

Figure labels: ACTIN BUNDLE; ADHESION PLAQUE; ACTIN BUNDLE; OTHER PROTEINS; p60src; VINCULIN; PLASMA MEMBRANE; ANCHOR PROTEIN; MATRIX PROTEINS

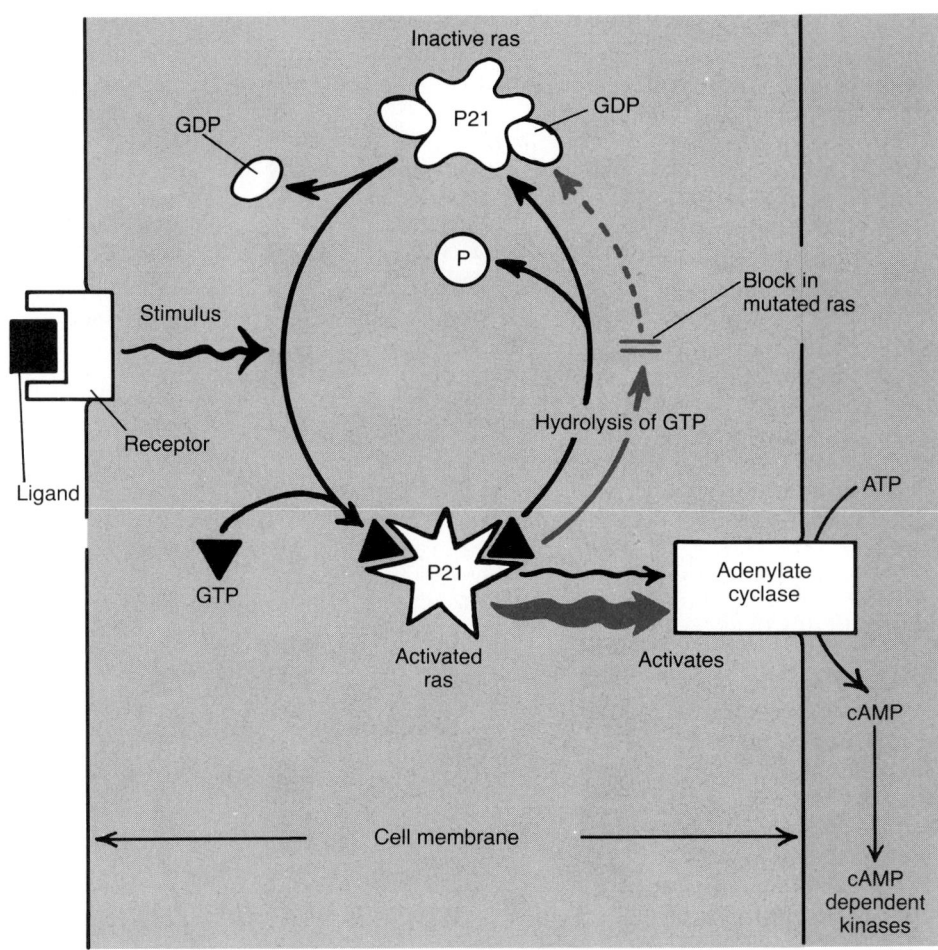

Figure 6–31. A model for action of *ras* genes. When a normal cell is stimulated through a receptor, inactive *ras* gene is activated, which in turn modulates the cellular activities by affecting cAMP levels. The mutant *ras* protein is permanently activated because of its inability to hydrolyze GTP, leading to continual stimulation of the cell without any external trigger.

cause sarcomas, carcinomas, and leukemias. Its cellular homolog c-*myc* has evoked much interest because of its association with Burkitt's lymphoma (p. 734). Two related genes, N-*myc* and L-*myc*, have been detected in human neuroblastomas and small cell lung carcinomas, but never in any retrovirus.

Many nuclear oncogenes are expressed during normal cell proliferation. For example, when cultured cells are stimulated to proliferate, say in response to a growth factor, c-*fos* transcripts increase dramatically within minutes and remain high for two to four hours. Within one to two hours of stimulation, c-*myc* RNA appears, but its levels decline prior to the entry of cells into the S-phase. Accordingly, transfection of quiescent cells with c-*myc* does not cause proliferation but renders them "competent" to receive growth signals from "progression factors" (p. 76). Thus it seems that the c-*myc* gene product substitutes for the signal delivered by competence factors such as PDGF. The orderly appearance and disappearance of c-*fos* and c-*myc* transcripts noted in vitro also occur in regenerating liver cells in vivo.[91] Because the products of these oncogenes are found only in the nucleus and some, such as the c-*myc* protein, bind to DNA, it is suspected that they interact with other genes that regulate mitosis. But much remains to be known about their normal functions and the mechanisms by which

they derail the orderly process of cell division in tumors.

ACTIVATION OF PROTO-ONCOGENES

In the preceding section we discussed some physiologic functions of the protein products of proto-oncogenes, and how changes in their activity could contribute to the development of cancer. Next we will focus on the mechanisms by which proto-oncogenes are transformed into oncogenes.

ACTIVATION BY POINT MUTATIONS.

The best example of a proto-oncogene activated by a point mutation is represented by the *ras* oncogene.[89] Most commonly, point mutations affect the 12th codon or 61st codon and sometimes 13th codon. These mutations lead to single amino acid substitutions in the *ras* protein (p21); remarkably in the case of the 12th codon, substitution for the normal amino acid glycine by any other amino acid except proline confers transforming ability in vitro.

Studies of human tumors have revealed that approximately 10 to 15% of all tumors tested carry mutated *ras* genes (H-*ras* and K-*ras*). However, with certain tumors the incidence seems to be higher. For example, in one recent study of lung tumors, mutant

K-*ras* gene was detected in 50% of adenocarcinomas but not in tumors of other histologic types.[92] Mutations in codon 12 of K-*ras* have also been noted in 30 to 40% of colonic tumors.[93] On the other hand, *ras* mutations are rarely encountered in tumors of breast or stomach. What causes *ras* mutations in humans is not known. However, it is interesting to note that in several chemically induced tumors in rats, the activating mutation in the *ras* oncogene has been correlated with the exact mutagenic change expected of the carcinogen.[94] For example, in mammary cancers induced by nitrosomethylurea (NMU), 87% carried an H-*ras* mutation in the 12th codon. The mutations consisted of a guanine to adenine transition that would be expected from the miscoding produced by the O^6-methyl guanosine, one of the major DNA adducts produced by NMU. These provocative findings suggest that at least some chemical carcinogens act by inducing mutations in proto-oncogenes.

ACTIVATION BY TRANSLOCATIONS. Chromosomal translocations occur at a high frequency in certain types of tumors (p. 260), suggesting that they may play a role in tumor development. This notion has gained credence since several translocations result in displacement of known proto-oncogenes (Table 6–12). *In their new locales, proto-oncogenes may become activated either because they are placed next to strong promoter/enhancer elements or because translocation removes them from the influence of normal regulatory sequences. Translocation can also affect the biochemical functions of proto-oncogenes by fusion with new genetic sequences.*

Alteration in the expression of a proto-oncogene resulting from translocation is best exemplified by Burkitt's lymphoma. All cases of this tumor carry one of three translocations, each involving chromosome 8q24, where the c-*myc* gene has been mapped. At its normal locus, the c-*myc* oncogene is tightly controlled and is expressed only during certain stages of the cell cycle. In Burkitt's lymphoma the most common translocation involves chromosomes 8 and 14, resulting in the movement of the c-*myc*–containing segment of chromosome 8 to 14q32 (Fig. 6–32). This places c-*myc* in close proximity to the immunoglobulin heavy chain (IgH) gene, a region with hectic transcriptional activity. Although the exact molecular

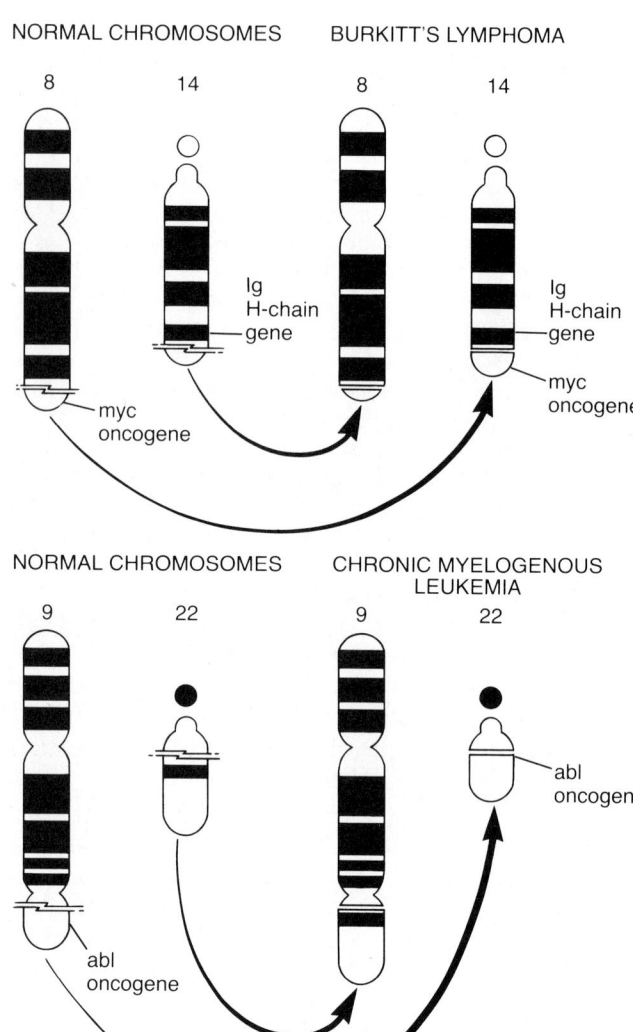

Figure 6–32. The chromosomal translocations with associated oncogenes in chronic myelogenous leukemia and Burkitt's lymphoma.

mechanisms by which such juxtaposition affects the transcription of c-*myc* gene is still not clear, it appears that in most cases the translocated *myc* gene is constitutively expressed at a high level. The variant translo-

Table 6–12. Leukemias and Lymphomas with Apparently Balanced Translocations and Associated Oncogenes

DISEASE	TRANSLOCATIONS	FREQUENCY (%)	ONCOGENE
Leukemias			
CML	t(9;22) (q34;q11)	>90	c-*abl* 9q34
AML (M2)	t(8;21) (q22;q22)	13	c-*mos* 8q22
AML (M3)	t(15;17) (q22;q11)	>90	c-*fes* 15q24
AML (M5)	t(9;11) (p22;q23)	22	None known
ALL	t(9;22) (q34;q11)	18	c-*abl* 9q34
ALL (B cell)	t(8;14) (q24;q32)	>90	c-*myc* 8q24
Lymphomas			
Burkitt's	t(8;14) (q24;q32)	>90	c-*myc* 8q24
Follicular (non-Hodgkin's)	t(14;18) (q32;q21)	>85	*bcl-2* 18q21

cations (accounting for 10% of all cases) involve the same region of chromosome 8 and either the immunoglobulin κ light-chain gene locus on chromosome 2 or the immunoglobulin λ chain locus on chromosome 22. In these translocations the c-*myc* gene remains on chromosome 8, but the transcriptionally active Ig light chain loci are inserted next to it. In either case the c-*myc* oncogene is activated, and the synthesis of its product (a DNA-binding protein) is greatly increased. This may deliver a sustained activating signal to the DNA and thereby contribute to neoplastic transformation.

The Philadelphia chromosome that is characteristic of chronic myelogenous leukemia typifies the second kind of genetic damage imposed by translocation. A reciprocal exchange between chromosomes 9 and 22 relocates a truncated portion of the proto-oncogene c-*abl* (from chromosome 9) to a newly recognized locus on chromosome 22 referred to as *bcr* (breakpoint cluster region). Although the normal c-*abl* proto-oncogene shares sequence homology with the tyrosine kinase family of oncogenes, its product does not exhibit enzyme activity. However, the c-*abl*-*bcr* hybrid gene codes for a chimeric protein that exhibits tyrosine kinase activity. Thus the translocation in chronic myeloid leukemia results in the generation of an enzyme activity that has been associated with several other proto-oncogenes (p. 285).

ACTIVATION BY GENE AMPLIFICATION. Increased expression of proto-oncogenes may occur following translocation, as in the case of c-*myc* gene in Burkitt's lymphoma, or by gene amplification. Amplification (reduplication) of genes can be detected by molecular studies or identified cytogenetically in the form of double minutes and homogeneous staining regions, as previously described (p. 262). The most interesting cases of amplification involve N-*myc* in neuroblastoma (Fig. 6–33), and c-*neu* in breast carcinoma. In neuroblastoma, multiple copies (3 to 300) of the N-*myc* gene are found in 38% of all tumors; furthermore, *there seems to be a strong correlation with advanced stage, poor prognosis, and* N-*myc amplification*.[95] The c-*neu* gene, whose product resembles epidermal growth factor receptor, was found to be amplified in 30% of breast cancers.[96] Once again, amplification of this gene was a significant predictor of overall survival and disease-free interval. In this context it is interesting to note that the expression of epidermal growth factor receptor on breast cancer cells (even in the absence of gene amplification) is also associated with poor prognosis. Presumably, the product of c-*neu* gene and EGF receptor binds to a common ligand that promotes the growth of tumor cells. Many breast carcinomas produce TGF-α, which bears significant homology to EGF and binds to EGF receptors. Tumor cells that express EGF receptor and the EGF receptor–like product of the *neu* gene may be subjected to autocrine stimulation by TGF-α.[97]

Amplification of many other proto-oncogenes, including members of the *myc* and *ras* gene family, has been noted in other cancers including those in-

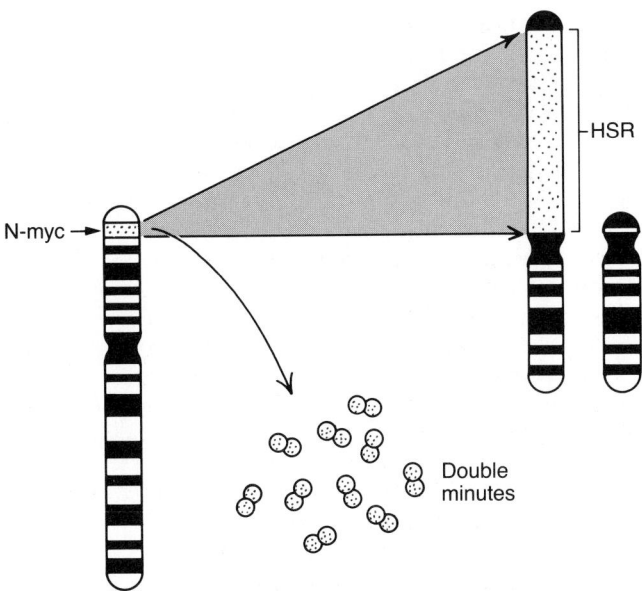

Figure 6–33. Amplification of the N-*myc* gene in human neuroblastomas. N-*myc* gene, present normally on chromosome 2p, becomes amplified and is seen either as extra chromosomal double minutes or as a chromosomally integrated homogeneous staining region. The integration involves other autosomes such as 4, 9, or 13. (Modified from Brodeur, G. M.: Molecular correlates of cytogenetic abnormalities in human cancer cells: Implications for oncogene activation. *In* Brown, E.B. (ed.): Progress in Hematology, Vol. XIV. Orlando, FL, Grune & Stratton, 1986, pp. 229–256.)

volving lung, bladder, pancreas, and colon. However, the significance of such amplification to the formation or progression of these tumors is much less clear.

CANCER SUPPRESSOR GENES (ANTI-ONCOGENES)

In our discussion thus far we have considered the involvement of proto-oncogenes in the pathogenesis of cancer. When activated (by either mutation or increased expression), proto-oncogenes are converted to oncogenes that promote excessive or inappropriate cell proliferation. To date, however, only 15 to 20% of human tumors have been found to contain activated oncogenes. It is possible that some tumors contain growth-promoting oncogenes that remain to be identified. *Alternatively, some cancers may arise not by activation of growth-promoting genes but by inactivation of genes that normally suppress cell proliferation.* The influence of such genes would be felt only when they are absent, and hence techniques such as transfection of tumor DNA would not be expected to reveal their existence. Indeed there is accumulating evidence that loss of certain "cancer suppressor" genes may be an important mechanism underlying malignant transformation.[98,99]

Like many discoveries in medicine, the cancer suppressor genes were excavated by digging among rare diseases, in this case retinoblastoma, a tumor that affects about 1 in 20,000 infants and children. Ap-

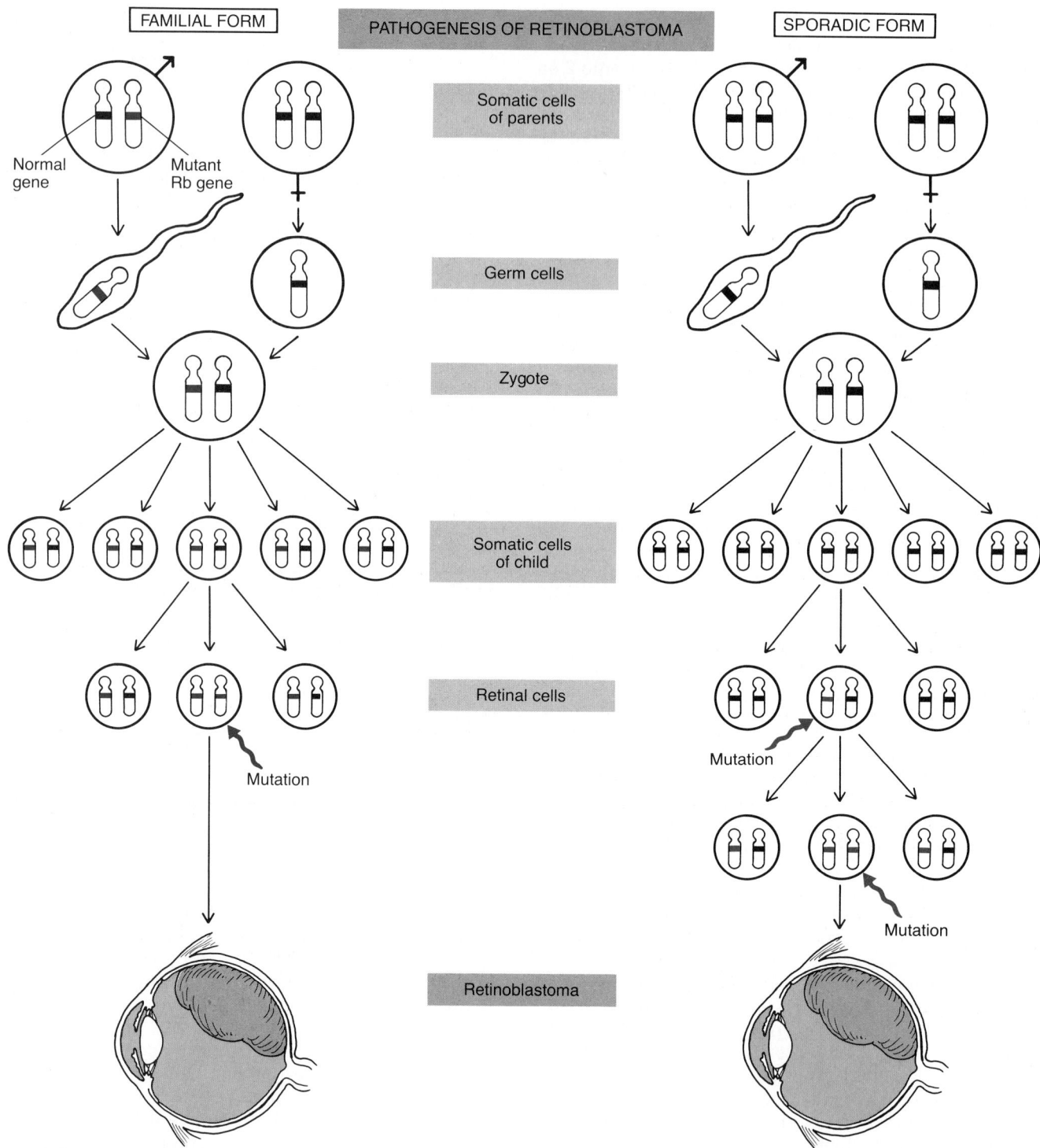

Figure 6–34. Pathogenesis of retinoblastoma. Two mutations at the Rb locus on chromosome 13q14 lead to neoplastic proliferation of the retinal cells. In the familial form, all somatic cells inherit one mutant Rb gene from a carrier parent. The second mutation affects the Rb locus in one of the retinal cells after birth. In the sporadic form, on the other hand, both mutations at the Rb locus are acquired by the retinal cells after birth.

proximately 60% of retinoblastomas are sporadic, and the remaining 40% are familial, with the predisposition to develop the tumor being transmitted as an autosomal dominant trait. To explain the familial and sporadic occurrence of an apparently identical tumor,

Knudson proposed his now famous "two hit" hypothesis of oncogenesis. He suggested that in hereditary cases one genetic change ("first hit") is inherited from an affected parent and is therefore present in all somatic cells of the body, whereas the second mutation ("second hit") occurs in one of the many retinal cells (which already carry the first mutation). In sporadic cases, however, both mutations (hits) occur somatically within a single retinal cell, whose progeny then form the tumor. Knudson's hypothesis has been amply substantiated by cytogenetic and molecular studies and can now be formulated in more precise terms:

- The mutations required to produce retinoblastoma involve the *Rb* gene, located on chromosome 13q14. In some cases the genetic damage is large enough to be visible in the form of a deletion of 13q14.
- Both normal alleles of the *Rb* locus must be inactivated ("two hits") for the development of retinoblastoma (Fig. 6–34). In familial cases, children are born with one normal and one defective copy of the *Rb* gene. They lose the intact copy in the retinoblasts through some form of somatic mutation (point mutation, interstitial deletion of 13q14, or even complete loss of the normal 13 chromosome). In sporadic cases, both normal *Rb* alleles are lost by somatic mutation in one of the retinoblasts. The end result is the same — a retinal cell that has lost both normal copies of the *Rb* gene gives rise to cancer.
- Recent studies indicate that patients with familial retinoblastoma are also at greatly increased risk of developing osteosarcoma and some other soft tissue sarcomas. Furthermore, inactivation of the *Rb* locus has been noted in some cell lines derived from cancers of the breast and lung.[100] Thus the loss of *Rb* genes may have greater implication than realized earlier.

At this point we should clarify some terminology. A child carrying an inherited mutant *Rb* allele in all somatic cells is perfectly normal (save for the increased risk of developing cancer). Since such a child is heterozygous at the *Rb* locus, it implies that heterozygosity for the *Rb* gene does not affect cell behavior. *Cancer develops when the cell becomes homozygous for the mutant allele or, put another way, loses heterozygosity for the normal Rb gene. Because the Rb gene is associated with cancer when both normal copies are lost, it is sometimes referred to as a "recessive cancer gene."* These findings with retinoblastoma have far-reaching implications. They support the idea that certain genes, of which *Rb* is one example, are dedicated to the down regulation of normal cell growth. Because their inactivation or loss is associated with development of cancer, they are also referred to as *"anti-oncogenes."*

The *Rb* gene stands as a paradigm for several other genes that act similarly. For example, a locus on the short arm of chromosome 11 plays a role in the formation of Wilms' tumor, hepatoblastoma, and rhabdomyosarcoma. Among the more common tumors, loss of heterozygosity for certain loci on chromosomes 13, 3, 5, 17, and 18 has been associated with cancers of the breast (13), lung (3), and colon (5, 17, 18).[40] Genes at these new tumor suppressor loci have yet to be identified, but given the rapid advances in molecular technology and the intense interest gen-

erated by these studies, the waiting period is not likely to be long.

While the concept of recessive cancer susceptibility genes seems established, we still do not know how these genes act. However, studies with the *Rb* gene have begun to provide some clues. The *Rb* gene has been cloned, and its protein product has been localized to the nucleus, where it binds to DNA and acts, most likely, as a repressor of DNA synthesis. The most telling data supporting the role of *Rb* protein as a natural anti-oncogene have come from work that was designed to study how DNA viruses transform cells. It had been known for some time that the transforming proteins of an adenovirus and SV40 virus bind to a nuclear protein in the host cell and that inactivation of this cellular protein represents a critical step in neoplastic transformation. What became evident recently was that the nuclear protein targeted by these oncogenic viruses is none other than the *Rb* protein.[81,82] These observations suggest that transforming activity of certain viruses may be related to their ability to absorb or neutralize the growth-inhibitory molecules exemplified by the *Rb* protein. It is likely that such growth-inhibitory proteins have some tissue specificity and that other regulatory proteins, each with its own target cells, will be found in the future.

PATHOGENESIS OF CANCER

A simplified scheme of cancer pathogenesis is depicted in Figure 6–35. Most elements of this flow

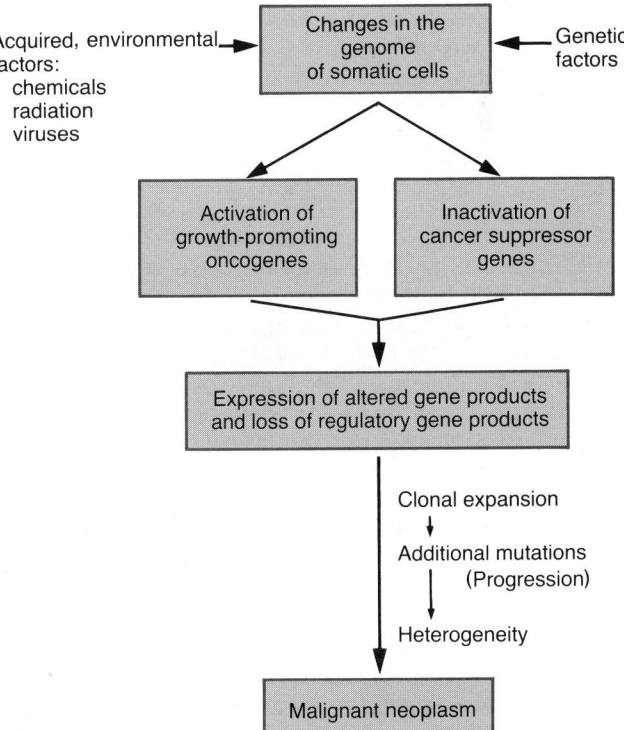

Figure 6–35. Flow chart depicting a simplified scheme of cancer pathogenesis.

chart have been addressed individually and hence only some salient and unifying themes will be emphasized.

1. Several lines of evidence suggest that cancer, in the final analysis, is a genetic disease that results when multiple mutations accumulate within the DNA of a cell:

• The cancerous phenotype is stably inherited.
• The majority of the agents—chemicals, ionizing radiation, viruses—that cause cancer in vivo or transform cells in vitro are mutagenic.
• Specific chromosomal abnormalities either predispose to cancer or are present in tumors.

Despite all the evidence pointing to genetic mechanisms in the induction of cancer, the role of abnormal gene expression caused by *epigenetic mechanisms* has to be considered. It is possible that some derangement of cellular differentiation and maturation imposed by abnormalities in epigenetic mechanisms, e.g., cytoplasmic regulatory products affecting transcription or translation, may give rise to cancer. Isolated pieces of evidence, such as the rare differentiation of a highly malignant neuroblastoma into a benign ganglioneuroma, support the primacy of epigenetic changes. However, cases such as these are the exception rather than the rule. In the vast majority of cases, it is far more likely that epigenetic changes are superimposed on initial mutagenic events.

2. Tumor cells may attain growth autonomy by two general pathways—activation of a growth-promoting oncogene or inactivation of a growth-inhibitory cancer suppressor gene. It is quite likely that both pathways operate in vivo and in the same cell. Very little is known about how cancer suppressor genes function, but much has been learned about the mechanisms by which oncogenes can confer growth autonomy. The multiple mechanisms by which activated oncogenes stimulate growth are illustrated in Figure 6–36 and are summarized below:

• Oncogenes (e.g., c-*sis*) may code for growth-promoting factors (PDGF) or deregulate genes that encode growth factors (such as TGF-α). As a result, tumor cells may produce large amounts of growth factors to which they can respond themselves.
• A second mechanism involves growth factor receptors. An oncogene may encode a defective receptor (e.g., v-*erb*B) that sends stimulatory signals to the cells even in the absence of the growth factor in the extracellular milieu. Alternatively, amplification and overexpression of growth factor receptor genes (e.g., c-*neu*) may render tumor cells exquisitely sensitive to low levels of growth factors that are below the threshold for stimulating normal cells.
• An oncogene may encode a protein that is a transducer of growth-promoting signals from an external receptor. The mutated version of the oncogene may produce a protein (e.g., c-*ras*) that continuously sends stimulatory signals into the cell even in the absence of any external trigger.

3. *Carcinogenesis is a multistep process.* This notion, derived initially from the study of chemical carcinogenesis (initiation and promotion), is widely applicable to all forms of cancer. Most cancers arise when two and possibly several mutations (acquired sequentially) accumulate within the DNA. Studies of oncogenes and anti-oncogenes fully support this view.

• DNA transfection experiments reveal that no single oncogene will transform primary cultures of normal cells. For example, when a *ras* or a *myc* gene is introduced singly into a normal fibroblast, the cells do not become tumorous. When both genes are introduced concomitantly, the fibroblasts acquire a fully transformed phenotype in vitro and also form tumors in vivo.
• These observations are buttressed by studies of human tumors in vivo. For example, Burkitt's lymphoma cells contain an activated *myc* gene and an activated N-*ras* gene. Conversely, some benign colonic tumors contain an activated *ras* gene,[40] indicating that additional events must be required for the *ras* oncogene–containing cell to become cancerous. The additional genetic events may involve activation of other oncogenes or inactivation of cancer suppressor genes.[101]

Given the fact that tumor cells must acquire a number of distinct traits, such as growth autonomy, invasiveness, and metastatic ability, it is not surprising that several oncogenes and cancer suppressor genes must conspire and collaborate to induce cancers. Each gene supplies one of the several attributes of a successfully growing tumor. Although not discussed earlier, there is emerging evidence that oncogenes are involved in conferring metastatic ability on tumor cells.[102]

4. Finally, it should be pointed out that *host factors may well play a role in the emergence of cancers.* The mere presence of transforming mutations does not necessitate their expression. In addition to the intracellular or local controls already discussed, systemic controls (e.g., the immune system) may exist. Many clinical observations, some cited earlier with respect to the acquired immune deficiency syndrome (p. 224), indicate that individuals suffering from an immunodeficiency are at greater risk of developing cancer. The interactions between the immune system and tumors will be considered next under the broad context of tumor-host interactions.

TUMOR-HOST INTERACTIONS

Neoplasms are essentially parasites. Some cause only trivial mischief, but others are catastrophic. Tumor-host interactions are, however, a two-way street, and the host impinges on the tumor as well. First we shall consider the effects of the tumor on the host, and then the converse.

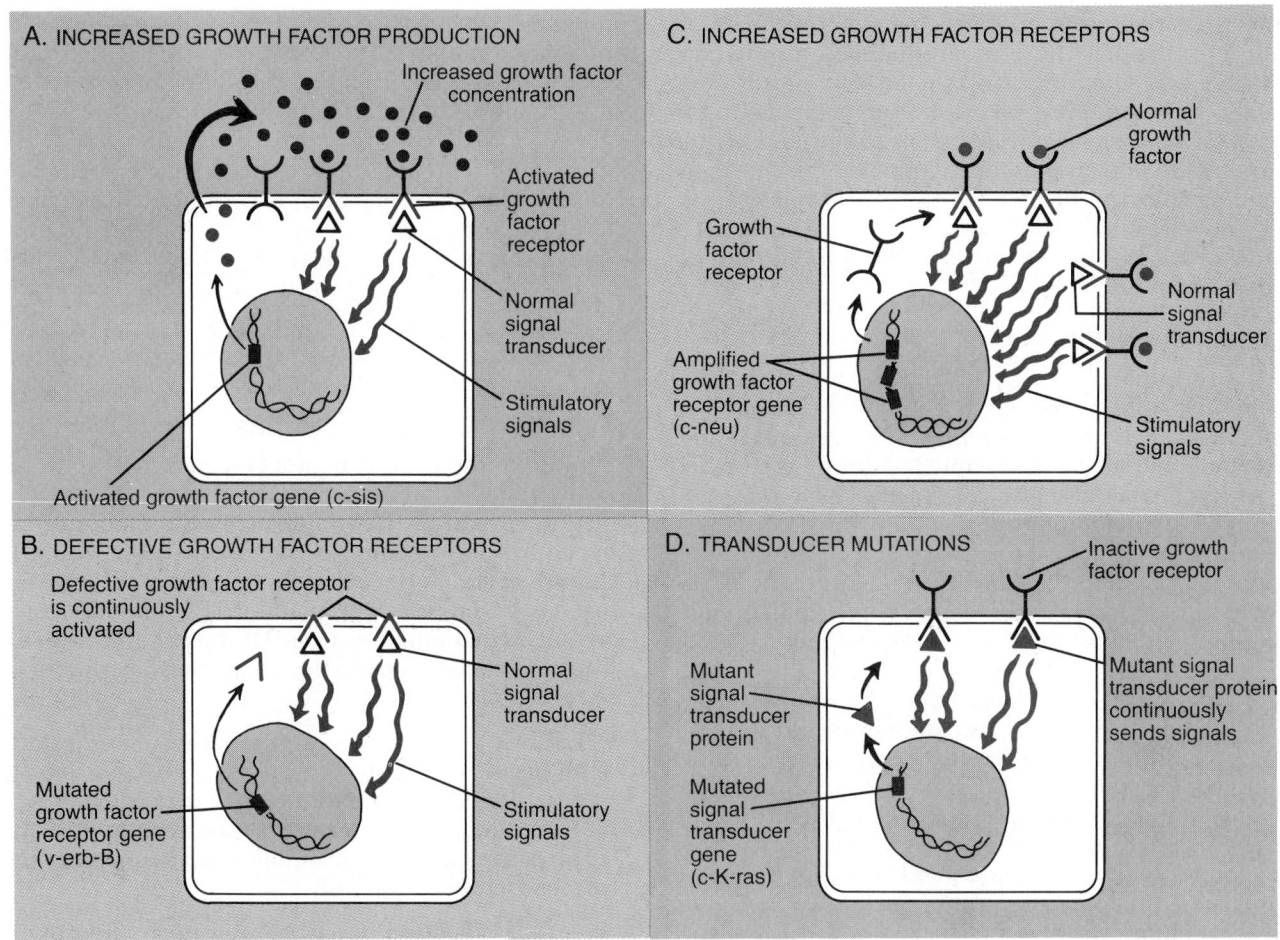

A. INCREASED GROWTH FACTOR PRODUCTION

Increased growth factor concentration

Activated growth factor receptor

Normal signal transducer

Stimulatory signals

Activated growth factor gene (c-sis)

B. DEFECTIVE GROWTH FACTOR RECEPTORS

Defective growth factor receptor is continuously activated

Normal signal transducer

Mutated growth factor receptor gene (v-erb-B)

Stimulatory signals

C. INCREASED GROWTH FACTOR RECEPTORS

Normal growth factor

Growth factor receptor

Normal signal transducer

Amplified growth factor receptor gene (c-neu)

Stimulatory signals

D. TRANSDUCER MUTATIONS

Inactive growth factor receptor

Mutant signal transducer protein

Mutant signal transducer protein continuously sends signals

Mutated signal transducer gene (c-K-ras)

Figure 6–36. Mechanisms by which an oncogene may promote cell growth. *A,* It may code for a growth factor and stimulate the tumor cell by autocrine mechanisms. *B,* It may produce a defective growth factor receptor that is constitutively activated (without interaction with a ligand). *C,* It may encode for a normal growth factor receptor, but oncogene amplification may increase the number of receptors on tumor cells. *D,* It may encode for defective signal transducers that transmit growth-promoting signals without any external trigger.

EFFECTS OF TUMOR ON HOST

Obviously, cancers are far more threatening to the host than benign tumors are. Nonetheless, both types of neoplasia may cause problems because of (a) location and impingement on adjacent structures, (b) functional activity such as hormone synthesis, (c) bleeding and secondary infections when they ulcerate through adjacent natural surfaces, and (d) initiation of acute symptoms caused by either rupture or infarction. Any metastasis has the potential to produce these same consequences. Cancers may also be responsible for cachexia (wasting) or paraneoplastic syndromes.

Local and Hormonal Effects

An example of disease related to critical location is the pituitary adenoma. Although benign and possibly not productive of hormone, expansile growth of the tumor can destroy the remaining pituitary and thus lead to serious endocrinopathy. Analogously, cancers arising within or metastatic to an endocrine gland may cause an endocrine insufficiency by destroying the

gland. Neoplasms in the gut, both benign and malignant, may cause obstruction as they enlarge. Infrequently, the peristaltic pull telescopes the neoplasm and its affected segment into the downstream segment, producing an obstructing intussusception (p. 881).

Neoplasms arising in endocrine glands may produce manifestations by elaboration of hormones. Such functional activity is more typical of benign tumors than of cancers, which may be sufficiently undifferentiated to have lost such capability. A benign beta-cell adenoma of the pancreatic islets less than 1 cm in diameter may produce sufficient insulin to cause fatal hypoglycemia. In addition, nonendocrine tumors may elaborate hormones or hormone-like products. The erosive destructive growth of cancers or the expansile pressure of a benign tumor on any natural surface, such as the skin or mucosa of the gut, may cause ulcerations, secondary infections, and bleeding. Indeed, melena (blood in the stool) and hematuria, for example, are characteristic of neoplasms of the gut and urinary tract, respectively. Neoplasms may cause disease in unusual ways. A mobile organ bearing a large tumor may, in some unknown manner, undergo torsion, thereby cutting off the venous drainage and sometimes also the arterial supply (Fig. 6–37). This complication most often occurs with benign ovarian neoplasms that become infarcted, and so cause acute lower abdominal pain and sometimes bleeding into the peritoneal cavity. Neoplasms, benign as well as malignant, may then cause problems in varied ways, but all are far less common than the cachexia of malignancy.

Cancer Cachexia

In the terminal stages of advanced cancer, patients commonly suffer progressive loss of body fat and lean body mass accompanied by profound weakness, anorexia, and anemia. This wasting syndrome is referred to as cachexia. Usually, an intercurrent infection brings a blessed end to the slow deterioration. There is, in general, some correlation between the size and extent of spread of the cancer and the severity of the cachexia. Small localized cancers therefore are generally silent and produce no cachexia, but there are rare exceptions.

The origins of cancer cachexia are obscure. Wasted patients with any form of chronic illness have impaired immune defenses and so are prone to infections, which could explain some of the debilitation and fever-induced hypermetabolism. Ulcerative lesions may bleed, accounting in some part for the anemia and weakness. Understandably, grief and depression affect the appetite. So there are many potential bases for manifestations. But these simplistic explanations are not sufficient for all cases, and more subtle metabolic abnormalities have been proposed. Patients with cancer cachexia appear to have higher rates of whole-body protein turnover than either non-cancer patients or starved normal subjects.[103] Con-

comitantly, there is a disproportionately increased rate of metabolism of all nutrients, often accompanied by a reduced food intake that has been related to abnormalities in the sensation of taste and in the central control of appetite.[104] Perhaps cachectin (TNF-α) is involved. This macrophage product acts to mobilize adipose tissue and may thus contribute to cachexia.[105] These metabolic abnormalities are not firmly established, but one fact is clear—cachexia is not caused by nutritional demands of the tumor. Cancers rarely grow as rapidly as the fetus, yet many a post-partal mother when getting on the scale laments that she did not suffer just a little bit of "cachexia"!

Paraneoplastic Syndromes

Symptom complexes in cancer-bearing patients that cannot readily be explained, either by the local or distant spread of the tumor or by the elaboration of hormones indigenous to the tissue from which the tumor arose, are known as *paraneoplastic syndromes*.[106] These occur in about 10% of patients with advanced malignant disease. Despite their relative infrequency, paraneoplastic syndromes are important to recognize.

• First, they may represent the earliest manifestation of an occult neoplasm.
• Second, in affected patients they may represent significant clinical problems and may even be lethal.
• Third, they may mimic metastatic disease and therefore confound treatment.

A classification of paraneoplastic syndromes and their presumed origins is presented in Table 6–13. A few comments on some of the more common and interesting syndromes follow.

The *endocrinopathies* are frequently encountered paraneoplastic syndromes. Because the native

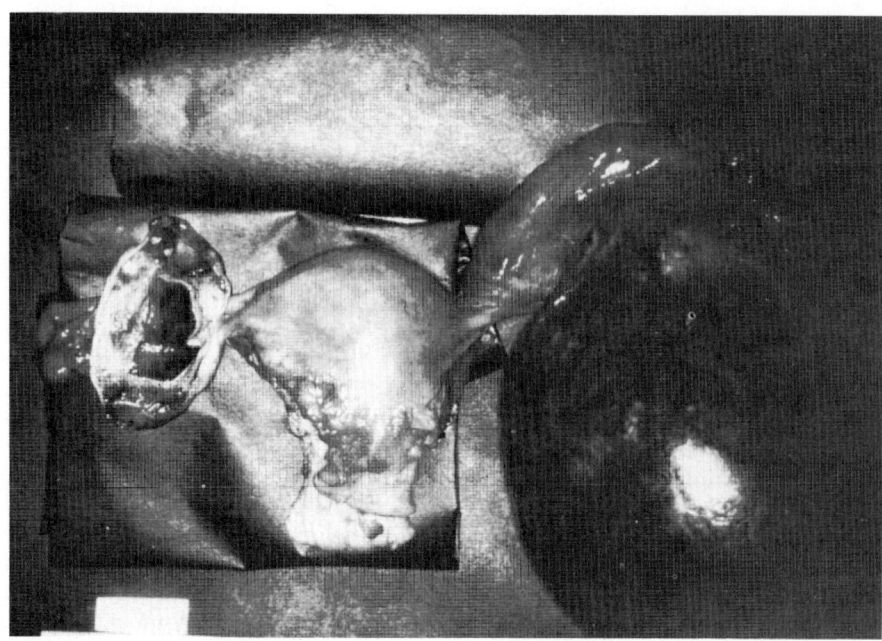

Figure 6–37. Torsion of a large, benign ovarian tumor (*right*) that has induced hemorrhagic infarction of the neoplasm. Compare the size of this tumor with the normal uterus and essentially normal hemisected ovary on the left. (Courtesy of Dr. Robert L. Ehrmann, Brigham and Women's Hospital.)

Table 6-13. Paraneoplastic Syndromes

CLINICAL SYNDROMES	MAJOR FORMS OF UNDERLYING CANCER	CAUSAL MECHANISM
Endocrinopathies		
Cushing's syndrome	Bronchogenic (small cell) carcinoma Pancreatic carcinoma Neural tumors	ACTH or ACTH-like substance
Hyponatremia	Bronchogenic carcinoma Intracranial neoplasms	Antidiuretic hormone or ADH-like substance
Hypercalcemia	Bronchogenic squamous cell carcinoma Breast carcinoma Renal carcinoma Adult T-cell leukemia/lymphoma	?Parathyroid hormone–like substance TGF-α
Hyperthyroidism	Blood dyscrasias Bronchogenic carcinoma Prostatic carcinoma	Thyroid-stimulating hormone or TSH-like substance
Hypoglycemia	Fibrosarcoma Other mesenchymal sarcomas Hepatocellular carcinoma	Insulin or insulin-like substance
Carcinoid syndrome	Bronchial adenoma (carcinoid) Pancreatic carcinoma Gastric carcinoma	Serotonin, bradykinin, ?histamine
Polycythemia	Renal carcinoma Cerebellar hemangioma Hepatocellular carcinoma	Erythropoietin
Nerve and Muscle Syndromes		
Myasthenia Disorders of the central and peripheral nervous systems	Bronchogenic carcinoma Breast carcinoma	?Immunologic, ?toxic
Dermatologic Disorders		
Acanthosis nigricans	Gastric carcinoma Lung carcinoma Uterine carcinoma	?Immunologic, ?toxic
Dermatomyositis	Bronchogenic, breast carcinoma	?Immunologic, ?toxic
Osseous, Articular, and Soft Tissue Changes		
Hypertrophic osteoarthropathy and clubbing of the fingers	Bronchogenic carcinoma	Unknown
Vascular and Hematologic Changes		
Venous thrombosis (Trousseau's phenomenon)	Pancreatic carcinoma Bronchogenic carcinoma Other cancers	?Hypercoagulability
Nonbacterial thrombotic endocarditis	Advanced cancers	Hypercoagulability
Anemia	Thymic neoplasms	Unknown
Leukemoid reaction	Thymic neoplasms	Unknown
Others		
Nephrotic syndrome	Various cancers	Tumor antigens, immune complexes

cells giving rise to the cancer are not of endocrine origin, the functional activity is referred to as *ectopic hormone production*. The elaboration of the hormone or hormone-like substance is attributed to derepression of genetic programs, as, for example, the formation of insulin by fibrosarcomas (usually retroperitoneal) or erythropoietin by renal cell carcinomas. Among the endocrinopathies, Cushing's syndrome is the most common. Approximately 50% of the patients with this endocrinopathy have carcinoma of the lung, chiefly the small cell type. It is caused by excessive production of ACTH or ACTH-like peptides. The precursor of ACTH is a large molecule known as pro-opiomelanocortin (POMC), which is widely distributed in many carcinomas and normal tissues. However, only a few tumors can cleave POMC to produce ACTH. An important question, therefore, is how the

processing of POMC is regulated (or dysregulated) in cancers that are associated with Cushing's syndrome. POMC is also the precursor of endorphin, met-enkephalin, and β-melanocyte stimulating hormone. It has been suggested that elaboration of these peptides with morphine-like activity may account for some of the poorly understood neurologic abnormalities in cancer patients.

Hypercalcemia is probably the most common paraneoplastic syndrome, and conversely, overtly symptomatic hypercalcemia is most often related to some form of cancer rather than to hyperparathyroidism. Two general processes are involved in cancer-associated hypercalcemia: (1) osteolysis induced by cancer, whether primary in bone, such as multiple myeloma, or metastatic to bone from any primary lesion; and (2) the production of calcemic humoral substances by extraosseous neoplasms. The nature of the calcium-mobilizing tumor products is still uncertain. One candidate is a PTH-like peptide that resembles the native hormone only in its amino-terminus. Although functionally related to PTH, it is a distinct molecule whose gene has been mapped to chromosome 12 (PTH gene is located on chromosome 11).[107] The other factor associated with the causation of hypercalcemia syndrome is TGF-α. It will be recalled that TGF-α shares sequence homology with EGF and is implicated in the autocrine growth of tumor cells. It stimulates osteoclasts in vitro and may well cause mobilization of calcium from the bones.[108] The most common neoplasm associated with hypercalcemia is the squamous cell bronchogenic carcinoma, rather than small cell cancer of the lung (more often associated with endocrinopathies). The recently recognized adult T-cell leukemia/lymphoma (p. 717) is also frequently associated with hypercalcemia.

The *neuromyopathic paraneoplastic syndromes* take diverse forms, such as peripheral neuropathies, cortical cerebellar degeneration, a polymyopathy resembling polymyositis (p. 207), and a myasthenic syndrome similar to *myasthenia gravis* (p. 1366). The etiology of these syndromes is poorly understood, and both immunologic reactions to tumor cells that cross react with target tissues and toxic products released by the neoplasm have been vaguely proposed.

Acanthosis nigricans is characterized by gray-black patches of verrucous hyperkeratosis on the skin (p. 1284). This disorder occurs very rarely as a genetically determined disease in juveniles or adults. In addition, particularly in those over the age of 35, the appearance of such lesions is associated in about 50% of cases with some form of cancer. Sometimes the skin changes appear before discovery of the cancer. It is important to remember, however, that in the remaining nongenetic cases there is no underlying cancer, but some endocrinopathy or, in fact, no associated disease may be present.

Clubbing of fingers and hypertrophic osteoarthropathy, described more fully on page 1333, are encountered in 1 to 10% of patients with bronchogenic carcinomas. Rarely, other forms of cancer are involved. Although the osteoarthropathy is seldom seen in noncancer patients, clubbing of the fingertips may be encountered in liver diseases, diffuse lung disease, congenital cyanotic heart disease, ulcerative colitis, and other disorders.

Several *vascular and hematologic manifestations* may appear in association with a variety of forms of cancer. As mentioned in the earlier discussion of thrombosis (p. 104), *migratory thrombophlebitis* (Trousseau's syndrome) may be encountered in association with deep-seated cancers, most often with carcinomas of the pancreas or lung. Disseminated intravascular coagulation (DIC) may complicate a diversity of clinical disorders, as pointed out on page 698. Among these is advanced cancer. In this setting hypercoagulability is postulated, attributed to the synthesis and/or release of platelet-aggregating fac-

tors and procoagulants (p. 100) from the tumor or its necrotic products. Bland, small, nonbacterial fibrinous vegetations sometimes form on the cardiac valve leaflets (more often on left-sided valves), particularly in patients with advanced cancer. These lesions are called *nonbacterial thrombotic endocarditis (NBTE)* or *marantic* (derived from marasmus) *endocarditis*. As the term marantic endocarditis indicates, these valvular vegetations are most often associated with the terminal phase of wasting disease. However, NBTE sometimes occurs in nonwasted, occasionally young individuals who do not have cancer; this is discussed in more detail on page 636. Whatever the setting, the vegetations are potential sources of emboli that assume increased importance in the young nonterminal patient.

HOST DEFENSE AGAINST TUMORS

It will be recalled that host defense systems can be broadly classified into two categories—adaptive and innate (p. 163). Each of these two effector systems could be involved in defensive reactions against tumors. The adaptive arm of the immune system includes antigen-specific T and B lymphocytes, which have the inherent capacity to distinguish "self" from "non-self." It follows that for tumors to be recognized by T or B lymphocytes, they must express unique "non-self" antigens. Because immunogenicity is central to the question of acquired tumor immunity, we will first focus our attention on tumor antigens.

TUMOR ANTIGENS. The issue of whether cancerous cells in humans bear antigens that are different from those of normal cells and can be recognized by the immune system of the host remains highly controversial. The controversy has its roots in the extrapolation of results obtained in animal model systems to humans. Nonetheless, a few generalizations can be made.

• Cancers induced in animals by oncogenic viruses and chemical carcinogens possess tumor antigens that evoke specific immune responses.
• Spontaneous tumors in animals are weakly, if at all, immunogenic, but more sensitive methods using highly specific monoclonal antibodies may modify this conclusion.
• There are hints that some cancers in humans evoke defensive reactions, but it is not clear whether these are specific immune responses.
• Such defensive reactions as can be demonstrated in humans are likely to be triggered by tumor-associated antigens (TAA) shared by histogenetically similar neoplasms.
• There is no unequivocal evidence that human cancers possess unique tumor-specific antigens.

In experimental model systems, tumor antigenicity is generally assessed by (1) the ability of an animal to resist a tumor implant following previous exposure to live or killed tumor cells; (2) the ability of a non–

tumor-bearing animal to resist a challenge when infused with immunocompetent cells from a tumor-bearing syngeneic host; and (3) the in vitro demonstration of tumor cell growth inhibition or destruction by cell-mediated or humoral effectors derived from tumor-bearing animals. Using these approaches it has been possible to document that viral and chemically induced cancers in experimental animals often have unique tumor-specific antigens (TSA), present only on tumor cells and different from those expressed by normal cells. Because these tumor antigens can induce resistance to a tumor implant, they are sometimes referred to as TSTA (tumor-specific transplantation antigens).

The evidence that human cancers express tumor-specific antigens is at best equivocal. It derives largely from the observations that certain cancers evoke significant lymphocytic infiltrates. These infiltrates are thought to be composed of immunocompetent cells, since in general these tumors carry a somewhat better prognosis than those neoplasms unassociated with lymphocytic responses. Until recently, it has been difficult to ascertain whether tumor-infiltrating lymphocytes contain specifically sensitized T cells. However, in preliminary studies it has been possible to demonstrate that some human melanomas are infiltrated with T cells that are specifically cytotoxic against autologous tumor cells.[109] The cancers yielding the strongest evidence for the existence of tumor antigens are melanocarcinomas, neuroblastomas, Burkitt's lymphoma, leukemia, osteogenic sarcomas, and cancers of the colon. But in most cases these tumor-associated antigens are shared by similar tumors in other hosts; i.e., they are associated with the histogenetic type of tumor rather than with the individual neoplasm. Furthermore, they appear to represent differentiation antigens particular to the differentiation stage at which the cancer cells are arrested. Normal embryonic cells bear similar antigens. Apparently, genetic programs repressed in differentiated cells are derepressed in the course of transformation. In this context certain cancers express embryonic antigens — e.g., germ cell and hepatocellular carcinomas often elaborate alpha-fetoprotein (p. 1114), and carcinomas of the colon as well as many other forms of cancer frequently produce carcinoembryonic antigen (p. 302). These oncofetal antigens are of little functional importance in the induction of a tumor rejection reaction but are of some value as tumor markers (p. 302). In conclusion, such antigens as may be expressed by spontaneous cancers in humans are, with few exceptions,[110] common antigens shared by other similar tumors and by differentiating normal cells. Since there is some evidence that they can evoke an immune response, we will next explore the following issues: (1) What is the nature of the host response to tumors in animals and possibly in humans? (2) Does a self-policing system that eliminates tumor cells (immunosurveillance) exist in humans? (3) Can the host defenses against tumors be exploited for immunotherapy?

NATURE OF HOST DEFENSES AGAINST TUMORS. Both humoral and cellular mechanisms may be involved in defense against tumors. The cells of the immune system have already been described, and so it is necessary here only to characterize them briefly. Three basic categories are arguably involved:

1. *Specifically sensitized cytotoxic T cells*, capable of recognition of membrane-associated tumor antigens in the context of class I histocompatibility antigens (p. 170).
2. *Natural killer (NK) cells* capable of destroying tumor cells without specific sensitization. As previously discussed, NK cells lyse tumor cells directly or by antibody-dependent cellular cytotoxicity (ADCC). The latter involves recognition and lysis of antibody-coated tumor cells through the Fc receptor on NK cells (see also Fig. 5–11, p. 177).
3. *Macrophages*, both nonspecifically activated (e.g., endotoxin) and activated by immune T cell–derived gamma interferon, may kill tumor cells by two mechanisms: (a) antibody-dependent cellular cytotoxicity (ADCC) and (b) the generation of cytotoxic products.

Uncertainty persists about which of these cell types, if any, contributes to tumor immunity in humans, as is discussed later.

Humoral mechanisms may also participate in tumor cell destruction, at least in animals. In experimental model systems, tumor antigens evoke specific antibodies. These immunoglobulins can exert antitumor effects by two mechanisms: (1) They can activate complement following binding to target cells to form the lytic C'8–9 complex; and (2) they can coat tumor cells and render them vulnerable to ADCC by NK cells or macrophages. An attempt to depict cellular mechanisms of tumor immunity is offered in Figure 6–38.

Paradoxically, both cell-mediated and humoral mechanisms may inhibit the defensive immune response to a tumor. T-suppressor cells have a central role in the regulation of both cellular and humoral immunity to all antigens, and tumors are no exception. Suppressor T cells inhibit tumor immunity in some experimental systems and may play a similar role in humans.[111] Humoral "blocking factors" may abrogate cell-mediated cytotoxicity. The nature of these factors is uncertain, but most of the evidence favors antigen-antibody complexes; circulating, shed tumor antigens may also play a role. Presumably, these factors operate by binding to and blocking either antigen sites on tumor cells or receptors on immunocompetent cells. In conclusion, it appears that the response of a host to its tumors may, on the one hand, be beneficial or, on the other hand, be detrimental by inhibiting any immune reactions.

IMMUNOSURVEILLANCE. To begin at the end, *there is no unequivocal evidence that humans enjoy a self-policing immune system.* The strongest argument for its existence is the increased frequency of cancers in immunodeficient hosts. About 5% of individuals

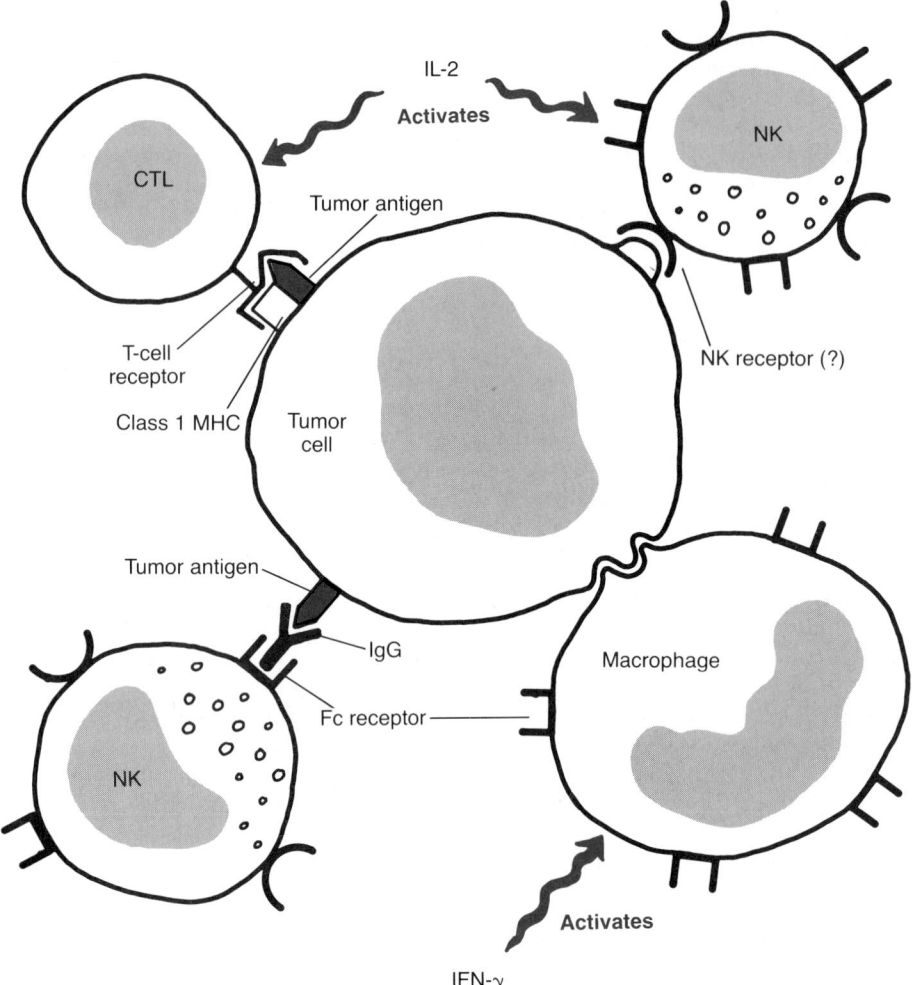

Figure 6–38. Cellular effectors of antitumor immunity and some cytokines that modulate antitumor activities.

with a congenital immunodeficiency develop cancers, about 200 times the expected rate. Analogously, immunosuppressed transplant recipients have an increased frequency of malignancies. It should be noted that most (but not all) of these neoplasms are lymphomas, often immunoblastic lymphomas. (There is a slight increase in the incidence of squamous cell carcinomas of the skin and lips as well.) Particularly illustrative is the X-linked, recessive immunodeficiency disorder termed XLP.[112] When affected boys develop an Epstein-Barr virus infection, it does not take the usual self-limited form of infectious mononucleosis but instead evolves into a chronic or sometimes fatal form of infectious mononucleosis or, even worse, a malignant lymphoma.

It has also been argued that the occurrence of cancers in otherwise immunocompetent humans occurs because mechanisms of tumor escape may exist:

• *Selective outgrowth of antigen-negative variants.* During tumor progression (p. 254), strongly immunogenic subclones may be eliminated, enriching the growing tumor with antigen-negative cells.
• *Loss or reduced expression of histocompatibility an-*

tigens. Tumor cells may fail to express normal levels of HLA class I antigens, thereby escaping attack by cytotoxic T cells.
• *Shedding or modulation of tumor antigens.* Sufficient shedding may inhibit tumor cell recognition.
• *Immunosuppression.* Many tumors can cause nonspecific suppression of immune response, often by secreting poorly defined soluble factors. As noted earlier, specific suppression of tumor immunity may be brought about by T-suppressor cells.

Each one of these mechanisms has been found to play a role in experimentally induced tumors. Furthermore, suppression of certain immune cells has been noted in patients with cancer.

An equally impressive roster of observations challenges the concept of immunosurveillance. The most common forms of cancers in immunosuppressed and immunodeficient patients are lymphomas, notably immunoblastic lymphomas, which could be the consequence of abnormal immunoproliferative responses to microbial infections or to the various therapeutic agents administered to these patients. An increased incidence of the most frequent forms of cancer — lung, breast, gastrointestinal tract — and multiple neoplasms might be anticipated in immunologic cripples but does not occur. Moreover, "nude" mice lacking a thymus gland and cell-mediated immunity have no increased incidence of spontaneous tumors, nor are they more susceptible to chemically induced tumors, although it should be noted that they have marked NK cell activity. So the uncertainty about immunosurveillance continues.

TUMOR IMMUNITY AND IMMUNOTHERAPY IN HUMANS. The issue of immune response to cancers in humans is a case of "the cup being half empty and half full." In view of the uncertainty surrounding expression of tumor-specific antigens on human tumor cells and consequently the relevance of "specific" immunity in immunosurveillance, much attention is focused on NK cells.[113] The concept that NK cells may be important in resistance against tumors is supported by several observations.

• NK cells do not require prior sensitization for efficient tumor cell lysis. Thus they can readily act as the "first line of defense" when tumor burden is low.
• Following activation with IL-2, NK cells can kill tumor cells from a wide variety of spontaneously arising human tumors. Such tumors are usually "nonimmunogenic" for the T- and B-cell systems.
• In animal models, NK cells have been convincingly demonstrated to have antitumor activity in vivo, especially in controlling hematogenous metastases.

In view of these observations, several strategies are currently being employed to harness IL-2 and NK cells for immunotherapy. According to one protocol, the peripheral blood lymphocytes of cancer patients are first cultured in vitro with IL-2 to activate them and expand their numbers (IL-2 is a mitogen for NK cells and T cells). Large numbers of lymphokine-activated killer (LAK) cells are then reinfused into the patient along with additional IL-2 to maintain the activity of transferred cells. In other protocols, IL-2 is infused either intermittently or continuously to activate cells in vivo, without prior culture in vitro. In a third approach (technically much more difficult), lymphoid cells isolated from the excised tumor are expanded in vitro with IL-2 and then reinfused into the patient. The efficacy of all these treatment modalities is still under investigation and carries with it the risk of toxicity caused by large amounts of IL-2 (e.g., pulmonary edema). However, results of early trials indicate partial or complete regression of metastases in some patients with renal cell carcinoma and malignant melanoma.[114]

In addition to IL-2, several other cytokines now available in pure form by recombinant DNA technology are being evaluated for antitumor activity. These include interferons (IFN) -α and -γ, and TNF-α. Interferon-α has been found to be of some benefit in hematologic malignancies, particularly hairy cell leukemia (p. 730). IFN-γ and TNF-α offer a promising approach, since they activate antitumor properties of macrophages and seem to act synergistically.

Although efforts to augment specific immunity have been generally frustrated owing to the weak immunogenicity of human tumors, there is renewed interest in the use of monoclonal antibodies for treatment of lymphoid malignancies. Neoplastic lymphoid cells, like their normal counterparts, bear unique antigen-specific receptors that carry idiotypic determinants (p. 189). Antibodies directed against the idiotype of the neoplastic clone can therefore be targeted specifically to the tumor cells. Such anti-idiotypic antibodies are conjugated with potent toxins (most commonly ricin) to deliver a lethal hit to the idiotype-positive tumor cells. The efficacy of such "magic bullets" in the treatment of leukemias and lymphomas of the immune cells is under active investigation.[115]

LABORATORY DIAGNOSIS OF CANCER

Every year the approach to laboratory diagnosis of cancer becomes more complex, more sophisticated, and more specialized. It may come as a rude surprise that, for virtually every neoplasm mentioned in this text, a number of subcategories have been characterized by the experts; but we must walk before we can run. Each of the following sections attempts to present the "state of the art," avoiding details of method.

HISTOLOGIC AND CYTOLOGIC METHODS. The laboratory diagnosis of cancer is, in most instances, not difficult. The two ends of the benign-malignant spectrum pose no problems; however, in the middle lies a "no man's land" where wise men tread cautiously. This issue was sufficiently emphasized earlier; here the focus is on the roles of the clinician (often a surgeon) and the pathologist in facilitating the correct diagnosis.

Clinicians tend to underestimate the important contributions they make to the diagnosis of a neoplasm. Clinical data are invaluable for optimal pathologic diagnosis. Radiation changes in the skin or mucosa can be similar to cancer. Sections taken from a healing fracture can mimic remarkably an osteosarcoma. Moreover, the laboratory evaluation of a lesion can be only as good as the specimen made available for examination. It must be adequate, representative, and properly preserved. Several sampling approaches are available: (1) excision or biopsy, (2) needle aspiration, and (3) cytologic smears. When excision of a small lesion is not possible, selection of an appropriate site for biopsy of a large mass requires awareness that the margins may not be representative and the center largely necrotic. Analogously with disseminated lymphoma (involving many nodes), those in the inguinal region draining large areas of the body often have reactive changes that may mask neoplastic involvement. Appropriate preservation of the specimen is obvious, yet it involves such actions as prompt immersion in a usual fixative (for example, formalin solution) or instead preservation of a portion in a special fixative (e.g., glutaraldehyde) for electron microscopy or prompt refrigeration to permit optimal hormone or receptor analysis. In the case of breast carcinoma, assays for estrogen and progesterone receptors provide guidelines for possible hormonal therapeutic interventions. Requesting "quick-frozen section" diagnosis is sometimes desirable, for example in determining the nature of a breast lesion or in evaluating the margins of an excised cancer to ascertain that the entire neoplasm has been removed. This method allows sectioning of a "quick-frozen" sample and permits histologic evaluation within minutes. In experienced, competent hands, frozen-section diagnosis is highly accurate, but there are particular instances in which the better histologic detail provided by the more time-consuming routine methods is needed—for example, when extremely radical surgery, such as the amputation of an extremity, may be indicated. Better to wait a few days despite the drawbacks than to perform inadequate or unnecessary surgery. Fortunately, except for the rare instances of rapidly growing sarcomas (usually in children), there is no evidence that cutting into a neoplasm followed by a few days' delay between biopsy and definitive surgery imposes any additional danger of dissemination of the tumor.

Fine needle aspiration of tumors provides another approach that is growing in popularity. The procedure involves aspirating cells and attendant fluid with a small-bore needle followed by cytologic examination of the stained smear. This method is employed most commonly for the preoperative assessment of readily palpable lesions in sites such as the breast, thyroid, lymph nodes, and, with the aid of a special needle, the prostate. Modern imaging techniques enable the method to be extended to lesions in deep-seated structures such as pelvic lymph nodes.[116,117] Fine needle aspiration is less invasive and more rapidly performed than are needle biopsies. In experienced hands it is an extremely reliable, rapid, and useful technique.

Cytologic (Papanicolaou) smears provide yet another method for the detection of cancer. This approach is widely used for the discovery of carcinoma of the cervix, often at an in situ stage, but it is also used with many other forms of suspected malignancy, such as endometrial carcinoma, bronchogenic carcinoma, bladder and prostatic tumors, and gastric carcinomas; for the identification of tumor cells in abdominal, pleural, joint, and cerebrospinal fluids; and, less commonly, with other forms of neoplasia.

As pointed out earlier, cancer cells have lowered cohesiveness and exhibit a range of morphologic changes encompassed by the term anaplasia. Thus, shed cells can be evaluated for the features of anaplasia indicative of their origin in a cancer (Figs. 6–39 and 6–40). In contrast to the histologist's task, judgment here must be rendered on the basis of individual cell cytology or (at most, perhaps) on that of a clump of a few cells without the supporting evidence of ar-

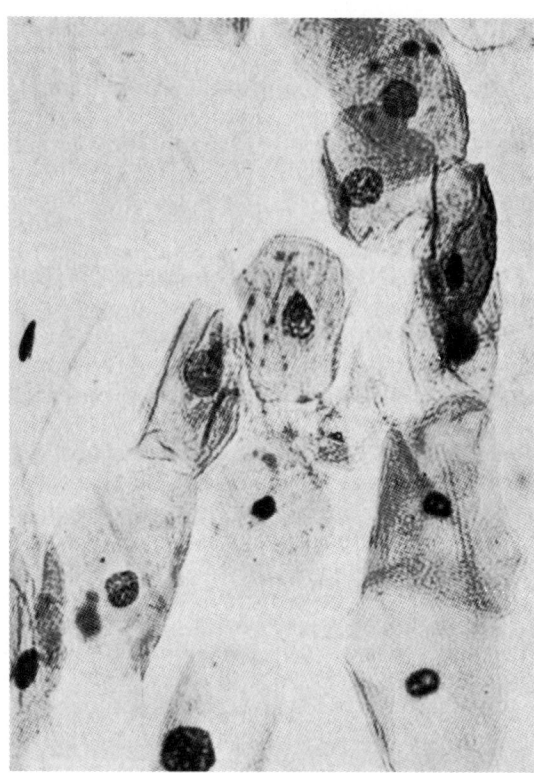

Figure 6–39. Exfoliative cell smear showing normal cytologic flora of the genital tract. Cells are largely flattened surface squamous epithelial cells.

chitectural disarray, loss of orientation of one cell to another, and (perhaps most important) evidence of invasion. This method permits differentiation among normal, dysplastic, and cancerous cells, and in addition permits the recognition of cellular changes characteristic of carcinoma in situ.

Cytologic interpretation requires a great deal of expertise but can yield with cervical smears nearly 100% correct positive diagnosis; i.e., false-positive results are rare. However, there is a significant fraction of false-negative diagnoses, owing largely to sampling errors. Smears for other types of tumors (e.g., lung, stomach, prostate) are more difficult to evaluate. Nonetheless, with all a positive finding almost always provides strong evidence of the existence of a cancer. It should be emphasized, however, that *all positive findings are best confirmed by biopsy and histologic examination before therapy is instituted.* A negative report does not exclude the presence of a malignancy. The gratifying control of cervical cancer is the best testament to the value of the cytologic method.

Although histology and exfoliative cytology remain the most commonly employed methods in the diagnosis of cancer, new techniques are being constantly added to the tools of the surgical pathologist. Some, such as immunocytochemistry, are already well established and widely utilized; others, including DNA probe analysis, are rapidly finding their way into the "routine" category. Only some highlights of these diagnostic modalities will be presented.

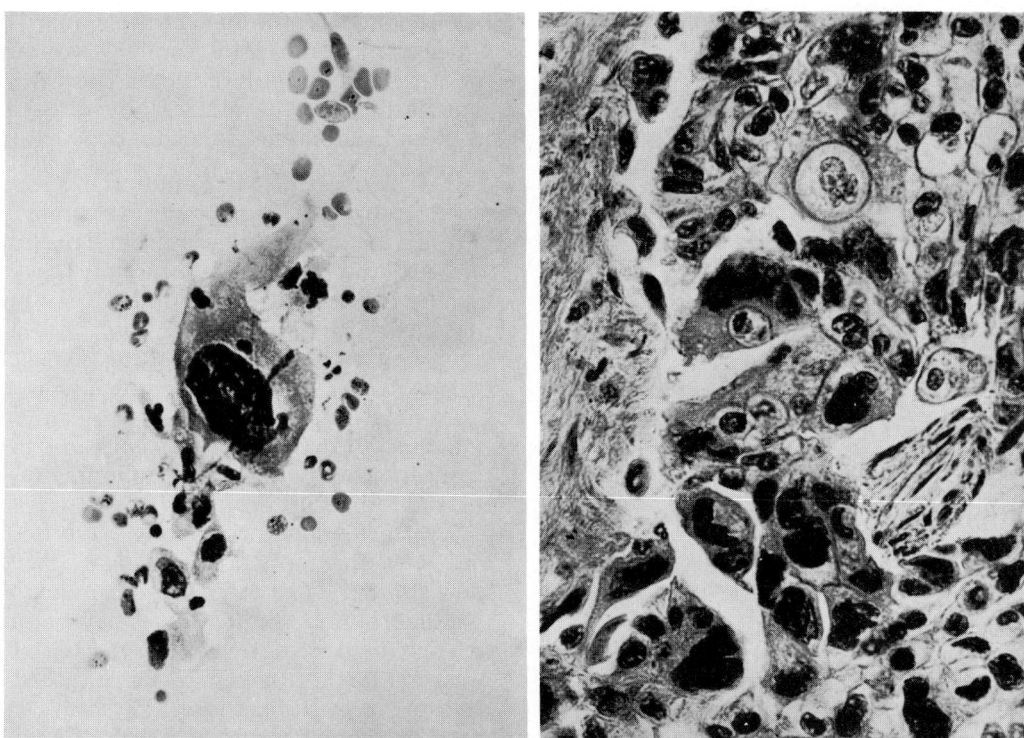

Figure 6–40. On the left is an exfoliative cell smear of vaginal secretions from a patient with a cervical cancer. Contrast the large, malignant anaplastic cell with the normal cells in Figure 6–39 (same magnification). On the right is a tissue section of the resected tumor showing the anaplastic cells in situ.

IMMUNOCYTOCHEMISTRY. The availability of specific monoclonal antibodies has greatly facilitated the identification of cell products or surface markers. For example, antibodies directed against intermediate filaments have proved to be of value in the classification of otherwise poorly differentiated tumors.[118] Table 6–14 lists the five major types of intermediate filaments and the types of tumors in which they are found. The presence of cytokeratin (detected by immunoperoxidase staining), for example, allows distinction between a poorly differentiated carcinoma and a large cell lymphoma. Both may look very similar by routine staining, but only carcinomas contain keratin (Fig. 6–41). Vimentin, the predominant intermediate filament of mesenchymal cells, is less specific because certain epithelial tumors (e.g., renal cell carcinomas) may coexpress keratin and vimentin. Desmin, on the other hand, is specific for neoplasms showing muscle differentiation.

Immunocytochemistry (in conjunction with immunofluorescence) has also proved useful in the identification and classification of tumors arising from T and B lymphocytes and from mononuclear-phagocytic cells. A list of monoclonal antibodies directed against various lymphohemopoietic cells was provided in Table 5–1 on page 165.

DNA PROBE ANALYSES. Molecular biology has moved from the research laboratory to the bedside. It is now possible to identify T- and B-cell neoplasms on the basis of clonal rearrangement of their receptor genes by employing Southern blot analysis (p. 167). Amplification of N-*myc* oncogene (neuroblastomas) and c-*neu* gene (breast carcinomas) has proved to be of prognostic value (p. 289). These oncogenes can be detected by Southern blot analysis of tumor DNA or in situ hybridization. Several other diagnostic applications of recombinant DNA technology will be cited with the discussion of specific tumors.

DNA FLOW CYTOMETRY. Flow cytometry can rapidly and quantitatively measure several individual cell characteristics, including the DNA content of tumor cells. It can be applied to specimens from a variety of sources such as fresh frozen surgical biopsies (from which nuclei can be extracted), pleural or peritoneal effusions associated with cancer, bone marrow aspirations, and cells obtained by irrigation of the urinary bladder. A relationship between abnormal DNA content and prognosis is becoming apparent for a variety of malignancies.[119,120] In general, aneuploidy seems to be associated with poorer prognosis in early-stage

Table 6–14. Intermediate Filaments and Their Distribution

Keratins	Carcinomas
	Mesothelioma
Desmin	Muscle tumors, smooth, striated
Vimentin	Mesenchymal tumors, some carcinomas
Glial filaments	Gliomatous tumors
Neurofilaments	Neuronal tumors

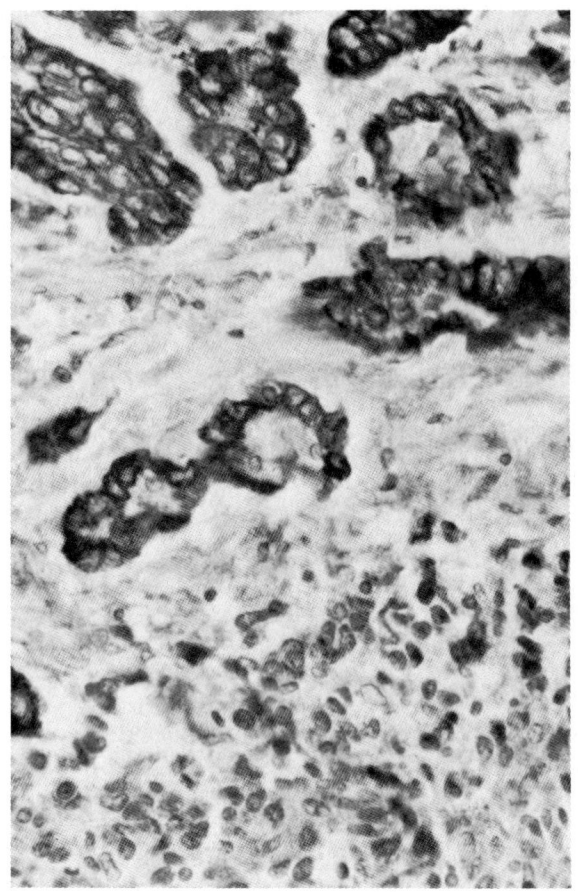

Figure 6–41. An antikeratin immunoperoxidase stain of a carcinoma of the lung. The atypical gland patterns above are stained dark, indicating a positive antikeratin reaction.

breast cancer, carcinoma of the urinary bladder, lung cancer, and colorectal cancer. Although measurement of DNA-ploidy is not a routine procedure in most institutions, it may well become a standard tool in the management of certain cancers in the future.

TUMOR MARKERS. Tumor markers are biochemical indicators of the presence of a tumor. They include cell surface antigens, cytoplasmic proteins, enzymes, and hormones. In clinical practice, however, the term usually refers to a molecule that can be detected in plasma or other body fluids. *Tumor markers cannot be construed as primary modalities for the diagnosis of cancer.* Their main utility in clinical medicine has been as a laboratory test to confirm the diagnosis. Some tumor markers are also of value in determining the response to therapy and in indicating relapse during the follow-up period.

A host of tumor markers have been described, and new ones appear every year.[121,122] Only a few have stood the test of time and proved to have clinical usefulness. The application of several markers listed in Table 6–15 will be considered with specific forms of neoplasia discussed in other chapters, so only a few examples will suffice here.

Carcinoembryonic antigen (CEA), normally produced in embryonic tissue of the gut, pancreas, and liver, is a complex glycoprotein that is elaborated by many different neoplasms. Depending on the serum level adopted as a significant elevation, it is variously reported to be positive in 60 to 90% of colorectal, 50 to 80% of pancreatic, and 25 to 50% of gastric and breast carcinomas. Much less consistently, elevated CEA has been described in other forms of cancer. CEA elevations have also been reported in many benign disorders, such as alcoholic cirrhosis, hepatitis, ulcerative colitis, Crohn's disease, and others. Occasionally levels of this antigen are elevated in apparently healthy smokers. Thus, CEA assays lack both specificity and the sensitivity required for the detec-

Table 6–15. Selected Tumor Markers

MARKERS	ASSOCIATED CANCERS
Hormones	
Human chorionic gonadotropin	Trophoblastic tumors, nonseminomatous testicular tumors
Calcitonin	Medullary carcinoma of thyroid
Catecholamine and metabolites	Pheochromocytoma and related tumors
Ectopic hormones	See *Paraneoplastic syndromes* (p. 295)
Oncofetal Antigens	
Alpha-fetoprotein	Liver cell cancer, nonseminomatous germ cell tumors of testis
Carcinoembryonic antigen	Carcinomas of the colon, pancreas, lung, stomach, and breast
Isoenzymes	
Prostatic acid phosphatase	Prostate cancer
Neuron-specific enolase	Small cell cancer of lung, neuroblastoma
Specific Proteins	
Immunoglobulins	Multiple myeloma and other gammopathies
Prostate-specific antigen	Prostate cancer
Mucins and Other Glycoproteins	
CA-125	Ovarian cancer
CA-19-9	Colon cancer, pancreatic cancer
CA-15-3	Breast cancer

tion of early cancers. Preoperative CEA levels have some bearing on prognosis because the level of elevation is correlated with body burden of tumor. In colon cancer the levels correlate with the widely used Dukes grading system (p. 901). In patients with CEA-positive colon cancers, the presence of elevated CEA levels six weeks after therapy indicates residual disease. Recurrence is indicated by a rising CEA level, with an increase in tumor marker level often preceding clinically detectable disease.

Alpha-fetoprotein (AFP) is another well-established tumor marker, discussed in some detail on page 1114. This glycoprotein is synthesized normally early in fetal life by the yolk sac and fetal liver. Abnormal plasma elevations are encountered in adults with cancer arising principally in the liver and germ cells of the testis. Elevated plasma AFP is also found less regularly in carcinomas of the stomach and pancreas. Like CEA, non-neoplastic conditions including cirrhosis, toxic liver injury, hepatitis, and pregnancy (especially with fetal distress or death) also may cause minimal-to-moderate plasma elevations of AFP. While there is, then, some problem with specificity, marked elevations of the plasma AFP level have proved to be a highly useful indicator of hepatocellular carcinomas and germ cell tumors of the testis (p. 961 and p. 1114). AFP levels decline rapidly after surgical resection of liver cell cancer or treatment of germ cell tumors. Serial post-therapy measurements of AFP (and human chorionic gonadotropin) levels in patients with germ cell tumors of the testis provide a sensitive index of response to therapy and recurrence.

Prostatic acid phosphatase is another widely utilized tumor marker. Prostatic carcinoma can be suspected when elevated levels of acid phosphatase are found in the blood. Regrettably, the levels become significantly raised only when the tumor is advanced (as is detailed on p. 1125) and so the false-negative rate is high. Prostate-specific antigen is a newly described serum marker which may prove useful in monitoring therapy and prognosis of prostatic carcinomas.[123]

This cursory overview suffices to indicate the many laboratory approaches in use for detection and diagnosis of tumors.

---

1. Cancer statistics, 1989. CA *39*:13, 1989.
2. Willis, R.A.: The Spread of Tumors in the Human Body. London, Butterworth & Co., 1952.
3. Everson T.C., and Cole, M.W.H.: Spontaneous Regression of Cancer. Philadelphia, W.B. Saunders Co., 1966.
4. Woodruff, M.F.A.: Tumor clonality and its biologic significance. Adv. Cancer Res.*50*:197, 1988.
5. Arnold, A.A., et al.: Monoclonality and abnormal parathyroid genes in parathyroid adenomas. N. Engl. J. Med. *318*:658, 1988.
6. Fearon, R.R., et al.: Clonal analysis of human colorectal tumors. Science *238*:193, 1987.
7. Ponder, B.A.J., et al.: Direct examination of the clonality of carcinogen-induced epithelial dysplasia in chimeric mice. J. Natl. Cancer Inst. 77:967, 1986.
8. Tannock, I.F.: Tumor growth and cell kinetics. *In* Tannock, I.F.,

and Hill, R.P. (eds.): The Basic Science of Oncology. New York, Pergamon Press, 1987, p. 140.
9. Folkman, J.: Tumor angiogenesis. Adv. Cancer Res. 43:175, 1985.
10. Folkman, J.: How is blood vessel growth regulated in normal and neoplastic tissue? Cancer Res. 46:467, 1986.
11. Folkman, J., et al.: A heparin-binding angiogenic protein-basic fibroblast growth factor is stored within basement membrane. Am. J. Pathol. *130*:393, 1988.
12. Foulds, L.: Neoplastic Development. New York, Academic Press, 1975.
13. Nicholson, G.L.: Tumor cell instability, diversification, and progression to the metastatic phenotype: from oncogene to oncofetal expression. Cancer Res 47:1473, 1987.
14. Fidler, I.J.: Review: biologic heterogeneity of cancer metastases. Breast Cancer Res. Treat. *9*:17, 1987.
15. Schnipper, L.E.: Clinical implication of tumor-cell heterogeneity. N. Engl. J. Med. *314*:1423, 1987.
16. Fidler, I.J.: The evolution of biologic heterogeneity in metastatic neoplasms. *In* Nicholson, G.L., and Milas, L. (eds.): Cancer Invasion and Metastases: Biologic and Therapeutic Aspects. New York, Raven Press, 1984, p. 5.
17. Liotta, L.A.: Editorial. H-*ras* p21 and the metastatic phenotype. J. Natl. Cancer Inst. 80:468, 1988.
18. Tryggvason, K., et al.: Proteolytic degradation of extracellular matrix in tumor invasion. Biochim. Biophys. Acta *907*:191, 1987.
19. Juliano, R.L.: Membrane receptors for extracellular matrix macromolecules: relationship to cell adhesion and tumor metastases. Biochim. Biophys. Acta *907*:261, 1987.
20. Liotta, L.A., et al.: Biochemical mechanisms of tumor invasion and metastases. Prog. Clin. Biol. Res. *256*:3, 1988.
21. Humphries, J.J., et al.: Investigation of the antimetastatic effects of agents that inhibit cell adhesion or protein glycosylation. J. Natl. Med. Assoc. 69:411, 1987.
22. Liotta, L.A., et al.: Biochemical interactions of tumor cells with the basement membrane. Annu. Rev. Biochem. 55:1037, 1986.
23. Pauli, B.V., and Knudson, W.: Tumor invasion: a consequence of destructive and compositional matrix alteration. Hum. Pathol. *19*:628, 1988.
24. Kalebic, T., et al.: A novel method for selection of invasive tumor cells: derivation and characterization of highly metastatic K1735 melanoma cell lines based on in vitro and in vivo invasive capacity. Clin. Exp. Med. *6*:301, 1988.
25. Zimmerman, A., and Keller, H.U.: Locomotion of tumor cells as an element of invasion and metastasis. Biomed. Pharmacother. *41*:337, 1987.
26. Kaminski, M., and Auerbach, R.: Tumor cells are protected from NK cell–mediated lysis by adhesion to endothelial cells. Int. J. Cancer. *41*:847, 1988.
27. Pauli, B.V., and Lee, C.: Organ preference of metastases: the role of organ-specifically modulated endothelial cells. Lab. Invest. *58*:379, 1988.
28. Bitter, M.A., et al.: Associations between morphology, karyotype, and clinical features in myeloid leukemias. Hum. Pathol. *18*:211, 1987.
29. Sandberg, A.A., et al: Chromosomes in solid tumors and beyond. Cancer Res. 48:1949, 1988.
30. Le Beau, M.M.: Chromosomal fragile sites and cancer-specific rearrangements. Blood 67:849, 1986.
31. Brodeur, G.M.: Molecular correlates of cytogenetic abnormalities in human cancer cells: implication for oncogene activation. Prog. Hematol. *16*:229, 1986.
32. Sandberg, A.A.: Editorial: The cytogenetic route of benign tumors. Cancer Genet. Cytogenet. *32*:11, 1988.
33. Cancer Facts and Figures. New York, American Cancer Society, 1987, p. 23.
34. Schneider, N.R., et al.: Genetic epidemiology of familial aggregation of cancer. Adv. Cancer Res. 47:1, 1986.
35. Hansen, M.F., and Cavenee, W.K.: Genetics and cancer predisposition. Cancer Res. 47:5518, 1987.
36. Rootman, J., et al.: Retinoblastomas. Perspect. Pediatr. Pathol. *10*:208, 1987.
37. Lambert, W.C.: Genetic diseases associated with DNA and chromosome instability. Dermatol. Clin. 5:85, 1987.

38. Knudson, A.G.: Genetics and cancer. In Burchenal, J.H., and Oettgen, H.F. (eds.): Cancer. Achievements, Challenges and Prospects for the 1980s. Vol 1. New York, Grune & Stratton, 1981, p. 381.

39. Doll, R., and Pet, R.: The causes of cancer: quantitative estimates of avoidable risks of cancer in the United States today. J. Natl. Cancer Inst. 66:1191, 1981.

40. Vogelstein, B., et al.: Genetic alterations during colorectal tumor development. N. Engl. J. Med. 319:525, 1988.

41. IARC Monographs. Evaluation of the carcinogenic risk of chemicals to humans. Supplement 4, Report of ad hoc working group, Lyons, February 8–12, 1982.

42. Pitot, H.C.: Fundamentals of Oncology. 3rd ed. New York, Marcel Dekker, 1986, p. 139.

43. Farber, E., and Sarma, D.S.R.: Hepatocarcinogenesis: A dynamic cellular perspective. Lab. Invest. 56:4, 1987.

44. Slaga, T.J. (ed.): Mechanisms of Tumor-Promotion: Tumor Promotion in Internal Organs. Boca Raton, CRC Press, 1983.

45. Farber, E.: Possible etiologic mechanisms in chemical carcinogenesis. Environ. Health Perspect. 75:65, 1987.

46. Weinstein, I.B.: The origins of human cancer: molecular mechanisms of carcinogenesis and their implications for cancer prevention and treatment—Twenty-seventh GHA Clowes Memorial Award Lecture. Cancer Res. 48:4135, 1988.

47. Miller, E.C., and Miller, J.A.: Searches for ultimate chemical carcinogens and their reaction with cellular macromolecules. Cancer 47:2327, 1981.

48. Pitot, H.C.: Fundamentals of Oncology. 3rd ed. New York, Marcel Dekker, 1986, p. 42.

49. Grunberger, D., et al.: Stabilization of Z-DNA conformation by chemical carcinogens. In Huberman, E., and Barr, S.H. (eds.): Carcinogenesis. Vol. 10. New York, Raven Press, 1985, p. 465.

50. Bell, J.C.: Oncogenes. Cancer Lett. 40:1, 1988.

51. Stowers, S.J., et al.: The role of oncogenes in chemical carcinogenesis. Environ. Health Perspect. 75:81, 1987.

52. Blumberg, P.C.: Protein kinase C as the receptor for the phorbol ester tumor promoters. Cancer Res. 48:1, 1988.

53. Nishizuka, Y.: Studies and perspectives of protein kinase C. Science 233:305, 1986.

54. Yuspa, S.H., and Poirier, M.C.: Chemical carcinogenesis: from animal models to molecular models in one decade. Adv. Cancer Res. 50:25, 1988.

55. Calabresi, P.: Leukemia after cytotoxic chemotherapy—a pyrrhic victory? N. Engl. J. Med. 309:1118, 1983.

56. Levin, W., et al.: Oxidative metabolism of polycyclic hydrocarbons to ultimate carcinogens. Drug Metab. Rev. 13:555, 1982.

57. Kleinfeld, M., et al.: Bladder tumors in a coal tar dye plant. Ind. Med. Surg. 35:570, 1966.

58. Pitot, H.C.: Fundamentals of Oncology. 3rd ed. New York, Marcel Dekker, 1986, p. 228.

59. Craighead, J.E., and Mossman, B.J.T.: The pathogenesis of asbestos-associated diseases. N. Engl. J. Med. 306:1446, 1982.

60. Pitot, H.C.: Chemicals and cancer: Initiation and promotion. Hosp. Pract. 18:100, 1983.

61. Henderson, B.E., et al.: Estrogens as a cause of human cancer. Cancer Res. 48:246, 1988.

62. Kohn, H.I., and Fry, R.J.M.: Radiation carcinogenesis. N. Engl. J. Med. 310:504, 1984.

63. Hall, E.J., and Hei, T.K.: Oncogenic transformation with radiation and chemicals. Int. J. Radiat. Biol. 48:1, 1985.

64. Fry, R.J.M., and Ley, R.D.: Ultraviolet carcinogenesis. In Slaga, T.J. (ed.): Mechanism of Tumor Promotion. Vol III. Tumor Promotion and Skin Carcinogenesis, Boca Raton, CRC Press, 1983, p. 73.

65. Kripke, M.L.: Immunological mechanisms in UV radiation carcinogenesis. Adv. Cancer Res. 34:69, 1981.

66. Fisher, M.S., and Kripke, M.L.: Suppressor T lymphocytes control the development of primary skin cancers in ultraviolet irradiated mice. Science 216:1133, 1982.

67. Elkind, M.M.: Repair processes in radiation biology. Radiat. Res. 100:425, 1984.

68. Kramer, K.H., et al.: DNA repair protects against cutaneous and internal neoplasia: evidence from xeroderma pigmentosum. Carcinogenesis 5:511, 1984.

69. Arlett, F.: Human DNA repair defects. J. Inherited Metab. Dis. 9(Suppl 1):69, 1986.

70. Fajardo, L.F.: Ionizing radiation and neoplasia. In Fenoglio-Preiser, C.M., et al.: (eds): New Concepts in Neoplasia as Applied to Diagnostic Pathology. Baltimore, Williams & Wilkins, 1986, p. 97.

71. Guerrero, I., et al.: Activation of a c-K-ras oncogene by somatic mutation in a mouse lymphoma induced by gamma radiation. Science 225:1159, 1984.

72. Ostrow, R.S., and Faras, A.J.: The molecular biology of human papilloma viruses and the pathogenesis of genital papillomas and neoplasms. Cancer Metas. Rev. 6:383, 1987.

73. Bonfiglio, T.A., and Stoler, M.H.: Human papillomavirus and cancer of uterine cervix. Hum. Pathol. 19:621, 1988.

74. Pfister, H.: Human papillomaviruses and genital cancer. Adv. Cancer Res. 48:113, 1987.

75. Howley, P.H.: On human papillomaviruses. N. Engl. J. Med. 315:1089, 1986.

76. Richart, R.M.: Causes and management of cervical intraepithelial neoplasia. Cancer 60:1951, 1987.

77. Richtsmeier, W.J., et al.: Epstein-Barr virus–associated malignancies. CRC Crit. Rev. Clin. Lab. Sci. 25:105, 1987.

78. Dillner, J., and Kallin, B.: The Epstein-Barr virus proteins. Adv. Cancer Res. 50:95, 1988.

79. Levine, A.J.: Oncogenes of DNA tumor viruses. Cancer Res. 48:493, 1988.

80. Cuzin, F., and Meneguzzi, G.: Stepwise transformation and cooperative interactions involving oncogenes of DNA tumor viruses. Adv. Viral Oncol. 6:21, 1987.

81. De Caprio, J.A., et al.: SV40 large tumor antigen forms a specific complex with the product of the retinoblastoma susceptibility gene. Cell 54:275, 1988.

82. Whyte, P., et al.: Association between an oncogene and an anti-oncogene: the adenovirus E1A proteins bind to the retinoblastoma gene product. Nature 334:124, 1988.

83. Bishop, J.M.: The molecular genetics of cancer. Science 235:305, 1987.

84. Kim, J.H., and Durack, D.T.: Manifestations of human T-lymphotropic virus type 1 infection. Am. J. Med. 84:919, 1988.

85. Ehrlich, G.D., and Poiesz, B.J.: Clinical and molecular parameters of HTLV-1 infection. Clin. Lab. Med. 8:65, 1988.

86. Nerenberg, M., et al.: The tat gene of human T-lymphotropic virus type 1 induces mesenchymal tumors in transgenic mice. Science 237:1324, 1987.

87. Weinberg, R.A.: The genetic origins of human cancer. Cancer 61:1963, 1988.

88. Deuel, T.F.: Polypeptide growth factors: roles in normal and abnormal cell growth. Annu. Rev. Cell Biol. 3:443, 1987.

89. Bos, J.L.: The ras gene family and human carcinogenesis. Mutat. Res. 195:255, 1988.

90. Guerrero, T., and Pellicer, A.: Mutational activation of oncogenes in animal model system of carcinogenesis. Mutat. Res. 185:293, 1987.

91. Thompson, N.L., et al.: Sequential proto-oncogene expression during rat liver regeneration. Cancer Res. 46:3111, 1986.

92. Rodenhuis, S., et al.: Mutational activation of the K-ras oncogene. N. Engl. J. Med. 317:929, 1987.

93. Bos, J.L., et al.: Prevalence of ras gene mutations in human colorectal cancers. Nature 327:293, 1987.

94. Barbacid, M.: ras genes. Annu. Rev. Biochem. 56:779, 1987.

95. Brodeur, G.M., et al.: Clinical implication of oncogene activation in human neuroblastomas. Cancer 58:541, 1986.

96. Slamon, D.J., et al.: Human breast cancer: Correlation of relapse and survival with amplification of the HER-2/neu oncogene. Science 235:177, 1987.

97. Sainsbury, J.R.C., et al.: Epidermal growth factor receptor status as predictor of early recurrence of and death from breast cancer. Lancet 1:1398, 1987.

98. Friend, S.H., et al.: Oncogenes and tumor-suppressing genes. N. Engl. J. Med. 318:618, 1988.

99. Klein, G.: The approaching era of the tumor suppressor genes. Science 238:1539, 1987.

100. Marx, J.L.: Eye cancer gene linked to new malignancies. (Research News.) Science 241:293, 1988.

101. Nowell, P.C.: Molecular events in tumor development. N. Engl. J. Med. 319:575, 1988.

102. Muschel, R., and Liotta, L.: Role of oncogenes in metastases. Carcinogenesis 9:705, 1988.

103. Jeevanandem, M., et al.: Cancer cachexia and protein metabolism. Lancet *1*:1423, 1984.

104. Editorial: Cancer cachexia. Lancet *1*:833, 1984.

105. Beutler, B.: The presence of cachectin/tumor necrosis factor in human disease states. Am. J. Med. *85*:287, 1988.

106. Ihde, D.C.: Paraneoplastic syndromes. Hosp. Pract. *22*:105, 1987.

107. Broadus, A.E., et al.: Humoral hypercalcemia of cancer. N. Engl. J. Med. *319*:556, 1988.

108. Abeloff, M.D.: Paraneoplastic syndromes. N. Engl. J. Med. *317*:1598, 1987.

109. Muul, L.M., et al.: Identification of specific cytolytic immune response against autologous tumor in humans bearing malignant melanoma. J. Immunol. *138*:989, 1987.

110. Real, F.X., et al.: Class I (unique) tumor antigens of human melanoma: identification of unique and common epitopes on a 90K Da glycoprotein. Proc. Natl. Acad. Sci. U.S.A. *85*:3965, 1988.

111. Schateen, S., et al.: Suppressor T cells and the immune response to tumors. CRC Crit. Rev. *4*:335, 1984.

112. Purtilo, D.T.: Biology of disease. Defective immune surveillance in viral carcinogenesis. Lab. Invest. *51*:373, 1984.

113. Ortaldo, J.R., and Longo, D.L.: Human natural effector cells: definition, analysis of activity, and clinical effectiveness. J. Natl. Cancer Inst. *80*:999, 1988.

114. Rosenberg, S.A., et al.: New approaches to the immunotherapy of cancer using interleukin-2. Ann. Intern. Med. *108*:853, 1988.

115. Vitteta, E.S., and Uhr, J.W.: Immunotoxins. Annu. Rev. Immunol. *3*:197, 1985.

116. Naylor, B.: Fine needle aspiration cytology of the breast: an overview. Am. J. Surg. Pathol. *12*(Suppl. 1) 54, 1988.

117. Lever, J.V., et al.: Fine needle aspiration cytology. J. Clin. Pathol. *38*:1, 1985.

118. Battifora, H.: Clinical applications of the immunohistochemistry of filamentous proteins. Am. J. Surg. Pathol. *12*(Suppl. 1):24, 1988.

119. Molenaar, W.M., et al.: DNA aneuploidy in rhabdomyosarcomas as compared with other sarcomas of childhood and adolescence. Hum. Pathol. *19*:573, 1988.

120. Merkel, D.E., et al.: Flow cytometry, cellular DNA content, and prognosis in human malignancy. J. Clin. Oncol. *5*:1690, 1987.

121. Virji, M.A., et al.: Tumor markers in cancer diagnosis and prognosis. CA *38*:104, 1988.

122. Carney, W.: Human tumor antigens and specific tumor therapy. Immunol. Today *9*:363, 1988.

123. Stamey, T.A., et al.: Prostate specific antigen as a serum marker for adenocarcinoma of the prostate. N. Engl. J. Med. *317*:909, 1987.

7

Infectious Disease

VIRAL, CHLAMYDIAL, RICKETTSIAL, AND BACTERIAL DISEASES

Franz von Lichtenberg, M.D.

INTRODUCTION

Ever since Pandora opened her mythical box, infectious diseases have plagued humanity, evolving with changing life conditions and population expansion. Populations in equilibrium with their endemic infectious diseases have been devastated by contact with infections of modern civilization; indeed, more American Indians may have died of measles than of the white man's bullets.[1] As urban populations expanded, unsanitary crowding invited the great medieval pandemics of plague and cholera, which now persist only in localized pockets. Even today, societies in densely populated developing countries are prey to tuberculosis, leprosy, malaria, filariasis, and schistosomiasis. Smallpox alone is back in Pandora's box, thanks to the only whole-hearted international preventive campaign ever undertaken. Other infections, in addition to smallpox, have been partly curbed by vaccines, including diphtheria, whooping cough, paralytic poliomyelitis, and measles.

*Infectious diseases of limited geographic distribution are marked by an asterisk.

Fungal, protozoal, and helminthic diseases are discussed on page 385.

Medical practices too have altered the panorama of infectious diseases. The discovery of penicillin by Fleming and the generations of new antibiotics and microbicidal drugs have radically changed not only the prevalence but also the course of most infectious diseases so that they now rarely appear in their classic forms. Yet for some, especially many viral infections, we still lack adequate prevention and treatment. Even preventable infectious disorders keep festering amid urban and rural squalor and during war and famine. Neither affluence nor improved medical technology has curbed the spread of venereal infections. In fact, medical technology itself is responsible for a new category of microbial diseases called "opportunistic infections." So-called altered hosts who receive cytotoxic and immunosuppressive therapy for tumors and tissue transplants become vulnerable to infections that are usually innocuous or dormant in normal adults. Invasive hospital procedures such as intubation, catheterization, or prosthetic implantation have provided new entry points for such infections.[2]

Still, the pace of these changes has been slow compared with the multiple mutations and genomic interchanges between viruses, phages, plasmids, and bacteria that have now become the ingenious tools of molecular biology. Genetic diversification helps to ensure microbial survival under selective pressure and thus facilitates the emergence of antibiotic-resistant bacterial strains.[3,4] Recently, Salmonella strains from antibiotic-reared cattle have been found to be responsible for outbreaks of human food poisoning. More suddenly and dramatically, "new" diseases have appeared from time to time: venereal syphilis was unknown before the siege of Naples in 1494; legionnaires' disease made its debut in Philadelphia in 1976; and the acquired immunodeficiency syndrome (AIDS) has quickly spanned the globe since its discovery in 1981. Even as investigators pursue the origins of human immunodeficiency virus (HIV-I) into the heart of Africa, new HIV variants and mutants are being discovered. Among other lessons, AIDS reminds us that in infectious disease, host factors require the same careful attention that has routinely been given to the identification of microbial agents. AIDS also tells us that battles against individual microbes are not easily won and that the war against human infection will continue as long as humankind endures.

In this age of international travel and vast population displacements, diseases are "exotic" only to the eye of the beholder, and the global view of infectious diseases is amply justified. For convenience, *geographically restricted diseases*, including those in the United States, are marked by an asterisk in this chapter. Some, however, will increasingly appear outside their known perimeters as global distances keep shrinking; others illustrate important pathogenic mechanisms and have therefore been referred to briefly.

Infectious diseases are the consequence of host-parasite interactions, and we shall first review the principles involved, together with the contributions of microbiology and immunology.

FACTORS RELATING TO PARASITE

Cooperation between microorganisms and higher phyla is the rule; disease is the exception.[5] No animal is free of smaller life except when reared as a germ-free laboratory artifact. Normal humans would be at risk of a vitamin K deficiency without their gut flora, which synthesize this essential nutrient. We are blissfully unaware of the Dermatonyssus mites that scavenge our hair follicles. Relationships that benefit both host and fellow passenger are termed *symbiotic*. *Commensals* share the host's food intake. *True parasites are those that interfere with the host's integrity and function, and the degree of such interference is a measure of their virulence or pathogenicity and of the adaptation of the host.* Long-standing human parasites tend to cause milder disease than those newly introduced, perhaps because sustained coexistence within a single host best subserves the perpetuation of the parasite — "selfish genes."

Human parasites belong to many plant and animal phyla, and range in size from the 20-nm poliovirus to the 10-m tapeworm *Taenia saginata*. Most are "microbes" (i.e., they are microscopic in size). Biochemically, the smallest viruses code for only three polypeptides, whereas the molecular complexity of helminths almost equals that of man. Speed of genetic variation depends on reproductive rate rather than size, and therefore fast-multiplying agents are better able to stay ahead of their host's defensive maneuvers. Some infectious organisms are *invariably pathogenic* for humans and their recovery in culture always signifies disease. Others must be regarded as *facultative pathogens* capable of either *colonization*, *invasion*, or both in succession; positive cultures of such organisms must therefore be interpreted cautiously, especially if the lesions in the host are incompatible with the particular agent found. The fungus *Candida albicans* offers a prime example. This organism is found in the oral cavity, gastrointestinal tract, and vagina of many normal individuals. Only in the predisposed host is it capable of producing invasive infections. Other organisms are almost entirely opportunists waiting to "pounce on" the particularly vulnerable host. With present-day methods of perpetuating life, the list and diversity of facultative human pathogens and opportunists keeps expanding, and few organisms colonizing humans can any longer be regarded as categorically innocuous.

Parasites vary with regard to the tissue and cellular microenvironment best suited to their survival and reproduction. For some, the skin provides the optimal habitat; for others, a mucosal surface; and for still others, the internal environment of the host. Some organisms are *extracellular parasites* and reproduce only outside of cells, but in this environment they are vulnerable to phagocytosis. Other *obligate intracellular parasites* require an intracellular microenvironment or must replicate in the nucleus of the host cell, as is the case with viruses. Some parasites can reproduce only within specific cell types or cellular organelles, which they seek out within the host. Still other organisms are *facultative intracellular parasites* that can survive and reproduce either outside of or within cells (Table 7–1).

Parasite entry into host cells can be *passive* (i.e., by phagocytosis, pinocytosis, or membrane fusion, as with coated viruses) or *active* and energy-requiring (as with rickettsiae or protozoa). The ability of microorganisms to convert from one state or habitat to another must always be kept in mind. Indeed, the higher parasite phyla have complex *life cycles* and must pass through alternate forms and hosts or environmental niches in order to infect man.

The preference of microorganisms for specific host tissues or cells is referred to as *tropism;* thus, gonococcal pili (Fig. 7–1) have ligand molecules that mediate adhesion to mucosal receptors,[6] and similar specific interactions are known for some of the viruses and intracellular parasites; however, preferential homing does not alone determine where disease will be expressed. Equally important are the permissiveness of the invaded tissue for microbial multiplication and its sensitivity to the adverse effects caused by the parasite (i.e., local vulnerability). A good example are the neurotropic viruses that colonize many tissues but damage mainly nerve cells (p. 1395).

TRANSMISSION OF INFECTIOUS AGENTS

Organisms causing infectious disease may be transmitted to vulnerable hosts through a variety of pathways:

1. *Direct spread* by contact or airborne particles from sick individuals to healthy hosts is characteristic of *contagious* infection, such as occurs in childhood measles or chickenpox. Such spread may result in epidemics. In some instances, short- or long-term asymptomatic carriers or shedders act as human reservoirs.
2. Spread may also occur by way of *contaminated water, food, or soil* from human or environmental reservoirs. The proverbial "Typhoid Mary," carrying *typhoid bacilli* in her gallbladder and stool, constituted such a human reservoir. *Legionella* may be disseminated from water tanks, cooling devices, even shower heads — places in which conditions for the proliferation of this bacterium are favorable. *Naegleria fowleri,* an ameboflagellate living in overgrown summer ponds, is an example of a free-living organism that can produce lethal meningoencephalitis in young healthy divers by penetrating the cribriform plate of the nasal roof.[7]
3. Infections can be acquired *prenatally,* passed from mother to fetus via the placenta, or *perinatally,* transmitted during or shortly after delivery. These forms of transmission are termed *vertical.*
4. Infections transmitted to humans from an animal host or reservoir are termed *zoonotic.* This occurs with all classes of parasites from viruses (e.g., equine encephalitis) to helminths (e.g., the pig roundworm, Trichinella). Zoonotic infections can be more or less pathogenic for humans than they are for their normal animal hosts. Some bat species harbor the lethal rabies virus with relative impunity, whereas the cowpox virus, causing disease in its natural host, is innocuous enough for man to serve as a vaccine against smallpox.

In sum, transmission of infection involves a number of factors including parasite biology, vector com-

Table 7–1. Classes of Human Endoparasites and their Habitats

TAXONOMIC CLASS	SIZE	SITE OF PROPAGATION	SAMPLE SPECIES AND ITS DISEASE	
Viruses	20–30 nm	Obligate intracellular	Poliovirus	Poliomyelitis
Chlamydiae	200–1000 nm	Obligate intracellular	C. trachomatis	Trachoma
Rickettsiae	300–1200 nm	Obligate intracellular	R. prowazekii	Typhus fever
Mycoplasmas	125–350 nm	Extracellular*	M. pneumoniae	Atypical pneumonia
Bacteria, spirochetes, mycobacteria	0.8–15 μm	Cutaneous	Staphylococcus epidermidis*	Wound infection
		Mucosal	Vibrio cholerae	Cholera
		Extracellular	Streptococcus pneumoniae	Pneumonia
		Facultative intracellular	Mycobacterium tuberculosis	Tuberculosis
Fungi Imperfecti	2–200 μm	Cutaneous	Trichophyton sp.	Tinea pedis (athlete's foot)
		Mucosal	Candida albicans*	Thrush
		Extracellular	Sporothrix schenkii	Sporotrichosis
		Facultative intracellular	Histoplasma capsulatum	Histoplasmosis
Protozoa	1–50 mm	Mucosal	Giardia lamblia	Giardiasis
		Extracellular	Trypanosoma gambiense	Sleeping sickness
		Facultative intracellular	Trypanosoma cruzi*	Chagas disease
		Obligate intracellular	Leishmania donovani	Kala-azar
Helminths	3 mm–10 m	Mucosal	Enterobius vermicularis	Oxyuriasis
		Extracellular	Wuchereria bancrofti	Filariasis
		Intracellular	Trichinella spiralis*	Trichinosis

* = Has alternate life stage, habitat, or disease form, described in text.

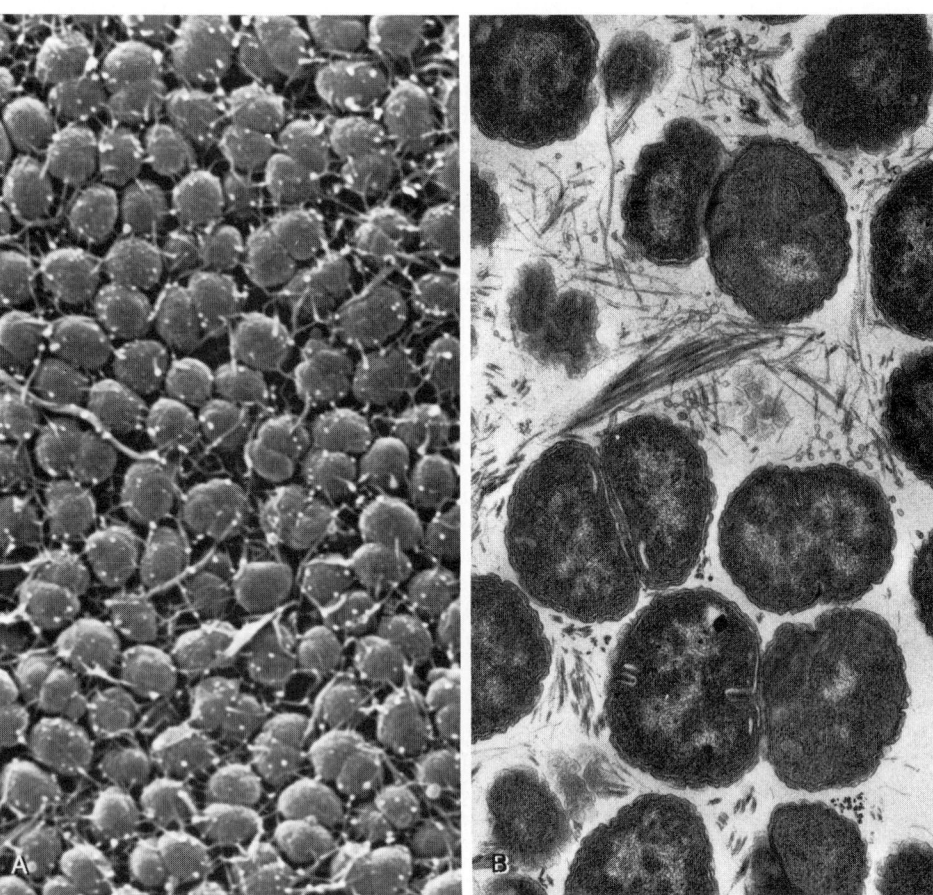

Figure 7–1. Gonococcal culture showing pili as seen by scanning electron microscopy *(A)*, and in clusters, as seen by transmission electron microscopy *(B)*. (Courtesy of Dr. John Swanson, Rocky Mountain Laboratories, Hamilton, Montana.)

petence, human behavior, and environmental conditions. Epidemiologic science analyzes all these factors in the hope of devising methods of preventing disease transmission, still by far the best way of controlling human infections.

FACTORS RELATING TO HOST

Fortunately there are many *host barriers to infection* that prevent access of parasites to their required environment or, failing that, can suppress infection or curtail its spread. These barriers and defenses take many forms, including (1) the intact integument and mucosal surfaces and secretions; (2) phagocytic white cells that are promptly marshaled to sites of entry; (3) the resident mononuclear-phagocyte (reticuloendothelial) system that effectively polices the internal environment for errant organisms; and (4) the all-important immune system. Phagocytosis (p. 48) and immunity (p. 163) have already been discussed. Overall, normal human barriers to infection are quite effective considering the ample opportunity that microbes have to consort with man. Only four of each ten exposures to gonococci actually result in gonorrhea, and it takes 10^8 vibrios, when ingested by human volunteers with normal gastric juices, to produce cholera.[8] However, normal barriers do occasionally fail, as is evident by the frequency of infectious disease.

The route by which infection enters may be (1) respiratory; (2) oral-fecal; (3) transmucosal; or (4) transcutaneous, usually aided by trauma, arthropod vectors, needles, or other contaminated devices. Most human pathogens follow a preferential route, but this does not preclude other possible entry sites. For instance, the bulk of tuberculous infections arise by droplet aspiration, but some may begin through the swallowing of infected milk or contaminated skin puncture. Moreover, the site of entry does not necessarily conform to the site of disease. The polioviruses first insensibly replicate in permissive host cells along the gastrointestinal tract, but then exert their destructive effects on neuronal targets, the anterior horn cells of the spinal cord. The tetanus bacilli may be confined to an inconspicuous contaminated skin wound but their toxin disrupts axonal transmission in the spinal cord. Usually, however, infection and disease localize and spread together.

HOST-PARASITE RELATIONSHIPS

Whether or not exposure to an infectious organism will result in disease is determined by the *virulence (or pathogenicity) of the invader* and by the *resistance of the host*. Although *infection* and *infectious disease* are words often used interchangeably, they are not synonymous. Infection refers to the ability of an organism to establish itself in a host, but its ability to produce an infectious disease relates to its *virulence.* The terms *resistance* and *virulence* are broad generalizations based on the complex host-parasite interplay that takes place at the molecular level. *High virulence implies the capability of causing disease in normally resistant people (i.e., in the majority of an exposed population). Low virulence denotes an agent effective only in hosts with low resistance, such as an opportunistic agent causing disease in hosts with impaired defense mechanisms, particularly impaired immune responses.*

The multiple parasite properties and products that, in their composite, determine virulence are only partly known; because of their variety and complexity they will be discussed as each microbial class is introduced. Host resistance, too, is clearly multifactorial, based on genetics, anatomy, and physiology as well as on the functions of the immune system. *Thus, poor circulatory or ventilatory status, debilitating systemic disease, or localized organ impairments can be equally predisposing to infectious disease as the better-known defects of phagocyte or immune function; several resistance factors can be simultaneously impaired in malnutrition, alcoholism, diabetes, and chronic hepatic or renal failure.*

The concept of *pathogenicity* involves all the following:

1. *The ability to establish infection and reproduce inside a host* by overcoming normal defenses or by taking advantage of defective host barriers.
2. *The generation of products* such as endotoxins, exotoxins, lytic enzymes, and other substances that *directly damage host tissue* beyond its normal repair capacity.
3. The *induction of host-cellular responses* that, although directed against the invader, may cause additional host damage. Thus, the immune response to the hepatitis viruses mediates the destruction of liver cells harboring viral or virus-directed antigens. Closely related is the phenomenon of cross reaction between microorganisms (nonself antigens) and self antigens, which constitutes a possible mechanism of the induction of autoimmune diseases (p. 190).

In the microbiologists' view, pathogenicity is linked to specific virulence factors such as the phage-induced exotoxin of *Corynebacterium diphtheriae*, without which this organism acts as a commensal. To the cell biologist and immunologist, host resistance is paramount. For example, during an epidemic of meningococcal infection, some contacts develop meningitis, but others carry the meningococcus in their nasal secretions for weeks without ill effect. Similarly, infections with *herpes simplex* virus I are common and may remain dormant indefinitely, detectable only by antibody titer. However, such infections also may generate "cold sores" episodically or may cause lethal pneumonia or encephalitis (p. 318).

Once introduced, pathogens may stay confined to their entry site or, if motile or reproducing beyond the capacity of host defenses to contain them, will spread, sometimes throughout the body. The routes of spread initially follow tissue planes of least resistance and the regional lymphatic and vascular anatomy. Thus, the virulent nonselective staphylococci may first induce a locally expanding skin abscess (furuncle). Depending on virulence and host resistance, this local infection may then lead to regional *lymphangitis* and *lymphadenitis*, followed by *bacteremia* (blood-borne infection) and colonization of distant organs. In the case of other, more fastidious pathogens, *tropism* determines the primary sites of tissue damage. Once a portal of entry has been gained, there is always the potential for spread to other sites. *Transient viremia, bacteremia, or parasitemia is common during the early stages of apparently localized infections, but it is usually curtailed as host leukocytic and immune responses come into play. When these are defective in an altered host or when the invader is highly virulent, spread will ensue. Major, sustained bloodstream invasion is obviously a feared consequence of any infection and is often fatal.*

HOST TISSUE RESPONSES TO INFECTION

In contrast to the almost unlimited molecular diversity of parasites, human cell types and their patterns of response are limited, as are the mediator mechanisms directing these responses. At the microscopic level, therefore, many pathogens evoke identical reaction patterns, and few of the features are unique to or pathognomonic of each agent.

Broadly speaking, there are five microscopic patterns of reaction:

1. *Exudative inflammation.* This is the familiar reaction to acute tissue damage described in Chapter 2, with increased vascular permeability and leukotaxis, predominantly of neutrophils. Massing of neutrophils results in the formation of pus. The rapidly dividing organisms that evoke this response, many of them bacteria of extracellular habit, are called "pyogenic." The chronic or healing phase of this pattern is often termed "nonspecific chronic inflammation."
2. *Necrotizing inflammation.* When tissue damage is initially severe, as in the case of highly virulent or toxic microorganisms, cell death can become the dominant feature, with relatively few reactive exudative components. These lesions may come to resemble ischemic necrosis. This reaction is also prone to appear when opportunistic pathogens acutely infect a host lacking cellular defenses.
3. *Granulomatous inflammation.* This pattern (p. 65) marked by aggregates of mononuclear phagocytes, is usually evoked by relatively slow-dividing infectious agents and by those of relatively large size, unmanageable by neutrophils alone; it is also common among the facultative intracellular organisms. Granulomas are among the more distinctive microscopic lesions and therefore suggest certain specific agents as their likely cause (e.g., mycobacteria, fungi, or parasites).

4. *Interstitial inflammation.* Diffuse, predominantly mononuclear interstitial infiltration is a common feature of all chronic inflammatory processes, but when it occurs acutely and in pure form, it is often a response to a viral agent. It also may arise in other infections that stimulate intense lymphocytic reactions, as in early treponemal diseases. This histologic pattern is often quite difficult to interpret in terms of its possible cause.

5. *Cytopathic-cytoproliferative inflammation.* When cell damage of a distinctive type precedes cell destruction, it may initiate cell replication and the formation of inclusion bodies or polykaryons. Such a reaction suggests an obligate intracellular parasite, usually a virus, even when the stromal inflammatory activity is relatively minor.

The aforementioned patterns of tissue reaction are useful as working tools in analyzing microscopic features of infective processes, but they rarely appear in pure form because they frequently overlap. More important, they are not exclusively due to infectious processes but can also be seen in tissue responses to physicochemical agents or in inflammatory diseases of unknown cause. Their most useful role is that of complementing a patient's clinical and microbiologic findings. If all three sets of observations are mutually compatible, diagnosis is assured; if not, the evidence must be reviewed for possible error or artefact. Histopathologic diagnosis, therefore, plays an important role in deciphering the nature of an infectious disease.

VIRAL DISEASES

Viruses are the most common causes of human illness, yet most human viral infections (> 400 species) are asymptomatic and go unrecognized; thus, the distinction between viral infection (replication within the host) and viral disease (replication with tissue damage) is critical. Moreover, different viruses can produce the same pathologic features (e.g., upper respiratory tract infections), and the same virus (e.g., cytomegalovirus [CMV]) can produce different diseases according to the host's resistance and age. Thus, although clinical findings can be distinctive, the role of the laboratory in viral diagnosis is all-important.[9,10]

Viruses depend on host cell metabolic and structural components for their replication—that is, *they are obligate intracellular parasites.* Each virion consists of a nucleic acid *genome* (single- or double-stranded; DNA or RNA; linear, circular, or segmented), surrounded by a *capsid* (protein coat). Single-stranded RNA may be "positive sense," serving as mRNA, or "negative sense," complementary to the positive strand (Table 7–2). The capsid is composed of one or several virus-encoded proteins arranged as repeated subunits into structures of icosahedral or helical symmetry. All helical animal viruses and some of the icosahedral type are covered by an *envelope* containing virus-specific proteins plus lipids and carbohydrates derived from host cell membranes as the virus buds through them.[9]

Viral replication cycles begin with viral *attachment* to the host cell via specific binding of viral proteins (e.g., influenza virus hemagglutinin, adenovirus fiber protein) to cellular surface receptors. Known receptors are the CD4 protein of helper lymphocytes for HIV, the C3D complement receptor for Epstein-Barr virus (EBV), and the acetylcholine receptor for rabiesvirus. Once attached, the entire virion or a portion containing the genome and essential polymerases *penetrates* the plasma membrane by receptor-mediated endocytosis, by envelope fusion with the plasma membrane, or by directly crossing the plasma membrane.

After or during penetration, the virus *uncoats* (i.e., it separates its genome from its structural components); it thus loses infectivity while entering the synthetic phase of *replication,* which is distinct for each virus family. Viral enzymes play an essential role here (e.g., RNA polymerase is needed by negative-strand RNA viruses to generate positive-stranded mRNA; reverse transcriptase is needed by retroviruses to generate DNA from their RNA template and to integrate that DNA into the host genome). Viral DNA synthesis occurs in the host nucleus, whereas RNA and protein synthesis usually takes place in the cytoplasm. Viral genomes and capsid proteins are synthesized and assembled into progeny virions and are either released directly or bud through the plasma membrane for release.

To induce systemic disease, a virus must successfully overcome natural host barriers and immune host defenses and must (1) enter the host and attach to nearby cells; (2) replicate within them; and (3) spread from the entry site to distant target cells.[11,12,13]

Viral entry can be via the respiratory, gastrointestinal, or genitourinary tract, or it can bypass the powerful skin or mucosal barriers by insect bite (arboviruses), animal bite (rabiesvirus), wound or minor abrasion (HIV), or needle (hepatitis B virus, HIV). The respiratory route is guarded by secretory IgA, alveolar macrophages, and natural killer (NK) cells and by an upward-gliding mucociliary blanket containing glycoprotein viral inhibitors. Specific receptors enable viruses to enter susceptible epithelia rather than be swept away. Thus, influenza viruses attach their hemagglutinin ligands to neuraminic acid–containing receptors of respiratory epithelial cells. Myxoviruses and paramyxoviruses use viral neuraminidase to lower the viscosity of mucus and free themselves from entrapment. Viral envelope and capsid proteins are determinants of viral infection routes (e.g., the gastrointestinal tract is defended by stomach acid, pancreatic proteolytic enzymes, and detergent bile salts, and few enveloped viruses can withstand that assault). By contrast, the capsid proteins of hepatitis A and other enteroviruses are acid-stable. Viruses may confine their pathologic attack to their primary replication site or spread systemically without causing local damage. Rotaviruses and other

Table 7-2. Human Viral Diseases and Their Pathogens

VIRAL PATHOGEN	VIRAL FAMILY	GENOMIC TYPE	DISEASE EXPRESSION
Respiratory			
Adenovirus	Adeno	DS DNA	Upper and lower respiratory tract infections (URI, LRI); conjunctivitis, diarrhea
Echovirus	Picorna	SS RNA*	URI, pharyngitis, skin rash
Rhinovirus	Picorna	SS RNA*	URI
Coxsackie virus	Picorna	SS RNA*	Pleurodynia, herpangina, hand-foot-and-mouth disease
Coronavirus	Corona	SS RNA*	URI
Influenza A, B	Orthomyxo	SS RNA†,‡	Influenza
Parainfluenza virus 1–4	Paramyxo	SS RNA†	URI, LRI, croup
Respiratory syncytial virus	Paramyxo	SS RNA†	Bronchiolitis, pneumonia
Digestive			
Mumps virus	Paramyxo	SS RNA†	Mumps, pancreatitis, orchitis
Rotavirus	Reo	DS RNA‡	Childhood diarrhea
Norwalk agent	Calici ?	SS RNA	Gastroenteritis
Hepatitis A virus	Picorna	SS RNA*	Acute viral hepatitis
Hepatitis B virus	Hepadna	DS DNA	Acute or chronic hepatitis
(Deltavirus)	?	RNA	With HBV, acute or chronic hepatitis
Non-A, Non-B hepatitis virus	?	?	Acute or chronic hepatitis
Systemic with Skin Eruptions			
Measles virus	Paramyxo	SS RNA†	Measles (rubeola)
Rubella virus	Toga	SS RNA*	German measles (rubella)
Parvovirus	Parvo	SS DNA	Erythema infectiosum Aplastic anemia
Vacciniavirus	Pox	DS DNA	Smallpox vaccine
Varicella-zoster	Herpes	DS DNA	Chickenpox, shingles
Herpes simplex virus I	Herpes	DS DNA	"Cold sore"
Herpes simplex virus II	Herpes	DS DNA	Genital herpes
Systemic with Hematopoietic Disorders			
Cytomegalovirus (CMV)	Herpes	DS DNA	Cytomegalic inclusion disease
Epstein-Barr (EBV) virus	Herpes	DS DNA	Infectious mononucleosis
HTLV I virus	Retro	SS RNA§	Adult T-cell leukemia; tropical spastic paraparesis
HTLV II virus	Retro	SS RNA§	Role still uncertain
HTLV V virus	Retro	SS RNA§	Mycosis fungoides
HIV I and II virus	Retro	SS RNA§	AIDS, ARC
Arboviral (Hemorrhagic) Fevers			
Denguevirus 1-4	Toga	SS RNA*	Dengue, hemorrhagic fever
Yellow fever	Toga	SS RNA*	Yellow fever
Colorado tick	Reo (Orbi)	SS RNA‡	Colorado tick fever
Regional hemorrhagic fever viruses	Arena	SS RNA†,‡	Bolivian, Argentinian, Lassa
	Bunya	SS RNA†,‡	Crimean-Congo, Hantaan, sandfly fever
	Filo?	SS RNA	Ebola, Marburg disease
Warty Growths			
Papillomavirus (HPV)	Papova	DS DNA	Condyloma; cervical carcinoma (HPV-16)
Molluscum virus	Pox	DS DNA	Molluscum contagiosum
Central Nervous System			
Poliovirus	Picorna	SS RNA*	Poliomyelitis
Rabiesvirus	Rhabdo	SS RNA†	Rabies
JC virus	Papova	DS DNA	Progressive multifocal leukoencephalopathy (opportunistic)
Arboviral Encephalitis viruses	Toga	SS RNA*	Eastern, Western, Venezuelan, St. Louis, California group
	Bunya	SS RNA†,‡	

HTLV, human T-cell leukemia virus; HIV, human immunodeficiency virus.

* Positive-sense genome (nucleotide sequences directly translated).

† Negative-sense genome (complementary to positive-sense strand).

‡ Segmented genome.

§ DNA step required in retroviral replication.

gastroenteritis agents both infect and damage intestinal epithelia, whereas reoviruses pass through mucosal M cells into the bloodstream without causing any detectable local injury. Herpesviruses, hepatitis B virus, HIV, and several papillomaviruses can enter through the genital mucosa. Again, some of these agents cause local pathology, others do not.

Viral spread can be via the bloodstream, lymphatics, or nerves. Hepatitis B (Dane) particles, picornaviruses, or togaviruses are transported free in the plasma, herpesviruses and HIV are carried by leukocytes, Colorado tick fever and Rift Valley fever viruses by red cells. Some viruses can replicate in macrophages traveling along lymph vessels, others find themselves inactivated. The neural route is obligatory for rabiesvirus and optional for varicella-zoster virus, which after its viremic phase hides in dorsal root ganglia, from whence it may emerge to travel along the nerves, causing painful shingles.

Infection of target cells distant from the site of entry, if not mediated by virus-specific receptors (p. 312), can be facilitated by tissue-specific proteases. Thus, paramyxoviruses are not infectious until their envelope glycoproteins undergo proteolytic cleavage. For some viruses (papillomaviruses, retroviruses) signals within the viral genome that stimulate gene transcription or translation within the host cell (enhancers, promoters, and transactivators) are important determinants of cell tropism.[14]

With respect to *virus–host cell interaction*, infection can be *abortive* (with incomplete viral replicative cycle), *latent* (the virus persists in cryptic form or is detectable only intermittently during disease episodes), or *persistent* (virions are synthesized continuously, with or without altered cell function). In *slow virus infection* there is persistent infection culminating in severe progressive disease after a long latency period. *Cell transformation* (p. 275) or, more commonly, *cell death* may also be the outcome of acute viral infection. Viral proteins inserted into the plasma membrane may damage its integrity or may promote cell fusion (paramyxoviruses, herpesviruses, HIV); viruses can inhibit cell DNA, RNA, or protein synthesis. As an example, poliovirus inactivates cap-binding protein, essential for translation of capped (cellular) mRNA while leaving translation of uncapped poliovirus mRNA unaffected. In *lytic infections*, some viruses (herpesvirus, measlesvirus) generate intranuclear or intracytoplasmic *inclusion bodies* (i.e., aggregates of virions or viral macromolecules). Because inclusions can be seen with the light microscope, they can be diagnostically useful; however, many viruses do not give rise to inclusions, and similar inclusions can have nonviral causes. Therefore, tissue culture and immunofluorescent, serologic, or molecular methods (e.g., probes for specific viral nucleic acid sequences) must often be resorted to for diagnosis.

In latent or persistent infections, both viral and host cell mutations are important. Reduction of the level of viral gene expression and avoidance of the host immune responses also play a role.[11,15] Some persistent viruses interfere with immune recognition by reducing the expression of viral polypeptides on the cell surface. They may also alter differentiated cell functions without interfering with "housekeeping functions," and this may lead to immune, neural, or endocrine deficiencies; for example, measlesvirus, influenzavirus, and CMV infect circulating leukocytes and can impair immunoglobulin synthesis and generation of cytotoxic T lymphocytes.

Because of their ability to replicate inside host cells, viruses challenge the host immune system in several unique ways.[11] Infected cells express virus-specific capsid proteins on their surface that become the target of immune defenses; in addition, viruses may infect the host's immunocompetent cells and alter their function. *Typically, viruses evoke inflammatory infiltrates composed of lymphocytes and macrophages; only with severe disease and tissue damage do neutrophils respond.*

Viral infection evokes *neutralizing antibodies*, which bind to specific epitopes on the viral capsid or envelope and can thus prevent viral attachment, penetration, or uncoating (or more than one of these); this highly specific immunity is the basis of antiviral vaccination, but it cannot protect against viruses with many antigenic variants (e.g., rhinoviruses). Specific agglutinins are formed as well and serve to enhance viral clearance by host phagocytes; activation of the alternate complement pathway in combination with antibody may result in direct lysis of enveloped viruses and of virus-infected cells. Moreover, infected cells may be killed by antibody- and complement-dependent cell-mediated cytotoxicity (ADCC).

Cellular immune responses are of critical importance in host resistance to viruses, and defects involving these immunocompetent cells can greatly aggravate viral disease, as in the case of children with the Wiskott-Aldrich syndrome (p. 223), who often die of measles pneumonia. NK cells are among the earliest antiviral defenses (with their numbers peaking at two to three days, long before antibodies), as are interferons, which either directly inhibit intracellular viral replication or boost cell-mediated responses. Next in order, activated macrophages can engulf and destroy some viruses while cytotoxic T cells (CTL) begin to recognize specific viral antigens in association with class I major histocompatibility complex (MHC) molecules and proceed to destroy host cells bearing these viral neoantigens. Because viral molecules can be expressed on cell surfaces early, prior to viral replication, CTL can limit viral spread and prevent further damage. Virus-specific T cells mediating delayed hypersensitivity and T-helper cells are instrumental in host cellular responses to viruses. Viral activation of T-helper cells may induce polyclonal B cell activation.

Immune responses to viruses can be both beneficial and damaging to the host.[11,15] Thus, antibodies may trigger immune complex disease, or they may cross react with normal cell components, resulting in direct cell injury. Anti-idiotypic antibodies (p. 189) may also be elicited and may produce abnormal cell activity by stimulating critical cell receptors. Virus-specific T cells can damage the host tissues they invade. Finally, viral infection of immunocompetent host cells (HIV, EBV) may severely impair overall host immune defenses. Despite the recent progress much remains to be learned about the role of viruses in causing and modifying the course of human disease.

VIRAL RESPIRATORY DISORDERS

Viral respiratory disorders are caused by many species and serotypes (Table 7–2). They are the most frequent and least preventable of all human infectious diseases and range in severity from the discomforting but self-limited common cold to life-threatening pneumonia, seen most often in debilitated, hospitalized, or immunosuppressed individuals. Moreover, viral infections of the lung predispose to bacterial superinfection; the rare cases of lethal bacterial pneumonia that originate outside hospitals are usually preceded by a respiratory viral prodrome. The basis of this viral-induced predisposition is not well understood but may involve breakdown of local host barriers, bronchial obstruction, and impairment of phagocyte competence.

Many agents are capable of causing respiratory disease, ranging from *upper respiratory tract infections (URIs)* such as rhinitis, sinusitis, otitis media, pharyngitis, and tonsillitis to *lower respiratory infections* (LRIs) named, as one descends the respiratory tree, laryngotracheobronchitis, bronchiolitis, interstitial pneumonia, and pleuritis. Each viral species may produce one or more of these patterns of disease:

1. Rhinoviruses remain strictly confined to the upper respiratory tract
2. Influenza mainly involves the upper and lower respiratory tracts but rarely other organs
3. Measles, rubella, and chickenpox "pass through" the respiratory tract but do not produce respiratory symptoms until secondary viremic spread has occurred

Coxsackie viruses are especially versatile: besides producing nonspecific URIs, certain A strains cause *herpangina*, a blistering inflammation of the pharynx that must be differentiated from herpes simplex or measles, and the mysterious *hand-foot-and-mouth disease.* Coxsackie B viruses can cause *pleuritis* (pleurodynia), *myocarditis*, or the *Guillain-Barré syndrome* and have been implicated in the possible causation of insulin-dependent diabetes mellitus.[15] Echoviruses characteristically produce a pharyngitis with a macular or petechial skin rash, and can also induce myocarditis. Types A and B influenza viruses are the dominating causes of lower respiratory tract infection marked by fever, myalgias, and headaches (the flu syndromes), but extrapulmonary complications may appear or even be lethal, as, for example, interstitial myocarditis or Reye's syndrome (p. 963) following aspirin therapy.[16,17] Rhinoviruses are the

major causes of the all-too-common *cold.* Their optimal growth temperature is 34°C, the temperature of nasal mucus! Respiratory syncytial viruses and parainfluenza viruses are especially important in infants and children, and can produce lethal *bronchiolitis* (croup) or *pneumonia.* Adenoviruses (31 known serotypes) can cause severe sporadic pneumonia, but are more frequently responsible for milder URI outbreaks. Some adenovirus serotypes cause *pharyngoconjunctival fever* (febrile pharyngitis with unilateral conjunctivitis); serotype B causes alarming epidemics of bilateral hemorrhagic *keratoconjunctivitis* without respiratory symptoms. Still other adenoviruses have been isolated during the occurrence of a whooping cough–like syndrome.

All these respiratory agents are contagious and are acquired largely by the respiratory route from a sick, incubating, or convalescing individual. An asymptomatic adenovirus carrier state is known among children. For all the agents the incubation time is generally brief, sometimes less than 24 hours.

MORPHOLOGY. The morphologic changes vary for each level of the respiratory tract affected. **URIs** are marked by mucosal hyperemia and swelling, with a nonspecific but predominantly lymphomonocytic and plasmacytic infiltration of the submucosa accompanied by overproduction of mucous secretions. The swollen mucosa and viscid exudate may plug the nasal channels, sinuses, or eustachian tubes and lead to suppurative secondary bacterial infection. Virus induced tonsillitis with enlargement of the lymphoid tissue within Waldeyer's ring is more characteristic of the young. Histologically, there is lymphoid hyperplasia, usually unassociated with suppuration or abscess formation such as is encountered with streptococci or staphylococci.

Laryngotracheobronchitis and bronchiolitis often accompanying the common "chest cold" are characterized by vocal cord swelling, abundant mucous exudation, and mucosal changes analogous to those encountered in the URI. Impairment of bronchociliary function invites bacterial superinfection with more marked suppuration. Plugging of small airways may give rise to focal lung atelectasis. In the more severe bronchiolar involvements, widespread plugging of secondary and terminal airways by cell debris, fibrin, and inflammatory exudate may, when prolonged, invite organization and fibrosis giving rise to so-called **viral obliterative bronchiolitis** and to permanent lung damage.

Viral pneumonias, like bacterial pneumonias, take a variety of anatomic forms. They may be patchy or disseminated, interstitial or consolidated, compatible with restoration of normal structure or responsible for permanent damage. In early and milder expressions of viral pneumonia, the involvement is patchy and restricted to an interstitial inflammatory reaction, with edema and mononuclear infiltration of the alveolar septa (p. 784). The air spaces remain clear save for scattered alveolar macrophages—**interstitial pneumonia.** The radiographic or clinical findings are not characteristic and may also be produced by *Mycoplasma pneumoniae.* With progression or in more severe involvements, the septal thickening and inflammatory infiltrate become more marked, and type II pneumocytes round up and desquamate into the alveolar spaces. Leakage of fibrinogen may disrupt the lining epithelial cells with the formation of hyaline membranes layering the septal walls (Fig. 7–2). These changes resemble those of the adult respiratory distress syndrome (diffuse alveolar damage, p. 760). In severe, fulminating, influenzal viral pneumonia, widespread fibrinohemorrhagic alveolar consolidation is superimposed on the changes described. Those viruses that have the power to cause necrosis (e.g., the adenovirus and herpesvirus families) can evoke neutrophilic responses. In many instances, however, the consolidative changes reflect bacterial superinfection. In the usual case, in the absence of parenchymal necrosis, the changes are entirely reversible, with restoration of the normal architecture. However, with protracted involvement or when there have been areas of necrosis, the inflammatory changes give way to interstitial fibrosis and organization of alveolar plugs that fuse with the septa. These changes produce the fine reticular or "ground-glass" pattern sometimes seen on chest radiography.

CLINICAL COURSE. Most URIs are transient or self-limited infections that produce manifestations too well known to merit repetition. The proverbial "take a couple of aspirins and give me a call tomorrow" is statistically sound advice. Nonetheless, these involvements require prompt attention in infants, the elderly, and persons with diabetes or preexisting chronic respiratory disease, as they impair ventilation and resistance to superimposed bacterial infection.

The LRIs such as bronchiolitis, atypical pneumonia, and the flu syndrome are far more serious. They may be associated with marked hypoxia even when there is only minimal clinical evidence of alveolar consolidation; often there are dramatic changes on the chest x-ray film without altered physical signs; hence, the designation *atypical pneumonia*. Regression of radiographic changes may lag behind improvement of the clinical status. Confusing clinical pictures

may also arise from bacterial or multiple opportunistic superinfections. Although recovery from influenza without sequelae is the rule, thousands died daily during the winter of 1918 (the year of the "swine flu"), frequently of bacterial pneumonia or sepsis. Outside the context of a known epidemic, etiologic diagnosis is difficult and is usually confirmed only during convalescence by rising serum antibody titers. In extreme cases, resort may be made to lung biopsy, but only the herpesvirus class, the measles viruses, and, rarely, the adenovirus produce diagnostic inclusion bodies by light microscopy (p. 319). Other viruses may be detectable by immunocytochemical or molecular hybridization methods. Vaccines and antiviral drugs have been only partially successful against respiratory viral infections, especially against established disease.

VIRAL DISORDERS OF DIGESTIVE TRACT

Mumps

Mumps is an acute, contagious childhood disease characterized by transient inflammation and swelling of the parotid glands and, less often, the other salivary glands. It may also involve the pancreas, testes, ovaries, and (rarely) the central nervous system or other systemic organs. Although usually mild, mumps occasionally causes acutely incapacitating, painful illness, especially in adult patients, or may leave permanent tissue destruction in its wake.

Mumps is caused by a paramyxovirus, usually acquired by respiratory droplet infection. Its peak incidence is in 5- to 15-year-olds. Asymptomatic or very mild infection is common; most but not all adults are immune. The usual duration of the acute illness is one or two weeks with gradual clinical improvement. Atypical presentations lacking parotid enlargement include abdominal pain, painful testicular swelling, or generalized lymphadenopathy and splenomegaly.

The parotitis is bilateral in about 70% of cases or unilateral in 20%, but in about 10% there is only sublingual involvement. Affected glands are enlarged, have a doughy consistency, and are moist, glistening, and reddish-brown on cross section. Testicular swelling may be spectacular, with parenchymal hemorrhage. **Microscopically,** at the peak of mumps parotitis, the gland interstitium is diffusely infiltrated by inflammatory edema and histiocytes, lymphocytes, and plasma cells, which compress acini and ducts. Sometimes there is focal necrosis and spillage of exudate into the epithelial structures. In the enzyme-rich pancreas, mumps lesions become more destructive, causing parenchymal and fat necrosis and polymorphonuclear cell infiltration. Similarly, in the testis, tightly contained by the tunica albuginea, tissue swelling may result in necrosis of seminiferous tubules with neutrophilic infiltration and focal hemorrhages and microinfarctions, thus accounting for the permanent fibrous scars sometimes left by mumps orchitis.[18]

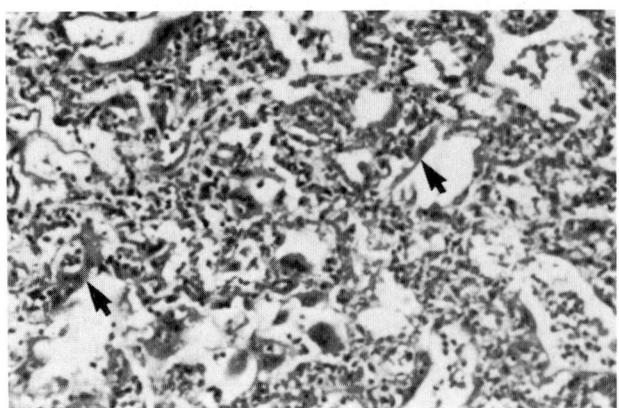

Figure 7–2. Interstitial viral pneumonia: Thickened, infiltrated septa; hyaline membranes *(arrows)*; pneumocyte desquamation; and syncytium formation.

Encephalitis or meningitis when it occurs, is usually mild and lacks distinctive pathologic features. The mumps virus does not produce characteristic cell inclusions in vivo.

Involvement of other organs may precede, accompany, or follow the parotitis. Orchitis, the most frequent (20%), is usually unilateral and is therefore rarely a cause of male sterility. Pancreatitis is detectable by elevation of the serum lipase level and by the other signs and symptoms of pancreatic necrosis (p. 983). It tends to be relatively mild and does not relapse. The diagnosis of mumps is usually made clinically, can be confirmed by convalescent serum titers, and, in the context of an outbreak, offers little difficulty. Sporadic deaths due to complicating myocarditis have been recorded. Mumps and measles live vaccines are now customarily administered together in childhood and should eventually make these infections vanish.

Viral Enteritis and Diarrhea

Viruses are major causes of acute diarrheal diseases previously attributed to uncertain causes (p. 867). Two major types of enteropathogenic viruses—rotaviruses and Norwalk agents—have now been characterized by immunoelectron microscopy, and more have been identified sporadically (e.g., astroviruses and caliciviruses). Adenoviruses are found in about 10% of diarrheas in children.

Rotaviruses are best visualized in negatively stained electron micrographs of stool ultrafiltrates, and thus far they have not been adapted to tissue culture; however, specific enzyme-linked immunosorbent assays (ELISAs) are now available.[19] Transmission is oral-fecal; children of weaning or older ages are most susceptible. Antibodies to rotavirus build up rapidly in normal humans, rendering most adults immune. The peak prevalence of disease is during the winter months in temperate climes, the dry season in the tropics. In the United States rotaviruses account for well over 50% of all childhood diarrheas; in developing countries, plagued by many diarrheal pathogens, they are responsible for between 12 and 38%. Fortunately, rotavirus diarrhea tends to be mild. Indeed, after its 48-hour incubation period, the diarrhea rarely lasts more than a few days (maximum, eight days), but fever, vomiting, and loss of appetite are frequent and induce dehydration and electrolyte imbalance, which can be lethal. *Animal studies and small bowel biopsies have shown mixed inflammatory infiltration of the lamina propria, shortening of villi, and cellular hyperplasia of mucosal crypts.*[20]

Norwalk agents (not yet fully classified) are also detectable by stool electron microscopy. Adults, as well as older children, are susceptible. Epidemics, usually local in scope, occur year-round. The incubation period can be as brief as 18 hours; the diarrhea is watery, without tenesmus, and usually abates in one or two days, although some patients may experience more prolonged and severe symptoms. Histologic findings in small bowel biopsies of human volunteers largely parallel those reported in rotavirus infection.[21] These changes last longer than do the clinical symptoms. Among the numerous causes of the adult diarrheal syndrome, Norwalk-type infections rank as relatively benign, and they require little more than bed rest and compensatory oral fluid intake.

VIRAL EPITHELIAL GROWTHS

These are listed in Table 7–2 and discussed in Chapter 27. Common features in the epithelial growths of viral origin are (1) exuberant but self-limited epithelial proliferation; (2) cytopathic changes in maturing epithelial cells (inclusion bodies or koilocytosis); and (3) predominantly mononuclear stromal and basal inflammatory infiltration.

VIRAL DISORDERS WITH EXANTHEMS OR SKIN RASHES

Measles (Rubeola)

For many centuries, rubeola was nearly universal among children 3 to 7 years old. It is an acute, febrile, systemic viral infection usually beginning with coryza and conjunctivitis, followed by typical spotty lesions inside the mouth, lymphoreticular hyperplasia, and a blotchy, generalized, erythematous (morbilliform) rash. Thanks to a 95% effective live attenuated vaccine, measles has become infrequent in the United States and Europe, and worldwide eradication is within reach.[22] However, with over 6000 cases reported in 1986, the disease seems to show potential for resurgence even in the United States.

The measles virus, an RNA paramyxovirus, is highly contagious by droplet aspiration and is transmissible via the placenta. Incubation averages ten days; fever and rash peak promptly within a few days and then gradually resolve over one or two weeks, barring complications. Photophobia and eye-burning are the first symptoms; a spotty enanthem that blisters and ulcerates deep in the cheek mucosa near the opening of Stensen's ducts (Koplik's spots) is diagnostic even before the rash begins. Swollen lymph nodes or splenic enlargement also occur early, and respiratory symptoms, especially dry cough, may be prominent; about one fifth of patients have lung opacities on chest radiograph. The rash is blotchy, reddish-brown, and barely elevated; begins behind the ears; travels down the neck, trunk, and extremities; and rarely becomes confluent. Except in severe, hemorrhagic "black measles," it blanches on pressure. The fever and symptoms usually abate as the rash blanches with mild epidermal scaling, and recovery is followed by immunity. Although generally benign in normal children, measles can be serious, especially in the very young, very old, and immunosuppressed, either by causing neural or visceral viral damage or, more commonly, because of bacterial superinfections. In children and adults in tropical countries, the illness can be fatal. Measles encephalomyelitis or interstitial, sometimes "giant cell," pneumonia can be a life-threatening acute complication. Moreover, measles has also been incriminated on varying evidence in subacute sclerosing panencephalitis (p. 1399), minimal disease nephrotic syndrome (p. 1036), and thrombocytopenic purpura (p. 692). Unlike German measles (see later), rubeola during pregnancy does not cause fetal congenital anomalies.

> Histologically, the rash is produced by dilated skin vessels, edema, and a moderate, nonspecific, mononuclear perivascular infiltrate. Ulcerated mucosal lesions in the oral cavity are marked by necrosis, neutrophils, and neovascularization. The lymphoid organs typically have marked follicular hyperplasia, large germinal centers, and randomly distributed multinucleate giant cells, called Warthin-Finkeldey cells, with eosinophilic nuclear and cytoplasmic inclusion bodies (Fig. 7–3). These are pathognomonic of measles, and on occasion permit its diagnosis from histologic examination of the lymphoid structures of an excised appendix.
>
> The milder forms of measles pneumonia show the same peribronchial and interstitial mononuclear infiltration seen in other nonlethal viral infections. In severe or neglected cases, bacterial superinfection may be a cause of death. Sometimes, diagnostic giant cells can be detected in the sputum. In debilitated children, especially those with mucoviscidosis, Wiskott-Aldrich syndrome, or lymphoreticular malignancies, measles pneumonia can be protracted and lead to respiratory failure and to pulmonary fibrosis. This picture is often referred to as "giant cell pneumonia." In such instances the virus may persist in respiratory secretions for months, long after the rash has disappeared. Uncommonly, postmeasles encephalomyelitis develops, caused, it is suspected, by an autoimmune reaction.

German Measles (Rubella)

Rubella, sometimes called "three-day measles," is a highly contagious but mild childhood systemic febrile viral infection characterized by a morbilliform (measles-like) rash and swelling of the posterior cervical lymph nodes. It is caused by a *togavirus* unrelated to the measles virus, and has a longer incubation period and a briefer, more benign course. Rubella tends to be more discomforting in adults, and is sometimes accompanied by joint pain and swelling reminiscent of rheumatic fever. The principal public health importance of rubella derives from its power to cause severe congenital malformations, mostly cardiac, when transmitted from mother to fetus (p. 520).

Smallpox (Variola)

The causative agent of smallpox, a 160-nm particle containing double-stranded DNA and terminal transcriptase, has finally been confined to cold storage in a few high-security reference centers. The last documented case of human smallpox occurred during a 1978 laboratory outbreak. All suspected cases since then have proved to be deceptive "look-alikes," some

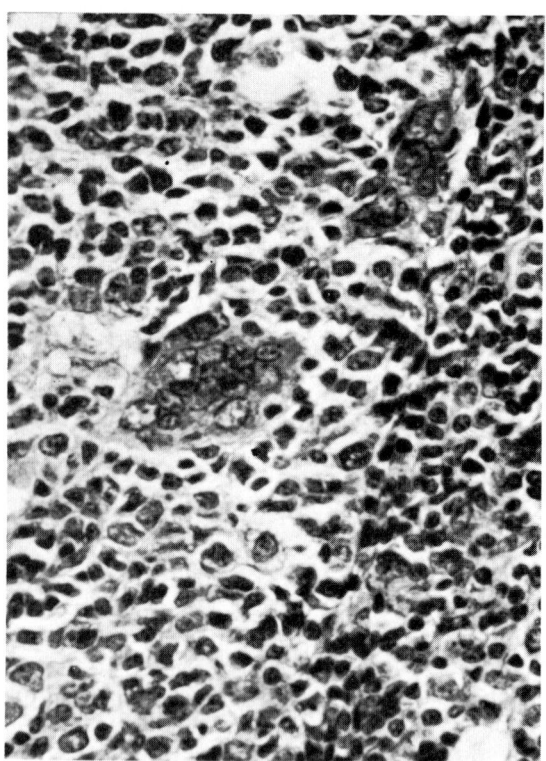

Figure 7–3. Measles giant cells in appendix.

due to the distantly related monkeypox virus or to hemorrhagic varicella.[23] Thus culminates the long and stormy history of cowpox vaccination, which began with Jenner's alertness to the well-known fact that milkmaids, unlike others of their time, rarely had their faces disfigured by pockmarks.

Should one be faced with a suspect case of smallpox today, the patient should be isolated and contacts limited to vaccinated health personnel. Expert examination of vesicle fluid is a critical step in confirming the diagnosis. Characteristic of active skin lesions are altered epidermal cells containing eosinophilic intracytoplasmic bodies *(Guarneri bodies)*. Immunofluorescence and electron microscopy should be carried out in a reference laboratory.

Other Skin Rashes

Erythema infectiosum and *roseola infantum* are two additional mild exanthematous eruptions of childhood; the former is caused by a parvovirus; the cause of the latter remains unknown. The diseases are virtually always nonfatal.

HERPESVIRUS DISEASES

The herpesviruses listed in Table 7–2 are responsible for a wide range of infections, from the trivial cold sore to lethal disseminated disease. Herpetic infections are widely prevalent throughout the world and their frequency increases with age from womb to grave; by maturity most adults carry one or another of these viruses or sometimes several, but the vast bulk of these infections are latent. Overt diseases then represent only the tip of the iceberg. Both newly acquired and activated latent infections can cause clinical disease. Whatever their clinical presentation, cutaneous or hemolymphopoietic, all herpetic infections must be considered systemic, and this is particularly true in immunodeficient and otherwise predisposed hosts. Patients treated for Hodgkin's disease or other lymphomas and recipients of bone marrow transplants are notoriously susceptible. The protean and grave systemic nature of these infections is most striking in a hospital setting, compared to the largely benign forms of disease seen in the community, such as chickenpox or infectious mononucleosis, which still make up the bulk of cases.

All the virions of the herpes family look similar by electron microscopy, just as their viral inclusions are indistinguishable by light microscopy, with the exception of those induced by the cytomegalovirus (p. 322). Yet each herpesvirus species is genetically and antigenically distinct and each differs in the disease spectrum it causes. Herpesviruses have marked host species specificity although, rarely, zoonotic infections by simian herpesviruses have induced severe illness in primate workers or fanciers.

Herpes Simplex (HSV I) and Herpes Genitalis (HSV II) Infections

Herpes simplex is transmitted by physical contact such as kissing, and is thus spread among family members and friends. About half of all babies in the United States are born with IgG antibodies to this agent transmitted across the placenta. As this immunity dissipates, new infections are acquired until, by age 45, close to 70% of people have become serologically positive—most without ever experiencing signs of disease, others after one or several episodes of fever blisters or cold sores. Only very few suffer major illnesses. By contrast, HSV II is transmitted by sexual contact or during birth; it is less prevalent overall but is likewise cumulative with age. Its incidence rises with the number of sexual partners and has therefore greatly increased in today's permissive society. Genital herpes has engendered considerable anxiety because there is tenuous evidence that it may contribute to the causation of cervical cancer, discussed in more detail on page 1142, and because of the risk of vertical transmission during childbirth inducing serious disease. Infections with both causative agents are difficult to prevent; there is as yet no vaccine.

The spectrum of both herpesvirus infections includes the following:

1. *Latency*—the virus slowly reproduces in trigeminal or other ganglia; diagnosis is made only by antibody titer.
2. *Skin or mucosal vesicles* (fever blisters, cold sores, gingivostomatitis, genital herpes).
3. *Severe vesicular eruption of the eye or skin* (herpes keratoconjunctivitis, eczema herpeticum, Kaposi's varicelliform eruption).

4. *Severe CNS lesions* (herpes simplex encephalitis, transverse myelitis).
5. *Opportunistic localized lesions of internal organs* (herpes esophagitis, herpes simplex pneumonitis).
6. *Overwhelming disseminated opportunistic infection* with focal necrosis of many organs in neonates and compromised adults.

Herpesvirus lesions, wherever located, are marked by cytopathic changes, principally the formation of Cowdry type A intranuclear inclusions. As the virions multiply within nuclei, the chromatin first fades to a lavender tinge on H and E staining and loses definition. Darkly stained chromatin clumps then cluster against the nuclear membrane and may herniate through it, imparting a spiked contour, while **the nuclear center, now containing live and dead virions is transformed into a large acidophilic inclusion separated from the nuclear rim by an artifactual cleft** (Fig. 7–4). Cell and nuclear size increase only slightly, in contrast to the striking enlargements induced by the CMV (p. 322). However, cell fusions may produce inclusion-bearing **polykaryons or giant cells,** which can also be found in smears of blister fluid **(Tzanck preparations),** confirming the diagnosis of a herpetic infection. More definitive identification of the herpesvirus within cells can be achieved by immunofluorescent methods or by DNA probes.

Fever blisters or cold sores favor the facial skin around mucosal orifices (lips, nares) but may occur in other

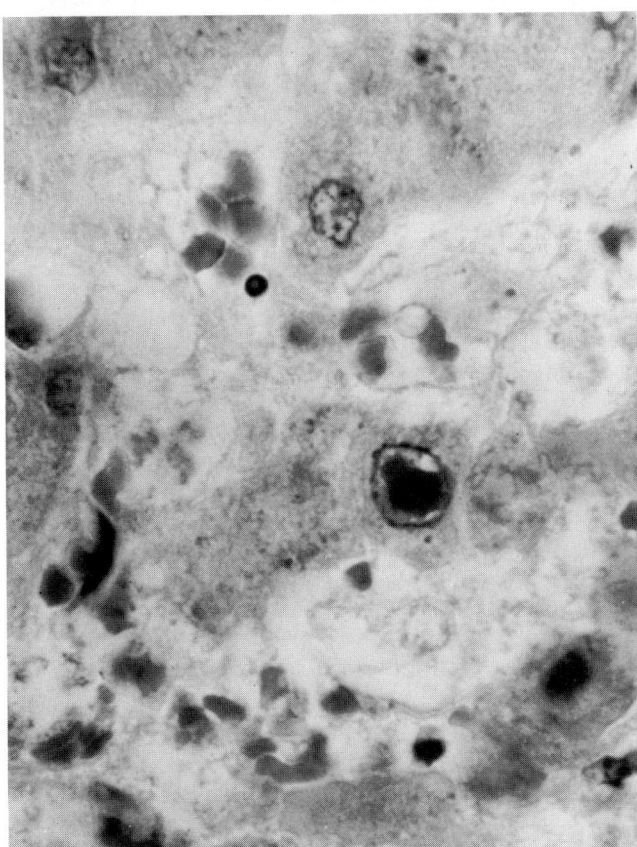

Figure 7–4. Herpes simplex inclusion body in a liver cell.

regions. Their distribution does not follow skin dermatomes, and bilateral lesions are common. Intraepithelial vesicles are created by intracellular edema and the ballooning degeneration of epidermal cells. The vesicles tend to burst, collapse, and crust promptly, but some may result in superficial ulcerations. Predisposing factors include old age, sunlight, respiratory infections, menstruation, and occasionally some underlying serious illness or hidden malignancy.

Genital herpes is characterized by vesicles on the genital mucous membranes as well as external genitalia. On moist mucosal surfaces the vesicles are transient and rapidly converted into superficial ulcerations, rimmed by an inflammatory infiltrate. The cellular changes are those already described. Large, solitary herpetic ulcers on the genitalia or lips, with swelling of satellite lymph nodes, may simulate a primary syphilitic chancre (p. 369).

Gingivostomatitis refers to a vesicular eruption that may extend from tongue to retropharynx, usually encountered in children and caused by HSV I. It must be differentiated from other vesicular eruptions in childhood, particularly that caused by Coxsackie virus, which tends to be milder and limited to the pharynx and tonsils. The herpetic infection may induce cervical lymphadenopathy and fever, but is self-limited.

Herpes keratoconjunctivitis of one or both eyes is similar to skin herpes but tends to ulcerate the delicate and gliding epithelia. It is frequently recurrent and is prone to bacterial superinfection; it may therefore cause corneal clouding, deep inflammation, and eventual blindness. Antiviral drugs, including acyclovir, can ameliorate this disorder.[24]

Kaposi's varicelliform eruption is a generalized vesiculating involvement of the skin occurring mainly in immunodeficient persons and those with previous dermatitis.

Eczema herpeticum is even more severe and is characterized by confluent, pustular, or hemorrhagic blisters. Bacterial superinfection is common, as is dissemination of the viral infection to internal viscera. Both these patterns of herpetic dermatitis can prove fatal.

Herpes simplex encephalitis is described on page 1397. This highly lethal involvement of the brain, usually by HSV I, appears in the absence of a skin rash. With state-of-the-art therapy, the salvage rate has increased modestly.

Visceral and disseminated herpes infections are usually encountered in particular clinical settings. Esophagitis almost always represents activation of a latent infection in hospitalized patients with some form of underlying cancer or under immunosuppressive treatment. The mucosal vesicles and ulcerations are no different from those already described, but they are readily superinfected by bacteria or fungi. Similarly, herpes bronchopneumonia, often necrotizing, is seen in predisposed individuals, particularly when an airway must be inserted through oral herpes territory.[25] Disseminated infection most often occurs in neonates, particularly premature babies, or those with abnormal immune systems. Usually, HSV II is transmitted during passage through the birth canal of infected mothers; this can be prevented by cesarean delivery when the risk is known. The disseminated disease in the neonate may be mild, but it is more often fulminating with generalized lymphadenopathy, splenomegaly, and necrotic foci throughout the lungs, liver, adrenals, and CNS. Brain damage may persist in the few infants who recover. Disseminated infections may also arise in adults, most often during cancer chemotherapy or immunosuppression following marrow and organ transplants. Necrotic foci may be present throughout the body, particularly in the liver and lungs, leading to hepatic failure or death from respiratory complications. In all these visceral and disseminated involvements, typical intranuclear inclusions often provide the etiologic diagnosis but may not be present in all of the lesions.

Chickenpox (Varicella) and Herpes Zoster

These two seemingly disparate disorders are both caused by the varicella-zoster virus (VZV) and are therefore closely related.

Chickenpox is an acute, highly contagious, but mild systemic viral infection with a vesicular, generalized skin eruption. It is today the most common infectious childhood rash, with a frequency hovering around 200,000 cases per year in the United States. It is usually of little consequence in normal children, but in those with immunodeficiencies it may cause pneumonitis, encephalitis, disseminated visceral lesions, and sometimes purpuric skin lesions. Severe neonatal disease may occur when the mother becomes infected shortly before delivery, but, *unlike German measles, infection during gestation rarely induces congenital malformations in the offspring.* In the usual childhood form of chickenpox the infection is acquired through the respiratory route, and after two to three weeks of silent incubation is followed by a viremia. A generalized rash appears, progressing rapidly from a macular to a vesicular stage without forming pustules. Each individual lesion resembles *"a dew drop on a rose petal."* Usually, several crops of lesions succeed each other, traveling from the trunk centrifugally to the face and extremities. *The lack of synchrony best differentiates this eruption from that caused by smallpox.* However, the rare, severe form may resemble hemorrhagic smallpox. Blistering may also occur on the buccal mucosa. Wherever they appear, the vesicles rupture, the rash crusts and scales, and the condition resolves within about a week. Lymph node swelling and calcified spots on chest x-ray may persist. The adult with varicella tends to be sicker than the child, with a greater tendency to develop pneumonitis or encephalitis. More often, infection with VZV remains latent in adults or else appears as herpes zoster.

Herpes zoster, also known as shingles, represents a reactivation of a latent VZV infection as shown by its greater frequency with advancing age. *Adults with shingles can transmit varicella to children, but not the converse.* The pathogenesis involves a previous attack of chickenpox followed by years of latency of the VZV in the sensory dorsal root ganglia. During an attack of shingles, reactivated virus travels centrifugally from the ganglia to the skin of the corresponding dermatomes, resulting in a localized vesicular eruption that is similar to that of chickenpox but differentiated by the often intense itching, burning, or sharp pain in the affected skin segment because of a simultaneous radiculoneuritis. Indeed, the pain may be disproportionate to the rash, especially when the trigeminal branches are involved; involvement of the geniculate ganglion may induce a facial paralysis (Ramsay Hunt syndrome). In more than 50% of cases, only a single unilateral thoracic dermatome is involved, but several crops of lesions may arise or recur after long intervals. Sometimes the eruptions are bilateral. Herpes zoster lesions are prone to appear in persons with advanced neoplastic disease, or, following immunosuppressive drugs, nearly one third of Hodgkin's disease patients treated with aggressive chemotherapy develop VZV lesions, usually within the first two years after treatment. In these circumstances, VZV may become disseminated and hemorrhagic, with widespread mucosal and visceral necrosis but only a feeble inflammatory response. In contrast, in the absence of a predisposing factor, shingles tends to follow a protracted but benign course.

> The herpes zoster skin vesicles are identical morphologically to those caused by HSV I and are replete with intranuclear inclusions. In chickenpox vesicles tend to remain intraepithelial, and healing therefore occurs by regeneration, leaving no scars. Traumatic rupture of the vesicles and bacterial superinfection lead to destruction of the basal epidermal layer, with a commensurately greater inflammatory response and a greater tendency to residual scarring. Hence, there is sound basis for the admonition "Don't scratch"! In severe varicella, focal hemorrhages may occur into and around the blisters.
>
> Herpes zoster is marked by a dense, predominantly mononuclear infiltrate into the sensory ganglia. Neurons and their supporting cells develop typical herpetic intranuclear inclusions, and occasional neurons may undergo necrosis with permanent loss. Interstitial pneumonia resembling that of other viral infections, encephalitis, and transverse myelitis are other potential sequelae of herpes zoster. Moreover, immunosuppressed patients may develop severe, necrotizing visceral lesions similar to those of disseminated herpes, often together with other opportunistic infections.

Cytomegalic Inclusion Disease (CID)

Cytomegalic inclusion disease is an exceedingly protean viral disease caused by the cytomegalovirus (CMV), a member of the herpesvirus group. Several serotypes of CMV have been isolated in humans that differ in antigenicity. Congenital infection contracted in utero bears little resemblance to the postnatally acquired disease in infants, which in turn differs from the infection in adults.

The infectious agent is spread through (1) intrauterine transmission to the fetus following a newly acquired infection or reactivation of a latent infection in the mother, (2) perinatal transmission to the fetus as it passes through the birth canal of a mother with a cervicovaginal infection, (3) respiratory droplet transmission among children and possibly between adults, (4) blood transfusions (in about 5% of blood donors the circulating leukocytes show latent CMV infections), (5) transplantation of virus-infected grafts from a donor with latent infection, (6) venereal transmission (virus has been isolated from both semen and vaginal fluid), and (7) transmission through mother's milk.[26]

By isolation of virus from secretions of the oral cavity or urine or by rising antibody titers, it has been shown that there are three peak periods of contraction of the virus. The first is in utero. Such infections may remain latent and have little effect on the fetus, or they may have a devastating impact on the brain and kill in utero or within the first weeks of life. The second peak occurs after birth and after the loss of maternal antibodies; thus, about 10% of all infants develop complement-fixing antibodies during the first year of life. Some of these infections may be acquired in the birth canal or during breast feeding. Most of these children, whatever the severity of the infection, continue to excrete virus for many months to years. There follows a period up to age 15 years during which the frequency of identifiable antibody increases more slowly, from approximately 10 to 20%. The third peak occurs after age 15, when the frequency of infection again rises. In the aggregate, between 50 and 80% of adults show evidence of exposure to CMV in the form of complement-fixing antibodies. Primary infection in adults is usually followed by only transient excretion of virus in the throat or urine for a few days to weeks. However, a pregnant woman acquiring a new infection will excrete virus from the throat, urine, and cervix throughout pregnancy and even in the breast milk for months afterward. *Despite the high frequency of infection in adults, it is almost always latent and asymptomatic unless the patient is immunocompromised (e.g., AIDS, p. 224) or debilitated.*[27] However, healthy adults who receive transfusions of large volumes of blood from multiple donors may acquire CID. Whether symptomatic infections in adults, or even in children, represent reactivation of endogenous latent virus or acquisition of a fresh infection often remains uncertain.

In neonates, full-blown, congenital, classic CID closely resembles erythroblastosis fetalis (p. 527). Affected infants are often premature or below average birth weight, and at birth or soon after manifest a hemolytic form of anemia, jaundice, thrombocytopenia, purpura, hepatosplenomegaly (due to extramedullary hematopoiesis), pneumonitis, deafness, chorioretinitis, and, most important, neurologic manifestations associated with extensive brain damage. At least half the infants with such severe disease die; some survive but are mentally retarded, whereas others with perhaps less overwhelming infection recover completely. However, it is now clear that *most congenital infections, perhaps as many as 90%, evoke no clinical manifestations at birth.* Despite this benign presentation, in rare cases, brain damage becomes evident over the span of the next few years. Between the extremes of classic CID and asymptomatic infections are those infants who suffer relatively minor illnesses, taking the form of hematologic derangements (often with purpura), mild respiratory disease, transient forms of hepatitis, or simply failure to thrive. Hepatosplenomegaly is often present in those with mild manifestations, and some have clinical evidence of neurologic involvement.

Congenital CID is therefore an unpredictable disease, and even those with mild or asymptomatic infections may suffer serious consequences years later, as shown in Figure 7–5.

In classic CID the most prominent and characteristic findings are markedly enlarged cells, with large pleomorphic nuclei harboring intranuclear inclusions. The inclusion may have a diameter half that of the nucleus and, like those of HSV, is surrounded by a clear halo, sharply demarcating it from the nuclear membrane. Smaller basophilic cytoplasmic inclusions are also seen and probably represent viral coat protein or complete viral units (Fig. 7–6). Cells so affected may not induce inflammatory reactions, but others die and evoke a leukocytic response. Inclusions and focal necroses may be found in virtually any organ, most often, in descending order of frequency, in the salivary glands, kidneys, liver, lungs, gut, pancreas, thyroid, adrenals, and brain. Cytomegalic inclusions are often abundant in the renal tubular epithelium and occasionally within endothelial cells of glomeruli. Desquamation of tubular cells sometimes permits diagnosis of this disease by examination of the urinary sediment. Similar cellular changes are often present in hepatocytes and almost always in the lining cells of portal bile ducts. Extramedullary hematopoiesis may induce marked hepatic as well as splenic enlargement. In some infants there are focal hepatic necroses. Lung changes take the form of an interstitial pneumonitis, accompanied by the characteristic intracellular inclusions in the alveolar lining cells and in endothelial cells of septal capillaries as well as in alveolar macrophages. Depending on the severity of the infection, intra-alveolar edema, proteinaceous exudate, and focal hyaline membranes may appear. Cytomegalic changes, focal necroses, or even sharply punched-out ulcerations may occur in the small and large intestines.

Damage to the brain is the most lethal aspect of classic CID. **Two types of lesions** are seen — focal acute inflammatory changes, with inclusion-bearing giant cells distributed principally in a narrow band in the subependymal and subpial tissue, and necrotic lesions irregularly scattered in the cerebrum. Most characteristic of CID is the tendency for these lesions to be located about the lateral ventricles and the aqueduct, down to the fourth ventricle. Frequently the foci of injury become calcified, and the location of these calcifications about the ventricles provides one of the most important clinical diagnostic clues to this infection. The neuronal cells within and about the areas of focal damage show all ranges of injury from chromatolysis to frank necrosis, and microcephaly or hydrocephalus sometimes develops.

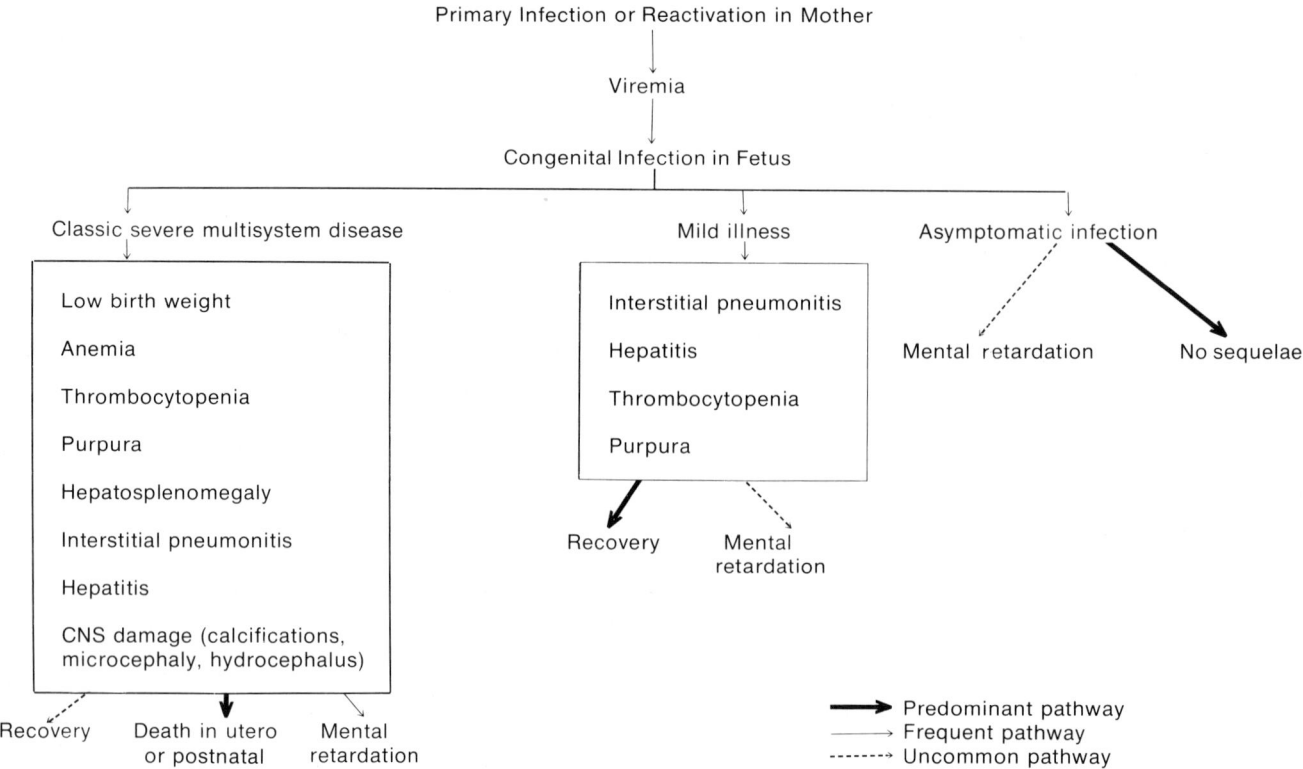

Figure 7–5. Potential pathways of congenital CID.

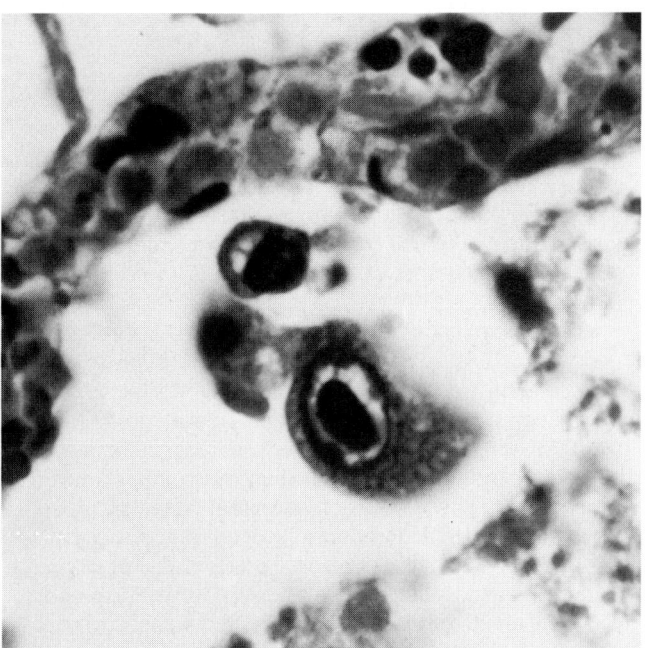

Figure 7-6. CMV nuclear and cytoplasmic inclusions in lung.

In less severe congenital CID, cytomegaly and inclusions are generally less frequent and less widely distributed. Sometimes, multinucleated giant cells appear in the liver, particularly in those children in whom the principal clinical manifestations are related to hepatitis.

Infections acquired postnatally tend, on the whole, to be asymptomatic but sometimes induce mild, transient illness. Symptoms and signs, when they appear, are extremely varied and include hepatosplenomegaly with or without evidence of hepatitis, interstitial pneumonitis, or enterocolitis secondary to ulcerative lesions in the intestines. Only rarely is the central nervous system obviously infected.

As unpredictable as CID is in childhood, it is even more so in adulthood. Much depends on the immunologic competence of the adult. In compromised hosts, e.g., AIDS, CID may produce an opportunistic infection, with involvement of organs as widespread as is seen in the classic congenital form of the disease, except that the CNS is rarely involved. Indeed, in such cases it is quite common to find concomitant invasion by other opportunists such as fungi and *Pneumocystis carinii* (p. 401). More often in adults, CID affects only the lungs and intestinal tract. The pulmonary changes are similar to those described in the congenital form of the disease.[28] In the small and large intestine, ulceroinflammatory lesions develop, often accompanied by the characteristic cytomegaly and inclusions within local endothelial and mucosal cells. Rarely, intestinal perforations may ensue. CMV chorioretinitis can occur alone or together with other organ involvements and, unless treated, will result in blindness.

Otherwise healthy children or adults may develop an infectious mononucleosis–like syndrome especially following transfusion of large volumes of blood from donors with latent CMV infections.[29] These patients manifest fever with lymphocytosis and atypical lymphocytes in the circulating blood, closely resembling infectious mononucleosis and distinguished from it only by the persistently negative heterophil tests (p. 325). Almost always this syndrome is self-limited and followed by complete recovery.

Infectious Mononucleosis (IM)

Infectious mononucleosis is a benign, self-limited lymphoproliferative disease caused by the Epstein-Barr virus (EBV), one of the herpesviruses.[30] *It is characterized by fever, generalized lymphadenopathy, sore throat, and the appearance in the blood of atypical activated T lymphocytes (mononucleosis cells.)* IM also affects the spleen, liver, and less often the heart, lungs, kidneys, hematopoietic system, and CNS. Thus, it may mimic other disorders, particularly viral hepatitis. Conversely, other viral agents, notably CMV, may produce clinical syndromes that can be differentiated from EBV disease only serologically. EBV is also strongly suspected of contributing to the causation of African (endemic) Burkitt's lymphoma and nasopharyngeal carcinoma, but it is not regularly found in patients with Burkitt's lymphoma outside of Africa (p. 715). Also, the role of EBV infection in triggering or complicating disease manifestations of AIDS is currently under discussion.

IM occurs principally in late adolescence or young adulthood, but may occasionally arise in children and the aged. It is more frequent in upper socioeconomic classes in developed nations. The reasons for this distribution are as follows: In most of the world, primary infection with EBV generally occurs in childhood and is usually asymptomatic. These infections confer immunity and eradicate the virus. Perhaps as many as 20% of the population in western countries harbor infected lymphocytes and shed infectious virus from the oropharynx.[31] In privileged societies, contact with such reservoir hosts may be delayed until late adolescence or young adulthood; in these delayed primary infections, symptomatic IM appears.

The EBV virus is transmitted from person to person, often by kissing, with transfer of virally contaminated saliva. In a susceptible seronegative host (lacking antibodies), the virions invade and replicate within salivary gland epithelial cells and then enter B cells in the lymphoid tissues, which possess receptors for the virus. A replicative virus cycle ensues, with dissemination of the agent either through the bloodstream or by the spread of the infected B cells themselves. In either event, death of the infected B cells with viremia produces an acute febrile reaction and specific immunologic responses. As antibodies appear, infectious virus disappears from the blood. IgM and later IgG antibodies to viral capsid antigen can be demonstrated. Virus neutralizing antibodies and antibodies to virus-directed B-cell membrane antigens also appear. These peak about two weeks after the infection and persist throughout life. Other virus-determined antibodies arise, and also transient heterophil (Paul-Bunnell) antibodies, whose association with EBV is still not well understood.

Although infectious B cells and free virions disappear from the blood following the humoral-antibody response, *EBV-transformed B lymphocytes carrying the virus genome integrated into their own DNA continue to be present in the circulation.* Such cells, if explanted in culture, are capable of indefinite reproduction ("in vitro immortality"), whereas cultures of normal B lymphocytes can be grown only for brief periods. In this latent form, the virus does not cause a full cytocidal replicative viral cycle. However, expression of at least some of the virus-determined antigens continues within these B cells, particularly a lymphocyte-detected membrane antigen. This membrane antigen is recognized by T-killer cells and stimulates their multiplication. *These T-killer cells are the atypical cells seen in the blood in mononucleosis,* and it is the stimulation of T cells throughout the body that is responsible for the lymphadenopathy and hepatosplenomegaly. The sore throat so typical of this disease in its early stage may be due to necrosis of B cells and possibly epithelial cells in the early virus replicative cycle in the oropharynx. The progressive increase in virus-specific antibodies and T-killer cells eventually brings the disease under control and eliminates the latently infected B cells.

Thus, in summary, the B cells in IM are infected and develop virus-directed membrane antigens that evoke a killer-cell (T-cell) response as the ultimate cause of the lymphoidal and visceral reaction throughout the body.

MORPHOLOGY. Anatomic studies have been confined largely to excised lymph nodes and liver biopsies, and to the rare patients who have died of rupture of the spleen or other complications.[32]

The **peripheral blood** usually shows an absolute lymphocytosis with a total white cell count between 12,000 and 18,000, 95% of which are lymphocytes. Many of these are atypical T lymphocytes approximately 12 to 16 μm in diameter, with an abundant, finely granular, basophilic cytoplasm. The nucleus is variable in shape and has no distinctive viral inclusion. The nuclear chromatin usually is finely divided but may be clumped. Nucleoli are generally absent. The most distinguishing features are small fenestrations or vacuolations in the cytoplasm. These abnormal cells are usually sufficiently distinctive to permit the diagnosis of IM on peripheral blood smear.

The **lymph nodes** are moderately enlarged throughout the body, principally in the posterior cervical, axillary, and groin regions. They show striking immunoproliferation of T cells in their paracortical zones, which become flooded by lymphocytes of varying size. There is, in addition, some B-cell reaction within the follicles. These become enlarged with prominent germinal centers, exhibiting many mitoses, or may become blurred as the follicular center cells intermingle with the perifollicular and paracortical cells. This lymphoproliferative reaction distorts but does not totally efface the normal architecture.[33] **Occasionally, large binucleate cells, Reed-Sternberg–like cells (p. 719), are found in these nodes,** and so the changes of IM must be differentiated from those of Hodgkin's disease (p. 717). Leukemia, too, must be ruled out by observing the normal but immunostimulated patterns of lymph node architecture characteristic of IM.

The **spleen** is usually enlarged to two to three times its normal size and is soft and fleshy with a hyperemic cut surface. The trabecular markings and follicular structure may become indistinct. Histologically, there may be prominence of the splenic follicles, or the architecture may be blurred by the heavy accumulation of immunostimulated lymphocytes. These cells sometimes infiltrate the trabeculae and the capsule, and they may contribute in this way to easy rupture, an important clinical complication of this condition. Increased numbers of plasma cells are often present.

The **liver** is sufficiently affected in most cases to cause elevated serum levels of glutamic pyruvic transaminase (SGPT) and other enzymes, but it is usually only mildly or moderately enlarged and is otherwise not unusual in its gross appearance. Histologically, there are three principal alterations: portal infiltrations, consisting almost entirely of abnormal mononuclear cells; invasion of the sinusoids by the same cells; and areas of scattered parenchymal necrosis filled with mononuclear cells. These changes may be difficult to differentiate from viral hepatitis.[34]

The **central nervous system** may be affected with congestion, edema, and perivascular mononuclear infiltrates in the leptomeninges. Focal aggregates of mononuclear cells may occur in the perivascular areas of the brain substance. Myelin degeneration and destruction of axis cylinders in the peripheral nerves are infrequent.

An interstitial "viral-type" pneumonitis has been observed in the lungs, and atypical lymphocytes have been described in the heart and bone marrow.

CLINICAL COURSE. Diagnosis of IM can be difficult because of its varied presentations and must be based on the sum of clinical, hematologic, and serologic findings. The disease often starts with chills, fever, malaise, sore throat, and painful enlargement of the cervical nodes. Pharyngitis and tonsillitis may be associated with a creamy exudate over these structures. Fine pinpoint petechiae in the palate are present at the height of the illness in somewhat fewer than half of the cases. Differential diagnosis must include streptococcal sore throat. A macular skin rash resembling rubella develops in 10 to 15% of cases. Splenomegaly may give rise to left upper quadrant pain or discomfort, and there may be tender hepatomegaly indigestion, and loss of appetite. The differential diagnosis in such cases is often infectious (viral) hepatitis. In other instances, the striking lymphocytosis associated with the lymphadenopathy raises the specter of leukemia. The clinical course is usually one of progressive improvement after two to four weeks of febrile illness, but the intercurrence of hepatic involvement or myocarditis with its associated T-wave abnormalities may prolong the disease. A rare, chronic form of IM has recently been documented.[35] Fatalities are rare in normal immunologic reactors and are attributable to rupture of the spleen or to such intercurrent infections as pneumonia and meningitis.

The hematologic findings (i.e., the elevated white count with a relative lymphocytosis and recognition of the atypical lymphocytes) are crucial to diagnosis. Abnormal levels of sheep red cell agglutinins (heterophil test) are usually present. Far more specific are the serodiagnostic procedures relating to the EBV antibodies discussed earlier.

Several kindreds of the X-linked recessive lymphoproliferative syndrome marked by an immunodeficiency state (described on p. 221) have been studied whose anomalous responses to the EBV included acutely lethal mononucleosis, development of autoimmune disease, and the delayed appearance of lymphomatous malignancies and leukemia (Fig. 7–7).[36] These observations and those on AIDS and on African Burkitt's lymphoma constitute a link between defective T-cell function, viral oncogenesis, and chromosomal translocations in the induction of neoplasia (p. 288).

ARBOVIRUS DISEASES*

Transmission of the arthropod-borne (ar-bo-) viruses depends on the geographic distribution of their specific insect vectors and animal reservoirs; globally such modes of spread cause only local outbreaks. However, human-to-human transmission by common mosquitoes can occur as happened historically during epidemics of yellow fever.[37] Future disasters of this kind are by no means unimaginable. Recently, Cuba and Puerto Rico have suffered dengue fatalities, and an efficient dengue vector mosquito has been detected in the southern United States. Arboviral disease manifestations range from a mild flulike syndrome to severe acute encephalitis (see p. 313) or to lethal hemorrhagic fever. Five domestic mosquito-borne encephalitis viruses have caused outbreaks in the United States (Table 7–2, p. 313). In addition, Colorado tick fever due to an arbovirus is endemic in that state. In its geographic distribution, tick vector, and clinical features it resembles Rocky Mountain spotted fever, a rickettsial infection (p. 332).

Although yellow fever has lately been confined to its monkey reservoir in the jungle, dengue fever remains widespread throughout the tropics. In its usual clinical form it resembles influenza but is characteristically accompanied by gnawing bone pain (breakbone fever). In severe, hemorrhagic dengue, seen mainly during Southeast Asian and Caribbean epidemics, a disseminated intravascular coagulation (DIC)–like syndrome is superimposed and the ensuing pulmonary and cerebral hemorrhages often prove rapidly fatal, especially in children.[38] Other fulminat-

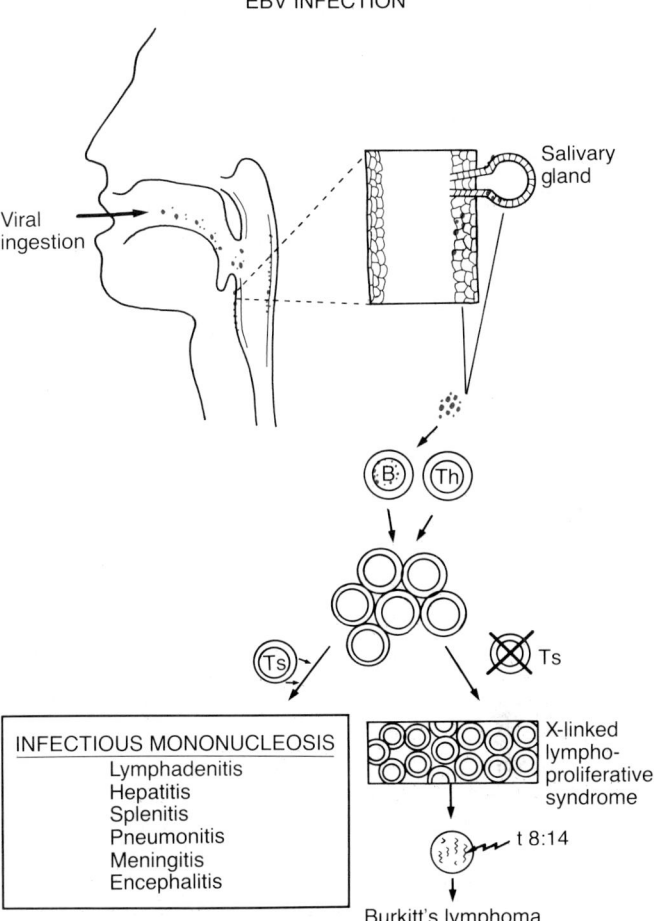

EBV INFECTION

Figure 7–7. The pathways of transmission of the Epstein-Barr virus leading in a normal individual to infectious mononucleosis or in those with a cell-mediated deficit to the X-linked lymphoproliferative syndrome and possibly to Burkitt's lymphoma when combined with an 8:14 autosomal translocation. Th = T helper cells. Ts = T suppressor/cytolytic cells.

ing hemorrhagic fevers (Table 7–2) can indiscriminately kill doctors, nurses, or laboratory workers, as happened during the well-publicized Lassa, Marburg, and Ebola virus disasters. There is no specific therapy to date, and these viruses must be handled with extreme caution.

VIRAL DISEASES OF THE CENTRAL NERVOUS SYSTEM

These diseases are described in detail in Chapter 29 and are listed in Table 7–2. It should be kept in mind that CNS manifestations may occur in many systemic viral infections not considered to be neuropathic and that *CNS damage may be direct or indirect, immediate or delayed.*

VIRAL HEART DISEASE

Viral heart diseases are discussed in Chapter 13. Of the viruses listed in Table 7–2, those most likely to damage the myocardium are the Coxsackie A and B viruses, echoviruses, poliovirsus, and influenza viruses.

VIRAL HEPATITIS

Infections caused by the human hepatitis viruses and their role in cirrhosis and liver cancer are discussed on page 959. Impairment of liver function may also occur in many other systemic viral infections, most commonly those of the herpesvirus family (Table 7–2). In addition, the yellow fever and hemorrhagic fever viruses can cause liver failure in previously normal persons.

RETROVIRAL DISEASES—HUMAN T-CELL LEUKEMIA, AIDS, KAWASAKI'S SYNDROME

Discovery of the retroviral causes of human T cell leukemia (HTLV-1, p. 734) and of the adult immuno-deficiency syndrome (AIDS, p. 224) has greatly expanded—no, transformed—our concepts of virus-induced diseases. The T-cell leukemia is the most solid link between a virus and a form of neoplasia in humans. And, as no one needs to be told, AIDS has already become a devastating pandemic. The recent finding of reverse transcriptase in lesions of Kawasaki's syndrome (Chapter 12) also points toward a possible viral causation.

AIDS is discussed in Chapter 5, HTLV-1 in Chapter 15, and Kawasaki's syndrome in Chapter 12.

CHLAMYDIAL DISEASES

Chlamydiae are obligate intracellular organisms, larger than viruses, which possess both DNA and RNA and form their own cell walls, much like bacteria. They also respond to wide-spectrum antibiotics, but not to the penicillins. Chlamydiae are passively taken up into phagocytic vacuoles of host cells in which they multiply, alternating between large (1000 nm) and small (200 to 300 nm) forms (*initial* vs. *elementary bodies*). Cytoplasmic chlamydial inclusions, important in microscopic diagnosis, consist of aggregates of these bodies in their vacuoles; they are best visualized by immunofluorescence or in Giemsa-stained cell smears. By an unknown mechanism, chlamydiae inhibit the fusion of lysosomes with primary phagosomes, and are thus protected from attack by proteases and oxygen-derived free radicals.

Chlamydiae synthesize their own nucleic acids but not their own ATP, and unlike viruses they cannot dictate host cell synthesis of new products. They have therefore served as unique models for analyzing parasite–host cell metabolic interactions.[39] Some human chlamydial infections such as inclusion body conjunctivitis and ornithosis are acute; others such as trachoma or venereal disease tend to be protracted, causing chronic inflammatory reactions, including granulomas. Both antibodies and cellular immunity are induced, but neither seems to cope effectively with established chronic infections. The subclassification of chlamydiae is still in a state of flux. Table 7–3 lists the known serotypes and corresponding human diseases.

Ornithosis (Psittacosis)

Ornithosis is caused by *Chlamydia psittaci*, transmitted to man by inhalation of dust-borne contaminated excreta from infected birds. Not just parrots, but many species of birds from canaries to seagulls, sick or ostensibly well, may harbor and transmit this infection.[40] Rarely, the disease is acquired through the bite of a bird or by direct contact with a patient. Household and larger epidemics have been reported. In man, *inhalation of the agent may lead to an asymptomatic infection, a transient flulike illness, or a serious, even fatal pneumonia.*

The incubation period varies from one to three weeks and is followed by the relatively sudden onset of fever and chills, malaise, headache, sore throat, and a nonproductive cough of variable severity. As in viral pneumonitis, dyspnea and hyperpnea may be pronounced at a time when cough, sputum, and chest physical signs are scarce or absent. X-ray findings do not always convey the extent of interstitial lung involvement. However, in the severest cases, there is pulmonary edema, alveolar damage, and consolidation; bacterial superinfection may further complicate the picture.

Table 7–3. Human Chlamydial Diseases and Species

SPECIES AND SEROTYPE	DISEASES	TRANSMISSION
Chlamydia psittaci	Ornithosis (psittacosis)	Aspiration of bird-contaminated particles
Chlamydia trachomatis		
A, B, Ba, C	Trachoma	Repeated contact, fomites, insects
D, E, F, G, H, I, J, K	Inclusion conjunctivitis	Birth canal infection (infants)
		Sexual contact, swimming (adults)
"	Nongonorrheal urethritis	Sexual contact
"	Postgonorrheal urethritis	Sexual contact
"	Proctitis, pharyngitis, cervicitis, arthritis	Sexual contact
L_1, L_2, L_3	Lymphogranuloma venereum	Sexual contact

The lung has focal, dusky areas of increased consistency and hyperemia and is increased in weight. The pleural surfaces are usually not affected. The bronchi and bronchioles show little change but in some cases considerable hyperemia, edema, and mucopurulent exudation are present. Histologically, there is edema and mononuclear leukocytic infiltration within the alveolar septa. Seroproteinaceous fluid or fibrin may accumulate in the air spaces, accompanied by mononuclear leukocytes. The alveolar septal cells are often hypertrophic and cuboidal. Occasionally, **intracytoplasmic bodies can be identified in these alveolar cells with the Giemsa or immunofluorescent technique.** They appear as coccoid bodies, 0.25 to 4.0 μm, dark blue on Giemsa stain of smears or sections. Necrosis of alveolar septa may lead to the formation of abscesses accompanied by neutrophilic infiltration or hemorrhages. There is focal variation in the severity of lung involvement. The hilar nodes are usually enlarged and edematous and show reticuloendothelial hyperplasia and acute lymphadenitis. **Lethal generalized disease,** seen mainly in epidemics, is marked by focal necroses in the liver and spleen and by diffuse mononuclear infiltrative changes in the kidneys, heart, and (sometimes) brain.

In the usual case, after two to three weeks of illness, the condition improves spontaneously or with therapy, and most patients recover. A fourfold rise in specific antibody to *C. psittaci* is considered diagnostic and can be confirmed by yolk sac or tissue culture inoculation. The prognosis is dependent on the virulence of the infective agent, and fatality rates ranging from 5 to 40% have been reported. It is important to note that immunity to this infection is incomplete, and that a carrier state may persist for years following recovery from active disease.

Chlamydial Urethritis and Cervicitis

These venereal infections are now the most frequent forms of chlamydial disease in the United States; more than half a million new cases of nongonorrheal urethritis are being reported annually, largely in males (p. 1095). These infections are often recognized by their persistence following treatment for gonorrhea (postgonococcal urethritis). Close to 50% are due to one of eight serotypes of *C. trachomatis* (Table 7–3). Chlamydiae can also be cultured from 30 to 50% of the asymptomatic female partners of these infected males, and from women with chronic cervicitis. Infants born to infected mothers may develop inclusion conjunctivitis or neonatal pneumonia.

Microscopically, in chlamydial infection one looks for inclusions in epithelial cells rather than for cocci in the leukocytes of the exudate. Former dependence on special stains for typical inclusions in cell smears has been eliminated by the use of fluorescent antibodies that reveal both inclusions and elementary bodies and provide greater diagnostic accuracy. Culture on McCoy cells and a microcomplement fixation test for type-specific chlamydial antibody are also available in specialized venereal disease centers and are applicable to secretions as well as to serum. For further detail, see page 1095.

Inclusion Conjunctivitis

Inclusion conjunctivitis is a benign, self-limited, suppurative conjunctivitis that occurs in newborns of mothers having *C. trachomatis* birth canal infections. Adults acquire this disease by contamination with genital secretions or by bathing in unchlorinated swimming pools (swimming pool conjunctivitis). *The chlamydial inclusions seen in the exudate are identical with those of trachoma,* but this more benign conjunctivitis is due to a different group of *C. trachomatis* serotypes (Table 7–3).

The incubation time, as assessed in newborns, varies from five to 12 days and the disease can last for several months if untreated. It is characterized by conjunctival hyperemia, edema, and a monocyte-rich purulent exudate, which diminishes after the first two weeks. In adult patients, lymphocytic infiltration is prominent, but lymph follicle formation is rare and the pannus (inflammatory membrane) and corneal scarring seen in trachoma do not occur. Certain differentiation from trachoma depends on type-specific antisera and on the immunoperoxidase and serologic methods employed for the diagnosis of urethral and cervical infections.

Trachoma*

Trachoma is a chronic suppurative eye disease with follicular keratoconjunctivitis caused by subtypes of *C. trachomatis* (Table 7–3). It is one of the leading global causes of blindness. Although the agent is widespread in many countries, *progressive trachoma is seen mostly in dry and sandy regions and among poor people and nomads.* In these endemic areas, the infection is acquired during childhood by repetitive exposures over months or years. The responsible chlamydial strains have been shown to enter cultured human cells only with difficulty.[41]

Trachoma is transmitted by direct human contact, by contaminated particles (fomites) and, very likely, by flies also. Infections can be either self-limiting or progressive; the latter type passes from a suppurative stage resembling inclusion conjunctivitis to deeper tissue involvement, with lymphoplasmacytic infiltration and formation of lymphoid cell follicles. The upper limbus of the cornea and the upper tarsal plate tend to be most severely involved by epithelial hyperplasia and follicular hypertrophy.[42] Soon, the conjunctiva ulcerates, and penetration into the cornea leads to pannus formation, fibroblast ingrowth, scarring, and eventual blindness. The scarring also hampers closure of the eyelids, in turn promoting bacterial superinfection. Furrowing of the mucosa overlying the tarsal plate and pitting of the upper rim of the limbus are characteristic late deformities of trachoma. *Tragically, despite the good response of this infection to sulfonamides and antibiotics, many young people in developing countries have lost their eyesight to trachoma for lack of access to medical care.*

Lymphogranuloma Venereum (LGV)

LGV is a venereally transmitted disease caused by the L-1, L-2, or L-3 serotype of *C. trachomatis*. It is not to be confused with *granuloma inguinale*, a bacterial venereal infection (p. 372). About 400 cases were reported in the United States in 1986, most imported from endemic tropical countries or transmitted among multiple sexual partners along with other venereal infections. A primary lesion — either genital, labial, anorectal, buccopharyngeal or even digital — is followed by rapid swelling of the regional lymph nodes (buboes), which become tender, matted, and fluctuant. In heterosexual males, inguinal lymphadenopathy is the rule; in females, spread is to the deep pelvic and perirectal lymph nodes. With rare exceptions, all lesions remain localized in these sites. If untreated, inflammation and scarring continue indefinitely. Late stages of neglected disease are sometimes seen — e.g., rectal stenosis in females due to pelvic scarring or chronic genital lymphedema (elephantiasis in the male, esthiomene in the female).[43]

In **stage I,** a small epidermal vesicle is formed that promptly bursts and ulcerates, oozing abundant neutrophilic exudate. Later, granulomas may form at the ulcer base but usually there is only nonspecific chronic inflammation. By specific immunofluorescence (sometimes also by Giemsa-stained smear), chlamydial inclusions can be demonstrated in these early lesions.

In **stage II,** a suppurative granulomatous lymphadenitis and perilymphadenitis ensues, matting the nodes together and sometimes converting them to fluctuant sacs, which discharge their pus through fistulae. Early on, the nodes appear fleshy and show diffuse reticulosis or scattered non-necrotizing granulomas, but soon these granulomatous lesions undergo central suppuration and become confluent, thereby forming irregularly shaped **stellate abscesses** (Fig. 7–8). These abscesses, rimmed by a layer of epithelioid macrophages, are near-diagnostic, but note that similar lesions may occur in cat-scratch fever and in some fungal or mycobacterial granulomatous infections. Again, diagnosis can sometimes be clinched by using special methods to demonstrate elementary bodies.

In late **stage III** lesions, chlamydiae are often too scarce for microscopic detection, and granulomas may be absent, leaving only chronic inflammatory infiltrates and dense fibrosis in their wake. Plasmacytic infiltration is usually dense, sometimes accompanied by systemic hyperglobulinemia. The histologic features thus are no longer distinctive but remain useful for differentiating rectal strictures due to LGV from neoplastic obstructions.

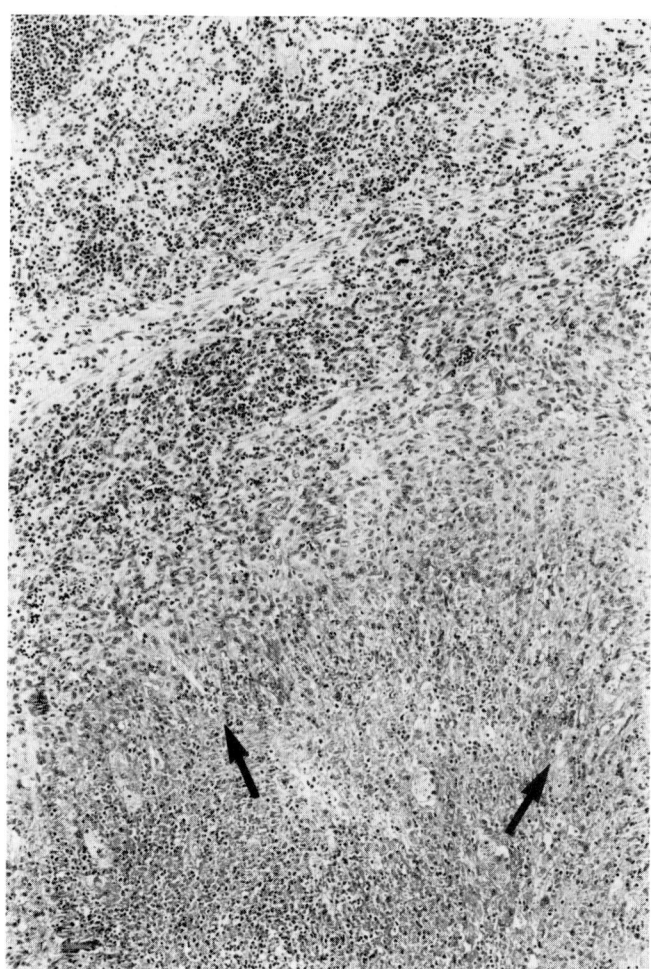

Figure 7–8. Lymphogranuloma venereum. The margin of a stellate abscess in a lymph node. The area of necrosis *(below)* is rimmed by a granulomatous reaction *(arrows).*

The diagnosis of LGV can usually be suspected by the clinical finding of large, fluctuant buboes or draining sinuses. Similarly, the combination of rectal stricture and perineal deformity in a young female is highly suggestive. *Characteristic histologic lesions with inclusion bodies confirm the diagnosis* (p. 327). A serotype-specific microimmunofluorescent test for L-type chlamydiae has recently been developed but is as yet available only in specialized centers. Definitive diagnosis can also be made from aspirates of buboes by growth of the agent in tissue culture. *It should not be overlooked that LGV patients frequently harbor other venereal diseases, including latent syphilis.*

RICKETTSIAL DISEASES

Rickettsiae are small, gram-negative, obligate intracellular bacteria that inhabit ticks, mites, fleas or lice; they seldom damage their natural arthropod hosts and are passed from generation to generation by transovarial infection. Many animals carry infected ectoparasites that can serve as "periodic augmentation hosts" for one rickettsial species or another. Rickettsial life cycles are designed to bridge long intervals between arthropod feedings and in no way depend on human contact; by the same token, these cycles are very difficult to interrupt by human intervention. When transmitted to humans, Rickettsiae multiply mainly in small vessel endothelia; therefore, the diseases they cause share many basic pathologic and clinical features. The tick-borne obligate intracellular bacteria of the genera Coxiella and Ehrlichia, which have traditionally been lumped with the rickettsiae, are biologically and genomically distinct. A listing of the species and diseases of this group is shown in Table 7–4.

Human rickettsial infections are usually acquired by accidental exposure to ticks, mites, or fleas in their natural habitats, but urban transmission also will occur and can reach epidemic proportions in communities infested by rats and lice. Infection is contracted either by an arthropod bite or by contact of arthropod excreta with abraded skin. Depending on rickettsial species, a dark, swollen, crusted skin lesion (eschar) may or may not appear at the inoculum site; its absence therefore does not rule out rickettsial infections, especially those of the typhus group (Table 7–4). Coxiella contrasts with other members of the group in being able to survive under dry environmental conditions; although transmitted to animals by ticks, its preferred route of human infection is by droplet aspiration to the lung.

How do rickettsiae cause disease? First, they must be rendered infectious for mammals by the arthropod's intake of a blood meal; this involves a rapid, temperature-dependent change in their surface molecules. Once inside the new host, they adhere to cholesterol-rich domains of the target cell membranes; a specific receptor molecule has not been identified. Rickettsiae enter the host cell by "induced endocytosis," are enveloped in phagosomal membranes, but soon escape into the cytosol and begin dividing by binary fission. In some rickettsial diseases, intracytoplasmic division proceeds until the host cell is loaded with organisms and literally bursts and dies; in others, rickettsiae are actively expelled by their host cells via elongated cytoplasmic projections, so that rickettsial cell loads stay moderate. All these successive rickettsia–cell membrane interactions — intake, cytosolic escape, and exocytosis — have been linked to the intracellular activation of phospholipase A_2, but it is not known whether that enzyme is of host or of rickettsial origin and how it alters its cellular substrates. Rickettsiae generate no distant-acting toxins and their gram-negative endotoxins are relatively feeble compared to those of enteric bacteria; in sum, there are still many unsolved questions about rickettsial damage to host cells and about their ultimate lethal effects.[44]

T-lymphocyte dependent immune responses are clearly important in the pathogenesis of rickettsial diseases; as in the case of viral infections, antigen-specific cytolytic T cells have been shown to recognize and destroy rickettsia-infected cells. Furthermore, interferon-gamma appears to be crucial for host defense against rickettsiae, and antibodies can convey passive protection. Both recovery from infection and vaccination confer lasting immunity; however, there

Table 7-4. Rickettsial Diseases and Pathogens

DISEASE	GEOGRAPHY	AGENT	TRANSMISSION	DISTINCTIVE FEATURES
Typhus Group (No eschar)				
Epidemic typhus	Worldwide (war, famine)	*R. prowazekii*	Louse feces	Endothelial infection; centrifugal-type rash
Brill-Zinsser disease	That of epidemic typhus	*R. prowazekii*	Late reactivation	Those of epidemic typhus, but generally milder
Flying squirrel typhus	Southeastern United States	*R. prowazekii*	Fleas, lice of flying squirrel	Similar to epidemic typhus, but mortality is lower
Murine typhus	Worldwide (rat-related)	*R. typhi (mooseri)*	Rat flea feces	Similar to epidemic typhus, but mortality is lower
Spotted Fever Group				
Rocky Mountain spotted fever	North and South America	*R. rickettsi*	Tick bite	Endothelia and vascular smooth muscle infected; rash is centripetal; eschar rarely seen
Bouttonneuse fever	Mediterranean, India	*R. conorii*	Tick bite	Prominent eschar, "tache noire"
North Asian and Queensland tick typhus	USSR, China, etc. Australia	*R. sibirica* *R. australia*	Tick bite	Both diseases are typical spotted fevers commonly with eschar
Rickettsial pox	United States, USSR, Korea, Africa	*R. akari*	Mite bite	Prominent eschar; papulovesicular rash (milder than RMSF)
Scrub Typhus	East Asia, Pacific	*R. tsutsugamushi*	Chigger bite	Frequent eschar and lymphadenopathy
Q Fever	Worldwide	*Coxiella burnetii*	Droplet inhalation	No eschar or rash; fever, pneumonia, ring granuloma
Ehrlichiosis	Not yet fully known	*Ehrlichia sennetsu, E. canis*	Tick bite	Fever, lymphadenopathy, no eschar or rash

are instances of rickettsial recurrence after long symptom-free intervals, and rickettsiae have been cultured from lymph nodes as late as one year after clinical recovery, suggesting that latent infections may not be uncommon.

It is now well known that *all human pathogenic Rickettsiae share an affinity for small vessel endothelia; some members of the spotted fever group additionally damage vascular smooth muscle; therefore, the pathology of the rickettsioses is dominated by focal vascular inflammation variably associated with a rash, or with vascular microthrombi, focal ischemia, or hemorrhage.* Characteristically, inflammatory responses are well circumscribed (nodular), relatively sparse, and predominantly mononuclear. Clotting and narrowing of vessels are confined to infected sites rather than systemic (as in DIC). Often the organs of victims show scant grossly visible evidence of the gravity of their illness. Coxiella infections sharply depart from this pattern. In Q fever, the primary target organ is the host lung; mononuclear phagocytes rather than endothelia are heavily parasitized. At the cellular level, coxiellae are lodged inside intracytoplasmic host membranes rather than free in the cytosol. Moreover, they carry plasmids that may serve as virulence factors; there is also indirect evidence of spore formation under adverse environmental conditions. Thus, Coxiella organisms in many ways resemble conventional gram-negative bacteria, especially Legionella, with which they may have been confused in the past (p. 347). Veterinary and human Ehrlichia infections (Table 7–4) have only recently been discovered.[45] The target cell is, once again, the host leukocyte, and microbial growth takes place inside phagosomes. Acute ehrlichiosis accompanied by lymph node swelling, leukopenia, and elevated liver enzyme levels can greatly resemble viral infections, especially mononucleosis.

The diagnosis of rickettsial diseases is easy only during epidemics. Isolated cases present the clinician with a long differential list of acute febrile illnesses and of rashes. Moreover, rickettsia-specific serum antibody titers, which must be relied on for definitive diagnosis, do not begin to rise until the second week of illness. Direct culture of rickettsiae requires special expertise and stringent safety devices available in only few laboratories. In this quandary, skin biopsy and immunofluorescent staining for rickettsial organisms have increasingly been resorted to for early diagnosis in recent years. Rickettsiae, like other intracellular bacteria, respond to appropriate wide-spectrum antibiotics, if given promptly; alert diagnosis and management can therefore be life-saving.

Typhus Fever

The pathology of *epidemic typhus* is typical of the entire typhus group, which also includes *Brill-Zinsser disease, murine typhus,* and *flying squirrel typhus* (Table 7–4); the latter three entities are therefore dealt with only briefly.

Epidemics of typhus occur when people become infested with lice, mainly in times of war, famine, or natural disaster[46]; millions succumbed to typhus in Europe during World War I. The most recent epidemics have been confined to strife-torn third-world countries, but an atomic war would surely bring on a new pandemic.

During epidemics, the typhus agent, *R. prowazekii*, is transmitted from man to man by human head and body lice (*Pediculus humanus*), mostly by scratching or rubbing of louse feces into the abraded human skin. Contaminated clothing free of lice can also transmit the rickettsiae. They are tiny (approximately 300 nm) intracellular organisms that can be visualized inside infected endothelial cells only by immunofluorescence or special stains. On Western blotting, numerous antigenic fractions have been resolved, several of which are currently being assayed for serodiagnostic purposes.

After an eight- to 15-day incubation period, headache, weakness, chills, and fever appear, followed in a few days by a generalized skin rash. During that period, hematogenous dissemination is taking place. At first the rash is maculopapular and pink to bright red, and pressure will blanch it, but during the second week lesions become darker and fixed. Characteristically, the rash begins on the trunk and extends centrifugally. In very severe cases, the individual macules and papules coalesce to produce irregular mottling and maplike blotches. During the second week, there is usually CNS involvement in the form of apathy, progressing to dullness, stupor, and even coma, sometimes punctuated by episodes of wild delirium. If the patient recovers, the rash begins to fade and the temperature begins to subside toward the end of the third week. Most fatalities occur during the second and third weeks of the illness.

In milder cases, the macroscopic changes are limited to the skin rash and small hemorrhages incident to the vascular lesions. In more severe cases there may be areas of necrosis of the skin with gangrene of the tips of the fingers, nose, ear lobes, scrotum, penis, and vulva. In such cases, irregular ecchymotic hemorrhages may be found internally, principally in the brain, heart muscle, testes, serosal membrane, lungs, and kidneys.

The microscopic findings in all cases tend to be far more widespread than the gross alterations would suggest. Most prominent are the small vessel lesions that underlie the rash, and the focal areas of hemorrhage and inflammation in the various organs and tissues affected. Endothelial proliferation and swelling in the capillaries, arterioles, and venules may narrow the lumina of these vessels. Surrounding the involved vessels, a cuff of inflammatory mixed leukocytes is usually present (Fig. 7–9). The vascular lumina are sometimes thrombosed but necrosis of the vessel wall is unusual in typhus, as compared with Rocky Mountain spotted fever. It is the vascular thromboses that lead to the gangrenous necroses of the skin and other structures.

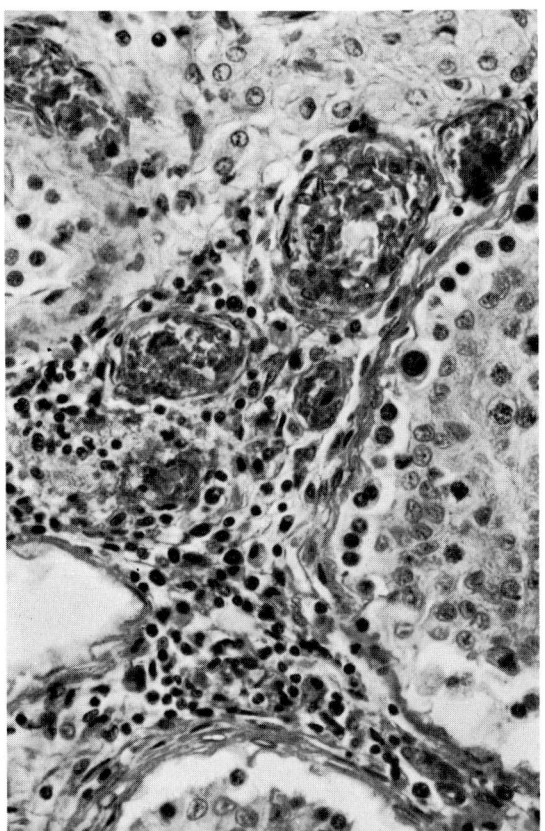

Figure 7 – 9. Testis in typhus fever with a focus of interstitial leukocytic infiltrate and acute vascular lesions.

contamination. Confirmation of the diagnosis by elevated titers of complement-fixing or agglutinating antibodies against *R. prowazekii* antigens can usually be obtained only during the second week and should not delay essential antibiotic treatment. The so-called Weil-Felix reaction, based on cross-reactive Proteus antigens, continues in use only in field settings where specific rickettsial antigens may be unavailable.

Brill-Zinsser disease is a recrudescent form of epidemic typhus, mysteriously arising years after the initial attack (which may already have been forgotten). In the United States, this disease occurs mostly in Eastern European immigrants. It is usually milder than epidemic typhus, and focal necrosis or gangrene is rarely encountered.

Flying squirrel typhus accounts for the sporadic occurrence of typhus fever in the Southern United States, remote from its usual setting. The causal agent is indistinguishable from *R. prowazekii.*

By contrast, *murine typhus* has remained endemic in enclaves of poverty all over the world, notably in those south of the Rio Grande. It is transmitted to man from murine reservoir hosts by rat fleas; its causal agent, *R. typhi (mooseri)* is biologically and serologically distinct from that of epidemic typhus. Murine typhus outbreaks tend to occur where least expected but are usually limited in their spread. About 60 cases per year are diagnosed in the United States. Mortality is lower both in flying squirrel and

> In the brain of untreated cases, the small vessel lesions tend to be limited to the gray matter and are often associated with focal microglial proliferations mixed with other leukocytes to produce the characteristic "typhus nodule" (Fig. 7 – 10). Microglial cells are also diffusely increased in numbers throughout the brain. Mononuclear cell meningitis, ring hemorrhages about the small vessels, and, occasionally, degenerative changes in neurones may occur. In addition, an interstitial pneumonitis may be present, sometimes accompanied by exudative consolidation of alveoli, most likely due to secondary bacterial invaders. Typically, there is also nonspecific lymphadenitis and splenitis. Foci resembling the typhus nodules of the brain may appear in the heart, kidney, testes, and liver.

The differential diagnosis of typhus includes other rickettsial infections as well as a long list of acute viral and bacterial disorders with prominent rashes ranging from enteroviral exanthema through meningococcemia to secondary syphilis. In addition, noninfectious entities such as thrombotic thrombocytopenic purpura and leukocytoclastic vasculitis must be considered. One should always inquire about rodents and arthropods in the patient's living environment. During physical examination, the physician, unless vaccinated or immune, must be on guard against self-

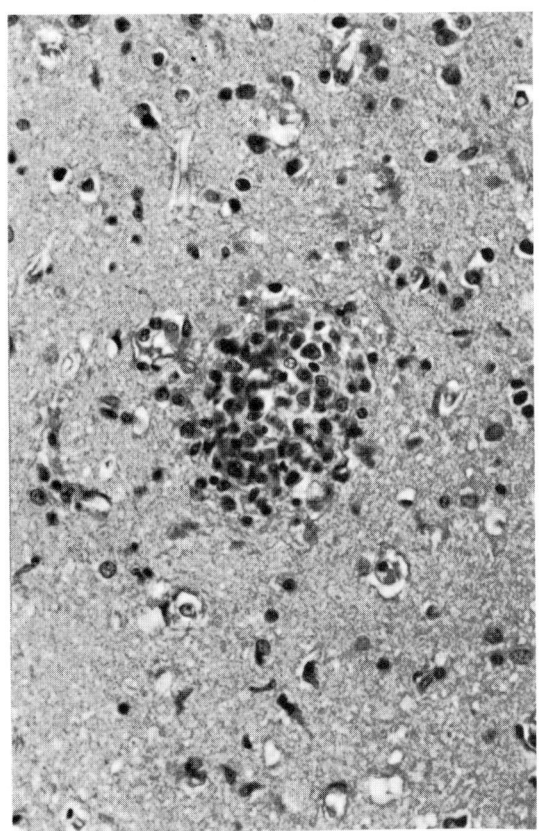

Figure 7 – 10. A typhus nodule in the brain.

murine typhus than in the epidemic form, for which estimates range to about 10% for treated cases, far below the awesome historical accounts of its toll.

Spotted Fevers*

The spotted fever rickettsial diseases (Table 7–4) are transmitted to man mostly by chance encounter with ticks in their natural habitat. Animal reservoir hosts, if they exist, have yet to be found. The exception is rickettsialpox, whose agent lurks in mites parasitic for urban rodents and accounts for outbreaks in places like New York or Moscow.

An eschar followed by a hemorrhagic rash is the hallmark of the spotted fevers, but both can sometimes be inconspicuous or absent, especially in mild infections; moreover, serologic studies have shown that rickettsial fevers can mimic a host of other common febrile diseases. In such cases, knowledge of the geography, transmission modes, and incubation times of rickettsiae together with a high index of suspicion can be helpful. Treatment of the spotted fevers has improved greatly in recent years, but their prevention remains a problem. Ticks cannot be eliminated from their vast habitat without inviting ecologic disaster; therefore, people must be trained to protect themselves from them.

Rocky Mountain spotted fever (RMSF) is native to the Americas and is described here as the prototype of the group; accounts of other spotted fevers (Table 7–4) are available elsewhere.[44] RMSF is caused by *R. rickettsii* and is transmitted by several species of hard ticks, mostly during the warm season. The numbers of cases reported in the United States in recent years have varied between 200 and 1100 per annum, with the highest attack rates per capita in Oklahoma, Tennessee, Arkansas, and Georgia. No age group is spared, but many adolescents and children become infected.

Patients with RMSF may or may not recall the infective tick bite; an eschar rarely forms to mark the site. After two to 12 days' incubation (mean six days), there is a two- to five-day interval without a rash marked by fever, headache, and muscle pain. Although treatment during this early stage will abort the disease, that opportunity is often missed. When the telltale rash begins, it is at first faint, pink, maculopapular, and predominantly peripheral in distribution; in fact it can be absent in 10% of cases. Later on, it extends both toward the trunk and over the palms of the hands and soles of feet and becomes dark and petechial. At this time, high fever and chills are common together with mental apathy and sometimes profound stupor. In the most severe cases, coalescence of skin lesions results in large, mottled ecchymoses or in maplike geographic patterns.

> Because the organisms penetrate deeply into the vessel walls, the vascular lesions that underlie the rash often lead to acute necrosis, fibrin extravasation, and thrombosis of the small blood vessels, including arterioles (Fig. 7–11). In

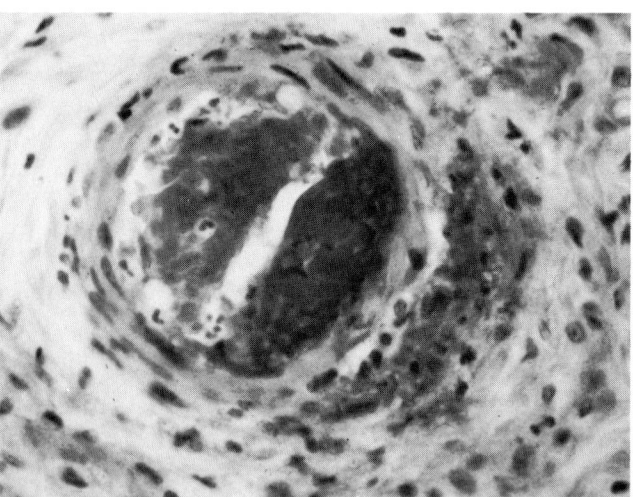

Figure 7–11. RMSF arteritis with mural thrombus and red cell extravasation.

> severe RMSF, foci of necrotic skin are thus induced, particularly on the fingers, toes, elbows, ears, and scrotum. Vascular necrosis and thrombosis are far more frequent with RMSF than with typhus and may mimic the necrotizing vasculitis of the collagen-vascular diseases. Despite frequent local thrombi, systemic DIC is rare, even in the most severe cases. The perivascular inflammatory response is similar to that of typhus, particularly in the brain, skeletal muscle, lungs, kidneys, testes, and heart muscle. The vascular necroses in the brain may involve larger vessels and produce focal areas of ischemic demyelinization or microinfarcts. A pneumonitis of primary rickettsial origin is present in severely affected patients and often predisposes to a secondary bacterial infection.

Antibiotic and supportive therapy has reduced the mortality rate to 3 to 10%. Deaths are due to shock, renal failure, and CNS damage. RMSF is especially severe in black patients with G6PD deficiency. The anatomic changes of RMSF resemble, to a considerable extent, those of typhus, meningococcemia, and other bacterial and viral diseases responsible for hemorrhagic rashes, and these conditions must be ruled out by appropriate laboratory tests. Diagnosis is urgent, because the prognosis depends on the duration of illness before therapy is instituted. Immunofluorescent staining of rickettsiae in skin biopsy specimens can be of help.

Scrub Typhus (Tsutsugamushi Fever)*

Scrub typhus, caused by *R. tsutsugamushi*, is a miteborne rickettsial disease endemic in countries of the Far East and Pacific rim, including China, Indonesia, Australia, Soviet Union, and India. Its territory thus extends over some of the world's most populous areas; nevertheless, reliable estimates of its frequency and health importance are lacking and biomedical information on scrub typhus is scanty.

In about half of the cases an eschar develops "right at the site of the bite of the mite" — more precisely the larval stage of the mite *(Leptothrombidium)*, whose adult stage feeds and mates only in the soil and transmits the rickettsia to its larvae by transovarial passage. The rash of scrub typhus is maculopapular, is usually mild, and may completely fail to appear. More often than in typhus or in spotted fever, there is lymphadenopathy or serosal inflammation of the pericardium, pleura, or peritoneum; by contrast, vascular necrosis and thrombosis or hemorrhage are rare. Otherwise, the gross and microscopic features resemble those of the typhus group of rickettsial diseases.[44]

Classic descriptions of scrub typhus, including those of fatal cases among the U.S. military, depict the disease as severe but, with the advent of effective serodiagnosis and antibiotic therapy, mild infections have become preponderant, and overall mortality is currently less than 2%.

Q Fever

Human Q fever, caused by *Coxiella burnetii,* is usually transmitted to man by the respiratory route from infected animals, especially sheep and cattle. *Q fever causes no eschar or skin rash* and can therefore mimic other infections that induce headache, cough, myalgia, swollen lymph nodes, or hepatosplenomegaly.[47]

In nature, this zoonosis is spread by ticks among many wild animal species, sheep, and cattle. Human infection is most frequently airborne; those handling pregnant or lactating cows or sheep, drinking unpasteurized milk, or working in slaughter-houses are at highest risk. Individuals residing even a mile distant from an infected herd are known to have become infected. *A negative occupational history, therefore, does not exclude this infection, although a positive one suggests it.*

The usual incubation period is three weeks; the onset of the disease with fever is sudden but in about ten days is followed by slow convalescence. Bradycardia, hepatosplenomegaly, and myalgias are among the more frequent findings. The mortality rate is less than 1% even without treatment. Respiratory involvement ranges from only a dry cough to severe interstitial pneumonitis resembling viral pneumonia, ornithosis, or "primary atypical pneumonia." Pulmonary bacterial superinfection or, rarely, infection of the heart valves or progressive liver failure (which may mimic that of viral hepatitis) accounts for the few deaths.

In fatal cases **there is an interstitial pneumonia virtually indistinguishable from viral pneumonia or primary atypical pneumonia.** Nearly confluent involvement of both lower lobes is characteristic. The alveolar walls are thickened by edema and a predominantly mononuclear infiltrate with focal exudation of fibrin and mononuclear, sometimes foamy, phagocytes. Necrosis of alveolar walls or extensive consolidation may develop, probably from bacterial superinfection. In severe prolonged disease, small granulomas may appear in the spleen, liver, or bone marrow, some with epithelioid cells radially arranged around a fat-containing vacuole ringed by fibrinoid material (ring granulomas).[48] These changes are suggestive but not diagnostic of Q fever. Focal perivascular inflammatory infiltrates may be seen in many other organs, and very rarely (in patients with immunodeficiencies) Coxiella endocarditis.

On Australian sheep farms and in California cattle-raising areas, Q fever is well known, but in areas of lower endemicity it is often not suspected until more common fevers have been ruled out. Sometimes it may be diagnosed only retrospectively. A complement fixation test using a *C. burnetii* antigen obtained from chick embryo cultures (phase 2 antigen) is available. A fourfold rise in titer or a single high titer should confirm the diagnosis after the second week. Although *C. burnetii* can be visualized in biopsies by immunofluorescent staining, this is rarely necessary except in prolonged and atypical cases.

MYCOPLASMAL DISEASES

Mycoplasmas are also called pleuropneumonia-like organisms (PPLOs) or Eaton agents. They are almost ubiquitous in nature both as saprophytes and as parasites, yet their biology and pathogenicity are perhaps the least well understood of any infectious agent.[49] They resemble the so-called L-forms of bacteria and are tiny organisms (125 to 350 nm) of polymorphous shape that form slow-growing, small, sometimes fried-egg–shaped colonies on special cell-free media. They can also be grown in yolk sac or tissue cultures. Not only are they the tiniest free-living organisms known, but they are also the cause of many important diseases of fowl and cattle; indeed, mycoplasmas have been isolated from a vast number of animals and plants, far down the evolutionary scale. Known human pathogenic mycoplasmas are listed in Table 7–5.

Mycoplasma pneumoniae is a frequent cause of primary atypical pneumonia (p. 784) and behaves as an extracellular human parasite. It incites epithelial damage in the airways.[50] *Ureaplasma urealyticum* and *M. hominis* cause purulent, acute, nongonococcal or "post-gonococcal" urethritis (p. 1095) as well as chronic pelvic inflammatory disease (p. 1132).[51] In addition, from time to time mycoplasmas are cultured from diseases of obscure cause for reasons equally obscure.

Mycoplasma Pneumonia

It is estimated that *M. pneumoniae* causes about 10 to 30% of primary interstitial pneumonias, mostly in adolescents and young adults. These infections are sometimes epidemic among military recruits and in closed institutions. The pulmonary involvement is very similar to that of viral pneumonia, described on pages 315 and 784. In the few cases studied,[50] the

Table 7-5. Human Mycoplasma Diseases

DISEASES	SPECIES*	IDENTIFICATION†
Tracheobronchitis, "primary atypical pneumonia"	M. pneumoniae	Culture, serotyping Cold hemagglutinin
Nongonococcal urethritis	Ureaplasma urealyticum, M. hominis	Culture, metabolism Serotyping

* Ten additional human mycoplasma species are known, but their pathogenicity remains uncertain.

† Special culture media are required, aerobic for M. pneumoniae, anaerobic for U. urealyticum.

pulmonary changes induced by the mycoplasma were sometimes complicated by bacterial superinfection. *Mycoplasma pneumoniae* elicits both 19S and 7S complement-fixing antibody. *It also elicits, in about 40% of infections, immunoglobulins that agglutinate human Group O red cells at 4°C—cold agglutinins—a test frequently used to confirm the diagnosis. It is also sometimes the cause of false-positive serologic tests for syphilis or streptococcal infections.* Although the mycoplasma pneumonia may last for weeks, even after the fever abates, mild infections detectable only by the cold agglutinin test are most common. Death is rare, and treatment with wide-spectrum antibiotics is effective.

BACTERIAL, SPIROCHETAL, AND MYCOBACTERIAL DISEASES

The extracellular bacterial pathogens of man must resist early engulfment by neutrophils in order to gain a foothold in host tissue, and many have remarkably effective mechanisms to favor their survival. Some generate toxins lethal for leukocytes and other host cells (e.g., the gas-forming anaerobes and anthrax bacilli). Others, such as the pneumococci, solve their survival problems by forming slippery hydrophilic capsules that resist attachment to wandering phagocytes. Pneumococcal capsules weakly activate the alternate complement pathway, but high-affinity binding via Fc receptors is delayed until macrophages have ingested sufficient numbers for effective antigen presentation and until opsonizing antibody is formed by specific B-cell clones. In addition, the pneumococci are capable of more than 80 permutations of their capsular polysaccharides, so that in repeated infection the host is unlikely to recognize the new serotype. *Borrelia recurrentis,* a spirochete, is programmed to repeatedly switch on new sets of antigenic surface determinants before each successive clone is exterminated by the host. This results in several clinical bouts of relapsing fever. Programmed antigenic variation and plasmid-induced antigenic variation are common among bacteria, and their full significance in human infection is still to be clarified.

Facultative intracellular bacteria such as the tubercle bacillus, Brucella, and other chronic infectious agents lack mucoid capsules and quick-acting toxins. *They counteract phagocyte aggression after being inte-*

riorized, either by inhibiting fusion of phagocytic vacuoles with lysosomes or by somehow shielding themselves from the free radicals and enzymes generated around them. Unlike viruses and rickettsiae, they cannot leave the phagosomes. Nonetheless, they have the potential of establishing latent foci of infection capable of long-term reactivation, often resulting in *granulomatous lesions.* Bacterial survival in the face of effective phagolysosome fusion is attributed to specific surface components, the best-known examples being the long-chain lipids and waxes of mycobacterial cell walls, such as *cording factor* (p. 375). In several important human diseases, foamy macrophages containing many large phagosomes replete with infectious organisms are featured (e.g., leprosy, leishmaniasis, rhinoscleroma, malakoplakia, and the so-called xanthogranulomatous infections.) This "foam cell" pattern is usually associated with poor host resistance to the proliferating agent.

Having established themselves, bacteria can damage host tissues directly in a number of ways:

1. Species capable of fast geometric multiplication soon reach sufficient numbers to compete with the nutritional requirements of host tissues; at the same time, their waste products may alter the local pH or oxygen tension or otherwise interfere with eukaryotic cell metabolism.

2. Many potentially harmful compounds are synthesized by bacteria, yet *relatively few bacterial products have been proved to have defined deleterious effects in vivo.* All the leukocidins, hemolysins, hyaluronidases, coagulases, fibrinolysins, and other miscellaneous enzymes extracted from bacterial cultures act on their respective substrates in vitro, but their role in human disease remains presumptive. By contrast, a few of *the so-called bacterial exotoxins directly determine disease manifestations by known molecular mechanisms.* Diphtheria toxin is a prime example; the structural gene coding for its production resides in a lysogenic bacteriophage that infects *Corynebacterium diphtheriae.* The toxin is a proenzyme protein composed of a C-terminal fragment essential for attachment and entry into cells and an enzymatically active N-terminal fragment that catalyzes the transfer of ADP-ribose from NAD into covalent linkage with elongation factor 2, thus halting the assembly of polypeptides on host cell ribosomes.[52] The toxic proenzyme of certain strains of *Pseudomonas aeruginosa,* named exotoxin-

A, acts in an identical manner. The heat-labile enterotoxins of *Vibrio cholerae* and of *Escherichia coli* are likewise ADP-ribosyl transferases, but these enzymes catalyze transfer from NAD to the guanyl-nucleotide–dependent regulatory component of adenylate cyclase, thereby generating excess cAMP. The two categories of toxins differ in their actions; release of cholera enterotoxin in the gut lumen activates the secretion of its mucosa, resulting in voluminous diarrhea and in loss of water and electrolytes; by contrast, wide dissemination of diphtheria toxin is first manifested by neural and myocardial dysfunction.

The gram-positive anaerobic clostridia are virtuosos of bacterial enzyme synthesis. *Clostridium perfringens*, the agent of gas gangrene, literally digests host tissues, including the relatively resistant collagens. Its alphatoxin is a lecithinase that disrupts plasma membranes, including those of red and white blood cells. More selective and subtle are the toxins of *C. tetani*, a wound contaminant, and of *C. botulinum*, which grows in poorly preserved food rather than in human tissue. Tetanospasmin finds its way to the presynaptic terminals of the spinal interneurons, where it interferes with the release of inhibitory transmitter substance, thus inducing the violent muscular contractions that characterize tetanic spasm. Botulinus toxins block the release of cholinergic neurotransmitters by intracellular Ca^{++}, particularly at the neuromuscular junctions, resulting in progressive paralysis of the limbs, breathing muscles, and cranial motor nerves. *Tetanus and botulinus toxins are so selective that the changes by which they kill can scarcely be visualized even by electron microscopy*, and their potency is such that a pinch of either would theoretically suffice to depopulate an entire megalopolis.

Toxin production by bacteria can be encoded by their own chromosomes as a stable species marker, but it can also be phage transmitted (as in diphtheria) or can be conveyed between bacterial strains or species by plasmids via the long sexual pili of these organisms. Thus, the enterotoxic ADP-ribosyl transferase of *E. coli* has proved to be plasmid transmissible. DNA hybridization methods are being developed to determine the presence or absence of toxin-encoding plasmids in isolates of enteric bacteria, having rich promise of clinical applications. The *bacterial cytogenetics of toxin production are analogous to those of antibiotic resistance;* here, too, resistance sometimes depends on a specific inactivating enzyme, such as a beta-lactamase (penicillinase) encoded within plasmids transmitted from one bacterial strain or species to another.[4]

3. *Bacterial cell walls, especially those of gram-negative organisms, contain lipopolysaccharide-protein complexes, the so-called endotoxins*, released mainly by disintegrating pathogens. The protein moiety of these molecules varies by species and can be discriminated by serotyping, but their lipopolysaccharide "business end" is shared between species and accounts for the striking systemic effects (such as high fever, increased capillary permeability, shock, and

DIC) seen in many severe infections. Some of the effects of endotoxins stem from disruption of neutrophils with release of enzymes and pyrogens but production of $TNF\alpha$ and IL-1 also may participate. Foci of necrosis in internal organs, including bilateral renal cortical necrosis (p. 1070), such as occur in endotoxemia, can be reproduced by repeated endotoxin injections or by blockade of the reticuloendothelial system prior to endotoxin challenge.

4. Bacteria contain many particulate and soluble antigens that evoke strong, often lasting host immune responses, both humoral and cellular. *Host defense against bacterial infections depends on phagocyte competence and on intact complement and immune systems* (Chapters 2 and 5). Acting in concert, they must overcome the evasive parasite maneuvers outlined earlier. In some instances, phagocyte competence bears the brunt of the defense; in others, the immune system does. Many extracellular bacteria are vulnerable to circulating antibodies and are readily opsonized, whereas intracellular organisms succumb mainly to macrophages activated by cellular immunity. Some infections can be efficiently prevented by vaccination: for example, immunization with modified bacterial toxins (toxoids) will provide a safeguard against tetanus or diphtheria. By contrast, previous exposure to staphylococci provides little protection against repeat challenge, and here resistance to infections depends largely on the host phagocytes. Antibodies cross reacting with other parasite species are not unusual and, in some chronic infections such as syphilis, antibodies to common cell antigens, called reagins, are formed, and are indeed used for serologic diagnosis.

In the altered host, any of the links in the chain of host defense can be weakened and, by analyzing these defects, critical effector systems for different pathogens can be defined. For example, patients with defective leukocyte granules, as in the Chédiak-Higashi syndrome (p. 51), suffer from recurrent acute bacterial infections, especially by staphylococci. Individuals deficient in the fifth and later components of complement are especially vulnerable to Neisseria bacteremia.[53] T-cell immunosuppressed patients frequently reactivate dormant infections by tubercle bacilli, herpesviruses, or other intracellular parasites.

Part of the abnormalities seen in acute infectious diseases can be host mediated. In acute infections, released IL-1 and $TNF-\alpha$ cause fever, and neutrophil proteases induce liquefaction necrosis and abscess formation. In chronic granulomatous infection due to facultative intracellular parasites such as the tubercle bacillus, the hypersensitivity mechanisms causing cell damage have been difficult to dissociate from those responsible for host resistance (p. 376). Thus, the defensive response of the host can be regarded as a two-edged sword. On the one hand, it is critical to overcoming an infection; on the other hand, it may itself contribute to the production of damage. Perhaps for that reason, in chronic infections immunomodulatory circuits[54] and anti-idiotypic antibodies come into play that spontaneously damp host inflammatory responses and render them more tolerable. In more practical terms, suppression of cell-mediated immunity by drugs is usually countervailing in chronic infection, although corticoid anti-inflammatory drugs have limited uses in reducing tissue responses when given concomitantly with specific antibiotics (e.g., in tuberculous meningitis).

When chronic infection becomes overwhelming, antigen-specific immunomodulation is sometimes replaced by a state of profound, nonselective host anergy in which there is unresponsiveness of T cells to common skin antigens (e.g., those of fungi or streptococci), loss of a previous reaction to tuberculin, and depressed lymphocyte response to mitogens. This can be accompanied by marked B-cell stimulation and hypergammaglobulinemia of a polyclonal type, a state best exemplified in late lepromatous leprosy.[55] The progressive downhill course that results from this anergy has been reported to be reversed by vaccination with mycobacterial antigens.

Table 7–6 provides a working classification of bacterial diseases that takes into account shared clinical and pathologic features likely to be considered in their differential diagnosis.

PYOGENIC COCCI

Organisms of this group evoke neutrophilic exudation and account for most of the suppurative lesions seen in medical practice, such as walled-off pus collections forming *abscesses,* or spreading suppurations, referred to as a *cellulitis* or *phlegmon.* These and other exudative lesions in various locations are described later. Similar suppurations can also be caused by other species or combinations of bacteria, especially by the gram-negative rods so widely prevalent in our hospitals today. Bacterial culture, therefore, is an indispensable tool for the correct diagnosis and treatment of all pyogenic infections.

Staphylococcal Infections

Coagulase-positive staphylococci (*S. pyogenes* var. *aureus*) can cause inflammation in any body site and hence can invade the lymphatics and bloodstream, giving rise to severe septicemia or endocarditis; moreover, some strains produce toxins that can damage tissues by local or remote action. Coagulase-negative "staph" (*S. epidermidis*) are less virulent and as a rule infect mainly previously damaged tissues and hosts, but lately infections caused by these organisms have been on a rise.[56]

Staphylococcus aureus is the commonest cause of skin abscesses (furuncles, carbuncles). In the lung, it causes severe, suppurative bronchopneumonia, and it frequently contaminates the wounds of surgical and trauma patients. Strains infecting only the keratinized skin layer cause a honey-colored, crusty dermatitis named *impetigo.* Rarely, *S. aureus* causes severe enteritis by direct invasion of the gut. More common and

less severe is diarrheal food poisoning due to staphylococcal enterotoxin. Staphylococcal toxins are also involved in the toxic shock syndrome of young women and in the scalded skin syndrome of children. By contrast, *S. epidermidis* infects mainly traumatic or surgical wounds or lodges on prosthetic implants, necessitating their removal. It causes life-threatening infections mainly in compromised and debilitated individuals. Consequently, in today's hospital populations its role has been increasing.[56] Moreover, *S. saprophyticus,* a coagulase-negative organism, has become recognized as a frequent cause of lower urinary tract infection in young women.

Staphylococci inhabit the nasopharynx and skin of most healthy people and pervade our homes and hospitals, but few belong to virulent strains. Some carriers, however, are periodically afflicted by mild skin or upper respiratory tract infections and spread their pathogens to others by contact or droplet emission. Carriers and their infective ambience can be monitored by cultures and phage typing. By these methods, hospital strains, often antibiotic resistant, can be distinguished from community imports and traced to infected individuals. Beta-lactamase producers were the first penicillin-resistant strains to achieve notoriety. Recently, methicillin-resistant staphylococci, unresponsive to most antibiotics, have emerged and have become a cause of great concern.

Staphylococci are infective only in large numbers; however, *once established, untreated infections frequently become invasive and progressive.* Even small skin lesions strategically located cannot be ignored (e.g., those of the upper lip or around the eye where the veins connect with dural sinuses). Walled-off abscesses near a body surface may heal uneventfully by spontaneous rupture or after surgical drainage. On the other hand, deep rupture into a serosal cavity induces a severe empyema, suppurative peritonitis, or pericarditis. Rather than causing abscess formation, highly virulent strains may produce poorly demarcated, spreading cellulitis or interstitial pneumonia, or may enter the bloodstream early, skipping lymphatic spread. *A sudden rise in body temperature in any person having a staphylococcal infection should therefore receive prompt medical attention because of the implicit danger of endocarditis and of metastatic abscesses.*

Regional lymphadenitis secondary to *S. aureus* infection is seldom as severe as the primary suppurative lesion it drains, but involvement of local veins may induce infected thrombi that can release pyemic bacterial clumps or septic emboli, likely to implant on heart valves or in distant organs such as the lung, brain, meninges, or kidneys. *Staphylococcus aureus endocarditis can be right- or left-sided and still ranks as the most frequent destructive, and lethal form of vegetative endocarditis* (p. 633). *Staphylococcus aureus* also may implant in large arteries, giving rise to mycotic aneurysms (p. 579). Staphylococcal septicemia originates, in order of frequency, from lesions of the skin, lungs, kidneys, intestinal tract, or bones. In

Table 7-6. Bacterial, Spirochetal, and Mycobacterial Diseases

CLINICAL OR MICROBIOLOGIC CATEGORY	SPECIES	FREQUENT DISEASE PRESENTATIONS
Infections by Pyogenic Cocci	Staphylococcus aureus, epidermidis	Abscess, cellulitis, pneumonia, septicemia
	Streptococcus pyogenes, beta hemolytic	URI, erysipelas, scarlet fever, septicemia
	Streptococcus pneumoniae (pneumococcus)	Lobar pneumonia, meningitis
	Neisseria meningitidis (meningococcus)	Cerebrospinal meningitis
	Neisseria gonorrhoeae (gonococcus)	Gonorrhea
Gram-Negative Infections, Common	* Escherichia coli	
	* Klebsiella pneumoniae	
	* Enterobacter (Aerobacter) aerogenes	Urinary tract infection, wound infection, abscess, pneumonia, septicemia, endotoxemia, endocarditis, etc.
	* Proteus spp. (mirabilis, morgagni, etc.)	
	* Serratia marcescens	
	* Pseudomonas spp. (aeruginosa, etc.)	Anaerobic infections
	Bacteroides sp. (fragilis, etc.)	
	* Legionella spp. (pneumophilia, etc.)	*Legionnaires' disease*
Gram-Negative Infections, Rare	Klebsiella rhinoscleromatis, ozenae	Rhinoscleroma, ozena
	Hemophilus ducreyi	Chancroid (soft chancre)
	Calymmatobacterium donovani	Granuloma inguinale
	Bartonella bacilliformis	Carrión's disease (Oroya fever)
Contagious Childhood Bacterial Diseases	Hemophilus influenzae	Meningitis, URI, LRI
	Hemophilus pertussis	Whooping cough
	Corynebacterium diphtheriae	Diphtheria
Enteropathic Infections	Enteropathogenic E. coli	
	Shigella sp.	
	Vibrio cholerae, etc.	Invasive or noninvasive gastroenterocolitis, some with septicemia
	Campylobacter fetus, jejuni	
	Yersinia enterocolitica	
	Salmonella spp. (1000 strains)	
	Salmonella typhi	Typhoid fever
Clostridial Infections	Clostridium tetani	Tetanus (lockjaw)
	Clostridium botulinum	Botulism (paralytic food poisoning)
	Clostridium perfringens, septicum, etc.	Gas gangrene, necrotizing cellulitis
	* Clostridium difficile	Pseudomembranous colitis
Zoonotic Bacterial Infections	Bacillus anthracis	Anthrax (malignant pustule)
	* Listeria monocytogenes	Listeria meningitis, listeriosis
	Yersinia pestis	Bubonic plague
	Francisella tularensis	Tularemia
	Brucella melitensis, suis, abortus	Brucellosis (undulant fever)
	Pseudomonas mallei, pseudomallei	Glanders, melioidosis
	Leptospira spp. (many groups)	Leptospirosis, Weil's disease
	Borrelia recurrentis	Relapsing fever
	Borrelia burgdorferi	Lyme borreliosis
	Rothia sp.	Cat-scratch disease
	Spirillum minus, Streptobacillus moniliformis	Rat-bite fever
Human Treponemal Infections	Treponema pallidum	Venereal, endemic syphilis (lues)
	Treponema pertenue	Yaws (frambesia)
	Treponema carateum (herrejoni)	Pinta (carate, mal del pinto)
Mycobacterial Infections	* Mycobacterium tuberculosis hominis, bovis (Koch's bacillus)	Tuberculosis
	M. leprae (Hansen's bacillus)	Leprosy
	* M. kansasii, avium, intracellulare, etc.	Atypical mycobacterial infections
	M. ulcerans	Buruli ulcer
Actinomycetaceae	* Nocardia asteroides	Nocardiosis
	Actinomyces israelii	Actinomycosis

* Important opportunistic infections.

its fulminant form (so-called gram-positive shock), it kills before subsidiary lesions develop, but when less fulminant it may permit the formation of metastatic abscesses. *Staphylococcus aureus sepsis constitutes a medical emergency and has a high mortality rate despite antibiotics; S. epidermidis sepsis tends to be more chronic and less dramatic. Culture is seldom falsely negative with staphylococcal infections and is the mandatory first diagnostic step in any suspected case.* It should be followed by antibiotic sensitivity tests to guide the therapy.

Coagulase and hemolysin production are markers of virulence although their role in the pathogenesis of lesions is unclear. Another S. aureus product, protein A, might inactivate host immunoglobulins by binding to the Fc fragment; *in any case, protective immunity against these infections is, for clinical purposes, negligible.* Staphylococci are catalase producers and are therefore particularly dangerous for patients with impaired phagocyte numbers or functions (p. 220). They are also frequent invaders of patients with granulomatous disease of childhood (p. 52). Strains producing specific toxins, such as shock syndrome toxin 1, enterotoxin B, epidermolytic toxin, or other "exfoliatins," are responsible for the distinctive gastrointestinal and cutaneous lesions described later.

FURUNCLE AND CARBUNCLE. *The furuncle, or boil, is a focal suppurative inflammation of the skin and subcutaneous tissue,* either solitary or multiple, or recurrent in successive crops. Beginning in a single hair follicle (folliculitis), a boil develops into a growing and deepening abscess that eventually "comes to a head" by thinning and rupturing the overlying skin. *A carbuncle causes deeper suppuration that spreads laterally beneath the deep subcutaneous fascia and then burrows superficially to erupt in multiple adjacent skin sinuses* (Fig. 7–12). Furuncles occur anywhere in the skin but are most common in moist, hairy areas such as the face, neck, axillae, groin, legs, and submammary folds. Carbuncles typically appear beneath the skin of the upper back and posterior neck, where fascial planes favor their spread. Persistent abscess formation of apocrine gland regions, most frequently of the axilla, is known as *hidradenitis suppurativa.* Those of the nailbed *(paronychia)* or on the palmar side of the fingertips *(felons)* are exquisitely painful. They may follow trauma or embedded splinters, and if deep enough may destroy the bone of the terminal phalanx

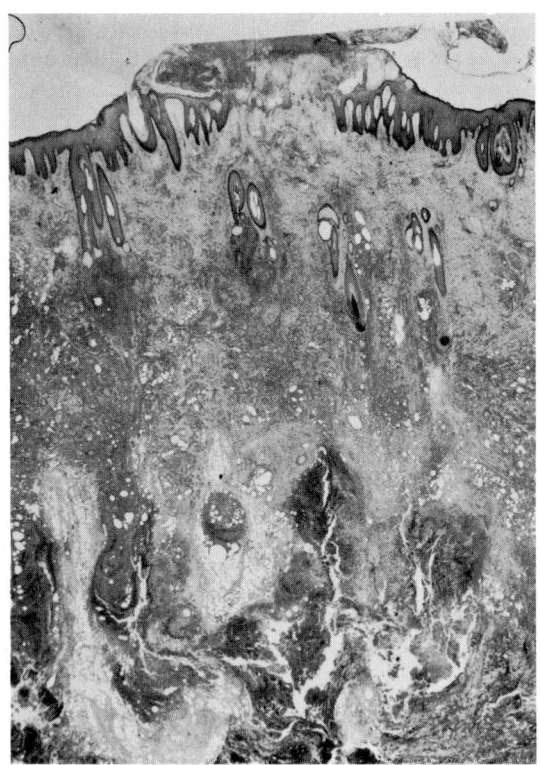

Figure 7–12. Staphylococcal carbuncle at low power showing deep-seated suppuration.

or detach the fingernail. The anatomic features of abscesses related to localized infections are detailed in Chapter 2. Although painful and disfiguring, most heal by themselves or after drainage, possibly leaving a small scar. However, spread and septic complications may occur, more often in diabetics or otherwise predisposed persons. Not all localized skin suppurations are caused by staphylococci; many other pyogenic organisms can cause similar lesions.

INFECTIONS OF SURGICAL WOUNDS. Postoperative wound infections are often but not always caused by staphylococci, including their antibiotic-resistant strains, sometimes traceable to carriers on the surgical team. Sutures and foreign bodies favor the persistence of such infections; inhalation anesthesia carries the risk of spread to the lungs. *Most surgical wound infections remain superficial, but only adequate drainage of all purulent pockets can stem their progress; antibiotics alone are not effective as long as sequestered pus remains.*

UPPER RESPIRATORY INFECTIONS. *Staphylococci are more likely to colonize than to infect the upper airways,* and this must be kept in mind when interpreting throat cultures, but patients with agranulocytosis or those severely debilitated can suffer severe, even necrotizing staphylococcal pharyngitis, tonsillitis, sinusitis, otitis, or retropharyngeal phlegmons. Trauma or impacted foreign bodies in these regions increase the risk. Unless treated, these infections may become life-threatening. *Suppurative sialoadenitis* occurs in dehydrated patients and in those with ductal obstruction by a sialolith as bacteria invade via the ducts and spread throughout the gland. None of these head and neck lesions is exclusively caused by staphylococci.

STAPHYLOCOCCAL BRONCHOPNEUMONIA. Although the anatomic changes conform to the general pattern described on page 780, *this bronchopneumonia is noted for its marked destructiveness.*[57] The mucosa of the secondary and tertiary bronchi is promptly ulcerated as purulent inflammation erodes their walls, branching out into multiple alveolar abscesses. Escape of air into the lung interstitium may occur in children and add to the ventilatory encroachment by forming air cysts that compress the surrounding lung. *Fulminant infections may spread through the lung septa as well as the airways to induce an interstitial pattern of inflammation.* More commonly, in adults, abscesses break into the pleura, resulting in empyema (p. 805) or bronchopleural fistulas; if untreated, septic spread and complications are likely. Staphylococcal pneumonia is a particular risk in patients with pulmonary viral infections. Other predisposing conditions include chronic pulmonary congestion and edema, chronic bronchiectasis, obstructive lung disease, bronchial asthma, and cystic fibrosis.

IMPETIGO. In contrast to the burrowing staphylococcal infections, those causing impetigo are strictly localized to the horny layer of the skin. Staphylococal and streptococcal impetigo are described on page 1308.

STAPHYLOCOCCAL FOOD POISONING. This disorder results from the ingestion of preformed enterotoxin in contaminated food and must not be confused with invasive staphylococcal enterocolitis or the food poisoning caused by *Clostridium botulinum* (p. 359). *An acute, self-limited gastrointestinal upset follows with nausea, vomiting, abdominal cramps, diarrhea, and prostration occurring within one to six hours of ingestion of the offending food,* usually custards, milk products, or unrefrigerated meat. Recovery is equally prompt and a fatal outcome is rare. As in other noninvasive enteritides, mucosal lesions are not demonstrable. The toxigenic staphylococcus must be recovered by culturing the food rather than the patient's excreta. Frequently, the correct diagnosis can be presumed on the simple basis of the brief incubation and duration of this disorder, compared with other food poisonings.

TOXIC SHOCK SYNDROME. *This sporadic, unexpected, and sometimes fatal febrile illness is characterized by volume-resistant shock, a diffuse macular rash, conjunctivitis, sore throat, and a pronounced gastrointestinal upset.* It can rapidly progress to renal and pulmonary failure and death.[58,59] It is often associated with the use of vaginal tampons during menstruation from which staphylococci with unique toxins have been cultured; highly absorbent tampons, left in longer than usual, seem to increase the risk. More rarely, toxic shock has followed surgical wound infections or staphylococcal superinfection of viral influenzal pneumonia and so may occur in children and men as well. *The toxic shock syndrome is easily confused with gram-negative endotoxemia and with acute infections of other causes,* such as leptospirosis (p. 365) or Rocky Mountain spotted fever (p. 332). Culture of the cervical secretions or the skin supports the diagnosis and permits selection of the appropriate antibiotic. During convalescence, scaling of the skin of the extremities is commonly seen.

SCALDED SKIN SYNDROME. Rapid subepidermal blebbing and exfoliation of skin with scant or no inflammatory change is seen in children of nursery school age and occasionally in vulnerable adults, most often caused by strains of *S. aureus* that generate an exfoliatin toxin. This lesion, also termed "toxic epidermal necrolysis," can be mistaken for scalded skin. It responds to appropriate antibiotics. In adults it is usually due to other causes and has a more ominous significance.

The versatility of *S. aureus* is depicted in Figure 7–13.

Streptococcal Infections

Although the morbidity related to these infections has decreased since the introduction of penicillin, streptococci still rank among the major human pathogens even where medical care is readily available and much more so among the underprivileged. Broadly speaking, *they cause two patterns of disease: (1) spreading suppurative infections, and (2) poststreptococcal hypersensitivity disease.* Suppurative inflammations may arise in any site; they are characterized by a thin, nonviscid exudate and a tendency to spread widely. The poststreptococcal syndromes comprise *rheumatic fever* (p. 629), *immune complex glomerulonephritis* (p. 1027), and *erythema nodosum* (p. 1299). The potential for poststreptococcal complications, sometimes following seemingly unimportant upper respiratory tract infections, makes prophylaxis and control a special concern.

A great many groups and subtypes of these organisms have been identified by cultural, biochemical, and immunologic criteria. The most common causes of disease in humans are the Lancefield group A beta-hemolytic streptococci, particularly *S. pyogenes*, of which 70 serotypes are known. Group B organisms are found in perinatal sepsis and infections of the newborn; rarely, groups C and G or others cause respiratory infections. "Untypable" alpha-hemolytic (green) organisms found in mouth flora, such as *S. viridans*, may cause endocarditis, usually in persons suffering from previous cardiac abnormalities (p. 633). More frequent today is bacterial endocarditis due to the D-group anaerobic *S. faecalis* (better known as the *enterococcus*), which is also an important cause of other infections, especially of the urinary tract. Septicemia and endocarditis by another D-group anaerobe, *S. bovis*, are commonly and mysteriously associated with a carcinoma of the colon, and this has led to the discovery of occult cancers on several occasions. Strains causing throat infections differ somewhat from those causing cutaneous infections.

The antigens and multiple virulence factors of streptococci are among the best studied in all of microbiology,[60] and comprise their *capsular polysaccharides*, the *M-proteins*, and the enzymes *streptokinase, streptodornase,* and *streptolysin A.* Strains with *erythrogenic toxin* account for the rash of scarlet fever, and all streptococcal strains have weakly endotoxic *peptidoglycans.*

With respect to host factors, many normal persons carry upper respiratory tract strains only potentially dangerous to others. Clinical infection is usually acquired from close contact with carriers or persons with active disease, and then only with inocula of millions of organisms. Therefore, outbreaks of *streptococcal pharyngitis* are most common in schools and among family members, peaking in wintertime. Relatively few among the many who are colonized develop disease. *Nevertheless, both persons with inapparent and those with overt streptococcal infections can develop antistreptolysin O (ASLO) titers and are at risk for subsequent poststreptococcal sequelae.* Skin infections such as *pyoderma, impetigo,* and *erysipelas* correlate with crowding, poor hygiene, and warm, moist tropical climates and sometimes follow minor trauma, cuts, and insect bites.

Natural and acquired, strain-specific resistance

STAPHYLOCOCCAL INFECTIONS

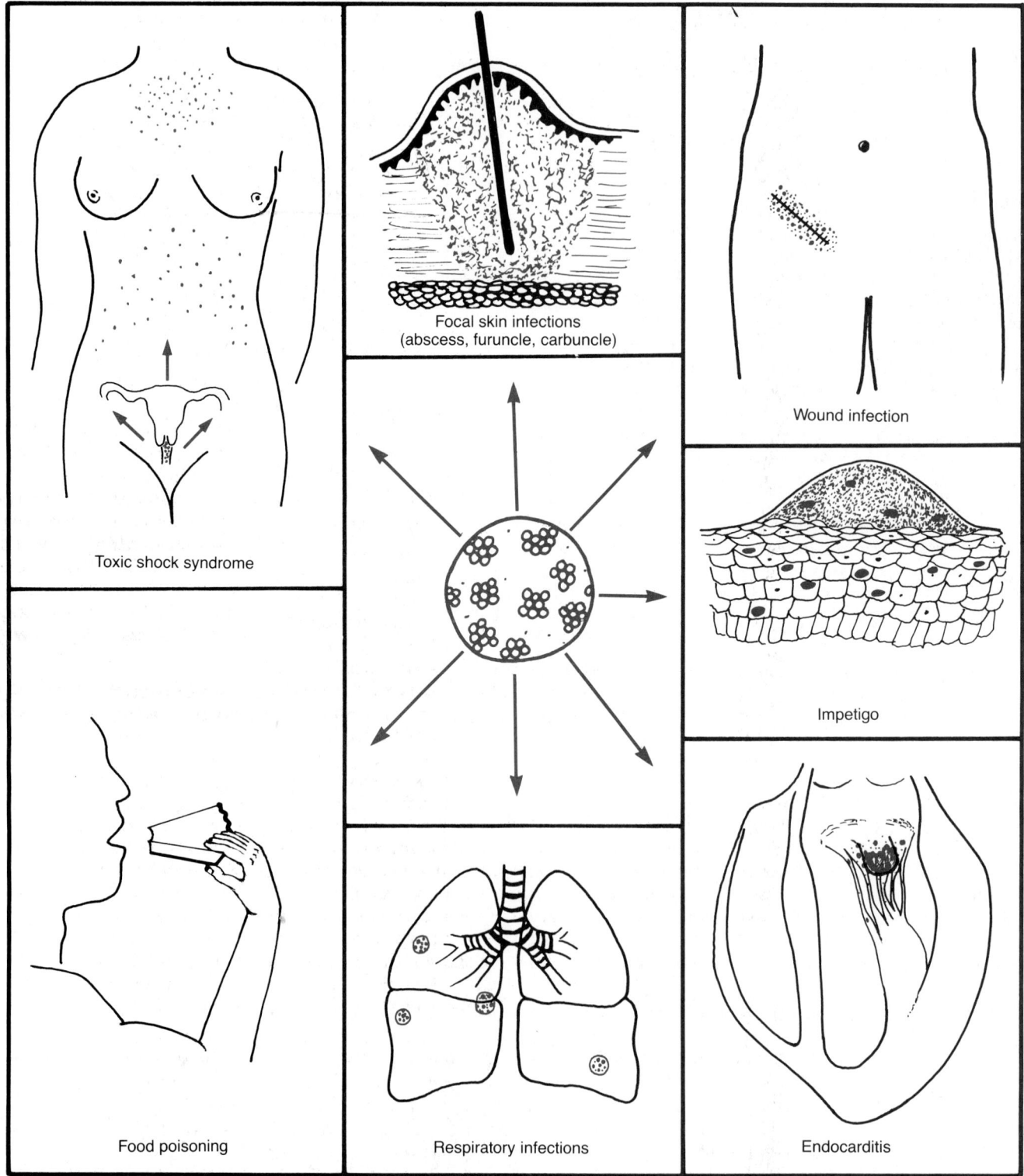

Toxic shock syndrome

Food poisoning

Focal skin infections
(abscess, furuncle, carbuncle)

Respiratory infections

Wound infection

Impetigo

Endocarditis

Figure 7–13. The many consequences of staphylococcal infection.

explains part of the epidemiologic pattern of streptococcal disease. The peak incidence of respiratory infection is in the 5- to 20-year-old age group. Younger children characteristically have milder infections; older people have fewer instances of both colonization and disease.

STREPTOCOCCAL UPPER RESPIRATORY TRACT INFECTIONS.
The intensity of nasopharyngeal lesions varies among individuals. Mild lesions, especially in toddlers, may resemble the common cold. Even older children and young adults often show only a reddened throat and mild pain on swallowing, indistinguishable from an adenovirus infection.

The more severe, typical case is marked by edema, pain, involvement of the epiglottis, and punctate abscesses of the tonsillar crypts, sometimes accompanied by cervical lymphadenopathy but usually in the absence of rhinitis. Because streptococcal infections have much greater potential for local and systemic complications than viral throat infections, throat culture is requisite in all such instances. With extension of the pharyngeal infection there may be encroachment on the airways, especially if there is peritonsillar or retropharyngeal abscess formation **(quinsy sore throat)**. These lesions are characterized by vasodilation, spreading edema, and intense diffuse neutrophilic exudation, often with a liberal admixture of mononuclear phagocytes, a pattern analogous to that of streptococcal cellulitis. Only rarely are there drainable collections of pus.

Fever, chills, and malaise are common systemic manifestations, hinting at bacteremia and possible spread to the heart, lung, or other viscera. Other complications, now rare in the penicillin era, are otitis media, mastoiditis, and spread to the meninges, dural sinuses, or brain. Always in the background is the threat of poststreptococcal complications.

SCARLET FEVER.
This febrile exanthematous disorder is *an acute streptococcal pharyngitis or tonsillitis accompanied by a rash due to the production of an erythrogenic toxin.* Scarlet fever is rare before the age of 3 years or over the age of 15. This upper age limit reflects previous exposure to, and the development of immunity to, the erythrogenic toxins, of which three variants are known.

The disease begins as a pharyngitis and tonsillitis as just described. Often, the tongue is bright red and the papillae are edematous—raspberry tongue—or, when the mucosa is coated and the papillae protrude—strawberry tongue. A punctate erythematous rash appears one to three days later and is diffuse, bright violaceous red, and most abundant over the trunk and inner aspects of the arms and legs. The face is also involved, but usually a small area about the mouth remains relatively unaffected, to produce the so-called circumoral pallor. Toward the end of the first week, the pharyngitis and rash begin to subside and the skin begins to scale and desquamate.

Microscopically, there is a characteristic acute, edematous, neutrophilic inflammatory reaction within the affected tissues (i.e., the oropharynx, skin, and lymph nodes). The inflammatory involvement of the epidermis is usually followed by hyperkeratosis of the skin, which accounts for the scaling during defervescence.

Scarlet fever has an incubation period of two to five days. Headache, nausea, vomiting, chills, and fever may appear early, ushering in the sore throat and diagnostic exanthem. Antibiotics have shortened the traditional one-week duration of the illness and prevented its invasive complications elsewhere in the head and neck; however, *scarlet fever is notorious for associated poststreptococcal sequelae, and timely treatment is therefore of the essence.* Rarely used today is the Dick test to determine susceptibility to infection; the appearance of local erythema following a skin injection of erythrogenic toxin indicates a lack of immunity.

STREPTOCOCCAL SKIN INFECTIONS.
Impetigo (p. 1308) can be caused by streptococci as well as by staphylococci; indeed, poststreptococcal diseases are increasingly being reported in children with this apparently benign infection. *Streptococcal folliculitis, pyoderma, wound infections, lymphatic spread, and sepsis* may be indistinguishable from analogous lesions of staphylococcal origin. However, *streptococcal infections more often induce lymphangitic "red streaks" along the course of draining lymphatics and less frequently cause focal tissue necrosis or abscess formation.* The exceptions are wound infections by microaerophilic (largely group D) streptococci, which may be complicated by gram-negative organisms. Such lesions are suppurative or gangrenous and undermining, and they may burrow deeply into subcutaneous tissues and muscles, forming multiple small pockets of pus to create a *phlegmon.*

Erysipelas is commonly seen in warm climates and is caused chiefly by the beta-hemolytic group A and occasionally by group C organisms. *It is manifested as a rapidly spreading, erythematous cutaneous swelling,* which may begin on the face or, less frequently, on the body or an extremity. The disease is uncommon before the age of 20 years and occurs chiefly in middle adult life. Certain individuals appear to be predisposed and suffer repeated attacks.

Anatomically, the disease is characterized by an irregular, spreading, maplike area of brawny erythema that has a sharp, well-demarcated, serpiginous border. A "butterfly" distribution is common on the face (Fig. 7–14). The skin of the affected part is thickened and has a consistency described as **tallow-like.** Gross areas of suppuration are uncommon. Red streaks of lymphangitis occasionally extend from the margins to the local nodes of drainage, and these nodes are often enlarged by acute lymphadenitis (p. 706). Histologically, there is a diffuse, acute edematous, neutro-

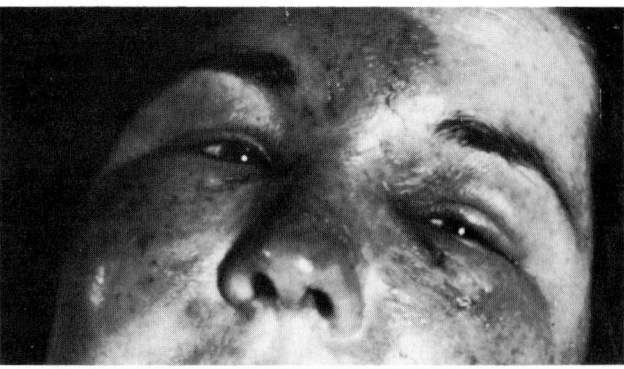

Figure 7-14. Streptococcal erysipelas.

philic, interstitial reaction in the dermis and epidermis extending into the subcutaneous tissues. The leukocytic infiltration is more intense about vessels and the skin adnexa. Microabscesses may be formed, but tissue necrosis is usually minor.

Because the inflammation rarely causes significant tissue destruction, resolution usually permits complete restitution of normal architecture. In addition to the local symptoms, regional lymphadenopathy, constitutional reactions, skin rash, bacteremia, and metastatic foci of infection may all follow, unless the disorder is treated promptly.

OTHER STREPTOCOCCAL INFECTIONS. Spread of the beta-hemolytic group A streptococci to the *lungs, heart valves, or meninges is rare* but can quickly become life-threatening. These organisms pose a particular hazard to splenectomized or splenic-dysfunctional patients in whom they tend to cause fulminant septicemia. *Puerperal sepsis* and perinatal *streptococcal disease,* caused by group A organisms, were formerly common on obstetric wards. Long ago, Semmelweiss discovered that these infections were transmitted by the doctors' own contaminated hands. Now these complications of childbirth and spreading pelvic lymphangitis have become rare, along with the classic *phlegmasia alba dolens,* and the bluish "phlegmasia cerulea," which resulted from secondary major vein thrombosis. Nonetheless, group **B** streptococci are still the most prominent cause of perinatal sepsis. Infections caused by the D-group of streptococci, including the *enterococci,* differ quite sharply from those related to the other strains discussed. Analogous to the gram-negative rods (p. 344), the D-group is sometimes responsible for cholecystitis; urinary, gastrointestinal, and postsurgical infections; endocarditis; and septicemia.

Pneumococcal Infections
(*Streptococcus pneumoniae*)

The pneumococcus has now been reclassified as a streptococcus. Pneumococci are responsible for most cases of *lobar pneumonia,* described on page 782, but can also cause bronchopneumonia, empyema, URIs (especially of the middle ear, sinuses, and mastoids), and severe meningitis or brain abscess. Less commonly they produce suppurative arthritis, endocarditis, or peritonitis. Severe infections may lead to pneumococcal bacteremia.

Pneumococci are found in the nasal secretions of up to 60% of normal adults during the winter months. Despite their almost undiminished sensitivity to penicillin, this endemicity makes them the leading cause of death from pneumonia even today, but now *most deaths occur among the aged, debilitated, and immunosuppressed.*[61]

The polysaccharides of pneumococcal capsules, already discussed as virulence factors (p. 334), elicit strain-specific protective antibodies. Over 80 antigenic serotypes are known; a combination of the 14 most frequent has proved satisfactory, but not uniformly effective, as a prophylactic vaccine.[62] The peptidoglycans of the pneumococcal cell wall have pyrogenic and weak endotoxic effects. Pneumococci are usually alpha-hemolytic and produce the enzyme L-alanine muramyl-amidase, but there is no certain evidence that they produce any diffusible toxins, and so there is as yet no satisfactory explanation for the "toxemic symptoms" and the DIC syndrome seen in bacteremic patients. In contrast to the exudate of other streptococci, pneumococcal pus tends to be thick and viscid because fibrin and nuclear DNA are not lysed. Drainage of pneumococcal empyema is notoriously difficult.

Lobar pneumonia is predominantly due to *S. pneumoniae,* but it also can be caused by strains of *Klebsiella pneumoniae, Hemophilus influenzae, Legionella pneumophila,* and *S. pyogenes.* Radiographic and clinical findings cannot reliably differentiate among these causes. *Smears of sputum or bronchial washings showing profuse gram-positive diplococci followed by culture are necessary to prove a pneumococcal origin.*

Pneumococcemia is in many ways similar to meningococcemia (p. 1253) and its outlook is of similar gravity; it is especially fulminant in asplenic patients. *Pneumococci are major causes of bacterial meningitis in the adult* (p. 1392), still one of the most lethal of meningeal infections *unless diagnosed and treated in the early stages. Pneumococcal peritonitis* is uncommon, except in patients with chronic ascites. It has repeatedly been described in association with the nephrotic syndrome.

Meningococcal Infections
(*Neisseria meningitidis*)

Neisseria meningitidis is a gram-negative diplococcus that colonizes the upper respiratory tract mucosae, but in susceptible individuals it may invade to cause purulent meningitis or bacteremia. A fulminant form of meningococcemia is the Waterhouse-Friderichsen syndrome (p. 1253), and there is also a chronic recurrent form. Involvement of the lung parenchyma, joints, endocardium, and pericardium and even of the conjunctivae and genitalia have all been sporadically observed, but *meningitis is the predominant manifestation in at least two thirds of all invasive meningococcal infections.*

Nine serogroups of *N. meningitidis* classified by antigens in their polysaccharide capsules are known. They possess proteases that cleave the heavy chain of IgA immunoglobulins, which may permit them to colonize the mucosa of the upper respiratory tract. Substrates poor in iron seem to enhance the virulence of strains of meningococci,[63] a possible factor in fulminant meningococcemia. Another virulence factor is the lipopolysaccharide of meningococcal cell walls, which has the properties of an endotoxin and can induce shock and DIC. Carrier rates and case rates of these organisms rank higher than those of pneumococci in persons between 1 month and 15 years of age, but the reverse is true in older individuals. Both rates rise precipitously during epidemics of cerebrospinal meningitis as a particular meningococcal strain gains dominance. Characteristically, clustered infections or small epidemics occur in families or institutions when one member develops meningitis. Both infection and colonization leave behind protective antibodies but not against a new strain.

Inflammation at the usual portal of entry, the nasopharynx, is often trivial and may be confused with a common cold. Invasion, possibly with bacteremia, may follow and result in (1) purulent meningitis; (2) meningococcal septicemia of moderate, fulminant, or chronic form; (3) both meningeal and septic involvement; or (4) any of the other, rarer localizations already enumerated.

The acute suppurative meningitis caused by meningococci is described on p. 1392 and the meningococcemia on p. 1253. About one quarter of all infections with these agents initially appear as septicemia with only a mild, rather nondescript febrile syndrome. One must therefore be aware of meningococcal bacteremia as a cause of fever, looking for skin lesions and petechiae (Fig. 7-15) and taking appropriate cultures. The proportion of meningococcal strains resistant to sulfonamides has now increased worldwide, but these and other antibiotics have improved mortality rates substantially. Even more important have been early diagnosis, contact tracing, and general hygiene, including isolation procedures.

Gonococcal Infections
(Neisseria gonorrhoeae)

Gonococci, pyogenic gram-negative diplococci, are well known as the cause of the common gonorrheal urethritis—popularly named "clap." Less commonly, the infection begins with gonococcal pharyngitis or proctitis, depending on sexual practices. Silent infection is widespread and favors easy transmission. Conjunctivitis may appear in adults from autoinoculation but is more common in neonates of infected mothers. Young girls cared for by infected adults or

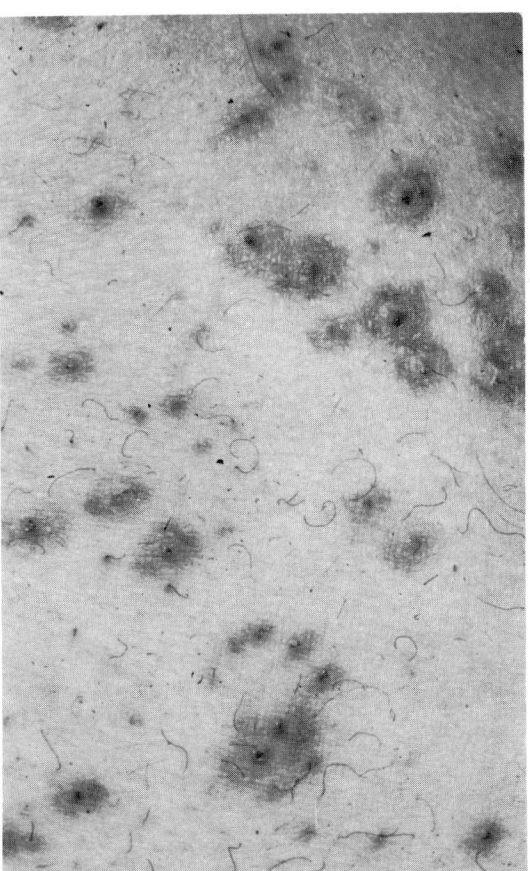

Figure 7-15. Close-up view of skin with the characteristic petechial rash of meningococcemia.

sharing their linen and towels may contract gonococcal vaginitis. Gonococci spread retrogradely from the anterior urethra to the male or female internal genitalia, where they produce chronic purulent inflammations or pelvic inflammatory disease. In the female, painful gonococcal perihepatitis may ensue; further spread in either sex can result in bacteremia-septicemia with prominent skin rash or arthritis, or in endocarditis or meningitis. Rarely, a skin wound may be the portal of entry.

In smears of exudate, *N. gonorrhoeae* is often seen inside host phagocytes. It lacks a true polysaccharide capsule but possesses pili that are important in mediating its attachment to columnar and transitional epithelial cells (Fig. 7-1). It does not attach to squamous epithelia. "Smooth" strains poor in pili are less virulent and are prone to cause asymptomatic urethritis or cervicitis. Gonococcal cell walls contain lipopolysaccharides with endotoxic properties. An IgA protease produced by these organisms may be of help in establishing the microbe in its mucosal habitat. Mucus and menstrual flow favor bacterial colonization and invasion; by contrast, normal human serum containing IgM and complement is bacteriostatic for some gonococcal strains. Convalescing patients generate specific opsonizing antibody, but it is not always protective, and reinfection by either the same or another strain of gonococcus is now so frequent that six-week follow-up cultures have become routine regardless of clinical course. Gonococci can serve as a prime example of constant, programmed genetic variation and it thus appears doubtful whether an effective vaccine can ever be devised. High-grade penicillin resistance in gonococci is usually due to one of two known beta-lactamase plasmids, and there also are now mutant strains with *relative* penicillin resistance, but 90% of all United States infections have remained penicillin sensitive. Given the frequency of low-grade and asymptomatic infections (50% in females),[64] culture on sensitive media (Thayer agar) is superior to other diagnostic procedures such as examination of stained smears of exudate. The presence of gonorrhea does not preclude concomitant syphilis or other venereal infections.

GONORRHEA. Gonorrhea may not be the most frequent infectious disease — that distinction belongs to the common cold — but it is still the most frequent reportable communicable disease in the United States. In 1979, at its peak, there were over one million reported cases and since then, they have plateaued at about 901,000 cases per year. Most cases are never diagnosed or reported, thwarting efforts to trace contacts. Individuals with inapparent gonococcal infection and multiple sexual partners play a large role in transmission.

Gonococci prosper best in warm, mucus-secreting epithelia such as the anterior urethra, accessory urethral glands, Bartholin's and Skene's glands, and uterine cervix. The infantile vagina is also susceptible, but not the squamous epithelium of the adult vagina. All gonococcal lesions are characterized at the outset by nonspecific exudative and purulent reactions followed by granulation tissue and scarring as chronicity increases; plasma cells are often prominent, but gonococci may be difficult to find microscopically, even on special staining.

In the male, the initial infection becomes manifest approximately two to seven days after an exposure by the appearance of suppurative exudation. There is first discharge of a mucopurulent exudate from the anterior urethra and meatus. The infection is limited largely to the superficial mucous membranes and accessory glands. The meatus becomes hyperemic, edematous, and obviously inflamed. Early gonorrhea is of little consequence if the disease is effectively treated at this stage and does not spread upward in the genital tract. However, **in untreated disease, it extends into the posterior urethra and to the major glands of the male genital tract.** Gonococcal epididymitis is characteristic of the neglected case, but the testis is remarkably resistant and orchitis rarely develops, save for a superficial reaction to the adjacent epididymal lesion. Secondary infections in the prostate, seminal vesicles, and epididymides are chronic, persistent, and suppurative, with abscess formation and destruction of the local structures. Urethral strictures and permanent sterility may result, a sequence rare in the penicillin era. **It is the asymptomatic male carrier who represents the greatest hazard to his female partners and is most likely to develop arthritis or gonococcemia.**

In the female, reddening and edema of the urethral meatus is often much less conspicuous, but abscess formation with bulging of Bartholin's and Skene's glands is common. **Cervicitis is the rule, but it gives rise to few specific symptoms. Gonococcal salpingitis may seal the tubes, resulting in pyosalpinx — pus-filled tubes, which may become hugely distended.** Bilateral tubal involvement obviously interferes with fertility. Tubo-ovarian abscesses and pelvic peritonitis result from further extension and may create multiple adhesions or points of blockage of the oviducts, later giving rise to sterility. **Gonococci are the most common cause of pelvic inflammatory disease (PID) in young women compared with gram-negative bacteria in older ones** (p. 1132).

Spread into the peritoneum in females can result in perihepatitis, manifested by stabbing right upper quadrant pain (the Fitz-Hugh-Curtis syndrome). *More important, gonococcal bacteremia is demonstrable by culture in up to 3% of infected persons,* many without symptoms, and can occur in patients with only pharyngitis or proctitis. Symptomatic gonococcemia is rarely as fulminant as meningococcemia, which it otherwise resembles, and generally skin lesions are less prominent (p. 1253). The hemorrhagic rash, when present, is found mostly on the extremities and is related to vasculitis of the dermal vessels. Two forms of gonococcal arthritis are known: (1) an acute polyarticular type free of culturable gonococci, clinically resembling active rheumatoid arthritis or Reiter's syndrome (p. 1096), which may coincide with bacteremic skin lesions; and (2) a more chronic form involving only one or a few joints, with purulent exudate and positive cultures. The frequency of gonococcemia and arthritis has lately been increasing in women, whereas that of gonococcal endocarditis and meningitis has become vanishingly low.

In sum, the clinical presentations of gonococcal infection range from the obvious (acute anterior urethritis following a sexual exposure) to the arcane (gonococcemia or arthritis, sometimes without a venereal history).

GRAM-NEGATIVE RODS

Here we deal with a miscellany of organisms (Table 7–6), formerly known mainly as causes of urinary and intra-abdominal infections and of rare pneumonias. All members of this group have lipid-rich cell walls, are nonsporulating, and, except for Enterobacter sp., are only facultative anaerobes. Drug resistance is frequent among these rods and difficult to predict owing to their liberal exchange of plasmids and resistance (R) factors acquired by conjugation and transduction. Since the therapeutic revolution of the 1950s and 1960s, these organisms have increasingly replaced the antibiotic-sensitive pyogenic cocci as causes of various septic and suppurative disorders. Together with the group D streptococci, they now account for the bulk of hospital-acquired and opportunistic bacterial infections, as well as for many terminal complications in advanced chronic diseases. At the same time, these gram-negative rods continue infecting normal hosts in the community, usually in more tractable forms than in the hospital setting. As in the case of the pyogenic cocci, their clinical and pathologic features overlap, and species identification by culture remains the cornerstone of diagnosis and management.

Escherichia coli Infections

This multitalented enteric gram-negative bacillus is best known as a noninvasive commensal that grows in mass culture in the human and animal gut lumen, perhaps keeping other, more harmful bacteria from proliferating. However, *E. coli* is also genetically the most versatile of bacteria and is both the recipient and source of many plasmid- and phage-mediated gene exchanges. Of the hundreds of *E. coli* serotypes arising from this genetic potpourri, only a few are virulent for normal humans and possess invasiveness or one of the other three mechanisms of enteropathogenicity discussed later (p. 866). Each of these disease roles is related to different *E. coli* plasmids and serotypes, and each can thus be acquired by an otherwise harmless *E. coli* strain. Here we are concerned only with *E. coli* as a urinary and septic pathogen.

Urinary tract infections with *E. coli* begin in the bladder (cystitis), with or without extension to the kidneys (pyelonephritis). *Indeed,* E. coli *accounts for the preponderance of primary uncomplicated urinary tract infections* (i.e., when there is no obvious cause for urinary stasis, such as an obstructing ureteral stone or enlarged prostate). Other gram-negative rods (Proteus, Enterobacter, Pseudomonas, etc.) become more prevalent with complicated, obstructive pyelonephritis. In most cases the organisms gain access to the bladder urine through the urethra, sometimes aided by catheterization or instrumentation (urethral dilation, cystoscopy, etc.). Here, they induce an acute inflammatory mucosal reaction. Retrograde spread up the ureters is the usual pathway of development of acute pyelonephritis, marked by focal suppuration within the renal parenchyma (p. 1051).

Escherichia coli is also a common cause (along with Enterobacter and Proteus organisms) of suppurative infections within the abdominal cavity. Thus, enteric organisms are found in acute appendicitis, acute cholecystitis, cholangitis, diverticulitis, and perforated gallbladder or peptic ulcer. In addition, *E. coli* is a common member of mixed wound infections and suppuration in and about the anus (ischiorectal abscess, pilonidal sinus). In a hospital setting, it is also found among the gram-negative organisms that invade the respiratory tract of debilitated patients, and may cause severe hemorrhagic bronchopneumonias. But the most feared consequence of infections with these organisms is the development of *gram-negative*

bacteremia. Once a rare clinical problem, its incidence has increased 20-fold over the past two decades. Fatality rates in gram-negative bacteremias approach 50%, and cause over 100,000 deaths annually in the United States. Death may be due to uncontrolled endotoxemic febrile reactions, metastatic dissemination of organisms, or endotoxic induction of DIC and shock (p. 335).

Many factors contribute to this growing clinical problem. The infections are difficult to eradicate because of microbial drug resistance. In the effort to control the local disease, administration of antimicrobial agents suppresses other drug-sensitive organisms, leaving the resistant gram-negatives to proliferate and spread into the blood. This unfortunate sequence is particularly liable to occur in predisposed hospitalized patients, such as the very young and very old, and those having diabetes mellitus, hematologic or neoplastic disorders, or some basis for depressed immunity. *Not all patients with gram-negative bacteremias have obvious local suppurative disease.* In fact, transient contamination of the blood is commonplace in daily life. In the normal individual this is of no consequence, but those with lowered resistance are at risk of developing gram-negative sepsis.

> Pathologic lesions caused by invasive *E. coli* are usually of the suppurative type and lack specific distinguishing features other than the occasional production of gas, which may mimic that of clostridial infection (p. 360) but differs in odor. *Escherichia coli* infections or mixed infections can indeed become gangrenous, especially those arising in abdominal viscera.

Rigors and spiking temperatures are seldom absent when *E. coli* sepsis ensues, and they are particularly frequent when there is gram-negative cholangitis or liver abscess formation.

Klebsiella and Enterobacter Infections

Klebsiella pneumoniae (also known as Friedländer's bacillus) and *Enterobacter aerogenes* are common enterobacteria, so closely related that they are, for practical purposes, indistinguishable. Their disease spectrum includes severe pneumonia, lobular or lobar; urinary tract infection; and miscellaneous septic lesions, but no enterotoxicity. *Klebsiella pneumoniae* is an aerobic lactose-fermenter with a thick mucoid capsule. It is rarely a commensal of the mouth and throat in normal individuals but is found there in about 20% of hospital patients. Lung infections probably come about by inhalation or aspiration, especially in patients who have difficulty swallowing, who are intubated, who have tracheostomies, or who have poor ciliary function due to alcoholism or chronic obstructive lung disease. *Klebsiella pneumoniae* is also a cause of urinary tract infections, particularly when there is urinary tract obstruction, and it is frequently present in mixed infections of the biliary tract. Uncommonly, suppuration in the sinuses, middle ears, mastoids, and meninges is attributable to this organism. It is important to identify this pathogen in all these settings because it is more resistant to antibiotics than *E. coli* and is therefore of graver significance.

Klebsiella pneumoniae usually produces a bronchopneumonia similar to that caused by other gram-negative bacilli, but distinguished by its tendency to abscess formation and pleural involvement, especially in the setting of aspiration or preexisting chronic lung disease. In some individuals, usually alcoholics acquiring their infection outside the hospital, Friedländer's bacillus causes a primary, lobar pneumonia quickly involving one or more lobes of the lung, indistinguishable clinically from pneumococcal lobar pneumonia (Fig. 7–16) (p. 782). Occasionally an acute pneumonia is followed by persistent chronic pulmonary infection, and Klebsiella sp. have been repeatedly cultured in chronic bronchitis, bronchiectasis, and lung abscesses.

Klebsiella pneumoniae septicemia, evidenced by chills, fever, malaise, and prostration, may occur in the course of the pneumonia or other localizations of this pathogen. Sometimes it appears without obvious focal infection. These gram-negative bacteremias can be extremely fulminating, and patients usually succumb without the development of metastatic tissue lesions.

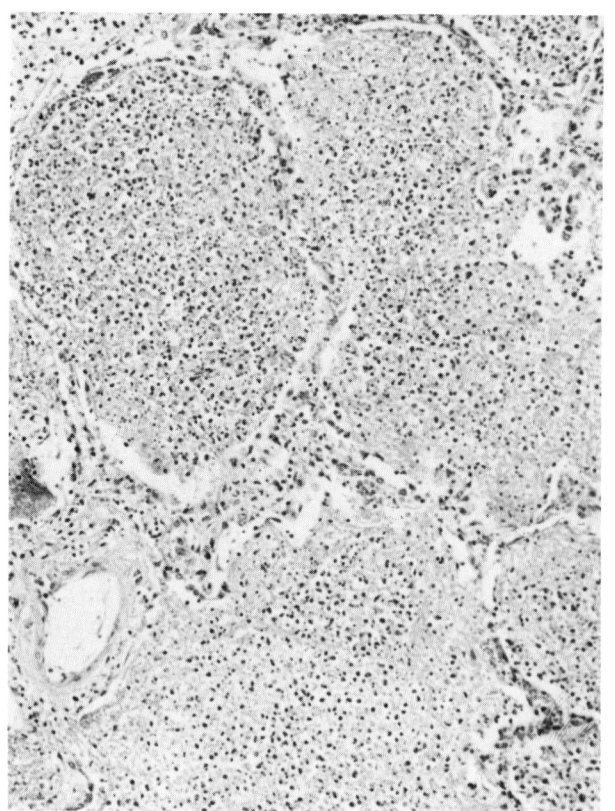

Figure 7–16. Klebsiella pneumonia. Note intra-alveolar exudate and destruction of alveolar septa.

Proteus and Serratia Infections

The spectrum of diseases caused by *Proteus mirabilis,* a motile gram-negative bacillus, is similar to that of *E. coli* and *K. pneumoniae.* It is most frequently a chronic urinary tract pathogen and is sometimes associated with xanthogranulomatous pyelonephritis, described on page 1057. Proteus pneumonia is uncommon and is usually found in debilitated hospitalized patients. The involvement tends to be lobular and most often in the posterior segment of an upper lobe, especially the right one, as in aspiration pneumonia. Abscess formation is frequent.

Serratia marcescens infection, likewise, is often manifested as a pneumonia, but it can involve many other organ systems, including the upper respiratory tract, normally a rare habitat of this organism. Infections are mostly limited to debilitated or immunosuppressed individuals, generally within hospitals. The simple practice of frequent hand washing by all hospital caregivers has greatly lowered their incidence. One claim to fame of this nosocomial pathogen is its former use as an "innocuous germ." It was commonly used for teaching medical students how to culture bacteria; on one occasion, it was even aerosolized throughout the New York subway system in a study of the logistics of germ warfare. Fortunately, no epidemic followed among the normal individuals placed at risk — an instructive, if involuntary, demonstration of the importance of host factors in the pathogenesis of gram-negative bacterial infections.[65]

Pseudomonas Infections

Pseudomonas aeruginosa is of low virulence for normal individuals owing to its poor resistance to natural host barriers, especially to neutrophilic phagocytosis. However, it commonly causes acute nosocomial and opportunistic gram-negative infections in the predisposed. Formerly known as *Bacillus pyocyaneus,* this microbe has become one of the most common and severe secondary invaders. It is widely distributed throughout hospitals and has been cultured from wash basins, respiratory tubing, nursery cribs, and even antiseptic-containing bottles. It also subsists on the moist skin or in the gut of some normal people, and it colonizes the pharynx of patients receiving antibiotics. From these multiple sources, it gives rise to miniepidemics in nurseries, intensive care units, and *particularly burn units, where it ranks first as a source of skin infections and generalized sepsis.* Indeed, the current practice of early coating of burn surfaces with antibacterial agents or grafting was devised primarily against surface contamination of the wound by Pseudomonas and other ambient organisms.[66] Premature infants, patients with neutropenia or any form of extensive wound, and immunosuppressed individuals are also at high risk. Once the organism is established, Pseudomonas pathogenicity is high. Several toxins have been isolated from its various strains, including the ADP ribosyl transferase named exotoxin A, a lethal toxin that shocks and kills rabbits in microgram amounts, and a leukocidin. Some strains of *P. aeruginosa* cause chronic infections of the urinary tract, external ear, and respiratory tree, especially in patients with mucoviscidosis and recurrent bronchopneumonias. *Pseudomonas maltophilia* and *P. cepacia* are similar in pathogenicity but are less commonly seen.

In addition to causing infections on the surface of the body, Pseudomonas may primarily involve the urinary tract or initially present as a pneumonia, in each case incurring the risk of bacteremia and disseminated gram-negative sepsis. Regardless of the source, the lung is frequently seeded and the resultant pneumonia then becomes a prominent part of the sepsis. Early lung involvement, whether by air or bloodstream, is thus an ominous sign; urinary Pseudomonas infections tend to be less rampant and may follow a chronic recurrent course. Successful therapy of these infections depends as much on host defenses (particularly, on a normal neutrophilic response) as on the appropriateness of the antibiotic. This gram-negative rod has the pernicious habit of replacing other pathogens as they are suppressed, so that persisting infections often turn out to be superinfections by Pseudomonas, for which the initial treatment is no longer appropriate—hence, the importance of follow-up cultures in hospitalized patients.

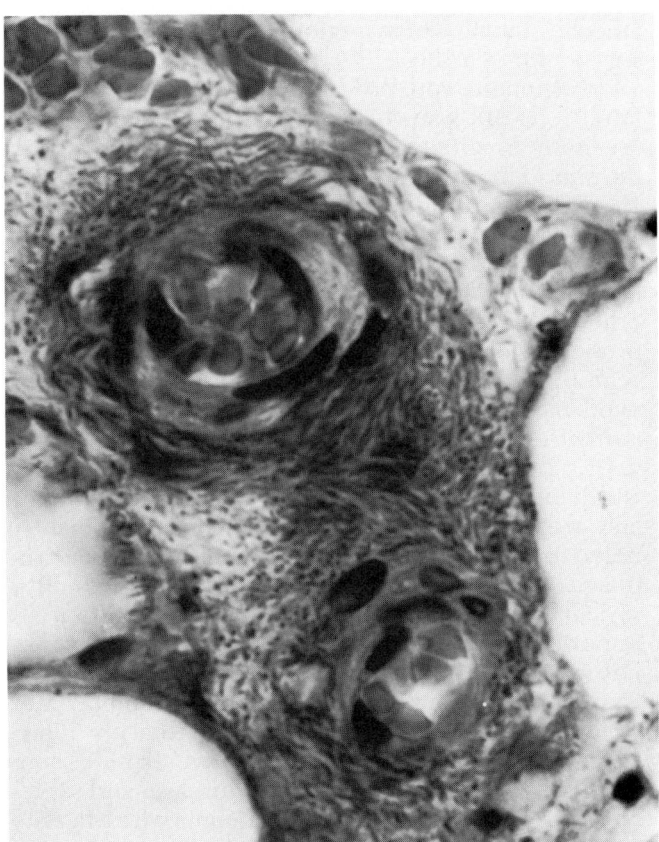

Figure 7–17. Pseudomonas vasculitis. The perivascular haze represents masses of organisms.

Microscopically, *P. aeruginosa* infection in the altered host is the prototype of a necrotizing inflammation. Masses of proliferating organisms cloud the host tissue with a bluish haze, concentrating in the wall of blood vessels, where host cells undergo coagulation necrosis and nuclei fade away (Fig. 7–17). This picture of gram-negative vasculitis accompanied by thrombosis and hemorrhage, although not pathognomonic, is highly suggestive of *P. aeruginosa*. The surprising scarcity of neutrophils in these sites is partly a function of previous systemic neutropenia, partly of violent necrosis. Grossly, Pseudomonas pneumonia distributes through the terminal airways in a "fleur-de-lis" pattern, with a striking alternation of whitish necrotic and dark red hemorrhagic areas. In skin burns, these organisms proliferate wildly, penetrating deeply into the veins to induce massive bacteremias. Well-demarcated necrotic and hemorrhagic skin lesions of oval shape often arise during these bacteremias and are named ecthyma gangrenosum. At their bases these lesions show the same Pseudomonas vasculitis seen in the lung. DIC is frequent with bacteremia. The heart valves may also become infected,[67] and when the brain is seeded cortical foci of necrosis may appear with inflammation of the leptomeninges.

Pseudomonas infections of persons with normal white cell defenses usually take the form of suppurative lesions, such as abscesses and streaky infiltrates in pyelonephritic kidneys (Chapter 21). Occasionally, pigment-producing strains of *P. aeruginosa* impart a bluish tinge to the accumulating pus (hence the term pyocyaneus). Suppurative meningitis may follow long-neglected otitis, particularly when other organisms have been suppressed by antibiotics.

With the more effective antibiotics now available, Pseudomonas mortality is abating but still is quite high; antibiotic choice is especially critical for hospital strains that exchange resistance plasmids with other bacteria.

Legionella Infections

When lethal pneumonia struck a group of participants at the 1976 convention of the American Legion in Philadelphia, the microbe hunt that ensued led to the unexpected finding of a hitherto unknown gram-negative bacterial pathogen, *Legionella pneumophila*. It was first visualized by silver staining in infected human tissue, then cultured on special media. Further study revealed that Legionella had been described as a "rickettsia-like organism" as early as 1947[68] and had been the unrecognized cause of sporadic cases of pneumonia for many years.[69] The new Legionella became identified as the type species of a family of gram-negative bacterial pathogens that includes *L. micdadei* (the "Pittsburgh pneumonia agent"), *L. bozemanii*, *L. dumoffii*, and *L. gormanii*, previously known only as scattered isolates. Finally, Legionella's transmission was found to be respiratory, and a major environmental source was found to be water reservoirs and cooling units of air-conditioning systems containing blue-green algae and free-living amebae, among which Legionella spp. can apparently survive for years.

Legionella spp. are small, gram-negative flagellated rods of somewhat polymorphous shape. They are best visualized by immunofluorescence, which permits identification of the various species. They can also be visualized (more easily on smears than in tissue) with the Dieterle silver stain, or by modified gram stains. *L. micdadei* is weakly acid-fast in tissue but not in culture. Legionella spp. release catalase and other enzymes, and their cell walls have endotoxic properties; none are encapsulated. Thus far, six serotypes of *L. pneumophila* have been identified; however, although some are more frequent pathogens than others, serotype bears no relation to disease severity. Indeed, the basis of Legionella pathogenicity is still uncertain. It is readily engulfed by neutrophils and mononuclear phagocytes, and it is efficiently killed by activated monocytes, but not by macrophages,[70] in whose phagosomes it may actually multiply early in the disease.[71] The role of host resistance is important, because most severe cases occur in immunosuppressed or compromised hospital patients.[68] Community outbreaks traceable to a common water source have been characterized by two sharply different patterns of disease: (1) Pontiac fever, a mild, nonfatal, self-limited systemic febrile disease; and (2) legionnaires' disease, a severe pneumonia with a fatality rate of 15 to 20% among patients not receiving appropriate antibiotic therapy. Overall, about 1000 cases per year are being reported in the United States.

After an incubation period of five days, legionnaires' disease is marked by the gradual onset of fever, dry cough, malaise, chest and abdominal pain, confusion, and sometimes diarrhea. As in typhoid fever, the pulse rate may be surprisingly slow relative to the fever and the leukocyte counts may not be impressive. Severe cases typically manifest scanty blood-streaked sputum, increasing respiration rate, high fever, and disproportionate systemic symptoms. Death may follow from respiratory failure or, in some cases, from a shocklike syndrome with DIC and renal failure. Erythromycin and other broad-spectrum antibiotics abbreviate the illness when given in a timely manner. *Legionella bozemanii* infections are the severest, and no survivors have yet been reported.

All Legionella species produce a lobular pneumonia of fibrinopurulent type that tends to be confluent, sometimes to the point of appearing lobar. Even early, a relatively high ratio of mononuclear phagocytes to neutrophils is characteristic. In the center of the lung lesions, phagocytes are destroyed and their nuclei broken up (leukocytoclasis), but intact macrophages congregate about the necrotic zone. Still more peripherally, pneumocyte proliferation, hyaline fibrin membranes lining alveolar spaces, and edema are present; in immunosuppressed or respirator-assisted patients, these changes may closely resemble diffuse alveolar damage and signal the development of DIC. Bacteria are copious in the leukocytoclastic areas and are seen inside large, intact, bubbly-appearing macrophages as well as in neutrophils. Secondary inflammation of the walls of small pulmonary arteries and veins is often intense and accompanied by thrombosis. Abscesses are frequent, but they tend to be small and rarely confluent. These destructive lesions explain the tendency to organization and scarring and account for the patient's prolonged convalescence. Fibrinous pleuritis is often relatively modest and the fluid in the pleural spaces is more often serous than purulent. The larger airways are only moderately affected compared with the bronchioles, which are largely plugged with exudate, perhaps explaining the scarcity of sputum. Even when the involvement is lobar, the lesions tend not to be all of the same stage, as is characteristic of pneumococcal pneumonia. In sum, the picture is one of a confluent bronchopneumonia of bacterial type, and it differs sharply from the interstitial pattern seen in viral and in some rickettsial infections.

Bacteremia has been repeatedly demonstrated in patients with pulmonary involvement. Organisms, and sometimes small foci of cell necrosis, can also be found in hilar nodes and in various parenchymal organs. Microscopic hematuria and unexplained renal failure are not uncommon in legionnaires' disease.

The sporadic appearance of Legionella pneumonia in vulnerable patients, its confluent lobular distribution, and its toxic symptoms all parallel the presentation of other gram-negative pneumonias but the sputum may be scanty and poor in leukocytes and may fail to yield a convincing, rich growth of organisms on routine media. Even on special media, growth is slow, and thus early diagnosis often requires invasive procedures such as lung aspiration or biopsy to identify the organisms. The radiographic changes parallel the distribution and diversity of the lung lesions, and they recede only slowly.

Anaerobic Gram-Negative Bacterial Infections

Of approximately 400 gram-negative anaerobic species found as commensals in the human bowel, vagina, and mouth, only a few become invasive. However, the frequency of this event is underestimated because, in lung abscesses formed by aspiration or in infections initiated by trauma or fecal leakage, these organisms are often present along with other bacteria and are revealed only by rigorously anaerobic methods of culture. The possible presence of anaerobes must therefore be remembered in abdominal sepsis, pelvic inflammatory disease, and lung abscesses and in septicemias arising from these and other conditions.

The genera Bacteroides, Fusobacterium, Peptococcus, and Peptostreptococcus are the most frequent anaerobic isolates other than clostridia (p. 358). The two dominant groups are *Bacteroides fragilis*, a gut-dwelling organism, and *Bacteroides mela-*

ninogenicus, a mouth commensal, also incriminated in periodontal disease. Both groups are composed of several species or subspecies and several hundred strains are known, but all seem to behave similarly. These organisms gain a foothold through a break in normal defense barriers, colonization along with another, more virulent bacterial invader, and proliferation in devitalized tissue. The virulence factors of Bacteroides are still only partly known. The cell-wall lipopolysaccharide endotoxin differs chemically from that of other gram-negative organisms and only rarely does *B. fragilis* bacteremia result in DIC or bleeding. On the other hand, pathogenic *B. fragilis* has a polysaccharide capsule that appears to facilitate its adhesion to peritoneal mesothelium.[72] It also elaborates a collagenase and a superoxide dismutase.

Bacteroides melaninogenicus, alone or in association with aerobic organisms, is found in abscesses and phlegmons mostly above the diaphragm (e.g., in the floor of the mouth, the retropharynx, and even the lung and brain). *Bacteroides fragilis* is typically a cause of, or a participant in, intra-abdominal and retroperitoneal sepsis and in pelvic peritonitis of women beyond their twenties; sometimes it infects surgical abdominal wounds. It may also be present in lung abscesses. In all these lesions, the pus is often discolored and foul smelling, especially in lung abscesses, and the suppuration is often poorly walled off. Otherwise, these lesions pathologically resemble those of the common pyogenic infections.

The outcome of Bacteroides infections depends on the patient's resistance; young women with pelvic infections do relatively well. Debilitated hosts have a high incidence of septicemia and a high mortality rate. *Bacteroides fragilis* is a collector of R factors and shows multiple and variable resistance to standard antibiotics. Surgical drainage is as essential as the use of combinations of antibiotics. Patients so treated have greatly reduced mortality rates in the range of 10%,[73] but it is likely that others in whom the anaerobes were not recognized have been recorded as therapy failures under miscellaneous diagnoses.

INFECTIONS OF CHILDHOOD

Three bacterial species, *Hemophilus influenzae, Bordetella pertussis,* and *Corynebacterium diphtheriae,* preferentially infect children after maternal antibody protection has been lost and before contact with these and other bacteria has generated some level of self-protection. Adults only occasionally suffer infection, largely those predisposed by viral illness, alcoholism, or chronic disease. At the turn of the century, 80% of all United States children contracted whooping cough; diphtheria was also quite common, with a 35% mortality rate. Routine administration of vaccine at 1 year of age has ended these pandemics but has not completely eradicated either disease. *Hemophilus influenzae* ("H. flu") is currently the biggest problem, especially in children under 1 year of age not pro-

tected completely by vaccine; it is also a true tissue invader, whereas *B. pertussis* and *C. diphtheriae* infect only luminal surfaces, causing disease mainly by their toxin production.

Hemophilus influenzae Infections

Hemophilus influenzae, an encapsulated coccobacillary or pleomorphic gram-negative organism, causes principally meningitis and upper respiratory infections, but sometimes also pneumonia, endocarditis, and miscellaneous suppurative infections. Many *H. influenzae* infections are of only moderate severity and are antibiotic-responsive, but *H. influenzae* meningitis, bronchiolitis, or obstructive epiglottitis in children can rapidly become life-threatening and currently impose about an 8% mortality rate.

More than 90% of human *H. influenzae* disease is accounted for by encapsulated type B strains, but other strains, even nonencapsulated ones, are occasionally pathogenic, as are two related species, *H. parainfluenzae* and *H. aphrophilus*. The organism's mucoid capsule, as with pneumococci, has an antiphagocytic role. With specific antisera it yields a *quellung* (swelling) reaction, useful for diagnosis. A limulus lysate assay for endotoxin is sometimes positive in cerebrospinal fluid during meningitis. A capsular polyribosphosphate, the B antigen, is the bacterium's principal seroreactant and is also the antigen used for vaccination. Unfortunately, the youngest children who need protection most are those who show weak antibody responses to B antigen. There is cross reactivity between antigens of Hemophilus and certain strains of *E. coli,* which may explain age-related immunity.

No more than 6% of healthy children carry type B *H. influenzae* organisms in their mouths, but many children carry other strains. The organism enters by the respiratory route and cases appear in small clusters or sporadically among members of day-care centers or families, rather than in meningococcus-like epidemics. The peak age of occurrence of meningitis is at one year, ranging from two months to seven years. The meningitis may appear suddenly or after a seemingly trivial prodrome mistaken for earache or for infant diarrhea. Neck stiffness or clear-cut neurologic signs of meningitis may not be evident. Because of endotoxin release by the bacteria, systemic manifestations are pronounced and, especially in young children, progression of the disease can be surprisingly fast. All too often, delayed treatment results in death or permanent neural damage. Patients with "flu" epiglottitis or respiratory or systemic infections tend to be somewhat older.

The diagnosis of an *H. influenzae* infection is often suggested by finding gram-negative coccobacillary forms in exudate or in the spinal fluid. Culture on special enrichment medium is effective, and rapid tests for B antigen by counterimmunoelectrophoresis, latex agglutination, or ELISA are available and are highly specific. Currently, most *H. influenzae* strains respond to antibiotics, but resistant beta-lactamase-bearing organisms are increasing in number.

> **Hemophilus influenzae lesions, like those of pneumococci, are exudative and rich in neutrophils and in fibrin, which gives the exudate a plastic quality and makes for slow resolution or sometimes organization and fibrous scarring. Respiratory infections** range from trivial involvements of the pharynx, middle ear, sinuses, or tonsils resembling viral URIs to severe febrile bacteremic illnesses sometimes resistant to routine antibiotics. **Acute epiglottitis** and related involvements are more frequently caused by *H. influenzae* than by any other pathogen. The uvula, epiglottic folds, and vocal cords rapidly become red and swollen, virtually suffocating the patient, sometimes within less than 24 hours, unless an airway is promptly established. **Descending laryngotracheobronchitis** may also result in airway obstruction as the smaller bronchi are plugged by dense, fibrin-rich exudate. These airway disorders are pediatric emergencies and have high mortality rates. **Hemophilus influenzae pneumonia** occurs in both children and adults; it either may follow an upper respiratory infection or bacteremia (i.e., may present as worsening of a previous respiratory disease) or may be a new complication of some other locus of infection. When it follows viral or other bacterial lung infection, it acquires special severity. Pulmonary consolidation is usually lobular and patchy, but when confluent and involving entire lung lobes it may be indistinguishable from pneumococcal pneumonia, except by microbiologic study.
>
> *Hemophilus influenzae* is the most common single cause of **suppurative meningitis** in children up to 5 years of age, after which the meningococcus takes over temporary primacy. Its pathology is described in detail on page 1392 but resembles that of other pyogenic infections. However, the meningeal exudate is usually tenacious because of its rich fibrin content.
>
> Other infections may be caused by this agent. An acute purulent conjunctivitis in children, "pink eye," long attributed to the Koch-Weeks bacillus, has now been proved to be due to *H. influenzae*. Like other gram-negative species, this organism can also cause septicemia, endocarditis, pyelonephritis, cholecystitis, and suppurative arthritis, usually in predisposed older individuals. All these lesions show the common anatomic characteristics of pyogenic infections.

Whooping Cough (*Bordetella pertussis*)

Whooping cough is an acute, highly communicable, usually self-terminating childhood disease characterized by violent coughing paroxysms followed by a loud inspiratory "whoop." It is caused by *B. pertussis*, a small, pleomorphic, gram-negative coccobacillus. Milder forms of the disease may resemble a trivial attack of acute bronchitis; conversely, whooping episodes occasionally occur during adenoviral infections or other URIs. Wide use of the diphtheria-pertussis-tetanus (DPT) vaccine has reduced the prevalence of whooping cough in the United States to less than 12,000 cases per year, but no one expects it to disappear entirely.

The causative organism, *B. pertussis*, has strong tropism for the brush border of the bronchial epithelium with which its growing colonies become entangled without actually invading tissue (Fig. 7–18). Diffusion of exotoxin from this source is thought to account for most of the characteristic disease manifestations (i.e., for the enhanced cough reflex, peripheral lymphocytosis, malaise, and frequent weight loss despite relatively mild fever).[74] These features may persist after the bacteria themselves have disappeared until all intracellular toxin is inactivated. The key to recovery and to immune protection is secretory antibodies of the IgA class that inhibit the adhesion step essential for bacterial proliferation.

> The respiratory lesions of established whooping cough resemble those of other forms of laryngotracheobronchitis. In severe cases there is bronchial mucosal erosion, hyperemia, and copious mucopurulent exudate but, unless superinfected, the lung alveoli remain open and intact. In parallel with the striking peripheral lymphocytosis (up to 90%), hypercellularity and enlargement of the mucosal lymph follicles and peribronchial lymph nodes have been observed.

After seven to ten days' incubation, the disease passes through a "catarrhal" period of coughing and sneezing, followed by the onset of the characteristic paroxysms. Violent coughing may cause leakage of air from distended airways, resulting in subcutaneous

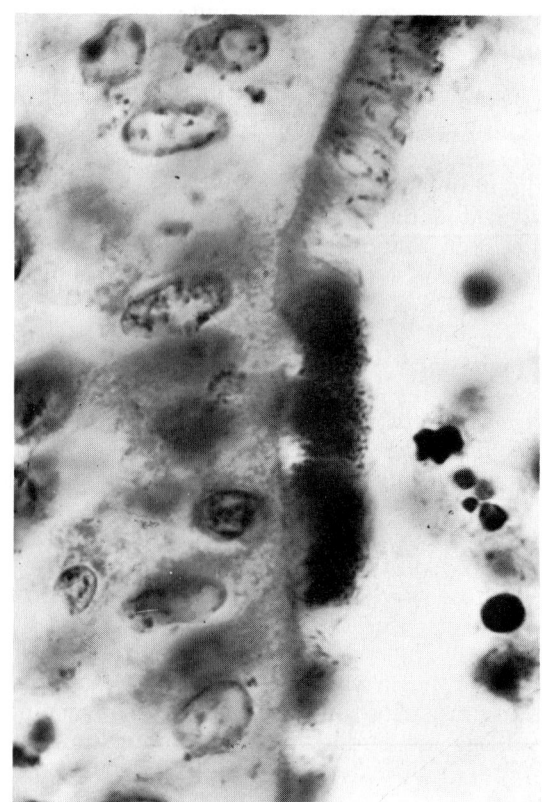

Figure 7–18. Whooping cough. High-power detail of columnar epithelium of a bronchus with bacilli entangled with the cilia.

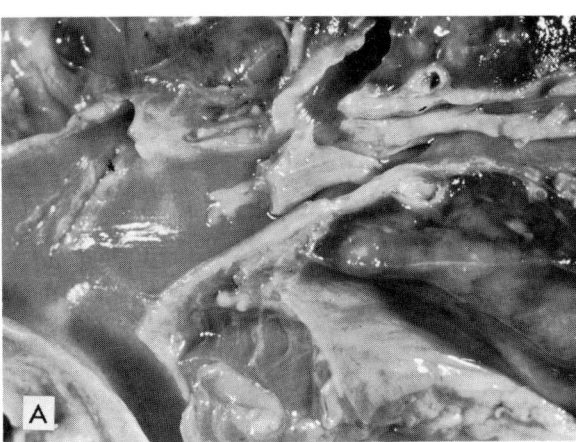 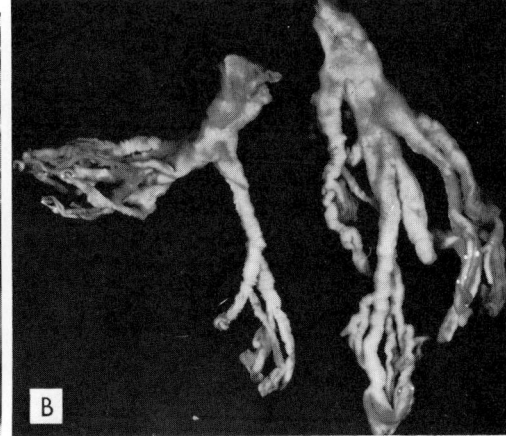

Figure 7–19. Membrane of diphtheria lying within transverse bronchus *(A)* and forming a perfect cast (removed from lung) of the branching respiratory tree *(B)*.

emphysema; more frequently, convulsions are set off by the hypoxia and by the constant, tiring coughing effort; coughing spells may drag on after fever subsides but in most cases, with or without treatment, normality gradually returns over several days. The role of whooping cough in promoting adult chronic obstructive lung disease (p. 766) has long been debated, but supporting evidence is scant. Usually, whooping cough leaves no sequelae.

Diphtheria (*Corynebacterium diphtheriae*)

Diphtheria is an acute communicable disease usually found in children from 2 to 15 years of age. Its agent, *C. diphtheriae*, localizes in the host's respiratory tree, ulcerates its mucosa, and induces the formation of an inflammatory membrane while phage-mediated diphtheria toxin (discussed on p. 334) damages remote organs, most prominently the myocardium and nerve tissue. The extent of respiratory involvement ranges from nasal diphtheria to deep, obstructive bronchitis (croup); rarely, the infection lodges in the adult human respiratory tract or skin. Depending on their toxin, strains of *C. diphtheriae* are designated *var. mitis* (mild) or *var. gravis*, but untreated diphtheria always carries a significant mortality and can leave behind serious sequelae. Formerly among the commonest childhood infections, it is today limited to children beyond the reach of normal school health services and to adults whose vaccine protection has decayed over the decades; in the United States, that risk is highest for children of illegal immigrants and for skid-row derelicts. A few hundred cases are reported each year.

During its one- to seven-day incubation period, *C. diphtheriae* proliferates at its site of implantation, usually the mucosa of the nasopharynx, oropharynx, larynx, or trachea. Reimplantation and satellite lesions in other sites (e.g., the esophagus or lower airways) are common. Edema and hyperemia of the affected epithelial surface appear

first. In the next few days, the elaboration of exotoxin causes necrosis of the epithelium, accompanied by an outpouring of large amounts of a dense fibrinosuppurative exudate. **The coagulation of this exudate on the ulcerated necrotic surface creates a tough, dirty gray-to-black, superficial membrane** (Fig. 7–19), **sometimes called a pseudomembrane.** This harbors sloughed necrotic epithelial cells as well as a profusion of the organisms. Neutrophilic infiltration in the underlying tissues becomes progressively more intense and is accompanied by marked vascular congestion, interstitial edema, and fibrin exudation. When the membrane is torn off its highly vascularized bed, oozing of blood occurs. Occasionally, inflammation and necrosis of the subjacent tissues permit spontaneous dislodgement and aspiration of the membrane, resulting in asphyxiation. With control of the infection, the membrane is either coughed up or is removed by enzymatic digestion, the inflammatory reaction subsides, and the local mucosal defect is closed by regeneration. The regional nodes of drainage respond with a nonspecific acute lymphadenitis, most dramatically expressed during the severe "bull's neck" type of diphtheria.

Although the bacterial invasion remains localized, generalized reticuloendothelial hyperplasia of the spleen and lymph nodes ensues, owing to the absorption of soluble exotoxin into the blood. **The exotoxin may cause fatty myocardial change with isolated myofiber necrosis, polyneuritis with degeneration of the myelin sheaths and axis cylinders, and (less commonly) fatty change or even focal necroses of parenchymal cells in the liver, kidneys, and adrenals.** Occasionally, in more severe cases, clustered cardiac muscle fibers show fatty change or necrosis.[75] These organ alterations are largely reversible and are rarely followed by permanent scarring, but both motor and sensory nerve fibers may fail to regenerate adequately, and minimal interstitial myocardial fibrosis may persist. Some long-lasting cardiac conduction defects may thus have originated during childhood diphtheria.[76]

Early pharyngeal diphtheria with its sore throat, fever, chills, and malaise may resemble a viral or streptococcal pharyngitis until the characteristic membrane is formed and dyspnea with crowing respiration or cyanosis gives rise to alarm; epidemics of the "gravis" strains of *C. diphtheriae* frequently cause croup, sudden asphyxiation, myocarditis, or neuritis. The onset of myocarditis usually lags a few days behind the development of respiratory symptoms; a slow heart beat in a febrile diphtheric patient is an indication for ECG study; if heart block is found, the prognosis must be guarded, even under intensive care. Neurologic symptoms can begin early or late in the course or during convalescence. Weakness or paralysis of the soft palate, of extraocular muscles of the eye, or even of the extremities occur in less than a quarter of cases and usually subside slowly, but sometimes they persist. All complications can be prevented by antitoxic serum only *before* diphtheria toxin has wrought its cell damage, but not thereafter. This urgency also applies to adult cutaneous diphtheria and should be kept in mind in the differential diagnosis of a skin ulcer lacking an obvious cause.

Culture of *C. diphtheriae* is essential for diagnosis because fungal or fusospirochetal infections sometimes cause similar membranous respiratory or cutaneous infections. Special fibrin-containing media are used for culturing *C. diphtheriae* because miscellaneous throat flora would otherwise overgrow that organism; in addition, positive cultures must be tested for toxigenicity by gel diffusion so as to avoid confusion with commensal mouth diphtheroids. Timely diagnosis of diphtheria can benefit not only the patient but also the community at risk by sounding the alert for preventive measures, including immunization!

ENTEROPATHOGENIC BACTERIA

Besides the bacterial species listed as common enteropathogens in Table 7–6 (p. 337), other organisms can involve the gut, most notably *Clostridium difficile* (p. 360) and the enterotoxin-producing or invasive staphylococci (pp. 335–336). Conversely, some enteropathogens can infect organs other than the gut. The diarrheal syndrome, a common denominator of enteric infections, also has many noninfectious causes and can vary greatly in severity. Thus far, *three mechanisms are known by which bacteria cause diarrhea:* (1) direct invasion of the gut wall, (2) the release of enterotoxins, and (3) the hypersecretory state elicited by bacterial adhesion to mucosal epithelial cells.[77] *Only invasive enteropathogens cause substantial leukocytic infiltration and exudation into the stool; adhesive or toxin-producing serotypes induce large diarrheal fluid losses in the absence of exudate or definable anatomic mucosal lesions.* This distinction is fundamental to the diagnosis and management of bacterial enteritis, and it makes direct microscopic stool examination for leukocytes an important aid in diagnosis. Also important is the use of culture media that permit the growth of fastidious enteric pathogens such as

Campylobacter. In some bacterial species, enteropathogenicity is stably transmitted by chromosomal DNA; in most, it is acquired via plasmids. It is often desirable, therefore, to go beyond cultural identification of the bacterial species. Serotyping, or the newer methods of DNA blotting or DNA-RNA hybridization, characterize the responsible organism far more specifically.

Enteric infection in the compromised host should be of special concern. Also, corticosteroids and immunosuppressive drugs sometimes used to treat idiopathic ulcerative colitis increase the pathogenicity of many enteric organisms; moreover, slowing of intestinal transit by antispasmodic drugs favors intraluminal bacterial proliferation and can thus aggravate and prolong enteric infection. The differential diagnosis between bacterial and idiopathic ulcerative colitis is especially crucial. Also of note — users of antacids lacking the barrier function of gastric acidity are at risk of infection by pH-sensitive enteric pathogens.

E. coli Enteric Infections

Although *E. coli* is a normal commensal of the human gastrointestinal tract, it has long been known as a cause of diarrhea and dysentery (painful bowel movements) in infants, children, and adults. Through plasmids, certain serotypes have acquired invasiveness, enteroadhesiveness, or enterotoxicity. *Invasiveness* has been associated mainly with the O-group of *E. coli* but is not limited to these strains. Most enteroinvasive epidemics in the United States occur in the Southwestern states among agricultural migrants or among children on Indian reservations. In developing countries these strains are frequent causes of dysentery. They produce inflammation and partial destruction of the colonic mucosa, similar to that of shigellosis, but milder as a rule (p. 356). After one to two days of incubation, enteroinvasive *E. coli* abruptly give rise to diarrhea, cramping pain, tenesmus, fever, and malaise of about one week's duration. Stools are watery and often contain flecks of mucus and neutrophilic exudate.

The *toxigenic E. coli* strains, also principally of the O-group, release a plasmid-acquired enterotoxin whose mode of action parallels that of *Vibrio cholerae* (p. 356). In this more common version of diarrheal disease, the mucosa, though severely deranged in its function, remains morphologically intact; stools have the rice-water quality seen in cholera. The disease in adults is usually mild, limited to three to seven days; in children, the diarrhea may be more severe and prolonged, and dehydration can lead to death without careful fluid management. The enterotoxin found in pediatric infections is heat stable, whereas that in adult traveler's diarrhea seems to be heat labile. Enterotoxic *E. coli* are widely disseminated in third-world countries, most of whose adult inhabitants become immune to the native flora. Nonimmune travelers are therefore vulnerable; perhaps one third of all cases of "Montezuma's revenge" are due to enterotoxic *E. coli,* thus emphasizing the benefits of prophylactic antibiotic use (others are due to calciviruses or to protozoal infections that fail to respond).

Escherichia coli enteroadhesive enteritis, first recognized in piglets (K88 strain), is being seen in humans. Activated by plasmids, the bacterial pili (normally initiating conjugation and DNA exchange) adhere instead to a receptor on the enteric epithelial cell membrane. On electron microscopy, bacteria are solidly anchored on the luminal surface of mucosal cells, which undergo cytoplasmic cupping and vacuolization. The mechanisms by which these organisms induce diarrhea are still poorly understood but appear to be distinct from those involved in the production of enterotoxin.[77]

Salmonella Infections

These gram-negative coliform organisms are among the foremost causes of food- and water-borne enteric infections in the world; about 50,000 cases are reported annually in the United States. Biochemical classification recognizes three human pathogenic species: (1) *S. typhi* (the cause of classic typhoid fever), (2) *S. cholerae-suis,* and (3) *S. enteritidis* (causing either acute enteritis or septicemia). However, well over 1000 serotypes of the *S. enteritidis* group have been identified, the most prevalent in the United States being *S. typhimurium, S. paratyphi, S. newport,* and *S. heidelberg.*

Salmonellae are versatile in antigenicity and disease manifestations, and may cause (1) typhoid fever; (2) enteric fevers, which basically resemble typhoid fever but are milder; (3) salmonella food poisoning, a form of acute gastroenteritis; (4) gram-negative septicemia; (5) localized abscesses and inflammatory foci in almost any organ of the body, including the bones and arteries; and (6) a chronic carrier state. They are acquired by ingestion of contaminated food or water. Small numbers of organisms will not produce disease, except in persons lacking gastric acidity. *Salmonella typhi* is shed in the feces, urine, vomitus, and oral secretions by infected humans, including convalescents, and by chronic carriers without overt disease who harbor the organisms in their gallbladders. Other salmonellae come principally from animals and their food products, which they widely contaminate; poultry and eggs are particular hazards. So many turtles carry salmonellae that they are banned as children's pets in the United States.

Salmonellae have flagellar, somatic, and outer coat antigens (named H, O, and Vi antigens, respectively). They lack enterotoxins but are capable of invading intestinal mucosal cells to cause degenerative changes in the brush border and apical cytoplasm.[78] They also induce luminal fluid accumulation in the isolated ileal loop prior to mucosal ulceration.[79] The manner in which salmonellae traverse the gut epithelium has not yet been adequately explained. After invasion they are taken up by neutrophils and macrophages within the lamina propria and can multiply for a time inside the phagosomes of these cells. Their ultimate destruction by phagocytes coincides with the onset of clinical convalescence.

TYPHOID FEVER. Luminal proliferation of *S. typhi,* mucosal penetration, uptake by macrophages, and dissemination to the lymphatic structures of the gut and mesentery are the earliest events in typhoid fever and are completed within the incubation period of one to two weeks. Bacteremia then ensues during the first week of clinical disease.

> The organisms cause enlargement of reticuloendothelial and lymphoid tissue throughout the body. Proliferation of phagocytes swells the lymphatic submucosal nodules of the entire gut, mainly Peyer's patches of the terminal ileum. These become sharply delineated, plateau-like elevations up to 8 cm in diameter, bulging into the intestinal lumen (Fig. 7-20). Concomitantly, the mesenteric lymph nodes, the spleen, and often the liver increase in size. In untreated cases, during the second week, the mucosa over the swollen ileal lymphoid tissue is shed, resulting in oval ulcers with their long axes in the direction of bowel flow (Fig. 7-21), a pattern seen only in typhoid fever and Yersinia infections (p. 866). (Intestinal tuberculosis, by contrast, produces circular or transverse ulcers.) Bleeding from typhoidal ulcers is usually scant, but it can sometimes become uncontrollable. Perforation, although rare, has been the cause of fatalities.

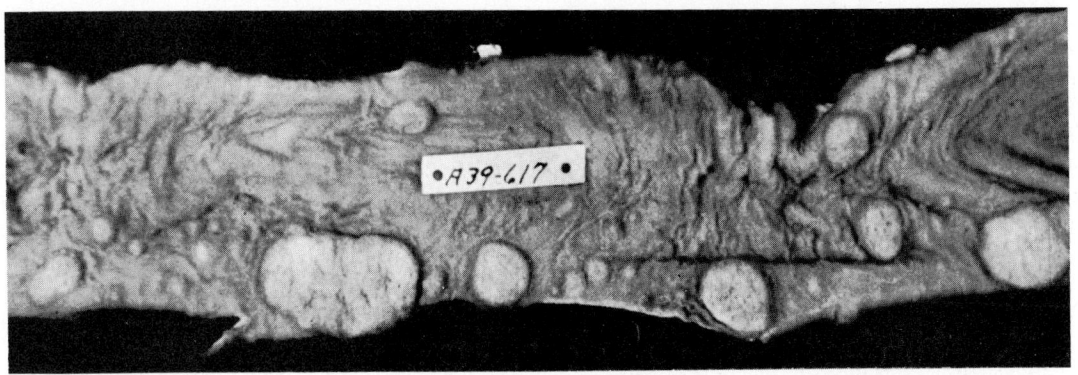

Figure 7-20. Typhoid fever. Gross view of markedly hyperplastic lymphoid follicles in opened ileum.

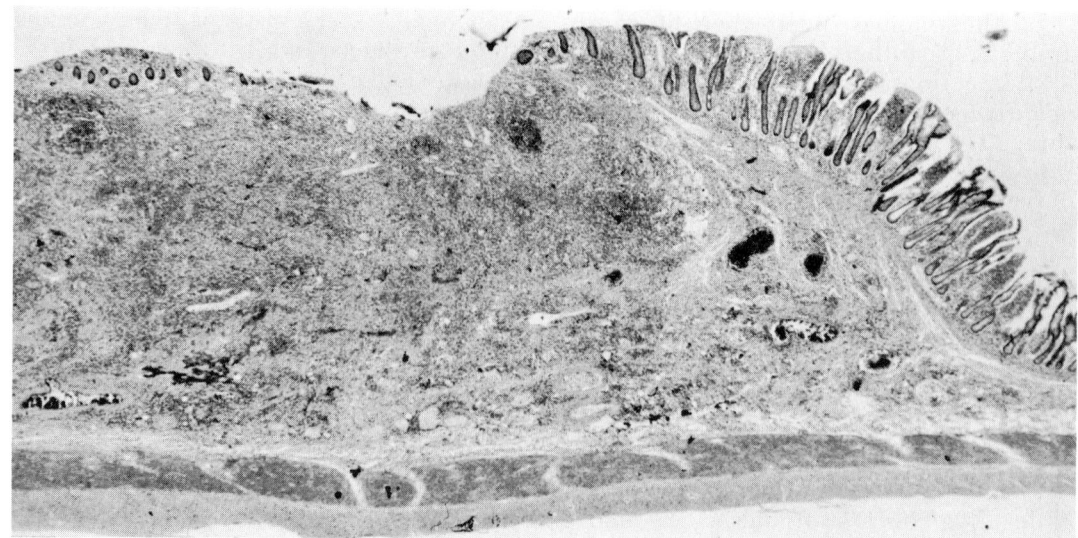

Figure 7–21. Typhoid fever. Low-power view of cross section of a markedly enlarged and disrupted lymphoid follicle in ileum, with necrosis of overlying mucosa.

Once past the peak of the disease, the ulcers heal slowly and the lymphatic structures amazingly regenerate without permanent scarring.

Histologically, there is both local and systemic mobilization and accumulation of mononuclear phagocytes. The macrophages form small nodular aggregates rather than full-fledged tuberculoid granulomas. They are filled with red cells (erythrophagocytosis) and nuclear debris, during the height of the disease (Fig. 7–22). The bacteria are sometimes scarce and are better stained with polychrome methylene blue than with Gram stain. Intermingled with the phagocytes are lymphocytes and plasma cells in liberal numbers, but granulocytes are typically quite scarce and congregate mainly near the ulcerated surface of Peyer's patches. There is also **neutropenia in the peripheral blood.**

The **spleen** is enlarged, soft, and bulging, with uniformly pale red pulp and obliterated follicular markings. Microscopically, it has marked sinus histiocytosis and reticuloendothelial proliferation, replicating the changes seen in the lymphoid tissues of the gut. Splenic rupture occurs but is uncommon. The liver shows small, randomly scattered foci of parenchymal necrosis in which the hepatocyte is replaced by a phagocytic mononuclear cell aggregate called a typhoid nodule; these distinctive nodules also occur in the bone marrow and lymph nodes. Treatment can, of course, arrest or modify all these classic lesions. Fatty change may appear in the liver of patients kept on prolonged liquid diets. Tetracycline treatment may result in microvesicular fatty liver change and in hepatic failure with jaundice (similar to the acute jaundice syndrome seen in pregnancy) (p. 916). A more frequent complication is pneumonia, generally due to intercurrent bacterial superinfection. Like other salmonellae, *S. typhi* can localize in many sites, including the con-

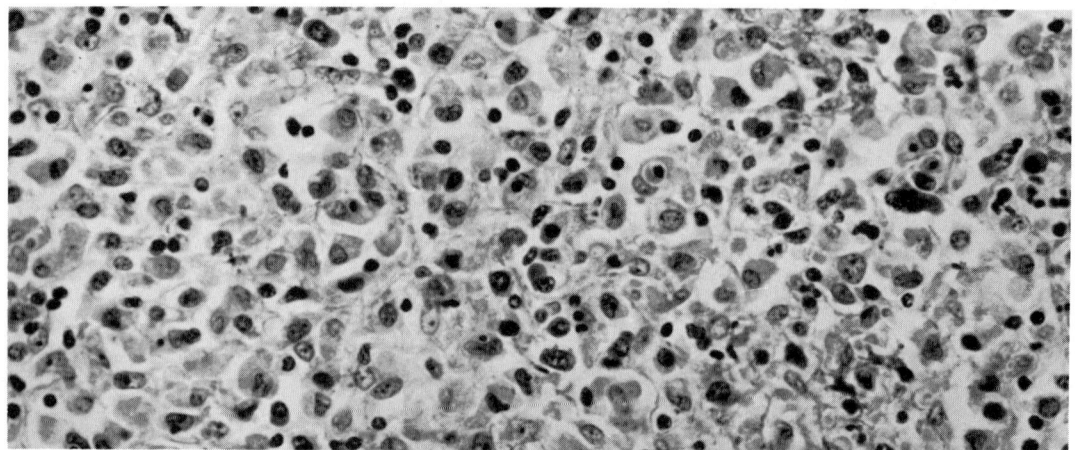

Figure 7–22. Typhoid fever. High-power detail of massed phagocytic cells in center of a reactive lymphoid follicle. Scattered cells contain phagocytized red and white cells.

junctivae, meninges, joints, kidneys, and gallbladder, but despite the early bacteremia of typhoid fever, only gallbladder infections attain a frequency of 3%, that of the carrier state. The gallbladder colonization may or may not be associated with gallstones and often requires cholecystectomy to eliminate bacterial shedding.

Classic typhoid fever is ushered in by malaise, headache, and fever with afternoon spikes that mount progressively each day. The fever stabilizes during the second week (the fastigium) and then gradually declines during the third and fourth weeks. A variety of abdominal symptoms (distention, colicky pain, or constipation alternating with diarrhea) point to the intestinal involvement.

During the second week, a characteristic skin rash, described as "rose spots" (1- to 5-mm red macules that blanch upon pressure), may appear, often on the lower anterior chest and upper abdomen. This eruption is rarely conspicuous and fades quickly. Characteristically, there is splenohepatomegaly, bradycardia, and leukopenia.

The diagnosis can be confirmed by *isolation of the organism from the blood* during the first week in about 90% of cases, falling to 50% by the third week. *Bacilli may appear in the stools early but are regularly recoverable only during the third to fifth weeks.* Urine cultures become positive during the third to fourth weeks in about one quarter of patients. Antibodies, as identified by the Widal reaction, are demonstrable during the second week of illness, with progressively rising titers during the subsequent two weeks.

Since typhoid fever fell to a frequency of 400 to 600 cases per year in the United States, almost all of them imported, its diagnosis has often been delayed, but appropriate antibiotics still abort its course. Resistance (R) factors have now appeared so that sensitivity testing and careful antibiotic selection have become mandatory. Infants, children, and the elderly are at highest risk, but death from intestinal perforation, intestinal hemorrhages, or intercurrent pneumonic infections still occurs in all age groups among the medically underserved.

OTHER SALMONELLA INFECTIONS. *Food poisoning* with vomiting and diarrhea represents the mildest expression of the Salmonella disease spectrum. Its incubation and duration are brief; its systemic effects relatively slight; complications are rare; and fatalities unknown. It often presents as a local epidemic traceable to a single food source. Little is known of its pathology except that lesions appear to be limited to the colon, are superficial, and heal promptly. Biopsies have shown mixed inflammatory cell infiltration of the lamina propria of the gut mucosa with superficial epithelial erosions; in a few cases, however, the lesions were severe enough to resemble those of idiopathic ulcerative colitis.[80]

Enteric fevers caused by *S. typhimurium, S. paratyphi, S. cholerae-suis*, and other miscellaneous *salmonellae* have features and severity intermediate between those of salmonella food poisoning and typhoid fever. Occasionally, however, *S. typhimurium* infection has proved fatal. *Salmonella bacteremia* can also occur in the absence of intestinal lesions or symptoms, as a febrile septic disease with or without localizing signs. Occasionally, the bacteremia recurs in an adult carrier who may only dimly recall having had enteric fever during childhood. Localized infections—pyelonephritis, cholecystitis, meningitis, pericarditis, mycotic aneurysm, endocarditis, and salpingitis—due to various Salmonella species may occur. Patients with hemoglobinopathies, especially with hemoglobin S disease (p. 666) are prone to prolonged Salmonella bacteremias and osteomyelitis. Patients, mostly in Egypt and Brazil, with Schistosoma infections may secondarily acquire chronic salmonellosis, arising from either urinary tract[81] or enteric lesions.[82] Treatment of both the helminthic and the Salmonella infection is necessary in such instances because the bacteria adhere to and symbiotically thrive on the parasite's tegument.[83]

Bacillary Dysentery

Dysentery means diarrhea with abdominal cramping and tenesmus from any cause, infectious or not. The term *bacillary dysentery* is reserved for infection by four *Shigella* species: *S. dysenteriae, S. flexneri, S. boydii*, and *S. sonnei*. These gram-negative coliform bacilli are facultative anaerobes; unlike the salmonellae, they are infectious only for man but can cause disease even when ingested in very small numbers. Transmission is fecal-oral; animal reservoirs or long-term human carriers play no significant role. Outbreaks occur frequently where food hygiene is poor (e.g., in third-world countries or in poorly run closed institutions). In the United States, reported cases have averaged about 18,000 per year.

Shigellae invade the colonic mucosa by traversing the epithelium and multiply in the lamina propria; thence they are carried to the intestinal lymph nodes but, unlike salmonellae, they do not cause bacteremia or localize in distant organs.[77] Stool culture on special enteric media is essential for diagnosis. Host tissue damage localizes to the colon and, sometimes, the terminal ileum. It is attributed largely to the release of endotoxin at the invaded sites, which results in mucosal necrosis; in addition, the strain *S. dysenteriae* I, known as the cause of great historical epidemics, produces Shiga neurotoxin, which elicits hindquarter paralysis in experimental animals. Most recent epidemics have instead been caused by *S. flexneri* or *S. sonnei* and have been comparatively mild and small; nevertheless, because of the danger bacillary dysentery poses to public health, all cases must be reported as well as treated. Because strains with antibiotic resistance have become an increasing problem, sensitivity testing should be done if possible.

In severe bacillary dysentery the colonic mucosa becomes hyperemic and edematous; enlargement of the lymphoid follicles creates small, projecting nodules. **Within the course of 24 hours a fibrinosuppurative exudate diffusely covers the mucosa and produces a dirty gray-to-yellow pseudomembrane.** The inflammatory reaction within the intestinal mucosa builds up, the mucosa becomes soft and friable, and irregular superficial ulcerations appear. If the infection is severe, large tracts may be denuded, leaving only islands of preserved mucosa (Fig. 7–23). Usually, all the ulcerations are superficial and rarely extend below the mucosal level. Macroscopically, they are not distinctive from the lesions of active idiopathic ulcerative colitis. Perforation is an uncommon complication (p. 886).

Histologically, there is a predominantly mononuclear leukocytic infiltrate within the lamina propria, but the surfaces of the ulcers are covered with an acute, suppurative, neutrophilic reaction accompanied by congestion, marked edema, fibrin deposition, and thromboses of small vessels. As the disease progresses, the ulcer margins are transformed into active granulation tissue. When the disease remits, this granulation tissue fills the defect, and the ulcers heal by regeneration of the mucosal epithelium.

The incubation period of bacillary dysentery is less than 48 hours. The severe case begins abruptly with watery diarrhea, nausea, and vomiting, often with crampy abdominal pain partly relieved by bowel movements, which may reach a frequency of 50 per day. The stools are scanty, mucoid, stained with blood, and flecked with pus. Numerous neutrophils can be seen microscopically; systemic manifestations include fever, headache, and, in severe untreated cases, dehydration, prostration, and clouded sensorium, sometimes even neck stiffness. Bacillary dysentery varies in its severity. Milder cases may resemble so-called food poisoning and, with appropriate electrolyte and water replacement, recovery is the rule. Severe bacillary dysentery is a harrowing experience for both patient and physician and can result in severe

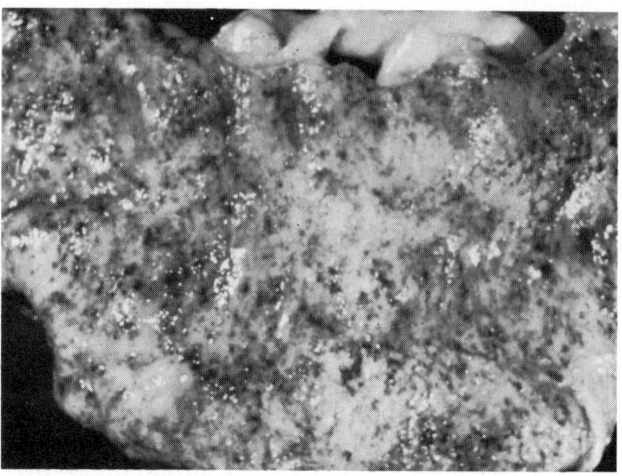

Figure 7–23. Shigella colitis with edema, ulceration, and pseudomembrane formation.

prostration or death, especially during major epidemics due to newly imported strains. The primary objective of antibiotic treatment is to prevent transmission; whether it shortens the course is uncertain.

Cholera (Vibrio cholerae)*

Vibrios are comma-shaped, gram-negative organisms, readily cultured on selective media and sometimes directly visible in stools by microscopy or immunofluorescence. *Vibrio cholerae* has been the cause of seven great pandemics of diarrheal disease, the latest one during the years 1961 to 1974. In addition to its three classic serotypes, the somewhat less pathogenic *V. cholerae el tor* has recently been spreading. The so-called *noncholera vibrios* such as *V. parahaemolyticus*, acquired from raw or poorly cooked seafood, cause milder diarrheal illness as a rule. *Vibrio alginolyticus* and the recently isolated *V. vulnificus* are seawater adapted and, unlike the enteropathogenic vibrios, cause skin infections and systemic sepsis.[84] Campylobacters are closely related to the Vibrios.

Cholera has been endemic as a childhood and adult disease in the watershed of the Ganges River for as long as can be remembered, and its pandemics have always traveled westward into Europe and Africa. In rural Bangladesh, India, and Indonesia, cholera, especially when inadequately treated, still takes a gigantic toll, particularly among children. The deaths are all the more tragic because the infection is more readily controlled than those caused by shigellae and other enteroinvasive pathogens. A minor outbreak was reported in the southwest of the United States in 1978, not traceable to any imported source.[85]

Vibrio cholerae is transmitted by the fecal-oral route, and its long-term excretion by convalescents and asymptomatic carriers contributes greatly to its spread. *Its pathogenicity is entirely attributable to an enterotoxin (Fig. 7–24), which activates the adenylate cyclase of the plasma membranes of the crypt epithelium of the small bowel.* Massive secretion of isotonic fluid ensues, overwhelming the reabsorptive function of the colon and resulting in the typical dilute rice-water or straw-colored diarrhea of cholera containing flecks of mucus, but few if any leukocytes.[86] Fortunately, the overall absorption of the gut remains intact so that the massive Na, K, HCO_2, and fluid losses can be replaced by oral formulas. The untreated adult patient presents a pitiful picture of dry mouth, sunken eyes, weak pulse, lethargy, and anuria. There may be bouts of vomiting and normal or even low body temperature. With fluid replacement and other supportive therapy, complete recovery is the rule, the mortality rate being now less than 1%; without adequate therapy, it ranges up to 50%. Deaths are mostly caused by dehydration, hypovolemic shock, and metabolic acidosis.

Vibrio cholerae **does not invade or damage the gut mucosa.** The vibrios, if stained by immunofluorescence, do not pass beyond the epithelial brush border. The mucosal

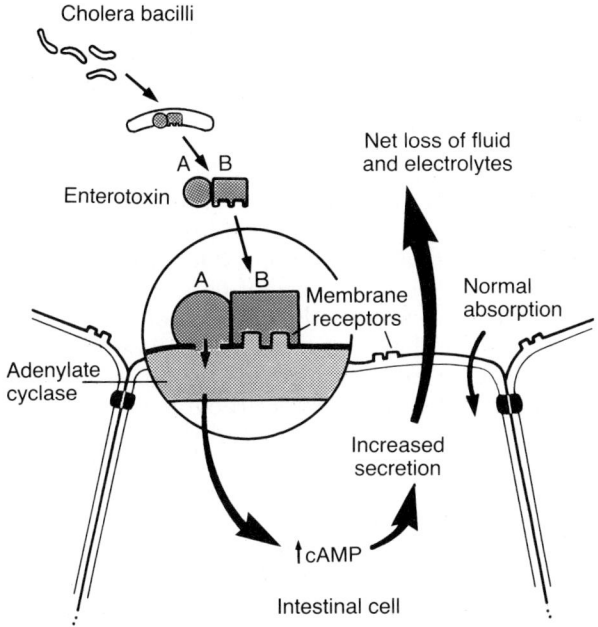

Figure 7–24. A schema of the mechanism of action of cholera enterotoxin in its induction of excessive mucosal secretory activity.

lamina propria usually shows congestion and a moderate infiltration of mononuclear inflammatory cells. Where cholera is endemic, such changes in the crypt-to-villus ratio (normally 1:3) as may appear in the jejunal mucosa are usually related to diet and chronic exposure to various enteric pathogens rather than to the vibrios. Interestingly, there is often hyperplasia of the lymphoid cells of Peyer's patches, and sometimes also of the mesenteric lymph nodes and spleen.[87] In sum, the few histologic alterations seen in biopsy specimens of cholera patients in no way reflect the dramatic functional effects of cholera toxin. Fatal cases may reveal the consequences of hypovolemic shock and electrolyte imbalance (e.g., lung edema with hyaline membranes and thickened alveolar septa, or focal myocardial necrosis); terminal bronchopneumonia may complicate the picture.

Immunity to cholera does not seem to be lasting, as reinfection is common and the currently available vaccine composed of killed vibrios protects only partially for three to six months, motivating a search for more effective immunogens.

Campylobacter Enteritis

Until recently, this comma-shaped, flagellated, gram-negative organism was classified with the vibrios. Only when special cultural conditions permitted its isolation did it become apparent that Campylobacter was an important cause of chronic gastritis, enterocolitis and septicemia in man that had frequently been missed by routine cultures for the coliforms and enterobacteria. The gastritis is discussed in detail on page 845; here our attention is directed to the enteritis. Currently, *Campylobacter jejuni* is responsible

for 5 to 11% of all cases of diarrhea and dysentery in United States hospitals, equaling or surpassing the salmonellae as an enteric pathogen.[88] Infection with Campylobacter spp. occurs by ingestion, most often of contaminated liquid or solid food, such as milk, poultry, or water. Epidemics are usually modest in size, affecting both children and adults. Sporadic infections may be derived from human or zoonotic sources; domestic dogs are frequent carriers.

Like salmonellae, *C. jejuni* causes disorders ranging from subclinical infection to incapacitating dysentery. Abdominal pain is a frequent complaint and may precede the diarrhea. Nausea, headache, myalgia, and fever are the most common symptoms; stools are foul-smelling, sometimes containing exudate and streaks or microscopic amounts of blood. Pain may persist after diarrhea ceases and the average duration of illness is about five days.

Campylobacter spp. may induce disease by three mechanisms, shared with other enteric pathogens. One is toxin-induced disease with watery diarrhea similar to cholera. Another type involves invasion and proliferation within the intestinal epithelium, leading to cell death. This is manifested clinically by bloody diarrhea and inflammatory cells in the stool. A third mechanism is termed translocation, whereby the organisms penetrate the intestinal mucosa and proliferate within the lamina propria and mesenteric lymph nodes. This may produce an enteric fever without frank dysentery. Variability in disease expression may thus be the result of different mechanisms. It is not clear whether such variation is due to inherent differences among strains of *C. jejuni* or to variable host response.[89]

Inflammation may involve the entire gut from the jejunum to the anus. In invasive infection, the colonic mucosa appears friable or superficially eroded on proctoscopy. By light microscopy, hyperemia, edema, and inflammatory infiltrates of neutrophils, lymphocytes, and plasma cells are seen. **There may be colonic crypt abscesses and ulcerations resembling those of chronic ulcerative colitis.** In the small bowel there is some decrease in the crypt-villus ratio.[90] Septicemia is uncommon and the infection has rarely been fatal, but correct identification of this agent and appropriate antibiotic regimens are obviously important as they can shorten the clinical course and prevent further transmission.

As noted, another member of the genus, *Campylobacter pylori*, has been identified in gastric isolates. This organism is significantly associated with histologic evidence of gastritis, especially of the antrum.[91] At present the role of these organisms in the production of the gastritis and peptic ulcer is under study.

Yersinia Enteritis

One relative of the plague bacillus, *Y. enterocolitica*, has now entered the constellation of enteropathogens and is now recognized as a major cause of bacterial enteritis in pediatric populations; it may infect adults as well. It too requires special media for identification. Both zoonotic and case-to-case transmission occur.

The organism may affect the upper as well as the lower digestive tract and sometimes causes pharyngitis or tonsillitis, along with cervical lymph node enlargement. Most frequently involved are the distal ileum and colon. The ulcerative intestinal lesions are not unlike those of typhoid fever. A more diffuse enteritis may also occur with villus shortening, crypt hyperplasia, and mucosal microabscesses.[92] Yersiniae traverse the intestinal mucosa and invade underlying tissues, producing characteristic microabscesses rimmed by activated mononuclear phagocytes in mesenteric lymph nodes. These granulomas resemble the stellate abscesses of lymphogranuloma venereum or cat-scratch disease. Mesenteric lymphadenitis is prominent in yersinia infection attributable to the necrotizing and suppurative lesions of the gut.

Because of its deeply invasive behavior, *Y. enterocolitica* belongs to the more severe and potentially lethal causes of dysentery. Its diarrheal syndrome varies from acute gastroenteritis or appendicitis to chronic relapsing ileocolitis, prompting surgical exploration.[93] Its destructive potential explains both the relatively prolonged disease caused by the agent and the urgency for appropriate antibiotic therapy.[94] Extraintestinal manifestations (arthritis, erythema nodosum, or glomerulonephritis) may complicate the clinical course. A hemagglutination test is available for diagnosis.

CLOSTRIDIA

The clostridia are a large family of gram-positive, sporulating anaerobes. They are inhabitants of the animal gut and their spores widely pervade pastures and garden soil. Only a few species are important causes of disease (Table 7–6, p. 337). Clostridia are better adapted to their gut-and-soil cycle than to mammalian tissue, which they invade only under conditions favorable for their growth: low oxygen tension, previous tissue damage, or poor phagocytic defense. Each human pathogenic species produces powerful specific toxins that can give rise to life-threatening illnesses, sometimes even in the absence of tissue invasion. Toxin release by clostridia requires germination of spores and proliferation without interference by competing flora. These conditions explain the relative rarity and severity of clostridial disease. Conversely, clostridial spores can be incidentally present in normal skin, clean wounds, and infections due to other pathogens; therefore, isolation of these organisms in anaerobic culture is not necessarily diagnostic of clostridial disease.

Tetanus (C. tetani)

Tetanus is a severe, acute disease characterized by convulsive contractions of voluntary muscles, in-

duced by the powerful neurotoxin *tetanospasmin*, elaborated by *C. tetani* (p. 335). The spores of the organisms, derived from the excreta of animals, are widely distributed and are often ingested but are incapable of germinating or generating toxin in the gut. Tetanus, therefore, usually results from spore contamination of wounds that permit the development of mixed infections providing both low oxygen tension and devitalized tissue necessary for germination of the spores; hence, the need for careful débridement of tissue injuries and for the opening of deep wounds suspected of harboring spores. Clean wounds such as needle or nail punctures provide less opportunity for spore germination but do not preclude tetanus. "Skin popping" or "mainlining" drug addicts are occasional victims. Newborn infants may be infected by fecal soiling of the umbilical cord stump, particularly when the squatting position or birthing chairs are used without proper attention to possible contamination. The incidence of neonatal tetanus has been greatly reduced by maternal vaccination during pregnancy, as maternal antibodies are passed to the infant.[95] In the United States the use of tetanus booster doses has lowered the annual incidence of tetanus to about 70 cases.

When released into the bloodstream, tetanospasmin attaches to the peripheral endings, mainly of motor neurons, then travels along nerves to bodies of origin situated in the CNS, but without affecting their function. *Only when it passes into the presynaptic terminals of inhibitory spinal interneurons do the symptoms of tetanus appear.* An increase in muscle tone results, giving rise to the spastic contractions characteristic of the disease. Loss of sympathetic inhibition induces an accelerated heart rate, hypertension, or other symptoms of cardiovascular instability. The toxin can be neutralized by antitoxin only before it combines with receptor nerve fibers; thereafter, its progressive effects are inexorable. Toxin cannot cross the blood-brain barrier and the patient's alertness and mentation remain tragically intact.

The usual incubation period is one to two weeks but may be shorter or even months long. The disease is ushered in by stiffness of voluntary muscles, usually first in the muscles of the jaw, followed by rigidity and tonic spasms of the facial muscles and then of the muscles of the trunk. As a consequence, there may be difficulty in opening the jaw (trismus), giving rise to the lay term "lockjaw." Facial involvement sometimes causes a sardonic smile (risus sardonicus), and contractions of the back muscles produce backward arching, or opisthotonos. Minimal stimuli, such as a noise or gentle moving of the patient, may set these affected muscles into violent, painful contractions. Dysphagia and respiratory difficulty develop with progression of the disease, and maintenance of an airway is routinely necessary to avoid asphyxiation.[96]

The morphologic changes are usually quite minimal. Examination of the local injury discloses only a nonspecific inflammatory reaction and tissue necrosis, due usually to a

mixed bacterial flora that may include gram-positive bacilli suggestive of *Clostridium tetani*. The neurologic changes are equally nonspecific and inconstant; they consist of swelling of the motor neurones of the spinal cord and medulla sometimes associated with nuclear swelling and chromatolysis.

Diagnosis depends largely on the clinical findings. Active immunization with tetanus toxoid protects against this disease, but the immunity fades within five to ten years. Prompt administration of antitoxin may block the development of clinical disease. At experienced intensive care centers the mortality rate from clinical tetanus has been lowered from about 60% to about 20% today. Once the attack passes, it leaves no permanent sequelae.

Botulism

The most common form of this severe paralyzing illness is *food poisoning caused by the ingestion of preformed* Clostridium botulinum *neurotoxin*. Rarely, botulism may be caused by *wound infection* or even more rarely by overgrowth of *C. botulinum* in the relatively germ-free intestines of infants. The usual source of *C. botulinum* spores in infants is contaminated honey.[97] Six specific subtypes of *C. botulinum* exotoxin have been identified; type A is the most lethal. The spores of the organisms are extremely resistant to drying and can withstand boiling for many hours. Appropriate anaerobic conditions for germination and toxin production are provided in processed or canned food kept without refrigeration, particularly when home-prepared and inadequately sterilized. The contaminated food may not appear to be spoiled. The preformed toxin is heat labile and is destroyed by boiling for ten minutes, but is resistant to gastric digestion and is readily absorbed into the blood.

Botulinus toxin (p. 335) attaches to the synaptic vesicles of cholinergic nerves, where it blocks the release of acetylcholine. This blockage is potentiated by nerve activity at the neuromuscular junction. The result is a descending form of paralysis from the cranial nerves down to the extremities.[98] Although the severest poisonings begin within a few hours, onset can be treacherously delayed for up to eight days. Cranial nerve palsies, ptosis, diplopia, dysphagia, and voice changes develop together with marked dryness of the mouth and, frequently, paralytic ileus. Paralysis of the respiratory muscles may precede that of the extremities. The patient remains mentally alert and afebrile, and cerebrospinal fluid is normal. Once the toxin has entered the synapses, it can no longer be inactivated by antitoxin, and only intensive supportive care is possible; this salvages close to 85% of victims. Recovery of motor function is slow but complete. Most deaths are caused by respiratory infections. Infant botulism occurs below 9 months of age; it may manifest itself as sudden infant death (SIDS) (p. 536) or as constipation, generalized weakness, respiratory difficulty, and lack of spontaneous movement. Appropriately treated babies have a lower mortality rate than adults.

Although depletion of acetylcholine in nerve endings is biochemically demonstrable, findings are poorly defined, nonspecific, and attributable largely to CNS and systemic hypoxia.

The diagnosis is supported by electromyographic studies and confirmed by demonstration of the toxin in the food, blood, or feces by inoculation into mice or rats. Botulism is as rare as it is difficult to eradicate. About ten adult outbreaks occur in the United States per year, each involving from one to seven people; infant cases number close to 100 per year. Awareness of the danger is the only practical preventive measure available. *Clostridium perfringens (welchii)* can also cause food poisoning with sudden vomiting and diarrhea, induced by its enterotoxin. This disorder develops within a few hours of contaminated food ingestion and is over within less than two days; it lacks the neurologic involvement of botulism but shares its noninvasive pathogenesis.

Septic Clostridial Infections

Clostridium perfringens (welchii) and *C. septicum, C. novyi, C. sordellii, C. bifermentans,* and other rare or untypable clostridia most frequently cause disease by invasion of traumatic or surgical wounds such as the amputation stumps of patients with gangrene of the leg. Clostridial sepsis is an ever-present threat when abortions are performed under unhygienic conditions. Rarely, peritoneal or generalized sepsis originating in ischemic or perforated bowel initiates infections.

In addition a severe, necrotizing (i.e., invasive) form of enteritis can be caused by *C. perfringens*, but it has been reported only in the malnourished (e.g., in World War II–impoverished children) and in vegetarian New Guinea natives after they have feasted on pigs (pigbel). This disease probably occurs in the United States but there are few well-documented reports.

Clostridium perfringens tissue invasion results either in *necrotizing cellulitis* in which gas is not formed and muscle necrosis is not extensive, or in outright *gas gangrene (clostridial myonecrosis)*, the most severe form of anaerobic infection.[99]

Clostridial cellulitis, which originates in wounds, differs from infections caused by the pyogenic cocci by its foul odor, its thin and discolored exudate, and the relatively prompt and wide tissue destruction that results in undermining edema and sloughing of the skin. Histologically, the amount of tissue necrosis is disproportional to the modest number of intact neutrophils, which increase only after these lesions begin to demarcate and build up granulation tissue along their edges. Very similar lesions can be caused by other organisms such as Enterobacter, the anaerobic streptococci, or enteric bacteria, including *E. coli*. Direct smears and cultures are helpful in making these distinctions and in instituting the correct therapy.

Gas gangrene usually begins in large traumatic wounds with pyogenic infections. Foreign bodies containing calcium or silicates may provide the appropriate lowering of oxygen tension for germination of spores. This is particularly prone to occur in compound fractures or around embedded debris or dirt. The clostridial collagenases aid in the spread of infections by destruction of the connective tissue framework (p. 335), and the clostridial lecithinases attack cell membranes. The destroyed tissue provides additional anaerobiosis for further microbial growth, with subsequent augmentation of the infection in a vicious cycle.

Gas gangrene usually becomes manifest within one to three days of injury and is characterized by marked edema and enzymic necrosis of involved muscle cells (Fig. 7–25). The extensive fluid exudation causes swelling of the affected region; the overlying skin becomes tense and pale from pressure. Necrosis or rupture of the skin may follow the formation of large bullous vesicles. The wound at this time contains large amounts of a serosanguineous exudate, but there is surprisingly little suppurative reaction.

Gas bubbles caused by fermentative reactions appear early in the gangrenous tissues, accompanied by the release of heme pigment into the exudate and affected tissues. The endothelial linings of the local blood vessels are stained by this hemolytic reaction, and injury to vascular walls may cause local thromboses. Numerous vegetative bacilli are present within the exudate. As the infection progresses, the inflamed muscles become soft, blue-black, friable, and sometimes almost semifluid as the result of the massive proteolytic action of the released bacterial enzymes. Absorption of the elaborated enzymes and invasion of the blood by the bacteria terminally induces hemolytic discoloration of the endothelial lining of the entire cardiovascular system and the formation of gas bubbles throughout the body, particularly in the liver, which create a "Swiss cheese" pattern. The bubbles are sometimes visible radiographically inside major veins or in the liver. Systemic changes are especially common and quick to develop in postabortion clostridial sepsis.

The initial clinical symptoms are pain and distention of tissues. Serosanguineous, slightly foul-smelling fluid exudes from the area of tissue injury, and very soon gas bubbles cause *crepitus* in the regions of bacterial growth. The absorbed toxins cause a rise in pulse rate often markedly out of proportion to the rise in temperature. Active hemolysis may cause *rapid drops in the red cell count and hematocrit,* accompanied by jaundice. At the time of death, no intact red cells may be left in circulation. Death is usually preceded by a period of prostration and shock. Treatment with polyvalent antitoxin and hyperbaric oxygen prevents the terminal complications and has

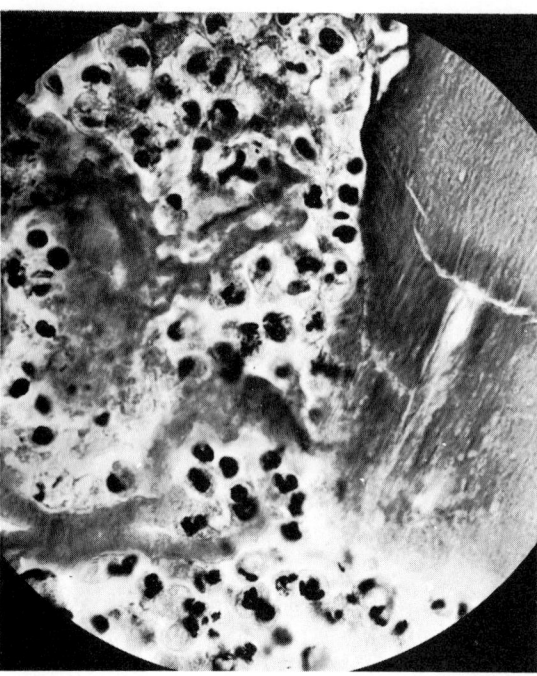

Figure 7–25. Gas gangrene. Histologic detail of enzymatic lysis of muscle cells with accompanying leukocytic exudation.

reduced the mortality rate to about 5 to 15%, but adequate débridement and cleansing of extensive tissue injuries is the proverbial "ounce of prevention worth a pound of cure."

Pseudomembranous Colitis (Clostridium difficile)

Severe colitis with pseudomembrane formation accompanied by diarrhea and clinical toxemia is caused by the enterotoxin of *C. difficile,* when this organism is able to proliferate in the gut.[100] Normally it is a minor commensal. Infection usually appears in severely ill patients, especially those receiving protracted, wide-spectrum antibiotic therapy. Particularly implicated are clindamycin, lincomycin, and more recently the cephalosporins, but the organism can be controlled by vancomycin, another potentially life-saving antibiotic. In some instances, pseudomembranous colitis has complicated Crohn's disease, ulcerative colitis, or ischemic bowel disease, and hence it must be suspected when a patient with these diseases takes a turn for the worse or fails to respond to ostensibly adequate treatment.[101] Infrequently, pseudomembranous colitis appears in otherwise healthy, sometimes quite young individuals (p. 889).

Macroscopically, patchy flecks of grayish-tan to black material composed of mucus, fibrin, inflammatory cells, and necrotic debris are adherent to the diffusely hyperemic colonic mucosa. These pseudomembranes, which may be small and punctate in some areas and confluent in others, are soft and easily wiped off, exposing superficial erosions in the underlying mucosa. Microscopically, the earliest change is focal necrosis of the surface epithelial cells in the glandular crypts, accompanied by an intense infiltration of neutrophils and fibrin plugging of capillaries in the lamina propria and by hypersecretion of mucus in adjacent crypts. This gives rise to the so-called "crypt abcesses"; involvement of adjacent crypts produces larger abscesses from which a mucus- and leukocyte-rich exudate erupts like a minivolcano to cover the surrounding mucosa, becoming adherent to the eroded superficial mucosa. With progression, there is necrosis and denudation of the mucosa, with a thick covering of fibrin, mucus, and inflammatory debris[102] (Fig. 7–26). Thrombosis of submucosal venules is a characteristic feature. The inflammation tends to remain relatively superficial and spreads laterally rather than deeply. However, exposure of the unprotected submucosa to the fecal stream may produce global dysfunction of the colonic musculature. The clostridia remain intraluminal.

Clostridium difficile colitis must be distinguished clinically from invasive Shigella, staphylococcal, or *C. perfringens* enteritis, each of which can be pseudomembranous. Early identification of this condition permits gratifyingly prompt control by appropriate antibiotic therapy. Several approaches are in use for diagnosis. The fecal extracts in suspected cases can be screened for *C. difficile* toxin, using antibodies cross reactive against a similar toxin of *C. sordellii*. Quantitative data can be obtained by titering stool filtrates for cytopathic effects on HeLa cell monolayers. Quantitative stool culture of *C. difficile* is also available but its results are necessarily delayed. Diagnostic clues may be a finely bosselated mucosal pattern on postevacuation x-ray contrast enema, or the typical early "explosive" colonic mucosal lesions on endoscopy. However, the clinical diagnosis of pseudomembranous colitis still remains relatively inaccurate, especially in the early stages when treatment would be most effective.

ZOONOTIC BACTERIA

The zoonotic bacteria are a varied group (Table 7–6, p. 337) having as a common denominator one or more animal reservoirs.[103] They are transmitted to humans from their animal hosts by direct contact, environmental contamination, insect vectors, or consumption of the animal products. The various resultant diseases, although very dissimilar, merit consideration together because their animal sources are traceable and their transmission can be and has been lowered by public health measures. Other bacteria not included here as zoonotic may also be harbored by animals (e.g., salmonellae, clostridia) but these organisms are widely disseminated in water, soil, or food and have therefore proved more difficult to control. Awareness of the rarer zoonoses can sometimes be lifesaving.

Anthrax (*Bacillus anthracis*)

Bacillus anthracis is a highly pathogenic, encapsulated, gram-positive, large, spore-bearing organism found in many species of animals. The spores persist in soil and in other sites for years, resist at least ten minutes of boiling, and withstand many of the common chemical disinfectants. When these bacilli grow in vivo they elaborate (1) a protective antigen having antiphagocytic activity, (2) an edema factor, and (3) a "lethal factor" having cytotoxicity.[104] In 95% of cases, human anthrax is contracted by skin contact with spore-bearing soil, contaminated hides, animal carcasses, or animal products (such as bone meal fertilizer). Textile workers, farmers, stevedores, and those in leather industries are at greatest risk. Spores can also be transmitted by contaminated instruments (e.g., in barber shops), but *man-to-man* transmission occurs infrequently, if at all. The local lesion is graphically described as a *malignant pustule.* However, the organism or its spores may also be airborne and inhaled, resulting in a diffuse pneumonic consolidation; this clinical variant is designated *woolsorter's disease.* The intestinal form of anthrax is extremely rare, but, in a recent Russian outbreak, its mortality was very high.[105] In all forms, bacteremia may ensue if the body defenses are overwhelmed.

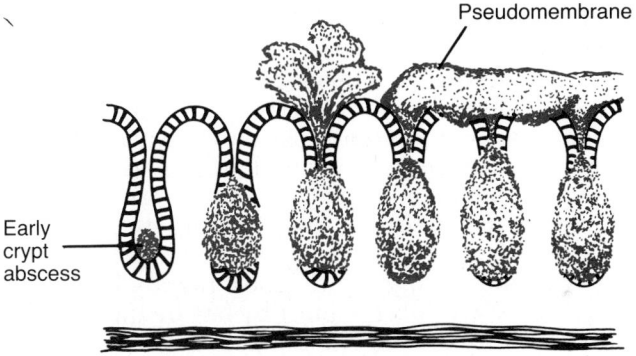

Figure 7–26. *Clostridium difficile* **pseudomembranous colitis. The schematic progression from a crypt abscess to its expansion and then eruption of the exudate onto the mucosal surface with formation by coalescence of a pseudomembrane.**

In **cutaneous anthrax** following an incubation period of several days, a small, red, macular lesion appears, resembling a flea bite. The macule enlarges and becomes edematous to create a papule and then a pustule that is filled with thin, bloody, purulent exudate, imparting a dark purple – black color to the skin. The surrounding tissues become edematous. **This combination of a relatively small hemorrhagic pustule with extensive brawny edema is the so-called malignant pustule.** In the course of the first week, the pustule ruptures and a black eschar forms, but the circumferential edema continues to expand. Satellite vesicles commonly appear about the primary lesion and the regional nodes become moderately enlarged owing to a nonspecific lymphadenitis. In contrast to the relatively painless malignant pustule, the nodes are very tender. Reddened lymphatics can often be found along the course of drainage. In mild infections, there may be only a blackish skin ulcer with little edema, and without microscopy or culture the diagnosis may be missed.

Histologically, the inflammatory reaction consists principally of intense edema, vascular congestion with hemorrhages, and necrosis of tissues resembling infarction. The leukocytic response is relatively deficient in contrast to the amount of tissue necrosis and consists of a mixture of neutrophils and mononuclear white cells. In the usual case, the inflammatory process slowly subsides, and the disease remains localized to the site of entry and the regional nodes. However, bacteremia may follow and give rise to meningitis or to localizations in the lungs, gut, or other tissues.

In **woolsorter's disease,** a diffuse pneumonia develops, characterized by extensive serofibrinous exudation that may produce total lobar consolidations. The characteristics of this pneumonia are its relative paucity of neutrophils, its tendency to develop hemorrhagic necrosis of alveolar septa, and the overwhelming abundance of the gram-positive bacteria within the inflammatory exudate. Thrombosis of small veins and arteries and profuse endothelial vascular damage are found in severe pulmonary anthrax.[104] Frequently, septicemia develops and causes death within a short time.

In acute human infections, *L. monocytogenes* evokes an exudative pattern of inflammation with numerous neutrophils. The **meningitis** it causes is macro- and microscopically indistinguishable from that caused by other pyogens (p. 1392); the finding of gram-positive, mostly intracellular bacillary rods in the CSF is virtually diagnostic. More varied lesions may be encountered in neonates and predisposed adults. Focal abscesses alternate with grayish or yellow nodules representing necrotic amorphous basophilic tissue debris. These can occur in any organ, including the lung, liver, spleen, and lymph nodes. In infections of longer duration, macrophages appear in large numbers, eventually to dispose of the necrotic remnants, but true epithelioid cell granulomas are rare.[108] Infants born live with Listeria sepsis often have a papular red rash over the extremities, and listerial abscesses can be seen in the placenta. A smear of the meconium will disclose the gram-positive organisms.

Systemic manifestations may be relatively mild in the cutaneous form, but the bacteremic and pneumonic forms are marked by high fever with signs of respiratory distress and severe prostration. There usually is only moderate elevation of the white cell count, and leukopenia sometimes develops. Electrolyte imbalances, hemoconcentration, and DIC may lead to death. Diagnosis rests on the identification of bacteria in the lesions or in the blood. With penicillin therapy, the fatality rate in cutaneous anthrax is now quite low (2 to 3%), but woolsorter's disease still has a high mortality, even if treated.

The discovery and culture of the anthrax bacillus and its spores, independently accomplished by Koch[106] and Pasteur,[107] was a true milestone in biology. These studies finally disposed of the theory of spontaneous generation and inspired Koch's postulates on which modern bacteriology is founded.

Listeriosis *(Listeria monocytogenes)*

Listeria monocytogenes is a gram-positive, microaerophilic, motile rod that grows well on ordinary media and, in tissue, often forms aggregates resembling Chinese letters. It occasionally causes community outbreaks of acute enteritis, traceable to contaminated milk or ice cream, but its major impact is on the fetus and on the immunosuppressed human adult.

In humans as in animals, amnionitis caused by Listeria may result in abortion, stillbirth, or neonatal sepsis; characteristically, the maternal infection is asymptomatic or mild, whereas that of the fetus is severe (granulomatosis infantiseptica). In opportunistic as well as in neonatal listeriosis, acute exudative leptomeningitis is often the predominant lesion; indeed, in hospitals with active organ transplant services, Listeria is one of the more frequent causes of meningitis today. The preferential occurrence of listeriosis in immunosuppressed patients and in utero suggests that undetected latent Listeria infection may be more widespread than is currently believed.

Mortality from listeriosis, despite its sensitivity to antibiotics, has remained high and seems to depend in part on the promptness with which therapy is instituted.

Plague *(Yersinia pestis)**

Yersinia pestis, the cause of plague, is a gram-negative bacillus, recognizable in smears stained with methylene blue by its safety pin appearance. It possesses a capsular glycoprotein with antiphagocytic properties and a potent gram-negative endotoxin, but its extraordinary lethal power probably derives from its massive proliferation in susceptible hosts.

Many wild animals are infected, especially rodents, which transmit plague to each other by arthropod bite or direct contact. Man is an accidental victim of this "sylvatic" cycle. Plague is an uncommon infection claiming less than 20 victims per year. The rare cases tend to occur in the western United States from Colorado to California. Squirrels are the principal reservoir. Similar sylvatic patterns persist in other endemic countries throughout the world, except in plague-free Australia.

Four forms of human plague are known: (1) "plague minor" with mild lymphadenopathy and constitutional symptoms; (2) bubonic plague with prominent lymph node swelling, the most frequent form; (3) pneumonic plague, either primary (i.e., droplet-transmitted) or complicating the bubonic pattern (5% of cases); and (4) septicemic plague without localizing symptoms, the most rapidly fatal form. All patients with plague must by law be quarantined and those with the pneumonic form require stringent precautions against airborne transmission. In recent years, all nascent epidemics of plague in Asia and Africa have been efficiently contained.

The distinctive histologic characteristics of plague are (1) the dramatic proliferation of the organisms; (2) the early appearance of a protein- and polysaccharide-rich effusion, with few inflammatory cells but with marked tissue swelling, followed by (3) necrosis of tissues and blood vessels with hemorrhage and thrombosis (Fig. 7–27); and (4) neutrophilic infiltrates that progressively accumulate in the demarcation zone around the necrotic areas as healing begins.[109]

In the **bubonic pattern** the site of entry is usually found on the legs and may be marked by a small pustule or ulceration; the nodes of drainage swell up dramatically within just a few days and become matted to form the characteristic "bubo." They are soft, pulpy, and plum-colored (hemorrhagic) and may undergo complete infarction or rupture through the skin. In the **pneumonic form** the picture is that of a severe, confluent, hemorrhagic, and necrotizing bronchopneumonia, often with fibrinous pleuritis. In **septicemic cases** the nodes throughout the body as well as the reticuloendothelial organs develop foci of necrosis, often resulting in hepatosplenomegaly. Fulminating bacteremia induces DIC with widespread hemorrhages and thrombi. In all forms of plague, the histologic lesions teem with organisms and the peripheral blood count shows a striking leukocytosis with neutrophilia.

Before the advent of antibiotics, mortality from the bubonic form varied between 50 and 90%, and the pneumonic or septicemic forms were almost invariably fatal. Today, with appropriate antibiotic therapy, mortality is about 5 to 20%. Although *Y.*

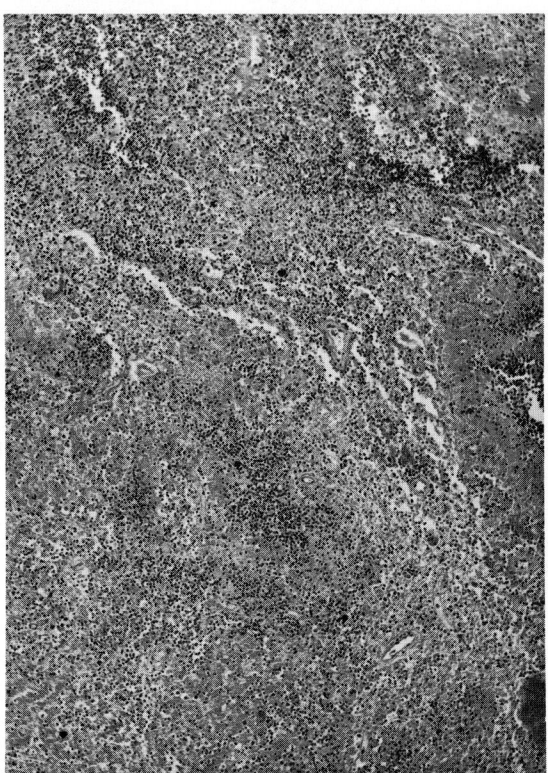

Figure 7–27. Plague. Low-power view of total hemorrhagic necrosis in a lymph node.

pestis has not developed resistance to antibiotics, the efficacy of these agents depends greatly on timing. When given later than 24 hours after onset of the pneumonic or septicemic forms of the disease, little benefit is noted. A vaccine offering six months' protection is available for workers likely to be exposed to *Y. pestis.*

Tularemia *(Francisella tularensis)*

Tularemia shares several key features with endemic plague: a wild animal source, transmissibility by arthropods, prominent lymph node swellings, and the occurrence of pneumonia. However, its agent, a small pleomorphic gram-negative coccobacillus, though equally infective, belongs to a different genus, is less virulent, has only a relatively feeble endotoxin, and is a facultative intracellular parasite. In contrast to *Y. pestis, F. tularensis* causes protracted, granulomatous lesions as the infection runs its long, debilitating, but rarely fatal course.

In the United States, between 140 and 310 infections are contracted yearly, most by persons handling rabbits or rabbit skins; worldwide, tularemia accounts for close to half a million cases per year. *Francisella tularensis* enters the host via the skin, the conjunctivae, or digestive or respiratory mucosae; infection comes about by contact, aspirated droplets,[110] or insect bite, but man-to-man transmission seems to play no role. Incubation time varies (1 to 21 days). In some cases, therefore, the source of infection is difficult to trace.

In the most common pattern, *ulceroglandular tularemia,* a local skin lesion first develops, usually on the hands, arms, or face (bubonic plague favors the legs). It changes from a rapidly growing papule to a pustule that ulcerates. Next, the draining lymph nodes enlarge and sometimes become fluctuant or ulcerate through the skin via sinus tracts. Within a week of onset, the bacteremic phase is ushered in by fever, chills, headache, digestive symptoms, and muscle and joint pains. Generalized lymphadenopathy and splenomegaly soon develop. However, in contrast to plague, there is seldom a brisk leukocytosis. In some patients, an erythematous maculopapular rash appears, thought to represent a hypersensitivity reaction. Bacteremia is usually curtailed within two to three weeks, but the infection may continue festering in local sites for months. Focal or confluent pulmonary opacities with hilar lymphadenopathy may appear on x-ray examination. Some patients develop involvements of the meninges, pericardium, heart valves, or bones. Patients with severe pneumonia and those with endotoxemic shock have the gravest forms of disease. The convalescence is protracted.[111]

The *oculoglandular* and *glandular* forms of tularemia are variants of the basic pattern in which the entry site either is in the conjunctiva or is simply inapparent. The *typhoidal form* presents with fever, hepatosplenomegaly, and toxemia, similar to Salmonella sepsis. Histopathologic lesions are similar in all four forms of tularemia.

The initial skin lesions resemble pyogenic ulcerations and are neutrophil-rich. Later, disseminated lesions undergo complete central necrosis, rimmed by epithelioid macrophages interspersed with giant cells to thus greatly resemble tubercles. As local lymph nodes begin to swell, they are at first firm and discrete owing to nonspecific lymphadenitis, but with the formation of abscesses they become soft, fluctuant, matted, and sometimes bubo-like. Grossly, they contain foci of purulent necrosis corresponding to the suppurative necrotic and granulomatous changes seen histologically. Similar, smaller lesions may also appear in more distant lymph nodes and organs, including the liver, lung, serosa, heart, or bones. By contrast, the enlarged spleen shows only nonspecific inflammatory infiltration and lymphoreticular hyperplasia. The focal necrotic lesions in the lung are often surrounded by alveolar consolidation and accompanied by serous or purulent pleuritis and hilar lymphadenopathy, mimicking primary tuberculosis. Healing of large tularemic lung foci or draining buboes often leaves deforming scars because of their destructive character, but the smaller lesions heal without sequelae.

The diagnosis can be established by several methods. Pleomorphic coccobacilli are readily visualized with methylene blue on smears of bubo aspirates. Isolation of the organism on special media should be attempted only by vaccine-protected personnel. Agglutinins take about two weeks to reach diagnostic levels. A skin test (Foshay's) is available but seldom used. Early antibiotic treatment is beneficial but less so during the chronic granulomatous phase, and it must be sustained in order to prevent relapse. Death from tularemia still occurs, especially in developing countries, but less frequently than the 1 to 6% of cases formerly reported. It should be noted here that an acute febrile disease resembling tularemia can be caused by *Pasteurella multocida*, usually following a dog or cat bite.

Brucellosis (Brucella spp.)

The most common form of brucellosis is an acute febrile systemic illness affecting workers employed in meat processing, animal husbandry, or veterinary medicine; others lacking occupational exposure occasionally become infected by consuming contaminated milk products. Subclinical and intermittent or chronic forms of brucellosis also exist, as well as lesions confined to a single site, but these are rarely seen or recognized. In fact, because of its varied clinical forms, brucellosis is suspected more often than it is diagnosed and reported. Fewer than 200 cases are registered yearly in the United States, compared to many thousands in other countries where uninspected meat and unpasteurized milk products continue to be consumed.

Four species of Brucella can infect humans; *B. melitensis* from goats, *B. abortus* from cattle, *B. suis* from pigs, and *B. canis* from dogs. *Brucella melitensis* infection may be more frequent globally, but the somewhat less virulent *B. abortus* predominates in the United States. All species are gram-negative aerobic coccobacilli and are notoriously difficult to culture or to stain and visualize in infected tissue. Brucellae are of intracellular habitat and macrophage activation is essential for halting their growth.

Inapparent brucella infection has been serologically demonstrated in many meat-packers and abattoir workers and presumably renders these individuals immune. *Acute brucellosis*, a self-terminating illness of less than a month's duration, may resemble viral disease, but relapses are common and pneumonia or localized lesions such as spondylitis, orchitis, or pyelonephritis may follow. *Chronic brucellosis*, although rare, must be considered a possible cause of transient fevers, obscure abdominal or musculoskeletal pains, and varied systemic symptoms including personality changes, all in the absence of clear-cut physical findings other than, perhaps, mild liver or splenic enlargement (approximately 10%).[112]

Following a brief bacteremic phase, Brucella diffusely colonizes the lymphoreticular system, with consequent proliferation of macrophages and lymphocytes. Soon, granulomas form; some of them are centrally necrotic, containing numerous neutrophils, especially in *B. suis* infection; others may lack necrosis and resemble sarcoid lesions[113] (p. 428). Granulomas and diffuse mononuclear infiltrates result in hepatosplenomegaly. Large, destructive localized lesions, at the sites mentioned earlier, resemble abscesses or focal infarcts. Sometimes they give a spotted appearance to the spleen. In some cases the lesions are all microscopic, but generally they are grossly visible as yellow foci, which riddle organs throughout the body. They may eventually calcify and become detectable radiographically. Extensive Brucella pneumonia, like that of tularemia, is focally destructive, granulomatous, and accompanied by hilar lymph node enlargement. It can be difficult to differentiate from tuberculosis. Most patients, however, have few or no focal pulmonary lesions.

Blood and bone marrow culture are the best diagnostic methods but are not always successful even if expertly done. A fourfold rise in IgM antibody titer or a single titer of 1/160 is strong presumptive evidence of recent Brucella infection but, in chronic cases there may only be elevated levels of IgG antibodies, which are less conclusive. Radioimmunoassays (RIA) and enzyme-linked immunosorption assays (ELISA) have recently come into use. It should however be noted that *B. canis* infected sera do not react with current standard antigens.

When liver biopsy is resorted to for diagnosis, small granulomas may be found and must be differentiated from those of sarcoidosis, miliary tuberculosis, or other chronic infections. Brucellae can seldom be visualized in such lesions, and culture of the biopsy material is therefore necessary. No human vaccine is available in the United States, but the infection responds to sustained treatment with antibacterial agents. United States mortality is now lower than the 2% formerly reported.

Glanders and Melioidosis*

Glanders, caused by *Pseudomonas mallei*, a small, gram-negative, nonmotile, nonsporing bacillus, either occurs as a severe acute disease or takes the form of a protracted infection resembling tuberculosis.[114] The organism is harbored by horses, mules, and donkeys and spreads on contact with broken skin or rarely is airborne. Uncommon but still endemic in South America, Asia, and Africa, the disease is very rare in the United States and the few cases seen are imported.

Acute glanders consists essentially of a rapidly developing, overwhelming pyemia. The incubation period of only one to five days is followed by the rather sudden onset of severe, prostrating infection with constitutional signs.

> A local papular abscess develops at the sites of inoculation, and the organism spreads from this site along the lymphatics to the regional nodes. Multiple satellite abscesses may occur along the pathways of drainage. The organism rapidly invades the blood to cause generalized pyemic abscesses in many organs and tissues, particularly in the lungs, liver, spleen, and muscles. Meningitis, osteomyelitis, and polyarthritis may all develop in the course of a few days. Diagnosis is frequently made by the demonstration of complement-fixing antibodies. Culture is hazardous and best left to reference laboratories.

Chronic glanders takes the form of a low-grade, febrile, infectious disease characterized by draining abscesses of the skin, lymphadenopathy, splenomegaly, and hepatomegaly. In time, the suppurative reaction becomes granulomatous. The lesions are not pathognomonic, and diagnosis rests on the serologic or cultural identification of the organism. Over half of these patients eventually die of their infection.

Melioidosis bears a marked similarity to glanders; its agent, *P. pseudomallei*, causes disease in rodents, dogs, cats, and horses, among others, and widely contaminates soil and water in the Southeast Asian countries of Kampuchea, Laos, Thailand, Malaysia, and Burma. Infection is acquired principally from soil or water. In the endemic foci, mild-to-inapparent as well as severe human melioidosis occurs. Moreover, although the incubation period can be as short as two days, latencies of several years' duration have been observed.[115] Among the United States military, melioidosis has been named the "Vietnamese time bomb." As in glanders, the acute lesions tend to be necrotic abscesses, and the chronic ones, granulomas.

Clinically, any organ or tissue can be involved, but in acute infections the lung is usually most prominently affected and shows a necrotizing, sometimes cavitating bronchopneumonia that tends to become confluent. Such infections, even with broad-spectrum antibiotic treatment, still carry a mortality rate approaching 50%; in the more chronic forms, combinations of antibiotics and surgical drainage have been reasonably effective.

Leptospirosis and Weil's Disease (*Leptospira interrogans*)

Mild or anicteric leptospirosis (90% of cases) is an acute, self-limited, febrile illness with protean symptoms; severe leptospirosis with jaundice, bleeding, and renal failure is called *Weil's disease*. Both disease forms tend to occur in warm and moist environments, inhabited by infected dogs or rodents. The causal agents are multiple variants of the species complex *Leptospira interrogans* (*L. icterohemorrhagiae*, *L. canicola*, *L. autumnalis*, and so forth). They are tightly wound spirochetes, up to 13 μm long, often shaped like a shepherd's crook; all can cause mild to severe disease.

Animal reservoirs bearing leptospirae exist both in the wild and in urban slums; the spirochetes survive when deposited in warm, alkaline soil or water and hence can infect humans by contact or by aerosol exposure. In the United States, fewer than 100 cases are reported yearly, mostly from southern locations, but probably many more pass unrecognized. Farmers, abattoir workers, trappers, and others in high-risk occupations constitute less than one third of cases; worldwide, the problem is huge but has not yet been reliably assessed.

Anicteric (mild) leptospirosis is typically a biphasic febrile disease.[116] During the initial *septicemic phase*, leptospirae can be cultured from the blood and cerebrospinal fluid; during the second, *immune phase*, they are found only in the urine. The incubation period ranges from five to 14 days and the disease from one to three weeks, but relapses are common. The temperature often rises abruptly, with chills, headache, and severe muscle pain or with nausea and vomiting. Within three to seven days the fever defervesces, only to recur one to three days later, this time at a lower level, but often accompanied by signs of meningeal irritation; it is at this stage that the true diagnosis may first be suspected. Cases with less typical courses are easily mistaken for viral meningitis. In the more severe *Weil's disease*, the biphasic course is obscured by the early advent of jaundice, renal failure, purpura, or hypotension, sometimes within two to three days of onset, peaking during the second week. Conjunctival irritation and hyperemia appear early in both mild and severe leptospirosis. In the army outbreak of "Fort Bragg fever," there was also a sentinel pretibial skin rash.

> During the early septicemic phase of **benign infection** leptospirae quickly disseminate and can be visualized by silver stain or immunofluorescence scattered through the liver, spleen, kidney, CNS, muscles, and other sites without apparent cellular reaction. Only later do mononuclear cell infiltrates become prominent, mostly in sites of focal cell necrosis such as striated muscle or kidney. Similarly, in

early disease, inflammatory cells are lacking in the cerebrospinal fluid, although leptospirae are present (sometimes in profusion); lymphocytes appear only during the immune phase, thus mimicking the picture of viral aseptic meningitis.

Weil's disease is characterized by hemolysis, jaundice, focal hemorrhages, cholestasis with mild, focal hepatocellular degeneration, interstitial nephritis with tubular necrosis, focal necrosis of voluntary muscles and generalized reticuloendothelial activation and hyperplasia.[117,118]

The finding of severe jaundice, hemorrhage, and fever in the face of only mild abnormalities of liver function tests and the early appearance of conjunctivitis should suggest Weil's disease rather than viral hepatitis, although these two infections can otherwise greatly resemble each other.

Early in the infection, the diagnosis can be confirmed by blood or cerebrospinal fluid culture; later, by urine culture using special media. More frequently it is confirmed by species-specific microagglutination tests. Complete recovery is the rule in mild leptospirosis. In Weil's disease the mortality rate has ranged from 15 to 40%, largely owing to renal failure, but dialysis, improved supportive care, and possibly early antibiotics should now substantially reduce this rate.

Relapsing Fever *(Borrelia recurrentis)*

Tick-borne relapsing fever is caused by several regional species of *Borrelia* and is transmitted to man from animal reservoirs in the wild by soft ticks of the genus Ornithodorus. Louse-borne disease, a more acute and severe malady, is due solely to *B. recurrentis* and is transmitted directly from human to human by body lice. Characteristic of both diseases is the occurrence of one or more sequential relapses separated by symptom-free intervals of about a week's duration.

Borreliae are loosely wound spirochetes up to 30 μm long. Unlike the treponemes of syphilis, they stain well with the Wright-Giemsa method and are readily visualized in blood smears or in other body fluids taken during febrile attacks. Microscopy is the usual means of diagnosis. Borreliae are difficult to culture, and they possess a slimy surface coat that changes its antigenic determinants during each relapse so that serologic tests are difficult to interpret.

The antigenic variability of borreliae, similar to that of African trypanosomes (p. 406), is achieved by preprogrammed shifts within the genome during reproduction.[119] By the time the host has generated sufficient antibodies to suppress the initial clone, a few borreliae have shifted to new surface antigens, and their proliferation will bring on the next relapse. The lessening severity of successive attacks of relapsing fever and its spontaneous cure in many untreated patients have been attributed to the limited genetic repertoire of borreliae, enabling the host to build up cross-reactive as well as clone-specific antibodies. When antibiotics kill many borreliae at once, this can bring on a dangerous abrupt rise in temperature with rigors, fall in blood pressure, and leukopenia, named

the *Herxheimer reaction*. This reaction usually abates within two hours, is followed by remission, and is believed to result from massive release of Borrelia endotoxin.[120]

In fatal louse-borne disease, the spleen is moderately enlarged (300 to 400 g), and histologically reveals focal necrosis and miliary collections of mixed leukocytes, including neutrophils. Numerous borreliae are seen about these foci. There is also congestion and hypercellularity of the red pulp with erythrophagocytosis. The liver may also be enlarged. It shows congestion and Kupffer cell prominence as well as scattered septic foci similar to those in the spleen, and these may also be present in other organs, including the heart, kidney, and meninges. Scattered hemorrhages resulting from DIC are frequently found in serosal and mucosal surfaces, skin, and viscera. Pulmonary bacterial superinfection is a frequent complication. Biopsy of the skin rash discloses vasodilatation with a dense perivascular inflammatory infiltrate of mononuclear leukocytes, but the intense endothelial reaction and necrotizing vasculitis of rickettsial lesions are missing. Exceptionally, both Borrelia and *R. rickettsii* can be transmitted simultaneously by the same vector.

Tick-borne relapsing fever occurs in the same settings as—and must be differentiated from—Rocky Mountain spotted fever or from other regional rickettsioses (p. 329), whose clinical features it tends to imitate, including sometimes a rash. Incubation averages one week and the first febrile episode lasts three to six days, ending sharply by crisis, only to relapse after a seven- to nine-day interval. Six or more relapses have occurred in untreated cases, each decreasing in intensity. The case fatality rate is 2 to 5% and wide-spectrum antibiotics are rapidly curative.

Louse-borne disease is stormier, more often complicated by CNS symptoms, hepatic failure, shock, or coma, but it usually involves fewer relapses. Its mortality among impoverished, disaster-stricken people has ranged from 4 to 50%, much of it due to intercurrent bacterial pneumonia.

Lyme Disease *(Borrelia burgdorferi)*

This new entity links together a set of protean manifestations previously described as separate diseases in Europe and in the United States, all of which are now known to be caused by infection with the spirochete *B. burgdorferi*. It is transmitted from animal reservoirs to humans by the nymphs and hard ticks of the genus Ixodes. At the time of this writing, Lyme borreliosis has been detected in rising numbers in 16 European countries, eastern and western United States, Canada, and Australia, with new transmission sites turning up yearly. In the United States alone, about 1500 cases per year are being reported. Moreover, the late tertiary stages and the intrauterine effects of Lyme disease have lately come under scrutiny. The clinical disease can be divided into a *primary stage* marked by a skin inoculation lesion; a *secondary stage* characterized by systemic dissemination; and finally a *tertiary stage* with joint, CNS, or cardiac involvement.

Both the European and the American form of Lyme disease begin with a characteristic lesion at the skin inoculation site, named *erythema chronicum migrans (ECM)* or *erythema migrans.* Intensive study over the course of a few years led to the discovery of the causative agent *B. burgdorferi.*[121,122] Since the identification of the causal spirochete, the United States and European disease forms have been found to overlap, although the former more often involves the joints and the latter the CNS and skin. Clearly, Lyme disease has long been masquerading under other disease labels and extends far beyond the environs of the Connecticut seaport for which it was named.[123]

Several tick species transmit *B. burgdorferi* vertically to their progeny by transovarial passage, among them *Ixodes dammini,* a parasite of white-tailed deer and field mice in the eastern United States whose accidental hosts, besides humans, include dogs and horses.[124] The western United States vector is *I. pacificus;* the European vector, *I. ricinus.* How many other hard tick vectors may exist throughout the world is not yet known.

The bite of the tiny nymphs often goes unnoticed. Three to 20 days later, one or several slowly spreading erythematous skin lesions appear. These continue expanding along their red, hot, prominent margins even as their central region blanches. Eventually the lesions of ECM fade away (sometimes after one or several relapses). Weeks to months later, some patients suffer facial palsy, or a stiff neck, or signs of meningoencephalitis, which in the European form can be quite severe. Other patients may present with myocardial involvement (e.g., atrioventricular block, rarely left ventricular dysfunction) or pericarditis; no valvular lesions have yet been reported. Most victims complain mainly of joint disease. Typically the knees or other large limb joints become swollen, hot, and painful in an asymmetric pattern similar to that of early rheumatoid arthritis. The disease may then abate slowly after several months of flareups and remissions, but some patients are left with permanent, disabling joint deformities or less often with cardiovascular or neural sequelae. Recently, reports of destructive tertiary neural and vascular lesions years after apparent cure of Lyme disease have begun to surface, together with reports of stillbirth due to maternal infection.

Few representative tissue samples have thus far been examined, mostly skin and synovial biopsy specimens. These have shown predominantly lymphoplasmacytic infiltrates with local edema or fibrin deposition lacking specific features. In synovial biopsies, early Lyme arthritis resembles early rheumatoid arthritis. Recently synovial arteritis with "onionskinning" has been reported to be a distinctive feature,[121] but it has not been found in biopsy specimens of skin or systemic lesions.

Survival of *B. burgdorferi* in host tissue during latent infection, as with the treponeme in syphilis, is strongly suspected but as yet unproved. There is however general agreement that appropriate tetracycline or penicillin treatment during the ECM stage of disease will prevent later systemic manifestations. Without treatment, the consequences can be serious, but mortality has thus far been minimal, attributable largely to superinfections. The diagnosis is likely to be missed when there is no fever, the ECM skin lesions are faded or atypical, joint or other pathologic features have turned chronic, and recollection of the early phases of the illness has been erased by time.

Borrelia burgdorferi is a 9 to 32 μm long, loosely coiled spirochete that can be grown in modified Kelly's medium. It is found in large numbers in ticks but is rarely demonstrable in human body fluids or tissue samples either by silver stains or immunofluorescence or by culture. Laboratory diagnosis therefore has to rely on the titers of serum antibodies against *B. burgdorferi* in ELISA or immunofluorescent slide assays. High IgM titers are indicative of a recent infection. Other laboratory findings frequent during active disease are hypergammaglobulinemia or cryoglobulinemia with circulating immune complexes and elevated sedimentation rates, but rheumatoid factor and antinuclear antibodies are characteristically absent. The scarcity of spirochetes in late Lyme disease and the polyclonal B cell activation noted during flareups suggest that host immune mechanisms play an important role in pathogenesis, but that role has yet to be defined.

Rat-Bite Fever

Two infections of similar presentation are associated with rat bites: that caused by *Spirillum minus* (sodoku) and that by *Streptobacillus moniliformis* (also named Haverhill fever). Both are obviously related to urban slum conditions and to lapses of pest control, and both present with swelling of the puncture site and local lymphadenopathy, followed by an acute febrile illness with a rash over the extremities resembling a viral infection. The incubation period of the spirillar form of rat-bite fever is longer (one to four weeks) than the streptobacillary form (one to two days). The former has a tendency to remit and exacerbate over a period of up to eight weeks. It is best diagnosed by animal inoculation of blood or by examination of blood under dark-field conditions or in Giemsa-stained smears. Streptobacillary infections average a briefer duration of one to two weeks, but often are accompanied by arthralgia or by symmetric swelling, heat, and redness of the large joints of the extremities, which may prolong the course of this infection. Diagnosis of streptobacillary infection is achieved by blood culture or agglutinin titers. No pathologic findings have been reported for either entity, except for one lethal case of *Streptobacillus* endocarditis.

Cat-Scratch Disease

This self-limited bacterial infection,[125,126] usually manifested by localized lymphadenopathy, is seen oftener in children (80% of cases) than in adults. It takes the form of regional lymphadenopathy, most frequently in the axilla and neck, one or more weeks usually following a feline scratch but occasionally after a splinter or thorn injury. A raised, inflammatory nodule, vesicle, or eschar may or may not appear at the site of skin injury. Cat-scratch disease is the commonest cause of the oculoglandular syndrome, or Parinaud's syndrome (i.e., swelling of the eye, jaw, and high cervical lymph nodes). Systemic manifestations are usually minimal, such as fever, mild neutrophilia or eosinophilia, and accelerated sedimentation rate. Uncommonly, neuroretinitis, pleurisy, arthritis, splenic abscess, or mediastinal masses — even focal osteomyelitis — have been reported, indicating systemic spread.

> The major anatomic changes involve the nodes of drainage, which may become significantly enlarged and sometimes fluctuant. Early in the condition there is a nonspecific reactive lymphadenitis (p. 705). Thereafter, sarcoid-like granulomas (p. 428) may develop throughout the lymph node, around its capsule, and in the walls of draining veins. Coalescence of these granulomas produces the most distinctive phase of the disease, with the formation of so-called **stellate abscesses** (i.e., irregular, central accumulations of vital and disintegrating neutrophils surrounded by a prominent rim of palisaded epithelioid macrophages). Although such abscesses are distinctive, they are not pathognomonic and are similar to the lesions of lymphogranuloma venereum.

A pleomorphic gram-negative bacterium has been found in primary lesions and lymph nodes. It is extracellular and can be visualized only by silver stains or electron microscopy. This organism has finally been cultured.[127,128] We can now look forward to better diagnostic tools. Until then, the diagnosis must be made on clinical grounds and confirmed by the morphologic findings.

TREPONEMES

Three pathogenic treponemes infect man — *Treponema pallidum*, *T. pertenue*, and *T. carateum*. *Treponema pallidum* is the cause of syphilis and is by far the most important and best studied of the treponemes. A variant of *T. pallidum* causes the rare bejel. *Treponema pertenue*, the cause of yaws, after nearing extinction as the result of an international eradication campaign, has since rebounded in several tropical countries. *Treponema carateum* continues to flourish in the remote corners of Latin America where pinta has always been a part of life. The treponemes are superbly adapted human parasites matching high infectivity, including transmission to the fetus, with low virulence, long periods of latency, and lifelong persistence in the untreated host. They produce no known toxins or tissue-destructive enzymes. Many of their lesions are linked to the host's immune responses, such as mononuclear cell infiltrates, proliferative vascular changes, and (sometimes) granuloma formation. Notwithstanding their slow progression the lesions may eventually become destructive, maiming, or lethal.

Human treponemes also pose peculiar diagnostic problems: they cannot be cultured in ordinary media or passed on to animal hosts other than primates; and they are often difficult to stain and detect in diseased tissues, requiring special procedures — silver stains, immunofluorescence, or dark-field examination. Chief reliance for diagnosis is placed on serologic tests that must be interpreted with caution.

Syphilis *(Treponema pallidum)*

Syphilis, also called lues, is a venereal disease of insidious and furtive habit. Neither the *primary chancre* nor the *secondary stage*, which takes the form of a rash, is accompanied by disturbing symptoms. The disease then enters a period of latency for years or decades, sometimes to be followed by the *tertiary stage* with its seriously disabling or fatal lesions. The late manifestations are localized principally to the cardiovascular and central nervous systems; other organs or structures are affected less frequently.

The chronicle of past peaks and valleys of syphilis transmission has some important lessons to offer: penicillin plus mass serologic testing and contact tracing had reduced the incidence of syphilis in the United States from its post–World War II peak of 70 cases to 3.5 per 10^5 population, but flagging control efforts and changes in sexual mores have brought on a slow resurgence to about 30 cases per 10^5 per year, particularly among urban teenagers and homosexuals. At the same time, ubiquitous use of antibiotics has made destructive tertiary and perinatal syphilitic lesions increasingly rare. The effect of the AIDS epidemic on transmission of syphilis appears to have been minimal or nil; in brief, syphilis in the United States is *down but not out* and, among fighting armies, conscripted labor, and prostitutes in other countries, it continues rampant.

The *causative agent* is a 10- to 13-μm slender, corkscrew-shaped spirochete, detectable only by silver impregnation, dark-field examination, or immunofluorescent techniques. Treponemas are readily killed by soap and antiseptics, cold, or drying. *Sexual intercourse is the usual mode of transmission*, although bacteria-laden secretions can also transfer the disease by other intimate contact. *Transplacental transmission occurs readily* and active disease during pregnancy results in congenital syphilis in the fetus.

Treponema pallidum has a double cell wall, and the outer one contains ligands for a wide variety of host cell membranes to which it is found to adhere, and from which it is capable of acquiring host proteins during infection.[129] Syphilis is one of the infections in which downward modulation of host lymphocyte responsiveness by a serum factor occurs,[130] and this early weakening of host immune reactivity may contribute to the latency and chronicity of ongoing infection. Yet even while treponemal infection actively proceeds, patients with syphilis develop immunity to challenge. About two weeks after the initial chancre, they become resistant to reinfection and, despite reexposure, do not develop a second chancre called "chancre immunity." Treatment very early in the disease may block this development.

Spirochetal antigens evoke host antibodies of two types: (1) *nonspecific antibodies, which react with a lipoidal antigen derived from beef heart* (cardiolipin); *and (2) specific antibodies to spirochetal antigens.* The nontreponemal antibodies (reagins) can be detected by readily performed, inexpensive complement-fixation or flocculation serologic tests for syphilis (STS), such as Wassermann, Kahn, Kline, Hinton, and VDRL. However, *because these serologic tests for syphilis do not detect specific treponemal antigens, they can also be positive in a great variety of nonluetic illnesses,* yielding what are known as *biologic false-positives* (BFP). BFP may be encountered in smallpox vaccination, infectious mononucleosis, leprosy, autoimmune diseases, viral hepatitis, and heroin addiction as well as in many acute febrile illnesses.

More specific than the STS are tests based on the detection of treponemal antigens. Among these the fluorescent treponemal antibody (FTA) test has been further refined by absorption of nonspecific spirochetal group antibodies from the patient's serum (FTA-ABS), and this test is now the standard method used. It is always advisable to follow up positive STS results with one of the more specific methods.

The natural course of acquired syphilis evolves in three stages. The *primary stage* follows an incubation period of 10 to 90 days (average, three weeks) and is marked by the development of the chancre at the site of treponemal invasion. Regional nontender adenopathy soon follows. Even before the chancre appears, a spirochetemia seeds tissues throughout the body, thus providing the basis for the later disseminated lesions of secondary and tertiary syphilis. The chancre usually heals in three to 12 weeks with or without therapy, and the patient then appears entirely well.

The *secondary stage* follows in approximately two weeks to six months (average, six to eight weeks). It is characterized by a generalized or, less often, a localized skin eruption. These manifestations too disappear spontaneously in about four to 12 weeks. The two early stages may be extremely subtle or occult. A chancre on the cervix or in the oropharynx would not be noted. The rash might be trivial and fleeting. *Many patients with unmistakable evidence of late syphilis recall no earlier manifestations.*

Following the secondary stage the patient again enters a period of apparent well-being referred to as *latent syphilis,* lasting years or decades. Only then may the lesions of *tertiary syphilis* appear. *These generally take one of three forms: (1) localized destructive lesions (gummas) of virtually any tissue, (e.g., liver, bones, testis, or skin); (2) cardiovascular lesions; or (3) CNS involvement.* However, many patients never develop tertiary lesions. Studies of untreated syphilitics

indicate that about one third achieve spontaneous cure with reversion of all serologic abnormalities. Another one third continue to have positive serologic tests but die of unrelated causes. Only the remaining one third develop the grave lesions of tertiary disease.[131,132]

Whatever the stage of the disease and location of the lesions, *histologic hallmarks of the inflammatory reaction are obliterative endarteritis and plasma cell infiltrates.* Small arteries and arterioles in the inflammatory reaction exhibit swelling and proliferation of endothelial cells to produce concentric "onionskin" layers that markedly narrow the lumen. About these vessels there is prominent perivascular cuffing by plasma cells.

Acquired Primary Syphilis

In the **primary stage the chancre usually occurs on the glans penis in males and on the vulva or cervix in females.** In approximately 10% of cases the chancre may be extragenital: lips, fingers, oropharynx, anorectum, or some other site. In about 50% of females and 30% of males, primary lesions either never develop or are not detected.

The chancre usually begins as a solitary, slightly elevated, firm, reddened papule that varies in size up to several centimeters in diameter. It then superficially erodes to create a clean-based, shallow ulceration on the surface of the slightly elevated papule. The contiguous induration characteristically creates a button-like mass directly subjacent to the eroded skin or mucosa, providing the basis of the designation **hard chancre.** Superimposed secondary bacterial infection may impart a suppurative exudation.

Histologically, the chancre is characterized by an intense mononuclear leukocytic infiltration, chiefly of plasma cells with scattered macrophages and lymphocytes (Fig. 7–28). Obliterative endarteritis, as described, is present within this inflammatory reaction.

Treponemes are not evident without special staining, but with silver impregnation or immunofluorescent techniques they can often be visualized in the surface layer of the ulceration or in the scant overlying exudate. The regional nodes are usually enlarged and may show nonspecific acute or chronic lymphadenitis (p. 707), may reveal a plasma cell-rich infiltrate, or may contain focal epithelioid cell granulomas.

Dark-field identification of treponemes provides the most definitive and earliest means of diagnosis. Treponemes can sometimes be aspirated from the enlarged regional nodes after they have disappeared from the chancre. *During the earliest weeks of syphilis the results from STS and specific tests for antitreponemal antibodies are usually negative.* Adequate treatment with penicillin during the primary stage prevents the development of secondary syphilis and, in most patients, maintains seronegativity or converts serodiagnostic tests to negative. In a few patients, despite adequate therapy, serologic tests remain positive, a phenomenon described as *serofastness.*

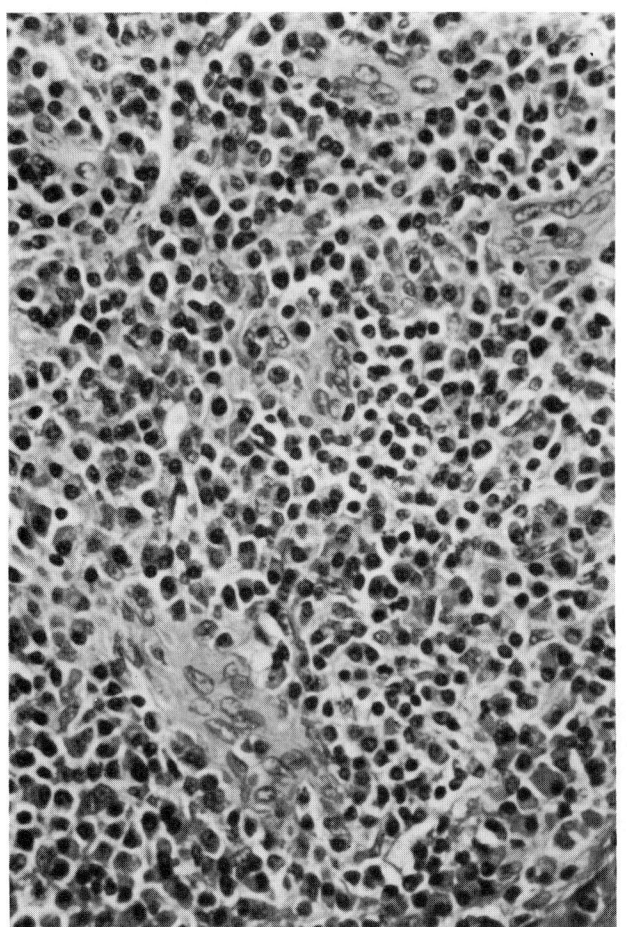

Figure 7–28. Syphilitic chancre: diffuse plasmacytic infiltration and endothelial proliferation.

Secondary Syphilis

The secondary stage is characterized by widespread mucocutaneous lesions that are often generalized over the entire body, including the mucous membranes of the oral cavity, palms of the hands, and soles of the feet. Most often the rash is macular, with discrete red-brown lesions, rarely over 5 mm in diameter. In other cases, follicular, pustular, annular, and scaling lesions may predominate.[133] Vesicular bullous and ulcerative lesions are uncommon. Reddened mucous patches may appear in the mouth or vagina. All the mucocutaneous lesions harbor organisms, but the most contagious are the wet types of mucous patches and skin lesions. Histologically, the inflammatory reaction in the foci of mucocutaneous involvement resembles that found in the chancre. However, there is less intensity to the plasma cell infiltrate and it is ordinarily confined to perivascular cuffing. When the rash is distinctly papular it is usually accompanied by thickening of the epithelium and elongation of the rete pegs. Occasionally, secondary syphilitic lesions are better localized. Thus, papular lesions in the region of the penis or vulva may become large, elevated, broad plaques. They sometimes also occur on the lips and perianal region. **These flat, red-brown elevations (up to 2 to 3 cm in diameter) are designated condylomata lata and are distinct from condylomata acuminata or venereal warts (p. 1100). The overlying epithelium is intact and hyperplastic unless secondarily traumatized or infected. Histologically, there is a characteristic plasma cell infiltrate, as well as the characteristic vascular obliterative endarteritis. Many spirochetes may be found in these condylomata.**

The lesions of secondary syphilis are not of themselves pathognomonic because there is such variability in their form. However, the diagnosis of syphilis must be suspected when a disseminated rash develops in a patient who appears to be relatively well except for generalized adenopathy, sore throat, or bone pain. In other bacteremic states associated with rashes, marked constitutional signs of fever, chills, malaise, and prostration usually accompany the skin lesions. A history of primary chancre cannot be relied on because in many patients the primary stage may have passed unnoticed. Thus, syphilis may be confused with noninfectious skin diseases having rashes.

A minority of patients with secondary syphilis develop a subacute meningitis, iritis, hepatitis, periostitis, or an immune complex glomerulopathy leading to the nephrotic syndrome (p. 1033). *At this stage of the disease the STS and treponemal tests are almost always positive.* Once again the opportunity is provided to treat these patients and prevent the development of tertiary syphilis.

Tertiary Syphilis

Late syphilitic disease has become very rare. The cardiovascular system is most commonly affected (80 to 85%). CNS involvement accounts for about 5 to 10%. Gummas in the liver and other sites make up the remainder. These localizations are not mutually exclusive.

Cardiovascular syphilis, principally involving the aorta, may become manifest years to decades after the initial infection. It causes inflammatory scarring of the tunica media (mesaortitis) with weakening and dilation (aneurysm formation), widening and incompetence of the aortic valve ring, and narrowing of the mouths of the coronary ostia (p. 580).

Central nervous system syphilis, or neurosyphilis (p. 1394), is another late manifestation and takes one of several forms, designated meningovascular syphilis, tabes dorsalis, and general paresis. In addition, patients with ataxia and sensory loss from tabes dorsalis may undergo a rapidly destructive degenerative arthritis of the knee joint (Charcot's joint).

The **syphilitic gumma** is characterized by a peculiar, rubbery, gummatous necrosis, most commonly found in the liver, bones, and testes. Gummas may occur singly or multiply, and they vary in size from microscopic defects resembling tubercles or sarcoid lesions to large tumorous masses of necrotic material. Erosion of a superficial cutaneous or submucosal gumma may yield a ragged ulcer that is extremely persistent and resistant to local therapeutic measures.

In the liver, scarring due to gummas may cause a distinctive hepatic lesion known as **hepar lobatum** (p. 957) (Fig. 7–29).

Histologically, active gummas consist of a center of a coagulated, necrotic material with faint persistence of the shadowy outlines of dead tissue cells and vessels. The margins of the gumma are composed of plump or palisaded macrophages and fibroblasts surrounded by large numbers of mononuclear leukocytes, chiefly plasma cells. Treponemes are scant in these gummas and are extremely difficult to demonstrate.

Congenital Syphilis

Congenital syphilis may be contracted by a fetus born up to five years after the mother first becomes infected, but the more recent the infection, the more certain the involvement of the fetus and the more florid the congenital disease; yet, adequate therapy early in pregnancy will completely protect the child. The treponemes do not invade the placental tissue or the fetus until the fifth month of gestation, and therefore syphilis is an uncommon cause of early abortion. Instead, it causes late abortion, stillbirth, or death soon after delivery, or it may persist in latent form to become apparent only during childhood or adult life.

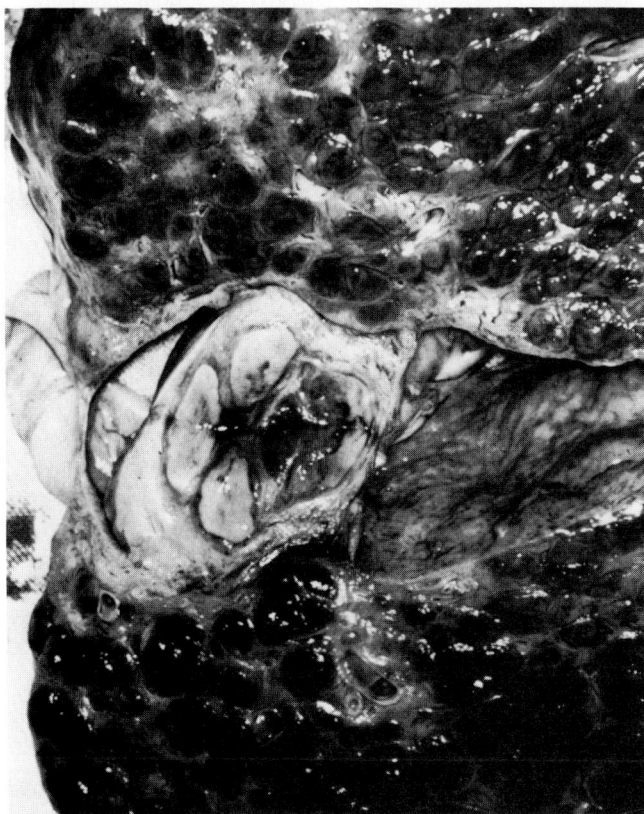

Figure 7–29. Syphilitic gumma of liver adjacent to the gallbladder bed with coarse scarring of the hepatic parenchyma (hepar lobatum).

In the **perinatal** and **infantile** forms of congenital syphilis, the most striking lesions affect the mucocutaneous tissues and bones. A diffuse rash develops, which differs from that of the acquired secondary stage in that there can be extensive sloughing of the epithelium, particularly on the palms and soles and about the mouth and anus. These lesions teem with spirochetes. There is also a generalized luetic osteochondritis and periostitis that affects all bones, most prominently the nose and lower legs. Destruction of the vomer causes collapse of the bridge of the nose and later on the characteristic saddle nose deformity. Periostitis of the tibia leads to excessive new bone growth on the anterior surfaces and produces anterior bowing, or saber shin. There is also widespread disturbance in endochondral bone formation. The epiphyses become widened as the cartilage overgrows. Cartilage is found as displaced islands within the metaphysis.

The **liver** usually is severely affected in congenital syphilis. Diffuse fibrosis permeates lobules to isolate hepatic cells into small nests, accompanied by the characteristic white cell infiltrate and vascular changes. Gummas are occasionally found in the liver, even in very early cases.

The **lungs** may be affected by a diffuse interstitial fibrosis that produces a marked increase in their consistency. In the syphilitic stillborn they appear as pale, virtually airless organs **(pneumonia alba).**

The generalized spirochetemia may lead to diffuse interstitial inflammatory reactions in virtually any other organ of the body (e.g., the pancreas, kidneys, heart, spleen, thymus, and endocrine organs). In the CNS meningovascular syphilis may develop. Eye changes consist of an interstitial keratitis or a choroiditis with focal or diffuse inflammatory scarring of the choroid. Abnormal pigment production in focal areas may produce the spotted retina of congenital syphilis.

The late-occurring form of congenital syphilis is distinctive in that *interstitial keratitis* is often accompanied by *periostitis, saber shins, and saddle deformity of the nose.* In addition, there are characteristic alterations in tooth formation due to spirochetal infection during development (Hutchinson's teeth). The incisor teeth are somewhat smaller than normal and have a screwdriver shape, or are pointed, to produce a peg-shaped or pumpkin-seed deformity. The defective formation of enamel results in notching of the biting margins of the incisors. Dental x-ray examinations show characteristic changes even before the teeth erupt. On the basis of the meningovascular involvement, eighth nerve deafness and optic nerve atrophy may develop. Among these many possible findings, most characteristic of delayed or "tardive" congenital syphilis is the triad of interstitial keratitis, Hutchinson's teeth, and eighth nerve deafness.

In contrast to many other bacteria, *T. pallidum* for many decades has remained sensitive to penicillin and to other antibiotics, and its prescribed treatment schedules have remained virtually unchanged.

Yaws, Bejel, and Pinta*

These three treponematoses are caused by spirochetes morphologically identical to *T. pallidum.* Yaws is a disease of the moist tropics, bejel one of desert zones, and pinta is limited to rural foci in Latin America. *All are transmitted by person-to-person contact but they are not venereal diseases.* Like syphilis, *bejel* is a chronic disorder with onset most often in childhood. The initial lesion involves the mucocutaneous surfaces. *Yaws* begins with a large, raised skin ulcer, the "mother yaw." Late in the course, bones may also be involved by gummatous lesions. However, CNS and cardiovascular lesions, which are the hallmark of tertiary syphilis, are rarely if ever seen. *Pinta,* unlike yaws and bejel, is purely a skin disease causing unsightly pigment changes, and it is therefore less serious. All the nonvenereal treponematoses evoke humoral antibodies that give positive serologic tests for syphilis and seem to protect the bearer from venereal lues.

UNCOMMON BACTERIA

Rhinoscleroma*

This is a destructive chronic infection of the nose and upper airways caused by an encapsulated, gram-negative bacillus related to *Klebsiella pneumoniae* (p. 782). In its endemic regions—parts of the Soviet Union, Europe, Latin America, and the Near East—rhinoscleroma is a well-known cause of facial deformity and of upper airway obstruction.[134] The agent, *K. rhinoscleromatis,* is readily cultured from rhinoscleroma lesions. Its transmission is not understood and its response to treatment is slow. The disease progresses insensibly from an initial stage resembling an ordinary cold to an atrophic stage in which the respiratory mucosa appears dry and granular, and finally to a nodular stage characterized by the growth of tumor-like submucosal masses caused by chronic inflammation. The pharynx and larynx may become involved, with consequent anosmia, dysphonia, and airway obstruction. Isolated laryngeal involvement is rare but dangerous.

Microscopically, the lesions are replete with foamy macrophages, some quite large or multinucleate (Mikulicz cells), and also contain lymphocytes and plasma cells. Within the cytoplasmic vacuoles of macrophages are encapsulated diplobacilli, best demonstrated by silver staining. The overlying epithelium shows proliferation, sometimes squamous metaplasia, or even pseudoepitheliomatous change.

Ozena

This disease is also a rare, severe, chronic rhinitis. However, instead of causing swelling it causes atrophy of the turbinates accompanied by a foul-smelling greenish exudate, nasal obstruction, and eventual anosmia. *Klebsiella ozaenae* is thought to be the responsible agent, but mixed cultures with other gram-negative bacilli have sometimes been isolated from these lesions. The histologic picture is one of nonspecific exudative and necrotizing inflammation.

Granuloma Inguinale (*Calymmatobacterium donovani*)

Granuloma inguinale—not to be confused with lymphogranuloma venereum (p. 328)—is a chronic, venereally transmitted disease with ulcerating and granulating lesions of the genital skin and mucosae that become quite disabling and deforming. The agent, *C. donovani,* is a tiny, encapsulated facultative, intracellular bacillus, sometimes referred to as a Donovan body. Granuloma inguinale is encountered worldwide, with the highest incidence in New Guinea and India. It is uncommon in Europe and the United States. The usual mode of transmission is by sexual contact, but for unknown reasons males are predominantly affected. Under highly endemic conditions nonvenereal transmission can also occur.[135]

After an incubation period of three days to several months, the initial lesion appears as a papule on genital, perineal, or more rarely extragenital sites (e.g., the lips). This enlarges, ulcerates, and begins spreading as an elevated, creeping sore with a necrotic center and an indurated, raised border. Satellite papules and ulcers may appear along the lymphatic drainage. In time, the ensuing fibrosis may cause dense scarring and sometimes keloid formation. Unlike lymphogranuloma venereum, however, the lymph nodes remain uninvolved and rectal strictures are not formed.

At the base of the ulcer and in the papillary dermis of the bordering skin or mucosa, microabscesses are formed, merging with the underlying, richly vascularized granulation tissue that constitutes the bulk of the lesion. In the most active, superficial sites, Donovan bodies can be seen in vacuolated macrophages. In H and E–stained sections, they appear as faintly bluish dots sticking to the contour of a vacuole. With Giemsa or silver stains, many more organisms are usually apparent, some in neutrophils but mostly in macrophages (Fig. 7–30). Deep to the granulation tissue, there is fibrosis and mononuclear cell infiltration. Along the expanding borders of the ulcer, the epidermis shows marked acanthosis and sometimes pseudoepitheliomatous hyperplasia. Granuloma inguinale usually remains localized wherever the lesion first appears but rarely, in pregnant women with involvement of the uterine cervix, metastatic dissemination to bones, joints, and other skin sites has been observed. Chemotherapy prevents the disfiguring lesions seen in neglected cases.

Chancroid, Soft Chancre (*Hemophilus ducreyi*)

Chancroid is an acute venereal disease characterized by the development of a necrotic ulcer, the *soft chancre,* at the site of inoculation of *H. ducreyi* on the genitals. This organism is highly infectious, and autoinoculation can lead to multiple chancres. The disease is transmitted by sexual intercourse, and infec-

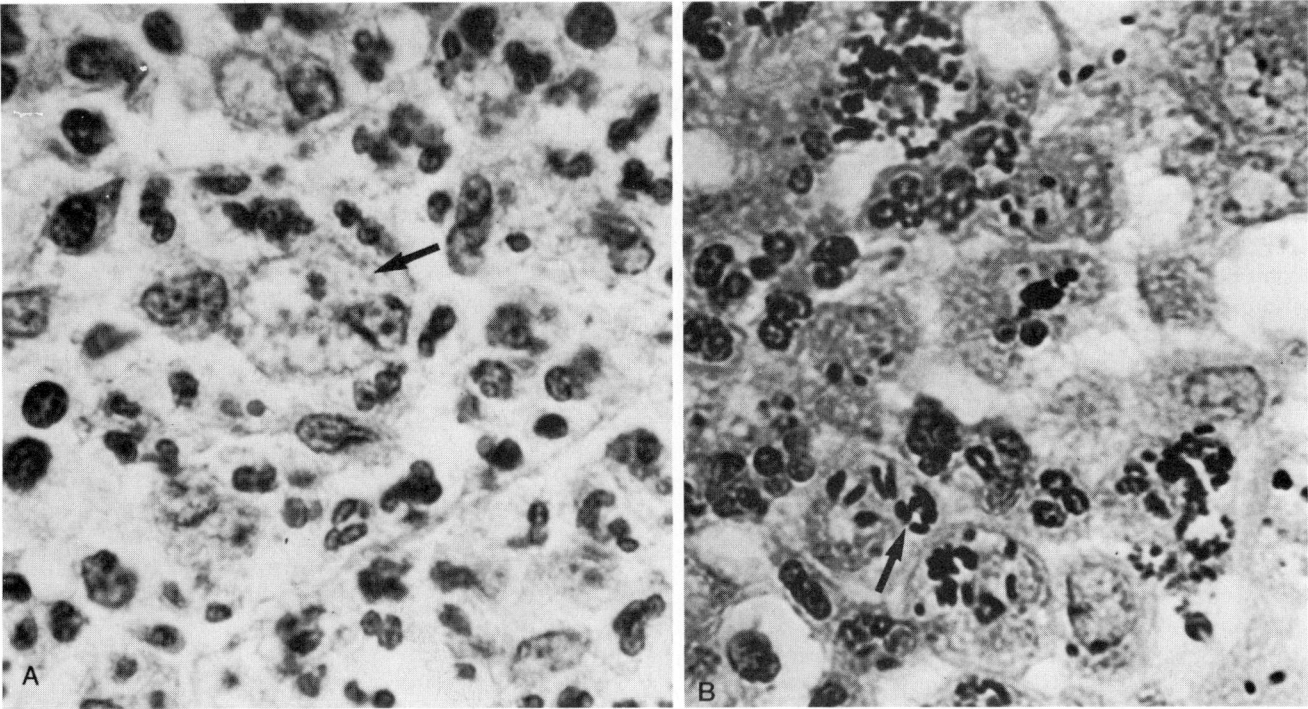

Figure 7–30. Granuloma inguinale. Donovan bodies as seen with H and E stain *(A)* and with silver stain *(B)*. (Courtesy of Dr. Jeffrey Goldstein, University of Florida, Gainesville.)

tion occurs through skin or mucous membrane abrasions. The organism has been isolated from the penile smegma and vaginal secretions of patients without manifestations of the disease. In the United States, cases have recently increased from about 800 per year to 3700 in 1986. The disease is more widely prevalent in the Orient, West Indies, and North Africa.

> The soft chancre usually occurs on the penis and about the labia minora and majora, approximately three to five days after infection. A small macule that becomes papular and then forms an intradermal abscess develops at the site of invasion. The overlying skin sloughs to produce a draining ulcer, which is at first shallow but may enlarge to 2 to 3 cm in diameter. The well-developed ulcer is covered with a necrotic, purulent slough and bears a resemblance to the chancre of syphilis, but it is less indurated as a rule. In about 50% of cases, the regional nodes undergo painful inflammatory hyperplasia over the course of one to two weeks. Suppuration may occur in these sites to produce fluctuant masses (buboes) that drain to the skin surface.
>
> Histologically, the soft chancre presents three zones. The surface of the ulcer is composed of disintegrating leukocytes and red cells. Deep to this level, there is a zone of granulation tissue with hyperplasia of the endothelial cells in the small vessels, as well as a mixed inflammatory reaction within and about the vessel wall. This vasculitis often leads to intravascular thrombosis or necrosis of the vessel wall. Beneath the granulation tissue, there is a third zone of more chronic inflammatory reaction with fibroblastic proliferation infiltrated with mononuclear leukocytes.

Clinically, the chancre is not particularly painful; however, the regional nodes of drainage are extremely tender, presumably owing to tension. The constitutional symptoms that accompany this disease are mild.[136]

The diagnosis of chancroid can be established by the isolation of *H. ducreyi.* A skin test for chancroid is available, and remains positive for several years after an acute infection.

Carrión's Disease (Hemobartonellosis)*

The endemic zone of *Bartonella bacilliformis* infection is limited to that of its sandfly vector, *Phlebotomus verrucarum,* which thrives in the Northern Andes at altitudes between 700 and 2500 m, largely within Peru. *Bartonella bacilliformis* is the prototype of hemophilic bacteria. It initially infects erythrocytes, causing an acute, febrile illness *(Oroya fever)* associated with hemolytic anemia and hepatosplenomegaly. This is followed by an eruptive phase in which the bartonellae localize in the skin, giving rise to numerous highly vascularized, nodular collections of inflammatory cells. The mortality rate is high in the initial hemolytic phase. The skin lesions usually develop after immunity is acquired and can be treated with chloramphenicol. Rarely, human infections with animal hemobartonellae have been reported in United States laboratory workers.[137]

MYCOBACTERIA

Mycobacteria share the basic structure of all bacterial organisms but have distinctive phosphoglycolipids, phospholipids, and waxes in their cell walls. Their family includes pathogens for many animals from mammals to mollusks, as well as free-living mycobacteria that sometimes contaminate laboratory samples and give rise to confusion with human pathogens. Besides the tubercle and leprosy bacilli, there are about 30 other human pathogenic species, called "atypical mycobacteria," which have been classified by their rate of growth, reaction to light, and production of pigment on artificial media. The most important human mycobacteria tend to be slow dividers and are facultative intracellular invaders, and some thrive best at low body temperatures. Their relatively modest infectivity contrasts with their marked ability to persist in tissues either in dormant form or as chronic, destructive pathogens. *Owing to their waxy cell components, many mycobacteria are acid fast* (i.e., they retain the red dye carbolfuchsin after rinsing with acid solvents).One of the pathogenic mycobacteria, the lepra bacillus, has never been cultured successfully. Others have special growth requirements, and even under optimal aerobic conditions they take several weeks to form colonies, so that cultures must be maintained and periodically monitored accordingly.

Tuberculosis

Tuberculosis is a worldwide, chronic, communicable disease caused by the "Koch bacillus," *Mycobacterium tuberculosis,* which usually affects the lungs but may cause lesions in any organ or tissue of the human body. It evokes focal granulomatous inflammatory reactions that typically undergo central caseous necrosis. *These "caseating granulomas" are the histologic hallmarks of tuberculosis, but because similar lesions can have other infectious and noninfectious causes, tubercle bacilli should always be demonstrated to confirm the histologic diagnosis of tuberculosis.*

Two species of tubercle bacilli infect humans: *M tuberculosis hominis* and *M. tuberculosis bovis.* Human tubercle bacilli are ordinarily transmitted by inhalation of infective droplets coughed or sneezed into the air by a patient with open lesions (i.e., tuberculous foci in communication with the airways). Bacilli remain viable in wet sputum for months and even in dried sputum particles for weeks. *Most infections are acquired by sustained exposure rather than casual contact.* Rarely, the conjunctivae or the abraded or punctured skin serves as a portal of entry. Bovine tubercle bacilli are transmitted by milk from diseased cows and first produce intestinal or tonsillar lesions. In developed countries, disease control in dairy herds and pasteurization of milk have virtually eradicated this mode of transmission, and in the United States, tuberculosis is now considered to be due to human bacilli unless proved otherwise. Elsewhere, extrapulmonary tuberculosis is sometimes due to bovine bacilli or to distinctive local human strains.[138]

INCIDENCE. Although tuberculosis is now both treatable and to some degree preventable, it is still the single most important bacterial infection worldwide.

Its true incidence cannot be precisely determined for the following reasons:

1. Only a fraction of persons with *M. tuberculosis* manifest clinical disease at any one time. *Most exposed individuals develop only an asymptomatic infection — and are converted to tuberculin reactors without necessarily developing disease.*
2. All infected persons remain indefinitely at risk of developing active disease.
3. Case reporting, even in developed countries, is always incomplete. In 1980, of a total United States population of 216 million, an estimated 15 million were *tuberculin reactors,* but only 30,000 *active* clinical cases were reported that year. In 1986, this number had leveled off at 22,800 — i.e., 9.4 cases per 10^5 population. Some of the cases were attributable to reactivation of tuberculosis in **AIDS** patients.

Thus, in terms of active disease, tuberculosis ranks behind venereal infections, but in terms of the total number of people infected, it retains its traditional primacy among bacterial infections. Worldwide there is much variation in the incidence and mortality associated with clinical tuberculosis. There are global pockets with a staggering incidence rate of 450 per 100,000 (Swaziland, Macau). Mortality rates too are many times higher in the developing countries. *Tuberculosis flourishes wherever there is poverty, malnourishment, and lack of adequate medical care.* Much of the decline of tuberculosis in the United States occurred before the advent of effective antibiotic therapy, owing to better living conditions. Unfortunately, those segments of the United States population that have benefited least from the improved quality of life (e.g., inner city minorities) continue to succumb to tuberculosis in unacceptably high numbers. In addition to socioeconomic factors, there also seem to be *racial or ethnic differences.* Africans, American Indians, blacks, and Eskimos are especially vulnerable, possibly because they have been unexposed until the recent past. Blacks in the U.S. Army have significantly higher morbidity rates from tuberculosis than do whites. However, no racial or economic *group* has proved resistant to sustained exposure, although susceptibility clearly differs among *individuals.* Thus, in the past, there has been a higher incidence of the disease in males than in females. Diabetes mellitus, alcoholism, malnutrition, congenital heart disease, chronic lung disease (particularly silicosis), and in fact any debilitating or immunosuppressive condition (e.g., Hodgkin's disease) predispose to active disease. Occupational hazards exist for physicians and hospital personnel.

A significant change in the age distribution of tuberculosis has occurred in the United States. Outside the inner city reservoirs of infection, where young adults are still at high risk, tuberculin reactivity and peak morbidity and mortality have all shifted from the 20-year-olds to the 50- and 60-year-olds. Childhood tuberculosis has declined most sharply —

fewer than 5% of teenagers now react to tuberculin. The peak mortality from tuberculosis in white males now occurs around age 54, and in white females after age 65. Thus, tuberculosis in the United States is today mainly a disease of the elderly who became infected early in life before transmission declined.[139]

CAUSATIVE ORGANISM. *Mycobacterium tuberculosis hominis* is a slender, delicately beaded rod averaging 4 μm in length when stained by the acid-fast (Ziehl-Neelsen) or fluorescent dye methods. It is undetectable by Gram stain or routine histologic techniques. Its dividing time is about 48 hours and growth in culture is slow; therefore, direct microscopic diagnosis in sputum, sediments, exudates, or biopsy specimens is time saving, although culture is still needed to rule out artifacts and verify the species. It should be remembered, however, that it takes between 10^5 and 10^6 bacteria per milliliter of tissue for them to be visually detectable. A gas chromatographic method for traces of tuberculostearic acids may prove helpful when microscopic examination fails to yield mycobacteria after painstaking search.[140] Even more sensitive are techniques for mycobacterial DNA hybridization, now available at state laboratories.[141]

Tubercle bacilli are strict aerobes; they thrive at a PO_2 of 140 mm Hg and this may explain their tendency to cause disease in the subapical portions of the lung ($PO_2 = 130$ mm Hg), and to become scarcer in necrotic tissue lacking blood-borne oxygen. Their growth is also inhibited by a pH lower than 6.5 and by long-chain fatty acids. On the other hand, *M. tuberculosis* can persist in dormant form in old necrotic and calcified lesions still capable of reinitiating growth.

PATHOGENESIS. The *pathogenesis* of tuberculosis involves four considerations: (1) the virulence of *M. tuberculosis*, (2) the role of induced hypersensitivity, (3) the role of immunity or resistance, and (4) the genesis of the granulomatous pattern of reaction so characteristic (but not necessarily diagnostic) of tuberculosis.

Mycobacterium tuberculosis has no known exotoxins, endotoxins, or histolytic enzymes. A variety of antigens (approximately 30) can be identified, but these seem to play no role in *virulence*. More important appears to be the microbial content of extractable *mycosides* (covalently linked complex lipids and carbohydrates). One derivative, called "cord factor" (trehalose 6–6 dimycolate), is essential for the in vitro growth of *M. tuberculosis* in a pattern of serpentine cords. Organisms growing in this fashion are virulent in animals. If cord factor is extracted from tubercle bacilli they are rendered avirulent. Cord-forming strains also possess a sulfated glycolipid (sulfatide), which prevents the fusion of phagosomes with the lysosomes and favors the intracellular survival of mycobacteria within macrophages.[142] Several of the mycobacterial cell wall constituents, including wax D (a glycolypid) and muramyl dipeptide (a small water soluble component), when injected with tuberculoprotein — itself weakly immunogenic — induce strong hypersensitivity to tuberculin and so act as adjuvants. Thus, *lipid fractions contribute both to virulence and to the sensitivity state associated with tuberculosis.*

The emergence of *hypersensitivity* to the tubercle bacillus plays a dominant role in the tissue destruction encountered in this disease. About two to four weeks after infection by the tubercle bacillus, sensitization appears as measured by the tuberculin test. The test antigen is purified protein derivation (PPD), derived from the culture medium in which tubercle bacilli have grown. In the widely employed Mantoux or Tine tests, an intradermal injection of PPD will evoke in the sensitized individual an area of induration (not simply erythema) at least 5 mm in diameter in 48 hours. Indeed, in the very sensitive, the site may become necrotic. *A tuberculosensitivity reaction signals infection in the host, but not necessarily disease.* It results from acquisition of delayed (cell-mediated) hypersensitivity (type IV) (p. 182).

Once an individual becomes tuberculin positive, he usually remains so for the rest of his life. The basis of such long-lasting sensitivity is uncertain but is thought to be the persistence of bacilli, either latent or actively multiplying. In support of this view, some sensitized individuals after an intensive course of chemotherapy become tuberculin negative, taken to mean eradication of all viable bacilli. Repeated PPD skin testing can itself be temporarily sensitizing, but permanent sensitivity is conferred only by intact bacilli, virulent or attenuated. *False-negative* reactions (about 5%), if not due to technical failure, may be caused by viral infection or vaccination, drugs, steroid hormones, malnutrition, neoplasms, sarcoidosis, immunosuppression, Hodgkins' disease, or other poorly understood interfering factors, including the waning of cellular immune responses in advanced age. Rarely, but most important, *true tuberculin anergy* can be due to overwhelming disseminated tuberculosis itself and may be accompanied by a nonselective suppression of skin responses to other antigens. *False-positive* tuberculin tests have resulted from previous host experience with atypical mycobacteria.

The appearance of tuberculin sensitivity heralds a change in the host's response to the bacilli. On first exposure, tubercle bacilli act as inert particulate matter and evoke a nonspecific neutrophilic inflammatory response. During this period, bacilli enter phagocytes (Fig. 7–31) but multiply unchecked and can drain via lymphatics and bloodstream to distant sites, where they may die, remain dormant, or later induce foci of disease. *Once sensitization appears the inflammatory reaction becomes granulomatous and, as cited earlier, the centers of the granuloma often undergo caseation necrosis, to form typical tubercles.* Thus, hypersensitization underlies the caseating destruction of tissue encountered in tuberculous lesions, but these damaging effects are counterbalanced by a concomitant increase in resistance to the infecting organisms, i.e., *increased capacity to phagocytose and inhibit the intracellular replication of bacilli.*

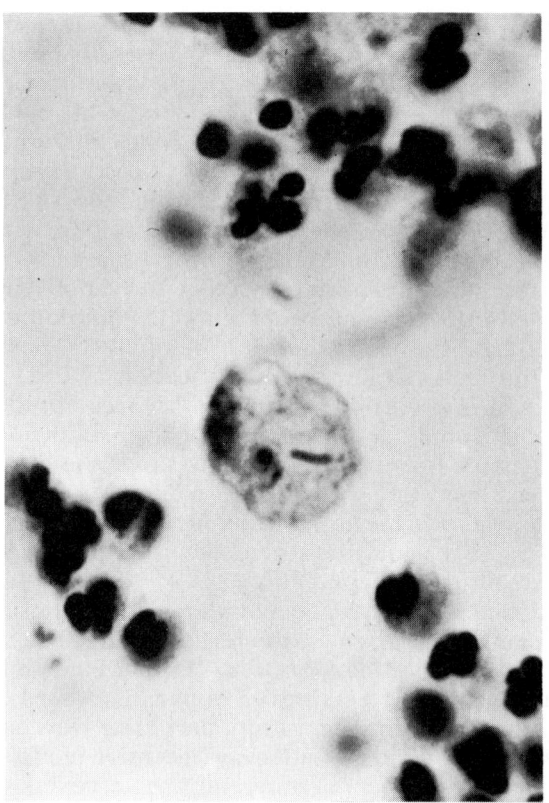

Figure 7–31. A mononuclear phagocyte with an engulfed tubercle bacillus.

Efforts have been made to determine whether hypersensitivity and immunity (resistance) are two concurrent phenomena or two expressions of a single process. When normal individuals are vaccinated with a preparation of avirulent tubercle bacilli—bacille Calmette Guérin (BCG)—the vaccinated individuals become tuberculin positive, but there is no agreement as to whether they also acquire resistance to a virulent infection. Estimates of the protective efficacy of BCG range from nil to 80%.[143] This issue is clouded by technical and epidemiologic complexities, and no firm conclusions have been reached about the relationship of hypersensitivity to increased resistance. In any event, most experts believe that BCG vaccination is inadvisable in areas with a low incidence of tuberculosis, where most young adults are tuberculin negative, because the opportunity is lost to detect the onset of infection.

Tuberculosis is the prototype granulomatous disease of humans. *Other granulomatous conditions include sarcoidosis, brucellosis, tularemia, syphilis, leprosy, glanders, lymphogranuloma venereum, cat-scratch fever, berylliosis, and some of the mycoses. Uncommonly, granulomas are found within neoplasms and as reactions to lipids or in diseases of obscure nature, such as Wegener's granulomatosis* (p. 574). The basic characteristics of granulomatous inflammation were discussed on page 65. Here it suffices to recall that *the tubercle comprises an organized microscopic aggregation of plump, rounded histiocytes (macro-*

phages) that vaguely resemble epithelial cells and are therefore called epithelioid cells. There may also be Langhans' multinucleate giant cells, formed by the fusion of macrophages or internal nuclear division without cytoplasmic division. About the granuloma, a peripheral collar of plump fibroblasts interspersed with lymphocytes is found. The description just given represents the *"hard" tubercle,* so designated because of the absence of central necrosis and softening. More often, the central region of the tubercle undergoes a characteristic form of granular, caseous necrosis. This *"soft" tubercle* is the hallmark of tuberculosis (Fig. 7–32). Although a variety of other inflammatory changes may also be present, such as purulent and fibrotic lesions, tubercles can always be found if properly sought.

With the electron microscope, epithelioid cells show highly ruffled, interdigitating cell membranes; well-developed endoplasmic reticulum; abundant mitochondria; and large Golgi complexes. Their cytoplasm contains numerous vesicles, but dense lysosome-like bodies are not typically seen. Thus, their ultrastructure suggests they are better equipped for secretory functions than for phagocytosis.[144] The mechanism of caseous necrosis, the other hallmark of a tuberculous granuloma, is poorly understood. Its appearance coincides with the acquisition of delayed hypersensitivity. Although there is little doubt that the formation of epithelioid cell granulomas in tuberculosis and several other infectious disorders is immunologically mediated, it should be pointed out that epithelioid cell transformation of macrophages can also be brought about by nonimmunologic mechanisms.[145]

In conclusion, although much remains unknown about the pathogenesis of tuberculosis, it is abundantly clear that the fundamental tissue reaction is granulomatous, frequently with central caseation necrosis, and that hypersensitivity and immunity both play major roles in the evolution of the disease.

Primary Tuberculosis

Primary tuberculosis is defined as infection of an individual lacking previous contact with tubercle bacilli. In primary lung infection, a single lesion (known as a Ghon focus) is usually found immediately subjacent to the pleura in the lower part of the upper lobes or upper part of the lower lobes of one lung, rarely elsewhere. These localizations reflect the areas receiving the greatest volume flow of inspired air. Bilateral or multiple foci are very infrequent. An active **Ghon focus** is a 1.0- to 1.5-cm area of gray-white inflammatory consolidation circumscribed from the surrounding lung parenchyma. The consolidated focus becomes granulomatous and then develops a soft, caseous, necrotic center by the second week. Tubercle bacilli, either free or within phagocytes, drain along the regional peribronchial lymphatic channels to the tracheobronchial **lymph nodes** and there evoke caseating granulomas. As a rule, the nodal involvement happens only on one side, that

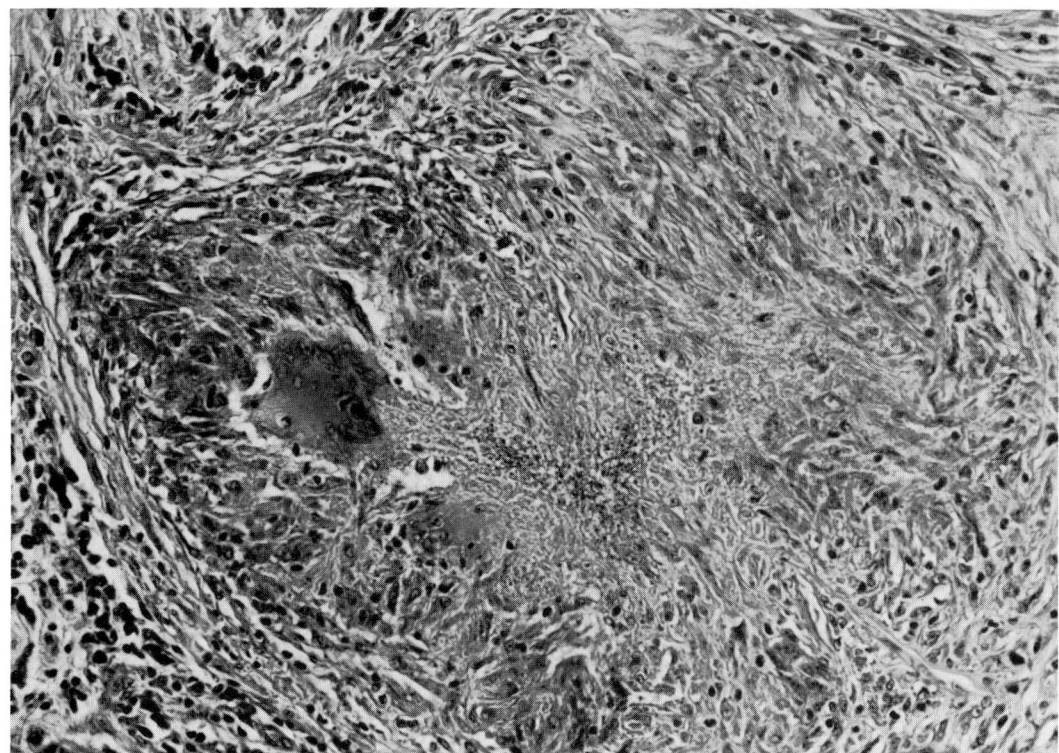

Figure 7-32. A tubercle with giant cell and central caseous necrosis.

of the lung focus. The combination of the primary lung lesion and lymph node involvement is referred to as the **Ghon complex** (Fig. 7-33).

In most cases, primary tuberculosis does not progress and undergoes shrinkage with fibrosis, calcification, and sometimes ossification, with fibrous scarring and puckering of the pleural surface. Occasionally, the pleural reaction may also become calcified. At the same time, fibrocalcific scarring replaces most of the tuberculous foci in the regional tracheobronchial nodes. Healed primary complexes are frequently quite small and may be hard to detect by either pathologic or x-ray studies. However, the infecting organisms are not totally eradicated, and bacilli may persist for years and perhaps for life.

Primary tuberculosis does not always follow a self-terminating course. *Progressive primary tuberculosis* is relatively rare and is more likely to affect children, although adult onset has become more frequent in those countries in which tuberculin conversion has shifted to the older age groups. In the so-called childhood form, the primary lung focus rapidly enlarges, erodes into the bronchial tree, and gives rise to new satellite lung lesions. This is accompanied and sometimes overshadowed by caseous enlargement of the hilar lymph nodes to the point of forming mediastinal masses that can encroach upon major bronchi and hamper air flow. At the same time, these highly active lesions may seed the bloodstream with tubercle bacilli, resulting in life-threatening *miliary dissemina-*

tion (or tuberculous meningitis) (p. 378). In adults, primary tuberculosis tends to pursue a less rampant course and therefore it is less readily distinguished from the secondary disease. It can be suspected in an adult when radiographs show the subapical lung portions to be spared of lesions in the presence of mediastinal lymph node enlargement, a rare distribution in the usual, secondary form of tuberculosis.

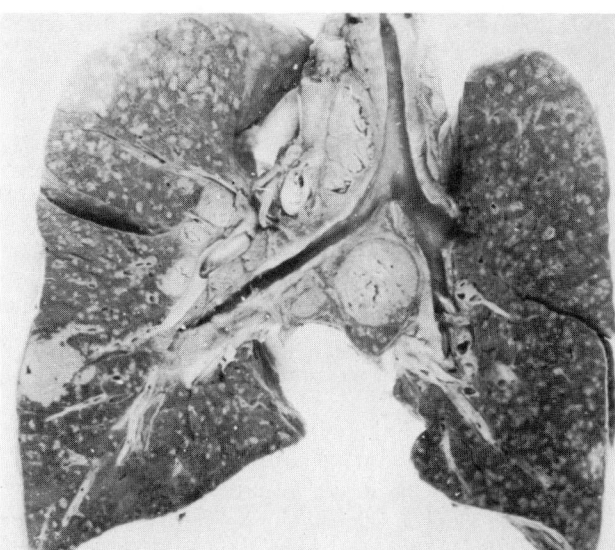

Figure 7-33. Progressive (childhood) primary tuberculosis: pneumonic focus (*left*, near pleura), massive caseous hilar lymphadenitis, and miliary tubercles throughout lung. Note tracheal displacement.

When primary tuberculous infection occurs at the less common portals of entry (gastrointestinal tract, oropharyngeal lymphoid tissue, skin), primary complexes, similar to those of the pulmonary form, evolve at these sites and in the corresponding draining nodes.

Secondary Tuberculosis

Secondary or postprimary tuberculosis is that phase of tuberculous infection that arises in a previously sensitized individual, whether the tubercle bacilli are derived from endogenous or exogenous sources. Most cases of secondary tuberculosis represent reactivation of asymptomatic primary disease and may occur at any time following a primary infection, sometimes many decades later, presumably whenever defenses are lowered. Less commonly, exogenous organisms may trigger the onset of secondary disease. This phase of the disease is sometimes inappropriately called "adult" or "reinfection" tuberculosis.

Secondary tuberculosis begins in the apical or posterior segments of one or both upper lobes, appearing close to the clavicle in chest x-ray films. Such lesions are referred to as Simon's foci and are believed to be seeded during the early period of tuberculosis bacteremia, favored by the high Po_2 of the region. The minimal pulmonary lesion in the apex consists of a 1- to 3-cm focal area of caseous consolidation, usually within 1 to 2 cm of the pleural surfaces. Less commonly, reactivation occurs in other parts of the lung. Perhaps because of the prompter phagocytosis and destruction of bacilli by activated macrophages in the partly resistant individual, satellite lesions in the regional nodes are distinctly rare and lung lesions are more apt to remain localized or progress slowly; however, at the same time, caseation occurs more rapidly, as does fibrotic walling off of the lesions.

Histologically, the usual reaction consists of tubercle formation with formation of epithelioid cells, Langhans' giant cells, caseation, fibrosis, and lymphocytic infiltration. However, when tuberculosis strikes immunosuppressed patients, there may be virtual absence of any reactive cells and the lesions may therefore be represented by cell-poor nondescript necrotic foci rich in mycobacteria. Conversely, the lesions may be rich in neutrophils, especially where cavities are formed from large coalescent caseous lesions, and have eroded into the airways.

The course of apical infection is extremely varied. (1) The pathologic process may undergo healing, scarring, and calcification to yield apical, **fibrocalcific "arrested" tuberculosis.** (2) The initial parenchymal infection may spread to the other areas of the lung through one of several pathways to create **progressive pulmonary tuberculosis** (p. 788). (3) It may extend to the pleura to produce pleural fibrosis, pleural adhesions, or inflammatory pleural effusions, or, by direct extension of the bacilli into the pleural cavity, lead to a **tuberculous empyema.** (4) When the pulmonary lesions erode into bronchi, the material may be coughed up and seed the mucosal lining of the bronchioles, bronchi, and trachea **(tracheobronchial tuberculosis),** or organisms may become implanted in the larynx to produce laryngeal tuberculosis. (5) Swallowed bacilli can become trapped by the lymphoid patches of the small and large bowel to cause **intestinal tuberculosis.**

(6) **Miliary tuberculosis** may result when the organisms gain access to the lymphatics and blood to seed distant organs. The term miliary is descriptive of the small, yellow-white, barely visible lesions, which resemble canary bird feed, or millet seeds. The miliary dissemination may be limited to the lungs when an **artery** is invaded, but when the seeding is heavy or when a caseous focus erodes into a **pulmonary vein,** systemic dissemination follows and miliary lesions may develop in virtually any organ of the body. However, certain tissues are remarkably resistant to tuberculous infection, and it is rare to find tubercles in the heart, striated muscle, thyroid, and pancreas. Favored sites of miliary localization are the bone marrow, eye grounds, lymph nodes, liver, spleen, kidneys, adrenals, prostate, seminal vesicles, fallopian tubes, endometrium, and meninges. Involvement of the eye grounds, bone marrow, and liver offers valuable clinical opportunities to diagnose miliary tuberculosis. The tubercles can be visualized in many instances in the eye grounds by simple funduscopic examination, and can often be identified in marrow and liver biopsies, even when there is no functional impairment of these organs. (7) **Progressive, isolated-organ tuberculosis** may occur in any one of the organs or tissues commonly affected by miliary dissemination. Most likely, in the course of lymphatic or hematogenous dissemination of bacilli, organisms are rapidly destroyed in all other sites save for the particular tissue involved in the isolated tuberculous process. The most common sites of such isolated-organ tuberculosis are the cervical lymph nodes (scrofula), meninges (tuberculous meningitis), kidneys (renal tuberculosis), adrenals (formerly an important cause of Addison's disease—p. 1252), bones (tuberculous osteomyelitis), and the fallopian tubes and epididymides (genital tuberculosis). From such focal lesions, further dissemination or seeding may occur and thus, in renal tuberculosis, it is common for infective material to drain through the urine and cause tuberculous cystitis. In the same way, tuberculous salpingitis is often followed by tuberculous endometritis and tuberculous pelvic peritonitis. Tuberculous epididymitis may be followed by extension of the tuberculous infection into the testes, and spread from the prostate and seminal vesicles may affect other organs in the genitourinary tract. In vertebral tuberculosis (Pott's disease), long fistulas may form along the psoas muscle to open and drain in the groin region. Long-lasting tuberculous lesions of all types may stimulate the reticuloendothelial system sufficiently to result in systemic secondary **amyloidosis** (p. 214), but this is rare in treated individuals.

Before this discussion is concluded, attention should once again be drawn to the need for positive identification of acid-fast tubercle bacilli in the anatomic lesions. Granulomatous lesions are not confined to tuberculosis, as pointed out earlier. Acid fastness is shared by other mycobacteria and by nocardiae

(p. 383). A diagnosis of tuberculosis should never be made definitively unless typical mycobacteria are seen in typical lesions or tubercle bacilli have been unmistakably identified by culture. Note that typing of mycobacterial cultures by DNA probes has increased both the speed and accuracy of laboratory diagnosis.[141]

Unfortunately, in all but the most rampant forms of tuberculosis, acid-fast bacilli in the diseased tissues are relatively scarce and therefore quite difficult to find. The most likely sites of their localization are recent necrotic foci still containing nuclear fragments and the walls of actively inflamed cavities; epithelioid cells rarely contain the bacilli. Even when they are not visible with the microscope, enough bacilli may be present in the tissues or in secretion such as sputum or gastric washings to be cultured successfully.

CLINICAL COURSE. The clinical signs and symptoms of pulmonary tuberculosis are as *varied* as the anatomic lesions. A minute focus of tuberculosis may be totally occult, whereas extensive tuberculosis is almost invariably accompanied by systemic reactions. Except in progressive primary disease, *primary tuberculosis is usually an entirely silent process.* In most cases, primary infection, past or present, is detected only by tuberculin testing or by routine roentgenography with visualization of a focus of scarring or calcification in the appropriate location in the lung parenchyma or tracheobronchial nodes. Occasionally the individual may have low-grade fever and lack of appetite.

Secondary tuberculosis may also be asymptomatic when the condition is confined to minimal lesions within the lung apices. *More often, however, these patients have insidious onset of fever (usually most marked in the midafternoon), night sweats, weakness, fatigability, and loss of appetite and weight.* As lung tissue is destroyed and bronchi are invaded, there is often productive cough, blood-streaked sputum, or hemoptysis. In other instances, pleural effusion may dominate the clinical picture. In advanced lesions, dyspnea and orthopnea may be present. When the process affects other organs the clinical manifestations are referable to these localizations: for example, meningitis or renal disease. When the disease is miliary in its dissemination and does not produce focalizing signs or detectable lesions, the symptom complex may be that of a fever of unknown origin (FUO). Because of their small size, miliary tubercles are often undiscovered by chest radiography. The many potential pathways of pulmonary tuberculosis are depicted in Figure 7–34.

The diagnosis of all forms of tuberculosis depends on identification or isolation of the causative organism. Tuberculin testing can be helpful in children or when recent conversion in an adult can be documented. Otherwise, skin reaction is of little diagnostic value. Neither does the failure to demonstrate tubercle bacilli in sputum or other secreta rule out the diagnosis of tuberculosis, because occasionally the lesions are not in contact with natural channels of drainage in the so-called "closed" case. Biopsy may have to be resorted to in such instances.

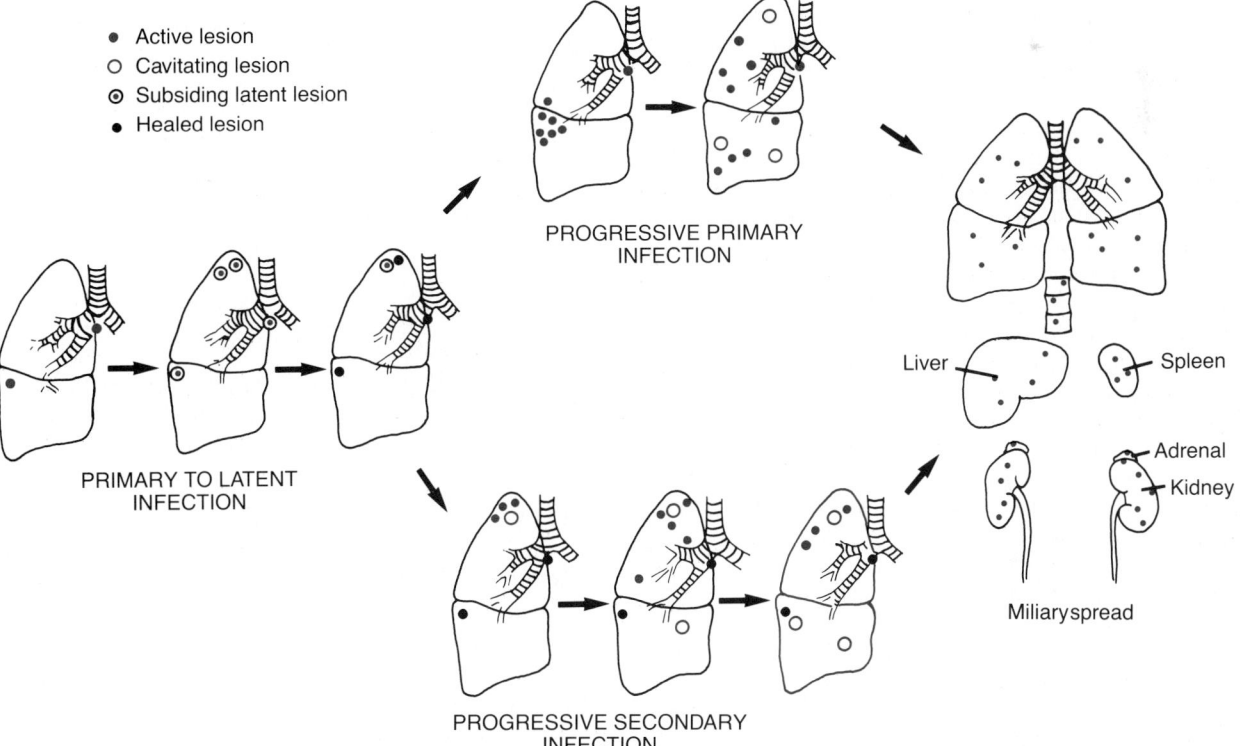

Figure 7–34. Potential progressions of pulmonary tuberculosis.

In recent years, the diagnosis of tuberculosis in North America has become more difficult since the number of classic cases has declined and more patients now present with "occult" or atypical disease.[146] Most common among the *atypical presentations* are late generalized infections in older people, some of which mimic hematologic syndromes, leukemoid reactions, or myelophthisic anemias. Reactivation of tuberculosis in the course of a preexisting major illness (e.g., malignancies or chronic renal failure and dialysis) also poses diagnostic problems. The same is true of AIDS patients, particularly those from developing countries, in whom tuberculosis is frequently rapidly progressive and atypical (Chapter 5). In all these clinical settings, one should remain alert to the possibility of tuberculosis, especially if the patient develops unexplained pyrexia. Fortunately, in all but those with advanced neglected disease, present methods of treatment with rifampicin, isoniazid, paraminosalicylates, or streptomycin can be expected to arrest progression and effect cure.

Atypical Mycobacterial Infections

The so-called atypical mycobacteria are related to *Mycobacterium tuberculosis* but differ significantly in their distribution and pathogenicity. Formerly uncommon, the prevalence of atypical mycobacterioses is on the rise because of their association with AIDS.

Atypical mycobacteria are widespread in the environment, in soil, water, plants, and animal excreta. Many are saprophytic or have very low pathogenicity. Skin test data in the southern United States suggest that many false-positive tuberculin reactors have been *exposed* to such organisms, but *progressive disease* caused by "atypicals" is less frequent and is predominantly opportunistic, affecting mainly those with reduced immunity or a pre-existing lung disease. In AIDS patients from developed countries, the role of *M. tuberculosis* is often taken by *M. avium-intracellulare*, causing rapidly progressing systemic infection (p. 224). There is also a significant association between hairy cell leukemia and infection with *M. kansasii* (p. 730). Human infections are derived directly from the environment and, unlike tuberculosis, there is no evidence for person-to-person transmission. The lesions associated with mycobacterioses vary considerably and range from granulomas to nodular foam cell lesions to purulent and necrotizing inflammation. In immunosuppressed individuals the entire reticuloendothelial system may be overrun by intracellular organisms, as in disseminated histoplasmosis (p. 394) or kala-azar (p. 409). Five patterns of disease may be seen:

1. *Pulmonary disease,* produced by *M. kansasii* or *M. avium-intracellulare,* mainly affects white males over the age of 45 years with pre-existing chronic bronchitis and emphysema; this is the most common form of atypical mycobacteriosis.[147]
2. *Lymphadenitis,* mainly affecting children, is produced by *M. avium-intracellulare* or *M. scrofulaceum.*

3. *Ulcerative skin lesions* caused by *M. ulcerans*[148] are endemic in Australia, parts of Africa, and Latin America. Similar skin lesions, caused by *M. marinum,* may be acquired in an aquarium setting.
4. *Injection abscesses* caused by *M. fortuitum* and *M. chelonei* occur sporadically all over the world.
5. In severely immunosuppressed patients, as in those with AIDS, life-threatening *bacteremias* may occur, based on widespread lymphoreticular involvement, principally by *M. avium-intracellulare.*

The diagnosis of mycobacterioses rests on culture in specialized media, differential biochemical tests, and DNA hybridization procedures. Because many of these organisms are free living or saprophytic, it is sometimes difficult to distinguish contamination or colonization from true infection. This difficulty arises mainly in patients with pulmonary fibrosis or cavitation resulting from previous tuberculosis or chronic obstructive airway disease. There is at present no satisfactory laboratory method of making this distinction; inoculation into hamsters may be resorted to in order to gauge the virulence of a given mycobacterial isolate, but in some cases therapeutic trial may be the only recourse. Unfortunately, some species respond only poorly or not at all to antituberculous drugs or antibiotics.

Leprosy (Mycobacterium leprae)

Leprosy, or Hansen's disease, is a slowly progressive mycobacterial infection affecting mostly the skin and peripheral nerves (i.e., the coolest parts of the body). If untreated, it often results in unsightly or disabling deformities. Despite its low communicability, leprosy remains endemic among an estimated 10.6 million people, most living in (or originating from) poor tropical countries. There is reason to believe that an even larger number of infections remain subclinical and undetected. At any rate, transmission has ceased in Europe and in the United States, but about 2500 patients continue to reside in a single specialized facility located in Carville, Louisiana. For thousands of years, victims of real or imagined leprosy were cruelly shunned by society, but better understanding and drug treatment have finally ended their ostracism.

Mycobacterium leprae is an acid-fast obligate intracellular organism whose optimal growth occurs at 36°C. Only humans and the nine-banded armadillo are naturally susceptible.[149] In thymus-deficient mice, *M. leprae* has a sluggish doubling time of 13 days. It has never been grown in cell-free media. None of its glycolipids and glycoproteins has toxic properties, but several elicit hypersensitivity in the form of skin reactions to lepromin (a bacterial extract) at 48 hours — the Fernandez reaction — and again at 3 to 4 weeks — the Mitsuda reaction. Antibodies are also formed, but host resistance to *M. leprae* is clearly linked to cellular immunity and not to antibody formation. In fact, no infectious disease shows a better correlation between T-lymphocyte reactivity and clinical course than is evident in the so-called polar (ends of the spectrum) forms of leprosy.

Patients with polar tuberculoid leprosy (the TT form) respond to *M. leprae* by mounting a vigorous T cell–mediated immunity, and, as in the case of tuberculosis, the sensitized T cells cause local aggregation and activation of macrophages, resulting in the formation of typical *tuberculoid granulomas with few surviving bacilli in the lesions.* The 48-hour lepromin skin test, an indication of delayed hypersensitivity to lepra bacilli, is strongly positive in TT. In sharp contrast, the polar lepromatous form (LL) is associated with lack of T cell–mediated immunity and therefore with poor host resistance. Enormous numbers of *M. leprae* can be seen within macrophages, which seem unable to destroy them or to limit bacterial growth, perhaps because of lack of activating signals derived from sensitized T cells (Fig. 7–35). Lepromatous lesions show nodular or diffuse aggregates of foamy macrophages rather than epithelioid cell granulomas, and their lepromin skin test is negative. As might be expected, in LL the disease is both much more extensive and progressive and more difficult to cure. The tissue reactions, bacillary load, and lepromin test results are variable in the intermediate forms and depend on their position within the spectrum of leprosy. The basis of immunologic failure is still a mystery. At onset it appears that the defect is selective for the lepra bacilli, because reactions to other T-cell antigens remain intact. In some fully developed cases, however, patients are anergic to several commonly used skin-test antigens.[150]

Patients with LL often have a polyclonal hypergammaglobulinemia. Obviously these antibodies offer little protection against the bacilli. On the contrary, the formation of antigen-antibody complexes may lead to erythema nodosum leprosum (ENL), a potentially life-threatening reaction. ENL is associated with vasculitis (responsible for erythematous skin nodules), arthralgias, fever, and sometimes glomerulonephritis. By contrast, tuberculoid patients may experience so-called borderline reactions (i.e., erythematous swellings of skin lesions, followed by clinical improvement and increased reactivity to lepromin).

Transmission of leprosy is direct from active cases, mostly LL. The tuberculoid form is not contagious. The mode of entry is unknown, but it probably involves droplet aspiration or skin contact. It has been suggested that subclinical infection may be far more common than currently believed.[151] Overt clinical infection requires prolonged close contact (years), such as occurs within a family, and once acquired the disease usually pursues an extremely slow course, spanning decades. Indeed, most patients die with leprosy rather than of it. The vital organs and CNS are rarely affected.

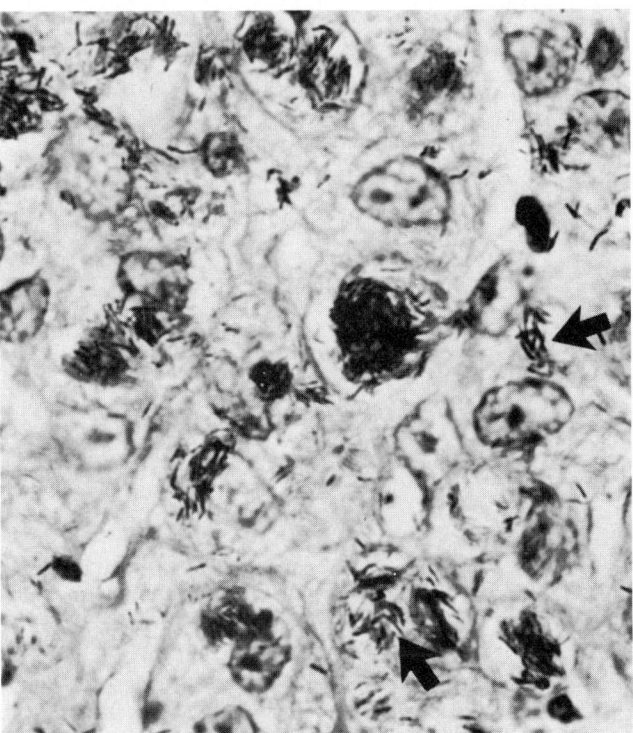

Figure 7–35. Leprosy. High-power view of acid-fast bacilli *(arrows)* proliferating in foamy macrophages.

In **LL,** once the organism invades, a bacteremia follows that often persists during the course of active disease. From the blood, organisms preferentially localize in the skin, peripheral nerves, anterior eye, upper airways (down to the larynx), testes, hands, and feet. This distribution reflects the fact that the organisms are able to proliferate only in cooler tissues. Wherever they localize they evoke an aggregation of lipid-laden macrophages **(lepra cells)**, often filled with masses of acid-fast bacilli **(globi)**. These reactions induce macular, papular, or nodular lesions in the skin, with a predilection for the face, ears, wrists, elbows, knees, and buttocks. The distribution of these skin lesions can be symmetric or even diffuse and thus difficult to notice. With progression the nodular lesions coalesce to yield a distinctive **leonine facies.** Most skin lesions are hypoesthetic or anesthetic. Lesions in the nose may cause persistent inflammation and bacilli-laden discharge. Airway obstruction may develop or sometimes the bridge of the nose may collapse or the septum may perforate. The peripheral nerves may be affected (usually symmetrically), especially the ulnar and peroneal nerves where they come near the skin surface. Loss of sensation and trophic changes in the hands and feet may follow the nerve lesions. Although the nerves are laden with bacilli, clinically evident neurologic involvement is not as prominent in LL as in the TT form, since there is less intraneuronal inflammation. Lymph nodes show aggregation of foamy histiocytes in the paracortical (T cell) areas, with enlargement of germinal centers. In advanced disease, similar aggregates of macrophages are also present in the splenic red pulp and in the liver. Testes are usually extensively involved, with destruction of the seminiferous tubules and consequent sterility. Gynecomastia is also a frequent finding.

TT begins with much more localized macular skin lesions. The macules, at first erythematous, enlarge and develop irregular shapes with indurated, elevated, hyperpigmented margins and depressed pale centers (central healing). The skin lesions are usually neither numerous nor bilaterally symmetric. Nerve involvement dominates this form of the disease, typically of the ulnar and peroneal nerves. The nerves are enclosed within granulomatous inflammatory reactions, and if small enough (e.g., the peripheral twigs) may be totally destroyed. The neural involvement thus often induces skin anesthesias and skin and muscle atrophy. The trophic changes render the patient liable to trauma of the affected parts with the development of indolent skin ulcers. When the neurologic and trophic involvements are advanced, contractures, paralyses, and autoamputation of fingers or toes may ensue. Facial nerve involvement can lead to paralysis of the lids, with keratitis and corneal ulcerations. Microscopically, all sites of involvement disclose granulomatous lesions closely resembling hard tubercles. As mentioned, bacilli are almost never identified in these lesions. The contrast between the lepromatous and tuberculoid forms of leprosy is highlighted in Figure 7–36.

The diagnosis of early or subtle forms of leprosy is sometimes difficult, especially in a nonendemic setting, and may involve skin biopsy, scraping of lesions or nasal smears, and the use of appropriate acid-fast stains. Lepromin testing is used as an adjunct to histologic analysis for the purpose of classifying the disease stage and planning the appropriate therapeutic regimen. Treatment with drugs has generally been successful but needs to be sustained, especially in lepromatous cases, to prevent resistance or relapse. An experimental vaccine is undergoing human trial; its results will not be known for several years.

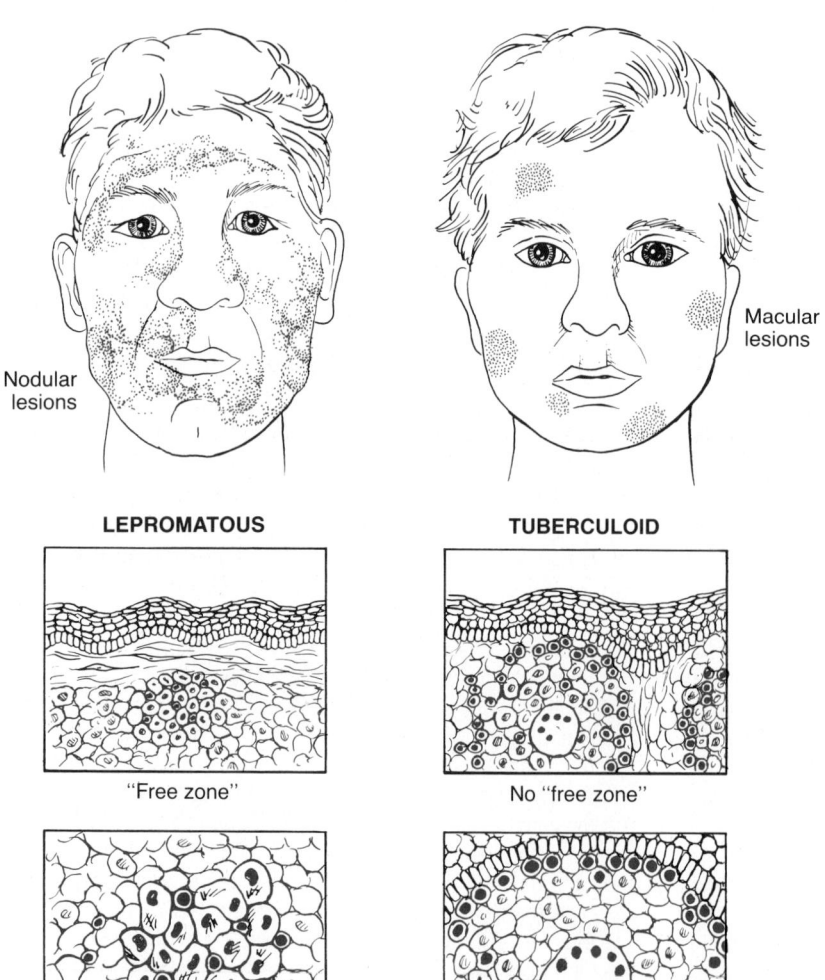

Nodular lesions

Macular lesions

LEPROMATOUS

"Free zone"

Foam cell lesions

TUBERCULOID

No "free zone"

Granulomatous lesions

Figure 7–36. A comparison of the polar extremes of leprosy. The nodular lepromatous form on the left demonstrates aggregates of lipid and bacilli-laden "lepra" cells deep to the epidermis (free zone). In contrast is the tubercular pattern on the right with macular skin lesions produced by a granulomatous reaction directly in contact with the epidermis (no free zone). Bacilli are extremely rare.

ACTINOMYCETES

Although traditionally discussed along with fungi, actinomycetes (Actinomycetales) are closely related to mycobacteria. They show some similarities to fungi, such as branching and the formation of a mycelial network, but the presence of muramic acid in their cell walls and the absence of a membrane-bound nucleus clearly aligns them with the bacteria. Of the several genera included in this group, Nocardia and Actinomyces are the most important human pathogens.

Nocardiosis

The nocardiae are long, filamentous, gram-positive, aerobic organisms that often aggregate in branching chains. They are weakly acid fast and can be stained with a modified acid-fast technique but not by the Ziehl-Neelsen stain for *M. tuberculosis.* They also differ from tubercle bacilli in their culture requirements, which are less fastidious, and by their extracellular habitat during infection. Approximately 1000 cases of nocardiosis are reported every year in the United States, but there are probably many more. Ninety per cent are caused by *N. asteroides* and the rest by *N. brasiliensis* and *N. caviae.* Most patients who develop nocardiosis are chronically ill or immunosuppressed; transplant rejection, corticosteroid therapy, and alveolar proteinosis (p. 795) are frequent antecedents.[152] In cases without a known predisposing condition (mostly skin infections), *N. brasiliensis* is the predominant pathogen.

Little is known of the transmission of nocardiae, which are widespread in soil and elsewhere in nature, and it is unclear whether the nosocomial form of nocardiosis represents *new* infection or reactivation. There is no evidence of person-to-person spread. The lung or skin is the usual primary site. In the United States, localized pulmonary disease is the most common form; second is severe, disseminated nocardiosis, including spread to the CNS. Localized skin infection, or mycetoma (p. 396), is uncommon in the United States, but it is endemic in Mexico and elsewhere in Latin America.

In the lung, nocardiae typically cause single or multiple, chronic, necrotizing, walled-off abscesses. Similarly, primary skin lesions are necrotizing or purulent, or both. Grossly nocardial lung abscesses are irregular in shape, with a soft purulent center surrounded by a broad rim of organizing pneumonia, much like the lesions caused by pyogenic bacteria. Fibrosis is seen only in long-standing lesions or during the healing stage, which is characteristically protracted. Pleural involvement is frequent, giving rise to fibrinous pleuritis or sometimes empyema. Microscopically there is widespread necrosis, with a fibrinous exudate rich in neutrophils. In contrast to tuberculosis, granulomas are not formed. The organisms do not stain with H and E and are therefore easily missed in routine sections. Gram staining and a modified acid-fast stain have to be utilized in suspected cases. Fragmentation of the filamentous nocardiae could cause confusion with tubercle bacilli, but staining and culture of the organisms differentiate the two. Nocardia grows out slowly on fungal and mycobacterial media, as well as on other media. In lung lesions, nocardiae appear as discrete filaments, but in mycetomas of the skin they form mycelial colonies not unlike those of Actinomyces except for their acid-fastness.

The clinical presentation of pulmonary nocardiosis can be confusing and the disease is often unsuspected until late in its course, after the common bacteria have been excluded and response to antibiotics has been disappointing. Dissemination can give rise to meningitis or symptoms of space-occupying lesions in the brain that are due to the formation of cerebral abscesses. In immunosuppressed patients, aggressive diagnostic evaluation for nocardiosis is warranted. If examination of sputum, pleural fluids, and bronchial washings is not helpful, open lung biopsy may be required. Most patients respond to appropriate drug therapy.

Actinomycosis

Actinomycosis is a chronic suppurative infection localized chiefly to the neck, lung, or abdomen. The lesions, which spread by contiguity, are markedly indurated and contain multiple abscesses that drain to the surface by sinuses. The discharge from the sinuses typically contains grossly visible yellowish colonies called sulfur granules. Most human infections are caused by *Actinomyces israelii*; other species, including *A. viscosus, A. odontolyticus,* and *A. naeslundii,* rarely produce disease. The actinomycetes are gram-positive, non–acid-fast, strictly anaerobic bacteria that are easily overgrown by other organisms and difficult to culture. They are commensals within the oral cavity (tonsillar crypts, tartar of teeth), alimentary tract, and vagina, invading only when the tissue is devitalized by trauma (e.g., dental surgery) or bacterial infections. Actinomycotic lesions often contain other bacteria including fusiform bacilli, gram-negative bacilli, and various streptococci. However, Actinomyces is capable of producing lesions in man and experimental animals without any synergistic bacterial flora. Unlike nocardiae, actinomycetes are pathogenic for normal hosts. They infect apparently healthy individuals when local conditions favorable for their growth are created by trauma or tissue devitalization and anaerobiosis. All infections are derived endogenously and there is no person-to-person spread. Three classic forms of actinomycosis are recognized—cervicofacial, abdominal, and thoracic—but the disease frequently presents in atypical fashion and can be confused with other infections or even neoplasms.[153]

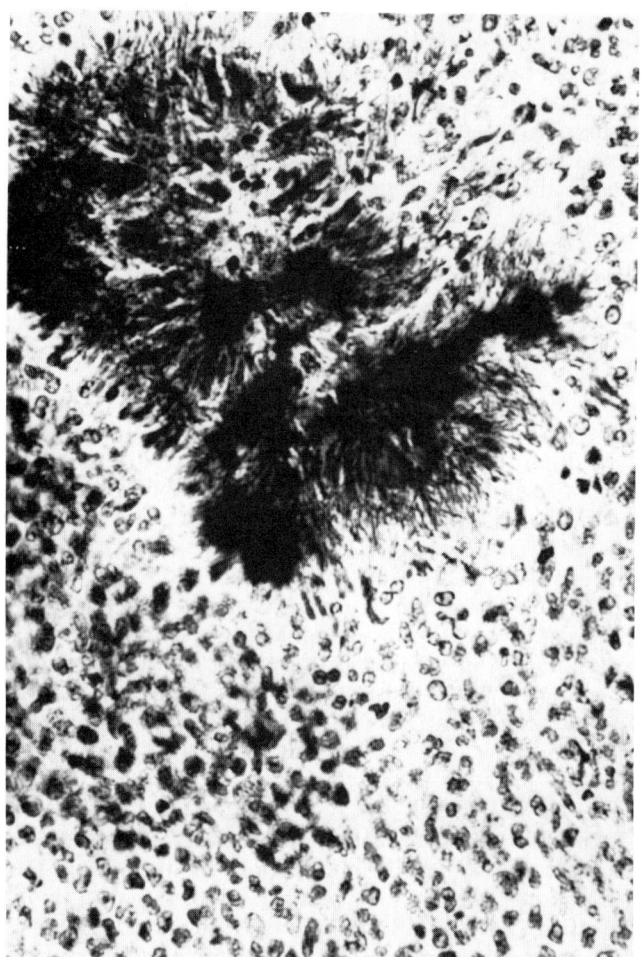

Figure 7–37. Actinomycotic abscess containing a colony or sulfur granule appearing as a black mass with radiating filaments.

Cervicofacial actinomycosis is the most frequent pattern. At first the gingivae and adjacent soft tissues become swollen and indurated, but the lesion is not extremely painful. In the course of time, a large, woody swelling develops, characteristically over the angle of the jaw, reminiscent of the actinomycotic infection in cattle—"lumpy jaw." These infections are characterized by great chronicity, burrowing, and invasive spread: thus, in the cervicofacial disease the **inflammation often extends to the skin to perforate and form multiple sinuses.** Periostitis and osteomyelitis with extensive destruction of bone (jaw or vertebrae) are common accompaniments. The histologic features can be briefly characterized as central suppurative necrosis surrounded by granulation tissue and intense fibrosis. Often included in the granulation tissue are many foamy histiocytes and plasma cells. The center of each abscess usually contains a bacterial colony consisting of intertwined radiating filaments (rays), capped by eosinophilic hyaline material (clubs), creating a sunburst pattern. These are the sulfur granules seen macroscopically (Fig. 7–37). Otherwise, the tissue response in actinomycosis is entirely nonspecific and the diagnosis must be made by identification of the causative agent. Sometimes an astute clinical observer will note diagnostic **sulfur granules** in the draining pus. For more certain identification, cultures may be required.

Abdominal actinomycosis arises from invasion of the intestinal mucosa, most commonly of the appendix or colon. There ensues an acute and chronic inflammatory reaction that penetrates the wall of the bowel to produce a localized peritoneal abscess, which then may extend into adjacent loops of bowel, the retroperitoneal tissues, and anterior abdominal wall and may sometimes dissect to the skin surface with the formation of draining external sinuses. Organisms may reach the liver either by the hematogenous route or by direct continuity, causing extensive liver abscesses. Further spread may then lead to subdiaphragmatic infections and eventual penetration of the diaphragm and intrathoracic infections. The increasing use of intrauterine contraceptive devices has led to the emergence of a pelvic form of the disease affecting the uterine cervix, fallopian tubes, ovary, and adjacent pelvic viscera.

Thoracic actinomycosis, either primary or following penetration of a subdiaphragmatic infection, causes lung abscesses that sometimes result in pulmonopleural fistulas or empyema. Further spread may erode the ribs and anterior chest wall or extend into the vertebral column and pericardial cavity.

Even in the presence of destructive local lesions, actinomycosis evokes few systemic symptoms, and the relative well-being of a patient bearing a large fistula-forming inflammatory mass is a valuable clinical clue. Actinomycoses respond well to sustained antibiotic treatment.

FUNGAL, PROTOZOAL, AND HELMINTHIC DISEASES AND SARCOIDOSIS

FUNGAL DISEASES
Deep Fungi
    Candidiasis (moniliasis)
    Mucormycosis (zygomycosis, phycomycosis)
    Aspergillosis
    Cryptococcosis
    Blastomycosis*
    Paracoccidioidomycosis*
    Coccidioidomycosis*
    Histoplasmosis*
    Unusual deep fungal infections*
Superficial Fungi (Dermatophytosis)

PROTOZOAL DISEASES
Luminal Protozoa
    Amebiasis
    Amebic meningoencephalitis
    Giardiasis
    Cryptosporidial and coccidial enteritis
    Trichomoniasis
    Pneumocystis pneumonia
Blood and Tissue Protozoa
    Malaria*
    Babesiasis
    African trypanosomiasis*
Intracellular Protozoa
    Chagas disease*

    Leishmaniasis*
    Toxoplasmosis
HELMINTHIC DISEASES
Intestinal Roundworms
    Ascariasis
    Trichuriasis
    Enterobiasis (oxyuriasis)
    Hookworm disease
    Strongyloidiasis
Tissue Roundworms
    Visceral larva migrans
    Guinea worm infection*
    Trichinosis
    Filariasis*
Cestodes, Tapeworms

    Intestinal tapeworm infections
    Cysticercosis
    Echinococcosis (hydatid disease)
Trematodes (Flukes)
    Fascioliasis
    Clonorchiasis and opisthorchiasis*
    Fasciolopsiasis*
    Paragonimiasis*
    Schistosomiasis (bilharziasis)
SARCOIDOSIS (OR BOECK'S SARCOID)

Some of the disorders covered in the following sections may be considered "exotic," but jet travel and the migration of individuals bring many of these conditions to countries where they are least suspected, making their diagnosis even more difficult. A working knowledge of these diseases has therefore now become the domain of every well-informed clinician if they are to be recognized and appropriately treated. The designation of "limited geographic distribution" must then be viewed as a guideline, not as an absolute.

FUNGAL DISEASES

Only a few fungal species commonly infect humans (Table 7–7), yet taken together they rank closely behind viruses and bacteria as causes of disease and are neither rare nor exotic. In tissues, fungi reproduce by simple division of round, yeastlike forms or of slender, tubular hyphae that form a mycelium. Rarely, fruiting bodies named conidia or sporangia are also formed, but the rich diversity of free-living and sexual reproductive stages is missing; in fact, some species form infective spores only in nature or in culture and these differ sharply from their tissue forms, which are noncommunicable (dimorphic fungi).

Fungal cells are relatively large (Table 7–1, p. 309) and their walls contain ergosterol and polysaccharides rather than the peptidoglycans of bacteria. Some species have slimy, antiphagocytic capsules; others have wall components resistant to phagolysosomal attack. *Fungi therefore can imitate the whole gamut of bacterial pathology from acute pyogenic to chronic granulomatous infection, and they may not reveal their presence until identified by laboratory methods.* Fortunately, their sturdy cell walls make fungi detectable microscopically (Fig. 7–38) even in the midst of necrosis; however, some are so adherent and tightly bound that they are rarely visible in body fluids or exudates, and tissue samples are required to find them. Fungal morphology can be distinctive enough for tentative microscopic species identification, but often culture is needed. Fungal pathogens grow well, if slowly, on appropriate media, but so do contaminating spores of free-living or commensal fungi. Therefore, *culture and tissue diagnosis combined provide the most useful information.*

Pathogenic fungi elaborate mycotoxins and enzymes but, with few exceptions, their role in human disease is still unclear. Their antigens, rich in polysaccharides, are sometimes diagnostically detectable; some can induce strong hypersensitivity responses of types III and IV (p. 178). Phagocytic competence plays a large role in antifungal defense,[154] and leukopenic patients are as vulnerable to fungi as to bacteria. *Corticosteroids and immunosuppressive drugs favor fungal infections of all varieties and species.* In altered hosts, fungal growth is often florid and widespread, with sparse cellular response. It extends into vessel walls to generate hemorrhage, thrombosis, and infarction. Thus, the combination of necrotic foci rimmed by hemorrhage and infarcts should arouse suspicion of a fungal cause.

Fungal pathogens are subdivided into those that remain *superficial* (i.e., restricted to the epidermal surface) and those that invade deep organs and tissues (*deep fungi*). Most important, some species are considered *opportunistic*, others truly *pathogenic* (i.e., capable of infecting normal persons) (see Table 7–7). Some pathogenic fungi are restricted geographically, and the diseases they cause are called *endemic mycoses*. (These are marked by asterisks in Table 7–7 and in the text.) Opportunistic fungi are cosmopolitan and owe their present high frequency largely to medi-

---

* Infectious diseases of limited geographic distribution are marked by an asterisk.

Table 7–7. Common Deep Fungal Infections

		WORLD-WIDE FUNGI		
Species	**Forms**	**Best Staining Methods***	**Portal of Entry**	**Distribution of Lesions**
Candida† (*albicans, krusei, glabrata, tropicalis, etc.*)	Nonbranching pseudohyphae; yeasts	Gram, PAS, MSS	GI, skin, intravenous	Superficial, deep, or systemic
Cryptococcus neoformans†	Encapsulated yeasts, single budding	Mucicarmine, PAS	Respiratory	Meninges, lung, systemic
Aspergillus (fumigatus, niger, etc.)	Branching hyphae; occ. conidia	PAS, MSS	Respiratory	(1) Endobronchial, noninvasive (2) Invasive: lung, upper respiratory, systemic
Genus Mucorales (Mucor, Absidia, Rhizophus)	Branching hyphae; rare sporangia	PAS, MSS	Respiratory	Upper respiratory, lung, systemic
Sporothrix schenkii†	Small yeasts	PAS, MSS	Skin	Skin; lymph nodes
		ENDEMIC FUNGI‡		
Blastomyces dermatitidis†	Yeasts with single broad-based budding	PAS, H&E	Respiratory	Lung, systemic with typical skin lesions
Paracoccidioides brasiliensis†	Yeast with multiple budding	PAS, H&E	Respiratory	Lung, systemic
Coccidioides immitis†	Spherule with endosporulation	PAS, H&E	Respiratory	Lung, systemic, meninges
Histoplasma capsulatum†	Small yeast with single budding	MSS	Respiratory	Lung, systemic, can involve any organ

* PAS = Periodic acid–Schiff; MSS = methenamine silver; H&E = hematoxylin and eosin.

† = Fungi that can infect hosts without known predisposing factors.

‡ = Limited in their geographic distribution, except *H. capsulatum.*

cal progress — maintenance of critically ill patients, immunosuppressive drugs, systemic chemotherapy and radiation for cancer, and antibiotics (themselves initially discovered in the Penicillium mold). Modern invasive hospital procedures and use of prostheses also favor fungal opportunism. Although the pathogenic fungi do not require such help, they can be roused from a dormant state or aggravated by similar factors and by AIDS.

Several fungal species do not conform neatly to the definitions just outlined. Thus, *Candida albicans,* usually considered an opportunist, can cause mild disease in ostensibly normal individuals. It can also progress from innocuous colonization to superficial and deep invasion, depending largely on diminishing host resistance (p. 308). In the case of the endemic mycoses, the number of infected persons detectable by skin testing with fungal antigens may be in the millions, but progressive disease is limited to only a fraction, probably those lacking a vigorous specific immune response (see coccidioidomycosis, p. 394). Thus, the dividing lines between fungal categories cannot be considered hard and fast. When host resistance is at its lowest ebb, specific chemotherapy can sometimes do no better than to induce a succession of opportunistic infections, each harder to eradicate than its predecessor. In such patients, even superficial dermatophytic fungi have become invasive (*Tricho-*

phyton beigeli)[155] and even tissue invasion by primitive algae (Prototheca sp.) has been observed.[156]

DEEP FUNGI

Candidiasis (Moniliasis)

Candidae are the most frequent causes of human fungal disease. *Candida albicans* is the most common species and can infect normal as well as altered hosts. In the latter, it is joined by other, less infective Candida species. All appear in tissues as nonbranching, boxcar-like chains of tubular cells, called pseudohyphae, from which small 2- to 4-μm yeast forms bud off, named blastospores. Either form or both may be seen in diseased tissues. Candida stains well with Gram, PAS, and silver stains (Fig. 7–39).

Candida albicans is found in the oral cavity, gastrointestinal tract, and vagina of a great many normal individuals. The normal bacterial microflora at these mucocutaneous surfaces has an inhibitory influence on the growth of Candida, and therefore its suppression (e.g., by antibiotics) or changes in pH may permit the fungus to proliferate. Three disease patterns are seen.

1. *Superficial proliferation* occurs at sites normally colonized by the fungus.

2. *Deep invasion* occurs from surface lesions when

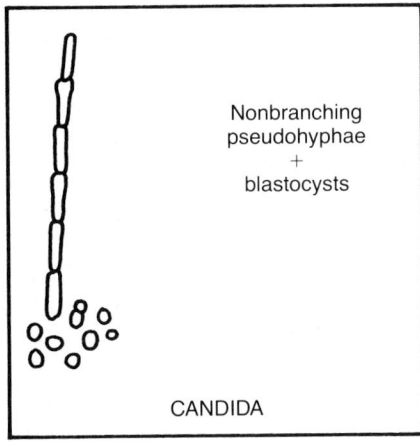

Nonbranching
pseudohyphae
+
blastocysts

CANDIDA

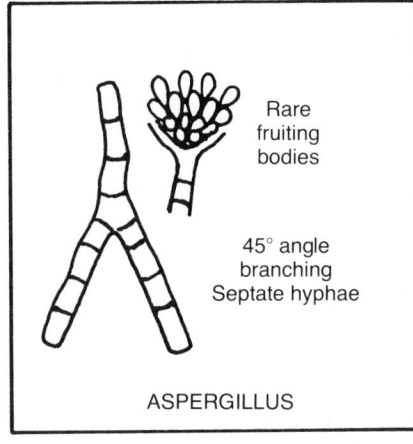

Rare
fruiting
bodies

45° angle
branching
Septate hyphae

ASPERGILLUS

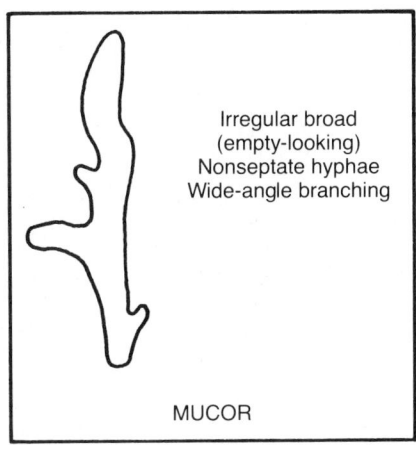

Irregular broad
(empty-looking)
Nonseptate hyphae
Wide-angle branching

MUCOR

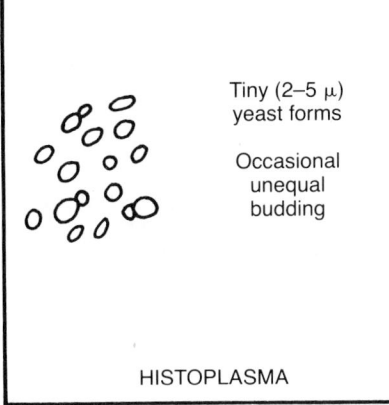

Tiny (2–5 μ)
yeast forms

Occasional
unequal
budding

HISTOPLASMA

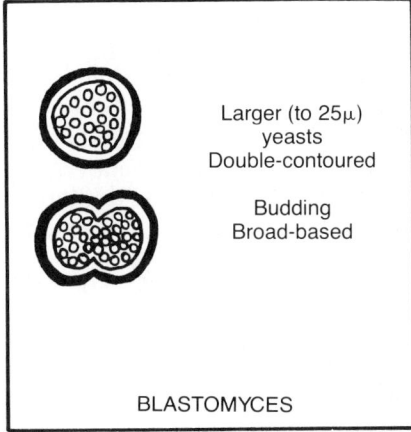

Larger (to 25μ)
yeasts
Double-contoured

Budding
Broad-based

BLASTOMYCES

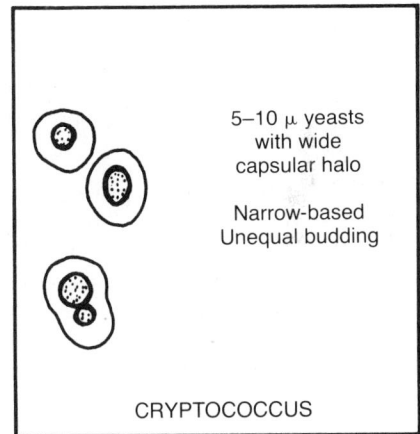

5–10 μ yeasts
with wide
capsular halo

Narrow-based
Unequal budding

CRYPTOCOCCUS

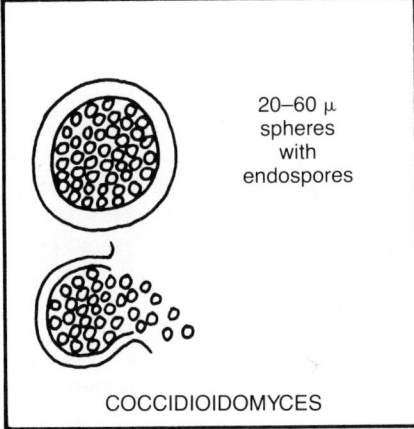

20–60 μ
spheres
with
endospores

COCCIDIOIDOMYCES

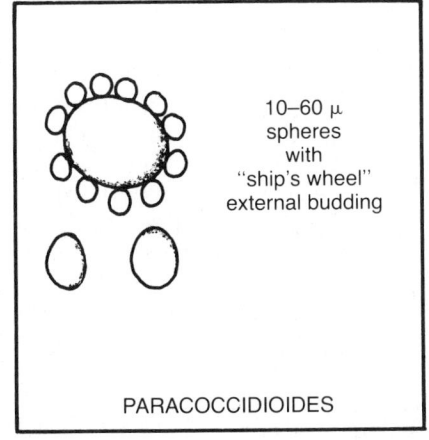

10–60 μ
spheres
with
"ship's wheel"
external budding

PARACOCCIDIOIDES

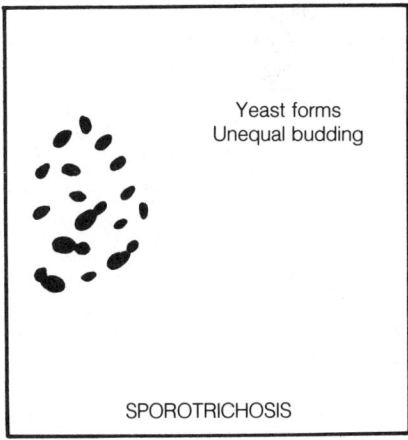

Yeast forms
Unequal budding

SPOROTRICHOSIS

Figure 7–38. Characteristic tissue forms of deep fungi.

there is a systemic impairment of host defenses; widespread dissemination of the fungus may follow.
3. *Direct inoculation into the bloodstream* can give rise to severe disseminated candidiasis in immunocompromised patients; the sources may be intravenous lines, catheters, peritoneal dialysis, or cardiac surgery or may be related to intravenous drug abuse with contaminated needles.

Thus, the disease spectrum of candidiasis ranges from the domain of office dermatology to that of the intensive care unit.

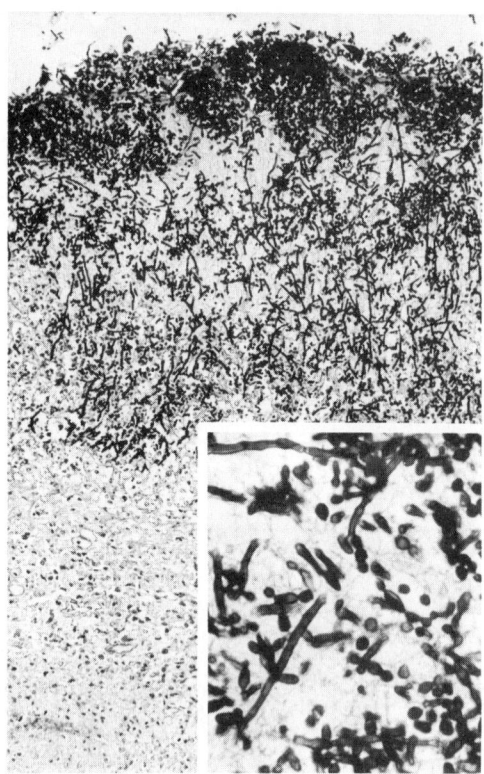

Figure 7–39. Candidal ulcer of esophagus with slender filamentous and yeast forms (silver stain).

The most common forms of candidiasis involve the mucosae of the oral cavity and vagina, producing superficial, curdy, white patches or large, almost fluffy, membranes that are easily detached, leaving a reddened, irritated underlying surface. Spread of oral candidiasis, as by a nasogastric tube, may lead to similar lesions in the esophagus.

Candidiasis of the oral cavity is known as **thrush.** It is most commonly encountered in newborns who are bottle-fed; as the normal microflora develops only after birth, oral candidiasis may resolve without any treatment. In adults, it is often seen during therapy with wide-spectrum antibiotics. In immunodeficient and immunosuppressed individuals, particularly those with depressed T-cell function, thrush is often the first indication of impending dissemination. Vaginal candidiasis in adults may also arise in any of the foregoing circumstances, but also **is commonly encountered in otherwise healthy young women taking oral contraceptives or during pregnancy.** The common forms of **oral** and **vaginal** candidiasis usually respond to topical therapy, but **cutaneous** eczematoid lesions may arise in moist areas of the skin (i.e., between the fingers and toes and in inguinal creases, inframammary folds, and the anogenital region). Microscopically, these lesions show nonspecific, acute, and chronic inflammation, with microabscesses, but in their chronic states granulomatous reactions may develop. Sometimes, hypersensitivity dermal reactions develop in sites remote from the infections, and these lesions are known as candidids or id reactions.

Candidiasis of the skin is often associated with diabetes mellitus or with exposure of the skin to excessive moisture. The fingernails may develop chronic onychia. Burn victims are also predisposed to cutaneous colonization and infection. In most of these instances the cutaneous disease responds readily to treatment of the underlying condition and to local therapy. On the other hand, *chronic mucocutaneous candidiasis,* lacking obvious antecedents, is quite persistent and difficult to treat. Some patients are found to have inherited or acquired defects in T cell–mediated immunity manifested by cutaneous anergy, impaired production of lymphokines, or poorly defined serum factors that inhibit lymphocyte activation; others have defects in neutrophil and monocyte functions. In yet another group, there are inherited polyendocrine deficiencies (hypoparathyroidism, hypoadrenalism, and hypothyroidism). Persistent mucocutaneous candidiasis therefore requires careful investigation of its multiple predisposing conditions.[157]

Severe, *invasive candidiasis* with visceral dissemination is indicative of a serious underlying disorder associated with immunosuppression or with phagocyte depletion. The portal of entry into the blood may be a destructive superficial lesion such as esophagitis (Fig. 7–39) or direct inoculation by needle or catheter. The course of candidal sepsis is somewhat less rampant than that of bacterial sepsis, but it eventually causes similar systemic manifestations, including shock and DIC. Although no organ is immune, the kidney, heart valves, lung, and liver are the most frequent targets of candidal sepsis.

Renal involvement, seen in over 90% of invasive cases, is characterized by the presence of innumerable microabscesses in both the cortex and the medulla. Microscopically, the yeast or pseudohyphal forms of the fungus can be seen to occupy the center of the lesion, with a surrounding area of necrosis and a polymorphonuclear infiltrate. Some fungal cells may be found inside glomerular capillary loops. **Candida endocarditis** resulting from direct inoculation of the fungi into the bloodstream gives rise to large, friable vegetations that frequently break off and occlude large arterial branches, sometimes those of an extremity. In the **lungs,** Candida lesions are often extensive and polymorphous; they may be spherical or irregular, and often they are hemorrhagic and partly infarct-like owing to invasion of vascular walls. Meningitis, intracerebral abscesses, enteritis, endophthalmitis, multiple subcutaneous abscesses, arthritis, and osteomyelitis are some of the other presentations of disseminated candidiasis. In any of these locations, the fungus may evoke little or no inflammatory reaction or may cause the usual suppurative response. In older or treated lesions, a granulomatous reaction is sometimes seen.

Candida glabrata (formerly called *Torulopsis glabrata*) can cause lesions like those of *C. albicans* but does not produce thrush or dermatitis. It can be distinguished by the tiny size of its blastospores (2 to 3 μm).

The diagnosis of Candida infection requires reasoned judgment. Candidae are normal inhabitants of the sputum and are often secondary invaders in other infections. Therefore, the mere culture of *Candida albicans* from oral or pulmonary lesions does not necessarily indicate a primary infection. The skin test with fungal antigens is of little diagnostic value because the organisms are so prevalent in the general population. Even candidemia and candiduria can be transient. Therefore, positive cultures must be interpreted in the light of patient status and the character of the lesions found. Similarly, humoral antibodies to candidal antigens are of little diagnostic value unless rising titers can be demonstrated. A diagnostic approach with some promise is the quantitative detection of fungal antigens in the circulation, but this is still in an experimental stage. Tissue diagnosis, of course, is definitive.

Mucormycosis (Zygomycosis, Phycomycosis)

Mucormycosis is an opportunistic infection caused by "breadmold fungi" of the genera *Mucor, Absidia, Rhizopus,* and *Cunninghamella,* also collectively referred to as the Phycomycetes. These fungi are widely distributed in nature but cannot harm immunocompetent individuals and infect even immunosuppressed persons less frequently than *Candida* or *Aspergillus* spp. Nevertheless, patients with potentially fatal diseases kept alive by modern medicine sometimes fall prey to these fungi and these infections have recently been increasing in frequency. Most Mucor infections occur in patients with diabetic ketoacidosis, advanced malignancy, leukemia, lymphoma, or immunodeficiency (including transplantation cases), and in those receiving wide-spectrum antibiotic, corticosteroid, or cytotoxic therapy. Many of these infections are hospital acquired (nosocomial).

The three primary sites of invasion are the nasal sinuses, lungs, and gastrointestinal tract, depending on whether the spores (widespread in dust and air) are inhaled or ingested. When spores implant in the nasal cavities, the fungus may spread into the sinuses, orbit, and brain, giving rise to **rhinocerebral mucormycosis.** This form of the disease is most commonly but not exclusively seen in association with diabetic ketoacidosis. The phycomycetes at first cause local tissue necrosis, simulating an ordinary sinusitis, but soon invade arterial walls and reach the periorbital tissues and cranial vault. A meningoencephalitis may follow or, in some cases, cerebral infarctions appear when arterial invasion induces thrombosis. At other times the cerebral hemispheres are directly invaded by the fungi. These localizations often lead to hematogenous dissemination. **The nonseptate, irregularly wide (6 to 50 μm) fungal hyphae with frequent right-angle branching are readily demonstrated in the necrotic tissues, stained with H and E or special fungal stains** (Fig. 7–40). **They look "empty" on ordinary stains.**

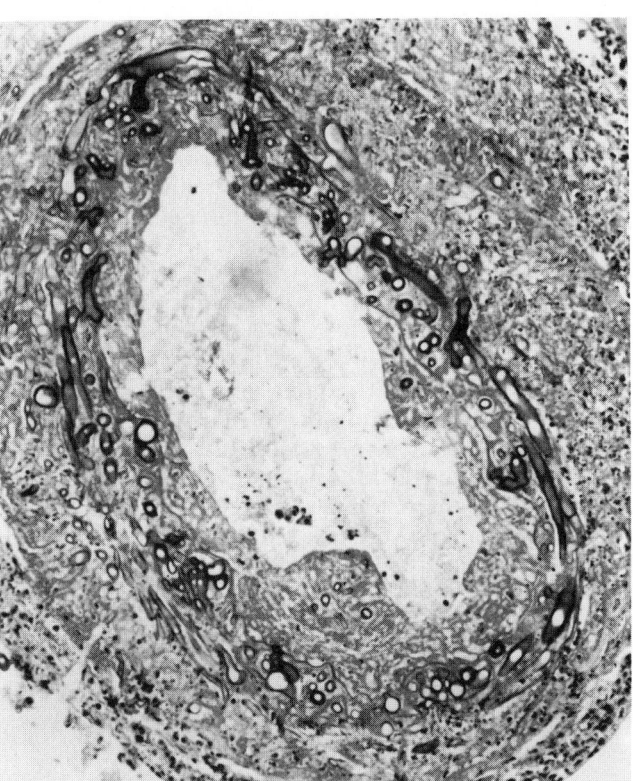

Figure 7–40. Mucormycosis with hyphae invading artery wall. Note irregular width and right-angle branching. (Courtesy of Dr. Jack Frenkel, University of Kansas, Kansas City, Mo.)

Lung involvement may be secondary to rhinocerebral disease, or it may be primary in patients with hematologic neoplasms. Again, the lung lesions combine areas of hemorrhagic pneumonia with vascular thrombi and with multiple distal infarctions. **Gastrointestinal mucormycosis** also can occur in severe malnutrition, particularly in children. In the lungs and gastrointestinal tract the organisms show the same propensity for invading arterial walls. Occasionally, they can be seen growing in tissues as if in culture medium without evoking an inflammatory reaction.

Mucormycosis is a grave disorder because it is an opportunistic disease in an already severely ill patient. Patients with nasal infections have recovered after early, high-dose antifungal therapy combined with surgical débridement. For the pulmonary, gastrointestinal, and disseminated forms, the outlook is still uniformly bleak.

Aspergillosis

Aspergillus fumigatus, A. niger, and other Aspergillus species rank closely behind *Candida* spp. in causing invasive fungal infections in hospitals, and these ubiquitous fungi can also cause hypersensitivity reactions in normal individuals either by inhalation of their spores or by noninvasive mycelial proliferation in the lumen of previously damaged airways; therefore, three classes of human aspergillosis must be distinguished: (1) allergic, (2) colonizing, and (3) invasive.

In addition, the toxin of *A. flavus,* a species not infective for humans, may be an important liver carcinogen when ingested with food (p. 959).

Allergic aspergillosis may manifest itself as *bronchial asthma,* similar clinically to other forms of extrinsic asthma. In nonatopic individuals, sensitization to the Aspergillus spores may produce an *allergic alveolitis* by inducing type III and type IV hypersensitivity reactions (p. 178). Both these forms of allergic aspergillosis result from inhalation of spores, without actual colonization of the respiratory mucosa. A third pattern, called *allergic bronchopulmonary aspergillosis,* is associated with hypersensitivity arising from superficial colonization of the bronchial mucosa. Often this occurs in previously asthmatic patients, whose symptoms become more severe and chronic. If untreated, persistent allergic aspergillosis may eventually result in chronic obstructive lung disease with peribronchial fibrosis and irreversible airway dilatation.

Colonizing aspergillosis (aspergilloma) implies growth of the fungus in pulmonary cavities with minimal or no invasion of the tissues. The cavities usually result from preexisting tuberculosis, bronchiectasis, old infarcts or abscesses. Proliferating masses of fungal hyphae called "fungus balls" can be seen as brownish masses lying free within the cavities. The surrounding reaction may be sparse or there may be chronic inflammation and fibrosis. Patients with aspergillomas usually have recurrent hemoptysis.

Invasive aspergillosis is an opportunistic infection confined to immunosuppressed and debilitated hosts (Fig. 7–41). The primary lesions are usually in the lung, but widespread hematogenous dissemination with involvement of the heart valves, brain, and kidneys is now increasingly common. The **pulmonary lesions** take the form of necrotizing pneumonia with sharply delineated, rounded gray foci with hemorrhagic borders, often referred to as **target lesions.** Because invasive aspergillosis is rapidly progressive, chronic granulomatous reactions are rarely seen. **In the tissues, Aspergillus appears as septate filaments of more uniform width than the phycomycetes, 5 to 10 μm thick, branching at more acute angles** (40 degrees). Its fruiting body resembles a holy-water sprinkler (aspergillus), hence its name. Like the Phycomycetes, Aspergillus has a tendency to invade blood vessels, and thus areas of hemorrhage and infarction are usually superimposed on the necrotizing, inflammatory tissue reactions.

In addition to life-threatening deep invasion of the lungs, Aspergillus can produce primary lesions localized to the eyes, paranasal sinuses, or external ear in apparently healthy individuals. Its rhinocerebral form, seen in immunosuppressed individuals, resembles that caused by phycomycetes.

Invasive aspergillosis is now a common and serious hospital problem. It is difficult to diagnose because aspergilli are rarely demonstrable in the patient's sputum or blood. It should be suspected in any severely debilitated person who suddenly takes a turn

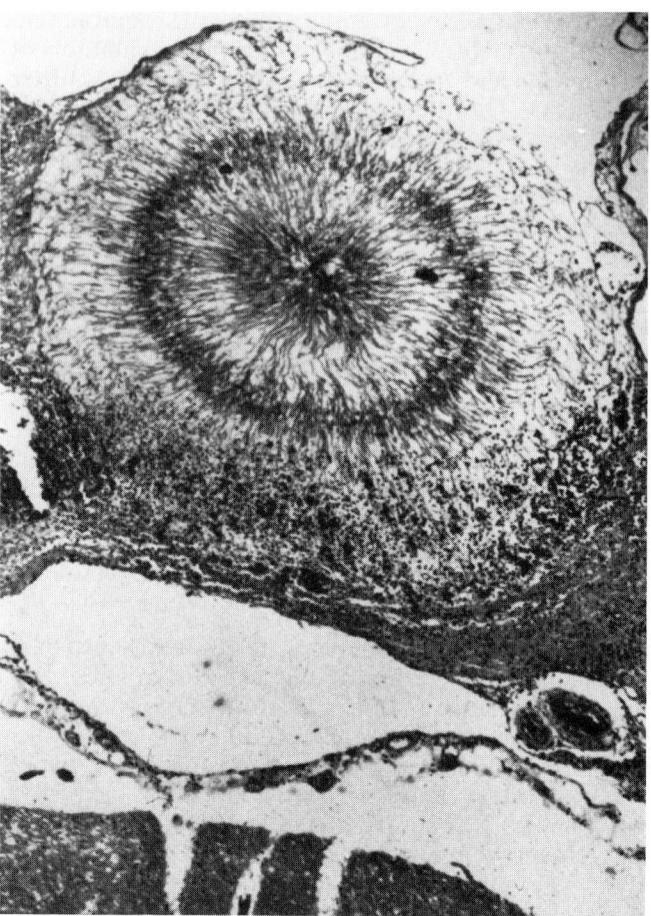

Figure 7–41. Aspergillus colony invading the basal leptomeninges in an immunosuppressed patient.

for the worse. The diagnosis usually depends on demonstration of the fungus in the tissues. Serology is of limited value, but recent attempts to demonstrate Aspergillus antigens appear promising. Aspergillus spores are widely distributed in the environment, especially in dust raised during the construction and renovation of buildings. The fungus is frequently cultured from hospital air. Contaminated rooms are difficult to disinfect and are an obvious hazard for immunosuppressed patients.

Cryptococcosis (*Cryptococcus neoformans*)

On massive exposure, cryptococcosis may arise in healthy individuals, but more commonly it occurs as an opportunistic infection, particularly in patients with leukemia, lymphoma, or Hodgkin's disease. It is today one of the most frequent superinfections seen in AIDS patients. The disease is caused by *Cryptococcus neoformans,* a round-to-oval yeast about 4 to 10 μm in diameter. Yeast forms are the only ones found in tissue. *They divide by unequal budding, and no hyphae or mycelia are seen.* Virulent strains have broad, slimy capsules appearing as empty haloes by routine histologic techniques. The mucicarmine method stains these capsules bright red and helps to differentiate cryptococci from other yeast forms of comparable size. Polysaccharide-rich capsular antigen diffuses into the spinal fluid and serum, where it can be detected by specific antibodies to facilitate early diagnosis. Somewhat less reliable is the use of India ink for visualizing the broad, shiny yeast capsule characteristic of this fungus by negative staining. However, it is difficult with this method to distinguish fungal cells from host leukocytes.

Birds, especially pigeons, excrete infective cryptococci without themselves suffering disease. Inhalation of the infective forms is the usual mode of infection, and therefore the lung is the primary site of localization. However, pulmonary infection may remain mild and asymptomatic even while the fungus is spreading to other organs, most notably the CNS. Clinically, therefore, *the most frequent manifestation of cryptococcal infection is meningitis.* Other forms, in order of severity, affect only the lung, or both lung and brain, or multiple widely distributed organs.

> The tissue response to cryptococci is extremely variable.[158] In immunosuppressed patients they may evoke virtually no inflammatory reaction, and gelatinous masses of fungi may develop as though in a culture medium. Thus, cryptococcal meningitis may disclose a pure culture of gelatinous organisms without accompanying white cells. In normal reactors or in those with protracted disease, the fungi often induce a chronic granulomatous reaction composed of macrophages, lymphocytes, and foreign body–type giant cells. Neutrophils and suppuration may also occasionally be seen. In about half the cases the infection extends into the brain substance about the perivascular spaces, and sometimes it enters the gray matter to produce small cysts filled with organisms and their mucinous secretions, the characteristic "soap-bubble" lesions (Fig. 7–42). Rarely, there is granulomatous arteritis of the circle of Willis.
>
> The lung involvement is equally variable. There may be one or more circumscribed foci or a diffuse pattern of infiltration. The lung nodules may be composed of "naked" masses of organisms, or, more likely in chronic cases, granulomatous infiltrate. Similar involvement of hilar lymph nodes may be evident. Chronic infection, especially in patients without underlying immunodeficiency, may produce solid lesions that remain stationary and may be mistaken for tumors (cryptococcomas). From their primary sites cryptococci may disseminate widely by the bloodstream to the skin, liver, spleen, adrenals, bones, or other tissues, usually in debilitated or severely immunosuppressed patients. Rarely, isolated lesions of the skin or of a joint are found without clear evidence of systemic invasion.

Pulmonary cryptococcosis can be differentiated from other lung infections by identification of the fungus in sputum or at biopsy. CNS cryptococcosis has an insidious onset, characterized by headache, dizziness, or cranial nerve impairments. Usually the patient has little fever and sometimes the picture is misinterpreted as tuberculous meningitis. Because

the capsular antigens are shed in body fluids, *their detection by the latex cryptococcal agglutinin test (LCAT) is an extremely valuable diagnostic tool.* This test is positive in the cerebrospinal fluid of over 90% of cases of cryptococcal meningitis and therefore has improved early diagnosis and treatment, without which the mortality rate of cryptococcal meningitis is high. Even with the latest antifungal drugs, immunosuppressed patients fare poorly, but the outlook is better for normal reactors; for instance, a pulmonary cryptococcoma, if surgically excised, may require no further treatment.

Blastomycosis *(Blastomyces dermatitidis)**

Blastomycosis is a chronic infection characterized by focal suppurative and granulomatous lesions, principally in the lungs and skin. The disease is virtually limited to North America, particularly in the Mississippi–Ohio River basins and the Middle Atlantic states, but sporadic cases have been reported in Central and South America, as well as in Africa. Males are affected nine times more often than females. The

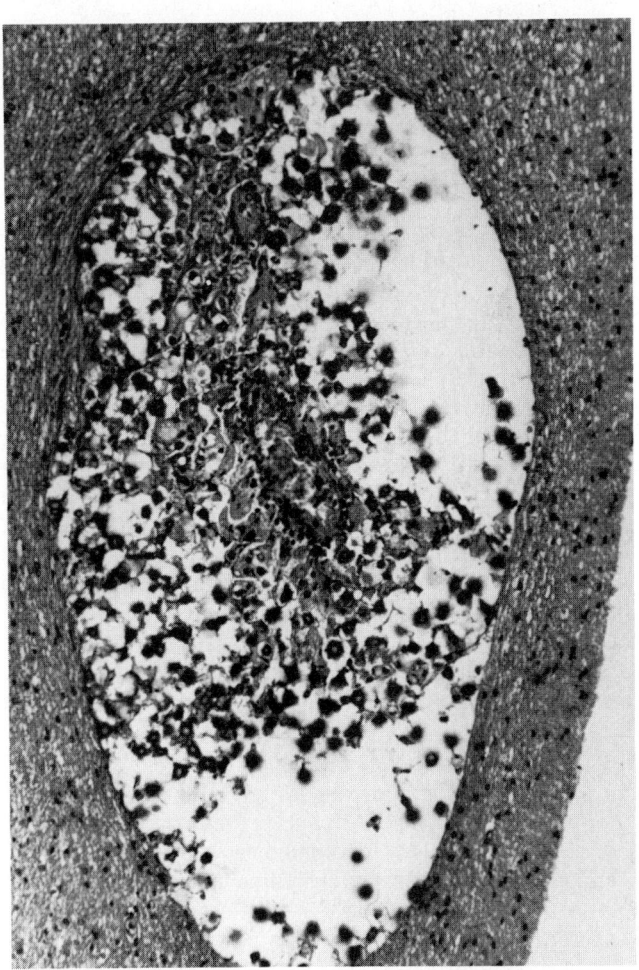

Figure 7–42. Cryptococcal proliferation in Virchow-Robin perivascular space of brain—a "soap-bubble" lesion (mucicarmine stain).

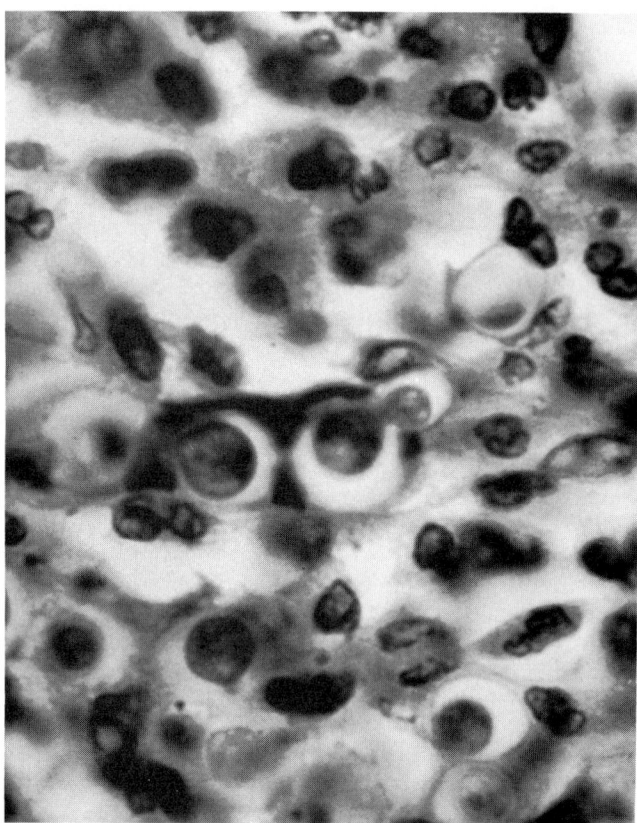

Figure 7–43. Blastomycosis with a cluster of organisms, one of which is in the process of reproduction by budding.

causative organism assumes a yeast form in tissue lesions and is round-to-oval, 5 to 25 μm in diameter with a thick, refractile (double-contoured) wall. *Budding forms generating daughter cells with a broad base (4 to 5 μm) are quite characteristic* (Fig. 7–43). The source of infection and route of transmission to humans are still somewhat uncertain. There are only a few reports of recovery of this agent in soil samples from farms or woods. Small epidemics have occurred among hunters. The disease is acquired by spore inhalation and therefore its primary localization is in the lung. From here, hematogenous fungal dissemination may occur, most commonly to the skin and sometimes to the bones, but virtually any organ may be involved. Cutaneous, osseous, or genital lesions are sometimes present without apparent pulmonary involvement, but in all cases the portal of entry is believed to be the lung.

Pulmonary blastomycosis may take one of several forms, most often that of a **solitary focus** of consolidation or of transient bilateral foci sometimes with involvement of regional nodes, simulating the Ghon complex of tuberculosis. These lesions usually heal, leaving behind a small fibrotic scar. Primary infection may be accompanied by erythema nodosum of the skin. Calcification of healed lesions, unlike those of tuberculosis or histoplasmosis, is uncommon. More rarely, **progressive lung disease** ensues, leading to miliary abscesses throughout the lung or to extensive focal consolidations with formation of cavities. Histologically, some of these lesions are rich in neutrophils and abscess-like; others show tubercle-like granulomas; most have a suppurative center surrounded by epithelioid macrophages and giant cells. Grumous caseation necrosis occurs less commonly than in tuberculosis or histoplasmosis, with which the lesions may otherwise be confused. **Histologic diagnosis depends on demonstration of characteristic double-contoured fungi, sometimes within giant cells.**

Skin involvement, with or without lesions in other organs, is frequent in the progressive form of blastomycosis. The cutaneous lesions tend to appear on the hands, face, feet, wrists, and ankles but eventually involve unexposed regions as well. They begin as indolent, chancre-like papules, but over the course of weeks or months become large, fleshy, fungating ulcers with raised, red, verrucous advancing margins. With healing the central regions may become scarred and depressed, while the disease activity continues at the periphery dotted by numerous microabscesses. Grossly, these skin ulcers have sometimes been confused with carcinomas. Histologically, too, the cutaneous lesion may be mistaken for malignancy owing to the striking **pseudoepitheliomatous hyperplasia,** which can mimic squamous cell carcinoma. The epithelium is extensively thickened, showing irregular cellular proliferation. The rete pegs are broadened, extend down into the underlying subepidermal connective tissue, and appear to anastomose deeply. However, there is no anaplasia or invasive growth, as in true neoplasia. Microabscesses, granulomas, and hybrids of both lesions are seen chiefly in the dermis, but may also extend up into the epidermis. They are surrounded by exuberant granulation tissue. Fungi are usually plentiful in the microabscess-studded ulcer base but may become sparse in healing skin lesions.

The symptoms of pulmonary blastomycosis are nonspecific and can resemble those of tuberculosis, other mycoses (especially histoplasmosis, which is endemic in the same regions), or lung tumors. The skin lesions may be confused with malignant ulcers. Diagnosis requires identification of the causative agent in exudates or tissue sections. When open lesions are present, diagnosis is best made by examination of KOH-treated sputum or bronchial aspirate.[159] Skin tests and serologic procedures, although available, are of doubtful reliability. Self-limited forms of blastomycosis do not require antifungal drugs. Late progressive stages respond poorly to available drugs and have a high mortality rate.

Paracoccidioidomycosis (South American Blastomycosis)*

This fungal infection is focally endemic in the area extending between Mexico to the north and Argentina to the south, with most cases occurring in Brazil, Venezuela, and Colombia. It predominantly affects male agricultural workers. The yeast form of *Paracoccidioides brasiliensis,* the causative fungus, is large (10 to 60 µm) and shows characteristic *multiple budding* around a mother cell, resulting in the formation of a fungal rosette or "ship's wheel image." The infection is acquired by inhalation, but pulmonary lesions are neither distinctive nor usually dominate the clinical picture. Much more commonly, extrapulmonary spread produces *a mucocutaneous lesion (often in the mouth, nose, or larynx), a spreading lymph node infection, or (sometimes) systemic dissemination.* Infection of mucous membranes may take the form of an inflammatory papilloma that resembles the early stages of blastomycosis. Extension of this lesion may give rise to a striking involvement of the regional nodes. Lymphadenopathy is sometimes encountered in patients who do not have a well-defined mucocutaneous lesion. When *P. brasiliensis* disseminates, the skin, gastrointestinal tract, lungs, liver, and other organs may be affected.[160] In all these sites, microabscesses or granulomatous inflammatory reactions develop, resembling those of blastomycosis. The chief differential diagnostic point is the demonstration of the large, double-contoured organisms that produce multiple buds.

Coccidioidomycosis (*Coccidioides immitis*)*

Coccidioidomycosis, caused by inhalation of the spores of *Coccidioides immitis*, is an acute or chronic infection that bears many similarities to tuberculosis. It commonly occurs as an acute, primary, self-limited pulmonary involvement with or without systemic manifestations, but in some cases it progresses to disseminated disease. The primary pulmonary lesion is usually asymptomatic or mild, but it induces delayed hypersensitivity to the fungal antigens. In a few cases, progression or reactivation of the primary infection leads to destructive lesions in the lungs or, more important, to disseminated disease throughout the body in a fashion reminiscent of progressive tuberculosis.

Coccidioidomycosis is most prevalent in the Southwest and far West of the United States and is particularly common in the San Joaquin Valley of California; in this locale, it is known as "valley fever." It also occurs in Mexico and parts of South America. Risk of infection is highest where bats and birds have their nests. *In tissue sections the fungus appears as a thick-walled, nonbudding spherule 20 to 60 µm in diameter, often filled with small endospores* (Fig. 7–44). Rupture of the spherule with release of endospores is the method of reproduction, but this form is noninfectious. In nature or artificial culture, reproduction is by boxcar-like arthrospores, easily detached and disseminated by air. Extreme caution is needed in handling this dimorphic fungus in the laboratory. Animals as well as man can be infected.

Approximately 60% of patients with primary coccidioidomycosis are unaware of the infection. Only skin sensitization to coccidioidin or spherulin (fungal antigens) discloses the existence of a past or present infection. Almost 80% of the population of the San

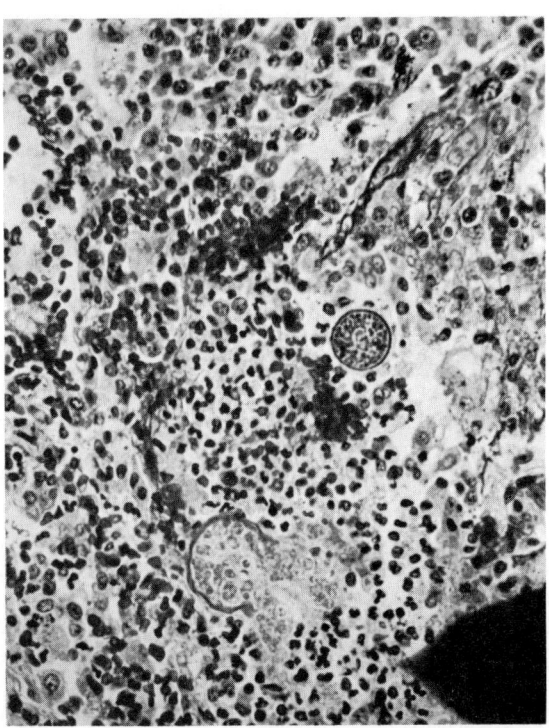

Figure 7–44. Coccidioidomycosis with several microorganisms filled with endospores. One has been caught at the moment of rupture with release of daughter spores.

Joaquin Valley are coccidioidin positive. In about 10% of patients the lung lesions evoke fever, cough, and pleuritic pains, accompanied by erythema nodosum or erythema multiforme (i.e., the "valley fever" complex).

> **Primary pulmonary coccidioidomycosis** most commonly takes the form of a solitary gray-white focus of consolidation, 2 to 3 cm in diameter, in the middle or lower lung fields. Occasionally a more diffuse pneumonic consolidation or multiple scattered foci of consolidation appear. Hilar lymphadenopathy may be present to mimic, with the parenchymal lesion, the Ghon complex of tuberculosis. More often, however, lymphadenopathy is absent.
>
> Histologically, two reaction patterns are seen. In cases in which there is florid proliferation of fungi, the response tends to be suppurative. More often, in instances with slower rates of fungal reproduction, granuloma production occurs, closely resembling tubercles. Fungal spherules usually are readily evident in the macrophages or giant cells within the granulomas. When the spherules rupture to release the endospores, a pyogenic reaction is superimposed (Fig. 7–44). Similar granulomas may appear in the draining lymph nodes. With time these active lesions fibrose and calcify. Thus, in many patients, only the telltale radiographic calcifications and positive skin reactions reveal the past existence of the infection.

In the great majority of patients, even those who are symptomatic, the primary pulmonary form of the disease is self-limited, like primary tuberculosis.

However, about 0.2% of infected white males and twice as many black or Asian males develop progressive coccidioidomycosis, possibly because they fail to mount an adequate cell-mediated immune response to the primary disease. Such individuals do not have dermal hypersensitivity at the time of the spread of the disease.

> Anatomically, the progressive disease usually takes the form of more extensive focal involvement of the lungs, frequently accompanied by spread to other sites of localization, principally the meninges, bones, adrenals, lymph nodes, spleen, and liver. In some patients, meningeal involvement may appear to be the sole localization. Progressive pulmonary coccidioidomycosis produces areas of gray-white consolidation, cavitation, scarring, and calcification, simulating progressive tuberculosis. A particularly "malignant" complication of this fungal infection is widespread miliary dissemination throughout the body. Coccidioidomycosis may involve the skin, possibly as a primary site, but more often as a manifestation of progressive disease in which the cutaneous involvement is only one site of hematogenous dissemination. At all these sites the inflammatory response may be purely granulomatous, pyogenic, or mixed. Purulent lesions dominate in patients with the least resistance and with widespread dissemination.

Most individuals with progressive disease have chills, fever, night sweats, weakness, and weight loss, accompanied by a cough productive of mucopurulent sputum. This sputum may harbor the pathognomonic microorganisms and thus permit a direct diagnosis. Unlike several of the previously discussed fungal diseases, *serologic tests are extremely valuable in establishing the diagnosis. With the reactive antibodies, precipitin, latex particle agglutination, or immunodiffusion tests are positive in virtually every symptomatic case.* Complement-fixing antibodies in the cerebrospinal fluid are diagnostic of coccidioidal meningitis. The skin tests with coccidioidin or spherulin are of value only in epidemiologic studies. The prognosis in coccidioidomycosis is generally favorable, but it becomes increasingly grave with the systemic dissemination of the organisms and the development of infections in the bones or CNS, which require long-term antifungal treatment, itself a cause of many complications.[161]

Histoplasmosis (*Histoplasma capsulatum*)*

Infection by the dimorphic fungus *H. capsulatum* is an endemic condition almost rivaling the frequency of tuberculosis in the United States today, especially in the Ohio-Mississippi River region. Far less frequently, it has been reported in other countries (e.g., Argentina). A related organism, *H. duboisii*, is found in central Africa. *Histoplasma capsulatum* is acquired by dust inhalation from soil contaminated with bird or bat droppings and has been spread widely by birds

such as nesting starlings. The organism grows in mycelial form in soil or on special media at room temperature, producing sprouting conidia of two sizes. The smaller ones (microconidia) are easily detached, windborne, and infectious; the larger, tuberculate ones (macroconidia) are diagnostic of *H. capsulatum* by their shape. AT 37°C on agar or in mammalian tissues there is conversion to a primitive 2- to 5-μm yeast form with a thin cell wall but lacking a true capsule (despite the organism's misleading name). These yeast forms are best visualized with the methenamine silver stain but are practically invisible in routine H and E sections. Neither they nor the patient bearing these forms can transmit the infection.

The clinical presentations and morphologic lesions of histoplasmosis strikingly parallel those of tuberculosis and coccidioidomycosis.[162] Depending on host resistance and immunocompetence, the fungus may induce (1) latent asymptomatic infection; (2) self-limited primary pulmonary involvement; (3) chronic, progressive, even cavitary pulmonary disease; (4) rapid, widely disseminated systemic involvement; and (5) localized lesions in one or more organs.

Latent or asymptomatic histoplasmosis can be discovered only by the finding of fibrocalcific residues at sites of past localization of the organisms, most often the lungs or hilar lymph nodes, accompanied by a positive histoplasmin skin test (analogous to the tuberculin test). In contrast to the Ghon complex of tuberculosis (p. 376), latent histoplasma foci are often multiple.

Primary pulmonary histoplasmosis is the most common clinical presentation. It occurs in otherwise healthy individuals (usually adults) as a mild, self-limited, febrile respiratory infection. Chest radiographs reveal hilar adenopathy with or without one or more focal pulmonary parenchymal shadows. Erythema nodosum or erythema multiforme sometimes appears, more commonly in females than in males. Rarely, this pattern is complicated by pericarditis arising by spread of the infection from adjacent involved nodes.

Chronic pulmonary histoplasmosis is the counterpart of secondary tuberculosis. It is characterized by unilateral or bilateral apical infiltrates that may progressively enlarge and cavitate as the disease spreads throughout the lung fields. Preexisting chronic lung disease favors the spread of infection. The most common clinical manifestations are cough, fever, night sweats, and weight loss. Death may occur from progression of the pulmonary lesions, dissemination of the infection, cor pulmonale, or bacterial superinfection. However, about one third of cases improve spontaneously, usually those with limited apical involvement.

Disseminated histoplasmosis may follow either primary or chronic pulmonary disease, but more often it appears as an acute, relentlessly progressive infection in the very old, the very young, or those with impaired cell-mediated immunity, such as AIDS patients. Characteristically, these patients have fever, generalized lymphadenopathy, abdominal symptoms, hepatosplenomegaly, wasting, anemia, leukopenia, and thrombocytopenia and may become jaundiced owing to extensive hepatic involvement. Often, meningitis becomes the dominant feature of the disease. This overwhelming dissemination of the fungi is often associated with anergy to histoplasmin.

In addition to these three classic clinical patterns, histoplasmosis sometimes presents in other ways. Rarely, extension of infection from mediastinal nodes gives rise to progressive scarring and contraction of the mediastinal structures — *sclerosing mediastinitis* — even as fungi become quite scarce. Compression of nerves, pulmonary veins, pulmonary arteries, superior vena cava, and esophagus may occur. More commonly, healing or healed, calcified or noncalcified, sometimes laminated pulmonary coin lesions or hilar lesions come to clinical attention on chest radiographs in the absence of other signs or symptoms. When solitary, these are called *histoplasmomas* and must be differentiated from other pulmonary granulomas and tumors (Fig. 7–45). Rarely, calcified histoplasmomas lacking viable fungi erode into a bronchus, and patients cough up the calcified debris (broncholithiasis). Diagnosis of such lesions is usually made after surgical excision by demonstration of the residual fungal cell walls on silver staining. Another uncommon presentation of histoplasmosis is the development of active localized disease in scattered organs. Thus, bilateral adrenal destruction may coexist with or follow only minor respiratory involvement and can lead to adrenal insufficiency (Addison's disease) (p. 1252). Endocarditis, chronic meningitis, granulomatous hepatitis, and gastrointestinal ulcerative involvement have all been reported.

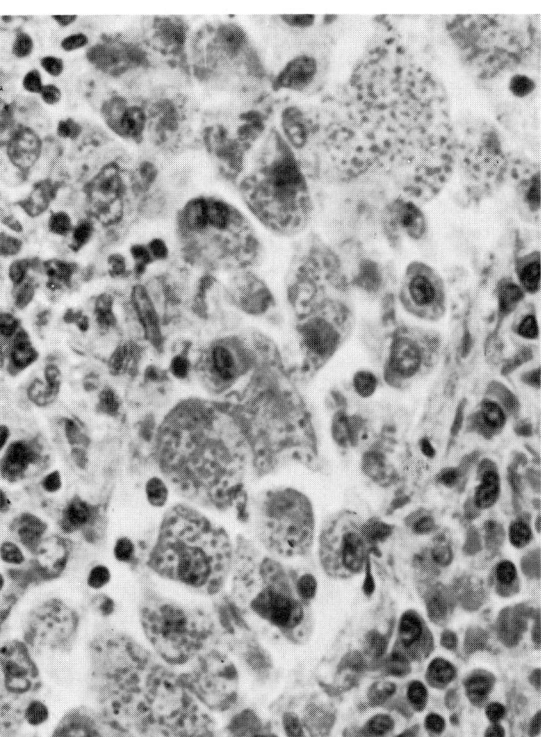

Figure 7–46. Disseminated histoplasmosis in a lymph node. The central phagocytes are stuffed with minute fungal yeast forms.

In otherwise healthy adults, histoplasmosis is characterized by the formation of epithelioid cell granulomas at the sites of localization of the fungus. These granulomas usually undergo coagulative necrosis and coalesce to produce larger areas of consolidation, but they may also liquefy to form cavities.[162] With spontaneous or drug control of the infection, the lesions undergo fibrosis and often calcification. Histologic differentiation from tuberculosis, sarcoidosis, and coccidioidomycosis requires identification of the yeast forms that persist in the lesions for many years even into the calcific stage. The macroscopic lesions of active **granulomatous histoplasmosis** in the lung and hilar lymph nodes appear as gray-white foci of consolidation and scarring. In the **chronic pattern of disease** these lesions are usually apical, with retraction and thickening of the apical pleura. Further progression involves more and more of the lung parenchyma, focally, sometimes with cavity formation, albeit somewhat less often than in tuberculosis. In **fulminant disseminated histoplasmosis,** epithelioid cell granulomas are not formed but instead there are focal accumulations of activated mononuclear phagocytes stuffed with fungal yeasts throughout the tissues and organs of the body. The cells of the reticuloendothelial system in particular become overloaded with yeast forms, reminiscent of kala-azar (Fig. 7–46) (p. 409).

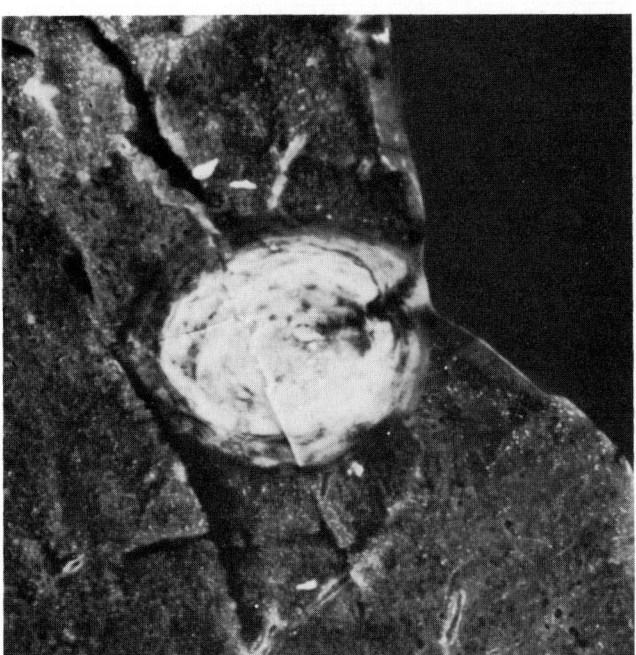

Figure 7–45. Histoplasmosis. Laminated granuloma of lung — a stationary disease form.

The clinical diagnosis of histoplasmosis depends largely on awareness of its protean presentations. The histoplasmin skin test is helpful but may be falsely negative in those with overwhelming infection. Tests for histoplasma antibodies, although available, suffer from a large proportion of false-positive and false-negative results. Definitive diagnosis is best made by culture (which may, however, require up to four weeks) or by direct demonstration of the characteristic small yeast forms in tissues or smears that must be differentiated from the yeast forms of candida and cryptococcus and from the protozoon *Pneumocystis carinii* (p. 402). Unlike the last two, histoplasma is frequently *intracellular*. Too often in the past, histoplasmosis has been mislabeled as tuberculosis.

Unusual Deep Fungal Infections*

Among the many rare and tropical deep fungal infections,[163] only two will receive brief mention here. *Mycetomas* are localized deforming tumefactions with multiple draining sinuses, most commonly of the foot (Madura foot). Many fungal species can cause these lesions, as well as some of the Actinomycetes, and their etiologic diagnosis is in the realm of specialized mycology. The commonest cause in Central and North America is *Nocardia brasiliensis* (p. 383). *Characteristic of mycetomas is the aggregation of fungi in masses or "grains" analogous to the sulfur granules of Actinomyces* (p. 384). By the time mycetomas are seen, the deep tissues and underlying bones and joints are usually involved and surgical therapy is necessary.

Chromomycosis causes large, warty, ulcerative skin lesions of the extremities with pseudoepitheliomatous epidermal hyperplasia. It occurs in warm, rural areas particularly in those of Mexico and Puerto Rico, and is due to a group of fungi forming pigmented spores and hyphae. This condition may be confused with a skin tumor.

SUPERFICIAL FUNGI (DERMATOPHYTOSIS)

These infections of the epidermis, hair, or nails by fungi that generally spare the deeper tissues are described in Chapter 27. They rarely are life-threatening but the unsightly skin lesions, hair loss, and itching can cause great distress to those affected. *In most cases, the causal fungus can be visualized if not identified by microscopic examination of skin scrapings and hair shafts.*

PROTOZOAL DISEASES

Parasitic protozoa (Table 7–8) are among the foremost causes of disease and death in developing countries. In industrialized countries, they are less often lethal but still widely prevalent. Yet only recently have the tools of immunology and molecular science been applied to protozoal diseases and opened new research horizons.[164] Eukaryotic parasites are vastly more complex than viruses or bacteria, and the rich diversity of their life cycles and pathogenetic mechanisms is difficult to fit into a brief outline.

Most parasitic protozoal life cycles revolve between a specific mammalian host and a specific vector

Table 7–8. Protozoa Pathogenic for Humans

SPECIES	ORDER	FORM, SIZE*	DISEASE
Luminal			
Entamoeba histolytica	Amebae	Trophozoite 15–50 μm	Amebic dysentery
			Liver abscess
Balantidium coli	Ciliates	Trophozoite 50–100 μm	Colitis
Naegleria fowleri	Ameboflagellates	Trophozoite 10–20 μm	Meningoencephalitis
Acanthamoeba sp.	Ameboflagellates	Trophozoite 15–30 μm	Same or ophthalmitis
Giardia lamblia	Mastigophora	Trophozoite 11–18 μm	Diarrheal disease
			Malabsorption
Isospora belli	Coccidia	Oocyst 10–20 μm	Chronic enterocolitis or malabsorption, or both
Cryptosporidium sp.	Coccidia	Oocyst 5–6 μm	
Trichomonas vaginalis	Mastigophora	Trophozoite 10–30 μm	Urethritis, vaginitis
Pneumocystis carinii	?	Trophozoite 6–8 μm, cyst 4–6 μm	Opportunistic lung infection
Bloodstream			
Plasmodium vivax	Hemosporidia	Trophozoites, schizonts, gametes (all small and inside red cells)	Benign, tertian malaria
P. ovale	Hemosporidia		Benign tertian malaria
P. malariae	Hemosporidia		Quartan malaria
P. falciparum	Hemosporidia		Malignant tertian malaria
Babesia microti, bovis	Hemosporidia	Trophozoites inside red cells	Babesiasis
Trypanosoma brucei, rhodesiense, gambiense	Hemoflagellates	Trypomastigote 14–33 μm	African sleeping sickness
Intracellular			
Trypanosoma cruzi	Hemoflagellates	Trypomastigote 20 μm	Chagas disease
Leishmania donovani	Hemoflagellates	Amastigote 2 μm	Kala-azar
Leishmania tropica, mexicana, brasiliensis	Hemoflagellates	Amastigote 2 μm	Cutaneous and mucocutaneous leishmaniasis
Toxoplasma gondii	Coccidia (Eimeriae)	Tachyzoite 4–6 μm (cyst larger)	Toxoplasmosis

* Found in human host.

or external environmental niche; each life stage must metamorphose or adapt its surface molecules to the next step in its cycle. Thus, *Leishmania* promastigotes, on completing their logarithmic divisions in the sandfly vector, become complement-resistant (i.e., infective for humans). Other protozoa cease reproducing under adverse conditions and change into hardier, semidormant forms; thus, amebic trophozoites give rise to cysts that can survive outside the gut. Some cycles are based on alternating sexual and asexual modes of reproduction (e.g., Toxoplasma gametes differentiate only in the gut of feline hosts that have fed on other host species bearing asexual parasite forms). One marvels at the ingenuity of design of the self-perpetuating protozoal life cycles. Only two human parasites (Pneumocystis and Trichomonas) lack known extrahuman life stages.

Following their entry into humans, protozoa must home to a site appropriate for their reproduction, which can be *luminal* (i.e., an epithelial surface), *hemic* (i.e., inside the bloodstream), or *intracellular* (Table 7–8). In a few cases, the receptor-ligand interactions that underlie the homing of protozoan parasites have been determined. Thus, the plasmodium of benign tertian malaria enters only red cells bearing the Duffy blood group determinant; Duffy-negative individuals are refractory to *P. vivax* malaria. The location of a parasite's "reproductive niche" determines many of its disease manifestations; thus, the behavior of *luminal parasites* is analogous to that of luminal bacteria. Both Giardia and Entamoeba can either colonize the human gut without causing disease or cause diarrheal illness, depending on the balance between the virulence of the parasite strain and the defense capacity of the host. Diseases caused by *hemic parasites*, such as malaria or African trypanosomiasis, resemble bacteremic conditions. They present with fever, rigors, and malaise; they activate the host lymphoreticular system, especially that of the spleen; and they can induce DIC if parasitemia keeps mounting without restraint. *Intracellular protozoa*, such as Leishmania, have features shared with obligate intracellular bacteria: chronicity, resistance to phagolysosomal attack, and a spectrum of clinical forms related to the status of host cellular immunity. However, it should be emphasized that there are at least as many differences between protozoal and bacterial diseases as there are analogies.

Our knowledge of the virulence factors of protozoan parasites remains incomplete. Certainly, motility aids parasites in their invasive and evasive maneuvers and can thus be regarded as a virulence factor. Luminal parasites kill host cells mainly by direct contact. Thus, virulent strains of *Entamoeba histolytica* generate a surface "ameobopore protein" that induces the formation of helical pores in host cell membranes, sufficient in size and charge to kill the cell via a sudden influx of solutes. Hemic and intracellular parasites kill cells only after entering them either actively, aided by penetration organelles as in Toxoplasma, or more often passively, by "induced endocytosis." Once

taken up, parasites usually damage host cells after multiplying sufficiently to interfere with cell metabolism or to destroy vital organelles. Thus, cultured cells loaded with *Trypanosoma cruzi* are seen to suddenly swell, burst, and die in a manner similar to cells overloaded with rickettsiae (p. 329). In addition to such direct effects, parasite invasion can trigger the same nonspecific inflammatory host mediators that potentiate bacterial tissue damage.

Host immune responses have the same importance in protozoal as in bacterial pathogenesis, as will be emphasized throughout this chapter; for example, malarial nephritis results from antibody complexes with malarial antigens, rather than from direct plasmodial kidney damage; in Chagas disease, chronic myocarditis continues progressing at a time when *T. cruzi* has virtually disappeared from heart tissue, but host immune reactivity against unrelated antigens continues high.

Host immunity also serves a pivotal protective function as witnessed by the fact that of the millions of people infected by protozoa, only a fraction show symptoms, usually individuals with the heaviest parasite loads or with impaired immune or phagocytic functions. Thus, Toxoplasma infection exists in up to 70% of the general population, detectable only by serology. Severe disease is limited to the newborn and to the immunosuppressed. Similarly, most adult inhabitants of holoendemic malarial zones have infections that have become inapparent over the years (though still capable of resurgence). These are examples of long-lasting, relatively stable, host-parasite equilibria favoring both host survival and perpetuation of the parasite life cycle.

In the service of that goal, protozoan parasites have developed diverse mechanisms that permit them to evade or subvert the immune responses of the host. For instance, successive clones of African trypanosomes undergo programmed variation of their surface antigens; plasmodia seek early refuge from host anti-sporozoite antibodies inside liver cells whence they emerge in a new form to initiate their erythrocytic cycle; and several of the chronic intracellular protozoa induce formation of suppressor cells so as to modulate the intensity of the host inflammatory responses. Evolving research to unravel this complex interplay makes stimulating reading,[165] but it can be referred to only briefly as we proceed to examine specific protozoal diseases.

LUMINAL PROTOZOA

Amebiasis (Entamoeba histolytica)

Amebiasis is primarily an infection of the colon, followed in some cases by spread to the liver, lungs, and brain. The disease is limited to human and nonhuman primates and ranges from mild chronic diarrhea to severe purging dysentery. Far more common than symptomatic amebiasis is the entirely asymptomatic carrier state, which constitutes the reservoir for transmission of the disease.

The responsible organism, *E. histolytica,* is a deceptively simple trophozoite (15 to 40 μm in diameter) with a relatively small nucleus, distinctive by its tiny central karyosome and aggregated RNA-DNA at the nuclear membrane and by its bubbly cytoplasm containing many glycogen rosettes. The outer cytoplasmic zone ("ectoplasm") is clear and forms pseudopods. The parasite derives its energy largely from anaerobic glycolysis. Mitochondria, typical lysosomes, Golgi bodies, and rough endoplasmic reticulum are lacking. Entamoebae kill host cells only on contact (see introduction, p. 397). Because *E. histolytica* is actively phagocytic and may contain red-cell or other cell debris, *it can be confused with host macrophages, but in its fresh state its motility is much more explosive; it also differs from the nonpathogenic intestinal amebae (E. coli, E. nana, and others) by its nuclear characteristics and its red cell ingestion* (Fig. 7–47). Under unfavorable conditions, *E. histolytica* forms a quadrinucleate cyst that survives in the outer environment. This is the infective form that reverts in the gut to the motile trophozoite after digestion of the cyst wall by gastric juice, thus completing the parasite's simple life cycle. Asymptomatic infected persons are called cyst-passers.

Entamoeba strains differ greatly in virulence; those with small, temperature-insensitive trophozoites are considered nonpathogenic. It therefore is not known what proportion of the population of cyst-passers is capable of transmitting amebic disease. In the United States and Europe, cyst-passers do not exceed 3 to 5% of adults and children. In 1986, only about 3600 cases of clinical intestinal amebiasis were reported in the United States (if indeed reliably identified).[166] The incidence is higher among travelers, refugees, immigrants, and urban homosexuals. High endemicity persists in many developing, although not necessarily tropical, communities. Mortality rates continue especially high in Mexico, Colombia, and India. Fecal contamination of food and water is the mode of transmission.

The cecum and ascending colon are affected most often, followed in order by the sigmoid, rectum, and appendix. However, in severe, full-blown cases the entire colon is involved. The amebae invade the crypts of the colonic glands and then burrow through the tunica propria, but they are usually halted in their progress by the muscularis mucosae. At this level, they fan out laterally to create a minute undermined ulceration having a flask shape (i.e., a narrow neck and broad base). As the undermining progresses, the overlying surface mucosa is deprived of its blood supply, and it sloughs. In this fashion, progressively larger ulcerations are produced that maintain their typical undermined shape and fairly clean bases.

The earliest amebic lesions seen in man and experimental animals are accompanied by neutrophilic responses, but **later ulcers are often notoriously poor in host inflammatory cells because the tissue destruction is due largely to liquefactive necrosis.** Yet, occasionally, advanced amebic gut lesions have vigorous inflammatory reactions, perhaps initiated by bacterial superinfection.[167] Only rarely do the ulcerations coalesce to denude entire segments of the bowel mucosa. The mucosa between ulcers is often normal or mildly inflamed, in contrast to chronic ulcerative colitis (p. 886). Penetration of the bowel wall is rare but may occur, especially in children or immunosuppressed patients. An amebic peritonitis ensues. Another, less common lesion is the ameboma, a napkin-like constrictive lesion that represents a profuse granulation tissue response sometimes confused grossly and radiologically with a tumor of the colon.[168]

In about 40% of defined cases, amebae penetrate vessels and are drained to the liver to produce solitary, or less often multiple, discrete abscesses, some exceeding 10 cm in diameter. They have a very scant inflammatory reaction in their margins and only a shaggy fibrin lining. Because of hemorrhage into the partially digested liver debris, the abscess cavities are sometimes filled with a chocolate-colored, relatively odorless, pasty material often likened to anchovy paste, but the abscess contents can be of any color, and secondary bacterial infection may convert these lytic lesions into frank suppurative abscesses. Solitary abscesses are most frequent in the right lobe. Following the development of hepatic lesions the lung may become involved, either by drainage of parasites through the blood vessels or by their direct penetration through the liver capsule, diaphragm, and pleural cavities to enter the lung parenchyma, again usually on the right side. Extension into the pericardial sac from a left-sided liver abscess or the formation of bronchopleural fistulas occurs in similar fash-

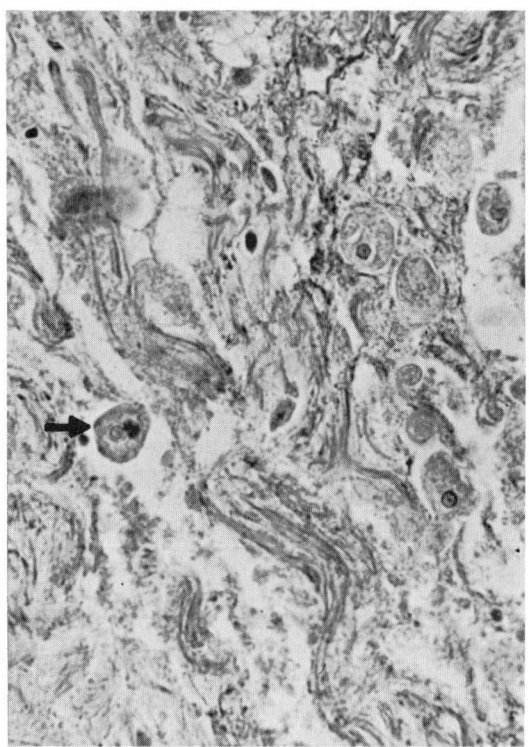

Figure 7–47. Amebiasis of colon. Histologic detail of vegetative parasites is shown. Arrow points to an ameba with a phagocytized red cell.

ion. In other cases, infection may spread into the kidney, stomach and duodenum or reenter the colon. One or several abscesses may develop in the brain by embolic dissemination of the amebae. **In all sites of localization the reaction is that of local lysis of tissues accompanied by a scant inflammatory infiltrate, principally of mononuclear cells.** Rarely, amebic cutaneous ulcers arise in the margins of a surgical wound of a patient who has had intestinal surgery during an active infection, or these may spontaneously arise in the perineum of a patient with neglected ulcerative rectal lesions. Rarely, they occur on the penis as the result of anal intercourse.

Important clinical features are as follows:

1. The intestinal manifestations of amebiasis range from acute to chronic, and from mild or no discomfort to classic dysentery with tenesmus and bloody stools. Invasive colonic amebiasis is rarely painless; usually there is cramping pain.

2. There may be long intervals between the travel that led to infection and the appearance of acute symptoms, during which the patient may either be symptom free or complain of only mild episodes of alternating constipation and diarrhea.

3. Liver, lung, or brain abscesses may present as solitary lesions in the absence of intestinal symptoms.

4. One of the clinical signs of an amebic liver abscess is exquisite tenderness at its point nearest the liver capsule.

5. Lung abscesses tend to evacuate via the bronchi, leading to massive coughing-up of chocolate-colored material lacking the repulsive malodorousness of anaerobic bacterial lung abscesses.

6. A high unilateral paralyzed diaphragm with basilar pleural effusion is a valuable radiographic sign of a liver abscess on that side.

7. Punctate ulcers of the lower colon in the face of intervening areas of normal mucosa may be a good proctoscopic clue, suggesting amebic colitis *but, in the final analysis, only the reliable identification of entamoebae in the lesions by an expert observer lends security to diagnosis.* A number of serologic tests, including immunofluorescence and complement fixation, have shown good sensitivity and specificity and can be of great help, but only in the invasive and extraintestinal forms of amebiasis.

Severe complications of amebiasis have followed surgical intervention for presumptive appendicitis or diverticulitis.[169] Cutting through the infected tissues will disseminate the parasite unless this is prevented by vigorous concurrent antiamebic drug treatment. Drug-resistant strains, however, have recently been spreading. *Similarly, amebic gut perforation or systemic infection can follow if a patient with active colitis is given corticosteroids for presumed idiopathic ulcerative colitis.*

Balantidium coli (Table 7–7) is a large, ciliate intestinal parasite prevalent in pigs, rats, and primates. It occasionally infects man, causing lesions very similar in type to those of acute *E. histolytica* infections.[170] Balantidiasis occurs mostly in the tropics, among malnourished individuals; in the United States, cases have been reported from prisons and institutions for the mentally retarded.

Amebic Meningoencephalitis

Only in 1965 did it become known that the free-living ameboflagellate *Naegleria fowleri* could cause an acute meningitis by entering the arachnoid space through the perforated cribriform plate of the nose.[7] *Acanthamoeba*, another free-living species able to induce cytopathic effects in accidentally contaminated tissue cultures, also has caused sporadic cases of human meningoencephalitis, mainly in immunosuppressed patients.[171] The aggregate yearly number of such cases in the United States is fortunately quite small, but Naegleria can kill a healthy youngster within a few days despite all medical efforts. In amebic meningoencephalitis there is usually a history of prolonged diving into stagnant waters. In the United States, lakes and impoundments from Virginia southward have been the main sources of infection, but in Europe, infections originating in unchlorinated swimming pools have also been reported. Currently it is not clear what factors induce virulence in Naegleriae, which are ordinarily innocuous and widely distributed in nature. Thermal pollution is suspected to be a factor, and if this is true the number of cases is likely to increase.

Incubation takes about five to six days. Neurologic deficit and coma progress rapidly, accompanied by fever, severe bifrontal headache, nausea, vomiting, and stiff neck. The cerebrospinal fluid shows elevated protein, normal or low sugar, and pleocytosis as in bacterial meningitis, but red cells are copious and *part of the cell count is often contributed by the proliferating amebae, which may not be recognized by the examiner or Coulter counter.*

In cerebrospinal fluid smears or tissue sections, these amoebae microscopically resemble human cells even more than do entamoebae. They have a relatively large nucleus and a small cytoplasmic mass, and may easily be mistaken for round cell infiltrates or tumor cells. However, in fresh preparations or cultures their motility is characteristic. Pathologic lesions are limited to the olfactory nerves and brain. There is clouding of the meninges with focal hemorrhages, often accompanied by extensive fibrinoid necrosis and thrombosis of blood vessels. There may also be necrosis of nerve tissue.

Several cases of chronic keratitis of the eye due to Acanthamoeba-induced ulceration have been reported in adult patients in the absence of CNS involvement and have proved difficult to cure. These infections have been traced to the prolonged, incautious use of soft contact lenses.[172]

Giardiasis *(Giardia lamblia)*

Intestinal flagellates of the Giardia group infect both animals and humans; infections of cats and beavers may possibly be transmitted to humans. The human parasite, *G. lamblia,* is the world's most prevalent pathogenic gut protozoan if both asymptomatic and symptomatic infections are counted. *Giardia trophozoites live in the duodenum and give rise to the only other life form, infective cysts that are only intermittently shed into the stools.* Estimates of prevalence based on the identification of cysts in the stool therefore err on the low side. Thus, 15% of random sera from residents of one city in the United States had antibodies specific for *G. lamblia.*[173] However, in Bolivia, where more than 50% of stools contain Giardia or its cysts, only a fraction of infected people concurrently experience diarrhea, and only a small segment of the latter develop prolonged or recurrent digestive troubles or the intestinal malabsorption syndrome. *Contaminated drinking water is the usual source of cysts.* In many cities such as Leningrad and Moscow, the tourist returns home with diarrhea, while the natives seem unaffected, whether shedding Giardia cysts or not. *Host factors are important in Giardia pathogenesis.*[174] Severe giardiasis is sometimes seen in patients with low serum IgA or with low overall immunoglobulin levels. Young children in day care centers or living in institutions have high Giardia infection rates, but again only 17% of the infected 1- to

3-year-olds have significant disease. Indeed, there is evidence that the youngest children derive protection from maternal breast-feeding, but not from cow's milk. In parts of Latin America where Giardia prevalence reaches 50% or more, diarrhea and malabsorption are in fact more common in older children and adults. Even normal persons in these areas show blunting of intestinal villi and hypercellularity of the lamina propria that would be interpreted as malabsorptive changes in the United States. In sum, our understanding of giardiasis remains quite limited, and the basic issue of how the parasite damages the host gut is still unresolved.

Giardia lamblia trophozoites, seen in smears *en face,* are pear shaped and binucleate, and look a bit like a cartoonist's drawing of a ghost. Their flagellae are rarely visible in routinely stained material. On cross section, however, they are sickle-shaped and their concavity holds a brushlike sucker plate best seen by electron microscopy. These plates are the parasite's means of epithelial attachment. Trophozoites appear in the stools only during diarrheal episodes. At other times they are replaced by smaller, quadrinucleate ovoid cysts, sometimes mistaken for parasite eggs. Diagnostic *duodenal aspiration is much more reliable than stool examination.* An ELISA test for Giardia antigens in stools has recently become available.

> Duodenal or jejunal biopsy specimens are often teeming with Giardia organisms lining the epithelial brush border (Fig. 7–48), but the intestinal morphology may range from virtually normal to markedly abnormal. Most commonly there is clubbing of villi and a decreased villus-crypt ratio, with a mixed inflammatory infiltrate of the lamina propria. The brush borders of the absorptive cells appear damaged on electron microscopy.[175] Sometimes there is virtual absence of villi, resembling the atrophic stage of gluten-induced enteropathy (p. 876). In giardiasis with immunoglobulin deficiencies, follicular hypertrophy of the mucosal lymphoid tissue has been a frequent finding, but the same syndrome can occur without such changes.[176] In some cases a scarcity or absence of plasma cells in the lamina propria has been noted.

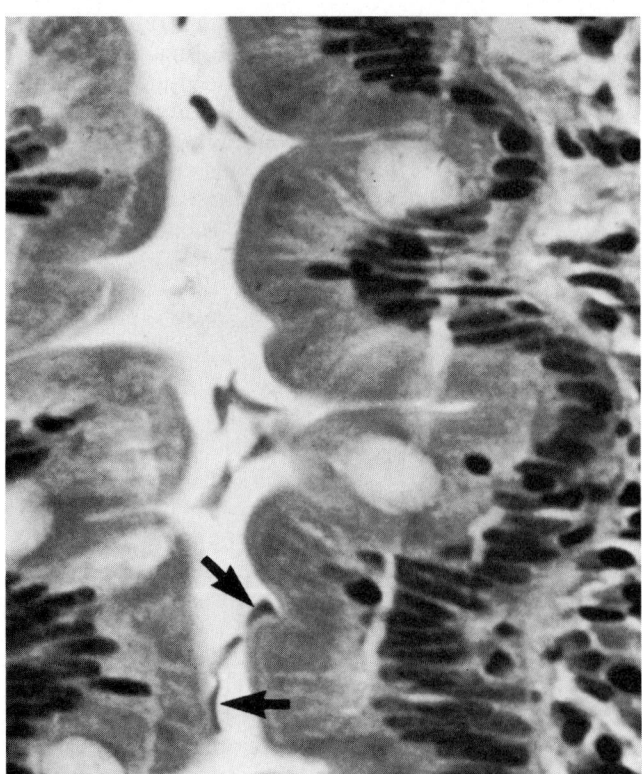

Figure 7–48. Giardiasis of jejunum. Parasites *(arrows)* show sickle-shaped profile; some are sitting on the epithelial brush border.

Mild indigestion or diarrhea may be the only symptoms of pathogenic Giardia infection; more suggestive is copious, watery diarrhea lasting days or weeks with flatulence and cramps followed by bulky, semisolid, malodorous stools, sometimes recurrent. Chronic giardiasis can cause malabsorption and weight loss or growth retardation as well as lactose intolerance and disaccharidase deficiency. Protein and fat loss can be considerable and vitamin B_{12} deficiency may occur, but the disease is virtually never fatal. All too often the diagnosis is delayed until empirical treatment for other presumed agents has proved ineffective. *Giardia lamblia* responds well to several antiparasitic drugs.

Cryptosporidial and Coccidial Enteritis

Cryptosporidium infection is one of the many causes of transitory diarrhea or dysentery in normal children. Outbreaks resemble those of giardiasis and occur mainly in daycare centers and in rural communities. By contrast, cryptosporidiosis in patients with AIDS gives rise to severe chronic malabsorption and diarrhea that can lead to death.

Ordinary stool examinations are relatively ineffectual for detecting microsporidia, as are ordinary histologic methods, and, for these reasons, the true frequency of this infection is not yet known. However, the use of a modified acid-fast staining technique for fecal specimens has revealed that normal animals as well as convalescent humans may shed cryptosporidial cysts in their feces for weeks or months and are thus potential sources of contamination.

Micro- and macrogametes of cryptosporidia adhere to the brush border of absorptive gut epithelia, enveloped by a host cell membrane (Fig. 7–49). Cysts are shed into the lumen. Diarrheal disease is associated with active protozoal proliferation and with mixed inflammatory infiltration of the lamina propia, but its pathophysiology and treatment remain to be fully elucidated.[177]

Coccidia are also important animal pathogens, but human infection is rare. Occasionally, in a diarrheal patient, *Isospora belli* cysts have been found in the stool. In patients with AIDS, Isospora cysts have even been observed outside the gut.[178]

Trichomoniasis *(Trichomonas vaginalis)*

The most frequent venereal parasitic infection is caused by *T. vaginalis*, a flagellate 15 to 18 μ in length, shaped like a turnip, with a single nucleus and three to four anterior flagellae. Its single posterior flagellum is provided with an axostyle and an undulating membrane, visible only on high magnification. This powerful motor system permits the organism to flit about actively when a fresh preparation from an inflamed urethra or vagina is examined microscopically. There is no cyst form; transmission is generally direct via sexual intercourse. Indirect transmission by contaminated articles is possible but unlikely, because the parasite cannot survive for long in the environment. *Optimal conditions for its long-term colonization exist in the vaginas of postpubertal women; in selected groups consulting the gynecologist, estimates have ranged up to 40%.*[179] *Immature female genitalia are refractory, probably by virtue of their fermentative bacterial flora. Infection of the male urethra, the second most common site, is less persistent but may be followed by involvement of the seminal vesicles and prostate.*

Trichomonas vaginalis is a near-commensal, producing symptoms only in a fraction of infected persons, mainly in those bearing recent infections. When genital inflammatory lesions are severe, interaction of *T. vaginalis* with bacterial pathogens must be suspected, even if many trichomonads are found. Burning, itching, and discharge are the most frequent symptoms in both males and females, especially before or during micturition. The discharge is typically described as scant and frothy, most often noticed in the morning. Sometimes there is increased frequency of voiding. Rarely, with involvement of the posterior male urethra, seminal vesicles, or prostate, there is perineal tenderness, and these organs may feel boggy on rectal examination.

Typically, there is spotty reddening and edema of the affected mucosa, sometimes with small blisters or granules, referred to as "strawberry mucosa." Histologically, the mucosa and superficial submucosa may be infiltrated by lymphocytes and plasma cells and polymorphonuclear leukocytes when lesions are intense. The discharge is rarely frankly purulent, as in gonorrheal or chlamydial infection. Aside from the presence of parasites, there are no specific pathologic features. The trichomonads are best seen in fresh preparations diluted with warm saline, but some authorities recommend smears stained by the Giemsa method. **When organisms are scarce, they are rarely the cause of disease.** Culture methods are available in specialized laboratories should visual inspection fail. **Trichomonads are only faintly stained on Papanicolaou smears and therefore are sometimes missed.**

Pneumocystis Pneumonia *(Pneumocystis carinii)*

Pneumocystis carinii is a ubiquitous opportunistic parasite of uncertain classification. It may in fact be more closely related to the fungi than to the protozoa.[179a] Nearly all normal children have acquired antibodies to *P. carinii* by their second birthday.[180] Only children with protein-calorie malnutrition and immunodeficient or immunosuppressed adults suffer pneumocystis pneumonia, a life-threatening condition if untreated. Among AIDS patients, pneumocystosis occurs so regularly that it is used as a diagnostic criterion. In experimental rats, *P. carinii* pneumonia can be readily elicited by repeated cortisone injec-

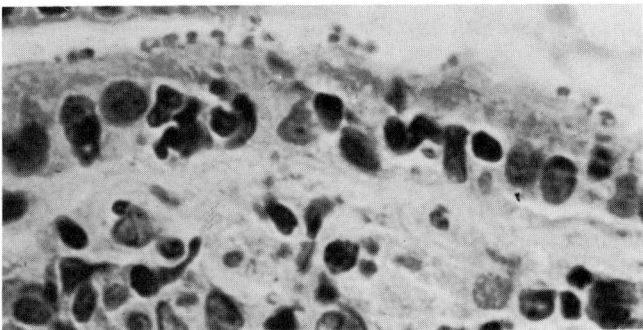

Figure 7–49. Cryptosporidium macro- and microgametes sitting on brush border of gut epithelium. Note inflammatory cells.

tions. Very likely, therefore, adult human disease also arises from activation of a latent infection.

Pneumocystis carinii trophozoites measure up to 6 μm with long filopodia. They attach to and graze on alveolar epithelial cells but do not invade them. Trophozoites are visible by electron microscopy and in toluidine blue– or polychrome-stained smears or sections, but not by routine histologic techniques. As they divide, some of them form cup-shaped or boat-shaped cysts whose cell walls are sharply outlined by methenamine-silver staining. Inside these cysts, reproduction proceeds and new trophozoites then continue the cycle. *Pneumocystis carinii* cysts must be differentiated from similarly sized (4 to 6 μm) fungal yeast forms also stainable by silver methods. Definitive diagnosis rests on microscopy; no reliable culture or antigen detection methods are yet available, although these are important research targets. Organisms are very rarely found in sputum. Bronchial washings are greater than 80% diagnostic in AIDS patients with pneumocystosis but are less sensitive in other immunosuppressed individuals. Frequently lung biopsy provides the only definitive answer.

Both clinically and pathologically, lesions are concentrated in but not limited to the lung. On x-ray examination, they often take the form of rapidly expanding perihilar shadows, but there is much variation in localizations and in radiologic and histologic appearances from case to case, and pneumocystosis is often clinically undistinguishable from other lung infections or from adult respiratory distress syndrome (ARDS) (p. 760).

Histologically, in the typical case, **the alveolar spaces are filled by an amphophilic, foamy, amorphous material resembling proteinaceous edema fluid, composed of proliferating parasites and cell debris** (Fig. 7–50). Usually there is an accompanying mild interstitial inflammatory reaction with widening of the septa, protein and fibrin exudation, pneumocyte proliferation, escape of red cells, and sometimes the formation of hyaline membranes. Affected lung appears airless, red, and beefy. Not infrequently there is concurrent infection by opportunistic bacteria, fungi, or viruses, especially CMV, which may overshadow the pathology caused by *P. carinii,* and exudative lesions or even granulomas may thus be found. Because pneumocystosis often supervenes as the terminal complication of other pulmonary infections or systemic diseases, **it can be diagnosed with certainty only by the direct demonstration of the parasite.** It should, however, be noted that the cyst form of *P. carinii* is relatively resistant to destruction and may persist even after treatment, when clinical signs have improved.

Typically, this disease presents as the sudden onset of fever, dyspnea, hypoxia, and a new lung shadow on x-ray films, leading to deterioration in the condition of a previously controlled but seriously ill patient. Less often there is also a cough. These nondescript features could herald a large variety of oppor-

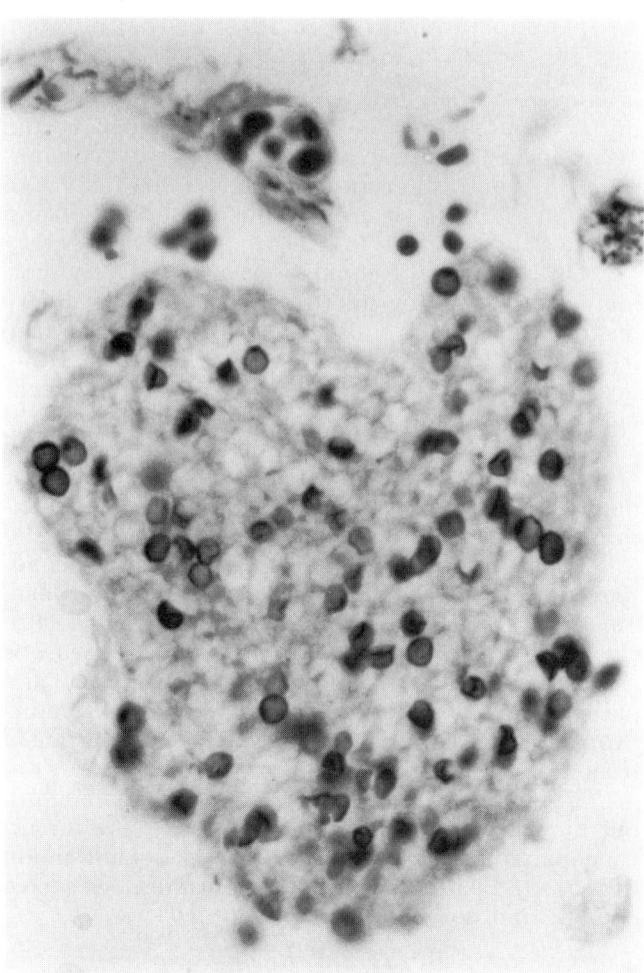

Figure 7–50. *Pneumocystis carinii.* A high-power detail of the foamy characteristic exudate lying within an alveolus containing numerous organisms highlighted by silver staining. Numerous characteristic "cup shapes" are evident.

tunistic lung infections besides *P. carinii.* Pneumocystosis, therefore, sometimes goes unrecognized, resulting in a high mortality. Early treatment can significantly improve the outlook for recovery. Nowadays, therefore, patients at risk frequently receive prophylactic drug combinations, most recently by aerosol inhalation, in an attempt to prevent pneumonia and thus avert open lung biopsy.[181] For these reasons, classic widespread pneumocystosis is becoming an increasingly rare condition at autopsy.

BLOOD AND TISSUE PROTOZOA

Malaria (Plasmodium spp.)*

Four species of plasmodia—*P. vivax, P. ovale, P. malariae,* and *P. falciparum*—are responsible for malaria, one of the most common ailments of mankind. Distributed throughout the tropics and subtropics, malaria is particularly prevalent in Africa and Asia, where millions are infected; the heaviest toll of mortality falls on children under 4 years of age. The disease is transmitted by more than a dozen species of

Anopheles mosquitos. Attempts to eradicate the infection have foundered, partly owing to socioeconomic factors and partly because of the unexpected proliferation of insecticide-resistant mosquitos and drug-resistant parasites. Nonetheless, vectorially transmitted malaria is now extremely rare in developed countries. In the United States, between 500 and 2000 cases have occurred annually in recent years. Meanwhile, malarial spread by worldwide jet travel continues, because the parasites invade the blood and can be transmitted by transfusion or among drug addicts. In such nonendemic settings, the lack of familiarity with malaria and its many clinical facets contributes to the danger of a missed diagnosis.

All four species of Plasmodium have complex sexual cycles in their insect vectors, ending with the production of sporozoites, which are inoculated into the mammalian host by mosquito bite. Only female anophelines take blood meals and transmit malaria. *Sporozoites* are antigenically distinct from all subsequent developmental parasite forms, and during their brief journey from the skin to liver cells they are vulnerable to specific antisporozoite antibodies. In an immune or vaccinated host, these antibodies may abort infection by coating the plasma membrane of the sporozoite

before it can invade the host liver cell. Within the hepatocyte the parasite transforms and divides (exoerythrocytic cycle), eventually to reenter the bloodstream in the form of merozoites capable of invading and multiplying in red cells. *Merozoites* are also antigenically distinct, and outside of red cells they are vulnerable to specific antibody. *They initiate the intraerythrocytic asexual cycle responsible for most of the anatomic and clinical features of malaria; merozoites grow to become trophozoites, which upon division form numerous schizonts. Released by rupture of the erythrocytes, these reenter other red cells to begin a new cycle.* After a few cycles, intraerythrocytic gametocytes (i.e., male and female offspring), are added to the cyclically generated asexual forms. Although *gametocytes* are not numerous, they are relatively long-lived and are the only forms capable of initiating the insect cycle when taken up by mosquitos Fig. 7–51).

Each species of Plasmodium produces a somewhat distinctive disease pattern related in part to the timing of its asexual intraerythrocytic cycle. *Plasmodium vivax* and *P. ovale* infections are rarely fatal and are marked by fever spikes roughly 48 hours apart — *benign tertian malaria.* With *P. malariae* the spikes occur at 72-hour intervals; this infection is prone to

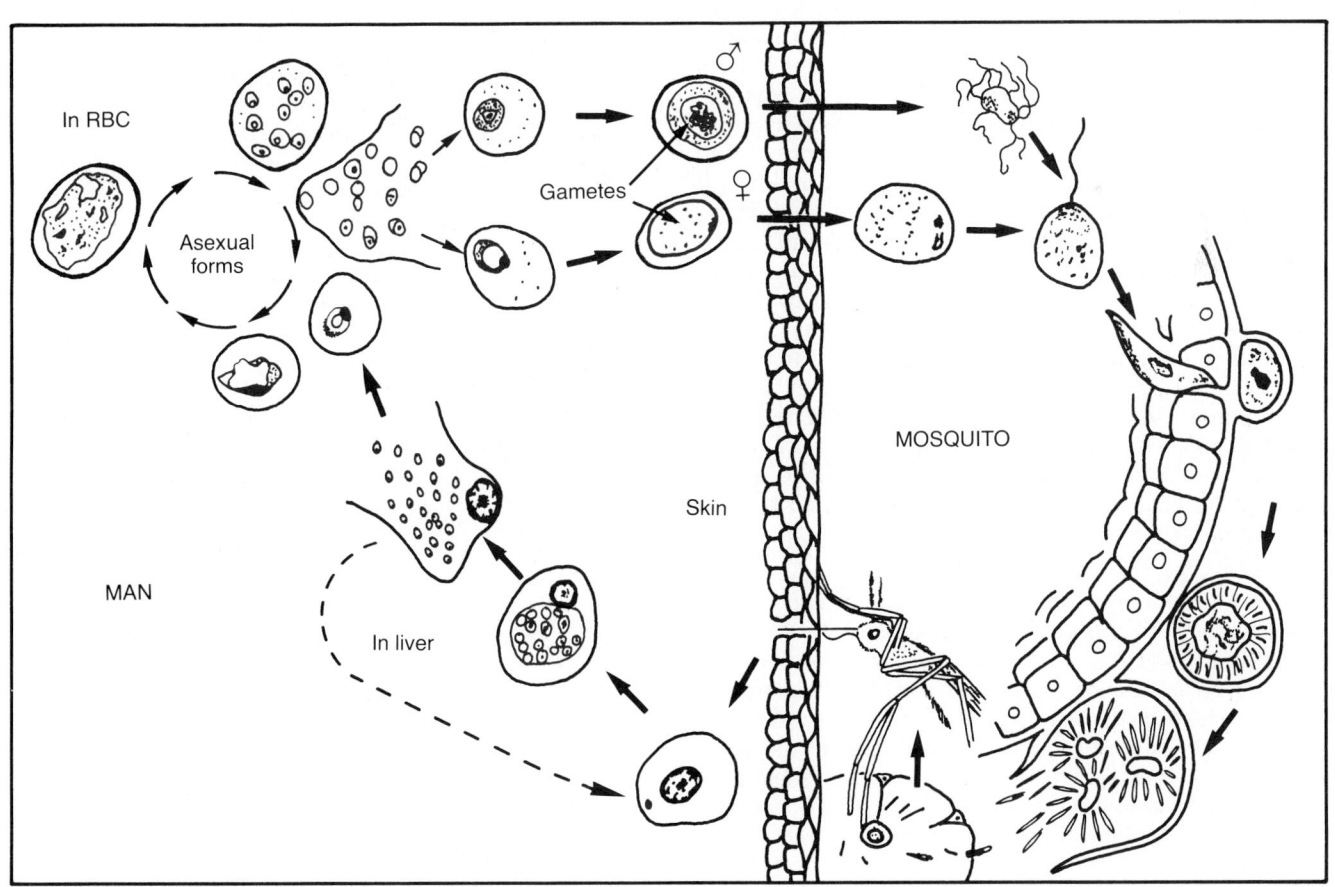

MALARIAL LIFE CYCLE

Figure 7–51.

long periods of latency—*benign quartan malaria.* *Plasmodium falciparum* is responsible for the highest parasitemias and for the bulk of mortality. The fever in this pattern of infection is sometimes irregular but often shows periodicity at 48-hour intervals—*malignant tertian malaria.* In all forms the red cell destruction causes anemia and, at the same time, malarial pigment produced by the parasite's digestion of heme is released. The damaged red cells and malarial pigment are removed from the blood by the monocyte-phagocyte reticuloendothelial system, inducing splenomegaly and hepatomegaly as well as the pigmentation seen in these enlarged organs and in the bone marrow. The "malignant" nature of *P. falciparum* may relate to several factors: unlike other plasmodia that prefer either young or older red cells, it indiscriminately parasitizes all red cells with glycophorin receptors, resulting in high and steeply rising parasitemias; it also induces sticky knobs in the erythrocyte membranes, which results in plugging of small vessels and tissue hypoxemia or ischemic necrosis. This process is particularly dangerous in the small vessels of the brain.[182]

Host factors also condition the occurrence and severity of malarial disease and even its geographic distribution. Protein-calorie malnutrition in African and Asian children compounds the systemic effects of malaria. However, cerebral malaria is less common among these partly immune children than it is among nonimmune visitors.[183] Blackwater fever, a form of hemoglobinuric renal failure seen in *P. falciparum* infection, is infrequent today and may have represented the concurrence of drug or alcohol toxicity. Sickle cell hemoglobin (HbS) tends to limit parasitemia, forcing the parasite to leave the red cell as its heme starts sickling. Endemic malaria is therefore less lethal in the HbS heterozygote (p. 666) and its geographic distribution reflects that of the sickle cell genes. There is suggestive evidence that G6PD deficiency may also offer some protection, although it also induces hemolysis when antimalarial drugs are given.[184] The Duffy blood group factor appears to be necessary for *P. vivax* red cell penetration, and black persons without that red cell receptor are therefore refractory to benign tertian malaria.[185]

Few observations are available on the morphologic changes in the nonfatal forms of malaria caused by *P. vivax,* *P. malariae,* and *P. ovale.* In *P. falciparum* infection, depending on its duration, **the spleen is markedly enlarged** and may exceed 1000 g. During the acute stage of the disease, the splenic enlargement is moderate and the substance congested or hemorrhagic. The capsule is thin and rupture of the spleen may occur but is rare. As the disease becomes more chronic there is increased cellularity and fibrosis, creating a solid enlargement. The capsule is thickened and on cross section the splenic substance is gray or black and brittle, traditionally described as "ague cake."

Histologically, in the acute stages there is marked splenic congestion along with hypertrophy and phagocytic activity of the reticuloendothelial cells and macrophages. Parasites may be seen within the trapped red cells. With chronicity, the phagocytic cells become more prominent, sometimes forming solid masses. They are laden with a finely divided **brown-black malarial pigment called hemozoin.** The pigment has a granular appearance, does not react with stains for ferrous iron, and is faintly birefringent. It resembles hematin, a product of red cell autolysis sometimes seen in congested organs. Accompanying the phagocytosis of pigment there is engulfment of parasites, leukocytic debris, and red cell debris. In the late stages of malaria, as the spleen continues to enlarge, the fibrous trabeculae thicken as the organ hardens and blackens.[186]

The liver is likewise enlarged in malaria. In acute malaria, this enlargement is only moderate and is accompanied by considerable hyperemia. As the infection becomes chronic or reinfections occur, the increase in size progresses and the organ becomes more firm and pigmented. The **Kupffer cells** are enlarged and hyperplastic; these become heavily laden with malarial pigment, parasites, and cellular debris (Fig. 7–52); some pigment may also be found in the parenchymal cells. The changes in the bone marrow and lymph nodes are of similar nature. Pigmented phagocytic cells may be found dispersed throughout the body in the subcutaneous tissues, lungs, and other sites, particularly when infection has saturated the principal reticuloendothelial organs.

The kidneys are often enlarged and congested. A dusting of pigment is often present in the glomeruli, and the tubules may contain hemoglobin casts, particularly in falciparum malaria.

In malignant falciparum malaria, there may be ex-

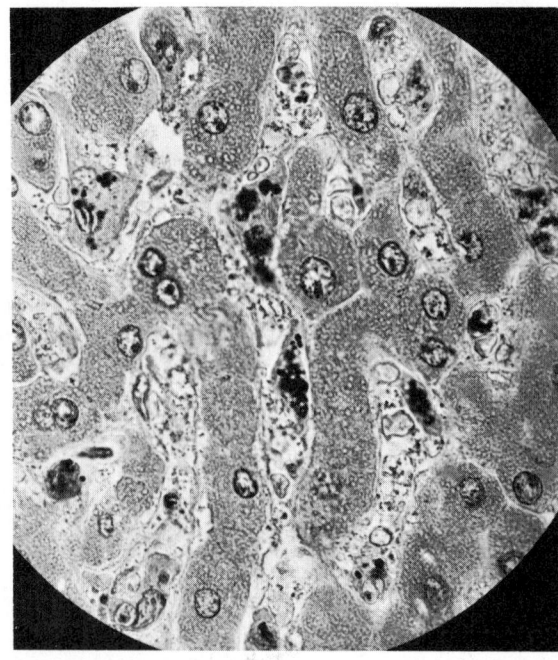

Figure 7–52. Malaria in liver with pigment-laden Kupffer cells.

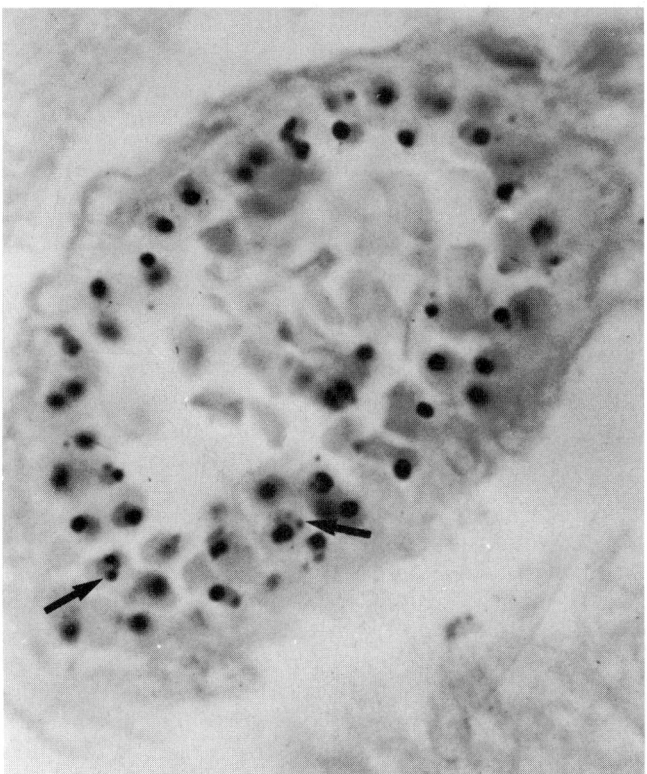

Figure 7–53. Cerebral malaria. Pigment dots *(arrows)* mark the parasitized red cells inside a vein. Note the margination of merozoite-containing red cells.

treme congestion of the brain vessels so that they become plugged with parasitized red cells, each cell containing a single dot of hemozoin pigment (Fig. 7–53). About these vessels, there are ring hemorrhages that are probably related to local hypoxia incident to the vascular stasis. Small focal inflammatory reactions (called malarial or Dürck's granulomas) may occur about these vessels. These granulomas consist of a small focus of ischemic necrosis surrounded by a microglial reaction. With more severe hypoxia, there is degeneration of neurons, focal ischemic softening, and occasionally a scant inflammatory infiltrate in the meninges. Nonspecific focal hypoxic lesions in the heart may be induced by the progressive anemia and circulatory stasis in chronically infected patients. In some, the myocardium also shows focal interstitial inflammatory infiltration.[186] Usually the pathophysiologic disturbances in malignant tertian malaria far outweigh the anatomic abnormalities found. Thus, in the nonimmune patient, pulmonary edema or shock with DIC is a frequent cause of death, sometimes in the absence of other characteristic lesions.

The popular image of malaria is limited to its classic, febrile paroxysms: After an incubation period of one to two weeks and three or four days of a nondescript malaise or fever, the disease declares itself by mounting fever to 40°C or higher, accompanied by chills and rigors. There is dry flushing of the skin,

restlessness, intractable headache, body aches, and sometimes delirium. A few hours later, sweating begins, the fever declines, and lassitude follows. After a day or two of respite another paroxysm begins. This classic pattern is largely seen in developed countries in returned travelers or in foreign visitors with severe acute *P. falciparum* infections (sometimes modified by ineffective previous drug prophylaxis). It may also occur with transfusion- or addict-derived malaria or during a late relapse of a previously treated chronic latent benign tertian or quartan malaria, especially after splenectomy.

Ironically, the classic clinical picture accounts for only a fraction of malarial disease. Latent endemic infection is far more frequent, particularly in the wet tropics where malaria transmission is constant, such as in West Africa.[183] Here, the survivors of early childhood infection have developed partial immunity and have low parasitemias, with or without hepatosplenomegaly or mild febrile episodes. In countries with alternating dry and rainy seasons, such as western Latin America, the disease attack rate increases along with the breeding mosquitos (the estivoautumnal pattern) even though few attacks are of the classic type. Overt disease in endemic areas may present in many ways. In young children it can easily be mistaken for pneumonia, diarrheal disease, or typhoid fever. Older children are the chief victims of the relatively rare nephrotic syndrome (p. 1033) associated principally with *P. malariae* infection.[187] Alternatively, endemic malaria may present as a chronic anemia with hepatosplenomegaly; as a protracted, febrile disorder of unknown cause; as renal shutdown; or as the insidious onset of jaundice and hepatic failure.

Catastrophic *P. falciparum* infection is most likely to develop in nonimmune teenagers or adults and in splenectomized individuals. This often lethal form of the disease is characterized by any or all of the following features: cerebral involvement with delirium progressing to coma; hypothermic shock (algid malaria); pulmonary edema; DIC; renal shutdown with hemoglobinuria; or liver failure.

Whatever the clinical pattern, the mainstay of diagnosis is identification of parasites in the blood smear. Indeed, there is a clear correlation between severity of illness and level of blood parasite count. Differentiation among the four species of Plasmodia is today a specialized skill that depends on subtle morphologic features of the parasites. Many drugs have been developed for the prevention and treatment of malaria, but the plasmodia have been equally adept at developing drug resistance. Recently a culture method for the blood forms of the plasmodia has been devised and is being used for the production of purified and cloned parasites and their antigens. This Trager culture method also permits sensitivity testing analogous to that employed with bacteria, but, with appropriate geographic information, effective therapy can often be started before drug sensitivities have been measured. Treatment of malaria is no longer the simple matter it was in the days before the development of drug-resistant strains. Malaria vaccine research has progressed, but its ultimate success still remains uncertain.[188]

Babesiasis (Babesia spp.)*

Babesia microti, a distant relative of the plasmodia, causes an acute, sometimes prolonged illness that may be incapacitating but is rarely fatal. It is seen mostly along the Eastern seaboard and on the islands of Nantucket and Martha's Vineyard. The cattle parasites *B. bovis* and *B. bigemina* can also sporadically infect asplenic humans to produce a rapidly fatal febrile infection with hemolysis and renal failure; these are rare infections, but they occur worldwide.

Over 100 symptomatic cases have been reported to date, all but a few in persons older than 40 years.[189] Serologic surveys indicate, however, that asymptomatic infection may be widespread among residents and visitors of all ages in the Northeastern summer resort areas. *Babesia microti* is transmitted by the bite of the tiny nymphal stage of the hard tick *Ixodes dammini*, whose adult stage feeds on deer and field mice. Ticks can transmit the parasite transovarially. Nymphs are active between May and September; human disease trails this timetable by about one month. Man is thus an accidental and often unaware victim of a natural cycle. *Babesia microti*, once introduced, invades the red blood cells and can be mistaken for *P. falciparum*, but it does not produce any pigment. Infections have been acquired by blood or platelet transfusion from asymptomatic donors. Because donors are currently not screened serologically for Babesia, the scope of babesiasis as a cause of post-transfusion fever is unclear.

Headache, fever, chills, myalgia, and fatigue suggesting a "summer flu" may be the only symptoms of babesiasis. The fever usually lasts no longer than one week and recovery is spontaneous but slow. Severe disease, mostly in splenectomized patients or in those debilitated by chronic diseases, can be prolonged or recurrent and can be accompanied by vomiting, hemolysis, jaundice, hemoglobinuria, renal failure, even coma. *The level of the* B. microti *parasitemia is a good indication of the severity of infection;* only 1% of erythrocytes are infected in mild cases, but rapidly rising parasitemia of more than 30% of red cells is seen in infections that become life-threatening. There is marked erythrophagocytosis associated with the red cell destruction. *Babesia bovis*, with its 60% or higher lethality, resembles severe *B. microti* infection. The combination of quinine and clindamycin has reversed rapidly rising parasitemias and is currently the treatment of choice.[190]

In fatal cases the anatomic findings have been those related to shock and hypoxia and include jaundice, hepatic necrosis, acute renal tubular necrosis, hemolysis, hemoglobinuria, anemia, and, sometimes, hemorrhagic manifestations. There is no rash or primary eschar that might suggest a tick connection. Diagnosis must be made microscopically by Giemsa-stained blood smears. The intraerythrocytic ring forms are tiny and difficult to see on routinely stained tissue sections.

African Trypanosomiasis (Trypanosoma rhodesiense, T. gambiense)*

African trypanosomal disease covers several clinical stages: (1) an acute febrile attack with purpura and DIC; (2) chronic, episodic fever with lymph node swelling and splenomegaly; and eventually (3) progressive brain dysfunction leading to "sleeping sickness," cachexia and death. All three disease stages may appear sequentially, or only the chronic stages may be apparent. *Trypanosoma rhodesiense* infection is often acute and virulent, and its tsetse fly *(Glossina)* vector prefers the savannah plains of East Africa; *T. gambiense* infection tends to be chronic and its vector thrives best in the West African bush. All the rare United States cases are imported. The vector species Glossina exists only in Africa, where its bite also transmits *T. brucei brucei*, which is prevalent among wild animals and cattle and is the ancestor species to which humans have become refractory. *Trypanosoma brucei* ravages cattle and sheep over millions of square miles of Africa. Wild animals can also serve as reservoirs for *T. rhodesiense*, whereas *T. gambiense* is largely carried from person to person. Tsetse flies seem to be angered by noisy Land Rovers, and safari hunters are known to be at risk.[191]

Bloodstream trypanosomes (trypomastigotes) are fusiform, flagellate, motile protozoa marked by an undulating membrane along the length of the organism. After inoculation of salivary forms by the tsetse, the parasites metamorphose and proliferate at the local site and gain entry to the lymphatics and bloodstream to induce a parasitemia. Within the blood they become vulnerable to opsonizing antibodies specific for their glycoprotein surface antigens. However, these parasites are able to generate a seemingly endless sequence of surface variant antigens, each composed of a single glycoprotein, so that a successor clone begins proliferating before antibody has eradicated its predecessors. This genetically programmed sequence[192] explains the persistent bouts of fever. The chronic assault on the host immune system, especially on the B cells, results in lymphoreticular hyperplasia with lymphadenopathy and splenomegaly. Concomitantly there is a striking IgM hypergammaglobulinemia. Only part of this immunoglobulin is directed specifically against trypanosomal antigens. Much of it may be an expression of polyclonal B-cell activation. Cellular immunity is also weakened.[193] Nonetheless, trypanosomes are vulnerable to neutrophil and macrophage destruction because they lack catalases and other scavengers of oxygen radicals produced by the phagocytes. The precise mechanism of trypanosome-induced tissue injury is unknown. Antigen-antibody complexes may release kinins and other mediators of inflammation, which may contribute. The release of lysosomal enzymes from degenerating phagocytes could also be a factor.

A large, red, rubbery chancre may form at the site of the insect bite; it is more frequently seen in Rhodesian trypanosomiasis. It teems with parasites and shows intense inflammatory infiltration, largely mononuclear, as well as vasodilatation and interstitial edema. With advancing chronicity of the disease, the lymph nodes and spleen enlarge owing to hyperplasia, accompanied by an infiltrate of lymphocytes, plasma cells, and macrophages that must ultimately dispose of the killed parasites. Trypanosomes are small and difficult to visualize except in "overstained" Giemsa sections. They tend to concentrate in capillary loops such as the choroid plexus and glomeruli. In time, and more often in prolonged Gambian disease, the parasites breach the blood-brain barrier and invade the CNS, to induce initially a leptomeningitis extending into the perivascular Virchow-Robin spaces and eventually a demyelinating panencephalitis. Particularly prominent in all sites of leukocytic infiltration are plasma cells containing glycoprotein globules, often referred to as flame cells or Mott cells (named after the first author to describe these brain changes). Severe acute trypanosomiasis may be followed by DIC, by an interstitial myocarditis, or by lethal bacterial superinfection. Chronic disease leads to progressive cachexia, and these patients, devoid of energy and normal mentation, literally waste away.

The onset of clinical manifestations is more frequently acute in the Rhodesian illness than in the Gambian variety, in which successive bouts of fever are spaced by latent periods of variable length, sometimes months to years. Until CNS manifestations appear, the disease is often confused with other chronic infections, but it can be diagnosed by visualizing the parasites. During early parasitemia these are easily seen on blood smears. In more chronic stages they may be detectable in the bone marrow, lymph nodes, and spleen, though usually not in great numbers. When parasites cannot be found, the characteristic IgM hyperglobulinemia is of some diagnostic value. Usually there is also anemia, granulocytopenia, and an elevated erythrocyte sedimentation rate. In most cases, if the patient with Gambian disease survives long enough, the meningoencephalitic phase makes its appearance. There is headache and lethargy that over the course of time progresses to a pathetic, vegetative state: drooping eyelids; open, mute mouth; total lack of response to external stimuli; and finally, death in coma. The devastating cerebral manifestations have been attributed to generation of phenylpyruvate and indol-3 ethanol by the trypanosomes in the brain.[194] Early African trypanosomiasis is treatable; in advanced sleeping sickness, di-fluoromethylornithine has recently shown some promise where none existed before.[195]

INTRACELLULAR PROTOZOA

Chagas Disease *(Trypanosoma cruzi)**

Also called American trypanosomiasis, Chagas disease is found from Texas to Argentina. Its acute stage may be asymptomatic or marked by fever and acute myocarditis. Its chronic phase results in progressive cardiac failure and is the most important cause of death from heart disease in several Latin American countries. In Brazil, but not elsewhere, chronic Chagas disease is also a cause of megaesophagus (p. 829) and megacolon (p. 883).

Dogs and wild animals, especially the opossum and armadillo, are hosts of *T. cruzi* strains, but humans are the principal source of human disease. The parasite is transmitted by "kissing bugs" (triatomidae) that hide in the cracks of rickety houses and feed on their sleeping inhabitants. Infection can also be acquired by transplacental passage, transfusion, or laboratory accident.

Trypanosoma cruzi, a fusiform hemoflagellate with an undulating membrane, circulates but does not multiply within the bloodstream. Rather, it invades tissue cells and assumes a leishmanial form, which then divides, eventually to reinvade the blood. Progressive multiplication within the parasitized cells produces intracellular pseudocysts packed with organisms (Fig. 7–54). As the disease progresses, parasitemia decreases but the tissue forms persist, causing either progressive acute infection, latent infection of indefinite duration, or latency followed by chronic infection.

In *acute disease*, damage results from direct invasion of cells by the parasites and from the consequent inflammatory changes. An erythematous swelling—the chagoma—may appear at the site of the bite, only to regress spontaneously. Rarely, the portal of entry may be the conjunctiva, producing unilateral edema, preauricular lymphadenopathy, and sometimes exophthalmos (Romaña's sign). Transient parasitemia undoubtedly follows all infections, including those with seemingly localized reactions, yet many individuals never show any further manifestations other than detectable antitrypanosomal antibodies. If acute Chagas disease does develop it is marked by high parasitemia and fever, principally with cardiac involvement, but sometimes with generalized lymphadenopathy or splenomegaly also. Acute chagasic myocarditis may be mild, detectable only by transient ECG changes, but in severe disease rapidly progressive cardiac dilatation and failure may ensue. Meningitis rarely occurs, mainly in newborns and young children. Death follows in about 5 to 10% of acute cases, generally from involvement of the heart. More often the febrile reaction and cardiac changes regress slowly as parasites virtually disappear from both the blood and tissues, and a latent period of variable duration follows.

Chronic disease usually arises in young and mature adults and presents mainly as the progressive onset of cardiac failure. At this late stage the parasite-

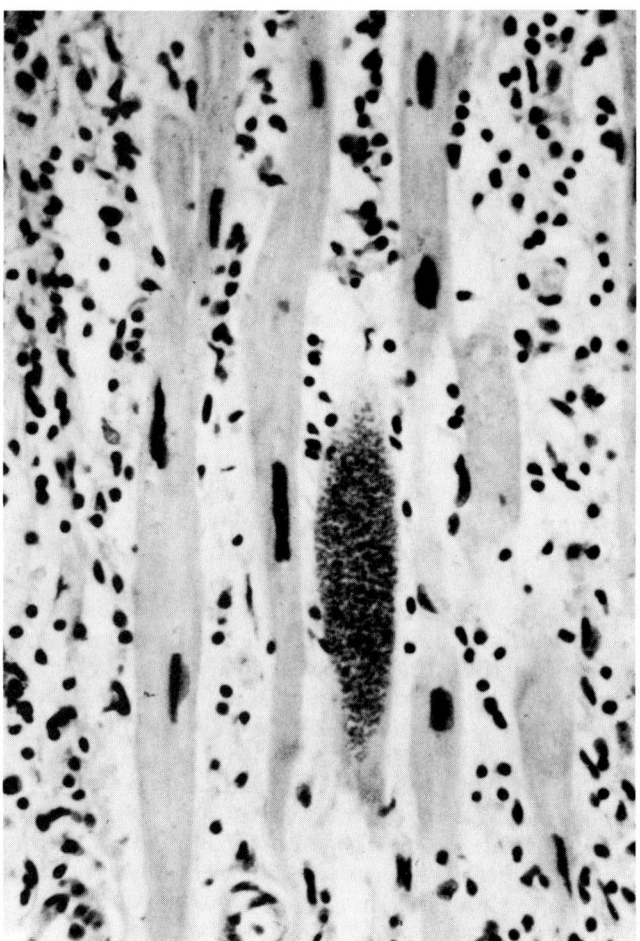

Figure 7–54. Chagasic myocarditis showing *T. cruzi*–filled pseudocyst, interstitial edema, and mononuclear infiltration.

mia remains scanty, and the organisms within the tissues are likewise often vanishing in number and difficult to find in histologic sections. Nonetheless, there is striking inflammatory infiltration of the myocardium and sometimes of the skeletal muscles, completely out of proportion to the number of parasites demonstrable. The pathogenesis of chronic Chagas disease is unknown. An autoimmune reaction mediated by cytotoxic T cells and by antibodies, reactive with human endocardial, myocardial, striated muscle cells and endothelium (EVI antibodies), has been postulated. However, it is not clear whether these immune reactions are the cause or the result of the tissue damage.[196]

> In **lethal acute chagasic myocarditis** the anatomic changes are diffusely distributed throughout the heart. Clusters of leishmanial forms swell individual myocardial fibers to create intracellular pseudocysts. There is focal myocardial cell necrosis accompanied by extensive, dense, acute interstitial inflammatory infiltration throughout the myocardium (Fig. 7–54), and there is often four-chamber cardiac dilatation.

> In **chronic Chagas disease** the heart is typically dilated, rounded in shape, and increased in size and weight. Often there are mural thrombi that, in about one half of autopsy cases, have given rise to pulmonary or systemic emboli or infarctions. Histologically, there is interstitial and perivascular inflammatory infiltration composed mainly of lymphocytes, plasma cells, and monocytes. It is heaviest in the right bundle branch of the cardiac conduction system.[197] Scattered foci of myocardial cell necrosis can sometimes be seen. There is also interstitial fibrosis, especially toward the apex of the left ventricle, which may undergo aneurysmal dilation and thinning (a suggestive, but not pathognomonic, feature of chronic chagasic myocarditis). In the Brazilian endemic foci, as many as one half of the patients with lethal carditis also have dilatation of the esophagus or colon, apparently related to damage to the intrinsic innervation of these organs. However, at the late stages when such changes appear, parasites cannot be found within these ganglia.

As many as 10% of the rural population in endemic foci suffer from chronic chagasic heart disease. Symptoms and signs range from right bundle branch block to progressive cardiac decompensation or thromboembolic manifestations to sudden death without previous warning. At this late stage organisms can rarely be identified in the blood, but complement-fixing antibodies can usually be demonstrated. A more laborious, but sometimes necessary, diagnostic measure is xenodiagnosis (i.e., identification of parasites in laboratory-bred triatomids two weeks after they have been allowed to feed on the patient's skin). New drugs have improved the outlook for patients with acute infection, but none have proved of value in chronic disease.[198]

Leishmaniasis (Leishmania spp.)*

All clinical forms of leishmaniasis are caused by a single parasite stage, the tiny ($<3\ \mu$), nonflagellated intracellular amastigote, recognizable in tissue sections or smears by two basophilic dots: the nucleus and the kinetoplast (i.e., a modified mitochondrial structure or "parabasal body" closely apposed to the dot-like blepharoplast). All leishmaniae are transmitted by the bite of sandflies (i.e., by diverse Phlebotomus spp. in the Old World, or by Lutzomyia spp. in the New). Nevertheless, *the disease manifestations caused by these organisms vary greatly by parasite species and endemic region of origin*. Until the taxonomy of the leishmania can be further defined,[199] the traditional classification will be followed here, which differentiates visceral *leishmaniasis or kala-azar* (caused by *L. donovani*) from *mucocutaneous leishmaniasis or espundia* (due to *L. brasiliensis*) and *major cutaneous leishmaniasis or tropical sore* (due to *L. major* and *L. mexicana*). All these infections occur largely in poor people in remote locations.

Kala-azar (Hindi for "black fever") results from the widespread invasion of the mononuclear-phagocyte system by *L. donovani*. It is an insidiously developing but severe systemic disease marked by hepatosplenomegaly, lymphadenopathy, pancytopenia, fever, and weight loss. The reticuloendothelial blockade produced by overloading the phagocytic cells with leishmaniae, coupled with pancytopenia, predisposes patients to intercurrent bacterial infections, the usual cause of death. Hemorrhages related to thrombocytopenia may also be fatal.

At autopsy the spleen, liver, and lymph nodes are all enlarged. Often the spleen reaches gigantic size (up to 3 kg); lymph nodes may achieve a diameter of 4 to 5 cm; the hepatomegaly is generally less extreme. In all these organs the phagocytic cells are markedly swollen and stuffed with leishmaniae (Fig. 7–55). The flooding of the spleen with infected macrophages, accompanied by marked plasmacytosis, obscures the organ's normal architecture. In the late stages of the disease the liver becomes increasingly and irreversibly fibrotic. Phagocytic cells crowd the bone marrow and may also be found in the lungs, gastrointestinal tract, kidneys, pancreas, testes, and other organs. Often there is hyperpigmentation of the skin in the extremities, accounting for the Indian designation of this condition. In the kidneys, immune complex deposition and mesangial proliferation are sometimes observed,[200] and in advanced cases amyloid deposition is frequent.

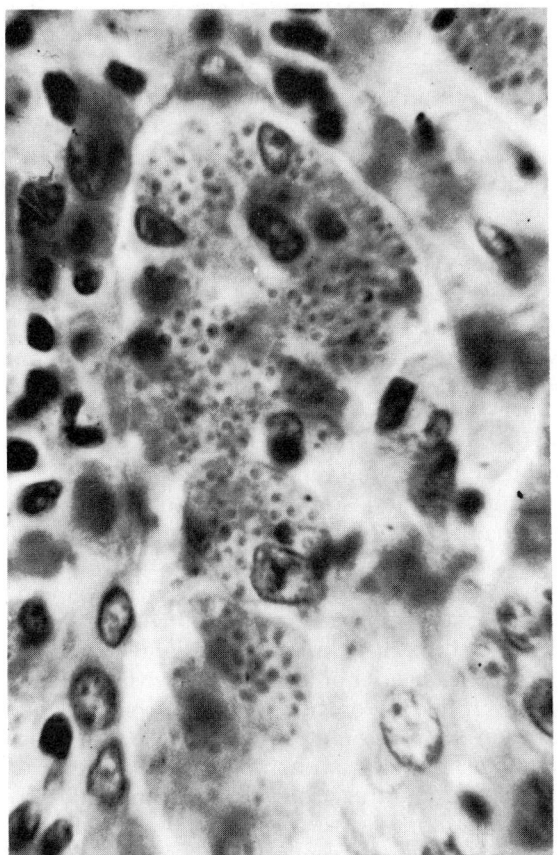

Figure 7–55. Visceral leishmaniasis (kala-azar). Phagocytes within a lymph node are laden with Leishmania.

Usually no local lesions occur at the site of the sandfly bite, but in African disease there may be a "primary chancre," which generally regresses before systemic manifestations develop insidiously, sometimes a year later. Periods of spiking fever ensue, followed by remissions and relapses. Most patients come to medical attention at an advanced stage of disease showing hepatosplenomegaly, lymphadenopathy, and pancytopenia. Serum albumin level is usually low, and *globulin concentration is markedly elevated, being predominantly the IgG fraction* (as opposed to IgM elevation in African trypanosomiasis). Clotting abnormalities are frequent. Patients who recover from systemic kala-azar, usually by treatment, may develop extensive skin involvement (post–kala-azar dermal leishmanoids) manifested as disfiguring papular or nodular lesions reminiscent of severe lepromatous leprosy. Histologically, these nodules contain numerous histiocytes stuffed with *L. donovani.* Unfortunately, such cases are among the worst responders to chemotherapy.

Diagnosis is best achieved by the demonstration of *L. donovani* in smears, tissue sections, or cultures in special biphasic media; skin testing with leishmanin is used to evaluate host reactivity, but may be negative in patients with advanced disease.

Mucocutaneous leishmaniasis is endemic in the hinterlands of several South American countries, including Brazil, and is caused by several species or strains of New World leishmania. It begins as a chronic skin ulcer (tropical sore) of the leg, forearm, trunk, or face. Before or after the ulcer regresses, sometimes even years later, *secondary moist, ulcerating, or nonulcerating lesions develop around or close to the mucocutaneous junctions;* these may localize in the larynx, nasal septum, anal zone, or vulva and can be destructive and disfiguring. These lesions undergo spontaneous exacerbations or remissions and usually last for a long time. Their histopathology varies with their activity and duration.[201]

Initially, a mixed inflammatory infiltrate with numerous parasite-containing histiocytes is seen together with many lymphocytes and plasma cells. Later the tissue reaction becomes granulomatous and the number of parasites declines; it is therefore important to sample for parasites at or near the raised growing border of ulcerated lesions where they are likeliest to persist.[202] Giemsa-stained impression smears prepared from biopsy specimens are likeliest to show leishmania.

Eventually, the lesions remit and scar. Even while a treated or untreated lesion seems to be healing, leishmaniae may remain present and reactivation may occur after long intervals. The role of host immunoregulation in leishmaniasis is less well understood than in leprosy, with which it otherwise shares many analogies.[203]

Cutaneous leishmaniasis exists in both the Old and New Worlds. Oriental tropical ulcer is caused by

Leishmania major and *is a relatively mild and localized disease compared with the mucocutaneous variant.* It is seen in much of Southern Asia and parts of Africa. An analogous chronic, self-healing cutaneous ulcer occurs in parts of Latin America, and typically affects the ear (i.e., the preferred biting site of the local sandflies). American cutaneous leishmaniasis is caused by *L. mexicana,* whose southernmost territory overlaps with that of *L. brasiliensis.* These two parasite species can now be distinguished by an ingenious new test involving hybridization of kinetoplast DNA.[199]

> Tropical ulcers are single and are usually located on exposed parts of the body; after a long incubation period, they begin as an itching papule surrounded by induration; this turns into a shallow, slowly expanding ulcer with irregular borders; healing is even slower than onset, but **most lesions involute within six months without requiring treatment.** Microscopically, the tissue reaction is granulomatous. Parasites are scarce in fully developed lesions, though detectable by culture, and cutaneous Leishmania hypersensitivity is strong.

Diffuse cutaneous leishmaniasis is the rarest form of dermal infection, thus far found only in Ethiopia and adjacent East Africa and in Venezuela, Brazil, and Mexico. *It too begins as a single skin nodule, but it continues spreading until the entire body may be covered by bizarre nodular lesions, some resembling keloids or large verrucae, some imitating the nodules of lepromatous leprosy.* These lesions do not ulcerate. Microscopically, they show vast aggregates of foamy macrophages containing myriads of leishmanial organisms. Characteristically, the patients are anergic not only to leishmanin but also to other skin antigens; because of their similarity to lepromatous patients, they are often erroneously sent to leprosaria. These infections have been notoriously difficult to cure by drug treatment. This form of leishmaniasis seems to be closely associated with impaired T-cell immunity, but whether it is causal or secondary is not clear. There is also some evidence that diffuse cutaneous leishmaniasis may be caused by specific strains.

Toxoplasmosis *(Toxoplasma gondii)*

Toxoplasma gondii is a coccidian parasite that infects many animal species. Its definitive hosts are domestic cats and some wild felines, in whose intestines sexual reproduction results in the formation of fertile oocysts. Shortly after being shed in the feces these oocysts are highly infective for most animals, including humans. The tissue forms of *T. gondii* are 3×6 μm, bow-shaped *tachyzoites* and larger *cysts* containing many *bradyzoites.* These can also transmit the infection to humans or animals, chiefly by ingestion of uncooked meat. The versatile life cycle of this parasite has made it prevalent throughout the animal world. Human infection is also worldwide and tends to be nearly universal in the humid tropics, but somewhat rarer in dry or cold climates. *In the United States, between 15 and 50% of the population have antibodies to T. gondii, with regional variations.*

Toxoplasma gondii is delicately adapted to intracellular survival in its many hosts and therefore rarely causes disease. In immunocompetent adult persons, toxoplasmosis is usually mild and self-terminating, and the bulk of infections remain subclinical. *Most of the toll is borne by fetuses, babies, and immunosuppressed individuals of any age.*[204,205] *In these predisposed groups toxoplasmosis can be devastating, causing severe CNS damage or blindness. For these reasons, pregnant women should avoid contact with infected or potentially infected cats and abstain from uncooked meat.* Entering through the gut, *T. gondii* spreads systemically, to penetrate into virtually any type of host cell, phagocytic or not. The parasite initially spreads from cell to cell as a tachyzoite; later it multiplies inside single cells to form microscopic cysts that can remain dormant for long periods. Small numbers of these cysts are formed in subclinical infections, detectable only by subinoculation into toxoplasma-free mice. *In infections of normal adults, it is therefore futile to look for parasites in tissue sections.* By contrast, in newborns and the immunosuppressed, as the infection mounts, myriad tachyzoites can usually be found in the lesions. Examined under oil, they reveal their characteristic tiny single nucleus, distinct from the double basophilic dots of the Trypanosoma-Leishmania family. Even more distinctive, but few in number, are the cysts that represent dead "nurse" cells filled with hundreds of bradyzoites. Toxoplasma is undetectable in blood or body fluids, but *high or rising antibody titers can be demonstrated by immunofluorescence or ELISA tests now widely in use.* In newborn infections, specific IgM antibodies are especially significant because they are less likely to have been passively transferred from the mother.

Several clinical forms of toxoplasmosis are recognized.

1. Acute infection in the normal adult commonly manifests itself as lymphadenopathy with or without fever, mimicking the onset of a lymphoma or a viral infection. The diagnosis is usually suggested by examination of an excised lymph node.
2. Found in infants and children, but rarely in normal adults, is the severe acute febrile form with evidence of pneumonia, liver dysfunction, or even myocarditis.
3. Maternal infection during early pregnancy may be entirely asymptomatic, but placental involvement can result in stillbirth or neonatal jaundice, pneumonia, myocarditis, or encephalitis, often with lethal results. Nonfatal infection of the fetus leads to brain damage, hydrocephalus, mental retardation, seizures, deafness, or other permanent neurologic deficits. These lesions may manifest themselves immediately or in delayed fashion.
4. Activation of a dormant Toxoplasma infection in an immunosuppressed individual most frequently expresses itself as an acute, progressive encephalitis

that, because of the rapidity of onset of coma, may remain clinically unrecognized.

5. Toxoplasma retinochoroiditis that can lead to blindness and glaucoma is a rare complication of chronic toxoplasmosis, sometimes seen in corticosteroid-treated individuals.

> **The morphologic pattern most often seen in otherwise normal adults is toxoplasma lymphadenitis. It is suggested by the triad of follicular hyperplasia, focal proliferation of transformed, "histioid" B cells, and scattered focal accumulations of small numbers of epithelioid-type macrophages not forming well-defined granulomas.** The disorder is more frequent in young women than in men, and cervical lymph nodes, especially those in the posterior neck, are most often affected.[205] Once suggested, the diagnosis can be confirmed by serologic titer. The disease is self-terminating. If the infection reverts to a chronic phase, the hazard to a fetus born later is minor compared with that of infection acquired during pregnancy.
>
> **Neonatal toxoplasmosis** is characterized by destructive lesions in multiple organs, notably the brain. Similar, but usually less destructive, lesions occur in the **severe form of acute adult toxoplasmosis.** In the CNS, microglial nodules with many tachyzoites appear, particularly about the ventricles and aqueduct, followed by extensive necrosis, vascular thrombosis, and intense inflammation. Obstruction of the aqueduct is frequent, resulting in hydrocephalus. If the infant survives long enough, these lesions eventually calcify. As the disease persists, Toxoplasma cysts frequently develop in the nerve tissue. In the infant, brain changes are often preceded by liver cell necrosis and sometimes by adrenal necrosis. The lung and heart may also be focally necrotic and inflamed. There is extramedullary hematopoiesis.
>
> Cysts in the brain are also a frequent feature in the **Toxoplasma encephalitis of immunosuppressed patients.** These cysts may rupture and release swarms of bradyzoites to incite a microglial nodular reaction. Multiple necrotic brain lesions, randomly distributed, may follow. Other organs, including the myocardium, may also show scattered parasites and focal inflammatory mononuclear infiltrates.
>
> In **Toxoplasma chorioretinitis,** destruction of the retina by tachyzoites is accompanied by a granulomatous reaction in the choroid and sclera.

Because of the huge disparity between the number of persons infected by Toxoplasma and the sporadic overt illnesses it causes, this parasite is rarely identified as the cause of its protean manifestations. Direct demonstration of *T. gondii* in tissue — the definitive diagnostic confirmation — is rarely achieved during the life of the patient when it is most needed. It is therefore prudent to obtain and compare the specific antibody titers at time of admission to the hospital, at the acute stage, and after some time interval for specific antibody titers whenever this infection is suspected. Adult toxoplasmosis is treatable by a combination of drugs, but the damage to the fetus is irreversible.

HELMINTHIC DISEASES

Helminths are the largest and most highly evolved endoparasites of man; they rely on the longevity of individual worms rather than on their multiplication inside the host. Procreation is by eggs or larvae, which must be cycled through the environment or through intermediate hosts before humans can be infected again. Helminths have strict host specificities either for a definitive species, in whom sexual reproduction takes place, or for their intermediate hosts or vector, in whom reproduction is asexual. They achieve only stunted development in unsuitable hosts (e.g., when humans are infected with animal filariae.)[206] Each species of parasitic helminth has its own intricately designed life cycle, seemingly fragile in its dependence on human or animal behavior, yet effective enough in some cases to maintain infections in millions of people. With few exceptions (e.g., Strongyloides) individual worm burdens in humans tend to be stable and long-lasting. Even reinfection does not often result in linear increases because the helminth-infected host builds up an immunity or because establishment of a single worm interferes with the development of others (e.g., the solitary pig tapeworm, *Taenia solium*). Under endemic conditions, most persons harbor a few worms and are free of disease; only a minority becomes heavily infected and ill. The enormous global prevalence figures reported — 400 million infections with Ascaris, and 250 million with schistosomes — must therefore be viewed as representing helminthic frequency and not necessarily helminthic disease.

Many helminthic disease manifestations depend on the worms' habitat or migration routes. On the basis of the habitat of the adult form, we can divide these parasites in an oversimplified manner into *intestinal* and *blood-tissue helminths*. However, several gut-dwelling worms have tissue-migrating larvae, and the tapeworms can be human gut or tissue dwellers, depending on whether man serves as their definitive or their intermediate hosts. The only intracellular form among the human parasitic helminths is the muscle larva of *Trichinella spiralis*, whose longevity compensates for the fleeting existence of its adult parent. Taxonomically, there are three major classes of helminths, the roundworms (Nematodes), flatworms (Cestodes), and flukes (Trematodes).

Intestinal helminths can behave as commensals (i.e., as "accidental pathogens"), as opportunists, or even, if sufficiently numerous, as virulent pathogens. *Adult worms can cause disease by (1) competing for essential host nutrients (e.g., vitamin B_{12} depletion by* Diphyllobothrium latum); (2) *mechanically obstructing or perforating the gastrointestinal tract* (Ascaris lumbricoides); (3) *blood-sucking (the hookworms,* Ancylostoma *and* Necator); (4) *inducing inflammatory* *and malabsorptive changes in the gut* (Strongyloides stercoralis); *or (5) inducing host hypersensitivity reactions (many helminths).* Hypersensitivity reactions are often caused by the migratory larval stages of those helminths that must invade tissues and undergo several molts in order to reach maturity in the gut. During that process, there is attrition of the less vigorous invasive larvae and shedding of surface antigens and somatic components. Although there is little evidence that these are toxic to the host, there is no doubt of their antigenicity and capacity to stimulate host antibodies and cellular immune responses. Nevertheless, the migratory schedules and antigenic variations of the developing forms permit a significant proportion to evade host defenses and reach the privileged gut environment. During reinfection, with host antibodies and memory cells poised to react to early helminth antigens, the number of developing forms able to reach their ultimate habitat is drastically reduced. Immunosuppression can dramatically abolish this protection. Similarly, *eosinophilia*, a hallmark of normal host immune responses to the richly glycosylated helminth antigens, can be abolished in an altered host.

Intestinal roundworms require only resistance to the host digestive juices as their condition of survival, but tissue-dwelling worms have developed elaborate mechanisms to evade host cellular defenses and antibodies.

1. In developing flatworms and flukes, antigenic variations occur in their cytoplasmic tegument analogous to those of molting helminth larvae.
2. There is surface acquisition of host-derived molecules such as red cell and histocompatibility antigens, which serve to partially disguise the parasite's identity.[207]
3. A general reduction in helminth surface antigenicity occurs, whose nature is still not fully understood.[208]
4. Enzymes of larval and adult blood flukes can cleave host immunoglobulins, leading to complement consumption and inactivation of clotting factors.
5. Cystic tapeworm larvae release sulfated polysaccharides, which inhibit mediators of inflammation and can generate their own lipoxygenase products, thus inhibiting platelet aggregation.
6. Leukocytes contacting the worm surfaces and phagocytosing their tegumental products soon detach themselves owing to the very high turnover of tegumental parasite glycoproteins and phospholipids.[209]
7. Some helminths generate products that directly suppress the host immunocompetent cells or elicit specific T-suppressor cells, damping immune responses.[210] As research continues, other ingenious evasive maneuvers of tissue helminths will probably be added to this compilation.[211]

Helminth challenge of an already infected host is always less likely to result in disease than primary infection, for the reasons already given, yet acquired resistance to a naturally occurring helminth infection is rarely complete. What generally ensues is the undisturbed survival of the established adult worms in the face of increased and accelerated attrition of the challenge-larvae, so that only a reduced number of new worms is added to the existing load. This "concomitant immunity"[212] is known to be T lymphocyte–dependent but its effector mechanisms are multiple and complex. In the schistosome experimental model, both antibodies and host effector cells are required for parasite killing. *Eosinophils are concentrated at the parasite-killing sites in vivo; in vitro,* they can kill early parasite forms in the presence of specific antibody by discharging reactive oxygen products, phospholipase A_2, and basic proteins damaging to the invader's tegument.[213] Similar evidence exists for other leukocytes, including macrophages.[214] It is thus still unclear whether eosinophils have a unique, protective role against helminth parasites or whether they simply act in concert with other leukocytes.[215]

Adult tissue-dwelling helminths generate eggs or larvae in volumes many times their own. Both parents and offspring are rich sources of excretory-secretory products, some functioning as proteolytic enzymes, others as powerful soluble or particulate antigens capable of evoking strong host immune responses. Circulating helminth antigens and antigen-antibody complexes can readily be detected and may play an important role in producing some of the lesions encountered (e.g., nephritis complicating schistosomiasis or filariasis). More important, helminth antigens can evoke various forms of local or systemic hypersensitivity reactions or, quite frequently, combinations of reactions, and it is generally agreed that the *disease potential of tissue helminths is largely due to their capacity to induce a spectrum of host hypersensitivities.* Tests for helminth-specific antibodies have been quite useful in epidemiologic studies and for clinical diagnosis, particularly when the parasites themselves are difficult to detect. The identification of antigens by monoclonal antibodies should further enhance their clinical value. By contrast, vaccination against helminths has thus far reached practical application only in the veterinary field.

INTESTINAL ROUNDWORMS
Ascariasis *(Ascaris lumbricoides)*

The largest (up to 35 cm long) and most common of the intestinal roundworms, *A. lumbricoides* is distributed worldwide and is indistinguishable from *A. suis,* the pig roundworm. It is spread between humans by fecal-oral transmission. In most infected persons, *A. lumbricoides* acts as a commensal, stays in the gut lumen, produces no disease, and eventually dies spontaneously and is shed. Infection is most common in children, becoming rarer from the second decade on. Eggs are excreted with the feces; larvae are liberated when Ascaris eggs are swallowed and reach the stomach. Following systemic tissue migration, they re-enter the gut from the lung via the larynx and trachea and then mature into adults.

Disease ensues under three circumstances:

1. Repeated seasonal entry of Ascaris larvae may result in allergic respiratory symptoms. (Ascaris polysaccharide antigen strongly stimulates IgE antibody formation.)
2. Heavy infection may obstruct a gut segment or sphincter.
3. Agitated worms may enter the appendix or common bile duct and cause perforation or bacterial infection with peritonitis, cholangitis, or sepsis.

Allergic ascariasis with hypereosinophilia, asthma, or urticaria is a seasonal phenomenon in parts of the Near East, especially the Arabian peninsula.[216] A more serious form has resulted from a massive oral load of pig ascaris eggs eaten during a college fraternity prank, inducing a spectacular allergic pneumonitis.[217] Pyloric obstruction by worms, best demonstrated by barium swallow, sometimes becomes an emergency in children, especially in the tropics, and can usually be alleviated without surgery. By contrast, appendiceal perforation requires emergency operation to avoid life-threatening bacterial and helminthic peritonitis. Near the perforated organ, Ascaris worms or eggs are found in the acute, fibrinopurulent exudate. Ascariasis of the common duct causes jaundice and gram-negative sepsis, and it can simulate severe hepatitis of other causes; fortunately, it is extremely rare. Although Ascaris infections have been linked to seizure disorders in children and to anemia or failure to gain weight, none of these charges has stood up to rigorous examination.

Trichuriasis (Trichuris sp.)

Trichuris trichiura, the whipworm, is a small intestinal roundworm up to 5.0 cm long with an attenuated anterior end (its "whip"). It is a very common, worldwide parasite whose life cycle lacks a tissue phase and it is simply transmitted by fecal contamination. It causes disease so rarely that the presence of its eggs in the stools serves largely as an indication to be alert for other parasites. However, poor children in the tropics or mentally retarded individuals sometimes acquire enough of these worms to make their cecum and colon appear villous. This comes about because the worms bury their anterior ends in the crypts of the mucosa, with their thicker half floating in the lumen. Massively infected persons may suffer from persistent diarrhea and tenesmus, and sometimes the load of worms combined with the edematous state of the mucosa produces sufficient obstruction and straining at stool to cause intussusception or rectal prolapse. Eosinophilia is common in heavy infections, the only ones meriting treatment with a vermifuge.

Enterobiasis (Oxyuriasis)

The pinworm, *Enterobius vermicularis*, is a tiny roundworm up to 13 mm long with prominent lateral ridges (alae), whose habitat is the gut. It causes the well-known night itch of children, and can be passed to siblings and sometimes to adults. Female worms migrate nightly to the anal skin for egg-laying, causing intense pruritus, insomnia, and irritability. Diagnosis can sometimes be made simply by inspection of the anus for worms. Enterobius eggs also stick to a piece of Scotch tape placed over the anus, which can then be directly examined under the microscope. The response of night itch to modern vermifuges is near miraculous, but reinfection is very common.

Intense, neglected enterobiasis can be complicated by spreading eczematous skin eruptions, and infection can be transferred to the nares. Enterobius has been suspect as a cause of symptoms simulating appendicitis and is regularly discovered in appendectomy specimens; however, its size is too small to obstruct the lumen and trigger bacterial superinfection (Fig. 7–56). Rarely, female worms migrate from the anus into the vagina to reach the fallopian tube and pelvic peritoneum. Egg-laying in these sites results in chronic granulomatous inflammation plus scarring, which may simulate bacterial or tuberculous pelvic inflammatory disease, thus producing a diagnostic conundrum when the pelvic lesions are discovered years after active enterobiasis has ceased.[218]

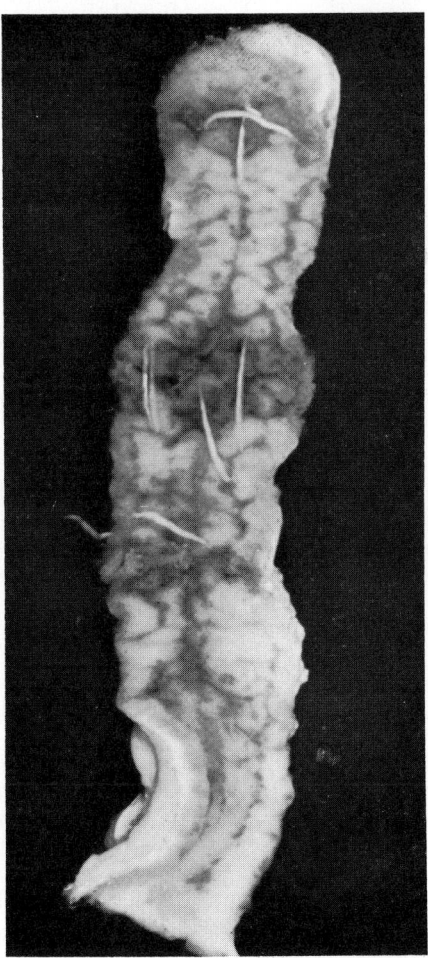

Figure 7–56. Pinworms in appendix.

Hookworm Disease (Necator, Ancylostoma spp.)

Unlike other intestinal roundworms, *Necator americanus* and *Ancylostoma duodenale*, with their sharp mouthplates, penetrate into the duodenal and jejunal mucosa and feed on blood. A considerable proportion of the blood is wastefully excreted into the intestinal lumen. Nevertheless, iron deficiency anemia due to hookworm alone is seen only in heavy infections, such as may still be found in some tropical countries and in the Appalachian region of the United States. In many instances of tropical anemia, hookworm disease potentiates the effects of malnutrition, malaria, or mixed parasitic infections of various kinds.

The parasite's life cycle requires hatching of infective larvae in the gut and fecal deposition in the soil. Penetrating the unshod skin of human feet, the larvae then migrate systemically and reach the lungs, from which they re-enter the gut by being coughed up and swallowed. Adult worms are up to 10 mm long and each can waste up to 43 μl of host blood per day.[219] Hookworm anemia is most common where human fecal contamination of the soil is heavy (e.g., in children of village communities in the tropics, especially those whose diet contains little iron). In such populations, one also sees hypoalbuminemia or intestinal malabsorption, or both, but this may be a combined effect of the parasites and poor nutrition. Treatment of the hookworms and iron supplementation may sometimes unmask an underlying macrocytic anemia due to folate deficiency. Children are known to increase their worm loads on reinfection, sometimes to huge proportions, but the declining frequency of hookworm infection in older persons in endemic areas suggests acquired immunity. Complete protection has been achieved in the dog by an irradiated live hookworm larval vaccine. The most effective measure against human hookworm anemia has been construction of rural latrines, as documented in Puerto Rico and the southern United States.[220]

> The lesions in the gut are relatively minor; punctate hemorrhages may be seen, but villous atrophy, when present, probably has other causes, and the biting defects caused by the worms are promptly regenerated after vermifuge treatment. Larval migration through the lung is generally silent.

Strongyloidiasis (*Strongyloides stercoralis*)

The mature parthenogenetic *S. stercoralis* female is small enough (up to 1 mm) to be almost entirely buried in an intestinal crypt of the duodenum or upper jejunum, where these worms reside. Thus, like other intestinal roundworms, *S. stercoralis* is a luminal dweller, but it more readily damages the absorptive surface of the gut, giving rise to chronic enteritis and the malabsorptive syndrome. Moreover, it is the only common human intestinal nematode whose life cycle permits larvae to become infective both in soil and in the host intestine itself, especially in malnourished and immunosuppressed individuals. This internal recycling of worms may result in sustained infection lasting for several decades following a single exposure, as occurred in World War II prisoners of war; or it may lead to Strongyloides hyperinfection (i.e., to a progressive, potentially lethal accumulation of worms and migratory larvae).[221] Strongyloides eggs mature high in the intestine, and the resulting larvae are easily missed on stool examination; duodenal aspiration or biopsy may sometimes be required for diagnosis. Transmission resembles that of hookworms and is more frequent in the rural tropics, but the disease is not limited to these locales. Strongyloidiasis occurs throughout the United States and is especially frequent in the Appalachian region. Severe cases occur in institutions for retarded or demented individuals, where fecal contamination is a fact of life. Elsewhere in the Americas, Brazil has been a major focus for many years.

In hypersensitive persons, larval skin penetration may give rise to an urticarial eruption that fades in a few days, but this is rarely recorded or remembered in the endemic setting. Similarly, larval lung migration at about seven days usually passes with a slight coughing episode, unless infection has been massive. The chronic, intestinal phase of infection may also remain asymptomatic but more often results in intermittent bouts of diarrhea, with or without evidence of malabsorption. Some patients, such as West Indian immigrants to Britain or the United States, manifest a spruelike syndrome with weight loss, fatty stools, and a protein-losing enteropathy, which gradually disappears after therapy. A similar syndrome found in the Philippines and Northeast Thailand is caused by *Capillaria philippinensis*. Endogenous Strongyloides hyperinfection, as seen in protein-deprived children or in cortisone-treated patients, is a grave illness, marked by nausea, fever, diarrhea, and (sometimes) paralytic ileus (an especially ominous sign). Concomitantly, there may be gram-negative sepsis, pneumonia, or meningitis, complications that tend to recur even after antibiotic treatment unless the underlying strongyloidiasis is also cured. Persistent eosinophilia is the rule in moderate infection, but this decreases in the hyperinfected, altered host.

> The lesions of strongyloidiasis mirror the clinical events. In mild, subclinical infection there may only be focal erythema and eosinophilia of the duodenal mucosa; females, eggs, and larvae are found burrowed in mucosal crypts (Fig. 7–57). In malabsorptive cases, the lamina propria is heavily infiltrated, the mucosal villi are blunted, the lacteals are dilated, and there is widespread mucosal edema. With hyperinfection, there is often ulceration of the small bowel; the invasive, filariform larvae of the worm, larger in size than the rhabdoid larvae of the lumen, are found in submucosal lymphatics and blood vessels of the small bowel, surrounded

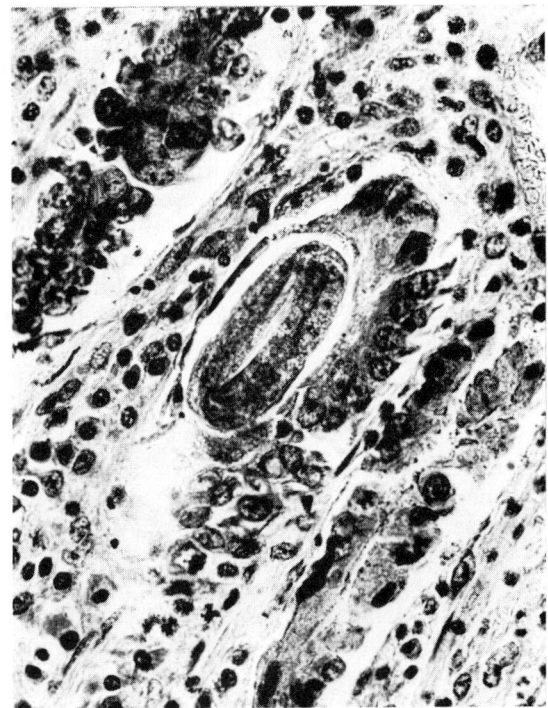

Figure 7–57. Strongyloidiasis in duodenal mucosa with a central, coiled rhabdoid larva.

by florid inflammation. Lower down, in the colon, they are seen mostly in the submucosa and muscularis, provoking focal accumulations of macrophages and lymphoid cells, but rarely well-defined epithelioid cell granulomas; the absence of a vigorous tissue response may be an indication of the depressed T-cell function found in such patients. In fatal infections the body is literally "riddled with worms." Migrating filariform larvae are most frequently seen in the lung, often associated with hemorrhage but with little focal inflammation. They may also appear in any other organ, including the liver and the CNS. Septic bacterial foci facilitated by the hyperinfection and depressed immunity are commonly seen at this stage, and hemorrhagic pneumonia is often the final insult.

Strongyloidiasis persists as a public health problem because of the same fecal contamination that permits other intestinal roundworms to prosper. It is, however, a more serious disease, as life-threatening as any severe bacterial or viral illness.

TISSUE ROUNDWORMS

Visceral Larva Migrans
(Toxocara canis, T. cati)

Toxocariasis is a *zoonotic* infection, acquired by children from puppies or kittens — the normal hosts — in whom the parasite undergoes full development. In man, the accidental host, worm development is stunted at the larval stage, but before these larvae die

in the various organs they have reached, they can cause significant tissue destruction and hypersensitivity reactions. A hypereosinophilic syndrome with fever and hepatosplenomegaly is the usual clinical presentation, at times with prominent gastrointestinal or respiratory symptoms or, rarely, visual impairment.[222] Unlike the intestinal roundworms, which are diagnosable by stool examination or duodenal aspirate, Toxocara larvae can be seen only in tissue samples. In the absence of such direct identification, serologic tests are helpful in dealing with this *occult parasitic infection.*

Toxocara, a large roundworm of the Ascaris family, is exquisitely adapted to canines or felines, which transmit the larvae transplacentally to their progeny; unless wormed early, these pets will shed many eggs into the environment in which children live and play. Ingested eggs liberate the larvae, which then enter the circulatory system and thus can reach any organ in the body.

The larvae are about 400 × 20 μm in size and provoke large, eosinophil-rich inflammatory foci with central necrosis, often containing numerous Charcot-Leyden crystals. Larvae, particularly disintegrating ones, may be difficult to locate in such foci and may require step-sectioning of the entire biopsy sample. During active infection the liver is generally enlarged and may appear studded with grayish-tan nodules up to 1 cm in diameter containing eosinophils, plasma cells, and scattered giant cells; there is also diffuse portal inflammatory infiltration with eosinophils and plasma cells. The lung may similarly show diffuse interstitial eosinophilia, resembling that seen in the acute allergic phase of human ascariasis or in Loeffler's syndrome (p. 794). Focal lung granulomas may appear around disintegrating Toxocara larvae.[223] Many other organs, including the heart, CNS, and rarely the eye, may show similar foci, and the consequent endophthalmitis may lead to retinal detachment and blindness, usually unilateral.

The active stage of toxocariasis begins suddenly or insidiously and lasts for several weeks or months, subsiding after two weeks in most cases. Manifestations are protean and include fever, cough, nausea, anorexia, body aches, weight loss, drenching sweats, asthma or urticaria, enlarged tender liver, lymphadenopathy, strabismus, and a host of other confusing complaints. Persistent eosinophilia of up to 40% of the differential count is an important clue, and there may be pronounced hyperglobulinemia. Eventually, if contact with infected pets is removed, the infection is self-terminating, but its course can be shortened and complications perhaps prevented by treatment.

Toxocariasis should be suspected in children living in crowded households with pets, in those with pica (compulsive dirt-eating), and in the presence of unexplained hepatomegaly, eosinophilia, or hyperglobulinemia. It is likely that subclinical infections are much more frequent than the overt.

Guinea Worm Infection
*(Dracunculus medinensis)**

The guinea worm, a long, thin tissue helminth up to 120 cm in length, belongs to a species distinct from the filariae of similar shape (p. 417). It causes disabling and painful inflammatory swellings of the skin. The ancient practice of removing the worm from its superficial location by winding it up on a stick is the probable origin of the caduceus, the emblem of medicine. *Guinea worm disease* is most common in parts of India and of West Africa, but occurs throughout the tropics. Buried in the human subcutaneous tissue, the adult worm discharges its larvae into water via skin blisters. The freshwater cyclops serves as the intermediary host, and new patients become infected by drinking from infested water. Provision of clean water breaks the cycle. Migration and maturation of worms may take as long as a year. Once in its final skin habitat, the worm causes swelling and blisters that often are located on the outer malleolus of the foot but also may appear in any other part of the skin. The lesions enlarge, becoming hard and edematous with the formation of multiple blisters and tracks that are prone to bacterial superinfection. The worm rears its ugly head where a blister has recently burst and thus becomes amenable to extraction. Death and degeneration of the worm lead to subcutaneous abscess formation and eventual calcification. Eosinophilia is found both in the blood and in the edematous granulation tissue that borders the local reaction to the worm. Some patients additionally manifest urticaria, and others become disabled by pain or inability to walk.

Trichinosis *(Trichinella spiralis)*

Trichinosis is a common disease throughout the world contracted by eating meat containing viable cysts of *Trichinella spiralis*. In man the parasite larva localizes principally within the striated muscles and therefore evokes generalized muscular aches and pains. However, during the early stage of infection the lungs, brain, heart, and other structures are also invaded. The disease is transmitted by the ingestion of inadequately cooked meat. Smoked meats are also dangerous because they are not cooked.

The larvae of the parasite encyst within the muscles of a wide variety of carnivores and omnivores. The chief reservoir for man is the infected pig (sometimes bear meat or other wild game). More stringent regulations—a decrease in garbage feeding of pigs, sterilization of garbage, and deep-freezing of pork—have markedly reduced the incidence of this disease in many countries, but no regulation is 100% fail-safe, and therefore trichinosis may prove difficult to eradicate completely. In the United States, reported cases have recently been ranging between 40 and 210 per year.

After ingestion of contaminated meat, the larvae are released in the stomach by proteolytic digestion of the cyst wall and attach themselves to the mucosa of the duodenum. As they mature into adult worms, they induce a mild transitory enteritis and malabsorption. About one week after copulation, a host of larvae are produced that penetrate the lacteals and eventually are drained into the blood. In this manner, they are disseminated and produce cell damage throughout the body (e.g., in the lung, heart, and brain). Meanwhile the adult worms die and are expelled. The larvae next invade striated skeletal muscle cells and modulate them to create an intracellular environment suitable for their own growth and maturation. This remarkable biologic coexistence of skeletal muscle cell and larvae has led to the muscle cell being called a "nurse cell."[224]

After the first week of their intracellular existence, the larvae become enclosed within a membrane produced by the host muscle cells (Fig. 7–58) which persists for the life of the larvae, possibly for years. Death of the larva and its "nurse" incites an inflammatory reaction characterized principally by lymphocytes and eosinophils. In time the dead larva calcifies. Therefore, infections in both animals and man can be recognized by microscopic identification of the viable or calcified larvae within striated skeletal muscle fibers. The most intense parasitization is encountered in the most active muscles of the body having the richest blood supply (i.e., the diaphragm, extraocular eye muscles, laryngeal muscles, and deltoid, gastrocnemius, and intercostal muscles). During active trichinosis there is often focal basophilic degeneration of muscle fibers. The calcified foci left

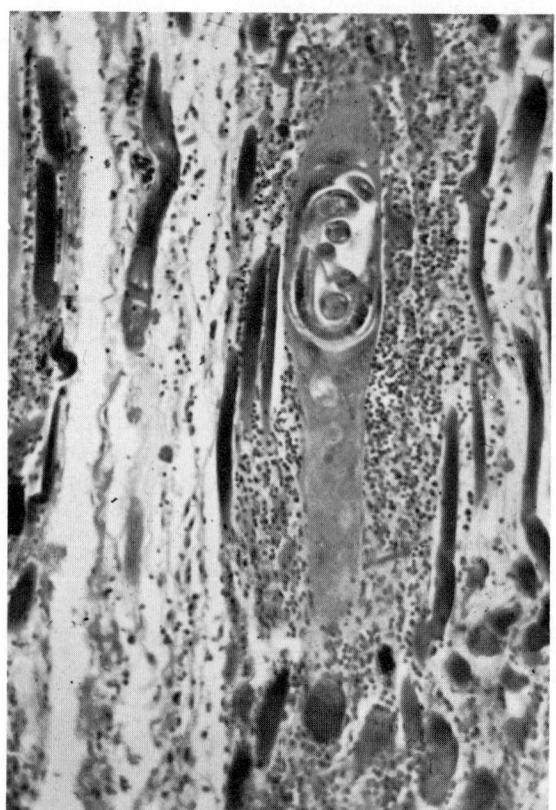

Figure 7–58. Trichinosis with a coiled, encysted parasite larva within skeletal muscle.

by dead larvae are characteristic enough to permit retrospective diagnosis even decades later.

During the invasive phase of trichinosis, cell destruction can be widespread and sometimes even lethal. Thus, in the heart, acute inflammatory changes are found during the early stages of the infection in the form of a patchy but widely scattered interstitial myocarditis, **but the larvae do not become encysted** within the myocytes. Instead they undergo necrosis and therefore cannot be identified. The inflammatory pattern in the myocardium is fairly nonspecific save for the prominence of eosinophils and some giant cells. Ultimately, fibrous scarring ensues. In the **lungs**, the reaction to the trapped larvae may consist only of edema and focal hemorrhages, but in some cases a marked leukocytic reaction with large numbers of eosinophils may appear, attributed to an allergic response. **Invasion of the CNS** is reflected by a diffuse lymphocytic and mononuclear infiltration in the leptomeninges and by the development of focal gliosis in and about the small capillaries of the brain substance, infiltrated with lymphocytes and eosinophils. Sometimes, necrotic larvae can be identified within these inflammatory nodules.

In most clinical cases, a history of the ingestion of improperly cooked pork products can be obtained. Trichinae are killed by cooking at a minimum temperature of 60°C for at least 30 minutes per pound of meat. Freezing the meat for 20 days at a temperature of −15°C (5°F) will also effectively destroy the trichinae. In United States locations, therefore, outbreaks of trichinosis occur mostly among ethnic groups processing their own traditional pork dishes for festive occasions or among fanciers of wild game and exotic meats. However, the disease may appear anywhere and may mimic a variety of other infections, as well as the collagen-vascular diseases and hematologic disorders. The period of invasion of the intestinal mucosa may be marked by vomiting and diarrhea, symptoms that suggest "food intoxication." During the hematogenous dissemination and the muscular invasion, widespread aches and pains and fever appear. Particularly characteristic are periorbital and facial edema. Eye movement and breathing and swallowing may be painful; patients often complain of backache and aching pain in the legs or joints. Often the invasion of the lung evokes cough and dyspnea, the latter materially contributed to by the involvement of the respiratory muscles. The CNS invasion may lead to headaches, disorientation, delirium, and a variety of other signs and symptoms strongly suggestive of a diffuse encephalitis. Cardiac failure may appear when the myocardial injury is severe. But the combination of fever, muscle tenderness, eosinophilia, and swelling of the eyelids is most typical.[225] The eosinophilia can account for 70% of the total white count. After the third week of the disease, serologic tests are positive except in overwhelming disease. A skin test is also available. Muscle biopsy, best taken near the tendinous insertion of the deltoids or gastrocnemius muscles, is definitive even earlier.

The mortality rate for trichinosis is low, but overwhelming infection may cause death when patients with severe involvement of the respiratory muscles develop intercurrent pulmonary bacterial infections or cardiac failure. Anti-inflammatory and symptomatic treatment will greatly reduce the severity of patient discomfort, but whether antihelminthic treatment is useful after larval invasion has occurred is debatable. Fortunately, mild and subclinical Trichinella infections are the rule, and severe ones the exception. Experimentally, even a minimal primary infection confers strong immunity to subsequent challenge, which may also be true of mild clinical infections. Several defensive mechanisms have been identified. At the time of adult worm development in the gut, a rapid rejection phenomenon is seen by which most female parasites are shed from the host mucosa before being able to deposit their larval progeny.[226] Newborn larvae, but not their later stages, are also susceptible to attack by eosinophilic and neutrophilic granulocytes in the presence of specific antibody.[227] Once ensconced in their nurse cells, however, Trichinella larvae are protected from both immune and phagocytic destruction.

Filariasis*

Human filarial infections are widely endemic in the insect-ridden lowlands and coastal plains of the tropics; animal filariae occasionally infect man in temperate as well as tropical zones. *Tropical filariasis* can be subdivided into (1) lymphatic filariasis, (2) onchocerciasis or "river blindness," and (3) the lesser tropical filarial infections. The best-known *zoonotic filariae* are those of dogs and raccoons.

It is estimated that 240 million people are infected by lymphatic filariae. Onchocerca infects about 40 million Africans. In the continental United States only scattered cases are seen among immigrants and returnees from endemic regions; a large epidemic arose in U.S. Marines during the World War II Pacific campaign.

Filariae are long, stringlike nematodes whose fertilized females release tiny microfilariae into the lymph, blood, or skin. When taken up by biting insects, these microfilariae molt and metamorphose into infective third-stage larvae, ready to infect a new host via the vector's proboscis. Migration from the biting site to their definitive habitat in the human body and maturation to the mating stage may take several months. Untreated human filariae survive for many years while maintaining steady microfilarial production. In lymphatic filariasis only part of the infected human population shows parasitemia at any one time; those with early infections and those with acquired immunity to microfilariae have "occult filariasis" (i.e., infection undetectable by blood concentration methods).[228] Infective larvae, adult worms, and microfilariae each have separate as well as shared antigens, and human immune responses vary individually and over the long duration of the disease. They range from virtual unresponsiveness to vigorous hypersensitivity,[229] and these variations account in part for the protean manifestations of filariasis, making its diagnosis and management difficult.

Lymphatic Filariasis (Wuchereria bancrofti, Brugia malayi)*

Wuchereria bancrofti measures up to 100 mm in length and is distributed worldwide in all tropical countries. *Brugia malayi*, somewhat smaller (25 mm long), is limited to Southeast Asia from Ceylon to the Philippines and is found as far north as central China. *Wuchereria bancrofti* has no known animal reservoir. *Brugia malayi* has strains that can infect monkeys and cats (potential reservoir hosts). Mosquito vectors vary by species; urban bancroftian filariasis found in the slums of many large tropical cities is transmitted mainly by *Culex fatigans*. As a rule, these infections are milder than those of rural filariasis, which is transmitted by any one of 80 mosquito species, depending on locality.

Most residents in endemic areas remain indefinitely asymptomatic, but newcomers to the tropics may develop acute symptoms several months after contracting infection. The acute phase manifests itself as bouts of fever, lymphangitic streaking of an extremity, transient intrascrotal pain and swelling, urticarial rashes, or tender lymphadenopathy, together with restlessness and apprehension. Eosinophilia is seen regularly, but microfilaremia may or may not be detectable. Acute symptoms often subside spontaneously but may recur or gradually shade into the chronic phase.

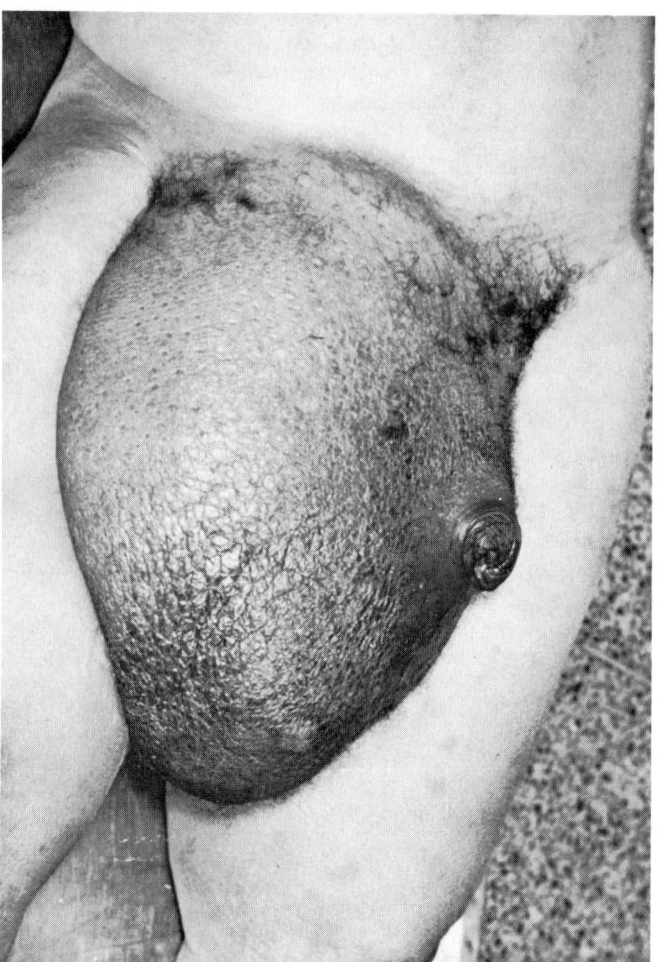

Figure 7–59. Elephantiasis of scrotum due to filariasis.

Chronic filariasis is characterized by persistent lymphedema of the scrotum, penis, or vulva, the leg, or even the breast or arm (the latter particularly in the Pacific focus). Frequently, there is hydrocele and lymph node enlargement. Rupture of a lymphatic varix may occur, leading to chyluria. Nodular inflammatory lesions or bacteriologically sterile abscesses may appear in the epididymis, along the spermatic cord, in an extremity, or around the external genital organs. In severe and long-lasting infections, chylous weeping of the enlarged scrotum may ensue (lymph scrotum) or a chronically swollen leg may develop tough subcutaneous fibrosis and epithelial hyperkeratosis, termed elephantiasis (Fig. 7–59). Elephantoid skin shows dilatation of the dermal lymphatics with widespread lymphocytic infiltrates and focal cholesterol deposits; the epidermis is thickened and hyperkeratotic.

Histologically, when adequately sought, adult filarial worms are found in lymphatics or nodes in all infections, either alive or dead and calcified. Some induce mild or no inflammatory reaction, although the lymphatics may be dilated and tortuous (lymphangiectasis). An intense eosinophil inflammation is seen in patients with recurrent filarial funiculoepididymitis, probably immunologically determined. In these lesions, lymphangitis extends far beyond the nesting points of the parasites themselves and may be hemorrhagic or fibrinous. The severest inflammatory lesions occur around disintegrating worms. Acute inflammation is followed by granulomatous foci that can be mistaken for mycobacterial lesions unless the parasite's cuticular remnants are recognized. Organization of the endolymphatic exudate results in polypoid infoldings of the vessel with persisting eosinophil and lymphocytic infiltration, a picture highly suggestive of lymphatic filariasis even if worms cannot be demonstrated. In endemic areas, filarial skin lesions often become superinfected by bacteria, with resulting cellulitis or abscess formation. In time the hydrocele fluid, which often contains cholesterol crystals, red cells, or hemosiderin, induces thickening and calcification of the tunica vaginalis. Microfilariae are difficult to find in histologic sections. Thus, the diagnosis frequently rests on combined clinical and pathologic criteria unless an adult parasite is found.

In Southeast India, Singapore, and sporadically elsewhere, occult filariasis may not be associated with microfilaremia or lymphatic obstruction. Instead there is a marked eosinophilia with asthma-like respiratory complaints or generalized lymphadenopathy (tropical eosinophilia or eosinophilic lung), related to high titers of antimicrofilarial antibody capable of triggering mast cell degranulation.[230] In tropical eosinophilia, besides eosinophil infiltration of the lung or lymphoreticular organs, dead microfilariae are found surrounded by stellate, hyaline eosinophilic precipitates embedded in small epithelioid cell granulomas (Meyers-Kouvenaar bodies).

Epidemiologic data suggest that filarial infection is cumulative over time and that chronic disease requires regular exposure. Prevention of mosquito-borne infection is clearly the best hope for controlling filariasis. Several drugs can suppress microfilaremia, but as yet there is no effective drug treatment for advanced filarial lesions.

Onchocerciasis*

Onchocerca volvulus, the largest of the human filariae, reaches up to 50 cm in length; it is transmitted by blackflies (Simulium sp.) rather than by mosquitos. The adult worm preferentially nests in the subcutaneous tissue and discharges its microfilariae into the interstitium of the skin rather than into the blood. The adult worms may eventually elicit unsightly subcutaneous nodules, but the most significant lesions of onchocerciasis are blindness and dermatitis caused by millions of microfilariae accumulated in the skin and in the eye chambers. The disease is often manifested only by pruritus. Onchocerciasis occurs in Africa and parts of Yemen and in an area ranging from Southern Mexico to Northern Brazil.

Severe infection results in chronic dermatitis with focal darkening or loss of pigment in the skin and scaling; later there is epidermal atrophy or subcutaneous edema with redundancy and thickening of the dermis. These stages of dermatitis have been graphically named "leopard skin," "lizard skin," and "elephant skin."[231] Lymph nodes, especially those of the groin, may show lymphocyte depletion and fibrosis and this may be followed by elephantiasis ("hanging groin"), seen mainly in Africa; in Yemen, onchocerciasis is associated with a marked papular dermatitis and with greatly enlarged lymph nodes, usually involving only one extremity.[232] Severe dermatitis is much less common in Latin America, and the nodules more frequently localize in the upper part of the body, often overlying bony prominences.

Histologic reactions to the adult worms are initially exudative, but later become granulomatous and fibrotic and eventually may calcify (Fig. 7–60). Reactions to live microfilariae are scanty and predominantly mononuclear and eosinophilic. At the later stages of dermatitis, there is subcutaneous edema, epidermal thickening, and hyperkeratosis with patchy pigment incontinence or hyperpigmentation, and finally fibrosis and dermal atrophy. The progressive eye lesions begin with punctate keratitis along with small, fluffy opacities of the cornea caused by degenerating microfilariae, which evoke an eosinophilic infiltration. This is followed by sclerosing keratitis, which opacifies the cornea, beginning at the scleral limbus. In addition, microfilariae in the anterior eye chamber give rise to iridocyclitis, sometimes ending in glaucoma; involvement of the choroid and retina, although less frequent, eventually results in atrophy and

irreversible loss of vision, sometimes affecting the optic nerve itself.[231] Unfortunately, antimicrofilarial drugs can cause an allergic flareup of the skin and eye lesions (Mazzotti reaction).

Microfilariae reach the inner organs as well and can sometimes be detected in the urinary sediment, but diagnosis is usually made by skin biopsy and direct microscopy.

Minor Tropical Filariae (Loa, Mansonella, Dipetalonema Spp.)*

These species rarely cause incapacitating illness. *Loa Loa* elicits transitory skin swellings caused by migrating adult worms, preferentially beneath the conjunctiva (it is sometimes called the "eye worm"). *Dipetalonema streptocerca* may cause itchy skin nodules or lesions that can be confused with leprosy or onchocerciasis.[233] All the species give rise to eosinophilia, and sometimes fever. Diagnosis and treatment are the domain of experienced consultants.

Zoonotic Filariasis (Dirofilaria immitis, D. tenuis, North American Brugia)

Few physicians recall that biting arthropods can inoculate man with filariae adapted to other mammalian

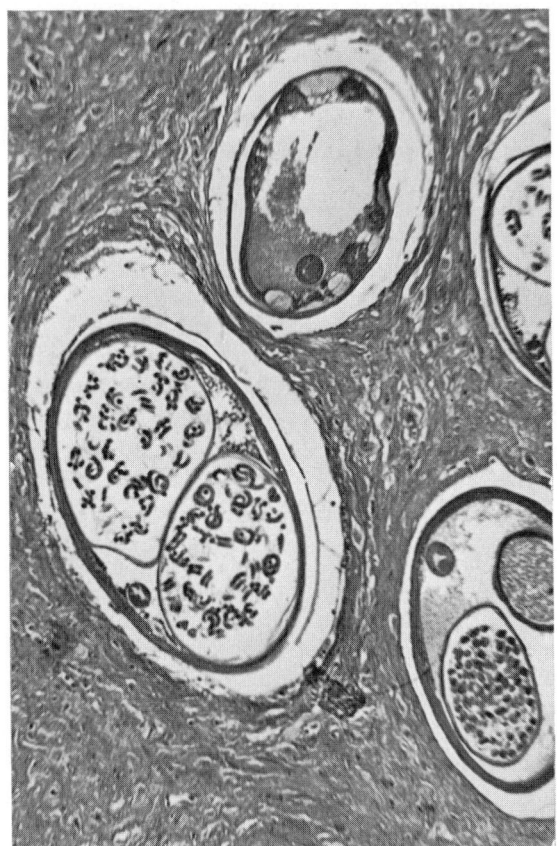

Figure 7–60. Onchocerciasis (Onchocerca volvulus) with gravid filaria enclosed in a subcutaneous fibrous nodule.

species. The dog heartworm, *D. immitis*, when transmitted to humans, develops only to its larval stage. Usually, a single larva is embolized from the right heart chambers into a pulmonary artery branch where it succumbs, giving rise to a small pulmonary infarct or coin lesion readily mistaken on x-ray examination for a tumor or other infection. Microscopically, such a lesion shows infarcted lung tissue in its center and granulomatous inflammation in its periphery; eosinophils may or may not abound in the specimen, and are rarely elevated in the blood. The causal worm in a feeding artery can easily be missed. The internal cuticular ridges of Dirofilaria, seen in cross section, are pathognomonic.[234]

Dirofilaria tenuis, a parasite of the raccoon, also causes abortive infections in man, in the form of either inflammatory subcutaneous nodules that come to surgery as presumed granulomas or dermatofibromas, or with other miscellaneous diagnoses. The conjunctiva has been a preferred site for *D. tenuis* larvae.[206] The larval worm occupies the center of the lesion, which is granulomatous and eosinophilic with marked peripheral fibrosis. *Dirofilaria immitis* is endemic throughout the United States, but *D. tenuis* infection prevails mostly in the South, especially in Florida.

North American Brugia, probably a parasite of the raccoon and the lynx, homes to lymph vessels and nodes. This infection has been reported along the Eastern seaboard from New York State to Quebec. The usual history is one of a single swollen lymph node, often in the neck or thoracic region, without any systemic manifestations. The differential diagnosis of lymphoma is often raised and the lymph node is then excised, resulting in cure. The correct diagnosis can be missed unless sufficient histologic sections are taken to discover a single, immature filaria, either intact or damaged, usually present at or near the lymph node hilus. The lymph node itself shows variable follicular hyperplasia, eosinophilia, or reticulosis. Peripheral eosinophilia is absent, and specific serologic tests are not yet available.[235]

None of the three animal filariae reviewed here is a common cause of disease nor do they cause serious human illnesses, but they can give rise to puzzling diagnostic problems.

CESTODES, TAPEWORMS

Tapeworms are intestinal parasitic flatworms (Platyhelminthes); some species may achieve lengths of 3 to 6 m. They possess a small head or scolex generating thousands of rectangular proglottids that articulate with each other and make up the bulk of the worm. *Human tapeworm infections take one of two forms:* (1) that in which the mature tapeworm is attached to the intestinal wall, and (2) that in which the larval forms invade the organs of the body to produce so-called larval cestodiasis.

Intestinal Tapeworm Infections

Among the many tapeworm species, four in particular may cause intestinal disease in man: *Taenia saginata* (beef), *T. solium* (pork), *Hymenolepis nana* (dwarf), and *Diphyllobothrium latum* (fish). Infection caused by these parasites is worldwide in distribution and is usually contracted by the ingestion of undercooked meat or fish. The meat of the intermediate host animals contains encysted larvae that excyst in the human intestinal tract and then mature into adults. These worms attach themselves to the bowel wall by their scolex, bearing hooks and sucker plates. The mature worm then progressively develops to the extraordinary lengths mentioned earlier. Adult tapeworms are well-adapted hermaphroditic parasites that seem to regulate their own numbers; thus, *T. solium* occurs singly as an example of "concomitant immunity." In many patients, tapeworms evoke no clinical signs or symptoms.

Clinical manifestations may arise, however, from (1) the physical mass of worms causing intestinal obstruction or (2) the competitive uptake of vitamin B_{12} to induce a megaloblastic anemia (p. 679). Systemic manifestations, including dizziness, restlessness, inability to concentrate on schoolwork, and others, have also been described.

The diagnosis of intestinal tapeworm infection is usually made by the finding of proglottids in the stools, more rarely by finding eggs, or by radiography (with contrast media) outlining the large tapeworms. Because all Taenia spp. eggs are similar, identification of the worm species depends on detailed examination of the proglottid. Careful stool examination is required after a vermifuge to make sure that the worm's scolex has been expelled, because otherwise the worm will regenerate. The scolex can be removed by colonoscopy,[236] but a good vermifuge can do the same job with less effort.

Cysticercosis

Man becomes the *definitive host* of the adult tapeworm, *T. solium*, by acquiring its *larvae* from pork meat. By contrast, unwitting ingestion of Taenia *eggs* deposited on fecally contaminated vegetables or self-contamination with such eggs converts man into the *intermediate host*. This is a more serious condition because each ingested egg spawns a hexacanth embryo, which penetrates the gut and is disseminated through the blood to develop into a cystic larva (cysticercus) in any body site, including the CNS or heart. Depending on the number and location of *cysticerci*, infections vary from inconsequential to life-threatening.

Cysticerci may be found in any organ, but preferred localizations are the brain, muscles, skin, and heart. They are ovoid, white-to-opalescent parasite cysts, rarely exceeding 1.5 cm in size, which contain an invaginated scolex bathed in clear cyst fluid (Fig. 7–61). The cyst wall is over 100 μm thick, is rich in glycoproteins, and evokes remarkably little host reaction as long as it remains intact. Once implanted, cysticerci endure in their dormant condition for many years, but eventually degenerate or break open and induce granuloma formation, focal scarring, and calcifica-

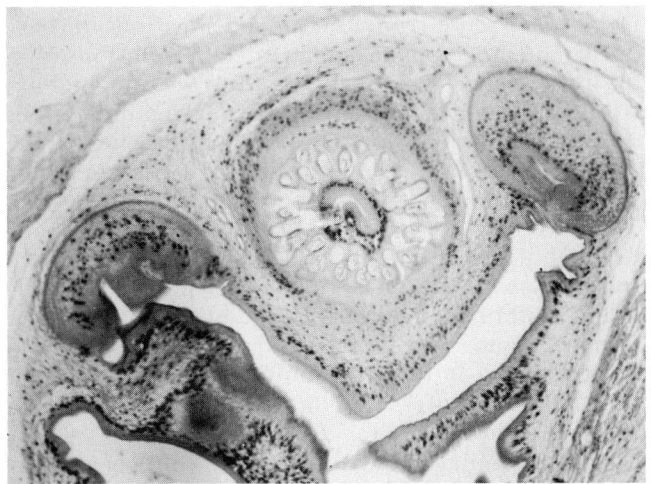

Figure 7–61. Cysticercus in subcutaneous tissue showing inverted scolex with sectioned hooklets *(center)* **and suction cups** *(both sides).*

tion, sometimes visible on radiographs as round, opaque densities. Rarely, a cysticercus may proliferate to larger size or to a branching, racemose stage.

Subcutaneous cysticerci form palpable nodules and are often removed by excision biopsy, after which the larvae can be visualized. Even degenerate cysticerci are recognizable by their many tiny, sharktooth-shaped birefringent hooklets, which are nearly indestructible. The finding of cutaneous cysts virtually guarantees CNS involvement, but the converse is not true. Cysts may involve the meninges, gray or white matter, sometimes even the sylvian aqueduct or ventricular foramina so as to block spinal fluid circulation.

Neurologic symptoms are protean, seizures being the most common. Occasionally, a cysticercus floating in a ventricle causes a rise of intracranial pressure and headache each time the patient lies down. Cysticerci of the psychomotor cortex may cause tumor-like localizing signs, but these are often absent even in heavy infections. Whether personality or psychiatric abnormalities can ensue from cysticercosis is controversial.[237] Bizarre symptoms also occasionally arise from myocardial cysticercosis. CT scans have greatly increased diagnostic accuracy and, in combination with x-ray studies, can detect both mild and severe CNS cysticercosis. An improved serologic test (ELISA) is also available. Thus, for the first time, large numbers of infected patients are now being found in the American Southwest and urban Northeast, many among Hispanics or Koreans. The problem is vastly greater in countries where there is fecal contamination of agricultural soil and where pork is a prized item in the diet. (The larvae of *T. saginata*, the cattle tapeworm, do not thrive in man.) Appropriate drug therapy with praziquantel effectively suppresses this parasite but has no effect on old or calcified foci.[238] Although infected persons show dermal hypersensitivity to cyst fluid, allergic or hypereosinophilic episodes are uncommon in cysticercosis.

Echinococcosis (Hydatid Disease)

Adult tapeworms of the genus Echinococcus are small and give their canine hosts little trouble. The intermediary hosts, including man, bear the brunt of the disease. Man becomes the accidental host by ingesting canine tapeworm eggs; these hatch in the duodenum, releasing invasive embryos that traverse the mucosa, enter portal branches, and are swept first into the liver, then to any other organ of the body. After long periods of silent growth, large parasitic cysts— *hydatids*—are formed in the liver and elsewhere; these can cause disease by compressing vital structures, by spilling allergenic cyst fluid, or by spawning proliferative "daughter cysts" that engage in tumor-like parasite growth. Bacterial superinfection converts the cyst into a large abscess. The disease, therefore, presents in many diverse clinical forms.

Echinococcus granulosus, causing unilocular hydatid cysts, is the most prevalent species. Its European strain cycles between dogs and sheep. Human infection is cosmopolitan, but is most common in the sheep-raising areas of the western United States, Australia, New Zealand, Argentina, the eastern Mediterranean, and the Near East. A Northern strain of this parasite has a wild-animal cycle involving wolves and deer; human cases are seen mainly in subarctic regions, including Alaska, Canada, and Siberia, and are usually quite severe. Two other echinococci are transmitted only by feral cycles. *Echinococcus multilocularis* is transmitted to moles and rodents by wild canines and sled dogs. In man, it causes *multilocular* (or alveolar) *hydatid cysts with unrestricted budding and without scolices,* which invade the liver much like a malignant tumor. This species shares the Arctic distribution of *E. granulosus*, but also exists in central and eastern Europe. *Echinococcus vogeli*, cycled between wild dogs and pacas, is responsible for multilocular hydatids in northern Latin America and Panama.[239]

About two thirds of human *E. granulosus* cysts are found in the liver, 5 to 15% in the lung, and the rest in bones, brain, or other organs. In the various organs, the larvae lodge within the capillaries and first incite an inflammatory reaction composed principally of mononuclear leukocytes and eosinophils. Many such larvae are destroyed, but others encyst. The cysts begin at microscopic levels and progressively increase in size, so that in five years or more they may have achieved dimensions over 10 cm in diameter. Enclosing an opalescent fluid is an inner, nucleated, germinative layer and an outer, opaque, non-nucleated layer. **The outer non-nucleated layer is quite distinctive and has innumerable delicate laminations** as though made up of many layers of gelatin. Outside this opaque layer, there is a host inflammatory reaction that produces a zone of fibroblasts, giant cells, and mononuclear and eosinophilic cells. In time, a dense fibrous capsule forms. When these cysts have been present for about six months, "daughter cysts" develop within them. These appear first as minute projections of the germinative layer, which develop central vesicles and thus form tiny "brood capsules."

Scolices of the worm develop on the inner aspects of these brood capsules and separate from the germinative layer to produce a fine, sandlike sediment within the hydatid fluid (Fig. 7–62).

This is the sequence followed in the soft tissues, such as the liver, that permit the progressive enlargement of the cyst. When the original implantation occurs in bone, the hydatid vesicle usually develops near the epiphyseal end or in vertebrae and flat bones. Fibrous adventitial encapsulation of the larva does not occur, and as it grows and develops it permeates the spongy trabeculation of the bone to produce multiple microcystic diverticula. The intervening fragments of bone undergo pressure atrophy and frequently the bone cortex is eroded, so that spontaneous fractures are not uncommon. Cysts that locate in the lung eventually erode into bronchi and are dramatically coughed up, fluid, membrane, and all; this sometimes results in spontaneous cure, but, rarely, freak penetration of a cyst into pulmonary vessels or heart chambers may cause lethal embolism. Liver and other abdominal cysts eventually become leaky, resulting in sterile inflammation or bacterial superinfection. This causes shrinkage, fibrosis, and eventual calcification of the cyst and destruction of the parasite structure, with only the pathognomonic, hooklet-bearing, degenerate scolices remaining intact amid the pastelike, yellow, cholesterol-rich debris. Cyst rupture into a large bile duct can result in acute cholangitis or cholecystitis.

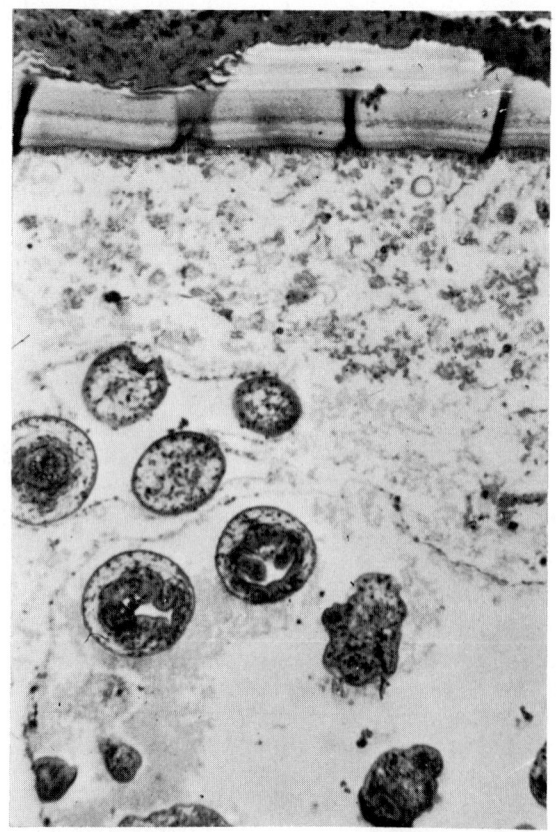

Figure 7–62. Echinococcosis. Wall of a cyst with laminated outer layer and inner germinative layer *(above)*. The cystic lumen contains many daughter "brood capsules."

As is evident from its many localizations, disease due to the dog tapeworm may present in various mystifying guises. The clinical symptoms of unilocular hydatid disease derive mainly from its complications (e.g., from compression of or rupture into vital structures). Except in the brain or heart, the parenchymal atrophy caused by the gradual expansion of the cyst can be remarkably silent. However, external leakage of cyst fluid caused by trauma or surgical spillage can spark an acute anaphylactic attack with severe allergic symptoms accompanied by hypereosinophilia. Surgical removal of these cysts is hazardous because spillage can also result in multiple cysts throughout the abdomen, unless they are sterilized by injection before excision.

Eosinophilia may or may not be present. Serologic tests for *E. granulosus* antigen and antibodies have been much improved, and CT scans have greatly increased the accuracy of diagnosis. Drug therapy is moderately successful in sterilizing the cysts, but some have to be surgically removed.

Echinococcus multilocularis larvae, which generate *alveolar cysts* with budding and invasive growth in the human liver, cause manifestations virtually indistinguishable from those of a primary liver cell tumor; the cysts can, in fact, invade the caval or portal veins or metastasize to the lung. Various combinations of drugs and surgery have been tried in this unusual infection with only moderate success. The untreated disease has been 100% lethal.

TREMATODES (FLUKES)

Fascioliasis (Liver Fluke, *Fasciola hepatica*)

Human fascioliasis is caused by the hermaphroditic flatworm *F. hepatica* (in Hawaii also *F. gigantica*), a trematode (fluke) normally adapted to sheep and cattle. The disease is acquired by eating watercress contaminated with the metacercarial form of the parasite. Its acute stage, marked by fever and abdominal pain, results from tissue migration and maturation of worms that eventually settle in the lumen of the gallbladder or bile ducts; the chronic stage is characterized by biliary obstructive symptoms. The disease is worldwide in both temperate and tropical zones; in the United States it is most frequent in Puerto Rico.[240]

The leaf-shaped adult parasites are up to 4 cm long; in the lumen of the biliary tree, they produce inflammation, intermittent obstruction, and dilatation with considerable thickening of the wall. *Fasciola hepatica* releases large amounts of proline, presumed to stimulate bile duct or gallbladder hyperplasia and fibrosis. The operculated Fasciola eggs, excreted via the feces, are diagnostic, although rarely present in large numbers.

In the United States, most cases are sporadic, but in European countries where family farms are more prevalent, larger community outbreaks have occurred, usually three months after consumption of contaminated watercress (the time needed for maturation of the flukes). The early symptoms of the acute disease are malaise, intermittent fever, night sweats, weight loss, and right upper quadrant pain and are not distinctive; not all patients show eosinophilia or urticarial rashes or elevated erythrocyte sedimentation rates. The acute phase is self-terminating, but treatment with drugs will shorten its course and prevent later biliary obstructive complications that include colicky pain, jaundice, and bacterial superinfection. Occasionally, ectopic migration of worms produces painful subcutaneous nodules.

> During the early migratory phase of fascioliasis, there is hepatomegaly with hemorrhagic-necrotic worm tracts, best seen in the subcapsular portion of the liver and sometimes resulting in peritoneal hemorrhage also. These lesions are replete with eosinophils and other inflammatory cells, but they ultimately heal, leaving only minor scars. Chronic Fasciola cholecystitis and cholangitis resemble the lesions caused by biliary calculi, but often show marked local eosinophilic infiltration, and there is hyperplasia of the bile duct epithelium, which is thrown into redundant infoldings. In the human liver, pericholangitis and periportal fibrosis are usually minimal.

With replacement of family farming by agribusiness in the United States, fascioliasis is destined to vanish. Meanwhile, it continues sporadically to pose a diagnostic and epidemiologic challenge.

Clonorchiasis and Opisthorchiasis*

These two smaller liver flukes (up to 1.5 cm long) differ from *F. hepatica* in many respects: (1) they are acquired by the eating of raw freshwater fish or crayfish that harbor metacercariae; (2) they commonly infect man, dogs, and cats in large numbers; (3) they colonize the small and large intrahepatic bile ducts and therefore produce chronic cholangitis with extensive liver damage and intrahepatic gallstones; and (4) they are associated with a high frequency of cholangiocarcinoma (p. 959).

Clonorchis sinensis is widespread in the Far East, ranging from Korea and Japan to the countries that were formerly termed Indochina, and is especially common in Hong Kong. *Opisthorchis viverrini* is hyperendemic in parts of Thailand and Laos. *Opisthorchis felineus* is reported mainly from Poland and the Soviet Union. Oriental liver fluke disease lacks an early tissue-invasive phase but instead develops in a chronic and insidious fashion. Persons infected by few worms may remain asymptomatic indefinitely. In heavier infections, anorexia, diarrhea, slight jaundice, and right upper quadrant discomfort are the most common complaints. Liver enlargement and eosinophilia may be present. Only by cholangiography or arteriography can the marked anatomic changes be appreciated: the hepatic vessels are stretched and narrowed, whereas the ducts show multiple irregularities and narrowings, often with berry-like dilations.

Sometimes the shadows caused by the leaf-shaped worms are also visible. Diagnosis is made by finding the tiny (30 μm), thick-walled, operculated eggs of these parasites in the stools.

> At autopsy, the liver is often enlarged; on section, it shows irregularly dilated bile ducts lined by fibrous tissue. The parasites can sometimes be flushed out and examined by compressing the organ, but more often they are found only microscopically. In complicated cases, there is often cholestasis, bacterial superinfection, or multiple stone formation. In the earliest lesions, microscopic evidence of inflammation of the bile ducts is usually modest, and eosinophilia is uncommon. Unlike schistosome eggs (p. 424), the tightly sealed eggs of the liver flukes cause little or no granulomatous inflammation. However, metaplasia and proliferation of the bile duct epithelium are marked and there is periductal fibrosis.[241] The gallbladder may also be parasitized and inflamed, especially in *O. viverrini* infection. In some cases the pancreatic ducts show epithelial metaplasia and partial obstruction, but the large, extrahepatic bile ducts are seldom abnormal. Cholangiocarcinoma, a rare tumor in the West, is a common form of cancer where Oriental liver flukes are endemic.

Therapeutic agents are available that are likely to diminish morbidity in the future; prevention of fecal contamination of fish ponds by humans and domestic animals is the long-term solution.

Fasciolopsiasis*

The large intestinal fluke *Fasciolopsis buski* (up to 7 cm long) localizes principally within the small bowel, where it usually causes rather mild inflammatory changes. For the most part these infections are found in India and China and other countries around the Indian Ocean. The pig is a major reservoir. When humans or animals deposit eggs in fresh water, a larval form, the miracidium, hatches and invades an appropriate snail. Within this host, the larvae are transformed to cercariae, which upon leaving the snail become encysted on water plants.

> Man contracts the infection by the ingestion of the contaminated plants or water. The cysts are dissolved in the upper intestinal tract, and the larval forms emerge, mature into adult worms, and become attached to the mucosa of the small bowel by means of their suckers. At the local sites of involvement, a hemorrhagic inflammation ensues which is at first fairly nonspecific, although characterized principally by eosinophils. As these focal injuries progress, actual abscesses may develop in the mucosa, with considerable destruction of the intestinal mucosa.

As a consequence of these anatomic lesions in the small bowel, patients often have abdominal pain and diarrhea. When the infection is very severe, a generalized, constitutional febrile reaction sometimes appears, accompanied by facial and periorbital edema.

Very infrequently, tangled masses of worms may produce acute intestinal obstruction. Diagnosis is made by identification of the characteristic eggs in the feces.

Paragonimiasis (Lung Fluke, Pulmonary Distomiasis)*

Flukes of the genus Paragonimus are small flatworms, 1.2 cm long, which cause cystic and inflammatory lesions mainly in the lung, more rarely in the brain and abdominal and other organs. Uncooked crabs and crayfish containing the metacercarial form are the main sources of human infection, and the parasite's life cycle is maintained by many hosts, including dogs, cats, and humans. Chronic cough, bronchiectasis, and hemoptysis are the most common manifestations. Formerly believed to be due to a single species (*P. westermani*) and limited to the Far East and Philippines, paragonimiasis caused by five other species has now been found in many parts of the tropics, including Central and South America and West Africa. In the United States clinical cases in Asian immigrants have recently increased in number.

Paragonimus eggs are coughed up, swallowed, and excreted with the feces. They hatch in water and release their miracidia, which then enter several susceptible snail species and develop into cercariae. When liberated, these attack various second intermediate crustacean hosts in which they encyst, to be eaten by man or other definitive hosts.

The ingested young flukes excyst and traverse the gut wall, peritoneum, and diaphragm on their way to the lung, usually without causing significant lesions or symptoms; however, parasites that die in ectopic locations can give rise to focal abscesses (e.g., in the gut wall, pancreas, or brain). Such ectopic lesions are most common in heavily infected individuals; cerebral paragonimiasis, simulating brain tumors, epilepsy, or meningitis, is therefore most common in highly endemic areas such as Korea, Japan, and parts of China, where local brain calcifications are frequent x-ray findings. Once arrived in their definitive habitat, the lung, the parasites incite an encapsulating inflammatory host reaction rich in eosinophils and then form multiple cysts, each a few centimeters in size. Here they lay large numbers of thick-shelled, operculated eggs, which add to the inflammatory process by inciting a granulomatous reaction. Sooner or later, Paragonimus cysts rupture into bronchioles, and their eggs, together with exudate and blood, begin to be expectorated or swallowed.[242] Chronic bronchial irritation by the long-lived worms and their eggs and by occasional dead parasites then leads to focal organizing pneumonitis and bronchiectasis. There frequently is bacterial superinfection. At this stage, the clinical picture often simulates tuberculosis, and in the Orient these two infections frequently coexist. Pure paragonimiasis less frequently involves the lung apices and subpleural parenchyma than does tuberculous infection. Abdominal symptoms are rarely present without significant pulmonary pathology.

Histopathologically, the lesions of paragonimiasis are varied. The cysts in the lungs (Fig. 7–63) form abscess-like collections of eosinophils mixed with Charcot-Leyden crystals. In the cyst wall and around eggs extruded from cysts, granulomas arise. Similar changes are seen in cerebral and ectopic Paragonimus lesions. Fibrous scarring then ensues, extending outward in radial fashion to further complicate the picture. Peripheral blood eosinophilia is inconstant, and diagnosis depends almost exclusively on identification of the parasite eggs in the sputum or feces.

The severity of the disease depends on the intensity of infection and ranges from mild to lethal. Clinical diagnosis is difficult, sometimes recognizable only when the characteristic lung cysts containing brownish material are visualized in a surgical or autopsy specimen, or when eggs are demonstrated on a smear of sputum or bronchial secretion.

Schistosomiasis (Bilharziasis)*

Man is the host of several species of schistosomes that reproduce sexually in the venous bloodstream. The adult parasites are well adapted to their human habitat and cause few changes, but the numerous eggs they lay elicit hypersensitivity granulomas in many

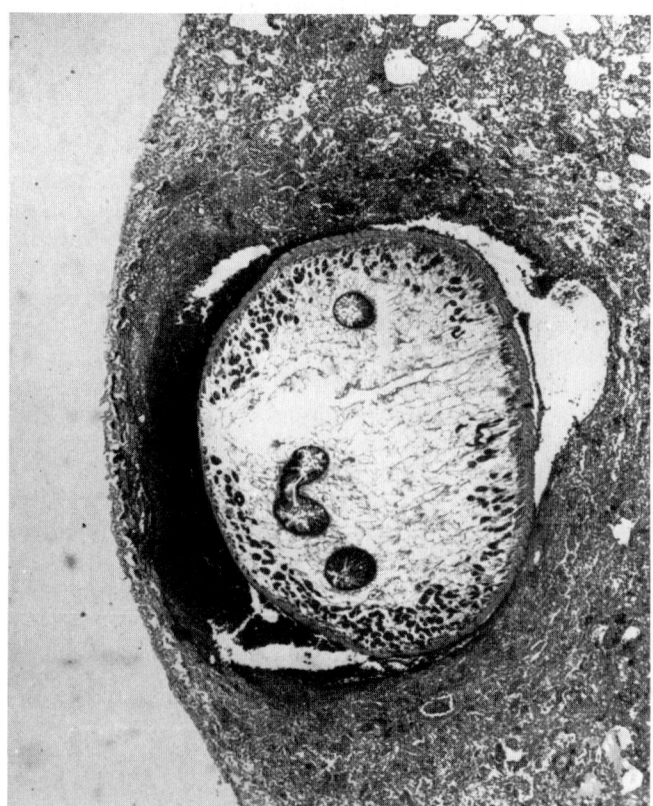

Figure 7–63. Paragonimiasis: adult worm in lung cyst, surrounded by acute hemorrhage. (Courtesy of Professor Muneo Yokogawa, Chiba University, Japan.)

organs; these ultimately result in fibrosis of the liver or in obstructive uropathy, and less frequently in lesions of other organs, including the CNS. The disease occurs throughout the tropics wherever the parasite's specific snail intermediate hosts are found. Of the 250 million people estimated to bear these infections, about 5% may suffer severe disease. Schistosomiasis therefore ranks high among the chronic endemic infections of mankind.[243]

Six schistosome species are known to infect man. The major ones are *Schistosoma mansoni* (Africa, Latin America, the Caribbean, parts of the Near East); *S. japonicum* (China, the Philippines, other parts of the Far East); and *S. haematobium* (Africa and parts of the Near East). Most species seek the portal vein branches as their habitat, but *S. haematobium* prefers the pelvic vena caval tributaries. Several species, but not *S. mansoni*, can also naturally infect animal reservoir hosts other than nonhuman primates, and several animal schistosomes can cause abortive human infections in which the parasites die largely in the skin, giving rise to a hypersensitivity dermatitis named "swimmer's itch" or cercarial dermatitis. This self-terminating disorder occurs in both temperate and tropical settings, including the United States.

Endemic human schistosomiasis is transmitted by water contact. The free-swimming, fork-tailed *cercariae* released by infected snails quickly burrow through the human epidermis, converting to young worms or *schistosomula*. These enter the bloodstream, pausing in the lung at four to 14 days, and continue recycling until they reach the intrahepatic portal radicles where they mature, finally descending into the mesenteric or pelvic venules where they begin their mating and egg-laying. Schistosome eggs measure up to 150 μm in length, too large to traverse capillaries; they are faintly yellow and translucent with a terminal *(S. haematobium)* or lateral *(S. mansoni)* spine, and contain a miracidial embryo. When mature eggs are deposited in water with human feces or urine, the miracidium hatches and seeks the specific intermediate snail host in which the asexual part of the life cycle is completed, culminating in the re-emergence of *cercariae* (Fig. 7–64). The early stages of infection are usually silent, but a fleeting rash may sometimes mark the penetration sites, and sometimes cough, fever, eosinophilia, and asthma-like symptoms appear. Each fertilized female can lay up to 500 eggs per day. The 1.5-cm long adults, wedged into a venule near the gut or urinary lumen, expel eggs, and these are either extruded into the feces or urine, caught in the wall of the conduit, or swept back by the bloodstream into the liver or lung. Although this early stage of the infection is usually asymptomatic, some individuals, often visitors from outside the endemic area, become febrile during this period, with high eosinophilia, hepatosplenomegaly, diarrhea, or allergic manifestations: this symptom complex is named acute schistosomiasis, toxemic schistosomiasis, or Katayama fever (in Japan). It, too, reverses spontaneously over several weeks and, as oviposition and egg excretion

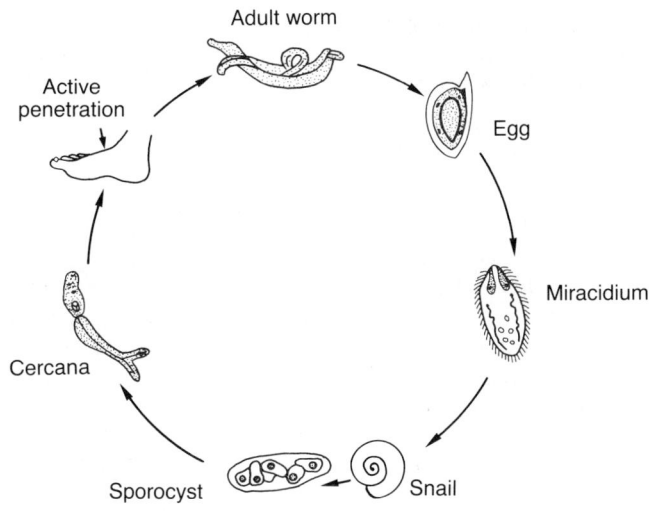

SCHISTOSOMAL LIFE CYCLE

Figure 7–64.

continue, the disease then enters a period of clinical latency. In most light infections, latency continues indefinitely; in severe ones, chronic disease makes its appearance years later.

PATHOGENESIS. Adult schistosomes do not incite significant host tissue reactions until they die or are killed by drugs. The dead parasites give rise to scattered, large, necrotic granulomas; there are too few in number to explain the manifestations of the disease. By contrast, the eggs, often numbered in millions, are known to release soluble antigens through their porous egg shells during their two- to three-week life span, thus inciting host cellular immunity and hypersensitivity. Those eggs that impact in small vessels are soon surrounded by granulomas containing macrophages and lymphoid and granulocytic elements, which are rich in eosinophils. Schistosome granulomas (Fig. 7–65) attain diameters of 500 μm or more, and thus they encroach on vessels and parenchymal tissues. However, as the infection turns chronic, granuloma sizes decrease through a complex regulatory process of immune modulation. After several weeks, schistosome eggs die and are destroyed. Each individual granuloma then heals with or without fibrous scarring, but new crops of granulomas continue appearing until the adult worms are killed or rendered infertile. Schistosome granulomas are immunologic and biochemical "factories" processing parasite egg antigens and somatic components and generating a host of enzymes, lymphokines, and other mediators.[244] They have served as useful experimental models of cell-mediated hypersensitivity; however, the manner in which the severe fibrotic lesions of chronic schistosomiasis derive from these focal lesions is still uncertain except for a clear relationship to the magnitude of worm and egg burdens.

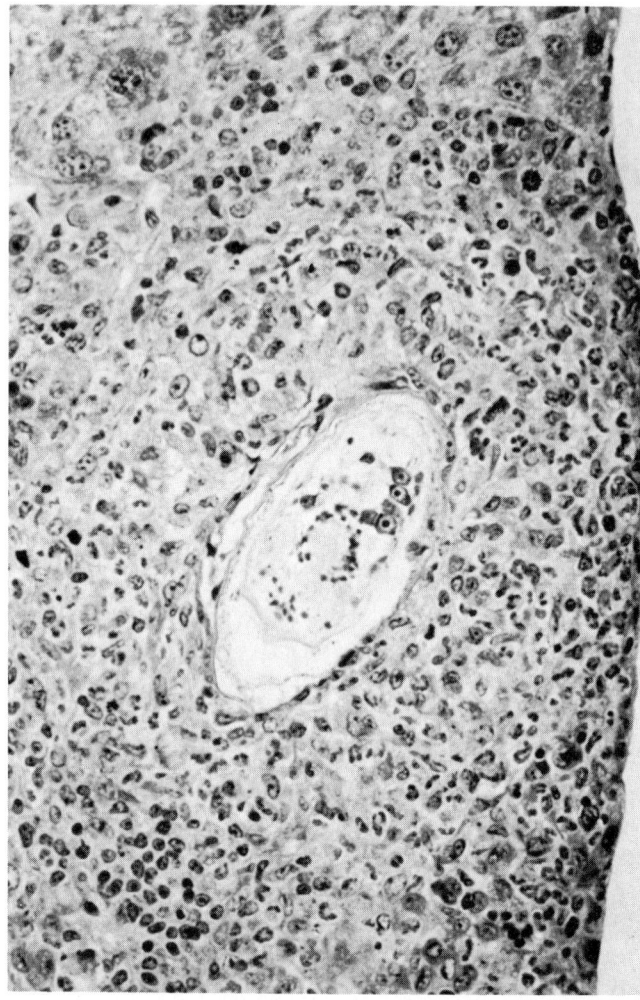

Figure 7-65. *Schistosoma mansoni* granuloma with miracidium-containing egg *(center)* and numerous scattered eosinophils.

brosis.''[245] Some portal triads may lack a perceptible vein lumen, and latex casts show widespread distortion and blockage of the portal vascular bed (Fig. 7-66). This accounts for pre-sinusoidal portal hypertension along with severe congestive splenomegaly, esophageal varices, superficial venous collaterals, and ascites. Jaundice, hepatocellular necrosis, and dysfunction tend to follow only after variceal hemorrhage has taken place.

Schistosome eggs diverted to the lung via portal collaterals, when large in number, may produce granulomatous pulmonary arteritis as they impact, leading to intimal hyperplasia, progressive arterial obstruction, and ultimately heart failure (cor pulmonale). Histologically, arteries in the lungs show disruption of the elastica layer by granulomas and scars, luminal organizing thrombi, and angiomatoid lesions similar to those of idiopathic pulmonary hypertension (p. 764). In addition, patients with hepatosplenic Manson's schistosomiasis have an increased frequency of mesangioproliferative or membranous glomerulopathy, and some glomeruli show deposits of immunoglobulin or complement, but rarely of schistosome antigen.[246]

In *S. haematobium* infection, the pathologic conditions differ sharply from those of Oriental and Manson's schistosomiasis. Bladder inflammatory patches due to massed egg deposition may appear early, and later they become rough sandy or fibrous patches. When these lesions become confluent, the entire bladder mucosa may become surrounded by a calcified egg layer, visible radiographically as a dense concentric rim (calcified bladder). Inflammation and fibrosis similarly invade the ureteral wall, leading to multiple ureteral stenoses or to irregular dilatation and hydronephrosis. Owing to their patchy distribution, *S. haematobium* eggs, even when small in number, can obstruct the lower ureters. During the early inflammatory stage, these

MORPHOLOGY. The lesions of schistosomiasis vary by species, intensity of infection, and stage. Asymptomatic subjects with light *S. mansoni* or *S. japonicum* infections may have only scattered eggs and granulomas in the gut, liver, and lung, with sporadic eggs elsewhere in the body. Pinhead-sized, white granuloma nodules are best seen beneath the liver capsule; often, the liver is darkened by regurgitated heme-derived pigment from the hematophagous schistosome gut. Like malaria pigment, schistosome pigment is Prussian blue-negative, and it accumulates in Kupffer cells and splenic macrophages without any known adverse consequences.

In severe **schistosomiasis mansoni** or **japonica,** inflammatory patches or pseudopolyps may form in the colon. The liver is dark in color, showing a bumpy but not a nodular surface, distinct from that of ordinary cirrhosis. In addition to granulomas, the cut surface of the organ shows widespread fibrous portal enlargement without distortion of the intervening parenchyma by regenerative nodules. The cut surfaces of the fibrous triads simulate the cross section of a clay pipe stem, giving rise to the term ''pipe-stem fi-

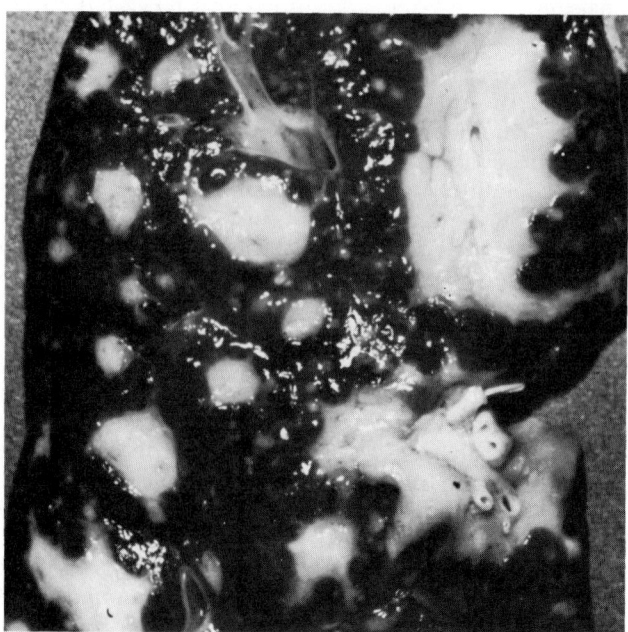

Figure 7-66. Liver pipe-stem fibrosis due to chronic *Schistosoma japonicum* infection.

lesions are reversible, but eventually reflux nephropathy (p. 1056) with interstitial inflammation, cortical atrophy, or bacterial superinfection may result in renal failure and death. This is common in hyperendemic Egypt but seen less often in subsaharan Africa. There is also a demonstrable association between urinary schistosomiasis and bladder cancer; the tumors occur in younger persons and are predominantly squamous rather than the transitional cell type (p. 1090).[247] By contrast, the severe liver and lung lesions of *S. mansoni* and *S. japonicum* infections are rare in urinary schistosomiasis.

Ectopic egg deposition has been reported in many organs, usually without major consequences, but *S. japonicum* infection of the brain or meninges can give rise to scattered or massed egg lesions and to miscellaneous neurologic symptoms. *Schistosoma mansoni* and, more rarely, *S. haematobium* eggs can mass in the spinal cord or cauda equina, with consequences ranging from transverse spinal cord necrosis to transient paralysis. These latter lesions are unrelated to the intensity or duration of schistosome infection and constitute a cogent argument for treating even lightly infected patients.

CLINICAL COURSE. Schistosomiasis mansoni is an insidious, chronic disease. In its endemic areas infected children may appear reasonably well, although they often have significant hepatomegaly. Albuminuria is somewhat more frequent in asymptomatic infected than in uninfected individuals. Hematuria is the first indication of *S. haematobium* infection, and it is so common in parts of Africa that it is regarded as a normal sign of puberty. The peak incidence of severe hepatosplenic schistosomiasis with portal hypertension and the obstructive uropathy of urinary schistosomiasis is during the early twenties, at a time when egg excretion may already have begun to decline. Superinfection with hepatitis B virus, frequent in the tropics, is known to aggravate and modify schistosomal liver disease. All too often, patients come to medical attention only after experiencing a life-threatening esophageal hemorrhage or when already showing a rising blood urea nitrogen (BUN) level. Others may present with anemia, hypersplenism, and retarded somatic development. Some are diagnosed and treated in their teens for protein-losing enteropathy due to schistosomal colonic polyposis, a disease form seen mainly in Near Eastern countries. The infection can also masquerade in other confusing ways.

Diagnosis is best made by finding the characteristic eggs in the feces or urine. Concentration methods are useful when eggs are scarce. Rectal biopsy, compressed between slide and coverglass and examined unstained, is sometimes necessary. Liver biopsy can be useful, but needle biopsy should not be used to determine whether pipe-stem fibrosis is present; that evaluation is best made by ultrasound study. A profusion of serologic tests for schistosomiasis exists; those employing egg antigens are the most reliable,[248] but parasitologic diagnosis is to be preferred because quantitative stool or urine egg counts render a useful estimate of the infection load. Treatment with newer drugs has been highly effective and often curative.

SARCOIDOSIS (OR BOECK'S SARCOID)

This very common condition, although not an infectious disease, is included here because of its histologic similarity to several infectious disorders, notably tuberculosis.

Sarcoidosis is a disease of unknown cause characterized by noncaseating granulomas in many tissues and organs.[249] Other diseases, including mycobacterial or fungal infections and berylliosis, can also produce "hard" granulomas; therefore, the histologic diagnosis of sarcoidosis must be made by exclusion. Sarcoidosis can involve many systems and organs and present in many clinical guises, but bilateral hilar lymphadenopathy or lung involvement is visible on chest radiographs in 90% of cases. Eye and skin lesions are next in frequency.

The prevalence of sarcoidosis is higher in females than in males but varies widely in different countries and populations. It has been estimated at 30 cases per 10^5 in New York City versus 64 per 10^5 in Stockholm. Among residents of North London, the prevalence per 10^5 population was 27 for United Kingdom natives, 97 for Irish, and 200 for West Indians. In the United States, the rates are highest in southeastern states; they are ten times higher in American blacks than in whites. By contrast, among Chinese and Southeast Asians, the disease is almost unknown.

ETIOLOGY AND PATHOGENESIS. The distinctive granulomatous tissue response seen in sarcoidosis suggests an immunologically mediated disease. Many causal agents have been proposed over the years (atypical mycobacteria, pine pollen, and so forth) and have fallen by the wayside, with current research being focused mainly on the possibility of an unknown virus. Meanwhile, several abnormal immunologic features have been found to be unique to sarcoidosis: Most patients manifest cutaneous anergy, not only to tuberculin but also to chemical cutaneous allergens, such as 2,3-dinitrochlorobenzene; peripheral blood T lymphocytes are sufficiently reduced in number to cause an absolute lymphopenia, and the proportion of circulating T-helper cells to T-suppressors is reduced from 2:1 to 0.8:1, whereas circulating B cells are normal in number and are in fact hyperreactive. All these findings indicate that patients with sarcoidosis have *deficient T-cell responses, but only in the peripheral blood.* When cell populations are obtained from *active lung lesions* by bronchoalveolar lavage and studied, the number of T cells at the site of the lesions is found to be *markedly increased with a ratio of 10 T-helpers to one T-suppressor* and these T cells are clearly activated. These uncontrolled T-helper cells and their lymphokines could well account for influx of monocytes, alveolitis, and noncaseating granuloma formation in the lung and for the resulting progressive fibrosis, all characteristic features of pulmonary sarcoidosis.[250] In sum, although the etiologic agent(s) of sarcoidosis remains unknown, there is evidence that patients who develop this disease show an inherently abnormal immunologic dissociation between local and peripheral T-cell responses.

MORPHOLOGY. Pathologic involvement of virtually every organ in the body has been cited at one time or another.[251]

Lymph nodes are involved in almost all cases. The most typical groups affected are the hilar and mediastinal nodes, but any other node in the body may be involved, particularly the cervical, epitrochlear, preauricular, and postauricular nodes. The tonsils are affected in about one quarter to one third of cases. The nodes are characteristically enlarged, discrete, and sometimes lobulated. When viewed on chest x-ray films, the bilateral hilar lymphadenopathy is referred to as "potato nodes." Typically, the affected nodes in the acute stages of the disease are soft and succulent, but in the more advanced, chronic stages they may become somewhat fibrotic. Histologically, all involved nodes show the classic **noncaseating granulomas** (Fig. 7–67). These are made up of an aggregate of tightly clustered epithelioid cells, often with Langhans' or foreign body–type giant cells. Rarely, some central nerosis is present.

In chronic disease, the granulomas may become enclosed within fibrous rims or eventually be replaced by hyaline fibrous scars. Two other microscopic features are often present in the granulomas: (1) laminated concretions com-

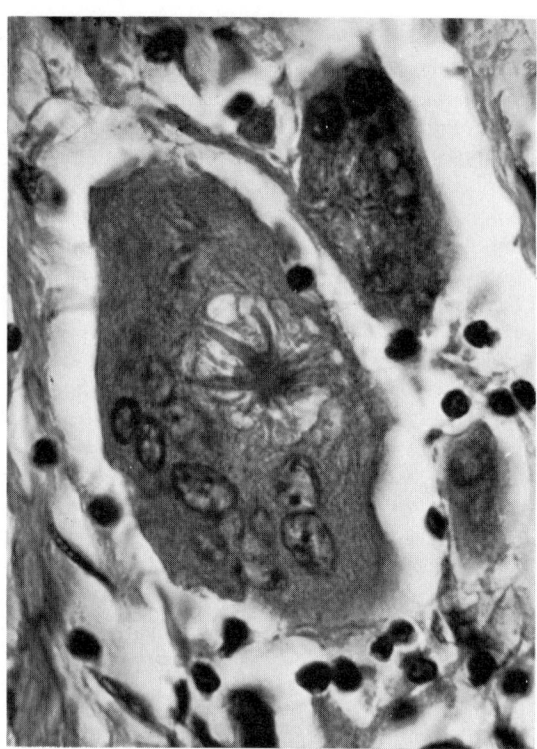

Figure 7–68. Characteristic asteroid body within a giant cell.

posed of calcium and proteins known as Schaumann bodies, and (2) stellate inclusions known as asteroid bodies enclosed within giant cells (Fig. 7–68). The latter are found in approximately 60% of the granulomas. None of these microscopic features is pathognomonic of sarcoidosis, because asteroid and Schaumann bodies may be encountered in other granulomatous diseases (e.g., berylliosis) (p. 67).

The **lungs** are common sites of involvement. Macroscopically, there is usually no demonstrable alteration, although at times the coalescence of granulomas may produce small nodules that are palpable or visible as 1- to 2-cm, noncaseating, noncavitated consolidations. Histologically, the lesions are distributed throughout the parenchyma, usually bilaterally, with some tendency to localize about blood vessels, bronchi, and lymphatics. In occasional cases cellular proliferative granulomas are present, but there appears to be a strong tendency for lesions to heal in the lungs, so that more often varying stages of fibrosis and hyalinization are found, causing interstitial pulmonary fibrosis (p. 789). There is, in fact, a strong suspicion that, in many cases of systemic sarcoidosis in which the lungs are not apparently involved at postmortem examination, previous lesions may have been present but have since disappeared. The pleural surfaces are sometimes involved.

The **spleen** is affected microscopically in about three quarters of the cases, but it is enlarged in only 18%. On occasion, granulomas may coalesce to form small nodules that are barely visible macroscopically. The capsule is not involved.

The **liver** is affected slightly less often than the spleen. It

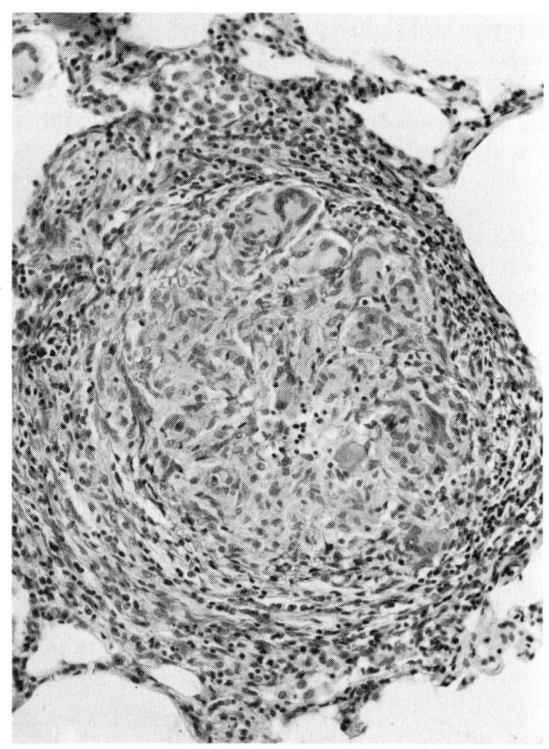

Figure 7–67. A characteristic sarcoid noncaseating granuloma in lung with many giant cells.

may also be moderately enlarged and may contain scattered granulomas, more in portal triads than in the lobular parenchyma. Needle biopsy may permit the identification of these focal lesions.

The **bone marrow** is an additional favored site of localization. Roentgenographic changes can be identified in about one fifth of cases of systemic involvement. The radiologically visible bone lesions have a particular tendency to involve phalangeal bones of the hands and feet, creating small circumscribed areas of bone resorption within the marrow cavity or a diffuse reticulated pattern throughout the cavity, with widening of the bony shafts and often new bone formations on the outer surfaces. Histologically, numerous characteristic sarcoid nodules are present in the marrow cavity.

Skin lesions are encountered in one third to one half of the cases. These are, in fact, the best-known lesions of sarcoidosis and were the ones first described by Boeck. Sarcoidosis of the skin assumes a variety of macroscopic appearances (e.g., discrete subcutaneous nodules; focal, slightly elevated, erythematous plaques; or flat lesions that are slightly reddened and scaling and resemble those of lupus erythematosus). Lesions may also appear on the mucous membranes of the oral cavity, larynx, and upper respiratory tract. In all instances, noncaseating granulomas are found histologically in the sites of involvement. Occasionally, deeply situated nodules, characteristic of erythema nodosum (p. 1299), have been described.

Involvement of the **eye, its associated glands, and the salivary glands** occurs in about one fifth to one half of the cases. The ocular involvement takes the form of iritis or iridocyclitis, either bilaterally or unilaterally. As a consequence, corneal opacities, glaucoma, and total loss of vision may occur. The posterior uveal tract is also affected, but less commonly, with resultant choroiditis, retinitis, and optic nerve involvement. These ocular lesions are frequently accompanied by inflammations in the lacrimal glands with suppression of lacrimation. Bilateral sarcoidosis of the parotid, submaxillary, and sublingual glands completes **the combined uveoparotid involvement designated as Mikulicz's syndrome (p. 821).**

Sarcoid granulomas occasionally occur in the heart, kidneys, CNS, and endocrine glands, particularly in the pituitary, as well as in other body tissues.

CLINICAL COURSE. Because of its varying severity and the inconstant distribution of the lesions, sarcoidosis is a protean clinical disease. In many patients, it is entirely asymptomatic and is discovered incidentally at autopsy. In still other instances, the disease is discovered unexpectedly on routine chest films as bilateral hilar adenopathy. Peripheral lymphadenopathy, cutaneous lesions, eye involvement, splenomegaly, or hepatomegaly may each be a presenting manifestation. In the great majority of cases, however, patients seek medical attention because of the insidious onset of respiratory abnormalities (shortness of breath, cough, chest pains, hemoptysis) or of constitutional signs and symptoms (fever, fatigue, weight loss, ano-

rexia, night sweats). Occasionally a systemic hypersensitivity reaction appears with the fairly acute onset of fever, erythema nodosum, and polyarthritis, associated with bilateral hilar adenopathy. Hyperglobulinemia, hypercalcemia, hypercalciuria, and resorptive or "punched-out" cystic lesions in the phalangeal bones are strongly supportive of the diagnosis, but any one or all of these features may be absent. Because of these variable and nondiagnostic clinical symptom complexes, resort is frequently made to lymph node or liver biopsy.

Sarcoidosis follows a fairly unpredictable course characterized by either progressive chronicity or periods of activity interspersed with remissions, sometimes permanent, that may be spontaneous or initiated by steroid therapy. Overall, 65 to 70% of affected patients recover with minimal or no residual manifestations. Twenty per cent have permanent loss of some lung function or some permanent visual impairment. Of the remaining 10%, some die of cardiac or CNS damage, but most succumb to progressive pulmonary fibrosis and cor pulmonale (p. 617). Patients presenting with hilar lymphadenopathy alone (stage I) have the best prognosis, followed by those with adenopathy and pulmonary infiltrates (stage II). Those presenting with pulmonary disease and no adenopathy (stage III) have few spontaneous remissions and are most likely to develop chronic pulmonary fibrosis.[252]

1. McNeill, W.H.: Plagues and Peoples. Garden City, NY, Anchor Press, Doubleday, 1976.

2. Meyerowitz, R.L.:The Pathology of Opportunistic Infection. With Pathogenetic, Diagnostic, and Clinical Correlations. New York, Raven Press, 1983.

3. Alford, R.H., and Hall, A.: Epidemiology of infections caused by gentamycin-resistant enterobacteriaceae over 15 years. Rev. Infect. Dis. *9*:1079, 1987.

4. O'Brien, T.F.: Resistance of bacteria to antimicrobial agents: Report of task force 2. Rev. Infect. Dis. *9(Suppl. 3)*:5244, 1987.

5. Thomas, L.: Thoughts for a countdown. *In* The Lives of a Cell; Notes of a Biology Watcher. New York, Viking Press, 1974, p. 6.

6. Swanson, J., et al.: Gonococcal pili variants in experimental gonorrhea. J. Exp. Med. *165*:1344, 1987.

7. Duma, R.L.: Primary amebic meningoencephalitis. CRC Crit. Rev. Clin. Lab. Sci. 2:163, 1972.

8. Hornick, R.B., et al.: The Broad Street pump revisited; response of volunteers to ingested cholera vibrios. Bull. N.Y. Acad. Med. *47*:1192, 1971.

9. Fields, B.N.: Virology. New York, Raven Press, 1985.

10. Evans, A.S.: Viral Infections of Humans: Epidemiology and Control. New York, Plenum Press, 1984.

11. Mims, C.A., and White, O.O.: Viral Pathogenesis and Immunology. Boston, Blackwell Scientific Publications, 1984.

12. Sharpe, A.H., and Fields, B.N.: Pathogenesis of viral infections: Basic concepts derived from the reovirus model. N. Engl. J. Med. *312*:486, 1985.

13. Notkins, A.L., and Oldstone, M.B.A.: Concepts in Viral Pathogenesis. New York, Springer-Verlag, 1984.

14. McKnight, S., and Tjian, R.: Transcriptional selectivity of viral genes in mammalian cells. Cell *46*:795, 1986.

15. Southern, P., and Oldstone, M.B.A.: Medical consequences of persistent viral infection. N. Engl. J. Med. *314*:359, 1986.

16. Heubi, J.E., et al.: Reye's syndrome: Current concepts. Hepatology *7*:155, 1987.

17. National Surveillance for Reye's Syndrome: Update: Reye's syndrome and salicylate usage. M.M.W.R. *31*:55, 1981.

18. Gall, E.: Mumps orchitis histopathology. Am. J. Pathol. *23*:637, 1947.

19. Zentner, B.S., et al.: Detection of rotavirus-specific antibodies by immunoperoxidase assay and enzyme-linked immunosorbent assay. J. Virol. Methods *11*:199, 1985.

20. Hall, G.A.: Comparative pathology of infection by novel diarrhea viruses. Ciba Found. Symp. *128*:192, 1987.

21. Schreiber, D.S., et al.: The small intestinal lesion induced by Hawaii agent acute infectious nonbacterial gastroenteritis. J. Infect. Dis. *129*:705, 1974.

22. Hinman, A.R.: World eradication of measles. Rev. Infect. Dis. *4*:933, 1982.

23. Fenner, F.: Can smallpox return? World Health Forum *8*:297, 1987.

24. Dorsky, D.I., and Crumpacker, C.S.: Drugs five years later: Acyclovir. Ann. Intern. Med. *107*:859, 1987.

25. Nash, G.: Necrotizing tracheobronchitis and bronchopneumonia consistent with herpetic infection. Hum. Pathol. *12*:283, 1972.

26. Weller, T.H.: The cytomegalovirus: Ubiquitous agents with protean clinical manifestations. N. Engl. J. Med. *285*:203, 267, 1971.

27. Betts, R.F.: Syndromes of cytomegalovirus infection. Adv. Intern. Med. *26*:447, 1980.

28. Craighead, J.E.: Cytomegalovirus pulmonary disease. Pathobiol. Annu. *5*:197, 1975.

29. Sterner, G., et al.: Acquired cytomegalovirus infection in older children and adults. Scand. J. Infect. Dis. *2*:95, 1970.

30. Epstein, M.A., and Achong, B.G.: Pathogenesis of infectious mononucleosis. Lancet *2*:1270, 1977.

31. Henle, W., et al: Epidemiologic aspects of Epstein-Barr virus and Epstein-Barr virus–associated disease. Ann. N.Y. Acad. Sci. *354*:326, 1980.

32. Kass, E.H., and Robbins, S.L.: Severe hepatitis in infectious mononucleosis: Report of a case with minimal clinical manifestations and death due to rupture of the spleen. Arch. Pathol. *50*:644, 1950.

33. Custer, R.P., and Smith, E.B.: The pathology of infectious mononucleosis. Blood *3*:830, 1948.

34. Sullivan, B.H., et al.: The liver in infectious mononucleosis. Am. J. Dig. Dis. *2*:210, 1957.

35. Schooley, R.T., et al.: Chronic Epstein-Barr virus infection associated with fever and interstitial pneumonitis. Clinical and serologic features and response to antiviral therapy. Ann. Intern. Med. *104*:636, 1986.

36. Grierson, H., and Purtilo, D.T.: Epstein-Barr virus infection in males with the x-linked lymphoproliferative syndrome. Ann. Intern. Med. *106*:538, 1987.

37. Strano, A.J.: Yellow fever. *In* Binford, C.H., and Connor, D.H. (eds.): Pathology of Tropical and Extraordinary Diseases. Washington, D.C., Armed Forces Institute of Pathology, 1976, p. 1.

38. Child P.L.: Viral hemorrhagic fevers. *In* Binford, C.H., and Connor, D.H. (eds.): Pathology of Tropical and Extraordinary Diseases. Washington, D.C., Armed Forces Institute of Pathology, 1976, p. 5.

39. Moulder, J.W.: The cell as an extreme environment. Proc. R. Soc. Lond. *204*:199, 1979.

40. Schachter, J.: Chlamydial infections. N. Engl. J. Med. *298*:428, 490, 540, 1978.

41. Gordon, F.B., and Quan, A.L.: Isolation of the trachoma agent in cell culture. Proc. Soc. Exp. Biol. Med. *118*:354, 1965.

42. Patton, D.L., and Taylor, H.R.: The histopathology of experimental trachoma: Ultrastructural changes in the conjunctival epithelium. J. Infect Dis. *153*:870, 1986.

43. Stewart, D.B.: The gynecological lesions of lymphogranuloma venereum and granuloma inguinale. Med. Clin. North Am. *48*:773, 1964.

44. Walker, D.H.: Pathology and pathogenesis of the vasculotropic rickettsioses. *In* Walker, D.H. (ed.): Biology of Rickettsial Diseases. Boca Raton, Fl, CRC Press, 1988, Chapter 9.

45. Maeda, K., et al.: Human infection with *Ehrlichia canis,* a leukocytic rickettsia. N. Engl. J. Med. *316*:853, 1987.

46. Zinsser, H.: Rats, Lice, and History. Boston, Atlantic Monthly Press, Little, Brown, and Company, 1935.

47. Sawyer, L.A., et al.: Q fever: Current concepts. Rev. Infect. Dis. *9*:935, 1987.

48. Walker, D.H.: Pathology of Q fever. *In* Walker, D.H. (ed.): Biology of Rickettsial Diseases, Boca Raton, Fl, CRC Press, 1988, Chapter 79.

49. Chanock, R.M.: Mycoplasma infections of man. N. Engl. J. Med. *273*:1199, 1257, 1965.

50. Rollins, S., et al.: Open lung biopsy in *Mycoplasma pneumoniae* pneumonia. Arch. Pathol. Lab. Med. *110*:34, 1986.

51. Taylor-Robinson, D.: The genital mycoplasmas. N. Engl. J. Med. *302*:1063, 1980.

52. Pappenheimer, A.M., and Gill, D.M.: Diphtheria. Science *182*:353, 1973.

53. Peter, G., et al.: Meningococcal meningitis in familial deficiency of the 5th component of complement. Pediatrics *67*:882, 1981.

54. Gerrard, T.L., and Fauci, A.S.: Activation and immunoregulation of antigen-specific human B lymphocyte responses: Multifaceted role of the monocyte. J. Immunol. *128*:2367, 1982.

55. Mehra, V., et al.: Lymphocyte suppression in leprosy induced by unique *M. leprae* glycolipid. Nature *308*:194, 1984.

56. Eykin, S.J.: Staphylococcal sepsis. The changing pattern of disease and therapy. Lancet *1*:100, 1988.

57. Wolleman, O.J., and Finland, M.: Pathology of staphylococcal pneumonia complicating clinical influenza. Am. J. Pathol. *19*:23, 1943.

58. Chesney, T.J., et al.: Clinical manifestations of toxic shock syndrome. J.A.M.A. *246*:741, 1981.

59. Abdul-Karim, S.W., et al.: Toxic shock syndrome: Clinicopathologic findings in a fatal case. Hum. Pathol. *12*:16, 1981.

60. Bimo, A.L.: *Streptococcus pyogenes*. *In* Mandell, G.L., Douglas, R.G., and Bennett, J.E. (eds.): Principles and Practice of Infectious Disease. 2nd ed. New York, John Wiley and Sons, 1985, p. 1124.

61. Austrian, R.: Pneumococcus; the first one hundred years. Rev. Infect. Dis. *3*:183, 1981.

62. Finland, M.: Conference on the pneumococcus. Summary and comments. Rev. Infect. Dis. *3*:358, 1981.

63. Brener, D., et al.: Increased virulence of *Neisseria meningitidis* after in vitro iron limited growth at low pH. Infect. Immun. *33*:59, 1981.

64. Barlow, D., and Phillips, I.: Gonorrhoea in women. Diagnostic, clinical, and laboratory aspects. Lancet *1*:761, 1978.

65. Yu, V.L.: *Serratia marcescens*. Historical perspective and clinical review. N. Engl. J. Med. *300*:887, 1979.

66. Order, S.A., and Moncrief, J.A.: The Burn Wound. Springfield, IL, Charles C Thomas, 1965.

67. Cohen, P.S., et al.: Infective endocarditis caused by gram-negative bacteria. A review of the literature, 1945–1977. Prog. Cardiovasc. Dis. *22*:205, 1980.

68. Blackmon, J.A., et al.: Legionnaires' disease. Pathological and historical aspects of a "new" disease. Arch. Pathol. Lab. Med. *102*:337, 1978.

69. Frenkel, J.K., et al.: Autopsy diagnosis of legionnaires' disease in immunosuppressed patients. Ann. Intern. Med. *90*:559, 1979.

70. Horwitz, M.A., and Silverstein, S.C.: Activated human monocytes inhibit the intracellular multiplication of legionnaires' disease bacteria. J. Exp. Med. *154*:1618, 1981.

71. Winn, W.C., and Meyerowitz, R.L.: The pathology of the Legionella pneumonias. Hum. Pathol. *12*:401, 1981.

72. Zaleznik, D.F., and Kasper, D.L.: The role of anaerobic bacteria in abscess formation. Annu. Rev. Med. *33*:217, 1982.

73. Gorbach, S.L., and Bartlett, J.G.: Anaerobic infections. N. Engl. J. Med. *290*:1177, 1237, 1289, 1974.

74. Nogimori, K., et al.: Dual mechanisms involved in the development of diverse biological activities of islet-activating protein (pertussis toxin) as revealed by chemical modification of the toxin molecule. Dev. Biol. Scand. *61*:51, 1985.

75. Boyer, N.H., and Weinstein, L.: Diphtheritic myocarditis. N. Engl. J. Med. *239*:913, 1948.

76. Butler, S., and Levine, S.A.: Diphtheria as a cause of late heart block. Am. Heart J. *5*:592, 1930.

77. Guerrant, R.L., et al.: Acute infectious diarrhea. I. Epidemiology, etiology, and pathogenesis. Pediatr. Infect. Dis. *5*:353, 1986.

78. Sprinz, H., et al.: Histopathology of the upper small intestine in typhoid fever. Am. J. Dig. Dis. *11*:615, 1966.

79. Rout, W.R. et al.: Pathophysiology of salmonella diarrhea in the rhesus monkey: Intestinal transport, morphological, and bacteriological studies. Gastroenterology *67*:59, 1974.

80. Mandal, B.K., and Mani, V.: Colonic involvement in salmonellosis. Lancet *1*:887, 1976.

81. Farid, Z., et al.: Chronic salmonellosis, urinary schistosomiasis, and massive proteinuria. Am. J. Trop. Med. Hyg. *21*:578, 1972.

82. Rocha, H., et al.: Prolonged Salmonella bacteremia in patients with *Schistosoma mansoni* infection. Arch. Intern. Med. *128*:254, 1971.

83. Melhem, R.F., and LoVerde, P.T.: Mechanisms of interaction of *Salmonella* and *Schistosoma* species. Infect. Immunol. *44*:274, 1984.

84. Kelly, M.T., and McCormick, W.F.: Acute bacterial myositis caused by *Vibrio vulnificus*. J.A.M.A. *246*:72, 1981.

85. Blake, P.A., et al.: Cholera—a possible endemic focus in the United States. N. Engl. J. Med. *302*:305, 1980.

86. Carpenter, C.C.J.: Mechanism of bacterial diarrheas. Am. J. Med. *68*:313, 1980.

87. Dammin, G.J.: Vibrio-caused diseases: Cholera. *In* Binford, C.H., and Connor, D.H. (eds.): Pathology of Tropical and Extraordinary Diseases. Washington, D.C., Armed Forces Institute of Pathology, 1976, p. 137.

88. Blaser, M.J., and Reller, L.B.: Campylobacter enteritis. N. Engl. J. Med. *305*:1444, 1983.

89. Walker, R.I., et al.: Pathophysiology of *Campylobacter* enteritis. Microbiol. Rev. *50*:81, 1986.

90. Colgan, T., et al.: *Campylobacter jejuni* enterocolitis. A clinicopathologic study. Arch. Pathol. Lab. Med. *104*:571, 1980.

91. Balzer, M.J.: Gastric campylobacter-like organisms, gastritis, and peptic ulcer disease. Gastroenterology *93*:371, 1987.

92. O'Loughlin, E.V., et al.: Clinical, morphological, and biochemical alterations in acute intestinal yersiniosis. Pediatr. Res. *20*:602, 1986.

93. Vantrappen, G., et al.: Yersinia enteritis and enterocolitis: Gastroenterologic aspects. Gastroenterology *72*:220, 1977.

94. Dammin, G.J.: Acute diarrhea and dysentery caused by *Yersinia enterocolitica*. *In* Binford, C.H., and Connor, D.H. (eds.): Pathology of Tropical and Extraordinary Diseases. Washington, D.C., Armed Forces Institute of Pathology, 1976, p. 162.

95. Berggren, G.G., et al.: Traditional midwives, tetanus immunization, and infant mortality in rural Haiti. Trop. Doct. *13*:79, 1983.

96. Weinstein, L.: Tetanus. N. Engl. J. Med. *289*:1129, 1973.

97. Feldman, R.A. (ed.): A seminar on infant botulism. Rev. Infect. Dis. *1*:612, 1979.

98. Simpson, L.L.: The action of botulinal toxin. Rev. Infect. Dis. *1*:656, 1979.

99. Darke, S.G., et al.: Gas gangrene and related infections: Classification, clinical features and aetiology, management, and mortality. A report of 88 cases. Br. J. Surg. *64*:104, 1977.

100. Triadofilopoulos, G., et al.: Differential effects of *Clostridium difficile* toxins A and B on rabbit ileum. Gastroenterology *93*:273, 1987.

101. Trnka, Y.M., and Lamont, J.T.: Association of *Clostridium difficile* toxin with symptomatic relapse of chronic inflammatory bowel disease. Gastroenterology *80*:693, 1981.

102. Price, A.G., and Davies, D.R.: Pseudomembranous colitis. J. Clin. Pathol. *30*:1, 1977.

103. Schultz, M.G.: Emerging zoonoses. N. Engl. J. Med. *308*:1285, 1983.

104. Dutz, W., and Kohout, E.: Anthrax. Pathol. Annu. *6*:209, 1971.

105. Wade, N.: Death at Sverdlovsk: A critical diagnosis. Science *209*:1501, 1980.

106. Koch, R.: Untersuchungen uber Bakterien. Die Aetiologie der Milzbrand Krankheit begrundet auf die Entwicklungsgeschichte des *Bacillus anthracis*. Beitr. z. Biol. d. Pflanzen (Breslau) *2*:277, 1877.

107. Pasteur, L.: Charbon et virulence. Bull. Acad. Med. (Paris) *7*:253, 1878.

108. Ishak, K.G.: Listeriosis. *In* Binford, C.H., and Connor, D.H. (eds.): Pathology of Tropical and Extraordinary Diseases. Washington, D.C., Armed Forces Institute of Pathology, 1976, p. 178.

109. Smith, J.H.: Plague. *In* Binford, C.H., and Connor, D.H. (eds.): Pathology of Tropical and Extraordinary Diseases. Washington, D.C., Armed Forces Institute of Pathology, 1976, p. 130.

110. Teutsch, S.M., et al.: Pneumonic tularemia on Martha's Vineyard. N. Engl. J. Med. *301*:826, 1979.

111. Evans, M.E., et al.: Tularemia: A 30-year experience with 88 cases. Medicine (Baltimore) *64*:251, 1985.

112. Young, E.J.: Human brucellosis. Rev. Infect. Dis. *5*:821, 1983.

113. Spink, W.W.: The Nature of Brucellosis. Minneapolis, University of Minnesota Press, 1956.

114. Sanford, J.: Pseudomonas species (including melioidosis and glanders). *In* Mandell, G.L., Douglas, R.G., and Bennett, J.E. (eds.): Principles and Practice of Infectious Disease. New York, John Wiley and Sons, 1979, p. 1720.

115. Piggott, J.A.: Melioidosis. *In* Binford, C.H., and Connor, D.H. (eds.): Pathology of Tropical and Extraordinary Diseases. Washington, D.C., Armed Forces Institute of Pathology, 1976, p. 169.

116. Jacobs, R.: Leptospirosis. Medical staff conference, University of California, San Francisco. West. J. Med. *132*:440, 1980.

117. Dooley, J.R., and Ishak, K.G.: Leptospirosis. *In* Binford, C.H., and Connor D.H. (eds.): Pathology of Tropical and Extraordinary Diseases. Washington, D.C., Armed Forces Institute of Pathology, 1976, p. 101.

118. Arean, V.M: The pathologic anatomy and pathogenesis of fatal human leptospirosis (Weil's disease). Am. J. Pathol. *40*:393, 1962.

119. Felsenfeld, O.: Borreliae, human relapsing fever, and parasite-vector-host relationships. Bacteriol. Rev. *29*:46, 1965.

120. Judge, D.M., et al.: Louse-borne relapsing fever in man. Arch. Pathol. *97*:136, 1974.

121. Lyme Disease and Related Disorders—2nd International Symposium, Vienna, Austria, September 17–19, 1985. Vienna, Hygiene Institute, University of Vienna, p. 75.

122. Johnson, R.C., et al.: *Borrelia burgdorferi* sp. nov.: Etiologic agent of Lyme disease. Int. J. Syst. Bacteriol. *34*:496, 1984.

123. Lastavica, C.C., et al.: Rapid emergence of a focal epidemic of Lyme disease in coastal Massachusetts. N Engl. J. Med. *320*:133, 1989.

124. Dammin, G.J.: Two new diseases and a new tick. Infect. Dis. Pract. *4*:1, 1980.

125. Wear, D.J., et al.: Cat-scratch disease: A bacterial infection. Science *221*:1403, 1983.

126. Margileth, A.M., et al.: Systemic cat-scratch disease: Report of 23 patients with prolonged or recurrent, severe bacterial infection. J. Infect. Dis. *155*:390, 1987.

127. Hadfield, T.L.: Is *Rothia dentocariosa* the cause of cat-scratch disease? (letter). Lancet *2*:720, 1985.

128. English, C.K., et al.: Cat-scratch disease. Isolation and culture of the bacterial agent. J.A.M.A. *259*:1347, 1988.

129. Alderete, J.F., and Baseman, J.B.: Surface-associated host protein on virulent *Treponema pallidum*. Infect. Immun. *26*:1048, 1979.

130. Freidman, P.S., and Turk, J.L.: A spectrum of lymphocyte responsiveness in human syphilis. Clin. Exp. Immunol. *21*:59, 1975.

131. Gjestland, T.: The Oslo study of untreated syphilis; an epidemiological investigation of the natural course of the syphilitic infection, based on a restudy of the Boeck-Bruusgaard material. Acta Dermatol. Venereol. (Oslo) *35*, Suppl. 34, 1955.

132. Rockwell, D.H., et al.: The Tuskegee study of untreated syphilis. Arch. Intern. Med. *114*:792, 1964.

133. National Centers for Disease Control (U.S. Public Health Service), Venereal Disease Program: Syphilis, a Synopsis. Washington, D.C., U.S. Government Printing Office, 1967.

134. Kerdel-Vegas, F., et al.: Rhinoscleroma. Springfield, IL, Charles C Thomas, 1963.

135. Kuberski, T.: Granuloma inguinale (donovanosis). Sex. Transm. Dis. *7*:129, 1980.

136. Hammond, G.W., et al.: Epidemiologic, clinical, laboratory, and therapeutic features of an urban outbreak of chancroid. Rev. Infect. Dis. *2*:867, 1980.

137. Dooley, J.R.: Haemotropic bacteria in man. Lancet *2*:1237, 1980.

138. Grange, J.M.: Tuberculosis. The changing tubercle. Br. J. Hosp. Med. *22*:540, 1979.

139. Slavin, R.E., et al.: Late generalized tuberculosis: A clinical pathologic analysis and comparison of 100 cases in the preantibiotic and antibiotic eras. Medicine *59*:352, 1980.

140. French, G.L., et al.: Diagnosis of pulmonary tuberculosis by detection of tuberculostearic acid in sputum by using gas chromatography–mass spectrometry with selected monitoring. J. Infect. Dis. *156*:356, 1987.

141. Shoemaker, S.A., et al.: Techniques of DNA hybridization detect small numbers of mycobacteria with no cross hybridization with nonmycobacterial respiratory organisms. Am. Rev. Resp. Dis. *131*:760, 1985.

142. Goren, M.B.: Immunoreactive substances of mycobacteria. Am. Rev. Respir. Dis. Suppl. *125*:50, 1982.

143. Luelmo, F.: BCG vaccination. Am. Rev. Respir. Dis. *125(Part 2)*:70, 1982.

144. Turk, J.L.: Delayed hypersensitivity. New York, Elsevier/North Holland, 1980, p. 275.

145. Tanaka, A., et al.: Epithelioid cell granuloma formation requiring no T cell function. Am. J. Pathol. *106*:165, 1982.

146. Enarson, D.A., et al.: Failure of diagnosis as a factor in tuberculosis mortality. Can. Med. Assoc. J. *118*:1520, 1978.

147. Tellis, C.J., and Putnam, J.S.: Pulmonary disease caused by nontuberculosis mycobacteria. Med. Clin. North Am. *64*:433, 1980.

148. Connor, D.H., et al.: Infections by *Mycobacterium ulcerans. In* Binford, C.H., and Connor, D.H. (eds.): Pathology of Tropical and Extraordinary Diseases. Washington, D.C., Armed Forces Institute of Pathology, 1976, p. 226.

149. Marchiondo, A.A., et al.: Naturally occurring leprosy-like disease of wild armadillos. Ultrastructure of lepromatous lesions. J. Reticuloendothel. Soc. *27*:311, 1980.

150. Bloom, B.R.: Learning from leprosy: A perspective on immunology and the third world. J. Immunol. *137*:1, 1986.

151. Reich, C.V.: Leprosy: Cause, transmission, and a new theory of pathogenesis. Rev. Infect. Dis. *9*:589, 1987.

152. Simson, G.L., et al.: Nocardial infections in the immunocompromised host: A detailed study in a defined population. Rev. Infect. Dis. *3*:492, 1981.

153. Brown, J.R.: Human actinomycosis: A study of 181 subjects. Hum. Pathol. *4*:319, 1973.

154. Diamond, R.D., et al.: Damage to pseudohyphal forms of *Candida albicans* by neutrophils in the absence of serum *in vitro.* J. Clin. Invest. *61*:349, 1978.

155. Yung, C.W., et al.: Disseminated *Trichosporon beigelii* (cutaneum). Cancer *48*:2107, 1981.

156. Sudman, M.S.: Protothecosis. A critical review. Am. J. Clin. Pathol. *61*:10, 1974.

157. Edwards, J.E., Jr. (Moderator): UCLA Conference. Severe Candida infections: Clinical perspective, immune defense mechanisms and current concepts of therapy. Ann. Intern. Med. *89*:91, 1978.

158. Baker, R.D., and Haugen, R.R.: Tissue changes and tissue diagnosis in cryptococcosis. Am. J. Clin. Pathol. *24*:14, 1955.

159. Sarosi, G.A., and Davies, S.F.: Blastomycosis. Am. Rev. Respir. Dis. *120*:911, 1979.

160. Franco, M.F., et al.: Paracoccidioidomycosis. A recently proposed classification of its clinical forms. Rev. Inst. Med. Trop. *20*:129, 1987.

161. Drutz, D.J., and Catanzano, A.: Coccidioidomycosis. Am. Rev. Respir. Dis. *117*:559, 1978.

162. Straub, M., and Schwarz, J.: Histoplasmosis, coccidioidomycosis and tuberculosis: A comparative pathological study. Pathol. Microbiol. *25*:421, 1962.

163. Binford, C.H., and Dooley, J.R.: Diseases caused by fungi and actinomycetes. *In* Binford, C.H., and Connor, D.H. (eds.): Pathology of Tropical and Extraordinary Diseases. Washington, D.C., Armed Forces Institute of Pathology, 1976, p. 551.

164. UNDP/WORLD BANK/WHO Special Programme for Research and Training in Tropical Disease: Tropical Disease Research: A Global Partnership, WHO Doc. ISBN92. Geneva, WHO, 1987, p. 192.

165. Rose, M.E., and McLaren, D.J.: Pathophysiologic responses to parasites. Parasitology *24(Suppl. 1)*:182, 1987.

166. Krogstad, D.J., et al.: Amebiasis. Epidemiological studies in the United States, 1971–1974. Ann. Intern. Med. *88*:89, 1978.

167. Brandt, H., and Perez-Tamayo, R.: The pathology of human amebiasis. Hum. Pathol. *1*:351, 1970.

168. Radke, R.A.: Ameboma of the intestine; an analysis of the disease as presented in 78 collected and 41 previously unreported cases. Ann. Intern. Med. *43*:1048, 1955.

169. McCoy, G.W., et al.: Epidemic amebic dysentery; the Chicago outbreak of 1933. N.I.H. Bulletin No. 166. Washington, D.C., U.S. Government Printing Office, 1963.

170. Arean, V.M., and Koppisch, E.: Balantidiasis. A review and report of cases. Am. J. Pathol. *32*:1089, 1956.

171. Martinez, A.J.: Is Acanthamoeba encephalitis an opportunistic infection? Neurology *30*:567, 1980.

172. Koenig, S.B., et al.: *Acanthamoeba* keratitis associated with gas-permeable contact lenses. Am. J. Ophthalmol. *103*:832, 1987.

173. Smith, P.D., et al.: IgG antibody to *Giardia lamblia* detected by enzyme-linked immunosorbent assay. Gastroenterology *80*:1476, 1981.

174. Moore, G.T., et al.: Epidemic giardiasis at a ski resort. N. Engl. J. Med. *281*:402, 1969.

175. Yardley, J.H., and Bayliss, T.M.: Giardiasis. Gastroenterology *52*:301, 1967.

176. Smith, P.D., et al.: Chronic giardiasis: Studies on drug sensitivity, toxin production, and host immune response. Gastroenterology *83*:797, 1982.

177. Soave, R., and Johnson, W.O., Jr.: *Cryptosporidium* and *Isospora belli* infections. J. Infect. Dis. *157*:225, 1988.

178. Restrepo, C., et al.: Disseminated extraintestinal isosporiasis in a patient with acquired immune deficiency syndrome. Am. J. Clin. Pathol. *87*:536, 1987.

179. Honigberg, B.M.: Trichomonads of importance in human medicine. *In* Kreier, J.P. (ed.): Parasitic Protozoa. Vol. 2. New York, Academic Press, 1978, p. 469.

179a. Edman, J.C., et al.: Ribosomal RNA sequence shows *Pneumocystis carinii* to be a member of the fungi. Nature *334*:519. 1988.

180. Meuwissen, J.H.: Parasitologic and serologic observations of infection with *Pneumocystis* in humans. J. Infect. Dis. *136*:43, 1977.

181. Young, L.S. (ed.): *Pneumocystis carinii* pneumonia. New York, Marcel Dekker, 1984.

182. Phillips, R.E., and Warrell, O.A.: The pathophysiology of severe falciparum malaria. Parasitol. Today *2*:271, 1986.

183. Edington, G.M.: Pathology of malaria in West Africa. Br. Med. J. *1*:715, 1967.

184. Marin, S.K., et al.: Severe malaria and glucose-6-phosphate dehydrogenase deficiency. A reappraisal of the malaria/G-6-P.D. hypothesis. Lancet *1*:524, 1979.

185. Miller, L.H., et al.: The Duffy blood group phenotype in American blacks infected with *Plasmodium falciparum* in Vietnam. Am. J. Trop. Med. Hyg. *27*:1261, 1977.

186. Spitz, S.: The pathology of malaria. Milit. Surg. *99*:555, 1946.

187. Hendrickse, R.G., et al.: Quartan malaria nephrotic syndrome. Collaborative clinicopathologic study in Nigerian children. Lancet *1*:1143, 1972.

188. Patarroyo, M.E., et al.: A synthetic vaccine protects humans against challenge with asexual blood stages of *Plasmodium falciparum* malaria. Nature *332*:158, 1988.

189. Dammin, G.J., et al.: The rising incidence of clinical *Babesia microti* infection. Hum. Pathol. *12*:398, 1981.

190. Wittner, M., et al.: Successful chemotherapy for transfusion babesiosis. Ann. Intern. Med. *96*:601, 1982.

191. Ashworth, T.G., and Goldsmith, J.: A reassessment of the epidemiology and clinicopathological features of human trypanosomiasis in Rhodesia. Centr. Afr. J. Med. Suppl. *21*:1, 1975.

192. Van der Ploeg, L.H.T.: Control of variant surface antigen switching in trypanosomes. Cell *51*:159, 1987.

193. Mansfield, J.M.: Immunobiology of African trypanosomiasis. Cell. Immunol. *39*:204, 1978.

194. Seed, J.R., et al.: Pathophysiological changes during African trypanosomiasis. *In* Mettrick, D.F., and Desser, S.S. (eds.): Parasites, Their World and Ours. Amsterdam, Elsevier Biomedical Press, 1982, p. 255.

195. Doua, F., et al.: Treatment of human late stage gambiense trypanosomiasis with α-difluoromethylornithine (Elflornithine). Am. J. Trop. Med. Hyg. *37*:525, 1987.

196. Hudson, L., and Britten, V.: Immune response to South American trypanosomiasis and its relationship to Chagas disease. Br. Med. Bull. *41*:175, 1985.

197. Andrade, Z.A., et al.: Histopathology of the conducting tissue of the heart in Chagas' myocarditis. Am. Heart J. *95*:316, 1978.

198. Marr, J.J., and Docampo, R.: Chemotherapy for Chagas disease: A perspective of current therapy and consideration for future research. Rev. Infect. Dis. *8*:884, 1986.

199. Wirth, D.: Rapid identification of Leishmania species by specific hybridization of kinetoplast DNA in cutaneous lesions. Proc. Natl. Acad. Sci. U.S.A. *79*:6999, 1983.

200. deBrito, T., et al.: Glomerular involvement in kala-azar. Am. J. Trop. Med. Hyg. *24*:8, 1975.

201. Neva, F.A.: Diagnosis and treatment of cutaneous leishmaniasis.

In Remington, J.S., and Schwartz, M.N. (eds.): Current Clinical Topics in Infectious Diseases. New York, McGraw-Hill Book Co., 1980, p. 364.

202. Connor, D.F., and Neafie, R.C.: Cutaneous leishmaniasis. *In* Binford, C.H., and Connor, D.H. (eds.): Pathology of Tropical and Extraordinary Diseases. Washington, D.C., Armed Forces Institute of Pathology, 1976, p. 258.

203. Ridley, D.S., and Ridley, M.J.: The evolution of the lesion in cutaneous leishmaniasis. J. Pathol. *141*:83, 1983.

204. Frenkel, J.K.: Toxoplasmosis. Pediatr. Clin. North Am. *32*:917,1985.

205. Remington, D.S., and Desmonti, G.: Toxoplasmosis. *In* Remington, D.S., and Klein, J.O. (eds.): Infectious Diseases of the Fetus and Newborn Infant. Philadelphia, W.B. Saunders Company, 1983, p. 143.

206. Beaver, P.C., and Orihel, T.C.: Human infection with filariae of animals in the United States. Am. J. Trop. Med. Hyg. *14*:1010, 1965.

207. Sher, A., et al.: Acquisition of murine major histocompatibility complex gene products by schistosomula of *Schistosoma mansoni*. J. Exp. Med. *148*:46, 1978.

208. Sher, A., and Moser, G.: Immunologic properties of developing schistosomula. Am. J. Pathol. *102*:121, 1981.

209. Samuelson, J.C., et al.: Schistosomula of *Schistosoma mansoni* clear concanavalin A from their surface by sloughing. J. Cell Biol. *94*:355, 1982.

210. Mahmoud, A.A.F.: Regulation of immunopathology in parasitic infections. *In* Ogra, P.L., and Jacobs, D.M. (eds.): Regulation of the Immune Response. Basel, Karger, 1983, p. 267.

211. MacInnes, A.J. (ed.): Molecular Paradigms for Eradicating Helminth Parasites. New York, Alan R. Liss, 1987, p. 576.

212. Smithers S.R., et al.: Host antigens in schistosomiasis. Proc. R. Soc. Series B *171*:483, 1969.

213. Butterworth, A.E., et al.: Damage to schistosomula of *Schistosoma mansoni* induced directly by eosinophil major basic protein. J. Immunol. *122*:221, 1979.

214. James, S.L., et al.: Macrophages as effector cells of protective immunity in murine schistosomiasis. II. Killing of newly transformed schistosomula by macrophages activated as a consequence of *Schistosoma mansoni* infection. J. Immunol. *128*:1535, 1982.

215. Capron, A., et al.: Immunity to schistosomes: Progress toward vaccine. Science *283*:1065, 1987.

216. Gelpi, A.P., and Mustafa, A.: Ascaris pneumonia. Am. J. Med. *44*:377, 1968.

217. Phills, J.A.: Pulmonary abnormalities and eosinophilia due to *Ascaris suum*. N. Engl. J. Med. *286*:965, 1972.

218. Symmers, W.St.C.: Pathology of oxyuriasis. Arch. Pathol. *50*:475, 1950.

219. Rep, B.H.: Pathogenicity of hookworms. The significance of population regression for the pathogenicity of hookworms. Trop. Geogr. Med. *32*:251, 1980.

220. Ashford, B.K.: Ankylostomiasis in Puerto Rico, 1900. *In* Kean, B.H., et al. (eds.): Tropical Medicine and Parasitology; Classic Investigations. Vol. 2. Ithaca, NY, Cornell University Press, 1978, p. 314.

221. Longworth, D.L., and Weller, P.F.: Hyperinfection syndrome with strongyloidiasis. *In* Remington, J.S., and Swartz, M.N. (eds.): Current Clinical Topics in Infectious Diseases. Vol. 7. New York, McGraw-Hill Book Co., 1986, p. 1.

222. Snyder, C.H.: Visceral larva migrans: Ten years' experience. Pediatrics *28*:85, 1961.

223. Kayes, S.G., and Oaks, J.A.: Development of the granulomatous response in murine toxocariasis. Am. J. Pathol. *93*:277, 1978.

224. Despommier, D.: Adaptive changes in muscle fibers infected with *Trichinella spiralis*. Am. J. Pathol. *78*:477, 1975.

225. Most, H.: Trichinosis—preventable yet still with us. N. Engl. J. Med. *298*:1178, 1978.

226. Castro, G.A.: Regulation of pathogenesis in disease caused by gastrointestinal parasites. *In* Johnson, R. (ed.): Physiology of the Gastrointestinal Tract. New York, Raven Press, 1982, p. 1381.

227. Kazura, J.W., and Grove, D.J.: Stage-specific, antibody-dependent, eosinophil-mediated destruction of *Trichinella spiralis*. Nature *274*:588, 1978.

228. Lie Kian, J.: Occult filariasis: Its relationship with tropical pulmonary eosinophilia. Am. J. Trop. Med. Hyg. *11*:646, 1962.

229. Piessens, W.F., et al.: Immunobiology of lymphatic filariasis. *In* Wyler, D., Pereira, M., and Wirth, D.F. (eds.): Biology of Parasitic Infections. New York, Scientific American Publishing Company, 1988.

230. Ottesen, E.A., et al.: Specific allergic sensitization to filarial antigens in tropical eosinophilia syndrome. Lancet *1*:1158, 1979.

231. Connor, D.H., and Neafie, R.C.: Onchocerciasis. *In* Binford, C.H., and Connor, D.H. (eds.): Pathology of Tropical and Extraordinary Diseases. Washington, D.C., Armed Forces Institute of Pathology, 1976, p. 360.

232. Bartlett, A., et al.: Variation in delayed hypersensitivity in onchocerciasis. Trans. R. Soc. Trop. Med. Hyg. *72*:372, 1978.

233. Meyers, W.M., et al.: Human streptocerciasis. A clinicopathologic study of 40 Africans (Zairians) including identification of the adult filaria. Am. J. Trop. Med. Hyg. *21*:528, 1972.

234. Ciferri, F.: Human pulmonary dirofilariasis in the United States: A critical review. Am. J. Trop. Med. Hyg. *31*:302, 1982.

235. Coolidge, C., et al.: Zoonotic Brugia filariasis in New England. Ann. Intern. Med. *90*:341, 1979.

236. Descombes, P., et al.: Endoscopic discovery and capture of *Taenia saginata*. Endoscopy *13*:44, 1981.

237. Brown, W.J., and Voge, M.: Neuropathology of Parasitic Infections. Oxford, Oxford University Press, 1982, p. 108.

238. Robles, C., et al.: Long-term results of praziquantel therapy in neurocysticercosis. J. Neurosurg. *66*:359, 1987.

239. D'Allessandro, R.L., et al.: *Echinococcus vogeli* in man with a review of polycystic disease in Colombia and neighboring countries. Am. J. Trop. Med. Hyg. *28*:303, 1979.

240. Bendezu, P., et al.: Human fascioliasis in Corozal, Puerto Rico. J. Parasitol. *68*:297, 1982.

241. Tansurat, P.: Opisthorchiasis. *In* Marcial-Rojas, R.A. (ed.): Pathology of Protozoal and Helminthic Diseases. Baltimore, Williams & Wilkins Co., 1971, p. 536.

242. Meyers, W.M., and Neafie, R.C.: Paragonimiasis. *In* Binford, C.H., and Connor, D.H. (eds.): Pathology of Tropical and Extraordinary Diseases. Washington, D.C., Armed Forces Institute of Pathology, 1976, p. 517.

243. Warren, K.S.: The relevance of schistosomiasis. N. Engl. J. Med. *303*:203, 1980.

244. Colley, D.G., et al.: Immunoregulatory cells and molecules in schistosomiasis. *In* MacInnes, A.J. (ed.): Molecular Paradigms for Eradicating Helminth Parasites. New York, Alan R. Liss, 1987, p. 116.

245. Symmers, W.St.C.: Note on a new form of liver cirrhosis due to the presence of the ova of *Bilharzia haematobia*. J. Pathol. Bacteriol. *9*:237, 1903.

246. Andrade, Z.A., and Rocha, H.: Schistosomal nephropathy. Kidney Int. *16*:23, 1979.

247. Cheever, A.W.: Schistosomiasis and neoplasia (editorial). J. Natl. Cancer Inst. *61*:13, 1978.

248. Mott, K.E., and Dixon, H.: Collaborative study on antigens for immunodiagnosis of schistosomiasis. Bull. WHO *60*:729, 1982.

249. Fanburg, B.C. (ed.): Sarcoidosis and Other Granulomatous Diseases. New York, Marcel Dekker, 1983.

250. Hunninghake, G.W., and Crystal, R.G.: Pulmonary sarcoidosis. A disorder mediated by excess helper T lymphocyte activity at sites of disease. N. Engl. J. Med. *305*:429, 1981.

251. Thrasher, D.R., and Briggs, D.D.: Pulmonary sarcoidosis. Clin. Chest Med. *3*:537,1982.

252. Romer, F.K.: Presentation of sarcoidosis and outcome of pulmonary changes. Dan. Med. Bull. *29*:27, 1982.

Nutritional Disease

Chronic undernutrition on which is superimposed periods of acute hunger continues to be a harsh reality of life throughout developing countries—recall the famines in Ethiopia, Somalia, Uganda, and elsewhere. At least 800 million people, mostly in Africa and Asia but also in the Americas, suffer such *primary malnutrition.*[1] Children under the age of five bear the brunt of this deprivation. In the majority of industrialized countries the death rate among children aged one to four years is about 1 per 1000; in drought-stricken Ethiopia it is 247 per 1000.[2] Some of this mortality is related to maternal malnutrition and premature delivery, but much is related to the impact of malnutrition on the body's defenses against infectious disease. Much as we would like to believe that steps have been taken to eradicate this problem, in the decade beginning in 1963 less than 50% of children four years of age were thought to have protein-calorie malnutrition in Asia (excluding the USSR and Northeast Asia), but currently the prevalence is over 60%.

Although these dietary deficiencies in the developing regions of the world involve mostly proteins and total calories, producing so called protein-energy malnutrition (p. 436), other specific nutrients are also usually lacking. In Africa, for example, large segments of the population suffer from anemia because of the lack of iron, have the eye condition xerophthalmia (p. 439) because of a deficiency of vitamin A, and have sufficiently severe lack of total calories and protein to produce marasmus-kwashiorkor (p. 436) as is depicted in Figure 8–1.

Malnutrition is common even in affluent societies. Some of it is the consequence, ironically, of an abundance of food—witness the frequency of obesity in the Western world. But in addition, primary malnutrition and *secondary, conditioned malnutrition* may be encountered under the following circumstances.

• *Poverty and ignorance.*[3] Those at particular risk of significant malnutrition are infants and children because of their increased growth requirements, and young multiparous women burdened with the increased demands of frequent pregnancies.

• *Acute and chronic illness.* Protein calorie undernutrition is thought to be present in one third of adult patients in United States hospitals owing to an inability to eat or absorb nutrients; the hypermetabolism of infection, fever or trauma; or abnormal intestinal nutrient losses.[4] Many of these influences are also prevalent in the surgical setting and postoperative period.

• *Genetic disease.* Certain deficiency states may arise despite an adequate dietary intake because of inborn errors of metabolism—for example, vitamin D–dependent rickets, in which an apparent lack of a hydroxylase blocks the conversion of vitamin D to its functionally active form.

• *Chronic alcoholism.* Reduced or imbalanced dietary intake and impairment in the uptake, utilization, or metabolism of nutrients are common in chronic alcoholics. Mainly involved are vitamin A, folate, thiamine, vitamin B_6, and sometimes protein and calories.[5]

• *Malabsorption syndromes* (p. 875). A variety of malabsorptive disorders may affect all nutrients (e.g., Crohn's disease), specific classes of nutrients (e.g., fats in biliary tract disorders or celiac disease), or specific nutrients (e.g., vitamin B_{12} in atrophic gastritis).[6]

• *Neonates and infants.* Nutritional requirements are greatest during early infancy, and the diet may be grossly inadequate as, for example, when the child is deprived of breast feeding by the birth of another infant, and adequate replacement is not instituted.[7]

• *The elderly.* Malnutrition is surprisingly common in those of advanced years for many reasons such as poverty, inadequate attention, loss of appetite, bizarre tea and toast diets, gastrointestinal disorders, and

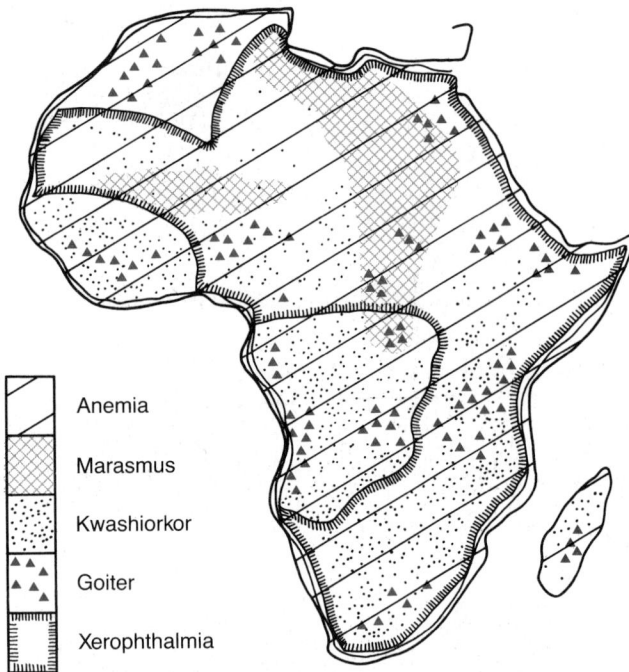

Figure 8 – 1. Malnutrition in Africa: five main deficiencies. (Reproduced with the kind permission of Dr. T.N. Maletnlema, Tanzania Food and Nutrition Center, Dar es Salaam, Tanzania. From Maletnlema, T.N.: The problem of food and nutrition in Africa. Wld. Rev. Nutr. Diet. 47:30, 1986.)

Legend for map:
- Anemia
- Marasmus
- Kwashiorkor
- Goiter
- Xerophthalmia

poorly understood bacterial overgrowth in the small bowel despite the absence of overt anatomic abnormalities.[8]

• *Restricted diets.* Although animal foods are not essential to health, vegetarian diets may be deficient in high-quality protein, vitamin B_{12}, and iron. Diets of this nature pose the greatest risk in actively growing children and during pregnancy.[9] Macrobiotic diets limited strictly to cereal grains are most likely to be imbalanced.

• *Drug-induced malnutrition.* A number of agents such as phenytoin, cholestyramine, and tetracycline, when employed for long periods of time, may interfere with the absorption or utilization of specific nutrients, chiefly the B vitamins and vitamin D.[10] Analogously, methotrexate is a folate agonist; isoniazid increases the requirement for pyridoxine; and antacids impair the absorption of copper and phosphate.

• *Total parenteral nutrition.* TPN, when prolonged, may lead to deficiencies of a variety of minerals (e.g., copper, zinc, phosphate) as well as inadequate supplies of phosphates, folates, and other nutrients.[4]

Whatever the nature of the nutritional disorder, whether primary or secondary, *overt morphologic lesions are relatively late manifestations*, save possibly for obesity. Long before anatomic changes become evident, functional deficits may appear. In addition, adaptive changes and bodily reserves to some extent mask the nutritional deficit. Even chronic protein-calorie deficit may not become evident for some time because it has been shown that reduction in physical activity and slowing of all metabolic processes may more or less balance the demand with the supply. Thus the first manifestation of chronic starvation may be merely listlessness or apathy. But in time, sooner in infants and children, the imbalance takes its toll on the growth rate and tissues and organs of the body. This "iceberg phenomenon" is even more applicable to deficiencies of specific nutrients, for example, iron deficiency. Reduced physical capacity, impaired learning ability, and deranged white cell function considerably antedate the appearance of the anemia. Thus, almost always, deficiency states are at first subclinical and can be discovered only by biochemical tests of the blood, plasma, or tissues.

PROTEIN-ENERGY MALNUTRITION

Marasmus-Kwashiorkor

Prolonged protein-calorie malnutrition, better known as protein-energy malnutrition (**PEM**), has its greatest impact on infants and children. It produces a range of clinical syndromes from kwashiorkor, at one end of the spectrum, related (not without some dispute) to a critical lack of protein despite a sufficient caloric intake, to marasmus, at the other end, caused by an overall lack of calories, or more bluntly, starvation. The term "kwashiorkor," derived from the Ga language of West Africa, means "the sickness that the older one gets when the next baby is born," i.e., when the older child is deprived of breast feeding and weaned to a diet largely of carbohydrate.

Kwashiorkor is characterized by apathy, peripheral edema, subcutaneous fat, moonface, enlarged fatty liver, and low serum albumin (Fig. 8 – 2). The edema may be generalized or localized to the upper or lower extremities. Although hypoalbuminemia must contribute to its causation, there is poor correlation between the severity of the edema and the serum albumin levels. Electrolyte disturbances, particularly potassium deficiency and sodium retention, may also play a role.[11] Characteristic of kwashiorkor but not always present are skin changes referred to as "flaky-paint" areas of depigmentation or hyperpigmentation, or in white infants, patches of dusky erythema. Hair changes may also be present, consisting of pallor, straightening (if the normal hair is curly), an abnormally fine texture, and loose attachment of the roots as evidenced by the ease with which the hair pulls out. A "flag sign" may appear as alternating bands of light (depigmented) and pigmented zones record periods of poor and more adequate nutrition (Fig. 8 – 3). Anemia is also frequently present owing to both iron and protein deficiency. Contributing to the anemia is insufficient synthesis of transferrin, the iron-transport protein of the blood, and of ceruloplasmin, the copper-transport protein.

Marasmus can be succinctly characterized as "wasting." These tragic infants and children have stunted growth; total loss of subcutaneous fat with atrophy of muscles producing broomstick arms and

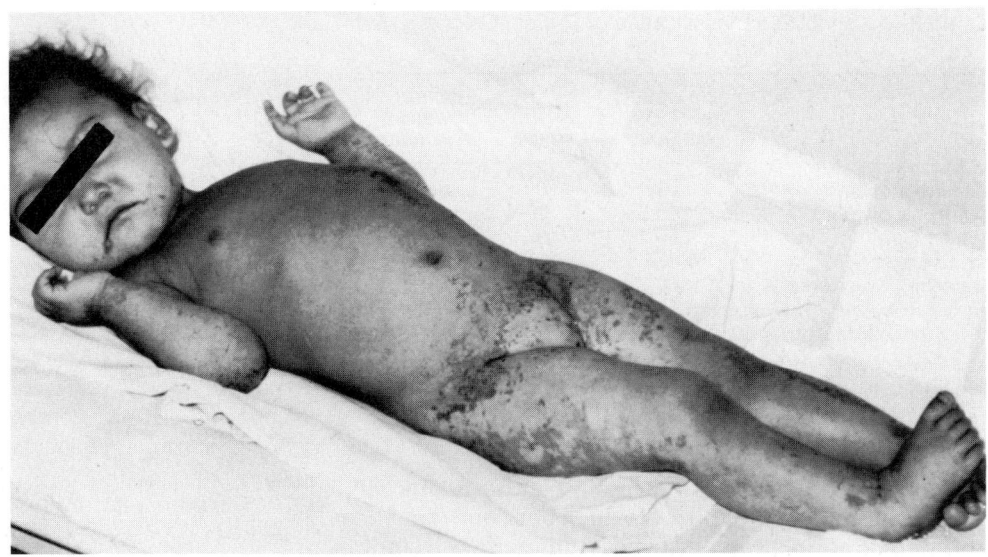

Figure 8–2. An infant with kwashiorkor revealing moonface, generalized edema, and skin rash over the extremities and lower trunk.

legs from which the skin hangs pathetically loose; and pinched, wizened faces imparting a prematurely aged appearance. In contrast to those with kwashiorkor, these children are alert and hungry and will eat ravenously if given food (Fig. 8–4). There is no edema or hepatic enlargement in the pure marasmic syndrome. *Between these two extremes is a range of hybrid syndromes such as "edematous marasmus" and* *"wasted kwashiorkor."* However, all PEM syndromes share to a greater or lesser extent some retardation in growth of the child (much more marked in marasmus), a general reduction in all physical and social activity, failure to thrive, and predisposition to infections, many of which are sufficiently severe to be lethal. A simplified overview of PEM in children is presented in Table 8–1.

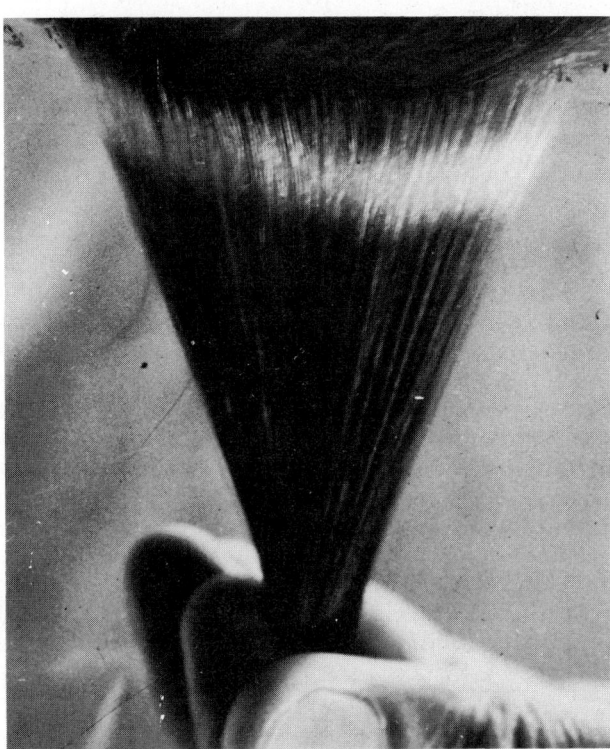

Figure 8–3. Kwashiorkor "flag sign." A tuft of hair in an infant showing a striking band of depigmentation, marking a period of severe malnutrition. (Courtesy of Dr. N. Scrimshaw, Massachusetts Institute of Technology; and the Institute of Nutrition of Central America and Panama.)

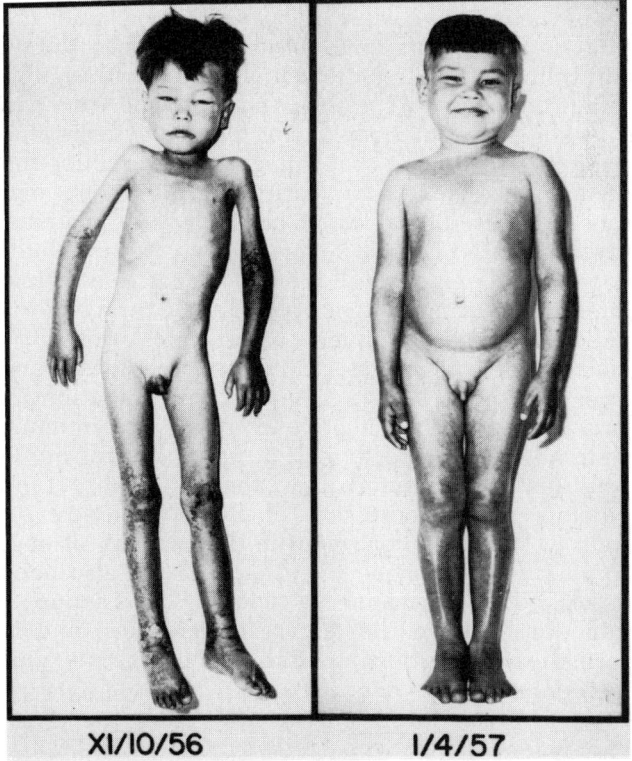

XI/10/56   1/4/57

Figure 8–4. Within every marasmic child *(left)* is a sturdy, smiling youngster; seen *(right)* after two months of adequate nutrition. (Courtesy of Dr. N. Scrimshaw, Massachusetts Institute of Technology; and the Institute of Nutrition of Central America and Panama.)

Table 8–1. Simplified Classification of Protein-Calorie Malnutrition

	BODY WEIGHT AS % OF STANDARD*	EDEMA	DEFICIT IN WEIGHT FOR HEIGHT
Underweight child	80–60	0	minimal
Nutritional dwarfing	<60	0	minimal
Marasmus	<60	0	++
Kwashiorkor	80–60	+	++
Marasmic kwashiorkor	<60	+	++

* Standard taken as 50th percentile of Harvard values.

Drawn from: WHO: Joint FAO/WHO Expert Committee on Nutrition, Eighth report. Food fortification and protein-calorie malnutrition. Tech. Rep. Ser. Wld. Hlth. Org., No. 477 (WHO, Geneva, 1971).

As pointed out, tragic protein-calorie malnutrition is endemic in the Third World. About one quarter of the total population of Africa is afflicted with some form of PEM.[12] However, marasmus is no stranger to industrialized countries, particularly among the infants and children of impoverished minority families.[13] Kwashiorkor, on the other hand, is largely restricted to Africa. "Formes frustes" of kwashiorkor are seen in chronic care hospitals and nursing facilities, among alcoholics, and during the postoperative period, when patients are maintained largely on intravenous glucose solutions without the addition of amino acids.

Although poverty, lack of food, and ignorance about the nutritive value of particular foods underlie PEM, other factors undoubtedly contribute. Intercurrent infections induce catabolic states with significant protein losses. They may thus predispose to kwashiorkor, sometimes converting a basically marasmic syndrome to kwashiorkor. Infections also reduce the dietary intake, increase nutritional requirements, and cause increased fecal losses, particularly of proteins. Children with PEM are bedeviled by parasites, childhood exanthems, and all manner of gastrointestinal infections. Recent surveys of children in rural Nigeria indicate that almost all have ascaris infestation, 60% malaria, 50% trichuriasis, 30% strongyloidiasis, and 12% amebiasis. The predisposition to infections is largely due to the effects of PEM on the immune system—premature thymic atrophy, depressed T-cell function mainly involving the CD-8 subset, and possibly some depression of B-cell antibody responses.[14] Some impairment in the capacity of neutrophils to kill phagocytized bacteria has also been described. In this manner, a vicious cycle is set up—infections worsen the dietary deficiencies, and in turn, the malnutrition impairs bodily defenses against infections.

MORPHOLOGY. The central anatomic changes in PEM are (1) growth failure, more marked in marasmus than in kwashiorkor; (2) peripheral edema in kwashiorkor; and (3) loss of body fat and atrophy of the muscle mass in marasmus. It has already been emphasized that the many hybrid syndromes blur the distinction between kwashiorkor and marasmus in some cases.

The **liver** in kwashiorkor, but not in marasmus, is enlarged and fatty, owing to decreased synthesis of carrier proteins. With restoration of an adequate diet the fat completely clears. Superimposed cirrhosis is a rarity.

The **small bowel** in kwashiorkor (rarely in marasmus) shows a decrease in the mitotic index in the crypts of the glands associated with mucosal atrophy and loss of villi and microvilli (Fig. 8–5). In such cases, there is concomitant loss of small intestinal enzymes, most often manifested as disaccharidase deficiency. Hence, these infants initially may not respond well to a full-strength, milk-based diet. An adequate diet and control of intercurrent intestinal infections permit restoration of the normal gastrointestinal mucosa.

The **bone marrow** in both kwashiorkor and marasmus may be hypoplastic owing mainly to depressed numbers of red cell precursors. How much of this derangement is due to a deficiency of protein, folates, or reduced synthesis of transferrin and ceruloplasmin is uncertain. Thus, anemia is usually present, most often hypochromic-microcytic, made worse by concomitant intestinal parasites such as hookworms. A concurrent deficiency of folates may lead to a mixed microcytic-macrocytic anemia. Adequate diet and control of infections promptly correct the hematologic abnormalities.

The **brain** in infants born to malnourished mothers and suffering PEM during the first one to two years of life is reported by some observers to show cerebral atrophy, a reduced number of neurons, and impaired myelinization of the white matter.[15,16] However, there is no universal agreement on the validity of these findings.

Many **other changes** may be present including thymic and lymphoid atrophy, more marked in kwashiorkor than in marasmus, the anatomic alterations induced by intercurrent infections, and deficiencies of other required nutrients such as iodine and vitamins.

There are still uncertainties in our understanding of PEM. Of particular concern is the impact of protein-energy malnutrition on the intellectual development of the child. Despite descriptions of putative regressive anatomic neurologic alterations, could genetic influences, cultural deprivation, and deficiencies of specific B vitamins underlie the impaired mental development so often encountered in these disadvantaged children? There is, however, complete agreement that an adequate diet, control of infections, and a reasonable lifestyle permit "catch-up growth" and restoration of a state of physical health and "intellectual health" in all but the terminally ill.

VITAMINS

The classic clinical features of a deficiency of a single vitamin are infrequently encountered today. In Third World countries the malnutrition tends to be more generalized, involving several vitamins and other mi-

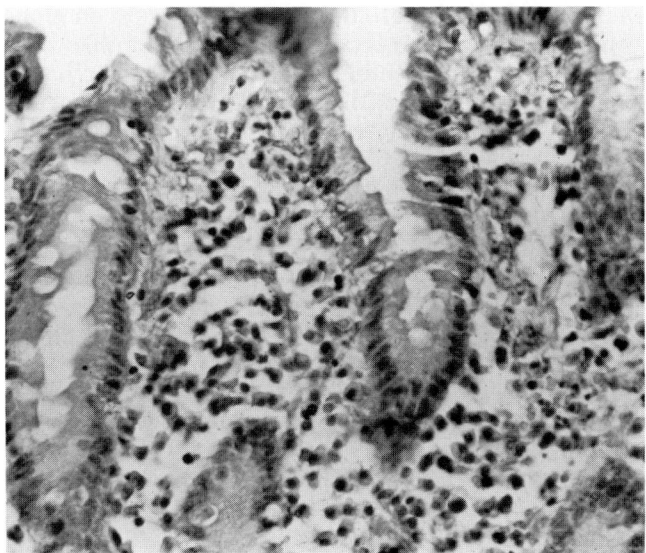

Figure 8–5. Kwashiorkor. Biopsy of small bowel revealing atrophy and blunting of villi and a nonspecific inflammatory infiltrate in the lamina propria.

cronutrients, proteins, and total calories as has already been noted. Thus the manifestations of the vitamin deficiencies are often submerged, or at least accompanied, by those related to the general undernutrition. In developed countries, similar generalized malnutrition occurs in the economically deprived. However, particular vitamin deficiencies still occur, principally in young children, adolescents, adult pregnant and lactating women, and among those of low socioeconomic status. Moreover, conditioned vitamin deficiencies develop in a variety of clinical situations affecting the absorption or metabolism of one or more vitamins, e.g., fat malabsorption.

FAT-SOLUBLE VITAMINS

Hypovitaminoses of the fat-soluble vitamins A and D on the basis of primary malnutrition occur throughout the world in economically deprived individuals, but hypovitaminoses of vitamins E and K are rare for reasons that will become apparent later. However, conditioned deficiencies of any one of the fat-soluble vitamins may arise even in affluent societies in the presence of biliary tract and pancreatic dysfunction and the intestinal malabsorption syndromes.

Vitamin A

Well-established deficiency states: Xerophthalmia (conjunctival keratinization); keratomalacia (corneal softening and ulceration); corneal scarring and blindness; impaired immune responses with increased mortality from infections (in children).

Possible consequences of a deficiency state: Impaired reproduction (in laboratory animals); impaired skeletal growth (in laboratory animals); increased predisposition to cancers of the skin, lungs, and other sites (in laboratory animals and possibly in humans).

A number of compounds have vitamin A activity. The most important and most active is retinol, an alcohol. Oxidation of retinol yields the aldehyde, retinal, and the acid, retinoic acid, also having vitamin A biologic activity. Retinyl esters are the storage form of vitamin A in the body. The important dietary sources of vitamin A are such animal-derived foods as eggs, butter, whole milk, and fish liver, which contain largely retinyl esters. There are also well over 2000 synthetic analogs of vitamin A having some, but not necessarily all, of its biologic activities. The term *retinoid* encompasses both naturally occurring and synthetic forms of vitamin A. There are, in addition, *provitamins, the carotenoids*, found in plants. The most important of these is beta-carotene consisting essentially of two linked molecules of retinol; rich sources of it are carrots, sweet potatoes, squash, pumpkins, mangoes, and spinach.

ABSORPTION, METABOLISM, AND TRANSPORT. Discussion of these processes will be limited to a few details relevant to the understanding of the normal function of vitamin A and the deficiency states. Excellent sources are available for more details.[17-19] As with all fats, the digestion and absorption of carotenes and retinoids requires bile, pancreatic enzymes, and some level of antioxidant activity in the food. Retinol, whether derived from ingested esters or from beta-carotene, is transported in chylomicrons to the liver for esterification and storage in hepatocytes and in the "fat-storing" Ito cells in the liver. More than 90% of the body's reserves are stored in the liver. In the normal individual on an adequate diet, the reserves of vitamin A in the liver are sufficient for at least six months of deprivation. Retinoic acid, on the other hand, can be absorbed unchanged; it represents a small fraction of vitamin A in the blood, active in epithelial differentiation and growth, but not in the maintenance of vision.

When the dietary intake of vitamin A is inadequate, the retinyl esters in the liver are mobilized and the released retinol is then bound to a specific retinol-binding protein (RBP) called transthyretin and synthesized in the liver. The uptake of retinol by the various cells of the body is dependent on membrane surface receptors specific for RBP, not for the retinol. The retinol is transported across the cell membrane, where it binds specifically to a cellular retinol-binding protein (CRBP), and the RBP is released.

BIOLOGIC FUNCTIONS OF VITAMIN A (RETINOL). In humans *the best defined functions of retinol are: (1) maintaining normal vision in reduced light, and (2) potentiating the differentiation of specialized epithelial cells, mainly mucus-secreting cells.* In laboratory animals, vitamin A deficiency produces sterility, fetal abnormalities, and impaired cartilaginous bone growth, but since analogous disturbances have not been documented in humans they will receive little further comment.[20,21] Later we shall return to a possible antiproliferative (anticancer) effect of vitamin A.

The *visual process* involves four kinds of vitamin A–containing pigments: rhodopsin in the rods, the most light-sensitive pigment and therefore important in reduced light; and three iodopsins in cone cells, each responsive to specific colors in bright light. The synthesis of rhodopsin involves oxidation of retinol derived from the blood to all-trans-retinal and then isomerization to 11-*cis*-retinal, which interacts with opsin, a protein in the rods, to form rhodopsin.[22] When a photon of light impinges on the dark-adapted retina, rhodopsin undergoes a sequence of configurational changes ultimately to yield all-trans-retinal and opsin. In the process, a nerve impulse is generated (by changes in membrane potential) that is transmitted via neurons from the retina to the brain. During dark adaptation some of the all-trans-retinal is reconverted to 11-*cis*-retinal, but most is reduced to retinol and lost to the retina, dictating the need for a continuous input of retinol. It is to the elegant studies of George Wald, for which he received a Nobel award, that we owe our understanding of the visual process.[23]

Less is known about the role of vitamin A in *cellular differentiation*, but it is clear that with a deficiency, mucus-secreting columnar epithelium in glands and mucosal surfaces is replaced by undifferentiating, nonsecreting, keratinizing squamous epithelium. Two hypotheses prevail. (1) The vitamin plays a role in the synthesis of specific glycoproteins involved in cell membrane structure and adhesion that may control cellular differentiation. (2) Vitamin A-CRBP complexes are transferred to the nuclei, where they affect gene expression by an as yet unknown mechanism because the binding is to nuclear membranes, not to DNA.

PREVALENCE AND CONSEQUENCES OF A DEFICIENCY STATE.

Vitamin A deficiency occurs worldwide. It is most prevalent on the basis of general undernutrition in Southeast Asia, Indonesia, and the Philippines, but it is also common in many regions of Africa and Central and South America.[24] In Asia as many as 5 million children develop xerophthalmia annually — one tenth having severe corneal involvement, and half of these becoming blind.[25] Even more tragic, among these children lacking vitamin A the mortality rate from infections such as measles, pneumonia, and infectious diarrhea is many fold greater than among those having no eye changes indicative of vitamin A deficiency.[26] Hypovitaminosis A is also seen sporadically in affluent societies among the economically deprived suffering from primary malnutrition, and as a conditioned deficiency among individuals having some cause for malabsorption of fats. In addition, extensive liver disease may lead to low circulating levels of vitamin A because of inadequate synthesis of RBP, just as the nephrotic syndrome may depress the levels of RBP because of excessive proteinuria. Not surprisingly then, hypovitaminosis A is a global problem.

> **MORPHOLOGY.** **Epithelial metaplasia,** as a consequence of impaired differentiation of specialized epithelial cells, is most evident in the mucous membranes of the eyes; the mucosa of the respiratory, gastrointestinal, and genitourinary tracts; and the lining epithelia of glandular ducts such as those in the pancreas. This metaplastic change has many adverse consequences. For example, in the upper urinary tract the desquamated keratinized squamae provide a nidus for stone formation. Desquamated squamous cells and cellular debris may obstruct small ducts in the pancreas (Fig. 8–6). The loss of mucus secretion leads to dryness of the conjunctival membranes in the eyes and serious injury to the cornea, as will be described later. When the respiratory airways are affected, the loss of mucus secretion and hence the defensive "mucociliary escalator," predisposes the lungs to infections. Squamous metaplasia in the sebaceous and sweat glands of the skin may cause **follicular hyperkeratosis** and predispose to acne, but such changes are uncommon in the young child.
>
> **The major target of vitamin A deficiency is the eye.** The first change is **xerosis** of the conjunctiva, characterized by dryness and wrinkling caused by replacement of mucus-secreting cells by squamous cells. This is followed by the formation of **Bitot's spots,** representing focal areas of opacity created by the accumulation of masses of desquamated cells and cell debris. Such changes may affect the cornea, so that it becomes dry, roughened, and sometimes edematous, impeding transmission of light. This predisposes to traumatic and infectious ulceration of the corneal surface, culminating sometimes in total erosion and liquefaction of the cornea — **keratomalacia.** Subsequent scarring or extrusion of the lens may then occur, leading to **blindness** (Fig. 8–7).

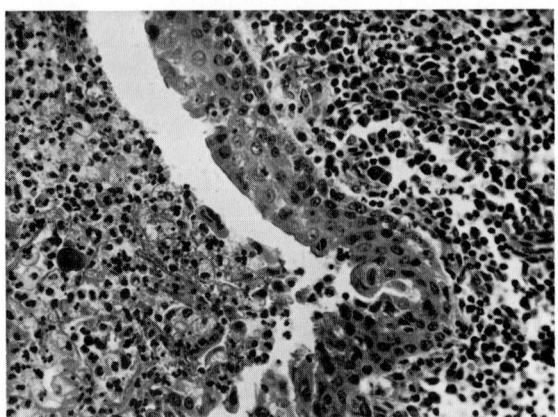

Figure 8–6. Squamous metaplasia of the epithelial lining of a duct in the pancreas.

RETINOIDS, CAROTENOIDS, AND CANCER.

The possibility that a deficiency of vitamin A may increase the predisposition to cancer has aroused great interest and has led to the hope that administration of vitamin A or its synthetic analogs might be preventive or beneficial in treatment. Despite the innumerable reports on these issues, firm conclusions have not been reached. A few of the more firmly based observations

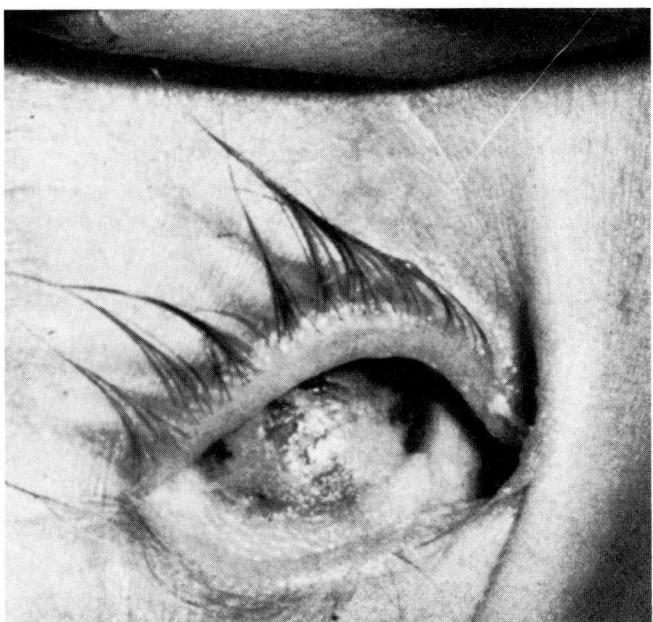

Figure 8–7. Advanced vitamin A deficiency with destruction of the eye. (Reproduced with the kind permission of Dr. Donald S. McLaren, Department of Medicine, Royal Infirmary, Edinburgh. From McLaren, D.: A Colour Atlas of Nutritional Disorders. London, Wolfe Medical Publications, Ltd., 1981, p. 26.)

VITAMIN A TOXICITY. Both acute and chronic excesses of vitamin A may produce toxic manifestations. Retinal esters or retinoic acid are more toxic than retinol, and synthetic analogs are less toxic. *Acute toxicity in children* from a single very large dose of retinyl ester or retinoic acid has produced headache, vomiting, stupor, and papilledema, all suggestive of a brain tumor. The *adult* may also develop acute neurologic changes similar to those seen in the child, but they are rarely so pronounced. *Chronic toxicity* in the child begins with anorexia, followed by weight loss, nausea, and vomiting; dryness of the mucosa of the lips; and dry skin with desquamation and itching. More protracted toxicity leads to hepatomegaly with parenchymal damage and fibrosis (sometimes associated with portal hypertension and ascites); periosteal neo-osteogenesis with painful bony exostoses; and in some instances visual and mental disturbances. Premature closure of the fontanelles has occurred, leading to prolonged increased intracranial pressure and possibly hydrocephalus. Chronic toxicity in the adult is also similar to that in the child save that bony changes are not prominent. Although synthetic retinoids are not associated with the syndromes just described, when administered for the treatment of acne during pregnancy they have induced an increased incidence of congenital malformations in the embryo (p. 521). Less disturbing is the appearance of yellowing of the skin, particularly of the palms, related to hypercarotenemia produced either by the consumption of monster amounts of carrots (rabbits and carrot freaks take note) or by an inborn error of metabolism. Although this benign pigmentation can be confused with jaundice, it does not produce yellowing of the sclerae.

follow. Vitamin A deficiency increases the susceptibility of laboratory animals to carcinogen-induced cancers of the oral cavity, lung, bladder, and colon. Conversely, retinoids have caused the regression or inhibited the development of a variety of experimentally induced cancers, such as those in the urinary tract and mammary gland of the rat and the skin of the mouse.[27]

Regrettably, the evidence derived from humans is more tenuous. Epidemiologic surveys have related a lower intake of vitamin A to an increased predisposition to lung cancer (the strongest association) and cancers of the oral cavity, larynx, esophagus, stomach, pancreas, gastrointestinal tract, bladder, prostate, and other sites.[28] However, the major sources of vitamin A in the diet of humans are vegetable carotenoids, and the putative anticancer effect of vitamin A may relate to the antioxidant action of beta-carotene rather than to its conversion to retinol. Nonetheless, retinoids, natural and synthetic, (as distinct from carotenoids) have been shown to be effective in causing regression of various premalignant diseases such as actinic keratosis, oral leukoplakia, bronchial metaplasia, laryngeal papillomatosis, cervical dysplasia, and metaplasia in the urinary bladder.[29] Evidence that they have reversed basal cell carcinoma and keratoacanthoma is more controversial. There is, however, no dispute that several nontumorous skin diseases, particularly severe acne, rosacea, psoriasis, and other keratinizing dermatoses are remarkably ameliorated or even cured by the new retinoids. An overview of the major features relating to vitamin A is offered in Figure 8–8.

Vitamin D

Well-established deficiency states: Rickets in children; osteomalacia in adults; and hypocalcemic tetany.

Possible consequences of a deficiency state: Disturbed immunoregulation; impaired control of cell proliferation and differentiation.

The major function of vitamin D, or more properly of its metabolites, is the maintenance of normal plasma levels of calcium and phosphorus. *It is therefore required for (1) the prevention of the bone diseases—rickets in growing children whose epiphyses have not already closed and osteomalacia in adults, and (2) the prevention of hypocalcemic tetany.* In passing it might be noted that calcium is also involved in blood clotting, maintenance of normal membrane permeability, and many important intracellular functions. Here our attention is focused on its role in bone formation. *The bone diseases produced by hypovitaminosis D are characterized basically by a failure of normal mineralization of newly laid-down osteoid.* In the case of rickets there is also defective mineralization of epiphyseal cartilage, necessary to control cartilaginous growth at the epiphyseal plate. With respect to the neuromuscular dysfunction termed hypocalcemic tetany, vitamin D maintains the

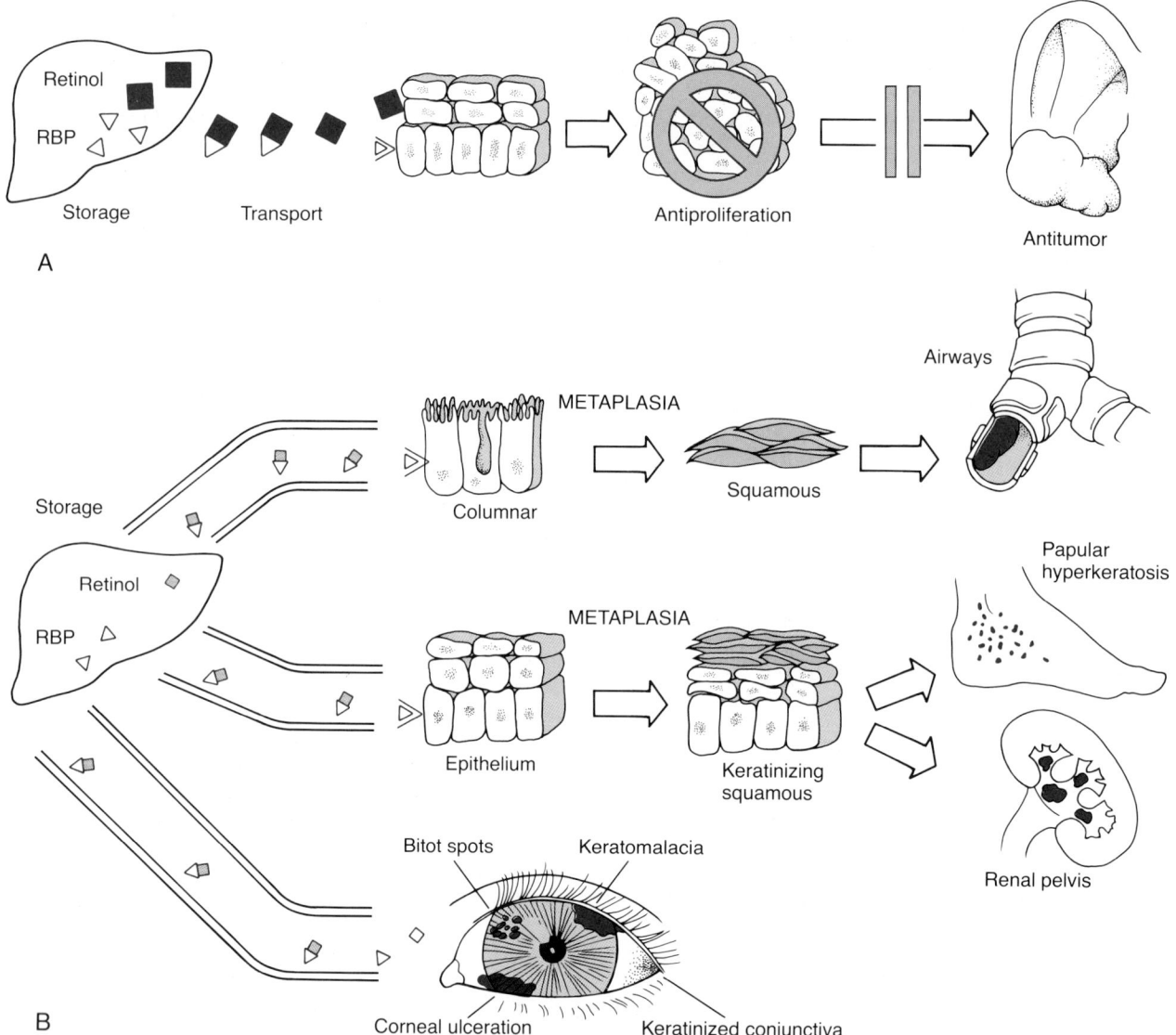

Figure 8–8. Vitamin A (retinol). *A,* The putative antiproliferative-antitumor action of normal levels of retinol delivered to epithelia from its storage site in the liver bound to retinol-binding protein (RBP). *B,* The deficiency state leads to (1) squamous metaplasia of columnar epithelia, e.g., in the airways; (2) hyperkeratinization of squamous epithelia, inducing papular hyperkeratosis of the skin and squamatization of the renal pelvis; and (3) keratinization of conjunctivae, leading to the many ocular changes shown.

normal concentration of ionized calcium in the extracellular fluid compartment requisite for normal neural excitation and relaxation of muscle. Insufficient ionized calcium in the extracellular fluid results in continuous excitation of muscle leading to the convulsive state, hypocalcemic tetany. Of recent date, a putative immunoregulatory function has been ascribed to vitamin D because receptors for one of its metabolites have been demonstrated in activated and malignant lymphocytes and in macrophages. Analogous receptors have been identified in some leukemic cell lines, raising the possibility that active metabolites of vitamin D play roles in cellular proliferation and differentiation.[30] Little is known yet about these newly described functions, and so they receive no further comment.

SOURCES AND METABOLISM OF VITAMIN D.

Humans have two possible sources of vitamin D — endogenous synthesis in the skin, and the diet. There are large amounts of the precursor 7-dehydrocholesterol in the skin; ultraviolet light in sunlight converts it to vitamin D_3. Depending on the skin's level of melanin pigmentation, which absorbs the UV light, and the amount of exposure to sunlight, about 80% of the body's need can be endogenously derived. The remainder is obtained from dietary sources such as deep-sea fish and ergosterol in plants and grains that is converted to vitamin D_2 in the body. In many countries, various foods are fortified with vitamin D_2. Since D_3 and D_2 undergo identical metabolic transformations and have identical functions, they will hereafter be referred to as vitamin D.

Before vitamin D becomes functionally active it must undergo metabolic conversion to 1,25-dihydroxyvitamin D (1,25-[OH]$_2$D), also known as *calcitriol*, which behaves, as will be seen, much in the manner of a hormone. The steps involved in the formation of this active metabolite have been well characterized.

1. Vitamin D, whether of endogenous or exogenous origin, is transported in the plasma bound to an alpha-1 globulin known as D-binding protein (DBP). In humans, the principal storage site of vitamin D is adipose tissue rather than the liver, as is the case with vitamin A.
2. Conversion to 25-hydroxyvitamin D (25-OH-D) occurs in the liver by the action of a 25-hydroxylase.
3. Subsequently, the 25-OH-D is converted in the kidney by a 1-alpha-hydroxylase into 1,25-(OH)$_2$D (calcitriol), which is at least 5 to 10 times more active than the parent vitamin.
4. The production of calcitriol by the kidney is regulated by the plasma levels of 1,25-(OH)$_2$D, calcium, and phosphorus. In a hormonal feedback loop, increased levels of calcitriol downregulate synthesis, and decreased levels do the converse. Hypocalcemia stimulates secretion of the parathyroid hormone that, in turn, augments the conversion of 25-OH-D to 1,25-(OH)$_2$D.[31] Hypophosphatemia directly increases the formation of 1,25(OH)$_2$D.
5. 25-OH-D may undergo alternative metabolic pathways, with the formation of functionally less active products such as 24,25-(OH)$_2$D or 25,26-(OH)$_2$D. These alternative conversions may represent a mechanism for the fine-tuning of plasma calcium levels.

NORMAL FUNCTIONS OF VITAMIN D. *The essential function of vitamin D — the maintenance of normal plasma levels of calcium and phosphorus — involves actions on the intestines, bones, and kidneys. To summarize, (1) it stimulates intestinal absorption of calcium and, independently, of phosphorus; (2) it collaborates with parathyroid hormone in the mobilization of calcium from bone; and (3) it stimulates the parathyroid hormone–dependent reabsorption of calcium in the distal renal tubules.* In addition, it is possible that vitamin D has other actions on cells of the immune system as noted previously.

How calcitriol stimulates *intestinal absorption of calcium and phosphorus* is still somewhat controversial. *At issue is whether it is a receptor- and gene-mediated function or a direct action on enterocytes augmenting uptake of the minerals from the intestinal lumen.* The weight of evidence favors the view that 1,25-(OH)$_2$D binds to receptors activating DNA-RNA synthesis of calcium and phosphorus transport proteins.[31] A genetic disorder, vitamin D–dependent rickets type II, is marked by target organ resistance to calcitriol and poor intestinal absorption, attributable to defective receptors, supporting the receptor-gene–mediated mechanism. However, still not ruled out is the possibility that calcitriol directly affects

membrane function, augmenting calcium and, independently, phosphorus uptake. Whatever the precise mechanism, vitamin D enhances calcium and phosphorus absorption.

Vitamin D has two opposing actions on bone depending on the plasma levels of calcium. *On the one hand, with hypocalcemia, 1,25-(OH)$_2$D collaborates with parathyroid hormone in the resorption of calcium and phosphorus from bone to support the blood levels. On the other hand, vitamin D is requisite for normal mineralization of epiphyseal cartilage and osteoid matrix.* It is still not clear how the resorptive function is mediated. Some studies suggest that vitamin D stimulates osteoclast-mediated bone resorption.[32] There is also evidence that the principal targets are the osteoblasts, and more specifically, inhibition of their synthesis of type I collagen, the major component of osteoid matrix, inevitably leading in the course of normal bone remodeling to net resorption. Whatever the mechanism, it is clear that the skeletal system is a major reservoir of calcium.

The precise details of mineralization of bone when the plasma levels of calcium and phosphorus are adequate are also uncertain. Two schools of thought prevail. One holds that the sole function of vitamin D is to maintain calcium and phosphorus at supersaturated levels in the plasma, although the precise manner of transfer of calcium from the plasma compartment to the mineralizing front is obscure.[33] The other view contends that calcitriol increases the synthesis in osteoid matrix of the calcium-binding proteins osteocalcin and osteonectin (analogous to fibronectin because they bind to both calcium and collagen).[34] Further studies are obviously needed.

Less well defined is the role of calcitriol in the renal reabsorption of calcium. Parathyroid hormone is clearly necessary, but it is believed that so is vitamin D. There is no substantial evidence that vitamin D participates in renal reabsorption of phosphorus. An overview of the normal metabolism of vitamin D and the consequences of a deficiency are offered in Figure 8–9.

PREVALENCE AND CONSEQUENCES OF A DEFICIENCY STATE. Rickets in growing children and osteomalacia in adults are worldwide skeletal diseases, but in developed countries they are rare on the basis of dietary deficiencies. However, both forms of skeletal disease may appear anywhere under conditions that derange vitamin D absorption or metabolism and in uncommon disorders that affect the function of vitamin D or disturb calcium or phosphorus homeostasis, as indicated in Table 8–2.[35]

NORMAL BONE DEVELOPMENT AND MAINTENANCE. An understanding of the morphologic changes in rickets and osteomalacia is greatly facilitated by a cursory review of normal bone development and maintenance. The skeleton is formed by *intramembranous ossification,* involving primarily the development of flat bones; and *endochondral ossification,* which accounts primarily for the formation of the

NORMAL VITAMIN D METABOLISM

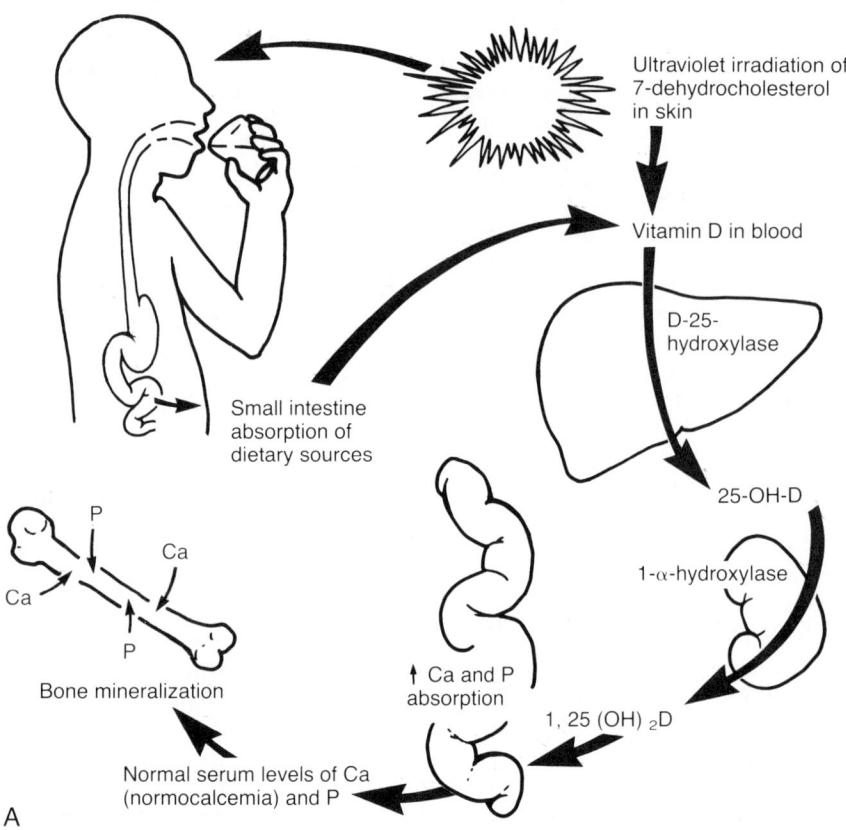

Ultraviolet irradiation of
7-dehydrocholesterol
in skin

Vitamin D in blood

D-25-
hydroxylase

25-OH-D

1-α-hydroxylase

Small intestine
absorption of
dietary sources

1, 25 (OH) $_2$D

↑ Ca and P
absorption

P   Ca

Ca

P

Bone mineralization

Normal serum levels of Ca
(normocalcemia) and P

A

VITAMIN D DEFICIENCY

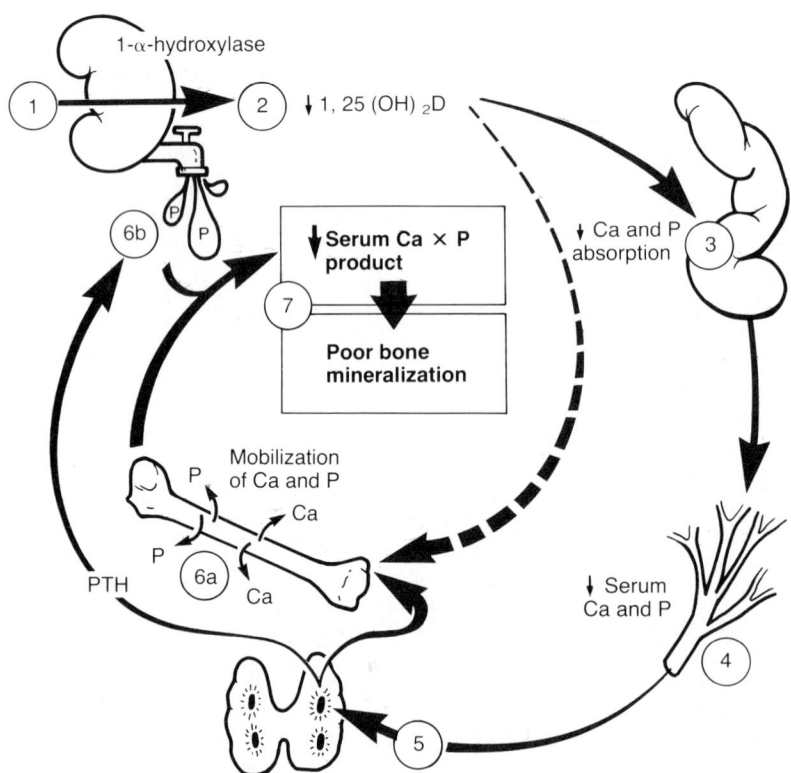

1-α-hydroxylase

① → ② ↓ 1, 25 (OH) $_2$D

6b   P   P

↓ Serum Ca × P
product

⑦

Poor bone
mineralization

↓ Ca and P
absorption

③

Mobilization
of Ca and P

P   Ca

P   ⑥a   Ca

PTH

↓ Serum
Ca and P

④

⑤

B

Figure 8–9. *A,* Schema of normal vitamin D metabolism. *B,* Hypovitaminosis
D. There is inadequate substrate for the
renal hydroxylase (1) yielding a deficiency of 1,25(OH)$_2$ (2) and deficient absorption of calcium and phosphorus
from the gut (3), with consequent depressed serum levels of both (4). The
hypocalcemia activates the parathyroid
glands (5), causing, along with the D deficiency, mobilization of calcium and
phosphorus from bone (6a). Simultaneously, the PTH induces wasting of
phosphate in the urine (6b). Consequently, the serum levels of calcium are
normal or near-normal, but the phosphate is low; hence, mineralization is
impaired (7).

Table 8–2. Pathophysiologic Mechanisms Associated with Rickets or Osteomalacia

INADEQUATE ENDOGENOUS SYNTHESIS AND DIETARY LACK[36]

In *developing countries* occurs because of varying combinations of dark skin, inadequate exposure to sunlight, and primary malnutrition. Infants predisposed by poor maternal nutrition and deficient postnatal reserves, and children because of increased demands of growth.

In *industrialized countries* occurs mainly in infancy and childhood. Contributory factors are: nonuse of fortified foods, e.g., vitamin D–supplemented milk; Northern hemisphere with little sunlight; poverty with general malnutrition; poor maternal nutrition. Osteomalacia apt to occur in *the elderly* because of such factors as avoidance of sunlight and restricted or bizarre diets.[37]

MALABSORPTION

Occurs with any disease that impairs intestinal absorption of fats, e.g., cholestatic liver disease or extrahepatic biliary tract obstruction, pancreatic insufficiency, celiac sprue, extensive small bowel disease, e.g., regional enteritis. Also occurs with abnormally rapid small intestinal transit following gastrectomy.

DERANGEMENTS IN METABOLISM OF VITAMIN D

Diffuse liver disease — interference with synthesis of the transport protein DBP.

Chronic renal failure — due to decreased conversion of 25-OH-D to 1,25-$(OH)_2D$ (p. 1017). Azotemia and acidosis also impair intestinal absorption of calcium. The osteomalacia in renal failure may be complicated by osteitis fibrosa related to secondary hyperparathyroidism producing so-called renal osteodystrophy.

Nephrotic syndrome — excessive excretion of vitamin D binding protein.

Drugs such as phenytoin, phenobarbital, and rifampin — induce P-450 enzymes accelerating the rate of degradation of sterols, among them vitamin D and its metabolites.

Vitamin D–dependent rickets type I (autosomal recessive) — genetic lack of or defect in 1,alpha-hydroxylase with an inability to convert 25-OH-D into 1,25-$(OH)_2D$.

END-ORGAN RESISTANCE TO VITAMIN D

Vitamin D–dependent rickets type II — attributed to defective receptors with inadequate calcium absorption in the intestine accompanied perhaps by deranged vitamin D function in other organs, e.g., bone.

OTHER RARE CAUSES

X-linked hypophosphatemic rickets, i.e., hypophosphatemia, normocalcemia, and low to normal plasma levels of calcitriol. Basic defects: renal phosphate wasting and possibly impaired intestinal absorption of calcium.

Tumor-induced osteomalacia, attributed to some tumor-produced product, causing impaired conversion of 25-OH-D into calcitriol and phosphate wasting.

Chronic use of antacids, e.g., Maalox, Mylanta — aluminum hydroxide binds to phosphate and interferes with absorption.

long tubular bones. With intramembranous bone formation, mesenchymal cells differentiate directly into osteoblasts, which synthesize the largely (90 to 95%) collagenous osteoid matrix. With endochondral formation, the growing cartilage at the epiphyseal plates is provisionally mineralized and then progressively resorbed and replaced by osteoid matrix, which then undergoes mineralization to create bone. With both pathways, once bone is formed it undergoes constant remodeling during life, involving continued osteoclastic resorption matched by osteoblastic activity. Indeed in young adults, the turnover rate of total skeletal calcium may reach 15 to 18% per year. In middle to late adult life, bone resorption dominates and with it skeletal mass is progressively lost. At sites of osteoblastic activity during both the development of the skeleton and its maintenance, about 1 μ of matrix osteoid is produced daily. Since mineralization lags by about 12 to 15 days behind matrix synthesis, *bone at virtually all ages contains osteoid matrix seams about*

12 to 15 μ in thickness. If mineralization is delayed or inadequate, as occurs in both rickets and osteomalacia, the osteoid seams thicken. In undecalcified microscopic sections with H and E stains, osteoid appears pink, whereas mineralized bone is more basophilic and has a blue cast. Special stains and tetracycline labeling more clearly delineate osteoid (p. 1317).[38]

MORPHOLOGY. The basic derangement in both rickets and osteomalacia, as already emphasized, is delayed and/or inadequate mineralization and hence an excess of unmineralized matrix. The changes in rickets, however, are complicated by inadequate provisional calcification of epiphyseal cartilage deranging endochondral bone growth. The following sequence then ensues in rickets.

—Overgrowth of epiphyseal cartilage due to failure of the cartilage cells to mature and disintegrate.

—Persistence of distorted, irregular masses of cartilage, many of which project into the marrow cavity.

—Deposition of osteoid matrix on inadequately mineralized cartilaginous remnants.

—Disruption of the orderly replacement of cartilage by osteoid matrix, with enlargement and lateral expansion of the osteochondral junction (Fig. 8–10).

—Abnormal overgrowth of capillaries and fibroblasts in the disorganized zone because of microfractures and stresses on the inadequately mineralized, weak, poorly formed bone.

—Deformation of the skeleton due to the loss of structural rigidity of the developing bones.

The conformation of the gross skeletal changes depends on the severity of the rachitic process, its duration, and in particular on the stresses to which individual bones are subjected. Age is therefore a particularly important factor, not only with respect to the rate of bone growth but also insofar as it conditions the type of stress. During the non-ambulatory stage of infancy the head and chest sustain the greatest stresses. The softened occipital bones may become flattened and the parietal bones can be buckled inward by pressure, but with the release of the pressure, elastic recoil snaps the bones back into their original positions—**craniotabes.** An excess of osteoid produces **frontal bossing** and a **squared appearance to the head.** Deformation of the chest results from overgrowth of cartilage and osteoid tissue at the costochondral junction producing the "**rachitic rosary.**" The weakened metaphyseal areas of the ribs are subject to the pull of the respiratory muscles and thus bend inward, creating anterior protrusion of the sternum—**pigeon-breast deformity.** The inward pull at the margin of the diaphragm creates **Harrison's groove,** girdling the thoracic cavity at the lower margin of the rib cage. The pelvis may become deformed. When the ambulating child develops rickets, deformities are likely to affect the spine, pelvis, and long bones (e.g., tibia) causing most notably **lumbar lordosis** and **bowing of the legs.**

Osteomalacia in the adult is much more subtle and is characterized by loss of skeletal mass or "too little" bone, referred to as **osteopenia.** It must therefore be differentiated, often with difficulty, from other osteopenias such as osteoporosis (p. 1324), osteitis fibrosa (p. 1326), and certain stages of Paget's disease of the bone (p. 1328). In these conditions there is no defect in mineralization and, in fact, an increased rate. In contrast, osteomalacia is marked by inadequate mineralization and hence an excess of unmineralized osteoid.[39] Skeletal deformities do not appear in osteomalacia—only apparent loss of bone density and cortical thickness as visualized by radiography or other techniques. Not surprisingly, with marked osteomalacia the "too-little bone" is subject to fractures, most often of the vertebrae, hips, wrists, and ribs, and to kyphoscoliotic deformity of the vertebral column as discussed on page 1325.

CLINICAL COURSE. In the growing child, full-blown rickets presents no clinical diagnostic challenge. In addition to the skeletal changes cited, the circulating levels of 25-OH-D and 1,25(OH)$_2$D are

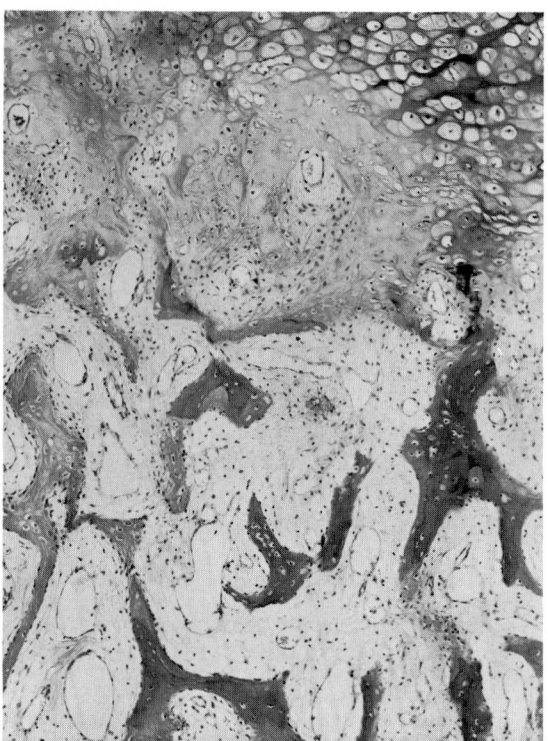

Figure 8–10. A detail of a rachitic costochondral junction. The palisade of cartilage is lost. Some of the trabeculae are old, well-formed bone, but the paler ones consist of unmineralized osteoid tissue.

low. The serum calcium may be low or normal. With severe depletion of bony reserves the serum calcium level may fall, with the appearance of hypocalcemic tetany. However, because of endogenous synthesis of vitamin D, forme fruste patterns are common and difficult to diagnose, particularly when accompanied by other nutritional deficiencies such as are common in underprivileged populations. Sometimes the only clue is a subnormal plasma level of 25-OH-D, but it should be recalled that there are forms of rickets in which the circulating levels of this metabolite are normal, e.g., vitamin D–dependent rickets type II and hypophosphatemic rickets.

The diagnosis of osteomalacia is even more difficult, particularly its differentiation from osteoporosis (p. 1324). It is beyond our scope to delve into this difficult diagnostic problem save to note that ultimately bone biopsy (usually transiliac) may be necessary to document the excess of unmineralized osteoid. The presence of some form of osteopenia should be suspected in elderly individuals having a predisposition to fractures with minimal trauma. In a series of elderly patients with hip fracture, osteomalacia was found in as many as 25%.[40] Less dramatic manifestations include proximal muscle weakness and bone pain most often localized to the pelvis, scapula, and ribs, related possibly to microfractures or pseudofractures commonly called milkman's fractures or Looser's zones. These are radiolucent lines several millimeters thick and sharply demarcated from the adjacent bone. They are attributed to resorption of the thin bone by overlying pulsating arteries. In the last analysis, the best way to make the diagnosis of osteomalacia in most instances is a therapeutic trial of vitamin D and calcium. The serum calcium and 25-OH-D levels are not usually helpful because they may be normal or low.

TOXICITY. Large excesses of vitamin D are well tolerated. Extreme acute overdosage is very uncommon but may cause hypercalcemia, which is transient unless the vitamin D excess is continued. Chronic toxicity with its increased levels of blood calcium may give rise to metastatic calcifications and renal stones as discussed on page 36.

Vitamin E

A group of eight closely related fat-soluble compounds—four tocopherols and four tocotrienols—all have vitamin E biologic activity. Among them, alpha-tocopherol is the most active and most widely available. For many years we have known that vitamin E deficiency in laboratory animals produced a variety of derangements including sterility and spontaneous abortion, muscular dystrophies, abnormal hemolysis, and encephalomalacia. However, as recently as 1977 it was said of vitamin E with reference to humans, "We are still faced with a vitamin looking for a disease with which it can have an honorable marriage."[41] But at long last it has found its mate—a well-defined neurologic syndrome.[42,43]

Vitamin E is so abundant in many foods—vegetables, grains, nuts and their oils, dairy products, fish, and meat—that a diet sufficient to sustain life is most unlikely to be insufficient in vitamin E. In animals a high dietary intake of polyunsaturated fatty acids (PUFA) increases the requirement for vitamin E; however, in humans, diets high in PUFA are also rich sources of vitamin E. The absorption of tocopherols, as with all fats, requires normal biliary tract and pancreatic function. After absorption vitamin E is transported in the blood in the form of chylomicrons, which rapidly equilibrate with the plasma lipoproteins, mainly low-density lipoproteins. Thus, disorders that derange fat absorption and chylomicron formation are the main causes of conditioned deficiencies of vitamin E (Table 8–3). Unlike vitamin A, which is stored mainly in the liver, vitamin E accumulates throughout the tissues of the body, mostly in fat depots, liver, and muscle.[44]

FUNCTION OF VITAMIN E. *This essential nutrient is one of a group of antioxidants (the only lipid-soluble antioxidant) that serve to scavenge free radicals formed in redox reactions throughout the body. It plays a role in termination of free radical–generated lipid peroxidation chain reactions, particularly in cellular and subcellular membranes that are rich in polyunsaturated lipids.* This action complements that of selenium, which as a constituent of glutathione peroxidase also metabolizes peroxides before they cause membrane damage. Why the nervous system is a particular target of vitamin E deficiency is not entirely

Table 8–3. Disorders Inducing Vitamin E Deficiency[43]

Abetalipoproteinemia	Autosomal recessive disorder characterized by inability to synthesize apoprotein B, an essential component of chylomicrons, low density and very low density lipoproteins leading to defective transport of vitamin E in the plasma.
Intrahepatic and extrahepatic cholestasis	Deficient delivery of bile to the small intestine with fat malabsorption.
Cystic fibrosis of the pancreas	Inadequate pancreatic enzymes and bile flow with fat malabsorption.
Small intestinal disorders	Celiac disease, extensive regional enteritis, radiation injury, and small bowel resection, for example, all may lead to steatorrhea and fat malabsorption.
Isolated vitamin E deficiency (rare)	No generalized fat malabsorption, but specific obscure defects of vitamin E absorption.
Low birth weight neonates	Physiologic immaturity of the liver and gastrointestinal tract, aggravated by formulas high in PUFA and low in alpha-tocopherol.

clear, but it is speculated that neurons with long axons are particularly vulnerable because of their large membrane surface area.[45] Mature red cells may also be particularly vulnerable because of the oxidative stress imposed by the generation of superoxide radicals during oxygenation of hemoglobin. Accordingly, vitamin E protects against peroxide-induced hemolysis along with glutathione peroxidase and other free radical scavengers.

PREVALENCE AND CONSEQUENCES OF A DEFICIENCY STATE. Hypovitaminosis E on a dietary basis is encountered uncommonly in the Western world for reasons already given. It occurs almost exclusively in association with disorders affecting its absorption and transport and in some premature and low birth weight infants as cited in Table 8–3. The most severe deficiencies are seen with abetalipoproteinemia, and even with this disorder clinical features relating to hypovitaminosis E rarely become evident before the end of the first decade of life.

The anatomic changes found in the nervous system depend on the duration and severity of the deficiency state. Most consistent is **degeneration of the axons in the posterior columns of the spinal cord with focal accumulation of lipopigment or complete loss of nerve cells in the dorsal root ganglia attributed to a dying-back type of axonopathy.**[42] Myelin degeneration in the sensory axons in peripheral nerves may also be present and, in more marked cases, degenerative changes in the spinocerebellar tracts as well. Neuronal pigmentation and loss have been observed in the sensory nuclei of the trigeminal, auditory, and vagus nerves.

In occasional cases, features of both primary and denervation muscle disease have been observed in skeletal muscle. The changes have taken the form mostly of cell atrophy with increased deposits of electron-dense inclusions, most likely lipofuscin and secondary lysosomes.

Retinal pigmentary degeneration similar to that seen in severe vitamin A deficiency has also been observed in patients with abetalipoproteinemia. Although it was at one time attributed to concomitant deficiencies of vitamins A and E, the retinopathy has developed in some patients receiving vitamin A supplementation, and conversely the changes have cleared following vitamin E administration.[46]

Whether vitamin E plays an important role in normal red cell survival continues to be a controversial issue. There is clear evidence that it is a specific erythropoietic factor for nonhuman primates and swine, but it has not been shown to be required for humans.[47] Nonetheless, vitamin E–deficient erythrocytes are more susceptible to oxidative stress and have a reduced half-life in the circulating blood. The life span of red cells in premature and small for gestational age infants is about two-thirds that of average full-term infants, ascribed (but not without dispute) to hypovitaminosis E.[48]

CLINICAL COURSE. The clinical manifestations of vitamin E deficiency depend on the distribution and severity of the neurologic lesions and vary somewhat among individuals. Most consistent are depressed or, more often, absent tendon reflexes, ataxia, dysarthria, loss of position and vibration sense, and loss of pain sensation. Muscle weakness is also common. In addition, there may be impaired vision and disorders of eye movement progressing sometimes to total ophthalmoplegia. Anemia is not a feature of the deficiency state in adults but is often found in premature infants and is probably multifactorial in origin.

Based on its antioxidant activity, vitamin E has been employed therapeutically in infants with the respiratory distress syndrome to counteract potential free radical injury induced by high levels of oxygen used for ventilatory support and in an effort to lower the incidence of retrolental fibroplasia (due to growth of immature retinal blood vessels) in premature infants exposed to high oxygen concentrations in incubators. In addition, megadose vitamin E supplementation has been touted by the manufacturers of vitamin pills to benefit such disparate conditions as muscular dystrophy, menopausal syndrome, diabetes, scleroderma, and infertility and to prevent cancer by reducing free radical–induced cell injury and proliferation.[27] There is no evidence that any of these uses are of any benefit save to those who sell vitamin E pills ("pill-poppers" should note).

TOXICITY. Although modest increases in the blood levels of tocopherol have not been shown to be harmful, massive overdosage has been associated with gastrointestinal disturbances (nausea, flatulence, or diarrhea), decreased platelet aggregation, prolongation of prothrombin time, interference with intestinal absorption of vitamins A and K, interference with wound healing, and necrotizing enterocolitis in vitamin E–treated infants.

Vitamin K

Deficiency state: Hypoprothrombinemia.

Vitamin K is a required cofactor for a hepatic microsomal carboxylase that converts specific glutamyl residues, in particular protein precursors, to gamma-carboxyglutamates (Gla). Four clotting factors require vitamin K for carboxylation: factor II (prothrombin), factor VII, factor IX, and factor X. The Gla residues are essential for the Ca^{++}dependent interaction of these proteins with a phospholipid surface involved in the rapid generation of thrombin.[49] In addition, three other plasma proteins having Gla residues are vitamin K dependent: proteins C, S and Z. Protein C is a circulating zymogen of a natural anticoagulant that is activated by thrombin in the presence of thrombomodulin. Activated protein C inhibits coagulation by inactivating factors VIIIa and Va.[50] This activity of protein C is enhanced by protein S. In addition, protein C has fibrinolytic activity related to its ability to neutralize a circulating inhibitor of tissue-type plasminogen activator. A function for protein Z has not yet been established. Gla-containing proteins are also found in many solid tissues, for example, osteocalcin in bone, possibly involved in calcification of osteoid matrix (p. 1315).

The precise biochemical events involved in the post-translational carboxylation of vitamin K–dependent proteins remain uncertain and will only be summarized (Fig. 8–11). In essence, *the reduced form of the vitamin in the presence of O_2 and CO_2 serves as a cofactor for the carboxylase present in liver microsomes in the conversion of glutamates to gamma-carboxyglutamates requisite for normal function of the vitamin K–dependent clotting factors.*[51] In the course of this reaction, vitamin K is converted to its 2,3 epoxide. Subsequently a vitamin K–epoxide reductase participates (solely or in concert with a second enzyme) in the reduction of the epoxide to the reduced form of vitamin K available to serve again in the carboxylase reaction. Since the vitamin can thus be efficiently recycled, the daily dietary requirement is very low.

Vitamin K can be synthesized endogenously by the intestinal flora. However, endogenous sources are inadequate for adults and fall far short of the needs of neonates. Exogenous sources are therefore necessary. The average diet in Western countries contains a large excess of fat-soluble vitamin K in a wide variety of plants, vegetables, and vegetable oils. Absorption in the small intestine requires adequate bile flow and pancreatic function. Moreover, the healthy adult has a reserve of vitamin K. Although said to be small, it is sufficient for weeks of a negative balance.[52] The sources of vitamin K are more precarious for neonates. The intestinal colonization has not yet fully developed; breast milk is a relatively poor source of vitamin K as compared with commercial formulas; and the

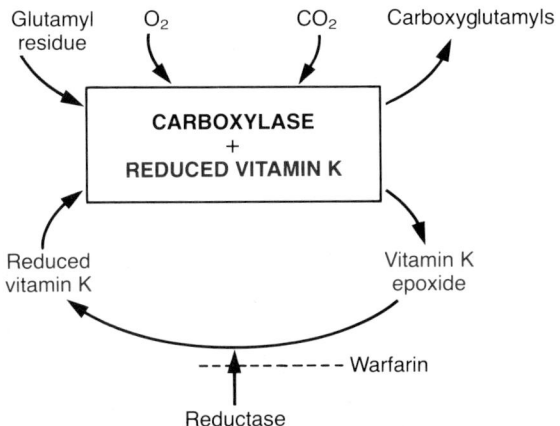

Figure 8–11. The biochemical events in the carboxylation of vitamin K–dependent proteins.

intestinal flora of the breast-fed infant produces less of the vitamin than the flora of the formula-fed infant. Moreover, the reserves of vitamin K in the postnatal period are uncertain and depend on the mother's vitamin K status.

PREVALENCE AND CONSEQUENCES OF A DEFICIENCY. Reliable data on the prevalence of vitamin K deficiency are not available because of a lack of sensitive and specific assays for the vitamin in the blood. Recourse has been made to the measurement of the one-stage prothrombin time (PT), a test that determines the plasma levels and activities of factors I, II, V, VII, and X by measuring the time required for clot formation in the test tube. You recall that factors II, VII, and X are vitamin K dependent. A deficiency of vitamin K or its antagonism by coumarin anticoagulants e.g., warfarin, prolongs the prothrombin time. More sensitive to small changes in vitamin K levels are factor VII assays. *More recently, the presence of and level of clotting factors completely or partially lacking carboxylated residues in the plasma are used as a measure of vitamin K deficiency; the abnormal prothrombins are variously referred to as des-gamma-carboxy-prothrombin or PIVKA-II (proteins induced in vitamin K absence).*

Because of its endogenous synthesis, vitamin K deficiency is uncommon. *It is most frequently encountered as a conditioned deficiency in (1) the newborn; (2) those suffering from some malabsorption syndrome, principally biliary tract disease; (3) patients on coumarin anticoagulation or receiving certain drugs; and (4) those with diffuse liver disease. Abnormal prothrombins can be detected in about 3% of full-term neonates, more often in those small for gestational age and particularly in premature infants.*[53] However, whether this is the consequence of a deficiency state or a reflection of physiologic immaturity of the liver remains uncertain. Whatever its origin, *the hypoprothrombinemia induces hemorrhagic disease of the newborn, the most serious manifestation of which is*

intracranial bleeding. Additional manifestations are bleeding from the umbilicus, ecchymoses, hematomas, and hematuria. In the full-term infant, the intestinal colonization develops sufficiently during the first week of life to correct the bleeding diathesis. The routine administration of vitamin K at birth continues to evoke controversy because of uncertainty about the need for it and the possible adverse effects of intramuscularly administered water-soluble synthetic analogs (e.g., hemolysis).[54]

In the adult, vitamin K deficiency and hypoprothrombinemia may lead to ecchymoses, gingival bleeding, hematomas, hematuria, and melena. The deficiency is usually secondary to one of the following.

Malabsorption syndromes and certain drugs (e.g., cholestyramine) impair absorption of vitamin K. The use of broad-spectrum antibiotics such as cephalosporins, sulfa drugs, and neomycin reduces the intestinal flora and endogenous synthesis of vitamin K, or inhibits the epoxide reductase to thus block the recycling of the vitamin.[55]

A number of *therapeutic agents* may lead to a deficiency state. The use of coumarin anticoagulants, say for thromboembolic disease, blocks the recycling of vitamin K by inhibition of the epoxide reductase, as indicated earlier. The long-term use of megadoses of vitamin E has also been reported to antagonize the carboxylation of vitamin K.

Diffuse parenchymal liver disease may impair the ability to utilize vitamin K in the biosynthesis of K-dependent clotting factors.

In passing, abnormal prothrombins (des-gamma-carboxyprothrombin) have been found in the plasma in about 75% of patients with hepatocellular carcinoma (p. 959) and in three infants with hepatoblastomas (p. 958).[56,57]

WATER-SOLUBLE VITAMINS

Included in this category are a complex of B vitamins (thiamine, riboflavin, niacin, B_6, folic acid, and B_{12}) and vitamin C (ascorbic acid). In addition, biotin and pantothenic acid are sometimes referred to as B vitamins, but they have not been associated with well-defined clinical deficiency states. Further comment on them, therefore, will be limited to the observation that excessive consumption of raw egg white, which antagonizes biotin, and prolonged parenteral alimentation have been reported to induce a scaly dermatitis and alopecia that responded to the administration of biotin.[58]

Most of the water-soluble vitamins are widely available and by and large are readily absorbed, chiefly in the small intestine. A variety of foods are rich sources of the B vitamins, principally cereals, leafy green vegetables, yeast, liver, and milk. Analogously, vitamin C, as is well known, is widely available in citrus fruits, vegetables, and some meats. Thus deficiency states of the water-soluble vitamins are not global problems, in comparison with vitamin A, for example. However, primary and conditioned deficiencies are encountered sporadically throughout the world.

Thiamine

Deficiency states: "dry" beriberi; "wet" beriberi; Wernicke-Korsakoff syndrome.

Thiamine is widely available in the diet, but refined foods such as polished rice, white flour, and white sugar contain very little.[59] Although the normal diet contains more than is required, some items such as raw fresh-water fish, strong tea, and coffee, and factors in myoglobin and hemoglobin act as antithiamines and reduce the dietary content of this vitamin. Reserves are relatively limited and are found mainly in skeletal muscle but also in heart, liver, kidney, and brain. Two mechanisms are involved in absorption: passive diffusion at high dietary concentrations and active energy-dependent transport at low concentrations. *During absorption, thiamine undergoes phosphorylation to produce thiamine pyrophosphate (TPP), the functionally active coenzyme form of the vitamin. Thiamine pyrophosphate has three major functions: (1) oxidative decarboxylation of alpha-ketoacids leading to the synthesis of ATP, (2) as a cofactor for transketolase in the pentose phosphate pathway, and (3) in a poorly understood manner it maintains neural membranes and normal nerve conduction, chiefly of peripheral nerves.[60]*

PREVALENCE AND CONSEQUENCES OF A DEFICIENCY.
In addition to many nonspecific manifestations to be detailed later, a deficiency of thiamine damages peripheral nerves ("dry" beriberi), the heart ("wet" beriberi), and the central nervous system (Wernicke-Korsakoff syndrome). In underdeveloped countries, when a large part of the scant diet constitutes polished rice, as occurs in many areas of Southeast Asia, thiamine deficiency sometimes develops. Beriberi has also been observed among maltreated prisoners of war. In developed countries clinically evident thiamine deficiency is uncommon on a strictly dietary basis, but surveys point to subclinical deficiencies among populations not having fortified foods available.[59]

In developed countries, overt thiamine deficiency is commonly encountered in chronic alcoholics, affecting as many as one quarter of those admitted to general hospitals in the United States.[60] Contributing to the impact of the hypovitaminosis B in this population is an apparent hereditary transketolase abnormality transmitted as an autosomal recessive trait, which seems to be common in chronic alcoholics, possibly only because special studies disclose it.[61] A deficiency state may also be seen as a result of pernicious vomiting of pregnancy, long-term unsupplemented parenteral nutrition, or debilitating illnesses that impair the appetite, predispose to vomiting, or cause protracted diarrhea. Because thiamine is required for carbohydrate metabolism, a subclinical deficiency state may be converted into overt disease by extended intravenous glucose therapy or refeeding of chronically malnourished individuals (e.g., alcoholics) unless adequate amounts of thiamine are administered concurrently.

The major targets of thiamine deficiency are (1) the heart, (2) the peripheral nerves, and (3) the brain.

The heart may be normal, have subtle changes, or be markedly enlarged and globular (owing to four-chamber dilatation) with pale, flabby myocardium. The dilatation thins the ventricular walls. Mural thrombi are often present, particularly in the dilated atria. The histologic changes are inconstant and unimpressive; they include interstitial myocardial edema, myofiber swelling and sometimes fatty change, and individual myofiber necrosis. Similar changes may occur in alcoholic cardiomyopathy (p. 644). The cardiac lesions in beriberi then are not pathognomonic (Fig. 8–12A).

In the peripheral nerves, the earliest changes are a symmetric, nonspecific polyneuropathy involving motor, sensory, and reflex arcs beginning particularly in the nerves of the feet and lower legs. With progression, the changes extend proximally while at the same time nerves of the upper extremities and trunk and even the vagus and phrenic nerves become involved. At the outset there is myelin degeneration, but depending on duration and severity of the deficiency, it may progress to disruption of axons. Sometimes the changes extend proximally to involve the associated anterior horn neurons and posterior columns of the spinal cord (Fig. 8–12B).

The central nervous system lesions of the Wernicke-Korsakoff syndrome take the form of focal, symmetric areas of grayish discoloration and sometimes softening with congestion and possibly punctate hemorrhages. These changes are particularly frequent in the paraventricular regions of the thalamus and hypothalamus; in the mammillary bodies (a favored location); about the aqueduct in the midbrain; in the floor of the fourth ventricle; and in the anterior region of the cerebellum. Histologically, there is variable hypertrophy and hyperplasia of small blood vessels, sometimes enclosed within fresh hemorrhage; degenerative changes in neurons extending to frank necrosis; and destruction of fibers in the locus accompanied by a surrounding glial reaction (Fig. 8–12C).

The reasons that the nervous system and the heart are the two major targets of thiamine deficiency are still poorly understood. With respect to the heart, it is theorized that the deficiency state impairs ATP synthesis, on which myocardial cell function is dependent. Conceivably, impaired glucose metabolism affects brain function, but how then to explain the focal nature of the lesions? In alcoholics the basis for the changes in the heart and nervous system is even more uncertain. Alcohol itself is known to damage the heart, peripheral nerves, and brain. Moreover, Korsakoff's psychosis (a feature of the deficiency state described below) responds poorly to the administration of thiamine. It is evident there is much yet to be learned about the pathophysiology of vitamin B_1.

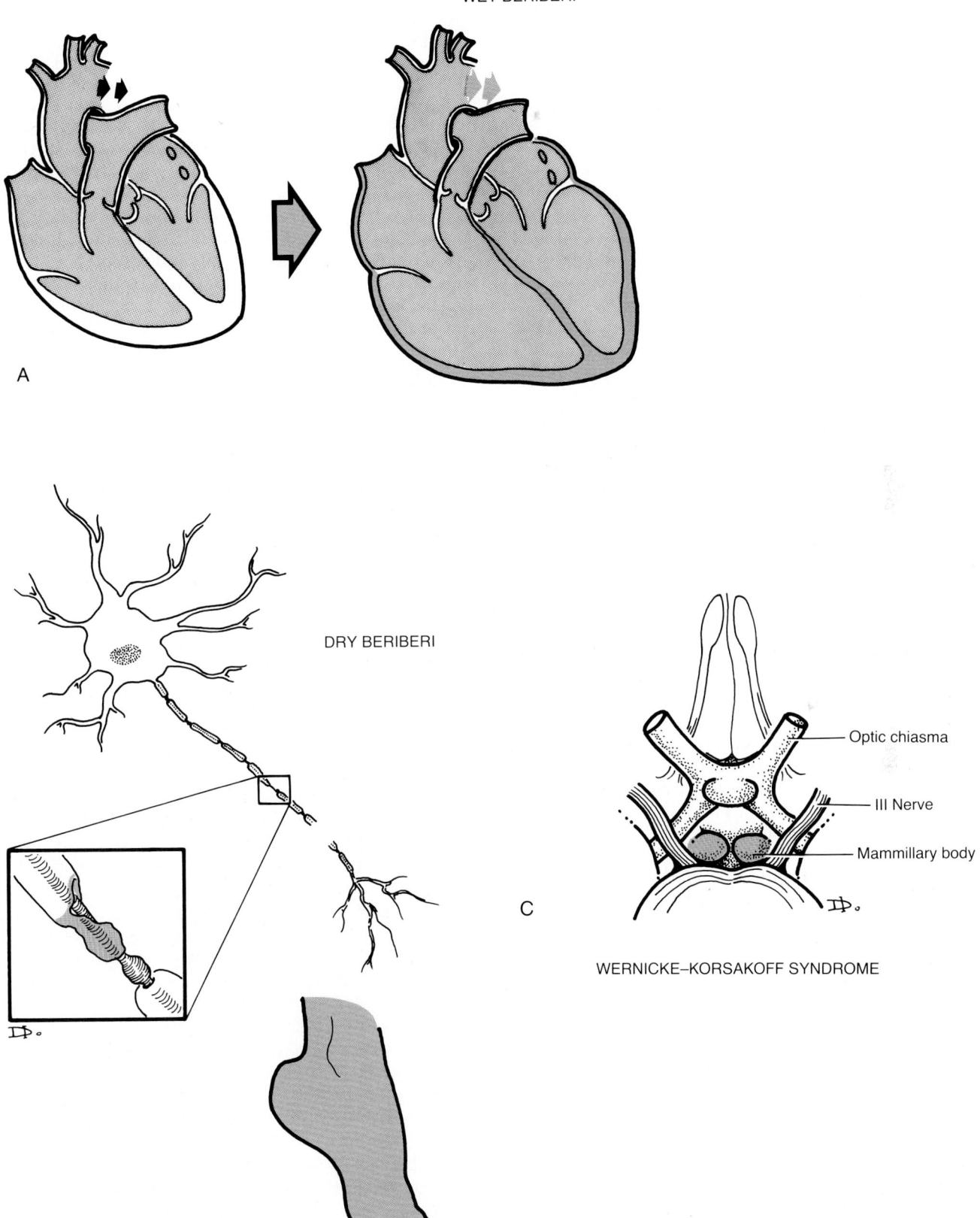

WET BERIBERI

A

DRY BERIBERI

Optic chiasma

III Nerve

Mammillary body

C

WERNICKE–KORSAKOFF SYNDROME

B

Figure 8–12. *A,* The flabby, four-chambered, dilated heart of "wet" beriberi. *B,* The peripheral neuropathy with myelin degeneration leading to foot drop, wrist drop, and sensory changes in "dry" beriberi. *C,* Hemorrhages into the mammillary bodies in the Wernicke–Korsakoff syndrome.

CLINICAL COURSE. The clinical manifestations of thiamine deficiency at the outset are very nonspecific, e.g., anorexia, weakness, weight loss, but as the condition progresses three distinctive syndromes can be recognized: (1) a polyneuropathy (dry beriberi), (2) a cardiovascular syndrome (wet beriberi), and (3) the Wernicke-Korsakoff syndrome. Typically, the three syndromes appear in the sequence given, but on occasion the deficiency state is manifested by only one of them. The polyneuropathy is manifested first by numbness and tingling of the feet and lower legs. Then the upper extremities may become involved. There is progressive sensory loss in affected parts accompanied by muscle weakness and hypo- or areflexia. Beriberi heart disease (wet beriberi) is associated with peripheral vasodilatation leading to more rapid arteriovenous shunting of blood, rapid circulation, and "high-output failure." With the onset of failure, decreased renal blood flow leads to vasoconstriction in the vascular bed of the kidney and retention of salt and water with the development of peripheral edema. When the deficiency state occurs particularly acutely, a fulminant form of heart failure may arise, referred to as *shoshin beriberi*.[62]

In protracted, severe deficiency states, most often encountered in chronic alcoholics in the Western world, Wernicke-Korsakoff syndrome may appear. In most instances, it develops against a background of peripheral neuropathy and cardiac insufficiency, but in some instances it is the presenting and only manifestation of thiamine deficiency. Wernicke's encephalopathy is marked mainly by opthalmoplegia, nystagmus, ataxia of gait and stance, and derangement of mental function characterized by global confusion, apathy, listlessness, and disorientation. About 10 to 20% of hospitalized patients die, usually of intercurrent infection, delirium tremens or liver failure (in alcoholics), or sudden cardiovascular collapse. In the remainder, however, these manifestations usually clear with thiamine administration, only to reveal in many instances an underlying Korsakoff psychosis taking the form of serious impairment of remote recall (retrograde amnesia), inability to acquire new information, and confabulation. Despite thiamine therapy, only about 20% of these patients recover completely, raising the possibility that the brain dysfunction is related more to alcohol toxicity than to vitamin deficiency.[63] Wernicke's encephalopathy and Korsakoff's psychosis are not distinct syndromes but rather successive stages of a single CNS disease having the same pathologic substrate.[64]

TOXICITY. Although the administration of thiamine sometimes produces dizziness and flushing, these manifestations are mild and transient. No serious untoward effects from massive doses have been recorded.

Riboflavin

Deficiency state: Ariboflavinosis.

Riboflavin is essential to normal cell metabolism. It is a critical component of the coenzymes flavin mononucleotide (FMN) and flavin adenine dinucleotide (FAD) that participate in a wide range of redox reactions. In addition, flavin in covalent linkage is incorporated into succinic dehydrogenase and monoamine oxidase as well as other mitochondrial enzymes. It is widely distributed in meat, dairy products, and vegetables as free riboflavin or riboflavin phosphate. Absorbed in the upper gastrointestinal tract through an active transport process, riboflavin is thought to be transported in the blood bound to specific proteins, with possibly some binding to IgG. Rare cases have been described of apparent riboflavin deficiency secondary to abnormal binding proteins.[65] The conversion of riboflavin into its coenzymes (FMN and FAD) is influenced by many factors, notably hormones and drugs. Thyroid hormone and adrenal steroids augment synthesis of the coenzymes, whereas phenothiazines such as chlorpromazine and tricyclic antidepressants (imipramine and amitriptyline) are inhibitory.[66]

PREVALENCE AND CONSEQUENCES OF A DEFICIENCY. Ariboflavinosis still occurs as a primary deficiency state among persons in economically deprived and developing countries. Under such circumstances, it is frequently accompanied by deficiencies of other vitamins and proteins. In industrialized nations, a deficiency is most likely to be encountered in alcoholics and in individuals with chronic infections, advanced cancer, or other debilitating diseases. Transient mild deficiency states may occur during pregnancy and lactation, and during the rapid growth of adolescence, when there is increased requirement for the vitamin.

MORPHOLOGY. Ariboflavinosis is associated with changes at the angles of the mouth (known as cheilosis or cheilitis), glossitis, and ocular and skin changes. In addition, some patients develop a normochromic, normocytic anemia caused by hypoplasia of the red cell precursors in the bone marrow.

CHEILOSIS. Cheilosis or, as it is sometimes called, cheilitis is usually the first and most characteristic sign of this deficiency state. However, identical lesions are found in aged individuals with poor dentition who are not vitamin deficient. It begins as areas of pallor at the angles of the mouth, with first a hyperkeratosis of the epidermis and a dermal inflammatory infiltrate. Cracks or fissures may appear, radiating from the corners of the mouth and tending to become secondarily infected and macerated. In far advanced cases, the oral mucous membrane at the angles of the mouth and the vermilion border of the lips are similarly affected.

GLOSSITIS. The tongue may take on a magenta hue, strongly resembling the red-blue coloration of cyanosis. Presumably this alteration reflects atrophy of the mucosa of the tongue (Fig. 8–13).

OCULAR LESIONS. The eye changes may be classified as superficial interstitial keratitis. In the earlier stages, the superficial layers of the cornea are invaded by capillaries. Interstitial inflammatory infiltration and exudation follow, to produce opacities and even ulcerations of the corneal surface. The lesion usually affects both eyes, but in certain instances it may be unilateral. Conjunctivitis is a common accompaniment.

DERMATITIS. A greasy, scaling dermatitis occurs over the nasolabial folds and may extend into a butterfly distribution to involve the cheeks and skin about the ears. Scrotal and vulvar lesions are common. In well-defined cases, atrophy of the skin may develop. It should be emphasized that the histologic changes are not in themselves distinctive or pathognomonic of ariboflavinosis; it is their distribution that suggests the diagnosis.

BONE MARROW. Erythroid hypoplasia is typically present but is usually not marked.

None of the findings just described is specific for riboflavin deficiency, since similar lesions are encountered with pyridoxine deficiency, for example, but in the aggregate they are highly suggestive. There is no clear understanding of why these specific target tissues are affected with the lack of a nutrient that has bodywide functions. Several reports indicate an important role for riboflavin in protein synthesis, but it is not clear that a derangement in this process accounts for the lesions described, save possibly for the erythroid hypoplasia and anemia.[67]

Niacin

Deficiency state: Pellagra.

Niacin is the generic designation for nicotinic acid and its functionally active derivatives (e.g., nicotinamide). Niacin in the form of nicotinamide is an essential component of two coenzymes—nicotinamide adenine dinucleotide (NAD) and nicotinamide adenine dinucleotide phosphate (NADP)—both having central roles in cellular intermediary metabolism. NAD functions as a coenzyme for a variety of dehydrogenases involved in the metabolism of fat, carbohydrate, and amino acids. NADP participates in a variety of dehydrogenation reactions, particularly in the hexosemonophosphate shunt of glucose metabolism.

PREVALENCE AND CONSEQUENCES OF A DEFICIENCY. Niacin can be derived from the diet or be endogenously synthesized. It is widely available in grains, legumes, and seed oils, with much lower quantities in meats. However, in some grains it is present in bound form and therefore not absorbable. The niacin in maize in particular is bound, and so pellagra has appeared with unexpected frequency among native populations subsisting largely on maize. *Niacin can also be synthesized endogenously from tryptophan.* Sixty mg of dietary tryptophan yields about 1 mg of niacin. However, a dietary excess of leucine, such as is found in millet (a cereal grain consumed in regions of Asia and Africa), blocks the conversion of tryptophan to niacin. *Thus, pellagra is not only a deficiency disease but also a disorder dependent on the specific amino acid content of the diet.* Awareness of this problem, more adequate diets, and food supplementation have greatly reduced the incidence of endemic pellagra, but it is still encountered among the Bantus of South Africa, in Egypt, and in the maize-eating populations of India. *In industrialized countries, pellagra is encountered sporadically, principally among alcoholics (usually in combination with other vitamin deficiencies) and those suffering from chronic debilitating illnesses such as tuberculosis, cirrhosis of the liver, and cancer.* It may also occur with protracted diarrheal states, with diets grossly deficient in protein, and with the chronic administration of drugs such as isoniazid and 6-mercaptopurine. *Two uncommon disorders affecting tryptophan metabolism may be complicated by pellagra: (1) the carcinoid syndrome, in which most of the tryptophan is usurped by the neoplasm for the formation of serotonin, and (2) Hartnup disease, in which several amino acids, including tryptophan, are poorly absorbed from the diet.*

MORPHOLOGY. The term pellagra, strictly speaking, refers to rough skin. The clinical syndrome, however, is classically identified by most clinicians as the three D's—dermatitis, diarrhea, and dementia.

The **dermatitis** occurs on the body symmetrically and, while it may affect any region, tends to be most severe in areas of exposure to chronic irritation or sunlight, such as the face, dorsa of the hands, wrists, elbows, and knees. The margins are usually sharply demarcated. The changes consist at first of redness and thickening of the skin with hyperkeratosis and scaling (Fig. 8–14). These early alterations are followed by increased vascularization and chronic inflammation with edema of the subepithelial dermal connective tissue, followed eventually by areas of depigmentation and increased pigmentation. At this stage a variegated dermatitis is present, with brown scaly areas alternating with areas of depigmented, shiny, atrophic skin. With chronicity, the skin may become markedly thickened by subcutaneous fibrosis and scarring. Lesions similar to these may occur in mucous membranes, particularly the

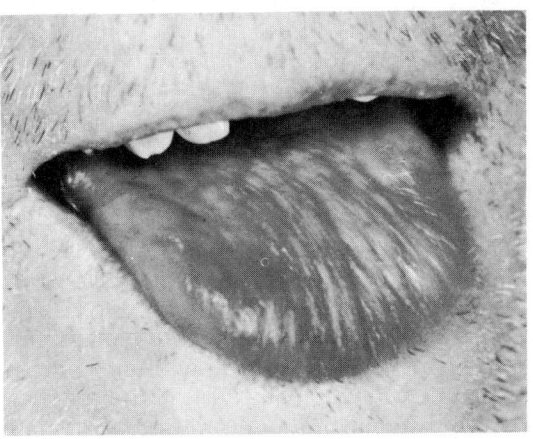

Figure 8–13. The glazed, shiny, atrophic tongue of riboflavin deficiency.

oral cavity and vagina. In the mouth, the early stages are marked by vascular congestion and edema of the tongue, and later by atrophy of the mucous membrane and ulceration, so that **the tongue becomes red, swollen, and beefy, a form of glossitis reminiscent of the black tongue found in animals.**

The **diarrhea** exhibited by patients with pellagra is presumed to be due largely to mucous membrane lesions similar to those in the skin. In experimental animals, the first histologic alterations represent vascularization, edema, and inflammation of the sub-mucosal connective tissue of the intestinal lining, which lead to atrophic mucosal glandular changes and eventual atrophy and ulceration of the overlying mucous membrane. These lesions may be found throughout all levels of the intestine but are most prominent in the esophagus, stomach, and colon.

The **dementia** is based on degeneration of the neurons in the brain, accompanied by degeneration of the tracts of the spinal cord. These spinal cord lesions bear a close resemblance to alterations in the posterior columns observed in pernicious anemia and raise the question of whether a deficiency of another factor in the B complex, such as B_{12}, may also be implicated. Macrocytic anemia may appear in some cases.

Two of the most dominant complaints of these patients are persistent fatigability and weakness, which have been misinterpreted as malingering or neurosis. Although the skin manifestations eventually appear, they may at times be delayed until significant involvement of the intestinal tract or central nervous system has already developed. Other less prominent clinical features include abdominal pain, dysphagia, proctitis, and vaginitis. It is difficult to explain the precise constellation of clinicoanatomic findings in pellagra on the basis of the known widespread functions of niacin. There is no reliable laboratory test for the diagnosis; recourse must be made to response to therapy.

TOXICITY. Large doses of nicotinic acid lower the plasma levels of low density and very low density lipoproteins and increase the levels of high density lipoproteins. There was hope that such therapy might protect against coronary heart disease, but large-scale studies have regrettably not been encouraging.[68] Moreover, long-term use of high doses has been associated with hepatic injury, activation of peptic ulcer, and arguably, induction of diabetes, dampening enthusiasm about the long-term therapeutic use of this vitamin.

Vitamin B_6 (Pyridoxine)

A primary, clinically overt deficiency of vitamin B_6 is rare in humans, but subclinical conditioned deficiency states, paradoxically, are thought to be quite common. Three naturally occurring substances (pyridoxine, pyridoxal, and pyridoxamine and their phosphates) possess vitamin B_6 activity and are generically referred to as pyridoxine. All are equally active metabolically, and all are converted in the tissues to the coenzyme form, pyridoxal 5-phosphate. The coenzyme participates as cofactor for a large number of enzymes involved in transaminations, carboxylations, and deaminations in the metabolism of lipids and amino acids, and in the immune response.[69] It is of particular importance in the metabolism of tryptophan, the trans-methylation of methionine, and the synthesis of delta-aminolevulinic acid (the heme precursor). Pyridoxal phosphate is also involved in stabilizing muscle phosphorylase and, in some poorly understood fashion, in the transmission of neural impulses.

The vitamin is abundantly available in the usual diet, since it is widely present in virtually all foods. However, food processing may destroy the pyridoxine, accounting for episodes of severe vitamin B_6 deficiency and convulsions in infants fed badly controlled dried milk preparations.[70] The neurologic manifestations probably stem from deficient amino acid decarboxylation (pyridoxine dependent) and thus insufficient synthesis of the inhibitory neurotransmitter gamma-aminobutyric acid. Decreased plasma levels of pyridoxine are fairly common among the elderly because of either inadequate dietary intake or increased need.[71]

Secondary hypovitaminosis B_6 may be precipitated by the increased requirement for the nutrient during pregnancy and lactation, by hyperthyroidism, and with high-protein diets. During pregnancy there is a marked gradient in the distribution of pyridoxine in favor of the fetus, thus depleting the mother. Breast-feeding by such mothers may lead to a deficiency state in the infants. Alternatively, interference with pyridoxine metabolism occurs in a variety of clinical circumstances. Pyridoxine deficiency is common in chronic alcoholics. Acetaldehyde, a metabolite of ethanol, displaces pyridoxal phosphate from proteins and thus increases the degradation of the coenzyme. Estrogens, including those contained in oral contraceptives, block the function of the coenzyme in tryptophan metabolism. Isoniazid, employed in the treatment of tuberculosis, combines with pyridoxal or pyridoxal phosphate to metabolically inacti-

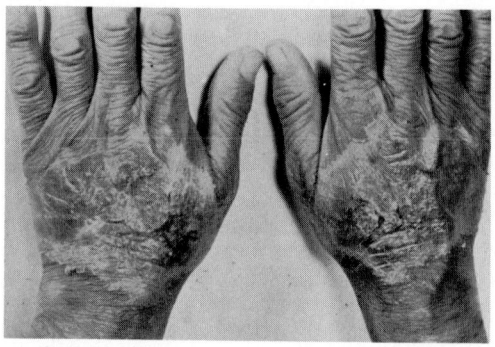

Figure 8–14. The sharply demarcated, characteristic scaling dermatitis of pellagra.

vate the vitamin. Penicillamine also forms an inactive product with pyridoxal phosphate.

The clinical manifestations of pyridoxine deficiency have been most clearly delineated in experimental subjects given the antagonist desoxypyridoxine, and include seborrheic dermatitis, cheilosis, glossitis, angular stomatitis, peripheral neuropathy, and sometimes convulsions. Impaired T-cell function and antibody synthesis have also been attributed to a deficiency of this vitamin. The anatomic changes underlying these findings are identical to those described with combined deficiencies of niacin and riboflavin. Infants born of vitamin-deficient mothers have suffered mental retardation. Rare cases of so-called hypochromic pyridoxine-responsive anemia have also been reported.

In closing, mention should be made of rare genetic disorders referred to as *vitamin B6 responsive syndromes.*[72] In one, a familial form of infantile convulsions and fatal brain damage, an apoenzyme for glutamic acid decarboxylase is defective in binding pyridoxal phosphate. Thus, there is decreased synthesis of the neurotransmitter gamma-aminobutyric acid. The pyridoxine-responsive anemia mentioned earlier may represent another genetic defect that requires increased levels of vitamin B6 for heme synthesis. Patients with homocystinuria, which is due to a deficiency of cystathione synthetase, are improved by the administration of large doses of vitamin B6. The same can be said of patients with xanthurenic aciduria related to a deficiency of the pyridoxal phosphate–dependent enzyme kynureninase. Thus, it is clear that an inadequacy of B6 involves more than merely a deficient diet.

Folic Acid (Folate)

Deficiency state: Megaloblastic anemia.

A deficiency of folic acid induces a megaloblastic anemia similar to that caused by a lack of cobalamin (vitamin B12). Since megaloblastic anemia and its origins are discussed on page 679, the present consideration of folic acid deficiency can be restricted to the nutritional origins of the deficiency state.

Folic acid is the generally used term for pteroylmonoglutamic acid, the precursor of a large family of folate compounds. The most important of the folates is tetrahydrofolic acid, which serves as an acceptor-donor of one-carbon fragments such as methyl and formyl groups. The pivotal importance of such transfers is presented in the later discussion of the anemia.

Humans are entirely dependent on dietary sources for their folic acid requirement, which is of the order of 50 to 200 μg daily.[73] Most normal diets contain ample amounts, the richest sources being green vegetables such as lettuce, spinach, asparagus, and broccoli. Certain fruits (e.g., lemons, bananas, melons), and animal proteins (e.g., liver) contain lesser amounts. The folic acid in these foods is largely in the form of folylpolyglutamates. *Despite their abundance in raw foods, polyglutamates (depending on the specific form) are very sensitive to heat; boiling, steaming, or frying of foods for five to ten minutes may destroy up to 95% of the folate content.* Intestinal conjugases split the polyglutamates into monoglutamates that are readily absorbed in the proximal jejunum. During intestinal absorption they are modified so that only 5-methyltetrahydrofolate enters the circulation as the normal transport form of folate. Once absorbed, the folate is probably transported by a specific folic acid–binding protein, the identity of which is still somewhat uncertain. The bodily reserves of folate are relatively modest, and a deficiency may arise with months of a negative balance. The functional role of folates and the many possible causes (other than dietary) and consequences of a deficiency state are presented in the later discussion (p. 684).

Vitamin B12 (Cobalamin)

Deficiency state: Megaloblastic anemia, neurologic damage, and male and female infertility.

The hematologic consequences of a deficiency of cobalamin are identical to those produced by a lack of folate; in addition, the deficiency damages peripheral nerves and the spinal cord and may be responsible for reduced fertility in women and men—hence the often used term "combined systems disease."

Cobalamin is a complex organometallic compound composed of a corrin ring (similar to the porphyrin ring) to which is attached a cobalt atom. The synthetic therapeutic form of vitamin B12 is a stable cyanocobalamin. Under normal circumstances, humans are totally dependent on dietary animal products in their diet for their vitamin B12 requirement. Microorganisms are the ultimate origin of cobalamin in the food chain. Plants and vegetables contain very little cobalamin save that contributed by microbial contamination; strictly vegetarian or macrobiotic diets then do not provide adequate amounts of this essential nutrient. The daily requirement is of the order of 2 to 3 μg, and the normal balanced diet contains significantly larger amounts. The reserves in the body, when fully maintained, are sufficient for years.

An ingenious and complex process has evolved for the absorption and transport of cobalamin while excluding functionally inactive analogs.[74] It involves a number of binding proteins, some of which are highly specific for cobalamin.[75] In the stomach, cobalamin is released from its dietary sources by peptic digestion. The gastric parietal cells in health secrete a large excess of intrinsic factor (IF) capable of binding the vitamin with great specificity. However, at the low pH of the stomach, most cobalamin is temporarily bound to salivary R protein. The complex then passes into the duodenum, where pancreatic proteases degrade the R protein, making the cobalamin available for intrinsic factor at a more favorable pH. The IF-cobalamin complex is resistant to proteolysis and passes into the distal ileum, where it binds to specific high-affinity receptors on ileal absorptive cells. The precise details of the subsequent passage of cobalamin across the plasma membrane of the enterocyte are unclear, but the process is energy dependent.[76] Whatever the pathway, newly absorbed cobalamin is found in the plasma bound to transcobalamin II (TCII) synthesized by the liver. All cells in the body have surface receptors specific for the TCII-cobalamin complex, providing for receptor-mediated endocytosis of the complex followed by lysosomal degradation of TCII with release of the cobalamin. However, 90% of cobalamin within the plasma is bound to two R proteins synthesized by white cells and possibly many other cell types as well. When found in the plasma, these R binders are called transcobalamins I (TCI) and III (TCIII). Their function is uncertain; conceivably they provide mechanisms for storage or clearance of excess cobalamin and its analogs.[77] An overview of this complex sequence of events is offered in Figure 8–15.

As the later discussion of the megaloblastic anemias (p. 679) will reveal, there are many potential causes of a vitamin B_{12} deficiency, the most important of which is inadequate synthesis of IF, producing what classically has been called pernicious anemia (p. 681).

Vitamin C (Ascorbic Acid)

Deficiency state: Scurvy.

Most mammals and even such humble forms as amphibians and reptiles have the talent to synthesize ascorbic acid from glucose via glucuronic acid because they possess a gluconolactone oxidase. Humans and even the more long-suffering guinea pigs, as well as other primates and some exotic flying mammals, lack this oxidase and so cannot synthesize ascorbic acid. The enzyme may well have been lost through an evolutionary mutation, and so we are all "walking inborn errors of metabolism" completely dependent on dietary sources of the vitamin. Ascorbic acid is present in milk and some animal products (e.g., liver, fish) and is abundant in a variety of fruits and vegetables. Some of the vitamin content is lost after long periods of storage of raw fruits and vegetables, but it is largely protected by most methods of food preservation and preparation. Thus all but the most restricted of diets provide adequate amounts of vitamin C.

Absorption of ascorbic acid in the small intestine involves an energy-dependent active transport system.[78] The mean body pool in healthy males is about 1500 mg, distributed in many organs with high concentrations in the adrenals and pituitary. About 50 mg is utilized daily. One would assume that a comparable intake of the vitamin would be sufficient, and indeed the Recommended Daily Allowance is 60 mg. Although such an intake will prevent scurvy, however, there is some evidence that larger daily amounts are required for optimal health—some would say 200 mg.[79] For example, emotional and physical stress increase the utilization of ascorbic acid. Analogously, cigarette smokers with vitamin C intakes comparable to those of nonsmokers have significantly lower serum levels of ascorbic acid.

Ascorbic acid functions in a variety of biosynthetic pathways by accelerating hydroxylation reactions. Best known is its function as a cofactor for prolyl hydroxylase requisite for the post-translational hydroxylation of proline in the cisternae of the rough endoplasmic reticulum. Procollagen having unhydroxylated proline is unstable and does not have the characteristic helical configuration. Deranged collagen synthesis is thought to underlie most of the manifestations of scurvy, but in experimental animals a deficiency of ascorbic acid leads also to suppression of collagen synthesis.[80] Vitamin C has many other functions, e.g., in the hydroxylation reactions involved in the synthesis of carnitine from lysine; in the hydroxylation of dopamine to form norepinephrine; by virtue of its reducing potential, in the prevention of oxidation of tetrahydrofolate to thus maintain the pool of folic acid; and by maintaining iron in its reduced state, enhancing absorption of non-heme iron, in the diet and the bioavailability of stored iron.[81]

PREVALENCE AND CONSEQUENCES OF A DEFICIENCY. As is well known, a deficiency of vitamin C will lead to scurvy. With the abundance of ascorbic acid in so many foods, this disorder has ceased to be a

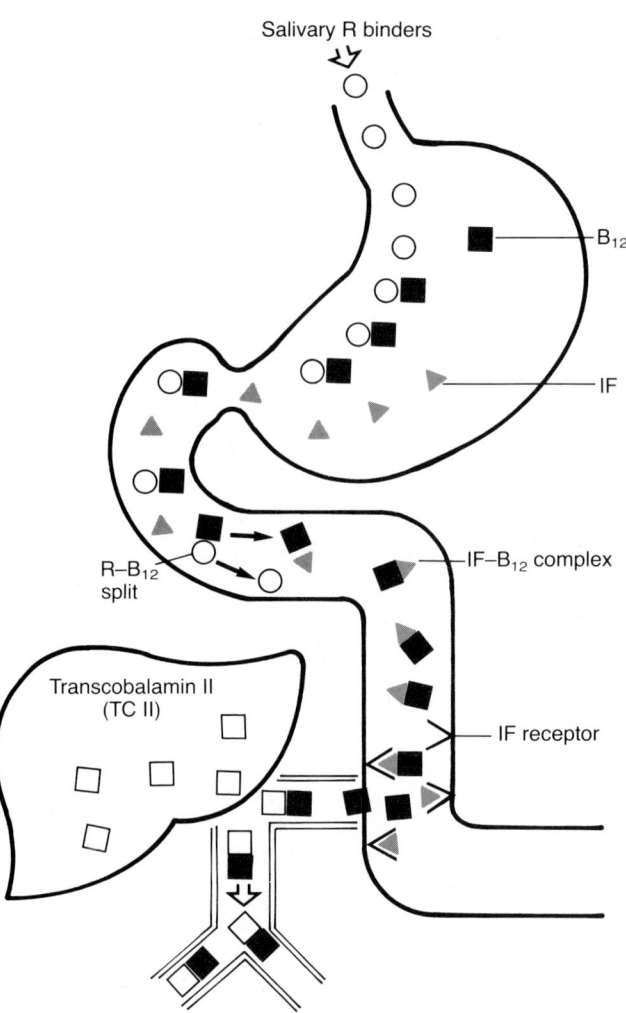

Figure 8–15. The metabolism of vitamin B_{12}.

global problem. However, it is sometimes encountered even in affluent populations as a conditioned deficiency, particularly among the elderly, those who live alone, and alcoholics, all of whom often have erratic and inadequate eating patterns. Occasionally scurvy appears in patients undergoing peritoneal dialysis and hemodialysis and among food faddists. Tragically the condition sometimes appears in infants who are maintained on formulas of processed milk without supplementation.

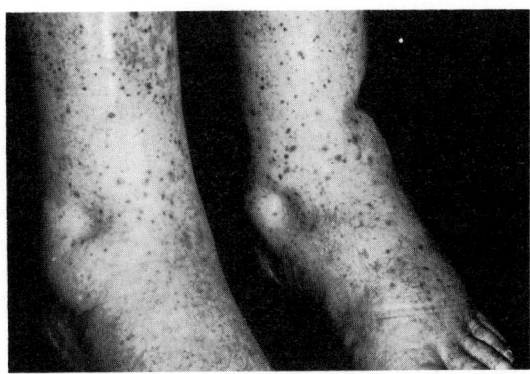

Figure 8–16. The lower extremities of a patient with marked malnutrition, nutritional edema, and petechial hemorrhages related to low levels of vitamin C.

Scurvy in the growing child is far more dramatic than in the adult. **Hemorrhages** constitute one of the most striking features. It is thought that the defect in collagen synthesis results in inadequate support of the walls of capillaries and venules. Thus **purpura and ecchymoses often appear in the skin, most prominently along the backs of the lower legs and in the gingival mucosa, particularly at the margins (Fig. 8–16).** Loose attachment of the periosteum and the hemorrhagic diathesis lead to extensive subperiosteal hematomas and bleeding into the joint spaces. Most threatening are retrobulbar, subarachnoid, and intracerebral hemorrhages, and indeed intracranial bleeding may prove fatal.

Skeletal changes may develop in the infant and child. **The primary disturbance is in the formation of osteoid matrix, not in mineralization or calcification such as occurs in rickets.** Both membranous and endochondral bone formation may be severely disrupted. In scurvy, the palisade of cartilage cells is formed as usual and is provisionally calcified. However, there is insufficient production of osteoid matrix by osteoblasts and what is laid down is unstable. Resorption of the cartilaginous matrix then fails or slows, and as a consequence there is cartilaginous overgrowth with long spicules and plates projecting into the metaphyseal region of the marrow cavity and sometimes widening of the epiphyses (Fig. 8–17). The unresolved cartilaginous spicules become patchily or completely mineralized (Fig. 8–18). Further disrupting the epiphyseal area are hemorrhages occasioned by poorly supported microvessels and by microfractures as well as subperiosteal hematomas. The poorly formed bone yields to the stresses of weight bearing and muscle tension with bowing of the long bones of the lower legs, and abnormal depression of the sternum with outward projection of the ends of the ribs creating a so-called **scorbutic rosary.** Further distorting the skeletal system are hematomas beneath and about the periosteum and into the joint spaces. The deranged bone formation also involves the jaws and alveolar bone. Thus the teeth are abnormally mobile and may be displaced or fall out.

Gingival swelling, hemorrhages, and secondary bacterial periodontal infection are common in severely scorbutic patients. The deficiency of vitamin C does not of itself cause the inflammation, but rather predisposes to excessive swelling and hemorrhages leading to prominent **gingival enlargement.**

A **distinctive, perifollicular, hyperkeratotic, papular rash** that may be ringed by hemorrhage often appears.

Wound healing and localization of focal infections are both impaired in scurvy because of the derangement in collagen synthesis. Thus there is poor healing of wounds and breakdown of recently healed wounds. **Anemia is a common finding.** Most often it is normochromic and normocytic, related to the bleeding into the various tissues and to the derangements in iron metabolism produced by a lack of ascorbic acid. Sometimes it is macrocytic, megaloblastic anemia due to folate deficiency. Folate is often found in the same foods as vitamin C, and scorbutigenic diets may well lack folate. In addition, however, you recall that vitamin C

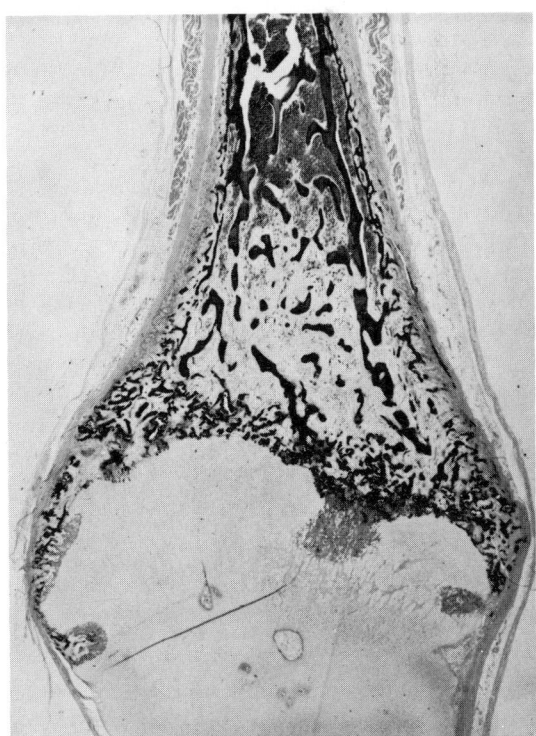

Figure 8–17. A longitudinal section of a scorbutic costochondral junction with widening of the epiphyseal cartilage and projection of masses of cartilage into the adjacent bone.

protects against oxidation of folic acid, and therefore the scorbutic individual is in double jeopardy of developing folate deficiency. The major features of scurvy in the child are summarized in Figure 8–19.

The **changes in the adult** are similar to those in the child, but skeletal deformation does not occur. Thus, the major anatomic changes relate to the bleeding tendency, skin rash, anemia, and often quite prominent, the hemorrhagic gingival enlargement accompanied by periodontal infection.

CLINICAL COURSE.   Because of its rarity, the diagnosis of scurvy can be made only by an awareness of the clinical settings in which the condition is likely to appear (cited earlier). The earliest manifestations at all ages are nonspecific and include lethargy, malaise, and weakness. The salient clinical findings in the adult have already been detailed, but particularly characteristic are skin purpura over the lower legs, easy bruisability, friable bleeding gums, and hematoma formation in virtually any site within the body, particularly those exposed to trauma, e.g., legs and arms. When unrecognized, the bleeding into the tissue may lead to severe anemia with apathy and listlessness, or even worse, an intracranial hemorrhage with convulsions, coma, and death.

Childhood scurvy is characterized by essentially the same findings as those found in later life, but they

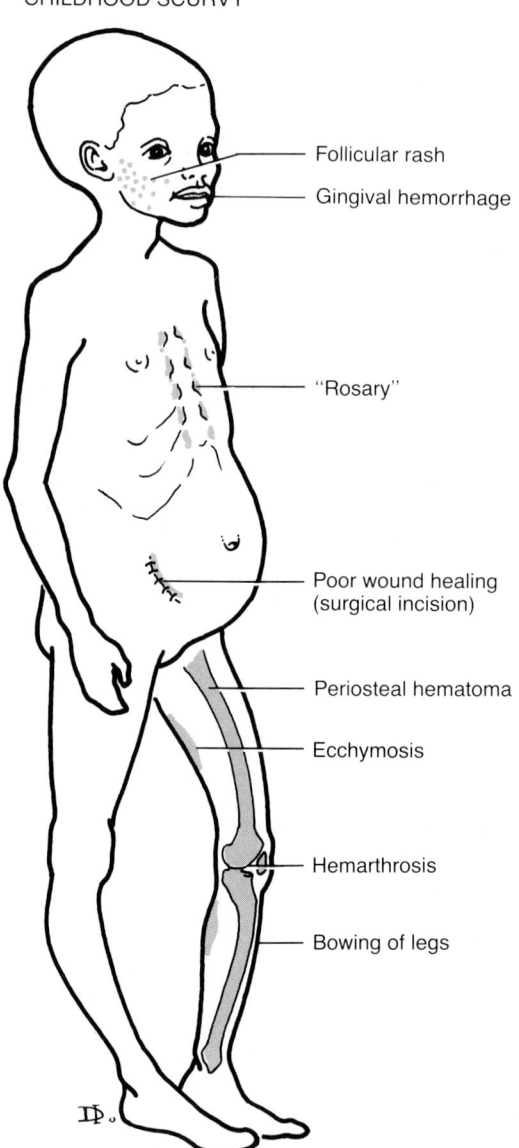

CHILDHOOD SCURVY

— Follicular rash
— Gingival hemorrhage

— "Rosary"

— Poor wound healing (surgical incision)

— Periosteal hematoma

— Ecchymosis

— Hemarthrosis

— Bowing of legs

Figure 8–19. Effects of childhood scurvy.

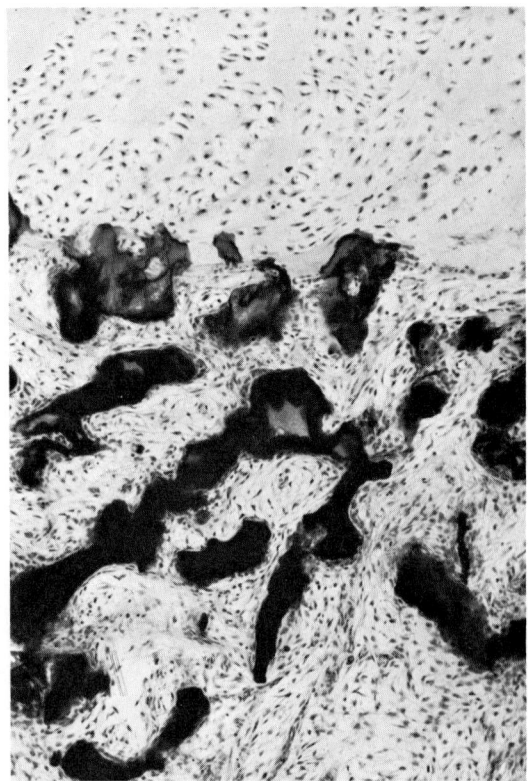

Figure 8–18. A detail of a scorbutic costochondral junction. The orderly palisade is totally destroyed. There is dense mineralization of the spicules present but no evidence of newly formed osteoid.

tend to occur against a background of skeletal system changes. *Subperiosteal hemorrhages with pain and swelling along the involved bones, and joint hemorrhages with pain and limitation of motion are particularly characteristic.* The skeletal hemorrhages tend to make the children lie quietly to spare unnecessary motion, with legs characteristically flexed onto the abdomen or in the frog position to relieve tension on the muscles, tendons, and fasciae. Growth retardation and skeletal deformities may appear in those with marked deficiency states. The blood loss and anemia cause listlessness, weight loss, irritability, and pallor. As in the adult, the course may suddenly take a downturn because of intracranial bleeding that may prove fatal.

Although the clinical findings may be highly suggestive, confirmation of the diagnosis usually requires documentation of abnormally low levels of ascorbic acid in plasma, white cells, or platelets.

THE MEGADOSE CONTROVERSY AND TOXICITY.

In the recent past a flurry of excitement was aroused by reports contending that megadoses of vitamin C (gram amounts) would increase resistance to the common cold and alleviate its symptoms.[82,83] A number of subsequent carefully controlled studies failed to demonstrate any significant benefit save possibly for mild alleviation of symptoms due to a mild antihistamine action of ascorbic acid. Subsequently, it was proposed that "increasing ascorbate intake would produce measurable benefits in both the prevention and the treatment of cancer."[84] Regrettably, subsequent studies failed to identify any benefit.[85]

Moreover, the doubtful benefits of megadoses of vitamin C must be placed in the perspective of possible untoward effects. Multigram amounts of ascorbic acid have induced uricosuria (with a low risk of stone formation); hemolysis in patients with red cell glucose-6-phosphate dehydrogenase deficiency; significantly increased absorption of non-heme iron with the potential of iron overload in predisposed individuals; and impaired bactericidal activity in leukocytes. Moreover, ascorbic acid may interfere with tests for fecal occult blood and urinary glucose as well as others.[79] Although none of these adverse effects is life threatening, all of them warrant consideration before ascorbic acid is confused with candy.

MINERALS

A number of minerals are no less essential for health than are the vitamins. Some, such as iron, calcium, and phosphorus, are required in large amounts. Others fall into the category of trace elements. Since calcium and phosphorus have already been considered in the discussion of vitamin D (p. 441), only iron and certain of the trace elements require further comment.

IRON

Deficiency states: Systemic impairments (see text); hypochromic microcytic anemia.

On a global basis, iron deficiency is more common than any other nutritional deficiency. It evolves through three identifiable stages: (1) depletion of iron stores indicated by a decline in serum ferritin; (2) a decrease in transport iron, when iron stores are depleted, characterized by abnormally low serum iron and a commensurate rise in the transferrin iron binding capacity (TIBC); and (3) the appearance of a hypochromic, microcytic anemia.[86] Although it is common to think of iron deficiency in terms of anemia, in fact it is a late manifestation and is preceded by disturbed function of many iron-dependent enzymes having wide-ranging clinical consequences.

The total iron content of the body, ranging from 2 gm in small women to 6 gm in large men, is an extremely closely guarded constant regulated by balancing absorption with losses through mechanisms discussed later (p. 685).[87,88] Here we are concerned with the nutritional aspects of iron deficiency. The normal Western diet contains approximately 10 to 20 mg of iron per day, most of which is found within the heme of animal products. The remainder is inorganic iron found in vegetables and grains. The bioavailability of dietary iron is as important as the overall content. About 20 to 25% of heme-iron is absorbable. In contrast, only about 1 to 2% of inorganic iron is assimilable. Ascorbic acid, citric acid, amino acids, and sugars in the diet enhance absorption of inorganic iron, but tannates (as in tea), carbonates, oxalates, and phosphates inhibit its absorption. The major site of absorption is the duodenum, but the stomach, lower levels of the small intestine, and colon may also participate to a small degree.

BASIS OF IRON DEFICIENCY.

An iron deficiency may result from: (1) dietary lack, (2) impaired absorption, (3) increased requirement, or (4) chronic blood loss (Fig. 8–20).

Dietary lack is a rare cause of iron deficiency in industrialized countries having abundant food supplies (including meat) and where about two thirds of the dietary iron is in the readily assimilable heme form. The situation is quite different in developing countries, where food is less abundant and diets are predominantly vegetarian, containing poorly absorbed inorganic iron. However, dietary inadequacy is still encountered in privileged societies under the following circumstances:

- *The elderly* often have very restricted diets with little meat for economic reasons or because of poor dentition.
- *The very poor,* often minority group, individuals are at risk for obvious reasons.
- *Infants* are also at high risk because the diet, predominantly milk, contains very small amounts of iron. Human breast milk, for example, provides only about 0.3 mg/L of iron, which, however, has a better bioavailability than cow's milk, which contains about twice as much iron but has poor bioavailability.
- *Children,* especially during the early years of life, as pointed out earlier, have a critical need for dietary iron to accommodate growth and expansion of the blood volume.

Impaired absorption is encountered in sprue, other causes of intestinal steatorrhea, and chronic diarrhea. Specific items in the diet, as is evident from the preceding discussion, may also affect absorption.

Increased requirement is an important potential cause of iron deficiency. It has already been emphasized that growing infants and children, adolescents, and premenopausal (particularly pregnant) women have a much greater requirement for iron than do nonmenstruating adults. Particularly at risk are eco-

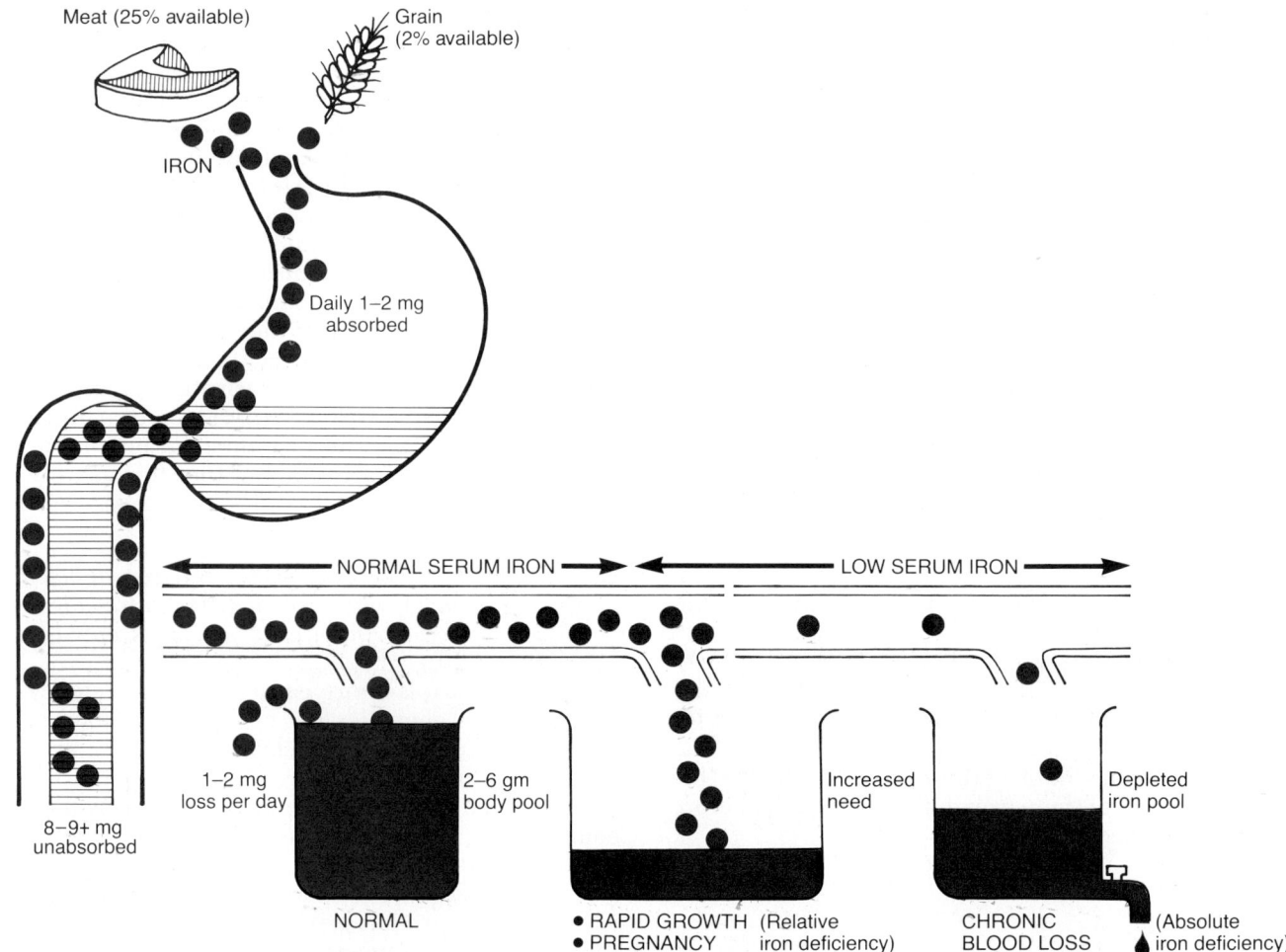

Figure 8–20. The causes of iron deficiency, including lack of dietary iron, impaired reabsorption, increased requirement for iron (as in rapid growth and pregnancy), and chronic blood loss.

nomically deprived women having multiple, frequent pregnancies.

Chronic blood loss is the most important cause of iron deficiency in the Western world. Bleeding within the tissues or cavities of the body may be followed by total recovery and recycling of the iron. However, external hemorrhage depletes the reserves of iron. Such depletion may occur from the gastrointestinal tract (e.g., peptic ulcers, hemorrhagic gastritis, gastric carcinoma, colonic carcinoma, hemorrhoids, or hookworm or pinworm disease), from the urinary tract (e.g., renal, pelvic, or bladder tumors), or from the genital tract (e.g., menorrhagia, uterine cancer).

When all the potential causes of an iron deficiency are taken into consideration, *deficiency in adult males and postmenopausal women in the Western world should be considered to be caused by gastrointestinal blood loss until proved otherwise. To prematurely ascribe an iron lack in such individuals to any of* *the other possible origins is to run the risk of missing an occult gastrointestinal cancer or other bleeding lesion.*

PREVALENCE AND CONSEQUENCES OF A DEFICIENCY. There is no consensus on the prevalence of iron deficiency because of the variable criteria employed for its diagnosis. Approximately 25% of infants in families of low socioeconomic status were found to have iron-deficiency anemia in a United States public health survey, but only 8% of those in more affluent families.[89,90] In Southeast Asia, 80% of pregnant women were found to be anemic.[91] When biochemical tests for serum iron or response to iron therapy were used as the criteria, the prevalence of iron deficiency reached almost 90% in menstruating adolescent girls and otherwise normal infants.[92,93] Whatever the precise frequency, it is evident that iron deficiency is widespread.

The *consequences of an iron deficiency*, as already emphasized, involve more than the development of hypochromic, microcytic anemia. Even in the absence of anemia, they constitute (1) *reversible alterations in cognitive function, particularly in children; (2) deficient immunologic and defensive responses to infectious disease* due to reduced bactericidal effectiveness of neutrophils and impaired cell-mediated immunity; (3) *abnormalities in thermoregulation*[94]; and (4) *reduced capacity for physical activity* related only in part to the lowered hemoglobin levels. Only the serum iron level or the iron-binding capacity of the serum would relate these manifestations to an iron lack. At this stage, a bone marrow aspirate stained with Prussian blue would reveal markedly reduced deposits of iron in macrophages. Persistence of the negative balance will in time lead to the iron deficiency—hypochromic, microcytic anemia—discussed on page 685.

TRACE ELEMENTS

Among the large number of inorganic elements found in cells, only four—zinc, copper, selenium, and iodine—have been associated with well-characterized deficiency states.[95] In theory, a deficiency of a trace element might occur for the same reasons as a lack of a vitamin. However, *three influences are particularly relevant: (1) total parenteral nutrition, (2) interference with absorption by dietary constituents, and (3) inborn errors of metabolism. Total parenteral nutrition* is a misleading term because, unless supplemented, it often lacks a number of critical elements. *Dietary interference* as a mechanism was first noted among inhabitants of Egypt and Iran who subsisted largely on unrefined cereals.[96] Sufficient phytic acid and fiber were present in the diet to bind and block zinc absorption. *Genetic malabsorption syndromes* involving a trace element are very rare. In one, failure to synthesize metallothionein (a metal-binding protein) in intestinal mucosal cells blocks absorption of both copper and zinc.

With these few general comments, the clinical effects of a lack of zinc, copper, and selenium will be described briefly. Iodine lack is discussed with the thyroid disorders (p. 1227).

ZINC DEFICIENCY. In the absence of such restricted diets as were responsible for a deficiency state in Iran and Egypt, a lack of zinc is very unusual, since it is reasonably abundant in meats, fish, shellfish, whole-grain cereals, and legumes. Most cases of zinc deficiency have been related to either total parenteral nutrition unsupplemented by zinc or a rare genetic syndrome that interferes with absorption.[97]

Zinc is an essential trace element for over 200 metalloenzymes and for normal nucleic acid, protein, and membrane metabolism. It has not been possible to neatly relate a particular clinical finding with a specific functional role of this element, but nonetheless a well-characterized deficiency syndrome has been identified.[98] The essential features are: *(1) a distinctive rash most often around the eyes, nose, mouth, anus, and distal parts, called acrodermatitis enteropathica (similar skin lesions may also occur in a variety of gastrointestinal diseases and chronic alcoholism); (2) anorexia often accompanied by diarrhea; (3) growth retardation; (4) depressed wound healing; (5) hypogonadism with impaired reproductive capacity; (6) altered immune function; (7) impaired night vision related to altered vitamin A metabolism; (8) depressed mental function; and (9) an increased incidence of congenital malformations in infants of zinc-deficient women capable of becoming pregnant.* The condition should be suspected in any case of obscure retarded growth or infertility associated with the characteristic rash. Oral zinc supplementation is promptly curative.

COPPER DEFICIENCY. Trace amounts of copper are critical to health, but an excess, such as is encountered in Wilson's disease (p. 956) has serious consequences. Copper is an essential component of many metalloenzymes, most of which are oxidases. As noted in the discussion of Wilson's disease, after absorption copper is transported to the liver, where it is bound to an alpha-2-globulin to produce ceruloplasmin, in which form it is nontoxic and available for distribution throughout the body. Ceruloplasmin is a ferroxidase that catalyzes the oxidation of ferrous to ferric iron, affecting the rate of uptake of iron by transferrin and hence its availability for heme synthesis (p. 686). Thus, anemia and sometimes neutropenia are features of copper deficiency. The metal and its enzymes are also involved in myelin synthesis or maintenance; hence, impaired myelination is encountered in animals with a lack of copper. Copper is critical to the function of several central nervous system enzymes, including dopamine-beta-hydroxylase, involved in the synthesis of neurotransmitters. The copper metalloenzyme—lysyl oxidase—is requisite for the formation of cross-linkages in elastin and collagen—hence the impairment of vascular integrity and skeletal growth and maintenance in deficient states. Tyrosinase is a copper-dependent enzyme, and with a deficiency little or no melanin is produced. Thus *infants and children lacking copper are characterized by: anemia, sometimes neutropenia, depigmentation of hair, osteoporosis, and various central nervous system abnormalities such as hypotonia and psychomotor retardation.*[99] *In adults the same changes may be present, but for less obvious reasons there may also be glucose intolerance and hypercholesterolemia.*[100]

The syndrome of copper deficiency is most often encountered in the following clinical settings: (1) prematurity; (2) generalized malnutrition and prolonged diarrhea in infancy; (3) persistent intestinal malabsorption; (4) infants or adults on long-term therapy with chelating agents; (5) long-term unsupplemented parenteral nutrition; and (6) the X-linked recessive condition known as *Menkes' kinky hair disease*. The outstanding clinical feature of this rare entity in infants is a strange steel-wool consistency to the hair, often accompanied by bone changes, abnormalities of the blood vessels, and progressive neurologic deterioration, ending most often in a very early death. The basis for this hereditary disorder appears to be some defect in the intestinal absorption of copper.[101]

SELENIUM DEFICIENCY. Selenium deficiency of dietary origin leading to muscle degeneration has long been recognized in ruminants and swine.[102] A comparable deficiency syndrome in humans first came to light in China with the recognition, mainly in children and young women, of a *congestive cardiomyopathy called Keshan disease* that was correctly attributed to a marked lack of selenium in soil, water, and food. An apparently identical cardiomyopathy occurred in an Occidental patient who had received nutritional support through parenteral supplementation.[103] To date, cardiomyopathy has not been identified in other patients on parenteral feeding, but skeletal myopathy has developed that responded to the administration of selenium. In addition, acne has in some patients been reported to respond to selenium supplementation. It has not been possible to correlate these clinical changes with specific known functions of selenium, e.g., a component of glutathione peroxidase that serves as an antioxidant (along with vitamin E). In passing, it should be noted that selenium has been shown to protect against chemically induced cancers in laboratory animals.[104] Regrettably, there is no evidence to date that it serves a similar role in humans.

NUTRITIONAL EXCESSES AND IMBALANCES

The well-defined nutritional diseases discussed thus far all stem from dietary deficiencies. However, overnutrition and dietary imbalances also may lead to diseases such as obesity, and predispose to many systemic diseases and possibly some forms of cancer. All three issues have evoked much controversy and are currently of considerable concern as will be pointed out in the following discussions.

OBESITY

Few subjects are more talked about, are less often corrected, and have supported more authors (of diet books) than obesity. Indeed, obesity has assumed near-epidemic proportions in many Western countries, particularly in the United States. It is the result of the intake of calories in excess of utilization, in essence the storage of unneeded energy in fat cells. Viewed in this way, obesity could have had evolutionary benefits permitting survival over periods of food deprivation. Regrettably the world is now divided into "haves," constantly surrounded by an excess of food and often obese, and the "have nots," largely in Third World countries, who die by the thousands from starvation.

The definition of obesity and how it is best determined are controversial. In clinical practice, obesity is generally gauged by body weight relative to height when compared with norm standards (categorized by sex, age, and approximate body frame). On this basis, *obesity is defined as a body weight 20% or more above the norm.* By these standards, it is estimated that about 20% of middle-aged males and 40% of middle-aged females in the United States are obese. Dissatisfactions with the norm standards (e.g., they have recently been revised upward) have led to an alternative definition — *the ideal weight for an individual represents his or her weight at the age of 25 years.* Here again, loss in muscle and skeletal mass that occurs with aging could well mask the accumulation of a good deal of adipose tissue. Thus, some prefer to compare the amount of subcutaneous fat as measured by the thickness of skin folds (conventionally in the triceps and subscapular areas) with norm standards. There are, then, difficulties with the clinical determination of obesity, particularly when it is not marked. It would be much easier and far more satisfying to define it as "any individual who is as fat as you are whom you do not like."

In the great majority of instances, two "pushing derangements" underlie the imbalance between caloric intake and utilization: most important, inadequate "pushing of oneself away" from the dining table to avoid overeating, and almost as important, insufficient "pushing of oneself out of the chair" to engage in physical activity. Other factors, however, may make small contributions. Diets composed largely of carbohydrates and fats require less energy for the assimilation and metabolism of the foodstuffs than do protein-rich diets. This differential can account over the years for a significant accumulation of excess calories. Another observation points to genetic predisposition. Children of overweight parents, when adopted by "lean" families, have a greater tendency to become obese than do adoptees from nonobese natural parents.[105] One of the factors may be a familial predisposition to "energy efficiency" — the ability to expend fewer calories for a given amount of activity.[105A] Nonetheless, taking into account all the variables, the harsh truth is — *obesity means too much food and too little activity.*

We come now to another issue — does obesity predispose to excess morbidity and mortality? On the one hand, obesity has been referred to as "adiposity in excess of that consistent with good health."[106] Indeed, life insurance studies propose that being overweight imposes a significant excess mortality (Table 8–4). On the other hand, it is pointed out that weight reduction is only rarely of benefit in the treatment of most diseases.[107] Another analysis also contends that there is no strong evidence that obesity shortens survival.[108] As is so frequently the case, the truth probably lies somewhere in the middle. Although mild obe-

Table 8-4. Relationship Between Weight and Life Span*

	EXCESS MORTALITY	
EXCESS WEIGHT	*Men*	*Women*
10% overweight	13%	9%
20% overweight	25%	21%
30% overweight	42%	30%

* Drawn from Build and Blood Pressure Study: Overweight: Its Significance and Prevention. 1959 Society of Actuaries, data from Metropolitan Life Insurance Company.

sity may not be harmful, marked obesity must be considered a health hazard and a predisposition to a number of clinical disorders, some of great importance.

Hypertension is unmistakably correlated with obesity.[109] In the long-term Framingham study, the risk of developing hypertension among previously normotensive individuals was proportional to the degree of over-weight. In those 20% overweight, the risk was eight times greater than among those 10% underweight. Furthermore, weight reduction lowers blood pressure in hypertensive individuals.

Type II (non-insulin-dependent) diabetes is strongly associated with obesity. Over 80% of patients with this disorder are more than 20% overweight. Indeed, the diabetes is often unmasked by the accumulation of excess fat and often reverts to a subclinical state with weight loss as is discussed on page 999.

Adiposity clearly predisposes to *hyperlipoproteinemia and atherosclerosis*. The association is relatively weak with the low density lipoproteins (LDL) carrying most of the cholesterol in the blood, but strong with the very low density lipoproteins (VLDL) containing most of the circulating triglycerides. With increasing stores of adipose tissue there is increased hepatic synthesis of VLDL, and in addition, increased mobilization of fatty acids, providing the substrate for increased hepatic triglyceride synthesis. However, as discussed on page 559, LDL is ultimately derived from VLDL and, as has been shown, there is a clear correlation between the serum LDL and cholesterol levels and atherogenesis.

Cholelithiasis (gallstones) is six times more frequent in obese than in lean subjects. The mechanism is mainly an increase in total body cholesterol, increased cholesterol turnover, and augmented biliary excretion of cholesterol in the bile, leading to supersaturation and the formation of gallstones.

Hypoventilation syndrome refers to a constellation of respiratory abnormalities encountered in the very obese. It has been called *pickwickian syndrome* after the fat lad who was constantly falling asleep in Dickens' "Pickwick Papers." Hypersomnolence both at night and during the day is characteristic and is often associated with apneic pauses during sleep, polycythemia, and eventual right-sided heart failure. The complete explanation of the hypoventilation syn-

drome is complex but is, at least in part, attributable to the increased burden on chest wall movement imposed by the subcutaneous fat.[110]

The association between obesity and *heart disease* is surprisingly complex. Clearly, significant obesity predisposes to atherosclerosis and coronary heart disease, and an increased mortality from myocardial infarction.[111] Most of the risk is the consequence of the associated hypertension, hyperlipoproteinemia, and diabetes. Nonetheless, a residual small increased risk can be ascribed directly to the obesity. For middle-aged men, modest increases in weight impose little or no danger and, according to epidemiologic data, may even protect against death from heart disease.[112,113] However, significant obesity causes an increase in heart size resulting from left ventricular hypertrophy; conversely, weight reduction is followed by a decrease in heart weight.[114] In addition, weight reduction lowers blood pressure, thus relieving the heart of an additional burden. *Obesity as an independent variable also increases the risk of sudden cardiac death.[114a] When all variables are taken into account, there can be little doubt that significant obesity per se predisposes to heart disease and to premature death from it.*

Stroke and obesity is another area in which the literature is filled with opposing viewpoints. One study contended that men who were overweight at 20 years of age and then gained 30 or more pounds thereafter had a twofold increase in the incidence of stroke.[115] Others deny any relationship and maintain that it is not the obesity per se, but the related hypertension.

Equally contentious is the relationship between adiposity and *cancer*, particularly cancers arising in the endometrium and breast. Here the problem is complicated by the role of particular foods, such as animal fats, which may have been consumed in excess in the production of obesity. This subject is explored in the following section on diet and cancer.

More clear-cut is the predisposing influence of marked adiposity on the development of *degenerative joint disease (osteoarthritis)*. This form of arthritis, which typically appears in older individuals, is attributed in large part to the cumulative effects of wear and tear. It is reasonable to assert that the greater the body burden of fat, the greater is the trauma to joints with decades of use. We may conclude by saying that obesity not only shortens the life span but also impairs its quality (Fig. 8-21).

DIET AND SYSTEMIC DISEASES

The composition of the diet, even in the absence of obesity, makes a significant contribution to the causation or progression of a large number of diseases. These interrelationships are detailed with the discussions of the various conditions, and so only a few examples will suffice here.

One of the most important and controversial issues today is the contribution of the diet to athero-

OBESITY

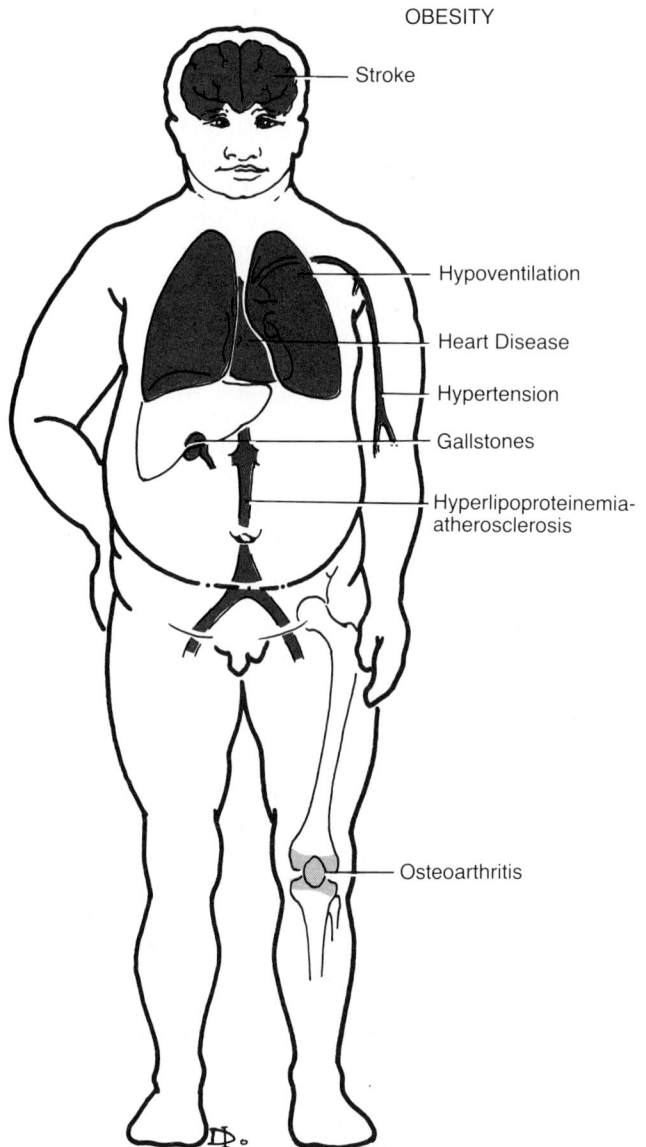

— Stroke

— Hypoventilation

— Heart Disease

— Hypertension

— Gallstones

— Hyperlipoproteinemia-
atherosclerosis

— Osteoarthritis

Figure 8–21. The major adverse consequences of obesity.

genesis. The central question is — can dietary modification, specifically reduction in the consumption of saturated animal fats (e.g., eggs, butter, and beef), reduce the serum cholesterol levels and prevent or retard the development of atherosclerosis, most importantly coronary heart disease? Without going into all of the evidence cited on page 558, the preponderant opinion is strongly affirmative based on the following findings. In experimental animals, cholesterol and fat must be added to their diets to produce atherosclerosis; when the atherogenic diets are stopped and the serum cholesterol level returns to baseline, the atherosclerotic lesions become smaller over the span of months.[116] Populations subsisting on diets low in saturated fat and cholesterol have significantly lower incidences of coronary heart disease and lower serum lipid levels than do populations consuming meat-rich Western diets containing large amounts of animal fats.

Dietary interventions aimed at reducing the intake of saturated fat and serum cholesterol-lowering drugs reduce the incidence of nonfatal and fatal myocardial infarction.[117]

The average adult in the United States consumes about 140 gm of fat per day and about 500 mg of cholesterol. The ratio of saturated fatty acids to polyunsaturated fatty acids in this fat is about 3 : 1. Lowering the saturates to the level of the polyunsaturates effects a reduction in the cholesterol content to about 200 to 300 mg, with a 10 to 15% reduction in the serum cholesterol level within a few weeks. Vegetable oils, such as corn and safflower oils, and fish oils contain highly polyunsaturated fatty acids. Fish oil fatty acids belonging to the "omega-3" or "N-3" family have more double bonds than the "omega-6" or "N-6" fatty acids found in vegetable oils. Substitution of a portion of the saturated fat with a fish oil for a four-week period induced a substantial reduction in serum lipid levels, particularly in triglycerides and very low density lipoproteins, which was greater than that induced by vegetable oils.[118] Significantly, a recent study of Dutch men whose usual daily diet contained 30 gm of fish revealed a substantially lower frequency of death from coronary heart disease than that among comparable controls.[119] The conclusion seems inescapable — animal fat with its cholesterol is no "friend of the heart."

To turn to other examples of the effect of the diet on disease, hypertension is beneficially affected by restricting sodium intake. A deficiency in dietary fiber or roughage resulting in decreased fecal bulk is thought to be responsible for or predispose to diverticulosis of the colon (p. 884). The effect of excess calories and obesity on diabetes was pointed out in a previous discussion (p. 999). Other examples could be cited, but it is clear that disease and the diet have many important interactions.

DIET AND CANCER

There is great concern today in governmental, scientific, and lay circles about the possibility that what we eat or fail to eat contributes to the causation of cancer.[120,121] While there are potentially carcinogenic influences prevalent in the environment, epidemiologic studies, attempting to control for the many variables, point to diet as a major factor. Support for this view comes from various sources but all the data are open to challenge. It is frequently contended that 80 to 90% of cancers in the United States and other industrialized nations can be attributed to lifestyle (including diet) and environmental influences.[122] Cancer of the stomach is about five times more frequent in Japan than in the United States, whereas the reverse holds true for cancer of the colon. Successive generations of Japanese families who migrated to the United States progressively acquire an incidence rate for both forms of cancer ever closer to that of their new home, attributed to change in diet (p. 264, Fig. 6–22).[123]

Even more convincing is the laboratory evidence from animals. Restriction of dietary intake lowers the spontaneous incidence of cancers in a variety of animals and also reduces the incidence and progression of experimentally induced neoplasms.[124]

Three aspects of the diet are of concern: (1) its possible content of exogenous carcinogens; (2) the potential that carcinogens might be endogenously synthesized from dietary components; and (3) a possible lack of protective factors.[125,126] *Relative to exogenous carcinogens,* it was pointed out in Chapter 6 (p. 272) that some naturally occurring carcinogens may be present in the diet, e.g., aflatoxins. The high incidence of hepatocarcinoma in Africa may be attributable in part to contamination of grains and nuts by aflatoxin B, resulting from the growth of *Aspergillus flavus.* Aromatic polycyclic hydrocarbons could be produced in the broiling and smoking of meats and fish (p. 271). Of great current interest is the controversy about the dangers of the artificial sweeteners saccharin and cyclamates (hence the search for natural, potentially safer agents). However, many analyses have failed to reveal any significant increase in the frequency of bladder cancer among users of saccharin and cyclamates.[127–130] Thus, although saccharin and cyclamates are probably not initiators of cancer, the possibility that they might enhance the action of concurrent carcinogenic influences has not been ruled out.

Concern about the *endogenous synthesis of carcinogens or promoters* from components of the diet relates principally to gastric, mammary, and endometrial carcinomas. With gastric carcinoma, nitrosamines and nitrosamides are in the spotlight. These compounds could be formed in the body from nitrites and amines or amides derived from digested proteins.[131] Sodium nitrite is added as a flavor and color preservative to foods such as processed meats, which are not heated sufficiently to destroy botulinal spores. Sodium nitrite is also present in some common vegetables. Nitrates are abundant in the soil and water and can be reduced to nitrites by bacterial action in the gut. There is, then, the potential for the endogenous production of carcinogenic agents from dietary components, which might well have an effect on the stomach exposed to the highest concentrations.

With carcinoma of the breast in postmenopausal women, several fairly recent epidemiologic studies implicate diets high in animal meats and fats, and overnutrition (obesity).[132,133] There is no shortage of theories to explain these associations. Dietary fat might serve as a vehicle for liposoluble carcinogens, cocarcinogens, or promoters. Estrogen metabolism might be altered in obese individuals with increased synthesis of the potentially more dangerous estrone (estradiol) and decreased synthesis of "antiestrogenic" 2-hydroxyestrone. Concomitantly, there might be increased conversion of androstenedione (of adrenal origin) to estrone in the mammary and peripheral fat depots. Indeed, the normal fat stores in the breast would increase local tissue levels. These hypothecations have been buttressed by animal studies showing an increased incidence of carcinogen-induced breast cancers when the fat level in the diet is raised.[134] Seductive as these observations may be, a large number of epidemiologic studies refute an association between breast cancer and dietary animal fats or obesity.[135,136] For the present, we must conclude that there is no solid evidence that diet plays a significant role in this form of cancer.

Low fiber and a high animal fat intake has been implicated in the causation of colonic cancer.[137] The most convincing attempt to explain these associations is the following. A high animal fat diet might have two effects. The high fat intake would increase the level of bile acids in the gut, which in turn would modify the intestinal flora, favoring the growth of microaerophilic bacteroides. It is then proposed that either the bile acids themselves, or metabolites of the bile acids produced by the bacteroides, might serve as carcinogens or promoters.[138] Furthermore, a low fiber content in the diet would decrease stool bulk and slow transit time, thereby exposing the mucosa to the putative offenders longer. Alternatively, certain types of fiber might bind carcinogens and thereby protect the mucosa. Reduction in stool bulk would also lessen the dilution of offending products. Unfortunately, attempts to document these theories in patients and experimental animals have on the whole led to contradictory results.[139,140]

There are many other ramifications to the story, e.g., the possible protective roles of vitamins A, C, and E; the contribution of a lack of selenium to a predisposition to cancer; and the growing anxiety (sometimes hysteria) about the use of food additives and agricultural pesticides and fungicides. Nevertheless, at present, while there are reasons for being cautious about the role of the diet in the development of certain forms of cancer, definitive proof or even persuasive evidence is still lacking.

1. Reutlinger, S., and Alderman, H.: The prevalence of calorie deficient diets in developing countries. World Dev. 8:239, 1980.

2. Ashworth, A.: International differences in child mortality and the impact of malnutrition. Hum. Nutr. Clin. Nutr. 36:279, 1982.

3. Massachusetts Department of Public Health: 1983 Massachusetts Nutrition Survey. Boston, 1983.

4. Rudman, D., and Williams, P.J.: Nutrient deficiencies during total parenteral nutrition. Nutr. Rev. 43:1, 1985.

5. Hoyumpa, A.M.: Mechanisms of vitamin deficiencies in alcoholism. Alcoholism Clin. Exp. Res. 10:573, 1986.

6. Cerda, J.J., and Artnak, E.J.: Nutritional aspects of malabsorption syndromes. Compr. Ther. 9:35, 1983.

7. Pereira, G.R., and Zucker, A.H.: Nutritional deficiencies in the neonate. Clin. Perinatol. 13:175, 1986.

8. Montgomery, R.D., et al.: Causes of malabsorption in the elderly. Age Ageing 15:235, 1986.

9. Helman, A.D., and Darnton-Hill, I.: Vitamin and iron status in *new* vegetarians. Am. J. Clin. Nutr. 45:785, 1987.

10. Roe, D.A.: Drugs and nutrient absorption. *In* Winick, M. (ed.): Nutrition and Drugs. New York, John Wiley & Sons, 1983, p. 129.

11. Waterlow, J.C.: Kwashiorkor revisited. The pathogenesis of oedema in kwashiorkor and its significance. Trans. R. Soc. Trop. Med. Hyg. 78:436, 1984.

12. Maletnlema, T.N.: The problem of food and nutrition in Africa. World Rev. Nutr. Diet. *47*:30, 1986.

13. Listernick, R., et al.: Severe primary malnutrition in United States children. Am. J. Dis. Child. *139*:1157, 1985.

14. Keusch, G.T. Host defense mechanisms in protein-energy malnutrition. Adv. Exp. Med. Biol. *135*:183, 1981.

15. Rosenthal, M.J., and Goodwin, J.S.: Cognitive effects of nutritional deficiency. *In* Draper, H.H. (ed.): Advances in Nutritional Research. Vol. 7. New York, Plenum Press, 1985, p. 71.

16. El-Tatawy, S., et al.: Cerebral atrophy in infants with protein-energy malnutrition. A.J.N.R. *4*:434, 1983.

17. Goodman, DeW. S.: Vitamin A and retinoids in health and disease. N. Engl. J. Med. *310*:1023, 1984.

18. Schoeff, L.: Vitamin A. Am. J. Med. Tech. *49*:447, 1983.

19. Olson, J.A.: Vitamin A. *In* Olson, R.E., Broquist, H.P., Chichester, C.O., Darby, W.J., Kolbye, A.C., Jr., and Stalvey, R.M. (eds.): Present Knowledge in Nutrition. 5th Ed. Washington, D.C., The Nutrition Foundation, 1984, p. 176.

20. Editorial: Vitamin A and retinol-binding protein in fetal growth and development of the rat. Nutr. Rev. *35*:305, 1977.

21. Wolf, G., et al.: Recent evidence for the participation of vitamin A in glycoprotein synthesis. Fed. Proc. *38*:2540, 1979.

22. Bowmaker, J.K., and Dartnall, H.J.A.: Visual pigments of rods and cones in a human retina. J. Physiol. *298*:501, 1980.

23. Wald, G.: Molecular basis of visual excitation. Science *162*:230, 1968.

24. Editorial: Vitamin A deficiency—a global disease. Nutr. Rev. *43*:240, 1985.

25. Sommer, A., et al.: Increased mortality in children with mild vitamin A deficiency. Lancet *2*:585, 1983.

26. Editorial: Vitamin A for measles. Lancet *1*:1067, 1987.

27. Bertram, J.S., et al.: Rationale and strategies for chemoprevention of cancer in humans. Cancer Res. *47*:3012, 1987.

28. Hennekens, C.H., et al.: Vitamin A, carotenoids, and retinoids. Cancer *58*:1837, 1986.

29. Lippman, S.M., et al.: Retinoids as preventive and therapeutic anti-cancer agents. Cancer Treat. Rep. *71*:391, 1987.

30. Editorial: Vitamin D: New perspectives. Lancet *1*:1122, 1987.

31. DeLuca, H.F.: Vitamin D–dependent calcium transport. *In* Graves, J.S. (ed.): Regulation and Development of Membrane Transport Processes. New York, John Wiley & Sons, 1985, p. 159.

32. Holtrop, M.F., et al.: 1,25-dihydroxycholecalciferol stimulates osteoclasts in rat bones in the absence of parathyroid hormone. Endocrinology *108*:2293, 1981.

33. DeLuca, H.F.: The metabolism and functions of vitamin D. Adv. Exp. Med. Biol. *196*:361, 1986.

34. Raisz, L.G., and Kream, B.E.: The regulation of bone formation. N. Engl. J. Med. *309*:29,83, 1983.

35. Audran, M., and Kumar, R.: The physiology and pathophysiology of vitamin D. Mayo Clin. Proc. *60*:851, 1985.

36. Belton, N.R.: Rickets—not only the "English disease." Acta Paediatr. Scand. (Suppl.) *323*:68, 1986.

37. Bouillon, R.A., et al.: Vitamin D status in the elderly: Seasonal substrate deficiency causes 1,25-dihydroxycholecalciferol deficiency. Am. J. Clin. Nutr. *45*:755, 1987.

38. Frost, H.M.: Tetracycline-based histological analysis of bone remodeling. Calcif. Tissue Res. *3*:211, 1969.

39. Bordier, P., et al.: Vitamin D metabolites and bone mineralization in man. J. Clin. Endocrinol. Metab. *46*:284, 1978.

40. Avioli, L.V.: Postmenopausal osteoporosis: Prevention versus cure. Fed. Proc. *40*:2418, 1981.

41. Mason, K.E.: The first two decades of vitamin E. Fed. Proc. *36*:1906, 1977.

42. Muller, D.P.R.: Vitamin E—its role in neurological function. Postgrad. Med. J. *62*:107, 1986.

43. Harding, A.E.: Vitamin E and the nervous system. C.R.C. Crit. Rev. Neurobiol. *3*:89, 1987.

44. Bieri, J.G., et al.: Medical uses of vitamin E. N. Engl. J. Med. *308*:1063, 1983.

45. Cavanaugh, J.B.: The problems of neurons with long axons. Lancet *1*:1284, 1984.

46. Muller, D.P.R., et al.: Long-term management of abetalipoproteinaemia: Possible role for vitamin E. Arch. Dis. Child. *52*:209, 1977.

47. Chow, C.K.: Vitamin E and blood. World Rev. Nutr. Diet. *45*:133, 1985.

48. Zipursky, A.: Vitamin A deficiency anemia in newborn infants. Clin. Perinatol. *11*:393, 1984.

49. Suttie, J.W.: Recent advances in hepatic vitamin K metabolism and function. Hepatology *7*:367, 1987.

50. Rappaport, E.S., et al.: Protein C deficiency. South. Med. J. *80*:240, 1987.

51. Friedman, P.A., and Prysiecki, C.T.: Vitamin K–dependent carboxylation. Int. J. Biochem. *19*:1, 1987.

52. Frick, P.G., et al.: Dose response and minimal daily requirement for vitamin K in man. J. Appl. Physiol. *23*:387, 1967.

53. Shapiro, A.D., et al.: Vitamin K deficiency in the newborn infant: Prevalence and perinatal risk factors. J. Pediatr. *109*:675, 1986.

54. Tripp, J.H., and McNinch, A.E.: Haemorrhagic disease and vitamin K. Arch. Dis. Child. *62*:436, 1987.

55. Creedon, K.A., and Suttie, J.W.: Effect of N-methyl-thiotetrazol on vitamin K epoxide reductase. Thromb. Res. *44*:147, 1986.

56. Soulier, J.P., et al.: A new method to assay des-gamma-carboxy-prothrombin. Results obtained in 75 cases of hepatocellular carcinoma. Gastroenterology *91*:1258, 1986.

57. Motohara, K., et al.: A carboxyprothrombin (PIVKA-II) as a marker of hepatoblastoma in infants. J. Pediatr. Gastroenterol. Nutr. *6*:42, 1987.

58. Mock, C.M., et al.: Biotin deficiency: An unusual complication of parenteral alimentation. N. Engl. J. Med. *304*:820, 1981.

59. Anderson, S.H., et al.: Adult thiamine requirements and the continuing need to fortify processed cereals. Lancet *2*:85, 1986.

60. Tanphaichitr, V., and Wood, B.: Thiamin. *In* Olson, R.E., Broquist, H.P., Chichester, C.O., Darby, W.J., Kolbye, A.C., Jr., and Stalvey, R.M. (eds.): Present Knowledge in Nutrition. 5th Ed. Washington, D.C., The Nutrition Foundation, 1984, p. 273.

61. Mukherjee, A.B., et al.: Transketolase abnormality in cultured fibroblasts from familial chronic alcoholic men and their male offspring. J. Natl. Cancer Inst. *79*:1039, 1987.

62. Pang, J.A.: Shoshin beriberi: An underdiagnosed condition. Intensive Care Med. *12*:380, 1986.

63. Wood, B., et al.: Wernicke's encephalopathy in a metropolitan hospital. Med. J. Aust. *144*:12, 1986.

64. Harper, C.G., et al.: Clinical signs in the Wernicke-Korsakoff complex: A retrospective analysis of 131 cases diagnosed at necropsy. J. Neurol. Neurosurg. Psychiatry *49*:341, 1986.

65. Chang, M.Y., et al.: Further studies on the riboflavin-binding immunoglobulin IgG. Equilibrium and kinetic aspects of the interaction. Biochemistry *20*:2922, 1981.

66. Rivlin, R.S.: Riboflavin. *In* Olson, R.E., Broquist, H.P., Chichester, C.O., Darby, W.J., Kolbye, A.C., Jr., and Stalvey, R.M. (eds.): Present Knowledge in Nutrition. 5th Ed. Washington, D.C., The Nutrition Foundation, 1984, p. 285.

67. Perry, G.M., et al.: The effect of riboflavin on red-cell vitamin B_6 metabolism and globin synthesis. Biomedicine *33*:36, 1980.

68. The Coronary Drug Project Research Group: Clofibrate and niacin in coronary heart disease. J.A.M.A. *231*:360, 1975.

69. Minns, R.: Vitamin B_6 deficiency and dependency. Dev. Med. Child. Neurol. *22*:795, 1980.

70. Molony, C.J., and Parmalee, A.H.: Convulsions in young infants as a result of pyridoxine deficiency. J.A.M.A. *154*:405, 1954.

71. Serfontern, W.J. et al.: Vitamin B_6 revisited. Evidence of subclinical deficiencies in various segments of the population and possible consequences thereof. S. Afr. Med. J. *66*:437, 1984.

72. Mudd, S.H.: Pyridoxine-responsive genetic disease. Fed. Proc. *30*:970, 1971.

73. National Research Council, Food and Nutrition Board: Recommended Daily Allowances. 9th Ed. Washington, D.C., National Academy of Sciences, 1980.

74. Kapadia, C.R., and Donaldson, R.M., Jr.: Disorders of cobalamin (vitamin B_{12}) absorption and transport. Annu. Rev. Med. *36*:93, 1985.

75. Seetharam, B., and Alpers, D.H.: Absorption and transport of cobalamin (vitamin B_{12}). Annu. Rev. Nutr. *2*:343, 1982.

76. Kapadia, C.R., et al.: Intrinsic factor–mediated absorption of cobalamin by guinea pig ileal cells. J. Clin. Invest. *71*:440, 1983.

77. Allen, R.H.: Human vitamin B_{12} transport proteins. Prog. Hematol. *9*:57, 1975.

78. Hornig, D.: Metabolism of ascorbic acid. World Rev. Nutr. Diet. *23*:225, 1975.

79. Levine, M.: New concepts in the biology and biochemistry of ascorbic acid. N. Engl. J. Med. *314*:892, 1986.

80. Chojkier, M., et al.: Specifically decreased collagen biosynthesis in scurvy dissociated from an effect on proline hydroxylation and correlated with body weight loss: *In vitro* studies in guinea pig calvarial bones. J. Clin. Invest. *72*:826, 1984.

81. Sauberlich, H.E.: Ascorbic acid. *In* Olson, R.E., Broquist, H.P., Chichester, C.O., Darby, W.J., Kolbye, A.C., Jr., and Stalvey, R.M. (eds.): Present knowledge in Nutrition. 5th Ed. Washington, D.C., The Nutrition Foundation, 1984, p. 260.

82. Pauling, L.: Vitamin C and the Common Cold. San Francisco, W.H. Freeman & Co., 1971.

83. Pauling, L.: Are recommended daily allowances for vitamin C adequate? Proc. Natl. Acad. Sci. U.S.A. *71*:4442, 1974.

84. Cameron, E., Pauling, L., and Leibowitz, B.: Ascorbic acid and cancer: A review. Cancer Res. *39*:663, 1979.

85. Creagan, E.T., et al.: Failure of high dose vitamin C (ascorbic acid) therapy to benefit patients with advanced cancer: A controlled trial. N. Engl. J. Med. *1*:687, 1979.

86. Reeves, J.D., et al.: Iron deficiency in health and disease. Adv. Pediatr. *30*:281, 1983.

87. Heubers, H.A., et al.: The significance of transferrin for intestinal absorption. Blood *61*:283, 1983.

88. Powell, L.W., and Halliday, J.W.: Iron absorption and iron overload. Clin. Gastroenterol. *10*:707, 1981.

89. Lane, M., and Johnson, C.L.: Prevalence of iron deficiency. *In* Oski, F.A., and Pearson, H.A. (eds.): Iron Nutrition Revisited—Infancy, Childhood, Adolescence: Report of the 82nd Ross Conference of Pediatric Research. Columbus, Ohio, Ross Laboratories, 1981, p. 31.

90. Picciano, M.F., and Deering, R.H.: The influence of feeding regimens on iron status during infancy. Am. J. Clin. Nutr. *33*:746, 1980.

91. A Report on the International Nutritional Anemia Consultative Group (INACG): Iron Deficiency in Women. Washington, D.C., The Nutrition Foundation, 1981, p. 68.

92. Sturgeon, P.: Studies of iron requirements in infants and children. II. The influence on normal infants of oral iron in therapeutic doses. Pediatrics *17*:341, 1956.

93. Vartiainen, E., et al.: Iron prophylaxis in menstruating teenage girls. Acta Obstet. Gynaecol. Scand. *46* (Suppl. 1):49, 1967.

94. Scrimshaw, N.S.: Iron deficiency and its functional consequences. Compr. Ther. *11*:40, 1985.

95. Nielsen, F.H.: Ultratrace elements in nutrition. Annu. Rev. Nutr. *4*:23, 1984.

96. Halsted, J.A., et al.: A conspectus of research on zinc requirements of man. J. Nutr. *104*:345, 1974.

97. Hambidge, K.M., et al.: Zinc and acrodermatitis enteropathica. *In* Hambidge, K.M., and Nichols, B.L. (eds.): Zinc and Copper in Clinical Medicine. New York, Spectrum, 1978, p. 81.

98. McClain, C.J., et al.: Functional consequences of zinc deficiency. Prog. Food Nutr. Sci. *9*:185, 1985.

99. Graham, G.C.E., and Cordano, A.: Copper deficiency in human subjects. *In* Prasad, A.S. (ed.): Trace Elements in Human Health and Diseases. Vol. 1. New York, Academic Press, 1976, p. 363.

100. Klevay, L.M.: Changing patterns of disease: Some nutritional remarks. J. Am. Coll. Nutr. *3*:149, 1984.

101. Danks, D.M., et al.: Menkes' kinky hair disease. Further definition of the defect in copper transport. Science *179*:1140, 1973.

102. Bruce, A.: Swedish views on selenium. Ann. Clin. Res. *18*:8, 1986.

103. Johnson, R.A., et al.: An occidental case of cardiomyopathy and selenium deficiency. N. Engl. J. Med. *304*:1210, 1981.

104. Clement, I.P.: Selenium inhibition of chemical carcinogenesis. Fed. Proc. *44*:2573, 1985.

105. Stunkard, A.J., et al.: An adoption study of human obesity. N. Engl. J. Med. *314*:193, 1986.

105a. Ravussin, E., et al.: Reduced rate of energy expenditure as a risk factor for body weight gain. N. Engl. J. Med. *318*:467, 1988.

106. Albrink, M.J.: Overnutrition and the fat cell. *In* Bondy, P.K., and Rosenberg, L.E. (eds.): Duncan's Diseases of Metabolism, 7th ed. Philadelphia, W.B. Saunders Co., 1974, p. 426.

107. Mann, G.V.: The influence of obesity on health. N. Engl. J. Med. *291*:178, 1974.

108. Andres, R.: Effect of obesity on total mortality. Int. J. Obes. *4*:381, 1980.

109. Dustan, H.P.: Obesity and hypertension. Compr. Ther. *6*:29, 1980.

110. Luce, J.M.: Respiratory complications of obesity. Chest *78*:626, 1980.

111. Sorlie, P., et al.: Body build and mortality. The Framingham Study. J.A.M.A. *243*:1828, 1980.

112. Keys, A.: Overweight, obesity, coronary heart disease and mortality. Nutr. Rev. *38*:297, 1980.

113. Editorial: Cardiopathy of obesity—a not so Victorian disease. N. Engl. J. Med. *314*:378, 1986.

114. MacMahon, S.W., et al.: The effect of weight reduction on left ventricular mass. A randomized control trial in young overweight hypertensive patients. N. Engl. J. Med. *314*:334, 1986.

114a. Editorial: Sudden cardiac death in obesity and hypertension. Lancet *1*:628, 1988.

115. Heyden, S., et al.: Weight and weight history in relationship to cerebrovascular and ischemic heart disease. Arch. Intern. Med. *128*:956, 1971.

116. Wissler, R.W.: Principles of the pathogenesis of atherosclerosis. *In* Braunwald, E. (ed.): Heart Disease: A Textbook of Cardiovascular Medicine, 2nd ed. Philadelphia, W.B. Saunders Co., 1984, p. 1183.

117. Frick, M.H., et al.: Helsinki Heart Study: Primary prevention trial with gemfibrozil in middle-aged men with dyslipidemia: Safety of treatment, changes in risk factors, and incidence of C.H.D. N. Engl. J. Med. *317*:1237, 1987.

118. Phillipson, B.E., et al.: Reduction of plasma lipids, lipoproteins, and apoproteins by dietary fish oils in patients with hypertriglyceredemia. N. Engl. J. Med. *312*:1210, 1985.

119. Kromhout, D.: The inverse relation between fish consumption and twenty-year mortality from coronary heart disease. N. Engl. J. Med. *312*:1205, 1985.

120. Editorial: Obesity: The cancer connection. Lancet *1*:1223, 1982.

121. Gori, G.B.: Dietary and nutritional implications in the multifactorial etiology of certain prevalent human cancers. Cancer *43*:2151, 1979.

122. Doll, R., and Peto, R.: The causes of cancer: Quantitative estimates of avoidable risks of cancer in the U.S. today. J. Natl. Cancer Inst. *66*:1191, 1981.

123. Haenszel, W., and Kurihara, M.: Studies of Japanese migrants. I. Mortality from cancer and other diseases among Japanese in the United States. J. Natl. Cancer Inst. *40*:43, 1968.

124. Clayson, D.B.: Nutrition and experimental carcinogenesis. A review. Cancer Res. *35*:3292, 1975.

125. Miller, A.B.: Nutrition and cancer. Prev. Med. *9*:189, 1980.

126. Habs, M., and Schmahl, D.: Diet and cancer. J. Cancer Res. Clin. Oncol. *96*:1, 1980.

127. Hoover, R.N., and Strasser, P.H.: Artificial sweeteners and human bladder cancer. Preliminary results. Lancet *1*:837, 1980.

128. Morrison, A.S., and Buring, J.E.: Artificial sweeteners and cancer of the lower urinary tract. N. Engl. J. Med. *302*:537, 1980.

129. Editorial: Saccharin and bladder cancer. Lancet *1*:855, 1980.

130. Cohen, S.M., et al.: Promoting effect of saccharin and DL tryptophan in urinary bladder carcinogenesis. Cancer Res. *39*:1207, 1979.

131. Tannenbaum, S.R.: Ins and outs of nitrites. Science *20*:7, 1980.

132. Vorherr, H.: Breast cancer in relation to overnutrition. Klin. Wochenschr. *58*:167, 1980.

133. Armstrong, B., and Doll, R.: Environmental factors and cancer incidence and mortality in different countries with special reference to dietary practices. Int. J. Cancer *16*:617, 1975.

134. Carrol, K.K., et al.: Dietary fat and mammary cancer. Can. Med. Assoc. J. *98*:590, 1968.

135. Enig, M.G., et al.: Dietary fat and cancer trends—a critique. Fed. Proc. *37*:2215, 1978.

136. Gaskill, S.P., et al.: Breast cancer mortality and diet in the United States. Cancer Res. *39*:3628, 1979.

137. Reddy, B.S.: Dietary fiber and colon cancer: Epidemiologic and experimental evidence. Can. Med. Assoc. J. *123*:850, 1980.

138. Weisburger, J.H., et al.: Nutrition and cancer—on the mechanisms bearing on causes of cancer of the colon, breast, prostate and stomach. Bull. N.Y. Acad. Med. *56*:673, 1980.

139. Graham, S.: Diet and cancer. Am. J. Epidemiol. *112*:247, 1980.

140. Burkitt, D.P.: Colonic-rectal cancer. Fiber and other dietary factors. Am. J. Clin. Nutr. *31*:S58, 1978.

9

Environmental Pathology

AIR POLLUTION
Tobacco smoking
Pneumoconioses
    Coal workers' pneumocon-
      iosis (CWP)—simple and
      complicated (progressive
      massive fibrosis)
    Silicosis
    Asbestosis and asbestos-re-
      lated lesions
    Berylliosis

Other dust diseases
CHEMICAL AND DRUG INJURY
Adverse drug reactions (ADRs)
    Predictable ADRs—relevant
      factors
    Unpredictable ADRs—
      relevant factors
    Halothane
    Isoniazid (INH)
    Acetaminophen (Tylenol)
    Aspirin (acetylsalicylic acid)

    Exogenous estrogens and
      oral contraceptives (OCs)
    Anticancer drugs
    Anti-infectives
    Immunosuppressants
Nontherapeutic agents
    Ethyl alcohol
    Methyl alcohol
    Lead
    Carbon monoxide (CO)
    Environmental and occupa-
      tional carcinogens

    Drug addiction
    Other nontherapeutic toxic
      agents
PHYSICAL INJURIES
Mechanical force
Changes in temperature
    Abnormally low temperatures
    Thermal burns
Changes in atmospheric pressure
Electrical injuries
Radiation injury
Non-ionizing radiation

Having a disease is a lot like having wealth—you either are born with it (or its seeds) or you must have acquired it. Since the number of congenital ("born with") and genetic disorders is limited, the preponderance are acquired and therefore are environmental in origin. Such a broad definition of environmental disease includes most ailments covered in this text. Here we are particularly concerned with those diseases related to specific hazards imposed on mankind by mankind itself. These environmental disorders are especially significant because most are preventable by readily available public health and personal measures.

It is clearly impossible to consider all the disorders encompassed within even our limited interpretation of the term "environmental pathology." A major subset is nutritional in origin; some of these are considered on page 434. The health consequences of inadequate water supplies and soil erosion are monumental but well beyond our scope. Here, then, our consideration will be restricted to the major disorders caused by air pollution, including the most pervasive form of air pollution, tobacco smoking; the diseases induced by chemicals including drugs; and those related to physical forces such as exposures to lightning, extreme heat or cold, marked variation in atmospheric pressure, and most important, ionizing radiation.

AIR POLLUTION

One of the dubious by-products of human existence is air pollution. The atmospheric "soup" that humans have generated is larded with all manner of undesirable gases, fumes, volatilized metals, and particulates. So many of these substances are present in various combinations in the ambient air that it has been impossible to segregate the effects of one pollutant from another.[1,2] Air pollution is, of course, worst in industrialized countries, particularly in urban centers such as Los Angeles, New York, and Mexico City, but the problem exists throughout the world, even in such unlikely locales as the Himalayas![3]

What are the health consequences of air pollution? There are varying levels of proof that air pollution in general, and tobacco smoking in particular, contribute to the causation and aggravation of many lung diseases. The evidence is fairly substantial that it contributes to or aggravates bronchitis, bronchiolitis, and emphysema (all three collectively referred to as chronic obstructive pulmonary disease or COPD; see p. 766). Irritants and toxins in the air also initiate or aggravate laryngeal inflammation, viral respiratory infections, and asthma. In addition, specific dusts, as will be pointed out, cause pneumoconioses. *But dwarfing all these ill effects are the health consequences of tobacco smoking.* COPD and respiratory disorders in general are discussed elsewhere. Remaining for consideration here are the hazards of tobacco smoking and the pneumoconioses.

TOBACCO SMOKING

Virtually everyone knows and agrees that smoking is a dirty, bad habit; it's expensive, addictive, burns holes in clothing and people, predisposes to or causes many illnesses, and even kills. Happily, the percentage of Americans who smoke has fallen from about 45% in 1958 to about 30% now. However, a very large problem remains; there are still about 40 to 50 million smokers in the United States.[4]

It is important to emphasize at the outset that *cigarette smoking is without doubt the most hazardous*

469

form of tobacco use. Pipe and cigar smoking, while less hazardous, are by no means totally innocent, and smokeless tobacco use (chewing, tobacco pouches, snuff-dipping) invokes its own set of dangers. Most of the data on dangers inherent in the use of tobacco are epidemiologic, and as a few dissenters and the tobacco manufacturers are at pains to point out, statistical association cannot prove causality. Nonetheless, the total body of evidence is quite compelling to most impartial observers and is best reviewed by division into the following considerations: (1) the contribution of cigarette smoking to disease; (2) the benefits of quitting; (3) the hazards of passive smoking; and (4) the consequences of smokeless tobacco.

The *contribution of cigarette smoking to disease* is well summarized in a recent report of the U.S. Department of Health and Human Services—"Today cigarette smoking is recognized as the single most preventable cause of death in our society, and the most important public health issue of our time."[5] The estimated annual excess mortality is about 350,000 —more than the total number of American lives lost in World War I, Korea, and Vietnam combined.[6] The sources of these premature deaths are depicted in Figure 9–1 and can be summarized as follows:

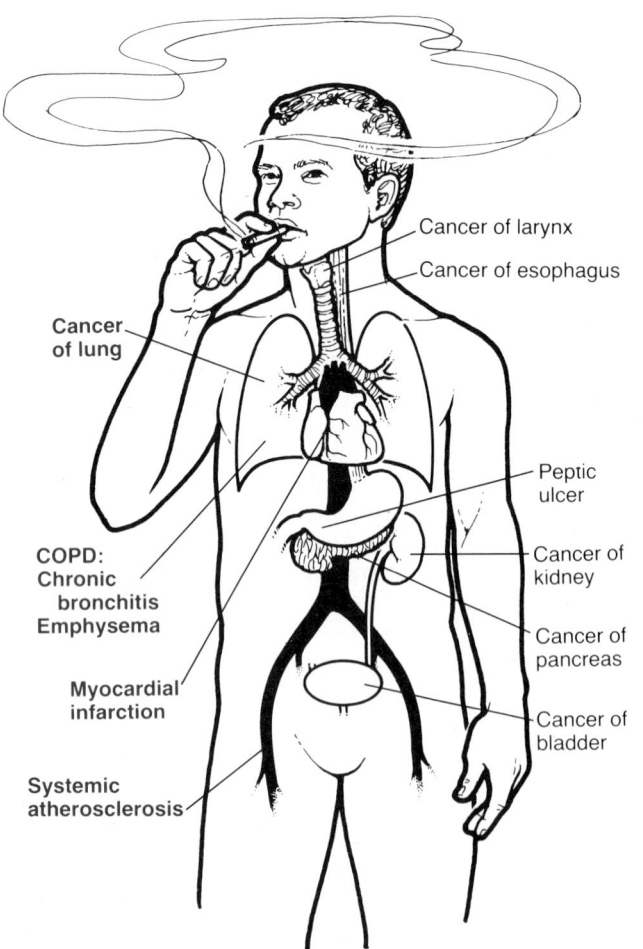

Cancer of larynx

Cancer of esophagus

Cancer of lung

Peptic ulcer

COPD: Chronic bronchitis Emphysema

Cancer of kidney

Cancer of pancreas

Myocardial infarction

Cancer of bladder

Systemic atherosclerosis

Figure 9–1. Adverse effects of smoking. The more common (on the left) and somewhat less common (on the right).

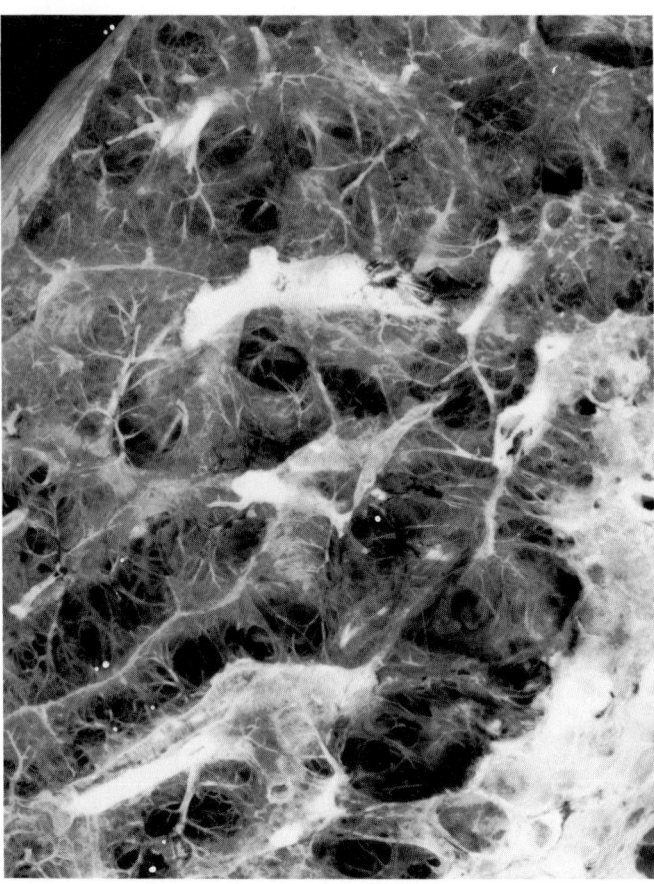

Figure 9–2. Pulmonary emphysema. A close-up of severe involvement with extensive destruction of pulmonary architecture, leaving only fibrotic strands and blood vessels traversing markedly distended airspaces.

• Cigarette smoking is a major cause of emphysema (Fig. 9–2) and chronic bronchitis, collectively referred to as COPD. These respiratory diseases account for about 62,000 deaths annually.
• It is a major risk factor for coronary atherosclerosis underlying coronary heart disease (CHD), especially myocardial infarction. CHD causes about 560,000 deaths annually, of which it is estimated that 30% or 170,000 are attributable to smoking. One pack of cigarettes per day increases the risk of CHD two fold.
• Bronchogenic carcinoma mortality has steadily increased in the United States over the past decades in both males and females. The rate of climb has begun to slow in males but is increasing in females. Currently lung cancer causes about 130,000 deaths annually in the United States, of which smoking is estimated to cause 100,000. The mortality from this form of cancer in those who have a long history of smoking over one pack per day is 10- to 14-fold higher than in nonsmokers, with a clear relationship between the amount smoked and the mortality rate.[7]
• Cigarette smoking increases the risk of cancer of the larynx, oral cavity, and esophagus by about seven fold and contributes to cancer of the kidney, urinary bladder, and pancreas.[8]
• Smoking during pregnancy is associated with an in-

creased risk of spontaneous abortion, perinatal mortality, and reduced birth weight.[9]
• It contributes to acute gastritis, probably peptic ulcers, and, as noted above, is a major risk factor for atherosclerosis.
• Cigarette smoking compounds the likelihood of cancer in those exposed to other carcinogenic influences, e.g., it increases by five fold the carcinogenicity of asbestos (p. 480).

The magnitude of the risk incurred by cigarette smokers is correlated with cumulative exposure, i.e., number of cigarettes smoked daily and years of smoking, usually quantitated in "pack-years," i.e., the number of packs smoked daily times the number of years. But other variables are also involved, such as age of onset of smoking, depth of inhalation, concomitant occupational exposure, and poorly understood individual, possibly genetic, factors. Particular note should be taken, the relationship is not linear— doubling the number of cigarettes smoked daily tripled the mortality rate from lung cancer among male British physicians.

It has not been possible to dissect the carcinogenity of cigarette smoke. It contains thousands of products, including carbon monoxide, nicotine, nitrosamines, and various polycyclic aromatic hydrocarbons. So-called safer cigarettes (low-tar-nicotine and filter tips) have been the industry's response to the growing public concern about these smoke-derived substances. Filter cigarettes now account for 60 to 90% of the sales market, and indeed early reports appeared to confirm their greater safety.[10] However, recent studies throw grave doubts on their benefits.[11] The "lowering" of the tar and nicotine content reported for these cigarettes has been accomplished by reducing the tobacco content and by interventions such as porous paper wrappers, lateral perforations in the filter, and other techniques that dilute the smoke drawn in by the machine.[12] But "men are not machines," and so some cigarette smokers inhale more deeply, for example, to compensate for the smoke dilution.[13] There are therefore reasons for questioning the benefit of so-called safer cigarettes. At present, the evidence indicates:

• They do *not* appear to lower the incidence of, or mortality from, coronary heart disease below that associated with the use of nonfilter cigarettes.[14]
• The risk of bronchogenic carcinoma *is reduced* in low-tar-nicotine and filter cigarette smokers as compared with those smoking high-tar-nicotine, nonfilter cigarettes.[15,16]
• There are no data yet on the impact of long-term use of "modified" cigarettes on the incidence of COPD.
• The lower mortality rates that "safer" cigarettes yield do not approximate those enjoyed by nonsmokers or exsmokers.
• Reported results are averages derived from cohort studies and may not be applicable to a particular smoker because of wide individual variability in smoking practices.

We must conclude that despite some putative improvements, the only "safe cigarette" is the discarded, unlit one.

BENEFITS OF QUITTING. The best parts of cigarette smoking are the benefits derived from quitting. They are:

• A relatively early reduction in the risk of coronary heart disease, particularly myocardial infarction. Smokers as compared with nonsmokers have a relative risk of myocardial infarction of about 3. With abstinence for 12 to 23 months the risk falls to about 2.0 and, after longer intervals, to baseline.[17]
• A fairly prompt alleviation of coughing, wheezing, and producing excess sputum. Even more important, after a long delay the mortality rate from COPD falls, as judged by the experience of a group of British physicians (Fig. 9–3). To be noted, the mortality rate continues to rise for the first nine years after cessation and never returns to the baseline of nonsmokers.
• A fall in mortality rate from bronchogenic carcinoma, which begins to appear in about five to nine years, and approaches basal nonsmokers' levels only after 14 years of abstinence (Fig. 9–3).
• A reduced predisposition to all other smoking-related diseases.

There can be no question then about the rewards of "kicking the habit."

PASSIVE SMOKING. One of the most disturbing aspects of tobacco smoking is its possible harmful effects on others. The consequences of smoke in the ambient air—passive smoking—have been studied for only a relatively few years, but the findings to date strongly suggest that it is detrimental and possibly carcinogenic.

The smoke drawn through the end of a cigarette, called "mainstream smoke," differs chemically from "sidestream smoke" produced by the burning cigarette between puffs. Sidestream smoke contains relatively more carbon monoxide, nitrosamines, and benzo(a)pyrene than does mainstream smoke. Related to the exposure, passive smokers may inhale the equivalent of about three actively smoked cigarettes per day.[18] As all nonsmokers know, the acute consequences of such exposure can be annoying (e.g., irritation of eyes, nasal stuffiness), but the chronic effects are of greater concern. A number of studies identified an increased incidence of respiratory illnesses and abnormal lung function in children under the age of two years whose mothers smoked, correlated with the amount smoked.[19] There is a further hint of growth retardation or impairment. Chronic passive smoking by adults has also been implicated in some abnormalities of lung function, pointing to irritative effects on the small airways, but further observation will be necessary to determine whether pulmonary emphysema or COPD follows.[20] But the major issue is—does passive smoking predispose to lung cancer? The verdict has not yet been rendered, but the weight of evidence suggests that nonsmoking women married to smokers

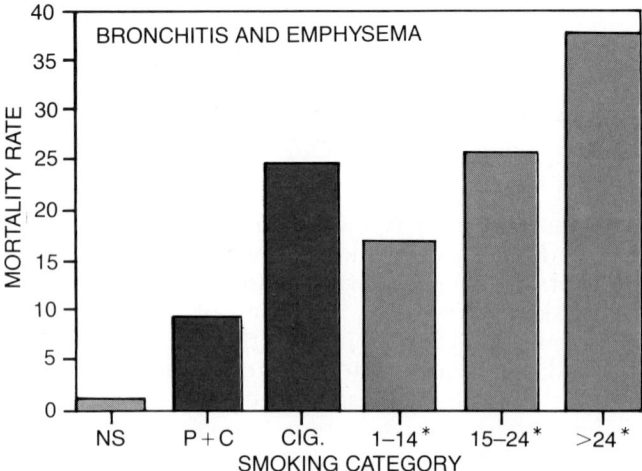

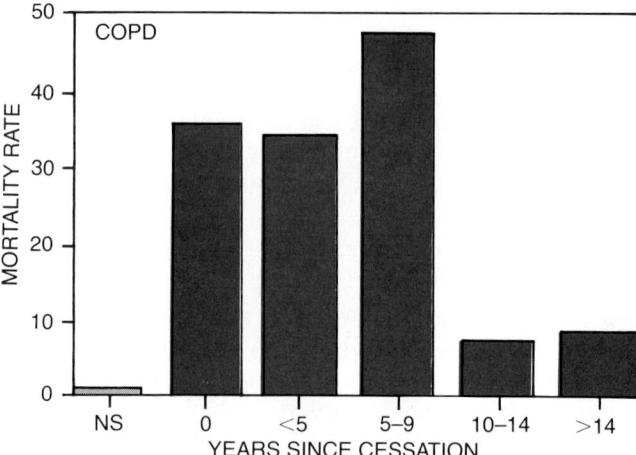

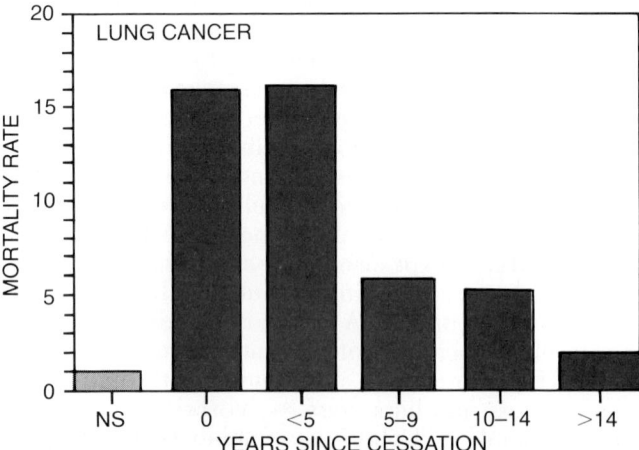

Figure 9–3. *Top,* Chronic bronchitis and emphysema mortality rates in male British physicians by smoking category. *Middle,* Mortality after smoking cessation due to COPD. *Bottom,* Mortality after cessation due to lung cancer. KEY: NS = nonsmokers; P + C = pipe and cigar smokers; CIG = all cigarette smokers; * = daily cigarette use; O = current smokers. (From Vial, W.C.: Southwestern internal medicine conference: Cigarette Smoking and Lung Disease. Am. J. Med. Sci. 291:130, 1986, based on data from Doll, R., and Peto, R.: Mortality in relation to smoking: 20 years' observation on male British doctors. Br. Med. J. 2:1525, 1976.)

have about a 30% greater chance of developing lung cancer than nonsmoking women with nonsmoking spouses.[21] The increased risk rises to about 70% when the spouse is a heavy smoker. Nonsmoking males are equally jeopardized by their spouses. While we wait for more definitive results, thousands of innocent bystanders may be exposed to premature death.[22]

HAZARDS OF SMOKELESS TOBACCO. The pressure to free the world of cigarette smoking has led to the re-emergence of smokeless tobacco as a cause of disease, namely cancer in the oral cavity.[23] It is not widely appreciated that in the United States there are at least 10 million users of smokeless tobacco — snuff, "tea bag" pouches containing tobacco, and chewing tobacco — 3 million of whom are under the age of 21![24] It is impossible to establish precise risk levels for any form of smokeless tobacco use because much depends on age at time of first exposure, exposure level, duration of use, and concurrent variables; however, analyses suggest a many-fold increased risk of cancer of the oral mucosa rising to about 50-fold among those with 50 or more years of use. The use of snuff is increasing at an alarming rate in the United States, especially among boys between 8 and 16 years of age, and the tragic consequences of this practice may not become evident for decades.[25] One can only conclude that to use tobacco is to risk "getting burned" even when the tobacco is not burning.

PNEUMOCONIOSES

The term "pneumoconiosis," originally applied to lung diseases caused by the inhalation of dust, now includes all disorders caused by the inhalation of any aerosol. Although there is a tendency to consider pneumoconioses as occupational disorders, in fact they are environmental diseases because they may involve the general population, particularly urban dwellers in the neighborhoods of industries that produce pollutants. Traces of asbestos, for example, are found in urban air. Happily, safety regulations have reduced the frequency of most of the pneumoconioses, but the long time lag involved in their emergence and progression makes them continue to be important causes of morbidity and mortality today. The most serious are those having the potential of progressing to irreversible nodular or diffuse fibrosis of the lung, i.e., coal worker's pneumoconiosis, silicosis, and asbestosis. There are, in addition, many other less common pneumoconioses such as berylliosis and those produced by less irritating dusts: siderosis (iron dust), stannosis (tin dust), and baritosis (barium dust), as well as a large number of pulmonary reactions caused by the inhalation of organic dusts and chemical fumes and vapors. A simplified classification is offered in Table 9–1. The specific changes caused by the more important dusts are presented in succeeding sections; however, certain pathogenetic principles apply to all.

The development of a pneumoconiosis is depen-

Table 9–1. Air Pollutant Lung Diseases

AGENT	DISEASE	EXPOSURE
Mineral Dusts		
Coal dust	Macules Progressive massive fibrosis Caplan's syndrome ? Gastric carcinoma	Coal mining (particularly hard coal)
Silica	Silicosis Caplan's syndrome	Foundry work, sandblasting, hard-rock mining, stone cutting, others
Asbestos	Asbestosis Pleural plaques Caplan's syndrome Mesothelioma Carcinoma of the lung, larynx, stomach, colon	Mining, milling, and fabrication, installation and removal of insulation
Beryllium	Acute berylliosis Beryllium granulomatosis ? Bronchogenic carcinoma	Mining, fabrication
Iron oxide	Siderosis	Welding
Barium sulfate	Baritosis	Mining
Tin oxide	Stannosis	Mining
Organic Dusts that Induce Extrinsic Allergic Alveolitis		
Moldy hay	Farmer's lung	Farming
Bagasse	Bagassosis	Manufacturing wallboard, paper
Bird droppings	Bird-breeder's lung	Bird handling
Organic Dusts that Induce Asthma		
Cotton, flax, hemp	Byssinosis	Textile manufacturing
Red cedar dust	Asthma	Lumbering, carpentry
Chemical Fumes and Vapors		
Nitrous oxide, sulfur dioxide, ammonia, benzene, certain insecticides (e.g., cyanate gases)	Bronchitis Asthma Pulmonary edema Respiratory distress syndrome Injury to exposed mucosal surfaces Fulminating poisoning	Occupational and accidental exposure

dent on: *(1) the amount of dust retained in the lung and airways; (2) the size, shape, and therefore buoyancy of the particles; (3) their solubility and physicochemical reactivity; and (4) the possible additional effects of other irritants, e.g., concomitant tobacco smoking.*

The amount of dust retained in the lungs is determined by its concentration in the ambient air, the duration of the exposure, and the effectiveness of clearance mechanisms. Most particles over 5 μ in diameter are either filtered out in the vibrissae of the nares or, after impaction on the linings of the airways, removed by the mucociliary escalator. Any influence, such as cigarette smoking, that affects the integrity of the mucociliary apparatus significantly predisposes to the accumulation of dust.

Small particles under 1 μ in diameter may remain suspended in the inspired air and be exhaled. Thus the most dangerous particles range from 1 to 5 μ in diameter because they may reach the terminal small airways and air sacs and settle on their linings. However, here is where macrophage clearance comes into play. Under normal conditions there is always a small pool of intra-alveolar macrophages that is expanded by recruitment of more macrophages when dust reaches the alveolar spaces. Phagocytosis of particles and emigration of the phagocytes provides a second line of defense. The *buoyancy of particles*, a function of shape relative to weight, also influences the likelihood of their reaching the distal air spaces. Certain particles such as asbestos fibers are long, slender, and light and so tend to be buoyant and stay in the central column of a rapidly moving stream of air; this permits them to escape clearance in the upper airways and to remain airborne until air flow slows in the smaller airways or alveolar sacs. Much of this understanding of the localization of dusts is owed to the use of whole-lung thin (Gough) sections. These allow an overall macroscopic and microscopic view of the precise distribution of dust collections and lesions and their relationship to the microscopic structure of the lung.[26]

The *solubility and cytotoxicity of particles*, influenced to a considerable extent by their size, modifies the nature of the pulmonary response. In general, the smaller the particle, the more likely and the more rapidly toxic levels will appear in the pulmonary fluids, depending, of course, on the solubility of the agent. Thus, finely divided dust may induce acute exudative reactions. In contrast, larger particles resist dissolution and so may persist within the lung parenchyma for years. They tend to evoke fibrosing collagenous pneumoconioses such as is characteristic of silicosis. The interplay of these variables is an important factor in determining whether or not a pneumoconiosis develops, and its nature. There is a relatively narrow margin between safety and danger. Against this background we turn to a consideration of the more common pneumoconioses.

Coal Workers' Pneumoconiosis (CWP) — Simple and Complicated (Progressive Massive Fibrosis)

In most industrialized nations, lung disease secondary to the inhalation of coal dust is uncommon because coal is no longer a widely used source of energy, and because engineering and health measures have lowered the level of air pollution in and about mines. *Simple coal workers' pneumoconiosis, which appears only after many years of underground mine work, is a relatively benign condition characterized by small, focal aggregations of coal dust–laden macrophages called coal macules within the lung parenchyma.*[27] In its milder expressions, this condition may produce a slight cough and some blackish sputum, but there is little or no dyspnea or disturbance in ventilatory function. Heavier accumulations of dust lead to larger macules and some ventilatory dysfunction accompanied by some dyspnea, but uncomplicated CWP is not often disabling.[28] With heavier pulmonary burdens of coal dust, fibrous scarring appears within the coal macules to produce clinically disabling *"complicated CWP,"* also referred to as *progressive massive fibrosis (PMF).*[29] It is important to note that *PMF is a generic term referring to progressive, disabling, sometimes fatal pulmonary scarring that may complicate any form of severe pneumoconiosis.*

There is no clear line demarcating advanced simple CWP from the milder forms of complicated CWP. Similarly, it is difficult to distinguish mild CWP from the banal accumulations of dust in the lungs *(anthracosis)* that are the almost inevitable consequence of cigarette smoking and life in the "dust bins" we call cities. In anthracosis, the macrophages in the alveoli and about the respiratory bronchioles become laden with dust and carbonaceous pigment. Drainage of the pulmonary accumulations sometimes leads to blackening of the regional lymph nodes, but otherwise they are harmless, causing no respiratory difficulty or radiographic changes; nor do they predispose to other forms of pulmonary disease. Thus, *anthracosis, simple CWP, and complicated CWP may be viewed as points along a spectrum of increasing accumulation of carbon dust within the lungs.*

The reported frequency of CWP among coal miners is extremely variable between countries and even among mines in a particular geographic area.[30] In the past, the majority of long-term workers in particular mines developed CWP; today the incidence is below 5%, and in some mines below 1%. There is similar variability in the reported frequency of transition of simple CWP into complicated CWP or PMF, but it is in the range of 2 to 8%. Much of this variability stems from differing criteria for the demarcation of the simple from the complicated disease. The factors predisposing to this transformation are still unknown, as will be pointed out.

MORPHOLOGY. In simple CWP, focal black pigmentations (macules) are scattered through the lung fields but are most numerous in the upper zones of the upper and lower lobes. They range up to 5 mm but are usually 1 to 2 mm in diameter. The airspaces in and about the macules may be enlarged, but the intervening parenchyma is unaffected. Similar pigmentations are seen over the pleura in distended lymphatics but without pleural puckering or reaction. Simultaneously, the regional lymph nodes become blackened. Histologically **the pigmented macules are composed of aggregations of coal dust–filled macrophages in close proximity to alveolar ducts and respiratory bronchioles (where the coal dust is first deposited).**[27] In time, in the more severe expressions of simple CWP, a delicate network of reticulin and collagen appears between the macrophages, and with it the respiratory bronchioles and subtended alveoli may become slightly dilated. Such dilatation has been referred to as centrilobular emphysema (p. 767), but some experts object to the use of the term "emphysema" because there is no destruction of alveolar walls.[31] Contributing significantly to the severity of the CWP is concomitant cigarette smoking. It adds a further element of bronchiolitis compounding respiratory deficits that the coal dust may have produced.

Complicated CWP (PMF) occurs on a background of simple CWP. It is characterized by large, sometimes massive, intensely blackened scars that exceed 2 cm in diameter and sometimes achieve dimensions of 5 to 10 cm.[32] The scarred areas are usually bilateral and may occur anywhere in the lungs but are most common in the upper parts of the lung. Larger lesions may extend across lobar fissures. When attached to the pleura, they may cause retraction and thickening of the pleura (Fig. 9–4).

Coalescence of the scars leads to large blackened areas of fibrosis, justifying the sometimes used designation "black lung disease." Occasionally the centers of scars are converted into cavities filled with a fluid to semifluid "India ink." The surrounding airspaces are usually markedly distended and may appear honeycombed, and the nodes of drainage are blackened, fibrotic, and often interadherent.

Microscopically, the massive scars comprise varying proportions of dense collagen and carbon pigment. The walls of respiratory bronchioles and pulmonary vessels trapped within the scar are thickened or their lumens are obliterated. Surprisingly, there is only a scant infiltrate of lymphocytes and plasma cells about the areas of fibrosis. Depending on the extent of the scarring and involvement of the pulmonary vasculature, right ventricular hypertrophy (cor pulmonale) may be present. In addition, miners who have rheumatoid arthritis and PMF sometimes develop apparent rheumatoid lesions in the lungs. They consist of rubbery-to-firm nodules, 0.5 to 2.0 cm in diameter, usually having foci of opaque necrosis and sometimes central liquefaction, cavitation, and calcification. On microscopic examination they strongly resemble subcutaneous rheumatoid nodules (p. 1351), with central fibrinoid necrosis and a characteristic enclosing inflammatory reaction. Caplan correctly related these lesions in miners to the concomitant rheumatoid arthritis, and hence the condition is sometimes called rheumatoid pneumoconiosis or **Caplan's syndrome**.[16] It may also be seen in silicosis, asbestosis, and other dust-caused pneumoconioses.[17] There are hints that the lung lesions are immunologic in origin, as is the arthritis.

PATHOGENESIS. In epidemiologic surveys the progression of simple CWP into the fibrosing complicated form PMF appears to be more common in older miners and in those with more marked severe expres-

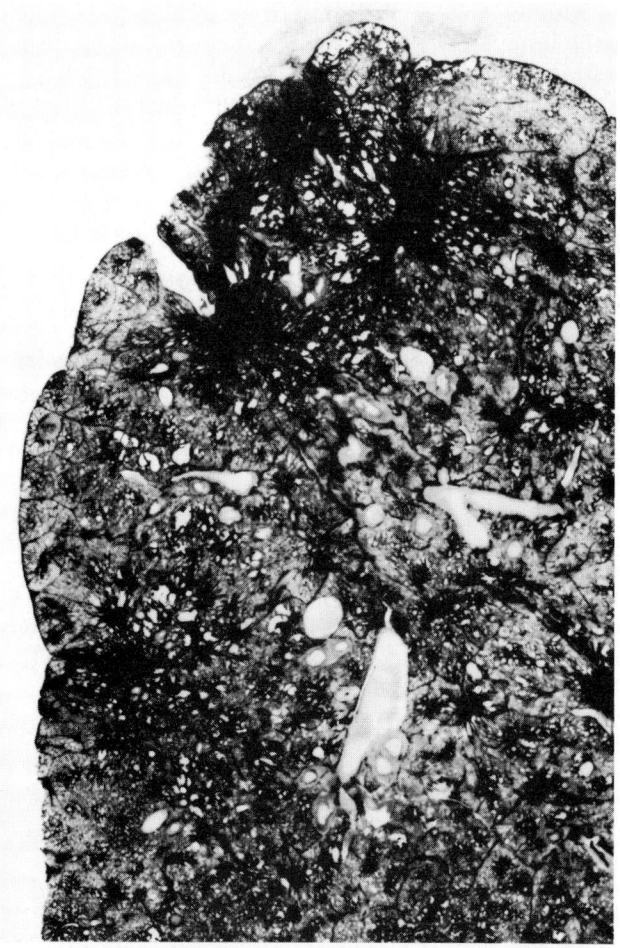

Figure 9–4. Complicated coal workers' pneumoconiosis (progressive massive fibrosis). The large blackened scars are principally located in the upper lobe. Note extensions of scars into surrounding parenchyma and retraction of adjacent pleura. (Courtesy of Dr. Werner Laquer, Dr. Jerome Kleinerman, and the National Institute of Occupational Safety and Health.)

sions of simple CWP.[33] These findings suggest that duration of exposure and magnitude of the coal dust burden are critical. However, the correlation is not perfect, and so other influences have been questioned. At one time, superimposed *tuberculosis* was thought to underlie fibrosing CWP, but it is clear that the two conditions are causally unrelated. *Silica dust* (derived from seams of quartz often found within coal deposits) was also once attributed causal significance in the development of PMF.[34] However, PMF has been observed in carbon-electrode makers and workers in similar occupations involving exposure to only pure volatilized carbon. *Lipid accumulation* resulting from dust-stimulated secretion of surfactant by type II epithelial cells may contribute to the fibrosis. The analogy is drawn between the fibrosis induced by the complex lipids in the walls of the tubercle bacilli and the fibrosing reactions in PMF.

Immunologic mechanisms are now favored. Miners with PMF sometimes develop rheumatoid disease and Caplan's syndrome accompanied by rheumatoid factor, antinuclear antibodies, and non–organ specific antibodies in the serum. However, in the absence of rheumatoid disease it has not been possible to document that autoantibodies are more prevalent in PMF than they are in CWP. Alternatively, cell-mediated mechanisms, and in particular *macrophages, are thought to be the pivotal effectors,* as shown in Figure 9–5. In brief, activation of these cells leads to the release of cytokines such as IL-1 and other growth factors for fibroblasts, inducing the progressive fibrosis in complicated CWP. Supporting this concept is the recent demonstration that human lung fibroblasts have high affinity receptors for IL-1.[35] In addition, the release of destructive enzymes and free radicals from macrophages may cause direct lung damage and contribute to the fibrosing reaction. We must leave it that, at the present time, the basis for the transformation of simple CWP into complicated CWP remains uncertain, although *most of the evidence suggests that the severity of the coal dust burden engulfed by macrophages is central.*

CLINICAL COURSE. CWP is usually asymptomatic and can be suspected only by the occupational history, possibly a cough productive of blackened sputum, or the finding of diffuse radiologic nodularities ("tattooing") on chest film. Such radiographic findings rarely appear before 30 years of work in coal mines. In cigarette-smoking miners, a chronic dry cough and exertional dyspnea may occur, but these symptoms are more likely to be related to the airway disease caused by cigarette smoke than to the CWP. However, uncommonly severe expressions of CWP may produce some loss of respiratory function, particularly in older men.[36]

PMF, by contrast, is a serious, disabling disease. At the outset it is manifested by dyspnea on effort, but as the pulmonary lesions advance the dyspnea worsens until it becomes evident at rest. The chronic cough produces coal dust–laden sputum, and some-

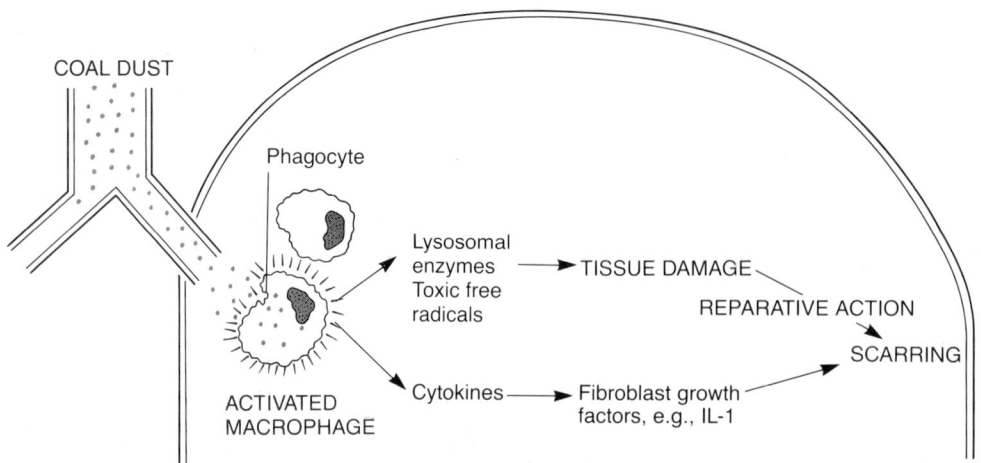

Figure 9–5. Potential pathways by which coal dust may induce pulmonary fibrosis.

times rupture of a lung cavity leads to an alarming release of jet-black sputum. Poorly localized chest pain is common, as is a purulent bronchitis related to intercurrent bacterial infection. In advanced cases, pulmonary hypertension and right ventricular hypertrophy may appear (p. 617). Still under study is the frequency of lung cancer in coal miners. Surprisingly, most studies find no increase in its prevalence when confounding influences, such as cigarette smoking, are carefully excluded.[37,38] There is a modest predisposition to carcinoma of the stomach, but to no other form of cancer. Suspected causes include swallowed coal dust with its potential carcinogens, or perhaps the common practice among coal miners of chewing tobacco (since smoking is forbidden within mines).

Silicosis

Prolonged inhalation of silica particles produces, after a long lag time (sometimes decades), a chronic, nodular, densely fibrosing pneumoconiosis that is insidious in onset and progressive in severity even after all further exposure has ceased. This fibrotic reaction is what is meant by the customary use of the term "silicosis." Silicosis is encountered in a diversity of industries including the mining of gold, tin, copper, and coal; in sandblasting, metal grinding, quarrying, and tunneling; and in the manufacture of ceramics and other refractory materials. Infrequently an acute silicosis is caused by intense exposure to fine dusts such as those produced by sandblasting and siliceous grinding wheels. This "accelerated silicosis" is characterized by areas of irregular fibrosis adjacent to alveolar spaces filled with a lipoproteinaceous exudate, producing a lesion closely resembling nonoccupational alveolar proteinosis (p. 795). Because this pattern is rare, the general term "silicosis" refers to the chronic disease, to which further comments are restricted.

Silicosis not only appears insidiously, but also evolves slowly over the span of decades and is compatible with long survival depending on many factors such as total dose, duration of exposure, type of silica

inhaled, and possibly individual factors. However, the early fibrosing reaction (simple silicosis) can progress to large areas of scarring—complicated silicosis, also called progressive massive fibrosis (PMF)—producing severe and sometimes fatal respiratory insufficiency. Moreover, the usual course of the disease may be suddenly worsened by the development of Caplan's syndrome (p. 475) or intercurrent tuberculosis (a 10- to 30-fold increased incidence).[39] There is, however, some good news—silicosis does not predispose to lung cancer or to any other form of cancer.

PATHOGENESIS. As is so often the case, there is more unknown than known about the pathogenesis of silicosis. The following points are reasonably well established.

• Crystalline silica, particularly quartz and cristobalite, is much more fibrogenic than amorphous (noncrystalline) silica, indicating that physical form and surface properties play some role.
• Scattered lymphocytes and alveolar macrophages are drawn rapidly to the sites of accumulation and engulf the particles.
• The dust-laden macrophages may clear the airspace of much of this pollution, but some macrophages with their silica "baggage" are trapped in the interstitial tissue or lymphatic channels about the airways. Some of the silica dust is transported into the subpleural and interlobular lymphatics as well as the hilar lymph nodes.
• Some silica particles may directly penetrate alveolar and airway lining cells to reach the interstitial tissues, where they are also engulfed by macrophages.
• The small fraction of retained silica dust leads to focal aggregations of resident and recruited macrophages, which are thought to be converted in time into the fibrosing nodules of silicosis.
• Silica dust may directly stimulate (irritate) type II alveolar lining cells to actively secrete surfactant. The complex lipids may be carried through the blood to the marrow, stimulating monopoiesis and thereby

augmenting the number of monocyte-macrophages available for recruitment.

From this point much is uncertain, in particular how the macrophage-particle interactions produce collagenous fibrosis. It is clear, however, that the macrophage plays a pivotal role. Until recently it was believed that the vengeful silica particles killed their macrophage hosts either by partial solution into silicic acid damaging lysosomal membranes or by hydrogen bonding to lysosomal membranes. There followed release of lysosomal hydrolases, which then induced lung injury and subsequent scarring. Studies of animal models embellished this theory, suggesting that macrophages also release chemotactins, such as leukotriene B_4, attracting neutrophils that contribute to the tissue injury by their release of degradative enzymes and possibly toxic free radicals.[40] However, this conception of the origin of the fibrosing reaction has been challenged on several scores: (1) Overt necrosis of pneumonocytes, macrophages, or neutrophils is not typically seen in silicosis; and (2) alveolar macrophages containing abundant dust particles, when recovered from bronchoalveolar lavages, have normal viability and function. For these reasons an alternative pathway has been suggested (Fig. 9–6).

Possibly the silica dust activates viable macrophages, with the secretion of macrophage-derived growth factors such as IL-1 and others producing the same fibrosing sequence proposed for the PMF of coal miners (p. 475). The intensity of the fibrosis may be up-regulated through the intervention of lymphocytes. T-helper cells activated by IL-1 release IL-2, a potent signal for the proliferation of T cells. Thus the lymphocyte population is expanded. Their production of macrophage migration inhibition factor, monocyte chemotactins, and gamma interferon would augment and activate macrophages at the local site and the amount of fibroblast growth factors. In this manner the collagenous reaction in silicosis is mediated by immunocompetent cells.[41] Simultaneously the activated T cells collaborate with B cells, leading to the production of elevated serum levels of IgG and IgM, antinuclear antibodies, rheumatoid factor, and circulating immune complexes so often seen in patients with silicosis.[42] Attractive as this conception of the pathogenesis of silicosis may be, it is still largely speculative.

MORPHOLOGY. Chronic silicosis (as distinct from accelerated silicosis) is characterized at the onset by tiny collagenous nodules, more palpable than visible. They tend initially to be located in the upper zones of the lungs, but with progression they extend throughout. The tiny nodules slowly enlarge, and some coalesce to produce minute areas of readily visible scarring (1 to 5 mm). In time the discrete nodules coalesce with the formation of stony-hard, large fibrous scars, usually in the upper lobes, causing contraction of the upper lobes and secondary expansion of the lower lobes (Fig. 9–7). Often the collagenous nodules or scars are blackened by concomitant accumulations of coal dust. The lung parenchyma between the scars may be compressed or emphysematous. Thus, honeycombing develops and is sometimes accompanied by subpleural bullae. Calcification may appear within the scarred areas. Similar collagenous nodules appear within the lymph nodes; peripheral involvement and subsequent calcification may produce so-called eggshell shadows on chest x-rays. Fibrous pleural plaques sometimes develop as well as adhesions that bridge and may even obliterate the pleural

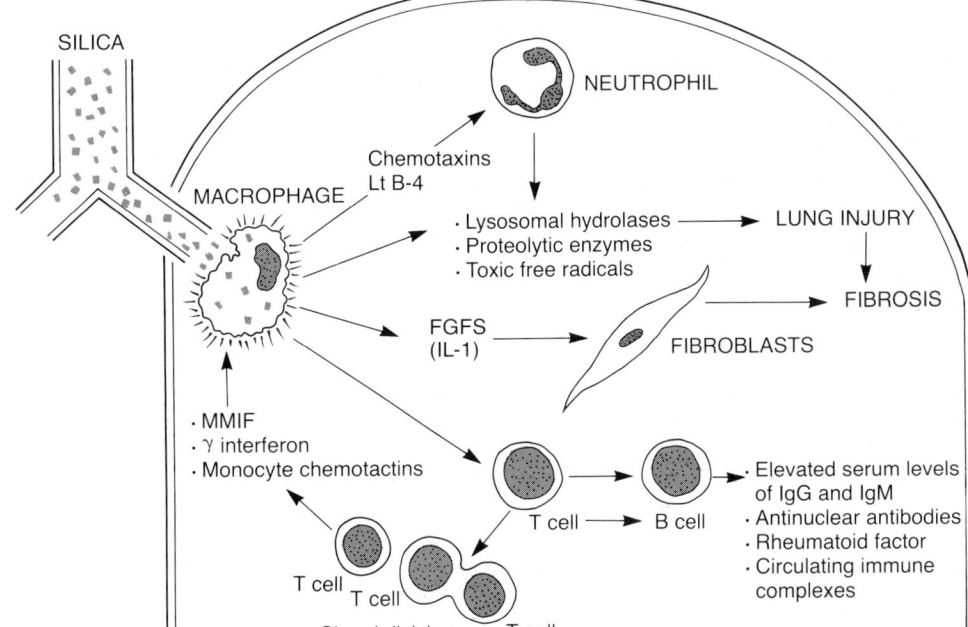

Figure 9–6. Suggested interactions of silica dust, pulmonary macrophage, neutrophils, and lymphocytes in the production of pulmonary fibrosis and elevated levels of circulatory immunoglobulins. FGFS = fibroblast growth factors; MMIF = macrophage migration inhibition factor.

cavities. These standard alterations may be complicated by tuberculous lesions with their foci of caseation and cavitation, or by the appearance of the gray-white necrotic lesions of Caplan's syndrome (p. 475).

Microscopically, discrete hyalinized collagenous nodules are seen about the respiratory bronchioles, associated alveoli, pulmonary arteries, and paraseptal and subpleural tissues. The collagen is laid down in concentric laminations, often separated by narrow, cleftlike spaces that may contain crystalline spicules presumably of silica. There is a surprisingly scant lymphocytic and occasionally plasma cell infiltrate about such foci. With enlargement, contiguous nodules are enclosed within encircling collagenous layers. In this fashion, the scarring extends and encroaches on respiratory bronchioles, contributing to bronchiolar obstruction and hyperinflation of alveoli (Fig. 9–8). Similar involvement of the pulmonary arteries adds an element of pulmonary hypertension to the disease. The intervening lung parenchyma is hyperinflated or emphysematous.

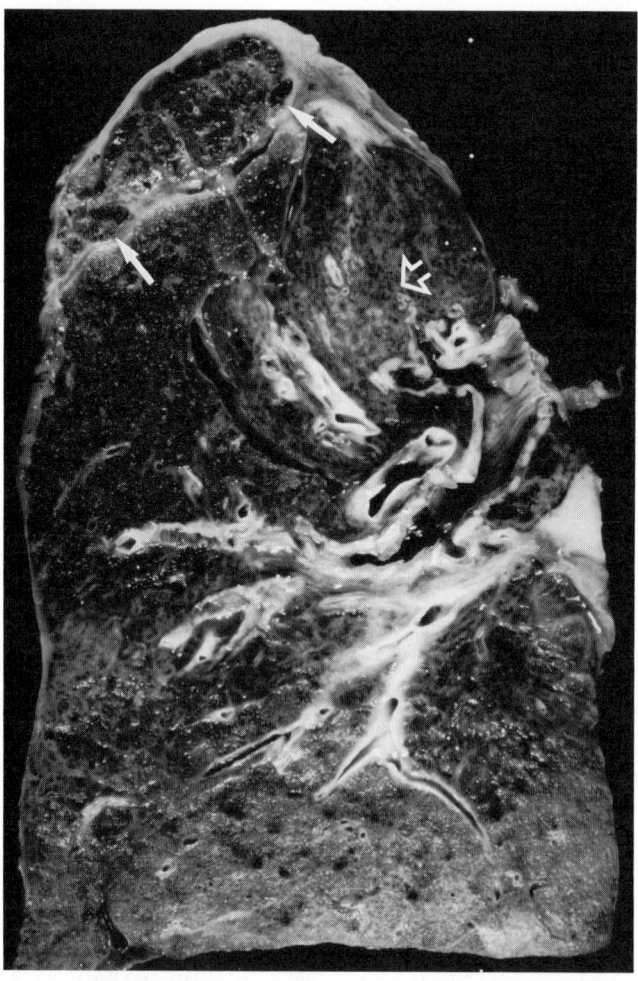

Figure 9–7. Advanced silicosis (right lung). There is marked fibrotic contraction of the upper lobe with partial fibrosis of the interlobar fissure *(single arrows)*. Fibrosis is evident in the contracted right middle lobe *(double arrow)*. Note pleural thickening in apical region. (Courtesy of Dr. John Godleski, Brigham and Women's Hospital.)

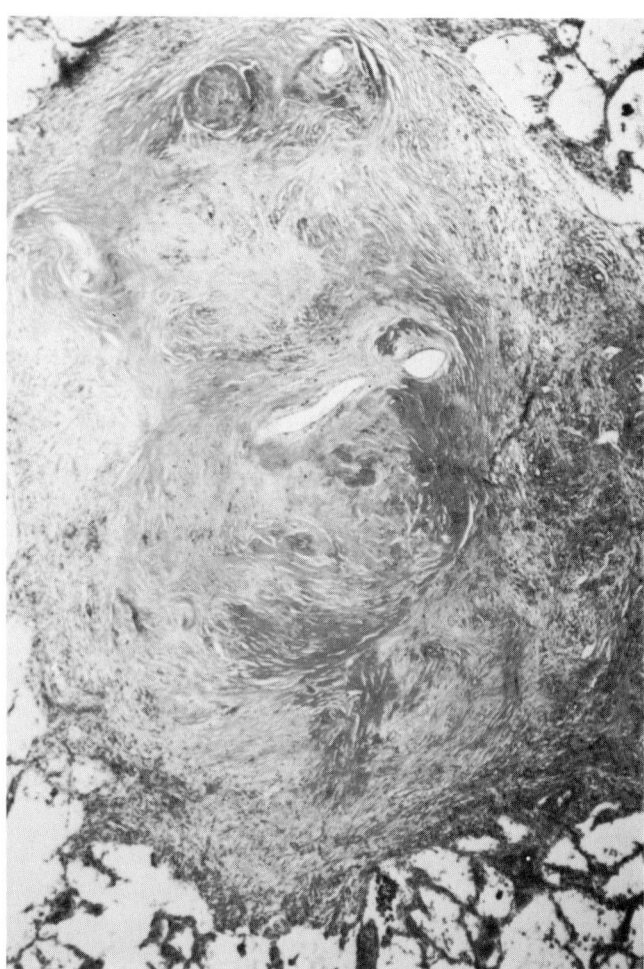

Figure 9–8. Several coalescent collagenous silicotic nodules. (Courtesy of Dr. John Godleski, Brigham and Women's Hospital.)

Helpful when present in the differentiation of chronic silicosis from other forms of collagenous pneumoconiosis is the polariscopic demonstration of numerous birefringent particles of silica and silicates within the fine, cleftlike spaces between the collagenous lamellae of the silicotic nodules. Cavitation may occur in uncomplicated silicosis, but when present, should raise the suspicion of intercurrent tuberculosis or Caplan's syndrome.

CLINICAL COURSE. Chronic silicosis is extremely insidious, and radiographic findings may appear years before there is any clinical evidence of respiratory dysfunction. Typically, the early phase of fine nodularity imparts a "snowstorm" appearance on chest radiograph. However, with progression the radiographic shadows become coarser and eventually coalescent (Fig. 9–9). At this stage there is marked decrease in lung compliance and in gas diffusion, and so dyspnea on exertion becomes evident. The breathlessness may at first be mild, but typical of silicosis is its relentless, slow progression, long after all further

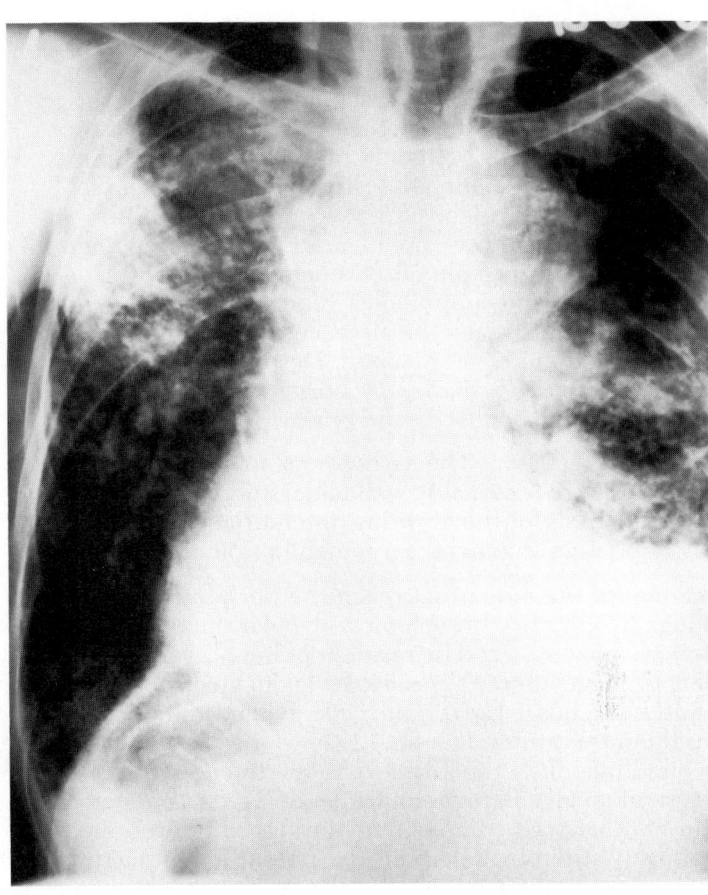

Figure 9–9. Advanced silicosis (chest film) with bilateral marked radiodensities in upper right and left midlung fields.

exposure has ceased. This clinical picture may be complicated by the development of rheumatoid arthritis (Caplan's syndrome) or other autoimmune diseases, chronic bronchitis, emphysema, cor pulmonale, or particularly pulmonary tuberculosis. The disease by itself is slow to kill, but it may make respiratory cripples of its victims. Obviously, an occupational history is of importance in establishing the diagnosis. As noted, there is no increased prevalence of bronchogenic carcinoma or other forms of cancer.

Asbestosis and Asbestos-Related Lesions

Overexposure to asbestos dust has been called "one of the worst industrial health tragedies in history."[43] It is estimated that this pollutant will cause 8000 to 10,000 deaths annually from now to the end of the century. *Inhalation of asbestos causes not only the pneumoconiosis—asbestosis—but also pleural effusions, pleural adhesions, parietal pleural fibrocalcific plaques, and an increased incidence of mesothelioma, bronchogenic carcinoma, and other forms of cancer.*[44,45] These various consequences occur singly or in combinations decades after exposure has ended.

Asbestos is a widespread air and water pollutant. The heaviest exposures are found in industries that mine, fabricate, and install asbestos and its more than 3000 products (such as flooring, ceiling, and roofing materials; insulation; sewer and water conduits; coat-ing compounds; brake linings, and clutch casings); asbestosis is encountered virtually exclusively among individuals having heavy occupational exposure. Even in hazardous occupations, asbestosis is very uncommon among those with less than 10 years of exposure.[46] However, significantly less exposure may be responsible for other possible consequences of this pollutant. Secretaries in mills, inhabitants of the immediate area around a mill, and asbestos workers' families have experienced an increased incidence of mesotheliomas, a form of neoplasia rarely encountered in nonexposed persons.[47] Little is known about variable susceptibility, but low-level pollution of the air in urban centers has engendered considerable concern in industrialized nations, especially in school-houses and buildings where asbestos has been used in ceilings and insulations.[48] Indeed, appropriate methods can reveal at autopsy a scattering of asbestos fibers in most urban dwellers' lungs. Even though asbestosis does not develop, pleural plaques may appear in lightly exposed individuals, such as spouses of asbestos workers and residents in proximity to a mine or factory. Analogously, potentially related cancers have appeared in individuals not having asbestosis but having an occupationally exposed family member.[49] Removal of asbestos insulation and ceilings from older buildings also imposes a risk.

Asbestos is a family of fibrous silicates divided into (1) curled, very slender, flexible serpentines, and

(2) brittle, straight amphiboles. The serpentine chrysotile accounts for over 90% of commercial use; two amphiboles—crocidolite and amosite—account for most of the remaining commercial use. Thus chrysotile is the major air pollutant, but these long, flexible fibers do not fragment, are resistant to air flow, and so tend to impact or deposit in the upper tracheobronchial tree, where they are cleared without reaching the vulnerable peripheral parenchyma. In contrast, the straight, stiff amphiboles tend to fracture and small fragments reach the airspaces, where some are also cleared but some retained. Despite these differences, *all types of asbestos are fibrogenic, but crocidolite is clearly the most carcinogenic.*

PATHOGENESIS. The early events in the origins of asbestosis are reasonably well understood but not the ultimate basis for the fibrosing, interstitial pneumonitis.[44,50] There is general agreement on the following:

• Some of the fibers that reach the periphery of the lungs (respiratory bronchioles, alveolar ducts, alveoli) are phagocytized by resident pulmonary alveolar macrophages. Some appear to be taken up directly by epithelial cells in the terminal airways and gain access to the interstitium.
• Simultaneously the asbestos fibers stimulate the release of an alveolar macrophage–derived chemotactin and activate complement through the alternate pathway, thereby releasing the potent chemotactin C5a. These chemoattractants augment the cellular response to the dust particles by recruiting both macrophages and neutrophils.
• Much of the engulfed dust is cleared by the macrophages, but some is carried by the phagocytes across the walls of the bronchioles and terminal air spaces to reach the interstitial tissue, lymphatics, pleura, and regional lymph nodes.
• Fibers phagocytized by macrophages are coated by complexes of hemosiderin and glycoproteins to create beaded, sometimes dumbbell-shaped *"asbestos bodies"* (Fig. 9–10), but most fibers are not engulfed and so remain uncoated. It should be noted that other types of fibers may also become coated, and so the generic term "ferruginous body" is applied to all types of coated fibers. Only ferruginous bodies having a core of asbestos are referred to as asbestos bodies.)

How does the asbestos dust evoke its fibrosing reaction? Several potential mechanisms have been proposed.[44,45]

1. *It is speculated that the macrophages and neutrophils accumulated at sites of fiber retention release lysosomal enzymes or generate toxic free radicals, injuring the pulmonary tissues and thereby evoking an inflammatory fibrosing reaction.*
2. *Partial solubilization of fibers and chemical injury might damage cell membranes, permitting the influx of Ca^{++} as the mediator of cell death.*
3. *Phagocytosis of asbestos particles by macrophages might initiate secretion of macrophage-derived growth*

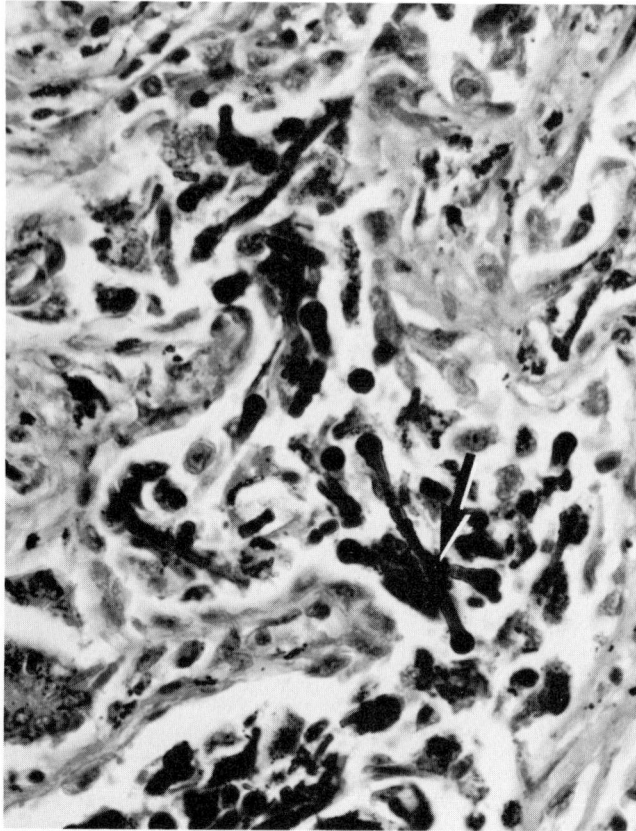

Figure 9–10. A high-power detail of asbestos bodies *(arrow)* with typical beading and knobbed ends.

factors including interleukin-1, accounting for the fibrosis (p. 477).
4. *Asbestos, particularly chrysotile, when added to cultures of fibroblasts in vitro, accelerates the rate of synthesis of reticulin and collagen. Conceivably the particles might have a similar effect in vivo.*
5. *Possibly all pathways have relevance and collaborate to produce the striking interstitial pneumonitis (Fig. 9–11).*

In addition, a variety of immunologic abnormalities have been reported in patients with asbestosis, but the roles, if any, of these abnormalities in the genesis of the disease remain unclear.[45] They could be merely epiphenomena.

In conclusion, it is evident that the basis for the lung's response to inhaled asbestos fibers is still uncertain. There is, however, little question about the central role of pulmonary alveolar macrophages.[51]

The pathogenesis of the other asbestos-related lesions is even more obscure. This is of particular concern with regard to the well-defined oncogenicity of these fibers. The relative risks of bronchogenic carcinoma are: nonexposed nonsmokers, 1; asbestos-exposed nonsmokers, 5; nonexposed smokers, 11; asbestos-exposed smokers, 55. *Clearly, in both nonsmokers and smokers, asbestos increases the likelihood of lung cancer fivefold, and equally clearly, smoking*

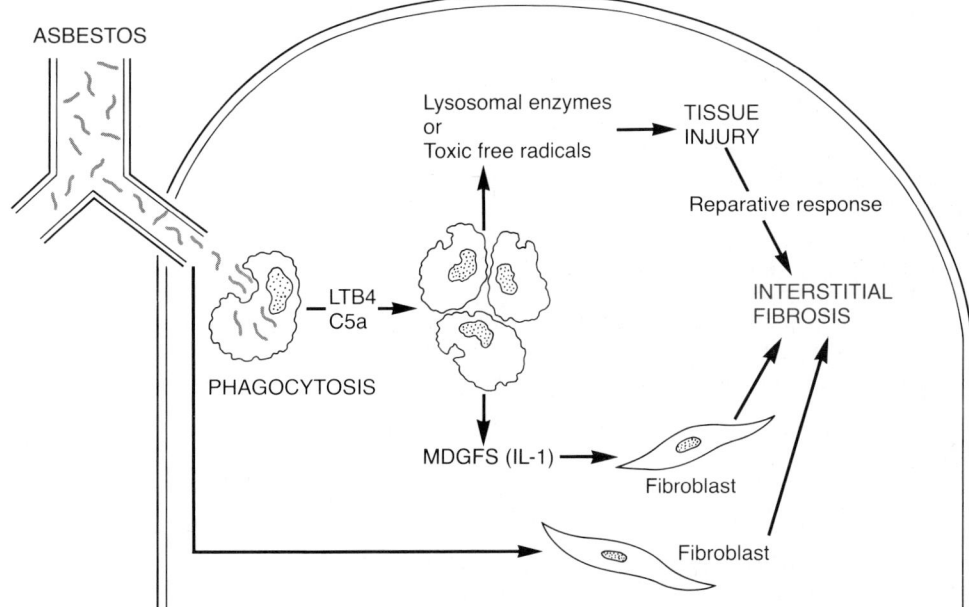

ASBESTOS

Lysosomal enzymes
or
Toxic free radicals → TISSUE INJURY

Reparative response

PHAGOCYTOSIS

LTB4
C5a

INTERSTITIAL
FIBROSIS

MDGFS (IL-1) → Fibroblast

Fibroblast

Figure 9–11. Potential mechanisms by which asbestos-laden macrophages may induce pulmonary interstitial fibrosis: (1) release of damaging enzymes or toxic radicals, (2) release of growth factors active on fibroblasts, or (3) direct stimulation of fibroblasts by asbestos dust. MDGFS = macrophage-derived growth factors including IL-1.

increases the risk of asbestos-induced cancer tenfold. Analogously, mesothelioma is a very rare form of cancer even among asbestos workers. Consequently, determining the precise level of risk imposed by these fibers has been difficult. But it can be said that a history of some type of hazardous occupation can be elicited in a large majority of all cases.

Two somewhat conflicting theories about the role of asbestos in the development of bronchogenic carcinomas have been advanced.[52] The first suggests that the fibers serve as tumor promoters, preparing the soil for other carcinogens. The fibers (particularly crocidolite, the most carcinogenic) have been shown to be cytotoxic to mammalian cells in vitro. Conceivably then, the fibers cause death of cells in the airways, stimulate cell replication, and render the proliferating epithelium particularly vulnerable to other environmental carcinogens, notably cigarette smoke. The second theory suggests that carcinogens such as polycyclic hydrocarbons derived from tobacco smoke are adsorbed onto the fibers and in this manner are concentrated at sites of asbestos retention.

The basis for the development of mesotheliomas is equally mysterious. It can be argued that the particles are carried through the lymphatics to the pleural mesothelium. But how to explain the occasional mesothelioma that arises in the peritoneal cavity? Could swallowing of fibers be involved? Unlike the case with bronchogenic carcinomas, cigarette smoke does not appear to be a factor with mesotheliomas.

In conclusion, it is evident that we "still have miles to go" before we understand why asbestos is so dangerous to man and why asbestos, but not silica, is such a potent carcinogen.

MORPHOLOGY. The anatomic changes of asbestosis will be discussed first, followed by the asbestos-related pleural lesions. Only a few comments concerning the related neoplasms will be made because bronchogenic carcinomas are discussed in detail on page 797 and mesotheliomas on page 807.

The hallmarks of **asbestosis** are: **(1) a diffuse interstitial fibrosis initially most marked in the periphery of the lower lobes, and (2) uncoated asbestos fibers and asbestos bodies within the areas of scarring.** The fibrosis begins about respiratory bronchioles and the alveolar ducts subpleurally and as the disease progresses extends inward and is accompanied by a fine fibrosis of the alveolar walls. This pattern of mild involvement is the most frequently encountered today because the recognition some years ago of the hazard of asbestos dust has reduced the intensity of the exposure. However, in persons exposed some decades ago the interstitial fibrosis extends centripetally, involves upper lobes, and destroys the overall alveolar architecture, inducing cystic spaces and honeycombing. In areas the fibrosis may become more dense, producing linear or even massive scars (Fig. 9–12). **The fibrosis is by and of itself nondistinctive, since other causes may result in similar changes; it is only the identification of asbestos bodies within the involved areas that permits the diagnosis of asbestosis.** Uncoated fibers can rarely be identified under the light microscope and require either phase microscopy or electron microscopy. The hilar nodes may be slightly fibrotic.

A number of complications may supervene. Marked emphysema may appear between the areas of interstitial fibrosis in patients with more severe expressions of asbes-

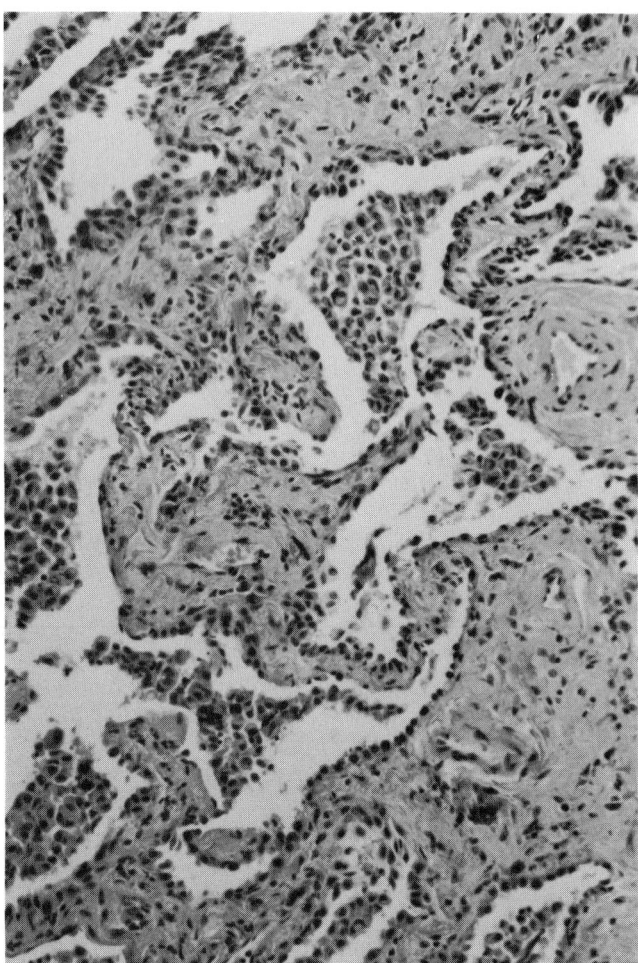

Figure 9–12. Asbestosis. Striking interstitial fibrosis with marked thickening of septal walls. Clusters of macrophages are present within air spaces. (Courtesy of Dr. John Godleski, Brigham and Women's Hospital.)

tosis. Secondary bronchiectasis or Caplan's syndrome (p. 475) may develop. The scarring may narrow or obliterate pulmonary arteries and arterioles, leading to pulmonary hypertension and cor pulmonale.

The **pleural reactions** to asbestos take one of three forms: (1) benign pleural effusions, (2) visceral pleural fibrosis (localized or diffuse), or (3) discrete fibrocalcific parietal pleural plaques. The pleural effusion is usually serous but may be bloody and is generally accompanied by subpleural asbestosis. In most cases it is not a forerunner of mesothelioma, but pleural effusion often antedates the development of this form of neoplasm. Fibrous thickening of the visceral pleura is a frequent accompaniment of asbestosis. It may, in advanced instances, encase the lungs and bind them into the thoracic cavity. **Dense fibrocalcific parietal pleural plaques are distinctive but not pathognomonic of asbestosis** (Fig. 9–13). They typically occur on the anterior and posterolateral aspects of the parietal pleura and over the domes of the diaphragms. The apices are rarely affected. The collagen deposits have distinct rounded or geographic margins and may reach 1 cm in

thickness. Sometimes they are minimally to heavily calcified, aiding their visualization on radiographs. They do not contain asbestos bodies, even in individuals having asbestosis, and as noted, they may appear in nonexposed individuals and in those having exposure but no asbestosis.

A number of forms of cancer have been associated with asbestos dust. Since all are described elsewhere, only a few comments will be made. First, it should be noted that there is no correlation between the severity of asbestosis and the development of malignancy. Indeed, lung cancers have developed in the absence of interstitial pulmonary fibrosis, and significantly, there is poor correlation between the intensity of exposure and the predisposition to cancer. *The most common form of associated malignancy is bronchogenic carcinoma,* as has been pointed out. Unlike those seen in the general population there is a preponderance of bronchogenic adenocarcinoma in asbestos-exposed individuals and relatively fewer squamous cell carcinomas. *Malignant mesotheliomas* are much less common than bronchogenic carcinomas, but the relationship to asbestos exposure is unmistakable. Although most occur in the pleural cavities, sometimes they arise in the peritoneal cavity in the absence of pleural involvement. Because these lesions do not

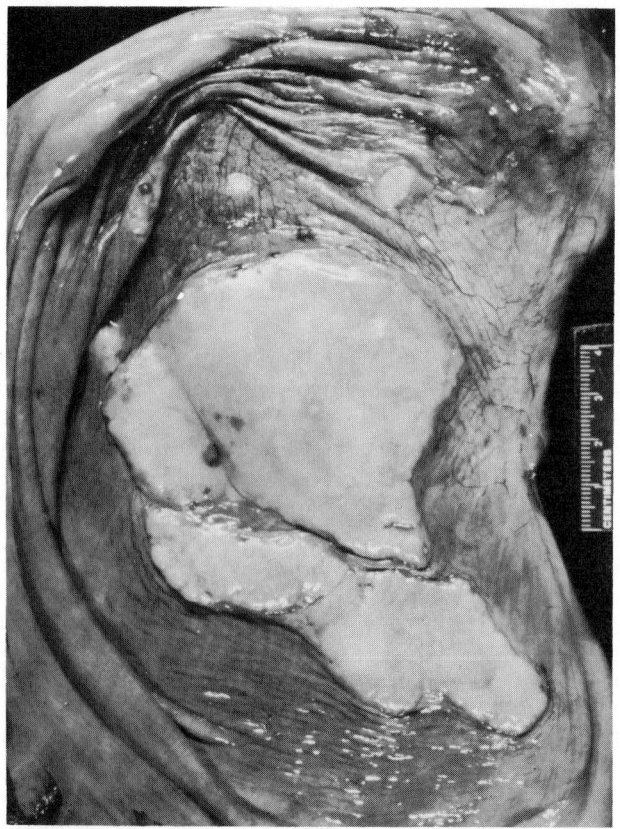

Figure 9–13. Asbestosis. Severe discrete, characteristic fibrocalcific plaques, on pleural surface of diaphragm. (Courtesy of Dr. John Godleski, Brigham and Women's Hospital.)

contain asbestos bodies and because they may occur in the absence of asbestos exposure, the implication of asbestos as a causal agent requires the identification of asbestos fibers in more than usual amounts in the pulmonary parenchyma. On less certain grounds, a predisposition to carcinomas of the esophagus, stomach, colon, and larynx and to a variety of lymphoid malignancies has been attributed to asbestos exposure.

CLINICAL COURSE. Asbestosis "sneaks up" on the patient. Quite often it is discovered in an asymptomatic individual on a routine chest film by the visualization of regular and linear opacities typically in the lower lung zones. Alternatively, previous exposure to asbestos may be brought to attention by the finding of a localized calcified pleural plaque with or without concomitant parenchymal changes. Eventually, after a long period of quiescence the interstitial fibrosis makes itself known by the insidious onset of dyspnea, at first related to effort but then even at rest. Typically the dyspnea is accompanied by a dry or productive cough, basilar inspiratory rales, and sometimes finger clubbing (p. 1333). With the passage of time the radiographic opacities involve ever greater lung fields, eventually leading to honeycombing. By this time the dyspnea may be severely incapacitating. Death usually occurs within 12 to 24 years of the onset of symptoms. This slow progressive downhill course may be speeded by the development of Caplan's syndrome, pulmonary hypertension, and cor pulmonale, or even worse, one of the forms of cancer mentioned earlier.

Berylliosis

Heavy exposure to airborne dusts or fumes of metallic beryllium or its oxides, alloys, or salts may induce an acute pneumonitis; more protracted exposure to lower levels of these pollutants may cause pulmonary and systemic granulomatous lesions very similar to those of sarcoidosis. However, recognition of these hazards and the imposition of occupational standards in 1948 have eradicated acute berylliosis and virtually ended the appearance of new cases of chronic berylliosis. Hence, only a few brief comments are indicated to aid in surveillance of these health hazards. Currently workers in the nuclear and aerospace industries, and in the fabrication of electrical and electronic equipment, have greatest potential for exposure. Their families are also somewhat at risk.[53] Beryllium-related disease has also reared its head in unsuspected locations such as dental laboratories, where technicians grind and polish beryllium alloy braces and the like.[54]

Acute berylliosis is basically an exudative, chemical pneumonitis marked by filling of the alveolar spaces with a protein-rich fluid. With survival the fluid may be resorbed, but in some cases it becomes organized.

Chronic berylliosis is thought to follow sensitization following long, protracted exposure to beryllium dust or vapors. The metal appears to act as a hapten to induce a cell-mediated immunologic response. The chronic disease is characterized by focal noncaseating granulomas, much like those of sarcoidosis, diffusely scattered in the interstitial tissue of the lung and particularly frequent in subpleural, septal, peribronchial, and perivascular locations. These granulomas may have three types of inclusions, usually enclosed within giant cells: (1) spiculated birefringent crystals up to 10 μm in length, (2) concentrically laminated Schaumann bodies (up to 50 μm in diameter), and (3) acidophilic, stellate asteroids identical to those seen in sarcoidosis (p. 428) (Fig. 9–14). Granulomas may also appear in the regional nodes and rarely in more remote nodes, kidneys, liver, and spleen. When beryllium gets into skin wounds, there may be a granulomatous reaction at the site of injury. In time, all the well-developed granulomas undergo progressive fibrosis, which, when the lung is significantly affected, leads to marked impairment of ventilatory function. The diagnosis depends on a history of exposure supported by the demonstration of beryllium-sensitized T cells (blast transformation, macrophage migration inhibition) and chemical assays for beryllium in the lung tissue, lymph nodes, and urine.[55]

Animal studies and epidemiologic surveys suggest an increased frequency of lung cancer in individuals having fairly heavy occupational beryllium exposure.[56]

Other Dust Diseases

There are many other forms of pulmonary dust disease in addition to those already discussed; however, most are less life-threatening than the collagenous pneumoconioses. They can be roughly segregated into three categories: (1) noncollagenous inorganic dust pneumoconiosis, (2) asthma, and (3) extrinsic allergic alveolitis.

The *noncollagenous inorganic dust pneumoconioses* include, in addition to uncomplicated coal workers' pneumoconiosis, such entities as siderosis, stannosis, baritosis, and other less common conditions. All of these noncollagenous pneumoconioses are characterized by focal accumulations of the particular dust in the lung to create macules resembling the coal-dust macule. Only very rarely are the pulmonary changes productive of respiratory difficulty, but in the exceptional instance with severe exposure any one of these disorders may prove fatal.

Asthma has many origins, as is evident in the full discussion on page 773. Whatever its origin, the disease is characterized by paroxysms of bronchospasm and bronchial changes that induce obstructive narrowing of the airways. One clinical pattern is known as occupational or industrial asthma because the attacks are triggered by a large variety of dusts — grain, wood dust, animal hair and dander, and others encountered in the workplace.

Extrinsic allergic alveolitis is a distinctive hypersensitivity pulmonary reaction to inhalation of one of a large number of organic dusts. It differs from asthma inasmuch as it takes the form of an interstitial inflammatory reaction, sometimes granulomatous, at the

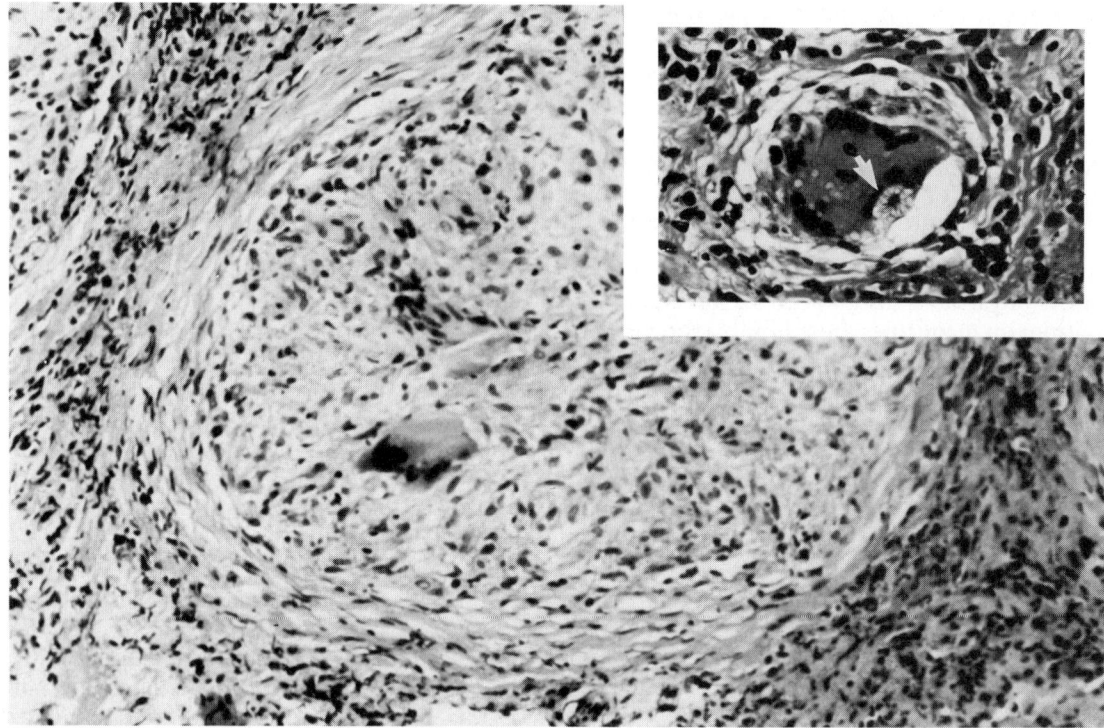

Figure 9-14. Chronic berylliosis. The well-developed noncaseating granuloma contains a central multinucleate giant cell. Inset is of a classic stellate asteroid within a giant cell *(arrow)*.

level of respiratory bronchioles and alveoli. Such inflammation is generally reversible but may progress to diffuse interstitial pulmonary fibrosis and permanent respiratory insufficiency. Various inhaled allergens are involved, such as spores of molds, pollens, animal and industrial particulates, and chemical fumes. The most important of these sensitivity disorders is *farmers' lung,* which typically appears within hours of inhalation of spores derived from a thermophilic actinomycete that grows on improperly dried and stored hay. More details on these dust-related hypersensitivity diseases are available on page 793 and in the literature.[57]

Byssinosis is an uncommon pulmonary disorder caused by organic dusts derived from cotton, flax, and hemp. It may first appear within weeks to months of onset of the occupational exposure, and takes more the form of an asthmatic bronchitis than involvement of the distal lung structures, such as occurs with the other organic dusts causing extrinsic allergic alveolitis. The basis for the lesions is not clear, but the evidence that they are hypersensitivity induced is not strong.

CHEMICAL AND DRUG INJURY

All chemicals, including therapeutic drugs, are capable of causing injury or even death. The most toxic are known as poisons; others are relatively innocuous, but, in sufficient quantity, even table salt can be damaging. In some instances the injury is the result of industrial exposure, perhaps accidental (recall Bhopal, India, where over 2000 were killed and over 200,000 injured). In other instances the injury is the consequence of self-administered (suicidal) or accidental overdosage. In still other instances it follows the nonmedical use of a "street drug," e.g., heroin, cocaine, "crack"; and in still others it is the unanticipated result of the self-administered or prescribed use of a standard medicine. The last category constitutes an adverse drug reaction (ADR).

In the overall perspective of diseases, chemical- and drug-related morbidity and mortality do not loom large, but nonetheless the deaths and illnesses caused by these substances are individual tragedies that might have been prevented or averted by prompt recognition and effective treatment. To place the problem in perspective, there are about 5000 to 6000 fatalities in the United States annually from self-administered overdoses of chemicals or drugs.[58] Many of the deaths involve teenagers and their use of illegal drugs.[59] Another large segment involves the deliberate action of those driven to take leave of this mortal coil. Most of the remainder are unintended and accidental and involve common household substances, (e.g., cleaning agents, bleaches, aspirin, and cosmetics). Tragically, some of these deaths befall very young children and are the consequence of busy, exploratory little hands. The accidental deaths are not surprising when viewed in the context of the estimated almost 2 million trivial to "hair-raising" poison exposures estimated to occur in the United States annually.[60] Adverse therapeutic drug reactions (ADRs), the great preponderance of which are nonfatal, constitute yet another large category of chemical and drug injury. The roster of implicated agents is almost limitless, and only a survey can be offered.

ADVERSE DRUG REACTIONS (ADRs)

An ADR is defined as "any response to a drug that is noxious and unintended and that occurs at doses used in humans for prophylaxis, diagnosis, or therapy excluding failure to accomplish the intended purpose." As ever more powerful drugs, such as the anticancer agents, have become available, the number of ADRs has increased. In a sense their increasing frequency is a testament to medical progress. In years past, without such agents many patients would have promptly succumbed to their primary disease, but today they survive, some to experience an ADR.

There are no satisfactory data on the precise frequency of ADRs. This lack provides an ideal climate for such headlines as "Bad prescriptions' kill thousands a year," implying thereby physician failures.[61] What do more sober analyses disclose? A detailed survey of a large number of so-called ADRs reported to a national registry in the United States revealed that in only 43% of 827 cases could the untoward reaction be reasonably attributed to a drug.[62] Moreover, if the suicidal or self-administered accidental overdoses were excluded, only about 25% of the 827 cases constituted true ADRs within the present definition of this term. Of these a relative handful (25) were the consequence of physician failures, e.g., inadequately monitored use or overuse of an agent, failure to recognize drug interactions, and ill-considered administration of a potentially dangerous drug. It is such disturbing misfortunes that Ingelfinger has aptly called "ADR's that count."[63] The great majority of ADRs constitute reactions to reasonably and appropriately used medicinals. Best estimates suggest that about 3 to 5% of all medicinal exposures cause adverse reactions, but the majority are self-limiting and of little consequence.[64] Happily, fatal ADRs are rare, and most occur in desperately ill patients requiring desperate measures. In an effort to halt the downward course of a patient with leukemia, potent chemotherapeutic agents are often employed. Regrettably, while the progression of the leukemia may be halted or at least slowed, often at the same time the normal marrow cells are destroyed. If then a fatal infection ensues because of a lack of white cells, is this an ADR that counts?

By what mechanisms do drugs produce ADRs? The great majority involve one of three pathways: (1) The drugs or their metabolites are directly toxic to cells; (2) they reduce the immunologic or hormonal defense of the host; or (3) they evoke immunologic or idiosyncratic reactions. The first two categories constitute more or less predictable reactions, whereas the last group are largely unpredictable.[65] Predictable ADRs are dose related, are well known to occur with the particular agent, and can usually be induced by the drug in experimental animals. None of these characteristics obtains in the case of unpredictable reactions. *Most ADRs (over 80%) are predictable, and those related to direct toxicity usually involve metabolic conversion of agents to toxic metabolities.*[66] A few details on predictable and unpredictable reactions follow.

Predictable ADRs — Relevant Factors

Age. The young and the old are particularly vulnerable.

Dose. Even though dosage is a recognized determinant, large doses may be necessary. Steroids are known to render individuals vulnerable to infections. They are also used to suppress rejection reactions in transplant recipients. Which risk is greater — a potentially fatal bacterial or fungal infection because of the use of large doses of steroids or cardiac transplantation rejection?

Route of administration. Parenteral therapy yields the highest blood levels and is therefore more likely to cause an ADR than is the oral route.

Ability to metabolize or excrete the drug. Impaired excretion would predictably lead to higher, potentially toxic levels in the blood and tissues, but ironically, increased ability to metabolize the drug may have the same effect. When prior exposure to an agent leads to increased activity of certain hepatic enzymes, more rapid metabolism of the drug produces higher, potentially toxic levels of metabolites.

Underlying disease. Pre-existing renal disease, for example, renders the patient particularly vulnerable to nephrotoxic agents.

Genetic factors. Uncommonly, these contribute to predictable ADRs. The best example is a genetic lack of glucose-6-phosphate dehydrogenase, rendering individuals vulnerable to hemolytic crises following exposure to oxidant drugs such as the antimalarials (primaquine and quinacrine).

Concurrent therapy. Cross reactions and interactions may lead to drug toxicity, e.g., aminoglycosides such as gentamicin or streptomycin given along with one of the cephalosporins enhance the likelihood of renal injury.

Pattern of reaction tends to be the same in all individuals.

Unpredictable ADRs — Relevant Factors

Dosage is irrelevant. Even minute doses may trigger reactions. Most are thought to be immunologic reactions, and severe anaphylactic reactions have followed trivial doses of penicillin (the metabolites of penicillin serve as haptens).

Route of administration. Certain agents are more immunogenic when applied topically.

Pattern of reaction is unpredictable. The same agent may cause different reactions in different individuals.

A few drugs tend to evoke particular patterns of response. For example, hydralazine and procainamide are the major drugs causing a lupus erythematosus–like syndrome.

Immunologic reactions are more likely or more se-

vere on second exposures to particular agents, but in some instances, desensitization can be produced.

Idiosyncratic reaction is the term applied to ADRs that are unpredictable, are not dose dependent, and are not clearly related to immunoreactions. Genetic or other poorly understood factors may underlie them. The best example is halothane hepatitis, appearing usually after a second or third exposure but occasionally after the first exposure. In the final analysis, all unpredictable ADRs are in some measure idiosyncratic.

It is impossible within the limitations of space to describe in detail the possible consequences of every drug, but an excellent source is available.[67] The two drugs arguably most often involved in *nonfatal* toxic ADRs are digoxin and aspirin, the former because the therapeutic and toxic doses are very close, and the latter because it is so widely used. The two agents probably responsible for most *fatal* ADRs are halothane (massive liver necrosis) and penicillin (severe allergic reactions). Some of the more common drug reaction patterns and implicated agents are presented in Table 9–2.

A few details on some of the more important agents follow.

Halothane

This rapidly acting anesthetic has produced hepatic necrosis that sometimes is massive and fatal but more often is centrilobular and self-limited. Although massive necrosis is rare, halothane and fulminant viral hepatitis constitute the two dominant causes of this catastrophe. The anatomic changes are indistinguishable from those produced by other hepatotoxins and can be connected to halothane only by historical data. When the liver destruction is widespread, the case fatality rate approaches 20 to 40%. The severity of the

Table 9–2. Some Common Drug Reactions and Causal Agents

REACTION	MAJOR OFFENDERS
Blood Dyscrasias (Occur in almost half of all drug-related deaths)	
Granulocytopenia	Ibuprofen
Thrombocytopenia	Quinidine
Hemolytic anemia	Methyldopa
Aplastic anemia	Phenacetin
Pancytopenia	Following chemotherapy of a primary cancer[68]
Leukemia	
Cutaneous Reactions	
Urticaria, macules, papules, vesicles, petechiae, exfoliative dermatitis, fixed drug eruptions	Antimitotics
	Antibiotics
	Hydantoin
	Phenindione
	Bromides
	Barbiturates
	Others
Renal Reactions	
Acute tubular necrosis	Cyclosporine
Tubulointerstitial nephritis	Sulfonamides
Glomerulonephritis	Penicillamine
Papillary necrosis	Phenacetin, aspirin
Pulmonary Reactions	
Diffuse alveolar damage	Bleomycin
Interstitial fibrosis	Nitrofurantoin
Edema	Amiodarone
	Busulfan
Hepatic Reactions (p. 962)	
Fatty change	Tetracycline
Hepatitis	Isoniazid
Cholestasis	Chlorpromazine (Fig. 9–15)
Focal to massive necrosis	Halothane
Systemic Reactions	
Anaphylaxis	Penicillin
Lupus erythematosus syndrome	Hydralazine
Vasculitis	Allopurinol
Hormonal Reactions	
Benign and malignant proliferations	Estrogens (diethylstilbestrol)
Thrombotic complications	Oral contraceptives (e.g., estrogens and progestins)
Adrenocortical insufficiency	Glucocorticoids

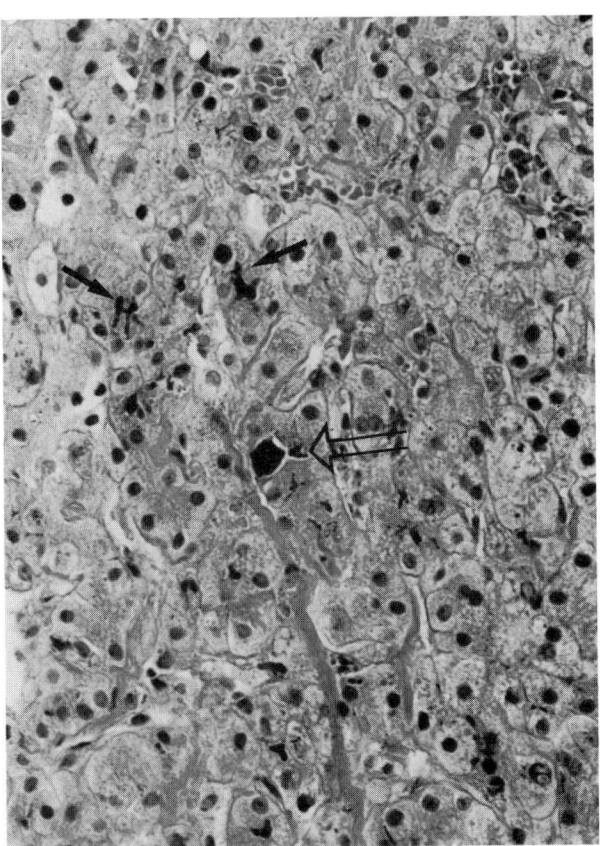

Figure 9–15. Cholestasis induced by chlorpromazine. Inspissated bile plugs can be seen in canaliculi between liver cells *(single arrows)* and in single ductule *(double arrow).*

necrosis tends to be greater in those who have had prior exposures, and so it has long been assumed that a hypersensitivity reaction to the drug or more likely to one of its metabolites, which serve as haptens, is responsible.[68] Some findings seem to confirm this mechanism, such as eosinophilia, apparent sensitized T cells, and antibodies that bind to rabbit hepatocytes.[69] However, the immunologic findings could equally well represent a reaction to hepatocytic antigens released by direct toxic drug injury. Indeed, halothane hepatitis has occurred after first use, particularly in individuals who have had significant hypoxic episodes during anesthesia or whose metabolism of the agent has been increased by prior exposure to other drugs metabolized by the same enzymes. Under hypoxic conditions, metabolites have been shown to bind to and inactivate hepatocytic macromolecules. Furthermore, there are suggestions of a genetic susceptibility to this toxicity. Thus halothane-induced injury is best viewed as an ADR in which individual susceptibility, toxicity, and hypersensitivity all play roles, perhaps of varying importance in individual instances.[70]

Isoniazid (INH)

Isoniazid is the drug of choice in the treatment of tuberculosis and the easiest to administer for long-term prophylaxis against the infection. However, two forms of ADRs are encountered. The most common is self-limited, is of little consequence, and resembles a mild viral hepatitis. Usually the symptoms and signs of the hepatic reaction appear a few weeks to months following the institution of therapy. Sometimes only a transient elevation of serum transaminase levels is seen. However in about 1% of cases, despite low dosages (under 5 mg/kg/day), the reaction progresses to produce focal liver cell necrosis or, rarely, submassive to massive fatal hepatic necrosis. The more severe attacks of liver injury tend to occur in older individuals. An acetylated metabolite of isoniazid appears to be the cause of the direct toxic injury, and accordingly, individuals who genetically are rapid acetylators are at increased risk.[71]

Infrequently, isoniazid induces an immunologic type reaction; urticaria, skin rash, and even a lupus erythematosus–like syndrome have been described, raising the possibility that the hepatic reaction may sometimes be immune-mediated.

Acetaminophen

This widely used (over-the-counter) analgesic and antipyretic, when taken in very large amounts, causes hepatic necrosis. The window between the usual therapeutic dose (0.5 gm) and the toxic dose (15 to 25 gm) is very large, and so the drug is ordinarily very safe. The massive toxic doses are generally suicidal in adults or teenagers, or accidental in children. Toxicity, when it appears, begins with nausea, vomiting, diarrhea, and sometimes shock, followed in a few days by evidence of jaundice; with the serious overdosages, liver failure ensues with centrilobular necrosis that may extend to entire lobules. In some cases there is concomitant evidence of renal and myocardial damage.

Acetaminophen toxicity is attributable to the formation of a toxic metabolite by the hepatic mixed-function oxidases. This metabolite is normally detoxified by binding to glutathione, but with extreme overdoses the glutathione is depleted and the reactive metabolite binds to hepatocytic macromolecules, resulting in the organ injury.

Aspirin (Acetylsalicylic Acid)

Despite its being popped into mouths as often as candy, and despite its potential toxicity, aspirin is associated with only sparse morphologic changes, meriting only brief commentary. The major untoward consequences of massive aspirin overdosage are metabolic. The ingestion of as little as 2 to 4 gm in children or 10 to 30 gm in adults may be fatal, but on the other hand, survival has been reported following doses fivefold larger. Usually such overdosage is accidental or suicidal. Fluid and electrolyte imbalances are produced. At first an alkalosis develops, followed by a metabolic acidosis that often proves fatal before anatomic changes can appear.

Chronic aspirin toxicity has followed the protracted consumption of 3 gm daily. This chronic salicylism is manifested by dizziness, nausea, vomiting, diarrhea, drowsiness, and indeed many of the characteristics of alcoholic intoxication. The central nervous system changes may progress to hallucinations, convulsions, and coma. The major morphologic consequences of chronic salicylism are varied. Most often there is an acute erosive gastritis (p. 842), producing overt or covert gastrointestinal bleeding. The damage to the gastric mucosa may lead to gastric ulceration, as is pointed out on page 850. Concomitantly, in chronic toxicity, a bleeding tendency may appear. You recall that aspirin inactivates cyclooxygenase and so impairs synthesis of prostacyclin and thromboxane A_2. The loss of these two contrary-acting agents has the net effect of a bleeding tendency. Petechial hemorrhages may appear in the skin and internal viscera. Together with bleeding from the gastric lesions, these hemorrhages add to the potential blood loss. Sometimes hypersensitivity reactions to aspirin cause urticaria, multiform skin rashes, exfoliative dermatitis, acute asthmatic attacks, or even anaphylaxis.

Proprietary analgesic mixtures of aspirin and phenacetin and possibly other agents, when taken over the span of years, have caused renal papillary necrosis referred to as analgesic nephropathy (p. 1058). This pattern of renal damage is uncommon in the United States but is still prevalent in Scandinavian countries, Australia, and New Zealand.

Exogenous Estrogens and Oral Contraceptives (OCs)

There is little disagreement about the importance of endogenous hyperestrinism in the development of endometrial carcinoma, and there is a strong suspicion that it predisposes to breast carcinoma. Thus there long has been concern about possible adverse effects of exogenous estrogens and their use to allay postmenopausal changes. Recently there has been a resurgence in the use of small doses of this hormone, sometimes coupled with progestins, to prevent or retard the progress of osteoporosis — an enormous health problem estimated to be responsible for over 1 million fractures in the United States annually.[72] But what are the other consequences of the administration of estrogenic agents? Much depends on dosage, the possible concomitant use of progestins, and the dose schedules of these two hormones. The following comments relative to exogenous estrogens represent generalizations.

• *Endometrial carcinoma* — Postmenopausal estrogens increase the incidence about threefold.[73] Sequential progestins appear to counteract this effect.[74]
• *Breast carcinoma* — Controversy persists; at the worst, exogenous estrogens induce a small increased risk, but concurrent progestins may neutralize this effect.[75]
• *Ovarian cancer* — Postmenopausal estrogen therapy may increase the risk two- to threefold, but more data are needed, especially on the effect of concomitant progestins.
• *Vaginal adenosis and subsequent superimposed vaginal clear-cell carcinoma* — Diethylstilbestrol during pregnancy increases the incidence of both conditions in the adolescent offspring (p. 1138).
• *Venous thrombosis and pulmonary embolism* — Postmenopausal estrogen therapy has induced a slight increase in the incidence of both vascular complications.
• *Whether protracted estrogen therapy protects against or contributes to the incidence of myocardial infarction remains uncertain.* Ironically, two studies with completely opposed viewpoints have appeared in the same journal.[76,77]

It is clear that estrogens can have adverse effects, but in postmenopausal women they have benefits, and so their use constitutes the proverbial "two-edged sword."

Oral contraceptives, despite their being in use for about 30 years and despite innumerable analyses of their effects, continue to evoke wide disagreement about their safety and adverse effects. Most of the available data relate to formulations used in the past containing much larger amounts of estrogens (both absolute and relative to their progestin content) than are used today. Without going into all of the details of the disagreement, it is possible to offer some reasonably supportable conclusions as follows.

• OCs, as used in the past, *increase the death rate from circulatory diseases fivefold.*
• Myocardial infarction and subarachnoid hemorrhage account for most of this excess cardiovascular mortality as is evident in Table 9–3.
• The risk of these cardiovascular complications is almost limited to women over 35 and is compounded by concurrent cigarette smoking. *There is virtually no increased risk in nonsmoking women under the age of 35.*
• *Breast carcinoma* — The issue is unresolved. Some studies indicate about a twofold increased risk, particularly with more than ten years of OC use and particularly when begun early in life and before the first pregnancy.[78] Other studies emanating from the

Table 9–3. Cardiovascular Effects of Oral Contraceptive Use — Analysis of 23,000 Users*

DISEASE	MORTALITY RATE PER 100,000 WOMAN YEARS (NO. OF DEATHS)		
	Current Users	Former Users	Controls
Ischemic heart disease	13.0	4.1	2.0
Subarachnoid hemorrhage	7.3	10.2	2.3
Cerebral thrombosis, hemorrhage, and embolism	2.7	8.1	2.7
Pulmonary embolism and venous thrombosis	2.8	2.2	0.0
Malignant hypertension	0.0	2.5	0.0

* Drawn from Royal College of General Practitioners Oral Contraception Study: Further analyses of mortality in oral contraceptive users. Lancet *1*:541, 1981.

Centers for Disease Control reveal no increased risk.[79] Possibly contributing to this conflict are variations in the estrogen content of the pill (both absolute and relative to the progestin content), duration of OC use, age at onset of use, and interval between first use and the time of the study. *With contemporary doses of estrogen and progestin, it is likely that there is little, if any, increased risk of breast cancer.*

• *Endometrial cancer* — No increased risk and very likely a protective effect.[80]

• *Cervical cancer* — Some increased risk, correlated with duration of use.[81]

• *Ovarian cancer* — Protects against; the longer the use, the greater the protection, which persists for some time after OC use has been stopped.[82]

• *Liver adenoma, focal nodular hyperplasia, and hepatocellular carcinoma* — Tenuous evidence that risk is slightly increased for all three, but only moderately convincing with adenoma.

• OCs are of benefit in the alleviation of rheumatoid arthritis and in lowering the incidence of benign proliferative disease of the breast and fibroadenomas of the breast but may predispose to gallstones.

The pros and cons of OC use must be viewed in the context of their wide applicability and acceptance as a form of contraception that protects against unwanted pregnancies with all their attendant hazards. Like all of us, OCs are neither all bad nor all good.

Anticancer Drugs

A large number of synthetic, natural plant, or microbe-derived drugs are currently available for the chemotherapy of cancer. All have as their primary function destruction or interference with the division or metabolism of cancer cells. Doxorubicin (Adriamycin), for example, is a potent cytotoxic antineoplastic agent. However, it also has cardiotoxicity when the cumulated dose reaches specific limits (Fig. 9–16). Those agents that impact on dividing cells also affect normal cells, such as those in the bone marrow and mucosa of the gastrointestinal tract. Thus, all forms of cancer chemotherapy tread the passage between Scylla and Charybdis — on the one side they can destroy cancer cells or at least make them falter, but on the other side they sometimes cause serious harm to vulnerable normal (most often marrow) cells. Unfortunately, too often, to achieve effective therapeutic doses some marrow injury is sustained, ranging from pancytopenia to anemia, leukopenia, or thrombocytopenia. In many patients the bone marrow recovers reasonably promptly, and regrettably, sometimes the cancer cells as well. However, during the period of marrow suppression, intercurrent infections (leukopenia) or bleeding episodes (thrombocytopenia) may appear, either of which may prove fatal.

When the patient survives these acute crises, sometimes months later a new ogre raises its head — a second malignancy. It may be a solid tissue tumor, but most often it takes the form of acute leukemia, which usually appears within about ten years of the treatment.[83] This tragedy is most common following the combined use of radiation and alkylating agents for the treatment of Hodgkin's disease but has also occurred with treatment of solid tumors. Both modalities of therapy are prone to induce mutations. Antimetabolite drugs, in contrast to alkylating agents, are less frequently associated with this tragic consequence. So it is that sometimes the successful control of a cancer ends up a Pyrrhic victory.[84,85]

Anti-Infectives

"Wonder drugs" have dramatically altered the frequency, severity, and mortality of infectious diseases, but they are also capable of causing mischief.

• Hypersensitivity reactions may result, ranging from trivial self-limited skin rashes to life-threatening anaphylaxis to exfoliative dermatitis.

• In the Darwinian struggle for survival, drug-resistant organisms have emerged, giving rise to drug-resistant, sometimes nosocomial, infections and to difficult-to-control epidemics in the community and hospitals.

• Eradication of the normal microflora of the body may give opportunists a field day, with the emergence of a disease more serious than the initial infection, e.g., a disseminated fungal infection. Secondary invaders may also proliferate (e.g., *Clostridium difficile*–induced colitis, p. 889).

All these potentials make understandable the wisdom of the judicious use of anti-infective drugs.

Immunosuppressants

The present era of organ transplantation and control of immunologically mediated diseases would not be possible without these agents, but they also involve risks. The major adverse reaction is predisposition to infection. It is well recognized that glucocorticoids, by suppressing the T-cell response, predispose to reactivation and spread of tuberculous and fungal infections.

In the immunocompromised patient who particularly lacks cell-mediated immunity, such microbes as cytomegalovirus, *Pneumocystis carinii*, and the fungi become serious threats to life — only recall the plight of patients with AIDS (acquired immunodeficiency syndrome). In addition, there is a well-defined increased risk of the development of lymphomas, principally immunoblastic lymphoma, in patients receiving long-term immunosuppressant therapy. It is conjectured that suppression of immunosurveillance potentiates the emergence of these neoplasms. Many immunosuppressants have toxicity for particular organs. Azathioprine is toxic to the lung and may produce diffuse interstitial pneumonitis.[86] Cyclosporine is a well-recognized cause of renal injury — interstitial fibrosis, tubular atrophy, focal glomerular sclerosis.[87] The liver and the myocardium may also have a toxic reaction to this agent, although much less often than the kidneys. The adverse reaction to an immunosuppressant is usually not fatal and is revers-

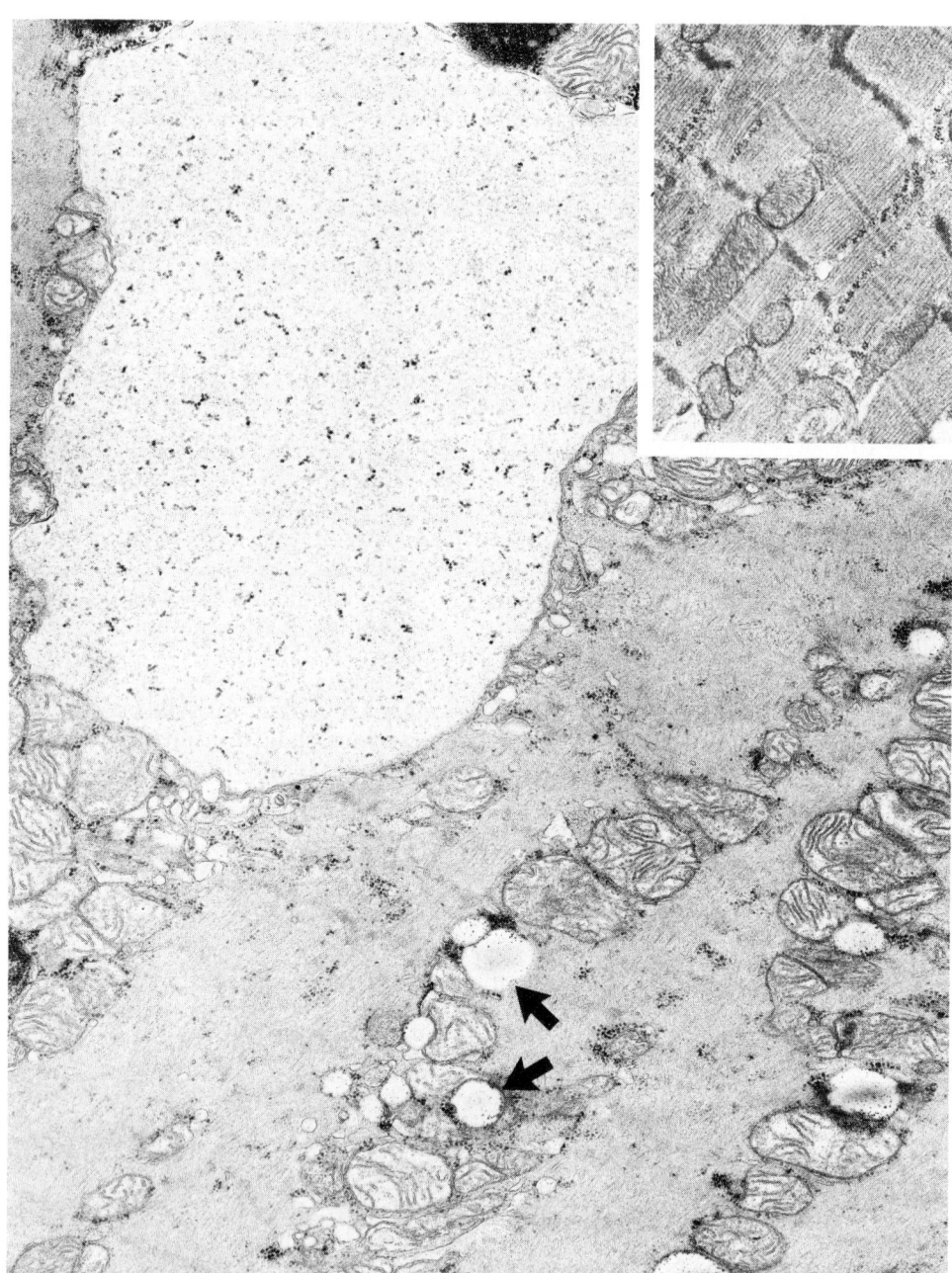

Figure 9–16. Doxorubicin (Adriamycin) cardiotoxicity. Electron micrograph reveals swelling of myofibers with loss of myofibrils (compare with normal in inset). There is also swelling of endoplasmic reticulum, producing small vacuoles (arrows) as well as large vacuole (upper left) (×17,000). (Courtesy of Dr. Frederick Schoen, Brigham and Women's Hospital.)

ible after withdrawal of the agent or substitution of another immunosuppressant, but sometimes infections by drug-resistant organisms such as fungi prove fatal. On balance, when the immunosuppressants are needed, as for example with organ transplantation, the benefit to risk ratio is clearly in favor of the drugs.

NONTHERAPEUTIC AGENTS

The particular environmental hazards discussed in the following sections were selected because of their clinical, public health, or societal importance.

Ethyl Alcohol

Consumption of ethanol now characterizes 80 to 90% of the adults in many populations in both developed and developing countries and so constitutes virtually a behavioral norm. Unfortunately, too often it becomes excessive, as occurs in 5 to 10% of adult males and about 5% of adult females in most privileged societies. It is estimated that in the United States there are over 10 million chronic alcoholics and an additional 7 million who drink sufficiently to have some adverse consequences. Of even greater concern is the growing problem of teenage alcohol abuse. It is fruitless to enter into the controversy of the definition of "alcohol abuse" and "heavy drinking," but operationally it can be characterized as alcohol consumption that adversely affects health, work performance, or psychologic and societal relationships. A simpler and less accurate definition is—anyone who drinks so much that they deny ever "touching the stuff." But more is involved in addiction to alcohol than psychopathology or inability to cope with "worldly slings and arrows." Studies of twins adopted in early childhood into separate families point to both genetic and environmental predisposition to chronic alcoholism. Alcoholics, to some extent then, are victims of their genes as well as their "urges."

The major effects of acute alcoholism are exerted on the CNS, but with chronic addiction other organs are also affected. Still uncertain is whether ethanol itself or its metabolites or by-products are responsible for its physical effects. Following ingestion, it is absorbed unaltered in the stomach and small intestine. Milk and fatty foods slow absorption. The alcohol is then distributed to all the tissues and fluids of the body in direct proportion to the blood level. Less than 10% of absorbed alcohol is excreted unchanged in the urine, sweat, and breath. The amount exhaled is in direct proportion to the blood level and forms the basis of the breath test employed by law enforcement agencies.

Most of the alcohol in the blood is metabolized in the liver through one major and two accessory pathways (Fig. 9–17). The microsomal P-450 oxidase pathway is inducible by alcohol and other agents.[88] A man of average size and weight metabolizes about 9.0 gm of alcohol (about 3/4 oz of whiskey) per hour irrespective of the blood level. You can't push it out of the pipeline by pouring more in! However, genetic polymorphisms of liver alcohol and aldehyde dehydrogenases have been identified, some capable of more rapid metabolism of substrate than others.[89] Moreover, chronic alcoholics develop some level of tolerance by virtue of enzyme induction leading to an increased rate of metabolism. In addition, they acquire some poorly defined adaptive capacity to perform motor and cognitive tasks at blood alcohol levels that would significantly affect the nonhabituated.[90] Thus there is some individual variability in the ability to handle alcohol, but the variations are confined to a narrow range. With this background we can turn to the effects of acute and then chronic alcoholism.

Acute alcoholism exerts its effects mainly on the central nervous system, but it may also remarkably quickly induce hepatic and gastric changes that are reversible in the absence of continued alcohol consumption. The hepatic changes were described on p. 944. The gastric changes constitute acute gastritis and ulceration (p 842). *In the central nervous system, alcohol itself is a depressant*, first affecting subcortical structures (probably the high brain stem reticular formation) that modulate cerebral cortical activity. Consequently, there is stimulation and disordered cortical, motor, and intellectual behavior so well known to every medical student. It should be sobering that acute alcoholism contributes significantly to over 50% of motor vehicle fatalities. At progressively higher blood levels, cortical neurons and then lower medullary centers are depressed, including those regulating respiration. Respiratory arrest may follow. These neuronal effects may relate to impaired mitochondrial function; structural changes are usually not evident in acute alcoholism. Occasionally, in fatal cases, there is cerebral edema, possibly secondary to hypoxia.

Blood alcohol levels and the degree of impairment of CNS function in nonhabituated drinkers are closely correlated. In individuals of average size, consumption of 180 ml (6 oz) of distilled spirits in a relatively brief time results in a blood alcohol level of approximately 100 mg/dl. This level will induce obvious ataxia and is considered by most jurisdictions as the legal upper limit of sobriety. Drowsiness occurs at about 200 mg/dl, stupor at 300 mg, and 400 to 500 mg will produce profound anesthesia, if not death. Fortunately, fatal levels are rarely encountered because "blessed stupor" intervenes. Even when large quantities are gulped rapidly with more bravado than brains, lifesaving vomiting due to gastric irritation often provides rescue.

Chronic alcoholism is responsible for morphologic alterations in virtually all organs and tissues in the body, particularly in the liver and stomach.[91] The precise basis for these widespread effects is not clear. As noted before, CNS, liver, and gastric changes are seen in short-term acute alcoholism. Only the gastric lesions that appear immediately after exposure can be related to the direct effects of ethanol on the mucosal vasculature.[92] The origin of the other chronic changes is less clear. Acetaldehyde, a major oxidative metabolite of ethanol, is a very reactive compound and has been proposed as the mediator of the widespread tissue and organ damage. Although the catabolism of

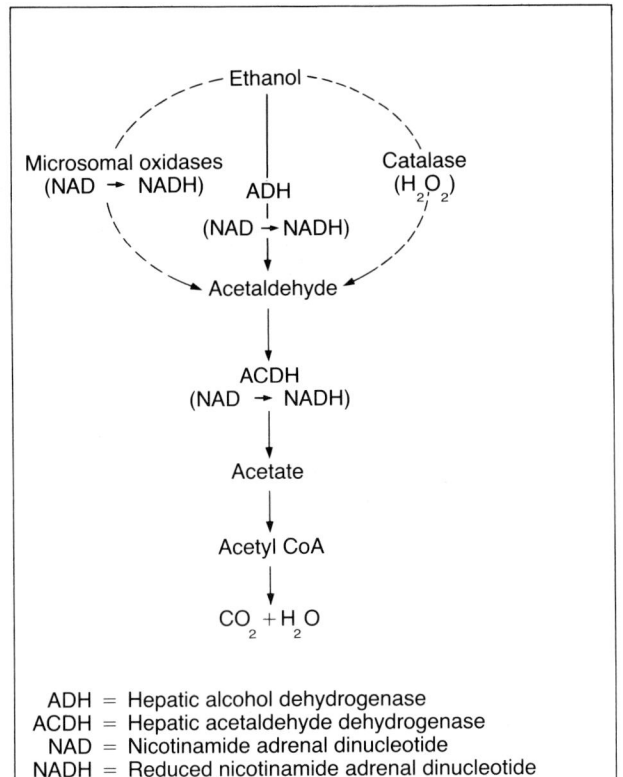

ADH = Hepatic alcohol dehydrogenase
ACDH = Hepatic acetaldehyde dehydrogenase
NAD = Nicotinamide adrenal dinucleotide
NADH = Reduced nicotinamide adrenal dinucleotide

Figure 9–17. Metabolism of alcohol the major (rate-limiting) pathway is via ADH.

acetaldehyde is more rapid than that of alcohol, chronic ethanol consumption reduces the oxidative capacity of the liver, raising the blood level of acetaldehyde, which is augmented by the increased rate of ethanol metabolism in the habituated drinker.[88] Increased free radical activity in chronic alcoholics has also been suggested as a mechanism of widespread tissue injury.[93] More recently, nonoxidative metabolism of alcohol, with the elaboration of fatty acid ethyl ester, has been proposed as the damaging agent as well as poorly defined immunologic mechanisms initiated by hepatocytic antigens released by acute injury. Still other proposals have been made, but in truth the "villain" has not yet been identified.

Whatever the basis, chronic alcoholics have a significantly shortened lifespan related principally to damage to the liver, stomach, brain, and heart. Alcohol is a well-defined cause of hepatic injury terminating in cirrhosis (p. 947). It is worthy of note that because of the epidemic proportions of alcohol abuse, cirrhosis of the liver has become the ninth leading cause of death in the United States. Massive bleeding from gastritis or gastric ulcer may prove fatal. In addition, chronic alcoholics suffer various damages to the nervous system. Some may be nutritional; a deficiency of vitamin B_1 is common in chronic alcoholics. The principal lesions of nutritional origin are peripheral neuropathies and the Wernicke-Korsakoff syndrome (p. 450). Cerebellar degeneration and optic neuropathy may appear, possibly directly related to alcohol or its products and uncommonly, cerebral atrophy. The cardiovascular consequences of alcohol abuse are also wide ranging. On the one hand, direct injury to the myocardium may produce a dilated congestive cardiomyopathy (p. 643). On the other hand, although still disputed, moderate amounts of alcohol may decrease the incidence of coronary heart disease and increase the levels of HDL. However, heavy consumption leading to liver injury results in lower levels of the HDL fraction of lipoproteins accompanied by an increased likelihood of coronary heart disease. Chronic alcoholism has a number of additional consequences, including an increased tendency to hypertension, a higher incidence of acute and chronic pancreatitis, and regressive changes in skeletal muscles — referred to as alcoholic myopathy.[95] Even more unhappily, the heavy use of ethanol during pregnancy can cause growth retardation and irreversible mental deficiency in the child.[96] Were these consequences not sufficient, alcohol abuse has also been implicated in an increased frequency of carcinoma of the oropharynx, larynx, esophagus, and possibly rectum and lung.[97] It is bad enough that acute alcoholism often unhinges the rudder of the ship; chronic alcoholism sometimes sinks it.

Methyl Alcohol

Methyl alcohol is more accessible than is generally appreciated. It may be used to denature ethanol and is found in solvents, Sterno, paint removers, and antifreezes. The toxic dose may be as small as 20 ml. Poisoning may also result from the inhalation of fumes in industry. When ingested, methyl alcohol causes patchy edema and hemorrhages in the stomach. On inhalation, edema and hemorrhage occur in the lung tissues, chiefly in the subpleural regions. However, methyl alcohol exerts its prime toxic effect after absorption by its oxidation to formaldehyde and formic acid. These toxic products are widely distributed in the body proportionate to the water content of the various tissues.[98] In sufficient amounts the toxic metabolites inhibit hexokinase activity. A metabolic acidosis follows, related in part to the formation of formic acid and in part to depressed hexokinase function. At the same time, the deranged glucose metabolism causes degeneration of the receptor cells of the retina with associated degeneration of the optic disc and nerve. *Degenerative neuronal changes, with swelling of the brain and brain stem, may develop in 12 to 24 hours, causing variable degrees of central nervous system depression to frank coma. The retina is the major target of methanol toxicity, and so retinal damage with visual impairment, and sometimes total blindness, constitute the major clinical features of the poisoning.* Both the eye and the brain changes are reversible with cessation of exposure if the injury is mild.

Lead

Lead is a furtive villain; it creeps in "on little cat's feet" as small daily increments silently accumulate to reach toxic levels. Sometimes in adults it announces itself relatively early with abdominal pain, fatigue, and arthralgia, but in infants and children it may remain unsuspected until it erupts in a catastrophic encephalopathic crisis. Poisoning by lead has proved to be one of the most difficult environmental health problems to control. Part of this difficulty is based on the lack of distinctive manifestations at an early phase in the process.

There are innumerable sources of lead in our environment. Some of the more important are listed below.

Occupational
Painting — especially spraying
Battery making and burning
Plumbing
Stained glass fabrication
Welding
Brass working
Foundry work
Lead smelting
Pottery work
Mining
Nonoccupational
Water supplies from lead pipes or lead-soldered joints
Dust and paint chips from older houses having lead paints
Air and soil pollution from leaded gasoline
Canned foods
Cooking in leaded pots
Newsprint — chewed or burned
Home-distilled wine/whiskey

It is evident that it is hard to avoid exposure to lead. Environmental lead is absorbed either through the gastrointestinal tract or through the lungs into the blood. In the United States, the acceptable upper limit of lead in the blood has been established by the Centers for Disease Control as 25 μg/dl.[99] The average range found in contemporary urban dwellers is 10 to 15 μg/dl. Contrast this level with that found in prehistoric man of 0.2 μg/dl.[100] Against this background, mass screening in the United States from 1976 to 1980 disclosed that 1.9% of the population from 6 months to 74 years of age had blood lead levels exceeding the acceptable limit. Even more significantly, *among children six months through five years old the blood lead levels were unacceptably elevated in 12.2% of black children usually living in older, lead-painted, peeling housing in city centers, as compared with 2.0% of white children usually living in middle-class circumstances.*[101] The principal contributors to this body burden are controversial and vary significantly with age.[102,103] Excluding occupational point sources, most agree that urban air, dirt, and food are the major offenders. Some years ago, automotive engines and industries emitted about 450,000 tons of lead per year into the air. Control measures (e.g., the use of unleaded gasoline) have significantly lowered the lead content of urban air and the level of lead in the blood. Volatilized lead is particularly hazardous, since most is absorbed in the lungs. By contrast, only a fraction of ingested lead is absorbed. Urban adults have a daily intake of 100 to 150 μg of lead in water and food, only about 10% of which is absorbed. Children have, on average, a lower intake but absorb about 50%. Flaking lead paint in older houses with soil contamination poses a major hazard to youngsters: Ingestion of up to 200 μg/day is possible.[104] Lead poisoning may, in fact, begin in utero; impaired cognitive development has been observed in infants having blood lead levels below 25 μg at birth, owing to maternal exposure to the pollutant.[105] So it is evident that even the so-called safe level of blood lead is not very safe.

Absorbed lead is mainly (80 to 85%) taken up by bone; the blood accumulates about 5 to 10%; and the remainder is distributed throughout the soft tissues. Although the soft tissue deposits have a half-life measured in hours to days, the skeletal deposits persist until the contaminated bone salts are recycled. In children, the bony deposits are located particularly in the epiphyses. In a sense this skeletal sequestration of lead protects the other tissues, but the slow turnover of bone mineral maintains elevated levels of lead in the blood for months to years.[106] Excretion occurs via the kidneys, thereby exposing these organs to potential damage.

Lead poisons enzymes by binding to disulfide groups and by denaturing proteins, altering their tertiary structure and thereby causes injury. The major anatomic targets of lead are the blood, nervous system, gastrointestinal tract, and kidneys (Fig. 9–18).

Blood changes are fairly early and characteristic.

Lead interferes with aminolevulinic acid dehydratase (ALA-D) and ferroketolase involved in the incorporation of iron into the heme molecule. As a consequence, the iron is displaced and zinc-protoporphyrin is formed. Thus, the level of zinc protoporphyrin or its product, free erythrocyte protoporphyrin, constitutes blood parameters of lead poisoning. *Typically, a microcytic, hypochromic, mild hemolytic anemia appears and, even more distinctive punctate basophilic stippling of the erythrocytes.*

Children are particularly vulnerable to brain damage, which may be very subtle and only functional, or massive and lethal.[107] In young children, sensory, motor, intellectual, and psychologic impairments have been described that can be encompassed within the terms reduced I.Q., learning disabilities, retarded psychomotor development, blindness, and in more severe cases, psychoses, seizures, and coma.[107a] Indeed the manifestations may mimic a space-occupying lesion with increased intracranial pressure. The anatomic changes underlying the more subtle functional deficits are ill defined and of obscure pathogenesis, but there is concern that some of the defects may be permanent. At the more severe end of the spectrum there is marked edema of the brain with flattening of the gyri and narrowing of the sulci (Fig. 9–19). Microscopically there may be demyelination of the cerebral and cerebellar white matter and death of cortical neurons with diffuse astrocytic proliferation. Often there is proliferation of the endothelium of small capillaries in the areas of damage. The neuronal loss has been tentatively attributed to lead-induced inhibition of mitochondrial oxidative phosphorylation. In the adult the central nervous system is less often affected, but *frequently a peripheral demyelinating neuropathy appears,* typically involving the motor innervation of the most commonly used muscles. Thus the extensor muscles of the wrist and fingers are often the first to be affected followed by paralysis of the peroneal muscles.

The gastrointestinal tract is a major source of clinical manifestations. *Lead "colic"* characterized by extremely severe, poorly localized abdominal pain is often associated with sufficient spasm and rigidity of the abdominal wall to create the impression of an acute "surgical abdomen." No intestinal morphologic changes have been identified, but often there is a "lead line" of precipitated lead sulfide along the gingival margins. It is rare in children and not seen in edentulous individuals. Moreover, although typical of lead poisoning, it may be encountered in other circumstances such as mercury poisoning.

The *kidneys* are affected less often than the blood or nervous system but nonetheless they may develop a chronic tubulointerstitial nephritis (p. 1051) or so-called Fanconi's syndrome marked by glycosuria, aminoaciduria, and phosphaturia secondary to altered tubular cell transport mechanisms. Often there is proteinuria, and reabsorption of the urinary proteins leads to large *eosinophilic droplets in the tubular epithelial cells.* As the poisoning progresses, the glo-

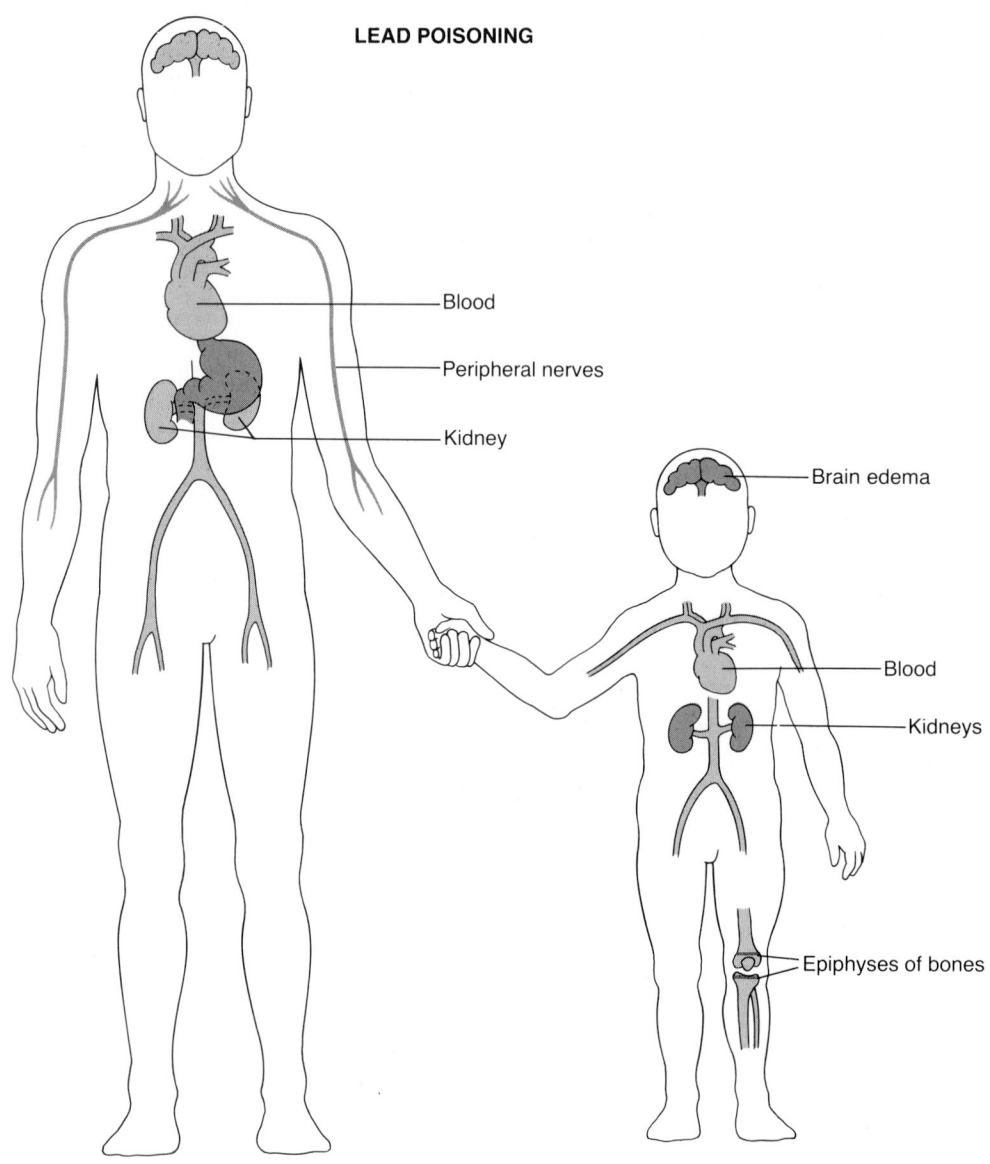

LEAD POISONING

- Blood
- Peripheral nerves
- Kidney
- Brain edema
- Blood
- Kidneys
- Epiphyses of bones

SOURCES

OCCUPATIONAL
Spray painting
Foundry work
Mining and extracting lead
Battery burning
Automotive exhaust

NONOCCUPATIONAL
Water supply
Paint dust and flakes
House dust
Urban soil
Newsprint

Figure 9–18. Lead poisoning. The major sites of lead-induced morphologic changes.

merular filtration rate falls and some patients develop renal failure.[108] The renal damage impedes normal excretion of uric acid and leads to hyperuricemia and so-called *saturnine gout.*

The diagnosis of lead poisoning requires a constant awareness of its prevalence. In children the only significant findings may be vague intellectual, behavioral, or motor abnormalities. In adults the abdominal pain, fatigue, and arthralgia are relatively nonspecific. Sometimes the first clue is anemia and basophilic stippling of the red cells. In some children, the intense radiopacity of the deposits in and about the epiphyses

of the growing bones raises the suspicion of lead poisoning (Fig. 9–20). Almost always, however, the diagnosis requires the confirmatory findings of elevated blood lead and free erythrocyte protoporphyrin (above 50 μg/dl) or, alternatively, zinc protoporphyrin levels. Other supportive findings are increased excretion of aminolevulinic acid in the urine and reduced erythrocyte aminolevulinic acid dehydratase activity. In view of all the potential consequences of advanced intoxication, it is hardly necessary to point out the importance of an early diagnosis before morphologic changes have developed.

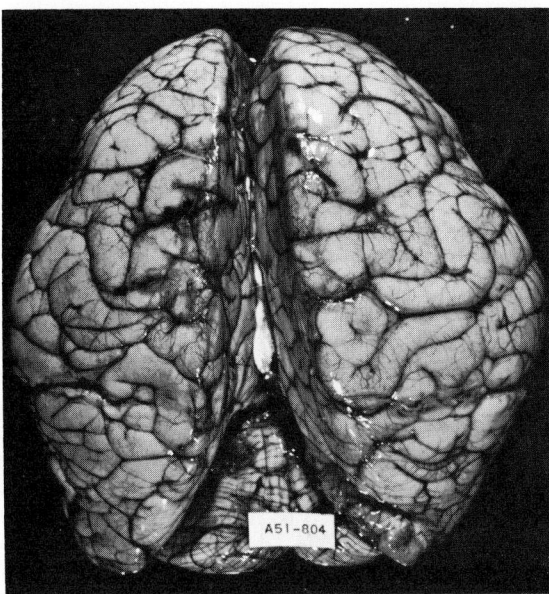

Figure 9–19. Cerebral edema in lead poisoning. The gyri are flattened and widened, and the sulci are narrowed and relatively inapparent.

Carbon Monoxide (CO)

This nonirritating, colorless, tasteless, odorless gas produced by the imperfect oxidation of carbonaceous materials continues to be a cause of accidental and suicidal death. It is widely available, being emitted from automotive engines and industrial processes using fossil fuels. Most heating and illuminating gases generated from fossil fuels (not natural gas) and cigarette smoke also contain it. The exhaust of automotive

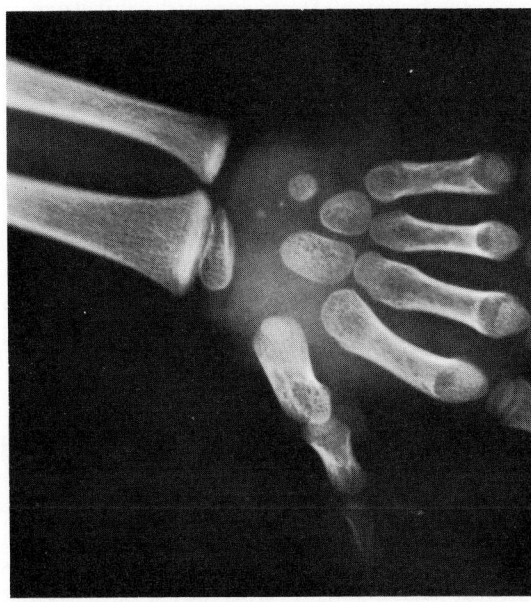

Figure 9–20. Lead deposits in epiphyses of wrist have caused a marked increase in their radiodensity so that they are as radiopaque as the cortical bone.

engines has about 5% CO; the average car in a small closed garage will induce lethal coma within five minutes. The CNS depression appears so insidiously that the victims may not be aware of their plight and indeed may be unable to help themselves.

CO acts as a systemic asphyxiant. Hemoglobin has a 200-fold greater affinity for CO than for oxygen. The resultant carboxyhemoglobin is incapable of carrying oxygen and furthermore interferes with the release of oxygen from oxyhemoglobin. Systemic hypoxia begins to appear when the hemoglobin is 20 to 30% saturated with CO, and unconsciousness and death are likely with 60 to 70% saturation. Depending on the rate of conversion to carboxyhemoglobin and the ultimate severity, two clinical patterns can be recognized.

Acute poisoning is marked by a characteristic cherry-red coloration to the skin and mucous membranes resulting from the carboxyhemoglobin. Depending on the rapidity of death morphologic changes may not be present, but with longer survival the brain may be slightly edematous and may have punctate hemorrhages and possibly hypoxic neuronal changes. Less commonly there is evidence of hypoxic damage to myocardial cells, renal tubular epithelial cells, and centrilobular hepatic cells. It should be noted that the morphologic changes are not specific for CO, since they simply imply systemic hypoxia; moreover, death often occurs so rapidly that the changes are not detectable by the light microscope and may or may not be discernible under the electron microscope. When the exposure has not been too long and the tissue hypoxia not too profound, complete recovery is possible. However, sometimes impairment of memory, vision, hearing, and speech remains.[109]

Chronic low-dose poisoning may appear because the carboxyhemoglobin, once formed, is remarkably stable and is displaced from hemoglobin over a period of days by the pressure and mass action of oxygen. So with low-level persistent exposure it may accumulate in the blood. The slowly developing hypoxia insidiously evokes changes in the central nervous system. Neuronal hypoxic injury is more or less widespread but is particularly marked in the basal ganglia and lenticular nuclei. In some instances demyelinating lesions develop in the cerebral white matter and may be followed by cystic rarefactions. Renal, hepatic, or cardiac dysfunction due to hypoxic injury may follow. Death may occur because of the brain and visceral damage, but in most instances of chronic poisoning the victim recovers, often with neurologic sequelae. The diagnosis of monoxide poisoning is critically dependent on the identification of significant levels of carboxyhemoglobin in the blood.

Environmental and Occupational Carcinogens

As was pointed out in Chapter 6, we virtually "swim in a sea of carcinogens," a few of which have been singled out in previous sections (cigarette smoke, asbestos). According to the Environmental Protection Agency, about 20% of the approximately 50,000 substances in current commercial use are putative carcinogens. The term "carcinogenic," however, is open to challenge, since it is often based on epidemiologic and animal studies of arguable relevance. Without getting mired in this highly controversial scientific and political morass, there can be no question that a large number of environmental and industrial substances are carcinogenic and indeed, when cigarette smoking is included, are directly or in part responsible for over half of all clinical cancers.[110] Some of the major implicated agents are listed in Table 9–4.

For further details, reference should be made to an authoritative review.[111]

Drug Addiction

Although AIDS dominates the headlines today, drug addiction is no less a contemporary epidemic. Indeed the two epidemics are closely related because, as you must know, drug abusers constitute a high risk group for AIDS. There are no precise data on the dimensions of the drug epidemic, but a few observations shed some light. A survey of a representative sample of young men in New York State with a mean age of 25 years revealed that 99% had used alcohol, 72% cannabis, 25% psychedelics, 30% cocaine, and 3% heroin.[112] It should be noted that the term "used" covers a wide range of exposure and should not be equated with "abused." But other studies indicate, for example, that approximately 5 million Americans use cocaine (or "crack") regularly, and each day another 5000 use it for the first time![113] In addition, it is estimated that in the United States there are over 800,000 heroin addicts taking heroin daily. Drug abuse is the leading cause of death in New York City among those 15 to 35 years of age, one third of these fatalities occurring in teenagers. There is then a major

epidemic that has shown no signs of yielding to efforts to control it.[114]

It has been difficult to segregate the adverse consequences of each of the agents in popular use.[115] Almost invariably, more than one has been used either simultaneously or sequentially. Some of the agents, particularly cocaine and heroin, are diluted ("cut") by a variety of substances, such as quinine, talc, or lactose, that themselves may induce pharmacologic, allergic, or foreign body reactions. Precise dosages are unknown — often to the user as well. With some of the agents such as heroin, the methods commonly employed for the preparation of a parenteral "shot" are less than fastidious. Unbelievably, in one study of heroin addicts, about one third had on occasion dissolved the drug in water from the toilet. Not surprisingly, "needle addicts" are prey to every type of infection known to medicine. There are then formidable difficulties in identifying the adverse effects of specific agents and distinguishing between their direct pharmacologic actions and the countless side effects caused by idiosyncratic reactions, adulterants, microbial contaminants, and other variables. Only brief comments will be made about a few relatively popular street drugs, followed by more detail about cocaine, heroin, and marijuana — the last because recent evidence indicates that it is more hazardous than formerly believed.[116]

Inhalants have achieved great popularity among the very young; surveys indicate that about 15% of the general urban population under 25 years of age (some less than 10 years of age) either experiment with or use them frequently. Favorites among the inhalants are glue, paint thinner, nail polish remover, and many substances in aerosol cans such as hairspray and room deodorizers. As a group the solvents and aerosolizers act as powerful central nervous system depressants; because they repress inhibitory pathways they produce a transient "high" much like that of acute alcoholism. Although for the most part their neurologic and psychologic effects, such as impairment in judgment, disorientation, and manic euphoria, are transitory, deaths from heart failure have been reported (the solvents and fluorocarbons in aerosol cans intensify the effects of epinephrine on the heart). On a happier note, "sniffing" does not lead to addiction and seems to lose its appeal in adult life.

Phencyclidine hydrochloride, also known as "angel dust" and "hog," was originally synthesized as a nonbarbiturate anesthetic agent. Once again the young discovered it as a hallucinogen, and it is estimated that over 5 million Americans between 12 and 25 years of age have smoked, snorted, ingested, or otherwise "tripped" with this substance. It acts variously as a depressant, a stimulant, and a hallucinogen — the most serious consequences being agitation, delirium, convulsions, and death. Most of the deaths are due to total loss of sensory and motor control leading to drowning, falling, or motor vehicle accidents. There is no evidence that the drug produces physical or psychologic dependence. However, numerous

Table 9–4. Some Major Environmental and Occupational Carcinogens

AGENT	TYPE OF CANCER
Arsenic (miners, insecticide manufacturers and users, chemical workers)	Skin, lung, liver carcinomas
Asbestos (p. 479)	Bronchogenic carcinoma, mesothelioma, others
Benzene (rubber cement workers, distillers, dye users)	Myelogenous leukemia
Beta-napthylamine (rubber, dye industries)	Bladder carcinoma
Cadmium (miners, processors)	Prostate, kidney carcinoma
Chromium (producers and processors)	Nasal cavity, sinus, lung, and laryngeal carcinomas
Cigarette smoke	Bronchogenic carcinoma, others
Nickel (miners and processors)	Nasal sinus, lung cancers
Nitrites (p. 465)	Stomach carcinoma
Uranium (miners and processors)	Lung carcinoma
Vinyl chloride (plastic industries)	Liver angiosarcoma

surveys indicate that users of phencyclidine have a significantly greater likelihood of becoming involved with "hard" drugs such as cocaine and heroin.[117]

Cocaine, although used by South Americans for millennia, has, along with its derivative "crack," become a major substance of abuse.[118] Cocaine, an alkaloid extracted from the leaves of the coca plant, is usually prepared in the form of a water-soluble powder—cocaine hydrochloride. As sold on the street it is liberally diluted with talcum powder, lactose, or some other look-alike. Extraction of the pure alkaloid from cocaine hydrochloride yields nuggets of "freebase" or "crack" (so called because of the cracking or popping sound it makes when heated.) The pharmacologic actions of cocaine and "crack" are identical, but the latter is far more potent. Both forms of the drug are absorbed from all sites and so can be "snorted," smoked when mixed with tobacco, ingested, or injected subcutaneously or intravenously.

Cocaine and its derivative do not produce true physical dependence in the manner of heroin, but continued "highs" create uncontrollable craving, and in this sense, addiction. The alkaloid also activates the sympathetic nervous system, resulting in dilated pupils, constriction of the small blood vessels, an acute rise in arterial pressure, tachycardia, and a predisposition to ventricular arrhythmias that have caused sudden death. The arrhythmias are attributed to a catecholamine-like action of cocaine on myocardial cells, leading to widespread myocardial contraction bands and myocyte necrosis (p. 610).[119] Diffuse myocardial damage may lead to congestive, dilated cardiomyopathy. In addition, in individuals with fixed coronary artery lesions, myocardial infarction has developed.[120] Infarctions have also occurred when the coronary arteries were apparently free of fixed lesions, raising the possibility of coronary spasm. Yet another hazard is nonspecific, severe, pulmonary edema either cardiac or anaphylactic in origin. These various disasters may occur with the use of usual recreational amounts of the drug. Thus, this once-thought relatively safe "highway to heaven" is now recognized to lead sometimes to the hospital or, even worse, to the grave.

Heroin, although not as widely used as cocaine, is the most hazardous. It is an addicting opioid (closely related to morphine) derived from the poppy plant. It is sold on the street "cut" with some agent, often quinine, so that the addict has no knowledge of the size of the dose he or she is taking. It is usually self-administered intravenously or subcutaneously along with an abundant "fauna and flora." It is short-acting, so it must be taken every few hours to avoid withdrawal symptoms. Its varied effects include euphoria, hallucinations, somnolence, and sedation. Heroin has a wide range of adverse physical effects from (1) the pharmacologic action of the agent; (2) reactions to the cutting agents or contaminants; (3) hypersensitivity reactions to the drug or its adulterants (quinine itself has neurologic, renal, and auditory toxicity), and (4) diseases contracted incident to the use of the needle.

Sudden death, usually related to overdosage, is an ever-present threat to the heroin addict. The doses self-administered are total unknowns because street samples range from 2% to 90% heroin. Understandably, most heroin sold by pushers is very dilute, but an easy way to dispose of a nonpayer is to provide an uncut preparation. Tolerance for the drug built up over time may be lost (as during a period of incarceration). Three overdose syndromes have been identified: (1) profound respiratory depression, (2) arrhythmias and cardiac arrest, and (3) severe pulmonary edema (Fig. 9–21).[121]

In addition to sudden death, heroin has a number of other unpleasant consequences.

- *Pulmonary complications* include moderate to severe edema, septic embolism, lung abscess, opportunistic infections, and foreign body granulomas from talc and other adulterants (Fig. 9–22).[122]
- *Granulomas* may occur in the lungs and are sometimes found in the mononuclear-phagocyte system, particularly in the lymph nodes draining the upper extremities, spleen, and liver. Examination under polarized light often highlights the trapped talc crystals (from the diluent), sometimes enclosed within foreign body giant cells.
- *Infectious complications* are extremely frequent. The four sites most commonly affected are the skin and subcutaneous tissue, heart valves, liver, and lungs. *Cutaneous lesions* are probably the most frequent telltale signs of heroin addiction—scarring at injection sites, hyperpigmentation over commonly used veins, thrombosed veins, and skin abscesses, cellulitis, and ulcerations usually secondary to subcuta-

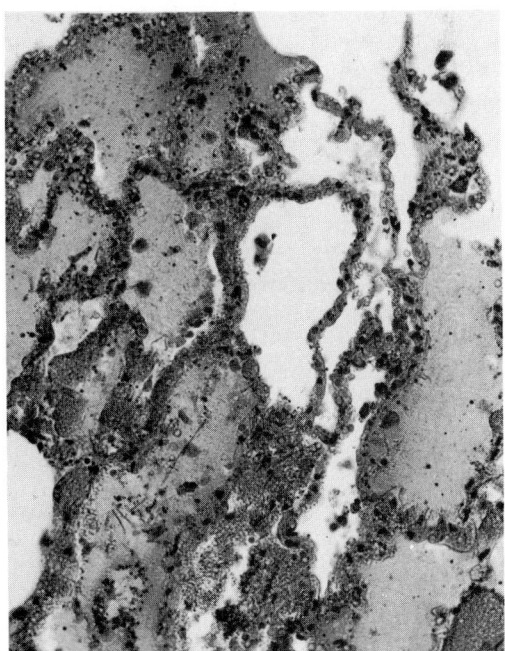

Figure 9–21. Lung of a heroin addict with patchy edema and atelectasis. Many of the alveolar spaces are filled with a proteinaceous fluid.

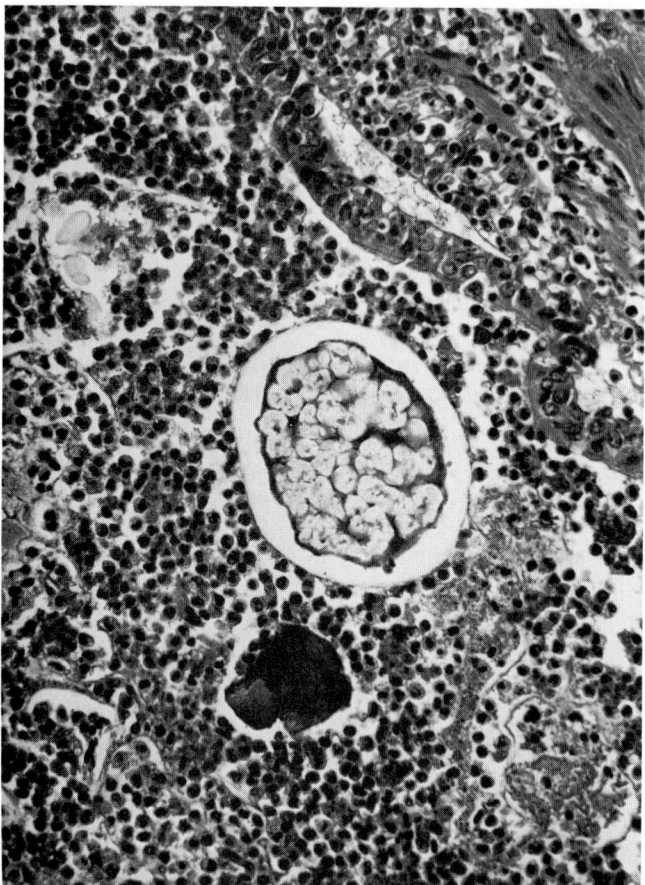

Figure 9–22. Aspiration pneumonia in a heroin addict. A small airway is filled with white cells among which are two large aspirated foreign bodies, the upper one probably of plant origin.

neous injections ("skin-popping"). The chronicity of these infections sometimes leads to systemic amyloidosis. In a series of addicts admitted to the hospital, over 10% had *endocarditis* (p. 633).[123] It takes a distinctive form often involving right-sided heart valves, particularly the tricuspid. Most cases are caused by *Staphylococcus aureus*, but fungi and every other organism in the "toilet" have been implicated. *Viral hepatitis* is the most common infection among addicts and is acquired by the casual interchange of needles. This practice has also led, as is well known, to addicts' having an incidence of *AIDS* second only to that of homosexuals. Finally, as mentioned, pulmonary infections also exact their toll and in many instances are caused by organisms of low virulence, e.g., opportunists such as *Pneumocystis carinii.*

• *Kidney disease* is a relatively common hazard. The two forms most frequently encountered are amyloidosis and focal glomerulosclerosis, and both induce heavy proteinuria and the nephrotic syndrome. The amyloidosis is attributed to the chronic skin suppuration mentioned earlier. The focal glomerulosclerosis resembles the idiopathic form and that seen with other conditions, and has a similar tendency to progress to end-stage renal failure (p. 1037).[124]

Were all these complications not sufficient, a miscellany of additional hazards face the heroin addict, including the risk of tetanus, peripheral neuropathy, acute and chronic myopathy, osteomyelitis, and acute disseminated vasculitis. The price of heroin addiction is clearly more than the cost of the drug. Some of the major consequences of heroin are presented in Figure 9–23.

Marijuana is the most widely used "illicit drug" (some would vehemently protest this designation) and the one that has evoked the greatest controversy about its safety. Marijuana is the dried flowering tops and leaves of the *Cannabis sativa* plant, containing the psychoactive substance delta-9-tetrahydrocannabinol (THC). When smoked in a "joint" about 50% of the THC is absorbed; when ingested, only about 5 to 10%. Hashish, the extracted resin, has five to ten times the potency of marijuana. According to several surveys, approximately 70% of 18- to 25-year-olds experiment with or regularly use "pot." Statistically, to not have used pot by age 25 must be considered deviant. However, this casual use is of concern for many reasons, not the least of which is the evidence that marijuana is frequently a stepping stone to deeper waters, although by itself it does not cause addiction.[125] Despite numerous studies, conflicting results still leave open the central question of whether the drug has persistent adverse physical and functional effects. Some of the untoward anecdotal events may be allergic or idiosyncratic reactions rather than being directly related to marijuana's pharmacologic effects. Yet another significant variable is the contamination of marijuana by herbicides and other sprays used by agencies to destroy the plantations. Paraquat, a favored spray, has strong toxicity for the lung. With all these variables, disagreement about the consequences of cannabis use persist, but recent findings have brought the pot to a boil.

Cell-mediated immunity may be impaired. Several in vitro studies point to a decrease in the number and function of T cells in humans, supported by animal studies. However, there is no clear evidence that the use of pot predisposes to infections or impairs the capacity to control the usual infections.[126] *Cannabis may induce chromosomal damage in somatic and germinal cells*, but here again the evidence is not incontrovertible.[127] Irregular mitoses, chromosomal translocations and breaks, and hypo- or hyperploidy have all been observed. Some of these observations were derived from in vitro exposure of growing human cells to THC, and, as is well known, any "foreign" substance (including aspirin) introduced into a culture adversely affects cell replication. Exposure of human sperm to THC resulted in decreased motility, and animal experiments suggest a reduction in fertility, litter size, and greater postnatal loss. Similarly, a large study involving many thousands of women who were marijuana users revealed lower birth weights, shorter gestation periods, and, significantly, an increased number of major malformations among the offspring.[128] Since the peak use of marijuana is among

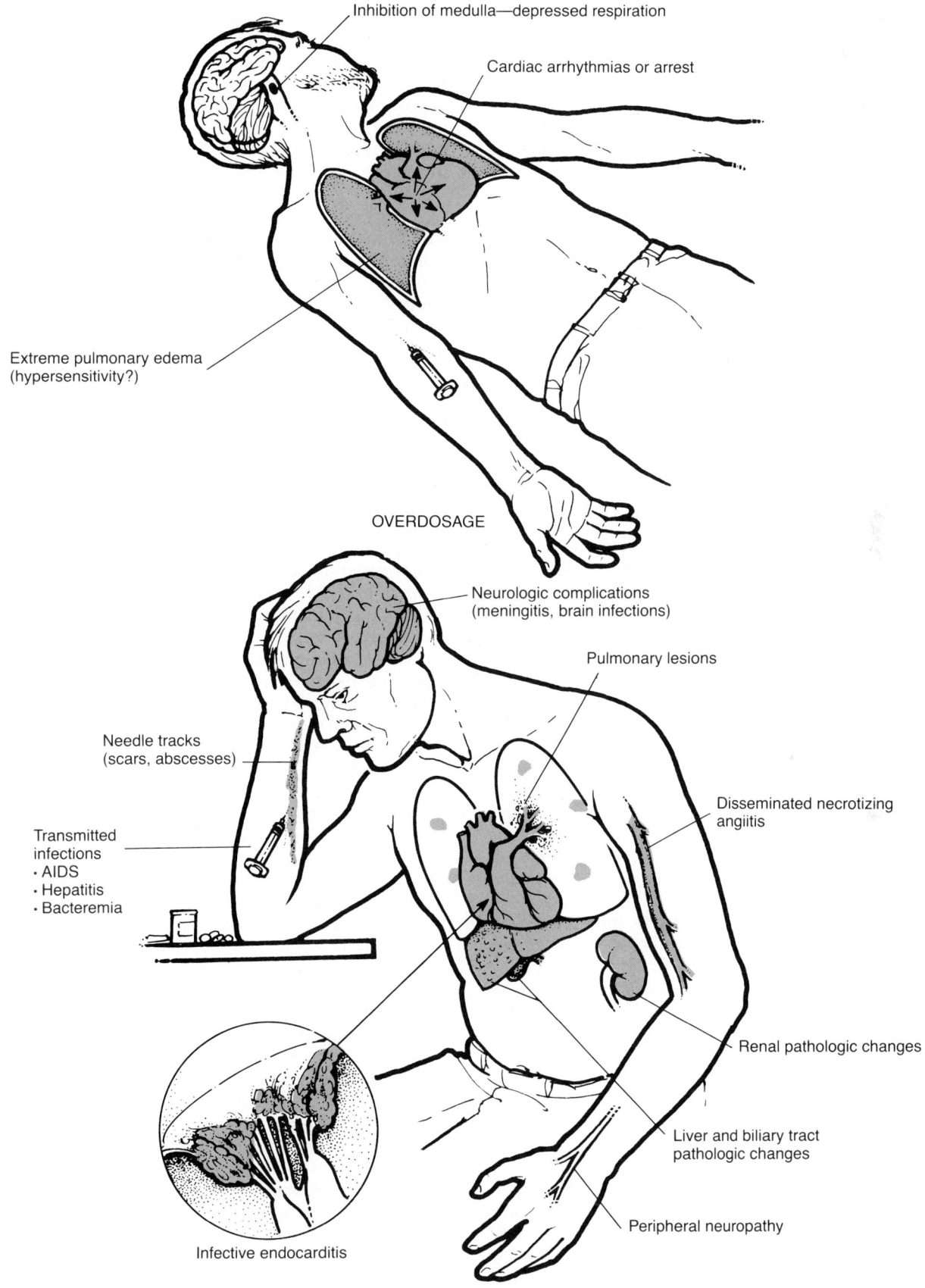

Inhibition of medulla—depressed respiration

Cardiac arrhythmias or arrest

Extreme pulmonary edema (hypersensitivity?)

OVERDOSAGE

Neurologic complications (meningitis, brain infections)

Pulmonary lesions

Needle tracks (scars, abscesses)

Transmitted infections
· AIDS
· Hepatitis
· Bacteremia

Disseminated necrotizing angiitis

Renal pathologic changes

Liver and biliary tract pathologic changes

Peripheral neuropathy

Infective endocarditis

HABITUAL USE

Figure 9-23. The major consequences of heroin addiction—overdosage *(above)* and less catastrophic consequences *(below).*

teenagers and young adults, these findings give one pause for thought.

Not unexpectedly, *the lungs are affected by chronic smoking of pot*; laryngitis, pharyngitis, bronchitis, cough and hoarseness, and asthma-like symptoms have all been described along with mild but significant airway obstruction. Smoking a cannabis reefer as compared with a cigarette is associated with a threefold increase in the amount of tar inhaled and retained in the lungs. The larger puff-volume, deeper inhalation, and longer breath-holding are presumably responsible.[116] To data cannabis has not been shown to increase the incidence of bronchogenic carcinoma; recall, however, that it took over 50 years to establish the carcinogenicity of tobacco. *Marijuana increases the heart rate and sometimes the blood pressure* and in the individual with fixed coronary narrowings may cause angina. *The functional and organic central nervous system consequences of cannabis* have received the greatest scrutiny. Clearly, the use of pot distorts sensory perception and impairs motor coordination, but these acute effects generally clear in four to five hours. More ominously, it has been reported that chronic smokers of cannabis have a sixfold greater risk of schizophrenia.[129] There are, then, disturbing findings, suggesting that the whole story is not known yet.[130] It should be evident there are reasons to "keep off the grass."

Other Nontherapeutic Toxic Agents

Literally hundreds of chemicals in addition to those already discussed have at one time or another caused toxic reactions in humans. Only a few of the more commonly encountered will be mentioned.

Chloroform and carbon tetrachloride are used at home in cleaning fluids and in industry mainly as degreasing agents. Inhalation of large amounts of fumes from these agents may cause profound central nervous system depression and death. Less extreme levels of exposure lead to centrilobular fatty change in the liver and, depending on dosage and individual susceptibility, possibly centrilobular to more extensive liver necrosis (p. 923).

Mushroom poisoning, caused usually by the ingestion of *Amanita phalloides*, may be fatal. Other species of mushrooms, particularly *Amanita muscaria*, may cause severe toxic reactions but are less often fatal. *A. phalloides*, known as the "angel of death," possesses a heat-resistant toxin — amanitin — that inhibits RNA polymerase. After a lag of 6 to 24 hours, nausea, vomiting, violent abdominal cramps, and diarrhea appear, often followed by cardiovascular collapse. In severe intoxications, headache, confusion, and convulsions may dominate the clinical presentation, to be followed by coma and death. The anatomic changes with less violent intoxications take the forms of centrilobular hepatic necrosis, renal tubular necrosis, and striated muscle focal necroses. If the victim survives, the hepatic destruction may be followed by

postnecrotic cirrhosis. When the CNS syndrome predominates, the victim rarely survives long enough to develop anatomic changes. *A. muscaria*, in contrast, possesses the parasympathomimetic muscarin. Toxic symptoms include pupillary constriction, sweating, nausea, vomiting, diarrhea, dyspnea, bradycardia, and hypotension. Although death may occur following these manifestations, recovery is the rule with supportive therapy.

Insecticides are not only toxic to plant pests but in sufficient amounts are also harmful to birds and beasts (including the human kind). They fall into two broad classes: (1) chlorinated hydrocarbons, e.g., chlordane, DDT, dieldrin, and lindane; and (2) organophosphorous compounds, e.g., malathion and parathion. Both types accumulate in fat stores, and so small daily increments may reach toxic levels. Moreover, most can be absorbed through the respiratory, skin, or gastrointestinal route; since they are very resistant to degradation in the environment, they persist in soil and water and contaminate all levels of the human food chain. Not surprisingly, DDT has been found in fruits, vegetables, meats, milk, and even infant foods.[131] The *chlorinated hydrocarbons* affect the central nervous system and induce at first hyperexcitability possibly followed by delirium and convulsions. More marked levels of toxicity are associated with central nervous system depression, paralysis, coma, and death. The toxic effects are expressed mainly in regressive changes in neurons within the brain and spinal cord, sometimes progressing to neuronal death. Fatty changes in the liver appear in more chronic poisoning. The *organophosphorous compounds* are basically inhibitors of acetylcholinesterase. Thus, acetylcholine accumulates at synaptic junctions and induces muscle twitching that progresses to flaccid paralysis and, more ominously, cardiac arrhythmias and respiratory depression, either of which may be fatal.

The *polychlorinated biphenyls (PCBs)* are dangerous pollutants because, once released into the environment, they are "forever," i.e., are resistant to natural processes of decay. They were used mostly in piping, hydraulic fluids, plasticizers, adhesives, and as filling agents in electrical transformers and capacitors. Recognition of their toxicity to humans led to legislation outlawing production of PCBs after 1977, but we are still left with the near-indestructible inheritance of prior years. Burning and incineration of industrial and municipal wastes disperses the PCBs into the environment. The PCBs have been implicated by animal studies in the production of hepatic, renal, and intestinal lesions; reproductive defects; and impaired immunity. In humans they have been associated with chloracne, impaired vision, impotence, and possibly infertility. These changes may not appear for many months after exposure. In addition, PCBs predispose to a deficiency of vitamin A and possibly other vitamins as well. Unfortunately, we are not likely to soon escape the potentially adverse effects of this unwanted resident of our environment.

PHYSICAL INJURIES

The many forms of physical energy that may give rise to injury can be classified into four groups: mechanical force, changes in temperature, changes in atmospheric pressure, and electromagnetic energy. Of the physical agents, mechanical force exemplified by the everyday occurrence of auto accidents is the most frequent cause of injury encountered in clinical practice. Much detail on mechanical injuries is unnecessary in general pathology, since only rarely do such cases necessitate pathologic study save for legal purposes. Changes in atmospheric pressure and hypothermia are relatively uncommon causes of injury, but hyperthermia (burn) is all too common. Radiation injuries, too, have assumed frightening importance as potential causes of widespread destruction.

MECHANICAL FORCE

Injury from mechanical force may occur whenever a mass hits the body, the body collides with a stationary mass, or, as sometimes occurs, both body and mass are in movement at the moment of impact. Several types of tissue injury or wounds may result, which can be grouped broadly into (1) soft tissue injuries, (2) bone injuries, and (3) head injuries. Injuries of the bones (p. 1322) and of the head (p. 1409) involve specialized problems best considered in the chapters dealing with these structures. Soft tissue injuries such as abrasions, lacerations, and contusions fall principally into the realms of surgery, inflammation, and repair and involve no special problems in anatomic pathology. A *contusion* is an injury caused by a blunt force that injures small blood vessels and causes interstitial bleeding, usually without disruption of the continuity of the tissue. A bruise of the skin is an example of a contusion. Sometimes deep-seated contusions of skeletal muscle, for example, may occur without evident injury to the skin or subcutaneous tissues. Analogously, laceration of the liver and spleen may be encountered in victims of an automobile accident without demonstrable damage to the abdominal wall. The possible systemic reactions to mechanical trauma are presented in the consideration of shock (p. 114).

CHANGES IN TEMPERATURE

As a homeothermic animal, man must maintain his internal temperature within the narrow range of 31° to 41°C, and even this upper limit can be tolerated only very briefly. Since abnormally high and low temperatures produce different patterns of tissue damage and have different pathogenetic mechanisms, they will be discussed separately.

Abnormally Low Temperatures

The effects of hypothermia depend on whether there is whole-body exposure or exposure only of parts. Death may result when the whole body is exposed, without inducing apparent necrosis of cells or tissues because the systemic homeostatic mechanisms are more vulnerable to hypothermia than are individual cells.

LOCAL REACTIONS. Chilling or freezing of cells and tissues causes injury in two ways:

1. Direct effects are probably mediated by physical dislocations within cells and the high salt concentrations incident to the crystallization of the intracellular water.
2. Indirect effects are exerted by microcirculatory changes. Depending on the rate at which the temperature drops and its duration, slowly developing chilling may induce vasoconstriction and some endothelial cell injury, followed by paralysis of vasomotor control and consequent vasodilation and increased permeability, leading to edematous changes. Such changes are typical of *"trench foot."* Atrophy and fibrosis may follow. Alternatively, with sudden sharp drops in temperature that are persistent, the vasoconstriction and increased viscosity of the blood in the local area may cause ischemic injury and degenerative changes in peripheral nerves. In this situation, only after the temperature begins to return toward normal do the vascular injury and increased permeability with exudation become evident. However, during the period of ischemia, hypoxic changes and infarction necrosis of the affected tissues may develop, for example, gangrene of toes or feet.

SYSTEMIC REACTIONS. When the entire body is exposed to excessively low temperatures (as now occurs too often among the homeless "lost souls"), there is at first marked vasoconstriction of the skin vessels, producing extreme pallor. As the hypothermia continues, peripheral vasodilation and hyperemia develop. Cooling of the peripheral blood soon causes depression of the temperature in the vital organs with slowing of metabolic processes, particularly in the brain and medullary centers. The usual cause of death appears to be circulatory failure. Sudden acute chilling may cause death in a relatively short time without apparent alteration of the body tissues. Under these circumstances, there may be no pathognomonic anatomic changes demonstrable at the time of postmortem examination. Fortunately, the reduction in metabolic rate that accompanies the hypothermia sometimes permits successful resuscitation of those in coma without significant damage to the brain and viscera — recall the children who have recovered totally after hours of submersion in icy waters. With more slowly developing, less severe hypothermia, the anatomic changes are usually limited to the superficial tissues and extremities and resemble the local reactions.

Thermal Burns

Of the approximately 5000 deaths caused by burns annually in the United States, a large proportion are particularly tragic because they involve children and young adults "with so much life left to live." Many factors affect the clinical significance of a burn.

• The percentage of total body surface involved.
• The depth of the burn.
• The possible development of internal injuries from inhalation of hot gases and fumes.
• The age of the patient.
• The immediacy and efficacy of the postburn therapy, in particular, fluid and electrolyte management, prevention of shock, and prevention or control of wound infection.

Surface and inhalational burn injuries are sufficiently different to require separate treatment.

SURFACE BURNS. The size of the burn wound and its depth are obviously of critical importance. Continuous improvement in therapy has almost invalidated the notion of an upper limit of body burn area compatible with survival. Nonetheless, any burn exceeding 50% of the total body surface, whether superficial or deep, is grave, and when it exceeds 70%, very often fatal.[132] As you would expect, the depth of the burn modifies this outlook. Many terms have been employed to attempt to express depth, but none is satisfactory, and so recourse has been made to the simple concept of *"partial"* and *"full-thickness"* burns. *Full-thickness burn* implies total destruction of the entire skin and dermal appendages, obviating the possibility of epithelial regeneration save from the margins (implying the need for skin grafting). The full-thickness burn may extend deep into the underlying muscles, viscera, and even bone, but with such penetration death is often immediate.

The *partial-thickness burn* implies preservation of some part of the skin, whether it be the epidermis itself or merely the dermal appendages from which epithelial regeneration may occur. Proteinaceous fluid seepage from a wound surface and the amount of cellular debris accompanying the burn injury are far greater with full-thickness than with partial burns. Partial-thickness burns imply a low intensity of heat and induce injury by accelerated metabolism of cells, by damaging cell membranes, by inactivation of temperature-critical enzymes, and by causing vascular injury. As is well known, the area becomes reddened as small blood vessels dilate, followed soon by increased capillary permeability with exudation of serous or protein-rich fluid, creating the typical "burn blister." The surface epithelial cells in the partial-thickness burn likewise give evidence of deranged membrane permeability with nuclear and cellular swelling. Depending on the variables of temperature and time, transepidermal necrosis may occur. If the skin has not been totally incinerated, the epithelial cells may disclose nuclear pyknosis and granular coagulation of the cytoplasm.[133] The dermal collagen takes on the appearance of a homogeneous gel. The cytologic changes just described may affect ever-deeper cells, including fibroblasts and endothelial and skeletal muscle cells. With intense heat there may be coagulation of the blood vessels and little evidence of exudation, but at the peripheral and deep borders between the nonviable and viable tissue, the described cellular and vascular changes will be evident as well as the inflammatory response.[134]

With burns of more than 30 to 40% of the body surface, systemic reactions become more important than the local injury. *Shock is the immediate postburn concern* (p. 114). It may be partly neurogenic in origin but soon thereafter is related to the massive outpouring of an exudate. *Progressive loss of plasma water induces hypovolemia and hemoconcentration.* Plasma proteins are simultaneously lost, and over the span of hours, with hemodilution, the plasma oncotic pressure falls to aggravate the fluid loss. In addition, *burns are frequently accompanied by acute gastroduodenal ulcerations* (Curling's ulcers) (p. 848). *Intravascular hemolysis* or DIC (p. 698) may occur and lead to renal tubular changes (ATN) or shock. Infection of the burn injury is, however, the most life-threatening complication.

Sepsis originating in burn wound infection is responsible for about 50 to 75% of postburn fatalities.[135] Despite strenuous preventive measures, the originally sterile burn wound often becomes secondarily infected; in the exudative outpouring and devitalized tissue, organisms proliferate as in a culture flask.[136] The predominant invader is *Pseudomonas*, and much less commonly other gram-negative bacilli and various other agents. Fungi, particularly *Candida* species, frequently supervene or predominate. This predisposition to infection involves more than merely a large open wound. Burn injury produces profound abnormalities in both local and systemic immunologic function. Cell-mediated and humoral reactions are both suppressed; complement, particularly through the alternative pathway, may be massively activated and then depleted, thereby depriving the body of a critical defense against the infections by gram-negative rods.[137] Phagocytic cell function is depressed, fibronectin levels reduced, and natural killer cell function suppressed.[138] Little is known about the precise origins of all these immunologic changes, circulating immunosuppressive factors have been suggested but not clearly identified. In sum, burned patients are not only grievously wounded but also rendered powerless to defend themselves. As a consequence, some wound infections run amok, producing regional thrombophlebitis, bacteremia, endocarditis, pneumonia, cellulitis, and contamination of every square inch of body surface, in particular the sites of intravascular lines (e.g., heparin locks). Blood-borne infection raises the specter of septic or endotoxic shock. For these reasons, much effort is now directed at methods to provide early temporary or definitive skin covers or grafts in the hope of avoiding life-threatening infections.

INTERNAL THERMAL INJURY. Individuals trapped in a burning building who inhale noxious fumes and heat may develop thermal injuries at any level of the respiratory tract from nose and mouth to the peripheral pulmonary parenchyma. The temperatures in burning rooms may reach 2000°C. At this level even so-called nonflammable objects ignite or melt. The release of inorganic and organic cyanides from plastics within the room and the rapidly developing hypoxia may kill within minutes. At less extreme levels of heat, oral cavity burns resemble surface burns — partial to full thickness. The epiglottis is often charred. The laryngeal and tracheobronchial mucosa may be severely injured, with secondary intense hyperemic edema that threatens the airway. For somewhat obscure reasons perhaps related to airstream dynamics, the sublaryngeal tracheal mucosa is often spared. Most distressing is the development, hours to days later, of the *acute respiratory distress syndrome* (p. 160) with severe pulmonary transudation and exudation. These pulmonary complications are present in 30% of patients dying within either the immediate resuscitative or the postresuscitative period. In addition to pulmonary edema, secondary infections with the development of bronchopneumonia, intra-alveolar hemorrhages, and atelectasis are common.

Thus, the severely burned patient confronts not only the effects of the direct injury but, even more important, its serious systemic consequences.

HEAT STROKE. Heat stroke may result from exposure to high ambient temperatures or from the inability to dissipate the metabolically generated heat produced by high fever or marked exertion. When the body temperature reaches 40°C or higher, generalized peripheral vasodilation occurs with sequestration of large volumes of blood, leading to a reduction in the effective circulating volume. When the heat stroke is basically febrile in origin, hypotension and CNS dysfunction progressing to coma dominate the clinical picture. In contrast, exertional heat stroke, with excessive sweating, is dominated by metabolic and fluid disturbances such as lactic acidosis, hyperkalemia, and with excessive exercise, myoglobinuria related to rhabdomyolysis. Whatever the origin, heat stroke may be complicated by DIC (p. 698), acute renal failure, adult respiratory distress syndrome, and hypoxic brain injury.

CHANGES IN ATMOSPHERIC PRESSURE

The direction of the pressure change (since in general the body withstands increases of pressure better than decreases), the magnitude of the change, and the rate of change all modify the extent, nature, and severity of the tissue damage. Changes in atmospheric pressure cause injuries in one of three ways: (1) Sudden increases or decreases of pressure may produce mechanical damage — blast injury; (2) with sudden decrease in pressure, free gaseous bubbles may be released in the blood and act as emboli, described earlier as caisson disease (p. 109); and (3) in low atmospheric pressures, lowered oxygen tension in the inspired air causes systemic hypoxia as is seen in high-altitude reactions. Only the first of these three forms of injury requires description here.

With *air blast* the compression wave impinges on the side toward the explosion and so may collapse the thorax, or violently compress the abdomen with rupture of internal organs. The pressure wave may enter the airways to damage the lungs. The following wave of decreased pressure may lead to sudden expansion of the abdomen and thorax with injury or rupture of intestines or lungs.

In *immersion blast*, the pressure is applied to the body from all sides. Individuals floating horizontally on the surface may simply be tossed out of the water virtually unharmed. Persons floating in an erect position are lifted slightly, if at all, and thus sustain pressure injuries to the lower half of the body resembling those described in air blast. Entrance of the water under pressure into the rectum or vagina is a particular hazard.

ELECTRICAL INJURIES

The passage of an electrical current through the body may be without effect; may cause sudden death by disruption of neural regulatory impulses, e.g., cardiac arrest; or may cause thermal injury to organs interposed in the pathway of the current. Many variables are involved: (1) the nature of the current (direct or alternating); (2) amperage; (3) voltage; (4) the path of the current through the body; (5) the resistance of the intervening tissues; and (6) the duration of exposure.

Each of these factors modifies the nature and extent of the injury. Alternating current is more dangerous than direct current because it induces tetanic muscular contractions "locking" the victim onto the electrical contact. The intensity of electrical flow through the tissues is a function of voltage, resistance of the tissues, and diffusion of the current. The pathway that the current takes is critical; electrical energy, as mentioned, disrupts normal neural impulses. Thus, if it should enter the top of the head, the flow of current through the brain may disrupt the normal cardiac and respiratory impulses from the medulla (the mechanism of death in electrocution). An equally strong current entering the lower part of the body and exiting through the foot might induce injury to tissues but not death. The pathway also determines the amount of diffusion of the current as explained below.

If critical neural pathways are not interrupted, the electrical energy may cause damage by generating heat. The current will disperse across the cross-sectional areas through which it flows. Hence in general, the trunk sustains less heat damage (other factors being equal) than the extremities, having smaller cross-sectional areas. Although all tissues of the body are conductors of electricity, their resistance to flow varies inversely to their water content. The greater the resistance of tissues and the voltage and amperage, the greater is the amount of heat generated. Bone and skin, especially thick skin, are particularly resistant, but wetting of the skin greatly reduces the resistance; an individual with sweaty palms may sustain a fatal internal injury, whereas in someone with dry hands, the same exposure might cause only skin charring. Sufficient ground contact permits the escape of electrical current and thereby reduces tissue damage. Other variables modify the extent of injury, such as size of the contact area permitting dispersion of electrical current over a wide area. A focal contact would produce a penetrating injury but a broader contact might not damage the skin.

The thermal effects of the passage of an electrical current vary from superficial skin burns to deep visceral lesions. High-intensity current, such as lightning coursing along the skin, produces linear arborizing burns known as lightning marks. Sometimes the intense current is conducted around the victim (so-called flashover), blasting and disrupting the clothing but doing little injury.[139] Less extreme voltages usually produce burn marks at the points of entry and exit of the current. However, currents transmitted through water or a good contact surface, as with moist skin, may cause little skin reaction and yet be of sufficient intensity to produce death by disturbing the cardiac or pulmonary rhythmic impulses. The heat generated internally causes variable damage depending on the voltage and amperage of the current. Lightning may produce sufficient heat and steam to explode solid organs, fracture bones, or char areas of organs. Focal hemorrhages from rupture of small vessels may be seen in the brain. Sometimes death is preceded by violent convulsions related to brain damage. Less intense voltage may heat, coagulate, or rupture vessels and cause hemorrhages; or in solid organs, such as the spleen and kidneys, cause infarctions or ruptures. The vagaries are almost limitless but in essence are permutations of interruption of neural pathways or burn injuries.

RADIATION INJURY

Few environmental influences can rival radiation in ubiquity. Cosmic rays of galactic and solar origin bathe the earth continuously and are the largest source of natural radiation. This radiation produces radionuclides such as tritium (^{3}H) and carbon 14 (^{14}C), which are incorporated into all living matter. A major consequence of cosmic radiation derives from its ultraviolet (UV) spectrum, and hence the great concern about the loss of our ozone shield.[140] Because of its short penetration, UV radiation affects mainly surface tissues such as the skin and eyes. It is a major cause of basal and squamous cell carcinomas of the skin among Caucasians[141] and contributes significantly to the development of malignant melanomas of the skin, cataracts, and possibly intraocular melanomas.[142] We are all at risk from cosmic radiation.

Radioactive elements in the earth's crust, such as uranium and radium, provide additional "natural" radiation that varies in quantity regionally. This source is particularly dangerous to miners of these ores. Under conditions of poor ventilation, mine air can become laden with radon emitted by the radioactive decay of uranium 238 and its daughter products. Inhalation of these pollutants accounted in years past for fatal lung malignancy in 50% to 70% of workers in particular mines in Germany and Czechoslovakia.[143] This type of mining hazard is far from resolved; a recent study of a group of uranium miners in the Colorado Plateau documented a lung cancer rate triple that for the general population of cigarette smokers.[144] Understandably, radon seepage into houses and water has raised concern.[145]

Radiation from the earth's crust or cosmic rays as described above is termed "background radiation." It is thought to account for 0.25 to 5% of naturally occurring genetic diseases.[146] In developed nations, human-generated radiation is responsible for much more radiation exposure than all sources of natural background radiation.[147] Medical, diagnostic, and therapeutic procedures account for most of this radiation exposure, but other possible sources are industrial products, nuclear power plants, and tragically in the past (we hope) the devastating intensity of nuclear weapons.

Being most concerned here with radiation's biologic potential, we leave the finer details of radiation physics to specialized texts.[148,149] It suffices for our purposes that radiation occurs in two forms: (1) electromagnetic waves (x-rays and gamma rays); and (2) energetic charged particles (alpha, beta—also known as electrons, protons, pi-mesons, and heavy ions) as well as neutral high-energy particles, e.g., neutrons. All these forms of radiation exert their effects on cells by the transfer of energy to the molecules and atoms within the cell. With sufficient energy transfer, orbiting electrons may be separated from the atomic nucleus, producing *ionization* of the atom or molecule. Transfer of less energy may only move the electron into an orbit more distant from the nucleus—*excitation*. Both the ionized and the excited states are unstable and have great potential for secondary reactions, but the biologic effect of radiation on cells is induced largely by ionization.

MECHANISMS OF ACTION. The precise details of how ionizing radiation exerts its biologic effects have remained elusive. Two proposals have been made: (1) the "*target theory,*" also known as the "direct hit," "quantum hit," or "direct action" theory; and (2) the "*indirect action*" theory.[150]

The "*target theory*" proposes that radiant energy acts by direct hits on target molecules within the cell. Models have been proposed invoking a single hit to one cell, single or multiple hits to many cells, or multiple hits to one cell; whatever the process, DNA, specifically the linkage and bonds within the molecule, is thought to be the key target of damage.[151,152]

The attack on the DNA may lead to mutations having genetic or cancerous potentials or to inhibition of cell division and cell death having acute somatic effects. However, macromolecules such as those within membranes and enzymes may also be damaged by radiation.

The *"indirect action theory"* proposes that radiant energy exerts its effect by producing free "hot" radicals within cells, according to the following sequence: Absorbed radiant energy leads to the radiolysis of cell water and the formation of the ionized water molecules H_2O^+ and H_2O^-. These dissociate to form the free radicals $H\cdot$ and $OH\cdot$, which in turn initiate a chain of reactions with themselves, their own reaction products, and tissue water to form other reactive radicals, such as H_2O_2 and HO_2. Ultimately, these free radicals interact with critical components, among which membranes, nucleic acids, and enzymes are the most important. In this sequential manner, a crucial biochemical change takes place, causing inhibition of cell division or cell death.

Radiant energy causes injury by both the "direct" and the "indirect" methods; gamma rays and x-rays act primarily by indirect action, whereas charged particulate radiation is more likely to act through "target," direct action.[146,153] The transfer of energy to a target atom or molecule from the incident source of radiant energy occurs within microfractions of a second, yet its biologic effect may not become apparent for minutes or even decades. *Radiation therefore has latency.*[154] During this latent period, it must be assumed (although the mechanism is poorly understood) that sequential reactions are occurring that ultimately exert a detectable functional or morphologic effect.

QUANTITATION OF RADIATION. Several units are used to quantify radiant energy. Strictly used, the "roentgen" (R) measures exposure to x- and gamma rays. One roentgen is the quantity of radiation that induces an emission equal to 1 electrostatic unit of charge in 1 cc of air. *Absorption* is a critical aspect of dose and is measured in *rads* (r) or *grays.* One *rad* is the dose resulting in the absorption of 100 ergs of energy per gram of target tissue for any type of radiation. For example, 1 roentgen delivered in air will lead to the absorption of about 87 ergs per gram by most tissues. A gray equals 100 rad; thus one centigray is the equivalent of a rad. Radionuclides are quantitated in terms of their instantaneous rates of disintegration measured in curies (ci) and their half-lives. One *curie* of radioactive isotope undergoes 3.7 times 10^{10} disintegrations per second. The *half-life* of an isotope defines the time during which one half of its unstable atoms will have disintegrated.

The relative effects of different types of radiation given at different doses can be compared in terms of their *"linear energy transfer"* (*LET*) and *"relative biologic effectiveness"* (*RBE*) or *"roentgen equivalent man"* (*REM*). LET expresses *energy loss per unit of distance traveled. The LET value of a form of radiation indicates the likelihood of its having an effect within a target area.* X-rays and gamma rays have low LET values. They penetrate tissues deeply but generate few interactions along their paths. On the other hand, charged particles or neutrons have a high LET with considerable ionization effect but shallow tissue penetration. There is a general relationship between LET value and type of injury—low-LET radiation is correlated with relatively minor, easily repaired chromosomal damage; and high-LET radiation with more severe, less easily repaired lesions.[147] *The RBE relates to the amount of cellular damage caused by a specific amount of radiant energy.*

BIOLOGIC EFFECTS OF RADIATION. The discussion of the impact of radiation on cells and tissues will be divided into the following: (1) general considerations, (2) effects on cells and tissues, (3) changes induced in certain specific organ systems, and (4) consequences of total body irradiation.

GENERAL CONSIDERATIONS. Radiant energy has substantial potential for serious injury to cells, since it attacks such critical components as DNA. Some cells and tissues of the body are more resistant to penetration by radiant energy than others; the outer keratinous shell of man is most radioresistant and so shields the more sensitive underlying tissues. In general, *cells are sensitive (in the short term) to radiant energy in direct proportion to their reproductive or mitotic activity and in inverse proportion to their level of specialization.*[155] This general thesis also applies to cancers, rapidly growing undifferentiated neoplasms being the most radiosensitive. However, some qualifications to this generalization are necessary. The terms "radiosensitive" and "radiocurable" are not synonymous. A tumor may virtually disappear with a single dose of radiation and be considered extremely radiosensitive. However, if all the target cells are not destroyed because the tumor is deeply situated or partially shielded by surrounding structures, it will recur. The tumor is then radiosensitive but not radiocurable. The volume of the tumor and its location in the body (superficial or deep) modify the extent of depletion of the cancer cells and the ultimate response to the radiation. Thus the term "radiosensitivity," as applied to cells and tissues, has an "acute" and "late" dimension. The acute reaction reflects the proliferative rate and vulnerability of the cells, whereas the late reactions also involve completeness of cell destruction and the damage to the vascular supply. With these cautionary notes, some broad generalizations about the sensitivity of some normal tissues and responsiveness of some tumors to radiation are offered in Table 9–5.

There are many exceptions to generalizations regarding the radiosensitivity of cells and their cancers. For example, normal kidney and lung are fairly radioresponsive. However, most tumors of these organs are difficult, if not impossible, to eradicate with radiation. Analogously, the testicular seminoma, which arises from primitive, proliferating germ cells, is ra-

Table 9–5. Radiosensitivity of Normal Tissues and Tumors

RADIOSENSITIVITY	NORMAL CELLS	TUMORS
High	Lymphoid, hematopoietic, spermatogonia, ovarian follicles	Leukemia-lymphoma, seminoma, dysgerminoma
Fairly high	Acute reactions for gastrointestinal and mucosal epithelium, hair follicles, and lung	Squamous cell carcinoma of skin, head and neck, and cervix
	Late reactions for lung, kidney	Adenocarcinoma of breast
		Neuroblastoma
Medium	Late reactions for gastrointestinal tract, endothelium, glandular epithelium of breast, glandular epithelium of pancreas, epithelium of bladder, growing cartilage, bone, and normal brain	Carcinoma of lung, esophagus, pancreas, bladder, medulloblastoma, ovarian cancer
Low	Bone, mature cartilage, muscle, peripheral nerves	Gliomas, large sarcomas, melanoma, renal cell cancer, osteosarcoma

With the gracious help of Dr. Norman Coleman, Harvard Medical School.

diosensitive but the more rapidly growing embryonal carcinoma, also of germ cell origin, is radioresistant. Other factors may play a role here, and perhaps the immune response (more evident in the case of the seminoma) cooperates to enhance the lethal effect of radiation. Such exceptions underscore the difficulties in making generalizations about the effectiveness of radiotherapy in particular cases. The only sure test is a therapeutic trial of radiation.

Dose is obviously important in determining the biologic effect of radiation. But in addition, when administered in divided doses (as is the usual practice in radiotherapy), *the rate of delivery significantly modifies the biologic effect.* Although the effect of radiant energy is cumulative, delivery in divided doses may allow cells to repair some of the damage in the intervals. The importance of repair of radiation damage is documented by genetic disorders such as *xeroderma pigmentosum*, discussed on page 274; individuals with this condition have a greatly increased vulnerability to skin cancers related to an inability to repair sunlight-induced dimers in the DNA of epidermal cells. *Thus, fractional dosages of radiant energy have a cumulative effect only to the extent that repair during the intervals is incomplete.* Radiotherapy of tumors exploits the fact that, in general, normal cells are capable of more rapid repair and recovery and so do not sustain as much cumulative radiation injury as tumor cells.

Oxygenation amplifies radiation damage to cells and tissues—"the oxygen effect." Radiant energy may interact with molecular oxygen to induce free radicals, such as superoxide, which can then interact with atoms and molecules to compound the cellular injury. The oxygen effect is significant in the radiotherapy of neoplasms. The center of rapidly growing tumors may be poorly vascularized and therefore somewhat hypoxic, making radiotherapy less effective.

EFFECTS ON CELLS AND TISSUES. Although radiant energy can affect cytoplasmic enzymes, macromolecules, and organelles, the most vulnerable target is nuclear DNA, with the following consequences:

In sufficient dosage radiation can inhibit indefinitely the cells' capacity to divide. This inhibition of cell proliferation is the usual mechanism by which radiation kills cells (except at extremely high levels of exposure). Selective inhibition of cell proliferation leading to cell killing during fetal development accounts for the somatic effects and teratogenicity of radiant energy.

Smaller doses of radiant energy may induce mutations and heritable or nonheritable alterations in metabolism that are compatible with cell survival and continued reproduction. When such injuries are heritable and involve germinal cells, overt or occult defects are transmitted to offspring.

Radiation is a potent cause of mutation and oncogenic transformation as was detailed in Chapter 6.

An overview of the mechanisms of action of radiation and its potential effects on cells is presented in Figure 9–24.

Cell killing by inhibition of proliferation is dependent on the life cycles of the various cell types in the body. Cells with a high turnover rate, such as the bone marrow and the mucosal epithelial cells of the stomach and small intestine, are understandably very vulnerable to cell death by inhibition of proliferation. At the other end of the spectrum are such nondividing cells as neurons or muscle cells which are consequently extremely radioresistant. Between these extremes, the more slowly dividing cells are particularly vulnerable to radiant energy during the G_2 phase (just prior to mitosis) and the M (mitotic) phase and are considerably less vulnerable during the S (synthetic) and G_1 (postmitotic) phases.

At the molecular level, the DNA sustains a variety of alterations depending on dosage, rate of delivery, and radiosensitivity of the cells. These include the formation of pyrimidine dimers, cross links, single-strand or double-strand breaks, and various rearrangements. Most DNA single-strand breaks are rapidly repaired, indeed within minutes. Double-strand breaks may also be joined promptly or more slowly, but some are irreparable. These alterations lead to a wide range of chromosomal and chromatid alterations including deletions, breaks, translocations, interad-

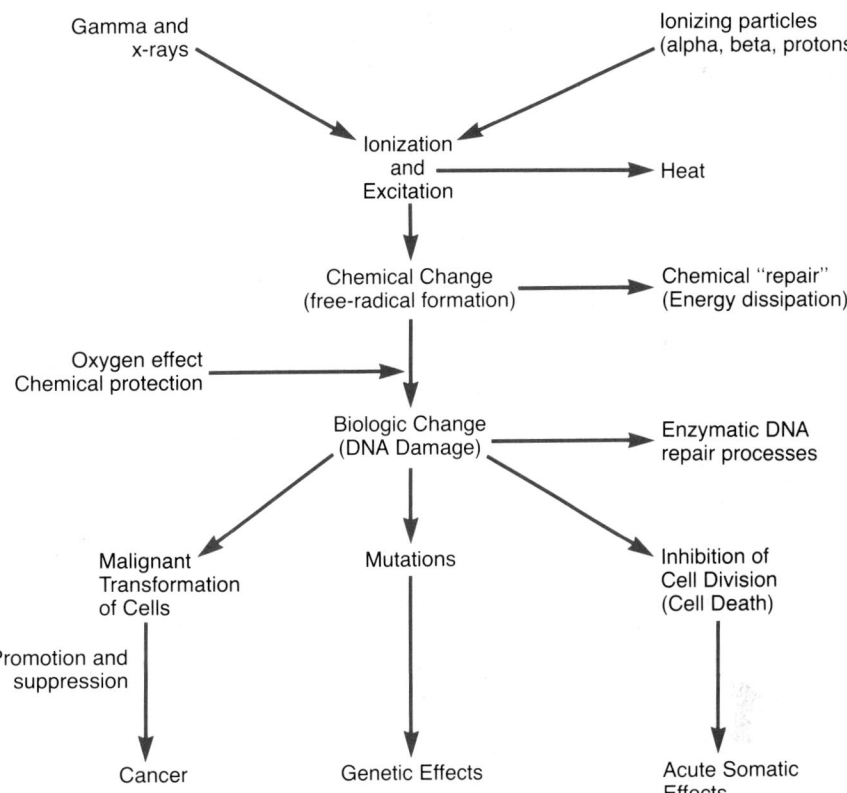

Figure 9–24. Development of radiation injury. (Reproduced with the kind permission of Dr. John B. Little, Harvard School of Public Health. From Little, J.B.: Biologic effects of low-level radiation exposure. *In* Taveras, J.M., and Ferrucci, J.T. (eds.): Radiology, Diagnosis — Imaging — Intervention. Vol. 1. Philadelphia, J.B. Lippincott Company, 1985.)

herence of chromosomes, fragmentation, and indeed all forms of abnormal chromosome morphology.[149] The mitotic spindle often becomes disorderly or even chaotic. Polyploidy and aneuploidy may be encountered. At the cellular level there may be nuclear swelling with condensation and clumping of the chromatin and sometimes nuclear membrane breaks. All forms of abnormal nuclear morphology may be produced. Giant cells with an extremely pleomorphic nucleus or more than one nucleus may appear and persist for years after exposure. At extremely high dosage levels of radiant energy, nuclear pyknosis or lysis appears quickly as a marker of early cell killing.

In addition to affecting DNA and nuclei, radiant energy may induce a variety of cytoplasmic changes including cytoplasmic swelling, mitochondrial distortion, and degeneration of the endoplasmic reticulum.[156] Plasma membrane breaks and focal defects may appear, and indeed some experts believe that cellular membranes constitute particularly sensitive targets to radiation.[157] To be noted: **The constellation of cellular pleomorphism, giant cell formation, conformational changes in nuclei, and mitotic figures creates a more than passing similarity between radiation-injured cells and cancer cells, a problem that plagues the pathologist when evaluating postirradiation tissues for the possible persistence of tumor cells.** Regrettably, there are no alterations at the level of the light or electron microscope that distinguish the effects of radiation from those caused by other damaging agents.

Vascular changes are prominent in all irradiated tissues (dose rate-dependent), be they normal or neoplastic. Endothelial cells are only moderately radioresponsive but, with the intensive therapy administered to tumors, radia-

tional changes are almost always seen in the vasculature of the neoplasm itself and in the normal tissues interposed between the source of the radiation and the neoplasm. During the immediate postirradiation period, vessels may show only dilatation, accounting for the erythema of the skin seen so often in radiotherapy. Later or with higher dosages, a variety of regressive changes appear, including endothelial cell swelling and vacuolation or even dissolution with total necrosis of the walls of small vessels (such as capillaries and venules). Affected vessels may rupture, yielding hemorrhages, or they may thrombose. For reasons unknown, these vascular changes are peculiarly spotty in their distribution along the course of a vessel and so, in the same tissue section, some channels are affected and others spared. In some part, the cancericidal effectiveness of radiation is attributable to such vascular damage. At a later stage, endothelial cell proliferation and collagenous hyalinization with thickening of the media are seen in irradiated vessels, resulting in marked narrowing or even obliteration of the vascular lumina.[158]

ORGAN SYSTEM CHANGES. The effect of radiation upon organs depends on the dose, type of tissue irradiated, and time lapse since irradiation. Injury may become apparent sometimes within days to months, or only after some time lapse (latency), which may be as long as many years.

The *skin* is in the pathway of all externally delivered radiation. The area of skin irradiated appears to be as critical as dose and type of radiation — the skin being more resistant to necrosis when only small areas

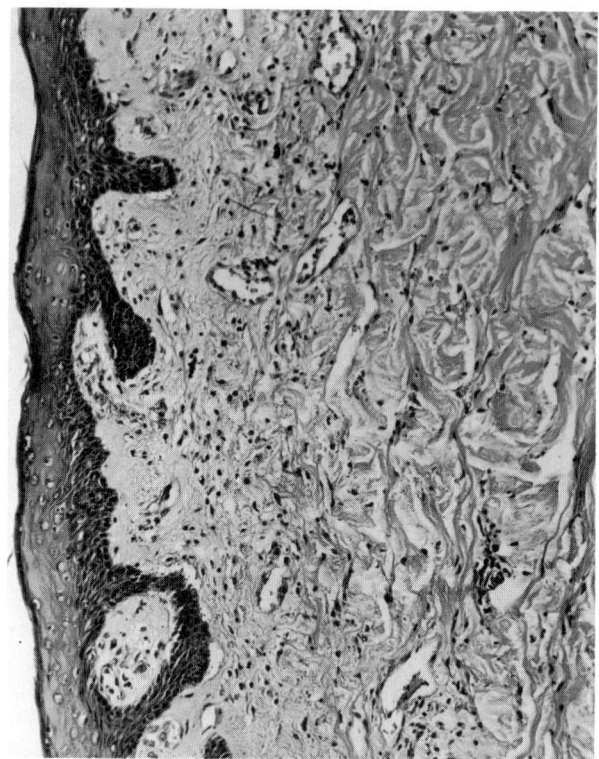

Figure 9–25. Chronic radiodermatitis. There is collagenous hyalinization of dermis, atrophy of skin appendages, and numerous dilated vascular telangiectases.

are exposed. Some regions of the skin are more susceptible than others, particularly those that are moist and subject to friction—the axilla, groin, and skin folds. Irradiated skin shows a range of changes from mild postirradiation erythema (two to three days), a postirradiation edema (two to three weeks), epithelial blistering and desquamation (four to six weeks), chronic radiodermatitis (months to years), to late-appearing cancers. Chronic radiodermatitis takes many forms, including blotchy increased pigmentation or depigmentation, hyperkeratosis, epilation (one to two months), skin atrophy, dermal and subcutaneous fibrosis, and in some instances, telangiectases and ulcerations (six months to five years) (Fig. 9–25). The epidermal cells may show any of the general cytologic alterations described previously, while the underlying dermis exhibits the characteristic radiation-induced vascular changes accompanied by hyaline collagenization of connective tissue and basophilic degeneration of elastic fibers. The atrophy, depigmentation, and telangiectasia commonly persist for decades.[159] Squamous cell cancers may appear as long as 56 years later but most commonly arise eight to ten years later.

The *hematopoietic and lymphoid systems* are extremely susceptible to radiant injury. With high dose levels and large exposure fields, severe lymphopenia may appear within hours of radiation, along with shrinkage of the lymph nodes and spleen. Radiation directly destroys lymphocytes, both in the circulating

blood and in tissues (nodes, spleen, thymus, gut) and causes all the cytologic disorganizations already described. With sublethal doses of irradiation, regeneration is prompt, however, from viable precursors, leading to restoration of the normal lymphocyte complement of the blood within weeks to months. The circulating granulocyte count may at first rise but begins to fall toward the end of the first week. Levels near zero may be reached during the second week. If the patient survives, recovery of the normal granulocyte counts may require two to three months. Platelets are similarly affected, with the nadir of the count occurring somewhat later than that of the granulocytes, while recovery is similarly delayed. The hematopoietic cells in the bone marrow are also quite sensitive to radiant energy, including the red cell precursors. The marrow may become virtually acellular weeks after heavy exposure and may contain only varying numbers of disintegrated cells. Erythrocytes are radioresistant, but anemia may appear after two to three weeks and be persistent for months because of marrow damage. Obviously, the severity of the blood and marrow depletion and its clinical significance depend on the dosage of radiation and the extent of marrow damage. Whole-body irradiation may be lethal. Localized exposure may have no effect on the circulating blood counts. The neutropenia and thrombocytopenia are responsible for increased susceptibility to infections and bleeding diatheses in the postirradiation period. If the patient survives these hazards and the hypoxic injury resulting from the anemia, regeneration from primitive precursors may yield complete recovery.

Studies of the survivors of the atomic bomb blasts have unmistakably demonstrated the leukemogenic effect of radiation (p. 511).

The *gonads* in both the male and the female, particularly the germ cells, are highly vulnerable to radiation injury, and sterility is a frequent residual of such damage. In the testis, spermatogonia, then spermatocytes, spermatids, and spermatozoa are radiosensitive in the order given. The cytologic changes to be observed are those already described (p. 506) but, as late residuals, there may be total atrophy and fibrosis with hyalinization of the testicular tubules. Sertoli cells and interstitial cells are radioresistant. Within the ovary, the germ cells and even more so the follicular granulosal cells are vulnerable. Indeed, for given dosages of the same form of radiation, sterility is more frequent in the female than in the male, principally because of radiation destruction of the ovarian follicles. Cessation of menses and menopausal changes may be temporary or permanent, depending on the dosage of radiation. In passing, it should be noted that the uterus and cervix are quite radioresistant and hence permit the installation of radioactive elements into the uterine cavity for the treatment of endometrial carcinomas.

The *lungs*, because of their rich vascularization, are vulnerable to radiation injury, and shortness of breath, coughing, and even acute fatal respiratory insufficiency may appear within weeks to months following sufficient exposure of large segments of the lung fields. During the acute phase, the endothelial cell changes described in the blood vessels are seen in the alveolar capillaries. The increased vascular permeability may lead to marked pulmonary congestion, edema, fibrin exudation, the formation of hyaline membranes, and even total filling of the air spaces by a rich proteinaceous and cellular debris, creating changes very similar to those seen in ARDS (p. 760). Later changes include fibrosis of the alveolar walls and the described vascular wall thickening and luminal narrowing (Fig. 9–26). The respiratory dysfunction may be crippling or fatal since the "radiation pneumonitis" creates a profound alveolocapillary block.

The *gastrointestinal tract* is quite radiosensitive and is frequently affected in all forms of deep radiation. Different portions of the gastrointestinal tract show differing sensitivities — the esophagus and rectum being relatively resistant while the midportions of the tract are quite sensitive. Soon after exposure, patients often have loss of appetite, nausea, and vomiting, and many develop severe diarrhea for a period of days. As might be expected, the intestinal epithelium is vulnerable because of its high turnover rate, and all forms of nuclear and cellular pleomorphism along with mitotic abnormalities are seen in mucosal cells in the postirradiation period. Mucosal edema,

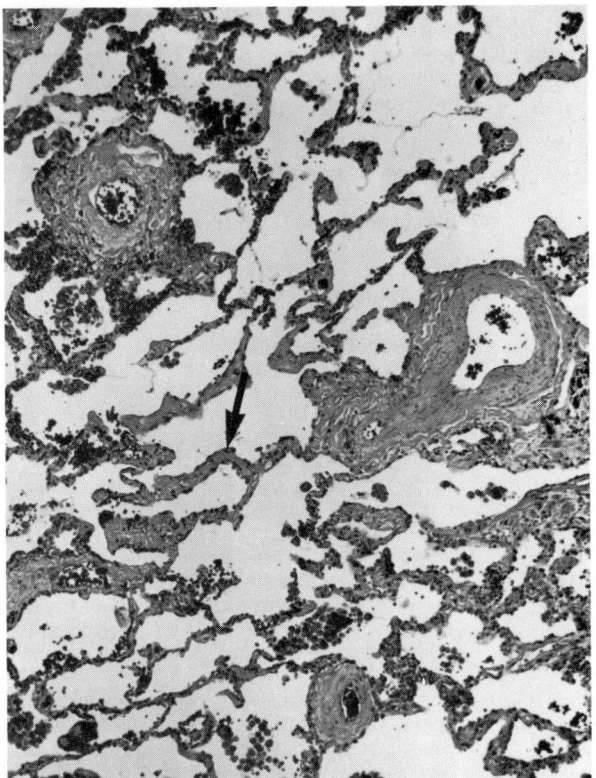

Figure 9–26. Chronic radiation damage to lungs. Note collagenous hyaline thickening of blood vessel walls and fibrosis of septal walls (arrow).

hyperemia, and ulcerations may appear, accompanied by vascular and connective tissue changes in the submucosa at all levels from the mouth to the anus. Later effects comprise mucosal and submucosal atrophy and fibrosis, accompanied sometimes by similar atrophy and fibrosis of the muscularis. These changes may indeed cause intestinal and esophageal strictures or even complete obstruction.

The *brain* in the adult is relatively radioresistant. It is quite radiosensitive during embryonic development when nerve cells and glial cells are especially affected; relatively small doses of radiation in animals have caused severe damage to the developing central nervous system. Adult nervous tissue, on the other hand, is relatively radioresistant. Sufficiently high doses even in the adult may damage astrocytes and cause late-appearing injury to neurons.[160] However, functional changes may appear during the immediate postirradiation period even though no morphologic changes are visible in the neurons. Necrosis of the brain and spinal cord has been reported following high dosages of radiation, presumably due to involvement of the small blood vessels.

A summary of the organs affected particularly often is presented in Figure 9–27, but ultimately, all organs and cells are vulnerable to sufficiently high levels of radiant energy. Those not already mentioned are relatively radioresistant, e.g., the thyroid, parathyroid, pituitary, and adrenal glands, the liver, mature bone, and cartilage. Growing bone and cartilage are, however, relatively radiosensitive, and development has been stunted in survivors of atomic bomb blasts who were exposed during childhood. Even though the kidneys are not very radiosensitive, they sometimes develop so-called radiation nephritis, following sufficient exposure.

TOTAL BODY RADIATION. Exposure of large areas of the body to even very small doses of radiation may have devastating effects.[161] As little as 100 to 300 rad of radiant energy in total-body exposure delivered in one dose may induce an "acute radiation syndrome." To place this radiation level in context, it must be appreciated that 4000 rad or more are often used in carefully shielded patients in the radiotherapy of tumors. Warren has provided an excellent summary of the significance of various levels of whole-body exposure (Table 9–6).[162] The lethal range for man begins at about 200 rad of total-body radiation, but is quite certain at 700 rad without medical intervention.[163] Based on these consequences, three often fatal acute radiation syndromes have been segregated: (1) hematopoietic, (2) gastrointestinal, and (3) cerebral.

The *hematopoietic syndrome* is encountered with the absorption of between 200 and 500 rad. It usually begins with mild gastrointestinal symptoms related to injury to the radiosensitive mucosal lining of the gut; these subside to be followed within days by lymphopenia, thrombocytopenia, neutropenia, and eventually anemia according to the sequence described on

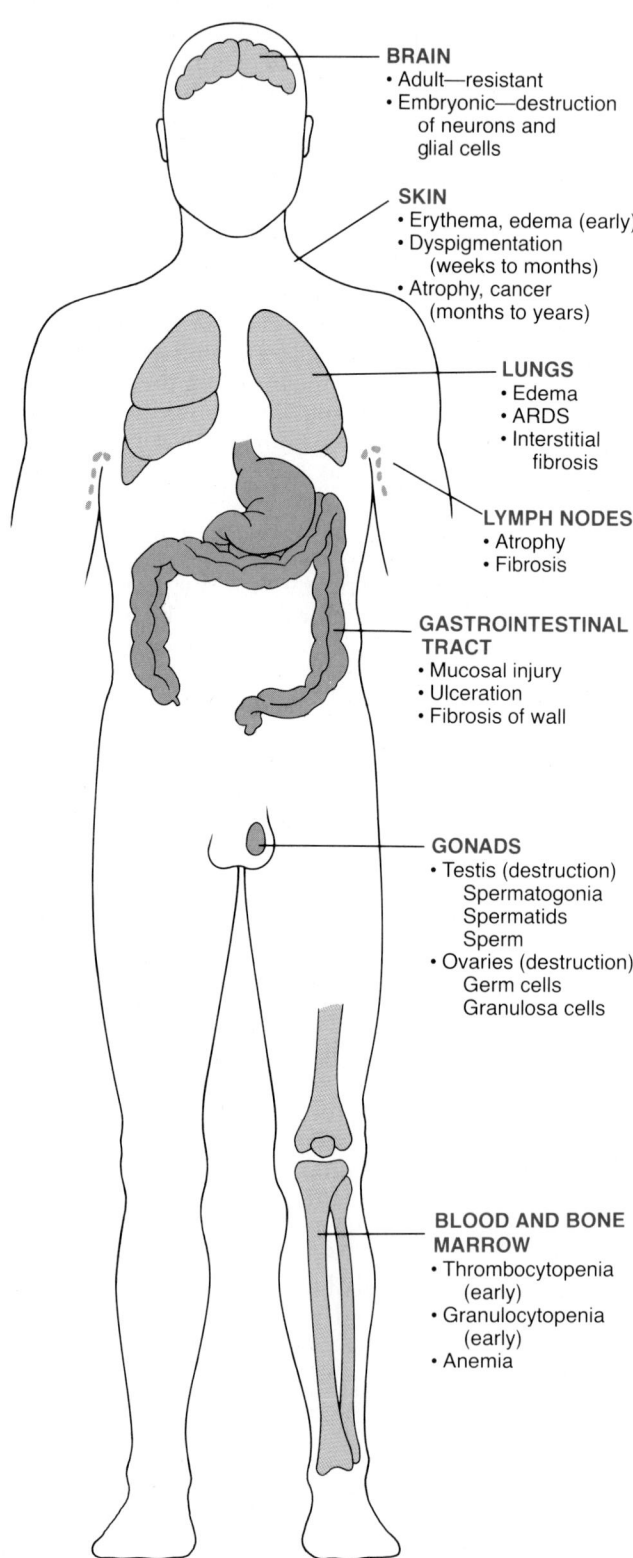

BRAIN
• Adult—resistant
• Embryonic—destruction
  of neurons and
  glial cells

SKIN
• Erythema, edema (early)
• Dyspigmentation
  (weeks to months)
• Atrophy, cancer
  (months to years)

LUNGS
• Edema
• ARDS
• Interstitial
  fibrosis

LYMPH NODES
• Atrophy
• Fibrosis

**GASTROINTESTINAL
TRACT**
• Mucosal injury
• Ulceration
• Fibrosis of wall

GONADS
• Testis (destruction)
  Spermatogonia
  Spermatids
  Sperm
• Ovaries (destruction)
  Germ cells
  Granulosa cells

**BLOOD AND BONE
MARROW**
• Thrombocytopenia
  (early)
• Granulocytopenia
  (early)
• Anemia

Figure 9–27. An overview of the major morphologic consequences of radiation injury.

page 508. As a consequence of these changes, bleeding problems or infections may make their appearance and are responsible for death in up to 50% of the victims.

The *gastrointestinal syndrome* occurs with a larger dose of absorbed radiation, on the order of 500 to 1000 rad. It is marked by nausea, vomiting, severe diarrhea, and sepsis. The loss of fluids may lead to dehydration, contraction of the effective circulating blood volume, vascular collapse, and death, usually within three to four days. These clinical signs and symptoms are related to widely scattered cell death throughout the body, particularly prominent in the bone marrow and actively replicating mucosal cells of the gastrointestinal tract. If the acute vascular collapse is effectively treated by massive plasma replacement, the hematopoietic syndrome almost always makes its appearance one to two days later.

The *cerebral syndrome* appears when the absorbed dose is greater than 5000 rad. It is always fatal and is characterized by listlessness and drowsiness, soon followed by convulsions, coma, and death within one to two hours.

Table 9–6. Expected Short-Term Effects from Acute Whole Body Radiation

DOSE IN RADS	PROBABLE EFFECT
10 to 50	No obvious effect except, probably, minor blood changes
50 to 100	Vomiting and nausea for about one day in 5 to 10% of exposed personnel. Fatigue, but no serious disability. Transient reduction in lymphocytes and neutrophils.
100 to 200	Vomiting and nausea for about one day, followed by other symptoms of radiatiion sickness in about 20 to 50% of personnel. No deaths anticipated. A reduction of approximately 50% in lymphocytes and neutrophils will occur.
200 to 350	Vomiting and nausea in nearly all personnel on first day, followed by other symptoms of radiation sickness, e.g., loss of appetite, diarrhea, minor hemorrhage. About 20% die within 2 to 6 weeks after exposure; survivors convalesce for about 3 months, although many have a second wave of symptoms at about 3 weeks. Up to 75% reduction in all circulating blood elements.
350 to 550	Vomiting and nausea in most personnel on first day, followed by other symptoms of radiation sickness, e.g., fever, hemorrhage, diarrhea, emaciation. About 50% die within one month; survivors convalesce for about 6 months.
550 to 750	Vomiting and nausea (or at least nausea) in all personnel within 4 hours after exposure, followed by severe symptoms of radiation sickness, as above. Up to 100% die, few survivors convalesce for about 6 months.
1000	Vomiting and nausea in all personnel within 1 to 2 hours. All die within days.
5000	Incapacitation almost immediately (minutes to hours). All personnel will die within one week.

From Warren, S.: Ionizing radiation. *In* Bioastronautics Data Book. 2nd ed. Washington, D.C., NASA, 1973.

In addition to these more or less "acute syndromes," total-body irradiation may result in a number of late-appearing sequelae. These have been graphically documented in the survivors at Hiroshima and Nagasaki; the tragic consequences of the atomic blasts will be briefly reviewed "lest we forget." Morgan has movingly detailed the events.[164] The great preponderance of the more than 100,000 immediate or relatively early fatalities at these cities were the result of the blast injuries and the following fire storms that engulfed these cities. Thousands more died from "acute radiation syndromes" and their sequelae. Months to years later a variety of forms of neoplasia began to appear, following the usual age distribution of each cancer but at higher rates than in nonexposed populations. A 20-fold increased incidence of acute leukemia has occurred in those who were less than 10 years or over 50 years of age at the time of the blasts. The latent period for the appearance of these leukemias in children was approximately five to ten years, whereas in adults it was 10 to 20 years. These disorders took the forms of acute lymphocytic, acute myelogenous, and chronic myelogenous leukemia but, for unknown reasons, chronic lymphocytic leukemia was rarely induced. In children under ten years of age at the time there has been an increased incidence of breast cancer (in females) and thyroid cancer as well as possibly lymphoma, multiple myeloma, and cancers of the stomach, esophagus, urinary tract, and salivary glands.[165,166] Individuals 50 years of age or older at the time of exposure have suffered a notable increase in the incidence of lung cancer. These postirradiation oncogenic changes are discussed in greater detail on page 274. In addition, atomic bomb survivors have developed lenticular opacities and persistent chromosomal aberrations in lymphocytes. Even those exposed in utero were not spared and have manifested an increased frequency of microcephaly and mental retardation.[167]

The atomic blasts make all too evident the injury-producing potential of radiant energy, albeit of enormous doses delivered within an instant in time. Studies of British patients with ankylosing spondylitis who were irradiated for treatment of their disease have documented the oncogenic potential of therapeutic exposure. Because of its cumulative effects there is understandably great concern about low-level radiation, as may be emitted from nuclear reactors and improper disposal of nuclear wastes. To date, clear documentation of carcinogenicity has not appeared, but the long latency is not comforting. There is ample evidence that low-level radiation may be carcinogenic. In few areas of medicine is the old dictum more applicable — be sure that the treatment is not worse than the disease.

NON-IONIZING RADIATION

It would be imprudent to conclude a chapter on environmental pathology without calling attention to the possible dangers of ultrasound, microwave, and laser energy. Although all of them find increasingly wide usage for medical, domestic, and industrial purposes, few data are available regarding their impact on man.[168] The cell destructiveness of laser beams is currently in the exploratory stage as a modality of therapy. Experiments in lower animals have shown that microwaves may cause cellular changes in the lens, bone marrow, and endocrine glands and may possibly have DNA-damaging potential. Unquestionably, some of this injury is due to the thermal effect, which is, of course, the virtue of microwave ovens. Ultrasound, too, has been shown to alter nerve transmission in lower animal forms, but once again it may relate to thermal effects. With the growing use of sonography in obstetrics and the widespread domestic and industrial use of ultrasonic cleaning devices and microwave ovens, we can only hope that these forms of energy will prove to have no late-appearing adverse effects.

1. Lippmann, M., and Lioy, P.J.: Critical issues in air pollution epidemiology. Environ. Health Perspect. *62*:243, 1985.

2. Environmental Quality — 1980. The 15th Annual Report of the Council on Environmental Quality. Washington, D.C., U.S. Government Printing Office, 1984, p. 11.

3. Davidson, C.I., et al.: Indoor and outdoor air pollution in the Himalayas. Environ. Sci. Technol. *20*:561, 1986.

4. National Center for Health Statistics: The National Health Interview Survey 1983. Hyattsville, Maryland, U.S. Department of Health and Human Services, 1983.

5. United States Department of Health and Human Services: Smoking and Health; a National Status Report. Rockville, Maryland, Public Health Service, Centers for Disease Control, 1986, p. 7.

6. Fielding, J.E.: Smoking: Health effects and control. N. Engl. J. Med. *313*:491,1985.

7. Hammond, E.C., and Horn, D.: Smoking and death rates. Report on 44 months of follow-up of 187,783 men. CA, A Cancer Journal for Clinicians *38*:28, 1988.

8. United States Department of Health and Human Services: The Health Consequences of Smoking: Cancer. A Report of the Surgeon General, 1982. DHHS publication No. (PHS)82-50179. Washington, D.C., Public Health Service, Office of Smoking and Health, U.S. Government Printing Office, 1982.

9. Reuben, D.H., et al.: Effect of passive smoking on birthweight. Lancet *2*:415, 1986.

10. Bross, I.D., and Gibson, R.: Risks of lung cancer in smokers who switched to filter cigarettes. Am J. Public Health *58*:1396, 1968.

11. Miller, G.H.: The "less hazardous" cigarette: A deadly delusion. N.Y. State J. Med. *85*:313, 1985.

12. Federal Trade Commission: Tar, Nicotine, and Carbon Monoxide of the Smoke of 207 Varieties of Domestic Cigarettes. Washington, D.C., U.S. Government Printing Office, January 1985.

13. Minty, B.D.: Some short term effects of changing to lower yield cigarettes. Chest *88*:531, 1985.

14. Castelli, W.P., et al. The filter cigarette and coronary heart disease: The Framingham Study. Lancet *2*:109, 1981.

15. Vutuc, C., and Kunze, M.: Tar yields of cigarettes and male lung cancer risk. J. Natl. Cancer Inst. *71*:435, 1983.

16. Lubin, J.H., et al.: Patterns of lung cancer risk according to type of cigarette smoked. Int. J. Cancer *55*:569, 1984.

17. Rosenberg, L., et al.: The risk of myocardial infarction after quitting smoking in men under 55 years of age. N. Engl. J. Med. *313*:1511, 1985.

18. Jarvis, M.J., et al. Absorption of nicotine and carbon monoxide from passive smoking under natural conditions of exposure. Thorax *38*:829, 1983.

19. Ferris, B.J., Jr., et al.: Effects of passive smoking on health of children. Environ. Health Perspect. *62*:289, 1985.

20. White, J.R., and Froeb, H.F.: Small airways dysfunction in non-smokers chronically exposed to tobacco smoke. N. Engl. J. Med. *302*:720, 1980.

21. Blott, W.J., and Fraumeni, J.F., Jr.: Passive smoking and lung cancer. J. Natl. Cancer Inst. *77*:993, 1986.

22. Fielding, J.E., and Phenow, K.J.: Health effects of involuntary smoking. N. Engl. J. Med. *319*:1452, 1988.

23. Connolly, G.N., et al.: The reemergence of smokeless tobacco. N. Engl. J. Med. *314*:1020, 1986.

24. Consensus Development Conference Statement: Health Implications of Smokeless Tobacco Use. Bethesda, Maryland, National Institutes of Health, 1986.

25. Editorial: Oral snuff: A preventable carcinogenic hazard. Lancet *2*:198, 1986.

26. Abraham, J.I.: Recent advance in pneumoconioses: The pathologist's role in etiologic diagnosis. Monogr. Pathol. *19*:96, 1978.

27. Green, F.H.Y., and Laqueur, N.A.: Coal workers' pneumoconiosis. Pathol. Annu. *15(pt.2)*:333, 1980.

28. Hurley, J.F., and Soutar, C.A.: Can exposure to coal mine dust cause a severe impairment of lung function? Br. J. Ind. Med. *43*:150, 1986.

29. Shennan, D.H., et al. Practice predisposing to the development of progressive massive fibrosis in coal miners. Br. J. Ind. Med. *38*:321, 1981.

30. Editorial: Coal and the lung. Thorax *38*:241, 1983.

31. Kockroft, A., et al.: Postmortem study of emphysema in coal workers and non-coal workers. Lancet *2*:600, 1982.

32. Kleinerman, J., et al.: Pathology standards for coal workers' pneumoconiosis. Arch. Pathol. Lab. Med. *103*:375, 1979.

33. Attfield, M., et al.: The incidence and progression of pneumoconiosis over 9 years in U.S. coal miners: No. 1, principal findings. Am. J. Ind. Med. *6*:407, 1984.

34. Seaton, A., et al.: Quartz and pneumoconiosis in coal miners. Lancet *2*:1272, 1981.

35. Chin, J., et al.: Identification of a high affinity receptor for native human interleukin 1-beta and interleukin 1-alpha on normal human lung fibroblasts. J. Exp. Med. *165*:70, 1987.

36. Soutar, C.A., and Hurley, J.F.: Relation between dust exposure and lung function in miners and ex-miners. Br. J. Ind. Med. *43*:307, 1986.

37. Ames, R.G.: Does coal workers' pneumoconiosis predict to lung cancer? Some evidence from a case-control study. J. Soc. Occup. Med. *33*:141, 1982.

38. Miller, B.G., and Jacobsen, M.: Dust exposure, pneumoconiosis, and mortality of coal miners. Br. J. Ind. Med. *42*:723, 1955.

39. Snider, D.E.: The relationship between silicosis and tuberculosis. Am. Rev. Respir. Dis. *118*:455, 1978.

40. Bowden, D.H., and Adamson, I.Y.R.: The role of cell injury and continuing inflammatory response in the generation of silicotic pulmonary fibrosis. J. Pathol. *144*:149, 1984.

41. Schmidt, J.A., et al.: Silica-stimulated monocytes release fibroblast proliferation factors identical to interleukin-1. A potential role of interleukin-1 in the pathogenesis of silicosis. J. Clin. Invest. *73*:1462, 1984.

42. Doll, N.J., et al.: Immunopathogenesis of asbestosis, silicosis, and coal workers' pneumoconiosis. Clin. Chest Med. *4*:3, 1983.

43. Editorial: New York Times, September 7, 1982.

44. Craighead, J.E., and Mossman, B.T.: The pathogenesis of asbestos-associated diseases. N. Engl. J. Med. *306*:1446, 1982.

45. Kagan, E.: Current perspectives in asbestosis. Ann. Allergy *54*:464, 1985.

46. Barkey, B.: Asbestos exposure. An update on pleural pulmonary hazards. Postgrad. Med. *74*:93, 1983.

47. Vianna, N.J., and Pola, A.K.: Nonoccupational exposure to asbestos and malignant mesothelioma in females. Lancet *1*:1061, 1978.

48. Warnock, M.L., et al.: The relation of asbestos burden to asbestosis and lung cancer. Pathol. Annu. *18(pt. 2)*:109, 1983.

49. Browne, K.: Is asbestos or asbestosis the cause of the increased risk of lung cancer in asbestos workers? Br. J. Ind. Med. *43*:145, 1986.

50. DeShazo, R.D.: Current concepts about the pathogenesis of silicosis and asbestosis. J. Allergy Clin. Immunol. *70*:41, 1982.

51. Lemaire, I., et al.: Alveolar macrophage stimulation of lung fi-broblast growth in asbestos induced pulmonary fibrosis. Am. J. Pathol. *122*:205, 1986.

52. Mossman, B., et al.: Asbestos: Mechanisms of toxicity and carcinogenicity in the respiratory tract. Annu. Rev. Pharmacol. Toxicol. *23*:595, 1983.

53. Tanaka, S., et al.: Beryllium disease. Necessity for continuing surveillance. Chest *84*:312, 1983.

54. Rom, W.N., et al.: Pneumoconiosis and exposures of dental laboratory technicians. Am. J. Public Health *74*:1252, 1984.

55. Constantinidis, K.: Acute and chronic beryllium disease. Br. J. Clin. Pract. *32*:127, 1978.

56. Wagoner, J.K., et al.: Beryllium: An etiologic agent in the induction of lung cancer, nonneoplastic respiratory disease, and heart disease among industrially exposed workers. Environ. Res. *21*:15, 1980.

57. Reynolds, H.Y.: Hypersensitivity pneumonitis. Clin. Chest Med. *3*:503, 1982.

58. National Institute of Mental Health: Mental Health, United States 1985. Taube, C.A., and Barrett, S.A. (eds.). Washington, D.C., U.S. Department of Health and Human Services, Public Health Service, Alcohol, Drug Abuse, and Mental Health Administration, 1985.

59. Trinkoff, A.M., and Baker, S.P.: Poisoning hospitalizations and deaths from solids and liquids among children and teenagers. Am. J. Public Health *76*:657, 1986.

60. Litovitz, T.L., et al.: 1985 annual report of the American Association of Poison Control Centers National Data Collection System. Am. J. Emerg. Med. *4*:427, 1985.

61. Rensberger, B.: Bad prescriptions kill thousands a year. New York Times, January 28, 1976.

62. Irey, N.S.: Adverse drug reactions and death. A review of 827 cases. J.A.M.A. *236*:575, 1976.

63. Ingelfinger, F.J.: Adverse drug reactions that count. N. Engl. J. Med. *294*:1003, 1976.

64. Jick, H.: Drugs—remarkably nontoxic. N. Engl. J. Med. *291*:824, 1974.

65. Hennigar, G.R.: Iatrogenic drug toxicity. *In* Scarpelli, D.G., et al. (eds.): The Pathologist and the Environment. Baltimore, Williams & Wilkins, 1985. p. 32.

66. Lawson, D.H.: Adverse drug reactions. Hum. Toxicol. *4*:122, 1985.

67. Dukes, M.N.G.: Meyler's Side Effects of Drugs. 9th Ed. Amsterdam, Excerpta Medica, 1980.

68. Brown, B.R., Jr.: Halothane hepatitis revisited. N. Engl. J. Med. *313*:1347, 1985.

69. Vergani, D., et al.: Antibodies to the surface of halothane-altered rabbit hepatocytes in patients with severe halothane-associated hepatitis. N. Engl. J. Med. *303*:66, 1980.

70. Farrell, G.C.: The hepatic side effects of drugs. Med. J. Aust. *145*:600, 1986.

71. Mitchell, J.R., et al.: Isoniazid liver injury. Clinical spectrum, pathology, and probable pathogenesis. Ann. Intern. Med. *84*:181, 1976.

72. Riggs, B.L., and Melton, L.J., III: Involutional osteoporosis. N. Engl. J. Med. *314*:1676, 1986.

73. Shapiro, S., et al.: Risk of localized and widespread endometrial cancer correlation to recent and discontinued use of conjugated estrogens. N. Engl. J. Med. *313*:969, 1985.

74. Judd, H.L., et al.: Estrogen replacement therapy: Indications and complications. Ann.. Intern. Med. *98*:195, 1983.

75. Greenberg, E.R., et al.: Breast cancer in mothers given diethylstilbestrol in pregnancy. N. Engl. J. Med. *311*:1393, 1984.

76. Stampfer, M.J, et al.: A prospective study of postmenopausal estrogen therapy in coronary heart disease. N. Engl. J. Med. *313*:1044, 1985.

77. Wilson, P.W.F., et al.: Postmenopausal estrogen use and cigarette smoking and cardiovascular morbidity in women over 50: The Framingham Study. N. Engl. J. Med. *313*:1038, 1985.

78. Meirik, O., et al.: Oral contraceptive use and breast cancer in young women. A joint national case-controlled study in Sweden and Norway. Lancet *2*:650, 1986.

79. Sattin, R.W., et al.: Oral contraceptive use and the risk of breast cancer: The cancer and steroid hormone study of the Centers for Disease Control and the National Institute of Child Health and Human Development. N. Engl. J. Med. *315*:405, 1986.

80. Editorial: Cancer risks of oral contraception. Lancet *1*:21, 1989.

81. Beral, V., et al.: Oral contraceptive use and malignancies of the genital tract. Lancet 2:1331, 1988.

82. Cancer and Steroid Hormone Study of the Centers for Disease Control and the National Institute of Child Health and Human Development: The reduction in risk of ovarian cancer associated with oral contraceptive use. N. Engl. J. Med. 316:650, 1987.

83. Blayney, D.W., et al.: Decreasing risk of leukemia with prolonged follow-up after chemotherapy and radiotherapy for Hodgkin's disease. N. Engl. J. Med. 316:710, 1987.

84. Calabresi, P.: Leukemia after cytotoxic chemotherapy—a pyrrhic victory. N. Engl. J. Med. 309:1118, 1983.

85. Bowin J.-F., et al.: Second primary cancers following treatment of Hodgkin's disease. J. Natl. Cancer Inst. 72:233, 1984.

86. Bedrossian, C.W., et al.: Azathioprine-associated interstitial pneumonitis. Am. J. Clin. Pathol. 82:148, 1984.

87. Palestine, A.G., et al.: Renal histopathologic alterations in patients treated with cyclosporine for uveitis. N. Engl. J. Med. 314:1293, 1986.

88. Lieber, C.S.: Biochemical and molecular basis of alcohol-induced injury to liver and other tissues. N. Engl. J Med. 319:1639, 1988.

89. Bosron, W.F., and Li, T.K.: Genetic polymorphism of human liver alcohol and aldehyde dehydrogenases and their relationship to alcohol metabolism and alcoholism. Hepatology 6:502, 1986.

90. Mendelson, J.H., and Mello, N.K.: Biologic concomitants of alcoholism. N. Engl. J. Med. 301:912, 1979.

91. Edmondson, H.A.: Pathology of alcoholism. Am. J. Clin. Pathol. 74:725, 1980.

92. Szabo, S.: Mechanisms of mucosal injury in the stomach and duodenum: Time sequence analysis of morphologic, functional, biochemical, and histochemical studies. Scand. J. Gastroenterol. 22(Suppl. 127):21, 1987.

93. Fink, R., et al.: Increased free radical activity in alcoholics. Lancet 2:291, 1985.

94. Laposata, E.A., and Lange, L.G.: Presence of nonoxidative ethanol metabolism in human organs commonly damaged by ethanol abuse. Science 231:497, 1986.

95. Editorial: Alcoholic cardiomyopathy. S. Afr. Med. J. 53:917, 1978.

96. Editorial: Alcoholic disease. Lancet 1:1105, 1982

97. Pollack, E.S., et al.: Prospective study of alcohol consumption and cancer. N. Engl. J. Med. 310:617, 1984.

98. Keeney, A.H., and Mellinkoff, S.M.: Methyl alcohol poisoning. Ann. Intern. Med. 34:331, 1951.

99. Centers for Disease Control: Preventing lead poisoning in young children. A statement by the Centers for Disease Control. Rockville, Maryland, Publications Office, Center for Environmental Health, January 1985.

100. Fergusson, J.E.: Lead: Petrol lead in the environment and its contribution to human blood lead levels. Sci. Total Environ. 50:1, 1986.

101. Mahaffey, K.R., et al.: National estimates of blood lead levels: United States, 1976–1980. Association with selected demographic and socioeconomic factors. N. Engl. J. Med. 307:573, 1982.

102. Neggers, Y.H., and Stitt, K.R.: Effects of high lead intake in children. J. Am. Diet. Assoc. 86:938, 1986.

103. Lenihan, J.: Hazards from lead in the environment. Practitioner 227:1373, 1983.

104. Duggan, M.J., and Inskip, M.J.: Childhood exposure to lead in surface dust and soil: A community health problem. Public Health Rev. 13:1, 1985.

105. Bellinger, D.: Longitudinal analyses of prenatal and postnatal lead exposure and early cognitive development. N. Engl. J. Med. 316:1037, 1987.

106. Bushnell, P.J., and Jaeger, R.J.: Hazards to health from environmental lead exposure. A review of recent literature. Vet. Hum. Toxicol. 28:255, 1986.

107. Chisolm, J.J.: The continuing hazard of lead exposure and its effects in children. Neurotoxicology 5:23, 1984.

107a. McMichael, A.J., et al.: Port Pirie cohort study: environmental exposure to lead and children's abilities at the age of four years. N. Engl. J. Med. 319:468, 1988.

108. Bennett, W.M.: Lead nephropathy. Kidney Int. 28:212, 1985.

109. Dalgaard, J.B.: Postmortem findings in carbon monoxide deaths. Acta Pathol. Microbiol. Scand. 154(Suppl.):186, 1962.

110. Ernst, P., and Theriault, G.: Known occupational carcinogens and their significance. Can. Med. Assoc. J. 130:863, 1984.

111. Haley, T.J.: Occupational cancer and chemical structure: Past, present, and future. Drug Metab. Rev. 15:919, 1984.

112. Editorial: Epidemiology of drug uses. Lancet 1:147, 1985.

113. Ableson, H.I., et al.: A decade of trends in cocaine use in the household population. Rockville, Maryland, National Institute of Drug Abuse Research Monograph, Series 61, 1985, p. 35.

114. Nicholi, A.M., Jr.: The nontherapeutic use of psychoactive drugs. A modern epidemic. N. Engl. J. Med. 308:925, 1983.

115. Kulberg, A.: Substance abuse: Clinical identification and management. Pediatr. Clin. North Am. 33:325, 1987.

116. Wu, T.-C., et al.: Pulmonary hazards of smoking marijuana as compared with tobacco. N. Engl. J. Med. 318:347, 1988.

117. Kandel, D.B., et al.: The epidemiology of adolescent drug use in France and Israel. Am. J. Public Health 71:256, 1981.

118. Crigler, L.L., and Mark, H.: Medical complications of cocaine abuse. N. Engl. J. Med. 315:1495, 1986.

119. Tazelaar, H.D., et al.: Cocaine and the heart. Hum. Pathol. 18:195, 1987.

120. Isner, J.M., et al.: Acute cardiac events temporally related to cocaine abuse. N. Engl. J. Med. 315:1438, 1986.

121. Ostor, A.G.: The medical complications of narcotic addiction. Med. J. Aust. 1:410,448,497, 1977.

122. Stern, W.Z., and Subbarao, K.: Pulmonary complications of drug addiction. Semin. Roentgenol. 18:183, 1983.

123. Blank, R.R., et al.: Infectious complications of illicit drug use. Int. J. Addict. 19:221, 1984.

124. Cunningham, E.E., et al.: Heroin nephropathy: A clinical pathologic and epidemiologic study. Am. J. Med. 68:47, 1980.

125. Johnston, L.D., et al.: Monitoring the future: Questionnaire from the nation's high school seniors 1979. Ann Arbor, Survey Research Center, University of Michigan, 1980.

126. Hollister, L.E.: Health aspects of cannabis. Pharmacol. Rev. 38:1, 1986.

127. Maykut, M.O.: Health consequences of acute and chronic marijuana use. Prog. Neuropsychopharmacol. Biol. Psychiatry 9:209, 1985.

128. Linn, S., et al.: The association of marijuana use with outcome of pregnancy. Am. J. Public Health 73:1161, 1983.

129. Andreasson, S., et al.: Cannabis and schizophrenia. A longitudinal study of Swedish conscripts. Lancet 2:1483, 1987.

130. Relman, A.S.: Marijuana and health. N. Engl. J. Med. 306:603, 1982.

131. Matsumura, F., and Madhukar, B.V.: Exposure to insecticides. Pharmacol. Ther. 9:27, 1980.

132. Anous, M.M., and Heimbach, D.M.: Causes of death and predictors in burned patients more than 60 years of age. J. Trauma 26:135, 1986.

133. Cuppage, F.E., et al.: Morphologic changes in rhesus monkey skin after acute burn. Arch Pathol. 195:402, 1975.

134. Cotran, R.S., and Remensnyder, J.P.: The structural basis of increased vascular permeability after graded thermal injury—light and electron microscopic studies. Ann. N.Y. Acad. Sci. 150:495, 1968.

135. Gelfand, J.A.: Infections in burned patients: A paradigm for cutaneous infection in the patient at risk. Am. J. Med. 76:158, 1984.

136. Teplitz, C.: Pathology of burns. In Artz, C.P., and Moncrief, J.A. (eds.): The Treatment of Burns. 2nd Ed. Philadelphia, W.B. Saunders Company, 1969, p. 22.

137. Stratta, R.J., et al.: Immunologic parameters in burned patients: Effect of therapeutic interventions. J. Trauma 26:7, 1986.

138. Blazar, B.A., et al.: Suppression of natural killer cell function in humans following thermal and traumatic injury. J. Clin. Immunol. 6:26, 1986.

139. Tribble, C.G., et al.: Lightning injuries. Compr. Ther. 11:32, 1985.

140. Jones, R.R.: Ozone depletion and cancer risk. Lancet 2:443, 1987.

141. Stern, R.S., et al.: Risk reduction for nonmelanoma skin cancer with childhood sunscreen use. Arch. Dermatol. 122:537, 1986.

142. Green, A., et al.: Sunburn and malignant melanoma. Br. J. Cancer 51:393, 1985.

143. Radford, E.P.: Potential health effects of indoor radon exposure. Environ. Health Perspect. 62:281, 1985.

144. Saccomanno, G., et al.: An epidemiological analysis of the relationship between exposure to Rn progeny, smoking, and bronchogenic carcinoma in the U-mining population of the Colorado Plateau — 1960–1980. Health Physics *50*:605, 1986.

145. Cross, F.T., et al.: Health effects and risks from ^{222}Rn in drinking water. Health Physics *48*:649, 1985.

146. Upton, A.C.: Radiation injury: Past, present, and future. *In* Hill, R.B., and Terzian, J.A. (eds.): Environmental Pathology, An Evolving Field. New York, Alan R. Liss, 1982, p. 9.

147. Lyon, J.L.: Radiation exposure and cancer. Hosp. Pract. *19*:159, 1984.

148. Johns, H.E., and Cunningham, J.R.: The Physics of Radiology. 3rd Ed. Springfield, Illinois, Charles C Thomas, 1969.

149. Pizzarello, D.J., and Witcofski, R.L.: Basic Radiation Biology. 2nd Ed. Philadelphia, Lea & Febiger, 1975.

150. Dalrymple, G.V., et al. (eds.): Medical Radiation Biology. Philadelphia, W.B. Saunders Company, 1973.

151. Hutchinson, F.: The molecular basis for radiation effects on cells. Cancer Res. *26*:2045, 1966.

152. Mettler, F.A., Jr., and Moseley, R.D., Jr.: Medical Effects of Ionizing Radiation. Orlando, Grune & Stratton, 1985.

153. Mettler, F.A., Jr., and Moseley, R.D., Jr.: Medical Effects of Ionizing Radiation. Orlando, Grune & Stratton, 1985, p. 5.

154. Rugh, R.: Damage to cells by ionizing radiation. Atompraxis *14*:13, 1968.

155. Anderson Hospital and Tumor Institute: Cellular Radiation Biology. Eighteenth Symposium on Fundamental Cancer Research, Houston, 1964. Baltimore, Williams & Wilkins Company, 1965.

156. Mettler, F.A., Jr., and Moseley, R.D., Jr.: Medical Effects of Ionizing Radiation. Orlando, Grune & Stratton, 1985, p. 18.

157. Chandra, S., and Stephani, S.: Plasma membrane as a sensitive target in radiation-induced cell injury and death: An ultrastructural study. Int. J. Radiat. Biol. *40*:305, 1981.

158. Benson, E.P.: Radiation injury to large arteries. 3. Further examples with prolonged asymptomatic intervals. Radiology *106*:195, 1973.

159. Cade, S.: Radiation-induced cancer in man. Br. J. Radiol. *30*:393, 1957.

160. Zeman, W.: Introduction to neuropathy related to physical forces. *In* Minckler, J. (ed.): Pathology of the Nervous System. Vol. 1. New York, McGraw-Hill Book Company, 1968, p. 862.

161. Conard, R.A., and Hicking, A.: Medical findings in Marshallese people exposed to fallout radiation. J.A.M.A. *192*:457, 1965.

162. Warren, S.: The Pathology of Ionizing Radiation. Springfield, Illinois, Charles C Thomas, 1961.

163. Mettler, F.A., Jr., and Mosely, R.D., Jr.: Medical Effects of Ionizing Radiation. Orlando, Grune & Stratton, 1985, p. 173.

164. Morgan, C.: Hiroshima, Nagasaki, and the RERF (Radiation Effects Research Foundation). Am. J. Pathol. *98*:843, 1980.

165. Finch, S.C.: The study of atomic bomb survivors in Japan. Am. J. Med. *66*:899, 1979.

166. Okita, T.: Review of 30 years of study of Hiroshima and Nagasaki atomic bomb survivors. II. Biological effects. J. Radiat. Res. (Suppl). *16*:49, 1975.

167. Troup, G.M.: Symposium: The delayed consequences of exposure to ionizing radiation. Pathology studies at the Atomic Bomb Casualty Commission. Hiroshima and Nagasaki, 1945–1970. II. Growth and development. Hum. Pathol. *2*:493, 1971.

168. Michaelson, S.M., et al.: Fundamental and Applied Aspects of Nonionizing Radiation. New York, Plenum Press, 1975.

Diseases of Infancy and Childhood

Children are not merely "little people," nor are their disorders merely variants of the diseases of adult life. Most childhood conditions are unique to or at least take distinctive forms in this stage of life, and so merit the designation pediatric diseases. Collectively they exact a heavy toll. Considering all ages from birth to senility, "certain conditions originating in the perinatal period" were reported to be the twelfth leading cause of death in the United States in 1986. As would be expected, the chances for survival of live-born infants improve with each passing week. The mortality rate in the first week of life is over ten times greater than in the second week. Ironically, this striking differential represents, at least in part, a triumph of improved medical care. Better prenatal care, more effective methods of monitoring the condition of the fetus, and more frequent resort to cesarean section before term when there is evidence of fetal distress all contribute to bringing onto this "mortal coil" live-born infants who in past years might have been stillborn. These represent, then, an increased number of "high-risk" infants. Nonetheless, the infant mortality rate in the United States has shown a gratifying decline from a level of 20.0 deaths per 1000 population in 1970 to 11.2 in 1985 (the latest year for which complete data are available).

Each stage of development of the infant and child is prey to a somewhat different group of disorders. The data available permit a survey of four time spans: (1) the neonatal period (the first four weeks of life), (2) infancy (the first year of life), (3) 1 to 4 years of age, and (4) 5 to 14 years of age. The single most hazardous period of life is unquestionably the neonatal period. Never again is the individual confronted with more dramatic challenges than in the transition from dependent intrauterine existence to independent postnatal life. From the moment the umbilical cord is severed, the circulation to the heart is radically rerouted. Respiratory function must take over the

role of oxygenation of the blood. Maintenance of body temperature and other homeostatic constants must now be borne alone by the fledgling organism. All these adaptations render the neonate particularly vulnerable.

The major causes of death in infancy and childhood are cited in Table 10–1. It is evident that congenital anomalies, respiratory distress syndrome, immaturity, birth trauma, birth asphyxia, complications of pregnancy, pneumonia, meningitis, diseases of the nervous system, and accidents represent the leading causes of death in the first 12 months of life.

Once the infant survives the first year of life, the outlook brightens measurably. However, it is sobering to realize that in the next two age groups — 1 to 4 and 5 to 14 — accidents have become the leading cause of death (Table 10–1). Among the natural diseases, in order of importance, congenital anomalies, malignant neoplasms, and pneumonia assume major significance. It would appear then that, in a sense, life is an obstacle course. Fortunately for the great majority of us, the obstacles are surmounted, or even better, bypassed. We can now take a closer look at the specific conditions encountered during the various stages of infant and child development.

BIRTH WEIGHT AND GESTATIONAL AGE

It has been known for many years that infants born before completion of the normal gestation period have higher morbidity and mortality rates than full-term infants. Understandably, the vital organs of preterm infants are immature and therefore unable to adapt readily to early extrauterine existence. As might be expected, infants who have failed to complete normal intrauterine growth weigh less than full-

Table 10-1. Selected Causes of Death in Infancy and Childhood*

CAUSES	UNDER 1 YR	1-4 YR	5-14 YR
All causes	1164.2	57.6	28.3
Certain conditions originating in perinatal period	562.0	0.6	0.0
Respiratory distress syndrome	109.7		
Disorders relating to short gestation and unspecified low birth weight	98.3		
Birth asphyxia	32.5		
Complications of placenta, cord, and membranes in newborns	26.4		
Birth trauma	16.8		
Hemolytic disease of newborn due to isoimmunization, and other perinatal jaundice	1.7		
All other conditions originating in perinatal period	276.6		
Congenital anomalies	247.8	7.5	1.6
Pneumonia	20.5	1.6	0.4
Diseases of respiratory system (excluding pneumonia)	12.8		
Diseases of nervous system and sense organs (excluding meningitis)	12.3		
Meningitis	9.1	1.4	0.1
Septicemia	7.5	0.6	0.1
Intestinal infectious diseases	3.8	0.1	0.0
Malignant neoplasms, including neoplasms of lymphatic and hematopoietic tissues	3.7	4.6	4.1
Intracerebral or intracranial hemorrhage	2.4	0.1	0.1
Cystic fibrosis	0.9	0.3	0.6
Accidents and adverse effects (including motor vehicle)	28.1	22.5	13.2
All other causes	253.3	18.3	8.1

* Death rates per 100,000 population in a specified group. Data for the year 1982. Modified from Vital Statistics of the United States, 1982, Vol. II, Mortality, Part A. DHHS publication No. (PHS) 86-1122, Public Health Service. Washington, D.C., U.S. Government Printing Office, 1986.

term infants. In view of this association between low birth weight and immaturity in preterm infants, birth weight has traditionally been used as a guidepost for fetal maturity. Thus, in the past, premature infants have been defined as those having birth weight less than 2500 gm, regardless of the age of gestation. Although birth weight is indeed an important predictor of neonatal mortality (Fig. 10-1), it is somewhat inaccurate to define prematurity by birth weight alone, because weight is but one of the several parameters of intrauterine growth. *Not in every case do fetal maturity and birth weight go hand in hand.* For example, an infant weighing 2300 gm but born at 34 weeks of gestation is likely to be more immature and therefore at greater risk of suffering the consequences of organ system immaturity (e.g., respiratory distress syndrome, RDS, p. 523) than the 2300 gm full-term infant with functional maturity of the lungs and little risk of developing RDS. As discussed later, these "small-for-dates" infants, who constitute a full one third of low-birth-weight infants, are also a high-risk group, but the underlying basis for their problems is somewhat distinct. In recent years, therefore, a system of classification that takes into account both gestational age and birth weight has gained acceptance. Infants are classified as being appropriate for gestational age (AGA), small for gestational age (SGA), and large for gestational age (LGA). Those whose birth weight falls between the 10th and the 90th percentiles for a given gestational age are considered AGA, whereas those who fall above or below these norms are classified as LGA or SGA, respectively. With respect to gestational age, infants born before 37 or 38 weeks are considered *preterm*, whereas those delivered after the 42nd week are considered *postterm*. Figure 10-1 presents several possible categories of

infants when both gestational age and birth weight are taken into account. It also demonstrates that the risk of neonatal mortality as well as morbidity is strongly influenced by both birth weight and gestational age. For example, infants born before the 34th week with birth weights between 1000 and 1500 gm have a 50% mortality and 90% morbidity; however, within the same weight category, birth after the 34th week reduces the risk of mortality to 13%, but the chances of morbidity remain high at 86%. These figures reflect the somewhat distinctive distribution of diseases within each of the birth weight-gestational age groups, which are discussed in specialized texts.[1] Here we will discuss briefly SGA infants to highlight the utility of this classification, because such infants make up a significant fraction of those with low birth weight.

SMALL-FOR-GESTATIONAL-AGE (SGA) INFANTS

Most experts agree that *at least one third of infants who weigh less than 2500 gm are born at term and that they are therefore undergrown rather than immature.* Impaired intrauterine growth underlies SGA. It may result from a variety of factors, which can be grouped broadly into three categories—fetal, placental, and maternal.

1. The factors associated with the fetus are those that reduce its growth potential despite an adequate supply of nutrients from the mother. Prominent among such fetal conditions are chromosomal disorders, congenital anomalies, and congenital infections. Although the higher incidence of congenital malforma-

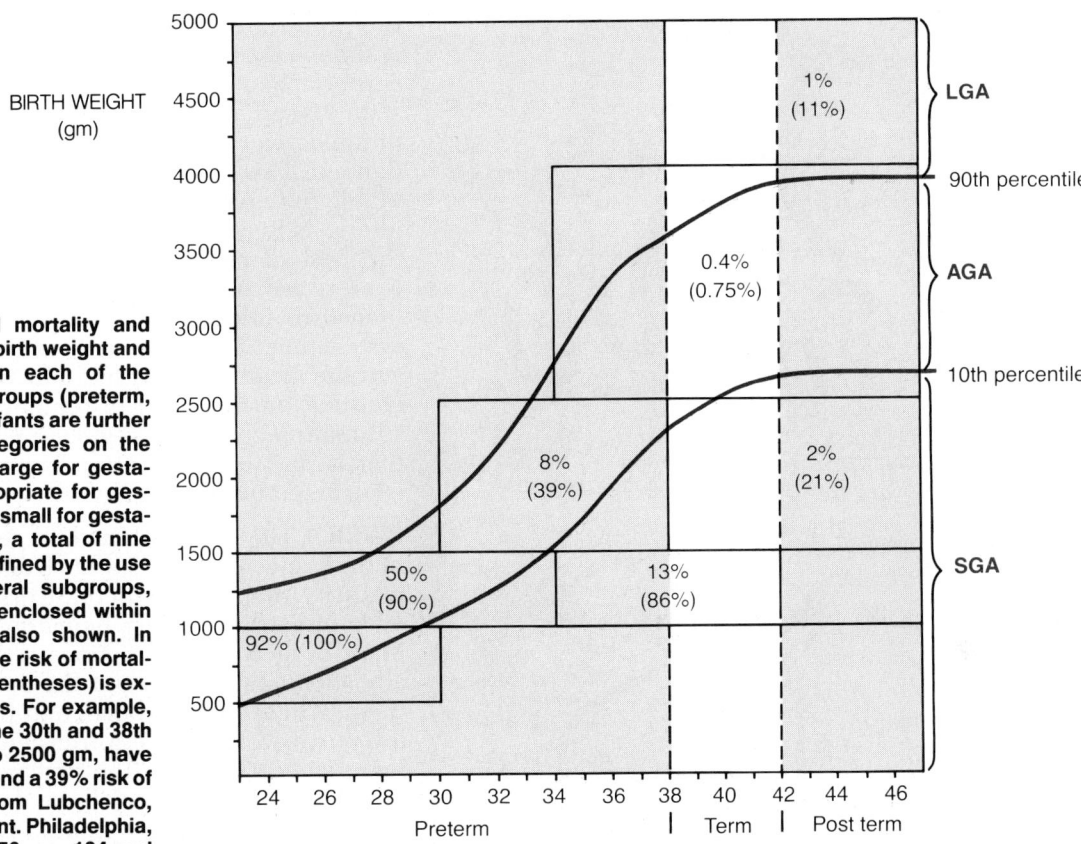

Figure 10-1. Neonatal mortality and morbidity according to birth weight and gestational age. Within each of the three gestational age groups (preterm, term, and post-term), infants are further divided into three categories on the basis of birth weight: large for gestational age (LGA), appropriate for gestational age (AGA), and small for gestational age (SGA). Thus, a total of nine major groups can be defined by the use of these criteria. Several subgroups, represented as boxes enclosed within continuous lines, are also shown. In each such subgroup, the risk of mortality and morbidity (in parentheses) is expressed as percentages. For example, infants born between the 30th and 38th week, weighing 1500 to 2500 gm, have an 8% risk of mortality and a 39% risk of morbidity. (Modified from Lubchenco, L.O.: The High Risk Infant. Philadelphia, W.B. Saunders Co., 1976, pp. 104 and 112.)

tions in small-for-dates infants is well established, the basis of this association is not clearly understood.[1a]

2. In the third trimester of pregnancy, vigorous fetal growth places heavy demands on the uteroplacental supply line. *Uteroplacental insufficiency,* therefore, is an important cause of growth retardation. This may result from infections, tumors, or vascular lesions such as infarctions. In some cases the placenta may be small without any detectable underlying cause.

3. By far the most common factors associated with SGA infants are *maternal*. Vascular diseases such as toxemia and chronic hypertension are often the underlying cause. Maternal undernutrition may also affect fetal growth, but the association between SGA and the nutritional status of the mother is complex. The list of other maternal conditions associated with SGA is long,[1] but some of the avoidable factors worth mentioning are maternal narcotic abuse, alcohol intake, and heavy cigarette smoking.

IMMATURITY OF ORGAN SYSTEMS

A major problem confronting the preterm infant regardless of birth weight is the functional and sometimes structural immaturity of various organs. Those who are also SGA are understandably the most seriously handicapped. Because immaturity may be the direct cause of death in very early preterm infants and

significantly biases the probable outcome in others, it is appropriate to consider the features of immaturity of the more vital organs.

LUNGS. During the first half of fetal life, the development of the lungs consists essentially of the formation of a system of branching tubes from the foregut that eventually give rise to the trachea, bronchi, and bronchioles. The alveoli only begin to differentiate at approximately the seventh month of gestation. They are at first imperfectly formed, with thick walls and large amounts of inter- and intralobular connective tissue. The vascularization is buried within this connective tissue and is not in immediate contact with the alveolar spaces (Fig. 10-2). The epithelium lining the airspaces at this time is cuboidal and not anatomically suited to effecting the rapid transfer of oxygen to the blood. Between the 26th and 32nd weeks of gestation, the cuboidal epithelium shows transition to the flat, type I alveolar epithelial cells as well as type II cells that contain lamellar bodies (see also p. 756). Further maturation of lungs leads to reduction in the interstitial tissues and increasing numbers of capillaries. However, even at full term the alveoli are small and the septa are considerably thicker than in the adult. Most of the cells lining the alveoli are type I cells. The type II cells appear in small clusters, mainly at the branching points of alveolar ducts. Develop-

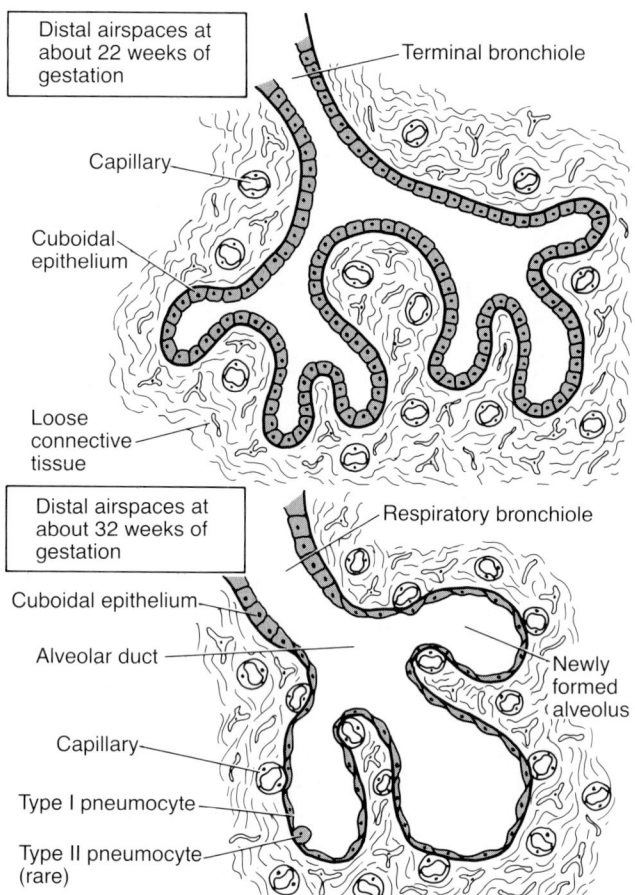

Distal airspaces at about 22 weeks of gestation

Terminal bronchiole

Capillary

Cuboidal epithelium

Loose connective tissue

Distal airspaces at about 32 weeks of gestation

Respiratory bronchiole

Cuboidal epithelium

Alveolar duct

Newly formed alveolus

Capillary

Type I pneumocyte

Type II pneumocyte (rare)

Figure 10-2. Schematic diagrams of fetal lung maturation.

ment of alveoli continues after birth, and the full adult complement of alveoli is reached at about 8 years of age.

The immature lungs, then, are grossly unexpanded, red, and meaty. The alveolar spaces are incompletely expanded and usually contain pink proteinaceous precipitate and occasional squamous epithelial cells. The presence of large amounts of amniotic debris, such as squames, lanugo hair, and mucus, usually indicates prenatal respiratory distress. Although lungs of stillborn infants usually sink when immersed in water, the "floating test" is not a critical index of postnatal respiration. Despite the fact that infants may have breathed prior to death, the very weak respiratory muscles and shallow respiration, with little exchange of air or resorption of the contained air, may both cause the lungs to sink when placed in water. Contrariwise, bacterial growth may produce gas that will create buoyancy in the lungs.

KIDNEYS. In the preterm infant the formation of glomeruli is incomplete. Primitive glomeruli can be seen in the subcapsular zone. These structures have an organoid, glandular appearance imparted by the presence of cuboidal cells in the parietal and visceral layers of Bowman's capsule. However, the deeper glomeruli are well formed and renal function is adequate to permit survival.

BRAIN. The brain is also incompletely developed in the preterm infant. The surface is relatively smooth and devoid of the typical convolutions found in the cerebral hemispheres of the adult. The brain substance is soft, gelatinous, and easily torn, and the definition between white and gray matter is somewhat ill defined. This lack of separation is in large part attributable to poorly developed myelination of the nerve fibers. Notwithstanding this underdevelopment, to the best of our present knowledge the vital brain centers are sufficiently developed even in the very immature infant to sustain normal central nervous system function. However, homeostasis is not perfect, and the preterm infant has difficulty in maintaining a constant normal level of temperature and has poor vasomotor control, irregular respirations, muscular inertia, and feeble sweating. None of these difficulties is incompatible with survival.

LIVER. The liver, although large relative to the size of the preterm infant, suffers from lack of physiologic maturity. Some of this increase in size is due to persistence of extramedullary hematopoiesis in this organ. Many or most of the functions of the liver are marginally adequate to carry out the demands placed upon them. Almost all newborns and particularly those of low birth weight have a transient period of physiologic jaundice within the first postnatal week. This jaundice stems from both breakdown of fetal red cells and inadequacy of the biliary excretory function of liver cells. Deficiencies of bilirubin glucuronyl transferase, hydroxylating enzymes, and protein synthetic capacity, to name only a few hepatic systems, all characterize the immature liver.

APGAR SCORE

The Apgar score, devised by Dr. Virginia Apgar, represents a clinically useful method of evaluating the physiologic condition and responsiveness of the newborn infant, and hence its chances of survival.[2] Table 10-2 indicates the five parameters to be scored and how they are quantitated. The newborn infant may be evaluated at one minute or at five minutes. A total score of 10 indicates an infant in the best possible condition. The correlation between the Apgar score and the mortality during the first 28 days of life is very impressive. Infants with a five-minute Apgar score of 0 to 1 have a 50% mortality within the first month of life. This drops to 20% with a score of 4, and to almost 0% when the score is 7 or better.[3]

BIRTH INJURIES

Birth injuries constitute important causes of illness or death in infants as well as in children during the first years of life. Understandably, LGA infants are at a greater risk of sustaining birth injuries, but no group is immune. Preterm AGA or SGA infants, although smaller, have higher associated morbidity as they are

Table 10–2. Evaluation of the Newborn Infant

SIGN	0	1	2
Heart rate	Absent	Below 100	Over 100
Respiratory effort	Absent	Slow, irregular	Good, crying
Muscle tone	Limp	Some flexion of extremities	Active motion
Response to catheter in nostril (tested after oropharynx is clear)	No response	Grimace	Cough or sneeze
Color	Blue, pale	Body pink, extremities blue	Completely pink

Sixty seconds after the complete birth of the infant (disregarding removal of the cord and placenta) the five objective signs are evaluated and each is given a score of 0, 1, or 2. A total score of 10 indicates an infant in the best possible condition.

Modified from Apgar, V.: A proposal for a new method of evaluation of the newborn infant. Anesth. Analg. *32*:260, 1953.

the least equipped to adapt. Anatomic immaturity may also increase the risk of some forms of birth injuries (e.g., intraventricular hemorrhage). These injuries may affect any part or any region of the body but most commonly involve the head, skeletal system, liver, adrenals, and peripheral nerves. Considering the violent expulsive forces to which the fragile fetus is exposed, it is quite surprising that birth injuries are so relatively uncommon. It is important to stress that although some birth injuries are avoidable, some are unavoidable even with optimal obstetric care. If the process of birth were not laborious to mother and infant, why would it have been termed "labor"?

Morbidity associated with birth injury may be acute (such as that due to fractures) or the result of later-appearing sequelae, such as following damage to nerves or the brain. The distribution of injuries (other than cephalhematoma, which is hardly to be considered an injury) in a large municipal hospital is as follows, in descending order of frequency: clavicular fracture, facial nerve injury, brachial plexus injury, intracranial injury, humeral fracture, and lacerations.[4] Among these, injuries involving the head are the most ominous. Discussion of the other birth injuries may be found in a review devoted to this subject.[5]

Caput succedaneum and *cephalhematoma* are so common even in normal uncomplicated births that they hardly merit the designation "birth injury." When the head is the presenting part, some portion of the scalp is exposed in the progressively dilating cervical os. As the fetus is subjected to the compressive forces of labor, fluid tends to accumulate in the small area of the scalp that presents in the cervical os and is not exposed to the increased uterine pressure. *The progressive accumulation of interstitial fluid in the soft tissues of the scalp gives rise to a usually circular area of edema, congestion, and swelling called a caput succedaneum.* Because the fluid accumulates in the subcutaneous tissue, it may extend across the suture lines. *Hemorrhage may occur into the scalp, producing a cephalhematoma.* Usually the blood accumulates subperiosteally, and therefore the overlying swelling does not cross the cranial sutures. Cephalhematoma thus is distinct from a caput succedaneum, which occurs more superficially in the soft tissues of the scalp. Both forms of injury are of little clinical significance and are of importance only insofar as they must be differentiated from skull fractures with attendant

hemorrhage and edema. In approximately 25% of cephalhematomas there is an underlying skull fracture.

The skull bones may be fractured or may override each other, particularly when there is some disturbance in the ordinary mechanism of labor. Precipitate or sudden delivery with incomplete molding of the head, inappropriate use of forceps, and prolonged intense labor with disproportion between the size of the fetal head and birth canal are some of the clinical circumstances that surround the occurrence of these skull injuries.

Intracranial hemorrhage is probably the most common important birth injury. These hemorrhages are generally thought to be related to excessive molding of the head or sudden pressure changes in its shape as it is subjected to the pressure of forceps or sudden precipitate expulsion. Prolonged labor, hypoxia, hemorrhagic disorders, or intracranial vascular anomalies are important predispositions. The hemorrhage may arise in tears in the dura, particularly in the falx cerebri and tentorium cerebelli; the dural sinuses may be stretched beyond their elastic limit and may rupture; the substance of the brain may be torn or bruised, leading to intraventricular hemorrhages or bleeding into the brain substance; or vessels that traverse the subdural space may be ruptured. Whatever their origin, intracranial hemorrhages are of great importance, as they cause sudden increases in intracranial pressure; damage to the brain substance; herniation of the medulla or base of the brain into the foramen magnum; and serious, frequently fatal depression of function of the vital medullary centers.

CONGENITAL MALFORMATIONS

Congenital malformations can be defined as structural defects that are present at birth, but some, such as cardiac defects and renal anomalies, may not become clinically apparent until years later. The term congenital does not imply or exclude a genetic basis for malformations. It is estimated that about 3% of newborns have a *major malformation*, defined as a malformation having either cosmetic or functional significance.[6] As indicated in Table 10–1, they are the leading cause of infant mortality.[7] Moreover, they continue to be a significant cause of illness, disability, and death throughout the early years of life. In a real sense, malformations found in live-born infants represent the less serious developmental failures in embryogenesis that are compatible with live birth. Perhaps 20% of fertilized ova are so anomalous that they are blighted from the outset. Less severe anomalies may be compatible with early fetal survival, only to lead to spontaneous abortion. As one descends the scale of severity, a level is reached that permits more prolonged intrauterine survival, with some disorders terminating in stillbirth, and those still less significant permitting live birth despite the handicaps imposed.

Here we should distinguish between malformations and deformations.[8] *Malformations represent primary errors in morphogenesis; deformations arise later in fetal life and represent alterations in form or structure resulting from mechanical factors.* We shall consider deformations at the end of this section. Malformations may present in several patterns. Some, such as congenital heart defects, involve single body systems, whereas in other cases multiple malformations involving many organs and tissues may coexist. Multiple congenital anomalies may have their origin in a single localized aberration in organogenesis leading to secondary ripple effects in other organs. For example, early urethral obstruction may secondarily affect renal morphogenesis as well as lead to defects in the lower limbs owing to compression of blood vessels. Such a pattern of cascade effects is called a *malformation sequence.* On the other hand, a patient may have several defects that cannot be explained on the basis of a single localized initiating malformation. These are called *malformation syndromes.* Most often they are caused by a single etiologic agent, e.g., viral infections that simultaneously affect several tissues.

ETIOLOGY. Known causes of human malformations can be grouped into two major categories — genetic and environmental (Table 10–3). Almost two thirds, however, have no recognized cause.

Malformations that are known to be genetic in origin can be divided into two groups: (1) those associated with chromosomal aberrations, and (2) those arising in single gene mutations. In addition many malformations are suspected to result from multifactorial inheritance, a term that implies the interaction of two or more genes of small effect with environmental factors. Because the precise environmental and genetic influences responsible for the malformations of this origin are largely unidentified, they are included in the unknown category (Table 10–3), to be discussed later.

Virtually all the *chromosomal syndromes* (Chapter 4) are characterized by congenital anomalies. Chromosomal abnormalities (p. 127) are present in approximately 4 to 5% of live-born infants with congenital malformations. Only one reaches the birth frequency of one in 1000 total births, namely, trisomy 21 (Down's syndrome) (p. 129). Next in order of frequency are Klinefelter's syndrome, Turner's syndrome, and trisomy 13 (Patau's syndrome). The re-

Table 10–3. Causes of Congenital Malformations in Humans

CAUSE	MALFORMED LIVE BIRTHS (%)
Genetic	
Chromosomal aberrations	5
Mendelian inheritance	15–20
(Familial and de novo mutations)	
Environmental	
Maternal infections	3
Rubella	
Toxoplasmosis	
Syphilis	
Cytomegalovirus	
HIV (human immune deficiency	
virus)	
Maternal disease states	4
Diabetes	
Phenylketonuria	
Endocrinopathies	
Drugs and chemicals	$\simeq 1$
Alcohol	
Folic acid antagonists	
Androgens	
Phenytoin	
Thalidomide	
Warfarin	
13-*cis*-retinoic acid	
Irradiation	$\simeq 1$
Unknown	65–70

Adapted from Brent, R.L.: The complexities of solving the problem of human malformations. Clin. Perinatol. *13*:491, 1986.

maining chromosomal syndromes associated with malformations are far more rare. The great preponderance of these cytogenetic aberrations arise as defects in gametogenesis and so are not familial. There are, however, transmissible chromosomal abnormalities, as for example the translocation form of Down's syndrome passed from one generation to the next, thus constituting a familial pattern of structural abnormalities.

Single gene mutations of large effect may underlie major malformations, which, as expected, follow mendelian patterns of inheritance. On the whole these are relatively uncommon and do not have a birth frequency of one in 1000 births. Among these rare entities are the relatively less serious limb malformations: polydactyly, syndactyly, and brachydactyly. However, there is still some question about the mode of transmission of some of these, and multifactorial inheritance cannot be totally excluded. In addition, there are a number of malformation syndromes in which multiple anomalies occur in disorders having mendelian modes of transmission, as for example Marfan's syndrome and the mucopolysaccharidoses.

Environmental influences such as viral infections, drugs, and irradiation to which the mother was exposed during pregnancy may induce malformations in the fetus and infant. Many viruses have been implicated, including the agents responsible for rubella, cytomegalic inclusion disease, herpes simplex, varicella-zoster infection, influenza, mumps, and enterovirus infections. To this list may now be added the human immunodeficiency virus (HIV), the causative agent of AIDS.[9] Among these, the rubella virus and the cytomegalovirus of cytomegalic inclusion disease are the most extensively investigated. With all viruses, the gestational age at which the infection occurs in the mother is critically important. *The at-risk period for rubella infection extends from shortly before conception to the 16th week of gestation,* the hazard being greater in the first eight weeks than in the second eight weeks. Various studies indicate that with infection in the first four-week period, approximately 50% of live-born infants will have malformations, a risk so great that abortion may be advised. The incidence of malformations is reduced to 20% or 7%, respectively, if infection occurs in the second or third month of gestation. The fetal defects are extremely varied, but the major triad comprises cataracts, heart disease, and deafness, referred to as "rubella syndrome." The cardiac lesions take many forms, particularly persistent ductus arteriosus, pulmonary artery hypoplasia, pulmonary valve stenosis, aortic stenosis, ventricular septal defect, and tetralogy of Fallot. Other possible concomitant defects are microphthalmia, microcephaly, mental retardation, hepatomegaly, splenomegaly, and retardation of both intrauterine and postnatal growth.

Intrauterine infection with the cytomegalovirus, mostly asymptomatic, is the most common fetal viral infection. Its prevalence is estimated to be 0.4 to 7.4%.[10] This viral disease is considered in detail elsewhere (p. 321), and it suffices here to indicate that the highest at-risk period appears to be the second trimester of pregnancy. Because organogenesis is largely completed by the end of the first trimester, congenital malformations occur less frequently than in rubella; nevertheless, the effects of virus-induced injury on the formed organs are often severe. Involvement of the central nervous system is a major feature, and the most prominent clinical changes are mental retardation, microcephaly, deafness, and hepatosplenomegaly. Several other abnormalities are detailed in the discussion of this condition on page 321. The other viral agents previously mentioned have at one time or another been implicated as infective causes of congenital malformations, but the number of reported cases is far fewer and the evidence less substantial.

A variety of drugs and chemicals have been suspected to be teratogenic. However, in view of the complex interactions between genetic and environmental factors in the pathogenesis of most common malformations, it is difficult to establish a definite role of a suspected teratogen. Furthermore, the more widely used a potential teratogen and the more common a suspected malformation, the more often will they be associated by chance. Perhaps fewer than 1% of congenital malformations are caused by drugs and chemicals. The list of chemicals and drugs definitely known to cause malformations includes thalidomide, folate antagonists, androgenic hormones, alcohol, anticonvulsants, warfarin (oral anticoagulant), and 13-*cis*-retinoic acid used in the treatment of acne. Here we will review the teratogenic action of two agents: thalidomide, which caused an epidemic of malformations in the early 1960s, and alcohol, which is widely used but poorly appreciated as a teratogenic agent. *Thalidomide,* once popular as a tranquilizer in Europe, is one of the few drugs that cause an extremely high frequency (50 to 80%) of malformations in those exposed to the drug during a vulnerable period. Although the characteristic anomalies of the thalidomide syndrome affect the limbs, several other organs may be affected, depending on the period of exposure during embryogenesis. The limb abnormalities range from severe, such as amelia (absence of limbs) and phocomelia ("seal limbs," absence of limb with hands or feet attached directly to the trunk), to minor, such as hypoplasia of the thumb. *Alcohol,* perhaps the most widely used agent today, has only recently been recognized as a teratogen. Although the exact frequency of alcohol-induced malformations is difficult to ascertain, estimates range from one to five live births per 1000.[11] Affected infants show growth retardation, microcephaly, atrial septal defect, short palpebral fissures, maxillary hypoplasia, and several other minor anomalies. These together are labeled the *fetal alcohol syndrome.* The level of alcohol consumption necessary to produce this has not been established with certainty. It is believed, however, that chronic consumption of 6 oz of alcohol per day constitutes a high risk, and fetal alcohol syndrome is unlikely to develop when the mother consumes less than 2 oz of alcohol per day.[12,12a]

Radiation, in addition to being mutagenic and carcinogenic, is teratogenic. Exposure to heavy doses of radiation during the period of organogenesis leads to malformations such as microcephaly, blindness, skull defects, spina bifida, and other deformities. Such exposure occurred in the past when radiation was used to treat cervical cancer. Similarly, exposure to radioactivity from atomic bomb explosions in Japan led to an increased incidence of malformations. Whether lower doses of radiation such as those used in diagnostic x-rays are also teratogenic is not known.[13]

The genetic and environmental factors just discussed can account for no more than one third of human congenital malformations. The causes of the vast majority of birth defects, including some relatively common disorders such as cleft lip and cleft palate, remain unknown. Multifactorial inheritance is believed to underlie the most common major malformations, particularly when the malformation is single, i.e., not associated with other malformations. You may recall from the earlier discussion in Chapter 4 that multifactorial inheritance is involved in many of the physiologic characteristics such as height, weight, and blood pressure. Such phenotypic characteristics fall on a continuous or gaussian distribution curve. Similarly, in the case of malformations, the liability to a disorder (determined by genetic and environmental factors) is a continuous variable, but there is in addition a "threshold" that divides individuals with and

Table 10–4. Approximate Frequency of the More Common Congenital Malformations in the United States

MALFORMATION	FREQUENCY PER 10,000 TOTAL BIRTHS
Hypospadias	28.23
Clubfoot without neural defects	25.61
Ventricular septal defect	15.23
Cleft lip with or without cleft palate	9.05
Congenital dislocation of hip without neural defects	8.92
Patent ductus arteriosus	7.50
Spina bifida without anencephaly	4.78
Anencephaly	3.14
Atrial septal defect	1.70
Cystic disease of kidney	1.30

Adapted from Edmonds, L.D., and James, L.M.: Temporal trends in the incidence of malformations in the United States: Selected years, 1970–71, 1982–83. MMWR (CDC Surveillance Summaries), *34*(No. 255): 155, 355, 1985.

without the disorder. Thus, it would appear that inheritance of a certain number of mutant genes and their interaction with the environment is required before the disorder is expressed. In the case of congenital dislocation of the hip, for example, depth of the acetabular socket and laxity of the ligaments are believed to be genetically determined, whereas a significant environmental factor is believed to be frank breech position in utero with hips flexed and knees extended. In most instances, however, the nature of genetic and environmental factors and their interplay are unknown. The approximate frequency of some common malformations in the United States is presented in Table 10–4.

PATHOGENESIS. The pathogenesis of congenital malformations is complex and still poorly understood. Certain general principles of developmental pathology that are relevant regardless of the etiologic agent will be discussed first. *The timing of the prenatal insult has an important impact on both the occurrence and the type of malformation produced.*[6]

The intrauterine development of humans can be divided into two phases: the embryonic period occupying the first nine weeks of pregnancy, and the fetal period terminating at birth. In the *early embryonic period* (first three weeks after fertilization), an injurious agent damages either enough cells to cause death and abortion, or only a few cells, presumably allowing the embryo to recover without developing defects. Between the third and ninth weeks the embryo is extremely susceptible to teratogenesis, and the peak sensitivity during this period is between the fourth and fifth weeks. It is during this period that organs are being created out of the germ cell layers. The process of organogenesis including the intricate morphogenetic movements is extremely susceptible to injury, regardless of its nature. The *fetal period* that follows organogenesis is marked chiefly by the further growth and maturation of the organs, with greatly

reduced susceptibility to teratogenic agents. Instead the fetus is susceptible to growth retardation or injury to already formed organs. For example, in the first trimester, viral infections such as rubella produce malformations by disrupting the developmental program, but later during pregnancy the result of virus infections is usually tissue injury accompanied by inflammation such as congenital encephalitis. Timing of the teratogenic insult is also important with respect to the specific malformation produced. During the period of morphogenesis, different organs are being formed both simultaneously and sequentially, but each organ has a critical period during which it is most susceptible to induction of malformation. It is therefore possible for a given agent to produce different malformations if exposure occurs at different times of gestation. In general, malformations resulting from incomplete morphogenesis usually have their origin when the development of the organ in question is not yet completed. For example, a ventricular septal defect may occur from exposure to a teratogen before six weeks of gestation, because the ventricular septum closes at this time. Similarly, cleft lip must occur before closure of the lip at 36 days. It must be remembered, however, that knowledge of embryologic timetables does not allow an estimate of the particular time when the malformation was produced; one can only say that the teratogen acted prior to a given time.

In producing malformations, *teratogens may act at several levels. These include cell proliferation, cell migration, differentiation, and in some instances damage to formed and differentiated organs.* Inhibition of cell proliferation or cell death occurring at critical points in development can lead to serious malformations. Failure or acceleration of planned cell death may also produce malformations such as syndactyly or cleft palate.[13a] As indicated earlier, cell migrations play an important role in morphogenesis. Orderly migrations take place in matrices, which may be disrupted by teratogenic agents. For example, in experimental animals, disturbance in collagen-matrix formation by cadmium produces major craniofacial anomalies because the migration of neural crest cells is inhibited. Anticonvulsant drugs, on the other hand, impair the appropriate differentiation of the mesenchyme and give rise to cleft palate in rodents. It must be remembered in this context that although a given teratogen may initiate its action primarily by affecting proliferation, migration, or differentiation, interference in any one of these mechanisms may lead to a cascade of effects in all three processes. Although the risk of malformations is reduced after morphogenesis is complete, differentiated tissues may also be affected by teratogens. For example, focal cell death in differentiated tissues caused by anoxia, chemicals, or virus infections can lead to formation of fluid- or blood-filled blebs that can result in significant local malformations.

Another important principle of teratology relates to the *role of heredity in the susceptibility to malformations.* Here we are concerned not with genetic factors in the causation of malformations but with the role of heredity in predisposition to the effects of known teratogens. The best example to illustrate this principle is cleft palate induced by cortisone in mice. A given dose of cortisol administered to the mother produces 100% incidence of cleft palate in the progeny of A strain mice but only 20% incidence in C57BL/6 mice. This has been related to the frequency of receptors for corticosteroids in the two strains of mice. Although no such clear example has been found in human teratogenesis, differences in susceptibility to drug-induced malformations has been noted. Thus, only 10 to 40% of offspring of mothers taking phenytoin (Dilantin) and only 25% of children of mothers exposed to warfarin develop congenital malformations. It has been suggested that such variations in teratogenic effects among individuals result from genetically determined differences in placental transport, absorption, metabolism, and distribution of the teratogenic agent.[12]

With this overview of some general mechanisms whereby congenital malformations may arise, we can now discuss deformations that represent the effects of abnormal mechanical forces on the developing fetus.

DEFORMATIONS

Deformations are common problems, affecting approximately 2% of newborn infants to varying degrees. Fundamental to the pathogenesis of deformations is localized or generalized compression of the growing fetus by abnormal biomechanical forces, leading eventually to a variety of structural abnormalities. In contrast to malformations, there is no intrinsic defect in morphogenesis, although fetal malformations may initiate a sequence of changes that ultimately lead to deformations. The most common underlying factor responsible for deformations is *uterine constraint*. Between the 35th and 38th weeks of gestation, rapid increase in the size of the fetus outpaces the growth of the uterus, and the relative amount of amniotic fluid (which normally acts as a cushion) also decreases. Thus, even the normal fetus is subjected to some form of uterine constraint. However, several factors increase the likelihood of excessive compression of the fetus, including maternal conditions such as first pregnancy, small uterus, malformed (bicornuate) uterus, and leiomyomas. Factors relating to the fetus, such as multiple fetuses, oligohydramnios, and abnormal fetal presentation, may also be involved. These and other details of deformations are discussed in specialized texts.[14]

Here we will present only one example of deformations resulting from relative lack of amniotic fluid, called the *oligohydramnios sequence*. A deficiency of amniotic fluid, with consequent increase in uterine constraint, may have a variety of causes, including chronic leakage of amniotic fluid due to rupture of the amnion, or uteroplacental insufficiency resulting from maternal hypertension or severe toxemia. Occasionally the oligohydramnios sequence may be initi-

ated by a fetal malformation such as renal agenesis, leading to lack of urine, which is a major constituent of amniotic fluid during pregnancy. The affected newborn presents with facial abnormalities including flattened nose and accordion ears. More serious are abnormalities of the limb joints, which are in aberrant positions and often stiff owing to poor mobility in utero. Hips may be dislocated. Growth of the chest wall and the contained lungs is compromised so that the lungs often achieve only a four- to five-month level of maturation. Several other less striking abnormalities are also apparent. Fortunately, deformations in general carry a much better prognosis than malformations and a much lesser risk of recurrence in subsequent infants.

RESPIRATORY DISTRESS SYNDROME IN NEWBORN

Respiratory distress is one of the most common and life-threatening complications to confront the newborn infant. It can have many origins, including (1) excessive sedation of the mother, with consequent depression of respiration in the infant; (2) brain injury, with failure of the central respiratory centers; (3) feeble respiratory efforts secondary to immaturity of the lungs and skeletal muscles (primary atelectasis); (4) aspiration during birth of blood clot and amniotic fluid when the amniotic debris (i.e., desquamated keratotic squames, mucus, lanugo hairs, proteinaceous precipitate, and blood) blocks ventilatory function; and (5) asphyxiating coils of umbilical cord about the neck of the infant. *But more important than all these by an order of magnitude is the idiopathic respiratory distress syndrome (RDS).* Despite the striking improvement in neonatal intensive care in the last two decades, RDS or its complications still take the lives of about 25,000 infants every year in the United States.

RDS is also known as hyaline membrane disease (HMD), highlighting one of the major pulmonary anatomic findings in this disease. In most cases this disorder presents in stereotyped fashion, which is best characterized by the following typical clinical setting. The infant is almost always preterm and appropriate for gestational age (p. 516), and there are strong, but not invariable, associations with diabetes in the mother and with delivery by cesarean section. Resuscitation may be necessary at birth, but usually within a few minutes rhythmic breathing and normal color are reestablished. However, soon afterward, often within 30 minutes, breathing becomes more difficult, there is retraction of the lower ribs and sternum on inspiration, and an expiratory grunt becomes audible. Over the span of the next few hours the respiratory distress becomes worse, the rate of breathing increases to over 100 breaths/min, and cyanosis becomes evident. Despite the labored breathing, little actual ventilation occurs, and fine rales can now be heard over both lung fields. A chest x-ray film at this time usually reveals uniform minute reticulogranular densities, producing a so-called "ground-glass" picture. At first the administration of 40 to 50% oxygen to the infant lessens the cyanosis; indeed, during the next 12 to 24 hours recovery may ensue, but in the fullblown condition the respiratory distress persists, cyanosis increases, and even the administration of 80% oxygen by a variety of ventilatory methods fails to improve the situation. Flaccidity, unresponsiveness, and periods of apnea may now appear and may presage death. However, if therapy staves off death for the first three or four days, the baby has an excellent chance of recovery.[15]

ETIOLOGY AND PATHOGENESIS. The pathogenesis of RDS is still incompletely understood, but a number of significant observations have been made. Immaturity of the lungs is the most important subsoil on which this condition develops. It may be encountered in full-term infants, but is much less frequent than in those "born before their time into this breathing world."[16] The incidence of RDS is inversely proportional to gestational age. It is estimated to occur in about 60% of infants born at less than 28 weeks of gestation, 15 to 20% of those born between 32 and 36 weeks, and less than 5% of those born after 37 weeks of gestation.[17] Although the point is still somewhat controversial, a good deal of evidence indicates that cesarean section, when performed before the 38th week of gestation, increases the risk of RDS—with a virtually exponential increase with each week of prematurity.[18] Infants of diabetic mothers, as contrasted with those of nondiabetic mothers, are at increased risk for development of RDS, especially if the maternal diabetes is not well controlled.[19,20] The sex of the infant is also a factor, males being affected 1.5 to 2 times more often than females.[21]

All the aforementioned clinical observations bear on what is now considered to be the *fundamental defect in RDS—a deficiency of pulmonary surfactant.* Surfactant is a generic name for surface active compounds synthesized by the lung. Surfactant consists predominantly of dipalmitoyl phosphatidylcholine and smaller amounts of phosphatidylglycerol. In addition to the phospholipids, surfactant contains at least two proteins that are thought to be important for normal surfactant function in vivo.[22] Surfactant reduces surface tension within the alveoli so that less pressure is required to hold alveoli open, and it maintains alveolar expansion by varying surface tension with alveolar size. It is synthesized by type II alveolar cells and can be visualized with the electron microscope as lamellar osmiophilic bodies. At birth, the first breath of life requires high inspiratory pressures to expand the lungs. With normal levels of surfactant the lungs retain up to 40% of the residual air volume after the first breath; thus, subsequent breaths require far lower inspiratory pressures. With a deficiency of surfactant the lungs collapse with each successive breath, and so the infant must work as hard with each successive breath as it did with the first. The problem of

"stiff" atelectatic lungs is compounded by the "soft" thoracic wall that is pulled in as the diaphragm descends. Progressive atelectasis and reduced lung compliance then lead to a train of events as depicted in Figure 10–3, resulting in a protein-rich, fibrin-rich exudation into the alveolar spaces with the formation of hyaline membranes. Built into the sequence of events are feedback loops, which constitute vicious circles that progressively increase the severity of the disease once it has begun. The fibrin-hyaline membranes constitute barriers to gas exchange, leading to CO_2 retention and hypoxemia, worsening the acidosis and subsequent events. The hypoxemia itself further impairs surfactant synthesis. Effective supportive therapy providing time for maturation and regeneration of the type II pneumocytes and increased surfactant synthesis can lead to recovery from this condition.

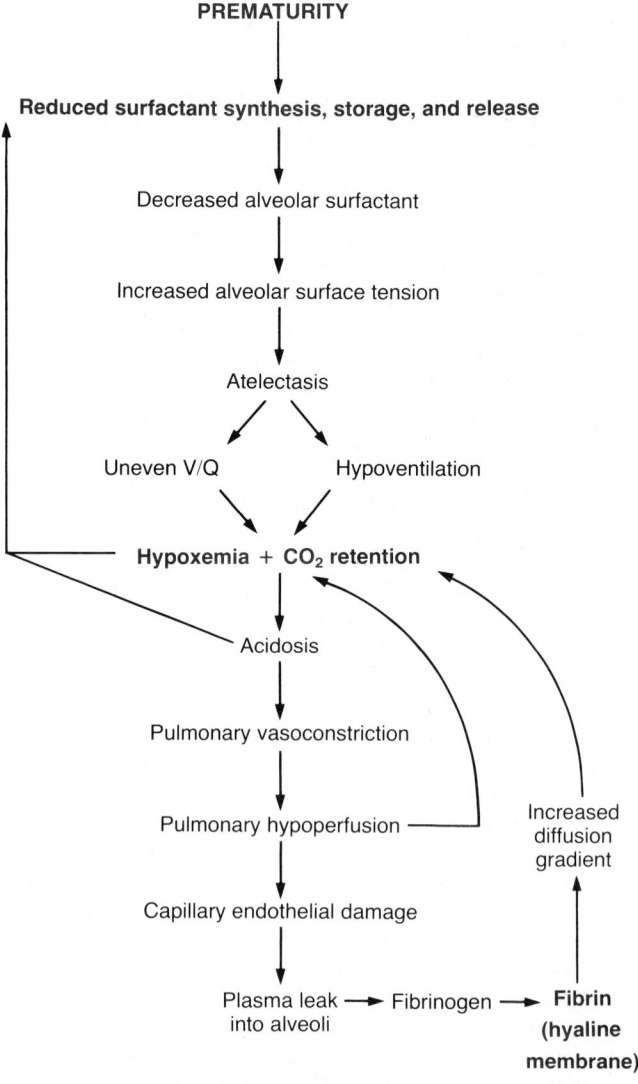

Figure 10–3. Schematic outline of pathophysiology of respiratory distress syndrome. V/Q = ventilation-perfusion ratio. (From Oh, W., and Stern, L.: Respiratory diseases of the newborn. *In* Stern, L., and Vert, P. (eds.): Neonatal Medicine. New York, Masson Publishing USA, 1987, p. 396.)

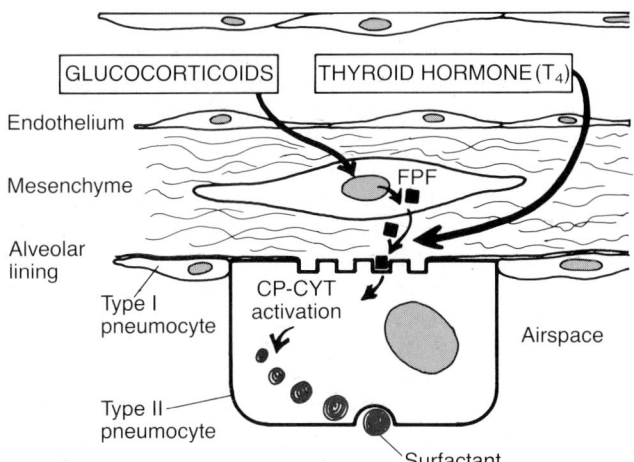

Figure 10–4. Schematic representation of events in surfactant production. Glucocorticoids (endogenous or exogenously administered) stimulate production of fibroblast pneumocyte factor (FPF) by acting on mesenchymal fibroblasts. FPF stimulates type II pneumocytes to produce choline-phosphate-cytidyl transferase (CP-CYT), the rate-limiting enzyme in the synthesis of phosphatidylcholine. Thyroxine is believed to synergize with FPF. The stimulatory effect of glucocorticoids on surfactant apoprotein synthesis is not depicted. (Modified from Start, A.R., and Frantz, I.P.: Respiratory distress syndrome. Pediatr. Clin. North Am. *33:*533, 1986; original figure drawn by Barry Smith, M.D.)

As noted immaturity of the fetal lung in preterm infants is the most major cause of surfactant deficiency. The production of surfactant increases gradually after the appearance of type II alveolar cells, but the largest increase occurs after 35 weeks of gestation. Surfactant synthesis is modulated by a variety of hormones including cortisol, insulin, prolactin, and thyroxine. The role of glucocorticoids is particularly important. The evidence is now convincing that corticosteroids induce the formation of surfactant lipids and apoprotein in fetal lung.[15,23] A schematic illustration of the mechanism by which phosphatidylcholine synthesis is augmented by cortisol is illustrated in Figure 10–4. Whereas thyroxine acts synergistically with cortisol, insulin is believed to antagonize glucocorticoid-induced stimulation of surfactant synthesis. The infant of a diabetic mother has hyperinsulinism as a compensatory reaction to the hyperglycemia in both mother and fetus. Thus, in these infants surfactant synthesis may be suppressed by the high blood levels of insulin, which counteract the effects of steroids. This may explain why infants of diabetic mothers have a higher risk of developing RDS. Why cesarean section should increase the risk of RDS is still an enigma. Indeed, there continues to be a debate in the literature as to whether this method of delivery is itself at fault or instead is indirectly involved because of the indication for cesarean section, e.g., antepartum hemorrhage and toxemia. Finally, the male preponderance has been related to the relatively early maturation of the female lung.

In closing, we should mention that RDS may also occur in adults (p. 760). Surfactant deficiency is the most common cause of RDS in newborns, but any agent capable of causing diffuse alveolar damage can result in similar respiratory problems in both infants and adults.

MORPHOLOGY. The lungs are extremely distinctive on gross examination. Although of normal size, they are solid, airless, and reddish purple like the liver, and they usually sink in water.[24] On low-power microscopic examination, they give the appearance of a solid tissue. The alveoli are poorly developed, and those that are present are collapsed. The atelectasis results from the clearance of fluid without its replacement by air.[25] When the infant dies early in the course of the disease, necrotic cellular debris is present in the terminal bronchioles and alveolar ducts. Later, the necrotic material becomes incorporated within pink hyaline membranes that line the respiratory bronchioles, alveolar ducts, and random alveoli, mostly the proximal alveoli (Fig. 10–5). The membranes stain for lipid, are Feulgen positive (indicative of nuclear debris), and give strong immunofluorescent reactions for fibrin. They are largely made up of fibrinogen and fibrin admixed with cell debris derived chiefly from necrotic alveolar-lining pneumocytes. The sequence of events that leads to the formation of hyaline membranes was depicted in Figure 10–3. To this sequence can be added necrosis of alveolar lining cells owing to hypoxia, a lesion that develops early and may be quite prominent.[26] There is a remarkable paucity of inflammatory reaction associated with these membranes. An ad-

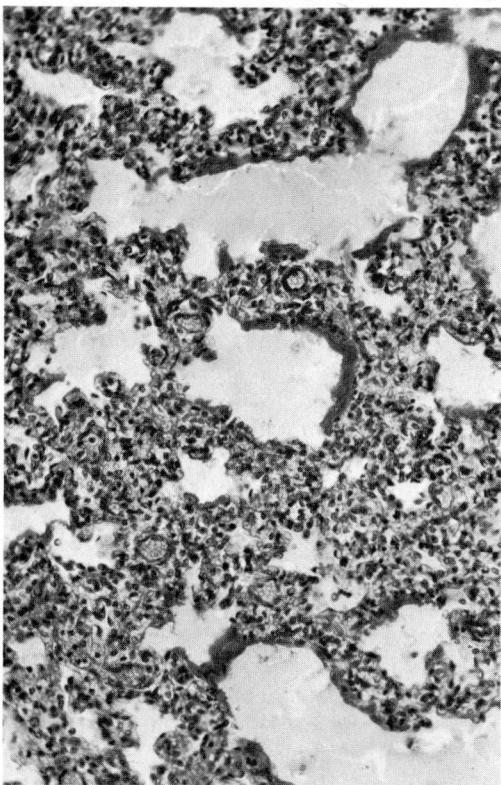

Figure 10–5. Hyaline membrane disease. There is alternating atelectasis and dilatation of the alveoli, and many airspaces are filled with fluid and lined by thick hyaline membranes.

ditional prominent feature is intense vascular congestion accompanied by distention of the lymphatics, which are often engorged with a protein-rich fluid. The lesions of hyaline membrane disease are never seen in stillborn infants or in those live-born babies who die within a few hours of birth.

In infants who survive more than 48 hours reparative changes are seen in the lungs. The alveolar epithelium proliferates under the surface of the membrane, which may be desquamated into the airspace, where it may undergo partial digestion or phagocytosis by macrophages. Concentric lamellar bodies within type II pneumocytes (morphologic markers of surfactant synthesis) can be found, but are decreased in number.

CLINICAL COURSE. It is difficult to express a clinical course and prognosis for this disease, as so much depends on the maturity and birth weight of the infant, the therapy employed, and the promptness of institution of the therapy. Overall, the mortality rate is approximately 20 to 30%, reaching levels exceeding 50% in infants in the range of 1000 gm body weight. The major threat to life is inadequate pulmonary exchange of oxygen and carbon dioxide, and with it a metabolic acidosis. The keystone of treatment is the delivery of oxygen to these severely hypoxic infants, usually accomplished by a variety of ventilatory assist methods, although as pointed out later there is promise in surfactant replacement therapy. In uncomplicated cases recovery begins to occur within three to four days. However, therapy carries with it the now well-recognized hazard of oxygen toxicity (p. 760). High concentrations of oxygen administered for prolonged periods have been proved to cause retrolental fibroplasia in the eyes and toxic changes in the lungs. Mechanical ventilation and oxygen toxicity may give rise to a subacute or chronic fibrosing condition called *bronchopulmonary dysplasia* (BPD). This complication may also occur in association with conditions other than RDS (e.g., viral pneumonia) if assisted ventilation and high concentrations of oxygen are utilized for treatment. Clinically BPD is characterized by persistence of respiratory distress for up to 3 to 6 months. Pathologically the larger airways show epithelial hyperplasia and squamous metaplasia. Alveolar walls are thickened and there is peribronchial as well as interstitial fibrosis. If oxygen toxicity is avoided and the infant can be kept alive for about three or four days, recovery can be anticipated without permanent sequelae.

Infants recovering from RDS are at increased risk of developing a variety of other complications as well. Most important among these are *patent ductus arteriosus, intraventricular hemorrhage,* and *necrotizing enterocolitis.* With the advent of neonatal intensive care that ensures better chances of recovery from the pulmonary problems, these complications are assuming increasing importance as causes of mortality and morbidity associated with RDS. We will discuss these briefly. You may recall that the *patent ductus* normally closes within a few hours after birth at full term (p. 623). However, because of immaturity, hypoxia, and acidosis, the closure of the ductus is delayed in infants with RDS. Early in the course of RDS, left-to-right shunt through the patent ductus is usually not significant because the presence of hypoxia in these infants causes pulmonary vasoconstriction and increased right-sided pressure. However, as hypoxia abates, reduced pulmonary blood pressure allows significant shunting, leading eventually to congestive heart failure and pulmonary congestion. This complication may be clinically significant in up to 30% of cases. Hypoxia and immaturity of the brain also provide the setting for *intraventricular hemorrhages,* which may afflict premature infants even in the absence of RDS.[27] In the premature infant a disproportionately large amount of cerebral blood flows through the periventricular circulation, where the vessel walls are fragile and poorly supported by the subependymal germinal matrix. In the presence of asphyxia, both cerebral blood flow and venous pressure increase, thus stretching the poorly supported delicate periventricular capillaries beyond their limits. Periventricular hemorrhage results, tracking its way into the ventricles in over 80% of cases. Often the hemorrhage assumes massive proportions because of excessive fibrinolytic activity in the periventricular region of the immature brain. Severe hemorrhage carries a toll of 50 to 65% mortality. RDS also provides the setting for a mysterious entity called *necrotizing enterocolitis* (p. 890), a dreaded complication in premature infants who are admitted to neonatal intensive care units. The cause and pathogenesis of necrotizing enterocolitis are poorly understood, but suspected factors include intestinal ischemia resulting from hypoxia, bacterial invasion, and hypertonic formula feeding. The lesions involve primarily the ileum and colon, which show extensive ulceration and necrosis, sometimes associated with perforation and peritonitis. Thus, although the high technology of today saves many infants with RDS, it also brings to the surface the exquisite fragility of the immature neonate.

A major thrust in the control of RDS focuses on prevention, either by delaying labor till the fetal lung reaches maturity or by inducing maturation of the lung in the fetus at risk. Critical to these objectives is the ability to assess fetal lung maturity accurately. Because pulmonary secretions are discharged into the amniotic fluid, analysis of amniotic fluid lecithin (phosphatidylcholine) provides a good estimate of the level of surfactant in the alveolar lining. Widely used for the assessment of fetal lung maturity is the relationship of amniotic fluid lecithin to sphingomyelin (the L/S ratio). In early pregnancy the concentration of sphingomyelin exceeds that of lecithin. At about 35 weeks of gestation the activity of type II pneumocytes increases greatly and hence the lecithin levels increase sharply, usually to more than twice that of sphingomyelin, and continue to increase while sphingomyelin levels decline. Clinical experience indicates that when the L/S ratio approximates 2 : 1, the threat of RDS is small. In recent years, measurement of phosphatidylglycerol and phosphatidylcholine phosphorus in the amniotic fluid has been found to provide important additional indicators of lung maturity. These phospholipids are detected after 36 weeks of gestation and increase progressively thereafter.

Because corticosteroids are known to accelerate maturation of fetal lung, prophylactic administration in women at risk for preterm delivery has been advocated. Success in reducing perinatal mortality from RDS has been documented in carefully selected cases.[28] The most exciting recent advance in the treatment of RDS has been the success of surfactant replacement therapy. Several clinical trials have confirmed that administration of aerosolized surfactant early in the course of RDS is associated with a reduction in morbidity and mortality.[29]

NEONATAL ASPHYXIA

Inadequate delivery of blood to the fetus may result in hypoxic damage manifesting as late gestational death, stillbirth, or a live-born infant with low Apgar scores, respiratory distress, and apnea. Disruption of oxygen delivery can originate in the umbilical cord, placenta, or the mother's systemic circulation. Occasionally direct injury may occur during the complex transitions that occur during delivery, which can contribute to hypoxia in the neonate. Although the underlying cause of neonatal hypoxia may not always be identified, several factors put the fetus at risk: placenta previa (implantation adjacent to the cervical os), abruptio placentae (premature separation), and umbilical cord compression or rupture. These may result in sudden death late in gestation or the syndrome of neonatal asphyxia. Other factors associated with asphyxia include toxemia, diabetes, extremes of maternal age, prolonged rupture of the membranes, chorioamnionitis, breech presentation, prolonged labor, prematurity, and multiple births.

The pathologic features of peripartum asphyxia vary depending on the time of survival after the hypoxic insult. A rapid prenatal demise may leave evidence only in the placental tissues, making their examination indispensable.[29a] Those infants resuscitated at birth and living for several days manifest changes due to the initiating insult with superimposed alterations induced by intensive therapy. On gross examination many of the infants are growth retarded and at autopsy are found to have numerous visceral hemorrhages. Areas of necrosis are often seen in the adrenal, renal papillae, and bowel. Those surviving long enough may have neuronal and cerebral white matter necrosis sometimes associated with hemorrhage. Such infants have a high probability of exhibiting long-term neurologic damage. In contrast to the microscopic changes in respiratory distress of prematurity, hyaline membranes when present line the distal alveoli rather than the terminal bronchioles. In

utero hypoxia may result in the passage of meconium with subsequent aspiration, further compromising respiratory function. Squamous cells, granular material, and yellow granules may be found in the alveoli. In addition meconium may be seen on the infant's skin, in the bronchi, and in macrophages in the fetal membranes. Neonatal asphyxia often necessitates the use of vigorous mechanical ventilation, which may result in alveolar tears, pneumothorax, and leakage of air into the interlobular septa, producing further damage.

ERYTHROBLASTOSIS FETALIS — HEMOLYTIC DISEASE OF NEWBORN

When the fetus inherits red cell antigenic determinants from the father that are foreign to the mother, a maternal immune reaction may occur, leading to hemolytic disease in the infant. Basic to such a phenomenon are leakage of fetal red cells into the maternal circulation and, in turn, transplacental passage of the maternal antibodies into the fetus. Any of the numerous red cell antigenic systems may theoretically be involved, but the major antigens known to induce clinically significant immunologic disease are the ABO and certain of the Rh antigens. The resultant fetal hemolytic reaction may cause mild-to-severe disease in the newborn, or even death. Thus, *erythroblastosis fetalis may be defined as a hemolytic disease in the newborn caused by blood-group incompatibility between mother and child.* The incidence of Rh erythroblastosis in urban populations has declined remarkably, owing largely to the current methods of preventing Rh immunization in "at-risk" mothers. Nevertheless, it is necessary to discuss Rh hemolytic disease in some detail because successful prophylaxis of this disorder has resulted directly from an understanding of its pathogenesis.

ETIOLOGY AND PATHOGENESIS. To explain the pathogenesis of Rh hemolytic disease, a few details of the Rh antigenic system will be reviewed. Of the approximately 25 Rh antigens, the D antigen is the major cause of Rh incompatibility. It is estimated that 15% of whites and 7% of blacks do not possess the D antigen and so are said to be Rh negative. Thus, among whites there is an approximately 12% chance of a mating between an Rh-positive male and an Rh-negative female. However, the frequency of manifest Rh erythroblastosis is much lower because several factors influence the maternal immune response to Rh-positive fetal cells. *Concurrent ABO incompatibility* protects the mother against immunization, presumably because leaked fetal red cells are promptly coated by circulating isohemagglutinins and then removed from the circulation by the mononuclear phagocytic system. Another critical factor that determines the magnitude of the antibody response is the *dose of the immunizing antigen.* Hemolytic disease develops in the newborn only when the mother has experienced a significant transplacental "bleed." It is generally thought that more than 1 ml of Rh-positive red cells is required to produce regularly a significant immune response in the mother. In the great majority of pregnancies transplacental hemorrhages of such magnitude occur only during delivery or abortions. *Previous sensitization* significantly alters the risk of development of erythroblastosis fetalis. The first exposure to Rh antigens initially stimulates an increase in IgM antibodies that do not cross the placenta. Subsequently there is a rise in IgG antibodies, small enough to cross the placenta. Because primary immunization usually occurs during labor, hemolytic disease rarely occurs during the first pregnancy unless, of course, the mother has experienced previous sensitization. In these days of meticulous blood typing, it is highly unlikely that an Rh-negative mother would be sensitized by an Rh-positive transfusion. However, a previous abortion or stillbirth of an Rh-positive fetus might induce prior sensitization. The greatest risk is encountered in second and subsequent pregnancies of Rh-positive infants because in presensitized women even a small transplacental bleed could trigger a brisk secondary IgG response. Administration of anti-D immunoglobulin to Rh-negative women within 72 hours of the birth of an Rh-positive infant is now a widely used practice that serves to prevent primary sensitization in the great majority of cases (p. 529). The success of this method of prophylaxis is based on the ability of the passively administered Rh antibody to coat the fetal cells in maternal circulation and thereby prevent exposure of the Rh antigens to the maternal lymphoid system.

Owing to the remarkable success achieved in prevention of Rh hemolytic disease, *fetomaternal ABO incompatibility is currently the most common cause of erythroblastosis fetalis.* Several features distinguish ABO hemolytic disease from that caused by Rh incompatibility. Although ABO incompatibility occurs in approximately 20 to 25% of pregnancies, only about one in ten of such infants develops laboratory evidence of hemolytic disease. Furthermore, because the immune reaction is much less severe than that encountered in Rh incompatibility, the hemolytic disease is severe enough to require treatment in only one in 200 cases of ABO incompatibility.[30] Several factors account for these observations. Most antibodies directed against A and B red cell antigens are of the IgM type and therefore do not cross the placenta. However, for reasons not well known, group O individuals often possess IgG, anti-A or anti-B (or both), without sensitization by previous pregnancy or blood transfusion. It is therefore not surprising that ABO hemolytic disease occurs almost exclusively in infants born to group O mothers and that the firstborn may also be affected. Fortunately, even in the presence of transplacentally acquired IgG antibodies, the lysis of infants' red cells is often minimal. The major factor responsible for this protection seems to be poor expression of blood group antigens A and B on neonatal red cells. In one study the strength of A antigen expression on cord blood cells was approximately 50% of that found on adult red cells.[31] An additional protective factor seems to be the presence of A and B antigens on cells other than red blood cells, thus sopping up some of the transferred antibodies. Only those few infants who express a relatively strong A antigen (usually A$_1$) suffer from ABO hemolytic disease. Because the antibodies are formed naturally, i.e., without obvious sensitization, there is no effective method of protection against ABO reactions.

The incidence of hemolytic disease due to incompatibilities of other blood groups is extremely small and a discussion of these may be found in published reviews.[30,32]

There are two major consequences of hemolytic disease of the newborn. Excessive destruction of red blood cells leads to reduction in the oxygen-carrying capacity of blood (anemia) on the one hand and accumulation of bilirubin (jaundice) on the other. However, the severity of these changes varies considerably. In the full-term infant, mild hemolytic reactions may induce neither anemia nor jaundice because marrow hyperactivity may compensate for the destruction of red cells, and the hepatic excretory system may be capable of handling the increased load of bilirubin. When the compensatory capacity of the marrow is exceeded, extramedullary hematopoiesis in the liver and spleen may suffice to maintain normal levels of red cells in the blood. More severe hemolytic destruction of red cells may exceed these compensatory mechanisms and lead to anemia, still unaccompanied by jaundice. If the hemolytic reaction is even more marked, the anemia is then associated with jaundice and, as will be seen, the development of moderate-to-massive anasarca. When the serum bilirubin exceeds 1 to 2 mg/dl, jaundice becomes clinically evident. Unconjugated bilirubin is water insoluble and has an affinity for lipids. In the infant with a poorly developed blood-brain barrier, the bilirubin may bind to the lipids in the brain and produce serious damage.

MORPHOLOGY. The anatomic findings in erythroblastosis fetalis vary with the severity of the hemolytic process. Infants may be stillborn, die within the first few days, or recover completely. In its mildest form, the anemia may be only slight, and the child may survive without further complication. More severe hemolysis gives rise to jaundice and other features associated with hemolytic anemias (p. 662). Hypoxic injury to the heart and liver may lead to circulatory and hepatic failure with resultant edema, sometimes so severe as to merit the designation of anasarca. The plasma protein levels sometimes drop to as low as 2.0 to 2.5 gm/dl because of reduced hepatic synthesis. This pattern is known as **hydrops fetalis.** In most cases the liver and spleen are enlarged, the degree depending on the severity of the hemolytic process and the compensatory extramedullary erythropoiesis.

The most serious threat in erythroblastosis is central nervous system damage known as **kernicterus.** In jaundiced infants, the unconjugated bilirubin appears to be particularly toxic to the brain tissue. The brain is enlarged and edematous and, when sectioned, is found to have a bright yellow pigmentation (kernicterus), particularly in the basal ganglia, thalamus, cerebellum, cerebral gray matter, and spinal cord. This pigmentation is evanescent and fades within 24 hours despite prompt fixation. It is therefore necessary to section the brain immediately in suspected cases to establish the diagnosis. It is worth noting that such pigmentation of the brain is not limited exclusively to erythroblastosis fetalis, as it has also been described in milder form in infants with severe physiologic jaundice of the newborn. This bile pigmentation of the brain is of considerable theoretical interest because, in the adult, some blood-brain barrier blocks the passage of bilirubin into the spinal fluid and substance of the brain even when there is severe jaundice. The precise blood level of bilirubin that will induce kernicterus is unpredictable, but neural damage rarely occurs if the serum bilirubin concentration is below 20 mg/dl. At lower levels, premature infants, especially, are at risk. The mechanism by which free (unconjugated) bilirubin enters the brain in the newborn is not clearly understood. The level of serum albumin (which binds bilirubin), pH of the blood, and hypoxia are all considered to be important factors in allowing the passage of bilirubin into the brain.[33]

Histologically, the diagnosis of erythroblastosis fetalis depends on the identification of abnormally increased erythropoietic activity in the infant. The red cell series in the marrow is hyperactive, and extramedullary hematopoiesis is almost invariably present in the liver (Fig. 10–6), spleen, and possibly other tissues, such as the lymph nodes, kidneys, lungs, and even the heart. This hematopoietic activity is sufficiently striking to account for increased numbers of reticulocytes, normoblasts, and erythroblasts in the circulating blood. Evidence of subcutaneous and visceral edema is present in the hydrops syndrome along with fluid in the peritoneal, pleural, and pericardial cavities.

CLINICAL FEATURES.

The clinical manifestations of erythroblastosis should be readily evident from the preceding discussion. They range from pallor, possibly accompanied by hepatosplenomegaly in the mildly affected infant (to which may be added jaundice with more severe hemolytic reactions), to the most gravely ill child with intense jaundice, widespread edema, and signs of neurologic involvement in the pattern referred to as hydrops fetalis.

In the last 15 years, remarkable success has been achieved in the prophylaxis of Rh hemolytic disease. As mentioned earlier, administration of anti-D immunoglobulin to Rh-negative (previously nonsensitized) women within 72 hours of delivery of an Rh-positive child prevents Rh immunization in the vast majority of cases. Obviously such treatment has to be employed not only after the first but also following each subsequent childbirth. Although experience has indicated that the use of immunoprophylaxis is highly successful in preventing Rh sensitization, it is not perfect. Approximately 2% of women at risk develop anti-D antibodies in the last trimester or within 72 hours

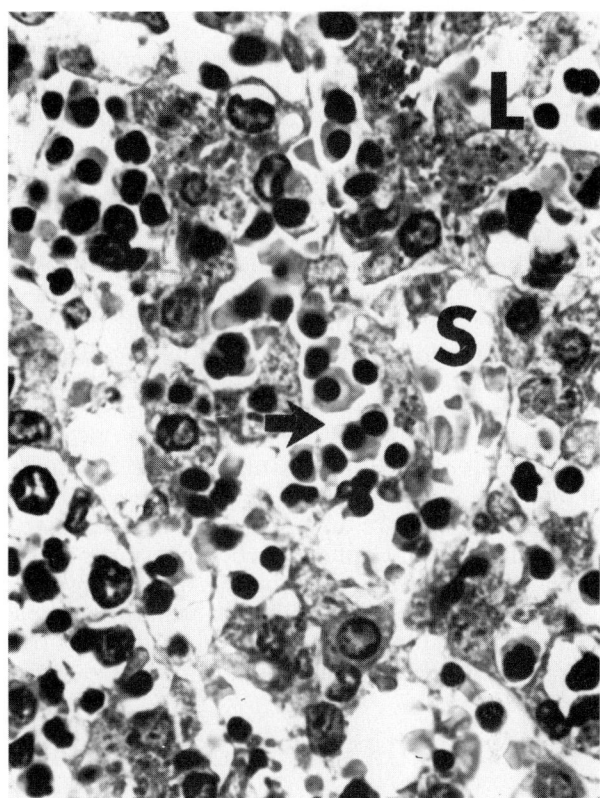

Figure 10–6. Liver in erythroblastosis fetalis with extramedullary hematopoiesis. L = liver cells; S = dilated sinusoid; arrow points to a cluster of nucleated red cells. (Courtesy of Dr. José Hernandez, Department of Pathology, Southwestern Medical School, Dallas, Texas.)

after labor, and thus fail to benefit from Rh immunoprophylaxis.[34] Some of these cases may result from unrecognized previous Rh-positive abortions, but many are believed to be due to significant transplacental bleeds during the early part of the third trimester. In principle, it should be possible to prevent sensitization in such women and thereby increase the success of Rh immunoprophylaxis if anti-D immunoglobulin is administered ante partum at 28 or 34 weeks of gestation as well as post partum. Although the success of such an approach has been documented in some studies, ante-partum administration of anti-D immunoglobulins is still not a widely accepted practice.[35]

Despite all efforts to prevent incompatibility reactions, it is still necessary to monitor the infant at birth for indications of impending disease. The most important clue to potential disease is a positive direct Coombs' test on fetal cord blood, which detects the presence of immunoglobulins coating the fetal red cells. In the *direct* Coombs' test, antiserum (Coombs' serum) against human gamma globulin induces agglutination of red cells coated with specific antibodies. An *indirect* Coombs' test employs normal red cells first exposed to the suspected serum and then treated with Coombs' serum, which then induces agglutination of the red cells if anti–red cell antibodies are present in the suspected serum. Postnatally, the severity of the hemolytic reaction can be monitored by the rapidity of the rise and the ultimate levels of the unconjugated bilirubin in the serum of the infant. The levels may be normal at birth because of placental clearance of the bilirubin, but in severe hemolytic disease they rise rapidly within the first day of life to reach extremely high levels (over 20 mg/dl). Premature or low-birth-weight infants are at greatest risk because their conjugating and excretory systems are less able to cope with the bilirubin overload.

The availability of tests to monitor the severity of the hemolytic reaction has opened a variety of avenues for the treatment of hemolytic disease of the newborn. When analysis of amniotic fluid discloses critical levels of bilirubin, premature delivery may be induced if the fetus is judged to be viable with regard to size. Earlier, fetal transfusion may be attempted.[36] Postnatally, a variety of supportive measures may be employed, including phototherapy (visual light oxidizes toxic unconjugated bilirubin to harmless, readily excreted, water-soluble dipyrroles) and, in severe cases, total exchange transfusion of the infant.

INBORN ERRORS OF METABOLISM

The number of now well-characterized inborn errors of metabolism has become astronomic and far beyond the scope of this chapter.[37] Most of these conditions are exceedingly rare. Some were discussed earlier, in the chapter on genetic disorders (p. 143). Only two, phenylketonuria and galactosemia, are selected for inclusion here because, in both, prompt recognition in the first days of life permits the institution of an appropriate dietary regimen that can prevent early death, or, even worse, survival with mental retardation.

PHENYLKETONURIA (PKU)

Phenylketonuria is an autosomal recessive disorder expressed in the homozygote, characterized by a lack of phenylalanine hydroxylase, which if untreated leads to hyperphenylalaninemia and usually mental retardation. The incidence of this disorder is one in 12,000 in the United States, being higher in those of Celtic origin and Central Europeans. This description applies to the great majority of patients said to have *classic PKU*, but several significant exceptions have been noted in recent years.[38] For example, it is quite clear that mere elevation of serum phenylalanine levels is not necessarily associated with the stigmata of PKU. Persons with so-called "benign hyperphenylalaninemia" do not develop mental retardation except in the few cases in which there is marked elevation of blood phenylalanine levels. At the other end of the spectrum are some patients in whom neurologic impairment occurs despite dietary control of phenylalanine intake. *These complexities are clearly significant because it can no longer be assumed that an infant with an elevated phenylalanine level requires the rigors of dietary restrictions, nor can the mere restriction of phenylalanine intake be considered adequate for every infant with hyperphenylalaninemia.* A detailed discussion of phenylalanine metabolism is beyond the scope of this book, but a brief overview is warranted to obtain some insight into the varieties of hyperphenylalaninemia.

In a normal child, less than 50% of the dietary phenylalanine is utilized for polypeptide and protein synthesis; most of that remaining is converted to tyrosine by means of hydroxylation. This reaction requires the phenylalanine hydroxylating system, which has several components in addition to the hepatic enzyme phenylalanine hydroxylase (PAH)[39] (Fig. 10–7). Two of the components, tetrahydrobiopterin (BH_4) and dihydropteridine reductase (DHPR), are relevant for our discussion. During the hydroxylation of phenylalanine to tyrosine, BH_4, which is the coenzyme for PAH, is converted to dihydrobiopterin (BH_2). The latter is then reduced back to BH_4 by the enzyme DHPR. As indicated in Figure 10–7, the regeneration of BH_4 is tightly coupled to the hydroxylation of phenylalanine. In addition to their role in phenylalanine metabolism, DHPR and BH_4 are involved in the hydroxylations of tyrosine and tryptophan, a fact that is relevant to the pathogenesis of the variant forms of PKU. With this background we can discuss the genetic and phenotypic variants of hyperphenylalaninemia.

The classic form of PKU is believed to result from

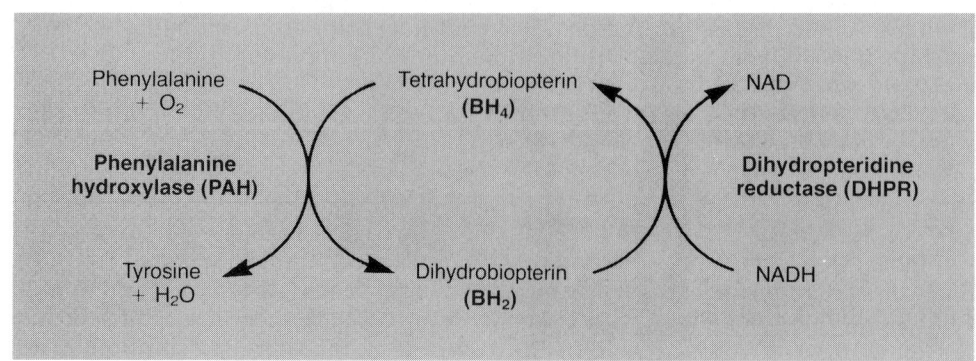

Figure 10–7. The phenylalanine hydroxylase system.

an almost complete lack (<0.27% of normal) of hepatic PAH, whereas a less severe deficiency of PAH may lead to benign hyperphenylalaninemia. In the latter condition hepatic PAH activity varies between 1.5 and 34.5% of normal. The levels of hydroxylase activity in turn determine the plasma phenylalanine levels. Persons with complete lack of hepatic PAH usually have sustained and marked hyperphenylalaninemia (>1 mM/liter; normal <0.12) when ingesting a normal diet, whereas phenylalanine levels range from 0.12 to 1.0 mM/liter in patients with benign hyperphenylalaninemia. Recent cloning of the PAH gene has shed considerable light on the genetic basis of these variations.[40] Molecular analyses have revealed the existence of several distinct mutations in the PAH gene (genetic heterogeneity). Different mutant forms of PAH are associated with a variable degree of reduction in the enzyme activity. Thus it seems that the PAH levels, and therefore the clinical severity of PKU, are conditioned by the specific combinations of mutant alleles that are inherited.[41]

Approximately 3 to 10% of patients with PKU have an underlying deficiency of enzymes other than PAH.[39] In one variant form the enzyme DHPR is lacking, whereas in another there is defective synthesis of BH_2 (see Fig. 10–7). As mentioned earlier, DHPR and BH_4 are required not only for phenylalanine metabolism but also for the hydroxylation of tyrosine and tryptophan, an essential step in the synthesis of their neurotransmitter metabolites. In such cases, the successful control of hyperphenylalaninemia by dietary measures fails to arrest the progressive neurologic damage because the synthesis of neurotransmitters remains impaired. At present the variant forms of PKU can be distinguished from classic PKU only in specialized laboratories.

With a block in the conversion of phenylalanine to tyrosine, several minor metabolites of phenylalanine are synthesized in excessive amounts. These include phenylpyruvic acid, phenyllactic acid, phenylacetic acid, and O-hydroxyphenylacetic acid, all of which are excreted in the urine. The peculiar musty or mouselike odor of untreated patients has been attributed to the presence of phenylacetic acid in the sweat. The basis of mental retardation in PKU is not entirely clear; excessive amounts of phenylalanine or its metabolites probably contribute to an impairment of lipid biosynthesis in the brain.[42] Although there is no straightforward or consistent relationship between plasma phenylalanine levels and brain development, it is generally considered that persons with plasma levels above 1 mM/liter (>16.5 mg/dl) are at a high risk of developing mental retardation. In variant forms of PKU, the additional lack of neurotransmitters (derived normally from tyrosine and tryptophan) contributes to the neurologic deterioration.

The only significant morphologic changes found in classic PKU are limited to the brain, and these are variable and nonspecific and cannot be related biochemically to the metabolic changes in these patients. Usually the brain decreases in weight. Defective development of myelin or the formation of an abnormal myelin produces spongy, focal lesions of the white matter.[43] With progression of the disorder, these defects become more evident, the demyelination becomes widespread, and the spongy foci are replaced by areas of gliosis.[44]

Infants with classic PKU are apparently normal at birth with no elevation of serum phenylalanine levels. Usually, however, by day 3 or 4 the serum phenylalanine levels begin to rise and in most cases exceed 1 mM/liter (>16.5 mg/dl). Manifestations of brain involvement in the form of abnormal electroencephalographic findings, seizures, and bizarre behavior become evident within three or four months in the untreated infant. Without dietary intervention, the cerebral damage progresses to reach its maximum at age 2 to 3 years. Most untreated patients have IQ values below 20, and fewer than 4% achieve scores greater than 50 to 60. Characteristically these infants develop the musty or mouselike odor previously mentioned and often eczema of the skin. Because of the deranged tyrosine metabolism, little or no melanin is synthesized, and therefore these patients frequently have unusually fair skin, blonde hair, and blue eyes even when the parents have very dark complexions.

With an appropriate special diet, free of phenylalanine and supplemented with tyrosine, blood levels of phenylalanine can be maintained at near-normal levels in the classic form and the mental retardation can be prevented. The IQ scores of treated children are near normal and the greatest benefit occurs if treatment is instituted within the first month of life and continued until six years of age. However, some recent studies indicate a fall in IQ several years after the cessation of treatment. Therefore, long-term dietary treatment is recommended and is of particular importance for female subjects with PKU who wish to have children, because high levels of phenylalanine have been proved to be teratogenic.[45,46]

In view of the disastrous but preventable effects of PKU in untreated individuals, great emphasis has been placed on early detection of affected infants. Neonatal screening for elevated blood phenylalanine levels is now widely practiced in the United States and several European countries. However, the screening procedures employed—the Guthrie bacterial inhibition assay and the fluorometric methods—cannot distinguish between various forms of hyperphenylalaninemias; hence a positive screening test must be followed by further metabolic testing. Antenatal diagnosis of PKU is not possible by the usual enzyme assays because PAH is not expressed in amniotic fluid cells. This hurdle has now been overcome by DNA analysis of fetal cells obtained by either amniocentesis or chorionic villus biopsy, since the mutant PAH gene is present in all cells.

GALACTOSEMIA

Two forms of galactosemia have been identified, each resulting from a hereditary deficiency of an enzyme involved in the metabolism of galactose. The more common form involves *a lack of galactose-1-phosphate uridyl transferase*, blocking the metabolism of galactose in Reaction 2 in Figure 10–8. The other form of galactosemia involves a deficiency of galactokinase, also transmitted as an autosomal recessive trait. In contrast to the transferase deficiency, this form is relatively benign and does not cause mental retardation but only the development of cataracts (opacification of the ocular lens); it will not be considered further here.

Estimates of the prevalence of the transferase deficiency range from one in 40,000 to one in 60,000.[47] With a total lack of transferase activity, infants cannot metabolize galactose-1-phosphate; when untreated, they develop progressive mental retardation and die early in infancy. Heterozygotes have half the normal level of transferase activity and are spared the consequences suffered by the homozygote.

With the rise in blood galactose levels, galactosuria appears, accompanied by generalized aminoaciduria resulting from impaired renal tubular reabsorption. *The diagnosis is suspected by the finding of reducing substances in urine that are not positive for glucose.* It can be readily established by a variety of tests. The transferase is normally found in liver cells, leukocytes, and erythrocytes, and sensitive enzyme assays permit identification of the enzyme lack in these cells. Similarly, antenatal diagnosis of this metabolic disorder is possible in cultured fibroblasts derived from amniotic fluid. Heterozygotes having a less severe deficiency in the transferase can also be detected. The elevated galactose levels in the blood and urine are less specific but are valuable clues to the existence of this condition.

In the untreated homozygous disease, infants appear normal at birth, but soon after milk feeding has been instituted develop listlessness, vomiting, diarrhea, and failure to thrive. Jaundice appears early and may seem to be a continuation of the neonatal physiologic jaundice. Soon thereafter, hepatomegaly, splenomegaly, and cataracts develop along with signs of hepatic failure. The liver damage may induce a prothrombin deficiency and a hemorrhagic tendency together with lowered glucose levels and attendant hypoglycemic symptoms. Mental retardation may now become evident. The downward course of the disease may be quite rapid with progressive motor and mental deterioration, leading to death from inanition or hepatic failure. White blood cells of galactosemic patients have reduced phagocytic and bactericidal activity, rendering these patients susceptible to serious bacterial infections. In particular, *Escherichia coli* septicemia is a dreaded complication that may be responsible for death within the first few weeks of life.

The involvement of the brain is surprisingly subtle. Nonspecific alterations appear in the central nervous system. Loss of nerve cells, gliosis, and edema are particularly prevalent in the dentate nuclei of the cerebellum and the olivary nuclei of the medulla. There is similar gliosis in the cerebral cortex and white matter, but only occasional damage in the basal ganglia.[48]

Although other organs such as the kidney and eyes are affected, the liver changes are most striking. The early hepatomegaly is due largely to fatty change, but in time cirrhosis supervenes (Fig. 10–9). Microscopically, there is extensive fat throughout the liver lobule as well as bile stasis, both within ductules at the periphery of the lobule and within biliary canaliculi. Often, liver cells are arranged in a rosette-like fashion about the bile plugs. With progression of the disease, a delicate fibrosis appears first in the periportal regions and eventually extends to produce scars bridging adjacent portal tracts. These liver changes have a remarkable resemblance to those found in patients with the cirrhosis of alcohol abuse. Occasionally, in addition to fat the liver cells contain an excess of glycogen.

The correlation of the morphologic changes in classic galactosemia with the metabolic derangement in galactose metabolism is not entirely clear. Currently it is proposed that, with the build-up of galac-

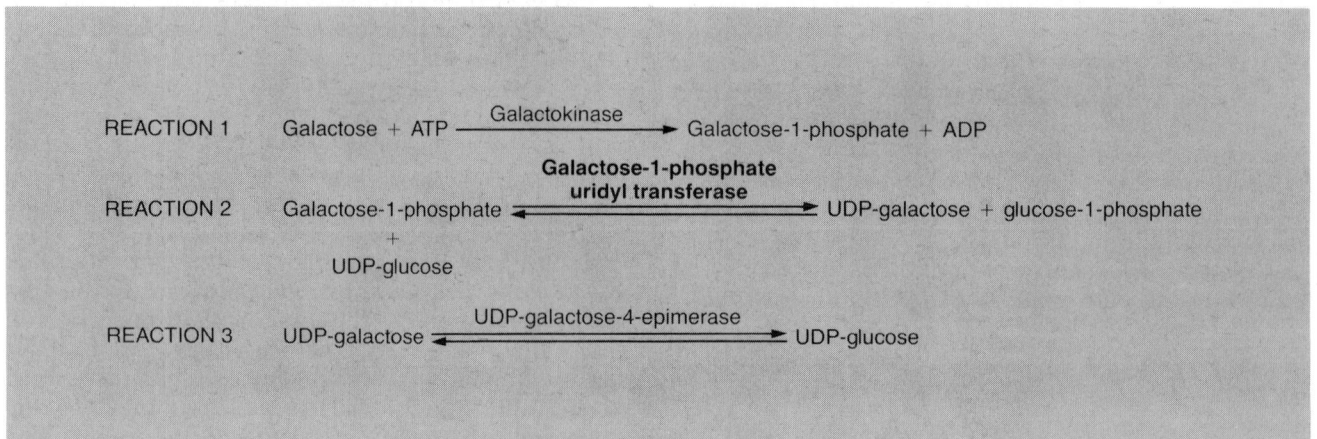

REACTION 1   Galactose + ATP $\xrightarrow{\text{Galactokinase}}$ Galactose-1-phosphate + ADP

REACTION 2   Galactose-1-phosphate $\underset{}{\overset{\textbf{Galactose-1-phosphate uridyl transferase}}{\rightleftharpoons}}$ UDP-galactose + glucose-1-phosphate

+ UDP-glucose

REACTION 3   UDP-galactose $\underset{}{\overset{\text{UDP-galactose-4-epimerase}}{\rightleftharpoons}}$ UDP-glucose

Figure 10–8. Pathways of galactose metabolism.

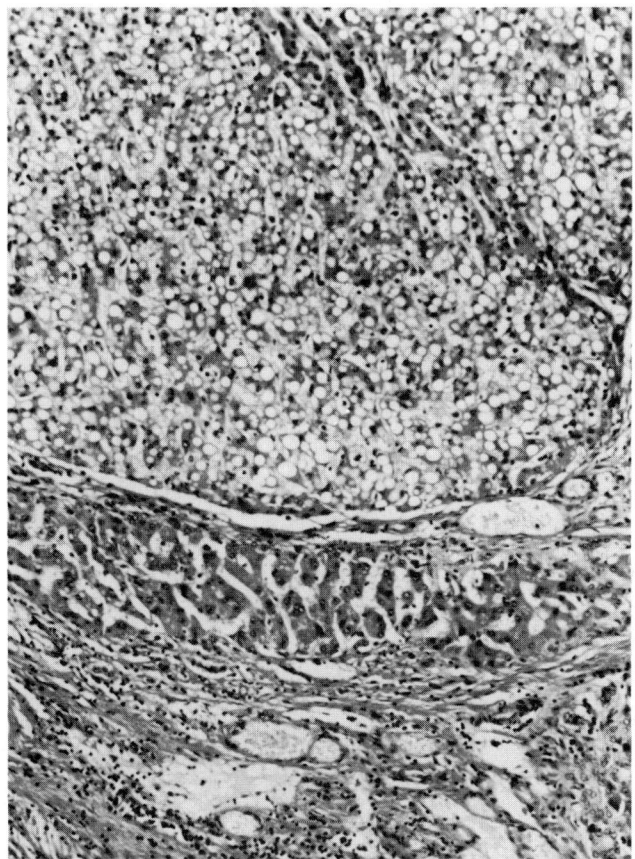

Figure 10-9. Galactosemia. Liver shows extensive fatty change and a delicate fibrosis. (Courtesy of Dr. Joe Rutledge, Southwestern Medical School, Dallas, Texas.)

tose-1-phosphate behind the transferase block, alternate metabolic pathways are activated with the formation of galactitol. It is postulated that the accumulation of galactitol within the lens leads to hyperosmolarity and excessive imbibition of water to induce the cataracts. The reason for the hepatotoxicity remains obscure.

Early recognition of the homozygous form of the disease, withdrawal of milk from the diet, and substitution of a galactose-free diet spare the infant the clinical and morphologic consequences, and normal development into adulthood may be expected. If treatment is delayed until the onset of symptoms, the neurologic damage seems to be irreversible, although improvements in cataracts and in liver functions may be noted. Delay in the institution of dietary treatment may produce other effects that may not be recognized for many years, such as ovarian atrophy.[49]

CYSTIC FIBROSIS (CF, MUCOVISCIDOSIS)

Among the genetic pediatric disorders, CF is probably the most important. It is very common and often fatal in childhood and young adult life. The cause is unknown, *but it is basically a disorder of exocrine glands affecting both mucus-secreting and eccrine sweat glands throughout the body.* The abnormally viscid mucous secretions in the excretory pancreatic ducts leading to their cystic dilatation and fibrous atrophy of the dependent exocrine glands first drew attention to this condition and gave rise to the designation *cystic fibrosis.* Later it became evident that the mucoid secretions throughout the body were abnormal, and thus this condition became known as *mucoviscidosis.* However, it was then recognized that elevation of sweat sodium chloride is characteristically present from birth and throughout life, making it evident that more than mucous glands are involved in this disorder, and so the less restrictive term cystic fibrosis is again favored. Nonetheless, the obstruction of organ passages by the abnormally behaving mucus leads to most of the clinical features of this disorder, i.e., chronic pulmonary disease, pancreatic insufficiency, steatorrhea, malnutrition, hepatic cirrhosis, intestinal obstruction, and other complications. These manifestations may appear at any point in life from before birth to much later in childhood or even in adolescence.[50]

INCIDENCE. Most of the evidence favors the view that cystic fibrosis follows simple autosomal recessive transmission. Homozygotes express this syndrome fully. Heterozygotes have no recognizable clinical symptoms. The frequency of cystic fibrosis in whites is approximately one in 2000. Orientals and blacks are seldom affected. On the basis of the frequency of affected homozygotes in the white population, it is estimated that one in 20 individuals must be heterozygous carriers.

ETIOLOGY AND PATHOGENESIS. Because CF is a mendelian disorder, it must result from mutation in a single gene, giving rise to changes in the structure or quantity of a single protein. Although the CF gene and its product have yet to be identified, we are at the threshold of major breakthroughs in unraveling its molecular basis. This optimism stems from several recent studies focused on two major areas: mapping of the CF gene and investigation of ion transport across epithelial cells of the affected organs.

THE CF GENE. There is little doubt that the CF gene is located on the long arm of chromosome 7. Analysis of DNA obtained from affected individuals and their family members has revealed several gene markers that are tightly linked to the CF gene. These linkage studies have narrowed the search for the culprit to an extremely small segment of chromosome 7, between bands q22 and q31.[51] Further molecular analysis of this region will, in all likelihood, lead to the identification of the CF gene. Although the CF gene product has not yet been identified, an immediate effect of these advances has been in the diagnosis of carriers and in antenatal detection of affected individuals. These applications will be described later in this section.

ION TRANSPORT IN CF. A series of electrophysiologic studies on sweat gland ducts and respiratory epi-

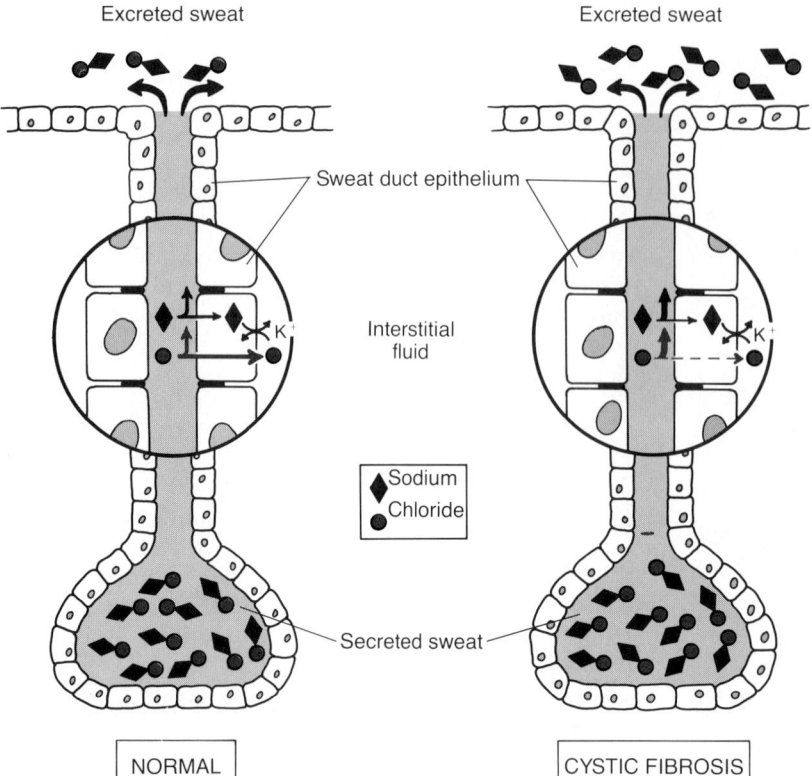

NORMAL

CYSTIC FIBROSIS

Figure 10-10. Schematic illustration of the defective Cl⁻ ion transport in cystic fibrosis sweat glands.

thelium point conclusively to a fundamental defect in the transport of chloride (Cl⁻) and possibly other anions across epithelia.[52-54] These observations provide the basis for a unifying hypothesis about the cellular defect in CF and the resulting alterations in exocrine secretions. As indicated in Figure 10-10, the concentrations of Na⁺ and Cl⁻ ions secreted into the *sweat glands* of CF patients are normal. However, unlike normal epithelial cells, those lining the CF *sweat ducts* are relatively impermeable to Cl⁻. Hence, as the sweat moves towards the surface, the reabsorption of Cl⁻ and the accompanying cation Na⁺ fails to occur. Not surprisingly, therefore, patients with CF excrete in their sweat an excess of sodium chloride, a finding that is highly characteristic of this condition. In the respiratory tract, transepithelial electrolyte transport controls the quantity and composition of the respiratory tract fluid. The normal airway epithelium actively transports Cl⁻ from the submucosal to mucosal surface. In CF there is a failure to secrete Cl⁻ ions into the lumen, which leads secondarily to reduced Na⁺ content in the luminal fluid. Because movement of water is driven by NaCl, the net effect of reduced Cl⁻ secretions is to lower the water content of the airway secretions, leading to their dehydration, which is responsible for the accumulation of hyperconcentrated, viscid secretions that obstruct the air passages and predispose to recurrent pulmonary infections.[55] In the pancreas, another important organ affected by CF, anion secretion also appears to be at fault. However, unlike respiratory fluids and sweat, the major anion secreted into the pancreatic ducts is

bicarbonate ion (HCO_3^-), not Cl⁻. Patients with CF have reduced bicarbonate (and water) content in their pancreatic secretions.[56] Since Cl⁻ and other anions such as HCO_3^- are transported across cell membranes through anion channels, deranged epithelial anion transport seems to be a generalized cellular defect in CF.[57] The mechanisms that regulate Cl⁻ transport are not fully understood, but there is emerging evidence that a calcium-binding protein that is an integral component of a regulatory complex may be at fault.[58,59]

To summarize, recent investigations have led to the localization of the CF gene on the long arm of chromosome 7. Although the gene product has not been identified, there are good reasons to believe that the CF gene is intimately related to the regulation of anion transport across epithelial cells. Reduced permeability of epithelial cell membranes to Cl⁻ and other anions seems to be the fundamental pathophysiologic feature of CF.

MORPHOLOGY. The anatomic changes are highly variable and depend on which glands are affected and on the severity of this involvement.[60] In some infants, the disease is quite mild and does not seriously disturb their growth and development, and they readily survive into adolescence or adult life. In others, the pancreatic involvement is severe and impairs intestinal absorption because of the pancreatic achylia, and so malabsorption, inanition, and stunted development not only seriously hamper life but also shorten survival. In others, the mucus secretion defect leads to obstruction of bronchi and bronchioles and crippling fatal pulmonary infections. Thus, cystic fibrosis may be compatible with long life or may cause death in infancy. Significantly, the sweat glands, producing a watery secretion, are morphologically unaffected.

Pancreatic abnormalities are present in approximately 85 to 90% of patients. In the milder cases, there may be only accumulations of mucus in the small ducts with some dilatation of the exocrine glands. In more advanced cases, usually seen in older children or adolescents, the ducts are totally plugged, causing atrophy of the exocrine glands and progressive fibrosis (Fig. 10–11). Because many of these children are being kept alive by appropriate therapy, it has become evident that the advance of the disease sometimes leads to total atrophy of the exocrine portion of the pancreas, leaving only the islets within a fibrofatty stroma. The total loss of pancreatic exocrine secretion impairs fat absorption, and so avitaminosis A may contribute to squamous metaplasia of the lining epithelium of the ducts in the pancreas, which are already injured by the inspissated mucus secretions. Thick viscid plugs of mucus may also be found in the small intestines of infants. Sometimes these cause small bowel obstruction known as **meconium ileus.**

The **liver involvement** follows the same basic pattern. Bile canaliculi are plugged by mucinous material. When this is of long duration, biliary cirrhosis (p. 953) with its diffuse hepatic nodularity may develop. Such severe hepatic involvement is encountered in only approximately 5% of patients, although minor hepatic alterations such as diffuse fatty change are fairly common.

The **salivary glands** are frequently involved with histologic changes similar to those described in the pancreas: progressive dilatation of ducts, squamous metaplasia of the lining epithelium, and glandular atrophy followed by fibrosis.

The **pulmonary changes** are seen in almost every case and are the most serious complications of this disease. These stem from the viscous mucous secretions of the submucosal glands of the respiratory tree with secondary obstruction and infection of the air passages. The bronchioles are often distended with thick mucus associated with marked hyperplasia and hypertrophy of the mucus-secreting cells. Superimposed infections give rise to severe chronic bronchitis and bronchiectasis (p. 777).[61] In many instances, lung abscesses develop. *Staphylococcus aureus* and *Pseudomonas aeruginosa* are the two most common organisms responsible for lung infections. For reasons not entirely clear, a mucoid form of *P. aeruginosa* seems to be emerging as the most frequent respiratory pathogen in CF. Once this organism is acquired, it seems to persist for long periods, presumably owing to its ability to escape phagocytosis and its impermeability to antibiotics. Even more sinister is the increasing frequency of infection with another pseudomonad, *P. cepacia.* This opportunistic bacterium is particularly hardy, and infection with this organism has been associated with fulminant illness.[62]

A variety of other morphologic changes may be present; important among these is the obstruction of wolffian duct derivatives, i.e., the epididymis and vas deferens, which is responsible for azoospermia and infertility in 95% of the males who survive to adulthood.

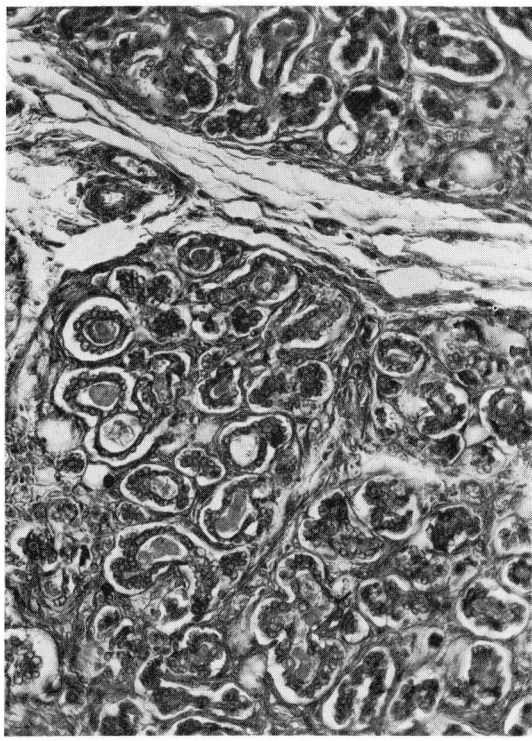

Figure 10–11. Cystic fibrosis of pancreas. Ducts are dilated and plugged with mucin, and parenchymal glands are totally atrophic and replaced by fibrous tissue.

CLINICAL COURSE. Few childhood diseases are as protean as cystic fibrosis in clinical manifestations. The symptomatology may range from mild to severe, from onset at birth to first becoming evident years later, and from syndromes that present essentially as chronic pulmonary disease to those that present as intestinal obstruction or as prolapse of the rectum owing to chronic constipation. In the classic case, the disorder is discovered in a child between the second and twelfth month of life who comes to attention because of malodorous steatorrhea and recurrent chronic pulmonary infections. Severely affected newborns may fail to regain their birth weight. In others (approximately 10 to 15%), the meconium ileus produces intestinal obstruction and, indeed, such may occur in utero and lead to perforation of the gut. The pancreatic insufficiency induces a malabsorption syndrome manifested principally as inanition, fat intolerance, steatorrhea, and deficient absorption of the fat-soluble vitamins A, D, and K (p. 439). Avitaminosis K may in turn lead to bleeding tendencies. In almost all instances, if the infant or child survives long enough, chronic cough, obstructive pulmonary disease, and persistent pulmonary infections develop and are responsible for approximately 80 to 90% of deaths.

Attention to the nutritional status of the patient and antibiotic control of pulmonary infections significantly prolong survival if the disease can be identified early. Most reliable is the detection of increased NaCl in the sweat. A positive sweat test in the presence of one or more of the major clinical features provides reasonable evidence of the disease. The recent mapping of the CF gene to chromosome 7, and the identification of tightly linked genetic markers that flank the CF gene, have made it possible to detect carriers and homozygous individuals prenatally. As discussed earlier (p. 158) prenatal diagnosis of CF and other disorders in which the affected gene itself has not yet been identified is based on the detection of DNA markers which are linked (coinherited) with the CF gene permitting RFLP analyses.[63]

Better medical care of these patients has produced heartening improvement in the outlook for this disease. Not more than two decades ago, most patients died in infancy; today the mean survival is approaching 25 years. Despite survival into adult life, most affected males are aspermic because of regressive changes in the epididymis, raising once again the puzzling problem of how the frequency of this serious deleterious gene or genes is maintained in the white population.

SUDDEN INFANT DEATH SYNDROME (SIDS)

The Second International Conference on Causes of Sudden Death in Infants formulated the most widely accepted definition of SIDS as follows: "the sudden and unexpected death of an infant who was either well or almost well prior to death, and whose death remains unexplained after the performance of an adequate autopsy."[64] Clearly, this definition reflects our ignorance of the very basis of this tragic disorder. Not surprisingly, therefore, the literature has been flooded with hypotheses, speculations, and conjectures, many of which have not stood the test of time. It may well be that the cause of SIDS is multifactorial. Thus SIDS may be considered a common tragic end point resulting from diverse influences acting singly, or more likely in concert at a particularly vulnerable period of growth and development. Here we will review the salient epidemiologic, anatomic, and pathophysiologic studies that have contributed to the formulation of some working hypotheses. A detailed discussion of these may be found in several reviews.[65-67]

Also called "crib death" or "cot death," this stunning family tragedy is by no means uncommon, as it is estimated to account for about 800 deaths annually in the United States. As infantile deaths due to nutritional problems and microbiologic infections have come under control in countries enjoying higher standards of living, SIDS has assumed greater importance and is now one of the major causes of mortality in 2- to 4-month-old infants. Around the world it causes from one to five deaths per 1000 live births.

Approximately 90% of all SIDS deaths occur dur-

ing the first six months of life, most between the ages of two and four months. This narrow window of peak susceptibility is a unique characteristic that is independent of other risk factors (to be described) and the geographic locale.[68] Most of these infants die at home, usually during the night after a period of sleep. Only rarely is the catastrophic event observed, but even when seen it is reported that the apparently healthy infant mysteriously and suddenly turns blue, stops breathing, and becomes limp without emitting a cry or struggle. Most have had minor manifestations of an upper respiratory infection preceding the fatal event.

In recent years the term "near-SIDS" has been applied to those infants who could be resuscitated after such an episode. There is little doubt that this term is diagnostically imprecise and that many such infants have definable underlying diseases. However, since some of the apparently normal "near-misses" have been reported to succumb later to SIDS, considerable interest is centered on the definition of potentially significant but subtle cardiovascular or pulmonary abnormalities in these infants.[69]

Circumstances surrounding SIDS have been explored in great detail and have yielded some observations, but the basic mystery has not been resolved. Based on epidemiologic studies a composite of factors that are associated with an increased risk of SIDS has been identified. These factors relate both to the mother and to the infant, as summarized in Table 10–5.

At autopsy a variety of findings have been recorded. They are usually subtle, of uncertain significance, and not present in all cases. An increase in the thickness of small pulmonary arteries due to medial smooth muscle hypertrophy and hyperplasia has been noted. This, along with gliosis in the brain stem, has been taken to indicate the presence of chronic hypoxia. Some investigators have reported that many of these infants have right ventricular hypertrophy, but whether this is primary or a consequence of pulmonary arterial changes is unresolved. Histologic abnormalities in the conduction system — the bundle of His and the sinoatrial node — have also been reported by some, but not confirmed by others. These infants also frequently exhibit retention of hepatic extramedullary hematopoiesis and periadrenal "brown" fat, and an increased volume of adrenal chromaffin cells. In a recent study elevated levels of fetal hemoglobin, sug-

Table 10–5. Factors Associated with SIDS

MATERNAL	INFANT
Young (less than 20 years of age)	Prematurity
Unmarried	Low birth weight
Short intergestational intervals	Male sex
Low socioeconomic group	Product of a multiple birth
Smoking	Not the first sibling
Drug abuse (e.g., methadone)	SIDS in a prior sibling
Risk greater for American blacks than whites (?socioeconomic)	

gesting a delay in the maturation of hematopoiesis, was noted.[70] It is tempting to speculate that all these changes relate to chronic hypoxemia, retardation of normal development, and chronic stress.[71] Petechiae in the pleura and epicardium as well as pulmonary congestion and edema compatible with hypoxic death are often found, but these could be agonal changes. There may also be some histologic evidence of recent respiratory infection, but these changes are generally considered not to be of lethal significance. Thus, autopsy fails to provide a clear cause of death and this may well be related to the possibility that SIDS is not a single entity.

For many years now, disturbed regulation of respiratory activity—"the apnea hypothesis"—has held center stage.[72] In favor of a primary respiratory dysfunction is the observation that, in some infants with episodes of "near-SIDS" that eventually culminated in sudden death, there is a history of repeated spells of apnea, some of which are prolonged (> 15 sec). Sleep could well be a predisposing factor, because it depresses central respiratory activity. Similarly, apneic episodes are more common with infection and in infants of low birth weight. Central hypoventilation is also associated with use of methadone by the mother, which, as indicated in Table 10–5, increases the risk of SIDS. The repeated episodes of hypoxia could be responsible for the changes in pulmonary vasculature and astrogliosis of the brain stem already mentioned. Seductive as this hypothesis is, it has been challenged by some recent studies,[73,74] which fail to show a causal relationship between episodes of apnea and subsequent development of SIDS. As is frequently the case with poorly understood disorders, softening of one hypothesis is usually accompanied by mushrooming of several others. To spare the reader "iatrogenic somnolence," only a sampling of the more recent hypotheses will be offered.

- *Inherited disorders of fat oxidation.* A subgroup of SIDS patients may have a genetic metabolic disorder characterized by a deficiency of medium-chain acyl CoA dehydrogenase. Such patients have fatty change in the liver at autopsy.[75]
- *Infections.* Focus has shifted from viral etiology to unsuspected intestinal infection with *Clostridium botulinum.*[76]
- *Defective control of body temperature.* Some preliminary studies indicate that SIDS may be related to a genetic defect that is manifested as acute (lethal) episodes of hyperthermia (malignant hyperthermia). Because SIDS victims when discovered have frequently been dead for several hours, such terminal hyperthermia would not be detected clinically.[77]

The litany of speculative hypotheses could be continued, but suffice it to say that none of these theories, alone or in combination, can at present explain these unexpected deaths. As mentioned at the outset further research is likely to reveal that SIDS is a heterogeneous, multifactorial disorder. Thus, it might be expected that further investigations will allow an increasing number of patients to be moved from the "unexplained" to "explained" category, permitting fewer "maybe's" and greater brevity.

TUMORS AND TUMOR-LIKE LESIONS OF INFANCY AND CHILDHOOD

Only 2% of all malignant tumors occur in infancy and childhood; nonetheless, cancer (including leukemia) is the leading cause of death from disease in the United States in children beyond infancy and up to 14 years of age. According to the Vital Statistics of the United States, in 1986 neoplastic disease accounted for approximately 8.7% of all deaths in this cohort; only accidents caused significantly more. Benign tumors are even more common than cancers. Most benign tumors are of little concern, but on occasion they cause serious disease or even death by virtue of their location or rapid increase in size.

It is surprisingly difficult to segregate on morphologic grounds true tumors or neoplasms from tumor-like lesions in the infant and child. Displaced cells and masses of tissue may be present from birth that are normal in appearance histologically but nonetheless grow at approximately the same rate as the growth of the fetus and infant. Indeed, few neoplasms grow as rapidly as the normal embryo. Should such displaced cells and masses be construed as new growths or simply as malformations that enlarge along with the child? In recognition of these intergrades between normal tissue growth and true neoplasia, several special categories of tumor-like lesions have been created.

CHORISTOMAS

The term choristoma has been applied to microscopically normal cells or tissues that are present in abnormal locations. Generally a choristoma is a cohesive mass of aberrant or heterotopic tissue, e.g., a rest of pancreatic tissue found in the wall of the stomach or small intestine, or a small mass of adrenal cells found in the kidney, lungs, ovary, or elsewhere. Rarely, choristomas take the form of scattered, normal-appearing cells found in inappropriate locations. The heterotopic rests are usually of only academic interest, but they can be confused clinically with neoplasms. Rarely, they are sites of origin of true neoplasms, producing the paradox of an adrenal carcinoma arising in the ovary.

HAMARTOMAS

The term hamartoma designates an excessive focal overgrowth of mature normal cells and tissues in an organ, composed of identical cellular elements. Although the cellular elements are mature and identical to those found in the remainder of the organ, they do not reproduce the normal architecture of the surrounding tissue. The line of demarcation between a hamartoma and a benign neoplasm is at best tenuous and is variously interpreted. Hemangiomas, lymphangiomas, rhabdomyomas of the heart, adenomas of the liver, and developmental cysts within the kidneys, lungs, or pancreas are construed by some as hamartomas and by others as true neoplasms. The frequency of these lesions in infancy and childhood gives credence to the belief that they are developmental aberrations, meriting the designation hamartoma. In support of this view, some of these tumors, principally hemangiomas, spontaneously regress and completely disappear. Whatever the interpretation, they are often present at birth, and for a time may rapidly enlarge along with the growth of the infant and child. In the course of such growth they can become bothersome clinical problems, as discussed later.

BENIGN TUMORS AND TUMOR-LIKE LESIONS

Reference has already been made to the difficulty in distinguishing benign tumors from hamartomas. The benign neoplasms are far more common in infancy and childhood than are cancers. Virtually any histologic pattern may be encountered, but within this wide array hemangiomas, lymphangiomas, and teratomas deserve special mention. They are described in greater detail in appropriate chapters, but here a few comments will be made about their special features in childhood.

Hemangiomas (p. 587) are the most common tumors of infancy. Architecturally they do not differ from those encountered in adults. In children most are located in the skin, particularly on the face and scalp, where they produce flat-to-elevated, irregular, red-blue masses; sometimes large lesions (considered by some to represent vascular ectasias, p. 590) are referred to as "port-wine stains." They may enlarge along with the growth of the child, but in many instances they spontaneously regress. In addition to their cosmetic significance, they can represent one facet of the hereditary disorder, von Hippel–Lindau disease. Very rarely, vascular tumors, particularly those in the liver and soft tissues, become malignant.

A wide variety of lesions are of lymphatic origin. Some of them—*lymphangiomas*—are hamartomatous or neoplastic in origin, whereas others appear to represent abnormal dilatations of preexisting lymph channels known as *lymphangiectasis*. The lymphangiomas (p. 593) are usually characterized by cystic and cavernous spaces. Lesions of this nature may occur on the skin but more importantly are encountered in the deeper regions of the neck, axilla, mediastinum, retroperitoneal tissue, and elsewhere (Fig. 10–12). Although histologically benign, they tend to increase in size after birth, both by the collection of fluid and by the budding of preexisting spaces. In this manner they encroach on vital structures such as those in the mediastinum or nerve trunks in the axilla to constitute serious clinical problems. Lymphangiectasis, in contrast, usually presents as a diffuse swelling of a part of or all of an extremity; considerable distortion and deformation may result as a consequence of the spongy, dilated subcutaneous and deeper lymphatics. However, the lesion is not progressive and does not extend beyond its original location. Nonetheless, it gives rise to difficult corrective cosmetic problems.

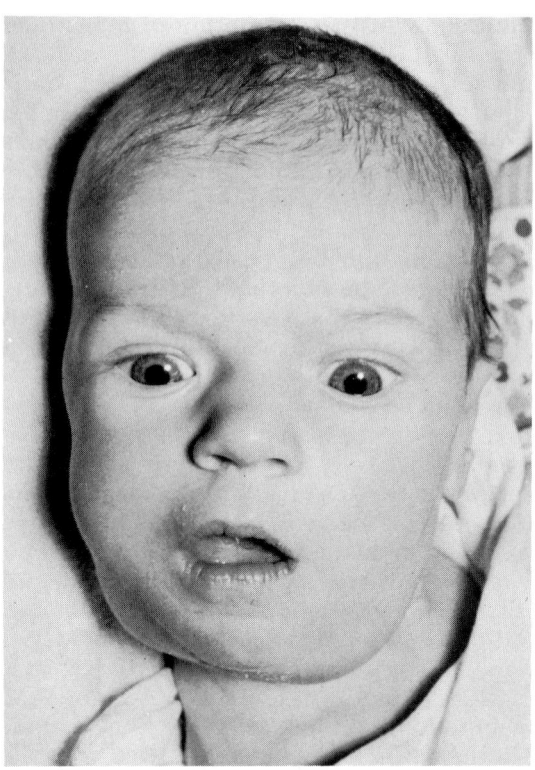

Figure 10–12. Infant with a submandibular lymphangioma causing irregular swelling beneath chin and in right buccal region.

Teratomas (p. 241) may occur as well-differentiated cystic lesions—dermoid cysts that are usually benign—or as solid malignant teratomas. They exhibit two peaks in incidence: the first at approximately two years of age and the second in late adolescence or early adult life. The first peak probably represents congenital neoplasms; the later-occurring lesions may merely be more slowly growing lesions of prenatal origin. Most teratomas of infancy and childhood arise in the sacrococcygeal region. Other sites include the gonads, mediastinum, base of the skull, roof of the pharynx, hard or soft palate, and base of the tongue. Sacrococcygeal teratomas occur in one of 20,000 to 40,000 live births and are noted four times more frequently in females than in males. Approximately 75% of these are histologically mature (p. 1112) with a benign course, and of the remainder about 12% are unmistakably malignant and lethal. Most of the benign teratomas are encountered in younger infants (below the age of four months), whereas children with malignant lesions tend to be somewhat older.[78]

MALIGNANT TUMORS

Cancers of infancy and childhood differ in many respects from those of later life.[79] Our purpose here is to point out these differential features rather than describe individual neoplasms, which are considered in later chapters dealing with the appropriate organs.

TYPES. Although any type of cancer may arise in the early years of life and indeed in utero, the distribution of common cancers of infancy and childhood differs sharply from that of adults. Carcinomas of the skin, lung, breast, prostate, and colon (to mention only some of the more common tumors) constitute the burden of neoplasia in adults, but these lesions are distinctly uncommon in childhood. Instead, the usual origins of childhood cancers are the hematopoietic system, nervous tissue (including the central and sympathetic nervous system, adrenal medulla, and retina), soft tissues, bone, and kidney. *Eight neoplasms exhibit sharp peaks in incidence in children under 5 years of age:* (1) leukemia (principally acute lymphoblastic leukemia), (2) neuroblastoma (Fig. 10–13), (3) Wilms' tumor, (4) liver cancer, (5) retinoblastoma, (6) rhabdomyosarcoma, (7) teratoma, and (8) ependymoma. Other forms of cancer are also common in childhood but do not have the same striking early peak. The age distribution of these cancers is roughly indicated in Table 10–6. Within this large array, leu-

Table 10–6. Common Malignant Neoplasms of Infancy and Childhood

0 to 4 YEARS	5 to 9 YEARS	10 to 14 YEARS
Leukemia	Leukemia	
Retinoblastoma	Retinoblastoma	
Neuroblastoma	Neuroblastoma	
Wilms' tumor		
Hepatoblastoma	Hepatocarcinoma	Hepatocarcinoma
Soft tissue sarcoma (especially rhabdomyosarcoma)	Soft tissue sarcoma	Soft tissue sarcoma
Teratomas		
CNS tumors	CNS tumors	
	Ewing's tumor	
	Lymphoma	Osteogenic sarcoma
		Thyroid carcinoma
		Hodgkin's disease

kemia alone accounts for more deaths in children under 15 years of age than all the other tumors collectively. In order of importance it is followed by neuroblastoma, Wilms' tumor, lymphoma, and osteogenic sarcoma. Collectively, these five forms of neoplasia account for almost three fourths of all tumor-related deaths in this age group.

GENETICS AND ORIGINS. As earlier discussions have noted (pp. 157 and 291), *genetic mutations underlie most tumors, including those that occur in childhood.*[80] In some instances the mutation produces both an increased predisposition to cancer and concomitant congenital malformations. These associations provide, in some instances, easily detected clinical syndromes having a strong potential for the later appearance of a neoplasm. For example, the child with congenital aniridia is vulnerable to Wilms' tumor. Usually the *A*niridia is also associated with *G*enitourinary malformations and mental *R*etardation (AGR complex). Hemihypertrophy (gross asymmetry of the body) carries with it an increased risk of Wilms' tumor, hepatoblastoma, and adrenocortical carcinoma.

Cancer-predisposing mutations may take the form of cytogenetic aberrations. A child with trisomy 21 (Down's syndrome) has about a one in 200 chance of developing leukemia, representing a ten- to 15-fold increased attack rate. Those with the chromosomal breakage syndromes have a high frequency of leukemias (p. 266).

Detailed genetic studies of two childhood tumors—retinoblastoma and Wilms' tumor—have provided new clues to the origin of human cancer, discussed earlier in Chapter 6 (p. 289).[81] These two tumors have been described in some detail on page 1462 and page 1077. However, because these studies have added a new dimension to our understanding of oncogenesis, they merit a brief recapitulation.

• Retinoblastoma and Wilms' tumor occur in both familial and sporadic forms. It has been estimated that

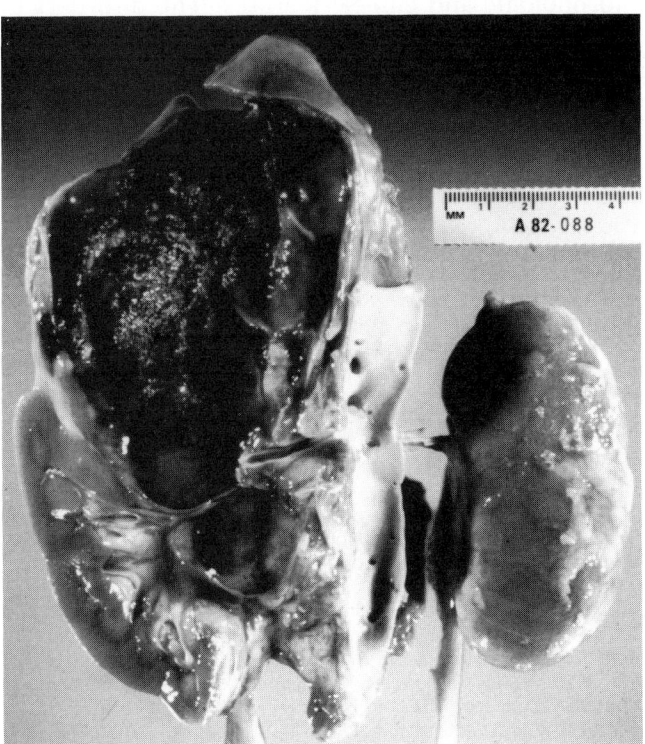

Figure 10–13. Adrenal neuroblastoma in a six-month-old child. The hemorrhagic, partially encapsulated tumor has displaced the opened left kidney and is impinging upon the aorta and left renal artery. (Courtesy of Dr. Joe Rutledge, Southwestern Medical School, Dallas, Texas.)

about 40% of all cases of retinoblastoma are inherited whereas familial Wilms' tumors are less common.

• Specific deletions involving chromosome bands 11p13 and 13q14 have been observed in a small proportion of the inherited and sporadic forms of Wilms' tumor and retinoblastoma, respectively. These data suggest that genes located within the deleted segments may play a role in tumorigenesis.

• More detailed molecular studies of tumor DNA have revealed subtle genetic alterations in the aforementioned chromosomal regions in virtually all patients with these tumors.

As discussed in Chapter 6, these studies have given rise to the concept of "recessive" cancer genes and provided a molecular basis for Knudson's two-hit theory of carcinogenesis[81] (p. 290).

Environmental influences also contribute significantly to the origin of childhood cancers. Best documented is the carcinogenic potential of radiant energy. The nuclear fallout of the atomic bombs has yielded a 1.5- to 1.8-fold increased incidence of cancer deaths (excluding leukemia) in survivors who received 200 rad or more of ionizing radiation. Chemical agents (including drugs) also contribute to the origin of malignant neoplasms. Vaginal adenosis—glandular inclusions thought to be precancerous—and vaginal adenocarcinoma have developed in children whose mothers received stilbestrol between the eighth and 18th weeks of pregnancy.[82] Most of these cancers occur late in the second decade or early in the third decade of life. Thus, it is evident that all the influences thought to have carcinogenic potential in adults may induce cancers in early life.

CLINICAL BEHAVIOR. Cancers of infancy and childhood behave quite differently from those of later life. They tend to be more rapidly growing and as a result often produce disproportionately large masses in the young. Bilateral neuroblastomas of the adrenals may induce a protuberant abdomen, as may other intra-abdominal masses. Often they are readily evident on visual inspection when the child is lying down. For unknown reasons, even large masses are not associated with early anemia, loss of weight, or cachexia in this age group. Instead, the clinical manifestations often resemble those of an infectious process, with fever and malaise. Many are responsive to irradiation and chemotherapy, and remarkable results have been achieved with these modalities in certain forms of cancer. For example, two-year survival rates of almost 95% have been reported after the combined use of surgery and chemotherapy in the treatment of Wilms' tumor in children in whom the tumor is limited to the kidney.

Spontaneous differentiation of some childhood tumors—for example, the embryonic neuroblastoma into the relatively benign ganglioneuroma—has been unmistakably documented in some patients. Spontaneous regression of neuroblastomas occurs most commonly in patients with limited disease, and remarkably in many with small primary tumors and extensive metastases involving liver, skin, and bone marrow (but not bone). Most of these patients are infants with a median age of 3 months, and according to some authors they should be classified into a special category called stage IV-S (special).[83] The basis of such spontaneous regression is not known, but possibilities include an immune response to the tumor or response to some endogenous growth and differentiation factor.

Depressing as the development of a cancer is in a child, the outlook is not entirely bleak. Moreover, clinical experience has shown that when metastases or recurrences have not taken place after a period of time represented by the patient's age at the time of removal of the lesion plus nine months, the probability is strong that a complete cure has been effected. In other words, cancers of infancy and childhood declare themselves early, and so both parents and patients can be reassured after an appropriate time interval that they no longer live under the sword of Damocles.

In this chapter, it must be apparent that we have only skimmed the surface of the large catalog of pediatric diseases. The disorders presented, however, are among the most common and important and rightfully belong within the scope of general medical knowledge. As stated at the outset, the major disorders of infancy and childhood are peculiar to the age group. Only a few, such as neoplasms and infections, also affect adults, and then they usually present different morphologic and clinical features. The disorders of children and of adults differ more than does the child from the adult.

1. Levene, M.I., and Dubowitz, V.: Intrauterine growth retardation. *In* Stern, L., and Vert, P. (eds.): Neonatal Medicine. New York, Masson Publishing USA, Inc., 1987, p. 107.

1a. Khoury, M.J., et al.: Congenital malformations and intrauterine growth retardation: A population study. Pediatrics 82:83, 1988.

2. Apgar, V.: A proposal for a new method of evaluation of the newborn infant. Curr. Res. Anesth. Analg. 32:260, 1953.

3. Drage, J.S., and Berendes, H.: Apgar scores and outcome of the newborn. Pediatr. Clin. North Am. 13:635, 1966.

4. Gresham, E.L.: Birth trauma. Pediatr. Clin. North Am. 22:317, 1975.

5. Andre, M., and Vert, P.: Birth injury. *In* Stern, L., and Vert, P. (eds.): Neonatal Medicine. New York, Masson Publishing USA, Inc., 1987, p. 176.

6. Shepard, T.H.: Human teratogenicity. Adv. Pediatr. 33:225, 1986.

7. Rosenthal, N., and Abramowsky, C.R.: The causes of morbidity and mortality among infants born at term. Arch. Pathol. Lab. Med. 112:178, 1988.

8. Spranger, J., et al.: Errors of morphogenesis: Concepts and terms. Recommendations of an international working group. J. Pediatr. 100:160, 1982.

9. Iosub, S., et al.: More on human immunodeficiency virus embryopathy. Pediatrics 80:512, 1987.

10. Hanshaw, J.B.: Cytomegaloviral Infection. *In* Beherman, R.E., and Vaughan, V.C. (eds.): Nelson's Textbook of Pediatrics. 13th ed. Philadelphia, WB Saunders Co., 1987, p. 668.

11. Golbus, M.D.: Teratology for the obstetrician: Current status. Obstet. Gynecol. 55:269, 1980.

12. Beckman, D.A., and Brent, R.L.: Mechanism of known environ-

mental teratogens: Drugs and chemicals. Clin. Perinatol. *13*:649, 1986.

12a. Jones, K.L.: The Fetal Alcohol Syndrome. Growth Genetics and Hormones. (BMI/McGraw Hill, New York) *4*:1, 1988.

13. Brent, R.L.: The effect of embryonic and fetal exposure to X-ray, microwaves, and ultrasound. Clin. Perinatol. *13*:615, 1986.

13a. Sulik, K.K., et al.: Teratogens and craniofacial malformations: relationship to cell death. Development *103* (Suppl):213, 1988.

14. Smith, D.W.: Recognizable patterns of human deformation. Identification and management of mechanical effects on morphogenesis. Major Probl. Clin. Pediatr. *21*:1, 1981.

15. Stark, A.R., and Frantz, I.D.: Respiratory distress syndrome. Pediatr. Clin. North Am. *33*:533, 1986.

16. Editorial: Born before their time into this breathing world. Br. Med. J. *2*:1403, 1976.

17. Oh, W., and Stern, L.: Respiratory diseases of the newborn. In Stern, L., and Vert, P. (eds.): Neonatal Medicine. New York, Masson Publishing USA, Inc., 1987, p. 395.

18. Usher, R., et al.: Respiratory distress syndrome in infants delivered by cesarean section. Am. J. Obstet. Gynecol. *88*:806, 1964.

19. Robert, M.F.: Association between maternal diabetes and the respiratory distress syndrome of the newborn. N. Engl. J. Med. *294*:357, 1976.

20. Mimouni, F., et al.: Respiratory distress syndrome in infants of diabetic mothers in the 1980s: no adverse effect of maternal diabetes with modern management. Obstet. Gynecol. *69*:191, 1987.

21. Perelman, R.H., et al.: Discordance between male and female deaths due to the respiratory distress syndrome. Pediatrics *78*:238, 1986

22. Weaver, T.E., and Whitsett, J.A.: Structure and function of pulmonary surfactant proteins. Semin. Perinatol. *12*:213, 1988.

23. Ballard, P.L., et al.: Regulation of pulmonary surfactant apoprotein SP 28-36 gene in fetal human lung. Proc. Natl. Acad. Sci. *83*:9527, 1986.

24. Lauweryns, J.M.: Hyaline membrane diseases: A pathological study of 55 infants. Pediatrics *50*:515, 1972.

25. Tomashefski, J.F., et al.: Pathologic observations on infants who do not survive the respiratory distress syndrome. In Nelson, G.H. (ed.): Pulmonary Development. Transition from Intrauterine to Extrauterine Life. New York, Marcel Dekker, Inc., 1985, p. 387.

26. de la Monte, S.M., et al.: Respiratory epithelial cell necrosis is the earliest lesion of hyaline membrane disease of the newborn. Am. J. Pathol. *123*:155, 1986.

27. Volpe, J.J., and Hill, A.: Periventricular-intraventicular hemorrhage. In Avery, G.B. (ed.): Neonatology. Pathophysiology and Management of the Newborn. Third edition. Philadelphia, J.B. Lippincott Co., 1987, p. 1105.

28. Avery, M.E., et al.: Update on prenatal steroid for prevention of respiratory distress. Am. J. Obstet. Gynecol. *155*:2, 1986

29. Taeusch, W., et al.: Surfactant for the treatment of respiratory distress syndrome: selected clinical issues. Semin. Perinatol. *12*:245, 1988.

29a. Naeye, R.L.: Functionally important disorders of the placenta, umbilical cord, and fetal membranes. Hum. Pathol. *18*:680, 1987.

30. Cherry, S.H.: Current concepts in hemolytic disease and blood group incompatibility. Mt. Sinai J. Med. *47*:454, 1980.

31. Grundbacher, J.F.: The etiology of ABO hemolytic disease of newborn. Transfusion *20*:563, 1980.

32. Editorial: Haemolytic disease of the newborn due to antibodies other than rhesus anti-D. Br. Med. J. *283*:514, 1981.

33. Harper, R.G., et al.: Kernicterus. Clin. Perinatol. *7*:75, 1980.

34. Nusbacher, J., and Bove, J.R.: Rh immunoprophylaxis: is antepartum therapy desirable? N. Engl. J. Med. *303*:935, 1980.

35. Tovey, L.A.D.: Hemolytic disease of the newborn — the changing scene. Br. J. Obstet. Gynecol. *93*:960, 1986.

36. Grannum, P.A., et al.: In utero exchange transfusion by direct intravascular injection in severe erythroblastosis fetalis. N. Engl. J. Med. *314*:1431, 1986.

37. Burton, B.K.: Inborn errors of metabolism: The clinical diagnosis in early infancy. Pediatrics *79*:359, 1987.

38. Kaufman, S.: Phenylketonuria and its variants. Adv. Hum. Genet. *13*:217, 1983.

39. Kaufman, S.: Unsolved problems in diagnosis and therapy of hy-

perphenylalaninemia caused by defects in tetrahydrobiopterin metabolism. J. Pediatr. *109*:572, 1986.

40. Guttler, F., and Woo. S.L.C.: Molecular genetics of PKU. J. Inher. Metab. Dis. *9* (Suppl. 1):58, 1986.

41. Guttler, F., et al.: Correlation between polymorphic DNA haplotypes at phenylalanine hydroxylase locus and clinical phenotypes of phenylketonuria. J. Pediatr. *110*:68, 1987.

42. Loo, Y.H., et al.: A biochemical explanation of phenylacetate neurotoxicity in experimental phenylketonuria. J. Neurochem. *45*:1596, 1985.

43. Malamud, N.: Neuropathology of phenylketonuria. J. Neuropathol. Exp. Neurol. *25*:254, 1966.

44. Salguero, I.F., et al.: Neuropathologic observations in phenylketonuria. Trans. Am. Neurol. Assoc. *93*:274, 1968.

45. Holtzman, N.A., et al.: Effect of age at loss of dietary control on intellectual performance and behavior of children with phenylketonuria. N. Engl. J. Med. *314*:593, 1986.

46. Guthrie, R.: Maternal PKU — a continuing problem. Am. J. Public Health *78*:771, 1988.

47. Kleigman, R.M., and Sparks, J.W.: Perinatal galactose metabolism. J. Pediatr. *107*:831, 1985.

48. Smetana, H.F., and Olen, E.: Hereditary galactose disease. Am. J. Clin. Pathol. *38*:3, 1962.

49. Kaufman, F.R., et al.: Correlation of ovarian function with galactose-1-phosphate uridyl transferase levels in galactosemia. J. Pediatr. *112*:754, 1988.

50. Fernald, G.W., and Boat, T.F.: Cystic fibrosis: Overview. Semin. Roentgenol. *22*:87, 1987.

51. Kane, K. Cystic fibrosis: recent advances in genetics and molecular biology. Ann. Clin. Lab. Sci. *18*:289, 1988.

52. Berschneider, H.M., et al.: Altered intestinal chloride transport in cystic fibrosis. FASEB J. *2*:2625, 1988.

53. Case, M.: Chloride ions and cystic fibrosis. Nature *322*:407, 1986.

54. Welsh, M.J., and Fick, R.B.: Cystic fibrosis. J. Clin. Invest. *80*:1523, 1987.

55. Knowles, M.R., et al.: Abnormal respiratory epithelial ion transport in cystic fibrosis. Clin. Chest Med. *7*:285, 1986.

56. Kopelman, H., et al.: Pancreatic fluid secretion and protein hyperconcentration in cystic fibrosis. N. Engl. J. Med. *312*:329, 1985.

57. Frizell, R.A.: Altered regulation of airway epithelial cell chloride channels in cystic fibrosis. Science *233*:558, 1986.

58. Dorin, J.R., et al.: A clue to the basic defect in cystic fibrosis from cloning the CF gene. Nature *326*:614, 1987.

59. Dubinsky, W.P.: The physiology of epithelial chloride channels. Hosp. Pract. *24*(1):69, 1989.

60. Oppenheimer, E.H., and Easterly, J.R.: Pathology of cystic fibrosis. Review of literature and comparison with 146 autopsied cases. Perspect. Pediatr. Pathol. *2*:241, 1975.

61. Friend, P.A.: Pulmonary infection in cystic fibrosis. J. Infect. *13*:55, 1986.

62. Goldman, D.A., and Klinger, J.D.: *Pseudomonas cepacia*: Biology mechanism of virulence, epidemiology. J. Pediatr. *108*:806, 1986.

63. Harris, A., et al.: Cystic fibrosis typing with DNA probes: experience of a screening laboratory. Hum. Genet. *79*:76, 1988.

64. Bergman, A., et al.: Sudden infant death syndrome. Proceedings of the Second International Conference on Causes of Sudden Death in Infants. Seattle, University of Washington Press, 1970.

65. Kraus, H.F.: Sudden infant death syndrome. Pathology and pathophysiology. Pathol. Ann. *19*(Pt 1):1, 1984.

66. Milner, A.D.: Recent theories on the cause of cot death. Br. Med. J. *295*:1366, 1987.

67. Williams, A.L.: Scientific research into the sudden infant death syndrome: An introduction to the first rotary health fund conference. Aust. Pediatr. J. (Suppl.):3, 1986.

68. Goldberg, J., et al.: Age at death and risk factors in sudden infant death syndrome. Aust. Pediatr. J. (Suppl.):21, 1986.

69. Simpson H., et al.: "Near miss" or "near-myth" for sudden infant death syndrome? Clinical observations in 57 infants. Aust. Pediatr. J. (Suppl.):47, 1986.

70. Giulian, G.G., et al.: Elevated fetal hemoglobin levels in sudden infant death syndrome. N. Engl. J. Med. *316*:1122, 1987.

71. Naeye, R.L., et al.: Cardiac and other abnormalities in the sudden infant death syndrome. Am. J. Pathol. *82*:1, 1976.

72. Shannon, D.C., and Kelly, D.H.: SIDS and near-SIDS. N. Engl. J. Med. *306*:959, 1023, 1982.

73. Davis, N., et al.: Epidemiological comparisons of sudden infant death syndrome with infant apnea. Aust. Pediatr. J. (Suppl.):29, 1986.

74. Consensus Statement: National Institute of Health Consensus development conference on infantile apnea and home monitoring. Sept. 29 to Oct. 1, 1986. Pediatrics 79:292, 1987.

75. Editorial: Sudden infant death and inherited disorders of fat oxidation. Lancet 2:1073, 1986.

76. Sonnabend, O.A.R., et al.: Continuous microbiological and pathologic study of 70 sudden and unexpected infant deaths: Toxigenic intestinal *Clostridium botulinum* infection in nine cases of sudden infant death syndrome. Lancet *1*:237, 1985.

77. Peterson, D.R., and Davis, N.: Sudden infant death syndrome and malignant hyperthermia diathesis. Aust. Pediatr. J. (Suppl.):33, 1986.

78. Bale, P.M.: Sacrococcygeal developmental abnormalities and tumors in children. Perspect. Pediatr. Pathol. *1*:9, 1984.

79. Hammond, G.D.: The cure of childhood cancers. Cancer *58*(Suppl):407, 1986.

80. Arthur, D.C.: Genetics and cytogenetics of pediatric cancers. Cancer *58*(Suppl.):534, 1986.

81. Knudson, A.G.: Genetics of human cancer. Annu. Rev. Genet. *20*:231, 1986.

82. Herbst, A.L., et al.: Clear cell adenocarcinoma of the genital tract in young females: Registry report. N. Engl. J. Med. *287*:1259, 1972.

83. Evans, A.E., et al.: A review of 17 IV-S neuroblastoma patients at the Children's Hospital of Philadelphia. Cancer *45*:833, 1980.

Diseases of Aging

Just as life is incurable, always ending in death, aging is inescapable, beginning at birth. Despite its universality, aging is difficult to define. Most widely accepted is — aging constitutes a decreasing ability to survive. There has been an enormous expansion of the "graying population" in all industrialized countries, and perhaps a less marked one in developing countries. In the United States in 1900 only 4% of the population was over the age of 65; in 1986 it was 11.6%; and in 2030 it is projected to rise to about 20%. In "people" numbers, there were about 26 million over the age of 65 in the United States in 1980, but that number will more than double by the year 2030. Even more remarkable are the substantial shifts occurring in the aging population. In this decade, there has been more than a 25% increase in persons 75 to 79 years old and over a 50% increase in those over the age of 85! These demographic trends reflect the "triumph of survivorship" and the deferment of death. In the 5000 years preceding 1900, the gain in life expectancy was about 26 years; since only the beginning of the present century the gain has been about 29 years! However, it is doubtful that life expectancy can be prolonged indefinitely. Comparative gerontologists have projected a maximum life span for humans in the range of 115 to 120 years, which is probably fortunate not only for society but also for the individual. By contrast, the maximum life span of the Indian elephant is 70 years, and that of the house mouse 3 years.[1] The considerably longer life span of humans is in some measure owed to the ability to control the ravages to which free-living animals are exposed, such as extremes of temperature, potential lack of food and water, and microbial attack (Fig. 11–1). The concept of a maximum life span suggests that even in the absence of disease the incredible "human machine" eventually wears out. Changes are occurring throughout life at the level of molecules, organelles, cells, organs, and systems, but what stops the

"clock of life" remains an enigma. A graphic overview of aging is provided by the *premature aging syndromes. Progeria,* for example, is characterized by marked growth deceleration, the external stigmata of aging (e.g., baldness, wrinkling of skin, atrophy of subcutaneous fat), and severe generalized atherosclerosis. Most of these unfortunates die of "old age" within the first two decades of life. Significantly, cell cultures from these individuals have the same morphologic and replicative characteristics of cells derived from normal-aged humans. Although the biology of senescence has functional, chemical, social, and psychologic dimensions, our consideration here will be limited to cellular aging, aging of organs and systems, and age-associated diseases.

CELLULAR AGING

Cellular function declines progressively with age. Aged mitochondria have a decreased ability to survive a hypoxic insult. Oxidative phosphorylation declines progressively, as does DNA and RNA synthesis of structural and enzyme proteins and membrane specializations such as receptors.[2] Senescent cells have a decreased capacity for uptake of nutrients and for repair of chromosomal damage. Concomitantly, there is a steady accumulation of senescent cell component residues in the form of lipofuscin, but whether this lipopigment deleteriously affects cell function remains unclear. Aged cells reveal other morphologic alterations including irregular and abnormally lobed nuclei, pleomorphic vacuolated mitochondria, decreased rough endoplasmic reticulum (ER), vesicular smooth ER, and distorted Golgi apparatus. A host of theories have been proposed to explain the biology of cellular aging. These can best be divided into the categories of "wear and tear" and "genome-based" concepts.

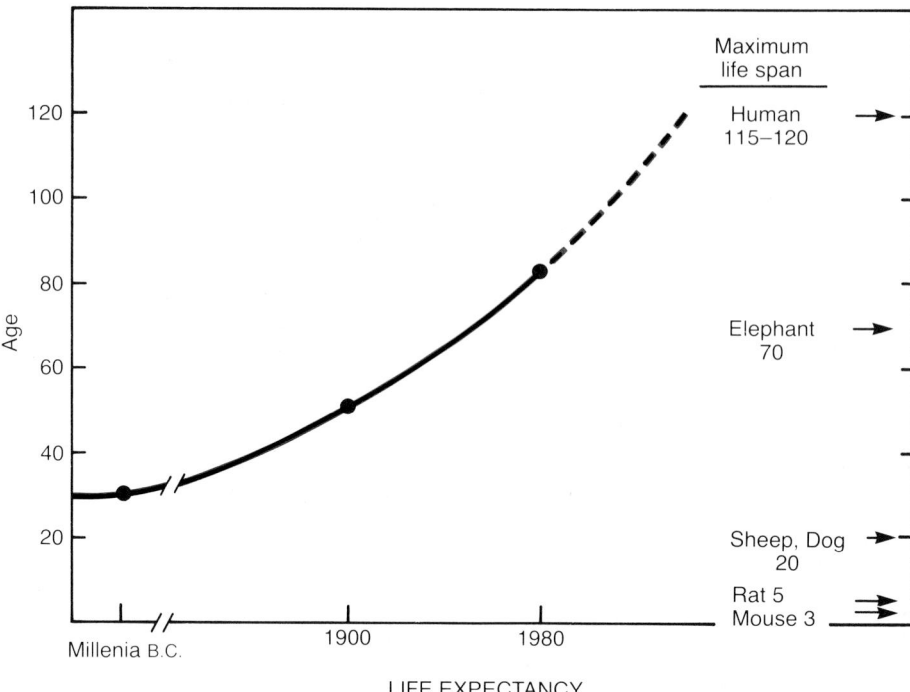

Figure 11–1. Comparative life spans.

"WEAR AND TEAR" THEORIES

These imply that the aging process in cells is the consequence of continual exposure throughout life to adverse exogenous influences leading to progressive encroachment on the cell's survivability. A schema of some of these theories is offered in Figure 11–2.

Free Radical Theory

A favored theory of cellular aging invokes the progressive accumulation of free radical damage throughout life. As you know, free radicals are formed either by exposure of cells and their organelles to ionizing radiation or by endogenous enzymatic reactions, mostly by the reduction of oxygen, with the production of the various radical species (discussed on page 9). They cause random damage to DNA, RNA, proteins, and enzymes; induce polymerization of membranes; and are capable of eventually causing cell death.[3] The accumulation of lipofuscin within cells, as detailed on page 24, is one manifestation of free radical action. Thus it has been proposed that "the aging process may be simply the sum of deleterious free radical reactions going on continuously throughout the cells and tissues."[4] According to this theory, much depends on defense mechanisms such as vitamin E, selenium-containing glutathione peroxidase, superoxide dismutase, and other antioxidants for the prevention or retardation of cellular senescence. Support for this theory comes from several sources. Dietary antioxidants increase life expectancy in rats, mice, and various nonmammalian species, but it is not clear that they act solely by reducing free radical injury, and they do not increase the maximum

life span. In primates, there is a correlation between the cellular levels of superoxide dismutase and life span. Appealing as the concept of free radical damage as the basis of cellular injury may be, it is uncertain that it is the fundamental mechanism of aging.

Post-translational Modifications (Cross-Linkage Theory)

Post-translational molecular changes are known to occur with age within both the extracellular and the intracellular compartments. Cerami and others have proposed that over the years nonenzymatic glycosylation of proteins is a universal phenomenon leading to the formation of "advanced glycosylation endproducts" capable of cross linking adjacent proteins.[5] Collagen is a major target; a progressive increase over time in cross-linkages in these molecules has been repeatedly demonstrated. Such linkages could decrease elasticity and permeability of the extracellular compartment and so impair flow of nutrients into, and waste products out of, cells. Analogously, glycosylations of other proteins, and in particular DNA and RNA, could result in impairment of cell metabolism or even crippling of cell function. One important post-translational modification—age-related glycosylation of lens proteins—underlies senile cataracts. A large number of intracellular agents have the capacity to induce such changes, including aldehydes, free radicals, sulfur cross-linkages, quinones, and polybasic acids and their esters as well as others. Although post-translational modifications in proteins, polypeptides, and other molecules have clearly been documented in aging cells, they have not been demonstrated to directly impair cell survivability.

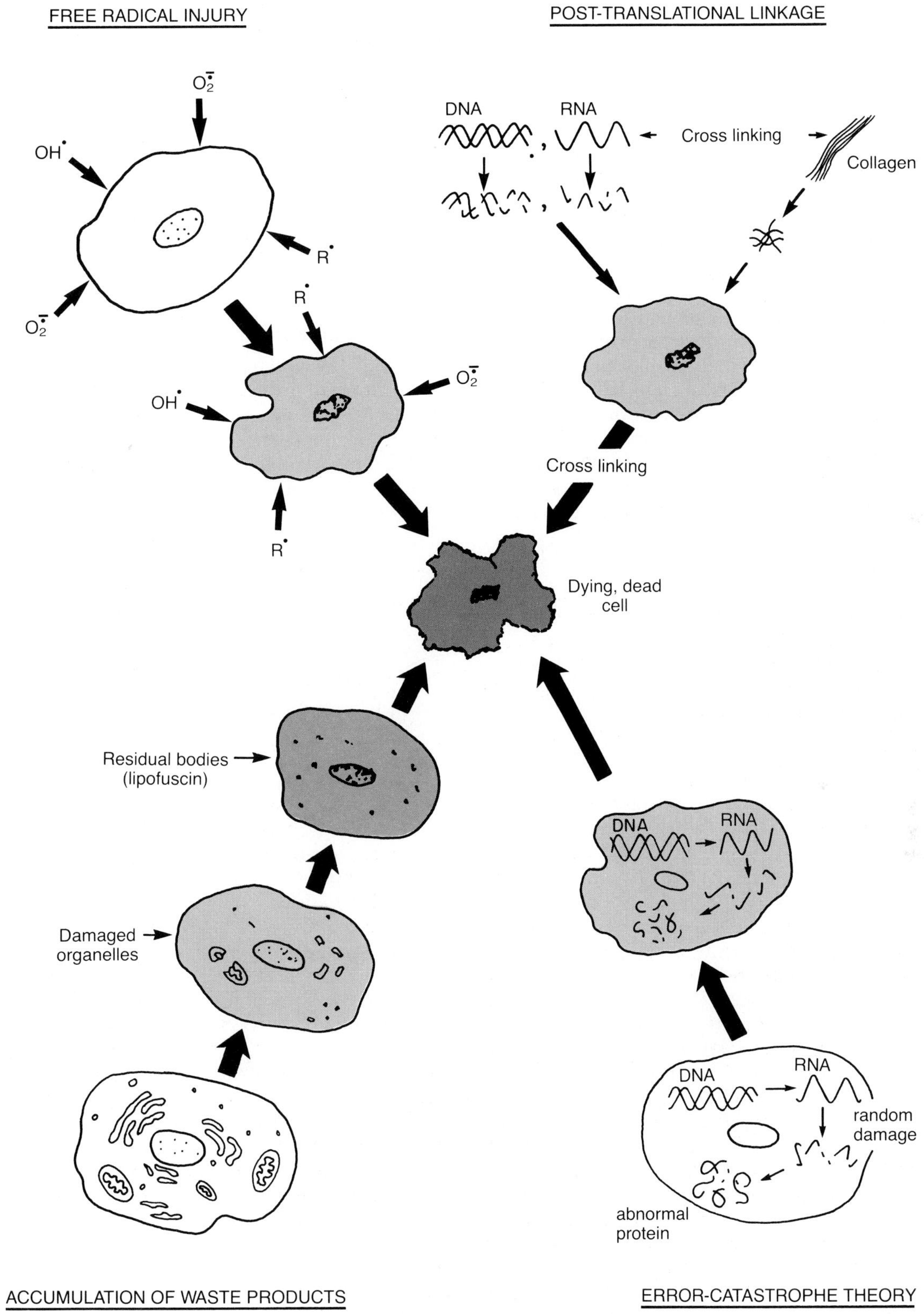

Figure 11–2. Wear and tear theories of cell death.

Accumulation of Waste Products Theory

As mentioned earlier, lipofuscin progressively accumulates with age in nondividing cells such as striated muscle cells (including cardiac myofibers and neurons. As you know, this age-associated pigment is probably the product of free radical peroxidation and polymerization of membrane lipoproteins. Although lipofuscin is known to accumulate with the passage of years, it has not been possible to correlate decreasing cell function or capacity to survive with the level of accumulation. However, the possibility of other toxic metabolic products has not been excluded.

Error-Catastrophe Theory

Random errors in translation or transcription could lead to the formation of abnormal proteins, which might accumulate to eventually impair cell function. Conceivably, critical proteins, such as RNA polymerase, might be involved and have a wide-ranging ripple effect. A major argument against this concept is that cellular function appears to decline slowly and progressively with aging rather than occurring sporadically and randomly. Moreover, mutations are a major feature of cancer cells, which unhappily live "forever."

GENOME-BASED THEORIES

It is widely believed that the best prescription for long life is to choose one's parents well. The difference in longevity between fraternal twins is, on average, much greater than that between identical twins. Analogously, the ancestors of centenarians tend to have been more long-lived than those of more short-lived individuals. There is then a body of evidence suggesting that longevity is under genetic control. As a consequence, a number of genome-based theories have emerged. These are diagrammed in Figure 11–3.

Finite Doubling Potential of Cells

Hayflick showed, many years ago, that the number of doublings of human fibroblast-like cells is fixed at about 50, presumably because of built-in genetic programs of senescence.[6] Introduction of senescent cells into young animals is without effect on this replicative potential, demonstrating that the limits are internal to the cell and are not a function of the environment.

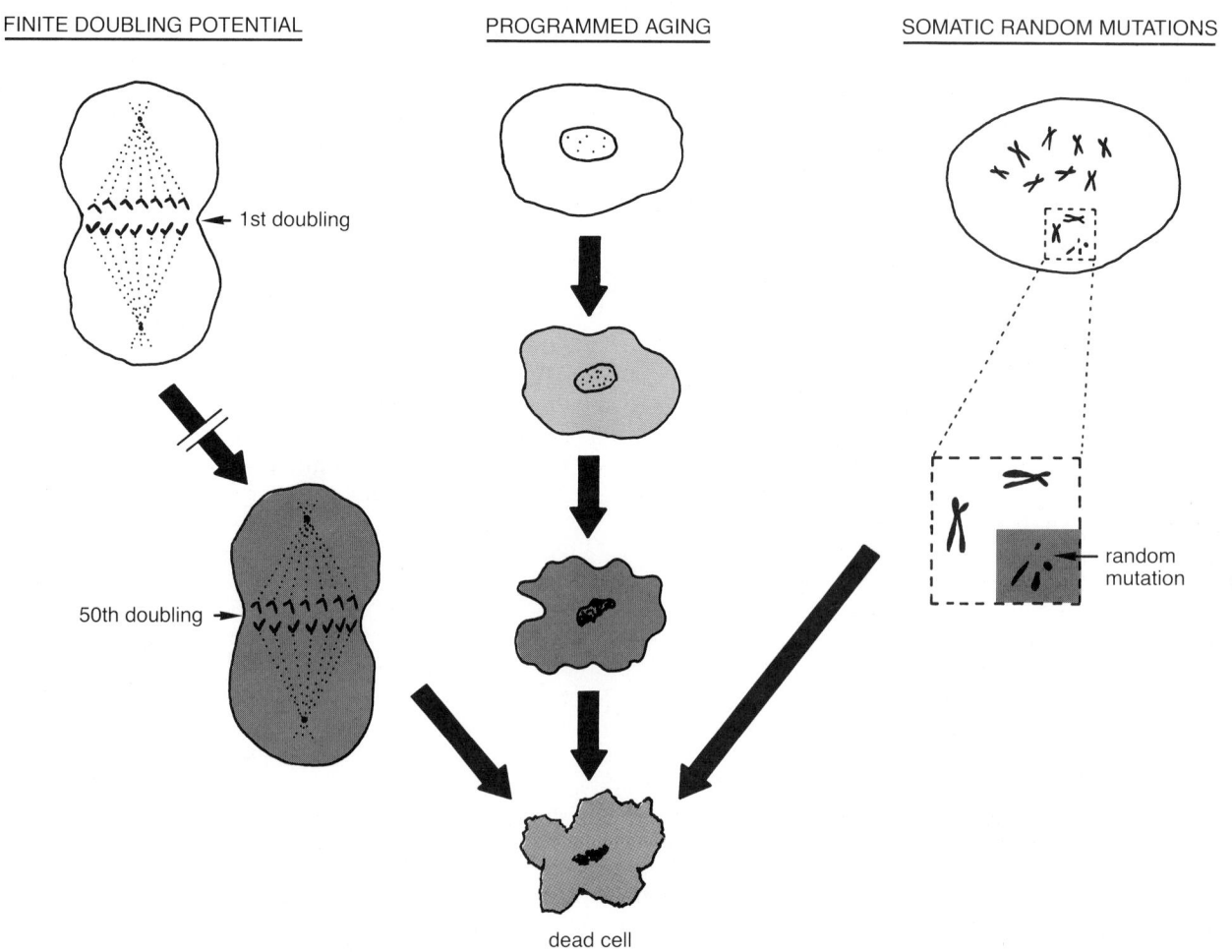

FINITE DOUBLING POTENTIAL   PROGRAMMED AGING   SOMATIC RANDOM MUTATIONS

1st doubling

50th doubling

random mutation

dead cell

Figure 11–3. Genome-based theories of aging.

Moreover, transplantation of the nucleus of an old cell into a young cytoplast yields a hybrid with a life span of the transplanted nucleus. The significance of the limit to cell doublings has, however, been questioned on the grounds that it may be an experimental artifact. Moreover, how this concept would apply to postmitotic cells, such as neurons or striated muscle cells, is unclear. Alternative explanations have been offered for Hayflick's observations. With replicating cells there is always a possibility that mitosis will give rise to cells that divide but are irreversibly committed to senescence and cell death (the commitment theory of cell aging).[7] Overgrowth of the cells committed to senescence may mask the existence or hamper the replicability of uncommitted immortal cells in culture. It is sufficient to say that finite replication can certainly not explain the aging of all cells in the body, such as the cardiac muscle cells and neurons.

Somatic Mutations

This theory proposes that errors of DNA replication that are not accurately repaired will ultimately impinge on the viability and survivability of cells. This concept is essentially a modification of the error-catastrophe theory. It proposes that instead of errors in translation or transcription being important, they must involve DNA directly. Conceivably, promoter or repressor sequences might be involved in altering the rate of synthetic genetic programs. Indeed, repair systems for DNA do slow in later life. However, somatic mutation implies a randomness to senescence, which is clearly a nonrandom phenomenon. Moreover, although mutations are readily produced in cells and experimental animals by irradiation, these aberrations in the genome do not consistently affect life span.

Programmed Aging

In place of the random events of genomic mutation or transcriptional errors, the "program theory" of aging assumes a predetermined sequence of events leading ultimately to senescence. The cells of the epidermis demonstrate beautifully genetic programs terminating in anucleate dead squames that are shed from the skin surface. Repression and derepression of genetic programs are presumably involved. Analogously, the same process may account for the senescence of other cells. Repression of genes encoding vital synthetic processes could be involved. Witness the incredible programmed senescence terminating in the death of the Pacific salmon after spawning. Attractive as this concept may be, it has been difficult to devise experimental strategies to prove or disprove it.

In conclusion, although there can be no doubt that cells age over time, the precise basis for this phenomenon remains elusive. The possibility must be entertained that senescence is multifactorial and that many pathways may contribute concurrently or sequentially.[8]

AGING CHANGES IN ORGANS AND SYSTEMS

There are well-delineated aging changes in the function of many organs and systems. Some systems —specifically the immune and neuroendocrine systems— are referred to as "aging hot spots" and the likely ultimate origin of the biologic process of senescence. In addition, aging changes have been observed in the cardiovascular and excretory (renal) systems as well as in others. These are not considered to be primary to the phenomenon of aging, and indeed it has been difficult to exclude the possibility that some or all may be the residuals of past disease rather than the pathophysiologic consequence of aging. Some of these systemic changes follow and along with them the changes with age in the composition of the body as a whole.

IMMUNITY AND SENESCENCE

Three important observations are consistent with the view that aging in the last analysis is the consequence of a decline in normal immune function. (1) In senescence there is a progressive quantitative and qualitative diminution in the capacity to produce antibodies. (2) There is a commensurate tendency for aggregates of lymphocytes to appear in the bone marrow and other sites and an increase in the development of autoimmune reactions and diseases.[9] (3) There is a profound decline in T-lymphocyte function with age. Underlying these phenomena is the age-related atrophy of the thymus that is often likened to an "organ clock" that eventually runs out. By age 50, the thymus is less than 15% of its maximum weight. At the same time, the number of population doublings of peripheral T cells progressively declines as a function of donor age, in parallel with the observations made by Hayflick on cultured human fibroblasts. The immune changes may be responsible for autoimmune injury to cells and tissues and may underlie the predisposition to infection seen in aged individuals and possibly the increasing incidence of cancer in the late years of life due to reduced immunosurveillance. Of interest, the two interventions that have been shown to prolong the life span of experimental animals, i.e., prepubertal malnutrition and hypothermia, also improve immune function. However, the immune system is clearly influenced by hormones (for example, adrenal steroids), and so it remains to be determined whether aging changes are a primary causative mechanism of senescence or merely secondary to other alterations.

NEUROENDOCRINE SENESCENCE

The neuroendocrine system has also been scrutinized as the possible "pacemaker" of aging. Some loss of neurons is associated with advanced age, and it can be speculated that if such losses occurred in the hypothalamus, they would have widely ramifying effects on the pituitary and endocrine target organs. Neuronal loss occurs in selective areas of the brain such as in the locus ceruleus, substantia nigra, hippocampus, caudate nucleus, putamen, and cerebral cortex, but age-related neuronal losses have not been documented in the critically important hypothalamus. Nonetheless, elderly individuals tend to develop hypertension possibly related to increased sympathetic system reactivity, impaired glucose tolerance, diminished thyroid function, and, of course, decline in gonadal function.[10] Despite all the decrements in neuroendocrine function, there is no substantial evidence that they are primary to the biology of senescence, because many lower organisms known to age over time have no well-developed neuroendocrine system.

THE BRAIN AND SENESCENCE

Although selective loss of isolated neurons occurs with senescence, as mentioned in the previous section, there is no evidence that the function of the brain significantly deteriorates with aging. Granted, with advancing years there are often mild loss in memory, some increased difficulty in learning new tasks, and some diminution in the speed of processing by the brain.[11] There is also a modest decrease of brain mass. But it should be noted that most brain functions involved in "intelligence" are remarkably preserved throughout life. The fact that the incidence of Alzheimer's disease increases steadily throughout life to affect about 5% of individuals over age 65 and 20% of those over age 80 has been taken to mean that senile dementia is a consequence of the aging process. This erroneous conception has been buttressed by the observation of senile plaques and neurofibrillary tangles typical of Alzheimer's disease in elderly "normal" individuals. However, the relationship of these findings to the later development of Alzheimer's disease remains unclear. Moreover, it is generally agreed that although Alzheimer's dementia may be an age-related disease, it is neither part of the process of senescence nor age-dependent. Witness the occasional cases that appear in the second and third decades of life and the many individuals who remain unaffected throughout a long life. In sum, there are some related changes in CNS function, but they do not impair the otherwise healthy individual's ability to live a long, productive, and vigorous life.

AGING AND THE CARDIOVASCULAR SYSTEM

A number of cardiovascular changes have been observed in elderly subjects, but many may be related to modifications in lifestyle (e.g., the elderly are more sedentary) or to intercurrent diseases, in particular atherosclerosis. In the Baltimore Longitudinal Study of Aging, it was shown that there is little or no decline in basal and exercise cardiac output related to aging alone.[12] There is a diminished heart rate owing to some diminution in the efficacy of beta-adrenergic stimulation of the heart, but cardiac output is maintained by adaptive mechanisms such as cardiac dilatation and greater stroke volume. Moreover, isolated cardiac muscle appears to suffer little age-dependent change in function, notwithstanding the possible accumulation of some lipofuscin.[13] Another aging change is a progressive rise in basal systolic blood pressure. This has been attributed to a loss of compliance of the aorta and major arteries with age.

> Arterial walls thicken and become stiffer. Some of this stiffness could be due to the glycosylation reactions cited earlier (p. 544). But, in addition, there is a progressive thickening of the intima owing to a gradual accumulation of smooth muscle cells and connective tissue (Fig. 11–4). The lipid content of the arterial wall, mainly cholesterol esters and phospholipids, increases. It has been estimated that between the second and sixth decades the arterial intima accumulates 10 mg of cholesterol per gm of arterial wall. These alterations are accompanied by a loss of elastin within the vessel walls and subsequent dilatation and tortuosity of the major arteries, including the aorta. All these diffuse changes are unrelated to the focal lesions of atherosclerosis.[14] In the heart, there is slight thickening of the valve cusps with increased prominence of the lines of closure. In addition, calcific deposits are frequent, but not universal, at the bases of the aortic cusps and mitral valve annulus.

There is a question — should atherosclerosis be construed as a disorder of aging or instead as a closely related but independent disease? As will be seen (p. 557), atherosclerosis is clearly age-related, and indeed few individuals in the Western world achieve adulthood free of atherosclerosis. Moreover, its severity generally increases with age, but it will become evident that other influences are even more important than age. So we must conclude — atherosclerosis is age-related but not age-dependent.

AGING AND THE KIDNEY

On average, there is a progressive decrease in renal blood flow and glomerular filtration rate over the life span of an individual. There may be as much as a 40% reduction in renal function in older persons as compared with healthy young adults.

> Changes in renal morphology have been described in elderly individuals, notably, scattered ischemic obsolescence and sclerosis of glomeruli. Although some of this glomerular loss may be due to disease-induced focal vascular occlusion, there is a linear relationship between the severity of the glomerular loss and age.[15]

However, when rigorous efforts are made to exclude previous renal disease and potentially damaging drug therapy as was done in the Baltimore Longitudinal Study of Aging, the surprising finding was that

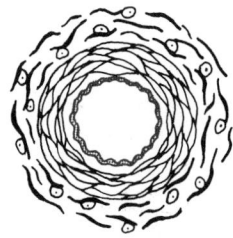

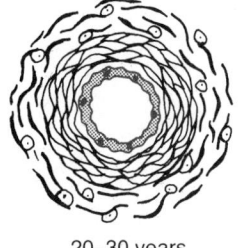

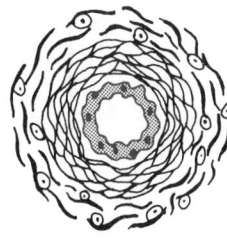

Figure 11-4. Intimal thickening with aging.

Normal artery   20-30 years   > 50 years

as many as one third of all subjects had no absolute decrease in renal function, and indeed a few had a statistically significant improved renal function over the span of 24 years.[16] The decline in renal function with age is not universal and may therefore reflect intercurrent damage to the kidney. Note should be taken, nonetheless, that in many elderly individuals there is often some reduction in renal function, whatever its origins, and with it possibly impaired excretion of drugs (discussed later).

AGING AND THE LUNGS

The lungs tend to become less elastic and compliant with aging and simultaneously tend to become expanded. This increased lung volume is attributed to qualitative changes in elastin and collagen without accompanying quantitative losses. Cross-linking glycosylation reactions may be involved.

> Grossly, the lungs appear overinflated; this change has been called "senile emphysema," but because there is no overt destruction of alveolar walls (necessary for the diagnosis of emphysema) the aging changes are better called **senile hyperinflation.** The alveolar ducts and respiratory bronchioles are somewhat enlarged, and the alveoli become somewhat smaller. Although loss of tissue elasticity may underlie these changes, an increasing kyphosis, so common in the elderly, with an increase in the anteroposterior depth of the thorax may contribute to the senile hyperinflation.

The pulmonary changes, unless complicated by other encroachments on lung function, usually cause little or no respiratory deficit.

AGING AND BODY COMPOSITION

The composition of the body changes substantially over the span of years, most notably with a loss of muscle and bone mass, often somewhat compensated for in terms of body weight by an increase in fat mass.[17] How much of the decrease in muscle mass is a consequence solely of aging or instead is related to reduction in physical activity is unknown, but it suffices that the elderly who remain physically active have only moderate loss of skeletal muscle, mainly type II "fast-twitch" fibers. Nonetheless, ligaments and tendons stiffen somewhat owing to the develop-

ment of collagen cross-linkages. Bone loss occurs in almost all postmenopausal women and elderly men, sometimes producing the condition known as osteoporosis (p. 1324) (Fig. 11-5). This decrement is almost certainly age-dependent, but the magnitude of the bone loss is affected by physical activity, nutrition, and hormonal changes, particularly reduction in the levels of estrogens and androgens. The *absolute* increase in fat mass with aging is maximal from young adult life until late middle age. Thereafter there is usually loss of subcutaneous fat but a continued *relative* overall increase. On the one hand, there is a clear correlation between obesity and impaired glucose tolerance and elevated blood pressure. On the other hand (ice cream freaks take note), a moderate increase in fat mass appears to lower the overall mortality rate. There are many changes in the body with aging, but other than slowing of motor function and reflex responses and particularly the ability to run a marathon, it is difficult to ascertain their significance.

AGING AND OTHER SYSTEMS

Senescent changes have been described in many other organs and systems, notably the liver, skin, and endocrine system. The liver mass decreases with age, a change that is attributed to dropout of individual cells. Hepatic blood flow in the average individual 70 years of age is about 50% that of a young adult. Does this loss of mass reflect repeated toxic insults during life to the much belabored liver, and is the reduced flow the consequence of primary cardiac dysfunction or atherosclerosis? Whatever the explanations, drug metabolism may be affected, as will be discussed later. Elderly people look old, in part, because of loss of melanocytes in the hair follicles, with loss of hair pigmentation and skin changes. Exposed skin becomes thin with diminution of epidermal proliferation; there is a random decrease in melanocytes with uneven pigmentation; and there is atrophy of subcutaneous fat. Most striking is the loss of elasticity, and wrinkling, reflecting loss of dermal elastin fibers while the collagen becomes less flexible and more insoluble and undergoes elastotic change. Surprisingly, these so-called aging skin changes are not seen in covered areas of the body and probably result from exposure to the elements, notably ultraviolet irradiation (the message to the young should not be lost).

It is evident that with aging there are alterations,

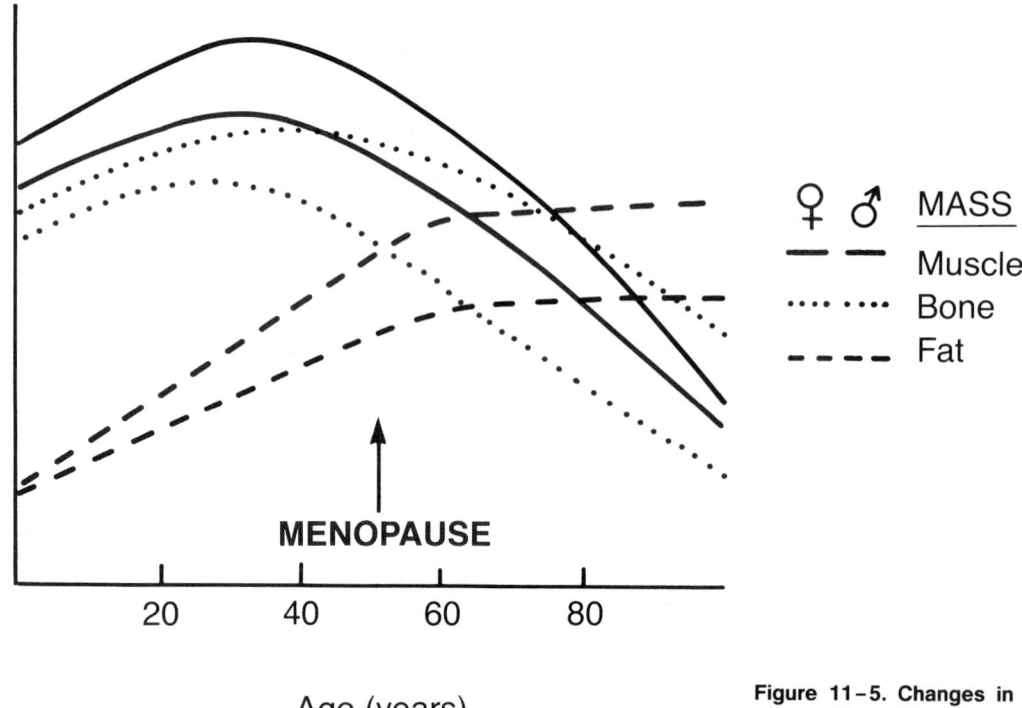

MENOPAUSE

Age (years)

Figure 11–5. Changes in body composition with aging.

whether physiologic or enviromental in origin, in many organ systems. Since these changes are not universal, it is unlikely that they are a consequence of physiologic senescence and in any event are of themselves not incapacitating. In clinical terms, the major consequence of aging may be "no change," a possibility that provides considerable comfort to antique writers of textbooks. Indeed, only about 5% of the elderly in the United States require nursing home care at any one time.

DISEASES OF AGING

Even pathologists know that the elderly are more vulnerable to disease than the young. Those over 65 in the United States spend, on average, three times as much on health care as those under 65. In the United States, after the first year of life the risk of dying is directly related to age. The curve begins to rise exponentially at about 50 years of age and does not plateau in the late years, contrary to the common myth about the survival of the fittest. At present only 2.3% of the population is aged 80 or over, but this group accounts for 17% of the mortality, underscoring the considerable increased burden imposed on the health care system as life has been prolonged.

A major issue for the gerontologist is the separation of those often fatal disorders that are a direct consequence of physiologic senescence (i.e., are "age-dependent") from those that are simply more prevalent in the advanced years of life and therefore "age-related." The issue is more than academic, since the term "age-dependent" implies that the condition

is an inevitable part of senescence, whereas age-related conditions offer the opportunity for prevention, control, or treatment. The distinction between these two categories is difficult and, in the last analysis, judgmental.[18] With recognition of the potential for disagreement, the major diseases encountered in the elderly are categorized in Table 11–1.

Whether age-dependent or age-related, it is clear that both categories of disease are age-associated and account for most of the morbidity and mortality in the "golden years of life." According to the United States Bureau of Vital Statistics, the five leading causes of death of those 75 to 84 years of age (expressed as approximate mortality rates per 100,000 of popula-

Table 11–1. Geriatric Disorders

AGE-DEPENDENT	AGE-RELATED
Cataracts	Systemic atherosclerosis
Hearing impairment	Acute myocardial infarction
Osteoporosis	Cerebrovascular disease
Osteoarthritis	Chronic ischemic heart disease
Vulvovaginal atrophy	Temporal arteritis
Nodular prostatic	Myelodysplastic syndrome
hyperplasia	Hypertension
? Parkinson's	Type II diabetes mellitus
disease	Vulnerability to infections
Senile hyperinflation	Alzheimer's disease
of lungs	Parkinson's disease
	Some cancers, e.g., prostate,
	breast, skin, colon
	Calcific aortic stenosis
	Paget's disease of bone
	Multiple myeloma
	Glaucoma

tion at risk) are heart disease, 7500; cancer, 2000; cerebrovascular disease, 1300; and influenza and pneumonia, 1000.

Another common geriatric problem is adverse drug reactions, which are significantly more common in the elderly. The rate of ADRs increases steadily after age 50; those over 60 have a twofold greater chance of developing an adverse reaction to medications than that seen in younger individuals, which rises to five- to eight-fold in those over 80. This increased risk has many origins. In part, it is due to the reduced renal clearance and hepatic metabolism noted in the advanced years of life. Also contributing are drug-drug interactions potentiated by the polypharmacy of senescence. There is, in addition, increasing sensitivity of the various tissues and organs of the body to particular drugs in the late years of life, e.g., the increased sensitivity of the central nervous system to narcotics and benzodiazepines. In the words of one pundit, "Old age ain't for sissies," [19] but to the brave in heart, it provides a broadened perspective on the changing scene and the opportunity to prove that senescence does not necessarily mean senility.

1. Kirkwood, T.B.L., and Holliday, R.: The evaluation of aging and longevity. Proc. R. Soc. Lond. (Biol.) *205*:531, 1979.
2. Scoggins, C.H.: The cellular basis of aging. West. J. Med. *135*:521, 1981.
3. Hayflick, L.: The aging process: Current theories. Drug Nutr. Interact. *4*:13, 1985.
4. Harman, D.: The aging process. Proc. Natl. Acad. Sci. U.S.A. *78*:7124, 1981.
5. Cerami, A., et al.: Glucose and aging. Sci. Am. *256*:90, 1987.
6. Hayflick, L.: Cell biology of human aging. Sci. Am. *242*:58, 1980.
7. Holliday, R., et al.: Cellular aging: Further evidence for the commitment theory. Science *213*:505, 1981.
8. Olson, C.B.: A review of why and how we age: A defense of multifactorial aging. Mech. Ageing Dev. *41*:1, 1987.
9. Weksler, M.: The senescence of the immune system. Hosp. Pract. *16*:53, 1981.
10. Hooyman, N., and Cohen, H.J.: Medical problems associated with aging. Clin. Obstet. Gynecol. *29*:353, 1986.
11. Katzman, R.: Aging and age-dependent disease: Cognition and dementia. *In* America's Aging: Health in an Older Society. Washington, D.C., National Academy Press, 1985, p. 129.
12. Rodeheffer, R.J., et al.: Exercise cardiac output is maintained with advancing age in healthy human subjects. Cardiac dilatation and increased stroke volume compensate for a diminished heart rate. Circulation *69*:203, 1984.
13. Lakatta, E.G., and Yin, F.C.P.: Myocardial aging: Functional alterations and related cellular mechanisms. Am. J. Physiol. *242*:H927, 1982.
14. Finch, C.E., and Schneider, E.L.: Handbook of the Biology of Aging, 2nd ed. New York, Van Nostrand Reinhold Co., 1985, p. 842.
15. Kaplan, C., et al.: Age-related incidence of sclerotic glomeruli in human kidneys. Am. J. Pathol. *80*:227, 1975.
16. Lindeman, R.D., et al.: Longitudinal studies on the rate of decline in renal function with age. J. Am. Geriatr. Soc. *33*:278, 1985.
17. Masoro, E. J.: Biology of aging. Current state of knowledge. Arch. Intern. Med. *147*:166, 1987.
18. Brody, J.A., and Schneider, E.L.: Diseases and disorders of aging: An hypothesis. J. Chronic. Dis. *39*:871, 1986.
19. Moore, H.: Sayings. *In* Alvarez, J., and Oldham, P. (eds.): Old Age Ain't for Sissies. Cameron, North Carolina, Crane's Creek Press, 1979.

NORMAL

In order to understand the diseases that affect the vessels, we should consider some of the distinctive anatomic and functional characteristics of these structures. *Arteries* are divided into three categories based on their size and certain histologic features: (1) large or elastic arteries, including the aorta; (2) medium-sized or muscular arteries, also referred to as distributing arteries; and (3) small arteries (usually less than 2 mm in diameter) that course, for the most part, within the substance of tissues and organs. All arteries characteristically possess three coats — *a tunica intima, a tunica media, and a tunica adventitia* — most clearly distinguished in the larger vessels (Fig. 12–1). As the vessels diminish in caliber, the three separable coats become progressively indistinct and eventually are no longer identifiable at the level of the arterioles.

The large elastic arteries of the body include the aorta and its major branches: the innominate, the subclavian, the beginning of the common carotid, and the origins of the pulmonary arteries. The *tunica intima* of these vessels is composed of the lining endothelial cells with their underlying subendothelial connective tissue. The latter consists of collagen, proteoglycans, elastin, and a number of other matrix glycoproteins. At birth, the tunica intima is quite thin, but throughout life it thickens by the progressive accumulation of connective tissue matrix as well as *myointimal cells*. The outer limit of the tunica intima is demarcated by a longitudinally dispersed layer of elastic fibers that create a thick felting of elastic tissue. These fibers are not compacted into a discrete *internal elastic lamina* in vessels of this caliber, as is the case in the muscular arteries (see later).

The *tunica media*, or muscular layer, is rich in elastic tissue in the large arteries, hence their designation as elastic arteries. The elastic fibers of the media are disposed in fairly compact fenestrated layers separated by alternating layers of smooth muscle cells. Condensation of the elastic tissue at the outer limit of the media produces a poorly defined external elastic membrane. The media is in general poorly vascularized. The inner smooth muscle layers depend largely on direct diffusion from the vessel lumen for their nutritional needs.

The *tunica adventitia* is a poorly defined layer of investing connective tissue in which elastic and nerve fibers and small, thin-walled nutrient vessels, the *vasa vasorum*, are dispersed. These nutrient vessels are derived from exiting arterial branches at points where they pass through the adventitia of the main vessel. In the aorta, vasa course back into the wall and can be identified in the outer third of the media. They ramify into minute, poorly defined channels but fail to enter the inner one third of the media or the intima.

The elastic content of the media of these large vessels provides great resilience, and their rebound following systole aids in the forward propulsion of the blood. In the aging process, the elastic fibers deteriorate and are replaced by fibrous tissue. With this loss of elasticity, these vessels expand less readily, particu-

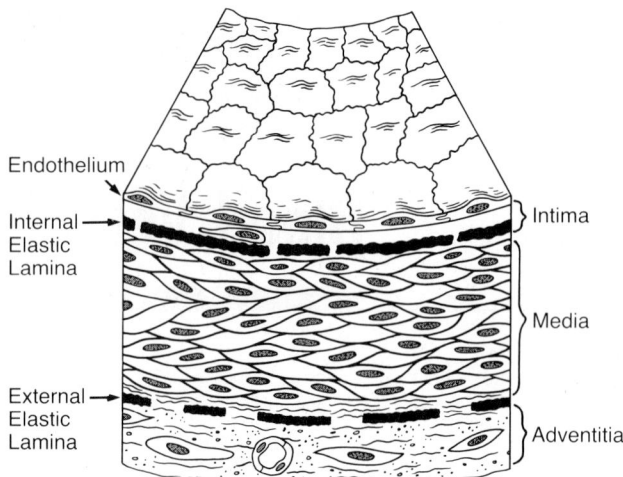

Endothelium

Internal
Elastic
Lamina

Intima

Media

External
Elastic
Lamina

Adventitia

Figure 12–1. Diagrammatic representation of the main components of the vascular wall, seen here in a muscular artery. (Redrawn from Ross, R., and Glomset, I.: The pathogenesis of atherosclerosis. N. Engl. J. Med. *295*: 369, 1976.)

larly when blood pressure is increased. The loss of elasticity further predisposes to stretching and elongation and accounts for the progressive development of tortuosity in these arteries in older age groups.

In the *muscular arteries of medium size,* the three coats are well defined and are derived by gradual transition from the layers in the larger elastic arteries. The outer limit of the *tunica intima* is clearly defined by a compact, wavy *internal elastic lamina.* Normally this lamina is a single discrete layer; occasionally, two layers may be present, but reduplication or fibrillation generally denotes an increased formation of elastic tissue incident to such abnormal stress as hypertension. *The internal elastic lamina is not a continuous structure but is interrupted by fenestrae, through which medial smooth muscle cells may migrate into the intima.*

The *tunica media* is largely made up of circular or spiral smooth muscle cells arranged in concentric layers. Fine elastic fibers can be visualized only with elastic tissue stains or on electron microscopy. The outer limit of this coat is marked by a well-defined external elastic membrane that is usually somewhat less well developed and delineated than is the internal membrane. The *tunica adventitia* resembles that in the large vessels but contains more abundant nerves, reflecting the role these vessels play in the autonomic regulation of blood flow.

In *small arteries* there is progressive loss first of the external elastic membrane and then of the internal elastic membrane so that, at the prearteriole level, the definition between the three coats is virtually lost. The tunica adventitia is of relatively greater thickness in these small vessels and approximately equals that of the tunica media. As the vessels approach the order of arterioles, the wall comprises an endothelial lining based on a scant subendothelial connective tissue, a layer of muscular media, and an investment of collagenous adventitia. The thickness of the wall is usually

about equal to the diameter of the lumen of the vessel. The arterioles are richly supplied by nervous connections with the autonomic nervous system, and these vessels constitute the major site of autonomic control of vascular flow. In this role, the small arteries and the arterioles bear the brunt of elevations of blood pressure and respond to these abnormal stresses by alterations in their structure (to be detailed later).

The differentiation of these three types of arteries is of considerable importance in pathology, as each class of vessel tends to be involved in specific disease processes and to have its own pattern of pathologic lesions. Thus, it will be shown that *atherosclerosis* is largely a disease of elastic and muscular arteries, whereas *hypertension* is associated with functional and structural changes in the small muscular arteries and arterioles that form the resistance vessels.

Veins in general are thin-walled vessels with relatively large lumina. The three separable coats seen in the arteries are not well defined in the veins. The tunica intima is composed largely of an endothelial lining based on a scant connective tissue layer. Internal elastic membranes delimiting the outer extent of the tunica intima can be well identified only in the largest veins. The media is poorly developed, is prominent only in the largest veins, and at best is unevenly distributed and provides very inadequate support in the thinned-out areas. Veins are thus predisposed to abnormal irregular dilation, compression, and easy penetration by tumors and inflammatory processes. Valves, essentially endothelial folds, are found in many veins, particularly those in the extremities. These valves break the column of blood and reduce the hydrodynamic load in the propulsion of blood back toward the heart.

The *lymphatics* are extremely thin-walled structures, difficult to identify in tissue sections because of their tendency to collapse under ordinary tissue pressures. Clear identification depends on the recognition of thin-walled, endothelium-lined channels devoid of blood cells. The major lymphatics, however, possess a thin supporting muscular wall as well as valves.

Although the major function of the lymphatics is as a protective drainage system, they also constitute an important pathway for the dissemination of disease by the conduction of bacteria and tumor cells to distant sites. The role that the lymphatics also play in the normal return of interstitial tissue fluid to the blood must not be overlooked and has been referred to previously (p. 60). Obstruction of these channels causes lymphedema.

Vascular endothelium and smooth muscle, the main components of the vascular wall (Fig. 12–2), play important roles in all types of vascular pathology. Much has been learned about the properties of the cells in these tissues, and a few points will be highlighted here.[1-3]

The single layer of continuous *endothelium* lining arteries and veins forms the unique thromboresistant layer between blood and potentially thrombogenic subendothelial tissues. The integrity of endothelium

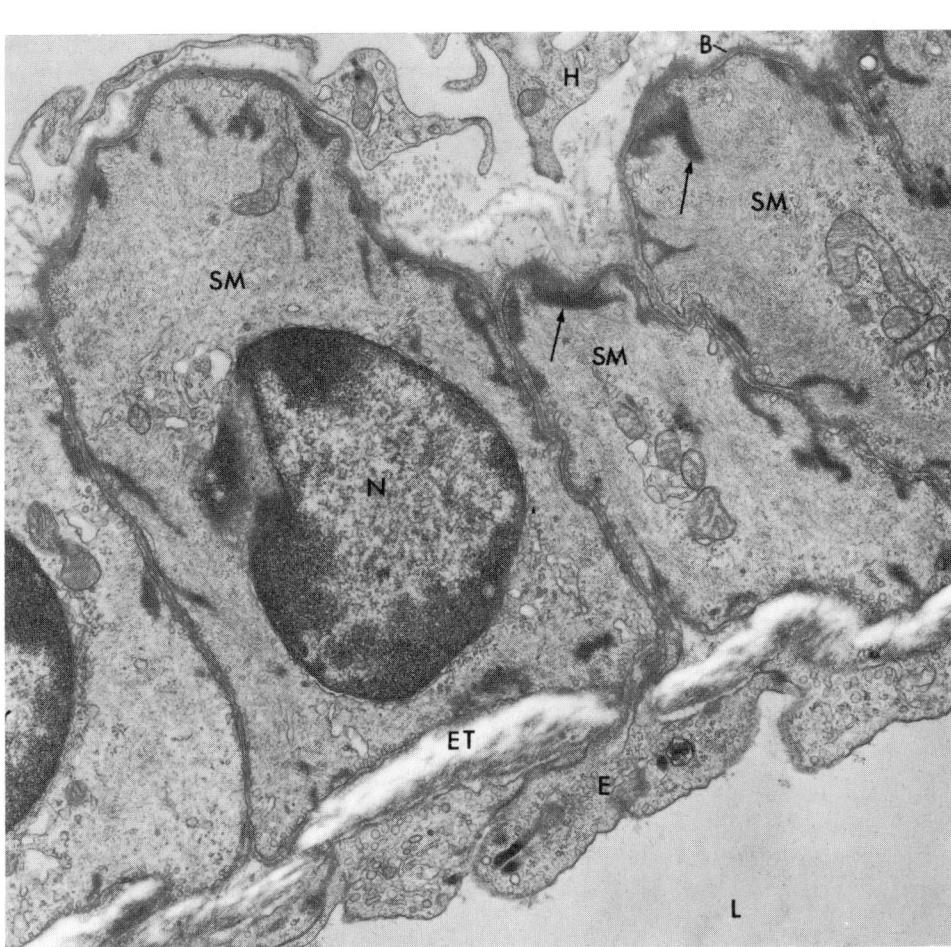

Figure 12-2. Wall of small artery in the myocardium. Continuous endothelium (E) is separated from smooth muscle layer (SM) by a thin elastica (ET)—unstained. Note peripheral bands in smooth muscle cells *(arrows)* and prominent external basement membrane (B). L = lumen; H = perivascular fibroblast; N = nucleus.

is a fundamental requirement for maintenance of normal structure and function of the entire vessel wall. Besides inducing the obvious thrombotic phenomena, endothelial injury may be responsible, at least in part, for the initiation of atherosclerosis and the vascular lesions of hypertension. Ultrastructurally, arterial endothelium resembles other continuous endothelia in its content of organelles and its rich supply of pinocytotic vesicles (Fig. 12-2). In addition, it contains unique, rod-shaped cytoplasmic organelles (the *Weibel-Palade bodies*), which serve as specific markers for endothelium.[4] Like other endothelia, normal arterial endothelium is a semipermeable membrane, controlling the transfer of small and large molecules into the arterial wall. It transports relatively slight amounts of proteins through pinocytotic vesicles. In most arterial regions, the intercellular junctions are normally impermeable to such molecules, but intercellular junctions are relatively labile structures that may widen under the influence of hemodynamic factors (such as high blood pressure) and possibly of vasoactive agents.

Despite its relatively simple structure, vascular endothelium is a versatile tissue having many synthetic and metabolic properties (Table 12-1).[1] Beyond their role as a permeability barrier, endothelial cells are involved in the maintenance of non-

thrombogenic blood-tissue interface (see p. 94; Fig. 3-6), in the modulation of blood flow and vascular resistance, in the regulation of immune and inflammatory reactions, and in the growth of other cell types. As mentioned earlier, endothelial cells can also actively contract. Thus, this thin cell, hardly visible in routine histologic sections, is not a simple passive membrane, as previously thought, but an active participant in the interaction between blood and tissues.

With regard to *vascular smooth muscle cells*, recent work has shown these to be capable of a great many functions.[5] In addition to their already established role in vasoconstriction and dilatation, smooth muscle cells are capable of synthesizing various types of collagen, elastin, and the proteoglycans of the extracellular space. As we shall see, these cells rather than fibroblasts are responsible for the intimal collagenization in atherosclerosis. They can also migrate and proliferate, and both these processes appear to be fundamental to the reaction of the vessel wall to injury. Like fibroblasts, smooth muscle cells also have receptors for low-density lipoprotein as well as the complement of enzymes that regulate intracellular cholesterol metabolism (p. 559). Finally, although not normally phagocytic, these cells can be stimulated to perform pinocytosis and phagocytosis and to develop a variety of hydrolytic enzymes, processes that may

Table 12–1. Endothelial Cell Properties and Functions

Maintenance of permeability barrier
Elaboration of anticoagulant and antithrombotic molecules
    Prostacyclin
    Thrombomodulin
    Plasminogen activator
    Heparin-like molecules
Elaboration of prothrombotic molecules
    Von Willebrand factor (Factor VIIIa)
    Tissue factor
    Plasminogen activator inhibitor
Modulation of blood flow and vascular reactivity
    Endothelium-derived relaxation factor, EDRF
    Endothelin (vasoconstrictor)
    Angiotensin converting enzyme (AI → AII)
    Prostacyclin
Regulation of inflammation and immunity
    Interleukin-1
    Adhesion molecules
Extracellular matrix production
Regulation of cell growth
    Growth stimulators (PDGF; CSF; FGF)
    Growth inhibitors (heparin, TGFβ)

PDGF = platelet-derived growth factor; CSF = colony-stimulating factor; FGF = fibroblast growth factor; TGFβ = transforming growth factor beta.

be important in lipid accumulation in the vessel wall during atherosclerosis.

PATHOLOGY

Although vessels are secondarily affected by lesions in adjacent structures, primary vascular disease is the major concern of this chapter. In general, all types of vascular diseases are significant because they may (1) weaken the walls of vessels and lead to dilatation or rupture, (2) narrow the lumina of vessels and produce ischemia, or (3) damage the endothelial lining and provoke intravascular thrombosis.

Vascular diseases may affect the arteries and, of these, the most prevalent and clinically significant is *atherosclerosis*. In the course of time, this disorder affects virtually every individual to some degree. The other arterial diseases are very much less common but, in the individual instance, may be responsible for considerable disability and even death. Certain of the venous disorders, such as varicose veins, are also very commonly encountered in clinical practice, in a frequency that almost approaches that of atherosclerosis. In general, however, these diseases of veins are more noteworthy for the disability they produce than for their importance as causes of death, but this should not imply that venous diseases are unimportant. Many are disabling to the point of being crippling, and certain disorders, such as phlebothrombosis, may lead to death by embolism. Diseases of arteries, veins, and

lymphatics will be discussed separately. Tumors of these vessels, however, will be considered as a group, because these neoplasms are for the most part quite similar clinically and anatomically.

ARTERIES

CONGENITAL ANOMALIES

The development of the far-flung complicated branching and anastomosing system of blood vessels and lymphatics results in a fairly standard or normal anatomic pattern. It is, however, not surprising that many aberrations departing from the classic pattern may be found. Most of the anomalies in the course and distribution of arteries are of importance only in surgical operative technique, in which recognition of the deviation is important to the surgical dissection. Occasionally, however, these minor anomalies have a greater significance in potentiating or even preventing disease. For example, a double renal arterial supply may prevent infarction of a kidney when one of the vessels is occluded by a thrombus or embolus. On the other hand, by crossing anterior to the ureter, the aberrant renal vessel may compress the ureter, obstruct the outflow of urine, and eventually cause urinary tract obstruction. In a somewhat analogous fashion, maldevelopment of a major coronary branch may predispose the myocardium to infarction. Among these diverse vascular anomalies, two have particular importance: *the developmental or berry aneurysm*, and *arteriovenous fistulas or aneurysms*. Berry aneurysms involve cerebral vessels and are discussed in Chapter 29.

ARTERIOVENOUS FISTULA OR ANEURYSM. Abnormal communications between arteries and veins may arise as developmental defects, from rupture of an arterial aneurysm into the adjacent vein, from penetrating injuries that pierce the wall of artery and vein and produce an artificial communication, and from inflammatory necrosis of adjacent vessels. The communication, therefore, is in only certain instances developmental in origin. The connection between artery and vein may consist of a well-formed vessel or a vascular channel formed by the canalization of a thrombus, or it may be mediated through an aneurysmal sac. Such lesions are extremely rare and are usually small. They are of some clinical significance, because they short-circuit blood from the arterial to the venous side and throw an increased burden upon the right side of the heart, predisposing to cardiac failure. Sometimes the very tortuous mass of vessels that presumably represents an arteriovenous aneurysm is designated as a *cirsoid aneurysm*.

ARTERIOSCLEROSIS

Arteriosclerosis literally means "hardening of the arteries," but more accurately it refers to a group of disorders that have in common thickening and loss of elasticity of arterial walls. Three distinctive morphologic variants are included within the term arteriosclerosis: *atherosclerosis*, characterized by the formation of atheromas (fibrofatty intimal plaques); *Mönckeberg's medial calcific sclerosis*, characterized by calcification of the media of muscular arteries; and *arteriolosclerosis*, marked by proliferative or hyaline thickening of the walls of small arteries and arterioles. These three forms are relatively easily distinguished by their morphologic appearance. More than one pattern can be identified in the same individual in different vessels or even in the same vessel. In particular, atherosclerosis and Mönckeberg's medial sclerosis often occur together, in the arteries of the legs of aged individuals. Because atherosclerosis is by far the most common and important form of arteriosclerosis, the terms are generally used interchangeably unless otherwise specified.

Atherosclerosis (AS)

Among the diseases in the Western world, atherosclerosis is overwhelmingly the prime disorder leading to death and serious morbidity. Global in distribution, it has reached alarming epidemic proportions in economically developed societies. Although any artery may be affected, the aorta and the coronary and cerebral systems are the prime targets, and so *myocardial infarcts* (heart attacks) and *cerebral infarcts* (strokes) are the two major consequences of this disease. Myocardial infarcts (MIs) alone account for 20 to 25% of all deaths in the United States, almost entirely attributable to AS. Atherosclerosis also causes a variety of other, less calamitous events that add to its toll, including *chronic ischemic heart disease, gangrene of the legs, mesenteric occlusion,* and *ischemic encephalopathy.* Despite a recent reduction in mortality from coronary heart disease, about 50% of all deaths in the

United States are still attributed to atherosclerosis-related diseases. Atherosclerosis is a slowly progressive disease that begins in childhood, but it does not become manifest until middle age or later, when the arterial lesions precipitate clinical manifestations by virtue of organ injury (Fig. 12-3). Its variable severity among nations, individuals, and social and ethnic groups is evidence that AS is not an inevitable consequence of life. An understanding of why some persons have only mild disease whereas others are severely affected, and discovery of the cause or causes of this rampant disorder, are two of the most urgently sought goals of medical research today.

DEFINITION. Atherosclerosis is a disease of large and medium-sized muscular arteries (e.g., coronary, carotid, arteries of the lower extremities) and the elastic arteries, such as the aorta and iliac vessels. *The basic lesion—the atheroma or fibrofatty plaque—consists of a raised focal plaque within the intima, having a core of lipid (mainly cholesterol, usually complexed to proteins, and cholesterol esters) and a covering fibrous cap.* These atheromas are sparsely distributed at first, but as the disease advances they become more and more numerous and sometimes literally cover the entire intimal surface of severely affected arteries. As the plaques increase in size, they progressively encroach on the lumen of the artery as well as on the subjacent media. Consequently, atheromas compromise arterial blood flow and weaken affected arteries. Many eventually undergo a variety of complications (e.g., calcification, ulceration, thrombus formation, and aneurysmal dilation) (p. 564). The lesions precipitate clinical manifestations by virtue of organ injury.

EPIDEMIOLOGY AND INCIDENCE. Much attention has been paid to the epidemiology and incidence of

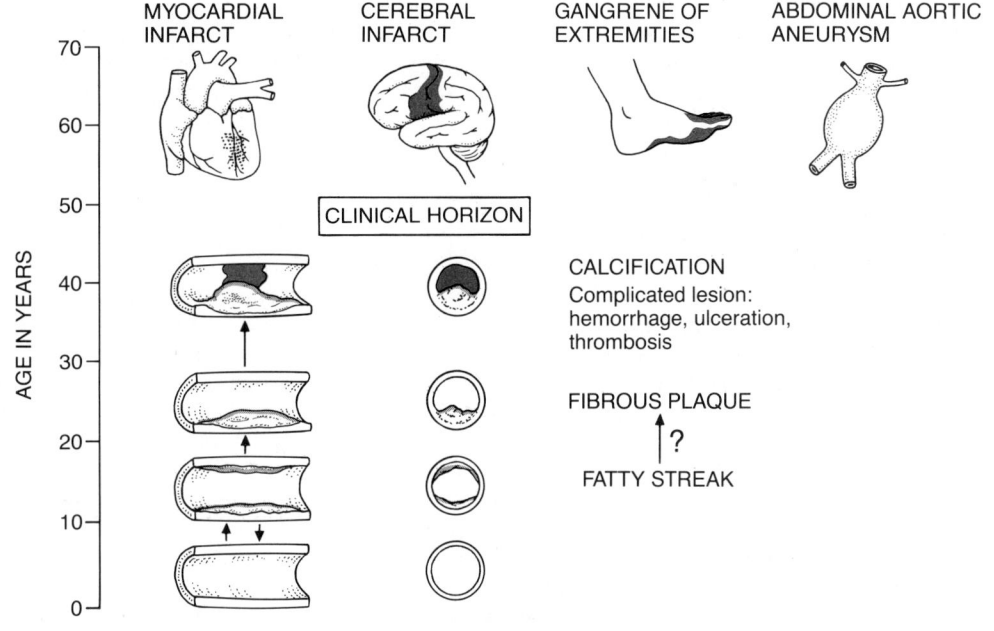

Figure 12-3. The natural history of atherosclerosis. Plaques usually develop slowly and insidiously over many years. As described in the text, they may progress from a fatty streak to a fibrous plaque and then to a complicated plaque that is likely to lead to clinical effects. (Modified from McGill, H.C., Jr., et al.: Natural history of human atherosclerotic lesions. *In* Sandler, M., and Bourne, G.H. [eds.]: Atherosclerosis and Its Origin. New York, Academic Press, 1963, p. 42; and Wissler, R.M.: *In* Braunwald, E. [ed.]: Heart Disease. Philadelphia, W.B. Saunders, 1984, p. 1188).

AS because the variable occurrence and severity of this disease among individuals and groups may provide important clues to its pathogenesis. Epidemiologic data are largely expressed in terms of ischemic heart disease (IHD), also called coronary heart disease (CHD), or by comparing the number of *deaths* caused by coronary heart disease. It must be stressed that this is not an entirely accurate reflection of AS, because other complex factors contribute to cardiac death (especially sudden death).

The deaths from cardiovascular disease (heart, brain, kidneys) in the United States rose from 14% of all deaths in 1937 to 54% in 1968, almost all cases being related to AS. But happily, they appeared to plateau in the late 1960s, and by 1975, for the first time, they showed a statistically significant decline.[6] From 1968 to 1984, there was a 38% decrease in the death rate from coronary heart disease and a 53% decrease in mortality from strokes (Fig. 12–4).[7] These downward trends, it is believed, are mediated largely by a reduction in atherosclerosis, influenced by changes in diet and life style, better control of hypertension, and improved therapy.

Nevertheless, the death rate from IHD in the United States is still among the highest in the world, lower than for Finland and Scotland, but above that of other well-developed, affluent countries, such as Canada, France, and the Scandinavian countries.[8] Conversely, the rates are remarkably lower in Asia, Africa, and South and Central America. Death rates from IHD in Japan are one sixth of those in the United States. Japanese who migrate to the United States and adopt the life styles and dietary customs of their new home acquire the predisposition to AS evident in the native American population. Thus, differences in diet, lifestyle, and personal habits are important in the pathogenesis and progression of this disease. Nevertheless, epidemiologic studies have not shown the reasons for differences between cultures that appear to be at least superficially similar. For example, why is the mortality rate from IHD for North American men under age 55 higher than that for Swedes of the same age group? Genetic factors may explain such differences, but no clear-cut patterns have emerged.

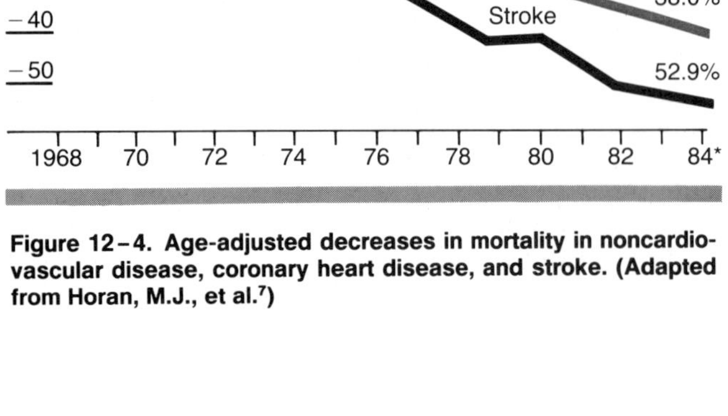

RISK FACTORS. Epidemiologic studies indicate that certain genetic or acquired factors increase the risk of AS.[9] Some of these, such as age, sex, and familial predisposition, are — alas — the irreversible accompaniments of our lives, but others are clearly or potentially reversible.

Age has a dominant influence on the development of clinically significant AS. Although some lesions of atherosclerosis may be present in childhood, clinically overt AS, as evidenced by death rates from ischemic heart disease, rises with each decade even up to age 85, although death from myocardial infarction seems to decline slightly after age 75.

There are striking *sex differences* in the incidence and severity of AS.[10] Death rates from IHD are significantly higher in males until age 75 to 85, when the incidences in males and females approach equality. Significantly, myocardial infarction is uncommon in premenopausal women, and in the age group of 35 to 55 the mortality rate of white males is over five times that of white females. Naturally, other risk factors influence the relative risk of IHD in females; the rate is increased in women with a history of heavy smoking, hypertension, or diabetes.

Some families suffer an increased frequency of heart attacks at an early age. This *familial predisposition* may represent the clustering of other risk factors within families rather than a unique genetic predisposition. In particular, hyperlipidemia (genetic or diet-induced), hypertension, and diabetes all tend to be familial. Nevertheless, there are families with high attack rates of IHD in which none of the known risk factors appears to operate.[11]

Granted that residency in certain affluent areas of the world, increasing age, and sex define the population at risk, not all members of this population develop clinically apparent AS. Other significant "risk factors" that predispose to AS and IHD have been identified by means of a number of prospective studies in well-defined population groups, such as the famed Framingham (Massachusetts) Study.[12] *Of the various risk factors, four are of prime importance: (1) hyperlipidemia, (2) hypertension, (3) cigarette smoking, and (4) diabetes.* Each will now be discussed.

Hyperlipidemia in Atherosclerosis. There is overwhelming evidence that hypercholesterolemia is a major risk factor in atherosclerosis. Here we shall review some of the evidence and some details of lipid metabolism as they relate to atherosclerosis. How lipids contribute to the development and progression of the lesion is discussed later under "Pathogenesis."

The evidence linking hypercholesterolemia and atherosclerosis takes many forms:[13,14]

1. The atherosclerotic plaques are rich in cholesterol and cholesterol esters, which are largely derived from the lipoproteins in the blood.

DECLINE IN AGE-ADJUSTED DEATH RATES
UNITED STATES, 1968-1984

Percentage decline from 1968 rate

Noncardiovascular disease 13.3%

Coronary heart disease 38.0%

Stroke 52.9%

Figure 12–4. Age-adjusted decreases in mortality in noncardiovascular disease, coronary heart disease, and stroke. (Adapted from Horan, M.J., et al.[7])

2. Full-blown atherosclerosis can be produced in most experimental animals, including subhuman primates, by feeding them diets that raise the plasma cholesterol level.

3. Genetic disorders causing severe hypercholesterolemia lead to premature atherosclerosis, often fatal in childhood, despite the absence of any other risk factor. Acquired diseases that cause hypercholesterolemia, such as the nephrotic syndrome and hypothyroidism, also increase risk for IHD.

4. With few exceptions, populations having relatively high levels of blood cholesterol have higher mortality from IHD.

There is no single level of plasma cholesterol that identifies those at risk. The higher the level, the higher the risk, although the risk rises significantly once a plateau level of 200 mg/dl is exceeded. The Framingham Study showed that in men and women 35 to 44 years of age, serum cholesterol levels of 265 mg/dl or over are associated with a five times higher risk of developing coronary artery disease than are levels below 220 mg/dl. *The most striking association is with elevated levels of low-density lipoprotein (LDL)*, the lipoprotein moiety richest in cholesterol; however, *hypertriglyceridemia* with increased concentrations of very-low-density lipoprotein (VLDL) also appears to increase risk. In contrast, serum levels of high-density lipoprotein (HDL) are *inversely* related to risk: the higher the level, the lower the risk.

There is a large body of evidence that a high dietary intake of cholesterol and saturated fats raises the plasma cholesterol level. Conversely, a diet low in cholesterol and low in the ratio of saturated to polyunsaturated fats lowers plasma cholesterol levels. Paradoxically, Greenland Eskimos, who have a high dietary fat consumption, have low rates of CHD. This is thought to be due to the high content of omega-3 fatty acids in their diets (present in fish and fish oils). Such fatty acids have a number of antiatherogenic effects, including the lowering of plasma LDL, increase of plasma HDL, and modification of prostaglandin/leukotriene production by blood and vascular cells (p. 54).[15]

5. Finally, recent prospective studies, such as the Lipids Research Clinics Coronary Primary Prevention Trial have shown that treatment with diet and cholesterol-lowering drugs reduces cardiovascular mortality in a selected group of patients with hypercholesterolemia.[16,17]

Lipid Metabolism. As is well-known, all lipids in plasma circulate in combination with protein. The plasma lipoproteins are a family of globular particles, each consisting of a core of neutral lipid (primarily triglyceride or cholesteryl ester) surrounded by a coat composed of polar lipids (phospholipid and free cholesterol) and apoprotein. Plasma lipoproteins can be divided into five types, depending on their electrophoretic mobility and sedimentation properties (Fig. 12–5): (1) *chylomicrons*, which have the lowest density, are composed primarily of triglyceride and are found in plasma only after a meal; (2) *very-low-density*

lipoproteins (VLDL), which mainly transport triglycerides that have been synthesized in the liver; (3) *intermediate-density lipoproteins* (IDL), which are remnants generated from the action of lipoprotein lipase on VLDL; (4) *low-density lipoprotein* (LDL); and (5) *high-density lipoprotein* (HDL). LDL and HDL function primarily in the transport of endogenous cholesterol to body cells. *About 70% of the total plasma cholesterol level in normal Americans is contained in LDL, the lipoprotein most strongly correlated with AS.* A relatively newly discovered variant of LDL, called *lipoprotein (a) [Lp(a)]*, possesses all the characteristics of LDL, but has its B apoprotein linked to a distinct lipoprotein (a) by disulfide bridges. Although its function is unknown, its plasma levels are correlated with increased risk of coronary artery disease.[17a]

Endogenous and exogenous cholesterol is transported by various lipoproteins via two separate pathways. In the *exogenous pathway* (Fig. 12–6), dietary triglycerides and cholesterol are incorporated into chylomicrons (containing apoproteins E, C11, and B48) in intestinal epithelial cells; via intestinal lymphatics, chylomicrons reach peripheral capillaries, to be hydrolyzed by an endothelial lipoprotein lipase, liberating fatty acids into adipose tissue and muscle. The resulting chylomicron remnants, rich in cholesterol, are then taken up by receptor-mediated pinocytosis and degraded in lysosomes by the liver. Thus chylomicrons transport exogenous cholesterol to the liver and triglycerides to the adipose tissue. Some of the cholesterol in the liver is excreted as free cholesterol or bile acids into the intestines.

In the *endogenous pathway* (detailed on p. 141, Fig. 4–11), VLDL, containing triglycerides and three apoproteins (E, C, and B100), is secreted by the liver and transported to adipose tissue and muscle, where a sequence of events occurs that transforms VLDL, via the formation of intermediate-density lipoprotein (IDL), to LDL. The core of LDL is composed almost exclusively of cholesteryl ester and the coat of only one protein, apoprotein B100. Two thirds of the resultant LDL is metabolized by liver cells and other cells in extrahepatic tissues (adrenal cells, fibroblasts, smooth muscle cells, lymphoid cells, endothelial cells) by the *LDL receptor pathway* (p. 142). This pathway is the means by which nonhepatic cells control the cholesterol needed for membrane synthesis; in the presence of low concentrations of extracellular LDL, more receptors are elaborated, and vice versa. The LDL receptor binds to apoproteins B and E. The remaining one third of LDL is degraded by LDL receptor–independent mechanisms. These include the scavenger cells of the mononuclear phagocyte system, which, as discussed later, have receptors for *modified LDL*. In addition, non–receptor-mediated fluid and adsorptive endocytosis also occurs in various cells, particularly in the presence of high LDL concentrations.

Unesterified cholesterol derived from normal turnover of cell membranes is transported by HDL into the plasma (Fig. 12–6). Through the action of the

	MAJOR LIPIDS	MAJOR APOPROTEIN(S)
Chylomicron 80–500 nm	80–95% TG (dietary)	C proteins, AI, AII, B48
VLDL 30–80 nm	45–65% TG (endogenous) 25% cholesterol	C proteins, B48, E
IDL 30 nm	45% cholesterol	B100, E
LDL 15–25 nm	70% cholesterol	B100
HDL 5–12 nm	<25% cholesterol	AI, AII

Figure 12–5. Characteristics of major plasma lipoproteins. Not shown is lipoprotein (a), a variant of LDL in which the apoprotein B100 is linked to apoprotein (a) by disulfide bonds.

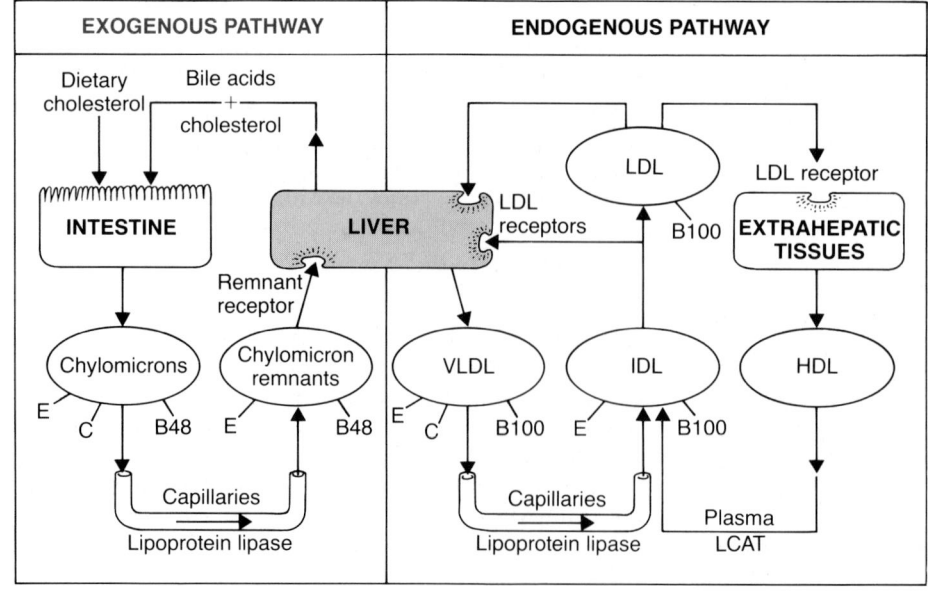

Figure 12–6. Pathways for receptor-mediated metabolism of lipoproteins carrying endogenous and exogenous cholesterol. HDL = high-density lipoprotein; LCAT = lecithin-cholesterol acyltransferase; LDL = low-density lipoprotein; IDL = intermediate-density lipoprotein; VLDL = very-low-density lipoprotein. The distinction between exogenous and endogenous cholesterol applies to the immediate source of the cholesterol in plasma lipoproteins. After the exogenous cholesterol has been delivered to the liver and has been secreted in VLDL, it is considered endogenous cholesterol. Note that HDL is the lipoprotein that removes cholesterol from extrahepatic cells. (From Goldstein, J.L., et al.: Defective lipoprotein receptors and atherosclerosis. N. Engl. J. Med. *309:*288, 1983. Reprinted, by permission, from The New England Journal of Medicine. Reprinted by permission of the copyright owner from The Role of Cholesterol in Atherosclerosis. Copyright © 1988 by Merck & Co., Inc., Rahway, New Jersey, U.S.A. All rights reserved.)

Table 12–2. The Hyperlipoproteinemias

TYPE	INCREASED LIPOPROTEIN CLASS	INCREASED LIPID CLASS	GENETIC DISORDERS	PRIMARY DEFECT	SECONDARY DISORDERS
1	Chylomicrons	Triglycerides	Familial lipoprotein lipase deficiency	Deficiency of lipoprotein lipase	SLE
2a	LDL	Cholesterol	Familial hypercholesterolemia (rarely 2b)	Deficiency of LDL receptor	Nephrotic syndrome; hyperthyroidism
2b	LDL and VLDL	Cholesterol and triglycerides	Familial combined hyperlipidemia (also 2a and 4)	Unknown	Nephrotic syndrome; stress, diet
3	Remnants (chylomicrons) and IDL	Triglycerides and cholesterol	Familial type 3 hyperlipoproteinemia	Abnormal apoprotein E	Hypothyroidism
4	VLDL	Triglycerides	Familial hypertriglyceridemia	Unknown	Diabetes mellitus; alcoholism
5	VLDL and chylomicrons	Triglycerides and cholesterol	Familial combined hyperlipidemia	Unknown; familial apoprotein CII deficiency (also CI)	Alcoholism; diabetes; oral contraceptives

plasma enzyme lecithin-cholesterol acyl transferase (LCAT) the cholesterol from HDL is delivered to IDL and eventually to LDL. Epidemiologic and experimental studies have shown an inverse relationship between the level of HDL and the development of AS. Although several mechanisms have been proposed for this protective action of HDL, none is proved. Probably the HDL fraction, usually low in cholesterol and rich in phospholipids, facilitates clearance of cholesterol from the atheromatous plaque and its transport to the liver, where it may be excreted rather than reutilized in further synthesis of LDL.

A number of genetic and acquired derangements influence both exogenous and endogenous pathways of cholesterol metabolism, result in hyperlipoproteinemia, and predispose to the development of AS. The hyperlipoproteinemias are classified as either primary genetic defects in lipid metabolism or secondary to some other underlying disorder, such as nephrotic syndrome or diabetes mellitus (Table 12–2). Some genetic disorders, such as familial hypercholesterolemia (p. 140), are single-gene dominant-recessive disorders, but many have a polygenic complex mode of inheritance and are markedly influenced by environmental factors, including diet. Although the most well-studied example of genetically induced hyperlipoproteinemia remains familial hypercholesterolemia caused by defects in the LDL receptor (p. 140), recent work has shown that *genetic defects in apoproteins may also be associated with hyperlipoproteinemia and accelerated atherosclerosis.*[18,19] For example, familial type III hyperlipoproteinemia, which is associated with premature atherosclerosis, is secondary to the presence of a variant apoprotein E that fails to bind normally to the LDL receptor. This defect has been traced to single amino acid substitutions (e.g., arginine for cysteine at residue 158) in the receptor binding site of the apoprotein E molecule.[18]

Hypertension. Elevated blood pressure unequivocally accelerates atherogenesis and increases the inci-

dence of IHD and cerebrovascular disease.[9] The higher the blood pressure, the greater the risk. In the Framingham Study, the incidence of IHD in men aged 45 to 62 with blood pressures exceeding 160/95 was more than five times that in normotensive men (blood pressure 140/90 or less). Diastolic hypertension is the more important correlate. The risk of IHD in individuals with diastolic pressures greater than 105 mm Hg is four times that of individuals with pressures 84 mm Hg or less. After age 45, the scales tip toward hypertension as a greater risk factor than hypercholesterolemia. Antihypertensive therapy reduces the incidence of strokes and possibly also of IHD.

Cigarette Smoking. In men who smoke one or more packs of cigarettes per day, the death rate from IHD is 70 to 200% higher than that for nonsmokers. Smoking is the major influence on the recent increases in incidence of CHD in women. At autopsy, the degree of aortic and coronary AS is greater in smokers than in nonsmokers. Smoking also increases the incidence of sudden death among victims of heart attacks. Cessation of cigarette smoking in high-risk men is followed by a reduction in the risk of dying from IHD.

Diabetes. Diabetes is associated with an increase in AS observed at autopsy, a twofold increase in incidence of myocardial infarction in diabetics as compared with nondiabetics, increased tendency toward cerebral thrombosis and infarction, and an eight- to 150-fold increased frequency of gangrene of the lower extremities.

Other Risk Factors. These are sometimes referred to as *"soft risk factors"* because they are associated with a less pronounced increased risk, which has been difficult to document in clear-cut statistical terms. These include (1) insufficient regular physical activity; (2) competitive, stressful lifestyle with type A personality behavior; (3) obesity; (4) the use of oral contraceptives; (5) hyperuricemia; and (6) high carbohydrate intake.

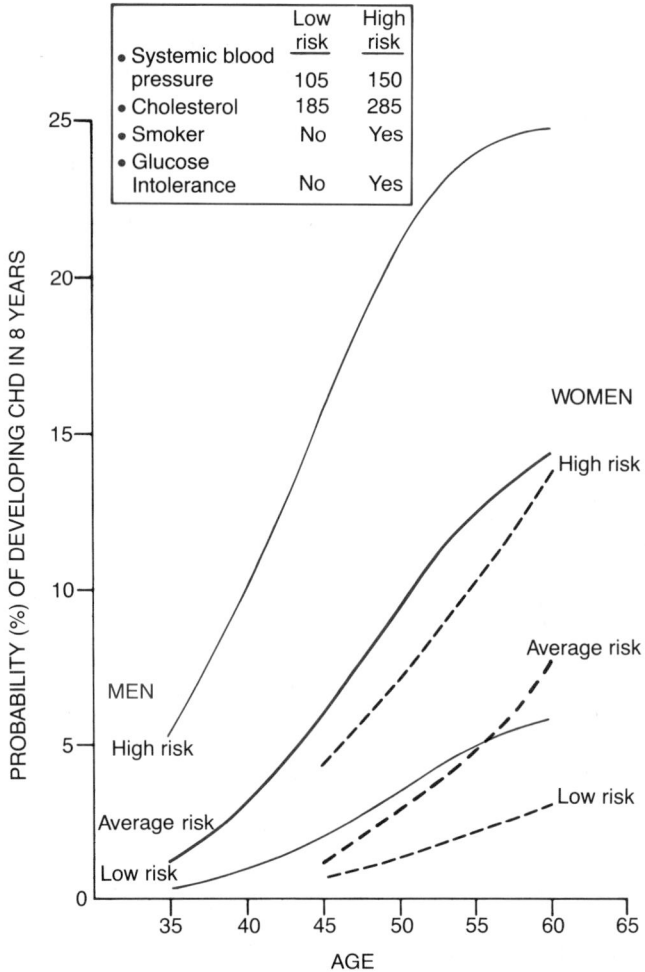

	Low risk	High risk
• Systemic blood pressure	105	150
• Cholesterol	185	285
• Smoker	No	Yes
• Glucose Intolerance	No	Yes

PROBABILITY (%) OF DEVELOPING CHD IN 8 YEARS

WOMEN

High risk

Average risk

Low risk

MEN

High risk

Average risk

Low risk

AGE

Figure 12–7. Graph depicting the influence of added risks. Probability of developing coronary heart disease in eight years according to age, sex, and risk category (The Framingham Heart Study). (From Braunwald, E. [ed.]: Heart Disease. A Textbook of Cardiovascular Medicine. Philadelphia, W.B. Saunders Co., 1984, p. 1209.)

Each of the major risk factors noted earlier contributes individually to the possible development of clinically significant AS, but multiple factors exert more than an additive effect. In the Framingham Study, for example, when three risk factors were present (hyperlipidemia, hypertension, and smoking), the rate of heart attacks was seven times greater than when none was present; when two risk factors were present, the risk was increased fourfold; and with one risk factor, the increase was twofold. These relationships are shown in Figure 12–7. *However, none of these factors is either necessary or sufficient for the development of AS*, and some patients have no obvious risk factor. Thus, the cause and pathogenesis of AS remain subjects of lively speculation and controversy. Before we delve into pathogenesis, however, it is desirable to understand the morphology of the lesions.

MORPHOLOGY. Descriptions of the morphology of atherosclerosis have been confounded by the heterogeneity of the histologic lesions present and the difficulty in assessing the relationship of one lesion to the other. Despite this, two well-accepted lesions can be described:[20-21] (1) the **atheromatous plaque,** which is by far the most important lesion, being the principal cause of arterial narrowing in adults, and (2) the **fatty streak,** which is present universally in children, even in the first year of life, and is important mainly as a possible precursor of the atheromatous plaque.

THE ATHEROMATOUS PLAQUE. This is the fundamental lesion of AS, also called the fibrous, fibrofatty, lipid, or fibrolipid plaque. **Macroscopically,** plaques are white to whitish-yellow in appearance, protrude into the lumen of the artery, and vary in size from 0.3 to 1.5 cm in diameter, but they sometimes coalesce to form larger masses (Figs. 12–8 and 12–9). On section, the luminal surface tends to be firm and white (the fibrous cap) and the deep portions yellow or whitish-yellow and soft. The center of larger plaques may contain a yellow, grumous fluid, from which the name **atheroma** — the Greek word for gruel — is derived.

The distribution of atherosclerotic plaques in humans tends to be quite constant and differs from the

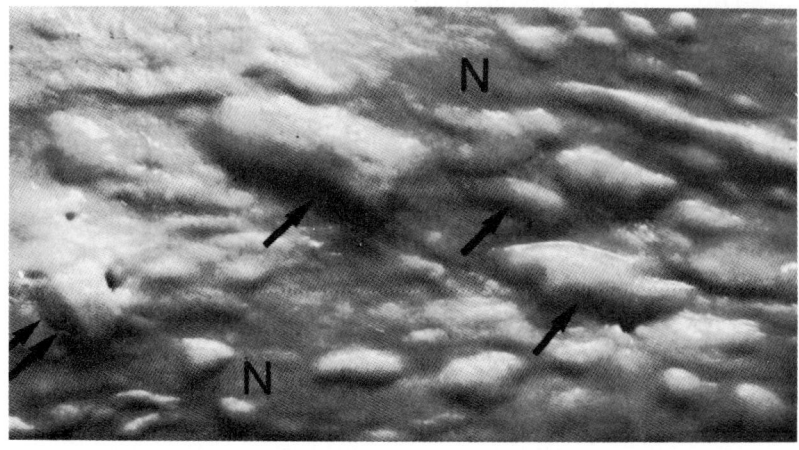

Figure 12–8. Close-up of atheromatous plaques as seen from luminal surface of aorta *(arrows)*. Note the plaque around the ostium of a branch vessel *(double arrow)* (×2.5). N = normal intima. (From Benditt, E.P.: The origin of atherosclerosis. Sci. Am. *236*:74, 1977. Copyright © 1977 by Scientific American, Inc. All rights reserved.)

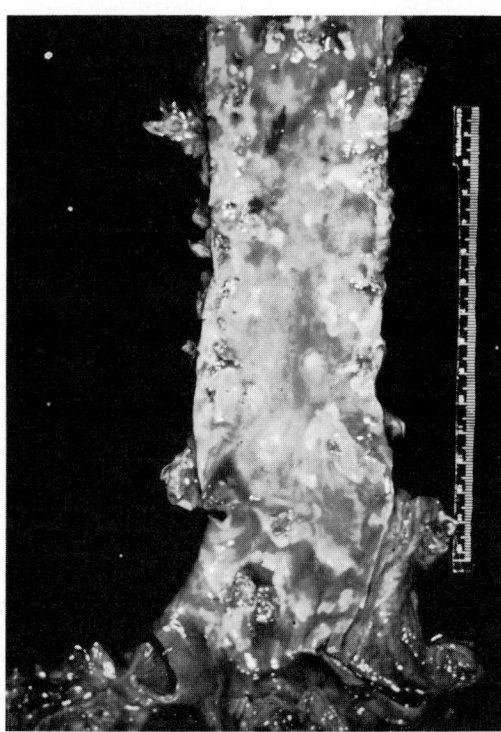

Figure 12-9. Atherosclerosis in the abdominal aorta. Note the extensive lesions covering the entire intimal surface.

distribution of fatty streaks. The abdominal aorta is much more involved than the thoracic aorta, and aortic lesions tend to be much more prominent around the ostia of its major branches. In descending order (after the lower abdominal aorta), the most heavily involved vessels are the coronary arteries (usually within the first 6 cm), the popliteal

arteries, the descending thoracic aorta, the internal carotid arteries, and the vessels of the circle of Willis. Vessels of the upper extremities are usually spared, as are mesenteric arteries and renal arteries, except at their ostia.

Histologically, the plaques have essentially three components: (1) cells, including smooth muscle cells, macrophages, and other leukocytes; (2) connective tissue, including collagen, elastic fibers, and proteoglycans; and (3) intracellular and extracellular lipid deposits (Fig. 12-10). These three components occur in varying proportions in different plaques, giving rise to a spectrum of lesions. Typically, the plaques are composed of a superficial part (the fibrous cap), made up of smooth muscle cells with a few leukocytes and relatively dense connective tissue; a cellular area beneath and to the side of the cap, consisting of a mixture of macrophages, smooth muscle cells, and T lymphocytes; and a deeper necrotic "core," in which there is a disorganized mass of lipid material, cholesterol clefts, cellular debris, lipid-laden "foam cells," fibrin, and other plasma proteins (Fig. 12-11). The lipid is primarily cholesterol and cholesteryl ester. Current studies indicate that the lipid-laden cells consist of both smooth muscle cells and blood-derived macrophages.[22] Finally, one can see—particularly around the periphery of the lesions proliferating small blood vessels—evidence of neovascularization of the plaques (Fig. 12-10).

Variations of the histologic features of plaques involve the relative numbers of smooth muscle cells, the amount of collagen and extracellular matrix, and especially the lipid content. The most typical atheromas contain relatively abundant lipid. Nevertheless, **many plaques are composed mostly of smooth muscle cells and fibrous tissue,** and coronary artery lesions are often largely fibrous.[23] In advanced AS, progressive fibrosis may convert the fatty atheroma to a fibrous scar.

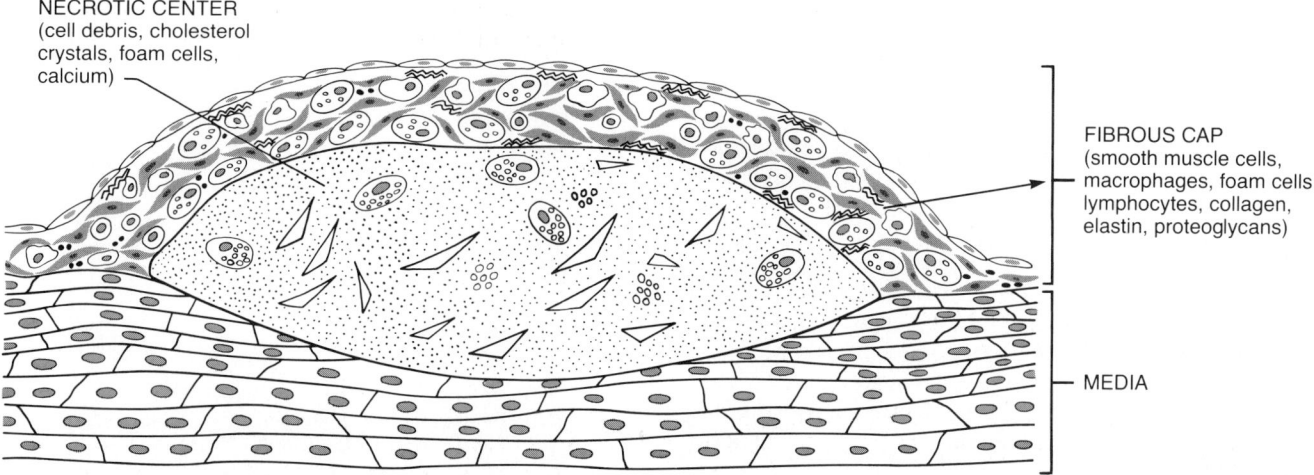

NECROTIC CENTER
(cell debris, cholesterol
crystals, foam cells,
calcium)

FIBROUS CAP
(smooth muscle cells,
macrophages, foam cells,
lymphocytes, collagen,
elastin, proteoglycans)

MEDIA

Figure 12-10. Major components of well developed atheromatous plaque: a cap composed of foam cells, proliferating smooth muscle cells, macrophages, lymphocytes, and extracellular matrix. The necrotic core consists of necrotic debris, extracellular lipid with cholesterol crystals, and foamy macrophages.

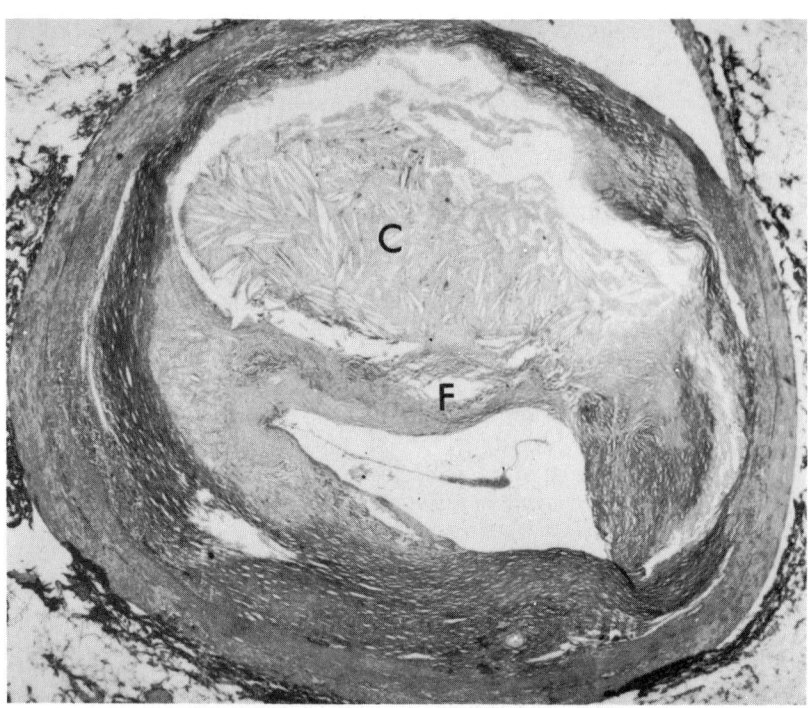

Figure 12–11. Histologic section of an atheromatous plaque. F = fibrous cap; C = central lipid core with typical cholesterol clefts. The lumen has been narrowed considerably. Note also that the media of the artery is thinned.

Fully developed atheromatous plaques may undergo a series of changes that result in so-called **complicated plaques**:

1. Almost always, atheromas in advanced disease undergo patchy or massive **calcification.** In severe atherosclerotic disease, arteries may be converted to virtual pipe stems, and the aorta may assume an eggshell brittleness.

2. **Ulceration** of the luminal surface and rupture of the atheromatous plaques may result in discharge of the debris into the bloodstream, producing microemboli **(cholesterol emboli).**

3. Superimposed **thrombosis,** the most feared complication, may occur on fissured or more often ulcerated lesions. Thrombi may either occlude the lumen or become incorporated within the intimal plaque (Fig. 12–12).

4. **Hemorrhage** into the plaque may occur, especially in the coronary arteries, from rupture of either the overlying endothelium or the thin-walled capillaries that vascularize the plaque. The resulting hematoma may remain localized within the intima or rupture into the lumen. Phagocytosis of this extravasated blood leads to the hemosiderin-laden macrophages frequently observed in plaques.

5. Although artherosclerosis is basically an intimal disease, in severe cases the underlying media undergoes considerable pressure atrophy and loss of elastic tissue, causing sufficient weakness to permit **aneurysmal dilation.** This process is discussed more fully on page 579.

Although any form of atheromatosis is serious, it is the "complicated lesion," in particular superimposed thrombosis, that gives this disease its grave clinical significance.

THE FATTY STREAK. Fatty streaks are important not because of any disturbance in blood flow that they may cause, but because they *may* be the precursors of the more ominous atheromatous plaques. The lesions begin as multiple yellow flat spots less than 1 mm in diameter and grow into elongated streaks, still no more than 1 to 2 mm wide but 1 cm long or even longer. The fatty streak (Fig. 12–13) is made up of a variable number of cells, of which some are elongated smooth muscle cells filled with intracytoplasmic

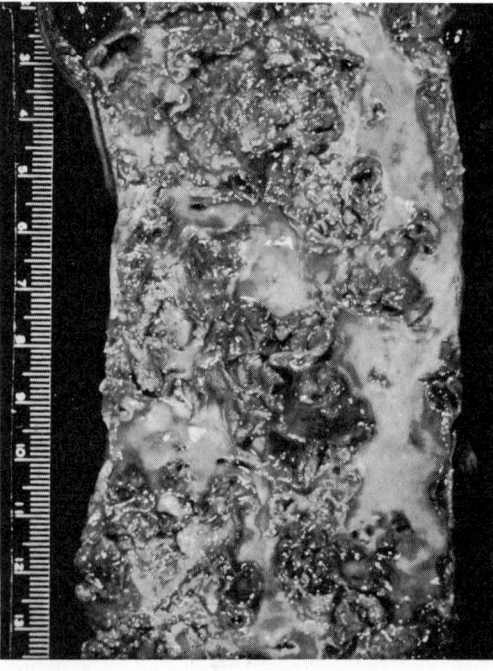

Figure 12–12. Close-up of intimal surface. Note the uneven surface caused by mural thrombi overlying atheromatous plaques.

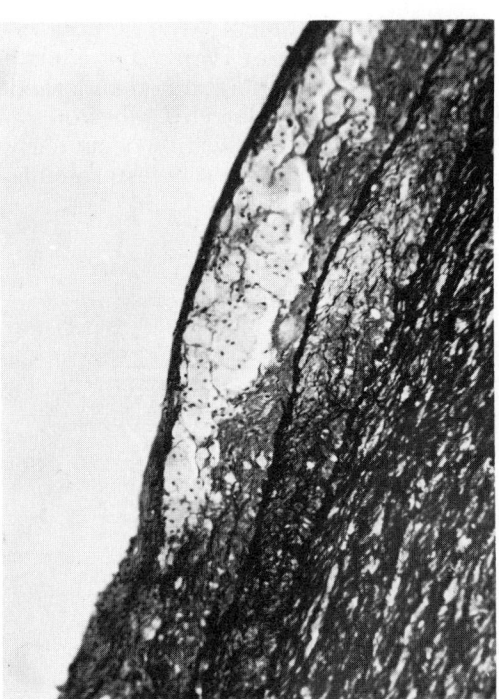

Figure 12 – 13. Fatty streak — a subintimal collection of foam cells. To the left is the lumen, and to the right, the muscularis.

lipid droplets and others are large and ovoid and represent blood-derived macrophages. T lymphocytes are also present. Lipid is also present extracellularly but in smaller amounts than in plaques, and proteoglycans, collagen, and elastic fibers are found in variable amounts.

Fatty streaks appear in the aortas of all children older than one year, regardless of geography, race, sex, or environment. The extent of aortic intimal surface covered by fatty streaks increases with age from about 10% in the first decade to 30 to 50% in the third decade. They subsequently decrease in number as atheromatous plaques begin to predominate.

The relationship of fatty streaks to atheromatous plaques is controversial.[24] Fatty streaks occur early in life in areas which are not particularly susceptible to developing atheromas later in life. In addition, fatty streaks frequently affect individuals in parts of the globe where plaques are relatively infrequent. However, fatty streaks do occur in coronary arteries at the same anatomic sites that are later prone to develop plaques.[24,25] Such fatty streaks in the coronary arteries continue to occupy increasing surface areas and seem to precede the formation of advanced lesions. Finally, some experimental evidence supports the concept of evolution of fatty streaks into plaques.[26]

It appears, then, that *fatty streaks are of universal occurrence and distribution, and most, especially those in the aorta, either disappear or remain harmless. In certain locations (e.g., in coronary arteries) and espe-* *cially in the predisposed individual, these streaks may conceivably evolve into plaques.*

An additional lesion that may bear a material relationship to atherosclerosis is the "intimal cushion" or "intimal pad." This is represented by small areas of white thickening at the site of arterial forks or ostia of branch vessels. Microscopically, the thickening is due to accumulation of smooth muscle cells and extracellular matrix in the intima, small but variable amounts of collagen, and virtually no lipid. When diffuse, the lesion is referred to as diffuse intimal thickening. In general, this thickening can be taken as normal, presumably as a result of hemodynamic or other stresses to the arterial wall with time. However, it has been noted that the intimal cushions occur in young males at the same sites that eventually develop plaques, suggesting a causal relationship,[27] but the issue is unsettled.

Having discussed the range of atheromatous lesions, *we should stress again that the most important lesion in terms of its pathologic consequences is the atheromatous plaque, in particular the complicated plaque.* In the capacious aorta, the important complications of these plaques are large mural thrombi that may dislodge and yield peripheral embolism, aneurysmal dilation due to impingement of the atheromatous plaques on the media, or rupture of cholesterol emboli into the bloodstream. Occlusion of the lumen of the aorta is unusual, as a rapidly moving bloodstream in the center usually prevents massive thrombi. However, in smaller arteries, particularly those in the brain and heart, the narrowing by atheromatous plaques, especially if accompanied by thrombosis or hemorrhage, will lead to occlusion and may be the ultimate event causing strokes and myocardial infarction.

PATHOGENESIS. The search for the cause and pathogenesis of AS, as for those of cancer, has become an insistent "golden grail." The subject has tantalized investigators from the days of Virchow. Here we can present only an overview of the various proposals that are of current interest.[13,28–32]

Any concept of the pathogenesis of AS should account for (1) the role of the important risk factors, particularly hyperlipidemia; (2) the focal nature of the lesions and their localization in the intima; (3) the presence of lipid in most lesions; and (4) the mechanisms of smooth muscle proliferation, which appears to be a fundamental and early event in the development of AS.

No single theory copes adequately with all these considerations. Historically, two hypotheses were dominant until recently. The first, originally termed the *"imbibition hypothesis"* by Virchow in 1856, held that cellular proliferation in the intima was a form of "low-grade inflammation" as a reaction to increased filtration of plasma proteins and lipids from the blood. Over the years, this concept has undergone modification to become the so-called "lipid," "insudation," or "infiltration" hypothesis. As we shall see later, this proposal has been incorporated in the more modern "reaction to injury" hypothesis dominant today. The second or *"encrustation theory,"* often ascribed to Rokitansky, postulated that small thrombi composed of platelets, fibrin, and leukocytes collected over foci of endothelial injury and that the organization of such thrombi and their gradual growth resulted in plaque formation. Few now believe that thrombus encrustation is the sole determinant of AS, but as we shall see, platelets, leukocytes, and fibrin clearly play a role in lesion formation.

We can now turn to some of the current theories of atherogenesis.

REACTION TO INJURY HYPOTHESIS. This theory, formulated by Ross and Glomset in 1976,[33] and modified in 1986,[29] states that *the lesions of atherosclerosis are initiated as a response to some form of injury to arterial endothelium*[13] (Fig. 12–14). The injury may be subtle or may be outright desquamation of endothelial cells. Focal sites of injury lead to increased permeability to plasma constituents, including lipids, and permit blood *platelets* and *monocytes* to adhere to endothelium or subendothelial connective tissue. Factors released from activated platelets or monocytes then cause migration of smooth muscle cells from media into the intima, followed by proliferation. Synthesis by smooth muscle cells of extracellular matrix components leads to accumulation of collagen, elastic fibers, and proteoglycans. Monocytes also enter the intima, transform into macrophages, accumulate lipid, and contribute to the evolution of the lesion. Single or short-lived injurious events are followed by regeneration of endothelium, restoration of endothelial function, and regression of the lesion. However, repeated or chronic injury finally results in the development of an atheromatous plaque.

Let us examine the various components of this hypothesis and how they may explain atherogenesis. There is considerable experimental support for *endothelial damage* as a cause of smooth muscle proliferation.[28,29,34] Endothelial injury induced in experimental animals by mechanical denudation, hemodynamic forces (arteriovenous fistula), immune complex deposition, irradiation, and chemicals causes intimal smooth muscle proliferation, and, in the presence of high-lipid diets, typical atheromas. Of importance is the possibility that chronic hyperlipidemia in itself may initiate endothelial injury, as we shall see (p. 567). Risk factors such as hypertension and cigarette smoking may also cause endothelial damage or increased endothelial permeability. Endothelial alterations induced by hemodynamic forces (shear stress or turbulent flow) can possibly explain the distribution of plaques at branch and fork points of arteries and in portions of the abdominal aorta.[35,36]

It should be stressed that frank endothelial denudation is not a necessary requirement for this theory. Nondenuding alterations in the functions of the versatile endothelial cell (Table 12–1, p. 556)—

referred to as endothelial "dysfunction"[37]—may well initiate a sequence of events that contribute to lesion formation. Foci of heightened endothelial permeability, increased leukocyte adhesion, and increased endothelial cell replication occur early in the course of experimental hypercholesterolemia, *without* overt endothelial desquamation.[28]

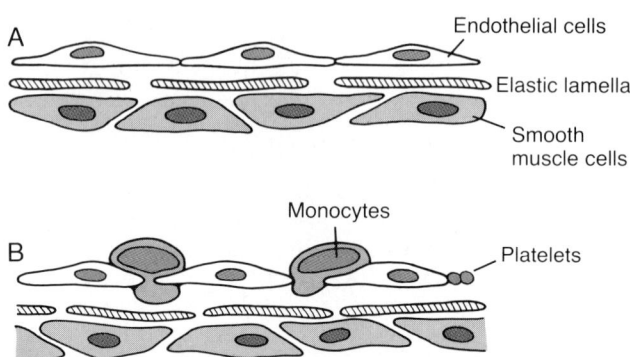

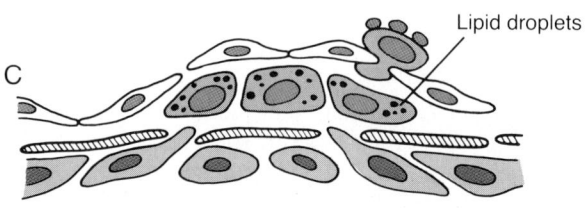

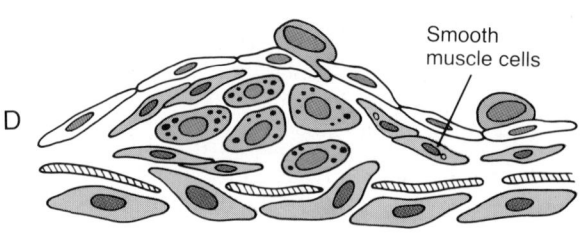

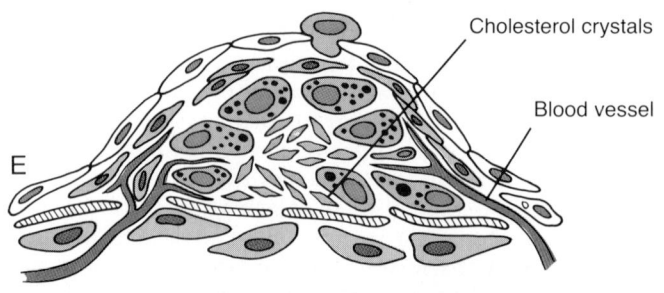

Figure 12–14. Processes in the response to injury hypothesis: *A*, Normal. *B*, Endothelial injury with adhesion of monocytes and platelets (the latter to denuded endothelium). *C*, Migration of monocytes (from lumen) and smooth muscle (from media) into intima. *D*, Smooth muscle proliferation. *E*, Well-developed plaque.

The second component of atherogenesis is *smooth muscle proliferation in the intima.* The proliferating cells originate from cells migrating from the media and possibly also from preexisting myointimal cells.[38] A number of smooth muscle mitogens derived from cells or serum have been implicated in such proliferation. Principal among these is the *platelet-derived growth factor* (PDGF) (p. 76),[39] present in the platelet alpha granules, and released after platelet adhesion to foci of injury. It is a likely candidate, as it is produced not only by platelets but also by macrophages,[40] endothelial cells,[41] and smooth muscle cells[42] — all involved in atherosclerosis. Other possible growth factors include fibroblast growth factor (FGF), epidermal growth factor (EGF), and transforming growth factor alpha (TGFα) (p. 77). In addition, growth stimulation can also be theoretically accomplished by loss of growth inhibitors, such as heparin-like molecules present in endothelial and smooth muscle cells,[43] or TGFβ, produced by macrophages or endothelial cells (see discussion of growth factors, p. 77). Whatever the stimulus, it is the smooth muscle cells that elaborate the extracellular components of the atheromatous plaque. Furthermore, the smooth muscle cells accumulate large amounts of cholesterol and cholesteryl esters and, together with infiltrating macrophages, give rise to the foam cells in the plaque.

The third component of the theory is the *role of macrophages.* Monocytes adhere to endothelium early in the course of experimental hypercholesterolemia, emigrate into the intima, and transform into lipid-laden macrophages.[26,43a,44] They are present in variable numbers in all stages of human atheromatous plaques.[22] In the lesions, macrophages are transformed into foam cells owing to the presence on their surface of at least two receptors: the beta-VLDL receptor, which recognizes VLDL from hypertriglyceridemic human serum,[45] and the modified LDL receptor (also called the scavenger receptor), which recognizes LDL that has been modified by acetylation, by treatment with malondialdehyde (a product of the platelet release reaction),[46] or by peroxidation.[47] Uptake by both of these receptors is followed by internalization, hydrolysis, and reesterification of cholesterol and its storage in lipid droplets, thus producing the foam cell.

In view of the large number of secretory products and biologic activities of macrophages, detailed in our discussion of inflammation (p. 61), it is likely that they play a role in the progression of the lesions. Macrophages, for example, produce interleukin-1 (IL-1) and tumor necrosis factor (TNF), (which increase adhesion of leukocytes) as well as chemotactic factors for leukocytes, and these may cause further recruitment of leukocytes into the plaque. They produce toxic oxygen species that cause *oxidation of the LDL* in the lesions.[48] Oxidized LDL, as we shall see, has many potential roles in lesion formation. Finally, the growth stimulators (e.g., platelet-derived growth factor) and growth inhibitors (e.g., TGFβ) elaborated by macrophages may modulate the proliferation of smooth muscle cells in the lesions.

The final aspect of the reaction to injury hypothesis is its relation to the *role of hyperlipidemia.* A number of mechanisms have been postulated, on theoretical grounds and from experimental studies, to account for the role of lipids in lesion formation.

1. Increases in plasma levels of LDL or some component of hyperlipidemic serum may *increase the rate of their penetration* into the artery wall.
2. The local conditions in the intima exposed to increased LDL concentrations may *promote formation of foam cells.* For example, LDL complexed to intimal proteoglycans is taken up avidly by macrophages.[49] As mentioned earlier, modification of LDL, perhaps through high concentrations of malondialdehyde produced by platelet release or through peroxidation, enhances its uptake by these cells via the scavenger receptor.
3. *Hyperlipoproteinemia may affect endothelial cells directly,* without leading to denudation, by causing foci of increased permeability, increased replication, and increased monocyte adhesion.[43,50]
4. *Oxidized lipoproteins* produced largely by the action of macrophage — derived oxygen metabolites —have several potential effects in lesion formation (Fig. 12–15).[13,48]
   a. They cause endothelial injury, thus further enhancing endothelial permeability.
   b. They result in smooth muscle injury, perhaps accounting for the central necrosis that occurs regularly in plaques.
   c. They promote foam cell formation, through their uptake by the scavenger receptor for modified LDL.
   d. They are chemotactic to peripheral blood monocytes but inhibit the motility of mature activated macrophages, thus favoring the recruitment and retention of macrophages in the lesions. That oxidized LDL may be important in vivo is suggested by recent studies showing a reduction in the number of lesions in hypercholesterolemic rabbits treated with antioxidant drugs.[51]

OTHER THEORIES OF ATHEROGENESIS. Although the concept of endothelial injury, coupled with the effects of hyperlipidemia, is an attractive explanation for atherogenesis, *the development of the atheromatous plaque could also be explained if smooth muscle proliferation was in fact the initial event.* Endothelial injury may then be a secondary phenomenon, or may indeed accentuate the lesion, but it would be neither the first nor a necessary event. There are several postulated mechanisms for such an occurrence:

1. It is possible that the amounts of lipid or oxidized lipids that would normally reach the smooth muscle layer in hypercholesterolemic individuals may somehow alter or injure smooth muscle cells and trigger proliferation.
2. There may be genetic or acquired aberrations of

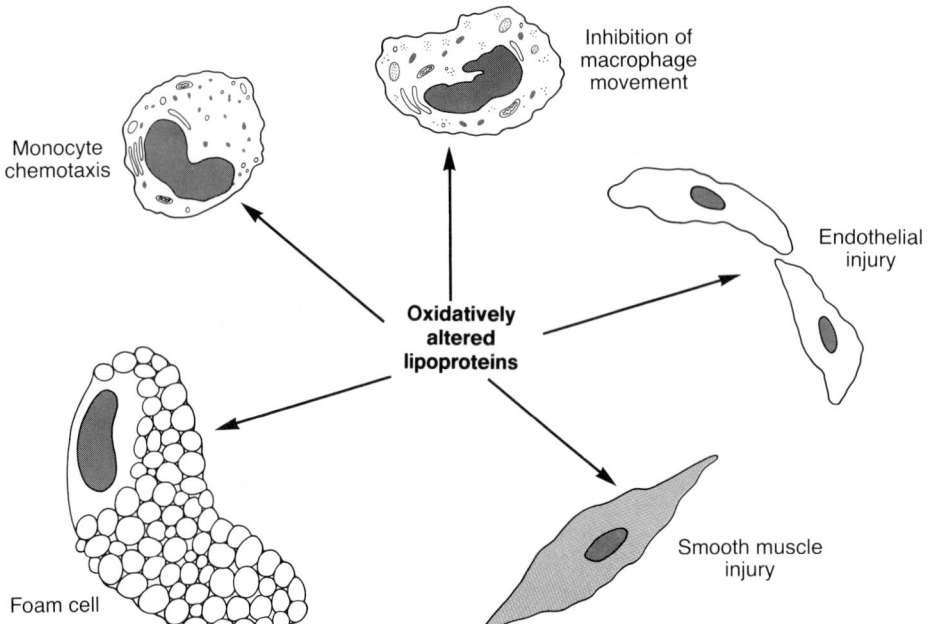

Figure 12–15. The possible effects of oxidized lipoproteins in atherogenesis (see text).

"growth control" of medial cells, leading to their proliferation. This idea is based on the *monoclonal hypothesis of atherogenesis,* which was given impetus by the observation that some human plaques appear to be composed of the progeny of a single cell (i.e., are monoclonal, or at the most oligoclonal). The monotypic nature of the smooth muscle cells in the plaque was interpreted by Benditt and Benditt[52] as evidence that plaques may be equivalent to benign monoclonal neoplastic growths (such as leiomyomas) and may be initiated by a mutation.[52a] The mutagenic effect may be from an exogenous chemical (e.g., hydrocarbons), an endogenous metabolite (e.g., cholesterol or some of its oxidants), or a virus. Although the universal monoclonal nature of the plaques has been questioned,[53] there is evidence in animals that certain oncogenic viruses (e.g., the agent of Marek's disease in chickens)[54] and carcinogens (anthracene derivatives) cause plaques in the aorta.[55] Herpesvirus mRNA has also been detected in human atheromatous plaques.[56]

Figure 12–16 summarizes some of the proposed mechanisms of atherogenesis. Although we are still far from understanding the complexities of AS, the current trend is to consider that atherosclerosis is a response of the vascular wall to a variety of initiating events that occur early in life, and that multiple pathogenic mechanisms contribute to the formation of the plaque and the progression of the lesions. *Clinically significant AS appears to be a disease of multiple origins.* In some individuals, severe or repeated endothelial injury may induce AS despite relatively normal cholesterol levels. In others, such as those with extreme hyperlipidemia, endothelial injury may not be necessary to trigger the same events. Perhaps the cumulative effect of many factors is involved, as seems evident from epidemiologic studies. At this stage, it is reasonable to attempt to halt AS during its progression rather than at its inception. The investigation of serum lipids, the study of risk factors and their manipulation, and the emphasis on prevention and treatment of thrombotic complications constitute attempts to approach the problem in this manner.

CLINICAL SIGNIFICANCE. The clinical manifestations of AS are as varied as the vessels affected and the extent of the atheromatous change. The lesions themselves do not cause symptoms or signs. They cause clinical disease only by (1) narrowing the vascular lumina to cause ischemic atrophy; (2) sudden occlusion of the lumen by superimposed thrombosis or hemorrhage into an atheroma, producing frank infarction; (3) providing a site for thrombosis and then embolism; or (4) weakening the wall of a vessel, followed by aneurysm formation or rupture. Although theoretically any organ or tissue in the body may be so involved, *symptomatic atherosclerotic disease is most often localized to the heart, brain, kidneys, lower extremities, and small intestine.* The importance of such vascular disease was amply documented by some of the epidemiologic data cited earlier in this discussion. It will be further documented throughout the remaining chapters of the book, because vascular disease constitutes a significant part of all organ and system pathology.

Given the fact that AS and CHD are virtually epidemic in affluent populations, methods of possible control are understandably major concerns of these groups. A number of clinical trials of prevention of AS and CHD have been instituted. All make the assumption that five factors capable of alteration are of cardi-

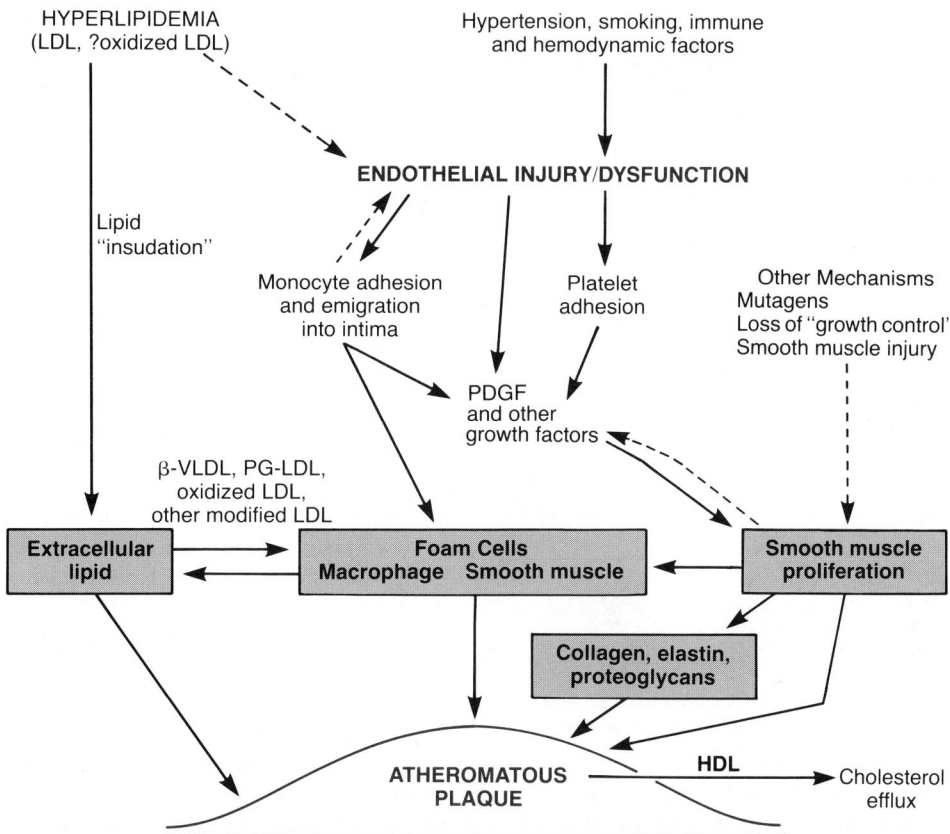

Figure 12–16. Schematic diagram of a hypothetical sequence of events and cellular interactions in atherosclerosis. Hyperlipidemia, as well as other risk factors, is thought to cause endothelial injury resulting in adhesion of platelets and monocytes and release of PDGF (and other growth factors), which lead to smooth muscle migration and proliferation. Smooth muscle cells produce large amounts of collagen, elastin, and proteoglycans, and these form part of the atheromatous plaque. Foam cells of atheromatous plaques are derived both from macrophages and from smooth muscle cells; from macrophages via the β-VLDL receptor and LDL modifications recognized by scavenger receptors (such as oxidized LDL); and from smooth muscle cells by less certain mechanisms. Extracellular lipid is derived from insudation from the lumen, particularly in the presence of hypercholesterolemia, and also from degenerating foam cells. Cholesterol accumulation in the plaque should be viewed as reflecting imbalance between influx and efflux, and it is possible that HDL is the molecule that helps clear the cholesterol from these accumulations. The diagram also depicts other postulated mechanisms for smooth muscle proliferation, bypassing primary endothelial injury: the action of mutagens, loss of growth control, and direct smooth muscle injury (such as by oxidized LDL). PG = Proteoglycan. (From Cotran, R.S., and Munro, J.M.: Pathogenesis of atherosclerosis: recent concepts. *In* Grundy, S.M., and Bearn, A.G. (eds.): The Role of Cholesterol in Atherosclerosis: New Therapeutic Opportunities. Philadelphia, Hanley and Belfus, 1988, p. 5.)

nal importance: diets high in cholesterol and saturated fat, hypercholesterolemia, hypertension, cigarette smoking, and diabetes. A review of clinical trials is beyond the scope of this book. Suffice it to say here that the evidence is good that control of hypertension and cigarette smoking diminishes the risk of CHD. Recent studies strongly suggest that treatment of hypercholesterolemia with diet and drugs reduces mortality from CHD.[17] Many, but not really all, investigators believe that *dietary* reduction of plasma cholesterol and cholesterol LDL levels would retard the progression of AS, but opinions on the strength of the probability vary widely, as CHD risk is multifactorial. However, experts on all sides of the controversy advocate a reduction in fat intake, avoidance of obesity,

moderation of salt intake, cessation of smoking, and the pursuit of physical activity as ways of life that are likely to reduce overall risk.

Mönckeberg's Arteriosclerosis (Medial Calcific Sclerosis)

Medial sclerosis is characterized by ringlike calcifications within the media of medium-sized to small arteries of the muscular type. Although Mönckeberg's medial calcific sclerosis may occur together with atherosclerosis in the same individual or even in the same vessel, *the two disorders are totally distinct anatomically, clinically, and presumably etiologically.* The vessels most severely affected are the femoral, tibial, radial, and ulnar arteries and the arterial supply of the

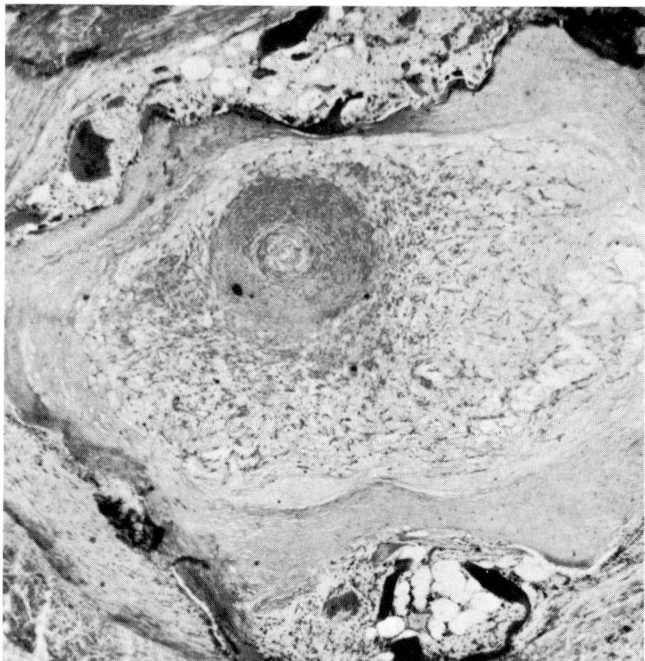

Figure 12–17. Mönckeberg's sclerosis. The lumen is narrowed by intimal atherosclerosis. Dark medial calcific deposits with bone and bone marrow in media (at 6 o'clock position).

genital tract in both sexes. Both sexes are affected indiscriminately. This disorder is rare in individuals under 50 years of age. Its genesis is still obscure, but according to prevailing concepts, medial calcification is related to prolonged vasotonic influences. In animals, analogous medial calcifications can be produced by the prolonged intravascular infusion of such vasoconstrictors as epinephrine and nicotine.

> The disorder is characterized by ringlike or plate calcifications within the wall of a vessel that create a "gooseneck lamp" nodularity on palpation. The calcification is not associated with any inflammatory reaction, and the intima and adventitia are largely unaffected. Commonly, bone and even marrow may form within the calcific plaques. Frequently, coexistent atheromas complicate the histologic changes (Fig. 12–17).

This disorder is of relatively little clinical significance. It accounts for roentgenographic densities in the vessels of the extremities in aged individuals.

Arteriolosclerosis

Included under this heading are two entities: hyaline arteriolosclerosis and hyperplastic arteriolosclerosis (Fig. 12–18). Although both lesions are clearly related to elevations of blood pressure, other causes may also be involved.

HYALINE ARTERIOLOSCLEROSIS. This condition is encountered frequently in elderly patients, whether normotensive or hypertensive, but it is more generalized and more severe in patients with hyper-

tension. The condition is also seen commonly in diabetes and forms part of the microangiography characteristic of diabetic disease (p. 1003). Whatever the clinical setting, the vascular lesion consists of a homogeneous, pink, hyaline thickening of the walls of arterioles with loss of underlying structural detail and with narrowing of the lumen.

It is believed that the lesions reflect leakage of plasma components across vascular endothelium and increasing extracellular matrix production by smooth muscle cells. Presumably, the chronic hemodynamic stress of hypertension or a metabolic stress in diabetes accentuates endothelial injury, thus resulting in leakage and hyaline deposition. The narrowing of the arteriolar lumina causes impairment of the blood supply to affected organs, particularly well exemplified in the kidneys. Thus, *hyaline arteriolosclerosis is a major morphologic characteristic of benign nephrosclerosis* in which the arteriolar narrowing causes diffuse renal ischemia and symmetric contraction of the kidneys (p. 1066).

HYPERPLASTIC ARTERIOLOSCLEROSIS. The hyperplastic type of arteriolosclerosis is generally related to more acute or severe elevations of blood pressure and is therefore characteristic of malignant hypertension (diastolic pressures usually over 110 mm Hg) (p. 1067). This form of arteriolar disease can be identified with the light microscope by virtue of its onionskin, concentric, laminated thickening of the walls of arterioles with progressive narrowing of the lumina (Fig. 12–18). With the electron microscope, these reduplicated cells have the appearance of smooth muscle cells. The basement membrane is likewise thickened and reduplicated. Frequently, but not invariably, these hyperplastic changes are accompanied by deposits of fibrinoid and acute necrosis of the vessel walls, referred to as *necrotizing arteriolitis.* The arterioles in all tissues throughout the body may be affected, favored sites being the kidney, periadrenal fat, gallbladder, peripancreatic, and intestinal arterioles.

INFLAMMATORY DISEASES — THE VASCULITIDES

Arteritis is encountered in a diversity of diseases and clinical settings.[57] The terms arteritis, vasculitis, and angiitis are used interchangeably because veins and capillaries may be involved in some of the conditions. In some instances, arteritis is produced when an artery is injured directly by a specific agent, such as by direct bacterial invasion, irradiation, mechanical trauma, and toxins. The most important entities, however, are the *noninfectious systemic necrotizing vasculitides.* Although all are characterized by inflammation and necrosis of blood vessels, they are segregated into a number of distinctive clinicopathologic syndromes affecting multiple organ systems. Many of these entities appear to have an immunologic basis. Vasculitis, also of immune origin, is a component of

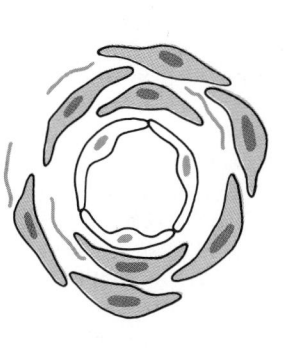
Normal

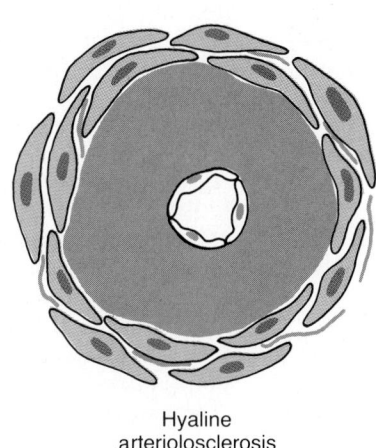
Hyaline
arteriolosclerosis

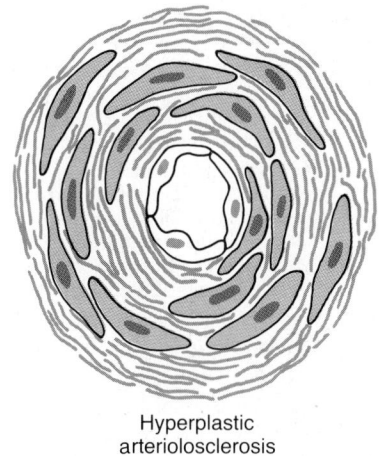
Hyperplastic
arteriolosclerosis

Figure 12–18. Diagram of two forms of arteriolosclerosis. Hyaline arteriolosclerosis, showing hyalin deposition in the intima and media. Hyperplastic arteriolosclerosis, showing concentric proliferation of smooth muscle cells in the vessel wall.

systemic lupus erythematosus (SLE) and sometimes complicates the other connective tissue disorders, such as scleroderma, polymyositis, rheumatoid arthritis, and rheumatic fever.

Before discussing some of the syndromes, we shall briefly review pathogenetic mechanisms that may be common to many vasculitides.

ETIOLOGY AND PATHOGENESIS OF VASCULITIS. Although little is known about etiologic agents, many types of vasculitis are thought to be induced by immune complexes, and the evidence for this can be summarized as follows:[57,58]

1. The vascular lesions resemble those found in experimental immune complex–mediated conditions, such as the local Arthus phenomenon and serum sickness.
2. Vasculitis is found in association with SLE and in this condition, DNA–anti-DNA immune complexes and complement are present in the vascular lesions.
3. In patients with mixed cryoglobulinemia, IgG, IgM (antibody to IgG), and complement components have been seen in involved vessels.
4. In some patients, viruses and other antigens have been localized in the lesions, together with the immunoglobulin and complement, and immune complexes are found in the circulation.
5. The most impressive evidence is the demonstration of a high incidence of hepatitis B antigenemia (HBsAg) and circulating HBsAg–anti-HBs immune complexes in the sera of some patients with vasculitis. Moreover, HBs antigen, immunoglobulins, and complement occur in the vascular lesions.

Other pathogenetic mechanisms should be considered. Cytotoxic antibodies to normal endothelial cells are seen in patients with active SLE and to "activated" endothelial cells in Kawasaki's disease.[59] Serum antineutrophil cytoplasmic autoantibodies are also present in polyarteritis and Wegener's granulo-matosis, and these *may* play a role in vascular injury.[60] The presence of mononuclear cells rich in T cells and of granulomas in some vasculitides suggests cell-mediated immunity, which may be directed against foreign antigens or endogenous components of the vessel wall. Defects in immunoregulation, well described in SLE (p. 196), may predispose to the development of vasculitis. Finally, it should be remembered that vasculitis may be caused by direct action of infectious organisms on vessel wall cells. Bacteria, viruses, mycoplasmas, rickettsiae, and fungi may all infect blood vessels directly and cause an infectious vasculitis (p. 578).

CLASSIFICATION. Many classifications of systemic vasculitis are available and depend on the size of the involved blood vessels, the anatomic site, the histologic characteristics of the lesion, or the clinical manifestations.[57,61,62] However, there is considerable clinical and pathologic overlap among these disorders, and some have thus been considered as "groups." Table 12–3 lists the most important groups of vasculitis as currently classified.

Polyarteritis Nodosa (PAN) Group

This group is characterized by systemic involvement with the vasculitic process and includes the first-recognized *classic* type of vasculitis, also called the *macroscopic* form of PAN, and certain variants thereof. *Classic PAN* is a disease of small or medium-sized muscular arteries, characteristically involving renal and visceral vessels and sparing the pulmonary circulation.

> **MORPHOLOGY.** Classic PAN may affect any artery of medium or small size in any organ, save possibly the lung. The more usual sites of involvement in autopsy series are the kidneys (85%), heart (75%), liver (65%), and gastrointestinal tract (50%), followed by the pancreas, testes, skel-

Table 12-3. Classification of Vasculitides

I. Polyarteritis nodosa group of systemic necrotizing vasculitides
  Classic polyarteritis nodosa
  Allergic angiitis and granulomatosis (Churg-Strauss variant)
  Systemic necrotizing vasculitis; "overlap syndrome"
II. Hypersensitivity angiitis
  Serum sickness and serum sickness–like reactions
  Henoch-Schönlein purpura
  Vasculitis associated with connective tissue disorders
  Essential mixed cryoglobulinemia with vasculitis
  Vasculitis associated with malignancy
III. Wegener's granulomatosis
IV. Temporal arteritis
V. Takayasu's arteritis
VI. Kawasaki's disease
VII. Thromboangiitis obliterans (Buerger's disease)
VIII. Miscellaneous (others)

etal muscle, nervous system, and skin. Grossly, the individual lesions involve sharply localized segments of vessel with a predilection for branching points and bifurcations. Intravascular thrombosis is a frequent sequel to the acute vasculitis. Ulcerations, infarctions, ischemic atrophy, or hemorrhages in the areas supplied by these vessels may provide the first clue to the existence of the underlying disorder.

Microscopically, the changes in the vessels may be divided into acute, healing, and healed stages. The **acute lesions** are characterized by fibrinoid necrosis, which may extend to involve the full thickness of the arterial wall, particularly in small arteries (Fig. 12–19). Numerous leukocytes, including neutrophils, eosinophils, and mononuclear cells, may be present in and often around the vessel wall. The necrosis may involve the entire circumference of the wall but is often localized to a segment. The affected portion may bulge in an aneurysmal fashion, and these aneurysms can frequently be demonstrated by arteriography. It is during this acute stage that the lumen becomes thrombosed (Fig. 12–20).

Healing lesions are characterized by fibroblastic proliferation in addition to the continuing necrotizing process. The leukocytic infiltrate will now exhibit large numbers of macrophages and plasma cells. The fibroblastic proliferation may extend into the surrounding adventitia, producing the firm nodularity that is sometimes grossly apparent. Thrombosis, if present, becomes organized.

The **healed lesions** consist merely of marked fibrotic thickening of the affected arterial wall. Elastic tissue stains are valuable in detecting healed polyarteritis, as they can disclose loss or fragmentation of the internal elastic lamina and its replacement by fibrous tissue (Fig. 12–21).

All stages may coexist in different loci, either within the same vessel or in different vessels. Only rarely are all lesions at one stage of inflammatory activity.

CLINICAL COURSE. Classic PAN is a disease of young adults, although it may occur in children and older individuals. It affects men more frequently than women, in the ratio of 2:1 to 3:1. Because the vascular involvement is widely scattered, it is obvious that the clinical signs and symptoms of this disorder may be varied and puzzling. Indeed, the dominant clinical characteristics of PAN are such nonspecific systemic reactions as low-grade fever, malaise, weakness, leu-

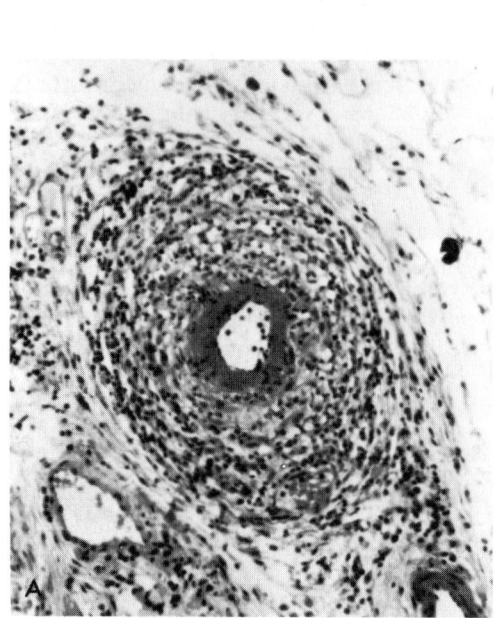
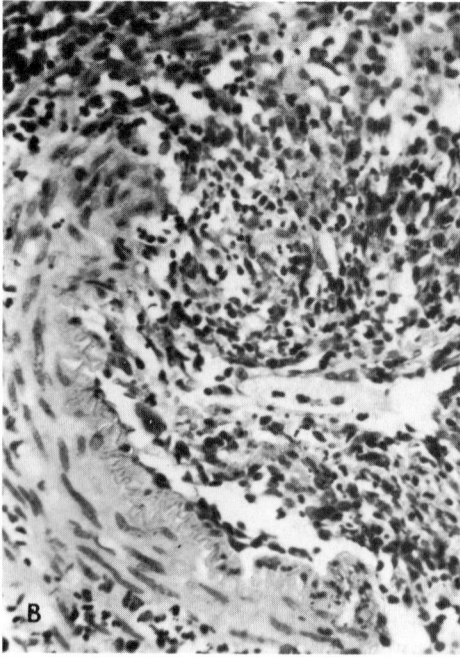

Figure 12–19. *A*, Polyarteritis nodosa. There is fibrinoid necrosis of intima and severe inflammatory infiltrate throughout the arterial wall. *B*, Higher-power view showing infiltrate of neutrophils and mononuclear cells in vessel wall.

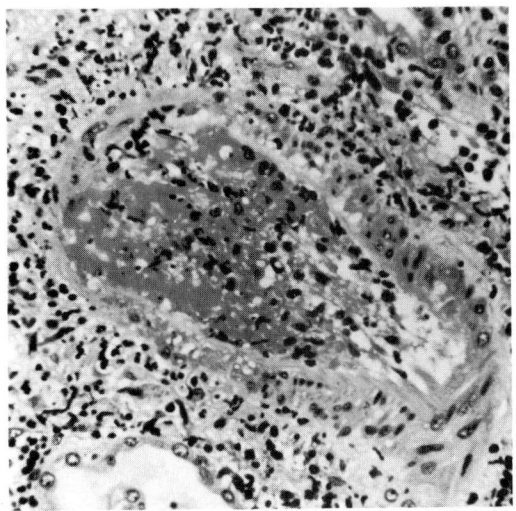

Figure 12–20. Polyarteritis nodosa. Small renal artery showing segmental fibrinoid necrosis of vessel wall and thrombotic occlusion of lumen. Note that part of vessel wall *(bottom right)* is uninvolved.

kocytosis, and symptoms referable to many systems. The course may be acute, subacute, or chronic and is frequently remittent, with long intervals of freedom from symptoms. The most common manifestations are *fever of unknown cause and weight loss; hematuria, albuminuria, and renal failure attributable to the renal involvement; hypertension, usually developing rapidly; abdominal pain and melena due to vascular le-*

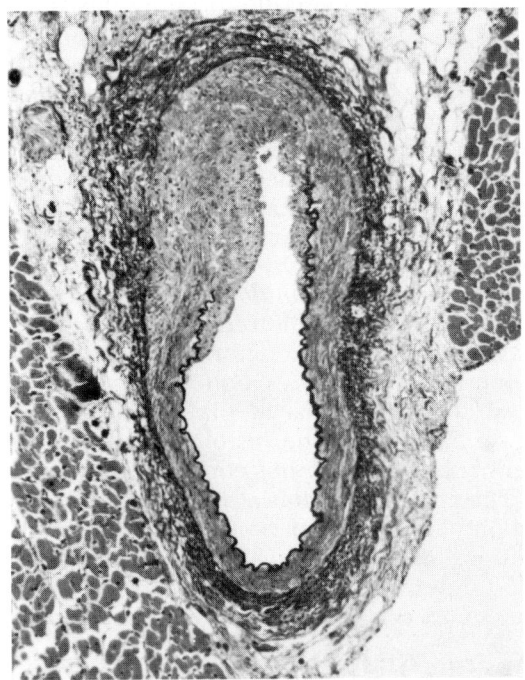

Figure 12–21. Elastic tissue stain of artery showing healed polyarteritis at upper left corner. The internal elastic lamina is destroyed and there is thickening of intima and media.

sions in the alimentary tract; diffuse muscular aches and pains; and peripheral neuritis, which is predominantly motor. About 30% of patients with PAN have underlying hepatitis B antigen in their serum. Antineutrophil antibodies are present in the serum and correlate with disease activity.[63]

The clinical diagnosis can usually be definitely established only by the identification of the vascular lesions. Clinically involved tissue is best for histologic examination, such as kidney and nodular skin lesions. Angiography shows vascular aneurysms in 50% of cases. Death may occur during an acute fulminant attack, but it may follow a protracted course. Untreated, the disease is fatal in most cases, but therapy with corticosteroids and cyclophosphamide results in remissions or cures in 90% of patients. Effective treatment of the hypertension is a prerequisite for a favorable prognosis.

Allergic granulomatosis and angiitis (the Churg-Strauss syndrome) has been distinguished from classic PAN because of a strong association with bronchial asthma and eosinophilia, the frequent involvement of pulmonary and splenic vessels, and the presence of intra- and extravascular granulomas. The vascular lesions, however, may be histologically identical to those of classic PAN. Vasculitis and granulomas occur in lungs, peripheral nerves, and skin, with a striking infiltration of vessels and perivascular tissues by eosinophils.[62]

Hypersensitivity (Leukocytoclastic) Angiitis

This group, also called microscopic polyarteritis, is differentiated from PAN because smaller vessels are affected (arterioles, venules, and capillaries). Furthermore, in a single patient, all lesions tend to be of the same age. It is a relatively frequently encountered type of vasculitis that typically involves the skin, mucous membranes, lungs, brain, heart, gastrointestinal tract, kidneys, and muscle. *The disease may be confined to the skin (cutaneous vasculitis),* in which it is manifested by palpable purpura (Fig. 12–22). In many cases a possible antigen can be traced as the precipitating cause. Drugs (e.g., penicillin), microorganisms (e.g., streptococci), heterologous proteins, and tumor antigens have been implicated as triggers of the disorder.

In general, muscular and large arteries are spared; thus, macroscopic infarcts similar to those seen in PAN are uncommon. Histologically, fibrinoid necrosis may be present, but in some lesions the change is limited to infiltration with neutrophils, which become fragmented as they flood the vessel wall. The term *leukocytoclastic angiitis* is given to such lesions, which are most common in postcapillary venules. Immunoglobulins and complement components are present in the vascular lesions of the skin, especially if these are examined within 24 hours of development. With the exception of those who de-

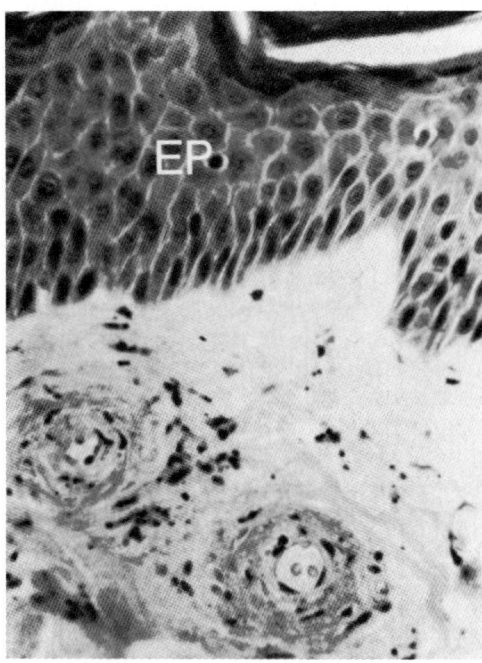

Figure 12–22. Hypersensitivity angiitis affecting skin. Note fragmented nuclei of neutrophils in vessel walls and perivascular spaces. EP = epidermis.

velop widespread renal or brain lesions, most patients respond well simply to removal of the offending agent.

Disseminated vascular lesions of hypersensitivity angiitis may appear in a number of relatively distinct syndromes. These include Henoch-Schönlein purpura, essential mixed cryoglobulinemia, vasculitis associated with some of the connective tissue disorders, and vasculitis associated with malignancy. These are discussed with the specific entities elsewhere in this book.

Wegener's Granulomatosis

This rare form of necrotizing vasculitis is characterized by (1) *acute necrotizing granulomas* of the upper and lower respiratory tract (nose, sinuses, and lung); (2) *focal necrotizing vasculitis*, most prominent in the lungs and upper airways but affecting other sites as well; and (3) renal disease in the form of focal or diffuse necrotizing glomerulitis.[64]

As with polyarteritis, males are more frequently affected than females, and the peak incidence is in the fifth decade. The typical clinical features include a persistent pneumonitis with bilateral nodular and cavitary infiltrates (95%), chronic sinusitis (90%), mucosal ulcerations of the nasopharynx (75%), and evidence of renal disease (80%). Other features include skin rashes, muscle pains, articular involvement, mono- or polyneuritis, and fever. Untreated, the course of the disease is malignant, 80% of patients dying within one year. *This grim prognosis is improved dramatically by the use of immunosuppressive drugs, such as cyclophosphamide; up to 90% of patients respond to such therapy.*

Involvement of the respiratory tract takes the form of focal acute necrosis in the nasal and oral cavities, paranasal sinuses, larynx, or trachea, as well as focal lesions scattered throughout the lung parenchyma. These areas are generally surrounded by a zone of fibroblastic proliferation with giant cells and leukocytic infiltrate, creating a more than superficial resemblance to a tubercle (Fig. 12–23A). These lesions undergo progressive fibrosis and organization. Some become cavitary. The vasculitis affects small arteries and veins and has been described in virtually every vessel and organ of the body, favored sites being the respiratory tract, kidneys, and spleen. These lesions are almost identical with those of the acute phase of polyarteritis nodosa (Fig. 12–23B), but often they contain granulomas, which may be within, adjacent to, or clearly separated from the vessel wall.

The renal lesions are of two types: in milder forms, or early in the disease, there is acute focal proliferation and necrosis in the glomeruli, with thrombosis of isolated glomerular capillary loops. This **focal necrotizing glomerulonephritis** (p. 1042) may resolve with therapy or may progress rapidly to the second type, in which there is diffuse proliferation and necrosis of the glomerulus, together with the formation of many glomerular crescents. Patients with focal lesions may have hematuria and proteinuria, whereas those with crescentic glomerulonephritis develop rapidly progressive renal failure.

Because of its striking resemblance to polyarteritis nodosa and serum sickness, it is thought that this disease represents some form of hypersensitivity, possibly to an inhaled infectious or other environmental agent, but no etiologic agent has been identified. Immune complexes have been seen in the glomeruli and vessel walls in occasional patients. The dramatic response to cyclophosphamide also strongly suggests an immunologic mechanism, perhaps of the cell-mediated type. The presence of serum autoantibodies against neutrophils appears to be a good marker for disease activity, but their role in the pathogenesis is unclear.[65]

Lymphomatoid granulomatosis[66] is an obscure entity that should be differentiated from Wegener's granulomatosis. It is characterized by pulmonary infiltration by nodules of lymphoid and plasmacytoid cells, often with cellular atypia. These infiltrates invade vessels, giving the histologic appearance of a vasculitis, but they do not constitute a true vasculitis.[61] The condition is initially localized to the lungs, but about one third of patients eventually show similar lesions in the kidneys, liver, brain, and other organs, and up to 50% develop malignant lymphoid tumors, most commonly non-Hodgkin's lymphoma.

Temporal (Giant Cell) Arteritis

Temporal arteritis is a focal granulomatous inflammation of arteries of medium and small size that affects principally the cranial vessels, especially the temporal arteries in older individuals.[67] In the more severe ex-

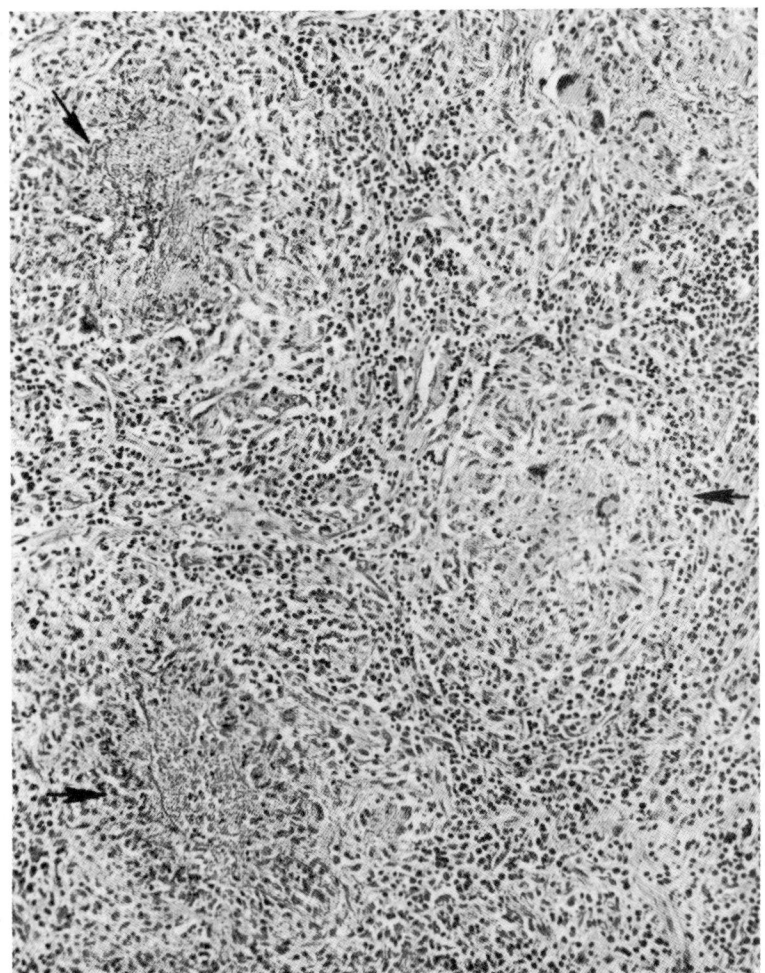

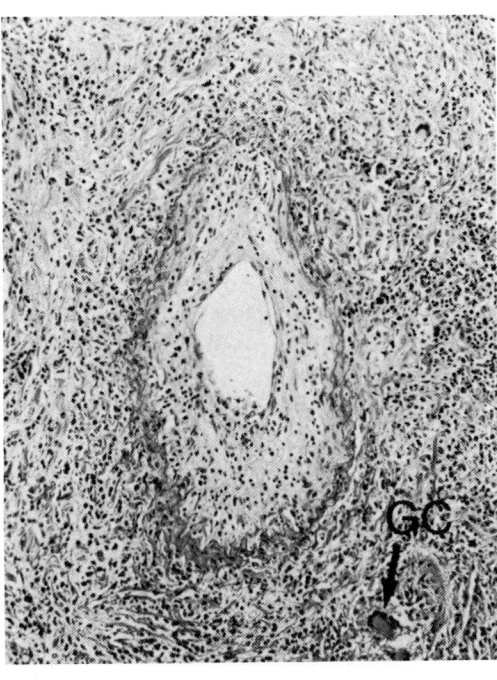

A

B

Figure 12–23. *A,* **Multiple granulomas in lungs in Wegener's granulomatosis *(arrows).* Note central necrosis and multinucleate giant cells.** *B,* **Small artery in lung in Wegener's granulomatosis. The wall is markedly thickened, fibrotic, and infiltrated with white cells. There is perivascular inflammation and a giant cell (GC).**

pressions of this disorder, lesions have been found in arteries throughout the body, and in some cases the aortic arch has been involved to produce so-called *giant cell aortitis.* Women are affected slightly more often than men, and the disease is rare in blacks.

Temporal arteritis is the most common of the vasculitides, its prevalence increasing significantly with age to about 850 per 100,000 population aged 80 years and over. Almost half of all patients with manifestations of temporal arteritis, such as headache, tenderness over the artery, visual loss, and facial pain, have systemic involvement and the syndrome of *polymyalgia rheumatica,* described later. However, 40% of biopsies of the temporal artery[68] are negative in patients with classic manifestations of this disease, and it must be assumed that the lesions were focal and were missed on biopsy.

The cause of this relatively common disease remains a puzzle. The morphologic alterations seem to suggest some sort of immunologic reaction against a component of the arterial wall. Some support for such a conception is provided by the finding of cell-mediated immunity to arterial antigen in some patients and by the response that is almost always achieved by corticosteroid treatment. There is a genetic predisposition, as evidenced by increased prevalence of HLA-DR4 antigen, and occasional familial clustering.

The histologic changes in arteries are quite variable and fall into three general patterns: (1) granulomatous lesions replete with giant cells, often in relation to fragments of the internal elastic membrane (Fig. 12–24); (2) nonspecific white cell infiltration (neutrophils and occasional lymphocytes and eosinophils) throughout the arterial wall; and (3) intimal fibrosis, usually with no morphologically apparent disruption of the internal elastic lamina. Giant cells are present in only two thirds of cases, and frequently many sections may have to be examined before one is detected. Thrombus formation commonly occurs in affected vessels and may be followed by either obliteration of the lumen or organization and recanalization. In healed phases, the artery is transformed into an obliterated fibrous cord. In addition to temporal arteries, involvement of vertebral and ophthalmic arteries is common, and some patients develop systemic lesions in any intermediate or large-sized muscular artery.

The disease may be insidious and vague in onset or may be heralded by the sudden onset of headache.

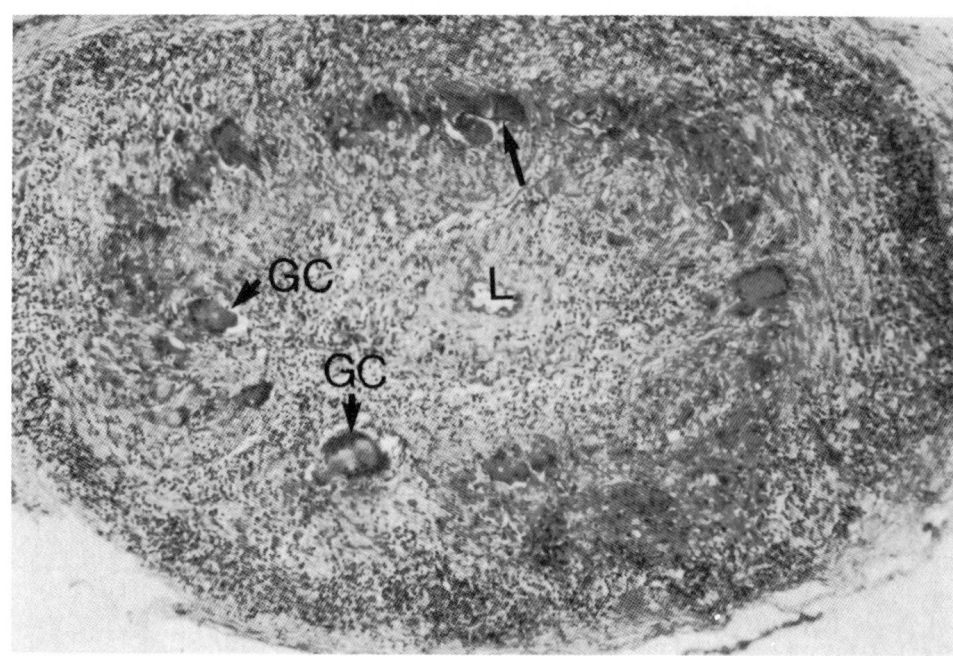

Figure 12–24. Temporal (giant cell) arteritis. Circumferential giant cells (GC) mark location of degenerated internal elastic membrane (*arrow*). L = lumen.

Often, the illness begins with a flulike syndrome and stiffness in the joints, an onset characterized as *polymyalgia rheumatica.*[67] There is often severe throbbing pain along the course of the artery; tenderness, swelling, and redness in the overlying skin; and claudication of the jaw. Visual symptoms (blurred or double vision or transient partial blindness) occur in 40% of patients.

The erythrocyte sedimentation rate (ESR) is markedly elevated in most cases. Biopsy may be diagnostic but may yield negative results when clinical syndromes are otherwise characteristic. In the absence of morphologic confirmation, it is often necessary to institute therapy on clinical grounds alone. In some instances, the disease is of acute and almost calamitous onset, and corticosteroid therapy must be instituted promptly to prevent visual impairment. Fortunately, the response to steroids is excellent. Involvement of visceral vessels may give rise to manifestations of myocardial ischemia, gastrointestinal disturbances, or neurologic derangements. When the aortic arch is involved, the symptoms may be identical to those of Takayasu's arteritis or aortic arch syndrome, discussed next.

Takayasu's Arteritis

This is a form of granulomatous vasculitis of medium and larger arteries, named after Takayasu. In 1908 he brought to attention a *clinical syndrome characterized principally by ocular disturbances and marked weakening of the pulses in the upper extremities (pulseless disease)*[69] *and related these findings to fibrous thickening of the aortic arch with narrowing or virtual obliteration of the origins of the great vessels arising in the arch.* It is most common in the Orient but has been reported in most areas of the world, including the United States. The illness is seen predominantly in females in the 15- to 45-year-old age group.

The cause and pathogenesis are unknown. There is an association with certain haplotypes (HLA-DR4) in the United States.

Although Takayasu's arteritis classically involves the aortic arch, in 32% of cases it also affects the remainder of the aorta and its branches, and in 12% it is limited to the descending thoracic and abdominal aorta. The gross morphologic changes comprise, in most cases, irregular thickening of the aortic wall with intimal wrinkling. When the aortic arch is involved, the orifices of the major arteries to the upper portion of the body may be markedly narrowed or even obliterated, accounting for the designation **pulseless disease.** Histologically, the early changes consist of an adventitial mononuclear infiltrate with perivascular cuffing of the vasa vasorum. In some cases, granulomatous changes appear within the media, replete with Langhans' giant cells and central necrosis. Later stages show extensive fibrosis of the media and marked acellular collagenous thickening of the intima. The fibrosing reaction thickens the wall of the aorta and extends into the proximal segments of the aortic branches, reducing their lumina to tiny, slitlike orifices.

The salient clinical features include weakening of the pulses of the upper extremities; a marked drop in blood pressure in the upper extremities; ocular disturbances, including visual defects, retinal hemorrhages, and total blindness; and various neurologic deficits, ranging from dizziness and focal weaknesses to complete hemiparesis. Hypertension is not infrequent and is due to involvement of the mouths of the renal arteries. The course of the disease is quite variable, and if the patient survives the first year or two of illness, the fibrotic quiescent stage may ensue and permit long survival, albeit with distressing neurologic and visual impairments.[70]

Kawasaki's Disease (Mucocutaneous Lymph Node Syndrome)

This acute illness of young children and infants is manifested by fever, conjunctival and oral erythema and erosions, a skin rash, and enlargement of lymph nodes.[71] The disease is known to be epidemic in Japan, but it has also been reported in Hawaii and is being described in increasing numbers in the United States. Although up to 70% of children may show clinical evidence of cardiac involvement, including coronary aneurysms (shown by angiography), the illness is self-limited in the vast majority of patients. Fatalities in 1 to 2% of patients are all due to coronary arteritis with superimposed thrombosis or ruptured coronary artery aneurysm. Iliac and other large arteries are involved less frequently. Histologically the vasculitis resembles PAN, consisting of necrosis and pronounced inflammation affecting the entire thickness of the vessel wall.

The cause is unknown, although a retroviral infection has been postulated.[72] Patients have a number of immunoregulatory disturbances, including T-cell activation, polyclonal B-cell activation, and circulating immune complexes.[73] Recently, lytic autoantibodies to cytokine-activated endothelial cells have been reported in patients with acute disease.[59] They disappear in convalescence and thus may contribute to the vascular injury in this disorder.

Thromboangiitis Obliterans (Buerger's Disease)

Thromboangiitis obliterans is a distinctive disease characterized by segmental, thrombosing, acute and chronic inflammation of intermediate and small arteries and veins of the extremities. Until recently the condition occurred almost exclusively in men who were heavy cigarette smokers.[74] Regrettably, there has been a recent increase in reported cases in women, reflecting increases in smoking by women in the past two decades.[62] The disorder must be differentiated from the other, more common causes of peripheral vascular disease, such as atherosclerosis, thromboembolism, and diabetic vascular disease. Buerger's disease begins before the age of 35 years in most patients and before 20 years in some. In many cases it affects the arms as well as the legs. Remissions and relapses correlate with cessation or resumption of smoking. Patients experience excruciating pain out of proportion to that found in other forms of peripheral vascular disease. Many times it is associated with migratory thrombophlebitis, but it is not associated with diabetes mellitus, hypercholesterolemia, or heart disease that might be the source of emboli.

ETIOLOGY AND PATHOGENESIS. The relationship to cigarette smoking is one of the most consistent aspects of this disease. Several possibilities have been postulated for this association, including direct endothelial toxicity induced by some tobacco products, increased sensitivity to such products, vasoconstriction induced by disturbances in catecholamine metabolism, and a hypercoagulability leading to thrombosis. None of these is proved. Cell-mediated hypersensitivity to types II and III collagen in these patients[75] raises the question of immunologic factors in the pathogenesis of this disease.[76]

This disease is rare in the United States and Europe, but is common in Israel, Japan, and India. Genetic predisposition is further suggested by the increased prevalence of HLA-A9 and HLA-B5 antigens in patients with Buerger's disease.[77] It may be, then, that certain susceptible genotypes are hypersensitive to tobacco products and that cell-mediated hypersensitivity contributes to vascular damage.

MORPHOLOGY. The lesions are sharply segmental and usually begin in arteries of small and medium size. It should be noted that, in contrast to atherosclerosis, Buerger's disease affects predominantly the medium and small arteries and only occasionally the larger arteries. Both upper and lower extremities are affected, in contrast to AS, which usually spares the upper extremities. After the arterial involvement, the accompanying veins and adjacent nerves are often secondarily affected, leading to progressive fibrous encasement of these three structures.

The acute involvements of either artery or vein are characterized by polymorphonuclear infiltration of all coats of the vessel wall, together with mural or occlusive thrombosis of the lumen. **Small microabscesses within the thrombus create a pattern quite distinct from the bland thrombosis of AS** (Fig. 12–25). These abscesses have a central focus of polymorphonuclear leukocytes surrounded by a fibroblastic, epithelioid-cell granulomatous enclosing wall that often contains Langhans'-type giant cells. In time, the thrombus undergoes organization and recanalization.

CLINICAL COURSE. The early manifestations are a superficial nodular phlebitis, cold sensitivity of the Raynaud type (p. 579) in the hands, and pain in the instep of the foot induced by exercise (so-called instep claudication). Eventually patients suffer from vascular insufficiency that often leads to gangrene of the extremities. Severe pain is common in the affected parts, in contrast to the relative painlessness of atherosclerotic occlusion. Abstinence from cigarette smoking is mandatory for these patients.

Vasculitis Associated with Other Underlying Disorders

Vasculitis may sometimes be associated with an underlying disorder, such as an immunologic connective tissue disease, a remote malignancy, or such systemic illnesses as mixed cryoglobulinemia and Henoch-Schönlein purpura. The vasculitis is usually of the hypersensitivity angiitis pattern (p. 573), but it may resemble classic PAN in some cases.

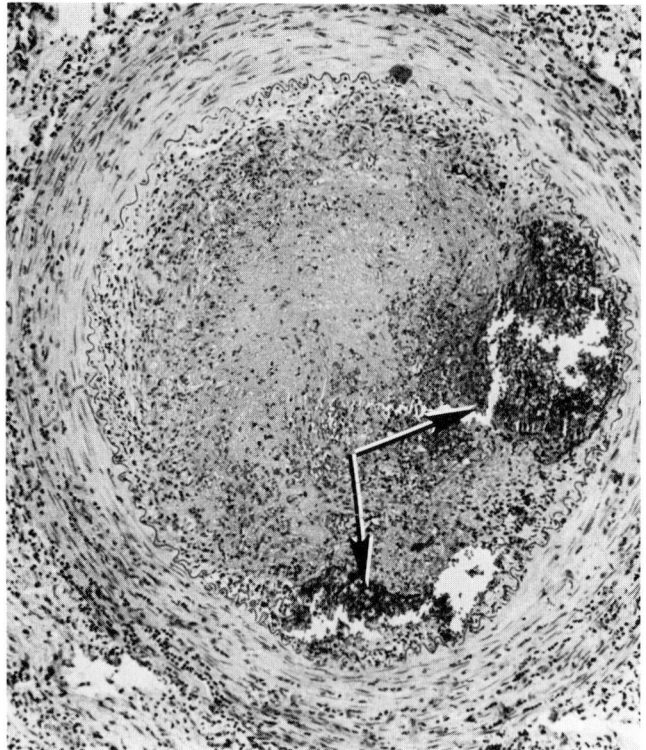

Figure 12–25. Thromboangiitis obliterans. Lumen (L) is occluded by a thrombus containing two abscesses (arrows). Vessel wall is infiltrated with leukocytes.

Of the *connective tissue disorders*, rheumatoid arthritis and SLE most commonly manifest a vasculitis. *Rheumatoid vasculitis* affects small and medium-sized arteries in multiple organs and may result in life-threatening visceral infarction. It occurs predominantly after long-standing rheumatoid arthritis in patients who also exhibit rheumatoid nodules, hypocomplementemia, and high titers of rheumatoid fac-

tor. Vasculitis in SLE is usually confined to smaller vessels of the skin, although immunoglobulin deposits can be demonstrated in vessels of many organs (see also p. 77). *Malignancies* associated with vasculitis are commonly of the lymphoproliferative type.

In concluding this discussion of the necrotizing vasculitides, it is obvious that they represent a heterogeneous group of syndromes that have in common, besides the vascular involvement, strong evidence for an immunologic basis. There is a great deal of overlap in morphologic and clinical manifestations among the disorders. Overlapping cases are sometimes referred to simply as "systemic necrotizing vasculitis." Proper recognition of some of the subsets of vasculitis is of therapeutic import, as exemplified by the dramatic response of Wegener's granulomatosis to specific therapy with cyclophosphamide. Table 12–4 provides salient features of the major forms of vasculitis.

Infectious Arteritis

Most instances of this condition are caused by the direct invasion of infectious agents — usually bacteria and fungi. Bacterial lesions are associated with necrotizing inflammation and are frequently encountered in bacterial pneumonia, adjacent to caseous tuberculous reactions, in the neighborhood of abscesses, and in the superficial cerebral vessels in cases of meningitis. Much less commonly, they arise from the hematogenous spread of bacteria, a pathway that presumably accounts for the seeding of the aortic wall in cases of septicemia or infective vegetative endocarditis. The lesions may cause rupture or produce weakening of the arterial walls and result in the formation of a *mycotic aneurysm.* Certain fungal infections, such as aspergillosis and mucormycosis, are particularly apt to cause vasculitis and thrombosis.

Clinically, infectious arteritis may be important

Table 12–4. Characteristics of Some Systemic Vasculitides

ANGIITIS	VESSELS INVOLVED	ORGAN OR TISSUE AFFECTED	PRINCIPAL MORPHOLOGIC FEATURES
Polyarteritis nodosa	Muscular arteries	Gastrointestinal tract, mesentery, liver, gallbladder, kidney, pancreas, muscles, other sites	Lesions of varying ages; all layers of vessels with acute fibrinoid necrosis and extensive periarterial inflammation
Hypersensitivity angiitis	Small venules, capillaries, arterioles	All organs and tissues (skin, muscles, heart, kidneys, lungs)	Acute necrotizing vasculitis with fibrinoid necrosis of entire wall; often thrombosis of lumen
Giant cell arteritis (temporal arteritis)	Muscular arteries	Usually temporal, ophthalmic, and cranial arteries; may be systemic	Disruption of elastic lamina with most intense reaction in intimal medial layers; giant cells engulf elastic fiber fragments; occasionally thrombosis of lumen
Takayasu's arteritis	Aorta, arteries	Extremities; head and neck; viscera	Granulomatous arteritis with fibrosis and marked narrowing
Kawasaki's disease	Arteries	Generalized; coronary arteries	Identical to polyarteritis (infantile polyarteritis)
Wegener's granulomatosis	Small arteries and veins	Lungs, kidneys, upper respiratory tract; occasionally systemic	Acute necrotizing vasculitis with fibrinoid necrosis of vessel wall; often proximate to granulomas in tissues
Buerger's disease	Arteries, veins, nerves	Extremities; viscera uncommonly	Thrombosis with microabscesses; acute inflammation permeates wall artery, but preserves underlying architecture

on several counts. By inducing thrombosis, it adds an element of infarction to tissues that are already the seat of inflammatory reaction and may therefore materially worsen the initial infection. In bacterial meningitis, for example, inflammation of the superficial vessels of the brain may predispose to vascular thromboses, with subsequent infarction of the brain substance and extension of the subarachnoid infection into the brain tissue. In tuberculous meningitis, it is the vascular involvement that leads to the most serious sequelae.

RAYNAUD'S DISEASE AND RAYNAUD'S PHENOMENON

Raynaud's disease is a *functional vasospastic disorder affecting the small arteries and arterioles of the extremities, occurring primarily in young, apparently healthy women.*[78] It affects the small arteries and arterioles of the extreme periphery of the body, most commonly the fingers and hands but occasionally the tip of the nose and the feet. Cold and emotional stimuli trigger the response, and the fingers become white, then blue, and finally red. The disease usually follows a benign course, but in long-standing, chronic cases tropic changes develop causing atrophy of the skin, subcutaneous tissue, and muscles. Ulceration and frank ischemic gangrene are rare. The cause is unknown but is postulated to be related to some form of hyperlability of the autonomic innervation of the affected vessels. *The symptoms are due to vasoconstriction; thus, true organic changes within the vessel wall are absent.* In long-standing cases, secondary intimal thickening and endothelial proliferation may occur.

It is important to distinguish Raynaud's disease from Raynaud's phenomenon. The latter is also characterized by cold sensitivity, pain, and color changes in the skin, but it is *always secondary to some underlying, often serious disorder causing an organic lesion in the arterial wall.* Raynaud's phenomenon is most often associated with arteriosclerosis, connective tissue diseases (scleroderma and SLE being the most common), thromboangiitis obliterans (Buerger's disease), cryoglobulinemia and multiple myeloma, ingestion of drugs (such as the ergotamine preparations), lead poisoning, primary pulmonary hypertension, and (rarely) cases of occult carcinoma. Raynaud's phenomenon may be the first manifestation of such underlying diseases. Tropic changes, ulcerations, and gangrene may develop.

The relationship of Raynaud's phenomenon to *scleroderma* deserves emphasis. Raynaud's phenomenon may precede the skin changes by months or even years. In some of these patients, Raynaud's phenomenon is associated with sclerosis of the fingers, together with ulceration developing on the digital pulp or along the side of the nail. This condition is called *acrosclerosis,* a form of *localized scleroderma* (p. 207). About 20% of these patients eventually develop systemic scleroderma.

AORTIC ANEURYSMS

One of the most striking results of all forms of vascular disease is the formation of an aneurysm. An *aneurysm* is a *localized abnormal dilatation of any vessel.* Aneurysms may occur in any artery or vein of the body, but the most common and most significant are in the aorta. Aortic aneurysms produce serious clinical disease and often cause death by rupture.[79]

The two most important causes are atherosclerosis and cystic medial necrosis, the latter to be described under the heading "Dissecting Aneurysms." Syphilis and trauma are two other causes of aortic aneurysms. Aneurysms of arteries can also be caused by polyarteritis nodosa; trauma leading to arteriovenous aneurysm; a congenital defect, such as that producing berry aneurysms in the brain; and infections that significantly weaken vascular walls, causing so-called *mycotic aneurysms.*

The classification of aneurysms by *gross appearance* attempts to characterize the macroscopic shape and size of the aneurysm (Fig. 12–26). A *berry* aneurysm refers to a small, spherical dilatation rarely exceeding a diameter of 1 to 1.5 cm. A *saccular* aneurysm might be described as a giant berry aneurysm. These dilatations usually are essentially spherical and vary in size from 5 to 20 cm in diameter. Characteristically, these aneurysms are partially or completely filled by thrombus (Fig. 12–27). In *fusiform* aneurysm there is gradual, progressive dilation of the vessel lumen. These aneurysms then take on a spindle shape, and the aneurysmal lumen is in direct continuity with the vascular lumen. The fusiform aneurysm varies in diameter (up to 20 cm) and in length; many involve the entire ascending and transverse portions of the aortic arch, whereas others may involve large segments of the abdominal aorta or even the iliacs. *Dissecting aneurysm* arises when blood enters the wall of the artery, dissecting between its layers and creating a cavity within the vessel wall (p. 582).

Arteriosclerotic (Atherosclerotic) Aneurysms

This type of aortic aneurysm is the most common form. Such aneurysms rarely develop before the age of 50 and are much more common in males. Fifty per cent of patients are hypertensive. These aneurysms usually occur in the abdominal aorta or common iliac arteries, but they occasionally affect the ascending arch and descending parts of the thoracic aorta. Syphilitic aneurysms are extremely infrequent in the abdominal aorta, and *all fusiform, cylindroid, or saccular aneurysms of the abdominal aorta should be considered to be arteriosclerotic until proved otherwise.*

Arteriosclerotic aneurysms are usually positioned below the renal arteries and above the bifurcation of the aorta (Fig. 12–26). Not infrequently, they are accompanied by smaller fusiform or saccular dilatations of the iliac arteries (Fig. 12–27). The genesis of these aneurysms is severe atherosclerosis, with consequent thinning and destruction of the

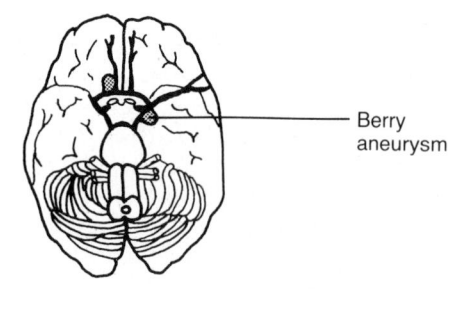

Berry aneurysm

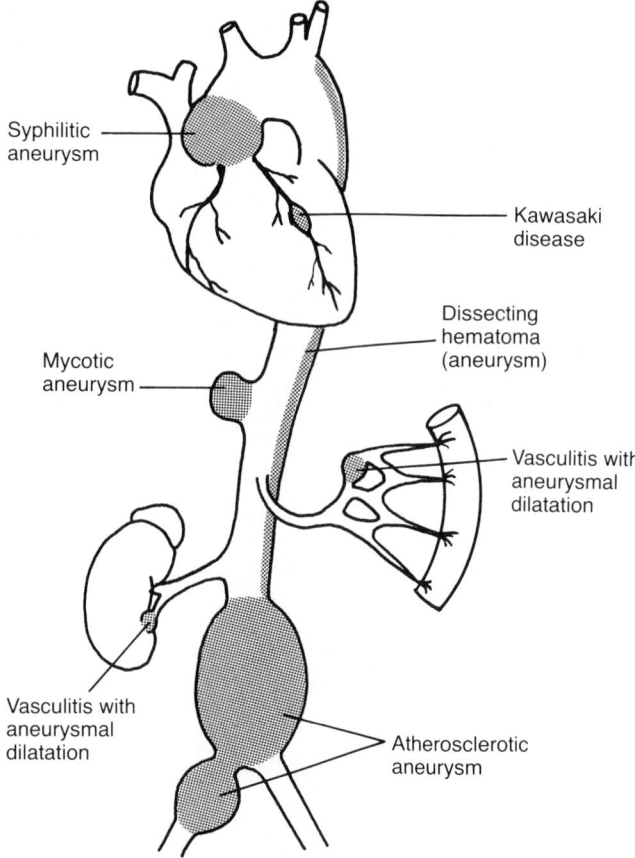

Syphilitic aneurysm

Kawasaki disease

Dissecting hematoma (aneurysm)

Mycotic aneurysm

Vasculitis with aneurysmal dilatation

Vasculitis with aneurysmal dilatation

Atherosclerotic aneurysm

Figure 12–26. Distribution and shape of various types of aneurysms.

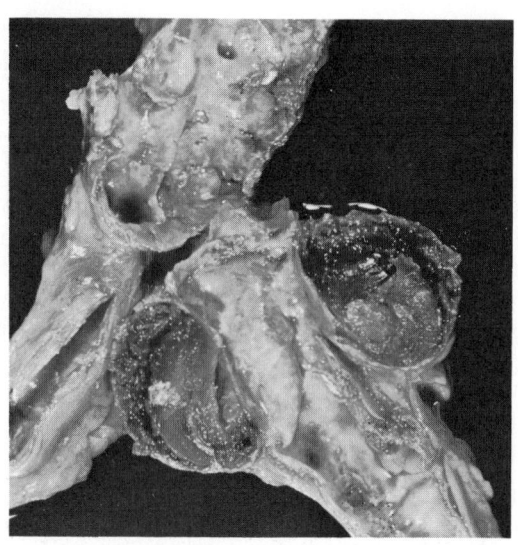

Figure 12–27. Arteriosclerotic saccular aneurysm of common iliac artery filled with laminated red (dark) thrombus.

media. With this severe atherosclerosis, it is very common to find atheromatous ulcers within the aneurysm, covered by mural thrombi. Sometimes the entire aneurysmal dilatation is filled with thrombus. Such mural thrombi are prime sites for the formation of emboli that lodge in the vessels of the lower extremity.

Occasionally the aneurysm may affect the take-offs of the renal, superior, and inferior mesenteric arteries, either by producing direct pressure on these vessels or by narrowing or occluding their ostia with mural thrombi.

Aneurysms give rise to clinical symptoms by various secondary effects: (1) rupture into the peritoneal cavity or retroperitoneal tissues, with massive or fatal hemorrhage; (2) impingement on an adjacent structure, such as compression of a ureter or erosion of vertebrae; (3) occlusion of a vessel by either direct pressure or mural thrombus formation, particularly of the vertebral branches that supply the spinal cord; (4) embolism from the mural thrombus; and (5) presentation as an abdominal mass that simulates a tumor.

Large arteriosclerotic aneurysms materially shorten longevity. Most fatalities result from rupture, a danger directly related to the size of the aneurysm. Patients with aneurysms less than 6 cm in diameter rarely die of rupture, whereas 50% of those with aneurysms 6 or more cm in diameter suffer fatal rupture within a ten-year period of follow-up. On this basis, most workers agree that, when discovered, large aneurysms should be replaced with prosthetic grafts. For abdominal aortic aneurysms, operative mortality for unruptured aneurysms is only 5%, whereas emergency surgery *after* rupture carries a mortality rate of more than 50%.

Syphilitic (Luetic) Aneurysms and Heart Disease

Syphilitic (luetic) aneurysms are almost always confined to the thoracic aorta and usually involve the arch. The ascending and transverse portions of the arch are favored sites, but the dilation may extend distally to the level of the diaphragm and, even more important, proximally to the level of the aortic valve. By virtue of dilation of the ring, the aortic valve may become incompetent, leading to luetic heart disease. At one time, syphilis accounted for the majority of

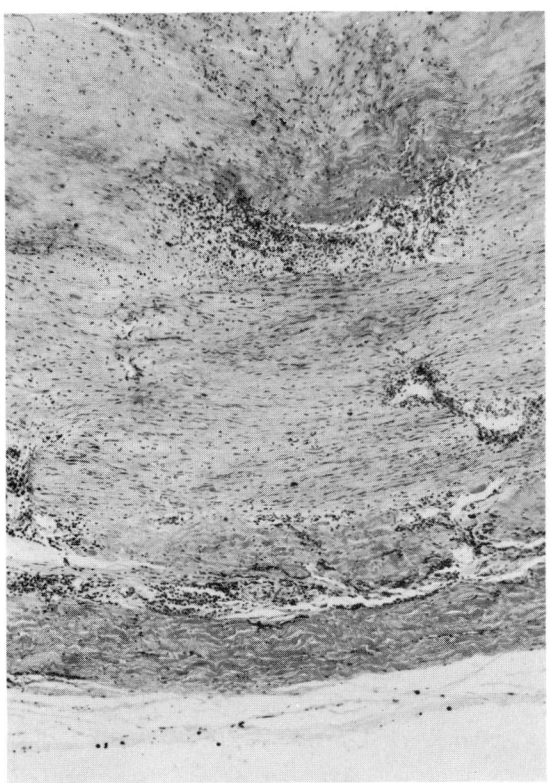

Figure 12–28. Syphilitic aortitis with scarring and vascularization of media. The intima is at the top.

Syphilitic aneurysms vary in gross appearance to encompass the saccular, fusiform, and cylindroid types. Their development is based on the medial destruction characteristic of tertiary luetic aortitis. The inflammatory involvement begins in the adventitia of the aorta, particularly involving the vasa vasorum with the production of obliterative endarteritis rimmed by an infiltrate of lymphocytes and plasma cells. The narrowing of the lumina of the vasa causes ischemic injury to the aortic media, with patchy uneven loss of the medial elastic fibers and muscle cells followed by inflammatory scarring and vascularization of the damaged media (Fig. 12–28). Contraction of fibrous scars may lead to wrinkling of intervening segments of aortic intima, producing what has been called "tree-barking." Luetic involvement of the aorta favors the development of superimposed atherosclerosis, inducing sometimes florid atheromatosis of the aortic root.

When luetic aortitis involves the aortic valve ring, it dilates, causing valvular insufficiency. The circumferential stretching of the valve leaflets narrows them and widens the interleaflet commissures. Over the course of time, the regurgitant turbulence produces thickening and rolling of the free margins, worsening the valvular incompetence (Fig. 12–29). As a consequence, the left ventricular wall undergoes volume overload hypertrophy, sometimes producing a massively enlarged heart (600 to 1000 g), descriptively referred to as "cor bovinum."

aneurysms of the thoracic aorta, but with the decline in cases of tertiary syphilis, the disorder is uncommon.

Thoracic aneurysms, both luetic and atherosclerotic, are much more prone to be associated with striking clinical manifestations than are the arterio-

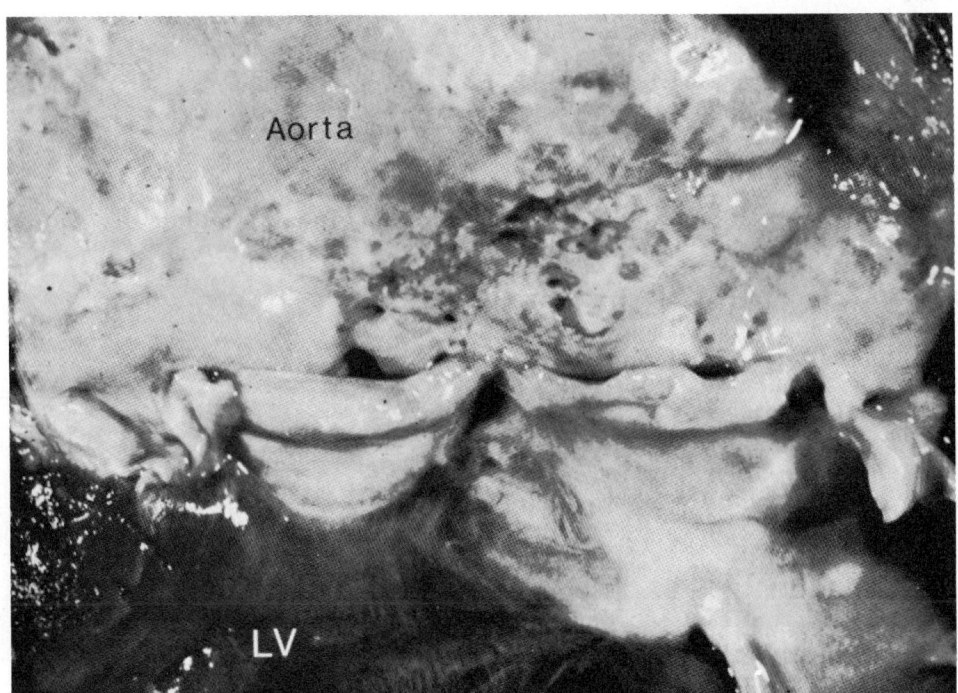

Figure 12–29. Syphilitic involvement of aorta and aortic valve. Valve leaflets are rolled and thickened. The commissures are widened. LV = left ventricle.

sclerotic abdominal aneurysms. Within the confined space of the thoracic cage, these enlargements give rise to signs and symptoms referable to (1) encroachment on mediastinal structures, (2) respiratory difficulties due to encroachment on the lungs and airways, (3) difficulty in swallowing due to compression of the esophagus, (4) persistent cough due to irritation of or pressure on the recurrent laryngeal nerves, (5) pain caused by erosion of bone (i.e., ribs and vertebral bodies), and (6) cardiac disease as the aneurysm leads to dilation of the aortic valve or narrowing of the coronary ostia. Many patients with luetic aneurysms die of cardiac decompensation secondary to the luetic involvement of the aortic valve, unless the incompetent valve is surgically replaced.

Dissecting Hematoma (Dissecting Aneurysm or Aortic Dissection)

Dissecting hematoma is the most common catastrophic illness involving the aorta. It is a dramatic illness in which, if untreated, the risk of death is 35% within 15 minutes after onset of symptoms and 75% by one week. Happily, these figures have improved considerably with early recognition and treatment.

As the name implies, these aneurysms are characterized by dissection of blood along the laminar planes of the aortic media, with the formation of a blood-filled channel within the aortic wall.[81] *They differ from the atherosclerotic and syphilitic aneurysms in that they are not usually associated with marked dilatation of the aorta.* For this reason, the terms "dissecting hematoma" and "aortic dissection" are preferred.[79-81] The condition most commonly occurs in the 40- to 60-year age group and is two or three times more frequent in men within this group. However, below age 40 the disease is not as rare in women, owing principally to the occurrence of dissections during pregnancy. Hypertension is almost invariably an antecedent (in 94% of cases) and may well play an important role in initiating the intramural hemorrhage.

The hemorrhage in dissecting hematomas occurs quite characteristically between the middle and outer thirds of the media (Fig. 12-30). The intimal tear, presumably the origin of dissection, is found in the ascending portion of the arch in 90% of cases, usually within 10 cm of the aortic valve. The tears are usually transverse or oblique, are 4 to 5 cm in length, and have sharp and clean but jagged edges (Fig. 12-31). The dissection then extends proximally toward the heart, as well as distally along the aorta to variable distances, sometimes all the way into the iliac and femoral arteries (Fig. 12-32). In some instances, the blood reruptures into the lumen of the aorta, producing a **second or distal intimal tear.** The site of such reentry is most often the iliac vessels, followed by neck vessels. **Five to 10% of dissecting aneurysms, however, do not have an obvious intimal tear,** either proximally or distally.

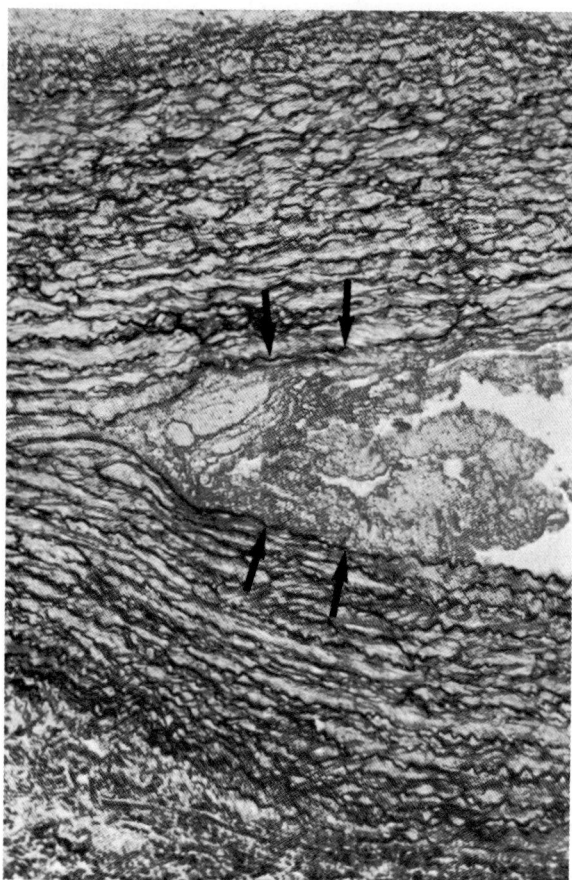

Figure 12-30. Dissecting aneurysm of aorta. The advancing dissection *(arrows)* is cleaving laminar planes of media.

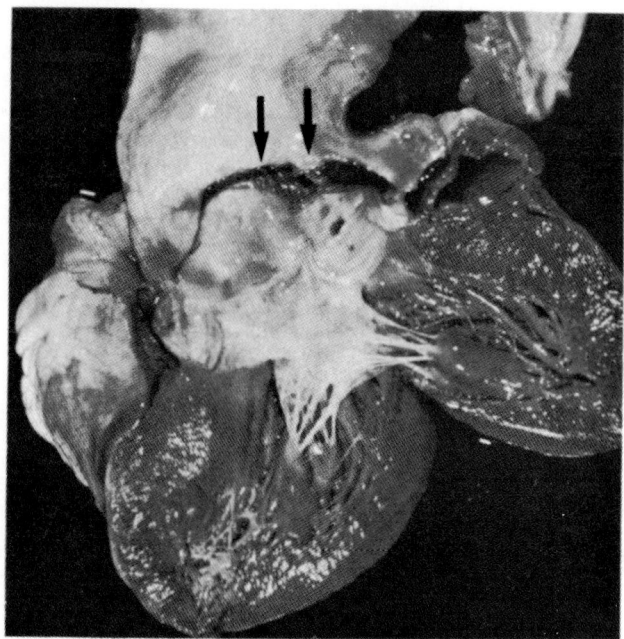

Figure 12-31. Irregular, jagged transverse tear in intima in a dissecting aneurysm *(arrows).*

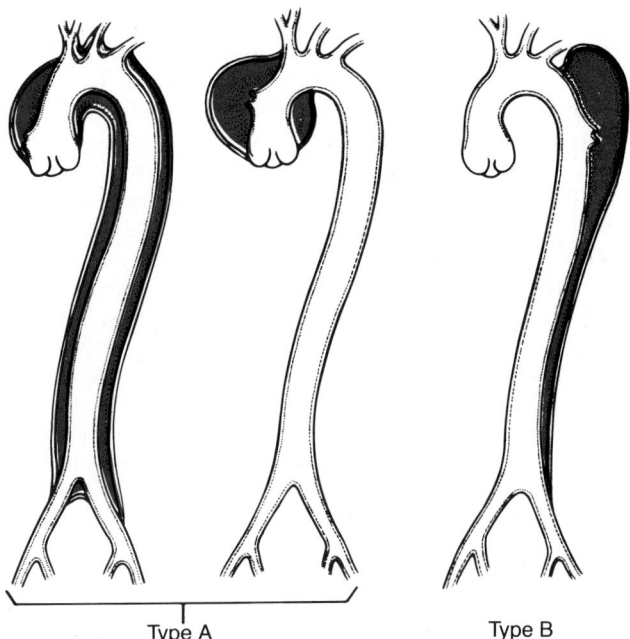

Figure 12-32. Classification of dissections into types A and B. Type A involves the ascending aorta and type B does *not* involve the ascending aorta.

Many times the dissection extends into the great vessels of the neck and, in other instances, into the coronary, renal, mesenteric, and iliac arteries (Fig. 12-33). The extravasation may completely encircle the aorta or may extend along one segment of the circumference. Infrequently the dissection is very short, and the extravasation penetrates the entire thickness of the aorta almost directly to cause immediate rupture. Eventually, **in almost all fatal dissections, external hemorrhage occurs into the periadventitial tissues or into surrounding structures or cavities.**

At postmortem examination, the most common precipitating cause of death is rupture of the dissection into any of the three body cavities (i.e., pericardial, pleural, or peritoneal). Quite rarely, cases are discovered in which a new vascular channel has apparently been formed within the media of the aortic wall that connects the proximal and distal intimal tear. It is assumed that in these **double-barreled aortas,** the two intimal tears have permitted the establishment of a through-and-through blood flow and thus averted a fatal extra-aortic hemorrhage. In the course of time, such false channels may become endothelialized.

Aneurysms are divided into two types on the basis of location and extent of dissection (Fig. 12-32): (1) *type A or proximal dissections* involve the ascending aorta or the ascending and descending aorta and are the most common and lethal type; (2) *type B or distal dissections* do *not* involve the ascending aorta and usually begin just distal to the subclavian artery, extending only downward into the descending and abdominal aorta.

PATHOGENESIS. Two questions arise concerning the pathogenesis of dissecting aneurysms. First, what causes the media of the aorta to weaken, allowing blood to dissect into the wall? Second, what causes the hemorrhage and intimal tears?[81]

In most patients with dissecting aneurysm, the media shows a variety of histologic changes that could conceivably weaken the wall, but uncertainty exists about the specificity of these lesions and their role in causing dissection. The most widely known lesion is so-called *cystic medial necrosis,* which consists of the accumulation of basophilic amorphous material in the media, often with formation of cystlike mucoid pools. The media in these focal areas may show loss of cells, hence the term necrosis, but there is no inflammatory response. *Elastic fragmentation* occurs in 95% of patients and medial fibrosis in 60%. These changes involve the musculoelastic media of the aorta and less commonly the coronary arteries and major branches of the aorta. These changes, however, *are also frequently present as a chance postmortem finding in patients who are free of dissection,* increasing in severity with age and possibly in the presence of hypertension. However, some of the changes, particularly the elastic fragmentation, are more severe and more widespread in patients with dissecting aneurysm.

The cause or causes of cystic medial necrosis are unknown. The frequent finding of focal medial lesions in the aorta proximal to aortic coarctation, where severe local hypertension exists, supports some causal relationship between hypertension and the development of lesions. Other explanations propose biochemical defects in the synthesis or maintenance of the

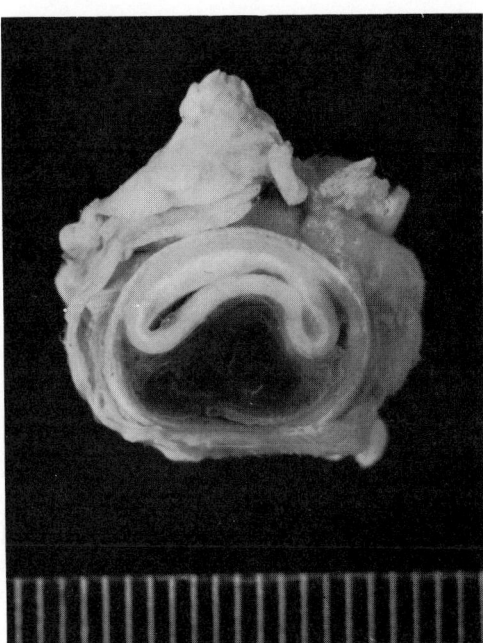

Figure 12-33. Cross section of common carotid artery with extension of a dissecting aneurysm and collapse of vessel lumen.

proteoglycans, collagen, and elastic fibers of the tunica media. *The relatively high incidence of cystic change and dissecting aneurysm in patients with the hereditary disorder Marfan's syndrome* supports such notions. As described earlier, these patients have a defect in forming stable collagen cross links, leading to structural defects involving the suspensory ligaments of the lens and the capsules of joints, excessive height, retinal detachment, and aortic regurgitation (p. 139).

Granted that some biochemical defect weakens the vessel wall, what causes the intimal tear and intramural aortic hemorrhage? *Favored today is the hypothesis that an intimal tear occurs owing to hemodynamic factors accentuated by the hypertension.* Hypertension is clearly the major risk factor in aortic dissection.[82] The intima overlying areas weakened by the medial degeneration *buckles into the lumen*, with the oncoming pressure wave creating a tendency for the buckled wall to be subjected to greater shearing force, thus inducing a luminal tear. Once the tear has occurred, the increased blood pressure present in most of these patients enhances dissection into the wall. Indeed, as discussed later, aggressive antihypertensive therapy is often effective in limiting dissection.

MORPHOLOGY. The gross morphology was described earlier. The characteristic microscopic lesion of **cystic medial necrosis** is that of focal separation of the elastic and fibromuscular elements of the tunica media by small cleftlike or cystic spaces filled with ground substance.[83,84] In the individual foci, the normal lamellar pattern of the elastic media is destroyed and is replaced by a poorly defined area of increased, slightly basophilic, amorphous material resembling the ground substance of connective tissue (Fig. 12–34). These foci are referred to as cystic. The lesions are haphazardly distributed throughout the thickness of the media. Elastic tissue stains are desirable to highlight focal areas of apparent destruction or separation of the normal lamellae of the medial wall. In addition to the myxoid cystic change, fragmentation of elastic tissue lamellae is frequently present, even outside areas of well-defined myxoid change. **Indeed, the severity of elastic fragmentation correlates more consistently with the presence of dissection than do the mucoid alterations.** Focal fibrosis of the media is a third type of histologic change, the significance of which is not well understood.

The clinical manifestations[85] of a dissecting aneurysm derive from (1) the dissection itself; (2) extension of the dissection into the great arteries of the neck or into the coronary, renal, mesenteric, or iliac arteries, causing obstruction of the vessels; (3) disruption of the aortic valvular apparatus, causing insufficiency; or (4) penetration of the thickness of the aorta, to cause rupture. The classic features related to the dissection are the sudden onset of excruciating pain, usually beginning in the anterior chest, radiating to the back, and moving downward as the dissection progresses. The intensity of this pain is readily confused with that of acute myocardial infarction. Helpful in this differentiation is the fact that, although patients with acute dissection may appear to be in shock, they generally have normal or elevated systemic arterial pressures, in contradistinction to the hypotension usually associated with myocardial infarction. Proximal dissections are the most lethal type, and death is due to through-and-through rupture of the aorta, near the site of the initial intimal-medial aortic tear, most commonly in the ascending portion. Extravasation of blood is usually into the *pericardial sac.* Extension of the dissection into the neck arteries leads to luminal narrowing, and this in turn causes arm or cerebral ischemia. Retrograde dissection may lead to extension into the media of a major coronary artery, with resultant severe myocardial ischemia. Dissection involving the aortic root leads to aortic regurgitation. The antemortem diagnosis of dissecting aneurysm and the differentiation of the types are based largely on aortic angiography.

At one time, the disease was almost invariably fatal, but the prognosis has markedly improved in recent years. Two major advances in treatment have been achieved: *the development of surgical procedures involving plication of the aortic wall, and the early institution of intensive antihypertensive therapy.* At present, immediate surgery is advocated in nearly all type A dissections, whereas hypotensive therapy is reserved for noncomplicated type B dissections and as an adjunct to surgery. Understandably, the prognosis for type A dissections is much poorer. Nevertheless, with these regimens, early recognition and treatment permit salvage of 65 to 75% of all dissections for two to four years, a remarkable achievement compared with the 5% one-year survival attained 20 years ago.

VEINS

Although diseases of veins are extremely common clinical problems, only a few entities are responsible for this high incidence. Varicose veins and phlebothrombosis together account for at least 90% of clinical venous disease.[86] In general, the diseases of veins are clinically significant on two accounts. First, most of these disorders predispose to intravascular thrombosis and potential embolism, and because the systemic veins are most often affected, pulmonary embolism and infarction are the potential serious sequelae. Second, intravascular thrombosis, narrowing, or abnormal dilation of veins with subsequent incompetence of the venous valves causes venous stasis. A fairly constant clinical pattern follows with passive congestion of the affected area, accompanied often by dusky cyanosis and edema. In many cases, venous drainage is restored by the opening of collateral bypasses. Often, however, the collateral channels create new clinical problems, well exemplified by the production of varices in the esophagus when the portal vein is obstructed. The possibility of rupture of the

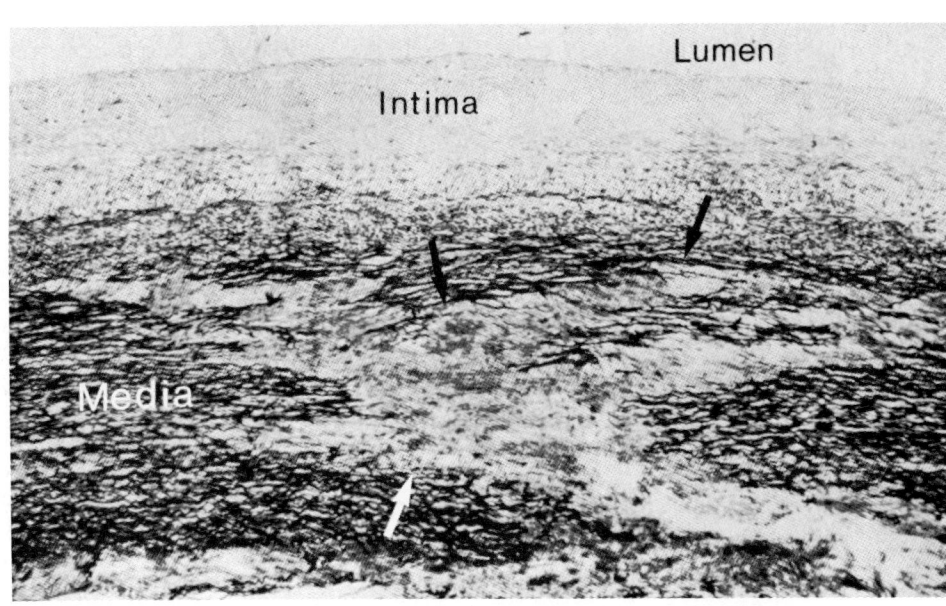

Figure 12–34. Cystic medial necrosis. Large defect in elastic lamellar pattern of media *(arrows)* **is highlighted by elastic tissue stain.**

esophageal varices is of far greater clinical importance than the underlying cause of the portal vein obstruction. On these two scores, diseases of veins take on great clinical significance.

VARICOSE VEINS

Varicose veins are abnormally dilated, tortuous veins produced by prolonged, increased intraluminal pressure. Although any vein in the body may be affected, the superficial veins of the leg are the preponderant site of involvement. One special type of varicosity is an important clinical problem; portal hypertension (usually due to cirrhosis of the liver) leads to varices in the esophageal and hemorrhoidal veins.

INCIDENCE. It is estimated that 10 to 20% of the general population eventually develop varicose veins in the lower legs. The condition is much more common in the age groups over 50, in which the incidence may reach a figure of 50%. Over the age of 30, females are affected four times more commonly than males, a reflection of the venous stasis in the lower legs caused by pregnancy.

PATHOGENESIS. Veins are frail structures that depend for their integrity on a thin media and the support of surrounding structures. A *familial tendency* toward the development of varicosities is postulated to be due to defective development of the walls of veins. *Obese* persons have a greater tendency to develop varicosities, probably because of the poor tissue support offered by the large accumulations of subcutaneous fat.

The most important influence on intraluminal venous blood pressure is posture. When the legs are dependent for long periods of time, venous pressures in these sites are markedly elevated (the increase has been measured to be ten times the normal). Therefore, occupations that require long periods of standing and long rides frequently lead to marked venous stasis and pedal edema, even in normal individuals with essentially normal veins *(simple orthostatic edema)*. Any condition that compresses or obstructs veins may cause marked increases of venous pressure distally, so that pregnancy, intravascular thrombosis, and tumor masses that impede return flow all promote the development of varicosities.

Varicosities occur principally in the superficial veins of the body, especially those of the lower extremities. The affected veins are dilated, tortuous, and elongated. There is marked variation in the thickness of the wall, with thinning at the points of maximal dilatation. When the disease is long-standing, compensatory hypertrophy of the medial muscle and fibrosis of the wall may produce a thick, opaque vessel wall.

Intraluminal thrombosis and valvular deformities (thickening, rolling, and shortening of the cusps) are frequently discovered when these vessels are opened. Microscopically, the changes consist of variation in the thickness of the wall of the vein caused by dilation on the one hand and by hypertrophy of the smooth muscle and subintimal fibrosis on the other hand. Frequently, there is degeneration of the elastic tissue in the major veins and spotty calcifications within the media **(phlebosclerosis).**

CLINICAL COURSE. Varicose dilation of veins renders the valves incompetent and leads to venous stasis, congestion, edema, and thrombosis. In the legs the distention of the veins is often painful, but most patients have no symptoms until marked venous stasis and edema develop. *Some of the most disabling sequelae are the development of persistent edema in the extremity and trophic changes in the skin that lead to stasis dermatitis and ulcerations* (Fig. 12–35). Because of the impaired circulation, the tissues of the affected part are extremely vulnerable to injury.

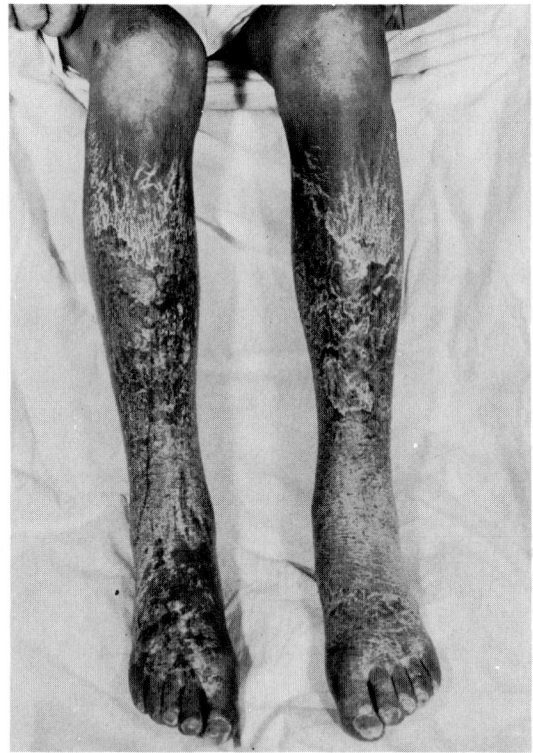

Figure 12–35. Stasis dermatitis in varicose veins of lower extremity.

Wounds and infections heal slowly or tend to become chronic *varicose ulcers.*

PHLEBOTHROMBOSIS AND THROMBOPHLEBITIS

According to current thought, phlebothrombosis and thrombophlebitis are two designations for a single entity caused by thrombus formation in veins. Thrombosis within a vein inevitably leads to inflammatory changes within the vein wall, hence the synonym thrombophlebitis.

The factors that predispose to venous thrombosis and the settings in which it is most often encountered have already been considered in the general discussion of thrombosis (p. 93). It need simply be reemphasized now that *cardiac failure* (particularly that associated with slowed venous return), *neoplasia, pregnancy, the postoperative state, and prolonged bed rest or immobilization are the five most important clinical settings predisposing to venous thrombosis.*

The deep leg veins account for over 90% of cases of thrombophlebitis. Specific mention should be made of the periprostatic plexus in the male and the pelvic veins in the female as additional moderately common sites for the appearance of thrombi. The large veins in the skull and the dural sinuses are possible sites of thrombosis when these channels become inflamed by bacterial infections of the meninges, middle ears, or mastoids. Similarly, infections in the abdominal cavity, such as peritonitis, acute appendicitis, acute salpingitis, and pelvic abscesses, may lead to inflammation and thrombosis of the portal vein or its tributaries.

CLINICAL COURSE. Thrombi in the legs tend, on the whole, to arise insidiously and to produce in the early stages few, if any, signs or symptoms. The local manifestations consist of edema distal to the occluded vein, dusky cyanosis, and dilatation of superficial veins. Sometimes local heat, tenderness, redness, swelling, and pain occur. However, even these signs may be absent, for when the patient is bedridden and the leg remains elevated, edema and congestion may be minimal or totally absent. Usually, however, in overt cases pain can be elicited by pressure over affected veins. In involvement of the lower extremities, squeezing the calf muscles or forced dorsiflexion of the foot evokes discomfort or pain. There are now several noninvasive methods (^{125}I-labeled fibrinogen; ultrasonography; plethysmography) that aid in the diagnosis, but venous angiography may have to be performed in some cases to establish the presence of deep vein thrombosis.

Not infrequently, the first manifestation of thrombophlebitis is the development of an embolic episode. Indeed, pulmonary embolism is one of the most common clinical problems, particularly in hospitalized patients.

The gravity of the possible consequence of phlebothrombosis strongly influences the management of all cardiac, postpartal, and postoperative cases. All such patients are urged to move about constantly in bed, perform muscle exercises to stimulate the venous flow in the legs, and become ambulatory as soon as is clinically feasible. In particularly vulnerable individuals, anticoagulant therapy may be administered when long-term bed rest is mandatory.

Bacterial infection of a thrombus may be a source of bacteremia and septic emboli. In the dural sinuses, such intravascular infections may spread to cause meningitis or abscess formations in the contiguous regions of the brain. Phlebitis of the portal veins may seed the liver with bacteria and produce multiple liver abscesses.

Phlegmasia Alba Dolens and Migratory Phlebitis

There are two special variants of primary phlebothrombosis, both of obscure nature. One is known as phlegmasia alba dolens and the other as migratory phlebitis. *Phlegmasia alba dolens* (painful white leg) refers to iliofemoral venous thrombosis occurring usually in pregnant women in the third trimester or immediately following delivery. Because of its association with pregnancy, this condition has also been called *"milk leg."* Classically, marked painful swelling of the lower extremity results, but experimental evidence suggests that venous stasis alone does not produce such severe edema. It is postulated that the thrombus initiates a secondary phlebitis, and the perivenous inflammatory response induces lymphatic blockage also. The predisposition to thrombosis here is attributed to the stasis of flow caused by the pressure of the gravid uterus and to the development of a hypercoagulable state during pregnancy.

Migratory thrombophlebitis is a term given to the appearance of venous thrombi, often multiple, which classically disappear at one site only to reappear elsewhere. This curious disorder is usually encountered in patients having a deep-seated visceral cancer, including pancreas, lung, and colon, and is one of the paraneoplastic syndromes (p. 296).

LYMPHATICS

Because of their widespread distribution and important role as drainage channels, involvement of the lymphatics is almost inevitable in all inflammations and whenever tumors metastasize through these vessels. In most of these instances, the lymphatic lesions are so small and focal as to have no significance. However, in some cases these secondary lesions represent serious complications that sometimes overshadow the primary disease.

LYMPHANGITIS

Bacterial infections may spread into and through the lymphatics to create acute inflammatory involvements in these channels. The most common etiologic agents are the group A beta-hemolytic streptococci, although any virulent pathogen may be responsible for an acute lymphangitis. Anatomically, the affected lymphatics are dilated and filled with an acute leukocytic exudate, chiefly neutrophils and histiocytes. The inflammation usually extends through the wall into the perilymphatic tissues. Sometimes the surrounding reaction is so extensive as to convert the process into a cellulitis or into multiple focal abscesses. The lymph nodes of drainage are almost inevitably involved, with changes characteristic of acute lymphadenitis.

Clinically, lymphangitis is recognized by painful subcutaneous red streaks that extend along the course of lymphatics, with painful enlargement of the regional lymph nodes. If the lymph nodes fail to block the spread of the bacteria, the infective material may eventually drain into the venous system and initiate a bacteremia or septicemia.

LYMPHEDEMA

Any occlusion of lymphatic vessels is followed by the abnormal accumulation of interstitial fluid in the affected part, referred to as *obstructive lymphedema*. The most common causes of such lymphatic blockage are (1) spread of malignant tumors with obstruction of either the lymphatic channels or the nodes of drainage; (2) radical surgical procedures with removal of regional groups of lymph nodes (e.g., axillary dissection of radical mastectomy); (3) postradiation fibrosis;

(4) filariasis; and (5) postinflammatory thrombosis and scarring of lymphatic channels. The morphologic changes consist of dilatation of lymphatics up to the points of obstruction, accompanied by increases of interstitial fluid. Persistence of the edema leads to an increase of interstitial fibrous tissue, most evident subcutaneously. Enlargement of the affected part, "peau d'orange" appearance of the skin, skin ulcers, and brawny induration are sequelae to such lymphedema. *Chylous ascites, chylothorax,* and *chylopericardium* are caused by rupture of obstructed, dilated lymphatics into the peritoneum, pleural cavity, and pericardium. Almost invariably, this is due to obstruction of lymphatics by an infiltrating tumor mass.

Other, rare types of lymphedema not secondary to any known obstructive disorder also occur, as discussed in the following paragraphs.

LYMPHEDEMA PRAECOX. This is an extremely uncommon condition affecting chiefly females between the ages of 10 and 25, characterized by the progressive onset of edema in one or both feet. The edema may remain localized to the feet or ankles or, with increasing severity of the condition, progress up the extremity into the lower trunk or other regions of the body. The edema is unremitting and slowly accumulates throughout life. The cause is obscure.

MILROY'S DISEASE. Milroy's disease resembles lymphedema praecox but is present from birth and is inherited as a mendelian trait. The condition is presumed to be caused by faulty development of lymphatic channels, possibly with poor structural strength, permitting abnormal dilation and incompetence of the lymphatic valves. In classic Milroy's disease, the lower extremities are the major, and frequently the only, site of involvement.

SIMPLE CONGENITAL LYMPHEDEMA. This disorder is distinguished from Milroy's disease by the fact that it affects only one member of the family, but it is present from birth. The anatomic distribution, histologic findings, and clinical significance are identical to those of Milroy's disease.

TUMORS

Vascular tumors are a heterogeneous group of neoplasms consisting of a spectrum of tumors—from the extremely benign hemangiomas, to intermediate lesions that are locally aggressive but infrequently metastasize, to relatively rare, highly malignant angiosarcomas.[88,89] In addition, congenital malformations such as those that occur in the Sturge-Weber syndrome may present as tumor-like lesions, as do some non-neoplastic inflammatory vascular proliferations, such as the *granuloma pyogenicum* of pregnancy. For these reasons vascular neoplasms are difficult to categorize clinically and histologically. Here we shall describe only those lesions that are common or clinically important.

Table 12–5. Tumors and Tumor-like Conditions of Blood Vessels

1. Benign
   Hemangioma
      Capillary
      Cavernous
      Epithelioid
      Granuloma pyogenicum
      Deep soft tissue hemangiomas
   Glomus tumor
   Vascular ectasias
2. Intermediate
   Hemangioendothelioma
   Epithelioid hemangioendothelioma
3. Malignant
   Angiosarcoma
   Hemangiopericytoma
   Kaposi's sarcoma

Vascular neoplasms are divided into benign and malignant on the basis of two major anatomic characteristics: (1) the degree to which the neoplasm is composed of well-formed vascular channels, and (2) the abundance and regularity of the endothelial cell proliferation. In general, benign neoplasms are made up largely of well-formed vessels with a significant amount of regular endothelial cell proliferation, whereas, on the opposite end of the spectrum, the frankly malignant tumors are solidly cellular and anaplastic and reproduce scant numbers of only abortive vascular channels. The endothelial nature of neoplastic proliferations that do not form distinct vascular lumina can sometimes be confirmed by finding the endothelium-specific Weibel-Palade bodies on electron microscopy or endothelium-specific markers by immunohistochemical techniques. The two most useful markers are Factor VIII–related antigens and a 1-fucose moiety present on the surface of endothelial cells which binds the lectin of *Ulex europaeus.*[90]

Table 12–5 lists the main types of vascular tumors.

BENIGN TUMORS AND TUMOR-LIKE CONDITIONS

Hemangioma

Hemangiomas are extremely common tumors, making up 7% of all benign tumors, and are most common in infancy and childhood. There are several histologic and clinical variants.

Capillary Hemangioma

Capillary hemangiomas are so designated because *they are composed of blood vessels that, for the most part, resemble capillaries*—narrow, thin-walled, and lined by relatively thin endothelium. They usually occur in the skin, subcutaneous tissues, and mucous membranes of the oral cavity and lips. They may also occur in internal viscera, such as the liver, spleen, and kidneys.

They vary in size from a few millimeters up to several centimeters in diameter. Characteristically, they are bright red to blue, on a level with the surface of the skin, or slightly elevated. Occasionally, pedunculated lesions are formed attached by a broad-to-slender stalk (Fig. 12–36). The covering epithelium is usually intact. The **"strawberry type"** of capillary hemangioma (juvenile hemangioma) of the skin of newborns grows rapidly in the first few months, begins to fade when the baby is 1 to 3 years old, and regresses by age 5 in 80% of cases.

Histologically, capillary hemangiomas are usually **well defined but unencapsulated.** They are made up of closely packed aggregations of thin-walled capillaries, usually blood-filled, separated by scant connective tissue stroma. The lumina may be partially or completely thrombosed and organized. Rupture of vessels causes scarring and accounts for the hemosiderin pigment found in occasional instances.

Cavernous Hemangioma

Cavernous hemangiomas are distinguished by the formation of *large, cavernous, vascular channels.* These hemangiomas often occur on the skin and mucosal surfaces of the body but are also found in many viscera, particularly the liver, spleen, pancreas, and occasionally the brain. In one rare entity, *Lindau-von Hippel disease,* cavernous hemangiomas occur within the cerebellum or brain stem and eye grounds, along with similar angiomatous lesions or cystic neoplasms in the pancreas and liver, as well as other visceral neoplasms. The dermal hemangiomas are present in childhood with a predilection for the head and neck.

Grossly, the usual cavernous hemangioma is a red-blue, soft, spongy mass 1 to 2 cm in diameter. Quite rarely, giant forms occur that affect large subcutaneous areas of the face, extremities, or other regions of the body. Histologically, the mass is sharply defined, but not encapsulated, and made up of large, cavernous, vascular spaces, partly or completely filled with fluid blood separated by a scant connective tissue stroma (Fig. 12–37). Intravascular thrombosis or rupture of channels may modify the histologic appearance.

In most situations, the tumors are of little clinical significance, although, when present in the brain, they are potential sources of increased intracranial pressure or hemorrhage.

Granuloma Pyogenicum (Granulation Tissue–Type Hemangioma)

Although the neoplastic nature of this lesion is uncertain, it is currently classified as a polypoid form of capillary hemangioma. The tumors appear as exophytic red nodules on the skin and gingival or oral mucosa, and they are often ulcerated. One third of le-

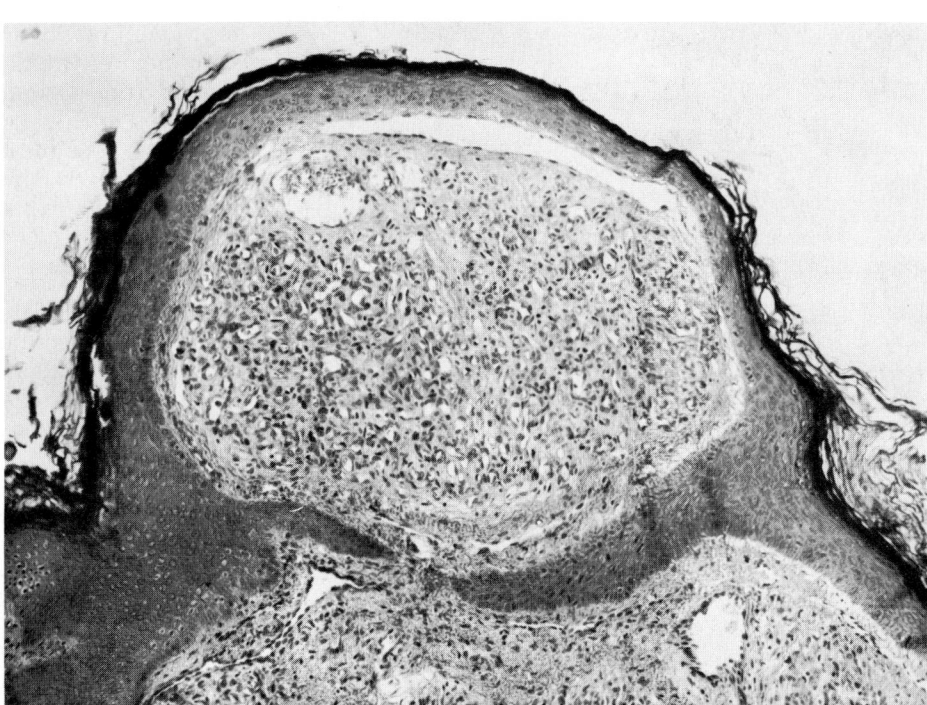

Figure 12-36. Capillary hemangioma of skin. Note slitlike spaces lined by endothelium.

sions develop after trauma, growing rapidly to reach a maximum size of 1 to 2 cm within a few weeks. Histologically, the proliferating capillaries are separated by extensive edema and an acute and chronic inflammatory infiltrate. Thus, the lesions bear a striking resemblance to exuberant granulation tissue. They are benign and most do not recur after excision.

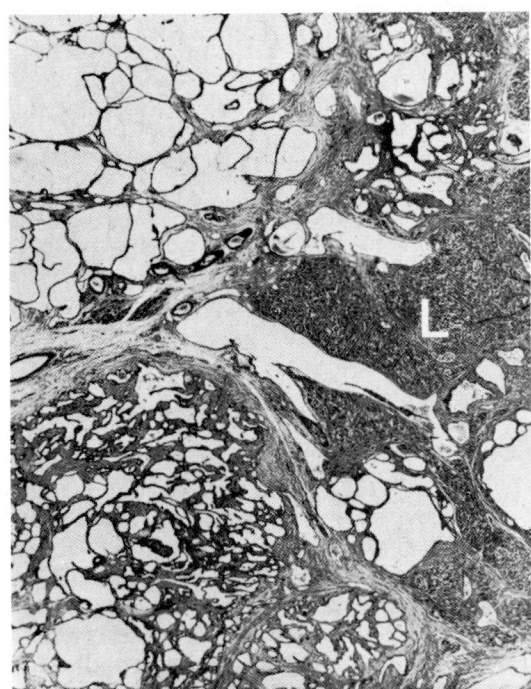

Figure 12-37. Cavernous hemangioma of liver. The dilated spaces are lined by endothelium. L = liver.

Pregnancy tumor (granuloma gravidarum) is a granuloma pyogenicum occurring in the gingiva of 1 to 5% of pregnant women. The lesions regress after delivery, and thus there is doubt whether they are true neoplasms.

Glomus Tumor (Glomangioma)

A glomangioma is a benign tumor that arises from the modified smooth muscle cells of the glomus body.[91] The normal glomus is a neuromyoarterial receptor that is sensitive to variations in temperature and regulates arteriolar flow. The glomus has an afferent artery, arteriovenous anastomosis, and efferent veins. Glomus bodies may be located anywhere in the skin but are *most commonly found in the distal portion of the fingers and toes*, especially under the nails. It is no surprise, then, that these are the common sites of glomus tumors (especially the fingers). These lesions can be almost positively identified by their extreme painfulness.

Grossly, the lesions are usually under 1 cm in diameter, and many are less than 3 mm in diameter. Tumors have been described that are productive of significant pain although they are smaller than the head of a pin. When present in the skin, they are slightly elevated, rounded, red-blue, firm, exquisitely painful nodules. Under the nail, they appear as minute foci of fresh hemorrhage. Histologically, *two components are present:* branching vascular channels separated by a connective tissue stroma that contains the second element — *aggregates, nests, and masses of the specialized glomus cells*. The individual cells are usually regular in size, round or cuboidal, and have scant cytoplasm (Fig. 12-38). On electron microscopy, they have features typical of smooth muscle cells.

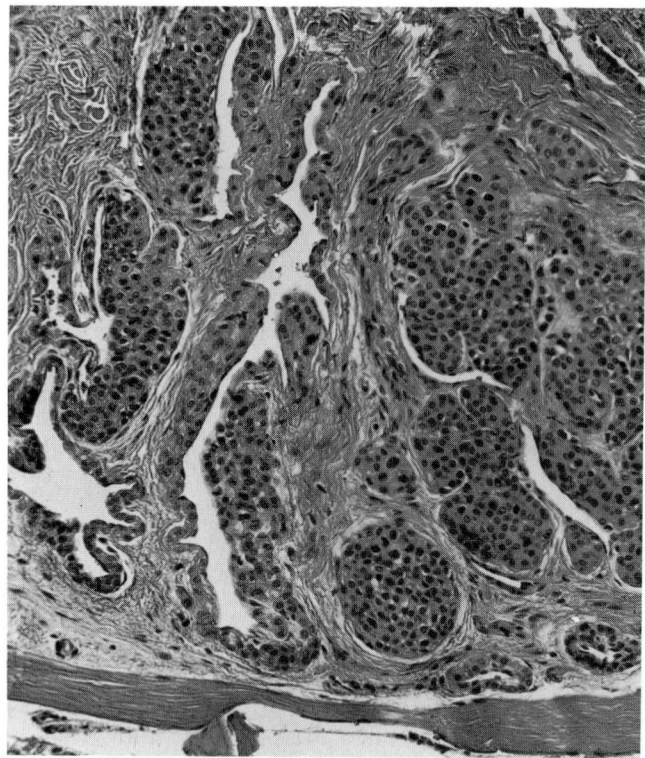

Figure 12-38. Glomus tumor. Note vascular channels and nests of cuboidal glomus cells. By electron microscopy, they resemble smooth muscle cells. (Courtesy of Dr. M.A. Venkatachalam.)

Excision produces prompt relief of pain. Typical glomus tumors also occur in the stomach and nasal cavity.

Vascular Ectasias (Telangiectases)

The term telangiectasis designates a group of abnormally prominent capillaries, venules, and arterioles that create small focal red lesions, usually in the skin and mucous membranes of the body. These dilatations probably represent congenital anomalies or acquired exaggerations of preexisting vessels and are therefore not true neoplasms.

Nevus Flammeus

This is a sophisticated name for the ordinary birthmark. The lesions are most common on the head and neck, range in color from light pink to deep purple, and are ordinarily flat. Histologically, they show only dilatation of vessels in the dermis. The vast majority ultimately fade and regress.

A special form of nevus flammeus, the so-called *port-wine stain*, may grow proportionately with the child, thicken the skin surface, and become unsightly. In addition, port-wine stains in the distribution of the trigeminal nerve may be associated with the *Sturge-Weber syndrome* (also called *encephalotrigeminal angiomatosis*). This is an extremely uncommon congenital disorder attributed to faulty development of certain mesodermal and ectodermal elements. It is characterized by venous angiomatous masses in the leptomeninges over the cortex and by ipsilateral port-wine nevi of the face, and it is often associated with mental retardation, seizures, hemiplegia, and radiopacities in the skull. The importance of this entity lies in the recognition that a large vascular malformation in the face may well be more than a coincidence in a child who exhibits some evidence of mental deficiency.

Spider Telangiectasia

The spider telangiectasis consists of a focal minute network of subcutaneous small arteries or arterioles arranged in a radial fashion about a central core. It is usually found on the upper parts of the body, particularly the face, neck, and upper chest, and is most common in *pregnant women* or in patients with liver disease, particularly *cirrhosis of the liver*. It is believed that the hyperestrinism found in these two conditions in some way evokes these vascular changes. Because these are composed of arterial vessels, they frequently pulsate, a useful diagnostic feature.

Hereditary Hemorrhagic Telangiectasia (Osler-Weber-Rendu Disease)

Osler-Weber-Rendu disease is characterized by multiple small aneurysmal telangiectases distributed over the skin and mucous membranes, present from birth and apparently of hereditary origin. It is a rare disorder, transmitted as a *dominant mendelian trait by either the male or the female and affecting both sexes equally*. However, about 20% of cases lack a family history.

The small (less than 5 mm) lesions are found directly beneath the skin or mucosal surfaces of the oral cavity, lips, alimentary tract, respiratory tract, and urinary tract, as well as in the liver, brain, and spleen.

Nosebleeds and bleeding into the intestinal, urinary, or respiratory tract are common clinical manifestations. This hemorrhagic tendency becomes more pronounced with increasing age. There is frequent hepatomegaly, most often caused by focal fibrovascular lesions throughout the liver lobules, but these patients are also prone to develop viral hepatitis B due to transfusion therapy. Usually, hemorrhages are readily controlled, and patients with this condition have a normal life expectancy.

INTERMEDIATE-GRADE TUMORS

Hemangioendothelioma

Hemangioendothelioma is used to denote a true neoplasm of vascular origin composed predominantly of masses of endothelial cells growing in and about vascular lumina. *The hemangioendothelioma represents an intergrade between the well-differentiated hemangiomas and the frankly anaplastic, totally cellular hemangiosarcomas.* It follows the pattern of distribution of the hemangiomas and is most frequently encountered in the skin but may affect the spleen and liver. Histologically, vascular channels are evident, but in addition there may be dominant masses and sheets of spindle-shaped cells. Occasionally, plump, somewhat larger cells and mitotic figures are encountered, producing a slight pleomorphism to the cell pattern.

The tumor's chief importance lies in its differentiation from the more ominous angiosarcoma. The clinical setting is critical. Borderline lesions that are present at birth often mature eventually, but in the setting of chronic lymphedema (p. 593) they should cause concern.

Epithelioid hemangioendothelioma is a unique vascular tumor occurring around medium-sized and large veins in the soft tissue of adults. Well-defined vascular channels are inconspicuous, and the tumor cells are plump and often cuboidal, thus resembling epithelial cells. They may occur in the lung as a so-called *intravascular bronchioalveolar tumor*. These tumors can thus be misdiagnosed as metastatic carcinomas. Their endothelial origin is confirmed by the presence of Weibel-Palade bodies and Factor VIII–associated antigens. Their clinical behavior is variable. Most are cured by excision, but up to 40% recur and 20% eventually metastasize.

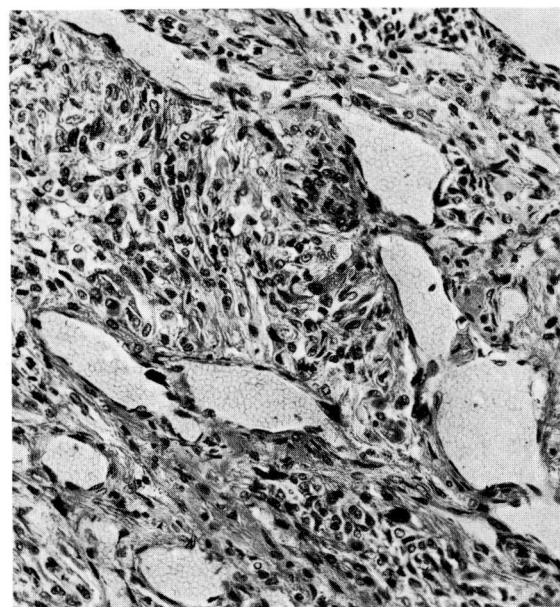

Figure 12–39. Hemangiosarcoma of low malignancy and only moderate anaplasia.

MALIGNANT TUMORS

Hemangiosarcoma (Angiosarcoma)

As the name indicates, this tumor is a malignant neoplasm of vascular origin, characterized by masses of endothelial cells displaying the cellular atypicality and anaplasia found in all malignancies. It may occur in both sexes and at all ages, anywhere in the body, but most often in the skin, soft tissue, breast, and liver. Grossly, cutaneous angiosarcomas may begin as deceptively small, sharply demarcated, asymptomatic red nodules, which may be multiple, but eventually most angiosarcomas become large, fleshy masses of pale gray-white, soft tissue.[90] The margins blend imperceptibly with surrounding structures. Areas of central softening, necrosis, and hemorrhage are frequent.

Microscopically, *all degrees of differentiation of these tumors may be found*, from those that are largely vascular with plump, anaplastic but recognizable endothelial cells to tumors that are quite undifferentiated, produce no definite blood vessels, and are markedly atypical (Fig. 12–39). In this more malignant variant, pleomorphism, tumor giant cells, and mitoses are characteristic.

Hepatic angiosarcomas are rare, but they are of interest because they are associated with distinct carcinogens: arsenic (exposure to arsenical pesticides), Thorotrast (a radioactive contrast medium widely used in radiology between 1928 and 1950), and polyvinylchloride (widely used in plastics).[92] The increased frequency of angiosarcomas among workers in the polyvinylchloride industry is one of the truly well-documented instances of chemical carcinogenesis in man. With all three agents, there is a very long latent period between exposure and the development of tumors, and there may be a premalignant phase in which diffuse sinusoidal hyperplasia occurs and cytologic abnormalities are seen in sinusoidal lining cells. The tumors are often multicentric and may arise concomitantly in the spleen.

Clinically, angiosarcomas have all the usual significance of a malignancy, with local invasion and distal metastatic spread. Some patients survive only weeks to months, whereas others may live for many years.

Hemangiopericytoma

Hemangiopericytoma, a rare neoplasm, may occur anywhere on the body but is most common on the lower extremities and retroperitoneum.[93] Electron microscopic studies clearly trace the origin of these tumors to pericytes, which are cells present in the walls of capillaries and venules, external to endothelial cells and enveloped by basement membrane. Most of these neoplasms are small, but rarely they achieve a diameter of 8 cm. They consist of numerous capillary channels surrounded by and enclosed within nests and masses of spindle-shaped cells, which occasionally can be ovoid or even round. Silver impregnation can be used to confirm that these cells are outside the basement membrane of the endothelium and hence are pericytes rather than endothelial cells. The tumors may recur, and as many as 50% metastasize to lungs, bone, and liver. Regional nodes are sometimes affected.

Kaposi's Sarcoma

Long considered to be an obscure tumor with an interesting epidemiology and an unknown histogenesis, Kaposi's sarcoma has recently come to the forefront because of its frequent occurrence in patients with acquired immune deficiency syndrome (AIDS).[94] Four forms of the disease are recognized:

1. *The classic, or European, form,* first described by Kaposi in 1862, was endemic to older men of Eastern European (especially Ashkenazic Jews) or Mediterranean descent. The tumor was uncommon in the United States, accounting for only 0.02% of all malignant tumors. Clinically, this form consists of multiple red to purple skin plaques or nodules primarily in the lower extremities, slowly increasing in size and number and spreading to more proximal sites. The tumors frequently remain localized to the skin and subcutaneous tissue but are locally aggressive, with an erratic course of relapses and remissions, rarely causing death of the patient. Visceral involvement occurs in only 10% of the cases and is usually clinically asymptomatic.

2. *African Kaposi's* is clinically similar to the European form, but occurs in younger men in equatorial Africa.[95] It has a very high prevalence in these regions, representing up to 10% of all tumors. In children aged 2 to 3 years in Africa, the disease is often associated with generalized involvement of lymph nodes, resembling lymphoma.

3. *Kaposi's sarcoma associated with renal transplant.* This form occurs in transplant recipients undergoing immunosuppressive therapy. It is reported in patients with Jewish or Mediterranean heritage, and it is either localized to the skin or results in widespread systemic involvement. The lesions often regress when immunosuppressive therapy is discontinued.

4. *Epidemic Kaposi's sarcoma, associated with AIDS,* is found in approximately one third of such patients, and it is more common in male homosexuals than in other groups at risk for AIDS. The cutaneous lesions have no predilection for the lower extremities, and they present as few or many pink-to-purple patches, plaques, or nodules with a propensity to become widely disseminated early in the course, involving mucous membranes, gastrointestinal tract, lymph nodes, and viscera. The tumors respond to cytotoxic chemotherapy and to therapy with α-interferon. Most patients eventually succumb to the infectious complications of AIDS rather than directly to the consequences of the tumor.

MORPHOLOGY. Histologically, all types of Kaposi's sarcoma are essentially similar. The early, or "patch," stage is characterized by jagged, thin-walled, dilated vascular spaces in the epidermis, with interstitial inflammatory cells and extravasated red cells (with hemosiderin deposition), a picture that may be difficult to distinguish from granulation tissue. The more characteristic features are seen in the later, nodular lesions and consist of plump, spindle-shaped stromal cells containing slit-like spaces filled with red cells, intertwined with vascular channels that are lined by recognizable endothelium (Fig. 12–40). The angiomatous elements tend to blend imperceptibly with the neo-plastic stromal cells, and thus the lesions eventually may resemble angiosarcomas or fibrosarcomas. Although the histogenesis of Kaposi's sarcoma is still a matter of some debate, the balance of evidence is that the cells are of endothelial origin.[96] There is also evidence of a lymphaticovenous differentiation of the endothelium, particularly in early lesions.[97]

The *pathogenesis* of Kaposi's sarcoma is unknown. A viral etiology is suggested by the epidemiologic features. Human immunodeficiency virus (HIV) itself is a cofactor in patients with AIDS, as suggested by the induction of Kaposi's sarcoma–like lesions in transgenic mice with the HIV transactivating gene.[98] Growth factors released by retrovirus-infected CD^{4+} T lymphocytes and from Kaposi's sarcoma cells themselves seem to play a role in the vascular proliferation and growth of stromal cells that characterize histologic lesions.[99]

Another unfortunate aspect of Kaposi's sarcoma is that about one third of patients subsequently develop a second malignancy, usually lymphoma, leukemia, or myeloma.[94] These considerations, as well as the association with AIDS and the increased frequency in immunocompromised hosts, suggest an interplay between viral infection and deficient immunoregulation in the pathogenesis of this disorder.

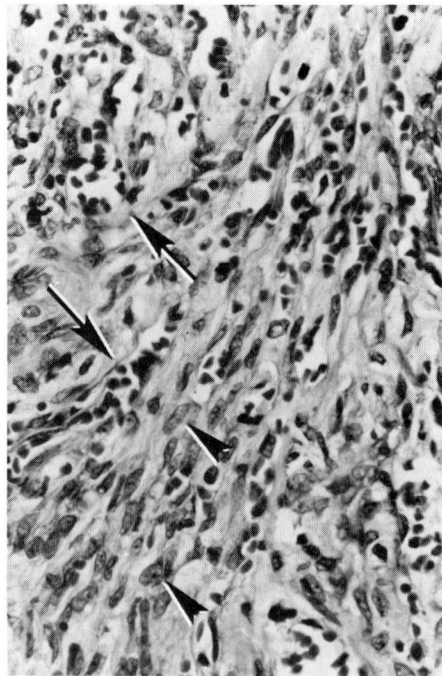

Figure 12–40. **Kaposi's sarcoma. High-power view showing vascular channels filled with red blood cells *(long arrows)* and spindle-shaped stromal cells *(arrowheads).***

TUMORS OF LYMPHATICS

Lymphangioma

Lymphangiomas are the lymphatic analog of the hemangiomas of blood vessels.

SIMPLE (CAPILLARY) LYMPHANGIOMA.

These masses are composed of small lymphatic channels. They tend to occur subcutaneously in the head and neck region as well as in the axilla. Rarely, they are found in the trunk, within internal organs, or in the connective tissue in and about the abdominal or thoracic cavities.

On body surfaces, they are slightly elevated or sometimes pedunculated lesions, 1 to 2 cm in diameter. In internal structures, they are sharply circumscribed, compressible, gray-to-pink lesions. Histologically, they are composed of a network of endothelium-lined lymph spaces that can be *differentiated from capillary channels only by the absence of blood cells.* Sometimes the lining cells hypertrophy, become cuboidal, and take on the appearance of glandular epithelium. A *lymphangiomyoma* is a variant that exhibits abundant smooth muscle in the wall of the lymphatic channels. These tumors are completely benign clinically.

CAVERNOUS LYMPHANGIOMA (CYSTIC HYGROMA).

These benign lymphatic tumors are composed of cavernous lymphatic spaces and therefore are analogous to the cavernous hemangioma. They almost invariably occur in the neck or axilla, and only rarely retroperitoneally. They occasionally achieve considerable size, up to 15 cm in diameter. Such large masses may fill the axilla or produce gross deformities in and about the neck. The tumors are made up of hugely dilated cystic spaces lined by endothelial cells and separated by a scant intervening connective tissue stroma. The margins of the tumor are not discrete, and these lesions are not encapsulated. Their removal is therefore difficult, and when bits of tumor are left in surgical resections, recurrence may be expected.

Lymphangiosarcoma (Lymphedema-Associated Angiosarcoma)

Lymphangiosarcoma is a rare tumor that develops after prolonged lymphatic obstruction and lymphedema. Most cases occur in the edematous arms of patients treated with radical mastectomy for carcinoma of the breast.[100] Clinically, the edematous arm may undergo acute swelling followed by the appearance of subcutaneous nodules, hemorrhage, and skin ulceration. The nodules are frequently multiple, but they later become confluent, forming a large mass. On the average, they appear about ten years after the mastectomy and have a very poor prognosis. They may also develop after prolonged lymphedema in the lower legs. Histologically, the tumor is composed of channels lined by anaplastic endothelial cells, and it resembles hemangiosarcoma, especially if hemorrhage has occurred.

1. Cotran, R.S.: Endothelial cells. *In* Kelley, W.N., Harris, E.D., Jr., Ruddy, S., and Sledge, C.B. (eds.): Textbook of Rheumatology, 3rd ed. Philadelphia, W.B. Saunders Co.,1989.
2. Simionescu, N., and Simionescu, M. (eds.): Endothelial Cell Biology. New York, Plenum Publishing Co., 1988.
3. Ryan, U. (ed.): Endothelial Cells. Boca Raton, Fl, CRC Press, 1988.
4. Weibel, E.R., and Palade, J.E.: New cytoplasmic components in arterial endothelium. J. Cell Biol. *23*:101, 1964.
5. Campbell, G.R., et al.: Arterial smooth muscle—a multifunctional mesenchymal cell. Arch. Pathol. Lab. Med. *112*:977, 1988.
6. Pells, S., and Fayerweather, W.E.: Trends in the incidence of myocardial infarction and in associated mortality and morbidity. N. Engl. J. Med. *312*:1005, 1985.
7. Horan, M.J., et al.: Progress against high blood pressure: A medical, scientific and public success story. *In* Forty Years of Achievement in Heart, Lung, and Blood Research. Washington, D.C., National Heart, Lung, and Blood Institute, 1987, p. 33.
8. Kuller, L.H.: Epidemiology of cardiovascular disease: Current perspectives. Am. J. Epidemiol. *104*:425, 1976.
9. Gotto, A.M., Jr., and Farmer, J.A.: Risk factors for coronary artery disease and their management. *In* Braunwald, E. (ed.): Heart Disease. A Textbook of Cardiovascular Medicine. 3rd ed. Philadelphia, W.B. Saunders Co., 1988, p. 1153.
10. McGill, H.C., Jr., and Stern, M.P.: Sex and atherosclerosis. Atheroscler. Rev. *4*:157, 1979.
11. Neufeld, H.N., and Goldbourt, V.: Coronary heart disease. Genetic aspects. Circulation *67*:943, 1983.
12. Kannel, W.B., et al.: A general cardiovascular risk profile. The Framingham Study. Am. J. Cardiol. *38*:46, 1976.
13. Steinberg, D.: Current theories of the pathogenesis of atherosclerosis. *In* Steinberg, D., and Olefsky, J.M. (eds.): Hypercholesterolemia and Atherosclerosis. Pathogenesis and Prevention. New York, Churchill-Livingstone, 1987, p. 5.
14. Eder, H.A., and Gidez, L.I.: The clinical significance of high density lipoproteins. Med. Clin. North Am. *66*:431, 1982.
15. Leaf, A., and Weber, P.: Omega 3 fatty acids and cardiovascular disease. *In* Braunwald, E. (ed.): Heart Disease Update. Philadelphia, W.B. Saunders Co., 1988, pp. 49–60.
16. Stamler, J., and Shekelle, R.: Dietary cholesterol and human coronary heart disease. Arch. Pathol. Lab. Med. *112*:1033, 1988.
17. Grundy, S.M., and Bearn, A.G. (eds.): The Role of Cholesterol in Atherosclerosis: New Therapeutic Opportunities. Philadelphia, Hanley and Belfus, 1988.
17a. Scanu, A.M.: Lipoprotein (a)—a potential bridge between the fields of atherosclerosis and thrombosis. Arch. Pathol. Lab. Med. *112*:1045, 1988.
18. Mahley, R.W.: Apolipoprotein E: Cholesterol transport protein with expanding role in cell biology. Science *240*:622, 1988.
19. Editorial: Apolipoprotein B and atherogenesis. Lancet *1*:1141, 1988.
20. Haust, D.: The natural history of human atherosclerotic lesion. *In* Moore, S. (ed.): Vascular Injury and Atherosclerosis. New York, Marcel Dekker, 1981, p. 1.
21. Tracy, R.E., et al.: Histometric components of aortic atherosclerosis which vary or remain constant among eight populations. Lab. Invest. *54*:314, 1986.
22. Gown, A.M., Tsukada, T., and Ross, R.: Human atherosclerosis. II. Immunocytochemical analysis of the cellular composition of human atherosclerotic lesions. Am. J. Pathol. *125*:191, 1986.
23. Roberts, W.C.: The coronary arteries in ischemic heart disease: Facts and fancies. Triangle *16*:77, 1977.
24. McGill, H.C., Jr.: Persistent problems in the pathogenesis of atherosclerosis. Arteriosclerosis *4*:443, 1984.
25. Stary, H.C.: Atheroma arises in eccentric intimal thickening from concurrent fatty streak lesions. Fed. Proc. *46*:418, 1987.
26. Faggiotto, A., and Ross, R.: Studies of hypercholesterolemia in

the nonhuman primate. II. Fatty streak conversion to fibrous plaque. Arteriosclerosis 4:341, 1984.

27. Velican, C., and Velican, T.: Intimal thickening in developing coronary arteries and its relevance to atherosclerotic involvement. Atherosclerosis 23:345, 1976.

28. Munro, J.M., and Cotran, R.S.: The pathogenesis of atherosclerosis: atherogenesis and inflammation. Lab. Invest. 58:249, 1988.

29. Ross, R.: The pathogenesis of atherosclerosis: An update. N. Engl. J. Med. 314:488, 1986.

29a. Ross, R.: The pathogenesis of atherosclerosis. In Braunwald, E. (ed.): Heart Disease. A Textbook of Cardiovascular Medicine. 3rd ed. Philadelphia, W.B. Saunders Co., 1988, p. 1135.

30. Mahley, R.W.: Development of accelerated atherosclerosis: Concepts derived from cell biology and animal model studies. Arch. Pathol. Lab. Med. 107:393, 1983.

31. Davies, P.F.: Vascular cell interactions with special reference to the pathogenesis of atherosclerosis. Lab. Invest. 55:5, 1986.

32. Schwartz, S.M., and Reidy, M.A.: Common mechanisms of proliferation of smooth muscle in atherosclerosis and hypertension. Hum. Pathol. 18:240, 1987.

33. Ross, R., and Glomset, J.A.: The pathogenesis of atherosclerosis. N. Engl. J. Med. 295:369, 420, 1976.

34. Stemerman, M.B., and Ross, R.: Experimental arteriosclerosis. I. Fibrous plaque formation in primates: An electron microscopic study. J. Exp. Med. 136:769, 1972.

35. Glagov, S., et al.: Hemodynamics and atherosclerosis. Insights and perspectives gained from studies of human arteries. Arch. Pathol. Lab. Clin. Med. 112:1018, 1988.

36. Davies, P.F., et al.: Turbulent fluid shear stress induces vascular endothelial cell turnover in vitro. Proc. Natl. Acad. Sci. U.S.A. 83:2114, 1986.

37. Gimbrone, M.A., Jr.: Endothelial dysfunction and the pathogenesis of atherosclerosis. In Gotto, A. (ed.): Atherosclerosis—V. Proceedings of the Vth International Symposium on Atherosclerosis. New York, Springer-Verlag, 1980, p. 415.

38. Thomas, W.A., et al.: Population dynamics of arterial cells during atherogenesis. VIII. Separation of the roles of injury and growth stimulation in early aortic atherogenesis in swine originating in pre-existing intimal smooth muscle cell masses. Exp. Mol. Pathol. 31:124, 1979.

39. Ross, R., Raines, E.W., and Bowen-Pope, D.F.: The biology of platelet-derived growth factor. Cell 46:155, 1986.

40. Shimokado, K., et al.: A significant part of macrophage-derived growth factor consists of at least two forms of PDGF. Cell 43:277, 1985.

41. Collins, T., et al.: Cultured human endothelial cells express platelet-derived growth factor A chain. Am. J. Pathol. 127:7, 1987.

42. Libby, P., et al.: Production of platelet-derived growth factor-like mitogen smooth muscle cells from human atheroma. N. Engl. J. Med. 318:1493, 1988.

43. Castellot, J.J.: Regulation of vascular smooth muscle growth by heparin and heparan sulfate. Semin. Thromb. Hemost. 13:489, 1987.

43a. Gerrity, R.G.: The role of the monocyte in atherogenesis. I. Transition of blood-borne monocytes into foam cells in fatty lesions. Am. J. Pathol. 103:181, 1981.

44. Joris, I., et al.: Studies on the pathogenesis of atherosclerosis. I. Adhesion and emigration of mononuclear cells in the aorta of hypercholesterolemic rats. Am. J. Pathol. 113:341, 1983.

45. Gianturco, S.H., and Bradley, W.H.: β-VLDL receptor pathway of macrophages. In Fidge, N.H., and Nestel, P.G. (eds.): Atherosclerosis VII. Amsterdam, Excerpta Medica, 1986.

46. Fogelman, A.M., et al.: Malondialdehyde alteration of low-density lipoproteins leads to cholesteryl ester accumulation in human monocyte-macrophages. Proc. Natl. Acad. Sci. U.S.A. 77:2214, 1980.

47. Parthasarathy, S., et al.: Macrophage oxidation of low-density lipoprotein generates a modified form recognized by the scavenger receptor. Arteriosclerosis 6:505, 1986.

48. Quinn, M.T., et al.: Oxidatively modified low-density lipoproteins: A potential role in recruitment and retention of monocyte/macrophages during atherogenesis. Proc. Natl. Acad. Sci. U.S.A. 84:2995, 1987.

49. Salisbury, B.G.J., et al.: Insoluble low-density lipoprotein-proteoglycan complexes enhance cholesteryl ester accumulation in macrophages. Am. J. Pathol. 120:6, 1985.

50. Gerrity, R.G.: Vesicular transport and intimal accumulation of macromolecules in atherosclerosis-susceptible areas is augmented by hyperlipidemia. Circulation 76:IV-295, 1987.

51. Kita, T., et al.: Probucol prevents the progression of atherosclerosis in Watanable heritable hyperlipidemic rabbit, an animal model for familial hypercholesterolemia. Proc. Natl. Acad. Sci. U.S.A. 84:5928, 1987.

52. Benditt, E.P., and Benditt, J.M.: Evidence for a monoclonal origin of human atherosclerotic plaque. Proc. Natl. Acad. Sci. U.S.A. 70:1753, 1973.

52a. Benditt, E.P.: Origins of human atherosclerotic plaque: the role of altered gene expression. Arch. Pathol. Lab. Med. 112:997, 1988.

53. Thomas, W.A., and Kim, D.N.: Atherosclerosis as a hyperplastic and neoplastic process. Lab. Invest. 48:245, 1983.

54. Fabricant, C.G.: Atherosclerosis: The consequence of infection with a herpes virus. Adv. Vet. Sci. Comp. Med. 30:39, 1985.

55. Majesky, M.W., et al.: Focal smooth muscle proliferation in the aortic intima produced by an initiation-promotion sequence. Proc. Natl. Acad. Sci. U.S.A. 82:3450, 1985.

56. Benditt, E.P., et al.: Viruses in the etiology of atherosclerosis. Proc. Natl. Acad. Sci. U.S.A. 80:6386, 1986.

57. Cupps, T.R., and Fauci, A.S.: The Vasculitides. Philadelphia, W.B. Saunders Co., 1981.

58. Kadison, P., and Haynes, B.F.: Vasculitis: Mechanism of vessel damage. In Gallin, J., et al. (eds.): Inflammation: Basic Principles and Clinical Correlates. New York, Raven Press, 1988, p. 703.

59. Leung, D.Y.M., et al.: Two monokines, IL-1 and TNF, render cultured vascular endothelial cells susceptible to lysis by antibodies circulating during Kawasaki's disease. J. Exp. Med. 164:1958, 1986.

60. Falk, R.J., and Jennette, J.C.: Antineutrophilic cytoplasmic autoantibodies with specificity for myeloperoxidase in patients with systemic vasculitis and idiopathic crescentic glomerulonephritis. N. Engl. J. Med. 318:1651, 1988.

61. Lie, J.T.: Coronary vasculitis. A review in the current scheme of classification of vasculitis. Arch. Pathol. Lab. Med. 111:224, 1987.

61a. Bacon, P.A.: Vasculitis. Acta Med. Scand. (Suppl.) 715:157, 1983.

62. Lie, J.T.: The classification of vasculitis and a reappraisal of allergic granulomatosis and angiitis (Churg-Strauss syndrome). Mt. Sinai J. Med. 53:429, 1986.

63. Savage, C.O.S., and Ng, Y.C.: The etiology and pathogenesis of major systemic vasculitides. Postgrad. Med. J. 62:627, 1986.

64. Fauci, A.S., et al.: Wegener's granulomatosis: Prospective clinical and therapeutic experience with 85 patients for 21 years. Ann. Intern. Med. 98:76, 1983.

65. Savage, C.O.S., et al.: Prospective study of radioimmunoassay with an autoantigen recognized by circulating anti-neutrophil antibodies in systemic vasculitis. Lancet 1:716, 1987.

66. Katzenstein, A.A., et al.: Lymphomatoid granulomatosis. A clinicopathologic study of 152 cases. Cancer 43:360, 1979.

67. Bengtsson, B.A., and Malmvall, B.E.: Giant cell arteritis. Acta Med. Scand. (Suppl.) 658:1, 1982.

68. Allsop, C.J., and Gallagher, P.J.: Temporal artery biopsy in giant cell arteritis. A reappraisal. Am. J. Surg. Pathol. 5:317, 1981.

69. Hall, S., et al.: Takayasu arteritis: A study of 32 North American patients. Medicine 64:89, 1985.

70. Lupi-Herrara, E., et al.: Takayasu's arteritis: study of 107 cases. Am. Heart J. 93:94, 1977.

71. Kawasaki, T., et al.: A new infantile acute febrile mucocutaneous lymph node syndrome (MCNS) prevailing in Japan. Pediatrics 54:271, 1974.

72. Burns, J., et al.: Polymerase activity in lymphocytes culture supernatants in patients with Kawasaki's disease. Nature. 323:814, 1986.

73. Hicks, R.V., and Melish, M.E.: Kawasaki syndrome. Pediatr. Clin. North Am. 33:1151, 1987.

74. Lie, J.T.: Thromboangiitis revisited. Pathol. Annu. 23(II):257, 1988.

75. Adar, R., et al.: Cellular sensitivity to collagen in thromboangiitis obliterans. N. Engl. J. Med. 308:1113, 1983.

76. Becker, C.G.: Immunologic aspects of vessel injury and thrombosis. In The New Dimension of Warfarin Prophylaxis. New York, Plenum Press, 1987, p. 131.

77. Greer, J.M., et al.: Vasculitis associated with malignancy. Medicine 67:220, 1988.

78. Brinstingl, M.: The Raynaud syndrome. *In* Harcus, A.W., et al. (eds.): Arteries and Veins. Edinburgh, Churchill-Livingstone, 1975, p. 32.

79. Eagle, A.E., and DeSanctis, R.W.: Diseases of the aorta. *In* Braunwald, E. (ed.): Heart Disease. A Textbook of Cardiovascular Medicine. Philadelphia, W.B. Saunders Co., 1988, p. 1546.

80. DeSanctis, R.W., et al.: Aortic dissection. N. Engl. J. Med. *317*:1060, 1987.

81. Anagnostopoulos, C.E.: Acute Aortic Dissections. Baltimore, University Park Press, 1975.

82. Larson, E.W., and Edward, W.P.: Risk factors for aortic dissection: A necropsy study of 161 cases. Am. J. Cardiol. *53*:849, 1984.

83. Klima, T., et al.: The morphology of ascending aortic aneurysms. Hum. Pathol. *14*:810, 1983.

84. Schlatmann, T., and Becker, A.: Pathogenesis of dissecting aneurysm of aorta. Comparative histopathologic study of significance of medial changes. Am. J. Cardiol. *39*:21, 1977.

85. Cambria, R.P., et al.: Vascular complications associated with spontaneous aortic dissection. J. Vasc. Surg. *7*:199, 1988.

86. Harcus, A.W., et al. (eds.): Arteries and Veins. Edinburgh, Churchill Livingstone, 1975.

87. Marder, V.J., and Sherry, S.: Thrombolytic therapy: current status (first of two parts). N. Engl. Med. *318*:1512, 1988.

88. Longtine, J., and Cotran, R.S.: Neoplastic disorders of blood vessels. *In* Loscalzo, J., et al. (eds.): Textbook of Vascular Medicine. Boston, Little Brown & Co. (in press).

89. Enzinger, F.M., and Weiss, S.W.: Soft Tissue Tumors. 2nd ed. St. Louis, C.V. Mosby Co., 1988, p. 489.

90. Ordonez, N.C., and Batsakis, J.G.: Comparison of *Ulex europeaus* 1 lectin and factor VIII–related antigen in vascular lesions. Arch. Pathol. Lab. Med. *108*:129, 1984.

91. Tsuneyoshi, M., and Enjogi, M.: Glomus tumor. A clinicopathologic and electron microscopic study. Cancer *50*:1601, 1982.

92. Popper, H., et al.: Development of hepatic angiosarcoma in man induced by vinyl chloride, Thorotrast, and arsenic: Comparison with cases of unknown etiology. Am. J. Pathol. *92*:349, 1978.

93. Enzinger, F.M., and Smith, B.H.: Hemangiopericytoma. An analysis of 106 cases. Hum. Pathol. *7*:61, 1976.

94. Safai, B.: Pathophysiology and epidemiology of epidemic Kaposi's sarcoma. Semin. Oncol. 14 (Suppl. 3):7, 1987.

95. Slavin, G., et al.: Kaposi's sarcoma in mainland Tanzania. A report of 117 cases. Br. J. Cancer 23:349, 1979.

96. Rutgers, J.L., et al.: The expression of endothelial cell surface antigens by AIDS-associated Kaposi's sarcoma: Evidence for a vascular cell origin. Am. J. Pathol. *122*:493, 1986.

97. Dictor, M., and Andersson, C.: Lymphaticovenous differentiation in Kaposi's sarcoma. Cellular phenotypes by stage. Am. J. Pathol. *130*:411, 1988.

98. Vogel, J., et al.: The HIV tat-gene induces dermal lesions resembling Kaposi's sarcoma in transgenic mice. Nature *335*:606, 1988.

99. Ensoli, B., et al: AIDS-Kaposi's sarcoma–derived cells express cytokines with autocrine and paracrine growth effects. Science *243*:223, 1989.

100. Woodward, A.M., et al.: Lymphoangiosarcoma arising in chronic lymphedematous extremities. Cancer *30*:149, 1976.

The Heart

This chapter opens with discussions of two points on the cardiac spectrum: certain normal features of the heart essential to understanding cardiac pathology and a brief review of congestive heart failure, the end point of most serious cardiac diseases.

NORMAL

ANATOMY. In the female, the average weight of the heart is 250 to 300 gm, and in the male, 300 to 350 gm, varying with height and skeletal structure. Normally the thickness of the wall of the right ventricle is 3 to 5 mm, and that of the left ventricle 1.3 to 1.5 cm. Greater weight or ventricular thickness indicates hypertrophy; below normal weight signifies atrophy of the heart; and below normal thickness of the ventricular walls implies dilatation. However, an apparently normal left ventricular thickness may be found in a markedly heavy, hypertrophied heart that has undergone cardiac dilation prior to death.

All cardiac valves act essentially as loose flap valves that balloon out to close the valvular orifice against regurgitation of blood. On gross inspection, normal valve leaflets are seen to be delicate and translucent, and without apparent vascularity. The lines of closure of the semilunar (pulmonic and aortic) leaflets are marked by linear thickenings, the centers of which

are occupied by small fibrous nodules, the corpora arantii. Round-to-oval fenestrations, 1 to 3 mm in diameter, frequently occur in the semilunar cusps close to the commissural attachments, but they do not compromise valve competence because they are located above the line of closure. The free margins of the tricuspid and mitral valves are tethered to the ventricular walls by delicate chordae tendineae, which are themselves attached to papillary muscles in the ventricular walls. In the case of the mitral valve, the ventricular attachments constitute two well-defined papillary muscles, the anterolateral representing a single, large, muscular column, and the posteromedial often divided into two or three smaller pillars. Thus, normal mitral valve function depends on the coordinated actions of cusps, chordae, papillary muscles, and associated left ventricular wall. In addition, the functional competence of all of the cardiac valves depends on the integrity of the basal attachments of the cusps. Thus, dilatation of the aortic root, as may occur with syphilis, renders the aortic valve regurgitant just as left ventricular dilatation may render the mitral valve incompetent. The histologic structure of the mitral valve assumes importance because, as will be seen, an important form of heart disease—mitral valve prolapse—is characterized by alterations in the composition of the cusps. Normally, in addition to an endothelial covering of exposed surfaces, there is a thin layer of collagen and elastic tissue on the atrial side of the cusps, a dense collagenous zona fibrosa along the ventricular surfaces, and a variable amount of loose myxoid connective tissue (zona spongiosa) interspersed between these layers.

No mechanical pump has the efficiency, durability, and reliability of the human heart. Basic to this function is the near-indefatigable cardiac muscle, about which a few points merit review. The myocardium comprises a syncytium of branching and anastomosing fibers divided into individual cells by modified, closely apposed cell membranes creating the *intercalated disks.* This apposition provides in essence a continuous "tight junction" with free passage of ions and action potentials such as an excitatory stimulus from cell to cell and throughout the syncytium. As you recall, the myocyte has a central nucleus (in contrast to skeletal muscle), is richly endowed with mitochondria so vital to the generation of the large amounts of ATP required for cardiac contraction, and has an abundant sarcoplasmic reticulum (comparable to endoplasmic reticulum) and an elaborate system of large T tubules that traverse adjacent to the Z lines and are continuous with the extracellular space. The T tubules provide a ready channel for ion fluxes, in particular Ca^{++} involved in cardiac contraction. The myocyte is divided into structural and functional subunits — sarcomeres — by transverse Z lines. Sarcomeres are marked by prominent central dark A bands (creating the cross-striations) attributable mostly to thick myosin filaments in register. The A band is flanked by lighter I bands made up of thin actin filaments in register. The thin actin filaments are attached at their outer ends to the Z lines and at their inner ends interdigitate partially between the myosin filaments. In the resting state, the actin filaments do not extend to the center of the sarcomere. Thus in truth the A band has partially overlapping myosin and actin filaments, but the I band has only actin filaments. Closely affiliated with the actin filaments are the regulatory proteins tropomyosin and troponin. The sarcomere ranges from 1.6 to 2.2 μm depending on the degree of contraction. In a greatly oversimplified view, when the heart contracts, it involves shortening of the collective sarcomeres by sliding of the actin filaments between the myosin filaments toward the center of the sarcomere. The optimal length of the sarcomere for forceful contraction is 2.2 μm. Shorter lengths result in overlap of actin filaments in the center of the A band and reduction in contractile force. Up to a point, longer lengths enhance contractility (Frank-Starling proposal). Thus, moderate dilation of the ventricle increases the force of contraction. However, there is a point with progressive dilation at which overlap of the actin and myosin filaments is reduced and the force of contraction turns sharply downward, as occurs so often in heart failure.

In addition, the cardiac muscle has specialized excitatory and conducting Purkinje fibers, which contain only few contractile myofilaments and conduct action potentials faster than contractile fibers. They are involved in the regulation of the rate and rhythm of the heart. These specialized myofibers make up (1) the sinoatrial (SA) pacemaker of the heart — the *SA node* — located in the posterior wall of the right atrium adjacent to the opening of the superior vena cava, (2) the *AV bundle* that conducts the impulse from the SA node to the AV node, (3) the *AV node* located at the junction of the median wall of the right atrium with the interventricular septum, and (4) the *bundle of His,* which traverses down the interventricular septum toward the apex to divide into right and left branches that further arborize in the respective ventricles. Lesions involving these specialized structures underlie many of the disturbances in cardiac rate or rhythm.

BLOOD SUPPLY TO HEART. *Functionally, the right and left coronary arteries behave as end arteries, although anatomically there are numerous intercoronary anastomoses in most normal hearts.* Most of the flow to the myocardium occurs during diastole, when the microcirculation is not compressed by the cardiac contraction. The subendocardial zone is most compressed and therefore less richly supplied with blood. Knowledge of the area of supply of the three major coronary trunks helps to explain the correlation between vascular lesions and myocardial infarctions. The anterior descending branch of the left coronary artery supplies most of the apex of the heart, the anterior surface of the left ventricle, the contiguous third of the anterior wall of the right ventricle, and the anterior two thirds of the interventricular septum. In most hearts the right coronary artery supplies the remainder of the anterior surface of the right ventricle, the posterior aspect of the right ventricle, the adjacent half of the posterior wall of the left ventricle, and the posterior third of the interventricular septum. To the circumflex branch of the left coronary artery remains only a small portion of the lateral aspect of the left ventricle extending slightly anteriorly and posteriorly. *Thus, occlusions of the right as well as the left coronary artery and their major branches may cause left ventricular damage.* The atria are supplied by branches from the arteries on the corresponding side. At the cellular level, individual muscle fibers are almost uniformly accompanied by several capillaries. This distribution may be important in hypertrophied hearts in which it is postulated that enlarged fibers may become so thick as to outgrow their blood supply.

In all or virtually all human hearts, there are numerous intercoronary anastomotic channels up to 40 μm in diameter. In the normal heart, little blood courses through these channels. However, when one trunk is narrowed, blood flows from the high to the low pressure system, and simultaneously the channels enlarge.[1] Thus, these anastomoses may play a role in supporting the blood flow to deprived areas of the myocardium, but, alas, they are not capable of compensating for sudden loss of a major coronary artery.

CONGESTIVE HEART FAILURE (CHF)

CHF will be considered at the outset because it is the potential end point of all forms of serious heart disease. *CHF can be defined as the pathophysiologic state resulting from impaired cardiac function rendering the heart unable to maintain an output sufficient for the metabolic requirements of the tissues and organs of the body.*[2] *CHF occurs either because of a decreased myocardial capacity to contract or because an excessive pressure-stroke-volume load is imposed on the heart.* Most instances of heart failure are the consequence of progressive deterioration of the myocardial contractile function (systolic dysfunction), as often occurs with ischemic injury. Sometimes the failure results from diminished outflow (pressure-volume overload), as caused by hypertension or by an inability of the heart to expand sufficiently during diastole (e.g., constrictive pericarditis) to accommodate the ventricular volume (diastolic dysfunction). Uncommonly, acute heart failure may occur with basically normal myocardial function, as, for example, massive pulmonary embolism and right heart strain (acute cor pulmonale). Whatever its basis, CHF is characterized by diminished cardiac output (sometimes called forward failure) or damming back of blood in the venous system (so-called backward failure), or both.

Although we speak of diminished myocardial contraction as the cause of heart failure, there is no clear understanding at the biomolecular level of the basis for the contractile failure.[3] In some instances — myocardial infarction, necrotizing inflammations — there is obvious death of myocytes and loss of vital elements of the "pump." In the absence of such acute losses, other mechanisms have been proposed, but none established — e.g., reduced adrenergic drive; reduction in beta-adrenergic receptor density[4]; decreased calcium availability, which is important in excitation-contraction coupling; impaired mitochondrial function; decreased ATPase function; and microcirculatory spasm. In the last analysis, we still do not understand why chronically overtaxed hearts eventually decompensate.

A variety of compensatory mechanisms come into play. The heart begins to dilate and according to Starling's law increases the force of contraction and size of the stroke volume. In time the increased stretching of fibers leads to hypertrophy. There is simultaneously expansion of the blood volume, further augmenting the stroke volume. Eventually, however, the compensatory mechanisms constitute an added burden. The myocardial hypertrophy may become detrimental because of the increased metabolic requirements of the enlarged muscle mass. Increased blood volume, which supports the cardiac output in the short term, also imposes an additional load on the failing heart. Ultimately, the primary cardiac disease and the superimposed compensatory burdens further encroach on the myocardial reserve until the cardiac dilation transgresses the point at which adequate myocardial tension can be generated. Then begins the downward slide of the stroke volume and cardiac output that often terminates in death. Thus, at autopsy the heart is often dilated and usually hypertrophied, but the extent of these changes varies from one patient to the next.

It is impossible from morphologic examination of the heart to differentiate the damaged but compensated organ from one that has decompensated. The amount of hypertrophy and dilatation does not permit a judgment, nor does the extent of the primary cardiac disease. *Many of the significant morphologic changes encountered in CHF are distant from the heart and are produced by the hypoxic and congestive effects of the failing circulation upon other organs and tissues.* It is important to recall that hypoxic or congestive changes, or both, may be produced in peripheral tissues and organs by states of circulatory insufficiency of noncardiac origin, e.g., hemorrhagic or septic shock. During shock, many organs suffer hypoxic injury because of hypoperfusion (p. 118).

Although the heart is a single organ, to some extent it acts as two distinct anatomic and functional units. Under various pathologic stresses, one side or, rarely, even one chamber may fail before the other(s) so that, from the clinical standpoint, left-sided and right-sided failure may occur separately. Because the vascular system is a closed circuit, failure of one side cannot exist for long without eventually producing excessive strain upon the other, terminating in total heart failure. The clearest understanding of the pathologic physiology is derived from a consideration of failure of each side separately.

LEFT-SIDED HEART FAILURE

As will be discussed, left-sided heart failure is most often caused by (1) ischemic heart disease, (2) hypertension, (3) aortic and mitral valvular diseases (rheumatic heart disease, calcific aortic stenosis), and (4) myocardial diseases. Except with obstruction at the mitral valve or other processes that restrict the size of the left ventricle, this chamber is usually dilated, sometimes quite massively. With left ventricular restrictive disorders and particularly with mitral stenosis, the dilatation is confined to the left atrium. The distant effects of left-sided failure are manifested most prominently in the lungs, although the function of the kidneys and brain may also be markedly impaired.

LUNGS. With the progressive damming of blood within the pulmonary circulation, pressure in the pulmonary veins mounts and is ultimately transmitted to the capillaries. Pulmonary congestion and edema result, as described in detail on page 759. It is sufficient to note here that the congestion first leads to the development of a perivascular transudate — "cuffing" — followed by progressive edematous widening of the alveolar septa, and in time by the accumulation of edema fluid, perhaps admixed with some red cells (related to microhemorrhages) in the alveolar spaces. Not infrequently, transudate accumulates within the pleural spaces, particularly on the left, producing a gross pleural effusion.

These anatomic changes produce striking clinical manifestations. *Dyspnea* (breathlessness) is usually the earliest and the cardinal complaint of patients in left-sided heart failure and is an exaggeration of the normal breathlessness that follows exertion. It is followed by *orthopnea*, which is dyspnea on lying down that is relieved by sitting or standing. Thus, the orthopneic patient employs several pillows and indeed may spend the night in a chair. *Paroxysmal nocturnal dyspnea*, also known as *paroxysmal cardiac dyspnea*, is an extension of orthopnea that consists of attacks of extreme dyspnea bordering on suffocation; these usually occur at night and force the patient to sit upright struggling for breath. Often the patient in panic opens a window in the hope of relieving the breathlessness. *Cough* is a common accompaniment of left-sided failure, and in severe cases may raise frothy, blood-tinged sputum.

KIDNEYS. With left-sided heart failure, the decreased cardiac output causes a reduction in renal perfusion, which has a number of consequences. The renin-angiotensin-aldosterone system is activated, inducing retention of salt and water with consequent expansion of the interstitial fluid volume and blood volume. This compensatory reaction contributes to the pulmonary edema in left-sided heart failure. In kidneys already suffering from hypoperfusion, whether related to the shock state or to hypertensive arteriolar narrowing, the reduced cardiac output may lead to ischemic acute tubular necrosis (p. 1048). If the perfusion deficit of the kidney becomes sufficiently severe, impaired excretion of nitrogenous products may cause azotemia, known as *prerenal azotemia*.

BRAIN. Cerebral hypoxia may give rise to hypoxic encephalopathy (p. 1403) and many symptoms, such as irritability, loss of attention span, and restlessness, and may even progress to stupor and coma. These symptoms, however, are encountered only in far-advanced congestive heart failure.

RIGHT-SIDED HEART FAILURE

Right-sided heart failure occurs in pure form in only a few diseases. Usually it is a consequence of left-sided failure, because any increase in pressure in the pulmonary circulation incident to left-sided failure must inevitably produce an increased burden on the right side of the heart. The causes of right-sided failure, then, must include all those that create left heart failure, particularly lesions such as mitral stenosis or congenital left-to-right shunts, which produce great increases in pulmonary pressure.

Pure right-sided failure most often occurs with *cor pulmonale*, i.e., right ventricular strain produced by intrinsic disease of the lungs or pulmonary vasculature. In these cases, the right ventricle is burdened by increased resistance within the pulmonary circulation. Dilatation of the heart is confined to the right ventricle and atrium. Other and less common causes of right-sided heart failure include the various forms of cardiomyopathy and diffuse myocarditis, which appear to affect the right ventricle more often than the left for reasons to be presented later. Rarely, right-sided failure is caused by tricuspid or pulmonic valvular lesions. Clinically, constrictive pericarditis simulates right-sided failure by damming blood back into the systemic venous system, although the right ventricle itself may be normal.

The major morphologic and clinical effects of pure right-sided failure differ from those of left-sided failure in that pulmonary congestion is minimal, whereas engorgement of the systemic and portal systems is more pronounced. It should be remembered, however, that in both instances the twin problems of systemic venous congestion and impaired cardiac output remain qualitatively the same. The major organs affected by right-sided heart failure are the liver, spleen, kidneys, subcutaneous tissues, and brain and the entire portal area of venous drainage.

LIVER. The liver is usually slightly increased in size and weight and on sectioning displays a prominent "nutmeg" pattern (Fig. 3–5, p. 92). This is composed of congestive red accentuation of the centers of the liver lobules surrounded by the paler, sometimes fatty, peripheral regions. The liver cells in the central region may become somewhat atrophic as a result of the congestive hypoxia related to the stagnant flow in the centrilobular sinusoids. Together, these changes are called *chronic passive congestion* (CPC) of the liver. In some instances the severe central hypoxia produces *centrilobular necrosis* along with the sinusoidal congestion.[5] If the right-sided failure is severe and rapidly developing, rupture of sinusoids will produce *central hemorrhagic necrosis*. If the patient does not die of the severe cardiac failure, the central areas in time become fibrotic, creating so-called *cardiac sclerosis*.

SPLEEN. Congestion produces an enlarged spleen that is tense and cyanotic. On section, blood freely exudes and the tissue collapses so that the capsule becomes wrinkled. Microscopically, there may be marked sinusoidal dilatation, accompanied by areas of recent hemorrhage and possible deposits of hemosiderin pigment. With long-standing congestion, the enlarged spleen may achieve a weight of 500 to 600 gm (normal, 150 gm), and the long-standing edema may produce fibrous thickening of the sinusoidal walls. The areas of previous hemorrhage are now transformed to hemosiderin deposits, to create the firm, meaty organ characteristic of *congestive splenomegaly* (p. 750).

KIDNEYS. Congestion and hypoxia of the kidneys are more marked with right-sided heart failure than with left, leading to greater fluid retention, peripheral edema, and more pronounced prerenal azotemia.

SUBCUTANEOUS TISSUES. Some degree of peripheral edema of dependent portions of the body occurs regularly. Indeed, ankle edema may be considered a hallmark of CHF. In severe or long-standing cases, edema may be quite massive and generalized, a condition termed *anasarca*. Of probable significance in the perpetuation of edema is the diminished clearing of plasma aldosterone by the congested liver. This contributes to the elevated levels of this hormone.

PLEURAL SPACES. Effusions may appear, particularly on the right.

BRAIN. Symptoms essentially identical to those described in left-sided failure may occur, representing venous congestion and hypoxia of the central nervous system.

PORTAL SYSTEM OF DRAINAGE. Splenic congestion has already been described. In addition, abnormal accumulations of transudate in the peritoneal cavity may give rise to *ascites.* Congestion of the gut may cause intestinal disturbances.

In summary, right-sided heart failure presents essentially as a venous congestive syndrome, with hepatic and splenic enlargement, peripheral edema, pleural effusions, and ascites. In contrast to left-sided failure, respiratory symptoms may be absent or quite insignificant. *The consideration of heart failure has been divided into two functional units. In the usual case of frank chronic cardiac decompensation, however, these early stages have already passed. Thus, the patient presents with the picture of full-blown CHF, encompassing the clinical syndromes of both right and left heart failure.*

TYPES OF HEART DISEASE

Heart disease is the predominant cause of disability and death in all industrialized nations. In the United States it accounts currently for about 700,000 to 750,000 deaths annually, almost 40% of the total mortality and just short of double the number of deaths caused by all forms of cancer together. In 1900, heart disease occupied fourth place among the ten leading causes of death. The reasons for the present preeminence of heart disease and some recent "heartening" trends are detailed on page 605.[6]

Four categories of cardiac disease account for about 85 to 90% of all cardiac deaths: (1) ischemic heart disease, (2) hypertensive heart disease and pulmonary hypertensive heart disease (cor pulmonale), (3) congenital heart disease, and (4) certain valvular diseases—calcific aortic valve sclerosis, mitral valve prolapse, infective endocarditis, and rheumatic heart disease. Because ischemic heart disease is responsible for the great majority of these deaths, this paramount condition is considered first, followed by the other major disorders. The remaining, less common cardiac diseases are grouped into endocardial-valvular, myocardial, and pericardial diseases, followed by a few entities that refuse to fit into any category.

ISCHEMIC HEART DISEASE (IHD)

IHD is the generic designation for a group of closely related syndromes resulting from an imbalance between the supply and demand of the heart for oxygenated blood. Although ischemia also invokes reduced nutrient substrates and inadequate removal of metabolites, the critical factor is the insufficiency of oxygen. Because coronary artery narrowing or obstruction underlies the myocardial hypoxia (anoxia) in the vast majority of cases, IHD has in the past been referred to as *coronary heart disease* (CHD). However, the International Classification of Diseases prefers the term *ischemic heart disease,* and so we bow to authority while frequently guilty of backsliding.

The heart may suffer a deficiency of oxygen when (1) an increase in demand (e.g., increased heart rate) outpaces the supply of oxygen, (2) oxygen transport in the blood is diminished (e.g., cyanotic congenital heart disease, severe anemia, carbon monoxide poisoning, advanced lung disease, cigarette smoking), but (3) *in over 90% of cases the root cause is reduction in coronary blood flow, owing largely to some complex dynamic interaction among fixed atherosclerotic narrowings of the subepicardial coronary arteries,[7] intraluminal thrombosis overlying a ruptured or fissured plaque, vasospasm, and platelet aggregation.[8]* Rarely, systemic hemodynamic deterioration (e.g., shock) or some form of nonatherosclerotic coronary disease (p. 604) contributes to the perfusion deficit.

Depending on the rate of development of the arterial narrowing(s) and its ultimate severity, four ischemic syndromes may result: (1) angina pectoris, of which there are three variants, the most threatening being unstable angina, (2) myocardial infarction, the most important form of IHD, (3) chronic ischemic heart disease, and (4) sudden cardiac death, which may be superimposed on any of the preceding three conditions. Which syndrome appears depends largely on the proportional contributions of fixed stenosis, thrombosis, platelet aggregation, and spasm. As might be expected, there is considerable overlap among them. Moreover, before any of these overt disorders become manifest, there is a long prodrome (decades) of silent, slowly progressive, coronary atherosclerosis. Thus, the syndromes of IHD are only the late manifestations of coronary atherosclerosis that likely began at birth (p. 565).

EPIDEMIOLOGY. IHD, in its various forms, is the leading cause of death in the United States and other industrialized nations and accounts for about 80% of all cardiac mortality. Annually, about 5 million individuals are diagnosed as having IHD, resulting in approximately 550,000 deaths, many more than all forms of cancer collectively.[9] Awesome as the data may be, they represent an improvement over those that prevailed several decades ago. Up to the late 1960s, the frequency of ischemic heart disease had progressively increased in most industrialized countries to almost epidemic proportions. At that time, the death rate from IHD began to fall in the United States and elsewhere. Since 1968, the overall mortality has fallen in the United States by almost 40%.[10] It is estimated that about 600,000 lives were saved in the United States between 1968 and 1977. A similar welcome trend has occurred in Switzerland, Italy, New Zealand, Australia, Belgium, Canada, and Finland, but not in Sweden, Denmark, the Soviet Union, and most Eastern European countries.[11] Japan too has enjoyed a decline in the mortality from IHD, but recent reports point to a possible upswing. These contrasts are attributed at least in part to differences in lifestyles and the prevalence of the major risk factors for atherosclerosis, (i.e., hypercholesterolemia, cigarette smoking, hypertension, and diabetes) (p. 558). Yet it is difficult to perceive significant differences between Sweden and Finland, so other factors may be involved as well. Some of the decline in mortality is due to improved therapy. Goldman has estimated that about 55% of the decline in mortality between 1968 and 1976 can be attributed to a fall in the incidence of IHD attributable to changed lifestyles, and the remaining 45% he attributed to improvements in the therapy of IHD (mainly acute myocardial infarcts) — for example, use of coronary care units, postinfarction thrombolysis, improved control of arrhythmias, coronary bypass surgery, and percutaneous, transluminal, coronary angioplasty.[12] Worthy of note, in one study of a large corporation the decline attributed to changed lifestyles was twice as great among salaried employees as among wage-earners, suggesting educational and socioeconomic influences.[13]

PATHOGENESIS. As already indicated, the imbalance between the supply of oxygen to the heart and its needs in the causation of the IHD syndromes may in some instances be related to increased myocardial demand or reduced oxygen carrying capacity of the blood, but the dominating influence is reduction in coronary perfusion. Five potential derangements may contribute: (1) first and foremost, stenosing coronary atherosclerosis, (2) platelet aggregation within the coronary system, (3) coronary vasospasm, (4) nonatherosclerotic coronary disease, and (5) hemodynamic derangements. Although there are still some areas of uncertainty, the following observations are reasonably well established.

ROLE OF CORONARY ATHEROSCLEROSIS[14]
• Over 90% of patients with one of the ischemic heart syndromes have advanced coronary atherosclerosis with one or more stenotic lesions causing at least 75% reduction of the cross-sectional area of at least one of the major subepicardial arteries. A 75% reduction will block the augmented coronary flow needed to meet even moderate increases in myocardial demand.
• Although only a single major coronary epicardial trunk may be affected, more often two or all three — left anterior descending (LAD), left circumflex (LC), right coronary (RC) — are involved[15] (Fig. 13–1). In general, about one third of patients have single-vessel, another third have two-vessel, and slightly more than a third have three-major-vessel disease.
• The clinically significant fixed stenosing plaques may be located anywhere within the three major trunks but tend to occur within the first 2 cm of the LAD and LC and the proximal and distal thirds of the RC. Sometimes the major secondary branches are also involved (i.e., the diagonal branches of the LAD, the obtuse marginal branches of the LC, or the posterior descending branch of the RC). Surprisingly, there is no strong correlation between the extent and severity of the stenosing coronary atherosclerosis and the various ischemic syndromes or their severity.[16]
• In the more serious forms of IHD — unstable angina, acute myocardial infarction, and sudden cardiac death — some combination of changes (an occlusive thrombus overlying an ulcerated or fissured plaque, platelet aggregation, or vasospasm) usually initiates the acute event, as will be discussed presently.

ROLE OF PLATELETS
• Rupture of an atherosclerotic plaque exposing subendothelial collagen may lead to platelet adherence, activation, and an autocatalytic chain reaction producing a large pool of activated platelets within the coronary system.[16]
• The aggregated platelets may contribute to the build-up of an occlusive thrombus or form microemboli to contribute to the perfusion deficit.
• Thromboxane, histamine, serotonin, and other vasoactive products are released by activated platelets, contributing to possible coronary vasospasm and reduced myocardial perfusion.
• Preliminary results of long-term use of small doses of aspirin suggest a reduction in death from IHD, attributed to inhibition of synthesis of thromboxane A_2, a potent aggregator of platelets and a vasoconstrictor.[17]
• Diets rich in fish with their polyunsaturated "omega-3" fatty acids substantially lower the incidence and mortality from ischemic heart disease attributed at least in part to reduced platelet aggregation (possibly also to induction of an antithrombotic state).[18]

ROLE OF VASOSPASM
• Vasospasm has been documented angiographically in large atherosclerotic epicardial arteries in some patients with angina or myocardial infarction.[19]
• In rare cases, coronary artery spasm has been associated with acute myocardial infarction in patients having *no* atherosclerotic coronary narrowings.
• Spastic narrowing of fixed coronary lesions may contribute to rupture or fissuring of plaques leading to thrombosis and platelet aggregation.
• The coronary arteries are well innervated, but in addition, platelet-derived products, such as thromboxane A_2, could initiate or aggravate coronary artery spasm.[20]

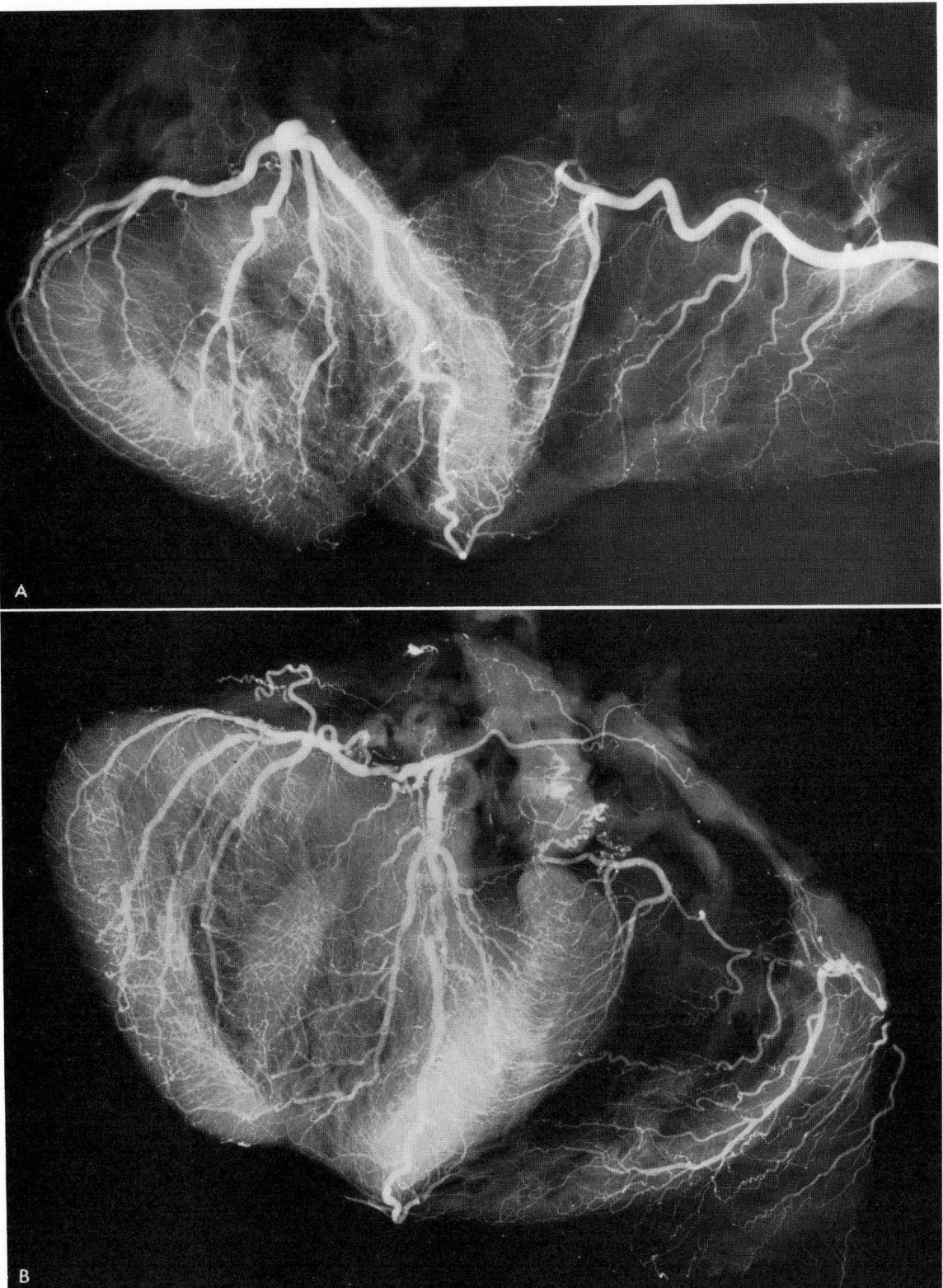

Figure 13–1. *A,* Angiogram of opened heart with normal coronary arteries filled with radiopaque mass. On right is the horizontal main right coronary artery with small descending twigs. On left is visualized the major left descending ramus and the horizontal major left circumflex ramus. Between these two are several large diagonal branches. The vessels show progressively diminishing lumina with no irregular narrowings or obstruction. *B,* Angiogram of an opened heart with severely narrowed and occluded atherosclerotic coronaries. The right coronary artery fails to fill over much of its length. The twigs of this vessel are filled by retrograde anastomotic collaterals. There is uneven narrowing and tortuosity of left descending ramus and left circumflex ramus. Compare with *A.*

ROLE OF NONATHEROSCLEROTIC LESIONS OF THE CORONARY ARTERIES

The following disorders, when they involve the coronary arteries, have all been associated with reduced perfusion and one or more of the IHD syndromes:

• Emboli to coronary arteries.
• Arteritis (e.g., Takayasu's disease, lupus erythematosus, Kawasaki's syndrome, polyarteritis nodosa, other forms).
• Cocaine abuse (arrhythmias, vasospasm).
• Trauma to coronary arteries.

ROLE OF HEMODYNAMIC ALTERATIONS

• Flow through the coronary system depends on the pressure differential between the blood at the levels of the coronary ostia and the coronary sinus.
• A significant drop in blood pressure as may occur in shock, massive hemorrhage, spinal anesthesia, or during an operation may severely reduce coronary perfusion, particularly in vessels already narrowed by fixed stenoses.
• Elevation in pressure in the right atrium and coronary sinus as occurs with marked tricuspid regurgitation lowers the differential in pressure and reduces perfusion.
• Left-sided heart failure reduces perfusion of the coronary system.

Certain of these various mechanisms are more important than others in the causation of the individual patterns of ischemic heart disease, as will be pointed out in the consideration of each. But various combinations are frequently involved in all.

ANGINA PECTORIS

Angina pectoris (AP) is a symptom complex of IHD characterized by paroxysmal attacks of substernal or precordial chest discomfort (variously described as constricting, squeezing, choking, knife-like) caused by myocardial ischemia that falls precariously short of inducing infarction. Often there is myocardial damage from previous old infarctions and usually evidence of long-standing marginal ischemia with interstitial fibrosis and myocyte atrophy. Because AP is basically a clinical syndrome, our consideration of it can be relatively brief.

There are three overlapping patterns of AP: (1) stable or typical angina, (2) Prinzmetal's or variant angina, and (3) unstable or crescendo angina. Although these subsets differ in some respects, individual patients may manifest features of one or all concurrently or at different times.[20] All are caused by varying combinations of fixed stenosing lesions, vasospasm, platelet aggregation, and increased myocardial demand. Although each of these mechanisms plays a greater role in certain subsets, all participate to some degree in the three patterns.

Stable angina is the most common form and is therefore called *typical AP.* This syndrome is charac-

teristically associated with electrocardiographic ST segment depression because the ischemia is most intense in the poorly perfused subendocardial region of the left ventricular myocardium compressed by the outer layers of myocardium. *The pathogenesis of typical AP appears to be stenosing coronary atherosclerosis that reduces the coronary perfusion to a critical level, rendering the heart vulnerable to further ischemia whenever there is increased demand, such as can be produced by physical activity, emotional excitement, or any other cause of increased cardiac workload.* In some instances, the attack of pain follows a level of exertion that would ordinarily be readily tolerated. It is possible, therefore, that in particular instances, vasospasm may contribute to the imbalance between supply and demand.[21]

Prinzmetal's variant angina refers to a pattern of angina that occurs at rest and has been documented to be due to coronary artery spasm. Usually there is elevation of the ST segment (in contrast to the ST segment depression in typical angina), indicative of transmural ischemia. Although individuals with this form of angina may well have significant coronary atherosclerosis, the anginal attacks are unrelated to physical activity, heart rate, or blood pressure and respond promptly to vasodilators such as nitroglycerin and calcium channel blockers. The pathogenesis of these vasospastic attacks is not known. One theory proposes atherosclerosis-induced hypercontractility of segments of the major epicardial coronary trunks. Another points to abnormal infiltrates of mast cells within the coronary adventitia and the possible release by them of humoral vasoconstrictants (e.g., histamine, serotonin, or PGD_2). In truth, the mechanism is not known.

Unstable or crescendo angina refers to a pattern that occurs with increasing frequency, is precipitated with progressively less effort, often occurs at rest, and tends to be of prolonged duration. In contrast to the other patterns, the ischemia in unstable angina appears to be precariously short of inducing infarction and so this syndrome is sometimes referred to as *"preinfarction angina"* or *"acute coronary insufficiency."* The basis for the perfusion deficit is not always clear and is likely to be multifactorial in origin and to involve the following:

1. Progressive atherosclerosis with increasingly stenotic fixed lesions.
2. Fissuring, ulceration, or rupture of an atherosclerotic plaque with superimposed thrombosis.
3. Platelet aggregation and activation in relation to a complicated atheromatous plaque worsening the luminal obstruction and releasing vasoconstrictor agents (e.g., thromboxane A_2).[22]
4. Vasospasm.

In most patients, rupture or fissuring of a fixed lesion with superimposed thrombosis is involved.[23] Usually, however, the occlusion involves a coronary branch rather than a main trunk, or coronary collaterals prevent infarction. There is, in addition, a growing body of evidence that either platelet activation and aggregation precede thrombus formation or that these alone are responsible for many attacks of unstable angina. Whatever the mechanism, unstable angina forewarns of the possibility of a subsequent acute myocardial infarction. In the spectrum of ischemic heart syndromes, then, it lies intermediate between stable angina on the one hand and myocardial infarction on the other.

MYOCARDIAL INFARCTION (MI)

As pointed out earlier, acute myocardial infarction (AMI) is overwhelmingly the most important form of IHD in industrialized nations, and alone is the leading cause of death in the United States and elsewhere. About 1,500,000 individuals in the United States suffer an AMI annually, resulting in about 500,000 deaths.[9] Over half of these fatalities occur before the patient reaches the hospital owing largely to the unfortunate onset of some form of fatal arrhythmia, such as ventricular fibrillation. In more personal terms a North American male has a one in five chance (some would say one in three chance) of having an MI or dying suddenly from an acute ischemic event before reaching the age of 65 years. There can be no doubt that MI is the number one clinical challenge in affluent societies.

There are in fact two types of myocardial infarction, having differing morphology and clinical significance. The more common and serious type is the *transmural infarct,* in which the ischemic necrosis involves the full or nearly full thickness of the ventricular wall and is at least 2.5 cm in greatest diameter. As will be seen, this pattern of infarction is usually associated with severe coronary atherosclerosis with superimposed thrombosis. In contrast, *subendocardial (nontransmural) infarcts* constitute areas of ischemic necrosis limited to the inner one third or at most one half of the ventricular wall. As was pointed out, the subendocardial zone is normally least well perfused and therefore most vulnerable to any reduction in coronary flow. The pathogenesis of these lesions is less clear, but in the great majority, there is diffuse stenosing coronary atherosclerosis but *no* superimposed thrombosis. However, the two types are closely interrelated because in experimental models and likely in humans the transmural infarct may begin with subendocardial necrosis that extends in a "wave front" across the full thickness of the ventricular wall.[24]

INCIDENCE. Because of the dominating importance of coronary atherosclerosis in its pathogenesis, the incidence of MI is the incidence of atherosclerosis (p. 558). The declining frequency of deaths from IHD, most caused by MI, in the United States and the geographic differences were discussed earlier (p. 558). *An MI may occur at virtually any age, but the frequency rises progressively with age.* MI may occur in the very elderly, as well as in younger individuals, even in the third decade of life, particularly when such predispositions to atherosclerosis as hypertension, cigarette smoking, diabetes mellitus, familial hypercholesterolemia, and other causes of hyperlipoproteinemia are present. Five per cent of "heart attacks" occur in people under age 40 and 45% under age 65. Blacks and whites are affected equally often. Throughout life, males are at significantly greater risk of dying of an MI than females, the differential progressively declining with advancing age. Only at age 80 and over does the gap close. White males under the age of 45 in the United States have a sixfold greater risk of MI than comparable females. In males 45 to 54 years of age, there is a four- to five-fold difference, which falls to about a two-fold difference in the eighth decade.[25] *Except for those having some predisposing atherogenic condition, women are remarkably protected against MI during reproductive life.* However, the use of oral contraceptives (OCs), *as formulated in the past,* increases the risk of MI. The general data were presented on page 488. Several studies have shown that users of OCs (as formulated in the past) have a 4.5-fold greater risk of sustaining an MI than nonusers. However, the risk is largely confined to those over the age of 35 who are smokers. Nonsmokers below this age incur no increased risk from the use of oral contraceptives. The newer formulations of OCs with their markedly reduced content of estrogen have reduced the risk at all ages by at least 80%.[26]

A number of other variables influence the risk and, therefore, the incidence of MI. Cigarette smoking is a major factor; the increased risk is linearly correlated with number of cigarettes smoked daily (Fig 13–2). Happily, the increased risk disappears within a few years of complete abstinence. More controversial are such influences as personality structure, regular exercise, and alcohol consumption. A number of studies have claimed that so-called type A individuals—hard-driving, impatient, competitive, compulsive—are coronary prone. However, recent studies do not reveal any increased risk in these "eager beavers."[27] Happily there is nearly universal agreement that an inverse relationship exists between regular exercise maintained for years and the risk of dying from IHD.[28] Moreover, physical activity appears to lessen the susceptibility to fatal cardiac arrhythmias following an MI. So it well may be that "the joggers shall inherit the earth." Moderate alcohol consumption has likewise been accorded a protective role. A recent study in women revealed that consumers of 1 to 2 drinks of liquor per day had about half the risk of myocardial infarction of abstainers.[29] Attractive as the idea may be of using martinis or other forms of alcohol for protection against coronary disease, there is evidence that heavy use of alcohol increases the risk of coronary heart disease.

PATHOGENESIS. First, the transmural infarct is considered, but the important point should be made at the outset: As the ischemic lesion develops, it

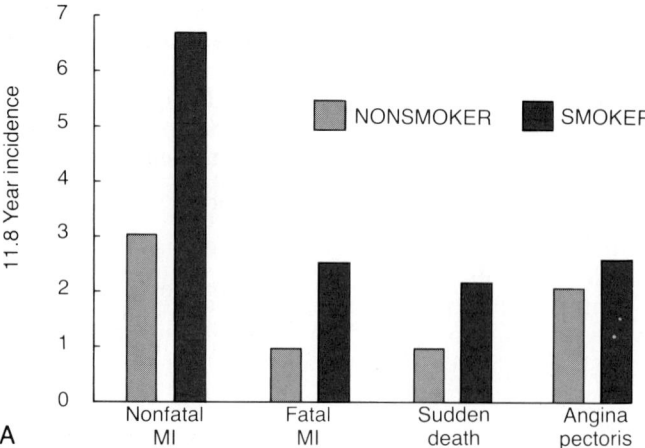

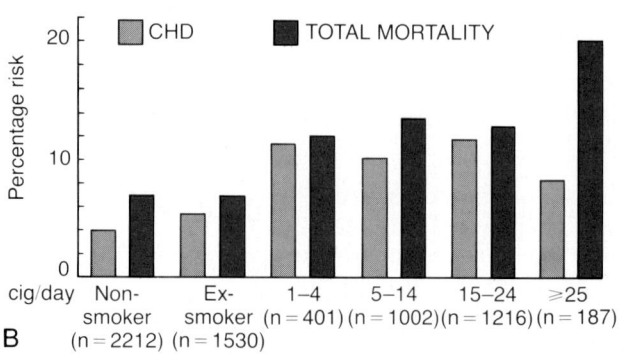

Figure 13–2. *A,* Smoking and risk for different manifestations of coronary heart disease among 7495 men, aged 47 to 55 years at the time of entry and followed up for 11.8 years. MI = myocardial infarction. *B,* Number of cigarettes smoked and risk for MI or sudden cardiac death and total mortality rate among 7495 men, aged 47 to 55 years at the time of entry and followed up for 11.8 years. (Modified from The Primary Prevention Study, Göteborg, Sweden.) (Redrawn from Wilhelmsen, L.: Coronary heart disease: Epidemiology of smoking and intervention studies of smoking. Am. Heart J. *115*:242, 1988.)

evolves in time and space (configuration). We consider the basis for the ischemia first and then the myocardial consequences of such ischemia. *There is growing consensus that about 90% of transmural acute myocardial infarctions (AMIs) are caused by an occlusive intracoronary thrombus overlying an ulcerated or fissured stenotic atheroma.*[30] Platelet aggregation and activation and vasospasm may contribute to the acute event, as is pointed out later, and infrequently by themselves may cause an AMI even in the absence of fixed critical stenoses. In addition, increased myocardial demand, as with tachycardia or hemodynamic problems, such as a drop in blood pressure, can worsen the situation and infrequently constitute the final blow in an already precarious situation. *Contrariwise, it is worth noting at this point that occlusive thrombosis may occur in markedly atherosclerotic coronary arteries without inducing infarction owing to collateral circulation.* As pointed out earlier (p. 598) there are numerous vascular intercommunications between major epicardial trunks and their ramifications. With stenosing or occluding disease, these collaterals may expand to provide perfusion from a relatively unobstructed trunk. Despite all these variables, *until proved otherwise, behind every AMI a dynamic interaction has occurred among several or all of the following: severe coronary atherosclerosis, an acute atheromatous change (fissuring, ulceration), superimposed thrombosis, vasospasm, and platelet activation.*[31] The interplay of all these variables and the interrelationships of the various forms of IHD are shown in Figure 13–3. In the typical case, the following sequence of events can be proposed:

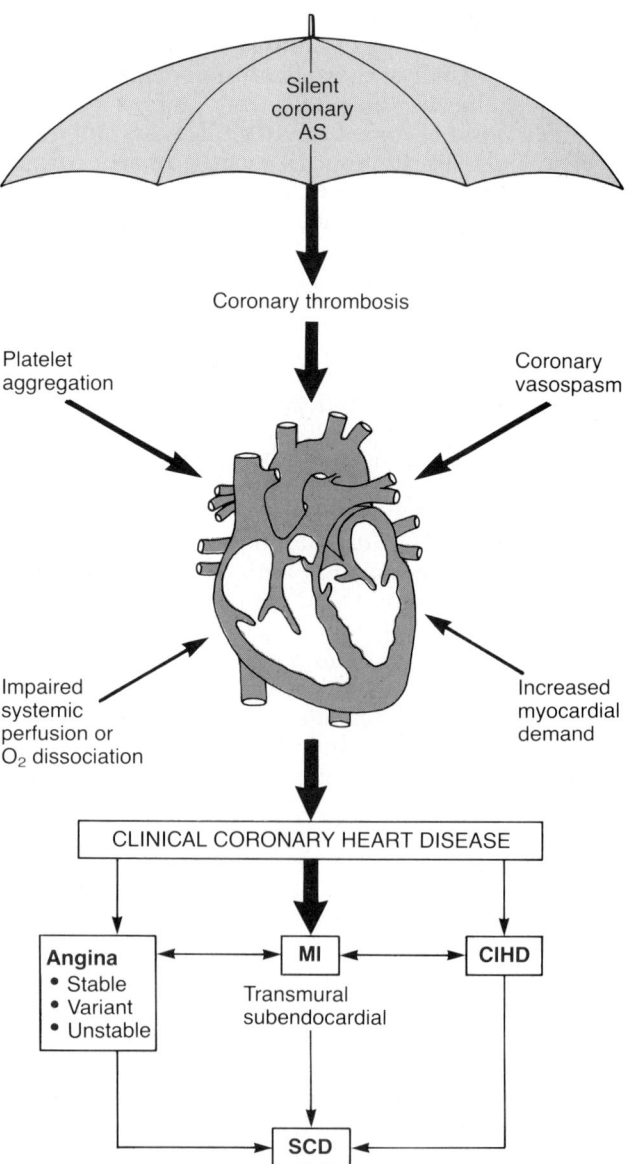

Figure 13–3. A schematic representation of the multiple mechanisms leading to clinical coronary heart disease and the interrelationships of the various clinical patterns. CIHD = chronic ischemic heart disease. SCD = sudden cardiac death.

• The initial event is a sudden change in the morphology of a stenosing atheroma, i.e., intraplaque hemorrhage, ulceration, or fissuring. Usually the atheroma had already caused more than a 75% reduction in luminal cross section. The mechanism of the atheromatous change is uncertain but may be an episode of vasospasm that fractures a calcific plaque, tachycardia imposing physical stresses, hypercholesterolemia, intraplaque hemorrhage with ballooning and rupture, or other mechanisms.[32]

• Platelets are exposed to subendothelial collagen with aggregation, activation, and release of adenosine diphosphate, a potent platelet aggregator, with build-up of the platelet mass. The platelet mass may give rise to emboli or initiate thrombosis.

• Simultaneously, tissue thromboplastin is released, activating the extrinsic pathway of coagulation.

• Adherent activated platelets release thromboxane A_2, serotonin, and platelet factors 3 and 4, predisposing to coagulation, favoring vasospasm, and adding to the mechanical build-up of the thrombus.

• Within the hour, perhaps in minutes, the thrombus evolves to become occlusive, triggering the transmural AMI.

If indeed thrombosis is the usual trigger event leading to AMI, how to explain past autopsy reports indicating coronary thrombosis in less than 50% of cases of myocardial infarction? The seminal observations of DeWood and coworkers offered a plausible explanation that has subsequently been confirmed by others. They demonstrated that when coronary angiography was performed within four hours of the onset of an apparent MI, a thrombosed coronary artery was found in almost 90% of cases, but that the incidence of acute occlusion fell to about 60% when the angiography was delayed until 12 to 24 hours following the infarction.[33] The implication was clear. With the passage of time, at least some occlusions clear spontaneously because of either lysis of the thrombus or relaxation of spasm, or a combination of the two. Numerous subsequent studies using intravenous or intracoronary infusion of fibrinolysins have documented the presence of thrombi by restoring flow to obstructed vessels in 75 to 95% of recent myocardial infarcts.[34] There can be little doubt then about the importance of thrombosis in the induction of most AMIs.

Relative to the 10% of transmural AMIs unassociated with atherosclerotic thrombosis, many mechanisms may be involved:

• In about one third of these cases, there is no significant atherosclerosis and indeed the coronary arteries appear normal angiographically.

• Vasospasm with or without coronary atherosclerosis may induce the acute perfusion deficit, perhaps in association with platelet aggregation.[35]

• Emboli from a left-sided mural thrombosis or vegetative endocarditis or paradoxic emboli from the periphery (through a patent foramen ovale) could cause the coronary occlusion.

• A nonatherosclerotic coronary lesion (e.g., some form of arteritis) with superimposed thrombosis may lead to coronary occlusion.

• Cocaine abuse with or without underlying coronary atherosclerosis has induced an AMI attributable to spasm and possibly superimposed thrombosis.[36]

As a group, patients with normal or relatively normal coronary arteries are young, have no history of antecedent angina, and have an excellent prognosis.

As mentioned at the outset, the development of an acute MI is a dynamic process. Ischemic myocardial cells do not die instantaneously, nor do all the cells at risk die simultaneously; the rates of cell death depend on variations in level of ischemia introduced by collateral flow. Acutely ischemic myofibers undergo the progressive sequence of changes cited in Table 13–1. The "window" between the onset of ischemia and irreversible injury is of obvious relevance to current methods of treatment of acute MIs using fibrinolytic agents and balloon angioplasty in an effort to establish reperfusion of the area of ischemia. Depending mostly on the duration of the period of complete ischemia, regions of the infarct partially (but inadequately) sustained by collateral flow may be salvaged. However, the "rescued" myocytes may have sustained sufficient biochemical injury to be dysfunctional ("stunned") for 1 to 2 days despite their viability.

In the experimental animal, about 20 to 40 minutes after complete occlusion of a major coronary artery a "wavefront" of ischemic necrosis of the dependent myocardium develops beginning in the subendocardial zone and progressing eventually across the thickness of the left ventricular wall. The subendocardium is the least well perfused zone of the left ventricular wall because its microcirculation is most subject to the compressive forces of the outer layers of myocardium during systole. Moreover, the collateral network is richest subepicardially and sparsest subendocardially. There is considerable evidence that transmural MIs in humans evolve in the same manner, beginning with subendocardial necrosis. The ultimate size of the infarct depends on: (1) the extent, severity, and duration of ischemia, (2) the magnitude of the collateral flow, and (3) the metabolic demands of the myocardium at risk. Depending on the interplay of these variables, the area of necrosis may well be surrounded by a margin of reversibly injured myofibers precariously sustained by flow from unaffected coronary networks and collaterals. Thus, the region of ischemic necrosis may well be an island in a larger area of patchy foci of necrosis, inter-

Table 13–1. Time Sequence of Changes in Acutely Ischemic Myocardial Cells

Beginning depletion of ATP	Almost immediate
Loss of contractility	1–2 minutes
50% depletion of ATP	10 minutes
Irreversible cell injury	20–40 minutes

mingled with reversibly injured myocytes. It is evident that the transmural MI is not from its beginning simply a defined focus of coagulative necrosis.

The *pathogenesis of the subendocardial infarct* differs somewhat from that of the transmural infarct. As pointed out, the subendocardium is most vulnerable to any reduction in coronary blood flow. Almost always there is advanced coronary atherosclerosis, but often no critical stenosis. Autopsy studies indicate coronary thrombosis in about 20% of instances,[37] but angiographic studies during life indicate greater frequency.[38] There is a suspicion then that often a thrombus initiates the process, but is then spontaneously lysed. In support of this hypothesis is the evidence that fibrinolytic treatment of patients with apparent recently developed subendocardial infarcts is of unmistakable benefit.[38] Be that as it may, at autopsy total occlusion of a major coronary artery or branch is uncommon, and so other possible scenarios have been proposed, such as diffuse atherosclerosis with global reduction of coronary flow transformed into critical insufficiency by increased demand, vasospasm, or platelet aggregation.

It is evident that many of the details of the sequence of events leading to both forms of MI are still uncertain, but at least the chaos has given way to mere confusion.

MORPHOLOGY.   Virtually all transmural infarcts involve the left ventricle (including the interventricular septum). When they affect the posterior free wall and posterior portion of the septum, they extend into the adjacent right ventricular wall in about 15 to 30% of cases.[39] Isolated infarction of the right ventricle occurs in 1 to 3% of cases, usually in association with chronic right ventricular strain and hypertrophy. Atrial infarction has been found to be present in 5 to 10% of cases of AMI when assiduously sought. Most often it occurs in conjunction with a large posterior left ventricular infarct that extends into the right ventricle and into one or both of the atria. Rarest of all is isolated atrial infarction, most often on the right. Atrial infarctions are worthy of note because they are almost always followed by mural thrombosis within the affected chamber and sometimes by cardiac rupture.[40]

The **transmural infarct** usually ranges from 4 to 10 cm in longest dimension, but may involve the entire circumference of the left ventricle. Almost always, there is a narrow rim of preserved subendocardial myocardium sustained by direct imbibition. As already emphasized, a related occlusive thrombus may or may not be identified at the time of postmortem examination, and indeed in rare instances the coronary arteries may be entirely normal when it is presumed that the causal mechanism was vasospasm. Despite these inconstancies, severe stenosing coronary atherosclerosis is generally present, and the frequencies of critical narrowing (and possibly thrombosis) of each of the three main arterial trunks and the associated myocardial lesions are as follows:

Left anterior descending coronary artery (40 to 50%)	Anterior wall of left ventricle near apex; anterior two thirds of interventricular septum
Right coronary artery (30 to 40%)	Posterior wall of left ventricle; posterior one third of interventricular septum
Left circumflex coronary artery (15 to 20%)	Lateral wall of left ventricle

Other locations are sometimes encountered, such as the left main stem coronary artery. One virtually never encounters stenosing atherosclerosis or thrombosis of a penetrating intramyocardial ramification of the epicardial trunks. Occasionally, a thrombus is present in the absence of an MI; intercoronary collaterals may provide sufficient flow to prevent ischemic necrosis. Alternatively, multiple severe stenoses or thromboses may be present with only a single transmural infarct owing to collateral circulation. Another variation on the collateral theme is the appearance of an infarction in the area of supply of the left anterior descending artery (LAD) in association with an acute thrombosis of the right coronary artery (RC) when the region of myocardium normally supplied by the LAD becomes dependent on collateral flow derived from the RC—"infarction at a distance."

Although most transmural infarcts occur singly, several of varying age in the same heart are not infrequently found. The patient may survive the initial insult only to succumb to a second weeks to years later. Indeed, recurrent infarctions are commonplace. Alternatively, extension of an infarct may lead to lesions of varying age—the "stuttering infarct." Examination of the heart in such cases often reveals a central zone of infarction that is days to weeks older than a peripheral margin of more freshly ischemic necrosis. An initial infarct may extend because of retrograde propagation of a thrombus, more proximal vasospasm, impaired cardiac contractility that renders more proximal stenoses critically insufficient, the development of platelet-fibrin microemboli, or the appearance of an arrhythmia.

Depending on the length of survival of the patient, the area of necrosis undergoes a progressive sequence of macroscopic changes.[41] Because of the time required for biochemical reactions to effect morphologic changes, myocardial infarcts **less than six to 12 hours old** are usually inapparent on gross examination. A slight pallor may be present. It is sometimes possible to highlight the area of necrosis within the first three to six hours by histochemical techniques. Because dehydrogenases are depleted in the area of ischemia, immersion of tissue slices in a solution of triphenyl-tetrazolium chloride (TTC) imparts a red-brown color to noninfarcted myocardium where the enzymes are preserved, revealing the infarcted areas as an unstained pale zone.[42,43] **By 13 to 24 hours,** the lesion can be identified either because of its pallor or because it has a red-blue cyanotic hue due to the stagnated, trapped blood. Progressively thereafter the infarct becomes a more sharply defined, yellow, well-demarcated, somewhat softened area that by the end of the first week is rimmed by a hyperemic, moist, narrow zone of highly vascularized reactive connective tissue (Fig. 13–4). Over the succeeding weeks, the necrotic muscle is progressively replaced by the ingrowth of fibrous vascularized scar tissue. In most instances, this scarring is well advanced by the end of the sixth week, but the time required for total replacement depends on the size of the original lesion.

There are many morphologic complications associated with transmural MIs, but even before these become apparent, the heart may decompensate because of the dysfunctional area of myocardium, and a variety of arrhythmias may appear, as will be pointed out later. The **anterior or posterior papillary muscle may undergo infarction** when the contiguous free wall is affected. The resultant loss of papillary muscle contraction may acutely induce incompetence of the mitral valve that can persist with fibrous healing of the infarct. Even worse, the **acutely infarcted papillary muscle may rupture transversely** to cause catastrophic gross incompetence of the mitral valve. A **fibrinous** or **fibrinohemorrhagic pericarditis** usually develops about the second or third day. This may be localized to the region overlying the necrotic area or it may be generalized. With healing of the infarct, the pericarditis usually resolves. Involvement of the ventricular endocardium often results in **mural thrombosis,** which produces a risk of **peripheral embolism,** and later dense fibrous thickening. **Rupture of the infarct** occurs in 1 to 5% of cases (Fig. 13–5). It may occur in the free wall of the left ventricle or less often, the IV septum. The median time to rupture is four to five days, when the ischemic focus is maximally soft.[44] However, rupture may occur within a day of infarction or, in other instances, as late as the end of the second week. Rupture of the free wall almost always causes massive pericardial hemorrhage and **cardiac tamponade.** Rupture of the interventricular septum produces a left-to-right shunt.[45] With large infarcts, the necrotic area may balloon out eventually to produce a **ven-**

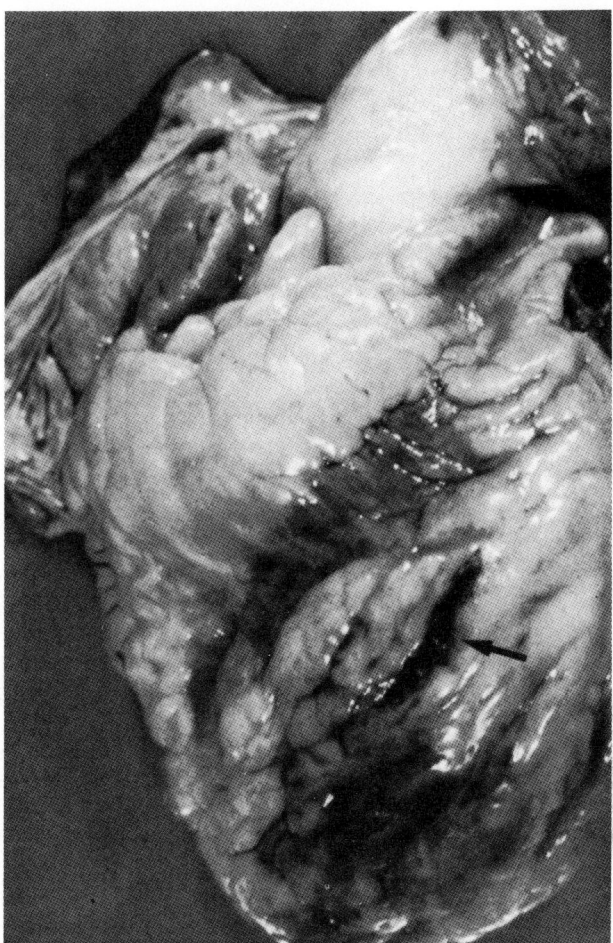

Figure 13–5. External surface of a heart with a three-day-old infarct. Dark linear tear *(arrow)* communicates with a rupture of anterior free wall of left ventricle.

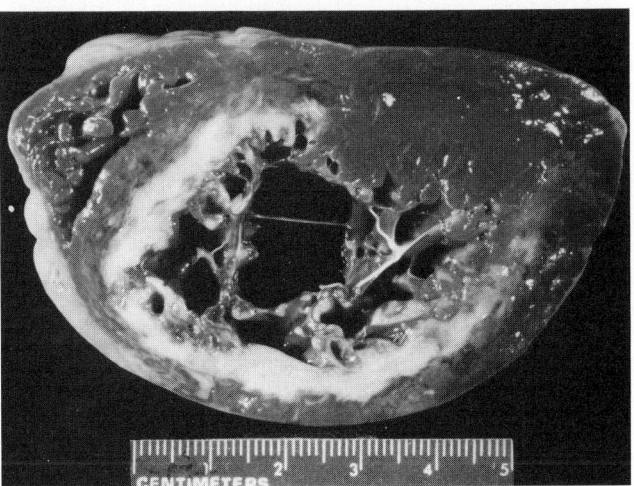

Figure 13–4. Acute myocardial infarction of the left ventricle of ten days' duration. The transection of the heart reveals the very large, almost circumferential, well-demarcated, pale, recent infarct. At points it traverses the wall.

tricular aneurysm. Mural thrombosis is common in such aneurysms.

The histopathologic changes also pursue a more or less predictable progression.[41,46] The irreversibly injured cells undergo typical ischemic coagulative necrosis followed eventually by fibrosis (Figs. 13–6 and 13–7). With the light microscope **using routine tissue stains the coagulative necrosis is not detectable for the first four to eight hours.** However, a number of more subtle changes may be seen at this time. There may be slight separation of the myocardial fibers by edema fluid. **Stretching and waviness of the myocardial fibers at the border of the infarct may appear an hour after the onset of ischemia.** It is thought that these changes result from the forceful systolic tugs by the viable fibers immediately adjacent to the non-contractile dead fibers, stretching and buckling them (Fig. 13–8). Two additional changes may be seen in the margins of infarcts: fine droplets of lipid in the viable cells adjacent to those that have died and large, cleared vacuolar spaces within cells, sometimes leaving only a peripheral rim of sarcoplasm harboring the displaced nucleus—so-called **vacuolar degeneration or myocytolysis.**[47] The vacuolar space is

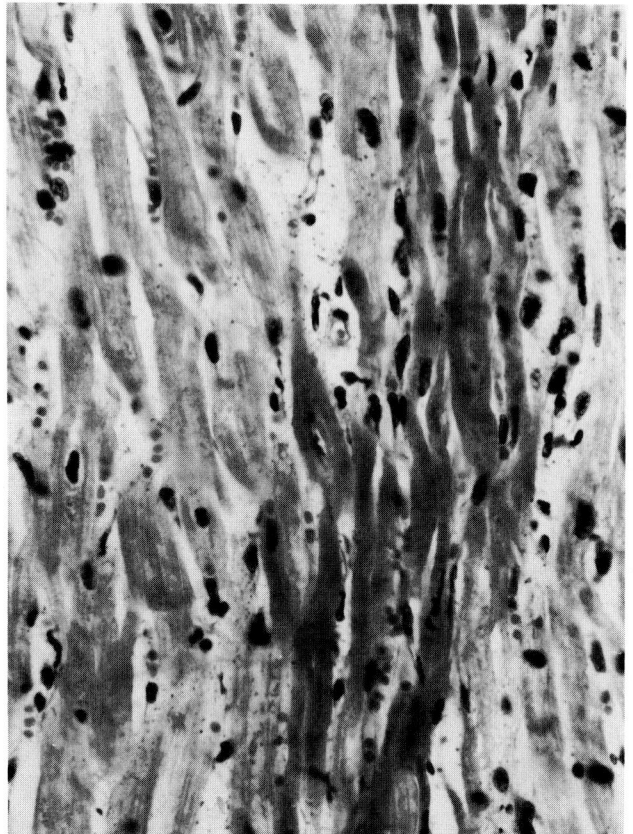

Figure 13–6. A small focus of acute infarction (two days old) on the margins of a large infarct. Dark coagulated myofibers with preserved outlines contrast with surrounding viable normal myocardial cells.

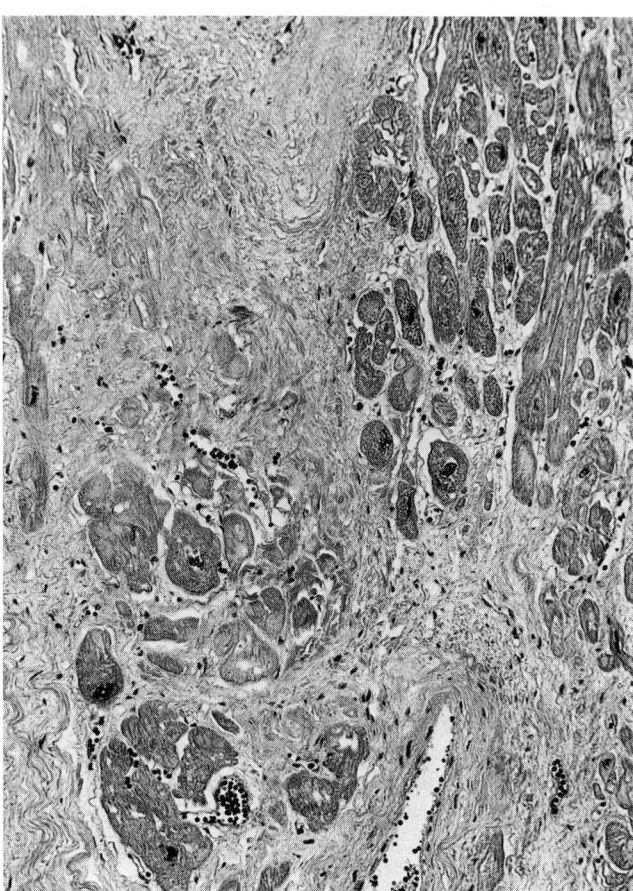

Figure 13–7. A well-healed myocardial infarct with replacement of the necrotic fibers by dense collagenous scar.

apparently filled with water but may contain traces of glycogen and lipids. It is a reversible alteration that is particularly frequent in the thin zone of viable subendocardial cells.

Early histologic recognition of acute MIs continues to be a problem of considerable importance, particularly when death has occurred within minutes to a few hours of the onset of the ischemic injury. No technique has proved infallible during the critical first hours following the onset of ischemia but some of the changes are collated in Table 13–2, in addition to the microscopic and macroscopic changes, which in the last analysis are the most dependable.

Many additional anatomic changes have been introduced by current methods of attempted prevention and treatment of an AMI. Virtually standard today is immediate thrombolytic therapy in an attempt to quickly reperfuse the infarct and possibly rescue the ischemic heart muscle or at least salvage the precarious margins. Occasionally, therefore, with fibrinolytic reperfusion within an hour, the heart may reveal no evidence of infarction; yet the "stunned," dysfunctional myocardium may not be capable of sustaining life. Sometimes there are focal areas of necrosis as markers of large surrounding zones of dysfunctional muscle.[48] With regard to the amount of tissue about the periph-

ery of an area of necrosis that might be salvaged by prompt intervention,[49] most of the evidence to date indicates that at best it is very limited. After an interval of complete ischemia lasting more than 1 to 2 hours the interface between viable and dead myocardium is quite sharply defined.[50] However, with early reperfusion of an area of ischemia, irreversibly injured myocytes may reveal **contraction band necrosis.**[50] It takes the form of intensely eosinophilic transverse bands that span the myofiber. They are produced by hypercontraction of myofibrils in the dying cell (Fig. 13–9). Thus ischemia followed soon thereafter by reperfusion may permit recovery of reversibly injured cells; but on the other hand, the rapid influx of Ca^{++} may irreversibly injure some precarious cells because of the abnormal permeability of their cell membranes[24] (Fig. 13–10).

Additional features introduced by current modes of therapy are coronary artery bypass grafts and intracoronary artery changes secondary to percutaneous transluminal balloon angioplasty.[51] Most commonly used for bypass grafts are segments of saphenous vein or the freed-up internal mammary artery, which retains its origin from the subclavian artery. When the venous grafts have been in place for 5 to 10 years they are likely to reveal fibrocollagenous intimal thickening and many develop atherosclerosis indistinguishable from that found in the native coronary

Table 13-2. Sequence of Changes in Myocardial Infarction

TIME	ELECTRON MICROSCOPE	HISTOCHEMISTRY	LIGHT MICROSCOPE	GROSS CHANGES
0–½ hr	*Reversible injury* Mitochondrial swelling; distortion of cristae; matrix densities; relaxation of myofibrils	↓Dehydrogenases ↓Oxidases ↓Phosphorylases ↓Glycogen ↓K and ↑ Na$^+$ and Ca^{++}	? Waviness of fibers at border	
1–2 hr	*Irreversible injury* Sarcolemmal disruption: mitochondrial amorphous densities			
4–12 hr	Margination of nuclear chromatin		Beginning coagulation necrosis; edema hemorrhage; beginning neutrophilic infiltrate	
18–24 hr			Continuing coagulation necrosis; Pallor (pyknosis of nuclei, shrunken eosinophilic cytoplasm), marginal contraction band necrosis	Pallor
24–72 hr			Total coagulative necrosis with loss of nuclei and striations; heavy interstitial infiltrate of neutrophils	Pallor, sometimes hyperemia
3–7 days			Beginning disintegration of dead myofibers and resorption of sarcoplasm by macrophages; onset of marginal fibrovascular response	Hyperemic border, central yellow-brown softening
10 days			Well-developed necrotic changes; prominent fibrovascular reaction in margins	Maximally yellow and soft vascularized margins, red-brown and depressed
7th wk				Scarring complete

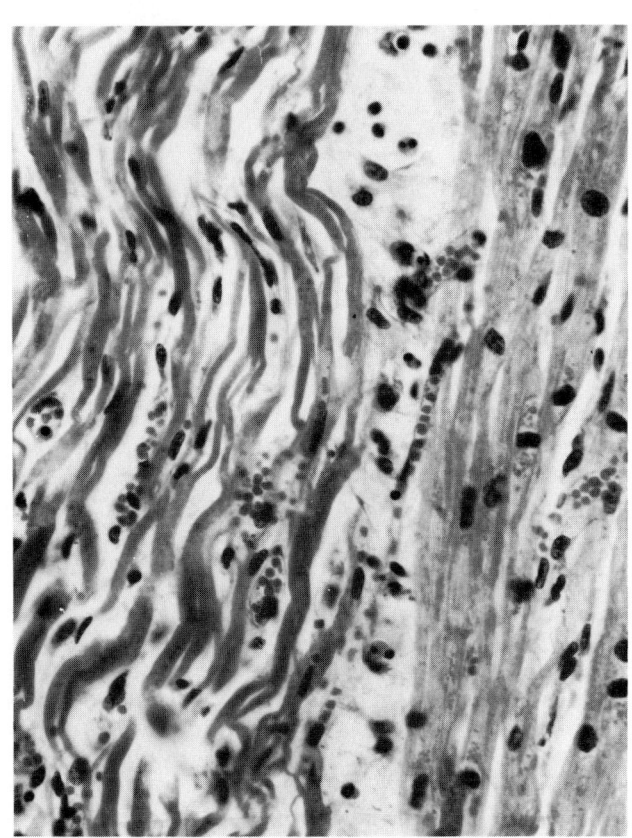

Figure 13-8. "Wavy fibers" in a two-day-old infarct showing coagulative changes, elongation, and narrowing, compared with normal fibers to right. Widened spaces between the dead fibers contain edema fluid and scattered neutrophils.

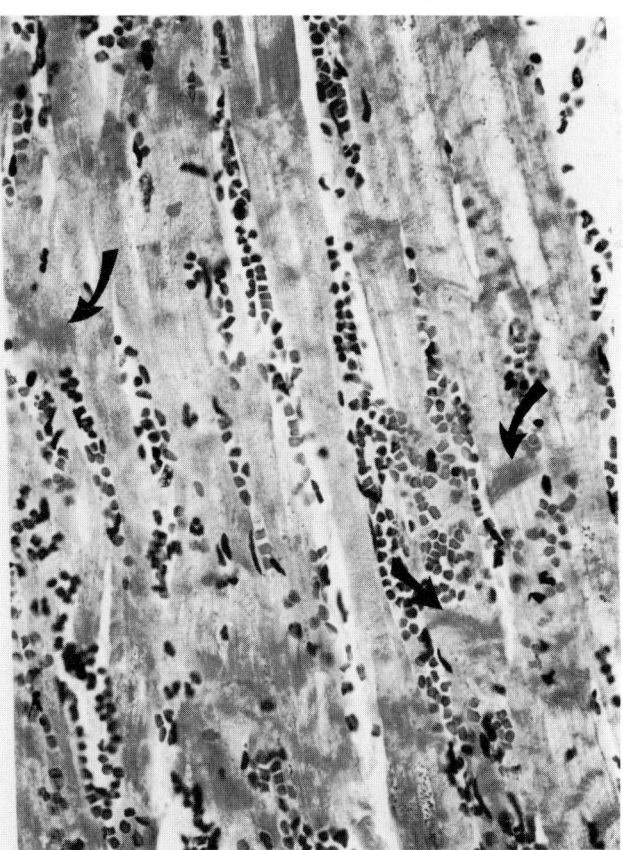

Figure 13-9. Contraction band necrosis *(arrows)* visible as dark bands spanning the myofibers. There is hemorrhage and neutrophilic infiltration between the fibers.

611

POTENTIAL OUTCOMES OF ISCHEMIA

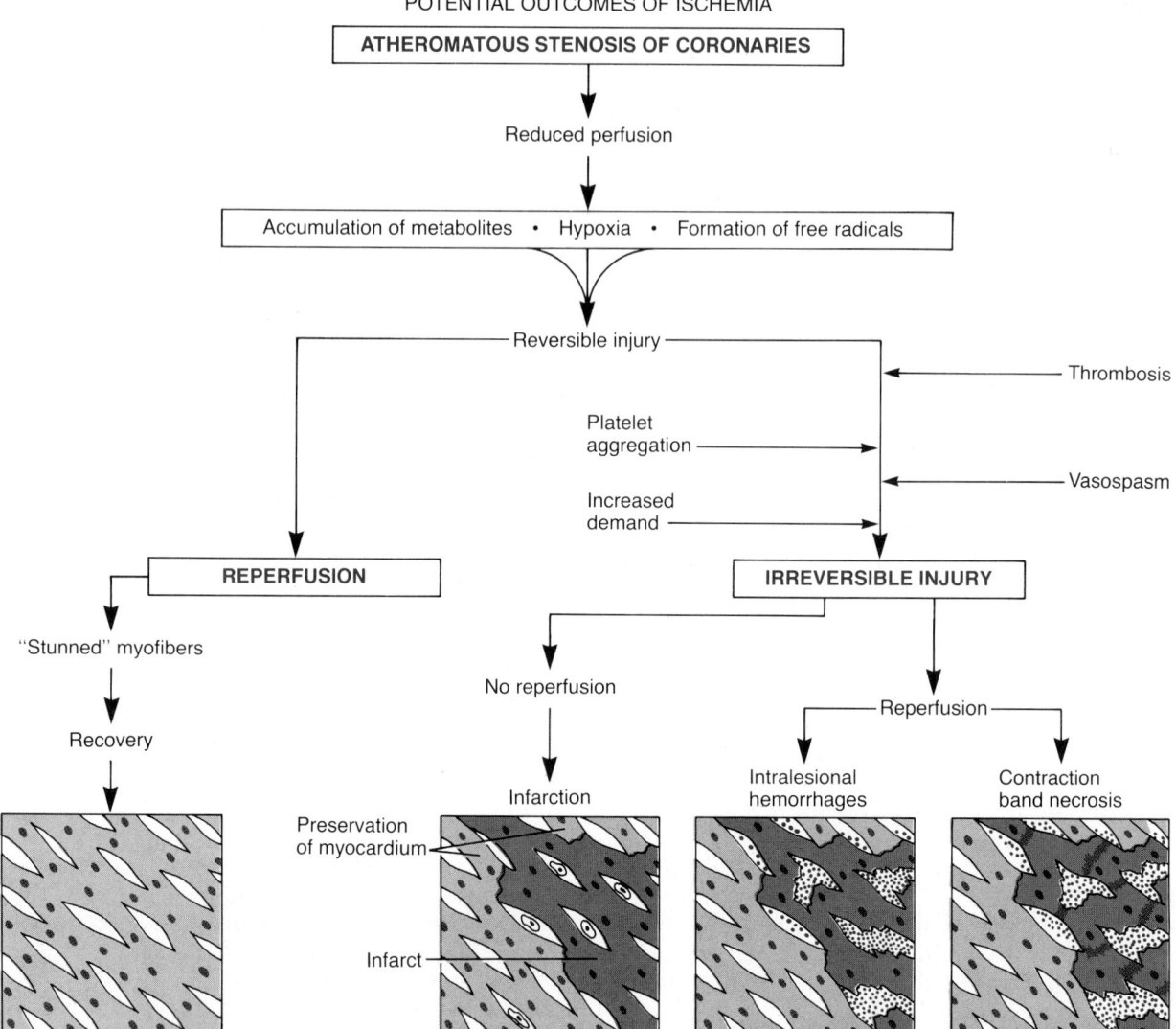

Figure 13–10. The many potential outcomes of reversible and irreversible ischemic injury to the myocardium.

arteries. In one study, 30% were completely occluded after 10 years.[52] These changes are present only to a minimal degree in internal mammary artery grafts of equivalent age. Angioplasty, in contrast, induces changes in the native atherosclerotic arteries. The process of balloon dilation characteristically causes plaque compression and fracture, often with accompanying localized hemorrhagic dissection or aneurysmal dilation of the adjacent arterial wall. Uncommonly, abrupt reclosure follows the angioplasty when a fragment or undermined flap suddenly closes the lumen to trigger an infarction. In about 30% of cases, restenosis develops in subsequent years.[53]

The morphology of the subendocardial infarct is analogous qualitatively to that of transmural lesions. By definition, however, the areas of necrosis are limited to the inner third of the left ventricular wall. The lesion may be multifocal, cover an arc of the circumference of the left ventricle, or sometimes totally encircle it. The temporal sequence of macroscopic and microscopic changes already described

for transmural MIs follows, save that the changes in gross appearance may not be as sharply defined as in larger lesions. Although mural thrombi may supervene over the endocardial surface of these lesions, pericarditis, ventricular aneurysms, and rupture rarely follow.

CLINICAL COURSE. The clinical diagnosis of acute MI is mainly based on three sets of data: (1) symptoms, (2) electrocardiographic (ECG) changes, and (3) elevations of specific serum enzymes, although other diagnostic modalities are available (e.g., radioisotope scanning). Typically, the onset is sudden and devastating with severe, constricting, crushing, burning, substernal or precordial pain that often radiates to the left shoulder, arm, or jaw. It is often accompanied by sweating, nausea, vomiting, or breathlessness. Occasionally, the clinical manifestations are much less specific and consist of burning substernal or epigastric discomfort that is interpreted as "indigestion" or "heartburn." In about 10 to 15% of patients the onset is entirely asymptomatic and the disease is only discovered later by routine ECG changes.[54]

The ECG changes usually become evident from the outset of the attack, although they may be nondiagnostic in 20 to 25% of patients, depending on the location of the infarct, its size, and the number of ECG leads examined. The precise changes that may be encountered are too complex to be discussed here in detail, but basically they consist of new Q waves associated with evolving ST-segment and T-wave changes in transmural infarction, or only ST-segment and T-wave changes in the subendocardial infarct. As the infarct evolves, the ST segment normalizes and the T waves invert. A variety of arrhythmias also may be present, as will soon be pointed out. These may be present from the outset or appear in the course of the next few hours.

Alterations of serum enzymes are more sensitive and reliable indicators of myocardial infarction than ECG changes. Serum glutamic-oxaloacetic transaminase (SGOT), lactic dehydrogenase (LDH), and creatine kinase (CK) levels are generally elevated following an infarct. All are soluble cytoplasmic enzymes that leak out of fatally damaged myocardial cells. The serum SGOT level begins to rise in about eight hours, peaks in 18 to 36 hours, and returns to baseline within three to four days. The LDH level does not begin to rise until about 24 hours, peaks in three to six days, and may not return to normal until the end of the second week. The CK serum level rises above baseline within four to eight hours and may peak very early or not for several days, falling to baseline in about four days. None of these enzymes, however, is entirely specific for an AMI. The most sensitive are the ratio of the LDH-1 isoenzyme to LDH-2, which is commonly above 1.0 in AMI. Analogously, elevation of the MB isoenzyme of CK (CK-MB) is quite specific. Although trace amounts of CK-MB are present in the small intestine, tongue, diaphragm, uterus, and prostate, diseases in these organs that might cause slight elevations of the MB isoenzyme are not likely to be confused with an MI.[55] Other diagnostic modalities such as echocardiography (for visualizing abnormalities of regional wall motion) and radioisotopic studies (such as radionuclide angiography, perfusion scintigraphy, and magnetic resonance imaging) are sometimes used in diagnostically difficult cases.

After the onset of an acute ischemic event, one of several pathways may be followed. Regrettably, one is very brief and marked by sudden cardiac death (SCD) (25% of patients).[56] Indeed, SCD accounts for about 60% of all deaths caused by IHD. However, mobile coronary care units and effective resuscitation teams now rescue many of these victims. If the patient develops an acute MI and reaches the hospital, the spectrum can be presented as follows:[*]

1. Uncomplicated cases (10 to 20%).
2. Complicated cases (80 to 90%).
   A. Cardiac arrhythmias occur in 75 to 95% of complicated cases.
   B. Left ventricular congestive failure with mild-to-severe pulmonary edema (60%).
   C. Cardiogenic shock (10%).
   D. Rupture of free wall, septum, papillary muscle (1 to 5%).
   E. Thromboembolism (15 to 40%).

Cardiac arrhythmias may appear at once and undoubtedly are responsible for many sudden deaths. Often they take the form of heart block, sinus bradycardia, sinus tachycardia, ventricular tachycardia, or ventricular premature contractions. Ventricular fibrillation and asystole are usually lethal, but prompt intervention by mobile and hospital coronary care units has succeeded in controlling arrhythmias in about one patient in four or five.

The next most important clinical problem in terms of both survival and frequency is left ventricular dysfunction, which varies from little or no contractile incompetence to severe "pump failure" — cardiogenic shock. Most often there is some degree of left ventricular failure with hypotension, pulmonary vascular congestion and transudation into the interstitial pulmonary spaces. This mild failure may be transient, but in other cases it progresses to a serious threat when intra-alveolar pulmonary edema causes marked respiratory embarrassment and even cyanosis. The most severe, extreme degree of "pump failure" usually becomes manifest when more than 40% of the left ventricle is infarcted. This is marked by a profound drop in cardiac output and blood pressure and the development of cardiogenic shock. Despite all heroic efforts to improve and sustain the circulation in these patients, severe cardiogenic shock has a nearly 70% mortality rate and accounts for two thirds of in-hospital deaths.

Were these hazards not enough, patients still confront the risk of myocardial rupture and mural thrombosis with peripheral embolization. Thromboembolism, especially when the brain is involved, constitutes an important in-hospital cause of death.

It is difficult to express a prognosis for AMI because of so many variables (e.g., age of patient, previous cardiovascular status, size and site of infarct, manner of treatment, and particularly delay between onset and treatment). Age over 65 years, female sex, history of diabetes mellitus, and a prior myocardial infarct all worsen the prognosis. The overall total mortality within the first year is about 35%. As indicated before, over half of these deaths occur before the individual reaches the hospital. An additional 15 to 20% of these deaths occur within the first six months, more than half before the patient leaves the hospital. Thereafter there is a late 10% mortality among the survivors with each passing year. Particularly important in improving the outlook has been the use of various fibrinolytic agents such as tissue-type

---

[*]Modified from Yu, P. N.: The acute phase of myocardial infarction. Cardiovasc. Clin. 7:45, 1975.

plasminogen activator within four hours of onset of the infarction. When used intravenously, this agent re-establishes the patency of the occluded coronary artery in about 70% of cases and significantly improves the survival rate.[34,57]

Far better than efforts to save people with an MI are attempts to prevent infarction in those who have never experienced one (primary prevention) or prevent reinfarction in those who have recovered from an AMI (secondary prevention). The gratifying decline in the incidence of death from ischemic heart disease, discussed earlier (p. 605), in effect is the consequence of some success with primary prevention, (i.e., control of the three major risk factors for atherosclerosis—hypercholesterolemia, hypertension, and cigarette smoking.[58] For the patient who has survived an acute infarct the same measures are appropriate, but in addition other forms of therapy may be employed, such as beta-blocker agents, antiplatelet agents, and anticoagulants to lower the likelihood of arrhythmias and thrombotic events. Clearly, although primary and secondary preventive measures have been major advances, there is much more to be accomplished if myocardial infarction is to be displaced as the number one killer in industrialized societies.

CHRONIC ISCHEMIC HEART DISEASE (CIHD)

CIHD is a somewhat controversial entity. The designation is used here for patients, usually elderly, who insidiously develop congestive heart failure, sometimes fatal, as a consequence of progressive ischemic myocardial damage. Many individuals with this condition die of other causes. In most instances there has been a history of angina and usually prior episodes of myocardial infarction, often 5 to 10 years before the onset of the congestive failure. In a few individuals, the progressive myocardial ischemia may be entirely silent save possibly for some readily managed arrhythmias, and the first indication of CIHD is congestive heart failure. Some experts contend that CIHD is merely postinfarction cardiac decompensation. Others stress the important contribution of slow myocyte degeneration and so prefer the designation "ischemic cardiomyopathy." Whatever the terminology, a significant number of individuals suffering from IHD eventually die of congestive heart failure as a consequence of slow, progressive ischemic atrophy and death of myocytes, sometimes punctuated by acute ischemic episodes.

The heart in CIHD may be normal, smaller than normal, or even hypertrophied. The pericardial surface is unaffected, but there may be some atrophy of subepicardial fat commensurate with the loss of subcutaneous adipose tissues encountered in aged individuals. Invariably there is moderate to severe stenosing atherosclerosis of the coronary arteries and sometimes total occlusions resulting from organized thrombi. The myocardium is generally browner than usual with patchy foci of gray-white fibrosis less than 1 cm in diameter, chiefly confined to the left ventricular myocardium. Well-healed gray-white scars of previous infarcts may or may not be present. The mural endocardium is generally normal, but there may be some light, patchy, fibrous thickenings. Similarly, the leaflets of the mitral valve may be slightly thicker than normal, with loss of their translucence, but the chordae tendineae are not thickened or fused as would be expected in healed rheumatic heart disease (p. 632). Heavy calcification of the mitral anulus behind the valve leaflets and piled-up masses of calcium within the sinuses of the aortic leaflets may both be present, but these valvular changes are accompaniments of the aging process and not clearly related to ischemic injury. **The major microscopic findings are a diffuse myocardial atrophy often with brown atrophy (p. 31) of myocytes; a diffuse, mainly perivascular, interstitial fibrosis; patchy (under 1 cm) foci of fibrous tissue; myocytolysis of single cells or clusters of cells (p. 609), and in some instances large healed scars of previous acute infarctions** (Fig. 13–11). It is the concurrence of atherosclerotic narrowing of the coronary arteries, myofiber atrophy, spotty myocytolysis, and diffuse, small myocardial scars that delineate the diagnosis of CIHD.[59]

CLINICAL COURSE. The clinical diagnosis of CIHD is made largely by the insidious onset of failure in patients who have had past episodes of MI or anginal attacks. In some instances, the failure is the first mani-

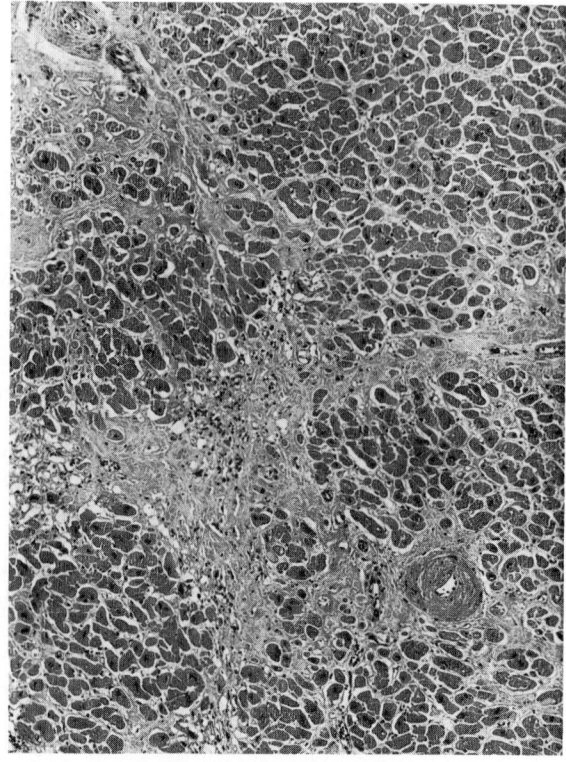

Figure 13–11. Patchy fibrous scarring principally about blood vessels of myocardium in CIHD.

festation of the progressive atherosclerotic encroachment on the cardiac reserve, and the diagnosis rests largely on the exclusion of other forms of cardiac involvement in patients of advanced age. There is, therefore, a tendency for overdiagnosis of CIHD in elderly individuals when other causes of failure are not discovered.

The electrocardiographic changes merely confirm diffuse myocardial disease, sometimes with conduction bundle-branch blocks. Such murmurs as may be present are more likely related to left-sided ventricular dilatation with subsequent valvular regurgitation or to concurrent but unrelated calcific valvular changes. Generally, the congestive failure progresses slowly over the course of many years. However, a serious cardiac arrhythmia or an infarction may supervene and cause death. Patients with this condition may die of entirely unrelated causes before the cardiac involvement becomes symptomatic. In this geriatric group, patients rarely have one disease, and most often the manifestations of CIHD are intermixed with those related to all the other problems of these "not-so-golden years."

SUDDEN CARDIAC DEATH (SCD)

Most commonly SCD is defined as unexpected death from cardiac causes within one hour of the onset of acute symptoms, but in some studies the time interval has been as long as 24 hours.[60] In the vast majority of cases in adults SCD is a complication of IHD. Sometimes it is the first clinical manifestation of IHD and unhappily the last. Less frequently it is caused by marked aortic valve stenosis, hereditary or acquired abnormalities of the cardiac conduction system, and electrolyte derangements. Even more rarely SCD strikes young people having some cardiac disorder such as myocarditis, mitral valve prolapse, or hypertrophic cardiomyopathy.[61] Although reported data vary widely based on the temporal definition of SCD, it is estimated that in the United States this catastrophe strikes about 300,000 to 400,000 individuals annually.

Recognizing the 10 to 20% of cases of non-atherosclerotic origin, marked coronary atherosclerosis with critical, greater than 75% stenosis involving more than one of the major vessels is present in 75 to 95% of victims. Frequently there is at least one stenosis greater than 85%.[62] The precise frequency of *acute coronary changes,* (i.e., thrombosis, plaque fissuring, intraplaque hemorrhage) has varied among the many relevant reports, but an average would be 40 to 50%.[63] However, this frequency may be spuriously low because of fibrinolytic resolution of thrombi and the possible contribution of vasospasm. A healed myocardial infarction is present in about 40%, but in those who have been rescued by prompt therapy from sudden cardiac arrest, new myocardial infarctions are found in 25% or less.[64] *The ultimate mechanism of death is almost always a lethal arrhythmia (e.g., asystole, ventricular fibrillation).* Long-standing coronary atherosclerosis with diffuse myocardial atrophy, interstitial fibrosis, and possibly healed infarctions impinge on the conduction system and create electromechanical cardiac instability. An acute event such as plaque fissuring or myocardial infarction might then induce further ischemia or encroach on the conduction system and trigger the fatal arrhythmia. Physical activity and increased myocardial demand could also lead to metabolic and electrolyte changes, potentiating the electrical instability. In addition, platelet aggregation and the release of vasoconstrictors such as thromboxane A_2 might contribute to ischemia-induced electrical instability.[65] It thus appears that *SCD is a multifactorial catastrophe involving in most instances an acute coronary artery change superimposed on the substrate of advanced coronary atherosclerosis.*

HYPERTENSIVE HEART DISEASE (HHD)

The minimal anatomic criteria for the diagnosis of HHD are the following: (1) left ventricular hypertrophy (usually concentric) in the absence of other cardiovascular pathology that might reasonably induce it, and (2) a history of hypertension. However, this definition requires considerable qualification. The study of animal models and clinical studies coupled with endomyocardial biopsies have revealed that demonstrable hypertrophy is a relatively late stage of hypertensive heart disease. Long before it becomes evident, there are more subtle biochemical and ultrastructural changes accompanied by functional alterations.[66] In addition, hypertension strongly predisposes to atherosclerosis and so most patients with elevated blood pressure have significant coronary atherosclerosis. Notwithstanding, the Framingham Study established unequivocally the relationship between hypertension alone and the development of left ventricular hypertrophy.[67]

Even mild hypertension (levels greater than 140/90) if sufficiently prolonged produces left ventricular hypertrophy.[68] Approximately 25% of the population of the United States suffers from hypertension of this degree, making hypertensive heart disease the second most common form of cardiac disease.[68]

PATHOGENESIS. Hypertrophy of the heart is an adaptive response to pressure overload or volume overload. In effect, it tends to normalize the systolic stress carried by individual myofilaments within myocytes. However, when the hypertrophy becomes marked it eventually leads to myocyte injury, heart failure, and cardiac dilatation. In hypertension, the pathogenesis of which is discussed on page 1062, the stimulus to hypertrophy is pressure overload. The pressure stress on the ventricular wall leads to the production within myocytes of new myofilaments, myofibrils, mitochondria, and ribosomes, and nuclear enlargement along with enlargement of the cell. Because mitotic division does not occur in adult muscle cells no new cells are produced.[69] There may, however, be replication of sarcomeres alongside existing sarcomeres, contributing to cell widening. Still not understood at the molecular level are the pathways by which physical stress induces the structural changes, but some studies suggest that stress alters the functional activity of protein kinase isoenzymes involved in synthesis of structural proteins. But more than stress may be involved in myofiber enlargement. In animal models, it can be shown that adrenergic stimulation by itself can lead to cardiac hypertrophy even with complete control of blood pressure — and, of even greater interest, it may do so by activation of the proto-oncogene c-myc.[70]

With ventricular hypertrophy, the heart may maintain an adequate output for decades despite the hypertension. What eventually ushers in the onset of cardiac decompensation remains a mystery. As the heart wall thickens, the oxygen demand is increased and the left ventricular compliance is reduced.[71] Ever-present coronary atherosclerosis undoubtedly adds an element of ischemia. Whatever the basis, diffuse interstitial fibrosis develops along with focal myocyte atrophy and degeneration. Moreover, the myofiber enlargement increases the distance for diffusion of oxygen and nutrients from adjacent capillaries. Other speculations have been offered, but ultimately the basis for cardiac failure in HHD remains unknown.

The essential morphologic evidence of compensated HHD is concentric hypertrophy (hypertrophy without dilatation) of the left ventricular wall without accompanying lesions that might account for it (e.g., aortic valve stenosis, coarctation of the aorta). The thickening of the left ventricular wall is more or less symmetric, increases the ratio of wall thickness to radius of ventricular chamber, and increases the weight of the heart disproportionately to the increase in size (Fig. 13–12). During the stages of compensated HHD, the left ventricular wall thicknesses may exceed 2.0 cm and the heart weight 500 gm. In time, the increased thickness of the left ventricular wall imparts a stiffness that impairs diastolic filling and consequently reduces the stroke volume output. The pericardium and valvular leaflets are unaffected. The myocardium is red-brown and homogeneous unless ischemic heart disease has introduced areas of scarring. With the onset of decompensation, there may be dilatation of the ventricular chamber with thinning of the wall and enlargement of the external dimensions of the heart.

Microscopically the changes in HHD are subtle and readily missed on routine evaluation. The earliest changes are myocyte enlargement with transverse diameters several times normal. As noted earlier, the enlargement reflects an increase in sarcoplasmic elements as well as nuclear enlargement possibly with hyperploidy. At a more advanced stage, the cellular enlargement becomes somewhat more irregular, with variation in the transverse diameter of individual cells and variation between adjacent cells. The disorganization becomes more marked with time and in the

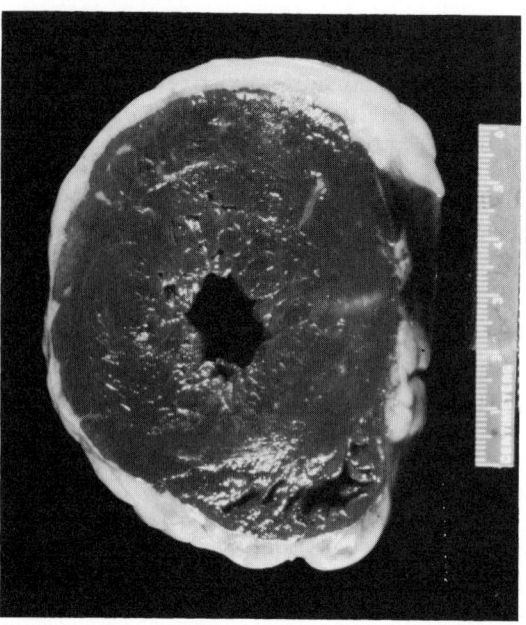

Figure 13–12. Hypertensive heart disease. Transection of heart revealing concentric marked thickening of left ventricular wall with reduction of lumen. Transected right ventricle is barely evident on lower right.

late stages is marked by regressive alterations with loss of myofibrils, disruption of Z bands, loss of the linear array of sarcomeres producing sharp angulations of the myocyte, random cell atrophy and death, and increased interstitial fibrosis.[72]

CLINICAL COURSE. Compensated HHD may be asymptomatic and suspected only in the appropriate clinical setting by electrocardiographic or echocardiographic indications of left ventricular enlargement. As already stressed, other causes for such hypertrophy must be ruled out. In many patients, however, it comes to attention by the onset of atrial fibrillation or cardiac decompensation with cardiac dilatation, or both. Often there are other manifestations frequently associated with hypertension (e.g., headache, dizziness, nosebleeds, and occasionally postural unsteadiness). Depending on the severity of the hypertension, its duration, the adequacy of therapeutic control, and the underlying basis for the hypertension (p. 1062), the patient may enjoy normal longevity to die of unrelated causes, may develop progressive ischemic heart disease owing to the effects of hypertension on coronary atherosclerosis, may suffer progressive renal damage or cerebrovascular "stroke," or may experience progressive heart failure. The risk of sudden cardiac death is also increased. Cardiac failure accounts for only about a third of all deaths among hypertensive subjects. There is substantial evidence that effective control of the hypertension will in time lead to regression of the cardiac hypertrophy.[73] Interestingly some antihypertensive agents such as direct-acting vasodilators do not lead to reduction in ventricular mass, but other agents such as the angiotensin-converting enzyme inhibitors appear to effectively reduce ventricular mass. Still uncertain is whether these "reborn" hearts will resume completely normal function.

COR PULMONALE (PULMONARY HEART DISEASE)

Cor pulmonale constitutes right ventricular enlargement secondary to pulmonary hypertension caused by disorders that affect either the structure or the function of the lungs. *The right ventricular enlargement and thickening caused by diseases of the left side of the heart and congenital heart diseases are excluded by this definition of cor pulmonale.* Increases in pulmonary blood pressure or pulmonary vascular resistance will both produce hypertension, but ultimately it is the pressure overload that leads to the right ventricular enlargement and so cor pulmonale is the right-sided counterpart of hypertensive heart disease. The major disorders that can lead to pulmonary hypertension are cited in Table 13-3.[74]

Based on the suddenness of development of the pulmonary hypertension, two forms of cor pulmonale may develop: acute and chronic. *Acute cor pulmonale* refers to the right ventricular dilatation that follows massive pulmonary embolization. *Chronic cor pulmonale* usually implies right ventricular hypertrophy secondary to prolonged pressure overload whether related to narrowings or obstructions of major ar-

Table 13-3. Disorders Predisposing to Cor Pulmonale

Diseases of the Lungs
Chronic obstructive pulmonary disease (COPD)
Diffuse pulmonary interstitial fibrosis
Extensive persistent atelectasis
Cystic fibrosis

Diseases of Pulmonary Vessels
Pulmonary embolism
Primary pulmonary vascular sclerosis
Extensive pulmonary arteritis (e.g., Wegener's granulomatosis)
Drug-, toxin-, or radiation-induced vascular sclerosis

Disorders Affecting Chest Movement
Kyphoscoliosis
Marked obesity (pickwickian syndrome)
Neuromuscular diseases

Disorders Inducing Pulmonary Arteriolar Constriction
Metabolic acidosis
Hypoxemia
    Chronic altitude sickness
    Obstruction to major airways
    Idiopathic alveolar hypoventilation

teries or compression of septal capillaries. In time, however, right-sided cardiac decompensation may develop with dilatation of the right heart. Whatever the disorder increasing the workload on the right side of the heart, the vasoconstrictive effects of hypoxemia and acidosis contribute significantly to the development of pulmonary hypertension (Fig. 13-13). The causative mechanisms of this vasoconstriction are not well known, but may be neurogenic or humoral in origin (local generation of vasoconstrictors such as thromboxane A_2, leukotrienes, epinephrine, and histamine.[75]

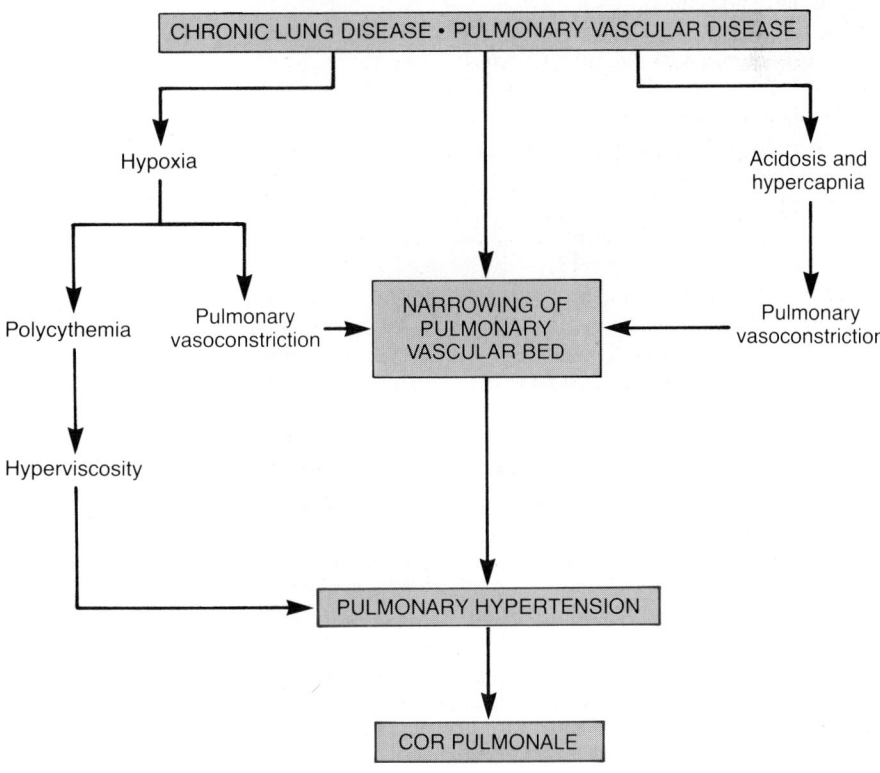

Figure 13-13. Pathogenesis of cor pulmonale. (Modified from Summer, W.R.: Acquired cor pulmonale, in Rubin, L.J.: Pulmonary Heart Disease. Boston, Martinus Nijhoff, 1984, pg. 285.

The anatomic changes are those that might be anticipated. In **acute cor pulmonale, there is marked dilatation of the right ventricle** and possibly of the right atrium. On cross section, the normal sickle shape of the right ventricle is replaced by a dilated ovoid possibly with thinning of the right ventricular wall (normal thickness, 0.3 to 0.5 cm). **In chronic cor pulmonale, the ventricular wall thickens, sometimes up to 1.0 cm or more, and may even come to approximate that of the left ventricle (Fig. 13–14).**[76] There is concomitant thickening of the trabeculae carneae and papillary muscles. Rarely, tricuspid regurgitation leads to slight fibrous thickening of the valves, but otherwise the remainder of the heart is essentially unchanged.

Chronic cor pulmonale is a surprisingly common condition because of its association with such widespread disorders as chronic bronchitis and emphysema (COPD) that affect perhaps 40 million or more individuals in the United States alone. Several studies suggest that cor pulmonale is responsible for 10 to 30% of admissions to hospitals for cardiac decompensation.[77] In most instances, the existence of cor pulmonale is overshadowed by the diseases leading to the

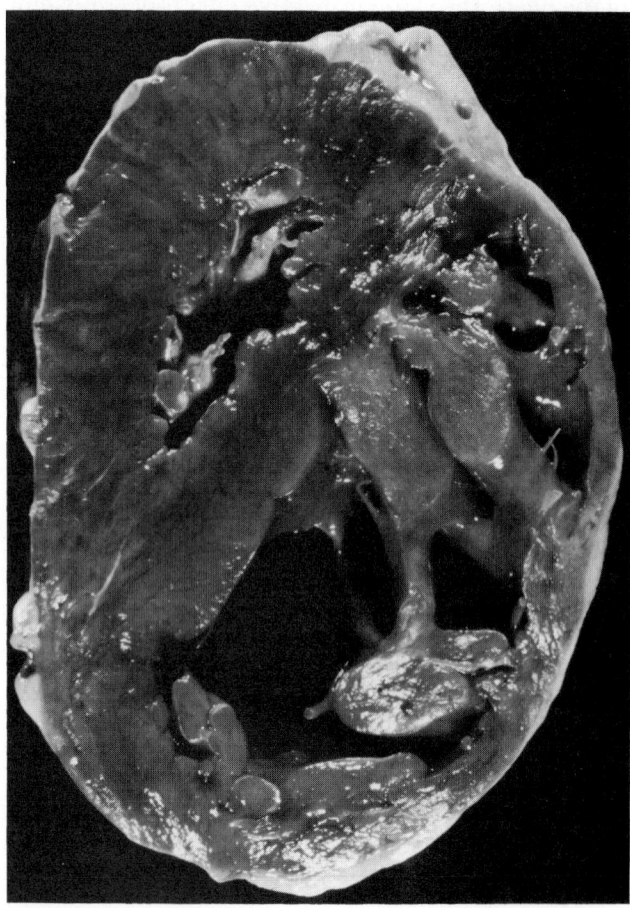

Figure 13–14. Chronic cor pulmonale. Transection of heart revealing a markedly dilated right ventricle below with thickened free wall and hypertrophied trabeculae. Transected left ventricle above has been compressed and dwarfed by right ventricular enlargement.

pulmonary hypertension. Thus, the cardiac diagnosis is heavily dependent on electrocardiography, echocardiography, pulmonary angiography, and radionuclide imaging. In the great majority of instances, when chronic cor pulmonale is present, the concomitant changes of pulmonary vascular sclerosis described on page 764 are also present.[78]

CONGENITAL HEART DISEASE

Congenital heart disease is most simply defined as an abnormality of the heart, present from birth. The more severe anomalies may be incompatible with intrauterine survival. When they permit live birth they may produce manifestations soon thereafter, along with the change from fetal to postnatal circulatory patterns. In some instances, the anomaly evolves postnatally: for example, a coarctation (narrowing) of the aorta may become more pronounced when the ductus arteriosus closes after birth. Some anomalies do not become evident until the adult years. The disorders that normally do not cause cardiac malfunction until adult life, such as the mitral prolapse or "floppy mitral valve" syndrome and bicuspid or unicuspid aortic valves, will not be included in our present consideration, nor the cardiovascular abnormalities encountered in a host of specific genetic disorders such as Marfan's, Ehlers-Danlos, and Hunter-Hurler syndromes, many of which are covered elsewhere.

INCIDENCE. Congenital heart disease is the most common type of heart disease among children; fortunately most forms are now amenable to surgical correction. Although figures vary, a generally accepted incidence of congenital heart disease is six to eight per 1000 live-born, full-term births. The incidence is higher in premature infants. This prevalence does not include perhaps the two most common cardiac abnormalities, bicuspid aortic valve and mitral valve prolapse, which often do not constitute functionally significant derangements in the early years of life.[79] There are even wider discrepancies in the reported frequencies of specific forms of congenital heart disease. The ten most common, accounting for about 85% of cases with approximate frequencies, are presented in Table 13–4. These more common anomalies will be described after some brief comments on etiology. For the less common lesions, reference may be made to specialized texts.[80,81]

ETIOLOGY. In over 90% of instances the cause of congenital heart disease is unknown. However, multifactorial inheritance with both genetic and environmental inputs is suspected.[82] About 5% of cases are associated with chromosomal abnormalities. The specific karyotypes involved are trisomies 21, 18, 13, 22, 9 (mosaic), and +14q–, and Turner's syndrome. About 2 to 3% of cardiovascular abnormalities are related to gene defects in a wide variety of autosomal dominant, autosomal recessive, and sex-linked hereditary syndromes (e.g., Ehlers-Danlos, Marfan's, mu-

Table 13-4. Approximate Frequencies of Cardiac Malformations

MALFORMATION	% OF CONGENITAL HEART DISEASE	MALE-FEMALE RATIO
Ventricular septal defect (VSD)	30	1:1
Patent ductus arteriosus (PDA)	10	1:2.5
Atrial septal defect (ASD)	10	1:3
Pulmonic stenosis	7	1:1
Coarctation of aorta	7	3-4:1
Aortic stenosis	6	3-5:1
Tetralogy of Fallot	6	1:1
Transposition of great arteries	4	3:1
Persistent truncus arteriosus	2	1:1
Tricuspid atresia	1.5	1:1

copolysaccharidoses, muscular dystrophies, and glycogenoses). Probably less than 1% can be clearly attributed to environmental influences. Best documented is maternal rubella in the first trimester of pregnancy, which may result in patent ductus arteriosus, pulmonic valvular or arterial stenosis or both, aortic stenosis, tetralogy of Fallot and ventricular septal defect, either singly or in combination, and sometimes also cataracts, deafness, and microcephaly.[83] A large number of other cardiac teratogenic influences have been identified in animals, such as hypoxia, ionizing radiation, and various drugs, but in humans, in addition to maternal rubella, there is substantial evidence implicating thalidomide and excessive alcohol consumption. Excessive cigarette smoking is also suspect.

The belief that the great majority (about 90%) of structural cardiac anomalies are multifactorial in origin is largely inferential.[84] On the one hand, there is a two- to ten-fold increase in the incidence of congenital heart disease in siblings of an affected patient or children of an affected parent, pointing to genetic influences. On the other hand, despite identical genes, monozygotic twins have only a 10% concordance for ventricular septal defects.[85] There is, as pointed out in Table 13-4, a well-defined sex preponderance for certain specific defects. Overall, males are more often involved. Thus, there are many hints of genetic influence, but the twin studies make clear that environmental influences, although rarely identifiable, must also contribute.

Several important observations relevant to genetic counseling should be mentioned at this point. The basic development of the heart occurs in the first 16 weeks of embryogenesis. Environmental insults, then, must occur during this vulnerable period to cause congenital heart disease. Most cardiovascular abnormalities clearly of genetic origin are associated with well-defined multisystem syndromes. The chromosomal syndromes (e.g., the trisomies) are largely the consequence of errors in gametogenesis and so most often are not familial. Only the cardiovascular abnormalities related to mutant genes (e.g., Marfan's, Ehlers-Danlos, and the mucopolysaccharidoses) are hereditary and familial. With these exceptions, parents of an affected child can be reassured that, although there is a somewhat increased risk for subsequent children, it is small (below 5%), and with a live-born infant the defect may well be amenable to surgical correction.[86] However, when more than one member of a family is affected, the risk rises sharply.

CLINICAL CONSEQUENCES. *The varied structural anomalies in hearts with congenital defects fall into two major categories: shunts or obstructions.*

A *shunt* denotes an abnormal communication between cardiac chambers or blood vessels or between chambers and blood vessels. The abnormal channels permit the flow of blood from left to right or the reverse depending on the pressure relationships. When blood from the right side of the heart enters the left side, cyanosis results as poorly oxygenated blood enters the systemic circulation. Certain congenital heart defects produce right-to-left shunts from early infancy and are known as *cyanotic congenital heart diseases* (e.g., tetralogy of Fallot, transposition of the great arteries, persistent truncus arteriosus, and tricuspid atresia). These abnormal communications also permit emboli arising in peripheral veins to bypass the normal filtration action of the lungs and thus enter the systemic circulation. Paradoxic embolism to the brain and brain abscess are potential consequences. Other abnormal communications constitute left-to-right shunts unassociated with cyanosis. However, in time, the overload of the right heart induces pulmonary hypertension and right ventricular hypertrophy. As the pressure on the right side of the heart rises, it comes to exceed that on the left and now the flow becomes right-to-left, creating what is called *cyanose tardive* or *late cyanotic congenital heart disease* (e.g., ventricular septal defect, atrial septal defect, and patent ductus arteriosus). Clinical findings frequently associated with severe, long-standing cyanosis are clubbing of the tips of the fingers and toes, hypertrophic osteoarthropathy (p. 1333) and polycythemia. Cerebral thrombosis in very young children sometimes occurs in these settings presumably related to the polycythemia, increased blood viscosity, and perhaps a febrile illness inducing dehydration.

Some developmental anomalies of the heart produce *obstructions to flow* because of abnormal narrowings. Prime examples are valvular stenoses or atresias. Obstructions do not generally cause cyanosis and therefore are called noncyanotic or *obstructive congenital heart disease* (e.g., coarctation of the aorta, aortic valvular stenosis, and pulmonary valvular stenosis).

Children with significant congenital cardiac defects may fail to thrive, suffer from retarded development, and are at greater risk of developing the diseases of childhood. Moreover, congenital anomalies producing jet streams — and therefore endothelial injury where the jet impinges — pose a particular risk for infective endocarditis (e.g., ventricular septal defect, patent ductus arteriosus, tetralogy of Fallot, and a tight aortic stenosis).

RIGHT-TO-LEFT SHUNTS — EARLY CYANOSIS

Tetralogy of Fallot

The four features of the tetralogy of Fallot are (1) ventricular septal defect (VSD), (2) an aorta that overrides the ventricular defect, (3) obstruction to the right ventricular outflow, and (4) right ventricular hypertrophy[87] (Fig. 13–15). The tetralogy is the most common form of cyanotic congenital heart disease that, even untreated, permits survival into adult life. Indeed, in an analysis of a large series of patients with this condition who died without ever having had cardiac surgery, about 10% had been alive at 20 years and 3% at 40 years. The severity of the clinical manifestations is directly related to the degree of obstruction to right ventricular outflow that determines the direction of blood flow.

> The heart is often enlarged and may be boot-shaped owing to marked right ventricular hypertrophy, particularly of the apical region. The VSD is usually large and often approximates the diameter of the aortic orifice. It often

> abuts on the aortic valve ring. The obstruction to right ventricular outflow is most often due to narrowing of the infundibulum of the right ventricle, but this alteration is sometimes associated with pulmonary valvular stenosis. Less commonly, the outflow obstruction is supravalvular. Sometimes there is complete atresia of the pulmonary artery or absence of a main branch, and only flow through a patent ductus or dilated bronchial arteries, or through both, permits survival. The aortic origin overrides or straddles the septal defect. Aortic valve insufficiency, atrial septal defect (ASD), tricuspid atresia, and endocardial cushion defect may also be present.

The clinical consequences of the tetralogy depend on its precise conformation. When the septal defect is large and the pulmonic stenosis is mild, there is a left-to-right shunt without cyanosis. *As the pulmonic stenosis increases in severity, there is commensurately greater resistance to right ventricular outflow, right-sided hypertension, and at some point reversal of the shunt to a right-to-left direction and along with it cyanosis.* As the fetus grows and the heart increases in size, the pulmonic orifice does not expand, making the obstruction ever worse. Thus, most infants with tetralogy are cyanotic from birth or soon thereafter. However, the pulmonic stenosis protects the lungs from volume and pressure overload and right ventricular failure is rare, because the right ventricle is decompressed into the left ventricle and aorta. Flow through the lungs may in some part be dependent on a patent ductus arteriosus. Surgical repair or at least partial correction is now possible and recommended, but the time of election remains somewhat controversial. Prolonged palliation carries with it the risk of infective endocarditis, usually involving the pulmonic stenosis. Other possible complications are polycythemia with a thrombotic diathesis, paradoxic embolism, and cerebral abscess.

Transposition of Great Arteries

Transpositions are a complex group of malformations in which there may be inversion of the aorta and pulmonary artery with respect to the ventricles, inversion of the atria with respect to the ventricles, ventricular inversion relative to the atria, or origin of both great vessels from a single ventricle. Only the most common form will be described, along with a few comments on two other variants. More details are available elsewhere.[88,89] *In the most common pattern, the aorta arises from the morphogenetic right ventricle and lies anterior to the pulmonary artery and toward the midline, while the pulmonary artery arises from the morphogenetic left ventricle (Fig. 13–16).* This malformation is particularly common in offspring of diabetic mothers. It causes cyanosis from birth. During intrauterine life, the patency of the foramen ovale and ductus arteriosus provide sufficient "mixing" of venous and systemic blood to permit survival. Postnatal survival requires continued "mixing," otherwise two separate circulations would exist, with the aorta

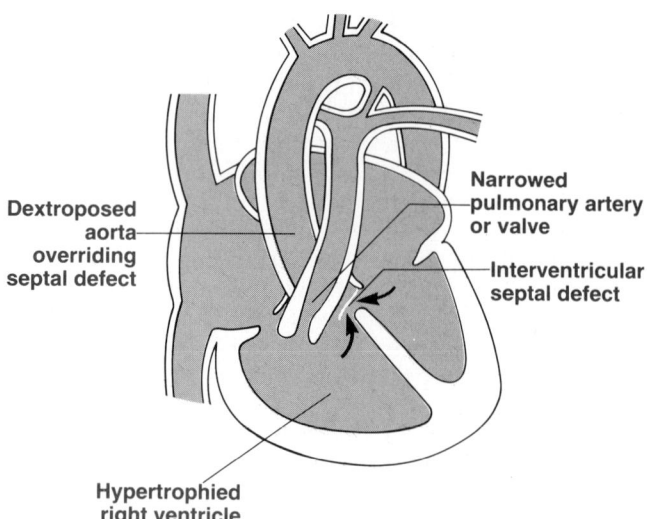

Dextroposed aorta overriding septal defect

Narrowed pulmonary artery or valve

Interventricular septal defect

Hypertrophied right ventricle

Figure 13–15. Tetralogy of Fallot. Origin of pulmonary artery has been displaced to the left to illustrate its stenosis.

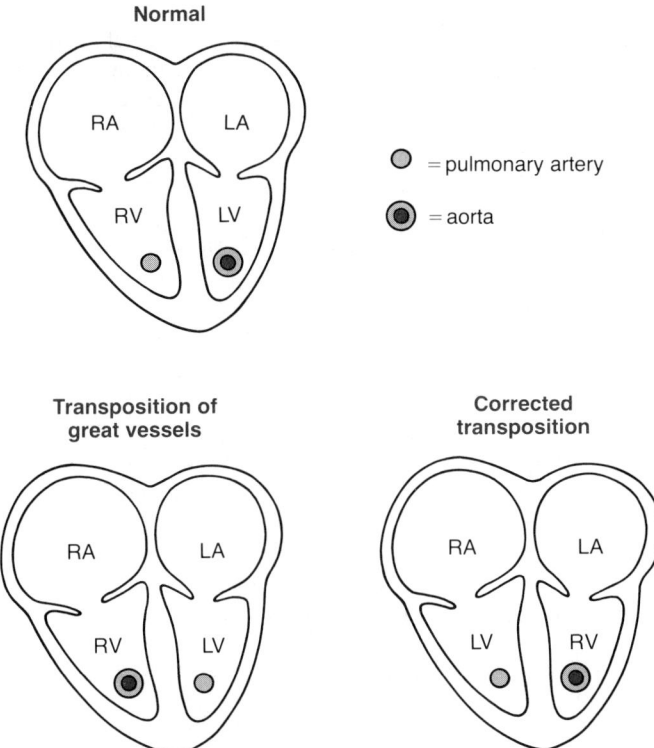

Normal

= pulmonary artery

= aorta

Transposition of great vessels

Corrected transposition

Figure 13–16. Diagrammatic representation of uncorrected and corrected transposition of the great vessels.

receiving unoxygenated blood from the systemic return and the pulmonary artery recycling oxygenated blood. Virtually all patients who survive the neonatal period have an interatrial communication; patent ductus is present in about 60% and a VSD in 30%. Right ventricular hypertrophy usually develops with survival for any period of time. This pattern of transposition is one of the common forms of cyanotic congenital heart disease and is a major cause of death in the first two months of life. Recognition of this entity requires correct differentiation of the morphogenetic, finely trabeculated left ventricle from the coarsely trabeculated right ventricle.

The outlook for infants with transposition of the great vessels depends on the degree of "mixing" of the blood, the magnitude of the tissue hypoxia, and the ability of the morphogenetic right ventricle to maintain the aortic outflow and systemic circulation. Without surgery, most patients die within the first months of life. Rare survivals into young adult life have been reported, usually when there is an associated large interatrial defect, a VSD with some pulmonic stenosis, or a single ventricle.

A variety of surgical approaches have been devised for increasing the intracardiac communication of the systemic and pulmonary circulations.

In so-called "corrected" transposition the ventricles are inverted relative to the atria. Thus, the morphogenetic right atrium communicates with the morphogenetic left ventricle that supplies a transposed pulmonary artery. On the other side of the heart, the left atrium communicates with the morphogenetic right ventricle that ejects into the transposed aorta. In the absence of other associated malformations, a functionally normal circulation would exist save that the systemic arterial supply is maintained by a morphogenetic right ventricle that usually undergoes marked hypertrophy. However, other malformations are usually present, particularly of the atrioventricular valves, and so a satisfactory physiologic circulation is rarely achieved.[90]

Another variant is the *Taussig-Bing malformation*. In this condition, the aorta comes off the right ventricle and there is a VSD directly beneath an "overriding" pulmonary artery that is situated in front of the aorta. Frequently, an associated coarctation of the aorta is present.

Truncus Arteriosus

The truncus arteriosus arises from a developmental failure of separation of the aorta from the pulmonary artery, resulting in a single large vessel receiving blood from both the right and left ventricles and an infundibular VSD. The coronary arteries of necessity take origin from the truncus a d a large tricuspid truncal valve is present that may be functional or anomalous. Truncus arteriosus is associated with a large number of concomitant defects including right aortic arch, hypoplastic pulmonary arteries, absence of ductus arteriosus, or an abnormally broad ductus arteriosus and, as mentioned, various defects in the truncal valve from gross insufficiency to stenosis. Because blood from the right and left ventricles mixes, there is early systemic cyanosis as well as increased pulmonary blood flow. In time, right ventricular hypertrophy appears and with it pulmonary vascular hypertensive changes. The prognosis for these infants is poor and so surgical correction is attempted at an early age sometimes with gratifying results.

Tricuspid Atresia

Complete absence of the tricuspid valve is known as atresia. It is almost always associated with underdevelopment of the right ventricle and an ASD. The circulation is maintained by a right-to-left shunt through the interatrial communication. Often the tricuspid atresia is associated with hypoplasia of the pulmonary artery and atresia or stenosis of the pulmonary valve. A VSD also is frequently present. Cyanosis is present virtually from birth and there is a high mortality in the first weeks or months of life. Palliative surgery may be possible, depending on the severity and number of associated anomalies.

LEFT-TO-RIGHT SHUNTS — LATE CYANOSIS

Ventricular Septal Defect

As pointed out earlier, VSD is the most common congenital cardiac anomaly. For reasons unknown, there has been a significant increase in the frequency of this defect in the United States. Frequently it is associated with other structural defects, particularly tetralogy of Fallot, but also patent ductus arteriosus, atrial septal defect, coarctation of the aorta, and transposition of the great arteries.[91] About 30% occur as isolated anomalies. Depending on the size of the defect, it may produce difficulties virtually from birth or, with smaller lesions, may not be recognized until later. In normal cardiac development between the fifth and sixth weeks of embryonic life, the common ventricular canal is divided by a septum. The basal portion of the septum close to the atrioventricular valves is membranous and derived from endocardial cushion tissue and the infundibular or conus septum. This membranous portion fuses with the cephalad growth of the muscular septum.

> VSDs vary enormously in size and location. They range from probe patencies to lesions sufficiently large to create virtually a single ventricle (cor triloculare biatriatum). About 90% lie within or immediately adjacent to the membranous septum and are therefore very close to the bundle of His (Fig.13–17). The remainder lie below the pulmonic valve (subpulmonic) or are located within the muscular septum. Most often single, those in the muscular septum may be multiple.[92]

The functional significance of a VSD depends on the size of the defect, level of pulmonary vascular resistance, and absence of pulmonary stenosis. Small defects (less than 0.5 cm in diameter) are known as Roger's disease. About 50% close spontaneously, and the remainder are generally well tolerated for years. However, they induce a loud murmur heard through-

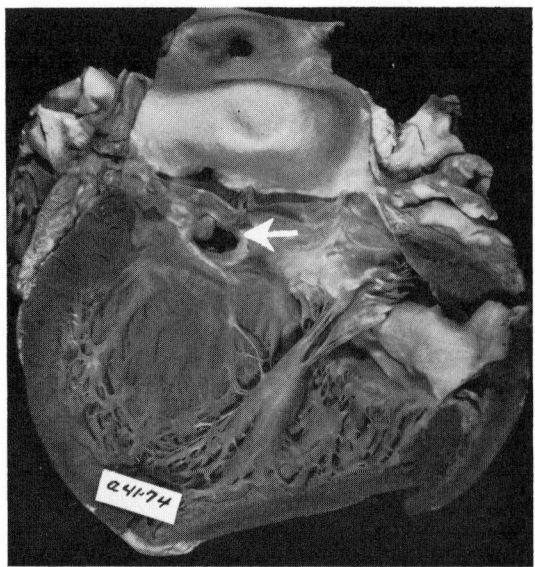

Figure 13–17. Ventricular septal defect high in membranous septum with fibrous thickening of margins of patency (arrow).

out systole, sometimes accompanied by a systolic thrill. Larger defects remain patent and permit a significant left-to-right flow. Right ventricular enlargement and pulmonary hypertension develop with reversal of flow and cyanose tardive, clubbing, and polycythemia. Large defects may become manifest virtually at birth because of signs of cardiac failure accompanying the murmur. There is, thus, a wide range in the behavior of VSD from spontaneous closure to fulminant cardiac failure.[93] A particular risk in those with small or moderate-sized defects is superimposed infective endocarditis, rarely encountered with large defects. Surgical closure of incidental VSDs is generally not attempted during infancy because of the possibility of spontaneous closure. However, correction is indicated in older children and adults when there is a moderate-to-large left-to-right shunt, before significant increased pulmonary vascular disease develops.

Atrial Septal Defect

With the exception of mitral valve prolapse (p. 628) and bicuspid aortic valve (p. 638), ASD is the most common congenital cardiac anomaly first recognized in adults, more frequently in females than in males. It usually passes unnoted in infants and children, only becoming manifest when reversal of flow through the shunt (due to development of increased pulmonary arterial pressure) induces cyanosis, or right-sided heart failure develops. *There are three types of ASD: ostium primum, ostium secundum, and sinus venosus.* Normally, at the end of the third or the beginning of the fourth week, the common atrial canal is divided by a septum primum contributed by the sinus venosus and endocardial cushion tissue. Two openings are left in the septum primum: an ostium primum, low and posteriorly in the neighborhood of the atrioventricular valve, and an ostium secundum, approximately where the foramen ovale will later be situated. At about the fifth week of embryogenesis, growth of the septum primum abolishes the low ostium primum. The ostium secundum, however, is partially closed by a newly formed septum secundum derived from the medial wall of the right atrium, which lies to the right of the septum primum. However, because this secondary septum is itself not complete, an aperture is left, known as the foramen ovale, which is juxtaposed to a more or less intact region of the septum primum lying to its left. Thus, a flaplike membrane covers the foramen ovale (Fig. 13–18). As long as pressure in the right atrium is higher than that in the left, the oxygenated blood in the right atrium flows into the left atrium. However, with birth and opening of the pulmonary circulation the pressure relationships are reversed, but flow from left to right is prevented by the flap valve covering the foramen ovale. Fusion of the membrane over the foramen normally follows. A nonfunctional oblique slit may persist, known as a *patent foramen ovale*, which permits little or no flow because of the flap valve arrangement.

PATENT FORAMEN OVALE

EMBRYOGENESIS

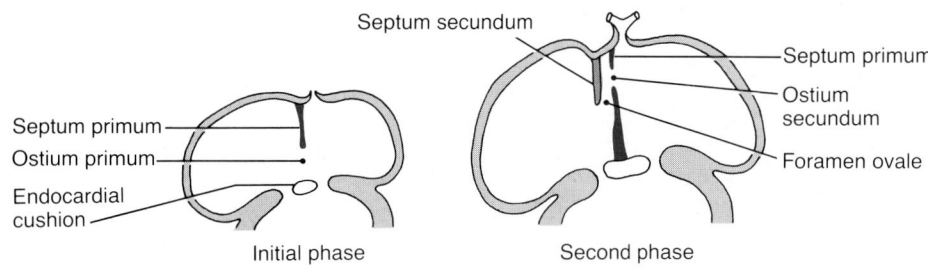

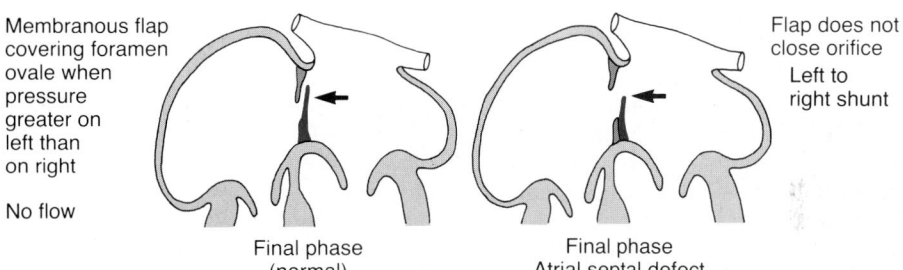

Figure 13–18. The embryogenesis of atrial septal defect.

Ostium primum anomalies represent only about 5% of ASDs. They occur low in the atrial septum adjacent to the atrioventricular valves and are sometimes associated with deformities of these valves. This type of ASD is common in Down's syndrome.

Ostium secundum occurs at the location of the foramen ovale because of juxtaposed defects in the primary and secondary septa. This pattern represents approximately 90% of all ASDs. It is sometimes associated with other defects—patent ductus arteriosus, VSD, pulmonary stenosis, transposition of the great arteries, and tetralogy of Fallot. The atrial aperture may be of any size: single, multiple, or sometimes fenestrated. A very large ostium secundum creates essentially a single atrial chamber.

Sinus venosus defects are located high in the atrial septum near the entrance of the superior vena cava. They account for about 5% of ASDs and are sometimes accompanied by anomalous connections of pulmonary veins from the right lung to the superior vena cava or right atrium.

ASDs are very well tolerated if small (less than 1 cm in diameter). Even larger defects do not constitute serious problems during the first decades of life when the flow is from left to right. A murmur is often present; it arises at the pulmonic valve as a result of excessive flow through the valve. Eventually, however, reversal of flow may occur as the right atrium and right ventricle hypertrophy, and pulmonary hypertension and arterial changes develop. Cyanosis, respiratory difficulties, and cardiac failure then ensue progressively. Rarely, a rheumatic, acquired mitral stenosis combines with an ASD (Lutembacher's syndrome) to greatly raise the left-sided pressure and hasten the development of pulmonary hypertension. Some would extend Lutembacher's syndrome to include the combination of ASD and pulmonary hypertension, whatever its cause (e.g., multiple pulmonary emboli or diffuse pulmonary vascular disease). Infective endocarditis is rare with ASDs because of the low pressure gradients and sluggish flow, but paradoxical embolism or brain abscess may appear. Operative closure of these defects is advised early in life to prevent anatomic changes in the pulmonary circuit incident to long-standing hypertension.

Patent Ductus Arteriosus (PDA)

The ductus arteriosus is a normal vascular channel during intrauterine life that courses between the bifurcation of the pulmonary artery and the aorta just distal to the origin of the left subclavian artery. In the full-term infant, the ductus closes functionally within the first day or two of life. More prolonged patency is generally permanent. In contrast, in the premature infant the ductus may remain patent for longer periods of time. The basis for abnormally persistent patency is not well understood. During fetal life, the relaxant effects of low oxygen tension and locally synthesized PGE appear to maintain its patency.[94] After birth, with left-to-right flow, the increased levels of oxygen stimulate muscular contraction. It is also possible that there is reduced synthesis of PGE. It should be evident why infants with the respiratory distress syndrome at birth often have prolonged patency of the ductus.

About 85 to 90% of PDAs occur as isolated defects. The remainder are most often associated with VSD, coarctation, or pulmonary or aortic stenosis. The length and diameter of the ductus vary widely. Sometimes it virtually consists of only a defect between the closely approximated pulmonary artery and aorta. In other instances, it is several centimeters in length. The diameter may range up to 1 cm. Commonly, the left ventricle is hypertrophied and the pulmonary artery dilated. In older children and adults, right ventricular hypertrophy appears when pulmonary hypertension supervenes.

Most often, PDA does not produce functional difficulties at birth. Indeed, a narrow ductus may have no effect on growth and development during childhood. However, its existence can generally be detected by a continuous harsh murmur described as machinery-like. Often it is accompanied by a systolic thrill. Because the shunt is at first left-to-right, there is no cyanosis. However, pulmonary hypertension and pulmonary vascular disease eventually ensue, with ultimate reversal of flow and all its associated consequences—right ventricular hypertrophy, cyanosis, clubbing, and polycythemia. Because the ductus empties into the aorta distal to the origin of the left subclavian artery, the cyanosis may affect the toes and lower extremities, but not the fingers.

There is general agreement that a PDA should be closed as early in life as is feasible. Up to the recent past, operative closure was recommended, but currently large-scale studies of pharmacologic closure (indomethacin to suppress prostaglandin E [PGE] synthesis) have proved promising.[95] On the other hand, preservation of ductal patency assumes great importance in the survival of infants with various forms of congenital heart disease restricting pulmonary blood flow, e.g., pulmonary valve atresia, transposition of the great arteries, and hypoplastic right heart. Paradoxically, then, the ductus may be either a threat to life or life saving.

OBSTRUCTIVE NONCYANOTIC CONGENITAL ANOMALIES

Coarctation of Aorta

Coarctation—narrowing or constriction—of the aorta ranks high in frequency among the common structural anomalies. Males are affected three to four times more often than females, although females with Turner's syndrome (p. 134) frequently have a coarctation. In the past, the narrowings have been subdivided into an "infantile" form with hypoplasia of the aortic arch proximal to the ductus and an "adult" postductal form, but there is little utility to this separation because clinical manifestations depend almost entirely on the location of the narrowing and its severity. Although coarctation may occur as the sole defect, in 50% of instances it is accompanied by other anomalies—patent ductus arteriosus, bicuspid aortic valve, congenital aortic stenosis, ASD, VSD, mitral regurgitation, and berry aneurysms of the circle of Willis.

Narrowing of the aorta may occur anywhere along its length, even below the diaphragm, but most coarctations are located just distal ("adult" form) or (less often) proximal to the ductus arteriosus or its obliterated ligamentum arteriosum ("infantile" form). The distal narrowings tend to be localized, ridge-like constrictions, whereas the preductal narrowings often involve large segments of the aortic root. The encroachment on the aortic lumen is also variable, sometimes leaving only a very small channel or, at other times, producing only minimal narrowing. With preductal coarctation, the ductus arteriosus is almost always open; in the postductal group, less than half have a patent ductus arteriosus (Fig. 13–19).

Preductal coarctation usually leads to manifestations early in life, and indeed it may cause signs and symptoms immediately after birth. Many infants with this anomaly do not survive the neonatal period. Much depends on the patency of the ductus arteriosus and its ability to supply sufficient blood to the aorta to sustain the circulation to the lower part of the body. With preductal coarctation, right ventricular hypertrophy develops in utero, and congestive heart failure may appear very early. In such cases the delivery of unsaturated blood through the ductus arteriosus produces cyanosis in the lower half of the body, whereas the head and arms are unaffected as their blood supply derives from vessels having origins proximal to the ductus.

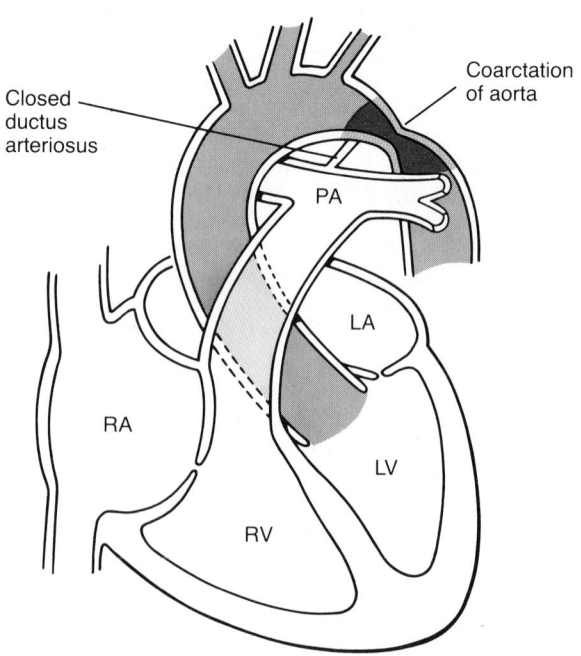

Figure 13–19. Diagram of major vessels showing a postductal coarctation of the aorta.

The outlook is much brighter with *postductal coarctation*, unless it is very severe. Most of the children are asymptomatic and the disease may go unrecognized until well into adult life. Typically, there is hypertension in the upper extremities, but weak pulses and a lower blood pressure in the lower extremities associated with manifestations of arterial insufficiency (i.e., claudication and coldness). Particularly characteristic in adults is the development of collateral circulation between the precoarctation arterial branches and the postcoarctation arteries. Thus, the intercostals may become enlarged and palpable. Radiographically visible erosions ("notching") of the inner surfaces of the ribs may be produced by abnormally dilated internal mammary arteries. The axillary arteries may also become dilated and obviously pulsatile.

With all significant coarctations, murmurs are often present throughout systole, and sometimes a thrill. Similarly, there is cardiomegaly. Ultimately, aortography is definitive. With uncomplicated coarctation, surgical resection and end-to-end anastomosis or replacement of the affected aortic segment by a prosthetic graft yields excellent results. Untreated, the mean duration of life is about 40 years. Deaths are caused by congestive heart failure, intracranial hemorrhage, infective aortitis at the point of narrowing, and rupture of the precoarctation aorta related to the hypertension and the development of cystic medial necrosis (p. 583).

Pulmonary Stenosis or Atresia with Intact Interventricular Septum

This is a relatively frequent cardiac malformation representing about 7% of all congenital heart diseases. It may occur as an isolated defect or as part of a more complex anomaly — tetralogy of Fallot or transposition. When the valve is entirely atretic it is commonly associated with a hypoplastic right ventricle and an ASD.

With atresia, there is no communication between the right ventricle and lungs, and so flow bypasses the right ventricle through an interatrial septal defect, thence entering the lungs through a patent ductus. Pulmonary stenosis, on the other hand, may be mild to severe. It is usually caused by fusion of the cusps, creating a dome-shaped structure surmounted by the valvular orifice. The thickness is created by an increase of myxomatous tissue. Right ventricular hypertrophy often develops and sometimes poststenotic dilatation of the pulmonary artery owing to jet-stream injury to the wall.

Mild stenosis may be asymptomatic and compatible with long life. The smaller the valvular orifice, the more severe is the cyanosis and the earlier its appearance. Isolated valvular stenosis is easily corrected with surgery, or in some cases by balloon dilation valvuloplasty.[96] When associated with right ventricular hypoplasia, the outlook is poor. It should be noted that obstruction to the pulmonary flow may be due also to subvalvular or supravalvular narrowings, or sometimes there are multiple sites of stenosis.

Aortic Stenosis and Atresia

The aortic valvular orifice may be narrowed or stenosed by acquired disease (rheumatic heart disease, degenerative calcific aortic stenosis), by anomalous development (atresia or stenosis), or by a combination of both (calcification of a congenitally malformed valve). The most common congenital anomaly is a bicuspid aortic valve, which is usually of little functional significance, but it is predisposed to secondary calcification in adult life, as will be pointed out later (p. 626). Rarely there is a single cusp, which surprisingly is compatible with survival. Here we are concerned with the narrowings and obstructions of the aortic valve present from birth.

Congenital aortic atresia is rare and is incompatible with neonatal survival. Congenital aortic stenosis, however, is compatible with survival depending on its severity. There are two types of stenosis, valvular and subvalvular. With valvular stenosis there is maldevelopment of the cusps to create essentially a thickened, fibrous diaphragm having a lumen of varying diameter. The subvalvular pattern comprises a thickened fibrous ring below the level of the cusps. With the exception of coarctation of the aorta and occasionally patent ductus arteriosus, other associated anomalies are uncommon. However, left ventricular hypertrophy frequently develops as a consequence of the pressure overload. Sometimes, poststenotic dilatation of the aortic root develops.

A prominent systolic murmur is usually detectable, and sometimes a thrill. It should be noted that there are other causes of obstruction to the left ventricular outflow, such as an unusually proximal coarctation (supravalvular obstruction) and hypertrophic cardiomyopathy (p. 644). In general, congenital stenoses are well tolerated unless very severe. Mild stenoses can be managed conservatively with antibiotic prophylaxis and avoidance of strenuous activity, but the threat of sudden death with exertion always looms. Surgical correction is usually indicated, however, with both mild and severe stenosis for hemodynamic reasons and to lessen the chance of infective endocarditis.

MALPOSITIONS OF THE HEART

Positional anomalies are, fortunately, uncommon. Some are extraordinary and are encountered in teratologic monsters such as the situation of the heart outside of the body (ectopia cordis) or within the abdomen with a diaphragmatic hernia. Other malpositions, such as dextrocardia, are of importance only as clinical diagnostic curiosities imposed upon unsuspecting medical students. In dextrocardia, the apex of the heart points to the right and is in the right hemithorax. Dextrocardia may be accompanied by inversion of all of the viscera in the recessively inherited condition "situs inversus totalis," thus creating a mirror image of the anatomic location of all viscera. The left-sided appendix and gallbladder can cause confusion for the unwary surgeon. Sometimes the situs inversus is accompanied by sinusitis and bronchiectasis, thus constituting *Kartagener's syndrome.* The basis for this curious complex of abnormalities is discussed on page 777. In most instances, the heart is otherwise normal and the individual may not even be aware of being a "walking medical curiosity." However, other cardiac malformations may be present.

Dextrocardia may not be accompanied by inversion of other viscera—isolated dextrocardia. Such hearts are almost always abnormal. Particularly common associations are transposition of the atria relative to the ventricles, or transposition of the great arteries, as has been described. Conversely, the viscera may be inverted with the heart in its normal position.[97] There is a well-defined association of asplenia or polysplenia with malpositions of the heart.

ENDOCARDIAL AND VALVULAR DISEASE

A number of acquired disorders are characterized principally by valvular involvement and dysfunction: mitral valve prolapse; rheumatic heart disease; calcific aortic valve stenosis; calcification of the mitral anulus; carcinoid heart disease and three forms of vegetative endocarditis; infective endocarditis; nonbacterial thrombotic endocarditis; and the endocarditis of systemic lupus erythematosus. The cardiac valvular ramifications of syphilis have already been discussed on page 580. Increasingly commonly today, diseased heart valves are replaced by prostheses. These interventions have engendered their own pathology, which will be considered later in this section. Before these disorders are presented, a discussion of a few general principles is in order.

Stenosis implies failure of a valve to open completely, thereby preventing forward flow. Isolated aortic stenosis and isolated mitral stenosis account for approximately half of all valve lesions encountered. *Insufficiency or regurgitation, in contrast, results from failure of a valve to close completely,* thereby allowing reversed flow. Stenosis and insufficiency often coexist in the same valve, but one of these defects usually predominates. More than one valve may be involved (combined disease). These dysfunctions vary in degree from slight and physiologically unimportant to severe and rapidly fatal. The degree of tolerable stenosis or insufficiency varies from valve to valve and with the rate of development. At one end of the spectrum, sudden destruction of an aortic valve cusp by infection (infective endocarditis) may cause rapidly fatal cardiac failure. In contrast, hemodynamically significant mitral stenosis usually is remarkably well tolerated over the several decades it takes to develop. Depending on degree, duration, and etiology, valvular stenosis or insufficiency may produce secondary

changes in the heart, blood vessels, and other organs, both proximal and distal to the valvular lesion. The abnormalities of flow also produce abnormal sounds (murmurs).

Valvular abnormalities may be caused by congenital disorders, as has been pointed out (p. 625), or by a variety of acquired diseases. *Although valvular insufficiency may result from either intrinsic disease of the valve cusps or damage to the supporting structures (e.g., the aorta, mitral anulus, chordae tendineae, papillary muscles) without primary changes in the cusps, and may appear acutely as with rupture of chordae, valvular stenosis almost always is due to a primary abnormality of the cusps and is virtually always a chronic process.* In contrast to the many potential causes of valvular insufficiency, only a relatively few conditions produce acquired valvular stenosis. The most important causes of heart valve dysfunction are summarized in Table 13–5 and are discussed in the specific sections below.[98]

CALCIFIC AORTIC VALVE STENOSIS

Aortic valve stenosis may occur as a congenital or an acquired lesion. *Congenital aortic stenosis* is discussed on page 625, where it was indicated that the valvular obstruction is present from birth. This definition excludes congenital bicuspid and the rare unicuspid valves that do not cause functional stenoses at birth. *Acquired aortic stenosis* may be rheumatic in origin (p. 632) or the consequence of calcification of either congenital bicuspid (or unicuspid) valves or calcification

Table 13–5. Major Etiologies of Acquired Valvular Heart Disease

MITRAL VALVE DISEASE	AORTIC VALVE DISEASE
Mitral Stenosis	**Aortic Stenosis**
Postinflammatory scarring (rheumatic heart disease)	Postinflammatory scarring (rheumatic heart disease)
	Senile calcific aortic stenosis
	Calcification of congenitally deformed valve
Mitral Regurgitation	**Aortic Regurgitation**
Abnormalities of leaflets and commissures	Intrinsic valvular disease
Postinflammatory scarring	Postinflammatory scarring (rheumatic heart disease)
Infective endocarditis	Infective endocarditis
Floppy mitral valve	Aortic disease
Abnormalities of tensor apparatus	Syphilitic aortitis
Rupture of papillary muscle	Ankylosing spondylitis
Papillary muscle dysfunction (fibrosis)	Rheumatoid arthritis
Rupture of chordae tendineae	Marfan's syndrome
Abnormalities of left ventricular cavity and/or anulus	
LV enlargement (myocarditis, congestive cardiomyopathy)	
Calcification of mitral ring	

From Schoen, F. J., Jr.: Symposium on cardiovascular pathology, part II. Surgical pathology of removed natural and prosthetic valves. Hum. Pathol. *18*:558, 1987.

of normal aortic valves in the aged.[99] With the decline in the incidence of rheumatic fever, rheumatic aortic stenosis now accounts for only about 10% of acquired aortic stenosis.[100] The overwhelming majority of cases represent, then, age-related degenerative calcifications that come to clinical attention in the sixth to seventh decades of life with preexisting bicuspid valves and not until the eighth and ninth decades with previously normal valves.

The morphologic hallmarks of nonrheumatic, calcific aortic stenosis are heaped-up, calcified masses within the aortic cusps protruding into the sinuses of Valsalva and distorting the cuspal architecture (Fig. 13–20). These changes are much more frequent in bicuspid aortic valves than in previously normal valves (Fig. 13–21). Notably in contrast to rheumatic aortic stenosis, there is no commissural fusion. When the process is not too far advanced, it may be possible to discern that in the congenitally bicuspid valves, the calcification begins at the free edges of the two cusps and progresses toward the base, whereas in the normal tricuspid valve it begins at the bases.

However, by the time these changes are seen at postmortem examination, the cusps are usually fibrosed and thickened in all cases. The fibrosis and calcification may so overwhelm the valve as to make difficult the identification of the preexisting architecture of the valve, but usually some vestiges of the commissures remain to permit differentiation of bicuspid from tricuspid valves. In passing, it should be noted that rarely heaped-up masses of calcification are present on the aortic leaflets as a vestige of prior infective endocarditis, but these tombstones of prior infection are not usually difficult to differentiate from senile calcific aortic stenosis.

The obstruction to left ventricular outflow leads to a pressure gradient across the calcified valve, which gradually increases over the course of years. The left ventricular output is maintained by the development of concentric left ventricular hypertrophy (pressure overload). Eventually, as the stenosis worsens, angina or attacks of syncope may appear, even during the years when cardiac compensation is maintained. The angina is probably a consequence of myocardial hypertrophy and higher left ventricular pressure hampering microcirculatory perfusion of the myocardium. The attacks of syncope are poorly understood but carry an increased risk of sudden death. Eventually, cardiac decompensation ensues. Because of the gravity of the prognosis in calcific aortic steno-

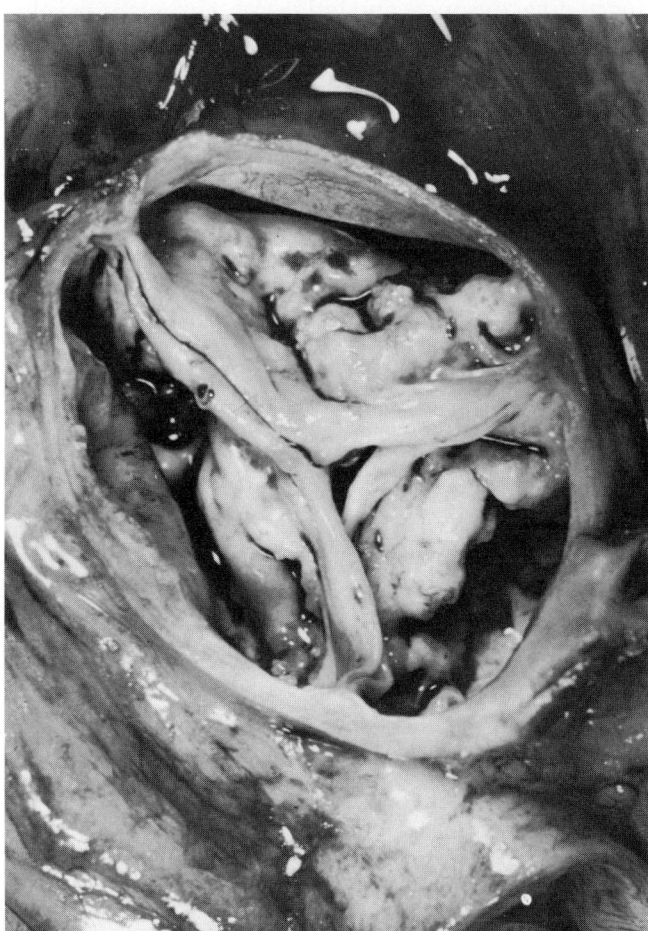

Figure 13–20. Degenerative calcific aortic stenosis in a 72-year-old woman with a previously normal valve having three cusps. Granular masses of calcium are heaped up within sinuses of Valsalva (view looking down at valve). Note that commissures are not fused as in postrheumatic aortic valve stenosis.

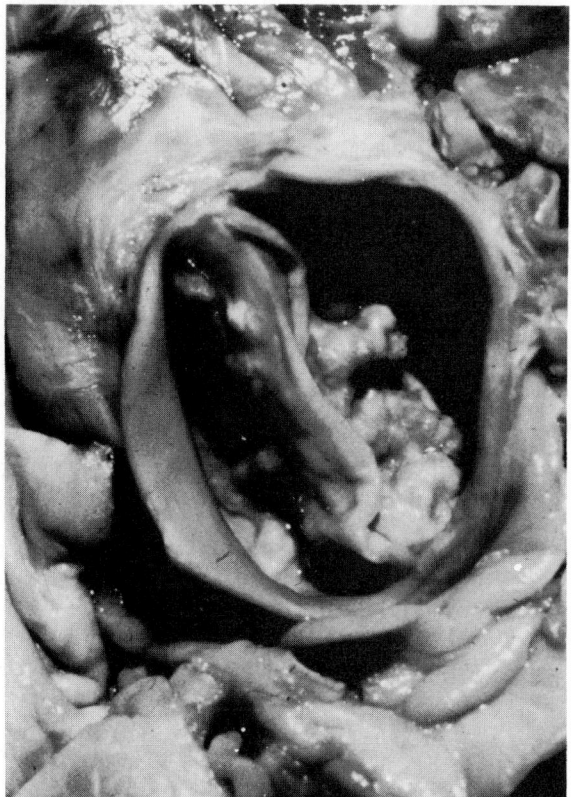

Figure 13–21. Calcific aortic stenosis superimposed on a bicuspid valve in a 52-year-old man.

sis, valve replacement or, in selected cases, balloon aortic valvuloplasty is recommended, in the appropriate setting, when the condition becomes symptomatic.[101]

MITRAL VALVE PROLAPSE

In this curious valvular abnormality, one or both "floppy" enlarged mitral leaflets prolapse, or balloon back, into the left atrium during systole. On auscultation only a midsystolic click or clicks may be heard, corresponding to snapping or tensing of an everted cusp, scallop, or chorda tendinea. Often, however, the valve becomes incompetent and the mitral regurgitation induces an accompanying late systolic or sometimes holosystolic murmur. Hence, this condition is also referred to as the "midsystolic click syndrome," "midsystolic click, late-systolic murmur syndrome," or variations on this theme. Other names based on anatomic changes include "billowing," "ballooning," "hooding," and "myxomatous" degeneration of the mitral valve. Whatever its name, it is an extremely common condition thought to be present in about 7% of the population of the United States, most often in women (female-to-male ratio, 6 : 4) between 20 and 40 years of age.[102] Usually it is an incidental finding on physical examination, but it may have serious import. Sometimes the valvular abnormality is one feature of Marfan's syndrome (p. 138).

The essential anatomic change in mitral valve prolapse is interchordal ballooning (hooding) of the mitral leaflets or portions of the leaflets.[103] Note should be taken that slight degrees of hooding are normal, particularly in elderly individuals, and so the differentiation between "normal" and "pathologic" is one of degree; Edwards suggests that hooding is pathologic when it projects more than 4 mm above the level of the base of the cusp[103] (Fig 13–22). Sometimes the chordae tendineae are elongated or attenuated, and occasionally they are ruptured. Concomitant involvement of the tricuspid valve is present in 20 to 40% of cases and of the pulmonary valve in about 10%[104] (Fig. 13–23). There is no commissural fusion, such as is seen in rheumatic heart disease.

Histologically, the essential changes are degeneration and attenuation of the zona fibrosa on which the structural integrity of the cusp depends, accompanied by compensatory thickening of the spongiosa layer. Normally the ratio of fibrosa to spongiosa is 1 : 1; in the well-defined floppy valve, the thickness of the spongiosa far exceeds that of the fibrosa. Encroachment by loose connective tissue on the collagen structure of the chordae tendineae accounts for their attenuation and occasional rupture.[105]

Secondary changes may appear subsequent to the stresses and injury incident to the billowing leaflets: (1) fibrous thickening of the valve leaflets particularly where they rub against each other, (2) fibrous deposits on the left ventricular surfaces, (3) thickening of the mural endocardium of the left ventricle as a consequence of friction-induced injury by the prolapsing leaflets, (4) thromboses on the atrial surfaces of the leaflets in the recesses behind the ballooned cusps, and (5) focal calcifications at the base of the posterior mitral leaflet.

The basis for the changes within the valve leaflets is unknown. Favored is the proposition of a developmental anomaly perhaps involving connective tissue throughout the body. You recall the previously mentioned association with Marfan's syndrome and occasionally with other hereditary disorders of connective tissue.[106] Even in the absence of these well-defined conditions, there are hints of extracardiac systemic structural abnormalities in some individuals with the floppy mitral valve syndrome, such as scoliosis, straight back, high arched palate, and others.

CLINICAL COURSE. Most patients with mitral valve prolapse are asymptomatic and the condition is discovered only on routine examination by the presence of a mid-systolic click. Echocardiography in such cases will usually reveal the mitral valve prolapse. A minority of patients present with chest pain mimicking angina, dyspnea, and fatigue or, curiously, psychiatric manifestations such as depression, anxiety reactions, and personality disorders. Although in some individuals these affective disorders may be related to excessive concern about their heart condition, frequently the individuals are totally unaware of any cardiac abnormality. The great majority of patients have no untoward effects related to the mitral valve prolapse. However, there are four principal concerns:[107]

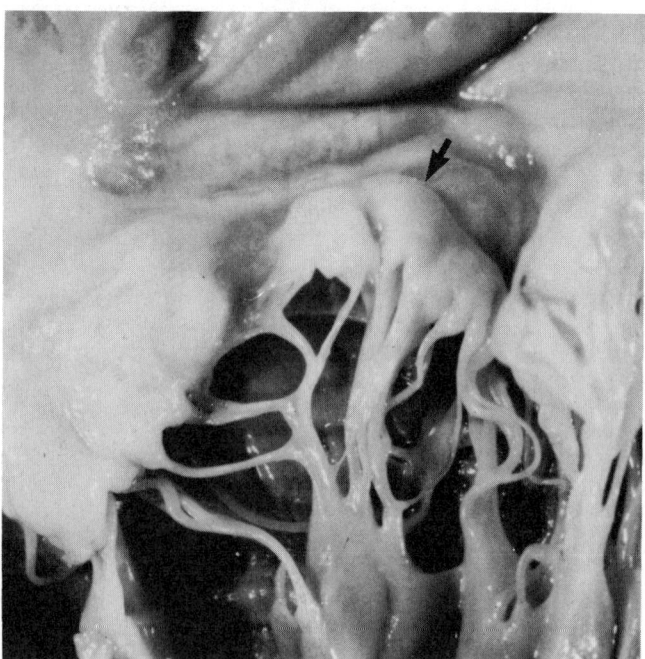

Figure 13–22. The mitral valve, when opened, revealing a prolapsed hooding of posterior leaflet *(arrow)* on right as compared with relatively normal anterior leaflet on left.

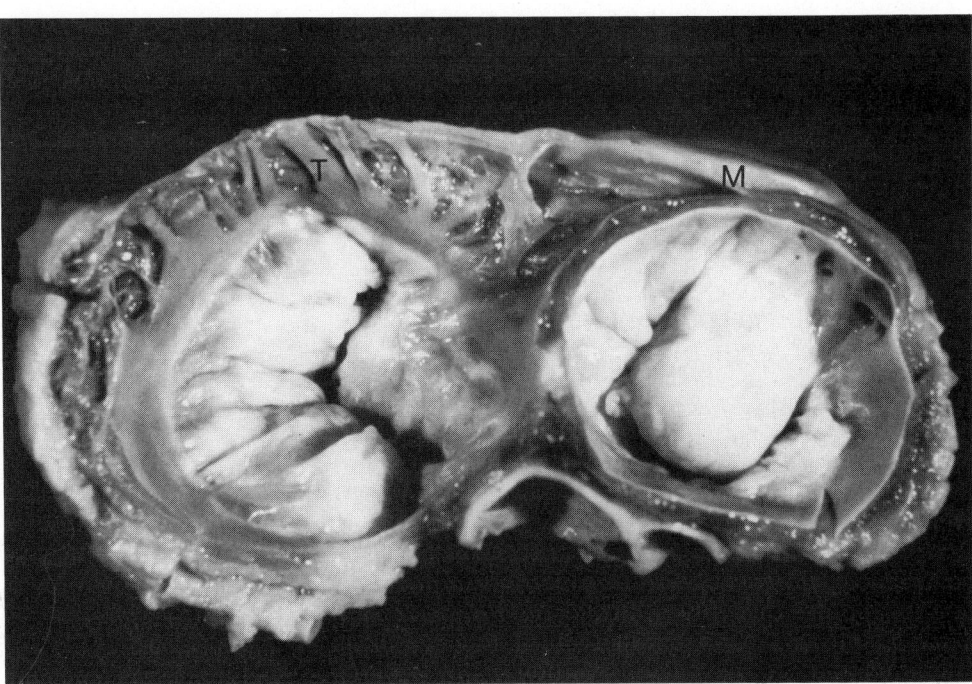

Figure 13–23. Prolapsed mitral (M) and tricuspid (T) valves as viewed from the atria.

1. Infective endocarditis, which is manyfold more frequent in these patients than in the general population.
2. The slow onset of mitral insufficiency, attributed to either dilatation of the mitral anulus or chordal lengthening. Infrequently the insufficiency appears suddenly, owing to chordal rupture. The regurgitation may become sufficiently marked to make replacement by an artificial valve necessary.
3. Arrhythmias, both ventricular and atrial, sometimes develop.
4. Sudden death is the most feared consequence of floppy mitral valves. It is fortunately an uncommon complication and is thought to be restricted to those patients having both mitral valve prolapse and some form of ventricular arrhythmia of uncertain origin. The risk of sudden death in the individual with a normal electrocardiogram is held to be remote.

RHEUMATIC FEVER (RF) AND RHEUMATIC HEART DISEASE (RHD)

Rheumatic fever is an acute, recurrent, inflammatory disease, principally of children, that follows a pharyngeal infection with group A streptococci. The evidence strongly suggests that it is the result of an immune response to streptococcal antigens inciting either a cross reaction to tissue antigens principally in the heart or an autoimmune reaction to tissue antigens. *The acute disease is characterized principally by (1) fever, (2) migratory polyarthritis of the large joints, (3) carditis, (4) subcutaneous nodules, (5) erythema marginatum of the skin, and (6) Sydenham's chorea—a neurologic disorder with involuntary purposeless, rapid movements.* Less commonly, the periarticular tissues, arteries, and lungs are also affected. Although the acute attack may induce arthritis and sometimes myocarditis, both resolve. In contrast, involvement of the cardiac valves has chronic sequelae that are most disabling. Chronic RHD is characterized principally by deforming fibrotic valvular disease (particularly mitral stenosis), which produces permanent dysfunction and severe, sometimes fatal, cardiac failure decades later. So it is said "rheumatic fever licks the joints but bites the heart."

INCIDENCE. The incidence of RF and therefore of its major sequela, RHD, has steadily declined in the United States and other developed countries. In 1940, the mortality rate from RHD in the United States was 20.6 per 100,000 population; in 1982, it was 2.2.[108] Nonetheless, periodically there is a resurgence of rheumatic fever in localized areas of the United States,[109] and the disease continues to be a global problem, with an estimated 15 to 20 million new cases a year.

ETIOLOGY AND PATHOGENESIS. There is near consensus that *RF results either from (1) heightened immunologic reactivity to streptococcal antigens that evoke antibodies cross reactive with tissue antigens or (2) some form of autoimmune reaction incited by a streptococcal infection.* Relative to the *cross-reactive theory:*

• There is a clear association between streptococcal pharyngitis and initial and recurrent attacks of RF.
• Depending on the time interval between the pharyngitis and RF, elevated serum titers of antistreptolysin O (ASO), antihyaluronidase, and others are almost always present.

• Direct bacterial invasion can be ruled out because the tissue lesions are sterile. Moreover, the time interval (one to five weeks) between the pharyngitis and the onset of RF favors an immune response.

• The more severe the streptococcal pharyngitis, the greater the likelihood of RF. The attack rate is approximately 3% following exudative epidemic streptococcal pharyngitis.

• Recurrent acute RF is preceded by a streptococcal infection. The frequency of such recurrence ranges from 5 to 50% and is also related to virulence of the reactivating infection.

• The decline in morbidity and mortality from rheumatic fever in the United States has been related to improved socioeconomic living conditions, better control of streptococcal infections by penicillin, and — for mysterious reasons — some apparent reduction in the virulence of the causative organisms.[110]

However, what determines which individual will develop RF and RHD following a provocative streptococcal infection remains unknown, as are the precise antigenic tissue targets of the putative cross-reactive antibodies. Individual susceptibility may be related to genetically determined immune response genes to streptococcal antigens. With respect to potential antigenic targets, the hyaluronate capsule of the streptococcus is identical to human hyaluronate, and antibodies to these targets cross react with glycoproteins in heart valves.[111] In addition, streptococcal membrane antigens evoke antibodies cross reactive with myocardial and smooth muscle sarcolemma. More recently, shared epitopes of streptococcal M proteins and cardiac myosin have been demonstrated.[112] Unfortunately, it has not been possible to prove to date that the cross-reactive antibodies are directly responsible for the tissue injury in RF.

Autoimmunity has also been invoked as a possible basis for RF.[113] In essence it is proposed that streptococcal infection in some way activates an autoimmune reaction to heart tissues. Anti-heart antibodies have been demonstrated in RF patients who develop carditis; they can be adsorbed by the patient's own atrial tissue; and immunofluorescent techniques demonstrate autoantibodies to heart tissue in focal lesions (Aschoff bodies). However, it has not been proved that these putative "autoantibodies" are *not* cross reactive with streptococcal antigens, and so to date, the cause of RF and RHD is not firmly established.

MORPHOLOGY. In acute rheumatic fever, widely disseminated, focal, inflammatory lesions are found in various sites. Within the heart they are most distinctive and are called **Aschoff bodies** (Fig. 13-24). They constitute foci of fibrinoid necrosis surrounded at first by lymphocytes and macrophages with an occasional plasma cell. As the Aschoff bodies reach full maturity, plump modified histiocytes appear in the inflammatory infiltrate called variously Anitschkow cells or Aschoff cells. These distinctive cells have abundant amphophilic cytoplasm and central round to ovoid nuclei in which the chromatin is disposed in a central, slender, wavy ribbon creating a resemblance to a caterpillar, hence the designation "caterpillar cells." Some of the larger altered histiocytes are multinucleated to form Aschoff giant cells. **This varied inflammatory infiltrate about the central focus of fibrinoid necrosis constitutes the full-blown Aschoff body that is pathognomonic of RF.** With time (years to decades), the Aschoff bodies eventually are replaced by fibrous scar, and so they are sometimes present in auricular biopsies from patients thought to have quiescent or chronic disease.[114]

During acute rheumatic heart disease, Aschoff bodies may be found in any of the three layers of the heart— pericardium, myocardium, or endocardium—hence the term pancarditis. **In the pericardium,** they are located in the subserosal fat and fibrous tissue, and they are accompanied by a fibrinous or serofibrinous pericardial exudate described as a "bread and butter" pericarditis (p. 649) (Fig. 13-25). Usually the pericarditis resolves in time, but it may leave delicate usually nonsignificant fibrous adhesions. The **myocardial involvement** takes the form of scattered Aschoff bodies within the interstitial connective tissue, often in relation to intramyocardial blood vessels. Adjacent myocytes may be damaged or killed.[115] Sometimes the inflammatory myocarditis leads to dilatation of the heart and ventricles, particularly the mitral valve ring. Although the myocarditis may not be accompanied by a pericarditis, there is usually concomitant involvement of the endocardium, mainly the left-sided valves. The **endocardial (i.e., valvular) involvement** is the most ominous aspect of rheumatic carditis and is responsible for the chronic disability decades after the acute disease. Aschoff bodies may be

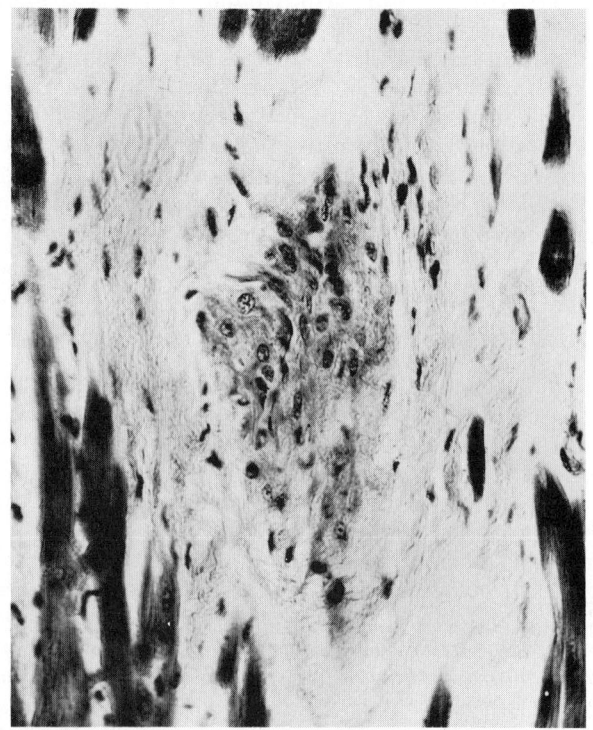

Figure 13-24. Aschoff body at medium power.

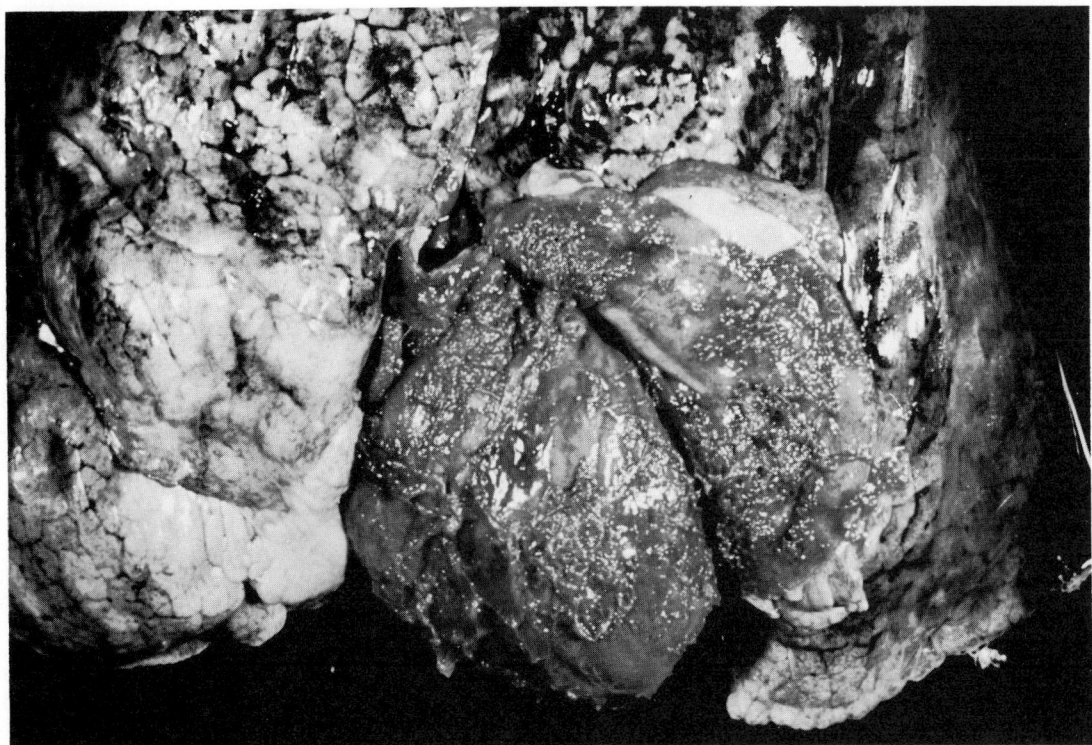

Figure 13-25. Acute rheumatic fibrinous pericarditis. Visceral pericardium (seen in center) and parietal pericardium to its right are shaggy. The lungs, still attached, are at left and right.

found below the mural endocardium, but much more important, inflammatory foci not replicating characteristic Aschoff bodies may also appear within the cardiac valves. Typically, there are foci of fibrinoid necrosis within the cusps overlaid by small (1 to 2 mm) friable vegetations—

verrucae—along the lines of closure (Fig. 13-26). These irregular warty projections probably result from the precipitation of fibrin at sites of erosion of inflamed endocardial surfaces where the leaflets impinge on each other. Similar verrucae may be seen along the chordae tendineae. These

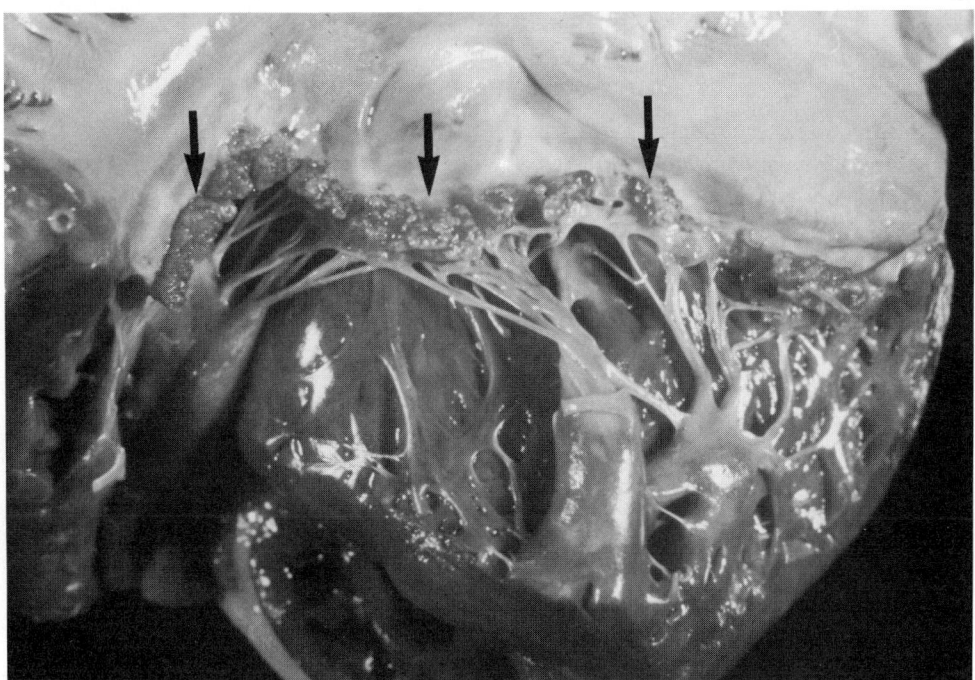

Figure 13-26. Acute rheumatic mitral valvulitis with a linear array of small vegetations along the line of closure of the leaflets *(arrows)*. (Courtesy of Dr. William Roberts, National Institutes of Health, Bethesda, MD, and the American Journal of Cardiology.)

acute valvular involvements cause less disturbance in cardiac function than the myocarditis with ventricular dilatation and consequent mitral insufficiency. The acute valvulitis may presumably resolve or induce only minimal fibrosis leaving little functional deficit, but, on the other hand, it may progress into chronic RHD. Subendocardial lesions may induce map-like thickenings called **MacCallum's plaques** usually in the left atrium.

Chronic rheumatic heart disease is characterized by permanent deformity of the valves involved in acute rheumatic disease. The frequency of this unfortunate sequence is more likely (1) when the first attack occurs in early childhood, (2) when the initial attack of rheumatic fever is severe, and (3) with recurrent attacks. Organization of the acute endocardial inflammation and subsequent fibrosing changes cause the valvular leaflets to become thickened, inelastic, shortened, and blunted. The mitral valve alone is involved in 65 to 70% of the cases, mitral and aortic in about 25%, to which infrequently is added tricuspid involvement and rarely pulmonic.[116] Fibrous bridging across the valvular commissures and calcification create "fish mouth" or "buttonhole" stenoses. Simultaneously the chordae tendineae become thickened, fused, and shortened (Fig. 13–27). In the aortic valve essentially the same cuspal process occurs and is often accompanied by prominent nodular calcifications in the sinuses of Valsalva behind the leaflets (Fig. 13–28). With a tight mitral stenosis, the left atrium and sometimes also the right atrium progressively dilate. The long-standing congestive changes in the lungs (p. 90) may in time lead to right ventricular hypertrophy. Often thrombi form within the auricular appendages. Similar, but less severe, fibrous thickenings and stenoses may occur in the tricuspid valve and rarely in the pulmonic. Chronic rheumatic heart disease usually does not appear until at least ten years after the initial acute attack, sometimes decades

later. At this late date, Aschoff bodies may well have disappeared, and so the recognition of chronic rheumatic valvulitis is more dependent on the characteristic gross alterations than on histologic evidence of rheumatic fever. Rarely, with recurrent acute attacks, the anatomic alterations of acute rheumatic carditis are superimposed on those of chronic RHD.

JOINTS. The likelihood of **acute arthritis** increases with age, appearing in about 90% of adults and less commonly in children. The large joints, such as the knees, are most often affected, but sometimes also the small joints of the hands and feet. Few histologic observations are available on the joints because the changes are transitory and resolve without sequelae. Histologically, there is a nonspecific mononuclear inflammatory infiltrate with edema, focal deposits of fibrinoid, and sometimes lesions resembling Aschoff bodies. The synovial membranes do not become ulcerated and the articular cartilage is unaffected. When changes appear on the radiograph or there is persistent joint deformity, intercurrent disease such as rheumatoid arthritis must be suspected.

SKIN. Lesions of the skin take the form of **subcutaneous nodules** or **erythema marginatum** and are present in 10 to 60% of cases, more often in children. The **subcutaneous nodules** are essentially giant Aschoff bodies with a large central area of fibrinoid enclosed by a cell population similar to that found in the cardiac lesions. The nodules are most often located overlying the extensor tendons of the extremities at the wrists, elbows, ankles, and knees. They sometimes are deeply situated over bony prominences, and rarely are located near the occiput. **Erythema marginatum** tends to have a bathing-suit distribution but may also occur over the thighs, lower extremities, and face. These lesions, which are quite distinctive, begin as flat-to-slightly elevated, slightly reddened maculopapules that progressively en-

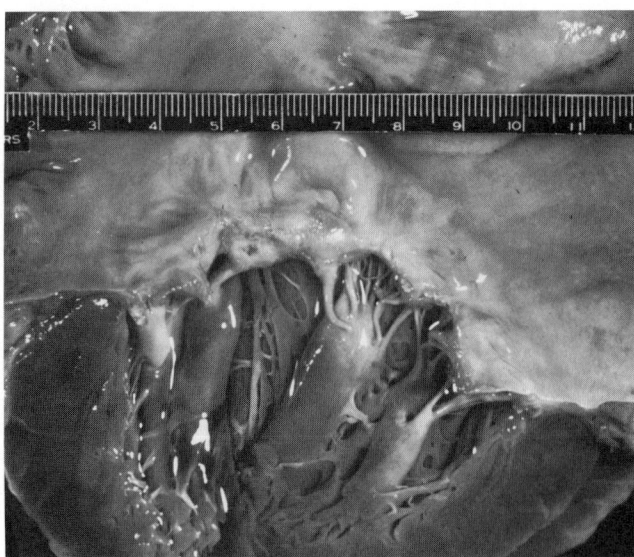

Figure 13–27. Chronic rheumatic mitral stenosis illustrating fibrous thickening and distortion of cusps, intercommissural scarring and fusion, and thickening and shortening of chordae tendineae. There is marked dilatation of the left atrium.

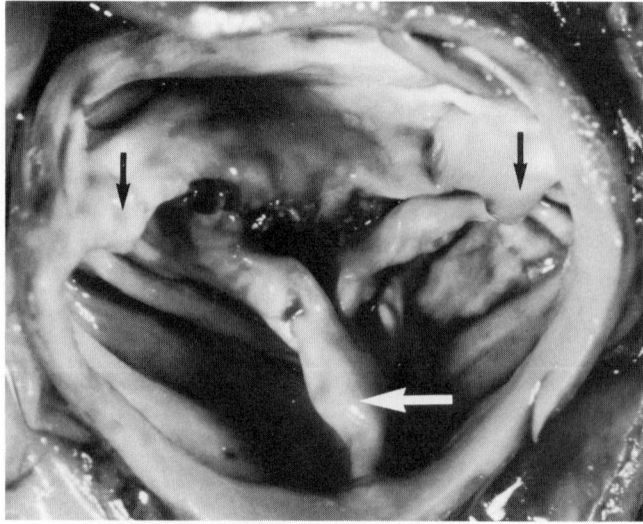

Figure 13–28. Chronic rheumatic aortic stenosis. The unopened valve seen from the aortic surface. The leaflets are thickened and distorted with marked intercommissural adhesion (arrows).

large. At the same time, the centers clear and may undergo slight pigmentation, but the peripheries continue to be reddened and elevated to create prominent erythematous margins.

ARTERIES. Rheumatic arteritis has been described in the coronary, renal, mesenteric, and cerebral arteries as well as in the aorta and pulmonary vessels during the height of an attack. The morphologic alterations are characteristic of hypersensitivity angiitis and were described on page 573.

LUNGS. Rheumatic pneumonitis and **pleuritis** are rare complications of the acute disease. The pulmonary changes consist largely of an interstitial reaction resembling viral pneumonitis (p. 784), sometimes accompanied by fibrinoid changes and an acute angiitis. A nonspecific serofibrinous pleuritis may be present. In the late chronic stages of RHD with mitral stenosis, congestive changes or dense interstitial fibrosis with siderotic nodules often appear.

CLINICAL COURSE. Acute rheumatic fever appears most often in children between the ages of 5 and 15. However, both younger and older individuals may be affected; about 20% of first attacks occur in middle to later life. The latent period between the streptococcal pharyngitis and the onset of the acute attack ranges from one to five weeks. Most attacks begin with migratory polyarthritis accompanied by fever. Typically one joint after another becomes painful and swollen for a period of days and then subsides spontaneously, leaving no residual disability. Acute carditis develops in about 50 to 75% of children between the ages of 2 and 16 years, but in only about 35% of adults having a single acute attack of RF.[117] Should a pericardial friction rub appear it usually clears in the course of days to weeks and leaves no sequelae. During the initial acute attack it is the myocarditis that is most threatening, causing arrhythmias (particularly atrial fibrillation) and prolongation of the electrocardiographic P–R interval. With fibrillation, auricular thrombi are prone to develop and constitute potential sources of emboli. Significant myocarditis may lead to cardiac dilation and murmurs of insufficiency principally of the mitral valve, but following the acute attack the insufficiency may resolve if there has been no acute valvulitis. Involvement of the valve cusps themselves is marked by an apical systolic murmur of mitral regurgitation or a basal diastolic murmur of aortic regurgitation, or both. Failure of clearance of these murmurs within the first three weeks is ominous, raising the likelihood of chronic progression. Overall the prognosis for the primary attack is generally good and only 1% of patients die from fulminant RF.

Following an initial attack, there is increased vulnerability to reactivation of the disease with subsequent pharyngeal infections, and the same manifestations are likely to appear with each recurrent attack. Thus, once carditis develops during the initial attack it is likely to be reactivated and to worsen with each recurrence. Conversely, if the heart is spared during the initial attack it may well go unscathed despite recurrences of RF. In the absence of cardiac involvement the patient may be entirely free from residuals and, spared recurrences, may live a normal life. However, because of the threat of recurrent disease it is now standard practice to administer prophylactic long-term antistreptococcal therapy to anyone who has had RF. When carditis has recurred, the outlook depends on the severity of the chronic valvular deformity. Females appear to be more vulnerable to mitral valve stenosis than males. The heart, even with damaged valves, may remain compensated for the duration of a long life, but usually, over the span of decades, decompensation and eventual full-blown cardiac failure develop. However, this course can now be altered by surgical replacement of damaged valves. Other hazards include embolization from mural thrombi within the atrial appendages and infective endocarditis superimposed on chronically deformed valves.

INFECTIVE ENDOCARDITIS (IE)

Infective endocarditis, one of the most serious of all infections, is characterized by colonization or invasion of the heart valves or the mural endocardium by a microbiologic agent, leading to the formation of friable vegetations laden with organisms—so-called infective vegetations. A similar phenomenon may occur within the aorta (infective endoaortitis), aneurysmal sacs, or other vessels. Virtually every form of microbiologic agent has at one time or another been responsible for these infections, but principally certain bacteria. IE has particular clinical importance because prompt diagnosis and effective treatment significantly alter the outlook for the patient.

On clinical grounds IE has been classified into acute and subacute forms. This subdivision expresses the range of severity of the disease and its tempo, conditioned in large part by the virulence of the infecting microorganism and the underlying cardiac status of the patient. A destructive, tumultuous infection, usually of a previously normal heart, with a highly virulent organism leads to death within days to weeks of 50 to 60% of patients.[118] On the other hand, with organisms of low virulence the heart is usually abnormal and the disease may appear insidiously and, even untreated, pursue a protracted course of many months. Following appropriate therapy for such infections, most patients recover. There is, however, no clear clinical delineation between acute and subacute IE; they are points along a spectrum. Similarly, the morphologic lesions make up a spectrum. Acute disease tends to be associated with highly virulent organisms that tend to produce necrotizing, ulcerative, invasive valvular infections, whereas in subacute disease the organisms are of lower virulence, and the vegetations are less destructive and often have evidence of healing. However, *the vegetations found in the heart in both clinical variants of the disease are more alike than different.* Nonetheless, the microbial flora and the pathogenetic influences responsible for the two clinical subdivisions are somewhat different.

EPIDEMIOLOGY AND PATHOGENESIS.

IE may develop in previously normal hearts, but a variety of cardiac abnormalities predispose to this form of infection. In years past, rheumatic heart disease was the major contributor, but now its primary position has been taken by congenital heart disease, particularly in children. The anomalies most often involved are those having small shunts or tight stenoses creating jet streams (e.g., a small interventricular septal defect — as compared with a large interatrial septal defect). A person with patent ductus arteriosus or tetralogy of Fallot is also at risk.[119] Additional major predispositions include mitral valve prolapse, degenerative calcific valvular stenoses, bicuspid aortic valve, and notably, at the present time, artificial valves and indwelling pulmonary artery catheters. Equally important as predisposing influences are neutropenia, immunodeficiency, immunosuppression, and IV drug abuse.

Virtually every bacterial species, as well as rarely fungi, rickettsae (Q fever), chlamydiae, and possibly viruses, have at one time or another been implicated in the causation of infective endocarditis. Overall about 65% of cases are attributable to various streptococci — viridans group, bovis, faecalis, and others.[120] These invasive, spreading organisms of relatively low virulence are the dominant causes of subacute disease because they are able to gain a foothold only in hearts having some underlying disease or predisposition. *Staphylococcus aureus* accounts overall for about 20 to 30% of cases; it is the leading cause of acute endocarditis and can implant on previously normal valves; it is the predominant agent in narcotic endocarditis; and it is a major cause of prosthetic valve endocarditis. Other significant etiologic agents include *Streptococcus pneumoniae*, gram-negative bacilli, particularly *Escherichia coli*, *Neisseria gonorrhoeae*, and uncommonly several concurrent organisms. In IV drug abusers the right-sided valves are commonly affected and the major offenders are *S. aureus*, Candida, and Aspergillus.[121] In several studies, this form of endocarditis accounts for about 10 to 15% of all cases. It also appears in 4 to 6% of patients with a prosthetic valve.[122,123] The major early offenders in such cases are staphylococcal skin contaminants (e.g., *S. aureus*, *S. epidermidis*), but later streptococci predominate.[124] In about 5 to 10% of all cases of endocarditis no organism can be isolated from the blood ("culture-negative" endocarditis) either because of prior antibiotic therapy, because of difficulties in isolation of the offending agent, or because they become deeply embedded within the enlarging vegetation and are not released into the blood.

Foremost among the factors predisposing to the development of endocarditis is seeding of the blood with microbes. The portal of entry of the agent into the bloodstream may be overt, as with an infection elsewhere, IV drug addiction, or a previous dental or surgical procedure. However, it may be covert. Transient bacteremias emanate frequently from the gut, oral cavity, and trivial injuries, seeding the blood with organisms usually of low virulence (e.g., viridans streptococci, *S. faecalis*, *E. coli*).

Granting the existence of blood-borne organisms, *three influences are thought to be important in the development of subacute endocarditis.*

• Most significant is the formation of sterile platelet-fibrin deposits (nonbacterial thrombotic endocarditis, or NBTE [p. 636]) at sites of impingement of eddy currents or jet streams created by the preexisting cardiac disease.[118]
• Agglutinating antibodies predispose to seeding of the sterile vegetations by creating clumps of organisms more likely to attach to evolving fibrinous deposits.
• Bacterial adhesion factors may also be important. Streptococci have been demonstrated to adhere to fibrin and platelet thrombi, whereas *E. coli* adhere poorly, perhaps explaining the striking difference in the frequency of these two organisms in the causation of endocarditis.

The events surrounding the development of acute IE are less well understood. Sometimes they are well defined, such as intravenous drug abuse with repeated contamination of the blood, or indwelling vascular catheters, or prosthetic valves that constitute foreign bodies inviting the localization of blood-borne agents. However, such special circumstances may not be necessary when the blood is seeded by highly virulent organisms such as *S. aureus*. Thus, it is believed that acute IE may develop in any individual when the organism is of sufficient virulence, the bacterial invasion is sufficiently large, and the resistance of the host is depressed.

MORPHOLOGY. The diagnostic findings in both the subacute and acute forms of the disease are friable, bulky, usually bacteria-laden vegetations most commonly on the heart valves. The vegetations in IE are bulkier than those produced by other forms of vegetative endocarditis (see Fig. 13–32, p. 638). They may occur singly or multiply on one or more valves on either side of the heart (Table 13–6). The individual vegetations vary from a few millimeters to several centimeters in greatest dimension. They can pile up or hang from the free margins of the leaflets as irregular, readily fragmented masses (Fig. 13–29). **The vegetations in acute endocarditis tend to be bulkier than those in subacute disease and moreover are situated more often on previously normal valves, cause perforation or erosion of the underlying valve leaflet, and sometimes erode into the underlying myocardium to produce abscess cavities (Fig. 13–30). In contrast, in the subacute form of the disease they less often erode or perforate the cusps and tend to produce smaller vegetations that often extend onto the adjacent mural endocardium.** With nonvalvular congenital defects, the vegetations tend to be

Table 13-6. Localization of Vegetations in Subacute, Acute, Narcotic, and Prosthetic Endocarditis

	SUBACUTE	ACUTE	NARCOTIC	PROSTHETIC
Left-Sided Valves	**85%**	**65%**	**40%**	**95%**
Aortic	15-25	20-25	25-30	45-50
Mitral	40-45	30-35	15-20	45-50
Aortic and mitral	20-30	15-20	15-20	Rare
Right-Sided Valves	**5%**	**20%**	**50%**	
Tricuspid	1-5	15	45-50	
Pulmonary	Rare	Rare	1-2	
Tricuspid and pulmonary	Rare	Rare	3	
Nonvalvular Congenital Defects	**10**	**10**	**5**	

Modified from Durack, D.T.: Infective and noninfective endocarditis. *In* Hurst, J.W. (ed.): The Heart, 6th ed. New York, McGraw-Hill Book Co., 1986, p. 1130.

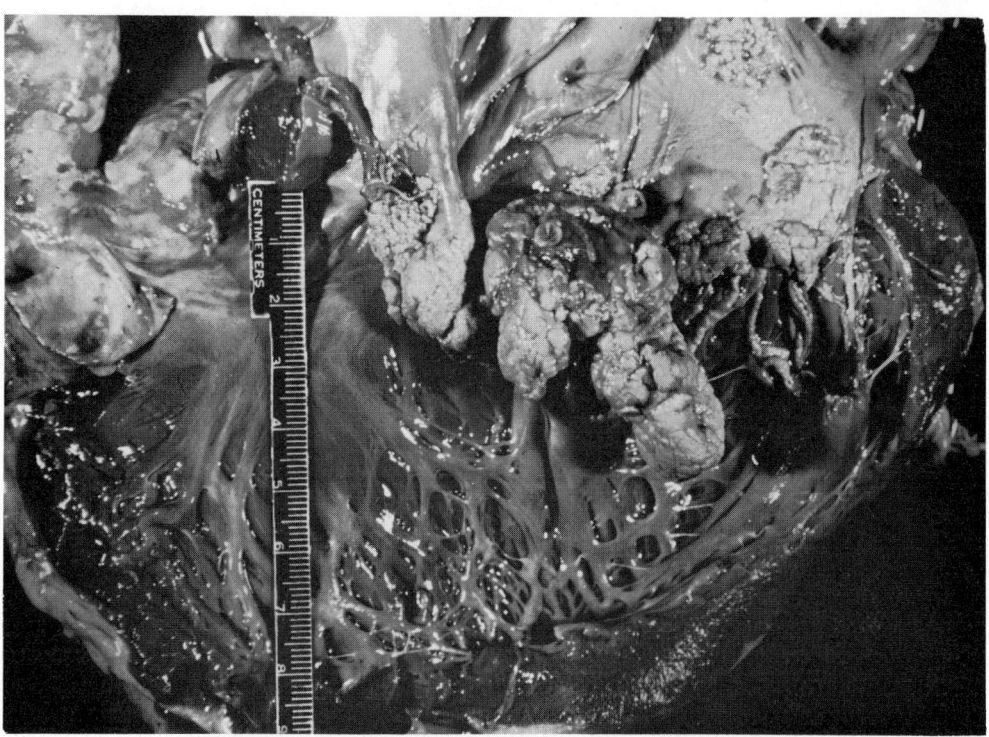

Figure 13-29. Infective endocarditis (bacterial) of mitral valve with extensive friable vegetations, obscuring valve leaflets, and extension of vegetations to atrial endocardium.

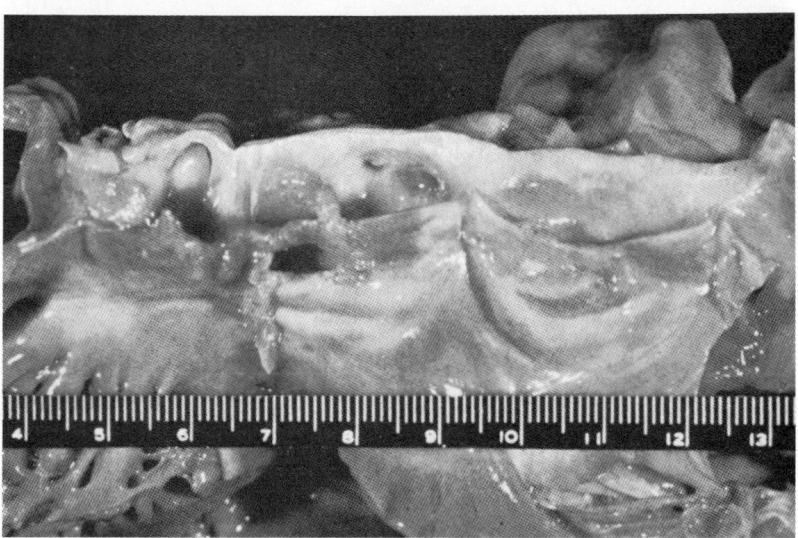

Figure 13-30. Acute infective endocarditis of aortic valve with through-and-through perforation of two cusps.

located on the "downstream" margin of the jet stream (e.g., on the right ventricular margins of an interventricular septal defect). With mechanical prostheses infections are usually located on the margin of the sewing ring, causing a ring abscess. Indeed with extension of the infection, a paravalvular perforation may develop, producing regurgitant leakage of blood — or, worse, the entire prosthesis may be dislocated from its attachments. Similar ring abscesses may develop with bioprostheses, but occasionally the vegetations involve the prosthetic valvular cusps themselves.

More and more cases are now identified with "healed endocarditis." The vegetations undergo progressive sterilization, fibrosis, and organization and eventually become calcified, leaving only irregular heaped-up fibrocalcific, nodular excrescences on the valve leaflets.

CLINICAL COURSE. Fever is the most consistent sign of infective endocarditis. But with *subacute disease*, particularly in the elderly, the fever may be slight or absent. Often the only manifestations of subacute endocarditis are nonspecific fatigue, loss of weight, and a flu-like syndrome. Indeed there may be little to point to the heart as the source of the problem. Murmurs may be present in patients with left-sided lesions but are absent in about 10% of patients with subacute disease and, moreover, may merely relate to the preexistent cardiac abnormality predisposing to IE. Only rarely are changing murmurs encountered in the subacute form of the disease. Petechiae, subungual hemorrhages, and Roth's spots in the eyes have now become uncommon clinical findings owing to the shortened clinical course of the disease as a result of antibiotic therapy.

In contrast, *acute endocarditis* has a stormy onset with rapidly developing fever, chills, weakness, and lassitude. One of the complications (to be described) generally makes its appearance within the first weeks of the onset of the disease. A murmur is more likely to be present with acute endocarditis because of the large size of the vegetations, and often it undergoes change as the vegetations fragment and embolize. The spleen is more often enlarged in the acute form of the disease than in the subacute.

Sometimes complications involving the heart or extracardiac sites call attention to the endocarditis, acute or chronic.[125] They include the following (Fig. 13–31):

- *Cardiac Complications*
  Valvular insufficiency or stenosis with cardiac failure
  Myocardial abscess with possible perforation of IV septum or free wall
  Suppurative pericarditis
  Dehiscence of artificial valve
- *Embolic Complications*
  With left-sided lesions
  To the brain, spleen, kidneys, other sites
  With right-sided lesions
  To the lungs

- *Metastatic Infections*
  With acute staphylococcal endocarditis to almost any organ or tissue (e.g., cerebral abscesses, meningitis, renal abscesses)
  With subacute streptococcal endocarditis (rare)
- *Renal Complications*
  Embolic infarction
  Focal glomerulonephritis — 50% of untreated cases and 15% of treated cases may lead to nephrotic syndrome or renal failure, or both (p. 1033)
  Diffuse glomerulonephritis — 50% of untreated cases and 10% of treated cases — leads to renal failure (p. 1029)
  Multiple abscesses — with acute staphylococcal endocarditis

Although the diagnosis can be suspected on the basis of the appearance of one or more of the complications mentioned, for confirmation a positive blood culture is required. With repeated blood samples, positive cultures can be obtained in 80 to 95% of cases. More important than the diagnosis of IE is its prevention by the prophylactic use of antibiotics in the patient with some form of cardiac anomaly or artificial valve who is about to have some dental or surgical procedure or other form of invasive intervention. With early diagnosis and appropriate treatment, the overall five-year survival is in the range of 50 to 90%, being best for streptococcus-induced subacute disease and worst for staphylococcal and fungal acute endocarditis. Intractable cardiac failure due to valvular destruction or uncontrolled infection is an indication for surgical valve replacement.

NONBACTERIAL THROMBOTIC ENDOCARDITIS (NBTE), MARANTIC ENDOCARDITIS

This disorder is characterized by the precipitation of small masses of fibrin and other blood elements upon the valve leaflets of either side of the heart. In contrast to IE, the vegetations in this condition are sterile and tend to be small (1 to 5 mm). They resemble those of acute rheumatic endocarditis and Libman-Sacks disease much more closely (Fig. 13–32). In NBTE, the vegetations may occur singly or less commonly multiply along the line of closure of the leaflet (Fig. 13–33). Infrequently, they occur at other sites on the leaflets and even on the pulmonic and tricuspid valves. In some instances, the affected leaflets have some form of previous damage, such as old inflammatory rheumatic changes or degenerative alterations due to vascular heart disease. Histologically, the vegetations are bland thrombi and there is no significant accompanying inflammatory reaction or organization. Consequently, they are only loosely attached to the underlying valve.

The significance and interpretation of these lesions are controversial. In most instances, the patients have died of some protracted debilitating disease such as metastatic cancer, renal failure, chronic sepsis, or

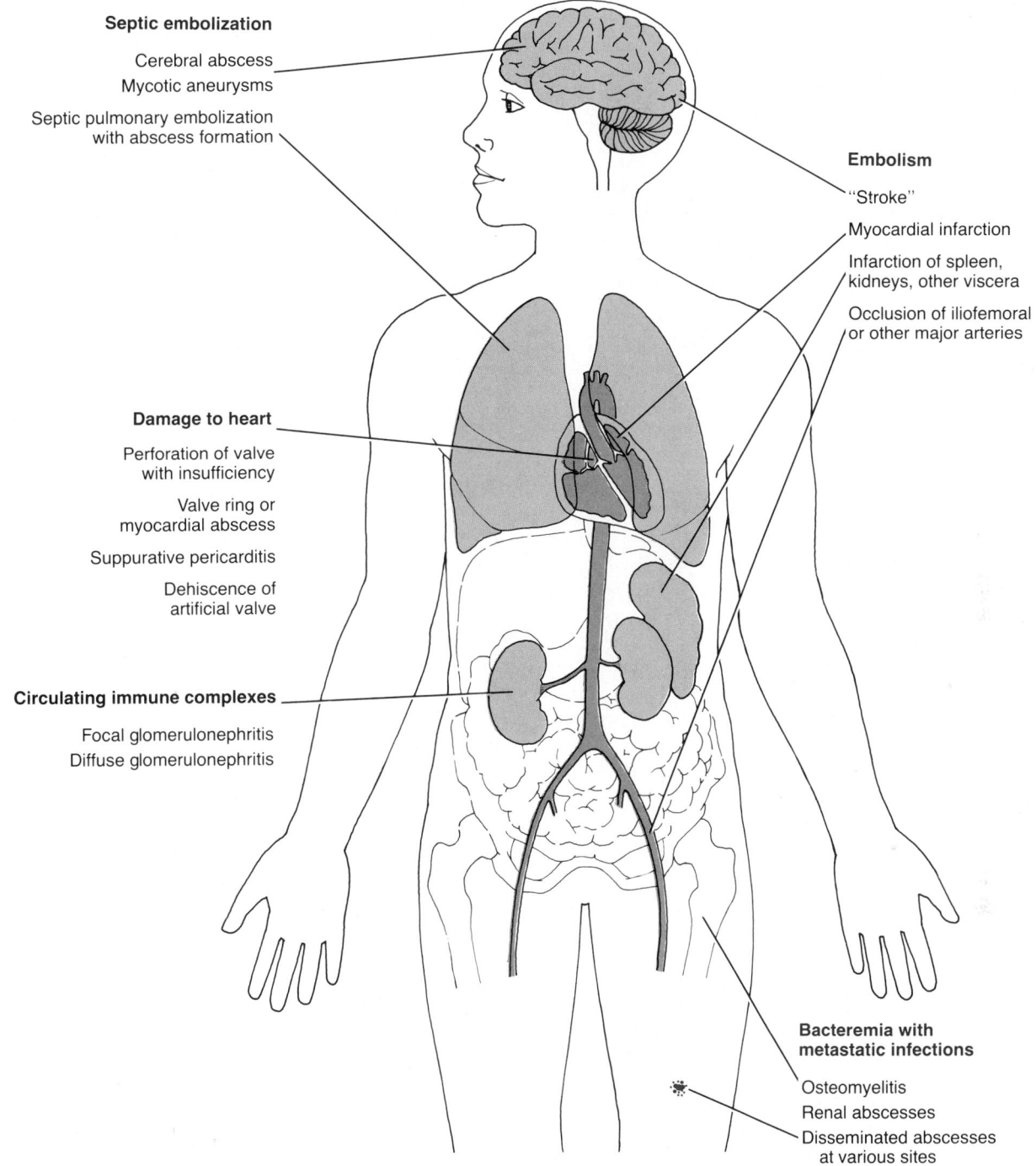

Septic embolization

Cerebral abscess
Mycotic aneurysms

Septic pulmonary embolization
with abscess formation

Embolism

"Stroke"

Myocardial infarction

Infarction of spleen,
kidneys, other viscera

Occlusion of iliofemoral
or other major arteries

Damage to heart

Perforation of valve
with insufficiency

Valve ring or
myocardial abscess

Suppurative pericarditis

Dehiscence of
artificial valve

Circulating immune complexes

Focal glomerulonephritis
Diffuse glomerulonephritis

**Bacteremia with
metastatic infections**

Osteomyelitis
Renal abscesses
Disseminated abscesses
at various sites

Figure 13–31. A schematic representation of the potential complications of infective endocarditis. (Modified from Bisno, A.L.: Staphylococcal endocarditis and bacteremia. Hosp. Pract. *21*:139, 1986.) (Illustration by Susan Tilberry.)

some other form of disease.[126] Sometimes they occur concomitantly with venous thromboses or in patients with pulmonary embolization, suggesting *a common origin in a hypercoagulable state perhaps related to the underlying disease, such as cancer.* Endocardial trauma as from an indwelling pulmonary artery (Swan-Ganz) catheter is a well-recognized predisposing condition. It should be noted, however, that *this form of thrombotic endocarditis has occurred in young*

individuals, even children, and sometimes in patients who are well nourished and distinctly not marantic.[127] Although the local effects on the valves are unimportant, the cardiac vegetations may be significant clinically because they are sometimes productive of emboli and infarctions in the brain, heart, kidneys, lungs, and elsewhere.[127] In addition, these bland vegetations could provide a soil for the implantation of microorganisms to yield IE (p. 633).

Comparison of vegetations

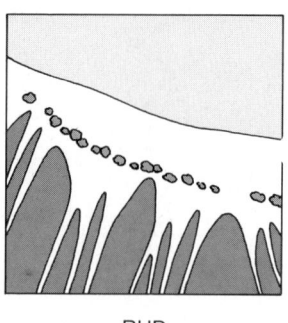 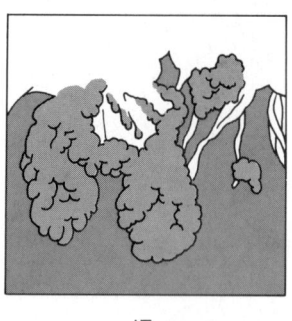 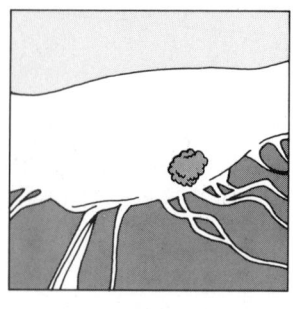 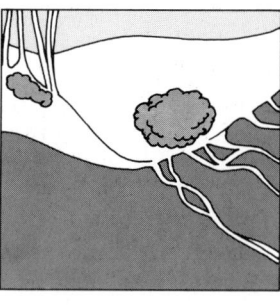

RHD   IE   NBTE   SLE

Figure 13-32. A diagrammatic comparison of the lesions in the four major forms of vegetative endocarditis. RHD (rheumatic heart disease) is marked by a row of warty small vegetations along the lines of closure of the valve leaflets. IE (infective endocarditis) is characterized by large irregular masses overhanging the free margins and extending onto the chordae and valve cusps. NBTE typically exhibits one or two small bland vegetations usually attached at the line of closure. SLE (Libman-Sacks endocarditis) may have small or medium-sized vegetations on either or both sides of the valve leaflets.

ENDOCARDITIS OF SYSTEMIC LUPUS ERYTHEMATOSUS (LIBMAN-SACKS DISEASE)

In systemic lupus erythematosus, mitral and tricuspid valvulitis is occasionally encountered. This form of endocardial involvement is one of the important components of this systemic immunologic disorder which sometimes requires surgery.[128] The connective tissue of the valves may become the site of mucoid pooling, fibrinoid necrosis, and subsequent collagenous fibrosis. Frequently, this type of valvulitis leads to the formation of small vegetations on the valve leaflets that sometimes can be confused with the much larger, friable vegetations of IE or with nonbacterial thrombotic endocarditis (Fig. 13-32). The characteristics and significance of Libman-Sacks disease have already been discussed (p. 201).

CALCIFICATION OF MITRAL ANULUS

In elderly individuals calcific deposits develop, often in association with ischemic heart disease, in the anulus of the mitral valve without significantly affecting the leaflets. They can often be visualized on gross inspection as an irregular, stony hard beading (2 to 5 mm in thickness) that lies behind the leaflets. There is virtually never any associated inflammatory change and it has been postulated that the calcium deposition reflects the degenerative changes of aging. It generally does not affect valvular function, but may lead to regurgitation by interference with systolic contraction of the mitral valve ring. Occasionally, the calcium deposits may penetrate sufficiently deeply to impinge on the conduction system and produce arrhythmias, and infrequently they provide a site for infective endocarditis.[129] Heavy calcific deposits are sometimes

Figure 13-33. *A,* Nonbacterial thrombotic endocarditis. A solitary dark vegetation *(arrow)* is seen on posterior mitral leaflet. *B,* Bland dark vegetation on low power *(arrow)* sits on top of noninflammatory leaflet, as seen on a transection of the valve.

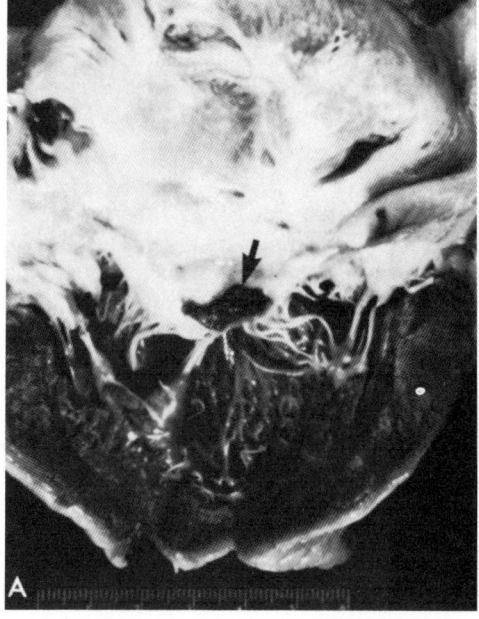 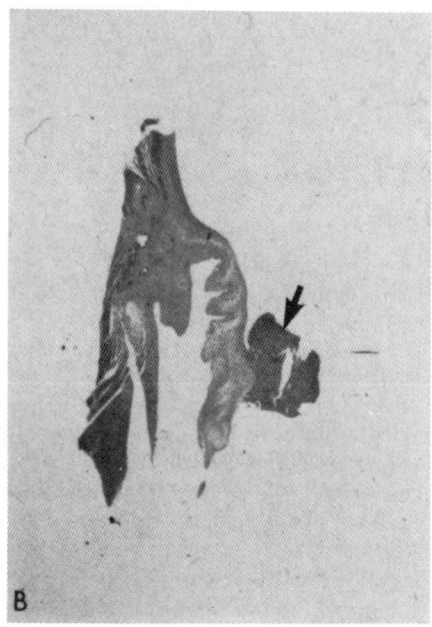

visualized on echocardiography or seen as a distinctive, ringlike opacity on chest radiographs.

CARCINOID HEART DISEASE

Cardiac involvement, principally of the endocardium and valves of the right heart, is one of the major features of the *carcinoid syndrome*, characterized by *distinctive episodic flushing of the skin, and cramps, nausea, vomiting, and diarrhea in almost all patients; bronchoconstrictive episodes resembling asthma in about one third of cases; and cardiac lesions in about one half* (p. 874). These clinical findings relate to the elaboration by argentaffinomas of a variety of bioactive products, including serotonin (5-hydroxytryptamine), kallikrein, bradykinin, histamine, prostaglandins, and newly described tachykinins P and K. However, which of the secretory products produces the various features of the syndrome is still not clear. The carcinoid syndrome is encountered in about 1% of all patients who have an argentaffinoma (whatever the primary site) and 10% of those with gastrointestinal carcinoids with hepatic metastases. In the absence of hepatic metastases, gastrointestinal carcinoids may not induce the syndrome because there is rapid metabolism of serotonin during traversal of the liver. In contrast, argentaffinomas primary in organs outside of the portal system of venous drainage (e.g., in the ovary or lung) may induce the carcinoid syndrome without antecedent hepatic metastases.

> The cardiovascular lesions associated with the carcinoid syndrome are unlike those produced by any other form of cardiac disease. In the majority of cases, plaquelike thickenings composed of an unusual type of fibrous tissue are superimposed on the endocardium of the cardiac chambers and valvular cusps, **mainly on the outflow tract of the right ventricle.** Occasionally, left-sided lesions are also encountered (Fig. 13–34). Histologically, the fibrous thickening bears a remarkable resemblance to the cellular atheromas described on page 563, but the changes involve larger areas of the mural endocardium.

The pathogenesis of the cardiac lesion is uncertain, but they are widely attributed to an elevated blood level of serotonin or bradykinin, although attempts to produce the cardiac changes by chronic infusions of serotonin or bradykinin in rats have failed. Recently attention has turned to the tachykinins—neuropeptide K and substance P.[130] A rough correlation was shown between the plasma levels of these tumor-derived substances and carcinoid heart disease. The fact that the cardiac changes are largely right-sided is explained by inactivation of both serotonin and bradykinin in the blood during passage through the lungs by the monoamine oxidase found in the pulmonary vascular endothelium. Incomplete inactivation of high blood levels might underlie the occasional occurrence of left-sided lesions.

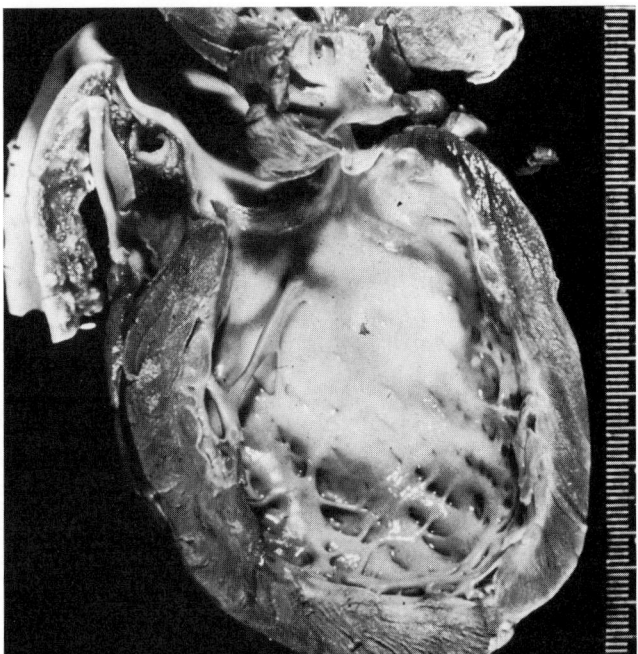

Figure 13–34. Carcinoid heart disease involving both sides of the heart. The left ventricular endocardium reveals marked fibromuscular pearly thickening.

Suffice it to say here that the basis of the morphologic changes in the carcinoid heart remains obscure.

COMPLICATIONS OF ARTIFICIAL VALVES

Replacement of damaged cardiac valves with prostheses has now become a common and often life-saving mode of therapy. In several large studies, the linearized rate of complications was 6 to 9% per patient year.[131] A large variety of artificial valves are in use; for our purposes it suffices to state that they fall into two categories—mechanical valves utilizing different types of occluders such as caged balls, tilting disks, or hinged flaps, and bioprostheses consisting of pretreated animal (usually porcine or bovine) valves. All prostheses, whether mechanical or biologic, are subject to complications, which can be categorized as follows.[132]

- Paravalvular leak
- Thromboembolism
- Infective endocarditis
- Structural or biologic deterioration
- Occlusion or dysfunction by tissue overgrowth
- Others

Paravalvular leaks on the whole are uncommon, often are insignificant, and result from either postsurgical separation of the sewing ring of the valve from the cardiac bed or from dehiscence of a stitch or other technical defect.

Thromboembolic complications are major sources of prosthesis-related morbidity and mortality, with a frequency of about 1 to 4% per patient year. These complications are generally more frequent with mechanical valves than with bioprostheses, dictating the greater need for anticoagulation with the use of mechanical prostheses. The thrombi may derange the function of mechanical valves and bioprostheses, embolize (most often to the brain), or become secondarily infected to produce infective endocarditis. In addition, hemorrhagic complications may arise secondarily because of the necessity of long-term anticoagulation in patients with artificial valves.

Infective endocarditis is an infrequent but serious potential complication developing in about 6% of patients within five years of valve replacement.[133] With mechanical valves, the endocarditis is usually located at the prosthesis-tissue interface, causing a ring abscess. With bioprostheses, it may be located similarly but may also involve the cuspal tissue. The pathogenetic flora and its relationship to the time interval since valve replacement are discussed on page 634.

Deterioration of mechanical valves is a relatively uncommon complication, but it is a major consideration with bioprostheses. Wear on mechanical occluders or related metal restraints or supports does occur but only rarely has it given rise to fatal complications. On the other hand, about 20 to 30% of glutaraldehyde-pretreated porcine aortic valves require replacement for sterile tissue degeneration, including calcification, within ten years.[133]

Many other complications such as hemolysis induced by mechanical obstruction to flow inherent in all artificial valves and dysfunction due to ingrowth of fibrous tissue may be serious in the individual instance, but overall do not constitute major problems. Valve replacement, life prolonging and life saving as it often is, incurs its own set of concerns. For this reason, there is active exploration of other approaches to the correction of valvular deformities such as catheter balloon valvuloplasty and cadaver-derived homografts.[133] What the long-term consequences of these newer treatment modalities will be only time will tell.

MYOCARDIAL DISEASE

Myocardial disease occurs in many of the major forms of heart disease, such as MI, rheumatic heart disease, and hypertensive heart disease, already discussed. Here our consideration is limited to two broad categories of myocardial involvement: (1) myocarditis, characterized by morphologic changes indicative of an inflammatory reaction, usually to some microbiologic agent; and (2) noninflammatory myocardial disease called cardiomyopathy. The noninflammatory involvements are further subdivided into cardiomyopathies of unknown cause, here referred to as "primary cardiomyopathy," and those of known cause — "secondary cardiomyopathy." Some authors would classify all forms of heart muscle disease as cardiomyopathy, identifying myocarditis as an infectious form of cardiomyopathy and those of known cause as spe-

cific heart muscle diseases. These taxonomic issues are not of great importance, but it is useful to segregate myocarditis from cardiomyopathy for clinical reasons. Myocarditis is often a primary heart disease. It is usually of sudden onset and often produces acute cardiac failure. It is generally characterized by a prominent inflammatory reaction, with necrosis of isolated cells or small groups of myocardial fibers, and it tends to pursue a relatively short course measured in weeks to a few months. In many instances, the prognosis is good. If the patient survives, it resolves, sometimes leaving little or no residual myocardial scarring. In contrast, in the primary cardiomyopathies, the myocardial alterations are associated with little inflammatory reaction. Most run a protracted course, and many never remit. For long periods of time, they usually evoke no symptoms until, for mysterious reasons and apparently without provocation, cardiac failure insidiously sets in. Such a clear separation into myocarditis or cardiomyopathy is not always possible, and many cases must be classified arbitrarily. However, endomyocardial biopsies obtained at cardiac catheterization promise to broaden our understanding of the nature and course of the conditions.[134]

MYOCARDITIS

Myocarditis is best defined as an inflammatory involvement of the heart muscle characterized by a leukocytic infiltrate and necrosis or degeneration of myocytes. It is an important form of heart disease because it may occur at any age, even in infancy, and occasionally with unexpected suddenness may induce cardiac failure or cause sudden death by arrhythmia. It is difficult to be certain of the precise clinical incidence of this condition because often the diagnosis is based on indirect evidence (e.g., fever and sudden appearance of ECG changes indicative of a diffuse myocardial lesion in the absence of other definable causes). It has been said to be present in from 1 to 4% of routine autopsies. In many of these cases, however, it was an incidental and chance finding, imparting in all likelihood an overestimate of the frequency of the clinically significant disease.[135,136]

The causes of myocarditis are legion and include virtually every known microbiologic agent, various forms of immunologically mediated damage, hypersensitivity reactions, and reactions to physical agents. The more important etiologies are present in Table 13-7, and a few comments are in order about some of these.

Most cases of well-documented myocarditis are of viral origin. Infants, immunosuppressed individuals, and pregnant women are particularly vulnerable. The most frequently implicated agents are Coxsackie A and B, ECHO, polio, influenza A and B, and HIV viruses, but many others may also be involved.[137] In most instances the cardiac involvement follows some days to a few weeks after a primary viral infection elsewhere, as in the lungs, upper respiratory tract, or

Table 13–7. Major Causes of Myocarditis

Viruses
Coxsackie A and B virus
ECHO virus, types 6, 7, 19, 22
Influenza virus
Poliomyelitis virus
Human immunodeficiency virus
Hepatitis virus
Epstein-Barr virus (infectious mononucleosis)
Cytomegalovirus

Chlamydia
C. psittaci

Rickettsia
R. typhi (typhus fever)
R. tsutsugamushi (scrub typhus)

Bacteria
Corynebacterium (diphtheria)
Salmonella
Mycobacterium (tuberculosis)
Streptococci (beta-hemolytic)
Neisseria (meningococcus)
Leptospira (Weil's disease)
Borrelia (relapsing fever)

Fungi and Protozoa
Trypanosoma (Chagas' disease)
Aspergillus
Blastomyces
Cryptococcus
Candida
Coccidioidomyces

Metazoa
Echinococcus
Trichinella

Immune-mediated Reactions
Poststreptococcal (rheumatic fever)
Systemic lupus erythematosus
Systemic sclerosis
Methyldopa
Sulfonamides
Penicillin
Para-aminosalicylic acid
Streptomycin
Transplant rejection

Physical Agents
Radiation
Heat stroke

Unknown
Sarcoidosis
Giant cell (Fiedler's) myocarditis
Kawasaki's disease

neuromuscular system (in poliomyelitis). Occasionally, the myocarditis is the sole or, at least, major focus of infection and so is referred to as *primary myocarditis*. The documentation of a viral etiology is almost always difficult. Most often, recourse is made to serologic demonstration of a rising antibody titer in the serum.

There is still uncertainty about the mechanisms involved in the production of cardiac damage by viral agents. Two possibilities exist.[138] There may be direct viral cytotoxicity. Alternatively, the specific agent may evoke a cell-mediated immune reaction, which then damages the cardiac myofibers harboring virus or virus-dictated antigens. The weight of evidence favors the latter mechanism. Infiltration of the myocardium by lymphocytes and macrophages is characteristic of most viral involvements of the myocardium. There is often a delay of days to a few weeks between the onset of an extracardiac viral infection and the appearance of the myocarditis. Immunoglobulins can often be demonstrated by immunofluorescent methods along the sarcolemmal sheaths of myofibers. In addition, activated macrophages, a defect in suppressor T-cell activity, and increased production of cytotoxic T-cells have been reported.[139]

Uncommonly, myocarditis is caused by one of the nonviral agents or their products cited in Table 13–7. A *particularly important form of infection is that caused by* Trypanosoma cruzi *producing Chagas' disease.* Although uncommon in the northern hemisphere, Chagas' disease affects up to one half of the population in endemic areas of South America, and myocardial involvement is found in approximately 80% of infected individuals. About 10% of patients die during an acute attack, or they may enter a chronic phase and develop progressive signs of cardiac insufficiency 10 to 20 years later. The importance of this cause of myocarditis is evident from the fact that it causes about 25% of all deaths in persons between the ages of 25 and 44 in endemic areas.[140] Trichinosis is the most common helminthic disease associated with localization of the causative agent in the heart muscle.

There are also noninfectious causes of myocarditis. Some are associated with systemic diseases of immune origin such as rheumatic fever and systemic lupus erythematosus. In other instances, hypersensitivity to a particular drug appears to be involved, as is the case with myocarditis related to allergic reactions to penicillin, sulfonamides, and other drugs. In some instances, the drug may have direct toxicity to the heart, (e.g., doxorubicin and others). Whether these toxicities should be considered instances of myocarditis is debatable, so later they are categorized as causes of cardiomyopathy (p. 648).

A special form of immune-mediated myocarditis is encountered during rejection of cardiac transplants. The reaction is characterized by myocardial interstitial edema and mononuclear infiltration, accompanied in the more severe rejections by focal myofiber necrosis. The level of immunosuppressive therapy needed is judged mainly by the severity of the rejection reaction seen in endomyocardial biopsies. Cyclosporine, a commonly used T-cell immunosuppressant, itself has cardiotoxicity, complicating the interpretation of the histologic picture.

Several forms of myocarditis are of idiopathic origin. Cardiac lesions were found at autopsy in about 20% of patients with sarcoidosis.[141] Although in many of these instances the involvement was of little clinical significance, sarcoidosis may cause sufficient myocardial damage to produce cardiac decompensation and arrhythmias, sometimes leading to sudden death. Another idiopathic disorder is so-called *giant cell myocarditis*. Morphologically and clinically it closely resembles yet another form of myocarditis—*Fiedler's*.

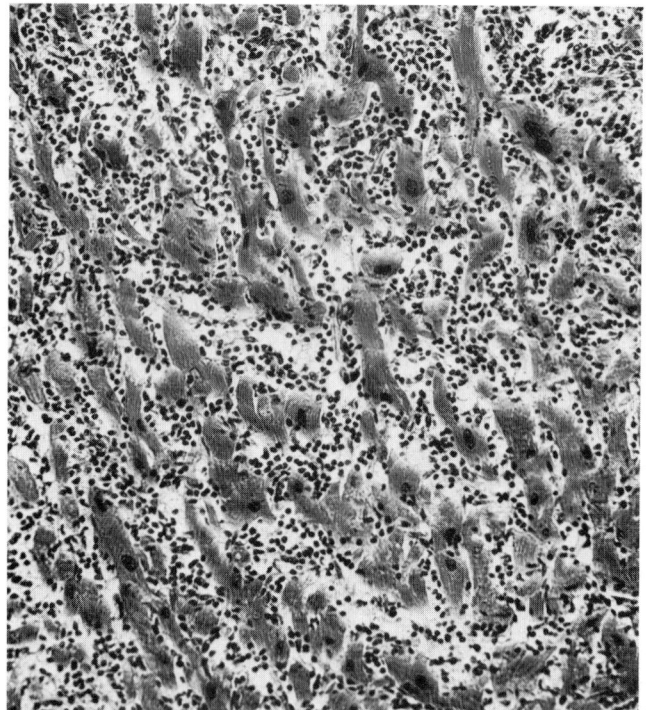

Figure 13–35. Viral myocarditis with marked interstitial edema and mononuclear inflammatory cell infiltration.

an interstitial edema that separates the individual myofibers (Fig. 13–35). The histologic pattern of reaction to bacterial invasion depends on the specific causative organism, but, in general, mirrors the changes produced by the same organism in extracardiac localizations. Thus, **pyogens induce more of a patchy, focal, suppurative reaction, and sometimes microabscesses with less prominence of the diffuse interstitial component.** Similarly larger parasites produce their typical tissue reactions within the heart muscle. You recall that, **in trichinosis, although the parasite often invades the heart, it rarely encysts within its myofibers.** Usually, therefore, only focal infiltrates of lymphocytes and eosinophils can be identified in foci of myocytolysis, but only rarely are larvae or fragments of larvae visible.[143] **The myocarditis of Chagas' disease is rendered distinctive by parasitization of scattered myofibers by trypanosomes accompanied by an inflammatory infiltrate of neutrophils, lymphocytes, macrophages, and occasional eosinophils** (Fig. 13–36).

Hypersensitivity reactions that involve the myocardium induce interstitial infiltrates that are principally perivascular, composed of lymphocytes, plasma cells, macrophages, and eosinophils. Occasionally, acute vasculitis can be seen similar to the small vessel lesions in hypersensitivity reactions within noncardiac tissues.

Both merit attention because they are often fatal.[142] The distinctive pathologic features of these entities are described later. Against this background we can turn to the anatomic changes seen in the various forms of myocarditis.

MORPHOLOGY. During the active phase of myocarditis the heart may appear normal or enlarged with dilatation of all chambers, but sometimes only the left or right ventricle. The lesions may be diffuse or patchy. The ventricular myocardium is typically flabby, and often mottled by either pale foci or minute hemorrhagic lesions. The endocardium and valves are unaffected except that mural thrombi may be present in any chamber. At some later date when the acute phase has passed, the heart may appear entirely normal or there may be residual dilatation or hypertrophy, or both. Indeed, there is a strong possibility that the late stages of viral myocarditis often present as so-called "dilated cardiomyopathy." In other instances, small foci of fibrosis may be evident throughout the myocardium.

The histologic changes are even more varied and, as would be expected, vary with the specific causative agent. Only some generalizations can be offered. It should be remembered that the involvement may be patchy and hence endomyocardial biopsies can be spuriously negative. During active disease, isolated myofiber lysis (myocytolysis) or patchy foci of necrosis are present and are accompanied by an inflammatory cell infiltrate. **With viral myocarditis there is a tendency for isolated fiber necrosis. The infiltrate is usually mononuclear—lymphocytes, macrophages, and occasional plasma cells—and is accompanied by**

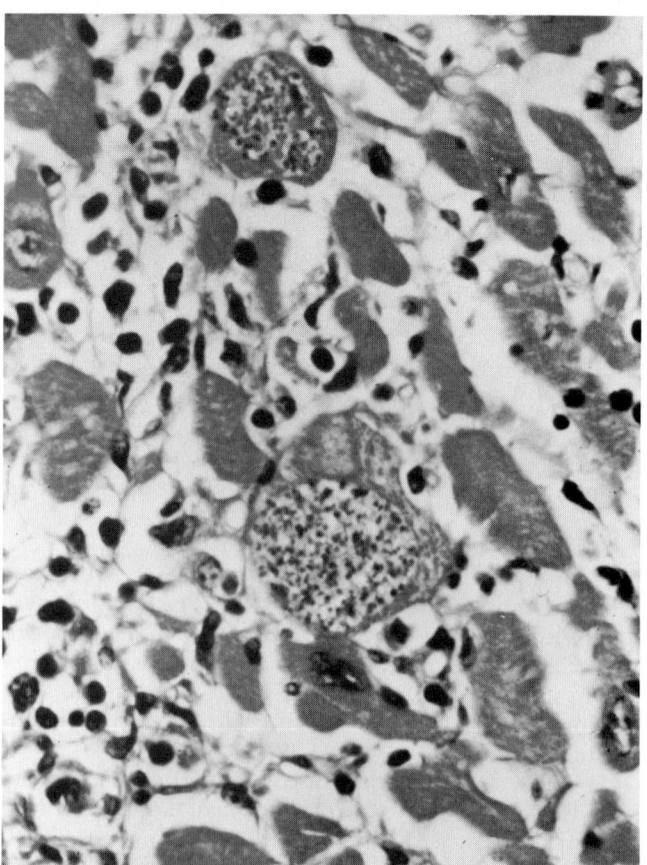

Figure 13–36. The myocarditis of Chagas' disease. Several myofibers are distended with trypanosomes. There is a surrounding inflammatory reaction and individual myofiber necrosis.

There remain two morphologically distinctive forms of myocarditis—**Fiedler's** and **idiopathic giant cell myocarditis.** Both are characterized by focal necroses associated with a granulomatous reaction containing multinucleate giant cells interspersed with lymphocytes, eosinophils, plasma cells, and macrophages.[116] There is a strong likelihood that both entities are, in fact, a single disease of unknown origin. A viral etiology is suspected, but the granulomatous nature of the reaction and the frequent presence of eosinophils suggest immune mediation.[142]

Whatever the pattern of histologic changes during the acute phase of the disease, all inflammatory lesions either resolve, leaving no residuals, or undergo progressive fibrosis, as mentioned earlier. Often the persistent connective tissue is sufficiently scattered and subtle to be virtually inapparent at a later date. With more severe damage, focal minute scars may remain; in extremely florid cases, they may become confluent and thus be grossly visible, particularly when subendocardial.

All forms of myocarditis evoke remarkably similar clinical manifestations that vary more in severity than in type. At one end of the clinical spectrum the disease is entirely asymptomatic and only suspected when ECG changes, particularly abnormalities of the ST segment and T wave, point to a myocardial lesion. At the other end of the spectrum the myocarditis announces itself by the sudden onset of congestive heart failure. In such cases, systolic murmurs related to dilatation of the atrioventricular valve rings may appear, and sometimes arrhythmias. Between these extremes are the many involvements associated with such symptoms as fatigue, dyspnea, palpitations, and precordial discomfort, sometimes accompanied by mild fever when the myocarditis is of infectious origin. Many patients recover completely without sequelae. The rare severe attack may pursue a rapidly downhill course to death in cardiac failure. Such fulminant progression is particularly characteristic of the giant cell myocarditides. Occasionally, years later, when an attack of myocarditis (particularly viral) is forgotten, the patient is diagnosed as having congestive cardiomyopathy of unknown cause. Endomyocardial biopsy is proving of great value in establishing the diagnosis and severity of the various forms of myocarditis.

CARDIOMYOPATHY (CMP)

Strictly speaking the term "cardiomyopathy" implies "heart muscle disease," but commonly it also implies "of a noninflammatory nature." Moreover, there is near consensus that myocardial disease related to hypertensive, congenital, valvular, or pericardial derangements should also be excluded from the category of cardiomyopathy. The World Health Organization also excludes ischemic injury and further limits the definition to "heart muscle diseases of unknown cause."[144] Thus, myocardial dysfunction of known origin (e.g., cobalt or lithium toxicity, hemochromatosis, and systemic muscular dystrophy) is excluded and is relegated to a separate category that some call "specific heart muscle disease." Here, along with other "middle-of-the-roaders," we shall adopt the classification of *primary CMP* to refer to heart muscle diseases of unknown cause and *secondary CMP* to refer to those myocardial disorders of known cause, excluding ischemic, hypertensive, valvular, pericardial, congenital, and inflammatory involvements.

Primary Cardiomyopathy

Because these conditions are by definition of unknown origin, they have traditionally been divided into pathophysiologic categories (Fig. 13–37).

1. Dilated (congestive) CMP
2. Hypertrophic CMP
3. Restrictive or obliterative CMP

Dilated (Congestive) CMP

Dilated CMP is characterized by the gradual development of cardiac failure associated with four-chamber dilatation of the heart of unknown cause.[145] Although the etiology is unknown, there is a strong suspicion that dilated CMP is the common end point of a variety of long-past insults to the myocardium. When first seen late in its course, the end result of these various injuries is the same.[137] Four pathogenetic pathways

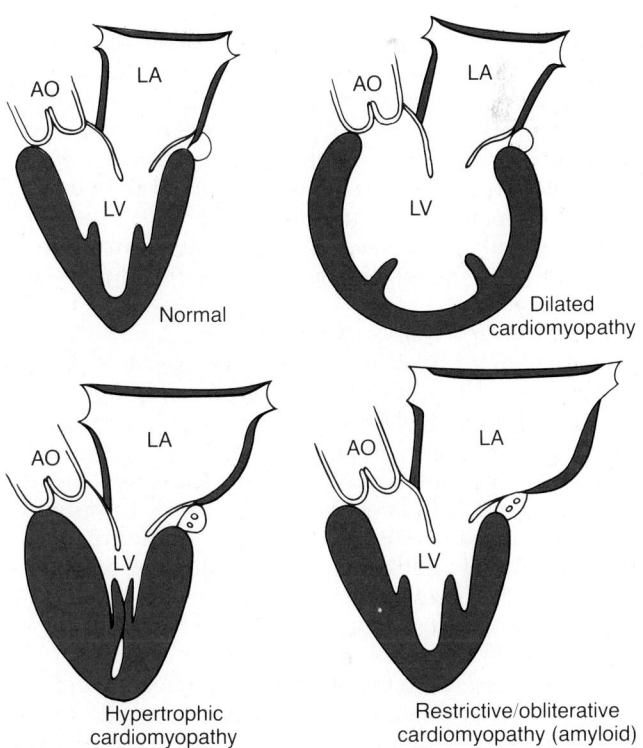

Figure 13–37. Representation of the three distinctive clinicopathologic forms of cardiomyopathy.

are suspected: (1) alcohol toxicity, (2) a pregnancy-associated nutritional deficiency, (3) a genetic defect, and (4) a postviral myocarditis.

Alcohol or one of its metabolites has a direct toxic effect on the myocardium. Moreover, chronic alcoholism may be associated with thiamine deficiency, introducing an element of beriberi heart disease (p. 450) (indistinguishable from dilated CMP). In addition, in years past, cobalt was added to beer before it was discovered that it had significant myocardial toxicity. That practice has now been discontinued. Even excluding all these variables, alcohol or its metabolites are widely acknowledged to be toxic to the myocardium, as was discussed on page 490. Furthermore, alcohol abuse is so widespread it offers a reasonable basis for most instances of dilated CMP.[146] Some would argue that such cases should be termed alcoholic CMP and therefore be excluded from the category of idiopathic disorders, but because the alcohol-myocardium link is still somewhat tenuous, it continues to be regarded as a possible basis for dilated CMP.

"Peripartum CMP" is the designation given to dilated CMP when it is discovered within the month before or after delivery. The basis for this relationship is uncertain, but because it most often occurs in impoverished women having frequent, multiple pregnancies, nutritional deficiency is suspected. Pregnancy also invokes the possibilities of hypertension, volume overload, or some metabolic derangement.[147] Whatever the basis, in about half of these patients, the dilatation of the heart disappears within months following delivery, unlike the classic course of dilated CMP. However, the other half of patients fail to recover and are at risk of dying with a subsequent pregnancy.

Genetic influences apply to only a few cases of dilated CMP when multiple members of a family are affected. Autosomal dominant, autosomal recessive, and, recently, X-linked inheritance have all been proposed for particular kindreds.[148] To date, no specific biochemical, functional, or structural abnormality of possible genetic origin has been identified in such cases.

A *postviral myocarditis* is a favored pathogenetic mechanism for dilated CMP.[149] Perhaps the strongest support for this theory comes from endomyocardial biopsies revealing changes suggestive of an inflammatory myocarditis in patients who otherwise have the classic features of dilated CMP. In addition, traces of humoral and cellular immune responses to potential viral agents have been found in some patients, raising the possibility that they are reflections of prior viral damage.[150] However, very few cases have been observed to progress from unequivocal myocarditis to unequivocal CMP.

Other possible mechanisms have been proposed, but at present dilated CMP remains a disorder of unknown cause. Indeed, it is in a sense a wastebasket term into which are placed dilated hearts usually in congestive failure having no well-defined origin.

The hearts are always increased in weight (up to 900 gm), but dilation of the ventricles may neutralize preexistent thickening of the ventricular walls. The poor cardiac contraction and stasis of blood in the cardiac chambers often leads to mural thrombi in the left ventricle, right ventricle, right atrial appendage, and left atrial appendage, in order of frequency.[151] The cardiac valves are usually normal, and most often the coronary arteries are normal or have minimal-to-moderate, nonobstructive atherosclerosis compatible with the patient's age.

Histologic examination of hearts at necropsy and of endomyocardial biopsies discloses only vague and nonspecific changes. Indeed, there may be no significant alterations in as many as one quarter of the cases.[152] Hypertrophy of occasional myocardial cells, atrophy of others, and occasionally some increase in interstitial fibrous tissue reminiscent of a past episode of a viral myocarditis are the most common changes.[153] Sometimes there is mild-to-moderate endocardial thickening, principally in the ventricles. Small interstitial foci of mononuclear inflammatory cells are sometimes observed. Neither the electron microscope nor histochemistry has contributed to the specificity of the changes, revealing only regressive alterations.[151]

This condition may occur at any age, including in childhood. It presents with slowly developing congestive heart failure that is progressive and unremitting in most cases. Only 25% of patients survive longer than five years. Regurgitant murmurs may be present owing to dilatation of the mitral or tricuspid valve rings or both. There are no other distinctive features and so the diagnosis is based largely on exclusion of other, better-defined forms of cardiac dilatation. Death is usually attributable to progressive failure, embolism from dislodgement of intracardiac thrombi, or a fatal arrhythmia. Because of the gravity of the prognosis, cardiac transplantation is sometimes recommended.

Hypertrophic CMP

This form of CMP is also known by such terms as asymmetric septal hypertrophy (ASH), idiopathic hypertrophic subaortic stenosis (IHSS), and hypertrophic obstructive cardiomyopathy. However, the name hypertrophic CMP seems preferable because the cardiac changes are not always obstructive and the hypertrophy is not always subaortic or asymmetric. The disorder is, however, characterized by a heavy muscular *hyper*contracting heart in striking contrast to the flabby, *hypo*contracting heart of dilated CMP. The etiology and pathogenesis of this condition are unknown, and so hypotheses abound.

The essential feature of hypertrophic CMP is cardiac enlargement with myocardial hypertrophy. The left ventricle is usually more involved than the right, and the atria may be slightly hypertrophied. Although the classic pattern is said to be disproportionate thickening of the interventricular septum as compared with the free wall of the left ventricle, in a substantial number of cases, the hypertrophy may be symmetric throughout the heart. In addition, the thickening of the wall may be remarkably variable with contiguous regions differing greatly in thickness. Sometimes the more apical regions of the left ventricle are affected, but more often the most marked thickening is in the basal septum. On cross section, the ventricular cavity loses its usual round to ovoid shape and may be compressed into a "banana-like" configuration by bulging of the interventricular septum into the lumen (Fig. 13–38). Of great importance in terms of the hemodynamics of hypertrophic CMP is the extent of thickening of the septum in the subaortic region. When the basal septum is markedly thickened at the level of the mitral valve and the mitral valve is positioned anteriorly, the outflow of the left ventricle at the end of systole may be markedly reduced to produce what is called **obstructive hypertrophic CMP.** With more apical thickening of the septum, the outflow tract is not obstructed and so there are also nonobstructive forms of hypertrophic CMP.[154] Sometimes also present are endocardial thickening or mural plaque formation in the left ventricular outflow tract, mitral valve thickening, and abnormal intramural coronary arteries.

The most distinctive feature microscopically, in addition to the changes of myocyte hypertrophy (p. 616), is disorganization of the hypertrophied myofibers so that adjacent cells are no longer oriented in parallel but are distributed in a haphazard pattern (Fig. 13–39). These cellular changes may be accompanied by disarray of the myofilaments within sarcomeres. This disorganization typically involves 25 to 50% of the septum and is somewhat less abundant in the left ventricular free wall. There is usually an overall delicate interstitial fibrosis. Several cautions should be noted: (1) Not all hearts with hypertrophic CMP reveal myofiber disorganization; (2) the change is not uniform from one area to the next; and (3) it is not unique to hypertrophic CMP and may also be seen with other forms of myocardial hypertrophy.[155] The small, intramural coronary arteries may have markedly thickened walls, particularly in the ventricular septum. Here again, these vascular changes may be encountered in all forms of myocardial hypertrophy.

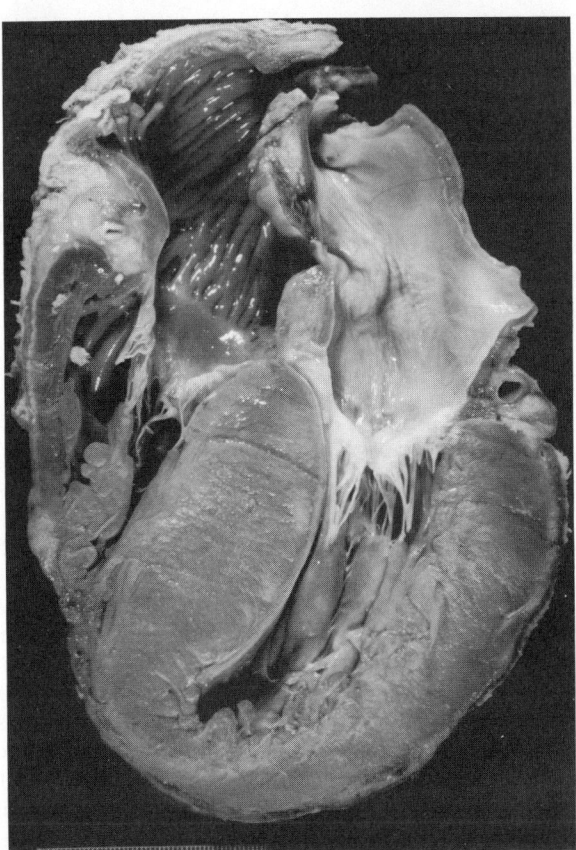

Figure 13–38. Hypertrophic cardiomyopathy with marked thickening of the left ventricular wall and particularly the interventricular septum. Note the reduced size of the ventricular cavity and the approximation of the basal septum to the mitral leaflet encroaching on the outflow tract.

There is substantial evidence that the disease is transmitted by autosomal dominant inheritance in over half the patients.[156] Although the remaining cases appear to be sporadic, it is possible that some represent new mutations or are the result of autosomal recessive transmission with reduced gene penetrance rendering kindred analysis difficult. In some instances, linkages to the HLA system have been proposed, but no consistent associations have yet been identified. Not clear, however, is how a genetic defect translates into myofiber and myocardial hypertrophy. The fiber disarray is likely a secondary phenomenon attributable to abnormal wall and cellular stresses. Many other etiologies have been suggested, such as (1) excessive responsiveness of the myofibers to circulating catecholamines, (2) myocardial ischemia incident to the abnormality in the intramyocardial arteries with secondary fibrosis and compensatory hypertrophy, or (3) a collagen disorder resulting in the diffuse fibrosis that impairs myofiber contraction and leads to the described hypertrophy.

Hypertrophic CMP occurs most often in young adults, but it may first appear in elderly patients. The condition is often asymptomatic, but nonetheless it incurs a high mortality rate from sudden death when affected individuals engage in strenuous physical activity. When the disease becomes symptomatic, the dominant manifestation is dyspnea sometimes accompanied by angina, dizziness, or evidence of congestive heart failure. As indicated, in some patients, the distal portions of the mitral valve come into contact with the markedly thickened basal ventricular septum to produce an outflow obstruction, but it has been pointed out that equally important, or perhaps more important, in the generation of clinical symptoms are increased wall thickness, reduced compliance, reduced volume capacity of the left ventricle, and consequent rapid emptying of a small stroke volume.[157] Paradoxically, then, congestive failure with dilation of the heart and impairment of systolic contractile function improves the situation and apparently accounts for the spontaneous improvement sometimes seen with this condition.

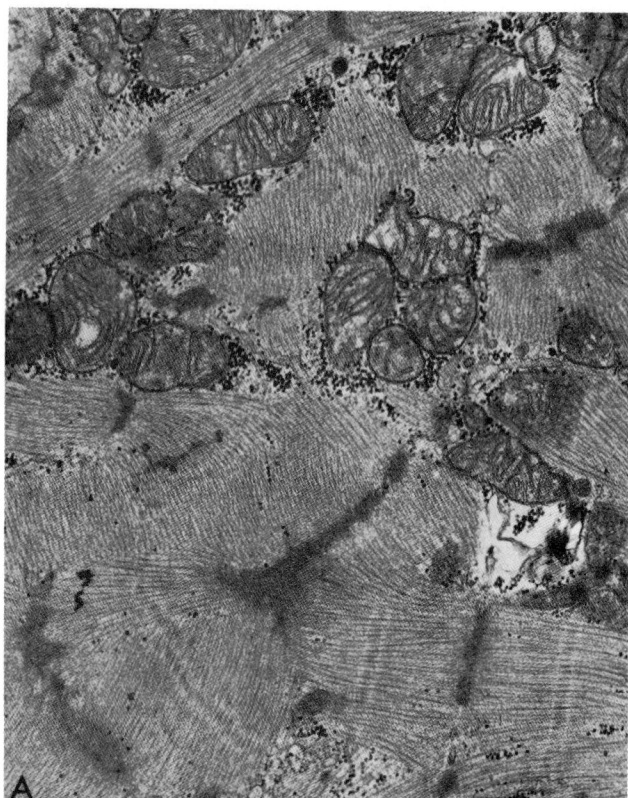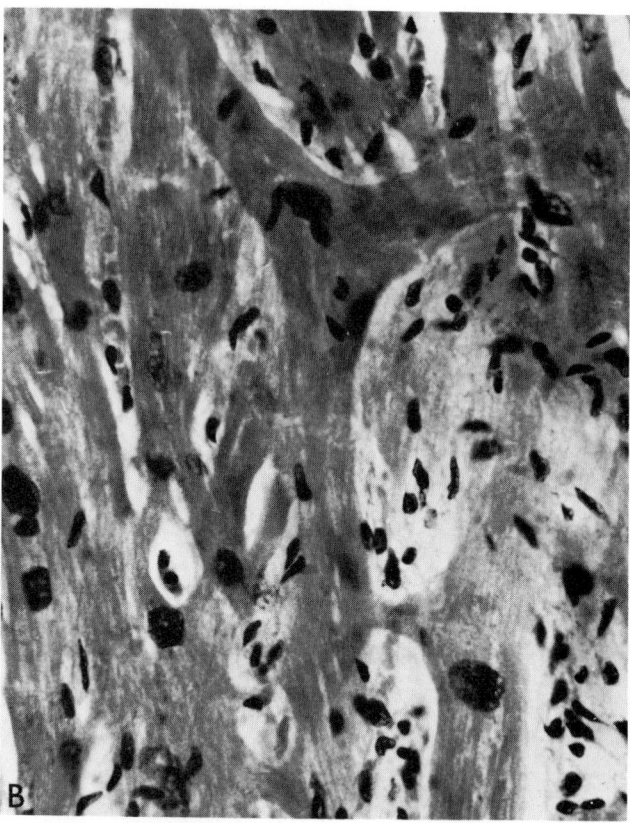

Figure 13–39. Electron micrograph *(A)* (courtesy of Dr. William Roberts, National Heart and Lung Institute, Bethesda, MD) and light microscopic section *(B)* of asymmetric septal hypertrophy revealing disarray and abnormal orientation of myofibers.

The course of hypertrophic CMP is extremely variable. Many patients remain the same over years of observation. A significant fraction improve, and only a minority become worse. Major problems are atrial fibrillation with mural thrombus formation, embolization from the mural thrombi, infective endocarditis on the mitral valve, intractable cardiac failure, and sudden death. With the recognition that obstructive symptoms are not due solely to thickening of the ventricular septum, thinning of the septum by surgery is done increasingly less often. Most patients can be significantly helped by medical therapy alone.

Restrictive/Infiltrative CMP

Restrictive/infiltrative CMP is both rare and diverse, having as a common denominator restriction of ventricular filling. A number of disparate entities induce this form of CMP, including cardiac amyloidosis, sarcoidosis (discussed elsewhere, p. 427), endocardial fibroelastosis, endomyocardial fibrosis, and Loeffler's endocarditis. Cardiac amyloidosis (p. 219), you recall, may appear along with systemic amyloidosis or may affect only the heart, particularly in the aged (so-called senile isolated cardiac amyloidosis). Indeed, senile cardiac amyloidosis has been identified in over 50% of individuals over the age of 70.[158] Although often an incidental finding, it may induce arrhythmias or restrictive CMP. Only brief comments about the last three entities follow.

Endomyocardial fibrosis and *Loeffler's endocarditis* (also called fibroplastic parietal endocarditis with blood eosinophilia) are rare entities that have sufficient morphologic features in common to raise the possibility that they are a single disorder at different stages of development.[159] *Endomyocardial fibrosis is principally a disease of children and young adults in Africa, characterized by fibrosis of the ventricular endocardium that extends from the apex toward the inflow tract of the right or left ventricle, or both.* Although largely subendocardial, the scarring may extend into the inner third of the myocardium. Varying degrees of inflammatory infiltrate, sometimes including eosinophils, may be found at the junction between the scarring and preserved myocardium. The fibrosis may also involve the tricuspid and mitral valves. Contraction of the fibrous tissue markedly diminishes the volume of affected chambers and so induces a restrictive CMP.[160] Ventricular mural thrombi sometimes develop and, indeed, there is a suggestion that the fibrous tissue results from the organization of mural thrombi. The etiology of this condition is unknown and, in addition to the usual speculations about viral infection, malnutrition, and autoimmune disease, heavy consumption of bananas and plantain has been implicated. These fruits are rich in serotonin, thought to induce the fibrotic changes similar to those of carcinoid heart disease (p. 639). *Loeffler's endocarditis is also marked by endo-*

myocardial fibrosis similar to that seen in the African disease. The original cases of this condition were confined to the temperate zones, but subsequently Loeffler's endocarditis has been reported in Africa and endomyocardial fibrosis in Scandinavia and Europe. Large mural thrombi are typically present in Loeffler's endocarditis. In addition to the cardiac changes there are often (1) an eosinophilic leukocytosis, (2) infiltration of various organs (especially the heart) by eosinophils, and (3) a rapidly fatal downhill course.[161] Sometimes, frank eosinophilic leukemia is present. In other cases there is no peripheral eosinophilia, and some form of cardiac hypersensitivity reaction to drugs, for example, is postulated.[162] The histologic evolution of Loeffler's endocarditis begins with foci of myocardial necrosis accompanied by an eosinophilic infiltrate that is most prominent in the inner third of the myocardium. It is followed by scarring of the necrotic areas and layering of the endocardium by thrombus. Organization of the thrombus produces the final stage of endomyocardial fibrosis. Unanswered is the question: Do the eosinophils in some way cause the myofiber necrosis or are they merely a reaction to injury of other origins? It is evident that there are many overlaps in the geographic distribution and morphologic changes of the African disease and Loeffler's disease.

Endocardial fibroelastosis is an uncommon heart disease of obscure etiology characterized by focal or diffuse, cartilage-like fibroelastic thickening of the mural endocardium. Most often only the left side of the heart is affected, but it occasionally involves both sides or (least commonly) only the right side. When we speak of EFE as an entity, there is the strong possibility that the cardiac changes are the final common outcome of a variety of forms of cardiac damage. This condition occurs in all age groups but is far more common in the first two years of life. From the pathogenetic standpoint, cases have been reported in identical twins, triplets, and siblings. The pattern of transmission is still uncertain, and both autosomal dominant inheritance with incomplete penetrance and autosomal recessive inheritance have been proposed as the genetic basis for the cardiac changes.[163] Not infrequently, congenital malformations are also present in the heart or elsewhere in the body, supporting the notion of some genetic disturbance. However, the overwhelming majority of cases occur in individual siblings, and so the concept that EFE is a hereditary malformation can at most apply to only a very few cases. About one third of all cases are accompanied by some form of congenital anomaly, most often patent foramen ovale, patent ductus arteriosus, anomalous left coronary artery, and aortic stenosis.[164]

Fibroelastosis of the endocardium appears as a diffuse or patchy opaque thickening of the mural endocardium predominantly of the left ventricle. However, the left atrium, right ventricle, and right atrium, in order of frequency, may also be involved. The thickening appears as a pearly-white, endocardial lining, sometimes having a depth ten times normal. It is usually covered by an intact endothelium. Mural thrombi overlying the fibrotic endocardium are present in a small percentage of cases. The trabeculae carneae are often flattened. Aortic stenosis, mitral stenosis, or both are present in some cases. The valves on the right are rarely affected. Cardiac enlargement is usually present, due mainly to left ventricular hypertrophy, dilatation, or both.

On histologic examination, the endocardial thickening can be resolved as a marked increase of collagenous and elastic fibers on the endocardial surface. This fibroelastic layer extends sometimes into the immediate subjacent myocardium.

The numerous theories of causation of EFE can be categorized as follows: (1) hypoxia (e.g., anomalous origin of coronary arteries from the pulmonary arteries); (2) hemodynamic pressure overload with excessive endocardial tension (e.g., septal defects, coarctation of the aorta); (3) myocardial metabolic or enzymatic defect; (4) autoimmune connective tissue disease; (5) congenital malformation; (6) lymphatic obstruction; and (7) fetal endomyocarditis, most likely viral. All are so speculative as not to merit further comment.

The significance of this lesion depends on the extent of involvement. When focal, it may have no functional importance and permit normal longevity. When diffuse, it may be responsible for cardiac decompensation and death. In infants, the cardiac failure may be rapid, progressive, and even fulminating. In older children and adults, however, there usually are signs and symptoms of cardiac decompensation for months to years, and death is occasioned by emboli arising in the mural thrombi or by chronic cardiac failure and its superimposed complications.

Secondary Cardiomyopathy

This designation refers to a constellation of myocardial involvements of presumed known etiology or associated with well-defined systemic diseases. The major etiologies and clinical associations are cited in Table 13–8. The myocardial lesions related to systemic and pulmonary hypertension, coronary artery disease, valvular heart disease, and congenital defects are excluded. For our purposes, the various forms of inflammatory myocarditis are also omitted as they were discussed earlier (p. 640). The morphologic changes found in most of the entities mentioned in Table 13–8 have been presented along with the parent condition. Only some comments on the toxic patterns not covered elsewhere are necessary.

Alcohol was discussed on page 490 and page 644 as a possible but unproved cause of dilated CMP. Cobalt too was discussed earlier (p. 644). Clearly it is a cardiotoxic agent disrupting pyruvate metabolism.[165]

Myocardial foci of apparent ischemic necrosis are frequently observed in patients having a pheochromocytoma with its elaboration of catecholamines. Similar changes have appeared in association with the

Table 13-8. Major Associations of Secondary CMP

Toxic
Alcohol
Cobalt
Catecholamines
Carbon monoxide
Lithium
Hydrocarbons
Arsenic
Cyclophosphamide
Doxorubicin (Adriamycin)
Daunorubicin

Metabolic Disease
Hyperthyroidism
Hypothyroidism
Hypokalemia
Hyperkalemia
Nutritional deficiency—thiamine, protein, other avitaminoses
Hemochromatosis

Neuromuscular Disease
Friedreich's ataxia
Muscular dystrophy
Congenital atrophies

Storage Disorders
Hunter-Hurler syndrome
Glycogen storage disease
Fabry's disease
Sandhoff's disease

Infiltrative
Leukemia
Carcinomatosis
Sarcoidosis

Immunologic
Post transplant

administration of large doses of vasopressor agents such as epinephrine. The mechanism of cardiotoxicity is uncertain, but it appears to relate to vasomotor constriction in the myocardial circulation in the face of an increased heart rate. The fact that aspirin, which blocks the cyclooxygenase of the arachidonic acid synthetic pathway, appears to offer some protection suggests that prostaglandins and platelets may contribute to the myocardial ischemia and cell death. Doxorubicin (Adriamycin) and daunorubicin are well recognized causes of myocardial injury. The hazard is dose dependent (total dose above 500 mg/m²) and attributed to lipid peroxidation of myofiber membranes.[166] Many other agents, such as lithium, phenothiazines, and lately cocaine, have been implicated in myocardial injury and sometimes sudden cardiac death (p. 615).

Common threads running throughout the cardiotoxicity of all chemicals and drugs (including diphtheria exotoxin) are myofiber swelling, fatty change, individual cell lysis (myocytolysis), and sometimes patchy foci of necrosis. Electron microscopy has revealed a variety of mitochondrial abnormalities, swelling and fragmentation of the endoplasmic reticulum, and lysis of myofibrils. With survival, these changes may resolve completely, leaving no apparent sequelae, but sometimes a subtle, interstitial fibrosis remains or, at most, small focal replacement scars.

PERICARDIAL DISEASE

Pericardial lesions are almost always associated with, or secondary to, some external disease (in other portions of the heart or in the surrounding structures) or a systemic disorder. Rarely, pericardial involvements may occur as primary, isolated processes. Despite the large number of etiologies of pericardial disease there are relatively few anatomic forms of pericardial involvement.[167]

ACCUMULATIONS OF FLUID IN PERICARDIAL SAC

PERICARDIAL EFFUSION. The term "pericardial effusion" is restricted to accumulations of noninflammatory fluids in the pericardial sac, as distinguished from collections of inflammatory exudate or blood (discussed later). Normally, there is about 30 to 50 ml of thin, clear, straw-colored, translucent fluid in the pericardial space. Under a variety of circumstances, effusions rarely larger than 500 ml may appear. The various types of effusion and their common causes are as follows:

Serous—congestive heart failure; hypoproteinemia (renal, hepatic, nutritional).

Serosanguineous—blunt chest trauma; cardiopulmonary resuscitation.

Chylous—lymphatic obstruction (benign or malignant mediastinal neoplasms).

Cholesterol—myxedema; idiopathic.

Most common is serous effusion in cardiac failure. The fluid is completely clear, watery, or straw-colored, and sterile. The serosal surfaces remain smooth and glistening. Because the fluid accumulates slowly it is usually without clinical significance save for producing a characteristic enlargement of the heart shadow on x-ray film. Rarely a large volume may embarrass diastolic filling of the heart, requiring withdrawal. Serosanguineous and chylous effusions—containing lipid droplets—rarely achieve sufficient volume to have clinical significance. Cholesterol effusions are exceedingly rare and are distinguished by the appearance of cholesterol crystals within the accumulated fluid. They are sometimes associated with myxedema, but more often are of unknown origin. It is speculated that breakdown of red cells in the past, with release of membrane lipids, may be the source of the crystals.

HEMOPERICARDIUM. The term hemopericardium should be limited to the accumulation of pure blood in the pericardial sac, and should be differentiated from hemorrhagic pericarditis, a condition in which there is an inflammatory exudate containing blood mixed with pus.

Hemopericardium is almost invariably due to traumatic perforation of the heart, rupture of the heart wall secondary to MI, or rupture of the intrapericardial aorta. Quite rarely, it may follow penetration of a myocardial abscess or tumor. Small, usually insignificant amounts of blood may extravasate from the trauma sometimes sustained during cardiopulmonary resuscitation. Rarely, however, marked hemorrhage occurs, clearly emphasizing the hazard entailed in such therapy. Hemorrhages in the bleeding diatheses, such as scurvy, leukemia, or thrombocytopenia, are rare causes of this condition.

The blood that escapes because of rupture of the heart or aorta rapidly fills the sac under greatly increased pressure and produces cardiac tamponade. As little as 200 to 300 ml may be sufficient to cause death. Although intracardiac injections may cause leakage of blood, death is usually already imminent when such measures are attempted and, under these circumstances, only small amounts of blood-tinged fluid appear in the pericardial sac.

PERICARDITIS

Inflammations of the pericardium are usually secondary to disorders in or about the heart, but sometimes they are caused by systemic disorders or by metastases from neoplasms arising in remote sites. Primary pericarditis is a rarity and almost always of viral origin. The major causes are presented in Table 13–9.

The various etiologies cited usually evoke an acute pericarditis, but a few, such as tuberculosis and fungi, produce chronic reactions. The acute and chronic reactions are morphologically nonspecific. Because many etiologies evoke identical anatomic changes and since it is usually impossible from pathologic examination to determine the etiologic basis for the reaction, a morphologic classification will follow, dividing the pericarditides into acute and chronic forms, and further subdividing the acute reactions on the basis of the character of the exudate. Sometimes, however, there is overlap among the categories. These subdivisions also have clinical relevance; to an extent, each induces somewhat distinctive signs and symptoms.

Table 13–9. Causes of Pericarditis

Infectious Agents
Viral
Pyogenic bacteria
Tuberculous
Fungal
Other parasites

Presumably Immunologically Mediated
Rheumatic fever
Systemic lupus erythematosus
Scleroderma
Postcardiotomy
Postmyocardial infarction
Drug-hypersensitivity reaction

Miscellaneous
Myocardial infarction
Uremia
Post cardiac surgery
Neoplasia
Trauma
Radiation

Acute Pericarditis

SEROUS PERICARDITIS. Serous inflammatory exudates are characteristically produced by nonbacterial inflammations, such as rheumatic fever, systemic lupus erythematosus, systemic scleroderma, tumors, and uremia. Similar effusions are also frequently encountered in the early stages of any form of bacterial pericarditis. Occasionally, a tuberculous infection of the pericardial sac or infections in the tissues contiguous to the pericardium evoke an inflammatory exudation that is principally serous in the early stages. For example, a bacterial pleuritis may cause sufficient irritation of the parietal pericardial serosa to cause a sterile serous effusion. In time, however, infection may extend across the anatomic barrier and the serous exudate is transformed into a frank suppurative reaction.

Occasionally, the Coxsackie A or B virus, adenovirus, or virus of influenza, ECHO virus type 8, and mumps virus, as well as others, is isolated from a serous exudate. In some instances a well-defined viral infection elsewhere — upper respiratory tract, pneumonia, parotitis — antedates the pericarditis to serve as the primary focus of infection. Infrequently, a viral pericarditis, most often related to Coxsackie and ECHO agents, occurs as an apparent primary involvement, usually in young adults. However, in many instances the etiology of apparent primary serous pericarditis remains unknown.

Morphologically, whatever the cause, there is an inflammatory reaction in the epi- and pericardial surfaces with scant numbers of polymorphonuclear leukocytes, lymphocytes, and histiocytes. Sometimes bacterial organisms or malignant tumor cells may be identified in the fluid, thus providing an indication of the etiology. Usually the volume of fluid is not large and varies between 50 and 200 ml. Because it represents a purely exudative phenomenon, it occurs slowly and therefore rarely produces sufficient increase in pressure to encroach upon the cardiac function. The fluid resorbs when and if the underlying disease remits. Organization or fibrous adhesions rarely develop.

FIBRINOUS AND SEROFIBRINOUS PERICARDITIS. These two anatomic forms are considered together because they represent essentially similar processes in which there is a more or less serous fluid mixed with a fibrinous exudate. This is the most frequent type of pericarditis. Common causes include MI, uremia, radiation to the chest, rheumatic fever, SLE, and trauma.[167] Bacterial, viral, and occasionally obscure myocardial inflammations may produce similar changes. Just as pneumonia or suppurative infections in the pleural cavities may produce serous pericarditis, in more severe cases they may cause the outpouring of fibrin. Fibrinous exudation may also follow cardiac surgery.

The gross morphologic alterations have already been described on page 69 (Fig. 13–40).

As is the case with all inflammatory exudates, *the*

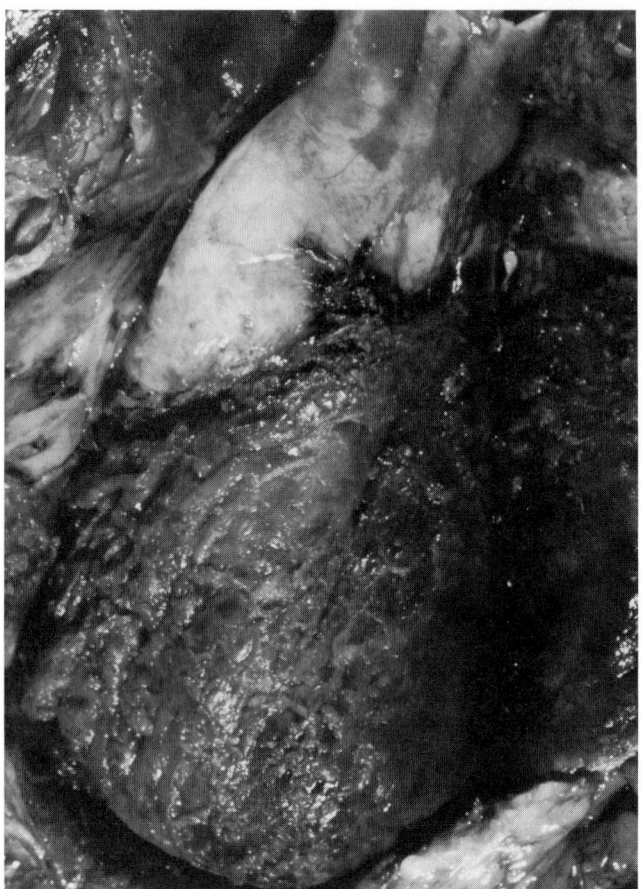

Figure 13–40. Fibrinous pericarditis, indicating the derivation of the term "bread and butter" pericarditis.

fibrin may be digested with resolution of the exudate, or may become organized. Organization and fibrous interadherence sometimes result in complete obliteration of the pericardial sac. This fibrosis yields a delicate, stringy type of adhesion, called *adhesive pericarditis,* which only rarely hampers or restricts cardiac action. With this type of pericarditis, the organization rarely extends to surrounding contiguous structures, such as the thoracic wall, diaphragm, or lungs, and therefore results only in obliteration of the space. In some cases, organization merely produces plaquelike fibrous thickenings of the serosal membranes.

From the clinical standpoint, *the development of a loud pericardial friction rub is the most striking characteristic of fibrinous pericarditis.* A collection of serous fluid may obliterate the rub by separating the two layers of the pericardium. Pain, systemic febrile reactions, and signs suggestive of cardiac failure may accompany the pathognomonic friction rub.

Fibrinous or serofibrinous pericarditis rarely leads to serious sequelae.

PURULENT OR SUPPURATIVE PERICARDITIS.

This form of pericardial inflammation almost invariably denotes the presence of bacterial, mycotic, or parasitic invasion of the pericardial space by orga-

nisms. It is most frequent in young males (male-to-female ratio, 3 : 1) between 10 and 40 years old. These organisms infect the pericardial cavity by (1) direct extension from neighboring inflammations, such as an empyema of the pleural cavity, lobar pneumonia, mediastinal infections, or, with infective endocarditis, bacterial invasion from the myocardium through the epicardium; (2) seeding from the blood; (3) lymphatic extension; or (4) direct introduction during cardiotomy. Immunosuppressive therapy potentiates all these pathways.

Quite rarely, a serosuppurative exudate may be produced by sterile inflammations, such as result from an MI or uremia. Rarely, severe viral infections of the heart, such as influenza or poliomyelitis, may cause suppurative pericarditis.

Morphologically, the exudate ranges from a thin to a creamy pus of up to 400 to 500 ml in volume. The serosal surfaces are reddened, granular, and coated with the exudate. Microscopically, there is a banal, acute, inflammatory reaction. Sometimes the inflammatory process extends into surrounding structures to induce a so-called *mediastinopericarditis.*

The clinical findings are essentially the same as those present in fibrinous pericarditis, but although a friction rub may be present, it is not usually so prominent as in the fibrinous variety. On the other hand, the signs of systemic infection are more marked; for example, spiking temperatures, chills, and fever.

Organization is the usual outcome of this inflammatory process, with resolution being infrequent. Because of the greater intensity of the inflammatory response, the organization produces *constrictive pericarditis.* Thus, suppurative pericarditis may lead to disabling consequences.

HEMORRHAGIC PERICARDITIS.

Hemorrhagic pericarditis denotes an exudate composed of blood mixed with a fibrinous or suppurative effusion. It is most commonly caused by tuberculosis or by malignant neoplastic involvement of the pericardial space, most often related to spread of lung and breast carcinomas, melanocarcinomas, lymphomas, and leukemias. It may also be found in bacterial infections or in cases of pericarditis occurring in patients with some underlying bleeding diathesis. Hemorrhagic pericarditis often follows cardiac surgery and sometimes is responsible for significant blood loss or even tamponade, requiring a "second look."

If the underlying cause is a tumor, neoplastic cells may be present in the effusion or in the pericardial or epicardial tissues. The clinical significance is that of a suppurative pericarditis, and resolution or organization with or without calcification is the eventual outcome.

CASEOUS PERICARDITIS.

Caseation within the pericardial sac is, until proved otherwise, tuberculous in origin. Infrequently, mycotic infections evoke a similar pattern. The tubercle bacilli usually involve the pericardium by direct spread from tuberculous foci within the tracheobronchial nodes. Often such direct continuity cannot be identified at postmortem and the possibility of lymphatic or of hematogenous dissemination from a noncontiguous focus cannot be excluded. The anatomic changes are typical of tuberculous infections elsewhere and need no further description. Caseous pericarditis is the most frequent antecedent of disabling fibrocalcific, chronic constrictive pericarditis.

Chronic or Healed Pericarditis

The term chronic pericarditis is a misnomer, because it refers in reality to a healed stage of one of the forms of pericardial inflammation already described. One pattern comprises the formation of pearly, thickened, nonadherent, epicardial plaques ("soldier's plaque"). Alternatively, thin, delicate adhesions may develop, which are termed diffuse or focal obliterative pericarditis according to their pattern. These rarely cause impairment of cardiac function, but they occur fairly frequently at autopsy and are often of obscure origin.

Two forms of healed pericarditis are of clinical importance: adhesive mediastinopericarditis and constrictive pericarditis.

ADHESIVE MEDIASTINOPERICARDITIS. This form of pericardial fibrosis may follow a suppurative or caseous pericarditis, but it can also be the consequence of previous cardiac surgery. Sometimes this pericardial reaction follows heavy irradiation to the mediastinum, as in radiotherapy for lymphomas or Hodgkin's disease. Only rarely is it a sequel to simple fibrinous exudation. The pericardial sac is obliterated, and adherence of the external aspect of the parietal layer to surrounding structures produces a great strain on cardiac function. With each systolic contraction, the heart is pulling not only against the parietal pericardium, but also against the attached surrounding structures. Systolic retractions of the rib cage and diaphragm, pulsus paradoxus, and a variety of other fairly pathognomonic findings may be observed clinically. *The increased workload causes cardiac hypertrophy and dilatation, which may be quite massive in more severe cases.*

CONSTRICTIVE PERICARDITIS. The heart may be encased in a dense, fibrous, or fibrocalcific scar that limits diastolic expansion and seriously restricts cardiac output. Sometimes there is a well-defined history of a previous suppurative or caseous pericarditis, but more often the cause is buried in the remote past (idiopathic).[168] Fibrinous or serofibrinous inflammatory reactions rarely lead to this form of damage. In constrictive pericarditis, the pericardial space not only is obliterated but is transformed into a dense layer of scar or calcification, many times 0.5 to 1.0 cm thick, which resists dissection. In extreme cases, it appears as if the heart were enclosed within a plaster mold *(concretio cordis)*. In less severe instances, only irregular calcific plates are produced.

Although the signs of cardiac failure may resemble those produced by mediastinopericarditis, the local findings in the heart are quite different. *Cardiac hypertrophy and dilatation cannot occur because of the dense enclosing scar,* and as a consequence the heart is described as a small, quiet heart with reduced minute volume output and reduced pulse pressure. Constriction of the venae cavae during the fibrotic process may block the venous return to the right side of the heart, simulating severe right heart failure.

RHEUMATOID HEART DISEASE

Rheumatoid arthritis is mainly a disorder of the joints, but it is also associated with many nonarticular involvements (e.g., subcutaneous rheumatoid nodules, acute vasculitis, and Felty's syndrome [p. 1353]). The heart is also involved in 20 to 40% of cases of severe prolonged rheumatoid arthritis. The most common finding is a fibrinous pericarditis that may progress to fibrous thickening of the visceral and parietal pericardium with dense fibrous adhesions. In the early stages of this process, rheumatoid inflammatory granulomatous nodules resembling those that occur subcutaneously (p. 1351) may be identifiable deep to the pericardial surfaces. Much less frequently, rheumatoid nodules involve the myocardium, endocardium, valves of the heart, and the root of the aorta[169] (Fig. 13–41). These inflammatory lesions are particularly damaging when they are located in the valves. Rheumatoid valvulitis can lead to marked fibrous thickening and secondary calcification of the cusps, producing changes resembling those of chronic rheumatic valvular disease, but intercommissural adhesion is rarely present.

TUMORS

Primary tumors of the heart are extremely rare, being found in one autopsy in 1000 to 10,000. In contrast, metastatic tumors to the heart occur in about 5% of patients dying of cancer. The most common primary tumors, in descending order of frequency, are myxomas, lipomas, papillary fibroelastomas, rhabdomyomas, angiosarcomas, and rhabdomyosarcomas. Note that the four most common are all benign and account collectively for about 70% of all primary tumors of the heart; the two sarcomas account for about 20%.

SECONDARY METASTASES

The major cancers associated with *cardiac metastases* (in descending order of frequency) are carcinoma of the bronchus and breast, malignant melanoma, lymphoma, and leukemia.[170] The metastatic tumors most often involve the pericardium and may be asymptomatic, produce manifestations of pericarditis, or penetrate the myocardium, leading to arrhythmias, congestive failure, or obstruction to the major inflow or outflow vessels sometimes worsened by superim-

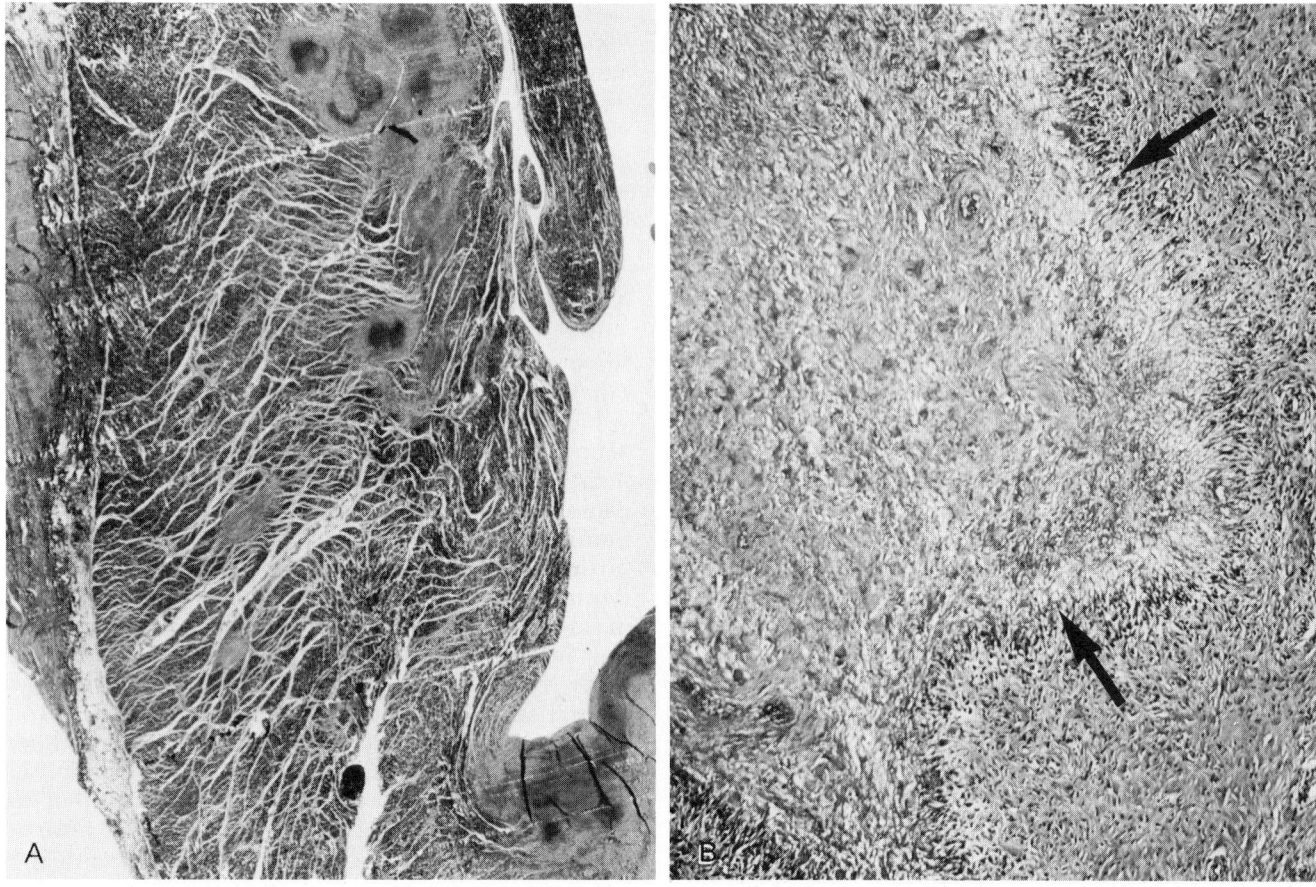

Figure 13–41. Rheumatoid heart disease. *A,* A transection of the left ventricular wall disclosing numerous intramyocardial granulomas seen *(B)* as having a peripheral inflammatory palisade *(arrows)* surrounding a central area of necrosis.

posed thrombosis. In other instances the metastases may directly seed the myocardium. The full spectrum of effects of metastases on the heart and pericardium is reviewed in Table 13–10, drawn from Schoen and colleagues.[171]

PRIMARY TUMORS

Myxomas are the most common primary tumor of the heart in adults. Although they may arise in any of the four chambers or, rarely, on the heart valves, about 90% are located in the atria, with a left-to-right ratio of approximately 4 : 1.[172] The tumors are almost always single, rarely multiple in several chambers. The region of the fossa ovalis is a favored site of atrial origin. They range from small (less than 1 cm) to large (up to 10 cm) sessile or pedunculated masses. In general, sessile lesions are globular, hard, mottled with hemorrhage, and easily confused with an organizing mural thrombus. Pedunculated myxomas tend to be soft, translucent, papillary, or villous lesions having a myxoid appearance. All are usually covered by an intact endocardium, but fragmentation and embolization of papillary lesions is sometimes encountered. The sessile pattern, when unfortunately located, and particularly the pedunculated form, is frequently sufficiently mobile to move into or sometimes through

the atrioventricular valves during diastole. Sometimes such mobility exerts a "wrecking ball" effect on the valve leaflets. Histologically, they are composed of stellate or globular myxoma cells, endothelial cells, macrophages, mature or immature smooth muscle cells, and a variety of intermediate forms embedded within an abundant acid mucopolysaccharide ground substance (Fig 13–42). Numerous small blood ves-

Table 13–10. The Spectrum of Direct Effects of Tumors on the Heart and Pericardium

SITE OF METASTASIS	FUNCTIONAL CONSEQUENCES	MOST LIKELY PRIMARY
Myocardium via hematogenous route	Arrhythmias Obstruction Restriction Infarction Dyskinesia	Any
Pericardium	Effusion Restriction	Lung or breast carcinoma, leukemia, lymphoma
Right atrial chamber	Obstruction	Renal adenocarcinoma, hepatoma, lung
Lung (multiple tumor emboli)	Cor pulmonale	Gastric, breast, hepatoma

Drawn from Schoen, F. J., et al.: Cardiac effects of noncardiac neoplasms. Cardiol. Clin. 2:657, 1984.

sels, sometimes having well-developed muscular walls, course through these lesions, and often hemosiderin pigment and macrophages laden with hemosiderin granules are present as stigmata of microhemorrhages. Ultrastructurally, the most prominent feature in some myxoma cells is an abundance of fine cytoplasmic fibrils similar to those of smooth muscle cells.[173] It has long been questioned whether cardiac myxomas are hamartomatous or organized thrombi, but the weight of evidence is on the side of benign neoplasia. All the cell types present are thought to derive from variable differentiation of primitive mesenchymal cells.

These neoplasms may be encountered at any age, even in infants, with a predominance in females. Because they may create ball-valve obstructions, they sometimes cause unanticipated syncopal attacks, cardiac insufficiency, and even sudden death, in apparently healthy young children and adults. Sometimes embolization, particularly to the brain, kidneys, or lungs, calls attention to these lesions. Present diagnostic techniques provide the opportunity to identify these masses, but differentiation from a mural thrombus is sometimes difficult despite all the newer diagnostic modalities. Surgical removal is usually curative, although sometimes the neoplasm recurs months to years later.

Lipomas may occur in the subendocardium, in

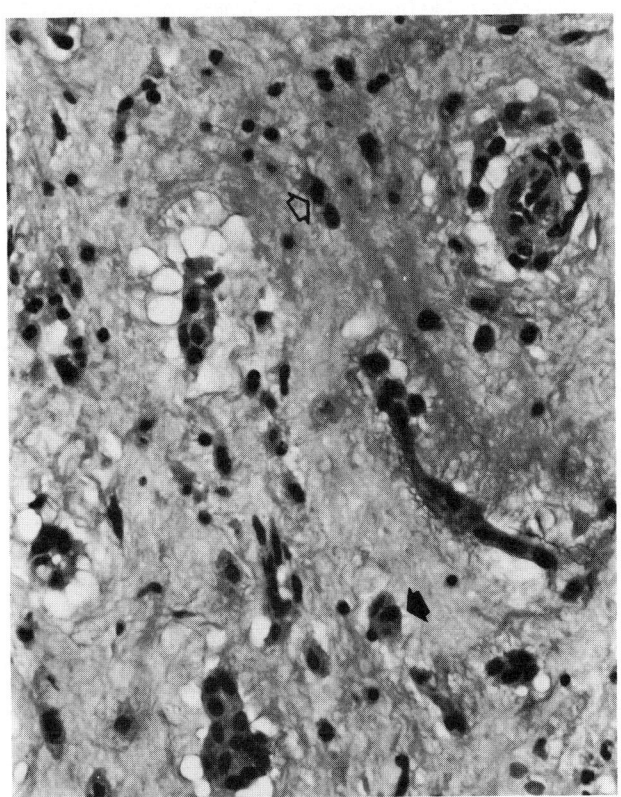

Figure 13-42. Atrial myxoma disclosing abundant ground substance in which are scattered mononuclear leukocytes, abnormal vascular formations, and a few myxoma cells (solid arrow), one with stellate processes (open arrow).

the subpericardium, or within the myocardium. They are well localized but poorly encapsulated, range in size up to 10 to 12 cm in diameter, tend to be polypoid, and depending on location may be asymptomatic, create ball-valve obstructions as with the myxomas described earlier, or produce arrhythmias. They are most often located in the left ventricle, right atrium, or interatrial septum. Some of these masses are very poorly encapsulated and appear to be infiltrative, raising the possibility that they (and possibly all lipomas) represent developmental hamartomatous accumulations of adipose tissue.

Papillary fibroelastomas are curious, usually incidental lesions most often identified at autopsy. Generally they are located on valves, particularly the ventricular surface of semilunar valves and the atrial surface of AV valves. For reasons that are unclear, the right-sided valves are most commonly involved in children and the left-sided valves in adults. They constitute a distinctive cluster of hairlike projections about 2 to 5 mm in length covering up to several centimeters in diameter of the endocardial surface. Larger lesions may sometimes be visualized by echocardiography. Histologically, these curiosities are covered by endothelium, deep to which is myxoid connective tissue containing abundant mucopolysaccharide matrix in which are dispersed smooth muscle cells, fibroblasts, and elastic fibers. Although called neoplasms, it is likely that the fibroelastomas represent organized thrombi. They should be differentiated from the much smaller, usually trivial, heaped-up *Lambl's excrescences* frequently found on heart valves at sites of endothelial damage.

Rhabdomyomas are much less common than myxomas. They are, however, the most frequent primary tumor of the heart in infants and children and are frequently discovered in the first years of life because of obstruction of a valvular orifice or cardiac chamber. They are generally small, gray-white myocardial masses up to several centimeters in diameter located on either the left or right side of the heart, protruding into the ventricular chambers. Histologically, they are composed of a mixed population of cells prominent among which are large, rounded or polygonal cells that have numerous glycogen-laden vacuoles separated by strands of cytoplasm running from the plasma membrane to the more or less centrally located nucleus — so-called *spider cells*. These cells can be shown to have myofibrils. In addition there may be spindle cells, histiocytic appearing cells, and an abundant mucopolysaccharide matrix. The nature of these lesions is in doubt, and it is highly likely that they are hamartomas rather than true neoplasms. There is a high frequency of tuberous sclerosis in patients with cardiac rhabdomyomas, lending credence to the belief that the cardiac lesions are malformational in origin.[174]

The *angiosarcomas* and *rhabdomyosarcomas* are not distinctive from their counterparts in other locations and so require no further comment here. In conclusion, the bad news about cardiac tumors is that they may be responsible for considerable morbidity and sometimes mortality, but the good news is that most are benign and many are amenable to resection when discovered by the alert cardiologist.

1. Newman, P.E.: The coronary collateral circulation: Determinants in ischemic heart disease. Am. Heart J. *102*:431, 1981.

2. Braunwald, E.: Pathophysiology of heart failure. *In* Braunwald, E. (ed.): Heart Disease: A Textbook of Cardiovascular Medicine. Philadelphia, W.B. Saunders Co., 1980, p. 453.

3. Bing, R.J.: The biochemical basis of myocardial failure. Hosp. Pract. *18*:93, 1983.

4. Bristow, M.R., et al.: Decreased catecholamine sensitivity and beta-adrenergic receptor density in failing human hearts. N. Engl. J. Med. *307*:205, 1982.

5. Arcidi, J.M., et al.: Hepatic morphology in cardiac dysfunction. A clinicopathologic study of 1000 subjects at autopsy. Am. J. Pathol. *104*:159, 1981.

6. Stamler, J.: Coronary heart disease: Doing the "right" things. N. Engl. J. Med. *312*:1053, 1985.

7. Reimer, K.A., and Jennings, R.B.: Myocardial ischemia, hypoxia, and infarction. *In* Fozzard, H.A., et al. (eds.): The Heart and Cardiovascular System. New York, Raven Press, 1986, p. 1133.

8. Brown, B.G.: Coronary vasospasm. Observations linking the clinical spectrum of ischemic heart disease to the dynamic pathology of coronary atherosclerosis. Arch. Intern. Med. *141*:716, 1981.

9. American Heart Association: 1988 Heart Facts. Dallas, American Heart Association National Center, 1988.

10. Gomez-Marin, O., et al.: Improvement in long-term survival among patients hospitalized with acute myocardial infarction, 1970–1980. The Minnesota heart survey. N. Engl. J. Med. *316*:1353, 1987.

11. Marmot, M.G.: Interpretation of trends in coronary heart disease mortality. Acta Med. Scand. Suppl. *701*:58, 1985.

12. Goldman, L.: Analyzing the decline in the CAD death rate. Hosp. Pract. *23*:73, 1988.

13. Pell, S., and Fayerweather, W.E.: Trends in the incidence of myocardial infarction and in associated mortality and morbidity in a large employed population, 1957–1983. N. Engl. J. Med. *312*:1005, 1985.

14. Roberts, W.C.: The coronary arteries in ischemic heart disease: Facts and fancies. Triangle *16*:77, 1977.

15. Lie, J.T.: Coronary thrombosis and acute MI. *In* Waller, B.F. (ed.): Contemporary Issues in Cardiac Pathology. Philadelphia, F.A. Davis Co., 1988, p. 23.

16. Buja, L.M., and Willerson, J.T.: The role of coronary artery lesions in ischemic heart disease: Insights from recent clinicopathologic, coronary arteriographic, and experimental studies. Hum. Pathol. *18*:451, 1987.

17. Steering Committee of the Physicians Health Study Research Group: Preliminary report: Findings from the aspirin component of the ongoing physicians' health study. N. Engl. J. Med. *318*:262, 1988.

18. Kromhout, D., et al.: The inverse relation between fish consumption and twenty-year mortality from coronary heart disease. N. Engl. J. Med. *312*:1205, 1985.

19. Buja, L.M., et al.: The role of coronary arterial spasm in ischemic heart disease. Arch. Pathol. Lab. Med. *103*:221, 1981.

20. Hillis, L.D., and Braunwald, E.: Coronary artery spasm. N. Engl. J. Med. *299*:695, 1978.

21. Ganz, P., et al.: Dynamic variations in resistance of coronary arterial narrowings in angina pectoris at rest. Am. J. Cardiol. *59*:66, 1987.

22. Willerson, J.T., et al.: Speculation regarding mechanisms responsible for acute ischemic heart disease syndromes. J. Am. Coll. Cardiol. *8*:245, 1986.

23. Vestrovec, G.W., et al.: Intracoronary thrombolysis in syndromes of unstable ischemia: Angiographic and clinical results. Am. Heart J. *104*:946, 1982.

24. Jennings, R.B., and Reimer, K.A.: Pathobiology of acute myocardial ischemia. Hosp. Pract. *24*:89, 1989.

25. Lerner, D.J., and Kannel, W.B.: Patterns of coronary heart disease, morbidity, and mortality in the sexes: A 26-year follow-up of the Framingham population. Am. Heart J. *111*:383, 1986.

26. Fortney, J.A., et al.: Oral contraceptives and life expectancy. Studies in Family Planning *17*:117, 1986.

27. Ragland, D.R., and Brand, R.J.: Type A behavior and mortality from coronary heart disease. N. Engl. J. Med. *318*:65, 1988.

28. Kannel, W.B., et al.: Epidemiological assessment of the role of physical activity and fitness in development of cardiovascular disease. Am. Heart J. *109*:876, 1985.

29. Stampfer, M.J., et al.: A prospective study of moderate alcohol consumption and the risk of coronary disease and stroke in women. N. Engl. J. Med. *319*:267, 1988.

30. Willerson, J.T., et al.: Conversion from chronic to acute coronary artery disease: Speculation regarding mechanisms. Am. J. Cardiol. *54*:1349, 1984.

31. Feldman, R.L.: Coronary thrombosis, coronary spasm, and coronary atherosclerosis and speculation on the link between unstable angina and acute myocardial infarction. Am. J. Cardiol. *59*:1187, 1987.

32. Davies, M.J., and Thomas, A.C.: Plaque fissuring — the cause of acute myocardial infarction, sudden aeschemic death, and crescendo angina. Br. Heart J. *53*:363, 1985.

33. DeWood, M.A., et al.: Prevalence of total coronary occlusion during the early hours of transmural myocardial infarction. N. Engl. J. Med. *303*:897, 1980.

34. Marder, V.J., and Sherry, S.: Thrombolytic therapy; current status. N. Engl. J. Med. *318*:1512, 1585, 1988.

35. Engel, H.J.: Coronary artery spasm as the cause of myocardial infarction during coronary arteriography. Am. Heart J. *91*:501, 1976.

36. Karch, S.B., and Billingham, M.E.: The pathology and etiology of cocaine-induced heart disease. Arch. Pathol. Lab. Med. *112*:225, 1988.

37. Woolf, N., and Davies, M.J.: Morphological variants of acute myocardial necrosis and their relationship to coronary artery thrombosis. Acta Med. Scand. (Suppl.) *642*:92, 1980.

38. Laffel, G.L., and Braunwald, E.: Thrombolytic therapy. A new strategy for treatment of acute myocardial infarction. N. Engl. J. Med. *311*:710, 770, 1984.

39. Ratliff, N.B., and Hackel, D.B.: Combined right and left ventricular infarction: Pathogenesis and clinicopathologic correlations. Am. J. Cardiol. *45*:217, 1980.

40. Gardin, J.M., and Singer, D.H.: Atrial infarction: Importance, diagnosis, and localization. Arch. Intern. Med. *141*:1345, 1981.

41. Mallory, G.K.: The speed of healing of myocardial infarction. A study of the pathologic anatomy in 72 cases. Am. Heart J. *18*:747, 1939.

42. Lie, J.T., et al.: Macroscopic enzyme-mapping verification of large homogeneous experimental infarcts of predictable size and location in dogs. J. Thorac. Cardiovasc. Surg. *69*:599, 1975.

43. Fallon, J.T.: Postmortem histochemical techniques. *In* Wagner, G.S. (ed.): Myocardial Infarction. Measurement and Intervention. The Hague, Martinus Nijhoff Publishers, 1981, p. 373.

44. Bates, R.J., et al.: Cardiac rupture — challenge in diagnosis and management. Am. J. Cardiol. *40*:429, 1977.

45. Radford, M.J., et al.: Ventricular septal rupture: A review of clinical and physiologic features and an analysis of survival. Circulation *64*:545, 1981.

46. Fishbein, M.C., et al.: The histopathologic evolution of myocardial infarction. Chest *73*:843, 1978.

47. Edwalds, G.M., et al.: Myocytolysis (vacuolar degeneration) of myocardium: Immunohistochemical evidence of viability. Hum. Pathol. *15*:753, 1984.

48. Schoen, F.J., et al.: Clinical temporary ventricular assist. Pathologic findings and their implications in a multiinstitutional study of 41 patients. J. Thorac. Cardiovasc. Surg. *92*:1071, 1986.

49. Hearse, D.J., and Yellon, D.M.: The "border zone" in evolving myocardial infarction: Controversy or confusion? Am. J. Cardiol. *47*:1321, 1981.

50. Reimer, K.A., and Ideker, R.E.: Myocardial ischemia and infarction: Anatomic and biochemical substrates for ischemic cell death and ventricular arrhythmias. Hum. Pathol. *18*:462, 1987.

51. Waller, B.F.: Pathology of transluminal balloon angioplasty used in the treatment of coronary heart disease. Hum. Pathol. *18*:476, 1987.

52. Campean, L., et al.: The relation of risk factors to the development of atherosclerosis in saphenous vein bypass grafts and the progression of disease in the native circulation. N. Engl. J. Med. *311*:1329, 1984.

53. Kent, K.M.: Coronary angioplasty. A decade of experience. N. Engl. J. Med. *316*:1148, 1987.

54. Epstein, S.E., et al.: Myocardial ischemia—silent or asymptomatic. N. Engl. J. Med. *318*:1038, 1988.

55. Lott, J.A.: Serum enzyme determinations in the diagnosis of acute myocardial infarction. Hum. Pathol. *15*:706, 1984.

56. Rissanen, V.: Sudden coronary death and coronary artery disease: A clinicopathologic appraisal. Cardiology *64*:289, 1979.

57. Guerci, A.D., et al.: A randomized trial of intravenous tissue plasminogen activator for acute myocardial infarction with subsequent randomization to elective coronary angioplasty. N. Engl. J. Med. *317*:1613, 1987.

58. Editorial: Primary prevention of ischaemic heart disease with lipid-lavering drugs. Lancet *1*:333, 1988.

59. Geer, J.C., et al.: Subendocardial ischemic myocardial lesions associated with severe coronary atherosclerosis. Am. J. Pathol. *98*:663, 1980.

60. Myerberg, R.J.: Sudden cardiac death: Epidemiology, causes, and mechanisms. Cardiology *74*(Suppl. 2):2, 1987.

61. Vermani, R., and Roberts, W.C.: Sudden cardiac death. Hum. Pathol. *18*:485, 1987.

62. Davies, M.J.: Pathological view of sudden cardiac death. Br. Heart J. *45*:88, 1981.

63. Davies, M.J., and Thomas, A.: Thrombosis and acute coronary artery lesions in sudden cardiac ischemic death. N. Engl. J. Med. *310*:1137, 1984.

64. Cobb, L.A., et al.: Sudden cardiac death. Modern Concepts Cardiovasc. Dis. *49*:31, 1980.

65. Hammon, J.W., and Oates, J.A.: Interaction of platelets with a vessel wall in the pathophysiology of sudden cardiac death. Circulation *73*:224, 1986.

66. Ferrans, V.J.: Morphology of the heart in hypertrophy. Hosp. Pract. *18*:67, 1983.

67. Levy, D., et al.: Echocardiographically detected left ventricular hypertrophy: Prevalence and risk factors. The Framingham heart study. Ann. Intern. Med. *108*:7, 1988.

68. Subcommittee of Definition and Prevalence of the 1984 Joint National Committee: Hypertension prevalence and the status of awareness, treatment, and control in the United States. Hypertension *7*:457, 1985.

69. Schoen, F.J., Jr.: Interventional Cardiovascular Pathology: Medical and Surgical Considerations. Philadelphia, W.B. Saunders Co., 1989, in press.

70. Starksen, N.F., et al.: Cardiac myocyte hypertrophy is associated with c-myc proto-oncogene expression. Proc. Natl. Acad. Sci. U.S.A. *83*:8348, 1986.

71. Grossman, W.: Cardiac hypertrophy: Useful adaptation or pathologic process? Am. J. Med. *69*:576, 1980.

72. Ferrans, V.J., and Butany, J.W.: Ultrastructural pathology of the heart. *In* Trump, B.F., and Jones, R.T. (eds.): Diagnostic Electron Microscopy. Vol. 4. New York, John Wiley and Sons, Inc., 1983, p. 319.

73. Frohlich, E.D.: The heart in hypertension. Unresolved conceptual challenges. Hypertension *11* (Suppl. 1):1, 1988.

74. Summer, W.R.: Acute cor pulmonale. *In* Rubin, L.J. (ed.): Pulmonary Heart Disease. Boston, Martinus Nijhoff, 1984, p. 285.

75. Bergofsky, E.H.: Humoral control of the pulmonary circulation. Annu. Rev. Physiol. *42*:221, 1980.

76. Edwards, J.E.: Pathology of chronic pulmonary hypertension. Pathol. Annu. *9*:1, 1974.

77. Intersociety Commission for Heart Disease Resources: Primary prevention of pulmonary heart disease. Circulation *41*:A–17, 1970.

78. Edwards, W.D.: Pathology of pulmonary hypertension. *In* Waller, B.F. (ed.): Contemporary Issues in Cardiovascular Pathology. Cardiovascular Clinics. Philadelphia, F.A. Davis Co., 1988, p. 321.

79. Higgins, I.T.: The epidemiology of congenital heart disease. J. Chronic Dis. *18*:699, 1965.

80. Nadas, A.S., and Fyler, D.C.: Pediatric Cardiology. 3rd ed. Philadelphia, W.B. Saunders Co., 1972.

81. Friedman, W.F.: Congenital heart disease in infancy and childhood. *In* Braunwald, E. (ed.): Heart Disease. A Textbook of Cardiovascular Medicine. Philadelphia, W.B. Saunders Co., 1980, p. 967.

82. Nora, J.J., and Nora, A.H.: The evolution of specific genetic and environmental counseling in congenital heart diseases. Circulation *57*:205, 1978.

83. Cooper, L.Z.: The history and medical consequences of rubella. Rev. Infect. Dis. 7 (Suppl 1):S-2, 1985.

84. Nora, J.J., et al.: Etiologic aspects of cardiovascular disease and predisposition detectable in the infant and child. *In* Friedman, W.F., et al. (eds.): Neonatal Heart Disease. New York, Grune & Stratton, 1973, p. 279.

85. Newman, T.B.: Etiology of septal defects: An epidemiologic approach. Pediatrics *76*:741, 1985.

86. Merrill, W.H., and Bender, H.W., Jr.: The surgical approach to congenital heart disease. Curr. Probl. Surg. *22*:1, 1985.

87. Page, G.G.: Tetralogy of Fallot. Rev. Crit. Care *15*:390, 1986.

88. Lev, M., et al.: Pathologic anatomy of complete transposition of the arterial trunks. Pediatrics *28*:293, 1961.

89. Elliot, L.P., et al.: Complete transposition of the great vessels. I. An anatomic study of 60 cases. Circulation *27*:1105, 1963.

90. Van Praagh, R.: What is congenitally corrected transposition? N. Engl. J. Med. *282*:1097, 1970.

91. Shankar, P.S.: Congenital heart disease. Q. Med. Rev. *32*:1, 1981.

92. Baker, E.J., et al.: The cross-sectional anatomy of ventricular septal defects: A reappraisal. Br. Heart J. *59*:339, 1988.

93. Hoffman, J.I.E., and Rudolph, A.M.: The natural history of ventricular septal defects in infancy. Am. J. Cardiol. *16*:634, 1965.

94. Gersony, W.M.: Patent ductus arteriosus in the neonate. Pediatr. Clin. North Am. *33*:545, 1986.

95. Peckham, G.J., et al.: Clinical course to one year of age in premature infants with patent ductus arteriosus: Results of a multicenter randomized trial of indomethacin. J. Pediatr. *105*:285, 1984.

96. Gikonyo, B.M., et al.: Anatomic features of pulmonary valvular stenosis. Pediatr. Cardiol. *8*:109, 1987.

97. Haroutunian, L.M., and Neill, C.A.: Dextrocardia: Analysis of 100 cases and family study of 40 cases. Circulation *24*:951, 1961.

98. Schoen, F.J., and Sutton, M.St.J.: Contemporary issues in the pathology of valvular heart disease. Hum. Pathol. *18*:586, 1987.

99. Selzer, A.: Changing aspects of the natural history of valvular aortic stenosis. N. Engl. J. Med. *317*:91, 1987.

100. Petersen, M.D., et al.: Types of aortic stenosis in surgically removed valves. Arch. Pathol. Lab. Med. *109*:829, 1985.

101. Khan, S.S., and Gray, R.: Recent developments in aortic stenosis. Compr. Ther. *14*:33, 1988.

102. Dean, G.A.: Mitral valve prolapse. Hosp. Pract. *20*:75, 1985.

103. Edwards, J.E.: Floppy mitral valve syndrome. *In* Waller, B.F. (ed.): Contemporary Issues in Cardiovascular Pathology. Philadelphia, F.A. Davis Co., 1988, p. 249.

104. Lucas, R.V., Jr., and Edwards, J.E.: The floppy mitral valve. Curr. Probl. Cardiol. *7*:1, 1982.

105. Baker, P.B., et al.: Floppy mitral valve chordae tendineae. Histopathologic alterations. Hum. Pathol. *19*:507, 1988.

106. Perloff, J.K.: Evolving concepts of mitral valve prolapse. N. Engl. J. Med. *307*:369, 1982.

107. Perloff, J.K.: Clinical and epidemiologic issues in mitral valve prolapse: Overview and perspective. Am. Heart J. *113*:1324, 1987.

108. Gillum, R.F.: Trends in acute rheumatic fever and chronic rheumatic heart disease. A national perspective. Am. Heart J. *111*:430, 1986.

109. Veasy, L.G., et al.: Resurgence of acute rheumatic fever in the intermountain area of the United States. N. Engl. J. Med. *316*:421, 1987.

110. Massell, B.F., et al.: Penicillin and the marked decrease in morbidity and mortality from rheumatic fever in the United States. N. Engl. J. Med. *318*:280, 1988.

111. Appleton, R.S., et al.: Specificity of persistence of antibody to the streptococcal group A carbohydrate in rheumatic valvular heart disease. J. Clin. Lab. Med. *105*:114, 1985.

112. Dale, J.B., and Beachey, E.H.: Epitopes of streptococcal M proteins shared with cardiac myosin. J. Exp. Med. *162*:583, 1985.

113. Stollerman, G.H.: Autoimmunity and rheumatic fever. *In* Cohen, I.R. (ed.): Perspectives in Autoimmunity. Boca Raton, FL, CRC Press, 1986.

114. Virmani, R., and Roberts, W.C.: Aschoff bodies in operatively excised atrial appendages and in papillary muscles. Frequency and clinical significance. Circulation 55:559, 1977.

115. Husby, G.H., et al.: Immunofluorescent studies of florid rheumatic Aschoff lesions. Arthritis Rheum. 29:207, 1986.

116. Roberts, W.C., and Virmani, R.: Aschoff bodies at necropsy in valvular heart disease. Evidence from an analysis of 543 patients over 14 years of age that rheumatic heart disease, at least anatomically, is a disease of the mitral valve. Circulation 57:803, 1978.

117. Chen, S., et al.: Rheumatic fever in children. A follow-up study with emphasis on cardiac sequelae. Jap. Heart J. 22:167, 1981.

118. Durack, D.T., and Beeson, P.B.: Pathogenesis of infective endocarditis. In Rahimtoola, S.H. (ed.): Infective Endocarditis. New York, Grune & Stratton, 1978, p. 1.

119. Johnson, C.M., and Rhodes, H.K.: Pediatric endocarditis. Mayo Clin. Proc. 57:86, 1982.

120. Sussman, J.I.: Viridans streptococcal endocarditis: Clinical, microbiological, and echocardiographic correlations. J. Infect. Dis. 154:597, 1986.

121. Haller, D.R.: Infections in intravenous drug abusers. Postgrad. Med. 83:95, 1988.

122. Schoen, F.J., and Levy R.J.: Bioprosthetic heart valve failure. Pathology and pathogenesis. Cardiol. Clin. 2:717, 1984.

123. Calderwood, S.B., et al.: Risk factors for the development of prosthetic valve endocarditis. Circulation 72:31, 1985.

124. Cowgill, L.D., et al.: Prosthetic valve endocarditis. Curr. Probl. Cardiol. 11:626, 628, 635, 646, 1986.

125. Weinstein, L.: Life-threatening complications of infective endocarditis and their management. Arch. Intern. Med. 146:953, 1986.

126. Rosen, P., and Armstrong, D.: Nonbacterial thrombotic endocarditis in patients with malignant neoplastic diseases. Am. J. Med. 54:23, 1973.

127. Young, R.S.K., and Zalneraitis, E.L.: Marantic endocarditis in children and young adults: Clinical and pathological findings. Stroke 12:635, 1981.

128. Galve, E., et al.: Prevalence, morphologic types, and evolution of cardiac valvular disease in systemic lupus erythematosus, N. Engl. J. Med. 319:817, 1988.

129. Fulkerson, P.K., et al.: Calcification of the mitral anulus: Etiology, clinical associations, complications, and therapy. Am. J. Med. 66:967, 1979.

130. Lundin, L., et al.: Carcinoid heart disease: Relationship of circulating vasoactive substances to ultrasound-detectable cardiac abnormalities. Circulation 77:264, 1988.

131. Hammond, G.L., et al.: Biological versus mechanical valves. Analysis of 1,116 valves inserted into 1,012 adult patients with a 4,818 patient-year and a 5,327 valve-year follow-up. Gen. Thorac. Cardiovasc. Surg. 93:182, 1987.

132. Schoen, F.J.: Modes of failure and other pathology of mechanical and tissue heart valve prostheses. In Bodnar, E., and Frater, R. (eds.): Replacement Cardiac Valves. New York, Pergamon Press. In press.

133. Schoen, F.J.: Cardiac valve prostheses. Pathological and bioengineering considerations. J. Cardiac Surg. 2:65, 1987.

134. Aretz, H.T., et al.: Myocarditis: A histopathologic definition and classification. Am. J. Cardiovasc. Pathol. 1:3, 1986.

135. Wenger, N.K.: Infectious myocarditis. Postgrad. Med. 44:105, 1968.

136. Gore, I., and Saphir, O.: Myocarditis: A classification of 1402 cases. Am. Heart J. 34:827, 1947.

137. Johnson, R.A., and Palacios, I.: Dilated cardiomyopathies of the adult. N. Engl. J. Med. 307:1051, 1119, 1982.

138. Woodruff, J.F.: Viral myocarditis: A review. Am. J. Pathol. 101:425, 1980.

139. Lowry, B.S.: Viruses and heart disease. A problem in pathogenesis. Ann. Clin. Lab. Sci. 16:358, 1986.

140. Fejfar, Z.: Cardiomyopathy: An international problem. Cardiologia (Basel) 52:9, 1968.

141. Roberts, W.C., et al.: Sarcoidosis of the heart. A clinicopathologic study of 35 necropsy patients (group I) and review of 78 previously described necropsy patients (group II). Am. J. Med. 63:86, 1977.

142. Davies, M.J., et al.: Idiopathic giant-cell myocarditis — a distinctive clinicopathological entity. Br. Heart J. 37:192, 1975.

143. Edwards, J.J., et al.: Studies on the pathogenesis of cardiac and cerebral lesions of experimental trichinosis in rabbits. Am. J. Pathol. 40:711, 1962.

144. Report of the WHO/ISFC Task Force on the Definition and Classification of Cardiomyopathies. Br. Heart J. 44:672, 1980.

145. Editorial: Natural history of dilated cardiomyopathy. Lancet 1:248, 1986.

146. Walsh, T.K., and Vacek, J.L.: Ethanol and heart disease: An underestimated contributing factor. Postgrad. Med. 79:60, 1986.

147. Homans, D.C.: Peripartum cardiomyopathy. N. Engl. J. Med. 312:1432, 1985.

148. Berko, B.A., and Swift, M.: X-linked dilated cardiomyopathy. N. Engl. J. Med. 316:1186, 1987.

149. Goodwin, J.F.: Mechanisms in cardiomyopathies. J. Molec. Cell Cardiol. 17:5, 1985.

150. Olsen, E.G.J.: Myocarditis — a case of mistaken identity. Br. Heart J. 50:303, 1983.

151. Roberts, W.C.: Cardiomyopathy and myocarditis; morphologic features. Adv. Cardiol. 22:184, 1978.

152. Olsen, E.G.J.: Special investigations of COCM: Endomyocardial biopsies (morphological analysis). Postgrad. Med. 54:486, 1978.

153. Baandrup, U., and Olsen, E.G.J.: Critical analysis of endomyocardial biopsies from patients suspected of having cardiomyopathy. Br. Heart J. 45:475, 1981.

154. Maron, B.J., et al.: Hypertrophic cardiomyopathy. Interrelations of clinical manifestations, pathophysiology, and therapy. N. Engl. J. Med. 316:780, 844, 1987.

155. Bulkley, B.H., et al.: Isometric cardiac contraction: A possible cause of the disorganized myocardial pattern of idiopathic, hypertrophic, subaortic stenosis. N. Engl. J. Med. 296:135, 1977.

156. Maron, B.J., and Mulvihill, J.J.: The genetics of hypertrophic cardiomyopathy. Ann. Intern. Med. 105:610, 1986.

157. Cryley, J.M., and Siegel, R.J.: Obstruction is unimportant in the pathophysiology of hypertrophic cardiomyopathy. Postgrad. Med. J. 62:515, 1986.

158. Westermark, P., et al.: Senile cardiac amyloidosis: Evidence of two different amyloid substances in the aging heart. Scand. J. Immunol. 10:303, 1979.

159. Baandrup, U.: Loeffler's endocarditis and endomyocardial fibrosis — a nosologic entity. Acta Pathol. Microbiol. Scand. 85:869, 1977.

160. Olsen, E.G.: Endomyocardial fibrosis and Löffler's endocarditis parietalis fibroplastica. Postgrad. Med. J. 53:538, 1977.

161. Solley, G.O., et al.: Endomyocardiopathy with eosinophilia. Mayo Clin. Proc. 51:697, 1976.

162. Olsen, E.G.J.: The pathology of cardiomyopathies. A critical analysis. Am. Heart J. 98:385, 1979.

163. Westwood, M., et al.: Heredity in primary endocardial fibroelastosis. Br. Heart J. 37:1077, 1975.

164. Schyrer, M.J.P., and Kamauchow, P.N.: Endocardial fibroelastosis. Etiologic and pathogenetic considerations in children. Am. Heart J. 88:557, 1974.

165. Kennedy, A., et al.: Fatal myocardial disease associated with industrial exposure to cobalt. Lancet 1:412, 1981.

166. Ferrans, V.J.: Overview of cardiac pathology in relation to anthracycline cardiotoxicity. Cancer Treat. Rep. 62:955, 1981.

167. Roberts, W.C., and Spray, T.L.: Pericardial heart disease. Curr. Probl. Cardiol. 2:1, 1977.

168. Kamaras, J., and Zaborsky, B.: Chronic constrictive pericarditis in children — etiology, clinical picture, and treatment. A report of 20 cases. Cor Vasa 23:66, 1981.

169. Bonfiglio, T., and Ativater, E.C.: Heart disease in patients with seropositive rheumatoid arthritis. A controlled autopsy study and review. Arch. Intern. Med. 124:714, 1969.

170. Kapoor, A.S.: Clinical manifestations of neoplasia of the heart. In Kapoor, A.S. (ed.): Cancer and the Heart. New York, Springer-Verlag, 1986, p. 21.

171. Schoen, F.J., et al.: Cardiac effects of noncardiac neoplasms. Cardiol. Clin. 2:657, 1984.

172. Wold, L.E., and Lie, J.T.: Cardiac myxomas. A clinicopathologic profile. Am. J. Pathol. 101:219, 1980.

173. Feldman, P.S., et al.: An ultrastructural study of 7 cardiac myxomas. Cancer 40:2216, 1977.

174. Fenoglio, J.J., et al.: Cardiac rhabdomyoma. A clinicopathologic and electron microscopic study. Am. J. Cardiol. 38:241, 1976.

Diseases of Red Cells and Bleeding Disorders

The bone marrow, lymph nodes, and spleen are all involved in hematopoiesis. Traditionally, these organs and tissues have been divided into *myeloid tissue*, which includes the bone marrow and the cells derived from it (e.g., erythrocytes, platelets, granulocytes, and monocytes), and *lymphoid tissue,* consisting of thymus, lymph nodes, and spleen. This subdivision is artificial with respect to both the normal physiology of hematopoietic cells and the diseases affecting them. For example, although bone marrow is not the site where most of the mature lymphoid cells are found, it is the source of lymphoid stem cells. Similarly, leukemias, which are neoplastic disorders of the leukocytes, originate within the bone marrow but involve the lymph nodes and spleen quite prominently. Some red cell disorders (hemolytic anemias) result from the formation of autoantibodies, signifying a primary disorder of the lymphoid tissues. Thus, it is not possible to draw neat lines between diseases involving the myeloid and lymphoid tissues. Recognizing this difficulty, we have somewhat arbitrarily divided diseases of the hematopoietic tissues into two chapters. In the first, we will consider diseases of red cells and those affecting hemostasis. In the second, we will discuss diseases affecting the leukocytes and the lymph nodes and disorders affecting primarily the spleen.

NORMAL

A complete discussion of normal hematopoiesis is beyond our scope, but certain features are helpful to an understanding of the diseases of blood.

NORMAL DEVELOPMENT OF BLOOD CELLS

In the human embryo, clusters of stem cells, called "blood islands," appear in the yolk sac in the third week of fetal development. At about the third month of embryogenesis some of these cells migrate to the liver, which then becomes the chief site of blood cell formation until shortly before birth, although the spleen, lymph nodes, and thymus make a small contribution during the last two trimesters. Beginning in the fourth month of development, hematopoiesis commences in the bone marrow. At birth, all the marrow throughout the skeleton is active and is virtually the sole source of blood cells. In the full-term infant, hepatic hematopoiesis has dwindled to a trickle but may persist in widely scattered small foci, which become inactive soon after birth. Up to the age of puberty, all the marrow throughout the skeleton is red and hematopoietically active. Usually by 18 years of age only the vertebrae, ribs, sternum, skull, pelvis, and proximal epiphyseal regions of the humerus and femur retain red marrow, the remaining marrow becoming yellow, fatty, and inactive. Thus, in adults, only about one half of the marrow space is active in hematopoiesis.

Several features of this normal sequence should be emphasized. By the time of birth, the bone marrow is virtually the sole source of all forms of blood cells and a major source of lymphocyte precursors. In the premature infant, foci of hematopoiesis are frequently evident in the liver, and rarely in the spleen, lymph nodes, or thymus. However, significant postembryonic extramedullary hematopoiesis is abnormal in the full-term infant. With an increased demand for blood cells in the adult, the fatty marrow may become transformed to red, active marrow. Moreover, this is accompanied by increased productive activity throughout the marrow. These adaptive changes are capable of increasing red cell production (erythropoiesis) seven- to eightfold. Thus, if the marrow precursor cells are not destroyed by metastatic cancer or irradiation, for example, and necessary substrate is available (e.g., adequate amounts of iron, protein, requisite vitamins, and so forth), such loss of red cells as may occur in hemolytic disorders produces anemia only when the marrow compensatory mechanisms are outstripped. Under these circumstances, extramedullary hematopoiesis may reappear, first within the liver and then in the spleen and lymph nodes.

ORIGIN AND DIFFERENTIATION OF HEMATOPOIETIC CELLS

There is little doubt that the formed elements of blood—erythrocytes, granulocytes, monocytes, platelets, and lymphocytes—have a common origin in a pluripotent hematopoietic stem cell.[1] This common precursor then gives rise to lymphoid stem cells and the trilineage myeloid stem cells, which are committed to produce lymphocytes and the myeloid cells, respectively (Fig. 14–1). The lymphoid stem cell, which has not been identified definitively, is believed to be the origin of precursors of T cells (pro–T cells) and B cells (pro–B cells), which differentiate into mature T cells and B cells under the inductive influence of the thymus and bursa-equivalent tissue, respectively. The details of lymphoid differentiation will not be discussed here, but it is worth pointing out that, unlike myeloid differentiation, there are no distinctive, morphologically recognizable stages. For definition, reliance must be placed on the detection of differentiation-specific antigens by monoclonal antibodies (p. 725). From the multipotent myeloid stem cell arise at least three types of committed stem cells capable of differentiating along the erythroid/mega-

karyocytic, eosinophilic, and granulocyte/macrophage pathways. Recent advances in cell culture techniques have made it possible to grow these committed stem cells in vitro with the production of colonies of differentiated progeny. Thus, the committed stem cells have been called colony-forming units (CFU). As indicated in Figure 14–1, granulocytes and macrophages have a common precursor, and hence colonies derived from CFU-G/M (colony-forming unit–granulocyte/macrophage) have a mixture of neutrophils and macrophages. In the erythroid pathway, two distinct committed stem cells can be recognized. Based on the morphology of the colonies, the more primitive of the two stages is called BFU-E (burst-forming unit–erythroid) and the later stage is called CFU-E (colony-forming unit–erythroid). From all these various committed stem cells, intermediate stages are derived, and ultimately the morphologically recognizable precursors of the differentiated cell lines, i.e., proerythroblasts, myeloblasts, megakaryoblasts, monoblasts, and eosinophiloblasts. These in turn give rise to mature progeny. Since the mature blood elements have a finite life span, it follows that their numbers must be constantly replenished. This can be realized if the stem cells possess the capacity not only to differentiate but also to renew themselves. *Thus, self-renewal is an important property of stem cells.* The pluripotent stem cells have the greatest capacity of self-renewal, but normally most of them are not in cell cycle. As commitment proceeds, self-renewal ability becomes limited, but a greater fraction of the stem cells are found to be in cycle. For example, very few trilineage myeloid stem cells are normally in cell cycle, but up to 50% of CFU-G/M are synthesizing DNA. This suggests that normally the pool of differentiated cells is replenished mainly by the proliferation of restricted stem cells. It is interesting to note that, although the earliest recognizable precursors (e.g., myeloblasts or proerythroblasts) are in active cell division, they cannot self-replicate, i.e., they differentiate and "die." By definition, then, they are not stem cells.

Since most forms of marrow failure or neoplastic disorders (e.g., aplastic anemias, leukemias, polycythemia) are disorders of stem cells, much interest is centered on the physiologic mechanisms that regulate the proliferation and differentiation of progenitor cells. Little is known about the factors that affect the proliferation of the most primitive stem cells, since clonal assays for their detection in vitro have not been fully developed. However, several regulatory factors that affect the committed stem cells have been identified. These include granulocyte-macrophage colony-stimulating factor (GM-CSF), which acts on CFU-G/M to produce granulocyte/macrophage colonies, and erythropoietin, which is essential for the differentiation of erythroid precursors. IL-3, or multi-CSF, is believed to be a growth factor for the trilineage myeloid stem cell, and it stimulates the more committed precursors (e.g., CFU-G/M, CFU-G, and CFU-M) as well. Many cells can give rise to hematopoietic

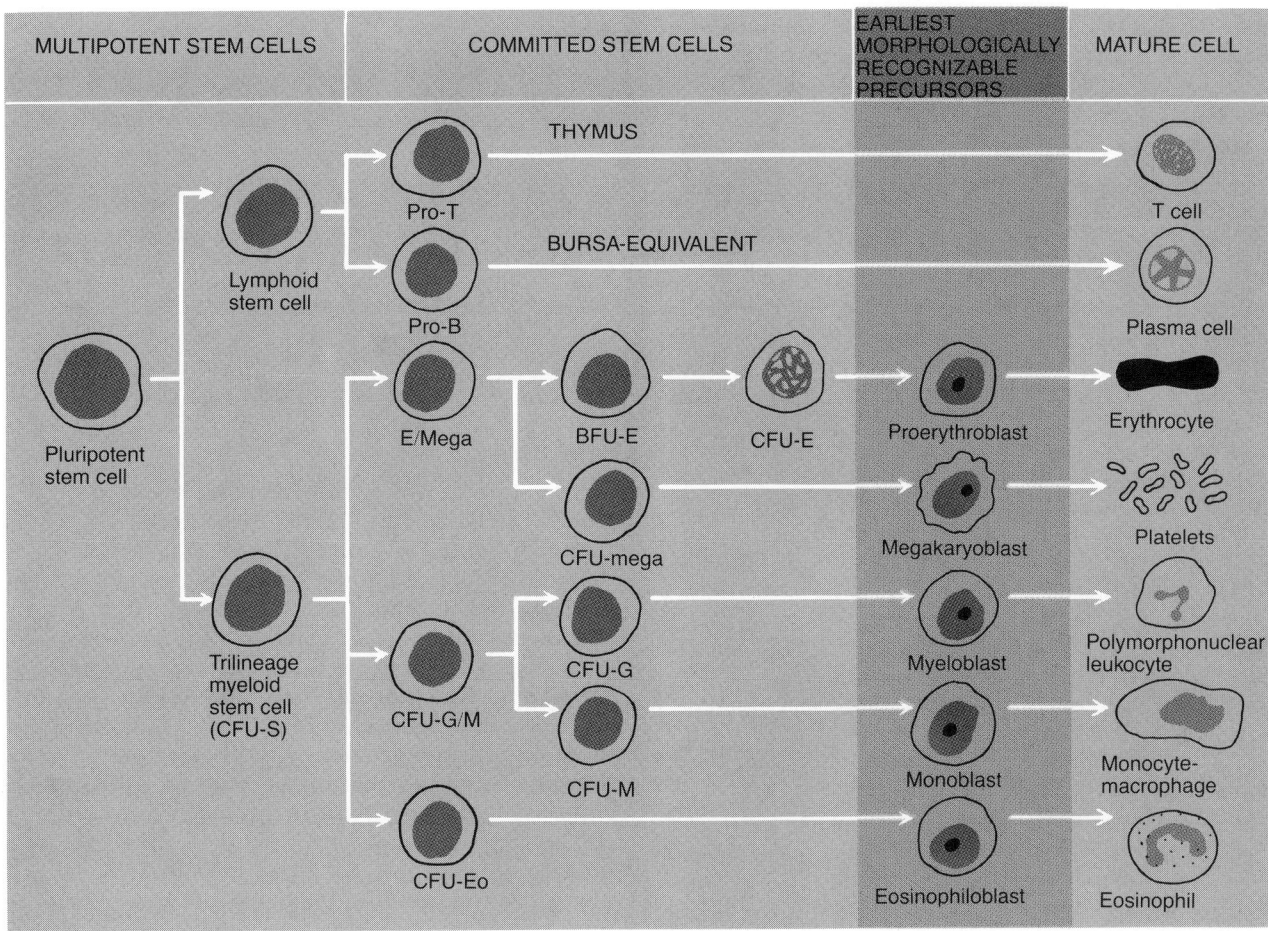

MULTIPOTENT STEM CELLS | COMMITTED STEM CELLS | EARLIEST MORPHOLOGICALLY RECOGNIZABLE PRECURSORS | MATURE CELL

Figure 14–1. Differentiation of hematopoietic cells. (Modified from Wyngaarden, J.B., and Smith, L. H. (eds.): Cecil Textbook of Medicine, 18th ed. Philadelphia, W.B. Saunders Co., 1988.)

growth factors: T cells produce IL-3 and GM-CSF, while fibroblasts and endothelial cells can (when stimulated by IL-1 or TNF-α) secrete GM-CSF. Erythropoietin is derived from the kidney but can also be produced by the liver. Although it has not been possible to develop an in vitro assay for the pluripotent stem cell, recent attempts to develop an assay for the trilineage myeloid stem cells have met with success. It has been possible to obtain mixed colonies containing erythroblasts, megakaryocytes, granulocytes, and macrophages, which could have arisen only from a multipotent stem cell. These exciting advances are interesting not only for developmental biologists but also for pathology students, since the pathogenesis of several hematologic disorders, including aplastic anemias, polycythemia, and leukemias, has already begun to be unraveled by the use of stem cell cultures. Furthermore, the availability of various recombinant colony-stimulating factors offers hope that they may be of clinical value in the treatment of conditions associated with impaired stem cell functions.[2]

NORMAL ANATOMY AND MORPHOLOGY OF BONE MARROW. The bone marrow not only is a reservoir of stem cells, but also provides a unique microenvironment in which the orderly proliferation and differentiation of precursor cells takes place. In addition, it regulates the release of fully differentiated cells into the circulation. The nature of the bone-marrow microenvironment and the factors that regulate the orderly release of blood cells are only beginning to be understood. In all likelihood, both structural (stromal) and humoral components of the bone marrow are involved in supporting hematopoiesis. Under the electron microscope, the marrow cavity appears to be a vast network of thin-walled sinusoids lined by a single layer of endothelial cells. Basement membrane and adventitial cells are present, but they form a discontinuous layer outside the endothelium. In between the sinusoidal network lie clusters of hematopoietic cells and fat cells, the latter being derived from accumulation of fat within the adventitial cells. Differentiated blood cells enter the sinusoids by transcellular migration through the endothelial cells. That this process is finely regulated is attested to by the fact that when hematopoiesis takes place at extramedullary sites, e.g., the spleen (p. 738), the peripheral blood contains all forms of abnormal as well as primitive blood cells that do not enter the blood in normal medullary hematopoiesis.

Although the morphology of the hematopoietic cells within the bone marrow is best studied in smears of marrow aspirates, useful information can also be obtained by studying the histology of bone marrow biopsies. For example, a reasonable estimate of marrow activity may be obtained by examining the ratio of fat cells to hematopoietic elements in bone marrow biopsies. In normal adults this ratio approaches 1 : 1, but with marrow hypoplasia (e.g., aplastic anemia) the proportion of fat cells is greatly increased, and conversely, fat cells may virtually disappear in diseases characterized by increased hematopoiesis (e.g., leukemias). When subjected to fixatives and tissue staining methods, the cells of the bone marrow and peripheral blood differ in appearance from those in air-dried Giemsa- or Wright-stained preparations. The maturational sequence of various cell types and their specific names are described in specialized texts.[3] The earliest identifiable myeloid cells, i.e., pronormoblasts, myeloblasts, and monoblasts, are all moderately large (10 to 20 μ in diameter), having abundant, deeply basophilic cytoplasm; round nuclei with coarsely clumped chromatin; and prominent nucleoli. It is extremely difficult, if not impossible, to differentiate in tissue sections the various "blast" forms. Often, tentative identification must be made on the basis of "the company they keep." Thus, a primitive cell found in relation to a focus of granulocytes is likely to be a myeloblast. Only when maturational differentiation appears can the various specific cell types be identified with assurance.

The relative proportion of cells in the bone marrow is almost always deranged in diseases of the blood and bone marrow. Normally, the marrow contains about 60% granulocytes and their precursors; 20% erythroid precursors; 10% lymphocytes and monocytes and their precursors; and 10% unidentified or disintegrating cells. Thus, the normal myeloid/erythroid ratio is 3 : 1. The dominant cell types in the myeloid compartment include myelocytes, metamyelocytes, and granulocytes. In the erythroid compartment the dominant forms are polychromatophilic and orthochromic normoblasts.

Under conditions of normal iron metabolism, approximately 30 to 40% of the normoblasts contain scattered ferritin granules, which are best visualized by special stains for iron (Prussian blue). Such cells are called **sideroblasts.** The ferritin granules presumably represent a reserve of iron on which the cell can draw for the synthesis of heme. The production of heme by the insertion of iron into protoporphyrin by heme synthetase and the production of globin are precisely balanced. When synthesis of either product is depressed, for whatever reason, excessive amounts of ferritin accumulate in sideroblasts (as occurs in sideroblastic anemia). With progressive accumulation of iron, mitochondria, the loci of heme synthetase, become stuffed with iron and rupture, producing distinctive **ring sideroblasts.** Thus, the state of iron reserves can be judged by the number of sideroblasts and their content of iron. If sideroblasts cannot be identified in the marrow, it signifies iron deficiency. However, an excess of sideroblasts, in particular ring sideroblasts, connotes an iron overload or the inability to utilize normal amounts of iron.

We now turn to consider the various disorders of the red blood cells.

PATHOLOGY

ANEMIAS

The function of red cells is the transport of oxygen into tissues. In physiologic terms, therefore, anemia may be defined as a reduction in the oxygen transport capacity of the blood. Since in most instances the reduced oxygen-carrying capacity of blood results from a deficiency of red cells, *anemia may be defined as a reduction below normal limits of the total circulating red cell mass.* This value is not easily measured, however, and therefore anemia has been defined as a reduction below normal in the volume of packed red cells, as measured by the hematocrit, or a reduction in the hemoglobin concentration of the blood. It hardly needs pointing out that fluid retention may expand plasma volume and fluid loss may contract plasma volume, creating spurious abnormalities in clinically measured values.

Innumerable classifications of anemia have been proposed. A highly acceptable one based on the underlying mechanism is presented in Table 14–1. Whatever the nature of anemia, the reduction in red cell mass and oxygen transport, when sufficiently severe, leads to certain changes throughout the body.

MORPHOLOGY. The pattern and severity of tissue changes depend, to a considerable extent, on the suddenness and quantity of blood loss and the duration of anemia. With sudden severe hemorrhage, red cells and circulating blood volume are lost proportionally, with the possible development of shock and its attendant clinical and morphologic changes (p. 118). When blood loss is slow, when red cell destruction outpaces production, or when some other impairment of red cell formation leads to an anemia, the resultant tissue hypoxia is characteristically reflected in certain morphologic alterations.

The skin is pale and usually becomes thin and inelastic as the epidermis and dermis atrophy. Frequently, the nails become brittle and lose their normal convexity to assume a concave spoon-shape (koilonychia), particularly in iron-deficiency anemia. Cells that are particularly vulnerable to hypoxia may undergo fatty change or even ischemic necrosis. Such damage is most frequently encountered in the muscle cells of the myocardium, the epithelial cells of the proximal convoluted tubules of the kidney, the centrilobular hepatic

Table 14–1. Classification of Anemia According to Mechanism of Production

I. BLOOD LOSS
  A. Acute: Trauma
  B. Chronic: Lesions of GI tract, gynecologic disturbances

II. INCREASED RATE OF DESTRUCTION (HEMOLYTIC ANEMIAS)
  A. Intrinsic (intracorpuscular) abnormalities of red cells
   Hereditary
    1. Red cell membrane disorders
      a. Disorders of membrane cytoskeleton: Spherocytosis, elliptocytosis
      b. Disorders of lipid synthesis: Selective increase in membrane lecithin
    2. Red cell enzyme deficiencies
      a. Glycolytic enzymes: Pyruvate kinase deficiency, hexokinase deficiency
      b. Enzymes of hexose monophosphate shunt: G6PD, glutathione synthetase
    3. Disorders of hemoglobin synthesis
      a. Deficient globin synthesis: Thalassemia syndromes
      b. Structurally abnormal globin synthesis (hemoglobinopathies): Sickle cell anemia, unstable hemoglobins
   Acquired
    1. Membrane defect: Paroxysmal nocturnal hemoglobinuria
  B. Extrinsic (extracorpuscular) abnormalities
    1. Antibody-mediated
      a. Isohemagglutinins: Transfusion reactions, erythroblastosis fetalis
      b. Autoantibodies: Idiopathic (primary), drug-associated, SLE, malignancies, mycoplasma infection
    2. Mechanical trauma to red cells
      a. Microangiopathic hemolytic anemias: Thrombotic thrombocytopenic purpura, DIC
      b. Cardiac traumatic hemolytic anemia
    3. Infections: Malaria
    4. Chemical injury: Lead poisoning
    5. Sequestration in mononuclear phagocytic system: Hypersplenism

III. IMPAIRED RED CELL PRODUCTION
  A. Disturbance of proliferation and differentiation of stem cells: Aplastic anemia, pure red cell aplasia, anemia of renal failure, anemia of endocrine disorders
  B. Disturbance of proliferation and maturation of erythroblasts
    1. Defective DNA synthesis: Deficiency or impaired utilization of vitamin B_{12} and folic acid (megaloblastic anemias)
    2. Defective hemoglobin synthesis
      a. Deficient heme synthesis: Iron deficiency
      b. Deficient globin synthesis: Thalassemias
    3. Unknown or multiple mechanisms: Sideroblastic anemia, anemia of chronic infections, myelophthisic anemias due to marrow infiltrations

cells, and the sensitive ganglion cells of the cortex and basal ganglia (p. 1403).

The increased demand for erythropoiesis in anemia causes the fatty marrow to become active and red if the marrow is capable of response. In some anemic states, such as aplastic anemia, the marrow cannot react. When the need is great, extramedullary hematopoiesis ensues, reverting to the fetal patterns of blood formation. Other more specific changes may also appear, determined by the particular type of anemia.

CLINICAL FEATURES. Attendant on the deranged physiology and morphologic alterations described, many nonspecific clinical signs and symptoms are seen in patients with anemia. Classically, these patients are pale and many have the nail deformity described. Weakness, malaise, and easy fatigability are common complaints. The lowered oxygen content of the circulating blood leads to dyspnea on mild exertion. If the fatty changes in the myocardium are sufficiently severe, cardiac failure may develop and compound the respiratory difficulty caused by reduced oxygen transport. Occasionally, the myocardial hypoxia manifests itself as angina pectoris, particularly when a pre-existing vascular disease has already rendered the myocardium partially ischemic. With acute blood loss and shock, oliguria and anuria may develop in the shock kidney. Central nervous system hypoxia may be evidenced by headache, dimness of vision, and faintness. Splenomegaly and hepatomegaly sometimes can be found, especially in infants with increased hematopoiesis in these organs. However, the most characteristic features of the anemia become evident only from laboratory studies of the peripheral blood.

ANEMIAS OF BLOOD LOSS

Acute Blood Loss

The clinical and morphologic reactions to blood loss depend on the rate of hemorrhage and whether the blood is lost externally or internally. With acute blood loss, the alterations reflect principally the loss of blood volume rather than the loss of hemoglobin. Shock and death may follow. If the patient survives, the blood volume is rapidly restored by shift of water from the interstitial fluid compartment. Restoration of blood fluid volume, which begins at once, reaches its full effect within 48 to 72 hours, when hematocrit values reach their lowest level and the full extent of the anemia becomes evident. Reduction in the oxygenation of tissues triggers the production of erythropoietin, and the marrow responds by increasing erythropoiesis. When the blood is lost internally, as into the peritoneal cavity, the iron can be recaptured, but if the blood is lost externally, the adequacy of the red cell recovery may be hampered by iron deficiency when insufficient reserves are present.

Soon after the acute blood loss the red blood cells appear normal in size and color (normocytic, normochromic). However, as the marrow begins to regenerate, changes occur in the peripheral blood. *Most striking is an increase in the reticulocyte count, reaching 10 to 15% after seven days.* The reticulocytes are seen as polychromatophilic macrocytes in the usual blood smear. These changes of red cell regeneration can sometimes be mistaken for an underlying hemolytic process. Mobilization of platelets and granulocytes from the marginal pools leads to thrombocytosis and leukocytosis in the period immediately following acute blood loss.

Chronic Blood Loss

Chronic blood loss induces anemia only when the rate of loss exceeds the regenerative capacity of the erythroid precursors or when iron reserves are depleted. In addition to chronic blood loss, any cause of iron deficiency such as malnutrition, malabsorption states, or an increased demand above the daily intake as occurs in pregnancy will lead to an identical anemia, discussed later (p. 685).

HEMOLYTIC ANEMIAS

The hemolytic anemias are all characterized by (1) shortening of the normal red cell life span, i.e., premature destruction of red cells; (2) accumulation of the products of hemoglobin catabolism; and (3) a marked increase in erythropoiesis within the bone marrow, in an attempt to compensate for the loss of red cells. These and some other general features will be briefly discussed before we describe the features of specific hemolytic anemias.

As is well known, the physiologic destruction of senescent red cells takes place within the mononuclear phagocytic cells of the spleen. In hemolytic anemias, too, the premature destruction of red cells occurs predominantly within the mononuclear phagocyte system (extravascular hemolysis). In only a few cases does lysis of red cells within the vascular compartment (intravascular hemolysis) predominate.

Intravascular hemolysis occurs when normal erythrocytes are damaged by mechanical injury (p. 678). For example, mechanical cardiac valves and thrombi within the microcirculation (disseminated intravascular coagulation, DIC) may disrupt erythrocytes and produce a form of hemolytic anemia referred to as microangiopathic hemolytic anemia (p. 679). Another major mechanism of intravascular hemolysis involves complement-induced lysis. Complement binding and activation may be mediated by antibodies, as occurs in a mismatched blood transfusion, or complement may lyse erythrocytes in the absence of antibody, in the rare disorder known as paroxysmal nocturnal hemoglobinuria (p. 676).

Whatever the mechanism, *intravascular hemolysis is manifested by (1) hemoglobinemia, (2) hemoglobinuria, (3) methemalbuminemia, (4) jaundice, and (5) hemosiderinuria.* When hemoglobin escapes into the plasma it is promptly bound by an α_2 globulin (haptoglobin) to produce a complex that prevents excretion into the urine, since the complexes are rapidly cleared by the reticuloendothelial system. A *decrease in serum haptoglobin level is characteristically seen in all cases of intravascular hemolysis.* When the haptoglobin is depleted, the unbound or free hemoglobin is in part rapidly oxidized to methemoglobin, and both hemoglobin and methemoglobin are excreted through the kidneys, imparting a red-brown color to the urine—hemoglobinuria and methemoglobinuria. Should the excretory capacity of the kidneys be exceeded, the free heme group derived from the retained methemoglobin complexes with albumin to produce methemalbuminemia, imparting a red-brown color to the blood. The renal proximal tubular cells may reabsorb and catabolize much of this filtered hemoglobin, but some passes out with the urine. Within the tubular cells, iron released from the hemoglobin produces hemosiderosis of the renal tubular epithelium, and shedding of such cells into the urine (where they can be identified by iron stains) constitutes the basis of the *hemosiderinuria.* Concomitantly, the heme groups derived from the complexes are catabolized within the mononuclear phagocyte system, leading ultimately to jaundice. In hemolytic anemias, the serum bilirubin is unconjugated (p. 913) and the level of hyperbilirubinemia depends on the functional capacity of the liver as well as on the rate of hemolysis. With a normal liver, the jaundice is rarely severe. Excessive bilirubin excreted by the liver into the gastrointestinal tract leads eventually to increased formation and fecal excretion (p. 915) of urobilin.

Extravascular hemolysis takes place whenever red cells are injured, are rendered "foreign," or become less deformable. For example, in hereditary spherocytosis an abnormal membrane cytoskeleton decreases the deformability of the red cell. Analogously, in sickle cell anemia, the abnormal hemoglobin "gels" or "crystallizes" within the erythrocyte, deforming it and reducing its plasticity. Since extreme alterations in shape are required for red cells to navigate the splenic sinusoids successfully, reduced deformability makes the passage difficult and leads to sequestration within the cords, followed by phagocytosis (Fig. 14–2). This is believed to be an important pathogenetic mechanism of extravascular hemolysis in a variety of hemolytic anemias. With extravascular hemolysis it is obvious that hemoglobinemia, hemoglobinuria, and the related intravascular changes do not appear. However, the catabolism of erythrocytes in the phagocytic cells induces anemia and jaundice

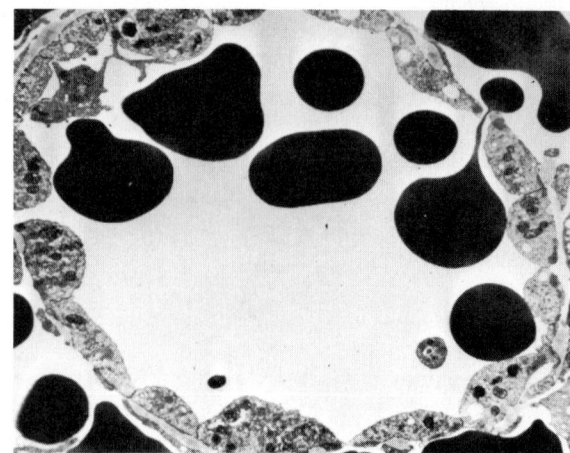

Figure 14–2. Splenic sinus (electron micrograph). An erythrocyte is in process of squeezing from cord into sinus lumen. Note degree of deformability required for red cell to pass through wall of sinus. (From Enriquez, P., and Neiman, R. S.: The Pathology of the Spleen: A Functional Approach. Chicago, The American Society of Clinical Pathologists, 1976, p. 7. Used by permission.)

that are otherwise indistinguishable from those caused by intravascular hemolysis. Furthermore, since some hemoglobin manages to escape from the phagocytic cells, plasma haptoglobin levels are invariably reduced. The morphologic changes that follow are identical to those in intravascular hemolysis, except that the erythrophagocytosis generally causes hypertrophy of the mononuclear phagocyte system of cells and this may lead to splenomegaly.

> Certain morphologic changes are standard in the hemolytic anemias, whether caused by intravascular or extravascular mechanisms. The anemia and lowered tissue oxygen tension stimulate increased production of erythropoietin, leading to an expansion of the erythron with **markedly increased numbers of normoblasts in the marrow** (Fig. 14–3); sometimes the expansion leads to extramedullary hematopoiesis. Unless there is some block in the formation of globin or heme, the accelerated compensatory erythropoiesis leads to a **prominent reticulocytosis in the peripheral blood.** Concomitantly, the expanded volume of the bone marrow causes pressure atrophy of the inner table of the cortical bone, resulting in neo-osteogenesis on the outer table. Such osseous changes are usually most evident in the ribs, facial bones, and calvaria. The elevated levels of bilirubin, when excreted through the liver, promote the formation of pigment gallstones (cholelithiasis). With chronicity, the phagocytosed red cells or hemoglobin will

> eventually lead to hemosiderosis, usually confined to the mononuclear phagocyte system. Thus, whatever the basis of the hemolysis, when sufficiently chronic, a common sequence of morphologic changes may be anticipated.

The hemolytic anemias can be classified in a variety of ways. One has already been suggested, namely division into intravascular and extravascular hemolytic disorders. However, since the number of disorders with predominantly intravascular hemolysis is limited, this classification is not entirely satisfactory. A pathogenetic classification could be based on whether the underlying cause of red cell destruction is extrinsic (extracorpuscular mechanism) or a defect inherent in the red cell (intracorpuscular defect). These anemias can also be divided into hereditary and acquired disorders. *In general, hereditary disorders are due to intracorpuscular defects and the acquired disorders to extrinsic factors such as autoantibodies.* Each of the classifications has value, but here we will follow the intrinsic-extrinsic outline given in Table 14–1, limiting consideration to the more common entities.

Hereditary Spherocytosis (HS)

This autosomal dominant disorder is characterized by an intrinsic defect in the red cell membrane that renders erythrocytes spheroidal, less deformable, and vulnerable to splenic sequestration and destruction. The prevalence of HS is highest in people of North European extraction, in whom rates of 1 in 5000 have been reported. Although most cases are related to autosomal dominant inheritance, approximately 20% of patients have unaffected parents, suggesting that the mutation often arises de novo.

PATHOGENESIS. The pathogenesis of the spheroidal shape of the erythrocyte is still somewhat uncertain, but recent studies come close to proposing a mechanism.[4] It appears that the fundamental defect is in the skeleton of the red cell membrane. Spectrin is the major skeletal protein of the basic filamentous framework. It consists of two polypeptide chains, alpha and beta, which are intertwined (helical) dimers, lying "flat" on the cytoplasmic aspect of the cell membrane (Fig. 14–4). The individual spectrin dimers are like segments of an extensive cable network that are linked to each other head to head to form tetramers. Lateral connections between spectrin tetramers are established through two additional proteins, actin and protein 4.1. The two-dimensional spectrin cable meshwork so formed is tethered to the inner surface of the cell membrane by yet another protein called ankyrin, which forms a bridge between spectrin and the cell membrane protein 3. Together these proteins are responsible for maintenance of the normal shape, strength, and flexibility of the red cell membrane. Although a deficiency of any one of the membrane skeletal proteins could adversely affect the red cells, a deficiency of spectrin seems to be the

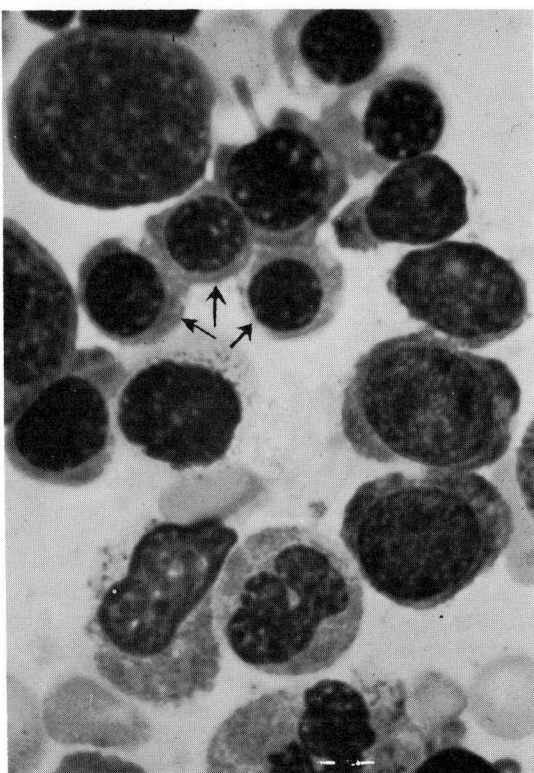

Figure 14–3. Marrow smear from one of the hemolytic anemias illustrating a proerythroblast *(upper left)* and normoblasts in various stages of differentiation. Arrows show late polychromatic normoblasts.

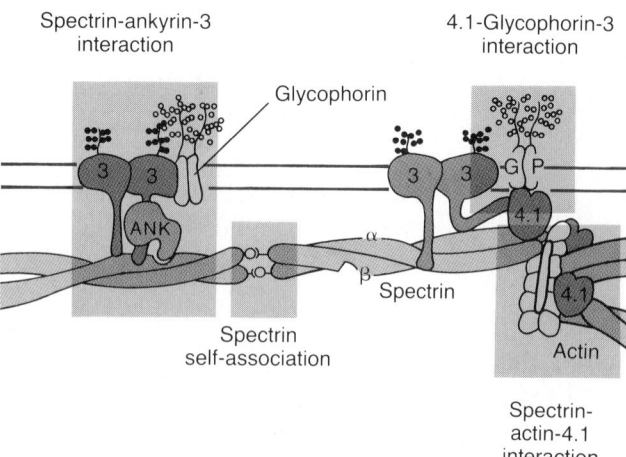

Figure 14–4. Schematic illustration of the organization of the major proteins of the red cell membrane and membrane skeleton. (Adapted from Wyngaarden, J.B., and Smith, L.H. (eds.): Cecil Textbook of Medicine. 18th ed. Philadelphia, W.B. Saunders Co., 1988.)

most common abnormality in patients with HS. The degree of spectrin deficiency varies from 75 to 90% of normal, and correlates closely with the severity of spherocytosis. In some kindreds a qualitative defect in red cell spectrin molecules has been found. The defect, expressed as reduced binding to protein 4.1, appears to involve approximately 50% of the spectrin molecules in heterozygotes. Red cells from these patients are also spectrin-deficient, possibly because the defective protein has a shorter half-life. *Spectrin deficiency is associated with reduced membrane stability and spontaneous loss of red cell membrane* (Fig. 14–5). The resulting reduction in cell surface-to-volume ratio "forces" the cells to assume the smallest possible diameter for a given volume, namely a sphere.

Although much remains to be learned about the molecular defects in HS, the travails of the red cells resulting from spheroidal transformation are fairly

well defined. In the life of the "portly" (and therefore inflexible) spherocyte, the spleen acts as the villain. As discussed earlier, the spleen serves as a watchdog ready to weed out the less-than-perfect erythrocytes as they traverse the red pulp. To enter the venous sinuses, normal red cells deposited into the cords of Billroth have to undergo extreme degrees of deformation (p. 662). Because of their spheroidal shape and reduced membrane plasticity, spherocytes have great difficulty in leaving the cords. As more and more spherocytes are detained, the already sluggish circulation of the cords stagnates further and the environment around the cells becomes progressively more hostile. Lactic acid accumulates and the extracellular pH falls, which in turn inhibits glycolysis and generation of ATP. Loss of ATP impairs the ability to extrude sodium, adding an element of osmotic injury. Stagnation in the cords also promotes contacts with macrophages, which are plentiful, and eventually the hapless spherocytes fall prey to the appetite of phagocytic cells. The few cells that manage to squeeze through the sinusoidal walls succeed at the expense of a portion of their cell membrane. These "bruised" cells are smaller and even less deformable, and are readily trapped in the cords when they re-enter the spleen. *The cardinal role of the spleen in the premature demise of the spherocytes is proved by the invariably beneficial effect of splenectomy. The spherocytes persist, but the anemia is corrected.*

MORPHOLOGY. Perhaps the most outstanding morphologic feature of this disease is the spheroidal shape of the red cells, apparent on smears as abnormally small cells lacking their central zone of pallor (Fig. 14–6). Spherocytosis, although distinctive, is not pathognomonic, since it is also seen in autoimmune hemolytic anemias. In addition to reticulocytosis and the general features of all hemolytic anemias, as previously detailed (p. 663), certain alterations are fairly distinctive. Moderate splenic enlargement is char-

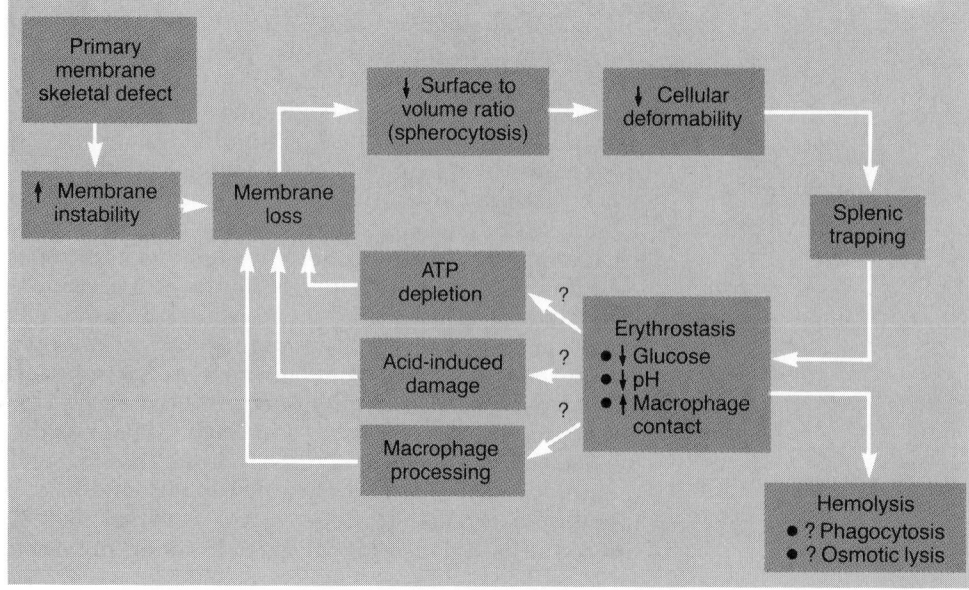

Figure 14–5. A model of the pathophysiology of hereditary spherocytosis. (Adapted from Wyngaarden, J.B., and Smith, L.H. (eds.): Cecil Textbook of Medicine. 18th ed. Philadelphia, W.B. Saunders Co., 1988.)

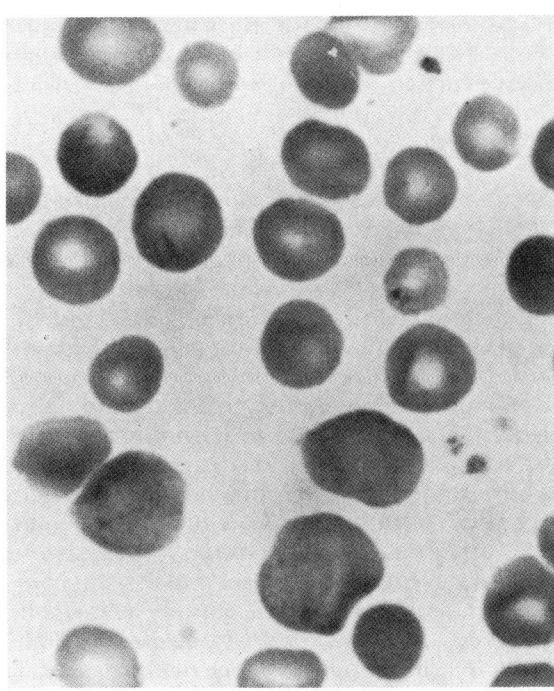

Figure 14–6. Peripheral blood smear from a patient with hereditary spherocytosis. Note the anisocytosis and several dark-appearing spherocytes with no central pallor. (Courtesy of Dr. Jose Hernandez, Department of Pathology, Southwestern Medical School, Dallas, Texas.)

acteristic of hereditary spherocytosis (500 to 1000 gm); in few other hemolytic anemias is the spleen enlarged as much or as often. It results from marked congestion of the cords of Billroth, leaving the sinuses virtually empty. Erythrophagocytosis can be seen within the congested cords. Typically present are the associated changes found in all hemolytic anemias, including increased erythropoiesis, bone changes, and hemosiderosis, as well as cholelithiasis (pigment stones) in 40 to 50% of the affected adults.

CLINICAL COURSE. The characteristic clinical features are anemia, splenomegaly, and jaundice.[5] The severity of the disease varies greatly from one patient to another. It may make its appearance at birth with marked jaundice, requiring exchange transfusion. In others, the mild red cell destruction is readily compensated for by expansion of the erythron. Only when this compensatory reaction is outpaced do symptomatic patients have a chronic hemolytic anemia, usually of mild-to-moderate severity. However, this more or less stable clinical course may be punctuated by "crises" of two kinds, often triggered by intercurrent infections. A *hemolytic crisis* may develop, characterized by the sudden onset of a wave of massive hemolysis accompanied by fever, abdominal pain, nausea, vomiting, jaundice, low blood pressure, tachycardia, and even shock. During active hemolysis, the patient classically becomes markedly jaundiced. Alternatively, an *aplastic crisis* (triggered usually by a parvovirus infection) may appear,

characterized by temporary suppression of red cell production, manifested by sudden worsening of the anemia, and the disappearance of reticulocytes from the peripheral blood. Transfusions may be necessary to support the patient, but eventually both these crises remit in most instances. Enlargement of the spleen, which is often progressive, is seen in 75 to 95% of the adults. Gallstones, found in many patients, may also produce symptoms (p. 969). Diagnosis is based on family history, hematologic findings, and laboratory evidence of spherocytosis, expressed as increased osmotic fragility. The spherocytes are particularly vulnerable to osmotic lysis, induced in vitro by solutions of hypotonic salt, since there is little margin for expansion of red cell volume without rupture.

Hemolytic Disease Due to Erythrocyte Enzyme Defects: Glucose-6-Phosphate Dehydrogenase Deficiency

The erythrocyte and its membrane are vulnerable to injury by exogenous and endogenous oxidants. Normally, intracellular reduced glutathione (GSH) inactivates such oxidants. *Abnormalities in the hexose monophosphate shunt or in glutathione metabolism resulting from deficient or impaired enzyme function reduce the ability of red cells to protect themselves against oxidative injuries and lead to hemolytic disease.* The most important of these enzyme derangements is a hereditary deficiency of glucose-6-phosphate dehydrogenase (G6PD) activity involved in the hexose monophosphate shunt pathway.[6] Millions of people throughout the world have such a deficiency. More than 150 G6PD genetic variants have been identified, but fortunately most evoke no clinical disorder or hemolytic anemia. Two variants, designated G6PD A⁻ and G6PD Mediterranean, lead to clinically significant hemolysis. The A⁻ type is present in about 10% of American blacks; G6PD Mediterranean, as the name implies, is found largely in populations in the Middle East. The basis of G6PD deficiency is somewhat different in the two genetic variants. In the A⁻ type of deficiency, a normal amount of the enzyme is synthesized in the red cell precursors, but it is more rapidly catabolized or inactivated during the life span of the red cell, so that older red cells become progressively more deficient in enzyme activity. Exposure to an oxidant, therefore, tends to induce hemolysis of older red cells but not the younger ones, and so the drop in hematocrit is mild or moderate. G6PD Mediterranean, on the other hand, is associated with markedly reduced activity throughout the entire life span of the red cell, suggesting that, in addition to rapid catabolism, impaired synthesis of the enzyme may be involved. In these individuals, the hemolytic crisis may produce profound drops in hematocrit and hemoglobin levels.

Inheritance of the mutant gene is X-linked. Thus, the defect is expressed in all erythrocytes of the affected male. In the heterozygous female, two populations of red cells, some deficient, others normal, are present owing to random inactivation of the X chromosomes. It follows that males are more vulnerable to oxidant injury than females, who usually have a smaller fraction of enzyme-deficient red cells. Only those carrier females who have an unusually large fraction of vulnerable red cells ("unfavorable lyonization") are susceptible to hemolytic anemia. It might be noted that the prevalence of such deleterious genes has in part been maintained because a deficiency of G6PD is thought to protect against malaria due to *Plasmodium falciparum.*

Numerous oxidant drugs may trigger hemolytic crises, principally the antimalarials — primaquine and quinacrine (Atabrine) — in addition to sulfonamides, nitrofurans, and others. Even more important are infections that presumably act by the generation of oxidant free radicals in macrophages.

The pathophysiology of hemolysis seems to involve the following sequence. Infection or exposure to oxidant drugs causes oxidation of GSH to glutathione, presumably through the production of H_2O_2. Since the regeneration of GSH is impaired in G6PD-deficient cells, hydrogen peroxide accumulates and injures other red cell constituents. Hemoglobin seems to be attacked on two fronts: oxidation of heme leading to formation of methemoglobin and, independently, oxidation of the sulfhydryl groups of the globin chains. The latter is particularly devastating, since it leads to denaturation of hemoglobin and formation of precipitates (Heinz bodies) within the cell. When attached to the cell membrane, Heinz bodies decrease erythrocyte deformability, thus rendering them susceptible to sequestration in the spleen. A remarkable phenomenon also follows: As the red cells pass through the splenic cords, phagocytic cells, principally macrophages, pluck out the Heinz bodies, a process referred to as pitting. The loss of membrane induces further membrane damage and simultaneously induces the formation of spherocytes. All these changes predispose the red cells to become trapped in splenic cords and destroyed by erythrophagocytosis (p. 664).

The clinical features of G6PD deficiency may be surmised from our discussion. Persons with the deficient enzyme do not have hemolysis unless exposed to the oxidant injuries alluded to above. After a variable lag period of two to three days, an acute hemolytic episode characterized by hemoglobinemia, hemoglobinuria, and decreased hematocrit levels is triggered. In patients with the G6PD A^- variant, since only the senescent red cells are lysed, the episode is self-limited and hemolysis stops when only the younger red cells remain in the circulation (despite continued administration of the oxidant drug). In contrast, the hemolytic episodes with the G6PD Mediterranean variant are much more severe, lasting for the duration of the oxidant injury. The peripheral blood smear shows Heinz bodies within the red cells as dark inclusions when stained with crystal violet. The recovery phase is heralded by reticulocytosis, as in the case of other hemolytic anemias. Since hemolytic episodes related to deficiencies of G6PD occur only on exposure to particular drugs, the morphologic changes encountered in most chronic hemolytic anemias are rarely present.

Sickle Cell Disease

Sickle cell disease is the classic prototype of a *hereditary hemoglobinopathy.* It results from a point mutation in the genetic code such that a single amino acid is substituted for another in one of the polypeptide chains of hemoglobin, transforming HbA into HbS. About 300 variant hemoglobins have been identified in which there is either an amino acid substitution or a deletion in one of the globin chains. Hemoglobin, as you recall, is a tetramer of four globin chains, comprising two pairs of similar chains, each with its own heme group. The hemoglobin in the adult is composed of 96% HbA ($\alpha_2\beta_2$), 3% hemoglobin A_2 ($\alpha_2\delta_2$), and 1% fetal hemoglobin (HbF, $\alpha_2\gamma_2$). The clinically significant variant hemoglobins involve β-chain abnormalities, among which the archetype is sickle hemoglobin (HbS). *Substitution of valine for glutamic acid at the sixth position of the β chain produces HbS.* About 8% of black Americans are heterozygous for hemoglobin S. If an individual is homozygous for the sickle mutation, almost all the hemoglobin in the erythrocyte is HbS. In the heterozygote, only about 40% is HbS, the remainder being normal hemoglobins. Where malaria is endemic, as many as 30% of black Africans are heterozygous. This frequency may be related in part to the slight protection against falciparum malaria afforded by HbS.

The HbS molecules upon deoxygenation undergo aggregation and polymerization, leading ultimately to distortion of the red cells, which acquire a sickle or holly-leaf shape (Fig. 14–7). *Sickling of the red cells has two major consequences:[7] (1) a chronic hemolytic anemia; and (2) occlusion of small blood vessels, resulting in ischemic tissue damage* (Fig. 14–8).

PATHOGENESIS. When exposed to low oxygen tensions, polymerization of HbS takes place, converting it from a freely flowing liquid to a viscous gel that is responsible for the distortion and reduced plasticity of the red cells.[8]

A number of factors that affect the rate and degree of sickling impact on the clinical expression of this disease. *Perhaps the most important of all is the amount of HbS and its interaction with the other hemoglobin chains in the cell.* In heterozygotes approximately 40% of the hemoglobin is HbS, the rest being HbA, which interacts only weakly with HbS during the processes of gelation. Therefore, the heterozygote has little tendency to sickle, except under conditions of severe hypoxia. Such an individual is said to have the *sickle cell trait,* and unless exposed to marked hypoxia has no hemolysis of red cells, nor an anemia. In contrast, the homozygote, with virtually undiluted hemoglobin of the S type, has full-blown *sickle cell anemia.* Beta-globin chains other than the normal

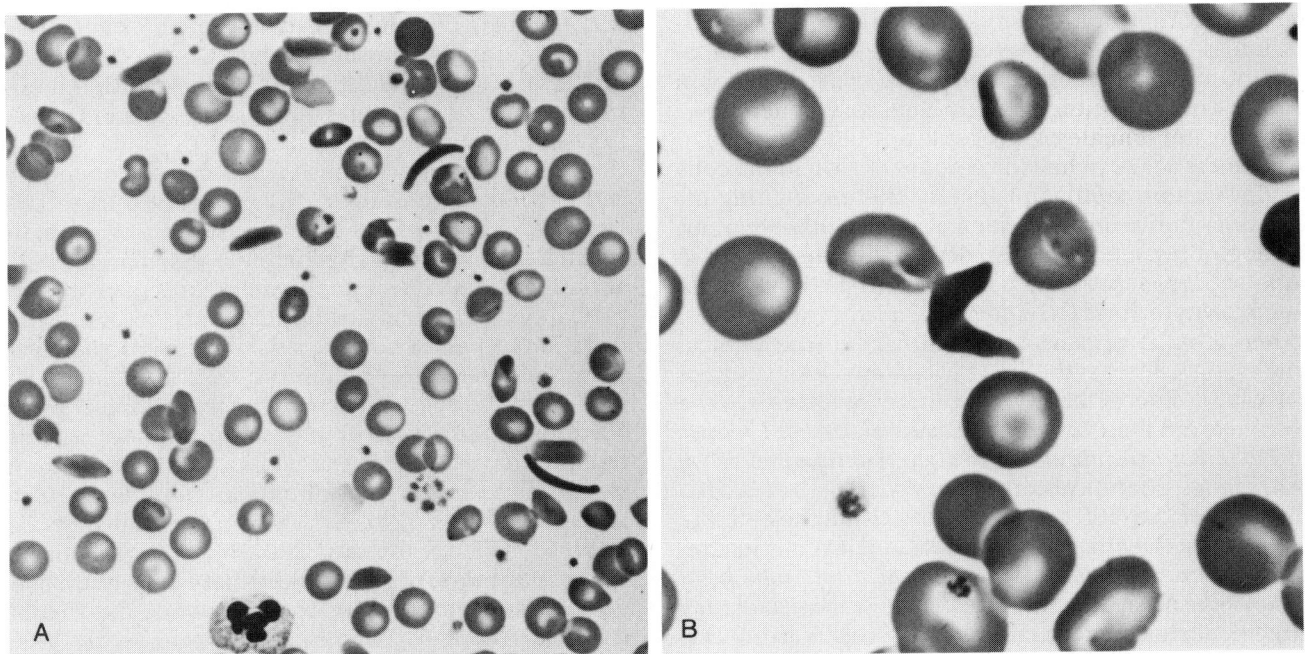

Figure 14-7. Peripheral blood smear from a patient with sickle cell anemia. On the left, low magnification shows sickle cells, anisocytosis, and poikilocytosis. The higher magnification on the right shows an irreversibly sickled cell in the center. (Courtesy of Dr. Robert W. McKenna, Department of Pathology, University of Texas, Southwestern Medical School, Dallas, Texas.)

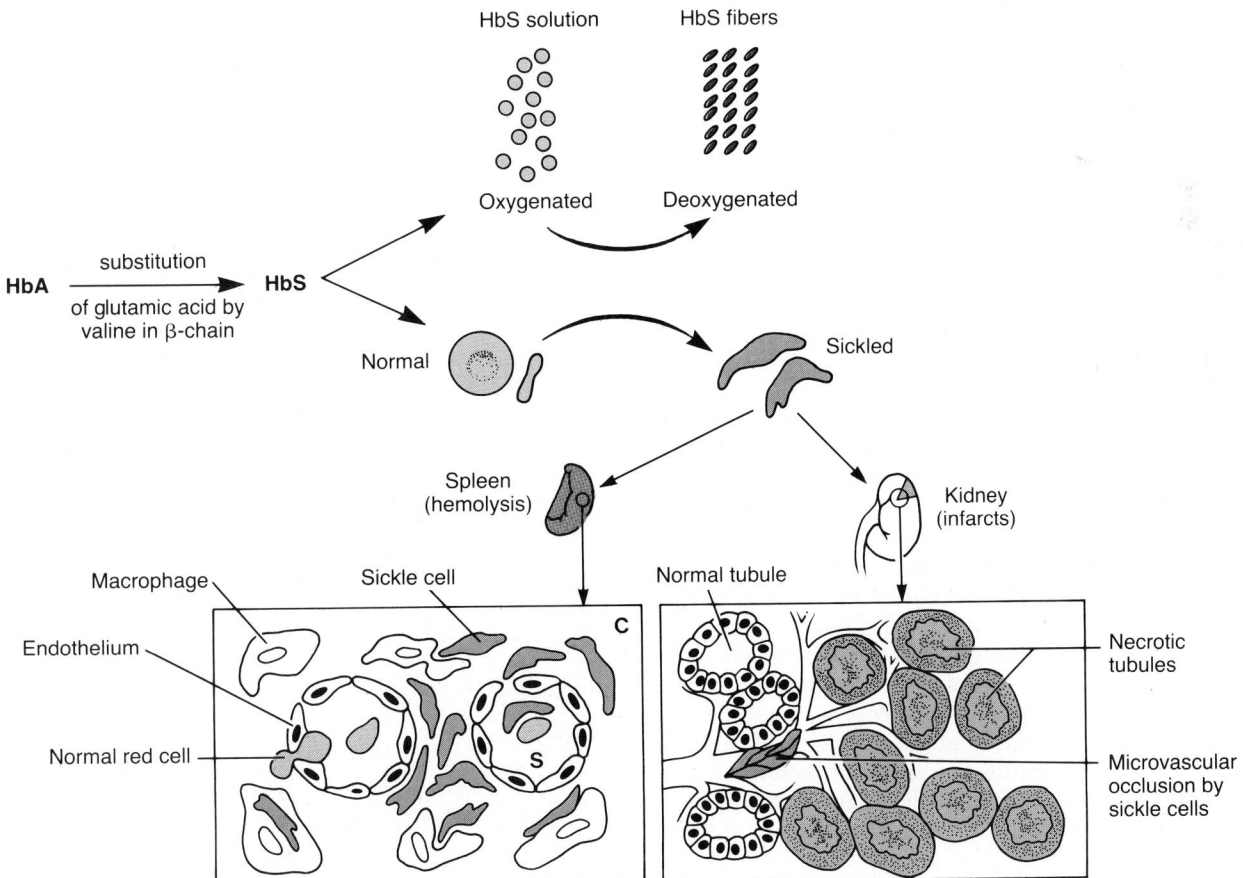

Figure 14-8. Pathophysiology and morphologic consequences of sickle cell anemia. Key: S, splenic sinusoids; C, splenic cords.

HbA and other non-α globins influence the crystallization of HbS and the severity of sickle cell anemia. For example, fetal hemoglobin (HbF) with its γ-globin chains does not interact with HbS, and hence newborns do not manifest the disease until they are five to six months of age, when the amount of HbF in the cells begins to approach adult levels. The modulating effect of β-globin chains is seen also with other mutant hemoglobins such as HbC and HbD. Either of these may be present along with HbS in red cells of a double heterozygote for HbS and the variant globin gene. When HbC is present along with HbS, the clinical features are less severe (than in patients homozygous for HbS), since HbS copolymerizes with HbC to a lesser extent than with other HbS molecules. *The rate of HbS polymerization is also significantly affected by the hemoglobin concentration per cell*, i.e., the MCHC. The higher the HbS concentration within the cell, the greater are the chances of contact and interaction between HbS molecules. Thus, *dehydration, which increases the MCHC, greatly facilitates sickling* and may trigger occlusion of small blood vessels (vaso-occlusive crisis). The hypertonic environment of the renal medulla can also initiate local sickling and infarction. Conversely, for a given amount of HbS per cell, conditions that decrease the MCHC would be expected to ameliorate the disease severity. This seems to be the explanation for the recent observation that, in patients with homozygous sickle cell anemia, the coexistence of thalassemia lessens the severity of the anemia. Thalassemia is characterized by reduced synthesis of globin chains (p. 670), which limits the total hemoglobin concentration per cell. Finally, *a fall in pH*, by reducing the oxygen affinity of hemoglobin, can increase sickling since it would enhance the amount of deoxygenated HbS.

Sickling of red cells is initially a reversible phenomenon; with oxygenation, HbS returns to the depolymerized state. However, with repeated episodes of sickling and unsickling, membrane damage ensues. Sickled cells lose potassium and water and at the same time gain calcium, which normally is rigorously excluded. The latter is considered particularly important in the genesis of *irreversibly sickled cells* (ISC), which retain their abnormal shape even when fully oxygenated and despite the deaggregation of HbS. Irreversibly sickled cells have very rigid and nondeformable cell membranes, and therefore have the same difficulty in negotiating the splenic sinusoids as do the spherocytes (p. 664). The sickled cells become sequestered in the spleen, where they are destroyed by the mononuclear phagocyte system. Some intravascular hemolysis may also occur owing to increased mechanical fragility of the severely damaged cells. The average red cell survival correlates with the percentage of ISC in circulation and is shortened to approximately 20 days. This finding supports the concept that the hemolysis results primarily from the lysis of ISC.

The pathogenesis of microvascular occlusions, a clinically important component of sickle cell anemia,

is much less certain. The well-known "vicious viscous" or kinetic hypothesis is based on the increase in blood viscosity brought about by the relative inelasticity of the sickled red cells. This results in retardation of blood flow, particularly in the microcirculation. As the capillary transit times are prolonged, the red cells are exposed to a longer period of relative hypoxia, which favors further sickling of cells upstream, leading finally to complete vascular occlusion and infarction. Although this scheme is plausible and probably correct in its basic tenets, an important question remains unanswered. Why is there no correlation between the frequency of ISC (which contributes to viscosity) and severity of organ involvement? Two studies address this issue. By using very sensitive techniques, Noguchi and Schechter found that in sickle cell anemia a small amount of polymerized HbS is present even in normal-appearing red cells exposed to 96 to 98% oxygen saturation.[8] Sickling, according to these authors, occurs only in those cells that have a very large amount of the polymer, while deformability and plasticity are impaired even with lesser amounts of polymerized HbS. According to this view, the amount and properties of the HbS polymer within normal-looking red cells, rather than the obviously sickled red cells, are the major determinants of abnormal flow, and therefore lack of correlation between the frequency of ISC and the incidence of vascular occlusion is not entirely surprising. Other explanations have concentrated on the possibility that vascular occlusion may be initiated by adhesions between red cells and capillary endothelial cells.[9] Increased adherence of normal-looking red cells from patients with sickle cell anemia and endothelial cells has been reported in culture, but the in vivo significance of this phenomenon remains to be established.

MORPHOLOGY. The anatomic alterations are based on the following three characteristics of sickle cell anemia: increased destruction of the sickled red cells with the development of anemia, increased release of hemoglobin and formation of bilirubin, and capillary stasis and thrombosis. Sickling of the red cells may be identified in tissue sections, particularly those fixed in formalin, because under these conditions anaerobiosis develops before complete fixation. However, sickling may not be evident when the section is quickly fixed. The consequences of the increased red cell destruction and anemia have already been detailed in the general consideration of all hemolytic anemias. Briefly, these involve pallor of the skin, systemic iron overload, and fatty changes in the heart, liver, and tubules of the kidney. Rarely, the erythrostasis in the liver leads to so-called sickle cell cirrhosis. The bone marrow is hyperplastic. This increased activity is due to expansion of normoblasts. The white cells and megakaryoctyes are unaffected. The expansion of the marrow may lead to resorption of bone with secondary new bone formation to produce the roentgenographic appearance in the skull of the "crew haircut." Extramedullary hematopoiesis may appear in the spleen or liver, and, rarely, in other sites.

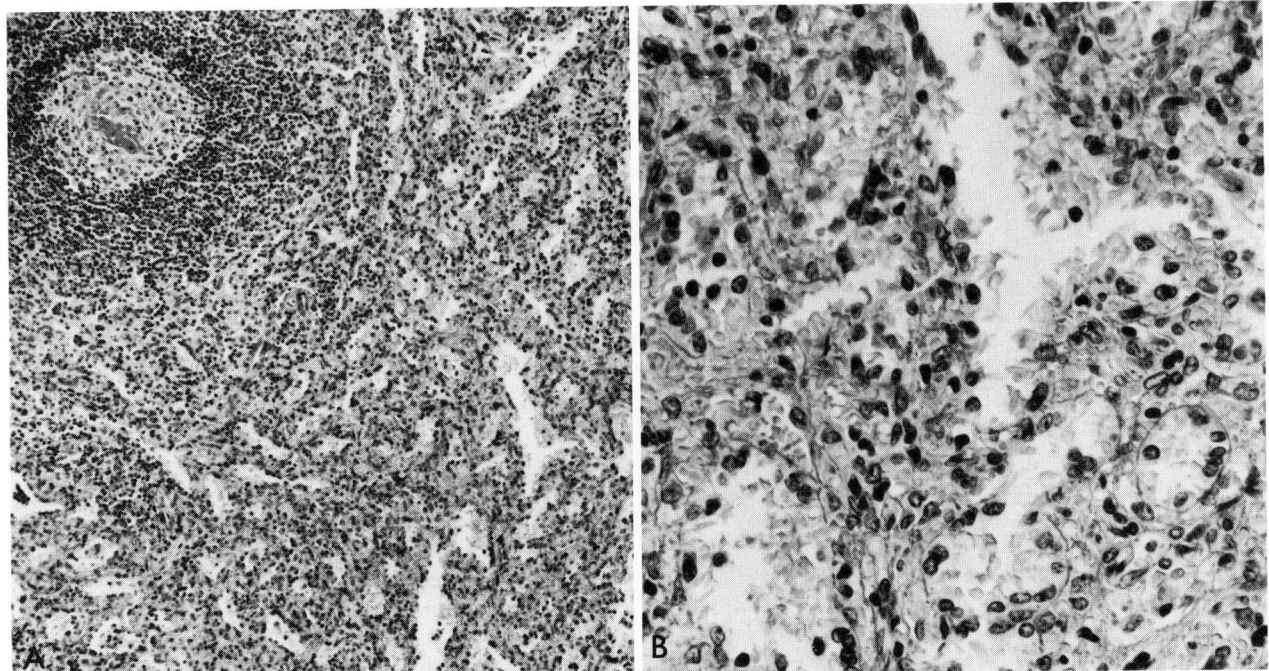

Figure 14–9. *A*, Spleen in sickle cell anemia (low power). White pulp on upper left is normal. Red pulp with its cords and sinusoids is markedly congested. *B*, Under high power, splenic cords are prominent owing to trapping of sickled red cells, which can also be seen in sinusoids. (Courtesy of Dr. Jose Hernandez, Department of Pathology, Southwestern Medical School, Dallas, Texas.)

In children, during the early phase of the disease, the spleen is commonly enlarged up to 500 gm. Histologically, there is marked congestion of the red pulp, due mainly to the trapping of sickled red cells in the splenic cords. However, sickling of cells may also occur in the sinuses, sometimes creating large lakes of red cells, sickled and jammed together in distended sinuses (Fig. 14–9). This erythrostasis in the spleen may lead to thrombosis and infarction or at least to marked tissue hypoxia. Sometimes the resulting focal fibrous scars contain deposits of hemosiderin and calcium, so-called **Gandy-Gamna bodies.** Continued scarring over the course of years causes progressive shrinkage of the spleen so that, in long-standing adult cases, only a small nubbin of fibrous tissue may be left; this is called **autosplenectomy** (Fig. 14–10). Infarctions secondary to

vascular occlusions and anoxia occur also in the bones, brain, kidney, liver, and retina.

Thrombotic occlusions have also been described in the pulmonary vessels, and many patients have cor pulmonale. Vascular stagnation in the subcutaneous tissue leads to leg ulcers in approximately 50% of adult patients, but is rare in children. The increased release of hemoglobin leads to pigment gallstones in some individuals, and all patients develop hyperbilirubinemia during periods of active hemolysis.

CLINICAL COURSE. *From the description of the disease to this point, it is evident that these patients are beset with problems stemming from (1) severe anemia, (2) vaso-occlusive complications, (3) predisposition to*

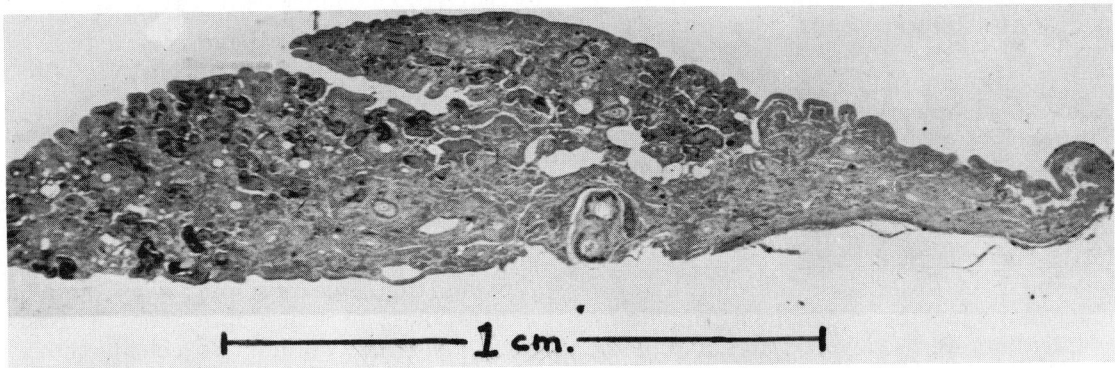

Figure 14–10. Sickle cell anemia. Cross section of a totally fibrotic spleen—autosplenectomy.

infections, and (4) chronic hyperbilirubinemia. In infants, there are impairment of growth and development and an increased tendency to serious infections. In adults, the chronic hemolytic disease induces a fairly severe anemia, with hematocrit values ranging between 18 and 30%. The chronic hemolysis is associated with striking reticulocytosis and hyperbilirubinemia. Irreversibly sickled cells can usually be seen in the peripheral smear. This protracted course is frequently punctuated by a variety of *"crises." Vaso-occlusive crises*, also called *painful crises*, represent episodes of hypoxic injury and infarction. Usually no predisposing causes can be identified, although an association with infection, dehydration, and acidosis (all of which favor sickling) has been noted. The pain can be extreme and may be referred to the abdomen, chest, or joints, depending on the site of vascular insufficiency. Sites most commonly involved by vaso-occlusive episodes are the bones, lungs, liver, brain, spleen, and penis. *In children, painful bone crises are extremely common and often difficult to distinguish from acute osteomyelitis.* Similarly, chest pain may be confused with infections that are also common. Central nervous system hypoxia may produce manifestations of a seizure or stroke. Although such crises are frequently reversible, they may be fatal. Leg ulcers are an additional reflection of the vaso-occlusive tendency. An *aplastic crisis* represents a temporary cessation of bone marrow activity, and it may be triggered by infections or folic acid deficiency, or both. Reticulocytes disappear from the peripheral blood, and there is sudden and rapid worsening of anemia. A so-called *sequestration crisis* may appear in children with splenomegaly and sometimes in adults whose spleens have not undergone autoinfarction. Massive sequestration of deformed red cells leads to rapid splenic enlargement, hypovolemia, and sometimes shock. With transfusion, this can be reversed. Male patients may suddenly develop painful priapism owing to vascular engorgement of the penis.

For reasons that are not clear, but possibly related to erythrophagocytosis and blockade of the mononuclear phagocyte system, splenic function in children is impaired even though splenomegaly is present. Later, splenic infarctions may significantly reduce the size and function of this organ. The *"functional splenectomy"* predisposes to blood-borne infections and, for unknown reasons, particularly predisposes to Salmonella osteomyelitis. These individuals are also unusually prone to infections caused by encapsulated organisms such as *Streptococcus pneumoniae* and *Hemophilus influenzae*, possibly related to an impairment of the alternate complement pathway normally activated by capsular polysaccharides. The infections in turn predispose to vaso-occlusive and aplastic crises.

In the course of the disease, chronic hypoxic organ damage may affect the spleen, heart, and lungs. The bones and joints are also favored sites of ischemic injury; microinfarctions may appear, or sometimes aseptic necrosis of the femoral head develops. Ocular lesions in the form of retinal infarcts, retinitis proliferans, and retinal detachment sometimes appear. Ischemic injury to the renal medulla may lead to loss of renal concentrating ability. The hyperbilirubinemia causes pigment stones in the gallbladder.

Diagnosis usually is readily made from the clinical findings and the appearance of the peripheral blood smear. It can be confirmed by various tests for sickling that, in general, are based on mixing a blood sample with an oxygen-consuming reagent, such as metabisulfite, to induce sickling. Hemoglobin electrophoresis can also demonstrate hemoglobin S on the basis of specific mobility. Prenatal diagnosis is possible by analysis of fetal DNA. As discussed earlier (p. 157), DNA obtained from cells in amniotic fluid is digested with the restriction enzyme Mst II and probed with a β-globin cDNA by Southern blot analysis. This technique can identify both homozygotes and heterozygotes.[10] Despite improvements in therapy, sickle cell anemia still markedly shortens longevity; many patients die before the age of 30. However, with supportive measures an increasing number survive well into adult life.

Thalassemia Syndromes

The thalassemia syndromes are a heterogeneous group of mendelian disorders, all characterized by a lack of or decreased synthesis of either the α- or the β-globin chain of hemoglobin A $(\alpha_2\beta_2)$. *Beta-thalassemia is characterized by deficient synthesis of the β chain, whereas α-thalassemia is characterized by deficient synthesis of the α chain. The hematologic consequences of diminished synthesis of one globin chain derive not only from the low intracellular hemoglobin (hypochromia) but also from the relative excess of the other chain.* For example, in β-thalassemia there is an excess of α chains. As a consequence, free α chains tend to aggregate into insoluble inclusions within erythrocytes and their precursors, causing premature destruction of maturing erythroblasts within the marrow *(ineffective erythropoiesis)* as well as lysis of mature red cells in the spleen *(hemolysis)*.

Beta-Thalassemia

The abnormality common to all β-thalassemias is a total lack or a reduction in the synthesis of structurally normal β-globin chains with unimpaired synthesis of α chains. However, the clinical severity of the anemia as well as the biochemical and genetic basis of β-globin chain deficiency is quite varied. We will begin our discussion with the molecular lesions in β-thalassemia and then integrate the clinical variants with the underlying molecular defects.

MOLECULAR LESIONS IN BETA-THALASSEMIA. A complex pattern of molecular defects underlying the thalassemias has emerged in recent years. To understand these, we must first review the structure and expression of normal globin genes. The adult hemoglobin, or HbA, contains two α chains and two β chains (coded by two β-globin genes each located on one of the two number 11 chromosomes). In contrast, two

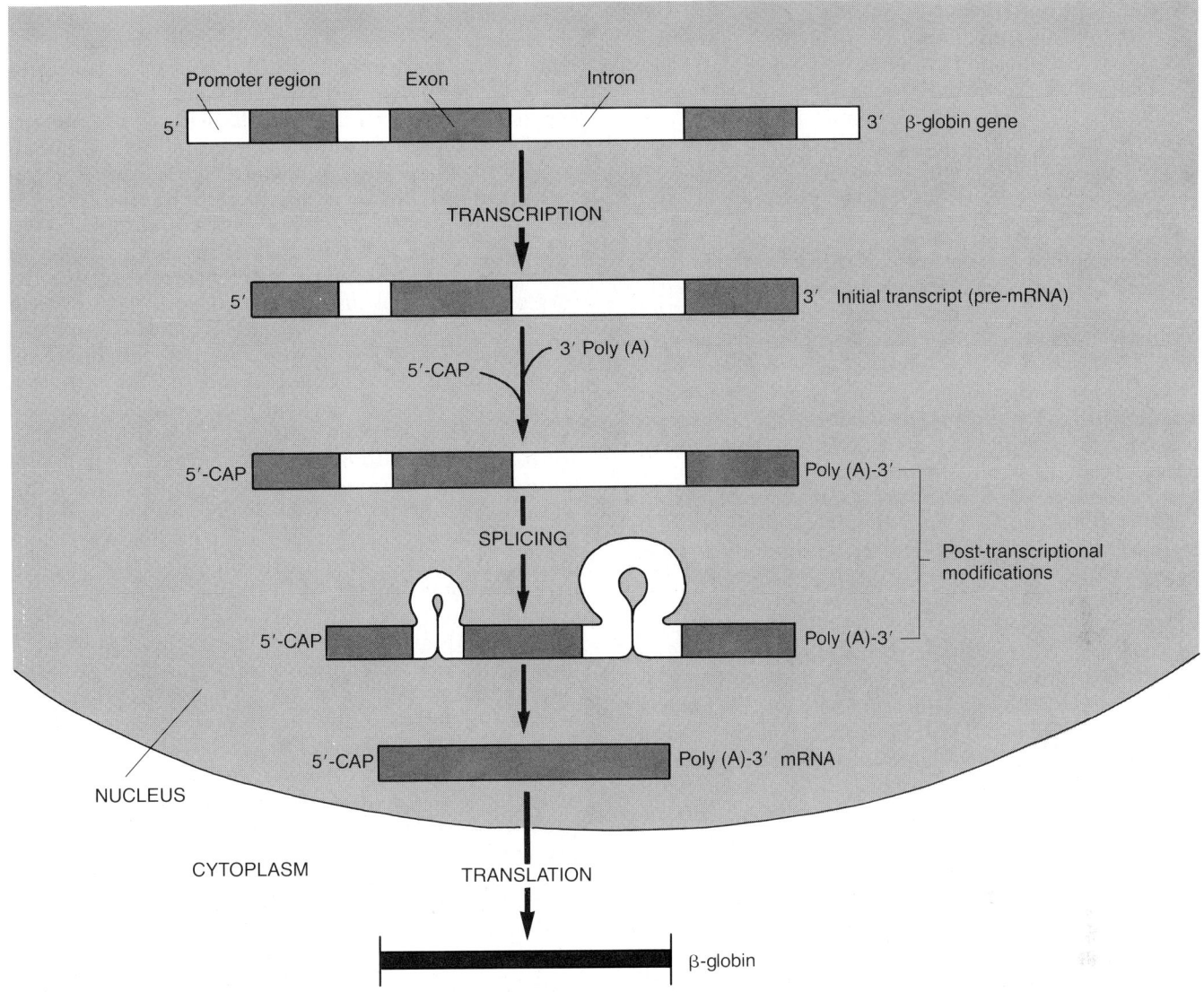

Figure 14–11. Diagrammatic representation of β-globin biosynthesis. Expression of β-globin gene begins in the nucleus with transcription of the entire gene, including introns and exons. During post-transcriptional processing, the intron transcripts are removed by splicing from pre-mRNA. The religated mRNA is transported to the cytoplasm, where it is translated to form β-globin.

pairs of functional α-globin genes are located on each number 16 chromosome. With recombinant DNA techniques it has been possible to clone all the human globin genes, and their nucleotide sequences have been determined. The basic structure of the α- and β-globin genes and the steps involved in the biosynthesis of globin chains are similar. These are depicted schematically in Figure 14–11. Each β-globin gene has three coding sequences, or *exons*, that are interrupted by two intervening sequences, or *introns*. Flanking the 5′ extremity of the globin gene are a series of untranslated *"promoter sequences"* that are required for the initiation of β-globin mRNA synthesis.

As with all eukaryotic genes, the biosynthesis of globin chains begins with the transcription of the globin genes within the nucleus. The initial mRNA transcript contains a copy of the entire gene, including all

the exons and introns. This large mRNA precursor undergoes several post-transcriptional modifications (processing) before it is converted into mature cytoplasmic mRNA ready for translation, i.e., splicing out the two introns and re-ligating the exons. The mature mRNA so formed leaves the nucleus and becomes associated with ribosomes, on which translation takes place. The pathway of α-globin gene expression is very similar. With this background we can discuss the molecular pathologic changes associated with β-thalassemias.

Beta-thalassemia syndromes can be classified into two categories: (1) *β⁰-thalassemia*, associated with total absence of β-globin chains in the homozygous state; and (2) *β⁺-thalassemia*, characterized by reduced (but detectable) β-globin synthesis in the homozygous state. Sequencing of cloned β-globin genes obtained from thalassemic patients has revealed over

38 different mutations responsible for β^0- or β^+-thalassemia.[11] Most of these result from single base changes. As opposed to the case with α-thalassemias, described later, gene deletions rarely underlie β-thalassemias.

Details of these mutations and their effects on β-globin synthesis can be found in specialized texts.[11,12] A few illustrative examples will be cited (Fig. 14–12).

• The promoter region controls the initiation and rate of transcription, and therefore mutations affecting promoter sequences usually lead to reduced globin gene transcription. Since some β-globin is synthesized, the patients develop β^+-thalassemia.

• Mutations in the coding sequences are usually associated with more serious consequences. For example, in some cases a single nucleotide change in one of the exons leads to the formation of a "termination" or "stop" codon, which interrupts translation of β-globin mRNA. Premature termination generates nonfunctional fragments of the β-globin, leading to β^0-thalassemia.

• Single nucleotide deletions or insertions may alter mRNA reading frames and introduce stop codons downstream that terminate protein synthesis. Such frameshift mutations also cause β^0-thalassemias.

• *Mutations that lead to aberrant splicing are the most common cause of β-thalassemia.* Most of these affect introns, but some have been located within exons. If the mutation alters the normal splice junctions, splicing does not occur and all of the mRNA formed is abnormal. Unspliced mRNA is degraded within the nucleus, and β^0-thalassemia results. However, some mutations affect the introns at locations away from the normal intron-exon splice junction. These mutations create new sites sensitive to the action of splicing enzymes at abnormal locations—within an intron, for example. Because normal splice sites remain unaffected, both normal and abnormal splicing occurs, giving rise to normal as well as abnormal β-globin mRNA. These patients develop β^+-thalassemia.[12]

PATHOPHYSIOLOGY OF ANEMIA. Two factors contribute to the pathogenesis of anemia in β-thalas-

semia (Fig. 14–13). Reduced synthesis of β-globin chains leads to lack of adequate HbA formation, so that the overall concentration of Hb in the cells (MCHC) is lower and the cells are hypochromic. Much more important, especially with severe impairment of β-globin synthesis, are the effects of imbalance between α- and β-chain synthesis. Since synthesis of α-globin chains continues unimpaired, most of the chains produced cannot find complementary β chains to bind. The free α chains form highly unstable aggregates that precipitate within the red cell precursors in the form of insoluble inclusions. *A variety of untoward effects follow, the most important being cell membrane damage leading to a loss of K^+ and impaired DNA synthesis. The net effect is destruction of the red cell precursors within the bone marrow, a phenomenon called ineffective erythropoiesis.* It is estimated that approximately 70 to 85% of the marrow normoblasts are destroyed in severely affected patients. The inclusion-bearing red cells derived from the nucleated precursors that escape intramedullary death are at an increased risk of destruction in the spleen. Because of poor deformability imposed by the intracellular aggregates, they are sequestered in the spleen, where macrophages attempt to "pluck out" inclusions from these erythrocytes, causing irreparable damage to the cell membranes in some cases. The damaged and defective red cells are eventually phagocytosed by the splenic macrophages, leading to a hemolytic state with considerable shortening of red cell survival. In severe β-thalassemia, marked anemia produced by ineffective erythropoiesis and hemolysis leads to several additional problems. Erythropoietin secretion is stimulated, which leads to extensive expansion of the erythron within the bone marrow and often at extramedullary sites. Massive erythropoiesis within the bones invades the bony cortex, impairs bone growth, and produces other skeletal abnormalities, described later. Extramedullary hematopoiesis involves the liver and spleen and in extreme cases produces extraosseous masses in the thorax, abdomen, and pelvis. *Another disastrous effect seen in severe β-thalassemia (as well as in other causes of ineffective erythropoiesis) is excessive absorption of dietary iron.* Coupled with

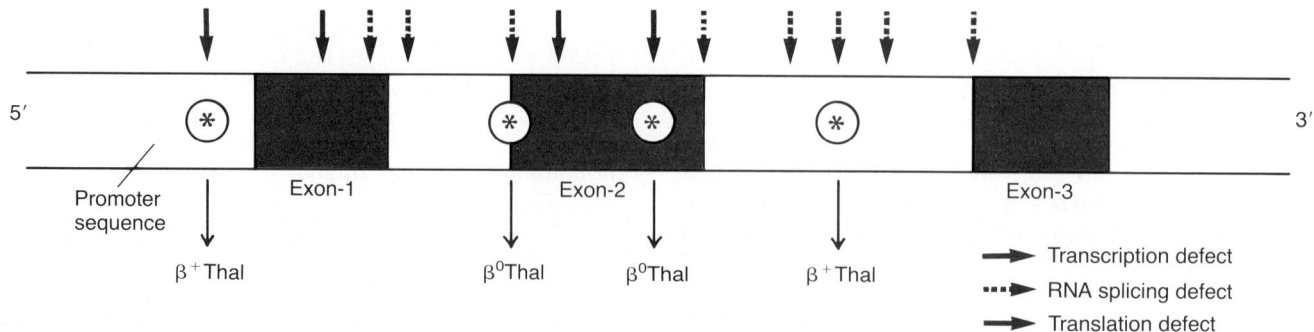

Figure 14–12. Diagrammatic representation of the β-globin gene and some sites where point mutations giving rise to β-thalassemia have been localized. (Modified from Wyngaarden, J.B., and Smith, L.H. (eds.): Cecil Textbook of Medicine, 17th ed. Philadelphia, W.B. Saunders Co., 1985.)

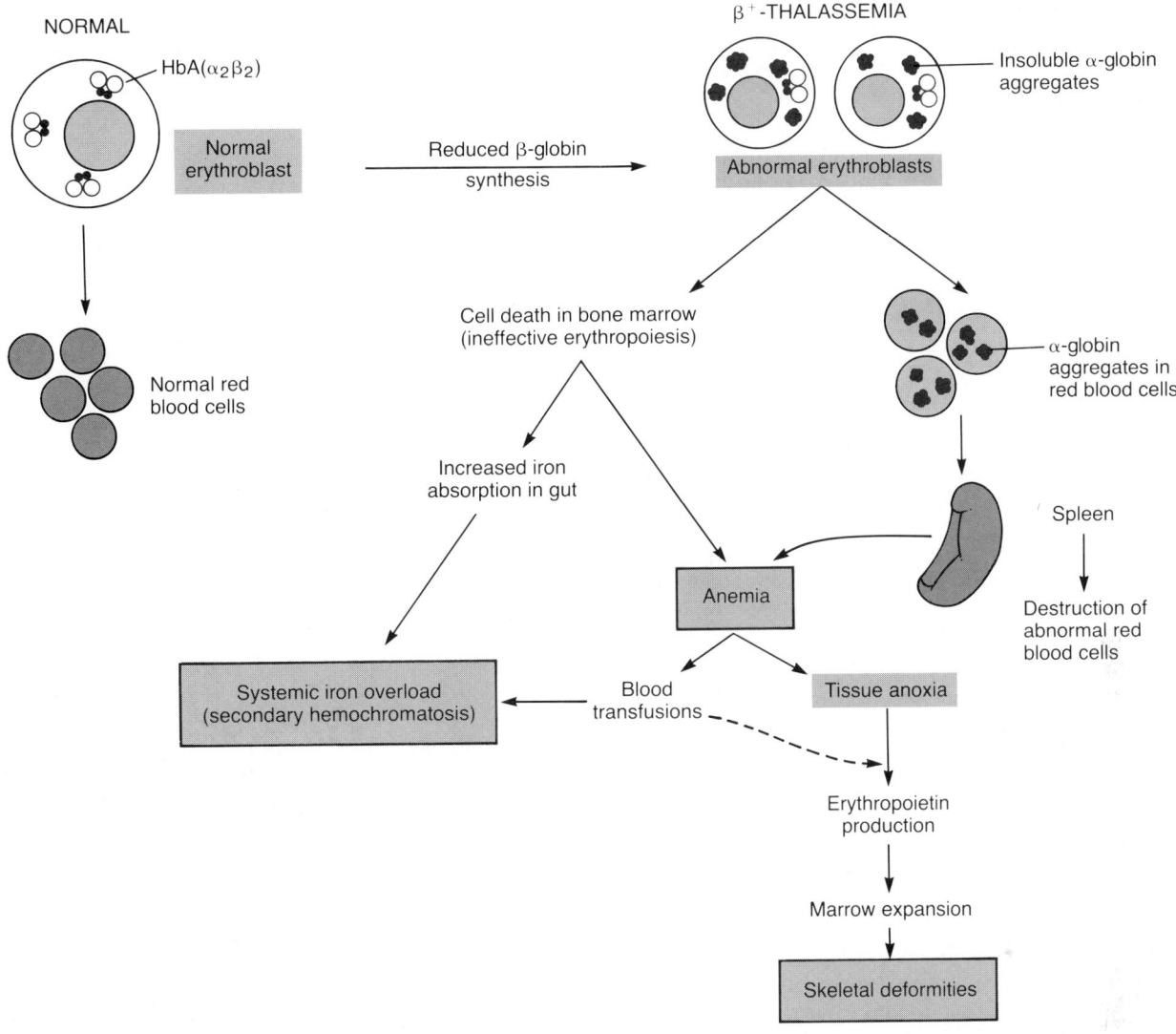

Figure 14–13. Pathogenesis of β-thalassemia major. Note that aggregates of excess α-globin are not visible on routine blood smears. Blood transfusions, on the one hand, correct the anemia and reduce stimulus for erythropoietin secretion and deformities induced by marrow expansion; on the other hand, they add to systemic iron overload.

the iron accumulation due to repeated blood transfusions required by these patients, a severe state of iron overload develops. Secondary injury to parenchymal organs, particularly the iron-laden liver, often follows and sometimes induces secondary hemochromatosis (p. 950).

CLINICAL SYNDROMES. The clinical classification of β-thalassemias is based on the severity of the anemia, which in turn is based on the type of genetic defect ($β^+$ or $β^0$) as well as the gene dosage (homozygous or heterozygous). In general, individuals who are homozygous for the β-thalassemia genes ($β^+$ or $β^0$) have very severe, transfusion-dependent anemia and are said to have *β-thalassemia major*. The presence of one normal gene in the heterozygotes usually leads to enough normal β-globin chain synthesis so that the affected individuals are usually asymptomatic with only a mild anemia. This condition is referred to as

β-thalassemia minor or *β-thalassemia trait*. A third clinical variant is characterized by an intermediate degree of severity, the so-called *β-thalassemia intermedia*. These patients have severe anemia, but not enough to require regular blood transfusions. Genetically, intermedia disorders are heterogeneous and include mild variants of homozygous $β^+$-thalassemia, some severe variants of heterozygous β-thalassemia ($β^0/β$ or $β^+/β$), and double heterozygosity for the $β^+$ and $β^0$ genes (genotype $β^+/β^0$). The clinical and morphologic features of thalassemia intermedia will not be described separately but may be surmised from the following discussions of thalassemia major and minor.

THALASSEMIA MAJOR. The β-thalassemia genes are most frequent, and thalassemia major is most common, in Mediterranean countries and parts of Africa and Southeast Asia. In the United States, the incidence is highest in immigrants from these areas.

Table 14–2. Clinical and Genetic Classification of Thalassemias

CLINICAL NOMENCLATURE	GENOTYPE	DISEASE	MOLECULAR GENETICS
A. Beta-Thalassemias			
I. Thalassemia major	1. Homozygous β^0-thalassemia (β^0/β^0) 2. Homozygous β^+-thalassemia (β^+/β^+)	Severe, requires blood transfusions regularly	1. Rare gene deletions in β^0/β^0 2. Defects in transcription, processing, or translation of β-globin mRNA
II. Thalassemia intermedia	β^0/β β^+/β^+	Severe, but does not require regular blood transfusions	
III. Thalassemia minor	β^0/β β^+/β	Asymptomatic with mild or absent anemia; red cell abnormalities seen	
B. Alpha-Thalassemias			
I. Silent carrier	$-\alpha/\alpha\alpha$	Asymptomatic; no red cell abnormality	Gene deletions mainly
II. Alpha-thalassemia trait	1. $--/\alpha\alpha$ (Asian) 2. $-\alpha/-\alpha$ (black African)	Asymptomatic, like β-thalassemia minor	
III. HbH disease	$--/-\alpha$	Severe, resembles β-thalassemia intermedia	
IV. Hydrops fetalis	$--/--$	Lethal in utero	

As indicated in Table 14–2, the genotype of these patients is usually β^+/β^+ or β^0/β^0. In some cases it is β^0/β^+ (double heterozygotes, if the two parents are carriers of β^+ and β^0 genes). With all these genotypes the anemia is very severe and first becomes manifest six to nine months after birth, as hemoglobin synthesis switches from HbF to HbA. In untransfused patients, Hb levels range between 3 and 6 gm per dl. The peripheral blood smear shows severe abnormalities; there is marked anisocytosis (variation in size) with many small and virtually colorless (microcytic, hypochromic) red cells. Abnormal forms, including target cells (so called because the small amount of hemoglobin collects in the center), stippled red cells, and fragmented red cells, are common. Inclusions representing aggregated α chains are usually not seen unless the spleen has been removed. The reticulocyte count is elevated but to an extent less than would be predicted from the severity of anemia. Variable numbers of normoblasts are usually seen in the peripheral blood. The red cells contain either no HbA at all (β^0/β^0 genotype) or very small amounts (β^+/β^+ genotype). HbF is markedly increased and indeed constitutes the major hemoglobin of red cells. HbA_2 levels are moderately elevated.

The major morphologic alterations, in addition to those characteristic of all hemolytic anemias, involve the bone marrow and spleen. In the typical patient there is striking expansion of the red marrow, virtually to the fetal level. The dominant change is a striking increase in the number of primitive nucleated erythroid precursors. The expansion of the marrow leads to thinning of the cortical bone, with new bone formation on the external aspect (Fig. 14–14). These changes are particularly evident in the maxilla and frontal bones of the face, sparing the mandible since it usually contains little marrow. Marked splenomegaly and hepatomegaly result both from reticuloendothelial cell hyperplasia secondary to active erythrophagocytosis and from extramedullary hematopoiesis. The spleen may increase up to 1500 gm in weight.

Hemosiderosis and even sometimes secondary hemochromatosis appear, related to a number of factors. Many of these patients have received numerous transfusions, providing a ready explanation for the iron overload. Ineffective erythropoiesis and possibly the chronic tissue hypoxia lead to increased intestinal absorption of iron. In any event, the hemosiderosis may have secondary consequences when the iron pigment accumulates in the myocardium, liver, or pancreas to induce organ injury.

The clinical course of β-thalassemia major is generally brief because, unless supported by transfusions, children suffer from growth retardation and die at an early age from the profound effects of anemia. Blood transfusions not only improve the anemia but also suppress secondary features related to excessive erythropoiesis. With transfusions, survival into the second and third decades of life is possible, but the overall outlook is grim. The clinical manifestations can largely be deduced from the hematologic and morphologic changes. In those who survive long enough the face becomes overlarge and somewhat distorted. Since the mandible is unaffected there is often malocclusion. Hepatosplenomegaly is usually present; the tissue hypoxia and systemic hemosiderosis may lead to delayed sexual development secondary to regressive changes in the gonads and other endocrine organs. Cardiac disease resulting from

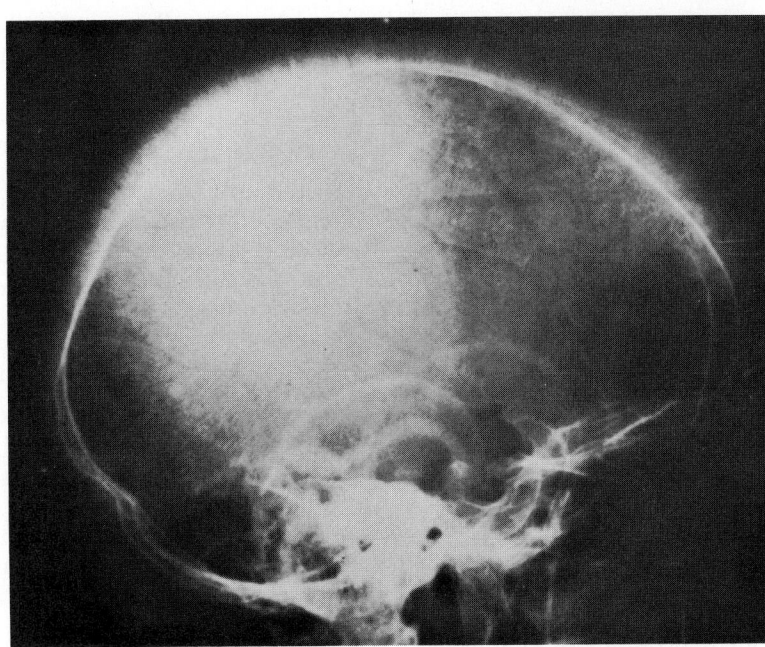

Figure 14–14. Thalassemia. X-ray of skull to show new bone formation on outer table producing perpendicular radiations characterized as a "crew haircut."

progressive iron overload and secondary hemochromatosis (p. 950) is an important cause of death even in patients who can otherwise be supported by blood transfusions. To reduce the amount of iron overload, most patients also receive iron-chelators. Nevertheless, the average age at death is 17 years. It is hoped that the recent remarkable success in cloning of globin genes will pave the way for gene therapy and eventual cure of these patients in the future. Prenatal diagnosis is possible by molecular analysis of DNA extracted from cells in the amniotic fluid. Two methods are employed: DNA restriction fragment length polymorphisms and oligonucleotide probe analysis. In the latter approach, synthetic oligonucleotides specific for the normal β-globin gene and for the mutant globin genes are used to discriminate between normal and mutant genes by Southern blot analysis. Details of the principles underlying these diagnostic techniques were discussed in Chapter 4 (p. 157).

THALASSEMIA MINOR. This is much more common than thalassemia major and understandably affects the same ethnic groups. In most cases these patients are heterozygotes for the $β^+$ or $β^0$ gene. Thalassemia trait is believed to offer resistance against falciparum malaria, accounting for its prevalence in those parts of the world where malaria is endemic. Almost invariably, individuals with the thalassemia trait are asymptomatic and anemia is very mild, if present. The peripheral blood smear usually shows some abnormalities affecting the red cells, including hypochromia, microcytosis, basophilic stippling, and target cells. Mild erythroid hyperplasia is seen in the bone marrow. The red cell survival may be slightly shortened or normal. A characteristic finding on hemoglobin electrophoresis is an increase in HbA_2,

which may constitute 4 to 8% of the total hemoglobin (normal $2.5 \pm 0.3\%$). HbF levels may be normal or slightly increased. Recognition of β-thalassemia trait is important on two counts: (1) its differentiation from the hypochromic microcytic anemia of iron deficiency and (2) genetic counseling. The importance of differentiating thalassemia trait from iron deficiency lies in the fact that the latter is benefited by iron therapy whereas the former may be worsened. In β-thalassemia trait there is a slight increase in iron absorption owing to modest ineffective erythropoiesis, and therefore iron administration contributes to possible iron overload during later years. The distinction can usually be made by measurement of serum iron, total iron-binding capacity, and serum ferritin (p. 688). Hemoglobin electrophoresis is also helpful.

Alpha-Thalassemias

These disorders are characterized by reduced synthesis of α-globin chains. Since there are normally four α-globin genes (one pair on each of the two number 16 chromosomes), the severity of the clinical syndromes shows a great variation, depending on the number of defective α-globin genes. As in the case of β-thalassemias, the anemia stems both from lack of adequate hemoglobin and from the effects of excess unpaired non-α chains (β, γ, δ). However, the situation is somewhat complicated by the fact that normally different non-α chains are synthesized at different times of development. Thus, in the newborn with α-thalassemia, there is an excess of unpaired γ-globin chains, resulting in the formation of $γ_4$-tetramers called Hb Barts, whereas in adults the excess β-globin chains aggregate to form tetramers called HbH. Since the non-α chains in general form more soluble and less toxic aggregates than those derived from α chains, the hemolytic anemia and ineffective erythropoiesis tend to be less severe than with β-thalassemias of similar degree of chain imbalance. All these factors make α-thalassemias somewhat distinctive, and we will briefly consider these below.

MOLECULAR PATHOLOGY. Unlike β-thalassemia, in which gene deletion has been detected only infrequently, the most common cause of reduced α-chain synthesis seems to be deletion of α-globin genes. As we shall discuss, from one to all four of the α-globin genes may be deleted, giving rise to a wide range of clinical severities. Two other less common causes of reduced α-globin synthesis have also been recognized. One nondeletional form resembles β-thalassemia in that the α-globin genes are present but they fail to be processed and expressed normally.

CLINICAL SYNDROMES. These are classified on the basis of the number and position of the α-globin genes deleted, which in turn determine the clinical syndrome. It will be useful at this point to recall that α-globin genes occur in linked pairs on each of the two chromosomes 16. Each α gene normally contributes approximately 25% of the α-globin chains and may be deleted independently of the other α-globin genes. The terminology of α-thalassemias is best considered along with Table 14–2, in which clinical terms and their genetic equivalents are presented along with the salient clinical features. Capsule descriptions follow.

SILENT CARRIER STATE. This is characterized by the deletion of a single α-globin gene and barely detectable reduction in α-globin chain synthesis. These individuals carrying three normal α-globin genes are completely asymptomatic and do not have anemia.

ALPHA-THALASSEMIA TRAIT. This is characterized by deletion of two α-globin genes. The involved genes may be from the same chromosome (with the other chromosome carrying the two normal genes), or one α-globin gene may be deleted from each of the two chromosomes (see Table 14–2). The former genotype is more common among Asian populations, whereas the latter is seen in those of African origin. Both these genetic patterns produce similar quantitative deficiencies of α-globin chains and therefore are identical clinically, but the position of deleted genes makes a big difference to the likelihood of severe α-thalassemia (HbH disease or hydrops fetalis) in the offspring. As is evident from Table 14–2, in black African populations in whom the two α genes are deleted from two separate chromosomes, mating of two individuals with the α-thalassemia trait would not result in progeny with HbH disease or hydrops fetalis.

The clinical picture in α-thalassemia trait is identical to that described for β-thalassemia minor, i.e., minimal or no anemia and no abnormal physical signs.

HEMOGLOBIN H DISEASE. This is associated with deletion of three of the four α-globin genes. As already discussed, HbH disease is seen mainly in Asian populations and rarely in those of African origin. With only one normal α-globin gene the synthesis of α chains is markedly suppressed and unstable tetramers of excess β globin are formed. These tetramers, called HbH, are considerably more soluble than the α-chain tetramers found in β-thalassemia. As such, the manifestations of HbH disease are milder than those of homozygous β-thalassemia and clinically resemble β-thalassemia intermedia. Inclusions of HbH can be demonstrated by incubation of red cells with brilliant cresyl blue in vitro. Oxidized HbH is precipitated by this procedure since it is unable to withstand oxidative stress. This property of HbH is the major cause of anemia, since older red cells with precipitates of oxidized HbH are removed by the spleen.

HYDROPS FETALIS. This is the most severe form of α-thalassemia, resulting from the deletion of all four α-globin genes. In the fetus, excess γ-globin chains form tetramers (Hb Barts) that have extremely high oxygen affinity but are unable to deliver the oxygen to tissues. Severe tissue anoxia associated with this condition invariably leads to intrauterine fetal death. The fetus shows severe pallor, generalized edema, and massive hepatosplenomegaly similar to that seen in erythroblastosis fetalis (p. 527).

Paroxysmal Nocturnal Hemoglobinuria (PNH)

This rare disorder of unknown etiology is characterized by chronic intravascular hemolysis that tends to get worse during the night. The basic mechanism causing hemolysis seems to be unusual sensitivity of the red blood cells to complement-mediated lysis. The increased sensitivity to complement results from the deficiency of a normal red cell membrane glycoprotein called decay accelerating factor (DAF). Normal levels of this protein limit the spontaneous in vivo activation of the alternative complement pathway by rapid inactivation of C3 convertase (C3bBb complex).[13] The membrane defect in PNH is not restricted to red blood cells, since platelets and granulocytes are also more sensitive to lysis by complement. In addition, nonlytic interactions between their cell membranes and complement produce functional abnormalities manifested by a striking predisposition to intravascular thromboses and infections.[14] In light of these findings, PNH is now considered to be a disorder of multipotent myeloid stem cells resulting from the proliferation of an abnormal clone of cells. This hypothesis is supported by the occasional transformation of PNH into other disorders of myeloid stem cells, including aplastic anemia (p. 688) and acute leukemia. The initiating event in all these cases may be a somatic mutation, but the nature of the mutagenic event remains mysterious.

Patients classically have intravascular hemolysis, which is paroxysmal and nocturnal in only 25% of cases. Most of the remaining patients have chronic hemolysis without dramatic hemoglobinuria. Over the long course of the disease, hemosiderinuria with loss of iron leads eventually to iron deficiency (Fig. 14–15). The other clinical manifestations include

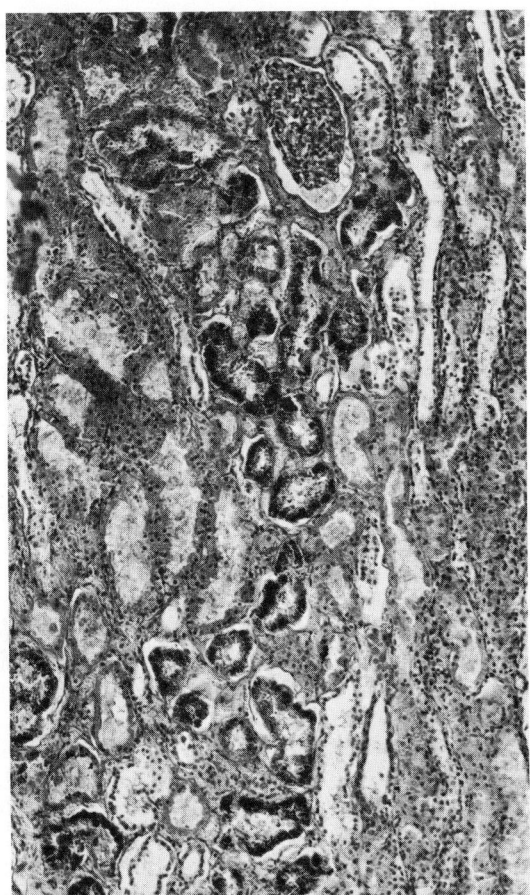

Figure 14–15. Paroxysmal hemoglobinuria. Dark renal tubules are heavily laden with hemosiderin in a 37-year-old patient with multiple recurrent hemolytic episodes.

multiple episodes of venous thromboses in the hepatic, portal, or cerebral veins, which are fatal in 50% of cases. Infection related to granulocytopenia or abnormal leukocyte functions is also prominent. The course of this disease is chronic, with a median survival of ten years.

Autoimmune Hemolytic Anemias (AHAs)

Hemolytic anemias in this category are caused by extracorpuscular mechanisms. Although these disorders are commonly referred to as autoimmune hemolytic anemias (AHAs), many prefer the designation *immunohemolytic anemias,* because in some instances the immune reaction is initiated by drug ingestion. They may occur as primary disorders in the absence of an underlying disease or may be secondary to some predisposing condition such as lymphoma, carcinoma, viral infection, or drug ingestion. In all instances, however, the hemolysis is related to the appearance of anti–red cell antibodies.[15] These immunohemolytic disorders have been classified in various ways but most commonly on the basis of the specific nature of antibody involved (Table 14–3).

Whatever the antibody, the differentiation of AHA from other forms of hemolytic anemia depends on demonstration of the existing antibodies. The major diagnostic criterion is the *Coombs antiglobulin test,* which relies on the capacity of the antibodies prepared in animals against human globulins to agglutinate red cells if these globulins are present on red cell surfaces. The temperature dependence of the autoantibody would further help specify the type of antibody. Quantitative immunologic methods to measure these autoantibodies directly are now available.

Warm Antibody AHA

In about 60% of patients, the condition is idiopathic and primary. In the remaining 40% there is an underlying predisposing condition, as mentioned in Table 14–3, or some drug exposure to thus produce a secondary form of AHA. Although autoantibodies are present in both groups (mainly IgG, although occasionally IgA) and may cause hemolysis within the bloodstream when present in high titers, most of the red cell destruction in this form of hemolytic disease is not due to intravascular hemolysis. Indeed, exposure of normal red blood cells to IgG antibodies and complement does not lead to hemolysis in vitro. In vivo, however, IgG-coated red cells are bound to Fc receptors on monocytes and splenic macrophages, and undergo spheroidal transformation. This process results from a partial loss of the red cell membrane by attempted phagocytosis of the IgG-coated cell. The ability to cause this interaction is greatest with IgG of subclasses 1 and 3 (the most common subclasses). *The spherocytes are then sequestered and removed in the spleen, the major site of red cell destruction in this disorder. Thus, moderate-to-severe splenomegaly is characteristic of this form of AHA.*

As is the case with most forms of autoimmunity, the cause of autoantibody formation in most cases is unknown. Factors discussed earlier in the general consideration of autoimmunity (p. 190) may apply. The mechanisms of hemolysis induced by the antibod-

Table 14–3. Classification of Autoimmune Hemolytic Anemias

I. ***Warm antibody AHA.*** Here the antibody is of the IgG type, does not usually fix complement, and is active at 37°C.
   A. *Primary* or idiopathic
   B. *Secondary* to:
     1. Lymphomas and leukemias
     2. Other neoplastic diseases
     3. Autoimmune disorder (particularly SLE)
     4. Drugs
II. ***Cold agglutinin AHA.*** Here the antibodies are IgM and are most active in vitro at 0–4°C. The antibody fixes complement at warmer temperatures, but agglutination of cells by IgM and complement occurs only in the peripheral cool parts of the body. Antibodies dissociate at 30°C or above.
   A. *Acute* (mycoplasma infection, infectious mononucleosis)
   B. *Chronic*
     1. Idiopathic
     2. Associated with lymphoma
III. ***Cold hemolysins*** (paroxysmal cold hemoglobinuria). In this condition, IgG antibodies bind to red cells at low temperature, fix complement, and cause *hemolysis* when the temperature is raised to 30°C.

ies are better understood. Three different immunologic mechanisms have been implicated.[16]

- *Hapten model.* The drugs — exemplified by penicillin and cephalosporins — may act as a hapten and combine with the red cell membrane to produce antibody directed against the red cell–drug complex, resulting in the destructive sequence cited above.
- *Immune complex model.* The drug serving as a hapten binds to a plasma protein and the drug-protein complex evokes antibodies. The resultant immune complexes nonspecifically attach to the red blood cell membrane, fixing complement and causing severe intravascular lysis. Here the red cells are "innocent bystanders." The red cell destruction, however, may also be extravascular. In the extravascular mechanism the immune complexes bind to monocytes and macrophages through Fc or C3b receptors, and spherocytosis and splenic sequestration ensue. Quinidine and phenacetin are prototype drugs responsible for this form of hemolysis.
- *Autoantibody model.* The drug, such as the antihypertensive agent α-methyldopa, in some manner initiates the production of antibodies that are directed against intrinsic red cell antigens, in particular the Rh blood group antigens. A typical positive IgG Coombs test without evidence of activation of complement makes these patients identical with those having the idiopathic, so-called autoantibody variety of AHA. In essence, the drug initiates an autoantibody reaction. Approximately 10% of patients taking methyldopa develop autoantibodies that can be detected in the Coombs test. However, only 1% develop clinically significant hemolysis.

Cold Agglutinin AHA

This form of immune hemolytic anemia is caused by IgM antibodies that bind avidly to red cells at low temperatures (0 to 4°C) and can remain immunologically reactive at temperatures that are achievable in vivo (30 to 32°C). Because they agglutinate red cells at low temperatures, they are referred to as cold agglutinins. These antibodies occur *acutely* during the recovery phase of certain infectious disorders such as Mycoplasma pneumonia and infectious mononucleosis. In the former, the antibodies are directed against the I antigen (closely related to the ABO antigens). In the latter, the antibodies are mainly targeted on the i antigen. This form of AHA is self-limited and rarely induces clinical manifestations of hemolysis. *Chronic cold agglutinins occur with lymphoproliferative disorders and as an idiopathic condition. The antibodies produced are monoclonal, suggesting that the underlying basis is similar to that of other monoclonal gammopathies (p. 739).* The clinical symptoms result from an in vivo agglutination of red cells and fixation of complement in distal body parts, where the temperature may drop to below 30°C. The antibody exerts its hemolytic effect predominantly by fixation of C3b to the surface of red blood cells, making them more susceptible to phagocytosis. For some obscure reason, the liver is more efficient in recognizing and sequestering the coated red cells than is the spleen; thus, splenomegaly is uncommon in this condition. The hemolytic anemia usually is of variable severity, and vascular obstruction by red cell agglutinates results in pallor, cyanosis of the body parts exposed to cold temperatures, and Raynaud's phenomenon (p. 579).

Cold Hemolysin AHA

Destruction of red cells in this variant occurs within the intravascular compartment. These autoantibodies are characteristic of the disease *paroxysmal cold hemoglobinuria* (PCH), which is noted for acute intermittent massive hemolysis, frequently with hemoglobinuria, following exposure of the affected patient to cold. Lysis is clearly complement dependent. The autoantibodies are IgG in nature and are directed against the P blood group antigen; they attach to the red cells and bind complement at low temperatures. When the temperature is elevated, the hemolytic action is mediated by the complement sequence, through activation of the lytic C5–9 complex. The antibody is also known as the Donath-Landsteiner (DL) antibody, previously associated with syphilis. Today, most cases of PCH follow various infections such as mycoplasma pneumonia, measles, mumps, and some ill-defined viral and "flu" syndromes. Some cases are idiopathic. Attacks are associated with hemoglobinuria, muscular pain, and fever, which disappear when the infections resolve. The idiopathic variety has a prolonged benign course, the patients being asymptomatic between attacks. The mechanisms responsible for the production of such autoantibodies are unknown.

Hemolytic Anemia Resulting from Trauma to Red Cells

Fragmentation of red blood cells when exposed to physical trauma may be severe enough to give rise to significant intravascular hemolysis. Clinically important are the hemolytic anemias associated with insertion of valve prostheses and diffuse deposition of fibrin in the microvasculature. In addition to immediate rupture, a wide variety of erythrocytic abnormalities are produced and are recognized in the peripheral blood film as burr cells, helmet cells, and triangle cells, as well as fragments of erythrocytes (schistocytes) (Fig. 14–16). *Hemolysis due to narrowing or obstructions in the microvasculature is called microangiopathic hemolytic anemia.* This form of anemia is encountered in disseminated intravascular coagulation (DIC), thrombotic thrombocytopenic purpura (TTP), the hemolytic-uremic syndrome, malignant hypertension, renal cortical necrosis, systemic lupus erythematosus (SLE), and metastatic adenocarcinoma. The common denominator is the presence of some vascular lesion. In DIC, the microthrombi constitute the point of impaction. In malignant hypertension, it is the markedly narrowed arterioles. In SLE, it is the necrotizing arteritis and arteriolitis. In patients with prosthetic heart valves, the red cells are damaged by the shear stress resulting from the turbulent

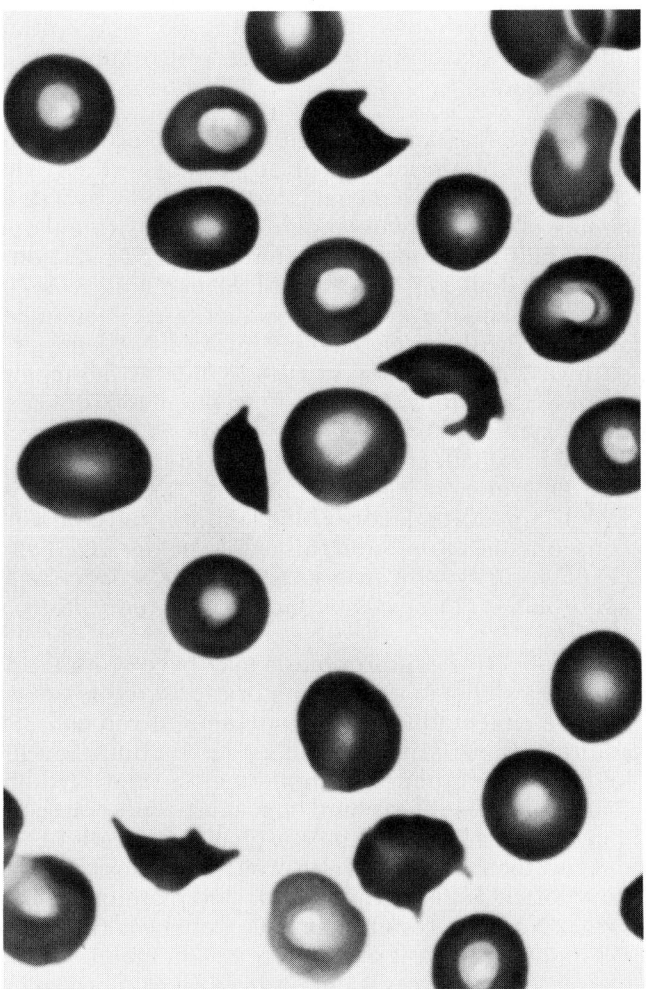

Figure 14-16. Microangiopathic hemolytic anemia. The peripheral blood smear shows several fragmented red blood cells. (Courtesy of Dr. Patrick Ward, Department of Pathology and Laboratory Medicine, University of Minnesota School of Medicine, Duluth, Minnesota.)

blood flow and abnormal pressure gradients caused by artificial heart valves.[17]

In most of these settings, the hemolysis is only a minor part of the clinical problem, and these patients rarely exhibit the morphologic changes encountered in the more chronic hemolytic diseases discussed earlier.

ANEMIAS OF DIMINISHED ERYTHROPOIESIS

It is astonishing to realize that in man approximately 9 billion red cells are normally destroyed hourly! Unless erythropoiesis can maintain this pace, anemia must develop. Diminished erythropoiesis can occur under a number of conditions. A major category constitutes a deficiency of some vital substrate that may lead to impaired proliferation or maturation of the erythroid cells. Included in this group are iron deficiency anemias in which heme synthesis is impaired, and anemia

of vitamin B_{12} and folate deficiency characterized by defective DNA synthesis (megaloblastic anemias). Another major category of decreased erythropoiesis can be loosely termed "marrow stem cell failure," which embraces such conditions as aplastic anemia, pure red cell aplasia, and anemia of renal failure. Aplastic anemias are associated with marrow hypoproliferation, but in nutrient deficiency anemias, even though the marrow is functionally hypoactive, it may be very cellular, as documented in the following discussion.

Megaloblastic Anemias

The following discussion will attempt first to characterize the major features of these anemias and then to discuss the two principal types of megaloblastic anemia: (1) pernicious anemia (PA), the major form of vitamin B_{12} deficiency anemia; and (2) folate deficiency anemia.

The megaloblastic anemias constitute a diverse group of entities, having in common a typical morphologic pattern in the blood and bone marrow. As the name implies, the erythroid precursors and erythrocytes are abnormally large, thought to be related to impairment of cell maturation and division. The peripheral blood reveals marked variation in the size and shape of red cells (anisocytosis), which are nonetheless normochromic. *Many erythrocytes are macrocytic and oval shaped (macro-ovalocytes) with mean corpuscular volumes (MCVs) over $100\,\mu^3$ (normal 82 to 92)*. Because they are thicker than normal and well filled with hemoglobin, most macrocytes lack the central pallor of normal red cells and may even appear

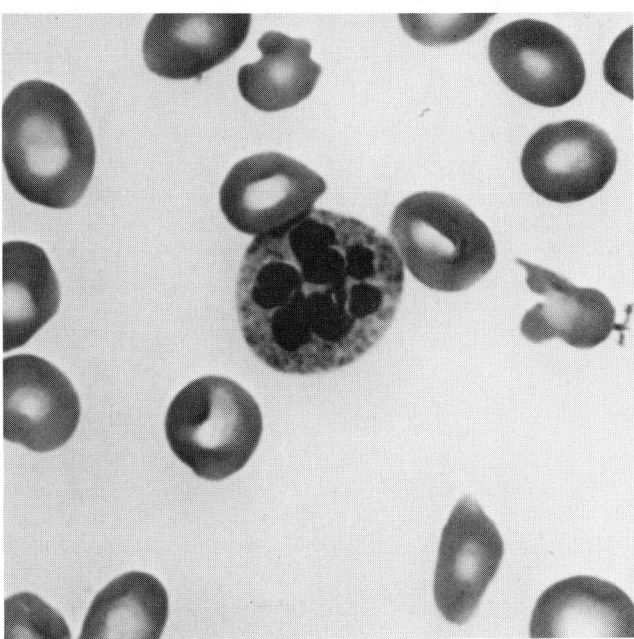

Figure 14-17. Megaloblastic anemia. Peripheral blood smear shows a neutrophil with seven-lobed nucleus (macropolycyte). (Courtesy of Dr. Robert W. McKenna, Department of Pathology, University of Texas, Southwestern Medical School, Dallas, Texas.)

"hyperchromic," but the mean corpuscular hemoglobin concentration (MCHC) is not elevated. The reticulocyte count is lower than normal and, occasionally with severe anemia, nucleated red cells appear in the circulating blood. *Neutrophils too are larger than normal (macropolymorphonuclear) and are hypersegmented, i.e., have five to six or more nuclear lobules* (Fig. 14–17). The marrow is hypercellular, and the megaloblastic change is detected in all stages of red cell development. The most primitive cells (promegaloblasts) are large, with a deeply basophilic cytoplasm and a distinctive fine chromatin pattern in the nucleus (Fig. 14–18). As these cells differentiate and begin to acquire hemoglobin, the nucleus retains its finely distributed chromatin and thus fails to undergo the chromatin clumping typical of the normoblast. Indeed, the development of a dense pyknotic nucleus, which occurs in the normal sequence of erythropoiesis, is delayed or fails to occur, creating an apparent *asynchronism* or *dissociation* between the cytoplasmic maturation and nuclear maturation. Analogously, the granulocytic precursors also reveal nuclear-cytoplasmic asynchrony, yielding giant metamyelocytes and band forms and hypersegmentation of the neutrophils, previously mentioned. Megakaryocytes, too, may be abnormally large and have bizarre, multilobate nuclei, but sometimes they appear relatively normal. With increased cellularity, much or all of the normally fatty marrow may be converted to red marrow. The erythroid/myeloid ratio, normally 1:3, may be transformed to 1:1. Nuclear-cytoplasmic asynchrony becomes apparent in all cells having a relatively rapid turnover, so megaloblastic and atypical cytologic alterations appear in the mucosal epithelium of the gastrointestinal tract, principally within the stomach.

PATHOPHYSIOLOGY. The fundamental causes of the megaloblastic change, or (to paraphrase Kass) why the megaloblast is a megaloblast at all and why a deficiency of B_{12} or folate should cause cells to enlarge and result in anemia, are still unanswered questions. Later we shall consider some of the metabolic roles of B_{12} and folate, but for here it suffices that vitamin B_{12} and folic acid are coenzymes in the DNA synthetic pathway. A deficiency of these vitamins or impairment in their utilization results in deranged or inadequate synthesis of DNA. The synthesis of RNA and protein is unaffected, however, so there is cytoplasmic enlargement not matched by DNA synthesis, which appears to delay or block mitotic division. Two consequences stem from this cytologic derangement: (1) *ineffective erythropoiesis* and (2) *the production of abnormal erythrocytes prone to hemolytic destruction.*[18]

Ineffective erythropoiesis may have several origins. The delay in nuclear maturation would reasonably be expected to slow production of red cells. In addition, there is intramedullary destruction of megaloblasts, which undergo autohemolysis more readily than do normoblasts and are more vulnerable to phagocytosis by mononuclear phagocytic cells in the marrow than are normal erythroid precursors. Premature destruction of granulocytic and platelet precursors also occurs, resulting in leukopenia and thrombocytopenia. The basis of the increased hemolysis of the mature erythrocytes is not entirely clear. Both an intracorpuscular defect, related perhaps to the defective red cells, and a poorly characterized plasma factor are believed to contribute. As in other hemolytic states, accelerated destruction of the red cells may lead to anatomic signs of mild-to-moderate iron overload after several years (p. 950).

The major causes of megaloblastic anemia are listed in Table 14–4.

It is evident that there are many bases for vitamin B_{12} deficiency, as pointed out on page 455. Inadequate diet is obvious but must be present for many years to deplete the reserves. Gastrectomy removes the source of intrinsic factor (IF). Ileal resection or diffuse ileal disease would remove or damage the site of IF-B_{12} complex absorption. Tapeworm infestation, by competing for the nutrient, could induce a deficiency state. Under some circumstances, e.g., pregnancy, hyperthyroidism, and disseminated cancer, the demand for vitamin B_{12} might be so great as to produce a relative deficiency, even with normal levels of absorption. As mentioned at the outset, pernicious anemia is an important cause of vitamin B_{12} deficiency. *The feature that sets pernicious anemia apart from the other vitamin B_{12} deficiency megaloblastic anemias is the cause of the B_{12} malabsorption: a lack of intrinsic factor.*

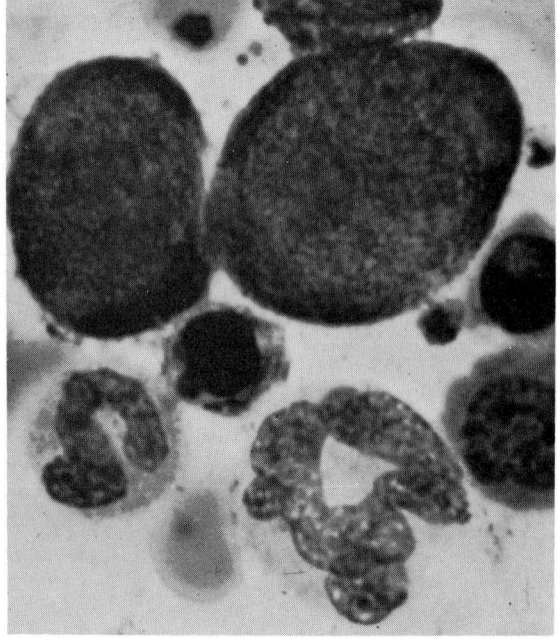

Figure 14–18. Marrow smear from a patient with pernicious anemia. Two megaloblasts are seen above.

Table 14-4. Causes of Megaloblastic Anemia

VITAMIN B$_{12}$ DEFICIENCY	
Decreased intake	Inadequate diet
	Impaired absorption
	Intrinsic factor deficiency
	Pernicious anemia
	Gastrectomy
	Malabsorption states
	Diffuse intestinal disease—lymphoma, systemic sclerosis, etc.
	Ileal resection, ileitis
	Competitive parasitic uptake
	Fish tapeworm infection
	Bacterial overgrowth in blind loops and diverticula of bowel
Increased requirement	Pregnancy, hyperthyroidism, disseminated cancer
FOLIC ACID DEFICIENCY	
Decreased intake	Inadequate diet—alcoholism, infancy
	Impaired absorption
	Malabsorption states
	Intrinsic intestinal disease
	Anticonvulsants, oral contraceptives
Increased loss	Hemodialysis
Increased requirement	Pregnancy, infancy, disseminated cancer, markedly increased hematopoiesis
Impaired utilization	Folic acid antagonists
UNRESPONSIVE TO VITAMIN B$_{12}$ OR FOLIC ACID THERAPY	
	Metabolic inhibitors, e.g., mercaptopurines, fluorouracil, cytosine, etc.
	Unexplained disorders
	Pyridoxine- and thiamin-responsive megaloblastic anemia
	Acute erythroleukemia (M6) (Di Guglielmo's syndrome)

Modified from Beck, W. S.: Megaloblastic anemias. *In* Wyngaarden, J. B., and Smith, L. H. (eds.): Cecil Textbook of Medicine. 18th ed. Philadelphia, W. B. Saunders Co., 1988, p. 900.

Pernicious Anemia (PA)

The basis of the defective absorption of vitamin B$_{12}$ in this form of megaloblastic anemia is *chronic atrophic gastritis* (p. 843) *with failure of production of IF.* In passing, it might be noted that "juvenile" PA encountered in childhood is not related to atrophic gastritis. The designation "pernicious" anemia is somewhat misleading, since the present availability of synthetic B$_{12}$ makes possible treatment and, to a large extent, control of this disease. Nonetheless, long historic usage and the need to set PA apart from the other B$_{12}$ deficiency states justifies the continued use of this name. It is well to discuss first the economy of vitamin B$_{12}$ in the body in order to place PA in perspective relative to the other forms of vitamin B$_{12}$ deficiency anemia.

Vitamin B$_{12}$ is a complex organometallic compound trivially known as cobalamin. The dietary sources and absorption of this vitamin were discussed on page 455 and therefore will be recapitulated only briefly. Absorption of vitamin B$_{12}$ requires IF, which is secreted by the parietal cells of the fundic mucosa along with HCl (Fig. 14–19). After peptic digestion of vitamin B$_{12}$-containing foods, the liberated vitamin is bound to salivary and gastric B$_{12}$-binding proteins, referred to as rapid (R) binders because of their electrophoretic mobility. Only a small amount is bound directly to IF. The R-B$_{12}$ complexes are transported to the duodenum, where they are broken down by the action of pancreatic proteases, and the released B$_{12}$ then attaches to IF. In this form IF-B$_{12}$ complex is transported to the ileum, where it adheres to IF-specific receptors on the ileal cells. By mechanisms that are still uncertain, B$_{12}$ traverses the plasma membrane to enter the mucosal cell. It is picked up from the cell by a plasma protein, transcobalamin II, which is capable of delivering it to the liver and other cells of the body, particularly the rapidly proliferating pool in the bone marrow and mucosal lining of the gastrointestinal tract.

There are only two reactions in man known to need B$_{12}$. *Methylcobalamin is an essential cofactor for the enzyme N^5-methyltetrahydrofolate-homocysteine methyltransferase, involved in the conversion of homocysteine to methionine* (Fig. 14–20). In the process, methylcobalamin yields its methyl group and is regenerated from N^5-methyltetrahydrofolic acid (N^5-methyl-FH$_4$), the principal form of folic acid in plasma, which is thus converted to' tetrahydrofolic acid (FH$_4$). The FH$_4$ is crucial since it is required (through its derivative N^{5,10}-methylene FH$_4$) for the conversion of deoxyuridine monophosphate (dUMP) to deoxythymidine monophosphate (dTMP), which is an immediate precursor of DNA. It has been postulated that the fundamental cause of impaired DNA synthesis in B$_{12}$ deficiency is the reduced availability of FH$_4$, since most of it is "trapped" as N^5-methyl-FH$_4$. Although the *methyltetrahydrofolate trap hypothesis* is supported by some experimental evidence, this issue is not resolved. Other investigators have suggested an alternative explanation that can best be dubbed the formate starvation hypothesis.[19] Accord-

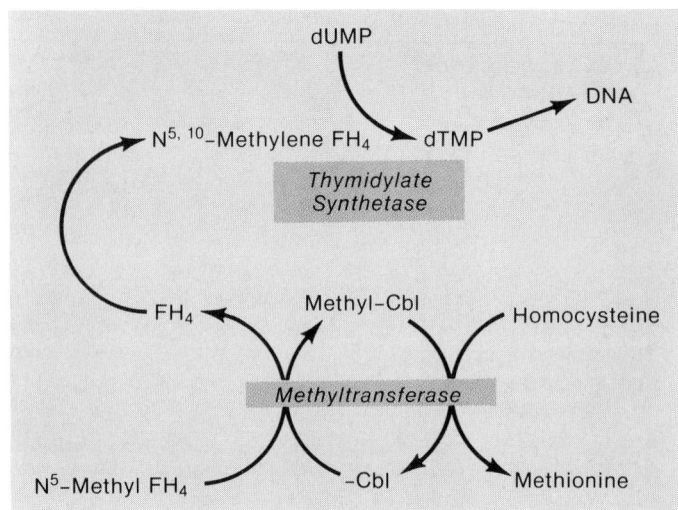

Figure 14–20. Diagram of relationship between N⁵-methyl FH₄: homocysteine methyltransferase and thymidylate synthetase. In cobalamin deficiency, folate is sequestered as N⁵-methyl FH₄. This ultimately deprives thymidylate synthetase of its folate coenzyme (N⁵,¹⁰-methylene FH₄) and thereby impairs DNA synthesis. (From Wyngaarden, J.B., and Smith, L.H. (eds.): Cecil Textbook of Medicine. 18th ed. Philadelphia, W.B. Saunders Co., 1988.)

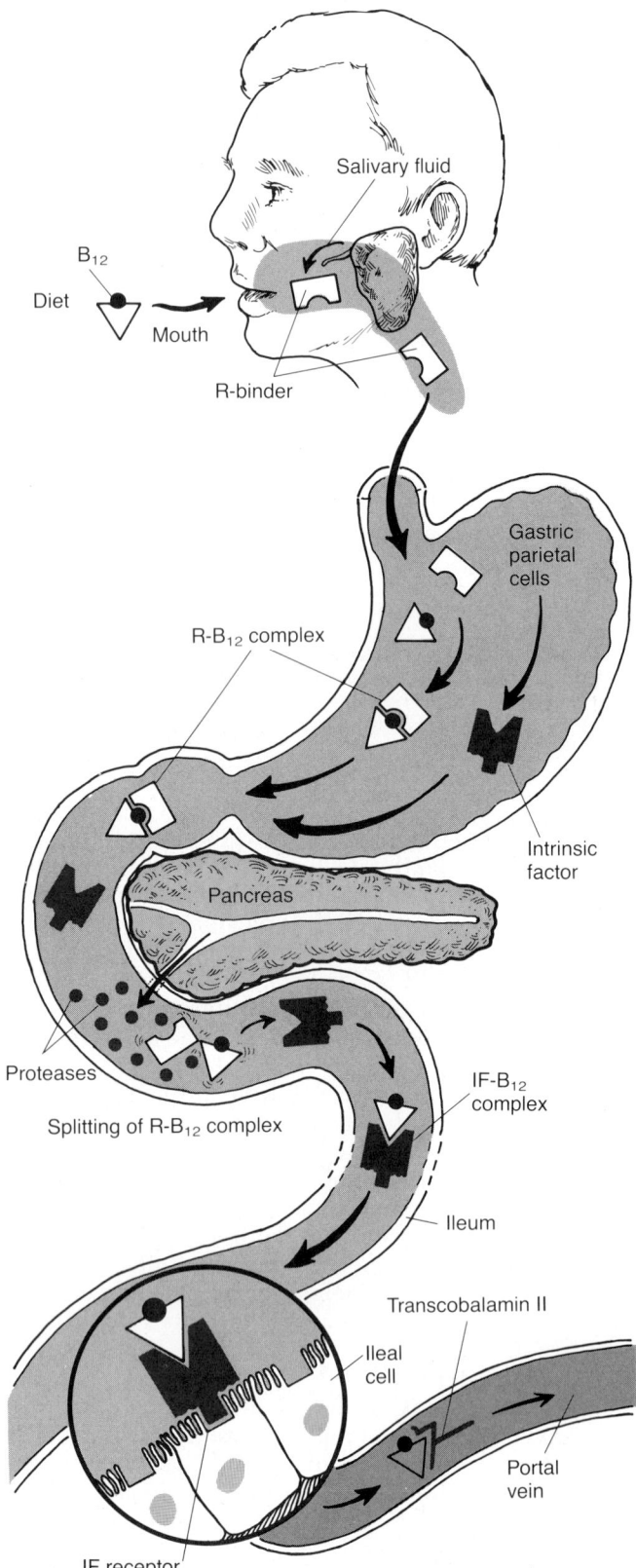

Figure 14–19. Schematic illustration of vitamin B₁₂ absorption.

ing to this view, the "internal" folate deficiency resulting from the lack of vitamin B_{12} is primarily due not to trapping of tetrahydrofolate but to failure to synthesize the metabolically active polyglutamate forms of folates. The synthesis of folate polyglutamates requires the single carbon formate groups derived from methionine, which in turn is generated by a B_{12}-dependent reaction (Fig. 14–20). In the formate starvation hypothesis, the importance of vitamin B_{12} is shifted from its role in the generation of FH_4 to the formation of methionine, which acts as the source of formate. Since the formation of both FH_4 and methionine is dependent on the availability of vitamin B_{12}, the two hypotheses are not mutually exclusive, but their relative contributions to the origins of megaloblastic anemia remain to be established.

Neurologic complications appear with vitamin B_{12} deficiency but are an even greater enigma.[20] Since the administration of folic acid, which relieves the megaloblastic anemia of B_{12} deficiency, fails to improve the neurologic deficit, internal folate deficiency must not be involved. It was stated earlier that only two reactions in man are known to require B_{12}. In addition to the transmethylation reaction discussed above, cobalamin is involved in the *isomerization of methylmalonyl coenzyme A to succinyl coenzyme A, requiring adenosyl cobalamin as a prosthetic group on the enzyme methylmalonyl-CoA mutase.* A deficiency of B_{12} thus leads to increased levels of methylmalonate, excreted in the urine as methylmalonic acid. Interruption of the succinyl pathway with the buildup of increased levels of methylmalonate and propionate (a precursor) could lead to the formation of abnormal fatty acids that may be incorporated into neuronal lipids. This biochemical abnormality may predispose to myelin breakdown and thereby produce some of the neurologic complications of B_{12} deficiency (p. 1434).

INCIDENCE. Although somewhat more prevalent in Scandinavian and "English-speaking" populations, PA occurs in all racial groups. It is slightly more common in males than in females and generally is diagnosed in the fifth to eighth decades of life. Whether or not there is a genetic predisposition to this disease is still unclear. Familial clusterings have been noted, but no definable genetic pattern of transmission has been discerned.

PATHOGENESIS. Chronic atrophic gastritis underlies the adult form of pernicious anemia, but its origin is still unknown. The mucosal atrophy is marked by a loss of parietal cells, a prominent infiltrate of lymphocytes and plasma cells, and megaloid and atypical nuclear changes in the mucosal cells similar to those found in the bone marrow. A number of immunologic reactions are associated with these morphologic changes. *Three types of antibodies are present in many, but not all, patients with PA.* About 75% of patients have an antibody that blocks B_{12}-IF binding, referred to as a *blocking antibody*. In the serum these are predominantly IgG, but may also be IgA. These are also found in the gastric juice, but here IgA antibodies predominate.[21] A second type, known as *binding antibody*, reacts with both IF and IF-B_{12} complex, and is found in about 50% of patients. It is present in the serum and gastric juice and can also be identified by immunofluorescent techniques in plasma cells in the gastric mucosa. It does not occur in the absence of the blocking antibody. The third type of antibody, present in 85 to 90% of patients, localizes in the microvilli of the canalicular system of the gastric parietal cell, sometimes referred to as *parietal canalicular antibody*. However, some patients with PA have none of these antibodies, and this has directed attention to possible cell-mediated immune reponses. Although in some patients there is evidence of T-cell reactions to IF (i.e., blast transformation and positive migration-inhibition tests), the frequency of these reactions has not been established.

In view of all the immunologic abnormalities it is considered quite likely that PA is an autoimmune disease and that the autoantibodies are causally related to vitamin B_{12} malabsorption. Several observations support this view.

• The majority of patients possess the gastric autoantibodies, discussed above.
• The parietal canalicular antibodies are complement fixing and therefore can damage the gastric parietal cells.
• The antibodies can be synthesized in the gastric mucosa and can inhibit absorption of vitamin B_{12}.
• There is a significant association between PA and autoimmune diseases affecting thyroid and adrenal glands.
• There is an increased frequency of serum antibodies

to intrinsic factor in patients with other autoimmune diseases.

It should be pointed out, however, that parietal canalicular antibodies are not absolutely specific for PA or other autoimmune diseases. They can be found in up to 50% of elderly patients with idiopathic chronic gastritis not associated with PA. Conceivably, in such cases they result from gastric injury, rather than cause it.

MORPHOLOGY. The major specific changes in PA are found in the bone marrow, alimentary tract, and central nervous system. Widespread nonspecific alterations incident to the generalized tissue hypoxia and abnormal hemolysis of blood may be present.

The bone marrow of untreated pernicious anemia is soft, red, jelly-like, and extremely hypercellular. Histologically, there is marked erythropoietic hypercellularity in which the erythroid elements sometimes equal or even outnumber the myeloid elements. **The most striking characteristic is the appearance of nests of megaloblasts** (Fig. 14–21). The earliest cells (promegaloblasts) are larger than pronormoblasts and have an abundant, deeply basophilic cytoplasm and a finely granular dispersion of chromatin within the nuclei. The nucleoli are large. As the megaloblasts differentiate, the immaturity of the nuclei contrasts with the apparent maturity of the cytoplasm. For example, **orthochromatic megaloblasts have a large amount of pink, well-hemoglobinized cytoplasm but the nucleus, instead of becoming pyknotic, remains relatively large and immature.** There may be a relative increase in the number of leukopoietic elements, but more striking is the presence of mature, large, polymorphonuclear leukocytes, the "macropolys." These cells characteristically have large nuclei, sometimes with six to seven individual lobes. Megakaryocytes may have similar changes.

With therapy, the megaloblasts, macrocytes, and macropolys disappear. Normal maturation and erythropoiesis reappear and are reflected in a great increase in the number of normoblasts and their descendants, as well as reticulocytes in the peripheral blood.

In the **alimentary system,** abnormalities are regularly found in the tongue and stomach. The tongue is shiny, glazed, and "beefy" **(atrophic glossitis).** The changes in the stomachs of adults are those of atrophic gastritis (p. 845). These atrophic changes are usually completely **absent** from juvenile patients with pernicious anemia. In the atrophic stomach, the submucosal vessels are readily visible and so produce a shiny red mucosal surface. The most characteristic histologic alteration is the atrophy of the fundic glands, affecting both chief cells and parietal cells. The parietal cells are virtually absent. The glandular lining epithelium is metaplastically replaced by mucus-secreting goblet cells that resemble those lining the large intestine, a change referred to as **intestinalization.** Some of the cells as well as their nuclei may increase to double the normal size. Presumably, these enlargements reflect the megaloid alterations discussed earlier. As will be seen, patients with pernicious anemia have a higher incidence of gastric

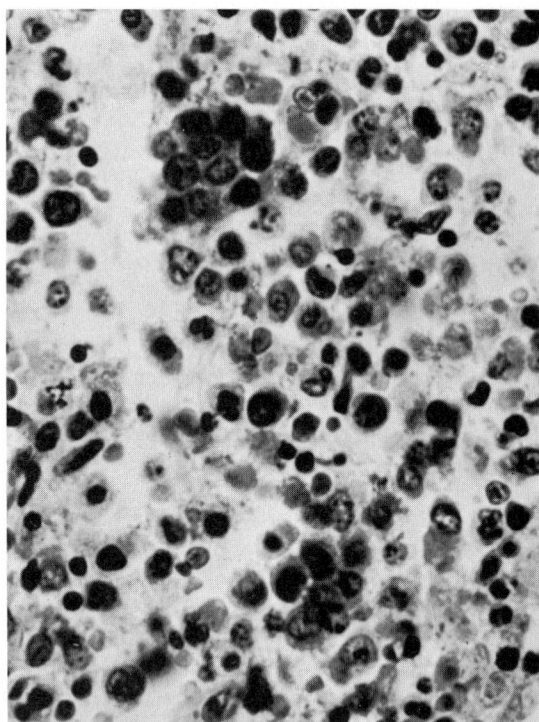

Figure 14–21. Pernicious anemia. Two nests of darkly stained megaloblasts in bone marrow.

cancer. It may be that these cellular alterations underlie the predisposition to malignancy.

Although parenteral administration of vitamin B$_{12}$ will correct the bone marrow changes in pernicious anemia, the gastric atrophy and achlorhydria persist unaffected. This exception is entirely compatible with the thesis that the gastric changes are primary and are not the effect of the B$_{12}$ deficiency.

Central nervous system lesions are found in approximately three-quarters of all cases of fulminant pernicious anemia, but it should be noted that in some cases neuronal involvement may occur in the absence of megaloblastic anemia. **The principal alterations involve the spinal cord, where there is myelin degeneration of the dorsal and lateral tracts,** sometimes followed by loss of axons. These changes give rise to spastic paraparesis, sensory ataxia, and severe paresthesias in the lower limbs. Less frequently, degenerative changes occur in the ganglia of the posterior roots and in the peripheral nerves (p. 1434).

Because of the hemolytic tendency and ineffective erythropoiesis in all megaloblastic anemias, hemosiderosis may be found in the liver, spleen, and bone marrow and in other elements of the mononuclear phagocyte system, but the spleen and liver usually are not significantly enlarged.

CLINICAL COURSE. Pernicious anemia is characteristically insidious in onset, so that by the time the patient seeks medical attention the anemia is usually quite marked. The usual course is progressive unless halted by therapy.

Diagnostic features include (1) a moderate-to-severe megaloblastic anemia; (2) leukopenia with hypersegmented granulocytes; (3) mild-to-moderate thrombocytopenia; (4) neurologic changes related to involvement of the posterolateral spinal tracts; (5) achlorhydria even after histamine stimulation; (6) decreased vitamin B$_{12}$ absorption; (7) low serum levels of vitamin B$_{12}$; (8) excretion of methylmalonic acid in the urine; and (9) most critically, a striking reticulocytic response and improvement in hematocrit levels following parenteral administration of vitamin B$_{12}$.

The cytologic aberrations in the gastric mucosa are associated with an increased risk of gastric cancer (p. 855). In addition, cardiac failure incident to hypoxic injury to the myocardium and intercurrent infections are hazards. However, with parenteral vitamin B$_{12}$ the anemia can be cured and the peripheral neurologic changes reversed, or at least halted in their progression. Obviously, death of brain cells cannot be reversed. Overall longevity may be restored virtually to normal.

"JUVENILE" PERNICIOUS ANEMIA. Childhood PA differs from the adult type inasmuch as there is no associated gastric abnormality. The mechanism of vitamin B$_{12}$ deficiency is not well understood and may be related to several hereditary derangements: (1) congenital inability to elaborate intrinsic factor, (2) synthesis of a biologically ineffective IF, and (3) some defect in the ileal mucosal receptors for the intrinsic factor–B$_{12}$ complex. Autosomal recessive inheritance has been identified within some families.

Anemia of Folate Deficiency

A deficiency of folic acid, more properly pteroylmonoglutamic acid, results in a megaloblastic anemia having the same characteristics as those encountered in vitamin B$_{12}$ deficiency. However, the neurologic changes seen in B$_{12}$ deficiency do not occur. Megaloblastic anemia secondary to folate deficiency is not common, but precarious folate levels in the body are surprisingly common: among the economically deprived of all countries who live on marginal diets; among pregnant women, in whom dietary inadequacies combine with increased metabolic requirements; and among alcoholics and drug addicts, with their well-known grossly inadequate diet. *The prime function of folic acid, specifically tetrahydrofolate (FH$_4$) derivatives, is to act as an intermediate in the transfer of one-carbon units such as formyl and methyl groups to various compounds* (Fig. 14–22). In this process, FH$_4$ acts as an acceptor of one-carbon fragments from compounds such as serine and formiminoglutamic acid (FIGlu), and the FH$_4$ derivatives so generated donate the acquired one-carbon fragments for the synthesis of biologically active molecules. FH$_4$, then, may be viewed as the biologic "middle man" in this trade. The most important metabolic processes dependent on such one-carbon transfers are (1) the synthesis of purines; (2) the synthesis of methionine from homocysteine, a reaction that also requires vitamin B$_{12}$ (p. 681); and (3) the synthesis of deoxythymid-

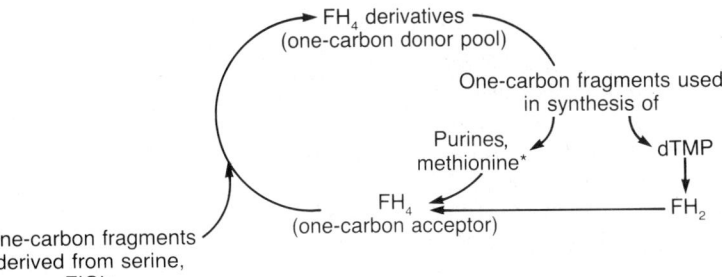

Figure 14–22. Schematic illustration of role of folate derivatives in transfer of one-carbon fragments for synthesis of biologic macromolecules. FH_4 = tetrahydrofolic acid; FH_2 = dihydrofolic acid; FIGlu = formiminoglutamate; dTMP = deoxythymidylate monophosphate; *synthesis of methionine also requires vitamin B_{12}.

ylate monophosphate (dTMP). In the first two reactions, FH_4 is regenerated from its one-carbon carrier derivatives and is available to accept another one-carbon fragment and re-enter the donor pool. In the synthesis of thymidylate, a dihydrofolate is produced that has to be reduced by dihydrofolate reductase to FH_4 to re-enter the pool. The reductase step is significant since this enzyme is susceptible to inhibition by various drugs. Among the biologically active molecules whose synthesis is dependent on folates, thymidylate is perhaps the most important. As discussed earlier in relation to pernicious anemia (p. 681), dTMP is required for DNA synthesis. It should be apparent from our discussion that suppressed synthesis of DNA, the common denominator of folic acid and B_{12} deficiency, is the immediate cause of megaloblastosis. A clinically insignificant biochemical effect of folate deficiency is the failure to metabolize formiminoglutamic acid (FIGlu), a breakdown product of histidine. With a deficiency of folate, FIGlu piles up and is excreted in the urine, providing a useful clinical indicator of folate deficiency.

The dietary source and absorption of folates were considered in an earlier chapter (p. 455). Here we need discuss only the three major causes of folic acid deficiency: (1) decreased intake, (2) increased requirements, and (3) impaired utilization (Table 14–4).

Decreased intake can result from either a nutritionally inadequate diet or impairment of intestinal absorption. A normal daily diet contains folate in excess of the minimal daily adult requirement of 50 to 200 μg. Inadequate dietary intakes are almost invariably associated with grossly deficient diets, particularly lacking vitamins, such as those in the "B group." Such dietary inadequacies are most frequently encountered in chronic alcoholics, the indigent, and the very elderly. In alcoholics with cirrhosis, other mechanisms of folate deficiency such as trapping of folate within the liver, excessive urinary loss, and disordered folate metabolism have also been implicated. Under these circumstances, the megaloblastic anemia is often accompanied by general malnutrition and manifestations of other avitaminoses, including cheilosis, glossitis, and dermatitis. Malabsorption syndromes such as nontropical and tropical sprue may lead to inadequate absorption of this nutrient. Similarly, diffuse infiltrative disease of the small intestine, e.g., lymphoma, may impair intestinal absorption. In addition, certain drugs, particularly the anticonvulsant phenytoin and oral contraceptives, impair absorption.

Despite adequate intake of folic acid, a *relative deficiency* can be encountered in states of increased requirement, such as pregnancy, infancy, hematologic derangements associated with hyperactive hematopoiesis (hemolytic anemias), and disseminated cancer. In all these circumstances, the demands of active DNA synthesis render normal intake inadequate.

Folic acid antagonists, such as methotrexate, 6-mercaptopurine, and cyclophosphamide, inhibit dihydrofolate reductase and lead to a deficiency of FH_4. With inhibition of folate function, all rapidly growing cells are affected, thus leading to ulcerative lesions within the gastrointestinal tract as well as megaloblastic anemia. Owing to their growth-inhibitory actions, these antimetabolites are used in cancer therapy.

As mentioned at the outset, *the megaloblastic anemia resulting from a deficiency of folic acid is identical to that encountered in B_{12} deficiency, in terms of the alterations both in the circulating blood and in the marrow precursors.* Thus, the recognition of folate deficiency requires the demonstration of (1) decreased folate levels in the serum or red cells and (2) increased excretion of FIGlu after an administered dose of histidine. The absence of neurologic changes and methylmalonic acid in the urine also rules against vitamin B_{12} deficiency as the cause of changes in the blood. Although prompt hematologic response heralded by the appearance of a reticulocytosis follows the administration of folic acid, it should be cautioned that, even in patients with a B_{12} deficiency anemia, a similar reticulocytosis may be produced by folic acid therapy. However, folic acid has no effect on the progression of the neurologic changes typical of the B_{12} deficiency states, and therefore the hematologic response to folate therapy cannot be used to rule out vitamin B_{12} deficiency.

Iron Deficiency Anemia

Deficiency of iron is probably the most common nutritional disorder in the world. Although the prevalence of iron deficiency anemia is higher in the developing countries, this form of anemia is also common in the United States. The factors underlying the iron deficiency differ somewhat in various population groups and can be best considered in the context of normal iron metabolism, some of which was also discussed in Chapter 8.[22-24]

IRON METABOLISM. Normally, the total body iron content is in the range of 2 gm in women and up to 6 gm in men. As indicated in Table 14–5, it is divided into functional and storage compartments. Approximately 80% of the functional iron is found in hemoglobin; myoglobin and iron-containing enzymes such as catalase and the cytochromes contain the rest. The storage pool represented by hemosiderin and ferritin contains approximately 15 to 20% of total body iron. It should be noted that even healthy young females have substantially smaller stores of iron than do males. They are therefore in much more precarious iron balance and are accordingly more vulnerable to excessive losses or increased demands associated with menstruation and pregnancy.

All storage of iron is in the form of either ferritin or hemosiderin. *Ferritin is essentially a protein-iron complex* that can be found in all tissues but particularly in liver, spleen, bone marrow, and skeletal muscles. In the liver, most of the ferritin is stored within the parenchymal cells, whereas in other tissues, such as spleen and bone marrow, it is mainly in the mononuclear phagocytic cells. The iron within the hepatocytes is derived from plasma transferrin, whereas the storage iron in the mononuclear phagocytic cells, including that in the Kupffer cells, is obtained largely from the breakdown of red cells. Within cells, ferritin is located both in the cell sap and in lysosomes, in which the protein shells of the ferritin are degraded and iron is aggregated into *hemosiderin* granules. With the usual cellular stains, hemosiderin appears in tissues as golden-yellow granules that vary somewhat in size and shape, presumably because of variation in the number of incorporated ferritin molecules. The iron is chemically reactive, and when hemosiderin is exposed to potassium ferrocyanide (Prussian blue reaction) in tissue sections, the granules turn blue-black. With normal iron stores only trace amounts of hemosiderin are found in the body, principally in reticuloendothelial cells in the bone marrow, spleen, and liver. In iron-overloaded cells, most of the iron is stored in the form of hemosiderin.

Very small amounts of ferritin normally circulate in the plasma. *Since the plasma ferritin is largely derived from the storage pool of body iron, its level is a good indicator of the adequacy of body iron stores.* Each microgram per liter of plasma ferritin is esti-

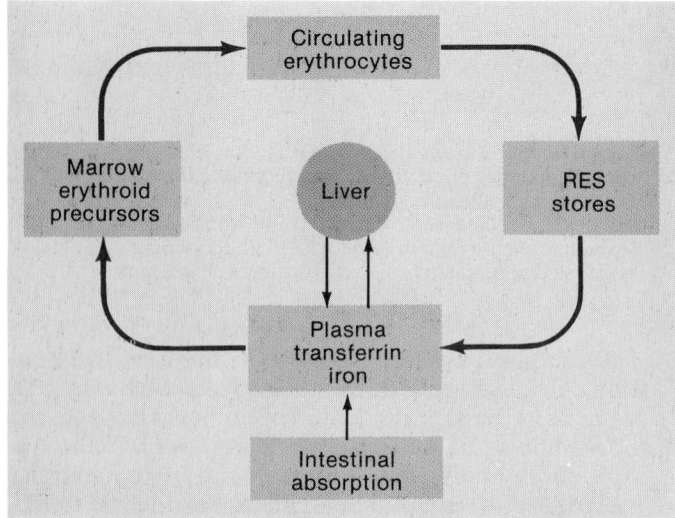

Figure 14–23. The internal iron cycle. In the plasma, iron bound to transferrin is transported to the marrow where it is transferred to developing red blood cells and incorporated into hemoglobin. The mature red blood cells are released into the circulation and after 120 days are ingested by macrophages in the reticuloendothelial system (RES). Here the iron is extracted from hemoglobin and returned to plasma, completing the cycle. (From Wyngaarden, J.B., and Smith, L.H. (eds.): Cecil Textbook of Medicine. 18th ed. Philadelphia, W.B. Saunders, 1988.)

mated to represent 8 mg of storage iron. In iron deficiency, serum ferritin is always below 12 μg per liter, whereas in iron overload very high values approaching 5000 μg per liter may be obtained. It should be noted, however, that the relationship between the degree of overload and serum ferritin levels is not linear. There are three circumstances under which serum ferritin cannot be used as a measure of body iron stores: in liver damage, in inflammatory states, and with some tumors. In these states, serum ferritin levels may be extremely high despite normal body iron stores. The physiologic importance of the storage iron pool is that it is readily mobilizable in the event of an increase in body iron requirements, as may occur following loss of blood.

Iron is transported in the plasma by an iron-binding glycoprotein called transferrin (Fig. 14–23). It is synthesized in the liver, having a molecular weight of 76,000 with two iron-binding sites. In the normal individual, transferrin is about 33% saturated with iron, yielding serum iron levels that average 120 μg per dl in men and 100 μg per dl in women. Thus, the total iron-binding capacity of serum is in the range of 300 to 350 μg per dl. The major function of plasma transferrin is to deliver iron to the cells, including erythroid precursors, where iron is required for hemoglobin synthesis. Immature red cells possess high-affinity receptors for transferrin, and iron is transported into erythroblasts by receptor-mediated endocytosis.[25] In the cytoplasm, iron is released within the endocytic vesicle and the transferrin-receptor complex is transported back to the surface,

Table 14–5. Iron Distribution in Healthy Young Adults (mg)

	MEN	WOMEN
Total	3450	2450
Functional		
Hemoglobin	2100	1750
Myoglobin	300	250
Enzymes	50	50
Storage		
Ferritin, hemosiderin	1000	400

where apotransferrin is released for another cycle of iron transport.

The absorption of iron and its regulation are complex and poorly understood. Some of the factors that affect iron absorption were discussed in an earlier chapter (p. 459). Here we will concentrate on the mucosal uptake of iron. The most active site of iron absorption is the duodenum, but the stomach, ileum, and colon may also participate to a small degree.

Mucosal uptake of iron occurs by two distinct pathways (Fig. 14–24). Approximately 25% of the heme iron derived from hemoglobin, myoglobin, and other animal proteins is absorbed. Released from its apoproteins by gastric acids, heme is taken up directly by the mucosal cells. Once inside the cells, heme is enzymatically degraded to release iron. In contrast, only 1 to 2% of non-heme iron is absorbed, by mechanisms that are complex and poorly understood. According to one widely accepted view, a mucosal transferrin is secreted into the lumen of the gut, where it binds iron and is then internalized by receptor-mediated endocytosis. Within the mucosal cell, iron is released and the transferrin and its receptor are recycled (Fig. 14–24). Iron absorbed by these two pathways appears to enter a common pool in the mucosal cell. Normally, a fraction of the iron that enters the cell is rapidly delivered to plasma transferrin. Most, however, is deposited as ferritin, some to be transferred more slowly to plasma transferrin, and some to be lost with exfoliation of mucosal cells. The extent to which the mucosal iron is distributed along these various pathways depends largely on the body's iron requirements. When the body is replete with iron, formation of ferritin within the mucosal cells is maximal, whereas in iron deficiency transport into plasma is enhanced.

Since body losses of iron are limited, iron balance is maintained largely by regulating the absorptive intake (mucosal block). The factors that regulate the absorption of available iron into the mucosal cell are largely unknown. It is, however, known that the rate and level of absorption are dependent on total body iron content and erythropoietic activity, more specifically the iron needs of the erythron. As body stores rise the percentage of iron absorbed falls, and vice versa. Some signal must be delivered to the mucosal cell, modifying its uptake and transfer of iron, and although there are many hypotheses, the nature of the signal remains unknown.[26]

ETIOLOGY. With this background of normal iron metabolism, we can discuss the causes and effects of iron deficiency.[27] The consequences of excess iron accumulation (iron overload) are considered on page 950. Negative iron balance and consequent anemia may result from (1) low dietary intake, (2) poor absorption, (3) excessive demand, or (4) chronic blood loss.

The iron requirements are best understood in the context of the fixed daily losses of iron, ranging between 1 and 1.5 mg. Thus to maintain a normal iron balance, approximately 1 mg of iron must be absorbed from the diet every day. Because only 10 to 15% of the ingested iron is absorbed, the daily iron requirement for adult males is 5 to 10 mg and for adult females 7 to 20 mg (p. 459). Since the average daily dietary intake of iron in the Western world is about 15 to 20 mg, most men ingest more than adequate iron, whereas many women consume just enough or marginally adequate iron. It is not surprising, therefore, *that iron deficiency resulting solely from poor dietary intake is rarely seen in the United States;* even in women, who have lower iron reserves and greater iron losses, other factors usually coexist. The situation is quite different in underdeveloped countries, where low intake as well as poor bioavailability of the iron exists, owing to a lack of meats and to predominantly vegetarian diets from which iron is poorly absorbed. *Malabsorption* of iron may occur in association with generalized malabsorption syndromes such as sprue and celiac disease, or after gastrectomy. The latter affects iron absorption by decreasing hydrochloric

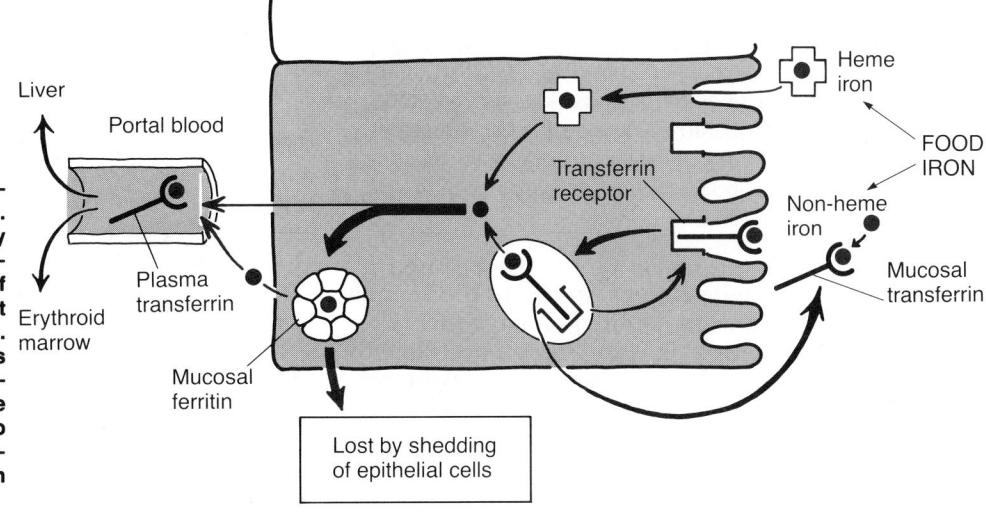

Figure 14–24. Diagrammatic representation of iron absorption. When the storage sites of the body are replete with iron and erythropoietic activity is normal, most of the absorbed iron is lost into the gut by shedding of the epithelial cells. Conversely, when body iron needs increase or erythropoiesis is stimulated, a greater fraction of the absorbed iron is transferred to plasma-transferrin, with a concomitant decrease in iron loss through mucosal ferritin.

Liver

Portal blood

Erythroid marrow

Plasma transferrin

Mucosal ferritin

Lost by shedding of epithelial cells

Transferrin receptor

Heme iron

FOOD IRON

Non-heme iron

Mucosal transferrin

acid and the transit time through the duodenum, the major site of iron absorption. *By far the most important cause of iron deficiency anemia in the Western world is chronic blood loss.* This may occur from the gastrointestinal tract (e.g., peptic ulcers, colonic cancer, hemorrhoids, hookworm disease, chronic aspirin ingestion) or the female genital tract (e.g., menorrhagia, malignancy). At the outset of chronic blood loss or other states of negative iron balance, the reserves in the form of ferritin and hemosiderin may be adequate to maintain normal hemoglobin and hematocrit levels as well as normal serum iron and transferrin saturation. Progressive depletion of these reserves will eventually lower the serum iron and transferrin saturation levels, but still may not be reflected in abnormalities in the erythron. Up to this stage of blood loss there is increased erythroid activity in the bone marrow and expansion of the erythron, but progressive disappearance of sideroblasts from the marrow. Thereafter, anemia will appear when all iron stores are depleted, now accompanied by low levels of serum iron and transferrin saturation as well as low serum ferritin. Pregnancy and infancy are two states that may be associated with iron deficiency owing to *increased demands* not met by normal dietary intake. *Whatever the basis, iron deficiency induces a hypochromic microcytic anemia.* Simultaneously, depletion of essential iron-containing enzymes in cells throughout the body may cause other changes, including koilonychia, alopecia, atrophic changes in the tongue and gastric mucosa, and intestinal malabsorption. Uncommonly, esophageal webs (p. 829) may appear, to complete the triad of major findings in the *Plummer-Vinson syndrome*: (1) microcytic hypochromic anemia, (2) atrophic glossitis, and (3) esophageal webs.

MORPHOLOGY. The bone marrow may disclose increased erythropoietic activity, predominantly at the level of normoblasts and their maturation forms. Specificity is lent to these changes by the absence of sideroblasts and the disappearance of stainable iron from the reticuloendothelial cells in the bone marrow. In the peripheral blood smear, red cells appear smaller (microcytic) and much paler (hypochromic) than normal. In many cells, hemoglobin is seen only in the form of a narrow peripheral rim (Fig. 14–25). Leukocytes and megakaryocytes are usually not affected. Changes may be encountered outside the bone marrow, the most important being atrophy of the tongue mucosa (atrophic glossitis) (p. 683), esophageal webs (p. 829), and gastric atrophy (p. 845).

The clinical manifestations related to the anemia are nonspecific and were detailed on page 661. Frequently, the dominating signs and symptoms relate to the underlying cause of the anemia, e.g., gastrointestinal or gynecologic disease, malnutrition, pregnancy, malabsorption, and so forth. The atrophic glossitis may be responsible for difficulty in swallowing. Gastrointestinal disturbances may be present associated with the disorder that led to the chronic blood loss (e.g., bleeding peptic ulcer or gastric carcinoma, diverticulitis, colonic cancer) or may emanate from the development of the atrophic gastritis.

The diagnosis of iron deficiency anemia ultimately rests upon laboratory studies. Both hemoglobin and hematocrit are depressed, usually to moderate levels, and are associated with hypochromia, microcytosis, and some poikilocytosis. *The serum iron and serum ferritin are low, and the total plasma iron-binding capacity (reflecting transferrin concentration) is high. Low serum iron with increased iron-binding capacity results in a reduction of transferrin saturation levels to below 15%.* Reduced heme synthesis leads to elevation of free erythrocyte protoporphyrin. Usually the leukocytes and platelets are not affected. The alert clinician who investigates an unexplained iron deficiency anemia occasionally discovers an occult lesion or cancer and thereby saves a life.

Aplastic Anemia

This somewhat misleading term is applied to pancytopenia, characterized by (1) anemia, (2) neutropenia, and (3) thrombocytopenia.[28] The basis for these changes is thought to be a failure or suppression of multipotent myeloid stem cells, with inadequate production or release of the differentiated cell lines. Less commonly, the stem cell defect is limited to the committed precursors, giving rise to pure red cell aplasia, or selective suppression of the white cell series. These will be considered later. The bone marrow in aplastic

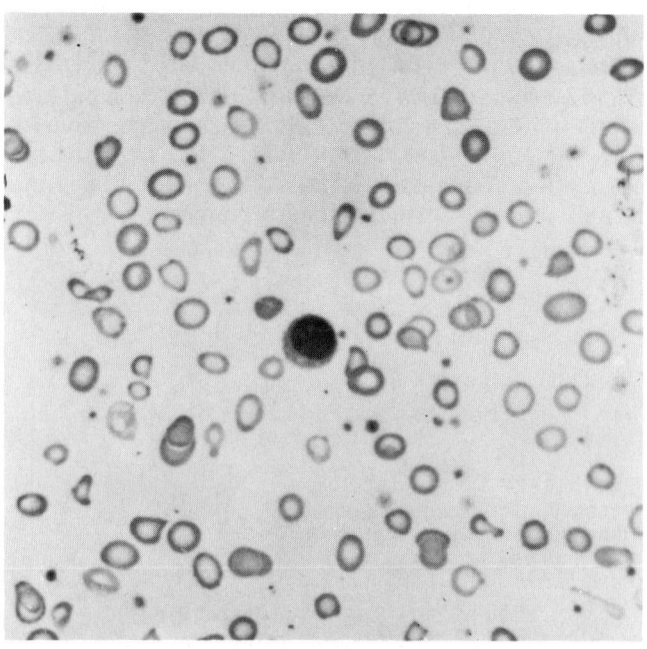

Figure 14–25. Hypochromic microcytic anemia of iron deficiency. Note that most red cells are smaller than lymphocyte nucleus seen in midfield. The small amount of hemoglobin is seen as a narrow rim at periphery of red cells. (Courtesy of Dr. Jose Hernandez, Department of Pathology, Southwestern Medical School, Dallas, Texas.)

Table 14-6. Major Causes of Aplastic Anemia

A. ACQUIRED
  I. Idiopathic
       Primary stem cell defect
       Immune-mediated
  II. Chemical agents
       Dose-related
            Alkylating agents
            Antimetabolites
            Benzene
            Chloramphenicol
            Inorganic arsenicals
       Idiosyncratic
            Chloramphenicol
            Phenylbutazone
            Organic arsenicals
            Methylphenylethylhydantoin
            Streptomycin
            Chlorpromazine
            Insecticides: e.g., DDT, parathion
  III. Physical agents (e.g., whole-body radiation)
  IV. Viral infections
       Non-A, non-B hepatitis
       CMV infections
       EBV infections
       Herpes varicella-zoster
  V. Miscellaneous
       Infrequently, many other drugs and chemicals
B. INHERITED—Fanconi's anemia

anemia is almost always markedly hypocellular, with a striking reduction in the precursors of red cells, granulocytes, and platelets.

ETIOLOGY. The major circumstances under which aplastic anemia may appear are listed in Table 14-6.

Most cases of aplastic anemia of so-called known etiology follow exposure to chemicals and drugs. With some agents the marrow damage is predictable, dose related, and, in most instances, reversible when the use of the offending agent is stopped. Best documented as known myelotoxins are benzene, chloramphenicol, alkylating agents, and antimetabolites, e.g., 6-mercaptopurine, vincristine, busulfan, and so forth. In other instances, the pancytopenia appears as an apparent idiosyncratic reaction to very small doses of known myelotoxins, e.g., chloramphenicol, or following the use of such drugs as phenylbutazone, methylphenylethylhydantoin, streptomycin, and chlorpromazine, which are generally without effect in other individuals. In such idiosyncratic reactions the aplasia may be severe and sometimes irreversible and fatal.

Whole-body *irradiation* is an obvious mechanism for destruction of hematopoietic stem cells. The effects of radiation are dose related. Persons at risk are those who receive therapeutic irradiation, radiologists, and individuals exposed to nuclear explosions or nuclear plant accidents.

Although aplastic anemia may appear in a variety of *infections*, it most commonly follows viral hepatitis of the non-A, non-B type.[29] Why certain individuals develop this hematologic complication in the course of their infection is not understood, but it is not related to the severity of infection. Direct injury to stem

cells could be postulated, but there are reasons for doubting such a simplistic explanation.

Fanconi's anemia is a rare familial form of aplastic anemia. In these patients the marrow hypofunction becomes evident early in life and is accompanied by multiple congenital anomalies such as hypoplasia of the kidney and spleen and hypoplastic anomalies of bone, particularly involving the thumbs or radii. Some of these individuals develop leukemia if they survive the hazards of the marrow hypofunction.

Despite all these possible causal influences, in fully 50% of the cases no provocating factor can be identified, and hence they are lumped into the *idiopathic* category.[30]

PATHOGENESIS. Although we speak of myelotoxic chemicals, drugs, and infections as causes of aplastic anemia, the precise mechanism of stem cell injury in these settings is poorly understood. Idiopathic cases are even more mysterious, and therefore numerous hypotheses have sprouted. Some of the most important clues regarding pathogenetic mechanisms have been obtained by evaluating various forms of treatment. The remarkable efficacy of bone marrow transplantation in the treatment of aplastic anemia suggests that *many cases of aplastic anemia result from defects in the number or function of stem cells.* With marrow transplants, defective stem cells are replaced by infusion of normal cells from HLA-matched donors. Because there is growing evidence that T cell–derived cytokines are intimately involved in the regulation of normal hematopoiesis,[31] much attention has focused on the possibility that marrow failure may result from immunologically mediated suppression of hematopoiesis. In support of the suppressor cell hypothesis is cited the ability of T lymphocytes from aplastic anemia patients to inhibit the in vitro growth of normal myeloid (CFU-G/M) or erythroid stem cells (BFU-E) obtained from healthy individuals.[32] The recovery of autologous marrow in some cases by administration of antilymphocyte globulin therapy is also consistent with an immunologic causation of aplastic anemia.[33]

In some patients with acquired or congenital aplastic anemia, there is subsequent development of acute leukemia. Such transformation suggests that, at least in a small proportion of cases, aplastic anemia may represent a preleukemic state.[34] Although much remains to be known, it is clear that aplastic anemia is not a single disease, but is a group of pathogenetically distinct disorders.

MORPHOLOGY. The bone marrow is markedly hypocellular and is composed largely of empty marrow spaces populated by fat cells, fibrous stroma, and scattered or clustered foci of lymphocytes and plasma cells (Fig. 14-26). In less extreme instances, scattered primitive precursor cells are found. Megakaryocytes are either absent or scant in number. A number of additional morphologic changes may accompany these marrow failures. Fatty

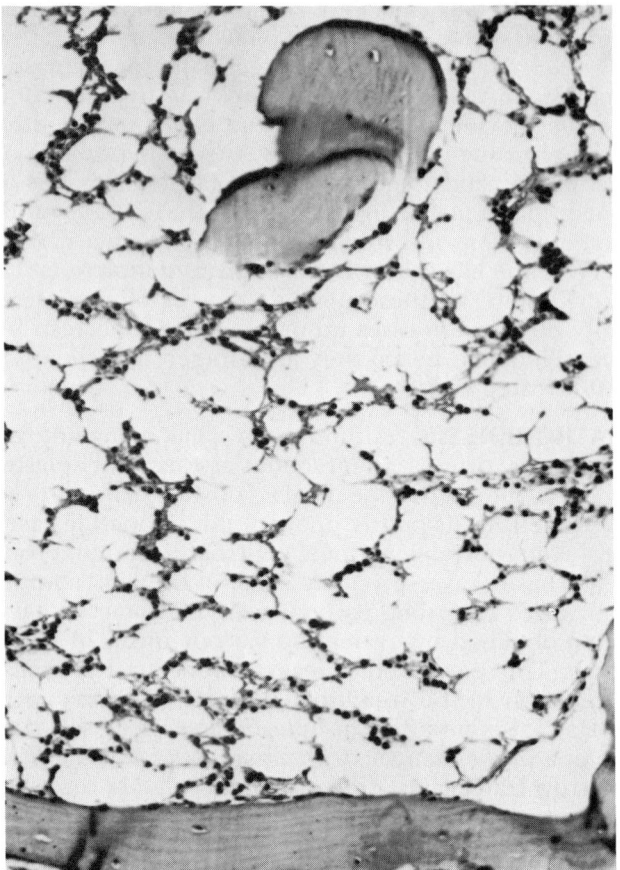

Figure 14-26. Aplastic anemia—bone marrow. The marrow is markedly hypocellular, composed largely of fat cells. (Courtesy of Dr. Robert W. McKenna, Department of Pathology, University of Texas, Southwestern Medical School, Dallas, Texas.)

changes may result from the anemia. Also evident may be the effects of bacterial infections or hemorrhagic diatheses secondary to the granulocytopenia or thrombocytopenia, respectively (p. 692). The toxic drug or agent may injure not only the bone marrow but also the liver, the kidneys, and other structures. Benzene, for example, may cause fatty changes in the liver and kidneys. In some instances, especially those with multiple transfusions, systemic hemosiderosis is present.

CLINICAL COURSE. Aplastic anemia may occur at any age and in either sex. Usually the onset is gradual, but in some cases the disorder strikes with suddenness and great severity. The initial manifestations vary somewhat, depending on the cell line predominantly affected. Anemia may cause the progressive onset of weakness, pallor, and dyspnea. Petechiae and ecchymoses may herald thrombocytopenia. Granulocytopenia may manifest itself only by frequent and persistent minor infections or by the sudden onset of chills, fever, and prostration. *Splenomegaly is characteristically absent, and if present, the diagnosis of aplastic anemia should be seriously questioned.* Typically, the red cells are normocytic and normochromic, although occasionally slight macrocytosis is present; *reticulocytosis is absent.*

The diagnosis rests upon examination of bone marrow biopsy and peripheral blood. It is important to distinguish aplastic anemia from other causes of pancytopenia, such as "aleukemic" leukemia and myelodysplastic syndromes (p. 728). Since pancytopenia is common to all these conditions, their clinical manifestations are often indistinguishable. However, with aplastic anemia the marrow is hypocellular owing to stem cell failure, whereas in leukemias and myelodysplasia the marrow is populated by abnormal and immature myeloid cells. The prognosis of marrow aplasia is quite unpredictable. As mentioned earlier, withdrawal of toxic drugs may lead to recovery in some cases. The idiopathic form has a poor prognosis. Bone marrow transplantation is an extremely effective form of therapy, especially in young (less than 40 years) patients.[35] Older patients benefit from immunosuppressive therapy with antithymocyte globulin.

Pure Red Cell Aplasia (PRCA)

Pure red cell aplasia is a rare form of marrow failure resulting from a specific aplasia of erythroid elements while granulopoiesis and thrombopoiesis remain normal.[36] It may occur in an acute form as an aplastic "crisis" during the course of some form of pre-existing hemolytic anemia or as a drug- or infectious disease–related disorder. PRCA may also appear insidiously in a chronic form, sometimes without apparent provocation, and at other times in patients having a thymoma. The latter association raises the question of some thymus-related immunologic mechanism and, indeed, in about half the patients, resection of the primary tumor is followed by hematologic improvement. Humoral or cellular autoimmunity against erythroid precursors can be demonstrated in some cases, and in such patients immunosuppressive therapy may be beneficial. In refractory cases, plasmapheresis has also been used with success.

Other Forms of Marrow Failure

Space-occupying lesions that destroy significant amounts of bone marrow or perhaps disturb the marrow architecture depress its productive capacity. This form of marrow failure is referred to as *myelophthisic anemia.* As would be anticipated, all the formed elements of the blood are concomitantly affected. However, characteristically immature forms of the red and white cells appear in the peripheral blood, a phenomenon attributed to a poorly defined "irritation effect." The most common cause of myelophthisic anemia is metastatic cancer arising from a primary lesion, most often in the breast, lung, prostate, thyroid, or adrenals. Multiple myeloma, leukemia, osteosclerosis, and lymphomas are less commonly implicated. Myelophthisic anemia has also been observed with myelofibrosis, a diffuse fibrosis of the marrow. Such cases are variants of the myeloproliferative syndrome (p. 737).

Diffuse liver disease, whether it be toxic, infectious, or a form of cirrhosis, is for obscure reasons often associated with an anemia attributed to bone marrow failure. Other contributing factors include folate deficiency and iron deficiency due to gastrointestinal blood loss (varices, hemorrhoids). In most of these instances, there is a pure erythropoietic depression and the red cells are normocytic, but if folate deficiency is significant, they are macrocytic. Depression of the white cell count and platelets has been described but is infrequent.

Chronic renal failure, whatever its cause, is almost invariably associated with anemia that tends to be roughly proportional to the severity of the uremia. The basis of the anemia is multifactorial. There is evidence of an extracorpuscular defect inducing chronic hemolysis. Some patients have an iron deficiency secondary to the bleeding tendency often encountered in uremia. Concomitantly, there is reduced red cell production, related most likely to advanced destruction of the kidneys, with inadequate formation of erythropoietin. Not surprisingly, therefore, recent trials of recombinant erythropoietin have demonstrated significant improvement of anemia in patients with renal failure.[37]

Significant chronic microbiologic infections and chronic inflammatory states such as rheumatoid arthritis and rheumatic fever are frequently associated with a mild-to-moderate normocytic normochromic anemia, although sometimes the red cells may be hypochromic and microcytic. The underlying mechanism is multifactorial. There is evidence for a hemolytic component with a shortened red cell survival time. The hemolysis may be related to nonspecific stimulation of reticuloendothelial cells. With respect to the iron metabolism, the serum iron levels are low, as is saturation of the iron-binding capacity. However, in contrast to iron deficiency, total iron-binding capacity is *reduced* (p. 688), and concomitantly, hemosiderosis is present in reticuloendothelial cells. This paradoxical combination has led to the conclusion that there is defective reutilization of iron due to some impediment in the transfer of iron from the mononuclear phagocyte system to the erythroid precursors. In many patients there also seems to be a defect in production of erythropoietin, because the levels of this factor are lower than expected for the degree of anemia. Whatever the pathophysiology of the anemia, it is reversible when the primary disease is controlled.

POLYCYTHEMIA

Polycythemia, or *erythrocytosis*, as it is sometimes referred to, denotes an increased concentration of red cells, usually with a corresponding increase in hemoglobin level. Such an increase may be *relative*, when there is hemoconcentration due to decreased plasma volume, or *absolute*, when there is an increase in total red cell mass. Relative polycythemia results from any cause of dehydration, such as deprivation of water,

Table 14–7. Pathophysiologic Classification of Polycythemia

RELATIVE	
	Reduced plasma volume (hemoconcentration)
ABSOLUTE	
Primary:	Abnormal proliferation of myeloid stem cells, normal or low erythropoietin levels (polycythemia vera)
Secondary:	Increased erythropoietin levels
	Appropriate: lung disease, high-altitude living, cyanotic heart disease
	Inappropriate: erythropoietin-secreting tumors (e.g., renal cell carcinoma, hepatoma, cerebellar hemangioblastoma)

prolonged vomiting, diarrhea, or excessive use of diuretics. It is also associated with an obscure condition of unknown etiology called stress polycythemia or Gaisböck's syndrome. *Absolute polycythemia* is said to be *primary* when the increase in red cell mass results from an intrinsic abnormality of the myeloid stem cells, and *secondary* when the red cell progenitors are normal but proliferate in response to increased levels of erythropoietin. Primary polycythemia (polycythemia vera) is one of several expressions of clonal, neoplastic proliferation of myeloid stem cells and is therefore best considered with other myeloproliferative disorders (p. 735). Secondary polycythemias may be caused by an increase in erythropoietin secretion that is physiologically appropriate or by an inappropriate (pathologic) secretion of erythropoietin (Table 14–7).

BLEEDING DISORDERS— HEMORRHAGIC DIATHESES

It is logical at this point to consider all the significant hemorrhagic disorders, whether they be related to platelet abnormalities or not. All have in common a tendency to spontaneous bleeding and excessive bleeding following trauma or a surgical procedure. Spontaneous bleeding usually takes the form of numerous small hemorrhages (petechiae, purpura) into the skin, mucous membranes, internal organs, joint spaces, or other tissues. Excessive bleeding following trauma may be triggered by such trivial provocations as bumping into the corner of a table or taking a misstep, followed by massive bleeding into the knee joint.

The causes of hemorrhagic diatheses can be divided into (1) increased fragility of vessels, (2) platelet deficiency or dysfunction, (3) derangements in the coagulation mechanism, and (4) combinations of these. Each of these categories is treated in successive sections.

HEMORRHAGIC DIATHESES RELATED TO INCREASED VASCULAR FRAGILITY

Disorders within this category, sometimes called nonthrombocytopenic purpuras, are relatively common but do not usually cause serious bleeding problems. Most often, they induce petechial and purpuric hemorrhages in the skin or mucous membranes, particularly the gingivae. On occasion, however, more significant hemorrhages may occur into joints, muscles, and subperiosteal locations or take the form of menorrhagia, nosebleeds, gastrointestinal bleeding, or hematuria. The platelet count, bleeding time, and coagulation time are usually normal. Sometimes, accompanying abnormalities in either platelet numbers or function contribute to the vascular instability by loss of the endothelial homeostatic role of platelets.

The varied clinical conditions in which hemorrhages can be related to abnormalities in the vessel wall include the following:

• *Many infections* induce petechial and purpuric hemorrhages, but especially implicated are meningococcemia, other forms of septicemia, severe measles, and several of the rickettsioses. The involved mechanism is presumably microbiologic damage (vasculitis) to the microvasculature or DIC (p. 698).
• *Drug reactions* sometimes induce abnormal bleeding. In many instances the vascular injury is mediated by the formation of drug-induced antibodies and the deposition of immune complexes in the vessel walls, with the production of a hypersensitivity (leukocytoclastic) vasculitis (p. 573).
• *Scurvy and the Ehlers-Danlos syndrome* represent examples of predisposition to hemorrhage related to impaired formation of the collagenous support of vessel walls. Essentially the same mechanism may be encountered in the very elderly, in whom atrophy of collagen is implicated. Similar is the predisposition to skin hemorrhages in *Cushing's syndrome,* in which the protein-wasting effects of excessive corticosteroid production cause loss of perivascular supporting tissue.
• *Henoch-Schönlein purpura* is a systemic hypersensitivity disease of unknown cause characterized by a purpuric rash, colicky abdominal pain (presumably due to focal hemorrhages into the gastrointestinal tract), polyarthralgia, and acute glomerulonephritis (p. 1043). All these changes are thought to result from the deposition of circulating immune complexes within vessels throughout the body and within the glomerular mesangial regions. A generalized vasculitis occurs, accompanied by an acute glomerulonephritis. With immunofluorescent techniques, deposits of IgA, C3, and fibrin can be seen within the mesangial regions of glomeruli. The trigger of the immunologic reaction is unknown, but there is some evidence suggesting activation of the alternate complement pathway because properdin is sometimes found in the glomeruli. In any event, the predisposition to hemorrhage resides in a hypersensitivity vasculitis.

In most of these conditions, the hemorrhagic diathesis does not cause massive bleeding but more often calls attention to the underlying disorder.

HEMORRHAGIC DIATHESES RELATED TO REDUCED PLATELET NUMBER: THROMBOCYTOPENIA

Reduction in platelet number constitutes an important cause of generalized bleeding. Depletion of the number of circulating platelets (thrombocytopenia) must be quite severe, to levels of the order of 10,000 to 20,000 platelets per mm^3 (normal range = 150,000 to 300,000 per mm^3) before the hemorrhagic tendency becomes clinically evident.

The important role of platelets in hemostasis was discussed in an earlier chapter (p. 95). It hardly needs reiteration that they are vital to hemostasis in that they form temporary plugs and participate in the clotting reaction. Thus, thrombocytopenia is characterized principally by bleeding, most often from small vessels. The common sites of such hemorrhage are the skin and mucous membranes of the gastrointestinal and genitourinary tracts, where the bleeding is usually associated with the development of small petechiae. Intracranial bleeding is another danger in thrombocytopenic patients with markedly depressed platelet counts.

The many causes of thrombocytopenia can be classified into the four major categories cited in Table 14–8.

A few comments about the less common causes are in order before we turn to the more common forms of thrombocytopenia. Generalized diseases of bone marrow may compromise the number of megakaryocytes. Thus, thrombocytopenia is seen in aplastic anemia and in the myelophthisic anemias related, for example, to metastatic cancer and leukemia.

Thrombocytopenia due to ineffective mega-

Table 14–8. Causes of Thrombocytopenia

I. DECREASED PRODUCTION OF PLATELETS
Generalized diseases of bone marrow
    Aplastic anemia: congenital and acquired (Table 14–6)
    Marrow infiltration: leukemia, disseminated cancer
Selective impairment of platelet production
    Drug-induced: alcohol, thiazides, cytotoxic drugs
    Infections: childhood rubella
Ineffective megakaryopoiesis
    Hereditary: Wiskott-Aldrich syndrome
    Acquired: Megaloblastic anemias

II. DECREASED PLATELET SURVIVAL
Immunologic destruction
    Autoimmune: idiopathic thrombocytopenic purpura, SLE
    Isoimmune: posttransfusion and neonatal
    Drug-associated: quinidine, heparin
    Infections: infectious mononucleosis, HIV infection
Increased consumption
    Disseminated intravascular coagulation
    Thrombotic thrombocytopenic purpura
    Giant hemangiomas
    Microangiopathic hemolytic anemias

III. SEQUESTRATION
    Hypersplenism

IV. DILUTIONAL

---

karyopoiesis may occur in Wiskott-Aldrich syndrome, a hereditary immunodeficiency state (p. 223). More commonly, this form of thrombocytopenia results from a deficiency of folate or vitamin B_{12} and is associated with ineffective erythropoiesis (p. 680).

As with hemolytic anemias, thrombocytopenia may be an acquired disorder related to increased destruction of platelets following drug ingestion or infections. The drugs most commonly involved are quinine, quinidine, methyldopa, thiazide diuretics, and heparin.[38] Immune reactions implicated in these drug reactions are essentially similar to those underlying drug-induced hemolytic anemias (p. 677). Thrombocytopenia is one of the most common hematologic manifestations of AIDS. It may occur early in the course of HIV infection and is believed to result from immune complex–mediated injury.

Just as red cells may be destroyed by *mechanical injury* in microangiopathic hemolytic anemia, so platelets may be destroyed by prosthetic heart valves, the narrowed microcirculation in malignant hypertension, and arterial disease associated with significant roughening of the endothelial surface.

Thrombocytopenia may appear unpredictably in any patient who has marked splenomegaly, or what has been referred to as *hypersplenism* (p. 749). Normally the spleen sequesters 30 to 40% of the mass of circulating platelets and, when enlarged, sequestrates as much as 90% of all platelets. Should the thrombocytopenia constitute an important part of the clinical problem, it can be cured by splenectomy.

Massive *transfusions* may produce a dilutional thrombocytopenia. Blood stored for longer than 24 hours contains virtually no viable platelets; thus, plasma volume and red cell mass are reconstituted by transfusion, but the number of circulating platelets is relatively reduced.

All these forms of thrombocytopenia are uncommon, compared with the following conditions.

Neonatal and Post-transfusion (Isoimmune) Thrombocytopenia

Both these disorders are examples of the development of antibodies directed against a specific platelet isoantigen. In addition to HLA and ABO antigens, platelets possess several antigenic determinants not present in other blood cells.[39] These include the Duzo, PL, and Bak antigen systems. Neonatal thrombocytopenia develops in a fashion exactly parallel to the hemolytic reaction in erythroblastosis fetalis (p. 527). A PL^{A1} antigen–negative mother carrying an antigen-positive fetus develops IgG antibodies against the PL^{A1} antigen, and the resulting antibodies cross the placenta to cause thrombocytopenia in the newborn. Anti-PL^{A1} antibodies are also believed to be responsible for the purpura associated with post-transfusional thrombocytopenia. In most cases the patient is PL^{A1}-negative and has been sensitized to PL^{A1}-positive blood by either a previous transfusion or pregnancy. When transfused with blood containing PL^{A1}-positive platelets, the anti-PL^{A1} antibody present in the recipient destroys not only the transfused PL^{A1}-positive platelets but also the autologous PL^{A1}-negative platelets, giving rise to thrombocytopenia. How the patient's own PL^{A1}-negative platelets are destroyed is not clear.

Idiopathic Thrombocytopenic Purpura (ITP)

There is a growing tendency to refer to ITP as autoimmune thrombocytopenia. However, the designation "idiopathic" seems more appropriate because it is not certain that the platelet destruction in all cases is autoimmune in origin. Nevertheless, there is general agreement that the thrombocytopenia is mediated by immunologic mechanisms, involving in most cases humoral antibodies or antigen-antibody complexes. Traditionally, ITP has been divided into acute and chronic forms, both of which are associated with increased platelet destruction and normal or increased megakaryocytes in the bone marrow. However, the pathogenesis of reduced platelet survival in the acute and chronic forms is probably quite distinct.

Acute ITP is a self-limited disorder seen most often in children following a viral infection, e.g., rubella, cytomegalovirus infection, viral hepatitis, and infectious mononucleosis. It is assumed without definite proof that the infection in some way stimulates an immune response that leads to platelet destruction. It may well be that antigen-antibody complexes directed against the virus are adsorbed onto platelets, predisposing to phagocytosis in the mononuclear phagocyte system. Thus, unlike chronic ITP (discussed below), acute ITP as currently understood does not represent direct antiplatelet, antibody-mediated thrombocytopenia.

Chronic ITP occurs most often in adults, particularly in women of childbearing age. It may appear as a primary disease but sometimes is associated with another immunologic disorder such as autoimmune hemolytic anemia or SLE, or occasionally with some form of lymphoproliferative disease.[40]

PATHOGENESIS. There is a great deal of indirect evidence that most patients with chronic ITP have autoantibodies directed against platelets:[41] (1) Infants born to mothers with ITP are often thrombocytopenic; (2) the plasma of patients with ITP causes a rapid fall in platelet count when transfused into normal recipients; (3) the serum factor responsible for thrombocytopenia can be localized to the IgG fraction of plasma and absorbed specifically to human platelets; (4) normal platelets are rapidly destroyed when administered to patients with ITP; and (5) ITP is sometimes encountered in patients with other forms of autoimmune disease such as SLE, autoimmune thyroiditis, and others. Nonetheless, direct evidence for the presence of circulating autoantibodies has been difficult to obtain, since conventional techniques for antibody detection, such as agglutination, are not easily adaptable for detection of antiplatelet antibodies. With some recently introduced refinements, however, it has been possible to detect and quantitate *platelet-associated immunoglobulins (PAIgG)*, which are elevated in more than 90% of the patients with ITP. More important, the levels of **PAIgG** are inversely related to the platelet count and the platelet survival, suggesting a pathogenetic role for these antibodies.[42] *However, it should be pointed out that the detection of PAIgG in a patient with thrombocytopenia does not necessarily imply that the platelets are coated by autoantibodies.* In certain clinical settings (e.g., drug-induced thrombocytopenia), the **PAIgG** may represent IgG-containing immune complexes bound to the platelet surface through its Fc-IgG receptor.

The exact nature of platelet antigens against which autoantibodies are formed in ITP has not been determined, nor is it clear what triggers autoantibody formation. One or more of the factors discussed previously in the general discussion of autoimmunity may be relevant (p. 190).

The mechanism of platelet destruction is similar to that seen in autoimmune hemolytic anemias (p. 677). Opsonized platelets are rendered susceptible to phagocytosis by the cells of the mononuclear phagocytic system. Lysis by complement fixation seems not to play a major role. About 75 to 80% of patients are remarkably improved or sometimes cured following splenectomy, which suggests that the spleen is the major site of removal of sensitized platelets. Since it is also the major site of autoantibody synthesis, the beneficial effects of splenectomy may in part derive from removal of the source of autoantibodies. Although destruction of sensitized platelets is the major mechanism of thrombocytopenia, there is some evidence that megakaryocytes may be attacked as well, since some antiplatelet antibodies also react with megakaryocytes.[43] In most cases, however, the megakaryocyte injury is not significant enough to deplete their numbers.

MORPHOLOGY. The principal morphologic lesions of thrombocytopenic purpura are found in the spleen and bone marrow. The secondary changes related to the bleeding diathesis may be found in any tissue or structure in the body.

The **spleen** is normal in size. Histologically, there is congestion of the sinusoids and hyperactivity and enlargement of the splenic follicles, manifested by the formation of prominent germinal centers. In many instances, megakaryocytes are found within the sinuses and sinusoidal walls. However, in most cases of thrombocytopenic purpura the splenic findings are not distinctive, and in all instances can hardly be considered as pathognomonic of this disorder.

The alterations in the bone marrow are equally disappointing. Most often the bone marrow appears quite normal and contains the usual numbers and types of erythropoietic and leukopoietic cells. An increased number of megakaryocytes is usually seen. Some are apparently immature with large, nonlobulated, single nuclei. These findings are not characteristic of ITP but merely represent accelerated thrombopoiesis. As such, they are seen in most forms of thrombocytopenia resulting from increased platelet destruction. The importance of the bone marrow examination is to rule out thrombocytopenias resulting from bone marrow failure. A decrease in the number of megakaryocytes virtually rules out the diagnosis of ITP.

The secondary changes relate to the hemorrhages that are dispersed throughout the body. The skin, serosal linings of the body cavities, epicardium and endocardium, lungs, and mucosal lining of the urinary tract are favorite sites for such petechial and ecchymotic hemorrhage (Fig. 14–27). Hemorrhages are also prone to occur in the brain, joint spaces, nasopharynx, and gastrointestinal tract.

The clinical manifestations of this disease are quite variable. Occasionally, the disease begins with a sudden shower of petechial hemorrhages into the skin without apparent antecedent injury or disease. More frequently, there is a long history of easy bruising, nosebleeds, bleeding from the gums, and extensive hemorrhages into soft tissues from relatively minor trauma. Also, the disease may become manifest first by the appearance of melena, hematuria, or excessive menstrual flow. Subarachnoid hemorrhages and intracerebral hemorrhages are serious consequences of thrombocytopenic purpura, but are fortunately rare

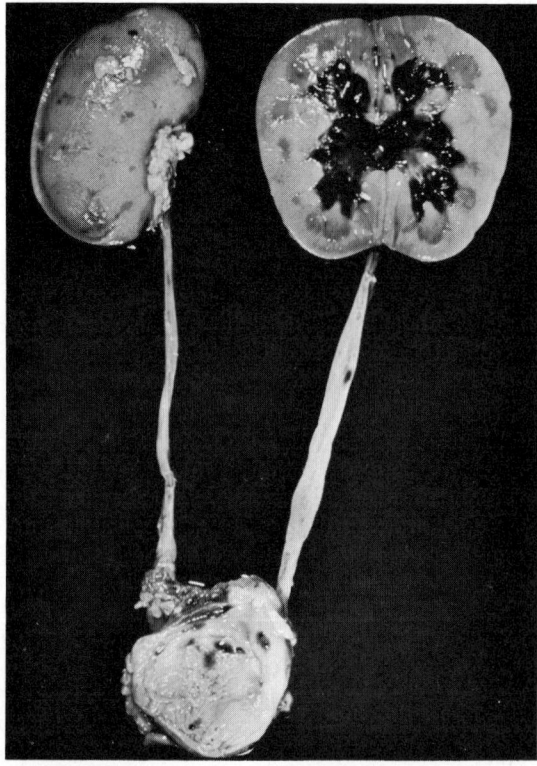

Figure 14–27. Thrombocytopenic purpura. Urinary tract with intrapelvic hemorrhages in kidneys and focal mucosal hemorrhages in urinary bladder.

in patients treated with steroids. Splenomegaly and lymphadenopathy are extremely uncommon in ITP, and their presence should lead one to consider other possible diagnoses.

The diagnosis can be only suspected by clinical features and must be supported by demonstration of thrombocytopenia with normal or increased mega-karyocytes in the bone marrow. Accelerated thrombopoiesis also leads to the formation of abnormally large platelets (megathrombocytes) detected easily in a blood smear. The prolongation of the bleeding time and the normal or relatively normal clotting time confirm the presence of thrombocytopenia. *A diagnosis of ITP, however, should be made only after all the possible known causes for platelet deficiencies, such as those listed in Table 14–8, have been ruled out.*

Thrombotic Thrombocytopenic Purpura (TTP)

This rare disorder of obscure nature is characterized mainly by *thrombocytopenia, microangiopathic hemolytic anemia, fever, transient neurologic deficits, and renal failure.*[44] Underlying most of these clinical manifestations are widespread hyaline microthrombi in the arterioles and capillaries, throughout all organs and tissues in the body. The intravascular thrombi are composed primarily of dense aggregates of platelets that are surrounded by fibrin.

The condition occurs more commonly in females than in males, with a peak incidence in the fourth decade. At one time it was regarded as almost invariably fatal, but it is now clear that with appropriate therapy (corticosteroids, platelet aggregation inhibitors, and, most recently, exchange transfusions) many patients survive.

The pathogenesis of this disorder is still a puzzle.[45] Unlike DIC (p. 698), activation of the clotting sequence is not of primary importance. There are suggestions that TTP is immunologically mediated. Complement components and immunoglobulins can sometimes be demonstrated in the vascular lesions. An IgG antibody cytotoxic for cultured human endothelial cells has also been reported in some cases. Thus, it has been proposed that this condition involves, for still unknown reasons, an immunologic reaction against endothelial cells predisposing to the aggregation of platelets. Alternatively, it has been proposed that the primary defect is formation of platelet aggregates in the circulation, which then lodge in the microcirculation. It is postulated that these patients synthesize a novel platelet agglutinating protein or abnormal forms of factor VIII–von Willebrand complex, which cause pathologic aggregation of platelets. This complex, as discussed later, is normally involved in the interaction of platelets with the subendothelial tissues (p. 696). A deficiency of prostacyclin, which normally prevents platelet aggregation, has also been suggested. At our present state of ignorance we can probe no farther into the pathogenesis of this condition. Only two facts seem reason-ably clear: The development of myriad platelet aggregates induces the *thrombocytopenia,* and the intravascular thrombi provide a rational explanation for a *microangiopathic form of hemolytic anemia* and organ dysfunctions resulting from widespread microvascular occlusions. These clinicopathologic features are shared by two closely related conditions, the hemolytic-uremic syndrome (p. 1069) and DIC (p. 698). Although the three may have diverse etiologies and somewhat differing patterns of organ involvement, common to all of them is widespread occlusion of the microvasculature due to deranged hemostasis.

HEMORRHAGIC DIATHESES RELATED TO DEFECTIVE PLATELET FUNCTIONS

Qualitative defects of platelet function may be congenital or acquired. Several congenital disorders characterized by prolonged bleeding time and normal platelet count have been described. The significance of these rare diseases lies mainly in the fact that they provide excellent model systems for investigating the molecular mechanisms of platelet functions.[46] On the basis of the predominant functional abnormality, congenital disorders of platelet function may be classified into three groups: (1) *defects of adhesion,* (2) *defects of aggregation,* and (3) *disorders of platelet secretion (release reaction).*

• Bleeding resulting from defective adhesion of platelets to the subendothelial collagen is best illustrated by the autosomal recessive *Bernard-Soulier syndrome.* In this disorder there is an inherited deficiency of a platelet membrane glycoprotein (GPIb) that is required for platelet-collagen interaction.
• Bleeding due to *defective platelet aggregation* is exemplified by *thrombasthenia,* which is also transmitted as an autosomal recessive trait. Thrombasthenic platelets fail to aggregate with ADP, collagen, epinephrine, or thrombin, possibly owing to a deficiency of two membrane glycoproteins (GPIIb and GPIIIa) that are involved in binding fibrinogen. In normal platelets these glycoproteins favor aggregation, presumably by creating fibrinogen "bridges" between adjacent platelets (Fig. 3–8, p. 97).
• *Disorders of platelet secretion* are characterized by normal initial aggregation with collagen or ADP, but the subsequent responses, such as secretion of prostaglandins and release of granule-bound ADP, are impaired. The underlying biochemical defects are varied, complex, and beyond the scope of our discussion.

Among the *acquired defects* of platelet function, two are clinically significant.[47] The first is related to ingestion of aspirin, which may significantly prolong the bleeding time. As you may recall, aspirin is a potent inhibitor of the enzyme cyclooxygenase and can suppress the synthesis of prostaglandins (p. 55), which are known to be involved in platelet aggregation and the subsequent platelet release reaction (p.

95). The antiplatelet effect of aspirin forms the basis of its use in the management of recurrent myocardial infarction (p. 614). In approximately 10% of healthy normal subjects, ingestion of even 1 gm of aspirin may prolong the bleeding time significantly and lead to increased bruisability. Clinically, significant postoperative oozing may occur in such patients if aspirin is used as an analgesic. It is suspected that these individuals have minor platelet function defects that are magnified by the intake of aspirin. *Uremia* (p. 1016) is the other condition that exemplifies an acquired defect in platelet functions. Although the pathogenesis of bleeding in uremia is complex and poorly understood, several abnormalities of platelet function have been found.[48]

HEMORRHAGIC DIATHESES RELATED TO ABNORMALITIES IN CLOTTING FACTORS

A deficiency of every one of the known clotting factors has been reported at one time or another as the cause of a bleeding disorder. The bleeding in these conditions differs somewhat from that encountered in platelet deficiencies. The apparent spontaneous appearance of petechiae or purpura is uncommon. More often the bleeding manifests as the development of large ecchymoses or hematomas following an injury, or as prolonged bleeding after a laceration or any form of surgical procedure. Bleeding into the gastrointestinal and urinary tracts, and particularly into weight-bearing joints, is a common manifestation. Typical stories describe the patient who continues to ooze for days following a tooth extraction or who develops a hemarthrosis after a relatively trivial stress on a knee joint. History may well have been changed by the presence of a hereditary coagulation defect in the intermarried royal families of Great Britain and Europe. Clotting abnormalities may occur as acquired defects, or, as mentioned, be hereditary in origin.

Acquired disorders are usually characterized by multiple clotting abnormalities. Vitamin K deficiency (p. 448) results in depressed synthesis of factors II, VII, IX, and X and protein C. Since the liver makes virtually all the clotting factors, severe parenchymal liver disease may be associated with a hemorrhagic diathesis. DIC (p. 698) produces a deficiency of multiple coagulation factors.

Hereditary deficiencies have been identified for each of the clotting factors. Deficiencies of factor VIII (classic hemophilia) and of factor IX (Christmas disease) are transmitted as sex-linked recessive disorders. Most of the others follow autosomal patterns of transmission. *Typically, these hereditary disorders involve a single clotting factor.*

The details of the diagnostic tests used to identify the specific clotting factor deficiency are beyond our scope and are readily available in specialized texts. In most cases, four screening procedures will localize the hemostatic abnormality: (1) bleeding time, (2) platelet count, (3) the prothrombin time, and (4) the partial thromboplastin time. Against this background we can turn to the more common of the coagulation disorders.

Deficiencies of Factor VIII-vWF Complex

Hemophilia and von Willebrand's disease, two of the most common inherited disorders of bleeding, are caused by qualitative or quantitative defects involving factor VIII-vWF complex. Before we can discuss these disorders it is essential to review the structure and function of factor VIII.[49,50]

Plasma factor VIII-vWF is a complex made up of two separate proteins (factor VIII and vWF factor) *that can be distinguished by functional, biochemical, and immunologic criteria.* One component, which is required for the activation of factor X in the intrinsic coagulation pathway, is called *factor VIII procoagulant protein,* or *factor VIII* (Fig. 14–28). Deficiency of factor VIII gives rise to classic hemophilia (hemophilia A). Through noncovalent bonds, factor VIII is linked to a much larger protein called the *von Willebrand's factor* (vWF). The latter, which forms approximately 99% of the complex, is not a discrete protein but exists in the form of a series of multimers that range in size from 4×10^5 to 12×10^6 daltons. *The most important function of vWF in vivo is to facilitate the adhesion of platelets to subendothelial collagen.* The vWF is crucial to the normal process of hemostasis (p. 94), and its absence in von Willebrand's disease leads to a bleeding diathesis. von Willebrand's factor can be assayed by immunologic techniques or by the so-called *ristocetin aggregation test.* Ristocetin (once used as an antibiotic) binds to platelets in vitro and activates vWF receptors on their surface. This leads to platelet aggregation if vWF is available to "bridge" the platelets (Fig. 14–28). Thus ristocetin-induced platelet aggregation can be used as a bioassay for vWF.

The two components of factor VIII-vWF complex are coded by separate genes and are synthesized by different cells. The vWF is produced by endothelial cells and megakaryocytes. It can be demonstrated in platelet granules. Factor VIII can be synthesized by several tissues, but in the absence of liver disease, hepatocytes are the major source of this protein.[50a] To summarize, *the two components of factor VIII-vWF complex, synthesized separately, come together and circulate in the plasma as a unit that serves to promote clotting as well as platelet–vessel wall interactions necessary to ensure hemostasis.* With this background we can discuss the diseases resulting from deficiencies of factor VIII-vWF complex.

von Willebrand's Disease

von Willebrand's disease is characterized clinically by spontaneous bleeding from mucous membranes, excessive bleeding from wounds, menorrhagia, and a prolonged bleeding time in the presence of *a normal platelet count.* In most cases it is transmitted as an autosomal dominant disorder, but several rare autosomal recessive variants have been identified.[51] Its

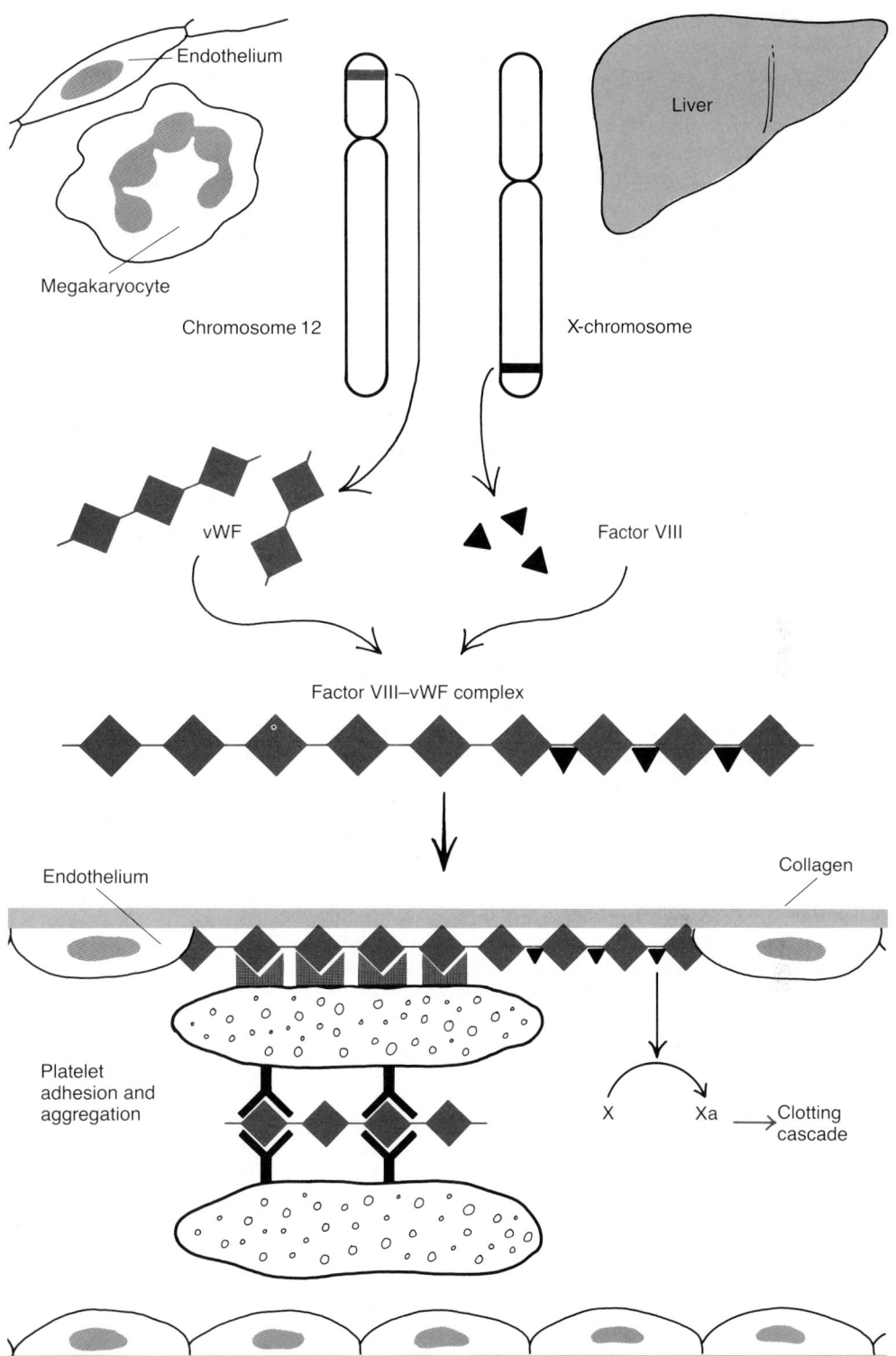

Figure 14-28. Synthesis, subunit structure, and functions of factor VIII-von Willebrand complex. von Willebrand's factor (vWF) is synthesized by endothelial cells and megakaryocytes; the vWF gene is located on chromosome 12. Factor VIII is synthesized in the liver and is encoded by a gene on the X-chromosome. vWF causes adhesion of platelets to the subendothelial collagen and promotes platelet aggregation. The adhesion and aggregation are mediated by two distinct receptors for vWF on platelets. Factor VIII takes part in the activation of factor X in the coagulation cascade.

precise incidence is difficult to estimate because in many instances the clinical manifestations are mild and variable, and the diagnosis requires sophisticated tests; thus the condition may pass unrecognized.

Without delving into great complexities, we can state that the *classic and most common variant (type I) of von Willebrand's disease is characterized by a re-*

duced quantity of circulating vWF. The synthesis of vWF is not impaired, but the release of vWF multimers is inhibited by some unknown mechanism. In the less common type II variant, multimer assembly is defective and hence the large and intermediate multimers, representing the most active form of vWF, are missing from plasma. Quite unexpectedly, levels of factor VIII, the procoagulant component of factor VIII-vWF complex, are also reduced in von Willebrand's disease. Even more curious is the observation that infusion of factor VIII–deficient (hemophilic) plasma (that contains vWF) causes an increase in the level of procoagulant activity. There is no satisfactory explanation for these findings, but it is suggested that vWF either protects factor VIII from degradation by acting as a "carrier," or in some way influences its synthesis or release. *To summarize, patients with von Willebrand's disease have a compound defect involving platelet function and the coagulation pathway.* However, except in the most severely affected (e.g., homozygous) patients, effects of factor VIII deficiency such as bleeding into the joints, which characterize hemophilia, are uncommon.

Factor VIII Deficiency (Hemophilia A, Classic Hemophilia)

This disease is caused by a reduced amount or activity of factor VIII. It is inherited as an X-linked recessive trait, and thus it occurs in males or in homozygous females. However, excessive bleeding has been described in heterozygous females, presumably caused by extremely "unfavorable lyonization" (inactivation of the normal X chromosome in most of the cells). The clinical syndrome develops only in the presence of severe deficiency (factor VIII levels less than 1% of normal). Mild or moderate degrees of deficiency (levels between 1 and 25% of normal) occur but are asymptomatic, although post-traumatic bleeding may be somewhat excessive. The variable degrees of deficiency in the level of factor VIII procoagulant are related to the type of mutation in the factor VIII gene. As with thalassemias, several genetic lesions (deletions, creation of stop codons, splicing errors) have been documented.[12] To add to the complexities, in about 10% of patients with hemophilia, levels of factor VIII appear normal by immunoassay, but the coagulant activity detected by bioassay is low. It is likely that in these patients a mutation causes the synthesis of an antigenically normal but nonfunctional protein. In any event, in all symptomatic cases there is a tendency toward massive hemorrhage following trauma or operative procedures. In addition, "spontaneous" hemorrhages are frequently encountered in regions of the body normally subject to trauma, particularly the joints, where they are known as hemarthroses. Recurrent bleeding into the joints leads to progressive deformities that may be crippling. *Petechiae and ecchymoses are characteristically absent. Although coagulation time is prolonged, bleeding time is normal.* At one time, about 50% of severely affected patients died before the age of five years. However, the recent use of factor VIII concentrates has substantially improved the prognosis.

Replacement therapy, however, is not an unalloyed blessing. It carries with it the risk of transmission of viral hepatitis. Until the mid-1980s, before routine screening of blood for HIV antibodies was instituted, thousands of hemophiliacs received factor VIII concentrates containing HIV. Many have subsequently developed AIDS (p. 225). With the current practice of using heat-treated factor VIII concentrates derived from the blood of HIV-seronegative donors, the risk of HIV transmission has been virtually eliminated. Although the gene for factor VIII has been cloned, genetically engineered factor VIII is not yet available for replacement therapy. A more immediate use of cloned factor VIII gene is for antenatal detection of carriers and affected individuals by utilizing RFLPs or oligonucleotide probes (p. 157).

Factor IX Deficiency (Christmas Disease, Hemophilia B)

Severe factor IX deficiency is a disorder that is clinically indistinguishable from hemophilia A. Moreover, it is also inherited as an X-linked recessive trait and may occur asymptomatically or with associated hemorrhage. In about 14% of these patients, factor IX is present but nonfunctional. *The coagulation time is prolonged; bleeding time is normal.* Identification of Christmas disease (named after the first patient with this condition and not the holy day) is possible only by assay of the factor levels.

DISSEMINATED INTRAVASCULAR COAGULATION (DIC)

Disseminated intravascular coagulation is an acute, subacute, or chronic thrombohemorrhagic disorder occurring as a secondary complication in a variety of diseases. It is characterized by activation of the coagulation sequence that leads to the formation of microthrombi throughout the microcirculation of the body, but often in a quixotically uneven distribution. Sometimes the coagulopathy is localized to a specific organ or tissue. *As a consequence of the thrombotic diathesis, there is consumption of platelets, fibrin, and coagulation factors and, secondarily, activation of fibrinolytic mechanisms* (p. 98). Thus, DIC may present with signs and symptoms relating to tissue hypoxia, and infarction caused by the myriad microthrombi, or as a hemorrhagic disorder related to depletion of the elements required for hemostasis (hence the term *consumption coagulopathy* is sometimes used to describe DIC). Activation of the fibrinolytic mechanism aggravates the hemorrhagic diathesis. Because of the consumption and secondary lysis of fibrin, DIC is also called *defibrination syndrome.*

ETIOLOGY AND PATHOGENESIS. At the outset it must be emphasized that DIC is not a primary disease. It is a coagulopathy that occurs in the course of a variety of clinical conditions. In discussing the general mechanisms underlying DIC, it would be useful to review briefly the normal process of blood coagulation and clot removal discussed earlier (p. 97). It suffices here to recall that clotting may be initiated by either of two pathways: (1) the *extrinsic pathway,* which is triggered by the release of tissue factor ("tis-

Table 14-9. Major Disorders Associated with DIC

OBSTETRIC COMPLICATIONS
Abruptio placentae
Retained dead fetus
Septic abortion
Amniotic fluid embolism
Toxemia

INFECTIONS
Gram-negative sepsis
Meningococcemia
Rocky Mountain spotted fever
Histoplasmosis
Aspergillosis
Malaria

NEOPLASMS
Carcinomas of pancreas, prostate, lung, and stomach
Acute promyelocytic leukemia

MASSIVE TISSUE INJURY
Traumatic
Burns
Extensive surgery

MISCELLANEOUS
Acute intravascular hemolysis, snakebite, giant hemangioma, shock, heat stroke, vasculitis, aortic aneurysm, liver disease

sue thromboplastin"); and (2) the *intrinsic pathway*, which involves the activation of factor XII by surface contact with collagen or other negatively charged substances. Both pathways, through a series of intermediate steps, result in the generation of thrombin, which in turn converts fibrinogen to fibrin. This process is regulated by *clot-inhibiting influences*, which include the activation of fibrinolysis involving generation of plasmin, and the clearance of activated clotting factors by the mononuclear phagocyte system or by the liver. From this brief review, it may be concluded that DIC may result from pathologic activation of the extrinsic and/or intrinsic pathways of coagulation or impairment of clot-inhibiting influences. Since the latter rarely constitute primary mechanisms of DIC, we will focus our attention on the abnormal initiation of clotting.[52]

There are two major mechanisms by which DIC may be triggered: (1) release of tissue factor or thromboplastic substances into the circulation; (2) widespread injury to the endothelial cells. Tissue factors initiate the extrinsic pathway and may be derived from a variety of sources, such as placenta in obstetric complications (Table 14-9) and the granules of leukemic cells in acute promyelocytic leukemia (p. 727). Mucus released from certain adenocarcinomas can also act as a thromboplastic substance by directly activating factor X, independent of factor VII. In gram-negative sepsis, bacterial endotoxins can cause release of thromboplastic substances contained within endothelial cells, and the lysosomes of granulocytes and monocytes. Endothelial injury, the other major trigger, can initiate DIC by causing release of tissue factor, promoting platelet aggregation, and by activating the intrinsic coagulation pathway. Widespread endothelial injury may be produced by deposition of antigen-antibody complexes (e.g., SLE), temperature

extremes (e.g., heat stroke, burns), or microorganisms (e.g., meningococci, rickettsiae).

Several disorders associated with DIC are listed in Table 14-9. Of these, DIC is most likely to follow *obstetric complications, malignancy, sepsis,* and *major trauma.* The initiating factors in these conditions are often multiple and interrelated. For example, in *infections,* particularly those caused by gram-negative bacteria, endotoxins released by the bacteria may activate both the intrinsic and the extrinsic pathways by producing endothelial cell injury and release of thromboplastins from inflammatory cells; furthermore, endotoxins inhibit the anticoagulant activity of protein C by suppressing thrombomodulin expression on endothelium.[53] Endothelial cell damage may also be produced directly by meningococci, rickettsiae, and viruses. Antigen-antibody complexes formed during the infection can activate the classic complement pathway, and the complement fragments can secondarily activate both platelets and granulocytes. Endotoxins as well as other bacterial products are also capable of directly activating factor XII. In *massive trauma, extensive surgery,* and *severe burns,* the major mechanism of DIC is believed to be autoinfusion of tissue thromboplastins. In *obstetric* conditions thromboplastins derived from the placenta, dead retained fetus, or amniotic fluid may enter the circulation. However, hypoxia, acidosis, and shock, which often coexist with the surgical and obstetric conditions, can also cause widespread endothelial injury. Supervening infection may complicate the problems further. Among *cancers,* acute promyelocytic leukemia and carcinomas of the lung, pancreas, colon, and stomach are most frequently associated with DIC. These tumors are associated with the release of a variety of thromboplastic substances including tissue factors, proteolytic enzymes, mucin, and other undefined tumor products.

The consequences of DIC are twofold. First, there is widespread deposition of fibrin within the microcirculation. This may lead to ischemia of the more severely affected or more vulnerable organs, and to a hemolytic anemia resulting from fragmentation of red cells as they squeeze through the narrowed microvasculature (microangiopathic hemolytic anemia, p. 678). Second, a hemorrhagic diathesis may dominate the clinical picture. This results from consumption of platelets and clotting factors as well as activation of plasminogen. Plasmin not only can cleave fibrin but can also digest factors V and VIII, thereby reducing their concentration further. In addition, fibrinolysis leads to the formation of fibrin degradation products, which inhibit platelet aggregation and fibrin polymerization, and have antithrombin activity. All these influences lead to the hemostatic failure seen in DIC (Fig. 14-29).

MORPHOLOGY. In general, thrombi are found in the following sites in decreasing order of frequency: brain, heart, lungs, kidneys, adrenals, spleen, and liver.[54] How-

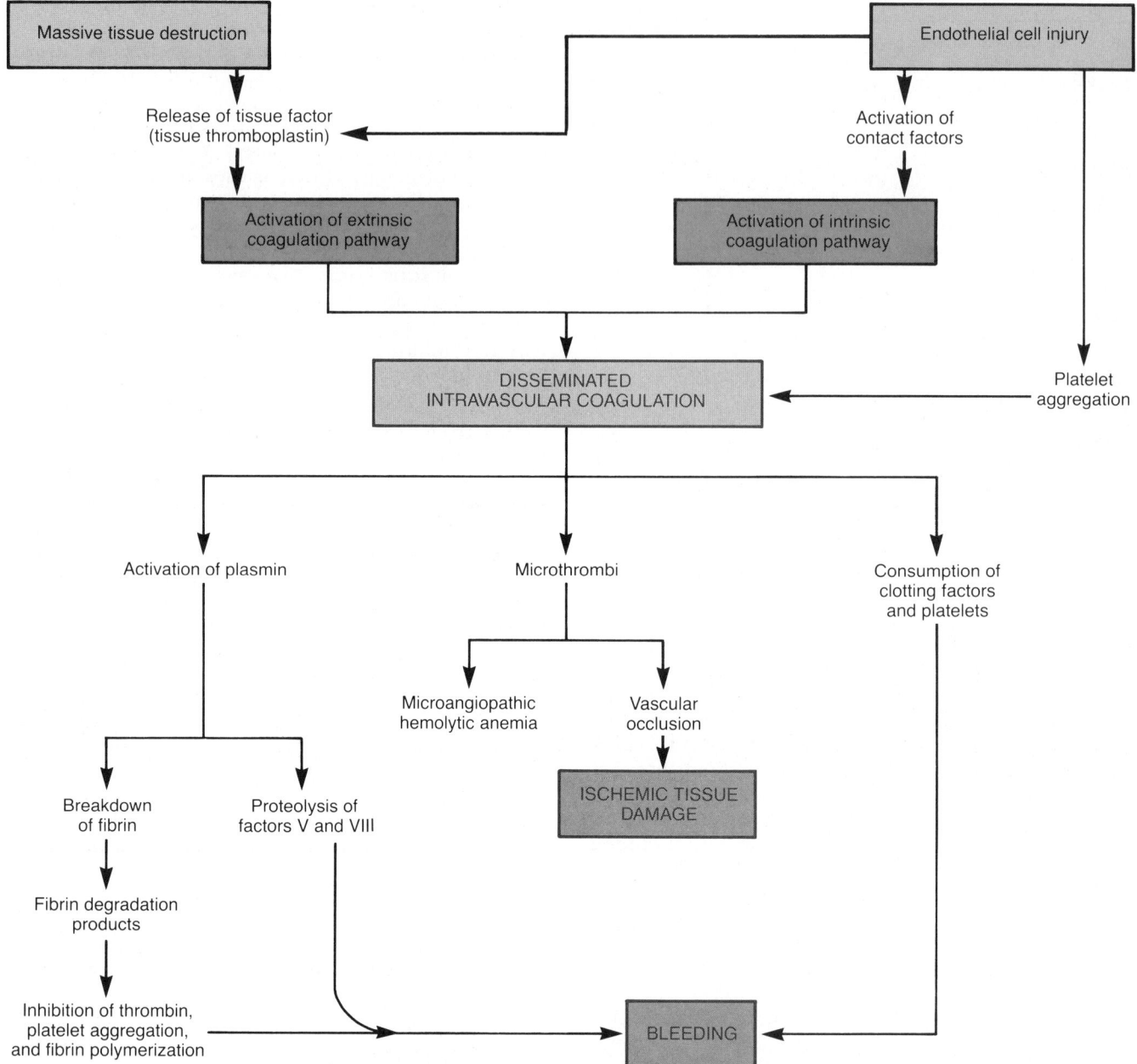

Figure 14–29. Pathophysiology of disseminated intravascular coagulation.

ever, no tissue is spared, and occasionally thrombi are found in only one or several organs without affecting others. In giant hemangiomas, for example, they are localized to the neoplasm. In this condition they are believed to result from local stasis and recurrent trauma to the poorly supported blood vessels.[55] The affected kidneys may reveal small thrombi in the glomeruli (Fig. 14–30) that may evoke only a reactive swelling of endothelial cells; however, in severe cases, microinfarcts or even bilateral renal cortical necrosis may result. Numerous fibrin thrombi may be found in the alveolar capillaries, sometimes associated with pulmonary edema and exudation of fibrin, to create "hyaline membranes" reminiscent of ARDS (p. 760). In the central

nervous system, microinfarcts may be caused by the fibrin thrombi, occasionally complicated by simultaneous fresh hemorrhage. Such changes are the basis for the bizarre neurologic signs and symptoms sometimes observed in this syndrome. Microthrombi may appear in the myocardium, but only rarely are they associated with infarction. The manifestations of DIC in the endocrine glands are of considerable interest. In meningococcemia, the massive adrenal hemorrhages of the Waterhouse-Friderichsen syndrome (p. 1253) are probably related to fibrin thrombi within the microcirculation of the adrenal cortex. Similarly, Sheehan's post-partum pituitary necrosis (p. 1211) may be one of the expressions of DIC. In toxemia of pregnancy (p.

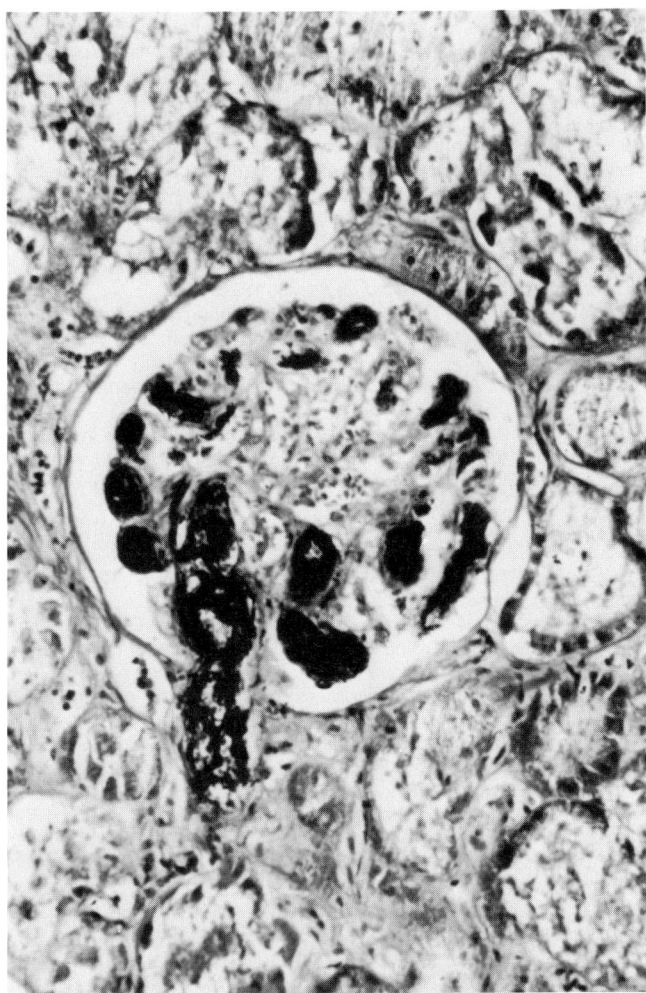

Figure 14-30. Disseminated intravascular coagulation. An affected glomerulus shows multiple darkly stained thrombi. (Courtesy of Dr. Patrick Ward, Department of Pathology and Laboratory Medicine, University of Minnesota School of Medicine, Duluth, Minnesota.)

1172), the placenta exhibits widespread microthrombi, providing a plausible explanation for the premature atrophy of the cytotrophoblast and syncytiotrophoblast encountered in this condition.

The bleeding manifestations of DIC are not dissimilar to those encountered in the hereditary and acquired disorders affecting the hemostatic mechanism discussed above.

CLINICAL COURSE. The onset may be fulminating, as in endotoxic shock or amniotic fluid embolism, or it may be insidious and chronic, as in cases of carcinomatosis or retention of a dead fetus. Overall, about 50% of individuals with DIC are obstetric patients having complications of pregnancy. In this setting, the disorder tends to be reversible with delivery of the fetus. About 33% of the patients have carcinomatosis. The remaining cases are associated with the varied entities previously listed.

It is almost impossible to detail all the potential clinical presentations, but a few common patterns may be cited. A microangiopathic hemolytic anemia may appear. Respiratory symptoms such as dyspnea, cyanosis, and extreme respiratory difficulty may predominate. Neurologic signs and symptoms represent another pattern including convulsions and coma. Renal changes such as oliguria and acute renal failure may dominate. Circulatory failure and shock may appear suddenly or develop progressively. In general, *acute DIC, associated for example with obstetric complications or major trauma, is dominated by bleeding diathesis, whereas chronic DIC such as may occur in a patient with cancer tends to present initially with thrombotic complications.* Accurate clinical observation and laboratory studies are necessary for the diagnosis. It is usually necessary to monitor the following: fibrinogen, platelets, prothrombin time, thrombin time, partial thromboplastin time, and fibrin degradation products.

The prognosis is highly variable and depends, to a considerable extent, on the underlying disorder. The management of these cases requires meticulous maneuvering between the Scylla of the thrombotic tendency and the Charybdis of the bleeding diathesis. Thus is posed the dilemma of whether to attempt to block coagulation or to control bleeding by the administration of coagulants. Each patient must be treated individually and, depending on the clinical picture, potent anticoagulants such as heparin and antithrombin III or coagulants in the form of fresh-frozen plasma may be administered. Platelet transfusions may sometimes be necessary. DIC is another of the therapeutist's nightmares.

1. Spangrude, G.J., et al.: Purification and characterization of mouse hematopoietic stem cells. Science *241*:58, 1988.

2. Neinhuis, A.W.: Hematopoietic growth factors. Biologic complexity and clinical practice. N. Engl. J. Med. *318*:916, 1988.

3. Wintrobe, M.M., et al.: Clinical Hematology. 8th ed. Philadelphia, Lea & Febiger, 1981.

4. Lux, S.E.: Disorders of red cell membrane. *In* Nathan, D.G., and Oski, F.A. (eds.): Hematology of Infancy and Childhood. 3rd ed. Philadelphia, W.B. Saunders Co., 1987.

5. Becker, P.S., and Lux, S.E.: Hereditary spherocytosis and related disorders. Clin. Hematol. *14*:15, 1985.

6. Valentine, W.N., et al.: Hemolytic anemias and erythrocyte enzymopathies. Ann. Intern. Med. *103*:425, 1985.

7. Embury, S.H.: The clinical pathophysiology of sickle cell disease. Annu. Rev. Med. *37*:361, 1986.

8. Schecter, A.N., et al.: Sickle cell disease. *In* Stamatoyannopoulos, G., et al. (eds.): Molecular Basis of Blood Diseases. Philadelphia, W.B. Saunders Co., 1987, p. 179.

9. Hebbel, R.P., et al.: The adhesive sickle erythrocyte: cause and consequence of abnormal interactions with endothelium, monocytes/macrophage and model membranes. Clin. Hematol. *14*:151, 1985.

10. Embury, S.H., et al.: Rapid prenatal diagnosis of sickle cell anemia by a new method of DNA analysis. N. Engl. J. Med. *316*:656, 1987.

11. Orkin, S.H.: Disorders of hemoglobin synthesis: The thalassemias. *In* Stamatoyannopoulos, G., et al. (eds.): Molecular Basis of Blood Diseases. Philadelphia, W.B. Saunders Co., 1987, p. 106.

12. Kazazian, H.H., and Antonarakis, S.E.: The varieties of mutation. Prog. Med. Genet. (New Series) *1*:43, 1988.

13. Fries, L.F., and Frank, M.M.: Molecular mechanism of complement action. *In* Stamatoyannopoulos, G., et al. (eds.): Molecular Basis of Blood Diseases. Philadelphia, W.B. Saunders Co., 1987, p. 450.

14. Rosse, W.F., and Parker, C.J.: Paroxysmal nocturnal hemogobinuria. Clin. Hematol. *14*:510, 1985.

15. Patten, E.: Immunohematologic diseases. J.A.M.A. *258*:2945, 1987.

16. Petz, L.D.: Drug induced hemolysis. N. Engl. J. Med. *313*:510, 1985.

17. Brain, M.D.: Microangiopathic hemolytic anemia. Annu. Rev. Med. *21*:133, 1970.

18. Herbert, V.: Biology of disease. Megaloblastic anemias. Lab. Invest. *52*:3, 1985.

19. Chanarin, I.: Megaloblastic anemia, cobalamin and folate. J. Clin. Pathol. *40*:978, 1987.

20. Beck, W.S.: Cobalamin and the nervous system. N. Engl. J. Med. *318*:1752, 1988.

21. Taylor, K.B., et al.: Gastrointestinal and liver diseases. *In* Stites, D.P., et al. (eds.): Basic and Clinical Immunology. 6th ed. Los Altos, Appleton and Lange, 1987, p. 462.

22. Conrad, M.E., and Barton, J.C.: Factors affecting iron balance. Am. J. Hematol. *10*:199, 1981.

23. Finch, C.A., and Heubers, H.: Perspectives in iron metabolism. N. Engl. J. Med. *306*:1520, 1982.

24. Aisen, P.: Current concepts in iron metabolism. Clin. Hematol. *11*:241, 1982.

25. Seligman, P.A., et al.: Molecular mechanisms of iron metabolism. *In* Stamatoyannopoulos, G., et al. (eds.): Molecular Basis of Blood Diseases. Philadelphia, W.B. Saunders Co., 1987, p. 219.

26. Powell, L.W., and Haliday, J.W.: Iron absorption and iron overload. Clin. Gastroenterol. *10*:707, 1981.

27. Scrimshaw, N.S.: Iron-deficiency and its functional consequences. Compr. Ther. *11*:40, 1985.

28. Rappaport, J.M., and Nathan, D.G.: Acquired aplastic anemia. Pathophysiology and treatment. Adv. Intern. Med. *27*:547, 1982.

29. Young, N.S., and Mortimer, P.P.: Viruses and bone marrow failure. Blood *63*:729, 1984.

30. Thomas, E.D., and Storb, R.: Acquired aplastic anemia. Progress and perplexity. Blood *64*:325, 1984.

31. Mangan, K.F.: Immune dysregulation of hematopoiesis. Annu. Rev. Med. *38*:61, 1987.

32. Mangan, K.F., et al.: In vitro evidence for disappearance of erythroid progenitor T suppressor cells following allogeneic bone marrow transplantation for severe aplastic anemia. Blood *71*:144, 1988.

33. Marsh, J.C.W., et al.: Survival after anti-lymphocyte globulin therapy for aplastic anemia depends on disease severity. Blood *70*:1046, 1987.

34. Orlandi, E., et al.: Adult leukemia developing after aplastic anemia: report of 8 cases. Acta Hematol. *70*:174, 1988.

35. Gordon-Smith, E.C.: Treatment of severe aplastic anemia by bone marrow transplantation. Hematol. Oncol. *5*:255, 1987.

36. Krantz, S.B., and Dessypris, E.N.: Pure red cell aplasia. *In* Golde, D.W., and Takaka, F. (eds.): Hemopoietic Stem Cells. New York, Marcel Dekker, 1985.

37. Erslev, A: Erythropoietin coming of age. N. Engl. J. Med. *316*:101, 1987.

38. Chong, B.H., and Castaldi, P.A.: Heparin-induced thrombocytopenia: further studies of heparin-dependent antibodies on platelets. Br. J. Haematol. *64*:347, 1986.

39. Klein, C.A., and Blajchman, M.A.: Alloantibodies and platelet destruction. Semin. Thromb. Hemost. *8*:105, 1982.

40. Brannan, D.P., and Guthrie, T.H.: Idiopathic thrombocytopenic purpura in adults. South. Med. J. *81*:75, 1988.

41. Kelton, J.G., and Gibbons, S.: Autoimmune platelet destruction: idiopathic thrombocytopenic purpura. Semin. Thromb. Hemost. *8*:83, 1982.

42. Kelton, J.G.: Advances in the diagnosis and management of ITP. Hosp. Pract. *20*:95, 1985.

43. Ballem, P.J., et al.: Mechanism of thrombocytopenia in chronic autoimmune thrombocytopenic purpura: evidence of both impaired platelet production and increased platelet clearance. J. Clin. Invest. *80*:33, 1987.

44. Kwaan, H.C.: Clinicopathologic features of thrombotic thrombocytopenic purpura. Semin. Hematol. *24*:71, 1987.

45. Lian, E.C-Y.: Pathogenesis of thrombotic thrombocytopenic purpura. Semin. Hematol. *24*:82, 1987.

46. Majerus, P.W.: Platelets. *In* Stamatoyannopoulos, G., et al. (eds.): The Molecular Basis of Blood Diseases. Philadelphia, W.B. Saunders Co., 1987, p. 689.

47. Harker, L.A.: Acquired disorders of platelet function. Ann. N.Y. Acad. Sci. *509*:188, 1987.

48. Remuzzi, G.: Bleeding in renal failure. Lancet *1*:1205, 1988.

49. Zimmerman, T.S., and Ruggeri, Z.M.: von Willebrand's disease. Hum. Pathol. *18*:140, 1987.

50. Hoyer, L.: Molecular pathology and immunology of Factor VIII (hemophilia A and Factor VIII inhibitors). Hum. Pathol. *18*:153, 1987.

50a. White, G.C., and Shoemaker, C.B.: Review: Factor VIII gene and hemophilia A. Blood *73*:1, 1989.

51. Ruggeri, Z.M., and Zimmerman, T.S.: Von Willebrand's factor and von Willebrand's disease. Blood *70*:895, 1987.

52. Carr, M.E.: Disseminated intravascular coagulation: pathogenesis, diagnosis, and therapy. J. Emerg. Med. *5*:311, 1987.

53. Moore, K.L., et al.: Endotoxin enhances tissue factor and downregulates thrombomodulin of human vascular endothelium in vivo. J. Clin. Invest. *79*:124, 1987.

54. Kim, H-S., et al.: Clinical unsuspected disseminated intravascular coagulation. Am. J. Clin. Pathol. *66*:31, 1976.

55. El-Dessouky, M., et al.: Kasabach-Merritt syndrome. J. Pediatr. Surg. *23*:109, 1988.

15

Diseases of White Cells, Lymph Nodes, and Spleen

WHITE CELLS AND LYMPH NODES

NORMAL

The origin and differentiation of white cells (granulocytes, monocytes, and lymphocytes) were briefly discussed in Chapter 14 along with the other formed elements of blood. Lymphocytes and monocytes not only circulate in the blood and lymph but also accumulate in discrete and organized masses, the so-called lymphoreticular system. Components of this system include lymph nodes, thymus, spleen, tonsils, adenoids, and Peyer's patches. Less discrete collections of lymphoid cells also occur in the bone marrow, lungs, and gastrointestinal tract and other tissues. Lymph nodes are the most widely distributed and easily accessible component of the lymphoid tissue and are hence frequently examined for the diagnosis of lymphoreticular disorders. It would therefore be advantageous to review the normal morphology of lymph nodes.

Lymph nodes, in general, are discrete structures, ovoid in shape, that vary from a few millimeters to 1 to 2 cm in length. Their consistency is soft and their cut surface is gray-white. They are surrounded by a capsule composed of connective tissue and a few elastic fibrils, perforated at various points by afferent lymphatics that empty into the peripheral sinus subjacent to the capsule. Branches of the sinus extend into the nodes and terminate at the hilus, where the efferent lymphatics emerge. All lymphatics are lined with mononuclear-phagocytic cells. Situated in the cortex or peripheral portion of the node are spherical aggregates of lymphoid tissue, the so-called primary follicles, which represent the B-cell areas. Upon antigenic stimulation, the primary follicles enlarge and develop pale-staining germinal centers composed of follicular center cells. Surrounding these germinal centers are mantles of small unchallenged B cells. The T cells occupy the parafollicular regions (p. 165). The medullary cords, occupying the central portion of the node, contain predominantly plasma cells and some lymphocytes. A delicate reticulin that connects peripherally with the capsule is the predominant supporting structure within the lymph nodes.

The morphologic description of the lymph node just given is highly idealized and falsely static. The size and morphology of lymph nodes are modified by stress, thyroid and adrenal function, and immune responses. As secondary lines of defense, they are constantly responding to stimuli, even in the absence of clinical disease. Trivial injuries and infections effect subtle changes in lymph node histology. More significant bacterial infections inevitably produce enlargement of nodes and sometimes leave residual scarring. For this reason, lymph nodes in the adult are almost never "normal," and they usually bear the scars of previous events, rendering the inguinal nodes particularly inappropriate for evaluative biopsies. Except in the child, it is difficult to find a "normal" node, and in histologic evaluations it is often necessary to distinguish changes secondary to past experience from those related to present disease.

PATHOLOGY

Disorders of white cells may be classified into two broad categories, *proliferative* and those characterized by a deficiency of leukocytes, i.e., *leukopenias.* Proliferations of white cells and lymph nodes may be reactive or neoplastic. Since their major function is host defense, reactive proliferation in response to an underlying primary, often microbial disease is fairly common. Neoplastic disorders, although less frequent, are much more important. In the following discussion, we will describe first the leukopenic states and summarize the common reactive disorders, and then consider in some detail malignant proliferations of the white cells that in many instances arise in the nodes.

LEUKOPENIA

The number of circulating white cells may be markedly decreased in a variety of disorders. An abnormally low white cell count *(leukopenia)* may occur because of decreased numbers of any one of the specific types of leukocytes, but most often involves the neutrophils *(neutropenia, granulocytopenia). Lymphopenias* are much less common, and in addition to the congenital immunodeficiency diseases (p. 221) they are associated with specific clinical syndromes (e.g., Hodgkin's disease, nonlymphocytic leukemias, following corticosteroid therapy, and occasionally in chronic diseases). Only the more common leukopenias involving granulocytes will be discussed here.

Neutropenia — Agranulocytosis

Reduction in the number of granulocytes in the peripheral blood — *neutropenia* — may be seen in a wide variety of circumstances. Frequently it is transient and of trivial significance. Sometimes the reduction in circulating neutrophils is marked and has serious consequences by predisposing to infections. When of this magnitude, it is referred to as *agranulocytosis.* The lymphocytes are not affected, so the percentage of lymphocytes is increased (relative lymphocytosis).

PATHOGENESIS. Considering first the broad topic of neutropenia, whatever its severity, a reduction in circulating granulocytes will occur if (1) granulopoiesis fails to keep pace with the normal turnover rate of neutrophils or (2) there is accelerated removal of neutrophils from the circulating blood. You recall that the neutrophil is a very short-lived cell having a half-life of only six to seven hours. Any impairment of granulopoiesis can therefore induce a neutropenia within hours to a few days.

Inadequate or ineffective granulopoiesis may be encountered with (1) suppression of pluripotent myeloid stem cells, as occurs in aplastic anemia (p. 688) and a variety of leukemias and lymphomas (p. 723) — in these conditions, granulocytopenia is accompanied by anemia and thrombocytopenia; (2) suppression of the committed granulocytic precursors, which occurs after exposure to certain drugs, as discussed below; or (3) megaloblastic anemias, due to vitamin B_{12} or folate deficiency (p. 679), in which defective DNA synthesis produces abnormal granulocytic precursors, rendering them susceptible to intramedullary death (ineffective granulopoiesis). Marrow granulopoiesis is increased, but the number of mature neutrophils entering the blood is decreased.

Accelerated removal or destruction of neutrophils is encountered with (1) immunologically mediated injury to the neutrophils, which may be idiopathic with no other abnormality, associated with a well-defined immunologic disorder (e.g., Felty's syndrome, p. 1353), or produced by exposure to drugs; and (2) splenic sequestration in which excessive destruction occurs secondary to enlargement of the spleen (p. 749), associated also with excessive destruction of red cells and platelets.

Among the many associations mentioned, *the most significant neutropenias (agranulocytoses) are produced by drugs.*[1] Certain drugs, such as alkylating agents and antimetabolites used in cancer treatment, produce agranulocytosis in a predictable, dose-related fashion. They cause a generalized suppression of the bone marrow, and therefore other cells are also affected (aplastic anemia). Agranulocytosis may also be encountered as an idiosyncratic reaction to a large variety of agents. The roster of implicated drugs includes aminopyrine, chloramphenicol, sulfonamides, chlorpromazine, thiouracil, and phenylbutazone. Although the mechanism of agranulocytosis here is obscure, both decreased production and increased destruction have been implicated. The neutropenia induced by chlorpromazine and related phenothiazines is of slow onset and is believed to result from the suppression of granulocytic precursors in the bone marrow. Chlorpromazine can inhibit DNA synthesis of marrow cells in vitro, and therefore it is postulated that certain individuals unusually sensitive to this effect develop agranulocytosis. Neutrophil production gradually becomes normal after the cessation of drug therapy. Agranulocytosis following administration of aminopyrine, thiouracil, and certain sulfonamides is believed to result from immunologically mediated destruction of mature neutrophils. Antibodies reactive against a complex between the drug or its metabolite (acting as the hapten) and leukocyte proteins may evoke a type II hypersensitivity reaction. Alternatively, neutrophils may be damaged as innocent bystanders by the adsorption of drug-antibody complexes on the surface and the subsequent activation of complement. In many cases, no antecedent cause of neutropenia can be detected but autoimmunity is suspected, since serum antibodies directed against neutrophil-specific antigens can be detected. Several recent reports indicate that severe neutropenia may occur in association with polyclonal or monoclonal proliferations of CD8+ large granular lymphocytes.[2] The mechanism of this neutropenia is not clear, but suppression of granulocytic progenitors in the bone marrow is considered most likely.

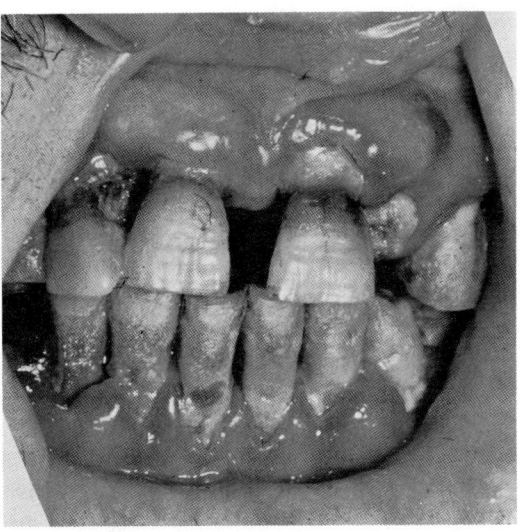

Figure 15–1. Agranulocytosis. Gingival margins show chronic suppurative necrotizing infection due to loss of protective white cells in circulation.

MORPHOLOGY. The anatomic alterations in the bone marrow depend on the underlying basis of the neutropenia. When it is caused by excessive destruction of the mature neutrophils, the marrow may be hypercellular with increased numbers of immature granulocytic precursors. Hypercellularity is also seen with ineffective granulopoiesis, as occurs in megaloblastic anemias. Agranulocytosis caused by agents that affect the committed granulocytic precursors are understandably associated with hypocellular marrow, resulting from greatly decreased leukopoietic elements. Erythropoiesis and megakaryocytes usually remain at normal levels, but with certain myelotoxic drugs all marrow elements may be affected. Occasionally, increased numbers of plasma cells and lymphocytes are found in the marrow, particularly as the marrow becomes acellular.

Infections are a characteristic feature of agranulocytosis. Ulcerating necrotizing lesions of the gingiva, floor of the mouth, buccal mucosa, pharynx, or anywhere within the oral cavity (agranulocytic angina) are quite characteristic of agranulocytosis (Fig. 15–1). These ulcers are typically deep, undermined, and covered by gray to green-black necrotic membranes from which numbers of bacteria or fungi can be isolated. Similar ulcerations may occur in the skin, vagina, anus, or gastrointestinal tract, but these sites are much less frequently involved. Severe necrotizing infections are also encountered, but less prominently, in the lungs, urinary tract, and kidneys. All these sites of infection are characterized by massive growth of bacteria (or other agents) with relatively poor leukocytic response. In many instances, the bacteria grow in colony formation (botryomycosis) as though they were cultured on nutrient media. The regional lymph nodes draining these infections are enlarged and inflamed. The spleen and liver are rarely enlarged.

CLINICAL COURSE. Agranulocytosis tends to follow a fairly characteristic clinical pattern. The initial symptoms are often malaise, chills, and fever, followed in sequence by marked weakness and fatigability, symptoms that stem from the severe infections characteristic of this disorder. In severe agranulocytosis with virtual absence of neutrophils, these infec-

tions may become so overwhelming as to cause death within a few days. Less extreme depression of the marrow may appear insidiously and come to light only during the investigation of frequent and persistent minor infections.

Characteristically, the total white cell count is reduced to 1000 cells per mm³ of blood and, in certain instances, to levels as low as 200 to 300 cells. Usually there is no associated anemia, save that caused by the infections, nor is there thrombocytopenia.

The prognosis is very unpredictable. Before the advent of antibiotics, the mortality rate ranged between 70 and 90%. At present the antibiotics, steroids, and supportive measures such as neutrophil transfusions allow better survival since, in many instances, the adverse effects of the toxic drug are discovered early and the depression of white cells eventually remits. The idiopathic form, too, may spontaneously remit or may progressively worsen, leading to death.

REACTIVE (INFLAMMATORY) PROLIFERATIONS OF WHITE CELLS AND NODES

Leukocytosis

Leukocytosis is a common reaction in a variety of inflammatory states. The particular white cell series affected varies with the underlying cause. In Chapter 2 we discussed *polymorphonuclear leukocytosis* (granulocytosis), which accompanies acute inflammation. Pyogenic infections are common causes of neutrophilic leukocytosis, but it may also result from nonmicrobial stimuli such as tissue necrosis caused by burns or myocardial infarction. In patients with severe, life-threatening sepsis, in addition to leukocytosis there may be morphologic changes in the neutrophils such as toxic granulations, Döhle bodies, and cytoplasmic vacuoles. *Toxic granules* are coarse and darker than the normal neutrophilic granules. Although their precise origin is not entirely clear, they are believed to represent abnormal forms of azurophilic granules. *Döhle bodies* are pale blue, round or oval inclusions that represent aggregates of the rough endoplasmic reticulum.

Eosinophilic leukocytosis is characteristic of allergic disorders such as bronchial asthma, hay fever (p. 776), parasitic infections, and some diseases of the skin. The latter include pemphigus, eczema, and dermatitis herpetiformis, all of which are probably immunologic in origin. In hospitalized adult patients the most likely cause of eosinophilia is an allergic drug reaction. *Elevations in monocyte count* may be seen in several chronic infections including tuberculosis, bacterial endocarditis, brucellosis, rickettsiosis, and malaria. Certain collagen vascular diseases such as systemic lupus erythematosus (SLE) and rheumatoid arthritis are associated with monocytosis, as are inflammatory bowel diseases such as ulcerative colitis and Crohn's disease. *Lymphocytosis* may accompany monocytosis in chronic inflammatory states such as brucellosis and tuberculosis, representing in these instances a sustained activation of the immune response. The lymphocyte count may also be increased in acute viral infections such as viral hepatitis, in cytomegalovirus infections, and particularly in infectious mononucleosis (p. 323).

In most instances, reactive leukocytosis is easy to distinguish from neoplastic proliferation of the white cells (i.e., leukemias) by the rarity of immature cells in the blood. However, in some inflammatory states, many immature white cells may appear in the blood and a picture of leukemia may be simulated *(leukemoid reaction)*. The distinction from leukemias may then be difficult, as discussed on page 729.

Infections and other inflammatory stimuli may not only cause leukocytosis but also involve the lymph nodes, which act as defensive barriers. The infections that lead to lymphadenitis (described below) are so numerous and varied that it is impossible to detail each, since it would be a virtual catalog of all systemic microbiologic diseases. Moreover, in most instances the lymphadenitis is of a banal variety and is entirely nonspecific, designated acute or chronic nonspecific lymphadenitis.

Acute Nonspecific Lymphadenitis

Lymph nodes undergo reactive changes whenever challenged by microbiologic agents or their toxic products, or by cell debris and foreign matter introduced into wounds or into the circulation, as in drug addiction.

Acutely inflamed nodes are most commonly caused by direct microbiologic drainage, and are seen most frequently in the cervical area in association with infections of the teeth or tonsil, or in the axillary or inguinal regions secondary to infections in the extremities. Similarly, acute lymphadenitis is found in those nodes draining acute appendicitis, acute enteritis, or any other acute infection. Generalized acute lymphadenopathy is characteristic of viral infections and bacteremia, particularly in children. The nodal reactions in the abdomen — mesenteric adenitis — may induce acute abdominal symptoms closely resembling acute appendicitis, a differential diagnosis that plagues the surgeon.

Macroscopically, the nodes become swollen, gray-red, and engorged. The capsules are generally intact, but permeation of infection may lead to inflammatory changes in the perinodal tissues. Histologically there is prominence of the lymphoid follicles and large germinal centers containing numerous mitotic figures. Histiocytes often contain particulate debris of bacterial origin or derived from necrotic cells (Fig. 15–2). When pyogenic organisms are the cause of the reaction, the centers of the follicles may undergo necrosis; indeed, the entire node may sometimes be converted into a suppurative mass. With less severe reactions, there is sometimes a neutrophilic infiltrate about the follicles, and numerous neutrophils can be found within the lymphoid sinuses. The cells lining the sinuses become hypertrophied and cuboidal and may undergo hyperplasia.

Clinically, nodes with acute lymphadenitis are enlarged because of the cellular infiltration and edema. As a consequence of the distention of the capsule, they are tender to touch. When abscess forma-

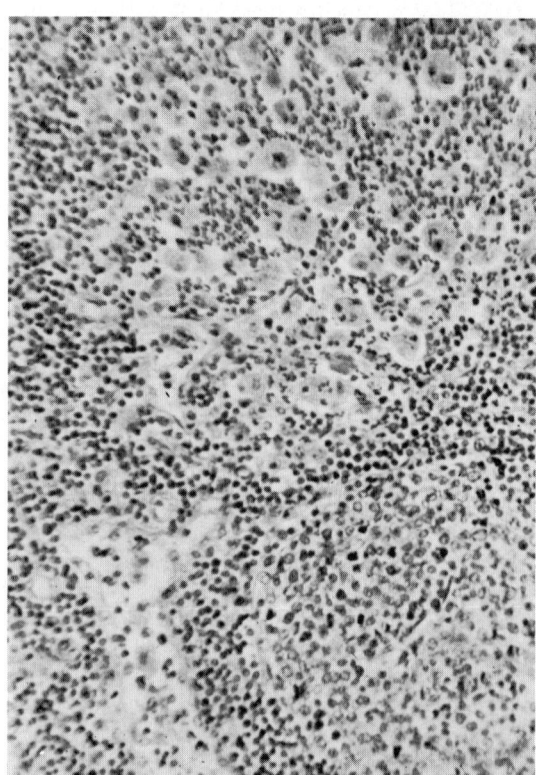

Figure 15–2. Acute lymphadenitis. High-power detail of germinal centers with large histiocytic cells showing phagocytic activity.

tion is extensive, they become fluctuant. The overlying skin is frequently red, and sometimes penetration of the infection to the skin surface produces draining sinuses, particularly when the nodes have undergone suppurative necrosis. With control of the infection, the lymph nodes may revert to their normal appearance or scarring may follow the more destructive disease.

Chronic Nonspecific Lymphadenitis

Chronic reactions assume one of three patterns, depending on their causation.[3] Most chronic infections caused by organisms that represent B-cell antigens induce follicular hyperplasia. Microbiologic agents or antigens that stimulate T cells produce a second type of pattern, called paracortical lymphoid hyperplasia. Drugs such as the anticonvulsant Dilantin (phenytoin) serving as haptens may induce this pattern of parafollicular hyperplasia. A third nonspecific pattern, referred to as sinus histiocytosis, is encountered in regional nodes draining a site of cancer.

Follicular hyperplasia is distinguished by prominence of the large germinal centers, which appear to bulge against the surrounding collar of small B lymphocytes (Fig. 15–3). Prominent within these germinal centers are lymphocytes in varying stages of "blast" transformation and large numbers of histiocytes containing phagocytized debris of bacterial or cellular origin. Plasma cells, histiocytes, and occasionally neutrophils or eosinophils may be found in the parafollicular regions, and there generally is striking hyperplasia of the mononuclear-phagocytic cells lining the lymphatic sinuses. Some specific causes of follicular hyperplasia include disorders such as rheumatoid arthritis, toxoplasmosis, and AIDS.

This form of lymphadenitis may be confused morphologically with follicular (nodular) lymphomas (p. 709). It is beyond our scope to go into all the subtle morphologic features in this differential, but several points may be noted. Favoring reactive follicular hyperplasia are (1) preservation of the lymph node architecture with presence of normal lymphoid tissue between germinal centers; (2) marked variation in the shape and size of lymphoid nodules; (3) a mixed population of lymphocytes in different stages of differentiation and histiocytes within germinal centers, i.e., reactive follicles are pleomorphic whereas lymphomatous nodules tend to be monomorphic; and (4) prominent phagocytic activity in germinal centers.[4]

Paracortical lymphoid hyperplasia is characterized by reactive changes within the T-cell regions of the lymph node, which encroach on, and sometimes appear to efface, the germinal follicles. In these regions, the T cells undergo progressive transformation to immunoblasts. These large cells, when viewed within a sea of smaller lymphocytes, impart a mottled appearance to the T-cell zones. In addition, there is hypertrophy of the sinusoidal and vascular endothelial cells and a mixed cellular infiltrate, principally of macrophages and sometimes of eosinophils. The striking increase in the number of immunoblasts may produce a pseudolymphomatous pattern, sometimes referred to as

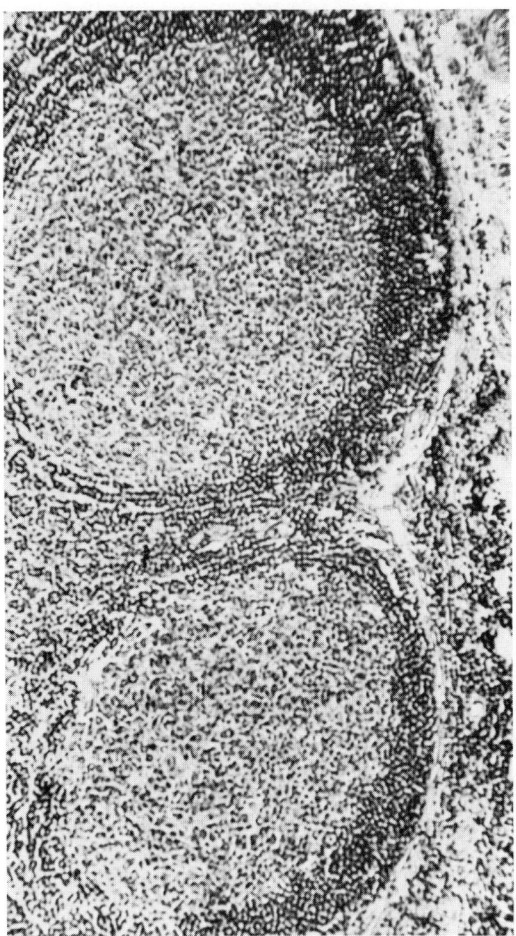

Figure 15–3. Chronic follicular hyperplasia, demonstrating marked enlargement and prominence of germinal follicles.

pseudolymphomatous lymphadenitis. Such changes are encountered particularly often in immunologic reactions induced by drugs (especially Dilantin) or following smallpox vaccination. Similar reactions have been described after the use of other vaccines.

Sinus histiocytosis refers to distention and prominence of the lymphatic sinusoids, encountered in lymph nodes draining cancers, particularly carcinoma of the breast. The lining endothelial cells are markedly hypertrophied, and the sinuses may be virtually engorged with histiocytes (Fig. 15–4). This pattern of reaction has been thought to represent an immune response on the part of the host to the tumor or its products. According to some, the presence of sinus histiocytosis is a sign of a favorable prognosis, but this issue is debatable.

Although the three patterns of reaction have been described separately, frequent combinations and intergrades are encountered. Characteristically, lymph nodes in chronic reactions are not tender, because they are not under increased pressure. Chronic reactions are particularly characteristic of inguinal and axillary nodes. Both groups drain relatively large areas of the body and so are frequently challenged, for

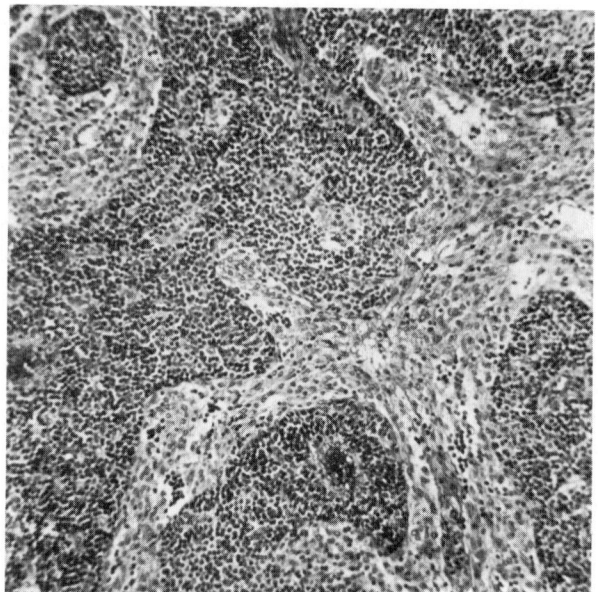

Figure 15–4. Sinus histiocytosis in an axillary node from a female patient with carcinoma of breast.

which reason these lymph nodes are inappropriate as biopsy specimens in the study of hematologic and lymphomatous disorders.

NEOPLASTIC PROLIFERATIONS OF WHITE CELLS

Malignant proliferative diseases constitute the most important white cell disorder. The several categories of these diseases can be briefly defined as follows:

1. *Malignant lymphomas* take the form of cohesive tumorous lesions composed mainly of lymphocytes and rarely of histiocytes that arise in lymphoid tissue anywhere in the body, most commonly within lymph nodes.
2. *Leukemias and myeloproliferative disorders* are neoplasms of the hematopoietic stem cells arising in the bone marrow that secondarily flood the circulating blood or other organs with transformed cells.
3. *Plasma cell dyscrasias and related disorders* usually arising in the bones take the form of localized or disseminated proliferations of antibody-forming cells. Thus, this category is marked by the appearance in the peripheral blood of abnormal levels of immunoglobulins or the light or heavy chains of the immunoglobulins.
4. The *histiocytoses* represent proliferative lesions of tissue macrophages or histiocytes. There is unfortunately much confusion in the terminology of histiocytic disorders. First, as indicated above, the rare neoplastic proliferations of histiocytes originating within the lymphoid tissue are grouped with the malignant lymphomas. Second, there is no evidence that some of the tumor-like proliferations—the so-called histio-

cytoses X, which are traditionally listed under this category—are indeed neoplastic. These complexities will be discussed further on page 745.

As can be seen, the neoplastic disorders of the white cells are extremely varied. In the following sections, each of the categories is treated separately.

MALIGNANT LYMPHOMAS

Lymphomas are malignant neoplasms characterized by the proliferation of cells native to the lymphoid tissues, i.e., lymphocytes, histiocytes, and their precursors and derivatives. Like other neoplasms, all lymphomas are of monoclonal origin, as can be documented by isoenzyme markers and clonal gene rearrangements. The term lymphoma is something of a misnomer, since these disorders are lethal unless controlled or eradicated through therapy.

Within the broad group of malignant lymphomas, *Hodgkin's disease* (Hodgkin's lymphoma) is segregated from all other forms, which constitute the *non-Hodgkin's lymphomas*. Although both have their origin in the lymphoid tissues, Hodgkin's disease is set apart by the presence of a distinctive unifying morphologic feature, the Reed-Sternberg giant cells. In addition, the nodes contain non-neoplastic inflammatory cells, which in most cases outnumber the neoplastic element represented by the Reed-Sternberg cell. Therefore, we will discuss non-Hodgkin's lymphomas and Hodgkin's disease separately.

NON-HODGKIN'S LYMPHOMAS (NHL)

The usual presentation of NHL is as a localized or generalized lymphadenopathy. However, in about one third of cases it may be primary in other sites where lymphoid tissue is found, e.g., in the oropharyngeal region, gut, bone marrow, and skin. Lymph node enlargement due to lymphomatous disease must be differentiated from that caused by the more frequent infectious and inflammatory disorders. Lymphomatous involvement often produces marked nodal enlargement, which is almost always nontender (Fig. 15–5). Although variable, all forms of lymphoma have the potential to spread from their origin in a single node or chain of nodes to other nodes, and eventually to disseminate to the spleen, liver, and bone marrow. Some, after becoming widespread, spill over into the blood, creating a leukemia-like picture in the peripheral blood. In such blood-borne dissemination, all lymph nodes throughout the body become flooded with lymphomatous cells. It may therefore be impossible to determine from microscopic examination of a lymph node alone whether it represents primary lymphomatous disease with involvement of the bone marrow and blood, or nodal changes incident to leukemia. This problem is encountered more often with certain cytologic forms of lymphoma than with

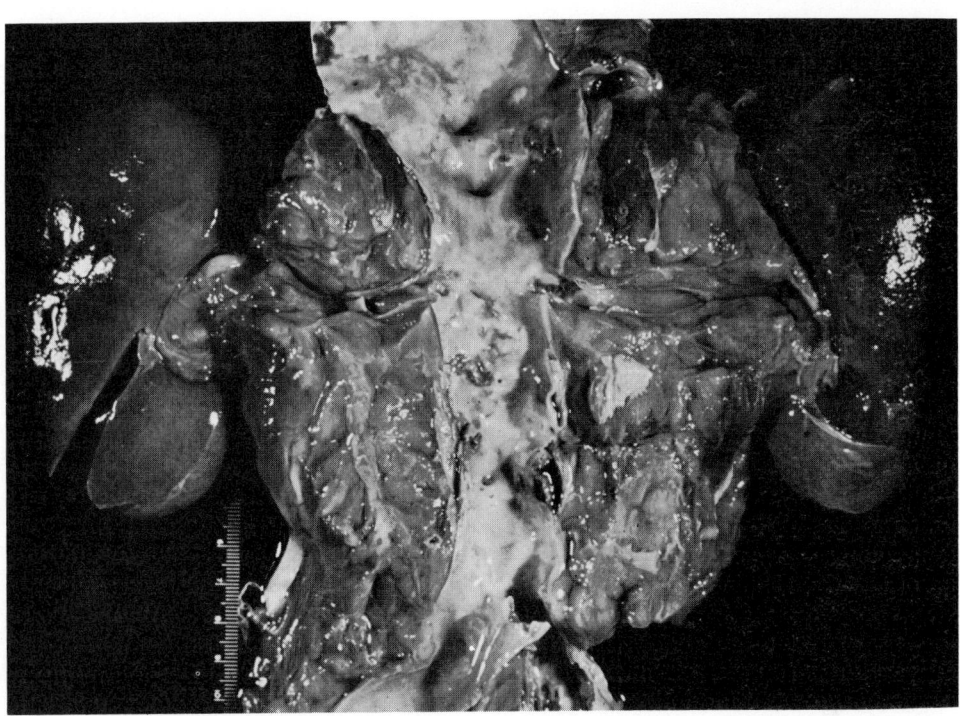

Figure 15–5. Lymphoma involving periaortic nodes.

others. Although we speak of NHL as a group, we should recognize that it encompasses a wide spectrum of disorders, differing in patient age at onset, the cells of origin, and response to therapy. It is therefore necessary to classify NHL into various subgroups.

Few areas of pathology have evoked as much controversy and confusion as the classification of NHL. Regrettably, even among expert "lymphomaniacs" there has been no unanimity regarding the best approach, and until the recent past there were more classifications than experts. In 1982, an international panel of experts decided to stem the growing tide of classifications by proposing yet another, possibly the ultimate, classification, entitled the Working Formulation of Clinical Usage,[5] which is now widely accepted. Before discussing the Working Formulation we will review the Rappaport and Lukes-Collins classifications—two conceptually different schemes that employ differing criteria and terminology for categorizing NHL.[6] It is necessary to start with this historical perspective, as it is essential for an understanding of the Working Formulation.

RAPPAPORT CLASSIFICATION. Proposed in 1966, this classification is based upon two morphologic features—the *cytologic appearance* of cells as seen with routine histology and the *growth pattern* of cells as nodular aggregates or diffuse infiltration throughout the node. When Rappaport presented his classification, knowledge about lymphocyte subsets, their activation, and their specific anatomic location within the lymph nodes was in its infancy. Therefore, the cytologic subdivision of NHL was based entirely on the following two criteria: (1) the apparent similarity of tumor cells to the two morphologically identifiable

units of the lymphoid system—lymphocytes and histiocytes; and (2) the "degree of differentiation" of the constituent cells. Tumors composed of cells similar in size and morphology to normal lymphocytes were considered well-differentiated lymphocytic lymphomas, whereas those composed of lymphocyte-like cells with irregular and angulated nuclei were considered to be poorly differentiated lymphocytic tumors. In contrast, if tumor cells were two to three times larger than small lymphocytes and had abundant cytoplasm, they were considered to resemble macrophages and were thus called histiocytic lymphoma. Lymphomas composed of cells intermediate in size and not clearly resembling lymphocytes or histiocytes were considered "undifferentiated."

Rappaport also observed that tumor cells were either spread diffusely or clustered into identifiable nodules throughout the lymph node, processes that destroyed lymph node architecture (Figs. 15–6 and 15–7). The nodular pattern was thought to reflect a cohesive tendency on the part of tumor cells, rather than an attempted recapitulation of normal lymph node follicles.

The Rappaport classification was widely employed in the United States because it was readily learned and highly reproducible and, more importantly, because it was clinically useful. For example, *a multitude of clinicopathologic studies have demonstrated that nodular architecture is associated with a prognosis that is significantly superior to that of the diffuse pattern.*[5,7]

However, in the early 1970s a better understanding of the normal immune system raised questions regarding the scientific validity of the Rappaport classification:

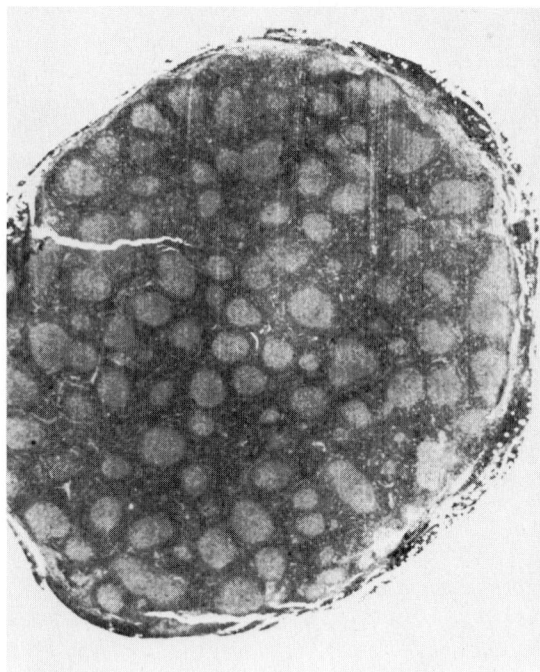

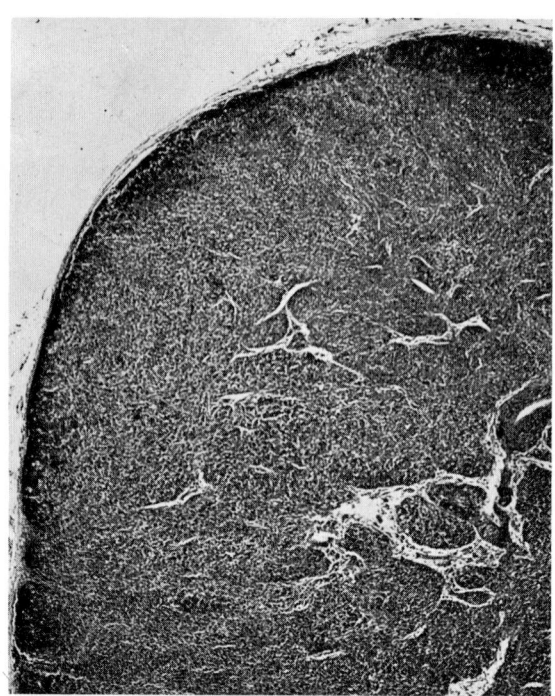

Fig. 15–6   Fig. 15–7

Figure 15–6. Non-Hodgkin's lymphoma, nodular pattern. Nodular aggregates of lymphoma cells are present throughout lymph node and in perinodal fat. (Courtesy of Dr. Jose Hernandez, Department of Pathology, Southwestern Medical School, Dallas, Texas.)

Figure 15–7. Non-Hodgkin's lymphoma, diffuse pattern. Nodal architecture is replaced by a diffuse sea of neoplastic lymphoid cells.

• First, it became clear that lymphocytes found to be identical by routine morphologic techniques were functionally heterogeneous. Two principal classes of lymphocytes (T and B cells) and several subpopulations were identified. The Rappaport classification did not relate the NHLs to these normal constituents of the lymphoid system.

• Second, the earlier view that the small lymphocyte is a static end-stage cell proved to be incorrect. Upon antigenic stimulation lymphocytes enlarge and undergo "blast transformation," acquiring an appearance that is conventionally associated with lack of differentiation. Furthermore, the transformed lymphocytes look deceptively similar to histiocytes. Indeed, the vast majority of the histiocytic lymphomas in the Rappaport scheme were later found to be related to transformed lymphocytes rather than macrophages.

LUKES-COLLINS CLASSIFICATION. In 1973–1974, two new classifications were proposed that attempted to address the scientific inaccuracies of the Rappaport scheme and to relate the NHLs to the normal immune system. Only the Lukes-Collins scheme will be reviewed here. The other, referred to as the Kiel classification,[5] is similar to the Lukes-Collins classification and will not be described.

On the premise that malignant lymphomas are neoplasms of the immune system, Lukes and Collins classified the NHLs on the basis of their cell of origin into three categories: tumors of T cells, B cells, or histiocytes.[8] Furthermore, Lukes and Collins sought correlations between the cytologic patterns in lymphomatous nodes and those evoked by antigenic challenge of lymphocytes. In the germinal centers of lymph nodes, four distinctive morphologic stages can be identified in the process of transformation of small resting B lymphocytes into immunoblasts. These stages include (1) small cleaved cells, (2) large cleaved cells, (3) small noncleaved cells, and (4) large noncleaved cells, as depicted in Figure 15–8. These cells differ with respect to cell size, nuclear configuration (clefts or folds), nuclear chromatin pattern, number of nucleoli, and degree of mitotic activity. All four of these cell types are referred to as follicular center cells (FCC). The large noncleaved follicular center cells leave the follicle and undergo further enlargement to become *immunoblasts*. Proliferation of immunoblasts produces daughter cells that eventually either become plasma cells or revert to the dormant state as small memory B lymphocytes. In the context of this scheme, Lukes-Collins proposed that B-cell tumors may be composed of cells that are apparently "frozen" anywhere along this differentiation pathway. According to Lukes, the nodular architecture seen in certain lymphomas is related to their origin from germinal center B cells (FCC). Their tendency toward nodularity is viewed as an attempt to reproduce (differentiate) a normal structure, analogous to gland formation by cells of an adenocarcinoma. The

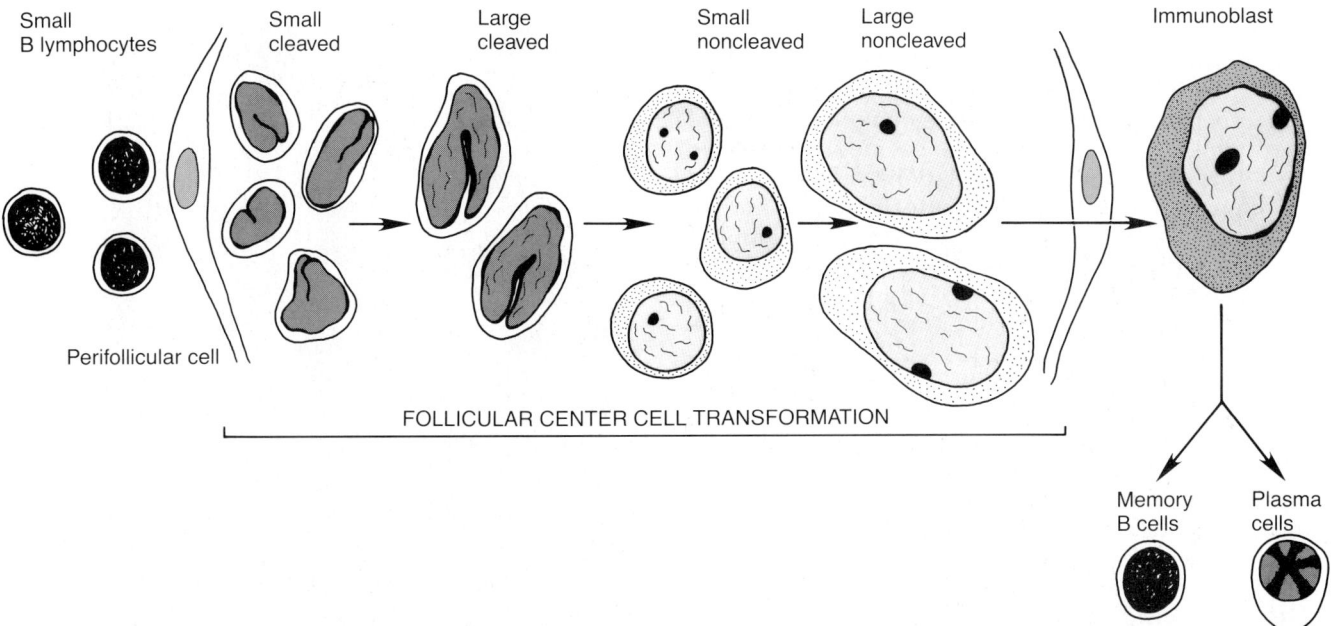

Small
B lymphocytes

Small
cleaved

Large
cleaved

Small
noncleaved

Large
noncleaved

Immunoblast

Perifollicular cell

FOLLICULAR CENTER CELL TRANSFORMATION

Memory
B cells

Plasma
cells

Figure 15–8. Schematic representation of normal antigen-induced transformation of B cells in the germinal centers of lymphoid follicles. (Drawn after Lukes, R.J., et al.: Immunologic approach to non-Hodgkin's lymphoma and related leukemias. Analysis of the result of multiparameter studies of 425 cases. Semin. Hematol. *15:*322, 1978.)

notion that nodular lymphomas are of B-cell origin was derived primarily from morphologic studies and has been amply confirmed by immunophenotyping and molecular analyses.

Conceptually, the immunologic approach is much more satisfying, as it places various lymphoid tumors into well-defined categories that can be related to specific normal B- or T-cell types of the immune system. However, are immunologically homogeneous categories associated with uniform clinical behavior? *The majority (65 to 70%) of NHLs are of B-cell origin,* but there is a great variation in their prognosis. At one extreme are follicular lymphomas, most of which are indolent tumors, and at the other extreme are highly aggressive immunoblastic lymphomas of B-cell origin. It is clear, therefore, that histogenetic similarity does not translate into uniform prognosis.

Working Formulation for Clinical Use

As the name indicates, this classification has a strong clinical bias. NHLs are divided into three major prognostic groupings: low, intermediate, and high grades based on survival statistics (Table 15–1). The five-

Table 15–1. A Working Formulation of Non-Hodgkin's Lymphomas for Clinical Usage (Equivalent or Related Terms of Rappaport and Lukes-Collins Classifications Are Shown)

WORKING FORMULATION	RAPPAPORT CLASSIFICATION	LUKES-COLLINS CLASSIFICATION
Low-Grade		
A. Small lymphocytic	Lymphocytic, well differentiated	Small lymphocyte and plasmacytoid lymphocytic
B. Follicular, predominantly small cleaved cell	Nodular, poorly differentiated lymphocytic	FCC, small cleaved
C. Follicular, mixed small cleaved and large cell	Nodular, mixed lymphocytic histiocytic	FCC, small cleaved and large cleaved
Intermediate-Grade		
D. Follicular, predominantly large cell	Nodular, histiocytic	FCC, large cleaved and/or noncleaved
E. Diffuse, small cleaved cell	Diffuse, poorly differentiated lymphocytic	FCC, small cleaved diffuse
F. Diffuse, mixed small and large cell	Diffuse, mixed lymphocytic and histiocytic	FCC, small cleaved, large cleaved, or large noncleaved
G. Diffuse, large cell	Diffuse histiocytic	FCC, large cleaved or noncleaved
High-Grade		
H. Large cell, immunoblastic	Diffuse histiocytic	Immunoblastic B- or T-cell type
I. Lymphoblastic	Lymphoblastic lymphoma	Convoluted T-cell lymphoma
J. Small noncleaved cell	Undifferentiated, Burkitt's and non-Burkitt's	FCC, small noncleaved
Miscellaneous		

year survival rate for tumors classified as low grade ranges from 50 to 70%, and for tumors of intermediate and high grade from 35 to 45% and 23 to 32%, respectively. Each prognostic group contains several morphologic categories. It will be evident from Table 15–1 that the Working Formulation uses a mixture of the Rappaport and Lukes-Collins terminology. Unlike the Lukes-Collins scheme, however, no attempt is made to segregate lymphomas on the basis of presumed cell of origin. The Working Formulation also contains a miscellaneous group that includes the rare histiocytic tumors, the HTLV-1–induced T-cell leukemia/lymphoma, and other T-lymphomatous disorders with prominent involvement of skin. With this background we will describe the clinicopathologic features of NHLs following the Working Formulation scheme. All morphologic types included in the Working Formulation will not be described in detail; instead we will select those most commonly encountered as well as some uncommon tumors that provide interesting insights into the biology of lymphomas. Details not included can be found in specialized reviews and monographs.[6,9]

Low-Grade Lymphomas

This category includes three tumors: small lymphocytic lymphoma; follicular, predominantly small cleaved cell lymphoma; and follicular mixed (small cleaved and large cell) lymphoma. The two follicular lymphomas will be discussed together, since they form a distinct clinicopathologic group.

SMALL LYMPHOCYTIC LYMPHOMA (SLL). This pattern makes up approximately 4% of all NHLs and is the only low-grade lymphoma that does not have a follicular architecture. It is, however, of B-cell origin, and the neoplastic B cells display surface IgM, IgD, and pan-B cell antigen CD19. This phenotype is similar to that of virgin B cells that have not yet encountered an antigen and are thought to be located at the periphery of the primary follicle. Morphologically the cell type consists of compact, small, apparently unstimulated lymphocytes with dark-staining round nuclei, scanty cytoplasm, and little variation in size (Fig. 15–9). Mitotic figures are rare, and there is little or no cytologic atypia. *Involvement of bone marrow is present in almost all cases, and in about 40% of patients the neoplastic cells spill over into blood, evoking a chronic lymphocytic leukemia–like picture.*[10] Conversely, in patients with the primary diagnosis of chronic lymphocytic leukemia (CLL), the nodes are invariably flooded with well-differentiated lymphocytes. Thus, it is impossible from a lymph node biopsy alone to differentiate CLL from SLL. Their clinical features are also similar. Both occur primarily in older age groups. Typically, these patients have generalized lymphadenopathy with mild-to-moderate enlargement of the liver and spleen; the associated symptoms are mild, and prolonged survival is usual. Some patients with a histologic picture closely resembling that of SLL also have monoclonal IgM immunoglobulin in the serum and a distinctive clinical syn-

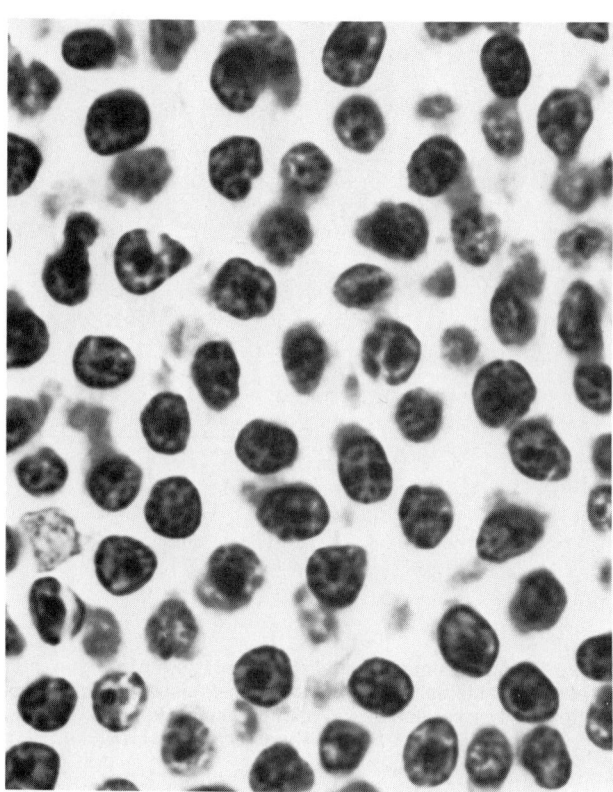

Figure 15–9. Non-Hodgkin's lymphoma, small lymphocytic type. Cytology is that of mature, uniform, unstimulated lymphocytes. (Courtesy of Dr. Jose Hernandez, Department of Pathology, Southwestern Medical School, Dallas, Texas.)

drome called Waldenström's macroglobulinemia (p. 743). In these patients the lymph nodes often contain variable numbers of plasma cells or "plasmacytoid lymphocytes," in addition to the well-differentiated lymphocytes described above. As discussed later, SLL, CLL, and Waldenström's macroglobulinemia represent different manifestations of the neoplastic proliferation of B lymphocytes, and as such are closely related to each other.

FOLLICULAR LYMPHOMAS. There are two cytologic subgroups of low-grade follicular lymphomas: follicular small cleaved cell and follicular mixed cell type. *Follicular small cleaved cell lymphoma* is the archetype of follicular lymphomas and the most common form of follicular NHL. The neoplastic B cells resemble small cleaved cells seen within normal germinal centers (see Fig. 15–8). They are slightly larger than normal lymphocytes, with scanty cytoplasm. *The most distinctive feature that differentiates the tumor cells from small normal lymphocytes is their irregular "cleaved" nuclear contour, characterized by prominent clefts, indentations, and linear infoldings (Fig. 15–10). The nuclear chromatin is coarse and condensed, and nucleoli are indistinct. Mitoses are infrequent, and there may be scattered large cleaved or noncleaved cells within the nodule, but they do not account for more than 20% of the cells. When the frequency of *large cells exceeds 20% but is less than 50%, the term follicular mixed small cleaved and large cell is used.* Follicular, mixed lymphomas constitute a small proportion of all follicular center cell tumors, and whether they form a distinct group is debatable. As might be expected from their morphologic similarity to germinal center cells, the neoplastic B cells in all follicular lymphomas express surface Ig and the pan-B cell antigen CD19.

Follicular lymphomas constitute approximately 40% of adult NHLs in the United States and are characterized by the following features:

- They occur predominantly in older individuals (rarely in persons under 20 years of age).
- They affect males and females equally.
- They present with painless lymphadenopathy, which is frequently generalized. Involvement of extranodal (e.g., visceral) sites is uncommon, but bone marrow is frequently involved (75% of cases) at the time of diagnosis.
- Peripheral blood involvement in the form of frank leukemia is less common than in SLL, but small clonal B-cell populations can be detected in most cases by flow cytometry or molecular techniques.
- In the majority of patients (about 85%), tumor cells reveal a characteristic translocation t(14;18). The break point on chromosome 18 involves 18q21,

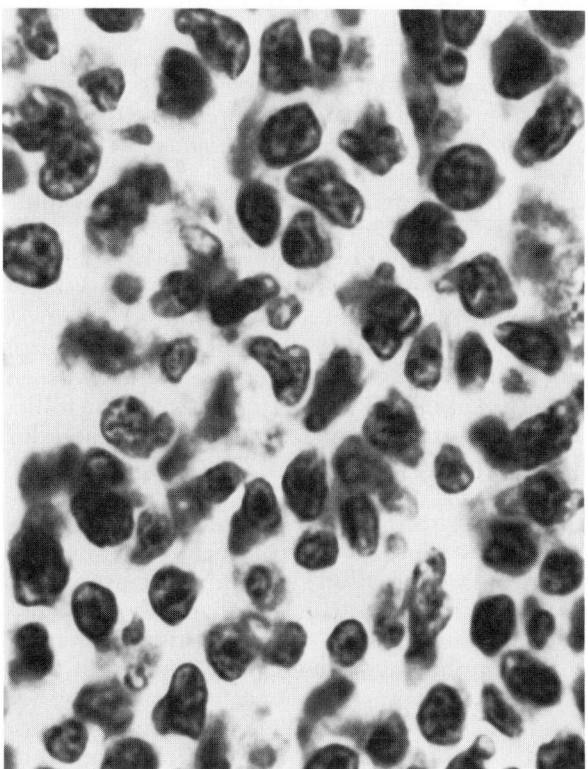

Figure 15–10. Non-Hodgkin's lymphoma, follicular small cleaved cell type. At this magnification the follicular architecture is not seen. Nuclei are irregular with indentations and marked angularity. (Courtesy of Dr. Jose Hernandez, Department of Pathology, Southwestern Medical School, Dallas, Texas.)

where a putative proto-oncogene *bcl–2* has been mapped.[11,12]

- Follicular lymphomas have a long natural history (median survival seven to nine years) that appears to be largely unaffected by treatment. It seems virtually impossible to eradicate these indolent tumors, and hence some authorities recommend that until better treatment protocols are devised, a "hands-off" approach is the best form of management.[13]
- In some patients with follicular lymphomas the tumors progress to a diffuse high-grade histologic type, with or without treatment. Such a transition usually occurs approximately eight years after diagnosis and in most cases represents the emergence of an aggressive subclone of the neoplastic B cells. Median survival is less than one year after such transformation.

Intermediate Grade Lymphomas

There are four tumors under this category of the Working Formulation, one with a follicular architecture and the other three with a diffuse pattern. The diffuse intermediate-grade lymphomas are distinguished on the basis of their cellular composition.

FOLLICULAR, PREDOMINANTLY LARGE CELL LYMPHOMA. This is an uncommon tumor and represents less than 15% of all follicular NHL. In contrast to the low-grade follicular lymphomas, the majority of the neoplastic cells are large, with cleaved or noncleaved nuclei. Mitotic figures are also more numerous. These tumors are prone to evolve into diffuse lymphomas early in their course and have a poorer prognosis than the vast majority of follicular lymphomas. Because in most series there are few tumors of this histologic type, an accurate evaluation of their natural history is difficult.[14]

DIFFUSE SMALL CLEAVED CELL LYMPHOMA. This type is composed of small cleaved cells that are similar to those that are present in the follicular small cleaved cell lymphoma. Briefly, the cells are somewhat larger than small lymphocytes and have an irregular cleaved nucleus with inconspicuous nucleoli and coarse chromatin. In contrast to follicular lymphomas of similar histologic type, these tumors have a higher male-to-female ratio and a median survival in the range of two to four years rather than seven to nine years. As compared with the United States, the incidence of these tumors is higher in Europe, particularly in Italy.

DIFFUSE MIXED SMALL AND LARGE CELL LYMPHOMA. These tumors contain a mixture of small cleaved cells already described and large cells that may be cleaved or noncleaved. The nuclei of *large cleaved cells* are irregular in contour, indented, and larger when compared with nuclei of normal histiocytes or endothelial cells (often used as a reference in evaluating size). The nuclear chromatin is slightly more dispersed than in a normal small lymphocyte, and nucleoli are inconspicuous. The cytoplasm is scant and pale. *Large noncleaved* cells are up to four times the size of normal lymphocytes, with a round or oval nucleus and one to two prominent nucleoli (Fig. 15–11). The nuclear chromatin is vesicular, and mitoses are prominent. The amount of cytoplasm is greater than in large cleaved cells and stains pale blue.

DIFFUSE LARGE CELL LYMPHOMA. This variant contains predominantly large cells of the cleaved and noncleaved types described above. It should be noted that the distinction between diffuse large cell lymphomas and the diffuse mixed variant is difficult and somewhat arbitrary. The two are merely different morphologic expressions within the spectrum of large cell lymphomas. Although classified as intermediate-grade lymphomas, these two variants have clinical features akin to those of the high-grade large cell immunoblastic lymphoma and will therefore be described in the next section.

High-Grade Lymphomas

Three lymphomas fall into this category: (1) large cell immunoblastic lymphomas; (2) lymphoblastic lymphoma, a tumor that occurs in adolescents and is associated with a characteristic clinical presentation; and (3) small noncleaved lymphomas, which include Burkitt's lymphoma and related B-cell neoplasms.

LARGE CELL IMMUNOBLASTIC LYMPHOMA. These lymphomas display a wide range of morpho-

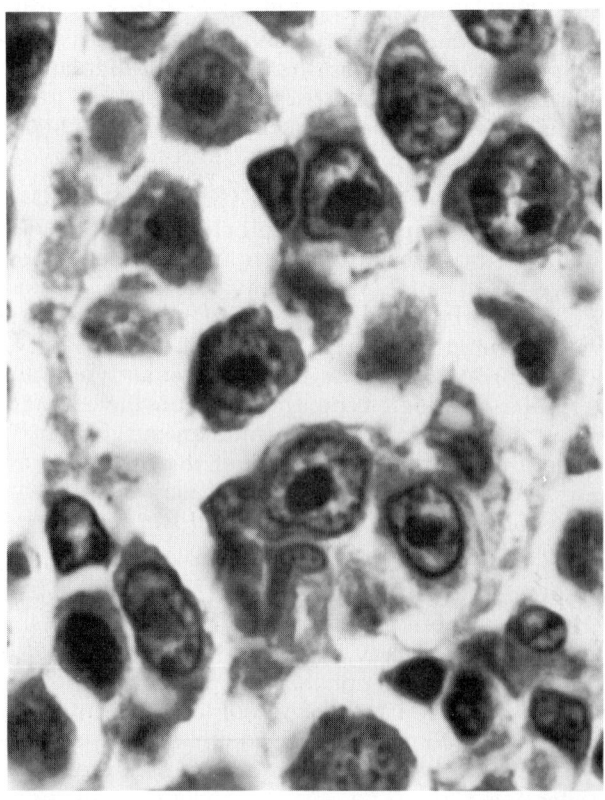

Figure 15–11. Non-Hodgkin's lymphoma, diffuse large cell type. Tumor cells in this example have large nuclei (compare with Figs. 15–9 and 15–10) and prominent nucleoli. (Courtesy of Dr. Jose Hernandez, Department of Pathology, Southwestern Medical School, Dallas, Texas.)

logic features. In some cases the tumor cells have plasmacytoid features and are therefore considered to be B immunoblasts. These cells are four to five times larger than a small lymphocyte and have a round or oval large nucleus that appears vesicular owing to margination of chromatin at the nuclear membrane. One or two centrally placed prominent nucleoli are usually seen. The cytoplasm is deeply staining, amphophilic, and pyroninophilic (increased affinity for the stain pyronin indicates accumulation of RNA in the cytoplasm in cells that are active in protein synthesis). In other cases, the tumor cells may contain large multilobated (polymorphous) nuclei, or the nucleus may be round with a clear cytoplasm. Some tumors have an admixture of large transformed cells and small atypical lymphocytes with contorted nuclei. Although features such as plasmacytoid appearance and clear cytoplasm or polymorphous nucleus are suggestive of B and T immunoblasts, respectively, most authors believe that there is a considerable morphologic overlap between B and T immunoblastic lymphomas[6]; therefore, a reliable distinction between the two types cannot be made without molecular or phenotypic studies. It is of interest to note that approximately 50% of B-immunoblastic lymphomas are associated with a previous history of an immunologic disorder such as Sjögren's syndrome or Hashimoto's thyroiditis, or with states of immunosuppression as in renal allograft recipients and patients with AIDS. This has relevance to the pathogenesis of lymphomas (p. 734).

Large cell immunoblastic lymphomas and the diffuse large cell and mixed lymphomas described earlier share several clinicopathologic features that differentiate them from follicular lymphomas.

• These tumors may arise from T or B cells, but numerically most are of B-cell origin. This can be demonstrated by immunophenotyping or by analyzing Ig gene rearrangements (Table 15–2).[15]
• They constitute 40 to 50% of adult NHLs; approximately one half have the diffuse large cell morphology. There is a slight male predominance with a median age of about 60 years. However, unlike follicular lymphomas, the age range is much wider, and diffuse NHLs constitute about 20% of childhood lymphomas.[16]
• In contrast to patients with follicular lymphomas, patients with these tumors typically present with a rapidly enlarging, often symptomatic mass at a single nodal or extranodal site. Localized disease and extranodal manifestations are more common than in follicular lymphomas. Indeed, involvement of the gastrointestinal tract, skin, bone, or brain may be the presenting feature. The Waldeyer's ring of oropharyngeal lymphoid tissue is involved in about 50% of these cases.
• Involvement of liver and spleen is not common at the time of diagnosis, but when it occurs, the lymphoma cells form large destructive masses, rather than forming the uniform miliary nodules that involve B-cell areas in low-grade follicular lymphomas.

Table 15–2. Techniques Used in the Diagnosis of Lymphoid Neoplasms

	TECHNIQUE		
CELL TYPE	*Immunologic**	*Molecular†*	*Histochemical*
T cells	Monoclonal antibodies	T-cell receptor gene rearrangement	—
B cells	Cell surface immunoglobulins‡	Immunoglobulin gene rearrangements	—
	Monoclonal antibodies		
Histiocytes	Monoclonal antibodies	—	Nonspecific esterases

*Immunologic techniques usually employ indirect immunofluorescence on frozen tissue sections or flow cytometry on cell suspensions. See Table 5–1 (p. 165) for listing of monoclonal antibodies specific for various cells.

†Molecular biologic techniques depend on demonstration of T-cell receptor or immunoglobulin gene rearrangements in the DNA extracted from tumor cells.

‡Clonal (neoplastic) proliferation of B cells is indicated by the presence of an immunoglobulin of a single light chain type. Cytoplasmic immunoglobulin, in the absence of surface immunoglobulin, is seen in pre-B cells.

- Bone marrow involvement is relatively uncommon in these patients, especially at the time of diagnosis. With progressive disease, however, the marrow may be involved, and, rarely, a leukemic picture may emerge.
- These three diffuse lymphomas are aggressive tumors that are rapidly fatal if untreated. However, with intensive combination chemotherapy, complete remission can be achieved in 60 to 80% of the patients and approximately 50% remain free of disease for several years and may be considered cured. This favorable response is related to the fact that these tumors have a high growth fraction, and most anticancer agents act on cells that are actively dividing (p. 253). In contrast, it should be recalled that although follicular lymphomas follow an indolent course, they are very difficult to cure.
- Despite impressive advances in accurate identification of the cell of origin and morphologic subclassification of these lymphomas, most studies have failed to show any significant correlation between cytologic subtype, immunologic phenotype, and response to therapy.[6,17] However, further stratification based on markers that identify T- and B-cell subsets may reveal differences. Some authors believe, for example, that large cell lymphomas exhibiting a post-thymic mature T-cell phenotype are the most aggressive of all diffuse lymphomas.[18]

LYMPHOBLASTIC LYMPHOMA (LL). This is a distinct clinicopathologic entity closely related to T-cell acute lymphoblastic leukemia (T-ALL). The tumor cells resemble the lymphoblasts of ALL. They are fairly uniform in size, with scanty cytoplasm and nuclei that are somewhat larger than those of small lymphocytes. The nuclear chromatin is delicate and finely stippled, and nucleoli are either absent or inconspicuous. In many, but not all, cases the nuclear membrane shows deep subdivision, imparting a convoluted (lobulated) appearance. In keeping with its aggressive growth, the tumor shows a high rate of mitosis, and as with other tumors having a high mitotic rate (e.g., Burkitt's lymphomas), a "starry sky" pattern is produced by the interspersed benign macrophages.

Lymphoblastic lymphoma predominantly affects males (2:1); most patients are under 20 years of age, although adults with this disease have been described. Although it constitutes less than 5% of all NHLs, approximately 40% of childhood lymphoma falls into this category.[16] A very characteristic clinical feature is the presence of a prominent mediastinal mass in 50 to 70% of patients at the time of diagnosis, suggesting a thymic origin. Indeed, the phenotype of the tumor cells resembles intrathymic T cells. Terminal deoxynucleotidyl transferase, an enzyme associated with primitive lymphoid cells, is expressed in all cases. In some patients the cells are CD2+, CD5+, and CD7+, as are early thymocytes, whereas in others CD4 and CD8 are coexpressed on tumor cells (see Fig. 15–18). The latter is noteworthy because CD4 and CD8 are never expressed together on mature peripheral T cells. The disease is rapidly progressive, and early dissemination to the bone marrow and thence to blood and meninges leads to the evolution of a picture resembling T-ALL. Until recently, the prognosis of this tumor was grim, but recent attempts to treat this tumor aggressively by utilizing protocols effective in ALL have produced encouraging results in some studies.[19]

SMALL NONCLEAVED CELL LYMPHOMA. Within this category fall Burkitt's lymphoma and related tumors seen outside Africa. It should be emphasized at the outset that the term "small" in the designation of these tumors is relative to the size of large noncleaved cells. As will be described below, the small noncleaved cells are intermediate in size between small lymphocytes and large noncleaved cells that are found in diffuse large cell lymphomas.

Burkitt's lymphoma was described initially in Africa, where it is endemic in some parts, but it also occurs sporadically in nonendemic areas including the United States. Histologically, the African and the nonendemic cases of Burkitt's lymphoma are identical, although there are some clinical and virologic differences. The relationship of these disorders to the Epstein-Barr virus (EBV) is discussed on pages 276 and 734. These tumors consist of a sea of strikingly monotonous cells, 10 to 25 μm in diameter, with round or oval nuclei containing two to five prominent nucleoli. The nuclear size approximates that of benign macrophages within the tumor. There is a moderate amount of faintly basophilic or amphophilic cytoplasm, which also is intensely pyroninophilic and often contains small, lipid-filled vacuoles (better appreciated on stained imprints of the tumor). A high mitotic index is very characteristic, as is cell death, accounting for the presence of numerous tissue macrophages with ingested nuclear debris. Since these benign macrophages, which are diffusely distributed among the tumor cells, are often surrounded by a clear space, they create a "starry sky" pattern (Fig. 15–12). Both the African and the non-African cases are found largely in children or young adults, accounting for approximately 30% of childhood NHLs in the United States. In both forms, the disease rarely arises in the lymph nodes. In African cases, involvement of the maxilla or mandible is the common mode of presentation (Fig. 15–13), whereas abdominal tumors (bowel, retroperitoneum, ovaries) are more common in cases seen in America. Leukemic transformation of Burkitt's lymphoma is uncommon, especially in African cases. These tumors respond well to aggressive chemotherapy, and long remissions have been reported. Although a relapse occurs in many cases, a 50% long-term survival rate can be expected with present methods of treatments.[19]

In the Working Formulation, a tumor distinct

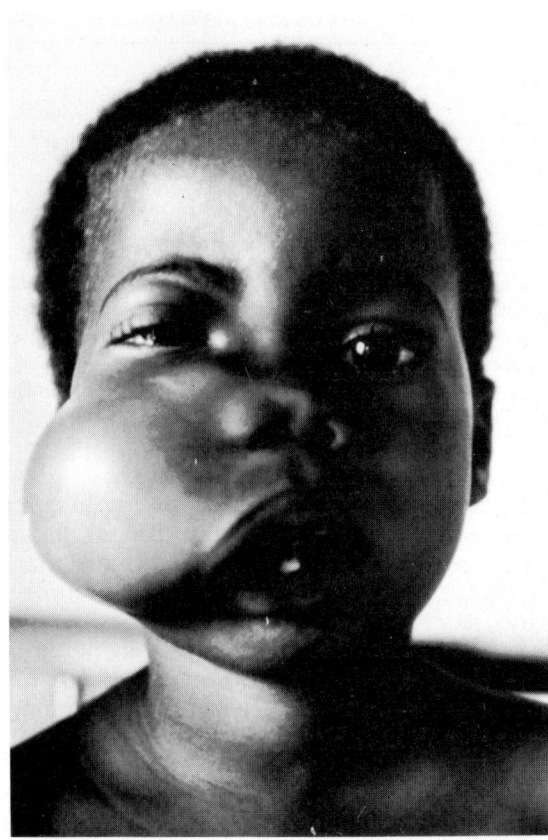

Figure 15–13. Burkitt's lymphoma in a nine-year-old child. The maxillary tumor mass is a characteristic presentation of this disease.

from Burkitt's lymphoma has also been included in the small noncleaved cell category. It commonly affects adults (median age 34 years) and is much less responsive to treatment. Histologically, the nuclei are approximately the same size as in Burkitt's tumor, but they show much greater variation in both shape and size, and occasional multinucleate cells are also seen. Because of the low frequency of this tumor, it has not been possible to determine whether it forms a distinct clinicopathologic entity.[6] Most investigators treat these tumors as aggressive large cell lymphomas.

Miscellaneous

This group includes several tumors such as the rare true histiocytic lymphomas and some that cannot be readily assigned to any one of the other categories. Only two, both of which are of T-cell origin, will be described here because each is associated with a rather distinct clinical presentation.

MYCOSIS FUNGOIDES AND SÉZARY SYNDROME. These are the best characterized of a group of disorders referred to as cutaneous T-cell lymphomas.[20] Involvement of skin is a hallmark of the tumors within this group. Clinically, the cutaneous lesions of *mycosis fungoides* show three somewhat distinct stages, discussed later (p. 1293). Briefly, mycosis fungoides presents with an inflammatory premycotic phase and progresses through a plaque phase

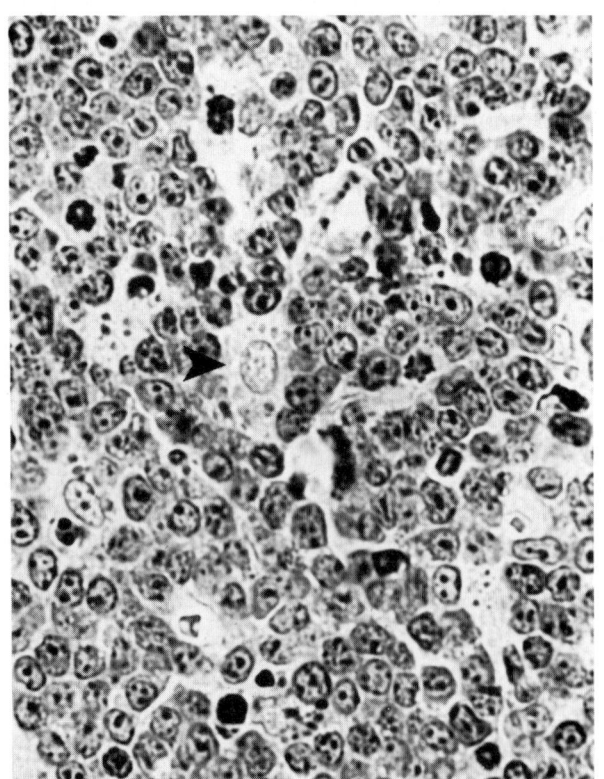

Figure 15–12. Burkitt's lymphoma. Tumor cells have multiple small nucleoli and high mitotic index. Lack of significant variation in nuclear shape and size lends a monotonous appearance interrupted by pale-staining, benign tissue macrophages *(arrow),* which impart a "starry sky" appearance better appreciated at a lower magnification. (Courtesy of Dr. Jose Hernandez, Department of Pathology, Southwestern Medical School, Dallas, Texas.)

to a tumor phase. *Histologically, there is infiltration of the epidermis and upper dermis by neoplastic T cells, which have an extremely unusual cerebriform nucleus.* This appearance results from marked and complex infolding of the nuclear membrane. In most patients with progressive disease, extracutaneous manifestations, characterized by nodal and visceral dissemination, appear. *Sézary syndrome* is a related condition in which skin involvement is manifested clinically as a generalized exfoliative erythroderma, but *in contrast to mycosis fungoides, the skin lesions rarely proceed to tumefaction.* Instead, there is an associated leukemia of "Sézary" cells that have the same cerebriform appearance noted in the tissue infiltrates of mycosis fungoides. Circulating Sézary cells can also be identified in up to 25% of cases of mycosis fungoides in the plaque or tumor phase, indicating that the two diseases have much in common. Fundamentally, both these disorders result from clonal proliferations of post-thymic CD4+ T lymphocytes. Although the prognosis in a given case depends on the extent of disease at the time of diagnosis, a median survival rate of eight to nine years is not unusual. In patients with disseminated disease associated with large numbers of tumor cells in the blood, a novel approach involving extracorporeal photochemotherapy seems to be promising.[21]

ADULT T-CELL LEUKEMIA/LYMPHOMA. This uncommon T-cell neoplasm has gained much prominence owing to its association with human T-cell leukemia virus-1 (HTLV-1), already discussed (p. 281). It is endemic in southern Japan and the Caribbean basin, but similar cases have been found sporadically in several countries including the southeastern United States.

Infection with HTLV-1 can give rise to a variety of clinical manifestations,[22] of which the most common is acute adult T-cell leukemia/lymphoma. This syndrome is characterized by skin lesions, generalized lymphadenopathy, hepatosplenomegaly, hypercalcemia, and an elevated leukocyte count with multilobed lymphocytes. Acute adult T-cell leukemia/lymphoma is an extremely aggressive disease with a median survival of about eight months. The tumor cells are CD4+, since HTLV-1 (like HIV-1) is tropic for T-helper cells. In addition, neoplastic lymphocytes express IL-2 receptor, although they are not dependent on IL-2 for their proliferation (p. 282).

In addition to tropism for CD4+ cells, HTLV-1 and HIV-1 share several other characteristics.[23]

• Both viruses can be transmitted by sexual intercourse or exposure to blood products or contaminated needles, or from a mother to her offspring.
• Both viruses can give rise to neurologic disorders. HTLV-1 infection has been associated with the syndrome of progressive spastic myelopathy in Japan.[24] The neurologic manifestations of HIV-1 infections are described in Chapter 29 (p. 1398).
• A long and variable latent period is characteristic of both viruses. It is estimated that the interval between infection (indicated by seroconversion) and development of T-cell lymphoma is years or possibly decades.

Since seroconversion following transfusion of blood from HTLV-1 seropositive donors has been documented, there is much concern regarding transmission of HTLV-1 infection by blood transfusions. Although no cases of adult T-cell leukemia/lymphoma have yet been attributed to blood transfusion, it is very likely that routine screening of donor blood for antibodies to HTLV-1 will be instituted in the near future.

ETIOLOGY AND PATHOGENESIS. The etiology of malignant lymphomas is as mysterious and puzzling as that of all neoplastic disorders. Because of the accumulating evidence that the etiology and pathogenesis of lymphomas and leukemias involve similar mechanisms, we will discuss them together later in this chapter (p. 733).

DIAGNOSIS AND STAGING. The diagnosis of NHLs can be suspected from the clinical features, but *histologic examination of the node is required for diagnosis.* Definite assignment of lymphomas to T- or B-cell lineage is accomplished by immunotyping and by analysis of T- and B-receptor gene rearrangements (Table 15–2). DNA hybridization studies also aid in the distinction between monoclonal (neoplastic) and polyclonal (reactive) proliferations of lymphocytes. Because neoplastic lymphocytes are associated with unique (clonal) gene rearrangements, the pattern of rearrangement can be used as a clonal tumor marker. This can be exploited to detect minimal residual disease after treatment or recurrences before they become clinically manifest.[25,26]

A form of clinical staging developed for Hodgkin's disease (see Table 15–4) is often used for NHL. However, it is much less useful in NHL since the correlation between the anatomic extent of the disease and the prognosis is less well established. For example, small lymphocytic lymphoma (SLL) is generally disseminated when the patient is first seen, but the prognosis in this case is excellent. Furthermore, the pattern of spread of NHL, unlike Hodgkin's disease, is less predictable and hence the utility of clinical staging is diminished.

A summary of the salient clinicopathologic features of NHLs is presented in Table 15–3.

HODGKIN'S DISEASE

Hodgkin's disease, like NHL, is a disorder involving primarily the lymphoid tissues.[27] It arises almost invariably in a single node or chain of nodes and spreads characteristically to the anatomically contiguous nodes. Nevertheless, it is separated from NHL for several reasons. First, it is characterized morphologically by the presence of distinctive neoplastic giant cells called Reed-Sternberg (RS) cells, admixed with a variable inflammatory infiltrate. Second, it is often associated with somewhat distinctive clinical fea-

Table 15–3. Summary of Non-Hodgkin's Lymphomas

LYMPHOMA TYPE OR GROUP	% (IN ADULTS)	SALIENT MORPHOLOGY	IMMUNOPHENOTYPE	COMMENTS
Small Lymphocytic Lymphoma (SLL)	3–4	Small unstimulated lymphocytes in a diffuse pattern	>95% B cells	Occurs in old age; generalized lymphadenopathy with marrow involvement and a blood picture resembling CLL; indolent course with prolonged survival
Follicular Lymphomas	40	Germinal center cells arranged in a follicular pattern	B cells	Follicular small cleaved-cell type most common; occur in older patients; generalized lymphadenopathy; associated with t(14;18); leukemia less common than in SLL; indolent course but difficult to cure
*Diffuse Lymphomas**	40–50	Various cell types; predominantly large germinal center cells; some mixed with smaller cells; others with immunoblastic morphology	~80% B cells ~20% post-thymic T cells	Occur in older patients as well as pediatric age group; greater frequency of extranodal, visceral disease; marrow involvement and leukemia very uncommon at diagnosis and poor prognostic sign; aggressive tumors but up to 60% are curable
Lymphoblastic Lymphoma	4	Cells somewhat larger than lymphocytes; in many cases nuclei markedly lobulated; high mitotic rate	>95% immature intrathymic T cells	Occurs predominantly in children (40% of all childhood lymphomas); prominent mediastinal mass; early involvement of bone marrow and progression to T-cell ALL; very aggressive
Small Noncleaved (Burkitt's) Lymphoma	<1	Cells intermediate in size between small lymphocytes and immunoblasts; prominent nucleoli; high mitotic rate	B cells	Endemic in Africa; sporadic elsewhere; predominantly affects children; extranodal visceral involvements presenting features; rapidly progressive but responsive to therapy; t(8;14) translocation characteristic
Mycosis Fungoides and Sézary Syndrome	Uncommon	Medium to large cells with markedly convoluted (cerebriform) nucleus	CD4 + T cells	Occur in older males; proclivity for involvement of skin in both forms; tumorous masses in mycosis fungoides; Sézary syndrome is leukemic variant
Adult T-Cell Leukemia/ Lymphoma	Rare	Very variable; cells may have cerebriform nuclei	CD4 + T cells	Associated with HTLV-1 infection; endemic in Japan and the Caribbean; cutaneous lesions, leukemia, spleen and lymph node involvement; rapidly fatal

*Includes diffuse large cell, diffuse mixed, and large cell immunoblastic lymphomas of the Working Formulation. Other NHLs with diffuse pattern, e.g., lymphoblastic lymphomas, that form distinct clinicopathologic categories not included.

tures, including systemic manifestations such as fever. Finally, the target cell of neoplastic transformation has yet to be identified with certainty. It accounts for 0.7% of all new cancers in the United States (which amounts to approximately 7400 new cases per year). Although overall it is an uncommon form of cancer, its importance stems from the fact that it is one of the most common forms of malignancy in young adults, with an average age at diagnosis of 32 years. Happily, tremendous progress has been made in the treatment of this disease in the last two decades, and it is now considered to be curable in most cases.

CLASSIFICATION. It should be some relief to the student to know that, unlike NHL, there is nearly universal acceptance of a single classification of Hodgkin's disease—the Rye classification.[28] Basically, there are four subtypes: (1) *lymphocyte predominance*, (2) *mixed cellularity*, (3) *lymphocyte depletion*, and (4) *nodular sclerosis*. Before delineating them, however, we should describe the common denominator among all—the RS cell—and the method used to characterize the extent of the disease in a patient—namely, the staging system.

A distinctive tumor giant cell known as the **Reed-Sternberg (RS) cell** is considered to be the essential neoplastic element in all forms of Hodgkin's disease, and its identification is essential for the histologic diagnosis. **Classically, it is a large cell (15 to 45 μm in diameter), most often binucleate or bilobed, with two halves often appearing as mirror images of each other (Fig. 15–14). At other times there are multiple nuclei, or the single nucleus is multilobate and polypoid. The nucleus is enclosed within an abundant amphophilic cytoplasm. Prominent within the nuclei are large, inclusion-like, "owl-eyed" nucleoli generally surrounded by a clear halo.** In typical RS cells the nucleoli are acidophilic or, at the least, amphophilic, and react strongly with RNA stains. Giant cells are sometimes found that have all the characteristics of the multinucleate cell just described and that contain only a single nucleus replete with large nucleolus. Although such cells may be biologic variants of the RS cell, they are not diagnostic of Hodgkin's disease. Other cells, uninucleate or multinucleate, may not have a nucleolus; these, too, are nondiagnostic. One additional variant, the so-called **lacunar cell,** is encountered primarily within one of the distinctive patterns of Hodgkin's disease called nodular sclerosis.

It is somewhat anticlimactic to report that cells closely simulating or identical with RS cells have been identified in conditions other than Hodgkin's disease. RS-like cells have been found in infectious mononucleosis and in solid tissue cancers, mycosis fungoides, lymphomas, and other conditions. Thus, although RS cells are requisite for the diagnosis, they must be present in an appropriate background of non-neoplastic inflammatory cells (lymphocytes, plasma cells, eosinophils). Stated another way, **the RS cell is necessary but not sufficient for the diagnosis.**

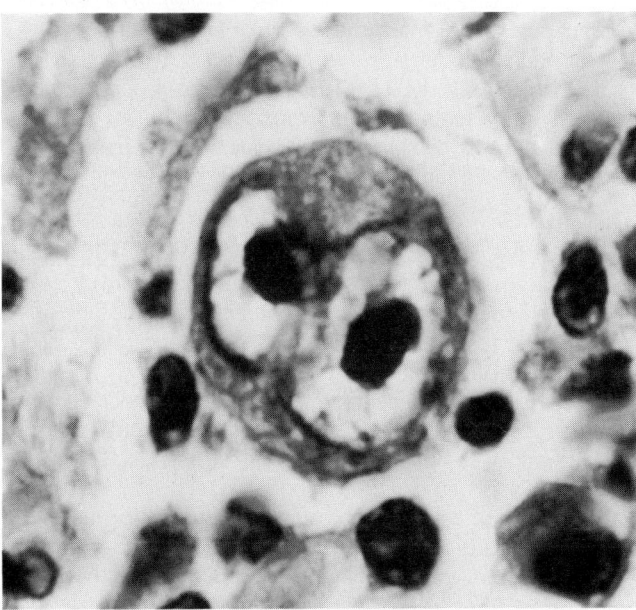

Figure 15–14. Reed-Sternberg cell. Note the prominent inclusion-like nucleoli with a clear halo around them. (Courtesy of Dr. Patrick Ward, Department of Pathology and Laboratory Medicine, University of Minnesota School of Medicine, Duluth, Minnesota.)

Table 15–4. Clinical Stages of Hodgkin's and Non-Hodgkin's Lymphomas (Ann Arbor Classification)*

STAGE	DISTRIBUTION OF DISEASE
I	Involvement of a single lymph node region (I) or involvement of a single extralymphatic organ or site (I$_E$).
II	Involvement of two or more lymph node regions on the same side of the diaphragm alone (II) or with involvement of limited contiguous extralymphatic organ or tissue (II$_E$).
III	Involvement of lymph node regions on both sides of the diaphragm (III), which may include the spleen (III$_S$) and/or limited contiguous extralymphatic organ or site (III$_E$, III$_{ES}$).
IV	Multiple or disseminated foci of involvement of one or more extralymphatic organs or tissues with or without lymphatic involvement.

*All stages are further divided on the basis of the absence (A) or presence (B) of the following systemic symptoms: significant fever, night sweats, and/or unexplained weight loss of greater than 10% of normal body weight.

From Carbone, P.T., et al.: Symposium (Ann Arbor): Staging in Hodgkin's disease. Cancer Res. *37*:1707, 1971.

The *staging of Hodgkin's disease* (Table 15–4) is of great clinical importance, since the course, choice of therapy, and prognosis are all intimately related to the distribution of the disease. Staging involves not only a careful physical examination but also several investigative procedures, including lymphangiography, chest x-ray, biopsy of the liver and bone marrow, scan of liver and spleen, and computed tomography. In selected cases, a laparotomy, which allows direct visualization of the intra-abdominal nodes, liver biopsy, and removal of the spleen are part of the staging protocol. It will become apparent that the more aggressive the variant of the disease, the greater the probability that it will be in a more advanced stage at the time of diagnosis.

With this background we can turn to the morphologic classification of Hodgkin's disease into its subgroups and point out some of the salient clinical features of each.[29] Later the manifestations common to all will be presented. The essential morphologic feature that serves to differentiate three subgroups (lymphocyte predominance, mixed cellularity, and lymphocyte depletion) is the frequency of the neoplastic elements (RS cells) relative to the reactive elements, represented by small lymphocytes. The extent of spread and the prognosis of Hodgkin's disease appear to be directly related to the ratio of RS cells to lymphocytes. The fourth subgroup, nodular sclerosis, appears to represent a special expression of the disease and has distinctive clinicopathologic features. The relative frequency of the four histologic subtypes may be gleaned from Table 15–5.

LYMPHOCYTE PREDOMINANCE HODGKIN'S DISEASE. This variant is characterized by a diffuse or sometimes vaguely nodular infiltrate of mature lym-

Table 15-5. Percentage of Patients in Each Pathologic Stage According to Histologic Subtype*

HISTOLOGIC SUBTYPE	NUMBER OF PATIENTS	PATHOLOGIC STAGE (%)		
		I and II	III	IV
Lymphocyte predominance	55	76	22	2
Mixed cellularity	215	44	47	9
Lymphocyte depletion	21	19	62	19
Nodular sclerosis	628	60	35	5

*From Desforges, J.F., et al.: Hodgkin's disease. N. Engl. J. Med. *301*:1212, 1979. Reprinted by permission of the New England Journal of Medicine.

phocytes admixed with variable numbers of benign histiocytes. Scattered among these cells are the distinctive RS cells, but these are almost always few in number (Fig. 15–15). Variants that lack the large "owl-eyed" nucleoli are somewhat more common but are not diagnostic. However, they serve as useful clues, since their presence warrants a careful search for typical RS cells. Other cells such as eosinophils, neutrophils, and plasma cells are scanty or absent, and there is little evidence of necrosis or fibrosis. A majority of patients are males, usually under 35 years of age, and they present with limited disease (Table 15–5). The prognosis is excellent. Without the identification of RS

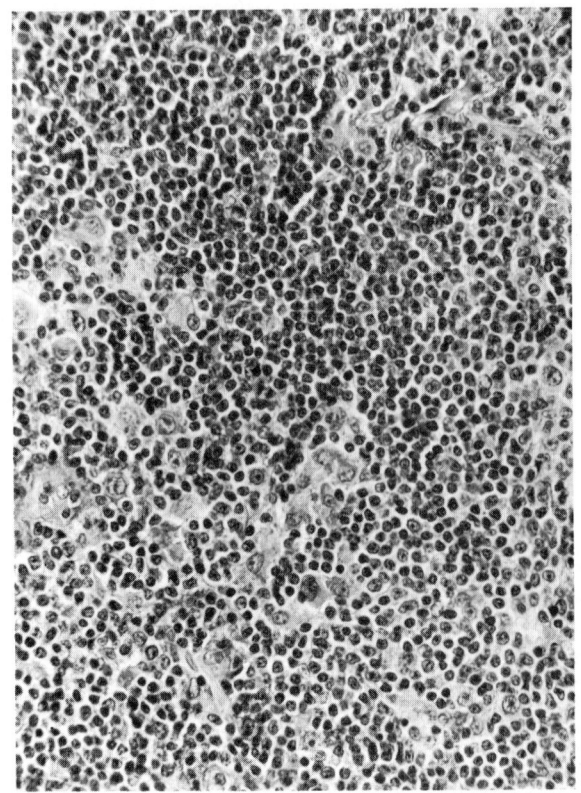

Figure 15-15. Lymphocyte-predominance Hodgkin's disease. (From Neiman, R.S.: Current problems in histopathologic diagnosis and classification of Hodgkin's disease. Pathol. Annu. *13:*289, 1978.)

cells, the lymphocyte predominance pattern could be readily mistaken for one of the lymphocytic forms of NHL. Indeed, several recent studies have raised the possibility that many cases classified as lymphocyte predominance Hodgkin's disease, especially those with a nodular infiltrate of lymphocytes, are in reality follicular non-Hodgkin's lymphomas.[30-32]

MIXED CELLULARITY HODGKIN'S DISEASE.

This form occupies an intermediate clinical position between the lymphocyte predominance and the lymphocyte depletion patterns. Typical RS cells are plentiful, but there are fewer lymphocytes than in lymphocyte predominance disease. The involvement of the lymph nodes is almost always diffuse. This pattern of Hodgkin's disease is rendered distinctive by its heterogeneous cellular infiltrate, which includes eosinophils, plasma cells, and benign histiocytes. Small areas of necrosis and fibrosis may be present, but they are usually not as prominent as in the lymphocyte depletion type. The mixed cellularity form of Hodgkin's disease is also more common in males.

Although the disease may be diagnosed in any of the clinical stages, as compared with the lymphocyte predominance pattern, more patients present with disseminated disease, and these patients more often have systemic manifestations (Table 15–5).

LYMPHOCYTE DEPLETION HODGKIN'S DISEASE.

This pattern is characterized by a paucity of lymphocytes and a relative abundance of RS cells or their pleomorphic variants. It presents in two morphologic forms, the so-called **diffuse fibrosis** and the **reticular variants.** In the former, the node is hypocellular and is replaced largely by a proteinaceous fibrillar material that represents a disorderly nonbirefringent connective tissue. Pleomorphic histiocytes, a few typical and atypical RS cells, and some lymphocytes are scattered within the fibrillar material (Fig. 15–16). The reticular variant is much more cellular and is composed of highly anaplastic, large, pleomorphic cells that resemble RS cells. Only a few typical RS cells can be recognized. A majority of patients with the lymphocyte depletion pattern are older, have disseminated involvement (Table 15–5), present with systemic manifestations, and have an aggressive form of the disease.

NODULAR SCLEROSIS HODGKIN'S DISEASE.

This pattern is distinct from the other three forms, both clinically and histologically. It is characterized morphologically by two features, including: (1) the presence of a particular variant of the RS cell, the **lacunar cell** (Fig. 15–17). This cell is large and has a single hyperlobated nucleus with multiple small nucleoli and an abundant, pale-staining cytoplasm with well-defined borders. In formalin-fixed tissue, the cytoplasm of these cells often retracts, giving rise to the appearance of cells lying in clear spaces or "lacunae." (2) The other feature seen in most cases is the collagen bands that divide the lymphoid tissue into circumscribed nodules (Fig. 15–17). The fibrosis may be scant or abundant, and the cellular infiltrate may show varying proportions of lymphocytes and lacunar cells. Classic RS cells are infrequent. In instances in which collagen bands are scanty, the diag-

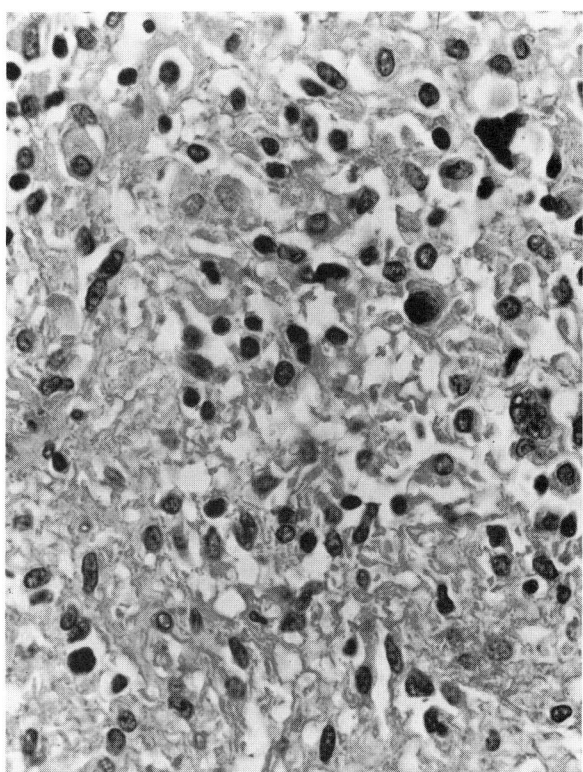

Figure 15–16. Lymph node in diffuse-fibrosis Hodgkin's disease. All cellular elements are greatly diminished, and granular, proteinaceous interstitial material is prominent. A few highly atypical polyploid cells that lack the cytologic features of Reed-Sternberg cells are present. (From Neiman, R.S.: Current problems in histopathologic diagnosis and classification of Hodgkin's disease. Pathol. Annu. *13*:289, 1978.)

nosis may rest with the identification of lacunar cells. Clinically, nodular sclerosis Hodgkin's disease has several distinctive features: It is the only form more common in women, and it has a striking propensity to involve the lower cervical, supraclavicular, and mediastinal lymph nodes. Most of the patients are adolescents or young adults, and they have an excellent prognosis, especially when seen in clinical stages I and II.

It is apparent that Hodgkin's disease spans a wide range of histologic patterns and that certain forms, with their characteristic fibrosis, eosinophils, neutrophils, and plasma cells, come deceptively close to simulating an inflammatory reactive process. **The diagnosis, then, of Hodgkin's disease rests solely on the unmistakable identification of the Reed-Sternberg cells in most variants and of the lacunar cells in the nodular sclerosis pattern.**

In all forms, involvement of the spleen, liver, bone marrow, and other organs and tissues may appear in due course and take the form of irregular, tumor-like nodules of tissue resembling that present in the nodes. At times the spleen is greatly enlarged and the liver is moderately enlarged by these nodular masses. At other times, the involvement is more subtle and becomes evident only on microscopic examination.

ETIOLOGY AND PATHOGENESIS. The origins of Hodgkin's disease are unknown. In the past it was believed that Hodgkin's disease was an unusual inflammatory reaction (possibly to an infectious agent) that behaved like a neoplasm. However, it is now widely accepted that Hodgkin's disease is a neoplastic disorder and that the RS cells represent the transformed cells. But the origin of RS cells remains an enigma. Virtually every cell of the lymphohematopoietic system has been blamed at one time or another.[33] The data relating to the origin of RS cells can be summarized as follows:

• Immunoenzymatic staining of RS cells on fresh lymph nodes has revealed staining with antigens specific for T cells (CD3, CD5, and CD2), or, in some cases, specific for B cells (CD19 and CD22).[34,35] In general, cells within the lymphocyte predominance type tend to stain with B-cell antigens. However, no single lineage-specific antigen has been found to mark RS cells in all cases.
• Molecular analysis of T-cell receptor (TCR) and Ig gene rearrangements has revealed a similar dichotomy. In some cases, RS cells and cell lines derived from these cells show clonal rearrangements of Ig genes; in others, TCRβ and TCRγ gene arrangements have been described.[36]

The general consensus from these studies seems to be that RS cells arise from lymphoid cells rather than from cells of the mononuclear-phagocytic series[33] and that Hodgkin's disease may be histogenetically heterogeneous. We must confess, however, that the present "state of the art" regarding the nature of RS cells can be best described as a "state of uncertainty."

Given that RS cells represent the malignant component of Hodgkin's disease, what causes neoplastic transformation? For years an infective etiology of Hodgkin's disease has been suspected, and some epidemiologists continue to incriminate Epstein-Barr virus as the culprit.[37] However, unlike African Burkitt's lymphoma, EBV viral DNA is found infrequently in lymph nodes of patients with Hodgkin's disease.[38,39] Interest in the infective etiology of Hodgkin's disease has nevertheless been sustained by reports that suggested a "clustering" of Hodgkin's disease among certain high school students.[40] Other studies, however, have failed to confirm the suggested horizontal spread of Hodgkin's disease.[41] The issue of an infectious origin therefore remains unresolved.

CLINICAL COURSE. Hodgkin's disease, like non-Hodgkin's lymphomas, usually presents with a painless enlargement of lymph nodes. Although a definitive distinction between Hodgkin's and non-Hodgkin's lymphomas can be made only by examination of a lymph node biopsy, several clinical features favor the diagnosis of Hodgkin's disease (Table 15–6). Younger patients, with the more favorable histologic types, tend to present in clinical stage I or II (see

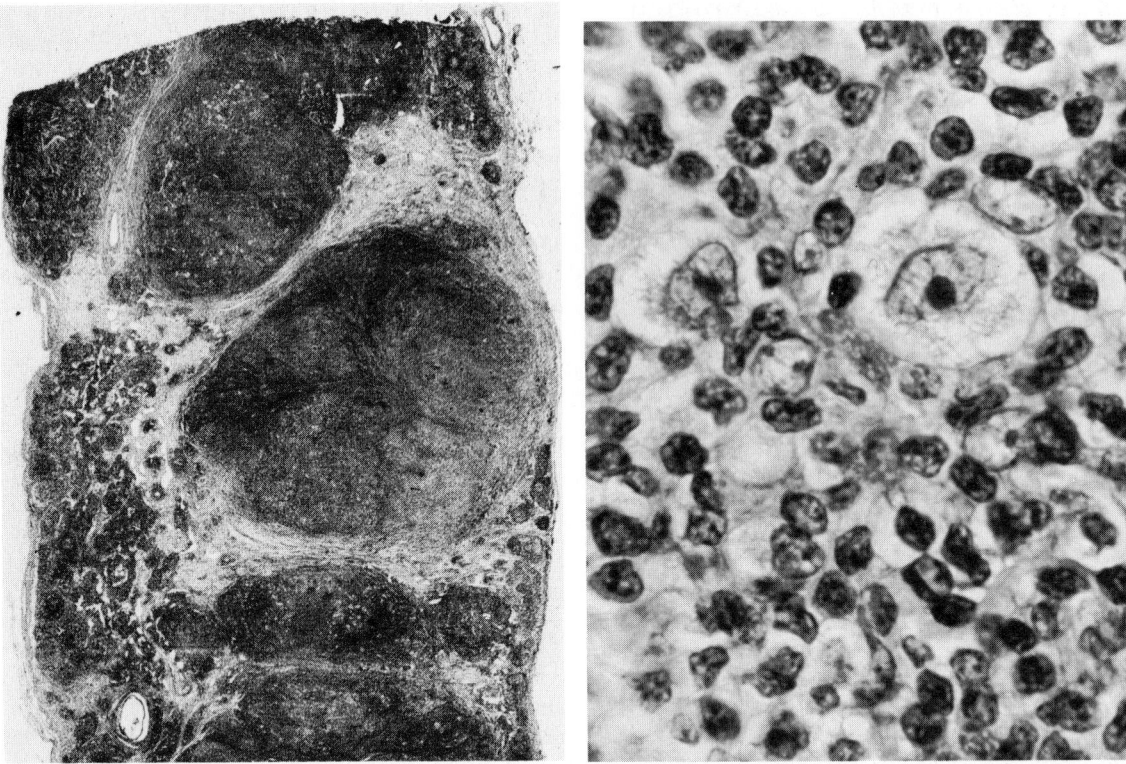

Figure 15–17. Hodgkin's disease—nodular sclerosis. The low-power view on the left shows well-defined bands of collagen enclosing nodules of abnormal lymphoid tissue. The high-power view on the right shows the distinctive lacunar cell, so called because the cell appears to lie within a cleared space. (Low-magnification photograph courtesy of Dr. Jose Hernandez, Department of Pathology, Southwestern Medical School, Dallas, Texas.)

Table 15 – 5) and are usually free of systemic manifestations. Patients with disseminated disease (stages III and IV) are more likely to present with systemic complaints such as fever, unexplained weight loss, pruritus, and anemia. As mentioned earlier (p. 719), these patients generally have the histologically less favorable variants. The outlook following aggressive radiotherapy and chemotherapy for patients with this disease, including those with disseminated disease, is changing rapidly. Currently the five-year survival rate of patients with stages I and IIA is close to 100%, and many can be cured. Even with advanced disease (stages IVA and IVB), 50% five-year disease-free survival can be achieved. As might be expected, the his-

tologic type affects the outcome of Hodgkin's disease. However, with current modalities of therapy, tumor burden (i.e., stage) is the most important prognostic variable.[42] Progress in the treatment of Hodgkin's disease has created a new set of problems. Long-term survivors of chemotherapy and radiotherapy have an increased risk of developing second cancers. Acute nonlymphocytic leukemia and lung cancer lead the list of second malignancies, but also included are non-Hodgkin's lymphoma, cancer of the stomach, and malignant melanoma.[43] The many therapeutic steps forward, in the light of this unhappy byproduct, may involve a few steps backward.

LEUKEMIAS AND MYELOPROLIFERATIVE DISEASES

The leukemias are malignant neoplasms of the hematopoietic stem cells, characterized by diffuse replacement of the bone marrow by neoplastic cells. In most cases, the leukemic cells spill over into the blood, where they may be seen in large numbers. These cells may also infiltrate the liver, spleen, lymph nodes, and other tissues throughout the body. Although the presence of excessive numbers of abnormal cells in the peripheral blood is the most dramatic manifestation of leukemia, it should be remembered that the leuke-

Table 15 – 6. Clinical Differences Between Hodgkin's and Non-Hodgkin's Lymphomas

HODGKIN'S DISEASE	NON-HODGKIN'S LYMPHOMA
More often localized to a single axial group of nodes (cervical, mediastinal, para-aortic)	More frequent involvement of multiple peripheral nodes
Orderly spread by contiguity	Noncontiguous spread
Mesenteric nodes and Waldeyer's ring rarely involved	Waldeyer's ring and mesenteric nodes commonly involved
Extranodal involvement uncommon	Extranodal involvement common

mias are primary disorders of the bone marrow. Indeed, some patients with a diffusely infiltrated bone marrow may present with leukopenia rather than leukocytosis.

CLASSIFICATION. Traditionally, leukemias are classified on the basis of the cell type involved and the state of maturity of the leukemic cells. Thus, *acute leukemias* are characterized by the presence of very immature cells (called blasts) and by a rapidly fatal course in untreated patients. On the other hand, *chronic leukemias* are associated, at least initially, with well-differentiated (mature) leukocytes and with a relatively indolent course. Two major variants of acute and chronic leukemias are recognized: *lymphocytic* and *myelocytic* (myelogenous). Thus, a simple classification would have four patterns of leukemia: acute lymphocytic leukemia (ALL), chronic lymphocytic leukemia (CLL), acute myelocytic (myeloblastic) leukemia (AML), and chronic myelocytic leukemia (CML). This simple and time-honored classification raises several difficulties when dealing with "chronic leukemias." Acute leukemias, despite differences in their cell of origin, share important morphologic and clinical features. They are associated with replacement of normal marrow elements by a sea of proliferating "blast cells" that do not seem to undergo normal maturation. Consequently, there is a loss of mature myeloid elements such as red cells, granulocytes, and platelets, and hence clinical features of acute leukemias are dominated by anemia, infections, and hemorrhages.

In contrast, the grouping together of chronic lymphocytic and myelogenous leukemias is problematic. A characteristic shared by these two disorders is that they are not rapidly fatal, but the clinical and morphologic features that seem to unite the acute leukemias are lacking. Furthermore, this traditional grouping of chronic leukemias has become less tenable with recent advances in our knowledge of the origins of chronic myelogenous leukemia and related disorders. *It is now widely accepted that CML, polycythemia vera, essential thrombocythemia, and myeloid metaplasia represent clonal neoplastic proliferations of the multipotent myeloid stem cells* (see Fig. 14–1). If the erythrocytic precursors dominate, the resulting clinical disorder is classified as *polycythemia vera;* on the other hand, the dominance of granulocytic series is manifested as *CML.* It seems that the term *chronic myeloproliferative disorders,* coined by Dameshek almost 40 years ago, best describes these neoplasms of the myeloid stem cell. Although the individual chronic myeloproliferative disorders have distinctive clinical features, interconversions and overlaps between some members of this group are well known and further attest to their relatedness. For example, a patient may present initially with polycythemia vera, but over the years this disorder may "convert" to myeloid metaplasia with myelofibrosis.

In analogy with chronic myeloproliferative disorders, it is possible to segregate chronic lymphoproliferative disorders. This group would include *chronic lymphatic leukemia* and *hairy cell leukemia,* both representing neoplastic proliferations of lymphoid cells, most often of B-cell lineage. It will be apparent that as proliferative disorders of lymphoid cells, they are related to the non-Hodgkin's lymphomas already discussed. Indeed, as already mentioned, there is very little clinical or anatomic difference between CLL and small lymphocytic lymphomas.

It should be obvious from the foregoing discussion that the heterogeneity of leukemias defies a rational classification that is scientifically accurate as well as clinically useful. In the ensuing discussion we will follow a clinically oriented approach of segregating the acute and chronic leukemias from the chronic myeloproliferative disorders such as polycythemia vera and myeloid metaplasia.

Our discussion will focus initially on the distinctive pathophysiologic and clinical features of different forms of leukemias; it will be followed by the description of morphologic changes that are common to most leukemias, and, finally, a discussion of the etiology and pathogenesis of leukemias and lymphomas.

ACUTE LEUKEMIAS

As with all leukemias, the acute ones have their origin in neoplastic monoclonal proliferation of hematopoietic stem cells. Acute leukemias are characterized by a paucity of mature cells and an accumulation of leukocyte precursors (leukemic blasts).

PATHOPHYSIOLOGY. Morphologic and cell kinetic studies have indicated that in acute leukemias there is a block in differentiation of leukemic stem cells and that the leukemic blasts have a prolonged rather than shortened generation time. *Thus, the accumulation of leukemic blasts in acute leukemia results primarily from a failure of maturation into functional end cells rather than from rapid proliferation of the transformed cells.* As the leukemic blasts accumulate in the marrow, they suppress normal hematopoietic stem cells by mechanisms that are incompletely understood. Suppression is in part related to physical replacement of normal precursor cells by the expanded clone of leukemic cells. However, in some patients the marrow is not completely replaced with malignant cells and indeed may be hypocellular. Thus, a simple hypothesis based on "crowding out" by malignant cells is insufficient to explain suppression of normal hematopoiesis. It is considered likely that leukemic cells actively inhibit normal stem cells by cellular or humoral mechanisms. Suppression of normal hematopoietic stem cells in acute leukemia has two important clinical implications: (1) The major manifestations result from the paucity of normal red cells, white cells, and platelets; and (2) therapeutically the aim is to reduce the population of the leukemic clone enough to allow recovery of normal stem cells. Quite unexpectedly, some recent molecular studies indicate that the normally differentiated cells found in the peripheral blood of some patients with therapy-induced remission are descendents of the leukemic stem cells.[44] These findings are of interest since they suggest that a block in maturation, the hallmark of acute leukemia, is not irreversible and that therapeutic strategies designed to favor differentiation of the leukemic clone may be useful adjuncts in the treatment of leukemia.[45]

Leukemic transformation may affect any stage during the differentiation of pluripotent hematopoietic stem cells (see Fig. 14–1, p. 659). Involvement of the lymphoid series gives rise to ALL, whereas neoplastic transformation of myeloid progenitor cells is expressed in the form of AML.

Acute Lymphoblastic Leukemia (ALL)

Acute lymphoblastic leukemia is primarily a disease of children and young adults. Approximately 1800 new cases are diagnosed each year in the United States in individuals under 15 years of age; this constitutes 80% of childhood acute leukemias. ALL occurs in adults, but much less frequently. Childhood ALL has a peak incidence at approximately four years of age. It is almost twice as common in whites as in nonwhites and is slightly more frequent in boys than in girls.[46]

CLASSIFICATION. ALL can be subdivided by morphologic and immunologic criteria. Morphologic subtypes designated L1, L2, and L3 have been defined in the French-American-British (FAB) classification of acute leukemias (Table 15–7). In approximately 85% of children with ALL, lymphoblasts are predominantly of the L1 subtype; fewer than 15% have L2 morphology, a subtype more commonly seen in adults. The L3 ALL usually equates with leukemic manifestation of Burkitt's lymphoma, and makes up approximately 1 to 2% of the lymphoblastic leukemias in children.[47]

An alternative immunologic subclassification is employed more widely and is based on the origin of the leukemic lymphoblasts and their stage of differentiation as defined by cell surface markers and antigen receptor gene rearrangements (Fig. 15–18). Because immunophenotyping has prognostic implications, it is detailed in Table 15–8 and summarized below:

• While the leukemic blasts express surface Ig in less than 2% of the patients, the vast majority of ALLs (80%) have proved to be of B cell origin.
• The leukemic blasts of almost every patient with B-cell ALL express the CD19 antigen (detected by anti-B4 antibody). Its expression is restricted to B cells; in some patients with early precursor B-cell ALL, CD19 is the only B-cell specific marker on the leukemic cells.
• T lymphoblasts in patients with T-cell ALL seem to be arrested at early intrathymic stages of maturation. Thus, T-cell ALL is related to lymphoblastic lymphoma (p. 715) but distinct from other T-cell neoplasms such as adult T-cell leukemia/lymphoma and Sézary syndrome, in which the neoplastic cells express the mature peripheral T-cell phenotype (p. 716).

Table 15–7. French-American-British (FAB) Classification of Acute Lymphoblastic Leukemias

LI	Small cells predominate but may vary, with some cells up to twice diameter of small lymphocytes. Nuclei are generally round and regular with occasional clefts. Nucleoli often are not visible. Cytoplasm is scanty. Cell population is homogeneous.
L2	Cells are heterogeneous in size, and share in features of both L1 and L3. Nuclei often show clefts. Nucleoli are often present.
L3	There is a homogeneous population of large cells (3 to 4 times the diameter of small lymphocytes). Nuclei are round-to-oval with prominent nucleoli. Cytoplasm is abundant and deeply basophilic.

• Prognostic differences exist among immunologic subtypes of ALL. The most favorable outcome is for patients with early precursor B-cell ALL, fortunately the largest group of all. The prognosis is intermediate for T-cell and pre–B-cell ALL, and it is the poorest for B-cell ALL. The latter, it should be noted, represents the leukemic phase of Burkitt's lymphoma.

CHROMOSOMAL CHANGES. Approximately 60% of patients with ALL have karyotypic abnormalities in their leukemia cells. Some of the cytogenetic changes contribute prognostic information that is independent of other variables such as sex, age, and immunophenotype. Hyperdiploidy (up to 60 chromosomes) is fairly common in early precursor B-cell ALL and is present in about 25 to 30% of all cases of ALL. There is a well-documented association between hyperdiploidy in the range of 51 to 60 chromosomes and good prognosis.[48,48a] Several other less common but prognostically important karyotypic abnormalities are listed below:

• A Philadelphia chromosome (Ph¹) that is microscopically indistinguishable from the Ph¹ seen in chronic myelogenous leukemia is found in about 15% of adult cases of ALL and about 5% of childhood cases. This translocation is associated with poor prognosis.
• About 20 to 25% of pre–B-cell ALLs have a t(1;19) translocation, associated with a poor prognosis.
• B-cell ALL of the FAB L3 type is almost invariably associated with the t(8;14) translocation characteristic of Burkitt's lymphoma. This subtype of ALL has a very poor prognosis.

Acute Myeloblastic Leukemia (AML)

Acute myeloblastic leukemias primarily affect adults between the ages of 15 and 39 years. They constitute only 20% of childhood leukemias. AML is extraordinarily heterogeneous, reflecting the complexities of myeloid cell differentiation.

PATHOGENESIS AND CLASSIFICATION. Acute myeloblastic leukemias are of diverse origin. Some arise by transformation of multipotent (trilineage) myeloid stem cells (see Fig. 14–1, p. 659), as evidenced by common cytogenetic abnormalities in granulocytic and erythroid precursors, even though myeloblasts dominate the blood and bone marrow. In

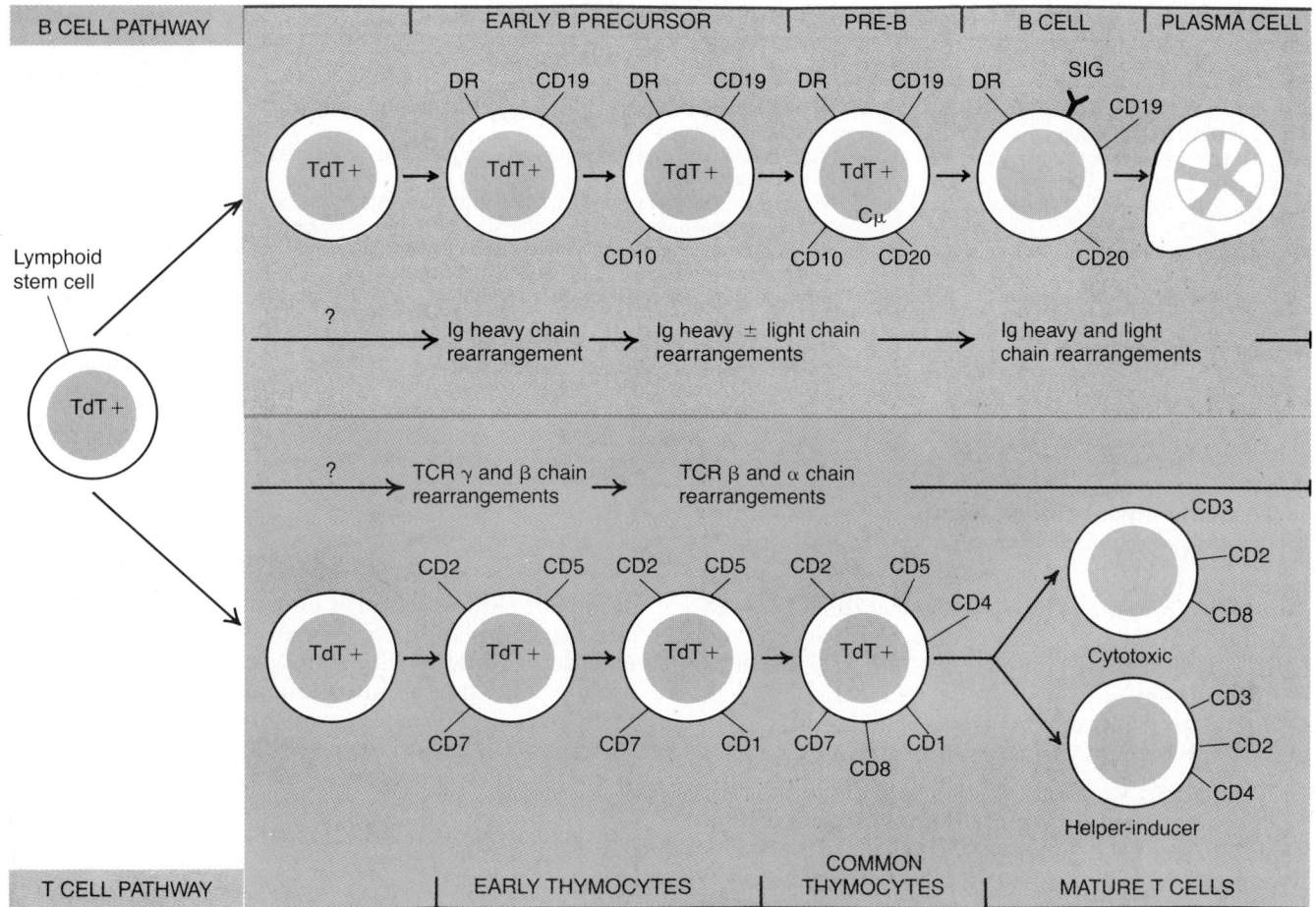

Figure 15–18. Schematic illustration of the phenotypic and genotypic changes associated with the differentiation of B cells and T cells. Not shown are some CD4+, CD8+ cells (common thymocytes) that also express CD3. CD = cluster designation. TdT = terminal deoxynucleotidyl transferase; Ig = immunoglobulin; TCR = T-cell receptor.

others the common granulocyte-monocyte precursor is involved, giving rise to myelomonocytic disease. In the widely used FAB classification (Table 15–9), AML is divided into seven categories. This scheme takes into account both the degree of maturation (M1 to M3) and the predominant line of differentiation of the leukemic stem cells (M4 to M7). In view of the marked heterogeneity of this group of leukemias, some authorities prefer to use the term "acute non-lymphocytic leukemia" to encompass the varied morphologic expressions. Monoclonal antibodies that recognize determinants on various myelomonocytic cells are available, but they are not widely utilized in the subclassification of acute nonlymphocytic leukemia.

Table 15–8. Immunologic Classification of ALL

	EARLY PRECURSOR B SUBTYPES		PRE-B	B	T	UNCLASSIFIED
	10%	*50%*	*20%*	*1–2%*	*15%*	*<5%*
Immunologic Markers						
HLA-DR	+	+	+	+	−	+
CD19 (B4)	+	+	+	+	−	−
CD10 (CALLA)	−	+	+	(−)	(−)	−
CD20 (B1)	−	±	+	+	−	−
Cμ	−	−	+	−	−	−
S Ig	−	−	−	+	−	−
Thymocyte* antigens	−	−	−	−	+	−
FAB Classification	L₁ L₂		L₁ L₂	L₃	L₁ L₂	Variable

Frequencies are approximations from several studies.

(−) Less than 10% of cases are positive for CD10.

*Markers for immature intrathymic T cells: CD2, CD5, CD7.

Table 15-9. FAB Classification of Acute Myeloblastic (Myelocytic) Leukemias (AML)

	FAB CLASS	% OF AML†	MORPHOLOGY	HISTOCHEMISTRY
M1	Acute myelocytic leukemia without differentiation	20	Myeloblasts predominate; distinct nucleoli; few granules or Auer rods	Myeloperoxidase +
M2	Acute myelocytic leukemia with differentiation	30	Myeloblasts and promyelocytes predominate; Auer rods may be present	Myeloperoxidase +++
M3	Acute promyelocytic leukemia	5	Hypergranular promyelocytes; often with many Auer rods per cell; may have reniform or bilobed nuclei	Myeloperoxidase +++
M4	Acute myelomonocytic leukemia	30	Myelocytic and monocytic differentiation evident; myeloid elements resemble M2; peripheral monocytosis	Myeloperoxidase ++ *Nonspecific esterase +
M5	Acute monocytic leukemia	10	Promonocytes or undifferentiated blasts	*Nonspecific esterase ++
M6	Acute erythroleukemia	5	Bizarre, multinucleated, megaloblastoid erythroblasts predominate; myeloblasts also present	Myeloperoxidase + (Myeloblasts) PAS + (Erythroblasts)
M7	Acute megakaryocytic leukemia	5	Pleomorphic undifferentiated blasts; react with antiplatelet antibodies; myelofibrosis or increased bone marrow reticulin	Platelet peroxidase + by electron microscopy

*Reaction inhibited by sodium fluoride.
†Percentages are approximations.

However, a panel of monoclonal antibodies (anti-My9, My7, and Mo1) directed against the CD33, CD 13, and CD11 determinants react with the leukemia cells in the majority (about 80%) of AMLs and are therefore helpful in distinguishing AML from ALL. Other features of value in providing diagnostic differentiation between AML and ALL are:

• *Morphologic features* of the leukemic blasts in Wright-Giemsa stained preparations. Myeloblasts are characterized by delicate nuclear chromatin, three to five nucleoli, and fine azurophilic granules in the cytoplasm (Fig. 15–19). In some cases, they possess distinctive red-staining intracytoplasmic rodlike structures referred to as Auer rods. In contrast, the nuclei of lymphoblasts have somewhat coarse and clumped chromatin and fewer nucleoli. Azurophilic granules and Auer rods are not present in the cytoplasm.
• *Cytochemistry.* In most cases of ALL, the blasts contain large aggregates of PAS-positive material, whereas myeloblastic leukemias are generally positive for myeloperoxidase. Monocytic differentiation is associated with staining for the lysosomal nonspecific esterases. *Terminal deoxynucleotidyl transferase (TdT), a DNA polymerase, is very useful in distinguishing ALL from AML, since this enzyme is present in 95% of cases of ALL and in less than 5% of AMLs.*

CHROMOSOMAL ABNORMALITIES. Special high-resolution banding techniques have revealed chromosomal abnormalities in approximately 90% of all AML patients. In 50 to 70% of the cases, the karyotypic changes can be detected by standard cytogenetic techniques. Many of the nonrandom chromosomal abnormalities have prognostic implications that are independent of other clinical prognostic factors.[49-51] These are summarized in Table 15–10.

CLINICAL FEATURES OF ACUTE LEUKEMIAS. Acute lymphoblastic and myeloblastic leukemias share several clinical features. Both forms have an abrupt, stormy onset, with most patients presenting within three months of the onset of symptoms. The dominant clinical features of acute leukemias are related to depression of normal marrow function and include (1) fatigue due mainly to anemia; (2) fever, usually reflecting an infection; and (3) bleeding (petechiae, ecchymoses, epistaxis, and gingival bleeding) secondary to thrombocytopenia. Generalized lymphadenopathy, splenomegaly, and hepatomegaly, the results of organ infiltration by leukemic cells, are characteristic of ALL but usually are not prominent

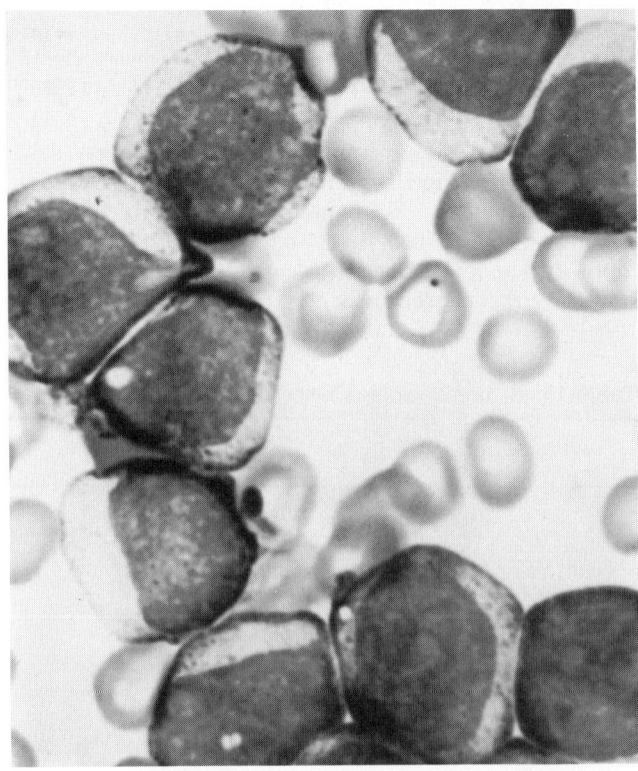

Figure 15–19. Acute myelocytic leukemia (M1). Myeloblasts flood the peripheral blood. (Courtesy of Dr. Robert W. McKenna, Southwestern Medical School, Dallas, Texas.)

Table 15–10. Chromosomal Abnormalities in AML and Their Significance

CHROMOSOME ABNORMALITY	FAB SUBGROUP	FREQUENCY	COMMENT
t(9;22) Ph¹ chromosome	M1	3%	Poor to intermediate prognosis
t(8;21)	M2	20%	Found more often in younger males; associated with good prognosis
t(15;17)	M3	70–100%	Unique to M3; intermediate prognosis
inv 16 or del 16q	M4	~25%	Good prognosis
del 11q or t(11;V*)	M5 (some M4)	30%	Intermediate prognosis
+8	M1, M2, M4, M5, M6	Variable	Most common abnormality in a wide variety of hematopoietic neoplasms; no prognostic association
−7 or del (7q)	—	—	Most frequently seen in patients older than 60 years in secondary
−5 or del (5q)			leukemias associated with exposure to environmental or occupational carcinogens

*V = Variable chromosomes.

(Courtesy of Dr. Nancy Schneider, Department of Pathology, Southwestern Medical School, Dallas, Texas.)

with AML. The marrow involvement in both disorders leads to subperiosteal bone infiltration, marrow expansion, and bone resorption, often resulting in bone pain and tenderness on palpation. CNS manifestations may appear with leukemic infiltration of the meninges, producing headache, nausea, vomiting, papilledema, cranial nerve palsies, and sometimes seizures and coma. Intracerebral or subarachnoid hemorrhages may result from thrombocytopenia and leukostasis, i.e., intravascular clumping of leukemic

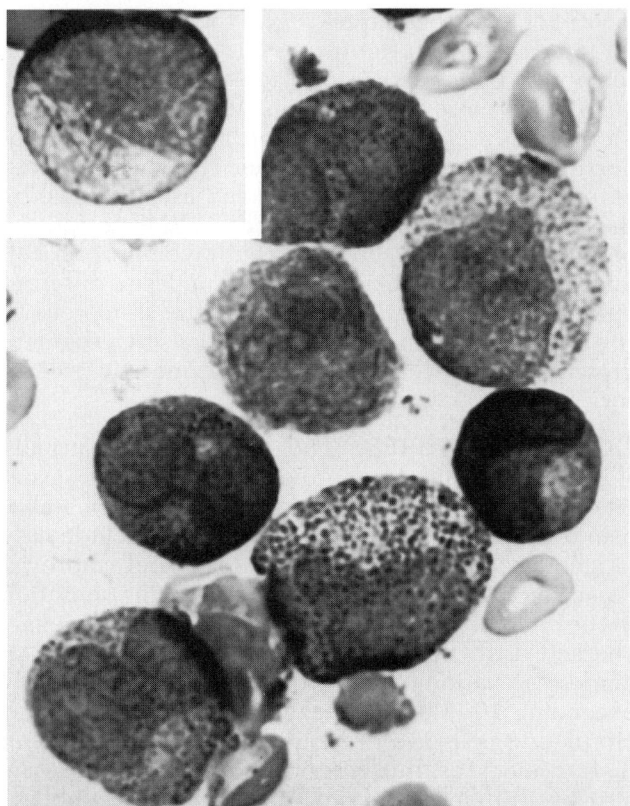

Figure 15–20. Acute promyelocytic leukemia (M3). Peripheral blood smear shows hypergranular promyelocytes. Inset (upper left) shows a cell with prominent Auer rods. (Courtesy of Dr. Robert W. McKenna, Southwestern Medical School, Dallas, Texas.)

blasts in the small blood vessels of the brain. Microvascular occlusions are seen most commonly in AML. Occasionally, DIC punctuates the course of the promyelocytic (M3) form of AML (p. 698), especially when cell lysis caused by therapy results in the release of thromboplastic substances from the granules (Fig. 15–20). As discussed earlier (p. 715), a mediastinal mass (reflecting involvement of thymus) is frequently seen in T-cell ALL. Although virtually any extramedullary site may be infiltrated by leukemic cells, testicular involvement is particularly common in ALL, and tumorous accumulations within soft tissues or bones, referred to as *chloromas* (owing to their green color), are seen most commonly in AMLs (M1 and M2). Infiltration of gums is characteristic of M4 and M5 AMLs. Several other less common but distinctive presentations of AML, associated for example with morphologically abnormal eosinophils or megakaryocytes, have also been described.[52]

Both forms of acute leukemia are characterized by distinctive laboratory findings. Anemia is almost always present. The white count in about half the patients is less than 10,000 cells per mm³ of blood, whereas in about 20% it is elevated above 100,000 cells per mm³. Much more important is the finding of immature white cells, including "blast" forms, in the circulating blood and the bone marrow, where they make up 60 to 100% of all the cells. The platelet count is almost always depressed and in a great majority of cases is less than 100,000 per mm³. Pancytopenia without any immature cells in the peripheral blood is found in a small percentage of cases and is referred to as aleukemic leukemia. Marrow examination in such cases helps to rule out aplastic anemia.

The prognosis for the two forms of acute leukemia is best considered individually because they differ so much. With modern chemotherapy (which includes prophylactic kill of leukemic cells that may find a sanctuary in the CNS), over 90% of children with ALL achieve complete remission and more than 60% are alive five years later. Most of them are likely to have been cured.[46] The prognosis is influenced by age, immunophenotype, and cytogenetic changes, as discussed. Briefly, ALL in children between two and ten years of age with early precursor B phenotype and hyperdiploidy in the range of 51 to 60 chromosomes has the most favorable outcome. Adults, or children with T-cell disease, fare much less well. The outlook for patients with AML is far less optimistic. Although 60 to 80% of patients achieve remission with intensive chemotherapy, relapse within 12 to 18 months is common and long-term disease-free survival can be expected in only 10 to 15% of cases. In view of such a grim prognosis, bone marrow transplantation is being attempted at many centers and is usually performed in young patients during first remission. Initial results in selected groups of patients are promising. It is being increasingly recognized that AML is a biologically heterogeneous group, and future studies are aimed at separating subgroups with differing natural histories.[53,54]

Myelodysplastic Syndromes

This term refers to a group of stem cell disorders characterized by maturation defects resulting in ineffective hematopoiesis and an increased risk of transformation to acute myeloblastic leukemias.[55,56] In patients with this syndrome, bone marrow is partly or wholly replaced by a clone of stem cells that retains the capacity to differentiate into red cells, granulocytes, and platelets, but in a manner that is both ineffective and disordered. As a result, the bone marrow is usually hypercellular or normocellular, but the peripheral blood shows pancytopenia. The abnormal stem cell clone in the bone marrow is genetically unstable, with a tendency to lose the ability for differentiation, thus giving rise to an acute leukemia.

Myelodysplastic syndromes have been classified into five categories on the basis of morphologic appearance of cells in the marrow and peripheral blood.[56] These will not be detailed here but include features such as megaloblastoid erythroid precursors, hypogranular myeloid precursors, increased proportion of blast cells in the marrow, micromegakaryocytes, agranular platelets, and unilobed or bilobed neutrophils. All these changes represent the morphologic expression of disordered hematopoiesis. Cytogenetic studies reveal chromosomal abnormalities in up to two thirds of the patients.[57] Some of the more common ones are loss of chromosomes 5, 7, or Y; deletions of parts of the long arms of chromosomes 5, 7, or 20; and trisomy 8.

Most patients with myelodysplasia are elderly males between 60 and 70 years of age. They present with weakness, infections, and hemorrhages, owing to pancytopenia. A sizable minority of patients are asymptomatic and are discovered following incidental blood tests. Although myelodysplasia is regarded as a preleukemic condition, only one third of the patients progress to frank AML; others are constantly threatened by infections and hemorrhages. The median survival is influenced by the specific form of myelodysplasia and by karyotypic abnormalities and varies from one to five years.[58]

CHRONIC MYELOID LEUKEMIA (CML)

This form of leukemia accounts for about 15 to 20% of all cases of leukemia. It is primarily a disease of adults between the ages of 25 and 60 years, with the peak incidence in the fourth and fifth decades of life. A slight male preponderance has been noted, but the clinical course of the disease is similar in both sexes.

PATHOPHYSIOLOGY. As mentioned earlier, CML is one of the four chronic myeloproliferative disorders. However, CML is associated with the presence of a distinctive chromosomal abnormality, the Ph^1 (Philadelphia) chromosome. *In approximately 90% of patients with CML, the Ph^1 chromosome, usually representing a reciprocal translocation from the long arm of chromosome 22 to another chromosome (usually the long arm of chromosome 9), can be identified in all the dividing progeny of multipotent myeloid stem cells (i.e., granulocytic, erythroid, and megakaryocytic precursors). This finding is firm evidence for the clonal origin of CML from the myeloid stem cells.* In some patients the Ph^1 chromosome can be seen in B cells as well, suggesting origin from the pluripotent hematopoietic stem cells. Interestingly, as you recall, the Ph^1 chromosome is sometimes seen in ALL. Although CML originates in the multipotent stem cells, granulocyte precursors constitute the dominant cell line. *Unlike the case in acute leukemias, there is no block in the maturation of leukemic stem cells.* Cell kinetic and in vitro culture techniques reveal that there is a 10- to 20-fold increase in the mass of granulocytic precursors in the bone marrow and spleen but that they do not divide more rapidly than normal stem cells.[59] Moreover, as compared with normal, a greater proportion of the expanded leukemic stem cells seem to enter the maturation compartment, as evidenced by the vast number of mature cells in the peripheral blood. The basis of the increased myeloid stem cell mass in CML, and its proclivity to undergo differentiation, seems to lie in a failure of the stem cells to respond to physiologic feedback signals that regulate growth and differentiation of hematopoietic precursors.

CLINICAL FEATURES. The onset of CML is usually slow, and the initial symptoms may be quite nonspecific. They are caused by anemia or by hypermetabolism due to increased cell turnover and include easy fatigability, weakness, weight loss, and anorexia. Sometimes the first symptom is a dragging sensation in the abdomen caused by the extreme splenomegaly characteristic of this condition. Usually, there is marked elevation of the leukocyte count, commonly exceeding 100,000 cell per mm^3 (Fig. 15–21). The circulating cells are predominantly neutrophils and metamyelocytes, but basophils and eosinophils may also be prominent. A small number of myeloblasts (<10%) can usually be detected in the peripheral blood. Because CML originates from the myeloid stem cell, it is not surprising that up to 50% of patients

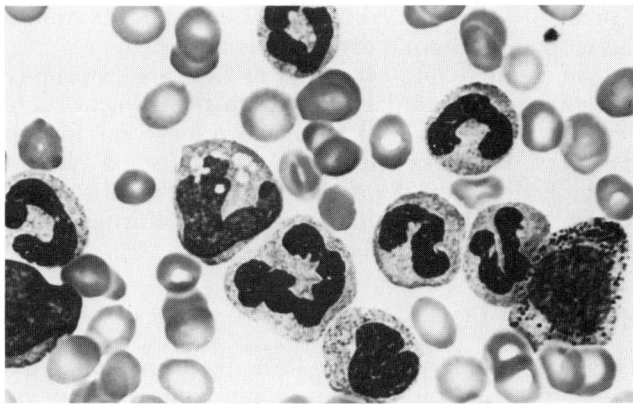

Figure 15–21. Chronic myeloid leukemia. Peripheral blood smear shows many mature neutrophils, some metamyelocytes, and a myelocyte. (Courtesy of Dr. Robert W. McKenna, Southwestern Medical School, Dallas, Texas.)

have thrombocytosis early in the course of their disease. *A characteristic finding in CML is the almost total lack of alkaline phosphatase in granulocytes. This serves to distinguish CML from a leukemoid reaction, which is also associated with a striking elevation of the granulocytic count* in response to infection, stress, chronic inflammation, and certain neoplasms. Other features that help to differentiate leukemoid reactions from CML are the presence of Ph[1] chromosome and increased numbers of basophils in the peripheral blood, both of which are quite typical of CML. The course of CML is one of slow progression, and even without treatment a median survival of three years can be expected.

After a variable period averaging three years, approximately 50% of patients enter an "accelerated phase," during which there is a gradual failure of response to treatment, increasing anemia and thrombocytopenia, acquisition of additional cytogenetic abnormalities, and finally, transformation into a picture resembling acute leukemia ("blast crisis"). In the remaining 50%, blast crises occur abruptly without an intermediate accelerated phase. In 70% of patients the blasts have the morphologic and cytochemical features of myeloblasts, but it is of interest to note that in 30% of patients the blasts contain the enzyme TdT, a marker of primitive lymphoid cells. The blasts in these cases belong to the B-cell lineage, as evidenced by the expression of CD10 and CD19 antigens and the presence of Ig gene rearrangements. This observation supports the notion that the target cell for transformation in CML may be the pluripotent stem cell capable of both myeloid and lymphoid differentiation.

The treatment of CML is unsatisfactory. Although it is possible to induce remissions with chemotherapy, the median survival (three to four years) is unaltered. The small number of CML patients who lack the Ph[1] chromosome seem to fare worse. Current efforts are directed toward "curing" CML with chemotherapy and bone marrow transplantation dur-

ing the chronic phase of the disease.[60] After the development of blast crisis, all forms of treatment become virtually ineffective.[61]

CHRONIC LYMPHOCYTIC LEUKEMIA (CLL)

CLL is the most indolent of all leukemias. It accounts for 25% of all cases of leukemia in the United States and Europe, occurring typically in persons over 50 years (median age 60 years); males are affected twice as commonly as females. It is distinctly uncommon in Japan and other Asian countries.

PATHOPHYSIOLOGY. CLL shows considerable overlap with small lymphocytic lymphoma. Like most other lymphoid malignancies, CLL is a neoplastic disorder of B cells. T-cell CLL is rare (<5% of all cases). The transformed B cells in CLL show the following characteristics:

• They possess surface immunoglobulin (IgM and IgD), express the pan–B cell antigens (CD19, CD20), and do not contain TdT or express the early B cell antigen CD10. Thus, their phenotype is quite distinct from lymphoblasts of most cases of ALL.
• They express either λ or κ light chain, indicating monoclonality.
• They are long-lived but are unable to differentiate into antibody-secreting plasma cells in vivo.
• Only a small fraction are proliferating at any given time.

Thus CLL is characterized by the accumulation of long-lived, nonfunctional B lymphocytes that infiltrate the bone marrow, blood, lymph nodes, and other tissues.[62,63]

CHROMOSOMAL ABNORMALITIES. Approximately 50% of the patients with CLL have abnormal karyotypes. Trisomy 12 is the most common, being seen in about one third of the patients; complex abnormalities involving chromosomes 14 and 11 are also found, usually in association with trisomy 12. Patients with cytogenetic changes require early treatment and have a significantly shorter survival.

CLINICAL FEATURES. Patients with CLL are often asymptomatic. When symptoms are present, they are nonspecific and include easy fatigability, loss of weight, and anorexia. Generalized lymphadenopathy and hepatosplenomegaly are present in 50 to 60% of the cases. Total leukocyte count may be increased only slightly or may reach 200,000 per mm³. In all cases there is absolute lymphocytosis of small, mature-looking lymphocytes (Fig. 15–22). Only a small fraction of lymphocytes are large ones with indented nuclei and nucleoli. Smudge cells (crushed nuclei of lymphocytes) are commonly seen in peripheral smears (Fig. 15–22). Because the leukemic B cells are nonfunctional, these patients often have hypogammaglobulinemia and increased susceptibility to bacte-

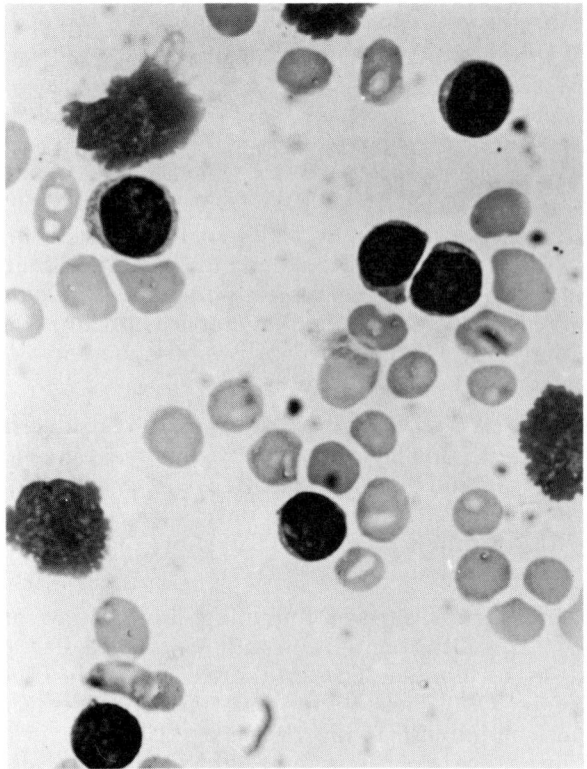

Figure 15–22. Peripheral blood smear from a patient with chronic lymphatic leukemia. Most leukemic cells have the appearance of unstimulated small or medium-size lymphocytes. Owing to excessive fragility, the neoplastic lymphocytes are often damaged, giving rise to several "smudge" cells. (Courtesy of Dr. José Hernandez, Department of Pathology, Southwestern Medical School, Dallas, Texas.)

rial infections. Paradoxically, some 10 to 15% of patients develop autoantibodies directed against red blood cells or platelets, resulting in autoimmune hemolytic anemia or thrombocytopenia. It is established that the autoantibodies are not produced by the ma-

Table 15–11. Staging Classification of CLL

STAGE	DESCRIPTION	MEDIAN SURVIVAL (YEARS)
A	Lymphocytosis with less than three areas of lymphoid enlargement*; no anemia or thrombocytopenia.	>10
B	More than three areas of lymphoid enlargement; no anemia or thrombocytopenia.	5
C	Anemia or thrombocytopenia regardless of the number of areas of lymphoid enlargement.	2

*Clinical enlargement of spleen, liver, cervical lymph nodes, axillary lymph nodes, and inguinal lymph nodes constitute five separate areas of involvement. Each of these five anatomic regions is considered one lymphoid area for the purpose of this classification. Modified from Binet, J.L., et al.: Chronic lymphocytic leukemia: proposal for a revised prognostic staging system. Br. J. Haematol. *48*: 305, 1981.

lignant B cell clone,[62] but why these patients should develop autoimmune disorders is unknown.

The course and prognosis of CLL are extremely variable and depend primarily on the clinical stage (Table 15–11). Overall, the median survival is four to six years. Whether the prognostic value of cytogenetic changes is independent of the clinical stage is not yet established. Unlike CML, transformation to acute leukemia with blast crisis is rare.

HAIRY CELL LEUKEMIA

This is a rare but distinctive form of chronic leukemia that derives its picturesque name from the appearance of the leukemic cells — fine hairlike projections, best recognized under the phase contrast microscope but also visible in routine blood smears.[64] This disease evoked much interest because hairy cells seem to express cell surface markers of T cells, B cells, and monocytes; therefore, their origin remained mysterious. However, molecular analyses leave little doubt that despite their somewhat unusual phenotype, hairy cells rearrange and express immunoglobulin genes, which firmly assigns them to the B-cell lineage. For routine diagnosis, however, it is not necessary to utilize DNA probe analysis, since there is one cytochemical feature that is quite characteristic of hairy cell leukemia, i.e., the presence of tartrate-resistant acid phosphatase (TRAP). The exceptions to this observation are few, and hence positive TRAP staining in leukemic cells endowed with "hair" is considered virtually diagnostic of hairy cell leukemia in the appropriate clinical setting.

Hairy cell leukemia occurs mainly in older males, and *its manifestations result largely from infiltration of bone marrow, liver, and spleen. Splenomegaly*, often massive, is the most common and sometimes the only abnormal physical finding. *Hepatomegaly* is less common and not as marked, and lymphadenopathy is distinctly rare. *Pancytopenia*, resulting from marrow failure and splenic sequestration, is seen in over half the cases. *Leukocytosis* is not a common feature, being present in only 25% of patients. Hairy cells can be identified in the peripheral blood smear in most cases. The course of this disease is chronic, and the median survival is four years. Splenectomy is of benefit in approximately two thirds of the patients. Recently, α-interferon has proved to be effective in this disease.[65]

MORPHOLOGY OF ALL LEUKEMIAS

There are two aspects to the morphologic features of leukemias: (1) the specific cytologic details of the leukemic cells seen in peripheral blood smears and bone marrow aspirates, and (2) the tissue changes produced by infiltrations of leukemic cells. The cytologic features specific for each form of leukemia have already been described. The tissue alterations produced by various leukemias are often similar and may be separated into primary changes, attrib-

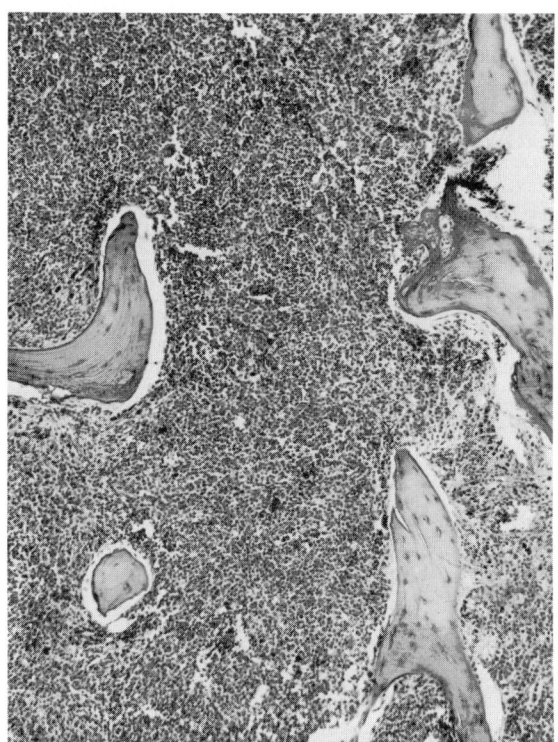

Figure 15–23. Myelogenous leukemia. Low-power view of bone marrow documents the flooding by leukemic cells.

uted directly to the abnormal overgrowth or accumulation of white cells; and secondary changes, caused both by the destructive effects of masses of these cells and by their relative ineffectiveness in protecting against infection.

Although the leukemic cells may infiltrate any tissue or organ of the body, the most striking changes are seen in the bone marrow, spleen, lymph nodes, and liver. In the full-blown case, the bone marrow develops a muddy, red-brown to gray-white color as the normal marrow is diffusely replaced by masses of white cells (Fig. 15–23). Sometimes these infiltrates extend into previously fatty marrow and encroach upon and erode the cancellous and cortical bone.

Massive **splenomegaly** is associated with CML and hairy cell leukemia. Splenic weights of 5000 gm or more are not unusual. Such spleens may virtually fill the abdominal cavity and extend into the pelvis. With CLL, enlargement of the spleen is less striking, and the weight of the spleen rarely exceeds 2500 gm. The acute forms of leukemia produce only moderate splenomegaly, usually between 500 and 1000 gm. On sectioning, the parenchyma is firm and muddy gray in color. When the splenomegaly is massive, as is most characteristic of CML, numerous areas of pale infarction may appear throughout the substance, caused presumably by infiltration and compression of vessels by leukemic cells (Fig. 15–24). In minimally enlarged spleens, the histologic appearance may be of focal leukemic infiltrates, with a background of fairly well-preserved normal architecture. In the lymphocytic forms, the white pulp is primarily involved. With more severe involvement the infiltrates become more diffuse. Ultimately, the underlying architecture is obliterated and replaced by a sea of homogeneous leukemic cells.

Whereas splenomegaly is more prominent with myelogenous than with lymphocytic leukemia, extreme **lymph node enlargement** is more characteristic of the lymphocytic forms (Fig. 15–25). Nevertheless, some degree of lymph

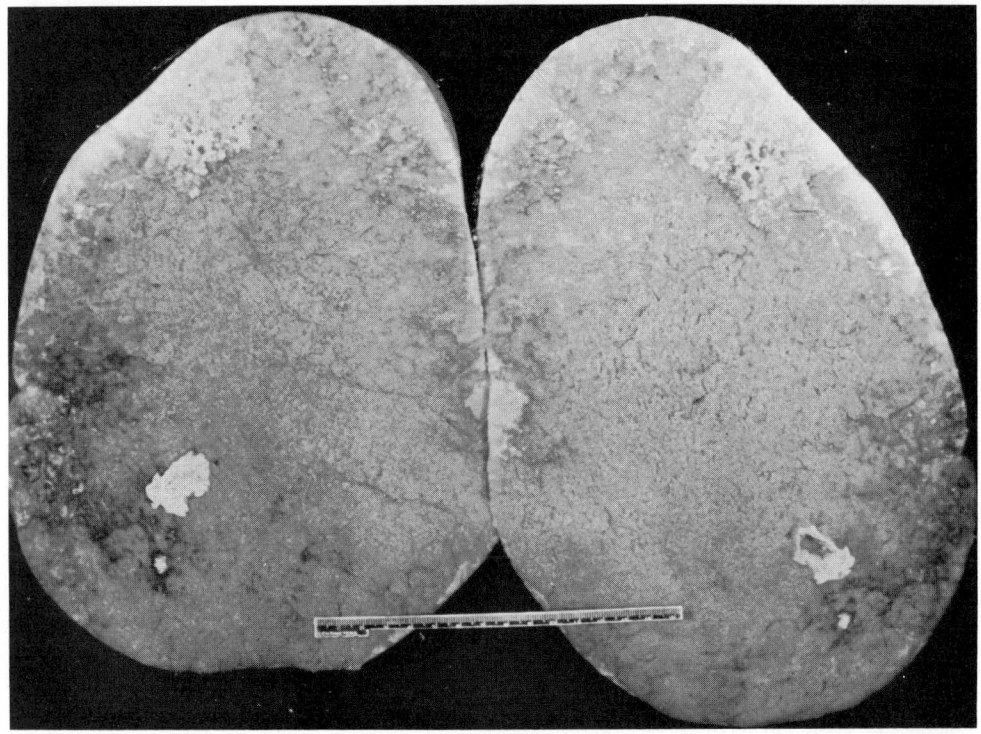

Figure 15–24. Spleen in chronic myelogenous leukemia. The massive enlargement dwarfs the 15-cm rule. Numerous small infarcts are dispersed through the cut surface.

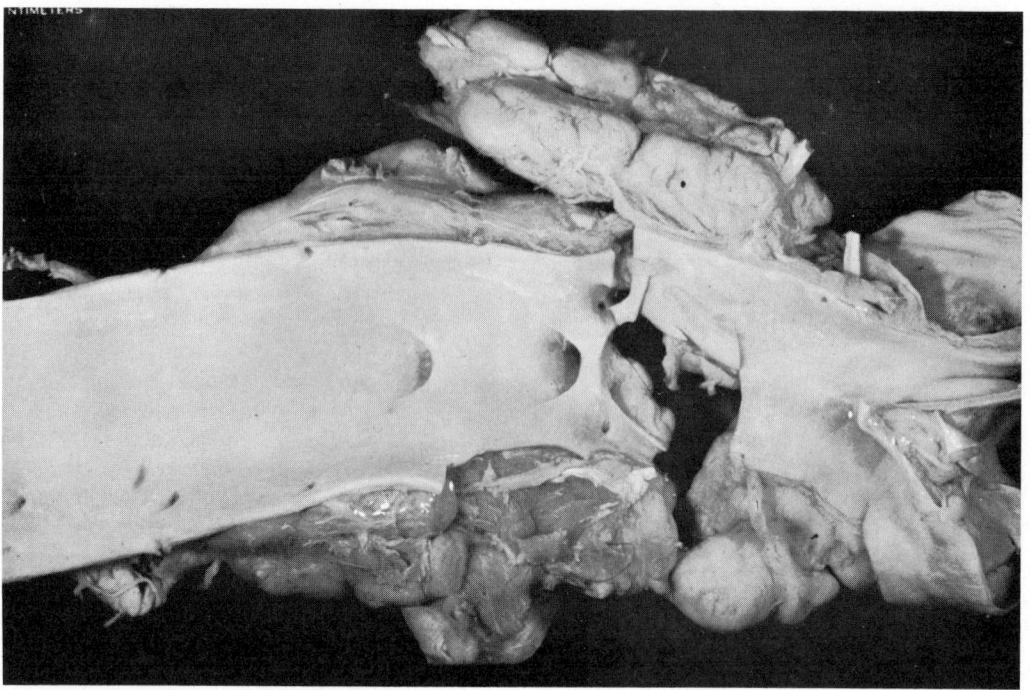

Figure 15–25. Periaortic lymph node enlargement in chronic lymphocytic leukemia.

node involvement is commonly present with all forms of leukemia. The affected nodes remain discrete, rubbery, and homogeneous. The cut section is soft and gray-white and tends to bulge above the level of the capsule. On histologic examination, severely involved nodes are seen to be dif-fusely flooded by the neoplastic cells. The underlying archi-tecture is obliterated, and sometimes the leukemic cells invade the capsule of the node and flood out into the sur-rounding tissues. With CLL, the histologic picture is identi-cal to that of a small lymphocytic lymphoma. With minimal

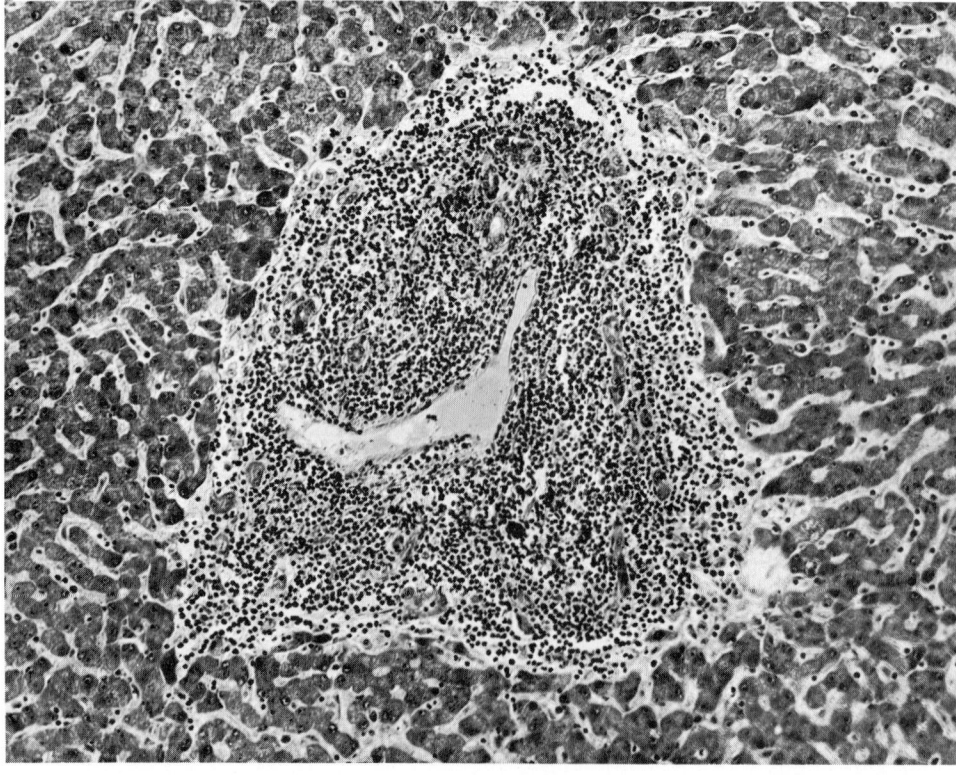

Figure 15–26. Chronic lymphocy-tic leukemia in liver. High-power detail of a periportal infiltrate. (From Jackson, H.J., Jr., and Parker, F., Jr. (eds.): Hodgkin's Dis-ease and Allied Disorders. New York, Oxford University Press, 1947.)

involvement in the myelogenous leukemias, the underlying architecture may be largely preserved.

Enlargement of the liver is somewhat more prominent with lymphocytic than with myelogenous leukemia. Histologically, the lymphocytic infiltrates are characteristically confined to the portal areas (Fig. 15–26), whereas infiltrates of myelogenous leukemia are not well defined and are present within the sinusoids throughout the lobule.

In addition to the principal sites of involvement, other tissues and organs may be affected. Leukemic infiltrates are frequently found in the kidneys, where they begin as small perivascular aggregates that progressively diffuse throughout the stroma. Similar changes may occur in the adrenals, thyroid, myocardium, testes, and, indeed, any tissue (Fig. 15–27). Of particular importance is the infiltration of the central nervous system by leukemic cells. This occurs most commonly in ALL. Protected by the blood-brain barrier from the effects of cytotoxic drugs, cells in the CNS may survive to eventually initiate a relapse unless prophylactic radiation or intrathecal chemotherapy is administered. **Infiltrates in the gingiva are particularly characteristic of monocytic leukemia.** Patients with this disorder have swelling and hypertrophy of the gingival margins, often with secondary infections.

The **secondary changes of all forms of leukemia** derive in large part from the pancytopenia that results from inhibition of normal hematopoiesis by leukemic cells. Anemia and thrombocytopenia are characteristic, especially of acute leukemia. Many times, the bleeding diathesis caused by the thrombocytopenia is the most striking clinical and anatomic feature of the disease. Petechiae and ecchymoses are seen in the skin. Hemorrhages also occur into the serosal linings of the body cavities and into the serosal coverings of the viscera, particularly of the heart and lungs. Mucosal hemorrhages into the gingivae and urinary tract are common. Intraparenchymal hematomas may develop, most frequently in the brain.

Although the total white blood cell count is usually markedly elevated, the defensive capacity of these abnormal cells is considerably less than normal. This is especially true of the acute forms. There is, then, a **functional** leukopenia with a resultant increased susceptibility to bacterial infection. These infections are particularly common in the oral cavity, skin, lungs, kidneys, urinary bladder, and colon, and they are often caused by "opportunists" such as fungi, *Pseudomonas,* and commensals.

ETIOLOGY AND PATHOGENESIS OF LEUKEMIAS AND LYMPHOMAS

As with all other cancers, the pathogenesis of neoplastic transformation of lymphohematopoietic cells is shrouded in mystery. However, in recent years there has been much excitement in this area of investigation, stemming from the convergence of research on *oncogenes, chromosomal abnormalities, and oncogenic viruses.*[66–68] Much of the evidence implicating alterations in structure and function of proto-oncogenes in the origin of cancer was discussed in Chapter 6; therefore, only a brief recapitulation, as it relates to neoplasms of the hematopoietic system, will be offered here. This will be followed by a discussion of the role of viruses in the pathogenesis of leukemias and lymphomas.

Omitting much detail, it can be stated that proto-oncogenes, present in all normal eukaryotic cells, play an important role in regulating their growth and differentiation. In many leukemias and lymphomas, karyotypic changes (usually translocations) shift the proto-oncogenes to new locations within the genome. Such chromosomal rearrangements may alter the function or structure of oncogenes in one of several ways:

• The translocation may place the oncogene next to a transcriptionally active area, which may lead to overexpression of the oncogene product, as exemplified by the c-*myc* gene in Burkitt's lymphoma (p. 288).
• During translocation, subtle mutations may be induced in the proto-oncogenes, leading to the transcription of a qualitatively different gene product.
• The proto-oncogene may fuse with another cellular gene normally located at the site to which it is translocated, resulting in the formation of a fusion gene. Such a hybrid gene may code for a new protein that affects cell growth. An example of this phenomenon is the c-*abl/bcr* gene formed in Ph[1] positive CML (p. 289).[69]

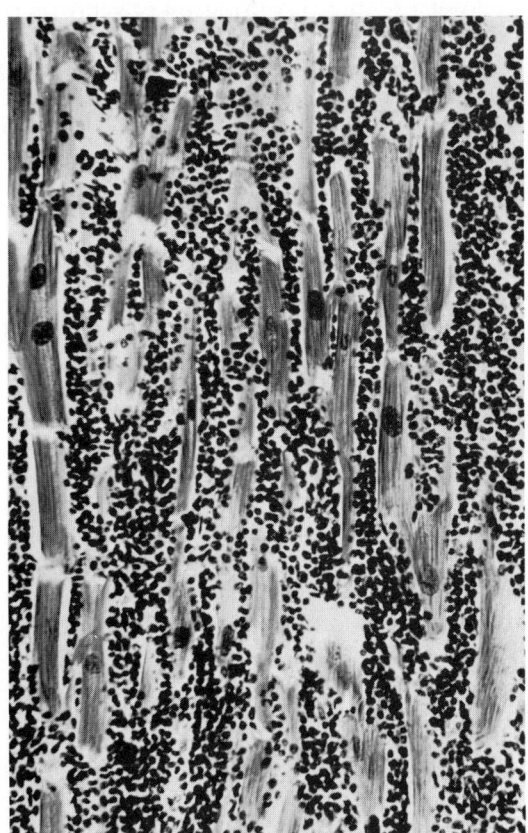

Figure 15–27. Chronic lymphocytic leukemia infiltrates in heart muscle. (From Jackson, H.J., Jr., and Parker, F., Jr. (eds.): Hodgkin's Disease and Allied Disorders. New York, Oxford University Press, 1947.)

In any event, overexpression or alteration of the oncogene product, brought about by one or more of the mechanisms listed above, somehow deranges growth regulation so as to produce a cell that is autonomous (p. 292). This schema of the pathogenesis of leukemias and lymphomas is supported by the following observations:

• With high-resolution banding techniques, nonrandom chromosomal abnormalities, most commonly reciprocal translocation, are noted in over 60% of all leukemias and lymphomas.[70]
• In many instances, proto-oncogenes have been located at or near the breakpoint of the chromosomes that are involved in the translocations (see Table 6–12, p. 288).
• In translocations associated with leukemias and lymphomas of the B-cell lineage, one of the two breakpoints almost always involves chromosome 14, particularly band q32, which contains the immunoglobulin heavy-chain locus (IgH). In contrast, the breakpoint in several T-cell lymphomas involves band q11 on chromosome 14, where the T-cell receptor α-chain gene is located. Since the IgH gene in B cells and the T-cell receptor gene in T cells are normally "turned on," it seems that translocations associated with B- or T-cell tumors uniquely involve those portions of the genome that are transcriptionally active in these cell types. Thus there is the potential for affecting the expression of a normal or mutated proto-oncogene that may come to lie next to these active sites.

Although much has been learned about the mechanisms by which products of normal or mutated oncogenes may transform cells (p. 282), the agents that *initiate* such disturbances (e.g., translocations) are largely unknown. As with many other cancers, *ionizing radiations* and *chemicals* have been implicated as mutagenic agents that "pull the trigger."[71,72] There is also suspicion that viruses are somehow involved, since virally induced leukemias and lymphomas are well known in laboratory animals. Although several viruses have been implicated in the causation of human cancer (p. 275), two deserve special mention in the context of leukemias and lymphomas—EBV and the human T-cell leukemia virus.

There is a substantial body of evidence linking EBV to the African Burkitt's lymphoma.[73] As was discussed previously, this tumor is almost always associated with the t(8;14) translocation, a change that may be critical to lymphomagenesis. What role then does the virus play in the pathogenesis of Burkitt's lymphoma? It is postulated that initially EBV acts as a B-cell mitogen and initiates a polyclonal B-cell proliferation (Fig. 15–28). In most individuals the lymphoproliferation is arrested, and either there is no disease or there is a self-limited episode of infectious mononucleosis (p. 323). However, in some individuals, presumably those with some overt or subtle immunologic defect, chronic polyclonal B-cell proliferation continues. The rapidly proliferating cells are at greatly enhanced risk of acquiring cytogenetic aberrations such as the t(8;14) translocation. This translocation may confer growth advantage on the affected cell owing to activation of the c-*myc* oncogene. Overexpression of the c-*myc* oncogene by itself is not sufficient for malignant transformation. In all likelihood it represents one of multiple steps in lymphomagenesis (p. 292). Additional mutations possibly affecting the N-*ras* oncogene occur in the B cells immortalized by the EBV. Together these changes lead to the emergence of a monoclonal B-cell neoplasm (Fig. 15–28). According to this view then, EBV itself is not directly oncogenic, but by acting as a polyclonal B-cell mitogen it sets the stage for the acquisition of the t(8;14) translocation and other mutations, which ultimately release the cells from normal growth regulation.

Although EBV is associated with only a few lymphomas, it has been postulated that the pathogenesis of other lymphoid malignancies may also involve a similar evolution from polyclonal to monoclonal proliferations.[74] This view has gained some credence from the observation that *the risk of developing malignant lymphomas is higher in those who are subjected to persistent antigenic stimulation, especially in association with defective immunoregulation.* Individuals in such high-risk categories include patients with the X-linked lymphoproliferative syndrome (p. 298), recipients of renal allografts, and patients with autoimmune diseases such as Sjögren's syndrome and AIDS.[75]

We come next to the role of HTLV-1 in the pathogenesis of acute T-cell leukemia/lymphoma. The evidence linking this virus with the causation of T-cell leukemia/lymphoma was discussed on page 281. It need only be emphasized that, as with Burkitt's lymphoma, the evolution of this tumor occurs in multiple steps. Initial polyclonal proliferation of HTLV-1 infected CD4+ cells (dependent on autocrine stimulation by IL-2) is followed by emergence of a growth factor–independent monoclonal neoplasm. These tumors are frequently associated with translocations involving chromosome 14 band 11q, the site of transcriptionally active T-cell receptor α-chain gene.[76] The significance of this translocation is not entirely clear, however.

MYELOPROLIFERATIVE DISORDERS

The concept that myeloproliferative disorders result from clonal neoplastic proliferations of the multipotent myeloid stem cells has already been discussed (p. 723). It was mentioned in our earlier presentation that four disorders—chronic myeloid leukemia, polycythemia vera, myeloid metaplasia with myelofibrosis, and essential thrombocythemia—are included in this group. CML was discussed along with other leukemias. Of the remaining three, only polycythemia vera and myeloid metaplasia with myelofibrosis will be presented here. Essential thrombocythemia occurs too infrequently to merit further discussion.

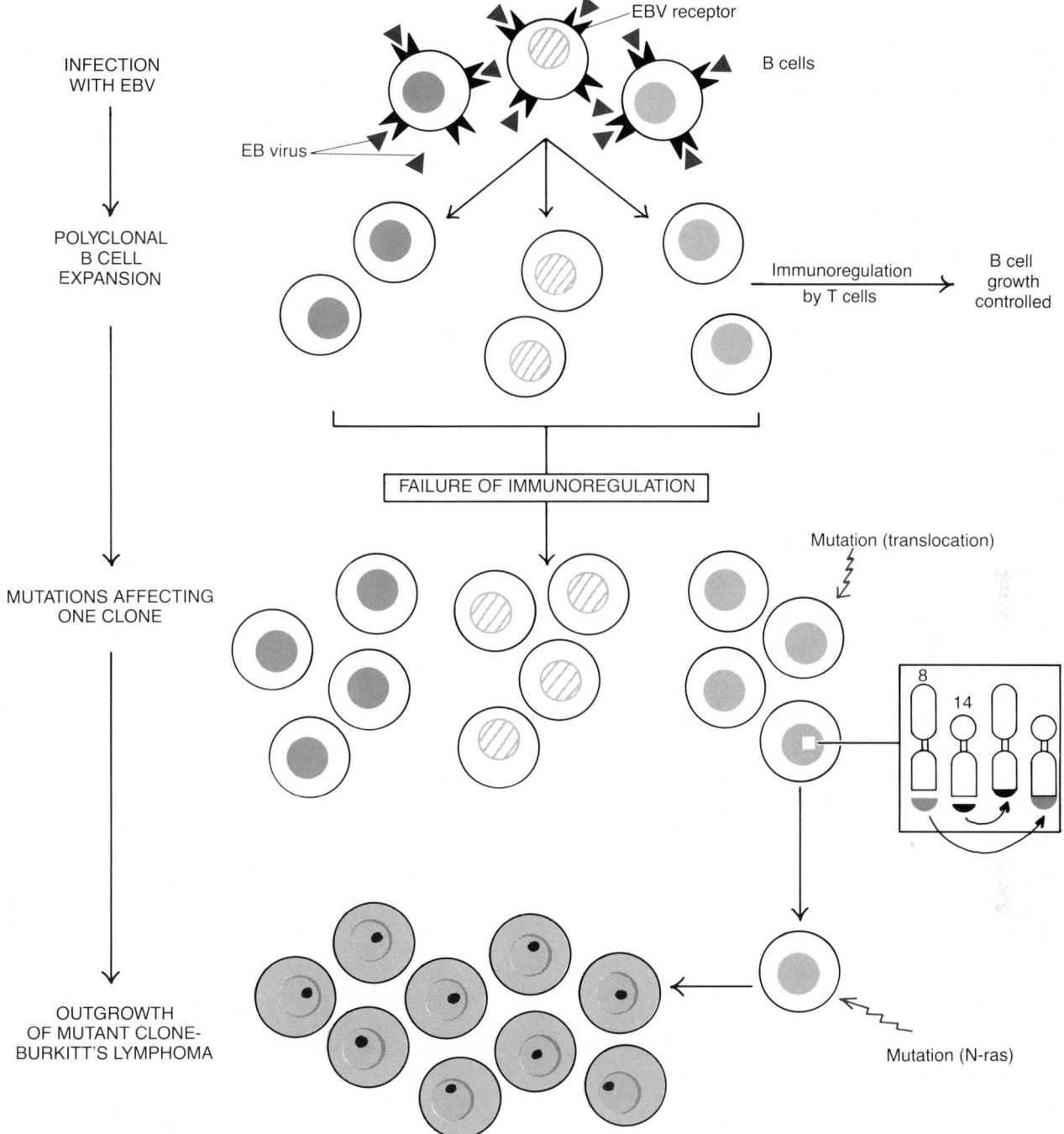

Figure 15–28. A scheme depicting the possible evolution of EBV-induced Burkitt's lymphoma.

Polycythemia Vera

As with all myeloproliferative disorders, polycythemia vera is associated with excessive proliferation of erythroid, granulocytic, and megakaryocytic elements, all derived from a single neoplastic stem cell. However, in *polycythemia vera the erythroid precursors dominate, and hence there is an absolute increase in red cell mass.* This should be contrasted with relative polycythemia, resulting from hemoconcentration (p. 691). Furthermore, unlike other forms of absolute polycythemia that result from an increased secretion of erythropoietin, polycythemia vera is associated with lower than normal levels of serum erythropoietin.[77]

In vitro culture of hematopoietic stem cells has provided important insights into the pathophysiology of polycythemia vera. In the blood and bone marrow of patients with this disorder there is an increase in the number of actively dividing myeloid stem cells that seem to require extremely small amounts of erythropoietin for erythroid differentiation. Although these abnormal erythropoietin-hypersensitive stem cells predominate, a small number of normal stem cells (which require much more erythropoietin) are also present. However, their proliferation and differentiation is suppressed, and normal red cells therefore constitute a minority in the peripheral blood. It seems that the erythrocytosis induced by the proliferation of the abnormal (neoplastic) stem cells suppresses the production of erythropoietin, thereby keeping the normal erythroid stem cells inactive. The number of normal stem cells seems to decline as the disease progresses. This observation has potential clinical significance because remission requires not only suppression of the neoplastic clones but also the re-emergence of the residual normal stem cells.

MORPHOLOGY. The major anatomic changes stem from the increase in blood volume and viscosity brought about by the erythrocytosis. Plethoric congestion of all tissues and organs is characteristic of polycythemia vera. The liver is enlarged and frequently contains foci of myeloid metaplasia. The spleen is also slightly enlarged, up to 250 to 300 gm, and quite firm. The splenic sinuses are packed with red cells, as are all the vessels within the spleen. Occasionally, extramedullary hematopoiesis can be seen within the red pulp. The major blood vessels are uniformly distended with thick, viscous blood.

Consequent to the increased viscosity and vascular stasis, thromboses and infarctions are common; they affect most often the heart, spleen, and kidneys. Hemorrhages occur in about a third of these patients, probably owing to excessive distention of blood vessels and abnormal platelet function. They usually affect the gastrointestinal tract, oropharynx, or brain. Although these hemorrhages are said on occasion to be spontaneous, more often they follow some minor trauma or surgical procedure. Peptic ulceration has been described in about a fifth of these patients.

The basic changes occur in the bone marrow, which is markedly hypercellular.[78] Typically, the marrow demonstrates hyperplasia of erythroid, granulocytic, and megakaryocytic elements. At the time of diagnosis, moderate to marked increase in marrow reticulin is seen in approximately 10% of the patients. As the disease changes its course, the marrow reflects the alterations and may become progressively fibrotic (myelofibrosis) or may be replaced by blasts (leukemic transformation), as discussed below.

CLINICAL COURSE. Polycythemia vera appears insidiously, usually in late middle age (40 to 60 years).[79] Males are affected somewhat more often than females, and whites are more vulnerable than blacks. The major clinical features of polycythemia stem from the increased blood volume and viscosity, vascular stasis, thrombotic tendency, and hemorrhagic diathesis. Most of the excess blood is trapped in the venous circulation, which is greatly distended. Classically, therefore, patients are plethoric and somewhat cyanotic owing to stagnation and deoxygenation of blood in peripheral vessels. Headache, dizziness, gastrointestinal symptoms, hematemesis, and melena are common. Splenic or renal infarction may produce abdominal pain. There is usually intense pruritus, possibly the result of an increased release of histamine from basophils. High cell turnover gives rise to hyperuricemia, and symptomatic gout is seen in 5 to 10% of cases.

The diagnosis is usually made in the laboratory. Red cell counts range from 6×10^6 to 10×10^6 per mm^3, with hematocrit values of 60% or more. Because there is hyperplasia of granulocytic precursors as well as megakaryocytes in the bone marrow, the white cell count may be as high as 80,000 per mm^3; the platelet count is greater than 500,000 per mm^3 in 50% of the patients at the time of diagnosis. In contrast to CML, granulocyte alkaline phosphatase levels are above normal. The platelets usually exhibit morphologic and functional abnormalities manifested as giant forms and megakaryocytic fragments and defective aggregation. As in all other myeloproliferative disorders, basophil and eosinophil counts may be increased. Histamine release from basophils may account for the pruritus as well as for the increased tendency for peptic ulceration.

About 30% of patients die from some thrombotic complication, affecting usually the brain or heart. An additional 10 to 15% die from some hemorrhagic complication. In patients who receive no treatment, death resulting from these vascular episodes occurs within months after diagnosis. However, if the red cell mass can be maintained near normal by phlebotomies, median survival of 10 years can be achieved.

Extended survival with treatment has revealed that the *natural history of polycythemia vera involves a gradual transition to a "spent phase," during which clinical and anatomic features of myeloid metaplasia with myelofibrosis develop.* Approximately 15 to 20% of patients undergo such a transformation after an average period of 10 years. This transition is brought about by creeping fibrosis in the bone marrow (myelofibrosis) and a shift of hematopoiesis to the spleen, which enlarges markedly. The peripheral blood picture changes to one that is characteristic of myelofibrosis. It is ironic that these patients, who may once have had to undergo repeated therapeutic phlebotomies, now require blood transfusions to correct their anemia. This is perhaps the most striking example of conversion of one myeloproliferative disorder to another. As with CML (another myeloproliferative disease), certain patients with polycythemia vera develop a terminal acute myeloblastic leukemia. However, the incidence of this transition is much lower than in CML. It is estimated to be about 2% in patients who are treated with phlebotomy alone[78] and about 15% in those who receive myelosuppressive treatment with chlorambucil or marrow irradiation with radioactive phosphorus. Presumably, the increase is related to the mutagenic effects of these therapeutic agents.

Myeloid Metaplasia with Myelofibrosis

In this chronic myeloproliferative disorder the proliferation of the neoplastic myeloid stem cells occurs principally in the spleen *(myeloid metaplasia)*, and in the fully developed syndrome the bone marrow is hypocellular and fibrotic *(myelofibrosis)*. Sometimes polycythemia vera and, less often, CML "burn out," as it were, and terminate in a myelofibrotic pattern. In many patients, however, extramedullary hematopoiesis in the spleen and marrow fibrosis arise insidiously without an identifiable preceding syndrome; hence the term *agnogenic (idiopathic) myeloid metaplasia* is sometimes used to describe this condition.

The cause of marrow fibrosis, which is characteristic of myeloid metaplasia, is not clear. Studies with G6PD isoenzymes indicate that the fibroblasts that replace the marrow do not belong to the neoplastic hematopoietic clone. No toxic cause for marrow destruction and subsequent scarring can be demonstrated, a feature that distinguishes this condition from myelophthisic anemias with extramedullary hematopoiesis, in which there are obvious mechanisms of marrow destruction such as metastatic tumors. It has been suggested that *marrow fibroblasts are stimulated to proliferate owing to an inappropriate release of platelet-derived growth factor and transforming growth factor-β (TGF-β) derived from the expanded pool of megakaryocytes and platelets.*[80] Functional and morphologic abnormalities of platelets are seen in myeloid metaplasia with myelofibrosis, and the two growth factors mentioned above are known to be mitogenic for fibroblasts. It is widely believed that the proliferation of neoplastic stem cells begins within the marrow and there is subsequent seeding of the spleen and other organs such as the liver. As the disease progresses, marrow fibrosis occurs secondary to the elaboration of fibroblast growth factors mentioned above. By the time the patient comes to clinical attention, fibroblasts have already taken over the marrow, and the spleen remains the major site of myeloproliferation. This scheme is supported by the finding of hypercellular bone marrow with prominent megakaryocytes early in the course of this disease.

MORPHOLOGY. The principal anatomic change is striking extramedullary hematopoiesis. The principal site of this is the spleen, which is markedly enlarged, sometimes up to 4000 gm (Fig. 15–29). The capsule is unaffected but occasionally shows underlying small infarcts. On section the spleen is firm, red to gray, and not dissimilar from that seen in CML. The lymphoid follicles are usually preserved. Histologically, the extramedullary hematopoiesis seems to be largely confined to the sinusoids in the red pulp. Typically, there is trilineage proliferation affecting normoblasts, granulocytic precursors, and megakaryocytes (Fig. 15–30). The last are usually prominent owing to their large size and nuclear morphology. The proliferating myeloid elements may diffuse into the splenic cords. The foci of myeloid metaplasia usually contain relatively normal proportions of immature red cells, white cells, and platelets, but certain cases show disproportionate activity in any one of the three major cell lines.

The liver is often moderately enlarged, with foci of extramedullary hematopoiesis. The lymph nodes may also be the site of blood formation but usually are not enlarged.

The classic bone marrow finding is diffuse fibrosis with obliteration of the normal myeloid elements (Fig. 15–31). On occasion, however, marrow biopsy discloses hypercellularity with proliferation of all the myeloid elements and sometimes prominent abnormal-looking megakaryocytes. Even in the early cellular phase, a telltale finding of the more extensive fibrosis to come is a delicate deposition of reticulin, evident only on special stains. Moreover, sequential studies have shown that the fibrosis appears first in centrally located bones, when the large bones of the extremities contain hyperplastic marrow.

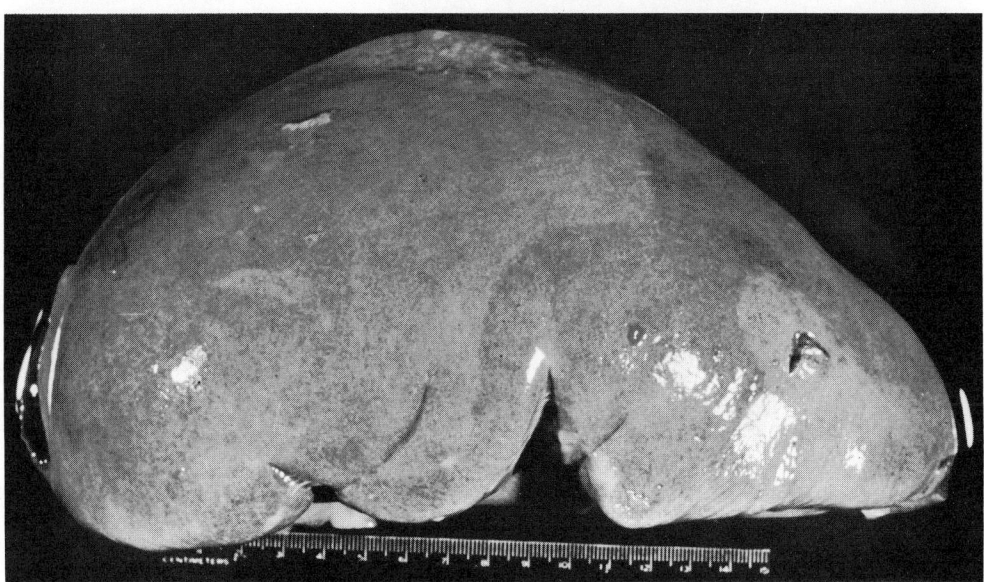

Figure 15–29. Myeloid metaplasia with myelofibrosis. Spleen is markedly enlarged and dwarfs the 15-cm rule. Irregular shading of capsule is an artifact.

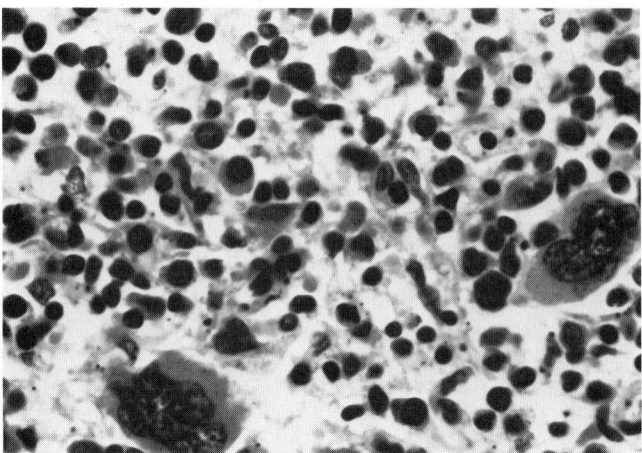

Figure 15–30. Myeloid metaplasia with myelofibrosis. Microscopic section of the spleen shows prominent megakaryocytes, normoblasts with dark compact nuclei, and some immature myeloid cells. (Courtesy of Dr. Jose Hernandez, Southwestern Medical School, Dallas, Texas.)

CLINICAL COURSE. Myeloid metaplasia is uncommon in individuals under 50 years of age. Except when preceded by polycythemia vera or CML, it usually comes to clinical attention because of either progressive anemia or marked splenic enlargement, producing a dragging sensation in the left upper quadrant. Some patients are asymptomatic. Most striking

are the laboratory findings. There is usually a moderate-to-severe normochromic normocytic anemia. Red cells show all manner of variation in size and shape, but *particularly characteristic are teardrop-shaped erythrocytes (poikilocytes)* (Fig. 15–32). In addition, numerous normoblasts and basophilic stippled red cells appear in the peripheral blood. The white cell count may be normal, leukopenic, or markedly elevated (80,000 to 100,000 per mm³), with a shift to the left. Basophils are usually prominent. Typically, myeloblasts, myelocytes, and metamyelocytes constitute a small fraction of the white cell population on peripheral smear. The platelet count is usually normal or elevated at the time of diagnosis, but thrombocytopenia supervenes as the disease progresses. Morphologic abnormalities of the platelets (giant forms) are frequent, and sometimes fragments of megakaryocytes may be detected in the peripheral blood. *To summarize, teardrop poikilocytes, leukoerythroblastic cells, and abnormal platelets in the peripheral smear are highly suggestive of myeloid metaplasia with myelofibrosis.* Biopsy of the marrow to detect the early deposition of reticulin or the more advanced fibrosis is essential for diagnosis. The differential diagnosis of CML frequently arises in these patients. In myeloid metaplasia, leukocyte alkaline phosphatase levels are often elevated, or at least normal, whereas in CML these levels are low or absent. Moreover, most patients with CML disclose the Ph¹ chromosome, which

Figure 15–31. Myelofibrosis. Marrow cavity is virtually replaced by fibrous tissue, totally obliterating normal hematopoietic elements.

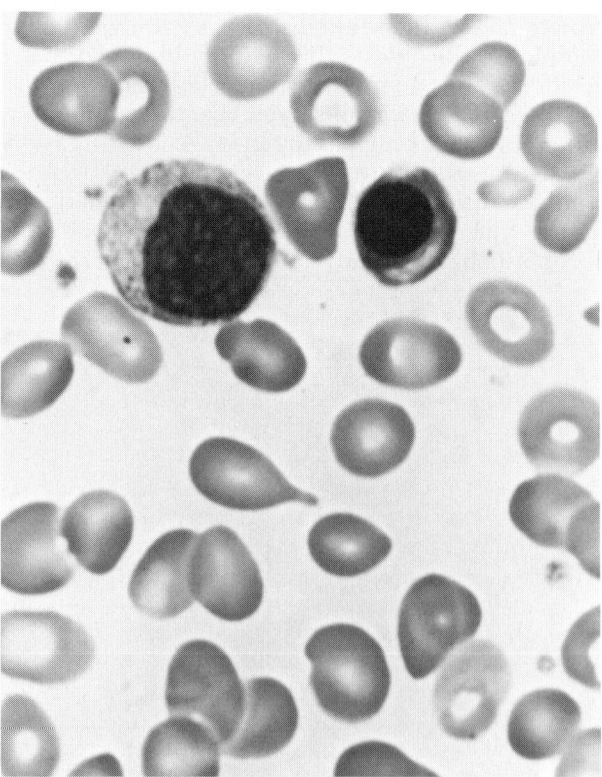

Figure 15–32. Myeloid metaplasia with myelofibrosis. Peripheral blood smear shows a teardrop red cell in the center field. An immature myeloid cell *(left)* and a nucleated red cell *(right)* are seen (Courtesy of Dr. José Hernandez, Southwestern Medical School, Dallas, Texas.)

is absent in agnogenic myeloid metaplasia. No unique cytogenetic abnormalities have been described in this disease. An equally difficult differential diagnosis is myelophthisic anemia secondary to an identifiable cause of marrow injury. In such cases the diagnosis of agnogenic myeloid metaplasia can be established only by careful history-taking to elicit the cause of marrow injury, or by morphologic detection of the underlying cause (e.g., cancer) in the marrow biopsy.

The course of this disease is difficult to predict. Despite weight loss attributed to the increased metabolism of the hyperproliferating cells, most patients can survive for years with transfusions. Sometimes the course is punctuated by episodes of acute left upper quadrant pain arising from splenic infarctions. Secondary gout may appear as a manifestation of the rapid turnover of blood cells. Threats to life are intercurrent infections, thrombotic episodes or bleeding related to platelet abnormalities, and in 5 to 10% of cases, transformation to acute leukemia.

PLASMA CELL DYSCRASIAS AND RELATED DISORDERS

The plasma cell dyscrasias are a group of disorders that have in common the *expansion of a single clone of immunoglobulin-secreting cells and a resultant increase in serum levels of a single homogeneous immunoglobulin or its fragments.* In almost all cases, these dyscrasias behave as malignant diseases, although occasionally monoclonal immunoglobulins are seen in otherwise normal elderly individuals. Collectively, these disorders account for about 15% of deaths from malignant white cell disease. As neoplasms of B cells, plasma cell dyscrasias are related to the non-Hodgkin's B-cell lymphomas. They differ, however, from the B-cell lymphomas discussed earlier by virtue of the fact that, in plasma cell disorders, the neoplastic B cells are differentiated enough to secrete immunoglobulins, and in most cases the clinical features are not dominated by lymphadenopathy. However, there are overlaps, as in the case of Waldenström's macroglobulinemia, to be described later.

The monoclonal immunoglobulin as identified in the blood is referred to as an M component in reference to *Myeloma*. Since complete M components have molecular weights of 160,000 or higher, they are largely restricted to circulating plasma and extracellular fluid. However, they may appear in the urine when there is some form of glomerular damage with heavy proteinuria. In some of these dyscrasias, excess light (L) or heavy (H) chains are also synthesized along with complete immunoglobulins, but the polypeptide chains are always identical to those found in the complete immunoglobulin, and thus the L chains are either kappa or lambda (never both) or the H chains of a single class (e.g., alpha, gamma, or mu), depending on the particular class of Ig. Occasionally only L chains or H chains are produced, without complete Ig. The *free L chains, known as Bence Jones proteins,* are sufficiently small to be rapidly excreted in the urine, and so may be totally cleared from the blood or persist only at very low levels. However, with renal failure or massive synthesis, they may appear in the blood in significant concentrations. Thus, *the common thread throughout this diverse group of entities is the appearance of excessive levels of complete or incomplete immunoglobulins in the plasma and/or urine. Hence, a variety of alternative designations have been applied to these dyscrasias, such as gammopathies, monoclonal gammopathies, dysproteinemias, and paraproteinemias.*[81]

A variety of clinicoanatomic patterns, cited below, can be differentiated among these gammopathies.

• *Multiple myeloma (plasma cell myeloma)* is the most important and most common syndrome. It is characterized by multiple neoplastic tumorous masses of more or less mature plasma cells, haphazardly scattered throughout the skeletal system and sometimes in soft tissues. *Solitary myeloma or solitary plasmacytoma* is an infrequent variant consisting of a solitary neoplastic mass of plasma cells found in bone or some soft tissue site.
• *Waldenström's macroglobulinemia* has been separated from the other gammopathies by virtue of the fact that it is characterized by the synthesis of IgM and a diffuse infiltrate of neoplastic B cells throughout the bone marrow as well as lymph nodes, liver, and spleen. Hence there is associated lymphadenopathy and hepatosplenomegaly, but the lytic bone lesions typical of myeloma are not present.
• *Heavy-chain disease* is a rare gammopathy distinguished by neoplastic medullary and extramedullary infiltrates of plasma cells, and precursors that synthesize only heavy chains.
• *Primary or immunocyte-associated amyloidosis* is also an expression of plasma cell dyscrasia. It may be recalled that this form of amyloidosis results from a monoclonal proliferation of plasma cells, with excessive production of free light chains that are deposited as amyloid (p. 213).
• *Monoclonal gammopathy of undetermined significance* (MGUS) refers to instances in which M components are identified in the blood of patients having no symptoms or signs of any of the better characterized monoclonal gammopathies. At one time this condition was termed benign monoclonal gammopathy, but this designation is misleading because some of these patients develop symptomatic multiple myeloma or other plasma cell dyscrasias after a variable interval.[82]

Against this background we can turn to some of the specific clinicoanatomic entities not discussed elsewhere in this text.

MULTIPLE MYELOMA

Multiple myeloma is basically a multifocal plasma cell cancer of the osseous system that in the course of its dissemination may involve many extraosseous sites. As pointed out, the neoplastic plasma cells synthesize complete and/or incomplete immunoglobulins. It is the most common of the gammopathies. Most patients are symptomatic when diagnosed. Clinical manifestations stem from the effects of (1) infiltration of organs, particularly the bones, by tumorous masses of plasma cells; and (2) the abnormal immunoglobulins secreted by the tumor cells.

In 99% of patients with multiple myeloma, electrophoretic analysis will disclose increased levels of one of the immunoglobulin classes in the blood and/or light chains in the urine (Bence Jones protein). In approximately 55% of patients, the M component is IgG, in 25% IgA, and rarely IgM, IgD, or IgE. In the remaining 20% of cases, Bence Jones proteinuria alone without serum M components is present. However, Bence Jones proteins are also present in the urine along with plasma M components in 60 to 70% of all myeloma patients.[81] *Identification of these proteins in the blood and urine constitutes one of the most important diagnostic features of this disease.* Electrophoresis of the serum or urine (paper, agar, cellulose acetate) is the most readily available and reliable procedure. When the serum electrophoretic pattern is analyzed, the M component yields a high spike, referred to as an M protein or M-component "spike." Immunoelectrophoresis, using appropriate monospecific antisera directed against the various heavy and light chains, is essential to establish the monoclonal nature of the M component. Bence Jones proteins in the urine are similarly detected by immunoelectrophoretic techniques.

ETIOLOGY AND PATHOGENESIS.

As was already pointed out, this group of disorders results from monoclonal proliferation of B cells in various stages of differentiation. The factors responsible for "turning on" a B-cell clone remain mysterious. It is postulated that prolonged antigenic stimulation may be the initial step in the pathogenesis of the plasma cell dyscrasias. This then provides the opportunity for spontaneous mutation, which might result in the neoplastic growth of the affected clone of B cells. As with many other B cell tumors, karyotypic abnormalities involving chromosome 14 band q32 have been detected in myeloma cells.[83] Although the specific translocations are different from the t(8;14) commonly found in Burkitt's lymphoma and B-cell ALL, they may be significant in the pathogenesis of multiple myeloma. Thus, according to this hypothesis, multiple myeloma requires two "hits" for its evolution—a prolonged antigenic stimulus and a mutation (see also p. 734).

MORPHOLOGY. Despite the abundance of abnormal biochemical findings, the ultimate diagnosis of plasma cell dyscrasias rests on the morphologic identification of the abnormal aggregates of plasma cells (Fig. 15–33). In most cases these cells make up more than 15%, and sometimes up to 90%, of all marrow cells. In many instances the neo-

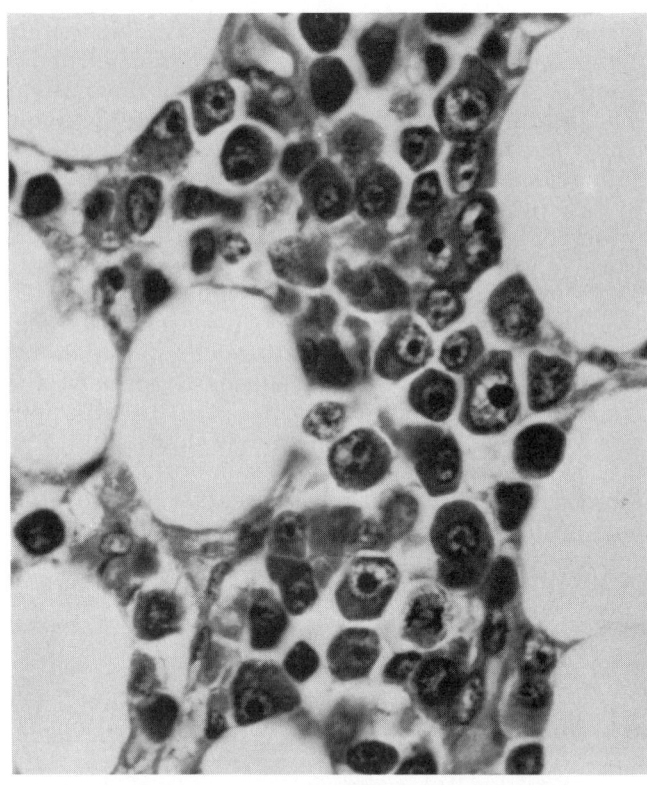

Figure 15–33. Multiple myeloma. Bone marrow biopsy reveals replacement of hematopoietic elements by aggregates of normal-looking plasma cells and some atypical variants with prominent nucleoli. (Courtesy of Dr. Patrick Ward, Department of Pathology and Laboratory Medicine, University of Minnesota School of Medicine, Duluth, Minnesota.)

plastic cells appear as mature plasma cells, but all ranges of immaturity may be encountered, including undifferentiated cells resembling lymphoid precursors as well as lymphocyte–plasma cell intermediates. It may be difficult to identify the neoplastic nature of the well-differentiated plasma cell lesions from the cytology of the individual cells; more important is their abnormal aggregation or evidence of their destructive potential in the form of infiltration, invasion, and erosion. Sometimes bi- or even trinucleate cells are seen in these lesions, essentially reproducing cancerous giant cells (Fig. 15–34). Electron microscopy has disclosed, in the myeloma cell, a highly developed endoplasmic reticulum, often stuffed with amorphous material compatible with immunoglobulin aggregates. Under the light microscope, the protein aggregates may appear as acidophilic inclusions known as **Russell bodies.** These, however, are not pathognomonic of myeloma, since they can also be seen in reactive plasma cells that are actively synthesizing immunoglobulins.

Multiple myeloma presents as multifocal destructive bone lesions throughout the skeletal system. The bone resorption results from the activation of osteoclasts by osteoclast-activating factors, such as lymphotoxin, secreted by the myeloma cells.[84] Although any bone may be affected, the following distribution obtains in large series of cases—vertebral column, 66%; ribs, 44%; skull, 41%;

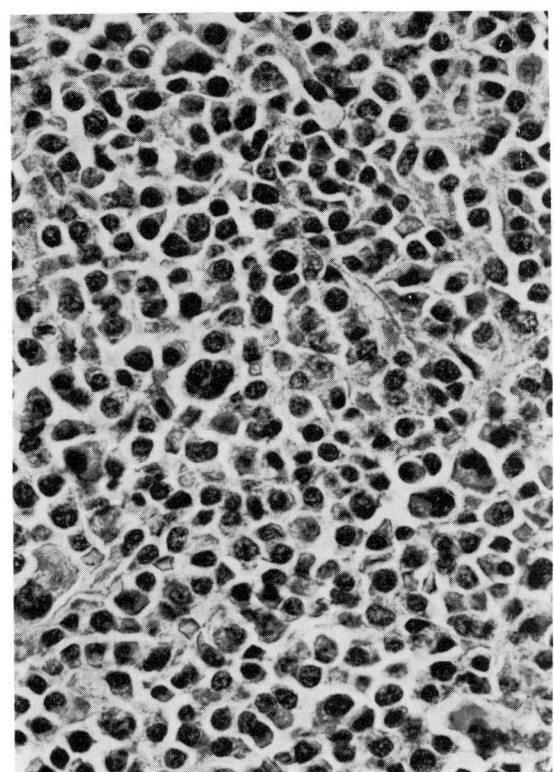

Figure 15–34. Multiple myeloma to show masses of plasma cells, mostly mature, but some with anaplasia and forming tumor giant cells.

pelvis, 28%; femur, 24%; clavicle, 10%; and scapula, 10%. These focal lesions generally begin in the medullary cavity, erode the cancellous bone, and progressively destroy the cortical bone. On section, the bony defects are filled with red, soft, gelatinous tissue. **Radiographically, the lesions appear as punched-out defects,** usually ranging between 1 and 4 cm in diameter (Fig. 15–35). In the late stages of multiple myeloma, plasma cell infiltrations of soft tissues may be encountered in spleen, liver, kidneys, lungs, and lymph nodes, or more widely.

Renal involvement, sometimes called **myeloma nephrosis,** appears in 60 to 80% of cases. Grossly, the kidneys may be normal in size and color, slightly enlarged and pale, or shrunken and pale because of interstitial scarring. The most distinctive features are microscopic.[85] Interstitial infiltrates of abnormal plasma cells or chronic inflammatory cell infiltrates may be encountered. However, the most prominent lesions are found in the distal convoluted and collecting tubules, which contain protein casts (Fig. 15–36). The casts are homogeneous and eosinophilic or polychromatic. Sometimes they are lamellar or granular. On immunofluorescent microscopy the casts reveal albumin, any class of immunoglobulin, and kappa or lambda light chains as well as Tamm-Horsfall protein.[86] In some cases the casts have the tinctorial and birefringent characteristics of amyloid (p. 210). The fact that amyloid fibrils can be produced in vitro by the proteolytic digestion of human Bence Jones protein makes this morphologic finding not surprising. The casts are usually surrounded by multinucleated giant cells, which were previously thought to be formed by the fusion of tubular epithelial cells. More recent studies suggest that the giant cells are derived from macro-

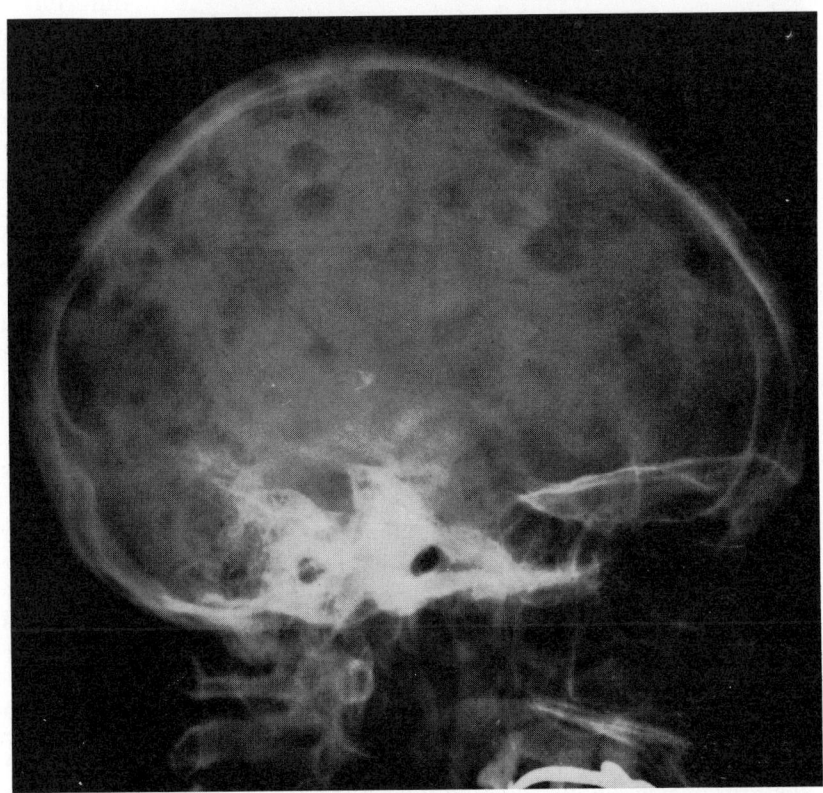

Figure 15–35. Radiograph of skull extensively involved by focal, sharply punched-out lesions of plasma cell myeloma.

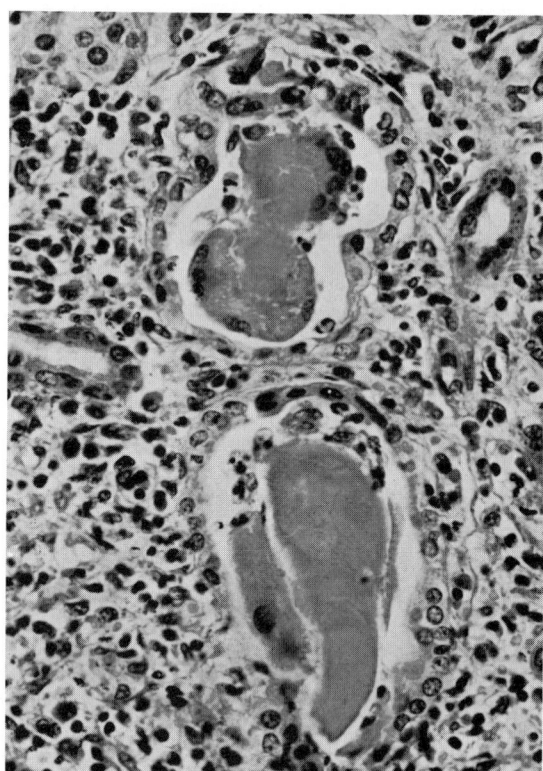

Figure 15-36. Proteinaceous casts surrounded by multinucleate giant cells in collecting tubules of kidney in myeloma nephrosis.

phages that migrate into the area through discontinuities in the tubular basement membrane.[87] The tubular atrophy associated with these lesions is accompanied by an increase of interstitial fibrous tissue. A number of other intercurrent changes may be present, including metastatic calcifications as a reflection of bone destruction and secondary hypercalcemia, pyelonephritis incident to the predisposition to infection in these patients, and systemic amyloidosis. All of these contribute to renal insufficiency.

A **myeloma neuropathy** may develop owing to tumorous infiltrations of nerve trunk roots. Vertebral fractures and compression of roots may add to these neurologic complications. Occasionally, a form of neuropathy occurs in the absence of obvious causes and may represent the nonspecific carcinomatous polyneuropathy discussed on page 1445. Pathologic fractures are sometimes produced by the plasma cell lesions; they are most common in the vertebral column but may affect any of the numerous bones suffering erosion and destruction of their cortical substance.

Systemic amyloidosis occurs in about 10% of patients. When this complication supervenes, it may introduce all the morphologic changes associated with the widespread deposits of amyloid described in an earlier chapter (p. 213).

CLINICAL COURSE. The peak age incidence of multiple myeloma is between 50 and 60 years. Both sexes are affected equally. As previously stated, the *clinical features of myeloma stem from the effects of (1) infil-*

tration of organs, particularly bones, by the neoplastic plasma cells; and (2) the production of excessive immunoglobulins, which often have abnormal physicochemical properties. Infiltration of bones is manifested by pain and pathologic fractures. Hypercalcemia resulting from bone resorption may give rise to neurologic manifestations such as confusion, weakness, lethargy, constipation, and polyuria. It also contributes to renal disease. *Recurrent infections with encapsulated bacteria (e.g., pneumococci) resulting from severe suppression of normal immunoglobulins pose a major clinical problem.* Cellular immunity is relatively unaffected. To explain the loss of normal immunoglobulins it is postulated that the myeloma cells secrete a factor capable of activating suppressor macrophages, which in turn inhibit normal B cells.[88] Excessive production and aggregation of myeloma proteins may lead to the hyperviscosity syndrome in approximately 7% of patients. Those with the IgA myeloma are particularly prone to this complication because of the tendency of IgA molecules to form polymers. Manifestations of the hyperviscosity syndrome including retinal hemorrhages, prolonged bleeding, and neurologic changes are much more common with Waldenström's macroglobulinemia and are therefore discussed later (p. 744). In some cases the M components may possess antibody activity against red cells or clotting factors, giving rise to hemolytic anemia and coagulation defects, respectively.[89] Amyloidosis of the AL type results from excessive imbalanced production of immunoglobulin light chains (p. 213). *Of great significance is renal insufficiency, which is second only to infections as a cause of death.* Renal failure develops in several different settings. In the more common form it develops insidiously and usually progresses slowly over a period of months or years. Another form occurs suddenly in the absence of obvious previous renal impairment and is manifested by acute renal failure. The pathogenesis of renal failure, which may occur in up to 50% of patients, is multifactorial and is discussed in Chapter 21 (p. 1061). The most important factor appears to be Bence Jones proteinuria, since the excreted light chains are believed to be directly toxic to the tubular epithelial cells.[90] In addition to these specific symptoms, some patients may present with anemia or weakness.

The clinical diagnosis of multiple myeloma rests on radiographic and laboratory findings and ultimately on biopsy of a lesion to reveal the tumorous aggregates of plasma cells. The radiographic changes are so distinctive that a reasonably certain diagnosis can usually be made. *Classically, the individual lesions appear as sharply punched-out defects, having a rounded soap-bubble appearance on x-ray film, but generalized osteoporosis may also be seen.* Almost all patients have a normochromic normocytic anemia, sometimes accompanied by moderate leukopenia and thrombocytopenia due to marrow failure. Rarely, neoplastic plasma cells flood the peripheral blood, giving rise to *plasma cell leukemia* (Fig. 15-37). The hyperglobulinemia leads to rouleaux formation on blood smear and an increased erythrocyte sedimentation rate. Hypercalcemia is frequently present. Most confirmatory of the diagnosis are M-protein spikes on blood or urine analysis. Quantitative analyses usually disclose more than 3 gm of Ig per dl of serum and more than 6 mg of Bence Jones proteins per dl of urine. The presence of the latter generally implies a graver prognosis.[91] As the disease progresses and the total mass of plasma cells expands, the level of M proteins increases. It should be remembered that, rarely, elevated serum immunoglobulins are absent in this disease (nonsecretory myeloma). Perhaps one third of the patients lack Bence Jones light chains. On the other hand, sometimes only Bence Jones proteins are present without increased serum gamma globulins (in so-called light-chain disease).

The prognosis for this condition depends on the stage of advancement at the time of diagnosis. Patients with multiple bony lesions, if untreated, rarely survive for more than 6 to 12 months. Chemotherapy in the form of alkylating agents induces remission in 50 to 70% of patients, but the median survival is still a dismal two to three years.

Solitary Myeloma (Plasmacytoma)

About 3 to 5% of monoclonal gammopathies consist of a solitary plasmacytic lesion, in either bone or soft tissue. The bony lesions tend to occur in the same locations as in multiple myeloma. Extraosseous le-

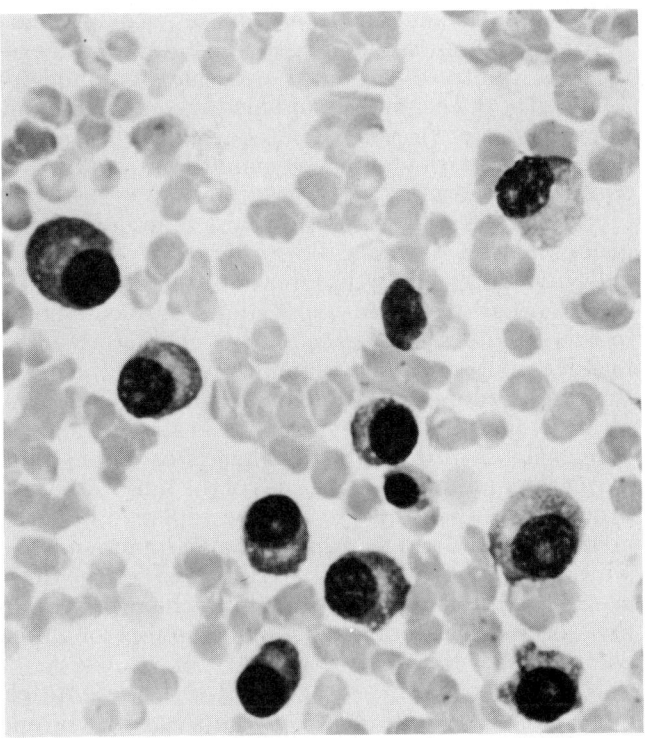

Figure 15-37. Multiple myeloma — plasma cell leukemia. The peripheral blood smear shows numerous plasma cells. (Courtesy of Dr. Patrick Ward, Department of Pathology and Laboratory Medicine, University of Minnesota School of Medicine, Duluth, Minnesota.)

sions are often located in the lungs, oronasopharynx, or nasal sinuses. Wherever they arise, they have the fleshy, red-brown appearance characteristic of the lesions in multiple myeloma. The cytologic detail is also similar. Elevated levels of M proteins in the blood or urine are found in approximately 25% of cases, but when present they are not as extreme as with multiple myeloma.[92] When patients with such localized disease are followed, *progression to classic multiple myeloma becomes manifest in most patients with osseous plasmacytoma, whereas extraosseous primaries rarely disseminate.* It appears that the solitary plasmacytoma involving the bones is an early stage of multiple myeloma, but in some individuals it may be present for 10 to 20 years without progression. Extraosseous plasmacytomas, particularly those involving upper respiratory tracts, represent limited disease that can usually be cured by local resection.

WALDENSTRÖM'S MACROGLOBULINEMIA

This dyscrasia, constituting about 5% of monoclonal gammopathies, *is marked by a diffuse, leukemia-like infiltration of the bone marrow by lymphocytes, plasma cells, and hybrid forms that synthesize a monoclonal IgM immunoglobulin, leading to macroglobulinemia.* Approximately half the patients have lymphadenopathy, hepatomegaly, or splenomegaly, alone or in combination. This disease may best be viewed as a cross between multiple myeloma and small lymphocytic lymphoma. As in myeloma, the neoplastic B cells secrete a monoclonal immunoglobulin. However, unlike myeloma but similar to lymphoma, the tumor cells diffusely infiltrate the lymphoid tissues, including bone marrow, spleen, and lymph nodes.

MORPHOLOGY. Typically, there is a diffuse, sparse-to-heavy infiltrate in the bone marrow of lymphocytes, plasma cells, lymphocytoid plasma cells, and other variants on this theme (Fig. 15-38). The infiltrate is rarely as heavy as that encountered in leukemia and does not occur in tumorous masses that are characteristic of plasma cell myeloma. Thus, there is no bone erosion or characteristic radiographic finding. Abnormal plasma cells are sometimes found. For example, "flame" cells have diffuse, intensely eosinophilic-staining cytoplasm. An increased number of mast cells may also be present.

A similar infiltrate may be present in the lymph nodes, spleen, or liver in patients having disseminated disease. Infiltration of the nerve roots, meninges, and cerebral substance by proliferating cells may also occur.

CLINICAL COURSE. Waldenström's macroglobulinemia is a disease of old age, presenting between the sixth and seventh decades. The dominant presenting complaints are weakness, fatigability, and weight loss — all nonspecific symptoms. As pointed out, lymphadenopathy, hepatomegaly, and splenomegaly are often present. The specific complaints stem largely

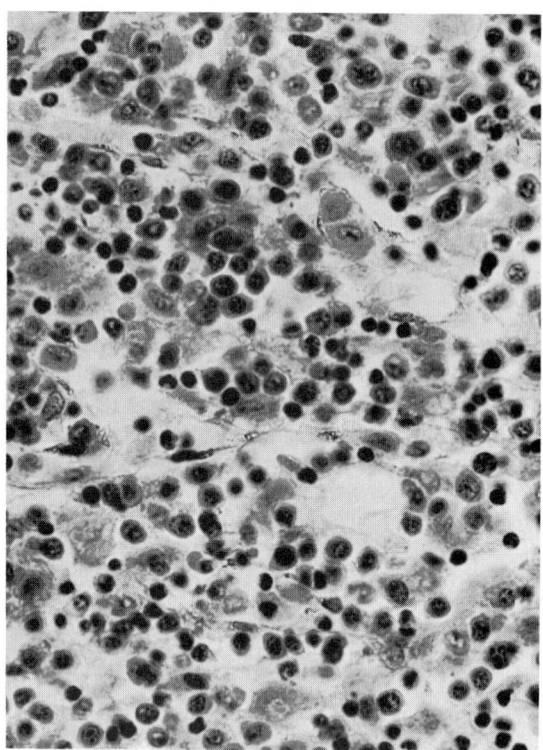

Figure 15–38. Waldenström's macroglobulinemia. Detail of marrow with pleomorphic cellularity containing recognizable lymphocytes and plasma cells admixed with many hybrid forms. (From Cabot Case Record 26–1964. N. Engl. J. Med. *270*:1190, 1964. Reprinted by permission from The New England Journal of Medicine.)

from the abnormal physicochemical properties of the macroglobulins. Because of their large size and increased concentration in blood, these paraproteins tend to form large aggregates that greatly increase the viscosity of blood. The resulting *hyperviscosity syndrome is characterized by visual impairment, neurologic signs, and excessive oozing from wounds.* The visual disturbances are related to the striking tortuosity and distention of retinal veins, with narrowing at arteriovenous crossings, producing what has been likened to a "sausage-link" pattern. Sometimes, retinal hemorrhages and exudates result from venous distention. The neurologic symptoms stemming from sluggish blood flow and sludging are protean; they include headache, dizziness, deafness, and even stupor in some cases. Excessive bleeding is related not only to hyperviscosity but also to interference in platelet function, as well as inhibition of clotting factors by macroglobulins. In some cases the abnormal globulins precipitate at low temperatures, giving rise to symptoms of *cryoglobulinemia* such as Raynaud's phenomenon and cold urticaria.

Despite the numerous clinical findings, diagnosis rests heavily on laboratory data. Unlike myeloma, there are no distinctive radiologic findings. Classically, the electrophoretic analysis of the serum discloses an M-protein spike, which is identified as IgM

by immunoelectrophoresis. Associated Bence Jones proteinuria occurs in 10 to 20% of cases; however, renal damage is much less common than in multiple myeloma, presumably because of the absence of other contributing factors such as hypercalciuria. A variety of other laboratory findings are present but are of less value diagnostically. These include anemia, an increased sedimentation rate, rouleaux formation, hyperviscosity, and cryoglobulinemia. Ultimately, *diagnosis rests on the typical bone marrow findings along with an M-protein spike, due to IgM, in the serum.* Differentiation of Waldenström's macroglobulinemia from malignant lymphoma is sometimes difficult. Since most lymphomas also have a B-cell origin, clinical forms intermediate between them and Waldenström's are not entirely unexpected. Differentiation, then, becomes largely a matter of semantics and is usually based on the predominant clinical symptoms.

The average survival in this disease is two to five years with appropriate chemotherapy.

HEAVY-CHAIN DISEASE

These extremely rare monoclonal gammopathies will be discussed only briefly. Three variants have been described, each characterized by elevated levels in the blood or urine of a specific heavy chain of immunoglobulins.[93] *Gamma-chain disease,* encountered most often in the elderly, resembles a malignant lymphoma more than a multiple myeloma. The manifestations consist of lymphadenopathy, anemia, and fever, often accompanied by malaise, weakness, and hepatomegaly or splenomegaly. Histologic study reveals an infiltrate of plasma cells and lymphocytes admixed with eosinophils and histiocytes. Lytic bone lesions are not present. The course can be rapidly downhill to death within a few months or may be protracted for years.

Alpha-chain disease, the most common in this group, may be viewed as a disorder of IgA-producing cells involving mainly the sites of normal IgA synthesis.[94] It occurs mainly in young adults, most commonly in the Mediterranean area, and is characterized by massive infiltration of the lamina propria of the intestine and abdominal lymph nodes by lymphocytes, plasma cells, and histiocytes. Villous atrophy and severe malabsorption with diarrhea, steatorrhea, and hypocalcemia are consequences of the infiltrate. With progression, the infiltrate may be replaced by large neoplastic cells and transform into an immunoblastic lymphoma of B cells (p. 714). Required for the diagnosis is the demonstration of alpha-chain protein in the serum. Occasionally, small amounts of alpha chains appear in the urine.

Mu-chain disease is the rarest of these entities, most often encountered in patients having chronic lymphocytic leukemia.[95] Characteristic are vacuolated plasma cells in the marrow. Immunoelectrophoresis reveals an excess of mu chains in the blood and sometimes also kappa-type light chains in the urine.

Hepatomegaly and splenomegaly are usually present, but in contrast to the usual case with CLL, peripheral lymphadenopathy is inconspicuous.

MONOCLONAL GAMMOPATHY OF UNDETERMINED SIGNIFICANCE

When large numbers of individuals above the age of 65 are screened by electrophoresis for M-protein serum spikes, about 5 to 10% are found to have elevated levels of IgG, IgA, or IgM, despite the fact that they are completely asymptomatic and clinical investigation does not disclose any of the well-defined immunoglobulin-producing diseases.[96] *To this dysproteinemia without associated disease, the term "monoclonal gammopathy of undetermined significance" (MGUS) is applied.* MGUS is much more common than previously appreciated; in one large study, over two thirds of the cases with a monoclonal serum protein belonged to this category.[97] Contrary to previous beliefs, the course of MGUS is not entirely benign. In a ten-year follow-up of 241 patients with MGUS, 18% developed a well-defined plasma cell dyscrasia (myeloma, macroglobulinemia, amyloidosis, or lymphoma). In another 9%, no overt disease appeared but a significant increase in the serum monoclonal protein suggested expansion of the abnormal plasma cell mass.[97] In general, patients with MGUS have less than 3 gm per dl of monoclonal protein, no Bence Jones proteinuria, and less than 5% plasma cells in the bone marrow. However, none of these criteria is absolutely reliable, and therefore the *diagnosis of MGUS requires careful exclusion of all the other specific forms of monoclonal gammopathies.* Whether a given patient with MGUS will follow a benign course, as most do, or develop a well-defined plasma cell neoplasm cannot be predicted, and hence periodic assessment of serum M component levels and Bence Jones proteinuria is warranted.

HISTIOCYTOSES

Several classifications of these disorders have been proposed. Some are based on segregation into reactive and neoplastic categories, others on the level of maturation of the histiocyte-macrophages involved. Still others include the histiocytic proliferations encountered in storage diseases such as Gaucher's and Niemann-Pick disease. Regardless of the nosologic scheme employed, it is relatively easy to segregate the clearly neoplastic proliferations such as the monocytic leukemias and the rare histiocytic lymphomas (p. 710) from the clearly reactive proliferations exemplified by tuberculosis and other infectious granulomas. Problems occur in trying to find a niche for certain rare proliferative disorders often described as *histiocytosis X. This term includes Letterer-Siwe syndrome, Hand-Schüller-Christian disease, and eosinophilic granuloma.* These three conditions are believed to represent different clinicoanatomic patterns of the same basic disorder. As will be described later, they differ with respect to the extent of organ involvement and the prognosis, but they are unified by the presence in the lesions of large, histiocyte-like cells that bear several similarities to Langerhans cells. These cells, you may recall (p. 168), are normally present within the epidermis and are believed to be related to the mononuclear phagocyte system. They have Fc receptors, bear HLA-D/DR antigens, and react with anti-CD1 antibody, which also binds to thymocytes but not to peripheral T cells. These immunologic markers are also present on the so-called histiocytosis X cells (HXC) that infiltrate the organs involved by these disorders.[98] The similarity between Langerhans cells and HXC extends also to the ultrastructural level. The cytoplasm of HXC contains characteristic inclusions called histiocytosis X (HX) bodies, which resemble Birbeck granules found in Langerhans cells (Fig. 15–39). *The HX body is seen as a pentalaminar, rodlike tubular structure with characteristic periodicity and sometimes a dilated terminal end (tennis-rac-*

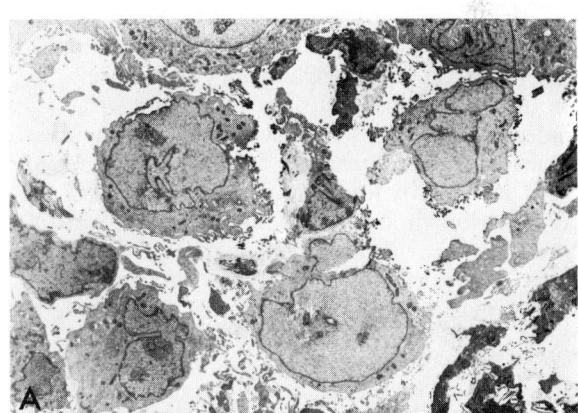

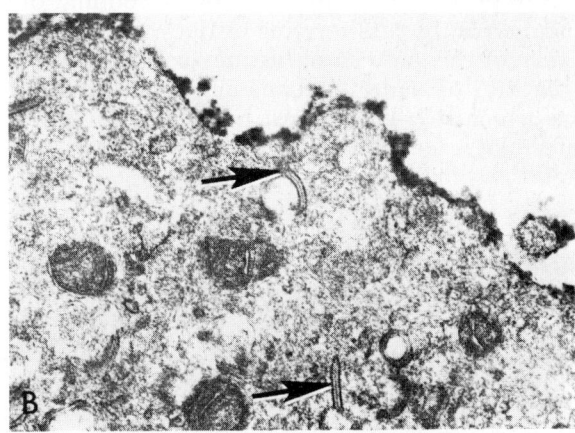

Figure 15–39. Langerhans cell histiocytosis. Infiltrate is composed of large, rounded cells containing reniform and infolded nuclei (A). At higher power (B), characteristic Birbeck granules *(arrows)* and membrane reactivity for thymocyte differentiation antigen CD1 (T6) (dense deposits along cell membrane) are observed. These features are also present in normal Langerhans' cells. (Courtesy of Dr. George Murphy, University of Pennsylvania School of Medicine, Philadelphia, Pennsylvania.)

quet appearance). Thus, histiocytosis X is viewed currently as a proliferative disorder of Langerhans cells or their marrow precursors, and hence the term "Langerhans cell histiocytosis" has been applied to them.[99] However, there is no unanimity regarding nomenclature. In recognition of their common origin, but somewhat distinctive clinicopathologic features, we will refer to the generalized fulminant form as acute disseminated Langerhans cell histiocytosis. The other two variants will be designated unifocal or multifocal Langerhans cell histiocytosis. Although the cell of origin seems to be reasonably well established, the pathogenesis of these disorders remains mysterious. The acute disseminated form behaves like a malignant tumor, whereas the unifocal and multifocal Langerhans histiocytoses appear to be non-neoplastic, rarely causing death. It is conceivable that they are all reactive disorders of variable severity, responding to unknown inciting agents.

Acute Disseminated Langerhans Cell Histiocytosis (Letterer-Siwe Syndrome)

This condition constitutes essentially an acute or subacute progressive systemic proliferation of mature and immature histiocytes. Classically, infants and young children under three years of age are affected. Sometimes the disease is present from birth. Occasional reports suggest that a closely similar disorder may also occur in adults.[100] In the very young the onset is marked by fever, sometimes related to a localized infection such as otitis media or mastoiditis, followed soon by a diffuse maculopapular eczematous or purpuric skin rash and subsequent enlargement of the spleen, liver, and lymph nodes throughout the body. Cystic, rarefied lesions may become apparent radiographically in the skull, pelvis, and long bones. Anemia, thrombocytopenia, and leukopenia are frequently present as manifestations of flooding of the bone marrow by proliferating histiocytes. The clinical picture of this pattern of histiocytosis shows several similarities to acute leukemia and a variety of infectious processes. These must be clearly excluded by morphologic and other appropriate criteria before diagnosis is made.

MORPHOLOGY. The characteristic microscopic feature of this disorder is proliferation of histiocytes throughout virtually all the organs and tissues of the body. The cells have abundant, often vacuolated cytoplasm, which is amphophilic-to-acidophilic, and vesicular oval, reniform, or indented nuclei. Nucleoli, when present, are small. Occasionally, multinucleated giant histiocytes are present, and in some cases, especially those involving adults, there may be some atypia and variation in histiocyte size and shape. With electron microscopy, occasional histiocytes can be seen to contain HX bodies (Fig. 15–39), described earlier. The histiocytic infiltrates can be seen in the skin lesions, lymph nodes, spleen, and liver and particularly within the bone marrow, where they may cause erosive defects visible on

x-ray film. In fatal cases, many other organs and tissues are affected, including the lungs, kidneys, gastrointestinal tract, and meninges.

The course of this condition is somewhat variable and appears to be related to age of onset and the degree of organ involvement. Up to the recent past, infants under six months of age generally pursued a rapid course to death within six months, and older children rarely survived more than one to two years. Intensive chemotherapy has remarkably improved this gloomy outlook. Currently, patients with organ dysfunction have a 40 to 50% chance of five-year survival, whereas a patient over two years of age without visceral involvement has approximately a 90% chance of living for five years.[101] Death is usually related to intercurrent infections and progressive anemia and debility.

Unifocal and Multifocal Langerhans Cell Histiocytoses (Eosinophilic Granuloma — Unifocal and Multifocal)

The distinctive morphologic lesions of both the unifocal and the multifocal variants consist of expanding, erosive accumulations of histiocytes usually within the medullary cavi-

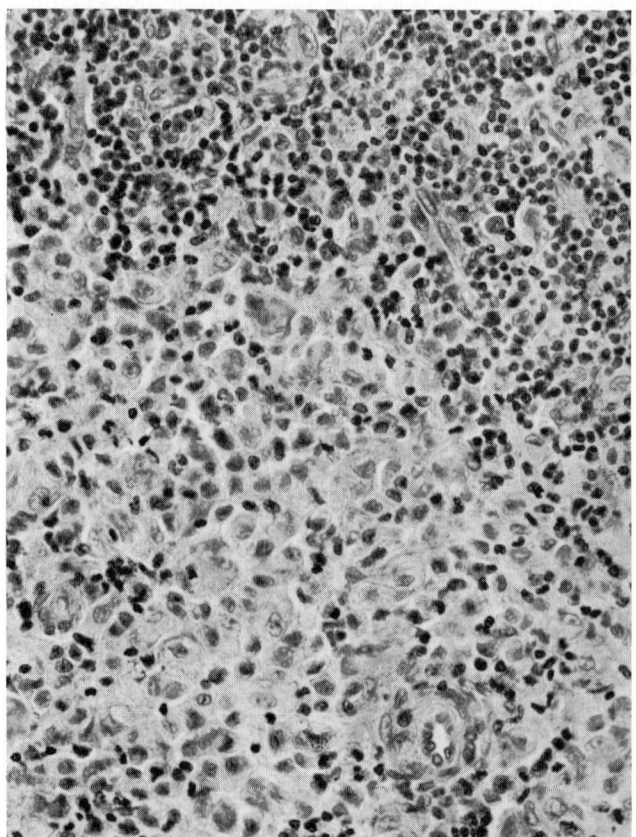

Figure 15–40. Langerhans cell histiocytosis (eosinophilic granuloma). The typical round and oval macrophages are most numerous below and are interspersed with scattered lymphocytes, plasma cells, and eosinophils.

ties of bones. Frequently, a few to many of the histiocytes are foamy and vacuolated. These are variably admixed with eosinophils, lymphocytes, plasma cells, and neutrophils (Fig. 15–40). Occasionally, there are areas of necrosis within these infiltrates, rimmed by a more intense infiltration of neutrophils and sometimes multinucleated histiocytes. The eosinophilic component ranges from scattered mature cells to sheetlike masses of cells. The foam cells, too, may be massed in some lesions, but since they merely reflect phagocytosis of lipid debris, they have no particular significance. Rod-shaped HX bodies may sometimes be present in the histiocytes within these lesions. Although virtually any bone in the skeletal system may be involved, favored localities are the calvarium, ribs, and femurs. Similar lesions are sometimes found in the skin, lungs, or stomach, either as unifocal lesions or as components of the multifocal disease.

Unifocal Langerhans cell histiocytosis (eosinophilic granuloma) is a benign disorder that occurs in children and young adults, especially males. The solitary lesions may be asymptomatic or may cause pain and tenderness as the lesion erodes the bone and in some instances leads to pathologic fractures. There are usually no systemic manifestations, such as fever, or involvement of the blood or viscera. Diagnosis is based on roentgenologic demonstration of a focal destructive bone lesion arising within the marrow cavity and on the characteristic morphologic findings. In some cases, spontaneous fibrosis and healing occur, usually in the span of a year or two. In other instances, curettage, excision, or local irradiation leads to a cure.

Multifocal Langerhans cell histiocytosis is a more disabling disease, with onset usually before the age of five years. Typically, patients have fever; a diffuse, scaly, seborrhea-like eruption, particularly on the scalp and in the ear canals; and frequent bouts of otitis media, mastoiditis, and upper respiratory infections as well as gingival inflammations. Mild lymphadenopathy, hepatomegaly, and splenomegaly due to infiltrates may be present. Pneumonitis with diffuse radiographic pulmonary opacities is sometimes present, perhaps related to granulomatous involvement of the lungs or to intercurrent microbiologic infections. About half the patients have granulomatous involvement of the posterior pituitary stalk or hypothalamus leading to diabetes insipidus. Orbital granulomas induce exophthalmos in about one third of patients. *The combination of calvarial bone defects, diabetes insipidus, and exophthalmos was referred to as the Hand-Schüller-Christian triad.* However, only a minority of patients with multifocal disease have the complete triad. It may be evident that the presentation of multifocal Langerhans histiocytosis with fever, skin rash, and multiple histiocytic lesions in bones and viscera bears considerable resemblance to acute disseminated histiocytosis, accounting for the belief that the two syndromes are variable expressions of a single disorder. However, in contrast to the acute disseminated form, the prognosis in multifocal Langerhans histiocytosis is good. In half the patients the lesions spontaneously resolve, and in the other half chemotherapy induces ultimate recovery.

SPLEEN

SPLENOMEGALY	**REACTIVE HYPERPLASIA OF**	**NEOPLASMS**
Hypersplenism	**SPLEEN**	**Primary Lesions**
CONGENITAL ANOMALIES	**CONGESTIVE SPLENOMEGALY**	**Secondary Lesions**
NONSPECIFIC ACUTE SPLENITIS	**SPLENIC INFARCTS**	**RUPTURE**

NORMAL

The spleen is to the circulatory system as the lymph nodes are to the lymphatic system. Among its functions are filtration from the bloodstream of all "foreign" matter including obsolescent and damaged blood cells, and participation in the immune response to all blood-borne antigens. Designed ingeniously for these functions, the spleen is a major repository of mononuclear phagocytic cells in the red pulp and of lymphoid cells in the white pulp. Normally in the adult it weighs about 150 gm and measures some 12 cm in length, 7 cm in width, and 3 cm in thickness.

It is enclosed within a thin, glistening connective tissue capsule that appears slate gray and through which the dusky red, friable parenchyma of the splenic substance can be seen. In man, unlike some animals, there is little if any smooth muscle in the capsule and therefore virtually no contractile function. The cut surface of the spleen is dotted with gray specks, the splenic or malpighian follicles that constitute the white pulp. In three dimensions this white pulp forms periarterial sheaths of lymphoid cells around the arteries, most abundant about the larger branches and progressively more attenuated as the arterial supply penetrates the splenic substance. A cross section of such an arrangement reveals a central artery surrounded eccentrically by a collar of T lymphocytes, the so-called periarteriolar lymphatic sheath. At intervals the lymphatic sheaths become expanded, usually on one side of the artery to form lymphoid nodules composed principally of B lymphocytes (Fig. 15–41). Upon antigenic stimulation, typical germinal centers form within these B-cell areas (p. 707). Eventually the arterial system terminates in fine penicilliary arterioles, which at first are enclosed within a thin mantle of lymphocytes but which then enter the red pulp, leaving behind their "fellow-travelers."

The red pulp of the spleen is traversed by numerous thin-walled vascular sinusoids, separated by the splenic cords or "cords of Billroth." The endothelial lining of the sinusoid is of the open or discontinuous type, providing passage of blood cells between the sinusoids and cords. The splenic cords are spongelike and consist of a labyrinth of macrophages loosely connected through long dendritic processes to create both a physical and a functional filter through which the blood can slowly seep.

It is widely believed that the blood, as it traverses the red pulp, takes two routes to reach the splenic veins.[102] Some of the capillary flow is into the splenic cords and is then gradually filtered out into the surrounding splenic sinusoids to reach the veins; this is the so-called open circulation, which is functionally the slow compartment. The other pathway involves direct passage from the capillaries to the splenic veins without the intervening stage of passage through the

cords. This, the "closed circuit," is understandably the more rapid compartment. According to current views, only a small fraction of the blood entering the spleen at any given time pursues the "open" route. Nevertheless, during the course of a day the total volume of blood passes through the filtration beds of the splenic cords, where it is exposed to the remarkably sensitive and effective phagocytic macrophages, which are able to screen the blood.

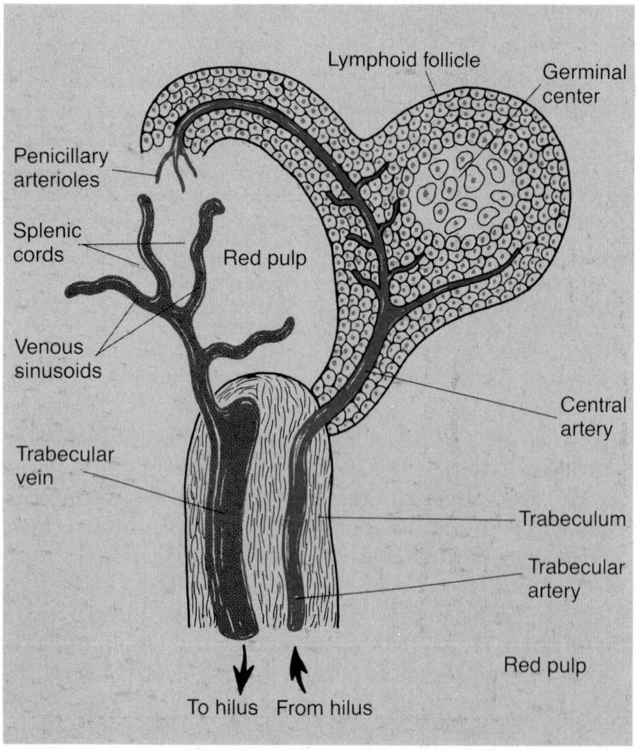

Most anatomic disorders of the spleen are secondary to some systemic disorder and thus are the consequence of normal splenic function. These can be segregated into four categories.

1. *Filtration of unwanted elements from the blood* by phagocytosis in the splenic cords is a major function of the spleen.[103] As you know, 1/120 of all red cells are destroyed daily by phagocytosis in the reticuloendothelial system. Engulfment by splenic macrophages accounts for approximately half this removal of obsolescent red cells from the circulation. The splenic phagocytes are also remarkably efficient in "culling" damaged red cells and leukocytes and red cells rendered foreign by antibody coating, as well as the abnormal red cells encountered in several of the anemias (e.g., hereditary spherocytosis, sickle cell anemia). As discussed earlier (p. 662), the red cells have to undergo extreme degrees of deformation during passage from the cords into the sinusoids. In several hemolytic anemias, the reduced plasticity of the red cell membrane leads to trapping of the abnormal red cells within the cords and subsequent phagocytosis by the cordal macrophages. In addition to removal of the red cells, splenic macrophages are also involved in "pitting" of red cells by which inclusions such as siderotic granules, Heinz bodies, and Howell-Jolly bodies are neatly excised without destruction of the erythrocytes. The phagocytes are also active in removal of other particulate matter from the blood, such as bacteria, cell debris, or abnormal macromolecules produced in some of the inborn errors of metabolism (e.g., Gaucher's disease, Niemann-Pick disease).

2. A second function of the spleen relates to its role as a *major secondary organ in the immune system*. The reticular network in the periarterial lymphatic sheaths traps antigen, permitting it to come into contact with effector lymphocytes.

3. The spleen is a *source of lymphoreticular cells and sometimes hematopoietic cells*. As you recall, splenic hematopoiesis normally ceases before birth, but in severe anemia, extramedullary splenic hematopoiesis may be reactivated.

4. Because of its rich vascularization and phagocytic function, the spleen also *constitutes a reserve pool and storage site*. In humans, the normal spleen harbors only about 30 to 40 ml of erythrocytes, but with splenomegaly this reservoir is greatly increased. The normal spleen also stores approximately 30 to 40% of the total platelet mass in the body. With splenomeg-

Figure 15–41. A schematic illustration of the normal splenic architecture. (Modified from Faller, D.V.: *Diseases of the spleen. In* Wyngaarden, J.B., and Smith, L.H. (eds.): *Cecil Textbook of Medicine.* 18th ed. Philadelphia, W.B. Saunders Co., 1988, p. 1036.)

aly this platelet storage may markedly increase, sometimes to up to 80 to 90% of the total platelet mass. Similarly, the enlarged spleen may trap a sufficient number of white cells to induce leukopenia.

In view of all these functions it is no wonder that the spleen becomes secondarily involved in a wide variety of systemic disorders.

PATHOLOGY

As the largest unit of the mononuclear-phagocytic system, the spleen is involved in all systemic inflammations and generalized hematopoietic disorders and many metabolic disturbances. It is rarely the primary site of disease. When the spleen is involved in systemic disease, splenic enlargement usually develops, and therefore splenomegaly is a major manifestation of disorders of this organ.

SPLENOMEGALY

Splenic enlargement may be an important diagnostic clue to the existence of an underlying disorder, but the condition itself may cause problems. When sufficiently enlarged, the spleen may cause a dragging sensation in the left upper quadrant and, through pressure on the stomach, cause discomfort after eating. In addition, its storage function may lead to the sequestration of significant numbers of blood elements, giving rise to a syndrome known as *hypersplenism* (described below). A listing, by no means exhaustive, of the disorders associated with splenomegaly is provided in Table 15–12.

The splenomegaly in virtually all the conditions mentioned has been discussed elsewhere. There remain only a few disorders that require consideration.

HYPERSPLENISM

Hypersplenism is encountered in only a minority of patients with splenic enlargement. In essence, this syndrome is characterized by the triad of (1) splenomegaly, usually caused by one of the disorders listed in Table 15–12; (2) a reduction of one or more of the cellular elements of the blood, leading to anemia, leukopenia, thrombocytopenia, or any combination of these, associated with hyperplasia of the marrow precursors of the deficient cell type; and (3) correction of the blood cytopenia(s) by splenectomy. The precise cause of this syndrome is still uncertain, but increased sequestration of the cells and the consequent enhanced lysis by the splenic macrophages seem to be the likely explanation for the cytopenias.

Table 15–12. Disorders Associated with Splenomegaly

I. **INFECTIONS**
Nonspecific splenitis of various blood-borne infections (particularly infective endocarditis)
Infectious mononucleosis
Tuberculosis
Typhoid fever
Brucellosis
Cytomegalovirus
Syphilis
Malaria
Histoplasmosis
Toxoplasmosis
Kala-azar
Trypanosomiasis
Schistosomiasis
Leishmaniasis
Echinococcosis

II. **CONGESTIVE STATES RELATED TO PORTAL HYPERTENSION**
Cirrhosis of liver
Portal or splenic vein thrombosis
Cardiac failure (right-sided)

III. **LYMPHOHEMATOGENOUS DISORDERS**
Hodgkin's disease
Non-Hodgkin's lymphomas
Histiocytoses
Multiple myeloma
Myeloproliferative syndromes (chronic myelogenous leukemia, polycythemia vera, myeloid metaplasia with myelofibrosis)
Chronic lymphocytic leukemia
Acute leukemias (inconstant)
Hemolytic anemias (autoimmune hemolytic anemia, hereditary spherocytosis, hemoglobinopathies)
Thrombocytopenic purpura

IV. **IMMUNOLOGIC-INFLAMMATORY CONDITIONS**
Rheumatoid arthritis
Felty's syndrome
Systemic lupus erythematosus

V. **STORAGE DISEASES**
Gaucher's disease
Niemann-Pick disease
Mucopolysaccharidoses

VI. **MISCELLANEOUS**
Amyloidosis
Primary neoplasms and cysts
Secondary neoplasms

CONGENITAL ANOMALIES

Complete absence of the spleen is rare and is usually associated with other congenital abnormalities such as situs inversus and cardiac malformations. *Hypoplasia* is a more common finding.

Abnormal lobulations, either shallow or deep, are another form of anomaly. These must be distinguished from depressed healed infarcts.

Accessory spleens (spleniculi) are common and have been encountered singly or multiply in one fifth to one third of all post-mortem examinations. They are usually small spherical structures that are histologically and functionally identical with the normal spleen, reacting to various stimuli in the same manner. They are generally situated in the gastrosplenic ligament or the tail of the pancreas, but are sometimes located in the omentum or mesenteries of the small or large intestine. Accessory spleens may have great clinical importance. In some hematologic disorders such as hereditary spherocytosis, thrombocytopenic purpura, and hypersplenism, splenectomy is a standard method of treatment. If a large accessory spleen is overlooked, the benefit from the removal of the definitive spleen may be lost.

NONSPECIFIC ACUTE SPLENITIS

Enlargement of the spleen, sometimes also called acute splenic tumor, occurs in any blood-borne infection. The nonspecific splenic reaction in these infections may be caused not only by the microbiologic agents themselves but also by the products of the inflammatory disease. Obviously, acute splenitis is also encountered in many specific infections, but these histologic changes usually provide some clue to the nature of the infection, as for example the striking reticuloendothelial hyperplasia and erythrophagocytosis in typhoid fever or the characteristic "mononucleosis cells" in infectious mononucleosis. In nonspecific acute splenitis it is impossible to identify the causative agent from the splenic changes.

Morphologically the spleen is enlarged (up to 200 to 400 gm) and soft. The color of the cut surface varies from grayish red to deep red; the white pulp is usually obscured. The splenic substance is often diffluent and may be sufficiently soft to literally flow out from the cut surface. Microscopically, the major change is acute congestion of the red pulp, which may encroach on and sometimes virtually efface the lymphoid follicles. Reticuloendothelial hyperplasia and numerous free macrophages are prominent within the sinusoids, and these phagocytic cells are often filled with viable and disintegrating bacteria as well as amorphous debris. An infiltrate of neutrophils, plasma cells, and occasionally eosinophils is sometimes present throughout the white and red pulp. At times there is acute necrosis of the centers of the splenic follicles, particularly when the causative agent is a hemolytic streptococcus. Rarely, abscess formation occurs. Infarcts, either bland or septic, may be present in those cases associated with infective endocarditis.

REACTIVE HYPERPLASIA OF SPLEEN

This rather vague designation refers to the splenic changes encountered in chronic inflammatory states, systemic antigenemia, immunologic-inflammatory conditions (rheumatoid arthritis, Felty's syndrome, bacterial endocarditis, SLE), systemic viremias (infectious mononucleosis, herpes simplex), and chronic graft rejections. In all these situations, the spleen along with the lymph nodes reacts as a component of the immune system, and so the spleen in these settings has been referred to by Enriquez and Neiman as an "activated spleen."[104]

The spleen is enlarged, sometimes up to 1000 gm, and generally is moderately firm. The splenic capsule is unaffected. The red pulp may be unusually congested, and on cut surface the splenic follicles are often prominent. Microscopically, the dominant changes are hyperplasia of the splenic follicles and marked reticuloendothelial hyperplasia, sometimes filling the sinusoids with phagocytic cells showing phagocytosis of debris (Fig. 15–42). Large germinal centers may be seen in the follicles, with prominent mitotic activity and transformation of many of the follicular center cells into "blasts." Macrophages, eosinophils, and numerous plasma cells are often present in both white and red pulp.

Should the underlying condition causing the splenic changes be amenable to control, the spleen in time generally reverts to normal or near-normal size.

CONGESTIVE SPLENOMEGALY

Persistent or chronic venous congestion may cause enlargement of the spleen, referred to as *congestive splenomegaly*. The venous congestion may be systemic in origin, may be caused by intrahepatic derangement of portal venous drainage, or may be due to obstructive venous disorders in the portal or

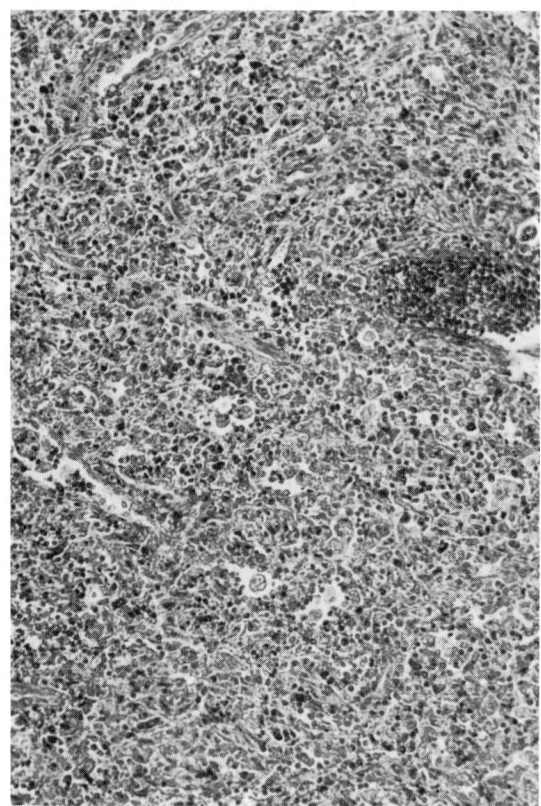

Figure 15–42. Chronic reactive hyperplasia of spleen. View of splenic substance. Sinuses are filled with macrophages and other white cells so that the low-power architecture is suffused with cells.

splenic veins. All these disorders ultimately lead to portal or splenic vein hypertension. *Systemic or central venous congestion* is encountered in cardiac decompensation involving the right side of the heart, and therefore is found in any type of long-standing cardiac decompensation. It is particularly severe in tricuspid or pulmonic valvular disease and in chronic cor pulmonale. In systemic venous stasis there are accompanying congestive changes in the liver and intestines, and frequently associated ascites and peripheral edema. Such systemic passive congestion produces only moderate enlargement of the spleen, so that it rarely exceeds 500 gm in weight.

The most common causes of striking congestive splenomegaly are the various forms of cirrhosis of the liver. The diffuse fibrous scarring of alcoholic cirrhosis and pigment cirrhosis evokes the most extreme enlargements. Less commonly, other forms of cirrhosis are implicated. In these conditions, there is sufficient impingement on the venous drainage through the liver to cause marked stasis within the portal system. At the same time, portohepatic artery shunts develop in the hepatic scars to raise the portal and splenic venous pressures even further.

Congestive splenomegaly is also caused by obstruction to the extrahepatic portal vein or splenic vein. The venous obstruction may be due to *spontaneous portal vein thrombosis.* Such thrombosis is usually associated with some intrahepatic obstructive disease, or may be initiated by inflammatory involvement of the portal vein *(pylephlebitis)* such as follows intraperitoneal infections. Thrombosis of the splenic vein itself may be initiated by the pressure of tumors in neighboring organs, e.g., carcinoma of the stomach or pancreas. Less often, it occurs as a splenic thrombophlebitis resulting from suppurative peritonitis, or as a bland thrombosis secondary to upper abdominal surgery or some disorder that predisposes to systemic venous thromboses.

Long-standing congestive splenomegaly produces marked enlargement of the spleen (1000 gm or more); the organ is firm and becomes increasingly so the longer the congestion lasts. The weight may reach 5000 gm. The capsule may be thickened and fibrous but is otherwise uninvolved. The cut surface has a meaty appearance and varies from gray-red to deep red, depending on the amount of fibrosis. Often the malpighian corpuscles are indistinct. Small gray-to-brown firm nodules scattered throughout the red pulp constitute the so-called **Gandy-Gamna** nodules described below. Microscopically, the pulp is suffused with red cells during the early phases but becomes increasingly more fibrous and cellular with time. The increased portal pressure causes deposition of collagen in the basement membrane of the sinusoids, which appear dilated owing to the rigidity of their walls (Fig. 15–43). The resulting impairment of blood flow from the cords to the sinusoids prolongs the exposure of the blood cells to the cordal macrophages, resulting in excessive destruction (hypersplenism).[105] Foci of recent or old hemorrhage may be present with deposition

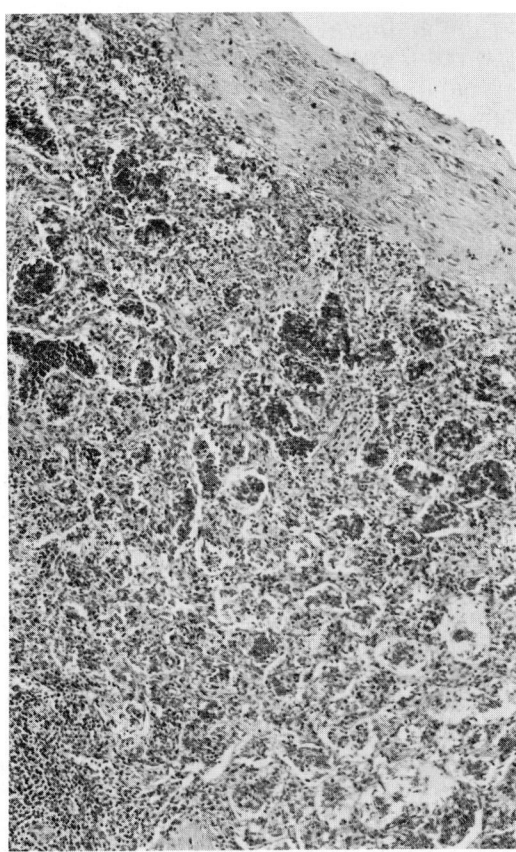

Figure 15–43. Congestive splenomegaly. Congestion of sinuses, fibrosis and widening of walls of sinuses, and fibrosis of capsule are the dominant features shown.

of hemosiderin in histiocytes. It is the organization of these focal hemorrhages that gives rise to the Gandy-Gamna nodules—foci of fibrosis containing deposits of iron and calcium salts encrusted on connective tissue and elastic fibers. The trabeculae are thickened and fibrous. In long-standing splenic congestion, foci of hematopoiesis appear, presumably as a response to the local vascular stasis and hypoxia.

SPLENIC INFARCTS

During the acute stages, infarcts of the spleen may cause enlargement, depending on the size and number of the lesions. The splenomegaly, however, is at most slight, and as the infarcts undergo fibrosis the spleen returns to normal size. Indeed, in the late stages, multiple splenic infarcts may cause loss of splenic substance. Splenic infarcts are comparatively common lesions. Caused by occlusion of the major splenic artery or any of its branches, they are almost always due to emboli that arise in the heart. The spleen, along with kidneys and brain, ranks as one of the most frequent sites of localization of systemic emboli. The infarcts may be small or large, multiple or single, or sometimes may involve the entire organ. They are usually of the bland, anemic type. Septic infarcts are found in infective endocarditis of the valves of the left side of the heart. Much less often, infarcts in the spleen are caused by local thromboses, especially in the myeloproliferative syndromes, sickle cell anemia, polyarteritis nodosa, Hodgkin's disease, and bacteremic diseases.

> Infarcts are characteristically pale and wedge-shaped, with their bases at the periphery where the capsule is often covered with fibrin (Fig. 15-44). Septic infarction modifies this appearance as frank suppurative necrosis develops. In the course of healing of these splenic infarcts, large, depressed scars may occur.

Splenic infarcts are an important clinical consideration in older cardiac patients who suddenly complain of left upper quadrant pain. This clinical accident is not an unusual accompaniment of bacterial infective endocarditis. Occasionally in these cases, the fibrinous perisplenitis leads to friction rubs that can be heard in the left upper quadrant. The destruction of splenic substance is not critically significant, and the major importance of these infarcts is their differentiation from other more serious intra-abdominal diseases that cause left upper quadrant pain: e.g., rupture of the spleen, perforation of the stomach or intestines, or rupture of an intra-abdominal aneurysm.

NEOPLASMS

Neoplastic involvement of the spleen, whether primary or secondary, may induce splenomegaly.

PRIMARY LESIONS

In general, primary tumors, either benign or malignant, are rare.

BENIGN. The following types of benign tumors may arise in the spleen: fibromas, osteomas, chondromas, lymphangiomas, and hemangiomas. The two last-named are the most common and are often cavernous in type. Undoubtedly, some of the hemangiomas are better classified as hamartomas than as neoplasms.

MALIGNANT. Any of the types of non-Hodgkin's lymphomas or Hodgkin's disease primary in the lymph nodes (p. 708) may be primary in the spleen, and in this organ they have the same characteristics as in the lymph nodes. In addition to these lesions, hemangiosarcomas with metastases, especially to the liver, do occur (p. 591).

SECONDARY LESIONS

Whether to call involvement of the spleen in Hodgkin's disease or disseminated non-Hodgkin's lymphomas a secondary lesion is largely a semantic issue; however, as you recall, splenic involvement in these conditions is by no means uncommon. Metastases of other types of tumors to the spleen have been reported to be rare, or present in 50% of cases when assiduously sought (especially with malignant melanomas). In either event, metastases appear in the spleen only when the primary lesion has disseminated widely, and are of little clinical consequence since the patients are almost always in a terminal stage.

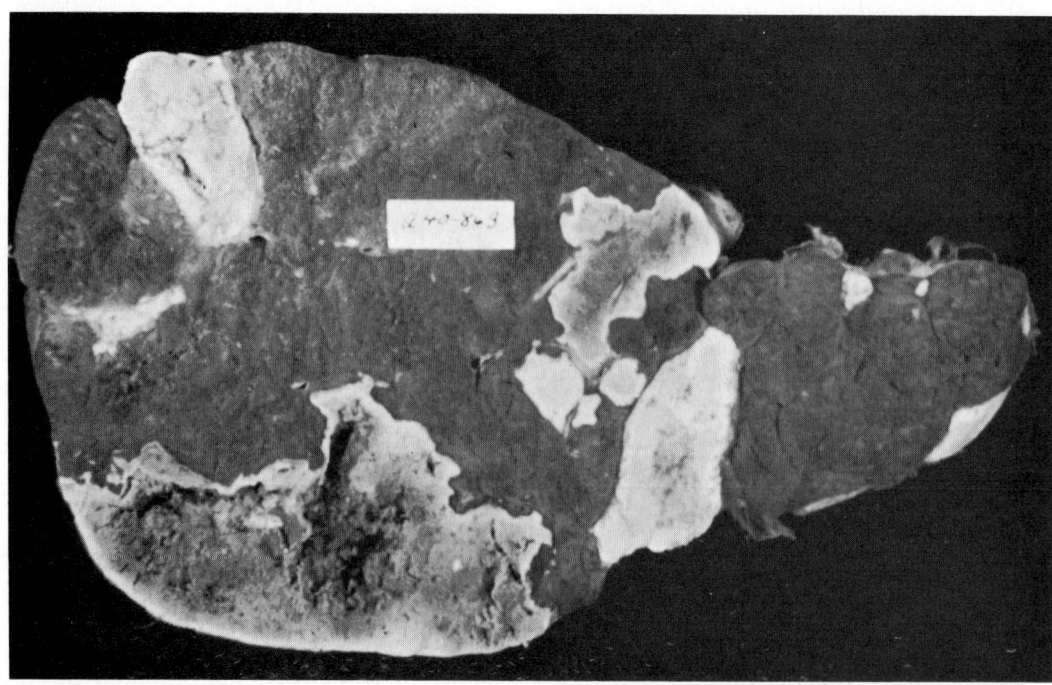

Figure 15-44. Splenic infarcts. Multiple wedge-shaped lesions are present, the largest having developed cystic softening.

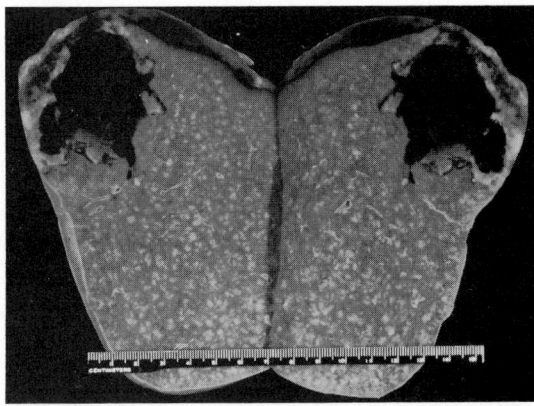

Figure 15–45. Large spontaneous hemorrhage into spleen of a 27-year-old patient with infectious mononucleosis. Hematoma ruptured through capsule and caused massive intraperitoneal hemorrhage.

RUPTURE

Rupture of the spleen is usually caused by a crushing injury or severe blow. Much less often, it is encountered in the apparent absence of trauma: this event is designated as spontaneous rupture. It is a clinical maxim that the normal spleen never ruptures spontaneously. In all instances of apparent nontraumatic rupture, some underlying condition should be suspected as the basis for the enlargement or weakening of this organ. Spontaneous rupture is encountered most often in infectious mononucleosis, malaria, typhoid fever, leukemia, and the other types of acute splenitis (Fig. 15–45). Rupture is usually followed by extensive, sometimes massive, intraperitoneal hemorrhage. The condition usually must be treated by prompt surgical removal of the spleen to prevent death from loss of blood and shock. In rare instances, clotting staunches the flow of blood. In some cases, following rupture, spleniculi may be found either localized or scattered throughout the peritoneal cavity, apparently transplants of splenic substance.

1. Young, G.A.R., and Vincent, P.C.: Drug-induced agranulocytosis. Clin. Hematol. *9:*483, 1980.

2. McKenna, R., et al.: Granulated T lymphocytosis with neutropenia: Malignant or benign chronic lymphoproliferative disorder? Blood *66:*259, 1985.

3. Schnitzer, F.: Reactive lymphoid hyperplasia. *In* Jaffe, E. (ed.): Surgical Pathology of the Lymph Node and Related Organs. Philadelphia, W.B. Saunders Co., 1985, p. 22.

4. Mann, R.B.: Follicular lymphoma and lymphocytic lymphoma of intermediate differentiation. *In* Jaffe, E. (ed.): Surgical Pathology of the Lymph Node and Related Organs. Philadelphia, W.B. Saunders Co., 1985, p. 167.

5. National Cancer Institute: Sponsored study of classifications of non-Hodgkin's lymphomas. Summary and discription of Working Formulation for Clinical Usage. Cancer *49:*2112, 1982.

6. Harris, N.L.: Lymphoma 1987. An interim approach to diagnosis and classification. Pathol. Annu. 22(Pt.2):1, 1987.

7. Matis, L.A., et al.: Nodular lymphomas: Current concepts. CRC Crit. Rev. Oncol. Hematol. *5:*171, 1986.

8. Lukes, R.J., et al.: Immunologic approach to non-Hodgkin's lymphomas and related leukemias. Analysis of the results of multiparameter study of 425 cases. Semin. Hematol. *15:*322, 1978.

9. Berard, C.W., et al. (eds.): Malignant Lymphoma. Baltimore, Williams & Wilkins, 1987.

10. Pangalis, G. A., et al.: Malignant lymphoma, well-differentiated lymphocytic: its relationship with chronic lymphocytic leukemia and macroglobulinemia of Waldenström. Cancer *39:*999, 1977.

11. Weiss, L.M., et al.: Molecular analysis of the t(14;18) chromosomal translocation in malignant lymphomas. N. Engl. J. Med. *317:*1185, 1987.

12. Yunis, J. J.: Multiple recurrent genomic defects in follicular lymphoma. A possible model for cancer. N. Engl. J. Med. *316:*79, 1987.

13. Gaynor, E. R., and Ultmann, J. E.: Non-Hodgkin's lymphomas: Management strategies. N. Engl. J. Med. *311:*1506, 1984.

14. Lieberman, P.H., et al.: Evaluation of malignant lymphomas using three classifications and the working formulation. Am. J. Med. *81:*365, 1986.

15. Aisenberg, A.C., et al.: Immunoglobulin gene rearrangements in adult non-Hodgkin's lymphoma. Am. J. Med. *82:*738, 1987.

16. Graham, M.: Non-Hodgkins' lymphomas. Pediatr. Annu. *17:*192, 1988.

17. Winter, J.N., et al.: Phenotypic analysis in diffuse, large cell lymphoma. Clinical and histologic association. Am. J. Clin. Pathol. *85:*425, 1986.

18. Hansen, C.A., et al.: Bone marrow manifestations of peripheral T-cell lymphoma. A study of 30 cases. Am. J. Clin. Pathol. *86:*449, 1986.

19. Magrath, I.T.: Malignant non-Hodgkin's lymphoma in children. Hematol. Oncol. Clin. North Am. *1:*477, 1987.

20. Knobler, R.M., and Edelson, R.L.: Cutaneous T cell lymphoma. Med. Clin. North Am. *70:*109, 1986.

21. Edelson, R., et al.: Treatment of cutaneous T-cell lymphoma by extracorporeal photochemotherapy. N. Engl. J. Med. *316:*297, 1987.

22. Kim, J.H., and Durack, D.T.: Manifestations of human T-lymphotropic virus type I infection. Am. J. Med. *84:*919, 1988.

23. Broder, S.: Pathogenic human retroviruses. N. Engl. J. Med. *318:*243, 1988.

24. Osome, M., et al.: Chronic progressive myelopathy associated with elevated antibodies to human T-lymphotropic virus 1 and adult T-cell leukemia-like cells. Ann. Neurol. *21:*117, 1987.

25. Cossman, J., et al.: Molecular genetics and the diagnosis of lymphoma. Arch. Pathol. Lab. Med. *112:*117, 1988.

26. Korsmeyer, S.J.: Antigen receptor genes as molecular markers of lymphoid neoplasms. J. Clin. Invest. *79:*1291, 1987.

27. Portlock, C.S.: Hodgkin's disease. Med. Clin. North Am. *68:*729, 1984.

28. Lukes, R.J., et al.: Report of the nomenclature committee. Cancer Res. *26:*1311, 1966.

29. Grogan, T.M.: Hodgkin's disease. *In* Jaffe, E.S. (ed.): Surgical Pathology of Lymph Nodes and Related Organs. Philadelphia, W.B. Saunders Co., 1985, p. 86.

30. Timens, W., et al.: Nodular lymphocyte predominance type of Hodgkin's disease is a germinal center lymphoma. Lab. Invest. *54:*457, 1986.

31. Trudel, M.A., et al.: Lymphocyte predominance Hodgkin's disease: a clinicopathologic reassessment. Cancer *59:*99, 1987.

32. Regula, D.P., et al.: Nodular and diffuse types of lymphocyte predominance Hodgkin's disease. N. Engl. J. Med. *318:*214, 1988.

33. Drexler, H.G., and Lever, B.F.: The nature of the Hodgkin's cell. Report of the First International Symposium of Hodgkin's lymphoma. Blut *56:*135, 1988.

34. Kadin, M., et al.: Expression of T-cell antigens on Reed-Sternberg cells in a subset of patients with nodular sclerosing and mixed cellularity Hodgkin's disease. Am. J. Pathol. *130:*345, 1988.

35. Falini, B., et al.: Expression of lymphoid-associated antigens on Hodgkin's and Reed-Sternberg cells of Hodgkin's disease. An immunocytochemical study on lymph node cytospins using monoclonal antibodies. Histopathology *11:*1229, 1987.

36. Roth, M.S., et al.: Rearrangement of immunoglobulin and T-cell receptor genes in Hodgkin's disease. Am. J. Pathol. *131:*331, 1988.

37. Mueller, N.: Epidemiologic studies assessing the role of Epstein-Barr virus in Hodgkin's disease. Yale J. Biol. Med. *60:*321, 1987.

38. Weiss, L.M., et al.: Epstein-Barr virus DNA in tissues of Hodgkin's disease. Am. J. Pathol. *129:*87, 1987.

39. Gallo, R.C., and Gelmann, E.P.: In search of a Hodgkin's disease virus. N. Engl. J. Med. *304:*169, 1981.

40. Vianna, N.J., and Polan, A.K.: Epidemiologic evidence for transmission of Hodgkin's disease. N. Engl. J. Med. *289:*499, 1973.

41. Gutensohn, N., and Cole, P.: Epidemiology of Hodgkin's disease. Semin. Oncol. *7:*92, 1980.

42. Spect, L., et al.: Tumor burden as the most important prognostic factor in early stage Hodgkin's disease. Cancer *61:*1719, 1988.

43. Tucker, M.A., et al.: Risk of second cancers after treatment of Hodgkin's disease. N. Engl. J. Med. *318:*76, 1988.

44. Fialkow, P.J., et al.: Clonal development, stem-cell differentiation and clinical remission in acute non-lymphocytic leukemia. N. Engl. J. Med. *317:*468, 1987.

45. Sachs, L.: Growth, differentiation and the reversal of malignancy. Sci. Am. *254*(1):40, 1986.

46. Poplack, D.G., and Reaman, G.: Acute lymphoblastic leukemia in childhood. Pediatr. Clin. North Am. *35:*903, 1988.

47. Favara, B.E.: The leukemias of childhood. Perspect. Pediatr. Pathol. *9:*75, 1987.

48. Look, A.T.: The cytogenetics of childhood leukemia: clinical and biologic implications. Pediatr. Clin. North Am. *35:*723, 1988.

48a. Uckun, F.M., et al.: Immunophenotype-karyotype associations in human acute lymphoblastic leukemia. Blood. *73:*271, 1989.

49. Dewald, G.W., and Pierre, R.V.: Cytogenetic studies in neoplastic hematologic disorders. Curr. Hematol. Oncol. *66:*231, 1988.

50. Schiffer, C.A., et al.: Prognostic impact of cytogenetic abnormalities in patients with de novo acute lymphocytic leukemia. Blood. *73:*263, 1989.

51. Second MIC Cooperative Study Group (1987): Morphologic, immunologic and cytologic (MIC) working classification of acute leukemia. Cancer Genet. Cytogenet. *30:*1, 1988.

52. Koeffler, H.P.: Syndromes of acute non-lymphocytic leukemia. Ann. Intern. Med. *107:*748, 1987.

53. Freireich, E.J.: Adult acute leukemia. Hosp. Pract. *21:*91, 1986.

54. Bitter, M.A., et al.: Associations between morphology, karyotype and clinical features in myeloid leukemias. Hum. Pathol. *18:*211, 1987.

55. Hamblin, R.J.: Myelodysplasia. Br. J. Hosp. Med. *38:*558, 1987.

56. Koeffler, H.P.: Myelodysplastic syndromes (preleukemia). Semin. Hematol. *23:*284, 1986.

57. Third MIC Cooperative Study Group (1987): Morphologic immunologic and cytogenetic working classification of the primary myelodysplastic syndromes and therapy related myelodysplasias and leukemias. Cancer Genet. Cytogenet. *32:*1, 1988.

58. Kerkhofs, H., et al.: Utility of the FAB classification for myelodysplastic syndromes: investigation of prognostic factors in 256 cases. Br. J. Hematol. *65:*73, 1987.

59. Strife, A., and Clarkson, B.: Biology of chronic myelogenous leukemia: Is discordant maturation the primary defect? Semin. Hematol. *25:*1, 1988.

60. Champlin, R.E., et al.: Bone marrow transplantation in chronic myelogenous leukemia. Semin. Hematol. *25:*74, 1988.

61. Kantarjian, H.M., et al.: Chronic myelogenous leukemia in blast crisis. Am. J. Med. *83:*445, 1987.

62. Gale, R.P., and Foon, K.A.: Biology of chronic lymphocytic leukemia. Semin. Hematol. *24:*209, 1987.

63. International Workshop on Chronic Lymphocytic Leukemia: Chronic lymphocytic leukemia: Recommendations for diagnosis, staging, and response criteria. Ann. Intern. Med. *110:*236, 1989.

64. Golomb, H.M. (ed.): Hairy cell leukemia. Semin. Oncol. *11:*1, 1984.

65. Golomb, H.M., and Ratain, M.J.: Recent advances in the treatment of hairy cell leukemia. N. Engl. J. Med. *316:*870, 1987.

66. Bishop, J.M.: The molecular genetics of cancer. Science *235:*305, 1987.

67. Weinberg, R.A.: The genetic origins of human cancer. Cancer *61:*1963, 1988.

68. Nowel, P.C.: Molecular events in tumor development. N. Engl. J. Med. *319:*575, 1988.

69. Kurzrock, R., et al.: The molecular genetics of Philadelphia chromosome-positive leukemias. N. Engl. J. Med. *319:*990, 1988.

70. Chaganti, R.S.K.: Cytogenetics of leukemia and lymphoma. *In* Berard, C.W., et al. (eds.): Malignant Lymphoma 1987. Baltimore, Williams & Wilkins, 1987, p. 184.

71. Rinsky, R.A., et al.: Benzene and leukemia. An epidemiologic risk assessment. N. Engl. J. Med. *316:*1044, 1987.

72. Moloney, W.C.: Radiogenic leukemia revisited. Blood *70:*905, 1987.

73. Pearson, G.R.: Recent advances in research on the Epstein-Barr virus and associated diseases. *In* Fairbanks, V.F. (ed.): Current Hematology and Oncology. Vol. 4. Chicago, Year Book Medical Publishers, 1986, p. 123.

74. Louie, S., et al.: Immunodeficiency and the pathogenesis of non-Hodgkin's lymphoma. Semin. Oncol. *7:*267, 1980.

75. Ioachim, H.L.: Neoplasms associated with immune deficiencies. Pathol. Annu. *22*(Pt.2):177, 1987.

76. Sadamori, N., et al.: Significance of chromosome 14 anomaly at band 14q11 in Japanese patients with adult T-cell leukemia. Cancer *58:*2244, 1986.

77. Silverstein, M.M.: Myeloproliferative disease. Curr. Hematol. Oncol. *6:*163, 1988.

78. Ellis, J.T., et al.: Studies of the bone marrow in polycythemia vera and the evolution of myelofibrosis and second hematologic malignancies. Semin. Hematol. *23:*144, 1986.

79. Conley, C.L.: Polycythemia vera. Diagnosis and treatment. Hosp. Pract. *22:*181, 1987.

80. Annotation: Fibrosis of the marrow: Content and causes. Br. J. Haematol. *59:*1, 1985.

81. Osserman, E.F., et al.: Multiple myeloma and related plasma cell dyscrasias. J.A.M.A. *258:*2930, 1987.

82. Kyle, R.A.: Benign monoclonal gammopathy—a misnomer? J.A.M.A. *251:*1949, 1984.

83. Cornwell, G.G.: Progress in multiple myeloma, amyloidosis, and related monoclonal dysproteinemias. Curr. Hematol. Oncol. *5:*121, 1987.

84. Garret, I.R., et al.: Production of lymphotoxin, a bone resorbing cytokine, by cultured human myeloma cells. N. Engl. J. Med. *317:*526, 1987.

85. Seney, F.D., and Silva, F.G.: Southwestern Internal Medicine Conference: plasma cell dyscrasias and the kidney. Am. J. Med. Sci. *293:*407, 1987.

86. Cohen, A.H., and Border, M.D.: Myeloma kidney. An immunomorphogenetic study of renal biopsies. Lab. Invest. *42:*248, 1980.

87. Start, D.A., et al.: Myeloma cast nephropathy: Immunohistochemical and lectin studies. Mod. Pathol. *1:*336, 1988.

88. Jacobson, D.R., and Zolla-Pazner, S.: Immunosuppression in multiple myeloma. Semin. Oncol. *13:*282, 1986.

89. Farhangi, M., and Merlini, G.: The clinical implications of monoclonal immunoglobulins. Semin. Oncol. *13:*366, 1986.

90. Defronzo, R., et al.: Renal function in patients with multiple myeloma. Medicine (Baltimore) *57:*151, 1978.

91. Hill, G.S., et al.: Renal lesions in multiple myeloma: Their relationship to associated protein abnormalities. Am. J. Kidney Dis. *2:*423, 1983.

92. Kyle, R.A.: Diagnosis and management of multiple myeloma and related disorders. Prog. Hematol. *14:*257, 1986.

93. Seligmann, M., et al.: Heavy-chain diseases: Current findings and concepts. Immunol. Rev. *48:*145, 1979.

94. Khojasteh, A., et al.: Immunoproliferative small intestinal disease. A "third world lesion." N. Engl. J. Med. *308:*1401, 1983.

95. Franklin, E.C.: Mu-chain disease. Arch. Intern. Med. *135:*71, 1975.

96. Crawford, J., et al.: Evaluation of monoclonal gammopathies in the "well" elderly. Am. J. Med. *82:*39, 1987.

97. Kyle, R.A.: Monoclonal gammopathy of undetermined significance (MGUS): A review. Clin. Hematol. *11:*125, 1982.

98. Jaffe, R.: Pathology of histiocytosis X. Perspect. Pediatr. Pathol. *9:*4, 1987.

99. The Writing Group of the Histiocytosis Society. Histiocytosis syndromes in children. Lancet *1:*208, 1987.

100. Wolfson, W.L., et al.: Systemic giant cell histiocytosis; report of a case and review of the adult form of Letterer-Siwe disease. Cancer *38:*2529, 1976.

101. Komp, D.M.: Langerhans cell histiocytosis. N. Engl. J. Med. *316:*747, 1987.

102. Weiss, L.: Red pulp of the spleen: structural basis of blood flow. Clin. Hematol. *12:*375, 1983.

103. Rosse, W.F.: Spleen as a filter. N. Engl. J. Med. *317:*704, 1987.

104. Enriquez, P., and Neiman, R.S.: The Pathology of the Spleen. A Functional Approach. Chicago, American Society of Clinical Pathologists, 1976, p. 11.

105. Bishop, M.B., and Lansing, L.S.: The spleen: A correlative overview of normal and pathologic anatomy. Hum. Pathol. *13:*334, 1982.

16

The Respiratory System

LUNG

NORMAL

The lungs are ingeniously constructed to carry out their cardinal function, the exchange of gases between inspired air and the blood. The present consideration of the normal lung is confined to re-emphasizing those features of the anatomy that are particularly pertinent to an understanding of the pathology of this organ.[1-3]

The weight of the normal adult lung averages 350 to 425 gm. The lungs are divided into lobes by fissures or clefts lined by visceral pleura. The right lung has three lobes: upper, middle, and lower; the left lung has only two lobes, its middle lobe being assumed by the *lingula*. The lung airways—the main right and left bronchi—arise from the trachea at the level of the 4th and 5th thoracic vertebrae and then branch dichotomously, giving rise to progressively smaller airways.

The right main stem bronchus is more vertical and more directly in line with the trachea than is the left. As a consequence, aspired foreign material, such as vomitus, blood, and foreign bodies, tends to enter the right lung rather than the left. The units of lung aerated by the branches of bronchi below the lobar bronchi, called *bronchopulmonary segments* (pyramidal in shape), can be surgically resected with little hemorrhage or air leakage.

In the trachea and major bronchi, the cartilage takes the form of C-shaped plates, leaving the posterior membranous portion free of cartilage. Smooth muscle is present only in the membranous portion. However, as the main bronchi enter the lungs, this organization changes; discontinuous plates of cartilage and muscle now encircle the entire wall. *Thus, only in the lung, where the muscle extends around the entire circumference of the bronchi, does bronchial constriction result in total obstruction of the airway lumen.*

Progressive branching of the bronchi forms *bronchioles*, which are differentiated from bronchi by the lack of cartilage and submucosal glands within their walls. Further branching of bronchioles leads to the *terminal bronchioles*, which are less than 2 mm in diameter. The part of the lung distal to the terminal bronchiole is called the *acinus*, or the *terminal respiratory unit*; it is approximately spherical in shape, with a diameter of about 7 mm. Acini contain alveoli and are thus the site of gas exchange (Fig. 16–1). An acinus is composed of (1) *respiratory bronchioles* (emanating from the terminal bronchiole), which give off from their sides several alveoli; these bronchioles then proceed into (2) the *alveolar ducts*, which imme-

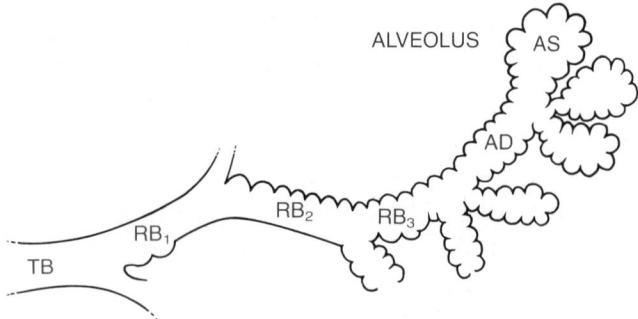

ALVEOLUS

Figure 16–1. This diagrammatic representation of an acinus shows a terminal bronchiole (TB); respiratory bronchioles of first (RB₁), second (RB₂), and third (RB₃) orders; an alveolar duct (AD); and an alveolar sac (AS). The acinus is the part of the lung distal to a terminal bronchiole, and emphysema is defined in terms of the acinus. (From Thurlbeck, W.M.: Chronic Airflow Obstruction in Lung Disease. Philadelphia, W.B. Saunders Co., 1976.)

diately branch and empty into (3) the *alveolar sacs*— the blind ends of the respiratory passages, whose walls are formed entirely of alveoli. It is important to note that the alveoli open into the ducts through large mouths. In the correct plane of section, therefore, all alveoli are open and have incomplete walls. A cluster of three to five terminal bronchioles, each with its appended acini, is usually referred to as the pulmonary *lobule*. As will be seen, this lobular architecture assumes importance in differentiation of the major forms of emphysema.

Attention should be called to the double arterial supply to the lungs, i.e., the pulmonary and bronchial arteries. In the absence of significant cardiac failure, the bronchial arteries of aortic origin can sustain the vitality of the pulmonary parenchyma when pulmonary arterial supply is shut off, as by emboli.

From the microscopic standpoint, it is well to remember that except for the vocal cords, which are covered by stratified squamous epithelium, the entire respiratory tree, including the larynx, trachea, and bronchioles, is lined by pseudostratified, tall, columnar, ciliated epithelial cells, heavily admixed with mucus-secreting goblet cells. The bronchial mucosa also contains neuroendocrine cells,[4] the bronchial counterparts of the argentaffin or Kulchitsky cells of the gastrointestinal tract. These cells exhibit neurosecretory-type granules; contain serotonin, calcitonin, and gastrin-releasing peptide (bombesin). Numerous submucosal, mucus-secreting glands are dispersed throughout the walls of the trachea and bronchi (but not the bronchioles).

The microscopic structure of the alveolar walls (or alveolar septa) consists, from blood to air, of the following (Fig. 16–2)[5]:

1. The *capillary endothelium* lining the intertwining network of anastomotic capillaries.
2. A *basement membrane and surrounding interstitial tissue* separating the endothelial cell from the alveolar lining epithelial cells. In thin portions of the alveolar septum, the basement membranes of epithelium and endothelium are fused, whereas in thicker portions they are separated by an interstitial space *(the pulmonary interstitium)*, containing fine elastic fibers, small bundles of collagen, a few fibroblast-like interstitial cells, smooth muscle cells, mast cells, and rare lymphocytes and monocytes.
3. The alveolar epithelium, a continuous layer made up of two principal cell types: flattened, platelike pavement *type I pneumocytes* (or membranous pneumocytes), covering 95% of the alveolar surface, and rounded *type II pneumocytes* (or granular pneumocytes), which exhibit surface microvilli and contain osmiophilic *lamellar bodies*. Type II cells are important for at least two reasons: (a) they are the source of *pulmonary surfactant* and (b) they are the main cell type involved in the repair of alveolar epithelium after destruction of type I cells. Loosely attached to the epithelial cells or lying free within the alveolar spaces are the *alveolar macrophages*. These are derived from blood monocytes and belong to the mononuclear phagocyte system. Often they are filled with carbon particles and other phagocytosed materials.

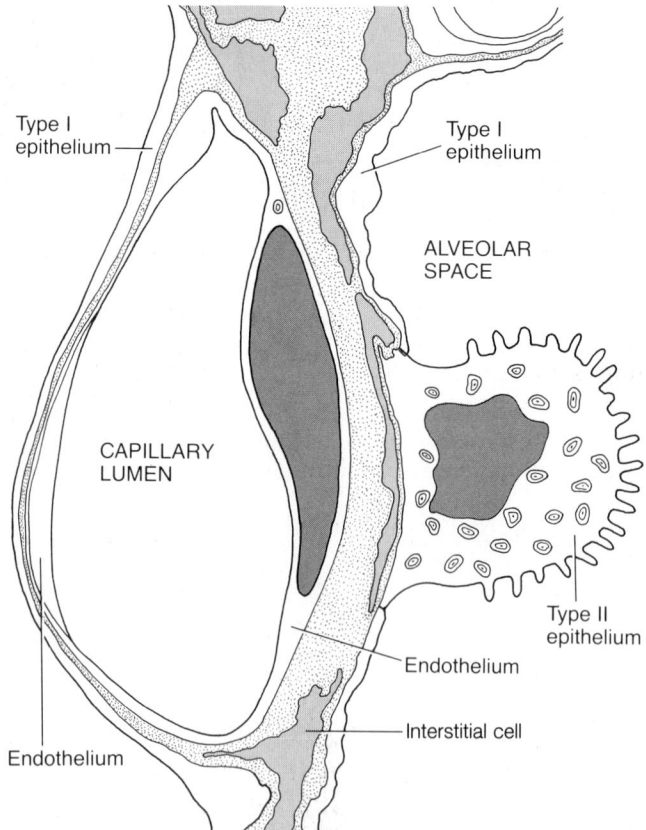

Type I epithelium

Type I epithelium

ALVEOLAR SPACE

CAPILLARY LUMEN

Type II epithelium

Endothelium

Interstitial cell

Endothelium

Figure 16–2. Microscopic structure of alveolar wall. Note that the basement membrane (stippled red) is thin on one side and widened where it is continuous with the interstitial space. Portions of interstitial cells are shown.

The alveolar walls are not solid but are perforated by numerous *pores of Kohn*, which permit the passage of bacteria and exudate between adjacent alveoli.

Adjacent to the alveolar cell membrane is the glycoprotein-containing cell coat upon which is a thin film of phospholipid, mostly phosphatidylcholine (lecithin), the *pulmonary surfactant.*[6] Lecithin is critical to the alveolar wall, as it serves to lower the surface tension of the alveolar lining and maintain the stability of the alveoli. Indeed, about half the normal compliance of the lung is due not to its elastic tissue but to these surface tension–lowering forces. Surfactant is synthesized in type II epithelial cells and stored in the osmiophilic lamellated bodies of such cells. Inadequate surfactant activity is believed to play a role in the respiratory distress syndromes of infants and adults (p. 760).

The structure of bronchioles (especially those less than 2 mm in diameter) is of special interest, because alterations in these "small airways" are important in the pathogenesis of chronic bronchitis and emphysema (p. 772). The structure of bronchioles differs in several respects from that of the alveolus on one hand and larger bronchi on the other. *The bronchiolar surface is covered with cilia, which are surrounded by a water-protein layer rich in lysozyme and immunoglobulins, but unlike the alveoli, the surface layer contains no surfactant and, unlike the bronchi, no mucus.* Indeed, there are no mucous cells in the walls of the bronchioles. Instead, nonciliated granulated *Clara cells* secrete the mucus-poor lining protein. In some inflammatory conditions of bronchioles, there is goblet cell metaplasia of the bronchiolar lining with an increase in mucus production and a diminution in the number of Clara cells.

PULMONARY DEFENSE MECHANISMS. Each day, the respiratory airways and alveoli are exposed to over 10,000 liters of air containing hazardous dusts, chemicals, and microorganisms. However, the normal lung is sterile, and although residents of most cities inhale several hundred grams of particles over their lifetimes, their lungs at autopsy show only a few grams of mineral ash. This is the result of efficient filtering and clearing mechanisms,[7,8] as follows (Fig. 16–3):

1. *Nasal clearance.* Particles deposited near the front of the airway on the nonciliated epithelium are normally removed by sneezing and blowing, whereas those deposited posteriorly are swept over the mucus-lined ciliated epithelium to the nasopharynx, where they are swallowed.
2. *Tracheobronchial clearance.* This is accomplished by the mucociliary action: the beating motion of cilia moves a film of mucus continuously from the lung toward the oropharynx; particles deposited on this film are eventually either swallowed or expectorated.
3. *Alveolar clearance.* Bacteria or solid particles deposited in the alveoli are phagocytosed by *alveolar macrophages,* which then eliminate the particle either by digesting it or by carrying it along to the ciliated

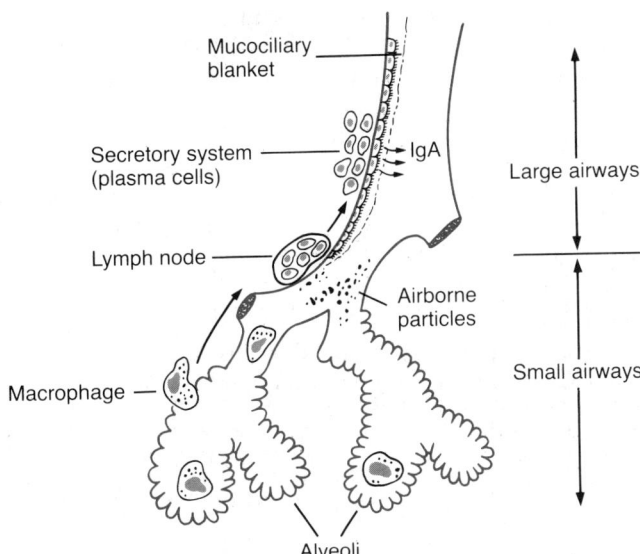

Figure 16–3. Components of lungs' defenses: mucociliary escalator in proximal bronchi and alveolar macrophages in distal airways. Arrows indicate possible routes alveolar macrophages may take in eliminating airborne particles. (From Daniele, R.P.: Immune defenses of the lung. *In* Fishman, A.P. [ed.]: Pulmonary Diseases and Disorders. New York, McGraw-Hill Book Co., 1988, p. 589. Used by permission of McGraw-Hill Book Company.)

bronchioles.[8] From here the macrophage is propelled to the oropharynx and then swallowed. Alternatively, the particle-laden macrophage may move through the interstitial space and either reenter the bronchioles or enter lymphatic capillaries. If the particle load is heavy and macrophage transport via the surface and alveolar pathways is overwhelmed, some particles may eventually reach the regional lymph nodes and, via the bloodstream, be carried elsewhere in the body.

Inhaled particles are deposited largely according to their size. Thus, particles over 10 μm are deposited largely in the turbulent air flow of the nose and upper airways; particles of 3 to 10 μm lodge in the trachea and bronchi by impaction; and smaller particles, about the size of most bacteria, 1.0 to 5.0 μm, are deposited in the terminal airways and alveoli. *Ineffective clearance of particles from these three sites is believed to be crucial to the pathogenesis of pulmonary infections (p. 778) and of the slowly developing pneumoconioses (p. 791).*

PATHOLOGY

It is impossible to overemphasize the importance of lung disease in the overall perspective of pathology and clinical medicine. Primary respiratory infections, such as bronchitis, bronchopneumonia, and other forms of pneumonia, are commonplace in clinical and pathologic practice. In this day of cigarette smoking and air pollution, chronic bronchitis and emphysema have become rampant, affecting large segments of the total population. Moreover, the lungs are secondarily involved in almost all forms of terminal disease, so that at virtually every autopsy some degree of pulmonary edema, atelectasis, or bronchopneumonia is found. Malignancy of the lungs has risen steadily in incidence, particularly in women, until it is now the most common form of visceral malignancy in both males and females. In the present consideration of the lung, emphasis will be placed on primary diseases that affect this important organ. For detailed descriptions of less common conditions, the reader is referred to current comprehensive books of pulmonary disease.[9-14]

CONGENITAL ANOMALIES

Developmental defects of the lung[5,13] include (1) agenesis or hypoplasia of both lungs, one lung, or single lobes; (2) tracheal and bronchial anomalies; (3) vascular anomalies; (4) congenital lobar overinflation (emphysema, p. 766); (5) congenital cysts; and (6) intralobar and extrapulmonary lobar sequestrations (p. 777). Only the last two anomalies will be discussed here.

Congenital cysts represent an abnormal detachment of a fragment of primitive foregut, and most consist of *bronchogenic cysts*. Bronchogenic cysts may occur anywhere in the lungs as single or, on occasion, multiple cystic spaces from microscopic size to over 5 cm in diameter. They are usually found adjacent to bronchi or bronchioles but may or may not have demonstrable connections with the airways. They are lined by bronchial-type epithelium, based on a thin layer of connective tissue, occasionally containing mucous glands or cartilage. In the uncomplicated case, the cavities are filled with mucinous secretion or with air. Infection of the secretions leads to suppuration, often associated with progressive metaplasia of the lining epithelium or even total necrosis of the wall of the cysts to create a lung abscess. Cysts may rupture into bronchi, which causes hemorrhage and hemoptysis; or they may rupture into the pleural cavity, resulting in pneumothorax or interstitial emphysema (p. 769).

Bronchopulmonary sequestration refers to the presence of lobes or segments of lung tissue *without a normal connection to the airway system*. Blood supply to the sequestered area arises not from the pulmonary arteries but from the aorta or its branches. *Intralobar sequestrations* are found within the pleural covering of the affected lobe and are usually associated with recurrent localized infection or bronchiectasis (discussed on p. 777). *Extralobar sequestrations* are separate from the pleural covering of the lung and may be found anywhere in the thorax or mediastinum. They are present most commonly in infants as abnormal mass lesions and may be associated with other congenital anomalies.

ALTERATIONS IN LUNG EXPANSION

ATELECTASIS

Atelectasis refers either to incomplete expansion of the lungs or to the collapse of previously inflated lung substance. This disorder may be present at birth, may arise during the first days of postnatal life, or may occur anytime thereafter. Whenever it occurs, it is characterized by areas of relatively airless pulmonary parenchyma. Significant atelectasis reduces oxygenation and predisposes to infection.

PATHOGENESIS. Acquired atelectasis, encountered principally in adults, may be divided into *obstructive (or absorptive)*, *compressive*, *contraction*, and *patchy atelectasis* (Fig. 16-4).

Obstructive atelectasis is the consequence of complete obstruction of an airway, which in time leads to *absorption* of the oxygen trapped in the dependent alveoli, followed by their collapse. There is, however, continued blood flow through the affected alveolar walls. The lung volume is diminished, and if a

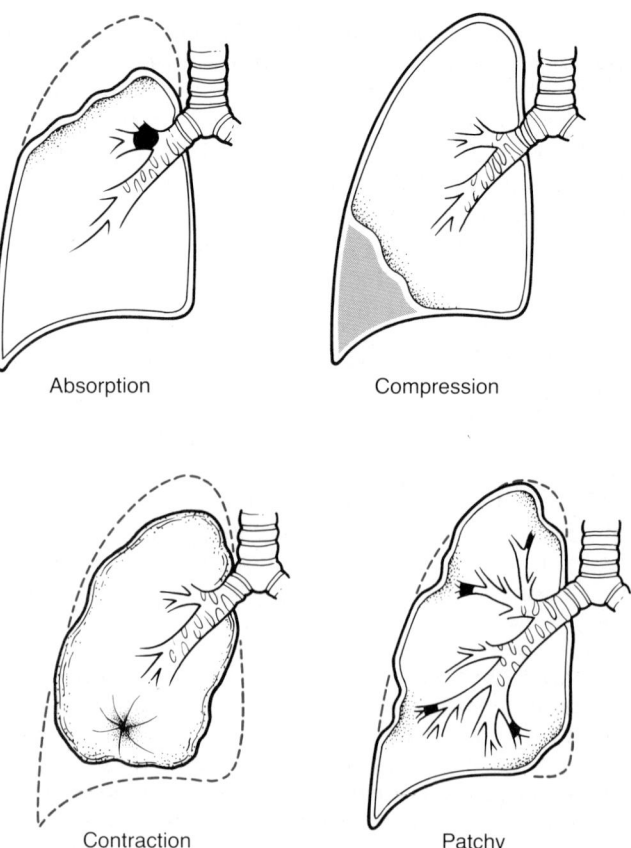

Absorption

Compression

Contraction

Patchy

Figure 16-4. Illustration of the various forms of atelectasis in the adult.

sufficient amount of parenchyma is affected the mediastinum shifts *toward* the atelectatic lung. This type of atelectasis is caused principally by excessive secretions or exudate within the second order and smaller bronchi, and it is therefore most often found in bronchial asthma, chronic bronchitis, bronchiectasis, postoperative states, and with aspiration of foreign bodies. Bronchial neoplasms are additional important causes of atelectasis, although in most instances they cause subtotal obstruction and produce localized emphysema.

Compressive atelectasis results whenever the pleural cavity is partially or completely filled by fluid exudate, tumor, blood clot, or air (the last-mentioned constituting *pneumothorax*) (p. 806). Compressive atelectasis is most commonly encountered in patients in cardiac failure who develop pleural fluid and in neoplastic effusions within the pleural cavities. It is also seen with rupture of a thoracic aneurysm causing hemothorax and in spontaneous or induced pneumothorax. Similarly, abnormal elevation of the diaphragm, such as that which follows peritonitis or subdiaphragmatic abscesses or which occurs in seriously ill postoperative patients, will induce basal atelectasis. With compressive atelectasis, the mediastinum shifts *away* from the affected lung.

Contraction atelectasis occurs when localized fibrotic changes increase recoil in a local area of the lung.

Patchy atelectasis develops when there is loss of pulmonary surfactant, as in the neonatal and adult respiratory distress syndromes, discussed elsewhere.

Because the collapsed lung parenchyma can be reexpanded, *atelectasis is a reversible disorder* that should not be permitted to contribute significantly to a fatal outcome. However, the atelectatic parenchyma is prone to develop superimposed infections.

DISEASES OF VASCULAR ORIGIN

PULMONARY CONGESTION AND EDEMA

A general consideration of edema is on page 87, and pulmonary congestion and edema were described briefly on page 91. Pulmonary edema can result from *hemodynamic* disturbances or from direct *increases in capillary permeability*, owing to microvascular injury (Table 16–1).[15,16]

HEMODYNAMIC PULMONARY EDEMA. The most common *hemodynamic* mechanism of pulmonary edema is that attributable to *increased hydrostatic pressure*, as occurs in congestive heart failure. Accumulation of fluid in this setting can be accounted for by Starling's law of capillary interstitial fluid exchange (p. 41). In short, the forces that move fluid out of the vessel wall are the mean intracapillary pressure and the small oncotic pressure of the interstitial

Table 16–1. Classification and Causes of Pulmonary Edema

HEMODYNAMIC EDEMA
Increased Hydrostatic Pressure
  Left heart failure
  Mitral stenosis
  Volume overload
  Pulmonary vein obstruction
Decreased Oncotic Pressure
  Hypoalbuminemia
    Nephrotic syndrome
    Liver disease
    Protein-losing enteropathies
Lymphatic Obstruction
EDEMA DUE TO MICROVASCULAR INJURY
Infectious agents
  Viruses, Mycoplasma, other
Inhaled substances
  Gases: Oxygen, nitrogen dioxide, sulfur dioxide, smoke
Liquid aspiration: Gastric contents, salt and fresh water
  drowning
Ingestants
  Chemotherapeutic agents: bleomycin, other
  Other medications: amphotericin B, colchicine, gold
  Other: heroin, kerosene, paraquat
Shock, trauma, and sepsis
Radiation
Miscellaneous
  Acute pancreatitis, cardiopulmonary bypass, fat or air embolism,
  uremia, heat
EDEMA OF UNDERTERMINED ORIGIN
High altitude
Neurogenic

fluid, and the forces moving fluid from the interstitium into the vessel lumen are the mean interstitial fluid pressure and the oncotic pressure of the plasma. In heart failure, there is an increase in pulmonary venous and capillary pressures and therefore in the forces moving fluid into the interstitium of the lung. Simultaneously, the interendothelial junctions stretch, are widened, and allow the increased movement of both fluid and macromolecules into the interstitium.[16] This results first in a marked increase in pulmonary lymphatic flow, which serves to drain off the accumulated fluid. *Only after lymphatic drainage has been increased by about tenfold does fluid accumulate.* At this stage, edema is purely "interstitial." It is only when critical elevations in interstitial pressure are reached or increased pressure is prolonged that the tight junctions between alveolar lining epithelial cells break and *alveolar edema* results.

Hemodynamic factors producing an imbalance in Starling forces also account for the pulmonary edema associated with volume overload and with hypoalbuminemia (e.g., the nephrotic syndrome). In the latter setting the principal derangement is a decrease in plasma oncotic pressure. Blockage of lymphatic drainage by tumors or inflammation is yet another mechanism leading to the accumulation of fluid within the lung owing to hydrostatic alterations.

Whatever the clinical setting, pulmonary congestion and edema are characterized by heavy, wet, subcrepitant lungs. Fluid accumulates in the basal regions of the lower lobes. Histologically, the alveolar

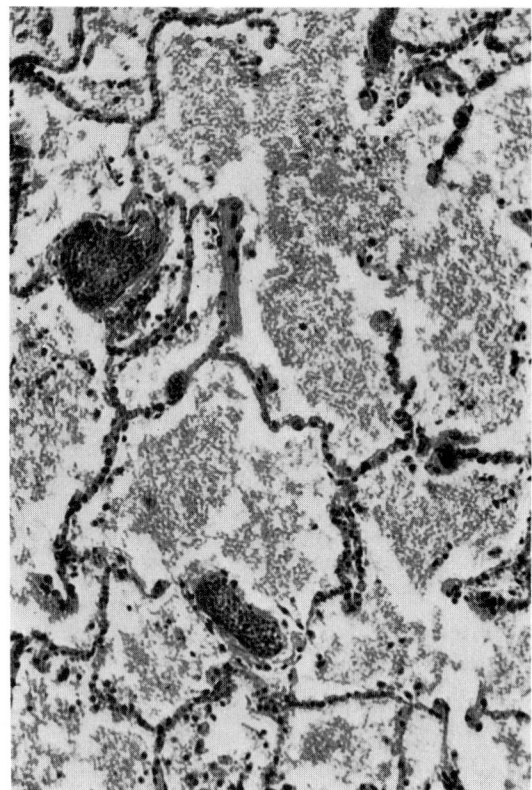

Figure 16–5. Pulmonary edema. Granular precipitate within alveolar spaces represents constituents of edema fluid.

ADULT RESPIRATORY DISTRESS SYNDROME

Synonyms for ARDS include adult respiratory failure, shock lung, diffuse alveolar damage (DAD), acute alveolar injury, and traumatic wet lungs. *ARDS and its many synonyms are descriptive terms for a syndrome caused by diffuse alveolar capillary damage and characterized clinically by the rapid onset of severe life-threatening respiratory insufficiency, tachycardia, cyanosis, and severe arterial hypoxemia that is refractory to oxygen therapy.*[17,18] In most patients there is evidence of severe pulmonary edema. Lung compliance is decreased, and chest radiographs usually show a diffuse alveolar infiltration.

The syndrome received attention during the Vietnam war as a complication of nonthoracic trauma with shock (hence the term shock lung), but it is now well-recognized as a complication of numerous other conditions seen in nonmilitary medicine.[17] The latter include (1) septic shock; (2) shock associated with trauma, hemorrhagic pancreatitis, burns, and complicated abdominal surgery; (3) *diffuse* pulmonary infections, mostly viral; (4) oxygen toxicity; (5) inhalation of toxins and other irritants (e.g., nitrogen dioxide); (6) narcotic overdose; (7) hypersensitivity reactions to organic solvents; (8) cardiac surgery involving extracorporeal cardiac pumps; and (9) aspiration pneumonitis. In many cases, a combination of the foregoing conditions — shock, oxygen therapy, and sepsis — is present.

capillaries are engorged and an intra-alveolar granular pink precipitate is seen (Fig. 16–5). Alveolar microhemorrhages and hemosiderin-laden macrophages (heart failure cells) are present. In long-standing cases of pulmonary congestion, such as those seen in mitral stenosis, hemosiderin-laden macrophages are abundant, and fibrosis and thickening of the alveolar walls cause the soggy lungs to become firm and brown. Changes such as these not only impair normal respiratory function but also predispose to infection. Thus, bronchopneumonia often terminates long-term congestive heart failure.

EDEMA DUE TO MICROVASCULAR INJURY. The second mechanism leading to pulmonary edema is *injury to the alveolocapillary membrane.* Here the pulmonary capillary hydrostatic pressure need not be elevated, and hemodynamic factors play a secondary role. The edema is initiated by injury to the vascular endothelium and frequently also to alveolar epithelial cells, resulting in leakage of fluids and proteins first into the interstitial space and, in more severe cases, into the alveoli. This is clearly the mechanism of locally occurring edema in bacterial or viral pneumonia. When it remains localized, as it does in most forms of pneumonia, the edema is overshadowed by the manifestations of infection. When diffuse, however, alveolar edema is an important contributor to a serious and often fatal syndrome — the *adult respiratory distress syndrome (ARDS) — which will be discussed next.*

PATHOGENESIS. ARDS is best viewed as the clinical and morphologic end result of acute alveolar injury caused by a variety of insults and probably initiated by different mechanisms. The initial and basic lesion is *diffuse damage to the alveolar wall*[10,19]; this is followed by a relatively nonspecific and usually predictable series of morphologic and physiologic alterations leading to respiratory failure (Fig. 16–6). The initial injury is to capillary endothelium, but eventually both endothelium and epithelium are clearly affected. Of interest is that type I epithelial cells are more vulnerable to most types of injury than are type II cells. Cellular damage leads to increased capillary permeability, interstitial and intra-alveolar edema, fibrin exudation, and formation of hyaline membranes.

What initiates endothelial or epithelial damage in these diverse conditions? The precise answer is unknown, but it seems likely that there is more than one initiating mechanism. For example, in toxicity induced by exposure to high concentrations (70 to 100%) of oxygen (oxygen toxicity), the injurious agents are almost certainly oxygen-derived free radicals (superoxide, hydroxyl ion, singlet oxygen), which directly affect cell membranes. Such may also be the case in ARDS induced by other toxins, such as the weed killer paraquat. Indeed, experimental oxygen toxicity can mimic most of the morphologic and functional features of ARDS.[20,21]

DIFFUSE ALVEOLAR DAMAGE

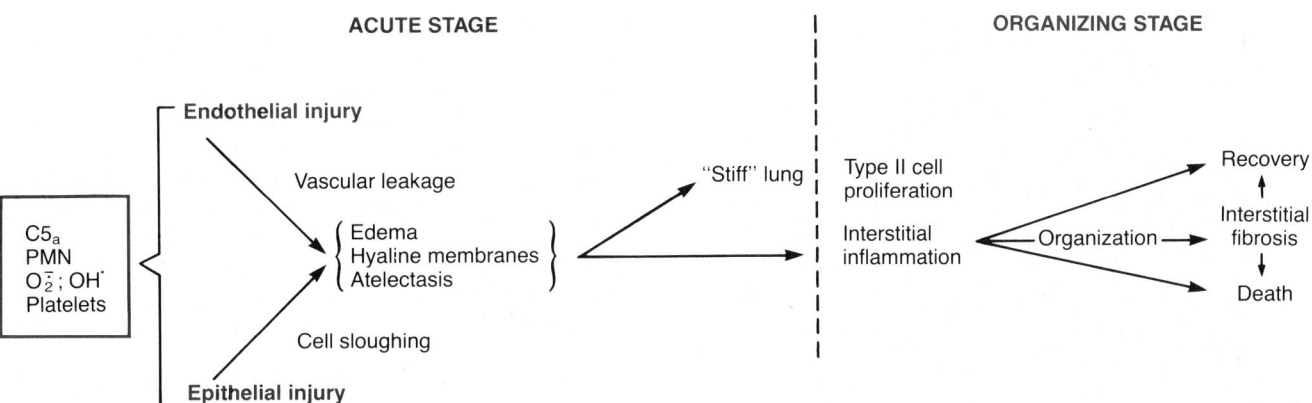

Figure 16–6. Pathogenesis of acute respiratory distress syndrome—a consequence of diffuse alveolar damage. PMN: polymorphonuclear leukocyte. (Modified from Katzenstein, A.-L.A., and Askin, F.B.: Surgical Pathology of Non-Neoplastic Lung Disease. Philadelphia, W.B. Saunders Co., 1982, p. 30.)

In most other conditions, such as septic or traumatic shock, the current evidence points to *pulmonary intravascular aggregation of leukocytes*, principally neutrophils, as an important early event in the process.[22] The scenario that emerges is that sepsis, trauma, cardiopulmonary bypass surgery, and other predisposing factors cause the liberation of mediators that induce leukocyte aggregation and activation in the lung. Activated complement components (C5a), platelet activating factor (PAF), and leukotriene B4 are examples of such mediators (p. 52). Stimulated neutrophils then secrete at least three classes of agents that may contribute to the alveolar injury: oxygen-derived free radicals, lysosomal enzymes (e.g., proteases), and products of arachidonic acid metabolism. The liberated oxygen-derived free radicals injure endothelium, causing increased permeability, and also probably epithelium, inducing alveolar edema. The liberated proteases destroy structural proteins, such as elastin and collagen. Products of arachidonic acid metabolism, such as thromboxane, are thought to result in the pulmonary vasoconstriction that also characterizes ARDS. Additional mechanisms postulated to play roles in ARDS include platelet aggregation with release of their vasoactive products, and intravascular coagulation.

The subsequent sequence of events is shown in Figure 16–6. In addition to the congestion, edema, and fibrin deposition, the alveolar walls become lined with waxy *hyaline membranes* such as are seen in hyaline membrane disease of neonates (p. 523). Such membranes consist of protein-rich edema fluid admixed with the cytoplasmic and lipid remnants of necrotic epithelial cells; they always reflect substantial epithelial cell injury. Loss of surfactant leads to atelectasis, and the combination of pulmonary edema and atelectasis result in the stiff (noncompliant) lung characteristic of ARDS. Subsequently, type II epithelial cells undergo proliferation in an attempt to regenerate the alveolar lining. There then is organization of the fibrin exudate, with resultant intra-alveolar fibrosis. Marked thickening of the alveolar septa ensues, caused by proliferation of interstitial cells and deposition of collagen. Not all patients follow this course. Recovery may take place at any stage, with resorption of the edema fluid and reexpansion of atelectatic areas.

MORPHOLOGY. The morphologic changes have already been discussed. In the acute edematous stage, the lungs are heavy, firm, red, and boggy. They exhibit congestion, interstitial and intra-alveolar edema and inflammation, fibrin deposition, necrosis of epithelial cells with formation of hyaline membranes, focal intra-alveolar hemorrhage, and patchy atelectasis (Fig. 16–7). In fatal cases there is usually terminal bronchopneumonia. In the later proliferative or organizing stages, alveolar spaces become lined by cuboidal or columnar type II epithelial cells, and there are variable degrees of interstitial and intra-alveolar fibrosis and inflammation.

CLINICAL COURSE. Patients who develop ARDS are usually hospitalized for one of the predisposing conditions listed earlier, and initially they have no pulmonary symptoms. ARDS is heralded by profound dyspnea and tachypnea, but the chest radiograph is initially normal. Subsequently there is increasing cyanosis and hypoxemia, respiratory failure, and the appearance of diffuse bilateral infiltrates on x-ray examination. Hypoxemia then becomes unresponsive to oxygen therapy, and respiratory acidosis develops. Progression from one phase to the next does not occur in all patients, and some recover completely. However, despite recent improvements in supportive respiratory therapy, the mortality rate among the 150,000 cases seen yearly in the United States is still about 50%.

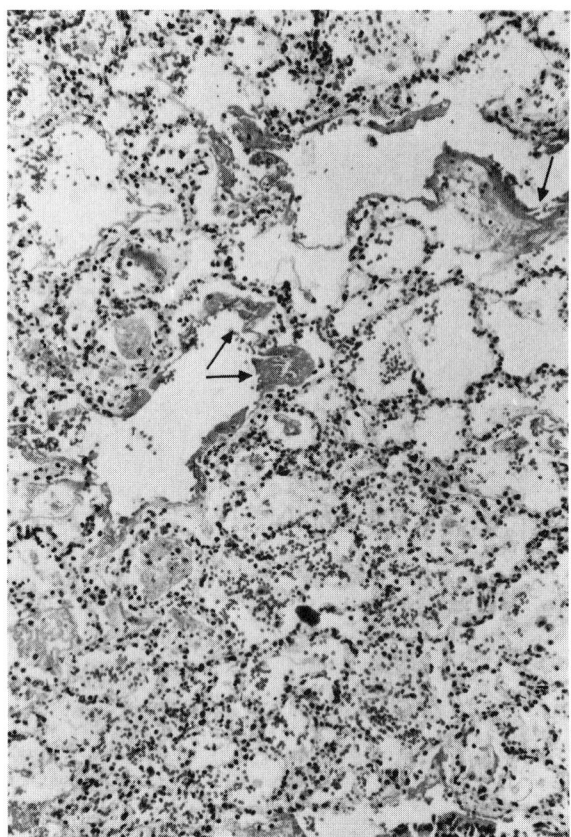

Figure 16–7. Adult respiratory distress syndrome. Some of the alveoli are collapsed, others distended. Many contain proteinaceous debris, desquamated cells, and, here and there, hyaline membranes *(arrows).*

PULMONARY EMBOLISM, HEMORRHAGE, AND INFARCTION

Occlusions of the pulmonary arteries by blood clot are almost always embolic in origin. In situ thromboses are rare and develop only in the presence of pulmonary hypertension and pulmonary atherosclerosis. However, thrombosis superimposed on a nonocclusive embolus may complete the arterial obstruction. The usual source of these emboli (thrombi in the deep veins of the leg) in over 95% of cases[23] and the magnitude of the clinical problem were discussed on page 105, where the awesome frequency of pulmonary embolism and infarction was emphasized. Suffice it to say here that pulmonary embolism causes more than 50,000 deaths in the United States each year. Its incidence at autopsy has varied from 1% in the general population of hospital patients to 30% in patients dying after severe burns, trauma, or fractures and 65% of hospitalized patients in one study in which special techniques were applied to discover emboli at autopsy.[24] It is the sole or major contributing cause of death in about 10% of adults dying acutely in general hospitals.

MORPHOLOGY. The morphologic consequences of embolic occlusion of the pulmonary arteries depend on the size of the embolic mass and the general state of the circulation. Large emboli may impact in the main pulmonary artery or its major branches or lodge astride the bifurcation as a **saddle embolus** (Fig. 16–8). Sudden death often ensues, owing to the block of blood flow through the lungs. Death may also be occasioned by acute dilatation of the right heart **(acute cor pulmonale).** In such sudden deaths, there may be no significant alterations in the lungs. Smaller emboli travel out into the more peripheral vessels where they may or may not cause infarction. **In patients with an adequate cardiovascular circulation, the bronchial artery supply can sustain the lung parenchyma despite obstruction to the pulmonary arterial system. Under these circumstances hemorrhages occur, but there is no infarction of the underlying lung parenchyma; only about 10% of human emboli actually cause infarction.** Although the underlying pulmonary architecture may be obscured by the suffusion of blood, **hemorrhages are distinguished by the preservation of the native pulmonary substance.** Resorption of the blood permits reconstitution of the preexisting architecture.

Pulmonary emboli cause infarction when the circulation is already inadequate, namely, in patients with heart or lung disease. For this reason, infarctions tend to be uncommon in the young. About three fourths of all infarcts affect the lower lobes, and in over one half they occur multiply. They vary in size from lesions barely visible to the naked eye to massive involvement of large parts of an entire lobe. Characteristically, they extend to the periphery of the lung substance with the apex pointing toward the hilus of the lung. The pulmonary infarct is classically **hemorrhagic** and appears as a raised, red-blue area in the early stages (Fig. 16–9). Often the apposed pleural surface is covered by a fibrinous exudate. If the occluded vessel can be identified, it will be found near the apex of the infarcted area. The red cells begin to lyse within 48 hours, and the infarct becomes paler and eventually red-brown as hemosiderin is produced. With the passage of time, fibrous replacement begins at the margins as a gray-white peripheral zone and eventually converts the infarct into a scar that is contracted below the level of the lung substance. Histologically, **the diagnostic feature of pulmonary infarction is the ischemic necrosis of the lung substance** within the area of hemorrhage. Such necrosis affects the alveolar walls, bronchioles, and vessels.

If the infarct is caused by an infected embolus, the infarct is modified by a more intense neutrophilic exudation and more intense inflammatory reaction. Such lesions are referred to as **septic infarcts,** and indeed some convert to abscesses.

CLINICAL COURSE. Pulmonary embolism is principally a complication in patients already suffering from some underlying disorder, such as cardiac disease or cancer, or who are immobilized for long periods. Younger women have an increased risk of suffering

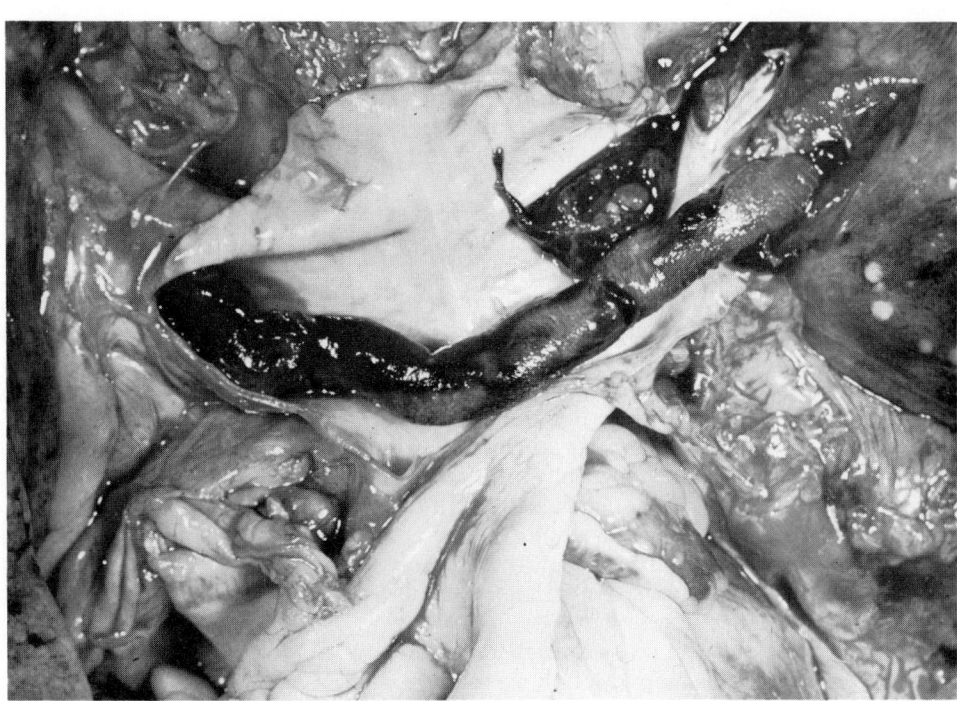

Figure 16-8. Large embolus from femoral vein lying astride main left and right pulmonary arteries.

pulmonary embolism in late pregnancy, following delivery, and with the use of contraceptive pills containing excesses of estrogens over progesterone.

The clinical significance of pulmonary embolism depends on the size of the occluded vessel, the number of emboli, and the overall status of the cardiovascular system. Emboli result in two main pathophysiologic consequences: *respiratory compromise* due to the nonperfused, though ventilated segment, and *hemodynamic compromise* due to increased resistance to pulmonary blood flow engendered by the embolic obstruction. The latter leads to pulmonary hypertension and acute failure of the right ventricle.

Large emboli are one of the few causes of virtually instantaneous death. If death occurs less suddenly, the clinical syndrome may mimic myocardial infarction with severe chest pain, dyspnea, shock, elevation of temperature, and increased levels of serum LDH. Smaller emboli sometimes cause acute right heart failure either by stimulating reflex vasoconstriction of pulmonary vessels or by releasing vasoconstrictor agents (e.g., thromboxane) from platelets.

Small emboli induce only transient chest pain and cough or possibly pulmonary hemorrhages without infarction in persons with a normal cardiovascular system. Only in the predisposed in whom the bronchial circulation itself is inadequate will they cause small infarcts. Such patients manifest dyspnea, tachypnea, fever, chest pain, cough, and hemoptysis. An overlying fibrinous pleuritis may produce a pleural friction rub.

The chest radiograph may disclose a pulmonary infarction, usually 12 to 36 hours after it has occurred, as a wedge-shaped infiltrate. In the absence of infarction, emboli can be detected by pulmonary perfusion

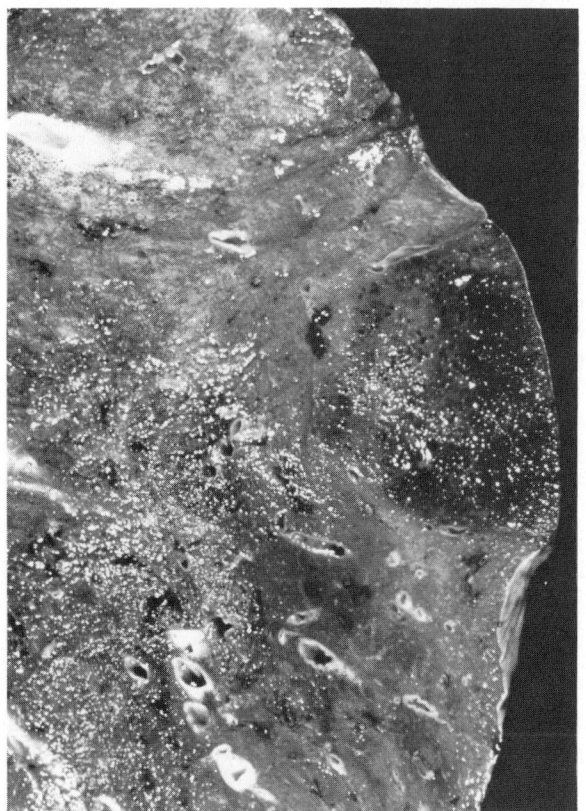

Figure 16-9. A relatively recent, small, roughly wedge-shaped hemorrhagic pulmonary infarct.

scintiphotography (photoscans) after parenteral injection of macroaggregates of albumin labeled with radionuclides such as technetium-99. Pulmonary angiography is the most definitive diagnostic technique, but entails more risk to the patient than do photoscans.

Emboli often resolve after the initial acute insult. The embolus contracts, as do all blood clots; fibrinolytic activity may then further reduce its size, and remarkable resolution with total lysis of the clot may follow. This happy outcome is the rule, rather than the exception, particularly in the relatively young. When unresolved, multiple small emboli over the course of time may lead to pulmonary hypertension, pulmonary vascular sclerosis, and chronic cor pulmonale. Perhaps most important is the fact that the small embolus may presage a larger one. In the presence of an underlying predisposing factor, patients with a pulmonary embolus have a 30% chance of developing a second embolus. The disease is fatal in only one of 10 treated patients.

Prevention of pulmonary embolism constitutes a major clinical problem for which there is no easy solution. Prophylactic therapy includes early ambulation in postoperative and postpartum patients, elastic stockings and isometric leg exercises for bedridden patients, and preventive anticoagulation in high-risk individuals. It is sometimes necessary to resort to insertion of a screen ("umbrella") into or ligation of the inferior vena cava—no small procedures in an already seriously ill patient.

PULMONARY HYPERTENSION AND VASCULAR SCLEROSIS

As should be well-known, the pulmonary circulation is one of low resistance; and pulmonary blood pressure is only about one eighth of systemic blood pressure. Pulmonary hypertension is caused largely by an increase in pulmonary vascular resistance, and (as reviewed in the discussion of cor pulmonale, p. 617) is most frequently *secondary* to (1) chronic obstructive or interstitial lung diseases, (2) recurrent pulmonary emboli, or (3) antecedent heart disease. Uncommonly, pulmonary hypertension is encountered in patients in whom all known causes of increased pulmonary pressure are excluded, and this is referred to as *primary* or *idiopathic pulmonary hypertension*.[25,25a] Distinction of primary hypertension from that caused by recurrent thromboembolism may be particularly difficult without morphologic examination, but it has been aided by angiography and radioisotope scanning.

PATHOGENESIS. Because most of the causes of secondary pulmonary vascular hypertension have already been considered, we are here concerned with the pathogenesis of primary pulmonary hypertension. Many theories have been proposed, which is another way of saying the problem is still unsettled.[25,27] One older theory proposed that multiple small repeated silent emboli are the cause of the pulmonary hypertension, and that their organization and incorporation within the arterial walls may be the cause of arterial thickening. *Most current theories, however, postulate neurohormonal vascular hyperreactivity as a central mechanism, in which chronic vasoconstriction induces pulmonary hypertension and, in time, intimal and medial vascular hypertrophy.* This concept is supported by the fact that patients with primary pulmonary hypertension often suffer from vasospastic disorders such as Raynaud's phenomenon (p. 579). In addition, pulmonary vascular resistance can be rapidly decreased in these patients with vasodilators. Such hyperreactivity, in turn, has several postulated mechanisms to explain its occurrence. One notion is that it results from an immune collagen-vascular disease, because both Raynaud's phenomenon and pulmonary hypertension occur in such disorders (scleroderma, SLE, rheumatoid arthritis): this is also in keeping with the prevalence of the disease in young women and its occasional occurrence in families.

Pulmonary hypertension has also been reported after ingestion of certain plants or medicines (dietary hypertension). A leguminous plant, *Crotalaria spectabilis*, indigenous to the tropics and subtropics and used medicinally in "bush tea," causes pulmonary hypertension in animals. Well-documented cases of pulmonary hypertension have been associated with the ingestion of the appetite depressant agent *aminorex* and adulterated olive oil.[11,25] It has been suggested that such substances may cause subtle injury to the endothelium, which then fails to inactivate vasoconstrictor substances that may be brought to the lungs, followed by vasoconstriction and hypertension.

MORPHOLOGY. A variety of vascular lesions occur in all forms of pulmonary hypertension,[26-28] whether primary or secondary, but few are specific. The presence of many organizing or organized thrombi favors recurrent thromboembolism as the cause of hypertension, and the coexistence of diffuse pulmonary fibrosis, or severe emphysema and chronic bronchitis, points to chronic hypoxia as the initiating event. The vessel changes involve the entire arterial tree from the main pulmonary arteries down to the arterioles (Fig. 16–10). In the main elastic arteries, the changes take the form of **atheromatous deposits** resembling atherosclerosis in the systemic arteries. However, they are rarely as marked as those found in advanced cases of atherosclerosis of the systemic arteries and are not often calcified or ulcerated. The medium-sized muscular arteries have striking **medial hypertrophy**. In milder cases, only **intimal thickening and fibrosis and some adventitial fibrosis** occur. In both medium- and small-sized arteries, the internal and external elastic membranes often undergo thickening and reduplication. **The arterioles and small arteries** (40 to 300 μm) **are most prominently affected, with striking increases in the thickness of the media, sometimes narrowing the lumina to pinpoint channels.** These changes are present in all forms of pulmonary hypertension but are best developed in the primary form. One extreme of the spectrum of pathologic changes, present most prominently in primary pulmonary hypertension, is **plexogenic pulmonary arteriopathy,** so-called because a tuft of cellular capillary formations resembling a vascular plexus is present within the lumina of dilated thin-walled arteries.[27]

CLINICAL COURSE. Although secondary forms can occur at any age, primary pulmonary hypertension is common in children around 5 years of age and in women of 20 to 40 years. Clinical signs and symptoms of both the primary and secondary forms of vascular sclerosis become evident only with advanced arterial disease. In cases of primary disease, the presenting features are dyspnea and fatigue, although occasionally syncopal attacks are the initial complaint. Some patients have chest pain of the anginal type and, indeed, develop severe respiratory distress and cyanosis. In the course of time, right ventricular hypertrophy occurs, and death from decompensated cor pulmonale usually ensues within two to eight years. However, continuous therapy with some of the more modern vasodilators appears to improve the outcome.

OBSTRUCTIVE VS. RESTRICTIVE PULMONARY DISEASE

Pulmonary physiologists have popularized the classification of *diffuse* pulmonary diseases into two categories: (1) *obstructive disease* (or *airway disease*), characterized by an increase in resistance to air flow owing to partial or complete obstruction at any level, from the trachea and larger bronchi to the terminal and respiratory bronchioles; and (2) *restrictive disease*, characterized by reduced expansion of lung parenchyma, with a decreased total lung capacity. Although many pathologic conditions have both obstructive and restrictive components, distinction of the two patterns of pulmonary dysfunction is useful in correlating the results of pulmonary function tests with the radiologic appearance of the lungs and the histologic findings in individual patients.

The major obstructive disorders (excluding tumor or inhalation of a foreign body) are *emphysema, chronic bronchitis, bronchiectasis,* and *asthma.* In patients with these diseases, pulmonary function tests show increased pulmonary resistance and limitation of maximal expiratory air flow rates during forced ex-

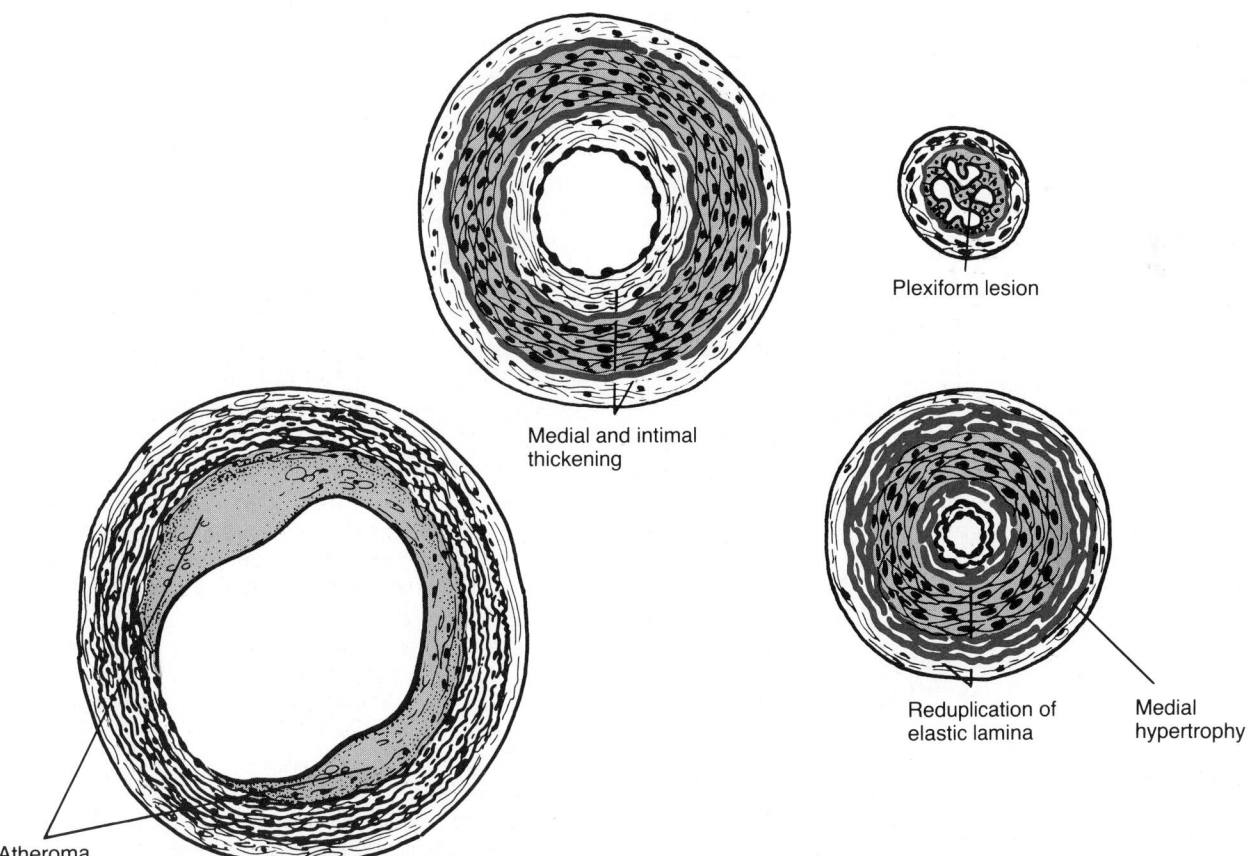

Plexiform lesion

Medial and intimal thickening

Reduplication of elastic lamina

Medial hypertrophy

Atheroma

Figure 16–10. Diagrammatic representation of patterns of pulmonary vascular sclerosis, based on the size of affected vessels. Atheroma formation is virtually limited to large vessels; medial and intimal thickening with reduplication of elastica is seen in medium-sized and somewhat smaller arteries; and the plexogenic lesion occurs in very small arteries and arterioles.

piration. Expiratory obstruction may result either from *anatomic airway narrowing*, such as is classically observed in asthma, or from *loss of elastic recoil* of the lung, which characteristically occurs in emphysema.

In contrast, restrictive diseases are identified by a reduced total lung capacity. The restrictive defect occurs in two general conditions: (1) *chest wall disorders in the presence of normal lungs* (e.g., neuromuscular diseases such as poliomyelitis, severe obesity, pleural diseases, and kyphoscoliosis), and (2) *acute or chronic interstitial and infiltrative diseases.* The classic acute restrictive disease is ARDS. Chronic restrictive diseases include the dust diseases or pneumoconioses, and most of the infiltrative conditions, discussed later (p. 789).

CHRONIC OBSTRUCTIVE AIRWAY DISEASE

The terms chronic obstructive airway disease (COAD) and chronic obstructive pulmonary disease (COPD) refer to a group of conditions—emphysema, chronic bronchitis, bronchial asthma, and bronchiectasis—that are accompanied by chronic or recurrent obstruction to air flow within the lung. Because of the increase in environmental pollutants, cigarette smoking, and other noxious exposures, the incidence of COPD has increased dramatically in the past few decades, and now ranks first as cause of activity restricting or bed-confining disability in the United States.[29]

EMPHYSEMA

Emphysema is a condition of the lung characterized by *abnormal permanent enlargement of the air spaces distal to the terminal bronchiole, accompanied by destruction of their walls.*[30] Enlargement of air spaces unaccompanied by destruction is termed *overinflation;* for example, the distention of air spaces in the opposite lung following unilateral pneumonectomy would be termed compensatory overinflation rather than emphysema.

The relationship between chronic bronchitis and emphysema is complicated, but fortunately the use of precise definitions has helped bring some order to what was once chaos. The definition of emphysema, as we have seen, is a morphologic one. Chronic bronchitis, on the other hand, is a disease that is defined in *clinical* terms as the condition characterized by chronic or recurrent excess mucus secretion in the bronchial tree. Indeed, the precise definition of chronic bronchitis states that "the sputum must be produced on most days for at least three months of the year and for at least two years.[30]

Emphysema and chronic bronchitis are best viewed as a spectrum (Fig. 16–11). At one end, for example, are patients with alpha-1-antitrypsin deficiency, who have almost pure emphysema with lungs

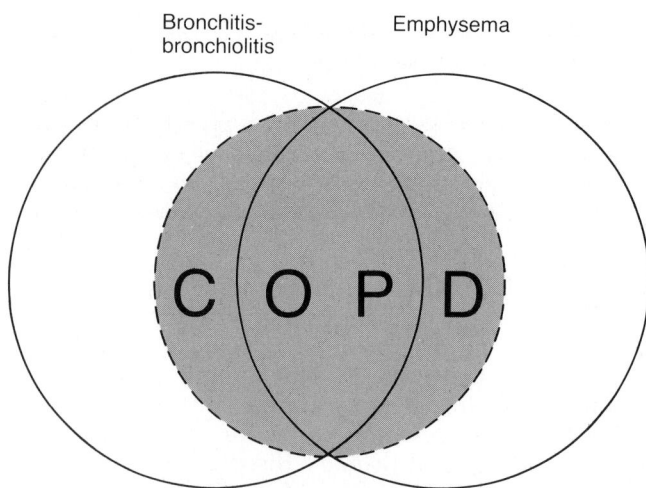

Figure 16–11. Interrelationships of bronchitis-bronchiolitis and emphysema in the production of chronic obstructive pulmonary disease (COPD). Note that when both conditions are present, the occurrence of COPD is virtually invariable. Less often, one or the other disorder alone induces COPD. One etiologic agent, cigarette smoking, is common to both.

full of enlarged airspaces. At the other end is virtually pure bronchitis with abundant sputum production and no organic alterations in the airways that cause obstruction. In the middle of the spectrum, the two coexist, almost certainly because one pathogenic mechanism—cigarette smoking—is common to both, as we shall see (p. 768). Although the clinical features and functional abnormalities in both conditions also overlap, it is often possible to distinguish between patients with predominant emphysema and those with predominant bronchitis, as shown in Table 16–2.[11]

TYPES OF EMPHYSEMA. Emphysema is not only defined in terms of the *anatomic* nature of the lesion, but it is also further classified according to its *anatomic distribution* within the lobule. Recall that the lobule is a cluster of acini, the alveolated terminal respiratory units. Although the term emphysema is sometimes loosely applied to diverse conditions, there are four types: (1) centriacinar, (2) panacinar,

Table 16–2. Emphysema and Chronic Bronchitis

	PREDOMINANT BRONCHITIS	PREDOMINANT EMPHYSEMA
Appearance	"Blue bloater"	"Pink puffer"
Age	40–45	50–75
Dyspnea	Mild; late	Severe; early
Cough	Early; copious sputum	Late; scanty sputum
Infections	Common	Occasional
Respiratory insufficiency	Repeated	Terminal
Cor pulmonale	Common	Rare; terminal
Airway resistance	Increased	Normal or slightly increased
Elastic recoil	Normal	Low
Chest radiograph	Prominent vessels; large heart	Hyperinflation; small heart

(3) paraseptal, and (4) irregular. Of these, the first two are the most important clinically.

CENTRIACINAR (CENTRILOBULAR) EMPHYSEMA. The distinctive feature of this type of emphysema is the pattern of involvement of the lobules; **the central or proximal parts of the acini, formed by respiratory bronchioles, are affected, while distal alveoli are spared** (Fig. 16–12). Thus, both emphysematous and normal airspaces exist within the same acinus and lobule (Fig. 16–13). The lesions are more common and usually more severe in the upper lobes, particularly in the apical segments. The walls of the emphysematous spaces often contain large amounts of black pigment. Inflammation around bronchi and bronchioles and in the septa is common. In severe centriacinar emphysema, the distal acinus may be involved, and differentiation from panacinar emphysema becomes difficult. Moderate-to-severe degrees of emphysema occur predominantly in male smokers, often in association with chronic bronchitis. In addition, so-called coal workers' pneumoconiosis (p. 474) bears a striking resemblance to centriacinar emphysema. These points suggest an important role for tobacco products and coal dust in the genesis of this type of emphysema.

PANACINAR (PANLOBULAR) EMPHYSEMA. In this type the **acini are uniformly enlarged from the level of the respiratory bronchiole to the terminal blind alveoli** (Fig. 16–13). It is important to emphasize that the prefix **pan** refers to the entire acinus but not to the entire lung (Fig. 16–12). In contrast to centriacinar emphysema, panacinar emphysema tends to occur more commonly in the lower zones and in the anterior margins of the lung, and it is usually most severe at the bases. It is the type of emphysema associated with **alpha-1-antitrypsin deficiency** (p. 769).

PARASEPTAL (DISTAL ACINAR) EMPHYSEMA. In this type the **proximal portion of the acinus is normal but the distal part is dominantly involved.** The emphysema is more striking adjacent to the pleura, along the lobular connective tissue septa, and at the margins of the lobules. It occurs adjacent to areas of fibrosis, scarring, or atelectasis and is usually more severe in the upper half of the lungs. The characteristic findings are of multiple, continuous, enlarged airspaces from less than 0.5 mm to more than 2.0 cm in diameter, sometimes forming cyst-like structures. This type of emphysema probably underlies many of the cases of spontaneous pneumothorax in young adults[1] (p. 806).

IRREGULAR EMPHYSEMA. Irregular emphysema, so named because the acinus is irregularly involved, is almost invariably associated with scarring. Thus, it may be the most common form of emphysema, as careful search of most lungs at autopsy would show one or more scars from a healed inflammatory process, such as tuberculosis. There is usually irregular enlargement of acini adjacent to such

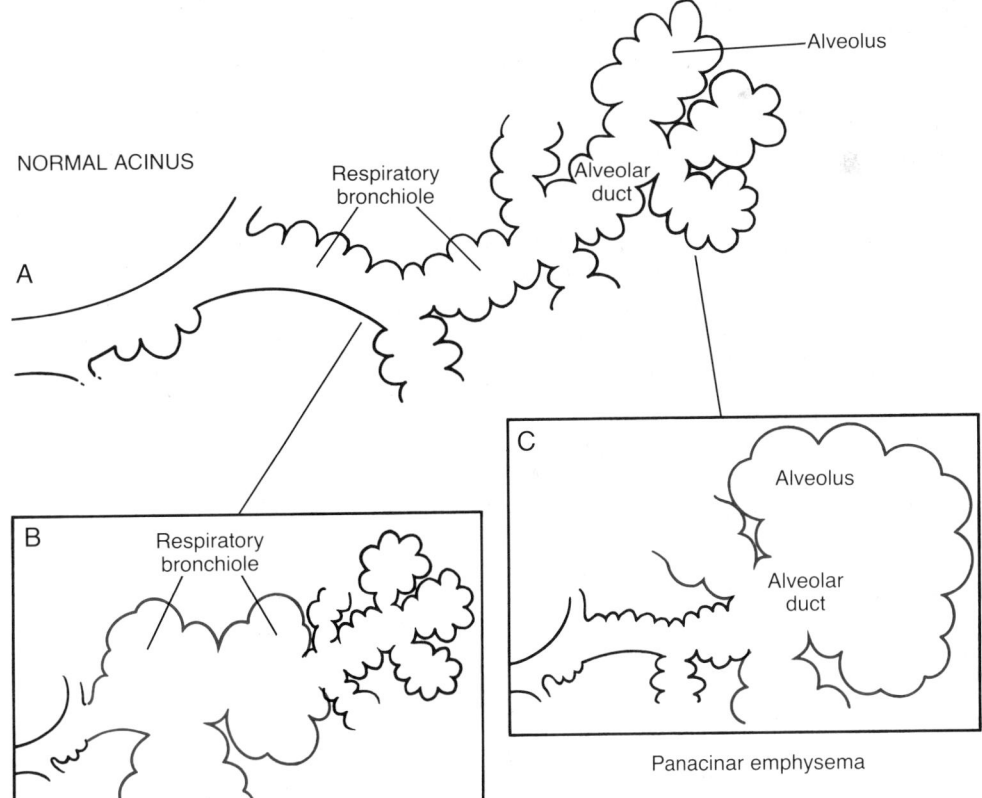

Figure 16–12. *A,* Diagram of normal structures within the acinus, the fundamental unit of the lung. *B,* Centrilobular (centriacinar) emphysema with dilatation that principally affects the respiratory bronchioles, at least at the outset. *C,* Panacinar emphysema with initial distention of the peripheral structures (i.e., alveolus and alveolar duct); the disease later extends to affect the respiratory bronchioles.

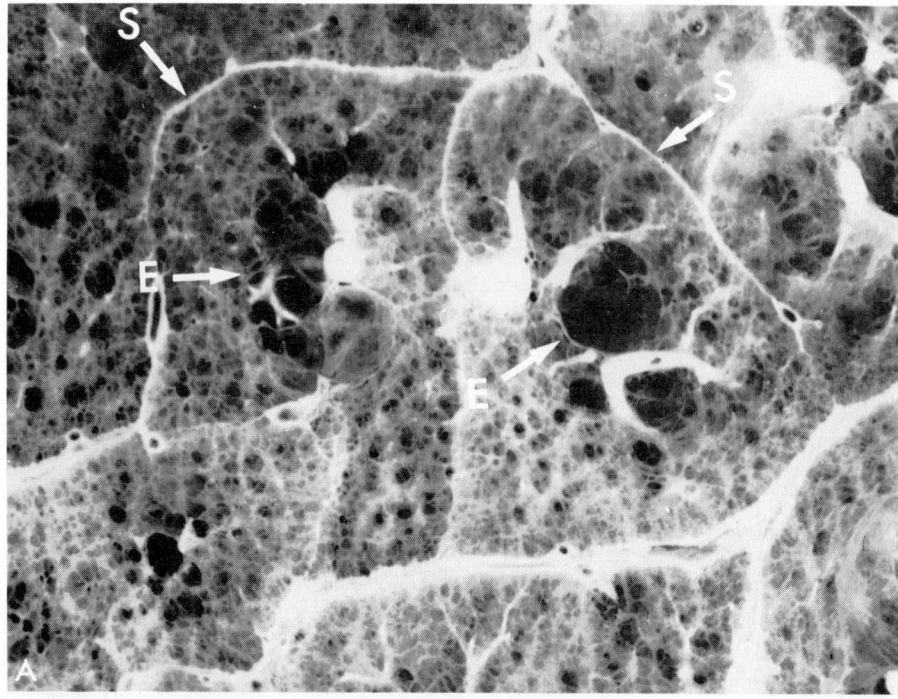

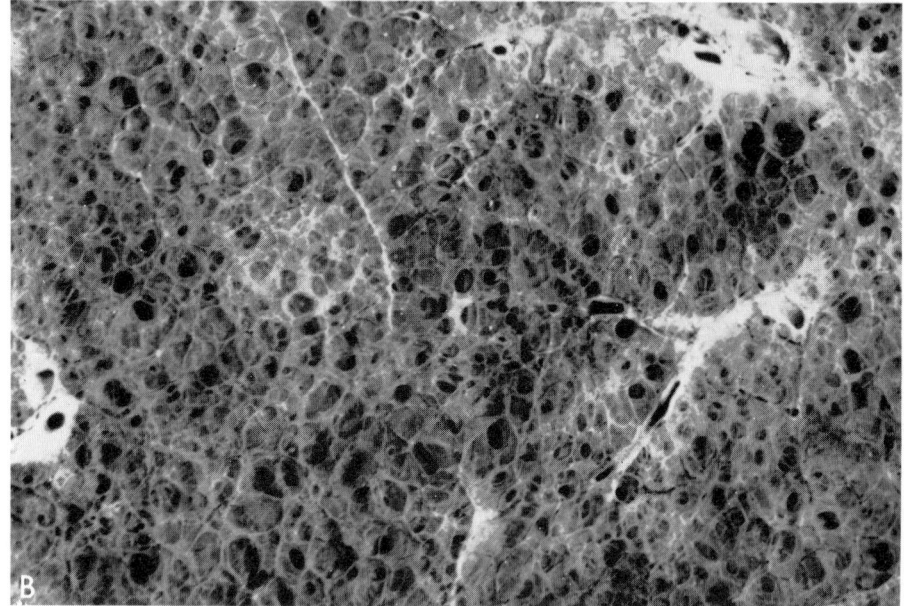

Figure 16–13. *A,* Centrilobular emphysema (magnification ×5). The pulmonary arteries contain a mass of injected barium gelatin. The emphysematous foci *(E)* abut on blood vessels and are removed from the septa *(S)* where the alveolar spaces cluster. *B,* Panacinar emphysema (×5) involving the entire pulmonary architecture. Compare with *A.* (From Bates, D.V., et al.: Respiratory Function in Disease. 2nd ed. Philadelphia, W.B. Saunders Co., 1971.)

scars, accompanied by destructive changes. In most instances, these foci of irregular emphysema are asymptomatic.

INCIDENCE. Emphysema is a common disease. Thurlbeck reports a 50% combined incidence of panacinar and centriacinar emphysema at autopsy. He considers the pulmonary disease to be responsible for the death of 6.5% of these patients.[1]

Emphysema, especially the centriacinar type, is much more common and more severe in men than in women. *There is a clear-cut association between heavy cigarette smoking and emphysema,* and the most se-

vere type occurs in males who smoke heavily. Although the emphysema does not become disabling until the fifth to eighth decades of life, it is well known clinically that ventilatory deficits may make their first appearance decades earlier in those destined to develop the full-blown disease. Indeed, emphysematous changes were found in the lungs of teenagers dying of accidental causes, who had been exposed to environmental air pollution.[31] Certain genetic and familial predispositions have been identified, as discussed later.

PATHOGENESIS. The genesis of the two common forms of emphysema — centriacinar and panacinar — is unsettled, and there is no reason why several etiologic and pathogenetic factors might not be involved. The three questions that need answers are (1) what is the relationship of emphysema to chronic bronchitis when both coexist?; (2) what is the cause of alveolar wall destruction, the sine qua non of emphysema?; and (3) what is the role of smoking or other pollutants in such destruction?

In answer to the first question, it is now thought that chronic bronchitis does *not* lead to the development of emphysema. In some cases of severe emphysema no bronchitis can be found, even on morphologic examination, and conversely, severe bronchitis is not necessarily associated with emphysema. *The frequent association of the two conditions reflects the common injurious link of tobacco smoke,*[32] which causes, as we shall see, increased mucus secretion in bronchial mucous glands, inflammation in the bronchioles, *and* destruction of alveolar walls.

There is now substantial evidence that the destruction of alveolar walls in emphysema develops independently of the bronchial changes. The most plausible current hypothesis to account for such destruction is the protease-antiprotease mechanism.[33] (Fig. 16–14)

This hypothesis is based on two important observations, one clinical and one experimental. The first is that homozygous patients with a genetic deficiency of the enzyme alpha-1-antitrypsin (α1-AT) have a markedly enhanced tendency to develop pulmonary emphysema, which is compounded by smoking.[34] You will recall (p. 57) that α1-AT—which is present in serum, tissue fluids, and macrophages—is a major inhibitor of proteases (particularly elastase) secreted by neutrophils during inflammation. The α1-AT is specified by the *proteinase inhibitor (Pi)* locus on chromosome 14 and is transmitted codominantly. Because of significant polymorphism of α1-AT, some 80 phenotypes have been identified.[35] The normal phenotype, called PiM, is present in 90% of the population. Of the several phenotypes associated with α1-AT deficiency, PiZ is the most common, being present in 0.012% of the United States population. Over 80% of PiZ phenotypes develop symptomatic emphysema. The second observation bearing on the protease-antiprotease hypothesis is that intratracheal instillation of the proteolytic enzyme papain, which degrades elastin, causes emphysema in experimental animals.[36]

The *protease-antiprotease theory*[33,36] holds that alveolar wall destruction results from an imbalance between proteases (mainly elastase) and antiproteases in the lung. Anything that decreases antielastase or increases elastase tips the balance in favor of proteolytic destruction of elastin and the development of emphysema. The principal antielastase activity in serum and interstitial tissue is α1-AT (other protease inhibitors are serum α1-macroglobulin and inhibitors in bronchial mucus), and the principal cellular elastase activity is derived from neutrophils (other elastases are formed by macrophages, mast cells, pancreas, and bacteria). Neutrophil elastase is capable of digesting human lung, and this digestion

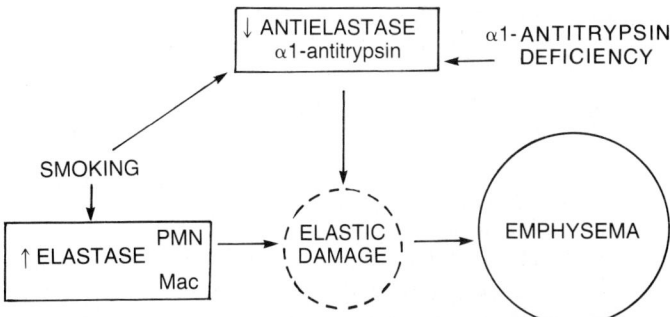

Figure 16–14. Protease-antiprotease mechanism of emphysema. Smoking inhibits antielastase and favors the recruitment of leukocytes and release of elastase. PMN = polymorphonuclear leukocytes; Mac = alveolar macrophages.

can be inhibited by α1-AT. Such elastase induces emphysema when instilled into the trachea of experimental animals.[37] Thus, the following sequence is postulated to explain the effect of α1-AT deficiency on the lung: neutrophils are normally sequestered in the lung (more in the lower zones than in the upper), and a few gain access to the alveolar space. Any stimulus that increases either the number of leukocytes (neutrophils and macrophages) in the lung or the release of their elastase-containing granules will increase elastolytic activity. Stimulated neutrophils also release oxygen free radicals, which, as we have seen (p. 57) inhibit α1-AT activity. With low levels of serum α1-AT, the process of elastic tissue destruction is unchecked, with consequent emphysema. *Thus, emphysema is seen to result from the destructive effect of high protease activity in subjects with low antiprotease activity.*

The protease-antiprotease hypothesis also explains the deleterious effect of cigarette smoking because both increased elastase availability and decreased antielastase activity occur in smokers (Fig. 16–14).[33,35] (1) Smokers have greater numbers of neutrophils and macrophages in their alveoli. The increased recruitment of neutrophils into the lung results, in part, from the release by activated alveolar macrophages of *neutrophil chemotactic factors*, this release being stimulated by smoking. In addition, nicotine is chemotactic for neutrophils, and cigarette smoke activates the alternate complement pathway.[33] (2) Smoking stimulates release of elastase from neutrophils. (3) Smoking enhances elastase activity in macrophages; macrophage elastase is not inhibited by α1-AT, and indeed can proteolytically digest this enzyme.[38] (4) Smoking causes mast cell activation, potentially resulting in the release of mast cell elastases as well as neutrophil chemotactic factors.[33] (5) Oxidants in cigarette smoke and oxygen free radicals secreted by neutrophils inhibit α1-AT and thus decrease net antielastase activity in smokers. *It is thus postulated that impaction of smoke particles in the small bronchi and bronchioles, with the resultant influx of neutrophils and macrophages, and increased elastase and decreased α1-AT activity, causes the centriacinar emphysema seen in smokers.* This can be contrasted with the panacinar emphysema of patients with generalized α1-AT deficiency. These concepts also explain the additive influence of smoking and α1-AT deficiency in inducing serious obstructive airway disease.

MORPHOLOGY. Important criteria for the diagnosis and classification of the emphysemas are derived from naked eye (or hand lens) examination of lungs fixed in a state of inflation. More detailed microscopic examination is necessary to visualize the abnormal fenestrations in the walls of the alveoli, the complete destruction of septal walls, and the distribution of damage within the pulmonary lobule. These septal changes are found in the walls of respiratory bronchioles, alveolar ducts, and alveolar spaces (Fig. 16–15). With advance of the disease, adjacent alveoli fuse to produce even larger abnormal airspaces and possibly blebs or bullae. Often the respiratory bronchioles and vasculature of the lung are deformed and compressed by the emphysematous distortion of the air spaces and, as mentioned, there may or may not be evidence of bronchitis or bronchiolitis.

The gross appearance of the lung in emphysematous disease depends on the form of emphysema and its severity. Panacinar emphysema, when well developed, produces voluminous lungs, often overlapping the heart and hiding it when the anterior chest wall is removed. The macroscopic features of centriacinar emphysema are less impressive. The lungs may not appear particularly pale or voluminous unless the disease is well advanced. Generally, the upper two thirds of the lungs are more severely affected. Large apical blebs or bullae are more characteristic of irregular emphysema secondary to scarring.

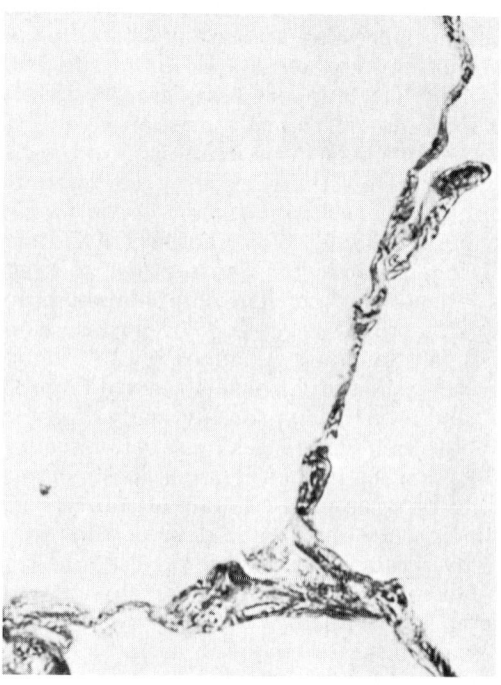

Figure 16–15. Panacinar emphysema in high-power detail, illustrating avascularity of septa.

CLINICAL COURSE. The clinical manifestations of emphysema do not appear until at least one third of the functioning pulmonary parenchyma is incapacitated. The panacinar form tends to be the most disabling because all alveoli are more or less affected. Dyspnea is usually the first symptom; it begins insidiously but is steadily progressive. In some patients, cough or wheezing is the chief complaint, easily confused with asthma. Cough and expectoration are extremely variable and depend on the extent of the associated bronchitis. Weight loss is common and may be so severe as to suggest a hidden malignant tumor. Classically, the patient is barrel-chested and dyspneic, with obviously prolonged expiration, and sits forward in a hunched-over position, attempting to squeeze the air out of the lungs with each expiratory effort. These unfortunate persons have a pinched face and breathe through pursed lips. *The only reliable and consistently present finding on physical examination is slowing of forced expiration.*

In patients with severe emphysema, cough is often slight, overdistention is severe, diffusing capacity is low, and blood gas values are relatively normal. Such patients may overventilate and remain well oxygenated, and therefore are euphoniously if somewhat ingloriously designated as *"pink puffers"* (Table 16–2). On the other hand, patients with chronic bronchitis more often have a history of recurrent infection, abundant purulent sputum, hypercapnia, and severe hypoxemia, prompting the equally inglorious designation of *"blue bloaters."* A hazard in severe emphysema, in addition to the respiratory difficulties, is the development of cor pulmonale and eventual congestive heart failure. Death in most of these patients is due to (1) right-sided failure, (2) respiratory acidosis and coma, and (3) massive collapse of the lungs secondary to pneumothorax.

OTHER TYPES OF EMPHYSEMA. Now we come to some conditions in which the term "emphysema" is applied less stringently and to some closely related conditions.

COMPENSATORY EMPHYSEMA. This term is sometimes used to designate dilatation of alveoli in response to loss of lung substance elsewhere. It is best exemplified by the hyperexpansion of the residual lung parenchyma that follows surgical removal of a diseased lung or lobe. In most instances, this constitutes compensatory **hyperinflation** as there is no accompanying destruction of septal walls.

SENILE EMPHYSEMA. Senile emphysema refers to the overdistended, sometimes voluminous lungs found in the aged. These changes result from age-related alterations of the internal geometry of the lung—**larger alveolar ducts** and **smaller alveoli.**[1] There is no significant loss of elastic tissue, and because there is no destruction of lung substance and the respiratory deficit is usually minimal, a better designation for such aging lungs would be **senile hyperinflation.**

OBSTRUCTIVE OVERINFLATION. Obstructive overinflation refers to the condition in which the lung expands because air is trapped within it. A common cause is subtotal obstruction by a tumor or foreign object. A classic example is **congenital lobar overinflation in infants.** This is a congenital anomaly, probably due to hypoplasia of bronchial cartilage, and is sometimes associated with other congenital cardiac and lung abnormalities. Overinflation in obstructive lesions occurs either (1) because of a ball-valve action of the obstructive agent, so that air enters on inspiration but cannot leave on expiration; or (2) because the bronchus may be totally obstructed, but ventilation through "collaterals" may bring in air from behind the obstruction. These collaterals are represented by the **pores of Kohn** and other direct accessory **bronchioloalveolar connections** (the canals of Lambert). Obstructive overinflation can be a life-threatening emergency because the affected portion extends sufficiently to compress the remaining normal lung.

BULLOUS EMPHYSEMA. Bullous emphysema refers merely to any form of emphysema that produces large subpleural blebs or bullae (spaces more than 1 cm in diameter in the distended state) (Fig. 16–16). They represent localized accentuations of one of the four forms of emphysema, are most often subpleural, and occur near the apex, sometimes in relation to old tuberculous scarring. On occasion rupture of the bullae may give rise to pneumothorax (p. 806).

INTERSTITIAL EMPHYSEMA. The entrance of air into the connective tissue stroma of the lung, mediastinum, or subcutaneous tissue is designated interstitial emphysema. In most instances, alveolar tears in pulmonary emphysema provide the avenue of entrance of air into the stroma of the lung, but rarely a wound of the chest that allows air to be sucked in or a fractured rib that punctures the lung substance may underlie this disorder. Alveolar tears usually occur when there is a combination of coughing plus some bronchiolar obstruction, producing sharply increased pressures within the alveolar sacs. Children with whooping cough and bronchitis, patients with obstruction to the airways (by blood clots, tissue, or foreign bodies), and individuals who suddenly inhale irritant gases provide classic examples.

Progressive accumulation of air may dissect through the fibrous connective tissue of the alveolar walls and into and along the fibrous septa of the lung to reach the mediastinum, and thence possibly the subcutaneous tissues. If the collection of air is small, it usually has no clinical importance. However, extensive insufflation of the lung may encroach upon the small blood vessels to create serious impairment of blood flow through the lungs. When the interstitial air treks into the subcutaneous tissue, the patient may literally blow up into an alarming, although usually harmless, "Walt Disney balloon" appearance with marked swelling of the head and neck and crackling crepitation all over the chest. In most instances such air is resorbed promptly as soon as the point of entrance is sealed.

CHRONIC BRONCHITIS

This disorder, so common among habitual smokers and inhabitants of smog-laden cities, is not nearly so trivial as was once thought. When persistent for years, it may (1) be associated with chronic obstructive airway disease, as discussed earlier; (2) lead to cor pulmonale and heart failure; and (3) cause atypical metaplasia and dysplasia of the respiratory epithelium, providing a possible soil for cancerous transformation. The widely accepted definition of chronic bronchitis is the clinical one — *chronic bronchitis is present in any patient who has persistent cough with sputum production for at least three months in at least two consecutive years.* The condition can be further characterized as *simple chronic bronchitis* or *obstructive chronic bronchitis;* in the latter there is physiologic evidence of airway obstruction. Both sexes and all ages may be affected, but chronic bronchitis is most frequent in middle-aged men. Ten to 25% of the urban adult population have chronic bronchitis[1]; country dwellers have a lower incidence.

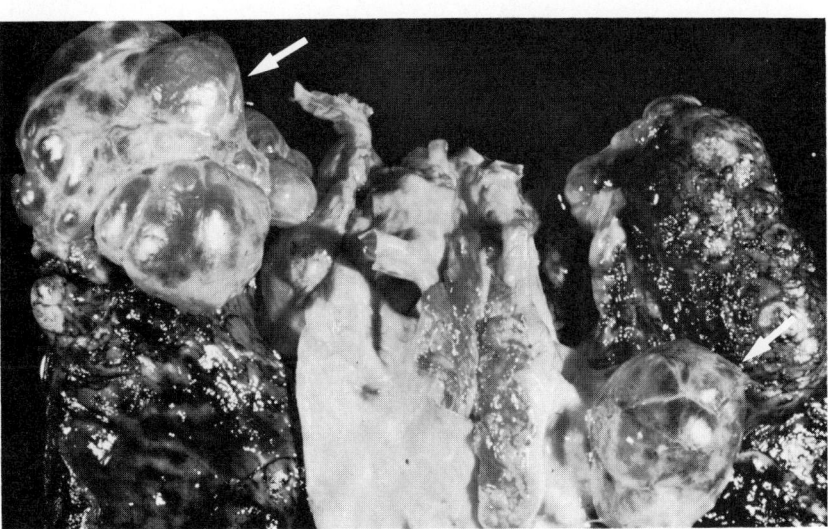

Figure 16–16. Bullous emphysema with large apical and marginal subpleural bullae *(arrows).*

PATHOGENESIS. Two sets of factors are important in the genesis of chronic bronchitis: (1) chronic irritation by inhaled substances and (2) microbiologic infections. Cigarette smoking remains the paramount influence. Chronic bronchitis is four to ten times more common in heavy smokers irrespective of age, sex, occupation, and place of dwelling.

The hallmark and earliest feature of chronic bronchitis is *hypersecretion of mucus,* which starts in the large airways and is associated with hypertrophy of the submucosal glands in the trachea and bronchi.[39] These changes contribute to excessive mucus production. As chronic bronchitis persists, there is also *a marked increase in goblet cells of small airways — small bronchi and bronchioles.* This excessive mucus production by goblet cells in small airways contributes to airway obstruction. It is thought that both the submucosal gland hypertrophy and the increase in goblet cells are caused by tobacco smoke or other pollutants (for example, sulfur dioxide, nitrogen dioxide); similar changes can be produced experimentally by inhalation of a variety of irritants. Mucosal secretion is under autonomic (vagal) control, but whether airway irritants cause mucus hypersecretion by stimulating neurohormonal pathways is unproved.[40]

Although mucus hypersection in large airways is the cause of sputum overproduction, it is now thought that *alterations in the small airways of the lung* (small bronchi and bronchioles, less than 2 to 3 mm in diameter) *are physiologically important and early manifestations of the chronic airway obstruction.*[40] Histologic studies of the small airways in young smokers disclose goblet cell metaplasia with mucous plugging of the lumen; clustering of pigmented alveolar macrophages; inflammatory infiltration; and (in a somewhat older group of patients) fibrosis of the bronchiolar wall.[41,42] It is postulated that smoking and other irritants, which cause the hypertrophy of mucous glands characteristic of chronic bronchitis, also cause the *bronchiolitis.*[43] Certain physiological studies suggest that this respiratory bronchiolitis is an important component in early and relatively mild air flow obstruction. *However, when bronchitis is accompanied by moderate to severe air flow obstruction, coexistent emphysema is the dominant lesion.*

The role of *infection* appears to be secondary. It is not responsible for the initiation of chronic bronchitis but is probably significant in maintaining it and may be critical in producing the acute exacerbations. Cigarette smoke predisposes to infection in more than one way: it interferes with ciliary action of the respiratory epithelium, may cause direct damage to airway epithelium, and inhibits the ability of bronchial and alveolar leukocytes to clear bacteria. Viral infections can also cause exacerbations of chronic bronchitis.

Following this review of the pathogenesis of both emphysema and chronic bronchitis, reference should be made to Figure 16–17, which attempts to follow the evolution of both conditions into chronic obstructive airway disease.

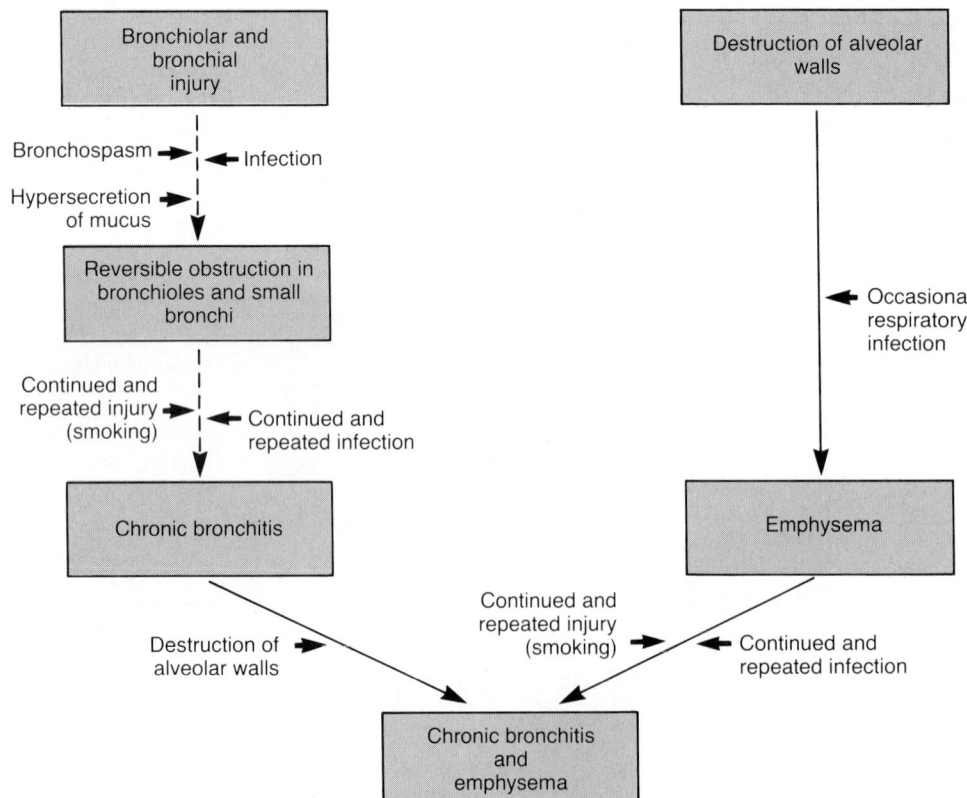

Figure 16–17. Schematic representation of evolution of chronic bronchitis *(left)* and of emphysema *(right).* Although both can culminate in chronic bronchitis and emphysema, the pathways are different, and either one may predominate. Dashed arrows on left indicate that, in the natural history of chronic bronchitis, it is not known whether there is a predictable progression from obstruction in small airways to chronic (obstructive) bronchitis. (From Fishman, A.P.: The spectrum of chronic obstructive disease of the airways. *In* Fishman, A.P. [ed.]: Pulmonary Diseases and Disorders, 2nd ed. 1988, p. 1164.

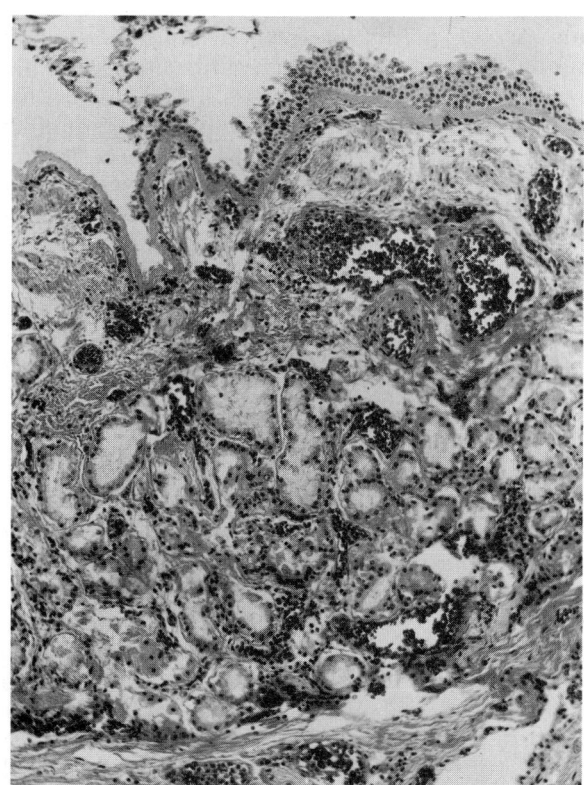

Figure 16–18. Chronic bronchitis. Lumen of bronchus is above. Note slight desquamation of mucosal epithelial cells and marked thickening of mucous gland layer (approximately twice normal). Vascular congestion is evident.

MORPHOLOGY. Grossly, there may be hyperemia, swelling and bogginess of the mucous membranes, frequently accompanied by excessive mucinous to mucopurulent secretions layering the epithelial surfaces. Sometimes, heavy casts of secretion and pus fill the bronchi and bronchioles.

The characteristic histologic feature of chronic bronchitis is enlargement of the mucus-secreting glands of the trachea and bronchi. Although the numbers of goblet cells increase slightly, the **major increase is in the size of the mucous glands** (Fig. 16–18). This increase can be assessed by the ratio of the thickness of the mucous gland layer to the thickness of the wall between the epithelium and the cartilage (Reid index).[44] The Reid index is increased in chronic bronchitis usually in proportion to the severity and duration of the disease. The bronchial epithelium may exhibit squamous metaplasia and dysplasia. There is marked narrowing of bronchioles caused by goblet cell metaplasia, mucous plugging, inflammation, and fibrosis. In the most severe cases there may be obliteration of lumina (**bronchiolitis fibrosa obliterans**). As discussed earlier, these bronchiolar changes probably contribute to the obstructive features in bronchitis patients.

The clinical sine qua non of chronic bronchitis is a persistent cough productive of copious sputum. For many years, no other respiratory functional impairment is present, but eventually dyspnea on exertion develops. With the passage of time, COPD may appear, accompanied by hypercapnia, hypoxemia, and mild cyanosis. Differentiation of this form of obstructive lung disease from that associated with emphysema can be made in the classic case (Table 16–2), but, as mentioned, many such patients have both conditions. Long-standing severe chronic bronchitis commonly leads to cor pulmonale and possible cardiac failure. Death may also result from further impairment of respiratory function incident to acute intercurrent bacterial infections.

BRONCHIAL ASTHMA

Asthma is a disease characterized by increased responsiveness of the tracheobronchial tree to various stimuli, potentiating paroxysmal constriction of the bronchial airways.[45]

It is a particularly distressing disease because those afflicted unpredictably experience disabling attacks of severe dyspnea and wheezing triggered by sudden episodes of bronchospasm. Between the attacks patients may be virtually asymptomatic, but in some persons chronic bronchitis or cor pulmonale often supervenes. Rarely, a state of unremitting attacks *(status asthmaticus)* proves fatal; usually such unfortunate patients have had a long history of asthma. In some cases, the attacks are triggered by exposure to an allergen to which the patient has previously been sensitized, but often no allergic trigger can be identified.

TYPES AND PATHOGENESIS. Asthma has traditionally been divided into two basic types — extrinsic (allergic, reagin-mediated, atopic) and intrinsic (idiosyncratic) — to which was added a third, mixed pattern in which both intrinsic and extrinsic factors are operative. However, it is probably more useful to classify asthma according to the principal stimuli that provoke the attacks. Table 16–3 lists the various groups, the precipitating factors, and the possible mechanisms involved in each group.[43]

Table 16–3. Types of Asthma

TYPES OF ASTHMA	PRECIPITATING FACTORS*	MECHANISM OR IMMUNOLOGIC REACTION
Atopic (allergic)	Specific allergens	Type I (IgE) immune reaction
Nonreaginic	Respiratory tract infection	Unknown; hyperreactive airways
Pharmacologic (e.g., aspirin-sensitive)	Aspirin	Decreased prostaglandins, increased leukotrienes
Occupational	Chemical challenge	Type I immune reactions
Allergic bronchopulmonary aspergillosis	Antigen (spores) challenge	Types I and III immune reactions

*All types may be precipitated by cold, stress, exercise. All have hyperreactive airways.

Atopic or allergic asthma: This is the most common type of asthma. The disease is triggered by environmental antigens such as dusts, pollens, animal dander, and foods, but potentially any antigen is implicated (Fig. 16–19A). A positive family history of atopy is common, and asthmatic attacks are often preceded by allergic rhinitis, urticaria, or eczema. Serum IgE levels are usually elevated. A skin test with the offending antigen results in an immediate wheal-and-flare reaction, *a classic example of type I IgE-mediated hypersensitivity reaction.*[44] IgE-mediated hypersensitivity elicits an *acute immediate response and a late phase reaction.*

You will recall that exposure of presensitized IgE-coated mast cells to the same or a cross-reacting antigen stimulates the release of chemical mediators from these cells. In the case of airborne antigens, the reaction occurs first on sensitized mast cells *on the mucosal surface* (Fig. 16–19B); the resultant mediator release opens the mucosal intercellular tight junctions and enhances penetration of antigen to the more numerous submucosal mast cells. In addition, direct stimulation of *subepithelial vagal* (parasympathetic) *receptors* provokes reflex bronchoconstriction. This occurs within minutes after stimulation and is called the *acute* or *immediate response.*[47] As detailed on page 174, the mediators of IgE-triggered reactions include both primary and secondary mediators. The primary mediators include (1) histamine, which causes bronchoconstriction by direct and cholinergic reflex actions, increased venular permeability, and increased bronchial secretions; it is probably important in the first few minutes of an asthmatic attack; and (2) eosinophilic (ECF) and neutrophilic chemotactic factors (NCF), which selectively attract eosinophils and neutrophils. The secondary mediators include (1) *leukotriene C_4, D_4, and E_4,* extremely potent mediators that cause prolonged bronchoconstriction as well as increased vascular permeability and increased mucus secretion; (2) *prostaglandin D_2 (PGD_2),* which elicits bronchoconstriction and vasodilatation; and (3) *platelet activating factor (PAF),* which causes aggregation of platelets and release of histamine and serotonin from their granules. The acute reaction is thus associated with bronchoconstriction, edema, mucus secretion, flushing, and in certain instances, hypotension. This is followed by the *late phase reaction* occurring several hours later and lasting for two days.[47,48]

The late phase reaction is caused by the recruitment of leukocytes—*basophils* (the circulating mast equivalents), *neutrophils,* and *eosinophils*—by the chemotactic factors derived from mast cells. These leukocytes release a second wave of mediators that stimulate the late reaction. Histamine releasing factors (HRF), produced by various cell types, induce release of histamine from basophils, causing bronchoconstriction and edema. In addition, neutrophils cause further inflammatory injury, and the *major basic protein of eosinophils causes epithelial damage.* The presence of both immediate and delayed reactions in IgE-mediated events, helps explain the prolonged manifestations of asthma and similar allergies.

Nonatopic asthma: The second large group is the *nonatopic* or *nonreaginic* variety of asthma, which is most frequently triggered by respiratory tract infection. Viruses (e.g., rhinovirus, parainfluenza virus) rather than bacteria are the most common provokers. A positive family history is uncommon, serum IgE levels are normal, and there are no other associated allergies. In these patients, skin test results are usually negative, and although hypersensitivity to microbial antigens may play a role, present theories place more stress on hyperirritability of the bronchial tree. It is thought that virus-induced inflammation of the respiratory mucosa lowers the threshold of the subepithelial vagal receptors to irritants.

Drug-induced asthma: Several pharmacologic agents stimulate asthma. *Aspirin-sensitive asthma* is a somewhat fascinating type occurring in patients with recurrent rhinitis and nasal polyps. These individuals are exquisitely sensitive to very small doses of aspirin, and they experience not only asthmatic attacks but also urticaria. It is probable that aspirin triggers asthma in these patients by inhibiting the cyclooxygenase pathway of arachidonic acid metabolism without affecting the lipoxygenase route, thus tipping the balance toward elaboration of the bronchoconstrictor leukotrienes (see Fig. 2–17, p. 56).

Occupational asthma is stimulated by fumes (epoxy resins, plastics), organic and chemical dusts (wood, cotton, platinum), gases (toluene), and other chemicals (formaldehyde, penicillin products).[45] Very minute quantities of chemicals are required to induce the attack, which usually occurs after repeated exposure. The underlying mechanisms vary according to stimulus and include type I IgG-mediated reactions, direct liberation of bronchoconstrictor substances, and hypersensitivity responses of unknown origin.

Allergic bronchopulmonary aspergillosis[49] is a special but well-studied type of asthma caused by the spores of *Aspergillus fumigatus.* When challenged with antigen intradermally or by inhalation, these patients develop *both an immediate type I IgE-induced reaction and a four- to six-hour type III IgE-mediated response.* It is thus thought that Aspergillus-induced, IgE-mediated mast cell degranulation causes bronchoconstriction and increased vascular permeability. The latter allows anti-Aspergillus antibodies to enter bronchi, combine with antigen, form immune complexes, and trigger inflammation and pulmonary damage.

Asthma can also be precipitated by cold, exercise, and emotional stress, but it is likely that these are nonspecific factors producing spasm in bronchi that have been rendered hyperirritable. Indeed, *an important feature of patients with asthma of all types— immunologic or otherwise—is the hyperreactivity of the airways to nonspecific irritants and bronchoconstrictor agents.* Several explanations have been ad-

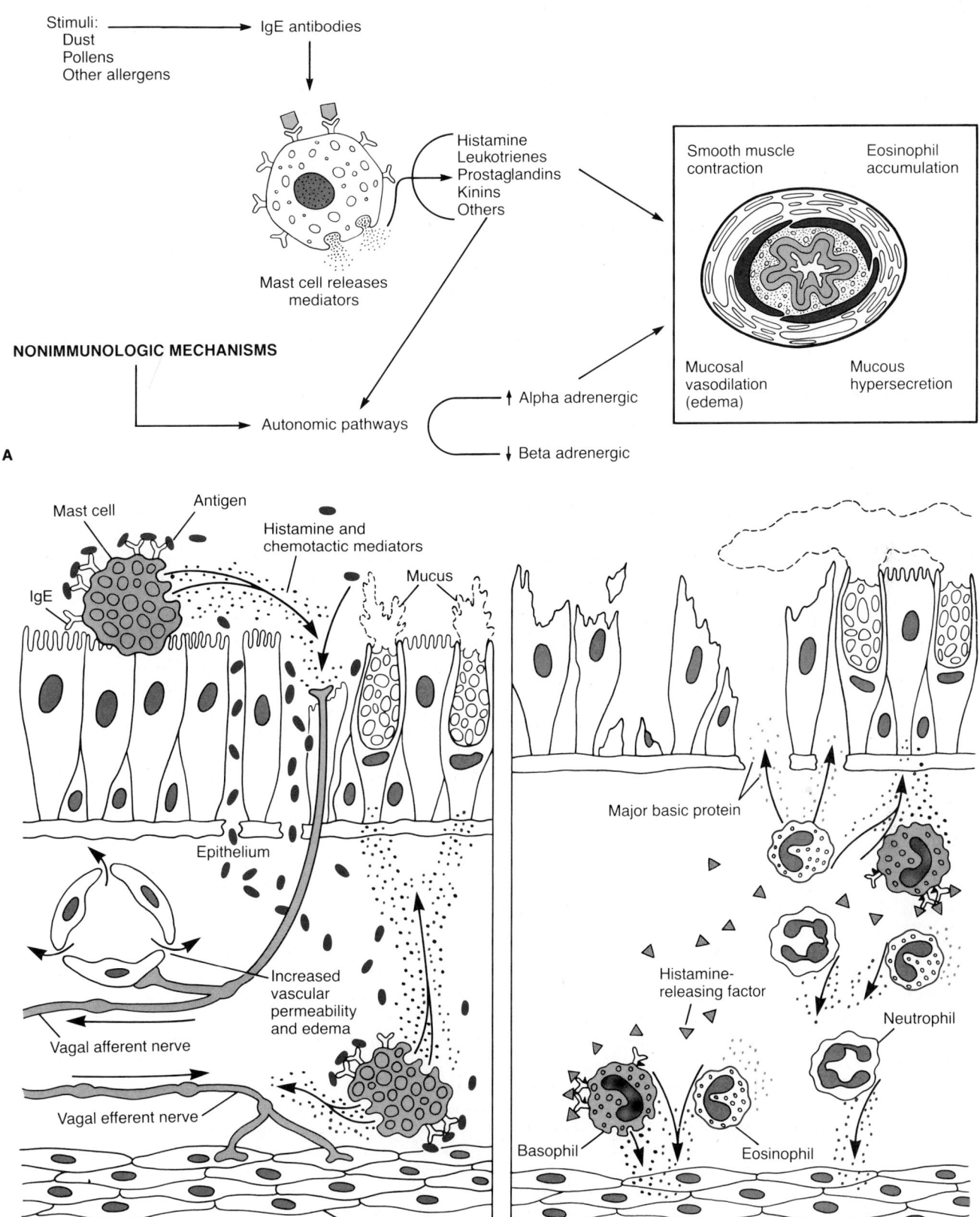

Figure 16–19. *A,* Allergic and nonimmunologic mechanisms in asthma.

B, Immediate *(left)* and late-phase *(right)* responses in allergic mucosal reactions. The immediate reaction is triggered by binding of antigen to IgE on the surface of superficial mast cells, which release histamine and other mediators. The latter open tight junctions between epithelial cells, allowing antigen to reach mast cells. Mediators increase vascular permeability and mucus production. Histamine and other mediators also interact with afferent nerves to initiate reflex responses. Mast cells also generate chemotactic factors and an influx of basophils, neutrophils, and eosinophils, which signals onset of the late-phase response (right panel). Histamine-releasing factors derived from a variety of cells act on basophils. Histamine and other mediators induce the late response. Major basic protein from eosinophils causes most of the epithelial damage. Modified from Lichtenstein, L.: The nasal late-phase response—an in-vivo model. Hosp. Pract. *23*(1):121, 1988. Illustration by Ilil Arbel.

vanced to explain such hyperirritability. Currently it is thought that *bronchial inflammation* may account for the hyperresponsiveness. Patients with asthma, even mild asthma, have a variety of inflammatory cells (mast cells, neutrophils, macrophages) in their bronchial walls, and mediators released from such cells (e.g., leukotrienes)[50,51] may be involved in the state of hyperirritability.

The role of *eosinophils* in asthma deserves mention. These cells are attracted by chemotactic factors released by mast cells. They themselves can release mediators, including leukotrienes and platelet activating factor. Eosinophils also produce the basic major protein (MBP) of their granules, and MBP has been shown to be toxic to respiratory epithelium and to accumulate in the lungs and sputum of patients with asthma.[52]

MORPHOLOGY. The morphologic changes in asthma have been described principally in patients dying of status asthmaticus, but it appears that the pathology in nonfatal cases is similar. Grossly, the lungs are overdistended because of overinflation, and there may be small areas of atelectasis. **The most striking macroscopic finding is occlusion of bronchi and bronchioles by thick, tenacious mucous plugs.** Histologically, the mucous plugs contain whorls of shed epithelium, which give rise to the well-known **Curschmann's spirals.** Numerous eosinophils and **Charcot-Leyden crystals** are present; the latter are collections of crystalloids made up of eosinophil membrane protein. The other characteristic histologic findings of asthma (Fig. 16–20) include (1) thickening of the basement membrane of bronchial epithelium; (2) edema and an inflammatory infiltrate in the bronchial walls, with prominence of eosinophils, which form 5 to 50% of the cellular infiltrate; (3) an increase in size of the submucosal mucous glands; and (4) hypertrophy of the bronchial wall muscle, a reflection of the prolonged vasoconstriction. Emphysematous changes sometimes occur, and if chronic bacterial infection has supervened, bronchitis (described earlier) may appear.

CLINICAL COURSE. The classic asthmatic attack lasts up to several hours and is followed by prolonged coughing; the raising of copious mucous secretions provides considerable relief of the respiratory difficulty. In some patients, these symptoms persist at a low level all the time. In its most severe form, *status asthmaticus,* the severe acute paroxysm persists for days and even weeks and, under these circumstances, the ventilatory function may be so impaired as to cause severe cyanosis and even death. The clinical diagnosis is aided by demonstration of an elevated eosinophil count in the peripheral blood and the finding of eosinophils, Curschmann's spirals, and Charcot-Leyden crystals in the sputum.

In the usual case, with intervals of freedom from respiratory difficulty, the disease is more discouraging and disabling than lethal. With appropriate therapy to relieve the attacks, these patients are able to maintain a productive life. Occasionally, the disease disappears spontaneously. In the more severe forms, the progressive hyperinflation may eventually produce emphysema. Superimposed bacterial infections may lead to chronic persistent bronchitis, bronchiectasis, or pneumonia. In some cases, cor pulmonale and heart failure eventually develop.

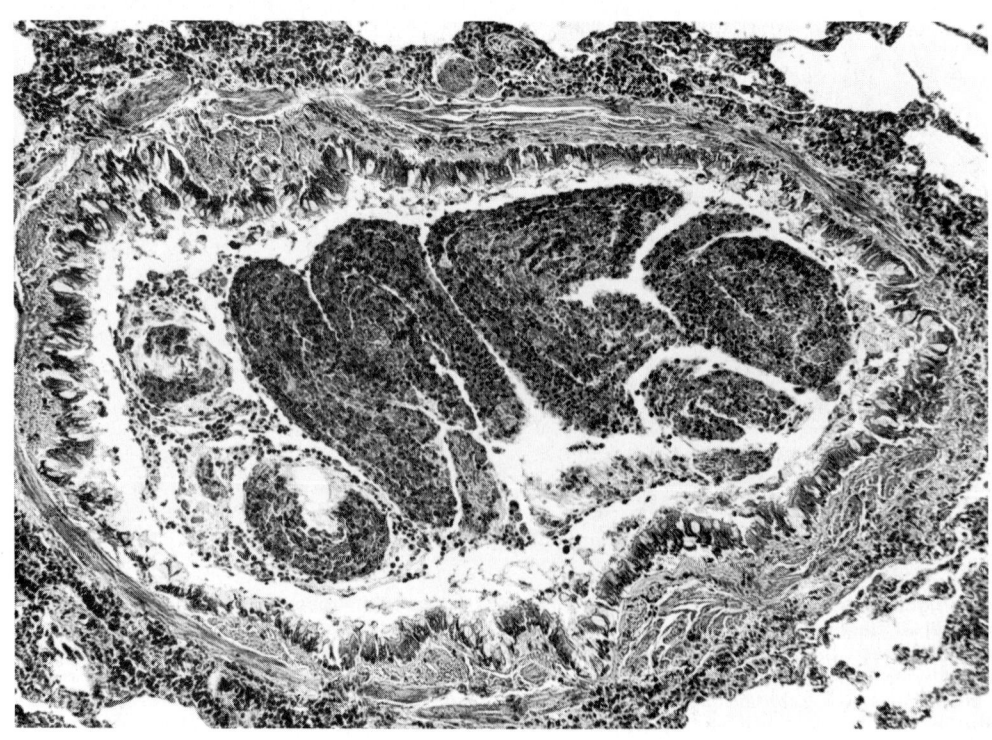

Figure 16–20. Bronchial asthma. A small bronchus containing plugs of mucin secretion as well as inflammatory cells within lumen. Note hypertrophy of mucin-secreting lining cells, hypertrophy of smooth muscle, and the peribronchial inflammatory infiltrate.

BRONCHIECTASIS

Bronchiectasis is a chronic necrotizing infection of the bronchi and bronchioles leading to or associated with abnormal dilation of these airways. It is manifested clinically by cough, fever, and the expectoration of copious amounts of foul-smelling, purulent sputum. To be considered bronchiectasis, the dilatation should be permanent; reversible bronchial dilatation often accompanies viral and bacterial pneumonia. Bronchiectasis has many origins and usually develops in association with the following conditions:[53]

1. *Bronchial obstruction.* Common causes are tumor, foreign bodies, and occasionally mucous impaction. Under these conditions, the bronchiectasis is localized to the obstructed lung segment. Bronchiectasis can also complicate diffuse obstructive airway diseases, most commonly atopic asthma and chronic bronchitis.
2. *Congenital or hereditary conditions.* These include
   a. *Congenital bronchiectasis.* This is caused by a defect in the development of bronchi and usually affects a whole lobe or entire lung.
   b. *Cystic fibrosis* (p. 553). Widespread severe bronchiectasis in this condition is a reflection of the generalized defects in exocrine gland secretion.
   c. *Intralobar sequestration of the lung* (see also p. 758). In this condition a part of the lung, usually in the left lower lobe, is supplied with blood not by a branch of the pulmonary artery but directly from one of the systemic arteries. Characteristically, the airways in the sequestered bronchiectatic lung tissue are separate from those in the adjacent normal lung. The affected part becomes infected and its airways dilate.
   d. *Immunodeficiency states.* These are associated with heightened susceptibility to repeated bacterial infections and localized or diffuse bronchiectasis.
   e. *Immotile cilia* and *Kartagener's syndromes.* A fascinating explanation for bronchiectasis is that which accounts for a curious disease called *Kartagener's syndrome* (bronchiectasis, sinusitis, and situs inversus). Patients with this syndrome have a *defect in ciliary motility, associated with structural abnormalities of cilia, most commonly absent or irregular dynein arms*—the structures on the microtubular doublets of cilia that are responsible for the generation of ciliary movement (Fig. 16–21).[54] The lack of ciliary activity interferes with bacterial clearance, predisposes the sinuses and bronchi to infection, and also affects cell motility during embryogenesis, resulting in the situs inversus. Males with this condition tend to be infertile, owing to ineffective mobility of the sperm tail. About half the patients with defective cilia have no situs inversus. The syndrome is inherited as an autosomal recessive trait. In some groups of patients the cilia are not immobile but have abnormal

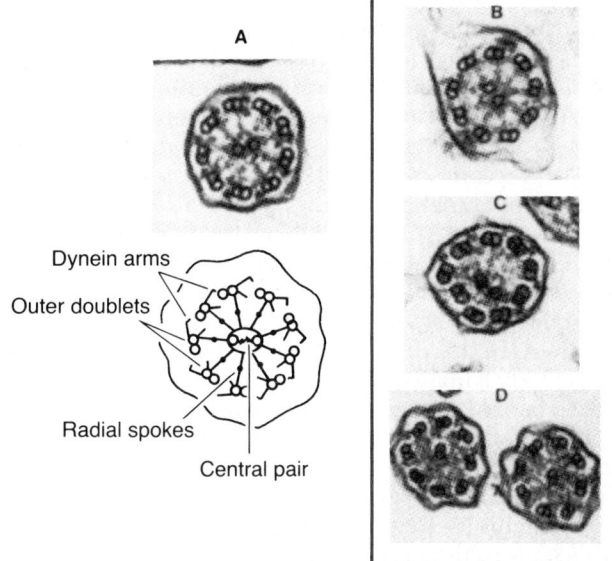

Figure 16–21. Ultrastructural abnormalities of cilia in immotile cilia syndromes. *A,* Normal cilium. *B,* Patient with Kartagener's syndrome. The dynein arms are absent. *C,* Radial spoke defect. *D,* transposition of microtubules. There are only eight peripheral doublets. The other peripheral pair of tubules has been transposed to center of cilium. The central pair is absent. Patients B, C, and D have immotile or poorly motile cilia. (From Katzenstein, A.-L.A., and Askin, F.B.: Surgical Pathology of Non-Neoplastic Lung Disease. Philadelphia, W.B. Saunders Co., 1982, p. 397. Courtesty of Dr. Jennifer Sturgess et al., Toronto, Ontario, Canada.)

movement (ciliary dyskinesia). The morphologic ciliary abnormalities are not entirely pathognomonic of the syndromes, since some abnormal cilia may be found in otherwise normal individuals or in patients with viral illnesses and bronchial inflammation.

3. *Necrotizing pneumonia.* Bronchiectasis occasionally follows necrotizing or suppurative pneumonias caused by the tubercle bacillus or staphylococcal or mixed infections; in past years it was considered to be a sequel to childhood necrotizing infections complicating measles, whooping cough, and influenza. This form of *postinfective bronchiectasis,* however, is no longer common in the United States.

ETIOLOGY AND PATHOGENESIS. *Obstruction* and *infection* are the most frequent influences associated with bronchiectasis, and it is likely that both factors are necessary for the development of the full-fledged bronchiectatic lesions. After bronchial obstruction (such as by tumors or foreign bodies), air is resorbed from the airways distal to the obstruction, with resultant atelectasis. With atelectasis, the elastic forces within the lobe disappear, so that the airways are no longer taut and they "relax," resulting in dilatation of the walls of those airways that are patent. These changes are reversible. *However, the changes will become irreversible* (1) *if the obstruction persists,* especially during periods of growth, because the airways will not be able to develop normally; and (2) *if there is added infection*. Infection plays a role in the pathogenesis of bronchiectasis in two ways: (a) it produces bronchial wall inflammation, weakening, and further dilation; and (b) the extensive bronchial and bronchiolar damage causes endobronchial obliteration, with atelectasis distal to the obliteration and subsequent bronchiectasis around atelectatic areas, as described earlier.

These mechanisms—infection and obstruction—are most readily apparent in the severe form of bronchiectasis associated with cystic fibrosis of the pancreas. In this disorder, there is squamous metaplasia of the normal respiratory epithelium with impairment of normal mucociliary action, infection, necrosis of the bronchial and bronchiolar walls, and subsequent bronchiectasis. In younger children, the changes take the form of bronchiolitis (occlusion of the bronchioles by granulation tissue), but older children tend to develop full-blown bronchiectasis.

MORPHOLOGY. Bronchiectatic involvement of the lungs usually affects the lower lobes bilaterally, particularly those air passages that are most vertical. When tumors or aspiration of foreign bodies lead to bronchiectasis, the involvement may be sharply localized to a single segment of the lungs. Usually the most severe involvements are found in the more distal bronchi and bronchioles. **The airways are dilated, sometimes up to four times normal size.** These dilatations may produce long, tubelike enlargements **(cylindroid bronchiectasis)** or, in other cases, may cause **fusi-**

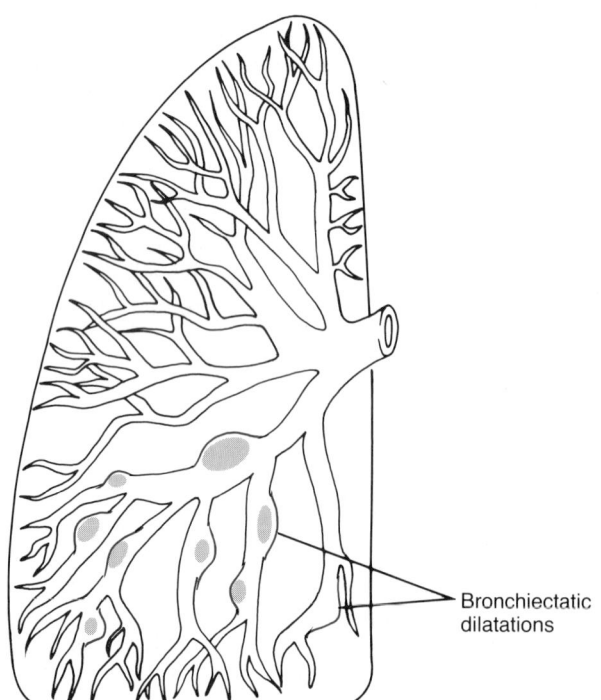

Figure 16–22. Diagram of bronchiectasis, showing saccular dilatations in the lower lobe.

Bronchiectatic dilatations

form or even sharply saccular distention **(saccular bronchiectasis)** (Fig. 16–22).

Characteristically, the bronchi and bronchioles are sufficiently dilated so that they can be followed, on gross examination, directly out to the pleural surfaces. By contrast, in the normal lung, the bronchioles cannot be followed by ordinary gross dissection beyond a point 2 to 3 cm removed from the pleural surfaces. In more severe involvements, the dilation may produce an almost cystic pattern to the cut surface of the lung (Fig. 16–23). Varying degrees of emphysema and atelectasis are also present.

The histologic findings vary with the activity and chronicity of the disease. In the full-blown, active case, there is an intense acute and chronic inflammatory exudation within the walls of the bronchi and bronchioles, associated with desquamation of the lining epithelium and extensive areas of necrotizing ulceration. There may be pseudostratification of the columnar cells or squamous metaplasia of the remaining epithelium. In some instances, the necrosis completely destroys the bronchial or bronchiolar walls and forms a lung abscess. Fibrosis of the bronchial and bronchiolar walls and peribronchiolar fibrosis develop in the more chronic cases. When healing occurs, there may be complete regeneration of the lining epithelium. However, usually so much injury has occurred that abnormal dilatation and scarring persist.

CLINICAL COURSE. The clinical manifestations consist of severe, persistent cough; expectoration of foul-smelling, sometimes bloody sputum; and dyspnea and orthopnea in severe cases. A systemic febrile reaction may occur when powerful pathogens are present. These symptoms are often episodic and are precipitated by upper respiratory tract infections or the introduction of new pathogenic agents. In the full-blown case, the cough is paroxysmal in nature. Such paroxysms are particularly frequent when the patient rises in the morning and the changes in position lead to drainage into the bronchi of the collected pools of pus. In the full-blown case, obstructive ventilatory insufficiency leads to marked dyspnea and cyanosis. Clubbing of the fingers sometimes develops in these patients. Cor pulmonale, metastatic brain abscesses, and amyloidosis are other, less frequent complications of bronchiectasis.

PULMONARY INFECTIONS

Respiratory tract infections are more frequent than infections of any other organ and account for the largest number of workdays lost in the general population. The vast majority are upper respiratory tract infections caused by viruses, but viral, mycoplasmal, bacterial, and fungal infections of the lung (pneumonias, bronchopneumonias, lung abscesses, and tuberculosis) still account for an enormous amount of morbidity and rank among the major immediate causes of death.[55] Many of these infections have been described in detail in Chapter 7. Here we shall review only those

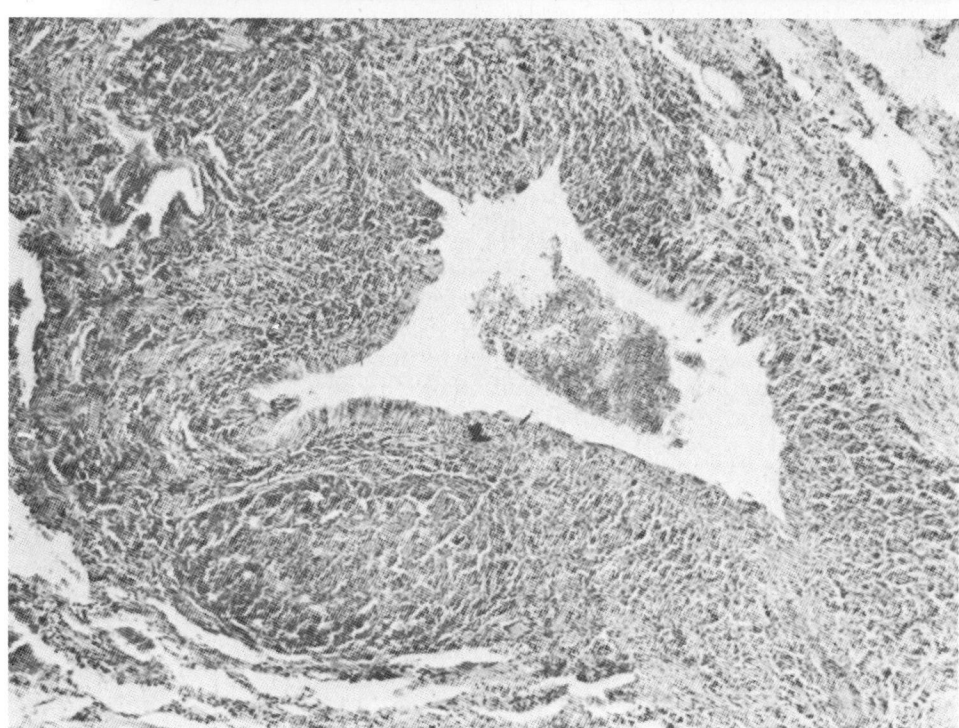

Figure 16-23. Bronchiectasis. *A,* Cut surface of basal region, showing transected, markedly distended peripheral bronchi. *B,* Bronchus is surrounded by an intense leukocytic infiltrate, and lining epithelium is eroded at the 9 to 12 o'clock positions. B

aspects of the pathology of pulmonary infections that need further discussion.

BACTERIAL PNEUMONIA

Bacterial invasion of the lung parenchyma evokes exudative solidification (consolidation) of the pulmonary tissue known as bacterial pneumonia. Many variables, such as the specific etiologic agent, the host reaction, and the extent of involvement, determine the precise form of pneumonia. Thus, classification may be made according to etiologic agent (e.g., pneu-mococcal or staphylococcal pneumonia), the nature of the host reaction (suppurative, fibrinous, and so forth), or the anatomic distribution of the disease (lobular [bronchopneumonia], lobar, or interstitial pneumonia). The anatomic but still classic categorization is often difficult to apply in the individual case, because patterns overlap. The lobular involvement may become confluent to produce virtually total lobar consolidation; in contrast, effective antibiotic therapy for any form of pneumonia may limit involvement to a subtotal consolidation. Moreover, the same organisms may produce lobular pneumonia in one patient, whereas in the more vulnerable individual a full-blown lobar involvement develops. *Most important, from the clinical standpoint, are identification of the causative agent and determination of the extent of disease.*

PATHOGENESIS. Although antibiotics have reduced the mortality rate from bacterial pneumonia, the disorder remains a major immediate cause of death in the terminal phase of many diseases. In addition, the use of antibiotics has resulted in an increased incidence of pneumonia caused by resistant organisms, which may be difficult to treat.

Recall first that the normal lung is free of bacteria and possesses a number of potent defense mechanisms that clear or destroy any bacteria inhaled with air or fortuitously deposited in the airway passages (p. 757). These defense mechanisms include (1) the filtering function of the nasopharynx, (2) the mucociliary action of the lower air passages, and (3) phagocytosis and elimination by the alveolar macrophages. In addition, immune mechanisms play a role in eliminating bacteria that reach the alveoli either through respiration or via the bloodstream. *Pneumonia results whenever these defense mechanisms are impaired or whenever the resistance of the host in general is lowered.*

The clearing mechanisms can be interfered with by many factors, such as the following:

1. *Loss or suppression of the cough reflex,* as a result of coma, anesthesia, neuromuscular disorders, drugs, or chest pain. This may lead to *aspiration* of gastric contents.
2. *Injury to the mucociliary apparatus,* by either impairment of ciliary function or destruction of ciliated epithelium. Cigarette smoke, inhalation of hot or corrosive gases, viral diseases, and genetic disturbances (e.g., the immotile cilia syndrome) all have this effect.
3. *Interference with the phagocytic or bactericidal action of alveolar macrophages.* Many factors have been shown to have this effect, including alcohol, tobacco smoke anoxia, and oxygen intoxication.
4. *Pulmonary congestion and edema.* Edema is one of the most common predispositions to terminal bronchopneumonia in patients with congestive heart failure or in debilitated patients with hypostatic pulmonary edema.
5. *Accumulation of secretions* in conditions such as cystic fibrosis and bronchial obstruction.

Factors that affect resistance in general include chronic diseases, immunologic deficiency, treatment with immunosuppressive agents, leukopenia, and unusually virulent infections.

Several other points need to be emphasized. First, one type of pneumonia sometimes predisposes to another, especially in debilitated patients. It is known, for example, that the most common cause of death in viral influenza epidemics is bacterial pneumonia. Second, although the portal of entry for most pneumonias is the respiratory tract, hematogenous spread from one focus to other foci can occur, and secondary seeding of the lungs may be difficult to distinguish from primary pneumonia. Finally, many patients with chronic diseases acquire terminal pneumonias while hospitalized. Thus, one must keep in mind the potential risks of *nosocomial infection:* bacteria common to the hospital environment may have acquired resistance to antibiotics; opportunities for spread are increased; invasive procedures such as intubations and injections are common; and bacteria may contaminate apparatus used in respiratory care units.

Bronchopneumonia

Patchy consolidation of the lung is the dominant characteristic of bronchopneumonia (Fig. 16–24). This parenchymal infection usually represents an extension of a preexisting bronchitis or bronchiolitis. It is an extremely common disease that tends to occur in the more vulnerable two extremes of life—infancy and old age. In the young, there is little previous experience with pathogenic organisms, rendering these patients susceptible to organisms of even low virulence. Resistance likewise falls in the aged, particularly in those already suffering from some serious disorder. Bronchopneumonia thus frequently provides the period at the end of a long sentence of progressive heart failure or disseminated tumor. On this account, it is a common finding on postmortem examinations.

ETIOLOGY. Although virtually any pathogen may produce these lung infections, the common agents are staphylococci, streptococci, pneumococci, *Hemophilus influenzae, Pseudomonas aeruginosa,* and the coliform bacteria.

> **MORPHOLOGY.** Foci of bronchopneumonia consist of consolidated areas of acute suppurative inflammation. The consolidation may be patchily distributed through one lobe but is more often multilobar and frequently bilateral and basal, because of the tendency for secretions to gravitate into the lower lobes. Well-developed lesions are 3 to 4 cm in

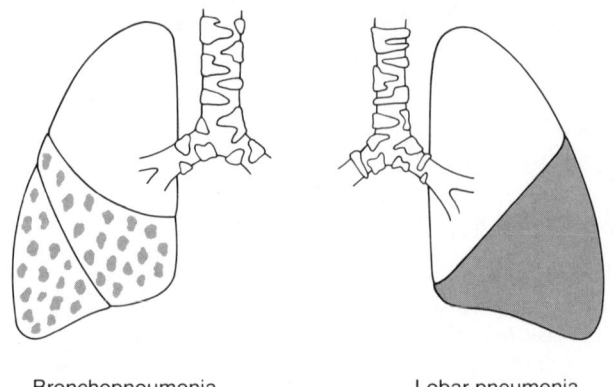

Bronchopneumonia   Lobar pneumonia

Figure 16–24. Comparison of bronchopneumonia and lobar pneumonia.

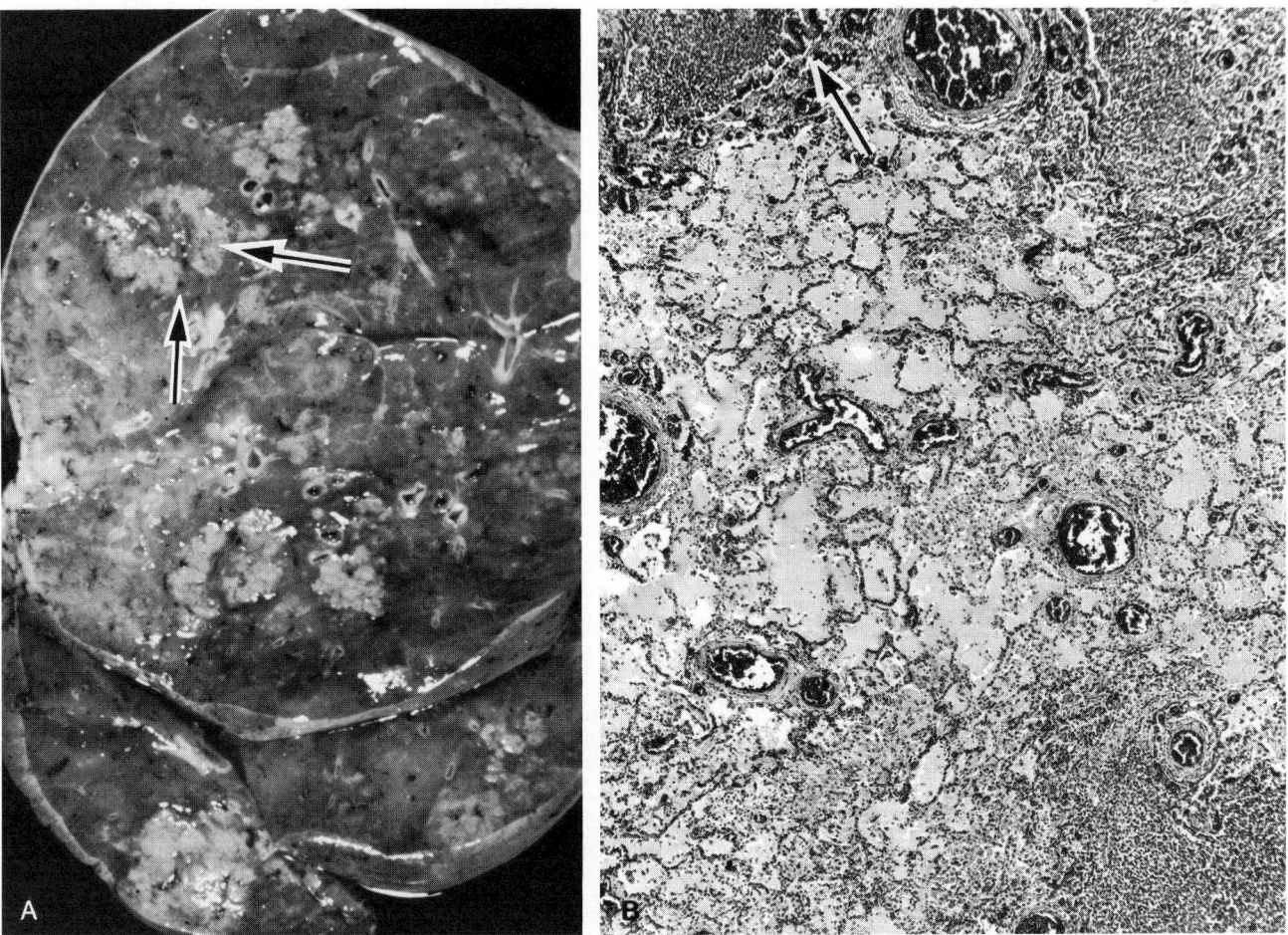

Figure 16-25. *A,* Bronchopneumonia. A gross section of lung showing patches of gray purulent consolidation *(arrows). B,* Histologic section to illustrate patchiness of inflammatory reaction in upper and lower parts of illustration. Note the edema fluid in less involved alveoli. Arrow points to bronchus with inflammation and ulceration.

diameter, slightly elevated, dry, granular, gray-red to yellow, and poorly delimited at their margins (Fig. 16-24). Confluence of these foci occurs in the more florid instances, producing the appearance of total lobar consolidation.

Histologically, the reaction usually comprises a suppurative exudate that fills the bronchi, bronchioles, and adjacent alveolar spaces (Fig. 16-25). Neutrophils are dominant in this exudation. Extremely aggressive organisms may lead to necrosis of the central regions of the lung lesions, to produce abscesses. Organization of the exudate may yield masses of fibrous tissue that constitute permanent residuals. Under happier circumstances, the exudate resolves, restoring the lung to its former state.

Particularly in infancy, the bacterial bronchopneumonia may remain interstitial within the alveolar septa, to produce an inflammatory reaction confined to the alveolar walls with little exudate in the airspaces, mimicking the interstitial pattern of viral pneumonia. **E. coli** and group B hemolytic streptococci are the most common causes for such a pattern.

CLINICAL COURSE. The clinical signs and symptoms of bronchopneumonia depend on the virulence of the invading agent and the extent of pneumonic involvement. The patient, usually elderly, has a temperature of 38° to 39.5°C, along with cough, expectoration, and expiratory rales in one or more lobes. Often there is a previous history of confinement to bed, malnutrition, some underlying serious disorder, aspiration of gastric contents, or an upper respiratory tract infection. Respiratory difficulty may be present but is usually not prominent. Chest radiographs may show focal opacities. When the pneumonia is caused by antibiotic-sensitive organisms, infection is readily controlled in patients not already mortally ill from some other cause.

The complications of bronchopneumonia are (1) the formation of lung abscesses; (2) spread to the pleural cavities, producing empyema; (3) spread to the pericardial cavity, producing suppurative pericarditis; and (4) the development of bacteremia with metastatic abscess formation in other organs.

Lobar Pneumonia

Lobar pneumonia is an acute bacterial infection of a large portion of a lobe or of an entire lobe, which tends to occur at any age but is relatively uncommon in infancy and in late life (see Fig. 16–24). Classic lobar pneumonia is now encountered much less often, owing to the effectiveness with which antibiotics abort these infections and prevent the development of full-blown lobar consolidation.

ETIOLOGY AND PATHOGENESIS. Ninety to 95% of all lobar pneumonias are caused by pneumococci *(Streptococcus pneumoniae)*. Most common are types 1, 3, 7, and 2. Type 3 causes a particularly virulent form of lobar pneumonia. About two thirds of pneumococcal pneumonias in hospitalized patients are bronchopneumonias, not lobar pneumonia. Occasionally, *Klebsiella pneumoniae*, staphylococci, streptococci, *Hemophilus influenzae,* and (in this day of antibiotic resistance) some of the gram-negative organisms, such as the Pseudomonas and Proteus bacilli, are also responsible for this lobar distribution of involvement.

The most common portal of entry is the air passages. A lobar distribution appears merely to be a function of the virulence of the organism and the vulnerability of the host. Heavy contamination by virulent pathogens may evoke this pattern in healthy adults, whereas organisms of lower virulence may accomplish the same in the predisposed patient. In lobar pneumonia there is more extensive exudation that leads to spread through the pores of Kohn. Moreover, the copious mucoid encapsulation produced by the pneumococci protects the organisms against immediate phagocytosis, and thus favors their spread.

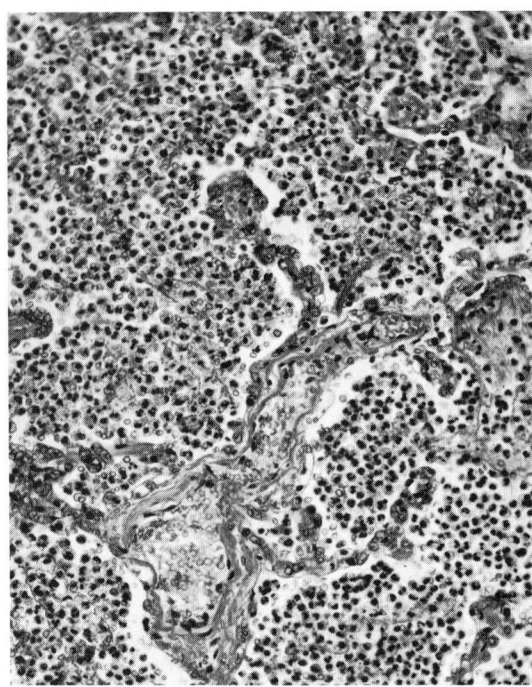

Figure 16–26. Lobar pneumonia. The stage of early red hepatization with congested septal capillaries and extensive white cell exudation into alveoli. Fibrin nets have not yet formed.

MORPHOLOGY. The histologic changes are presented first, as they make the gross alterations understandable.

Lobar pneumonia consists, in essence, of a widespread fibrinosuppurative consolidation of large areas and even whole lobes of the lung. In its evolution, the pneumonic involvement follows the basic pattern of all inflammations and begins with serous exudation and accompanying vascular engorgement, followed by a fibrinocellular exudation, culminating ultimately in either resolution of the exudate or, less happily, its organization.

Four stages of the inflammatory response have classically been described: congestion, red hepatization, gray hepatization, and resolution. But present-day effective antibiotic therapy frequently telescopes or halts the progression, so that often at autopsy the anatomic changes do not conform to the older classic stages.

The first **stage of congestion** represents the developing bacterial infection and lasts for about 24 hours (and thus is rarely seen histologically). It is characterized by vascular engorgement, intra-alveolar fluid with few neutrophils, and often the presence of numerous bacteria. Grossly, the involved lobe is heavy, boggy, red, and subcrepitant.

The **stage of red hepatization** that follows is characterized by increasing numbers of neutrophils and the precipitation of fibrin to fill the alveolar spaces (Fig. 16–26). The massive confluent exudation obscures the pulmonary architecture. Extravasation of red cells causes the coloration seen on gross examination. In many areas, the fibrin strands stream from one alveolus through the pores of Kohn into the adjacent alveolus. The white cells contain engulfed bacteria. An overlying fibrinous or fibrinosuppurative pleuritis is almost invariably present. On gross examination, the lobe now appears distinctly red, firm, and airless with a liver-like consistency, hence the term hepatization.

The **stage of gray hepatization** follows with a continuing accumulation of fibrin associated with the progressive disintegration of inflammatory white cells and red cells. This exudate contracts somewhat to yield a clear zone adjacent to the alveolar walls. In the usual case, the alveolar septa are preserved. The progressive disintegration of red cells and the persistence of fibrinosuppurative exudate give the gross appearance of a grayish-brown, dry surface (Fig. 16–27). Sometimes, when the bacterial infection extends into the pleural cavity, the intrapleural fibrinosuppurative reaction produces what is known as **empyema.**

The final **stage of resolution** follows in the great preponderance of cases with a favorable outcome. The consolidated exudate within the alveolar spaces undergoes progressive enzymic digestion to produce a granular, semifluid debris that is either resorbed, ingested by macrophages, or coughed up. In such favorable cases, the normal lung parenchyma is restored to its normal state. The pleural reaction may similarly resolve, but more often it undergoes organization, leaving fibrous thickening or permanent adhesions.

Many **complications** may supervene during this classic evolution. (1) The type 3 pneumococcus and the Klebsiella bacillus characteristically produce an **abundant mucinous secretion.** (2) These same organisms and the staphylococci frequently cause **abscess formation.** (3) **Organization of the exudate** may convert the lung into a solid tissue (Fig. 16–28). (4) **Bacteremic dissemination** to the heart valves, pericardium, brain, kidneys, spleen, and joints may cause metastatic abscesses, endocarditis, meningitis, or suppurative arthritis.

CLINICAL COURSE. In the classic pattern of lobar pneumonia the onset of the disease is sudden, with malaise, shaking chills, and fever. Cough appears with expectoration of at first a slightly turbid, watery sputum indicative of the stage of congestion, followed by a frankly purulent, hemorrhagic, so-called "rusty" sputum characteristic of the stage of red hepatization. The temperature elevation may be very marked, up to 40° or 41°C. If the causative organism is the type 3 pneumococcus or Klebsiella bacillus, the sputum has

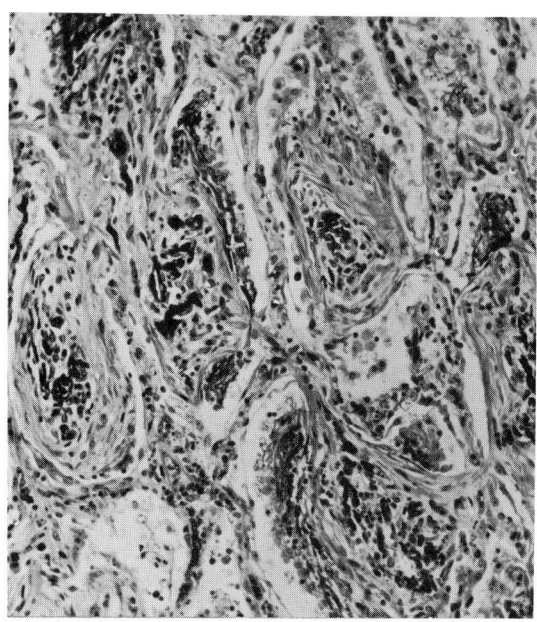

Figure 16–28. Organization of lobar pneumonia. Alveolar spaces are virtually filled with connective tissue that can be seen in areas to be streaming through pores of Kohn (in center of picture).

the same tenacious, mucinous quality as does the exudate in the lungs. Shortness of breath, orthopnea, and cyanosis may appear when there has been encroachment upon the vital capacity of the lung parenchyma. The fibrinosuppurative pleuritis is accompanied by pleuritic pain and pleural friction rub. The physical findings vary with the stage of pneumonia. Within the first few days, limitation of breath sounds and fine crepitant rales herald the development of the stage of congestion. Two or three days after onset, more fully developed dullness, increased tactile and vocal fremitus, and bronchial breath sounds reflect the solidification of the lung. As resolution occurs, moist rales reappear, the dullness diminishes, and the bronchial breath sounds and tactile and vocal fremitus gradually subside. The characteristic radiologic appearance is that of a radiopaque, usually well-circumscribed lobe.

This classic progressive symptom complex is, however, totally modified by the administration of antibiotics. Treated patients may be relatively afebrile with few clinical signs 48 to 72 hours after the initiation of antibiotics. The identification of the organism and the determination of its antibiotic sensitivity are the keystones to appropriate therapy. Fewer than 10% of patients with lobar pneumonia now succumb and, in most such instances, death may be attributed either to a complication such as empyema, meningitis, endocarditis, or pericarditis or to some predisposing influence such as debility or chronic alcoholism.

PNEUMONIA IN IMMUNOCOMPROMISED HOST

The appearance of a pulmonary infiltrate and signs of infection (e.g., fever) is fast becoming one of the most

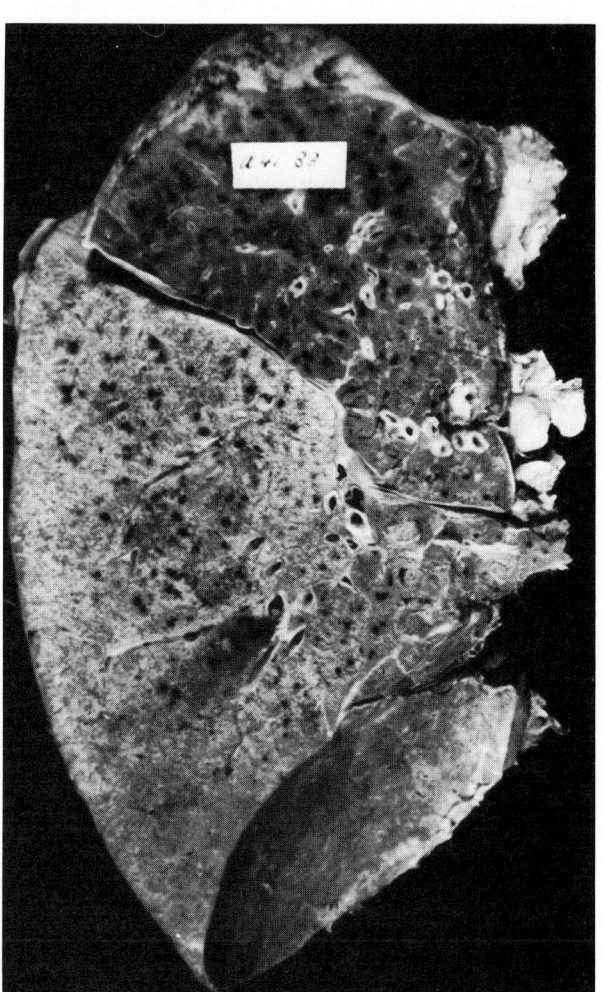

Figure 16–27. Lobar pneumonia—gray hepatization. The lower lobe is uniformly consolidated creating a "plaster-cast" impression of the dome of the diaphragm. Note exudate (pleuritis) layering the diaphragmatic surface.

Table 16-4. Causes of Pulmonary Infiltrates in Immuno-compromised Hosts

DIFFUSE INFILTRATE	FOCAL INFILTRATE
Common	*Common*
Cytomegalovirus	Gram-negative rods
Pneumocystis carinii	*Staphylococcus aureus*
Drug reaction	Aspergillus
	Candida
	Malignancy
Uncommon	*Uncommon*
Bacteria	Cryptococcus
Aspergillus	Mucor
Cryptococcus	*Pneumocystis carinii*
Malignancy	*Legionella pneumophila*

Modified from Fanta, C. H., and Pennington, J. L.: Fever and new lung infiltrates in the immunocompromised host. Clin. Chest Med. 2:19, 1981.

common and serious complications of patients whose immune and defense systems are suppressed by disease, chemotherapy for organ transplants and tumors, or irradiation.[56] A wide variety of so-called opportunistic infectious agents, many of which rarely cause infection in normal hosts, can cause these pneumonias, and often more than one agent is involved.[57] Mortality from these opportunistic infections is high. In the case of acquired immunodeficiency syndrome (AIDS), nearly 100% of patients will suffer from an opportunistic infection, most commonly caused by *Pneumocystis carinii*.[58] Table 16-4 lists some of the agents according to their prevalence and to whether they cause local or diffuse pulmonary infiltrates. It is well to remember that such infiltrates may also be due to drug reactions or to involvement of the lung by tumor. The specific infections are discussed in Chapter 7.

VIRAL AND MYCOPLASMAL PNEUMONIA (PRIMARY ATYPICAL PNEUMONIA)

The term primary atypical pneumonia (PAP) was initially applied to an acute febrile respiratory disease characterized by patchy inflammatory changes in the lungs, largely confined to alveolar septa and pulmonary interstitium. The term "atypical" denotes the lack of alveolar exudate, but a much more accurate designation is *interstitial pneumonitis*. The pneumonitis is caused by a variety of organisms, the most common being *Mycoplasma pneumoniae*. Other etiologic agents are viruses, including influenza virus types **A** and **B**, the respiratory syncytial viruses (RSV), adenovirus, rhinoviruses, rubeola and varicella viruses; Chlamydia (psittacosis); and *Coxiella burnetii* (Q fever).[59] In some cases, the cause is undetermined.

Any one of these agents may cause merely an upper respiratory tract infection, recognized as the common cold, or a more severe lower respiratory tract infection. The circumstances that favor such extension of the infection are often mysterious but include malnutrition, alcoholism, and underlying debilitating illnesses.

MORPHOLOGY. All causal agents produce essentially similar morphologic patterns. Because the patients with mild cases recover, our understanding of the anatomic changes is necessarily based on the more severe, fatal expressions of these infections. The pneumonic involvement may be quite patchy or may involve whole lobes bilaterally or unilaterally. The affected areas are red-blue, congested, and subcrepitant. There is no obvious consolidation such as is encountered in lobar pneumonia. The pleura is smooth, and pleuritis or pleural effusions are infrequent.

The histologic pattern, too, depends on the severity of the disease. Predominant is the interstitial nature of the inflammatory reaction, virtually localized within the walls of the alveoli. The alveolar septa are widened and edematous and usually have a mononuclear inflammatory infiltrate of lymphocytes, histiocytes, and occasionally plasma cells. In very acute cases, neutrophils may also be present. The alveoli may be free of exudate, but in many patients there are intra-alveolar proteinaceous material, a cellular exudate, and characteristically pink hyaline membranes lining the alveolar walls, similar to those seen in hyaline membrane disease of infants (Fig. 16-29). These changes reflect **alveolar damage** similar to that seen diffusely in the adult respiratory distress syndrome (p. 761).

Superimposed bacterial infection modifies the histologic picture by causing ulcerative bronchitis and bronchiolitis, and may yield the anatomic changes already described under bacterial pneumonia. Subsidence of the disease is followed by reconstitution of the native architecture.

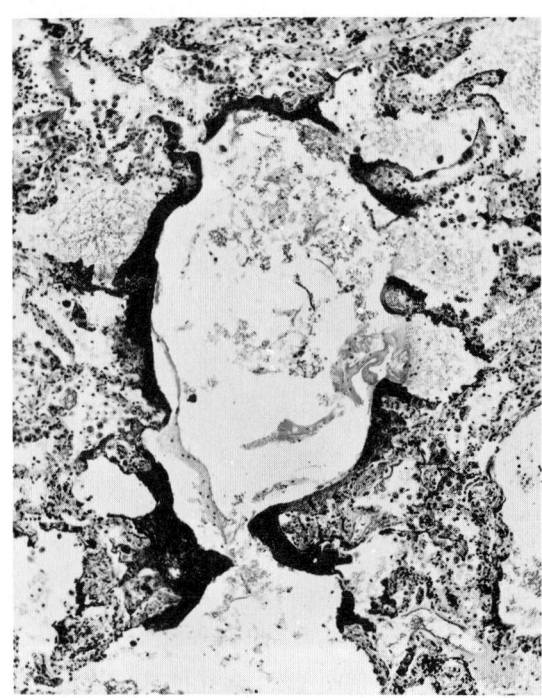

Figure 16-29. Primary atypical (viral) pneumonia with prominent hyaline membranes and interstitial inflammatory infiltration.

Some viruses such as herpes simplex, varicella, and adenovirus may be associated with necrosis of bronchial and alveolar epithelium and acute inflammation. Epithelial giant cells with intranuclear or intracytoplasmic inclusions may be present in cytomegalic inclusion disease. Other viruses produce cytopathic changes, as described in Chapter 7.

CLINICAL COURSE. As indicated, the clinical course is extremely varied. Many cases masquerade as severe upper respiratory tract infections or as "chest colds." Even patients with well-developed atypical pneumonia have few localizing symptoms. Cough may well be absent, and the major manifestations may consist only of fever, headache, muscle aches, and pains in the legs. Cough, when present, is characteristically dry, hacking, and unproductive of sputum. The edema and exudation are both strategically located to cause an alveolocapillary block and thus evoke symptoms out of proportion to the scanty physical findings. One of the useful laboratory aids in differentiating viral atypical pneumonia from the *M. pneumoniae* form is the detection of elevated cold agglutinin titers in the serum. These are present in about half of patients with Mycoplasma and in 20% of adenovirus infections, and are absent in other viral pneumonias. Isolation of the causative agent, whether viral or Mycoplasma, requires fairly fastidious technical methods.

The ordinary sporadic form of the disease is usually mild with a low mortality rate, below 1%. However, interstitial pneumonia may assume epidemic proportions with intensified severity and greater mortality, as all too grimly documented in the highly fatal influenzal pandemics of 1915 and 1918 and the many smaller epidemics since. Secondary bacterial infection by staphylococci or streptococci is common in such circumstances.

LUNG ABSCESS

The term pulmonary abscess describes a local suppurative process within the lung characterized by necrosis of lung tissue. Lung abscesses may develop at any age and are especially frequent in young adults. Oropharyngeal surgical procedures, sinobronchial infections, dental sepsis, and bronchiectasis play important roles in their development. Males are affected somewhat more often than females.

ETIOLOGY AND PATHOGENESIS. Although under appropriate circumstances any pathogen may produce an abscess, the commonly isolated organisms include aerobic and anaerobic streptococci, *Staphylococcus aureus*, and a host of gram-negative organisms. Mixed infections occur very often because of the important causal role that inhalation of foreign material plays. *Anaerobic organisms* normally found in the oral cavity, including members of the Bacteroides, Fusobacterium, and Peptococcus species, are the exclu-

sive isolates in about 60% of cases.[60] The causative organisms are introduced by the following mechanisms:

1. *Aspiration of infective material* (the most frequent cause). This is particularly common in acute alcoholism, coma, anesthesia, sinusitis, gingivodental sepsis, and debilitation in which the cough reflexes are depressed. Aspiration of gastric contents is serious because the gastric acidity adds to the irritant role of the food particles, and, in the course of aspiration, mouth organisms are inevitably introduced.
2. *Antecedent primary bacterial infection.* Postpneumonic abscess formations are usually associated with *Staphylococcus aureus*, *Klebsiella pneumoniae*, and the type 3 pneumococcus. Fungus infections and bronchiectasis are additional antecedents to lung abscess formation.
3. *Septic embolism.* Infected emboli from thrombophlebitis in any portion of the systemic venous circulation or from vegetative bacterial endocarditis on the right side of the heart are trapped in the lung.
4. *Neoplasia.* Secondary infection is particularly common in the bronchopulmonary segment obstructed by a primary or secondary malignancy. This sequence is typical of bronchogenic carcinoma in which impaired drainage, distal atelectasis, and aspiration of blood and tumor fragments all contribute to the development of sepsis.
5. *Miscellaneous.* Direct traumatic penetrations of the lungs; spread of infections from a neighboring organ, such as suppuration in the esophagus, spine, subphrenic space, or pleural cavity; and hematogenous seeding of the lung by pyogenic organisms may all lead to lung abscess formation.

When all these causes are excluded, there are still cases in which no reasonable basis for the abscess formation can be identified. These are referred to as *"primary cryptogenic"* lung abscesses.

MORPHOLOGY. Abscesses vary in diameter from a few millimeters to large cavities of 5 to 6 cm. They may affect any part of the lung and be single or multiple. Pulmonary abscesses due to aspiration are more common on the right (the more vertical main bronchus) and are most often single. Abscesses that develop in the course of pneumonia or bronchiectasis are usually multiple, basal, and diffusely scattered. Septic emboli and pyemic abscesses, by the haphazard nature of their genesis, are multiple and may affect any region of the lungs.

The cavity may or may not be filled with suppurative debris, depending on the presence or absence of a communication with one of the air passages. When such communications exist, the contained exudate may be partially drained to create an air-containing cavity. Superimposed saprophytic infections are prone to flourish within the already necrotic debris of the abscess cavity. Continued infection leads to large, fetid, green-black, multilocular cavities with poor margination, designated **gangrene of the** lung. **The cardinal histologic change in all abscesses is suppurative destruction of the lung parenchyma within the central area of cavitation** (Fig. 16–30). In chronic cases, considerable fibroblastic proliferation produces a containing fibrous wall.

CLINICAL COURSE. The manifestations of pulmonary abscesses are much like those of bronchiectasis and are characterized principally by cough, fever, and copious amounts of foul-smelling purulent or sanguineous sputum. If the abscess is solitary, respiratory difficulty may be minimal. Fever, chest pain, and weight loss are common. Clubbing of the fingers and toes may appear within a few weeks after onset of an abscess. Diagnosis of this condition can only be suspected from the clinical findings and must be confirmed by roentgenography and bronchoscopy. Often the fluid levels can be demonstrated by radiographs. Whenever an abscess is discovered, it is important to rule out an underlying carcinoma, as this is present in 10 to 15% of cases.

The course of abscesses is variable. With antimicrobial therapy, most resolve with no major sequelae. Surgery is rarely necessary to remove the abscess. Complications include extension of the infection into the pleural cavity, unusual hemorrhage, the development of *brain abscesses* or *meningitis* from septic emboli, and (rarely) reactive secondary amyloidosis.

PULMONARY TUBERCULOSIS

A general discussion of tuberculosis is in Chapter 7. Here we shall only briefly describe the effects of this infection on the lungs.[61]

As indicated earlier, the overwhelming preponderance of tuberculous infections affect the lungs and, indeed, begin there. Pulmonary involvement is still the major cause of tuberculous morbidity and mortality. The prevention and control of these pulmonary, infections accounts for tuberculosis being a relatively uncommon cause of death today, although a leading cause in 1900 in the United States. The present U.S. death rate from tuberculosis is about 2 per 100,000 population as compared with a death rate of 200 in 1900. Regrettably, in many parts of the world, underprivileged populations still suffer from death rates 20 times those of industrialized nations, and indeed, high-incidence pockets of infection are found among the poor in the most affluent countries.

Primary Pulmonary Tuberculosis

Except for the rare intestinal (bovine) tuberculosis, and the even more uncommon skin, oropharyngeal, and lymphoidal primary sites, the lungs are the usual location of primary infections. As detailed earlier (p. 376), the initial focus of primary infection is the *Ghon complex*, which consists of (1) a parenchymal subpleural lesion, either just above or just below the interlobar fissure between the upper and lower lobes; and (2) enlarged caseous lymph nodes draining the parenchymal focus (Fig. 16–31).

The course and fate of this initial infection are variable, but in most cases patients are asymptomatic and the lesions undergo fibrosis and calcification. Exceptionally, particularly in infants and children or immunodeficient adults, *progressive spread with cavitation, tuberculous pneumonia, or miliary tuberculosis* may follow a primary infection. However, even in

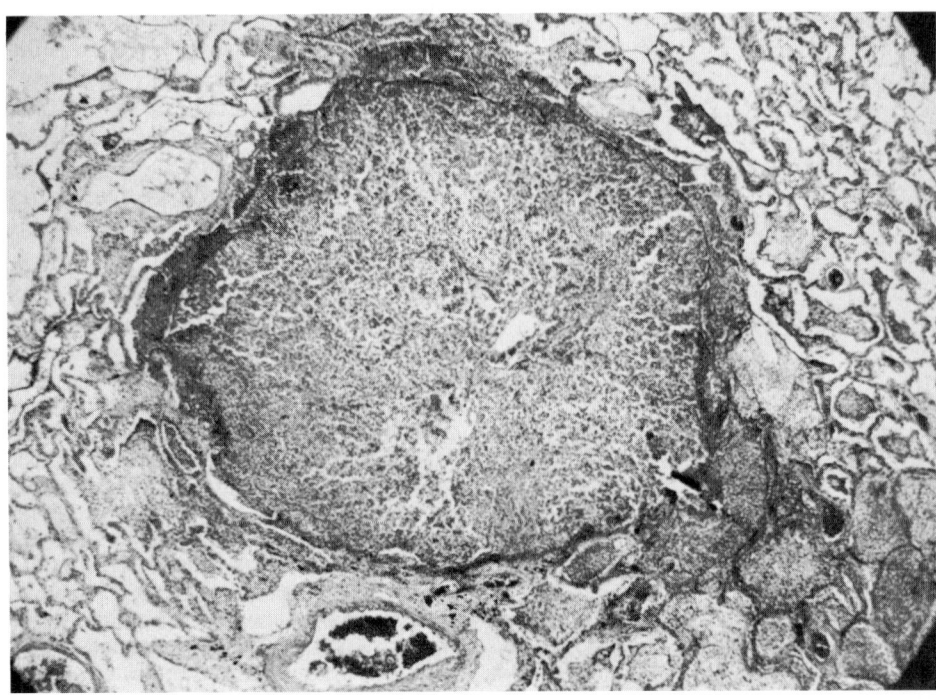

Figure 16–30. Pyemic lung abscess with complete destruction of underlying parenchyma within focus of involvement.

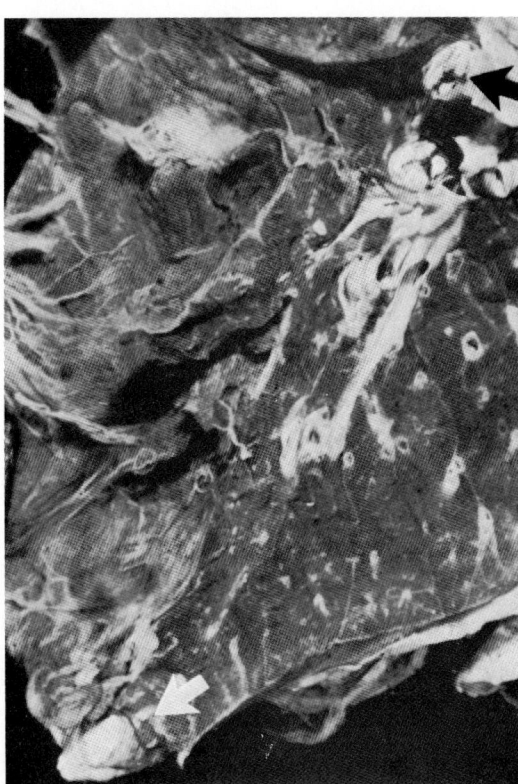

Figure 16–31. Primary pulmonary tuberculosis. Parenchymal focus of white caseation is present in lower left corner *(arrow)*, and caseated lymph nodes of drainage can be seen in upper right *(arrow)*.

In the favorable case, the initial parenchymal focus develops a small area of caseation necrosis that does not cavitate, because it fails to communicate with a bronchus or bronchiole. The usual course is one of progressive fibrous encapsulation, leaving only fibrocalcific scars that depress and pucker the pleural surface and cause focal pleural adhesions. Sometimes these fibrocalcific scars become secondarily blackened by anthracotic pigment.

Histologically, coalescent granulomas are present, composed of epithelioid cells surrounded by a zone of fibroblasts and lymphocytes that usually contains one or more

these progressive cases the infection may be halted at any stage, followed by fibrous encapsulation, scarring, and calcification, leaving only fibrocalcific residues.

Secondary (Reactivation) Pulmonary Tuberculosis

Most cases of secondary pulmonary tuberculosis represent reactivation of an old, possibly subclinical infection. You will recall that during primary infection bacilli may disseminate, without producing symptoms, and establish themselves in sites with high oxygen tension, particularly the lung apices. Reactivation in such sites occurs in no more than 5 to 10% of cases of primary infection. However, secondary tuberculosis tends to produce more damage to the lungs than does primary tuberculosis. The contributions of immunity as opposed to hypersensitivity to the development of lesions have been discussed earlier.[62]

MORPHOLOGY. The **secondary pulmonary tuberculosis lesion** is located in the apex of one or both lungs (Fig. 16–32). It begins as **a small focus of consolidation, usually less than 3 cm in diameter.** Less commonly, initial lesions may be located in other regions of the lung, particularly about the hilus. In almost every case of reinfection, the regional nodes develop foci of similar tuberculous activity.

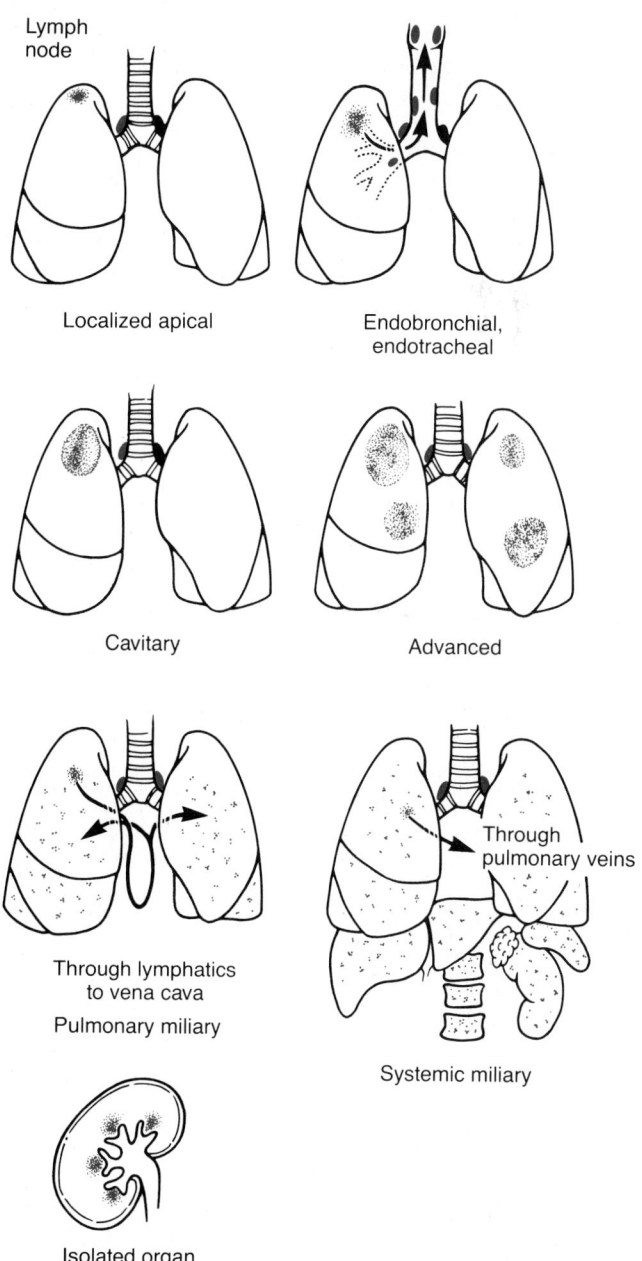

Figure 16–32. Diagrammatic representation of the many patterns of secondary tuberculosis, ranging from initial apical localization to miliary dissemination to isolated involvement of an organ (kidney).

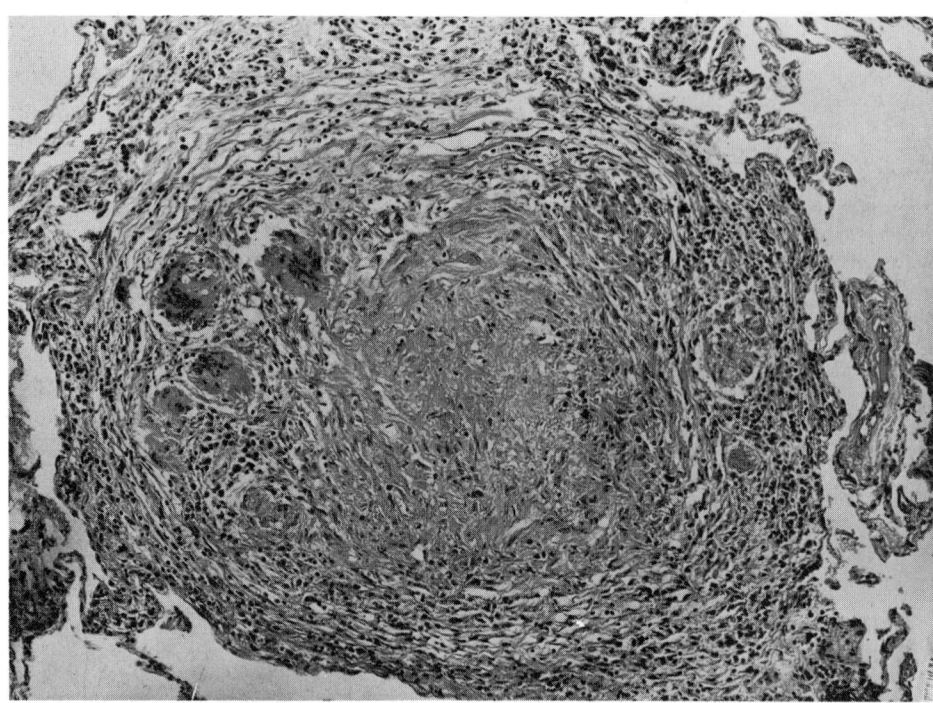

Figure 16–33. A characteristic tubercle in detail to illustrate central granular caseation and epithelioid and giant cells.

Langhans' giant cells. Some caseation is usually present in the centers of these tubercles, the amount being entirely dependent on the sensitization of the patient and the virulence of the organisms (Fig. 16–33).

As the lesion progresses, more tubercles coalesce to create a confluent area of consolidation. In the favorable case, either the entire area is eventually converted to a fibrocalcific scar, or the residual caseous debris becomes totally and heavily walled off by hyaline collagenous connective tissue. In these late lesions, the multinucleate giant cells tend to disappear. Tubercle bacilli can be demonstrated in the early exudative and caseous phases, but it is usually impossible to find them in the late fibrocalcific stages. However, it cannot be assumed that their absence in histologic sections is tantamount to their total destruction, because in many of these instances culture of the lesions or inoculation of this material into guinea pigs yields the organisms.

The subsequent course of the secondary lesions is variable. They may either heal spontaneously or with therapy, resulting in a fibrocalcific nodule, or progress along the many pathways discussed next under Progressive Pulmonary Tuberculosis (Fig. 16–32).

Progressive Pulmonary Tuberculosis

A variable, undetermined number of active lesions continue to progress over a period of months to years, causing further pulmonary and even distant organ involvements. The resultant clinicopathologic consequences include cavitary fibrocaseous tuberculosis (apical and advanced); miliary tuberculosis; and tuberculous bronchopneumonia (Fig. 16–32).

CAVITARY FIBROCASEOUS TUBERCULOSIS. The name fairly well describes this stage of disease. By erosion into a bronchiole, drainage of the caseous focus transforms it into a cavity. Growth and multiplication of the tubercle bacilli under these conditions are favored by the increased oxygen tension. In most cases, the cavity remains localized to the apex (apical cavitary fibrocaseous tuberculosis).

The cavity is lined by a yellow-gray caseous material and is more or less walled off by fibrous tissue. Not uncommonly, thrombosed arteries may traverse these cavities to produce apparent fibrous bridging bands. When such cavitation occurs in the apices, the pathways for further dissemination of the tuberculous infection are prepared. The infective material may now disseminate through the airways to other sites in the lung or upper respiratory tract. Spread may also occur to the lymph nodes via the lymphatics, and thence retrogressively through other lymphatics to other areas of the lung or other organs. Miliary dissemination through the blood is a further hazard.

Cavitary fibrocaseous tuberculosis may affect one, many, or all lobes of both lungs in the form of isolated minute tubercles, confluent caseous foci, or large areas of caseation necrosis (**advanced fibrocavity tuberculosis**).

In the progress of this disease, the pleura is inevitably involved and, depending on the chronicity of the disease, serous pleural effusions, frank tuberculous empyema, or massive obliterative fibrous pleuritis may be found. In the course of extensive fibrocaseous tuberculosis, it is almost inevitable that tubercle bacilli become implanted on the mucosal linings of the air passages, and that **endobronchial and endotracheal tuberculosis** develop. These lesions may later become ulcerated to produce irregular, ragged, necrotic, mucosal ulcers. Accompanying the endobronchial tuberculosis, **laryngeal seeding and intestinal tuberculosis** may occur. Fortunately these complications of tuberculosis are now uncommon.

MILIARY TUBERCULOSIS. Lymphohematogenous dissemination may give rise to miliary tuberculosis, confined only to the lungs or involving other organs also. The distribution of miliary lesions depends on the pathways of dissemination. Tuberculous infection may drain via the lymphatics through the major lymphatic ducts into the right side of the heart, and thence spread into a diffuse, blood-borne pattern throughout the lungs **alone.** Because most of the bacilli are filtered out by the alveolar capillary bed, the infective material may not reach the arterial systemic circulation. However, such limitation to the lungs usually is not complete, and some bacilli pass through the capillaries to enter the systemic circulation and produce distant organ seedings. In other circumstances, a tuberculous focus may erode directly into a pulmonary **artery** and thence be spread only in the pattern of supply of this single vessel to produce a localized miliary dissemination within the alveolar parenchyma. On the other hand, extension into a pulmonary **vein** is likely to be followed by disseminated miliary tuberculosis throughout the body or isolated organ tuberculosis.

In all instances of the miliary type of distribution, the individual lesions vary from one to several millimeters in diameter and are distinct, yellow-white, firm areas of consolidation that usually do not have grossly visible central

caseation necrosis or cavitation at the time of examination (Fig. 16–34). Histologically, however, these present the characteristic pattern of individual or multiple confluent tubercles having microscopic central caseation.

TUBERCULOUS BRONCHOPNEUMONIA. In the highly susceptible, highly sensitized individual, the tuberculous infection may spread rapidly throughout large areas of lung parenchyma to produce a **diffuse bronchopneumonia,** or lobar exudative consolidation, at one time descriptively referred to as "galloping consumption." Sometimes, with such overwhelming disease, well-developed tubercles do not form, and it may be difficult to establish on histologic grounds the tuberculous nature of the pneumonic process. However, numerous bacilli are usually present in such exudates.

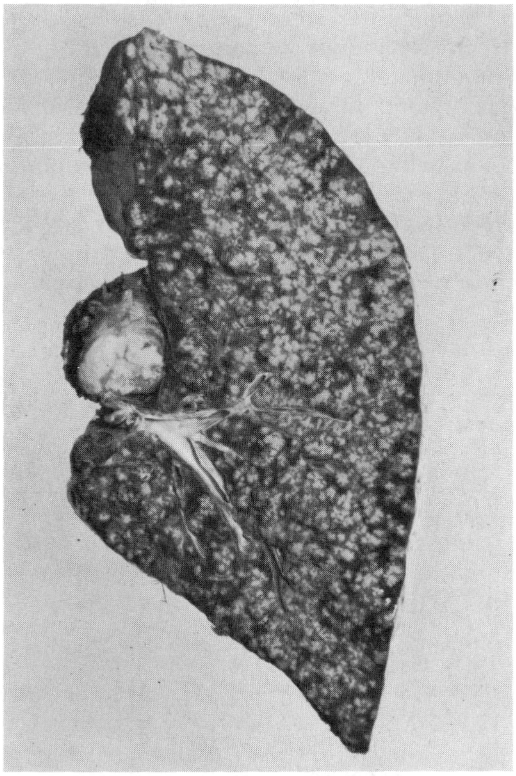

CLINICAL COURSE. In cases of suspected tuberculous tissue changes, the diagnosis is confirmed by acid-fast smears and cultures. The clinical course of pulmonary tuberculosis depends entirely on the activity, extent, and pattern of distribution of the tuberculous pulmonary infection and is extremely variable (p. 378).

The great majority of cases respond to present-day chemotherapeutic measures unless the disease is very advanced or intercurrent problems such as diabetes mellitus or reactive amyloidosis complicate the outlook.

Figure 16–34. Advanced miliary tuberculosis of lung. Foci of caseation have coalesced to produce large nodules of consolidation.

DIFFUSE INTERSTITIAL (INFILTRATIVE, RESTRICTIVE) DISEASES OF THE LUNG

This heterogeneous group of diseases is characterized predominantly by diffuse and usually chronic involvement of the pulmonary connective tissue, principally the most peripheral and delicate interstitium in the alveolar walls. Recall that the interstitium consists of the basement membrane of the endothelial and epithelial cells (fused in the thinnest portions), collagen fibers, elastic tissue, proteoglycans, fibroblasts, mast cells, and occasionally lymphocytes and monocytes.

There is no uniformity regarding terminology and classification of these diseases.[63,64] Many of the entities are of unknown cause and pathogenesis, some have an intra-alveolar as well as an interstitial component, and there is frequent overlap in histologic features among the different conditions. Nevertheless, their similar clinical signs, symptoms, radiologic alterations, and pathophysiologic changes justify their consideration as a group. These disorders account for about 15% of noninfectious diseases seen by pulmonary physicians.

In general, the clinical and pulmonary functional changes are those of *restrictive rather than obstructive lung disease* (p. 765). Patients have dyspnea, tachy-

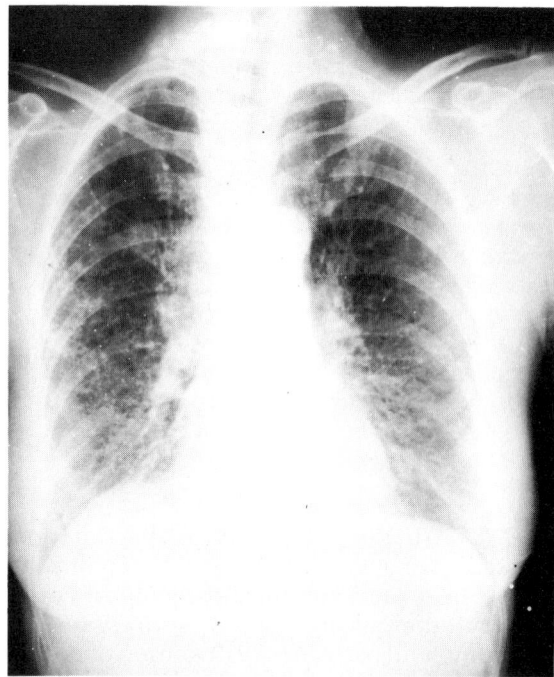

Figure 16–35. Diffuse interstitial pneumonitis. Note bilateral "ground-glass" densities. (Courtesy of Dr. G. Balikian, Brigham and Women's Hospital, Boston.)

pnea, and eventual cyanosis, without wheezing or other evidence of airway obstruction. The classic physiologic features are reductions in oxygen-diffusing capacity, lung volumes, and compliance. *Chest radiographs show diffuse infiltration by small nodules, irregular lines, or "ground-glass" shadows* (Fig. 16–35), hence the term "infiltrative." Eventually, right-sided heart failure with cor pulmonale may result. Although the entities can often be distinguished in the early stages, the advanced forms are hard to differentiate, as they result in scarring and gross destruction of the lung, often referred to as "end-stage lung" or "honey-comb lung."

CLASSIFICATION. Diffuse infiltrative disease can be divided into two broad categories (Table 16–5): those with known causes and those of unknown cause, some of which can be defined either as clinicopathologic syndromes or as having characteristic histology.[64] Most of these entities are discussed in other sections of this book. Here we shall briefly review current concepts of pathogenesis that may be common to all and discuss those in which lung involvement is the primary or major problem. In terms of frequency, the most common conditions are environmental diseases (24%), sarcoidosis (20%), idiopathic pulmonary fibrosis (15%), and the collagen-vascular diseases (8%). The remainder have over 100 different causes and associations.

PATHOGENESIS. It is now thought that regardless of the type of interstitial disease or specific cause, the earliest common manifestation of most of the interstitial diseases is *alveolitis,*[65,66] i.e., an accumulation within the alveolar structure of inflammatory and immune effector cells (Fig. 16–36). Under normal conditions these cells account for no more than 7% of the total lung cell population, and consist of macrophages (93%), lymphocytes (7%), and neutrophils and eosinophils (less than 1%). In alveolitis there is a marked increase in the number of these cells, and a change in their relative proportions. The accumulation of leukocytes has two consequences: it distorts the normal alveolar structures *and* results in the release of mediators that can injure parenchymal cells and stimulate fibrosis. The final result is an end-stage fibrotic lung in which the alveoli are replaced by cystic spaces separated by thick bands of connective tissue interspersed with inflammatory cells. This is the picture of the "end-stage lung" in which there is widespread loss of function of alveolocapillary units.

Let us briefly examine the various components of the scheme shown in Figure 16–36. The initial stimuli for the alveolitis are as heterogeneous as the causes outlined in Table 16–5. Some of these stimuli, such as oxygen-derived free radicals and some chemicals, are

Table 16–5. Diffuse Interstitial Lung Diseases

Known Cause	Unknown Cause

1. Occupational and environmental inhalants
   a. Inorganic dusts (silicosis, asbestos, coal workers' pneumoconiosis (Chapter 9)
   b. Organic dusts (hypersensitivity pneumonitis)
   c. Gases, fumes, aerosols (oxygen toxicity, sulfur dioxide, toluene)
2. Drugs and toxins
   Chemotherapeutic agents (busulfan, bleomycin)
   Antibiotics (nitrofurantoin)
   Other drugs (gold, penicillamine)
   Toxins (paraquat)
3. Infections
   Viral (influenza, cytomegalovirus)
   Bacterial (widespread tuberculosis)
   Fungal
   Parasitic *(Pneumocystis carinii)*
	1. Sarcoidosis
	2. Associated with collagen-vascular disorders and vasculitis (e.g., rheumatoid arthritis, systemic lupus erythematosus, Wegener's granulomatosis)
	3. Goodpasture's syndrome
	4. Idiopathic pulmonary hemosiderosis
	5. Eosinophilic pneumonia
	6. Histiocytosis X
	7. Alveolar proteinosis
	8. Desquamative interstitial pneumonitis
	9. Idiopathic pulmonary fibrosis

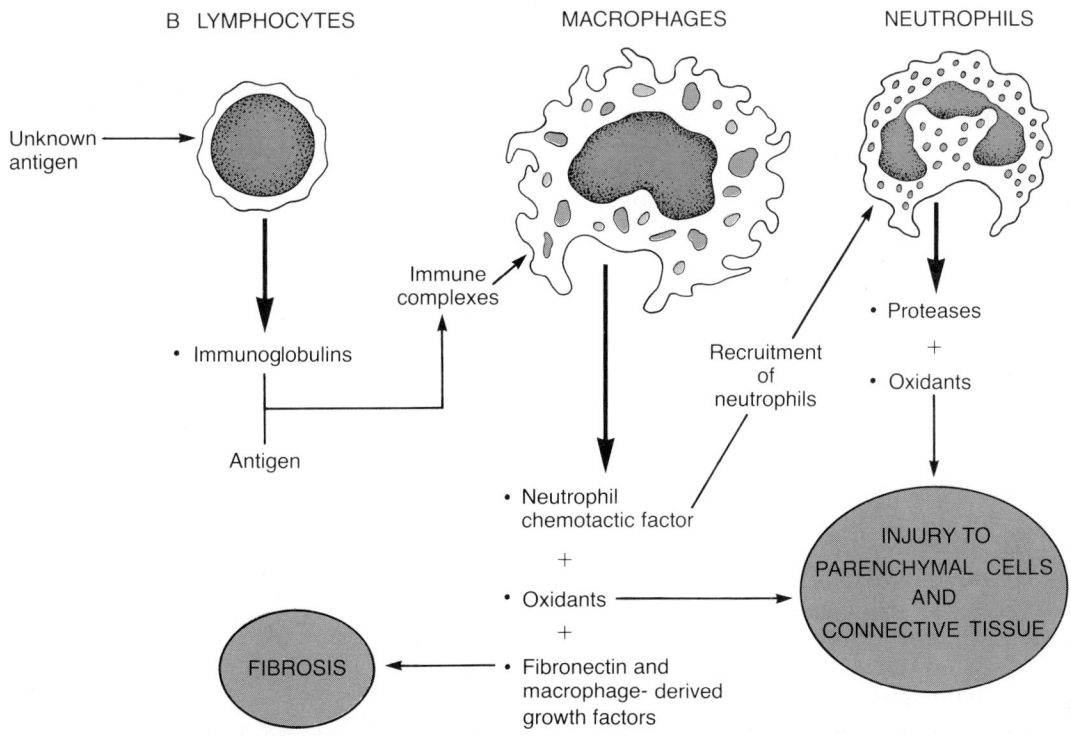

Figure 16-36. Current concepts of the pathogenesis of idiopathic pulmonary fibrosis, in which immune complexes to some undetermined antigen may be the initial trigger to macrophage and neutrophil accumulation and activation. In other conditions, T cell–mediated reactions may predominate. The end result is lung damage and fibrosis.

directly toxic to endothelial cells, epithelial cells, or both. But beyond direct toxicity, the critical event is the *recruitment and activation of inflammatory and immune effector cells.* Neutrophil recruitment can be caused by complement activation in some immune-mediated disorders, but in addition the alveolar macrophages, which increase in number in all interstitial diseases, release a *chemotactic factor* that is relatively specific for neutrophils (NCF). Asbestos particles and immune complexes (through the Fc receptor on the macrophage) stimulate the release of NCF. NCF also "activates" the neutrophils, causing them to secrete proteases and toxic oxygen free radicals, which contribute further to tissue damage and provide a mechanism for maintenance of the alveolitis. In diseases such as sarcoidosis, *cell-mediated* immune reactions result in the accumulation of monocytes and T lymphocytes, and formation of granulomas. It is thought that interactions among lymphocytes and macrophages and the release of lymphokines and monokines are responsible for the slowly progressive pulmonary fibrosis that ensues. The alveolar macrophage, in particular, plays a central role in the development of fibrosis. As reviewed in the discussion of chronic inflammation (p. 62), macrophages elaborate several factors that can cause tissue destruction (e.g., oxygen-derived free radicals, proteases) and promote fibroblast proliferation and collagen deposition (e.g., platelet-derived growth factor [PDGF], fibroblast growth factor [FGF], and interleukin-1 [IL-1]).

PNEUMOCONIOSIS

This term designates a disease of the lungs caused by the inhalation of dust. Policard defines it far more elegantly: "The conflict of living matter with the mineral world: the pneumoconioses."

The variety of clinically and anatomically described pneumoconioses appears to grow with each year. As environmental diseases, they have been covered in Chapter 9, with principal attention to coal workers' pneumoconiosis, silicosis, and berylliosis, asbestosis.

IDIOPATHIC PULMONARY FIBROSIS

This term refers to a poorly understood pulmonary disorder characterized histologically by diffuse interstitial inflammation and fibrosis, which in the advanced case results in severe hypoxemia and cyanosis. There are at least 20 synonyms for this entity (e.g., chronic interstitial pneumonitis, Hamman-Rich syndrome), and in Britain it is known as *diffuse* or *cryptogenic* (i.e., *idiopathic*) *fibrosing alveolitis.* The term *usual interstitial pneumonitis (UIP)* is employed by some to differentiate this condition from the desquamative type (desquamative interstitial pneumonia, or DIP) described later and from other, rarer examples of so-called giant cell and lymphocytic interstitial pneumonitis.[64,68] It should be stressed that similar pathologic findings may occur as the result of well-defined entities, such as the pneumoconioses, hypersensitivity pneumonitis, oxygen toxicity pneumonitis, scleroderma, and irradiation injury. In about half the cases of interstitial fibrosis, however, there is no known underlying disease, and the term *idiopathic* is applied.

Males are affected more often than females, and although the disease may occur at any age, most patients are between 30 and 50 years old.

It is now thought that this disorder represents a stereotyped inflammatory response of the alveolar wall to injuries of different types, durations, and intensities. The proposed sequence of events, described earlier (p. 790), begins with some form of alveolar wall injury, which results in interstitial edema and accumulation of inflammatory cells (alveolitis). The type I membranous pneumocyte is particularly susceptible to injury. Subsequently there is hyperplasia of type II pneumocytes in an attempt to regenerate the alveolar epithelial lining. Fibroblasts then proliferate, and progressive fibrosis and collagenization of both the interalveolar septa and the intra-alveolar exudate result in obliteration of normal pulmonary architecture.

Immune mechanisms may trigger this sequence of events.[65] There are high levels of circulating immune complexes or cryoimmunoglobulins in the serum of patients with idiopathic interstitial pneumonia, particularly in cases in which biopsy shows significant cellular infiltration rather than interstitial fibrosis. Granular deposits of IgG can be seen in the alveolar walls, suggesting that immune complexes may play a pathogenetic role, but the nature of the antigens within the complexes is unknown.

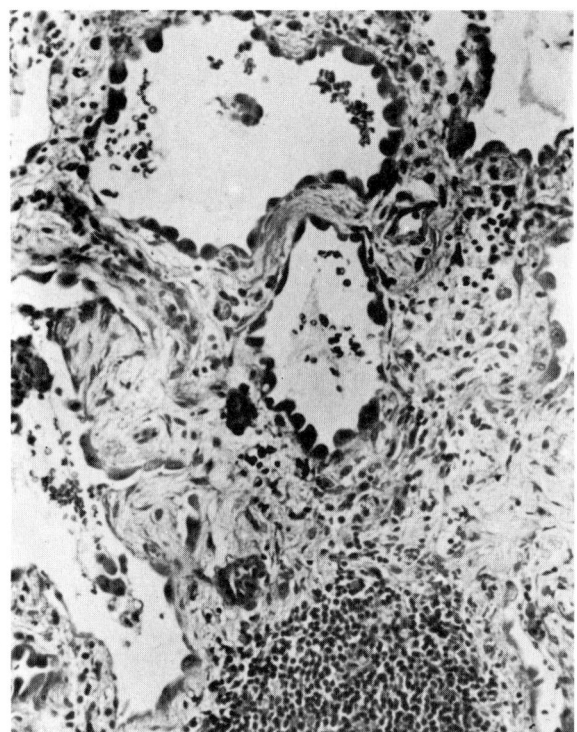

Figure 16–37. Diffuse interstitial fibrosis. Note marked interstitial fibrosis, focal chronic inflammation, and dilated spaces lined by cuboidal type II epithelial cells.

> The morphologic changes vary according to the stage of the disease. In early cases, the lungs grossly are firm in consistency and microscopically show pulmonary edema, intra-alveolar exudation, hyaline membranes, and infiltration of the alveolar septa with mononuclear cells. There is hyperplasia of type II pneumocytes, which appear as cuboidal or even columnar cells lining the alveolar spaces. With advancing disease, there is organization of the intra-alveolar exudate by fibrous tissue, as well as thickening of the interstitial septa owing to fibrosis and variable amounts of inflammation. At this stage the lungs become solid, with alternating areas of fibrosis and more normal-appearing lung. In the end stages of the disorder, the lung consists of spaces lined by cuboidal or columnar epithelium and separated by inflammatory fibrous tissue (Fig. 16–37). This gives the typical appearance of the **honeycomb lung.** Small cysts are often seen, and there is also intimal thickening of the pulmonary arteries and lymphoid hyperplasia. As mentioned earlier, this advanced picture can result from any of the disorders listed in Table 16–5. Thus it is necessary to exclude the known causes of interstitial fibrosis by clinical, radiologic, or serologic means before the diagnosis of idiopathic interstitial fibrosis is made.

As would be expected, patients exhibit varying degrees of respiratory difficulty and, in advanced cases, hypoxemia and cyanosis. The septal fibrosis constitutes a significant physiologic alveolocapillary block. Cor pulmonale and cardiac failure may result. The progress in the individual case is unpredictable. In some patients the disease remits spontaneously. In a few the process progresses very rapidly, leading to fibrosis in a matter of weeks, whereas in others it develops over many years. In most cases, death occurs in about two years.

DESQUAMATIVE INTERSTITIAL PNEUMONITIS (DIP)

In some patients with interstitial pneumonitis there is prominent aggregation of mononuclear cells within the alveoli, presumably desquamated from the alveolar walls.[69] These patients usually present with the slow development of cough and dyspnea, eventually leading to marked respiratory embarrassment, cyanosis, and clubbing of the fingers. Classically, the radiologic picture is that of bilateral lower-lobe ground-glass infiltrates.

> The most striking histologic finding is the accumulation in the airspaces of a large number of macrophages containing lipid and PAS-positive granules. Some of the macrophages contain lamellar bodies (surfactant) within phagocytic vacuoles, presumably derived from necrotic type II pneumocytes. There is often an interstitial pneumonitis and

an accompanying hyperplasia of the septal lining epithelial cells and desquamation of these cells into the airspaces (Fig. 16–38).

The cause is unknown. Patients are benefited by steroid therapy, which often leads to clearing of the lungs. Some patients with DIP have or subsequently develop significant interstitial fibrosis; for this reason, many authors object to the term DIP and consider the entity an early stage of idiopathic interstitial fibrosis, discussed earlier. Nevertheless, the presence of a prominent desquamative component has practical implications because such patients apparently have a better response to steroid therapy than those with the usual interstitial fibrotic pattern.[64]

HYPERSENSITIVITY PNEUMONITIS

The term hypersensitivity pneumonitis describes a spectrum of immunologically mediated, predominantly interstitial lung disorders caused by intense and often prolonged exposure to inhaled organic dusts and related occupational antigens.[64,70] Affected individuals have an abnormal sensitivity or heightened reactivity to the antigen, which, in contrast to that occurring in asthma, involves primarily the *alveoli*. It is important to recognize these diseases early in their course, as progression to serious chronic fibrotic lung disease can be prevented by removal of the environmental agent.

Most commonly, hypersensitivity results from the inhalation of organic dust containing antigens made up of spores of thermophilic bacteria, true fungi, animal proteins, or bacterial products. Numerous specifically named syndromes are described, depending on the occupation or exposure of the individual. *Farmer's lung* results from exposure to dusts generated from harvested, humid, warm hay that permits the rapid proliferation of the spores of thermophilic actinomycetes. *Pigeon breeder's lung* (bird fancier's disease) is provoked by proteins from serum, excreta, or feathers of the birds. *Humidifier* or *air-conditioner lung* is caused by thermophilic bacteria in heated water reservoirs. There is also a mushroom picker's lung, a maple bark disease, and duck fever (from duck feathers).

The clinical manifestations are varied. Acute attacks, which follow inhalation of antigenic dust in sensitized patients, consist of recurring attacks of fever, dyspnea, cough, and leukocytosis. Diffuse and nodular infiltrates appear in the chest radiograph, and pulmonary function tests show an acute restrictive effect. Symptoms usually appear four to six hours after exposure. If exposure is continuous and protracted, a chronic form of the disease supervenes that no longer features the acute exacerbations on antigen reexposure. Instead, there are signs of progressive respiratory failure, dyspnea, and cyanosis and a decrease in total lung capacity and compliance—a picture hard to differentiate from other forms of chronic interstitial disease.

Histologic descriptions come from biopsies of patients with subacute and chronic forms, rather than from those with acute attacks. The alterations include interstitial pneumonitis consisting primarily of lymphocytes, plasma cells, and macrophages (some of the latter having a foamy cytoplasm); interstitial fibrosis; obliterative bronchiolitis; and outright granuloma formation. In over half the patients there is also evidence of an intra-alveolar infiltrate.

The evidence from experimental and human studies strongly suggests a type III immune complex pathogenesis for the early lesions, followed by a type IV delayed hypersensitivity reaction for the granulomatous components.

Byssinosis is an occupational lung disease of textile workers that is apparently induced by the inhalation of airborne fibers of cotton, linen, and hemp. Acute effects include cough, wheezing, and airway obstruction, a picture that resembles bronchial asthma. Prolonged exposure leads to disabling chronic lung disease characterized by chronic bronchitis, emphysema, and interstitial granulomas. Evidence for an immunologic hypersensitivity in this disorder is not as clear as in the other conditions described under this heading.

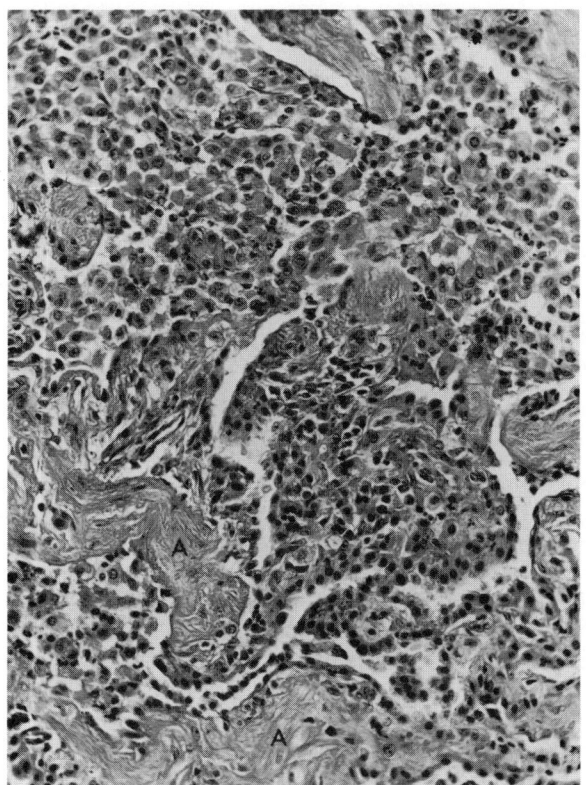

Figure 16–38. Desquamative interstitial pneumonitis. High-power detail of lung to demonstrate fibrous thickening of alveolar walls (A) and accumulation of large numbers of mononuclear cells within alveolar spaces.

PULMONARY EOSINOPHILIA (PULMONARY INFILTRATION WITH EOSINOPHILIA)

A number of clinical and pathologic pulmonary entities are characterized by an infiltration of eosinophils. The cause and pathogenesis of these disorders are diverse. They have been divided into the following categories:[71] (1) *simple pulmonary eosinophilia,* or Loeffler's syndrome; (2) *tropical eosinophilia,* caused by infection with *microfilariae* (p. 417); (3) *secondary chronic pulmonary eosinophilia* (which occurs in a number of parasitic, fungal, and bacterial infections; in hypersensitivity pneumonitis; in drug allergies; and in association with asthma, allergic bronchopulmonary aspergillosis, or polyarteritis nodosa); and (4) so-called idiopathic *chronic eosinophilic pneumonia.* The mechanisms that lead to eosinophilia in these conditions are almost certainly immunologic, although the sequence of events for each is far from clear.

Loeffler's syndrome is characterized by transient pulmonary lesions, eosinophilia in the blood, and a benign clinical course. Roentgenograms are often quite striking, with shadows of varying size and shape in any of the lobes suggesting irregular intrapulmonary densities. The lungs show alveoli whose septa are thickened by an infiltrate composed of eosinophils and occasional interspersed giant cells. There is also focal hyperplasia of the alveolar epithelial lining cells, but no vasculitis, fibrosis, or necrosis.

Chronic eosinophilic pneumonia is characterized by focal areas of cellular consolidation of the lung substance distributed chiefly in the periphery of the lung fields. Prominent in these lesions are heavy aggregates of lymphocytes and eosinophils within both the septal walls and the alveolar spaces. Clinically there is high fever, night sweats, and dyspnea, all of which respond to corticosteroid therapy. Obviously, this rare entity can be diagnosed only when other causes of chronic pulmonary eosinophilia are excluded.

DIFFUSE PULMONARY HEMORRHAGE AND GOODPASTURE'S SYNDROME

Hemorrhage from the lung is a dramatic complication of some interstitial lung disorders. Among these so-called *pulmonary hemorrhage syndromes*[72] are (1) Goodpasture's syndrome; (2) idiopathic pulmonary hemosiderosis; and (3) vasculitis-associated hemorrhage, which is found in conditions such as hypersensitivity angiitis, Wegener's granulomatosis, and lupus erythematosus.

Goodpasture's syndrome is an uncommon but intriguing condition characterized by the *simultaneous appearance of a form of proliferative, usually rapidly progressive glomerulonephritis and a necrotizing hemorrhagic interstitial pneumonitis.* The evidence is quite substantial that the renal and pulmonary lesions are the consequence of antibodies evoked by antigens common to the glomerular and pulmonary basement membranes.[73] The immunopathogenesis of the syndrome and the nature of the Goodpasture's antigens are described on page 1031, in the discussion of glomerulonephritis. Most cases begin clinically with respiratory symptoms, principally hemoptysis, and radiographic evidence of focal pulmonary consolidations. Very soon, manifestations of glomerulonephritis appear, leading to rapidly progressive renal failure. The common cause of death is uremia. Most cases occur in the second or third decade of life and there is a preponderance among males.

In the classic case, the lungs are heavy and contain focal areas of red-brown apparent consolidation. Histologically, there are acute focal necroses of alveolar walls associated with intra-alveolar hemorrhages, fibrous thickening of the septa, and hypertrophy of lining septal cells. Depending on the duration of the disease, there may be organization of blood in the alveolar spaces. Often the alveoli contain hemosiderin-laden macrophages (Fig. 16-39). Immunofluorescent studies reveal linear deposits of immunoglobulins along the basement membranes of the septal walls. The kidneys reveal the characteristic findings of focal proliferative glomerulonephritis in the early cases, or crescentic glomerulonephritis in patients with rapidly progressive glomerulonephritis. Immunofluorescent linear deposits of immunoglobulins and complement are also seen along the glomerular basement membranes, similar to those in the alveolar septa.

Although it is clear that antibasement antibodies are associated with this disease, the trigger initiating the autoimmune disorder is still unknown. In experimental animals, concomitant toxic pulmonary injury by toxic oxygen species or hydrocarbons increases fixation of antibodies onto basement membranes and induces pulmonary hemorrhage. In humans, virus infection, exposure to hydrocarbon solvents (used in the dry-cleaning industry), and smoking have been implicated as cofactors in the causation of the syndrome and may act by a similar mechanism.

The once dismal prognosis for this disease has been markedly improved by intensive *plasma exchange.* This procedure is thought to be beneficial by removing circulating anti-basement membrane antibodies as well as chemical mediators of immunologic injury. Simultaneous immunosuppressive therapy inhibits further antibody production. Both the lung hemorrhage and the glomerulonephritis improve with this form of therapy.

IDIOPATHIC PULMONARY HEMOSIDEROSIS

This uncommon pulmonary disease of obscure nature usually presents with an insidious onset of productive

/>

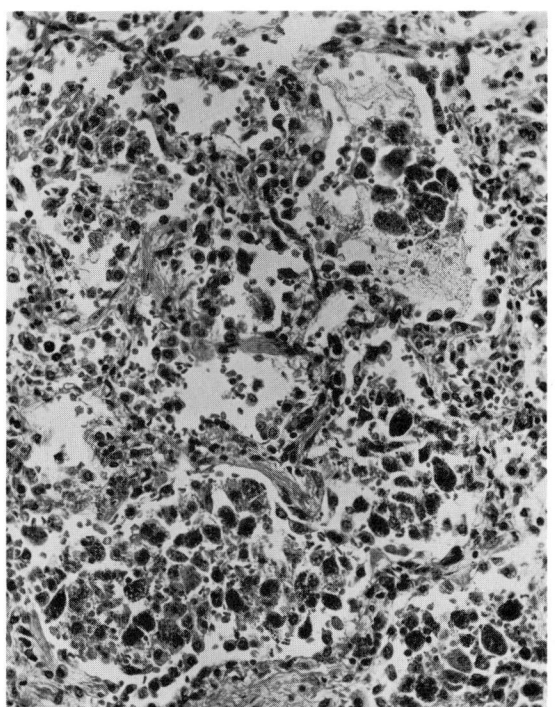

Figure 16–39. Lung in Goodpasture's syndrome. Alveolar walls are thickened with focal areas of necrosis. Alveolar spaces contain hemosiderin-laden macrophages secondary to intra-alveolar hemorrhages.

cough, hemoptysis, anemia, and weight loss associated with diffuse pulmonary infiltrations similar to Goodpasture's Syndrome. However, it tends to occur in younger adults and children. The cause and pathogenesis are unknown, and no anti–basement membrane antibodies are detectable in serum or tissues.

The lungs are moderately increased in weight, with focal areas of consolidation that are usually red-brown to red. The cardinal histologic features of pulmonary hemosiderosis are reported as "striking degeneration, shedding and hyperplasia of alveolar epithelial cells, and marked localized alveolar capillary dilatation." There are varying degrees of pulmonary interstitial fibrosis; hemorrhage into the alveolar spaces; and hemosiderosis, both within the alveolar septa and in macrophages lying free within the pulmonary alveoli.

Idiopathic pulmonary hemosiderosis runs the gamut from mild to severe disease. Some patients have recurrent, not severe, episodes of hemoptysis with intervening periods of good health (save for anemia) and may have a normal life span. Some develop progressive pulmonary fibrosis and run an erratic progressive course with advancing cardiac failure; others may die suddenly of massive pulmonary hemorrhage. Patients follow a chronic remittent course over a period of years, and then improve spontaneously or with treatment and have no further recurrences.

PULMONARY ALVEOLAR PROTEINOSIS

This is a disease of obscure cause and pathogenesis, characterized radiologically by diffuse pulmonary opacification and histologically by accumulation in the intra-alveolar spaces of a dense granular, strongly PAS-positive material that contains abundant lipid.[74] This entity is discussed here because the radiographic picture is one of diffuse infiltrative disease, but its histologic alterations are intra-alveolar rather than alveolar and it does not usually progress to chronic fibrosis. Patients, for the most part, present with nonspecific respiratory difficulty of insidious onset, cough, and abundant sputum that often contains chunks of gelatinous material. Some have symptoms lasting for years, often with febrile illnesses. Progressive dyspnea, cyanosis, and respiratory insufficiency may occur, but some patients tend to have a benign course, with eventual resolution of the lesions.

Morphologically, the disease is characterized by a peculiar, homogeneous, granular precipitate within the alveoli, causing focal-to-confluent consolidation of large areas of the lungs (Fig. 16–40). On section, turbid fluid exudes from these areas. As a consequence, there is a marked increase in size and weight of the lung. The alveolar precipitate is PAS-positive and also contains finely divided lipid. Biochemically, the material is similar to surfactant but fails to show surfactant properties. By electron microscopy, the

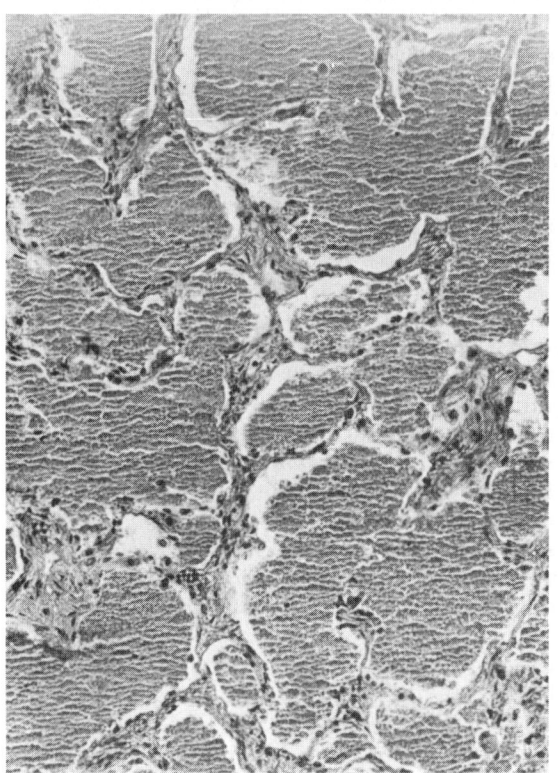

Figure 16–40. Pulmonary alveolar proteinosis. Alveoli are filled with a dense amorphous protein-lipid granular precipitate.

alveolar contents consist of necrotic alveolar macrophages and type II pneumocytes, amorphous precipitate, with considerable numbers of lamellar osmiophilic bodies morphologically resembling surfactant material. The involved alveoli are often lined with hyperplastic pneumocytes, and focal areas of necrosis of these cells are seen with the light microscope. There is a surprising absence of any inflammatory reaction in the affected alveoli.

Some patients suffering from this disease may have an occupational exposure to irritating dusts (including silica dust) and other chemicals. This disease also occurs in immunosuppressed patients and in association with hematolymphoid malignancies and opportunistic infections.[75] Theories of pathogenesis suggest either excessive production of surfactant-like material by hyperplastic type II epithelial cells or, more likely, a defect in the macrophage clearance of intra-alveolar accumulations of surfactant.

PULMONARY INVOLVEMENT IN COLLAGEN-VASCULAR DISORDERS

These diseases are discussed in other chapters but are listed here, since they can lead to a picture of chronic interstitial fibrosis.[76]

Diffuse interstitial fibrosis occurs classically in progressive systemic sclerosis (*scleroderma*), discussed on page 206. Less commonly, patchy and transient parenchymal infiltrates are noted in *lupus erythematosus*, and occasionally severe lupus pneumonitis may occur and may be one of the major clinical problems in such patients. In *rheumatoid arthritis*, pulmonary involvement is common and may occur in one of five forms: (1) chronic pleuritis, with or without effusion; (2) diffuse interstitial pneumonitis and fibrosis; (3) intrapulmonary rheumatoid nodules; (4) rheumatoid nodules with pneumoconiosis (Caplan's syndrome); and (5) pulmonary hypertension. Thirty to 40% of patients with classic rheumatoid arthritis have abnormalities in pulmonary function. In certain patients the disorder progresses to end-stage lung disease. Lung involvement is also common in the vasculitides[77] (p. 573), particularly in allergic angiitis and granulomatosis (the Churg-Strauss syndrome).

Wegener's granulomatosis, considered on page 574, represents an acute necrotizing vasculitis with granuloma formation, affecting particularly the lungs, kidneys, and upper respiratory tract. In the lung, there are necrotizing granulomas and a prominent vasculitis. *Lymphomatoid granulomatosis* is a disorder characterized by an aggressive pleomorphic cell infiltrate composed of lymphocytes, large macrophages, and plasma cells; vascular involvement; and destruction of lung parenchyma. Although it may remain confined to the lung, the disease can affect the skin, nervous system, and kidney, and in 15 to 50% of cases it may evolve into a malignant lymphoma.

OTHER FORMS OF PULMONARY DISEASE

LIPID PNEUMONIA

This term refers to patchy pneumonic consolidation associated with accumulation of lipid, usually within "foamy" macrophages.

In *endogenous or obstructive* lipid pneumonia, the lipid is derived from degenerating cells, including surfactant from type II pneumocytes.[13] The most frequent causes are obstruction by bronchogenic cancer, tuberculosis, abscess formation, and bronchiectasis. Grossly, the pneumonic foci show a characteristic yellow color ("golden pneumonia") caused by accumulation of foamy, fat-filled macrophages, which fill the alveoli. Cholesterol clefts surrounded by giant cells are often also present histologically.

Exogenous lipid pneumonia is caused by aspiration of a variety of oils. This is usually encountered in weak infants and in those with congenital malformations in whom the swallowing reflex may be deranged. In adults, lipid pneumonia usually follows the protracted use of mineral oil as a laxative or the use of oily nose drops or hairsprays. In general, the more unsaturated the oil, the greater is its toxicity. Some of the most reactive oils are those found in lard and peanuts. When aspirated, even milk and cream are capable of evoking an inflammatory response.

MORPHOLOGY. In general, the lesions are bilateral, but in the exogenous form they tend to affect the right lung more than the left because of the direct drainage path of the right main stem bronchus. The aspirated oil is emulsified once it reaches the alveoli, and the fine droplets are phagocytized by large numbers of macrophages called out in response to this foreign material (Fig. 16–41). Multinucleate giant cells are often present. With progression of the lesion, fibroblasts invade the cellular lipid exudate. Multinucleate giant cells may develop within the alveolar organization, to form granulomas.

Lipid pneumonia may be discovered as an incidental finding at autopsy. However, symptomatic manifestations may be occasioned by superimposed bronchitis, bronchiolitis, bronchiectasis, and bronchopneumonia.

DRUG-INDUCED PULMONARY DISEASE

Drugs can cause a variety of respiratory alterations in structure and function,[64,78] including bronchospasms, pulmonary edema, chronic pneumonitis with fibrosis, and hypersensitivity pneumonitis (Table 16–6). For example, cytotoxic drugs used in cancer therapy (e.g., bleomycin) cause pneumonitis and pulmonary fibrosis as a result of direct toxicity of the drug and by

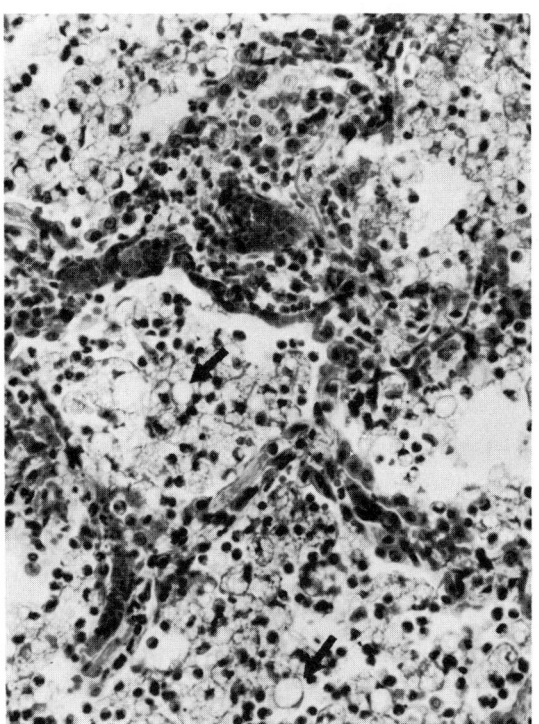

Figure 16-41. Lipid pneumonia. Alveoli contain the characteristic lipid-laden macrophages with large, clear cytoplasmic vacuoles (arrows).

stimulating the influx of inflammatory cells into the alveoli. Amiodarone, a drug that controls resistant cardiac arrhythmias, is preferentially concentrated in the lung and causes significant pneumonitis in 5 to 15% of patients receiving the drug. The point to make is that drug-induced pulmonary disease may mimic pulmonary changes due to other causes and must therefore be considered in the differential diagnosis of pulmonary dysfunction.

TUMORS OF LUNG

A variety of benign and malignant tumors may arise in the lung, but the vast majority (90 to 95%) are bronchogenic carcinomas.[79,80] About 5% are bronchial carcinoids, and 2 to 5% are mesenchymal and other miscellaneous neoplasms. The term "bronchogenic" is used for most lung cancers, but it is somewhat mis-

Table 16-6. Examples of Drug-Induced Pulmonary Disease

DRUG	PULMONARY DISEASE
Cytotoxic drugs:	
bleomycin	Pneumonitis and fibrosis
methotrexate	Hypersensitivity pneumonitis
Amidarone	Pneumonitis and fibrosis
Nitrofurantoin	Hypersensitivity pneumonitis
Aspirin	Bronchospasm
Beta-antagonists	Bronchospasm

leading in that it implies a bronchial origin for all lung cancers, despite the fact that adenocarcinomas, which are peripheral in location, are most often bronchiolar in derivation.

BRONCHOGENIC CARCINOMA

In industrialized nations, public enemy number one among cancers is bronchogenic carcinoma. It is the most common visceral malignancy in males; it alone accounts for approximately one third of all cancer deaths in males and one twentieth of all deaths in both sexes. Although females are affected less frequently, the incidence is increasing dramatically, and lung cancer has passed breast carcinoma as a cause of cancer death in women.[81]

INCIDENCE. The annual number of deaths from lung cancer in the United States increased from 18,000 in 1950 to an estimated 125,000 in 1988.[81] The age-adjusted death rate from cancer of the lung since 1950 has more than trebled in males, rising from 19.9 to an outstanding 74 per 100,000 population. The death rate in females since 1950 has risen from 4.5 to 25 per 100,000. Cancer of the lung now accounts for 20% of all cancers in males and 11% in females. In 1988 there were an estimated 150,000 new cases of lung cancer.

Cancer of the lung occurs most often between ages 40 and 70 years, with a peak incidence in the sixth or seventh decade. Only 2% of all cases appear before the age of 40. The male-female death rate and incidence ratio for lung cancer among whites reached a peak of approximately 7:1 in 1960, but in 1988 it had fallen to 2:1 — almost certainly the delayed consequence of increased cigarette smoking among women.

ETIOLOGY AND PATHOGENESIS

TOBACCO SMOKING. The evidence establishing a positive relationship between tobacco smoking and lung cancer is well-nigh incontrovertible. The collective evidence is of three kinds: statistical, clinical, and experimental.[82,83]

Statistical evidence is most compelling. In numerous retrospective studies of patients who died of bronchogenic carcinoma compared with controls, there was an invariable statistical association between the frequency of lung cancer and (1) the amount of daily smoking, (2) the tendency to inhale, and (3) the duration of the smoking habit. Compared with nonsmokers, average smokers of cigarettes have a tenfold greater risk of developing lung cancer, and heavy smokers (over 40 cigarettes per day for several years) have at least a 20-fold greater risk. Eighty per cent of lung cancers occur in smokers. Cessation of smoking for 10 years reduces risk to control levels. The epidemiologic studies also show an association between cigarette smoking and the following cancers, in decreasing order of frequency: lip, tongue, floor of mouth, pharynx, larynx, esophagus, urinary bladder, and pancreas.[83] Cigar and pipe smoking increases risk, though much more modestly than smoking of unfiltered cigarettes.

Clinical evidence is largely obtained through observing histologic changes in the lining epithelium of the respiratory tract in smokers. A systematic study of bronchial epithelium of smokers showed atypical and hyperplastic changes in about 10% of smokers, 1 to 2% of those smoking filter-tipped cigarettes, and 15% of patients who died of lung cancer; 96.7% of cigarette smokers showed some atypical cells in the bronchial tree, whereas 0.9% of controls had similar cells.[84,85]

The *experimental work* has focused mainly on attempts to induce cancer in experimental animals with extracts of tobacco smoke.[86] Over 1200 substances have been counted in cigarette smoke, and many of these are potential carcinogens. They include both initiators (polycyclic aromatic hydrocarbons, such as benzo[a]pyrene) and promoters such as phenol derivatives. Radioactive elements may also be found (polonium-210, carbon-14, potassium-40) as well as other contaminants, such as arsenic, nickel, molds, and additives. Protracted exposure of mice to these additives induces skin tumors. However, efforts to produce lung cancer by exposing animals to tobacco smoke have been unsuccessful. The few cancers that have been produced have been bronchioloalveolar carcinomas, a type of human tumor not associated with smoking in humans.

INDUSTRIAL HAZARDS. Certain industrial exposures increase the risk of development of lung cancer. All types of *radiation* may be carcinogenic.[87] There was an increased incidence of lung cancer among survivors of the Hiroshima and Nagasaki atomic bomb blasts. *Uranium* is weakly radioactive, but lung cancer rates among nonsmoking uranium miners are four times higher than those of the general population, and among smoking miners they are about ten times higher.

Asbestos has now become a universally recognized carcinogen, particularly when coupled with smoking.[88] Asbestos workers who do not smoke have a five times increased risk, and those who smoke have a 50 to 90 times greater risk of developing lung cancer than do nonsmoking controls. The latent period before the development of lung cancer is 10 to 30 years. Among asbestos workers, one death in five is due to bronchogenic carcinoma, one in ten to pleural or peritoneal mesotheliomas (p. 857), and one in ten to gastrointestinal carcinomas.

There is also an increased risk of respiratory cancer among persons who work with *nickel, chromates, coal, mustard gas, arsenic, beryllium,* and *iron* and in newspaper workers, African gold miners, and haloether workers.[82]

AIR POLLUTION. Unquestionably, we all "swim" in a sea of carcinogens, and it is conceivable that atmospheric pollutants may play some role in the increased incidence of bronchogenic carcinoma today. However, there is a difference of opinion as to whether urban as opposed to rural areas have an increased risk *after* populations are corrected for smoking. Although most authorities acknowledge the existence of a small *urban factor* in lung cancer incidence, the main culprit, far and away, is cigarette smoking.[89]

GENETIC FACTORS. Occasional familial clustering has suggested a genetic predisposition to lung cancer, as has the variable risk even among very heavy smokers. However, attempts at defining markers of genetic susceptibility have proved elusive.

SCARRING. The *pathogenesis* of lung cancer has been discussed in the chapter on neoplasia. Recent studies have shown the occurrence of activated oncogenes in lung cancer tissue.[90] These include amplification of *myc* genes in small cell cancers, point mutations in coding regions of *ras* oncogenes in several types of cancer cell lines, and specific mutational activation of *K-ras* oncogene in adenocarcinomas.[91] Whether increases or alterations in the proteins expressed by these activated genes play a role in the pathogenesis of lung cancer is now under study.

Finally some lung cancers arise in the vicinity of pulmonary scars and are termed "scar cancers." Histologically, these tumors are usually adenocarcinomas. Among the scars incriminated are old infarcts, metallic foreign bodies, wounds, and granulomatous infections such as tuberculosis. In most instances of scarring in cancers, however, the fibrosis is secondary to the cancer, rather than being a pre-existing lesion.

HISTOLOGIC CLASSIFICATION. Numerous histologic classifications of bronchogenic carcinoma have been proposed, but the currently popular ones, based on classifications of the World Health Organization (Table 16–7),[92] divide these tumors into four major categories: squamous cell carcinoma, making up 35 to 50%; adenocarcinoma, 15 to 35%; small cell carcinoma, 20 to 25%; and large cell carcinoma, 10 to 15%.[93] The range of incidences reflects different populations (autopsy or surgical series) and the use of

Table 6–7. Histologic Classification of Bronchogenic Carcinoma

---

Squamous cell (epidermoid) carcinoma
Adenocarcinoma
   Bronchial derived
     (acinar; papillary; solid)
   Bronchioloalveolar
Small cell carcinoma
   Oat cell (lymphoycyte-like)
   Intermediate cell (polygonal)
   Combined (usually with squamous)
Large cell carcinoma
   (undifferentiated; giant cell; clear cell)
Combined squamous cell carcinoma and
   adenocarcinoma

varying histologic criteria among different pathologists. In addition, there may be mixtures of the histologic pattern, even in the same cancer.[93] Thus, combined types of squamous cell carcinoma and adenocarcinoma or of small cell and squamous cell carcinoma are not infrequent.

From a histogenetic point of view, it seems most likely that all histologic variants of bronchogenic carcinoma, including small cell carcinoma as well as the bronchial carcinoid, to be described later, are derived from entoderm—a view consistent with the frequency of tumors with mixed histologic patterns.[93]

MORPHOLOGY. Bronchogenic carcinomas arise most often in and about the hilus of the lung. About three fourths of the lesions take origin from first-, second-, and third-order bronchi. A small percentage have a more peripheral origin but are still not located far out near the pleura. A small number of primary carcinomas of the lung arise in the periphery of the lung substance from the alveolar septal cells or terminal bronchioles. These are predominantly adenocarcinomas, including those of the bronchioloalveolar type, to be discussed separately.

In its development, **carcinoma of the lung begins as an area of in situ cytologic atypia that, over an unknown interval of time, yields a small area of thickening or piling up of bronchial mucosa.** With progression, this small focus, usually less than 1 cm in area, assumes the appearance of an irregular, warty excrescence that elevates or erodes the lining epithelium (Fig. 16–42). The tumor may then follow one of a variety of paths. It may continue to fungate into the bronchial lumen to produce an intraluminal mass. At other times, it rapidly penetrates the wall of the bronchus to infiltrate along the peribronchial tissue (Fig. 16–43) into the adjacent region of the carina or mediastinum. In other instances, the tumor grows along a broad front to produce a cauliflower-like intraparenchymal mass that appears to push lung substance ahead of it. In almost all patterns, the neoplastic tissue is gray-white and firm to hard. Especially when the tumors are bulky, focal areas of hemorrhage or necrosis may appear to produce yellow-white mottling and softening. Sometimes these necrotic foci cavitate.

Extension may occur to the pleural surface and then within the pleural cavity or into the pericardium. Spread to the tracheal, bronchial, and mediastinal nodes can be found in most cases. The frequency of such nodal involvement varies slightly with the histologic pattern, but averages over 50%.

More distant spread of bronchogenic carcinoma occurs through both lymphatic and hematogenous pathways. These tumors have a distressing habit of spreading widely throughout the body and at an early stage in their evolution. Often the metastasis presents as the first manifestation of the underlying occult bronchogenic lesion. No organ or tissue is spared in the spread of these lesions, but the adrenals, for obscure reasons, are involved in over half the cases. The liver (30 to 50%), brain (20%), and bone (20%) are additional favored sites of metastases.

SQUAMOUS CELL CARCINOMA. This type is most commonly found in men, and it is most closely correlated with a smoking history. The microscopic features are familiar in the form of production of keratin and intercellular bridges in the well-differentiated forms, but many less well-differentiated squamous cell tumors are encountered that begin to merge with the undifferentiated large cell pattern. This

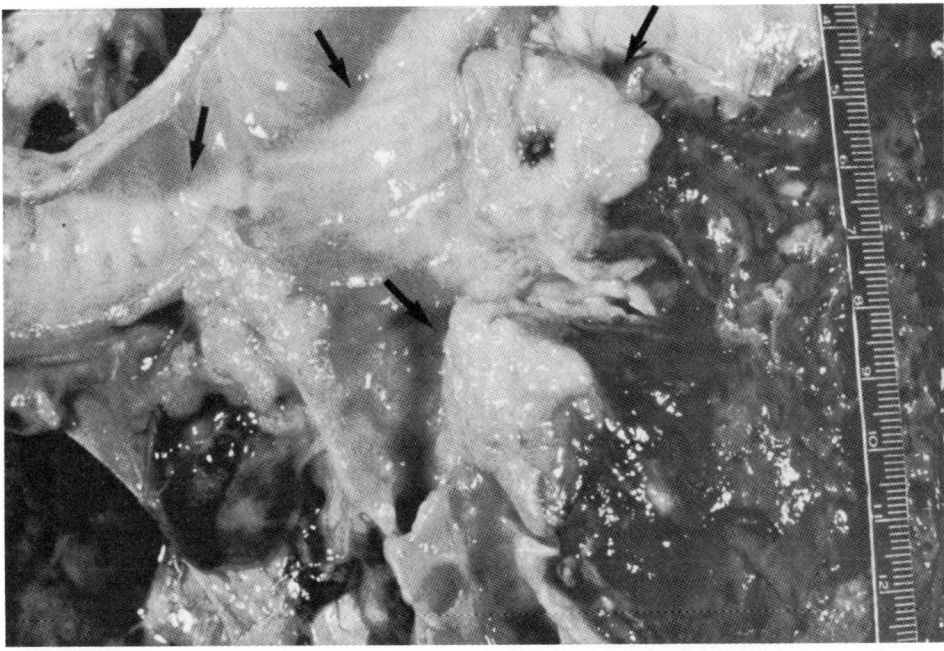

Figure 16–42. Extensive bronchogenic carcinoma arising at bifurcation of trachea. Note white tumor *(arrows)* in the mucosa *(upper left arrows)* and nodular neoplasm invading wall of trachea and main right stem bronchus at several points *(arrows)*.

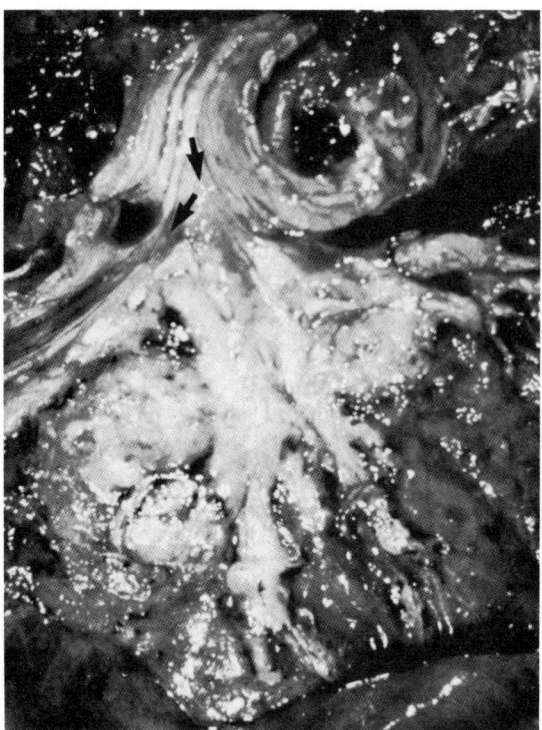

Figure 16–43. Bronchogenic carcinoma infiltrating peribronchial lung substance. Arrows point to bronchial lumen.

tumor tends to spread locally and metastasize somewhat later than the other patterns, but its rate of growth in its site of origin is usually more rapid than that of other types. Squamous metaplasia, epithelial dysplasia, and foci of frank carcinoma in situ are sometimes present in bronchial epithelium adjacent to the tumor mass.

ADENOCARCINOMA. Histologic classifications of adenocarcinomas include at least two forms: (1) the usual bronchial-derived adenocarcinoma; and (2) a somewhat distinctive type termed **bronchioloalveolar carcinoma,** which probably arises from terminal bronchioles or alveolar walls. There may be overlap between these two forms, but the bronchioloalveolar carcinoma has sufficiently distinctive gross, microscopic, and epidemiologic features to be discussed separately.

The regular bronchial adenocarcinoma occurs with about equal frequency in males and females, unlike the small cell or squamous carcinomas, in which there is a preponderance among males. The lesions are usually more peripherally located; tend to be smaller, and vary histologically from well-differentiated tumors with obvious glandular elements to papillary lesions resembling other papillary carcinomas, to solid masses with only occasional mucin-producing glands and cells. About 80% contain mucin. Adenocarcinomas grow more slowly than squamous cell carcinomas. Peripheral adenocarcinomas are sometimes associated with areas of scarring (scar carcinoma). In most cases, the scar is a desmoplastic response to the tumor,[94] but occasionally the scar undoubtedly precedes the cancer.[95] Adenocarcinomas are less frequently associated

with a history of smoking than are squamous cell carcinomas.

SMALL CELL CARCINOMA. This is a highly malignant tumor of a somewhat distinctive cell type. The epithelial cells are generally small, have little cytoplasm, are round or oval, and occasionally lymphocyte-like (though about twice the size of a lymphocyte). This is the classic "oat cell" (Fig. 16–44). Other small cell carcinomas have spindle-shaped or polygonal cells and may be thus classified (spindle or polygonal small cell carcinoma). The cells grow in clusters that exhibit neither glandular or squamous organization.

Electron microscopic studies show dense-core neurosecretory granules in some of these tumor cells.[4,96] The granules are similar to those found in the neuroendocrine argentaffin (Kulchitsky) cells present along the bronchial epithelium, particularly in the fetus and neonate. The occurrence of neurosecretory granules, the ability of some of these tumors to secrete polypeptide hormones, and the presence by immunohistochemical stains of neuroendocrine markers such as neuron-specific enolase, parathormone-like, and other hormonally active products suggest derivation of this tumor from neuroendocrine-programmed cells of the lining bronchial epithelium.

Small cell carcinomas have a strong relationship to cigarette smoking. Most often hilar or central, they are the most aggressive of lung tumors, metastasize widely, and are essentially incurable by surgical means. They are the most common pattern associated with ectopic hormone production.

LARGE CELL CARCINOMA. These anaplastic carcinomas have larger, more polygonal cells and vesicular nuclei. They probably represent those squamous cell carcinomas and adenocarcinomas that are so undifferentiated that they can no longer be recognized. Some of these large cell carcinomas contain intracellular mucin, some exhibit large numbers of multinucleate cells **(giant cell carcinoma),** some have cleared cells and are termed **clear**

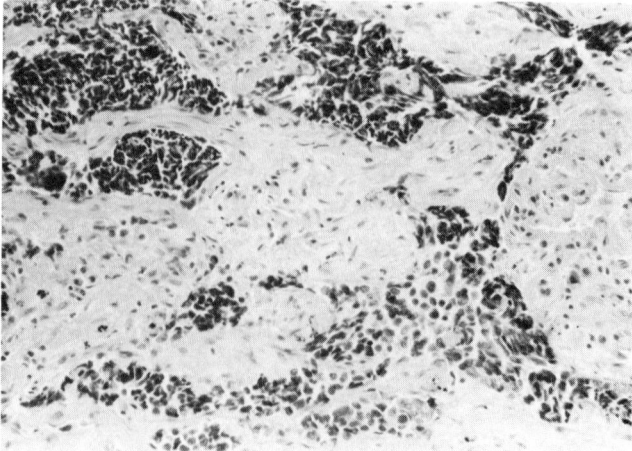

Figure 16–44. Small cell carcinoma. Note islands of small, round, oval or spindly, deeply basophilic cells (Courtesy of Dr. Marcel Seiler, Boston.)

cell carcinoma, and some have a distinctly spindly histologic appearance **(spindle cell carcinoma).**

SECONDARY PATHOLOGY. Bronchogenic carcinomas cause related anatomic changes in the lung substance distal to the point of bronchial involvement. **Partial obstruction may cause marked focal emphysema; total obstruction may lead to atelectasis.** The impaired drainage of the airways is a common cause for **severe suppurative** or **ulcerative bronchitis** or **bronchiectasis. Pulmonary abscesses** sometimes call attention to a silent carcinoma that has initiated the chronic suppuration. Compression or invasion of the superior vena cava may lead either to marked venous congestion or to the full-blown **superior vena caval syndrome.** Extension to the pericardial or pleural sacs may cause **pericarditis** or **pleuritis** with significant effusions.

STAGING. A uniform TNM system for staging cancer according to its anatomic extent at the time of diagnosis is extremely useful for many reasons, chiefly for comparing treatment results from different centers.[97] The following scheme groups tumors according to the TNM classification into four stages:

OCCULT. Bronchopulmonary secretions contain malignant cells, but there is no other evidence of lung cancer (TX NO MO).

STAGE I. A tumor classified as 3 cm or less in greater diameter (T1), with or without involvement of the ipsilateral hilar nodes, or a tumor over 3 cm in diameter without any nodal involvement (T1 NO MO, T1 N1 MO, or T2 NO MO).

STAGE II. A tumor classified over 3 cm with involvement of the ipsilateral hilar nodes (T2 N1 MO).

STAGE III. Any tumor invading the pleura and adjacent structures, or involving the contralateral mediastinal nodes, or exhibiting distant metastases.

CLINICAL COURSE. Lung cancer is one of the most insidious and aggressive neoplasms in the whole realm of oncology.[98] In the usual case, it is discovered in the sixth decade of life in patients whose symptoms are of approximately seven months' duration. The major presenting complaints are cough (75%), weight loss (40%), chest pain (40%), and dyspnea (20%). Not infrequently, the tumor is discovered by its secondary spread in the course of investigation of an apparent primary neoplasm elsewhere.

Despite all efforts at early diagnosis by frequent radioscopic examination of the chest, cytologic examination of sputum, bronchial washings or brushings, and the many improvements in thoracic surgery, radiotherapy, and chemotherapy, the overall five-year survival rate is on the order of 9%.[99] In many large clinics, not more than 20 to 30% of lung cancer patients have lesions sufficiently localized to permit even an attempt at resection. In general, the adenocarcinoma and squamous cell patterns tend to remain localized longer and have a slightly better prognosis than the undifferentiated cancers, which usually are advanced lesions by the time they are discovered. The overall five-year survival rate of males is approximately 10% for squamous cell carcinoma and adenocarcinoma, but only 3% for undifferentiated lesions. Surgical resection for *small cell carcinoma* is so ineffective that the diagnosis essentially precludes surgery. Untreated, the survival time for small cell cancer is six to 17 weeks. But this cancer is particularly sensitive to radiation and chemotherapy, and indeed potential cure rates of 15 to 25% for limited disease have been reported in some centers. Unfortunately most patients have distant metastases upon diagnosis. Thus, even with treatment, the mean survival after diagnosis is about one year.

Despite this discouraging outlook, it must never be forgotten that many patients have been cured by lobectomy or pneumonectomy, emphasizing the continued need for early diagnosis and adequate prompt therapy. Indeed, in the uncommon but happy instance of *localized solitary tumors less than 4 cm in diameter, surgical resection results in up to 40% five-year survival for squamous cell carcinoma and 30% for adenocarcinoma and large cell carcinoma.*

Bronchogenic carcinoma can be associated with a number of paraneoplastic syndromes (p. 294), some of which may antedate the development of a gross pulmonary lesion. The hormones or hormone-like factors elaborated include (1) *antidiuretic hormone,* inducing hyponatremia due to inappropriate ADH secretion; (2) *ACTH,* producing Cushing's syndrome; (3) *parathormone or prostaglandin E,* inducing hypercalcemia; (4) *calcitonin,* causing hypocalcemia; (5) *gonadotropins,* causing gynecomastia; and (6) *serotonin,* associated with the carcinoid syndrome. Any one of the histologic types of tumors may occasionally produce any one of the hormones, but tumors producing ACTH and ADH are predominantly small cell carcinomas, whereas those producing hypercalcemia are mostly squamous cell tumors.[100] The carcinoid syndrome is associated rarely with small cell carcinoma but is more common with the bronchial carcinoids, described later.

Other systemic manifestations of bronchogenic carcinoma include a *myopathy,* characterized by muscle weakness; *peripheral neuropathy,* usually purely sensory; dermatologic abnormalities, including *acanthosis nigricans* (p. 284); hematologic abnormalities such as *leukemoid reactions;* and finally a peculiar abnormality of connective tissue called *hypertrophic pulmonary osteoarthropathy,* associated with clubbing of the fingers.

Apical lung cancers in the superior pulmonary sulcus tend to invade the neural structures around the trachea, including the cervical sympathetic plexus, and produce a group of clinical findings that includes severe pain in the distribution of the ulnar nerve and *Horner's syndrome* (enophthalmos, ptosis, miosis, and anhidrosis) on the same side as the lesion. Such tumors are also referred to as *Pancoast's tumors.*

There is much yet to be learned about the biology of these neoplasms, but most important is an understanding of their causes. Until we know more, cigarette smoking must stand indicted as the major villain.

BRONCHIOLOALVEOLAR CARCINOMA

As the name implies, this form of lung cancer occurs well out in the pulmonary parenchyma in the terminal bronchioloalveolar regions.[101,102] It represents, in various series, 1.1 to 9.0% of all lung cancers. Changes are very similar histologically to an apparently infectious disease of South African sheep known as *jagziekte*. However, numerous efforts to identify an infectious agent in humans or to transmit the disease to sheep with cell-free extracts of human carcinoma have been unavailing.

Histologically, the tumor is characterized by distinctive, tall, columnar-to-cuboidal epithelial cells that line up along alveolar septa and project into the alveolar spaces in numerous branching papillary formations (Fig. 16–45). The tumor cells often contain abundant mucinous secretions. The degree of anaplasia is quite variable, but most tumors are well differentiated and tend to preserve the native septal wall architecture. Ultrastructurally, bronchioloalveolar carcinomas are a heterogeneous group, consisting of mucin-secreting bronchiolar cells, Clara cells or (rarely) type II pneumocytes.

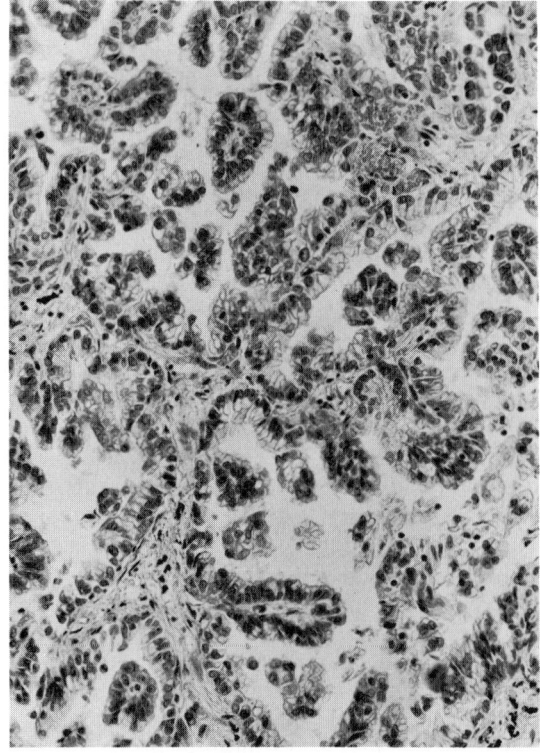

Figure 16–45. Terminal bronchiolar (alveolar) carcinoma with characteristic tall columnar cell papillary growth.

Macroscopically, the tumor almost always occurs in the peripheral portions of the lung either as a single nodule, or more often as multiple diffuse nodules that sometimes coalesce to produce a pneumonia-like consolidation. The parenchymal nodules have a mucinous gray translucence when secretion is present and otherwise appear as solid gray-white areas, which can be confused with pneumonia on casual inspection. Because the tumor does not involve major bronchi, atelectasis and emphysema are infrequent accompaniments. Metastases are not widely disseminated or large, nor do they occur early, but they eventually appear in up to 45% of cases.

Clinically, these tumors occur in patients of all ages from the third decade to advanced years of life. They are equally distributed among males and females. The symptoms, which usually appear late, are much like those of bronchogenic carcinoma, with cough, hemoptysis, and pain the major presenting findings. Occasionally they may produce a picture of diffuse interstitial pneumonitis. Solitary lesions are surgically resectable, resulting in 50 to 75% five-year survival, but the overall survival rate is about 25%.

BRONCHIAL CARCINOID

Bronchial carcinoids represent 1 to 5% of all lung tumors.[103] They make up over 90% of a group of bronchial tumors formerly classified as "bronchial adenoma," but now known to be often locally invasive or occasionally capable of metastasis.[104] The remaining 10% of the group includes *adenoid cystic carcinoma* and *mucoepidermoid carcinoma*—tumors with histologic patterns reminiscent of similar tumors in salivary glands (p. 824). Most patients with carcinoid tumors are under 40 years of age, and the incidence is equal for both sexes. There is no known relationship to cigarette smoking or other environmental factors. Bronchial carcinoids show the neuroendocrine differentiation of the Kulchitsky cells of bronchial mucosa and resemble intestinal carcinoids, described in detail on page 873. They contain dense-core neurosecretory granules in their cytoplasm, secrete hormonally active polypeptides, and occasionally occur as part of multiple endocrine neoplasia.

Histologically, the tumor is composed of nests, cords, and masses of cells separated by a delicate fibrous stroma. In common with the lesions of the gastrointestinal tract, the individual cells are quite regular and have uniform round nuclei and infrequent mitoses (Fig. 16–46). Occasional carcinoid adenomas display variation in the size and shape of cells and nuclei and, along with this pleomorphism, tend to demonstrate a more aggressive and more invasive behavior. On electron microscopy the cells exhibit the dense-core granules characteristic of other neuroendocrine tumors (Fig. 26–36), and by immunochemistry are found to contain serotonin, neuron-specific enolase, bombesin, calcitonin, or other peptides.

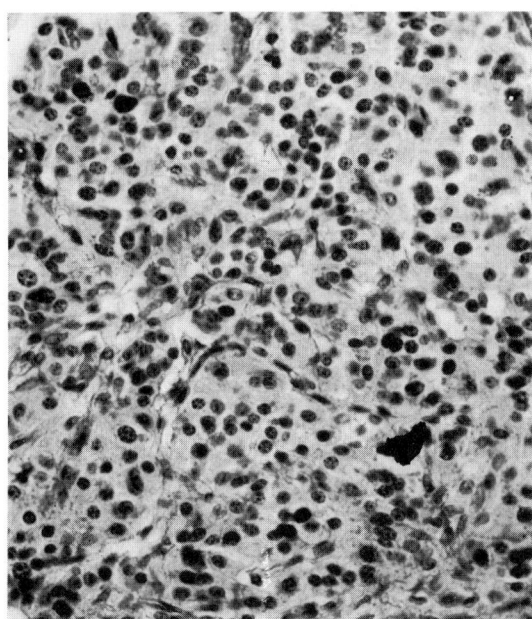

Figure 16-46. Bronchial carcinoid with small rounded uniform cells.

On gross examination, the tumors grow as finger-like or spherical polypoid masses that commonly project into the lumen of the bronchus and are usually covered by an intact mucosa. They rarely exceed 3 to 4 cm in diameter. Most are confined to the main stem bronchi. Others, however, produce little intraluminal mass but instead penetrate the bronchial wall to fan out in the peribronchial tissue, producing the so-called "collar-button" lesion (Fig. 16-47).

The clinical manifestations of bronchial carcinoids emanate from their intraluminal growth, their capacity to metastasize, and the ability of some of these lesions to elaborate vasoactive amines. Persistent cough, hemoptysis, impairment of drainage of respiratory passages with secondary infections, bronchiectasis, emphysema, and atelectasis are all by-products of the intraluminal growth of these lesions.

About 40% of these tumors metastasize to regional nodes and cause enlargement of the hilar nodes; 5 to 10% also metastasize to the liver to produce hepatomegaly. Most interesting, however, are those functioning lesions of the argentaffinoma pattern capable of producing the classic carcinoid syndrome, i.e., intermittent attacks of diarrhea, flushing, and cyanosis. Overall, most bronchial carcinoids do not have secretory activity and do not metastasize, but follow a relatively benign course for long periods and are therefore amenable to resection. The reported 5 to 10 year survival rates are 50 to 95%.

MISCELLANEOUS TUMORS

The complex category of benign and malignant mesenchymal tumors, such as fibroma, fibrosarcoma, leiomyoma, leiomyosarcoma, lipoma, hemangioma, hemangiopericytoma, and chondroma, may occur but such tumors are rare. Benign and malignant lymphoreticular tumors and tumor-like conditions, similar to those described in other organs, may also affect the lung, either as isolated lesions or more commonly as part of a generalized disorder. These include non-Hodgkin's and Hodgkin's lymphoma, lymphomatoid granulomatosis, pseudolymphoma, and plasma cell granuloma.

The relatively common *hamartoma* merits a brief description. It is usually discovered as an incidental, rounded focus of radiopacity on a routine chest film, giving rise to what the roentgenologist calls a "coin lesion." These neoplasms are rarely over 3 to 4 cm in diameter and are principally composed of mature hyaline cartilage. Occasionally, the cartilage contains cystic or cleftlike spaces, and these may be lined by characteristic respiratory epithelium. At other times, there are admixtures of fibrous tissue, fat, and blood vessels, making it clear that these lesions probably represent a hamartoma of the lung.

Tumors in the mediastinum either may arise in mediastinal structures or may be metastatic from the lungs or other organs. They may also invade or compress the lungs. Table 16-8 lists the most common tumors in the various compartments of the mediastinum. Specific tumor types are discussed in appropriate sections of this book.

METASTATIC TUMORS OF LUNG

The lung is more often affected by metastatic growths than it is by primary neoplasms. Both carcinomas and sarcomas arising anywhere in the body may spread to the lungs via the blood or lymphatics or by direct

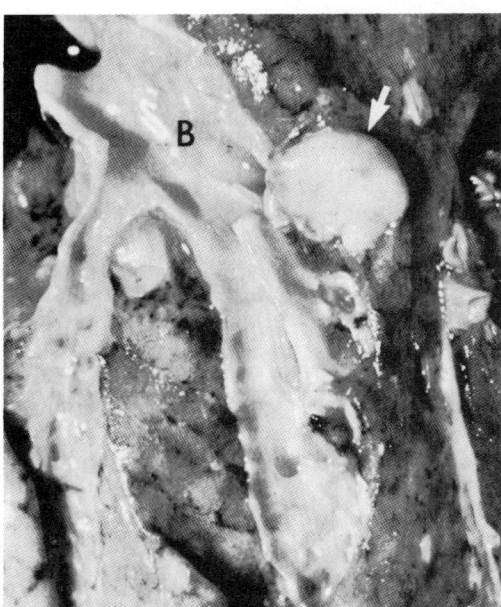

Figure 16-47. Bronchial carcinoid growing as a spherical pale mass (*arrow*) apparently external to lumen of bronchus (B).

Table 16-8. Mediastinal Tumors

SUPERIOR MEDIASTINUM	POSTERIOR MEDIASTINUM
Lymphoma	Neurogenic tumors
Thymoma	(schwannoma;
Thyroid lesions	neurofibroma)
Metastatic carcinoma	Lymphoma
Parathyroid tumors	Gastroenteric hernia
ANTERIOR MEDIASTINUM	**MIDDLE MEDIASTINUM**
Thymoma	Bronchogenic cyst
Teratoma	Pericardial cyst
Lymphoma	Lymphoma
Thyroid lesions	
Parathyroid tumors	

continuity. Growth of contiguous tumors into the lungs occurs most often with esophageal carcinomas and mediastinal lymphomas.

The pattern of metastatic growth within the lungs is quite variable. In the usual case, multiple discrete nodules are scattered throughout all lobes (Fig. 16–48). These discrete lesions tend to occur in the periphery of the lung parenchyma rather than in the central locations of the primary bronchogenic carcinoma.

As a second macroscopic variant, metastatic growths may confine themselves to peribronchiolar and perivascular tissue spaces, presumably when the tumor has extended to the lung through the lymphatics. Here the lung septa and connective tissue are diffusely infiltrated with the gray-white tumor. Least commonly, the metastatic tumor is totally inapparent on gross examination and only becomes evident on histologic section as a diffuse intralymphatic dissemination dispersed throughout the peribronchial and perivascular channels. The subpleural lymphatics may be outlined by the contained tumor producing an anatomic pattern referred to as *lymphangitis carcinomatosa*. In certain instances, microscopic tumor emboli fill the small pulmonary vessels and may result in life-threatening pulmonary hypertension.

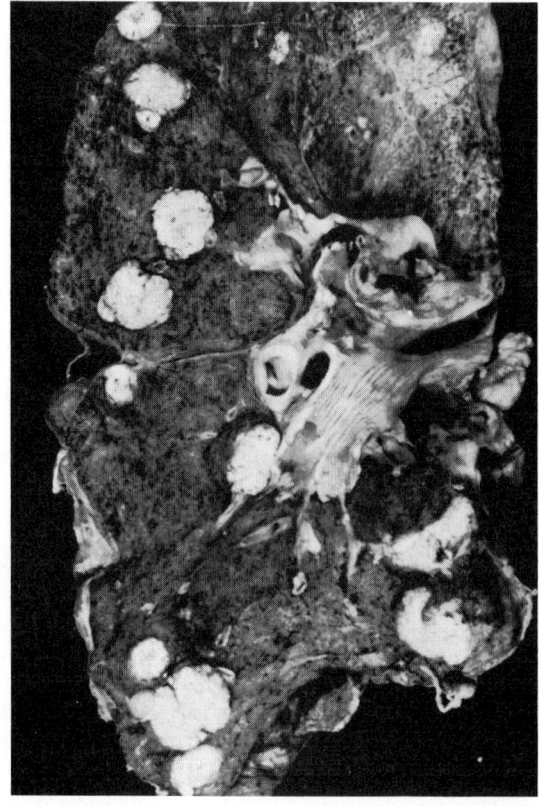

Figure 16–48. Metastases in lung from a breast carcinoma in a 56-year-old woman.

PLEURA

INFLAMMATIONS
NONINFLAMMATORY PLEURAL
EFFUSIONS
PNEUMOTHORAX
TUMORS OF PLEURA
Benign Mesothelioma (Pleural Fibroma)
Malignant Mesothelioma

Pathologic involvement of the pleura is, with rare exceptions, a secondary complication of some underlying disease. The only primary disorders that are reasonably common are (1) primary intrapleural bacterial infections that imply seeding of this space as an isolated focus in the course of a transient bacteremia and (2) a primary neoplasm of the pleura—mesothelioma. With these exceptions, pleural diseases usually follow some underlying disorder, most often pulmonary. Secondary infections are extremely common, however, and pleural adhesions or other forms of pleural involvement are present in at least two thirds of all postmortem cases. Occasionally, the secondary pleural disease assumes a dominant role in the clinical problem, as occurs in bacterial pneumonia with the development of empyema.

Pleural effusion is a common manifestation of both primary and secondary pleural involvements.[105] Normally, no more than 15 ml of serous, relatively acellular, clear fluid lubricates the pleural surface. Increased accumulation of pleural fluid occurs under five settings: (1) increased hydrostatic pressure, as in congestive heart failure; (2) increased vascular permeability, as in pneumonia; (3) decreased oncotic pressure, as in nephrotic syndrome; (4) increased intrapleural negative pressure, as in atelectasis; and (5) decreased lymphatic drainage, as in mediastinal carcinomatosis. The character of the pleural effusion under these circumstances is variable, as we shall see.

Diseases of the pleura can be divided for convenience into inflammations, noninflammatory pleural effusions, and neoplasms.

INFLAMMATIONS

Inflammations of the pleura (pleuritis), depending on their stage and causative agent, can be divided on the basis of the character of the resultant exudate into serous, fibrinous, serofibrinous, suppurative (empyema), and hemorrhagic pleuritis.

SEROFIBRINOUS PLEURITIS. Serous, serofibrinous, and fibrinous pleuritis are all caused by essentially the same processes. Fibrinous exudations generally reflect a later and more severe exudative reaction that, in an earlier developmental phase, might have presented as a serous or serofibrinous exudate.

The common causes of such pleuritis are inflammatory diseases within the lungs, such as tuberculosis, pneumonia, lung infarcts, lung abscess, and bronchiectasis. Rheumatoid arthritis, disseminated lupus erythematosus, uremia, the diffuse systemic infections, and other systemic disorders also cause serous or serofibrinous pleuritis. Occasionally, metastatic involvement of the pleura produces a pure serous or serofibrinous pleuritis. Irradiation used in therapy of tumors in the lung or mediastinum often causes a serofibrinous pleuritis.

In most instances the serofibrinous reaction is only minimal, and the fluid exudate is resorbed with either resolution or organization of the fibrinous component. Accumulation of large amounts of fluid may sometimes be responsible for considerable encroachment upon lung space and give rise to respiratory distress.

SUPPURATIVE PLEURITIS (EMPYEMA). A purulent pleural exudate usually implies bacterial or mycotic seeding of the pleural space. Most commonly, this occurs by contiguous spread of organisms from intrapulmonary suppuration, but occasionally it occurs by lymphatic or hematogenous dissemination from a more distant infection. Rarely, suppurative infections below the diaphragm, such as the subdiaphragmatic or liver abscess, may extend by conti-

nuity through the diaphragm into the pleural spaces, more often on the right side.

Empyema is characterized by yellow-green creamy pus that may accumulate in large volumes (up to 500 to 1000 ml), but usually in smaller amounts than the serous reactions described. The exudate is made up of masses of polymorphonuclear neutrophils admixed with other leukocytes. Although it may be difficult to visualize microorganisms on smears of the exudate, it should be possible to demonstrate them by culture. Empyema may resolve, but this fortunate outcome is less common than organization of the exudate, with the formation of dense, tough fibrous adhesions that frequently obliterate the pleural space. Sometimes a thick, dense connective tissue layer is formed that envelops the lungs and seriously embarrasses pulmonary expansion.

HEMORRHAGIC PLEURITIS. True sanguineous inflammatory exudates must be differentiated from bloody or traumatic contamination of serous or serofibrinous exudates. The slight bleeding that often occurs in the course of fluid withdrawal is the most frequent cause of confusion. Hemorrhagic exudates are infrequent and are found in hemorrhagic diatheses, rickettsial diseases, and neoplastic involvement of the pleural cavity. The sanguineous exudate must be differentiated from whole blood that may fill the pleural cavity when an aneurysm ruptures. When hemorrhagic pleuritis is encountered, careful search should be made for the presence of exfoliated tumor cells.

NONINFLAMMATORY PLEURAL EFFUSIONS

HYDROTHORAX. Noninflammatory collections of serous fluid within the pleural cavities are called hydrothorax. The fluid is clear and straw-colored and has the other characteristics already mentioned. Hydrothorax may be unilateral or bilateral, depending on the underlying cause. The most common cause of hydrothorax is cardiac failure, and for this reason it is usually accompanied by pulmonary congestion and edema. In cardiac failure, hydrothorax is usually, but not invariably, bilateral. Transudations may collect in any other systemic disease associated with generalized edema, and are therefore found in renal failure and cirrhosis of the liver.

In most instances, hydrothorax is not loculated, but, in the presence of pre-existent pleural adhesions, local collections may be found walled off by bridging fibrous tissue. Except for these localized collections, the fluid usually collects basally, when the patient is in an upright position, and causes compression and atelectasis of the inundated regions of the lung. If the underlying cause is alleviated, hydrothorax may be resorbed, usually leaving behind no permanent alterations. Highly satisfying relief of respiratory distress is accomplished by the withdrawal of large pleural transudates.

HEMOTHORAX. The escape of blood into the pleural cavity is known as hemothorax. It is almost invariably a fatal complication of a ruptured aortic aneurysm. Pure hemothorax is readily identifiable by the large clots that accompany the fluid component of the blood. Because this calamity often leads to death within minutes to hours, it is uncommon to find any response within the pleural cavity. Rarely, leakage of smaller amounts may not prove fatal promptly and provides a stimulus to organization and the development of pleural adhesions.

CHYLOTHORAX. Chylothorax is an accumulation of milky fluid, usually of lymphatic origin, in the pleural cavity. Chyle is milky white because it contains finely emulsified fats. When it is allowed to stand, a creamy, fatty, supernatant layer separates. True chyle should be differentiated from turbid serous fluid, which does not contain fat and does not separate into an overlying layer of high fat content. Chylothorax may be bilateral but is more often confined to the left side. The volume of fluid is variable but rarely assumes the massive proportions of hydrothorax.

Chylothorax is most often encountered in malignant conditions arising within the thoracic cavity, usually malignant lymphomas that cause obstruction of the major lymphatic ducts. More distant cancers may metastasize via the lymphatics and grow within the right lymphatic or thoracic duct to produce obstruction. Presumably obstruction causes rupture of these ducts, with the escape of the milky-white chylous fluid.

PNEUMOTHORAX

Pneumothorax refers to air or gas in the pleural cavities, and may be spontaneous, traumatic, or therapeutic. Spontaneous pneumothorax may complicate any form of pulmonary disease that causes rupture of an alveolus. An abscess cavity that communicates either directly with the pleural space or with the lung interstitial tissue may also lead to the escape of air. In the latter circumstance, the air may dissect through the lung substance or back through the mediastinum, eventually to enter the pleural cavity. Pneumothorax is most commonly associated with emphysema, asthma, and tuberculosis. Traumatic pneumothorax is usually caused by some perforating injury to the chest wall, but sometimes the trauma pierces the lung to provide two avenues for the accumulation of air within the pleural spaces. Therapeutic pneumothorax was once a commonly practiced method of deflating the lung to favor the healing of tuberculous lesions. Such induced pneumothorax subsides slowly, however, because of absorption of the introduced air, and requires constant replenishment. The same is true for spontaneous and traumatic pneumothorax, provided the original communication seals itself.

Of the various forms of pneumothorax, the one that attracts greatest clinical attention is so-called *spontaneous idiopathic pneumothorax.* This entity is encountered in relatively young people; appears to be due to rupture of small, peripheral, usually apical subpleural blebs; and usually subsides spontaneously as the air is resorbed. Recurrent attacks are common and may be quite disabling.

Pneumothorax can be identified anatomically only by careful opening of the thoracic cavity under water to detect the escape of gas or air bubbles. This technique is best performed by creating a pocket of a skin flap that can be filled with water before the thorax is opened. By puncturing the pleural cavity with some instrument under water, it is possible to note the escape of bubbles. Pneumothorax may have as much significance as a fluid collection within the lungs, as it also causes compression, collapse, and atelectasis of the lung and may be responsible for marked respiratory distress. Occasionally, the lung collapse is marked: when the defect acts as a flap valve and permits the entrance of air during inspiration, but fails to permit its escape during expiration, it effectively acts as a pump that creates *tension pneumothorax.*

TUMORS OF PLEURA

The pleura may be involved in primary or secondary tumors. Secondary metastatic involvement is far more common than are primary tumors. The most frequent metastatic malignancies arise from primary neoplasms of the lung and breast. Advanced mammary carcinomas frequently penetrate the thoracic wall directly to involve the parietal and then the visceral pleura. They may also reach these cavities through the lymphatics and, more rarely, the blood. In addition to these cancers, malignancy from any organ of the body may spread to pleural spaces. Ovarian carcinomas are the major offenders, as these tumors tend to cause widespread implants in both the abdominal and the thoracic cavities. In most of these metastatic involvements, a serous or serosanguineous effusion follows that may contain desquamated neoplastic cells. For this reason, careful cytologic examination of the sediment is of considerable diagnostic value.

BENIGN MESOTHELIOMA (PLEURAL FIBROMA)

There are two types of mesotheliomas, benign and malignant. The benign mesothelioma (called pleural fibroma) is a localized growth that is often attached to the pleural surface by a pedicle. The tumor may be small (1 to 2 cm in diameter) or reach an enormous size, but always remains confined to the surface of the lung. These tumors do not usually produce a pleural effusion. Grossly, they consist of dense fibrous tissue with occasional cysts filled with viscid fluid; microscopically, the tumors show whorls of reticulin and collagen fibers among which are interspersed spindle cells resembling fibroblasts. For this reason, these mesotheliomas are also termed "fibromas." The benign mesothelioma has no relationship to asbestos exposure.

MALIGNANT MESOTHELIOMA

Malignant mesotheliomas are rare tumors that arise from either the visceral or the parietal pleura.[106,107] Although uncommon, they have assumed great importance in the past few years because of their increased incidence among persons with heavy exposure to asbestos.[108] In coastal areas with shipping industries in the United States and Britain, and in Canadian and South African mining areas, up to 90% of reported mesotheliomas are asbestos related. The lifetime risk of the development of mesothelioma in heavily exposed individuals is as high as 7 to 10%. There is a long latent period of 25 to 45 years for the development of asbestos-related mesothelioma, and there seems to be no increased risk in asbestos workers who smoke. *This is in contrast to asbestos-related bronchogenic carcinoma, in which the risk of cancer is markedly magnified by smoking.* Thus, for asbestos workers (particularly those who are also smokers), the risk of dying of lung carcinoma far exceeds that of developing mesothelioma.

Asbestos bodies are found in increased numbers in lungs of patients with mesothelioma, and mesotheliomas can be induced readily in experimental animals by intrapleural injections of asbestos.[107] There is little doubt about the carcinogenicity of asbestos; the mechanisms of cancer induction are discussed on page 471.

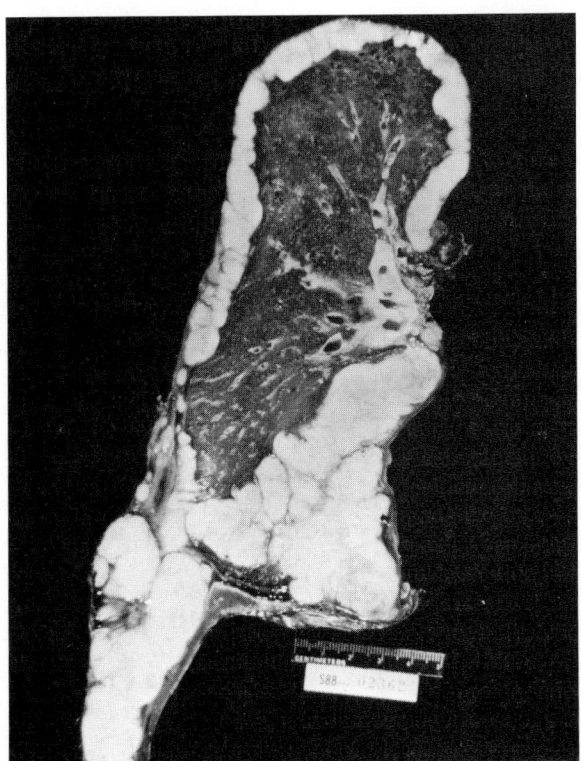

Figure 16–49. Malignant mesothelioma. Note thick, firm, white, pleural tumor tissue that ensheathes this bisected lung. *(arrows).*

Malignant mesothelioma is a diffuse lesion that spreads widely in the pleural space and is usually associated with extensive pleural effusion and direct invasion of thoracic structures. The affected lung is ensheathed by a thick layer of soft, gelatinous, grayish-pink tumor tissue (Fig. 16–49). Microscopically, malignant mesotheliomas consist of a mixture of two types of cells, one of which might predominate in an individual case. Mesothelial cells have the potential to develop as either mesenchymal stromal cells or epithelium-like lining cells. The mesenchymal type of mesothelioma appears as a spindle cell sarcoma, resembling fibrosarcoma **(sarcomatoid type)**, whereas the papillary type consists of cuboidal, columnar, or flattened cells forming a tubular and papillary structure **(epithelial type)**, resembling adenocarcinoma (Fig. 16–50). Indeed, epithelial mesothelioma may at times be difficult to differentiate from pulmonary adenocarcinoma. Special features that favor mesothelioma include the following: positive staining for acid mucopolysaccharide, which is inhibited by previous digestion by hyaluronidase; strong staining for keratin proteins, with accentuation of perinuclear rather than peripheral staining; lack of staining for carcinoembryonic antigen (CEA); and, on electron microscopy, the presence of long microvilli and abundant tonofilaments, but absent microvillous rootlets and lamellar bodies (Fig. 16–51). The mixed type of mesothelioma contains both epithelial and sarcomatoid patterns.

The presenting complaints are chest pain, dyspnea, and, as noted, recurrent pleural effusions. Concurrent pulmonary asbestosis (fibrosis) is present in only 20% of patients with pleural mesothelioma. Fifty per cent of those with pleural disease die within 12 months of diagnosis, and very few survive longer than two years. The lung is invaded directly, and there is metastatic spread to the hilar lymph nodes and eventually to liver and other distant organs.

Mesotheliomas also arise in the peritoneum, pericardium, tunica vaginalis, and genital tract (benign adenomatoid tumor, see p. 1116). *Peritoneal mesotheliomas* are particularly related to very heavy asbestos exposure; 50% of such patients also have pulmonary fibrosis. Although in about 50% of cases the disease remains confined to the abdominal cavity, intestinal involvement frequently leads to death from intestinal obstruction or inanition.

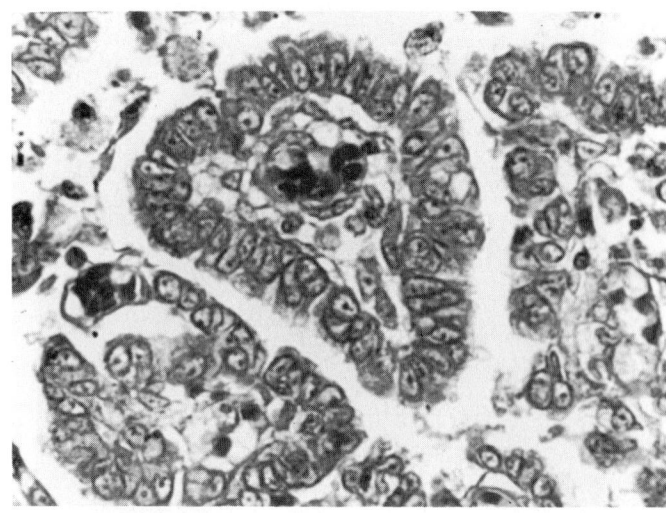

Figure 16-50. Mesothelioma, papillary epithelial type. Note resemblance to papillary adenocarcinoma.

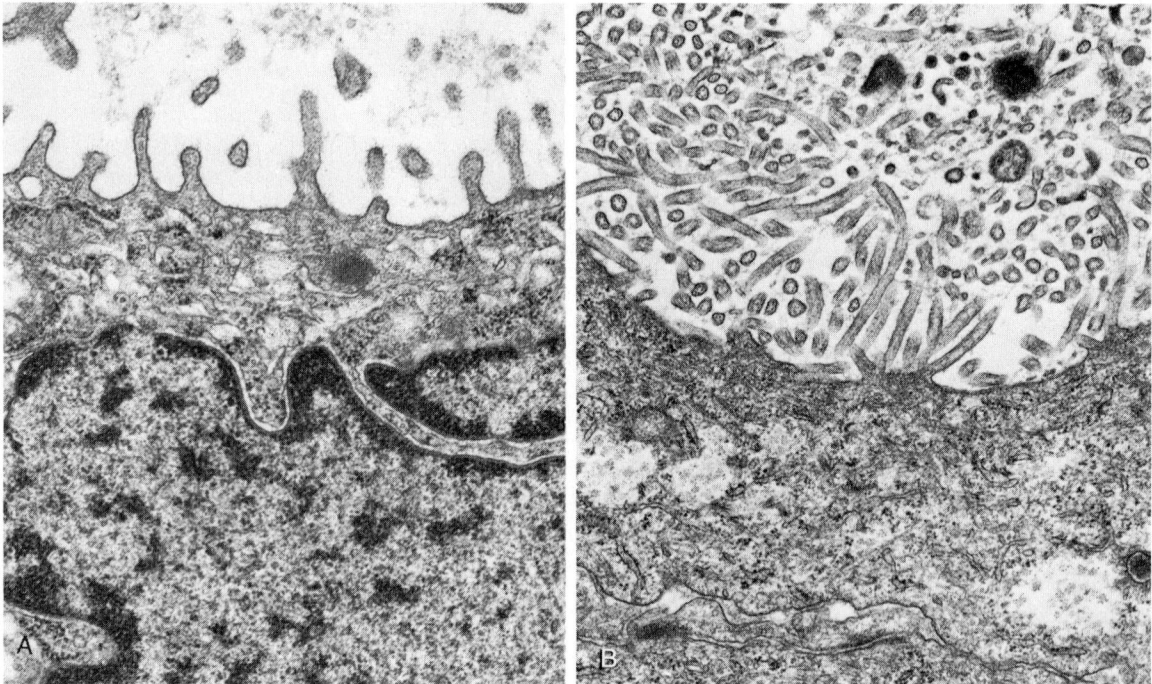

Figure 16-51. Ultrastructural features of pulmonary adenocarcinoma *(A)*, characterized by short plump microvilli, contrasted with those of mesothelioma *(B)*, in which microvilli are numerous, long, and slender. (Courtesy of Dr. Noel Weidner, Brigham and Women's Hospital, Boston.)

1. Thurlbeck, W.M.: Chronic Airflow Obstruction in Lung Disease. Philadelphia, W.B. Saunders Co., 1976.

2. Murray, J.F.: The Normal Lung: The Basis for Diagnosis and Treatment of Pulmonary Disease. Philadelphia, W.B. Saunders Co., 1976.

3. Kuhn, C., III: Normal anatomy and histology. *In* Thurlbeck, W.M.: Pathology of the Lung. New York, Thieme Medical Publishers, 1988, p. 13.

4. Gould, V.E., et al.: Neuroendocrine components of the bronchopulmonary tract: Hyperplasias, dysplasia, and neoplasms. Lab. Invest. *49*:519, 1983.

5. Weibel, E.R.: Design and structure of the human lung. *In* Fishman, A.P. (ed.): Pulmonary Disease and Disorders. Second edition. New York, McGraw-Hill Book Co., Vol. 1, 1988, p. 61.

6. Kikkawa, Y., and Smith, F.: Cellular and biochemical aspects of pulmonary surfactant in health and disease. Lab Invest. *49*:122, 1983.

7. Brain, J.D., et al. (eds.): Respiratory Defense Mechanisms. New York, Marcel Dekker, 1977.

8. Green, G.M., et al.: Defense mechanisms of respiratory membranes. Am. Rev. Respir. Dis. *115*:495, 1977.

9. Spencer, H.: Pathology of the Lung Excluding Pulmonary Tuberculosis. Third edition. New York, Pergamon Press, 1977.

10. Katzenstein, A.-L.A., and Askin, F.B.: Surgical Pathology of Non-Neoplastic Lung Disease. Philadelphia, W.B. Saunders Co., 1982.

11. Fishman, A.P. (ed.): Pulmonary Diseases and Disorders. Second edition. New York, McGraw-Hill Book Co., 1988.

12. Dunnill, M.S.: Pulmonary Pathology. New York, Churchill Livingstone, 1982.

13. Thurlbeck, W.M. (ed.): Pathology of the Lung. New York, Thieme Medical Publishers, 1988.

14. Dail, D.H., and Hammar, S.P. (eds.): Pulmonary Pathology. New York, Springer-Verlag, 1988.

15. Ayres, S.M.: Mechanisms and consequences of pulmonary edema. Am. Heart J. *103*:97, 1982.

16. Hogg, J.C., and Katzenstein, A.-L.: Pulmonary edema and diffuse alveolar injury. *In* Thurlbeck, W.M. (ed.): Pathology of the Lung. New York, Thieme Medical Publishers, 1988, p. 263.

17. Hyers, T.M., and Fowler, A.A.: Adult respiratory distress syndrome: Causes, morbidity and mortality. Fed. Proc. *45*:25, 1986.

18. Hawley, M.E., and Bone, R.C.: Acute respiratory failure. Pathophysiology, causes and clinical manifestations. Postgrad. Med. *79*:166, 1986.

19. Rinaldo, J.E., and Rogers, R.M.: Adult respiratory distress syndrome. Changing concepts of lung injury and repair. N. Engl. J. Med. *315*:578, 1986.

20. Balentine, J.D.: Pathology of Oxygen Toxicity. New York, Academic Press, 1983.

21. Pratt, P.C.: Pathology of adult respiratory distress syndrome. *In* Thurlbeck, W.M., and Abell, M.R. (eds.): The Lung: Structure, Function and Disease. Baltimore, Williams & Wilkins Co., 1978, p. 43.

22. Simon, R.H., and Ward, P.A.: Adult respiratory distress syndrome. *In* Gallin, J., et al. (eds.): Inflammation: Basic Principles and Clinical Correlates. New York, Raven Press, 1987, p. 815.

23. Goldhaber, S.Z. (ed.): Pulmonary Embolism and Deep Venous Thrombosis. Philadelphia, W.B. Saunders Co., 1985.

24. Freiman, D.G., et al.: Frequency of pulmonary thromboembolism in man. N. Engl. J. Med. *272*:1278, 1965.

25. Fishman, A.P., and Pietra, G.G.: Primary pulmonary hypertension. Annu. Rev. Med. *31*:421, 1980.

25a. Hughes, J.D., and Rubin, L.J.: Primary pulmonary hypertension. Medicine *65*:56, 1986.

26. Heath, D., and Smith, P.: Disorders of the vascular system. *In* Thurlbeck, W.M. (ed.): Pathology of the Lung. New York, Thieme Medical Publishers, 1988.

27. Edwards, W.D.: Pathology of pulmonary hypertension. Cardiovasc. Clin. *18*:321, 1988.

28. Wagenvoort, E.A., and Wagenvoort, E.: Pathology of Pulmonary Hypertension. New York, John Wiley & Sons, 1977.

29. U.S. Vital Health Statistics. Disability Days. U.S. Series 10 #158, p. 61, 1983.

30. American Thoracic Society: Chronic bronchitis, asthma and pulmonary emphysema. Statement by the Committee on Diagnostic Standards for Nontuberculous Respiratory Disease. Am. Rev. Respir. Dis. *85*:762, 1962.

31. Kleinerman, J., et al.: The occurrence and incidence of emphysematous lesions in men from 15 to 44 years of age. Am. Rev. Respir. Dis. *98*:152, 1968.

32. Thurlbeck, W.M.: Chronic airflow obstruction. *In* Thurlbeck, W.M. (ed.): Pathology of the Lung. New York, Thieme Medical Publishers, 1988, p. 519.

33. Janoff, A.: Emphysema: Proteinase-antiproteinase imbalance. *In* Gallin, J., et al. (eds.): Inflammation: Basic Principles and Clinical Correlates. New York, Raven Press, 1988, p. 803.

34. Laurell, C.B., and Eriksson, S.: The electrophoretic alpha-1-antitrypsin deficiency. Scand. J. Clin. Lab. Invest. *15*:132, 1963.

35. Senior, R.M., and Kahn, C.: The pathogenesis of emphysema. *In* Fishman, A.P. (ed.): Pulmonary Diseases and Disorders, 3rd ed. New York, McGraw-Hill, 1988, p. 1209.

36. Gross, P., et al.: Enzymatically produced pulmonary emphysema: A preliminary report. J. Occup. Med. *6*:481, 1964.

37. Senior, R.M., et al.: The induction of pulmonary emphysema with human leukocyte elastase. Am. Rev. Respir. Dis. *116*:469, 1977.

38. Werb, Z., et al.: Elastases and elastin degradation. J. Invest. Dermatol. *79*(Suppl.):154s, 1982.

39. Reid, L.M., et al.: Pathophysiology of bronchial hypersecretion. Eur. J. Respir. Dis. (Suppl.) *153*:19, 1987.

40. Petty, D.L.: Chronic Obstructive Pulmonary Disease. Second edition. New York, Marcel Dekker, 1985.

41. Hogg, J.C., et al.: Site and nature of airway obstruction in chronic obstructive lung disease. N. Engl. J. Med. *276*:1355, 1968.

42. Cosio, M., et al.: The relations between structural changes in small airways and pulmonary-function tests. N. Engl. J. Med. *298*:1277, 1978.

43. Lumsden, A.B., et al.: Goblet and Clara cells of the human distal airways: Evidence for smoking induced changes in their number. Thorax *39*:844, 1984.

44. Reid, L.: Chronic obstructive pulmonary diseases. *In* Fishman, A.P. (ed.): Pulmonary Diseases and Disorders. New York, McGraw-Hill Book Co., 1988, p. 1247.

45. Hogg, J.C.: Bronchial asthma. *In* Thurlbeck, W.M., and Abell, M.R. (eds.): The Lung: Structure, Function and Disease. Baltimore, Williams & Wilkins Co., 1978, p. 180.

46. McFadden, E.R., Jr.: Asthma: General features, pathogenesis and pathophysiology. *In* Fishman, A.P. (ed.): Pulmonary Diseases and Disorders, 2nd ed. New York, McGraw-Hill Book Company, 1988, p. 1295.

47. Kaliner, M.A.: Late phase reactions. N. Engl. Reg. Allergy Proc. *7*:236, 1986.

48. Lichtenstein, L.M.: The nasal late-phase response—an In vivo model. Hosp. Pract. *23*:119, 1988.

49. Greenberger, P.A., and Patterson, R.: Allergic bronchopulmonary aspergillosis. Model of bronchopulmonary disease with defined serologic, radiologic, pathologic and clinical findings from asthma to fatal destructive lung disease. Chest *91*:165S, 1977.

50. Adelroth, E., Morris, M.M., Hargreave, F.E., and O'Byrne, P.M.: Airway responsiveness to leukotrienes C4 and D4 and to methacholine in patients with asthma and normal controls. N. Engl. J. Med. *315*:480, 1986.

51. Bigby, T.D., and Nadel, J.A.: Asthma. *In* Gallin, J., et al. (eds.): Inflammation: Basic Principles and Clinical Correlates. New York, Raven Press, 1988, p. 679.

52. Gleich, G.J., and Adolphson, C.R.: The eosinophilic leukocyte. Adv. Immunol. *39*:177, 1986.

53. Swartz, M.N.: Bronchiectasis. *In* Fishman, A.P. (eds.): Pulmonary Diseases and Disorders. Second edition. New York, McGraw-Hill Book Co., 1988, p. 1553.

54. Wilton, L.J., et al.: Kartagener's syndrome with motile cilia and immotile spermatozoa: Axonemal ultrastructure and function. Am. Rev. Respir. Dis. *134*: 1233, 1986.

55. Pennington, J.E.: Respiratory Infections: Diagnosis and Management. New York, Raven Press, 1988.

56. Fanta, Ch.H., and Pennington, J.E.: Fever and new lung infiltrates in the immunocompromised host. Clin. Chest Med. *2*:19, 1981.

57. Myerowitz, R.L.: The Pathology of Opportunistic Infections with Pathogenetic, Diagnostic, and Clinical Correlations. New York, Raven Press, 1983.

58. Macher, A.M.: The pathology of AIDS. Public Health Rep. *103*:246, 1988.

59. Miller, R.: Mycoplasma, Chlamydia and coxiella infections of the respiratory tract. *In* Thurlbeck, W.M.: Pathology of the Lung. New York, Thieme Medical Publishers, 1988, p. 181.

60. Johanson, W.G., et al.: Aspiration pneumonia, anaerobic infections and lung abscess. Med. Clin. North Am. *64*:385, 1980.

61. Auerbach, O., and Dail, D.H.: Mycobacterial infections. *In* Dial, D.H., and Hammer, S.P. (eds.): Pulmonary Pathology. New York, Springer-Verlag, 1988, p. 173.

62. Collins, F.M.: The immunology of tuberculosis. Am. Rev. Respir. Dis. *125*:42, 1982.

63. Fulmer, J.D.: An introduction to the interstitial lung diseases. Clin. Chest Med. *3*:457, 1982.

64. Colby, T.V., and Carrington, C.B.: Infiltrative lung disease. *In* Thurlbeck, W.M.: Pathology of the Lung. New York, Thieme Medical Publishers, 1988, p. 425.

65. Crystal, R.G., et al.: Interstitial lung diseases of unknown cause: Disorders caused by chronic inflammation of the lower respiratory tract (Parts I and II). N. Engl. J. Med. *310*:154, 235, 1985.

66. Reynolds, H.Y.: Lung inflammation. Normal defense mechanism or a complication of some diseases. Ann. Rev. Med. *38*:295, 1987.

67. Snider, G.L.: Interstitial pulmonary fibrosis. Chest *89*:1115, 1986.

68. Liebow, A.A., and Carrington, C.B.: The interstitial pneumonias. *In* Simon, M., et al. (eds.): Frontiers in Pulmonary Radiology. New York, Grune & Stratton, 1969.

69. Liebow, A.A., et al.: Desquamative interstitial pneumonia. Am. J. Med. *39*:369, 1965.

70. Stankus, R.P., and Salvaggio, J.E.: Hypersensitivity pneumonitis. Clin. Chest Med. *4*:55, 1983.

71. Schatz, M., et al.: Eosinophils and immunologic lung disease. Med. Clin. North Am. *65*:1055, 1981.

72. Leatherman, J.W., et al.: Alveolar hemorrhage syndromes. Medicine 63:343, 1984.

73. Salant, D.J.: Immunopathogenesis of crescentic glomerulonephritis and lung purpura. Kidney Int. 32:408, 1987.

74. Smith, F.B.: Alveolar proteinosis: Atypical pulmonary response to injury. N.Y. State J. Med. 80:1372, 1980.

75. Bedrossian, C.W.M., et al.: Alveolar proteinosis as a consequence of immunosupression. A hypothesis based on clinical and pathologic observations. Hum. Pathol. 11:527, 1980.

76. Eisenberg, H.: The interstitial lung disease associated with collagen-vascular disorders. Clin. Chest Med. 3:564, 1982.

77. Dreisin, R.B.: Pulmonary vasculitis. Clin. Chest Med. 3:607, 1982.

78. Cooper, J.A.D.: Mechanisms of drug-induced pulmonary disease. Annu. Rev. Med. 39:395, 1988.

79. Carter, D., and Eggleston, J.C.: Tumors of the lower respiratory tract. Atlas of Tumor Pathology. Second Series. Fascicle 17. Washington, D.C., Armed Forces Institute of Pathology, 1980.

80. Churg, A.: Tumors of the Lung. In Thurlbeck, W.M. (ed.): Pathology of the Lung. New York, Thieme Medical Publishers, 1988.

81. Silverberg, E., and Lubera, U.J.: Cancer statistics. CA 38:2, 1988.

82. Frank, A.L.: The epidemiology and etiology of lung cancer. Clin. Chest Med. 3:219, 1982.

83. Smoking and Health — A National Status Report. A Report to Congress. Washington, D.C., Department of Health and Human Services, 1987. Publication No. HHS/PHS/CDC 87-8396.

84. Auerbach, O.: Changes in bronchial epithelium in relationship to cigarette smoking, 1955–1960 vs. 1970–1977. N. Engl. J. Med. 300:295, 1979.

85. Auerbach, O., et al.: Changes in bronchial epithelium in relationship to sex, age, residence, smoking and pneumonia. N. Engl. J. Med. 267:111, 1962.

86. Wynder, E.L., and Hoffman, D.: Tobacco and Tobacco Smoke: Studies in Experimental Carcinogenesis. New York, Academic Press, 1967.

87. Cihak, R.W.: Radiation and lung cancer. Hum. Pathol. 25:25, 1971.

88. Selikoff, I.J., et al.: Asbestos-associated disease in United States shipyards. Ann. N.Y. Acad. Sci. 330:295, 1979.

89. Wynder, E.L., and Hoffman, D.: Tobacco. In Schottenfeld, D., and Fraumeni, J.F. (eds.): Cancer Epidemiology and Prevention. Philadelphia, W.B. Saunders Co., 1982, p. 277.

90. Salmon, D.J.: Protoncogenes and human cancers. N. Engl. J. Med. 317:955, 1987.

91. Rodenhuis, S., et al.: Mutational activation of the K-ras oncogene: A possible pathogenetic factor in adenocarcinoma of the lung. N. Engl. J. Med. 317:929, 1987.

92. Yesner, R., et al. (eds.): International Histological Classification of Tumors. No. 1: Histological Typing of Lung Tumors. Second edition. Geneva, World Health Organization, 1982.

93. Yesner, R., and Carter, D.: Pathology of carcinoma of the lung: Changing patterns. Clin. Chest Med. 3:257, 1982.

94. Madri, J.A., and Carter, D.: Scar cancers of the lung: Origin and significance. Hum. Pathol. 15:625, 1984.

95. Barsky, S.H., et al.: The extracellular matrix of pulmonary scar carcinomas is suggestive of a desmoplastic origin. Am. J. Pathol. 124:412, 1986.

96. Carter, D., and Yesner, R.: Carcinomas of the lung with neuroendocrine differentiation. Semin. Diagn. Pathol. 2:235, 1985.

97. Cohen, M.H.: Natural history of lung cancer. Clin. Chest Med. 3:229, 1982.

98. Carney, C., et al.: Cancer of the Lung. In Fishman, A.P. (ed.): Pulmonary Diseases and Disorders. Second edition. New York, McGraw-Hill Book Co., 1988.

99. Jett, J.R., et al.: Lung cancer: Current concepts. CA 33:74, 1983.

100. Carney, D.N., and Minna, J.D.: Small cell cancer of the lung. Clin. Chest Med. 3:389, 1982.

101. Clayton, F.: The spectrum and significance of bronchioalveolar carcinomas. In Rosen, P.P., and Fechner, R.E.: Pathology Annual: 1988. Norwalk, Appleton & Lange, 1988, p. 361.

102. Bolen, J.W., and Thorning, D.: Histogenic classification of pulmonary carcinomas. Peripheral adenocarcinomas studied by light microscopy, histochemistry, and electron microscopy. Pathol. Annu. 17:77, 1982.

103. Sayler, D.C., and Eggleston, J.C.: Bronchial carcinoid tumors. Cancer 36:15, 1975.

104. Hurt, R., and Bates, M.: Carcinoid tumors of the bronchus. Thorax 39:617, 1985.

105. Sahn, S.A.: Pleural manifestations of pulmonary disease. Hosp. Pract. 16:73, 1981.

106. Corson, J.M.: Pathology of malignant mesothelioma. In Antman, K., and Aisner, J. (eds.): Asbestos-Related Malignancy. Orlando, Grune & Stratton, 1987, p. 179.

107. Roggli, V.L., et al.: Pathology of human mesothelioma: etiologic and diagnostic considerations. Hum. Pathol. 22(II):91, 1987.

108. Antman, K., and Aisner, J. (eds.): Asbestos-Related Malignancy. Orlando, Grune & Stratton, 1987.

Diseases of the Head and Neck*

This chapter is concerned with diseases of the ear, upper respiratory tract (including nasal cavities, paranasal sinuses, nasopharynx, and larynx), oral cavity, and salivary glands. These disorders include some of the most common ailments of mankind. They run the gamut from diseases that are annoying but relatively harmless, such as the common cold; to those that are unique to individual organs and cause considerable suffering, such as the various forms of deafness; to those that have characteristics in common with lesions of other organs, such as infections and tumors. Here we shall briefly review those disorders in which a knowledge of the pathology is of clinical importance.

THE EXTERNAL EAR

The skin of the ear may be involved by any of the dermatologic conditions—inflammations, tumors, and tumor-like conditions—discussed in Chapter 27. The ear develops from the branchial arches and clefts, and numerous deformities and anomalies in shape and structure can occur during development; most are innocuous. However, certain deformities are associated with other serious congenital disorders, such as renal agenesis, described in Chapter 21 (p. 1018).

CAULIFLOWER EAR. This term is used to describe an acquired deformity of the auricle secondary to cartilage degeneration (chondromalacia) induced by trauma. It is commonly observed in boxers and wrestlers. Histologically, there is a loss of chondrocytes resulting in a homogeneous matrix with perichondral and intrachondral fibrosis. Loss of the cartilage rigidity results in contractures and deformity.

CHONDRODERMATITIS NODULARIS HELICIS. This entity, also termed "painful nodule of the ear,"

presents as a small nodular lesion of the helix occurring in late middle or old age. It has a raised center containing a crust or scale[1] and thus can be confused with basal cell carcinoma or squamous cell carcinoma. Histologically it is characterized by epithelial hyperplasia with underlying collagen degeneration, chronic inflammatory cell infiltration, vascular proliferation, and fibrosis. There may be focal degeneration of cartilage adjacent to the lesion. The lesion is cured by excision and has no premalignant connotation. The etiology is unknown.

RELAPSING POLYCHONDRITIS. This is a rare chronic disease of unknown etiology characterized by destruction of cartilage.[2] It is often associated with manifestations of systemic connective tissue disease. The acute lesions frequently involve the auricles bilaterally, which swell and become erythematous, but spare the tragus. Histologically, the lesions show acute inflammatory cell infiltrates of the perichondral areas, associated with focal degeneration and vascularization of cartilage. The chronic inactive lesions show chronic inflammatory cells and fibrous replacement of the cartilage. Cartilage of the nose, trachea, and ribs may be involved.[3] The etiology is unknown, but autoimmune reactions to collagen have been postulated.

MALIGNANT EXTERNAL OTITIS. This is a necrotizing inflammation of the external canal, often with bone involvement, caused by *Pseudomonas aeruginosa* infection.[4] It is observed predominantly in older diabetic patients. Unless aggressive debridement and antibiotic therapy are instituted, the patients die from meningitis or brain abscesses due to extension of the infection to these structures. Histologically the lesion is characterized by acute inflammatory cell infiltration in all of the involved tissues, with focal tissue necrosis and microabscess formation.

TUMORS. Tumors and tumor-like conditions of the external ear include a variety of cutaneous cysts (e.g.,

* With gratitude to Dr. Max Goodman for his contributions in the section on diseases of the ear.

epidermal inclusion cysts), benign neoplasms (e.g., squamous cell papilloma, nevi), and malignant lesions (e.g., basal cell carcinoma, squamous cell carcinoma, malignant melanoma). Special neoplasms arise from the modified cerumen-secreting apocrine sweat glands of the external auditory canals.[5] These are either adenomas or adenocarcinomas and resemble the sweat gland adenomas (hidradenoma) and adenocarcinoma of skin appendages (p. 1285). Mixed tumors (pleomorphic adenoma) and adenoid cystic carcinomas similar to those in salivary glands (p. 822) may also arise from the accessory glands in the ears.

MIDDLE EAR

OTITIS MEDIA. This term refers to inflammation of the middle ear, sometimes associated with an upper respiratory tract infection.[6] It may be *acute, chronic,* or *serous. Acute otitis media* may be caused by viral or bacterial infections, or bacterial infection complicating a viral illness.[7] *Acute suppurative otitis media* is most frequently caused by *Streptococcus pneumoniae* or *Haemophilus influenzae.* Clinically it is characterized by a bulging, hyperemic tympanic membrane, the result of accumulation of fluid in the middle ear, as well as ear pain and tenderness. Incision of the tympanic membrane releases the exudate, reduces pressure, and eliminates the pain. Mastoid air cells may become infected, producing mastoiditis, but this complication is now rare as the infection responds rapidly to antibiotics.

Chronic otitis media manifests as persistent drainage from the ear associated with tympanic membrane perforation and some degree of hearing impairment. Polypoid granulation tissue may be present in the external canal *(aural polyps)* attached to the tympanic membrane or middle ear structures. Persistent inflammation in the middle ear may lead to resorption of ossicles and disarticulations, resulting in marked conductive hearing loss. Granulomatous lesions such as those caused by tuberculosis and fungal infection are also causes of chronic otitis media.

Serous otitis refers to nonsuppurative fluid accumulation in the middle ear. It is frequently associated with dysfunction or obstruction of the eustachian tube, such as may result from tonsillar hyperplasia or recurrent infection. This condition is an important cause of hearing problems in children that are not recognized for a period of time. Treatment is aimed at removing obstructive lesions of the eustachian tube and establishing aeration of the middle ear.

TUMORS. Middle ear tumors are uncommon.[8] The most frequent is *cholesteatoma.* This tumor is most often found in the middle ear or mastoid area; grossly it resembles a pearl. It is thought to be a postinflammatory, non-neoplastic condition. Histologically the tumor consists of an epidermal cystic structure filled with desquamated fibrillar layers of keratin debris admixed with cholesterol crystals (Fig. 17–1). The le-

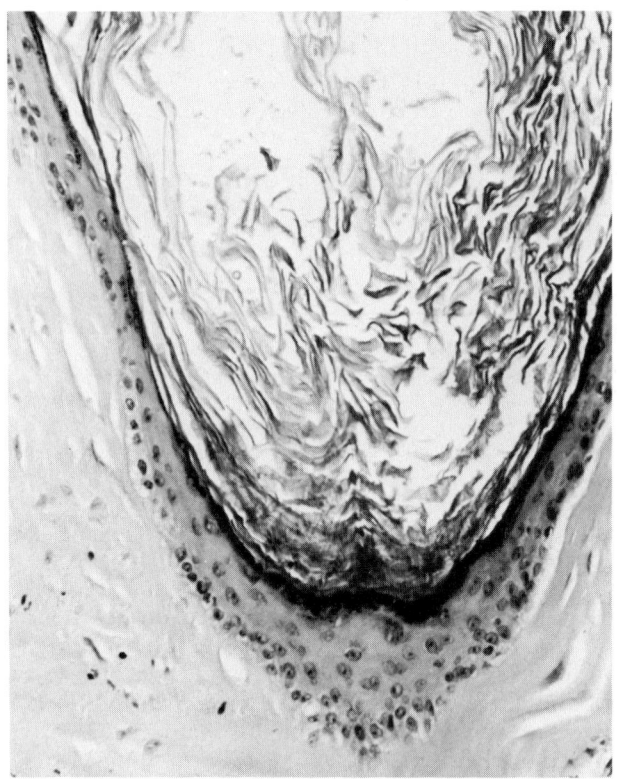

Figure 17–1. Cholesteatoma. A high-power detail of the epidermal lining and keratinous debris within the cystic lesion.

sion is thought to arise from ingrowth of squamous epithelium from the external ear into the middle ear following an otitis media which perforates the drum. As the cysts increase in size they produce hearing impairment and erode into adjacent structures, e.g., mastoid bone. Cholesterol granulomas may be present in ears with cholesteatoma, but are not required to establish the diagnosis of cholesteatoma. Treatment is thorough surgical removal.

True middle ear neoplasms are rare and include nonchromaffin paraganglioma (p. 1263) and squamous cell carcinoma.

INNER EAR

Inner ear lesions are usually associated with a loss of vestibular and cochlear functions, resulting in varying degrees of hearing impairment and dizziness. These problems may relate to neuronal degeneration, nerve compression, or inflammatory conditions.

OTOSCLEROSIS. This disorder is characterized by bone deposition in the annulus around the stapes footplate, resulting in ankylosis of the footplate and conductive hearing loss. It is the most common cause of hearing loss in young adults and is inherited as an autosomal dominant trait with variable penetrance. Histologically the lesions vary according to the stage of development at the time of biopsy. Early lesions show fibrosis and vascular proliferation with woven bone deposits. Late lesions show irregular bone deposits simulating localized Paget's disease of bone (p. 1328). Clinically the hearing loss can be compensated by various interventions aimed at the establishment of fluid movement in the vestibule.

MENIERE'S DISEASE. This is a rather common entity manifested clinically by attacks of vertigo, nystagmus, nausea, tinnitus, and hearing loss. Morphologically there is hydropic dilatation of the endolymphatic system of the cochlea, and Reissner's membrane is frequently ruptured. The cause is unknown.

INFECTIOUS AND POSTINFECTIOUS LABYRINTHITIS. A variety of viruses may cause inflammation of the labyrinth and manifestations of vestibular and cochlear dysfunction—including hearing loss. Mumps, cytomegalovirus, and rubella are causes of such viral labyrinthitis.

Occasionally, symptoms of vertigo, nausea, and tinnitus resembling Meniere's disease follow upper respiratory viral infections. This so-called *postinfectious labyrinthitis* may last for several weeks but eventually disappears spontaneously.

ACOUSTIC NEUROMA. This is a neoplasm of Schwann cells arising in the eighth cranial nerve. The lesions are usually located in the internal auditory canal area and cerebellopontine angle regions. They are described on page 1445, but it should be noted here that they cause compression of the vestibular nerve and result in deafness. It is important to recognize these tumors as early as possible to prevent permanent nerve damage. Computerized tomography and magnetic resonance imaging can establish this diagnosis when the tumors are small.[9]

NASAL CAVITIES AND ACCESSORY AIR SINUSES

Inflammatory diseases are the most common disorders to affect the nose and accessory nasal sinuses. These inflammations are as frequent and as commonplace as the "common cold." Most are more discomforting than serious. However, persistent bacterial infections occasionally give rise to clinically significant disease, and in these instances spread of the infection may lead to dangerous sequelae. Not to be forgotten is the occasional instance of destructive inflammatory nasal disease, which represents one facet of the systemic entity Wegener's granulomatosis (p. 796). Tumors may arise in either the nasal cavity or the sinuses, but these are infrequent.

INFLAMMATIONS

RHINITIS. This designation is given to inflammation of the nasal cavities. *Acute rhinitis* is almost invariably initiated by one of the many viruses now proved to cause upper respiratory infections. Several of the better studied adenoviruses produce nasopharyngitis, pharyngotonsillitis, and many other clinical variants that are all included under the category of the "common cold" or upper respiratory infection. These viral agents usually evoke a profuse catarrhal discharge that is familiar to all and the bane of the kindergarten teacher. During the initial acute stages of rhinitis, the nasal mucosa is thickened, edematous, and red; the nasal cavities are narrowed and the turbinates are enlarged. Secondary bacterial infection modifies the character of the discharge and produces an essentially mucopurulent to sometimes frankly suppurative exudate.

Allergic rhinitis (hay fever) is initiated by sensitivity reactions to one of a large group of allergens, perhaps most commonly the plant *pollens.* As described for the pathogenesis of asthma (p. 773), allergic rhinitis is an IgE-mediated immune reaction and consists of an *acute response* mediated by mast cell degranulation and release of mediators, followed by a *late persistent response* caused by infiltration of leukocytes—eosinophils, basophils, neutrophils, and macrophages.[10,11] Both responses are associated with considerable edema. Recurrent allergic rhinitis eventually leads to focal enlargements of the mucosa giving rise to *"nasal polyps,"* which are merely inflammatory hypertrophic swellings but not true neoplasms (Fig. 17–2A). Recurrent allergic nasal polyps can reach dimensions of over 5 cm in diameter. Histologically, polyps consist of a loose edematous stroma exhibiting scattered accumulations of inflammatory cells—including neutrophils, eosinophils, and plasma cells with occasional clusters of lymphocytes (Fig. 17–2B).

SINUSITIS. This inflammatory condition is closely related to rhinitis. Almost invariably, acute inflammatory involvement of the nasal cavities precedes and leads to infections and inflammations of the air sinuses by obstructing the drainage orifices of the sinuses. The edema of the lining epithelium may completely obstruct the drainage orifice of the sinus and, if the sinus fills up with mucus, may lead to a *mucocele.* In the stages of secondary bacterial or mycotic infection, frank suppuration replaces the watery discharge. The accumulation of such pus is sometimes designated an *empyema* of the sinus.

Suppurative infections within the sinuses are of somewhat greater significance than those in the nose because of the close relationship of these structures to the cranial vault. The spread of these infections is more prone to produce osteomyelitis and the intracranial infections listed in the above discussion of rhinitis. A serious fungal infection by the *mucormycoses* (p. 389) is particularly seen in patients with diabetic acidosis. Chronic sinusitis is also a component of *Kartagener's syndrome,* which (together with bronchiectasis and situs inversus) is caused by defective ciliary action (p. 777).

NECROTIZING GRANULOMATOUS SINUSITIS. Necrotizing ulcerative lesions of the upper respiratory tract include three groups of disorders: *We-*

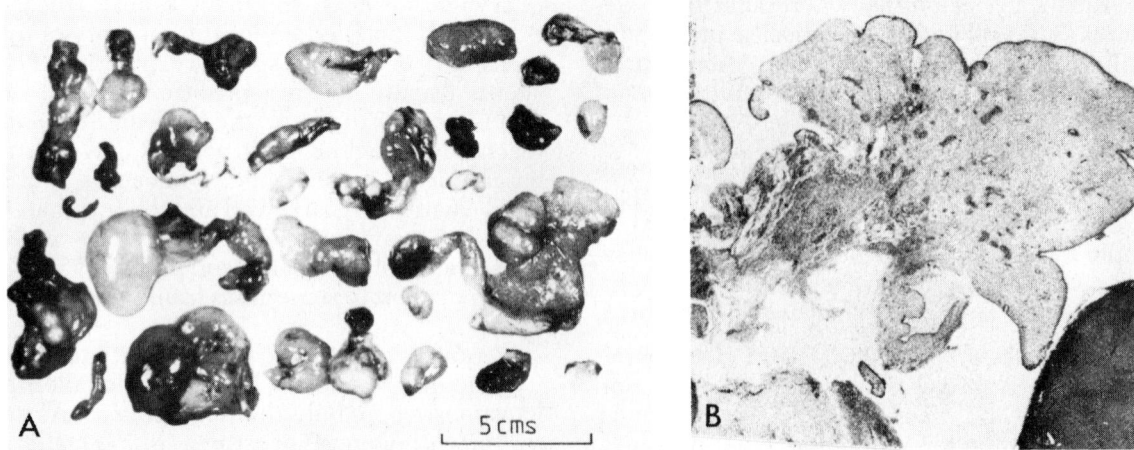

Figure 17–2. *A*, Multiple benign allergic polyps removed from nose of an old man. *B*, Low-power histology of an allergic polyp exhibiting marked submucosal edema. (Both from Friedman, I., and Osborn, D. A.: Pathology of Granulomas and Neoplasms of the Nose and Paranasal Sinuses. New York, Churchill Livingstone, 1982, p. 30. Reproduced with permission.)

gener's granulomatosis, discussed on page 796, *mucormycosis,* discussed in Chapter 7, and *polymorphic reticulosis* (lethal midline granuloma).

POLYMORPHIC RETICULOSIS (LETHAL MIDLINE GRANULOMAS).[12]
These present as ulcerating mucosal lesions of the upper respiratory tract unresponsive to antibiotic treatment. There is destruction of cartilage and extensive necrosis of tissue. Viable tissue in the ulcerated lesions shows vascular thrombosis associated with a dense lymphoid cell infiltrate. The lymphoid infiltrates are pleomorphic and consist of aggregations of large atypical cells, small lymphocytes, plasma cells, eosinophils, and macrophages. Many of the atypical lymphoid cells exhibit immunologic markers common to T-cell lymphomas (p. 718), and indeed the lesions are now considered to be variants of peripheral T-cell lymphoma. The disorder is frequently lethal, death being due to bacterial infection, pneumonia, or hemorrhage from ruptured vessels. Chemotherapeutic agents used for T-cell lymphomas have given beneficial results.

TUMORS OF THE NOSE, SINUSES, AND NASOPHARYNX

Tumors in these locations are infrequent but include the entire category of mesenchymal and epithelial neoplasms.[8] Brief mention may be made of somewhat distinctive types.

Isolated plasmacytomas may arise in the lymphoid structures adjacent to the nose and sinuses. These may protrude within these cavities as polypoid growths, varying from 1 cm to several centimeters in diameter, covered usually by an intact overlying mucosa. The histology is that of a malignant plasma cell tumor and is identical to that described on page 740. Only rarely do these lesions progress into multiple myeloma.

Olfactory neuroblastomas (esthesioneuroblastomas) are highly malignant tumors composed of small round cells and are exquisitely sensitive to radiation therapy. They are of neural crest origin and arise from the olfactory mucosa covering the superior third of the nasal septum and the cribriform plate. The recent report of an 11-22 translocation in these tumors, a translocation also associated with Ewing's tumor of bone (p. 1342) and peripheral neuroectodermal tumors, suggests a common histogenesis to these small, round cell tumors.[13]

Nasopharyngeal angiofibroma is a highly vascular tumor that occurs almost exclusively in adolescent males. Despite its benign nature, it may cause serious clinical problems because of its tendency to bleed profusely during surgery.[14]

The *inverted papilloma* is a benign but locally aggressive neoplasm occurring in both the nose and the paranasal sinuses. As the name implies, the papillomatous proliferation of squamous epithelium, instead of producing an exophytic growth, extends into the mucosa, i.e., is inverted (Fig. 17–3). If not adequately excised, it has a high rate of recurrence, with the potentially serious complication of invasion of the orbit or cranial vault; rarely, frank carcinoma may also develop.

Carcinomas in these locations are keratinizing or nonkeratinizing squamous cell carcinomas. They are insidious malignant lesions that produce the characteristic ulcerating, fungating growth typical of these tumors elsewhere. Some are closer in histologic detail to *transitional cell carcinoma,* characterized by strands and masses of polygonal-to-spindle cells growing within a fibrous stroma. The cell boundaries are poorly defined, and often the masses of cells take on the appearance of a syncytium. In some of these epithelial growths, there is an abundant lymphoid infiltrate within the fibrous stroma, and the tumor is hence designated *lymphoepithelioma* (Fig. 17–4).

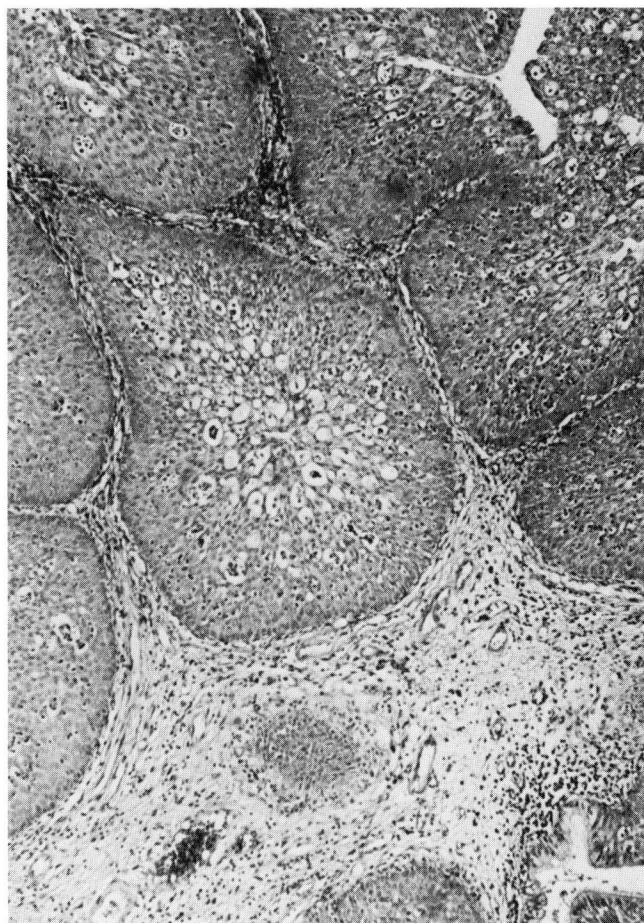

Figure 17–3. Inverted papilloma. Surface of lesion is at right. The masses of squamous epithelium are growing inward, hence the term "inverted." (Courtesy of Dr. Gilbert Brodsky, Brigham and Women's Hospital, Boston, Massachusetts.)

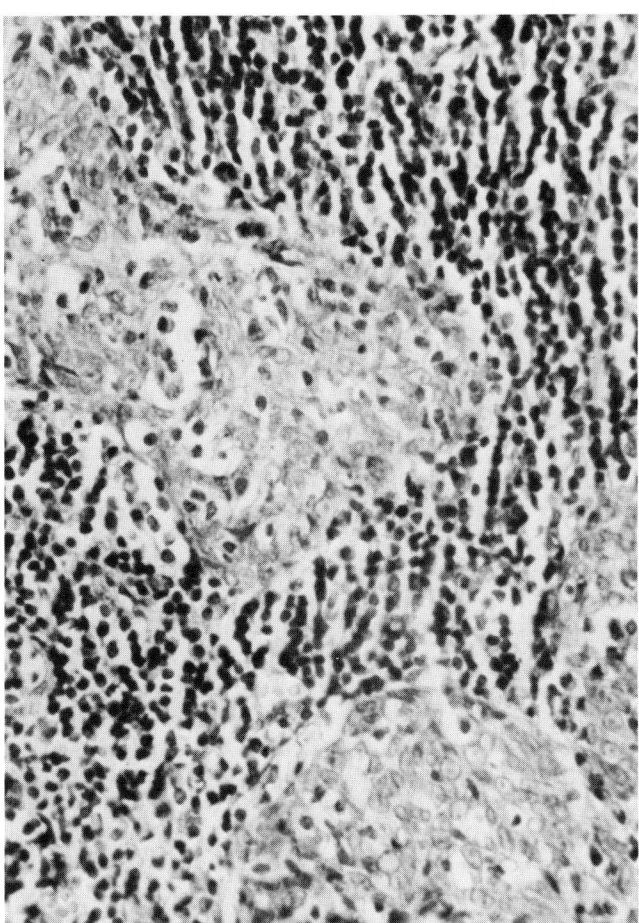

Figure 17–4. Lymphoepithelioma. The syncytium-like nests of epithelium are surrounded by masses of lymphocytes. (Courtesy of Dr. Gilbert Brodsky, Brigham and Women's Hospital, Boston, Massachusetts.)

The Epstein-Barr virus has been identified in many of these tumors.[15] Nasopharyngeal carcinomas are common malignancies in the southern Chinese population. All these malignancies progressively invade and destroy, spread to cervical nodes, and, in late cases, metastasize to distant areas. i.e., lungs, pleural cavities, liver, and remote chains of lymph nodes. Many are radiosensitive, and five-year cure rates of 80% for localized cancer and 50% for advanced cancer have been reported.[16]

LARYNX

There are only two reasonably common forms of disease of the larynx: inflammations and tumors.

INFLAMMATIONS

Inflammation of the larynx, *laryngitis*, usually occurs as a part of inflammatory disorders of the upper or lower respiratory air passages. Occasionally, most often in heavy smokers, the larynx is affected alone without involvement of the lower air passages. How-

ever, the larynx may be affected in many systemic infectious diseases, such as tuberculosis and diphtheria, and it may also be secondarily involved in inflammations that begin in the oral cavity, such as streptococcal sore throat, moniliasis, or any of the nonspecific bacterial disorders of the oral cavity or accompanying lymphoid structures. Laryngeal inflammation, although usually of slight clinical significance, may at times be serious, especially in infancy or childhood when the marked exudation or edema may cause laryngeal obstruction. In particular, *acute epiglottitis*, usually caused by *Haemophilus influenzae* or beta-hemolytic streptococci, results in marked edema and enlargement of the epiglottis sufficient to produce airway obstruction that is life-threatening in infants. Tracheotomy is a lifesaving measure in these cases. Adults have a larger margin of safety owing to the larger size of the larynx and the better development of the accessory muscles of respiration.[17]

TUMORS

Neoplasms of the larynx are, on the whole, uncommon. These tumors may be either benign or malignant, and the malignant forms are almost invariably squamous cell carcinomas.

BENIGN TUMORS. The benign tumors run the gamut of every cell type found within this structure and accordingly include polyps, papillomas, chondromas, and leiomyomas. With the exceptions of the polyp and the papilloma, the benign tumors are extremely uncommon and follow the identical pattern of growth of these tumors situated anywhere in the body.

Polyps of the larynx are smooth, rounded, sessile, or pedunculated nodules no more than 1 cm in diameter and occur most often on the true vocal cords.[18] They usually are totally covered by squamous epithelium that may become ulcerated when the nodules are exposed to the trauma of the opposing vocal cord. Microscopically, the polyp is composed largely of a core or stroma of connective tissue, varying from a loose myxomatous network to a dense, collagenous, hyaline mass. When the lesions are ulcerated, there is considerable inflammatory reaction.

Polyps occur chiefly in adults and predominantly in males. They are most often found in heavy smokers or in individuals who impose great strain upon their larynx *(singers' nodes)*. Because of their strategic location, they characteristically cause modification of the character of the voice and progressive hoarseness.

The *papilloma* is a true neoplasm that grows as a soft, succulent, raspberry-like, friable excrescence or nodule, usually on the true vocal cords. Papillomas rarely exceed 1 cm in diameter, are frequently ulcerated because of their fragility, and bleed readily on manipulation. On histologic inspection, papillae are composed of multiple finger-like projections consisting of a central core of fibrous tissue covered by stratified squamous epithelium. In many cases, protracted trauma to these masses produces marked epithelial atypicality and proliferation. In most instances, the gross morphology is sufficiently distinctive to distinguish these lesions from carcinomas (Fig. 17–5).

These lesions occur at any age and, although usually single in adults, may be multiple in children. The multiple juvenile papillomas often regress at puberty; they are known to be caused by one of the human papilloma viruses (HPV11).[19] These childhood tumors are responsible for progressive hoarseness and, if large, encroachment on the airway, with respiratory difficulty. Malignant transformation is rare.

MALIGNANT TUMORS. Although any type of malignancy, carcinomatous or sarcomatous, may arise in the larynx from the native cell population, all are extremely uncommon save for carcinomas arising in the surface epithelium. The squamous carcinomas are usually found in adults beyond the fourth decade of life and are considerably more common in males than in females. Cigarette smoking and other environmental factors play roles in their development.[20] An increased incidence of exposure to asbestos has also been reported in patients with laryngeal cancer.

Most carcinomas of the larynx occur directly on

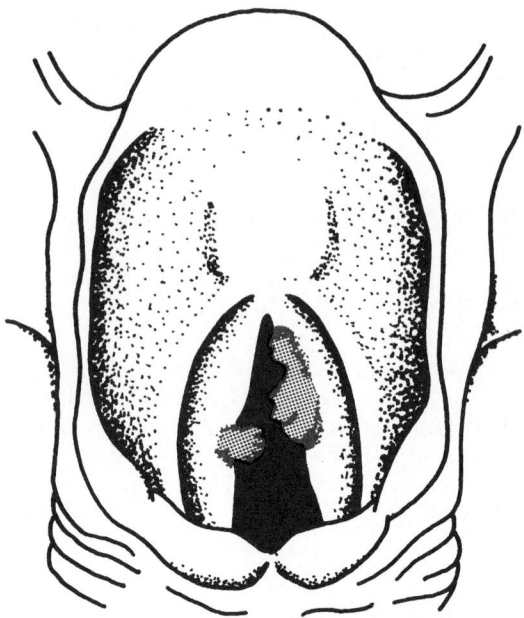

Figure 17–5. A representation of the larynx. On the left vocal cord there is a discrete, small, protruding papilloma, to contrast with the more extensive irregular invasive squamous cell carcinoma on the right cord.

the vocal cords, but they may also be found above and below the cords, on the epiglottis and aryepiglottic folds, and in the piriform sinuses. Those arising within the larynx are termed *intrinsic;* those that extend or arise outside are designated *extrinsic.* These begin as in situ lesions that later yield pearly gray wrinkling and thickening of the epithelium to become plaque-

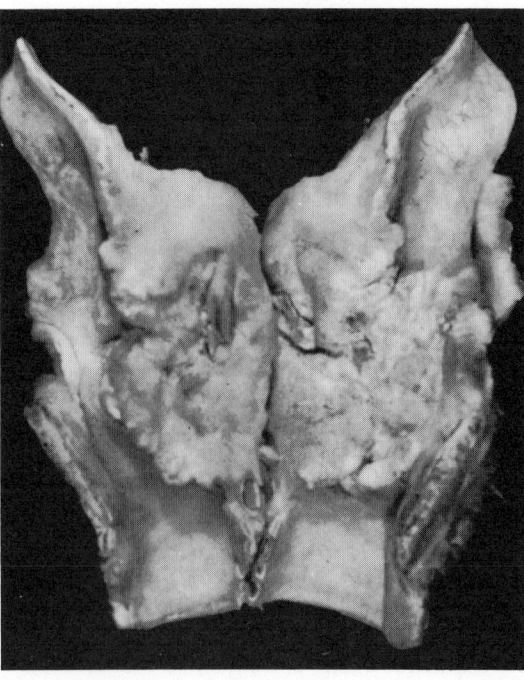

Figure 17–6. Invasive carcinoma of larynx, transected to illustrate intraluminal growth of neoplasm.

like lesions, which then ulcerate, fungate, and extend centrifugally (Figs. 17–5 and 17–6).[21] Histologically, 95% are squamous cell carcinomas, either keratinizing or nonkeratinizing. The degree of anaplasia of the squamous cell pattern is variable. The rare adenocarcinomas are presumed to originate in mucus-secreting glands.

Clinically, cases usually first become apparent with the onset of resistant, progressive hoarseness, followed possibly by pain, difficulty in swallowing, hemoptysis, and eventually even respiratory distress. Irradiation, often combined with laryngectomy, has increased the five-year survival rate of such patients to over 50%. The tumors kill by direct extension associated with ulceration, bacterial infection, and resultant debilitation; by widespread metastasis; and by secondary bacterial infections of the lower respiratory air passages and lungs.

ORAL CAVITY

The oral cavity is more than merely an orifice into which food can be stuffed (intermittently or constantly as the case may be). It is a complex portal to the digestive and respiratory tracts, lined by nonkeratinized epithelium save in the regions bound to bone (i.e., palate and gingiva) where it is keratinized. Scattered throughout the mucosa are minor salivary glands and sebaceous glands in the lips and buccal mucosa. These adnexal structures are rarely sites of origin of tumors. Its teeth and periodontal tissues are exceedingly common sites of woe, but these disorders are better left to specialized texts. Frequently, systemic diseases such as hereditary telangiectasia (Osler-Weber-Rendu disease), leukemia, scurvy, scarlet fever, and diphtheria involve the oral cavity, but these changes require no repetition here. Our present consideration is limited to the more common congenital anomalies, distinctive inflammatory lesions of the oral mucosa, and preneoplastic changes, as well as tumors and tumor-like proliferations.

CONGENITAL ANOMALIES

The complex embryologic development of the oral cavity and its associated structures not surprisingly results in a large variety of developmental anomalies involving the lips, palate, uvula, tongue, and jaws. Among the more common are *cleft upper lip (harelip)* sometimes accompanied by *cleft palate.* Although most of these clefts occur as isolated defects, rarely they call attention to more complex congenital disorders related to a chromosomal abnormality (e.g., trisomy 13 and 4p- syndromes). Other less common anomalies include an abnormally large tongue *(macroglossia)*, as for example in trisomy 21, *microglossia*, *ankyloglossia* (tongue-tie), and *fissuring.* Equally uncommon are *branchial cleft cysts.* These appear as subcutaneous, 1- to 3-cm cystic lesions in the antero-lateral aspect of the neck, filled with a serous or slightly mucinous secretion and lined by squamous epithelium sometimes with focal areas of pseudostratified, columnar respiratory epithelium. Subepithelial aggregates of lymphoid tissue are frequently present.

INFLAMMATIONS

Despite the fact that the oral cavity harbors myriad microorganisms luxuriating in the nutritious environment of the mouth, the oral mucosa is highly resistant to its indigenous flora. The relative rarity of significant oral infections is owed to many factors, including competitive suppression of overgrowth of potential pathogens by the organisms of low virulence; the secretion of secretory IgA and other immunoglobulins by local subepithelial collections of lymphocytes and plasma cells; the antibacterial effects of saliva; and the diluting and irrigating effects of food and drink. Nonetheless, any lowering of the individual's resistance or immunity, or disturbance of the microbiologic flora by antibacterial therapy predisposes to inflammations of the oral cavity. Only a few of the more common and distinctive inflammatory disorders are presented, excluding oral lichen planus, a common condition in the mouth that is discussed on page 1301.

APHTHOUS ULCERS (CANKER SORES). These extremely common superficial ulcerations of the oral mucosa affect up to 40% of the population. They are more common in the first two decades of life and may have a familial component since they tend to be prevalent within particular families. The individual lesions appear as single or multiple shallow fibrin-coated ulcerations created by denudation of the squamous mucosa. The underlying inflammatory infiltrate is largely mononuclear, but when secondary bacterial infection supervenes, numerous neutrophils appear in the inflammatory infiltrate. Typically, the ulcers are less than 1 cm in size, but occasionally they may coalesce to produce larger, extremely painful lesions. They tend to appear in successive crops sometimes related to episodes of stress, fever, or ingestion of certain foods. The underlying etiology is unknown; viruses, mycoplasma, hypersensitivity, and autoimmune reactions have all been implicated but are unproved.

Aphthous ulcers by and of themselves are more painful than serious, but they may be associated with inflammatory bowel disease and Behçet's syndrome. Typically, the frequency of outbreaks decreases with advancing age.

HERPETIC STOMATITIS. Herpes simplex types I and II may cause both orofacial and genital infections, but HSV-I is more frequently responsible for lesions in and about the mouth ranging from the relatively trivial *cold sore* to a vesiculoinflammatory eruption involving large areas of the oral mucosa and lips (gingivostomatitis). In addition, as noted on page 320, HSV may involve the membranes of the eye (keratoconjunctivitis) and in neonates or immunocompromised adults may involve visceral organs (e.g., lungs, liver) or produce encephalitis or fatal disseminated disease.[22] These viruses are virtually ubiquitous in the general population; over 90% of adults have antibodies to HSV by the fourth decade of life. Once an individual is infected, the virus spreads intraneurally to regional ganglia (e.g., the trigeminal ganglion), where it remains latent but can be reactivated whenever conditions are appropriate.

The "cold sore" or "fever blister" (herpes labialis), as is well known to all, constitutes a vesicular lesion usually located around mucosal orifices such as the lips and nares. Often several lesions appear simultaneously or in quick succession. There is frequently a history of previous respiratory infection or fever, exposure to sunlight or cold, or trauma to the area, but whether these influences in fact activate the virus remains unclear.

The vesicular lesion begins with a focus of intracellular and intercellular edema followed by ballooning degeneration of epidermal cells and acantholysis (separation of cells) with the formation of an intraepithelial vesicle (blister). Individual epidermal cells in the margins of the vesicle or lying free within the fluid develop intranuclear inclusions composed of live and dead virions. Sometimes several cells fuse to produce polykaryons or giant cells that can be identified in smears of blister fluid (Tzanck preparations). The vesicles are prone to burst to produce superficial ulcerations, and in most cases, in the course of a few days are covered with a fibrinous coagulum and progressively heal.

Primary herpetic gingivostomatitis is a more florid form of herpetic infection of the oral cavity that occurs in the compromised host (debilitation, impaired immunity, immunosuppressive therapy, and in the very young who lack antibodies). The lips and gingival and buccal mucosae are involved but sometimes also the tongue and retropharynx. The individual lesions may begin as vesicles but may extend into the mucosa and deep cutaneous layers, favoring systemic dissemination. Coalescence of the lesions leads to denudation of large areas of the mucosa. There is a commensurate greater inflammatory reaction and consequent edema and erythema.

ORAL CANDIDIASIS (MONILIASIS, THRUSH).

Candida albicans is the most frequent cause of fungal human disease in general and very much the most common cause of oral fungal involvement. The organism is a normal inhabitant of the oral cavity in 30 to 40% of the population. When the bacterial flora of the oral cavity is perturbed by antibiotic therapy, or in individuals who have diabetes mellitus, xerostomia, impaired immunity (e.g., AIDS), or severe debilitation, this otherwise harmless commensal proliferates to cause overt lesions. On obscure grounds, similar monilial lesions may appear in the vagina, not only in those who are predisposed but also sometimes in apparently healthy young women, particularly those who use oral contraceptives.

Typically, thrush takes the form of a superficial, curdy, gray to white membrane that can be readily scraped off to reveal an underlying erythematous inflammatory base. In the milder expressions, there is minimal ulceration of the mucosal surface and only a superficial subepithelial inflammatory infiltrate. More severe oral infections may produce mucosal ulceration and a correspondingly greater inflammatory reaction.

In the debilitated, compromised host, the oral candidal infection may be spread into the esophagus by the introduction of a nasogastric tube. Even more threatening, in the vulnerable individual, is more widespread mucocutaneous infection with invasion of the fungi into the deeper tissues of the oral cavity, increasing the potential for bloodstream dissemination. Uncommonly, and also in the vulnerable individual, oral candidiasis is followed by widespread mucocutaneous infection that has greater potential for invasion and dissemination.

PREMALIGNANT LESIONS

LEUKOPLAKIA AND ERYTHROPLASIA. The term "leukoplakia" simply means "white plaque." Several conditions such as white sponge nevus, lichen planus, and thrush may produce white plaques, but increasingly the term "leukoplakia" is restricted to areas of epithelial thickening (hence white) that range from completely benign to highly atypical and precancerous cell changes. Erythroplasia (dysplastic leukoplakia), in contrast, is the term applied to red velvety areas that usually remain level with, or may be slightly depressed in relation to, the surrounding mucosa, but tend to have greater epithelial atypia incurring a higher risk of malignant transformation.[23] Occasionally an intermediate type of lesion is encountered, having the characteristics of both leukoplakia and erythroplasia and termed "speckled leukoplakia."

Leukoplakia may occur anywhere in the oral mucosa. It appears as a sharply circumscribed, whitish yellow or gray plaque(s) slightly elevated above the surrounding uninvolved mucous membrane (Fig. 17-7A-B). The lesions range from less than 1 cm to large lesions many centimeters in greatest dimension. The surface may be smooth or wrinkled. **Histologically, they fall into two general categories: (1) those in which the mucosal thickening is occasioned by orderly, banal, epidermal hyperplasia accompanied by hyperkeratosis on the surface; and (2) disorderly epidermal hyperplasia (dysplasia of varying severity ranging up to carcinoma in situ)** (Fig. 17-7C-D) (p. 1288). Usually there is an inflammatory infiltrate in the subepithelial tissues composed largely of lymphocytes and occasional macrophages.

In **erythroplasia**, there is a greater tendency for atypicality of the epidermal cells and marked dysplasia. Hyperkeratosis such as is seen in leukoplakia is infrequent. The

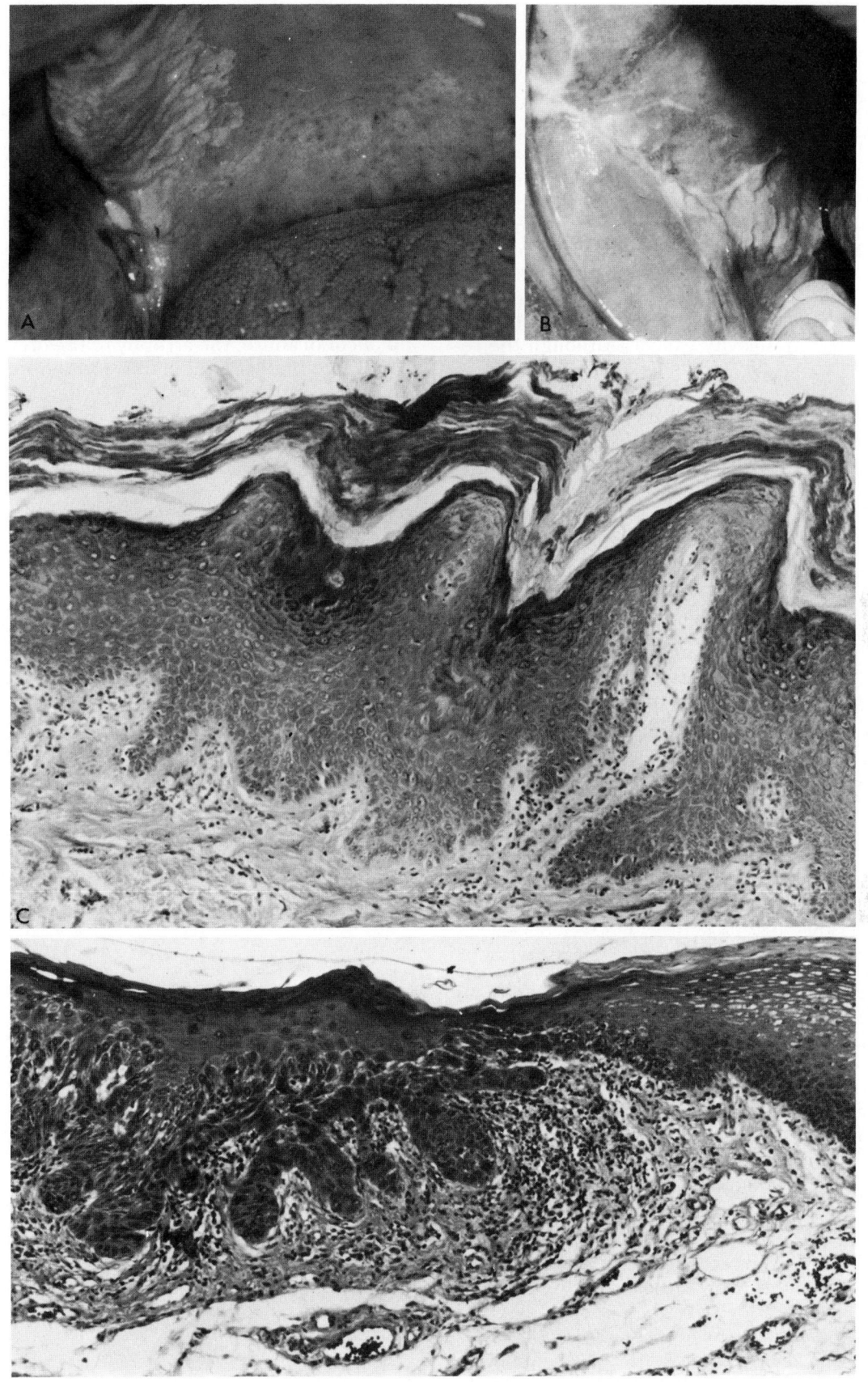

Figure 17–7. *A,* Leukoplakia of palate in a heavy smoker. *B,* Leukoplakia of buccal mucosa in a smoker. *C,* Microscopic appearance of simple leukoplakia showing hyperkeratosis. *D,* Microscopic appearance of erythroplasia (dysplastic leukoplakia) showing cellular pleomorphism bordering on carcinoma in situ. (Courtesy of Dr. Gilbert Brodsky, Brigham and Women's Hospital, Boston, Massachusetts.)

red coloration is imparted by a more intense subepithelial inflammatory reaction with vascular dilatation and a heavier infiltrate of mononuclear cells.[24]

The cause of leukoplakia and erythroplasia is unknown but chronic friction (as with ill-fitting dentures or jagged teeth), smoking, alcohol abuse, and persistent exposure to potential irritants (lovers of hot pizza take note) are thought to contribute. Whatever their origins, the clinical significance of leukoplakia and erythroplasia is their relationship to the subsequent development of oral cavity cancer. Although the reported data vary widely, *leukoplakia has about a 1 to 15% transformation rate depending on histologic criteria, whereas erythroplasia incurs up to a 50% malignant transformation rate.*[25] Ultimately, the risk correlates with the degree of atypia in the lesion, whatever its designation. *Hairy leukoplakia* is an interesting lesion associated with the acquired immunodeficiency syndrome (AIDS). It usually occurs on the lateral margin of the tongue as white confluent patches having a corrugated or "hairy" surface.[25a] Histologically, there is marked acanthosis, hyperkeratosis, and focal koilocytosis but little atypia. HIV, human papilloma virus, and EBV antigens are present in the lesions, and replicating herpes-type (EBV) particles are frequently present within the epithelial cells. Over 50% of lesions are superinfected with candida. The lesion is not precancerous. It may, however, precede the development of overt AIDS by two to three years.

TUMORS AND TUMOR-LIKE CONDITIONS

Benign tumors and tumor-like lesions of the oral cavity are uncommon. A few of the more interesting are hemangiomas (p. 588) and granular cell myoblastomas (p. 1371). Hemangiomas may develop anywhere in the oral mucosa, as sporadic lesions or sometimes in profusion in hereditary hemorrhagic telangiectasia (Osler-Weber-Rendu syndrome). Granular cell myoblastomas, usually benign, sometimes arise in the tongue. Both these neoplasms occur in many other locations and so are described elsewhere. A few additional lesions encountered more frequently will be described later. The most significant and prevalent neoplasm is the squamous cell carcinoma.

SQUAMOUS CELL CARCINOMA. Cancers of the oral cavity represent about 5% of all malignant tumors in humans; fortunately, many can be cured and so they cause a relatively smaller share of cancer deaths. Over 90% of these malignancies are squamous cell carcinomas arising in the oral mucosa; the remainder include malignant melanomas, exceedingly rare cancers arising in the subepithelial lymphoid tissues and minor salivary glands, and sarcomas.

Squamous cell carcinomas may occur anywhere in the oral cavity but, in descending order of frequency, are located on the lip (principally lower), anterior floor of the mouth, mobile tongue, palate, and posterior tongue (Fig. 17–8). Males are affected more often than females, the ratio varying from 8 : 1 for carcinoma of the lips down to parity for carcinoma arising on the gingiva. The etiology of these neoplasms is as obscure as it is for all forms of cancer, but thought to contribute are smoking; smokeless tobacco use (chewing, buccal pouches); protracted irritation as from ill-fitting dentures or jagged teeth; chronic dental and oral infections; exposure to sunlight (for lips); heat (pipe smoking) for carcinoma of the lower lip; alcohol abuse; the atrophy of the oral mucosa encountered in the Plummer-Vinson syndrome; and radiation exposure. Many of these same influences are thought to be important in the development of leukoplakia and erythroplasia, the precancerous lesions discussed previously. A regional predisposing influence is the chewing of betel nuts in India and parts of Asia.

In its earliest stages, squamous cell carcinoma of the oral mucosa appears either as a raised, firm, pearly plaque or as an area of irregular, roughened, mucosal thickening. Often these changes appear on a background of erythroplasia or leukoplakia. As the cancerous areas enlarge they undergo central ulceration. With progression, shaggy necrotic ulcerations appear rimmed by elevated, hyperemic, firm, rolled borders. With time the ulcers become larger and deeper, with extension into surrounding tissues and possibly fixation to adjacent structures. Histologically, these cancers begin as in situ lesions, sometimes with surrounding areas of epithelial atypicality or dysplasia characteristic of some forms of leukoplakia and erythroplasia. With progression, the carcinoma in situ breaks through the base-

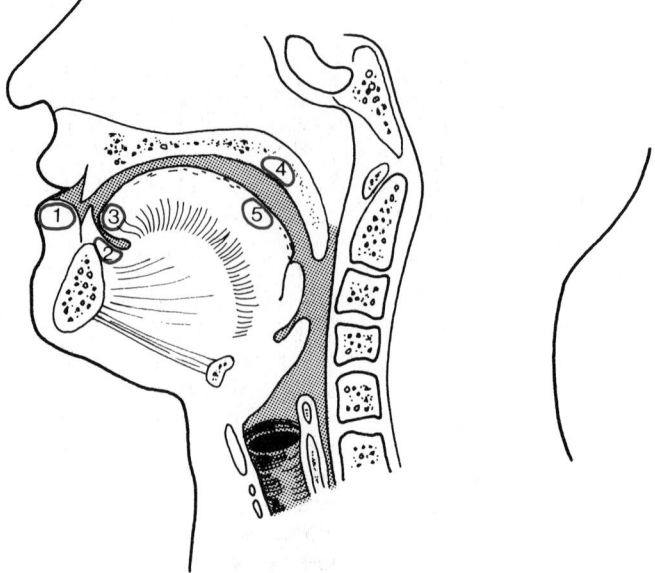

Figure 17–8. A schematic representation of the sites of origin of squamous cell carcinoma of the oral cavity in numerical order of frequency.

ment membrane and invades the subepidermal connective tissue as tongues or islands of cancer usually surrounded by a prominent inflammatory infiltrate. These neoplasms range from well-differentiated keratinizing carcinomas to highly undifferentiated lesions.

When unrecognized, these cancers eventually spread typically first to the submandibular nodes and high jugular nodes and then to more distant sites. Carcinoma of the lower lip tends to metastasize late and therefore offers the best five-year survival (approximately 85 to 90%). In contrast, cancers in the floor of the mouth, anterior tongue, and base of the tongue metastasize comparatively early and yield five-year survivals ranging from 25 to 65%. The level of differentiation of the neoplasm and its extent (stage) significantly modify the likelihood of metastases and therefore the outlook for the patient. All these neoplasms take months to years to progress through the stages of marked dysplasia to carcinoma in situ to overt carcinoma and are readily accessible to cytologic or biopsy diagnosis before they have reached the stage of incurability. Every death caused by an oral cavity cancer must then be viewed as a health education or clinical failure, since the presence of "some lesion" has almost always been known long before its true nature is established.

SQUAMOUS CELL PAPILLOMA. Papillomas, very similar to condylomata acuminata of the skin, sometimes appear on the buccal mucosa, gingivae, palate, lips, and tongue. There is presumptive evidence that they are, like their skin counterparts, caused by human papilloma viruses, but the specific implicated serotypes have not been identified.[26] They appear as papillated exophytic growths, usually less than 1.5 cm in diameter, resembling cutaneous warts. Histologically, they are made up of numerous slender papillae having fibrovascular cores covered by keratinized, stratified squamous epithelium. Superficial ulceration and infection are sometimes superimposed and incite more active epithelial hyperplasia with more frequent mitoses, but dysplastic changes are rare and malignant transformation even more rare.

TUMOR-LIKE LESIONS. The *peripheral giant cell granuloma,* also termed an *epulis,* is not a neoplasm but an unusual inflammatory lesion ranging up to 1.5 cm in diameter that characteristically protrudes from the gingiva in close relationship to the teeth. These lesions usually arise in young to middle-aged adults but sometimes in the very young and very old. Typically they are 1- to 1.5-cm hemispheric masses that may be covered by intact or ulcerated mucosa. On transection, they range from gray to brown and are nondistinctive. However, histologically they are composed of a striking aggregation of multinucleate, "foreign body–like" giant cells separated by a scant fibroangiomatous stroma. There may be foci of hemosiderin deposition as a consequence of prior hemorrhages or an inflammatory infiltrate secondary to mu-

cosal ulceration. Although not encapsulated, they are usually well delimited and readily excised. Their chief importance is in their differentiation from true central giant cell tumors, which sometimes arise within the jaws (p. 1343), or from intraosseous reparative giant cell granulomas ("brown tumors") seen in hyperparathyroidism (p. 1327).

The *pyogenic granuloma* takes the form of a red, friable, soft mass of proliferating capillaries covered by an intact or ulcerated mucosa. Most patients are pregnant, and indeed this lesion is sometimes termed *"pregnancy tumor."* However, these lesions may occur in nongravid females and in males. On the one hand, they are viewed as polypoid hemangiomas, but on the other hand, they are thought to result from a persistent inflammatory stimulus such as debris or calculus lodged in the gingival sulcus.

Subepithelial fibrovascular proliferation may give rise to so-called *gingival hyperplasia* about the teeth in epileptics on long-term phenytoin (Dilantin) therapy. Finally, obstruction to the outflow ducts of the myriad mucous glands found in the oral mucosa and lips by impacted food debris or some form of injury (as by repeated biting of the cheeks or lip) may produce small (usually less than 1 cm) cysts filled with mucinous secretion called *mucoceles.*

SALIVARY GLANDS

There are three major salivary glands — parotid, submandibular, and sublingual — as well as innumerable minor salivary glands distributed throughout the mucosa of the oral cavity. All these glands, particularly the major ones, are subject to inflammation or to the development of neoplasms.

INFLAMMATION (SIALADENITIS)

Sialandenitis may be of viral, bacterial, or autoimmune origin. The most common form of viral sialadenitis is mumps, in which usually the major salivary glands, particularly the parotid, are affected (epidemic parotitis). This condition is discussed on page 316, where it is pointed out that other glands, e.g., the pancreas and testes, may also be involved. Autoimmune disease underlies the inflammatory salivary changes of Sjögren's syndrome, discussed on page 202. In this condition, the widespread involvement of the salivary glands and the mucus-secreting glands of the nasal mucosa induces *xerostomia* — dry mouth; associated involvement of the lacrimal glands produces dry eyes — *keratoconjunctivitis sicca.* The combination of salivary and lacrimal gland inflammatory enlargement with xerostomia is sometimes called *Mikulicz's syndrome,* a noncommittal term to include all forms of involvement of these glands, including sarcoidosis, leukemia, lymphoma, and other tumors, that are sometimes accompanied by xerostomia. Xerostomia may also be secondary to radiation-induced salivary gland atrophy or to drugs, e.g., antihistamines, phenothiazines.

SIALOLITHIASIS AND NONSPECIFIC SIALADENITIS. Nonspecific sialadenitis most often involving the major salivary glands, particularly the submandibulars, is an uncommon condition encountered in a variety of circumstances. Sometimes it is secondary to ductal obstruction produced by stones (*sialolithiasis*) in the major excretory ducts. Possible pathogenetic mechanisms of stone formation are obstruction to the orifices of the salivary glands by impacted food debris and edema about the orifice following some injury. Neither hyperparathyroidism nor a particular diet is involved; frequently the stones are of obscure origin.

The ductal obstruction, even in the absence of secondary bacterial invasion, dilates the arborizing ductal system and induces a periductal reactive inflammation. In time, however, secondary bacterial invasion is prone to occur and induce more marked sialadenitis. For somewhat obscure reasons, bacterial or suppurative parotitis sometimes also develops in elderly patients with a recent history of major thoracic or abdominal surgery. Here dehydration with decreased secretory function may predispose to secondary bacterial invasion. Supporting such a potential sequence is the development of sialadenitis in patients receiving long-term phenothiazines that suppress salivary secretion.

Whatever the origin, the obstructive process and bacterial invasion lead to a nonspecific inflammation of the affected glands that may be largely interstitial, or when induced by staphylococcal or other pyogens, may be associated with overt suppurative necrosis and abscess formation. Unilateral involvement of a single gland is the rule. The inflammatory enlargement causes painful enlargement and sometimes a purulent ductal discharge.

NEOPLASMS

In view of their relatively undistingished normal morphology, the salivary glands give rise to a surprising variety of benign and malignant tumors (Table 17–1). Fortunately, only a relatively few of these neoplasms make up over 95% of salivary gland tumors, and so our consideration can be restricted to them. Overall, salivary gland neoplasms are relatively uncommon and represent less than 2% of tumors in humans. About 85% arise within the parotid. Most of the remainder occur in the submandibular gland, with a very small residual occurring in the sublingual and minor salivary glands. Curiously, the great preponderance of lesions in the parotid glands (65 to 80%) are benign, but in the other major and minor salivary glands, between 35% and 50% are malignant. Even when malignant these tumors tend to pursue a slow course characterized by local recurrence and eventual invasion of adjacent structures. Metastases tend to occur late, and therefore curative excision or radiation is more possible for these cancers than for most.

Table 17–1. Classification of Salivary Gland Tumors

EPITHELIAL TUMORS
Adenoma
  Pleomorphic adenoma
  Monomorphic adenoma
    Adenolymphoma
    Oxyphilic adenoma
    Other types of adenoma
Mucoepidermoid tumor
Acinic cell tumor
Carcinoma
  Carcinoma in pleomorphic adenoma
  Adenocystic carcinoma
  Adenocarcinoma
  Epidermoid carcinoma
  Undifferentiated carcinoma

OTHER PRIMARY TUMORS
Fibroma
Fibrosarcoma
Lipoma
Hemangioma
Neurilemmoma
Lymphoma
Melanoma

All salivary gland neoplasms, whether benign or malignant, present as nonpainful, palpable masses. Those in the parotids produce distinctive swellings in front of and below the ear. Generally, when first diagnosed they range between 2 and 6 cm in diameter and are mobile on palpation except in the neglected cancer, which becomes adherent to surrounding structures. Nonetheless, *whether benign or malignant, total excision of parotid tumors is hampered by their proximity to the facial nerve, accounting for frequent recurrences,* as will be pointed out in the following discussion. Because of this relationship to the facial nerve, in time enlarging neoplasms often induce pain, numbness, paresthesias, or facial paralysis. While such symptoms are more characteristic of invasive parotid cancers, they may also be produced by benign tumors that in their slow expansion impinge on the facial nerve.[27] The average duration of symptoms with benign tumors before they come to clinical attention is approximately 24 months, as compared with 9 to 10 months for cancers. However, there are ultimately no reliable criteria to differentiate on clinical grounds the benign from the malignant lesion; morphologic study, possibly of fine needle aspirates, is requisite.[28]

PLEOMORPHIC ADENOMA. Because of their remarkable histologic diversity, these neoplasms have in the past been called *mixed tumors.* They constitute 65 to 80% of tumors in the major salivary glands. In essence, they are composed of epithelial elements dispersed throughout a matrix of mucoid, myxoid, and chondroid tissue. In some lesions, the epithelial elements predominate, but in others the reverse obtains. They may appear at any age, most frequently in the fifth and sixth decades, with a small but distinct female preponderance. The great majority arise in the parotids and only rarely in the other major and minor salivary glands. Single tumors are the rule, but rarely two or more lesions appear simultaneously on the same or both sides.

Grossly, these tumors are encapsulated, somewhat lobulated masses ranging up to 6 cm in greatest dimension. Expansile growth produces tonguelike protrusions that may be left behind at surgical excision, accounting for the recurrence rate of 5 to 50%.[29] The cut surface is gray-white with variegated myxoid areas and areas of blue translucence representing chondroid.

Microscopic examination reveals the heterogeneity mentioned (Fig. 17–9). The epithelial elements form ducts, acini, irregular tubules, or strands or sheets of cells. They are of ductal and myoepithelial origin. The cells lining ductal or glandular formations are cuboidal or columnar, and often there is PAS-positive secretion within the glandular or ductular spaces. Often small, dark, spindled, myoepithelial cells underlie the cuboidal epithelium to create distinctive double strands of epithelial cells. In addition, the myoepithelial elements may be dispersed in islands or strands, often embedded within a loose connective tissue or myxoid tissue. Typically there are areas of loose myxoid tissue, sometimes enclosing islands of apparent chondroid matrix or rarely bone. The epithelial and apparent mesenchymal elements are randomly intermixed, but in some areas the epithelial formations may be dominant while in other areas the mesenchyme-like elements are dominant. The histologic diversity is almost limitless, but it is precisely this feature that characterizes the pleomorphic adenoma.

Excision of these neoplasms may be difficult because of their proximity to the facial nerve and because small projections may extend well beyond the main mass. Recurrences may not appear until years, sometimes decades, later. Because of the scattering of tumorous protrusions that are left behind, recurrent lesions tend to be multifocal, in contrast to primary tumors, which are almost always unifocal. Despite such behavior the recurrent tumors are almost always benign. The issue of whether long persistence of a pleomorphic adenoma or previous surgery contributes to malignant transformation is controversial, as is discussed next.

CARCINOMA ARISING IN PLEOMORPHIC ADENOMA.

In large series of pleomorphic adenomas, approximately 2% reveal areas of unequivocal malignancy.[29] These cancers may appear in the primary neoplasm or in recurrences. The average age of the patient harboring a carcinoma in a pleomorphic adenoma is about 60 years, which is one to two decades older than the average age of patients with a benign neoplasm. This fact has been taken to mean that long persistence of a pleomorphic adenoma increases the risk of malignant transformation. The possibility that these neoplasms were cancerous from the outset cannot be ruled out, but it is unlikely that a cancer would remain dormant for decades. Moreover, in many if not most instances the focus of cancer is found within a benign pleomorphic adenoma. Whether incomplete excision of a benign lesion and subsequent recurrence favors transformation remains uncertain, but clearly in some instances the cancer appears as a primary lesion before any surgical intervention.

These cancers take the form of adenocarcinoma, undifferentiated carcinoma, adenocystic carcinoma, or mucoepidermoid tumor. Foci of squamous metaplasia are occasionally encountered. The prognosis depends on the extent of the malignant change. When the focus is delimited, cure can still be effected by surgical excision, sometimes combined with radiotherapy. Larger cancers invade surrounding structures and may eventually metastasize to regional

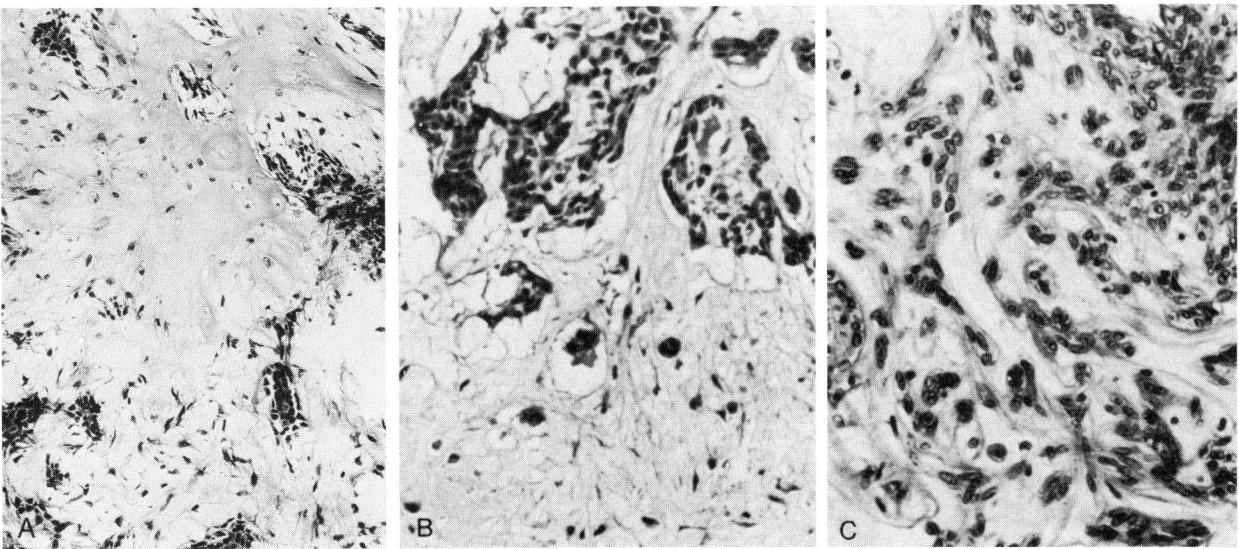

Figure 17–9. *A,* Low-power view of a pleomorphic adenoma showing abundant myxoid stroma with areas of chondroid and osteoid cells and interspersed islands of epithelial cells. *B,* The epithelial acinar formations scattered through a loose myxoid stroma. *C,* Islands and strands of myoepithelial cells with small, darkly staining nuclei.

nodes and more distant sites, resulting in about a 50% mortality rate within five years. One study tentatively suggests that activation of an oncogene (H-ras, K-ras, or myc) may be involved in the malignant transformation.[30]

ADENOLYMPHOMA (PAPILLARY CYSTADENOMA LYMPHOMATOSUM).

This tumor is composed of cystic or cleftlike spaces lined by tall columnar cells overlying an abundant lymphoid tissue. Sometimes it is referred to as *Warthin's tumor*. These neoplasms account for about 5 to 10% of all parotid gland tumors. Origin in other salivary glands is exceptional.

> The usual neoplasm is a round to oval encapsulated mass 5 to 6 cm in diameter. The transected surface is pale gray and typically reveals cystic or cleftlike spaces filled with a mucinous gray or sometimes pale brown secretion. Microscopically, these lesions are very characteristic. The spaces are enclosed by a regular palisade of tall columnar or cuboidal epithelial cells having a finely granular, markedly eosinophilic cytoplasm and small round or vesicular nuclei. Typically, there is an underlying layer of smaller cuboidal or polygonal cells. Directly beneath these epithelial elements is the lymphoid tissue, often with germinal centers. Nodular masses of lymphoepithelial elements typically protrude into the cystic spaces to convert them into narrow clefts (Fig. 17–10). Mucus-secreting cells are dispersed between the tall columnar epithelial cells, accounting for the secretion found within the lumina. Occasionally there are foci of squamous metaplasia.

The histogenesis of the adenolymphoma has long been disputed. On the one hand, it is proposed that it arises in vestigial embryonic remnants of bronchial cleft origin, accounting for the epithelial and lymphoid elements. The fact that these lesions arise only in the parotids and are not seen in other salivary glands lends support to this thesis. On the other hand is the view that these neoplasms arise from usual parotid duct epithelium that undergoes oncocytic change (i.e., the accumulation of numerous giant mitochondria producing abundant granular eosinophilic cytoplasm), and that the lymphoid tissue is essentially a reactive accumulation of non-neoplastic B and T cells. Whatever their origin, adenolymphomas are slowly growing, benign tumors that are readily cured by excision.

MUCOEPIDERMOID TUMOR.

These neoplasms are composed of variable mixtures of squamous cells, mucus-secreting cells, and intermediate hybrids. They represent about 5 to 10% of all salivary gland tumors and occur preponderantly in the parotids. Uncommonly, they arise in the submandibular glands or minor salivary glands. In the latter they represent the second most common form of malignant neoplasm.

> These tumors range up to 6 to 8 cm in diameter; they may be poorly encapsulated or completely lack a capsule so that the tumor margin infiltrates surrounding tissues.

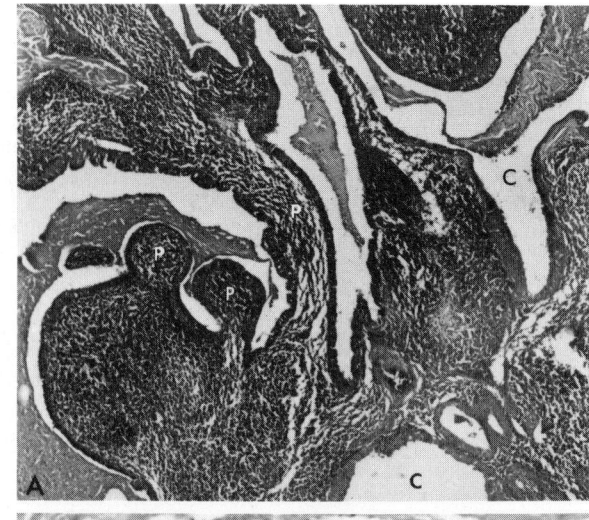

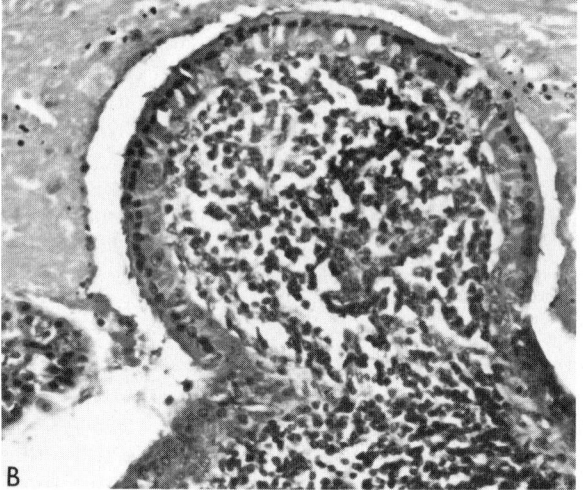

Figure 17–10. *A,* Low-power view of adenolymphoma (Warthin's tumor) showing cystic spaces (C) and papillary projections (P). *B,* High-power view of papillary projection showing double-layered epithelium (best seen to left) and lymphoid tissue in central portion.

> The transected surface is gray-white and frequently punctuated by mucin-containing cysts. Histologically, the basic pattern is that of cords, sheets, or cystic configurations of squamous, mucous, or intermediate cells. The hybrid cell types often have squamous features in which small to large mucus-filled vacuoles are present, best brought out by PAS stains. The cytologic appearance ranges from well-differentiated cells with small regular nuclei to less well differentiated cells with variably sized nuclei, hyperchromatism, and occasional mitotic figures. The squamous cells may form intercellular bridges or keratin pearls. In one common pattern, well-defined squamous cells about the periphery of a nest of cells merge imperceptibly into polygonal, well-defined, mucus-secreting cells within the center of the nest (Fig. 17–11). In some tumors, there are cells with cleared cytoplasm that is PAS negative.

It is difficult to confidently predict the biologic behavior of a tumor from its histology. Since mucoepidermoid tumors range all the way from benign to

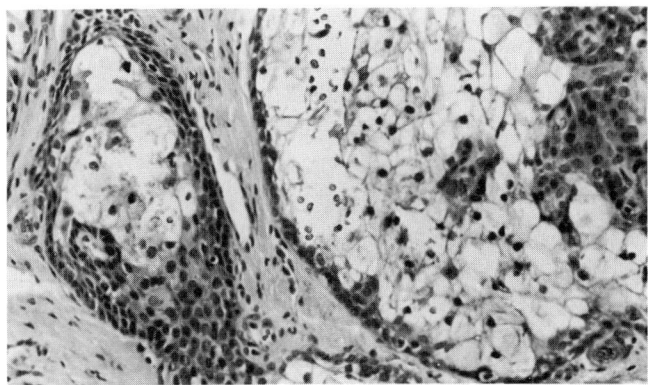

Figure 17–11. Mucoepidermoid carcinoma showing islands having squamous cells at the margins gradually merging into central masses of mucous and clear cells.

overtly malignant, the two ends of the spectrum can be reasonably well differentiated. At the benign end are well-differentiated mucus-secreting and squamous cells with little variation in cell and nuclear size and few mitoses, whereas at the malignant end the tumors are composed largely of squamous cells having considerable pleomorphism and mitotic activity. In the large middle area fall the neoplasms of indeterminate clinical behavior. Overtly malignant mucoepidermoid tumors metastasize to regional nodes and distant sites such as bone, lung, and brain. The five-year survival with the well-differentiated lesions is about 90%, falling to about 20 to 30% with those having unmistakable anaplasia.[27]

OTHER SALIVARY GLAND TUMORS. Two relatively uncommon tumors merit brief characterization — the acinic cell tumor and the adenoid cystic carcinoma.

The *acinic cell tumor* is composed of cells resembling the normal serous cells of salivary glands. It is a slowly growing neoplasm that despite an apparent benign appearance may recur and rarely metastasize. These are generally small lesions that are often encapsulated but may be poorly defined. The principal cell type is a large rounded or polygonal cell with finely granular basophilic or cleared cytoplasm. These are disposed in glandular or sheetlike patterns (Fig. 17–12A). There is usually little anaplasia and few mitoses. Some tumors are slightly more pleomorphic and in about 10% of instances metastasize, usually to regional nodes. Even these more aggressive

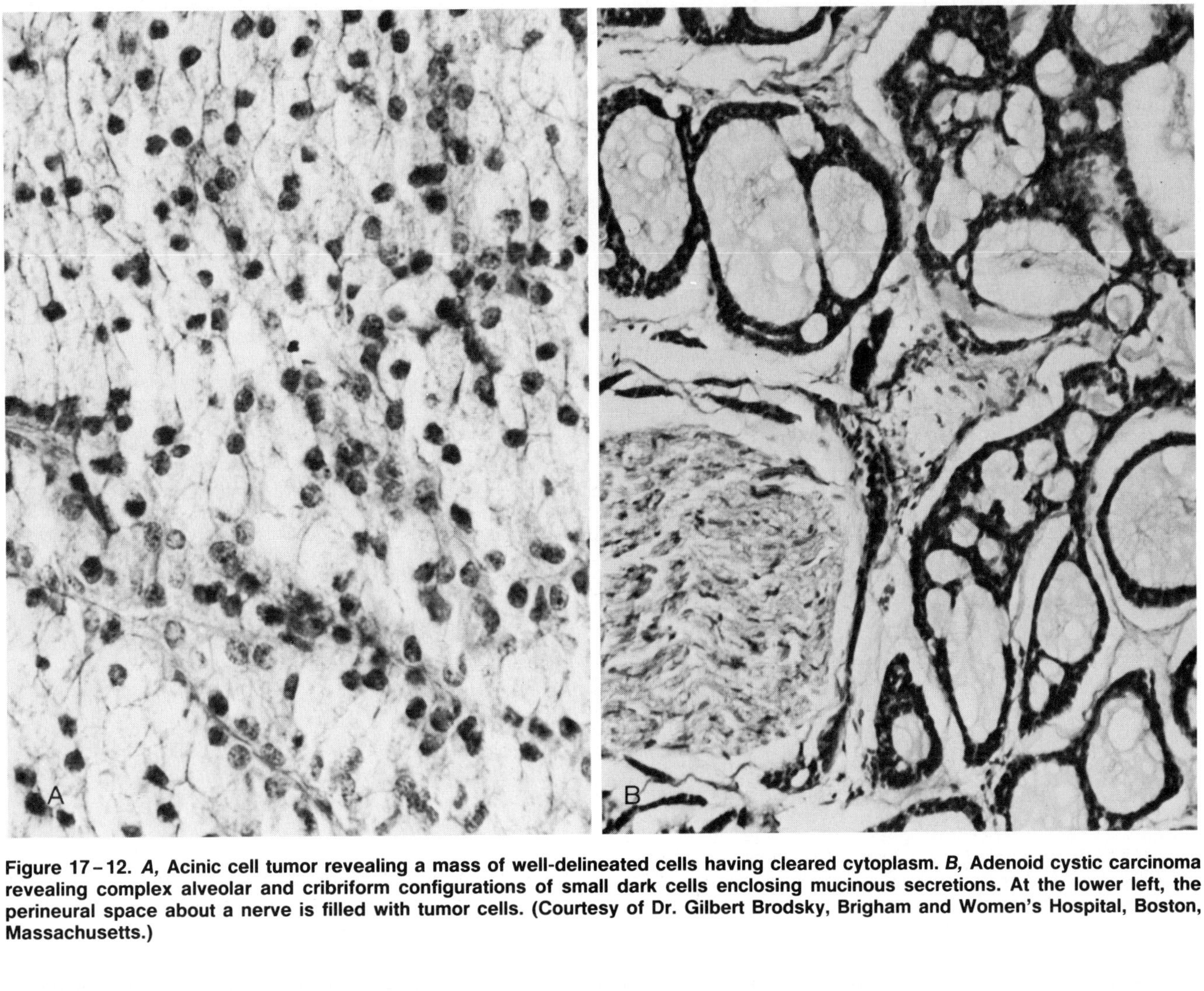

Figure 17–12. *A,* Acinic cell tumor revealing a mass of well-delineated cells having cleared cytoplasm. *B,* Adenoid cystic carcinoma revealing complex alveolar and cribriform configurations of small dark cells enclosing mucinous secretions. At the lower left, the perineural space about a nerve is filled with tumor cells. (Courtesy of Dr. Gilbert Brodsky, Brigham and Women's Hospital, Boston, Massachusetts.)

lesions run a prolonged course; thus there is about 90% five-year survival, falling to about 60% at 20 years. These tumors may be encountered at any age, more often in women.

Adenoid cystic carcinomas (cylindromas) are uncommon neoplasms in the major salivary glands, but they represent about one fifth of all tumors in the minor salivary glands. Although they may arise at any age, most patients are middle-aged, and there is a female preponderance. Grossly, cylindromas are indistinguishable from pleomorphic adenomas. Histologically they are composed of small cells having dark compact nuclei and scant cytoplasm; these cells tend to form cystic or alveolar spaces, producing a so-called cribriform pattern. In some areas the cells produce solid nests. As in the pleomorphic adenoma, the cells lining the cystic spaces tend to be cuboidal and resemble duct cells; immediately beneath these are small, dark, myoepithelial-appearing elements. Within the cystic spaces there is often eosinophilic granular material that may appear hyalinized or in other areas may appear mucinous and strongly PAS positive (Fig. 17–12*B*). Generally, there is a scant stroma separating the epithelial configurations, which ultrastructurally can be shown to contain basement membrane–like material. As with most salivary gland neoplasms, the prognosis depends on the adequacy of surgical excision. Overall, these lesions are slowly growing with a strong propensity to invade nerves; are stubbornly recurrent; and have a greater tendency to hematogenous dissemination (about 45%) than most other forms of salivary gland tumors. Thus they metastasize more often to distant sites, e.g., bone, liver, and brain, than to regional nodes. The five-year survival rate is about 60 to 70%, but drops to about 30% at ten years and 15% at fifteen years.

As is shown in Table 17–1, there are still other more rare salivary gland tumors, such as adenocarcinomas, melanomas, and mesenchymal tumors, but all are too seldom encountered to warrant detailed description.

1. Metzger, S.A., and Goodman, M.L.: Chondrodermatitis helicis. A clinical evaluation and pathologic review. Laryngoscope *86*:1402, 1976.

2. McAdam, L.P., et al.: Relapsing polychondritis: Perspective study of 23 patients and a review of the literature. Medicine (Baltimore) *55*:193–215, 1976.

3. McCaffrey, T.V., et al.: Head and neck manifestations of relapsing polychondritis: Review of 29 cases. Otolaryngology *86*:473, 1978.

4. Meandez, G., Jr., et al.: Malignant external otitis: A radiographic-clinical correlation. Am. J. Roentgenol. *132*:957, 1979.

5. Hicks, G.W.: Tumors arising from the glandular structures of the external auditory canal. Laryngoscope *93*:326, 1983.

6. Paparella, M.M.: Current concepts of otitis media. Henry Ford Hosp. Med. J. *31*:30, 1983.

7. Henderson, F.W., et al.: A longitudinal study of respiratory viruses and bacteria in the etiology of acute otitis media with effusion. N. Engl. J. Med. *306*:1377, 1982.

8. Hyams, V.J., et al.: Tumors of the upper respiratory tract and ear. Armed Forces Institute of Pathology Atlas of Tumor Pathology. Second Series. Fascicle 25, 1988.

9. Harner, S.G., and Laws, E.R., Jr.: Clinical findings in patient with acoustic neuroma. Mayo Clinic Proc. *58*:721, 1983.

10. Nacerio, R.M., et al.: Inflammatory mediators and late antigen-rhinitis. N. Engl. J. Med. *313*:65, 1985.

11. Lichtenstein, L.M.: The nasal late-phase response—an in-vivo model. Hosp. Pract. *23*:119, 1988.

12. Harrison, D.F.M.: Mid-line destructive granuloma: Fact or fiction? Laryngoscope *97*:1049, 1987.

13. Whang-Penn, J., et al.: Translocation t (11 : 22) in esthesioneuro-blastoma. Cancer Genet. Cytogenet. *1*:155, 1987.

14. Jones, G.C., et al.: Juvenile angiofibroma. Arch. Otolaryngol. Head Neck Surg. *112*:1191, 1986.

15. Purtilo, D.T., and Sakamoto, K.: Epstein-Barr virus and human disease: Immune responses determine the clinical and pathologic expression. Hum. Pathol. *12*:677, 1981.

16. Costa, J.: Nasopharyngeal carcinoma. Hum. Pathol. *12*:386, 1981.

17. Nayo Smith, M.F., et al.: Acute epiglottitis in adults. N. Engl. J. Med. *314*:1133, 1986.

18. Cambic, V., et al.: Vocal cord polyps: Incidence, histology, and pathogenesis. J. Laryngol. Otol. *95*:609, 1981.

19. Byrne, J.C., et al.: Human papillomavirus-11 DNA in a patient with chronic laryngotracheobronchial papillomatosis and metastatic squamous-cell carcinoma of the lung. N. Engl. J. Med. *317*:873, 1988.

20. Moore, C.: Cigarette smoking and cancer of the mouth, pharynx and larynx. JAMA *218*:553, 1971.

21. Decker, J.W., et al.: Advanced laryngeal cancer. Arch. Otolaryngol. Head Neck Surg. *112*:1163, 1986.

22. Corey, L., and Spear, P.G.: Infections with herpes simplex viruses. N. Engl. J. Med. *686*:749, 1986.

23. Cawson, R.A.: Premalignant lesions in the mouth. Br. Med. Bull. *31*:164, 1975.

24. Lucas, R.B.: Pathology of Tumours of the Oral Tissues, 4th ed. Edinburgh, Churchill-Livingstone, 1984, p. 111.

25. Crissman, J.D., et al.: Preinvasive lesions of the upper aerodigestive tract: Histologic definitions and clinical implications (a symposium). Pathol. Annu. *22*:311, 1987.

25a. Lumerman, H.S., et al.: The oral cavity. *In* Harawi, S., and O'Hara, C.J. (eds.): Pathology and Pathophysiology of AIDS and HIV-Related Diseases. St. Louis, C.V. Mosby, 1989, p. 353.

26. Scully, C., et al.: Papilloma viruses: Their possible role in oral disease. Oral Surg. Oral Med. Oral Pathol. *60*:166, 1985.

27. Illes, R.W., and Brian, M.B.: A review of the tumors of the salivary gland. Surg. Gynecol. Obstet. *163*:399, 1986.

28. Sismanis, A., et al.: Diagnosis of salivary gland tumors by fine needle biopsy. Head Neck Surg. *3*:482, 1981.

29. Lucas, R.D.: Pathology of Tumours of the Oral Tissue, 4th ed. Edinburgh, Churchill-Livingstone, 1984, p. 297.

30. Field, J.K., and Spandidos, D.A.: Expression of oncogenes in human tumours with special reference to the head and neck region. J. Oral Pathol. *16*:97, 1987.

The Gastrointestinal Tract

ESOPHAGUS

Yogeshwar Dayal M.D., and Ronald A. DeLellis, M.D.

CONGENITAL ANOMALIES
Atresia, Fistulas, and Stenosis
LESIONS ASSOCIATED WITH
MOTOR DYSFUNCTION
Achalasia
Esophageal Rings and Webs

Hiatal Hernia
Lacerations (Mallory-Weiss
Syndrome)
INFLAMMATIONS
Esophagitis
VASCULAR LESIONS

Varices
TUMORS
Benign
Malignant
Squamous cell carcinoma
Adenocarcinoma

NORMAL

The normal esophagus is a hollow, highly distensible muscular tube that extends from the pharynx, at about the level of the C6 vertebra, to the gastroesophageal junction at the level of the T11 or T12 vertebra. Measuring between 10 and 11 cm in the newborn, it grows to a length of about 25 cm in the adult. Three points of luminal narrowing can be identified along its course —proximally at the cricoid cartilage, midway in its course where the left main bronchus crosses it anteriorly, and distally where it pierces the diaphragm. Each of these sites is prone to trauma or perforation by impacted foreign bodies. Manometric recordings of intraluminal pressures in the esophagus have identified two "high-pressure" areas that remain relatively contracted in the resting phase. A 3 cm segment in the proximal esophagus at the level of the cricopharyngeus muscle is referred to as the upper esophageal sphincter (UES); another 2 to 4 cm segment in the intra-abdominal portion just proximal to the anatomic gastroesophageal junction is referred to as the lower esophageal sphincter (LES). Each of these sphincters is physiologically important, since abnormalities in their function frequently lead to clinical disease.

In keeping with the structural organization of the gastrointestinal tract, the wall of the esophagus consists of mucosa, submucosa, muscularis propria, and an adventitia. The mucosa is composed of a nonkeratinizing stratified squamous epithelial layer that overlies a lamina propria. In addition, a small number of specialized cell types, such as melanocytes, endocrine cells, and Langerhans cells (p. 1277), have been described in the basal layers of the esophageal epithelium. The submucosa consists of loose connective tissue containing blood vessels, a rich network of lymphatics, a sprinkling of chronic inflammatory cells, an occasional lymphoid follicle, and scattered mucus-producing glands that open onto the mucosal surface. The muscularis propria, as in other portions of the gastrointestinal tract, consists of an inner circular and an outer longitudinal coat of smooth muscle with an intervening, well-developed myenteric plexus. The muscularis propria of the proximal 6 to 8 cm of the esophagus also contains striated muscle fibers from the cricopharyngeus. The relative proportion of these skeletal fibers decreases distally, and in the adult they normally do not extend beyond the initial 10 to 12 cm. This feature explains why skeletal muscle disorders cause esophageal dysfunction. In sharp contrast to the rest of the gastrointestinal tract, the esophagus is mostly devoid of a serosal coat. Only small segments of the intra-abdominal portion are covered by serosa; elsewhere the esophagus is covered by a coat derived from periesophageal adventitia. This lack of serosal coat, together with the intimate anatomic proximity to important thoracic viscera, is of significance in promoting ready and widespread dissemination of infections and tumors of the esophagus into the posterior mediastinum. Such spread is further facilitated by the rich network of mucosal and submucosal lymphatics that run longitudinally along the esophagus.

The functions of the esophagus, as is well known, are to conduct food and fluids from the pharynx to the stomach and to prevent reflux of gastric contents into the esophagus. These functions require coordinated motor activity, namely a wave of peristaltic contraction in response to swallowing or to esophageal distention, relaxation of the lower esophageal sphincter in anticipation of the peristaltic wave, and closure of the lower esophageal sphincter after the swallowing reflex. The mechanisms governing this motor function are surprisingly complex and still imperfectly understood. It suffices for our purposes that they involve both extrinsic and intrinsic innervation, myogenic properties, and humoral substances.

The control of lower esophageal sphincter (LES) function is poorly understood.[1] LES relaxation in anticipation of peristaltic waves may be mediated by adenosine triphosphate or vasoactive intestinal peptide but is dependent on an intact vagal trunk to the esophageal plexus. Maintenance of sphincteric closure of the LES is necessary to prevent reflux of gastric contents, which, relative to the esophagus, are under positive pressure. Many substances increase LES tone, e.g., gastrin, acetylcholine, serotonin, prostaglandin $F_{2\alpha}$, motilin, substance P, histamine, and pancreatic polypeptide. Which of these agents are of importance in the normal physiologic function of the LES is uncertain, but at present gastrin is accorded only a minimal role.[2] The rather banal anatomy of the esophagus and the LES belies their complex physiology.

PATHOLOGY

Lesions of the esophagus run the gamut from highly lethal cancers to less life-threatening, but nonetheless disabling, neuromuscular disturbances, inflammations, and vascular abnormalities. Because they are fatal, carcinomas of the esophagus are the most important disorders of this level of the gut, making up about 10% of all cancers of the alimentary tract. Second in importance are esophageal varices, which are mostly associated with portal hypertension and cirrhosis. Their rupture is frequently followed by massive hematemesis (vomiting of blood) and exsanguination. Other lesions such as achalasia, webs, esophagitis, and hiatal hernias are more frequent but less threatening to life. Distressing to the gastroenterologist is the fact that all disorders of the esophagus tend to produce similar symptoms. Dysphagia (subjective difficulty in swallowing) and "heartburn" are major symptoms of all forms of esophageal pathology. Pain and hematemesis are sometimes evoked, particularly by those lesions associated with ulceroinflammatory changes in the esophageal wall. The clinical differential diagnosis of disorders of the esophagus is difficult and often requires specialized procedures such as cineradiography, manometry, and esophagoscopy.

CONGENITAL ANOMALIES

Developmental defects in the esophagus are uncommon. Because they cause immediate regurgitation when feeding is attempted, they are usually discovered soon after birth. They must be corrected early, since they are incompatible with life.

ATRESIA, FISTULAS, AND STENOSIS

Absence (agenesis) of the esophagus is extremely rare and may affect the entire length or only a portion of it. Much more common are atresia and fistula formation. In embryologic development, the gut and respiratory tract begin as a single tube; thus, developmental anomalies frequently involve both tracts.

In *atresia,* a segment of the esophagus is represented by only a thin, noncanalized cord with the resultant formation of an upper blind pouch connected to the pharynx and a lower pouch leading to the stomach. Most commonly, the atresia is located at or near the tracheal bifurcation. In about 80 to 90% of cases, the lower pouch communicates with the trachea or main stem bronchi through a tracheo- or bronchoesophageal *fistula.* Much less commonly, a fistula exists between the blind upper esophageal pouch and the respiratory tree (Fig. 18–1).

Excessive salivation, vomiting, coughing from regurgitated aspirated mucus, and paroxysmal suffocation from food that passes directly from the upper pouch into the respiratory tree are the prominent clinical manifestations. Even cyanosis and asphyxia may result. When the lower pouch communicates with the respiratory tract, the stomach tends to fill with air. Death may occur from asphyxia, aspiration pneumonia, and fluid and electrolyte imbalances.

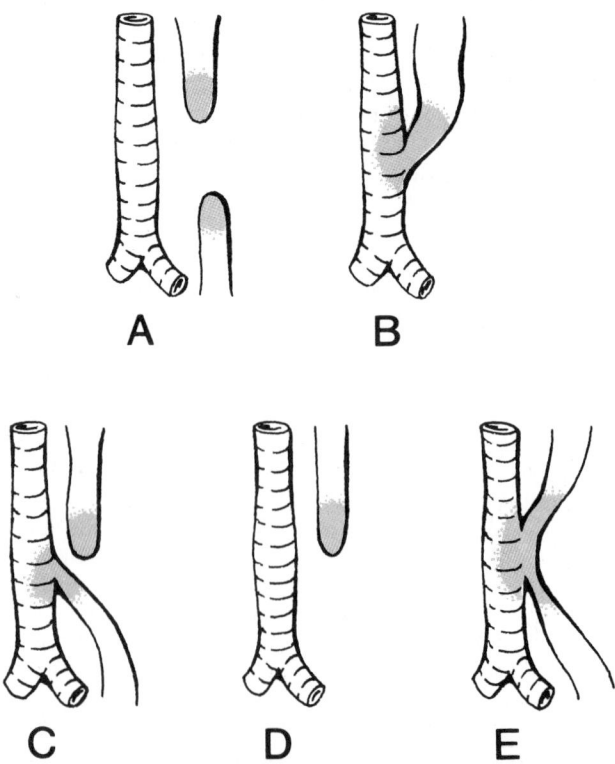

Figure 18–1. Esophageal atresia and tracheoesophageal fistula. Type C, in which the proximal esophagus ends in a blind pouch while the distal segment communicates with the trachea or a main stem bronchus, is the most common variety. (Adapted from Morson, B.C., and Dawson, I.M.P. (eds.): Gastrointestinal Pathology. Oxford, Blackwell Scientific Publications, 1972.)

Often associated with such anomalies are congenital heart disease and malformations of other portions of the gastrointestinal tract.

Stenosis of the esophagus may occur as a developmental defect, or it may be an acquired lesion resulting from involvement of the esophagus in scleroderma or inflammatory scarring secondary to esophagitis (p. 832). When present as a congenital defect, stenosis is manifested by feeding difficulty from birth. Acquired stenoses usually first become manifest in adult life. The anatomic changes consist of fibrous thickening of the esophageal wall with atrophy of the muscularis. Secondary to esophagitis, the fibrosis is accompanied by chronic inflammatory infiltrates, principally in the submucosa and periesophageal fibrous tissue. The lining epithelium is usually thin and sometimes ulcerated. In severe acquired stenoses, virtually total obstruction may result.

LESIONS ASSOCIATED WITH MOTOR DYSFUNCTION

Dysphagia is encountered both with derangements in motor function of the esophagus and with diseases that narrow or obstruct the lumen, such as fibrous stenoses or cancerous lesions. True dysphagia can be mimicked by the psychologic disturbance *globus hystericus*, which produces the sensation of uncomfortable fullness or a "lump in the throat" not necessarily associated with swallowing. This section directs our attention to four entities that are caused by or that induce motor dysfunction of the esophagus: achalasia, esophageal rings and webs, hiatal hernias, and lacerations of the esophagus.

ACHALASIA

Achalasia (failure of relaxation) is characterized clinically by progressive dysphagia and regurgitation, which usually become manifest in young adulthood but may appear in infancy or childhood. Manometric studies show three major abnormalities in achalasia: (1) aperistalsis, (2) partial or incomplete relaxation of the LES, and (3) increased basal tone of the LES.[3]

The pathogenesis of these motor dysfunctions is still not understood but appears to involve some derangement in the innervation of the esophagus and its lower sphincter. However, the locus of the neural defect is uncertain because anatomic studies have yielded inconstant findings. Most studies, but not all, reveal a loss of myenteric ganglion cells in the body of the esophagus.[4,5] There is less agreement as to whether the ganglion cells in the lower sphincter are normal, reduced, or absent. The etiology of the neural changes is usually obscure. In only one situation is the etiology of achalasia known, namely Chagas' disease caused by *Trypanosoma cruzi*. This infection causes destruction of the myenteric plexus, not only in the wall of the esophagus but also in the duodenum, colon, and ureter. Thus, patients with Chagas' disease may also have megaduodenum, megacolon, and megaureter. These extraesophageal involvements are not seen in the nontrypanosomal cases of achalasia.

Classically, in the usual sporadic form of achalasia there is progressive dilatation of the esophagus above the level of the lower sphincter. The wall of the esophagus may be of normal thickness, thicker than normal owing to hypertrophy of the muscularis, or thinned out by dilatation. The myenteric ganglia are usually absent from the body of the esophagus but may or may not be reduced in number in the region of the lower sphincter. The lining of the esophagus may be unaffected, but sometimes ulceroinflammatory lesions with fibrotic thickening are seen just above the lower sphincter. Leukoplakia may appear in the inflammatory regions, and rarely these mucosal thickenings progress to cancer.

The classic clinical symptom of achalasia is progressive dysphagia. Regurgitation and aspiration of undigested food may occur at night, leading possibly to aspiration pneumonia. The most serious aspect of this condition is the hazard of development of carcinoma of the esophagus, said to occur in 2 to 7% of affected patients. These cancers usually appear at a younger age than in individuals without this disease, sometimes as early as the third decade of life.

ESOPHAGEAL RINGS AND WEBS

Rings and webs are uncommon lesions encountered in a variety of clinical circumstances. *Those in the upper esophagus (above the aortic arch) are often designated "webs" to differentiate them from lower esophageal "rings."* Most patients are over the age of 40 years. Webs are generally, although not exclusively, seen in women. In the past, great emphasis was placed on the fact that these women often had a concomitant iron deficiency anemia and sometimes atrophic chronic glossitis as well (*Plummer-Vinson or Paterson-Kelly syndrome*). Recent studies indicate, however, that esophageal webs may be seen without an associated anemia and that the concurrence of webs, anemia, and glossitis is probably coincidental.

Lower esophageal (Schatzki's rings) usually occur close to the squamocolumnar junction and are not associated with iron deficiency anemia or confined to women. The gastroenterologic literature suggests that they are more frequent than pathologic studies would indicate. Undoubtedly, they might be missed by the pathologist, since normal LES tone contributes to their prominence, and once the esophagus is opened, they could virtually disappear. About 15% of patients with this anatomic condition have an accompanying hiatal hernia.

Well-developed esophageal webs appear as smooth mucosal ledges in the opened esophagus. Virtually all lower rings are found in the caudal 5 cm and mostly at the squa-

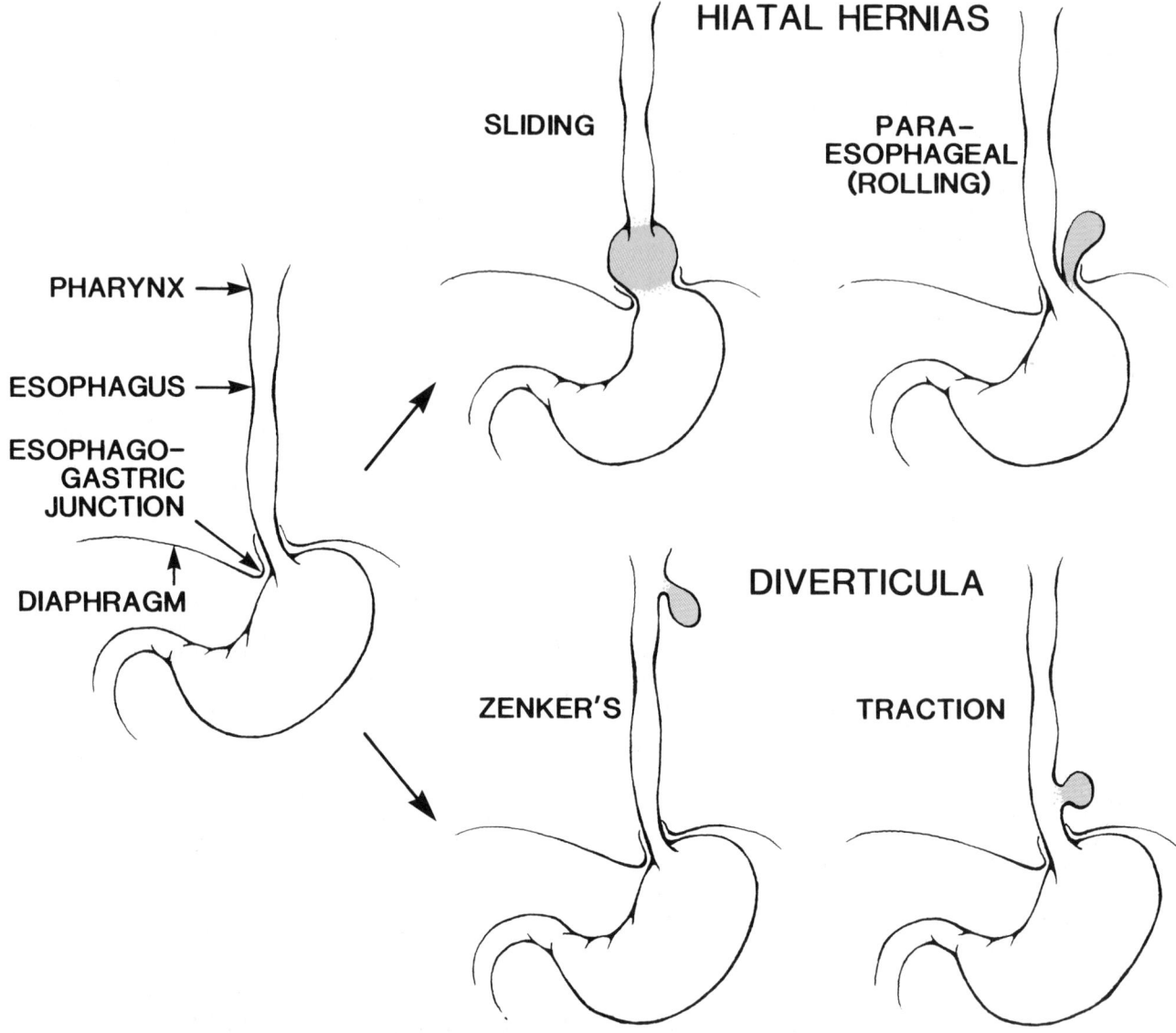

Figure 18-2. Comparison of various forms of hiatal hernias and esophageal diverticula.

mocolumnar junction. They rarely protrude into the lumen more than 5 mm and have a thickness of 2 to 4 mm. Histologically, the upper surface is covered by stratified squamous epithelium and the undersurface by columnar gastric-type epithelium. The central core is composed of a vascularized fibrous tissue often containing scattered inflammatory cells.

Dysphagia, usually provoked when an individual bolts solid food, is the main symptom associated with esophageal rings or webs. Pain is infrequent. Often the discomfort is episodic, with long symptom-free intervals. In some patients, the discomfort progressively worsens with the years and is elicited even by soft food; in others, the condition constitutes only a nonprogressive annoyance that persists throughout life.[6]

HIATAL HERNIA

Hiatal hernia is a disorder of the gastroesophageal junction that results in a saclike dilatation of the stomach protruding above the diaphragm.

Two anatomic patterns can be recognized, but only with difficulty because relaxation of tissue tone after death obscures both forms of hiatal hernia. In the first, the esophagus ends above the diaphragm, creating a symmetric, bell-like dilatation of that portion of the stomach within the thoracic cavity. The dilatation is bounded below by the diaphragmatic narrowing. This abnormality may result from a congenitally short esophagus or may be an acquired defect secondary to long-standing fibrous scarring of the esophagus. Whatever the basis, traction on the stomach pulls a portion of it into the thorax. About 90% of all hiatal hernias are of this type.[7] The supradiaphragmatic herniation of the stomach is accentuated by muscular contraction of the esophagus during the act of swallowing, and so this traction pattern is called a **sliding hernia** (Fig. 18–2).

The second pattern is designated **"paraesophageal hiatal hernia."** A portion of the cardiac end of the stomach dissects alongside the esophagus through a defect in the diaphragmatic hiatus to produce an intrathoracic sac. It is usually small and is found alongside the normally positioned lower end of the esophagus. Because the stomach rolls up alongside the esophagus, this form is sometimes called a **rolling hernia.** Less than 10% of hiatal hernias are of this type. More extreme forms of paraesophageal hernia are encountered following traumatic rupture of the diaphragm. It is important to differentiate these two forms; only the paraesophageal type is vulnerable to strangulation and infarction.

Enthusiastic roentgenologists report hiatal hernias in 4 to 7% of otherwise normal individuals,[8] over half of whom have no symptoms whatsoever. Only about 9% (usually those with a sliding hernia) suffer from such disturbances as retrosternal burning pain ("heartburn") and sometimes regurgitation of gastric juices into the mouth. These manifestations are attributed to incompetence of the esophagogastric sphincter and are accentuated by positions favoring reflux, e.g., bending forward or lying supine. Such symptoms are more common in elderly obese women, and it is not certain that they are related to the hiatal hernia. It should be cautioned that gastroesophageal reflux or heartburn can occur without a hiatal hernia; conversely, hiatal hernia can be present without these symptoms. Bleeding is sometimes seen but very likely is associated with the development of secondary esophagitis or gastritis.[9]

LACERATIONS (MALLORY-WEISS SYNDROME)

Small tears in the esophagus are fairly uncommon lesions that usually occur as a result of prolonged vomiting. These lesions are encountered most commonly, but not exclusively, in chronic alcoholics with a history of hematemesis following a bout of excessive vomiting. Normally, a reflex relaxation of the musculature of the gastrointestinal tract precedes the antiperistaltic wave of contraction. One pathogenetic concept speculates that during episodes of prolonged vomiting, this reflex relaxation fails to occur.[10] The refluxing gastric contents suddenly overwhelm the contraction of the sphincter of the cardia, and massive dilatation and tearing of the stretched wall ensue at the esophagogastric junction. Since these tears may also occur in persons who have no history of vomiting, other mechanisms must exist. Several studies have related these tears to underlying inapparent hiatal hernias.

The linear irregular lacerations are oriented in the axis of the esophageal lumen and are several millimeters to several centimeters in length. **They usually are found astride the esophagogastric junction or in the proximate gastric mucosa** (Fig. 18–3). The tears may involve only the mucosa or may penetrate deeply enough to perforate the wall.

The histology is not distinctive. The early lesion is a nonspecific traumatic defect accompanied by fresh hemorrhage into the margins of the defect. A nonspecific inflammatory response follows. Infection of the defect may lead to an inflammatory ulcer or to mediastinitis.

Esophageal lacerations account for 5 to 10% of all cases of massive hematemesis, but more often the

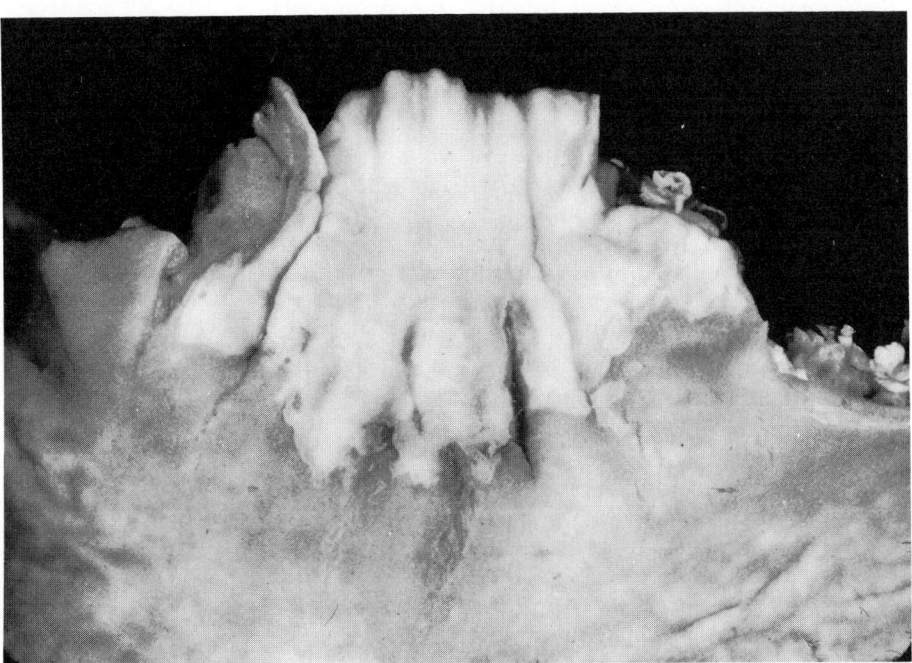

Figure 18–3. Esophageal laceration. Gross view demonstrating longitudinal lacerations extending from esophageal mucosa into stomach mucosa.

bleeding is not profuse and ceases without surgical intervention; supportive therapy such as vasoconstrictive medications and transfusions, or sometimes balloon tamponade, is usually all that is required.[11] Clinical evidence suggests that complete healing may occur, since a previous episode may leave no residua.

INFLAMMATIONS

Inflammatory lesions of the esophagus are relatively common autopsy findings, but only rarely do they cause clinical symptoms. Indeed, in most cases they represent agonal changes appearing within the last days of life, presumably reflecting profound debility and deranged sphincteric control mechanisms at the cardioesophageal junction. Significant inflammation is encountered in a wide variety of clinical circumstances and may be responsible for disturbing symptoms and even death.

ESOPHAGITIS

The following are the more important circumstances under which inflammations of the esophagus (esophagitis) may appear:

1. Reflux of gastric contents, so-called reflux esophagitis.
2. Prolonged gastric intubation.
3. Ingestion of irritants such as alcohol, corrosive acids, or alkalis (in suicide attempts); excessively hot fluids, such as tea; and heavy smoking.
4. Uremia.
5. Bacteremia or viremia with direct infection of the esophageal wall or contiguous structures. Herpes simplex virus and cytomegalovirus are the more common offenders.
6. Fungal infections (candidiasis, mucormycosis, aspergillosis) in debilitated patients, in those with an immunologic deficiency or receiving immunosuppressive therapy, and in association with broad-spectrum antibiotic therapy.
7. Radiation.
8. Cytotoxic anticancer therapy, with or without superimposed fungal infection.
9. In association with such systemic desquamative dermatologic conditions as pemphigoid and epidermolysis bullosa.
10. Graft-versus-host disease.

PATHOGENESIS. Among these associations, reflux of gastric contents is the first and foremost cause of esophagitis. The origins of reflux esophagitis are more obscure than the term would imply. Reflux of small amounts of acid-peptic gastric juice is a common event in normal individuals and is not productive of esophagitis. *The development of inflammatory changes in the esophagus is thought to require multiple concurrent influences*[12]: (1) *Frequent and protracted reflux is requisite*—thus, incompetence of the lower esophageal sphincter is an important predisposition;

(2) *disordered esophageal motility* permits the refluxed gastric contents to remain in contact longer with the esophageal mucosa; and (3) *elevated acid-peptic levels of the regurgitated fluid as well as of bile acids and lysolecithin* derived from regurgitated duodenal contents are additional contributing factors.

There are many other origins of esophagitis, as has been indicated. With some, such as intubation, radiation, and direct microbial seeding, the cause of injury is obvious. *Candidal esophagitis* has increased in frequency with the growing use of immunosuppressive, broad-spectrum antibacterial and antineoplastic drugs. The fungal infections are usually encountered in terminally ill patients, who become particularly vulnerable to fungal opportunists. Exogenous damaging influences, such as smoking and consumption of alcohol and excessively hot fluids, may also play causal roles. Esophagitis is more frequent among chronic alcoholics and heavy cigarette smokers. In Northern Iran, where alcohol is not consumed, the drinking of copious quantities of hot tea is suspected; esophagitis was observed in 86% of the population.[13] But often the pathogenesis is obscure, as it is in the case of uremia.

The anatomic changes depend on the causative agent and on the duration and severity of the exposure. Simple hyperemia may be the only alteration. More severe degrees of injury result in edema and thickening of the wall, sometimes pseudomembrane formation, or areas of superficial necrosis and ulceration. Typically, candidiasis produces large, gray-white inflammatory pseudomembranes or ulcerative lesions teeming with the causative fungus. If the inflammatory process has been severe, fibrosis and stricture formation may follow. Histologically, the reaction depends on the intensity of the injury. Thickening of the epithelium, largely by widening of the basal layer; thinning of the surface layers so that submucosal pegs reach the lumen; and inflammatory cell infiltrates particularly in areas of ulceration have been recorded.[14]

The histologic changes in **reflux esophagitis** are characterized by basal zone hyperplasia exceeding 20% of the epithelial thickness, papillae extending into the superficial third of the epithelium, and the presence of intraepithelial eosinophils with or without polymorphs (Fig. 18–4).[14] The presence of intraepithelial eosinophils is a sensitive and specific marker for gastroesophageal reflux, and since such infiltrates may occur even in the absence of basal zone hyperplasia, they are believed to be the earliest histologic abnormality in reflux esophagitis. The intraepithelial polymorphs, on the other hand, are markers of ulceration (and hence severity) rather than the presence of reflux esophagitis.

In patients with persistent gastroesophageal reflux, the distal esophagus may become lined with columnar secretory epithelium rather than the usual stratified squamous epithelium. In 1957 Barrett referred to this morphologic change as **lower esophagus lined by columnar epithelium.**[15] Although this designation has gained wide acceptance, the entity is more often referred to as **Barrett's**

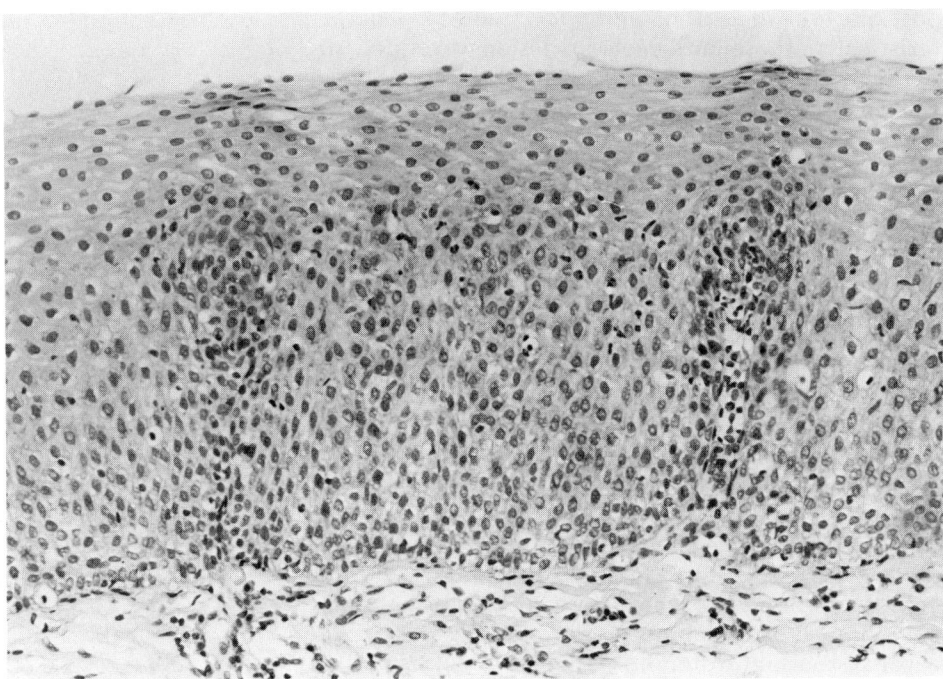

Figure 18-4. Reflux esophagitis. The expanded regenerative zone occupies more than half the epithelial thickness, and the elongated papillae reach close to the epithelial surface.

esophagus. Barrett's esophagus is thus a condition in which a gastric or intestinal type of mucosa lines the distal esophagus above the LES. Although it may rarely be congenital in origin, Barrett's esophagus is most often an acquired condition and represents an important complication of long-standing gastroesophageal reflux. Although more common in adults, it is also seen in children and even in infants under two years of age.

The pathogenesis of Barrett's esophagus is as follows: Prolonged recurrent gastroesophageal reflux leads to inflammation and eventually to ulceration of the squamous epithelial lining. Healing occurs by re-epithelialization and ingrowth of immature pluripotent stem cells, which in the microenvironment of a low pH in the distal esophageal lumen differentiate into a gastric type (cardiac or fundic) or intestinal type (specialized) epithelium that is more resistant to injury from refluxing gastric contents. Such a metaplastically derived mucosal lining may replace the esophageal mucosa circumferentially or in irregularly dispersed patches. The longitudinal extent and pattern of mucosal replacement is related to the severity of the reflux. The clinical significance of Barrett's esophagus is related to such secondary complications as the development of ulcers (Barrett's ulcer), strictures, and adenocarcinoma (Fig. 18-5).[16] The ulcers resemble gastric ulcers in their biologic behavior and frequently give rise to bleeding.

The clinical manifestations of esophagitis consist principally of dysphagia, retrosternal pain, and sometimes hematemesis or melena.

Esophagitis must be differentiated from agonal or

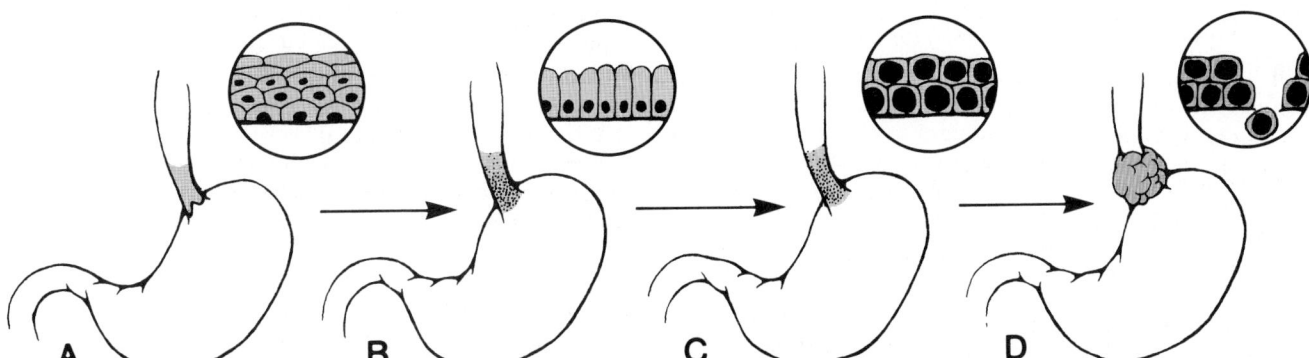

Figure 18-5. The normal esophagus (A) is lined by a stratified squamous epithelium. Prolonged gastroesophageal reflux leads to a metaplastic replacement of the squamous epithelium in the distal esophagus by a columnar type of epithelium (B) that is referred to as Barrett's epithelium. In patients with long-standing Barrett's esophagus, the columnar epithelium may become dysplastic (C) and eventually lead to the development of invasive adenocarcinoma (D).

post-mortem digestion—*esophagomalacia.* Characteristically, these post-mortem lesions produce superficial discolorations or autolysis of the esophageal wall, which is brown-black owing to acid digestion of hemoglobin. A spotted or bizarre maplike pattern, often called leopard spotting, is produced. The ultimate criterion of the nature of such post-mortem lesions is the absence of an inflammatory process.

Adenocarcinomas represent the most ominous complication of Barrett's esophagus, since it has been estimated that patients with Barrett's esophagus are at about 30 to 40 times higher risk of developing adenocarcinoma than the general population.[16]

VASCULAR LESIONS

VARICES

Regardless of cause, portal hypertension, when sufficiently prolonged or severe, induces the formation of collateral bypass channels wherever the portal and caval systems interdigitate. The pathogenesis of portal hypertension and the locations of these bypasses are considered in some detail on page 942. Here we are concerned with the collaterals that develop in the region of the lower esophagus when portal flow is diverted through the coronary veins of the stomach into the plexus of esophageal submucosal veins, thence into the azygous veins, and eventually into the systemic circulation. The increase in pressure in the esophageal plexus produces dilated tortuous vessels called varices. *Portal hypertension is most commonly caused by cirrhosis,* although rarely it may be produced by portal vein thrombosis, hepatic vein thrombosis (Budd-Chiari syndrome), pylephlebitis, or tumorous compression or invasion of the major portal radicles. Varices occur in approximately two thirds of all cirrhotic patients and are most often associated with alcoholic cirrhosis. They are less commonly found in association with pigment cirrhosis and postnecrotic scarring of the liver and are rarely produced by biliary or cardiac cirrhosis. Very infrequently, varices are encountered in systemic amyloidosis and sarcoidosis. Furthermore, rare cases have been described without evident cause for the portal hypertension.

Varices are difficult to visualize in surgical or post-mortem material, because when the veins are transected, the varices collapse. Under optimal conditions, they appear as tortuous dilated veins that protrude directly beneath the mucosa or in the periesophageal tissue along the distal esophagus (Fig. 18-6).

When the varix is unruptured, the overlying mucosa may be normal, but often it is eroded and inflamed because of its exposed position. If rupture has occurred in the past, thrombosis or superimposed inflammation may be seen (Fig. 18-7).

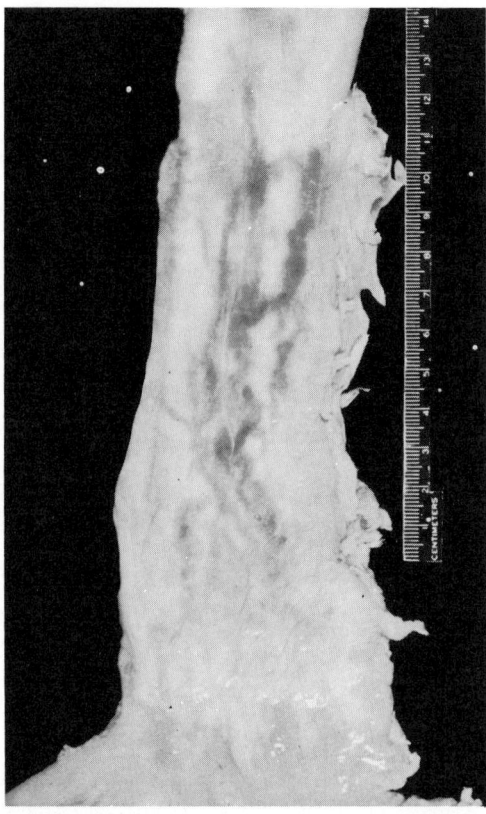

Figure 18-6. Esophageal varices. Gross view demonstrating tortuous dilated submucosal varices in middle and lower thirds of esophagus.

Varices produce no symptoms until they rupture, when massive hematemesis ensues. Among patients with advanced cirrhosis of the liver, half the deaths result from rupture of a varix. Some patients die as a direct consequence of the hemorrhage and others of hepatic coma triggered by the hemorrhage. Once begun, the hemorrhage rarely subsides spontaneously. Rupture of the varix may occur spontaneously when there has been silent inflammatory erosion of the overlying thinned mucosa. On the other hand, in many of these patients, vomiting with presumed increase of hydrostatic pressure within the varix is antecedent to the rupture. Even when varices are present, they account for only half of all episodes of massive hematemesis. In the remainder the bleeding arises from concomitant gastritis, esophageal laceration, or peptic ulcer. However, when varices bleed, 40% of patients die after the first episode. In those who survive, rebleeding occurs in about half, with an approximate 40% mortality rate following each episode.

TUMORS

BENIGN

A variety of benign tumors occur in the esophagus. These rarely exceed 3 cm in diameter and occur

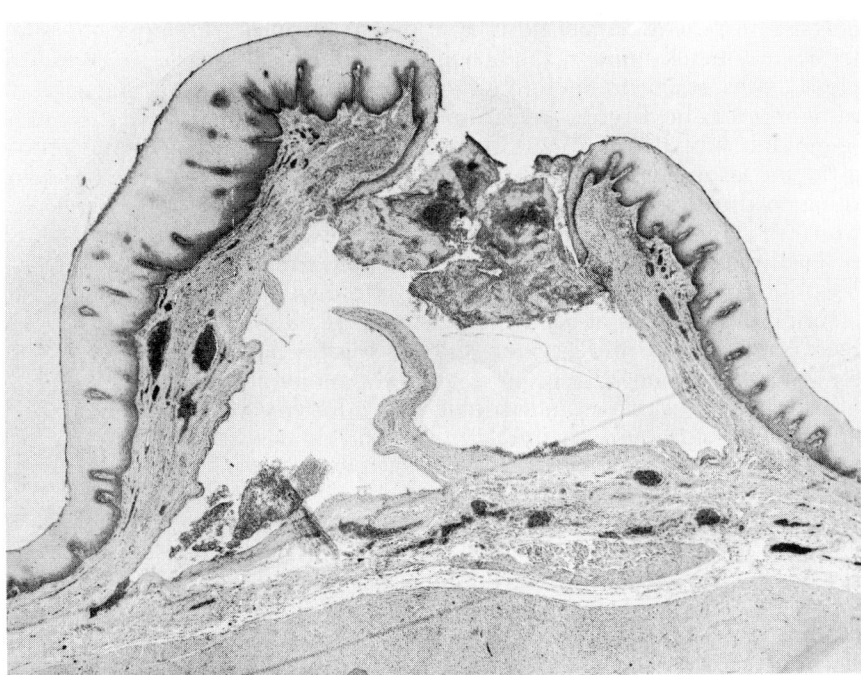

Figure 18-7. Esophageal varix. Low-power cross section of a dilated submucosal varix that has ruptured through the mucosa. A small amount of thrombus is present within the point of rupture.

mostly as intramural, solid, gray masses. The most common is the leiomyoma, but fibromas, lipomas, hemangiomas, neurofibromas, lymphangiomas, and squamous papillomas may also arise in this location. The first two are sometimes referred to collectively as stromal or spindle cell tumors. They are rarely large enough to cause symptoms.

MALIGNANT

Malignant stromal tumors (formerly called leiomyosarcomas and fibrosarcomas) of the esophagus are so rare as to be medical curiosities. Carcinomas represent the vast majority of malignant esophageal tumors. These are classified according to their cell type. Squamous cell carcinomas constitute between 80 and 85% of esophageal cancers, adenocarcinomas make up about 5 to 10%, and the remainder comprise undifferentiated or rarer cancers. Only the squamous cell and "adeno" lesions will be described.

Squamous Cell Carcinoma

In the United States, carcinomas of the esophagus represent about 10% of all cancers of the gastrointestinal tract, but they cause a disproportionate number of cancer deaths. They remain asymptomatic during much of their development and so are often discovered too late to permit cure. Most in the United States occur in adults over the age of 50; children are seldom affected.

EPIDEMIOLOGY. While squamous cell cancer of the esophagus occurs throughout the world, its incidence varies considerably not only between countries but occasionally also within the same country. Thus, areas with a particularly high incidence of esophageal

cancer have been noted in Northern China, Iran, the USSR, and South Africa. Much of our current knowledge about the demographic and etiologic aspects of this cancer is derived from epidemiologic studies conducted in these regions. In the United States, a country with a low incidence of esophageal cancer, it affects between 2 and 8 per 100,000 persons yearly and is predominantly a disease of adult males (M:F = 4:1). Blacks throughout the world are at higher risk than are whites; in the United States, both black males and females have a roughly fourfold higher incidence than do whites.

ETIOLOGY AND PATHOGENESIS. Squamous cell cancer of the esophagus is believed to have a multifactorial origin, with some factors being highly significant (Table 18-1). Of importance in its pathogenesis are (1) the consumption of foods contaminated by

Table 18-1. Factors Associated with the Development of Squamous Cell Carcinoma of the Esophagus

DIETARY
Fungal contamination of foodstuffs
High content of nitrites/nitrosamines
Deficiency of vitamins (A, C, riboflavin, thiamine, pyridoxine)
Deficiency of trace metals (zinc, molybdenum)

ESOPHAGEAL DISORDERS
Achalasia
Diverticula

LIFESTYLE
Alcohol consumption
Tobacco abuse

GENETIC PREDISPOTION
Long-standing celiac disease, ectodermal dysplasia, epidermolysis bullosa

certain fungi, e.g., Aspergillus, and diets rich in nitrites and nitrosamines; (2) chronic nutritional deficiency of certain vitamins (e.g., vitamins A, C, and members of the B complex group) or trace metals (e.g., zinc, molybdenum); (3) the presence of esophagitis and esophageal stasis; (4) chronic alcohol and tobacco abuse; and (5) a racial or genetic predisposition (e.g., among blacks or patients with long-standing celiac disease, ectodermal dysplasia, and epidermolysis bullosa).[17,18] Thus, in the Western Hemisphere, alcohol and tobacco abuse represent significant risk factors for this form of cancer. Earlier studies have shown a more than 40-fold increase in the incidence of esophageal cancer in individuals with a history of alcohol intake of more than 80 gm/day, and cigarette smoking of more than 40 pack-years.[19] United States veterans with a history of significant alcohol abuse and cigarette smoking represent a particularly high risk group.[20] The risk is related not only to the duration and severity of the abuse but, also at least for alcohol, to the type of alcoholic beverage consumed, being higher for hard liquor than for beer or wine. Some alcoholic drinks contain significant amounts of such carcinogens as polycyclic hydrocarbons, fusel oils, and nitrosamines along with other mutagenic compounds. Furthermore, since certain nutritional deficiencies are commonly associated with chronic alcohol abuse, these may act as promoters or potentiators of carcinogenesis.

In other areas of the world particularly in Iran and Northern China, where alcohol and tobacco are *not excessively consumed*, a variety of environmental factors and dietary deficiencies appear to play more significant roles. In these areas, the following have been implicated: (1) microbial contamination of food and water; (2) low molybdenum content in soil and in food grown in such soils; (3) a diet rich in corn, millet, and wheat and poor in vegetables, fruits, and animal protein, which predisposes to zinc deficiency; and (4) the consumption of pickled vegetables, which during the pickling process get heavily contaminated by certain fungi.[21,22] These factors in combination lead to a synthesis of increased amounts of nitrosamines or their precursors—compounds known to induce tumors in a variety of target organs.

In summary, therefore, it appears that environmental and dietary factors perhaps act synergistically and that nutritional deficiencies possibly act as promoters for the tumorigenic effects of certain unidentified carcinogens. It has even been suggested that the chronic esophagitis so commonly observed in persons living in areas of high incidence of squamous cell carcinoma is itself the result of continuous low-grade exposure to such carcinogens rather than the result of ingestion of indigenously brewed "teas."[18,23] This chronic esophagitis results in an increased epithelial cell turnover, which, over a length of time in an environment of ongoing carcinogen exposure and combined nutritional deficiencies, progresses to dysplasia and eventually to carcinoma.[18] The rate of progression along the chronic esophagitis–dysplasia–cancer

sequence may well be modified or modulated by genetic and racial factors. Be it as it may, the fundamental pathway to carcinogenesis would be related to both the concentration and the solubility of the carcinogenic agent(s), its permeation through the mucosa to the basal zone, and the proliferation kinetics of the target cells located there.[18]

MORPHOLOGY.   Like squamous cell carcinomas arising in other locations, those of the esophagus begin as inapparent in situ lesions. When they become overt, about 50% of these tumors are located in the middle third, 30% in the lower third, and 20% in the upper third of the esophagus. Early overt lesions are usually discovered accidentally and appear as small, gray-white, plaque-like thickenings or elevations of the mucosa. These extend with time along the long axis of the esophagus and, in months to years, eventually encircle the lumen. From this point, three morphologic patterns may evolve. **The most common one (60%) is that of the polypoid fungating lesion that protrudes into the lumen. The second gross pattern (25%) is a necrotic cancerous ulceration that excavates deeply into surrounding structures** and may erode into the respiratory tree and the aorta or permeate the mediastinum and pericardium (Fig. 18–8). **The third morphologic variant is a diffuse infiltrative form that tends to spread within the wall of the esophagus, causing thickening, rigidity, and narrowing of the lumen** with ulceration of the mucosa (Fig. 18–9).

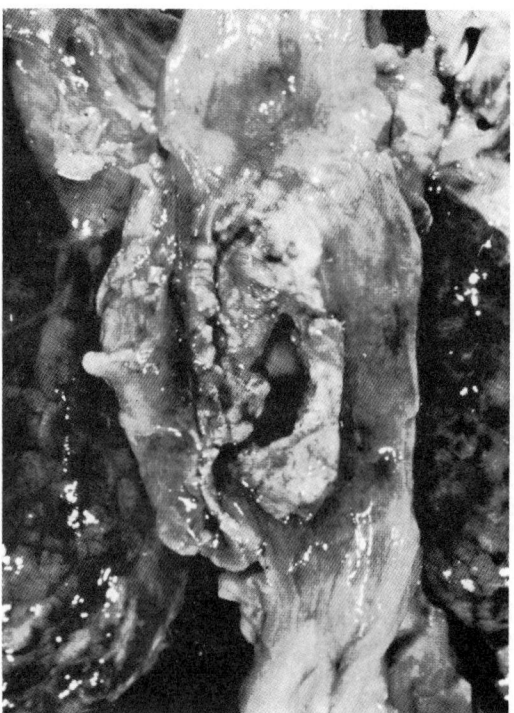

Figure 18–8. Carcinoma of esophagus viewed from esophageal aspect, showing a large defect in central necrotic portion. Tumor has directly invaded trachea to produce an esophagotracheal fistula.

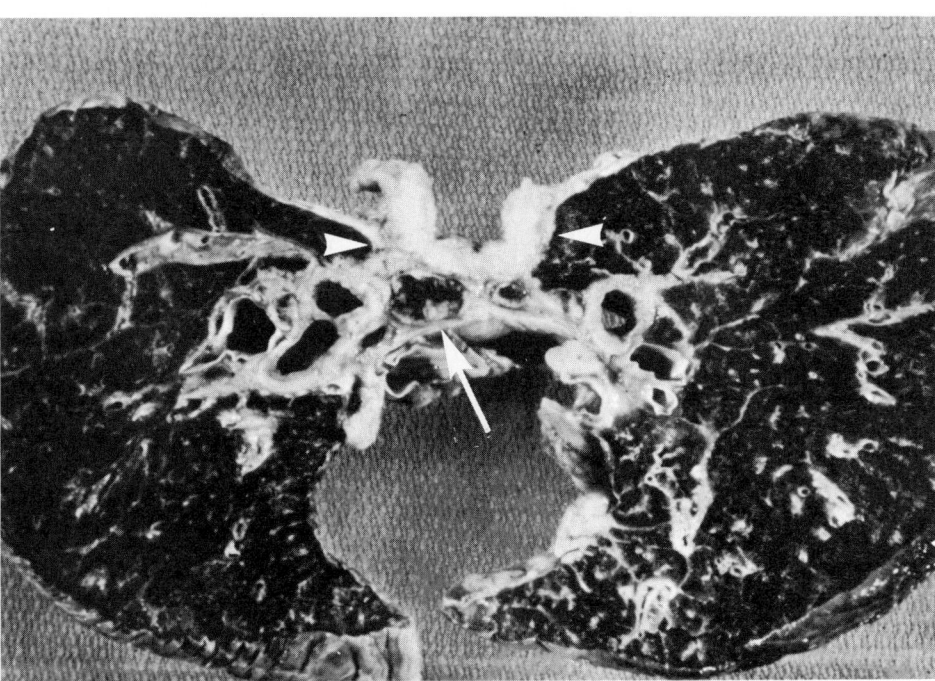

Figure 18–9. Esophageal carcinoma on transverse sectioning of esophagus and lungs. There is a diffuse thickening of the esophageal wall *(arrowheads)* by the infiltrating tumor cells. These cells have extended into the tracheobronchial tree, leading to dense adhesions and expansion of the surrounding connective tissues. An anthracotic lymph node also contains metastatic tumor *(arrow)*.

Most squamous cell carcinomas are moderately to well differentiated. Irrespective of the degree of their differentiation, most tumors are quite large by the time they are diagnosed and have already invaded the wall or beyond. The rich lymphatic network in the submucosa promotes extensive circumferential and longitudinal spread, and intramural tumor cell clusters may often be seen several centimeters away from the main mass. Local extension into adjacent mediastinal structures occurs early and often in this disease and seriously limits the chance of curative resection. Tumors located in the upper third of the esophagus metastasize to cervical lymph nodes; those in the middle third to the mediastinal, paratracheal, and tracheobronchial nodes; and those in the lower third most often spread to the gastric and celiac group of nodes.

Carcinoma of the esophagus has been staged as follows:

Stage I: Limited to esophagus; less than 5 cm in length.

Stage II: Limited to esophagus; greater than 5 cm in length, with resectable nodes.

Stage III: Lesion greater than 10 cm in length; extension through esophagus into adjacent structures; inoperable nodes or inoperable lesion.

Stage IV: Lesion as in stage III; evidence of perforation, fistula, or distant metastases.

CLINICAL COURSE. Esophageal carcinoma is insidious in onset and produces dysphagia and obstruction gradually and late. Patients subconsciously adjust to their increasing difficulty in swallowing by progressively altering their diet from solid to liquid foods. Extreme weight loss and debilitation result from both the impaired nutrition and the effects of the tumor itself. Hemorrhages and sepsis may accompany the ulcerative changes. Occasionally, the first alarming symptom is the aspiration of food that enters the respiratory tree through a cancerous tracheoesophageal fistula. It should be noted that such fistula formation is almost always caused by carcinoma of the esophagus. Bronchogenic carcinoma rarely invades the esophagus and hence rarely produces fistulous tracts. The insidious invasive growth of these neoplasms usually leads to large lesions by the time a diagnosis is established, making resection difficult if not impossible. Generally, resection is possible in less than half the cases. Even with standard methods of therapy, such as surgical resection or supervoltage irradiation, 70% of patients are dead within one year of the diagnosis, and the five-year survival rate is 5 to 10%.

Adenocarcinoma

Adenocarcinomas of the esophagus are most often located in its middle or lower third, and some of the more distally located tumors may even extend into the stomach. Adenocarcinomas have been estimated to account for between 5 and 10% of all esophageal cancers.[24] While some series mention a range of up to 15% for its incidence, this higher figure most likely reflects inclusion of gastric carcinomas that straddle the gastroesophageal junction.

Although these tumors were once thought to arise from the submucosal glands in the esophageal wall, it is now believed that the vast majority arise on a background of Barrett's mucosa. A high proportion of these tumors, when critically evaluated for the presence of Barrett's epithelium, show foci of gastric or intestinal type lining both in their immediate vicinity and elsewhere in the distal esophagus. Furthermore, areas of low- and high-grade dysplasia identified in such foci of Barrett's mucosa are often (93%) seen to blend with the tumors. Thus, the concept that adenocarcinomas in Barrett's mucosa evolve through a series of sequential changes within the mucosa, ranging from Barrett's epithelium to dysplastic Barrett's epithelium to carcinoma in situ to invasive carcinoma, is now increasingly accepted.[25,26]

Clinical studies too have reported an increased risk of adenocarcinoma in patients with Barrett's mucosa, and a prevalence ranging from under 5% to over 46% has been reported in patients with these changes. The higher figure most likely reflects a selection bias, and about 8 to 10% appears to be a more reasonable estimate of the risk of adenocarcinoma developing in Barrett's mucosa.[24]

MORPHOLOGY.   Most adenocarcinomas present as a mass or as nodular elevations of an otherwise intact distal esophageal mucosa. Since tumors arising in Barrett's mucosa are frequently multicentric, several such nodules may be detectable radiologically or at endoscopy.

Histologically, they have been classified as intestinal type, diffuse or adenosquamous, although an adenoid cystic (cylindromatous) variant histologically similar to that arising in the salivary glands has occasionally been described. The intestinal type of adenocarcinoma is characterized by well-formed glands lined by clearly neoplastic cells and is histologically identical to the intestinal type of adenocarcinoma arising in the stomach and intestines. The adenosquamous type is composed of an admixture of adenocarcinoma and squamous cell carcinoma and may show predominance of one or the other component. The diffuse type of carcinoma is seen as mucin-producing neoplastic cells diffusely infiltrating the esophageal wall.

Most adenocarcinomas of the esophagus are moderately to poorly differentiated tumors that have often invaded beyond the esophageal wall and metastasized to the regional lymph nodes by the time they are diagnosed. Pathologic staging of the disease is similar to that for squamous cell carcinomas.

CLINICAL COURSE.   Adenocarcinomas arising in Barrett's esophagus chiefly occur late in life, and patients are generally over 40 years of age (median age 50 years). This may be due to the fact that dysplastic and malignant transformation occurs only in long-standing cases of Barrett's esophagus. The disease is almost unknown among blacks, and there is a strong male predominance ($M:F = 5-6:1$).

As in squamous cell carcinomas, patients usually present because of progressive dysphagia but on close questioning will also admit to long-standing symptoms of heartburn, regurgitation, and epigastric pain that are related to their concurrent gastroesophageal reflux disease. Some patients, interestingly, reveal a history of such symptoms only in the remote past but deny having any of these symptoms for the past several years. Patients may have had corrective surgery for the gastroesophageal reflux disease in the past. It should be noted that while such procedures relieve symptoms of reflux, at least in adults, they do not cause regression of Barrett's epithelium and therefore do not appear to influence the risk of developing a subsequent carcinoma.

STOMACH

NORMAL

The stomach is a complex glandular digestive and endocrine organ that is divided into three major anatomic regions (Fig. 18–10). The glands of the cardia are mucin secreting, while those of the body and fundus contain both acid-secreting parietal cells and pepsinogen-secreting chief cells. In addition to hydrochloric acid, the parietal cells also produce intrinsic factor, which is essential for vitamin B_{12} absorption. The glands in the antrum are rich in gastrin-secreting G cells. The histology of the various glands is presented below, but some general comments are necessary for an understanding of gastric pathology.

The entire mucosal surface as well as the lining of the gastric pits is composed of so-called surface cells that are tall, columnar, and mucin secreting. They have basal nuclei and crowded, small, relatively clear mucigen-containing granules in the supranuclear regions. With appropriate fixation the mucigen granules can be stained with mucicarmine or the PAS reaction. Ultrastructurally, the surface mucous cells have

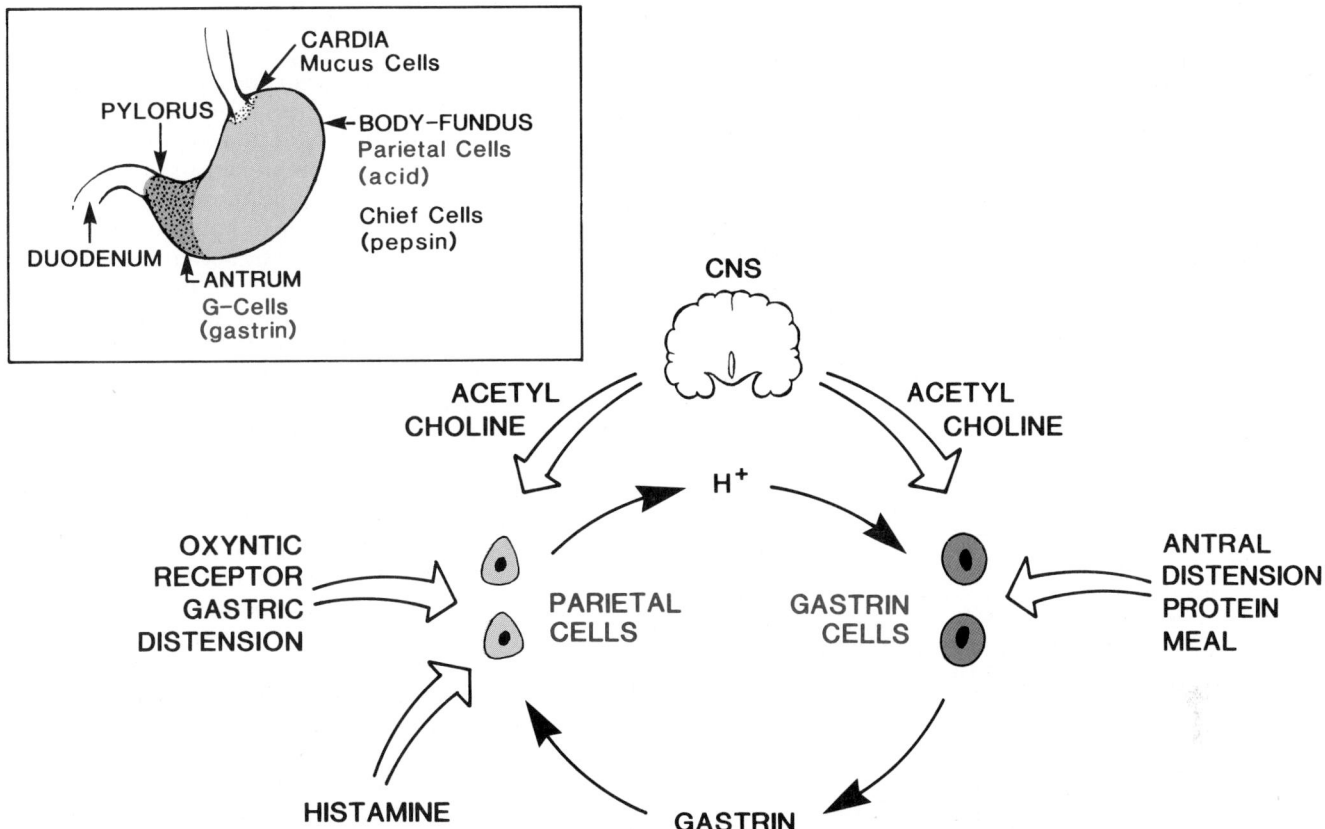

Figure 18–10. Anatomy and physiology of the stomach. In the cephalic phase, impulses originating in the CNS travel along cholinergic pathways and lead to the release of acetylcholine in the mucosa. Acetylcholine stimulates the acid-secreting parietal cells and the gastrin-producing G cells. In the gastric phase, distention of the stomach wall leads to acid secretion from the parietal cells, while antral distension and presence of protein in the stomach both stimulate gastrin secretion from the G cells. (Adapted from Gray, G.M.: Peptic ulcer disease. *In* Rubenstein, E., and Federman, D.D. (eds.): Gastroenterology (4), Scientific American Medicine. Section 4, II, Peptic Ulcer Disease. New York, Scientific American, Inc., 1988, p. 3 © Scientific American, Inc. All rights reserved.)

short microvilli and a thin coating of fine filamentous glycocalyx on their free surfaces. Deep within the gastric pits, where the various glands empty into these pits, the surface epithelial cells are somewhat modified into so-called neck cells. These neck cells are thought to be the progenitors of both the surface epithelium and the cells of the gastric glands. Mitoses are extremely common in these neck cells, and the entire gastric mucosal surface is totally replaced every two to six days.

The *cardiac* glands in the gastric cardia are lined by cells indistinguishable from the neck cells of the gastric glands. Scattered individual argentaffin cells (described below) may be present among the mucous cells.

The *gastric (oxyntic) glands* in the body or the fundus of the stomach are composed in their upper regions of mucous neck cells, below which are chief cells. The chief cells are rendered distinctive by their large, pale, zymogen granules, most prominent apically. The parietal cells are quickly recognized in H and E preparations by their bright eosinophilia. Ultrastructurally they reveal numerous mitochondria and prominent intracellular canaliculi into which the gastric acid is secreted.

Pyloric (antral) glands are made up largely of cells resembling those of the neck regions of the gastric glands. They may contain granules similar to those found in the chief cells or the surface epithelium. Numerous endocrine cells producing gastrin are also present.

Endocrine cells, characterized by a granular or pale pink cytoplasm, are widely distributed in the mucosa throughout the gastrointestinal tract. Although the existence of such cells was first reported in 1870 by Heidenhain, credit for their discovery has generally been assigned to Kulchitsky — hence they are often referred to as *Kulchitsky cells.* Because of an apparent similarity to the chromaffin cells of the adrenal medulla, they also came to be referred to as *enterochromaffin cells.* In keeping with the adrenal medulla, they were believed to have an endocrine function. On account of their morphologic similarities under light microscopy, these cells were originally regarded as a homogeneous population. However, it was soon shown that the intracytoplasmic granules in some of these cells had the special property of reducing silver salts (argentaffin cells), whereas the granules of other cells took up silver but could not reduce it unless exogenous reducing substances were added (argyrophil cells). This "histochemical heterogeneity" was shown to be related to certain peptides and biogenic amines stored within the cytoplasmic granules.[27] Ultrastructural studies also confirmed the heterogeneous nature of these cells by showing that the granules of the various cells differed in size, shape, and electron density. Immunohistochemical techniques using antibodies to various gastrointestinal hormones have permitted an accurate identification of the cell of origin for the various hormones and mapping of their anatomic distribution in the gut. The human gut is currently believed to have at least 19 different endocrine cell types. Their present nomenclature, secretory product (when known), and anatomic distribution are schematically depicted in Figure 18–11.

The various secretory products, some of which are also present in the intramural autonomic nerve terminals, act as chemical messengers and modulate normal digestive functions by a combination of endocrine, paracrine, and neurocrine mechanisms. Each endocrine cell type, therefore, is normally dispersed in different locations of the gut in numbers tailored to meet physiologic needs pertinent to that site. Thus the proximal small bowel (duodenojejunal segment), normally the site of a number of complex integrated secretory, absorptive, and motor activities, is heavily populated with large numbers of different cell types, while the colon, a comparatively less active site for absorption or secretion, is only sparsely populated by such cells. By virtue of the large numbers of the various functionally heterogeneous cell types present in it, the mammalian gut has also come to be regarded as a very versatile endocrine organ—and perhaps the largest one of them all!

Despite their functional heterogeneity, the gut endocrine cells share a number of histochemical and ultrastructural characteristics not only among themselves but also with other endocrine cell types such as the C cells of the thyroid, the chromaffin cells of the adrenal medulla, the corticotrophs and melanotrophs of the pituitary, and certain cells in the carotid body, the bronchi, the hypothalamus, and the sympathetic ganglia. The most important histochemical property common to several of these cells is their ability to take up aromatic amines or their precursors and decarboxylate them. The term APUD—an acronym for this characteristic—was adopted as a generic name for the entire family of these widely dispersed endocrine cells. Originally believed to be of neural crest origin, the APUD cells have now been shown by detailed embryologic studies to be of endodermal derivation.[28] The term APUD is no longer in vogue, and the peptide- and amine-producing cells of the gut and other sites are now referred to as neuroendocrine cells.

The process of gastric acid secretion is relevant to the later consideration of peptic ulcer disease. The capacity to secrete hydrochloric acid is directly proportional to the total number of parietal cells in the glands of the body and fundus of the stomach, i.e., *the parietal cell mass*. The most important physiologic stimulus to these cells is food in the stomach, but its effect is mediated by humoral and neural mechanisms. *The secretory process is best considered by dividing it into its three traditional phases—cephalic, gastric, and intestinal.* The *cephalic phase* is initiated by the sight, taste, smell, chewing, and swallowing of palatable food. This phase is largely mediated by direct vagal stimulation of parietal cells but may also involve vagal stimulation of gastrin release. The *gastric phase* involves stimulation of mechanical and chemical receptors in the gastric wall. Mechanical stimulation occurs with gastric distention and appears to be mediated by vagal impulses. The chemical stimuli, the most important of which are digested proteins and amino acids, induce the release of gastrin, the most potent mediator of acid secretion. Fat and glucose in the stomach do not stimulate gastric acid se-

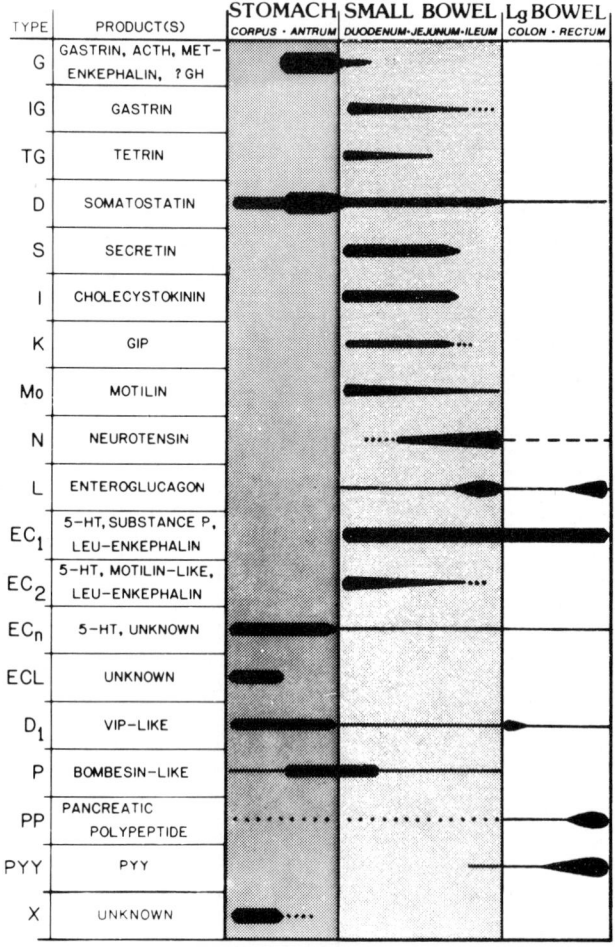

Figure 18–11. Chart depicting nomenclature, secretory products, and anatomic distribution of the various endocrine cells of the gastrointestinal tract. The width of the horizontal lines indicates their numbers relative to each other, while the extent of the lines depicts their presence in different segments of the gut. (Modified from O'Briain, D.S., and Dayal, Y.: The pathology of the gastrointestinal endocrine cells. *In* DeLellis, R.A. [ed.]: Diagnostic Immunohistochemistry. New York, Masson Publishing U.S.A., Inc., 1981, p. 75.)

cretion. Gastrin, produced by the G cells in the antropyloric and duodenal mucosa, occurs chiefly in two molecular forms — either as a peptide with 17 amino acids (G-17, or "little" gastrin) or as one with a 34 amino acid sequence (G-34, or "big" gastrin). Other variants have also been identified. G-34 has the longest half-life in the circulation and so is the major form present in the blood. However, G-17, having a much shorter circulating half-life, is the most potent stimulus to gastric acid secretion. These details make it clear why assay of the gastrin level in the blood may not accurately reflect the acid secretory drive unless radioimmunoassay is employed using antibodies specific for the G-17 form of gastrin, which do not cross react with smaller and larger peptides. The *intestinal phase* is initiated when food containing digested proteins enters the proximal small intestine. The stimulation of acid secretion that occurs at this time is thought to be related to the elaboration in the small intestine of a polypeptide quite distinct from gastrin.

Histamine is a potent acid secretagogue and exerts its influence on the parietal cells by activating adenylate cyclase, thereby increasing intracellular levels of cyclic AMP. Thus acetylcholine, gastrin, and histamine stimulate the K^+, H^+-ATPase located on the luminal surface of the parietal cell and evoke secretion. The importance of histamine as a physiologic stimulant of acid secretion remains uncertain. Inhibition of acid secretion by parietal cells can be achieved by antagonists to histamine H_2 receptors, such as cimetidine and ranitidine, or by blocking the K^+, H^+-ATPase activity by agents such as omeprazole.

How does the normal stomach resist the corrosive effects of acid-peptic-gastric secretion? At maximal secretory rates the intraluminal concentration of hydrogen ion in the stomach is *3 million times*(!) greater than that of the blood and tissues. Most important is the so-called gastric mucosal barrier. Normally, the mucosal luminal epithelial cells are bound to each other by intercellular tight junctions, and so the intact surface epithelial layer provides a barrier to back-diffusion of hydrogen ions. Adding to this barrier is secretion of acid buffer by the surface cells, since there is a pH gradient across the layer of mucus secretion attached to the surface cells. Any impairment of this mucosal barrier permits penetration of hydrogen ions into the mucosa, which ironically stimulates further secretion of gastric acid and pepsinogen. Thus, while acid is diffusing into the mucosa, the luminal hydrogen ion concentration is simultaneously rising. *A number of agents have been shown to damage the mucosal barrier, including alcohol, cigarettes, bile acids, corticosteroids, lysolecithin, and particularly aspirin.* All disrupt the continuity of the epithelial surface and so induce increased shedding of surface cells, to contribute possibly to the development of gastric mucosal erosions or ulcers. A variety of other influences, all imperfectly understood, conduce to the protection of the gastric mucosa, at least in animals.[29] Adequate mucosal blood flow, normal levels in mucosal cells of carbonic anhydrase (which participates in the forma-

tion of bicarbonate and so protects cells to an extent against excessive drops in pH), and prostaglandins all serve to defend the mucosa against the erosive action of acid-peptic secretion.[30] Gastric mucin must play some role in protection of the mucosa; therapeutic agents that stimulate mucus output have been shown to favor the healing of peptic ulcers and to protect against recurrences.[31] Dilution and neutralization of gastric acid by protein foods and refluxed bicarbonate from the duodenum also make some contribution. Imperfect as our understanding of the defensive mechanism(s) may be, it is obviously a physiologic marvel, or our gastric walls would suffer the same fate as a piece of swallowed meat.

PATHOLOGY

The stomach is an important segment of the alimentary tract from the standpoint of its diseases. Peptic ulcers have become almost a hallmark of so-called civilized life and are found in up to 10% of the general population in North America. In this day of cigarette smoking, alcohol consumption, and stress, gastritis is one of the everyday causes of "indigestion." Gastric cancer, despite its decreasing incidence in the United States, still remains a leading cause of death from cancer.

CONGENITAL ANOMALIES

DIAPHRAGMATIC HERNIAS

Weakness or partial-to-total absence of a region of the diaphragm, usually on the left, may permit the abdominal contents to herniate into the thorax. These hernias differ from hiatal hernias only insofar as the defect in the diaphragm does not involve the hiatal orifice. The hernial wall in these lesions is most often composed only of peritoneum and pleura. Usually, the stomach or a portion of it insinuates into the pouch, but occasionally small bowel and even a portion of the liver accompany it (Fig. 18–12).

PYLORIC STENOSIS

Narrowing of the pyloric lumen may be encountered in infants as a congenital defect or in adults as an acquired disease secondary to inflammatory fibrosis or tumorous invasion. Rarely, in adults, the condition represents a previously unrecognized congenital defect.

Congenital hypertrophic pyloric stenosis is an apparently familial malformation characterized by hypertrophy and possibly hyperplasia of the circular muscle of the muscularis propria of the pylorus. The narrowing may lead to edema or inflammatory

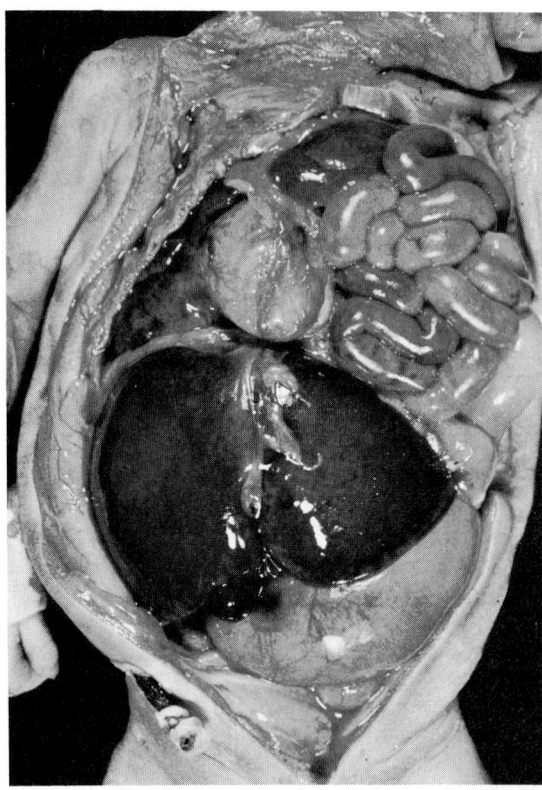

Figure 18–12. In situ view of opened trunk of an infant with a diaphragmatic hernia. Numerous loops of small bowel and portions of the colon are evident in the left pleural cavity. The markedly displaced lung can be seen at the very apex of the cavity.

changes within the mucosa and submucosa, which aggravates the narrowing. It is reported to occur in from 1 in 300 to 1 in 900 live births and affects males and females in a ratio of 4 : 1. The genetic mode of transmission is not firmly established, but multifactorial inheritance is suspected. Monozygotic twins have a high rate of concordance of the condition.

Regurgitation and vomiting usually appear in the second or third week of life. Physical examination reveals visible peristalsis and a firm ovoid palpable mass that represents the hypertrophied pyloric musculature. A full-thickness muscle-splitting incision (pyloromyotomy) in the region of the pylorus is curative.

Acquired pyloric stenosis is one of the long-term risks of patients with antral gastritis or peptic ulcers close to the pylorus. Carcinomas of the pylorus or head of the pancreas, or lymphomas, are more ominous causes of acquired disease. Whatever the cause, resection of the involved segment of bowel or some form of bypass procedure may be necessary as a curative or palliative measure.

MISCELLANEOUS LESIONS

Gastric dilatation may arise because of organic or functional obstruction of the pylorus. Organic causes include gastric outlet obstruction, e.g., pyloric steno-

sis, either congenital or secondary to ulcer disease. The functional basis appears to be atony of the stomach and intestines (paralytic ileus), which may appear in patients with generalized peritonitis. The stomach may contain as much as 10 to 15 liters of fluid. On account of enormous dilatation, the gastric wall may be markedly thinned—even to the point of translucency.

Gastric rupture is a rare but devastating event. It may follow blunt trauma to the abdomen, or consumption of enormous quantities of beer, with apparent release of sufficient carbon dioxide to bring the beer-drinking spree to an unhappy end; and it may complicate cardiac resuscitation with mouth-to-mouth breathing and inflation of the stomach. When external cardiac massage is applied gastric rupture may occur. It has also been associated with the strain of labor. Whatever the basis, it is a calamitous event followed rapidly by shock or death, unless immediately recognized and treated surgically.

INFLAMMATIONS

GASTRITIS

Although gastritis is an unquestioned clinical and anatomic disorder, it is a much abused medical term. It is commonly used to explain such transient or seemingly trivial complaints as "sour stomach," "dyspepsia," and "indigestion" without substantiating clinical or anatomic evidence. On the other hand, gastritis may be present anatomically without inducing clinical symptoms. Thus, gastritis is both an overused term and an underdiagnosed clinical condition.

Acute Gastritis

There is no general agreement on the classification of various forms of gastritis. Depending on the extent of destruction, acute inflammations have been divided into several types—acute gastritis, acute hemorrhagic gastritis, acute erosive gastritis, and acute stress erosions. These terms encompass an anatomic continuum that is discussed below; stress ulcers are reviewed in a later section.

Acute gastritis is an acute mucosal inflammatory process, usually of a transient nature. The inflammation may be accompanied by hemorrhage into the mucosa and, in more severe instances, by concomitant erosions to produce acute erosive or acute hemorrhagic erosive gastritis. The severe erosive form of the disease is an important cause of acute gastrointestinal bleeding.

PATHOGENESIS. The pathogenesis of these lesions is poorly understood. Acute gastritis frequently is associated with (1) chronic use of aspirin; (2) excessive alcohol consumption; (3) heavy smoking; (4) treatment with cancer chemotherapeutic drugs; (5) uremia; (6) systemic infections (e.g., salmonellosis); (7) staphylococcal food poisoning; (8) severe stress, such as extensive burns, trauma, or surgery; (9) shock; and (10) gastric irradiation or freezing. One or more of the following influences are thought to be operative in these varied settings: increased acid secretion with back-diffusion; decreased production of bicarbonate buffer; reduced blood flow, which permits acid ions to accumulate; and damage to the barrier itself. Reference was made earlier to the important role of the intact mucosa (p. 841) in preventing back-diffusion of hydrogen ion. Aspirin breaks this mucosal barrier and causes increased turnover of surface mucosal cells. Alcohol also damages the surface epithelial cells, but this occurs secondary to subepithelial hemorrhages due to vascular injury. Increased back-diffusion has also been demonstrated in critically ill patients and in animals subjected to hemorrhagic shock, so stress also may play some role.

Mucosal hypoperfusion is another major contributory mechanism leading to mucosal injury. Diminished blood flow to the mucosa would reasonably be expected in any form of shock and might also occur from the vasoconstrictive effects of nicotine with heavy smoking. The acute gastritis following gastric irradiation or freezing might also, at least in part, be mediated by mucosal hypoperfusion. Concomitantly, mucosal ischemia would impair the barrier function of the mucosa. Thus, ischemic injury would synergize the deleterious effects of back-diffusion of hydrogen ions. Other mucosal insults have been identified in experimental animals, such as regurgitation of bile acids and lysolecithin, and inadequate mucosal synthesis of prostaglandins, but what role these play in the acute gastritis of humans is unknown.[29]

MORPHOLOGY. Depending on the severity of the insult, the mucosal response may vary from only moderate edema and slight hyperemia to hemorrhagic erosion of the gastric mucosa. In the milder forms, the surface epithelium may be intact and the lamina propria may contain only occasional, scattered leukocytes. In the extreme pattern, best referred to as **acute hemorrhagic erosive gastritis**, there is superficial sloughing of the mucosa, accompanied by hemorrhage into the lamina propria and an acute inflammatory infiltrate. Large areas of the gastric mucosa may be denuded, but the involvement, as stated, is superficial and rarely affects the entire depth of the mucosa, sparing the underlying wall.

CLINICAL COURSE. The wide range of morphologic changes embraced by the term "acute gastritis" is paralleled by the range of clinical manifestations. Undoubtedly, minor involvements occur that produce no symptoms. At the other end of the spectrum are cases with massive hematemesis and acute abdominal pain. In between are those cases manifested by epigastric pain, nausea, and vomiting. In some instances, the first indication of gastritis is the sudden onset of hematemesis or melena. In Great Britain, 25% of all cases of hematemesis and melena arise in severe gastritis related to the heavy use of aspirin.[32]

Chronic Gastritis — Fundal and Antral

The unqualified term "chronic gastritis" encompasses a range of lesions extending from superficial gastritis to atrophic gastritis to gastric atrophy. These forms are poorly delineated from each other since *they make a morphologic continuum of increasingly intense inflammatory infiltration of the mucosa accompanied by progressively more marked atrophy of the mucosal glands. The glandular atrophy is often accompanied by metaplasia, dysplasia, and atypia of the surface epithelium.* These changes underlie the major clinical consequences of chronic gastritis: (1) the possible loss of parietal cells and their synthesis of intrinsic factor (IF), resulting in inadequate absorption of vitamin B_{12} and pernicious anemia (PA); (2) an increased predisposition to gastric carcinoma; and (3) a possible contribution to peptic ulceration (p. 850).

Chronic gastritis is currently viewed as a histologic abnormality shared by a number of different diseases, each producing mucosal inflammation by a different etiology or mechanism. These pathogenetic differences are, in turn, reflected in a number of different biologic characteristics, such as variable distribution of the lesions in the stomach; differences in the acid secretory status and the degree of associated hypergastrinemia; propensity to lead to gastric atrophy, polyps, and cancer; and association with pernicious anemia or peptic ulcer disease. The earlier pathologic differentiation into fundal and antral types has now more or less been superseded by the clinicopathologic grouping of chronic gastritis into types A, B, and AB. This classification has served to clarify some of the confusing and otherwise conflicting data. *Type A corresponds to fundal gastritis of the earlier classification, while types B and AB are subcategories of antral gastritis.*

Type A (fundal) gastritis characteristically involves the body-fundic mucosa preferentially. Although the antral mucosa is commonly said to be spared in this form of gastritis, it is not invariably so; the antral mucosa usually shows a significant — but less intense — degree of chronic gastritis. Most patients with type A gastritis have circulating antibodies to parietal cells and intrinsic factor (IF), which may lead to immunologic destruction of parietal cells as is discussed on page 683. These patients, therefore, have hypo- or achlorhydria, a high intragastric pH, and hypergastrinemia. The loss of parietal cells from the proximal gastric mucosa leads to a significant degree of gastric atrophy and intestinal metaplasia. On account of the impaired secretion of IF, a small subset (10%) of these patients go on to develop overt pernicious anemia after a period of several years. Because of the absence of acid in the gastric secretions bathing the antral mucosa, these patients develop a secondary hyperplasia of gastrin-producing G cells in the antral mucosa and significant hypergastrinemia. This type of gastritis is frequently associated with autoimmune disorders such as Hashimoto's thyroiditis and Addison's disease and is therefore also referred to as autoimmune gastritis.[33]

Type B or antral gastritis not surprisingly affects the antral mucosa. In contrast to the fundal or type A pattern this form of gastritis is not associated with parietal cell antibodies, pernicious anemia, or any other autoimmune diseases and is therefore regarded as nonimmune in type. It represents the most common form of chronic gastritis and outstrips the type A 4 : 1 in frequency. On account of the heterogeneous patient population and variations in clinicopathologic features, antral gastritis is now believed to include two subtypes referred to as *hypersecretory gastritis* and *environmental gastritis.* The hypersecretory type is restricted to the antrum and usually is not associated with any significant gastric atrophy or intestinal metaplasia. *Patients invariably secrete excess acid, have a low intragastric pH, and frequently have an associated duodenal ulcer.* Serum gastrin levels are usually within normal limits. A small proportion of individuals have associated gastric ulcers. Patients with this type of gastritis, because of the gastric hypersecretion and the associated ulcer disease, are frequently symptomatic, but the symptoms are related to the hypersecretion and peptic ulcer disease and hardly ever to the gastritis per se.

Environmental gastritis is so designated because it has a worldwide distribution and in any given country is the most common form of gastritis in all age groups — particularly in the elderly. Its etiology and pathogenesis are therefore believed to be related to environmental factors that have yet to be clearly defined. There is a strong association, however, with such mucosal lesions as gastric atrophy, intestinal metaplasia, gastric polyps, and gastric cancer. Clinical and epidemiologic studies conducted in Europe and Japan have shown that environmental gastritis starts with a patchy, irregularly focal involvement of the antral mucosa. With age, the lesions not only become confluent but also extend proximally into the body-fundic region, especially along the lesser curvature.[33,34] In early lesions the inflammation is confined to the superficial gastric mucosa (superficial gastritis); it gradually extends deeper into the mucosa to damage the glands and cause mucosal atrophy (chronic atrophic gastritis) with intestinal metaplasia. This sequential progression of superficial gastritis to chronic atrophic gastritis is now recognized as a well-established continuum. However, since chronic gastritis represents a dynamic process, all stages may coexist in a given stomach at any one time. A Finnish study of patients with normal mucosa or superficial gastritis followed for 23 to 27 years showed that of those with normal mucosa, 58% had developed superficial gastritis and 14% had chronic atrophic gastritis; among those with superficial gastritis initially, 42% had progressed to atrophic gastritis.[34] It is of interest that the incidence of environmental gastritis not only varies from one country to another but also shows considerable differences within the same country. Furthermore, in countries with a high incidence of gastric cancer, such as Japan, and in those with areas of both high and low rates of gastric carcinoma, such as Colombia, the incidence of this form of gastritis closely parallels that of gastric cancer.[35] In areas with a high incidence of gastric cancer, environmental gastritis makes its appearance earlier in life; thus in Japan its occurrence among asymptomatic teenagers lies between 15 and 22%, increasing to around 90% in those 60 years of age.[36] A similarly high incidence (75%) has been reported for Colombians over the age of 45. Comparable figures for the United States population are not yet available.

Since environmental gastritis is closely associated with chronic atrophic gastritis and the lesions affect both the antral and the fundic mucosa, it is synonymously referred to as chronic atrophic gastritis and gastritis type AB. Clinically, individuals with this type of gastritis are usually asymptomatic (at least in the early stages) and often hypochlorhydric owing to parietal cell damage and atrophy of the body-fundic mucosa. However, since parietal cells are never completely destroyed, these patients do not develop achlorhydria or pernicious anemia. Serum gastrin levels too are usually within the normal range or only modestly elevated. A small subset of patients may have associated gastric ulcers. Patients with environmental gastritis do not have circulating antibodies to parietal cells or IF and no associated autoimmune diseases.

ETIOLOGY AND PATHOGENESIS. Since chronic gastritis represents a common histologic endpoint of mucosal injury produced by a variety of mucosal insults, its etiology is multifactorial, and environmental factors, yet to be clearly delineated, appear to be particularly important. Among the various factors suspected are some altered immunologic mechanism, alcohol, and duodenal reflux. Although a causative role for both humoral and cell-mediated immune injury has been accepted for type A gastritis, there is little evidence of an immunologic mechanism in a majority of patients with type B or AB.

Reflux of duodenal contents into the stomach appears to be of importance in the pathogenesis of chronic gastritis seen in patients who have undergone partial gastrectomy or pyloroplasty. In those with an anatomically intact pyloric sphincter, the sphincter tone may be either inherently weak or decreased by local hormonal influences, e.g., gastrin. In the duodenal lumen, lecithin, a normal constituent of bile, is converted into lysolecithin in the presence of bile acids, trypsin, and phospholipase A secreted in the pancreatic juice. The lysolecithin-rich duodenal contents, when refluxed into the stomach, are cytotoxic to the gastric mucosal epithelium and cause back-diffusion of acid. Local release of histamine from intramucosal mast cells may also participate to a significant degree in the pathogenesis of the lesions, since H_2 antagonists are known to promote healing in gastritis.

Although earlier reports had stated that alcohol did not cause gastritis, more recent studies comparing the frequency of chronic gastritis in alcoholics and nonalcoholics have shown that alcoholics have a higher prevalence of chronic gastritis.[37] Furthermore, the lesions appear at an earlier age and are more severe with ingestion of increasingly larger amounts of alcohol.

MORPHOLOGY. Irrespective of the type of chronic gastritis (A, B, or AB), the histologic changes are closely similar. In the early phases **(chronic superficial gastritis),** there may be some flattening of the mucosa, but it is generally not marked. An inflammatory infiltrate of lymphocytes and plasma cells is typically present within the lamina propria, usually limited to the upper third of the gastric mucosa (Fig. 18–13). In the **chronic atrophic gastritis stage,** the mucosa is more obviously thinned and flattened, with extension of the infiltrate in the lamina propria to the deeper glandular layer. It may appear reddened as the submucosal vessels become more apparent. There is often atrophy of the glands and a variety of cytologic changes in the surface epithelial cells, as described below. In type A (fundal) gastritis the gastric glands are atrophic; those that persist often undergo cystic dilatation and are lined by gastric mucous cells of the type seen in the antral region (antropyloric metaplasia) or metaplastic intestinal cells (intestinal metaplasia).

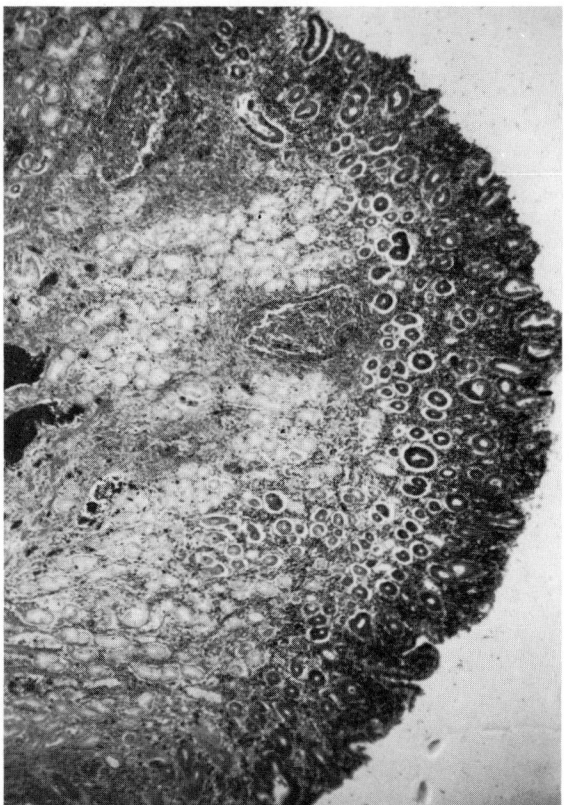

Figure 18–13. Chronic superficial gastritis with an intense inflammatory infiltrate and some disorganization of glands involving upper one third of gastric mucosa.

There is a conspicuous paucity of parietal cells. The antral mucosa in type A gastritis is never completely normal and shows a milder form of inflammation and intestinal metaplasia. In type B gastritis the inflammatory and glandular changes are largely limited to the antrum but, save for location, resemble those already described for type A gastritis.

The morphologic alterations of **chronic gastric atrophy** are an extension of the atrophic changes encountered in atrophic gastritis. Rugal folds are flattened or absent, and the mucosa takes on a shiny, glazed appearance. The glandular atrophy is now almost complete save for scattered, shortened, sometimes cystically dilated glands. The surface epithelium as well as that lining the gastric pits takes the form of mucus-secreting goblet cells interspersed with cells characteristic of intestinal epithelium-bearing microvilli. Occasionally, abortive, villus-like projections may appear. **In type A gastritis, parietal cells are almost totally absent from such atrophic glands as persist.** In contrast, in type B or AB the parietal cells in the body and fundus of the stomach persist. **Whatever the distribution of the mucosal involvement, the surface epithelium undergoes a variety of metaplastic and dysplastic alterations,** including variation in size, shape, and orientation of the epithelial cells, often accompanied by nuclear enlargement and atypicality. These cytologic aberrations possibly reflect the persistence of damaging influences responsible for the development of the gastric mucosal atrophy. **The cellular atypia tends to be most marked in long-standing type A gastritis associated with PA.** In this setting, it is tempting to speculate that the deficient absorption of vitamin B_{12} impairs DNA synthesis and so inhibits cell replication, with the formation of abnormally large, atypical cells, as discussed on page 680. Whatever their origin, the cytologic changes may become so severe as to mimic in situ carcinoma; indeed, they probably account for the increased incidence of gastric cancer in atrophic forms of gastritis, particularly in association with PA.

Campylobacter Gastritis

Only within the recent past has the pathogenetic importance of *Campylobacter pyloris* been discovered. In humans, this curved, spiral, or S-shaped organism has been demonstrated only in the stomach, where it is seen characteristically within the mucous layer overlying the mucosa or along the luminal surfaces of the mucosal epithelial cells, the mucous neck cells, and the epithelial cells lining the gastric pits. Although it is rarely seen within the gastric surface epithelial cells, no extension into the deeper tissues has been documented so far.

The clinical significance of *C. pyloris* lies chiefly in its ubiquitous worldwide distribution; its prevalence in 20% of the adult population, a frequency that rises with advancing age; and a strong association between its presence in the stomach and such diverse conditions as antral (type B) gastritis (Fig. 18–14), gastric and duodenal ulcer disease, gastric cancer, and nonulcerous dyspepsia.[38–40] Although on gastric biopsy these organisms are present in less than 10% of

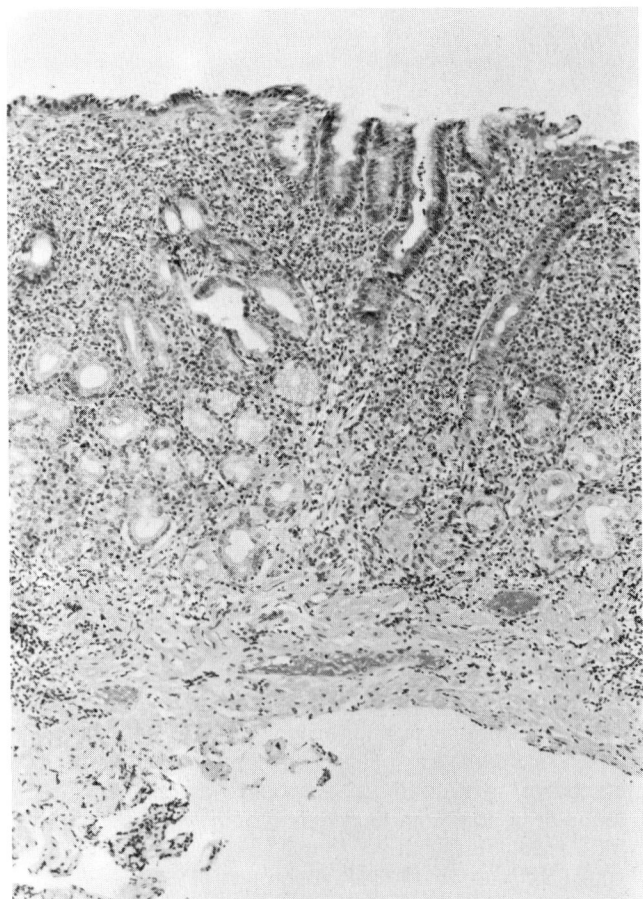

Figure 18–14. Campylobacter gastritis. Note that the inflammatory infiltrate is preferentially located in the lamina propria of the superficial one third of the mucosal thickness.

normal healthy volunteers, they have been demonstrated in over 60% of those with chronic gastritis, in 65% of those with gastric ulcers, and in 85 to 100% of those with duodenal ulcers.[41] However, on account of the absence of any microbial invasion of the inflamed tissues, their pathogenetic significance is controversial. Characteristic of *C. pyloris*–induced gastritis are polymorphonuclear leukocytes on a background of an otherwise chronic gastritis, typically limited to the superficial lamina propria and the epithelial lining of the surface and the gastric pits. In contrast, the polymorphs in other types of gastritis, e.g., that induced by aspirin, alcohol, or bile reflux, are scattered throughout the mucosal thickness. The distribution of these organisms in the stomach can be very patchy and irregular, with areas of heavy colonization adjacent to those with no organisms. Even in heavily colonized stomachs, the organisms are absent from areas with *intestinal metaplasia*. In the duodenum too, these organisms are exclusively confined to foci of *gastric metaplasia*, such as those seen in the duodenal cap region in patients with duodenal ulcers. This distributional pattern has led to speculation that the presence of certain surface receptors is essential for tissue colonization by *C. pyloris* and that such receptors are

present only in gastric epithelial cells. The presence of *C. pyloris* in antral biopsies strongly correlates with active (95%) and quiescent (65%) gastritis. This type of gastritis is invariably present in patients with active gastric or duodenal ulcers and persists even after the ulcers have healed, and so it appears that the organisms are more likely to be related to the associated gastritis than to the ulcer disease per se.[40] Perhaps the recurrence of peptic ulcers in such patients may even be related to the persistent colonization of the gastric mucosa by these organisms.

C. pyloris organisms have adapted themselves to colonizing the gastric mucosal surface within the protective covering of the mucus layer (Fig. 18–15). Their urease activity enables them to generate enough ammonia locally to adequately buffer any minor fluctuations in the pH of their proximate microenvironment. These organisms also elaborate a protease that *breaks down glycoproteins* in the gastric mucus, which may explain the mucus depletion seen histologically in areas of heavy colonization. Damage to the protective mucus layer exposes the underlying epithelial cells to the damaging influence of acid-pep-

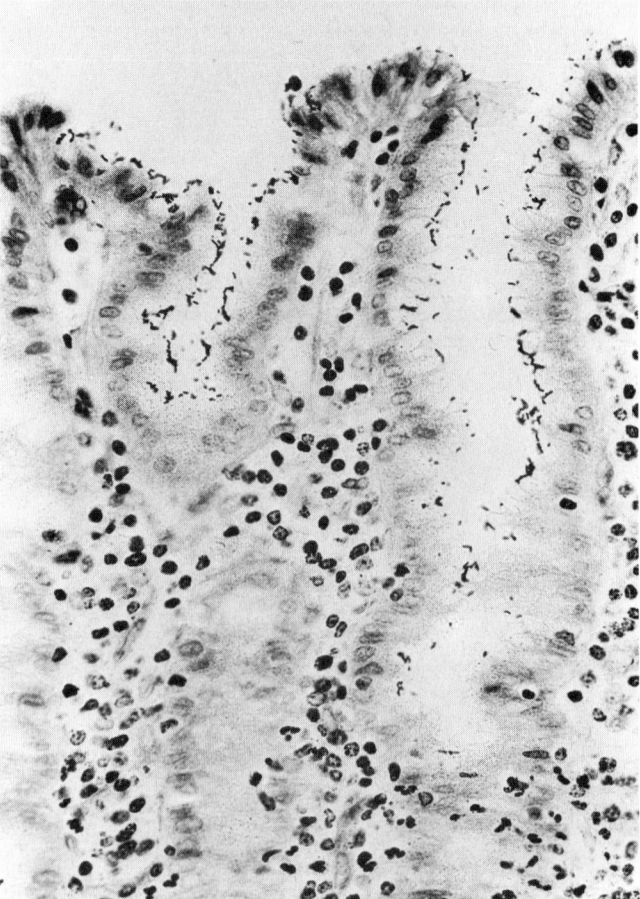

Figure 18–15. Campylobacter gastritis. A Warthin-Starry stain showing large numbers of Campylobacter organisms along the luminal surface of the gastric epithelial cells. Note that no tissue invasion is present.

tic digestion and leads to inflammation (acute gastritis and perhaps some dyspepsia). Persistence of organisms in the stomach leads to development of an active chronic gastritis. The development of antibodies to *C. pyloris* leads to clearing the organisms from the body-fundic region, but colonization of the antropyloric mucosa and any areas of metaplastic mucosa in the duodenal bulb may persist. The chronically inflamed mucosa is more susceptible to acid-peptic injury and is thus more prone to peptic ulceration. This sequence of events may explain why gastric and duodenal ulcers are so frequently located in the antrum and the duodenal bulb.

Hypertrophic Gastritis

This designation encompasses a group of uncommon conditions, all characterized by giant cerebriform enlargement of the rugal folds of the gastric mucosa (Fig. 18–16). The term hypertrophic gastritis, although firmly fixed in medical practice, is a misnomer since the rugal enlargement is caused neither by inflammatory gastritis nor by hypertrophy, but by hyperplasia of the mucosal epithelial cells. *Three variants are rec-*

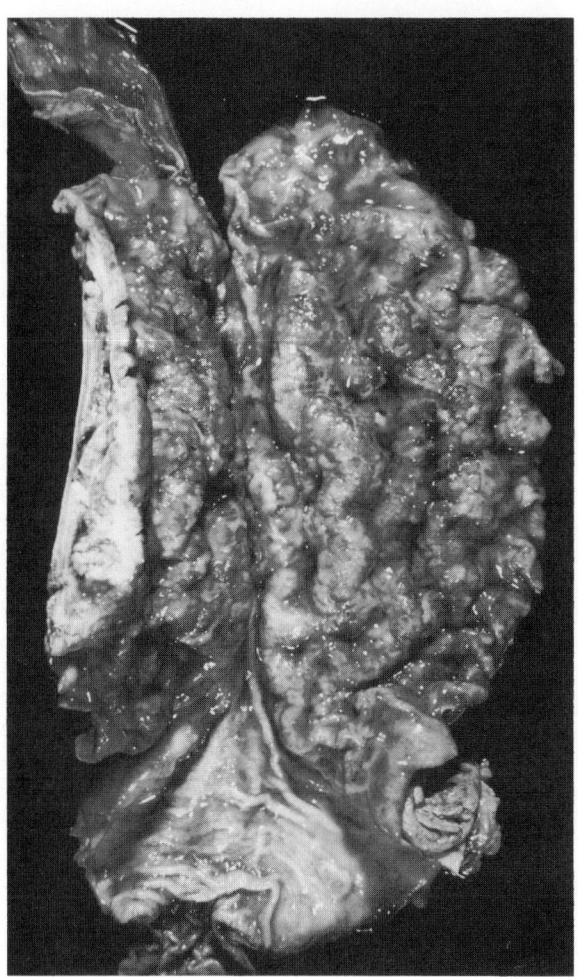

Figure 18–16. Hypertrophic gastritis of stomach, sparing antral region below. Marked thickening of rugal folds simulates diffuse neoplastic infiltration.

ognized: (1) Ménétrier's disease related to hyperplasia of the surface mucous cells; (2) hypersecretory gastropathy associated with hyperplasia of the parietal and chief cells within the gastric glands; and (3) gastric gland hyperplasia secondary to the excessive gastrin secretion by a gastrinoma in the Zollinger-Ellison syndrome (p. 1007). The first two may be variations of a single entity, differing only in the amount of parietal and chief cell hyperplasia and, therefore, in the levels of gastric acid secretion. All three conditions are of clinical importance because on x-ray examination or endoscopy they mimic infiltrative cancer or lymphoma of the stomach. They may also be associated with significant clinical morbidity.

Ménétrier's disease, an idiopathic condition, is most often encountered in patients in their fourth to sixth decade, and occasionally in children. Although the condition may be asymptomatic and discovered only on radiography, it often produces epigastric pain, nausea, vomiting, and sometimes bleeding related to superficial rugal erosions. As would be expected, the gastric secretions contain excessive mucus and in many instances little or no hydrochloric acid when the parietal cells undergo atrophy. In some patients, there is excessive protein loss in the gastric secretion sufficient to produce hypoalbuminemia and peripheral edema, thus constituting a form of *protein-losing gastroenteropathy*. Infrequently the mucosal hyperplasia becomes metaplastic, to provide a soil for the development of gastric carcinoma.

Other Forms of Gastritis

A *granulomatous gastritis* may occur in patients with sarcoidosis and regional enteritis but more often appears as an isolated disorder. Isolated granulomatous gastritis tends to occur in persons 40 years of age or older, whereas the other two variants generally are found in younger individuals.

Another rare variant is *eosinophilic gastritis*. Here there is prominent infiltration of the mucosa, and sometimes of the deeper layers of the stomach wall, by eosinophils. This distinctive infiltrate may be accompanied by granuloma formation (allergic granulomatosis) and occasionally by acute vasculitis of the small arteries within the stomach wall (reminiscent of the changes in the allergic granulomatosis of Churg and Strauss [p. 573]).

ACUTE GASTRIC EROSIONS AND ULCERATIONS

Focal, acutely developing gastric mucosal defects may appear following severe stress, whatever its nature—hence, the often used designation *stress ulcers*. Generally, there are multiple lesions located mainly in the stomach but occasionally also involving the duodenum. They range in depth from mere shedding of the superficial epithelium to deeper lesions that involve the entire mucosal thickness. The shallow erosions are then, in essence, an extension of acute erosive gastritis (p. 842). The deeper lesions comprise well-defined ulcerations but are not precursors of chronic peptic ulcers, having a totally different pathobiology.

Stress erosions and ulcers are most commonly encountered in patients with shock, extensive burns, sepsis, or severe trauma; in any intracranial condition that raises intracranial pressure, e.g., trauma, brain tumors; and following intracranial surgery. Those associated with intracranial problems are referred to as *Cushing's ulcers.*

The genesis of the acute mucosal defects in these varied clinical settings is poorly understood. Acid-peptic secretions are requisite for their appearance, but hypersecretion of gastric acid is clearly documented only with Cushing's ulcers. Here, direct stimulation of vagal nuclei by increased intracranial pressure is proposed, and indeed the acid hypersecretion can be blocked by parenteral administration of anticholinergic drugs. In contrast, low-to-normal levels of gastric acid are present in the other clinical settings. Mucosal hypoxia, related to either neurogenic or catecholamine-induced vasoconstriction, is perhaps the leading pathogenetic hypothesis for such lesions. The ischemic hypoxia may (1) damage the mucosal barrier and permit back-diffusion of hydrogen ions, rendering the mucosa more vulnerable to acid-peptic attack; or (2) directly injure mucosal cells by oxygen or metabolic deprivation.[42] Systemic acidosis, a common finding in shock states, may also contribute to erosive lesions in the stomach, presumably by lowering the intracellular pH levels of mucosal cells already rendered hypoxic by stress-induced vasoconstriction.

A number of exogenous agents, such as alcohol, smoking, caffeine, and certain drugs (aspirin, corticosteroids, indomethacin, and phenylbutazone), are widely thought to be ulcerogenic and may potentiate the appearance of stress ulcers. Best documented is the damaging effect on the mucosa of unbuffered aspirin, as pointed out on page 843, but what role it plays in the induction of acute stress ulcers is uncertain.[43] Chronic ethanol consumption and smoking may induce gastric hypersecretion and injure the mucosal barrier, but it is not certain that they produce mucosal defects. Similarly, corticosteroids and indomethacin have been associated with gastric complaints and even evidence of gastric bleeding, and although they may potentiate stress ulceration, their pathogenetic role is far from clear. In the last analysis, the pathogenesis of acute gastric stress lesions in man is unknown.

MORPHOLOGY. The morphologic differentiation between an acute erosion and an acute stress ulcer is poorly defined. The term erosion is applied to lesions confined to the gastric or duodenal mucosa. When these lesions penetrate the muscularis mucosae, they are called acute gastric or stress ulcers. They may occur singly or, more often, multiply throughout the stomach and duodenum. Typically they are found anywhere in the stomach and do not have

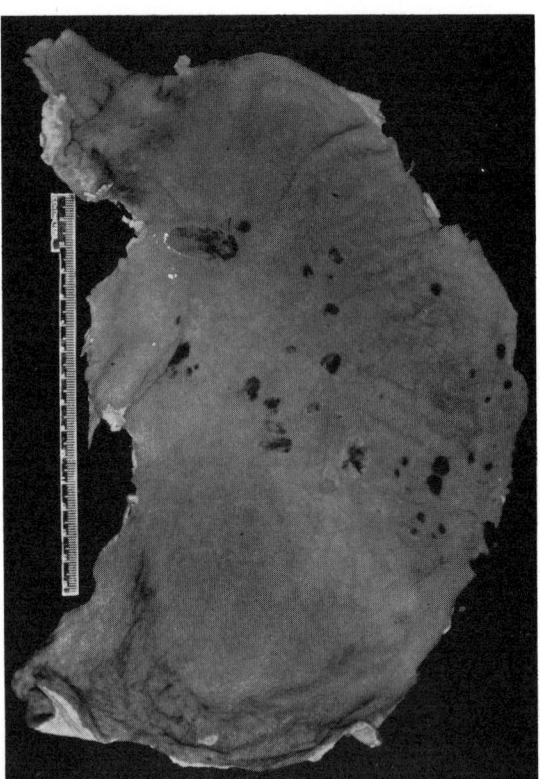

Figure 18–17. Acute gastric ulcers occurring in a patient dying of severe burns. The dark brown staining is produced by digestion of exuded red cells.

the predilection for the antral region and lesser curvature exhibited by chronic peptic ulcers. Circular and small, they are usually less than 1 cm in diameter. The ulcer base is frequently stained a dark brown by the acid digestion of the accompanying bleeding (Fig. 18–17). The margins, which rarely show significant hyperemic reaction, are poorly defined because the ulcer is superficial in nature. The rugal pattern is not affected, and the margins and base of the ulcer are not indurated.

Depending on the duration of the ulceration, there may be some inflammatory infiltration in the margins and base. Red blood cells and fibrin often coat the base. There is usually conspicuous absence of underlying scarring or thickening of blood vessel walls such as is seen in the more chronic forms. Healing with complete re-epithelialization occurs after the causative factors are removed. This regrowth of epithelium may be quite active and demonstrate many mitotic figures. The time required for complete healing varies from days to several weeks. Most often these lesions produce few symptoms, but sometimes they bleed massively to cause death.

PEPTIC ULCERS

Peptic ulcers are chronic, most often solitary, lesions that occur in any level of the gastrointestinal tract exposed to the aggressive action of acid-peptic juices. They are so common in industrialized nations that, as noted earlier, they virtually represent "stigmata of

Table 18–2. Distribution of Peptic Ulcers

Duodenum (first portion)
Stomach (usually antrum)
Barrett's esophagus
Gastroenterostomy stoma
Duodenum, stomach, jejunum (Zollinger-Ellison syndrome)
Meckel's diverticulum with ectopic gastric mucosa

civilization.'' Approximately 98 to 99% of peptic ulcers occur in either the duodenum or the stomach in a ratio of about 4 : 1. About 10 to 20% of patients with a gastric ulcer have a concurrent duodenal lesion. The distribution of peptic ulcers is summarized in Table 18–2.

Wherever they occur, chronic peptic ulcers have a fairly standard, virtually diagnostic gross and microscopic appearance (Fig. 18–18). Despite this uniform morphology, gastric and duodenal ulcers may represent two somewhat distinctive diseases. Different influences are thought to be involved in their pathogenesis, and there are further contrasts in their genetic linkages. Nonetheless, gastric and duodenal ulcers will be considered together, highlighting these variables.

EPIDEMIOLOGY. Peptic ulcers are remitting-relapsing lesions that are most often diagnosed in middle-aged to older adults, but they may first become evident in young adult life. They often appear without obvious precipitating influences and may then, after a period of weeks to months of active disease, heal with

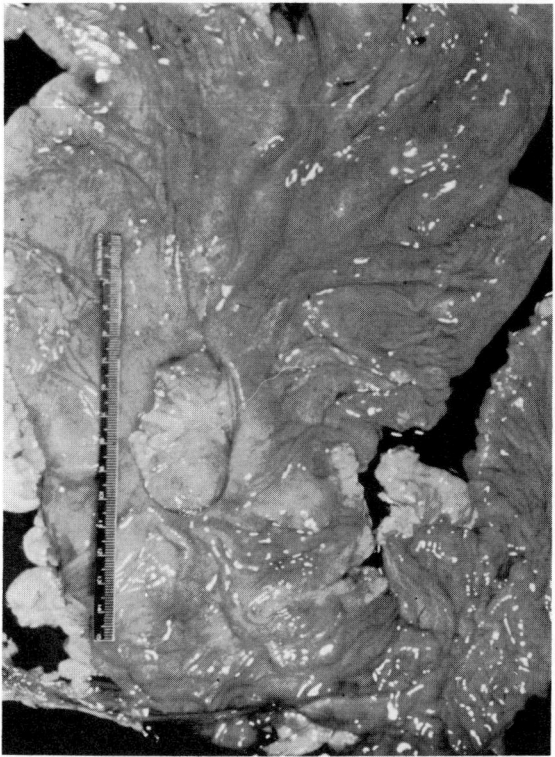

Figure 18–18. A large, deeply excavated peptic ulcer occurring in prepyloric region of stomach along lesser curvature.

or without therapy. However, ''once a peptic ulcer patient, always a peptic ulcer patient.'' Thus, it is difficult to express accurate data on the frequency of active disease. The best estimates of gastroduodenal ulcer frequency from autopsy studies and surveys of patients indicate a range of 6 to 14% for men and 2 to 6% for women.[44] The male : female ratio for duodenal ulcers is about 3 : 1, and for gastric ulcers around 1.5 to 2 : 1. Women are most often affected at, or after, the menopause. In more individual terms it is estimated that an adult male in the United States has about one chance in ten of developing an ulcer before the age of 65. It is of interest that half a century ago, duodenal ulcer was much more common than it is now; the reasons for its decline are obscure, but no such welcome trend has been observed for the gastric ulcer.[45]

Genetic influences are important in the predisposition to duodenal ulcer but appear to play no role with gastric ulcer. Duodenal ulcers are about three times more common in first-degree relatives of ulcer patients than in the general population. A 50% concordance for duodenal ulcers has been observed in monozygotic twins as compared with 14% in dizygotic twins.[46] Individuals of blood group O are about 37% more likely to develop these lesions than those of other blood groups. Another genetic trait is the capacity to secrete mucopolysaccharide blood group substances into salivary and gastrointestinal secretions. ''Nonsecretors'' are 50% more prone to duodenal ulcers than are ''secretors.'' An increased incidence of HLA-B5 antigen has also been identified in white males with duodenal ulcer.[47] An elevated serum level of immunoreactive pepsinogen I has been observed in several kindreds having multiple members with duodenal ulcers.[48] The genetic trait for pepsinogen hypersecretion segregates as an autosomal dominant and is hailed as a ''marker'' for a predisposition to duodenal ulcer. The absence of similar genetic findings in patients with gastric ulcers underscores the previously expressed suspicion that duodenal and gastric ulcers may represent different diseases, sharing only ''a hole in the gastroduodenal mucosa.''

Duodenal ulcer is more frequent in patients with alcoholic cirrhosis, chronic renal failure, chronic obstructive pulmonary disease, and hyperparathyroidism. Numerous explanations have been offered to explain these associations, but all are tenuous. All that can be said with any certainty is that increased serum calcium levels, whatever the cause, stimulate gastrin secretion and, therefore, acid secretion in the stomach.

PATHOGENESIS. Although significant advances have been made in the clinical management of peptic ulcer disease, very few inroads have been made in our understanding of its pathogenesis. Certain broad generalizations, made several years ago, are just as valid now as then.

Some level of acid-pepsin secretion is requisite for the development of duodenal and gastric ulcers — ''no acid, no ulcer.''[49]

• All peptic ulcerations probably arise because of an imbalance between the aggressive action of acid-pepsin secretion and the normal defenses of the gastroduodenal mucosa.

• For duodenal ulcers the major causal influence appears to be exposure of the duodenal mucosa to excessive amounts of acid and pepsin.

• For gastric ulcers the major causal influence appears to be some breakdown in gastric mucosal defenses against acid and pepsin.

It would be simplistic, however, to ascribe duodenal ulcerogenesis solely to excessive gastric acid, and gastric ulcers solely to impaired defenses. Both sides of the equation are probably relevant for all peptic ulcers. Moreover, other influences must exist to explain the facts that peptic ulcers are usually focal, solitary lesions and have a predilection for specific locations within the duodenum and stomach. Peculiarly, localized forces must be at work, but their nature is unknown. Within this framework of uncertainty we can turn first to a consideration of duodenal ulcer.

DUODENAL ULCERS. In general, *duodenal ulcer patients have (1) an increased capacity to secrete acid and pepsin, (2) increased responsiveness to stimuli of acid secretion, and (3) more rapid gastric emptying.*[50] However, not all these characteristics are present in every patient.

In general, duodenal ulcer patients have a higher mean basal acid output and maximal acid output than do normal controls, and significantly higher levels than are present in patients with gastric ulcers. However, in almost half the patients with duodenal ulcer the hypersecretion is not very marked, and there is considerable overlap between the duodenal ulcer and normal groups. The acid hypersecretion can be directly correlated with an increased parietal cell mass, on average twice normal.[51] Here again, there is overlap with normal individuals and those with gastric ulcer. The basis for the elevated number of parietal cells is unknown but likely is constitutional.

Increased responsiveness to all known stimuli of gastric acid secretion is usually present in patients with duodenal ulcers.[52] This is not merely a function of their greater parietal cell mass, since the maximal secretory output is disproportionate to the basal acid output. The mechanism of this increased responsiveness is unknown. It does not appear to be due to increased vagal tone, since vagotomy reduces the acid secretion in duodenal ulcer patients no more than in those with gastric ulcers. The weight of evidence points to increased gastrin drive. Although patients with duodenal ulcers have only modestly elevated serum gastrin levels, they do tend to have increased amounts of gastrin in their antral mucosa,[52] and some have even been shown to have increased numbers of gastrin-producing cells in the antral mucosa.[53-55] However, this is not a universal finding, since other workers have observed such increases only in a small subset of duodenal ulcer patients.[56,57]

Abnormally rapid gastric emptying is another frequent finding in patients with duodenal ulcer. As a consequence, gastric contents are emptied into the duodenum before the buffering capacity of a meal has effectively neutralized the gastric acidity. Thus, the duodenal mucosa is exposed to a greater acid load.[51]

Many more pathogenetic influences have been reported, but all are of uncertain significance. The prevailing wisdom that ulcers, both duodenal and gastric, tend to occur in individuals having certain personalities — hard-driving, achievement-oriented "ulcer types" — can be neither confirmed nor denied. There are, however, numerous instances in which stress, anxiety, and fatigue have reactivated or perpetuated ulcer disease. Concern has been expressed about the ulcerogenic potential of cigarette smoking, corticosteroids, and certain drugs (principally unbuffered aspirin), but substantial evidence that they induce duodenal ulceration is lacking. These agents have also been incriminated in the reactivation of duodenal ulcer, but once again the evidence is unconvincing. In conclusion, current evidence indicates that *the production of a duodenal ulcer is the consequence of excess exposure of the duodenal mucosa to the aggressive actions of gastric–acid–pepsin that overwhelm the normal defenses.* The facts that most ulcers occur in the first portion of the duodenum with its unbuffered acid and that histamine (H_2) antagonists, which reduce gastric acidity, promote healing support a causal role for excess gastric acid in the production of duodenal ulcers. Still unresolved is the contribution of *C. pyloris*–induced duodenitis in the pathogenesis of these lesions (p. 845).

GASTRIC ULCERS. On the average, *patients with gastric ulcers have low-to-normal levels of gastric acid,* but never true achlorhydria.[58] *Most of the accumulated data favor the existence of some primary defect in gastric mucosal resistance.*[49] Two influences that might explain the lowered resistance have been observed with some regularity: (1) an increased tendency to back-diffusion of hydrogen ions, suggesting some derangement in the gastric mucosal barrier; and (2) the frequent association of chronic antral gastritis with the ulcer.

In 60 to 80% of instances, gastritis is present in association with gastric ulcerations. It invariably involves the antrum (chronic antral gastritis) but sometimes also the body of the stomach. It is significant that in most cases the gastritis persists after the ulcer heals, suggesting that it is primary and the ulcer secondary.[59] The gastritis may be related to pyloric sphincter incompetence and reflux of bile into the stomach. Lower basal sphincter pressure has been observed in patients with gastric ulcer than in normal individuals or those with duodenal ulcers. Moreover, the sphincter pressure apparently does not increase in response to such normal stimuli as secretin, cholecystokinin, or intraduodenal amino acids or fat. Cigarette smoking also decreases the resting sphincter pressure and thus increases bile reflux. Thus, it is possible that bile acids and possibly lysolecithin diffuse back into the stomach, damage the mucosal barrier, and thus lead to chronic gastritis and simultaneously to increased acid penetration, with its ulcerogenic potential.[60]

Chronic exposure to exogenous damaging agents, such as unbuffered aspirin, alcohol, and certain drugs (e.g., nonsteroidal anti-inflammatory agents), has been invoked as another possible basis for gastric ulceration. *The minority of patients who do not have gastritis often are habitual users of aspirin.* It is proposed, then, that aspirin-induced back-diffusion may cause ulceration with or without producing gastritis, but this remains to be proved.[61] Chronic ethanol consumption, corticosteroids, indomethacin, and phenylbutazone have also been implicated in the development of gastric peptic ulcers, but solid evidence has not yet been presented.

Yet another postulation for the pathogenesis of gastric ulcer invokes some deficiency — quantitative or qualitative — in gastric mucus. The supportive evidence derives largely from the healing effects of a variety of drugs that promote mucus output.[62] You recall that *Campylobacter pyloris* breaks down the glycoproteins within the gastric mucus, favoring the development of chronic gastritis and possibly gastric ulceration. *There is the suggestion, then, that gastric mucus is protective, and that lowering of this defense favors gastric ulceration.*

If one accepts the concept of lowered gastric mucosal resistance, the problem remains: Why are ulcerations almost always solitary with specific preferential localizations? *Most gastric ulcers occur in the antral mucosa adjacent to the acid-secreting fundic mucosa.* Furthermore, they are almost always located in an area crossed by a broad band of circular muscle.[63] It is speculated that, in this location, peristaltic muscular contractions reduce mucosal blood flow and thus lower defenses in the non–acid-secreting antral mucosa against the load of acid elaborated by the body and fundus.

In summary, therefore, *ulcer subjects, for unknown reasons, are prone to mucosal injury by virtue of a defective mucosal barrier to back-diffusion of hydrogen ions. They are also predisposed to pyloric reflux and the development of chronic antral gastritis. In some, exogenous agents (in particular, unbuffered aspirin) may produce a level of mucosal damage that would not occur in normal individuals having normal mucosal barriers. Mucosal ischemia governs the localization of the ulcer when these injury-producing influences are present.*

MORPHOLOGY. The gross appearance of a chronic peptic ulcer, whether gastric or duodenal, is quite characteristic. In at least 80% of cases they are solitary lesions. In about 10 to 20% of patients with gastric ulceration there is a coexistent duodenal ulcer. About 90% of duodenal ulcers occur in the first portion of the duodenum, generally within a few centimeters of the pyloric ring. The anterior wall of the first portion of the duodenum is more often affected than the posterior wall. Gastric ulcers are predominantly located along the lesser curvature, in or around the border zone between the corpus and the antral mucosa. Less commonly, they may occur on the anterior or posterior walls of the stomach as well as on the greater curvature.

Peptic ulcers are usually small; well over 50% are less than 2 cm in diameter, and 75% are less than 3 cm. However, about 10% of benign ulcers are greater than 4 cm in diameter. Almost all these larger lesions occur in the stomach. Some carcinomatous ulcers are less than 4 cm in diameter. **Size, therefore, does not differentiate a benign from a malignant ulcer.**

The classic peptic ulcer is a round-to-oval, sharply punched-out defect with relatively straight walls. The mucosal margin may overhang the base slightly, particularly on the upstream portion of the circumference. The margins are usually level with the surrounding mucosa or only slightly elevated (Fig. 18–19). Heaping-up of these margins is extremely rare in the benign ulcer but is characteristic of the malignant lesion. The depth of these ulcers varies from superficial lesions, involving only the mucosa, down to deeply excavated, penetrating ulcers having their base in the muscularis. Penetration of the entire wall may occur, and occasionally the base of the ulcer may be formed by the adjacent pancreas, omental fat, or adherent liver. The base of all peptic ulcers is smooth and clean, owing to peptic

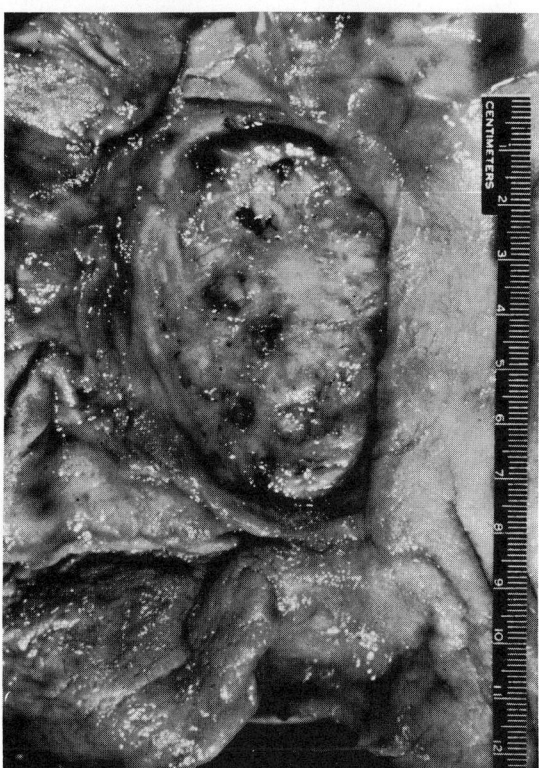

Figure 18–19. A large, benign peptic ulcer illustrating sharply defined margins, which overhang on proximal aspect *(right)* and shelve on distal aspect. Note absence of beading of margin and apparent absence of necrotic tissue in clean-appearing base. Despite the 7-cm diameter, no malignancy is present.

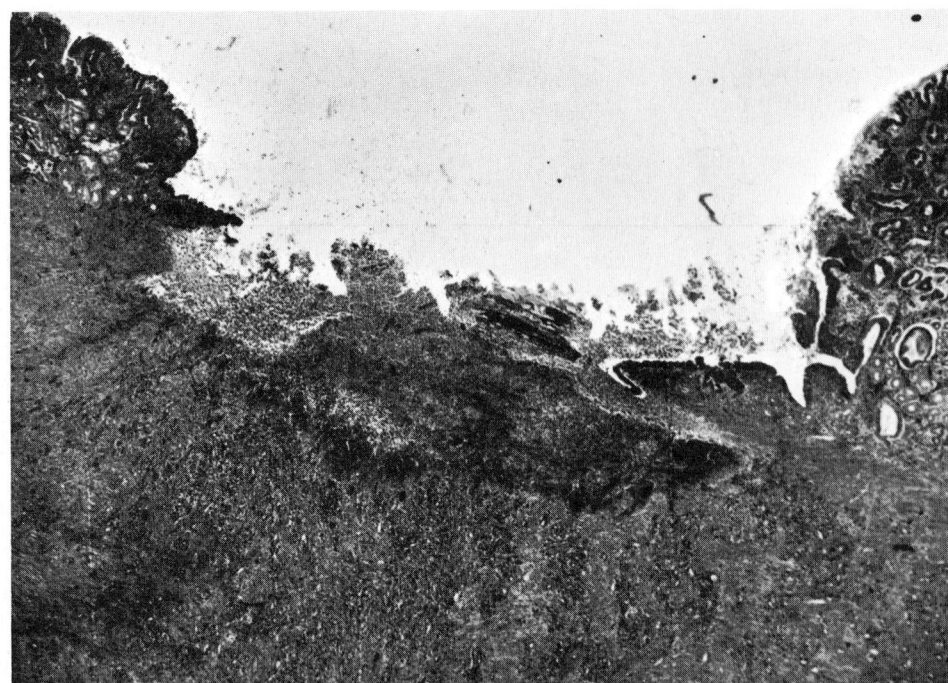

Figure 18–20. Low-power view of a peptic ulcer to illustrate depth of lesion.

digestion of any exudate. At times, thrombosed or even patent vessels that provided the source of a fatal hemorrhage project into the base. In most peptic ulcers, underlying scarring causes puckering of the surrounding mucosa, so that the mucosal folds radiate from the crater in spoke-like fashion. The gastric mucosa surrounding an ulcer is somewhat edematous and reddened, owing to the almost invariable gastritis.

The histologic appearance varies with the activity, chronicity, and amount of healing. In the stage of active necrosis, four zones are classically demonstrable: (1) The base and margins have a superficial thin layer of necrotic fibrinoid debris not visible to the naked eye; (2) beneath this layer is the zone of active nonspecific cellular infiltrate with neutrophils predominating; (3) in the deeper layers, especially in the base of the ulcer, there is active granulation tissue infiltrated with mononuclear leukocytes; and (4) the granulation tissue rests on a more solid fibrous or collagenous scar (Figs. 18–20 and 18–21). The scarring characteristically fans out widely and may extend to the serosal surface. The vessel walls within the scarred area are characteristically thickened by the surrounding inflammation and occasionally are thrombosed. The lamina propria of the mucosa surrounding the gastric ulcer is infiltrated by plasma cells, lymphocytes, and a few neutrophils.

CLINICAL COURSE. Gastric and duodenal ulcers represent chronic and recurrent lesions. They may heal, but there is always the risk of recurrence in the same focus or of the development of another ulcer elsewhere. Some ulcer patients are virtually asymptomatic, but much more often they experience pain, usually epigastric, which is variably described as burning, gnawing, or boring. The pain is intermittent; with duodenal ulcers, it classically begins 90 minutes

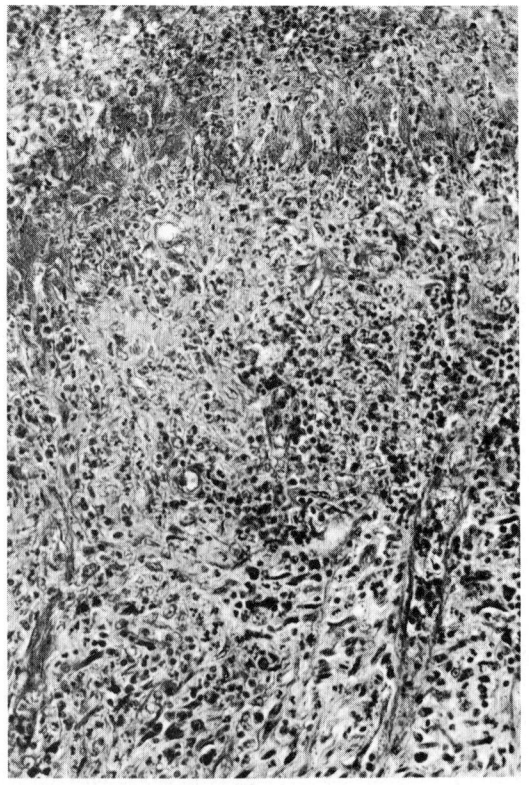

Figure 18–21. High-power detail of base of an ulcer demonstrating some of the zones that constitute the inflammatory response. The zone of fibrinoid necrosis is above.

to three hours after a meal and is relieved by milk, food, antacids, or vomiting. With gastric ulcers, about one fifth of patients experience pain within the first 30 minutes after eating, and it is not relieved by eating. About half the patients with either gastric or duodenal ulcer have pain or discomfort one to two hours after going to bed. Occasionally with penetrating duodenal ulcers, particularly those on the posterior wall, the pain may be steady, severe, and referred to the back or right upper quadrant, whereas with penetrating gastric ulcers the pain is more often referred to the left upper quadrant, thorax, and back. Uncommonly, the first manifestation of an ulcer is hematemesis. The "bleed" may be small and recurrent or may be massive, sometimes leading to shock. Other less common symptoms include anorexia, nausea, and vomiting. Weight loss is not uncommon with benign peptic ulcers, perhaps related to self-imposed dietary restrictions.

Under appropriate management, including regulated diet, antacids, and drugs to reduce acid secretion (e.g., H_2 antagonists) or to increase mucus output, the pain abates and indeed may not recur if the ulcer heals. However, a recurrence of symptoms may follow dietary indiscretions or stress.

The diagnosis and localization of peptic ulcers involve a variety of techniques, including gastric analyses for acidity; upper gastrointestinal radiographic studies; endoscopy; and cytologic examinations of gastric aspirate or brushings to rule out the presence of an ulcerative carcinoma. The diagnosis of duodenal ulcer can usually be made readily by radiographic studies. With gastric peptic ulcers it is more difficult, because the lesion may be small and difficult to visualize in the capacious stomach. In most reported series, roentgenologic examination detects 90% of all gastric lesions and correctly interprets approximately 90% of detected lesions. The same data apply to gastroscopy, but x-ray studies and gastroscopy together accurately detect and diagnose 95 to 98% of gastric lesions.

The complications of peptic ulcer disease are (1) bleeding, (2) perforation or penetration into an adjacent viscus, (3) obstruction from edema or from scarring of the pylorus or duodenum, and (4) perhaps, malignant transformation. Significant massive bleeding occurs in about one fourth to one third of patients. Malignant transformation is unknown with duodenal ulcers but is said to have occurred with gastric lesions. More likely, the "ulcer" was malignant from the outset. "Cancers ulcerate, but ulcers rarely cancerate." Thus, most patients with ulcer disease struggle through life perhaps chained to a bottle of antacid or H_2 antagonists, coddling their delicate entrails.

TUMORS

BENIGN

Benign gastric tumors have variously been reported to be present in 5% to almost 25% of autopsies, which must reflect differences in the vigor and enthusiasm devoted to their quest.[64,65] However, they are very uncommon *clinical* problems, since most are incidental curiosities discovered at autopsy. They comprise spindle (stromal) cell tumors, polyps, lipomas, neurogenic tumors, hemangiopericytomas, hemangiomas, granular cell tumors, and heterotopic pancreatic rests. Only two lesions—spindle cell tumor and polyp, merit further consideration.

Stromal Cell Tumors

Spindle cell, also called stromal cell, tumors include a broad variety of lesions, such as leiomyomas, neurofibromas, schwannomas, and so forth, that are composed of spindle-shaped cells. They are well-demarcated, firm nodules (almost always less than 4 cm in diameter) arising within the muscularis. Thus, they are submucosal and, being small, do not erode the overlying mucosa. Morphologically, they exactly resemble their counterparts in other locations (p. 872). Rarely, they grow to larger size (up to 5 cm in diameter) and produce hemispheric elevation of the mucosa with ulceration over the dome of the tumor. Such larger lesions may produce symptoms resembling those of peptic ulcer, particularly bleeding that is sometimes massive. Most often, discovery before death is incidental to radiographic or endoscopic examination of the stomach for other reasons. Malignant transformation has been reported.

Polyps

Polyps are among the more common benign neoplasms of the stomach, but they are nonetheless rarities, found in about 0.5% of autopsies and in between 2 and 6% of patients who undergo an upper endoscopy study. Histologically, *the great majority are either hyperplastic (inflammatory) polyps or neoplastic (tubular adenomas or villous adenomas), which differ greatly in their clinical significance.*[66,67]

Hyperplastic polyps are by far the most common type (90%). They result from an exaggerated regenerative response to mucosal injury.

Since they appear to reflect a field effect, these polyps are usually multiple and occur as smooth, soft, pale gray mucosal elevations (Fig. 18–22). Most are under 1 cm and are sessile, but the larger ones may be pedunculated and show hemorrhages and ulcerations on their bulbous tips. Microscopically, they appear to be composed predominantly of hyperplastic glands lined by cells similar to those seen in gastric pits. Tubules and microcysts are formed, which are lined by a single layer of regularly arrayed cells. The intervening stroma is often inflamed.

Hyperplastic polyps are regenerative non-neoplastic lesions that have no malignant potential per se. However, since the frequency with which such polyps are seen in stomachs resected for carcinoma is significantly high (20 to 28%), the presence of hyperplastic

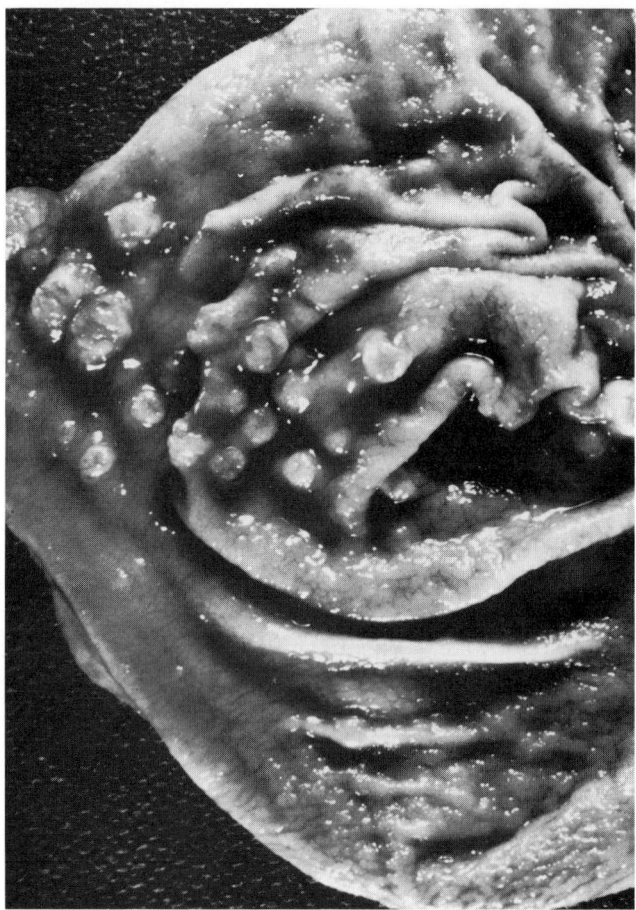

Figure 18–22. **Multiple hyperplastic polyps of stomach. There are multiple sessile polyps situated on the mucosal folds. Most of the polyps are smooth-surfaced, small, and uniform in size. (From Kasimer, W., and Dayal, Y.: Gastritis, gastric atrophy, and gastric neoplasia.** *In* **Chopra, S., and May, R.J. (eds.): Pathophysiology of Gastrointestinal Disorders. Boston, Little, Brown, and Co., 1989. Used by permission.)**

gastric polyps should prompt a search for carcinoma elsewhere in the stomach.[66] Generally asymptomatic, these polyps are most commonly detected during a radiologic, endoscopic, or gross examination of a stomach resected for some other disease.

Neoplastic polyps are true neoplasms and account for nearly 10% of all gastric polyps. Also referred to as adenomas or adenomatous polyps, these lesions are usually single and may grow up to 3 or 4 cm in size (Fig. 18–23). The larger polyps are usually pedunculated and have a lobulated, cauliflower-like head that is frequently inflamed and ulcerated. Microscopically, they display closely packed glandlike, tubular structures or villous processes that are lined by neoplastic cells. The morphologic features are similar to those of neoplastic polyps seen in the colon (p. 893). Varying degrees of atypia and dysplasia may be present, and frankly malignant foci can be present in such polyps, particularly in the larger ones.

Neoplastic polyps have an overall risk of between 40 and 60% of undergoing malignant change. They are also associated with a high risk (40%) of a coexistent carcinoma elsewhere in the stomach. Simple polypectomy is not sufficient in their treatment, since carcinomatous glands may invade the cores of these lesions and extend into the underlying wall. Indeed, 10 to 15% of frank carcinomatous lesions have metastasized by the time of discovery.

Infrequently, multiple polyps occur in the stomach as part of the diffuse gastrointestinal polyposis of familial multiple polyposis or the Peutz-Jeghers syndrome (p. 892).

MALIGNANT

Among the malignant tumors that occur in the stomach, carcinoma is overwhelmingly the most important and the most common (approximately 90 to 95%). Next in order of frequency, but far less common, are the lymphomas (4%) and malignant spindle cell tumors (2%). In addition, carcinoid tumors sometimes occur in the stomach, accounting for nearly 3% of all gastric malignancies.

Carcinoma

Gastric cancer is a worldwide disease. Its incidence, however, varies widely, being particularly high in Japan, Chile, Costa Rica, Colombia, China, Portugal, Iceland, Finland, and Scotland and considerably lower in the United States, United Kingdom, Canada, Australia, New Zealand, Greece, Nicaragua, Honduras, and Sweden. In most countries, there has been

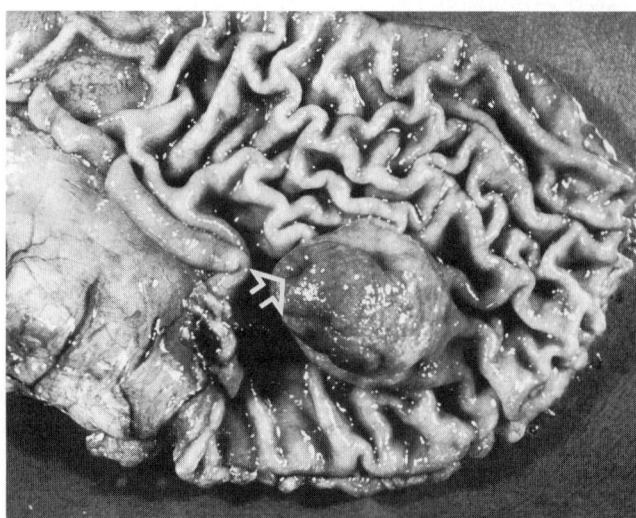

Figure 18–23. **Adenomatous polyp of stomach. Note the considerably larger size of the polyp and its lobulated configuration. A small ulceration** *(arrow)* **can be identified on its surface. (From Kasimer, W., and Dayal, Y.: Gastritis, gastric atrophy, and gastric neoplasia.** *In* **Chopra, S., and May, R.J. (eds.): Pathophysiology of Gastrointestinal Disorders. Boston, Little, Brown, and Co., 1989. Used by permission.)**

a steady decline in both the incidence and the mortality of gastric cancer during the past five decades. Thus, during the last 50 years, the mortality rate from gastric cancer in the United States has dropped from about 30 to 6 per 100,000 for men, and from 21 to 4 per 100,000 for women.[68] Nonetheless, gastric cancer remains a formidable challenge, since its overall five-year survival rate still continues to be dismally poor (5 to 15% in the United States).[69] It continues to be a leading cause of all cancer-related deaths in countries where its incidence is high.

ETIOLOGY AND PATHOGENESIS. While many factors have been incriminated in the etiology of gastric cancer, most of the epidemiologic evidence suggests that environmental (chiefly dietary) factors are the most important. However, genetic and racial factors may play some role.[70] Certain racial and ethnic groups (such as blacks, American Indians, and native Hawaiians in the United States, and Maoris in New Zealand) have a high risk of developing gastric cancer, as do individuals with blood group A.[70] But since only about 4% of patients with gastric cancer have a family history of this disease, genetic factors are unlikely to be major influences in the vast majority of cases. A study of Japanese immigrants to the United States has shown that although the first generation had the same high incidence of gastric cancer as in Japan, subsequent generations acquired an incidence rate comparable to that of native Americans.

Other observations highlight the importance of dietary factors as significant determinants of risk for gastric cancer. Numerous studies from various countries have reported that ingestion of certain foodstuffs or adherence to certain culinary practices is associated with a high risk of gastric cancer. The food may contain a carcinogen or be converted into one either during preparation and preservation or in the stomach after ingestion. Salted meats, fava beans, and corn are the staple diet in areas of Colombia where gastric cancer is very common[71]; likewise, in Japan, pickled raw vegetables, salty sauces, dried salted fish, and rice dusted with asbestos-containing talc all have been implicated. High quantities of 3,4-benzopyrene have been identified in the smoked foods consumed in the high-incidence areas of Iceland. A high intake of nitrate in food and drinking water has been associated with an increased risk of gastric cancer in several countries.[72,73] In this regard, it should be mentioned that the practice of adding nitrites as a preservative for certain meats (sausages, frankfurters) may have a contributory role. It is of interest that green, leafy vegetables and citrus fruits that act as antioxidants are protective for gastric cancer; a negative correlation has indeed been demonstrated between the high intake of fresh vegetables and gastric cancer.[74] A high intake of animal fat has also been considered a protective factor against gastric cancer.[74]

In sum, populations at high risk for gastric cancer have the following dietary characteristics in common[71]: *(1) a high intake of salt, (2) a low intake of animal fat and protein, (3) a high intake of complex carbohydrates chiefly derived from grains and tuberous roots, (4) a high intake of nitrate, and (5) a low intake of green, leafy vegetables and fruits.*

In addition to putative roles for dietary factors, host factors appear to be related to the development of gastric cancer. Certain diseases or pathologic states that produce hypo- or achlorhydria, e.g., *chronic gastritis types A and AB, and pernicious anemia*, are associated with an increased risk for gastric cancer. The gastric mucosa in each of these conditions shows a prominent degree of glandular atrophy and intestinal metaplasia, which are frequently the basis for dysplastic changes that lead to a long-term 7 to 10% risk of gastric cancer. Patients who have had *partial gastrectomies* are also believed to have a higher risk of gastric cancer in the residual gastric stump. The hypo- or achlorhydria in the postgastrectomy state and the associated chronic gastritis occurring secondary to bile reflux together encourage bacterial colonization in the gastric stump and promote the conversion of dietary nitrates and nitrites into nitrosamines. *Gastric neoplastic polyps*, particularly those arising on a background of chronic gastritis, are also known to turn malignant and may represent a final common pathway by which gastric cancer may arise.

EVOLUTION OF GASTRIC CANCER. Without knowledge of its etiology, the only hope for improving the outlook for patients with gastric carcinoma is earlier diagnosis while curative resection is still possible. It has been found that *all gastric carcinomas arise as in situ lesions confined to the mucosal epithelium alone.* The in situ lesion, confined within the basement membrane of the glands, may represent a solitary focus, but in one half of cases multiple foci, perhaps closely adjacent, arise simultaneously. The in situ lesion then breaks through the epithelial basement membrane and invades the lamina propria of the mucosa and eventually the submucosa, and, with time, ultimately the deeper layers. Metastases may appear at any stage of this evolution. *When the local lesion is still limited to the mucosa and submucosa, without penetration of the muscularis propria, it is referred to as early gastric carcinoma (EGC).*[69] Tumors that have penetrated into or beyond the muscularis propria are referred to as advanced gastric carcinomas. This distinction is of great clinical significance, since the prognosis following surgery of these two groups is vastly different (see below). Elaborate classifications of the gross morphology of EGC have been developed, dividing the lesions into protruding, flat, and depressed categories as well as others. However, here it suffices to note that in most instances EGC produces sufficient alteration of the mucosa to enable recognition of the lesion on barium study or endoscopy, permitting confirmatory biopsy. In Japan, remarkable results were achieved when these diagnostic procedures were included in annual clinical examinations of middle-aged to older adults. The five-year survival rate for patients with EGC after surgical resection was 93 to 99%, in comparison with 5 to 15% in the usual case mix.[69] Ample opportunity exists for discovery of early gastric carcinomas because they evolve very slowly and, in some instances, have been found to take eight years to become more invasive.[75]

MORPHOLOGY. Gastric carcinomas have been divided into a bewildering array of subsets based on gross patterns, extent of invasion, and histogenesis. Remarks here will be restricted to the major categories. The localization of tumors within the stomach is as follows: pylorus and antrum, 50 to 60%; cardia, 25%; and the remainder in other areas. The lesser curvature is involved in about 40% and the greater curvature in 12%, the remainder being found on the anterior or posterior walls. **Thus, a favored location is the lesser curvature of the antropyloric region.** Ulcerative cancers in this location may closely mimic, both radiologically and on inspection, chronic peptic ulcers, but most have nodular raised margins. By contrast, a pyloroantral ulcerative lesion on the greater curvature is more likely to be malignant. Carcinomas at the time of discovery range from relatively small tumors (about 10% are less than 2 cm in diameter) to lesions that involve virtually the entire stomach; about 80% are between 2 and 10 cm in diameter. They have been segregated into many patterns.

The frequency of **early gastric carcinoma** (10 to 35%) is obviously dependent on the intensity of the diagnostic effort to uncover asymptomatic disease. In Japan, EGC constitutes about 35% of all newly diagnosed gastric cancers. In the United States, the figures are closer to 10% but will surely increase as more experience is acquired in recognizing these lesions endoscopically. They appear as flat areas of mucosal thickening and induration or may be protuberant, ulcerated, or excavated. Some tumors may cover large areas of the gastric mucosa and yet show no extension into the muscular coat.

Advanced gastric carcinomas, i.e., those that have penetrated into the muscularis propria or beyond, were traditionally categorized as ulcerative, ulcerated-infiltrative, polypoid, and diffusely infiltrative (linitis plastica). Such a classification has now fallen into disfavor because a large proportion of tumors have mixed features that make it difficult to categorize them accurately. More importantly, however, this classification had limited usefulness, since the gross features of the lesions did not appear to correlate with the specific histologic subtypes or their depth of invasion and provided no information as to their prognosis.[76] A more recent classification divides gastric cancers into (1) **expanding carcinomas** and (2) **infiltrative carcinomas.**

Expanding carcinomas are characterized by an apparently cohesive mass of tumor cells that grow along broad fronts, creating a "pushing" invasive margin. With this type of invasion the extent of the lateral spread can generally be appreciated by the surgeon, to permit adequate margins of resection. In the more ominous **infiltrative pattern,** the tumor cells do not appear to be cohesive and so penetrate individually and in small clusters, resulting in poorly defined invasive margins and generally more diffuse involvement of the stomach.

Histologically, all gastric carcinomas are composed of basically two cell types: metaplastic intestinal cells and gastric mucous cells. Sometimes, mixtures of these cell types are found. The metaplastic intestinal cells contain large apical vacuoles (goblets) of mucus that usually can be shown to be, in part, acidic intestinal mucin, but sometimes neutral gastric mucin. Microvillous striated borders may be found along the luminal surface of some cells. In addition, these cells contain alkaline phosphatase, amino peptidase, and beta-glucuronidase enzymes not usually observed in normal gastric mucosal cells. In well-differentiated tumors, these two types of cells are readily identified, but with loss of differentiation and progressive anaplasia, both mucin secretion and distinctive cell characteristics disappear.

Either cell type may form well-defined neoplastic glands (adenocarcinomas), occasionally with papillary ingrowths (papillary adenocarcinomas). In less well differentiated neoplasms, the cells tend to be disposed in disorderly masses, islands, or small clusters, or sometimes singly. In addition, the amount of mucin secretion varies, irrespective of the cell type. Numerous mucin vacuoles may distend cells or may coalesce and compress the flattened nucleus against the plasma membrane to create "signet-ring cells" (Fig. 18–24). In other instances, the mucus may lie within neoplastic glands. Sometimes, large lakes of secretion, in which isolated tumor cells or glands appear to float, literally dissect through cleavage planes. In diffuse infiltrative cancers the tumor cells are often accompanied by an abundant fibrous stroma. This desmoplasia accounts for much of the thickening of the gastric wall, and it may be so florid as to render identification of the cancerous cells difficult. The diffuse thickening of the gastric wall has given rise to the term "leather-bottle" stomach, also called **linitis plastica.**

Gastric cancers have also been divided by some experts into "intestinal type" and "gastric-infiltrative" categories based on the predominant cell type in the neoplasm.[77] This classification has pathogenetic and clinical significance. Intestinal type lesions are more often of the expanding variety associated with chronic gastritis and the consequent intestinal metaplasia seen in chronic gastritis. This pattern has a better prognosis than does the gastric infiltrative type and appears to be more closely correlated with environmental influences; it is the form predominantly encountered in high-incidence locales and countries.

One additional variant of gastric carcinoma merits mention: a so-called **undifferentiated carcinoma** composed of sheets of small cells with round-to-ovoid, deeply hyperchromatic nuclei. On electron microscopy, cytoplasmic secretory granules are evident in these cells, and some are argentaffin positive. Such tumors are presumably derived from endocrine cells found in the gastric mucosa as well as throughout the gut.[78] Because these neoplasms are capable of elaborating a variety of amine or polypeptide hormones, e.g., histamine, 5-hydroxytryptamine, and ACTH, they belong to the category of neuroendocrine tumors (p. 872).

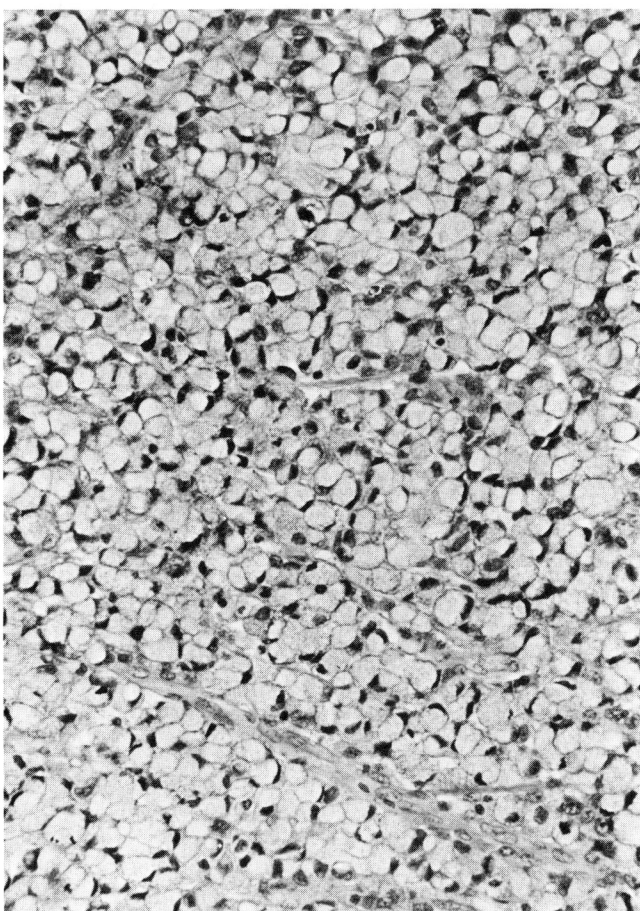

Figure 18-24. Infiltrating carcinoma of stomach. The uniform-sized tumor cells seen infiltrating the gastric wall show abundant intracellular mucin that pushes the nucleus to one side, giving the cells their typical "signet ring" appearance. (From Kasimer, W., and Dayal, Y.: Gastritis, gastric atrophy, and gastric neoplasia. *In* Chopra, S., and May, R.J. (eds.): Pathophysiology of Gastrointestinal Disorders. Boston, Little, Brown, and Co., 1989. Used by permission.)

In time, gastric carcinomas progressively penetrate the stomach wall to appear as small, gray-white, subserosal nodules. They extend laterally, sometimes to invade the entire stomach and occasionally the duodenum. Interestingly, the duodenal invasion is generally subserosal, without involvement of the mucosa. Metastases to regional lymph nodes are present in 80 to 90% of specimens obtained from total gastrectomy. Widespread peritoneal seedings and metastases to the liver or lungs, as well as to other organs, are encountered in 20 to 40% of necropsies on patients who have died of this disease. One pattern of metastatic dissemination deserves special citation. Dissemination of tumor cells to the ovaries is encountered in about 10% of fatal cases of gastric carcinoma. The ovarian masses have been called **Krukenberg tumors** (Fig. 18-25). These are discussed more completely on page 1170, but we may note here that Krukenberg tumors of the ovaries may also arise by spread of other mucinous adenocarcinomas such as those of the breast, pancreas, and

gallbladder. Typically, the enlarged ovaries contain signet-ring, mucin-secreting cells in an abundant fibrous stroma. There have been remarkable cases in which clinical recognition of the ovarian mass(es) led to the identification of the primary gastric cancer, and at the time of laparotomy there was no evidence of metastases in other organs.

CLINICAL COURSE. Gastric carcinoma is an insidious disease that is generally asymptomatic until late in its course. At present the five-year survival rate in the United States ranges between 5 and 15%, and this prognosis has not improved in the last 40 years.[69] The discovery of "early gastric carcinoma," with its much better prognosis, is totally dependent on early recognition by endoscopy and radiographic barium studies. In individuals with more advanced cancer, the frequency of symptoms is as follows:

Symptom	% of Cases
Weight loss	80
Abdominal pain	72
Anorexia	57
Vomiting	44
Changed bowel habit	35
Dysphagia	14
Anemic symptoms	12
Hemorrhage	10

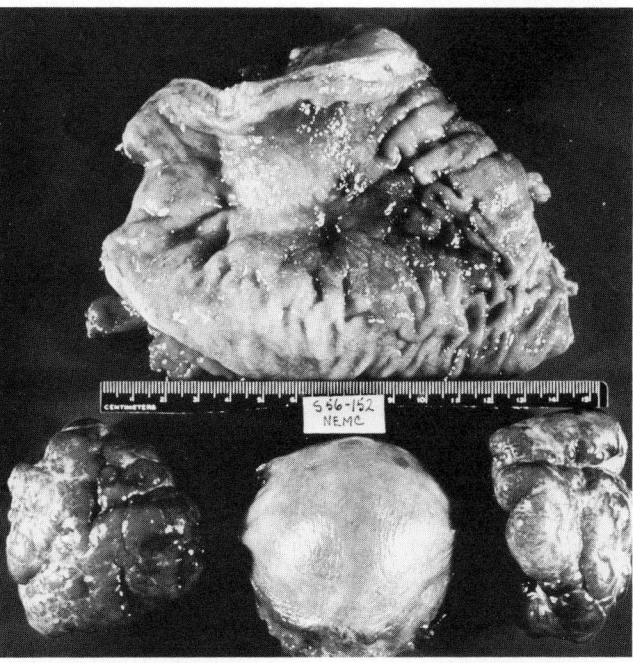

Figure 18-25. Infiltrating carcinoma of the stomach with bilateral ovarian metastases (Krukenberg tumors). Note that the wall of the stomach is diffusely thickened and that the ovaries are enlarged and bosselated. This is rather characteristic of Krukenberg tumors. (From Kasimer, W., and Dayal, Y.: Gastritis, gastric atrophy, and gastric neoplasia. *In* Chopra, S., and May, R.J. (eds.): Pathophysiology of Gastrointestinal Disorders. Boston, Little, Brown, and Co., 1989. Used by permission.)

Most of these symptoms are nonspecific, rendering early diagnosis of this form of cancer difficult. The abdominal pain is usually referred to the epigastrium but is often vague and intermittent. Occult bleeding is frequent, sometimes producing "coffee-grounds" vomitus, but more often is associated only with guaiac-positive stools. Some patients (10%) experience massive hematemesis, sufficient to cause shock. Achlorhydria or hypochlorhydria is noted in about half the patients. Abnormally low levels of gastric acid are infrequent in young individuals and those with superficial carcinoma. When the achlorhydria is histamine- or pentagastrin-fast, one can assume that an ulcerative lesion is cancerous.

In view of the nonspecific presentation of this form of cancer, the diagnosis and, in particular, the differentiation of a benign from a malignant ulcer require careful evaluation, involving radiographic, endoscopic, cytologic, and finally biopsy studies (Table 18–3).

All too often the primary lesion comes to attention because of metastatic disease. Hepatomegaly due to metastases is already present at the time of first diagnosis in about 10% of cases. It may be accompanied by ascites and, less frequently, jaundice. Spread to remote lymph nodes sometimes heralds the existence of the gastric primary. *For uncertain reasons, the supraclavicular (Virchow's) nodes and scalene nodes are often involved and enlarged relatively early in the course of the disease.* Metastases to the ovaries (Krukenberg tumors) are sometimes discovered on pelvic examination, even before gastric symptoms appear. The tumor mass may seed the peritoneal cul-de-sac, producing a so-called rectal shelf on rectal examination. Thus, the prognosis for this disease to date has been bleak. On the basis of past practices of case finding, only about half the lesions at the time of discovery are sufficiently localized to permit an attempt at resection, accounting in large part for the poor overall five-year survival rate.[69]

Endocrine Cell Tumors (Carcinoids)

Although these stomach lesions are rare, they tend, like those in the small and large intestine, to be infil-trative, aggressive tumors that metastasize in about one third of cases. These are described in detail on page 872.

Gastrointestinal Lymphomas

Lymphomas in the course of their systemic dissemination may secondarily involve any segment of the gastrointestinal tract, but they may also arise as primary neoplasms anywhere in the lymphoid elements found throughout the gut. In all sites of origin, in the gut they have similar morphologic characteristics and thus are all considered here as a group. *Most arise in the stomach and small intestine.*[79] The gastric primaries represent only 3 to 5% of all gastric malignancies. The ileum, colon, and jejunum are the other sites of involvement in descending order of frequency. Primary gastrointestinal lymphomas are defined as lymphomas arising anywhere in the gut with no evidence of systemic (liver, spleen, or bone marrow) involvement at the time of presentation. Secondary gastrointestinal lymphomas, on the other hand, involve the gut *after* initial presentation elsewhere and do so as part of their systemic spread.[80]

Primary gastrointestinal lymphomas may be categorized into three major types: (1) the Western or sporadic type, (2) the sprue-associated type, and (3) the Mediterranean type. The *Western type,* as the name suggests, is the most common type in the Western hemisphere. Its etiology is unknown, and no specific association with any predisposing diseases or pathologic lesions has been reported. This type of lymphoma usually affects adults, lacks a predilection for either sex, and may arise anywhere in the gut: stomach in approximately 55 to 60% of cases; small intestine in about 25 to 30%; proximal colon in from 10 to 15%; and distal colon in up to 10%. The appendix and esophagus are so infrequently involved that accurate figures are hard to obtain.

The *sprue-associated lymphoma* is relatively uncommon in the United States; its prevalence in Europe appears to be higher—possibly reflecting a higher incidence of sprue. It arises in some patients with a long-standing malabsorption syndrome that is not necessarily a gluten-sensitive enteropathy. It

Table 18–3. Clinical Features of Benign and Malignant Gastric Ulcers

	BENIGN ULCER	MALIGNANT ULCER
Age of patient	Tends to occur in younger individuals	Tends to occur in older individuals
Duration of symptoms	Varies from weeks to many years	Varies from weeks to months but rarely for years
Sex	Marked male preponderance	Slight male preponderance
Gastric acidity	May be normal or increased—anacidity rare	May be normal but can be totally absent
Location of lesion	Usually lesser curvature of pyloric or prepyloric region—however, may be on greater curvature or anterior or posterior wall	Greater curvature of pyloric and prepyloric regions—however, may be on lesser curvature or in other sites in stomach
Size of lesion	Usually is less than 2 cm in diameter and rarely over 4 cm	Usually greater than 4 cm in diameter but may be smaller
Response to medical therapy	Usually shows prompt evidence of healing on adequate treatment	May respond to medical therapy but usually is refractory
X-ray	Demonstrates a small punched-out niche without involvement of surrounding wall	Demonstrates defect with irregular or heaped-up margins and possible involvement of surrounding wall and mucosa

occurs in relatively younger individuals (30 to 40 years of age) and is usually preceded by a 10- to 20-year history of symptomatic malabsorption. The lesions occur predominantly in the proximal small bowel with about two thirds arising in the duodenojejunal segment—an area that is more severely involved by the malabsorption process itself. The distal small bowel may be involved in about 10% of cases. Lesions are, however, uncommon in the stomach and large bowel.[81] *Mediterranean lymphomas* were so named because the initial cases of this type of gastrointestinal lymphoma were diagnosed along the Mediterranean coast. Although similar cases were subsequently reported from the Western world, most patients have at least had a Mediterranean ancestry.[82] The diagnosis is made most commonly in children and young adults, and both sexes appear to be affected equally. The lesions, like those in the sprue-associated lymphomas, most often arise in the proximal small bowel on a background of diffuse mucosal plasmacytosis in the affected segment. Usually such a plasmacytosis is of long standing, and a high proportion of patients have malabsorption preceding the development of the lymphoma. A small subset of cases occur in patients with alpha–heavy-chain disease (p. 744).

The lesions can assume any of a large variety of gross characteristics depending on their location. Thus some diffusely infiltrating lesions may produce localized mural thickening with effacement of the overlying mucosal folds and focal ulceration, whereas others may appear polypoid, protruding into the lumen, or as large, fungating, ulcerated masses. Nodal involvement occurs frequently; the disease may, in fact, be primarily nodal in origin. Since all the intramural lymphoid tissue in the gut is mucosal and submucosal, the early lesions appear as a plaque-like expansion of the mucosa and submucosa. With gradual enlargement over a period of time, the overlying mucosa may become ulcerated, allowing the lesion to infiltrate into the muscular coat. Tumor infiltration splays the muscle fibers, gradually destroying them. Because of this feature, these lesions frequently cause motility problems with secondary obstruction. Large tumors sometimes perforate because of lack of stromal support.

Histologically most sporadic gastrointestinal lymphomas are B-cell lesions. Those associated with sprue have now been classified as genuine histiocytic lesions. The histogenesis of Mediterranean lymphomas, commonly referred to as immunoproliferative small intestinal disease (IPSID), is controversial. The vast majority of sporadic gastrointestinal lymphomas are derived from follicle center cells (FCCs) and, like lymphomas elsewhere, consist of a mixture of FCCs (both cleaved and noncleaved) and immunoblasts in varying proportion (p. 710). In the Mediterranean type, plasma cell differentiation, uncommon in nodal FCC lymphomas, occurs frequently.

Primary gastrointestinal lymphomas are said to have a better prognosis than do those arising in other sites, which may be due to the overall earlier stage at which they are discovered. The prognosis is better for gastric lymphomas (40 to 50% five-year survival) than for those located distally in the small or large bowel (15 to 25% survival). In general, depth of local invasion, size of the tumor, and extension into adjacent viscera are important determinants of prognosis.

Sarcomas

The most frequent malignant stromal tumors of the stomach are leiomyosarcomas, fibrosarcomas, and endothelial sarcomas. Both individually and collectively they are rare. Since these tumors are quite similar histologically as well as clinically, with few features of specific differentiation, they are currently all grouped under the umbrella of malignant stromal (spindle) cell tumors.

They may appear at any age and in either sex. Grossly, either they produce large, bulky, intramural masses that eventually fungate and ulcerate into the gastric lumen, or they project subserosally. On cross section they have a typical soft, fish-flesh appearance, are somewhat lobulated, and frequently have areas of hemorrhage, necrosis, or cystic softening. Histologically they resemble leiomyosarcomas found elsewhere (p. 1155). Because they tend to grow as cohesive masses without the diffuse infiltrative characteristics of gastric carcinomas, many are amenable to surgical removal, yielding a 50 to 60% five-year survival rate. Metastases, however, are present in about one third of cases (Fig. 18–26).

Leiomyoblastomas are uncommon histologic variants of malignant spindle (stromal) cell gastric tumors that rarely arise elsewhere. Nonetheless, their recog-

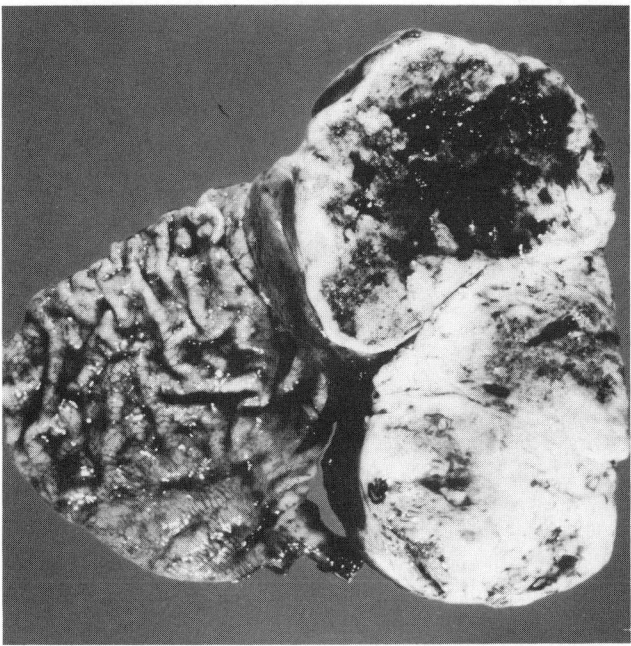

Figure 18–26. Malignant spindle cell tumor of stomach. The cut section of this large, well-circumscribed tumor shows extensive areas of hemorrhagic necrosis. Note that this large tumor mostly protrudes outside the stomach rather than into the lumen.

nition is important because, despite their ominous gross and microscopic appearance, many are biologically benign. Their malignant potential is intermediate between that of benign spindle cell tumor and that of the malignant counterpart. Grossly, they are usually large, fairly well-circumscribed intramural masses that project into the gastric lumen, sometimes with ulceration of the gastric mucosa over the dome of the mass. Microscopically, they are characterized by large pleomorphic cells having central nuclei that are variable in size and shape. The cells have an abundant eosinophilic or clear cytoplasm that sometimes leaves distinct, clear perinuclear halos. Ultrastructural studies in some cells reveal microfilaments typical of smooth muscle cells, which, with the immunoperoxidase technique, can be shown to be myosin. Special stains for reticulin (silver, gold techniques) disclose an abundant reticulum that encloses individual cells. Mi-

toses may be scant or abundant, and the biologic behavior appears to be related to the number of mitoses. When five or more are present in ten high-power fields, the neoplasm is very likely to be malignant and to have metastatic potential.[83,84]

Metastatic Carcinoma

Metastatic involvement of the stomach is a rarity. Although such spread may be produced by carcinomas arising elsewhere, particularly breast carcinomas and malignant melanoma, the most common sources of gastric metastases are generalized lymphomatosis and leukemia. Most lesions are multiple and differ from primary tumors in that they usually affect the submucosa and muscularis primarily, and only secondarily invade the mucosa. Central ulceration of these masses may occur.

SMALL INTESTINE

CONGENITAL ANOMALIES	CROHN'S DISEASE (REGIONAL	MALABSORPTION SYNDROMES	OBSTRUCTIVE LESIONS
ISCHEMIC BOWEL DISEASE	ENTERITIS)	Celiac Sprue	Hernias
Transmural Infarction	TUMORS	**Tropical Sprue**	**Intestinal Adhesions**
Mucosal and Mural Infarction	**Benign**	**Whipple's Disease**	**Intussusception**
INFECTIVE ENTEROCOLITIS	**Malignant**	**Bacterial Overgrowth Syndrome**	**Volvulus**
Bacterial Enterocolitis	Carcinoid tumors	**Disaccharidase Deficiency**	
Nonbacterial Gastroenterocolitis	Carcinoma	**Abetalipoproteinemia**	

NORMAL

The arterial supply of the small intestine is largely derived from the superior mesenteric artery, which progressively divides as it approaches the gut. A small lesion, then, in the root of the mesentery may compromise the vascular integrity of yards of small intestine. However, the arterial branches are richly interconnected by arching arcades. Thus, obstructive lesions of a secondary branch of the superior mesenteric artery may be without effect. When vascular lesions occur close to the gut in the intramural end-arteries, small ischemic lesions result. Since the lymphatic drainage essentially parallels the vascular supply but does not have the intricate patterns of arcades, involvement of a small focus of lymph nodes or lymphatics produces a rather large segment of intestinal lymphedema.

The histologic identification of the small bowel rests on the recognition of villi. Between their bases and extending into the deeper levels of the mucosa are the pitlike crypts. The height of the villi is three times greater than the depth of the crypts, a point of some

importance in the interpretation of small bowel biopsies. Distinctive of the duodenum are the elaborately branched Brunner's glands, which penetrate the muscularis mucosae into the submucosa. The lamina propria in the small intestine contains not only phagocytic cells but also lymphocytes (in great abundance in the ileal Peyer's patches) as well as plasma cells. Immunoglobulins, particularly IgA, are synthesized by these cells and probably serve an important protective function against bacterial invasion.

The epithelium lining the crypts differs from that covering the villi. Four types of crypt epithelial cells have been identified: (1) Paneth cells, (2) undifferentiated cells, (3) goblet cells, and (4) endocrine cells.[85] *Paneth cells* have a basophilic cytoplasm that contains large secretory granules. Studies suggest that these cells contain lysozyme, IgG, and IgA.[86] *Undifferentiated cells* are the most numerous in the crypts. *Goblet cells* are packed with mucigen granules, creating large apical vacuoles, which, when seen in the light microscope, give these cells some fanciful resemblance to brandy goblets. The goblet cells are obviously the source of the mucus secretion of the small intestine. The endocrine cells of the gut have already been described (p. 840).

The surface covering of the villi is made up of

three types of cells, principally absorptive cells interspersed with goblet cells and a few endocrine cells. These are bound together by "tight junctions," which maintain a virtually impermeable barrier between the luminal contents and the subepithelial lamina propria. All molecules save the smallest, such as sodium, chloride, and water, which diffuse to some degree between cells, must pass through the surface mucosal cells. The absorptive cells are highly specialized on their luminal surface by microvilli, expanding their luminal surfaces by perhaps 30 fold. They, in turn, are covered by a firmly attached, filamentous-appearing glycoprotein coat that is secreted by the absorptive cells. This microvillous, membrane–fuzzy coat complex provides an ideal milieu for the terminal digestion of foodstuffs by amylases and proteases. The microvillous membrane also contains disaccharidases and certain peptidases involved in the terminal degradation of saccharides and polypeptides to their monosaccharide and amino acid residues; it also contains other enzymes and carrier proteins involved in sugar and amino acid transport.[87] The membrane possesses specific receptors, such as those in the ileum for intrinsic factor–vitamin B_{12} complexes.

The regenerative capacity of the small intestine epithelium is remarkable. Cellular proliferation is confined to the basal portions of the crypts; from here, the cells migrate in an escalator-like fashion to the tip of the villus, where they are eventually shed into the lumen. This journey takes between 72 and 96 hours. Thus the surface epithelial lining of the small bowel is renewed every three to four days. During this migration the cells undergo differentiation, with the progressive acquisition of intramembrane particles (probably representing membrane-associated enzymes) and the development of the tight junctions, which are better organized in villous cells than in crypt cells.[88] The looser junctions in the crypts suggest that this region is more involved in absorption of ions and water than is the surface of the villi. The rapid renewal of the small intestinal epithelium provides a remarkable capacity for repair, but in another sense renders the small intestine particularly vulnerable to agents that interfere with cell replication, as, for example, radiation or cancer chemotherapeutic drugs.

PATHOLOGY

The principal types of pathologic conditions in this segment of the gut are inflammatory disorders and derangements that lead to malabsorption. Because the lumen is narrow, intestinal obstruction is a frequent complication of some of the lesions. In contrast to the stomach and colon, primary tumors are relatively uncommon in the small intestine despite the enormous surface area of the epithelium at risk and its constant replicative activity.

CONGENITAL ANOMALIES

Numerous developmental defects of rotation and reduplication occur in the small intestine, but they are rare. Anomalies that are encountered sufficiently often to merit description include atresia and stenosis, diverticula, and pancreatic rests.

Atresia implies noncanalization of the developing gut. In atresia, either a segment of the bowel is entirely missing, leaving a proximal segment with a blind end separated at some distance from the distal bowel, or the upper and lower segments are united by a solid fibrous cord. *Stenosis*, on the other hand, implies narrowing of an already canalized bowel, e.g., by fibrosis or stricture. It may be either mild and of little consequence or severe and obstructive. Atresias and stenoses may occur singly or multiply, involving any level of the jejunum or ileum. These lesions may at times be associated with a variety of congenital anomalies.

In the muscular wall of the jejunum and ileum, the points at which mesenteric vessels and nerves enter provide foci of weakness where the mucosa and submucosa may herniate into the mesentery (Fig. 18–27). Such *diverticula* occur about one tenth as

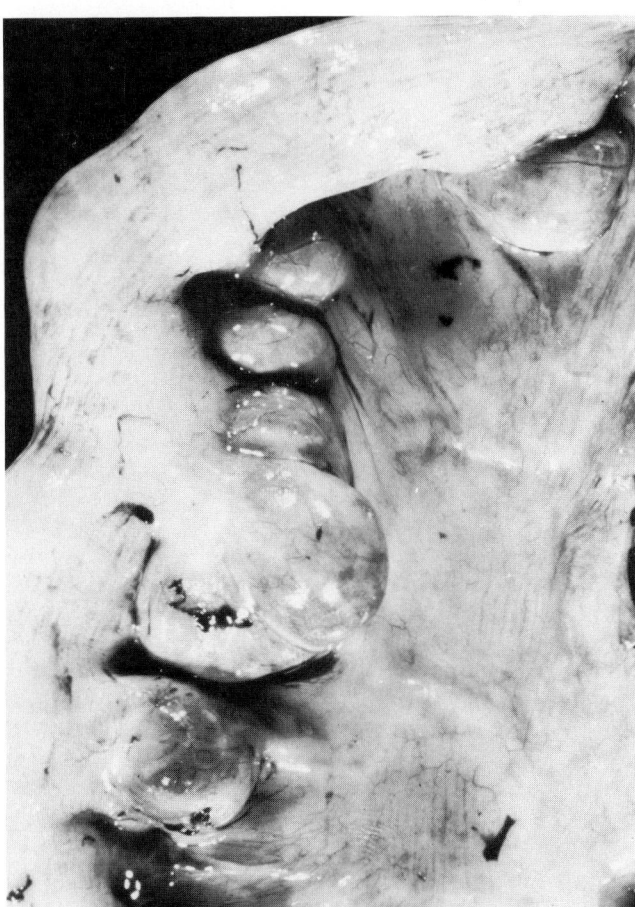

Figure 18–27. Multiple jejunal diverticula. Note that these diverticula are on the mesenteric side of the jejunum. Such diverticula typically have wide ostia communicating with the intestinal lumen, and they frequently contain myriad proliferating aerobic and anaerobic bacteria in their lumina.

often as do duodenal diverticula and are therefore exceedingly rare. Histologically, the muscular coats of the diverticula are absent or thinned, leaving only the mucosa and submucosa. Intestinal stasis in the diverticula leads to considerable overgrowth of both aerobic and anaerobic bacteria. This may occasionally produce malabsorption of essential nutrients and vitamins through a variety of mechanisms discussed later (p. 880). Very rarely, the diverticula are the sites of intestinal bleeding or inflammatory perforation.[89] Those of the duodenum may impinge on the biliary and pancreatic ducts and may sometimes be obstructive.

Persistence of a vestige of the omphalomesenteric duct may give rise to a solitary diverticulum, usually within 12 inches of the ileocecal valve (*Meckel's diverticulum*) (Fig. 18–28). Rarely, it occurs in more proximal locations, sometimes up to 2 to 3 feet from the ileocecal valve.

These diverticula vary in conformation from a fibrotic cord to a pouch having a lumen greater than that of the ileum and a length as great as 5 to 6 cm. The composition of the wall is similar to that of the small bowel, but there are several points of difference. Het-

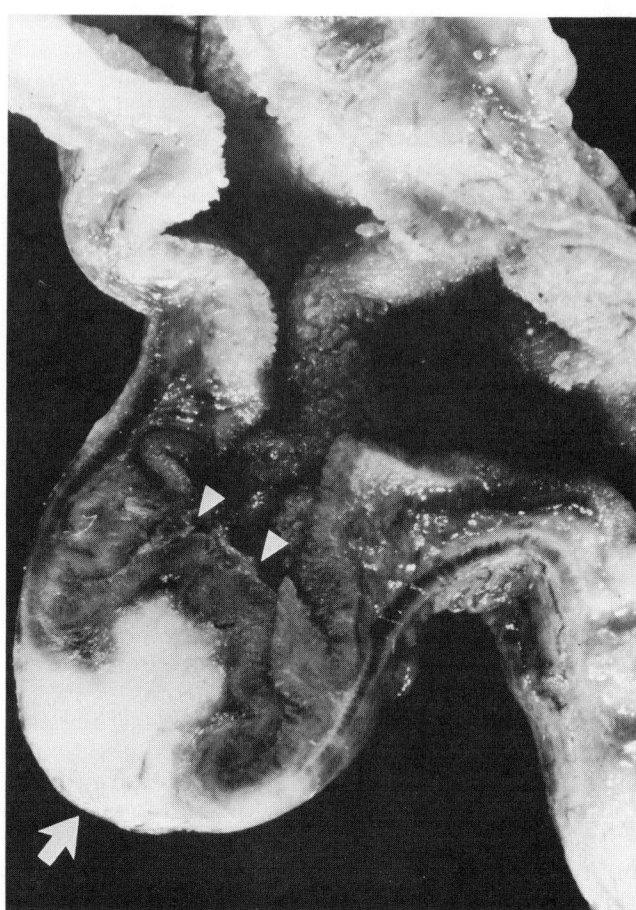

Figure 18–29. Meckel's diverticulum. The cut section of the same diverticulum as in Figure 18–28 shows the diverticulum communicating with the intestinal lumen. The tip of the diverticulum *(arrow)* contains ectopic pancreas, while the mucosal lining shows ectopic gastric mucosa *(arrowheads).*

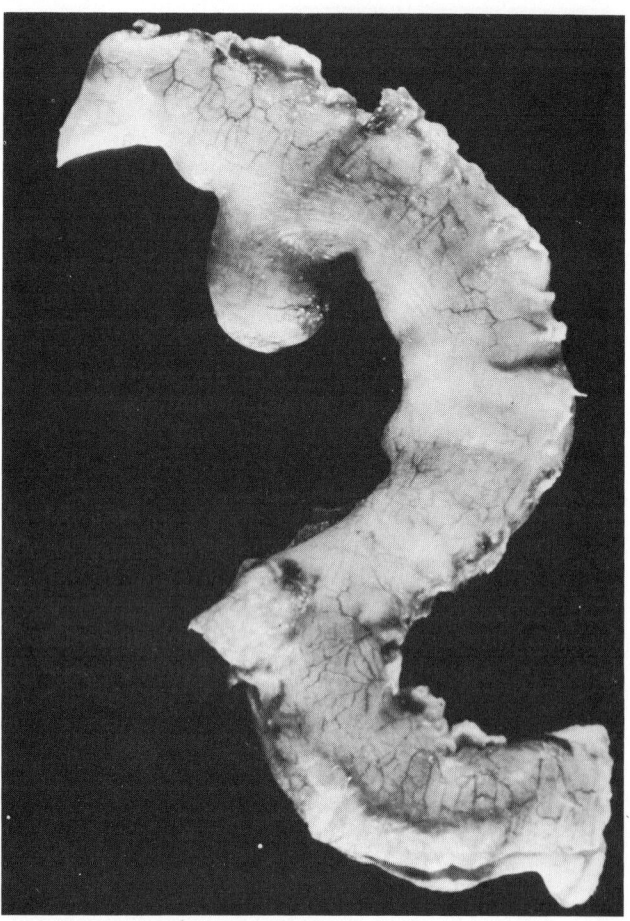

Figure 18–28. Meckel's diverticulum. Derived from an abnormal persistence of the omphalomesenteric duct, this diverticulum is most often located in the terminal ileum. Note that it is situated on the antimesenteric side of the bowel wall.

erotopic rests of gastric mucosa are found in about one half of all Meckel's diverticula. Peptic ulceration sometimes occurs in the mucosa of the diverticulum adjacent to the island of gastric mucosa (Fig. 18–29). Mysterious intestinal bleeding or symptoms resembling those of an acute appendicitis may result.

Rests of essentially normal pancreatic tissue, appearing as small, 1 to 2 cm sized mucosal elevations, can occur anywhere in the small bowel, least often in the jejunum. They are of interest to the surgeon and endoscopist, since they can be confused with a primary tumor of the bowel. On cut surface, they show the typical yellow, lobulated appearance of normal pancreatic tissue.

ISCHEMIC BOWEL DISEASE

The small intestine alone, the colon alone, or sometimes both may sustain hypoxic injury related to various causes of vascular compromise. Collectively, all these lesions are designated *mesenteric ischemias.* The lesions of the colon are sometimes referred to as *ischemic colitis.*[90] Depending on the severity of the reduction in blood flow, three morphologic patterns are somewhat arbitrarily segregated as follows: (1) *infarction or gangrene of the bowel,* implying transmural ischemic necrosis due to the absence of or a marked reduction in blood perfusion; (2) *hemorrhagic gastroenteropathy,* characterized by hemorrhage and necrosis limited to the mucosa and submucosa with sparing, usually of the deeper layers, related to less extreme reduction in blood flow; and (3) *chronic ischemia,* leading in time to fibrotic narrowing of affected bowel. Classically, these categories have implied that infarction is the result of total mesenteric occlusion by a thrombus or embolus; that hemorrhagic gastroenteropathy follows acute nonocclusive hypoperfusion; and that chronic ischemia is the consequence of severe organic vascular narrowing inducing a persistent perfusion deficit. Because there is no sharp line dividing infarction from severe hemorrhagic enteropathy, a more descriptive simplified terminology has been proposed: (a) *transmural infarction*; (b) *mural infarction* — if the injury extends from the mucosa into the submucosa and muscularis; and (c) *mucosal infarction* — if the lesion extends no deeper than the muscularis mucosae.[91] Here we shall adopt the newer terminology.

TRANSMURAL INFARCTION

Transmural infarction is more common in the small intestine probably because of differences in the patterns of blood supply. The small intestine is totally dependent on its mesenteric vessels, but the large intestine throughout much of its course is closely applied to the posterior abdominal wall, from which it may derive accessory blood supply and venous drainage. Transmural infarction usually involves one (often long) segment of gut, although rarely several discontinuous areas are affected.

PATHOGENESIS. The basic patterns of transmural infarction are *thrombosis* or *embolism of the superior mesenteric artery* affecting only the small bowel (about 50% of acute mesenteric ischemias); *mesenteric venous thromboses* involving the small or large bowel, or both (25% of cases); and *partial narrowing of arteries or veins with superimposed reduced flow* affecting the small or large bowel, or both (25% of cases).

Arterial thromboses are most often triggered by advanced atherosclerosis. The superior mesenteric artery is commonly involved, close to its origin, but sometimes also the celiac axis and/or the inferior mesenteric artery. Because of the rich anastomotic communications between these three major arterial trunks, critical reduction of flow may require compromise of at least two. Sometimes cardiac failure or a hypotensive crisis in a patient with marked atherosclerotic narrowing (without total occlusion) may suffice to cause infarction. Vasospasm of uncertain cause superimposed on vascular narrowing is another potential pathogenetic mechanism.[92] Other causes of arterial narrowing, usually with superimposed thrombosis, include dissecting aortic aneurysm, tumorous invasion of the root of the mesentery, and *fibromuscular hyperplasia of the intestinal arteries.* Most individuals with this last-mentioned form of vascular disease are elderly, have cardiac failure, and are on digitalis therapy. Digitalis toxicity or sensitivity reaction to the drug may play some role in the induction of the fibromuscular lesion. Arterial thrombosis has also been reported in association with the use of oral contraceptives having a high estrogenic content. More often, oral contraceptives induce venous thromboses. Acute arteritis, such as may be encountered in polyarteritis nodosa, systemic lupus erythematosus, and rheumatoid disease, is a rare cause of arterial thrombosis.

Embolic arterial occlusion involves most often the branches of the superior mesenteric artery, but sometimes one of the other major trunks. The origin of the inferior mesenteric artery from the aorta is oblique and this may spare it somewhat from more frequent embolic occlusion. The emboli arise from intracardiac mural thrombi, infective endocarditis, nonbacterial thrombotic endocarditis, thrombi superimposed on valvular prostheses, atrial myxomas, or ulcerated atherosclerotic plaques, particularly during intraaortic diagnostic or therapeutic procedures (angiography, balloon pumping). As with thrombosis, the embolus must lodge in the proximal segments of the arteries to induce sufficient restriction of the blood supply to cause ischemic injury. More distal lodgment may be compensated for by anastomotic channels.

Venous thrombosis accounts for a minority of bowel infarctions. Some instances follow upper abdominal surgery. Venous thromboses may also be associated with cardiac failure, polycythemia, portal stasis, external pressure on veins by tumors or aneurysms, and the hypercoagulable state. Ischemic lesions of the bowel secondary to venous thrombosis have also been encountered in young women using oral contraceptives, but the causal relationship is still in some doubt.[93]

Gangrene of the bowel may also result from occlusion of arterial or venous vessels by strangulated hernias, torsions, and intestinal adhesions. Despite the multiplicity of possible causes, there remains a significant percentage of cases in which no well-defined underlying or antecedent basis for the vascular insufficiency can be identified.

MORPHOLOGY. Transmural infarction of the small bowel may involve only a short segment but more often involves a substantial portion of the total length. Colonic infarction tends to occur at the splenic flexure, which represents the watershed between the distribution of the superior and inferior mesenteric arteries (Fig. 18–30). **Regardless of whether the arterial or the venous side is occluded, the infarction always appears grossly hemorrhagic.** In the early stages, the segment of bowel appears intensely congested and dusky to purple-red, with small

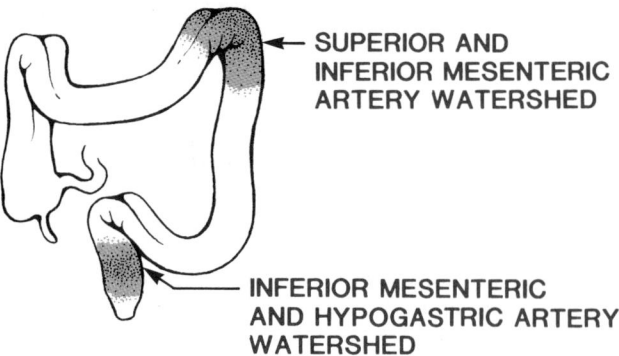

SUPERIOR AND
INFERIOR MESENTERIC
ARTERY WATERSHED

INFERIOR MESENTERIC
AND HYPOGASTRIC ARTERY
WATERSHED

Figure 18–30. Ischemic bowel disease. Although any area of the bowel may be involved, the stippled area of the splenic flexure is more commonly affected, since it is not retroperitoneal as is the rectum, and it is the watershed area between the major arteries.

and large foci of subserosal and submucosal ecchymotic discoloration (Fig. 18–31). Later the wall becomes edematous, thickened, rubbery, and hemorrhagic. Commonly at this stage, the lumen contains sanguineous mucus or frank blood. In arterial occlusions the demarcation from normal bowel is usually sharply defined, but in venous occlusions the area of dusky cyanosis fades gradually into the adjacent segments of normal bowel, leaving no clear-cut definition between viable and nonviable bowel. Histologically, there is often suffusion of the bowel wall masking the underlying ischemic necrosis of the native structure. If death occurs within 24 hours, little cellular response may be demonstrable. Later, lesions may show characteristic inflammatory infiltrations and ulcerations. Ulceration of the mucosa, com-

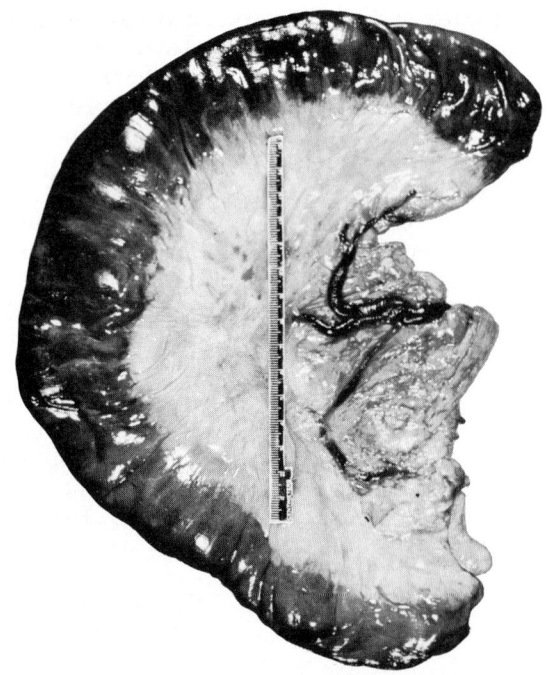

Figure 18–31. A loop of infarcted small intestine showing dark hemorrhagic discoloration. A large branching thrombus is evident in the arterial supply.

plicated by inevitable secondary bacterial contamination, and perforation of the wall are likely to occur within three to four days. Identification of the vascular occlusion is often difficult, and indeed may be impossible when the critical ischemia is caused in part by spasm or a low perfusion state.

CLINICAL COURSE.   Bowel infarction is an uncommon but grave disorder that imposes a 50 to 75% mortality rate.[94] It tends to occur in older individuals, usually in their sixth or seventh decade, when cardiac and vascular diseases are most prevalent. Older diabetics are at particular risk. Pre-existent intra-abdominal disease with the potential of adhesions or torsion also increases the risk. The onset is heralded by the development of signs and symptoms clinically indistinguishable from those encountered in all "acute abdomens," whatever the cause. Characteristically, there is sudden onset of severe abdominal pain, nausea, vomiting, or sometimes diarrhea that may progress rapidly (within 24 to 48 hours) to shock. Soon after, peristaltic sounds diminish or disappear, and spasm to boardlike rigidity of the abdominal wall becomes evident, secondary to the development of acute peritonitis, as bacteria permeate the necrotic bowel wall. Because there are far more common causes for these manifestations, such as acute appendicitis, perforated peptic ulcer, and acute cholecystitis, the diagnosis of intestinal gangrene is frequently delayed or missed.

MUCOSAL AND MURAL INFARCTION

Mucosal and mural infarction (also called hemorrhagic gastroenteropathy) may involve any level of the gut from stomach to anus. *Unlike outright infarction, this ischemic injury appears to relate to hypoperfusion, damaging only the inner layers of the gut while sparing the deeper levels of the muscularis and the serosa.*[94]

The lesions may be multifocal or continuous and widely distributed throughout the gastrointestinal tract. Affected areas of bowel may appear dark red or purple owing to the accumulated luminal hemorrhage. Notable, however, is the absence of hemorrhage, necrosis, or inflammatory exudation involving the serosal surface, changes that are more typical of transmural infarction of the bowel wall. On opening the bowel lumen, there is hemorrhagic, edematous thickening of the mucosa, sometimes with superficial ulceration. Edema and hemorrhages may in some cases penetrate more deeply into the submucosa and muscular layers. As expected, the histologic findings range from vascular dilatations, associated with a few extravasated red cells, to hemorrhagic necrosis of the mucosa, more often superficial but sometimes extending into the submucosa and superficial muscularis.

As the terms "mucosal" and "mural infarction" are used here, the hypoxic damage may extend deeply, but by

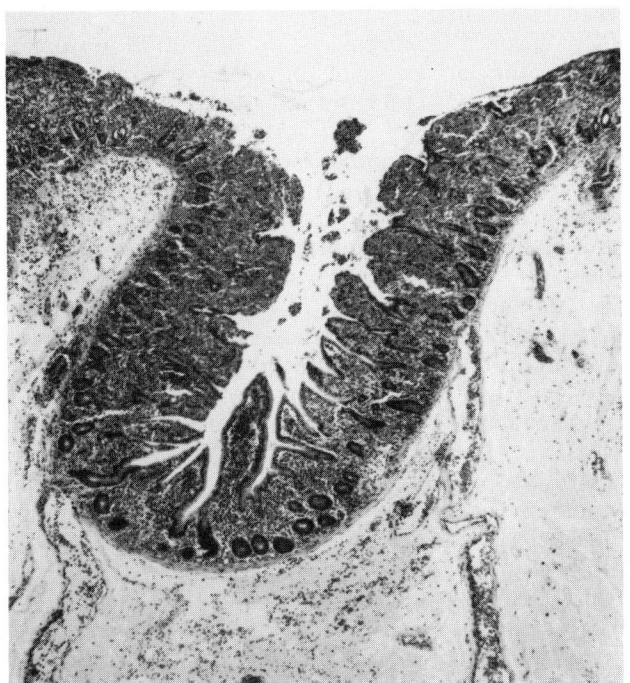

Figure 18–32. Mucosal infarction of small intestine with hemorrhagic suffusion of lamina propria and superficial sloughing of surface at upper left. There is marked edema but no hemorrhage in noninfarcted submucosa.

definition the serosa is spared (Fig. 18–32). Bacterial superinfection and the formation of enterotoxic bacterial products (p. 889) may induce superimposed pseudomembranous inflammation, particularly in the colon.[95] Thus the anatomic changes of mucosal and mural infarction, in some cases, may mimic ulceroinflammatory enterocolitis (p. 867) or pseudomembranous enterocolitis (p. 889) of nonvascular origin.

The pathogenesis of mucosal and mural infarction involves nonocclusive hypoperfusion of the intestinal tract. Why the resultant lesions are segmental and patchy remains unexplained. Shock and cardiac failure are major factors. The common denominator in these settings is a reduction in the effective circulating blood volume, with shunting of blood to vital organs and away from the splanchnic bed.[95] Infections may contribute by inducing vasomotor changes such as have been described in endotoxic shock (p. 115). Many patients have received digitalis and norepinephrine, and since both agents have vasoconstrictive effects, they may contribute to the perfusion deficit. In some cases, minute intramural thrombi have been found, possibly representing causative mechanisms. Alternatively, these vascular thromboses may be only secondary to the surrounding inflammatory reaction.

The clinical onset is marked by abdominal pain, cramps, and bloody diarrhea, often with worsening of the shock state. Should the low perfusion state be correctable, acute mucosal and submucosal infarction is reversible and complete restoration of the bowel wall can occur, as evidenced by failure to find residual changes at a later date. Deeper levels of damage may be irreversible.

INFECTIVE ENTEROCOLITIS

Inflammatory diarrheal diseases of the bowel make up a veritable Augean stable of entities. Some are caused by microbiologic agents, including bacteria, viruses, fungi, protozoa, and helminths.

Insights have been gained recently about the basic mechanisms by which coliform enteropathogens cause diarrhea. Three attributes are of importance: (1) the capacity to invade; (2) enterotoxins, some of which are heat labile while others are heat stable; and (3) an adherence mechanism providing for binding of organisms to the mucosal lining. Invasive organisms often induce mucosal ulcerations accompanied by white cells or pus in the stool. In contrast, organisms (*E. coli* and *Vibrio cholerae*) that release toxins cause diarrhea by activation of membrane-associated adenylate cyclase stimulating fluid and electrolyte secretion, inducing a watery diarrhea ("rice-water" stools). With organisms capable of adherence, the pathogenesis of the diarrhea is obscure, but electron microscopy reveals a virtual carpeting of the mucosal surface by the causative agent. *It is possible, therefore, to divide the diarrheal syndromes into two large pathogenetic categories: (1) those associated with enteroinvasive organisms in which mucosal ulcerations often occur; and (2) those resulting from enterotoxins or adhesion not associated with mucosal ulcerations.*

Some of the microbial causes of diarrhea principally affect the small intestines (enteritis) and others principally the colon, but in most instances there is considerable overlap. Whatever the main location, the intestines respond with a limited range of reactions. Thus, many microbiologic agents produce nondistinctive morphologic changes that can be characterized as ulceroinflammatory, with the exception of the enterotoxigenic agents (serotypes of *E. coli* and *V. cholerae*). *Morphologic examination of the lesions, then, is of limited value in establishing the specific etiology.* From the clinical standpoint also, virtually all forms of inflammatory disease of the bowel produce similar manifestations, principally diarrhea, some with associated fever whereas others are afebrile. Although a history of travel to areas endemic for particular agents may provide diagnostic leads, identification of the agent responsible for the diarrheal inflammatory disease requires isolating the bacterial or viral organism from the lesion and/or the stool. Radiologic or endoscopic procedures do not provide any specific information in this regard.

Bowel infections may occur in previously healthy individuals but are particularly serious in immunocompromised patients, in whom intestinal colonization by organisms of even low virulence occurs quite readily. Common settings are uremia, hypoperfusion states such as shock and cardiac failure, nonenteric

Table 18–4. Microbial Causes of Diarrheal Disease

Bacterial invasive enterocolitis
    Campylobacter jejuni
    Escherichia coli (particular serotypes)
    Salmonella
    Shigella
    Tuberculosis
    Yersinia enterocolitica
    Aeromonas hydrophila
Bacterial toxigenic enterocolitis
    Vibrio cholerae
    E. coli (particular serotypes)
Viral (nonbacterial) enterocolitis
Fungal enterocolitis
    Candidiasis
    Mucormycosis
Enterocolitis caused by protozoa and metazoa
    Entamoeba histolytica
    Giardia lamblia
    Schistosoma mansoni
    Cryptosporidia

infections requiring broad-spectrum antibiotic therapy, cancer under treatment by radiation or cytotoxic drugs, and conditions associated with immunologic incompetence or suppression, notably **AIDS.** The premature infant also is often predisposed to its own intestinal flora. Although in otherwise healthy adults these infections are disturbing but not usually threatening incursions on the "joie de vivre," in the predisposed they may lead to disseminated lesions in other organs and even death.[96]

The major microbiologic offenders are listed in Table 18–4. With some, the bowel disease is only one component of a systemic disorder. In other instances the gastrointestinal involvement is the primary feature, sometimes having systemic ramifications. All these agents are discussed in detail in Chapter 7 and so only some general comments are offered, followed by a survey of the morphologic lesions.

BACTERIAL ENTEROCOLITIS

At the outset, food poisonings related to the ingestion of preformed bacterial toxins should be differentiated from enteric infections. Improperly stored foods contaminated by *Clostridium botulinum* and *Staphylococcus aureus* permit the elaboration in vitro of potent enterotoxins that may cause a violent and sometimes fatal gastroenterocolitis or a self-limited mild disease, depending on the amount of food ingested. Although the mucosal inflammatory changes may mimic the early invasive stage of bacterial infections, *they are the result of extremely acute intoxications.* Usually they are not accompanied by ulcerations and promptly regress if the subject survives. Somewhat analogous toxigenic bacteria that colonize the gut may induce acute, sometimes severe, diarrheal syndromes despite the absence of mucosal defects.

Among the invasive organisms, *Campylobacter jejuni* has emerged in recent years as a major cause of enterocolitis. In one analysis of patients hospitalized

for diarrheal disease, *C. jejuni* was identified in about 8% of cases.[97] Outbreaks of this infection in humans have mainly arisen from ingestion of contaminated food or water.[98] The reservoir of infection is the gastrointestinal tract of wild and domesticated animals that man either eats or contacts directly or indirectly. The severity of the disease ranges from a self-limited mild enterocolitis to severe recurrent disabling diarrhea that may mimic ulcerative colitis or Crohn's disease.

Specific serotypes of *E. coli* cited on page 345 have been identified as causes of diarrhea in infants and in adults who are exposed to organisms during foreign travel ("Montezuma's revenge") to which they have not developed immunity. Specific serotypes possess one or more of the three pathogenetic capabilities mentioned earlier.[99] Some organisms penetrate the surface glycocalyx, disrupt the microvillous brush border, and may cause blunting of the villi as well as a mild histiocytic infiltrate in the lamina propria, but it is not clear whether the diarrheal disorder is functional or due to damage to surface epithelial cells. Other gram-negative enteropathogens are the well-known *V. cholerae*, Salmonella, and Shigella. These all produce food- and water-borne infections that are frequently characterized by marked involvement of the small and large intestine. They are discussed in detail in Chapter 7.

Tuberculosis may involve the bowel as a primary gastrointestinal infection from ingestion of contaminated milk or milk products in areas where control of bovine tuberculosis is not rigorous. More often, enteric infections are secondary to the swallowing of organisms coughed up from a caseating pulmonary focus.

Yersinia enterocolitica is a gram-negative coccobacillus that uncommonly produces enteric disease, principally in infants and children, that is very severe and potentially lethal.[100] Extraintestinal infection may appear with the enteric involvement, such as pharyngitis, pericarditis, and peritonitis.

Some pathogens preferentially involve the small intestine, others the colon, and still others both levels. The macroscopic alterations with all enteric pathogens are extremely variable, ranging from focal areas of mucosal edematous hyperemia to enlargement of lymphoid tissues to excavated ulcerations (Fig. 18–33). Sometimes the inflammation is marked by pseudomembrane formations that range from yellow-gray to more hemorrhagic exudates that thus mimic clostridial pseudomembranous enterocolitis (p. 889). The distribution of such focal lesions is extremely variable. On occasion, only one rather long segment of bowel is affected. More often, there are multiple scattered lesions with intervening areas of uninvolved mucosa. The ulcerations may therefore be dispersed or sometimes virtually coalescent to denude large areas, reminiscent of severe ulcerative colitis (p. 886). The serosal surfaces juxtaposed to these lesions may be entirely normal or covered by serous, fibrinous, or hemorrhagic exudate.

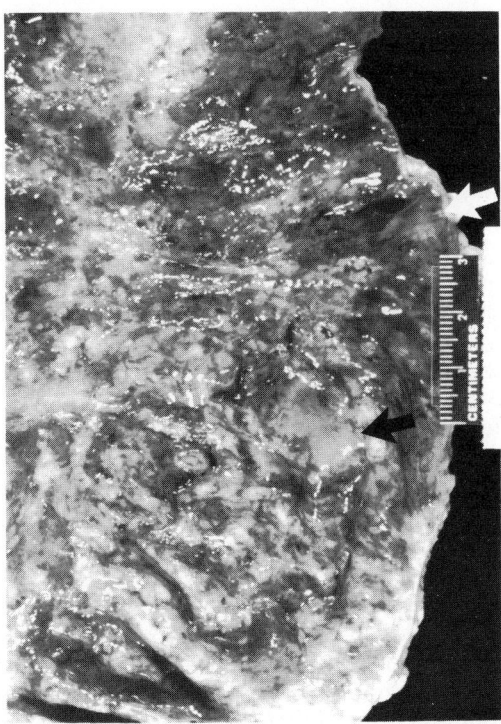

Figure 18–33. Infective enterocolitis. Segment of colon showing pale granular inflamed mucosa with patches of coagulated exudate *(black arrow)*. Compare with relatively normal mucosa *(white arrow)*.

Some subtle microscopic differences may be noted among the various causative agents, but basically all induce acute-to-chronic inflammatory changes. Salmonella infection is associated with prominent lymphoid aggregates produced by striking hypertrophy of mononuclear phagocytes that sometimes reveal phagocytized red cells. Campylobacter tends to produce granulomatous stellate ulcers. Nonetheless, more evidence must be derived from identification of the offending pathogen by culture of the stool or tissue lesions.

On occasion the ulceroinflammatory changes are confined to the anorectal region; this pattern of proctitis is particularly common among male homosexuals. The causative agents include *Treponema pallidum*, gonococci, chlamydia, and herpes simplex virus. The enteric disease is distinctive by virtue of its localization, but other forms of inflammatory bowel disease also may induce only proctitis without involvement of more proximal levels of the gut.

Whatever the causative agent, these involvements are marked by abdominal cramps, diarrhea, and sometimes fever. Notably, ulceroinvasive infections may give rise to blood and pus in the stools.

NONBACTERIAL GASTROENTEROCOLITIS

Microbiologic agents other than bacteria—viruses, fungi, protozoa, and helminths—may induce clinical gastroenteric diseases, some of which are very common in underdeveloped parts of the world.[101] *Viral gastroenteritis* is said to be second only to the common cold as a cause of illness in the United States. Several groups of viral enteric pathogens are responsible for what is clinically termed *acute infectious nonbacterial gastroenteritis.* Parvovirus-like agents may produce disease in adults, and reovirus-like agents can cause illness in infants. More recently, the rotavirus has emerged as another cause of diarrheal disease, principally in infants and children, in whom rotaviral infection is so severe that strenuous efforts are being made to develop a preventative vaccine.[102] Although viral diarrheal diseases are generally transient and only temporarily incapacitating, they may be more serious and indeed fatal in infants and the malnourished, particularly when concomitant bacterial or protozoal enteric infections are present.

Knowledge of the virus-induced morphologic changes is derived largely from biopsy studies of otherwise healthy individuals, since fatal illnesses are usually complicated by bacterial infections. In nonfatal cases, frank necrosis and ulceration of the mucosa have not been observed. The major findings consist of shortening of the villi of the small intestine accompanied by an inflammatory infiltrate of neutrophils and mononuclear cells within the lamina propria. The surface absorptive cells have revealed a variety of abnormalities, including vacuolation, shortening or loss of microvilli, and accumulation of increased numbers of lysosomes. Viral particles have not been identified within affected tissues in infections caused by the parvovirus-like agent, but they have been seen in disease caused by the reovirus-like agent.[103]

Fungi—Candida and mucormycetes—may invade the mucosa of the small or large intestine, but almost always as a consequence of fungemia in a terminally ill patient either immunosuppressed or dying of some debilitating disease. The *protozoa*—*Entamoeba histolytica* and *Giardia lamblia* (p. 397)—are also well-known causes of intestinal disease. Amebiasis (p. 400) in particular preferentially causes extensive ulcerations in the large bowel, and these may require differentiation from nonspecific ulcerative colitis and bacteria-induced ulcerations.

CROHN'S DISEASE (REGIONAL ENTERITIS)

Crohn's disease is perhaps best described as an idiopathic, chronic, ulceroconstrictive inflammatory bowel disease that is characterized pathologically by sharply delimited and typically transmural involvement of all layers of the bowel wall by a noncaseating granulomatous process. Any segment of the gastrointestinal tract, from the mouth to the anus, may be involved, although the disease most commonly affects the terminal ileum and/or colon. Although primarily an enteric disorder, it appears to be systemic in distribution. Lesions of Crohn's disease have been observed in the skin, femur, striated muscle, and lung.[104] Moreover, many complications may accompany the bowel involvement, such as arthritis, uveitis, erythema nodosum, and various inflammatory changes in the liver.[105] When first described in 1932 by Crohn and colleagues, it was thought that the bowel involvement was limited to the terminal ileum, and it was thus designated *terminal ileitis.* Later it was appreciated that sharply delineated segmental areas of the small bowel might be affected, leaving intervening unaffected ("skip") segments — hence the designation *regional enteritis.* Since that time it has become apparent that any level of the enteric tract may be involved. Indeed, there is epidemiologic evidence that the intestinal distribution of the disease is shifting, with increased involvement of the large bowel.[106] Analyses of large series of patients reveal that *the terminal ileum is affected in 65 to 75% of cases, with concurrent involvement of the colon in half of these. The colon alone is involved in 20 to 30% of cases.*[107,108] The colonic involvement is often referred to as *granulomatous colitis.*

Typically, Crohn's disease is characterized by a granulomatous inflammatory reaction with through-and-through involvement of the thickness of the bowel wall. In approximately 40% of cases, however, granulomas are either poorly developed or totally absent. In contrast, ulcerative colitis is an inflammatory response limited largely to the colonic mucosa and submucosa.

EPIDEMIOLOGY. Crohn's disease occurs throughout the world. There are, however, striking differences in incidence; for example, it is much more frequent in the United States, Great Britain, and Scandinavia than in Japan, the USSR, and the South American nations. Moreover, the incidence is on the increase in high-risk countries. It occurs at any age but most often is first detected in the second decade of life. A minor peak occurs in the elderly. Females are affected slightly more often than males. Whites develop the disease two to five times more often than do nonwhites, but diagnostic facilities and case finding may play some role. In the United States, regional enteritis occurs three to five times more often among Jews than among non-Jews.

Because there are many hints that immunologic mechanisms play a role in the initiation or perpetuation of Crohn's disease (and ulcerative colitis), an intensive search has been made for genetic markers. No well-defined HLA associations have been identified. An older observation that patients with Crohn's disease complicated by a form of vertebral arthritis known as ankylosing spondylitis have an increased frequency of HLA-B27 is now recognized to relate to the ankylosing spondylitis alone. Occasional reports documenting the occurrence of the disease in monozygotic twins suggest a genetic predisposition, but the findings are inconclusive.

ETIOLOGY AND PATHOGENESIS. Since the origins of Crohn's disease and ulcerative colitis have revealed a great many similarities, it is reasonable to consider the etiology and pathogenesis of both conditions together, employing the commonly used term "inflammatory bowel disease" (IBD).

Theories about the origins of IBD can be divided into three groups: (1) those invoking an infectious agent; (2) those contending that immunologic mechanisms initiate or perpetuate the condition; and (3) an assortment of concepts implicating psychosomatic, dietary, vascular, traumatic, hormonal, and other mechanisms. Currently favored theories fall within the first two groups.

Many microorganisms have been hailed as putative causes of IBD, but to date none has been confirmed.[104,109,110] Impetus for a microbiologic etiology was provided by a report in 1970 that cell-free filtrates prepared from Crohn's tissue, when inoculated into the footpads of mice, would induce granulomas.[111] It appears likely, however, that the inflammatory reactions are secondary to xenotropic tissue antigens, since inoculation of rabbits with *normal* human bowel homogenate has been shown to produce inflammatory changes resembling the granulomas of Crohn's disease.

Viruses — rotavirus, Epstein-Barr virus, and uncharacterized RNA intestinal cytopathic viruses — continue to be favored candidates.[112] Some ultrafiltrates of tissue of Crohn's disease and ulcerative colitis have been cytopathic in tissue cultures of mucosal epithelial cells, and virus-like particles have been observed in the dying cells.[113] Attempts to isolate the cytopathic agent suggest that it is a small RNA virus variously classified as ECHO-27, reovirus, rotavirus, or uncertain. Electron and immune electron microscopic studies, however, have failed to reveal viral particles in lesions,[114] and attempts to culture viruses from diseased bowel have largely failed or revealed merely passenger agents.

Bacteria have also been implicated in the causation of IBD, including Pseudomona-like organisms, enteric anaerobes, cell wall–defective *Mycobacterium kansasii,* chlamydia, and *Yersinia enterocolitica,* but proof of their roles is still lacking.[109,115] The search for an infectious etiology for IBD continues, but at present no organism has been convincingly implicated.

A mountain of evidence points to immunologic derangements in IBD, but whether they are causal or secondary phenomena is unclear. Antibody-mediated mechanisms, cell-mediated reactions, and immunologic deficiencies all have their champions. A specific anticolon antibody that does not cross react with *E. coli* has been described in diseased tissues, and increased synthesis of IgG has been documented in mucosal lymphoid cells derived from diseased segments of bowel.[116,117] However, there does not appear to be any clear correlation between the level of these antibodies and the activity of the underlying disease.

Moreover, IBD may occur in individuals with agammaglobulinemia, and ultimately none of these antibodies is regularly with effect in tissue culture.

Attempts to relate circulating immune complexes to the intestinal lesions have also been discouraging. However, they may play some role in the causation of the extraintestinal lesions associated with IBD. Attention has also been directed to the possibility that an anaphylactoid hypersensitivity reaction mediated by IgE might release vasoactive substances from mast cells in the bowel wall, and thus cause edema of the bowel wall to impair the normal barrier function of the mucosa. However, the case for such a mechanism is at best not strong.

Cell-mediated immunologic damage is an attractive hypothesis because lymphocytes and macrophages are so numerous in the lesions of IBD. Various studies have documented circulating T cells sensitized to a number of colonic and bacterial antigens, but it remains to be proved that the T cells are cytotoxic to bowel epithelium.[118] Collaboration between humoral antibodies and K cells might induce so-called antibody-dependent cellular cytotoxicity (ADCC). The K cells are cytotoxic in vitro to colonic epithelial cells in the presence of IgM. However, there is poor correlation between antibody-dependent cellular cytotoxicity and the activity of the disease. A slightly different approach suggests that some immunologic deficiency leads to uncontrolled exaggerated reactions to a variety of bowel antigens, resulting in mucosal damage. Indeed, there are hints of some immunodeficiency with Crohn's disease, such as impaired synthesis of IgA in the bowel mucosa or macrophage incompetence.[119] The current status of the pathogenetic role of immune mechanisms is perhaps best summarized by Sachar: "We can conclude that IBD probably induces immune aberrations in the host and that the inflammatory reactions may even be mediated in part via immune effector pathways. To date, however, the case for the primary pathogenetic role of immunologic factors in IBD remains unproved."[109]

The many *other etiologic theories* are all too poorly substantiated to merit detailed mention. Psychosomatic factors have long been invoked because certain personality types—immature, dependent, passive—often suffer from a so-called irritable colon. But there is no evidence that such emotional bowel disturbances lead to organic disease. Food allergies, primary vascular disease within mural small arteries or arterioles, and chronic trauma have all received their share of attention but at present are not given credence as pathogenetic mechanisms. Prostaglandins have come to the forefront with reports of elevated PGE_2 levels in colonic venous blood and rectal mucosa in patients with ulcerative colitis.[120] However, prostaglandins are known to be mediators of inflammatory reactions, and thus the increased levels might merely be epiphenomena. Therefore, despite the plethora of theories, the causation of IBD remains unknown.

MORPHOLOGY. One of the most distinctive macroscopic features of Crohn's disease is the **sharp demarcation of the segmental bowel involvement, which may occur, as mentioned, in any level of the enteric tract.** In its classic form, 15 to 25 cm of the terminal ileum is affected. Sometimes, several sharply demarcated diseased segments are separated by normal bowel, producing what are called "skip" lesions, a distribution not found in ulcerative colitis. Early Crohn's disease is marked by rubbery, edematous, hyperemic thickening of the small intestinal wall. At this stage the mucosa may show only minute hyperemic ("aphthoid") ulcerations closely resembling canker sores. **As the disease evolves to the classic stage, the affected segment becomes thickened and inflexible and has been likened to a lead pipe or rubber hose** (Fig. 18–34). The serosal surface is granular and dull gray, and often the mesenteric fat "creeps up" over the bowel surface, so that the gut may seem virtually buried. The mesentery of the involved small intestinal segment is also thickened, edematous, and sometimes fibrotic. The lumen is almost always narrowed; this is evidenced on x-ray as the "string sign," a thin stream of barium. Varying degrees of mucosal edema, ulceration, and sloughing are found. Commonly, the ulcers are long and serpentine (Fig. 18–35). **Often they are extremely narrow fissures** and can be virtually hidden between the folds of the mucosa. In chronic cases, the ulcers or fissures may penetrate deeply to form fistulous tracts with other loops of bowel. In other in-

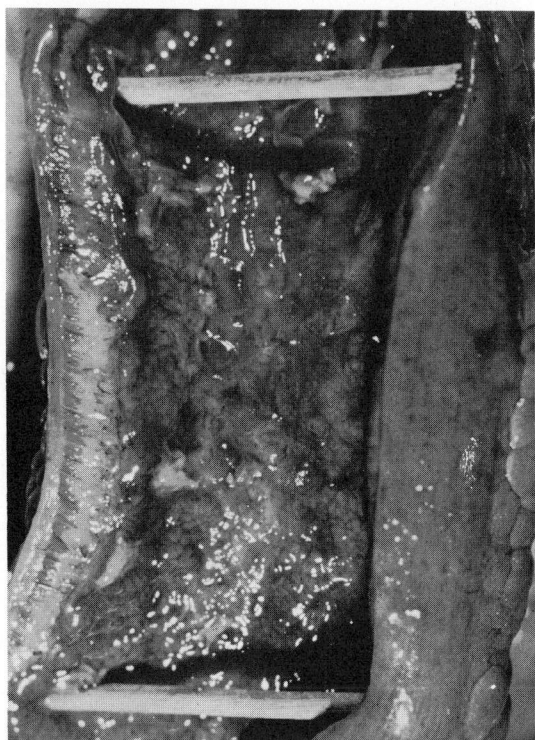

Figure 18–34. Crohn's disease of ileum. Close-up of a segment of thickened bowel wall. Note wooden pegs required to keep lumen exposed.

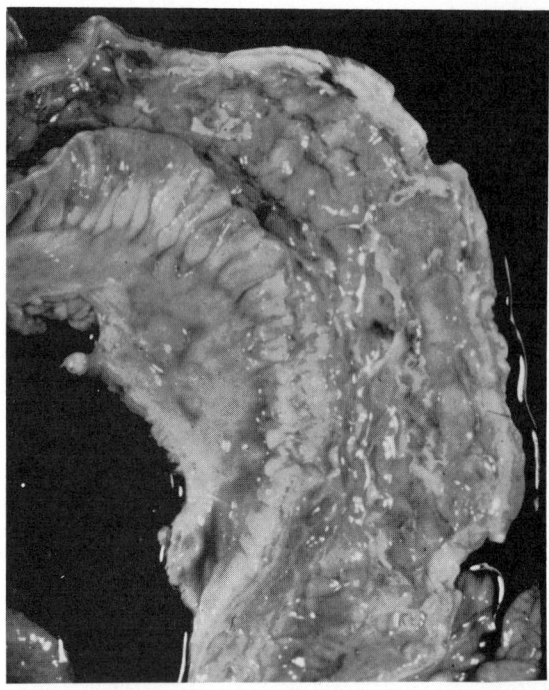

Figure 18–35. Regional enteritis of distal ileum demonstrating fibrosis and thickening of wall as well as long, serpentine, pale ulcerations of mucosa.

tulas, pericolonic abscesses, and perianal and perirectal sepsis.

The most characteristic histologic features of Crohn's disease are (1) transmural inflammation (in the form of chronic inflammatory infiltrates and fibrosis) affecting all layers to the serosa, (2) noncaseating granulomas resembling those of sarcoidosis, (3) dilatation or sclerosis of lymphatic channels, and (4) lymphoid aggregates (sometimes with germinal centers) in all levels of the bowel wall. The granulomas, however, are absent or not well developed in approximately 40% of cases. There is variable ulceration and destruction of the mucosa, marked submucosal fibrosis with chronic inflammatory reaction, relative preservation of the muscularis, and again, marked subserosal fibrosis with chronic inflammatory changes (Fig. 18–36). The inflammatory response in the mucosal ulcerations is entirely nonspecific and is largely composed of neutrophils, lymphocytes, macrophages, and plasma cells. The preserved mucosa between the ulcers often shows a diffuse nonspecific inflammation with flattening of the villi and active goblet cell secretion (Fig. 18–37). More important, atypical metaplasia and dysplasia of epithelial cells may be present not only close to ulcerations but also in intervening areas. Within the submucosal and subserosal zones, the inflammatory foci of mononuclear cells are often aggregated into lymphoid follicles, and some of these con-

stances, penetration of the wall of the small intestine may create abscesses, either within the peritoneal cavity or within the mesenteric fat.

When present, the distribution of the colonic involvement, referred to as **granulomatous colitis**, is extremely variable.[121] Most often the cecum and a portion of the right colon are affected in continuity with ileal involvement. In other instances, isolated or multiple segments are diseased, sometimes producing "skip" lesions similar to those in the small bowel. The colitis may be limited to the descending colon, sometimes extending into the sigmoid. It should be particularly noted that the rectum is diseased in about half of all patients with colonic involvement—either in continuity with left-sided colitis or sometimes as a "skip" lesion. In a small percentage of patients the involvement is restricted to the anorectal region, and in the most severe expression of granulomatous colitis the entire large bowel is affected. Typically, the macroscopic changes are almost identical with those described in the small intestine, complete with transmural fibrosing inflammation, linear fissures, thickening of the bowel wall, and sometimes narrowing of the lumen. **It is the "skip" lesions, the thickening of the bowel wall, and the tendency for the ulcerations to form fissures that most sharply distinguish granulomatous colitis from ulcerative colitis macroscopically.** However, in some instances there is less fibrotic thickening and the inflammation is more limited to the mucosa and submucosa, closely mimicking ulcerative colitis. Indeed, most experts concede that in 10 to 20% of cases it is impossible to discriminate granulomatous from ulcerative colitis.[122] Whatever the gross appearance, the colonic changes in Crohn's disease may be complicated by perforation, fis-

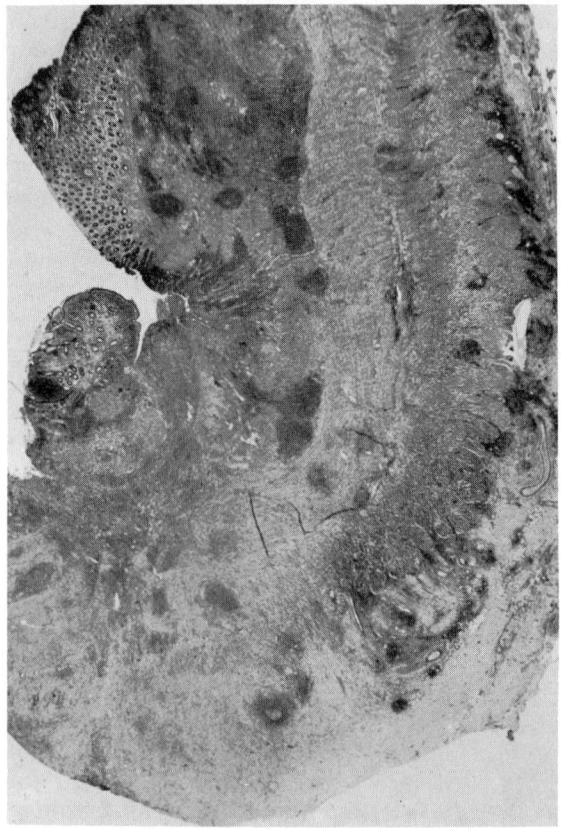

Figure 18–36. Low-power view of marked inflammation, thickening, and ulceration caused by regional enteritis. Foci of inflammatory cells are evident at points distant from the ulceration. Note width of submucosa.

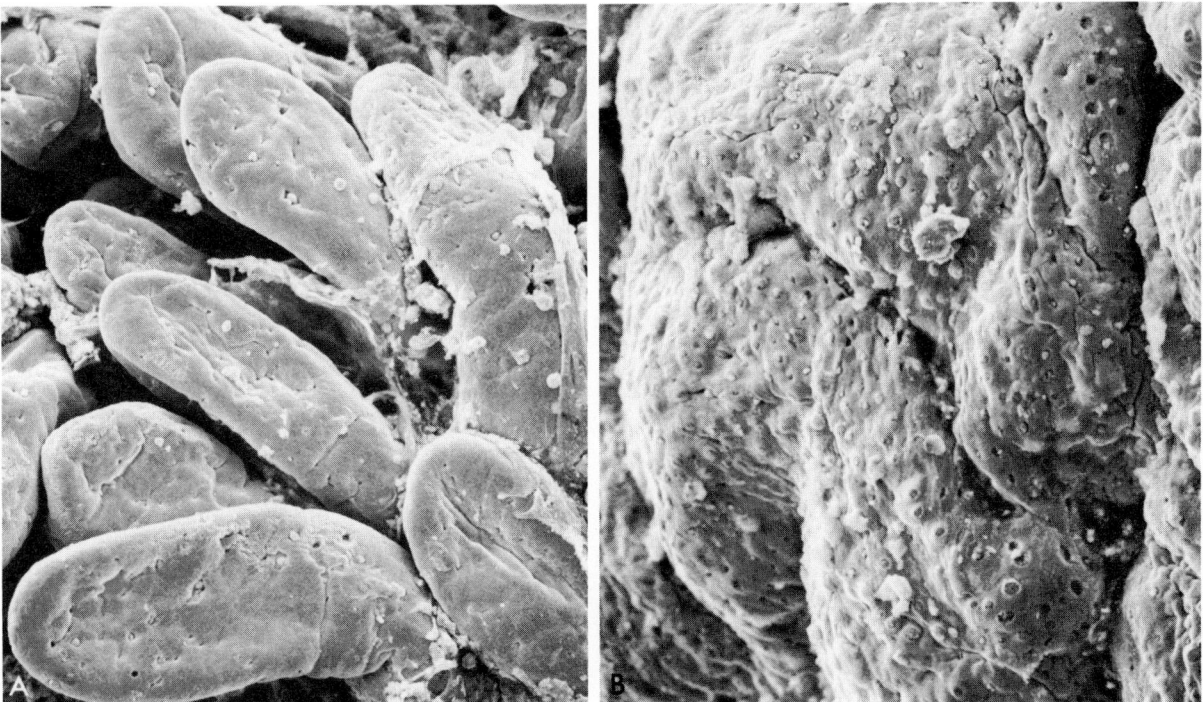

Figure 18–37. *A,* Scanning electron micrograph of normal ileal mucosa with thin, finger-shaped villi and mucus secretion exuding from goblet cell orifices. *B,* Uninvolved, nonulcerated mucosa of Crohn's disease with complete flattening and fusion of surface villi. More goblet cell orifices are visible, actively secreting mucosa. (Courtesy of Dr. A. M. Dvorak, Beth Israel Hospital, Boston.)

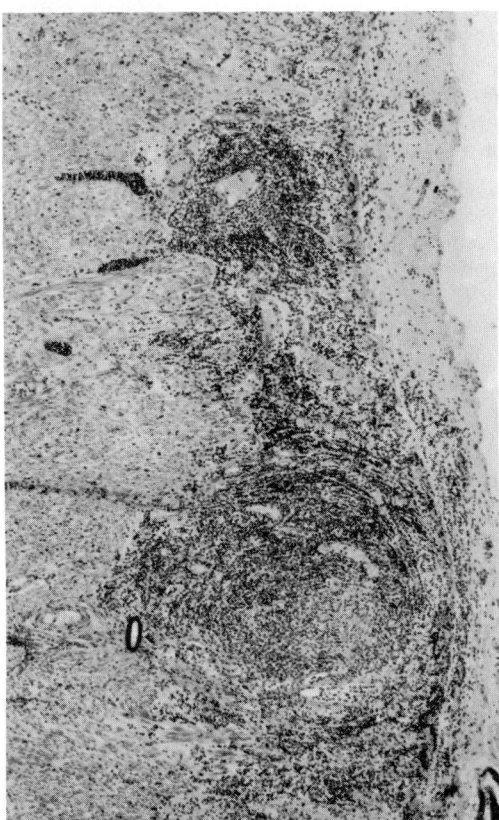

Figure 18–38. Serosal surface of a segment of bowel involved by regional enteritis, illustrating foci of chronic inflammatory cells, which sometimes contain central granulomatous responses resembling sarcoid.

tain well-formed, sarcoid-like granulomas (Fig. 18–38). Similar chronic inflammatory changes, often replete with granulomas, affect the regional nodes of drainage. The precise stimulus to this granuloma formation remains unclear.

CLINICAL COURSE. The clinical manifestations of Crohn's disease are extremely variable. The disease usually begins with intermittent attacks of relatively mild diarrhea, fever, and right lower quadrant or sometimes periumbilical abdominal pain. These attacks are spaced by asymptomatic periods lasting for weeks to many months. In those with colonic involvement, the pain may be localized to the left lower quadrant or lower abdomen. The manifestations are often present for several years before the diagnosis is established. Often the attacks are precipitated by periods of physical or emotional stress. As pointed out earlier, emotional influences are not thought to have any role in the initiation of the disease, but they may contribute to flare-ups. Occult or overt (in those with colonic involvement) blood in the stool may lead to anemia over the span of time, but massive bleeding is uncommon. In about one fifth of the patients the onset is more abrupt, with acute right lower quadrant pain, fever, and diarrhea sometimes suggesting acute appendicitis or an acute bowel perforation. The course of the disease includes bouts of diarrhea with fluid and electrolyte losses, weight loss, and weakness. *During this lengthy, chronic disease, fibrosing strictures,* particularly of the terminal ileum, may lead to intestinal obstruction. *Fistulas* — to other loops of the bowel, to the urinary bladder, perirectal, or into a peritoneal abscess — develop in about 10 to 15% of cases. *Extensive involvement of the terminal ileum may cause marked loss of albumin (protein-losing enteropathy); generalized malabsorption; specific malabsorption of vitamin B$_{12}$, with consequent pernicious anemia; or malabsorption of bile salts, leading to steatorrhea.* Migratory polyarthritis, sacroiliitis, ankylosing spondylitis, erythema nodosum, or clubbing of the fingertips may sometimes precede small bowel involvement. Uveitis, nonspecific mild hepatic pericholangitis, and renal disorders secondary to trapping of the ureters in the inflammatory process sometimes develop. An increased incidence of gallstones has also been noted in these patients. Rarely (1%), systemic amyloidosis is a late consequence. Overshadowing all these complications is the now well-documented increased incidence of cancer of the gastrointestinal tract (about 3%) in patients with long-standing progressive Crohn's disease. Such carcinomas may arise in the small intestine or the colon. Sometimes these tumors arise in nondiseased segments of the gut. However, the risk of colonic cancer in Crohn's disease, though increased, is somewhat less than that in patients with chronic ulcerative colitis.

TUMORS

It is one of the enigmas of medicine that tumors of the small intestine, both benign and malignant, are such rarities. Although the small bowel represents 75% of the length of the entire gastrointestinal tract, neoplasms in this location account for only 3 to 6% of all gastrointestinal tumors. In most series, malignant tumors are slightly more common than benign, in a ratio approximating 1.5 : 1.

BENIGN

Most benign tumors of the small intestine are discovered only at post-mortem examination, or incidentally in the course of radiographic studies of the small bowel for other reasons. However, large lesions may produce partial or intermittent obstruction, bleeding, intussusception, and volvulus. *Benign stromal cell tumors (p. 853) are the most common form, followed in descending order of frequency by adenomas and angiomas.* Adenomatous polyps may occur singly or multiply, most often in the duodenum and ileum. Morphologically, they resemble those occurring in the stomach and colon (p. 893), and range from pedunculated adenomas to sessile villous adenomas with the full spectrum of intergrades.[123] The larger adenomas, particularly those having villous features like those in the colon, often undergo malignant transformation; in one series of 51 pedunculated and sessile adenomas, 33 contained foci of carcinoma.[123] Thus,

sporadic polyps of the small intestine, although rarities, are ominous lesions. Multiple pedunculated polyps may appear in the small intestine in familial multiple polyposis (p. 896) and in the Peutz-Jeghers syndrome (p. 892).

MALIGNANT

As stated earlier, cancers are very uncommon in the small intestine, but they are more prevalent than benign tumors. More than half arise in the ileum.[124,125] Endocrine cell tumors (carcinoids) and lymphomas are the most frequent forms of cancer in the small intestine, followed in order by adenocarcinomas and leiomyosarcomas. Lymphomas in the small intestine are identical both morphologically and clinically to those encountered in other segments of the gastrointestinal tract, and are described on page 858.

Carcinoid Tumors

The term "carcinoid" is used as a generic name for neoplasms arising from endocrine cells (or their precursors) dispersed along the gastrointestinal mucosa. Formerly these cells were known as Kulchitsky cells or enterochromaffin cells (because of an affinity for chrome salts). The secretory granules in these endocrine cells often have an affinity for soluble silver salts — hence the tumors are sometimes called argentaffinomas. The cells in some neoplasms can directly deposit silver salts and are termed argentaffin positive. Some cells require an exogenous reducing agent to deposit the silver salts and are termed argyrophil positive. Since carcinoids can arise anywhere in the gastrointestinal tract, they have been classified as fore-, mid-, or hindgut, based on the embryologic derivation of the site of their origin. Between 60 and 80% of these tumors arise in the midgut (most often in the appendix and terminal ileum). About 10 to 20% arise in the hindgut (mostly in the rectum), while the remainder are located in the foregut-derived structures — stomach, duodenum, and esophagus, in that order of frequency. Similar neoplasms may arise outside the gastrointestinal tract, e.g., in the lungs, biliary tract, ovaries, and elsewhere.

All carcinoids are potentially malignant tumors; the tendency for aggressive behavior correlates with such factors as the site of origin, the depth of local intramural penetration by the tumor, and the size of the tumor. Appendiceal and rectal carcinoids are seldom malignant, and even though they may show extensive local spread, metastatic dissemination is infrequent. Ileal, gastric, and colonic carcinoids, on the other hand, are frequently malignant, and a high proportion of these have already metastasized by the time they are detected. Similarly, deep local invasion up to or beyond halfway through the wall in the case of extra-appendiceal carcinoids, is associated with a high incidence (90%) of nodal and distant metastases. As for size, more than 66% of carcinoids greater than 2 cm show metastases when first detected, whereas less than 5% of those under 1 cm do so.[27]

HISTOGENESIS. Although certain tumors designated as argentaffinomas, gastrinomas, and somatostatinomas were initially believed to be derived from the normal EC_1, G, and D cells, respectively, it has been impossible to assign a specific lineage to the carcinoids on account of the heterogeneity in their various characteristics. Argentaffinomas, gastrinomas, and somatostatinomas frequently contain other hormones as well and are therefore "multihormonal" in nature.[126-128] Some of these additional products, such as insulin, calcitonin, ACTH, and so forth, may not even be normally produced by the gut endocrine cells. Ultrastructurally, too, the secretory granules in the tumor cells resemble those of immature endocrine cells more closely than those of the functionally mature endocrine cells of the corresponding type, suggesting that carcinoids arise from immature, functionally uncommitted endocrine cells that subsequently undergo further differentiation.

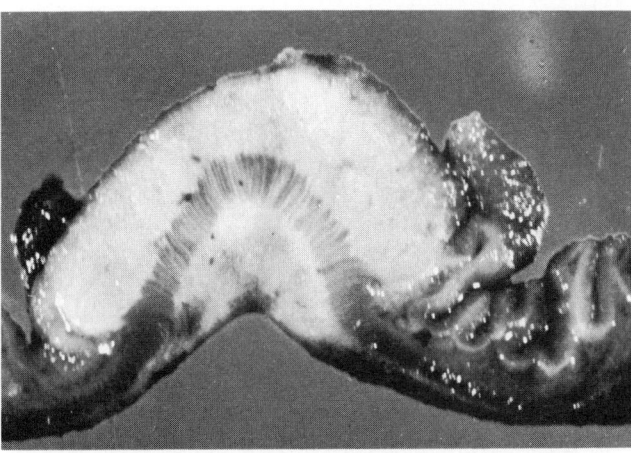

Figure 18-39. Carcinoid tumor of ileum. Cut section of this tumor shows a circumscribed plaque-like elevation of the mucosa and the tumor cells diffusely infiltrating the full thickness of the bowel wall. Note that the bowel wall is slightly buckled in the region of the tumor and the muscle coat is hypertrophied. This is a rather common feature in ileal carcinoids.

MORPHOLOGY. Irrespective of their location in the gut, carcinoids usually appear as small, round, or plaque-like submucosal elevations (Fig. 18-39). In the smaller tumors the overlying mucosa may be intact, but ulceration occurs when the tumor protrudes into the lumen in a polypoid fashion. Gastric and ileal carcinoids are frequently multicentric in origin, while those arising elsewhere are usually solitary. Appendiceal carcinoids are most often located distally or at the tip of the appendix and are usually small, nodular masses. Classically, all gastrointestinal carcinoids are bright yellow or yellowish gray on transection and are typically deeply infiltrative.

Histologically, these tumors may show any of a variety of architectural patterns that have been referred to as insular, trabecular, glandular, mixed, or undifferentiated. **The tumor cells are monotonously similar to each other and are characterized by a pale pink or granular cytoplasm and a round to oval nucleus with stippled chromatin. Generally, there is minimal mitotic activity, cytologic atypia, or nuclear pleomorphism, except in the undifferentiated tumors.** However, these latter tumors can be readily identified as carcinoids on account of their argyrophilic properties. An interesting type is the so-called goblet cell carcinoid, which shows abundant mucus-producing signet-ring type cells. This pattern is most often seen in appendiceal and gastric carcinoids. All variants permeate the underlying wall and often penetrate between muscle bundles down to the serosa.

Foregut carcinoids most commonly arise in the stomach and duodenum and show a trabecular or mixed architectural pattern. Gastric carcinoids often arise on a background of pre-existing endocrine cell hyperplasia and are therefore frequently multicentric in origin. Although most foregut carcinoids are hormonally nonfunctional, secretory products, including gastrin, somatostatin, glucagon, ACTH, and serotonin, have been demonstrated in these tumors.[127] On rare occasions, gastric carcinoids have produced Zollinger-Ellison syndrome, Cushing's syndrome, or an atypical carcinoid syndrome. Secretory granules of varying size can be related to specific secretory products by immunoreactive methods. In general, foregut tumors are argyrophilic (p. 840) or nonreactive.

Midgut carcinoids are readily recognized by their characteristic insular growth pattern (Figs. 18-40 and 18-41). While serotonin is the dominant secretory product of midgut carcinoids, nearly 80% of these tumors are multihormonal in nature; products such as gastrin, ACTH, calcitonin, glucagon, and substance P also have been identified in these tumors.[127,128] Most of these tumors are composed of cells bearing secretory granules that are both argentaffin and argyrophil positive (p. 840).

Hindgut carcinoids most often arise in the rectum, which is the third most common site for gastrointestinal carcinoids. These tumors show either a pure trabecular or a mixed architectural pattern. An impressive array of secretory products, such as glucagon, pancreatic polypeptide, somatostatin, insulin, and serotonin, has been identified in rectal carcinoids.[128-130] As with their counterparts in "loftier locations," the secretory products are associated with cytoplasmic granules immunoreactive to appropriate antibodies. Hindgut tumors are variably argentaffin or argyrophil positive.

CLINICAL COURSE. Most gastrointestinal carcinoids are asymptomatic tumors that are discovered incidentally during surgery or autopsy. A small proportion may cause obstruction or bleeding secondary to intussusception or to a sharp angulation of the bowel wall (especially in the small intestine) at the site of the tumor. Although appendiceal carcinoids are often detected incidentally in appendices removed for appendicitis, this association is fortuitous. Being of endocrine origin, carcinoid tumors are capable of producing a variety of syndromes or endocrinopathies as a direct result of the overproduction of a par-

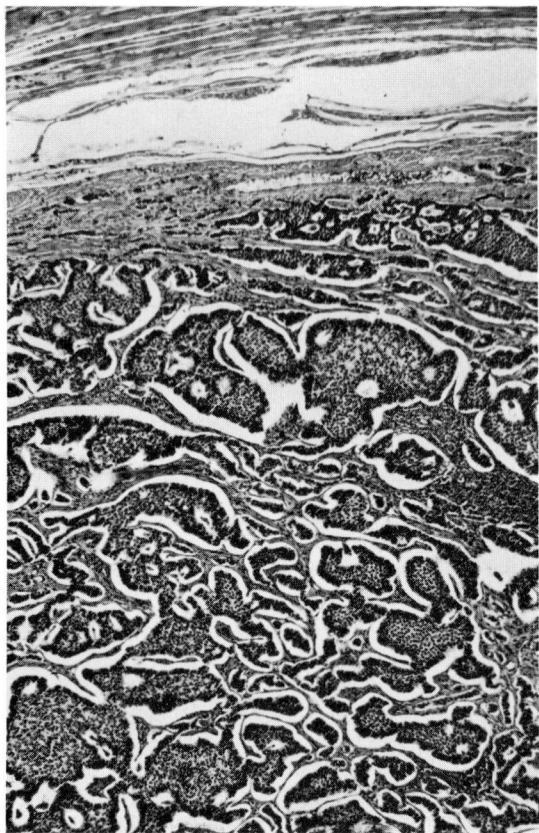

Figure 18–40. Endocrine cell tumor of appendix. Low-power view taken from one margin of tumor in contact with muscularis. Characteristic pattern of growth and invasion of wall is evident.

ticular biogenic amine or peptide hormone. Some tumors are "hormonally functional," while others are "nonfunctional." Functional neoplasms give rise to a variety of syndromes, including the carcinoid syndrome, Zollinger-Ellison syndrome, Cushing's syndrome, and others.

Some of these neoplasms (detailed earlier) are associated with a distinctive *"carcinoid syndrome" characterized by paroxysmal flushing, episodes of asthma-like wheezing, right-sided heart failure (p. 639), attacks of explosive watery diarrhea, abdominal pain, edema, and pellagra-like lesions of the skin and oral mucosa.* Although several secretory products, such as serotonin (5-hydroxytryptamine; 5-HT), 5-hydroxytryptophan (5-HTP), histamine, kallikrein, and bradykinin, have been identified, the principal agent in the production of the syndrome appears to be serotonin, while others, such as substance P, histamine, bradykinin, kallikrein, and perhaps prostaglandins, play a minor contributory role.[131]

The normal EC cells in the gut, on account of their biosynthetic capacities (see p. 840), take up tryptophan to synthesize serotonin. This serotonin, when released into the portal circulation, is promptly taken up by the platelets, metabolized by the liver and lungs into 5-hydroxyindole–acetic acid (5-HIAA), and excreted in the urine. Normally less than 1% of

the dietary tryptophan is converted into serotonin, the rest being utilized for protein synthesis or incorporated into nicotinamide. In patients with the carcinoid syndrome, both the primary and the metastatic tumors take up disproportionately large amounts (up to 60%) of tryptophan. This is first hydroxylated to 5-hydroxytryptophan (5-HTP) and then decarboxylated to 5-HT and 5-HIAA. Foregut carcinoids, on the other hand, have a partial or complete absence of the decarboxylating enzymes and are therefore unable to decarboxylate all the 5-HTP. These tumors therefore produce large amounts of 5-HTP and small quantities of 5-HT and 5-HIAA. The 5-HTP released by the tumors is then converted to 5-HT and 5-HIAA by the decarboxylases in other viscera. Thus patients with midgut carcinoids and the classic carcinoid syndrome have elevated levels of 5-HT and 5-HIAA in their blood and urine, whereas those with foregut tumors have elevated levels of 5-HTP, 5-HT, and 5-HIAA.

Although this syndrome is classically associated with ileal carcinoids, it has also been described in association with gastric, pancreatic, appendiceal, cecal, colonic, and rarely, rectal carcinoids as well as with those in such extraintestinal locations as the lungs and ovaries.[131-133] The syndrome occurs in about 1% of all patients with carcinoids, in 10% of those with gastrointestinal carcinoids, and in 20% of those with widespread metastases. *For gastrointesti-*

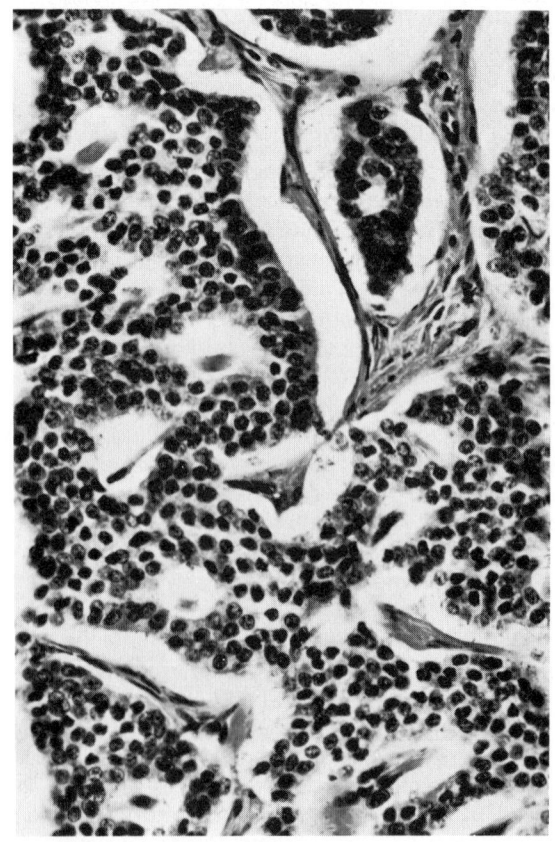

Figure 18–41. Close-up of cellular detail in Figure 18–40 to show uniformity of nuclear size and shape and growth pattern.

nal carcinoids, the development of the syndrome requires the presence of hepatic metastases, but they are not required for extraintestinal carcinoids for reasons cited below. Hepatic metastases frequently reach sizes several times that of the primary tumor, and thus produce enormous amounts of 5-HT and 5-HTP. Moreover, the products of the metastases are released directly into the systemic circulation via the hepatic veins without being subjected to any metabolic degradation. It should be emphasized that functioning carcinoids that produce the carcinoid syndrome are morphologically identical to other functioning and nonfunctioning tumors arising in comparable sites.

Carcinoma

Adenocarcinomas, despite the rapid turnover of the small intestinal mucosa, are very uncommon. They grow in a napkin-ring encircling pattern or as polypoid fungating masses, recapitulating in a sense left-sided or right-sided colonic cancers (p. 898), respectively (Fig. 18–42). Most small bowel carcinomas arise in the duodenum—which, inch for inch, represents the site of greatest predilection for these tumors. Cramping pain, nausea, vomiting, and weight loss are the common presenting signs and symptoms, but as pointed out, such manifestations generally ap-

pear late in the course of these cancers. Most have already penetrated the bowel wall, invaded the mesentery or other segments of the gut, spread to regional nodes, and sometimes metastasized to the liver and more widely by the time of diagnosis. Despite these problems, wide "en bloc" excision of these cancers yields about a 70% five-year survival rate.[134] Duodenal lesions located in the periampullary region may lead to obstructive jaundice early in their course.

MALABSORPTION SYNDROMES

The malabsorption syndrome is characterized by abnormal fecal excretion of fat (steatorrhea) and variable malabsorption of fats, fat-soluble vitamins, other vitamins, proteins, carbohydrates, minerals, and water. *At the most basic level, it is the result of disturbance, in most cases, of at least one of three functions: (1) digestion of nutrients to smaller molecules that can be absorbed or transported across the intestinal mucosal cell; (2) a reduction in the absorptive capacity of the bowel, principally the small intestine; or (3) abnormal transport of absorbed products.*[135] Most of the digestive process begins in the stomach, with its content of acid and pepsin, and continues in the small intestine, under the influence of bile and pancreatic and small intestinal enzymes. Absorption, although it may occur throughout the small intestine and, indeed, to a minimal degree in the colon as well, takes place chiefly in the upper small intestine, namely the duodenum and jejunum. Vitamin B_{12} and bile acids are notable exceptions and are absorbed in the lower small intestine. The absorptive surface of the small intestine is enormously expanded by the villi and the microvilli, which are estimated to number 2×10^8 per cm². Any disorder reducing the absorptive surface of the gut will lead to malabsorption.

The diseases and disorders causing malabsorption are both numerous and variably classified. An all-inclusive classification is presented in Table 18–5, from which it is apparent that malabsorption may be caused by a number of dissimilar mechanisms. Some affect mainly intraluminal digestion of nutrients. Others involve principally the transport and absorption of foodstuffs across the intestinal mucosal cells. Still others, such as lymphatic obstruction, impinge principally on the transport of fats once they have traversed the mucosal cell membrane. However, in many of the categories mentioned, the basis for the malabsorption is poorly understood or is a consequence of multiple defects. Malabsorption may not be associated with morphologic abnormalities when it is functional in origin. Moreover, such changes as are present may at times be secondarily induced by malabsorption itself. Recent refinements in endoscopic techniques have permitted biopsies of the small bowel mucosa to be obtained with relative ease. These biopsies not only permit elegant evaluations of mucosal changes but also can be used for biochemical, histochemical, and organ culture techniques. Some

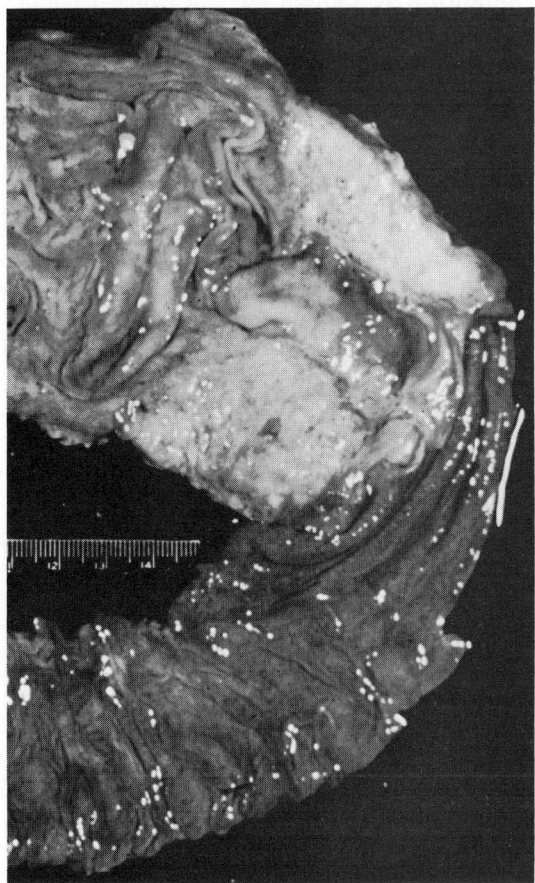

Figure 18–42. Carcinoma of small intestine growing in an annular encircling fashion.

Table 18-5. Classification of Malabsorption Syndromes

CATEGORY I: DEFECTIVE INTRALUMINAL HYDROLYSIS OR SOLUBILITY
  A. Primary pancreatic insufficiency
  B. Secondary pancreatic insufficiency
  C. Deficiency of conjugated bile salts, including intestinal resection
  D. Bacterial overgrowth (bile salt deconjugation)
    1. Blind loops
    2. Multiple strictures and jejunal diverticula
    3. Fistulas
    4. Postgastrectomy
    5. Scleroderma and pseudo-obstruction

CATEGORY II: MUCOSAL CELL ABNORMALITY AND INADEQUATE SURFACE
  A. Primary mucosal cell disorders
    1. Disaccharidase deficiency and monosaccharide malabsorption
    2. Abetalipoproteinemia
    3. Vitamin B_{12} malabsorption
    4. Cystinuria and Hartnup's disease
  B. Small bowel disease
    1. Celiac disease
    2. Whipple's disease
    3. Allergic and eosinophilic gastroenteritis
    4. Nongranulomatous ileojejunitis
    5. Crohn's disease (transmural enteritis)

CATEGORY III: LYMPHATIC OBSTRUCTION
  A. Lymphoma
  B. Tuberculosis and tuberculous lymphadenitis
  C. Lymphangiectasia

CATEGORY IV: MULTIPLE DEFECTS
  A. Subtotal gastrectomy
  B. Distal ileal resection, disease, or bypass
  C. Radiation enteritis

CATEGORY V: UNEXPLAINED
  A. Hypogammaglobulinemia
  B. Carcinoid syndrome
  C. Diabetes mellitus
  D. Mastocytosis
  E. Hyperthyroidism, hypothyroidism, hypoadrenocorticism, and hypoparathyroidism

CATEGORY VI: INFECTION
  A. Tropical sprue
  B. Acute infectious enteritis
  C. Parasitoses

CATEGORY VII: DRUG-INDUCED MALABSORPTION
  A. Cholestyramine
  B. Colchicine
  C. Irritant laxatives
  D. Neomycin
  E. *p*-Aminosalicylic acid
  F. Phenindione

From Sleisenger, M.H., and Brandborg, L.L.: Malabsorption, Vol. 13. Major Problems in Internal Medicine, Philadelphia, W. B. Saunders Co., 1977, p. 130.

concept of the usefulness of intestinal biopsy can be gained from Table 18-6, which presents some of the typical findings and their specificity in many of the malabsorptive conditions.

Clinically, all the malabsorption syndromes resemble each other more than they differ. Particularly common are weight loss, anorexia, abdominal distention, borborygmi, muscle wasting, and passage of abnormally bulky, frothy, greasy, yellow or gray stools. More specific manifestations appear in particular categories. When there is inadequate protein absorp-

tion, edema and ascites may be superimposed. Severe disturbances of fat absorption may lead to signs and symptoms of avitaminosis A, avitaminosis K, and avitaminosis D. In turn, malabsorption of vitamin D and calcium may lead to skeletal changes, bone pain, and predisposition to fracture. Hypocalcemia may also result in paresthesias or even tetany, convulsions, and coma. Inadequate absorption of folate and vitamin B_{12} produces signs and symptoms related to megaloblastic anemia. When the malabsorption syndrome is associated with profuse diarrhea and significant loss of fluids, sodium, and potassium, it may be life threatening.

Among the many disorders that give rise to such syndromes, those most commonly encountered in the United States are celiac sprue, regional enteritis, and chronic pancreatitis. A second category of importance would include Whipple's disease, small intestinal diverticulosis, tropical sprue, disaccharidase deficiency, abetalipoproteinemia, amyloidosis, intestinal scleroderma, postgastrectomy states, and blind-loop syndromes (related to surgical procedures or congenital reduplication of the ileum).[135] Many of these more or less common entities have been discussed elsewhere; only a few remain to be considered.

CELIAC SPRUE

This condition is known by a variety of names— *gluten-sensitive enteropathy, nontropical sprue, and adult and childhood celiac disease.* It is related to dietary gluten and is very likely an immune reaction to a constituent (gliadin) of this protein. Celiac disease is characterized by a striking loss of villi in the small intestine and, with it, a marked reduction in the absorptive surface area. Although the disease is usually diagnosed in early childhood, it may not be detected until years later. Females are affected more frequently than males. There are many suggestions pointing to a hereditary background. Familial clustering has been noted; as many as 80% of patients are HLA-B8, and over 90% D/DR3 or D/DR7, which may have relevance to the pathogenesis of this condition in terms of inherited specific immune response genes.[136]

There is now unmistakable evidence that celiac disease can be cured by placing patients on a gluten-free diet. Gluten and the derivative gliadin are proteins found particularly in wheat, barley, and rye grains. *The preponderance of data points to a hypersensitivity reaction to antigenic determinants within gliadin as the cause of the intestinal changes.*[137] The small intestinal mucosa, when exposed to gluten, accumulates a large number of B cells sensitized to gliadin.[138] Circulating antibodies to gliadin are present in all patients under two years of age and in many who are older. It would appear that with antigenic challenge by gliadin there is local synthesis of immunoglobulins in the small bowel mucosa.[139] On gluten-free diets the titers of circulating antibodies fall or disappear.[140] However, antibodies cannot be demonstrated in all patients with this condition, and more-

Table 18–6. Malabsorption Syndromes—Abnormalities in Small Intestinal Biopsies

DISORDERS WITH CHARACTERISTIC FINDINGS
1. *Celiac and tropical sprue:* Blunted or absent villi, abnormal surface epithelium, lengthened crypts, increased mononuclear cell infiltrate in lamina propria
2. *Whipple's disease:* Lamina propria stuffed with glycoprotein-containing macrophages, villous abnormality of variable severity, bacilli demonstrable in macrophages during active disease in ultrathin sections or on electron microscopy
3. *Abetalipoproteinemia:* Mucosal absorptive cells vacuolated by lipid inclusions, villous structure normal
4. *Agammaglobulinemia:* Flattened or absent villi, absence of plasma cells, increased lymphocytic infiltrate
5. *Amyloidosis:* Demonstration of amyloid in and about vessels of lamina propria with Congo red staining and birefringence
6. *Regional enteritis:* Noncaseating granulomas
7. *Parasitic infections:* Identification of parasite in biopsy sections, e.g., giardiasis, strongyloidiasis, schistosomiasis, histoplasmosis, cryptosporidiosis
8. *Mastocytosis:* Mast cell infiltrates of lamina propria
9. *Intestinal lymphoma:* Possible foci of malignant lymphoid cells in lamina propria, villous abnormality of variable severity
10. *Allergic and eosinophilic gastroenteritis:* Infiltrates of excessive numbers of eosinophilic leukocytes, lesion patchy, villous structure may be normal or severely deranged
11. *Tuberculosis and tuberculous lymphadenitis:* Chance finding of caseating granuloma or margin of tuberculous ulcer

DISORDERS IN WHICH BIOPSY MAY BE ABNORMAL BUT IS NOT NECESSARILY DIAGNOSTIC
1. *Folate deficiency:* Shortened villi, megalocytes in blood vessels, decreased mitoses in crypts
2. *Vitamin B$_{12}$ deficiency:* Similar to folate deficiency
3. *Radiation enteritis:* Similar to folate deficiency
4. *Systemic scleroderma:* Increased fibrosis in lamina propria, possible derangement in villous structure
5. *Lymphangiectasia:* Dilated lacteals and lymphatics in lamina propria, blunted and clubbed villi

over there is often a poor correlation between the severity of the disease and the level of the antibodies.

In a typical untreated case of celiac disease, the mucosa appears flat or convoluted, and histologic examination reveals marked atrophy or virtually complete loss of villi. The surface epithelium shows degeneration and flattening of the normally tall columnar cells and an increased number of lymphocytes in the epithelial layer (Fig. 18–43A). At times, though, the surface epithelium may be normally columnar. The crypts, on the other hand, are elongated, hyperplastic, and tortuous. Typically there is increased mitotic activity, with mitoses occasionally seen high in the crypts. The lamina propria has an overall increase in plasma cells, lymphocytes, macrophages, eosinophils, and mast cells. With immunoperoxidase staining, large numbers of immunocytes bearing IgA antigliadin antibodies are seen in the small bowel mucosa, with some increase in IgM-bearing cells. Electron microscopy discloses that the microvilli are markedly distorted and shortened, while the mitochondria have unusual sizes and shapes and show changes in their cristae. The ribonucleoprotein granules are abnormally abundant. All these structural changes are more marked in the proximal small intestine than in the distal, since it is the proximal jejunum that is exposed to the highest concentration of dietary gluten. It should be mentioned, however, that although these changes are characteristically seen in celiac sprue, they can be mimicked by other diseases, most notably by tropical sprue. Although in the United States, nearly 85% of patients with these histologic features in their small bowel biopsy will turn out to have celiac disease, this diagnosis ultimately rests on reversal of these changes following a period of gluten exclusion from the diet (Fig. 18–43B).

Individuals with long-term untreated celiac sprue may suffer a number of complications. Faulty absorption of iron, folates, calcium, and vitamin D may lead to anemia, paresthesias, muscle cramps, and osteoporosis. Neurologic symptoms related to patchy demyelination have also been reported. However, the most unpleasant consequence of long-term celiac disease is a 10 to 15% chance of developing cancer within eight to ten years. Over half are gastrointestinal lymphomas, now referred to as B-cell lymphomas, and the remainder are carcinomas distributed throughout the gastrointestinal tract but disproportionately in the small intestine.[141] Whether strict adherence to a gluten-free diet reduces the risk of developing malignancies is still unclear.

TROPICAL SPRUE

This condition is so named because this celiac-like disease occurs almost exclusively in people living in or visiting the tropics. In the latter case, symptoms may appear several months or years after the visit. However, it has been suggested that tropical sprue is inappropriately named because, save for the similarity of the mucosal changes to those of celiac disease, there is little commonality between these two entities. Tropical sprue is of unknown etiology, although there are suggestions that it may be caused by enterotoxigenic *E. coli*.[142] It has a curious geographic distribution: Although common in the Caribbean, it has not been reported from Jamaica, and it does not occur in Africa south of the Sahara. In certain tropical areas, as in South India, the disease has been known to occur in endemic form. Furthermore, epidemic outbreaks of tropical sprue have occasionally been reported, but even in such outbreaks the affected individuals do not always have identifiable enteric pathogens. Thus, no specific causal microbiologic agent has been clearly associated with tropical sprue, although specific strains of *E. coli* are currently favored candidates. Despite the etiologic uncertainties, most patients are

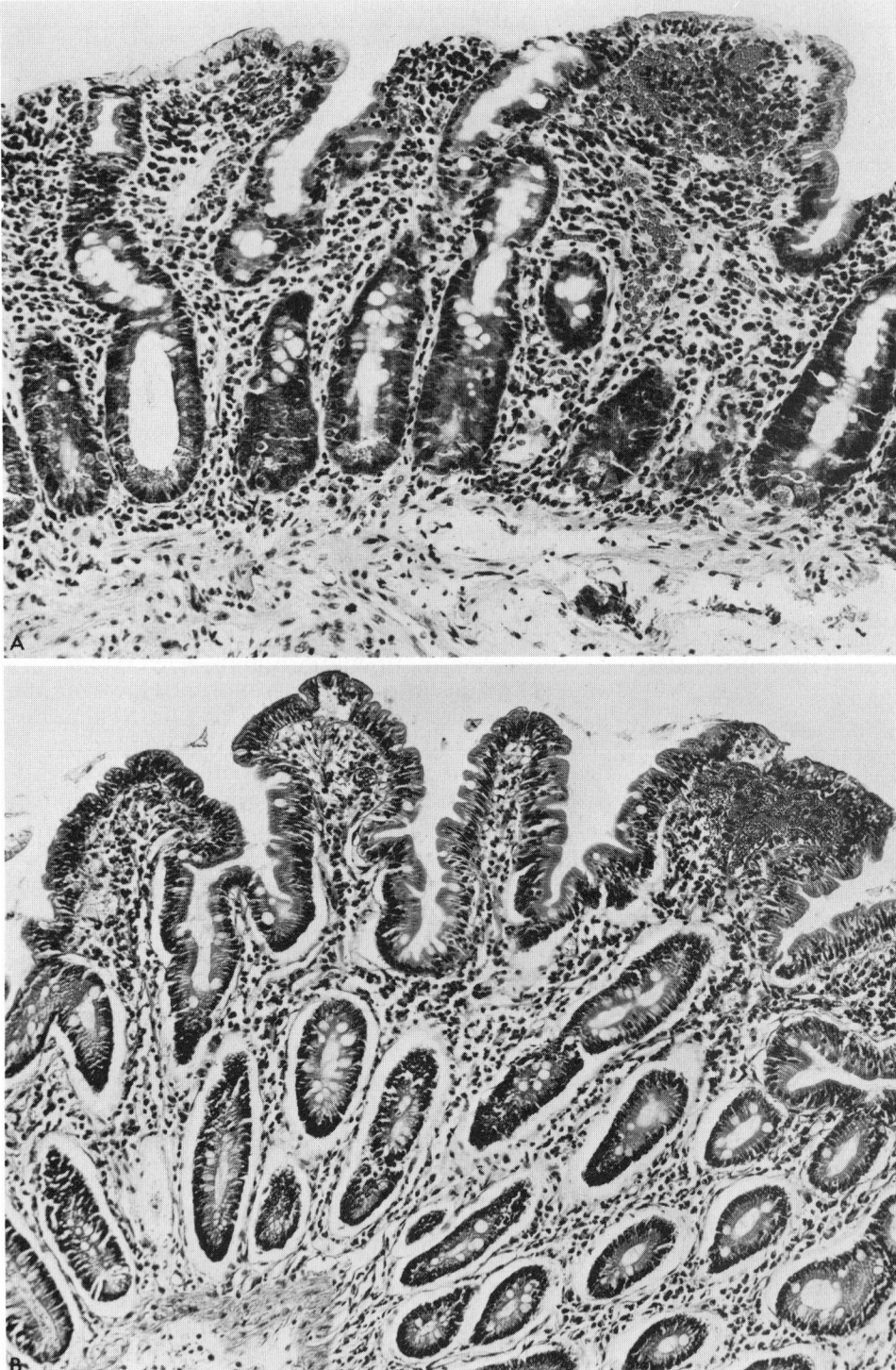

Figure 18–43. *A*, Celiac disease — a jejunal peroral biopsy of gluten enteropathy with atrophy and blunting of villi and an inflammatory infiltrate in lamina propria. *B*, Celiac disease — same patient as in *A* after five days on a gluten-free diet.

benefited or cured by long-term broad-spectrum antibiotic therapy.

Intestinal changes are extremely variable. In some patients the mucosal histology is not abnormal, whereas in others the changes are similar to those of celiac disease. It should be emphasized that in sharp contrast to celiac disease, in which the brunt of the disease is borne by the proximal small bowel mucosa, injury in tropical sprue is predominantly seen in the distal bowel, and the proximal jejunal mucosa may be uninvolved except in severe cases. Furthermore, although the histologic changes in tropical sprue closely mimic those seen in celiac disease, the relatively large numbers of lymphocytes and the presence of eosinophils in the lamina propria help distinguish it from celiac disease. On account of mucosal injury to the terminal ileum in tropical sprue, patients frequently have folate and/ or vitamin B_{12} deficiency, leading to marked atypical enlargement of the nuclei of epithelial cells characteristic of the nuclear changes seen, for example, in pernicious anemia.

WHIPPLE'S DISEASE

This uncommon multisystem disease is intriguing and frustrating. *Apparent rod-shaped bacilli can be readily visualized under the electron microscope within and between glycoprotein-laden, PAS-positive macrophages in many organs throughout the body, principally the small bowel mucosa. The organism cannot be isolated, however, and so no specific causal agent has yet been identified.* The PAS-positive glycoprotein granules within the macrophages are thought to be bacterial products. Numerous microbiologic studies of patients with Whipple's disease have yielded over 25 different microorganisms, many not bacilliform.[143] Immunologic and histochemical studies of lesions have been equally frustrating, yielding positive results with antisera for Streptococcus groups A, B, C, and G and *Shigella flexneri*.[144] Superimposed on all these complexities is the lack of an inflammatory response at the sites of localization of the apparent bacilli in the various tissues. Nevertheless, Whipple's disease responds promptly and dramatically to antibiotic therapy, often with permanent remission. The tangle is yet to be unraveled.

Whipple's disease was once thought to be solely an intestinal disorder characterized by malabsorption, but it is now apparent that it is a systemic disease, involving not only the small intestine but also the skin, central nervous system, joints, heart, blood vessels, kidney, lung, serosal membranes, lymph nodes, spleen, and liver.[145] Indeed, a migratory polyarthritis is often the presenting manifestation. Occasionally, patients develop neurologic disturbances without manifestations of intestinal disease.[146] This condition has presented as cardiac disease before intestinal, articular, or systemic involvement was apparent.[147] Whether intestinal involvement would eventually have developed with these unusual presentations is not clear.

The hallmark of this condition is the macrophage laden with PAS-positive granules and occasional rod-shaped organisms. In the classic case these cells crowd the lamina propria of the small intestinal mucosa (Fig. 18–44). Distention of the villi imparts a shaggy, "bearskin rug" gross appearance to the intestinal mucosal surface. In untreated cases the bacillary bodies may also be seen lying free in the interstitial spaces in the lamina propria of the small bowel, in neutrophils, and sometimes within the mucosal epithelial cells (Fig. 18–45). Thus, the "organism" has the capacity to invade cells. Accompanying all these changes within the intestinal mucosa is dilatation of the lymphatics, which sometimes contain lipid droplets, suggesting some lymphatic obstructive process. Occasionally, rupture of these

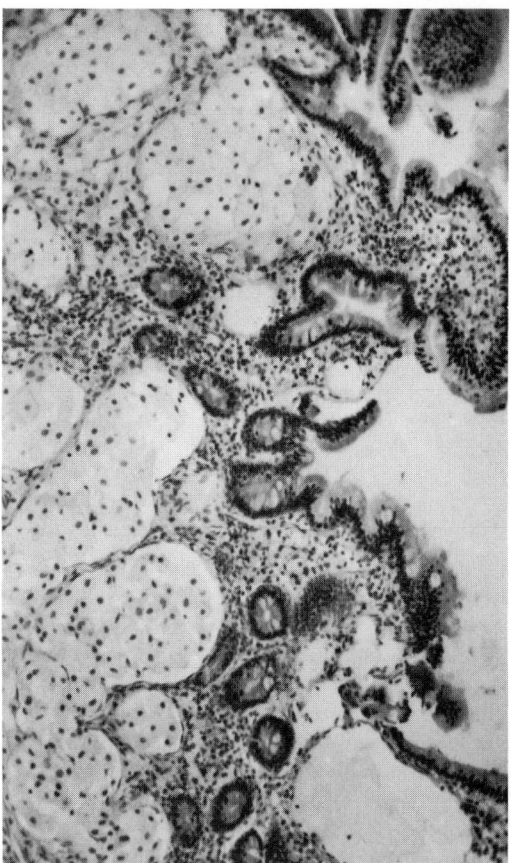

Figure 18–44. Whipple's disease with clusters of distended macrophages lying within lamina propria of intestinal mucosa.

channels may give rise to lipogranulomas. The draining mesenteric lymph nodes of affected segments of the gut reveal the same microscopic changes. Characteristic macrophages containing bacillary bodies may be found in other levels of the gastrointestinal tract as well as in various other organs. For example, they can be found in the synovial membranes of affected joints, but damage to the articular surface is rarely present. They may also diffusely infiltrate the central nervous system, cardiac valves, subendocardium, and myocardial interstitial tissue, sometimes collecting into focal aggregates.[143] With antibiotic therapy the bacillary bodies disappear, only to reappear if the patient suffers a relapse.[145]

Whipple's disease usually presents as a form of malabsorption with diarrhea, steatorrhea, abdominal cramps, distention, fever, and marked weight loss. It is principally encountered in Caucasians in the fourth to fifth decades of life, with a strong male predominance in the ratio of 10:1. As pointed out, atypical presentations are quite frequent; indeed, Whipple's disease must be suspected, even in the absence of intestinal symptoms, as a cause of polyarthritis, obscure CNS complaints, focal hyperpigmentations of the skin, and numerous other symptom complexes. The diagnosis rests on light microscopic recognition

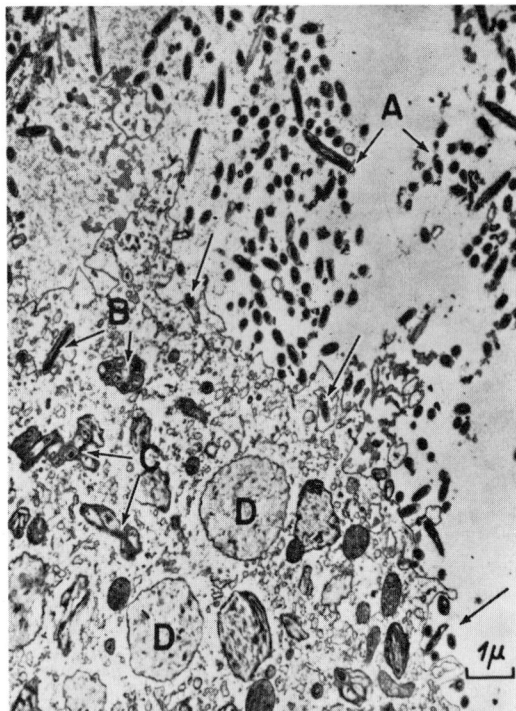

Figure 18–45. Electron micrograph of an involved histiocyte in Whipple's disease. A = bacilliform bodies outside cell with arrows pointing to loci where they appear to be penetrating cell boundaries. B and C = distorted forms. D = uninvolved lysosomes.

of PAS-positive macrophages that can be shown to contain rod-shaped organisms under the electron microscope. This once usually fatal condition can now be cured promptly by appropriate antibiotic therapy, and thus its recognition is crucial.

BACTERIAL OVERGROWTH SYNDROME

For purposes of this discussion, this syndrome is perhaps best described as a pathologic colonization of the jejunal lumen by an abnormally large population of both anaerobic and aerobic organisms qualitatively similar to those present in the colon.[148] The small bowel lumen is not normally sterile, and its bacterial population is held in check by a number of physiologic factors. Important among the "surveillance" mechanisms are the continuous peristaltic activity of the gut, the normal gastric acidity that imparts a low pH to the luminal contents of the proximal small bowel, and the presence of immunoglobulins secreted into the lumen by the mucosal cells.[148,149]

As a corollary, therefore, bacterial overgrowth can be expected to occur in patients with intestinal lesions that predispose to luminal stasis (strictures, fistula, jejunal diverticula, blind loops or pouches, reduplications, and motility disorders of the gut) and in postoperative states associated with secondary hypo- or achlorhydria, long afferent loops, and segments of denervated bowel. It may additionally occur in patients with immune deficiency or mucosal dis-

ease of the small bowel. A wide spectrum of absorptive defects, including malabsorption of proteins, fats, carbohydrates, vitamins, water, and electrolytes, ensues as a result of complex interrelated pathophysiologic mechanisms. The etiology of the malabsorption in this syndrome is multifactorial and related to (1) the excessive bacterial load competing for essential nutrients; (2) deconjugation of bile salts and dehydroxylation of fatty acids by the bacteria, resulting in impaired micelle formation and fat absorption; (3) bacterial inactivation of lipase; or (4) mucosal damage induced secondarily by volatile fatty acids liberated from bacterial fermentation of carbohydrates, by the hydroxy fatty acids produced by bacterial breakdown of fats, and by bacterial proteases damaging the brush border of the epithelial cells.[148,149]

Although small bowel mucosal biopsies may show nonspecific increases in inflammatory infiltrates in the lamina propria, it is uncertain that these are due to bacterial overgrowth per se. Demonstration of increased numbers of aerobic and anaerobic organisms in jejunal aspirates is therefore a more pertinent diagnostic procedure.[148,149] A proper recognition of this syndrome is important since malabsorption can be cured in patients with surgically correctable lesions, but whatever the circumstance, treatment with appropriate antibiotics usually yields prompt clinical improvement.[149]

DISACCHARIDASE DEFICIENCY

The disaccharidases, of which the most important is lactase, are localized to the apical cell membrane of villous absorptive epithelial cells. Congenital lactase deficiency is a very rare condition, but acquired lactase deficiency is common, particularly among North American blacks. With insufficient lactase, the disaccharide lactose cannot be broken down into its monosaccharides, glucose and galactose. The unabsorbed lactose exerts an osmotic pull, leading to watery diarrhea and malabsorption. A deficiency of this enzyme may occur early in life as a familial inborn error of metabolism or may apparently develop in adult life as an acquired disorder. When hereditary, malabsorption becomes evident with the initiation of milk feeding. The infants develop explosive, watery, frothy stools and abdominal distention. When exposure to milk or milk products is terminated, the malabsorption is promptly corrected.

In the adult, lactose intolerance may appear with viral and bacterial infections of the gastrointestinal tract as well as in other disorders of the gut. Despite the clinical manifestations, neither light nor electron microscopy has disclosed abnormalities of the mucosal cells of the bowel in either the hereditary or the acquired form of the disease.

The diagnosis can be suspected with the breath hydrogen test. Bacterial fermentation of the unabsorbed sugars leads to the production of increased amounts of hydrogen, which can be measured readily by gas chromatography.[150]

ABETALIPOPROTEINEMIA

This form of malabsorption is familial and transmitted by autosomal recessive inheritance. It fundamentally constitutes an inborn error of metabolism, characterized by an inability to synthesize apoproteins required for the export of lipoproteins from mucosal cells. Free fatty acids and monoglycerides resulting from hydrolysis of dietary fat enter the absorptive epithelial cells and are re-esterified in the normal fashion but cannot be synthesized into chylomicrons. As a consequence, triglycerides are stored within the cells creating lipid vacuolation, which is readily evident under the light microscope, particularly with special fat stains. Concomitantly, there is severe hypolipidemia related largely to depressed levels of chylomicrons, prebetalipoproteins (VLDL), and betalipoproteins (LDL). The failure to absorb certain essential fatty acids leads to a defective lipid membrane of the red cells and accounts for their characteristic "burr cell" appearance.[135] The disease becomes manifest in infancy and is dominated by failure to thrive, diarrhea, and steatorrhea.

OBSTRUCTIVE LESIONS

Obstruction of the gastrointestinal tract may be caused by lesions at any level, but the narrow lumen of the small intestine makes obstruction most common at this location. The causes of such obstruction are classified in Table 18–7. Tumors and infarction, although the most serious, account for only about 10 to 15% of small bowel obstructions. Four of the entities — hernias, intestinal adhesions, intussusception, and volvulus — account collectively for 80%.

HERNIAS

A weakness or defect in the wall of the peritoneal cavity may provide an area where persistent intraperitoneal pressure will eventually push out a pouch-like, serosa-lined sac called a hernial sac. The usual sites of such weakness in the anterior abdominal wall are the areas of the inguinal and femoral canals, at the umbilicus, and in surgical scars. More rarely, similar retroperitoneal defects occur in the posterior wall of the abdominal cavity, chiefly about the ligament of Treitz. Hernias are of interest chiefly because segments of viscera frequently protrude and become trapped in them. This is more apt to occur in inguinal than in femoral hernias, since the former tend to have narrow orifices and large sacs. If the small bowel is involved, partial or complete obstruction of its lumen may follow. Pressure by the neck of the pouch may impair the venous drainage of the trapped viscus. The venous stasis and edema increase the bulk of the contents of the hernial sac, so that the intestinal loops are permanently trapped or *incarcerated*. With time, the increased volume may seriously compromise the venous drainage and arterial supply to the viscus (*strangulation*) and lead to infarction or gangrene of the trapped segment.

If strangulation does occur, the gross and microscopic picture of the affected gut exactly resembles that previously described for bowel infarction. Not only the small bowel but also portions of the omentum, and sometimes segments of the large bowel, tend to become trapped in these hernial sacs.

INTESTINAL ADHESIONS

As peritonitis heals, adhesions may develop. These fibrous bridges can create closed loops through which other viscera may slide and eventually become trapped, just as in a hernial sac. Intestinal obstruction, partial or complete, ensues and may be complicated by infarction of the trapped segment of bowel. This sequence of events occurs most commonly in postoperative patients who develop peritoneal adhesions to the wound in the abdominal wall and within the operative site. Quite rarely, adhesions may occur without previous peritoneal inflammation from fibrous bands arising as congenital defects. Intestinal obstruction and strangulation must be considered, then, even without a previous history of peritonitis or surgery.

INTUSSUSCEPTION

This is an uncommon but intriguing disorder (in part because of its euphonious name), most often encountered in infants and children, in which one segment of small intestine, constricted by a wave of peristalsis, suddenly becomes telescoped into the immediately distal segment of bowel. Once trapped, the invaginated segment is propelled by peristalsis farther into the distal segment, pulling its mesentery along behind it (Fig. 18–46). The trapped bowel is referred to as the intussusceptum, and the segment that envelops it is known as the intussuscipiens. The pathogenesis of this lesion in children and infants is obscure. There is usually no underlying anatomic lesion or defect in the bowel to explain such an occurrence. Intussusception also occurs in adults when an intraluminal mass or tumor acts as the point of traction and pulls along the

Table 18–7. Major Causes of Intestinal Obstruction

MECHANICAL OBSTRUCTION
Strictures, congenital and acquired; atresias
Meconium in mucoviscidosis
Imperforate anus
Obstructive gallstones, fecaliths, foreign
  bodies
Adhesive bands or kinks
Hernias
Volvulus
Intussusception
Neurogenic paralytic ileus
Tumors

VASCULAR OBSTRUCTION
Bowel infarction

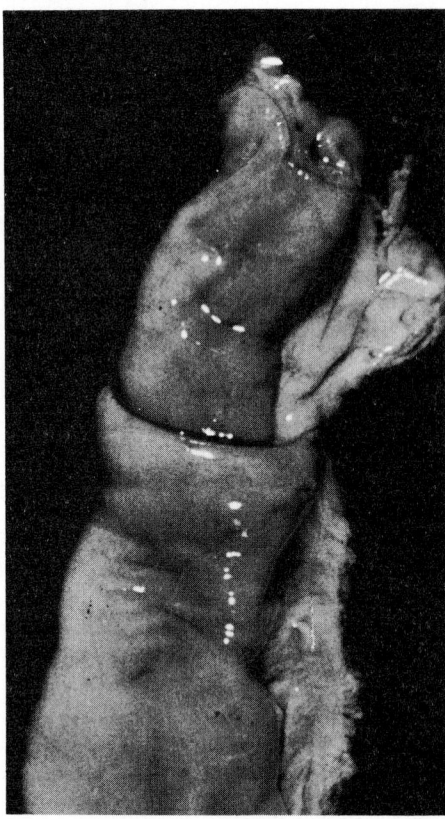

Figure 18–46. Intussusception of small intestine viewed from external aspect.

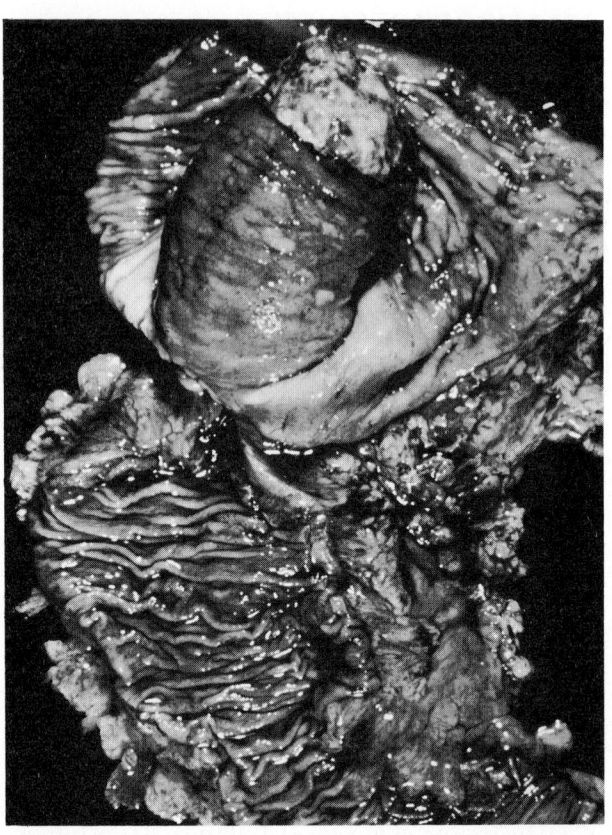

Figure 18–47. Intussusception of small intestine. Bowel has been opened to demonstrate necrotic tip of intussusceptum.

segment of gut as it telescopes into the distal segment. Intestinal obstruction ensues, and because of trapped mesenteric vessels, infarction supervenes (Fig. 18–47).

VOLVULUS

Complete twisting of a loop of bowel about its mesenteric base of attachment provides another mechanism for producing intestinal obstruction and infarction. This lesion occurs most often in the small bowel; however, large redundant loops of sigmoid are sometimes involved. Recognition of this seldom encountered lesion demands a constant awareness of its possible occurrence.

Having successfully traversed the small intestine, we perforce arrive at the colon.

COLON

CONGENITAL ANOMALIES	**VASCULAR LESIONS**	**Necrotizing Enterocolitis**	Relationship of neoplastic
Megacolon — Hirschsprung's	**Hemorrhoids**	**Collagenous Colitis**	polyps to carcinoma
Disease	**Angiodysplasia**	**TUMORS**	Familial polyposis syndromes
IDIOPATHIC DISORDERS	**INFLAMMATIONS**	**Polyps and Polyposis Syndromes**	**Malignant Tumors**
Diverticular Disease	**Idiopathic Ulcerative Colitis**	Non-neoplastic polyps	Carcinoma
Melanosis Coli	**Pseudomembranous Colitis**	Neoplastic polyps	Other tumors
	(PMC)		

NORMAL

The colon in man is both a storage and an absorptive organ. The subdivisions of the large bowel into the cecum, ascending colon, transverse colon, and descending colon are well known. Perhaps somewhat less well understood are the exact limits of the sigmoid colon and rectum. The former begins at the pelvic brim, includes the sigmoid flexure, and connects below with the rectum at approximately the level of the third sacral vertebra. The rectum is the portion distal to the sigmoid; it is approximately 6 inches long. The proximal portion is within the peritoneal cavity, and the distal segment is extraperitoneal. The reflection of the peritoneum from the rectum over the pelvic floor produces a cul-de-sac known as the pouch of Douglas. This space is a favored site for the implantation of spreading intra-abdominal tumors, which produce a perirectal mass called a rectal shelf. These masses are within 3 inches of the anus and are therefore within reach of the examining finger.

The blood supply to the right side of the colon up to the transverse colon is derived from the superior mesenteric artery. Occlusion of the superior mesenteric artery therefore causes infarction of the small bowel and may also infarct the ascending colon. Almost the entire remainder of the intra-abdominal colon is supplied by the inferior mesenteric artery. The lower rectum receives its supply from the hemorrhoidal branches of the internal iliac or internal pudendal artery, the upper level by the superior hemorrhoidal branch of the inferior mesenteric. The venous drainage follows essentially the same distribution. Therefore, within the rectal vasculature there is an anastomotic capillary bed between the superior hemorrhoidal veins draining through the portal system and the inferior hemorrhoidal veins, which drain through the inferior vena cava. In portal hypertension, these capillaries can become distended and provide a bypass for portal venous obstruction. Since for most of its extent the colon is a fixed retroperitoneal organ, it derives considerable accessory blood supply and lymphatic drainage from a wide area of the posterior abdominal wall, making infarction and obstructive lymphedema most uncommon at this level of the bowel.

Microscopically, in contrast to the small intestine, the colon has no villi. The absorptive surface itself is flat but is punctuated by numerous straight tubular crypts that extend into the underlying lamina propria. The crypts are lined mainly by goblet mucous cells with occasional endocrine cells. The mucosal surface is covered mainly by absorptive cells that bear on their luminal surfaces microvilli that are less abundant than those found in the small intestine. Intimately attached to these microvilli is an elaborate fibrillar glycoprotein extraneous coat similar to that found in the small intestine. Paneth cells, found mostly in the lower crypts, are dispersed throughout the right colon. Scattered within the mucosa are lymphoid foci covered by somewhat flattened cells that are thought to engulf and transfer antigens to the underlying immunocytes. Cell renewal in the colon and rectum essentially follows the pattern described in the small intestine, with most of the cell replication occurring in the base of the crypts. The intrinsic innervation of the colon comprises Auerbach's plexus within the muscular layer and Meissner's submucosal plexus. Both consist of nests of ganglion cells interconnected by unmyelinated postganglionic fibers that extend through the thickness of the bowel wall to provide communications between the plexuses.

PATHOLOGY

Certain lesions that affect the colon constitute some of the most frequently encountered diseases in clinical practice, particularly surgical practice. Cancer of the large bowel is the second most common cause of cancer death. The extremely common hemorrhoid, a comparatively trivial lesion, may produce in the aggregate more clinical discomfort than almost any other affliction to which humans are heir. In addition, inflammatory disorders such as ulcerative colitis and functional derangements such as spastic and mucous colitis are by no means uncommon. In terms of clinical and pathologic importance, then, the colon and stomach are the two areas of major importance in the gastrointestinal tract.

CONGENITAL ANOMALIES

Congenital anomalies of the colon are encountered infrequently. *Malrotations* may occur in which the cecum fails to descend to its definitive adult position in the right lower quadrant. Such malpositioning may confuse the diagnosis of acute appendicitis. *Reduplications* of the colon have been described rarely, with the occasional formation of entire double large bowels.

MEGACOLON— HIRSCHSPRUNG'S DISEASE

Marked dilatation of the colon, or megacolon, occurs both as a congenital and as an acquired disorder. Although the mode of transmission of congenital megacolon, also known as *Hirschsprung's disease*, is unclear, about 4% of siblings of an index patient may be expected to have the disease. It is ten times more frequent in patients with Down's syndrome than in the general population.

The origin of *congenital megacolon* is a failure during embryogenesis of development of Meissner's and Auerbach's plexuses. Normally, neuroblasts migrate in a cephalocaudal direction in the gut to reach the rectum at about 12 weeks of development. If the migration falls short, some portion of the distal colon lacks ganglion cells and there is a consequent functional loss of peristalsis—in effect, a colonic obstruction. Thus, in all patients, ganglion cells are lacking at the anorectal junction, but the extent of more proximal involvement depends on the severity of the migratory defect. In the vast majority of patients the proximal border of the aganglionic segment is located within the rectum or sigmoid. In only 10 to 20% of patients is a longer segment affected, and only very rarely the entire colon (aganglionosis of the colon).

Hirschsprung's disease is characterized by the absence of ganglion cells and erratic proliferation of nonmyelinated nerve fibers in the nondilated segment of colon. Since the rectum is always affected, it is the optimal site for biopsy, but the distal 2 to 3 cm should be avoided since ganglia are normally sparse here. Both Meissner's and Auerbach's plexuses develop more or less contemporaneously in the embryo; colonoscopic biopsies that include only the mucosa and submucosa are therefore usually sufficient to reveal ganglion cells if they are present.[151] However, if they are not found, transmural biopsy at the time of surgery may be necessary to confirm their absence.

In the common pattern in which both rectum and rectosigmoid are affected, the descending colon undergoes dilatation and hypertrophy first. Eventually, however, the entire colon may become involved, and in extreme cases the functional obstruction may cause dilatation of the small intestine. The appendix, too, may become dilated and in some cases has perforated. The wall of the dilated bowel may undergo hypertrophy and thickening. Sometimes, however, the distention outruns the hypertrophy, leading to thinning and potentiating rupture, particularly of the distended cecum, which has the thinnest wall. The mucosal lining may be intact throughout, but the functional obstruction may predispose to an inflammatory enterocolitis, or impacted feces may induce stercoral ulcerations.

Hirschsprung's disease usually manifests itself in the immediate neonatal period by failure of passage of meconium followed by obstructive constipation. In some instances, when only a short segment of the rectum is affected, the build-up of pressure may permit occasional passage of stools, or even intermittent bouts of diarrhea. Abdominal distention (when a sufficiently large segment of colon is involved) confirms the presence of an intestinal obstruction. The diagnosis can be suspected on the basis of the clinical findings, and is firmly established if a biopsy documents the absence of ganglion cells in the nondilated colon. The major threats to life in this disorder are superimposed enterocolitis with fluid and electrolyte disturbances, and perforation of the colon or appendix with peritonitis.[152]

Acquired megacolon is encountered with chronic organic obstruction such as narrowing of the bowel due to inflammatory disease, with neoplasia, or as an apparent functional disorder. Emotional problems may underlie some of these functional disturbances, but in other instances there appears to be a motility dysfunction. Nevertheless, the intrinsic innervation of the bowel is normal. However, in the megacolon of Chagas' disease (p. 407) it is destroyed.

Imperforate anus results when the membrane that separates the entodermal hindgut from the ectodermal anal dimple fails to perforate. An intact membranous septum may completely close the anal canal. This type of anomaly occurs in 1 in 5000 births. Occasionally, the occlusion may take the form of agenesis, atresia, or stenosis of the rectal canal. When unrecognized, colonic distention may develop. In a significant number of these developmental failures, fistulous communications occur with the genital tract in the female or with the urinary tract in either sex.

IDIOPATHIC DISORDERS

DIVERTICULAR DISEASE

Saccular outpouchings of the colon are prone to develop with advancing age, particularly in the rectosigmoid, and are referred to as *diverticular disease.* At one time this condition was called *diverticulosis* and was thought to be of importance principally because it predisposed to the development of inflammatory changes — *diverticulitis* — which then led to clinical symptoms. It is now clear that diverticulosis in the absence of inflammatory changes may produce symptoms indistinguishable from those of diverticulitis, mainly lower abdominal discomfort with intermittent cramping pain or sometimes continuous pain. Making the similarity even more complete, in about half the instances, diverticulitis is not associated with fever or leukocytosis.[153]

The prevalence of this condition in Western societies has risen remarkably since the turn of the century. It is much less frequent in nonindustrialized tropical countries and in Japan. Diverticula are rare in persons under 30 years of age; in those over the age of 60 the prevalence is about 50% in high-risk locales. Thus, a progressive rise in the mean age of certain populations may explain at least some of the increased frequency of this condition.

Most diverticula (95%) are located in the sigmoid colon. However, the descending colon, and indeed the entire colon, may also be affected. Hypertrophy of the musculature of affected segments of colon is commonly seen. The taeniae coli are unusually prominent and have an almost cartilaginous consistency. The circular muscles are also thicker than normal. In most specimens, **small flasklike or spherical outpouchings, usually 0.5 to 1 cm in diameter, can be identified along the margins of the taeniae.** In the absence of secondary inflammation they are elastic, compressible, and easily emptied of fecal contents. Characteristically, these sacs dissect into the appendices epiploicae and may therefore be missed on casual inspection.

When inflammatory changes supervene, they tend to extend about the diverticula, producing peridiverticulitis, and to dissect into the immediately adjacent pericolic fat. Perforation of diverticula usually initiates the inflammatory process. Over the course of time, the numerous foci of inflammatory reaction may cause marked fibrotic thickening in and about the colonic wall, producing sufficient narrowing to resemble remarkably a colonic cancer. Extension of the infection may lead to pericolic abscesses, sinus tracts, and sometimes pelvic or generalized peritonitis.

Histologic examination of uninflamed diverticula discloses a remarkably thin wall composed of a flattened or atrophic mucosa, compressed submucosa, and attenuated or totally absent muscularis (Fig. 18–48).

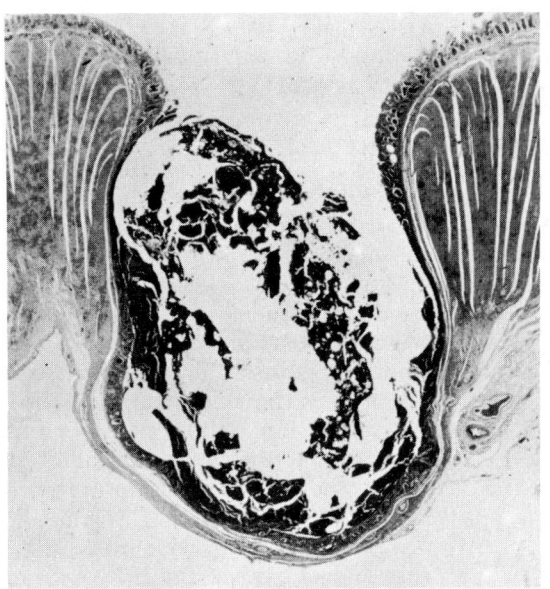

Figure 18–48. Low-power view of diverticulum of colon indicating marked thinning of wall and absence of muscularis.

PATHOGENESIS. The morphology of diverticula strongly suggests that *two factors are important in their genesis: (1) foci of muscular weakness in the colonic wall, and (2) intraluminal pressure.*[154] Thus, *diverticula represent herniations of the mucosa and submucosa at points of muscular weakness.* Angiographic studies indicate that such weaknesses occur wherever the arterial vasa recta penetrate the muscularis to ultimately ramify in the submucosa and mucosa. The connective tissue sheaths that surround these perforating vessels provide avenues devoid of muscularis for the development of herniations.

Whether especially high intraluminal pressure is requisite for the formation of these herniations remains controversial.[155] To explain the epidemiologic data cited earlier, it has been proposed that diets low in fiber content reduce the stool bulk. This, in turn, leads to increased peristaltic activity, particularly within the sigmoid colon.[156] However, it has been shown that asymptomatic patients with diverticula do not necessarily have increased intraluminal pressure or decreased stool weight.[157] Nonetheless, increased intraluminal pressure leading to *exaggerated peristaltic contractions sequestering segments of the bowel (segmentation) is correlated with symptomatic disease whether inflammation is present or not.* Thus, we may conclude that *a low-fiber diet, hyperactive peristalsis with segmentation, and increased intraluminal pressure are not requisite for the development of diverticula; however, such deranged motility accounts for most of the symptomatology of this condition.*

CLINICAL COURSE. Most individuals with diverticular disease remain asymptomatic throughout their lives. Indeed, the lesions are most often discovered as incidental findings during barium studies for other reasons or at post-mortem examination. Only about 20% of those affected ever develop manifestations.

These are intermittent, cramping, or sometimes continuous lower abdominal discomfort; constipation; distention; and a sensation of never being able to empty the rectum completely. Sometimes there is alternating constipation and diarrhea. Patients with this condition may have minimal chronic or intermittent bleeding or rarely massive hemorrhages, but before such blood loss is attributed to diverticular disease, other more likely causes must be excluded.

Longitudinal studies have shown that diverticula can regress in the early stages of their development or, conversely, become more numerous with time. Whether a high-fiber diet prevents such progression or protects against superimposed diverticulitis is still unestablished. In most instances patients live comfortably with their diverticula, although some require high-fiber diets such as supplementation with unprocessed bran—leading one improved but revolted patient to grumble: "The treatment may be worse than the disease."[158] Even when diverticulitis supervenes, it most often resolves spontaneously. Only a relatively few patients with symptomatic disease severe enough to lead them to seek hospitalization require surgery for obstructive or inflammatory complications.

MELANOSIS COLI

This curious brown-black discoloration of the mucosa, involving either a large segment or the entire large bowel, is of anatomic interest only, since it never produces clinical symptoms. The mucosal surface is intact and unaltered other than for the pigmentation, which histologically is associated with brown-black pigment granules within large mononuclear cells or macrophages in the lamina propria. Histochemical studies indicate that the pigment has some characteristics of both melanin and lipofuscin. The pigment accumulation has been attributed to the use of cathartics of the anthracene type, including cascara sagrada, senna, aloe, and rhubarb, and indeed can be induced in individuals by the chronic use of these agents. The pigmented lysosomal granules represent phagocytized debris of mucosal cells damaged by the toxic action of the cathartics.[159]

VASCULAR LESIONS

Ischemic injury to the colon, often somewhat inappropriately referred to as ischemic colitis, was discussed on page 862.

HEMORRHOIDS

Hemorrhoids are variceal dilations of the anal and perianal venous plexuses. These extremely common lesions affect about 5% of the general population and are rarely encountered in persons under the age of 30, except in pregnant women. They develop secondary to persistently elevated venous pressure within the hemorrhoidal plexus. The most frequent predisposing influences are constipation with straining at stool and the venous stasis of pregnancy. More rarely, but much more importantly, hemorrhoids may reflect collateral anastomotic channels that develop as a result of portal hypertension.

> The varicosities may develop in the inferior hemorrhoidal plexus and be located below the anorectal line (external hemorrhoids), or they may develop from dilatation of the superior hemorrhoidal plexus and produce internal hemorrhoids (Fig. 18–49). Commonly, both plexuses are affected, and the varicosities are referred to as combined hemorrhoids.
>
> Histologically, these lesions consist only of thin-walled, dilated, typical varices that protrude beneath the anal or rectal mucosa. In their exposed, traumatized situation, they tend to become thrombosed and, in the course of time, canalized. Superficial ulceration, fissure formation, and hemorrhagic infarction with strangulation complicate the histologic picture and clinical problem.

ANGIODYSPLASIA

Tortuous, abnormal dilations of the submucosal veins in the cecum and ascending colon are recognized as a frequent cause of lower gastrointestinal bleeding in the aged.[160] These vascular lesions escaped detection in the past because they were so hard to identify clinically with then-available diagnostic methods.[161] Barium studies do not reveal the vascular dilatations since they are almost entirely intramucosal. The pathologist, too, may miss them as the blood drains out during dissection. Only when colonoscopy and selective mesenteric angiography became available was it possible to identify these lesions.

> Angiodysplasia is most often located within the cecum, but the right colon may also be affected. The vascular alterations range from small, focal, mucosal, vascular ectasias to large, dilated, tortuous, submucosal veins associated with extensive dilatation of thin-walled mucosal venules and capillaries.[162] Rupture of one or more of these abnormal vessels accounts for the colonic bleeding.

The incidence of this condition is not known, but it has been referred to as one of the major causes of unexplained anemia or gastrointestinal bleeding in the aged.[160,163] Most authors believe that they are acquired vascular ectasias that rarely appear before the seventh decade of life. Partial, intermittent obstruction of the submucosal veins where they traverse the muscularis may underlie their development. According to Laplace's law, tension in the wall of a cylinder is a function of intraluminal pressure and diameter. Because the cecum has the widest diameter of the colon, it develops the greatest wall tension. Intermittent occlusion of thin-walled veins then occurs where they pass through the muscularis, raising pressures in the submucosal and mucosal tributaries. Vascular degenerative changes related to aging may also play some role.[160]

INFLAMMATIONS

Certain forms of colitis caused by specific infectious agents were considered together with the involvements of the small intestine on page 865, since inflammations of the small bowel and colon are so closely related. Others are discussed in Chapter 7. There remain to be considered idiopathic ulcerative colitis, pseudomembranous colitis, necrotizing enterocolitis, and so-called collagenous colitis.

IDIOPATHIC ULCERATIVE COLITIS

This form of colitis is a recurrent acute and chronic ulceroinflammatory disorder of unknown etiology af-

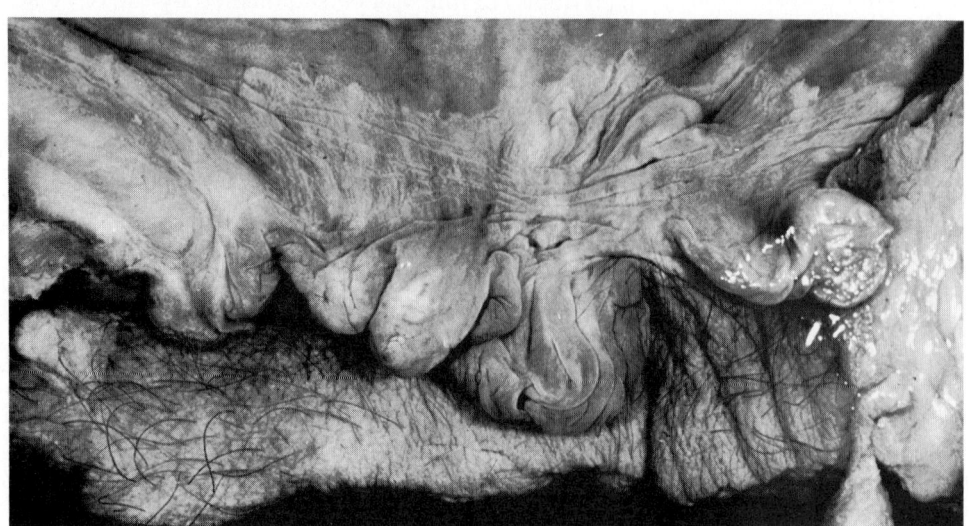

Figure 18–49. Hemorrhoids. External mucosal protrusions containing markedly dilated veins.

fecting principally the rectum and left colon, but sometimes the entire large bowel.[104] Like Crohn's disease, ulcerative colitis is a systemic disorder associated in some patients with migratory polyarthritis, sacroiliitis, ankylosing spondylitis, uveitis, various forms of hepatic involvement, and skin lesions. As mentioned previously, there are many other similarities between the two conditions (p. 868). Thus, there is a growing tendency to refer to both as a single entity— "inflammatory bowel disease" (IBD). However, unlike the granulomatous inflammatory changes in Crohn's disease, well-developed granuloma formation rarely, if ever, appears in ulcerative colitis.

EPIDEMIOLOGY. Ulcerative colitis is global in distribution despite previous misconceptions that it was principally a disease of Western nations. In the United States, Great Britain, and Scandinavia the incidence is about 4 to 6 per 100,000 population. It is much less common in the USSR, Japan, and the South American nations. The incidence of this condition in high-risk locales has risen significantly in the past few decades.[164] In the United States it is more common among whites than among blacks. Females are affected more often than males. The onset of the disease peaks between the ages of 20 and 25 years, but the condition may arise in both younger and considerably older individuals. As with Crohn's disease, there are hints of genetic influences. About 25% of families of patients have other members with ulcerative colitis and/or Crohn's disease.[165] Individuals with both ulcerative colitis and ankylosing spondylitis have an increased frequency of HLA-B27, but this association is related to the spondylitis and not to the ulcerative colitis. The etiology and pathogenesis of IBD have been considered earlier (p. 868).

MORPHOLOGY. Ulcerative colitis invariably begins in the rectum and gradually extends along the colon in a retrograde fashion. It is a disease of continuity, and "skip" lesions such as occur in Crohn's disease are not found (Fig. 18–50). Sometimes one segment of the colon

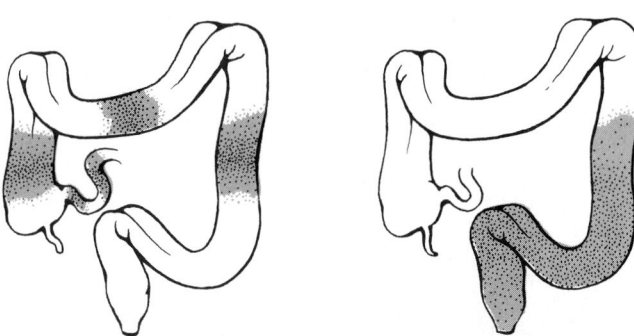

Figure 18–50. Crohn's disease *(left)* **and ulcerative colitis** *(right).* While Crohn's disease typically involves the small and large intestine in a segmental manner with intervening "skip" areas, ulcerative colitis is generally a disease of contiguity that starts in the rectum and progresses in a retrograde fashion to involve varying lengths of the colon.

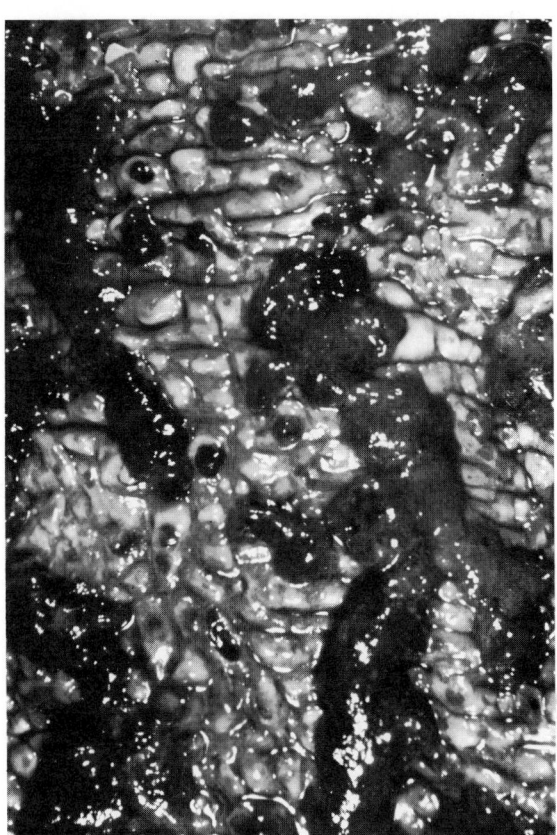

Figure 18–51. Ulcerative colitis. The dark, irregular pattern comprises ulcerations that have in many instances coalesced, leaving virtual islands of residual, paler mucosa. A tendency toward pseudopolyp formation is already evident.

shows active inflammatory ulceration while another segment may be healing, creating the false impression of discontinuous lesions on endoscopic examination. However, such areas invariably show microscopic evidence of inflammation. In severe expressions of ulcerative colitis, with involvement of the entire colon, a "backwash ileitis" may develop in about 10% of patients, but the small intestinal involvement is never as extensive as with fully evolved regional enteritis.[121]

An acute and a chronic phase can be recognized. The hyperemic, edematous mucosa in the acute stage may reveal the absence of the usual mucous secretions. More apparent in the acute disease is the development of small focal mucosal hemorrhages, many of which develop suppurative centers **(crypt abscesses)** that may give rise to small ulcerations. With progression these small ulcers coalesce to become irregular in shape, but rarely do they replicate the linear serpentine fissuring of Crohn's disease (Fig. 18–51). In the usual acute-to-chronic disease the ulcerations are confined to the mucosa and submucosa and do not erode the muscularis. Often the undermined edges of adjacent ulcers interconnect to create tunnels covered by tenuous mucosal bridges (Fig. 18–52). Expansion and coalescence of the ulcers can denude large tracts of the involved colon, and sometimes in severe cases they become deeper to extend into the muscularis. Virtually the entire

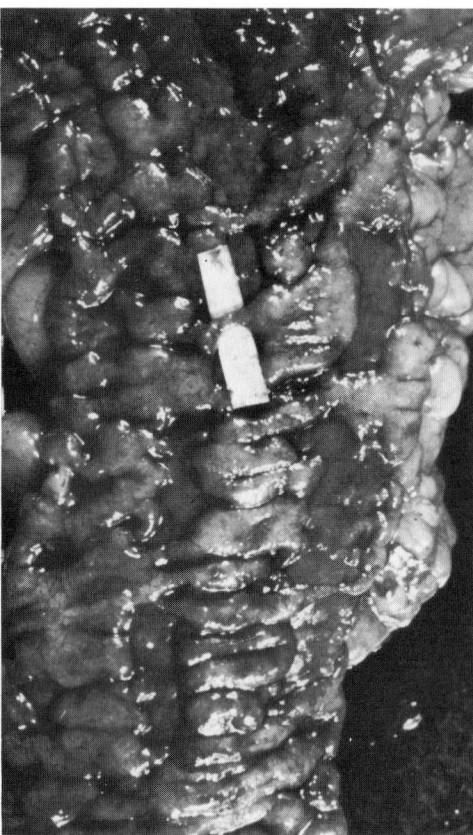

Figure 18–52. Chronic nonspecific ulcerative colitis. The irregular, elongated, seemingly smooth-based ulcers are separated by transversely corrugated strands of persisting mucosa. Coalescence of undermined margins of closely adjacent ulcers has left a bridge of mucosa, seen over the central paper tab.

mucosa may be destroyed, often leaving residual islands of edematous hyperemic mucosa. Swollen, inflammatory tags of mucosa may bulge upward to create inflammatory **"pseudopolyps."** Sometimes, in the very acute severe disease, there is marked "toxic" dilatation of the colon. Indeed, the inflammatory process may create microfissures to penetrate the colonic wall, producing pericolic abscesses, but gross fistulous tracts such as are seen in Crohn's colitis are very rare.

Over the long chronicity of recurring attacks, the ulceroinflammatory disease leads to fibrosis and thickening of the bowel wall, but rarely sufficiently to cause obstruction. With remission the ulcers heal, but the pseudopolyps may remain as well as such residual fibrosis and thickening of the wall as have developed. Particularly important is the possible superimposition of colonic carcinoma, as discussed later.

Histologically, the active phase of disease is characterized by crypt abscesses and ulcerations extending down to the muscularis and surrounded by a prominent mucosal infiltrate of inflammatory cells (Fig. 18–53). The inflammatory process appears to begin within the depths of scattered crypts; as the disease continues and becomes chronic, rupture of the crypts into the lamina propria and into the submucosa permits the process to expand laterally.

In this way the surrounding mucosa is undermined and sloughs to produce an ulceration. The contiguous lamina propria is heavily infiltrated with neutrophils, lymphocytes, plasma cells, and occasionally mast cells. Sometimes the small vessels immediately underlying an ulceration disclose acute vaculitis, raising the possibilities that the ulcerations are the consequence of ischemic necrosis of the mucosa followed by secondary infection, and that the basic process in ulcerative colitis is an immunologically mediated diffuse vasculitis. Important features that help to differentiate ulcerative colitis from Crohn's colitis are as follows: (1) The ulcerations rarely extend significantly into the muscularis, and hence there rarely is fistula formation; (2) the inflammatory reaction is nonspecific and there is no granuloma formation; (3) there are no "skip" lesions as in Crohn's disease; and (4) the inflammatory tags of mucosa, the pseudopolyps, are not seen in Crohn's disease.

Particularly significant in this condition is the spectrum of epithelial changes seen in the inflamed segment of colon, collectively referred to as low- to high-grade dysplasia to overt carcinoma.[166] Sometimes these cytologic changes are present in uninflamed mucosa, some distance from active disease. The severity of the dysplasia and risk of carcinoma are directly related to the extent and duration of the disease in the colon. With extensive involvement or so-called universal (entire colon) involvement, the incidence of carcinoma is about 1% at under 10 years, 3.5% at 15 years, 10 to 15% at 20 years, and over 30% at 30 years.[167] With only left- or right-sided colitis, the risk with long-standing disease is in the range of 3 to 5%. When the involvement is

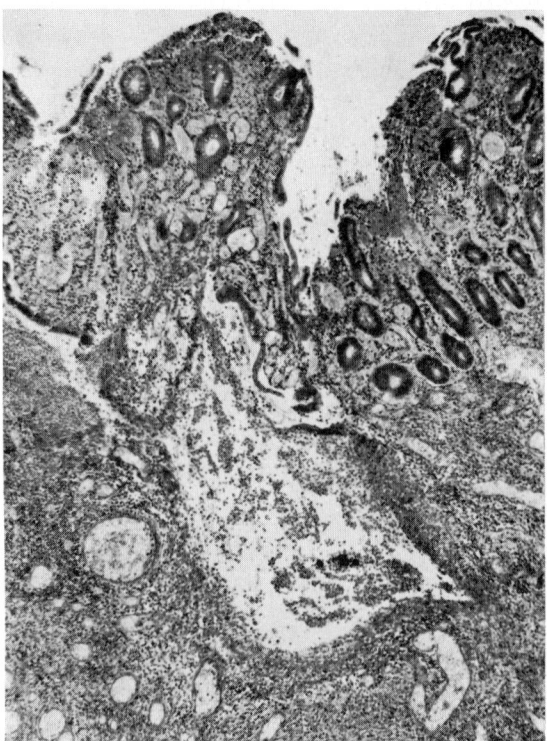

Figure 18–53. A deeply situated mucosal abscess in early developmental stage of acute ulcerative colitis.

Table 18–8. Relative Frequency of Morphologic Findings in Ulcerative Colitis (UC) vs. Crohn's Disease of Colon (CD)

	UC	CD
GROSS FEATURES		
Total colonic involvement	+ + +	+
Distal predominance	+ + + +	+
Right colon predominance	0	+ + +
"Skip" lesions	0	+ + +
Broad-based ulcers	+ + +	+
Serpentine fissures	+	+ + + +
Transmural fibrous thickening	+	+ + + +
Pseudopolyps	+ + +	0 to +
MICROSCOPIC FEATURES		
Granulomas	0	+ +
Nonspecific acute and chronic inflammation	+ + + +	+ +
Crypt abscesses	+ + + +	+
Transmural inflammation	+	+ + +

Modified from Yardley, J.H., and Donowitz, M.: Colorectal biopsy in inflammatory bowel disease. *In* Yardley, J.H., et al. (eds.): The Gastrointestinal Tract. Baltimore, Williams & Wilkins Co., 1977, p. 50.

limited to the rectum, there is less danger of cancer. Ulcerative colitis is typically a recurrent disease. During remissions the mucosa may regenerate, often with the production of a more primitive epithelium lining cystically dilated and atypical glands. The precancerous epithelial changes may persist, however, as does the risk, and so the statement "ten years' duration" does not necessarily imply unremitting active disease.

Although repeated reference has been made to anatomic features that help to differentiate ulcerative colitis from Crohn's disease, experts point out that in about 10 to 20% of resected colonic specimens the colitis is "indeterminate."[168,169] Some of the overlaps and differential features are summarized in Table 18–8.

CLINICAL COURSE. Ulcerative colitis typically presents as a relapsing disorder marked by attacks of bloody mucoid diarrhea that may persist for days, weeks, or months and then subside, only to recur after an asymptomatic interval of months to years or even decades. In the fortunate patient, the first attack is the last. At the other end of the spectrum, the explosive initial attack may lead to such serious bleeding and fluid and electrolyte disturbance as to constitute a medical emergency. In most patients, bloody diarrhea containing stringy mucus as well as lower abdominal pain and cramps, usually relieved by defecation, are the first manifestations of the disease. These appear insidiously but become progressively worse. Often this first attack is preceded by a stressful period in the patient's life. Persistence of the manifestations for even a short time is usually followed by fever and weight loss. Spontaneously, or more often after appropriate therapy, these symptoms abate in the course of days to weeks. An asymptomatic interval of varying length follows, after which, typically, stress (emotional or physical) may cause a flare-up of the

clinical manifestations. Sometimes, concurrent intraluminal growth of *Clostridium difficile* with its enterotoxin provokes the recurrent attack. Sudden cessation of bowel function with production of toxic dilatation of the colon, called toxic megacolon, may appear with any acute attack.

The outlook for patients with this condition depends on two factors: (1) the severity of the disease and (2) its duration. About 60% of patients have what can be called mild disease. In these individuals, the bleeding and diarrhea are not severe, and systemic signs and symptoms are absent. Medical management is usually effective in controlling the manifestations, and the development of colonic cancer is much less frequent than in the severe forms of the disease. About 25% of patients have "fulminant ulcerative colitis." The sudden onset may be characterized by intractable diarrhea, severe bleeding, high fever, and serious electrolyte and fluid disturbances. This toxic form of the disease, unless controlled, can lead to death soon after onset.

As must now be obvious, the most feared long-term complication is cancer.[170–172] There is a greater tendency for carcinomas to arise in multiple sites in these patients than in those without pre-existing colitis. Moreover, the underlying inflammatory disease tends to mask the symptoms and signs of carcinoma, so that these cancers are extremely insidious and inoperable twice as often as those in patients without colitis.[171,172]

PSEUDOMEMBRANOUS COLITIS (PMC)

This entity (also described on p. 360) constitutes an acute form of colitis characterized by pseudomembrane formation overlying sites of mucosal injury. It is usually, if not always, caused by the toxin of *Clostridium difficile*, a normal gut commensal.[173] However, this brief characterization requires qualification. Infrequently, the small intestine is involved, and so the condition sometimes is truly "pseudomembranous enterocolitis." Pseudomembrane formation is not restricted to *C. difficile*; it may result from ischemic injury or other enteric infections with staphylococci, Shigella, and sometimes Candida. *C. difficile* has also been implicated in initiating relapses of chronic IBD.[174] *More often, this organism induces an acute diarrheal colitis in patients without a background of chronic enteric disease who have received broad-spectrum antibiotics, particularly clindamycin and lincomycin.*[175] However, the condition may appear in the absence of antibiotic therapy, typically after surgery or superimposed on some chronic debilitating illness. It has also been recorded as a spontaneous infection in young adults without predisposing influences.[176]

Fully evolved PMC is marked by patchy areas of mucosal inflammation in the large intestine to which are attached dirty, gray-yellow membranous coagula constituting the pseudomembranes. The underlying mucosal surface may reveal very shallow to well-defined ulcerations of the mucosa. Milder expressions may reveal only hyperemia, edema, and thickening of the mucosa without pseudomembrane formation. Microscopically, the pseudomembrane is composed of coagulum of fibrin and mucin containing recognizable inflammatory cells, as well as a potpourri of cellular debris derived from leukocytes and mucosal epithelial cells. Typically, the fibrinomucinous exudate appears to erupt in volcano-like fashion from crypt abscesses in the mucosa. It is the coalescence of the extruded exudate that creates the membranes. There is an intense infiltrate of neutrophils admixed with mononuclear cells in the lamina propria of affected areas.

The diagnosis can be established clinically by identification of the toxin in the stools.

NECROTIZING ENTEROCOLITIS

Necrotizing enterocolitis (NEC), an acute necrotizing inflammation of the small and large intestine, is the most common acquired gastrointestinal emergency of neonates.[177] Although it is said to affect about 10% of infants born at term, its incidence is higher in those born prematurely or with a low birth weight. It may occur at any time during the first three months of life, but its peak incidence is around the time (two to four days) when infants are started on oral foods. Whereas earlier studies had implicated intestinal ischemia as an important contributory factor, subsequent observations documented a high prevalence of NEC in formula-fed infants and a correspondingly low frequency among the breast fed. This suggested that NEC may be caused by a combination of factors, including ischemic injury, microbial agents, the functional immaturity of the immune apparatus in the neonatal gut, and the absence from commercial formulas of certain immunoprotective factors normally present in human milk. Human breast milk is known to contain certain specific (secretory IgA or immunocompetent cells) and nonspecific factors that protect the neonate against gastrointestinal infections.[178,179]

The disease may manifest with a variety of symptoms such as abdominal distress, tenderness, ileus, diarrhea, and frank gastrointestinal bleeding; intestinal perforation, gangrene, peritonitis, or sepsis and shock may supervene. Radiologic evidence of ileus and the presence of gas in the bowel wall (pneumatosis intestinalis), under the diaphragm, or in the biliary passages are ominous signs usually seen in well-established cases.[177] The disease most commonly affects the terminal ileum, cecum, and ascending colon, but in severe cases the entire bowel may be involved. The histologic changes are quite variable depending on the stage of the disease and are characterized by mucosal edema, hemorrhage, and necrosis in the early phases, with the formation of a pseudomembrane of fibrinous exudate, polymorphonuclear

leukocytes, and necrotic cellular debris covering the necrotic mucosa and submucosa. As the disease progresses, the involvement spreads longitudinally to involve larger areas and transmurally to involve the muscle coats as well, sometimes leading to perforation and peritonitis.

While treatment in the early stages is directed at correction of the fluid and electrolyte imbalance, maintenance of blood pressure, and reversal of the shocklike state, the onset of gangrene and perforation of the diseased bowel require prompt surgical intervention. Long-term complications developing in these patients include malabsorption, strictures, short bowel syndrome secondary to ileal resection, and recurrence of the disease.

COLLAGENOUS COLITIS

This recently recognized form of colitis is a distinct clinicopathologic entity characterized clinically by a history of chronic or episodic watery diarrhea, and pathologically by the presence of a distinct collagenous band beneath the colonic surface epithelium.[180] This form of colitis almost always occurs in patients 30 years or older (mean age 60 years) and affects women about four times as commonly as men.[181] Although an occasional patient may have bloody diarrhea or mild steatorrhea, most patients characteristically present with a watery diarrhea that is never so severe or protracted as to cause dehydration. Of particular interest, patients with collagenous colitis very often also have a variety of autoimmune and other diseases (e.g., thyroiditis and hypothyroidism, arthritis, rheumatic fever, myasthenia gravis, temporal arteritis, chronic hepatitis, atrophic gastritis type A, diabetes mellitus, duodenal ulcer, and obstructive pulmonary disease), and a high proportion of those tested show a positive rheumatoid factor and antinuclear antibody.[181,182]

Radiologically the colonic mucosa is generally unremarkable, and it may be deceptively "normal" on endoscopy even when florid changes are present on histologic examination. This underscores the need for obtaining mucosal biopsies and securing histologic confirmation in suspected cases. Furthermore, since both the intensity of the inflammatory (colitis) component and the distribution and thickness of the subepithelial collagenous band may vary from area to area, it is imperative that such biopsies be obtained from multiple sites.[183]

The histologic features in a full-blown case of collagenous colitis include damage to the surface epithelium, which may become detached as a layer from the underlying lamina propria. The surface epithelial cells show varying degrees of cuboidalization, loss of mucin content, cytoplasmic vacuolation, and an infiltration of large numbers of lymphocytes, polymorphs, and eosinophils. The immediate subepithelial zone shows the deposition of a hypocellular collagenous band in which congested capillaries can occasionally be identified.[183] The lamina propria contains increased numbers of acute and chronic inflammatory infiltrates. In sharp contrast to the extensive degenerative changes seen in the surface epithelial cells, the crypt epithelium is well preserved; although occasional crypt abscesses may be present, they are never as numerous or prominent a feature as in ulcerative colitis. It should be noted that while the presence of a subepithelial collagenous band is the histologic hallmark of collagenous colitis, it is often discontinuous in its distribution and is often indistinct. Furthermore, similar, although considerably thinner, collagenous bands have been observed in ulcerative colitis and Crohn's colitis. Thus differential diagnosis between these conditions, so important for patient management, can be difficult if the characteristic collagenous band is absent, indistinct, or thin.[183] The absence of a significant degree of crypt distortion or crypt atrophy and the paucity of crypt abscesses despite severe damage to the surface epithelium are histologic features that favor a diagnosis of collagenous colitis.

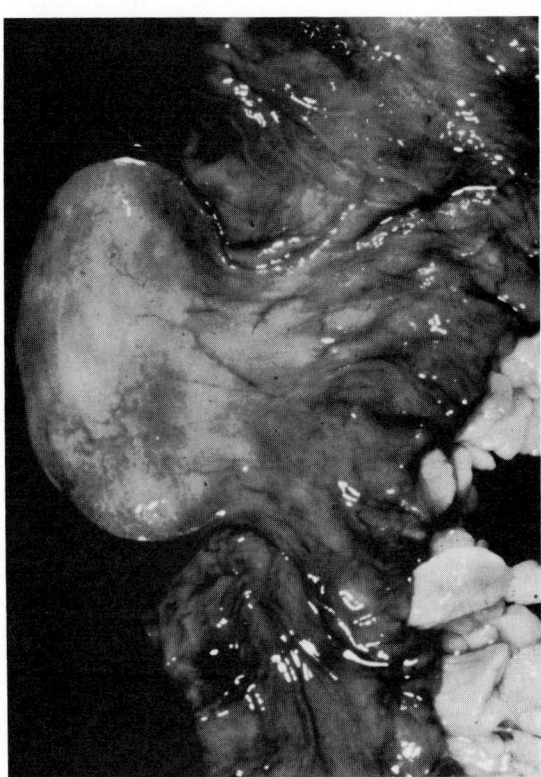

Figure 18–54. Submucosal lipoma in colon, which has been pedunculated by traction of intestinal peristalsis.

The exact mechanism for the watery diarrhea remains unresolved. While some workers have proposed that it is secretory in nature, others believe that the diarrhea is related to the damaged surface epithelium and represents a "malabsorption of water and electrolytes." Similarly, the etiology of collagenous colitis continues to elude us. Based on its strong female predominance and its strong association with a number of different autoimmune disorders, current opinion suggests that collagenous colitis may be another autoimmune disease.[181]

TUMORS

The colon (as used here to include the rectum) is the segment of the gastrointestinal tract most frequently affected by tumors. Bronchogenic cancer "holds the grisly trophy" for being the leading cancer killer, but colonic carcinoma is second; the respective number of deaths in the United States in 1988 were estimated at 139,000 and 61,500. Benign tumors such as lipomas, leiomyomas, angiomas, and mesenchymal lesions may occur here (Fig. 18–54), but the great majority of benign tumors are epithelial polyps. These are even more common than cancers and are present in as many as 25 to 50% of older adults.[184] Many are non-neoplastic and are referred to as hyperplastic polyps, hamartomatous polyps, inflammatory polyps, or lymphoid polyps. However, some are true neoplasms and are generically referred to as adenomas. These have great importance because they represent precursors of colonic cancer.[185] Both adenomatous polyps and colonic carcinomas represent a challenge to clinical medicine, since diagnostic modalities are widely available for their early discovery when cure can be achieved by resection. Thus, each death from colonic cancer in the United States must be viewed as a preventable tragedy.

POLYPS AND POLYPOSIS SYNDROMES

Polyps and polypoid lesions are essentially protruding space-occupying lesions within a hollow viscus. When used in a pathologic sense, *the term "polyp" is usually restricted to mucosal growths—both benign and malignant*—whereas others, including inflammatory masses, hamartomas, and tumors arising from the submucosa or the muscle coats should be referred to as polypoid lesions.

Polyposis signifies the presence of multiple polyps, whereas "polyposis syndrome" is an expression applied to a variety of different syndromes characterized by the presence of multiple pedunculated or sessile tumors of the mucosa in the stomach, duodenum, small bowel, colon, or rectum. Although polyposis most frequently involves the entire gastrointestinal tract, it may be confined to a single segment, most often the large bowel. Although these conditions can be detected by clinical, endoscopic, and radiologic examination, the various syndromes are in most instances differentiated only after a histologic examination of one or more polyps, since each of the syndromes is associated with a specific type of polyp.

Colorectal polyps are conventionally categorized into two major groups—the *non-neoplastic* and the *neoplastic* polyps (Table 18–9). Each category includes polyps of different histologic appearance that, at least in the non-neoplastic category, reflects their

Table 18–9. Classification of Colorectal Polyps

NON-NEOPLASTIC POLYPS	NEOPLASTIC POLYPS
Hyperplastic polyp	Benign
Hamartomatous polyp	Tubular adenoma
Inflammatory polyp	Tubulovillous adenoma
Lymphoid polyp	Villous adenoma
	Malignant
	Polypoid carcinoma

mode of origin. The various types of neoplastic polyps, however, represent a histologic continuum that extends from tubular adenomas at one end of the spectrum to polypoid carcinoma at the other. Each of the polyps and their associated syndromes, if any, will be discussed in the following sections.

All epithelial polyps arise from the cells deep in the crypts of the colonic mucosal glands. *Normally, cell division in the colonic mucosa is restricted to the deepest third of the crypt.* Presumably, in the formation of epithelial polyps the controlling mechanisms of cell division are deranged, and lead to the formation of hyperplastic or neoplastic lesions.[186] Thus, it is proposed that *some loss of growth control in a slightly expanded zone of crypt cells leads to a hyperplastic polyp. A more complete loss of controls along the entire crypt results in a neoplastic polyp.* In the course of such changes, the cells along the entire depth of the crypt (including the upper two thirds) retain their capacity to divide. It would appear that mechanisms that normally shut off DNA synthesis in the upper two thirds of the crypt are to a greater or lesser extent lost. The ultimate size of the neoplastic polyp may be a function of time, the extent of loss of growth controls, the adequacy of the blood supply, or other factors still unknown.

Non-neoplastic Polyps

HYPERPLASTIC POLYPS. These represent 90% of all epithelial polyps in autopsy surveys, but account for only 15 to 20% of surgically removed polyps because most are asymptomatic and removed only when discovered in the course of investigations for other reasons. They may arise at any age but are usually diagnosed in the sixth and seventh decades.

About 60 to 80% are located in the rectosigmoid, 20% in the ascending colon, and the remainder in other colonic locations.[187] Typically, they are smooth, moist, round, dewdrop-sized, sessile lesions sitting on top of a mucosal fold. They may occur singly, but multiple polyps are very frequent. In autopsies 90% are less than 5 mm in diameter, but surgical specimens tend to be larger because with enlargement they are more likely to be symptomatic. Large lesions may have a short broad stalk and thus resemble the pedunculated tubular adenoma. Histologically, they are composed of well-formed glands and crypts lined by non-neoplastic epithelial cells, most of which show differentiation into either mature goblet or absorptive cells. Owing to

infoldings of the crowded epithelial cells, the linings often develop a serrate or sawtooth luminal profile. The glands and crypts are separated by connective tissue resembling the lamina propria. Larger hyperplastic polyps sometimes develop foci of adenomatous change, described below.

The major clinical significance of these lesions is their differentiation from the more ominous adenomatous polyps. The small, sessile, moist lesions are reasonably distinctive. The rare hyperplastic polyp with a stalk may be diagnosed as such only after a histologic examination. While *pure hyperplastic polyps have no malignant potential in general, a small proportion of those with adenomatous foci may undergo neoplastic transformation.*

JUVENILE POLYPS. Representing developmental malformations affecting the glands and lamina propria, these lesions consist of essentially normal mucosal components arranged abnormally, and hence they are categorized as *hamartomatous polyps.* They may occur sporadically or be associated with a *juvenile polyposis syndrome* transmitted by autosomal dominant inheritance. The vast majority of juvenile polyps, whether sporadic or in the polyposis syndrome, occur in children below the age of five years; the frequency tapers sharply thereafter. Nearly 80% of sporadic juvenile polyps occur in the rectum, while the rest may be scattered anywhere throughout the colon. Usually single or few in number, these polyps give rise to painless rectal bleeding after defecation and may occasionally lead to iron deficiency anemia.

Typically, they are large, rounded, smooth or faintly lobulated lesions with a stalk that may reach up to 2 cm in length. The larger lesions undergo secondary ulceration, inflammation, and bleeding. The large "head" on a stalk frequently causes the lesions to undergo torsion, infarction, and autoamputation, when they may be passed in the stool. Histologically, they are characterized by mucus-filled, cystically dilated tubules lined by normal or inflamed mucosa. The intervening lamina propria is rather abundant, forms the bulk of the polyp, and is usually inflamed. The surface may be congested or ulcerated.

These polyps merely represent a developmental aberration and have no malignant potential. When associated with the *juvenile polyposis syndrome*, multiple polyps occur throughout the gastrointestinal tract but are most numerous in the colon and stomach. However, the number of colorectal polyps in these patients may decrease with age as the polyps undergo autoamputation. The gross and microscopic features of the polyps in the polyposis syndrome are identical to those seen in the more common solitary lesion.

PEUTZ-JEGHERS POLYPS. These lesions are also hamartomatous polyps. They may occur singly or multiply in the *Peutz-Jeghers syndrome.*

The Peutz-Jeghers syndrome is characterized by autosomal dominant inheritance: multiple Peutz-Jeghers polyps scattered throughout the entire gastrointestinal tract, and melanotic mucosal and cutaneous pigmentation around the lips, oral mucosa, face, genitalia, and palmar surfaces of the hands.[188-190] The distribution of polyps in patients is said to be stomach 25%, colon 30%, and small bowel 100%. Regardless of whether they occur as solitary or as multiple lesions in the Peutz-Jeghers syndrome, the polyps tend to be large and pedunculated with a firm lobulated contour. They may occur anywhere in the gastrointestinal tract but most often arise in the small bowel. Histologically, they consist of a branching framework of connective tissue and smooth muscle lined by normal intestinal epithelium rich in goblet cells. The polyp has an arborizing pattern of growth, and the glands are elongated and convoluted.

While these hamartomatous polyps themselves do not have malignant potential, patients with the Peutz-Jeghers syndrome have an increased risk of developing carcinomas of the pancreas, breast, lung, ovary, and uterus. When these patients develop gastrointestinal cancer, it appears to arise not from the hamartomatous polyps but from coexistent adenomas.

INFLAMMATORY POLYPS. These polyps occur in patients with long-standing inflammatory bowel disease, and are most commonly observed in chronic ulcerative colitis and rarely in Crohn's disease with extensive colonic involvement. They result from reepithelialization of ulcers and overgrowth of the overhanging margins, and usually appear as blunt-tipped, wormlike mucosal tags without any distinction between the head and stalk. Histologically they show a central cylindrical connective tissue core with an inflammatory infiltrate and a superficial covering of distorted regenerating intestinal epithelium with a few cystically dilated glands. Since these lesions represent an exuberant reparative response to long-standing full-thickness mucosal injury rather than true epithelial proliferations, they have in the past also been referred to as *pseudopolyps*. These lesions are usually multiple and may occur in a segmental or diffuse distribution in the colon. They have no malignant potential and are not associated with any syndrome. Carcinomas occurring in inflammatory bowel disease arise from areas showing dysplastic changes and *not* from these polyps.

LYMPHOID POLYPS. These polyps occur as a mucosal protrusion secondary to a reactive hyperplasia of the mucosal and submucosal lymphoid tissues. Since such lymphoid tissue is normally dispersed throughout the gastrointestinal tract, and particularly in the terminal ileum and the rectum, these polyps may involve the gut in a localized or diffuse fashion (polyposis). The diffuse form is uncommon and occurs in children and young adults, whereas the more common localized form affects the rectum in elderly individuals. Invariably small and asymptomatic, lymphoid polyps in both the solitary and the diffuse forms show an orderly arrangement of enlarged lymphoid follicles with prominent germinal centers occupying the mucosa and submucosa. The overlying epithelium shows some inflammation but is otherwise unremarkable. The lesion has no malignant potential but needs to be distinguished from malignant lymphoma involving the bowel wall. A familial incidence has been described, but this does not appear to be genetic in origin.

Neoplastic Polyps

This group of polyps, generically referred to as adenomas, includes the tubular adenomas, villous adenomas, tubulovillous adenomas, and polypoid carcinomas. While the polypoid carcinoma is clearly a malignant lesion and the others are its benign counterparts, all are neoplastic proliferations of epithelial origin and protrude into the lumen as space-occupying lesions. Each type may be pedunculated (i.e., have a stalk) or sessile and may be solitary or multiple. In the context of neoplastic polyps, it should be borne in mind that while tubular adenomas and villous adenomas have distinctly different gross and microscopic appearances, they merely represent different growth patterns of the same neoplastic process. Tubulovillous adenomas have features common to both and occupy an intermediate position in this scheme. Neoplastic polyps, especially the tubular adenomas, are associated with specific polyposis syndromes that are characterized by an increased risk for developing colon cancer.

TUBULAR ADENOMA. About 75% of all neoplastic polyps are tubular adenomas. Because of this predominance they are sometimes referred to as adenomatous polyps. Tubular adenomas occur sporadically in the general population but are also encountered in certain well-defined hereditary syndromes. In one large series, the average age of patients having sporadic tubular adenomas was 60 years, with a male preponderance of $2:1$.[191] The frequency progressively increases after 30 years of age. These are the lesions that sit in the center of the "adenoma-carcinoma sequence" controversy.

Tubular adenomas are found mainly in the distal colon and rectum (75%). About 50 to 60% arise in the rectosigmoid and are accessible to sigmoidoscopic examination. **More than 50% of sporadic tubular adenomas occur singly. In about 30 to 40% of cases two or more are present simultaneously, and one sixth of patients have more than five.**[192,193] In practical clinical terms, when a single tubular adenoma is present, there is a 20% chance of finding an additional one or more within five years; this increases to 40% when multiple polyps are present. Most often the polyps have slender stalks and raspberry-like heads. Occasionally they are sessile, ovoid, or hemispheric lesions or, rarely, flat and plaque-like. The heads of the pedunculated lesions range in size from a few millimeters to many centimeters in diameter, and the stalks from 1 cm to several centimeters in length.[193] Transection discloses a central core of fibrovascular tissue that arises in the submucosa and extends in continuity through the center of the stalk and head (Fig. 18–55). The stalk is usually covered with normal colonic mucosa, but in the head of the lesion the polypoid epithelium is clearly neoplastic and composed of closely aggregated, elongated tubules and glands separated by a scant connective tissue stroma. The epithelial cells lining these configurations show poor differentiation into the two normal cell types, although scattered goblet cells may persist. **The cytologic atypia of the neoplastic cells and their lack of differentiation into specialized cell types most clearly separate neoplastic polyps from hyperplastic polyps.** The cells are tall and crowded and have pseudostratified nuclei, giving the appearance of a "picket fence." It should be noted that while most tubular adenomas are made up entirely of uniform-sized tubules or glands, a small proportion contain areas with villous features. By generally accepted convention, when up to 20 or 25% villous areas are present, the lesions are still referred to as tubular adenomas. In most instances, when carcinomatous change occurs in a tubular adenoma, it does so in the villous areas.[194] In such areas marked nuclear hyperchromasia and an increase in the nuclear-cytoplasmic ratio are usually present. A range of dysplasia and atypia is encountered. At one end of the spectrum, in the tubular adenomas the cells lining the tubules and glands have oc-

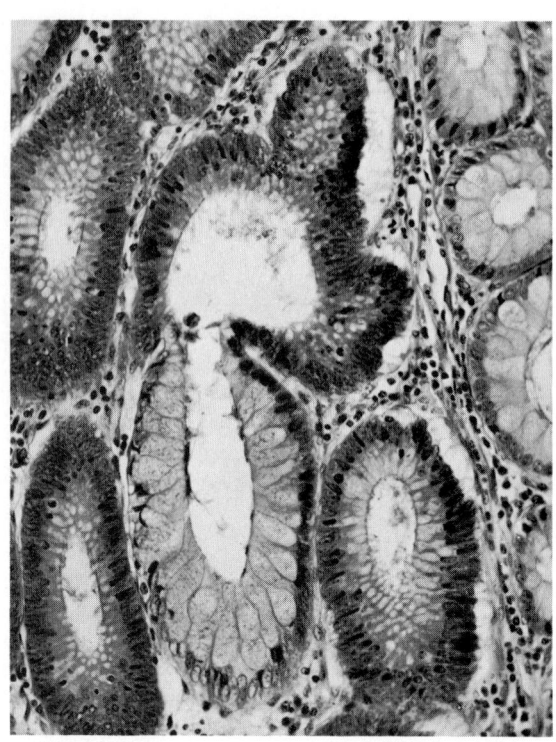

Figure 18–56. High-power detail of a junctional group of glands at point of transition between normal colonic mucosa and polypoid atypicality. A striking comparison is evident between regular, columnar, mucus-secreting epithelium and atypical, but not cancerous, polypoid epithelium.

casional mitoses and some hyperchromasia, but anaplasia is absent (Fig. 18–56). As would be expected of a benign lesion, there is no evidence of penetration of glands or cells into the central fibrovascular core. From this clearly innocent end of the spectrum all degrees of cytologic atypia and dysplasia may be encountered, to the extreme of unmistakable anaplasia indicative of carcinoma. Glands crypts tend to be more closely packed and sometimes "back to back." In these areas there is cell crowding and increase in nuclear size as well as hyperchromasia; the cells lose their normal palisaded array and pile up upon one another. Mitotic figures become more numerous and abnormal. **The atypical epithelium may remain restricted within the glandular basement membranes (carcinoma in situ) or invade the fibrovascular core.** It is now generally agreed that as long as the carcinoma is entirely intramucosal it has little, if any, metastatic potential. Resection of such lesions along with a peripheral rim of uninvolved mucosa and submucosa (such as is present in the stalk of a pedunculated lesion) is regarded as curative. When, on the other hand, the highly dysplastic cells and glands are seen invading beyond the muscularis mucosae into the submucosa, the lesion is invasive and has metastatic potential.

The diagnosis of carcinoma in a tubular adenoma can be treacherous and ultimately is subjective, accounting for the great variability in the reported frequencies of cancer in tubular ademonas. Clear-cut

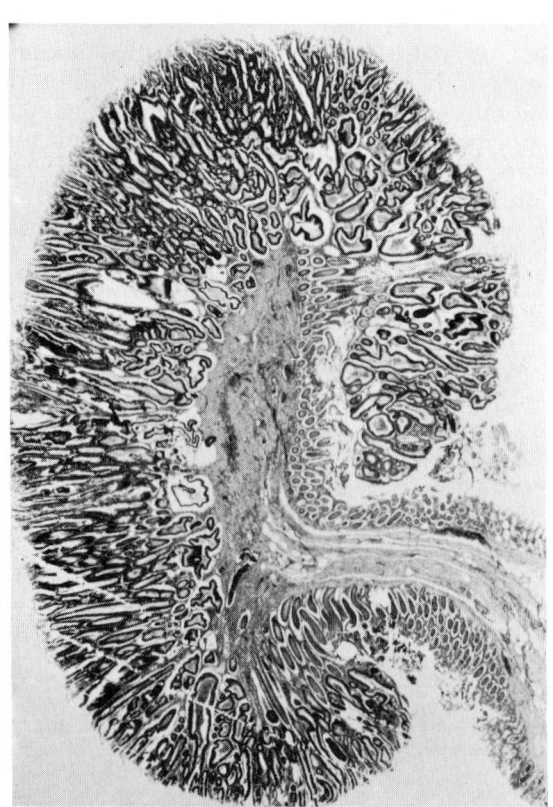

Figure 18–55. Low-power view of a slender-stalked colonic polyp indicating increased chromaticity and height of glands covering head of lesion.

invasion of the fibrovascular core, particularly when it extends through the muscularis mucosae, is the most reliable criterion. The following generalizations are relevant. *Tubular adenomas less than 1 cm in diameter, which make up between 60 and 70% of all adenomatous polyps in the colon, have a 1% chance of containing invasive tumor. In those 1 to 2 cm in size, the risk of cancer rises to 10% in parallel with the proportion of villous architecture. In those greater than 2 cm in diameter, the risk of cancer is even higher (45%). Overall, because most of these lesions are small when discovered, the incidence of carcinoma is about 3 to 5%.*[195,196]

Recent genetic linkage studies indicate that an inherited susceptibility to adenomatous polyps and colorectal cancer is common with a gene frequency of 19%.[197]

VILLOUS ADENOMA. Any colonic adenoma that is more than 50% villous in architecture is called a villous adenoma. These are the least common, the largest, and the most ominous of the epithelial polyps. They are usually first identified in patients 60 to 65 years of age; uncommonly they occur under the age of 50. Males and females are affected almost equally.

The distribution of these lesions in the colon closely parallels that of colon cancer. The vast majority (75%) are located in the rectum and rectosigmoid area; the cecum and ascending colon are the next most common sites, while the remainder are scattered elsewhere in the colon. They range in size from less than 1 cm to 10 cm in diameter. The great

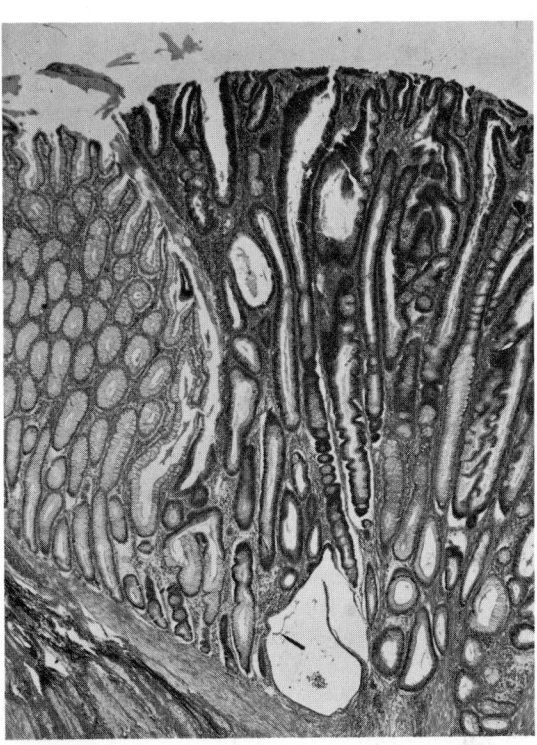

Figure 18–58. Junction between normal colonic mucosa on left and sessile polyp on right. Polypoid area reveals crowded papillae covered by hyperchromatic epithelium with loss of mucus secretion, sometimes containing cross sections of glands representing a tubuloadenomatous component.

preponderance are broad, sessile, slightly lobular, velvety gray-tan lesions projecting along a broad front about 1 to 3 cm above the surrounding mucosa (Fig. 18–57). Focal areas of hemorrhage or surface ulcerations are sometimes present. Infrequently, they have a broad, short stalk.

Histologically, at least half of the villous adenoma is composed of finger-like, or sometimes branching, papillae covered by polypoid epithelium. The residual portion may have tubular features. **There is an almost linear correlation between the size of the polyp and its proportion of villous features.**[196] Each papilla is composed of a fibrovascular core covered by epithelium ranging (among the various lesions) from a single layer of regularly aligned, tall columnar cells to unmistakably anaplastic cells having a disorderly multilayered arrangement (Fig. 18–58). In the anaplastic areas, the individual cells have large hyperchromatic nuclei, and mitoses may be numerous. Carcinoma in situ, without invasion of the underlying fibrovascular core or submucosa of the colon, is present in about 10% of villous adenomas, with frank invasive carcinoma in an additional 25 to 40% (average among series, 30%).[198]

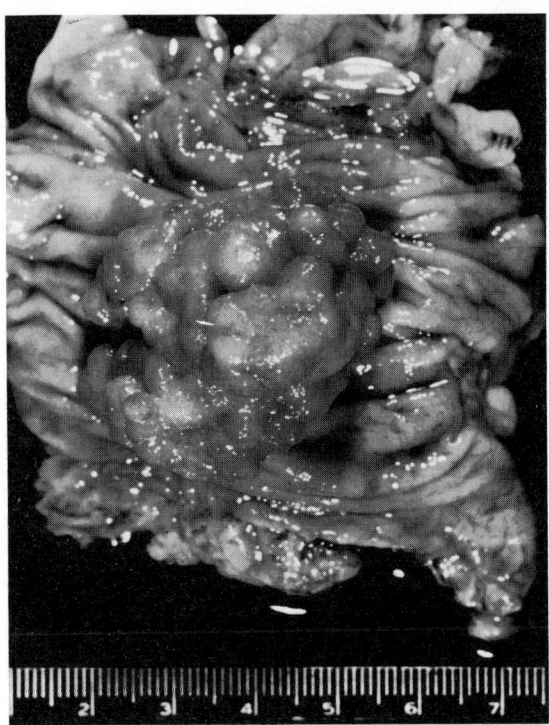

Figure 18–57. Close-up of villous sessile polyp of colon that, on histologic examination, proved to be benign.

Villous adenomas are symptomatic much more frequently than are tubular adenomas. Most commonly they cause rectal bleeding, but they infrequently may hypersecrete copious amounts of mucoid material that is sufficiently rich in protein to produce hypoproteinemia, particularly hypoalbuminemia, constituting in effect a protein-losing enteropathy. In addition, the mucous secretion may cause hypokalemia. Rarely, the villous lesions may induce persistent diarrhea and significant loss of fluid and other electrolytes.

There is no dispute that *villous adenomas are precancerous lesions that harbor invasive cancers in about one third of cases.* Thus, diagnosis at the earliest possible moment and adequate resection are imperative, especially so in the larger lesions that have a considerably higher risk of harboring a malignancy.

TUBULOVILLOUS ADENOMA. Tubulovillous adenomas, as the name implies, combine features of both tubular and villous adenomas. By definition, the villous component ranges between 20–25 and 50%. As already noted, lesions with less than 20 to 25% villous architecture are defined as tubular adenomas, and those with more than 50% as villous adenomas. With their proportion of villous elements, the malignant potential of tubulovillous adenomas is about halfway between the other two types.[196]

The distribution of these lesions in the colon is the same as that of tubular adenomas. They range in diameter from 0.5 to 5 cm and thus are intermediate between tubular and villous adenomas. Most have a stalk and are macroscopically indistinguishable from tubular adenomas, but they have a slightly greater tendency to sessile growth. The histologic appearance covers a wide spectrum from that of the clearly benign tubular adenoma to all levels of atypia and anaplasia, extending to invasive carcinoma in the villous areas. Differentiation of tubulovillous lesions from the other two forms can be accomplished only microscopically.

Relationship of Neoplastic Polyps to Carcinoma

It has already been emphasized that all neoplastic polyps have malignant potential, greatest with the villous adenoma and least with the pure tubular adenoma. *Studies have shown that the probability of carcinoma occurring in a neoplastic polyp is related to (1) the size of the polyp, (2) the relative proportion of its villous component, and (3) the presence of significant cytologic atypia (dysplasia) in the neoplastic cells.*[196] It is, however, important to remember that these three features are interrelated. Thus, large polyps tend to be made up of a higher proportion of villous elements, and such areas in turn frequently show a higher degree of dysplasia than is seen in the nonvillous component. Since evaluation of both the villous component and the degree of dysplasia in a polyp requires histologic examination (and hence excision) of the entire polyp, size of the polyp appears to be the only helpful preoperative guideline for predicting the presence or absence of cancer within a polyp. *Thus, it has been shown that the incidence of cancer in polyps under 1 cm in diameter is very low indeed; between 1 and 2 cm the incidence rises to about 10%; those above this size are cancerous in up to 45% of instances.* Molecular biologic studies are consistent with a model of colorectal tumorigenesis in which the steps required for the development of a cancer from a polyp involve the mutational activation of an oncogene coupled with the sequential loss of several tumor suppressor genes. Thus, colorectal carcinomas frequently exhibit mutations of the *ras* oncogene together with allelic deletions of chromosomes 5, 17, and 18.[199] Current evidence thus suggests that the vast majority of colonic cancers arise in pre-existing neoplastic polyps. However, in view of the foregoing discussion it must be emphasized that the risk for cancer lies not so much in having a polyp but in whether the polyp will turn malignant. It is clear that not all neoplastic polyps will turn malignant, and even the few that do take several years, perhaps a decade or more, to do so.[196]

Familial Polyposis Syndromes

In a few instances, the tendency to develop neoplastic polyps of the colon is familial, most often with an autosomal dominant mode of transmission.[188–190] In many cases, the polyps are associated with developmental abnormalities outside the intestinal tract. The three more important of this group are familial multiple polyposis of the colon, Gardner's syndrome, and Turcot's syndrome. You recall that in the Peutz-Jeghers syndrome the multiple polyps are hamartomatous (p. 892).

Familial polyposis coli (FPC) is characterized by the presence of innumerable neoplastic polyps in the colon (Fig. 18–59). Virtually carpeting the entire colon, these polyps are sometimes so closely packed that they are too numerous to count. Radiologically this imparts a furry appearance to the mucosa. The disease is inherited as an autosomal dominant trait. While there is considerable variation in the age at which polyposis is first diagnosed, most cases are identified in the second and third decades of life, and nearly 20% are diagnosed after the age of 40. It is thus impossible to estimate at what age a patient ceases to be at risk of developing the disease.

Patients with FPC have an average of about 1000 polyps in their colons, with most having between 500 and 2500. Occasionally, they may have as few as 150 polyps. Thus, a patient has to have more than 100 neoplastic polyps in the colon before a diagnosis of FPC can be considered. Occasionally, similar neoplastic polyps may also appear in the stomach, duodenum, or small intestine.

Histologically, the vast majority of the polyps in FPC are tubular adenomas, although occasional ones may also show villous features admixed within them. There is a very high incidence of malignant transformation of polyps in this condition. Some patients already have cancer of the colon or rectum at the time of diagnosis. It has been estimated that unless the diseased colon is removed, the risk of colorectal cancer developing in FPC is 100%. The longer the adenomas are permitted to remain in the colon, the greater is the risk of malignancy.

Once a diagnosis of FPC has been made, a pro-

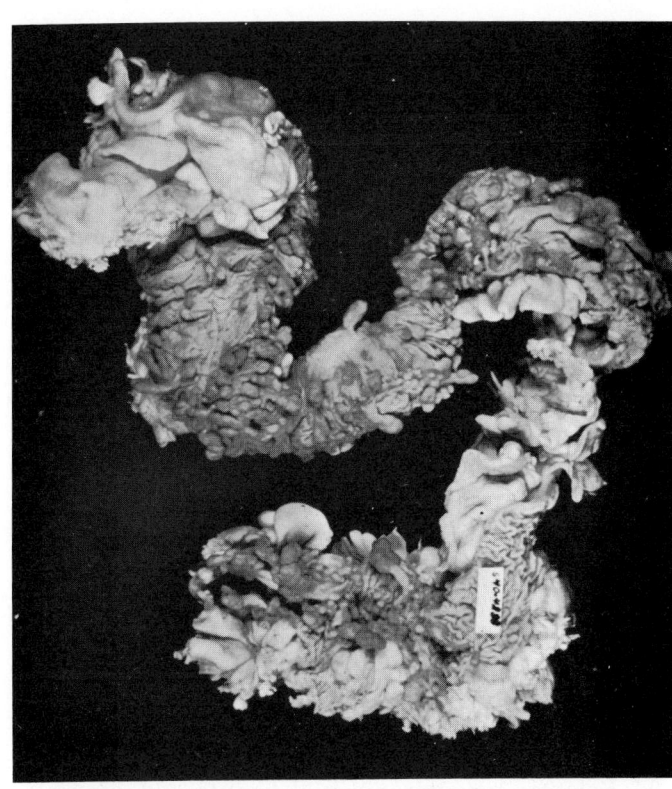

Figure 18–59. Heredofamilial polyposis of colon. Bowel is studded with numerous small polyps.

phylactic colectomy or proctocolectomy is usually recommended. Follow-up studies on patients with FPC who did not undergo colectomies for various reasons have shown a 10% incidence of colon cancer at 10 years, 50% at 20 years, and 100% at 30 years. Cancer-preventive measures in FPC thus include a prophylactic colectomy as soon as possible, and the early detection of the disease in other siblings and first-degree relatives at risk. These individuals should be evaluated radiologically and endoscopically, beginning at age 15 or so and at periodic two- to three-year intervals if the initial examinations are negative. Such a surveillance program to intercept the progress of FPC has reduced the incidence of colon cancer from 66% to 7.5% in those called up for examination because they were at risk.[200]

Gardner's syndrome consists of a combination of polyposis coli (identical to that in FPC), multiple osteomas, epidermal cysts, and fibromatosis. Also present, but not as frequently, are abnormalities of dentition, such as unerupted and supernumerary teeth, and a higher frequency of duodenal and thyroid cancer.[188,190,201] The syndrome is transmitted as an autosomal dominant trait with variable expressivity, and patients have the same high risk of developing colon cancer as those with FPC. Most workers believe that Gardner's syndrome and FPC are essentially one and the same disease caused by an abnormality of a pleiotropic gene. The basic manifestation is the colonic polyposis; the wider spectrum of abnormalities seen in Gardner's syndrome is due to variable penetrance of the genetic mutation. Thus, the term Gardner's syndrome is reserved for those cases with extracolonic manifestations.[201]

Turcot's syndrome is a rare variant marked by the combination of multiple colonic polyposis and tumors of the central nervous system.[190,201,202]

MALIGNANT TUMORS

Carcinoma

Virtually 98% of all cancers in the large intestine are carcinomas. They represent one of the prime challenges to the medical profession, because they arise in polyps and produce symptoms relatively early and at this stage are generally curable by resection. Too often, these early symptoms are largely ignored by the patient and sometimes insufficiently investigated by the physician.

Colorectal cancer is the second most common form of visceral cancer (after lung) in the United States. With nearly 150,000 new cases being diagnosed each year and about 60,000 deaths caused by it, this disease accounts for nearly 15% of all cancer-related deaths in the United States.

EPIDEMIOLOGY, ETIOLOGY, AND PATHOGENESIS. The incidence of colorectal cancer shows marked variation throughout the world—being high in the United States, Saskatchewan in Canada, the United Kingdom, New Zealand, Australia, Denmark, and Sweden, and relatively low in Colombia, Japan, India, South Africa, Israel, Finland, Poland, and Puerto Rico. Except in Japan, where its incidence is low, colorectal cancer appears to be a "disease of affluence," since its incidence closely parallels the socioeconomic standards of the various countries. These geographic variations in incidence are also associated with significant differences in the distributional pattern of the tumors within the colon. Thus, in the low-incidence countries, the lesions tend to be more frequently located in the cecum and ascending colon, whereas in the high-incidence locales they are most frequently concentrated in the rectum and sigmoid colon. It is of interest that in the United States and other developed countries, this distributional pattern is slowly changing, toward an increase in the incidence of carcinoma of the right colon.[203,204] A study from a Boston area hospital has shown that between 1928 and 1967 the relative incidence of right colon cancer rose from 7% to 22%, while the relative frequency of rectal, rectosigmoid, and sigmoid cancers fell from 80% to 62%.[205] A similar decrease in the relative frequency of rectal and sigmoid carcinomas has been reported from the Philadelphia area.[206] This decreasing incidence of rectosigmoid carcinomas is most likely related to the increasing use of flexible sigmoidoscopic instruments and the more aggressive removal of "suspicious-looking" adenomatous polyps within reach of the instrument.[205]

Relative to environmental factors and dietary practices, studies on Japanese and Polish immigrants to the United States have shown that although these groups came from low-incidence areas, within a period of 20 years they acquired an incidence comparable to that of native Americans.[207,208] It is noteworthy that both groups, for the most part, had turned to the dietary practices of their adoptive country, significantly different from those in their countries of birth.

Some of the most significant dietary factors that appear to predispose to a higher incidence of colorectal cancer are (1) a low content of unabsorbable vegetable fiber, (2) a high content of refined carbohydrates, and (3) a high fat content. It has been shown that a reduced dietary intake of vegetable fiber is generally linked to a compensatory increased consumption of refined sugars. The reduced fiber content results in decreased stool bulk, increased transit time in the bowel, and an altered bacterial flora of the intestinal contents. The degradative products of the carbohydrate-rich foods are therefore present in higher concentrations in the small stools and are held in contact with the colonic mucosa for longer periods of time. The altered bacterial flora with increased numbers of clostridial and Bacteroides organisms and lower numbers of enterococci and other anaerobic bacteria in the colon brings about a more complete breakdown of bile salts and sterols in the stools (both related to high-animal-fat diets) — perhaps leading to the formation of a carcinogen or cocarcinogen that might initiate, promote, or potentiate the development of cancer.

It is of interest that the geographic incidence of colorectal cancer parallels that of diverticular disease, appendicitis, neoplastic colorectal polyps, and inflammatory bowel disease. A lack of adequate dietary fiber has been implicated in the pathogenesis of both diverticulosis coli and appendicitis, while neoplastic colorectal polyps and inflammatory bowel disease represent a pool of lesions from which such cancers arise.

Some interesting and highly speculative trends have emerged over the past three or four decades.[241] Although the mortality rate for this form of neoplasia for whites in the United States has remained the same over this time span, i.e., about 20 per 100,000 population (an improved prognosis has counterbalanced the 50% increase in incidence), the mortality rate for blacks has doubled. For the first time since data have been available, colorectal cancer may be relatively more common among blacks than among whites. There are other striking comparisons, such as significant differences in mortality rates in different regions of the same country. There is a well-defined higher mortality rate for colorectal cancer in urban areas than in rural areas in the United States and many other countries. This is most striking in Africa, where colonic cancer is extremely rare in rural blacks and is two to three times more frequent in urban blacks. Could these contrasts reflect dietary influences?

Carcinoma of the large bowel has its peak incidence in the seventh decade of life. Less than 20% of cases are diagnosed in persons under the age of 50, and undoubtedly some of these younger patients are accounted for by the hereditary polyposis syndromes. In such individuals the tumor may appear as early as the third or fourth decade of life. When the neoplasm occurs in the rectum, there is a male : female ratio of approximately 2 : 1; in more proximally located tumors there is no sex preponderance.

MORPHOLOGY. About 60 to 70% of colorectal carcinomas are located in the rectum, rectosigmoid, or sigmoid colon. The remainder are fairly evenly distributed all the way back to the cecum. Infrequently, multiple carcinomas arise concurrently, most often in patients with familial multiple polyposis or ulcerative colitis.

Although all colorectal cancers begin as in situ carcinomas, on the left side when discovered, they tend to become annular, encircling lesions that produce so-called napkin-ring constrictions of the bowel with early symptoms of obstruction (Fig. 18–60). **On the right side, the tumors tend to grow as polypoid fungating masses that extend along one wall of the more capacious cecum and ascending colon.** Obstruction is uncommon. Thus, from the standpoint of morphology and clinical behavior, carcinomas of the left and right colon behave as two distinct tumor types.

The **early lesion on the left side** appears as a small elevated button or as a small polypoid mass. As the tumor grows, it forms a raised plaque that continues to increase in size (Fig. 18–61). It eventually extends to encircle the wall, and it has been estimated that it takes approximately one to two years for such a lesion to encircle the lumen totally. The deeper layers are invaded slowly, and for a long time the

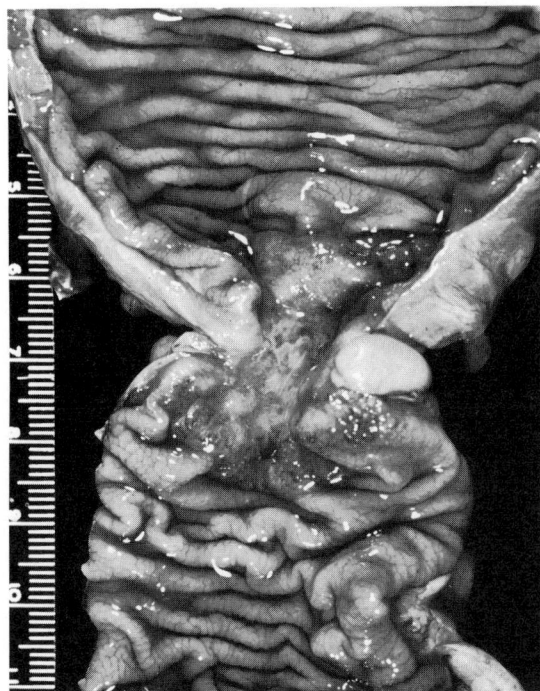

Figure 18–60. Carcinoma of left colon that has completely encircled lumen. Dilation of proximal bowel lumen is evident.

frequently, left-sided lesions produce little luminal growth but instead infiltrate the bowel wall and cause flattening and small ulcerations of the mucosa. All patterns extend in time through the bowel wall into the pericolic fat and regional lymph nodes. The penetration of the bowel wall may, on occasion, produce pericolic abscesses or even peritonitis. Eventually these cancers metastasize, but not before a considerable period of growth. Rarely, right-sided lesions assume this annular pattern.

The **cancers of the right colon** begin as sessile lesions similar to those of the left but progressively assume a polypoid fungating appearance (Fig. 18–62). They frequently become bulky, cauliflower-like masses or large, irregular spreading papillomatous lesions that protrude into the lumen. Plaque-like or ulcerative lesions of the right side are infrequent. Right-sided lesions eventually penetrate the wall and extend to the mesentery, regional nodes, and more distant sites. Because the lesions occur in the capacious cecum and do not cause obstruction, they may remain clinically silent for long periods of time. Quite uncommonly, colonic carcinomas of the right side grow in an invasive, infiltrating fashion with mucosal flattening and ulceration without luminal projections.

neoplasm tends to remain superficial. Eventually, ulceration takes place in the middle of the ring as penetration of the bowel wall encroaches on the blood supply. At this time, the annular constriction characteristically shows heaped-up margins with a central ringlike ulceration or excavation. In-

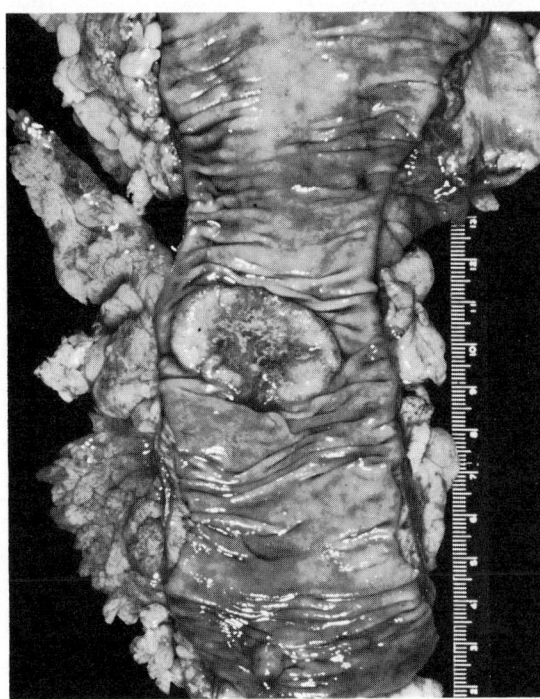

Figure 18–61. An elevated, plaque-like adenocarcinoma of colon.

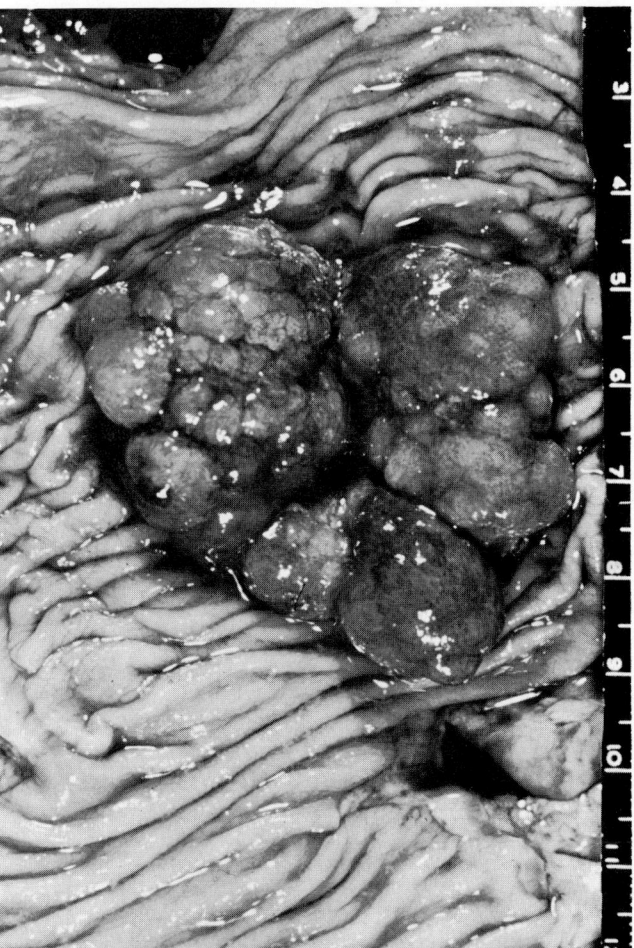

Figure 18–62. A polypoid fungating carcinoma of right colon in a 56-year-old male.

Unlike the gross pathology, the microscopic characteristics of right- and left-sided colonic carcinomas are similar. **Ninety-five percent of all carcinomas of the colorectum are adenocarcinomas,** many of which produce mucin (Figs. 18-63 and 18-64). Commonly this mucin is secreted extracellularly either within gland lumina or within the interstitium of the gut wall. Because this secretion dissects the wall, it aids the extension of the malignancy and worsens the prognosis.

Certain exceptions to the described patterns should be cited. Some cancers, particularly in the distal colon close to the anus, have foci of squamous cell differentiation and are therefore referred to as adenosquamous carcinomas. Another infrequent variant is the small cell undifferentiated carcinoma presumably arising from neuroendocrine cells. Such neoplasms, as you may surmise, elaborate a variety of hormonal or bioactive secretory products. Another variant is the infiltrative, poorly differentiated carcinoma that tends to produce long, tapered strictures. It may occur in the absence of ulcerative colitis but is particularly associated with inflammatory bowel disease. The lack of exophytic growth renders radiographic identification difficult, particularly when it is against a background of ulcerative colitis.

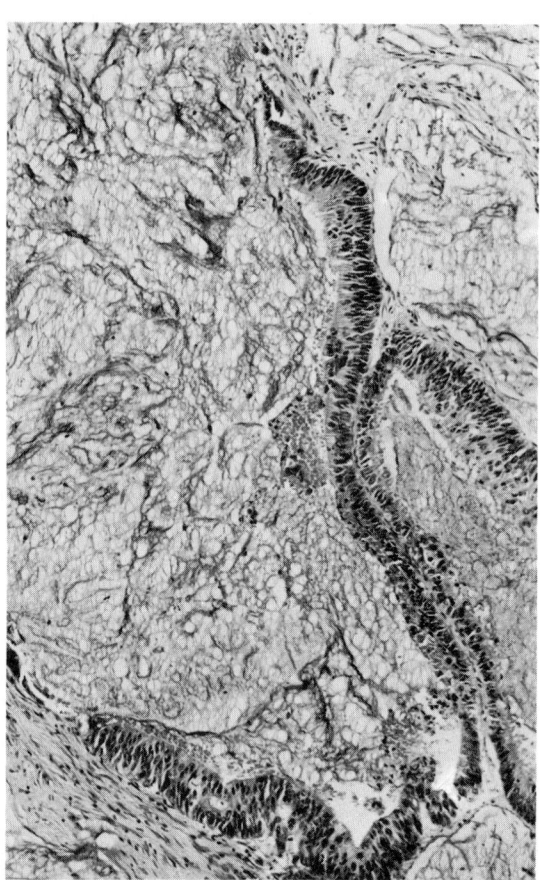

Figure 18-64. Low-power field of an invasive cancer of colon illustrating extensive mucin formation, which appears in the illustration as stringy coagulated material.

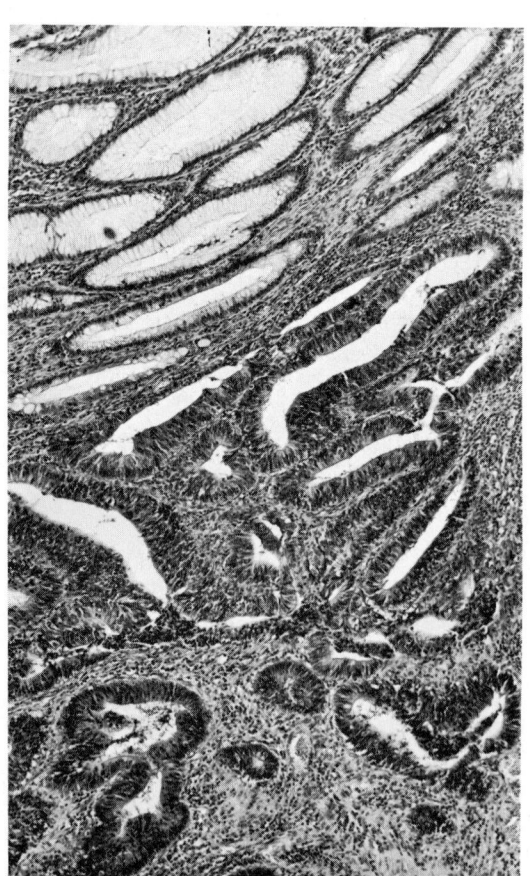

Figure 18-63. Transition zone between anaplastic glands of an adenocarcinoma of colon and the normal colonic epithelium.

CLINICAL COURSE. It is now appreciated that carcinoma of the colorectum is present for a considerable time before it produces clinical symptoms. However, inconstant occult bleeding and/or change in bowel habit are present for many months, perhaps years, before diagnosis. In theory, the chance for early discovery and successful removal should be greater with lesions of the left side because these patients usually have prominent disturbances in bowel function such as melena, diarrhea, and constipation. It would be suspected, therefore, that rectosigmoid lesions would yield a better survival rate. However, cancers of the rectum and sigmoid tend to be more infiltrative than those of the proximal levels of colon, and therefore have a somewhat poorer prognosis. Cecal and right colonic cancers are most often called to clinical attention by the appearance of weakness, malaise, weight loss, and unexplained anemia. These lesions bleed readily, and investigation of occult gastrointestinal bleeding or unexplained anemia sometimes leads to their discovery at an early stage.

All colorectal tumors spread by direct extension into adjacent structures and by metastasis through the lymphatics and blood vessels. In order of preference, the favored sites of metastatic spread are the regional lymph nodes, liver, lungs, and bones, followed by

Table 18-10. Modified Dukes Classification of Carcinoma of the Colon

DUKES TYPE	STAGE OF NEOPLASM
A	Limited to mucosa
B1	Extending into muscularis propria but not penetrating through it with uninvolved nodes
B2	Through entire wall with uninvolved nodes
C1	Limited to the wall with involved nodes
C2	Through all layers of the wall with involved nodes
D	With distant metastatic spread

From Astler, V.B., and Coller, F.A.: The prognostic significance of direct extension of carcinoma of the colon and rectum. Ann. Surg. *139*:846, 1954.

many other sites including the serosal membrane of the peritoneal cavity, brain, and others. In general, the disease has spread beyond the range of curative surgery in 25 to 30% of patients.

The diagnosis of colorectal cancer relies on a large variety of techniques, including tests for blood in the stool, digital examination, proctoscopy, sigmoidoscopy, colonoscopy, contrast radiographic studies, and CT scans. Colonic cancers produce a variety of tumor antigens that can be detected in the blood and provide potential methods of diagnosis. In longest use as a diagnostic aid is carcinoembryonic antigen (CEA), but many other new markers are under study.[209] The serum levels of CEA are directly related to the size of the primary tumor and its extent of spread. Thus, in early favorable lesions, CEA "positivity" is found in 19 to 40% of patients. In contrast, in

Table 18-11. AJC Postsurgical Pathologic Assessment

Primary tumor (T)
TX — Depth of penetration not specified
T0 — No clinically demonstrable tumor
TIS — Carcinoma in situ (no penetration of lamina propria as shown by biopsy or histological examination of the resected specimen)
T1 — Clinically benign lesion or lesion confined to the mucosa or submucosa
T2 — Involvement of muscular wall or serosa; no extension beyond
T3 — Involvement of all layers of colon or rectum, with extension to immediately adjacent structures or organs; no fistula present
T4 — Fistula present along with any of the above degrees of tumor penetration
T5 — Tumor spread by direct extension, beyond the immediately adjacent organs or tissues
( )T — Multiple primary carcinoma
Regional nodal involvement (N)
NX — Nodes not assessed or involvement not recorded
N0 — Nodes not believed to be involved
N1 — Regional nodes involved (distal to origins of the ileocolic, right colic, middle colic, and inferior mesenteric arteries)
Distant metastasis (M)
MX — Not assessed
M0 — No (known) metastasis
M1 — Distant metastasis present (including extra-abdominal nodes, intra-abdominal nodes proximal to mesocolon and inferior mesenteric artery, peritoneal implants, liver, lungs, and bones)

From Stearns, M.W., Jr.: Staging colonic and rectal cancer. Int. Adv. Surg. Oncol. *4*:189, 1981.

those with large metastatic neoplasms, there is virtually 100% CEA positivity. Overall, in all unselected series of preoperative patients, the test is positive in 60 to 70%.[210] However, positive CEA tests may also be produced by cancers of the lung, breast, ovary, urinary bladder, and prostate as well as a number of non-neoplastic disorders, including alcoholic cirrhosis, pancreatitis, and ulcerative colitis. Because elevated levels have little specificity, they are of greatest use to assess possible recurrence following resection of the primary tumor. If total removal has been accomplished, the CEA levels disappear. Return of CEA positivity is a highly reliable indicator of recurrence of the primary neoplasm. Similarly, the CEA test can provide a rough quantitation of the effectiveness of chemotherapy.

The prognosis for patients with colorectal carcinoma, as might be expected, is dependent on (1) the extent of bowel involvement, (2) the presence or absence of spread to lymph nodes or more distant sites, (3) the histologic differentiation of the lesion, and (4)

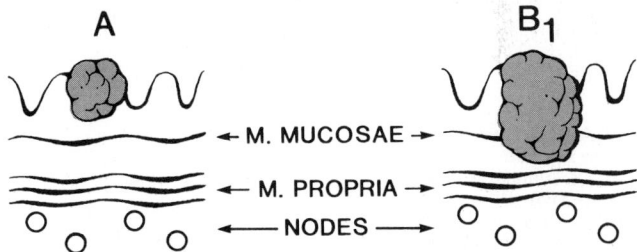

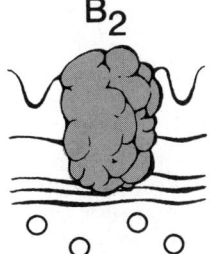 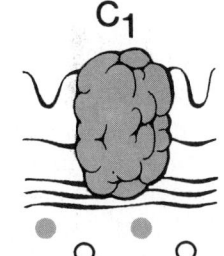

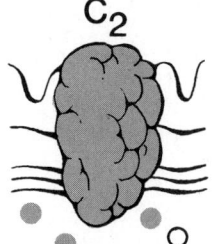 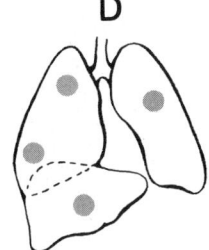

Figure 18-65. Pathologic staging of colorectal cancer. This Astor-Coller modification of Dukes' classification for grading colorectal cancer is based on the extent of local spread of the tumor (stages A through C) and the presence of distant visceral metastases (stage D). This scheme of staging has significant prognostic implications in that the five-year mortality figures progressively increase with the stage of the tumor.

to some extent its location within the colon. Among these variables, the extent of the neoplasm and its potential metastases clearly are of greatest importance. Several staging systems are now in use. The modified Dukes proposal is presented in Table 18–10. It is, however, a postoperative staging system based on morphologic examination of the specimen (Fig. 18–65). The American Joint Committee (AJC) for Cancer Staging and End-Result Reporting has proposed a classification based on the TNM system (Table 18–11).[211] Overall, if all patients, even those whose lesions prove to be inoperable, are included, the five-year survival rate is in the range of 35 to 49%. These data are particularly discouraging in light of the earlier remarks about the potential for early diagnosis and cure of this disease.

Other Tumors

Malignant spindle cell tumors arising from stromal elements and malignant lymphomas may develop within the colon. These tumors are grossly and microscopically similar to those arising in other portions of the gastrointestinal tract. Additionally, carcinoid tumors may also arise within any area of the colon, most commonly in the rectum.

Squamous cell carcinomas are largely limited to the anal canal. These tumors initially present as plaque-like thickenings of the mucosa. Later, they may fungate and become ulcerated. Another tumor that arises within the anal canal from the region of the transition of the squamous and glandular epithelium has been referred to as a transitional cell carcinoma. These tumors, which have also been called cloacogenic or basaloid carcinomas, are three or four times less common than is squamous carcinoma. Both squamous cell and transitional cell carcinomas are locally invasive and metastasize to regional nodes and distant sites. Extramammary Paget's disease (p. 1198) may involve the anal region, and rarely, malignant melanomas may originate in this site.

APPENDIX

INFLAMMATIONS
Acute Appendicitis
MUCOCELE OF APPENDIX AND
  PSEUDOMYXOMA PERITONEI
TUMORS OF APPENDIX
Carcinoma and Other Tumors

NORMAL

The appendix is a mysterious structure with no known function, at least in adults. Histologically, the appendix has the same four layers as the remainder of the gut. The distinguishing feature of this organ is the extremely rich lymphoid tissue present in the mucosa and submucosa, which, in young individuals, forms an entire layer of germinal follicles and lymphoid pulp. This lymphoid tissue underlying the mucosal epithelium and glands undergoes progressive atrophy during life to the point of complete disappearance in advanced age. In the elderly the appendix, particularly the distal portion, sometimes undergoes fibrous obliteration.

PATHOLOGY

Diseases of the appendix loom large in surgical practice. Appendicitis is the most common acute abdominal condition the surgeon is called on to treat. It is, under different conditions, one of the best recognized clinical entities and one of the most difficult diagnostic problems that confront the clinician. A differential diagnosis of the disease must include virtually every acute process that can occur within the abdominal cavity as well as some of the emergencies that affect the organs of the thorax.

INFLAMMATIONS

ACUTE APPENDICITIS

Acute appendicitis is mainly a disease of adolescents and young adults, but it may occur in any age group. Almost half a century ago, Wangensteen and coworkers demonstrated that obstruction to the appendiceal lumen predisposed to the development of acute appendicitis.[212] Obstruction, usually in the form of a fecalith and, less commonly, a calculus, tumor, or ball of worms (oxyuriasis vermicularis), can be demonstrated in 50 to 80% of inflamed appendices. It should be comforting to grape addicts that seeds have not yet been implicated. Presumably, with obstruction and continued secretion of mucinous fluid the intraluminal pressure builds up in the obstructed segment to cause eventual collapse of the veins of drainage. Ischemic injury then favors bacterial invasion to add an element of inflammatory edema and exudation, further embarrassing the blood supply. Thus, a vicious circle is created, leading to inflammatory changes in the appendix related to both bacterial invasion and ischemic injury. However, a significant minority of inflamed appendices have no demonstrable luminal obstruction, and the pathogenesis of the inflammation remains unknown.

In the earliest recognizable acutely inflamed appendix, there is usually a scant neutrophilic exudation throughout the mucosa, submucosa, and muscularis. Occasionally, the mucosal involvement is most prominent. At this phase of the reaction the subserosal vessels are congested, and often there is scant, perivascular, neutrophilic emigration. This serosal reaction transforms the normal glistening serosa into an infected, dull, granular, red membrane. This external appearance is recognized by the surgeon as **early acute appendicitis.** At a later stage, the neutrophilic exudation through the wall is more advanced, with numerous polymorphonuclear leukocytes within the muscularis and a layered fibrinopurulent reaction over the serosa (Fig. 18–66). As the inflammatory process worsens, there is abscess formation within the wall, along with ulcerations and foci of suppurative necrosis in the mucosa. At this stage, the serosa usually is heavily layered with fibrinosuppurative exudate, and the state of the appendix might be termed **acute suppurative appendicitis.** Further worsening of the reaction leads to large areas of hemorrhagic green ulceration of the mucosa, along with similar green-black gangrenous necrosis throughout the wall, extending to the serosa. This level of severity is the immediate antecedent to rupture due to an **acute gangrenous appendicitis.**

The histologic criterion for the diagnosis of acute appendicitis is polymorphonuclear leukocytic infiltration of the muscularis. Usually, neutrophils and ulcerations are also present within the mucosa. Since drainage of an exudate into the appendix from a focus of infection in a higher level of bowel may also induce some scant neutrophilic infiltrate in the mucosa, it is believed that evidence of the inflammation within the muscularis is requisite for the diagnosis.

Classically, acute appendicitis produces the following, in the sequence given: (1) pain, at first periumbilical but then localizing to the right lower quadrant; (2) nausea and/or vomiting; (3) abdominal tenderness, particularly in the region of the appendix; (4) mild fever; and (5) an elevation of the peripheral white cell count up to 15,000 to 20,000 cells/mm³. Regrettably, this classic presentation is more often absent than present. The pain, nausea, and vomiting are most consistently present, but tenderness may be deceptively absent or maximal in atypical locations, e.g., right flank or midline pelvis. The white cell count may not be elevated, or at other times may be so high as to suggest alternative diagnoses. These nonclassic presentations are encountered more often in young children and the very elderly.

There is general agreement that highly competent surgeons make about 10 to 30% false-positive

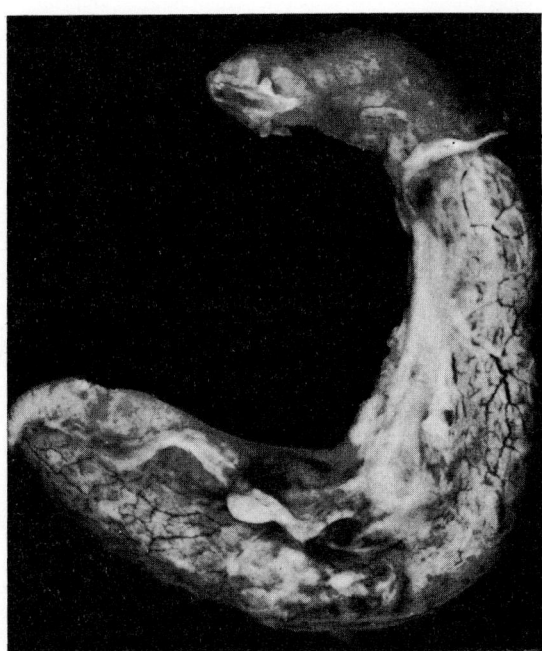

Figure 18–66. A suppurative exudate covering serosa of appendix. Uneven dilatation is produced by impacted fecaliths.

diagnoses of acute appendicitis.[213] The most common conditions that mimic it are mesenteric lymphadenitis, usually secondary to an enterocolitis (often unrecognized) caused by Yersinia or some virus; a systemic viral infection; acute salpingitis; ectopic pregnancy; "mittelschmerz" (pain caused by trivial pelvic bleeding at time of ovulation); and Meckel's diverticulitis. But most often, when the abdomen is explored and the appendix is uninvolved, no disease of any kind is found, leaving the surgeon mumbling such vagaries as "cecitis" or "appendiceal colic." The penalty for undue delay is perforation followed by a periappendiceal abscess and/or peritonitis. Other potential but uncommon complications of appendicitis include pylephlebitis with thrombosis of the portal venous drainage, liver abscess, and bacteremia. *The discomfort and risks associated with an exploratory laparotomy and discovery of "no disease" are far outweighed by the morbidity and mortality (about 2%) associated with perforation.*

True *chronic inflammation* of the appendix is rare. Much more frequently, recurrent acute attacks may be inappropriately referred to as chronic appendicitis. In some patients, the appendix from birth is a mere fibrous cord. It must not be assumed, therefore, that extensive fibrosis of the appendiceal architecture implies a chronic inflammatory reaction or the end stage of a previous inflammation.

MUCOCELE OF APPENDIX AND PSEUDOMYXOMA PERITONEI

Dilatation of the appendiceal lumen by mucinous secretion is designated *mucocele* (Fig. 18–67). Traditionally, two forms of mucocele were described: (1)

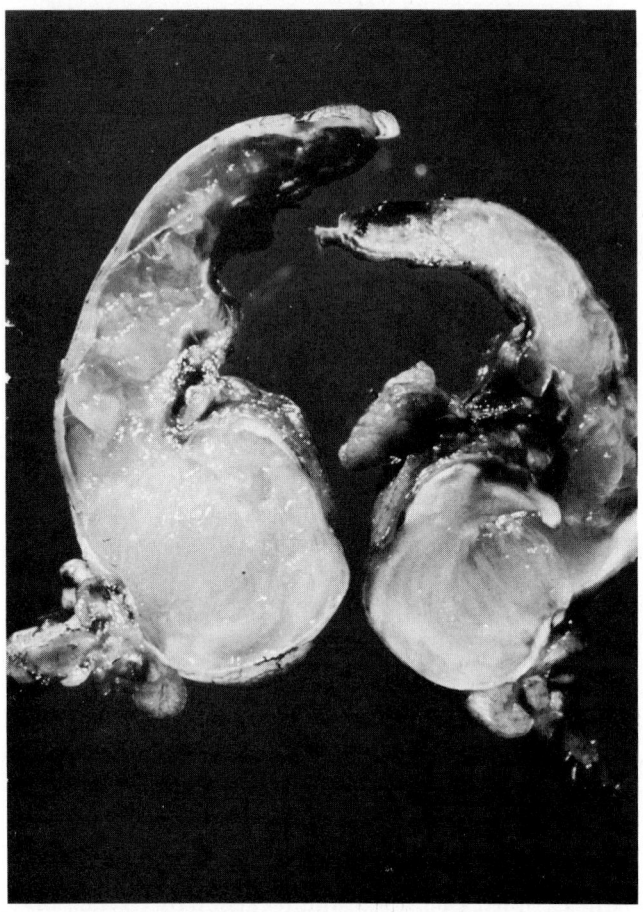

Figure 18–67. Hemisected mucocele of the appendix. Note the distention due to the mucus accumulated in the lumen.

obstructive and (2) neoplastic. This view assumed that obstruction of the appendiceal lumen by a fecalith might not lead to inflammatory changes, but instead permit mucinous secretions to accumulate in the sequestered lumen.[258] This hypothesis, however, is no longer tenable. It is now recognized that mucocele of the appendix is caused by one of three patterns of epithelial proliferation: (1) mucosal hyperplasia remarkably similar to the changes seen in hyperplastic polyps of the colon; (2) mucinous cystadenoma (by far the most common form); or (3) mucinous cystadenocarcinoma.[214]

The histologic features of cystadenomas and cystadenocarcinomas closely mimic their ovarian counterparts, as described on page 1160. All three lesions are associated with appendiceal dilatation secondary to mucinous secretions. With **mucosal hyperplasia** there is no evidence of appendiceal rupture or of peritoneal mucinous implants. With **cystadenomas** the luminal dilatation is more striking and is associated with appendiceal perforation in 20% of instances. In such cases, localized collections of mucus are present, either attached to the serosa of the appendix or lying free in the peritoneal cavity. Histologic examination of the mucus, however, reveals no neoplastic cells. Follow-up of these patients after removal of the appendix, and sometimes the right colon, has shown that none had any complications related to the appendiceal lesion or the extravasated mucus. **Mucinous cystadenocarcinomas** are one fifth as common as cystadenomas. Macroscopically, they produce mucin-filled cystic dilation of the appendix indistinguishable from that associated with the benign tumors. However, penetration of the bowel wall by neoplastic cells and spread beyond the appendix in the form of peritoneal implants is frequently present. In its fully developed state the peritoneal cavity becomes distended with tenacious, semisolid mucin—**pseudomyxoma peritonei**—in which anaplastic cystadenocarcinomatous cells can be found.[214] **The feature that differentiates pseudomyxoma peritonei from mucinous spillage is the presence of cancerous cells within the mucin, not seen with the nonmalignant lesions producing mucocele. Thus, in reality, pseudomyxoma peritonei is a form of intraperitoneal spread of mucin-secreting cancer.** Spread of the neoplasm above the diaphragm or invasion of abdominal viscera is exceptional. Ovarian mucinous cystadenocarcinomas may produce an identical picture (p. 1161).

TUMORS OF APPENDIX

Tumors of the appendix such as those described above are very rare. The most common is the endocrine cell tumor (carcinoid), which was discussed on page 872 along with similar lesions of the entire gut. This neoplasm most frequently involves the distal tip of the appendix, where it produces a solid bulbous swelling 2 to 3 cm in diameter, which on section is yellow and firm. The lumen and architecture of the wall are obliterated in the area of involvement. Histologically, these tumors are identical to other midgut carcinoids. Despite their benign cytologic appearance, tumors frequently show intra- and transmural extension locally. Nodal metastases are very infrequent and occur only with tumors greater than 2 cm in size.[215] Distant spread is very rare. A simple appendectomy is adequate treatment for the localized tumors less than 2 cm in diameter, while a more radical approach may be adopted for the larger ones.[215]

CARCINOMA AND OTHER TUMORS

On rare occasions, non–mucin producing carcinomas of the appendix may cause a typical neoplastic enlargement of the organ. Benign and malignant mesenchymal growths in this organ, resembling their counterparts in other areas, are reported as medical curiosities.

INFLAMMATIONS

Peritonitis may be due to either bacterial invasion or chemical irritation. The most common causes of sterile peritonitis in order of frequency are bile, pancreatic enzymes, and surgically introduced foreign material.

Perforation or rupture of the biliary system evokes a highly irritating peritonitis. In the early stage, it is usually limited to the right upper quadrant, and on examination the peritoneal exudate is bile-stained. Later the biliary discoloration is masked by the progressive suppuration that ensues concomitantly with superimposed bacterial contamination.

Acute hemorrhagic pancreatitis is a calamitous disorder characterized by hemorrhage and necrosis of the pancreas (p. 983). Concomitantly, pancreatic enzymes leak into the peritoneal cavity. These proteolytic and lipolytic ferments evoke a striking peritoneal reaction and, at the same time, digest fat tissue. With the release of fatty acids, saponification with calcium salt (formation of soaps) produces chalky white precipitates in focal areas of fat wherever it is exposed to these enzymes. At the same time, globules of free fat may be found floating in the peritoneal fluid that accumulates. After 24 to 48 hours, however, bacterial permeation of the bowel wall usually leads to a frank suppurative exudation.

The reaction to surgically introduced foreign materials such as talc is usually localized and minimal. No clinical symptoms may result, and the only significance of such disease lies in the possible development of foreign-body type granulomas, followed by fibrosis and adhesions.

BACTERIAL PERITONITIS

Bacterial peritonitis is almost invariably secondary to extension of bacteria through the wall of a hollow viscus or to rupture of a viscus. The common primary disorders leading to such bacterial disseminations are *appendicitis, ruptured peptic ulcer, cholecystitis, diverticulitis, strangulation of bowel, and acute salpingitis.* Virtually every bacterial organism has been implicated, most commonly *E. coli,* alpha- and beta-hemolytic streptococci, *Staphylococcus aureus,* enterococci, gram-negative rods, and *Clostridium perfringens.* The last organism is a frequent inhabitant of the gut and therefore a frequent contributor to peritonitis. However, it rarely causes true gas gangrene in the abdominal cavity. Much less common than these secondary forms of bacterial peritonitis is so-called spontaneous bacterial peritonitis that sometimes appears in cirrhotics. The usual causal agent is *E. coli,* but the manner by which it invades the peritoneal cavity is unknown (possibly blood-borne). Spontaneous pneumococcal peritonitis is a curiosity occasionally encountered in children with renal disease. Both the source of the organism and the mode of spread are obscure.

Depending on the duration of the peritonitis, the membranes show the following changes. Approximately two to four hours after involvement, there is loss of the gray, glistening quality of the peritoneal surface, and it becomes dull and lusterless. There is, at this time, a small accumulation of essentially serous or slightly turbid fluid. Later the exudate becomes creamy and obviously suppurative. In some cases, it may become extremely thick and plastic and even inspissated, especially in dehydrated patients. The volume of such exudate varies enormously. In many cases, it may be localized by the omentum and viscera to a small area of the peritoneal cavity, particularly as in an appendiceal abscess; or it may become generalized to involve the entire abdominal cavity. In generalized peritonitis, it is important to remember that exudate may accumulate under and above the liver to form **subhepatic** and **subdiaphragmatic abscesses.** Collections in the lesser omental sac may likewise create residual persistent foci of infection.

The inflammatory process is typical of an acute bacterial infection anywhere and produces the characteristic neutrophilic infiltration with fibrinopurulent exudation. The reaction usually remains superficial and does not penetrate deeply into the visceral structures or abdominal wall. **Tuberculous peritonitis** tends to produce a plastic exudate studded with minute, pale granulomas.

These inflammatory processes can heal either spontaneously or with therapy. In the course of healing, the following may obtain: (1) *The exudate may be totally resolved, leaving no residual fibrosis; (2) residual, walled-off abscesses may persist, eventually to heal or serve as foci for new infection; or (3) organization of the exudate may occur, with the formation of fibrous adhesions.*

SCLEROSING RETROPERITONITIS

Dense fibromatous overgrowth of the retroperitoneal tissues may sometimes develop, designated sclerosing retroperitonitis or retroperitoneal fibromatosis. In some instances the mesentery is also involved. The fibrous overgrowth is entirely nondistinctive and, although infiltrative, does not display frank anaplasia. There is usually an accompanying inflammatory infiltrate of lymphocytes, plasma cells, and neutrophils, suggesting inflammatory rather than neoplastic disease. The fibrosis is particularly important because it often encroaches on the ureters and may produce hydronephrosis. The fibrous tissue insinuates itself into the retroperitoneal fat and about the retroperitoneal organs, and in some ways is the analog of the desmoid tumor (p. 1380). The cause of this curious condition is obscure, but as pointed out on page 1085, may be a reaction to certain drugs (e.g., ergot derivatives) or may be an autoimmune reaction.

MESENTERIC CYSTS

Large-to-small cystic masses are sometimes found within the mesenteries in the abdominal cavity or attached to the peritoneal lining of the abdominal wall. These cysts are usually of obscure nature and origin, and sometimes offer difficult clinical diagnostic problems because they present on palpation as abdominal masses. Many classifications have been proposed that attempt to designate groups according to common pathogenetic origins. On this basis, it has been suggested that mesenteric cysts be divided into (1) those arising from sequestered lymphatic channels; (2) those derived from pinched-off enteric diverticula that usually arise during the early development of the fore- and hindgut; (3) those derived from the urogenital ridge or its derivatives, i.e., the urinary tract and male and female genital tracts; (4) those derived from walled-off infections or following pancreatitis, more properly called *pseudocysts;* and (5) those of malignant origin.

TUMORS

Virtually all tumors of the peritoneum are malignant and can be divided into primary and secondary forms.

Primary tumors of the peritoneum are extremely rare and are called mesotheliomas (p. 807). These exactly duplicate the tumors found in the pleura and the pericardium. Like the supradiaphragmatic tumors, peritoneal mesotheliomas are associated with asbestos exposure in at least 80% of cases. How inhaled asbestos induces a peritoneal neoplasm is a mystery.

Secondary tumors of the peritoneum are, in contrast, quite common. In any form of advanced cancer, penetration to the serosal membrane or metastatic seeding may occur. The most common tumors producing diffuse serosal implantation and sometimes pseudomyxoma peritonei are ovarian and pancreatic carcinomas. However, any type of intra-abdominal malignancy may be implicated, and occasionally tumors in extra-abdominal locations within the body.

Additional mention might be made of the very uncommon tumors that may arise from retroperitoneal tissues, i.e., fat, fibrous tissue, blood vessels, lymphatics, nerves, and the lymph nodes alongside the aorta. These native structures may give rise to benign or malignant tumors derived from any of the indigenous mesenchymal cell types that resemble their counterparts arising elsewhere in the body.

1. Cohen, S.: Motor disorders of the esophagus. N. Engl. J. Med. *301:*184, 1979.
2. Cohen, S., et al.: Gastrointestinal motility. Int. Rev. Physiol. *19:*107, 1979.
3. Fisher, R., and Cohen, S.: Disorders of the lower esophageal sphincter. Annu. Rev. Med. *26:*373, 1975.
4. Adams, W.M., et al.: Ganglion cells in achalasia of the cardia. Virchows Arch. [Pathol. Anat.] *372:*75, 1976.
5. Cohen, S., et al.: The site of denervation in achalasia. Gut *13:*556, 1972.
6. Schatzki, R., and Gary, J.E.: The lower esophageal ring. Am. J. Roentgenol. *75:*246, 1956.
7. Hagarty, G.: A classification of esophageal hiatus hernia with special reference to sliding hernia. Am. J. Roentgenol. *84:*1056, 1960.
8. Editorial: Asymptomatic hiatus hernia. Lancet *1:*870, 1969.
9. Palmer, E.D.: Hiatus hernia and hemorrhage. Am. J. Med. Sci. *249:*417, 1963.
10. Weiss, S., and Mallory, G.K.: Lesions of cardiac orifice of the stomach produced vomiting. J.A.M.A. *98:*1353, 1932.
11. Editorial: Mallory-Weiss through the endoscope. Lancet *1:*1294, 1978.
12. Dodds, W.J., et al.: Pathogenesis of reflux esophagitis. Gastroenterology *81:*376, 1981.
13. Crespi, M., et al.: Oesophageal lesions in Northern Iran: A premalignant lesion. Lancet *2:*217, 1979.
14. Jamieson, G.G., and Duranceau, A.: The pathology of gastroesophageal reflux. In Duranceau, A., and Jamieson, G.G.: Gastroesophageal Reflux. Philadelphia, W.B. Saunders, 1988, p. 46.
15. Barrett, N.R.: The lower esophagus lined by columnar epithelium. Surgery *41:*881, 1957.
16. Spechler, S.J., and Goyal, R.K.: Barrett's esophagus. N. Engl. J. Med. *315:*362, 1986.
17. Enterline, H., and Thompson, J.: Pathology of the Esophagus. New York, Springer-Verlag, 1985, p. 145.
18. Munoz, N., and Crespi, M.: High-risk conditions and precancerous lesions of the esophagus. In Sherlock, P., Morson, B.C., Barbara, L., and Veronisi, U. (eds.): Precancerous Lesions of the Gastrointestinal Tract. New York, Raven Press, 1983, p. 53.
19. Tuyns, A.J., et al.: Role of diet, alcohol and tobacco in esophageal cancer as illustrated by two contrasting high-incidence areas in the North of Iran and West of France. Front. Gastrointest. Res. *4:*101, 1979.
20. Rogers, E.L., et al.: Increasing frequency of esophageal cancer among black male veterans. Cancer *49:*610, 1982.
21. Yang, C.S.: Research on esophageal cancer in China: a review. Cancer Res. *40:*2633, 1980.
22. Mingxin, L., et al.: Recent progress in research on esophageal cancer in China. In Klein, G., and Weinhous, S. (eds.): Advances in Cancer Research. New York, Academic Press, 1980, p. 173.
23. Oelette, G.J., et al.: Esophagitis in a population at risk for esophageal carcinoma. Cancer *57:*2222, 1986.
24. Haggitt, R.C., and Dean, P.J.: Adenocarcinoma in Barrett's epithelium. In Spechler, S.J., and Goyal, R.K. (eds.): Barrett's Esophagus: Pathophysiology, Diagnosis and Management. New York, Elsevier, 1985, p. 153.
25. Haggitt, R.C., et al.: Adenocarcinoma in the columnar epithelium–lined lower (Barrett) esophagus. Am. J. Clin. Pathol. *70:*1, 1978.
26. Reid, B.J., et al.: Endoscopic biopsy can detect high-grade dys-

plasia or early adenocarcinoma in Barrett's esophagus without grossly recognizable neoplastic lesions. Gastroenterology *94:*81, 1988.

27. Dayal, Y.: Endocrine cells of the gut and their neoplasms. *In* Norris, H.T. (ed.): Contemporary Issues in Surgical Pathology, Vol. 2. New York, Churchill Livingstone, 1983, p. 267.

28. LeDouarin, N.M.: The embryological origin of cells associated with the digestive tract. *In* Bloom, S.R. (ed.): Gut Hormones. Edinburgh, Churchill Livingstone, 1978.

29. Kivilaakso, E., and Silen, W.: Pathogenesis of experimental, gastric mucosal injury. N. Engl. J. Med. *301:*364, 1979.

30. Miller, T.A., and Jackobson, E.D.: Gastrointestinal cytoprotection by prostaglandins. Gut *20:*75, 1979.

31. Editorial: Acid reduction or mucosal protection for peptic ulcer? Lancet *2:*473, 1982.

32. Valman, H.B., et al.: Lesions associated with gastroduodenal hemorrhage in relation to aspirin intake. Br. Med. J. *4:*661, 1968.

33. Barwick, K.W.: Chronic gastritis, the pathologists' role. Pathol. Annu. *22:*223, 1987.

34. Ihamaki, T., et al.: Long term observation of subjects with normal mucosa and superficial gastritis. Results of 23–27 years follow-up examination. Scand. J. Gastroenterol. *13:*771, 1978.

35. Owen, D.A.: Gastritis and duodenitis. *In* Appelman, H.D. (ed.): Contemporary Issues in Surgical Pathology, Vol. 4. New York, Churchill Livingstone, 1984, p. 37.

36. Kimura, K.: Chronological transition of the fundic pyloric border determined by step-wise biopsy of the lesser and greater curvatures of the stomach. Gastroenterology *63:*584, 1972.

37. Parl, F.F., et al.: Histologic and morphometric study of chronic gastritis in alcoholic patients. Hum. Pathol. *10:*45, 1979.

38. Goodwin, C.S.: Duodenal ulcer, Campylobacter pylori and the"leaking roof" concept. Lancet *2:*1467, 1988.

39. Drumm, B., et al.: Association of Campylobacter pylori on the gastric mucosa with antral gastritis in children. N. Engl. J. Med. *316:*1557, 1987.

40. Blaser, M.J.: Gastric campylobacter-like organisms, gastritis and peptic ulcer disease. Gastroenterology *93:*371, 1987.

41. Yardley, J.H., and Paull, G.: Campylobacter pyloridis: a newly recognized infectious agent in the gastrointestinal tract. Am. J. Surg. Pathol. (Suppl. 1) *12:*89, 1988.

42. Menguy, R.: The prophylaxis of stress ulceration. N. Engl. J. Med. *302:*461, 1980.

43. Rees, W.D., and Turnberg, L.A.: Reappraisal of the effects of aspirin on the stomach. Lancet *2:*410, 1980.

44. Watkinson, G.: The incidence of chronic peptic ulcer found at necropsy. Gut *1:*14, 1960.

45. Mendeloff, A.I.: What has been happening to duodenal ulcer. Gastroenterology *67:*1020, 1974.

46. Eberhard, G.: Peptic ulcer in twins. A study in personality, heredity and environment. Acta Psychiatr. Scand. *44* (Suppl.):205, 1968.

47. Rotter, J.I., et al.: HLA-B5 association with duodenal ulcer. Gastroenterology *73:*438, 1977.

48. Grossman, M.I., et al.: Peptic diseases. Gastroenterology *69:*1071, 1975.

49. Chapman, M.L.: Peptic ulcer. A medical perspective. Med. Clin. North Am. *62:*39, 1978.

50. Cox, A.J.: Stomach size and its relation to chronic peptic ulcer. Arch. Pathol. *54:*407, 1952.

51. Fordtran, J.S., and Walsh, J.H.: Gastric acid secretion rate and buffer content of the stomach after eating. J. Clin. Invest. *52:*647, 1973.

52. Ferguson, D.J.: Studies on gastrin from human stomachs. Surg. Forum *84:*1951, 1950.

53. Dayal, Y., and Wolfe, H.J.: Antropyloric G-cell population in gastric and duodenal ulcer disease: a morphometric analysis. Lab. Invest. *38:*341, 1978.

54. Keuppens, F., et al.: Estimation of the antral and duodenal gastrin cell population removed by gastrectomy from patients with peptic ulcer. Surg. Gynecol. Obstet. *146:*400, 1978.

55. Takahashi, T., et al.: G-cell population in resected stomachs from gastric and duodenal ulcer patients. Gastroenterology *78:*498, 1980.

56. Creutzfeldt, W., and Arnold, R.: Endocrinology of duodenal ulcer. World J. Surg. *3:*605, 1979.

57. Polak, J.M., et al.: D-cell pathology in duodenal ulcers and achlorhydria. Metab. Clin. Exp. *28* (Suppl. 1), 1239, 1978.

58. Grossman, M.I.: A new look at peptic ulcer. Ann. Intern. Med. *84:*57, 1976.

59. Gear, M., et al.: Gastric ulcer and gastritis. Gut *12:*639, 1971.

60. Thomas, W.E.G.: Duodeno-gastric reflux. A common factor in pathogenesis of gastric and duodenal ulcer. Lancet *2:*1166, 1980.

61. Piper, D.W., et al.: Analgesic ingestion and chronic peptic ulcer. Gastroenterology *80:*427, 1981.

62. Spiro, H.M.: Clinical Gastroenterology. 3rd ed. New York, Macmillan, 1983, p. 304.

63. Oi, M., et al.: A possible dual control mechanism in the origin of peptic ulcer. Gastroenterology *57:*280, 1969.

64. Beard, R.J., et al.: Non-carcinomatous tumors of the stomach. Br. J. Surg. *55:*535, 1968.

65. Ming, S.-C.: Tumors of the esophagus and stomach. Atlas of Tumor Pathology. Fascicle #7, 99. Washington, D.C., Armed Forces Institute of Pathology, 1973.

66. Ming, S.-C., and Goldman, H.: Gastric polyps. A histogenetic classification and its relation to carcinoma. Cancer *18:*721, 1965.

67. Ming, S.-C.: The adenoma-carcinoma sequence in the stomach and colon. II. Malignant potential of gastric polyps. Gastrointest. Radiol. *1:*121, 1976.

68. Silverberg, E., and Lubera, J.: Cancer statistics. CA *36:*9, 1986.

69. Antonioli, D.A.: Current concepts in carcinoma of the stomach. *In* Appelman, H.D. (ed.): Contemporary Issues in Surgical Pathology, Vol. 4. New York, Churchill Livingstone, 1984, p. 121.

70. van Wayhen, R.G.A., and Linschoten, H.: Distribution of ABO and rhesus blood groups in patients with gastric carcinoma with reference to its site of origin. Gastroenterology *65:*877, 1973.

71. Correa, P., et al.: Diet and gastric cancer: Nutrition survey in a high risk area. J. Natl. Cancer Inst. *70:*673, 1983.

72. Hill, M.J., et al.: Bacteria, nitrosamines and cancer of the stomach. Br. J. Cancer *28:*562, 1973.

73. Zaldivar, R., and Robinson, H.: Epidemiological investigation of stomach cancer mortality in Chileans: Association with nitrate fertilizer. Z. Krebrosch. Klin. Onkol. *80:*289, 1972.

74. Joossens, J.V., and Geboers, J.: Epidemiology of gastric cancer: A clue to etiology. *In* Sherlock, P., Morson, B.C., Barbara, L., and Veronisi, U. (eds.): Precancerous Lesions of the Gastrointestinal Tract. New York, Raven Press, 1983, p. 97.

75. Fugita, S.: Biology of early gastric carcinoma. Pathol. Res. Pract. *163:*297, 1978.

76. Ming, S.-C.: Gastric carcinoma. A pathobiological classification. Cancer *39:*2475, 1977.

77. Lauren, P.: The two histological main types of gastric carcinoma: Diffuse and so-called intestinal-type carcinoma. An attempt at a histoclinical classification. Acta Pathol. Microbiol. Scand. *64:*31, 1965.

78. Chejfec, G., and Gould V.E.: Malignant gastric neuroendocrinomas. Ultrastructural and biochemical characterization of their secretory activity. Hum. Pathol. *8:*433, 1977.

79. Henry, K., and Farrer-Brown, G.: Primary lymphomas of the gastrointestinal tract. I. Plasma cell tumours. Histopathology *1:*53, 1977.

80. Weingrad, D.N., et al.: Primary gastrointestinal lymphomas. Cancer *49:*1258, 1982.

81. Isaacson, P., et al.: Malignant histiocytosis of the intestine: report of three cases with immunological and cytochemical analysis. J. Clin. Pathol. *35:*510, 1982.

82. Lewin, K.J., et al.: Primary intestinal lymphoma of "Western" and "Mediterranean" type, alpha chain disease and massive plasma cell infiltration. Cancer *38:*2511, 1976.

83. Appelman, H.D.: Stromal tumors of the esophagus, stomach and duodenum. *In* Appelman, H.D. (ed.): Pathology of the Esophagus, Stomach and Duodenum. New York, Churchill Livingstone, 1984, p. 195.

84. Appelman, H.D.: Smooth muscle tumors of the gastrointestinal tract: what we know now that Stout did not know. Am. J. Surg. Pathol. *10* (Suppl. 1):83, 1986.

85. Trier, J.S.: Studies on small intestinal crypt epithelium. I. The fine structure of the crypt epithelium of the proximal small intestine of fasting humans. J. Cell Biol. *18:*599, 1963.

86. Rodning, C.B., et al.: Immunoglobulins within human small-intestinal Paneth cells. Lancet *1:*984, 1976.

87. Isselbacher, K.J.: The intestinal cell surface. Some properties of normal, undifferentiated and malignant cells. Ann. Intern. Med. *81:*681, 1974.

88. Madara, J.L., et al.: Structural changes in the plasma membrane accompanying differentiation of epithelial cells in human and monkey small intestine. Gastroenterology *78:*963, 1980.

89. Thomas, C.S., Jr., et al.: Jejunal diverticula as a source of massive gastrointestinal bleeding. Arch. Surg. *95:*89, 1967.

90. Ottinger, L.W.: Acute mesenteric ischemia. N. Engl. J. Med. *307:*535, 1982.

91. Swerdlow, S.H., et al.: Intestinal infarction. A new classification (Letter). Arch. Pathol. Lab. Med. *106:*218, 1981.

92. Boley, S.J.: Early diagnosis of acute mesenteric ischemia. Hosp. Pract. *16:*63, 1981.

93. Civetta, J.M., and Kolodny, M.: Mesenteric venous thombosis associated with oral contraceptives. Gastroenterology *58:*713, 1970.

94. Marshak, R.J., et al.: Ischemia of the colon. Mt. Sinai J. Med. *48:*180, 1981.

95. Norris, H.T.: Ischemic bowel disease: Its spectrum. *In* Yardley, J.H., Morson, B.C., and Abell, M.R. (eds.): The Gastrointestinal Tract. Baltimore, Williams & Wilkins, 1977, p. 15.

96. Editorial: Traveller's diarrhea. Lancet *1:*77, 1982.

97. Colgan, T., et al.: Campylobacter jejuni enterocolitis. Arch. Pathol. Lab. Med. *104:*571, 1980.

98. Blazer, M.J., and Reller, L.B.: Campylobacter enteritis. N. Engl. J. Med. *305:*1444, 1981.

99. Guerrant, R.L.: Yet another pathogenic mechanism for *Escherichia coli* diarrhea. N. Engl. J. Med. *302:*113, 1980.

100. Bradford, W.B., et al.: Pathologic features of enteric infection with *Yersinia enterocolitica.* Arch. Pathol. *98:*17, 1974.

101. Trier, J.S., et al.: The pathology of acute nonbacterial gastroenteritis. *In* Yardley, J.H., Morson, B.C., and Abell, M.R. (eds.): The Gastrointestinal Tract. Baltimore, Williams & Wilkins, 1977, p. 36.

102. Kapikaian, A.Z.: Approaches to immunization of infants and young children against gastroenteritis due to rotaviruses. Rev. Infect. Dis. *2:*459, 1980.

103. Suzuki, H., and Konno, T.: Reovirus-like particles in jejunal mucosa: a Japanese infant with acute infectious nonbacterial gastroenteritis. Tohoku J. Exp. Med. *115:*199, 1975.

104. Kirsner, J.B., and Shorter, R.G.: Recent developments in "non-specific" inflammatory bowel disease. N. Engl. J. Med. *306:*775, 837, 1982.

105. Greenstein, A.J., et al.: The extraintestinal manifestations of Crohn's disease and ulcerative colitis: A study of 700 patients. Medicine *55:*401, 1976.

106. Janowitz, H.D.: Crohn's disease—50 years later. N. Engl. J. Med. *304:*1600, 1981.

107. Janowitz, H.D., and Sachar, D.B.: New observations in Crohn's disease. Annu. Rev. Med. *27:*269, 1976.

108. Selby, W.S., et al.: Crohn's disease. A review of 122 cases. Aust. N.Z. J. Med. *9:*145, 1979.

109. Sachar, D.B.: Aetiologic theories of inflammatory bowel disease. Clin. Gastroenterol. *9:*231, 1980.

110. Kirsner, J.B.: Inflammatory bowel disease; considerations of etiology and pathogenesis. Am. J. Gastroenterol. *69:*253, 1978.

111. Mitchell, D.N., and Rees, R.J.W.: Agent transmissible from Crohn's disease tissue. Lancet *2:*168, 1970.

112. Gitnick, G.L.: Etiology of inflammatory diseases: Are we making progress? Gastroenterology *78:*1090, 1980.

113. Gitnick, G.L., et al.: Evidence for the isolation of a new virus from ulcerative colitis patients: Comparison with virus derived from Crohn's disease. Dig. Dis. Sci. *24:*609, 1979.

114. Dvorak, A.M., et al.: Absence of virus structures in Crohn's disease tissues studied by electron microscopy. Lancet *1:*328, 1978.

115. Gorback, S.L.: Intestinal microflora in inflammatory bowel disease. *In* Kirsner, J.B., and Shorter, R.G. (eds.): Inflammatory Bowel Disease. Philadelphia, Lea & Febiger, 1980, p. 55.

116. Das, D.M., et al.: Isolation and characterization of colonic tissue-bound antibodies from patients with idiopathic ulcerative colitis. Proc. Natl. Acad. Sci. U.S.A. *9:*4528, 1978.

117. Bookman, M.A., and Bull, D.M.: Characteristics of isolated intestinal mucosal lymphoid cells in inflammatory bowel disease. Gastroenterology *77:*503, 1979.

118. Falchuk, Z.M., et al.: Human colonic lamina propria lymphocytes mediate mitogen-induced but not spontaneous cell-mediated cytotoxicity (Abstract). Gastroenterology *76:*1129, 1979.

119. Brooks, M.: Crohn's disease. A functional deficiency of IgA? Lancet *1:*158, 1981.

120. Gould, S.R., et al.: Increased prostaglandin production in ulcerative colitis. Lancet *2:*98, 1977.

121. Price, A.B., and Morson, B.C.: Inflammatory bowel disease: The surgical pathology of Crohn's disease and ulcerative colitis. Hum. Pathol. *6:*7, 1975.

122. Lee, K.S., et al.: Indeterminate colitis in the spectrum of inflammatory bowel disease. Arch. Pathol. Lab. Med. *103:*173, 1979.

123. Perzin, K., and Bridge, M.F.: Adenomas of the small intestine: A clinicopathologic review of 51 cases and a study of their relationship to carcinoma. Cancer *48:*799, 1981.

124. Sager, G.F.: Primary malignant tumors of the small intestine, a 22-year experience with 30 patients. Am. J. Surg. *135:*601, 1978.

125. Wilson, J.M., et al.: Primary malignancies of the small bowel: A report of 96 cases and review of literature. Ann. Surg. *180:*175, 1974.

126. DeLellis, R.A., et al.: Carcinoid tumors: Changing concepts and new perspectives. Am. J. Surg. Pathol. *8:*295, 1984.

127. Dayal, Y., and Wolfe, H.J.: Regulatory substances in clinically non-functioning gastrointestinal carcinoids. *In* Falkmer, S., Hakanson, R., and Sundler, F. (eds.): Evolution and Tumor Pathology of the Neuroendocrine System. Amsterdam, Elsevier Science, 1984, p. 497.

128. Solcia, E., et al.: Endocrine cells of the gastrointestinal tract and related tumors. *In* Ioachim, H.L. (ed.): Pathobiology Annual, Vol. 9. New York, Raven Press, 1979, 163.

129. O'Briain, D.S., et al.: Rectal carcinoids as tumors of the hindgut endocrine cells. Am. J. Surg. Pathol. *6:*131, 1982.

130. Falkmer, S., et al.: Occurrence of pancreatic polypeptide, somatostatin, glucagon, insulin, enkephalin, β-endorphin and substance P cells in rectal carcinoids. *In* Miyoshi, A. (ed.): Gut Peptides: Secretion, Function and Clinical Aspects. Amsterdam, Elsevier/North Holland, 1979, p. 351.

131. Creutzfeldt, W., and Stockmann, F.: Carcinoids and carcinoid syndrome. Am. J. Med. *82* (Suppl. 5B):4, 1987.

132. Saegesser, F., and Gross, M.: Carcinoid syndrome and carcinoid tumors of the rectum. Am. J. Proctol. *20:*27, 1969.

133. Chatterjee, K., and Heather, J.C.: Carcinoid heart disease from primary ovarian carcinoid tumors. Am. J. Med. *45:*643, 1968.

134. Coutsoftides, T., and Shibata, H.R.: Primary malignant tumors of the small intestine. Dis. Colon Rectum *22:*24, 1979.

135. Trier, J.S.: Intestinal malabsorption: Differentiation of cause. Hosp. Pract. *23:*195, 1988.

136. Keuning, J.J., et al.: HLA-DW3 associated with coeliac disease. Lancet *1:*506, 1976.

137. Ashkenezi, A., et al.: An in vitro immunological assay for the diagnosis of coeliac disease. Lancet *1:*627, 1978.

138. Rosekrans, P.C., et al.: Long-term morphological and immunohistochemical observations on biopsy specimens of small intestine from children with gluten-sensitive enteropathy. J. Clin. Pathol. *34:*138, 1981.

139. Savilahti, E., et al.: IgA antigliadin antibodies: A marker of mucosal damage in childhood coeliac disease. Lancet *1:*320, 1982.

140. Congdon, P.: Small bowel mucosa in asymptomatic children with celiac disease. Am. J. Dis. Child. *135:*118, 1981.

141. Swinson, C.M., et al.: Coeliac disease malignancy. Lancet *1:*111, 1983.

142. Klipstein, F.A., et al.: Enterotoxigenic intestinal bacteria in tropical sprue. Ann. Intern. Med. *79:*632, 1973.

143. Keren, D.F.: Whipple's disease. A review emphasizing immunology and microbiology. CRC Crit. Rev. Clin. Lab. Sci. *14:*75, 1981.

144. Kent, S.P., and Kirkpatrick, P.M.: Whipple's disease. Immunological and histochemical studies of 8 cases. Arch. Pathol. Lab. Med. *104:*544, 1980.

145. Dobbins, W.O. III: Whipple's disease. *In* Berk, J.E., et al. (eds.): Bockus Gastroenterology. 4th ed. Vol. III, The intestine. Philadelphia, W.B. Saunders, 1985.

146. Feurle, G.E., et al.: Cerebral Whipple's disease with negative jejunal histology. N. Engl. J. Med. *300:*907, 1979.

147. Bostwick, D.G., et al.: Whipple's disease presenting an aortic insufficiency. N. Engl. J. Med. *305:*995, 1981.

148. Bjorneklett, A.: Small bowel bacterial overgrowth syndrome. Scand. J. Gastroenterol. *18* (Suppl. 85):83, 1983.

149. Losowsky, M.C., et al.: Causes of steatorrhea. *In* Losowsky, M.S., Walker, B.E., and Kelleher, J. (eds.): Malabsorption in Clinical Practice. London, Churchill Livingstone, 1974, p. 143.

150. Littman, A.: Lactose deficiency, diagnosis and management. Hosp. Pract. *22:*111, 1987.

151. Andrassy, R.J., et al.: Rectal suction biopsy for the diagnosis of Hirschsprung's disease. Ann. Surg. *193:*419, 1981.

152. Gryboski, J.D.: The enterocolitis of Hirschsprung's disease. J. Clin. Gastroenterol. *1:*248, 1979.

153. Larson, D.M., et al.: Medical and surgical therapy in diverticular disease: A comparative study. Gastroenterology *71:*734, 1976.

154. Almy, T.P., and Howell, D.A.: Diverticular disease of the colon. N. Engl. J. Med. *302:*324, 1980.

155. Weinreich, J., and Anderson, D.: Intraluminal pressure of the sigmoid diverticula and related conditions. Scand. J. Gastroenterol. *11:*581, 1976.

156. Painter, N.S.: Diverticular disease of the colon: A bane of the elderly. Geriatrics *31:*89, 1969.

157. Eastwood, M.A., et al.: Colonic function in patients with diverticular disease. Lancet *1:*1181, 1978.

158. Editorial: Keep taking your bran. Lancet *1:*1175, 1979.

159. Walker, N.I., et al.: Melanosis coli: A consequence of anthraquinone-induced apoptosis of colonic epithelial cells. Am. J. Pathol. *131:*465, 1988.

160. Boley, S.J., et al.: On the nature and etiology of vascular ectasias of the colon; degenerative lesions of aging. Gastroenterology *72:*650, 1977.

161. Editorial: Angiodysplasia. Lancet *2:*1086, 1981.

162. Mitsudo, S.M., et al.: Vascular ectasias of the right colon in the elderly. A distinct pathologic entity. Hum. Pathol. *10:*585, 1979.

163. Howard, O.M., et al.: Angiodysplasia of the colon; experience of 26 cases. Lancet *2:*16, 1982.

164. Garland, C.F., et al.: Incidence rates of ulcerative colitis and Crohn's disease in 15 areas of the U.S. Gastroenterology *81:*1115, 1981.

165. Farmer, R.G., et al.: Studies of family history among patients with inflammatory bowel disease. Clin. Gastroenterol. *9:*271, 1980.

166. Riddell, R.H., et al.: Dysplasia in inflammatory bowel disease: Standardized classification with provisional clinical applications. Hum. Pathol. *14:*931, 1983.

167. Greenstein, A.J., et al.: Cancer in universal left-sided ulcerative colitis: Factors determining risk. Gastroenterology *99:*290, 1979.

168. Price, A.B., and Morson, B.C.: Inflammatory bowel disease; the surgical pathology of Crohn's disease and ulcerative colitis. Hum. Pathol. *6:*7, 1975.

169. Lee, K.S., et al.: Indeterminate colitis in the spectrum of inflammatory bowel disease. Arch. Pathol. Lab. Med. *103:*173, 1979.

170. Sachar, D.B., and Greenstein, A.J.: Cancer in ulcerative colitis: Good news and bad news. Ann. Intern. Med. *95:*462, 1981.

171. Ritchie, J.K., et al.: Prognosis of carcinoma in ulcerative colitis. Gut *22:*752, 1981.

172. Kleinman, M.S., and Listensky, C.: Inflammatory bowel disease and cancer. Hosp. Pract. *19:*56, 1984.

173. Bartlett, J.G.: Antibiotic-associated colitis. Viewpoints Dig. Dis. *16:*9, 1984.

174. Bolton, R.P., et al.: Clostridium difficile–associated diarrhoea—a role in inflammatory bowel disease. Lancet *1:*383, 1980.

175. Bartlett, J.G., et al.: Antibiotic-associated pseudomembranous colitis due to toxin-producing clostridia. N. Engl. J. Med. *298:*531, 1978.

176. Moskowitz, M., and Bartlett, J.G.: Recurrent pseudomembranous colitis unassociated with prior antibiotic therapy. Arch. Intern. Med. *141:*663, 1981.

177. Kleigman, R.M., and Fanaroff, A.A.: Necrotizing enterocolitis. N. Engl. J. Med. *310:*1093, 1984.

178. Gotoff, S.P.: Neonatal immunity. J. Pediatr. *85:*149, 1974.

179. Head, J.R.: Immunobiology of lactation. Semin. Perinatol. *1:*195, 1977.

180. Lindstrom, C.G.: "Collagenous colitis" with watery diarrhoea—a new entity? Pathol. Eur. *11:*87, 1976.

181. Bayless, T.M., et al.: Collagenous colitis (Editorial). Mayo Clin. Proc. *62:*740, 1987.

182. Giardiello, F.M., et al.: Collagenous colitis: physiologic and histopathologic studies in seven patients. Ann. Intern. Med. *106:*46, 1987.

183. Jessurun, J., et al.: Chronic colitis with thickening of the subepithelial collagen layer (collagenous colitis): histopathologic findings in 15 patients. Hum. Pathol. *18:*839, 1987.

184. Chapman, I.: Adenomatous polyps of large intestine: Incidence and distribution. Ann. Surg. *157:*223, 1963.

185. Fenoglio, C.M., and Lane, N.: The anatomic precursor of colorectal cancer. Cancer *34:*819, 1974.

186. Maskens, A.P.: Histogenesis of adenomatous polyps in the human large intestine. Gastroenterology *77:*1245, 1979.

187. Estrada, R.G., and Spjut, H.J.: Hyperplastic polyps of the large bowel. Am. J. Surg. Pathol. *4:*127, 1980.

188. Bussey, H.J.R.: Gastrointestinal polyposis. Gut *11:*970, 1970.

189. Bulow, S.: Colorectal polyposis syndrome. Scand. J. Gastroenterol. *19:*289, 1984.

190. Erbe, R.W.: Current concepts in genetics: inherited gastrointestinal-polyposis syndromes. N. Engl. J. Med. *294:*1101, 1976.

191. Spjut, H.J., and Estrada, R.G.: The significance of epithelial polyps of the large bowel. Pathol. Annu. *12* (Part 1):147, 1977.

192. Shinya, H., and Wolff, W.I.: Morphology, anatomic distribution and cancer potential of colonic polyps. Ann. Surg. *190:*679, 1979.

193. Kent, T.H., and Mitros, F.A.: Polyps of the colon and small bowel, polyp syndromes and polyp-carcinoma sequence. *In* Norris, H.T. (ed.): Contemporary Issues in Surgical Pathology, Vol. 2. New York, Churchill Livingstone, 1983, p. 167.

194. Bussey, H.J.R.: Multiple adenomas and carcinomas. *In* Morson, B.C. (ed.): The Pathogenesis of Colorectal Cancer. Philadelphia, W.B. Saunders Co., 1978, p. 72.

195. Muto, T., et al.: The evolution of cancer of colon and rectum. Cancer *36:*2251, 1975.

196. Day, D.W., and Morson, B.C.: The adenoma-carcinoma sequence. *In* Morson, B.C. (ed.): The Pathogenesis of Colorectal Cancer. Philadelphia, W.B. Saunders Co., 1978, p. 58.

197. Cannon-Albright, L.A., et al.: Common inheritance of susceptibility to colonic adenomatous polyps and associated colorectal cancers. N. Engl. J. Med. *319:*533, 1988.

198. Coutsoftides, T., et al.: Malignant polyps of the colon and rectum. A clinicopathologic study. Dis. Colon Rectum *22:*82, 1979.

199. Vogelstein, B., et al.: Genetic alterations during colorectal tumor development. N. Engl. J. Med. *319:*525, 1988.

200. Bussey, H.J.R.: Polyposis syndromes. *In* Morson, B.C. (ed.): The Pathogenesis of Colorectal Cancer. Philadelphia, W.B. Saunders Co., 1978, p. 81.

201. Watne, A.L., et al.: Gardner's syndrome. Surg. Gynecol. Obstet. *141:*53, 1975.

202. Gardner, E.J.: Familial polyposis coli and Gardner's syndrome—is there a difference? *In* Ingall, J.R.F., and Mastromarino, A.J. (eds.): Prevention of Hereditary Large Bowel Cancer. New York, Alan R. Liss, 1983, p. 39.

203. Eisenberg, H. (ed.): Cancer in Connecticut, Incidence and Rates, 1935–1962. Hartford, Connecticut State Dept. of Health, 1966.

204. Liechty, R.D., et al.: Adenocarcinoma of the colon and rectum. Review of 2261 cases over a 20 year period. Dis. Colon Rectum *11:*201, 1968.

205. Cady, B., et al.: Changing patterns of colorectal carcinoma. Cancer *33:*422, 1974.

206. Rosato, F.E., and Marks, G.: Changing site distribution patterns of colorectal cancer at Thomas Jefferson University Hospital. Dis. Colon Rectum *24:*93, 1981.

207. Haenszel, W., and Kurihara, M.: Studies of Japanese migrants. 1. Mortality from cancer and other disease among Japanese in the United States. J. Natl. Cancer Inst. *40:*43, 1968.

208. Staszewski, J., and Haenszel, W.: Cancer mortality among the Polish born in the United States. J. Natl. Cancer Inst. *35:*291, 1965.

209. Ferrands, P.A., et al.: Radioimmunodetection of human colorectal cancer by an anti-tumour monoclonal antibody. Lancet *2:*297, 1982.

210. Neville, A.M.: Carcinoembryonic antigen, the current status. Arch. Pathol. Lab. Med. *105:*281, 1981.

211. Stearns, M.W.: Staging colonic and rectal cancer. Int. Adv. Surg. Oncol. *4:*189, 1981.

212. Wangensteen, O.H., and Dennis, T.: Experimental proof of the obstructive origin of appendicitis in man. Ann. Surg. *110:*629, 1939.

213. Law, D., et al.: The continuing challenge of acute and perforated appendicitis. Am. J. Surg. *131:*533, 1976.

214. Gray, G.F., Jr., and Wackym, P.A.: Surgical pathology of the vermiform appendix. Pathol. Annu. *21* (Pt. 2):111, 1986.

215. Moertel, C.G., et al.: Carcinoid tumor of the appendix: treatment and prognosis. N. Engl. J. Med. *317:*1699, 1987.

The Liver and Biliary Tract

LIVER

NORMAL

The liver, quite rightly, has been called "the custodian of the milieu intérieur." Hepatic disorders, therefore, have far-reaching consequences on the body's homeostasis that are best understood from the perspective of normal structure and function. Only a few salient features can be reviewed. The normal adult liver weighs 1400 to 1600 gm and is nonpalpable under the costal edge unless displaced downward by the right diaphragm, when a smooth nonpulsatile edge may "peek out."

Microscopically and functionally, the liver has been subdivided classically into roughly hexagonal *lobules*, 1 to 2 mm in diameter, oriented about a central vein (a tributary of the hepatic vein). The blood supply to the liver parenchyma flows from the portal triads to the central veins; about 30 to 40% is provided by the terminal ramifications of the hepatic artery and the remainder by the portal vein radicles.

It has been argued that the liver cells about the central vein are most remote from the blood supply and therefore are at the periphery of the "metabolic lobules" referred to as *acini*. These are centered about portal vein and hepatic artery *branches* that leave the portal tracts at intervals and run along the sides of the classic lobule to serve pie-shaped segments of contiguous lobules.[1] The parenchyma of the acinus is divided into three zones, zone 1 being closest to the arterial and portal supply, zone 3 abutting the central vein, and zone 2 being intermediate. This may explain why many forms of toxic injury to the liver are most severe in the periphery of the *classical lobule*, because zone 1 is exposed to the greatest concentration of blood-borne hepatotoxins. Analogously, hypoxic injury such as occurs with shock or cardiac failure, although referred to as central necrosis, is actually located at the periphery of the acinus in zone 3, most remote from the arterial and portal supply. Despite the many virtues of the acinus conception, the classical lobule is an "old soldier" that will not die and so persists as the standard hepatic unit.

There is little disagreement about the internal architecture of the lobule or acinus. Oversimplified for the sake of brevity, it comprises cribriform, branching, or anastomosing sheets or plates of hepatocytes seen in microscopic sections as cords of cells radially disposed about the central vein. The lineup of hepatocytes about the portal tracts is referred to as the limiting plate. There is relatively little variation in liver cell size but considerable variation in nuclear size, number, and ploidy. Some nuclei are considerably larger than others, and their karyotypes may

911

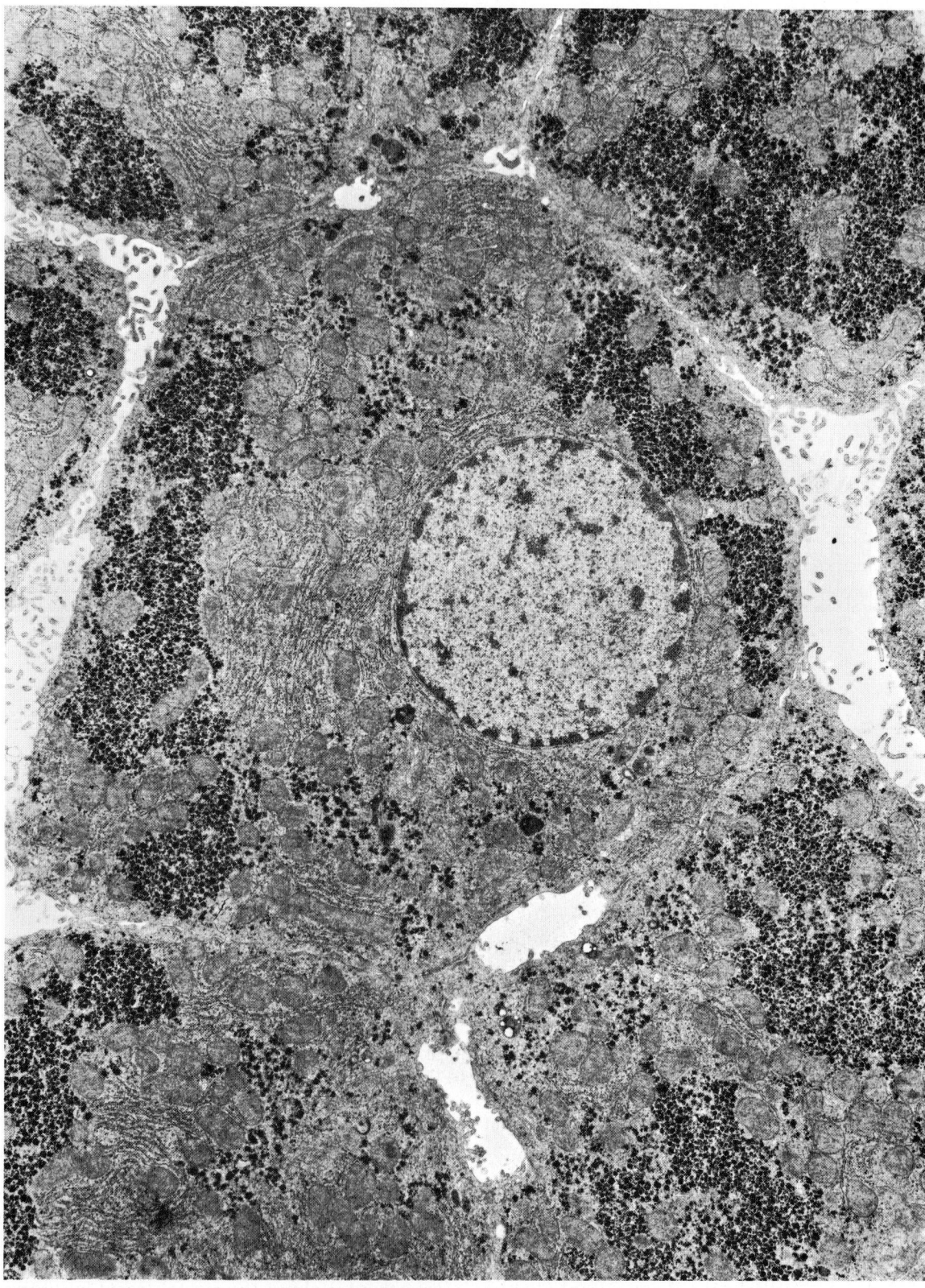

Figure 19–1. Low-power electron micrograph of normal rat liver cell. Dark granules are glycogen. The large lateral spaces are vascular sinusoids. Above and below are biliary canaliculi sandwiched between liver cells. Note microvilli in sinusoids and canaliculi. (Courtesy of Dr. H. D. Fahimi, Mallory Institute of Pathology.)

range up to octaploidy. In addition, although uninucleate cells are the rule, a significant fraction are binucleate. The cytoplasm is equally variable, reflecting to some extent the functional activity of the cell. In the previously normal individual who dies suddenly of extrahepatic causes, abundant glycogen can be visualized in PAS stains as aggregates or rosettes closely associated with the smooth endoplasmic reticulum (SER) (Fig. 19–1). Normally there are only scattered, fine vacuoles of lipid.

Interposed between the radial cords of hepatocytes are vascular sinusoids receiving blood from both the portal and the arterial systems and draining into the central veins. The sinusoids are lined by fenestrated and discontinuous endothelial cells, attached to which are scattered the Kupffer cells of the reticuloendothelial or monocyte phagocyte system. Between the sinusoids and liver cell cords are the narrow spaces of Disse, into which protrude hepatocytic microvilli and in which are found scattered fat-containing lipocytes (Ito cells) of mesenchymal origin, thought to play some role in fat transport and storage of vitamin A. The dual blood supply through the portal vein and hepatic artery provides a great deal of, but not total, protection against infarctions.

The biliary system begins in the centrilobular regions as an elaborate network of canaliculi interposed between abutting hepatocytes. These progressively join toward the periphery of the lobule, to drain eventually into the intermediate canals of Hering close to the portal tracts, which become the interlobular bile ducts within the portal triads. The interhepatocytic biliary canaliculi are channels, 1 to 2 μm in diameter, formed merely by grooves along the external surfaces of abutting liver cells. Thus, the walls of these channels are the plasma membranes of the liver cells punctuated by numerous microvilli that protrude into the lumina of the canaliculi (Fig. 19–2). Membrane-associated actin and myosin microfilaments within the hepatocytes are particularly abundant about the canalicular walls as well as in the microvilli. The microfilaments, as will be seen, are thought to play some role in transport of bile through the canaliculi.[2] It is within the canals of Hering that specialized, somewhat flattened bile duct epithelial cells first appear.

The liver has enormous reserve and regenerative capacity. When the remaining hepatic parenchyma is normal, patients have survived resection of about 80% of the liver. With partial hepatectomy, subsequent regenerative activity occurs throughout the residual liver with enlargement of the remaining lobules and disorderly proliferation of hepatocytes at the cut surfaces, restoring to a considerable extent mass and function. The disordered parenchyma may not restore functioning biliary channels and so cannot efficiently participate in bile production. However, the newly formed hepatocytes can participate in most of the remaining hepatic anabolic and catabolic functions. When hepatotoxic substances such as carbon tetrachloride destroy only some of the hepatocytes within the lobule, leaving the connective tissue framework intact, almost perfect reconstitution can occur.

BILIRUBIN FORMATION AND SECRETION. Only bilirubin metabolism and bile secretion will be briefly reviewed to facilitate the understanding of hyperbilirubinemia (jaundice).[3,4] Bile production can be conveniently divided into (1) bilirubin formation, (2) transport in the blood, (3) uptake and intracellular transport, (4) glucuronidation, and (5) excretion (secretion) into the canaliculus (Fig. 19–3). *Bilirubin formation* involves selective cleavage of the heme ring. About 70% is derived from the breakdown of

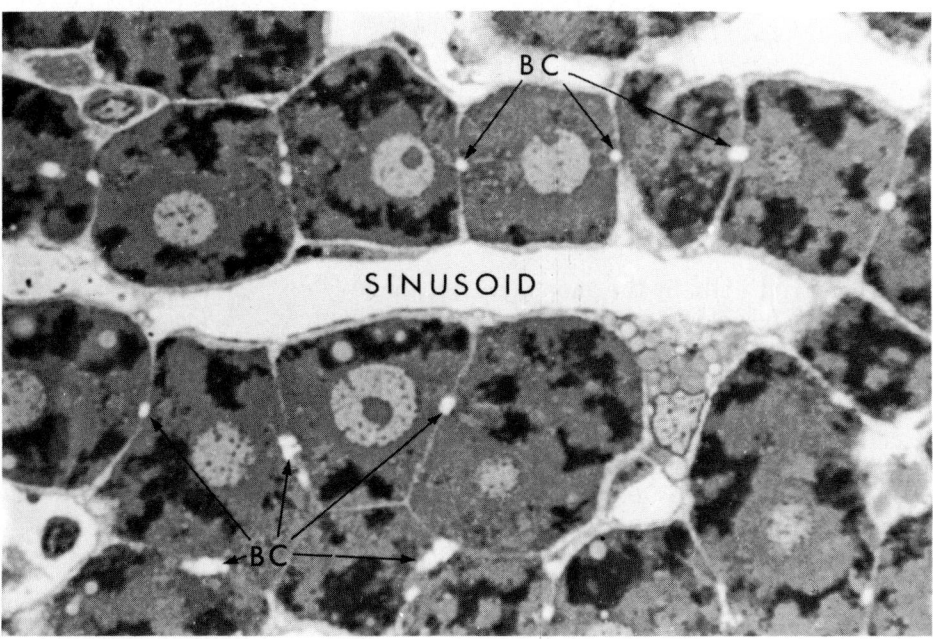

Figure 19–2. Low-power photomicrograph of liver fixed by vascular perfusion. Liver cords are oriented on both sides of vascular sinusoid. BC marks biliary canaliculi between adjacent liver cells. (Courtesy of H.D. Fahimi, M.D., University of Heidelberg. Reproduced with permission from Lab. Invest. 16:736, 1967. Copyright 1967, The Williams and Wilkins Company, Baltimore.)

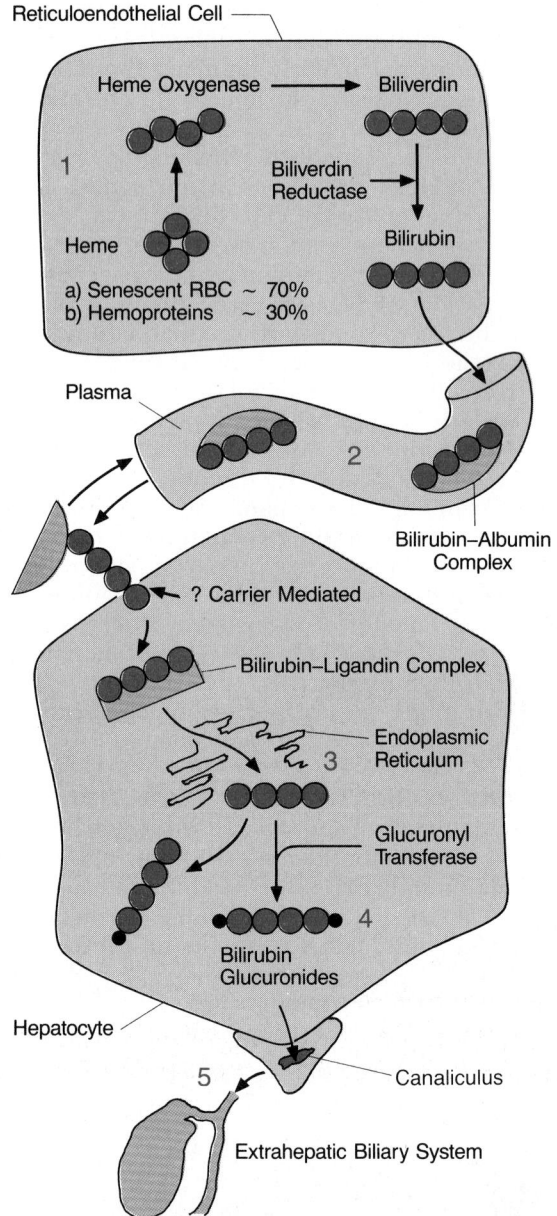

Figure 19–3. Schematic of bilirubin metabolism indicating types of derangements leading to jaundice: (1) excessive release of heme pigment (hemolytic anemia); (2) reduced hepatic uptake; (3) impaired conjugation of bilirubin; (4) deranged intrahepatic bilirubin excretion; (5) extrahepatic bilirubin obstruction.

senescent red cells in the mononuclear phagocyte (RE) system (especially in the spleen, liver, and bone marrow). Increased breakdown of red cells, as occurs with intravascular hemolysis or resorption of extravascular blood in the gut or a hematoma, provides a greater load of heme for bilirubin production. Most of the remainder is derived from the turnover of hepatic heme or hemoproteins, e.g., the p-450 cytochromes. A minor contribution comes from premature destruction of newly formed red cells in the bone marrow (ineffective erythropoiesis). The heme is converted into biliverdin through the stages depicted in Figure 19–3.

Transport of bilirubin in the plasma from its various sites of formation, e.g., spleen, to the liver requires that it be bound tightly to albumin, since the nascent unconjugated bilirubin is virtually insoluble in aqueous solutions at the pH of blood. A very small fraction of the bilirubin in the plasma is unbound. In severe hemolytic disease, this unbound fraction may be of great importance because it may be able to cross the incompletely developed blood-brain barrier in infants to damage the brain (kernicterus) (p. 528).[5]

The *uptake and intracellular transport* of bilirubin is still incompletely understood. It appears that the albumin of the bilirubin-albumin complex binds to a specific membrane receptor.[6] A conformational change in albumin releases it from the receptor and bilirubin; the latter then binds to specific domains (?receptors) on the hepatocytic membrane and is transferred across the plasma membrane by a carrier mechanism. This transfer mechanism is shared by other organic anions such as sulfobromophthalein (BSP) (used for a liver excretory function test). Once across the plasma membrane, the bilirubin is presumably bound to a cytosolic protein — ligandin — and in some manner is transferred to the endoplasmic reticulum for further metabolism.

Glucuronidation is required to convert bilirubin into a water-soluble, nontoxic pigment that can be secreted by the liver cell. First, the bilirubin is esterified with probably one molecule of glucuronic acid by glucuronyl transferase to form bilirubin monoglucuronides. Most (80 to 90%) is then converted into diglucuronides; the remainder persists as monoglucuronides. There are several transferases, but only one form appears to be involved in the glucuronidation, because a genetic deficiency of this particular transferase underlies some of the hereditary disorders of bilirubin metabolism discussed later. A small fraction of the glucuronides perversely undergoes deconjugation. Thus in patients with hyperbilirubinemia related to an excretory defect with so-called regurgitation of bilirubin into the blood, although most is in the form of conjugated bilirubin, a small fraction is unconjugated.

There are important pathophysiologic differences between unconjugated and conjugated bilirubin. *Unconjugated bilirubin is toxic to tissues, is not soluble in aqueous solutions, and is tightly complexed to albumin, in which form it cannot be excreted in the urine even when the blood levels are high. As noted earlier, a small amount of unconjugated bilirubin is unbound, and therefore when present in excess, may cause toxic injury to tissues, particularly the brain. In contrast, conjugated bilirubin is water-soluble, nontoxic, and under normal conditions only loosely bound to albumin. Because of the solubility and weak association with albumin, when present in excess it is excreted in the urine (bilirubinuria).*

Excretion or secretion of bilirubin into the biliary apparatus is largely a mysterious phenomenon involving transfer of the glucuronides from within the endoplasmic reticulum into the lumen of the bile canaliculus. The transport across the canalicular membrane appears to be carrier mediated and is the rate-limiting step in the removal of bilirubin from the cell. Other organic anions, such as BSP and radiopaque agents used in gallbladder visualization, utilize this same pathway, but bile acids appear to have an independent carrier pathway. Nonetheless, excretion of bile acids augments the rate of bilirubin clearance; either the bile salts directly stimulate bilirubin (and anion) excretion or the two excretory pathways are somehow linked.

Once in the canaliculus the bilirubin flows through ever larger intrahepatic ducts, eventually to reach the extrahepatic biliary tract and the intestinal tract. Most of the bilirubin is converted by the intestinal flora into urobilinogen, and the residue is excreted. A small amount of urobilinogen is also excreted in the stool, but most is absorbed into the blood to be returned to the liver through the portal system to be again excreted into the bile. During this enterohepatic circulation, a small amount is lost in the urine.

To complete the consideration of bilirubin metabolism, *bile formation and flow* should be briefly addressed. Bile is essentially formed in the canaliculi of the hepatic lobules and is then modified downstream in the larger ductules and ducts by reabsorption or secretion of solutes and water.[7] The most abundant substances secreted in bile are the bile salts, representing mostly conjugates of cholic and chenodeoxycholic acids with glycine and taurine. Bile also contains substantial amounts of bilirubin, cholesterol, phospholipids (mainly lecithin), and the electrolytes found in plasma, notably sodium. *The driving force for canalicular bile formation and flow is active transport of solutes, producing an osmotic gradient along which water flows.* Two somewhat overlapping mechanisms are thought to exist. The first and more important is called bile acid–dependent bile formation, which proposes that the major osmotic force is derived from the active secretion of bile acids. The other, somewhat analogous mechanism is designated bile acid–independent bile formation. Here, less importance is attached to the bile acids, and Na^+, K^+-ATPase–mediated active sodium transport is postulated as the driving osmotic force. The flow of water along the osmotic gradient creates the driving force for biliary flow. In addition, circumcanalicular microfilaments of actin and myosin have been identified in hepatocytes. Conceivably, contraction of these "miniscule muscles" may also contribute to bile flow. In sum, *bile formation (including flow) is energy dependent, whether it be the energy required for active transport of bile salts and sodium into the canaliculi or the energy required for the contraction of hepatocytic microfilaments.*

The bile acids are also important in maintaining in solution the hydrophobic cholesterol secreted by hepatocytes, by incorporating it into micelles along with the bile acids and phospholipids. It might be noted that this pathway of excretion of cholesterol accounts for the hypercholesterolemia often associated with disorders obstructing the outflow of bile. When the bile reaches the small intestine, the micelles are disassociated and some of the bile salts are excreted but most are reabsorbed. The relevance of these details of bilirubin and bile metabolism will become evident in the later consideration of hyperbilirubinemia.

PATHOLOGY

Vulnerable to a wide variety of metabolic, circulatory, toxic, microbial, and neoplastic insults, the liver is one of the most frequently injured organs in the body. In some instances the disease is primary in the liver: for example, viral hepatitis and hepatocellular carcinoma. More often the hepatic involvement is secondary, often to some of the most common diseases of man, such as cardiac decompensation, disseminated cancer, alcoholism, and extrahepatic infections. Many liver disorders are more reasonably discussed elsewhere and receive no further consideration here, e.g., fatty change (Fig. 19–4) (p. 20), glycogen accumulation in diabetics (p. 24), storage diseases (p. 144), and amyloidosis (p. 210).

Various forms of pigment may accumulate in the liver, the two most important being hemosiderin and

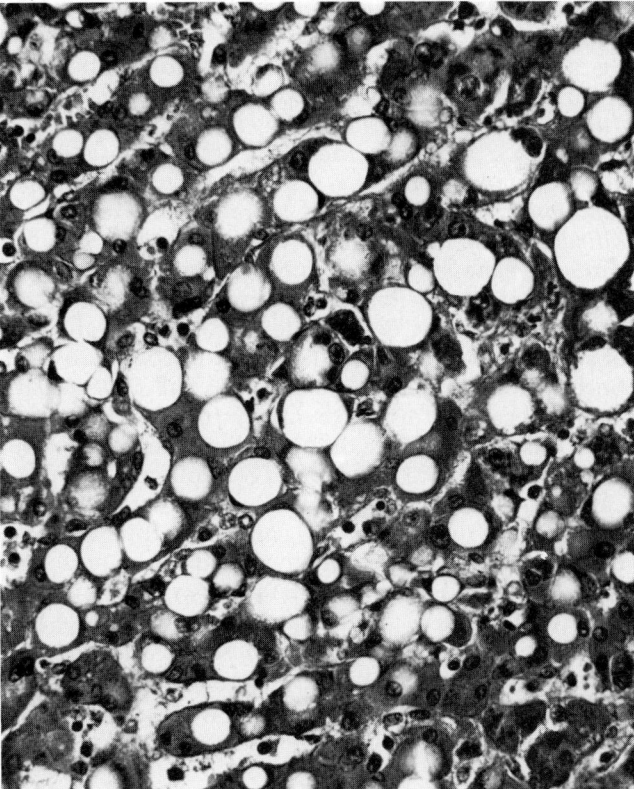

Figure 19–4. Fatty liver. High-power detail revealing large vacuoles compressing cytoplasm and nuclei to the periphery.

lipofuscin. The latter was described on page 24, and details on hemosiderosis were given on page 686 and will also be considered later. You may recall that the appearance of lipofuscin within cells is a marker of atrophy, and so is encountered in livers that have decreased in size and undergone what is called "brown atrophy." With these few reminders, further discussions can be limited to involvements not covered elsewhere.

Whether primary or secondary, all hepatic derangements tend to cause similar signs and symptoms; because of the liver's considerable reserve, however, manifestations appear only when the injury is significant and diffuse or strategically located so as to obstruct biliary outflow. Ultimately, hepatic failure may ensue. Because jaundice and hepatic failure are common to so many forms of liver disease, they will be discussed at the outset.

JAUNDICE

Jaundice, also called *icterus*, refers to yellow-green pigmentation of the skin or sclerae by bilirubin. It is particularly noticeable in the eyes because of the high scleral content of elastin, which has a special affinity for bilirubin. *Jaundice always signifies hyperbilirubinemia*, but it does not become clinically evident until the serum bilirubin level exceeds 2 mg/dl (normal 0.5 to 1 mg).

Many clinical disorders are associated with jaundice, but ultimately they fall within one or more of the following four pathogenetic categories: (1) *overproduction of bilirubin by increased breakdown of red cells;* (2) *impaired uptake of bilirubin from the blood due to intrahepatocytic derangements;* (3) *decreased conjugation either because of a genetic lack of glucuronyl transferase or some acquired disturbance in its function;* and (4) *impaired secretion or excretion of bilirubin, either intrahepatic or extrahepatic.* The first three mechanisms yield mainly unconjugated hyperbilirubinemia. The last mechanism, whether it relates to an intrahepatic cellular defect or an extrahepatic obstructive process, results mainly in conjugated hyperbilirubinemia and cholestasis. The intrahepatic category can be further divided into (a) excretory defects associated with diffuse liver disease affecting perhaps all functions of the liver cell and therefore called *hepatocellular cholestasis;* and (b) cholestasis related to a disturbance in canalicular bile flow but unassociated with parenchymal disease and thus sometimes called *"pure" cholestasis.*[8] Admittedly, this subdivision is somewhat arbitrary because persistent bile retention within the liver cell, as may occur in pure cholestasis, in time leads to liver cell damage, and so the two patterns merge. Against this background the major clinical disorders associated with jaundice are cited in Table 19–1.

Virtually all the conditions cited in Table 19–1 are described elsewhere in this text; only a few comments are required here on two uncommon entities.

Table 19–1. Pathophysiologic Classification of Jaundice*

PREDOMINANTLY UNCONJUGATED HYPERBILIRUBINEMIA
Overproduction
  Intravascular hemolysis—hemolytic anemias
  Extravascular hemolysis—resorption of blood from large hematomas, large internal hemorrhages (e.g., gastrointestinal bleeds), hemorrhagic infarcts (e.g., lung)
  Ineffective erythropoiesis
Decreased Hepatocellular Uptake
  Drugs
  Sepsis
  Markedly reduced caloric intake (near-starvation)
Decreased Hepatocellular Conjugation (hereditary lack or impaired function of glucuronyl transferase)
  Gilbert's syndrome
  Crigler-Najjar syndrome
  Neonatal jaundice
  Drug inhibition, e.g., chloramphenicol
  Diffuse hepatocellular disease, e.g., hepatitis, cirrhosis
PREDOMINANTLY CONJUGATED HYPERBILIRUBINEMIA (CHOLESTASIS)
Impaired Hepatocellular Secretion
  "Pure" cholestasis
    Dubin-Johnson and Rotor syndromes
    Congenital atresia or strictures of the intrahepatic ducts
    "Early" biliary cirrhosis
    Fibrocystic disease of pancreas
    Drugs, e.g., oral contraceptives, estrogens, methyl testosterone
    Benign familial recurrent cholestasis
    Recurrent jaundice of pregnancy
  Hepatocellular cholestasis
    Some cases of viral hepatitis ("cholangiolitic" viral hepatitis)
    Some cases of alcohol-induced fatty liver or hepatitis
    Some forms of chemical or drug-induced injury
Extrahepatic Obstruction to Biliary Apparatus (approximate order of frequency)
    Obstructive gallstones
    Carcinoma of head of pancreas
    Obstructive carcinoma of extrahepatic ducts or papilla of Vater
    Inflammatory stenosing strictures usually related to previous biliary surgery
    Congenital atresia of the extrahepatic ducts

* The disorders cited are illustrative and not a complete listing.

Benign familial recurrent cholestasis is an obscure nonprogressive form of conjugated hyperbilirubinemia that, as indicated, tends to run in families and usually has an early age of onset. For these reasons it is vaguely attributed to a congenital derangement in canalicular bile flow. There are no histologic changes in the liver (other than the features of cholestasis) or obstructive lesions in the biliary apparatus, despite the persistence of the disease or the number of recurrences. *Recurrent jaundice of pregnancy* most often appears during the last trimester. The biochemical changes mimic those of extrahepatic obstructive disease, but they promptly clear after delivery and sometimes recur with subsequent pregnancies. The condition is thought to be related to an abnormal sensitivity to increased levels of estrogens, analogous to the jaundice caused in some individuals by exogenous female sex hormones.

The morphologic features of cholestasis depend somewhat on its severity, duration, and underlying cause. In general, the intrahepatic disorders tend to produce milder degrees of cholestasis than the extrahepatic disorders. **The most distinctive features of intrahepatic disorders are elongated green-brown plugs of bile in dilated canaliculi, most prominent toward the centers of the lobules, accompanied by droplets of bile pigment within liver cells and sometimes Kupffer cells** (Fig. 19–5). In "pure" cholestasis the liver cells at the outset appear morphologically normal by light microscopy, but they soon develop wispy cytoplasm referred to as **feathery degeneration,** attributed to retention of bile acids. This cytoplasmic change may also appear with extrahepatic obstructive disease but is rarely as marked. The cytoplasmic appearance is created by numerous aqueous microvacuoles. Ultrastructural examination reveals a variety of organellar changes such as mitochondrial swelling, and distention of the ER and Golgi complex, but perhaps most relevant is disorganization of the pericanalicular membrane-associated actin filaments. Similar changes appear in hepatocellular cholestasis but are superimposed on those of the underlying disease. Eventually **the canalicular bile stasis, whatever its origin, leads to proliferation of intralobular ductules and portal tract bile ducts, sometimes accompanied by mild periportal fibrosis, mimicking biliary cirrhosis** (p. 953).

In contrast to the intrahepatic cholestatic syndromes, **extrahepatic obstructions induce a pattern of cholestasis that begins with distention of the extrahepatic biliary apparatus by bile, with progressive retrograde extension of the bile stasis into the intrahepatic duct system.** The bile stasis in the duct radicles within the portal triads leads to proliferation of the epithelial lining cells, sometimes accompanied by an increase in surrounding fibrous tissue. Eventually the canaliculi become distended with bile, and pigment can be seen within liver cells and Kupffer cells, recapitulating the changes of intrahepatic cholestasis. **The most helpful differential feature of extrahepatic obstruction is rupture of canaliculi with extravasation of bile, producing so-called bile lakes surrounded by injured or necrotic liver cells.** Because stasis of bile predisposes to ascending bacterial infections, extrahepatic cholestasis may be complicated by ascending cholangitis and cholangiolitis marked by intraductal and intraductular accumulations of neutrophils.

Whatever the underlying disorder, cholestasis itself is regularly associated with distinctive clinical changes—there is conjugated hyperbilirubinemia with jaundice, bilirubinuria, and even more characteristic, elevation of the serum level of bile acids, producing one of the most distressing features of cholestasis—itching (pruritus). Often the rise in serum bile acids and the pruritus precede the appearance of jaundice. Hyperlipidemia also sometimes appears, with the formation of skin xanthomas related to impaired excretion of cholesterol but also to increased synthesis of cholesterol. Another characteristic finding is an elevated serum level of alkaline phosphatase. This enzyme is normally present in many other tissues, e.g., bone, and so the increased levels must be determined to be hepatocytic in origin. The increased phosphatase levels are a more sensitive

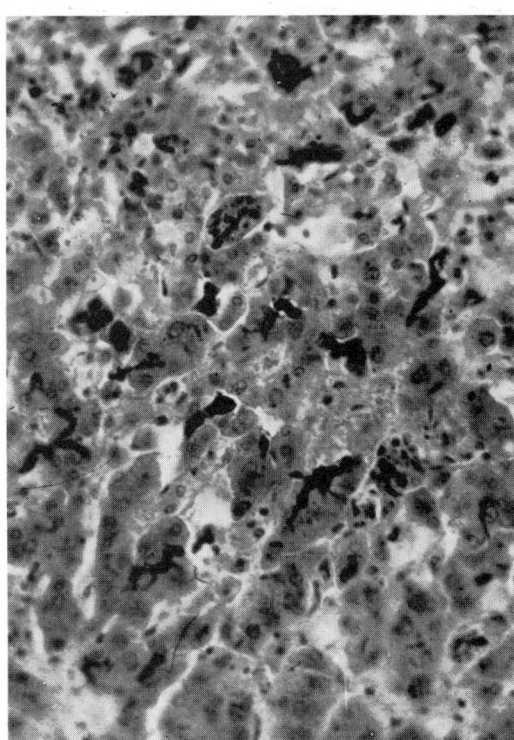

Figure 19–5. Liver-bile stasis. Bile canaliculi distended with inspissated bile. Kupffer cells contain phagocytized bile.

marker of cholestasis than is hyperbilirubinemia, often preceding it. Many other changes may accompany the reduced bile flow into the intestines, including malabsorption of fat and fat-soluble vitamins, and so steatorrhea and manifestations related to a deficiency of vitamins A, D, or K sometimes develop, principally hypoprothrombinemia (vitamin K deficiency). *Thus come about the major clinical markers of "pure" cholestasis: conjugated hyperbilirubinemia, elevated levels of serum bile acids and alkaline phosphatase, hyperlipidemia, and hypoprothrombinemia with a consequent bleeding diathesis. When the cholestasis arises because of diffuse injury to liver cells causing so-called hepatocellular cholestasis, the laboratory findings also include many of the changes associated with liver failure, for example, elevated serum levels of the aminotransferases as pointed out on page 918.*

The differentiation of intrahepatic (so-called medical) jaundice from that due to extrahepatic lesions (often referred to as surgical or sometimes obstructive jaundice) can often be critical. Extrahepatic biliary obstruction can sometimes be surgically alleviated, since it is most often produced by impaction of a gallstone in the common bile duct or ampulla of Vater. In contrast, intrahepatic "medical" jaundice cannot be benefited by surgery, and indeed the patient's condition may be worsened by the operation. It is beyond our scope to delve into this difficult diagnostic problem except to point out that, as mentioned, with time the intrahepatic and extrahepatic derangements tend to merge and so there is urgency to make the correct diagnosis as soon as possible. Although a variety of diagnostic modalities are available, such as liver function tests, cholecystography, cholangiography, ultrasonography, scintigraphy, CT, and MRI scan, ultimately it may be necessary to biopsy the liver to establish the diagnosis.

HEPATIC FAILURE

Like a sand castle on the shore, the liver's functional capacity may crumble grain by grain in the sun, be more rapidly undermined by the oncoming tide, or be suddenly obliterated by a massive wave. Thus hepatic failure may result from the slow deterioration of liver function by some chronic progressive disorder, or more rapid worsening liver function may be caused by repeated acute injuries or a catastrophic event such as massive necrosis.[9] The major disorders having these potentials can be divided into three categories:

1. Ultrastructural lesions that do not necessarily produce overt liver cell necrosis: Reyes' syndrome, acute fatty liver of pregnancy, tetracycline toxicity.
2. Chronic liver disease (acute or chronic failure): chronic active hepatitis, cirrhoses (most types), Wilson's disease.
3. Massive hepatic necrosis (fulminant failure): fulminant viral hepatitis, drugs and chemicals, e.g., halothane, acetaminophen, antidepressants; industrial agents, e.g., carbon tetrachloride phosphorus; mushroom poisoning, e.g., *Amanita* species.

Whatever the underlying condition, the clinical features of hepatic failure are much the same, but because of the liver's innumerable functions hepatic failure has many dimensions. Certain signs, symptoms, and biochemical changes are characteristic and readily understood (Table 19–2).

Many disorders may lead to hepatic failure, but the great preponderance of cases are related to overwhelming viral hepatitis, alcoholic liver disease, and

toxic drug injury as by halothane. The liver functional insufficiency may appear within days of the acute assault despite the absence of pre-existing liver damage. A variety of forms of stress contribute to the onset of failure, whatever the basic disorder. For example, gastrointestinal bleeding, acute infections, electrolyte disturbances, and any form of severe stress such as major surgery, heart failure, or shock may serve as the final straw when the hepatic functional reserve is already precarious. Unfortunately, there is no satisfactory treatment for hepatic failure and coma when there is massive hepatic necrosis save for liver transplantation. With less disastrous events (e.g., Reye's syndrome, viral submassive necrosis), recovery has occurred. Overall the mortality rate is 80%. A few words about the hepatorenal syndrome and the encephalopathy are in order.

HEPATORENAL SYNDROME

Few terms in medicine are more misunderstood than *hepatorenal syndrome.* When used appropriately it refers to the appearance of *renal failure in patients with severe liver disease or in those undergoing surgery for biliary tract obstruction in the absence of intrinsic morphologic or functional cause for the renal failure.* Excluded by this definition is concomitant damage to both organs, as might occur with carbon tetrachloride toxicity, for example. Also excluded are those instances of advanced cirrhosis complicated by gastroesophageal varices, massive bleeding, and shock leading to acute tubular necrosis and renal failure. Indeed, in the hepatorenal syndrome kidney function promptly improves if the liver function can be restored (sometimes by liver transplantation). Preservation of the structure of the kidneys is further attested to by the few cases in which they were used for transplantation.[10]

Typically the appearance of this syndrome in a patient with liver failure is heralded by a drop in renal

Table 19–2. Major Clinical Features of Hepatic Failure

CLINICAL FEATURE	BASIS
Jaundice	Although total bilirubin metabolism is deranged, liver cell secretion is the rate-limiting step, and so conjugated hyperbilirubinemia predominates.
Hypoalbuminemia	Reduced synthesis of albumin
Coagulopathy (worsened by malabsorption of vitamin K)	Reduced synthesis of clotting factors—II, V, VII, IX, and X
Disseminated intravascular coagulation	Activation Hageman factor, inadequate clearance of activated factors
Hyperammonemia	Urea cycle defects
Fetor hepaticus (a musty sweet-and-sour odor to breath)	Inconstant, related to the formation of mercaptans by bacterial action on sulfur-containing amino acid methionine
Increased serum levels of hepatic cytosolic enzymes, i.e., lactic dehydrogenase (LDH), alanine aminotransferase (ALT) (glutamic pyruvic transaminase—GPT), and aspartate aminotransferase (AST) (glutamic oxalacetic transaminase—GOT)	Seen only with active liver cell necrosis; level of increase more or less correlated with extent of liver destruction. LDH relatively nonspecific
Gynecomastia, testicular atrophy, palmar erythema, and spider angiomas of the skin	Putatively related to impaired estrogen metabolism and consequent hyperestrogenism
Hepatorenal syndrome	To be discussed
Hepatic encephalopathy	To be discussed
Coma	Usually follows encephalopathy and precedes death

output associated with a rising BUN and creatinine value. Despite hyperosmolarity, the urine sodium is low but the urine is otherwise devoid of proteins and abnormal sediment. The pathogenesis of this syndrome remains mysterious. The favored theory postulates reduction of renal blood flow (more marked in the cortex than in the medulla) due to cortical vasoconstriction, but the basis for this reduced perfusion is uncertain. Numerous hypotheses have been offered, including (1) increased production of the vasoconstrictive thromboxane A_2 and decreased synthesis of the vasodilator PGE_2[11]; (2) reduced effective circulating volume secondary to the appearance of ascites leading to increased levels of renin and aldosterone; and (3) vasoconstriction produced by gut-derived bacterial endotoxins that escape normal clearance in the liver.[12] Attractive as these ideas may be, the hepatorenal syndrome remains a pathogenetic enigma.

HEPATIC ENCEPHALOPATHY

Hepatic encephalopathy, also called *hepatic coma*, is another feared feature of acute and chronic liver failure.[13] It may also appear with portosystemic shunting and is sometimes referred to as portosystemic encephalopathy. *Basically, it is a metabolic disorder of the central nervous system and neuromuscular system. This conclusion is supported by the fact that in the great majority of instances there are only minor morphologic changes in the brain, such as edema and inconstant changes in astrocytes (p. 1435). Even more important, if hepatic function can be restored, the encephalopathy is reversible without residual complications. Functionally it is characterized by nonspecific electroencephalographic changes, disturbed consciousness progressing to coma, fluctuating neurologic signs, a distinctive "flapping tremor" known as asterixis, and in most cases, progressive confusion, drowsiness, coma, and often death.*[14] Particularly distinctive is the *asterixis*, a series of nonrhythmic, rapid extension-flexion movements of the head and extremities, best seen when the arms are held in extension with dorsiflexed wrists.

The genesis of the CNS manifestations is still uncertain, but whatever the causative agent, there is circumstantial evidence that it represents some toxic product not metabolized by the liver and apparently derived from protein degradation in the intestines. Consistent with this view is the encephalopathy with portosystemic shunting, whether spontaneous in advanced cirrhosis or surgical (portacaval anastomosis), bypassing hepatic metabolism of putative toxins. In addition, a high protein intake worsens the encephalopathy and, conversely, a low protein diet is often beneficial. Analogously, gastrointestinal bleeding with resorption of the blood products may precipitate the syndrome, whereas antibiotics to reduce the intestinal flora are effective in treatment. Four hypotheses are still under active investigation.[15]

1. The *ammonia hypothesis*—impaired hepatic function blocks the degradation of ammonia to urea, and the hyperammonemia constitutes a neurotoxin.

2. The *synergistic neurotoxin hypothesis*—the combined actions of ammonia, mercaptans, and short-chain fatty acids derange neuronal function or transmission of signals.
3. The *false neurotransmitter hypothesis*—normal neurotransmitters, e.g., dopamine, are displaced by such false neurotransmitters as gamma-aminobutyric acid (GABA) and octopamine.
4. The *amino acid hypothesis*—elevated plasma levels of tryptophan and its metabolites, e.g., serotonin, may be toxic to the brain or may lead to decreased production of excitatory neurotransmitters and increased production of weak neurotransmitters.

It is fruitless to go into more detail on any one of these hypotheses because, to date, there is no convincing evidence to indict any one as the basic cause of the syndrome. Conceivably, several may act in concert, or each may be capable of inducing the neurologic syndrome in particular patients.[16]

HEREDITARY HYPERBILIRUBINEMIAS

A small group of rare familial disorders is characterized by jaundice, ranging from mild to severe, caused by genetic defects in the metabolism of bilirubin. Most of these conditions are relatively benign, but one, Crigler-Najjar syndrome Type I, is invariably lethal and fortunately rare. All these disorders have interesting features in common:

1. Despite the presence of jaundice, conventional liver function tests are almost always normal, except for BSP clearance in most individuals with Gilbert's syndrome.
2. There are no well-defined anatomic changes in any of the conditions except for striking obscure pigmentation of the liver in the Dubin-Johnson syndrome.
3. Clinical recognition is of great importance because in all, save the Crigler-Najjar I syndrome, the individuals "are more yellow than sick," and so the jaundice should not be construed as a manifestation of a serious hepatic disease.

The salient features of the various syndromes are presented in Table 19–3. It is evident that both Crigler-Najjar and Gilbert's syndromes constitute nonhemolytic unconjugated hyperbilirubinemias, whereas the Dubin-Johnson and Rotor syndromes are conjugated hyperbilirubinemias. Only a few additional comments will be made.[3]

CRIGLER-NAJJAR SYNDROME TYPE I

This rare autosomal recessive cause of unconjugated hyperbilirubinemia is almost uniformly fatal during the neonatal period because of the progressive development of kernicterus. The basic defect is a complete absence of glucuronyltransferase activity. A few indi-

Table 19–3. The Hereditary Hyperbilirubinemias

DISORDER	INHERITANCE	DEFECTS IN BILIRUBIN METABOLISM	SERUM BILIRUBIN PATTERN	
			Unconjugated	*Conjugated*
Crigler-Najjar syndrome type I	Autosomal recessive	Absent glucuronyltransferase activity	Usually > 20 mg/dl	Absent or minimal
Crigler-Najjar syndrome type II	Autosomal dominant with variable penetrance	Decreased glucuronyltransferase activity	Usually < 20 mg/dl	Absent or minimal
Gilbert syndrome	? Autosomal dominant	Decreased glucuronyltransferase activity, with decreased conjugation, ? decreased hepatic uptake	Usually < 6 mg/dl	Absent or minimal
Dubin-Johnson syndrome	Autosomal recessive	Impaired biliary secretion (? canalicular membrane-carrier defect)	Minimal	Usually < 5 mg/dl
Rotor syndrome and hepatic storage syndrome	Autosomal recessive	? Decreased hepatic uptake and storage ? Decreased biliary secretion	Minimal	Present (usually < 5 mg/dl)

Modified from Gollan, J.L., and Knapp, A.B.: Bilirubin metabolism and congenital jaundice. Hosp. Pract. *20:*83, 1985.

viduals, perhaps with a less extreme enzyme lack, survive into adolescence only to die of progressive encephalopathy related to the accumulation of unconjugated bilirubin in the CNS. Only trace amounts of conjugated bilirubin, largely monoglucuronides, are secreted in the bile, and so it is virtually colorless. The only inconstant morphologic change in the liver is canalicular cholestasis. The inbred Gunn rat provides an excellent model of this disorder, even to the point of developing kernicterus.

CRIGLER-NAJJAR SYNDROME TYPE II

This form of unconjugated hyperbilirubinemia differs from type I in many respects: (1) It appears to follow autosomal dominant transmission with variable penetrance.[17] (2) There is a deficiency of glucuronyltransferase activity, but it is not profound and varies in severity from one patient to another. Thus there is some production of monoglucuronides. (3) The unconjugated hyperbilirubinemia is generally mild. (4) *Kernicterus appears only rarely, and indeed with milder deficiencies of the transferase the longevity may be normal.* (5) In most cases the liver is entirely normal. (6) Clinical improvement has been achieved by treatment of the child with phenobarbital, which induces the synthesis of increased amounts of glucuronyltransferase and so augments the conjugation of bilirubin.

GILBERT'S SYNDROME

Affecting up to 7% of the population, *Gilbert's syndrome constitutes a form of unconjugated hyperbilirubinemia that is mild and compatible with normal longevity.* The condition is most often recognized during the second and third decades of life, when some unrelated hemolytic event emphasizes the jaundice. However, abnormal hemolysis is not intrinsic to the condition. The precise nature of the metabolic defect is not clear because no single defect can explain all the observed abnormalities. Virtually all patients have re-

duced glucuronyltransferase activity in the liver, and with it, reduced hepatic bilirubin clearance. Most patients have a moderately reduced rate of bilirubin uptake, a finding that cannot be readily explained by the transferase deficiency. Thus this syndrome probably embraces more than one genetic error. Not surprisingly then, the mode of transmission is still uncertain. The liver is morphologically normal save possibly for some increased lipofuscin pigment, mainly in the centrilobular hepatocytes. The importance of recognizing this benign condition and not making these chronically jaundiced individuals "hepatic cripples" is obvious.

DUBIN-JOHNSON SYNDROME

Unlike the previously described hereditary conditions, *the Dubin-Johnson syndrome is a benign disorder characterized by (1) chronic or intermittent conjugated hyperbilirubinemia, (2) a genetic defect in the canalicular transport of organic anions, including conjugated bilirubin; and (3) a grossly pigmented liver.* The dark gray discoloration of the liver is caused by numerous coarse granules within the cytoplasm of hepatocytes that can be resolved as lysosomes (Fig. 19–6). Despite intensive investigation, the precise nature of the pigment remains obscure; although it has been called melanin-like, it has biophysical characteristics unlike those of melanin. Neither is the pigment a porphyrin or lipofuscin, nor is it related to bilirubin; indeed, there is no cholestasis in the liver.[18] Interestingly, with acute hepatocellular injuries such as acute viral hepatitis, the pigment disappears from the liver and is excreted through the urine, only to reaccumulate when the viral infection clears. Thus the nature of the pigment remains obscure, but it appears to be a product in active turnover because in "the sick liver" it rapidly disappears. Although fluctuating jaundice is characteristic, most patients are otherwise asymptomatic. However, because of the transport defect they are unable to excrete such organic anions as BSP, and so the gallbladder and bile

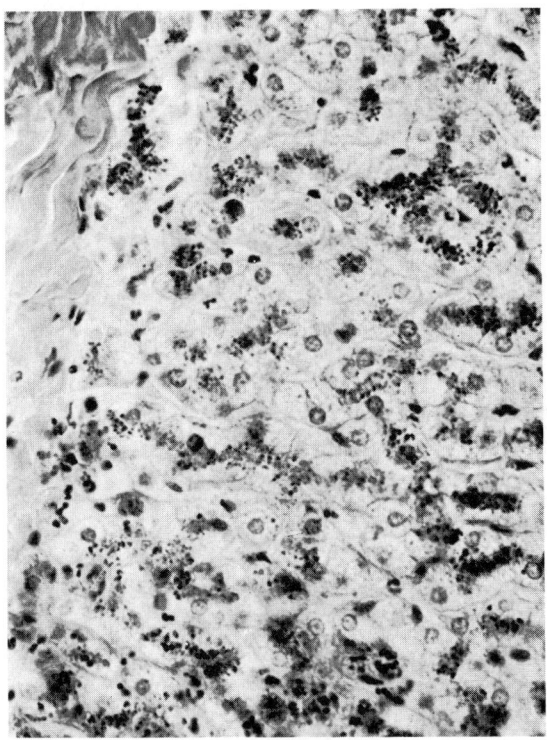

Figure 19–6. Dubin-Johnson disease, showing fine dustlike pigmentation of liver cells.

ducts cannot be visualized by oral cholecystography. Corriedale sheep have an analogous hepatic defect.

ROTOR SYNDROME

Much less common than the Dubin-Johnson syndrome, *the Rotor syndrome also represents a form of asymptomatic conjugated hyperbilirubinemia, but the liver is not pigmented.* The gallbladder can usually, although not invariably, be visualized on oral cholecystography. The nature of the metabolic defect is unclear, although derangements in hepatic uptake and storage of organic anions are suspected.

CIRCULATORY DISORDERS

Disturbances in the vascular supply or venous drainage of the liver are extremely common, but the great preponderance of these disturbances, such as venous congestive changes, do not produce clinically significant liver dysfunction. At the other extreme are the rare but often fatal hepatic vein thromboses.

ACUTE AND CHRONIC PASSIVE CONGESTION AND CENTRAL HEMORRHAGIC NECROSIS OF LIVER

These hepatic alterations are considered together because they represent essentially a morphologic continuum.

Acute and chronic passive congestion (CPC) of the liver in the great majority of instances reflects acute or slowly developing cardiac decompensation, particularly right-sided failure. Because there is an element of preterminal circulatory failure with virtually every death, congestive hepatic changes are commonplace at autopsy. The morphologic changes with acutely developing congestion constitute slight enlargement of the liver, which is typically tense and cyanotic with rounded edges. Microscopically there is marked centrilobular congestion, as described on page 92 and page 600.

Central necrosis, sometimes called *ischemic* hepatitis, is a more significant alteration. Central necrosis may appear with all forms of hepatic hypoperfusion, as was discussed on page 92.[19] When associated with right heart failure, constrictive pericarditis, or hepatic vein thrombosis, central congestive changes play a role in the pathogenesis of the lesion, producing what is called *central hemorrhagic necrosis (CHN)* (p. 600). The anatomic changes of centrilobular necrosis and CHN may closely resemble those of CPC, but close inspection on reflected light usually discloses slight depression of the necrotic lobular centers, which are congested in CHN, imparting a nutmeg appearance. The distinctive microscopic features were presented in the earlier discussion.

With marked central necrosis, the parenchymal damage may be sufficient to induce mild to moderate jaundice, elevated serum aminotransferases, and minimal derangement of other liver function tests.

CARDIAC SCLEROSIS

This uncommon complication of severe cardiac failure basically represents the fibrosing reaction that follows long-standing severe CPC and/or centrilobular necrosis. Presumably the protracted central hypoxia prevents hepatocellular regeneration, resulting in scarring. Sometimes this condition has been called *cardiac cirrhosis* but, as will be evident (p. 941), the pattern of liver fibrosis and damage rarely fulfills the accepted criteria for the diagnosis of cirrhosis.

The scarring of cardiac sclerosis is delicate, subtle, and easily missed on both gross and microscopic examination. Typically, the liver is slightly reduced in size and has a fine pigskin grain on its external surface. On transection there is a subtle depression of the centers of the lobules, creating a resemblance to CHN, but the congestive features are less prominent. There is often some increased resistance to finger-fracture of the hepatic substance. Microscopically, there is a subtle increase in fibrous tissue about the central veins, from which delicate strands fan out into the surrounding liver substance. The fibrosis is often sufficiently subtle to require special stains to highlight the collagen. Interconnection of the fibrous strands to produce tracts of fibrous tissue bridging with those of adjacent lobules (cardiac cirrhosis) is seen only in extreme examples, usually in association with tricuspid insufficiency.

The clinical consequences of cardiac sclerosis are either negligible or identical to those of CHN. The chronic liver damage rarely induces portal hypertension or the other accompaniments of well-defined cirrhosis of the liver.

INFARCTS OF LIVER

The double blood supply to the liver undoubtedly accounts for the rarity of infarcts. Infrequently, however, thrombosis or compression of an intrahepatic branch of the hepatic artery caused by polyarteritis nodosa, embolism, neoplasia, or sepsis results in a localized infarct that is usually anemic or sometimes hemorrhagic when small (due to suffusion of portal blood). It is often difficult to identify the arterial occlusion. It should be noted that occlusion of an intrahepatic branch of the portal vein does not cause ischemic infarction, but instead a sharply demarcated area of red-blue discoloration inappropriately referred to as an *infarct of Zahn*. Microscopically there is no necrosis, only hepatocellular atrophy secondary to marked sinusoidal congestion. Occasionally, thromboses are evident in the portal vein branches within the affected parenchyma.

Accidental or intentional interruption of the main hepatic artery does not always produce ischemic necrosis of the organ if the liver is otherwise normal and the point of arterial interruption is proximal to one of its major or large accessory branches. The retrograde arterial flow through these vessels, when coupled with the portal venous supply, may be sufficient to sustain the vitality of the liver parenchyma.

HEPATIC VEIN THROMBOSIS BUDD-CHIARI SYNDROME)

The Budd-Chiari syndrome originally was characterized by hepatomegaly, ascites, and abdominal pain caused by thrombosis of the hepatic veins. In most instances the syndrome appeared suddenly and was usually fatal. Since that time the definition has been expanded to include acute to chronic syndromes possibly caused by constrictive pericarditis, right atrial myxoma, and hepatic veno-occlusive disease (see next section).[20] However, the purists, whom we eagerly join, point out that attempts to compare end results of treatment are confused by combining "apples and oranges," and so *here we restrict our discussion to thromboses within the hepatic vein, including the adjacent inferior vena cava. Analysis of a large series of patients with such lesions revealed that about half the cases were associated with (in order of frequency) polycythemia vera, pregnancy, the post-partum state, the use of oral contraceptives, paroxysmal nocturnal hemoglobinuria, and intra-abdominal cancers, particularly hepatocellular carcinoma.* All these conditions produce thrombotic tendencies, or in the case of liver cancers, sluggish flow. Uncommon causes include myeloproliferative disorders, infections, trauma, and membranous webs of obscure origin (probably orga-

nized, recanalized thrombi) in the major hepatic veins or inferior vena cava. For unknown reasons, so-called membranous webs constitute a very common cause of the syndrome globally but are relatively uncommon in the United States.[21] After all these potentiating conditions are excluded, about 30% of cases are idiopathic in origin.

With acutely developing thrombosis of the major hepatic veins or inferior vena cava, the liver is swollen and red-purple and has a tense capsule. Sometimes only the right or the left hepatic vein is affected, producing subtotal involvement. On transection, the affected hepatic parenchyma reveals severe centrilobular congestion and necrosis, with marked distention of the central sinusoids, which sometimes rupture into the spaces of Disse. In instances in which the thrombosis is more slowly developing, as with membranous webs, the liver may show the changes of cardiac sclerosis (p. 921). The major veins may reveal totally occlusive fresh thrombi, subtotal occlusion, or in chronic cases, organized thrombi. Almost always, ascites is also present.

The majority of patients with the Budd-Chiari syndrome present with evidence of rapidly developing abdominal pain, hepatomegaly, and ascites with abdominal distention. The pain is presumably caused by distention of the liver capsule or abdominal distention. Jaundice is usually absent or at most is mild, and routine liver function studies are only modestly abnormal. In a minority of cases, the patients present with the subtle and insidious onset of intractable ascites without significant hepatomegaly or abdominal pain. The diagnosis, when suspected, can be confirmed by angiography, scintiscan, or MRI scan. Untreated, the mortality of the acutely developing condition is extremely high. Prompt surgical intervention and the creation of portosystemic venous shunts, permitting reverse flow through the portal vein, considerably improve the prognosis. The chronic form of the condition is far less lethal and about half the patients are alive after five years.[22]

HEPATIC VENO-OCCLUSIVE DISEASE (VOD)

This condition is sufficiently rare to justify inclusion only as a differential diagnosis for Budd-Chiari syndrome. It comprises subendothelial sclerosis with thickening and obliteration of the smaller and central veins within the liver (Fig. 19–7). Sometimes the narrowed veins undergo thrombosis that may extend into the major outflow veins, thus approximating the Budd-Chiari syndrome. The basis for VOD is somewhat obscure, but it has been associated with hepatotoxic alkaloids found in medicinal teas (Jamaica "bush tea"), antineoplastic drugs, immunosuppressants, hepatic irradiation, and bone marrow transplantation followed by graft-versus-host disease (many of these patients also received immunosuppressants). It is ap-

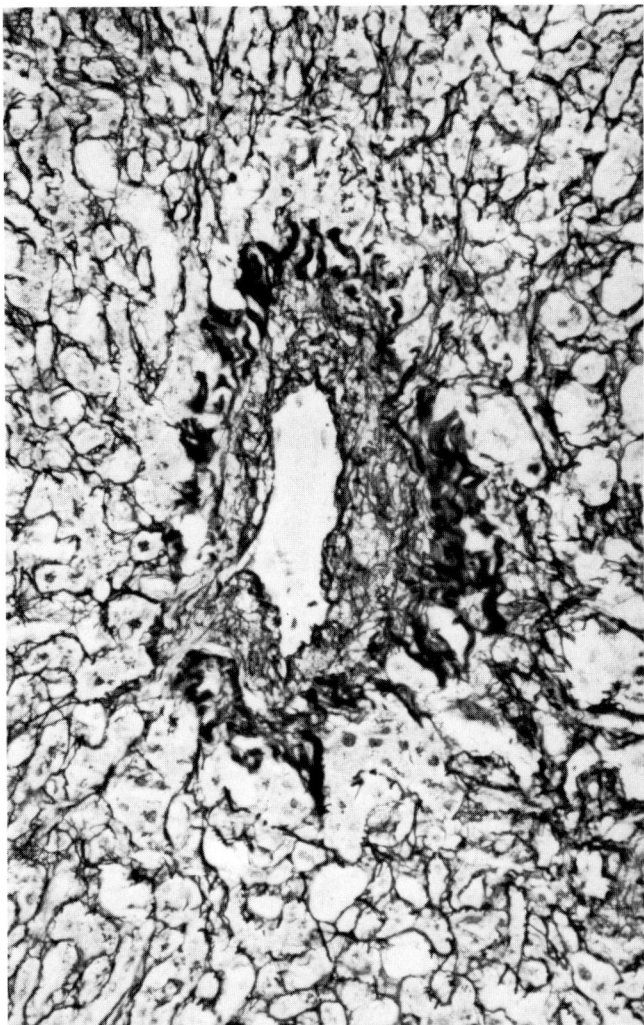

Figure 19–7. Veno-occlusive disease. A reticulin stain revealing the parenchymal framework of the lobule and the significantly thickened wall of the central vein.

parent that the hepatic outflow obstruction in VOD develops insidiously and produces manifestations virtually indistinguishable from the chronically developing Budd-Chiari syndrome. Differential diagnosis usually requires biopsy of the liver and/or imaging techniques to rule out thrombosis of the major hepatic veins.[23]

PORTAL VEIN OBSTRUCTION AND THROMBOSIS

Blockage of the portal vein is much better tolerated than obstruction of the hepatic vein. The occlusive process may arise within the extrahepatic course of the portal vein or within its intrahepatic distribution. *Extrahepatic causes* include (1) cancers arising within abdominal organs; (2) peritoneal sepsis, e.g., acute diverticulitis, appendicitis, initiating *pylephlebitis* within the portal vein itself or its major radicles with propagation into ever larger channels; (3) pancreatitis that initiates thrombosis within the splenic vein fol-

lowed by propagation into the portal vein; and (4) postsurgical thromboses following upper abdominal procedures. Rarely, agenesis or aplasia of the portal vein is found. The most common *intrahepatic cause* is cirrhosis of the liver followed, in terms of frequency, by intravascular invasion by primary or secondary cancer in the liver.

Occlusive disease of the portal vein or its major radicles typically produces abdominal pain and, in most instances, ascites and other manifestations of portal hypertension, principally esophageal varices (prone to rupture). The ascites, when present, is often massive and intractable. Impairment of the visceral blood flow often leads to bowel infarction. When the condition is secondary to pylephlebitis, spread of the infection may yield multiple liver abscesses. The diagnosis can sometimes be made by CT scan or angiography, but often surgical exploration is required not only to attempt to relieve the venous obstruction by shunting procedures but also possibly to resect infarcted bowel.[24]

A comparison of the Budd-Chiari syndrome, veno-occlusive disease, and portal vein occlusion is offered in Figure 19–8.

NECROSES

Virtually any significant insult to the liver, whether it be traumatic, toxic, microbiologic, or vascular, may kill liver cells. Depending on the magnitude and nature of the insult, the necrosis may be limited to some of the cells within the hepatic lobules, or it may destroy entire lobules or even the whole liver. *Submassive to massive necrosis* is most commonly caused by chemical and drug toxicity and viral hepatitis; it is discussed in more detail on page 937. The less severe injuries are divided into (1) *focal ("spotty," random) necrosis* and (2) *zonal necrosis* when it tends to involve particular regions of the lobule, i.e., centrilobular, midzonal, or peripheral.

Focal (random) necroses are most characteristic of microbiologic infections. Some of the major diseases producing such changes are viral hepatitis, miliary tuberculosis, typhoid fever, tularemia, and brucellosis, but all bacteremias, viremias, or fungemias may produce focal necroses. In some instances, as for example viral hepatitis, the necroses may be very random, involving individual cells or small clusters of cells. Other conditions such as typhoid fever, tularemia, and brucellosis tend to destroy somewhat larger clusters of cells. Indeed the focal necrosis may expand into macroscopic abscesses as occurs, for example, with staphylococcal or gram-negative sepsis. The precise patterns of histologic change vary with the causative agent.

The three patterns of *zonal necrosis* are each associated with particular causative influences. *Centrilobular necrosis* (p. 920) is characteristic of ischemic injury such as occurs with the low-flow states produced by shock and left ventricular failure.[19] This

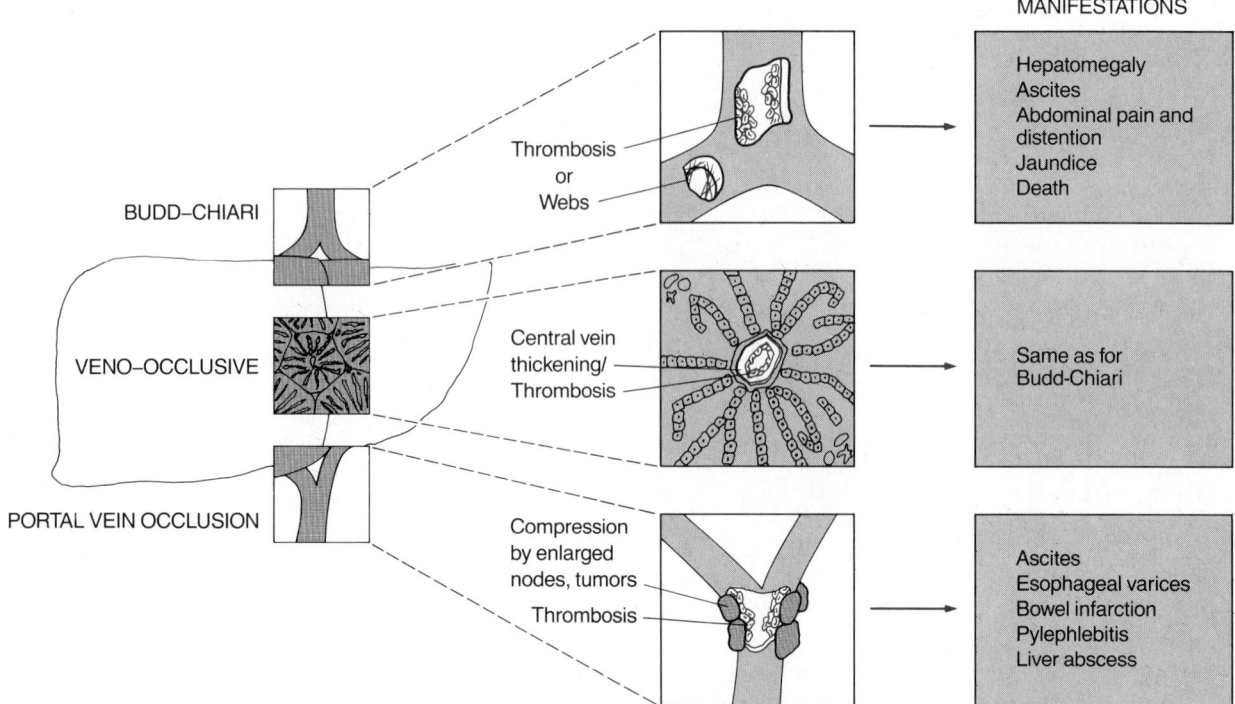

Figure 19-8. The anatomic changes and clinical manifestations of Budd-Chiari syndrome, veno-occlusive disease, and portal vein occlusion are contrasted.

pattern of liver damage is sometimes called "ischemic hepatitis," a regrettable usage since it is not basically an inflammatory process. Concomitant marked venous congestion produces so-called central hemorrhagic necrosis as was described on page 92). Many drug and chemical toxic reactions, e.g., chloroform and carbon tetrachloride (p. 500) poisoning, cause mainly centrilobular necrosis. *Midzonal necrosis* is an unusual pattern seen in yellow fever. The basis for this localization is unknown. Often the dying cells undergo a peculiar form of condensation and are transformed into acidophilic rounded "Councilman bodies," seen also in viral hepatitis. *Peripheral necrosis* is seen in phosphorus poisoning and eclampsia. In the latter, there may also be fibrin thrombi within the vascular sinusoids in the necrotic zone and sometimes hemorrhages. The vascular thromboses may produce microinfarcts and hemorrhagic mottling of the liver surface (p. 1172).

INFECTIONS

The liver is almost inevitably involved in all bloodborne infections, whether systemic or arising in the abdominal cavity. Virtually all have been considered elsewhere, but some of the more common implicated infections are military tuberculosis, malaria, staphylococcal bacteremia, infectious mononucleosis, the salmonelloses, and amebiasis. Indeed, needle liver biopsy is often employed in occult infections for telltale evidence of the causative agent, particularly

when miliary tuberculosis is suspected. There are, in addition, several primary hepatic infections that require detailed consideration: the important and common viral hepatitis, and the less common but distinctive ascending cholangitis (leading often to abscesses) and primary sclerosing cholangitis.

VIRAL HEPATITIS

A number of systemic viral infections may involve the liver. A generally mild hepatitis is common during the acute phase of infectious mononucleosis. The cytomegalovirus may produce hepatitis; it can be quite severe in the newborn or in the immunosuppressed adult. Yellow fever was a major and serious cause of hepatitis in tropical countries. Infrequently, and primarily in children, significant liver disease appears in the course of rubella, adenovirus, and enterovirus infections.[25] However, *unless otherwise specified, the term "viral hepatitis" is generally reserved for infection of the liver caused by a small group of hepatotropic viruses.* Two of these agents, hepatitis A virus (HAV) and hepatitis B virus (HBV) have been isolated and cloned and so are well delineated. Another, hepatitis delta virus (HDV), although it has not been isolated and cloned, has been well delineated. It is a defective virus that can cause disease only when there is concomitant HB infection. In addition, there are clinically and morphologically indistinguishable instances of viral hepatitis caused by yet-to-be-defined agents (there appears to be more than one involved); these are referred to as non-A, non-B viruses (NANBV).

All the hepatotropic viruses cause virtually the same clinicomorphologic patterns of acute hepatitis. Only virologic or serologic markers, or the absence of them in NANB hepatitis, distinguish the various etiologies. However, they vary in their potential to produce chronic and fulminating disease or the carrier state. Thus it is possible to describe later (p. 931) the various patterns of disease with little regard for etiology — but first each virus must be characterized.

Hepatitis A Virus (HAV)

Hepatitis A, at one time called infectious hepatitis, is usually a benign, self-limited disease (incubation period 14 to 45 days).[26] In the developing world, HA accounts for about 20 to 25% of cases of acute hepatitis, but the percentage is much smaller in developed countries. In adults, acute HA is usually an overt febrile illness; however, in childhood, when most infections are incurred in developing countries, the disease tends to be mild or asymptomatic.[27] *HAV does not cause chronic hepatitis or the carrier state and only very rarely fulminant hepatitis, and so the fatality rate associated with HAV is about 0.1%.*[28] *Moreover, because the viremia of the acute disease is remarkably transient, HAV is rarely implicated in transfusion-acquired hepatitis.*

EPIDEMIOLOGY AND BIOLOGY. Typically in Western countries HA occurs as sporadic disease in susceptible adults, the agent being spread by oral ingestion of contaminated water supplies and foods. However, close personal contact during the incubation period with an infected individual and fecal-oral contamination accounts for about 25% of all cases. Spread of infection is prone to occur among men living in military camps, inmates of mental institutions, male homosexuals having oral-anal contact, and during travel into foreign countries where the disease is endemic. The virus has on occasion been responsible for common-source epidemics, for example, within a household or among members of a day-care center. Induced disease in primates permits the observation of early events and the extremely transient period of the viremia and fecal shedding. In humans, only rarely is the virus detectable in the stool or blood; presumably these events have passed by the time overt disease appears. Since transmission of the virus is by the fecal-oral route, the peak period of infectivity occurs during the incubation period and first few symptomatic days.

HAV is a small, nonenveloped, single-stranded RNA virus, which by electron microscopy is a roughly spherical particle about 27 nm in diameter having icosahedral symmetry. Its RNA genome has been transcribed into complementary DNA (cDNA) that has been cloned and sequenced.[29] With the use of a cDNA probe, it is possible to identify HAV, for example in liver cells, in both experimental and clinical hepatitis by molecular hybridization techniques.[30]

The virus has been successfully propagated in cell cultures of human and primate origin and, significantly, it replicates and is released from infected cells without adverse effect on them. How then does it cause hepatitis? Proposed is an immunologic response. Although the inflammatory infiltrate in the liver is dominantly mononuclear, cytotoxic T cells for virally infected hepatocytes have not been documented. On the other hand, in vitro, normal peripheral lymphocytes (presumably natural killer cells) destroy HAV-infected monkey kidney cells. In sum, although an immunologic mechanism is suspected as the cause of the liver injury, it is far from established.

It is impossible to identify the particular causative agent responsible for an attack of acute hepatitis from the clinical signs and symptoms alone; reliance must be placed on virologic and serologic markers. An overview of the appearance and disappearance of HAV markers is offered in Figure 19–9. A few points should be underscored. Specific antibody against the HAV initially of the IgM type appears in the blood at the onset of symptoms, constituting a reliable marker of acute infection. Fecal shedding of virus ends as the IgM titer rises. The IgM response begins to decline in a few months but can sometimes be identified in very low titer for as long as 6 to 12 months. IgG anti-HAV can be detected in the serum soon after the IgM antibody appears. It persists for years, perhaps for life, providing protective immunity against reinfection with HAV. Elevated levels of IgG antibody do not indicate acute infection, only exposure to HAV.

Hepatitis B Virus (HBV)

HBV, a DNA virus, is the most versatile of the hepatotropic viruses. It can produce (1) an asymptomatic carrier state, (2) acute hepatitis, (3) chronic hepatitis, (4) progression of chronic disease to cirrhosis, and (5) fulminant hepatitis with massive liver necrosis. Furthermore, HBV plays some important role in the development of hepatocellular carcinoma (p. 959). The approximate frequencies of these variable outcomes are depicted in Figure 19–10. This agent also collaborates with the defective delta hepatitis virus, conferring on it the capacity to replicate and cause delta virus disease. Infection with HBV is a global problem, and an enormous effort is being made to develop vaccines to bring the oncogenicity and mortality of this agent under control.[31]

EPIDEMIOLOGY AND BIOLOGY. HB is spread mainly by parenteral routes. There are close to 200 million carriers of the virus in the world and about 1.5 million in the United States alone. Moreover, the virus is present in the blood during the last stages of the incubation period (30 to 180 days) of acute infection. *Thus it can be transmitted by transfusion, blood products, needle-stick accidents, and obviously among IV drug addicts.* Dialysis patients and health workers are also at increased risk. However, a significant fraction of individuals with hepatitis B provide no history of parenteral exposure, and so spread by other modes is suspected; the viral genome has been shown in body fluids including saliva, semen, and vaginal fluid. Thus

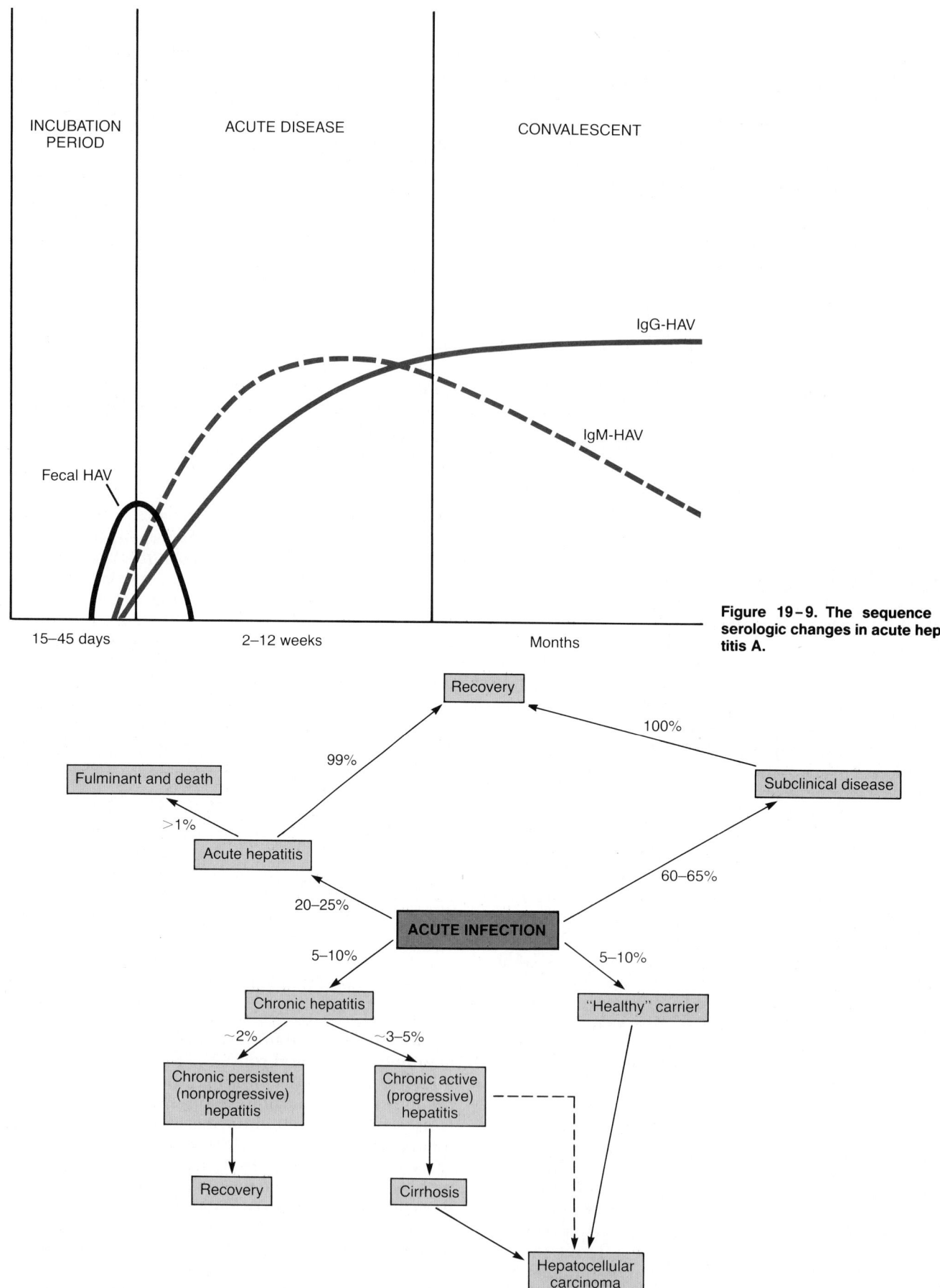

INCUBATION
PERIOD

ACUTE DISEASE

CONVALESCENT

IgG-HAV

IgM-HAV

Fecal HAV

15–45 days

2–12 weeks

Months

Figure 19–9. The sequence of serologic changes in acute hepatitis A.

Recovery

100%

99%

Fulminant and death

Subclinical disease

>1%

Acute hepatitis

20–25%

60–65%

ACUTE INFECTION

5–10%

5–10%

Chronic hepatitis

"Healthy" carrier

~2%

~3–5%

Chronic persistent
(nonprogressive)
hepatitis

Chronic active
(progressive)
hepatitis

Recovery

Cirrhosis

Hepatocellular
carcinoma

Figure 19–10. Schematic of the potential outcomes with their approximate frequencies of hepatitis B acute infection in adult life.

926

close intimate or sexual contact with an infectious individual may transmit the disease, which explains the increased risk within families and among homosexuals. In endemic regions such as Africa and Southeast Asia, spread from an infected mother to a neonate during birth (vertical transmission) is common. These neonatal infections often lead to the carrier state for life.

More is known about the molecular biology of HBV than about any other pathogenic virus.[32] It is a DNA virus, closely related to viruses that infect woodchucks, ground squirrels, and ducks. The complete human virion (also called a Dane particle) is spherical and has a diameter of about 42 nm. It has an outer envelope of protein, lipid, and carbohydrate enclosing an electron-dense, 27 nm, slightly hexagonal inner core. Hepatitis B surface antigen (HBsAg) is found in the envelope. There are several antigenic subtypes of HBsAg, useful only in epidemiologic tracing of sources of infection. Of interest, it was the chance discovery of an unusual antigen in an Australian aborigine that led to the identification of HBV (hence the synonym "Australia antigen"). During infection with HBV, not only are infectious complete virions replicated but also a massive excess of HBsAg that appears in the cells and the serum as spheres and tubules approximately 22 nm in diameter (Fig. 19–11). These particles are not infectious, but they can be harvested and used to induce a protective antibody

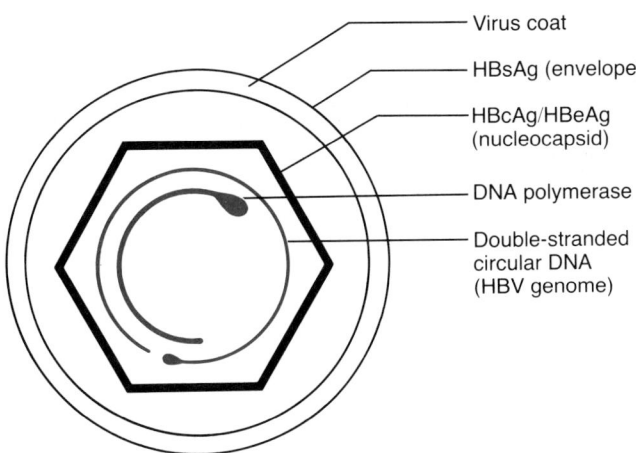

Figure 19–12. Diagrammatic representation of structure and components of hepatitis B. (Drawn from Gerber, M.A., and Thung, S.N.: Molecular and cellular pathology of hepatitis B. Lab. Invest. 52:572, 1985.)

response that can neutralize the virus. The viral nucleocapsid contains HBV-DNA, DNA-polymerase, hepatitis B core antigen (HBcAg), and HBeAg, which appears to be integral to HBcAG. The genome of HBV is a partially double-stranded circular DNA molecule having 3200 nucleotides (Fig. 19–12). The outer long strand of the genome is almost complete but is nicked; it carries four potential genes and all of the genomic information.[33] One gene, the S gene, codes for the major polypeptide of HBsAG. A pre-S segment of the genome or the combined pre-S segment and S gene encode for an envelope receptor for polymerized human serum albumin (pHSA).[33a] Significantly, hepatocytes appear to have pHSA receptors as well. *Thus viral entry into liver cells may depend on pHSA serving as a linkage between the putative receptors on the HBV and the endogenous receptors for polymerized albumin on hepatocytes.* Interestingly, the receptors on the viral envelope are specific for human and chimpanzee pHSA, explaining the limited range of infectivity of the HBV.

After exposure to the virus, there is a relatively long asymptomatic incubation period ranging from 4 to 26 weeks (average 1.5 to 2 months), followed by acute disease lasting many weeks to months. The natural course of the disease can be followed by the serologic markers in the serum (Fig. 19–13). Several significant points should be noted.

HBsAg is the earliest to appear. It is an indicator of active HBV infection, either acute or chronic. It appears before the onset of symptoms, peaks during the overt disease, and then usually declines to undetectable levels in three to six months.

HBeAg and, along with it, HBV-DNA and DNA polymerase appear in the serum soon after HBsAg is detectable and also before the onset of symptoms. All these markers are evidence of active viral replication. HBeAg peaks during the acute disease and disappears before HBsAg is cleared from the serum. *Persistence*

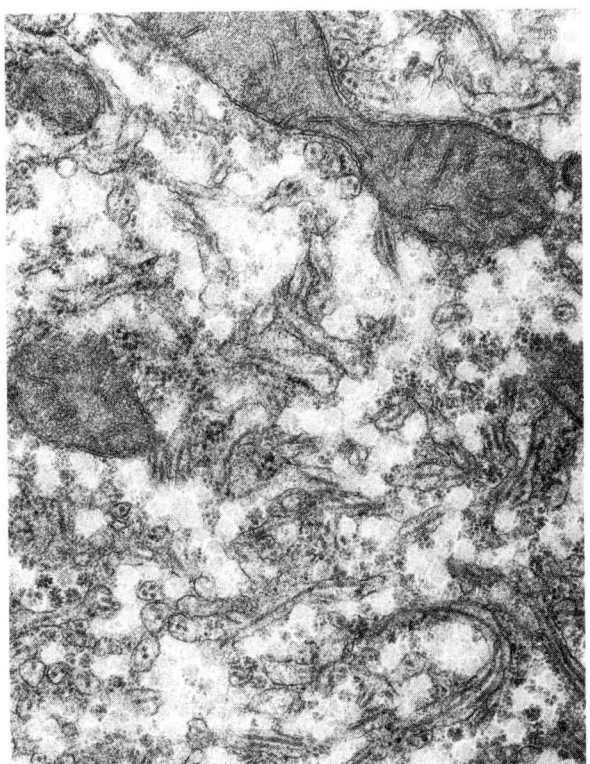

Figure 19–11. Electron micrograph of hepatitis B surface antigen in the form of spherules and tubules within hepatocytic cytoplasm (× 21500). (Courtesy of Drs. M.A. Gerber and S.N. Thung, Mount Sinai School of Medicine.)

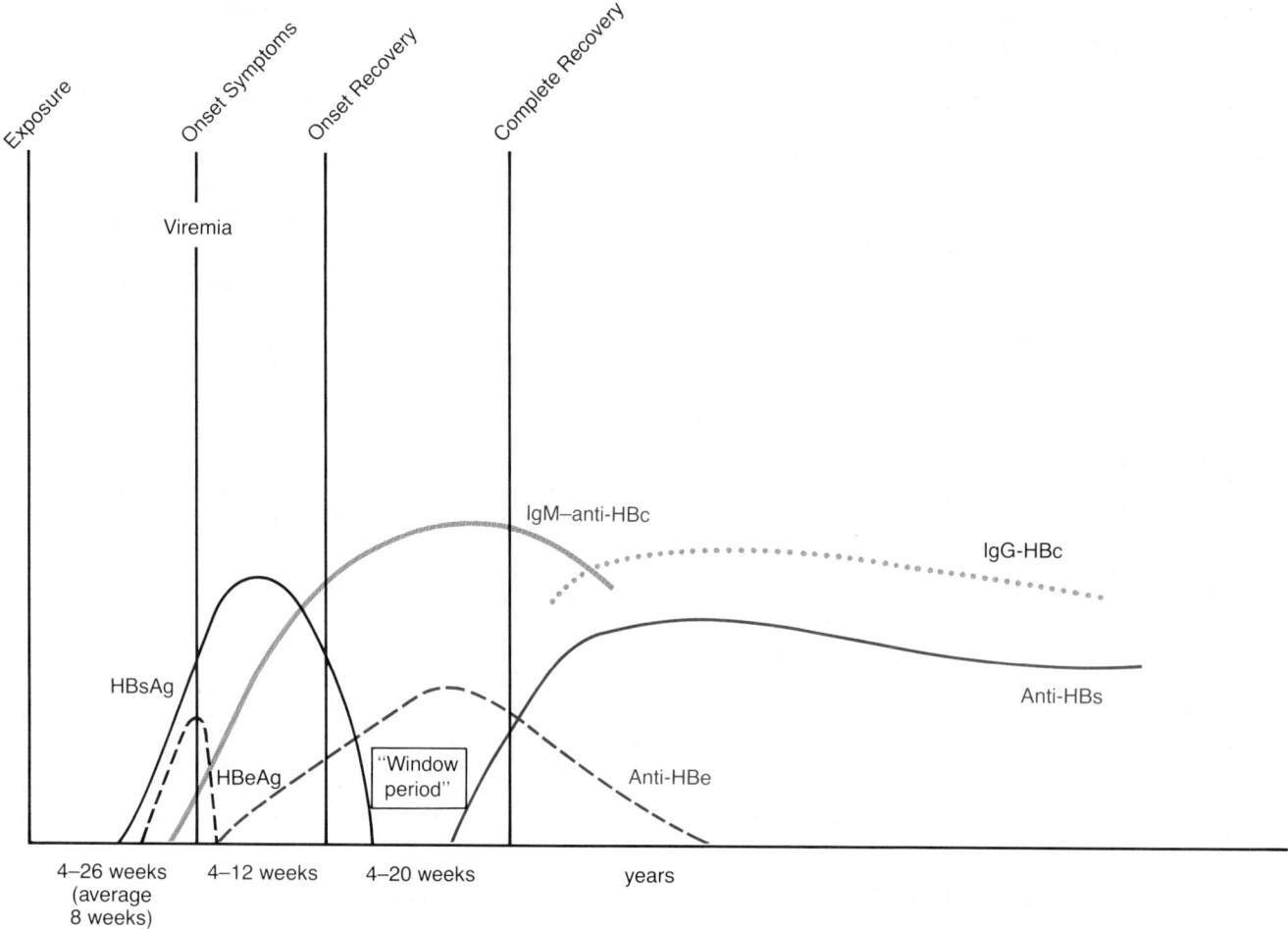

Figure 19–13. Sequence of serologic changes in acute hepatitis B.

of HBeAg is an important clinical indicator of continued active viral replication, continued infectivity, and probable progression to chronic hepatitis.

HBV-DNA in the serum is the most certain indicator of hepatitis B infection. It is transiently present during the presymptomatic phase of the incubation period and for a brief time during the acute overt disease.

Anti-HBe is detectable shortly after the disappearance of HBeAg. This seroconversion implies that the acute infection has reached its peak and the disease is on the wane.

IgM anti-HBc begins to be detectable in the serum shortly before the onset of symptoms and concurrent with the onset of elevated transaminase levels indicative of hepatic injury. Over the span of months the IgM antibody is replaced by IgG anti-HBc, and so an elevated level of IgM anti-HBc indicates a recent acute infection.

Anti-HBs does not begin to rise until the acute disease is over and convalescence has begun. In most cases, anti-HBs is not detectable for a few weeks to several months after the disappearance of the HBsAg. This interval is often referred to as the "window period," during which neither HBsAg nor anti-HBs is

detectable in the serum, making anti-HBc and anti-HBe the only markers of the disease. Anti-HBs persists in the great majority of patients for life, conferring protection against subsequent infection.

PATHOGENESIS. Most of the evidence suggests that immunologic mechanisms rather than direct viral cytotoxicity cause the hepatocellular damage. Arguing strongly against a direct viral cytopathic effect is the fact that hepatocytes containing complete virions or viral antigens in "healthy" HBV carriers have no evidence of injury. On the other hand, *a strong case can be made for immune mechanisms and specifically sensitized cytotoxic T cells as the mediators of the hepatic injury.*[33,34]

1. HBV infections pass through two phases. The first proliferative phase constitutes a period of viral replication, during which **HBV-DNA** is present in episomal form in the liver cells with complete formation of virions and all associated antigens.

2. During this phase, T cells sensitized to membrane-associated HBsAg and, particularly HBcAg, are found at sites of liver cell damage.[35]

3. T8 (cytotoxic/suppressor) lymphocytes are localized to the areas of cell necrosis.[36]

4. The proliferative phase is followed by an integrative phase. Virions are no longer produced, and the viral DNA is incorporated into the genome of the host cell. With the disappearance of antigens and antigenic challenge to T cells, and the appearance of antibodies to the various antigens, infectivity ends and active liver damage subsides.

The immunologic hypothesis, however, does not explain the extraordinary variation in the course and outcome of HBV infections. Therefore, recourse has been made to a variety of possible modifying influences, including antibody-mediated modulation of viral antigens, genetic host responsiveness, enhancement of the T-cell reaction by antibody-dependent cellular cytotoxicity, and possible concurrent infection with another hepatotropic virus, to name the most favored notions. It is evident that many penetrations have been made into the biology of the HBV, but areas of uncertainty persist.

Delta Hepatitis Virus (HDV)

HDV is a very small, defective RNA virus that can replicate and cause infection only when it is encapsidated by HBsAg. Hence delta hepatitis can develop only when there is concomitant hepatitis B infection. This unique dependence restricts the clinical distribution of delta hepatitis to basically two settings:

1. Acute *coinfection* occurs when a single exposure to a serum contains both HDV and HBV. The HBV must become established first to provide the HBsAg necessary for the pathogenicity of the HDV.

2. *Superinfection* of a chronic carrier of HBV with HDV results in combined disease about 30 to 50 days later. The carrier may have been previously "healthy" with no apparent hepatic dysfunction, or may have had underlying chronic hepatitis, indolent or active (p. 931).[37]

There are differing clinical consequences with these two patterns of combined infection. Simultaneous coinfection with HBV and HDV results in hepatitis ranging from mild to fulminant, but fulminant disease is more likely (about 3 to 4%) than with HBV alone. On the other hand, chronicity rarely develops. When HDV is superimposed on chronic HBV infection it significantly worsens the outlook, and any one of the following courses may eventuate. (1) Acute hepatitis is likely to erupt in the previously healthy HBV carrier; (2) it may convert mild HBV hepatitis into fulminant disease; and (3) there is a strong tendency (10 to 40%) to chronic progressive disease, often terminating in cirrhosis.[38] Depiction of these possible outcomes is presented in Figure 19–14. In addition, there is inferential evidence that HDV infection may persist as a carrier state.

EPIDEMIOLOGY AND BIOLOGY. Infection by the delta agent is worldwide, but the prevalence varies

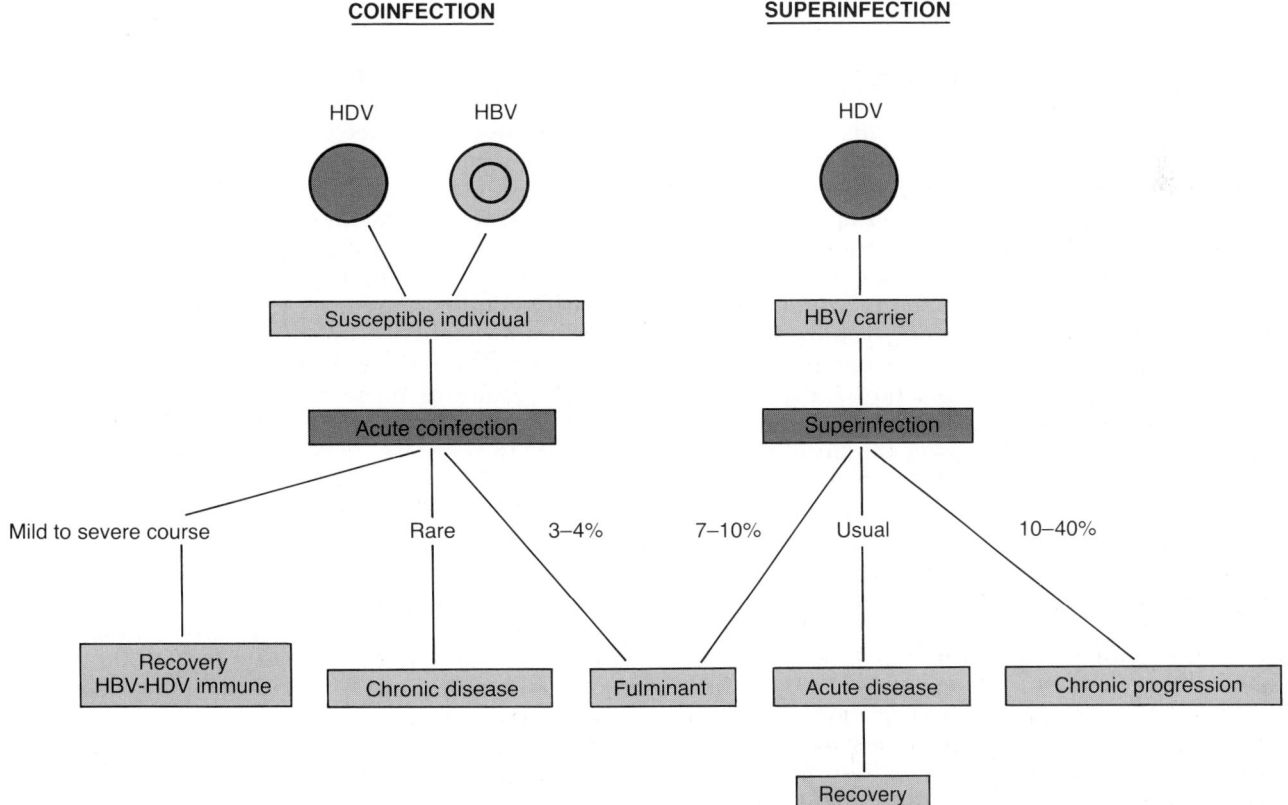

Figure 19–14. The differing clinical consequences of two patterns of combined HDV and HBV infection. (© US & Canadian Academy of Pathology, Inc., 1985.)

greatly. In Africa, the Middle East, and southern Italy, for example, about 50% of HBsAg carriers have anti-HDV. In these endemic regions the mode of spread is unclear. In the United States, delta infection is relatively uncommon and is largely restricted to drug addicts and male homosexuals. The prevalence in drug addicts in the United States indicates that spread can occur through percutaneous routes. However, there is a low incidence of infection in the general population of the United States; point-source, small outbreaks suggest that transmission also may occur by close and prolonged contact.[39] It is believed that 3 to 12% of apparently asymptomatic American blood donors with HBsAg have antibodies to the delta virus, suggesting the possibility of subclinical delta infection or an asymptomatic carrier state that creates a pool of HDV.[40]

HDV, without the HBsAg envelope, has a diameter of about 36 nm. The entire RNA genome has not been isolated; however, overlapping segments have been cloned, making it possible to deduce that the complete agent is about 1700 nucleotides in length.[41] Both subhuman primates and woodchucks are susceptible to HDV provided that there is coinfection with HBV, yielding reasonable models of the human disease. In the experimental animal, several weeks after inoculation with HBV or HDV, intranuclear proliferation of HDV can be detected in liver cells. Several weeks thereafter the HDV is detectable in the serum, but the viremia is transient and is usually completed by the time symptoms appear. Thus maximal infectivity precedes the onset of clinical manifestations of illness.

Both virologic and serologic methods are available to detect delta infection. A cDNA probe for the HDV permits identification of the virus in the blood and liver just prior to and in the early days of acute symptomatic disease. More widely available are radioimmunoassays for HDAg. It can also be demonstrated by immunoperoxidase methods in frozen as well as in fixed liver specimens. With chronic HBV-HDV infection, the delta antigen is present at very low levels for months or even longer, but more often anti-HD is used as a marker of chronic infection. As with all forms of hepatitis, IgM anti-HD is the most reliable indicator of acute infection; it begins to appear about one month following the onset of symptoms. In time the IgM anti-HD is replaced by IgG anti-HD, the levels of which persist for years to confer protection.

PATHOGENESIS. *The delta virus, in contrast to HBV, is believed to have a direct cytopathic effect on hepatocytes.* Support for this view comes from experimental disease in chimpanzees showing a direct relationship between viral dose and severity of liver injury. On the other hand, there are blood donors with no history of a prior attack of hepatitis or evidence of hepatic disease who have transmitted HDV, suggesting that the virus is not always cytopathic.[42] The complex relationship between HBV and HDV makes it difficult to unravel the pathogenesis of HDV-induced liver injury.

Non-A, Non-B (NANB) Hepatitis Viruses

Cases of hepatitis, mostly transfusion-associated, in which there are no virologic or serologic markers to point to any of the well-defined viral etiologies are attributed to putative NANB viruses. Three and possibly more viruses are thought to be involved. NANB hepatitis can be transmitted by both percutaneous and nonpercutaneous routes, including water-borne epidemic spread, and there are suggestions that the agents implicated in these various modes of spread differ.[43,44] As many as 60% of transfusion-associated cases of acute NANB hepatitis progress to chronic hepatitis. Alternatively, the acute attack may flare into fulminant or subfulminant liver failure. Indeed, the NANB viruses are responsible for at least 30% of cases of fulminant viral hepatitis.[45] Infection may also give rise to an asymptomatic carrier state. Estimates have been made that perhaps 2 to 3% of the general population of the United States are asymptomatic carriers of NANB hepatitis. Thus, the NANBV has the same potential as the HBV save that it does not appear to be implicated in hepatocellular carcinoma.[46]

EPIDEMIOLOGY AND MOLECULAR BIOLOGY. About 90 to 95% of cases of transfusion-associated hepatitis are attributable to NANBV. It is believed that 1 to 2% of volunteer blood donors and up to 5% of commercial donors are carriers. About 7 to 10% of multitransfused patients in the United States develop hepatitis; indeed, any percutaneous exposure to blood or blood products carries risk. Not surprisingly, an increased incidence of NANB hepatitis is encountered in drug addicts, hemodialysis and renal transplant patients, health workers because of accidental needle sticks or cuts, and those with coagulation disorders requiring plasma products such as factor VIII (for hemophilia), particularly when derived from multiple donor sources. NANBV are also thought to account for 20 to 30% of cases of sporadic hepatitis in the general population. The mechanism of transmission in many of these cases is obscure, and so the possibility has been raised of direct person-to-person spread. In addition, several epidemics of apparent NANB hepatitis in India have been attributed to fecal contamination of water supplies by NANBV.

There are significant differences in the clinical consequences of the disease based on modes of transmission.[47] Blood-transmitted disease is rarely fulminant but has a tendency to progress to chronic disease. Epidemic water-borne disease tends to be more severe and more often fulminant than coagulation factor–transmitted disease. There is a wide range in the incubation periods of these various modes of transmission from 14 to 180 days. Possibly this range is the consequence of differing causative agents. Indeed, putative viral particles of widely varying size (at least 20 to date), cytoplasmic tubules, and other ultrastructural changes compatible with an RNA virus have been described. But it is by no means certain that any has etiologic significance. Most convincing has been a report of 32 nm virus-like particles (distinct from HAV) in the stools of those suffering from enterically transmitted disease.[47a] Clarification of the NANB viruses must await isolation of the agents and identification of their markers.

A comparison of the salient features of the various hepatitis viruses is offered in Table 19–4.

Clinical Syndromes

Only the HAV is dependable; it produces solely acute hepatitis, usually relatively benign. Its only deviation from this behavior is the rare instance (0.1% of cases) of fulminant disease. All of the remaining hepatotropic viruses are more unpredictable and are capable of inducing the various syndromes listed below:

Carrier state: (a) without clinically apparent disease—"healthy carrier"; (b) with chronic hepatitis.

Acute hepatitis: (a) icteric; (b) anicteric.

Chronic hepatitis: (a) chronic persistent hepatitis; (b) chronic active hepatitis.

Fulminant hepatitis: with massive to submassive hepatic necrosis.

Before each of these clinicomorphologic patterns is discussed, two points should be made. (1) The evidence implicating particular viruses in this spectrum of syndromes is stronger for HBV than for other agents, and (2) the HBV also appears to be oncogenic or to at least contribute significantly to the development of primary hepatocellular carcinoma (p. 959).

Carrier State

Generically the term "carrier" denotes an individual without manifest symptoms who harbors and therefore can transmit an organism. Based on this definition, there are two types of carriers of the hepatotropic viruses: (1) The first includes those who harbor one of the viruses but are suffering little or no adverse effects from their "fellow traveler." These persons are often called "healthy carriers." (2) The second category refers to those who have chronic disease but have few or no symptoms and may not be disabled by their infection. Both constitute reservoirs of infection.

Recall, the HAV does not produce the carrier state. In contrast, 0.1 to 1.0% of blood donors in North America and Western Europe are HBV carriers, and in certain Asian and African populations as many as 5 to 15%.[48] The two factors bearing most heavily on the likelihood of a person's becoming an HBV carrier are age at time of infection and immune status. Infection early in life, as by vertical transmission from mother to offspring during childbirth, usually (90 to 95%) produces a carrier state. This mode of spread is very common in Asia and Africa and accounts for the very high carriage rate in those regions. In contrast, in adults, only 1 to 10% of HBV infections yield the carrier state. *Also likely to become carriers are individuals who have impaired immunity, whether constitutional or related to therapy; have received multiple transfusions or plasma products; are on hemodialysis; are drug addicts; or are institutionalized, mentally retarded patients.* Indeed, among these vulnerable populations the carrier rate may reach 10 to 15% even in Western countries.

The situation is less clear with the HDV because of its dependence on the HBV. On the one hand, when both HBV and HDV are present in an individual the infection is almost always overt, often progressive, and the virus is thought to be cytopathic and not likely to lead to an asymptomatic carrier state. On the other hand, there is a well-defined low risk of post-transfusion hepatitis D, indicative of a carrier state.[39,40]

There are no satisfactory data on the prevalence of the NANBV carrier state because of the lack of serologic markers. However, based on the frequency of transfusion-associated hepatitis, 90 to 95% of which is NANB hepatitis, it is calculated that about 2 to 3% of the general population of the United States harbor NANBV.

Table 19–4. Salient Features of Hepatitis Viruses

	AGENT	MAJOR ANTIGENS	ANTIBODIES	TRANSMISSION	INCUBATION PERIOD	CARRIER STATE	CHRONICITY
HAV	27 nm RNA	HAAg	anti-HAV	Fecal-oral	15–45 days	None	None
HBV	42 nm DNA	HBsAg HBcAg HBeAg	anti-HBs anti-HBc anti-HBe	Parenteral; close personal contact	30–180 days	0.1–1.0% of blood donors in U.S. and Western world	5–10% acute infections
HDV	36 nm DNA (defective)	Delta antigen	anti-delta	Parenteral; close personal contact	30–50 days (in superinfection)	In U.S. mainly drug addicts, male homosexuals	10–40% in superinfection
NANBV (parenteral)	Unknown	Unknown	Unknown	Transfusion	14–180 days	2–3% of blood donors in U.S. and Western world	40–60%
NANBV (epidemic)	? 27–32 nm particle	Unknown	Unknown	Water-borne	Unknown	Unknown	Rare

Only the HBV carrier state is associated with distinctive morphologic changes, although it may be possible to identify HDV carriers as well. The liver biopsy in the "healthy" HBV carrier reveals more or less normal morphology except for evidence of the virus in occasional cells. Viable isolated cells or clusters of hepatocytes have **"ground-glass,"** **finely granular, eosinophilic cytoplasm** (with H and E staining) (Fig. 19–15). The granules are better seen after staining with orcein or aldehyde fuchsin.[49] By electron microscopy, the granules can be resolved as spheres and tubules that immunoperoxidase methods prove to be HBsAg. Other cells have **"sanded" nuclei** imparted by their being stuffed with HBcAg.[50] Cells with "sanded" nuclei are less numerous than those with "ground-glass" cytoplasm. In situ hybridization and radioautography will sometimes disclose HBV viral DNA sequences in scattered hepatocytes that fail to provide immunohistochemical evidence of antigens.[51] cDNA probes for the HDV and immunocytochemical methods for HDAg or anti-HD have been used successfully in primate models and will likely prove to be of value in humans.

As mentioned previously, some carriers have chronic hepatitis, and in such livers there is scant evidence of viral footprints. In general, there is an inverse relationship between the number of viral- and antigen-bearing hepatocytes and the severity of liver injury.

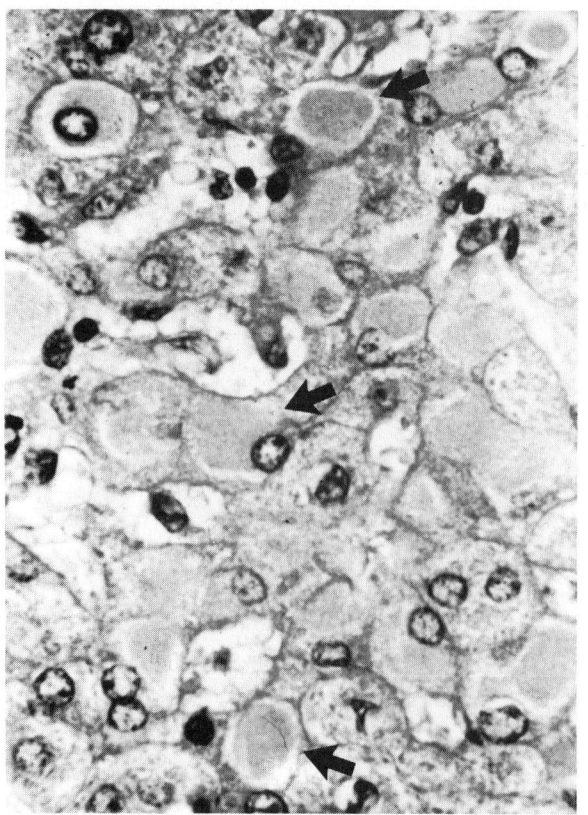

Figure 19–15. Ground-glass hepatocytes (*arrows*) in HBV infection (H and E). (Courtesy of Dr. Hans Popper, The Mount Sinai Medical Center.)

Clinical recognition of carriers is obviously of importance, particularly in donor selection. For HBV the marker most widely used is the presence of HBsAg in the serum. When HBeAg is also detectable, the level of infectivity is high. Conversely, seroconversion of an individual to anti-HBe implies that viral replication has been controlled and along with it the risk of transmission. The clinical identification of HDV in HBV carriers depends largely on the demonstration of anti-HD.[52]

Acute Viral Hepatitis

Acute viral hepatitis can be caused by any one of the hepatotropic viruses. Whatever the agent, *the disease is more or less the same and can be subdivided into four phases: (1) an incubation period, (2) a symptomatic preicteric phase, (3) a symptomatic icteric phase, and (4) convalescence.* Not all acute attacks proceed through all these phases. For example, many acute infections, as for example HA in very young children and NANB hepatitis in adults, are virtually asymptomatic or are readily overlooked because they are anicteric. Nonetheless, consideration of the four overlapping phases permits an overview of the most common course of acute hepatitis.

The *incubation period* varies significantly among the several viruses: For HA it is about 28 days (range 15 to 45); for HB the mean is 75 days (range 30 to 180); for HD, 15 to 90 days; and for NANB, extremely variable from 14 to 180 days. During the incubation period the individual is usually unaware of viral exposure, but as was indicated in the discussion of the individual viruses, peak infectivity for all occurs during the last asymptomatic days of the incubation period and the early days of acute symptoms.

The *preicteric phase* of acute hepatitis is marked by nonspecific, constitutional symptoms. Malaise is the most characteristic initial complaint; it is followed in a few days by general fatigability, nausea, loss of appetite, and sometimes weight loss. Typically there is a particular distaste for coffee or smoking. Low-grade fever, headaches, muscle and joint aches, and pains and diarrhea are inconstant manifestations. About 10% of patients with acute hepatitis, most often those with hepatitis B, develop a serum sickness–like syndrome in the preicteric stage, consisting of fever, rash, and arthralgias. This syndrome is attributed to circulating immune complexes. In the typical case, even before jaundice appears (if it does), elevated serum levels of ALT (alanine aminotransferase) or AST (aspartate aminotransferase) documenting hepatocytic injury provide the first specific clue to the nature of the illness.

The *icteric phase*, if it appears, is caused mainly by conjugated hyperbilirubinemia. It is usual in adults (but not in children) with hepatitis A, but may be absent in about half the cases of hepatitis B and the majority of NANB hepatitis. In these anicteric cases, the illness may be dismissed as flu-like unless its true nature is revealed by elevated serum aminotransferase levels. In icteric patients the urine turns darker (bilirubinuria), and in some the stools become lighter owing to cholestasis (cholestatic hepatitis). Distressing itching caused by retention of bile salts can be a problem. The liver may be mildly enlarged and moderately tender to percussion. Curiously, with the onset of the icteric phase, the constitutional symptoms begin to clear and the patient feels better. In a few weeks to perhaps several months, usually sooner with HA and NANB than with the other forms of acute hepatitis, the jaundice and most of the systemic symptoms clear as convalescence begins.

Integral to the diagnosis of acute hepatitis are liver function tests and serologic studies. In addition to the elevated levels of bilirubin (in some cases) and aminotransferases, markers of hepatocytic injury include prolonged prothrombin time, and hyperglobulinemia. In contrast, the serum level of alkaline phosphatase is usually only mildly elevated. Most definitive are the serum levels of antigens or antibodies. A sample of some typical profiles is offered in Table 19–5.

MORPHOLOGY. The changes in acute viral hepatitis are virtually the same irrespective of the causative agent, although very subtle differences have been described.[53,54] It is important to note that these viral changes can be mimicked by drug reactions. Grossly, the liver is slightly enlarged and more or less green depending on the phase of the acute disease and the level of jaundice.

Histologically, **the major findings are (1) diffuse liver cell injury with lobular disarray; (2) necrosis of random, isolated liver cells or small clusters of cells; (3) reactive changes in Kupffer cells and sinusoidal lining cells; (4) an inflammatory infiltrate in the portal tracts; and (5) evidence of hepatocytic regeneration during the recovery phase.**[55]

The **liver cell injury** is manifested by swelling, sometimes with partial clearing of the cytoplasm secondary to hydropic distension of endoplasmic reticulum, producing what is called **ballooning degeneration.** Fatty change is unusual in acute viral hepatitis except with NANBV. **Lobular disarray** results from the cellular swelling, necrosis, and regeneration of cells producing compression of the vascu-

lar sinusoids and loss of the normal, more or less radial array (Fig. 19–16). Two patterns of **liver cell necrosis** appear. In one, the cells appear to undergo fragmentation and condensation; the cytoplasm becomes intensely eosinophilic and the nuclear fragments dark and shrunken. The dead fragments are then phagocytized or extruded into the adjacent space of Disse or biliary canaliculus.[56] These red (in H and E stains) refractile "mummies" are called **Councilman bodies** and are distinctive features of, but not pathognomonic of, viral hepatitis. In the other pattern of necrosis, isolated or clustered cells undergo apparent lysis (**"dropout necrosis"**). Notably, there are no "ground-glass" cells or "sanded" nuclei in acute hepatitis unless the disease is in transit to chronic hepatitis. Another prominent feature is **marked hypertrophy and probable hyperplasia of Kupffer cells and sinusoidal lining cells,** both of which are often laden with lipofuscin pigment. **The portal tracts are usually infiltrated with inflammatory cells,** mainly lymphocytes admixed with macrophages and rare eosinophils and neutrophils. Plasma cells are uncommon in the usual case. The portal infiltrate is said to be slightly more pronounced in hepatitis A. The inflammatory infiltrate may in some cases permeate the lobule in the form of sinusoidal accumulations of mainly mononuclear cells. Eventually, during the **recovery phase,** scattered bi- and trinucleate liver cells and mitotic figures provide evidence of regeneration. Mentioned last, because of its inconstancy and variability, is **bile stasis,** which may be entirely absent in anicteric hepatitis. Conversely, in some cases a typical cholestatic picture may appear (as is described on page 916), often accompanied by inflammatory changes in the bile ducts within the portal triads.

Necrosis of confluent areas of hepatocytes may merely reflect a severe attack of acute viral hepatitis, but may herald progression to chronic or fulminant hepatitis. Particularly with hepatitis B, these foci of necrosis may interconnect adjacent areas of necrosis to bridge central to portal, central to central, or portal to portal areas, referred to as **bridging necrosis. Bridging necrosis and "piecemeal" necrosis** of cells (described later in the consideration of chronic hepatitis [p. 936]) when present in acute hepatitis were at one time thought to portend impending chronic or fulminant disease.[57] Although these changes may have

Table 19–5. Diagnostic Tests in Acute Hepatitis

IgM-Anti-HAV	HBsAg	IgM-Anti-HBc	IgG-Anti-HBc	IgM-Anti-HDV	
+	−	−	−	−	Acute hepatitis A
−	+	−	−	−	Early acute hepatitis B
−	+	+	−	−	Acute or chronic hepatitis B or chronic carrier
−	−	−	+	−	Past exposure to hepatitis B
−	+	+	−	+	Acute coinfection with HBV and HDV
−	+	−	+	+	Acute hepatitis D superimposed on chronic carriage of hepatitis B
−	−	−	−	−	Probably NANB hepatitis

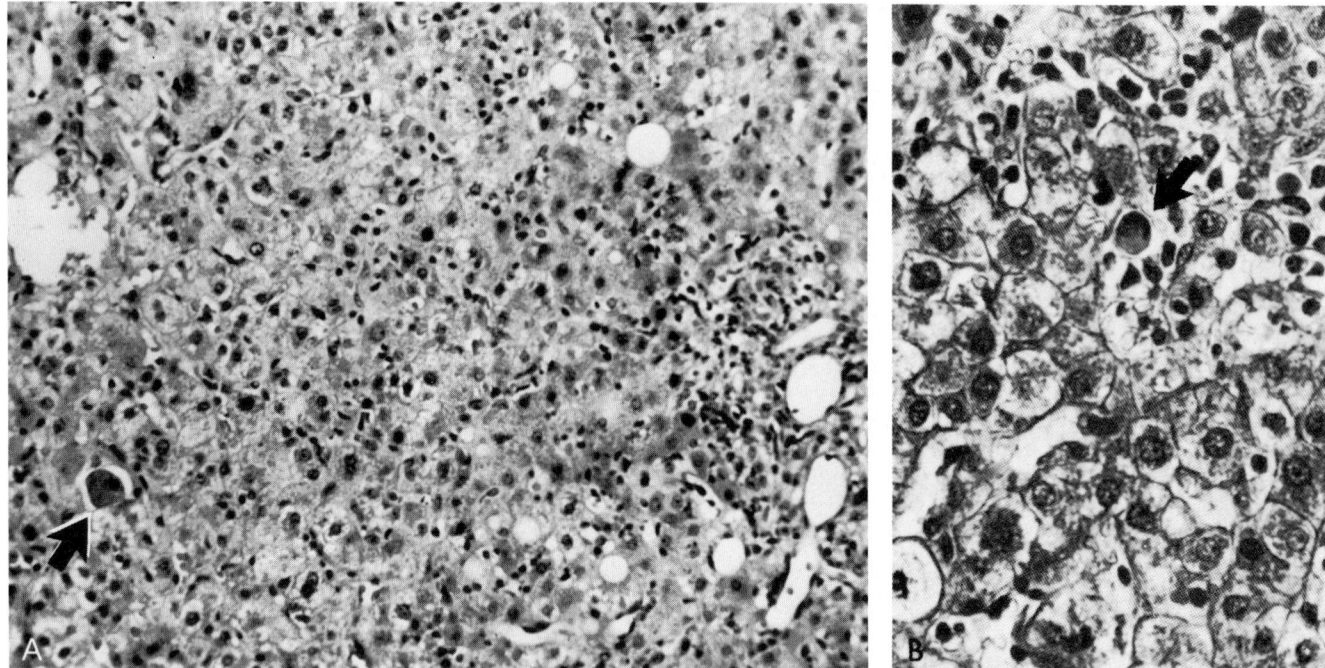

Figure 19–16. A, Acute viral hepatitis showing lobular disarray, mild periportal infiltrate at right, and Councilman body *(arrow)*. B, High-power detail of acute viral hepatitis with cellular disarray, ballooning, inflammatory cells in sinusoids, and Councilman body *(arrow)*. (Courtesy of Dr. Hans Popper, The Mount Sinai Medical Center.)

some prognostic value in the elderly, in young adults they may not be ominous.[58] Ultimately, prognostication by histopathology is hazardous.

Not all cases of acute viral hepatitis have a happy ending. About 1% or less of acute infections flare into fulminant, usually fatal hepatitis with submassive to massive necrosis of the liver. While more details are given in subsequent sections, this tragic complication is rare with HAV and more frequent with HBV (especially if there is concurrent HDV infection) and NANBV. More frequent is the development of chronic disease seen in 5 to 10% of cases of acute hepatitis, save those caused by HAV.

Chronic Hepatitis

Symptomatic, biochemical, or serologic evidence of continuing inflammatory hepatic disease for more than six months without steady improvement is taken to mean chronic hepatitis. *There are several variants of chronic hepatitis, but the principal subtypes are (1) chronic persistent hepatitis (CPH), and (2) chronic active hepatitis (CAH), sometimes called chronic aggressive hepatitis. These two patterns have very different clinical implications. CPH is a relatively benign smoldering infection that may persist for many months to years without seriously impairing the hepatic function. This pattern of chronic hepatitis sometimes underlies the carrier state described earlier. In contrast, CAH implies progressive liver damage leading often to cirrhosis, hepatic failure, and death.* The differentiation of these two types of chronic hepatitis may be diffi-

cult, particularly because there are intermediate cases in which even interpretation of the liver biopsy is precarious. Moreover, occasional cases of chronic persistent hepatitis have episodes of apparent activation suggesting conversion to chronic active hepatitis, and conversely, quiescent chronic active hepatitis may be misinterpreted as chronic persistent hepatitis.[59] Nonetheless, liver biopsy usually provides welcome reassurance to those with chronic persistent hepatitis.

Although the hepatitis viruses are responsible for most cases of chronic hepatitis, there are many other etiologies: Wilson's disease, alpha-1-antitrypsin deficiency, chronic alcoholism, drug reactions (isoniazid, methyldopa, methotrexate), and autoimmunity. The last-mentioned produces what has been called "lupoid" hepatitis, to be described later. The frequency of the development of chronic hepatitis when of viral origin varies with the particular agent.

• *HAV*—Does not produce chronic hepatitis.
• *HBV*—About 5% of infections become chronic, approximately one-third chronic persistent hepatitis, and two-thirds chronic active hepatitis.
• *HDV*—Adequate data on the frequency of chronic HDV infection are not available. In general, coinfection with HBV and HDV produces a severe but self-limited disease that clears. In contrast, HDV infection superimposed on the chronic carrier state of HBV imposes a significant (10 to 40%) risk of chronicity.
• *NANBV*—With post-transfusion hepatitis, the frequency of chronicity is 40 to 60%, most cases conforming to chronic active hepatitis. In the absence of

an identifiable percutaneous inoculation the frequency is 10% or less.

What factors lead to the development of chronic viral hepatitis? Such information as is available relates almost entirely to HBV. The basic proposal is — *some impairment or defect in the host immune response results in failure to control continued HBV replication.*[33] The inadequate immune response may stem from (1) a defective hepatitis B viral genome yielding incomplete expression of viral antigens, which therefore evoke an inadequate immune response; (2) a defect in function or number of cytotoxic T cells; (3) increased T-suppressor cell function; (4) antiviral antibodies that mask or modulate viral antigens; and (5) dissociation of viral antigens and HLA-antigens on the plasma membrane with failure to provide a recognizable immune signal. Other factors may also affect the adequacy of the immune response, including genetic responsiveness, hormones (e.g., steroids), and drugs. Much is uncertain, but it is clear that chronicity is more frequent in neonates and the very elderly, in males, in association with immunoincompetence or immunosuppression, in Down's syndrome, in patients on hemodialysis, in recipients of multiple transfusions, and in homosexuals.[60]

CHRONIC PERSISTENT HEPATITIS (CPH).

This sequel to acute hepatitis caused by HBV, by NANBV, or rarely by combined HBV and delta infection is a relapsing, remitting condition that is usually benign and eventually self-limited. It is not associated with progressive liver damage. *In most instances, it can be viewed as delayed recovery from the acute episode, but it may take as long as several years to clear.*[61] During this long recovery period, the individual may be symptom free, and the only evidence of persistent abnormality is an elevated serum level of one of the aminotransferases — hence, the facetious designation "transaminitis." However, fatigue, malaise, and loss of appetite may wax and wane, sometimes with bouts of mild jaundice. HBsAg is found in the serum of 20 to 60% of these patients, and much less often evidence of a combined HBV-HDV etiology. When all viral markers are negative, NANBV or a nonviral etiology must be assumed.

The mild morphologic changes are not pathognomonic and can be summarized as **chronic triaditis.** An inflammatory infiltrate of lymphocytes, macrophages, and occasional plasma cells, with possibly a rare neutrophil or eosinophil, is present in the portal tracts. Follicular aggregates may be formed. Importantly, **the infiltrate is limited to the portal tracts and does not spill out into the hepatic parenchyma.** The liver architecture is usually well preserved but sometimes reveals vestiges of the acute disease. With CPH related to the HBV, "ground-glass" hepatocytes (p. 932) are sometimes present and may be numerous.[62] **Notably absent are significant hepatocyte necrosis or the important hallmarks of chronic active hepatitis (CAH), i.e., piecemeal necrosis of the liver cells at the limiting plate and bridging necrosis.** The alterations of CPH are then quite nonspecific and can be mimicked by drug injury, systemic infections, and early primary biliary cirrhosis.

In some cases, the morphologic changes are equivocal, suggesting transition from CPH to CAH.[63] Conversely, treatment of CAH has led to conversion of the liver biopsy to apparent CPH, but with cessation of the therapy the morphologic changes often revert.[64] Thus, persistent hepatitis and active hepatitis in a sense represent the two ends of a spectrum of chronicity; there are cases that swing one way or the other, depending apparently on the response of the host.

CHRONIC ACTIVE HEPATITIS (CAH).

Generically, chronic active hepatitis may be defined as a chronic necrotizing and fibrosing hepatic disease of varied etiology. It is in most instances a serious progressive disorder, as noted earlier. Although the HBV is responsible for most cases of CAH, the frequency of this untoward event is greater with NANBV and combined HBV-HDV. In addition, there are nonviral causes, such as an autoimmune reaction, drugs, or a metabolic disorder.[64a] When all known etiologies have been excluded, a substantial residuum of unknown origin remains.

At this point it is well to characterize *chronic autoimmune hepatitis.*[65] Its major features include:

1. Female predominance, particularly young and perimenopausal women.
2. The absence of serologic markers of a viral etiology.
3. Elevated serum IgG levels.
4. High serum titers of non–organ-specific autoantibodies, e.g., antinuclear, anti–smooth muscle, and antimitochondrial antibodies. Because there is often a positive LE test, autoimmune hepatitis has in the past been called "lupoid" hepatitis.
5. High serum levels of organ-specific autoantibodies, e.g., to liver-specific protein (LSP), liver membrane antigen (LMA), and liver microsomes (LKM).
6. A genetic predisposition marked by HLA B8 or DRw3.
7. A prominence of plasma cells in the periportal inflammatory infiltrate.

Additional features supporting a possible autoimmune basis for this form of CAH include the frequent concurrence of other forms of autoimmune disease, such as thyroiditis, arthritis, vasculitis, and Sjögren's syndrome, and the beneficial response in many (but not all) patients to the administration of steroids, in marked contrast to viral CAH. As with most autoimmune diseases, the trigger event and pathogenesis of the reaction against "self" are obscure. Both cytotoxic T cells and antibody-dependent cellular cytotoxicity have been implicated, with most of the evidence favoring the latter.[66]

The morphologic changes of CAH in general must be divided into those general features found in all cases whatever the etiology, and specific features relating to the particular cause. The distinctive general features are **(1) an exuberant portal inflammatory infiltrate that spills out of the portal tracts, (2) piecemeal necrosis, (3) bridging necrosis, and (4) progressive fibrosis extending from the portal tracts into the hepatic parenchyma, leading in many cases to fully developed cirrhosis.**[67]

In contrast to classic acute hepatitis in which the inflammatory reaction is more or less limited to the portal tract, in CAH it spills out into the periportal parenchyma (Fig. 19–17). It is composed mainly of lymphocytes and macrophages but is often heavily admixed with plasma cells. Sometimes, the infiltrate forms lymphoid follicles. Depending on the activity of the disease, there may or may not be ballooning of hepatocytes. **The two most distinctive features of CAH are piecemeal necrosis and bridging necrosis.** In the former, the spreading inflammatory infiltrate comes into direct contact with liver cells that undergo a peculiar condensation and fragmentation (apoptosis) lending a "moth-eaten" appearance to the usual regular array of the limiting plate. **Bridging necrosis** is the consequence

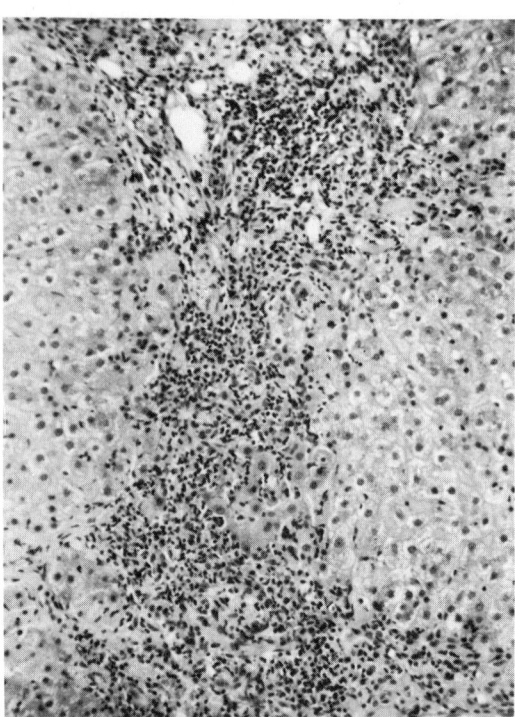

Figure 19–18. Chronic active hepatitis with bridging necrosis. (Courtesy of Dr. Hans Popper, The Mount Sinai Medical Center.)

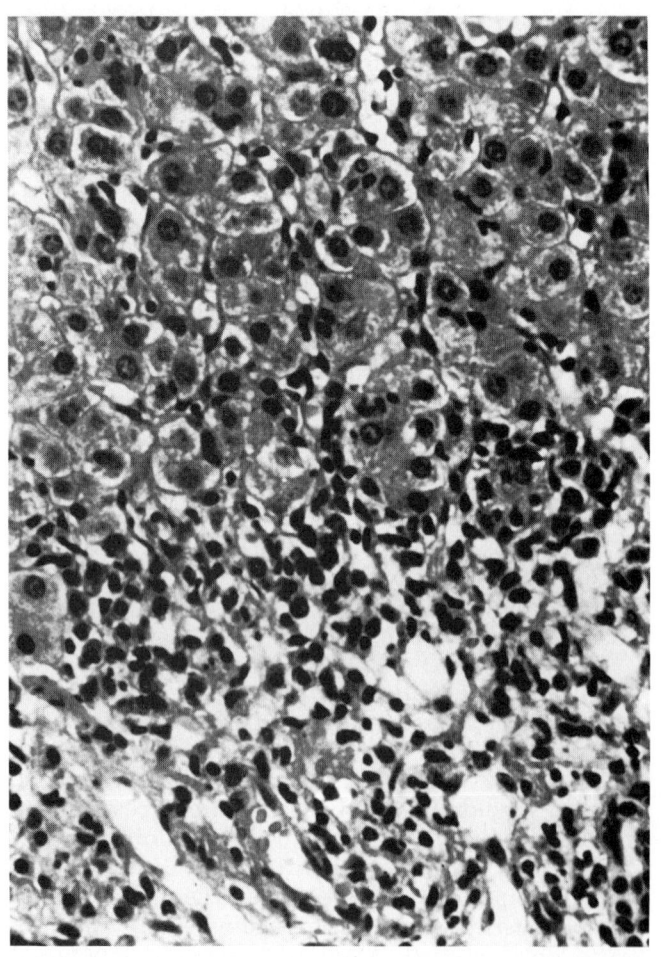

Figure 19–17. Chronic active hepatitis. The portal inflammatory infiltrate below is spilling out into the parenchyma, destroying the limiting plate.

of lytic destruction of numerous clusters of hepatocytes with coalescence of these foci to create tracts where all hepatocytes are missing, leaving only the collapsed reticulin network. These tracts may bridge central-to-portal, central-to-central, or portal-to-portal areas, hence the term "bridging necrosis" (Fig. 19–18). Although piecemeal necrosis and bridging necrosis do not imply inevitability of progression to CAH, they are ominous findings in acute disease, strongly suggesting that scarring is likely to follow, and possibly cirrhosis. A schematic comparison of the morphologic changes in acute and chronic active hepatitis is offered in Figure 19–19.

In many cases, HBV and HDV can be identified in biopsies by immunocytochemical or in situ hybridization methods.[51] You recall that continued viral replication is characteristic of CAH, caused by hepatitis B. Histologic evidence of the virus is often present, but it should be noted that it is more subtle than in "healthy" carriers, in whom the specific cytologic changes seen with HBV were described (p. 932). Unfortunately, in many cases of HBV- and HDV-induced disease, traces of persistent virus may be lacking or extremely scanty at the time of morphologic study. There still remains the dilemma of differentiating NANBV-induced CAH (for which there are no markers) from CAH of autoimmune origin. In last analysis, it is frequently impossible to identify the etiology of CAH in tissue samples, and so great reliance must be placed on clinical, virologic, and serologic observations.

The clinical findings in CAH are highly variable. Some cases are marked by the features seen in acute

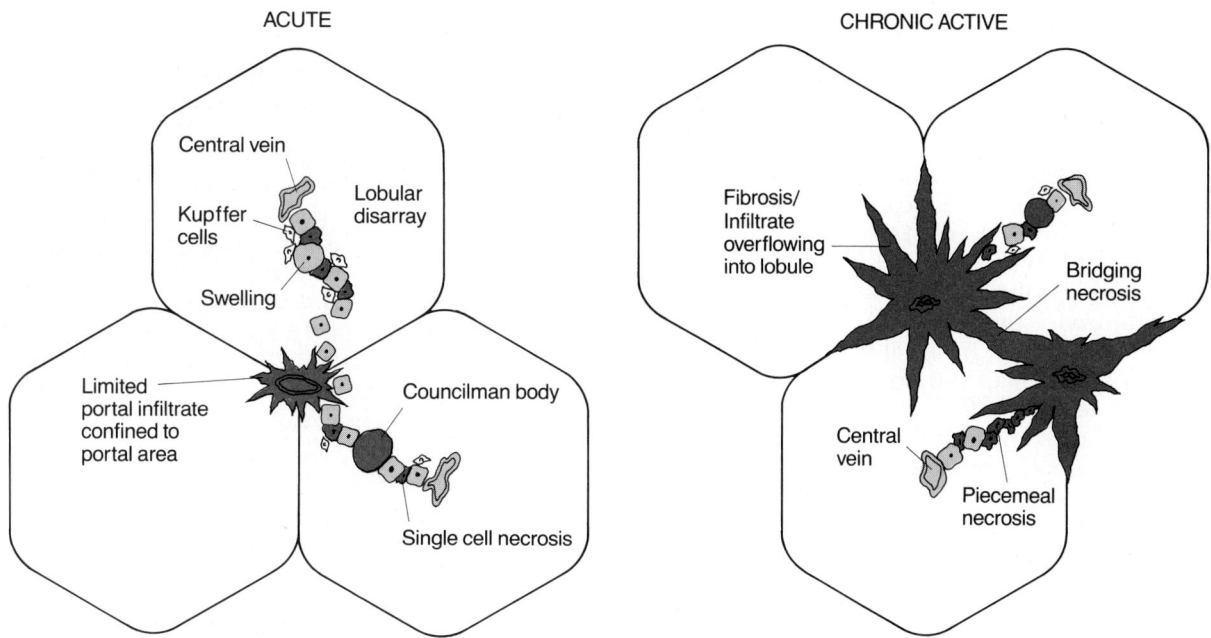

Figure 19-19. A schematic comparison of acute and chronic active hepatitis.

hepatitis, i.e., fatigue, malaise, mild fever, and sometimes jaundice. Occasionally in cases of HBV or autoimmune origin, immune-complex diseases, such as disseminated vasculitis (polyarteritis nodosa) and glomerulonephritis, appear. On the other hand, the patient may be virtually asymptomatic, and the underlying liver disease comes to attention only by the appearance of ascites and other manifestations of portal hypertension, when the scarring and cirrhosis are already well developed (p. 942). Laboratory studies in almost all cases will reveal elevated serum transaminase levels, prolongation of the prothrombin time, and in some instances, hyperglobulinemia and hyperbilirubinemia.

The clinical course is unpredictable. Some patients have rapidly progressive disease, particularly those with combined HBV-HDV infections, and develop cirrhosis within a few years. Conversely, those with disease of NANB or autoimmune origin may experience spontaneous remission. Overall, the five-year mortality is about 25 to 50%. The major causes of death are liver failure with hepatic encephalopathy, cirrhosis with massive hematemesis from esophageal varices, and in the case of those who acquired the HBV early in life, hepatocellular carcinoma.

Submassive to Massive Necrosis (Fulminant Hepatitis)

When hepatic insufficiency progresses from onset to death (or hepatic transplantation) within two to three weeks, it is termed fulminant liver failure. A less rapid course, extending up to three months, is called submassive failure. Both patterns are fortunately uncommon and are caused mainly by rampant to fulminant viral hepatitis and drug (or chemical) toxicity. However, as Table 19-6 indicates, there are many other

possible etiologies and ultimately some cases of unknown etiology.

Viral hepatitis accounts for 50 to 65% of all cases.[45] Young female drug addicts and homosexual and bisexual males are disproportionately repre-

Table 19-6. Causes of Fulminant or Subfulminant Liver Failure

Acute viral hepatitis
  Acute hepatitis A
  Acute hepatitis B
  Acute hepatitis D (delta)
    Coinfection
    Superinfection
  Acute non-A, non-B hepatitis
    Epidemic
    Sporadic
  Acute hepatitis due to infection with herpes viruses
Acute drug-induced hepatitis
Acute hepatitis due to poisoning
Other causes
  Ischemic liver cell necrosis
  Obstruction of the hepatic veins
    Budd-Chiari syndrome
    Veno-occlusive disease of the liver
  Massive malignant infiltration of the liver
  Wilson's disease
  Microvesicular steatosis
    Acute fatty liver of pregnancy
    Reye's syndrome
    Drug-induced microvesicular steatosis
  Autoimmune chronic active hepatitis
  Reactivation of chronic hepatitis B
  Hyperthermia
  Liver transplantation
  Partial hepatectomy

From Bernau, J., Rueff, B., and Benhamou, J-P.: Fulminant and subfulminant liver failure: definitions and causes. Semin. Liver Dis. 6:97, 1986. Thieme Medical Publishers, Inc. Reprinted by permission.

sented among these victims. Among those cases of viral origin, HBV accounts for about 35 to 45% and NANBV for about the same proportion. Combined HBV-HDV is responsible for fewer cases, and HAV is involved only rarely. However, combined HBV-HDV and NANBV infections incur substantial risks.

Various drugs and chemicals are responsible for about 25 to 30% of all cases of massive to submassive destruction of the liver. Principally implicated are isoniazid, antidepressants (particularly monoamine oxidase inhibitors), nonsteroidal anti-inflammatory drugs, acetaminophen, halothane and its derivatives (p. 486), methyldopa, and the mycotoxins of the mushroom *Amanita phalloides*. Obviously, chemicals such as phosphorus and chlorinated hydrocarbons are also hepatotoxic, as are many other drugs, but are encountered less frequently.

No comment will be made on the many other potential causes of hepatic failure, but the extent and rapidity of the destructive process is extremely variable. The previous condition of the liver naturally influences the outcome as does the patient's age. Otherwise healthy young adults fare better than the aged. Whatever the primary insult, reduced perfusion of the liver, as in cardiac decompensation or shock and serious systemic infection, further burdens the liver, compounding the likelihood of serious damage. In most cases of HBV etiology, the principal determinant of the severity of injury is the strength of the immune response; the stronger the immunologic reaction, the greater the destruction.

All causative agents produce essentially identical morphologic changes that vary with the severity of the necrotizing process (submassive to massive) and duration of sur-

vival. With all, the distribution of liver destruction is extremely capricious. **The entire liver may be involved or sometimes, for completely obscure reasons, only random areas.** For example, the left lobe may be virtually totally destroyed, with the right lobe curiously spared, or patchy large areas may be dispersed haphazardly throughout the liver. During the early phase there is progressive loss of liver substance with depression of affected areas. With massive involvement of the entire liver, it shrinks in size over the course of days to as little as 500 to 700 gm and is transformed into a red, limp organ covered by a wrinkled, too-large capsule (Fig. 19–20). Blotchy green bile staining may be present. On transection, necrotic areas have a muddy red, mushy appearance with patchy bile staining.

Histologically, the necrosis may wipe out entire lobules or be less extreme, destroying the central and midzonal regions and sparing the periphery of the lobule. Presumably, the most hypoxic zones are most vulnerable to further insult. Most often, there is complete destruction of innumerable contiguous lobules with liquefaction of hepatocytes, leaving only a collapsed reticulin framework and preserved portal tracts (Fig. 19–21). With loss of the hepatic parenchyma and shrinkage of the liver, the reticulin framework becomes more condensed and the portal tracts appear to converge. There may be surprisingly little inflammatory reaction in the viable margins save possibly for an increase in lymphocytes, macrophages, and occasional neutrophils within the portal tracts.

A number of secondary changes appear when the patient survives for more than a week. Regenerative activity appears in surviving hepatocytes. With zonal necrosis, the framework is preserved and the regeneration is orderly; in time the native architecture may be virtually restored, but proliferating narrow cords of epithelial cells derived from the

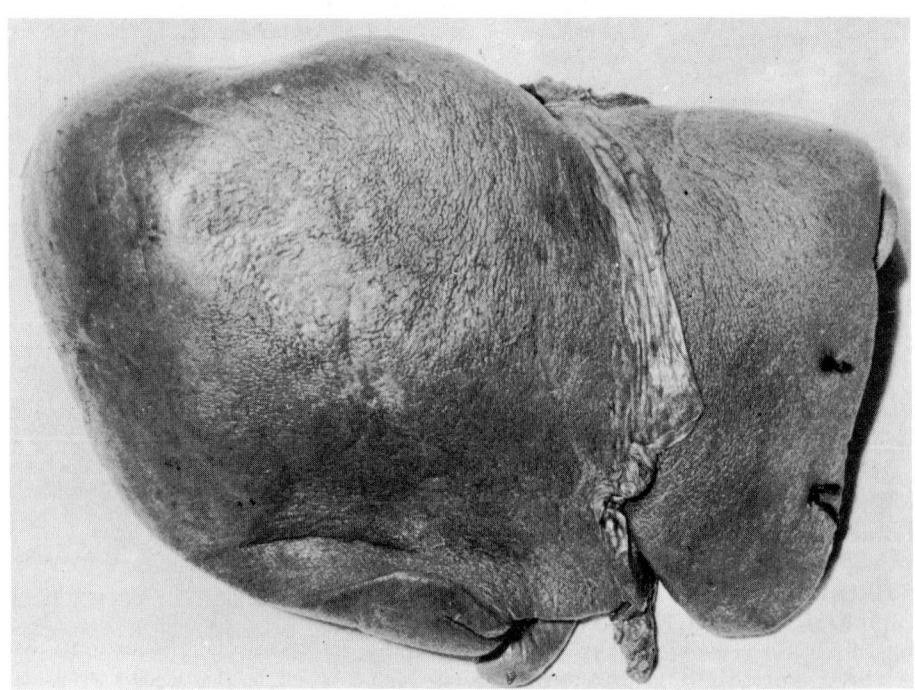

Figure 19–20. Massive necrosis. Liver is small (700 gm), pale, and soft in consistency. Capsule is wrinkled.

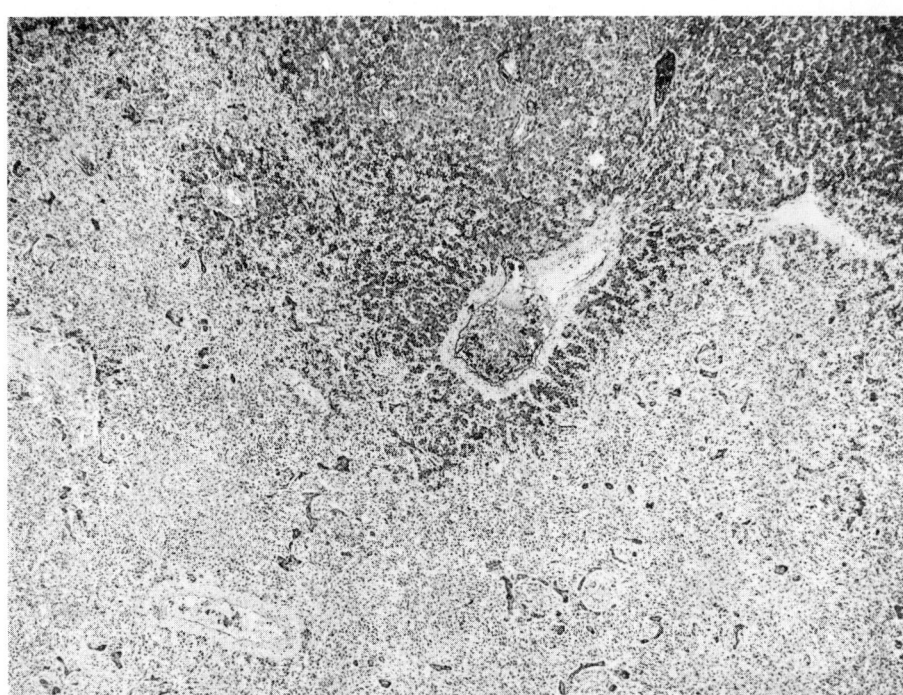

Figure 19-21. Massive necrosis. In lower portion of field, complete necrosis is apparent, with removal of all liver cells in many adjacent liver lobules.

cholangioles may appear in the periportal region. The Kupffer cells that survive the necrotizing process also undergo hypertrophy and hyperplasia, and in the course of time become laden with lipofuscin and cellular debris. With more extensive destruction of entire lobules the regeneration is more disorderly, yielding nodular masses of liver cells. There very often is little or no scarring following massive necrosis; the patient either succumbs or is kept alive by virtue of restoration of pre-existing architecture. To anticipate a later discussion, **massive necrosis is then an infrequent antecedent to postnecrotic cirrhosis.** Scarring is much more likely in those with chronic active hepatitis or a protracted course of submassive or patchy necrosis.

The clinical features of hepatic failure were described on page 918. It suffices here to point out that depending on the magnitude of the insult and the resistance of the host, the mortality rate ranges from 25 to 90% (in the absence of liver transplantation). The only happy aspect of this very grave condition is that survivors of massive necrosis related to viral infections almost never become carriers and have lifelong immunity to the particular causative virus.

PERICHOLANGITIS AND CHOLANGITIS

An increase in inflammatory cells within the portal tracts (principally about the bile ducts), when unaccompanied by evidence of intraductal inflammatory or parenchymal injury, is referred to as *pericholangitis*. It consists solely of a portal triaditis marked principally by lymphocytes and macrophages with occasional plasma cells, neutrophils, and eosinophils.

This is an extremely common anatomic finding and is usually of little or no clinical significance. Infrequently it is associated with fever, mild pruritus, mild jaundice, and modest elevations of alkaline phosphatase.

The genesis of *pericholangitis* is obscure. Its strongest clinical association is with inflammatory bowel disease.[68] It is also encountered in association with blood-borne infection, abdominal sepsis, and pancreatitis. Antibiotic therapy is usually without benefit, arguing against direct bacterial infection. It is assumed, therefore, without proof, that drainage of bacterial products underlies the inflammatory changes. The principal importance of this condition is that it offers a possible explanation for mild jaundice and elevated alkaline phosphatase levels in patients with inflammatory bowel disease or significant extrahepatic infections.

Cholangitis implies intraductal inflammation of the extrahepatic or intrahepatic ducts, or more often both. It is marked anatomically by suppuration within the ducts, usually accompanied by bile stasis (Fig. 19-22). Almost always, it is related to some obstructive lesion within the major extrahepatic ducts, usually a gallstone impacted in the common bile duct. Infrequently, cholangitis complicates carcinomas arising in the extrahepatic bile ducts, papilla of Vater, or head of the pancreas; acute pancreatitis; and benign strictures of the bile ducts.[69] With these origins, infection by enteric organisms, such as *E. coli*, Klebsiella, and Enterobacter, are most common. Less frequently, staphylococcal and streptococcal species, and anaerobes, e.g., bacteroides and clostridia, are also present. Almost always the infection begins in the common bile duct or hepatic ducts and progressively

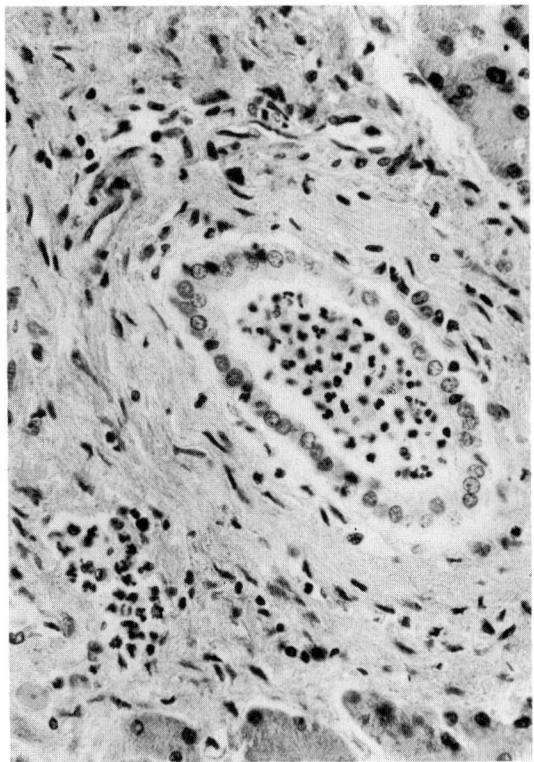

Figure 19–22. Acute cholangitis with neutrophils within a bile duct and in a focus on lower left outside of duct.

ascends into the intrahepatic ramifications *(ascending cholangitis)*. Acute cholangitis has also been reported as a complication of toxic shock syndrome (p. 339), ascribed to circulating exotoxin. Whatever the origin, the patient typically has high fever, chills, jaundice, and often marked leukocytosis. Surgical drainage of the duct system is generally necessary for relief of symptoms, control of infection, and prevention of subsequent liver abscesses.[70]

PRIMARY SCLEROSING CHOLANGITIS (PSC)

This uncommon condition merits brief citation because it produces a cholestatic syndrome characterized by pruritus, mainly conjugated hyperbilirubinemia, and marked elevation of serum alkaline phosphatase that must be differentiated from the more common causes of obstructive jaundice, e.g., obstructive gallstones or carcinoma of the pancreas or common bile duct. It is of unknown etiology, occurs mainly in males under 45 years of age, and is most often associated with chronic ulcerative colitis and various autoimmune diseases, although it may appear in the absence of any pre-existing condition.[71] As the name indicates, *it is marked by a segmental, random and uneven chronic fibrosing inflammatory reaction involving single or varying combinations of the extrahepatic and intrahepatic bile ducts, and less commonly the pancreatic duct. The intrahepatic ductal lu-*

mina may be entirely obliterated, leaving only a fibrous scar, or in the regions proximal to the narrowings, there may be ductal dilatation. A mononuclear inflammatory infiltrate accompanied by occasional neutrophils and eosinophils may be present in the fibrous tissue. As visualized on cholangiography, the ducts may appear beaded or show haphazard narrowings and dilatations. The involvement may be diffuse, segmental, or relatively limited in distribution, but it tends to be most restrictive at the confluence of the right and left hepatic ducts. The condition is progressive, leading to biliary cirrhosis and ultimately liver failure usually within four to five years.

LIVER ABSCESSES

In developing countries, liver abscesses are common; most represent parasitic infections, e.g., amebic, echinococcal, and (less commonly) other protozoal or helminthic organisms. In developed countries, liver abscesses are becoming uncommon and most are bacterial in origin, but a continuing low prevalence of amebic abscesses (p. 398) is still encountered, usually in immigrants from endemic regions.[72] Most liver abscesses represent a secondary complication of an infection elsewhere. The organisms reach the liver through one of the following pathways: (1) portal vein, (2) arterial supply, (3) ascending infection in the biliary tract (ascending cholangitis), (4) direct invasion of the liver from a nearby infection, or (5) a penetrating injury. Once, the majority of hepatic abscesses in the United States resulted from portal spread of organisms from an infection within the abdominal cavity, e.g., appendicitis, diverticulitis, colitis. Understandably, the major offenders were *E. coli*, Pseudomonas, *Klebsiella* species, Enterobacter species, group D streptococci, and a variety of anaerobes such as Bacteroides species.[73] Early recognition of abdominal sepsis and effective antibiotic treatment have reduced the importance of this pathway. Currently the two major modes of spread are (1) biliary tract disease with ascending cholangitis, and (2) arterial blood-borne spread of a primary infection elsewhere in the body in those suffering from some form of immune deficiency, e.g., old age with debilitating disease, immunosuppression, or cancer chemotherapy with marrow failure.[74] In these settings, enteric organisms, streptococcal species, fungal infections (notably Candida species) and antibiotic-resistant organisms, e.g., staphylococci, Pseudomonas, and *Enterobacter aerogenes*, have come to assume greater importance. In about one third of the cases, the abscesses are cryptogenic and appear in the absence of a primary focus elsewhere. Sometimes organisms cannot be recovered, for technical reasons or because of antibiotic suppression of the causal agents.[75]

Depending on their pathogenesis, pyogenic hepatic abscesses may occur as solitary or multiple lesions ranging in size from millimeters to massive lesions many centimeters in diameter. Bacteremic spread through either the arterial or the portal system and ascending cholangitis tend to produce multiple small abscesses, whereas direct extension and trauma usually cause solitary large abscesses. The gross features and histologic changes are those to be anticipated in any abscess formation and are not distinctive save in the cases of fungal or amebic origin, in which it may be possible to visualize the offending agents in histologic sections. On rare occasion, abscesses, particularly amebic, located in the subdiaphragmatic region of the liver burrow through the diaphragm into the thoracic cavity to produce empyema or a lung abscess. Rupture of subcapsular liver abscesses has also led to peritonitis or subhepatic or subdiaphragmatic abscesses.

Liver abscesses, whatever their origins, are associated with fever, and in many instances, right upper quadrant pain, tender hepatomegaly, and uncommonly jaundice. These manifestations are indistinguishable from those of ascending cholangitis, which indeed may have led to the hepatic lesions. The diagnosis of larger (over 0.5 cm) lesions can usually be made by ultrasonography, CT, MRI scan, or scintiscans singly or in combination. Although antibiotic therapy may suffice to control smaller lesions, surgical drainage is often necessary and indicated when there is a solitary lesion or a few large lesions. Without drainage, the mortality rate with large liver abscesses approaches 70 to 80%, but with early recognition and appropriate management, it has been reduced to 20 to 30%.[74]

CIRRHOSIS

Cirrhosis is a generic term for hepatic disease of varied etiology (e.g., alcohol abuse, iron overload, drugs, chronic active hepatitis), having the following characteristics:[76]

1. *The architecture of the* total *liver is disorganized* by interconnecting fibrous scars formed in response to hepatocytic injury and loss.
2. The *fibrosis* may take the form of delicate bands (portal-central, portal-portal, or both) but may constitute broad scars replacing multiple adjacent lobules.
3. *Parenchymal nodules are created by the regenerative activity and network of scars.* The nodules vary in size, depending on causation, from micronodules (less than 3 mm in diameter) to macronodules (3 mm to several centimeters in diameter).
4. The *vascular architecture* is reorganized by the parenchymal damage and scarring, with the formation of abnormal arteriovenous interconnections.

Several features should be underscored. The parenchymal injury and consequent fibrosis extend throughout the liver. Focal injury with scarring does not constitute cirrhosis. Nodularity, micro- or macro-,

is requisite for the diagnosis. The fibrosis, once developed, is irreversible even though some regression has been observed in experimental animals and putatively in humans with hemochromatosis (discussed later). The vascular interconnections between the arterial and portal systems in cirrhosis impair the perfusion of the parenchyma and at the same time contribute to portal hypertension.

In many countries of the Western world, including the United States, cirrhosis is one of the ten leading causes of death. It achieved this unenviable prominence by a dramatic increase in frequency between 1950 and 1973 from 8.5 to 15.0 per 100,000 population, most of the increase attributable to alcohol abuse. Even though rampant alcoholism has not been curtailed, the mortality rate from alcoholic cirrhosis has fallen in recent years to 10.2 for reasons that are not clear but may include improved medical care, and conceivably a growing public awareness of the "evils of the bottle."[77]

There is no satisfactory classification of cirrhosis. Thus, it has been proposed that *cirrhosis be divided simply into two large categories: (1) micronodular, in which the preponderance of parenchymal nodules are less than 3 mm in diameter; and (2) macronodular, in which most of the nodules exceed 3 mm in diameter.* Appealing as such simplification may be, it is purely descriptive and offers no guidelines for clinical management. Accordingly, resort will be made to the historically sanctified classification drawing on both putative etiologies and presumed pathogenesis. An approximate frequency of each category in the Western world is included.[78]

Alcoholic cirrhosis	60–70%
Postnecrotic cirrhosis	10%
Biliary cirrhosis (primary and secondary)	5–10%
Pigment cirrhosis (in hemochromatosis)	5%
Cirrhosis associated with Wilson's disease	rare
Cirrhosis associated with alpha-1-antitrypsin deficiency	rare
Cryptogenic cirrhosis	10–15%

Not included in the above classification are the very infrequent types of cirrhosis associated with chronic right heart failure (cardiac cirrhosis); galactosemia; glycogen storage disease IV; diffuse infiltrative cancers of the liver (carcinomatous cirrhosis); and syphilis (congenital and tertiary). Also not included is *Indian childhood cirrhosis*, encountered principally in India, Southeast Asia, and the Middle East, which partakes of the morphologic features of cirrhosis associated with chronic active hepatitis and alcoholic cirrhosis.[79]

All forms of cirrhosis may be clinically silent. When symptomatic they lead to certain clinical manifestations that are usually most marked in the alcoholic form. Typically there is anorexia, weight loss, weakness, and in advanced disease, frank debilitation. Some of the weight loss may be masked by the not trivial amounts of "empty" calories provided by alcohol. Nonetheless, the "pasty" obesity cannot mask the muscle wasting, most evident in the extremities. Palmar erythema, spider angiomas (usually most visible over the chest), gynecomastia, gonadal atrophy, amenorrhea, and changes in the distribution of body hair may appear, all attributed to hyperestrinism secondary to impaired hepatic metabolism of estrogens. Dupuytren's contracture of the palmar fascia and finger clubbing develop infrequently, for poorly understood reasons. When the liver disease is advanced there is impaired synthesis of not only albumin, but also fibrinogen, prothrombin, and coagulant factors V, VII, IX, and X. Although some of these changes may have serious consequences such as a bleeding diathesis, they are significant for the most part as clinical clues to the presence of advanced liver disease and cirrhosis. Sometimes renal failure (the hepatorenal syndrome) complicates the course. In other rare instances, patients develop the nephrotic syndrome (p. 1033). It is now appreciated that "silent" glomerular lesions are common in cirrhotics. The changes comprise glomerular deposits of IgA and sometimes IgG, IgM, and/or C3, accompanied in some cases by mesangial or membranous changes.[80] Were these problems not sufficient, the alcoholic with or without cirrhosis also has an increased frequency of acute gastritis and peptic ulcers. The ultimate mechanism of most deaths is (1) progressive liver failure, (2) a complication related to the development of portal hypertension (see below), or (3) the development of hepatocellular carcinoma. Before describing the various types of cirrhosis, we should consider one of the serious consequences of cirrhosis — portal hypertension.

PORTAL HYPERTENSION

Increase in pressure in the portal system may develop in a variety of clinical circumstances, but the great majority of instances are related to cirrhosis. *The various causative conditions can be divided into three categories: (1) posthepatic, (2) prehepatic, and (3) intrahepatic.* Common to almost all is an increased resistance to portal flow. In a few, there is also some increased inflow into the portal system. The major *posthepatic causes* of portal hypertension are severe right-sided heart failure, Budd-Chiari syndrome (p. 922), and constrictive pericarditis. The major obstructive *prehepatic conditions* constitute thrombosis and narrowing (as by cancers or enlarged portahepatic nodes) of the portal vein before it ramifies within the liver (p. 923). Prehepatic portal hypertension may also occur because of increased inflow in hematologic disorders marked by massive splenomegaly, creating in essence an arteriovenous fistula that shunts blood into the splenic vein. The dominant *intrahepatic cause* is cirrhosis. Far less frequent intrahepatic causes are schistosomiasis, veno-occlusive disease, massive fatty change, diffuse fibrosing granulomatous disease such as sarcoidosis and miliary tuberculosis, and focal nodular hyperplasia. There are, in addition, rare cases of idiopathic portal hypertension. Despite all these possible causes, *portal hypertension means cirrhosis until proved otherwise.*

The basis for the portal hypertension in cirrhosis is mainly increased resistance to portal flow at the level of the sinusoids due to perisinusoidal deposition of collagen with narrowing of the sinusoidal channels, and compression of central veins by perivenular fibrosis and expansile parenchymal nodules. Arteriovenous anastomoses in the fibrous scars (presumably imposing arterial pressure on the low-pressure venous system) may also play a role.[81] *Whatever the mechanism, four major clinical consequences follow: (1) ascites; (2) the formation of portosystemic venous shunts, particularly in the gastroesophageal plexus; (3) congestive splenomegaly; and (4) occasionally hepatic encephalopathy (p. 919) secondary to the diffuse parenchymal damage and portosystemic shunting (Fig. 19–23).*

ASCITES. *Ascites refers to the collection of excess fluid in the peritoneal cavity.* It usually becomes clinically detectable when at least 500 ml has accumulated, but many liters may collect and cause abdominal distention. It is generally a serous fluid having less than 3 gm/dl of protein (largely albumin) as well as the same concentrations of solutes such as glucose, sodium, and potassium as the blood. Thus, withdrawal of large volumes of ascitic fluid for relief of symptoms invokes a substantial loss of protein and solutes. The fluid may also contain a scant number of mesothelial cells and mononuclear leukocytes. The presence of significant numbers of neutrophils suggests secondary infection, whereas red cells point to possible disseminated intra-abdominal cancer. In about 20% of cases of long-standing ascites, the peritoneal fluid seeps through transdiaphragmatic lymphatics to produce hydrothorax, more often on the right side.

The *pathogenesis of ascites* is complex and not entirely understood, but two mechanisms probably play major roles.

— *Increased hepatic lymph formation* — The discontinuous endothelial lining of the hepatic sinusoids does not restrain plasma proteins, and so the portal hypertension leads to the formation of a protein-rich transudate that weeps through the hepatic capsule accounting for the protein content of the fluid.[82]

— *Renal retention of sodium and water* — During the development of ascites there is sodium retention despite a total body sodium that is greater than normal. Controversy continues as to whether the sodium and water retention is a renal response to reduced effective circulating volume due to sequestration of fluid in the peritoneal cavity ("underfilling theory"), or instead is a primary response (for obscure reasons) marked by salt and water retention with expansion of the blood volume ("overfilling theory").[83,84]

Minor contributions to the genesis of the ascites may be made by increased intraperitoneal lymphatic seepage and reduced peritoneal reabsorption.

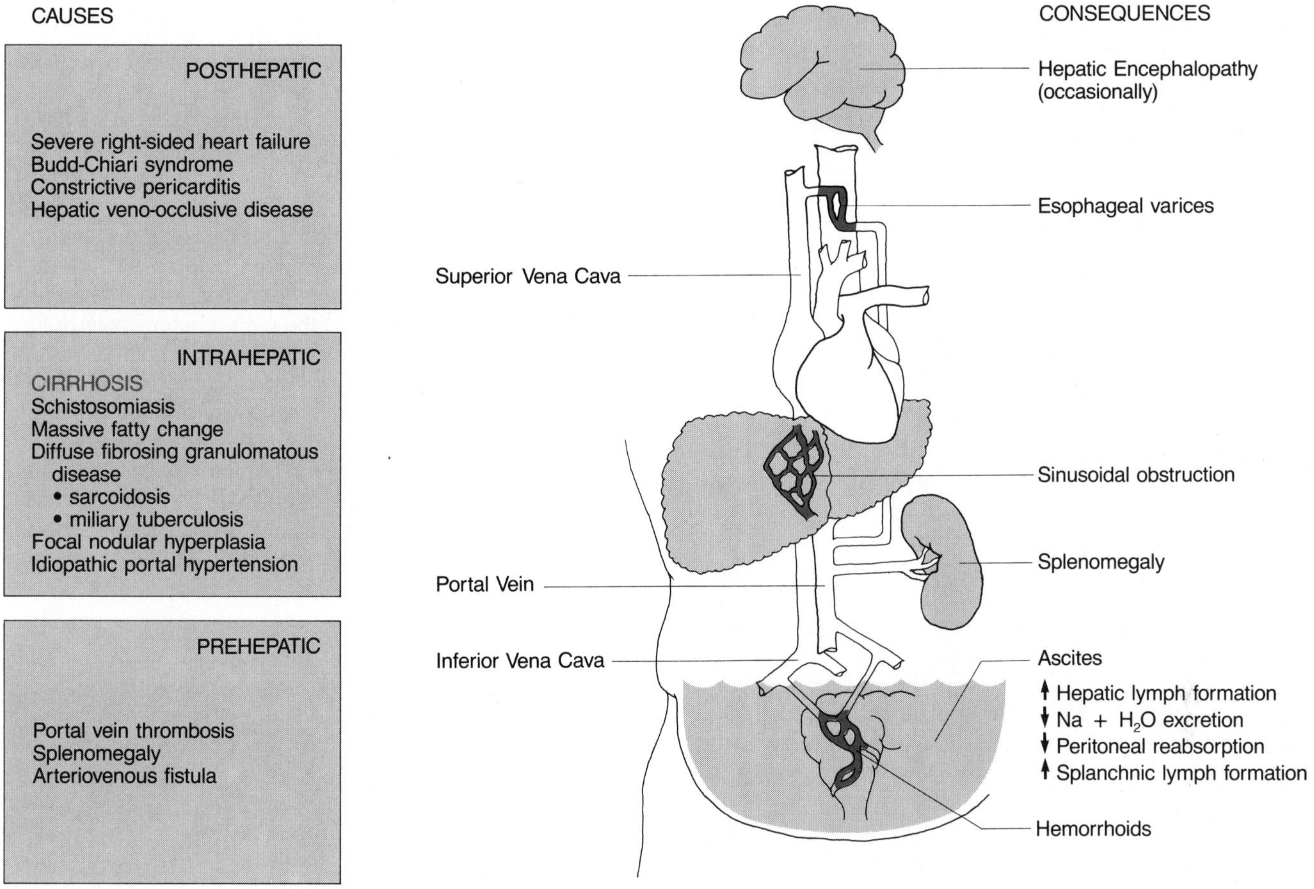

CAUSES

POSTHEPATIC

Severe right-sided heart failure
Budd-Chiari syndrome
Constrictive pericarditis
Hepatic veno-occlusive disease

INTRAHEPATIC

CIRRHOSIS
Schistosomiasis
Massive fatty change
Diffuse fibrosing granulomatous
  disease
  • sarcoidosis
  • miliary tuberculosis
Focal nodular hyperplasia
Idiopathic portal hypertension

PREHEPATIC

Portal vein thrombosis
Splenomegaly
Arteriovenous fistula

CONSEQUENCES

Hepatic Encephalopathy
(occasionally)

Esophageal varices

Superior Vena Cava

Sinusoidal obstruction

Splenomegaly

Portal Vein

Inferior Vena Cava

Ascites
↑ Hepatic lymph formation
↓ Na + H_2O excretion
↓ Peritoneal reabsorption
↑ Splanchnic lymph formation

Hemorrhoids

Figure 19-23. The three categories of portal hypertension and the major anatomic consequences.

PORTOSYSTEMIC SHUNTS (COLLATERAL CHANNELS). With the rise in pressure, portal vein bypasses develop wherever the systemic and portal circulations share common capillary beds. Principal sites are: veins around and within the rectum (hemorrhoids); the cardioesophageal junction (esophagogastric varices) (Fig. 19-24); the retroperitoneum; and the falciform ligament of the liver (periumbilical or abdominal wall collaterals). The hemorrhoids are indistinguishable from those encountered in noncirrhotic persons but serve as a possible clinical clue to the liver disease. Hemorrhoidal bleeding may occur but is rarely massive or life-threatening. Much more important are the esophagogastric varices (see p. 834) that appear in about 65% of patients with advanced cirrhosis of the liver, and cause massive hematemesis and death in about half of them. Abdominal wall collaterals appear as dilated subcutaneous veins that extend from the umbilicus toward the rib margins *(caput medusae)*. These tortuous dilated channels constitute an important clinical hallmark of portal hypertension.

SPLENOMEGALY. Long-standing congestion may cause congestive splenomegaly (p. 750). The degree of enlargement varies widely up to 1000 gm and is not necessarily correlated with other features of portal hypertension. Massive splenomegaly may secondarily

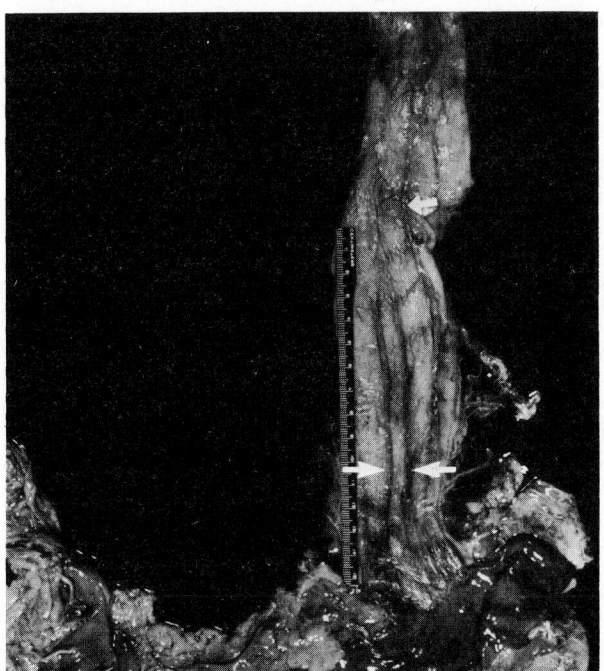

Figure 19-24. Esophageal varices. Dilated submucosal veins (*arrows*) in lower portion of esophagus in a patient with advanced alcoholic cirrhosis.

induce a variety of hematologic abnormalities attributed to hypersplenism (p. 749).

HEPATIC (METABOLIC) ENCEPHALOPATHY.

This serious neurologic disorder has already been described (p. 919). Although it may appear with hepatic failure from any cause, it is particularly associated with advanced cirrhosis because of the diffuse parenchymal damage and portosystemic shunting.

After this general overview of the clinical consequences of cirrhosis we can turn to the specific types.

ALCOHOLIC LIVER DISEASE (ALD) AND CIRRHOSIS

Chronic consumption of alcohol often leads to three distinctive, albeit overlapping, forms of liver disease; (1) hepatic steatosis, (2) alcoholic hepatitis, and (3) cirrhosis, collectively referred to as alcoholic liver disease (ALD).[85,86] The relationship of these three patterns of liver damage to each other is still somewhat controversial, but in most cases the alcoholic who continues to imbibe progresses from fatty change to bouts of alcoholic hepatitis to alcoholic cirrhosis in the course of 10 to 15 years. On the other hand, argument continues as to whether fatty change by and of itself predisposes to cirrhosis. Moreover, in animal models and some individuals, alcoholic cirrhosis may appear without apparent preceding episodes of alcoholic hepatitis. Did the sequential biopsies miss it?[87] So the relationship of these three forms of ALD to each other is still open to question, as will be pointed out in the following discussions.

Alcoholic Steatosis (Fatty Liver)

Within a few days of administration of alcohol to well-nourished nonalcoholic volunteers, fat appeared within liver cells.[88] The origin of the fat was discussed in detail on page 21. Suffice it here that it represents mainly (1) increased synthesis of triglycerides because of increased delivery of fatty acids to the liver, as well as enhanced synthesis of fatty acids; (2) decreased fatty acid oxidation; and (3) decreased formation and release of lipoproteins. However, what underlies this deranged metabolism is not clear. Years ago, malnutrition (so characteristic of chronic alcoholism) was thought to play a role. Then malnutrition as a factor was discounted as it became evident that ethanol itself or one of its metabolites (e.g., acetaldehyde) is a hepatotoxin, as is discussed more fully on page 491.[89] Currently, malnutrition has again been raised as a possible cofactor in ethanol-induced injury. Clinical signs of ALD have been shown to abate with vitamin-protein supplements despite continued alcohol consumption.[90]

At the outset, lipid accumulates in a microvesicular form within the cytoplasm of the liver cells, predominantly in the perivenular (centrilobular) zone. With further accumulation the small vacuoles coalesce, creating large clear **macro-**

vesicular spaces that virtually transform the cell into a lipocyte with a compressed, peripherally displaced nucleus. Entire liver lobules may now be affected (Fig. 19–25). Concomitant retention of proteins (and water) adds to the cellular enlargement.[91] The liver may be enlarged to 4 to 6 kg with a soft, yellow, greasy cut surface. The capsule remains smooth and glistening. Rupture and coalescence of adjacent expanded cells may produce so-called fatty cysts. Uncommonly, **lipogranulomas** appear, marked by focal aggregates of lymphocytes, macrophages, and sometimes multinucleated giant cells. At the ultrastructural level, mitochondria are swollen and distorted and sometimes reveal disrupted membranes along with proliferation of the SER.[92] Such alterations underscore the toxicity of ethanol.

In a minority of cases, perivenular fibrosis appears and may be accompanied by perisinusoidal fibrosis.[93] At first very delicate and subtle, the perivenular fibrosis eventually rims and may even narrow the central veins. Many experts believe that the appearance of the delicate fibrosis augurs

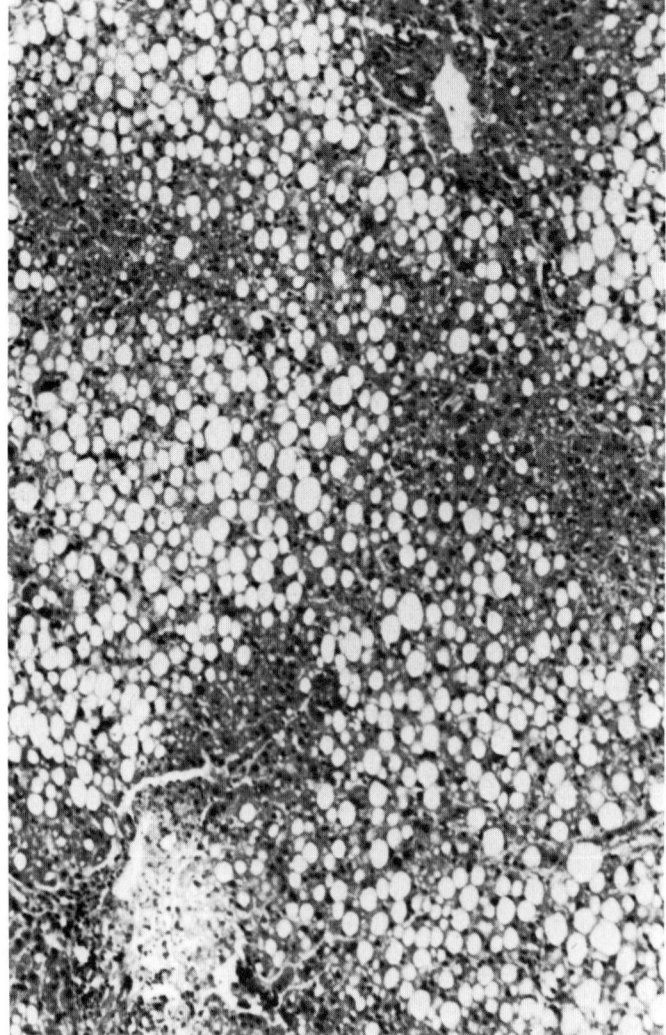

Figure 19–25. Alcoholic hepatic steatosis. Virtually all the hepatocytes contain large lipid vacuoles.

the eventual development of alcoholic cirrhosis unless complete abstinence is observed.[93] Occasionally, cholestasis is present in the fatty liver and is accompanied by focal liver cell necrosis; such changes are particularly prominent in impending hepatic failure.

Hepatic steatosis may develop without clinical or biochemical evidence of liver disease. On the other hand, when the involvement is severe it may be associated with malaise, anorexia, nausea, abdominal discomfort, tender hepatomegaly, sometimes jaundice and elevated aminotransferase levels, or hepatic failure or even sudden death (probably caused by alcohol-related cardiac arrhythmias).[94]

The relationship of simple fatty liver to alcoholic hepatitis and alcoholic cirrhosis continues to be controversial. On the one hand, it should be emphasized that *in the absence of perivenular and pericellular fibrosis, the fat can be completely cleared from the liver, restoring normal structure and function,* if further ingestion of alcohol is discontinued and an adequate diet maintained. On the other hand, follow-up studies of patients with steatosis having the fibrotic changes described indicate that with continued alcohol consumption a large majority will develop progressive fibrosis, sometimes culminating in overt cirrhosis. There is evidence that nonalcoholic fatty livers, such as may develop in diabetic or overweight persons, or following jejunoileal bypass (for the treatment of obesity), or because of drug ingestion (estrogens, amiodarone), may rarely develop a so-called fatty liver hepatitis or cirrhosis.[87] We must conclude, therefore, that *fatty change by and of itself is a benign condition, but that under some circumstances, at present poorly understood, it may constitute a precursor to cirrhosis of the liver even in the nonalcoholic.* Perhaps severity of the fatty change or its duration or individual susceptibility determines the outcome.

Alcoholic Hepatitis

This form of ALD (alcoholic liver disease) is characterized mainly by acute liver cell necrosis. It tends to appear relatively acutely, usually following a bout of heavy drinking superimposed on steatosis or already-developed cirrhosis. With avoidance of alcohol and establishment of adequate nutrition, it may subside within weeks to months only to recur with further alcohol abuse. In some patients, despite abstinence, the hepatitis persists and progresses to cirrhosis. Whatever the circumstances, it represents the relatively sudden loss of hepatic reserve, and may precipitate hepatic failure or sometimes the hepatorenal syndrome (p. 918). When it appears in a fatty liver, it almost always (some would say always) is followed within a few years by cirrhosis. It is frequently superimposed on fatty change, but the relationship of the two is still mysterious and best discussed after its morphology and pathogenesis.

MORPHOLOGY. The main features of alcoholic hepatitis are:—**Liver cell necrosis**—Single or scattered foci of cells marked by clusters of neutrophils undergo lytic or coagulative necrosis mainly in the perivenular region of the lobule (Fig. 19–26). The overall extent of the necrosis is variable. By electron microscopy, hepatotoxic changes are seen in the forms of swollen, giant mitochondria and hyperplasia of the SER.

—**Mallory bodies**—Scattered hepatocytes have eosinophilic cytoplasmic inclusions that take the form of "candle drippings" or haphazard coalescent perinuclear skeins (Fig. 19–27). Usually they are found in ballooned degenerating hepatocytes. These inclusions are sometimes called **alcoholic hyalin,** but this designation is misleading because they are also seen in primary biliary cirrhosis, Wilson's disease, Indian childhood cirrhosis, chronic cholestatic syndromes, focal nodular hyperplasia, and hepatocellular carcinoma. Although they are present in the great majority of cases of alcoholic hepatitis, rarely there are none. Composed of aggregates of intermediate filaments of prekeratin (cytokeratin) that permit the use of immunoperoxidase methods for their visualization, they also possess non-prekeratin antigens of uncertain nature and origin.[95,96]

—**Inflammatory cell infiltrate**—Mostly neutrophils with scattered mononuclear leukocytes are found within and about degenerating liver cells, particularly those having Mallory bodies. The greater the liver cell necrosis, the more abundant the neutrophils. The inflammatory infiltrate may permeate the lobule in some cases, and occasionally the portal tracts, with spillover into the adjacent parenchyma.

—**Fibrosis**—In the great majority of instances, alcoholic hepatitis is accompanied by pericellular and perivenular fibrosis. With persistent or repeated bouts of alcoholic hepatitis, fibrous spurs projecting into the hepatic parenchyma may appear (lending credence to the belief that alcoholic hepatitis is a forerunner of cirrhosis). To be noted, the combination of portal and periportal inflammation and fibrosis creates a remarkable resemblance to chronic, active viral hepatitis.

PATHOGENESIS. The pathogenesis of Mallory bodies and of the hepatocyte necrosis is uncertain, and so theories abound. Liver cells normally produce prekeratin (cytokeratin). A favored concept invokes depolymerization of tubulin by the toxic action of alcohol or one of its metabolites (?acetaldehyde). Disorganization of the cytoskeleton might then lead to aggregation or possibly decreased catabolism of prekeratin filaments (Fig. 19–28).[97] However, other mechanisms must also be involved because identical structures may appear in the other conditions mentioned not associated with alcohol toxicity. There is not even a single favored theory to explain the liver cell necrosis.[98] Some of the current proposals are:

1. Ethanol or its major metabolite, acetaldehyde, induces damage by covalent binding to hepatocyte proteins as well as by initiating free radical formation and lipid peroxidation of cell membranes.[99]

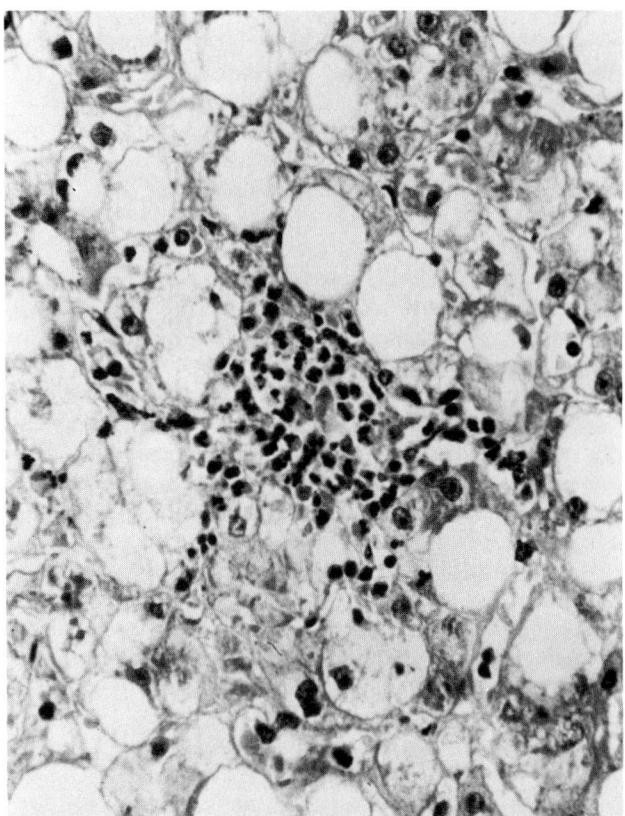

Figure 19–26. Alcoholic hepatitis. The central cluster of neutrophils marks the site of a necrotic hepatocyte.

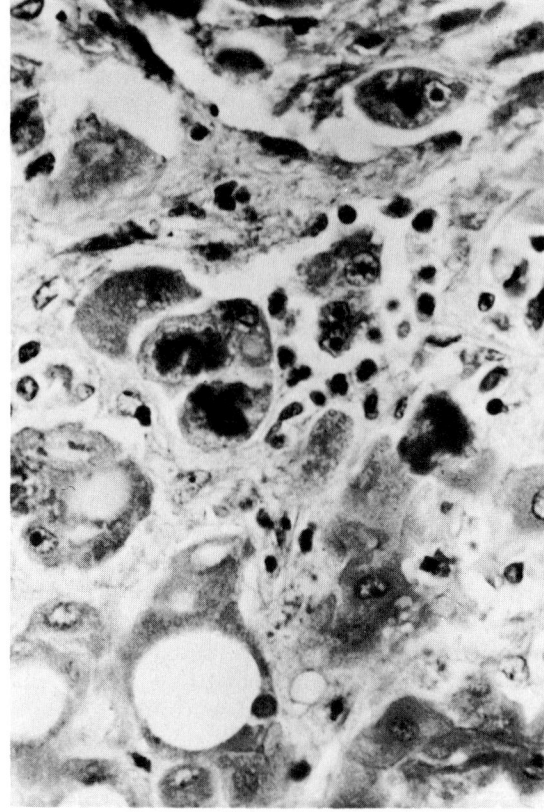

Figure 19–27. Alcoholic hepatitis. Numerous dark Mallory bodies are seen within both vital and disintegrating hepatocytes.

2. The increased metabolism of hepatocytes imposed by the blood levels of ethanol produces a greater requirement for oxygen delivery to the liver, and with the perisinusoidal fibrosis creating a barrier, leads to hypoxic damage.

3. Ethanol may modify membrane permeability, exposing liver cells to toxins otherwise well tolerated.

4. The damage may be mediated by antibodies and sensitized T cells directed against liver cells or against Mallory body antigens.

5. Concomitant malnutrition may increase the vulnerability of liver cells to a variety of hepatotoxins.[90]

Still other notions could be cited, but morphologic changes indistinguishable from alcoholic hepatitis may be encountered in a variety of nonalcoholic circumstances, including jejunoileal bypass, diabetes mellitus, and morbid obesity and in adverse reactions to a variety of drugs, including glucocorticoids and amiodarone, and so it must be admitted that the basis for the liver cell necrosis is still unclear.

The role of alcoholic hepatitis in the production of cirrhosis is a favored subject for disagreement among hepatologists. On the one hand is the view that repeated bouts of alcoholic hepatitis excite inflammatory fibrosing reactions that ultimately lead to cirrhosis. On the other hand, Popper and Lieber reported that some baboons, after chronic exposure to alcohol, developed alcoholic cirrhosis without apparent episodes of hepatitis.[100] Moreover, alcoholic hepatitis is quite uncommon in Japanese who develop cirrhosis, suggesting that it is not an integral part of the progressive disease. So at present, although the role of hepatitis is still being debated, no one can doubt that continuation of alcohol abuse in the face of hepatitis carries with it about a 30 to 35% risk of the development of cirrhosis, particularly in women (for obscure reasons).[101]

CLINICAL COURSE. Alcoholic hepatitis may be asymptomatic or may produce fulminant hepatic failure. Between these two extremes is a range of severity of malaise, anorexia, weight loss, upper abdominal discomfort, tender hepatomegaly, and often jaundice with elevated aminotransferase levels. These same symptoms, you recall, may also be produced by alcoholic steatosis. More distinctive of hepatitis are fever and a neutrophil leukocytosis. An acute cholestatic syndrome may appear, similar to large bile-duct obstruction; these are the patients who are apt to develop liver failure, sometimes leading to death in hepatic coma. The outlook is as unpredictable as the drinking habits of the individual. Each bout of hepatitis incurs about a 10 to 20% risk of death. If the patient survives repeated bouts, cirrhosis is likely to appear in about one third within a few years. With proper nutrition and total cessation of alcohol consumption, however, the alcoholic hepatitis may slowly clear.

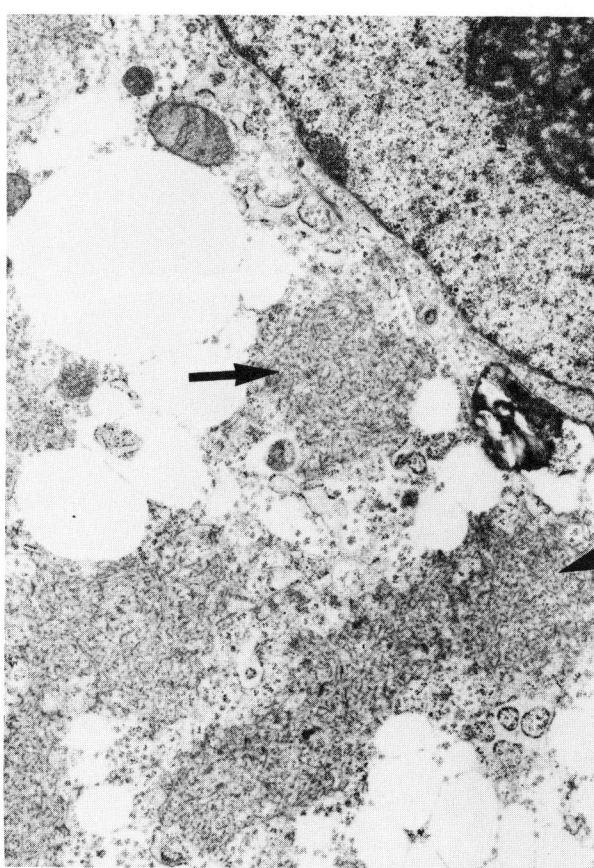

Figure 19–28. Electron microscopic detail of a liver cell, revealing closely packed filaments of alcoholic hyalin (*arrows*) as well as large, cleared lipid vacuoles. (Courtesy of Dr. Marcel Seiler, Pathology Department, West Roxbury VA Hospital, Harvard Medical School, Boston.)

Alcoholic Cirrhosis

Even though alcohol is the most common cause of cirrhosis in the Western world and is responsible there for 60 to 70% of all cases of cirrhosis, it may be comforting, albeit enigmatic, to members of the "cocktail circuit" that only about 10 to 15% of "devotees of the still" ever get cirrhosis. Numerous attempts have been made to define a "safe" upper limit of daily alcohol consumption, with, as might be expected, markedly varying results. Although all such generalizations must of necessity often be wrong, it is widely proposed that a daily alcohol intake in excess of 60 to 80 gm for men and 20 gm for women (male sexists must have set such a low limit) for ten or more years incurs a significant risk of cirrhosis.[102] In real-life terms, 8 to 10 ounces of "neat" liquor a day will likely turn the trick. Not surprisingly, the incidence of this form of ALD more or less parallels the average per capita consumption of alcohol.

PATHOGENESIS. The basis for the liver cell necrosis that precedes the fibrosis, i.e., the nature of the specific toxic agent, still is uncertain as has been amply emphasized. Two additional issues in the pathogenesis of alcoholic cirrhosis are (1) the cells that produce the collagenous fibrous septa that characterize the cirrhotic liver, and (2) the mechanisms that activate them. Once again, uncertainty prevails, but the fibrosis involves mainly an increase in collagen types I and III, which are normal elements of the framework of the liver. Currently favored as the source of this collagen are myofibroblasts normally present in blood vessel and sinusoidal walls.[103] It is proposed that ethanol in some way stimulates their synthesis of collagen. Fibroblasts, ubiquitously present in the structural framework of the liver, may also participate as well as ethanol-induced depression of collagen turnover.

The proposed signals that "turn on" increased synthesis of collagen are too elusive to merit more than passing mention, but two schools of thought exist. One holds that the fibrosis is the natural response to the cell death and that inflammation occurs with repeated bouts of alcoholic hepatitis. The "nonhepatitis school" raises one of the following possibilities: (1) direct stimulation of collagen-forming cells by ethanol or one of its metabolites, (2) alcohol-induced liver cell injury that evokes immunologic reactions leading to activation of macrophages or T cells that elaborate growth factors, or (3) ethanol-induced increased activation of synthetic enzymes, e.g., prolyl hydroxylase. In the last analysis, the pathways leading to the scarring of alcoholic cirrhosis remain unknown, but some concept of the interrelationships among alcohol-induced steatosis, hepatitis, and cirrhosis is offered in Figure 19–29.

Alcoholic cirrhosis begins as a large, fatty, micronodular liver (usually weighing over 2 kg) that is transformed, over the span of years, into a shrunken, nonfatty, macronodular cirrhotic liver (sometimes less than 1 kg in weight) (Fig. 19–30). **There is generally an inverse relationship between the amount of fat and the amount of fibrous scarring.** Early in the course of the cirrhogenic process, the fibrous septa are delicate and extend from central vein to portal regions as well as from portal tract to portal tract. The parenchyma within the nodules is extensively fatty and disorganized as regeneration transforms the normal liver cords into irregular aggregates. Because of their fat content, the nodules and the liver are tawny-yellow, from which the term "cirrhosis" derives. The changes of alcoholic hepatitis (in particular, liver cell necrosis and Mallory bodies) and bile stasis may or may not be present.

As the scarring increases with time, the nodularity becomes more prominent, and scattered nodules enlarge because of regenerative activity, creating a so-called hob-nail appearance on the surface. The amount of fat is reduced. Now the fibrous septa dissect and surround lobules and often have a modest infiltrate of lymphocytes with some reactive bile duct proliferation. The liver shrinks progressively in size, becomes more fibrotic, loses fat, and is converted into a macronodular pattern as parenchymal islands are engulfed by ever wider bands of fibrous tissue (Fig. 19–31). Bile stasis often develops and sometimes a modest increase in cytoplasmic hemosiderin due to enhanced

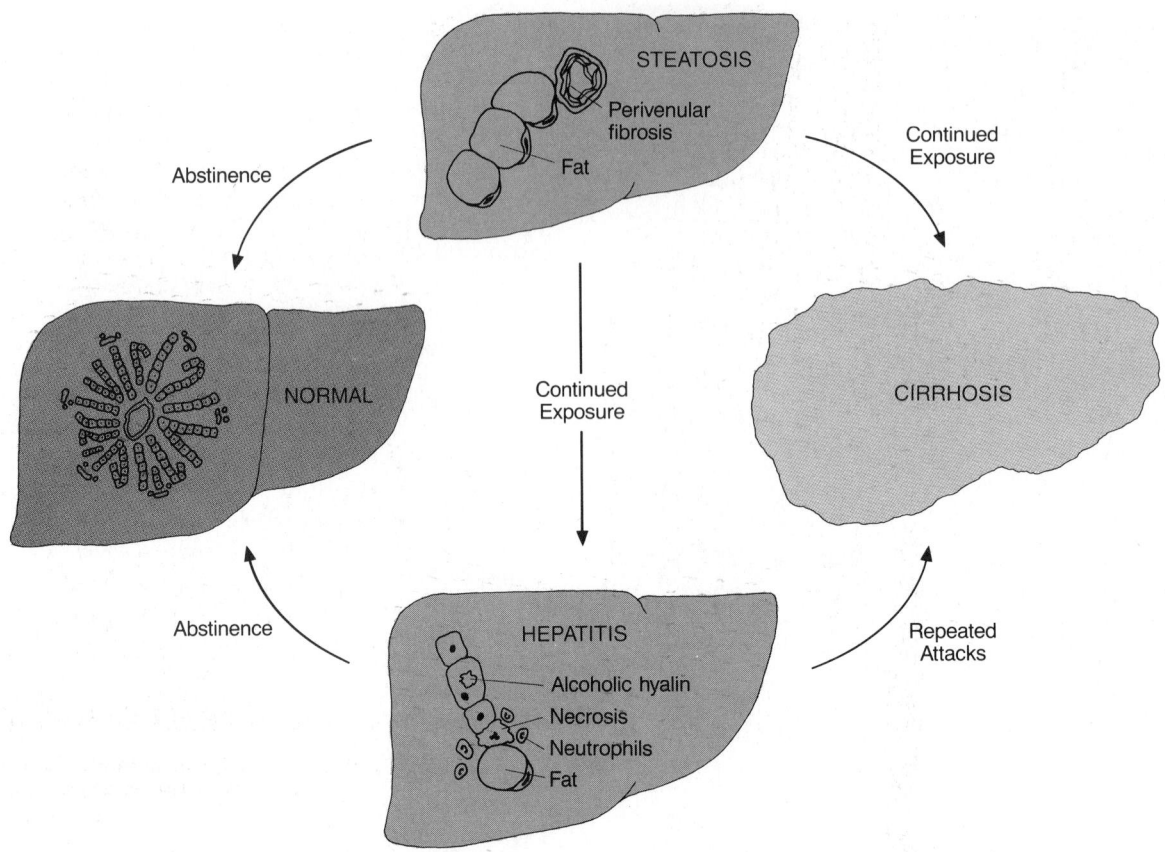

Figure 19–29. The interrelationships among alcoholic steatosis, hepatitis, and cirrhosis.

iron absorption in the alcoholic. Mallory bodies are only rarely evident in this late stage, and there would be no clue to the etiology of the cirrhosis. Thus, **end-stage alcoholic cirrhosis comes to resemble, both macroscopically and microscopically, postnecrotic cirrhosis** (to be described).

CLINICAL COURSE. The general manifestations of all forms of cirrhosis were presented on page 941. Like the others, alcoholic cirrhosis may remain entirely submerged (about 10%) and be discovered only at autopsy. Men usually in their fifth and sixth decades of life are more frequently affected than women, but changing mores have led to an increasing frequency of this condition in younger males and in females. In the typical case, after such symptoms as malaise, weakness, weight loss, and loss of appetite appear, the patient develops jaundice, ascites, and peripheral edema, the latter due to impaired synthesis of albumin. The slow downhill course may be hastened by a bout of hepatic decompensation triggered by intercurrent stress, infection, a gastrointestinal bleed, or a wave of alcoholic hepatitis.

The laboratory findings early in the course may be entirely unremarkable. However, as the disease progresses and worsens there are elevated serum aminotransferase levels, hyperbilirubinemia, variable elevation of serum alkaline phosphatase, and possibly anemia and hypoproteinemia with reversal of the albumin/globulin ratio. In some instances, liver biopsy may be indicated because experience teaches that in about 10 to 20% of cases of presumed alcoholic cirrhosis, another disease is found on biopsy.

Unless the patient avoids alcohol and maintains a nutritious diet, the usual course over a period of years is progressively downhill, with deteriorating hepatic

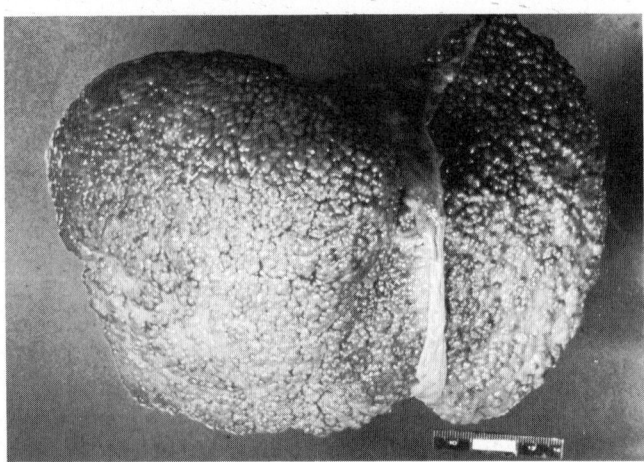

Figure 19–30. Alcoholic cirrhosis, showing the characteristic micronodular pattern.

previous viral infection (hence the synonym posthepatitic cirrhosis). In about 20 to 25% of cases it evolves from chronic active hepatitis B infection. How many additional cases are related to non-A, non-B or to delta chronic active hepatitis is not known. In a small number of instances there is a well-documented history of acute liver damage caused by some hepatotoxin such as phosphorus, carbon tetrachloride, mushroom poisoning, or a drug such as acetaminophen, oxyphenisatin, or alpha-methyldopa. Undoubtedly, some cases represent end-stage alcoholic cirrhosis, readily misinterpreted as macronodular postnecrotic cirrhosis in the absence of a history of chronic alcoholism. After all these possibilities have been excluded, there remains a large residual of uncertain origin. *A single attack of massive hepatic necrosis only infrequently gives rise to postnecrotic cirrhosis,*[104] because either it is fatal or regeneration of the liver cells permits survival with little or no residual scarring. However, submassive necrosis, whether caused by viruses or other hepatotoxins, may produce diffuse scarring, meriting the designation "postnecrotic cirrhosis."

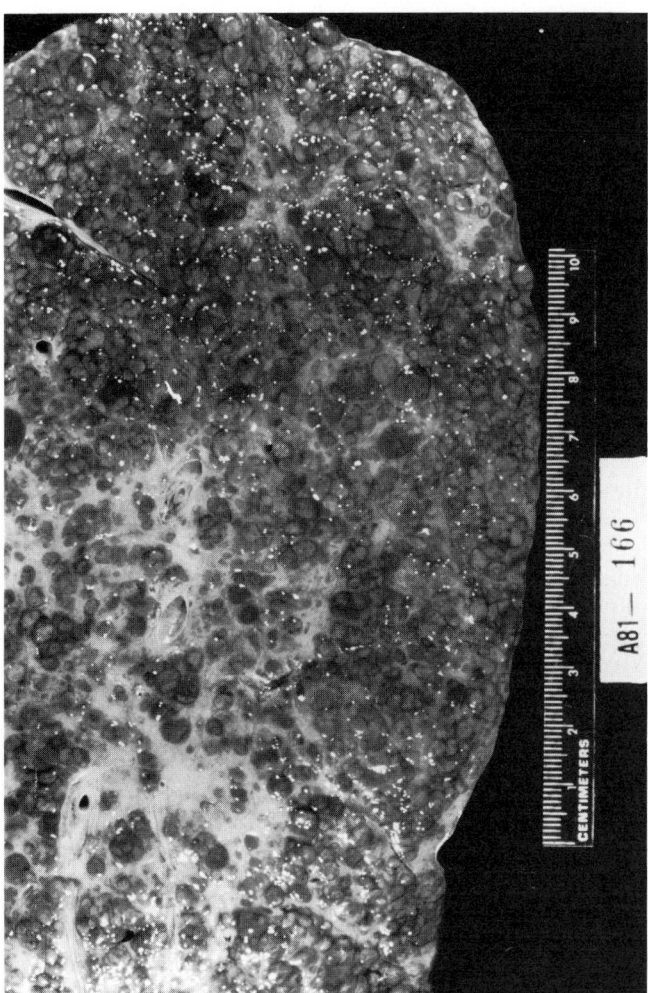

Figure 19–31. Advanced alcoholic cirrhosis with large areas of scarring and variability in size of the nodules.

function and the development of portal hypertension with its sequelae, e.g., ascites, gastroesophageal varices, and hemorrhoids. The five-year survival of abstainers is almost 90% in those free of jaundice, ascites, and hematemesis but drops to 50 to 60% in those who revert to former ways. The immediate causes of death are (1) hepatic coma; (2) a massive gastrointestinal hemorrhage from esophageal varices or, less often, peptic ulceration or gastroesophageal laceration; (3) an intercurrent infection (to which these patients are predisposed); or (4) hepatorenal syndrome following a wave of alcoholic hepatitis. In about 3 to 6% of the cases, death is related to the development of a hepatocellular carcinoma, a frequency well below that seen with postnecrotic cirrhosis.

POSTNECROTIC CIRRHOSIS

This is a macronodular pattern of cirrhosis of varied and sometimes unknown origin. It is characterized by large irregular nodules separated by variable but mostly broad scars. The most common known cause is

MORPHOLOGY. Typically, some time after the acute event, the liver is small, weighing less than 1 kg with nodules of varying size some several centimeters in diameter and broad bands or areas of depressed scarring. Microscopically, the fibrous scars are typically infiltrated with lymphocytes and macrophages and, in places where entire lobules have been destroyed, they may contain distorted portal triads along with irregular strands and nests of bile duct epithelium resulting from replication of bile ducts and cholangioles. Characteristically the portal triads are closely approximated where the hepatocytes of entire lobules have been destroyed with collapse of the reticular framework. In end-stage disease, active liver cell necrosis is inconspicuous. Fat may or may not be present within surviving hepatocytes, but it is rarely prominent and bile stasis is equally variable. **Ultimately, the diagnosis rests on excluding other bases for a macronodular cirrhosis (e.g., end-stage alcoholic disease), the coarseness of the scars, and the size and irregularity of the parenchymal nodules** (Fig. 19–32).

The clinical course is as varied as the origins of this form of cirrhosis. In many cases the cirrhosis is asymptomatic and is discovered only at laparotomy or autopsy, or by the chance finding of abnormal liver function tests. Sometimes splenomegaly or other manifestations of portal hypertension, such as a massive gastrointestinal bleed or ascites, call attention to the hepatic involvement, or such stigmata of cirrhosis as spider angiomas, gynecomastia, or amenorrhea constitute the presenting features of the disease. Also, there may be prominent signs and symptoms suggestive of progressive chronic active hepatitis, described earlier (p. 935). In such instances the disease may pursue a relentless course to death within a year or more, but some patients have a more indolent, prolonged

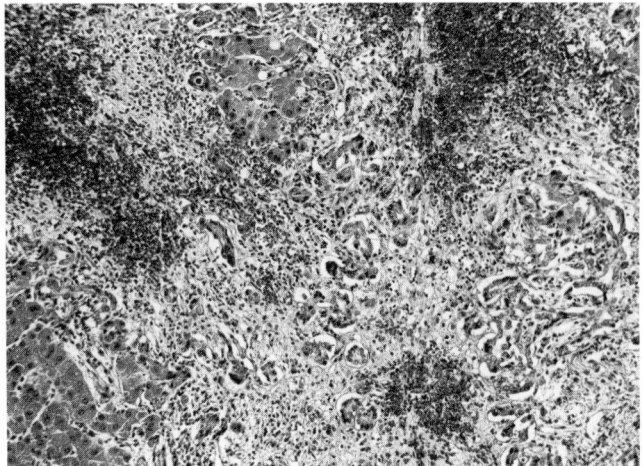

Figure 19–32. Postnecrotic scarring. An island of preserved parenchyma is visible at lower left. Remainder of field represents a broad area of scarring.

course. The ultimate cause of death is usually hepatic failure, sometimes with encephalopathy, or massive hemorrhage from a ruptured gastroesophageal varix. This form of cirrhosis, particularly when related to hepatitis B virus infection early in life, often leads to hepatocellular carcinoma (15 to 30% of cases). If, however, the hepatitis B infection was acquired later in adult life, the risk of hepatic cancer is much lower (p. 959). In all analyses, macronodular cirrhosis is more frequently complicated by hepatocellular carcinoma than any other form of cirrhosis.[105]

PIGMENT CIRRHOSIS— HEMOCHROMATOSIS

Hemochromatosis is an iron overload disorder that in years past could not be diagnosed until the progressive accumulation of iron, mainly in the form of ferritin and hemosiderin, caused organ injury, particularly to the liver and pancreas. The disease was then diagnosed on the basis of the classic triad: (1) a micronodular pigment cirrhosis in all cases, (2) diabetes mellitus in about 75 to 80% of cases, and (3) skin pigmentation in about 75 to 85% of cases. The last two features accounted for the older designation *"bronze diabetes."* However, the disease can now be discovered much earlier by biochemical studies of the blood (p. 952) before cirrhosis and other organ injuries have developed.[106]

You recall from the earlier discussion (p. 686) that the total body iron pool ranges from 2 to 6 gm in adults. In hemochromatosis, the accumulation may reach 50 to 60 gm, enough to set off the metal detector alarm at airports! The most common and the most severe overload is found in a genetic disorder in which the basis for the excess iron accumulation is obscure; it is called *idiopathic (primary, genetic) hemochromatosis.* The other forms, having more or less obvious sources of the excess iron, are called *secondary he-*

mochromatosis. They generally have less marked iron overload and therefore less evidence of functional or morphologic damage to sites of deposition (Table 19–7).

Most of the following comments relate to idiopathic hemochromatosis.

About 70% of individuals with this condition are HLA-A3, but only 28% of the general population are. Closely linked to HLA-A3 and therefore also present in many patients with the idiopathic form of the disease is B7, B14, or Bw35.[107,108] A "susceptibility gene" is believed to be located on chromosome 6 in close linkage with the HLA locus. Family studies suggest autosomal recessive inheritance of the susceptibility gene. Individuals homozygous for this mutant gene absorb a large excess of iron and develop hemochromatosis; heterozygotes have a less pronounced metabolic aberration and are spared the disease but often have biochemical evidence of mild iron overload (discussed later). There is a strong male predominance in a ratio of 5 to 7:1, attributed to the protection against iron overload afforded by menstrual losses and the drains of pregnancy. However, iron balance studies suggest that intestinal absorption in women far exceeds these losses, and so the female genotype may in some way suppress the expressivity of the gene.

PATHOGENESIS. As you know, the total body content of iron is normally a closely guarded constant maintained by balancing gastrointestinal intake and losses. As pointed out on page 459, the average diet in the United States and other Western countries contains much more iron than should be absorbed because mechanisms of excretion are limited to about 1 mg a day. Iron balance therefore requires rigorous control of absorption, but regrettably the mechanisms that effect this control are still obscure. The precise basis for the iron overload in primary hemochromatosis is unknown, hence the designation "idiopathic." Numerous proposals have been made, among which the following are favored.[109]

1. The defect resides at the level of the mucosal cells in the duodenum and jejunum, where iron is absorbed from the diet. It may involve specific membrane re-

Table 19–7. Causes of Hemochromatosis*

Idiopathic (primary, hereditary) hemochromatosis
Secondary hemochromatosis
    Secondary to anemia and ineffective erythropoiesis
        Thalassemia, major
        Sideroblastic anemia
    Secondary to liver disease
        Alcoholic cirrhosis
        Following portacaval anastomosis
    Secondary to high iron intake
        Prolonged ingestion of medicinal iron
        Prolonged consumption of iron-laden wine, Kaffir beer, etc.
        Multiple transfusions

* Based on Powell, L.W., et al.: Hemochromatosis: 1980 update. Gastroenterology 78:374, 1980.

ceptors, iron-ligand complexes, or intracellular transport proteins (transferrin), all of which are involved in the movement of iron across enterocytes into the plasma.[110]

2. There may be a genetic defect in the immediate postabsorptive excretion of iron, leading to excess retention.[111]

3. The defect may reside in the loss of regulatory signals delivered to the intestinal mucosa by mononuclear phagocytes (RE cells) controlling absorption. Conceivably, there is some genetic inability of the phagocytes to take up iron, because despite overloading of parenchymal cells they are spared.

The excess iron in idiopathic hemochromatosis accumulates preferentially in the cytoplasm of parenchymal cells, such as those in the liver, pancreas, and endocrine glands, disturbing the structure and function of the involved organs. In contrast, when iron is liberated from red cells, as in hemolytic anemias and following multiple transfusions, it is deposited largely in the mononuclear phagocyte system. This pattern of accumulation, you recall, is referred to as *systemic hemosiderosis*; it is not associated with organ dysfunction or injury. However, in some instances, massive systemic hemosiderosis appears to lead to "spillover" of iron into parenchymal cells, producing a hybrid condition that some would call a form of secondary hemochromatosis.

The pathogenesis of secondary hemochromatosis is less obscure than that of the idiopathic form of the disease. In the anemias cited in Table 19–7, the excess iron results not only from transfusions but also from the increased absorption of iron that accompanies ineffective erythropoiesis. More vexed is the question of whether prolonged consumption of iron can produce iron overload. For example, since alcohol enhances iron absorption, does prolonged consumption of considerable amounts of iron with alcohol, e.g., in wine, lead to iron overload? This phenomenon is well exemplified by "Bantu siderosis" produced by the consumption of large amounts of traditional beer home-brewed in steel drums.[112] Analogously, a modest increase in hemosiderin is often seen in the liver cells in alcoholic cirrhosis (p. 947), but whether this iron accumulation is sufficient to cause secondary hemochromatosis is still disputed. The consensus is that when the iron overload in alcoholics causes organ injury, the individual probably has the "susceptibility gene."

Granted the cytoplasmic overload of iron in parenchymal cells, how does it cause injury? There are only theories. One hypothesis is that iron in the cells leads to the formation of free radicals such as superoxide and hydroxyl radical, which then cause lipid peroxidation and membrane damage to cells and subcellular components. Another proposition invokes the deposition of excess iron in lysosomes increasing their fragility, with lysosomal disruption and cell injury.[113] Whatever the action of iron, it is reversible if the cell is not fatally injured because, as pointed out later,

removal of excess iron from the body, as by venesection, mobilizes the hemosiderin and ferritin from parenchymal cells, followed by improved function.

As pointed out, the definition of hemochromatosis has been broadened to include marked iron overload as judged by the serum iron, transferrin saturation, and ferritin levels irrespective of whether there is evidence of organ injury (as for example cirrhosis). The morphologic common denominator therefore becomes the increased amounts of ferritin and hemosiderin in the parenchymal cells of many organs and tissues throughout the body. Organ injury is a time-quantity function of the iron accumulation. Thus, the development of pigment cirrhosis and other parenchymal damage is a relatively late consequence of a large load of excess iron. In this context, the "early" changes will not be described, only the anatomic changes of fully evolved "advanced" hemochromatosis.

The principal features of classic idiopathic hemochromatosis are:

1. Excessive deposits of ferritin (p. 686) and hemosiderin in the liver, pancreas, myocardium, joint linings, endocrine glands, and skin, in decreasing order of severity.

2. Micronodular pigment cirrhosis of the liver (Fig. 19–33).

3. Pigmentation, atrophy, and fibrosis of the pancreas, mainly the pancreatic islets.

4. Hemosiderin deposition in many other sites, e.g., muscle

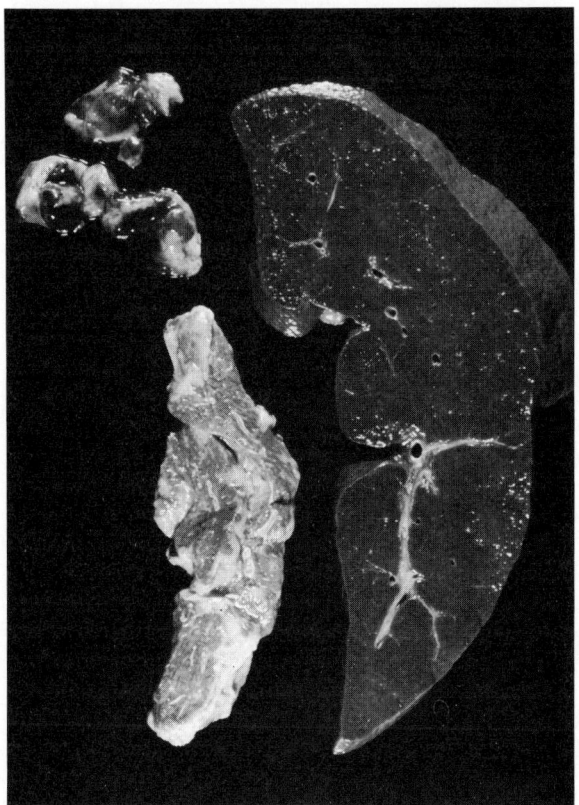

Figure 19–33. Hemochromatosis. Darkly pigmented micronodular liver is seen on right, slightly pigmented transected pancreas at lower left, and pigmented lymph nodes at upper left.

and endocrine glands, generally unaccompanied by fibrosis.

Liver biopsies indicate that the iron accumulation first becomes evident as increased amounts of ferritin and then golden-yellow granules of hemosiderin in the cytoplasm of all hepatocytes, with some predilection for the periportal areas. Bile duct epithelium and Kupffer cell pigmentation is less marked. At this early stage, the liver is characteristically slightly larger than normal, dense, and chocolate brown. As the pigmentation becomes heavier, there is slowly evolving liver damage and development of fibrous septa in a pattern resembling that in alcoholic cirrhosis, leading ultimately to a micronodular cirrhosis. Now there may be some reduction in liver size, but rarely is it marked. The Prussian blue reaction can be used on both gross tissue slices and sections to highlight the hemosiderin (Fig. 19–34). Fat is usually absent, as is overt cell necrosis. Biochemical determination of the hepatic iron concentration (particularly valuable as a diagnostic aid in liver biopsies) will almost always reveal over 400 μg of iron/100 mg of wet liver (normal less than 30 μg). In years past, before the institution of iron-draining therapy, primary carcinoma of the liver appeared in 15 to 20% of cases.

The **pancreas** is intensely pigmented, has a diffuse interstitial fibrosis, and may be somewhat decreased in size because of atrophy and loss of parenchymal cells. Hemosiderin is found in both the acinar and the islet cells, and

sometimes in the interstitial fibrous stroma. There is some correlation between the intensity of the iron deposits in the pancreatic islets and the occurrence and severity of the diabetes.

The **heart** is often enlarged and has hemosiderin granules within the myocardial fibers. The pigmentation may induce a striking brown coloration to the myocardium. A delicate interstitial fibrosis may or may not be present.

The **endocrine glands** (thyroid, parathyroid, pituitary, and, in particular, adrenals) also reveal a brownish coloration related to the accumulation of hemosiderin in the parenchymal cells.

The **skin** has increased pigmentation in 80 to 90% of patients. This is mainly due to increased amounts of melanin (seen with various forms of cirrhosis), which imparts a golden-brown color. There is also a distinctive, metallic, slate-gray pigmentation related to accumulation of hemosiderin in dermal macrophages and fibroblasts.

The **joint synovial linings** have hemosiderin pigmentation in 30 to 50% of cases. An acute synovitis may follow. There is also excessive deposition of calcium pyrophosphate, which damages the articular cartilage and sometimes produces disabling polyarthritis, referred to as pseudogout.

The **testes** may be small and atrophic but are not usually significantly pigmented. It is thought that the atrophy is secondary to some derangement in the hypothalamic-pituitary axis.

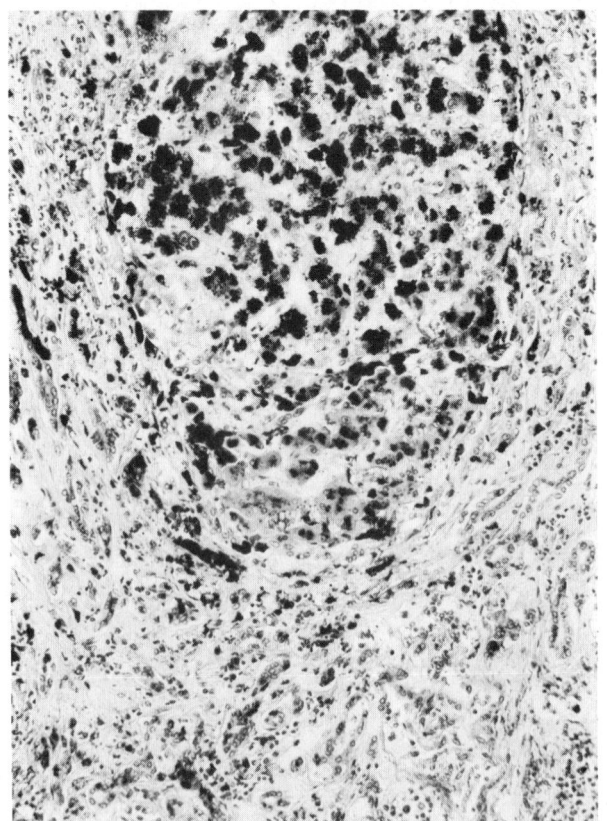

Figure 19–34. Pigment cirrhosis with well-developed scarring. The hemosiderin principally within hepatocytes appears black in Prussian blue reaction.

CLINICAL COURSE. Every disease should be diagnosed early in its course, but with hemochromatosis, early diagnosis provides the rare opportunity of preventing the damaging effects of the iron overload, e.g., cirrhosis. Unfortunately, at this early stage the diagnosis is most difficult and usually depends on screening of family members of patients for biochemical evidence of iron overload. In the great majority of homozygotes, the serum iron is above 250 μg/dl (normal 50 to 150), serum ferritin is above 500 ng/ml (normal below 150), and transferrin saturation approaches 100% (normal 25 to 50%). Heterozygotes may be spared the organ injury but nevertheless have laboratory values intermediate between normal levels and those of homozygotes.

The principal manifestations of developed idiopathic hemochromatosis include hepatomegaly, abdominal pain, skin pigmentation, diabetes mellitus or deranged glucose metabolism, cardiac dysfunction (arrhythmias, cardiomyopathy), and atypical arthritis. In some patients, the presenting complaint is hypogonadism, e.g., amenorrhea in the female, and loss of libido and impotence in the male. As mentioned, the classic triad of pigment cirrhosis with hepatomegaly, skin pigmentation, and diabetes mellitus may be absent. Moreover, the so-called bronze pigmentation is most prominent in the sun-exposed areas and resembles a suntan.

Although the diagnosis can be suspected from the signs and symptoms, laboratory evidence of iron overload is requisite. Should these values be equivocal, liver biopsy may be necessary with the demonstration of excessive stainable iron and an iron concentration above 400 μg/100 mg wet weight. An additional, less definitive finding is urinary excretion of significant amounts of iron following the administration of the iron chelator desferrioxamine.

The natural course of the disease can be substantially altered by a variety of interventions, mainly phlebotomy and the use of iron chelators to drain off the excess iron. With this treatment, the abdominal pain and skin pigmentation clear relatively promptly. The cardiac manifestations, such as decompensation and arrhythmia, and the deranged glucose metabolism significantly improve or disappear in about half the patients.[114] However, the arthritis (p. 1360), which can be mild or destructive, the hypogonadism, and the cirrhosis are not improved despite rare reports of some reversal of the fibrosis. The five-year mortality rate is 11% for those receiving intensive iron-draining therapy, but 67% in the untreated group. The presence of cirrhosis materially worsens the outlook.[115] The major causes of death today are hepatocellular carcinoma, cardiac disease, and liver failure. Carcinoma of the liver has not been reported in hemochromatosis in the absence of cirrhosis. Even when cirrhosis is present, the frequency of this fatal neoplasm is greater in those not receiving treatment for the iron overload than in those depleted of iron. Now it should be apparent why early diagnosis and appropriate control of the patient's iron stores are critical.

BILIARY CIRRHOSIS

There are two distinctive forms of biliary cirrhosis. One, *primary biliary cirrhosis, is thought to be an autoimmune disorder focused on interlobular bile ducts and cholangioles, and so is best remembered as destructive sclerosing cholangitis and cholangiolitis. The other variant, secondary biliary cirrhosis, results from obstruction to the major extrahepatic ducts.* Both forms, however, are characterized morphologically by a micronodular cirrhosis resulting from fibrous septa that emanate from the portal tracts to eventually enclose individual lobules.

Secondary Biliary Cirrhosis

Secondary biliary cirrhosis is the simpler to characterize. It follows any of the disorders that cause prolonged extrahepatic obstructive jaundice (p. 916). The outflow obstruction produces bile stasis throughout the entire biliary tree until eventually the inspissated impacted bile damages the interlobular bile ducts and cholangioles. A secondary inflammatory reaction initiates the scarring, leading to the cirrhosis. Secondary bacterial infection (ascending cholangitis and cholangiolitis) may contribute to the damage. Sometimes an ascending infection, even in the absence of marked bile stasis, produces a so-called infectious variant of secondary biliary cirrhosis. Enteric organisms such as coliforms and enterococci are the common culprits. With this form of secondary biliary cirrhosis, there may be little or no bile stasis.

Primary Biliary Cirrhosis (PBC)

A progressive, often fatal cholestatic condition of unknown etiology, PBC is marked by chronic inflammation of the intrahepatic ducts, leading to their destruction and, in time, cirrhosis. Clinically, it must be differentiated from large duct obstruction with consequent secondary biliary cirrhosis.[116] It is largely a disease of women, with a female to male ratio of approximately 9 : 1; the average age of onset is 50 to 55 years with a range of 20 to 80 years. Some genetic influence is suggested by the occurrence of the disease in more than one family member, but no mendelian pattern has been identified. A recent report calls attention to an increased frequency of HLA-DR8 in individuals with this disorder.[117] The pathogenesis is best considered after the morphology.

Four histologic stages have been described.[118]

Stage I — florid duct lesion. There is random, florid, focal destruction of the septal and interlobular bile ducts, which are surrounded by a dense infiltrate of lymphocytes, histiocytes, plasma cells, and perhaps a few eosinophils. The lymphocytes infiltrating the bile ducts have been shown to be T-8 suppressor/cytotoxic cells, and those surrounding the ducts T-4 helper/inducer cells (features suggestive of immune-mediated damage). The inflammatory reaction is largely confined to the portal triads. Granulomas within the lymphoid infiltrates are sometimes present. Typical cholestasis begins to appear.

Stage II — ductular proliferation. The ductal involvement is now more global, with a reduction in the number of normal bile ducts and an increase in the number of bizarre-shaped ducts. The inflammatory infiltrate extends beyond the portal triads into the surrounding parenchyma with destruction of some cells in the limiting plates (highly reminiscent of chronic active hepatitis). **In the periportal regions, ductular proliferation creates tangled knots and strands of epithelium devoid of lumina** (Fig. 19–35). Granulomas are now less frequent, but cholestasis within the canaliculi and hepatocytes is more evident. Mallory bodies (p. 945) are sometimes found in damaged liver cells.

Stage III — fibrosis. The inflammatory infiltrate is less prominent and is replaced by fibrous septa that may in places interconnect portal areas to create micronodules. There is a distinct reduction in the number of bile ducts and in the frequency of granulomas, but the cholestasis is more marked.

Stage IV — cirrhosis. The fibrous septa have now fairly uniformly bridged portal areas enclosing individual lobules to thus create an overt micronodular cirrhosis. There is a scant, inflammatory lymphocytic infiltrate within the fibrous strands as well as persistent disordered aggregations of ductular epithelium. Larger bile ducts have virtually disappeared. The cholestasis impairs the excretion of copper, which sometimes can be visualized as fine cytoplasmic granules with rhodanine or rubeanic acid stains. The levels

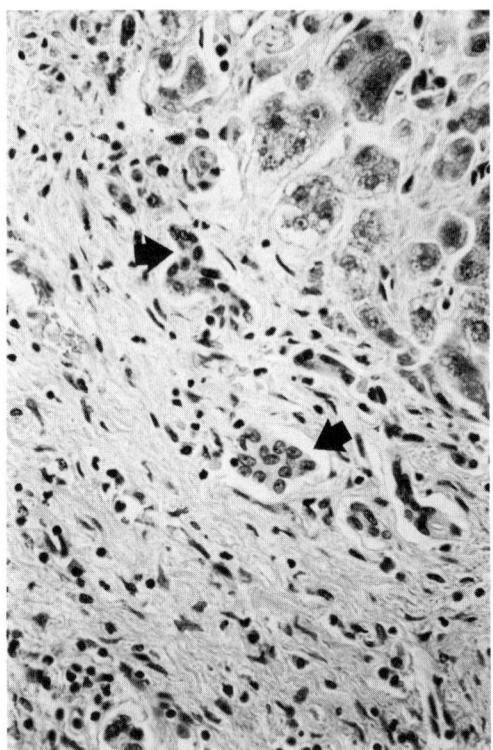

Figure 19–35. Primary biliary cirrhosis. A fibrous scar traversing liver (hepatocytes at upper right). Note tangled knots of bile duct epithelial cells *(arrows)* within scar.

of copper in the liver may approach those of Wilson's disease.

It is evident from the foregoing that, at the outset, the liver does not appear abnormal to the naked eye. As the disease progresses, bile stasis stains the liver green but the capsule is still smooth and glistening. The weight may now be normal but is often increased owing to the inflammation. Over the span of years, a fine granularity appears until eventually there is a slight decrease in liver weight and size and a well-developed, uniform micronodularity.

PATHOGENESIS. *A large number of immunologic abnormalities have been observed in patients with PBC, but direct proof that the destruction of the ductal epithelium is immune-mediated is lacking.*[119,120] The epithelial cells sometimes express increased amounts of class I histocompatibility antigens HLA-A, B, and C and also class II HLA-DR antigens, making them prime targets for immune reactions. Thus, it is proposed that PBC is an autoimmune disease. Patients with this condition have an increased incidence of scleroderma, Sjögren's syndrome, arthropathy resembling rheumatoid arthritis, and particularly some variation of the sicca syndrome in the great majority of cases, suggesting some autoimmune diathesis. The most prominent immunologic abnormalities are (1) increased levels of serum immunoglobulins, particularly IgM; (2) a variety of circulating autoantibodies, but particularly antimitochondrial antibody in 95% of

patients; (3) increased levels of circulating immune complexes; (4) a decreased number of circulating T cells (both helper and suppressor); and (5) a chronically activated complement system with abnormally rapid turnover of complement components.

Along with these abnormalities, there are the histologic inflammatory changes and granuloma formation (resembling those in graft-versus-host disease) that offer further support to the notion of immune mediation. However, to date it has not been possible to document either humoral or cellular cytotoxic attack on the ductal epithelium. Other etiologies therefore cannot be excluded, such as abnormal copper metabolism, viral infection, genetic susceptibility to an environmental agent, or a hepatic variant of sarcoidosis.

CLINICAL COURSE. PBC is basically a cholestatic disorder. It is, however, extremely insidious in onset; many patients are asymptomatic, having only a markedly elevated serum alkaline phosphatase value. The serum bilirubin level may still be normal, and the serum levels of aminotransferases normal or slightly elevated. Inevitably, over the course of many months, these laboratory values begin to rise as does the serum cholesterol level, and the disease becomes symptomatic with fatigue, jaundice, pruritus (itching of the skin), and abdominal discomfort due to either hepatosplenomegaly or concurrent cholelithiasis (about 15% of cases). Eventually, marked jaundice, hepatic decompensation, and manifestations of portal hypertension, e.g., variceal bleeding, appear.

The physical findings are extremely variable and depend on the stage of the disease when diagnosed. Whereas, at one time, virtually all patients had hepatomegaly, it is present in less than half now. Analogously, splenomegaly has become much less common. In addition to jaundice, there may be hyperpigmentation of the skin (of obscure nature), or in some cases, xanthelasma, or xanthomas related to the hyperlipoproteinemia often seen in this condition. Additional complications may appear, including steatorrhea, osteomalacia (related largely to malabsorption), and/or osteoporosis.

The outlook for the patient depends on the stage of the condition when discovered. The survival of asymptomatic patients after diagnosis does not differ from that of matched controls, but with more advanced symptomatic disease the average length of survival from the onset of symptoms is approximately 12 years. Liver biopsy is therefore often employed to confirm the diagnosis and to evaluate the stage of the hepatic disease. The presence of granulomas is a favorable finding, since these are most often present early in the course, but the presence of fibrosis or cirrhosis considerably darkens the horizon. The major cause of death is liver failure, followed in order by massive variceal hemorrhage, intercurrent infection (to which these patients are particularly susceptible), or the development of a related cancer. Hepatocellular carcinoma appears in about 3 to 4% of patients, and curiously there is an almost equal incidence of breast cancer, for obscure reasons.[121]

CIRRHOSIS ASSOCIATED WITH ALPHA-1-ANTITRYPSIN (A1AT) DEFICIENCY

A1AT deficiency is an autosomal allelic (codominant) condition marked by abnormally low serum levels of this major protease inhibitor in homozygotes. As a consequence, pulmonary disease (emphysema) or hepatic disease, or sometimes both, may develop. A1AT is a glycoprotein synthesized in mononuclear phagocytes and hepatocytes whose major function is the inhibition of proteases, including elastases, released at sites of cell injury and inflammation. A deficiency permits destructive enzymes to run amok.

A large number of protease inhibitor (pi) gene mutations (identified alphabetically) encode for a variety of abnormal enzyme proteins, resulting in a range of functional deficiencies of A1AT (p. 769).[122] The normal phenotype is pi-MM; Pi-SS homozygotes have approximately 50% of normal A1AT function, while pi-ZZ homozygotes have only 10%. A rare variant termed pi-null has no detectable functioning serum A1AT. With most mutant genes the mRNA is translated, and a protein (differing from the normal by a single amino acid substitution) is produced but *not* secreted by the liver cells or mononuclear phagocytes. Thus the abnormal A1AT accumulates within its cells of origin rather than being released into the serum.[123] *It creates round-to-oval cytoplasmic globular inclusions in hepatocytes, which in routine H and E stains are acidophilic and indistinctly demarcated from the surrounding cytoplasm.* They are strongly PAS positive and diastase resistant (Fig. 19–36). Characteristically, these inclusions are scattered throughout the cytoplasm and do not displace the nucleus, but when numerous, they may coalesce into a single, large globule pushing the nucleus to one side. By electron microscopy they lie within smooth, and sometimes rough, endoplasmic reticulum.[124] The globules are also present in diminished size and number in intermediate deficiency states. In contrast, in the null-null genotype, no A1AT is produced and so does not accumulate within the cells.

The hepatic syndromes associated with pi-ZZ homozygosity are extremely varied. They range from neonatal hepatitis to childhood cirrhosis to cirrhosis that becomes apparent only late in life, when the liver scarring is well advanced.[125]

Neonatal hepatitis is described later (p. 964), and it is sufficient to note that the histologic manifestations vary from active inflammatory disease to a form of almost "pure" cholestasis resembling biliary tract obstruction.

Childhood cirrhosis may appear with or without an antecedent history of neonatal hepatitis. It takes the form of a micronodular cirrhosis, but in a few cases, with progression

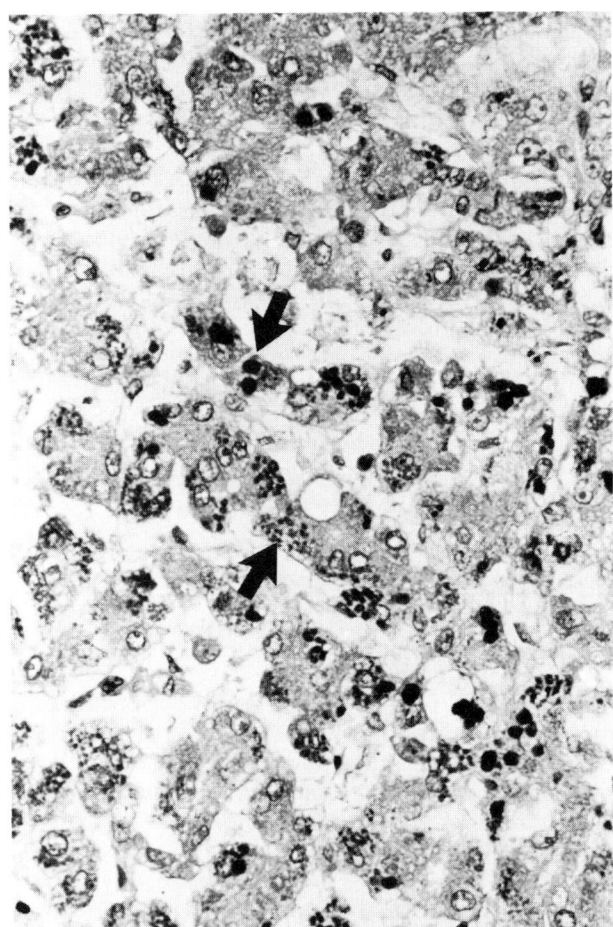

Figure 19–36. Alpha-1-antitrypsin deficiency. PAS stain of liver. The characteristic cytoplasmic granules *(arrows)* vary markedly in size. (Courtesy of Dr. R.A. DeLellis, Pathology Department, Tufts Medical School, Boston.)

of the condition a macronodular pattern emerges. The diagnostic feature is the characteristic A1AT globules within hepatocytes.

Adult cirrhosis may be micronodular, but in most cases, presumably because of advanced disease, it is macronodular. The fibrous scarring is irregular, expanding and interconnecting portal tracts, sometimes isolating individual lobules or at other times enclosing many adjacent lobules. Frequently, piecemeal necrosis reminiscent of hepatitis B can be identified in the periportal regions, where the globules are most prominent. Infrequently, fatty change and Mallory bodies are present. Rarely, hepatocarcinoma complicates the liver disease in adults.

A1AT deficiency, as pointed out earlier, may present with respiratory disease owing to the development of panlobular emphysema, or it may become apparent as liver disease any time from birth to adulthood. At birth or a few months thereafter it may be discovered because of laboratory evidence of abnormal liver function or overt hepatitis with cholestatic jaundice; later in adolescence it may take the forms of hepatitis or cirrhosis, but in other instances it remains silent until cirrhosis appears in middle to later life.[126] Attacks of hepatitis may subside with apparent complete recovery, or they may become chronic to lead progressively to cirrhosis.[127]

The role of the accumulation of A1AT in the induction of the liver disease is not clear. It is significant that patients who are pi-null have no detectable A1AT in the plasma or characteristic globules within hepatocytes and have no evidence of liver disease. Although this would suggest that the accumulation of antiprotease within hepatocytes is damaging, numerous inclusions may be present in completely viable cells, arguing against direct cytotoxicity. Moreover, globules may not be evident in individuals with a deficiency state and well-developed hepatic disease. Much remains to be learned.

CIRRHOSIS OF WILSON'S DISEASE (HEPATOLENTICULAR DEGENERATION)

This autosomal recessive disorder of copper metabolism is marked by the accumulation of toxic levels of copper in many tissues and organs, principally the liver, brain, and eye—hence the designation "hepatolenticular degeneration." Other sites may also be affected but with less serious consequences.

To understand Wilson's disease, we should briefly review normal copper absorption and transport. Approximately 30 to 40% of ingested copper is absorbed in the stomach and duodenum, followed by rapid transport to the liver loosely complexed with albumin. The complexes are dissociated at the plasma membrane of liver cells, and the free copper is transferred into the hepatocytes, where it is bound to apoceruloplasmin in which form it is secreted into the serum. Ceruloplasmin accounts for 90 to 95% of plasma copper, and normally it is recycled to the liver, where it is degraded within lysosomes with release of the copper, which is then excreted in bile. The remainder of the plasma copper is loosely bound to albumin, some of which is excreted in the urine. The amount excreted by the kidney, however, is minuscule as compared with biliary excretion.

In Wilson's disease the initial steps of copper absorption and transport to the liver are normal. However, the absorbed copper fails to enter the circulation in the form of ceruloplasmin. Thus serum ceruloplasmin levels are characteristically low. The absorbed copper continues to accumulate in the liver in excess of the metallothioneine-binding capacity, causing toxic liver injury. Usually by five years of age, nonceruloplasmin-copper spills over into the circulation, causing pathologic changes at other sites such as brain, cornea, kidneys, bones, joints, and parathyroids. Concomitantly, urinary excretion of copper, which is a minor route of copper loss in normal individuals, is markedly increased.

The nature of the metabolic error in Wilson's disease is still unknown. At one time it was thought that reduced hepatic synthesis of apoceruloplasmin was the basic defect, allowing free ("toxic") copper to escape into the circulation. However, this possibility seems to have been ruled out; the apoceruloplasmin gene has been mapped to chromosome 3, whereas the gene for Wilson's disease has been assigned to chromosome 13.[128] According to current thought, *there is a defect in the mobilization of copper from hepatocellular lysosomes for excretion via the bile.* The resulting accumulation damages liver cells and secondarily suppresses apoceruloplasmin synthesis. The basis of impaired biliary copper excretion remains mysterious. *In any event, biochemically Wilson's disease is characterized by a decrease in serum ceruloplasmin, increase in hepatic copper, and increased urinary excretion.* Serum copper levels are of no diagnostic value, since they may be low, normal, or elevated, depending on the stage of evolution of the disease.

The pathogenesis of the copper-induced injury is still unresolved. Favored theories include (1) heavy metal poisoning of hepatic enzymes; (2) copper binding to cytosolic proteins such as tubulin (perhaps accounting for the formation of Mallory bodies) or binding to sulfhydryl groups in proteins; and (3) the formation of free radicals. Against this background we can turn to the morphologic consequences.

The hepatic changes range from relatively minor to massive damage as follows.[129]

Fatty change—mild to moderate with vacuolated nuclei (glycogen or water) and occasionally focal necroses.

Acute hepatitis—The changes closely mimic those of acute viral hepatitis (p. 932) save possibly for the accompanying fatty change. A small amount of copper can sometimes be visualized with rhodanine or rubeanic acid stains in peripheral (zone 1) hepatocytes either as a reddish cytoplasmic blush or in the form of distinct granules of varying size (lysosomal accumulations).

Chronic active hepatitis—The changes resemble those of chronic active viral hepatitis, but again sometimes have such distinguishing features as fatty change and vacuolated nuclei. The copper accumulation, when present, tends to be more prominent than in the stage of acute hepatitis. Infrequently, Mallory bodies (p. 945) are present.

Cirrhosis—The changes range from a micronodular to a macronodular cirrhosis. Often there is active necrosis of hepatocytes, documenting the progression of the hepatic disease. Fatty changes and vacuolated nuclei may be seen, but more distinctive are the Mallory bodies found in about half the cases and the copper deposit.

Massive liver necrosis—a rare manifestation and indistinguishable from that caused by viruses or drugs.

Save for the massive necrosis, which is an uncommon presentation, the other patterns of hepatic involvement probably represent stages in the evolution of full-blown cirrhosis. It is evident that none of the anatomic changes is pathognomonic because even the copper accumulation may be found in primary biliary cirrhosis and Indian childhood cirrhosis.

Kayser-Fleischer rings appear in the cornea in almost all patients with neurologic involvement. These are green to brown deposits of copper in Descemet's membrane close to the limbus of the cornea.

The neurologic changes comprise toxic injury to neurons, most marked in the basal ganglia, particularly the putamen, sometimes leading to grossly visible cavitations.

Although most patients come to clinical attention in childhood or adolescence with manifestations of liver disease, e.g., jaundice and hepatomegaly, when neurologic changes have not yet developed, the reverse is true in about 40% of cases.[130] The disease may appear as early as the fourth or fifth year of life as acute or chronic hepatitis. The liver disease may apparently clear only to surface years later as fully developed cirrhosis, or the hepatitis may pursue a relentless course to liver failure. In adults, the hepatic injury usually appears insidiously when the cirrhosis has already fully evolved. When the hepatic involvement remains subclinical, the condition comes to attention as a Parkinson-like movement disorder, as a psychiatric disturbance ranging from behavioral disorders to frank psychosis or because of the eye changes. Early recognition permits the use of copper chelators, e.g., penicillamine, to prevent the accumulation of copper, thereby sparing the liver, brain, and other organs from damage, and, not incidentally, the life of the patient.

OTHER FORMS OF CIRRHOSIS

Infrequently, cirrhosis appears in certain clinical settings not previously mentioned. *Infants and children with the inborn metabolic errors galactosemia and tyrosinosis may develop cirrhosis if they survive long enough.* Uncommonly, severe *cardiac sclerosis* (p. 92) becomes sufficiently marked to justify the designation "cardiac cirrhosis." Even more uncommonly, the desmoplastic reaction excited by a diffusely infiltrative cancer of the liver (primary or secondary) creates a *carcinomatous cirrhosis* or pseudocirrhosis disease. *Congenital syphilis,* happily now a rare disease, causes diffuse interstitial scarring of the liver that may mimic cirrhosis. In the adult, *multiple hepatic gummas in tertiary syphilis* may, in time, give rise to contracted scars that produce deep creases in the surface of the liver. This pattern of involvement is called *hepar lobatum,* but does not constitute a valid form of cirrhosis. Infections caused by liver flukes, which preferentially invade the larger bile ducts within the liver, may cause sufficient obstruction to mimic or induce secondary biliary cirrhosis.

After all the major categories of cirrhosis of presumed known causation have been excluded, there remain a substantial number of cases (ranging around the world from 10 to 60%) of completely obscure origin, referred to as *cryptogenic cirrhosis.*[131,132] The magnitude of this "wastebasket" and its variable size in reported series speak eloquently to the differences in criteria employed in the categorization of diverse forms of cirrhosis and the general lack of understanding of the origins of many cases of cirrhosis.

BENIGN PROLIFERATIONS AND TUMORS

Benign tumorous lesions of the liver have come to assume greater importance because they now sometimes appear as masses on CT or MRI scans performed for other reasons, requiring differentiation from a metastasis or primary carcinoma of the liver. However, most of these benign conditions are uncommon or of little clinical significance, and so comments will be limited to the relatively more frequent.

Cavernous hemangiomas, identical to those occurring in other parts of the body, sometimes produce discrete red-blue, soft nodules, usually less than 2 cm in diameter. They often occur directly beneath the capsule, are sometimes multiple, and are composed of cavernous endothelium-lined, blood-filled channels.

Cysts may occur singly or multiply. They have been subdivided into several categories.[133] (1) *Simple cysts* may occur singly or as clusters of small lesions (microhamartomas) ranging up to several centimeters in diameter, lined by flattened atrophic biliary epithelium. They are rarely associated with polycystic kidney disease. (2) *Congenital intrahepatic biliary dilatations may appear in a condition known as Caroli's disease.* Although it is suspected to be genetic in origin, the mode of inheritance is unknown. The importance of this form of cystic disease derives from the connection of the cysts to the biliary tree and therefore their vulnerability to intrabiliary spread of infection. The individual cysts are usually less than 1 cm in diameter, are lined by biliary epithelium, and sometimes contain inspissated bile or inflammatory exudate (Fig. 19–37). In about one quarter of the cases, they are associated with polycystic kidneys. (3) *Choledochal cysts,* representing large dilatations of the common bile duct, usually in children, may achieve a diameter of 5 to 6 cm. They have significance because they predispose to biliary tract obstruction and gallstone formation and, rarely, have been the site of origin of carcinoma. (4) *Polycystic liver disease,* suspected of autosomal recessive inheritance in children and autosomal dominant inheritance in adults, is marked by multiple cysts ranging up to several centimeters in diameter. This pattern of cystic disease of the liver is often associated with polycystic kidneys.

FOCAL NODULAR HYPERPLASIA

These lesions appear as well-demarcated but poorly encapsulated nodules, ranging up to many centimeters in diameter. Generally they are tan to yellow and somewhat variegated on cross section, but they may be bile-stained. Typically there is a central gray-white

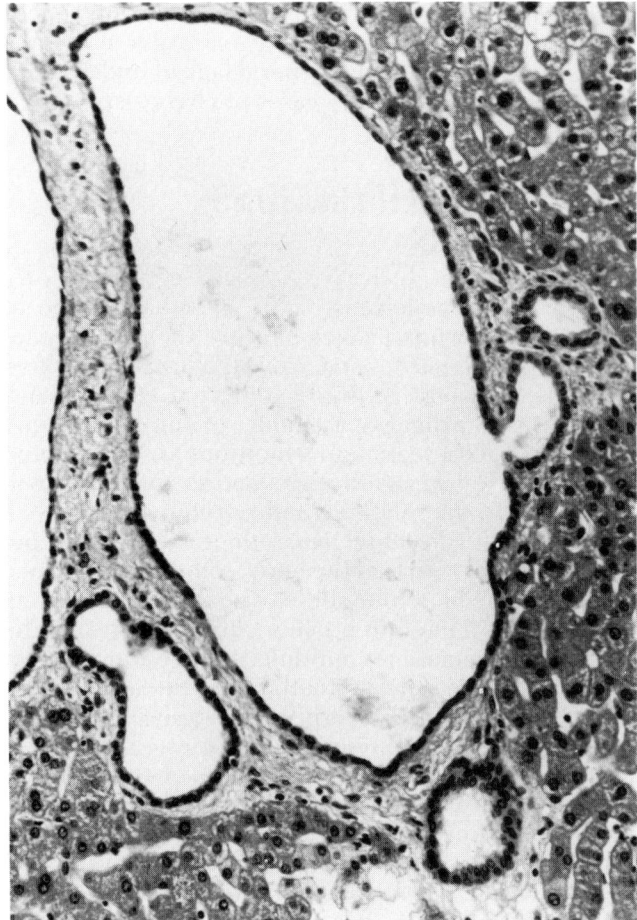

Figure 19–37. Congenital biliary cysts (Caroli's disease) lined by apparent epithelial cells.

stellate scar from which radiate fibrous septa to the periphery. The parenchyma between the septa is composed of glycogen- or lipid-rich, otherwise normal hepatocytes. Distinctive are the numerous bile ducts and an intense lymphocytic infiltrate within the fibrous septa. These lesions are more common in women than in men and are thought by some (but denied by others) to be associated with the use of oral contraceptives.[134] Although generally considered to be innocent hamartomas, they are sometimes viewed as one end of the spectrum of proliferations of liver cells terminating in hepatocellular carcinoma.

ADENOMA

There are two types of adenoma: (1) those of bile duct origin, and (2) those composed of liver cells. *Bile duct adenomas* are firm, pale, discrete nodules rarely over 1 cm in diameter. Unlike the liver cell adenoma, they are almost never bile-stained. Histologically, they are composed of epithelium-lined channels or ducts separated by a scant-to-abundant connective tissue stroma. They are generally considered to be hamartomas. Because of their small size, they are usually found as incidental lesions at post-mortem examination.

Liver cell adenomas tend to occur in young women who have used oral contraceptives. Their increased frequency since the advent of this form of contraception supports a causal association, as do reports of regression of these neoplasms following discontinuance of their use.[135,136]

Liver cell adenomas are pale yellow-tan, frequently bile-stained nodules, found anywhere in the hepatic substance but often beneath the capsule. They range from several centimeters up to 30 cm in diameter. Although they are usually well demarcated, encapsulation may not be grossly evident. On occasion, peripheral pseudopods project into the normal liver substance, creating the false impression of malignant invasion. Histologically, adenomas are composed of sheets and cords of cells that may entirely resemble normal hepatocytes or have some variation in cell and nuclear size. Sometimes the cells have cleared cytoplasm. Prominent in these tumors are abnormally disposed, dilated vascular sinusoids, but bile ducts are usually absent. A capsule that ranges from delicate collapsed reticulin to well-defined connective tissue usually separates the lesion from the surrounding normal parenchyma, but it may be deficient in places and indeed be entirely lacking in some adenomas.

Liver cell adenomas have clinical significance for two reasons: (1) When they present as an intrahepatic mass, they are readily mistaken for the more ominous hepatocellular carcinoma; and (2) subcapsular adenomas have a tendency to rupture, particularly during pregnancy, and cause severe intraperitoneal hemorrhage.[137] The rare reports of their conversion to hepatocellular carcinomas may well represent diagnostic confusion rather than neoplastic conversion.

MALIGNANT TUMORS

The liver and lungs share the dubious distinction of being the visceral organs most often involved in the metastatic spread of cancers. Thus, the overwhelming majority of cancers in the liver are metastases, most commonly from carcinomas of the breast, lung, and colon. By contrast, primary carcinomas of the liver are relatively uncommon in North America and Western Europe. However, these primary malignant neoplasms are very prevalent in other countries and, on a global basis, primary liver cell carcinoma is probably the most common visceral malignant tumor in males.[138] Two additional forms of primary liver cancer—the hepatoblastoma and angiosarcoma—are very rare and merit only brief description.

The *hepatoblastoma* is a tumor usually of infancy that is capable of metastasis but sometimes permits successful resection. There are two anatomic variants: (1) the *epithelial type*, composed of small, compact, dark embryonal or fetal hepatocytes bearing only a vague resemblance to mature liver cells; and (2) the *mixed type,* composed of more or less similar cells admixed with those having a slightly greater resemblance to mature liver cells, interspersed with foci of mesenchymal differentiation, e.g., striated muscle, cartilage, osteoid. Unless successfully resected, both variants are usually fatal within a few years.

The *angiosarcoma* is a highly aggressive neoplasm resembling those occurring elsewhere (p. 591). However, it is of interest because in the past it was associated with exposure to vinyl chloride, arsenic, or Thorotrast. The latent period between exposure to the putative carcinogen and the appearance of the neoplasm has ranged up to several decades. These highly aggressive neoplasms metastasize widely and generally kill within a year.

PRIMARY CARCINOMA OF LIVER

There are basically two types of primary carcinoma of the liver: One is the *hepatocellular carcinoma* (HCC) or *liver cell carcinoma;* the other, composed of bile duct epithelium, is designated *cholangiocarcinoma.* Very infrequently a neoplasm appears to share characteristics of both lines—the hepatocholangiocarcinoma. HCC, grievously sometimes still called a hepatoma, accounts for over 90% of all primary liver cancers. Virtually all the remainder are cholangiocarcinomas; the mixed pattern is very uncommon. Understandably, most of the following remarks relate to the HCC. There has been an upsurge of interest in HCC for several reasons: (1) the striking differences in its worldwide distribution; (2) the existence of new insights into potential causative influences; and (3) the possibility that interventions now available could reduce the incidence of this form of cancer.

EPIDEMIOLOGY. The global distribution of HCC is closely linked to the distribution of hepatitis B virus (HBV) infection. The prevalence of HCC in autopsies in the United States and Europe is about 0.4% (where HBV carriers are less than 1%), whereas in Africa and Southeast Asia the prevalence of HCC is 2 to 8% (where the carrier rate is tenfold higher). Moreover, in the cancer high-incidence regions the carrier state begins in infancy because of vertical transmission of the virus from infected mothers. In the high-incidence locales, HCC constitutes almost 40% of all cancers, making it the most common form of malignant neoplasia in males and one of the most common in females, but in the United States and Western Europe, HCC represents only 2 to 3% of all cancers.[139] Another strong influence on the distribution of HCC is cirrhosis. Worldwide, HCC is associated with cirrhosis in 60 to 90% of cases, most often the macronodular postnecrotic type, itself closely associated with HBV. In the Western world, where HBV carriage is not prevalent, cirrhosis is present in 85 to 90% of cases of HCC; where HBV carriage is much more prevalent, however, HCC has a less strong association

with cirrhosis. In the United States and Western Europe, these cancers are seldom encountered before age 60, with a male : female ratio of about 6 to 8 : 1. In Africa and Southeast Asia, where HBV carriage usually begins soon after birth, this form of cancer occurs in younger individuals, often between 20 and 40 years of age, with a male : female ratio of about 3 to 4 : 1.[140]

ETIOLOGY AND PATHOGENESIS. There is a large body of evidence linking protracted infection with HBV to the genesis of HCC.[141] In Taiwan, for example, where maternal-infant spread of infection is common, the relative risk of developing HCC is over 200 times greater among carriers than among noncarriers.[141] In contrast, infection acquired in adult life, as is characteristic in the Western world, only infrequently leads to HCC. More direct pathogenetic evidence has been the documentation of integration of HBV-DNA into the genome of HCC tumor cells derived from humans.[142] A variety of genotypic alterations have been identified, including integration of multiple viral copies, deletions of sequences flanking the site of viral integration, and in some instances, rearrangements and translocations of the cellular genome. No transforming protein has been identified, such as is associated with most acutely transforming oncogenic viruses. A sequence of pathogenetic events has thus been proposed. *Infection with the HBV at first is productive. When the virus persists, as in chronic active hepatitis or the carrier state, integration of viral DNA into the hepatocellular genome occurs, followed possibly by cellular transformation and the emergence of HCC.*[143]

The apparent involvement of HBV infection does not preclude a role, albeit a poorly understood role, for other possible influences such as cirrhosis. Chronic regenerative activity in cirrhosis may serve as a promoter for other carcinogenic influences. Alternatively, the damaged liver may be rendered more vulnerable to carcinogens. It should be noted, however, that HCC may arise in the absence of cirrhosis, as it often does in Africa and Asia and even in Western countries (10 to 15%), particularly in children and young adults. A number of environmental carcinogens have at one time or another also been incriminated as possible hepatocarcinogens. Foremost among them is aflatoxin B_1 produced by the fungus *Aspergillus flavus* (p. 272). It is known to produce liver cancers in rats, fowl, and fish. The mycotoxin is suspected to be a significant contributor to the unusually high prevalence of HCC in Africa and Southeast Asia.[144] High levels of aflatoxin B_1 have been shown to bind to mitochondrial DNA, providing further support for the possibility that it is carcinogenic.[145] Oral contraceptives have also come under scrutiny, but the implicating evidence is very tenuous.[146]

None of the influences related to HCC has any bearing on the development of cholangiocarcinoma. No causal role has been established for HBV, cirrhosis, or the exogenous putative carcinogens mentioned above. The only recognized causal influences are previous exposure to Thorotrast (formerly used in radiography of the biliary tract) and invasion of the biliary tract by the liver flukes—*Opisthorchis sinensis*—and its close relatives.

MORPHOLOGY. The HCC, the cholangiocarcinoma, or the mixed pattern—may appear grossly as (1) a **unifocal,** usually large mass; (2) **multifocal,** widely distributed nodules; or (3) a diffusely **infiltrative** cancer, permeating widely or sometimes involving the entire liver. All three patterns may cause liver enlargement (2000 to 3000 gm), particularly the unifocal massive and multinodular patterns, which also often produce clinically palpable irregularity of the liver edge. When discrete masses can be seen, they are basically yellow-white, punctuated sometimes by areas of hemorrhage or necrosis (Fig. 19–38). The diffuse pattern may blend in deceptively with the cirrhotic background. **Hepatocellular carcinomas sometimes take on a green hue when composed of well-differentiated hepatocytes capable of secreting bile. Cholangiocarcinomas are rarely bile stained,** because differentiated bile duct epithelium does not synthesize bile. Infrequently with HCC, but very often with cholangiocarcinoma, the tumor substance is extremely firm and gritty, related to a dense desmoplasia. **All patterns of HCC have a strong propensity for invasion of vascular channels.** Sometimes the intravascular neoplasm extends in a long, snakelike mass into the portal vein or hepatic vein, and even into the inferior vena cava and right side of the heart.

The histology of **HCC** is given first. These cancers range from well-differentiated to highly anaplastic undifferentiated lesions. The well- and moderately well-differentiated forms are composed of tumor cells, recognizable as hepatocytic in origin (Fig. 19–39). In these neoplasms, the cells are disposed either in a trabecular (sinusoidal) or an acinar (tubular) pseudoglandular pattern. The trabeculae are made up of several layers of tumor cells, separated by vascular channels (bearing some resemblance to sinusoids) embedded within a connective tissue sheath. In the acinar or pseudoglandular pattern, the differentiated tumor cells are often disposed about lumina. Sometimes these lumina contain plugs of inspissated bile. An uncommon variant of the well- to moderately well-differentiated HCC is made up of "clear cells" because of the high content of cytoplasmic glycogen. Such tumors bear a strong resemblance to clear-cell renal carcinomas.

Poorly differentiated forms can be characterized as pleomorphic giant cell or small, completely undifferentiated cell or spindle cell. The giant cell neoplasm may be totally anarchic with sheets of wild-looking cells having abundant cytoplasm and often bearing multiple nuclei and atypical mitoses. Areas of ischemic necrosis are frequent in such lesions. The spindle cell variant may mimic a sarcoma, and indeed often has an abundant fibrous stroma separating the parenchymal cells. Sometimes the stroma is sufficiently vascularized to resemble an angiosarcoma. Bile formation in such undifferentiated lesions is uncommon. Vascular invasion is a common finding in all forms of HCC.

A number of additional features may be present in HCC, more often in the well-differentiated variants. Occasionally cytoplasmic inclusions, typical of Mallory's alcoholic hyalin, are found. When persistent hepatitis B infection is present, the tumorous hepatocytes may have hepatitis B surface antigen by immunoperoxidase methods. Immunohistochemical staining also reveals A1AT in tumor cells in 70 to 75% of cases.[147] Alphafetoprotein (AFP) can be identified in 60 to 80% of tumors, and carcinoembryonic antigen in 30%. The most reliable features of HCC are bile pigment within tumor cells or, on electron microscopic examination, the formation of bile canaliculi.

A distinctive clinicopathologic variant has been described—**the fibrolamellar carcinoma.**[148] It usually constitutes a single large, sometimes apparently encapsulated, mass that on transection appears multinodular (vaguely resembling focal nodular hyperplasia; p. 957). This variant most often arises in the absence of cirrhosis. Histologically it is composed of acidophilic polygonal cells growing in nests or cords separated by fibrous stroma.[149] Sometimes bands of fibrous tissue radiate from a central focus, creating the nodularity seen on the gross. Hyalin globules and PAS-positive inclusions may be present within the cytoplasm of the tumor cells. Recognition of this type of HCC is important because of its distinctly better prognosis, as will be pointed out later.

Cholangiocarcinomas have a more limited histologic range. Most are well-differentiated sclerosing adenocarcinomas with clearly defined glandular and tubular structures lined by somewhat anaplastic cuboidal-to-columnar epithelial cells. These neoplasms are often desmoplastic, so that dense collagenous stroma separates the parenchymal elements. Mucus is frequently present within cells and the lumina, but not bile. Thus, in needle biopsies these neoplasms may be extremely difficult to differentiate from metastatic adenocarcinomas. Vascular invasion is less common with cholangiocarcinomas than with HCC and, when present, takes the form of lining of vessels by cancer cells rather than the solid cords of neoplasm seen with

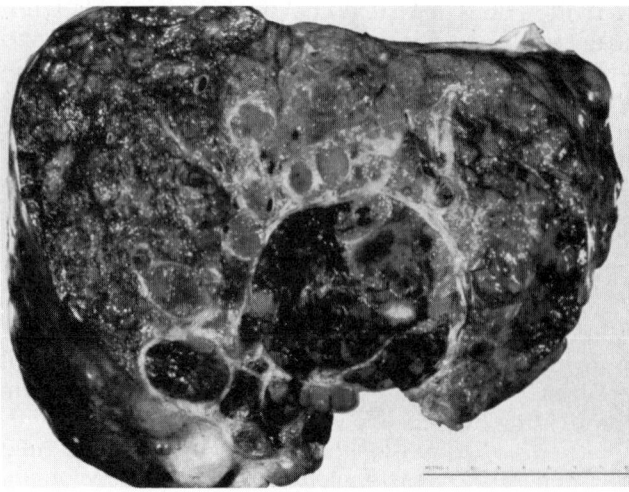

Figure 19–38. Hepatocellular carcinoma extensively replacing the liver substance. In areas, the neoplasm is hemorrhagic and necrotic.

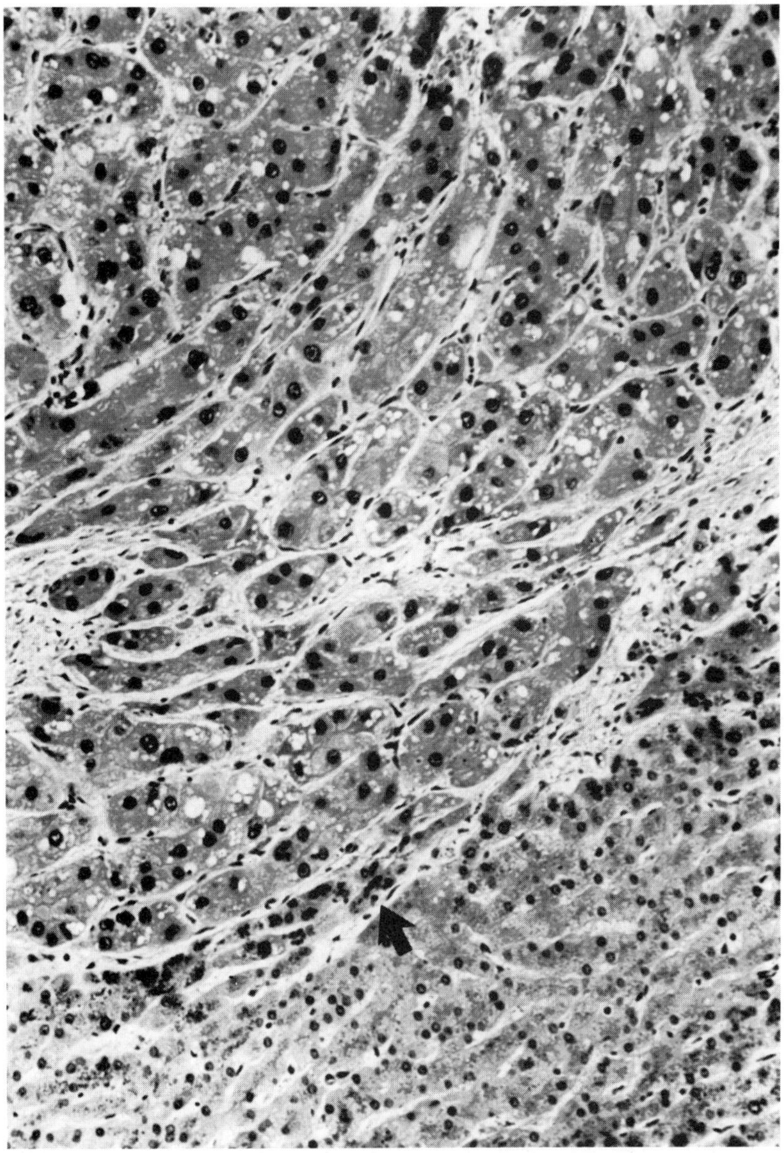

Figure 19-39. Hepatocellular carcinoma occupying the upper left. The residual normal hepatic parenchyma is seen below on the right. The arrow marks the junction. Tumor cells have moderate variation in cell and nuclear size and shape but retain their resemblance to normal liver cells.

HCC. There is no association other than coincidence with pre-existing cirrhosis, nor with HBV antigens or AFP.

The HCC and the cholangiocarcinoma differ somewhat in their patterns of spread. Hematogenous metastases to the lungs, bones (mainly vertebrae), adrenals, brain, or elsewhere are present at autopsy in about 50% of cases of cholangiocarcinoma. Hematogenous metastases are less frequent with HCC and may not be present despite clear evidence of venous invasion until late in the course of the disease, when the lungs are most frequently involved. Lymph node metastases to the perihilar, peripancreatic, and para-aortic nodes above and below the diaphragm are found in about half of all cholangiocarcinomas and less frequently with HCC.

CLINICAL COURSE. The clinical manifestations of primary liver cancer are seldom characteristic and often are masked by those related to the background cirrhosis or chronic hepatitis. Most patients have ill-defined upper abdominal pain, malaise, fatigue, weight loss, and in less than half the cases, awareness of an abdominal mass or abdominal fullness. However, in 70 to 85% of cases, enlargement of the liver can be felt on palpation, with sufficient irregularity or nodularity of the anterior edge to permit differentiation from cirrhosis. Sometimes the liver is tender. Jaundice, fever, and gastrointestinal or esophageal variceal bleeding are inconstant findings.

Laboratory studies may be helpful but are rarely conclusive. Elevated levels of serum alpha-fetoprotein are found in 60 to 75% of patients with HCC. However, these findings are likely to be negative with small, neoplasms; moreover, false positive results are encountered with yolk-sac tumors and many nonneoplastic conditions including cirrhosis, massive liver necrosis, chronic hepatitis, normal pregnancy, fetal distress or death, and fetal neural tube defects such as anencephaly and spina bifida. The CEA levels are less often elevated but are even more nonspecific

(p. 302). Recently a promising new test has been reported; des-gamma-carboxyprothrombin was shown to be detectable in the serum of 75 to 90% of patients with HCC.[150] Apparently carcinoma cells synthesize this precursor of prothrombin, but cannot carboxylate the glutamic acid residues. However, all these biochemical tests often fail to detect small lesions, when curative resection might be possible. Most valuable for small tumors are ultrasonography, hepatic angiography, CT and MRI scans.

The natural course of this aggressive neoplasm is progressive enlargement of the primary mass until it encroaches on hepatic function or metastasizes, generally first to the lungs and then to other sites. Overall, death usually occurs within six months from (1) cachexia, (2) gastrointestinal or esophageal variceal bleeding, or (3) liver failure with hepatic coma.[151] The only ray of light in this otherwise dismal scene is the possibility of significantly reducing the global mortality from HCC by immunization of high-risk populations, in whom infections are commonly acquired early in life, against the HBV. In several controlled trials to date, mostly on high-risk homosexual men, a vaccine prepared from harvested HBsAg has demonstrated an 85 to 90% protective efficacy.[152] Since then, synthetic and recombinant vaccines of HBsAg, which are devoid of the risk of viral transmission have been developed; the results of their use are beginning to appear.[152a]

The fibrolamellar variant of HCC is associated with a far less grim outlook. It arises most often in children, adolescents, and young adults in the absence of underlying liver disease and may be discovered while still amenable to surgical resection. Thus the average survival is one to three years, and about 60% of patients are alive at five years.[149]

METASTATIC TUMORS

Metastatic involvement of the liver is far more common than primary neoplasia. Although the most common primaries producing hepatic metastases are those of the breast, lung, and colon, any cancer in any site of the body may spread to the liver. Typically, multiple nodular implants are found that often cause striking hepatomegaly (Fig. 19–40). The liver weight may exceed several kilos. There is a tendency for metastatic nodules to outgrow their blood supply, producing central necrosis and umbilication when viewed from the surface of the liver.

Always surprising is the amount of metastatic involvement that may be present in the absence of clinical or laboratory evidence of hepatic functional insufficiency. Often the only clinical telltale sign is hepatomegaly, sometimes with nodularity of the free edge. However, with massive or strategic involvement (obstruction of major ducts), jaundice and abnormal liver function tests may appear.

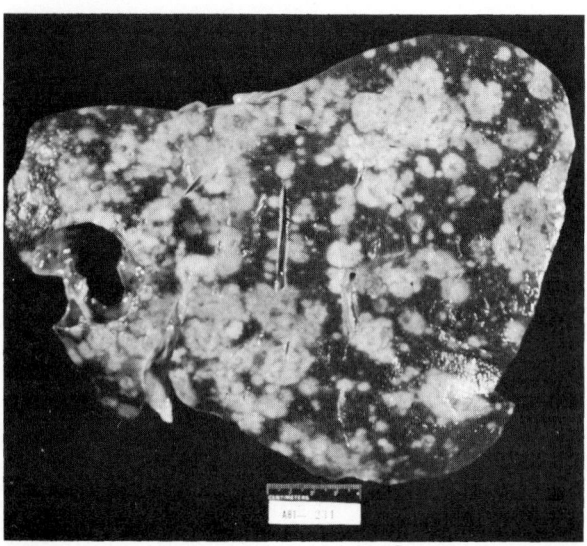

Figure 19–40. Multiple hepatic metastases from a primary gastric carcinoma.

MISCELLANEOUS DISORDERS

A few hepatic conditions do not fit well into any of the previous categories and so are included here.

DRUG-RELATED INJURY

Adverse drug reactions (ADRs), as noted on page 485, have wide-ranging consequences, one of which is liver injury. They are said to be responsible for about 2 to 5% of all cases of jaundice in general hospital populations[153] and for many more in hospitalized geriatric populations. Moreover, they grow ever more frequent. In one study in Japan, ten times as many cases of drug-related hepatic injury were reported in the years 1964 to 1973 as in the previous decade — perhaps the price that must be paid for medical progress.[154] No attempt will be made to provide a compilation of all implicated drugs; comments instead will be limited to general principles and common reaction patterns. Far more complete coverage is readily available.[155–157]

PATHOGENESIS. The hepatotoxicity of therapeutic agents involves several independent but perhaps at times collaborative mechanisms: (1) *The drug or one of its metabolites is directly toxic to the liver; (2) the drug reduces the immunologic or hormonal defense of the host; (3) the drug or, more likely, one of its metabolites becomes a hapten to convert an intracellular protein into an immunogenic signal.* The first two pathways are responsible for "direct," "predictable," dose-dependent hepatotoxicity, and the last one for "indirect," "unpredictable" hepatotoxicity, as was discussed on page 485.

Although many agents can be categorized as predictable or unpredictable hepatotoxins, very often the basis for the ADR is uncertain. Halothane (an in-

halant anesthetic) is a case in point, as was discussed on page 486. Most adverse reactions have appeared following repeated use of the anesthetic compatible with the development of drug sensitization. However, in a minority of cases, the reactions have occurred after the first use of halothane when prior sensitization cannot be invoked. *The present consensus is that the formation of toxic metabolites causes the liver cell injury in predisposed individuals, followed in some cases by an immune response to released hepatic proteins, adding to the injury.*[158] Thus halothane partakes ambiguously of the characteristics of a "direct" and an "indirect" hepatotoxin.

ADRs induce an astonishing range of hepatic changes that virtually recapitulate all types of hepatic disease.[159] Because of these similarities, it is not necessary to describe the particular patterns of reaction. They are briefly presented in Table 19–8 along with some of the implicated agents. Drugs frequently involved in direct predictable reactions are acetaminophen, isoniazid, alpha-methyldopa, chlorpromazine, methotrexate, halothane, and

Table 19–8. Major Hepatic Drug Reactions and Some Implicated Agents

TISSUE REACTION	EXAMPLES
Microvesicular fat	Tetracycline Salicylates
Macrovesicular fat	Methotrexate Perhexiline Ethanol
Cholestasis (with or without hepatocellular injury)	Chlorpromazine Sex steroids, including oral contraceptives
Centrilobular necrosis	Acetaminophen Halothane
Massive necrosis	Halothane Acetaminophen Alpha-methyldopa
Hepatitis, acute to chronic	Isoniazid Oxyphenisatin Alpha-methyldopa Nitrofurantoin Phenytoin Cinchophen
Fibrosis-cirrhosis	Methotrexate Cinchophen Amiodarone
Granuloma formation	Sulfonamides Alpha-methyldopa Quinidine Phenylbutazone Hydralazine Allopurinol
Veno-occlusive disease	Cytotoxic drugs
Hepatic or portal vein thrombosis	Estrogens, including oral contraceptives
Focal nodular hyperplasia	?C-17 alkylated steroids, including oral contraceptives
Adenoma	Oral contraceptives
Hepatocellular carcinoma	?Anabolic steroids, oral contraceptives

tetracycline. Those most commonly implicated in hypersensitivity reactions are sulfonamides, alpha-methyldopa, quinidine, phenylbutazone, hydralazine, and allopurinol. Not surprisingly, these are the same agents that often produce granulomatous reactions in the liver.

Only a few comments will be made about some of the patterns of reactions (Table 19–8). Unpredictable hepatotoxic reactions may be identical to those caused by direct toxic reactions. While there is some relationship between the type of hepatotoxin and the pattern of reaction, it is not inviolate. The same agent may in one instance cause only centrilobular necrosis, or in another massive necrosis, as is the case with halothane. Analogously, methyldopa may induce a range of changes from acute to chronic hepatitis to massive necrosis. The drug reaction may be indistinguishable from non–drug-related disease.

The microvesicular fatty change produced by tetracycline is indistinguishable from that associated with Reye's syndrome and aspirin toxicity. Tetracycline toxicity has on occasion produced necrotizing reactions, rarely massive, sometimes with rapid deterioration of liver function. Cholestasis produced as a hypersensitivity reaction to sex steroids and chlorpromazine often poses a difficult diagnostic problem because it can be indistinguishable from the many other causes of conjugated hyperbilirubinemia cited on page 916. Although a mild hepatitic reaction generally accompanies the chlorpromazine-induced cholestasis, occasionally there is cholestasis alone, which could be misinterpreted as obstructive in origin. Focal nodular hyperplasia, adenoma, and hepatocellular carcinoma have been cited as possible adverse reactions to C-17 alkylated steroids, such as are present in some oral contraceptives and androgenic agents. The substantiating data are fragmentary but are strongest with adenomas, as noted on page 489. It should be evident that ADRs must be considered in the differential diagnosis of all forms of hepatic disease.

REYE'S SYNDROME (RS)

RS is an acute postviral illness, largely of children, characterized by encephalopathy, microvesicular fatty change of the liver, and widespread mitochondrial injury. Rare cases have been reported in adults.[160] The typical patient is a child between 6 months and 15 years of age who about three to five days following a viral illness (most often influenza A or B or varicella) has the onset of pernicious vomiting. Initially there is little change in consciousness save for some lethargy. Serum bilirubin, ammonia, and aminotransferase levels are essentially normal at this time. About three quarters of the cases progress no further save possibly for a brief period of obtundation or excitability, and then progressively improve thereafter with no residual effects.[161] The remaining 25% of patients have more serious illness with progressively deeper levels of coma accompanied by elevations in the serum levels of bilirubin, aminotransferases, and particularly ammonia. With this more serious illness, survivors may be left with permanent neurologic impairments. The fatality rate ranges from 10 to 40% depending on the number of mild cases included in the data base. Death is most commonly related to profound depression of central nervous system function, but rare patients die of liver failure.

The hepatic abnormalities comprise:

1. Microvesicular hepatic steatosis during the first three to seven days of illness (Fig. 19–41).
2. Hepatic mitochondrial injury evidenced by pleomorphic enlargement with disruption of cristae and electron lucent matrices. There are concomitant reductions in mitochondrial enzymes involved in the citric acid cycle and urea formation.
3. Cerebral edema is typical of all cases; severity of the edema corresponds to the severity of the neurologic dysfunction. Histologically there is swelling of astrocytes. Myelin blebs and mitochondrial alterations appear in neurons but are less pronounced than those in the liver.[162]
4. Skeletal muscles, kidneys, and heart may also reveal microvesicular fatty change and mitochondrial alterations, although more subtle than those of the liver.

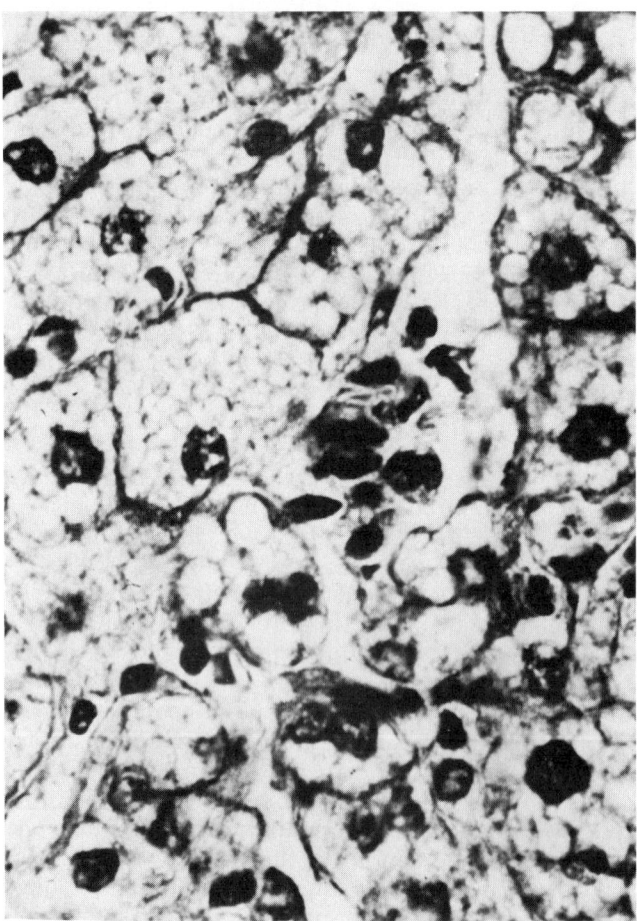

Figure 19–41. Reye's syndrome with microvesicular hepatic steatosis (fatty change).

The pathogenesis of Reye's syndrome is incompletely understood, but it is generally believed to involve biochemical derangements alone or in combination with viral infection. *Greatest interest is focused on (1) hyperammonemia, (2) elevated serum free fatty acids, and (3) salicylate (e.g., aspirin) toxicity or synergism.*[163] Hyperammonemia, probably related to reduced function of mitochondrial enzymes, correlates with the severity of the coma, but the vomiting and lethargy predate the development of significant hyperammonemia. Free fatty acidemia and lactic acidosis have been shown in experimental animals to profoundly affect mitochondrial function and morphology and secondarily lead to hyperammonemia; in most patients with Reye's syndrome, elevated serum free fatty acids and acidosis are present even in mild cases. However, is the acidemia the cause or the consequence of mitochondrial injury of other origins? The role of salicylates is equally controversial. In most surveys of Reye's syndrome, 90 to 95% of children have received some form of salicylates (usually aspirin) in the course of their febrile viral illness.[164] Control subjects with similar illnesses who did not develop Reye's syndrome have, on average, received salicylates less frequently.[165] In addition, salicylate intoxication alone produces hepatic dysfunction and encephalopathy, and in many instances, microvesicular fatty changes in the liver. However, mitochondrial abnormalities are not present, and the salicylate levels in children with RS do not approach toxic levels. Because of a lack of a satisfactory pathogenetic theory, exploration of other factors and influences continues, such as the roles of endotoxin, interferon, and tumor necrosis factor. Significantly, however, the number of reported cases of RS in the United States has declined along with the decreased use of aspirin during febrile illnesses in children.[166] The major features of RS are shown in Figure 19–42.

NEONATAL CHOLESTASIS

Prolonged conjugated hyperbilirubinemia in the neonate poses a serious and difficult clinical diagnostic problem for reasons that will become clear. The major conditions causing it are *extrahepatic biliary atresia* (EHBA) and a variety of forms of hepatoparenchymal injury, collectively referred to as *neonatal hepatitis.* Although these two categories have been segregated, there is a possibility that both are different anatomic expressions of a common etiologic agent (e.g., reovirus type 3). Hence both have been encompassed within the term *"infantile obstructive cholangiopathy."*[167] Justification for this usage comes from some similarity in the morphologic changes produced by atresia of bile ducts and direct involvement of parenchymal cells. Nonetheless, morphologic differentiation between EHBA and the primary hepatoparenchymal causes of jaundice in the newborn is important and usually possible.

EHBA refers to complete obstruction of at least some of the hepatic ducts or common bile duct in the

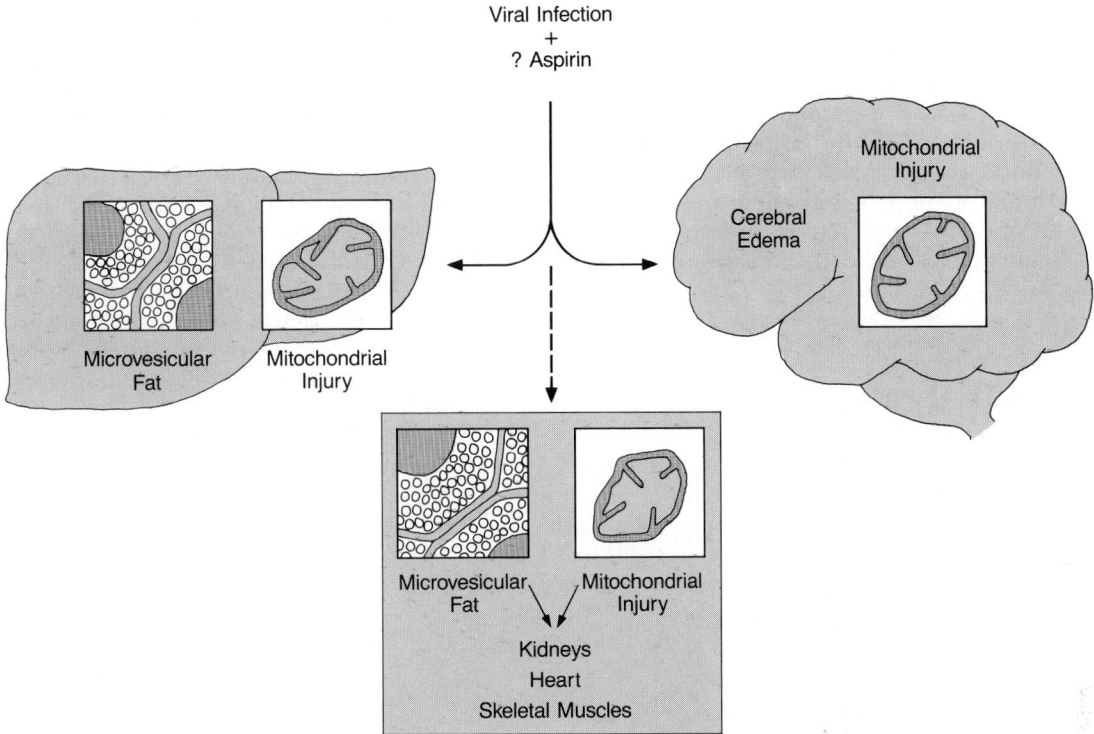

Figure 19–42. Reye's syndrome. A schematic presentation of the presumed pathogenesis and morphologic consequences.

absence of trauma. It is an uncommon condition encountered most often in normal-weight, full-term, female infants who sometimes have associated polysplenia or, rarely, concurrent congenital anomalies suggesting a genetic defect. The laboratory studies are those anticipated with an obstructive jaundice and often do not differentiate the condition from diffuse parenchymal disease. *Salient features include (1) inflammation and fibrosing stricture of the hepatic or common bile ducts; (2) periductular inflammation of intrahepatic ductules and cholangioles; (3) proliferation of smaller bile ducts, with possibly some disappearance of larger interlobular ducts; and (4) when unrecognized for several months, the development of periportal fibrosis and cirrhosis.* Cholestasis is evident (p. 916) and possibly some changes in the hepatic parenchyma resembling those of "neonatal hepatitis." Due note should be made that alpha-1-antitrypsin deficiency may mimic **EHBA** on biopsy.

Neonatal hepatitis is not a specific entity, but instead a generic term for a variety of hepatic parenchymal disorders causing conjugated hyperbilirubinemia in the neonate. Regrettably, many of the conditions subsumed under this rubric are not inflammatory, but there is the saving grace that irrespective of the etiology (when known) the morphologic changes are remarkably constant.[168] The major conditions included under neonatal hepatitis are cited in Table 19–9.

Despite the diversity of etiologies, *the major morphologic features of neonatal hepatitis are (1) lobular disarray with focal liver cell necrosis, (2) prominent giant cell transformation, (3) mononuclear infil-*

tration of the portal areas, (4) reactive changes in the Kupffer cells, and (5) cholestasis.[169] Other specific changes may be present, such as the intracytoplasmic inclusions of **A1AT**, intranuclear inclusions of **CMV**, and fatty change (and possibly cirrhosis) in galactosemia and tyrosinemia. It should be noted that in some cases there is proliferation of cholangioles accompanied by some portal fibrosis, recalling the changes of **EHBA**. Thus, although the differential diagnosis can be made morphologically in about 90% of cases, some involvements constitute "nasty" differential problems. Clinically, infants with neonatal hepatitis are more likely to be male, have low birth weight, and have, in about one third of cases, other congenital anomalies.

In the overall spectrum of causes of neonatal cholestasis, 50 to 60% of cases represent idiopathic neonatal hepatitis, about 20% EHBA, and perhaps 15% alpha-1-antitrypsin deficiency. Differentiation of the

Table 19–9. Major Origins of Neonatal Hepatitis

I. Idiopathic neonatal hepatitis	III. Genetic and metabolic
II. Known infectious etiologies	disorders
Hepatitis A and B	Alpha-1-antitrypsin deficiency
Echo viruses 11, 14, 19	Cystic fibrosis
Coxsackie virus B	Tyrosinemia
Cytomegalovirus	Galactosemia
Herpes simplex virus	Niemann-Pick disease
Syphilis	Total parenteral nutrition
Gram-negative sepsis	
Toxoplasmosis	
Endotoxemia	

two most common causes assumes great importance. Some with **EHBA** can be benefited by various surgical procedures aimed at bypassing the extrahepatic bile duct obstruction. Failure to recognize such patients will almost certainly lead within months to years to fatal liver cirrhosis. In contrast, the great majority of instances of idiopathic hepatitis are benign and spontaneously remit with supportive therapy. Liver biopsy has been said to make the discrimination in about 90% of cases.[170]

POST-MORTEM CHANGES

It is necessary to mention briefly the morphologic changes that may occur after death, to avoid confusion with ante-mortem liver disease. Depending on the adequacy and promptness of the methods used to preserve the body, such as refrigeration, the liver may undergo post-mortem autolysis. Usually it begins to become evident about 24 hours after death, and produces progressive mushy softening and enzymic disintegration of cells in the complete absence of reactive inflammatory changes. The nuclei progressively fade and the cells fall away from the reticular framework. Often, bacterial proliferation can be seen within the autolytic parenchyma. In some instances, gas-forming organisms such as *Clostridium welchii* are borne from the gastrointestinal tract to the liver through the portal system during the agonal stage of life. Growth of these organisms and the release of gas may produce visible or palpable gaseous bubbles— *foamy liver*. Obviously, no inflammatory response accompanies the bacterial invasion.

Appropriately, the description of post-mortem changes brings to an end the consideration of the liver.

BILIARY SYSTEM

CONGENITAL ANOMALIES	MISCELLANEOUS DISORDERS	Carcinoma of Gallbladder
CHOLELITHIASIS (GALL-STONES)	OF THE GALLBLADDER	Carcinoma of Bile Ducts and
ACUTE CHOLECYSTITIS	TUMORS	Ampulla of Vater
CHRONIC CHOLECYSTITIS	**Papilloma, Adenoma, and**	
	Adenomyoma of Gallbladder	

Although diseases of the biliary tract do not occupy a central place in medicine, some are very common (cholecystitis and cholelithiasis) and others are too often fatal (carcinomas). Before discussing the major conditions of this system, a few comments may be helpful on some possibly less well known normal features of the structure and function of the biliary apparatus.

In approximately 60 to 70% of individuals the pancreatic duct joins the common bile duct to drain through a common channel; in the remainder the ducts enter separately. This detail, as will be seen, has some relevance to the possible pathogenesis of acute cholecystitis and pancreatic necrosis. Histologically, the gallbladder, unlike the gastrointestinal tract, lacks a muscularis mucosae and submucosa and therefore is composed of (1) a mucosal lining of a single layer of tall columnar cells; (2) a fibromuscular layer of smooth muscle cells and elastic fibrils; (3) a layer of subserosal fat with arteries, veins, lymphatics, nerves, and paraganglia; and (4) a peritoneal covering save where the gallbladder is embedded in the liver substance. The mucosal epithelium is thrown up into numerous interlacing tiny folds, creating a honeycombed surface. In the neck of the gallbladder, these folds form the spiral valves of Heister, between which gallstones love to snuggle. Sometimes small tubular inclusions (*ducts of Luschka*) are found buried within the gallbladder wall, having no communication with the lumen. In addition, small outpouchings of the mucosa of the gallbladder may penetrate into the wall (*Rokitansky-Aschoff sinuses*). Whether they represent acquired herniations or developmental deviations remains unknown, but in either event they are possible sites for gallstone nucleation and inflammation.

As it is secreted by the liver, bile is composed of about 3% solutes, the remainder being water. The relative proportions of various solutes are depicted in Figure 19–43. Although the liver secretes 0.5 to 1.0 liter of bile daily, the gallbladder capacity is only about 50 ml. Some of this accommodation is achieved by drainage of bile into the duodenum, but in addition the gallbladder concentrates bile five- to tenfold.

The bile acids, chenodeoxycholic acid and cholic acid, are produced in the liver by catabolism of cholesterol; linkage to taurine or glycine creates the major bile salts. You may recall that a large fraction of the bile salts drained into the duodenum is reabsorbed in the small intestine and colon and returned to the liver via the portal blood to again be recycled (the enterohepatic circulation). The phospholipid is lecithin, presumably synthesized within liver cells. Cholesterol may in part be synthesized de novo in liver

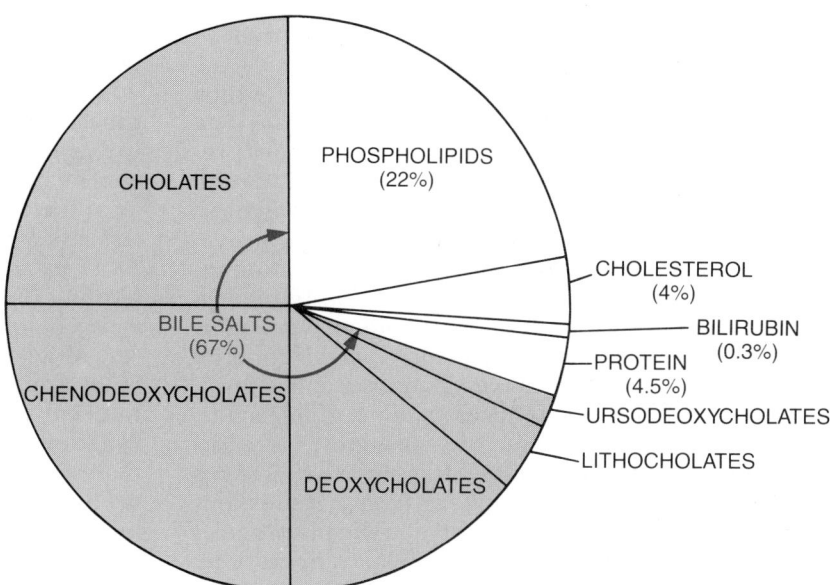

Figure 19–43. Typical solute composition of gallbladder and hepatic bile in health. (From Carey, M.C.: Biliary lipids and gallstone formation. In Csomos, G., and Thaler, H. (eds.): Clinical Hepatology. Berlin, Springer Verlag, 1983, pp. 52–69. Used by permission.)

cells, but most is derived from plasma lipoproteins returned to the liver and then secreted into the bile. Cholesterol is not soluble in aqueous bile but is maintained in solution by incorporation into micelles along with the bile acids and lecithin, as will be discussed later. The relative concentrations of cholesterol, bile salts, lecithin, and protein in bile are critically important to the pathogenesis of gallstones.

CONGENITAL ANOMALIES

A large number of developmental anomalies of the gallbladder and bile ducts have been described; most are uncommon, are rarely of clinical significance, and are of interest largely to the surgeon and embryologist. A few are sufficiently common to mention because they produce curious cholecystograms and show up on ultrasonography, CT, and MRI scans. The gallbladder may be *congenitally absent*, or at the other extreme, there may be *duplication* of the gallbladder with joined or independent cystic ducts. A longitudinal septum may create a *bilobed gallbladder*. *Aberrant locations* occur in 5 to 10% of the population, most commonly partial or complete embedding of the gallbladder in the liver substance. A *folded fundus* is the most common anomaly, creating the so-called *phrygian cap*. If the fold is sufficiently acute, it may create a terminal saccule that empties incompletely on gallbladder contraction to provide a site for stasis and concentration of bile with the potential for gallstone formation. *Agenesis* of all or any portion of the hepatic or common bile ducts or *atretic* narrowing of these channels is a serious anomaly that may cause extrahepatic biliary obstruction, requiring surgical intervention to prevent the development of obstructive biliary cirrhosis.

CHOLELITHIASIS (GALLSTONES)

About 20 million Americans are said to have gallstones, leading to some 500,000 cholecystectomies annually.[171] Whether "silent" stones justify surgery and whether all these cholecystectomies are necessary constitute major controversies to which we shall return later. Nonetheless, the importance of cholelithiasis as a clinical problem cannot be doubted because annually perhaps 10,000 individuals die of gallstone disease and its complications.

There are two main types of gallstones. *About 85% are composed predominantly of cholesterol,* although usually there are minor contributions of bile salts, bilirubin, protein, and inorganic salts, mainly calcium. *The remainder are composed predominantly of bilirubin and are commonly called pigment stones.* Some of these contain other components such as bile acids, fatty acids, and inorganic salts, while others are virtually pure calcium bilirubinate. Between the "pure" cholesterol and "pure" pigment stones there is a broad spectrum of so-called mixed stones, in essence "deviant" cholesterol stones.

The major driving forces in lithogenesis are the cholesterol saturation of the bile and hemolysis. It is important to note that both cholesterol and unconjugated bilirubin are virtually insoluble in water. The amount of cholesterol solubilized in bile is about 2 million times greater than its aqueous solubility. This solubilization is accomplished and dependent (as will be discussed) on the level of bile salts, and to a lesser extent, lecithin. Accordingly, *any supersaturation of the bile by cholesterol relative to the bile salts and any increase in the unconjugated bilirubin content are lithogenic.*

INCIDENCE AND RISK FACTORS. Certain groups are far more prone than others to develop gallstones.

The major risk factors and therefore distribution of gallstones are cited in Table 19–10.

Comments about some of these influences as they relate to *cholesterol stones* follow.[172]

Ethnic-heredity (genetic). Cholesterol stones predominate in Northern Europe and North and South America, but pigment stones are more prevalent in the rural Orient. In American Indian tribes, the prevalence of cholesterol stones approaches 75%, but pigment stones are rare. This predisposition to cholesterol stones, particularly among Indian women, is believed to be the consequence of a racial (?genetic) tendency to secrete excessive amounts of cholesterol, and concomitantly, inadequate amounts of bile acids.

Age. The prevalence of gallstones increases throughout life. In the United States less than 5 to 6% of the general population under 40 have stones, but about 25 to 30% of those over 80 do. The influence of age is attributed to increasing cholesterol secretion.

Sex. Females are at least twice as "lithogenic" as males. In autopsy studies, about 8% of men and 20% of women in the United States have gallstones. Thought to underlie this predisposition are estrogen-related inhibition of bile acid synthesis and possibly some increased formation of cholesterol. Multiple pregnancies may enhance the predisposition.

Diet and obesity. Although obviously interrelated, a high-calorie diet and obesity as independent variables both increase cholesterol secretion by the liver. Keep your spirits up, however; a moderate intake of alcohol appears to be protective. Moreover, high-cholesterol diets do not make a significant contribution. The old but somewhat ungracious "four F's"—fat, female, fertile (multiparity), and forty—well characterizes the individual at particular risk.

Drugs. Clofibrate, used to lower blood cholesterol, appears to increase cholesterol secretion by the liver. Exogenous estrogens have a double effect, decreasing the level of bile salts by suppressing bile acid synthesis and increasing secretion of cholesterol. Endogenous estrogens have a similar effect as can be documented by the change in bile composition at the time of puberty in girls, presumably accounting for the female preponderance mentioned earlier. Oral contraceptives, one would assume, would have a similar effect, but recent studies have failed to confirm this risk.[173]

Gastrointestinal disorders. Any condition such as Crohn's disease that impairs reabsorption of bile salts is an obvious predisposing influence.

Much less is known about the risk factors for pigment stones. In general, "mixed" pigment stones tend to occur in Orientals, and "pure" pigment stones in Occidentals.[174] Disorders that are associated with hemolysis of red cells, such as the hemolytic anemias, predispose to an increased content of unconjugated bilirubin in the bile. In addition, pigment stones are more common among patients with cirrhosis, for unknown reasons. Unlike the case with cholesterol gallstones, pigment stones are not associated with the four "F's."

PATHOGENESIS. Three stages are involved in the formation of gallstones: (1) supersaturation of bile, (2) nucleation or initiation of stone formation, and (3) growth by accretion. *Critical to the formation of cholesterol stones is supersaturation of bile with cholesterol.* Cholesterol is maintained in solution by incorporation within micelles in which an array of bile salts constitute the outer face with their hydrophilic hydroxyl groups in contact with the aqueous solution, while their hydrophobic steroid groups provide an internal milieu in which cholesterol is soluble. The addition of lecithin, a polar phospholipid, to the external array of bile salts increases the ability of the micelles to solubilize cholesterol. *Thus, supersaturation of bile with cholesterol or deficient secretion of bile acid (salts) or lecithin is lithogenic.*[175] Gallbladder stasis with increased reabsorption of water may contribute to the supersaturation of cholesterol.[176]

Although cholesterol supersaturation is necessary for gallstone formation, it is not sufficient; normal control subjects free of gallstone disease may also have cholesterol supersaturation. *What then initiates nucleation?* Here the evidence is more tenuous. Two influences are proposed: (1) a deficiency of an antinucleating factor and (2) an increased secretion of mucinous glycoproteins. The precise nature of the antinucleating factor has not been identified, but it may be composed of apoproteins of serum lipoproteins.[177] Mucin, on the other hand, appears to serve as a nucleating agent in cholesterol supersaturated bile. In combination with bilirubin, it may form a sludge serving as "seed crystals" that initiate crystallization of cholesterol. Prostaglandins may play some role in stone formation by stimulating mucin secretion, because the administration of aspirin reverses the lithogenicity of supersaturated bile.[178] In summation, *cholesterol stone formation may occur when there is supersaturation of gallbladder bile with cholesterol*

Table 19–10. Risk Factors for Gallstones

CHOLESTEROL STONES

Demography: Northern Europe, North and South America; American Indians; Mexican Americans; probable familial predisposition
Obesity
High-calorie diet
Clofibrate therapy
Gastrointestinal disorders; ileal (e.g., Crohn's) disease, resection, or bypass; cystic fibrosis with pancreatic insufficiency
Female sex hormones; female preponderance after puberty; estrogenic medications; ?oral contraceptives
Advancing age
Probable but not well established: pregnancy, multiparity, diabetes mellitus, and polyunsaturated fats

PIGMENT STONES

Demography: Oriental more than Occidental; rural more than urban
Chronic hemolysis
Alcoholic cirrhosis
Biliary infection
Advancing age

due either to increased secretion of it or to decreased secretion of bile acids and lecithin accompanied by a deficiency of an antinucleating factor or an increased secretion of pronucleating mucin and biliary sludge (Fig. 19–44). Added to this equation are the potential nucleating influences of calcium salts and bacteria (when the bile is infected).[179]

Much less is known about pigment stone formation. Critical is an increased concentration of unconjugated bilirubin in the bile.[180] However, most of the bilirubin secreted into the bile is conjugated. Conceivably, when there is hemolysis of red cells and an increased bilirubin load presented to the hepatocyte, more bilirubin is secreted in unconjugated form. Alternatively, glucuronidase, which deconjugates bilirubin, may be secreted into the bile, but these notions are somewhat speculative. In Orientals, infection of the biliary tract by liver flukes—*Opisthorchis sinensis*—is an additional influence favoring formation of pigment stones.

> **MORPHOLOGY.** Although gallstones may form anywhere in the biliary system, the great preponderance of cholesterol stones arise in the gallbladder. They vary from "pure" to "mixed." **Pure cholesterol stones** are pale yel-

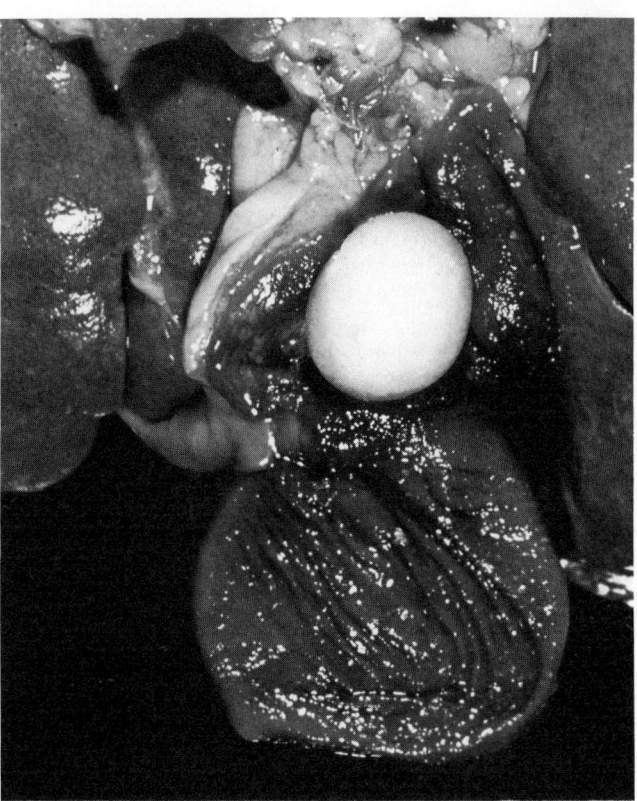

Figure 19–45. A pure cholesterol gallstone—pale yellow and semitransparent.

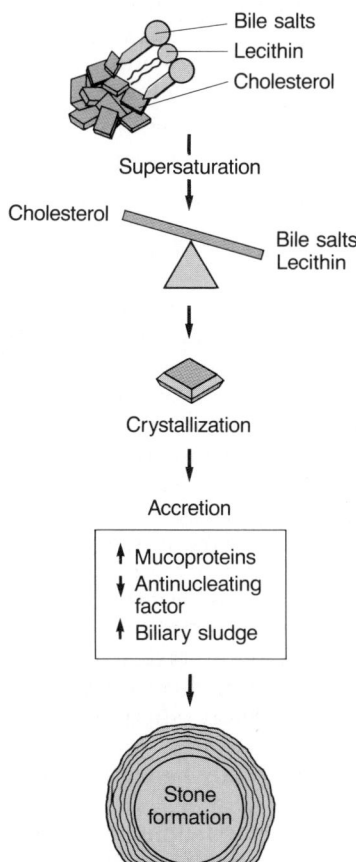

Figure 19–44. A schematic representation of the three stages in cholelithiasis: (1) supersaturation, (2) crystallization, (3) accretion.

low, are round to ovoid, and have a finely granular external surface (Fig. 19–45). Most often, multiple stones are present that range up to several centimeters in diameter. Rarely, there is a single much larger stone that may virtually fill the fundus. Transection of all "pure" stones usually reveals a glistening crystalline radiating palisade. **It should be noted that such stones are radiolucent.** More often, cholesterol stones contain varying proportions of calcium carbonate, phosphates, and bilirubin. Such "mixed" stones tend to occur in great numbers and are classically 1 to 3 cm in diameter, having rounded or faceted exteriors owing to tight apposition. The larger the calculi, the less likely they are to enter the cystic or common ducts to produce obstruction either to the cystic duct or, more seriously, to the common bile duct. It is the very small stones—"gravel"—that are more dangerous. On transection, "mixed" stones may appear lamellated and be variable gray-white to black depending on the proportions of cholesterol, bilirubin, and inorganic salts. Sufficient calcium carbonate is found in 10 to 20% of **"mixed" stones** to render them radiopaque. **Pigment stones** composed of "pure" calcium bilirubinate often appear as jet black ovoids. They are rarely greater than 1.5 cm in diameter and almost invariably are present in great number (Fig. 19–46). Sometimes they take the form of "jack-stones."

CLINICAL IMPLICATIONS. The clinical significance of gallstones has been disputed for decades. Specifically at issue is: Should gallstones be removed

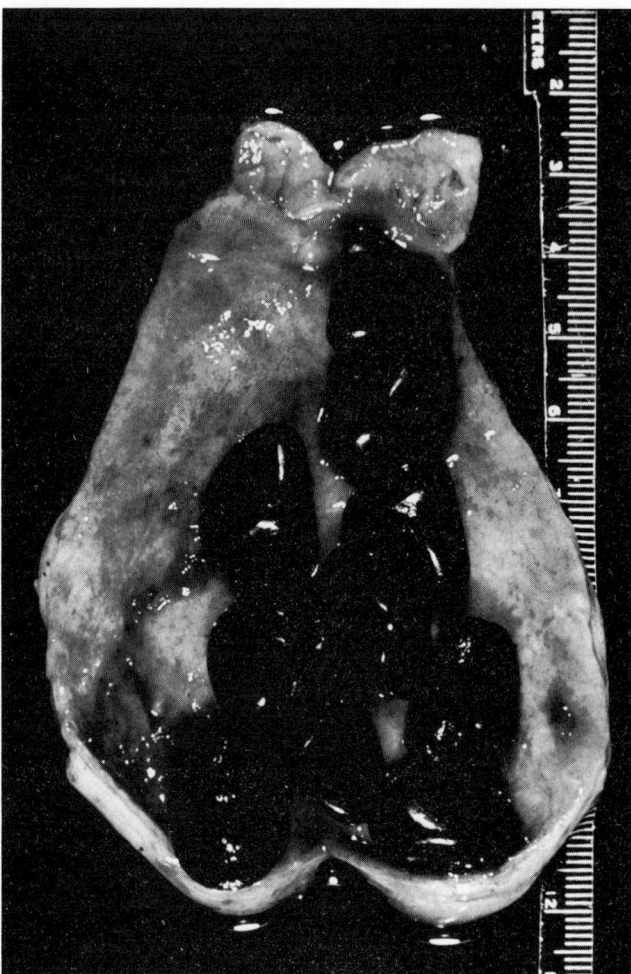

Figure 19–46. Pigment gallstones. They are jet black and are set against the background of a thickened fibrotic gallbladder with marked atrophy of the mucosa.

as soon as discovered? Most often, this means cholecystectomy. Although pure cholesterol stones can sometimes be dissolved by medical treatment such as the administration of chenodeoxycholate, this agent must be taken for one to two years, and it is effective in only about one third of cases with a 50% recurrence rate after cessation of therapy. Arguments in favor of cholecystectomy as soon as is feasible are:

• They may pass into and obstruct the common duct (recall that smaller stones are more threatening than large ones).
• When they enter the cystic or common bile duct, they often produce excruciating biliary colic. Whether stones in the gallbladder alone may cause symptoms is uncertain. Frequently these individuals complain of indigestion, intolerance of fatty foods, and episodes of nausea and vomiting, but such manifestations cannot be positively ascribed to the stones because they are also encountered in those lacking stones.
• Stones predispose to cholecystitis when they ob-

struct the neck of the gallbladder or cystic duct. Infrequently, obstruction of the gallbladder does not lead to infection, but instead to filling of the gallbladder by clear mucinous secretion referred to as *hydrops* or *mucocele* of the gallbladder. This constitutes one basis for nonvisualization of the gallbladder on oral cholecystography.
• By causing partial obstruction of the common bile duct, they may predispose to ascending suppurative cholangitis.
• Rarely, larger stones, after inducing cholecystitis, have eroded through the wall of the gallbladder and an adherent loop of intestine to obstruct the lumen of the small intestine (*"gallstone ileus"*).
• Most controversial of all, they may predispose to development of carcinoma of the gallbladder (p. 974).

It is said that symptomatic cholelithiasis incurs about a 30% risk of producing some complication requiring surgery within five years. On the other hand, about 50% of all gallstones are asymptomatic or "silent."[181] In one study with a 15-year follow-up, only 15% of individuals with "silent stones" developed symptomatic disease, and less than 3% had serious complications requiring cholecystectomy on an emergency basis. None died because of their gallstone disease. Thus the controversy continues, with one school advocating "watchful waiting" because of the low incidence of complications and because doubt still remains about the role of stones in the induction of gallbladder carcinoma, and the other school replying—"To wait is to play Russian roulette." Regrettably, as is so often the case, there are no certain guidelines.

ACUTE CHOLECYSTITIS

Cholecystitis may be acute, chronic, or acute superimposed on chronic. Chronic cholecystitis is far more common than acute disease, but the latter is more important because it often produces a surgical emergency. Acute cholecystitis in 90% of cases is initiated by impaction of a gallstone within the neck of the gallbladder or the cystic duct, and so is referred to clinically as *calculous acute cholecystitis*. In the remaining minority of cases, stones are not present— hence, *"acalculous acute cholecystitis."*

Acute calculous cholecystitis is one of the major clinical complications of cholelithiasis. Because of its relationship to gallstones, its distribution in the population follows that of cholelithiasis (p. 967), i.e., older, obese, female. It usually appears with remarkable suddenness and constitutes, in many instances, an acute surgical emergency because of its potential for rupture.

The precise events leading to the acute inflammation are little understood. Only this much is known: The process begins with calculous obstruction to the gallbladder neck or cystic duct. Bacteria—*E.*

coli, other gram-negative aerobic rods, enterococci, or a variety of anaerobes (chiefly clostridria) — can be identified in the bile in about 80% of cases early in the course.[182] Salmonella is a rare invader. This bacterial invasion is thought to be a secondary event, since it is not present in the remaining 20%. Other factors then must initiate the acute reaction. *Without substantial proof, the formation of inflammatory mediators such as lysolecithin and prostaglandins, and increased intraluminal pressure with compromise of the blood supply, in concert with chemical irritation of bile acids, have been invoked.* In a few cases, enzymes of pancreatic origin, such as phospholipase, have been identified in the bile during the acute phase of the disease, but their pathogenetic significance has been doubted because they can also be identified sometimes in normal post-mortem gallbladders. It is clear that much remains uncertain, but *there is fairly general agreement that bacterial infection is a secondary and not a triggering event.*

Acalculous acute cholecystitis is much less common (10%) than the variant associated with stones. Unlike its "calculated" cousin, acute acalculous cholecystitis tends to occur somewhat more often in males (especially over the age of 65) and in children. Notable associations are previous surgery, prolonged labor, severe trauma (including burns), systemic arteritis (particularly polyarteritis nodosa), bacteremia, diabetes mellitus, and intravenous hyperalimentation.[183] Uncommon predisposing conditions include salmonellosis, cholera, and parasitic infestation of the gallbladder. Common to most of these predispositions is the likelihood of transient invasion of the bloodstream by organisms, with seeding of the gallbladder. Favoring this localization of organisms is evidence suggesting that despite the absence of gallstones, cystic duct obstruction is frequently present, but its mechanism remains unclear.[184] Functional obstruction and distention of the gallbladder might compromise the vascular supply to the mucosa and provide a favorable environment for bacterial seeding. *Save for the absence of stones, acalculous cholecystitis is the same morphologically as the calculous variant.*

In **acute calculous cholecystitis,** the gallbladder is usually enlarged (two- to threefold) and tense, and often assumes a bright red or blotchy, violaceous to green-black discoloration, imparted by subserosal hemorrhages. The serosal covering is frequently layered by fibrin and, in the very intense reaction, by a definite suppurative, coagulated exudate. In the calculous variety, an obstructive stone is almost always present in the neck of the gallbladder or cystic duct. The gallbladder lumen, in addition to other possible gallstones, is tensely filled with a cloudy or turbid bile that may contain large amounts of fibrin and frank pus, as well as hemorrhage. When the contained exudate is virtually pure pus, the condition is referred to as **empyema of the gallbladder.** The gallbladder wall is thickened and edematous. The mucosa may be merely patchily or totally

hyperemic in the milder cases, transformed to a green-black necrotic surface in more severe cases **(gangrenous cholecystitis),** or have small-to-large ulcerations. In this fashion infections may penetrate the wall to give rise to pericholecystic, subhepatic, or subdiaphragmatic abscesses or generalized peritonitis, or worse, the gallbladder may rupture.[185] Other possible complications are ascending cholangitis, liver abscess, and septicemia.

Histologically, the inflammatory reactions are not distinctive and consist of the usual patterns of acute inflammation, i.e., edema, leukocytic infiltration, vascular congestion, frank abscess formation, or gangrenous necrosis, when vascular stasis complicates the edematous inflammatory response.

The inflammatory reaction may subside and the neutrophils then are replaced by scattered lymphocytes, macrophages, and occasional eosinophils. Alternatively, in other cases, the deposition of calcium within the gallbladder wall gives rise to the so-called calcified gallbladder or **porcelain gallbladder.** In an unknown number of instances, the subsidence of the acute response leads to chronic cholecystitis.

The signs and symptoms of acute calculous cholecystitis and acalculous cholecystitis are much the same. Most patients present with right upper quadrant pain, tenderness, leukocytosis, and sometimes a palpably enlarged, exceedingly tender gallbladder. The pain often radiates to the right shoulder, right scapula, or interscapular area. Fever and mild jaundice may or may not be present. In patients with stones there may be a history of past episodes of biliary colic, fatty food intolerance, and other manifestations of previous chronic cholecystitis with cholelithiasis.[186] In some instances, the acalculous disease is far more insidious because these patients tend to already have some previous serious condition such as prior surgery, severe trauma, and bacteremia, whose manifestations tend to submerge those related to the gallbladder disease.

Ultimately the diagnosis rests on the documentation of abnormal gallbladder function, enlargement of the gallbladder, thickening of its walls, and in most instances associated cholelithiasis. The diagnostic modalities in widest use are oral and infusion cholecystography, ultrasonography, and CT scan. Even when the diagnosis is established, the difficult question arises: Should the inflamed gallbladder be removed as soon as is feasible to lessen the likelihood of pericholecystic spread of infection or rupture, or can the patient be managed medically for a period of time with antibacterial therapy so that surgery can be performed on a nonemergent basis? Large-scale studies indicate that approximately 75% of patients treated medically have remission of acute symptoms, but in the remaining 25% a complication such as spreading infection or rupture necessitates prompt surgical intervention. Even those who have a remission are likely to have a recurrence within the next few years.

However, the mortality for emergent surgery is of the order of 3 to 5%, but for elective surgery, after some control of the crisis situation has been achieved, it is less than 1%. There are no comforting landmarks as to which approach should be followed, and each clinician "walks his own wilderness."[187]

CHRONIC CHOLECYSTITIS

Chronic cholecystitis may be a sequel to repeated bouts of mini-acute cholecystitis, but in most instances it develops in the apparent absence of antecedent attacks of acute inflammation. *Virtually always it is associated with cholelithiasis and so is encountered most often in middle-aged and older obese females (female:male ratio, 3:1).* The evolution of chronic cholecystitis is even more obscure than that of acute cholecystitis. Although virtually always associated with gallstones, it is doubtful that they play a direct role in the initiation of inflammatory disease within the gallbladder wall. More likely, supersaturation of the bile predisposes to both the inflammation and the stone formation. Thus, bile acids and lysolecithin may cause chemical injury, but proof is lacking. Microorganisms, usually *E. coli* and enterococci, or rarely salmonella, can be cultured from the bile in only about one third of the cases. It is evident that the cause of chronic cholecystitis is little understood.

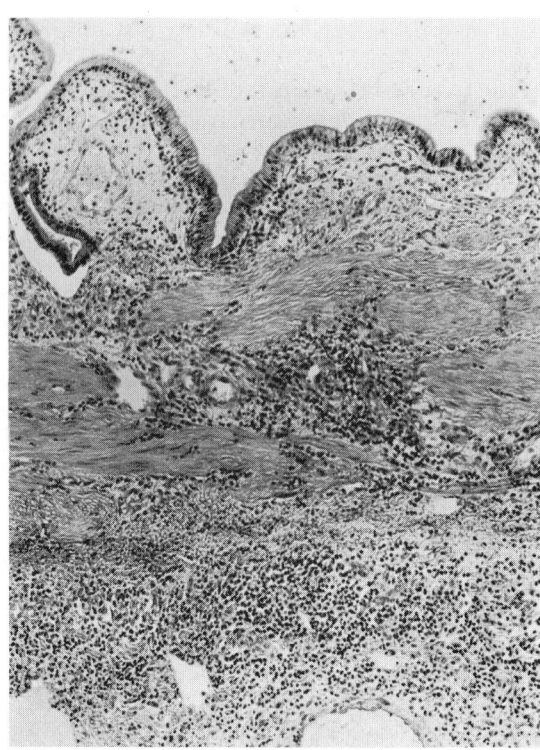

Figure 19–47. Chronic cholecystitis with increased subepithelial fibrosis and marked leukocytic infiltration. Mucosal folds are somewhat flattened.

The morphologic changes in chronic cholecystitis are extremely variable. Generally the mere presence of stones within the gallbladder, in the absence of acute inflammation, is taken as sufficient justification for the diagnosis, and in such circumstances there may be only minimal evidence of mural chronic inflammation. The gallbladder may be contracted, normal in size, or enlarged. The size of the organ depends on the balance between the development of fibrosis in the wall and the element of obstruction in the genesis of the inflammation. The serosa is usually smooth and glistening, but often it is dulled by subserosal fibrosis. In other instances, dense fibrosis adhesions may remain as sequelae of pre-existent acute inflammation. On section, the wall is variably thickened, rarely to more than three times normal. It has an opaque gray-white cut section and may be less flexible and translucent than normal. In the uncomplicated case, the lumen usually contains fairly clear, green-yellow, mucoid bile. Stones are present in almost all cases (Fig. 19–47). The mucosa itself is usually preserved and has no loss of the usual mucosal folds that create the normal honeycombed pattern. In other instances, when the lumen of the gallbladder is partially or totally obstructed, the gallbladder contents may be under sufficient pressure to cause flattening of the mucosal folds and thinning and atrophy of the mucosa.

Histologically, the degree of inflammatory reaction is quite variable. In the mildest cases, only scattered lymphocytes, plasma cells, and macrophages are found beneath the columnar lining epithelium and in the subserosal fibrous tissue. In better developed cases, there is some increase of fibrous tissue subepithelially and subserosally, accompanied by a mononuclear cell infiltration. Inflammatory proliferation of the mucosa and fusion of the mucosal folds may give rise to buried crypts of epithelium within the gallbladder wall, designated as **cholecystitis glandularis.** Dystrophic calcification within the gallbladder wall may yield a **"porcelain gallbladder"** identical to that which follows acute cholecystitis.

Sometimes the anatomic changes of acute cholecystitis are superimposed upon the chronic changes just described, implying acute exacerbation of a previously chronically injured gallbladder. This pattern of reaction is called **acute on chronic cholecystitis.**

Chronic cholecystitis is more a morphologic than a clinical entity. Although heartburn, belching, intolerance to fatty foods, and vague epigastric discomfort are frequently attributed to chronic cholecystitis, these manifestations occur with equal frequency in patients having no gallstones and presumably no inflammatory involvement of the gallbladder. Nonetheless, the condition may be discovered in the course of the investigation of such complaints. Thus, chronic cholecystitis is a diagnosis that is sometimes made only after the gallbladder has been removed or at autopsy. Its clinical significance derives from the accompanying gallstones.

MISCELLANEOUS DISORDERS OF THE GALLBLADDER

Cholesterolosis of the gallbladder is virtually without clinical significance, but it is an entity that delights the pathologist. It refers to focal accumulations of lipid-laden macrophages within the tips of mucosal folds directly beneath the columnar epithelium (Fig. 19–48). When viewed from the surface, the mucosa is studded with minute yellow flecks having some fancied resemblance to the surface of a strawberry — hence the synonym *"strawberry gallbladder."*[188] The origin of this fascinating change is uncertain, but it has been attributed without proof to imbibition of cholesterol from supersaturated bile. As far as is known, it causes no symptoms and does not predispose to cholecystitis or functional derangement.

Inflammatory polyps constitute sessile mucosal projections, with a surface of columnar epithelial cells covering a fibrous stroma infiltrated with chronic inflammatory cells. Sometimes the stroma is composed of lipid-laden macrophages analogous to those seen in cholesterolosis. Rupture of these fatty macrophages may produce xanthogranulomas. These lesions are of

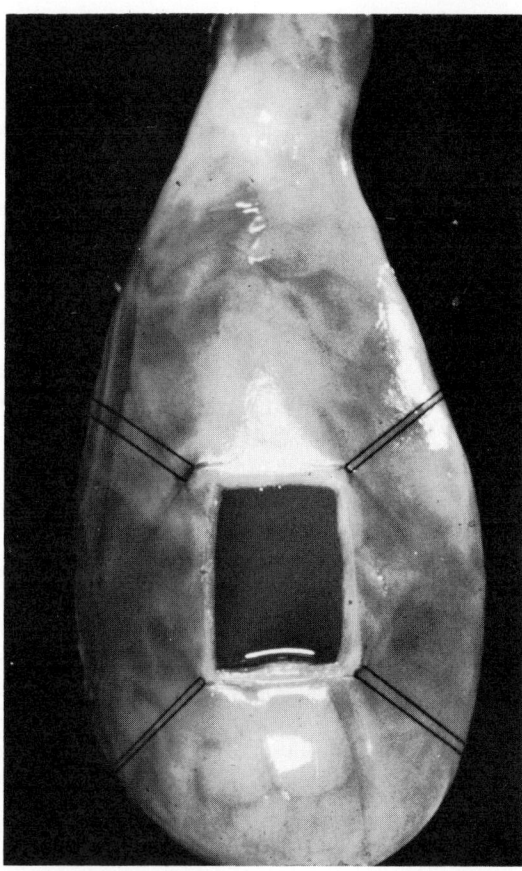

Figure 19–49. Hydrops of gallbladder. A window has been cut out to reveal the clear, translucent, mucoid contents.

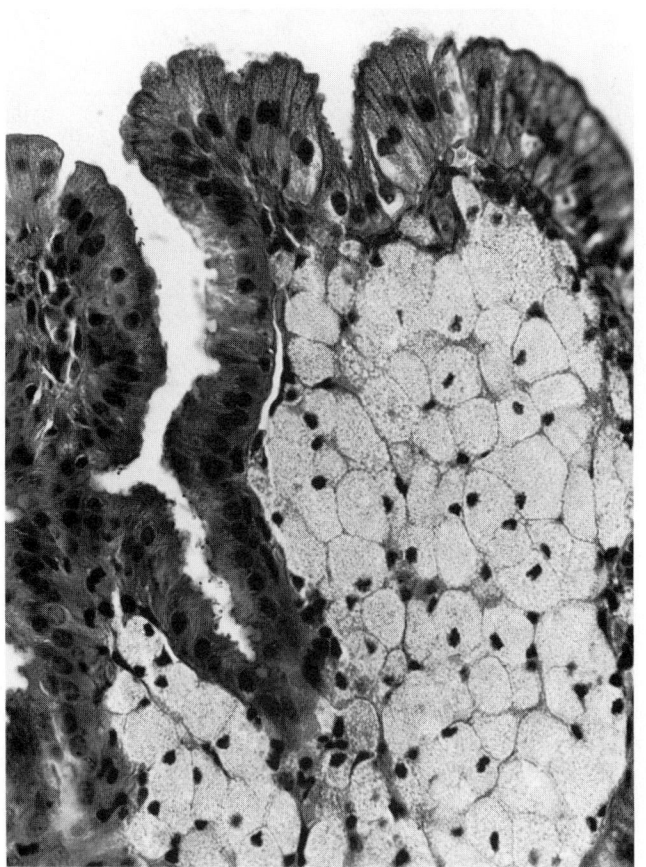

Figure 19–48. Cholesterolosis of the gallbladder. Beneath the epithelial mucosa are aggregates of lipid-laden histiocytes.

clinical significance only because they must be differentiated from neoplasms when visualized on cholecystograms, ultrasonography, or CT scans. On occasion, the overlying epithelium may be somewhat hyperplastic, but there is no evidence that they predispose to the development of tumors.

Hydrops or mucocele of the gallbladder was mentioned earlier (p. 970) as distention of the gallbladder by a clear, watery, mucinous secretion when the neck of the gallbladder or cystic duct becomes totally obstructed, usually by an impacted stone (Fig. 19–49). Stones are usually present within the lumen of the gallbladder. Presumably the trapped bile is resorbed, and the gallbladder becomes filled with secretions derived from the lining mucosal cells. Indeed, the gallbladder may become quite distended, with an extremely thin atrophic wall and virtual total atrophy of the lining epithelium. Occasional individuals have manifested epigastric pain, discomfort, nausea and vomiting, and other features suggestive of cholelithiasis or chronic cholecystitis, but it is highly likely that these signs and symptoms relate more to the deranged gallbladder function caused by the calculous obstruction than to the hydrops itself.

TUMORS

Although fibromas, myomas, neuromas, hemangiomas, and the malignant counterparts of these lesions as well as carcinoids have been described in the biliary tract, the only neoplasms of sufficient frequency and clinical importance to merit description are the papilloma, adenoma, and adenomyoma of the gallbladder; carcinoma of the gallbladder; and carcinoma of the bile ducts and ampulla of Vater.

PAPILLOMA, ADENOMA, AND ADENOMYOMA OF GALLBLADDER

Papillomas and adenomas of the gallbladder are very infrequent, benign epithelial tumors. They both represent localized overgrowths of the lining epithelium. Although these lesions are small and easily missed, there is a greater tendency to overdiagnose these conditions, since inflammatory polyps or edema of the wall may create local projections that can be interpreted as benign neoplasms. The papilloma may occur singly or multiply as small, branching, pedunculated masses less than 1 cm in diameter that project into the lumen of the gallbladder. They are usually connected to the underlying wall by a slender stalk. In contrast, the adenoma is a broad-based, hemispheric elevation, again less than 1 cm in diameter, that is firmly attached to the underlying wall.

Both are composed histologically of a vascularized connective tissue stroma covered by a single layer of well-oriented, well-differentiated columnar lining epithelial cells. The adenoma also has contained glands in the stroma. Rarely, there is concomitant proliferation of the smooth muscle cells to create a leiomyomatous tumor enclosing nests of ductules lined by columnar epithelial cells—the so-called *adenomyoma*. These benign neoplasms may be detected on cholangiography or CT scan and then require differentiation from more ominous malignancies. A recent study suggests a close relationship between adenomyomas and carcinomas.[189] Papillomas, by fragmentation, may provide a nidus for the formation of a gallstone.

CARCINOMA OF GALLBLADDER

Among cancers of the extrahepatic biliary tract, carcinoma of the gallbladder is much more prevalent than cancer arising in the ducts (2 to 4:1). It is an uncommon form of neoplasia but nonetheless constitutes a

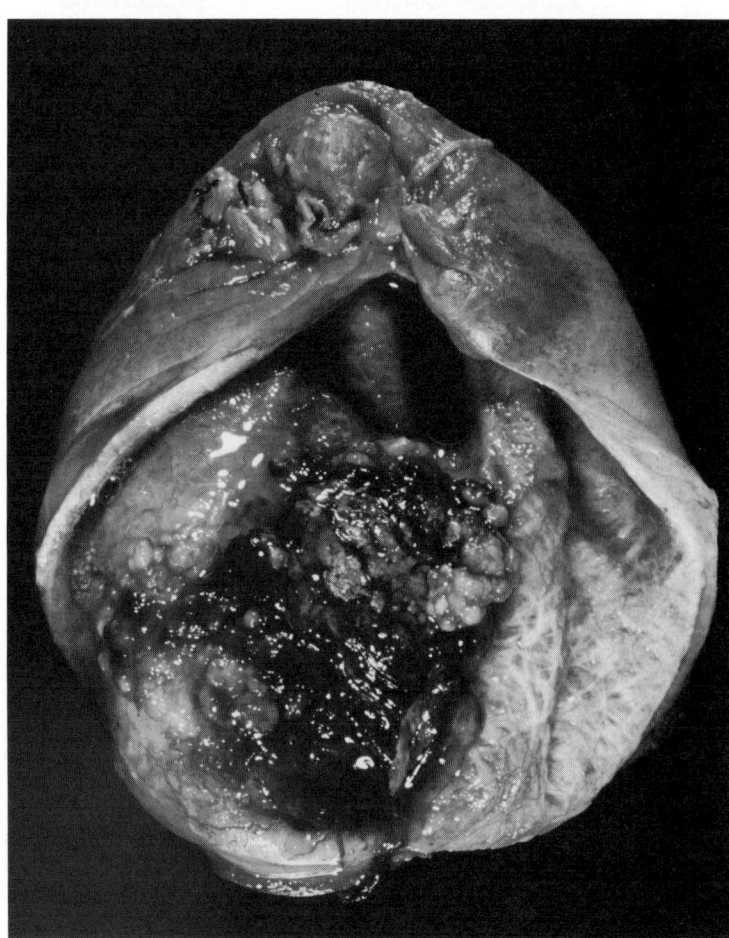

Figure 19–50. Carcinoma of the gallbladder as seen with the opened fundus. The neoplasm has fungated into the lumen and is partially hemorrhagic.

major medical challenge; only rarely is it discovered at a resectable stage, and so the mean five-year survival (whether surgery is performed or not) has remained for many years at the disappointing level of about 1%.[190] It is about twice as common in women as in men, with a peak incidence in the seventh decade of life.

A number of influences are thought to predispose to this form of cancer. Most important, but still poorly understood, are gallstones and the associated inflammation. Cholelithiasis and chronic cholecystitis are present in 75 to 90% of cases of carcinoma of the gallbladder.[191] Conversely, carcinomas of the gallbladder are found in about 0.5% of patients with gallstones. However, it is not clear whether the stones and inflammation directly predispose to the carcinomatous change, or are the consequence of influences that also predispose to the development of cancer. It may be significant that derivatives of cholic acid are powerful experimental carcinogenic agents.

Morphologically, carcinomas of the gallbladder are usually divided into two gross patterns, infiltrating and fungating. The most common sites of involvement are the fundus and neck; about 20% involve the lateral walls. The **infiltrating type** is more common and usually appears as a poorly defined area of diffuse thickening and induration of the gallbladder wall that, when discovered, may cover several square centimeters or may involve the entire gallbladder or large portions of it. Deep ulceration may cause direct penetration of the gallbladder wall or fistula formation to adjacent viscera into which the neoplasm has grown. These tumors are scirrhous and therefore have an extremely firm consistency. Often the tumor extends beneath the serosa in small, irregular, nodular projections, or it may directly penetrate the gallbladder wall to invade the liver bed.

The **fungating pattern** grows into the lumen as an irregular, small cauliflower mass, but at the same time invades the underlying wall. The luminal portion may be necrotic, hemorrhagic, and ulcerated (Fig. 19–50). By the time these neoplasms are discovered, **most have invaded the liver centrifugally,** and many have extended to the cystic duct and adjacent bile ducts and portahepatic lymph nodes. These neoplasms are entirely asymptomatic and can thus grow for a long time until discovered by their extension into surrounding structures. If the cystic duct is occluded, the trapped bile is resorbed, producing hydrops of the gallbladder.

The great preponderance are adenocarcinomas. Some are papillary and others are infiltrative and poorly differentiated or undifferentiated (Fig. 19–51). About 5% are squamous cell carcinomas (arising in metaplastic epithelium) or have adenosquamous differentiation. Not surprisingly, the poorly differentiated adenocarcinomas tend to be associated with the widest metastatic dissemination; in contrast, those with squamous differentiation produce few metastases. Overall, the liver, perihilar and more distant lymph nodes, peritoneum, gastrointestinal tract, and lungs are the most frequent sites of seeding.

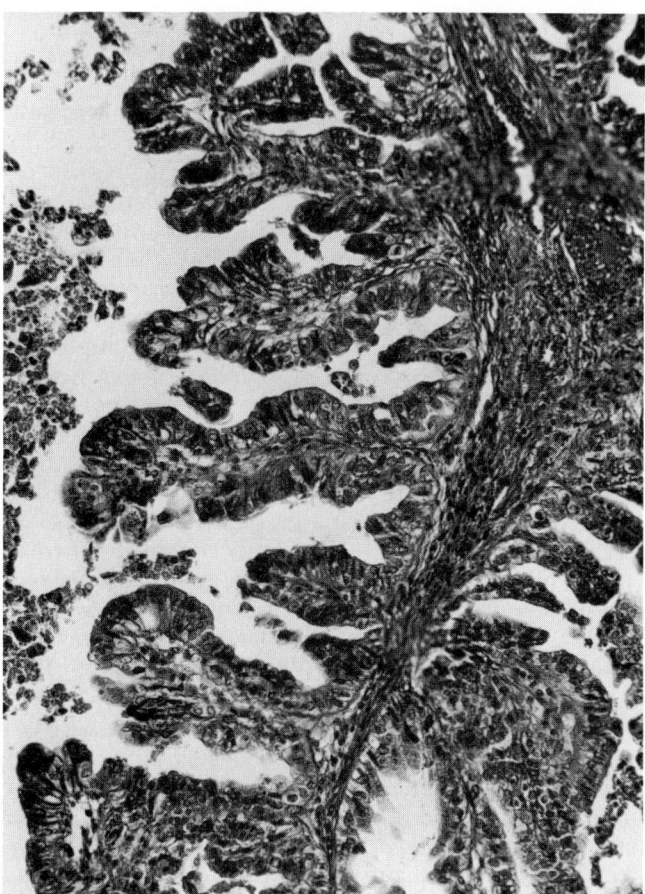

Figure 19–51. A detail of carcinoma of the gallbladder, showing well-developed papillary formations.

These carcinomas are extremely insidious and frequently asymptomatic until brought to attention by their spread into bile ducts. Thus, neoplasms are sometimes found unexpectedly either at laparotomy for other disease or in gallbladders removed for cholelithiasis. Occasionally, hepatic enlargement due to metastases is the first indication of the neoplasm. The most frequent presenting symptom is abdominal pain, followed by jaundice, anorexia, weight loss, palpable gallbladder, and nausea and vomiting, but none of these manifestations is present in a significant number of patients.[192] The lucky symptomatic patient develops a palpable gallbladder and acute cholecystitis secondary to extension of the tumor into the cystic duct before it has spread elsewhere. The diagnosis rests largely on cholecystography documenting gallstones in addition to abnormalities of the gallbladder wall profile. Ultrasonography to identify dilated bile ducts and CT scans are also helpful. Because present methods of treatment, i.e., surgical resection perhaps followed by radiation or chemotherapy, are rarely curative, some contend that earlier cholecystectomy for gallstones would have prevented the development of this form of carcinoma in one patient in 200 (0.5% incidence with gallstones)—but which one?

CARCINOMA OF BILE DUCTS AND AMPULLA OF VATER

The designation carcinoma of the bile ducts is meant to include involvement of any of the extrahepatic bile ducts as well as the intraduodenal segment. The latter form is usually distinguished as *carcinoma of the peri-ampulla of Vater*. These malignancies are uncommon but far outnumber in frequency all the other rare benign neoplastic involvements of these structures (papilloma and adenoma). The same age range is affected as in carcinoma of the gallbladder, but, although this last-mentioned neoplasm is more common in females, carcinomas of the bile ducts are slightly more frequent in males.[193] There is no convincing association between gallstones and bile duct cancer, since they are found in only 35 to 50% of cases. On the other hand, there is a suggestion that chronic inflammation within the ducts and bile acids may constitute predisposing influences. In the Orient, infections by *Ascaris* and *Opisthorchis sinensis* are thought to constitute significant predispositions.[194] For unknown reasons, patients with ulcerative colitis are at slightly increased risk.

The sites of biliary tract tumors differ among reported series, but in general, in descending order of frequency, are gallbladder, ampulla of Vater, common duct, hepatic ducts, and junction of the hepatic and common ducts (Klatskin tumor)[194] (Figure 19–52). Carcinomatous involvement of ductal structures

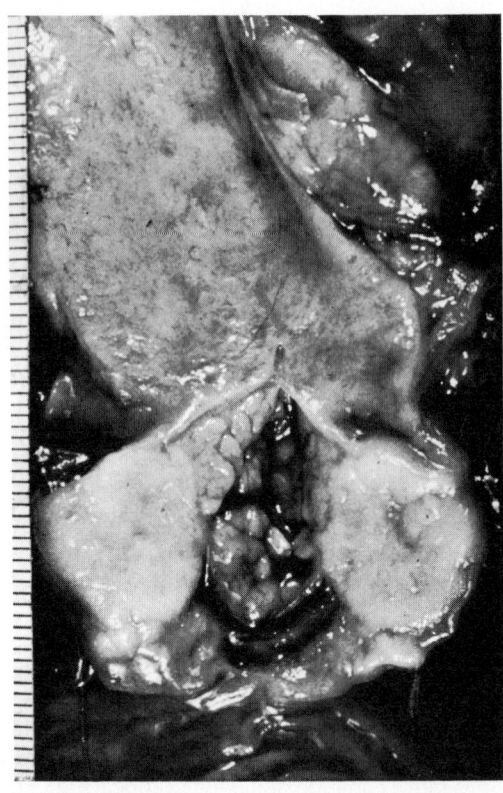

Figure 19–53. Carcinoma of papilla of Vater. Widened common bile duct comes down from above. Neoplasm has been split open to demonstrate 1.5 cm size of mass.

in the aggregate occurs less often than carcinoma of the gallbladder. Although these tumors, because of their strategic location, would be expected to come to clinical attention early, about 75% have invaded contiguous structures, e.g., liver, or metastasized to liver, lungs, regional nodes, and elsewhere by the time they are discovered.

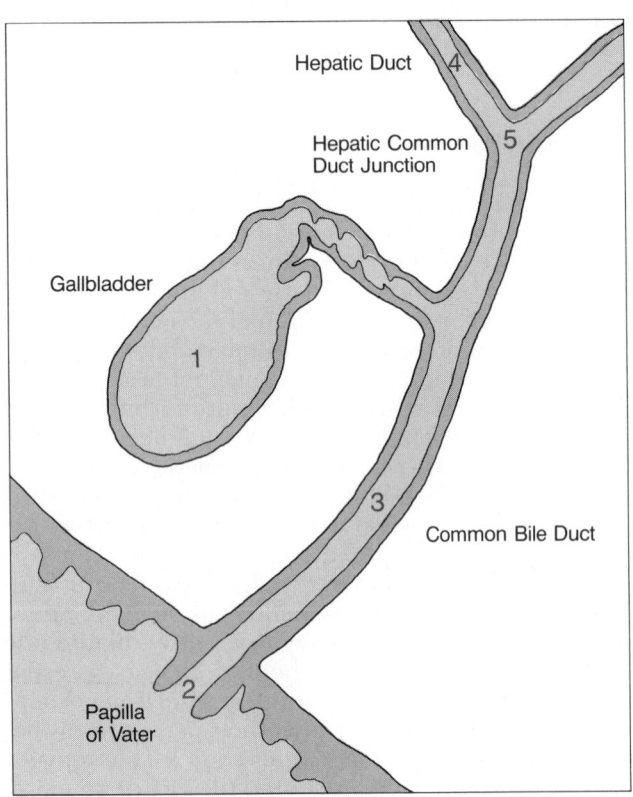

Figure 19–52. The rank order of frequency of cancer in the biliary apparatus.

They take one of three forms: (1) papillary fungating, (2) intraductal nodules, and (3) diffuse infiltrative lesions of the wall of the ducts. In the region of the papilla they generally take the form of small hemispheric masses narrowing the orifice and protruding into the duodenal lumen. Only rarely do they exceed 2 to 3 cm in diameter and 1 cm in height (Fig. 19–53). In most instances the overlying duodenal mucosa is intact, but occasionally permeation of the duodenal wall may cause ulcerations and, for this reason, is associated with melena. Whatever the location, obstruction may give rise to dilatation of the more proximal biliary structures. Cancers arising in the cystic duct may produce hydrops of the gallbladder.

Histologically, most of these neoplasms are adenocarcinomas that may or may not be mucin secreting. Some have papillary characteristics and, uncommonly, squamous metaplasia gives rise to squamous cell carcinomas or adenosquamous lesions. For the most part, an abundant fibrous stroma accompanies the epithelial proliferation.

When symptoms appear with these neoplasms, they are usually related to ductal obstruction (85 to 100% of cases), namely, obstructive jaundice, often preceded by decolorization of the stools, nausea and vomiting, and weight loss. Hepatomegaly is present in about 50% and a palpable gallbladder in about 25%.[190] Associated changes are elevated levels of serum alkaline phosphatase, bile-stained urine, elevated serum aminotransferase, and prolonged prothrombin time.

The differentiation of obstructive jaundice due to neoplasia from calculous disease is a major clinical problem. In this differential diagnosis it is important to rule in or out the presence of stones in the gallbladder or ducts, using one of the many diagnostic modalities mentioned. However, the mere presence of gallstones does not preclude the existence of concomitant neoplasia. The cancers can sometimes be diagnosed by transhepatic or retrograde cholangiography, ultrasonography, and, in some cases, CT scan or MRI, but most often all that can be established is abnormal dilatation of ducts (ultrasonography is said to be 95% accurate).[195] Examination of duodenal drainage for tumor cells or for crystalline debris accompanying gallstones is sometimes of use in the differential diagnosis. Ultimately, however, surgical exploration may be necessary. Most of these ductal cancers are not surgically resectable at the time of clinical diagnosis. The average postoperative survival is six months to one year. Cancer of the periampullary region, however, offers a somewhat better prognosis. Depending on the extent of invasion, the five-year survival following surgical resection (Whipple procedure) is 85% for localized lesions and falls to 10 to 25% for more infiltrative neoplasms.

1. Rapaport, A.M.: The structural and functional units of the human liver (liver acinus). Microvasc. Res. *6:*212, 1973.

2. Adler, M., et al.: Pericanalicular, hepatocytic, and bile ductular microfilaments in cholestasis in man. Am. J. Pathol. *98:*603, 1980.

3. Gollan, J.L., and Knapp, A.B.: Bilirubin metabolism and congenital jaundice. Hosp. Pract. *20:*83, 1985.

4. Spivak, W.: Bilirubin metabolism. Pediatr. Annu. *14:*451, 1985.

5. Hauser, S.C., and Gollan, J.L.: Recent developments in hyperbilirubinemia and bilirubin metabolism. *In* Gitnick, G. (ed.): Current Hepatology. 4th Ed. New York, John Wiley & Sons, 1984, p. 453.

6. Fevery, J., et al.: New clinical aspects of bilirubin metabolism. Acta Gastroenterol. Belg. *48:*258, 1985.

7. Paumgartner, G., and Paumgartner, D.: Current concepts of bile formation. *In* Popper, H., and Schaffner, F. (eds.): Progress in Liver Diseases. Vol. 7. New York, Grune & Stratton, 1982, p. 207.

8. Zimmerman, H.J.: Intrahepatic cholestasis. Arch. Intern. Med. *139:*1038, 1979.

9. Nachbauer, C.A., and Fischer, J.E.: The failing liver. Surg. Clin. North Am. *61:*221, 1981.

10. Koppel, M.H., et al.: Transplantation of cadaveric kidneys from patients with hepatorenal syndrome: Evidence for the functional nature of renal failure in advanced liver disease. N. Engl. J. Med. *280:*1367, 1969.

11. Zipser, R.D., et al.: Urinary thromboxane D_2 and prostaglandin E_2 in the hepatorenal syndrome: Evidence for increased vasoconstriction and decreased vasodilator factors. Gastroenterology *84:*697, 1983.

12. Editorial: Hepatorenal syndrome or hepatic nephropathy. Lancet *1:*801, 1980.

13. Schenker S., and Hoyumpa, A.M., Jr.: Pathophysiology of hepatic encephalopathy. Hosp. Pract. *19:*99, 1984.

14. Sherlock, S.: Hepatic encephalopathy. *In* Csomos, G., and Thaler, H. (eds.): Clinical Hepatology. Berlin, Springer-Verlag, 1983, p. 291.

15. Jones, E.A., and Shafer, D.F.: Hepatic encephalopathy: A neurochemical disorder. *In* Popper, H., and Schaffner, F. (eds.): Progress in Liver Diseases. Vol. 8. Orlando, Grune & Stratton, 1986, p. 525.

16. Fraser, C.L., and Arieff, A.I.: Hepatic encephalopathy. N. Engl. J. Med. *313:*865, 1985.

17. Odell, G.B., and Childs, B.: Hereditary hyperbilirubinemias. *In* Steinberg, A.G., et al. (eds.): Progress in Medical Genetics. Vol. 4. Philadelphia, W.B. Saunders Company, 1980, p. 103.

18. Wolkoff, A.W.: Inheritable disorders manifested by conjugated hyperbilirubinemia. Semin. Liver Dis. *3:*65, 1983.

19. Arcidi, J.M., et al.: Hepatic morphology in cardiac dysfunction. A clinicopathologic study of 1,000 subjects at autopsy. Am. J. Pathol. *104:*159, 1981.

20. Milliken, W.G.: Approach to the spectrum of Budd-Chiari syndrome: Which patients require portal decompression. Am. J. Surg. *149:*167, 1985.

21. Rector, W.G., et al.: Membranous obstruction of the inferior vena cava in the United States. Medicine *64:*134, 1985.

22. Gupta, S., et al.: Budd-Chiari syndrome: Long term survival and factors affecting mortality. Q. J. Med. (New Series) *60:*781, 1986.

23. Woods, W.G., et al.: Fatal veno-occlusive disease of the liver following high dose chemotherapy, irradiation, and bone marrow transplantation. Am. J. Med. *68:*285, 1980.

24. Witte, C.L., et al.: Protean manifestations of pylethrombosis, a review of 34 patients. Ann. Surg. *202:*191, 1985.

25. Soltis, R.D.: New concepts in viral hepatitis. Geriatrics *36:*62, 1981.

26. Lemon, S.M.: Type A viral hepatitis. New developments in an old disease. N. Engl. J. Med. *313:*1059, 1985.

27. Kao, H.W., et al.: The persistence of hepatitis A IgM antibody after acute clinical hepatitis A. Hepatology *4:*933, 1984.

28. Lešničar, G.: A prospective study of viral hepatitis A and the question of chronicity. Hepatogastroenterology *35:*69, 1988.

29. Feinstone, S.M.: Hepatitis A. *In* Popper H., and Schaffner, F. (eds.): Progress in Liver Diseases. Vol. 8. Orlando, Grune & Stratton, 1986, p. 299.

30. Ticehurst, J.R.: Hepatitis A virus: Clones, cultures, and vaccines. Semin. Liver Dis. *6:*46, 1986.

31. Grady, G.F.: The here and now of hepatitis B immunization. N. Engl. J. Med. *315:*250, 1986.

32. Standring, D.N., and Ritter, W.J.: The molecular analysis of hepatitis B virus. *In* Popper H., and Schaffner, F. (eds.): Progress in Liver Diseases. Vol. 8. Orlando, Grune & stratton, 1986, p. 311.

33. Gerber, M.A., and Thung, S.N.: Molecular and cellular pathology of hepatitis B. Lab. Invest. *52:*572, 1985.

33a. Thung, S.N., and Gerber, M.A.: Hepatitis B virus and polyalbumin receptors. *In* Popper, H., and Schaffner, F. (eds.): Progress in Liver Diseases. Vol. 8. Orlando, Grune & Stratton, 1986, p. 335.

34. Desmet, V.J.: Liver lesions in hepatitis B viral infection. Yale J. Biol. Med. *61:*61, 1988.

35. Mondelli, M., and Eddleston, A.L.W.F.: Mechanisms of liver cell injury in acute and chronic hepatitis B. Semin. Liver Dis. *4:*47, 1984.

36. Govindarajan, S., et al.: Identification of T lymphocytes and subsets in liver biopsy cores of acute viral hepatitis. Liver *3:*13, 1983.

37. Rizzetto, M.: The delta agent. Hepatology *3:*729, 1983.

38. Craig, J.R., et al.: Delta viral hepatitis. Histopathology and course. Pathol. Annu. *21:*1, 1986.

39. Bonino, F., and Smedile, A.: Delta agent (type D) hepatitis. Semin. Liver Dis. *6:*28, 1986.

40. Rosina, F., et al.: Risk of post-transfusion infection with the hepatitis delta virus: A multicenter study. N. Engl. J. Med. *312:*1488, 1985.

41. Wang, K.S.: Structure, sequence, and expression of the hepatitis delta viral genome. Nature *323:*508, 1986.

42. Rizetto, M.: The clinical significance of delta agent in liver disease. *In* Brunner, H., and Thaler, H. (eds.): Hepatology: A Festschrift for Hans Popper. New York, Raven Press, 1985, p. 153.

43. Dienstag, J.L., and Alter, H.J.: Non-A, non-B, hepatitis: Evolving epidemiologic and clinical perspective. Semin. Liver Dis. *6:*67, 1986.

44. Tabor, E.: The three viruses of non-A, non-B hepatitis. Lancet 1:743, 1985.

45. Bernau, J., et al.: Fulminant and subfulminant liver failure: definitions and causes. Semin. Liver Dis. 6:97, 1986.

46. Shih, J. W.-K., et al.: Non-A, non-B hepatitis: Advances and unfulfilled expectations of the first decade. In Popper, H., and Schaffner, F. (eds.): Progress in Liver Diseases. Vol. 8. Orlando, Grune & Stratton, 1986, p. 433.

47. Tremolada, F., et al.: Blood-transmitted and clotting-factor-transmitted non-A, non-B hepatitis. Clinical differences and evolution. J. Clin. Gastroenterol. 10:413, 1988.

47a. Bradley, D.W. and Balayan, M.S.: Virus of externally transmitted non-A, non-B hepatitis. Lancet 1:819, 1988.

48. Szmuness, W.: Recent advances in the study of the epidemiology of hepatitis B. Am. J. Pathol. 81:629, 1975.

49. Kostich, N.D., and Ingram, C.D.: Detection of hepatitis B surface antigen by means of orcein staining of liver. Am. J. Clin. Pathol. 67:20, 1977.

50. Bianchi, L., and Gudat, F.: Sanded nuclei in hepatitis B: Eosinophilic inclusions in liver cell nuclei due to excess in hepatitis B core antigen formation. Lab. Invest. 35:1, 1976.

51. Naoumov, N.V.: In situ hybridisation in formalin fixed, paraffin wax embedded liver specimens: Method for detecting human and viral DNA using biotinylated probes. J Clin. Pathol. 41:793, 1988.

52. Arico, S., et al.: Clinical significance of antibody to the hepatitis delta virus in symptomless HBsAg carriers. Lancet 2:356, 1985.

53. Kryger, P., and Christofferson, P.: Liver histopathology of the hepatitis A virus infection. A comparison with hepatitis type B and non-A, non-B. J. Clin. Pathol. 36:650, 1983.

54. Okuno, T., et al.: Pathology of acute hepatitis A in humans. Comparison with acute hepatitis B. Am. J. Clin. Pathol. 81:162, 1984.

55. Huang, S.-N., Fisher, M.M.: Pathology of viral hepatitis. In Farber, E., et al. (eds.): Pathogenesis of Liver Disease. Baltimore, Williams & Wilkins, 1987, p. 153.

56. Searle, J., et al.: The significance of cell death by apoptosis in hepatobiliary disease. J. Gastroenterol. Hepatol. 2:77, 1987.

57. Boyer, J.L., and Klatskin, G.: Pattern of necrosis in acute viral hepatitis. Prognostic value of bridging (subacute hepatic necrosis). N. Engl. J. Med. 283:1063, 1970.

58. Peters, R.L.: Viral hepatitis: A pathologic spectrum. Am. J. Med. Sci. 270:17, 1975.

59. Reynolds, T.B.: Chronic hepatitis: Current dilemmas. Am. J. Med. 69:485, 1980.

60. Gerber, M.A.: Immunopathology of chronic hepatitis. In Farber, E., et al. (eds.): Pathogenesis of Liver Diseases. Baltimore, Williams & Wilkins, 1987, p. 54.

61. Dietrichson, O.: Chronic persistent hepatitis. A clinical, serologic, and prognosis study. Scand. J. Gastroenterol. 10:249, 1975.

62. Deodhar, K.P., et al.: Orcein staining of hepatitis B antigen in paraffin sections of liver biopsies. J. Clin. Pathol. 28:66, 1975.

63. Celle, G., et al.: Morphologic evaluation of CAH with and without therapy. A two-year follow-up. Hepatogastroenterology 27:283, 1980.

64. Czaja, A.J., et al.: Corticosteroid-treated chronic active hepatitis in remission. Uncertain prognosis of chronic persistent hepatitis. N. Engl. J. Med. 304:5, 1981.

64a. Olsson, R., et al.: Chronic active hepatitis in Sweden. The etiologic spectrum, clinical presentation, and laboratory profile. Scand. J. Gastroenterol. 23:463, 1988.

65. Schaffner, F.: Autoimmune chronic active hepatitis: Three decades of progress. In Popper, H., and Schaffner, F. (eds.): Progress in Liver Diseases. Vol. 8. Orlando, Grune & Stratton, 1986, p. 485.

66. Paronetto, F.: Cell-mediated immunity in liver disease. Hum. Pathol. 17:168, 1986.

67. Ruebner, B.H., and Montgomery, C.K.: Hepatitis. In Pathology of the Liver and Biliary Tract. New York, John Wiley & Sons, 1982, p. 33.

68. Dordal, E., et al.: Hepatic lesions in chronic inflammatory bowel disease. I. Clinical correlations with liver biopsy diagnoses in 103 patients. Gastroenterology 52:239, 1967.

69. Chock, E., et al.: Acute suppurative cholangitis. Surg. Clin. North Am. 61:885, 1981.

70. O'Connor, M.J., et al.: Acute bacterial cholangitis. Arch. Surg. 117:437, 1982.

71. Weisner, R.H., et al.: Diagnosis and treatment of primary sclerosing cholangitis. Semin. Liver Dis. 5:241, 1985.

72. Thompson, J.E., Jr., and Glasser, A.J.: Amebic abscess of the liver. J. Clin. Gastroenterol. 8:550, 1986.

73. Miedema, B.W., and Dineen, P.: The diagnosis and treatment of pyogenic liver abscesses. Ann. Surg. 200:328, 1984.

74. Bertel, C.K., et al.: Treatment of pyogenic hepatic abscesses. Arch. Surg. 121:554, 1986.

75. Editorial: Pyogenic liver abscess—a continuing problem of management. Lancet 1:1170, 1976.

76. Anthony, P.P., et al.: The morphology of cirrhosis: Definition, nomenclature, and classification. Bull. W.H.O. 55:521, 1977.

77. Leads from the MMWR: Trends in mortality from cirrhosis and alcoholism—United States, 1945–1983. J.A.M.A. 256:3337, 1986.

78. Riepe, S.P., and Galambos, J.T.: Cirrhosis. In Gitnick, G. (ed.): Current Hepatology. Vol. IV. New York, John Wiley & Sons, 1984, p. 117.

79. Popper, H., et al.: Cytoplasmic copper and its toxic effects. Studies in Indian childhood cirrhosis. Lancet 1:1205, 1979.

80. Kawaguchi, K., and Koike, M.: Glomerular lesions associated with cirrhosis. An immunohistochemical and clinicopathologic analysis. Hum. Pathol. 17:1137, 1986.

81. Groszman, R.J., and Atterbury, C.E.: The pathophysiology of portal hypertension: A basis for classification. Semin. Liver Dis. 2:177, 1982.

82. Witte, C., et al.: Lymph imbalance in the genesis and perpetuation of the ascites syndrome in hepatic cirrhosis. Gastroenterology 78:1059, 1980.

83. Rocco, V.K., and Ware, A.J.: Cirrhotic ascites. Ann. Intern. Med. 105:573, 1986.

84. Ring-Larsen, H., and Henriksen, J.H.: Pathogenesis of ascites formation and hepato-renal syndrome: Humoral and hemodynamic factors. Semin. Liver Dis. 6:341, 1986.

85. Hall, P.: Pathology and pathogenesis of alcoholic liver disease. In Hall, P. (ed.): Alcoholic Liver Disease. New York, John Wiley & Sons, 1985, p. 41.

86. Pimstone, N.R., and French, S.W.: Alcoholic liver disease. Med. Clin. North Am. 68:39, 1984.

87. Schaffner, F., and Thaler, H.: Nonalcoholic fatty liver disease. In Popper, H., and Schaffner, F. (eds.): Progress in Liver Diseases. Vol. 8. Orlando, Grune & Stratton, 1986, p. 283.

88. Rubin, E., and Lieber, C.S.: Alcohol-induced hepatic injury in nonalcoholic volunteers. N. Engl. J. Med. 278:1869, 1968.

89. Lieber, G.S.: Metabolism and metabolic effects of alcohol. Med. Clin. North Am. 68:3, 1984.

90. Mitchell, M.C., and Herlong, H.F.: Alcohol and nutrition: Caloric value, bioenergetics, and relationship to liver damage. Annu. Rev. Nutr. 6:457, 1986.

91. Baraona, E., et al.: Alcohol hepatomegaly: Accumulation of protein in the liver. Science 190:794, 1975.

92. Bruguera, M., et al.: Giant mitochondria in hepatocytes: A diagnostic hint for alcoholic liver disease. Gastroenterology 73:1383, 1977.

93. Worner, T.M., and Lieber, C.S.: Perivenular fibrosis as precursor lesion of cirrhosis. J.A.M.A. 254:627, 1985.

94. Randall, B.: Fatty liver and sudden death. Hum. Pathol. 11:147, 1980.

95. Barbatis, C., et al.: Disorganization of intermediate filament structure in alcoholic and other liver diseases. Gut 27:765, 1986.

96. Ray, M.B.: Distribution patterns of cytokeratin antigen determinants in alcoholic and nonalcoholic liver diseases. Hum. Pathol. 18:61, 1987.

97. Denk, H., et al.: Pathology of the cytoskeleton of hepatocytes. In Popper, H., and Schaffner, F. (eds.): Progress in Liver Diseases. Vol. 8. Orlando, Grune & Stratton, 1986, p. 237.

98. Mezey, E.: Alcoholic liver disease. In Popper, H., and Schaffner, F. (eds.): Progress in Liver Diseases. Vol. 7. New York, Grune & Stratton, 1982, p. 555.

99. Lieber, C.S.: Alcohol and Liver: 1984 update. Hepatology 4:1243, 1984.

100. Popper, H., and Lieber, C.S.: The histogenesis of alcoholic fibrosis and cirrhosis in the baboon. Am. J. Pathol. 98:695, 1980.

101. Pares, A., et al.: Histological course of alcoholic hepatitis: Influence of abstinence, sex, and extent of hepatic damage. J. Hepatol. 2:33, 1986.

102. Lieber, C.S.: Pathogenesis and early diagnosis of alcoholic liver injury. N. Engl. J. Med. 298:888, 1978.

103. Lieber, C.S., and Leo, M.A.: Interaction of alcohol and nutritional factors with hepatic fibrosis. *In* Popper, H., and Schaffner, F. (eds.): Progress in Liver Diseases. Vol. 8. Orlando, Grune & Stratton, 1986, p. 253.

104. Popper, H., and Schaffner, F.: Chronic hepatitis: Taxonomic, etiologic, and therapeutic problems. *In* Popper, H., and Schaffner, F. (eds.): Progress in Liver Disease. Vol. 5. New York, Grune & Stratton, 1976, p. 535.

105. Kew, M.C., and Popper, H.: Relationship between hepatocellular carcinoma and cirrhosis. Semin. Liver Dis. *4:*136, 1984.

106. Crosby, W.H.: Hemochromatosis: Current concepts and management. Hosp. Pract. *22:*173, 1987.

107. Fairbanks, V.F., and Baldus, W.P.: Hemochromatosis: The neglected diagnosis. Mayo Clin. Proc. *61:*296, 1986.

108. Simon, M., et al.: The genetics of hemochromatosis. Prog. Med. Genet. *4:*135, 1980.

109. Bassett, M.L., et al.: Genetic hemochromatosis. Semin. Liver Dis. *4:*217, 1984.

110. Cox, T.M., and Peters, T.: The kinetics of iron uptake *in vitro* by human duodenal mucosa: Studies in normal subjects. J. Physiol. *289:*469, 1979.

111. Bjorn-Rasmussen, E.: Iron absorption: Present knowledge and controversies. Lancet *1:*914, 1983.

112. Gordeuk, V.R., et al.: Dietary iron overload persists in rural sub-Saharan Africa. Lancet *1:*1310, 1986.

113. Powell, L.W., and Halliday, J.W.: Iron, ferritin, and the liver. *In* Popper, H., and Schaffner, F. (eds.): Progress in Liver Diseases. Vol. 7. New York, Grune & Stratton, 1982, p. 599.

114. Rakko, P.S., et al.: Successful reversal by chelation therapy of congestive cardiomyopathy due to iron overload. J. Am. Coll. Cardiol. *8:*436, 1986.

115. Niederau, C., et al.: Survival and causes of death in cirrhotic and in noncirrhotic patients with primary hemochromatosis. N. Engl. J. Med. *313:*1256, 1985.

116. Dabaghi, R.E., and Lester, R.: Primary biliary cirrhosis. Am. Fam. Physician *33:*155, 1986.

117. Gores, G.J., et al.: Primary biliary cirrhosis: Associations with major histocompatibility complex class II antigens. Hepatology *7:*889, 1987.

118. Kaplan, M.M.: Primary biliary cirrhosis. N. Engl. J. Med. *316:*521, 1987.

119. Kaplan, M.M.: Primary biliary cirrhosis. Adv. Intern. Med. *32:*359, 1987.

120. MacFarlane, I.G.: Autoreactivity against biliary tract antigens in primary biliary cirrhosis. Mol. Aspects Med. *8:*249, 1985.

121. Wolke, A.M., et al.: Malignancy in primary biliary cirrhosis: High incidence of breast cancer in affected women. Am. J. Med. *76:*1075, 1984.

122. Fagerhol, M.K., and Cox, D.W.: The pi polymorphism: Genetic, biochemical, and clinical aspects of human alpha-1-antitrypsin. Adv. Hum. Genet. *11:*1, 1981.

123. Callea, F., et al.: Alpha-1-antitrypsin (ATT) and its stimulation in the liver of pi MZ phenotype individuals: A "recruitment-secretory block" ("R-SB") phenomenon. Liver *4:*325, 1984.

124. Yunis, E.J., et al.: Fine structural observations of the liver in alpha-1-antitrypsin deficiency. Am. J. Panthol. *82:*265, 1976.

125. Millward-Sadler, G.H.: Alpha-1-antitrypsin deficiency and liver disease. Acta Med. Port. (Suppl. 2), 91, 1981.

126. Sveger, T.: Liver disease in alpha₁-antitrypsin deficiency detected by screening of 200,000 infants. N. Engl. J. Med. *294:*1316, 1976.

127. Editorial: Alpha₁-antitrypsin deficiency and liver disease. Br. Med. J. *283:*807, 1981.

128. Frydman, M., et al.: Assignment of the gene for Wilson's disease to chromosome 13: Linkage to the esterase D locus. Proc. Natl. Acad. Sci. U.S.A. *82:*1819, 1985.

129. Stromeyer, F.W., and Ishak, K.G.: Histology of the liver in Wilson's disease. A study of 34 cases. Am. J. Clin. Pathol. *73:*12, 1980.

130. Scheinberg, I.H., and Sternlieb, I.: Wilson's disease. *In* Major Problems in Internal Medicine. Vol. 23. Philadelphia, W.B. Saunders Company, 1984, p. 78.

131. MacSween, R.N.M., and Scott, A.R.: Hepatic cirrhosis: A clinicopathologic review of 520 cases. J. Clin. Pathol. *26:*936, 1973.

132. Purtilo, D.T., and Gottlieb, L.S.: Cirrhosis and hepatoma occurring at Boston City Hospital (1917–1968). Cancer *32:*458, 1973.

133. Summerfield, J.A., et al.: Hepatobiliary fibropolycystic diseases. J. Hepatol. *2:*141, 1986.

134. Mays, E.T., et al.: Focal nodular hyperplasia of the liver. Possible relationship to oral contraceptives. Am. J. Clin. Pathol. *61:*735, 1974.

135. Mettlin, L., and Natarajan, N.: Studies of the role of oral contraceptive use in the etiology of benign and malignant tumours. J. Surg. Oncol. *18:*73, 1981.

136. Edmondson, H.A., et al.: Regression of liver cell adenomas associated with oral contraceptives. Ann. Intern. Med. *86:*180, 1977.

137. Hayes, D., et al.: Hepatic cell adenoma presenting with intraperitoneal haemorrhage in the puerperium. Br. Med. J. *2:*1394, 1977.

138. London, W.T.: Primary hepatocellular carcinoma—etiology, pathogenesis, and prevention. Hum. Pathol. *12:*1085, 1981.

139. Szmuness, W.: Hepatocellular carcinoma and hepatitis B virus. Evidence for a causal association. Prog. Med. Virol. *24:*40, 1978.

140. Editorial: Hepatocellular cancer: Differences between high and low incidence regions. Lancet *2:*1183, 1987.

141. Beasley, R.P.: Hepatitis B virus. The major etiology of hepatocellular carcinoma. Cancer *61:*1942, 1988.

142. Beasley, R.P., and Hwang, L.-Y.: Epidemiology of hepatocellular carcinoma. *In* Vyas, G.H., et al. (eds.): Viral Hepatitis and Liver Disease. Orlando, Grune & Stratton, 1984, p. 209.

143. Lieberman, H.M., and Shafritz, D.: Persistent hepatitis B virus infection and hepatocellular carcinoma. *In* Popper, H., and Schaffner, F. (eds.): Progress in Liver Diseases. Vol. 8. Orlando, Grune & Stratton, 1986, p. 395.

144. Patten, R.C.: Aflatoxins and disease. Am. J. Trop. Med. Hyg. *30:*422, 1981.

145. Niranjan, B.G., et al.: Preferential attack of mitochondrial DNA by aflatoxin B₁ during hepatocarcinogenesis. Science *215:*73, 1982.

146. Genton, C.Y.: Oral contraception and cancer risk. Schweiz. Med. Wochenscher. *111:*1742, 1981.

147. Thung, S.N., et al.: Distribution of five antigens in hepatocellular carcinomas. Lab. Invest. *41:*101, 1979.

148. Berman, M.A.: Fibrolamellar carcinoma of the liver: An immunohistochemical study of nineteen cases and a review of the literature. Hum. Pathol. *19:*784, 1988.

149. Berman, M.M., et al.: Hepatocellular carcinoma. Polygonal cell type with fibrous stroma—an atypical variant with favorable prognosis. Cancer *46:*1448, 1980.

150. Soulier, J.-P., et al.: A new method to assay des-gamma-carboxyprothrombin. Results obtained in 75 cases of hepatocellular carcinoma. Gastroenterology *91:*1258, 1986.

151. Nagasue, N., et al.: The natural history of hepatocellular carcinoma. A study of 100 untreated cases. Cancer *54:*1461, 1984.

152. Eder, G., et al.: Hepatitis B vaccine. *In* Popper, H., and Schaffner, F. (eds.): Progress in Liver Diseases. Vol. 8. Orlando, Grune & Stratton, 1986, p. 367.

152a. Bruckstein, A.H.: Immunoprophylaxis of viral hepatitis. Postgrad. Med. *84:*85, 1988.

153. Koff, R.S., et al.: Profile of hyperbilirubinemia in three hospital populations. Clin. res. *18:*680, 1970.

154. Sameshina, Y., et al.: Clinical statistics on drug-induced liver injuries. Drug-induced liver injuries in Japan in the last thirty years. Jpn. J. Gastroenterol. *71:*799, 1974.

155. Zimmerman, H.J.: Hepato-toxicity. New York, Appleton-Century-Crofts, 1978.

156. Davis, M., Tredger, J.M., and Williams, R. (eds.): Drug Reactions and the Liver. London, Pitman Medical Ltd., 1981.

157. Ishak, K.G.: The liver. *In* Riddell, R.H. (ed.): Pathology of Drug-Induced and Toxic Diseases. New York, Churchill Livingston, 1982, p. 457.

158. Crawford, J.S.: Halothane and the liver. Br. Med. J. *293:*334, 1986.

159. Sherlock, S.: The spectrum of hepatotoxicity due to drugs. Lancet *2:*440, 1986.

160. Meythaler, J.N., and Varma, R.R.: Reye's syndrome in adults. Diagnostic considerations. Arch. Intern. Med. *147:*61, 1987.

161. Holtzhauer, F.J., et al.: Reye's syndrome. An epidemiologic analysis of mild disease. Am. J. Dis. Child. *140:*1231, 1986.

162. Partin, J.C., et al.: Brain ultrastructure in Reye's syndrome (en-

cephalopathy and fatty alteration of the viscera). J. Neuropathol. Exp. Neurol. *34:*425, 1975.

163. Heubi, J.E., et al.: Reye's syndrome: Current concepts. Hepatology *7:*155, 1987.

164. Editorial: Reye's syndrome and aspirin: Epidemiological associations and inborn errors of metabolism. Lancet *2:*429, 1987.

165. Centers for Disease Control: Reye's syndrome: United States, 1985. M.M.W.R. *35:*66, 1986.

166. Remington, P.L., et al.: Decreasing trends in Reye syndrome and aspirin use in Michigan, 1979–1984. Pediatrics *77:*93, 1986.

167. Landing, B.H.: Considerations on the pathogenesis of neonatal hepatitis, biliary atresia, and choledocal cyst — the concept of infantile obstructive cholangiopathy. Prog. Pediatr. Surg. *6:*113, 1974.

168. Balistreri, W.F.: Neonatal cholestasis. J. Pediatr. *106:*171, 1985.

169. Spivak, W., and Grand, R.J.: General configuration of cholestasis in the newborn. J. Pediatr. Gastroenterol. Nutr. *2:*381, 1983.

170. Brough, A.J., Bernstein, J.: Congenital hyperbilirubinemia in early infancy. Hum. Pathol. *5:*507, 1974.

171. Smith, B.F., and LaMont, J.T.: The pathogenesis of gallstones. Hosp. Pract. *19:*93, 1984.

172. Bennion, L.J., and Grundy, S.M.: Risk factors for the development of cholelithiasis in man. N. Engl. J. Med. *299:*1221, 1978.

173. Royal College of General Practitioners Oral Contraceptive Study: Oral contraceptives and gallbladder disease. Lancet *2:*957, 1982.

174. Trotman, B.W., and Soloway, R.D.: Pigment gallstone disease: Summary of the National Institutes of Health — International Workshop. Hepatology *2:*879, 1982.

175. Weisberg, H.F.: Pathogenesis of gallstones. Ann. Clin. Lab. Sci. *14:*243, 1984.

176. Roslyn, J.L., et al.: Enhanced gallbladder absorption during gallstone formation: The roles of cholesterol saturated bile and gallbladder stasis. Am. J. Med. Sci. *292:*75, 1986.

177. Holzbach, R.T., et al.: Biliary proteins: Unique inhibitors of cholesterol crystal nucleation in human gallbladder bile. J. Clin. Invest. *73:*35, 1984.

178. Smith, B.F., and LaMont, J.T.: The central issue of cholesterol gallstones. Hepatology *6:*529, 1986.

179. Whiting, M.J., and Watts, J.M.: Cholesterol gallstone pathogenesis: A study of potential nucleating agents for cholesterol crystal formation in bile. Clin. Sci. *68:*589, 1985.

180. Ostrow, J.B.: Bilirubin solubility and etiology of pigment gallstones. Prog. Clin. Biol. Res. *152:*53, 1984.

181. Gracie, W.A., and Ransohoff, D.F.: The natural history of silent gallstones. The innocent gallstone is not a myth. N. Engl. J. Med. *307:*798, 1982.

182. Claesson, B.E.B., et al.: Microflora of the gallbladder related to duration of acute cholecystitis. Surg. Gynecol. Obstet. *162:*531, 1986.

183. Lin, K.Y.-K.: Acute acalculous cholecystitis: A limited review of the literature. Mt. Sinai J. Med. *53:*305, 1986.

184. Stephenson, S.E., et al.: Acute cholecystitis: An experimental study. Ann. Surg. *157:*687, 1963.

185. Hallendorf, L.C., et al.: Gangrenous cholecystitis: A clinical and pathologic study of 100 cases. Surg. Clin. North Am. *28:*979, 1948.

186. Seal, M.L.: Cholecystitis occurring without stones. Postgrad. Med. *79:*151, 1986.

187. Reiss, R., et al.: A new look at acute cholecystitis. Mt. Sinai J. Med. *53:*103, 1986.

188. Feldman, M., and Feldman, J., Jr.: Cholesterolosis of the gallbladder. Gastroenterology *27:*641, 1954.

189. Yamaguchi, K., and Enjoji, M.: Carcinoma of the ampulla of Vater. A clinicopathologic study and pathologic staging of 109 cases of carcinoma and 5 cases of adenoma. Cancer *59:*506, 1987.

190. Anderson, J.B., et al.: Adenocarcinoma of the extrahepatic biliary tree. Ann. R. Coll. Surg. *67:*139, 1985.

191. Sons, H.U.: Autopsy findings in 287 cases of gallbladder carcinoma. J. Surg. Oncol. *28:*199, 1985.

192. Shukla, V.K., et al.: Primary carcinoma of the gallbladder: A review of a 16-year period at the University Hospital. J. Surg. Oncol. *28:*32, 1985.

193. Roberts, J.W.: Carcinoma of the extrahepatic bile ducts. Surg. Clin. North Am. 66:751, 1986.

194. Sons, H.U., and Borchard, F.: Carcinoma of the extrahepatic bile ducts: A postmortem study of 65 cases and review of the literature. J. Surg. Oncol. *34:*6, 1987.

195. Bruggen, J.T., et al.: Primary adenocarcinoma of the bile ducts. Clinical characteristics and natural history. Dig. Dis. Sci. *31:*840, 1986.

THE EXOCRINE PANCREAS

NORMAL

In its posterior location in the upper abdomen, the pancreas is one of the "hidden" organs in the body. It is virtually impossible to palpate clinically. Diseases that impair its function evoke signs or symptoms only when far advanced, because there is such a large reserve of both endocrine and exocrine function. Some lesions are manifested only by encroachment on neighboring structures. For example, carcinoma of the pancreas may be discovered only when it invades the vertebral column, occludes the biliary system, or causes disturbances in the stomach or colon.

The pancreas arises from two duodenal buds that are referred to, respectively, as the dorsal and ventral pancreas.[1] Fusion of the two creates the adult organ, after which the two contributions can no longer be distinguished. The ductal drainage systems anastomose, and the definitive pancreatic duct is formed by fusion of the ventral duct with the distal portion of the dorsal duct (the duct of Wirsung). Occasionally, the proximal portion of the dorsal duct persists as the *accessory duct of Santorini*. However, there is much variability in this ductal system. In two thirds of adults the major pancreatic duct does not empty directly into the duodenum but into the common bile duct just proximal to the ampulla of Vater, thus providing a common channel to the pancreatic and biliary drainage.

In the adult the average pancreas is about 15 cm in length, weighs 60 to 140 gm, and consists of a head, body, and tail. Its gross anatomic relationships include immediate proximity to the duodenum, ampulla of Vater, common bile duct, superior mesenteric artery, portal vein, spleen and its vascular supply, stomach, transverse colon, left lobe of the liver, and lower recesses of the lesser omental cavity (Fig. 20–1). Inflammatory and neoplastic processes within the pancreas may cause secondary involvement of many adjacent structures that produces, in many cases, the characteristic signs and symptoms of pancreatic disease.

Histologically, the pancreas has two separate components, the exocrine and endocrine glands. The endocrine pancreas is described on page 992. The exocrine portion, constituting 80 to 85% of the organ, is made up of numerous small glands (acini) aggregated into lobules. The epithelial cells are columnar to truncated pyramids radially oriented about the gland circumference. Small microvilli project from the apical surfaces of the secretory cells into the lumen. The cells are deeply basophilic because of their abundance of granular endoplasmic reticulum and ribosomes. The Golgi complex is well developed in these cells and, along with the endoplasmic reticulum, appears to be oriented toward the basal region. The apical regions of the cells contain abundant membrane-bound zymogen granules.

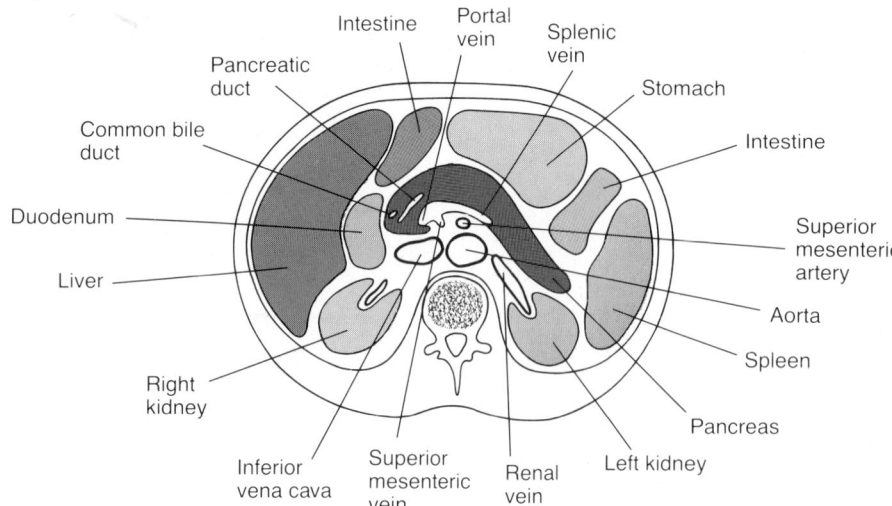

Figure 20-1. Anatomic relationships of the pancreas seen in a cross section of the abdomen at the level of the upper lumbar vertebrae. (From Go, V.W., et al.: The Exocrine Pancreas. Biology, Pathobiology and Diseases. New York, Raven Press, 1986.)

The ductal system of the pancreas is produced by progressive anastomosis of the extremely fine radicles that begin within the secretory acini. These small ducts eventually drain into the main pancreatic ducts. At first cuboidal, their lining epithelium becomes progressively higher to produce tall, columnar, mucus-secreting cells. About the larger ducts, there are numerous accessory branching ducts and mucous glands.

It is hardly necessary here to reiterate the secretory functions of the pancreas and the regulatory mechanisms that control such activity. Several points, however, are directly pertinent to disease processes and merit reemphasis.[2] The pancreas secretes 1.5 to 3 liters per day of an alkaline fluid containing enzymes and zymogens. Secretion is adjusted to the workload that it is called on to handle, i.e., the volume and character of the intestinal contents. The regulation of this secretion is a complex process that involves humoral and neural factors. The most important of these regulators are the hormones *secretin* and *cholecystokinin*, produced in the duodenum. The former stimulates water and bicarbonate secretion by duct cells, and the latter enhances the discharge of enzyme-containing zymogen granules by acinar cells. When the pancreas is stimulated to secretory activity, the zymogen granules, enclosed within membranous sacs originating from the Golgi complex, migrate to the apical region of the cell. Here the sac becomes attached to the plasma membrane, and rupture at the point of attachment releases the enzyme-rich zymogen granules into the acinus of the gland (Fig. 20-2). Fats and alcohol are particularly active stimulators of secretin production, and therefore indirectly of the pancreas.

A second point of interest relates to the elaboration of the enzymes.[3] These include trypsin, chymotrypsin, aminopeptidases, elastase, amylases, lipases, and phospholipases. Trypsin itself is a key enzyme, as it triggers activation of other enzymes. Self-digestion of the pancreas is prevented by several means: (1) These enzymes are elaborated as inactive precursors that are activated only in the duodenum; (2) they are sequestered in membrane-bound granules within acinar cells; (3) protease inhibitors are normally present within acini and pancreatic secretion; and (4) intrapancreatic release of trypsin activates an enzyme that degrades other zymogens to inert products. One of the most important pancreatic diseases, acute pancreatic necrosis, is initiated by activation of these enzymes within the pancreatic parenchyma.

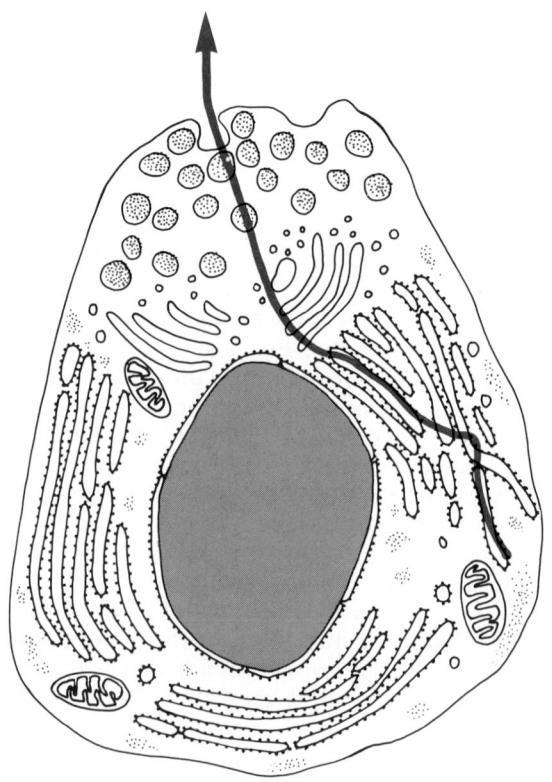

Figure 20-2. Ultrastructural characteristics of the acinar cell and pathway *(red line)* of synthesis and secretion of zymogens.

PATHOLOGY

The most significant disorders of the exocrine pancreas are cystic fibrosis (p. 533), acute and chronic pancreatitis, and tumors.[4] It should be emphasized that, from the standpoints of both morbidity and mortality, diabetes mellitus (a disorder of endocrine metabolism) overshadows all the other pancreatic disorders. However, a knowledgeable alertness to exocrine pancreatic disease is most necessary, since almost all these disorders are difficult to diagnose because of the hidden position and large reserve function of this organ, and because they appear under such diverse guises as a catastrophic "acute abdomen" or the silent growth of a carcinoma.

CONGENITAL ANOMALIES

The pancreas is subject to a variety of congenital disorders that, with the exception of fibrocystic disease, are either quite uncommon or of little clinical significance.[1] The gland may be totally absent (agenesis). Complete agenesis is quite regularly associated with widespread severe malformations that are incompatible with life. The endocrine and exocrine elements may be *hypoplastic*. The gland may exist as two separate structures representing the persistence of the dorsal and ventral pancreas. The head of the pancreas may encircle the duodenum as a collar *(annular pancreas)* and sometimes may cause subtotal duodenal obstruction and consequent clinical symptoms. Two additional anomalies occur with sufficient frequency or have sufficient clinical significance to merit separate consideration.

ABERRANT PANCREAS

Aberrant, or ectopic, displaced pancreatic tissue is found in about 2% of all routine post-mortems. The favored sites for such ectopia follow the order of the descent of the intestinal tract; i.e., they are most common in the stomach and duodenum with about equal frequency, next in the jejunum, then in Meckel's diverticulum, and then in the ileum. Usually, the masses vary from a few millimeters to 3 to 4 cm in diameter. They appear as single or multiple, firm, yellow-gray nests within the wall of the gut subjacent to the mucosa, lying usually within the submucosa (Fig. 20–3). They are composed histologically of glands that appear completely normal, and not infrequently islets of Langerhans are also present.

In such locations, they may be discovered accidentally in the course of a laparotomy, visualized radiographically as sessile lesions that project slightly into the lumen of the bowel, or seen on endoscopy in the course of studies for gastrointestinal symp-

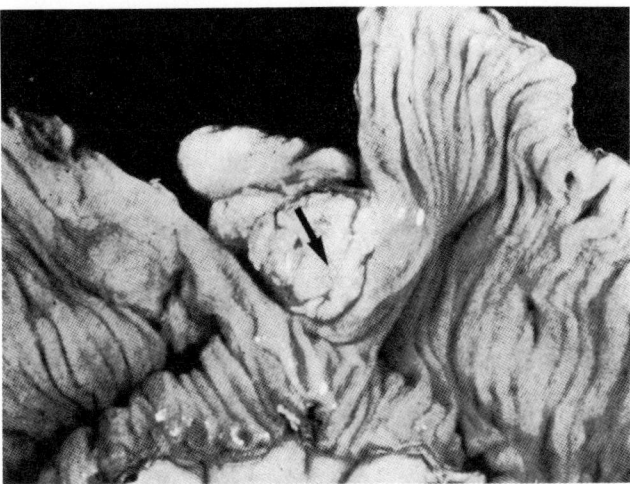

Figure 20–3. Aberrant pancreas. Mucosa of jejunum has been incised to disclose the rest of the pale yellow-white, submucosal, lobulated pancreatic tissue *(arrow)*.

toms. About 2% of islet cell tumors arise in ectopic pancreas.[5]

ANOMALIES OF DUCTS

Anomalies of the pancreatic duct represent a second type of congenital defect that is sometimes of clinical importance. The ducts of Wirsung and of Santorini may both persist as totally separate structures. The major excretory pancreatic duct, the duct of Wirsung, may drain into the common bile duct or may drain through an abnormally high orifice in the duodenum. These variations seem to be of little importance except for two considerations: (1) Unless recognized, they may potentiate ligation or severance of ducts during surgery around the ampulla, causing serious sequelae; and (2) one of these anomalies, *pancreas divisum*, predisposes to recurrent pancreatitis (p. 987).

PANCREATITIS

Inflammation of the pancreas, almost always associated with acinar cell injury, is termed pancreatitis.[6] Clinically and histologically, pancreatitis presents as a spectrum, dependent on duration and severity. *Acute pancreatitis* includes a mild, self-limited form termed *interstitial or edematous pancreatitis*, and a more serious severe type, *acute hemorrhagic* (necrotizing) *pancreatitis*. In *chronic relapsing pancreatitis*, there is persistence or recurrence of episodes of active pancreatitis, eventually leading to chronic pancreatic insufficiency *(chronic pancreatitis)*.

ACUTE PANCREATITIS

Acute pancreatitis is defined as an acute condition, typically presenting clinically with abdominal pain asso-

ciated with raised pancreatic enzymes in blood or urine, and caused by inflammation, and (commonly) necrosis of pancreatic tissue.[6] In its severe form, called *acute hemorrhagic pancreatitis* or *acute pancreatic necrosis*, there is extensive fat necrosis in and about the pancreas and in other fatty depots in the abdominal cavity and hemorrhages into the parenchyma of this organ.

Acute hemorrhagic pancreatitis occurs about once in every 500 to 600 medical and surgical admissions to a general hospital. Although by no means common, it may be a dramatic, life-threatening illness. Acute pancreatitis occurs most often in middle life. About 80% of cases are associated with two conditions: *biliary tract disease* and *alcoholism.* Acute pancreatitis often follows an alcoholic debauch or an excessively large meal. The male : female ratio is 1 : 3 in those with biliary tract disease and 6 : 1 in those with alcoholism.

ETIOLOGY. As mentioned, the two leading conditions associated with acute pancreatitis are biliary tract disease (especially cholelithiasis) and excessive alcohol intake.[7] Gallstones are present in 35 to 60% of cases of pancreatitis, and about 5% of patients with gallstones develop pancreatitis. The proportion of cases of acute pancreatitis caused by alcoholism varies in different countries: It is 65% in the United States, but 20 to 25% in Sweden and 5% or less in southern France and England.[7] Other less common causes of pancreatitis (Table 20–1) include trauma; extension of inflammation from adjacent peptic ulcers or abdominal infections; blood-borne bacterial infections; viral infections such as mumps and hepatitis; acute ischemia induced by vascular thrombosis, embolism, polyarteritis nodosa, and shock; hypothermia; and drugs (azathioprine, thiazides, sulfonamides, and oral contraceptives).[8] Pancreatitis is also occasionally associated with hyperlipoproteinemia (especially types I and V) and with hyperparathyroidism and other hypercalcemic states.[9] A hereditary predisposition to pancreatitis has been identified in some families, transmitted apparently as an autosomal dominant trait.[10] However, such familial disease more commonly takes the form of chronic relapsing pancreatitis

Table 20–1. Conditions and Etiologic Agents Associated with Pancreatitis

CHOLELITHIASIS
ALCOHOLISM
Trauma
Extension from adjacent tissues
Blood-borne bacterial infection
Viral infections
Ischemia
Vasculitis
Drugs
Hyperlipidemia
Hypercalcemia
Hereditary/familial

(p. 987) rather than acute pancreatitis. Although relatively rare, familial pancreatitis is the most common type encountered in children. In many patients the etiology of acute pancreatitis is unknown; in various studies this so-called *idiopathic pancreatitis* accounts for 9 to 50% of all patients with the disease.

PATHOGENESIS. The anatomic changes in this disease suggest that the acute pancreatic necrosis is caused by the destructive effects of pancreatic enzymes, which run amok within the pancreatic parenchyma.[11–13]

It will be well to remember that the exogenous pancreas secretes at least 22 enzymes: 15 proteases (including elastase), three to six amylases, lipase, and phospholipase. These are normally present in acinar cells in the proenzyme form and need to be activated to fulfill their enzymatic potential. Proteolysis, lipolysis, and hemorrhage account for the three major morphologic features of pancreatitis. Thus, it would be natural to assume that proteases (trypsin, chymotrypsin), lipase and phospholipases (which degrade lipids and membrane phospholipids), and elastase (which breaks down the elastic tissue of vessels) are the keys to such pancreatic destruction. *Trypsin could play a key role, as it is able to activate the other proenzymes taking part in the process of autodigestion,* such as proelastase and prophospholipase. Indeed, trypsin, chymotrypsin, elastase, and phospholipase activity is present in human pancreatic juice, ascitic fluid, and blood in human and experimental acute pancreatitis.[14] Trypsin also converts prekallikrein to kallikrein, thereby activating the kinin system and indirectly, through activation of Hageman factor, the clotting and complement system (p. 54). These mediators then contribute to the local inflammation, thrombosis, tissue damage, and hemorrhage characteristic of acute hemorrhagic pancreatitis, as well as to the systemic manifestations of the disease. Thus, *the activation of trypsinogen is an important triggering event in pancreatitis.*

But how are these enzymes activated and released within the pancreas? Theories abound, largely based on animal models, but it is likely that more than one pathway may lead to such activation.[15] Some of the postulated mechanisms, depicted in Figure 20–4, are as follows:

1. *Acinar cell injury.* Viruses, endotoxin, drugs, ischemia, and trauma[11,16] result in direct acinar cell damage, with intrapancreatic activation and release of enzymes.

2. *Duct obstruction.* Since the main pancreatic duct joins the common bile duct in two thirds of normal individuals, gallstones impacted in the ampulla of Vater can presumably cause pancreatic duct obstruction. Indeed, 70 to 85% of patients with biliary disease–associated pancreatitis have evidence of gallstones either in the ampulla or in the stools,[17] and there is an association between the migration of gall-

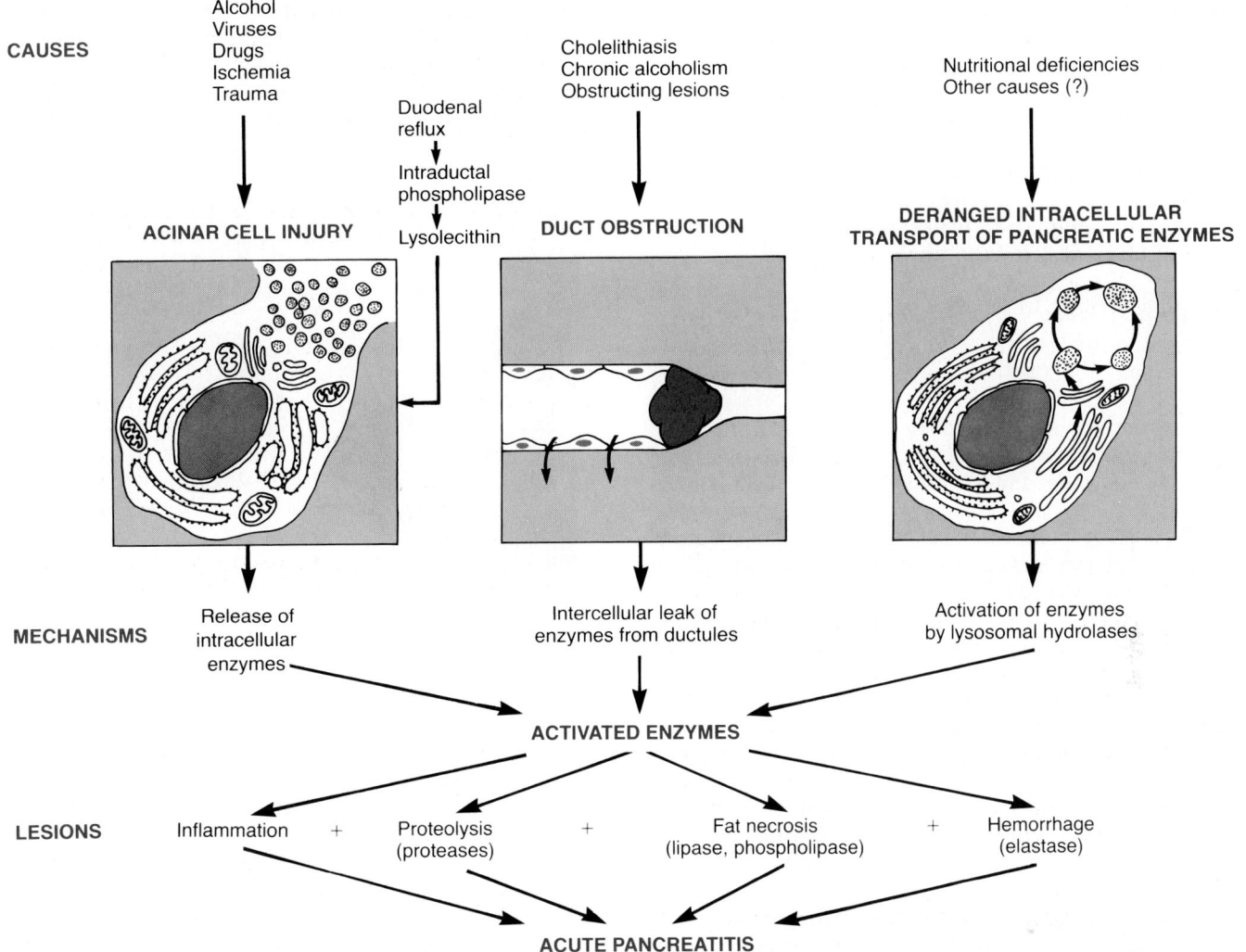

CAUSES

Alcohol
Viruses
Drugs
Ischemia
Trauma

Cholelithiasis
Chronic alcoholism
Obstructing lesions

Nutritional deficiencies
Other causes (?)

Duodenal
reflux

Intraductal
phospholipase

Lysolecithin

ACINAR CELL INJURY

DUCT OBSTRUCTION

**DERANGED INTRACELLULAR
TRANSPORT OF PANCREATIC ENZYMES**

MECHANISMS

Release of
intracellular
enzymes

Intercellular leak of
enzymes from ductules

Activation of enzymes
by lysosomal hydrolases

ACTIVATED ENZYMES

LESIONS

Inflammation + Proteolysis
(proteases) + Fat necrosis
(lipase, phospholipase) + Hemorrhage
(elastase)

ACUTE PANCREATITIS

Figure 20–4. Three pathways in the pathogenesis of acute pancreatitis—acinar cell injury, duct obstruction, and a derangement in lysosomal traffic. See text. (Adapted from Longnecker, D.S.: Am. J. Pathol. *107*:103, 1982; and Steer, M.L., and Meldolisi, J.: Annu. Rev. Med. *39*:95, 1988.)

stones and the onset of the disease.[18] It is *postulated* that increased intraductal pressure leads to intercellular leakage of enzymes from small ducts into the interstitium. However, it must be stated that clear-cut evidence of obstruction in clinical pancreatitis is lacking,[19] and experimental work indicates that obstruction alone is insufficient to cause hemorrhagic pancreatitis. One factor that may contribute to pancreatic necrosis in this setting is *duodenal reflux*. This occurs owing to damage to the sphincter of Oddi by the chronic biliary disease, allowing duodenal contents to enter the pancreas. Lecithin in duodenal contents is converted by phospholipase A into the highly toxic lysolecithin, which contributes to acinar cell necrosis. 3. *Derangements of intracellular transport of enzymes, with activation by lysosomal hydrolases.* In normal acinar cells the digestive enzymes and the lysosomal hydrolases are transported in separate pathways after their synthesis in the endoplasmic reticu-

lum and packaging in the Golgi apparatus. The digestive enzymes, as we have seen in Figure 20–2, make their way through zymogen granules to the cell surface, while lysosomal hydrolyses are transported into the lysosomes.[20] In experimental pancreatitis induced by a choline-deficient diet supplemented by ethionine, or by infusion of a secretagogue, there is evidence that the pancreatic enzymes are activated *intracellularly*, as a result of a *derangement in their intracellular transport such that they localize within the lysosomes and are then activated by the lysosomal hydrolases* (Fig. 20–4).[12,13] A blockage in exocytosis seems to contribute to this deranged transport. Whether this mechanism is relevant to human pancreatitis is now under study.

The manner by which alcohol precipitates pancreatitis is unknown. Increased transient pancreatic exocrine secretion, contraction of the sphincter of

Oddi, and direct toxic effects on acinar cells have all been postulated from experimental studies. It must be stated that many authorities now feel that *most cases of alcoholic pancreatitis are acute exacerbations of chronic asymptomatic pancreatitis rather than acute pancreatitis.* According to Sarles,[21] chronic alcohol ingestion causes secretion of protein-rich pancreatic fluid leading to deposition of inspissated protein plugs and *obstruction of small pancreatic ducts,* followed by degeneration of acini and fibrosis.

MORPHOLOGY. The histologic changes are presented first because they can be predicted, to a considerable extent, from the presumed pathogenesis of this disease. The basic alterations are four in number: **proteolytic destruction of pancreatic substance, necroses of blood vessels with subsequent hemorrhage, necrosis of fat by lipolytic enzymes, and an accompanying inflammatory reaction.** The extent and predominance of each of these alterations depend on the duration and severity of the process. In the very early stages, only interstitial edema is present. Soon after, focal and confluent areas of frank necrosis of endocrine and exocrine cells are found. Neutrophilic infiltration and interstitial hemorrhage eventually ensue.

The most characteristic histologic lesions of acute pancreatic necrosis are the focal areas of *fat necrosis* (p. 8) that occur in the stromal, peripancreatic fat, and fat depots throughout the abdominal cavity (Fig. 20–5). These lesions consist of enzymatic destruction of fat cells, in which **the vacuolated fat cells are transformed to shadowy out-**

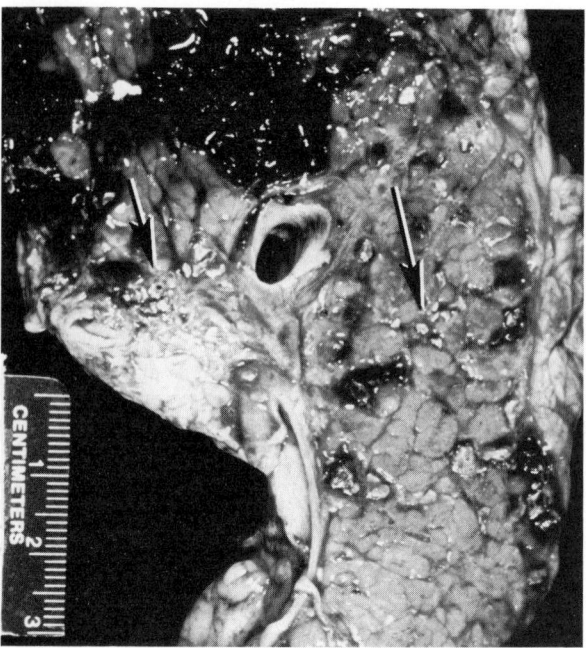

Figure 20–6. Acute hemorrhagic pancreatitis. Note the hemorrhage *(top)* and foci of chalky fat necrosis in pancreas and fat *(arrows).*

lines of cell membranes filled with pink, granular, opaque precipitate. Amorphous basophilic calcium precipitates may be visible within the necrotic focus.

Macroscopically, the dominant characteristics of acute pancreatic necrosis are **areas of gray-white proteolytic destruction of parenchymal substance, hemorrhage, and chalky white areas of fat necrosis.** In the typical case there is an extremely variegated, maplike patterning in the pancreas, with areas of blue-black hemorrhages and other areas of gray-white necrotic softening, alternating with sprinkled foci of yellow-white, chalky fat necrosis (Fig. 20–6).

Characteristically, the peritoneal cavity contains a serous and slightly turbid, brown-tinged fluid in which globules of oil can be identified (so called chicken-broth fluid). Foci of fat necrosis may be found in any of the fat depots, such as in the omentum, mesentery of the bowel, and properitoneal deposits. If the patient survives, the acute necrotizing damage may resolve slowly and be replaced by diffuse or focal parenchymal or stromal fibrosis, calcifications, and irregular ductal dilatations. Occasionally, liquefied areas are walled off by fibrous tissue to form small or large cystic spaces, known as **pseudocysts.**

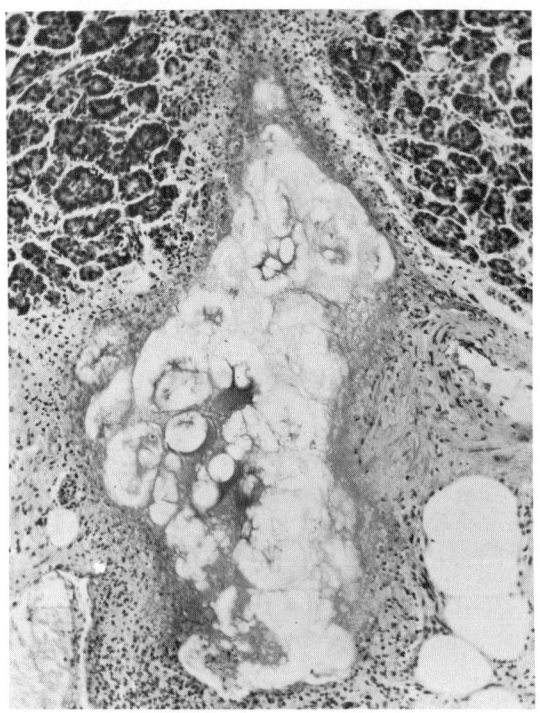

Figure 20–5. Acute pancreatic necrosis. Central focus of necrotic fat is surrounded by a rim of leukocytic infiltration.

CLINICAL COURSE. Full-blown, acute pancreatic necrosis is a medical emergency of the first magnitude.[5] These patients usually have the sudden calamitous onset of an "acute abdomen" that must be differentiated from diseases such as acute appendicitis, perforated peptic ulcer, acute cholecystitis with rupture, and occlusion of mesenteric vessels with infarction of the bowel. Characteristically, the pain appears without prodromal symptoms, usually soon after a large meal or an alcoholic binge. The pain is constant and intense, and is often referred to the upper back. In many cases, peripheral vascular collapse and shock occur. Many explanations have been offered for this rapid development of shock. Loss of blood, when severe, and electrolyte disturbances clearly contribute to the hypotension. There is increasing evidence, however, that release of vasodilatory agents such as bradykinin and the prostaglandins may be the cause of shock in acute pancreatitis. Endotoxemia with complement activation has also been implicated.[22]

Jaundice sometimes appears after the first day and is presumed to be due to edematous narrowing of the common bile duct. The laboratory may provide direct support for the diagnosis. Characteristically, there is an elevation of the serum amylase level within the first 24 hours and the serum lipase level somewhat later (72 to 94 hours). Both fall to basal levels two to five days after the acute phase passes. Elevated serum amylase may occur in other acute abdominal catastrophes, but elevated serum lipase is more specific for pancreatic disease. Glycosuria occurs in 10% of cases. In patients with fat necrosis, hypocalcemia is frequent and, if persistent, is a poor prognostic sign.

Therapy for acute pancreatitis is supportive and aimed at "giving the pancreas a vacation," i.e., inhibition of pancreatic secretion. This is accomplished by stopping oral intake of food and fluids, withdrawal of gastric secretions by nasogastric suction, and intravenous fluid replacement. About 5% of these patients die from shock during the first week of the clinical course. Acute adult respiratory distress syndrome and acute renal failure are particularly ominous complications. If patients survive, a variety of sequelae may follow, including *pancreatic abscess, pseudocyst* (p. 989), and *duodenal obstruction* (Fig. 20–7).

CHRONIC PANCREATITIS

This entity might be more appropriately termed *chronic relapsing pancreatitis* because it often represents progressive destruction of the pancreas by repeated flare-ups of a mild or subclinical type of acute pancreatitis.[23] The disease occurs in the same type of patient likely to develop acute pancreatitis—most commonly the alcoholic, and less frequently, the pa-

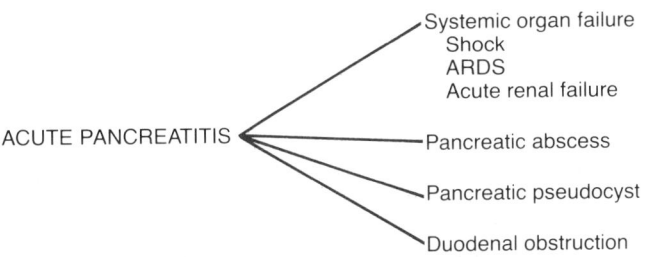

ACUTE PANCREATITIS
- Systemic organ failure
- Shock
- ARDS
- Acute renal failure
- Pancreatic abscess
- Pancreatic pseudocyst
- Duodenal obstruction

Figure 20–7. Complications and sequelae of acute pancreatitis.

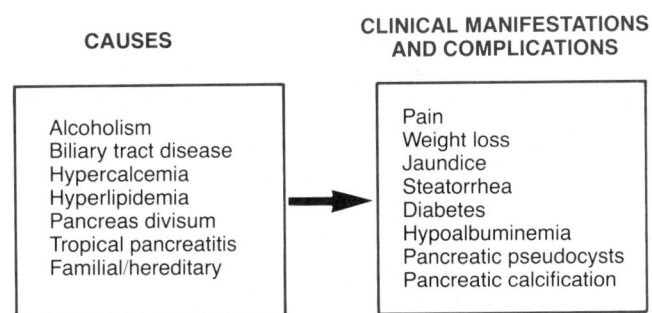

CAUSES	CLINICAL MANIFESTATIONS AND COMPLICATIONS
Alcoholism Biliary tract disease Hypercalcemia Hyperlipidemia Pancreas divisum Tropical pancreatitis Familial/hereditary	Pain Weight loss Jaundice Steatorrhea Diabetes Hypoalbuminemia Pancreatic pseudocysts Pancreatic calcification

Figure 20–8. Causes and consequences of chronic pancreatitis.

tient with biliary tract disease (Fig. 20–8). Hypercalcemia and hyperlipidemia also predispose to chronic pancreatitis. In up to 12% of patients, recurrent pancreatitis is associated with *pancreas divisum*, a developmental anomaly of the pancreatic duct resulting from incomplete fusion of the ventral and dorsal pancreatic anlage.[24] There are relatively rare special forms of chronic pancreatitis, such as *nonalcoholic tropical pancreatitis* and *familial hereditary pancreatitis*. Familial pancreatitis begins in childhood and predisposes to the development of pancreatic carcinoma in later years. Up to 40% of patients have no recognizable predisposing factor.

The pathogenesis of chronic pancreatitis is as varied as that of acute pancreatitis.[25,26] *However, chronic pancreatitis is not usually preceded by an attack of classic acute hemorrhagic pancreatitis,* and usually patients with acute hemorrhagic pancreatitis who recover develop "pseudocysts" rather than chronic fibrosing pancreatitis. In chronic alcoholic pancreatitis, Sarles[21] believes that chronic alcohol intake causes increased protein secretion by the pancreas, and that the subsequent obstruction of ducts by protein-rich plugs contributes to the damage. Genetic factors appear to operate in certain cases. Protein-calorie malnutrition probably plays a role in the tropical pancreatitis present in southeast Asia and parts of Africa, where alcohol consumption is extremely low.

Morphologically there are several patterns of chronic pancreatitis. The most common type is **chronic calcifying pancreatitis,** most frequently seen in alcoholics.[25] The lesions have a lobular distribution, and all components of the involved lobule are affected. There is atrophy of the acini, marked increase in interlobular fibrous tissue, and a chronic inflammatory infiltrate around lobules and ducts (Fig. 20–9). The interlobular and intralobular ducts are dilated and contain protein plugs in their lumina. The ductal epithelium may be atrophied or hyperplastic, or may show squamous metaplasia (Fig. 20–10). The islets appear remarkably unaltered, even though they are enmeshed in sclerosed tissue or severely damaged lobules. **Grossly,** the gland is hard and exhibits foci of calcification and fully developed pancreatic calculi. Pancreatic calculi vary from concretions invisible to the naked eye to stones 1 cm to several centimeters in diameter. **Pseudocyst formation is common in this type of pancreatitis.**

A second morphologic form of pancreatitis is **chronic obstructive pancreatitis;** here, the distribution of lesions is not lobular, and the ductal epithelium generally is less severely damaged. There may be protein plugs in the ducts, but this is a rare finding, and calcified stones are exceptional. The most common cause of this type appears to be stenosis of the sphincter of Oddi associated with **cholelithiasis.** The lesions are more prominent in the head of the pancreas, and regress after sphincterotomy of the sphincter of Oddi. Any other obstructive lesion of the pancreatic ducts may result in this morphologic change, such as carcinoma or accidental ligation of the duct during gastrectomy.

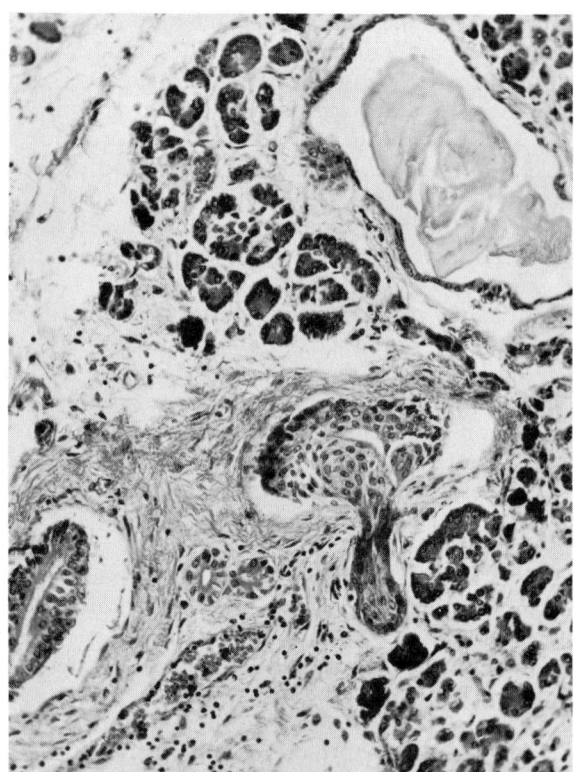

Figure 20–10. Pancreas with squamous metaplasia of one of the small ducts virtually obliterating its lumen. Note dilated duct above filled with inspissated secretion.

Both morphologic forms of the disease are characterized by recurrent attacks of pain at intervals of months or years. The intervals between episodes may shorten progressively until the attacks are almost constant. The attacks may be precipitated by alcohol abuse, overeating, or the use of opiates and other drugs. In an acute attack there may be mild fever and slight jaundice, upper abdominal tenderness, mild or moderate elevations of serum amylase, and alkaline phosphatase. Abdominal radiography may show calcification in the region of the pancreas. Diabetes, steatorrhea, and pancreatic pseudocysts occur so frequently that they may perhaps be considered late features rather than complications of chronic pancrea-

titis. Profound weight loss and hypoalbuminemic edema are present in end-stage pancreatic insufficiency. Between attacks during the early stages of the disease, patients may be entirely asymptomatic. For this reason and because of the wide spectrum of the clinical manifestations and the recurrent nature of this condition, chronic relapsing pancreatitis is a difficult diagnosis to make clinically. Ultrasound and CT scanning are most helpful in such settings; they can detect cysts, calcifications, and enlarged ducts and can exclude tumors.

TUMORS

The heading "tumors" is used to include a variety of non-neoplastic and neoplastic masses that involve this organ. The non-neoplastic masses almost invariably take the form of cysts, whereas the neoplasms are of both benign and malignant and primary and secondary types.

CYSTS

Cysts are infrequent findings in the pancreas, but are of considerable clinical significance, since they may present as abdominal masses that are suspected of being malignant.

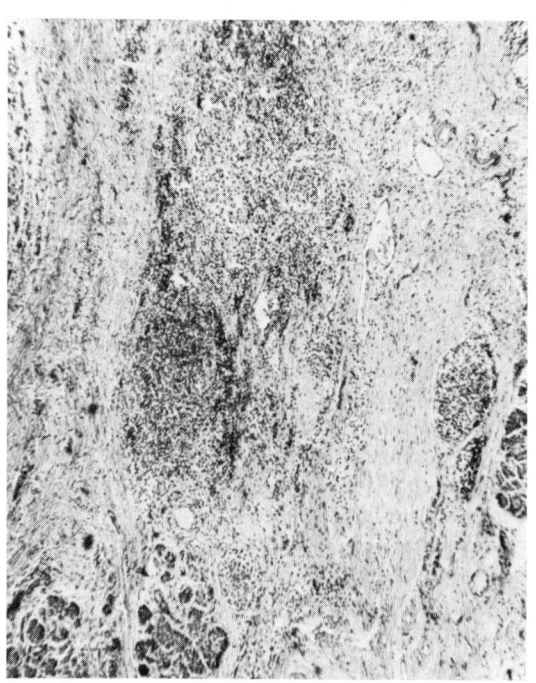

Figure 20–9. Chronic pancreatitis. A focus of chronic inflammation and fibrosis in the center. Remaining acini are at lower left.

Congenital Cysts

Congenital cysts are believed to result from anomalous development of the pancreatic ducts. *Congenital cystic disease of the pancreas, liver, and kidney not infrequently coexists.* These cysts are usually multiple, but occasionally occur singly. They range in size from microscopic lesions to larger spaces up to 3 to 5 cm in diameter. They are lined by a smooth, glistening membrane that may, on histologic section, have total atrophy of the lining epithelial cells or may show preservation of flattened pavement or low cuboidal epithelial cells. They are usually enclosed in a thin fibrous capsule and are filled with a clear-to-turbid mucoid or serous fluid.

In one rare entity, *Lindau–von Hippel disease*, angiomas are found in the retina and cerebellum or brain stem in association with cysts in the pancreas, liver, and kidney.

Pseudocysts

This term is applied to a collection of fluid that arises from loculation of inflammatory processes, necroses, or hemorrhages.[27] *This type represents the overwhelming majority of clinically important cysts and is almost always associated with pancreatitis.* Pseudocysts may also follow traumatic injury to the abdomen with direct damage and hemorrhage in the pancreas. Acute pancreatitis or trauma precedes the clinical discovery of a pseudocyst in nine of ten cases.

These cysts are usually solitary and most measure 5 to 10 cm in diameter. They may be situated within the pancreatic substance, but more often they are found adjacent to the pancreas, particularly in the region of the tail of the pancreas. The cyst walls may be thin, or thick and fibrous (Fig. 20–11). Character-

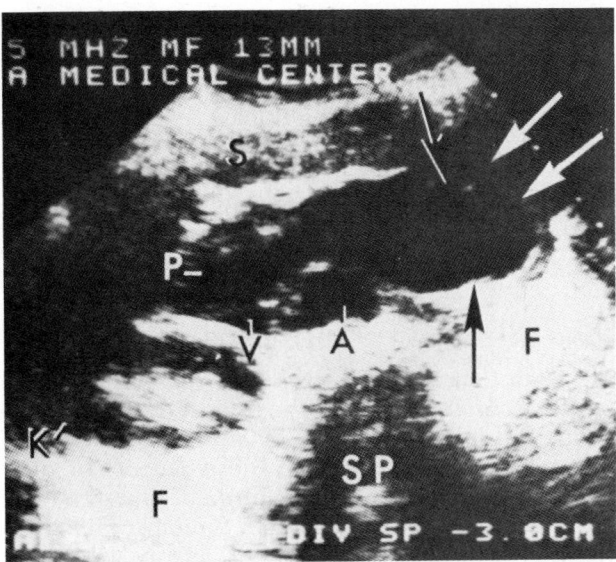

Figure 20–12. Ultrasound of transverse section of abdomen showing a large pancreatic cyst *(arrows).* **Anterior abdominal wall is on top. A = aorta; V = inferior vena cava; SP = spine; K = kidney; F = fat; S = stomach; P = splenic vein–portal vein confluence.**

istically, they do not have an epithelial lining and have no connection or communication with surrounding ductal systems. There may be a marked inflammatory reaction in the fibrous capsule, and often, organizing blood clot, old blood pigment, precipitates of calcium, and cholesterol crystals. The cyst fluid is usually serous and turbid.

Pseudocysts produce abdominal pain and intraperitoneal hemorrhage, and if infected, may cause generalized peritonitis. However, their clinical significance lies in their being discovered as an abdominal mass in a location that strongly suggests a primary intra-abdominal malignancy.

The diagnosis is made by ultrasonography or CT scanning (Fig. 20–12). With ultrasound, the pseudocysts are evident as sonolucent areas with relatively smooth, well-circumscribed outlines. They are usually unilocular; multiloculation suggests a neoplastic cyst. CT scanning adds to the specificity of ultrasound in this setting.

Benign Tumors

Benign pancreatic tumors are rare.[28] Two deserve attention because they are usually cystic and need to be differentiated from benign cysts. The *serous cystadenomas* are usually large multiloculated cysts, most common in elderly women, that are incidental findings either at autopsy or during investigation of other abdominal conditions. They constitute 4 to 10% of all pancreatic cysts. Histologically, the cysts are lined by flattened cuboidal epithelium with clear, glycogen-rich cytoplasm. One variant, named *microcystic*

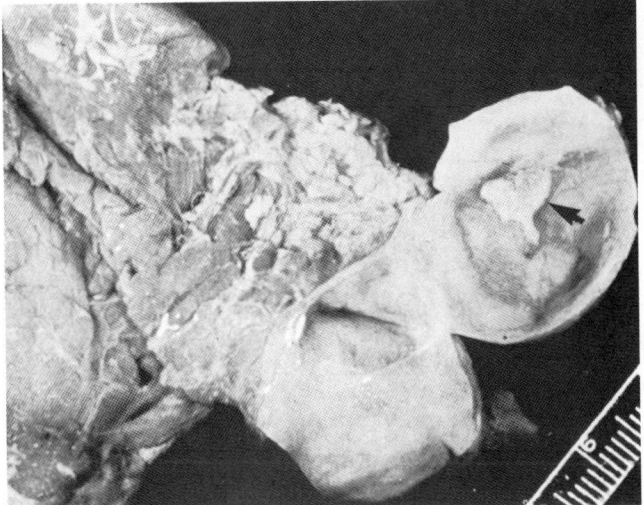

Figure 20–11. Pseudocyst of pancreas. Cyst has been opened and the contents drained. A small plaque of white calcium is visible in wall *(small arrow).*

tumor, consists of many small cysts. The *solid-cystic (papillary-cystic) tumor* is predominantly seen in adolescent girls and women under age 35. It is a large, rounded, well-circumscribed mass that has solid and cystic zones. Histologically, the tumor cells are small and uniform and have a finely granular eosinophilic cytoplasm. They grow in solid sheets or papillary projections. The tumors cause abdominal discomfort and pain and are usually cured by resection.

CARCINOMA OF PANCREAS

The term "carcinoma of the pancreas" is meant to imply carcinoma arising in the exocrine portion of the gland. Although duct cells make up only 4% of all pancreatic cells, virtually all these cancers begin in the ductal epithelium; the acini themselves give origin to less than 1% of malignant tumors.[29,30] Tumors that arise from the islets of Langerhans are specifically designated as islet cell tumors and will be considered later (p. 1005).

Pancreatic cancer continues to be a depressingly difficult problem.[31] These highly fatal cancers have a deceptively silent growth habit, so that by the time they are diagnosed they are rarely curable. Pancreatic cancer accounts for 5% of all cancer deaths in the United States. There are 26,000 new cases and 24,000 deaths from the disease each year.[32] The incidence has increased threefold in the last 40 years; this has been ascribed to smoking, diet, and chemical carcinogens.[33] The risk of pancreatic cancer among heavy smokers is about 2 to 2.5 times that of nonsmokers. There is also a positive but unexplained correlation between mortality from cancer of the pancreas and per capita consumption of fats, and possibly calories. There is a higher risk of pancreatic cancer among

chemists, and particularly in those exposed to industrial agents such as beta-naphthylamine and benzidine. Both ductal and acinar cancers can be induced by chemicals (e.g., nitrosamines) in animals.[34] The incidence rates are higher in blacks than in whites, in males than in females, in diabetics than in nondiabetics, and in the presence of hereditary chronic pancreatitis.[35,36] These tumors occur most often in the sixth, seventh, and eighth decades of life, although about 10% of patients are much younger.

These lesions may arise anywhere in the pancreas, but most studies show a fairly standard distribution: head of pancreas, 60%; body of pancreas, 15% to 20%[29]; and tail of pancreas, 5%.[29] In 20% the tumor either is diffuse or has spread so widely as to preclude localization of its site of origin. Tumors of the head of the pancreas are in a strategic location to impinge upon the ampulla of Vater, common bile duct, and duodenum and thus cause obstructive biliary symptoms relatively early in their life history. These lesions, therefore, tend to be discovered while still small and before widespread metastasis has occurred. In contrast, cancers in the body and tail may grow silently for longer periods and become manifest only by extension to adjacent structures and by metastatic dissemination.

Grossly, carcinomas in the **head of the pancreas** are fairly small lesions that frequently cause little or only moderate expansion of the pancreatic tissue. Sometimes they are totally inapparent on external examination of the organ and create only the impression of some increased consistency and irregular nodularity. Other lesions create masses up to 8 to 10 cm in diameter. The gray-white, scirrhous, homogeneous tumor infiltrates and replaces the lobular architecture

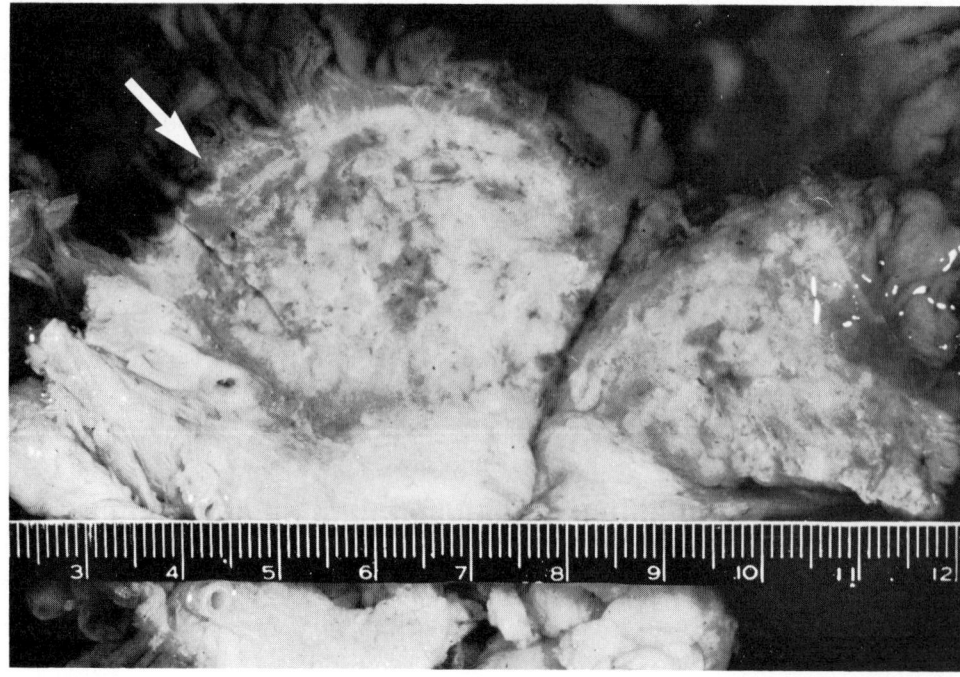

Figure 20–13. Carcinoma of head of pancreas. Mottled invasive lesion has grown into wall of duodenum, which appears at upper extent of tumor *(arrow).*

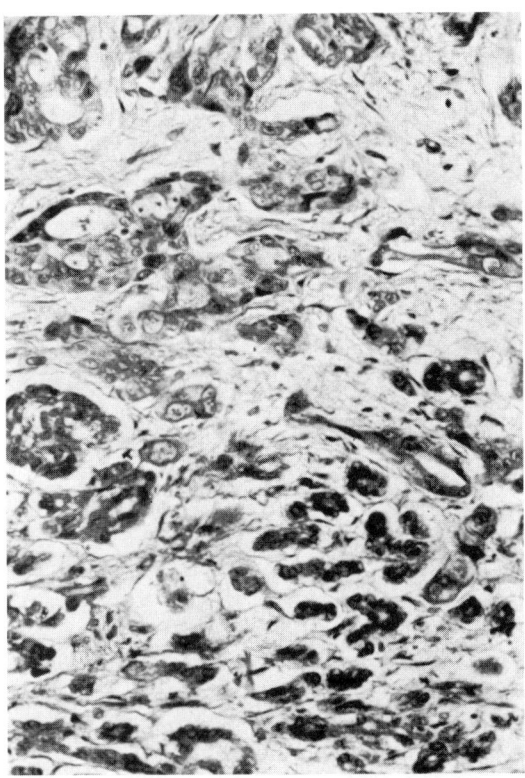

Figure 20–14. Adenocarcinoma of pancreas. Malignant glands are invading pancreatic substance seen at bottom of photograph.

of a normal pancreas. Characteristically, such lesions have poorly defined, obviously infiltrative margins (Fig. 20–13). The tumor usually extends to the margin of the duodenum and invades the wall as well as the common bile duct. In a small percentage of cases, it extends directly through the wall to produce either a small fungating lesion or an irregular ulceration. In this infiltrative growth, it surrounds and compresses the common bile duct or ampulla of Vater, causing biliary obstruction. Extension to peripancreatic and portohepatic nodes with isolated small metastases in the liver is not uncommon. But because these tumors produce biliary tract obstruction and jaundice at an early date, they usually have not had a long history before discovery, and patients die of the hepatobiliary dysfunction before the tumor has become widely disseminated.

Carcinomas of the body and tail are usually large, hard, irregular masses that sometimes wipe out virtually the entire tail and body of the pancreas. On cross section, the tumors exactly resemble those of the head of the gland, but **frequently extend more widely than those of the head.** They impinge upon the adjacent vertebral column, extend through the retroperitoneal spaces inferiorly and superiorly, and occasionally invade the adjacent spleen or adrenal. They may extend into the transverse colon or stomach. Peripancreatic, gastric, mesenteric, omental, and portohepatic nodes are involved, and the liver is strikingly seeded with tumor nodules to produce hepatic enlargement. Massive hepatic metastases are quite characteristic of carcinoma of the tail and body of the pancreas, and are attrib-

uted to invasion of the splenic vein that courses directly along the margins of this organ.

Histologically, most carcinomas of the pancreas grow in more or less well-differentiated glandular patterns and are thus **adenocarcinomas** (Fig. 20–14). The tumors may be mucinous or non–mucin secreting. The glands are atypical, irregular, small, and bizarre and are usually lined by anaplastic cuboidal-to-columnar epithelial cells. Other variants grow in an undifferentiated pattern. About 10% assume either an **adenosquamous pattern** or the uncommon pattern of extreme anaplasia with **giant cell formation,** numerous mitoses, and bizarre pleomorphism; 0.5% arise in cysts and are termed **cystadenocarcinoma.** Rarely, carcinomas arise from acinar cells **(acinar cell carcinoma),** particularly in children.

CLINICAL COURSE. Carcinomas of the pancreas, even those of its head, are insidious lesions that undoubtedly are present for months and possibly years before they produce symptoms referable to their expansive growth.[37] The major symptoms include weight loss, abdominal pain, back pain, anorexia, nausea, vomiting and generalized malaise, and weakness. Jaundice is present in about 90% of patients with carcinomas of the head, and in 10 to 40% of those with cancer of the body or tail.

The diagnosis and localization of pancreatic tumors are aided by ultrasonography, which can differentiate cysts from solid tumors, and CT scan of the pancreas (Fig. 20–15). Percutaneous needle biopsies from tumors specifically localized by these

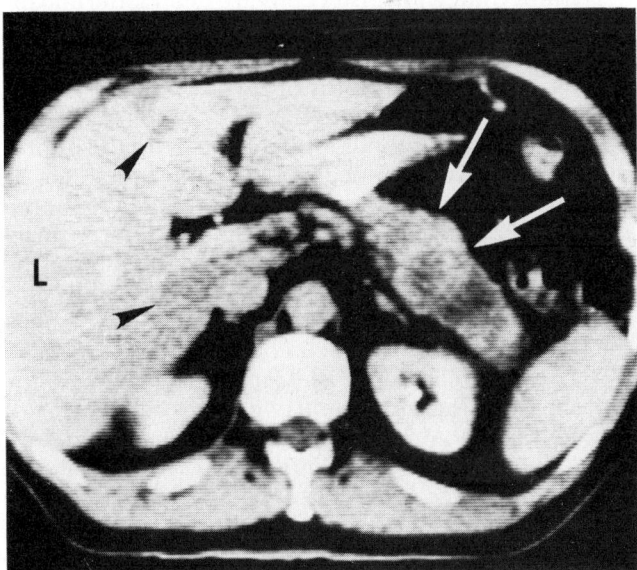

Figure 20–15. CT scan at midabdominal level demonstrating pancreatic carcinoma. Compare with Figure 20–1 to localize the other organs. Pancreatic tail is enlarged and heterogeneous *(long arrows).* Liver (L) contains multiple focal lucencies, corresponding to metastatic deposits *(arrowheads).* Stomach, spleen, and kidneys are also visible. (Courtesy of Dr. S. Seltzer, Brigham and Women's Hospital, Boston.)

techniques may obviate the need for exploratory laparotomy.

Migratory thrombophlebitis, known clinically as *Trousseau's syndrome,* occurs in 10% of patients. Ironically, Trousseau diagnosed his own fatal disease as cancer of the pancreas when he developed migratory thrombophlebitis. These spontaneously appearing and disappearing thromboses are also encountered in other forms of cancer, but the two highest levels of correlation are with pancreatic and pulmonary neoplasms (see p. 296).

The symptomatic course of pancreatic carcinoma is typically brief and progressive. Only 20% of the tumors are resectable at the time of diagnosis. The average duration from diagnosis until death is six months. One-year survival is 10% and five-year survival is 1 to 2%.

THE ENDOCRINE PANCREAS

DIABETES MELLITUS
Morphology of Diabetes and
**   Late Complications**
Clinical Course

ISLET CELL TUMORS
Beta-Cell Tumors (Insulinoma)
Zollinger-Ellison Syndrome
**   (Gastrinoma, Ulcerogenic Islet**
**   Cell Tumor)**

Other Rare Islet Cell Tumors
Multiple Endocrine Neoplasia
**   (MEN) Syndromes**

NORMAL

The endocrine pancreas consists of about 1 million microscopic cellular units — the islets of Langerhans — and a few scattered cells within the small pancreatic ducts.[38,39] In the aggregate the islets in the adult human weigh only 1 to 1.5 gm.

Embryologically, islet cells are of endodermal origin, and form at many points along the pancreatic tubuloductal system. The first evidence of islet formation in the human fetus occurs at 9 to 11 weeks, with the appearance, on H and E sections, of dark, deeply eosinophilic cells interspersed with the lighter duct cells. Insulin and glucagon, however, can be measured and visualized earlier immunocytochemically. The dark cells subsequently proliferate, forming clusters that evaginate and then detach from the tubuloductal system to form discrete islets. The islets are then invaded by capillaries that separate the cluster into the typical islet cell cords.

In the human adult, islets measure 50 to 250 μm and consist of four major and two minor cell types.[38,39] The four main types are *B (beta), A (alpha), D (delta),* and *PP (pancreatic polypeptide) cells.* These make up about 70, 20, 5 to 10, and 1 to 2%, respectively, of the islet cell population. They can be differentiated morphologically by their staining properties with certain dyes, by the ultrastructural morphology of their granules, and (most important) by their hormonal content in immunohistochemical studies that employ specific antibodies to individual hormones.

The *B cell* (beta) (Fig. 20–16) produces *insulin.* The description of insulin secretion by beta cells is detailed in the discussion of diabetes (p. 995). The granules have rectangular profiles and a crystalline matrix and are surrounded by a halo (Fig. 20–17). Hyperplasia and neoplasia of these cells are responsible for the important clinical syndrome of hyperinsulinism. *A cells* (alpha) secrete *glucagon,* which induces hyperglycemia by its glycogenolytic activity in the liver. Alpha-cell granules are round, with closely applied membranes and a dense center (Fig. 20–18). *D cells* (delta) contain somatostatin, which suppresses both insulin and glucagon release. Delta cells have large, pale granules with closely applied membranes (Fig. 20–18). *PP cells* have small, dark granules and are not only present in islets but also scattered in the exocrine pancreas. They contain a unique pancreatic polypeptide that exerts a number of gastrointestinal effects such as stimulation of secretion of gastric and intestinal enzymes and inhibition of intestinal motility. The two rare cell types are *D1 cells* and *enterochromaffin cells.* D1 cells have distinctive granules by electron microscopy and elaborate *vasoactive intestinal peptide* (VIP), a hormone that induces glycogenolysis and hyperglycemia and also stimulates gastrointestinal fluid secretion and causes secretory diarrhea. *Enterochromaffin cells* synthesize serotonin and are the source of pancreatic tumors that induce the carcinoid syndrome (p. 1007).

We now turn to the two main disorders of islet cells: diabetes mellitus and islet cell tumors.

PATHOLOGY

Despite the minute size of the islets of Langerhans, even collectively, the endocrine pancreas is responsi-

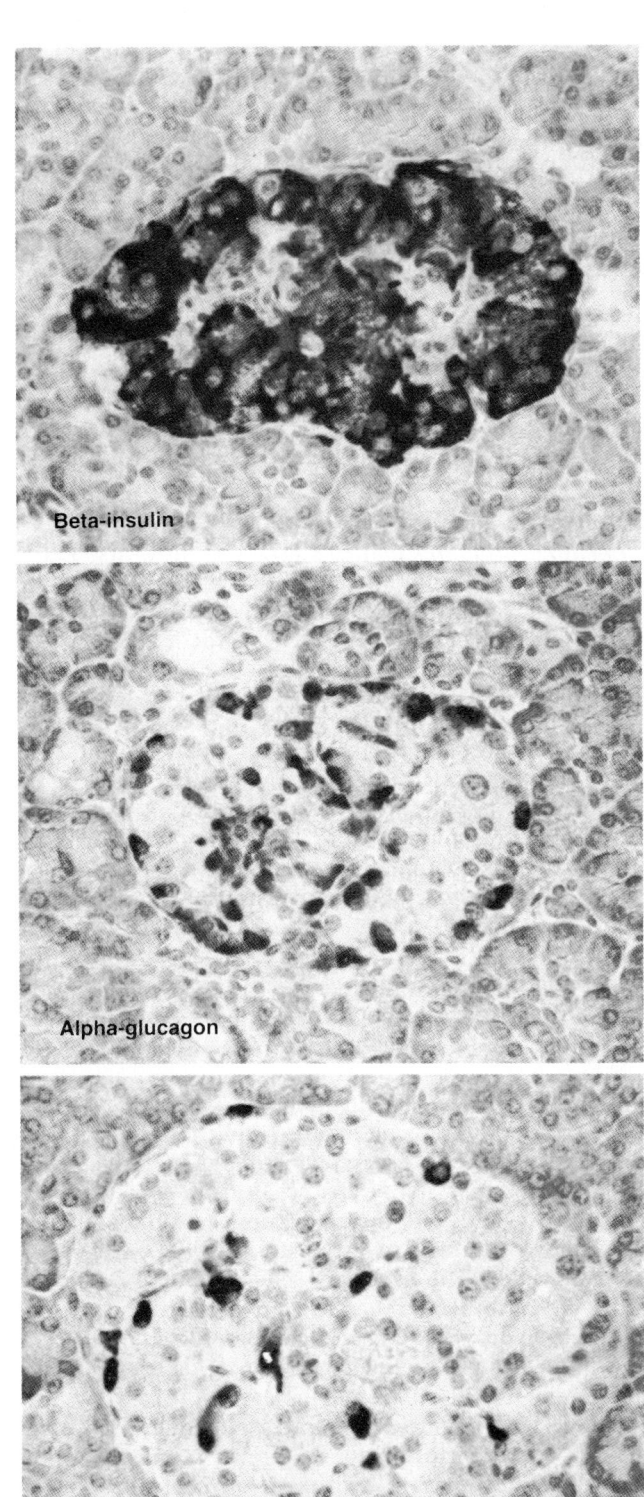

Beta-insulin

Alpha-glucagon

Delta-somatostatin

Figure 20–16. Islets stained by immunoperoxidase technique for insulin *(top),* glucagon *(middle),* and somatostatin *(bottom).* The dark reaction product identifies beta, alpha, and delta cells, respectively. (Courtesy of Dr. A. Like, University of Massachusetts School of Medicine.)

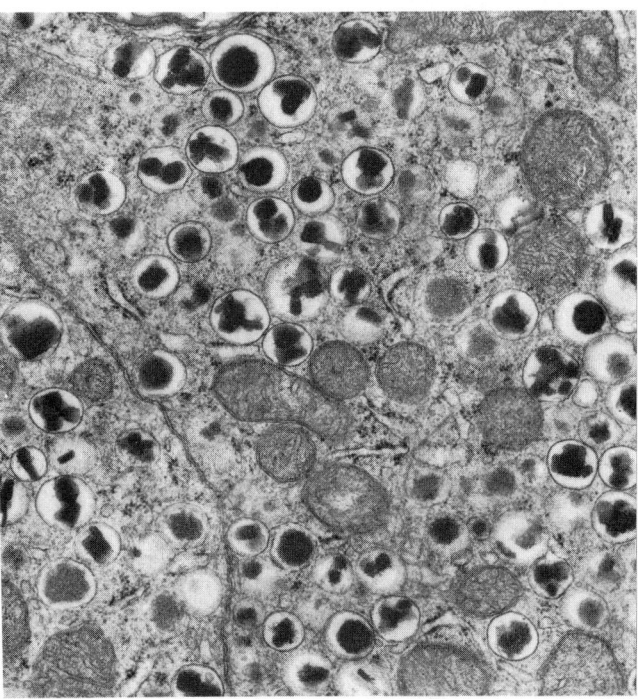

Figure 20–17. Electron micrograph of a portion of a beta cell with characteristic membrane-bound granules, each containing a dense, often rectangular core and a distinct halo. (Courtesy of Dr. A. Like, University of Massachusetts School of Medicine.)

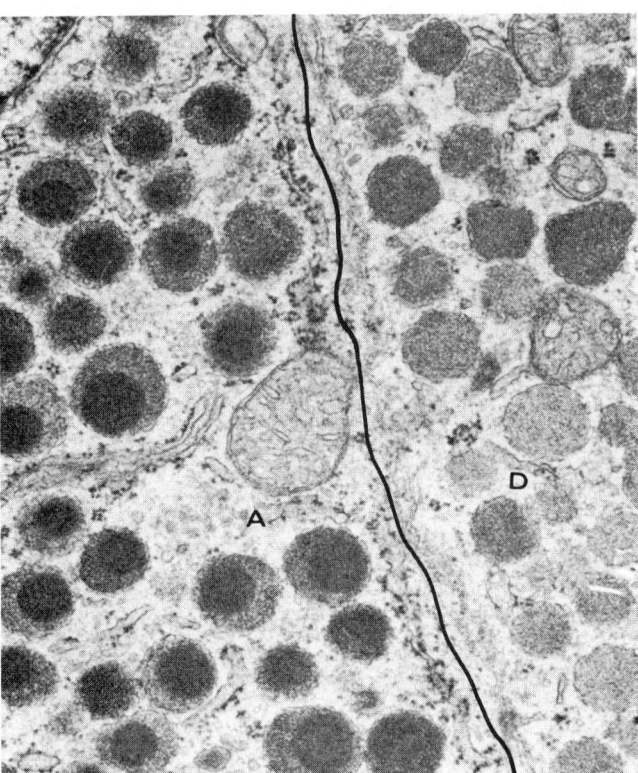

Figure 20–18. Portions of an alpha cell *(left, A)* and a delta cell *(right, D).* Granules in both cells have closely apposed membranes, but the alpha cell granule exhibits a dense, round center. (Courtesy of Dr. A. Like, University of Massachusetts School of Medicine.)

Table 20-2. Types of Diabetes

PRIMARY (IDIOPATHIC) DIABETES
Type I (Insulin-dependent diabetes mellitus, IDDM)
Type II (Non-insulin dependent diabetes mellitus, NIDDM)
Nonobese NIDDM
Obese NIDDM
Maturity-onset diabetes of the young (MODY)
SECONDARY DIABETES
Chronic pancreatitis
Postpancreatectomy
Hormonal tumors (e.g., pheochromocytoma, pituitary tumors)
Drugs (corticosteroids)
Hemochromatosis
Genetic disorders (e.g., lipodystrophy)

ble for a disproportionate amount of morbidity and mortality. Diabetes mellitus alone ranks among the top ten causes of death in Western nations, and despite important improvements in its clinical management, to date it has not been possible to control significantly its lethal consequences. The various forms of neoplasia arising in the islets, although far less common, produce some fascinating, often difficult to diagnose endocrinopathies. The endocrine pancreas is therefore a source of significant clinical disease.

DIABETES MELLITUS

Diabetes mellitus is a chronic disorder affecting carbohydrate, fat, and protein metabolism. A characteristic feature of diabetes mellitus is *hyperglycemia*, a reflection of impaired carbohydrate (glucose) utilization resulting from a defective or deficient insulin secretory response.[40]

CLASSIFICATION AND INCIDENCE. In this section, we will deal principally with *primary or idiopathic diabetes mellitus*, which is by far the most common and important entity. Primary diabetes must be distinguished from *secondary diabetes*, which includes forms of hyperglycemia associated with identi-

fiable causes in which destruction of pancreatic islets is induced by inflammatory pancreatic disease, surgery, tumors, certain drugs, iron overload (hemochromatosis), and certain acquired or genetic endocrinopathies (Table 20-2).

Primary diabetes mellitus probably represents a heterogeneous group of disorders having hyperglycemia as a common feature. Until recently, several classifications have existed based on differing criteria, some using clinical features, others etiology, and some the presumed natural history of diabetes. In an attempt to overcome problems in classification, the National Diabetes Data Group of the National Institutes of Health developed a classification (Table 20-3); this basically divides primary diabetes into two variants that differ in their pattern of inheritance, insulin responses, and origins.[41] The first is *insulin-dependent diabetes mellitus (IDDM)*, now also called *type I diabetes,* and previously known as juvenile-onset and ketosis-prone diabetes. This variant accounts for 10 to 20% of all cases of idiopathic diabetes. The remaining 80 to 90% of patients have the second variant, designated *non-insulin dependent diabetes mellitus* (NIDDM), also called *type II diabetes* and previously referred to as adult-onset diabetes. Type II diabetes is further divided into obese and nonobese types, and a third rare form, known as *maturity-onset diabetes of the young* (MODY). MODY is manifested by mild hyperglycemia and is transmitted as an autosomal dominant trait. It should be stressed that while the two major types of diabetes have different pathogenetic mechanisms and metabolic characteristics, the chronic, *long-term complications in blood vessels, kidney, eye, and nerves occur in both types and are the major causes of morbidity and death in diabetes.*

With an annual toll of about 35,000, diabetes mellitus is the seventh leading cause of death in the United States. It is estimated that 1 to 2% of the adult population have diabetes mellitus. The prevalence of type I diabetes varies widely around the world,[42,43] probably as a reflection of some as yet obscure environmental factors in the pathogenesis of the disease,

Table 20-3. Type I vs. Type II Diabetes

	TYPE I (IDDM)	TYPE II (NIDDM)
Clinical	Onset <20 years	Onset >30 years
	Normal weight	Obese
	Decreased blood insulin	Normal or increased blood insulin
	Islet cell antibodies	No islet cell antibodies
	Ketoacidosis common	Ketoacidosis rare
Genetics	50% concordance in twins	90-100% concordance in twins
	HLA-D linked	No HLA association
Pathogenesis	Autoimmunity	Insulin resistance
	Immunopathologic mechanisms	Relative insulin deficiency
	Severe insulin deficiency	
Islet Cells	Insulitis early	No insulitis
	Marked atrophy and fibrosis	Focal atrophy and amyloid
	Beta cell depletion	Mild beta cell depletion

as we shall see. In the United States, the prevalence of type I diabetes is 0.25% by age 20.

PATHOGENESIS

The pathogenesis of the two types will be discussed separately, but first we will briefly discuss normal insulin metabolism, since some aspects of insulin release and action are important in the discussion of pathogenesis.

NORMAL INSULIN METABOLISM. The chemical structure, molecular biology, biosynthesis, and secretory pathways of insulin are now understood in elegant detail.[43,44] Indeed, the human insulin gene was one of the first human genes to be cloned. It is encoded on the short arm of chromosome 11 and is expressed in the beta cells of the pancreatic islets, where mature insulin mRNA is transcribed. Translation of the message occurs in the rough endoplasmic reticulum, yielding preproinsulin. There follows proteolytic cleavage of the prepeptide sequence to yield proinsulin, and in the Golgi apparatus, cleavage of the C-peptide to yield insulin sequences. Both insulin and C-peptide are then stored in secretory granules and secreted together after physiologic stimulation (Fig. 20–19). Release from beta cells occurs as a biphasic process involving two pools of insulin. A rise in the blood glucose levels, for example, calls forth an immediate release of insulin, presumably that stored in the beta-cell granules. If the secretory stimulus persists, a delayed and protracted response follows, which in-

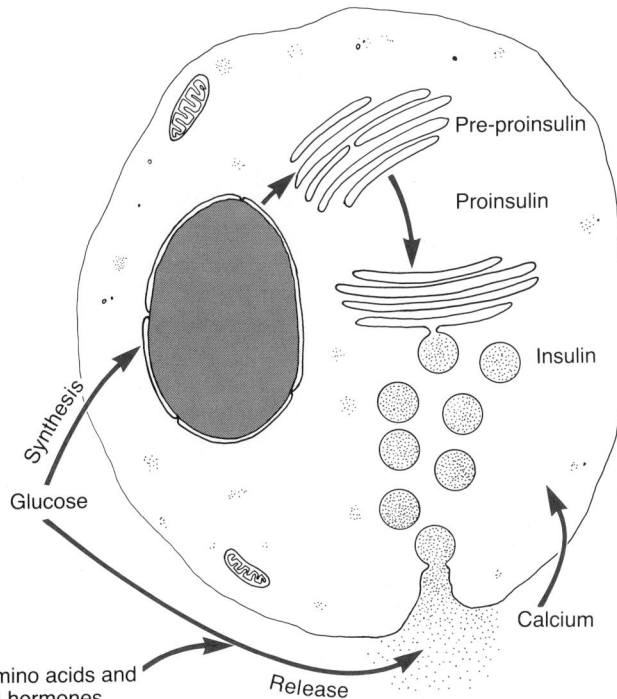

Figure 20–19. Insulin synthesis and secretion. Note that glucose stimulates both synthesis and secretion, while other agents— amino acids and certain GI hormones— induce only secretion.

volves active synthesis of insulin. *The most important stimulus that triggers insulin release is glucose, which also initiates insulin synthesis.* Other agents, including intestinal hormones and certain amino acids (leucine and arginine), as well as the sulfonylureas stimulate insulin release but not synthesis. Calcium influx into the cells, alpha-adrenergic agents, and cAMP are involved in insulin secretion.

Insulin is a major anabolic hormone.[43] It is necessary for (1) transmembrane transport of glucose and amino acids, (2) glycogen formation in the liver and skeletal muscles, (3) glucose conversion to triglycerides, (4) nucleic acid synthesis, and (5) protein synthesis. *Its prime metabolic function is to increase the rate of glucose transport into certain cells in the body.* These are the striated muscle cells, including myocardial cells, fibroblasts, and fat cells, representing collectively about two thirds of the entire body weight. In addition to these metabolic effects, *insulin and insulin-like growth factors initiate DNA synthesis in certain cells and stimulate their growth and differentiation.*[45]

Insulin interacts with its target cells by first *binding to the insulin receptor,* composed of two glycoprotein subunits α and β (Fig. 20–20).[46,47] The number and function of these receptors are important in regulating the action of insulin. Insulin binds to the extracellular portion of the α-subunit, and this in turn activates the tyrosine-specific protein kinase activity of the cytoplasmic portion of the β-subunit. The β-subunit tyrosine kinase then catalyzes phosphorylation of the β-subunit itself as well as other intracellular proteins. This is followed by a number of cellular responses, including activation or inhibition of insulin-sensitive enzymes in mitochondria, protein synthesis, and DNA synthesis. One of the important early effects of insulin that is likely to be mediated by protein phosphorylation involves translocation of *glucose transport units* from the Golgi apparatus to the plasma membrane, thus facilitating cellular uptake of glucose.

PATHOGENESIS OF TYPE I DIABETES. *This form of diabetes results from a severe, absolute lack of insulin, caused by a reduction in the beta-cell mass.* Type I diabetes usually develops in childhood, becoming manifest and severe at puberty. Patients *depend on insulin for survival.* Without insulin, they develop acute metabolic complications, such as acute ketoacidosis and coma.

A great deal has been learned about the pathogenesis of type I diabetes.[48–54] Three interlocking mechanisms are responsible for the islet cell destruction: *genetic susceptibility, autoimmunity, and an environmental insult.* A postulated sequence of events involving these three mechanisms is shown in Figure 20–21. It is thought that a *genetic susceptibility* to altered immune regulation, linked to specific alleles in the class II major histocompatibility complex (HLA-D), predisposes certain individuals to the development of *autoimmunity to islet beta cells.* The au-

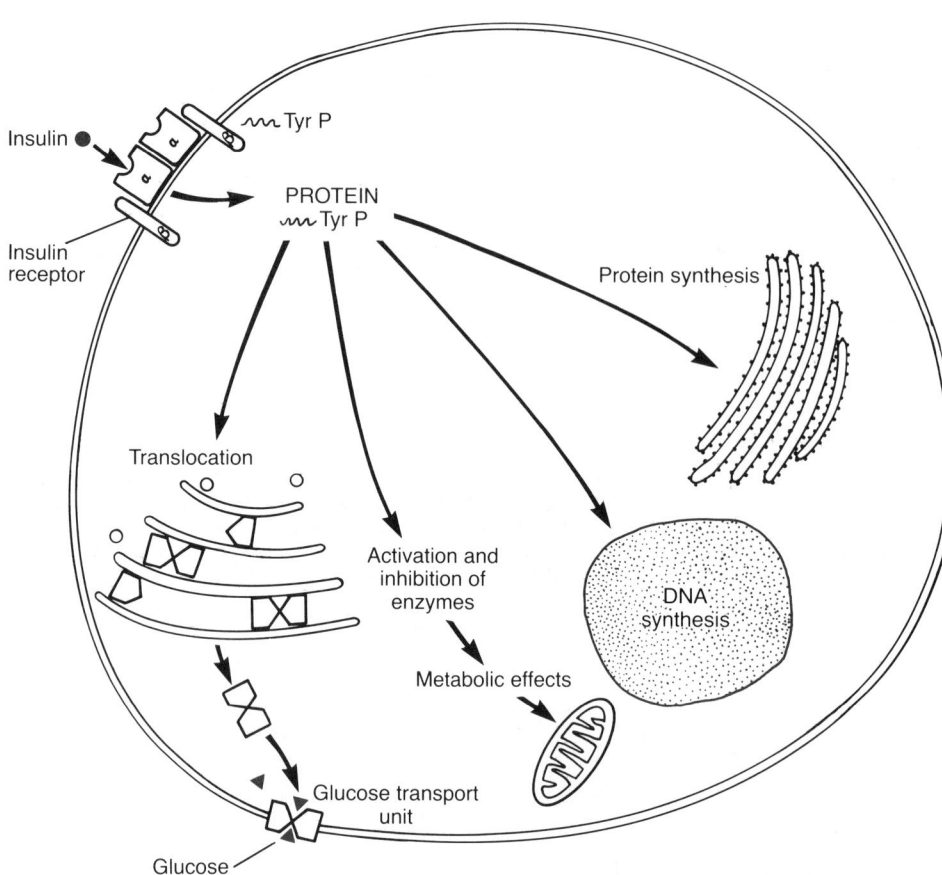

Insulin

Insulin receptor

Tyr P

PROTEIN
Tyr P

Protein synthesis

Translocation

Activation and inhibition of enzymes

DNA synthesis

Metabolic effects

Glucose transport unit

Glucose

Figure 20–20. Schematic model of insulin action on an insulin-responsive cell. Insulin binds to the α-subunit of the insulin receptor, and activates tyrosine-specific protein kinase autophosphorylation (of the β-subunit) as well as phosphorylation of other intracellular proteins. This is followed by DNA synthesis, protein synthesis, altered mitochondrial metabolism, and translocation of glucose transport units from the Golgi apparatus to the plasma membrane.

toimmunity either develops spontaneously or, more likely, is triggered by an environmental agent (a virus, chemical, or unknown toxin), resulting in acute *insulitis* and damage to B cells. An autoimmune reaction directed against B cells then causes further beta-cell injury and eventually, when most of the cells are destroyed, overt diabetes mellitus appears (Fig. 21–21A). Let us briefly discuss the three important mechanisms in the sequence.

Genetic Susceptibility. It has long been known that diabetes mellitus can aggregate in families. However, the precise mode of inheritance of the susceptibility genes for type I diabetes remains unknown. Among identical twins, the concordance rate (i.e., both twins affected) is only approximately 50%. Only 5 to 10% of children of first-order relatives with type I diabetes develop the disease. Environmental factors must therefore play an important role in this type of diabetes, as we shall see.

At least one of the susceptibility genes for type I diabetes resides in the genes encoding the class II antigens of the major histocompatibility region of chromosome 6 (HLA-D).[55] You will recall (p. 170) that the HLA-D region contains three subregions—DP, DQ, and DR—, that the class II molecules are highly polymorphic, and that each has numerous alleles. About 80% of patients with type I diabetes have either HLA-DR3 or HLA-DR4 alleles, whereas in the general population the prevalence of these antigens is only 30 to 50%. Individuals who are HLA-DR3 positive have a fivefold greater risk of developing diabetes, and those with HLA-DR4, a seven times increased risk, compared with those who are HLA-DR3 or -4 negative. DR3/4 heterozygotes have an approximately 14.3 increased risk. Recently, a still stronger association was made with certain alleles in the DQ locus, which are in "linkage disequilibrium" with HLA-DR.[56] Indeed, analysis of DNA sequences from the DQβ locus of diabetics and nondiabetics has shown that *simple differences in the structure of the DQ molecule*—for example, replacement of the normal Asp amino acid at position 57 by Ser, Ala, or Val—*confers increased susceptibility to type I diabetes in Caucasians.* Position 57 faces the antigen-binding cleft of the class II molecule, fueling speculation that polymorphism at this site could alter beta cell antigen presentation and in some way predispose to autoimmunity.[57]

Whether a second diabetogenic allele, not linked to the HLA region, is required for the development of diabetes (as is the case in a genetic model of diabetes [NOD] in mice) is now under investigation.[58]

Autoimmunity. Autoimmunity and immunopathologic mechanisms clearly play a role in type I diabetes.[59] Some of the evidence is as follows:

1. Lymphocytic infiltration of the islets, often intense (insulitis), is frequently observed in type I diabetes of

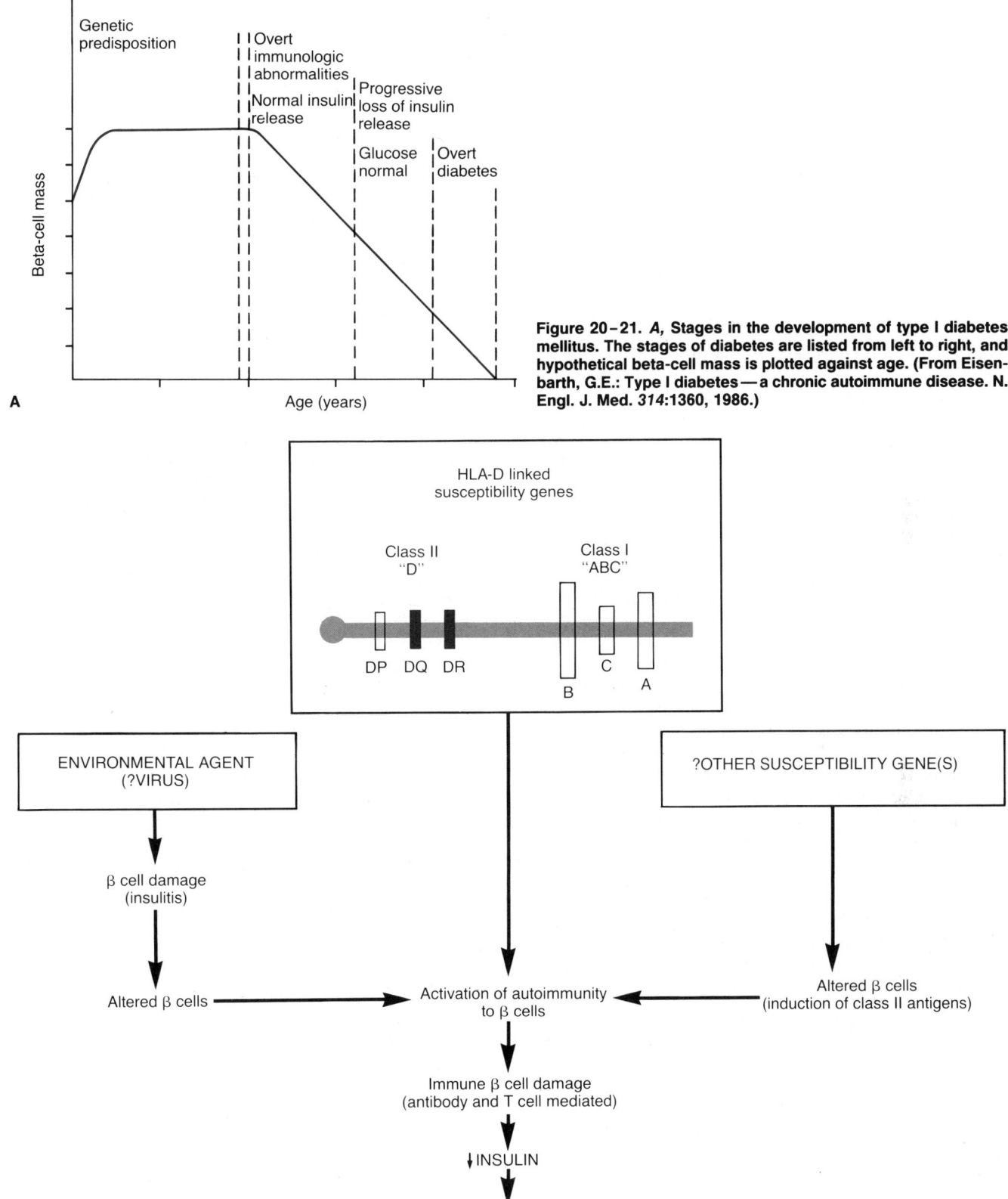

Figure 20–21. *A,* Stages in the development of type I diabetes mellitus. The stages of diabetes are listed from left to right, and hypothetical beta-cell mass is plotted against age. (From Eisenbarth, G.E.: Type I diabetes—a chronic autoimmune disease. N. Engl. J. Med. *314*:1360, 1986.)

Figure 20–21. *B,* Postulated mechanisms in the pathogenesis of type I diabetes. Susceptibility to the development of diabetes is enhanced by HLD-D linked genes (HLA DR/DQ), which serve to activate or amplify autoimmune reactions to beta cells. Either environmental agents (? virus) or other susceptibility genetic determinants are thought to alter beta cells and make them antigenic. Autoimmune reactions to beta cells result in antibody and T cell–mediated damage to cells, which in the absence of beta cells regeneration, results in insulin depletion and diabetes.

recent onset.[60,61] In animal models of type I diabetes, T and B lymphocytes infiltrate the islets with the development of diabetes.

2. Up to 90% of patients with type I diabetes have islet cell antibodies, when tested within one year of diagnosis. Asymptomatic individuals who have a higher than normal risk of developing type I diabetes develop islet cell antibodies *months to years before the clinical onset of diabetes.* About half of first-degree relatives of diabetic children positive for complement-fixing islet cell antibodies (ICA) eventually become insulin-dependent, as opposed to 0.3% of ICA-negative subjects.[62] There is also evidence for cell-mediated autoimmunity against islet cells in humans.

3. In two experimental models of type I diabetes, the **BB** rat and **NOD** mouse, there is substantial evidence of autoimmunity and a lymphocytic insulitis, in which helper/inducer and cytotoxic/suppressor subsets of T lymphocytes, as well as natural killer cells, are present. Eventually, when the inflammatory cells disappear, the islets are depleted of beta cells.[48]

4. In approximately one fifth of cases of type I diabetes, other endocrine disorders suspected to be of autoimmune origin are also present. These include Addison's disease, hypothyroidism, and Graves' disease.

5. In experimental animals and in humans, *the insulitis is associated with aberrant expression of class II MHC molecules on the surface of beta cells* (but not other endocrine cells in the islets) *and increased expression of class I molecules.*[61] Normal beta cells do not possess class II molecules on their surface. Class II MHC molecules, it will be recalled, are essential for the recognition by helper T-cells of a foreign or autologous antigen, and class I molecules are recognized by cytotoxic T cells. It is not clear, whether this aberrant MHC expression is a primary or secondary event.[63] One view holds that a primary immune defect results in aberrant class II molecules on beta cells, which leads to recognition of normal beta-cell antigens by specific T-helper cells, and lymphocytic infiltration (Fig. 20–21B, right). Cytokines (such as γ interferon) in the infiltrate then cause increased class I expression, leading to recognition and destruction of beta cells by cytotoxic cells. The other view is that the lymphocytic infiltration and an immune response to beta cells, initiated by some virus infection, occurs first and the resultant cytokines then stimulate class I and class II expression of cells (Fig. 20–21B, left).[64] In vitro, the actual destruction of islet cells can result from the synergistic effects of cytokines, including gamma interferon, tumor necrosis factor, lymphotoxin, and interleukin-1 on the islet cells.[65]

To summarize, there is overwhelming evidence implicating autoimmunity and immune-mediated injury as causes of beta-cell loss in type I diabetes mellitus. Indeed, immunosuppressive therapy with cy- closporine has recently been shown to prevent the development of or to ameliorate type I diabetes in experimental animals and in children with this disease.[66,67]

Environmental Factors. Granted that a genetic susceptibility, leading to autoimmune destruction of islet cells, is the cause of insulin deficiency in type I diabetes, what triggers the autoimmune reaction? One answer, as we have discussed, is that a non–HLA linked second diabetogenic gene, similar to that which occurs in the BB rat and NOD mice, induces so-called *primary autoimmunity,* in which an immune response occurs against normal unaltered beta cells, causing the initial insulitis. Although such an "insulitis" allele may in fact exist, most authorities now believe that the initial trigger for the development of insulitis is an environmental factor.

The epidemiologic data on type I diabetes clearly point to environmental factors. For example, Finnish children have a 60- to 70-fold increased risk of type I diabetes compared with Korean children. In the Northeastern United States, over the last 30 years there has been a tripling of type I diabetes in children under the age of 15. In three studies in Japan, Israel, and Canada, emigrants assume a risk of type I diabetes closer to that of their destination country than of their country of origin.[68] *These and other results suggest that diabetes is a rare outcome of some relatively common viral infection, delayed by a long latency period necessary for the progressive autoimmune loss of beta cells to occur, and dependent on the modifying effects of alleles in the major histocompatibility region.*[47] One good example of such an occurrence is the development of type I diabetes in patients with congenital rubella. In these individuals, infection occurs in utero, but type I diabetes does not develop until childhood or puberty in about 20% of infected patients, almost always in those with HLA-DR3 or DR4 antigens.[69] A variety of other viral infections have been implicated as triggers, including mumps, measles, coxsackie B virus, cytomegalovirus, and infectious mononucleosis.[70] Certain viruses can cause beta-cell loss by direct destruction of the islets, but in most of the models, immunopathologic processes associated with humoral- or cellular-mediated mechanisms are more important. The most likely scenario is that viruses trigger an immune response to beta cells in individuals with HLA-linked susceptibility.

Experimentally, a number of chemicals, including streptozotocin, alloxan, and pentamidine, also induce islet cell destruction. In particular, pentamidine, a drug used for the treatment of parasitic infections, has been occasionally associated with the development of abrupt-onset diabetes, and cases of diabetes have also been reported after accidental or suicidal ingestion of Vacor, a pharmacologic agent used as a rat exterminator.[70] These chemicals act either directly on islet cells or by triggering an immune mechanism. Viruses, chemicals, and environmental toxins are thus being actively sought as culprits in the genesis of type I diabetes, and the disease once called the "geneticists's nightmare" is now considered an "epidemiologist's dream."[42]

Figure 20–21B summarizes the postulated pathways in the pathogenesis of type I diabetes mellitus and the contribution of genetic, immunologic, and environmental factors.

PATHOGENESIS OF TYPE II DIABETES. Much less is known, unfortunately, about the pathogenesis of non–insulin dependent diabetes, which, it should be re-emphasized, is by far the most common type. Genetic factors are of even greater importance than in type I diabetes, and among identical twins, the concordance rate is over 90%.[71] However, except for the maturity-onset type of diabetes of the young (MODY), described earlier, the mode of inheritance is unclear. Unlike type I, the disease is not linked to any HLA haplotype, and there is no evidence that autoimmune mechanisms are involved. Obesity and overeating play important roles in type II diabetes, and there is a correlation between the disease and increasing age.

Two metabolic defects characterize type II diabetes: (1) *a derangement in insulin secretion* that is delayed or that is insufficient relative to the glucose load, and (2) an inability of peripheral tissues to respond to insulin–*insulin resistance*. The primacy of one or the other of these defects is a matter of continuing debate.[72] The issue is complicated by the frequent occurrence of obesity in patients with type II diabetes. Obesity, even in the absence of diabetes, is characterized by insulin resistance and hyperinsulinemia. However, when obese type II patients are compared with weight-matched nondiabetics, it appears that the insulin levels of obese diabetics are below those observed in obese nondiabetics, suggesting a relative insulin deficiency. Furthermore, in patients with moderately severe type II diabetes (fasting plasma glucose level of 200 to 300 gm/ml), it is possible to demonstrate an absolute deficiency of insulin. Recent studies also show that abnormalities in the usual pattern of pulsatile or oscillatory insulin secretion is an early phenomenon in type II diabetes.[73] *We can conclude, therefore, that most patients with type II diabetes have a relative or absolute deficiency of insulin*, which, however is much milder than that of type I diabetes.[74] The cause of this insulin deficiency is unknown. One view is that it represents the progressive, age-related loss of beta-cell function, which is accelerated in subjects with genetically predetermined diabetes.[72]

There is also substantial evidence for *insulin resistance* in type II diabetes.[72] Although obesity is emphasized as a factor in insulin resistance, the latter is

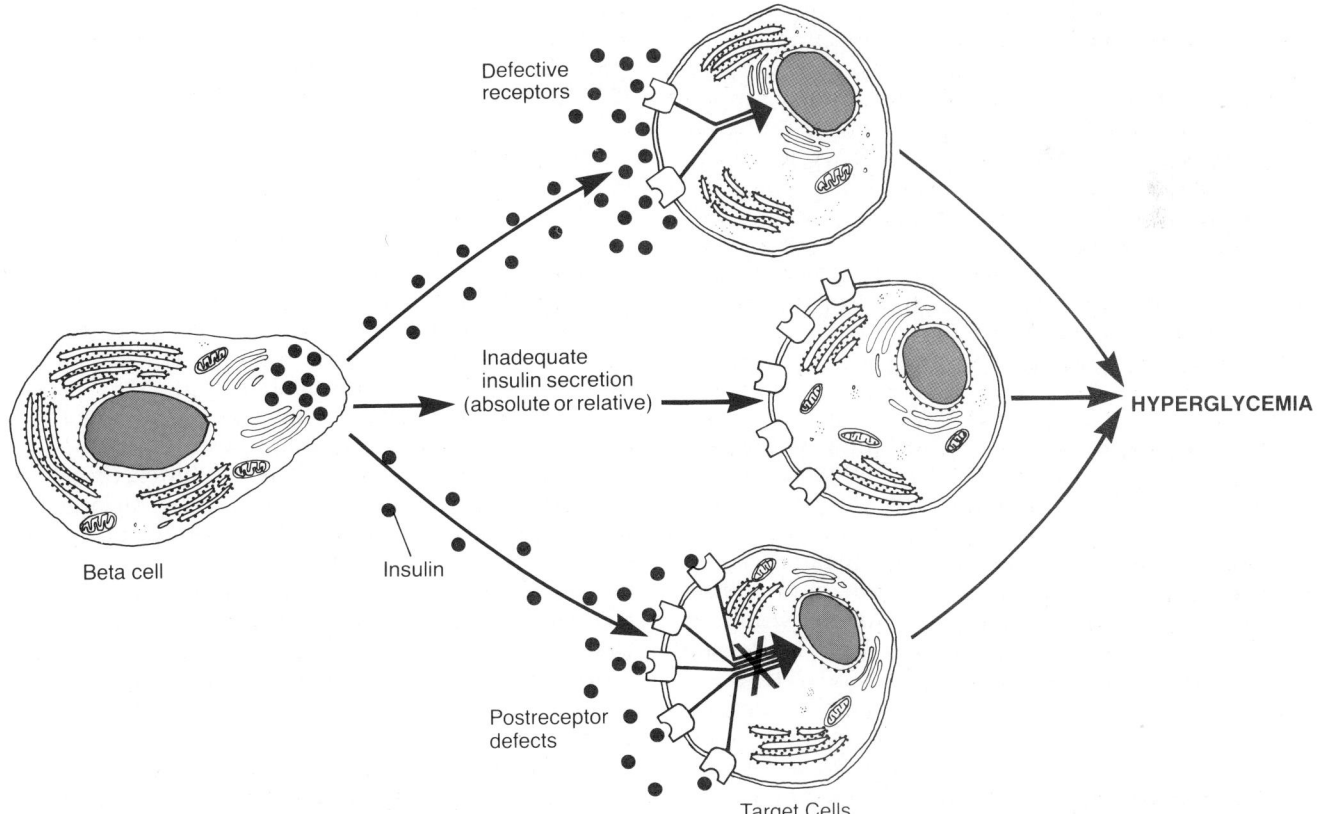

Figure 20–22. Pathogenesis of type II diabetes: a derangement in insulin secretion and insulin resistance. The latter can be due to decreased or abnormal insulin receptors or a postreceptor defect.

also encountered in nonobese patients with type **II** diabetes. The cellular bases for insulin resistance are multiple (Fig. 20–22). There is a *decrease in the number of insulin receptors* as well as additional deficits in the insulin receptor's tyrosine kinase activity. In addition, it is now thought that there is a *postreceptor defect* associated, in some patients, with *reduced numbers and impaired activity of glucose transport units.*[75] You will recall (Fig. 20–20) that these are intracytoplasmic proteins that enhance transmembrane diffusion of glucose and are normally activated by the binding of insulin to its receptor.

To summarize, type **II** diabetes is a complex, multifactorial disorder involving both impaired insulin release and end-organ insensitivity. Insulin resistance, frequently associated with obesity, produces excessive stress on beta cells, which may fail in the face of sustained need for a state of hyperinsulinism. A genetic factor is involved, perhaps leading to accelerated age-related loss of beta-cell function.

PATHOGENESIS OF THE COMPLICATIONS OF DIABETES. The pathogenesis of the complications of long-standing diabetes, such as microangiopathy, retinopathy, nephropathy, and neuropathy, are currently the subject of a great deal of research. Although there are some who feel that these complications are a genetic concomitant unrelated to the metabolic abnormalities, *most of the available evidence suggests that the complications of diabetes mellitus are a consequence of these metabolic derangements.*[76] The most telling evidence comes from the finding that kidneys, when transplanted into diabetics from nondiabetic donors, develop the lesions of diabetic nephropathy within three to five years after transplantation. Conversely, kidneys with lesions of diabetic nephropathy demonstrate a reversal of the lesion when transplanted into normal recipients. Since hyperglycemia is the most obvious and consistent metabolic abnormality in diabetes mellitus, many mechanisms linking hyperglycemia to the complications of long-standing diabetes have been explored. Currently, two such mechanisms are being investigated.

1. *Nonenzymatic glycosylation.* This refers to the process by which glucose chemically attaches to the amino group of proteins without the aid of enzymes.[77,78] Glucose forms chemically reversible glycosylation products with protein (named Schiff bases), which may rearrange to form more stable Amadori-type early glycosylation products, which are also chemically reversible (Fig. 20–23). The degree of enzymatic glycosylation is directly related to the level of blood glucose. Indeed, *the measurement of glycosylated hemoglobin (HbA1C) levels in the blood is a useful adjunct in the management of diabetes mellitus,* since the nonenzymatic glycosylation of Hb continues over the 120-day life span of the red cell. It has recently been shown that some of the early glycosylation products on collagen and other long-lived

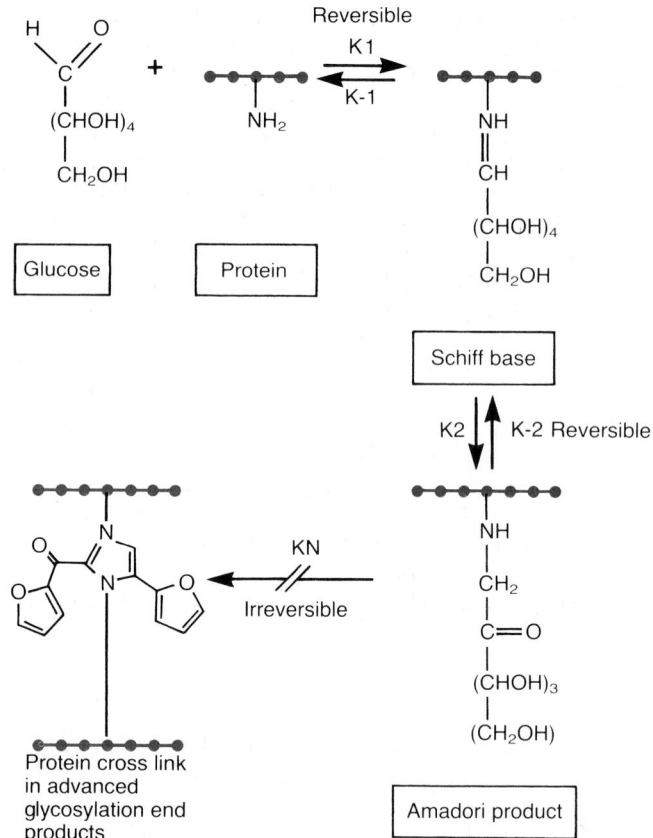

Figure 20–23. Nonenzymatic glycosylation of proteins. The advanced glycosylation product involves protein-protein cross linking. Note that while the early glycosylation products are reversible, advanced end products are irreversible. (Modified from Brownlee, M., et al.: N. Engl. J. Med. *318*:1315, 1988.)

proteins of the vessel wall, rather than dissociating, undergo a slow series of chemical rearrangements to form *irreversible advanced glycosylation end products* (AGE), which accumulate over the lifetime of the vessel wall. There is evidence that such AGEs, particularly on collagen, correlate with the severity of diabetic complications (retinopathy).[79]

Several mechanisms for the pathogenicity of these AGE products have been postulated[78]:

(a) *AGEs* attached to collagen in blood vessel wall irreversibly cross link to plasma proteins. In large vessels, cross linking to low-density lipoprotein (LDL), for example, retards its efflux from the vessel wall and enhances the deposition of cholesterol in the intima, thus accelerating atherogenesis (p. 567). In capillaries, including those of renal glomeruli, plasma proteins such as albumin would bind avidly to the glycosylated basement membrane, accounting in part for the increased basement membrane thickening characteristic of diabetic microangiopathy.

(b) AGE cross-linked collagen and other proteins are resistant to enzymatic degradation. Thus, cross linking decreases protein removal while enhancing protein deposition.

(c) Cross linking of insoluble basement membrane components, such as collagen type IV, *to each other* through AGE products may impair the interaction with other basement membrane components (laminin, proteoglycans). Reduction in basement membrane proteoglycans, in particular, increases capillary permeability, particularly in the glomerulus (p. 1044).

(d) Binding of AGE product proteins with specific receptors on macrophages stimulates the secretion by such macrophages of interleukin-1 and tumor necrosis factor.[80] As we have seen, these two monokines have profound influences on endothelial cells and fibroblasts (Fig. 2–20, p. 59), which may contribute to diabetic microangiopathy.

Evidence that AGE products are pathogenic in vivo is derived from studies in an experimental model of diabetes, in which basement membrane thickening was prevented by treatment with aminoguanidine, a pharmacologic agent that binds preferentially to the active precursors of AGE products (Fig. 20–23) and therefore prevents their cross linking to collagen.[78]

2. *Intracellular hyperglycemia with disturbances in polyol pathways.*[81,82] In some tissues (such as nerves, lens, kidney, and blood vessels), which do not require insulin for glucose transport, hyperglycemia leads to an increase in intracellular glucose. The excess glucose is metabolized to *sorbitol*, a polyol, by the enzyme aldose reductase, and eventually to fructose (Fig. 20–24). The accumulated sorbitol and fructose lead to increased intracellular osmolarity and influx of water, and eventually, to osmotic cell injury. Sorbitol accumulation is decreased associated with a decrease in *myo-inositol content*, resulting in decreased phosphoinositide metabolism, diacylglycerol, protein kinase C and NA^+/K^+ ATPase activity. This mechanism may be responsible for damage to Schwann cells and to pericytes of retinal capillaries, with resultant peripheral neuropathy and retinal microaneurysms, respectively. In the lens, osmotically imbibed water causes swelling and opacity. That this pathway may contribute to the ocular and neurologic complications of diabetes is supported by experimental studies in which pharmacologic inhibition of aldol reductase prevented the fall in *myo*-inositol content and decrease in ATPase activity, as well as the development of cataracts and neuropathy. In addition, *myo*-inositol has been shown to improve the manifestations of neuropathy in human diabetics.

METABOLIC DERANGEMENTS. Diabetic patients exhibit a wide spectrum of deranged carbohydrate metabolism, from those having mild or asymptomatic disease without fasting hyperglycemia to those having severe fasting hyperglycemia in the fully expressed clinical disease.[83] *Although attention is focused on the disordered carbohydrate metabolism, we should not overlook the important fact that all pathways of intermediary metabolism are disrupted.* Insulin is a major anabolic hormone in the body. Derangement of insulin function affects not only glucose metabolism but also fat and protein metabolism.

The most profound deficiency of insulin, and therefore the most severe derangements in metabolism, are usually encountered in type I diabetes. The assimilation of glucose and other insulin-sensitive sugars into muscle and adipose tissue is sharply diminished or abolished. Not only does storage of glycogen in liver and muscle cease, but reserves are depleted by glycogenolysis. Fasting hyperglycemia may reach levels many times greater than normal, and when the level of circulating glucose exceeds the renal threshold, glycosuria ensues. The excessive glycosuria induces an osmotic diuresis and thus polyuria, causing a profound loss of water and electrolytes (Na, K, Mg, P) (Fig. 20–25). This obligatory water loss combined with the hyperosmolarity resulting from the increased levels of glucose in the blood tends to deplete intracellular water, as, for example, in the osmoreceptors of the thirst centers of the brain. In this manner, intense thirst (polydipsia) appears. Through poorly defined pathways, increased appetite (polyphagia) develops, thus completing the classic triad of diabetic findings—*polyuria, polydipsia, and polyphagia.* With a deficiency of insulin, the scales swing from insulin-promoted anabolism to catabolism of proteins and fats. Proteolysis follows, and the glucogenic amino acids are removed by the liver and used as building blocks in gluconeogenesis, worsening the deranged carbohydrate metabolism.

Two important acute metabolic complications of diabetes mellitus follow, *diabetic ketoacidosis* and *nonketotic hyperosmolar coma.*

Diabetic ketoacidosis occurs almost exclusively in type I diabetes, and is stimulated by *severe insulin deficiency coupled with absolute or relative increases of glucagon* (Fig. 20–25). The insulin deficiency

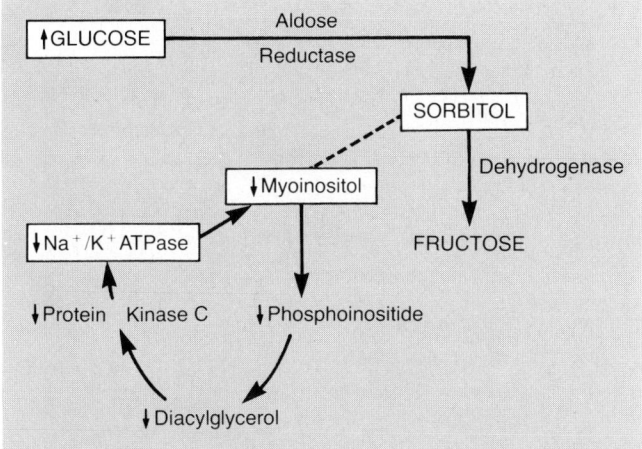

Figure 20–24. Intracellular hyperglycemia, the sorbitol pathway, and effects on myoinositol. See text. (Adapted from Greene, D.A., et al.: N. Engl. J. Med. 316:599, 1987.)

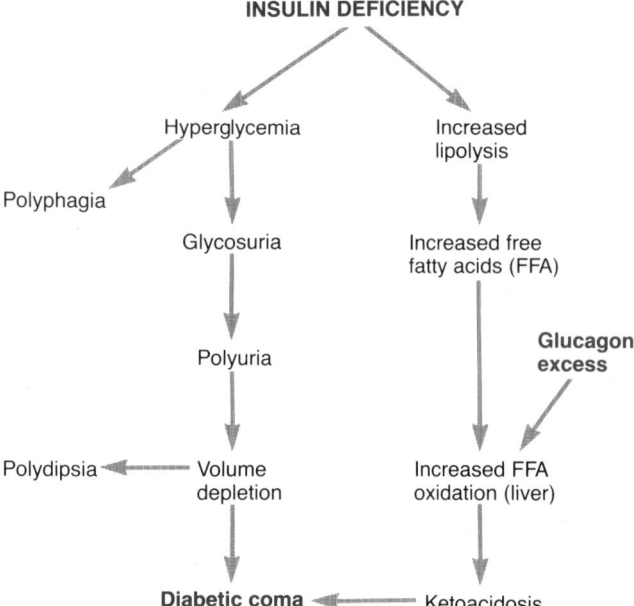

Figure 20–25. Sequence of metabolic derangements in diabetes mellitus.

causes excessive breakdown of adipose stores, resulting in increased levels of free fatty acids. Oxidation of such free fatty acids within the liver through acetyl CoA produces ketone bodies. *Glucagon* is the hormone that accelerates such fatty acid oxidation. The rate at which ketone bodies are formed may exceed the rate at which acetoacetic acid and beta-hydroxybutyric acid can be utilized by muscles and other tissues. Ketogenic amino acids aggravate the derangements in lipid metabolism. Ketogenesis thus increases, leading to ketonemia and ketonuria. If the urinary excretion of ketones is compromised by dehydration, the plasma hydrogen ion concentration increases, and *systemic metabolic ketoacidosis* results.

In type II diabetes, polyuria, polydipsia, and polyphagia may accompany the fasting hyperglycemia, but ketoacidosis is rare. Adults, particularly elderly diabetics, develop *nonketotic hyperosmolar coma*, a syndrome engendered by the severe dehydration resulting from sustained hyperglycemic diuresis, which is coupled with the inability of these patients to drink water. The absence of ketoacidosis and its symptoms (nausea, vomiting, respiratory difficulties) delays the seeking of medical attention in those patients until severe dehydration and coma have occurred.

MORPHOLOGY OF DIABETES AND ITS LATE COMPLICATIONS

The important morphologic changes in diabetes are related to its many late systemic complications, since they are the major causes of morbidity and mortality. There is extreme variability among patients in the time of onset, the severity of these complications, and

the particular organ or organs involved. In most patients, regardless of the type of diabetes, when the disease has been present for 10 to 15 years, morphologic changes are likely to be found in the basement membranes of small vessels *(microangiopathy)*, arteries *(atherosclerosis)*, kidneys *(diabetic nephropathy)*, retina *(retinopathy)*, nerves *(neuropathy)*, and other tissues, and clinical evidence of dysfunction in these organs is present.

ISLET CHANGES. Surprisingly, lesions in the pancreas are neither constant nor necessarily pathognomonic.[84,85] They are more likely to be distinctive in type I than in type II. One or more of the following alterations may be present: (1) **Reduction in the size and number of islets.** This is most often seen in type I diabetes, particularly with rapidly advancing disease. Most of the islets are small, inconspicuous, and not easily detected in routinely stained sections. They are composed of thin cords of cells intermingled with fibrous stroma. Careful morphometric studies performed with special stains show reduction in beta cells even in type II disease, but this change is subtle and not easily detected. (2) **Increase in the size and number of islets.** This may be seen in diabetic or nondiabetic infants of diabetic mothers. Presumably the maternal hyperglycemia leads to fetal hyperglycemia and compensatory hyperplasia of the fetal islets. (3) **Beta-cell degranulation.** This is most often encountered in the insulin-dependent variant and is thought to represent depletion of secretory stores of insulin in already damaged cells. (4) **Fibrosis of islets.** (5) **Amyloid replacement of islets** by an amorphous substance having

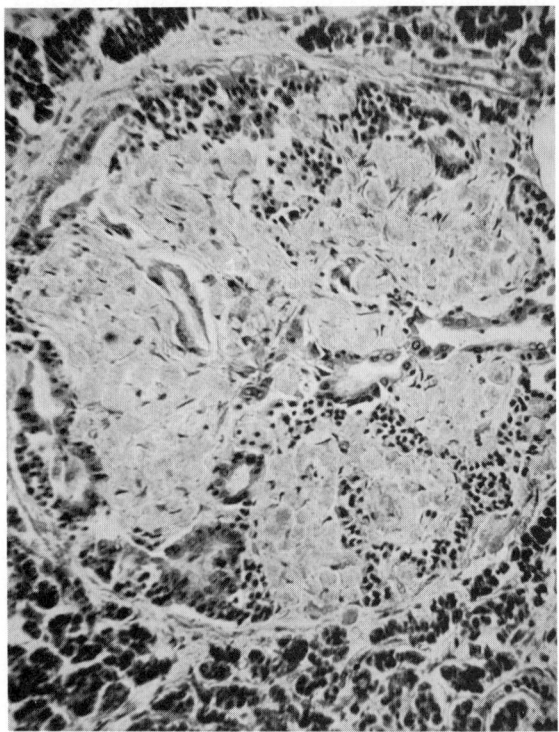

Figure 20–26. Amyloid deposition in an islet in pancreas of a diabetic.

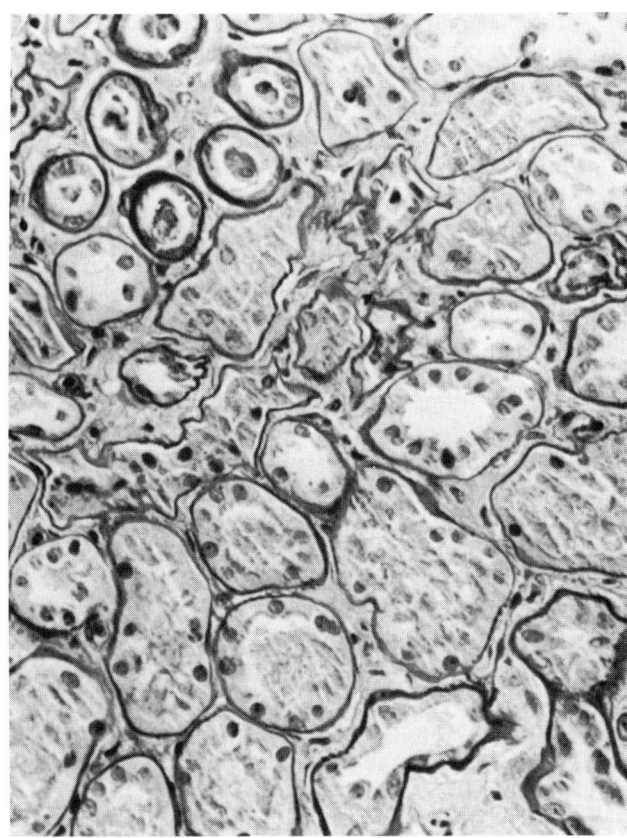

Figure 20-27. PAS stain of renal cortex showing thickening of basement membrane in a diabetic.

the fibrillar substructure characteristic of amyloid (Fig. 20-26). Both the collagenous and the amyloid deposits occur at first about the microcirculation within the islets and progressively extend to obliterate the surrounding cells. These changes may be found in type I but are more characteristic of the late chronic stages of type II. Neither change is diagnostic of diabetes, since both are sometimes found in elderly nondiabetic patients with advanced atherosclerosis and presumably ischemic injury to islets. (6) **Leukocytic infiltrations** may take one of two forms. The most common pattern is a heavy lymphocytic infiltrate within and about the islets, referred to as **insulitis.** Insulitis is most frequent in young diabetics with a brief history of symptomatic diabetes. The possible autoimmune significance of such an inflammatory infiltrate has already been discussed (p. 998). Eosinophilic infiltrates may also be found, particularly in diabetic infants who fail to survive the immediate postnatal period.

DIABETIC MICROANGIOPATHY. One of the most consistent morphologic features of diabetes is diffuse thickening of basement membranes.[39] The thickening is most evident in the capillaries of the skin, skeletal muscles, retina, renal glomeruli, and renal medulla, giving rise to the characteristic *diabetic microangiopathy* of these organs. However, it may also be seen in

such nonvascular structures as renal tubules, Bowman's capsule, peripheral nerves, and placenta.

By light microscopy, the thickening appears as widening of the basement membrane by a homogeneous, sometimes multilayered hyaline substance, which is strongly positive with the PAS stain (Fig. 20-27). Under the electron microscope the thickening either may be homogeneous (Fig. 20-28) or, particularly in the skin, may consist of several laminated circumferential layers.[86] Despite the increased thickness of basement membranes, diabetic capillaries are **more** leaky than normal to plasma proteins. As will be seen, the microangiopathy has far-reaching implications, inducing serous lesions in the renal glomeruli and retina and possibly contributing to the increased vulnerability of the diabetic individual to neuropathy. It should be noted that similar microvascular lesions can be found in aged nondiabetic patients, but rarely to the extent seen in those with long-standing diabetes.[86]

The pathogenesis of diabetic microangiopathy is still uncertain, although it is clearly related to the hyperglycemia. A number of biochemical basement membrane alterations occur,[87] including increased amounts and synthesis of collagen type IV,[88] and decreases in proteoglycans.[89] The latter can account for the increased glomerular permeability characteristic of diabetic nephropathy. As explained earlier, there is some evidence that *advanced glycosylation end products play a role in the pathogenesis of these changes.*

Hyaline arteriolosclerosis, the vascular lesion associated with hypertension (p. 570), is both more prevalent and more severe in diabetics than in nondiabetics. However, it is not specific for diabetes and may be seen in elderly nondiabetics without hypertension. It takes the form of an amorphous, hyaline thickening of the wall of the arterioles, which causes narrowing of the lumen (Fig. 20-29).

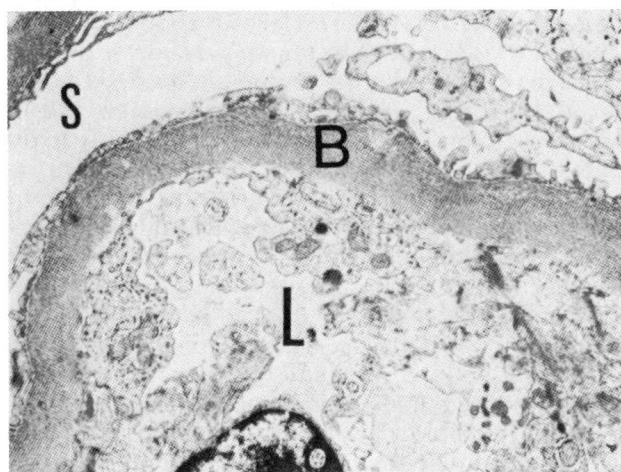

Figure 20-28. Markedly thickened glomerular basement membrane (B) in a diabetic. L is the glomerular capillary lumen and S is the urinary space.

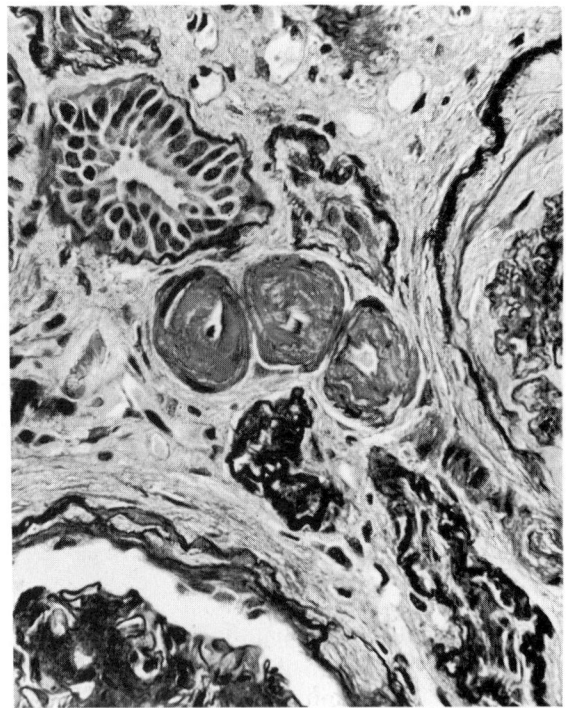

Figure 20-29. Hyaline arteriosclerosis. Note a markedly thickened, tortuous afferent arteriole (cut in three planes). The amorphous nature of the thickened vascular wall is evident.

Not surprisingly, in the diabetic it is related not only to the duration of the disease but also to the level of the blood pressure. Although at one time it was attributed to hypertension, so common among diabetics, it can also be seen in diabetics who do not have hypertension.

ATHEROSCLEROSIS. Atherosclerosis begins to appear in most diabetics, whatever their age, within a few years of onset of both type I and type II diabetes. Less than 5% of nondiabetics as opposed to approximately 75% of diabetics below the age of 40 have moderate to severe atherosclerosis. Diabetic atherosclerotic lesions tend to be numerous and florid and to undergo the constellation of changes leading to complicated lesions, i.e., ulceration, calcification, and superimposed thromboses. Thus, relatively early in the diabetic's life, atherosclerosis may result in arterial narrowings or occlusions and attendant ischemic injury to organs; alternatively, it may induce aneurysmal dilatation, seen most often in the aorta, with the grave potential of rupture. *This large vessel disease accounts for the heavy toll exacted by myocardial infarction, cerebral stroke, and gangrene of the lower extremities in these patients.* Whereas myocardial infarction is uncommon in nondiabetic females during reproductive life, it is almost as common in diabetic females as in diabetic males. Gangrene of the lower extremities is 100 times more common in diabetics than in nondiabetics.

The susceptibility of the diabetic to atherosclero-

sis is due to several factors. *Hyperlipidemia* occurs in one third to one half of patients, but even those with normal lipids have severe atherosclerosis. *HDL levels are reduced* in type II diabetes, possibly enhancing susceptibility to atherogenesis. *Nonenzymatic glycosylation* (see p. 1000) of LDL renders it most recognizable by the LDL receptor, while glycosylated HDL is more readily degradable than normal HDL — both these effects enhance atherogenesis.[90] LDL cross linked to collagen increases with the degree of glycosylation of the collagen molecule, thus retarding cholesterol efflux from the arterial wall.[91] Diabetics have *increased platelet adhesiveness* and response to aggregating agents. These changes are also likely to favor atherogenesis. Most patients with type II diabetes also tend to be *obese* and *hypertensive,* so that other contributing influences are present. Whatever the mechanism(s), all diabetics who have had the disease for at least ten years, irrespective of the age of onset, are likely to have clinically significant atherosclerosis.

DIABETIC NEPHROPATHY. The kidneys are usually the most severely damaged organs in the diabetic. Renal failure, usually due to renal microvascular disease, accounts for many diabetic deaths in both juveniles and adults. Any one or any combination of the following major lesions may be found: (1) *glomerular involvement* with three distinctive patterns: diffuse glomerulosclerosis, nodular glomerulosclerosis, and exudative lesions — these result in proteinuria, and in time progress to chronic renal failure; (2) *arteriolosclerosis,* including so-called benign nephrosclerosis and frequently associated with hypertension; (3) bacterial urinary tract infection, with *pyelonephritis* and sometimes *necrotizing papillitis.*

The glomerular and arteriolar lesions are the most important and are intimately linked to the overall diabetic microangiopathy. Since diabetic renal disease is one of the major causes of renal morbidity and mortality, the subject will be discussed in detail in Chapter 21 (p. 1044).

DIABETIC OCULAR COMPLICATIONS. One of the most threatening aspects of diabetes mellitus is the development of visual impairment consequent to retinopathy, cataract formation, or glaucoma. Diabetic retinopathy is the fourth leading cause of all legal blindness (visual acuity of 20/200 or worse) in the United States today. In the development of diabetic retinopathy, the duration of disease appears to be a very important determinant. It has been estimated that if a patient is diagnosed as a diabetic at age 30, there is a 10% chance he will have some degree of diabetic retinopathy by age 37, a 50% chance by age 45, and a 90% chance by age 55. However, it should be appreciated that diabetic retinopathy does not always impose a visual handicap, depending on whether the macula is involved or not. The lesions are described in detail in Chapter 30, p. 1460.

DIABETIC NEUROPATHY. Peripheral nerves, brain, and spinal cord may all be damaged in long-standing diabetes. Most commonly encountered is *symmetric peripheral neuropathy* affecting both motor and sensory nerves of the lower extremities. It is characterized by Schwann cell injury, myelin degeneration, and also axonal damage. Damage to the Schwann cells or possibly axons is believed to be the primary event. The peripheral neuropathy is sometimes accompanied by disturbances in the neural innervation of the pelvic organs *(autonomic neuropathy)* leading to sexual impotence and bowel and bladder dysfunction.

The cause of the neuropathy is somewhat uncertain, and several explanations have been offered. It may be related to diffuse microangiopathy affecting the nutritional maintenance of the peripheral nerve. This mechanism seems to be the most likely explanation for *diabetic mononeuropathies* affecting, for example, obturator, femoral, or sciatic nerves. Disordered glucose metabolism, rather than vascular insufficiency, is believed to be the cause of polyneuropathies.

Accumulation of sorbitol, described earlier, appears to be responsible for the Schwann cell injury in this condition. Neuronal degeneration in the brain and spinal cord may also appear. In addition, the diabetic has some predisposition to cerebral infarctions and brain hemorrhages, the latter related to the hypertension seen so often in these patients. It is worth noting that neurons are vulnerable to the hypoglycemia encountered in insulin reactions and to the ketoacidosis of the uncontrolled diabetic state.

CLINICAL COURSE

It is difficult to sketch with brevity the diverse clinical presentations of diabetes mellitus, because the disease may appear as silently as a cat or storm in like an enraged bull.[76,92] Only a few stereotypical responses can be presented.

Type I diabetes, which begins by age 20 in most patients, is dominated largely by signs and symptoms emanating from the disordered metabolism discussed earlier—polyuria, polydipsia, polyphagia, and ketoacidosis. The plasma insulin is low or absent, and glucagon levels are increased. Glucose intolerance is of the unstable or brittle type and is quite sensitive to administered exogenous insulin, deviations from normal dietary intake, unusual physical activity, infection, or other forms of stress. Inadequate fluid intake or vomiting may rapidly lead to significant disturbances in fluid and electrolyte balance. Thus, these patients are vulnerable, on the one hand, to *hypoglycemic episodes* and, on the other, to *ketoacidosis.* Infection may precipitate these conditions, and indeed may precede the first manifestations of diabetes in some patients. Fortunately, these metabolic hazards are more avoidable than the long-term sequelae.

Type II diabetes mellitus may also present with polyuria and polydipsia, but unlike type I diabetes, the patients are often older (over 40 years) and frequently obese. In some cases medical attention is sought because of unexplained weakness or weight loss. Frequently, however, the diagnosis is made by routine blood or urine testing in asymptomatic individuals. Although patients with type II diabetes also have metabolic derangements, these are usually relatively mild and controllable, and so this form of the disease is not often complicated by ketoacidosis unless intercurrent infection or stress imposes new burdens. *In both forms of long-standing diabetes, atherosclerotic events such as myocardial infarction, cerebrovascular accidents, gangrene of the leg, and renal insufficiency,* as well as the microangiopathic complications, are the most threatening and most frequent concomitants.

Diabetics are also plagued by an enhanced susceptibility to infections such as tuberculosis, pneumonia, pyelonephritis, and those affecting the skin. Collectively, such infections cause the deaths of about 5% of diabetic patients. The basis for this susceptibility is probably multifactorial; impaired leukocyte functions (p. 51) as well as poor blood supply secondary to vascular disease are involved. A trivial infection in a toe may be the first event in a long succession of complications (gangrene, bacteremia, and pneumonia) that ultimately lead to death. The diabetic's life expectancy has not significantly improved over the past three decades and, as mentioned at the outset, this disease continues to be one of the top 10 "killers" in the United States. It is hoped that islet cell transplantation, which is still in the experimental stage, will lead to the cure of diabetes mellitus. Even then, the full benefit of islet cell replacement can be derived only early in the course of diabetes, before the myriad vascular complications have set in. Certain current studies show that good, early control of the hyperglycemia will prevent or ameliorate some of the complications of diabetes,[92] but convincing prospective studies on the issue are still not in hand.[93]

ISLET CELL TUMORS

Islet cell tumors[39] are rare in comparison with tumors of the exocrine pancreas. They are most common in adults and can occur anywhere along the length of the pancreas. They may be hormonally functional or entirely nonfunctional. The tumors may be single or multiple and benign or malignant, the latter metastasizing to lymph nodes and liver. When multiple, each tumor may be composed of a different cell type.

The three most common and distinctive clinical syndromes associated with hyperfunction of the islets of Langerhans are (1) *hyperinsulinism and hypoglycemia,* (2) *the Zollinger-Ellison syndrome (gastrinoma), and* (3) *multiple endocrine neoplasia.* Each of these may be caused by (1) diffuse hyperplasia of the islets of Langerhans, (2) benign adenomas that occur singly or multiply, and (3) malignant islet tumors.[39]

BETA-CELL TUMORS (INSULINOMA)

Beta-cell tumors (insulinomas) are the most common of islet cell tumors and may be responsible for the elaboration of sufficient insulin to induce clinically significant hypoglycemia. There is a characteristic clinical triad resulting from these pancreatic lesions: (1) Attacks of hypoglycemia occur with blood sugar levels below 50 mg/dl of serum; (2) the attacks consist principally of such central nervous system manifestations as confusion, stupor, and loss of consciousness and are clearly related to fasting or exercise; (3) the attacks are promptly relieved by the feeding or parenteral administration of glucose. There are other causes for hypoglycemia when a patient manifests this classic triad, but the cause should first be sought in the pancreas.

Analysis of pancreatic islet lesions inducing hyperinsulinism indicates that about 70% are solitary adenomas, approximately 10% are multiple adenomas, 10% are metastasizing tumors that must be interpreted as carcinomas, and the remainder are a mixed group of diffuse hyperplasia of the islets and adenomas occurring in ectopic pancreatic tissue.[93] The **insulinomas** vary in size from minute lesions that are difficult to find even on the dissecting table to huge masses of over 1500 gm (Fig. 20–30).[93] Most occur singly, but sometimes multiple adenomas are found scattered throughout the pancreas. They are usually encapsulated, firm, yellow-brown nodules, histologically composed of cords and nests of well-differentiated beta cells that do not differ from those of the normal islet (Fig. 20–31). On electron microscopy, the tumor cells exhibit the typical beta cell granules, and by immunohistochemistry, insulin can be readily visualized in tumor cells.

Five per cent of insulinomas are malignant. Histologically these tumors display little evidence of anaplasia and may be impossible to differentiate from benign tumors. The diagnosis is made in the presence of metastasis or local invasion beyond the substance of the pancreas.

Hyperinsulinism may also be caused by diffuse hyperplasia of the islets.[94] This change is found occasionally in adults but is characteristic of infants born of diabetic

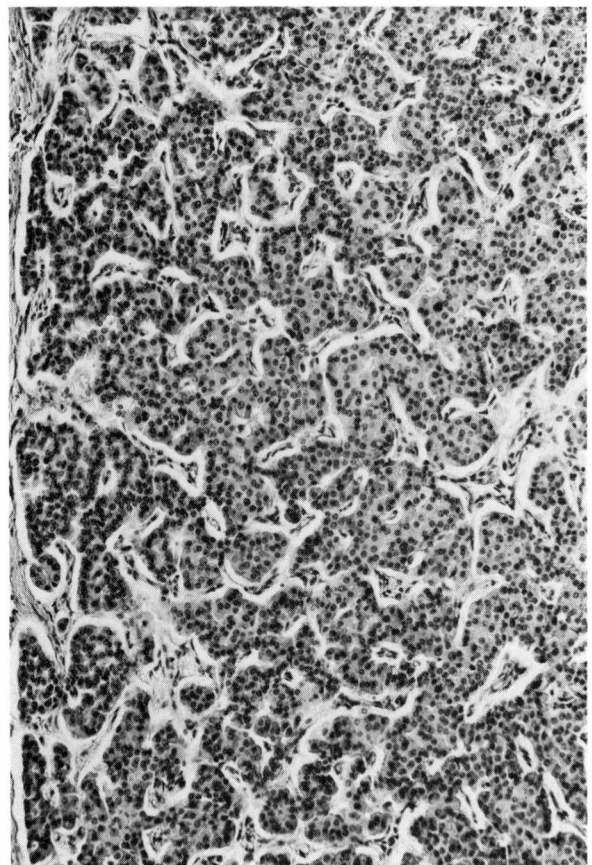

Figure 20–31. Islet cell adenoma of pancreas. The well-defined margin of an islet cell tumor. Note resemblance of tumor cells to normal islet cells.

mothers. Long exposed to the hyperglycemia of the maternal blood, the infant responds by an increase in the size and number of its islets. In the postnatal period, these hyperactive islets may be responsible for serious episodes of hypoglycemia.

Although, with newer evaluation procedures, up to 80% of islet cell tumors may show excessive insulin secretion, the hypoglycemia is mild in all but 20%, and many never become clinically symptomatic. The critical laboratory findings in insulinomas are high circulating levels of insulin and a high insulin to glucose ratio. Surgical removal of the tumor is usually followed by prompt reversal of the hypoglycemia.

It is important to note that there are a variety of functional and organic disorders, in addition to the beta-cell lesions, that cause hypoglycemia. Such functional hypoglycemia is sometimes encountered quite mysteriously in patients without apparent underlying cause, and may here be referred to as idiopathic hypoglycemia. It is also found in so-called insulin-sensitivity states, early diabetes mellitus, after partial gastrectomy, in starvation, and in certain leucine-sensitive states. The organic causes for hypoglycemia include, in addition to beta-cell lesions already de-

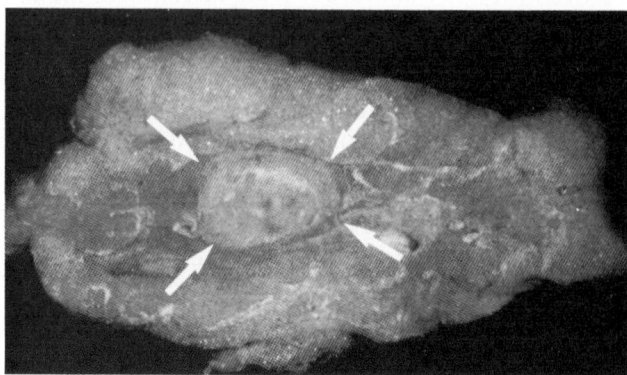

Figure 20–30.   Islet cell adenoma of pancreas. Small, pale tumor is seen on transection of pancreas *(arrows)*.

scribed, diffuse liver disease, the glycogenoses, hypofunction of the anterior pituitary and adrenal cortex, and a variety of extrapancreatic neoplasms.

ZOLLINGER-ELLISON SYNDROME (GASTRINOMA, ULCEROGENIC ISLET CELL TUMOR)

This syndrome is classically composed of the triad of recalcitrant peptic ulcer disease, gastric hypersecretion, and pancreatic islet cell tumor. Fundamental to the peptic ulcerations is gastric hypersecretion.[95] The stimulus to such hypersecretion has been clearly established as gastrin, so the tumor is also known as a *gastrinoma.* Gastrin has been demonstrated in these tumors by radioimmunoassay and has been elaborated in cultures of tumor cells. Although most common in the pancreas, 10 to 15% of gastrinomas occur in the duodenum. Serum gastrin levels are elevated, and indeed *hypergastrinemia can point to the presence of early gastrinomas before the development of ulcer disease.*

A definitive gastrin-producing cell in the *normal* human pancreas has not been identified. However, gastrin-producing cells in some of the more well-differentiated islet cell tumors have ultrastructural features similar to those of normal intestinal and gastric G cells, the latter known to be the source of gastrin in these tissues.

> **Approximately 60% of gastrinomas are malignant, and 40% are benign.** Only spread to lymph nodes or metastasis marks the tumors as malignant. Some of the benign adenomas occur multiply and in association with endocrine adenomas elsewhere, justifying their being classified as examples of multiple endocrine neoplasia.[95] Seventy-five per cent of the ulcers occur in the usual sites within the stomach or, more often, in the first and second portions of the duodenum. Abnormally located peptic ulcers in the distal portions of the duodenum and jejunum occur in 25% of cases. In one of ten patients, there are multiple ulcerations. The stomach also shows hyperplasia of the acid-secreting parietal cells.[96]

Patients with the Zollinger-Ellison syndrome present formidable problems in clinical management. They have striking gastric hypersecretion, which presumably produces the intractable ulcers. In addition, diarrhea is often sufficiently extreme to cause serious problems in fluid and electrolyte control, and many patients develop malabsorption syndromes. Moreover, the lesions in the pancreas not only may be malignant but also, even when benign, may be very small or multiple and difficult to discover at surgical exploration. It is not uncommon, therefore, for symptoms to be recurrent following removal of any apparent solitary lesion, with later discovery of additional lesions within the pancreas.

OTHER RARE ISLET CELL TUMORS

Alpha-cell tumors (glucagonomas) are associated with increased serum levels of glucagon and a syndrome consisting of mild diabetes mellitus, a characteristic migratory necrotizing skin erythema, and anemia.[97] They occur most frequently in peri- and postmenopausal women and are characterized by extremely high plasma glucagon levels.

Delta-cell tumors (somatostatinomas) are associated with diabetes mellitus, cholelithiasis, steatorrhea, and hypochlorhydria. They are exceedingly difficult to detect preoperatively. High plasma somatostatin levels are required for diagnosis.

Vipoma (diarrheogenic islet cell tumor) is an islet cell tumor that induces a characteristic syndrome of *watery diarrhea, hypokalemia,* and *achlorhydria* (the **WDHA** syndrome) caused by release of *vasoactive intestinal peptide* (VIP) from the tumor.[98] Some of these tumors are locally invasive and metastatic. Neural crest tumors, such as ganglioneuroma, neuroblastoma, neurofibroma, and pheochromocytoma, can also be associated with the vipoma syndrome.

Pancreatic *carcinoid tumors* producing serotonin and an atypical carcinoid syndrome are exceedingly rare. *Pancreatic polypeptide–secreting* islet cell tumors are endocrinologically asymptomatic, despite the presence of high levels of the hormone in plasma.[99]

Some pancreatic and extrapancreatic tumors produce two or more hormones, usually simultaneously and occasionally in sequence. In addition to insulin, glucagon, and gastrin, islet cell tumors produce ACTH, MSH, vasopressin, norepinephrine, and serotonin. These are called *multihormonal tumors* to distinguish them from the multiple endocrine neoplasias described before, in which a multiplicity of hormones are produced by several different glands.

MULTIPLE ENDOCRINE NEOPLASIA (MEN) SYNDROMES

These fascinating syndromes, as first described, comprised the common association of "multiple endocrine adenomas" of the pituitary, pancreas, and parathyroid glands. Wermer[100] expanded this entity when he noted the frequent occurrence of peptic ulcers in these patients. He further postulated a familial distribution, now defined as an *autosomal dominant mode of transmission with incomplete penetrance.* Since these original descriptions, the Zollinger-Ellison syndrome has been noted in individuals with multiple endocrine tumors, and families have been identified in which one member had the Zollinger-Ellison syndrome while others had multiple adenomas.[101]

The MEN syndromes have been subdivided into several types, depending on the organs involved and the presence or absence of peptic ulcerations (Table 20–4). MEN I (Wermer syndrome) consists of tumors or hyperplasias of the parathyroid glands, pituitary, adrenal cortex, pancreatic islets, and thyroid, to-

Table 20-4. Multiple Endocrine Neoplasia Syndromes

LESIONS	MEN I	MEN IIa	MEN IIb or III
Pituitary	+ + +	0	0
Medullary carcinoma of thyroid	+	+ + + +	+ + + +
Parathyroid	+ + +	+ +	+
Adrenal cortex	+ + +	+	+
Pheochromocytoma	0	+ + + +	+ + + +
Pancreas	+ + + +	0	0
Peptic ulcer	+ + + +	0	0
Mucocutaneous neuromas	0	0	+ + + +

gether with peptic ulcerations and gastric hypersection. In contrast, **MEN II** (Sipple syndrome) is characterized by multiple pheochromocytomas (tumors of the adrenal medulla), medullary carcinoma of the thyroid (p. 1238), and parathyroid hyperplasia or adenoma, *but not pancreatic islet cell tumors or peptic ulceration.* In some families with **MEN II** there is, in addition to the tumors described, a distinctive constellation of mucocutaneous lesions, including neuromas of the eyelids, tongue, lips, intestines, bronchus, and bladder. To these, the term **MEN IIb** or **MEN III** has been given, to differentiate them from **MEN IIa**, in which mucocutaneous neuromas are not present. Table 20-4 indicates the areas of overlap of **MEN I** and **MEN II**. It is evident that **MEN I** comprises, in essence, polyendocrine involvement associated with peptic ulcers. In contrast, **MEN II** is better remembered as the medullary carcinoma-pheochromocytoma syndrome not associated with peptic ulcers. Both patterns of **MEN** are familial. The **MEN I** gene has recently been mapped to chromosome 11[101] and the **MEN IIa** locus to chromosome 10.[102] In the **MEN I** studies, there is evidence that tumor formation is associated with loss of the gene, possibly unmasking a recessive mutation at this locus (as is the case with the retinoblastoma gene, p. 289).

The range of clinical presentations that may be encountered in **MEN I** and **MEN II** is highly heterogeneous. In the individual patient, one or two of the functioning lesions usually overshadow the others. Among the more frequent presentations are (1) intractable peptic ulcer disease; (2) evidence of hyperparathyroidism; (3) manifestations arising in the pancreatic islet lesions, such as hyperinsulinism; (4) Cushing's syndrome; and (5) hypertension related to the pheochromocytoma.

1. Go, V.W., et al.: The Exocrine Pancreas. Biology, Pathobiology and Diseases. New York, Raven Press, 1986, pp. 1–9, 775–783.

2. Meyer, J.H.: Pancreatic physiology. *In* Sleisenger, M.H., and Fordtran, J.S. (eds.): Gastrointestinal Disease. Pathophysiology, Diagnosis, Management. 4th ed. Philadelphia, W.B. Saunders Co., 1989.

3. Rindernecht, H.: Pancreatic secretory enzymes. *In* Go, V.W., et al.: The Exocrine Pancreas. Biology, Pathobiology and Diseases. New York, Raven Press, 1986, pp. 163–184.

4. Fitzgerald, P.J., and Morrison, A.B. (eds.): The Pancreas. Baltimore, Williams & Wilkins Co., 1980.

5. Douglas, H.D., et al.: The significance of pancreatic heterotopia in relation to cancer of the head of the pancreas. Gastroenterology 59:860, 1970.

6. Singer, M.V., Gyr, K., and Sarles, H.: Revised classification of pancreatitis. Gastroenterology 89:683, 1985

7. Ranson, J.H.C.: Risk factors in acute pancreatitis. Hosp. Pract. 20:69, 1985.

8. Mallory, A., and Kern, F.: Drug-induced pancreatitis: A critical review. Gastroenterology 78:813, 1980.

9. Bess, N.A., et al.: Hyperparathyroidism and pancreatitis. Chance or a causal association? J.A.M.A. 243:246, 1980.

10. Stafford, R.J., and Grand, R.J.: Hereditary disease of the exocrine pancreas. Clin. Gastroenterol. 11:141, 1982.

11. Longnecker, D.S.: Pathology and pathogenesis of diseases of the pancreas. Am. J. Pathol. 107:103, 1982.

12. Steer, M.L., and Meldolisi, J.: The cell biology of experimental pancreatitis. N. Engl. J. Med. 316:144, 1987.

13. Steer, M.D., and Meldolisi J.: The pathogenesis of acute pancreatitis. Annu. Rev. Med. 39:95, 1988.

14. Dubick, M.A., et al.: Digestive enzymes and protease inhibitors in plasma from patients with acute pancreatitis. Pancreas 2:187, 1987.

15. Soergel, K.H.: Acute pancreatitis. *In* Sleisinger, M.H., and Fordtran, J.S. (eds.): Gastrointestinal Disease. 4th ed. Philadelphia, W.B. Saunders Co., 1989, pp. 1814–1839.

16. Longnecker, D.S.: Environmental factors and disease of the pancreas. Environ. Health Perspect. 20:105, 1977.

17. Kelly, T.R., and Swaney, P.: Gallstone pancreatitis: The second time around. Surgery 92:571, 1982.

18. Farinon, A.M., et al.: Physiopathologic role of microlithiasis in gallstone pancreatitis. Surg. Gynecol. Obstet. 164:252, 1987.

19. Editorial: Obstruction or reflux in gallstone-associated pancreatitis. Lancet 1:915, 1988.

20. Kornfield, S.: Trafficking of lysosomal enzymes in normal and diseased states. J. Clin. Invest. 77:1, 1986.

21. Sarles, H.: Epidemiology and pathophysiology of chronic pancreatitis and the role of pancreas stone formation. Clin. Gastroenterol. 13:895, 1984.

22. Foulis, A.K., et al.: Endotoxemia and complement activation in pancreatitis. Gut 23:656, 1982.

23. Vennes, J.A.: Chronic pancreatitis. Gastroenterology 82:1471, 1982.

24. Richter, J.M., et al.: Association of pancreas divisum and pancreatitis, and its treatment by sphincteroplasty of the accessory ampulla. Gastroenterology 81:1104, 1981.

25. DiMagno, E.P., and Clain, J.E.: Chronic pancreatitis. *In* Go, V.W., et al.: The Exocrine Pancreas. Biology, Pathobiology and Diseases. New York, Raven Press, 1986, pp. 541–576.

26. Grendell, J. H., and Cello, J.P.: Chronic pancreatitis. *In* Sleisinger, M.H., and Fordtran, J.S. (eds.): Gastrointestinal Disease. 4th ed. Philadelphia, W.B. Saunders Co., 1989, pp. 1842–1867.

27. Winship, D., et al.: Pancreatitis: Pancreatic pseudocysts and their complications. Gastroenterology 73:593, 1977.

28. Kloppel, G., and Fitzgerald, P.G.: Pathology of non-endocrine pancreatic tumors. *In* Go, V.W., et al.: The Exocrine Pancreas. Biology, Pathobiology and Diseases. New York, Raven Press, 1986, pp. 649–678.

29. Cubrilla, A., and Fitzgerald, P.J.: Tumors of exocrine pancreas. *In* Atlas of Tumor Pathology. Tumor Fasicle Series. Washington, D.C., Armed Forces Institute of Pathology, 1983.

30. Chen, J., and Baithun, S.: Morphological study of 391 cases of exocrine pancreatic tumours with special reference to the classification of exocrine pancratic carcinoma. J. Pathol. 146:17, 1985.

31. Cello, J.P.: Carcinoma of the pancreas. *In* Sleisinger, M.H., and Fordtran, J.S. (eds.): Gastrointestinal Disease. 4th ed. Philadelphia, W.B. Saunders Co., 1989, pp. 1884–1896.

32. Silverberg, E., and Lubera, J.: Cancer statistics, 1987. Cancer 37:2, 1987.

33. Wynder, E.L., et al.: Epidemiology of cancer of the pancreas. J. Natl. Cancer Inst. 50:645, 1973; Cancer Res. 35:228, 1977.

34. Pour, P., et al.: Current knowledge of pancreatic carcinogenesis and its relevance to human disease. Cancer 47:1573, 1981.

35. Gordis, L., and Gold, E.: Epidemiology and etiology of pancreatic

cancer. *In* Go, V.W. et al.: The Exocrine Pancreas. Biology, Pathobiology and Diseases. New York, Raven Press, 1986, pp. 621–636.

36. Levin, D.C., et al.: Demographic characteristics of cancer of the pancreas: mortality, incidence and survival. Cancer *47*: 1573, 1981.

37. Beazley, R.M., and Cohn, R.I.: Pancreatic cancer. Cancer *31*: 346, 1981.

38. Mendelsohn, G.: The endocrine pancreas and diabetes mellitus. *In* Medelsohn, G. (ed.): Diagnosis and Pathology of Endocrine Diseases. Philadelphia, J.B. Lippincott Co., 1988, p. 273.

39. Bloodworth, J.M.B., and Creider, M.H.: The endocrine pancreas and diabetes mellitus. *In* Bloodworth, J.M.B., Jr. (ed.): Endocrine Pathology. Baltimore, Williams & Wilkins Co., 1982, pp. 556–720.

40. Volk, B.W., and Arquilla, E.R. (eds.): The Diabetic Pancreas. 2nd ed. New York, Plenum Medical Publishing, 1985.

41. Bennett, P.H. The diagnosis of diabetes: New internal classification and diagnostic criteria. Annu. Rev. Med. *34*:295, 1983.

42. Raymond, C.A.: Insulin dependent diabetes mellitus called epidemiologist's dream. J.A.M.A. *259*:1614, 1988.

43. Kahn, R.: Molecular mechanisms of insulin action. Annu. Rev. Med. *36*:429, 1985.

44. Seldin, R.F., et al.: Regulation of insulin-gene expression. N. Engl. J. Med., *317*:1067, 1987.

45. Hollenberg, M.D.: Receptors for insulin and growth factors: a rationale for common and distinct mechanisms of cell activation. Clin. Invest. Med. *10*:457, 1987.

46. Truglia, J.A., et al.: Insulin resistance: receptor and post-binding deficits in human insulin and non–insulin dependent diabetes mellitus. Am. J. Med. *79*(Suppl. 2B):13, 1985.

47. Kahn, R.C., and White, M.F.: The insulin receptor and the molecular mechanism of insulin action. J. Clin. Invest. *82*:1151, 1988.

48. Craighead, J.E.: The pathogenetic basis for Type I diabetes mellitus. Adv. Pathol. *1*:157, 1988.

49. Krolewski, A.S., et al.: Epidemiologic approach to the etiology of type I diabetes mellitus and its complications. N. Engl. J. Med. *317*:1390, 1987.

50. Rossini, A.A.: Special speculations on etiology of diabetes mellitus. Diabetes *37*:257, 1988.

51. Bosie, E., et al.: Mechanisms of autoimmunity: relevance to the pathogenesis of type I insulin-dependent diabetes mellitus. Diabetes/Metabolism Reviews *38*:93, 1987.

52. Eisenbarth, G.S.: Type I diabetes: Clinical implications of autoimmunity. Hosp. Pract. *22*:135, 1987.

53. Rossini, A.A., et al.: Immunology of insulin dependent diabetes mellitus. Annu. Rev. Immunol. *3*:289, 1985.

54. Rotter, J.I., and Rimoin, D.L.: The genetics of diabetes. Hosp. Pract. *22*:120, 1987.

55. Bell, G.I., et al.: The molecular genetics of diabetes mellitus. Ciba Found. Symp. *130*:167, 1987.

56. Todd, J.A., et al.: A molecular basis for MHC Class II–associated autoimmunity. Science *240*:1083, 1988.

57. Todd, J.A., et al.: HLA-DQ B gene contributes to susceptibility and the resistance to insulin dependent diabetes mellitus. Nature *329*:599, 1987.

58. Hatori, T., et al.: Thy-1 linked diabetogenetic gene but not MHC-linked gene causes the primary destruction of B-cells of the N.O.D. mouse. Diabetes *36*(Suppl. 1):82A, 1987.

59. Eisenbarth, G.S.: Type I diabetes mellitus: a chronic autoimmune disease. N. Engl. J. Med. *314*:1360, 1986.

60. Gepts, W.: Pathologic anatomy of the pancreas in juvenile diabetes mellitus. Diabetes *14*:619, 1965.

61. Foulis, A.K.: The pathogenesis of beta cell destruction in Type I diabetes mellitus. J. Pathol. *152*:141, 1987.

62. Tarn, A.C., et al.: Predicting insulin-dependent diabetes. Lancet *1*:845, 1988.

63. Parham, P.: Intolerable secretion in tolerable transgenic mice. Nature *333*:500, 1988.

64. Baird, J.D., et al.: MHC expression in the pancreas. Nature *239*:493, 1987.

65. Pukel, C., et al.: Destruction of rat islet cell monolayers by cytokines: synergistic interactions of gamma interferon, tumor necrosis factor, lymphotoxin, and interleukin-1. Diabetes *37*:133, 1988.

66. Bougneres, P.F., et al.: Factors associated with early remission of Type I diabetes in children treated with cyclosporin. N. Engl. J. Med. *318*:663, 1988.

67. Herold, K.C., and Rubenstein, A.H.: Immunosuppression for insulin-dependent diabetes. N. Engl. J. Med. *318*:701, 1988.

68. Rewers, M., LaPorte, R.E., et al.: Apparent epidemic of insulin-dependent diabetes mellitus in Midwestern Poland. Diabetes *36*:(1) 106, 1987.

69. Rubenstein, P., et al.: The HLA system in congenital rubella. Patients with and without diabetes. Diabetes *31*:1088, 1982.

70. Craighead, J.E.: Viral diabetes. *In* Volk, B.W., and Arquilla, E.R. (eds.): The Diabetic Pancreas. New York, Plenum Medical Publishing, 1985, pp. 439–466.

71. Barnett, A.H., et al.: Diabetes in identical twins: A study of 200 pairs. Diabetologica *20*:57, 1981.

72. Cahill, G.F.: Beta cell deficiency, insulin resistance or both? N. Engl. J. Med. *318*:1268, 1988.

73. O'Rahilly, S.: Impaired pulsatile secretion of insulin in relatives of patients with non-insulin dependent diabetes. N. Engl. J. Med. *318*:1225, 1988.

74. Truglia, J.A., Olefsky J.M., et al.: Mechanisms of insulin resistance in non–insulin dependent diabetes. Am. J. Med. *79*(Suppl. 3B):12, 1985.

75. Garvey, W.T., et al.: Role of glucose transporters in the cellular insulin resistance of Type II non–insulin dependent diabetes. J. Clin. Invest. *81*:1528, 1988.

76. Clements, R.S., and Bell, D.H.S.: Complications of diabetes: Prevalence, detection, current treatment, and prognosis. Am. J. Med. *79*(Suppl.5A):2, 1985.

77. Brownlee, M., et al.: The pathogenic role of non-enzymatic glycosylation in diabetic complications. *In* Crabbe, M.J.C. (ed.). Diabetic Complications: Scientific and Clinical Aspects. London, Churchill Livingstone, 1987, pp. 94–139.

78. Brownlee, M., et al.: Advanced glycosylation end products in tissue and the biochemical basis of diabetic complications. N. Engl. J. Med. *318*:1314, 1988.

79. Monnier, V.M., et al.: Relation between complications of Type I diabetes mellitus and collagen-linked fluorescence. N. Engl. J. Med. *314*:403, 1986.

80. Vlassara, H., et al.: Cachectin, TNF and IL-2 synthesis and secretion are induced by glucose-modified binding to a high affinity macrophage receptor. Science. In press.

81. Greene, D.A., et al.: Sorbitol, phosphoinositides and sodium potassium ATPase in the pathogenesis of diabetic complications. N. Engl. J. Med. *316*:599, 1987.

82. Weingrad, A.I.: Does a common mechanism induce the diverse complications of diabetes? Diabetes *36*:396, 1987.

83. Foster, D.W.: Diabetes mellitus. *In* Braunwald, E., et al. (eds.): Harrison's Textbook of Internal Medicine. 11th ed. New York, McGraw-Hill, 1987, p. 1778.

84. Gepts, W., and LeCompte, P.M.: The pancreatic islets in diabetes. *In* Skyler, J.S., and Cahill, G.F. (eds.): Diabetes Mellitus. New York, Yorke Medical Books, 1981, p. 1.

85. Wellmann, K.F., and Volk, B.: Islets of Langerhans structure and function in diabetes. Pathobiol. Annu. *5*:105, 1980.

86. Vracko, R.: A comparison of the microvascular lesions in diabetes mellitus with those of normal aging. J. Am. Geriatr. Soc. *30*:201, 1982.

87. Martinez-Hernandez, A., et al.: The basement membrane in pathology. Lab. Invest. *48*:656, 1983.

88. Shimomura H., and Spiro, R.G.: Studies on macromolecular components of diabetes: decreased levels of heparan sulfate and laminin. Diabetes *36*:374, 1987.

89. Rohrbach, D.H., and Martin, G.R.: Structure of basement membrane in normal and diabetic tissue. Ann. N.Y. Acad. Sci. *401*:203, 1982.

90. Brownlee, M., et al.: Nonenzymatic glycosylation products on collagen covalently trap low density lipoprotein. Diabetes *34*:938, 1985.

91. Symposium on diabetes. Am. J. Med. *79*(Suppl. 5A):1, 1985.

92. Hanssen, K.F., et al.: Diabetic control and microvascular complications: the near normoglycemic experience. Diabetologica *29*:667, 1986.

93. The Diabetes Control and Complications Trial Research Group: Diabetes control and complications trial. Are continuing studies of metabolic control and microvascular complications in insulin dependent diabetes mellitus justified? N. Engl. J. Med. *318*:246, 1988.

94. Freisen, S.R.: Tumors of the endocrine pancreas. N. Engl. J. Med. *306*:580, 1982.

95. Ellison, E.H., and Wilson, S.D.: The Zollinger-Ellison syndrome: Reappraisal and evaluation of 260 registered cases. Ann. Surg. *160*:512, 1964.

96. Solcia, E., et al.: Pathology of the Ellison-Zollinger syndrome. Prog. Surg. Pathol. *1*:119, 1980.

97. Bloom, S.R., and Polak, A.M.: Glucagonoma syndrome. Am. J. Med. *82*:25, 1987.

98. Krejs, G.J.: Vipoma syndrome. Am. J. Med. *82*:37, 1987.

99. Tomita, T., et al.: Pancreatic polypeptide–secreting islet-cell tumors. A study of three cases. Am. J. Pathol. *113*:134, 1983.

100. Wermer, P.: Endocrine adenomatosis and peptic ulcer in a large kindred: Inherited multiple tumors and mosaic pleiotropism in man. Am. J. Med. *35*:205, 1963.

101. Larsson, C., et al.: Multiple endocrine neoplasia type I gene maps to chromosome 11 and is lost in insulinoma. Nature *332*:85, 1988.

102. Simpson, N.E., et al.: Assignment of multiple endocrine neoplasia type 2A on chromosome 10 by linkage. Nature *328*:528, 1987.

21

The Kidney

NORMAL

What is man but an ingenious machine designed to turn, with "infinite artfulness, the red wine of Shiraz into urine"? So said the story teller in Isak Dinesen's *Seven Gothic Tales.* More accurately but less poetically, human kidneys serve to convert over 1700 liters of blood per day into about 1 liter of a highly specialized concentrated fluid called urine. In so doing, the kidney excretes the waste products of metabolism, precisely regulates the body's concentration of water and salt, maintains the appropriate acid balance of plasma, and serves as an endocrine organ, secreting

such hormones as erythropoietin, renin, and prostaglandins. The physiologic mechanisms that the kidney has evolved to carry out these functions require a high degree of structural complexity.

Each human adult kidney weighs about 150 gm. As the ureter enters the kidney at the hilus, it dilates into a funnel-shaped cavity, the *pelvis,* from which derive two to three main branches, the *major calyces*; the latter subdivide again into about three to four *minor calyces.* There are about 12 minor calyces in the human kidney. On cut surface, the kidney is made up of a *cortex* and a *medulla,* the former 1.2 to 1.5 cm in thickness. The medulla consists of *renal pyramids,* the apices of which are called *papillae,* each related to a calyx. Cortical tissue extends into spaces between adjacent pyramids as the *renal columns of Bertin.* From

1011

the standpoint of its diseases the kidney can be divided into four components: blood vessels, glomeruli, tubules, and interstitium.

BLOOD VESSELS. The kidney is richly supplied by blood vessels, and although both kidneys make up only 0.5% of the total body weight, they receive about 25% of the cardiac output. Of this, the cortex is by far the more richly vascularized, receiving 90% of the total renal circulation. The main renal artery divides into anterior and posterior sections at the hilus. From these, *interlobar arteries* emerge, course between lobes, give rise to the *arcuate arteries*, which arch between cortex and medulla, in turn giving rise to the *interlobular arteries*. From the interlobular arteries, *afferent arterioles* enter the glomerular tuft where they progressively subdivide into 20 to 40 capillary loops arranged in several units or lobules. Capillary loops ultimately merge together to exit from the glomerulus as *efferent arterioles*. From the efferent arterioles, the subsequent course of capillaries varies considerably. In general, efferent arterioles from superficial nephrons form a rich vascular network that encircles cortical tubules *(peritubular vascular network)*, while deeper juxtamedullary glomeruli give rise to the *vasa recta*, which descend as straight vessels to supply the outer and inner medulla. These descending arterial vasa recta then make several loops in the inner medulla and ascend as the *venous vasa recta*.

The anatomy of renal vessels has several important implications. First, because the arteries are largely end arteries, occlusion of any branch results in infarction of the specific area it supplies. It must also be evident that glomerular disease that interferes with blood flow through the glomerular capillaries must have profound effects on the tubules, within both the cortex and the medulla, because all tubular capillary beds are derived from the efferent arterioles. The peculiarities of the blood supply to the renal medulla render them especially vulnerable to ischemia; the medulla is relatively avascular and the blood in the capillary loops in the medulla has a remarkably low hematocrit value. Thus, any minor interference with the blood supply of the medulla may result in medullary necrosis. The renal cortex, on the other hand, is more vulnerable to hypertensive changes, as the normal pressure in glomerular capillaries is higher than in other capillary beds, and elevations of blood pressure in the aorta are transmitted to the afferent arterioles.

GLOMERULUS. The glomerulus is a vascular-epithelial organ designed for the ultrafiltration of plasma (Fig. 21–1). Embryologically, it is formed by an invagination of a capillary-containing mesenchymal mass into an epithelium-lined sac, Bowman's space.[1] The epithelium that invests the capillary network (visceral epithelium) is incorporated into and becomes an intrinsic part of the filtration membrane, whereas the parietal epithelium lines Bowman's space, the cavity in which plasma filtrate first collects. From the capil-

lary lumen to the urinary space (Figs. 21–1 and 21–2), the glomerular filtering membrane consists of the following structures:[2]

- A thin layer of fenestrated *endothelial cells*, each fenestrum being about 70 to 100 nm in diameter.
- A *glomerular basement membrane* (GBM) about 320 nm wide in the human adult, with a thick central electron-dense layer, the *lamina densa*, and peripheral thinner electron-lucent layers, the *lamina rara interna and lamina rara externa*.

The *visceral epithelial cells* (podocytes). Podocytes are structurally complex cells that possess interdigitating processes embedded in and adherent to the lamina rara externa of the basement membrane. Adjacent *foot processes* (pedicels) are separated by 20 to 30 nm wide *filtration slits*, which are bridged by a thin diaphragm.

Several biochemical components are present in the GBM.[3]

1. *Collagen type IV* occupies all three layers and accounts for about 50% of dry weight of GBM; collagen is presumably responsible for the structural strength of the capillary wall.

2. *Laminin* is present throughout the GBM but concentrated in both laminae rarae; it plays a role in the adhesion and attachment of endothelial and epithelial cells to the matrix.

3. *Polyanionic proteoglycans*, particularly heparan sulfate, are distributed in clusters, spaced at 50 to 60 nm intervals, along both laminae rarae. As we shall see, they are thought to account—at least in part—for the so-called *glomerular polyanion* responsible for the charge-dependent glomerular filtration barrier.

4. *Entactin* is a glycoprotein of uncertain role.

5. *Fibronectin* is distributed in small amounts in the laminae rarae.

6. Other glycoproteins of uncertain composition, are also found. In addition to these components, an anionic sialoglycoprotein layer coats the surface of endothelial and visceral epithelial cells.

The main function of the glomerulus is filtration. Two characteristics distinguish glomerular filtration from transcapillary exchange in other organs: (1) the glomerulus almost completely excludes plasma proteins of the size of albumin (molecular weight ± 70,000, radius 3.6 nm) and larger from the filtrate; and (2) it exhibits an extraordinarily high permeability to water and small solutes. The latter can be accounted for by the highly fenestrated endothelium and the presence of the epithelial slits, both of which allow free passage of fluid.

The filtration of macromolecules across the glomerulus decreases with increasing effective molecular radius, approaching zero at a radius of approximately 3.5 nm.[4] There is thus a *size-dependent permeability barrier in the glomerulus. The GBM is the principal structure responsible for this size discrimina-*

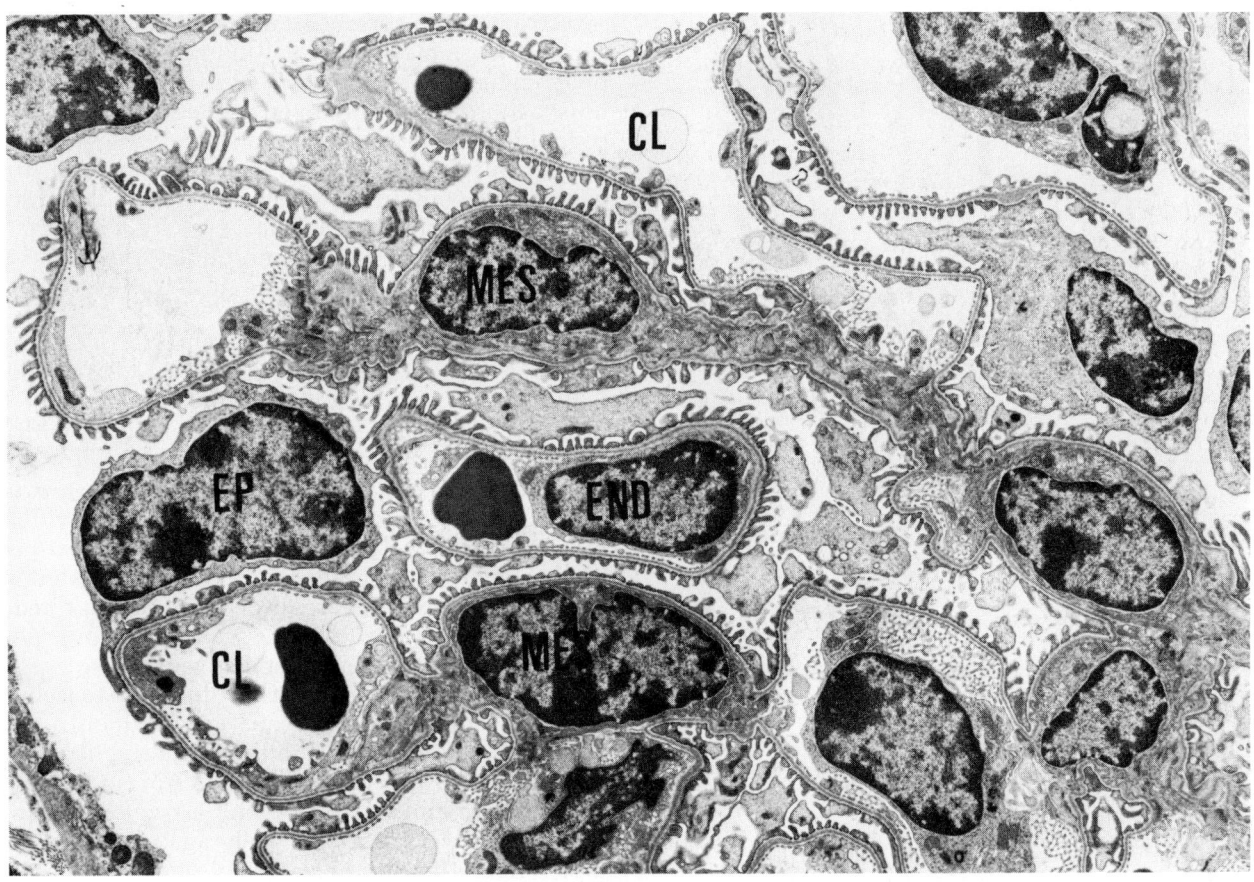

A

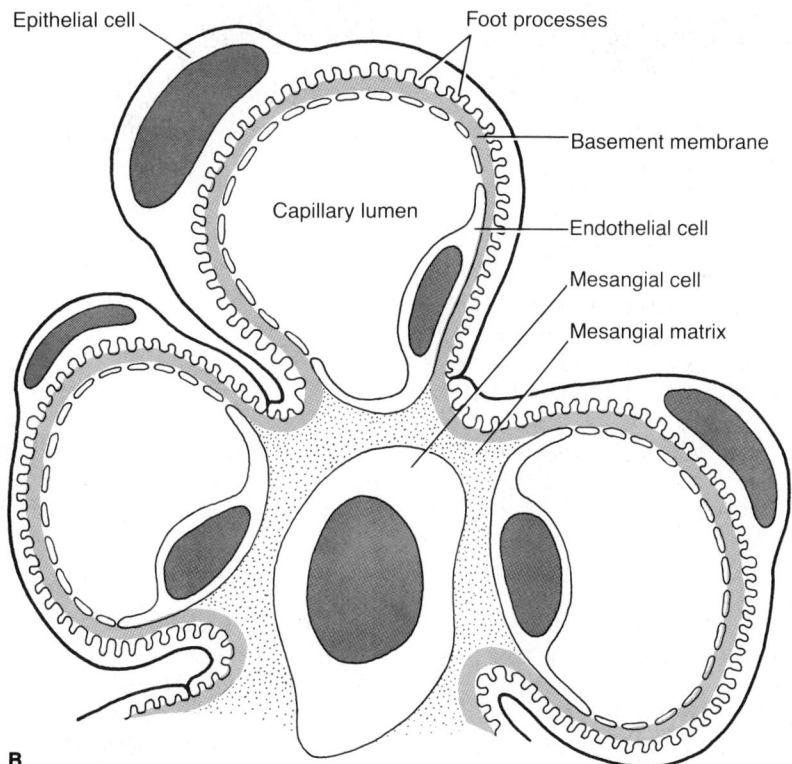

Epithelial cell

Foot processes

Basement membrane

Capillary lumen

Endothelial cell

Mesangial cell

Mesangial matrix

B

Figure 21–1A. Low-power electron micrograph of renal glomerulus. CL = capillary lumen; MES = mesangium; END = endothelium; EP = visceral epithelial cells with foot processes. (Courtesy of Dr. Vicki Kelley, Brigham and Women's Hospital.) B, Schematic representation of glomerular ultrastructure.

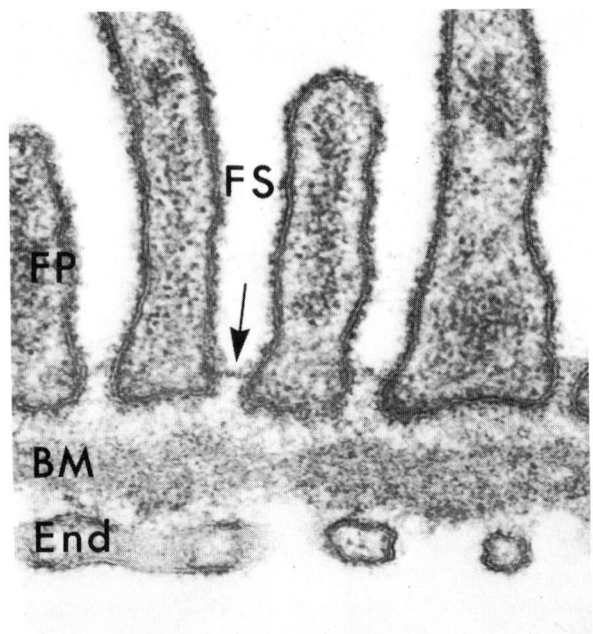

Figure 21–2. Glomerular filter consisting of fenestrated endothelium (End), basement membrane (BM), and foot processes (FP). FS = filtration slit. Arrow indicates the slit diaphragm. Note that the BM consists of a central lamina densa, labeled BM, sandwiched between two looser layers, the lamina rara interna and lamina rara externa.

tion.[5] Alterations in the structure and composition of the GBM are thus central to the leakage of proteins and blood cells characteristic of glomerular injury.

In addition to size, the *glomerulus can discriminate among molecules according to their charge,* allowing greater penetration of neutral and cationic molecules than of anionic molecules of the same size.[2,6] This charge-dependent restriction is important in the virtually complete exclusion of albumin from the filtrate, because albumin is an anionic molecule of a pI ±4.5. Charge selectivity is dependent on the presence of the negatively charged glomerular polyanions described previously, including heparan sulfate proteoglycan.[5] It follows, therefore, that loss of glomerular polyanion may result in increased filtration of proteins.[7]

Another important component of the glomerulus is the *mesangium,* also called the centrilobular or axial region (Fig. 21–1).[8] The mesangium forms a branching supportive framework around which the anastomosing capillaries of individual glomerular lobules ramify. It is continuous at the hilus with the lacis cells of the juxtaglomerular apparatus. It consists of stellate *mesangial cells* embedded in a basement membrane–like PAS-positive glycoprotein—the *mesangial matrix.* The mesangial matrix is composed of similar biochemical components as the GBM. Mesangial cells are clearly contractile[9]; by their contraction in response to neurohormonal agents they are thought to modulate intraglomerular blood flow under physiologic conditions. Mesangial cells are also endocytic and serve to ingest macromolecules that may have leaked across the glomerulus. Small numbers of Ia-positive phagocytic cells are present in the normal rat glomerulus[10]; these may be involved in phagocytosis of larger particles and in local immune reactions within the glomerulus. In normal glomeruli the mesangial area is narrow and contains a small number of cells and scant matrix. However, mesangial cell hyperplasia, increased mesangial matrix, and infiltration of the mesangium by circulating leukocytes are seen in a variety of glomerular diseases.

TUBULES. The structure of renal tubular epithelial cells varies considerably at different levels of the nephron and, to a certain extent, correlates with the functional capacity of the tubular segment. For example, the highly developed structure of the *proximal tubular cells,* with their abundant long microvilli, numerous mitochondria, apical canaliculi, and extensive intercellular interdigitations, may be correlated with their major functions: reabsorption of two thirds of filtered sodium and water as well as glucose, potassium, phosphate, amino acids, and proteins. The proximal tubule is particularly vulnerable to ischemic damage. Furthermore, toxins are frequently reabsorbed by the proximal tubule, rendering it also susceptible to chemical injury.

A remarkable structure, the *juxtaglomerular apparatus* (JG),[11] snuggles closely against the glomerulus where the afferent arteriole enters it. The JG apparatus consists of (1) the *juxtaglomerular cells,* modified granulated smooth muscle cells in the media of the afferent arteriole that contain the hormone renin; (2) the *macula densa,* a specialized region of the distal tubule as the latter returns to the vascular pole of its parent glomerulus—here the tubular cells are more crowded and the cells are somewhat shorter and possess distinct patterns of interdigitation between adjacent membranes; and (3) the *lacis cells* or *nongranular cells,* which reside in the area bounded by the afferent arteriole, the macula densa, and the glomerulus. They resemble mesangial cells and appear to be continuous with them. The JG apparatus is a small endocrine organ, the JG cells being the principal sources of renin production in the kidney.

INTERSTITIUM. The renal *interstitium* is an important component of the kidney, as it appears to be the primary site of reactivity in a variety of renal diseases. In the normal cortex, the interstitial space is compact, being occupied by the fenestrated peritubular capillaries and a small number of fibroblast-like cells.[12] Any obvious expansion of the cortical interstitium is usually abnormal; this expansion can be due to edema or infiltration with acute inflammatory cells, as in acute interstitial diseases, or may be caused by accumulation of chronic inflammatory cells and fibrous tissue, as in chronic interstitial diseases. The amount of mucopolysaccharide in the interstitial tissue of the medulla increases with age and in the presence of ischemia.

PATHOLOGY

INTRODUCTION

Disorders primary in the kidneys are responsible for a great deal of morbidity but fortunately are not major causes of mortality. To place the problem in some perspective, approximately 35,000 deaths are attributed yearly to renal disease in the United States, in contrast to about 750,000 to heart disease, 400,000 to cancer, and 200,000 to stroke. Morbidity, however, is by no means insignificant. Millions of persons are affected annually by nonfatal kidney diseases, most notably infections of the kidney or lower urinary tract, kidney stones, and urinary obstruction. Twenty per cent of all women suffer from infection of the urinary tract or kidney at some time in their lives, and at least 1% of the United States population develop renal stones. Similarly, dialysis and transplantation keep many patients alive who would formerly have died of renal failure, adding to the pool of renal morbidity.[13] The cost of such programs now exceeds 2 billion dollars annually. Renal disease also has special importance to the clinician because so many of the deaths occur in young people.

Traditionally, diseases of the kidney have been divided into those that affect the four basic morphologic components: glomeruli, tubules, interstitium, and blood vessels. This is generally a useful approach, since the early manifestations of disease affecting each of these components tend to be distinct. Further, some components appear to be more vulnerable to specific forms of renal injury; for example, *glomerular diseases are most often immunologically mediated, whereas tubular and interstitial disorders are more likely to be caused by toxic or infectious agents.* Nevertheless, the anatomic interdependence of structure in the kidney implies that damage to one almost always secondarily affects the others. Disease primary in the blood vessels, for example, inevitably affects all the structures dependent on this blood supply. Severe glomerular damage impairs the flow through the peritubular vascular system; conversely, tubular destruction, by increasing intraglomerular pressure, may induce glomerular atrophy. Thus, whatever the origin, there is a tendency for all forms of chronic renal disease ultimately to destroy all four components of the kidney, culminating in chronic renal failure and what has been called *end-stage kidneys.* The functional reserve of the kidney is large, and much damage may occur before there is evident functional impairment. For these reasons, the early signs and symptoms are particularly important to the clinician.

The widespread use of renal biopsy has changed our concepts of renal disease, particularly of the various types of glomerulonephritis. A number of special stains and techniques are used to highlight morphologic and immunologic details in such biopsies. These include:

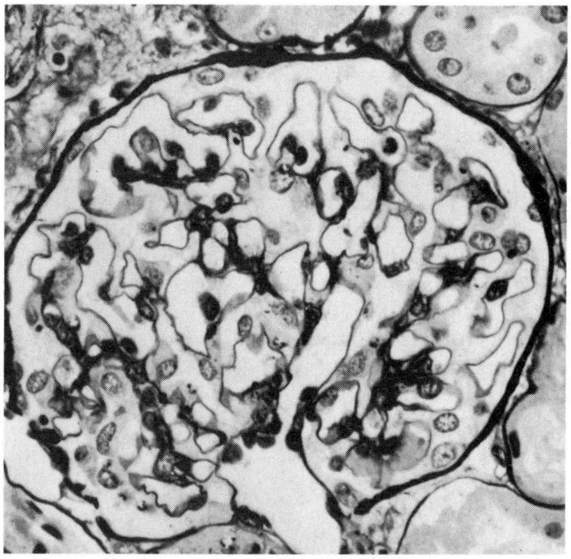

Figure 21–3. Glomerulus, stained with silver impregnation method. Note silver-positive (black) thin basement membranes of glomerulus and tubules.

1. The **periodic acid–Schiff stain** (PAS), which outlines the basement membranes of glomeruli and tubules and highlights the mesangial matrix.

2. **Silver impregnation** stains, which also mark the glomerular and tubular basement membranes (Fig. 21–3).

3. **Immunofluorescence and immunoperoxidase studies,** which localize various types of immunoglobulins, antigens, complement, fibrin-related compounds, and cell surface markers.

4. **Electron microscopy,** which is frequently essential in resolving the fine details of glomerular lesions.

5. **Other special stains,** such as those for fibrin, amyloid, and lipids.

CLINICAL AND PATHOPHYSIOLOGIC CONSIDERATIONS

THE MAJOR SYNDROMES

Clinical manifestations of renal disease vary according to the component of the kidney primarily affected, the acuteness of development of the disorder, and, to a certain extent, the mechanism of renal injury. In general, however, the clinical presentations can be grouped into eight reasonably well defined syndromes.[14] Some of these are peculiar to glomerular diseases (p. 1023); others are present in diseases that affect any one of the components.

1. *Acute nephritic syndrome* is a glomerular syndrome dominated by the acute onset of usually grossly visible hematuria (red blood cells in urine), mild-to-moderate proteinuria, and hypertension; it is the classic pre-

sentation of acute poststreptococcal glomerulonephritis.

2. The *nephrotic syndrome* is characterized by heavy proteinuria (over 3.5 gm per day), hypoalbuminemia, severe edema, hyperlipidemia, and lipiduria (lipid in the urine).

3. *Asymptomatic hematuria or proteinuria*, or a combination of these two, is usually a manifestation of subtle or mild glomerular abnormalities.

4. *Acute renal failure* is dominated by oliguria or anuria (no urine flow), with recent onset of azotemia (p. 1048). It can result from glomerular injury (such as crescentic glomerulonephritis), interstitial injury, or acute tubular necrosis.

5. *Chronic renal failure*, characterized by prolonged symptoms and signs of uremia, is the end result of all chronic renal diseases.

6. *Renal tubular defects* are dominated by polyuria (excessive urine formation), nocturia, and electrolyte disorders (e.g., metabolic acidosis). They are the result of either diseases directly affecting tubular structure (e.g., medullary cystic disease, p. 1021) or defects in specific tubular functions. The latter can be inherited (e.g., familial nephrogenic diabetes, cystinuria, renal tubular acidosis) or acquired (e.g., lead nephropathy).

7. *Urinary tract infection* is characterized by bacteriuria and pyuria (bacteria and leukocytes in the urine). The infection may be *symptomatic* or *asymptomatic*, and it may affect the kidney (*pyelonephritis*) or the bladder (*cystitis*) only.

8. *Nephrolithiasis* (renal stones) is manifested by renal colic, hematuria, and recurrent stone formation (p. 1073).

In addition to these renal syndromes, *urinary tract obstruction* (p. 1072) and *renal tumors* (p. 1075) represent specific anatomic lesions with often varied manifestations.

RENAL FAILURE

Acute renal failure implies a rapid and frequently reversible deterioration of renal function. As a characteristic syndrome with a complex pathogenesis, it is discussed separately on page 1048. Here the discussion is limited to *chronic renal failure*, which is the end result of a variety of renal diseases and is the major cause of death from renal disease.

Some terminology must first be clarified. *Azotemia* is, strictly speaking, a biochemical abnormality that refers to an elevation of the blood urea nitrogen (BUN) and creatinine levels and is largely related to decreased glomerular filtration rate (GFR). Azotemia may, of course, be produced by many renal disorders, but it may also arise from extrarenal disorders. *Prerenal azotemia* is encountered when there is hypoperfusion of the kidneys, as occurs in congestive heart failure, shock, volume depletion, and hemorrhage, all of which impair renal function without causing parenchymal damage. Similarly, *postrenal azotemia* is seen whenever there is obstruction to urinary flow below the level of the kidney; if the obstruction is severe and protracted, it will inevitably produce renal lesions. Until such time, however, relief of the obstruction will be followed by prompt correction of the azotemia.

When azotemia becomes associated with a constellation of clinical signs and symptoms and biochemical abnormalities, it is termed uremia. Thus, uremia is a clinical syndrome, not merely a biochemical abnormality. It is characterized not only by failure of renal excretory function but also by a host of metabolic and endocrine alterations incident to renal damage. There are, in addition, secondary gastrointestinal, neuromuscular, and cardiovascular involvements, which are usually necessary for the diagnosis of uremia. *Uremia* is thus the sine qua non of symptomatic chronic renal failure.

Although exceptions abound, the evolution from normal renal function to symptomatic chronic renal failure progresses through four stages that merge into one another.

• *Diminished renal reserve.* In this situation the GFR is about 50% of normal. Serum BUN and creatinine values are normal and the patients are asymptomatic. However, they are more susceptible to developing azotemia with an additional renal insult.
• *Renal insufficiency.* The GFR is 20 to 50% of normal. Azotemia appears, usually associated with anemia and hypertension. Polyuria and nocturia occur, as a result of decreased concentrating ability. Sudden stress (e.g., with nephrotoxins) may precipitate uremia.
• *Renal failure.* The GFR is less than 20 to 25% of normal. The kidneys cannot regulate volume and solute composition, and patients develop edema, metabolic acidosis, and hypocalcemia. Overt uremia may ensue, with neurologic, gastrointestinal, and cardiovascular complications.
• *End-stage renal disease.* The GFR is less than 5% of normal; this is the terminal stage of uremia.

The details of the pathophysiology of chronic renal failure are beyond the scope of this book and are well covered in various nephrology texts.[14-17] Here we shall mention only briefly the principal clinical abnormalities and their presumed cause.

FLUID, ELECTROLYTE, AND ACID-BASE DISTURBANCES. These are directly related to the role of the kidney in volume and electrolyte homeostasis. *Dehydration* tends to appear early in the course of some forms of renal disease in which there is impairment of concentrating ability and consequent excretion of large volumes of water. With progression, glomerular filtration is ultimately impaired, with retention of both salt and water. Moreover, in most forms of chronic renal disease, an activated renin-angiotensin system leads to hyperaldosteronism, which further compounds the retention of salt and water and results in *edema.*

Metabolic acidosis is largely due to a reduction in

NH_3 production, resulting in insufficient buffering of H^+ ions in the urine. There also is commonly a decreased serum bicarbonate level, a lowered blood pH, and variable degrees of compensatory hyperventilation. Occasionally, the sighing respiration through somewhat pursed lips demonstrates the classic *Kussmaul breathing*.

ABNORMALITIES IN CALCIUM PHOSPHATE AND BONE METABOLISM. Classically, the patient with chronic renal failure exhibits an increase in serum phosphate when the GFR falls below 25% of normal. This hyperphosphatemia enhances calcium entry into bones, causing hypocalcemia, which in turn leads to compensatory activity in the parathyroid glands, increased serum parathormone levels, and progressive hypertrophy and hyperplasia of the parathyroid glands (p. 1246). There are other causes for the hypocalcemia. The diseased kidney fails to synthesize 1,25-dihydroxyvitamin D_3, the active metabolite of vitamin D that normally enhances absorption of calcium from the gastrointestinal tract; thus, diminished calcium absorption by the gut contributes to hypocalcemia. In addition there is some evidence that parathormone fails to mobilize calcium salts from bone adequately in patients with chronic renal failure. Thus, in long-standing uremia, skeletal abnormalities characteristic of hyperparathyroidism and hypocalcemia may appear, sometimes referred to as *renal osteodystrophy*. Morphologically, these changes resemble those seen in *osteomalacia* or *osteitis fibrosa cystica*. Impaired bone growth in children and a tendency to spontaneous fractures are further manifestations of such renal osteodystrophy.

CARDIOPULMONARY ABNORMALITIES. Congestive heart failure, probably in part secondary to salt retention, is one of the most common manifestations. *Hypertension* is often present and is caused largely by the hypervolemia. There is also evidence of increased renin production in uremia. *Uremic pericarditis* is a frequent complication of chronic uremia. Characteristically, it takes the form of a marked fibrinous exudate and is sometimes accompanied by a fibrinous pleuritis. To the clinician, these are manifested as pericardial and pleural friction ribs. Both have been shown to clear with adequate dialysis, and only rarely do they give rise to significant fibrous adhesions. *Pulmonary edema* is usually secondary to congestive heart failure or overhydration. Occasionally uremia is associated with the presence of hyaline membranes along alveolar walls (p. 761), suggesting a direct increase in pulmonary capillary permeability *(uremic pneumonitis)*.

HEMATOPOIETIC MANIFESTATIONS. *Anemia* is generally normochromic and normocytic, but it is sometimes hypochromic. The anemia is due to decreased production of erythropoietin by the diseased kidney, bone marrow depression caused presumably by uremic plasma, uremic hemolysis due to a poorly defined extracorpuscular defect, blood loss from gas-

troenteritis, and some degree of hypersplenism. Some uremic patients develop a *bleeding diathesis*. This is due in part to abnormal platelet aggregation and decreased platelet factor 3 release.

GASTROINTESTINAL SIGNS AND SYMPTOMS. These may consist of only nausea and vomiting, but some patients have gastrointestinal bleeding. The hemorrhage arises in diffuse or patchy ulcerations that may affect virtually any level of the gut, from the oral cavity to the anus. Uremic *esophagitis, gastritis,* and *colitis* are the more common localizations of the gastrointestinal lesions.

DERMATOLOGIC CHANGES. These consist principally of a peculiar sallow coloration to the skin and itching. The skin color is in part the consequence of anemia, but it may also result from the accumulation in the skin of urinary pigment, principally urochrome (which normally gives urine its characteristic color). The origin of uremic itching remains unexplained, but it can be very distressing to the patient.

NEUROMUSCULAR DISTURBANCES. These are common manifestations of the uremic state that, although often mild, may sometimes be incapacitating. They include myopathy, encephalopathy, and peripheral neuropathy (p. 1443). Most of these are reversed by dialysis. Seizures, stupor, and coma are common in terminal uremia.

Having discussed the manifestations of uremia, we should ask what produced them.[18] One observation appears to be well established: although the severity of uremic signs and symptoms correlates roughly with the blood concentration of urea, this product is not the prime cause. Other compounds suspected of causing the uremic syndrome are the guanidino compounds, urates and other metabolic end products of nucleic acid metabolism, aliphatic amines, and the so-called "*middle molecules.*" The latter are polypeptides of 300 to 3500 daltons that produce prominent abnormal "uremic peaks" in uremic plasma subjected to a variety of chemical separation procedures. It has been suggested that elevated levels of *parathormone* may be directly toxic to cells and may also contribute to uremic toxicity by augmenting catabolism and the resultant plasma accumulation of nitrogenous waste products.[18] *It is thus likely that the far-reaching manifestations of uremia are caused by a diverse number of retained compounds rather than a single molecule.* Against this background of the clinical syndrome of chronic renal failure, we can turn to consider the renal diseases that cause it.

CONGENITAL ANOMALIES

About 10% of all persons are born with potentially significant malformations of the urinary system. Renal dysplasias and hypoplasias account for 20% of chronic renal failure in children. Polycystic kidney disease (a congenital anomaly that becomes apparent in adults) is present in one in 3000 hospital admissions and is responsible for about 10% of chronic renal failure in humans.

Congenital renal disease is most often a result of a developmental defect that arises during gestation and does not have a hereditary basis. However, some developmental defects, notably polycystic kidney disease and medullary cystic disease, are clearly hereditary. As a rule, developmental abnormalities involve structural components of the kidney and urinary tract. However, enzymatic or metabolic defects in tubular transport, such as cystinuria and renal tubular acidosis, also occur. Here we shall restrict the discussion to structural anomalies involving primarily the kidney. Anomalies of the lower urinary tract are discussed in Chapter 22.

AGENESIS OF THE KIDNEY.

Total bilateral agenesis of the kidneys, which is incompatible with life, is usually encountered in stillborn infants. It is often associated with many other congenital disorders, (limb defects, hypoplastic lungs), and leads to early death. Unilateral agenesis is an uncommon anomaly that is compatible with normal life, if no other abnormalities exist. The opposite kidney is usually enlarged as a result of compensatory hypertrophy. Some patients eventually develop progressive glomerular sclerosis in the remaining kidney, probably as a result of the adaptive changes in hypertrophied nephrons (p. 1029), and in time chronic renal failure.

HYPOPLASIA.

Renal hypoplasia refers to failure of the kidneys to develop to a normal size. This anomaly may occur bilaterally, resulting in renal failure in early childhood, but it is more commonly encountered as a unilateral defect. True renal hypoplasia is extremely rare, most cases reported probably representing not an underlying developmental failure but acquired scarring due to vascular, infectious, or other parenchymal diseases. Differentiation between congenital and acquired atrophic kidneys may be impossible, but *a truly hypoplastic kidney should show no scars and should possess a reduced number of renal lobes and pyramids:* six or fewer. In one form of hypoplastic kidney, *oligomeganephronia,* the kidney is small but the nephrons are markedly hypertrophied.

ECTOPIC KIDNEYS.

The development of the definitive metanephros may occur in ectopic foci, usually at abnormally low levels. These kidneys lie either just above the pelvic brim or sometimes within the pelvis. They are usually normal or slightly smaller in size, but otherwise are not remarkable. Because of their abnormal position, kinking or tortuosity of the ureters may cause some obstruction to urinary flow, which predisposes to bacterial infections.

HORSESHOE KIDNEY.

Fusion of the upper or lower poles of the kidneys produces a horseshoe-shaped structure continuous across the midline anterior to the great vessels. This anomaly is quite common and is found in about one in 500 to 1000 autopsies. Ninety per cent of such kidneys are fused at the lower pole, and 10% are fused at the upper pole.

MISCELLANEOUS ANOMALIES.

There is a heterogeneous group of developmental anomalies that affect the kidney, most of which are of no clinical significance. A double or an extrarenal pelvis may occur with otherwise normal kidneys. These are of interest only insofar as they may produce modifications in the patterns of the pyelogram. Anomalous renal arteries may arise either directly from the aorta or as branches from the renal artery. Sometimes such vessels are of benefit, since they maintain the blood supply to a portion of the kidney if the main renal artery is occluded. However, some of these anomalous vessels to the lower pole may cause ureteral obstruction when they cross anterior to the ureter and compress it.

CYSTIC DISEASES OF THE KIDNEY

Although not all cysts of the kidney are congenital, all types of cysts are discussed here for convenience.

Cystic diseases of the kidney are a heterogeneous group comprising hereditary, developmental but nonhereditary, and acquired disorders. As a group, they are important for several reasons: (1) they are reasonably common and often represent diagnostic problems for clinicians, radiologists, and pathologists; (2) some forms, such as adult polycystic disease, are major causes of chronic renal failure; (3) they can occasionally be confused with malignant tumors. A useful classification of renal cysts is as follows:[19,20]

1. Cystic renal dysplasia
2. Polycystic kidney disease
   a. Adult (autosomal dominant) polycystic disease
   b. Childhood (autosomal recessive) polycystic disease
3. Medullary cystic disease
   a. Medullary sponge kidney
   b. Nephronophthisis–uremic medullary cystic disease (UMCD) complex
4. Acquired (dialysis-associated) cystic disease
5. Simple renal cysts
6. Miscellaneous parenchymal renal cysts
   a. Associated with infection (tuberculous, echinococcal cyst)
   b. Associated with tumor (cystic degeneration of carcinoma)
   c. Traumatic intrarenal hematoma
7. Perihilar renal cysts (pyelocalyceal cysts, hilar lymphangitic cysts)

Only the more important types of cystic disease will be discussed.

Many theories have been suggested to explain the genesis of polycystic kidneys.[21] Current studies, based largely on spontaneous and drug-induced cystic disease in animals, suggest three mechanisms (Fig. 21–4): (1) partial intratubular obstruction, causing

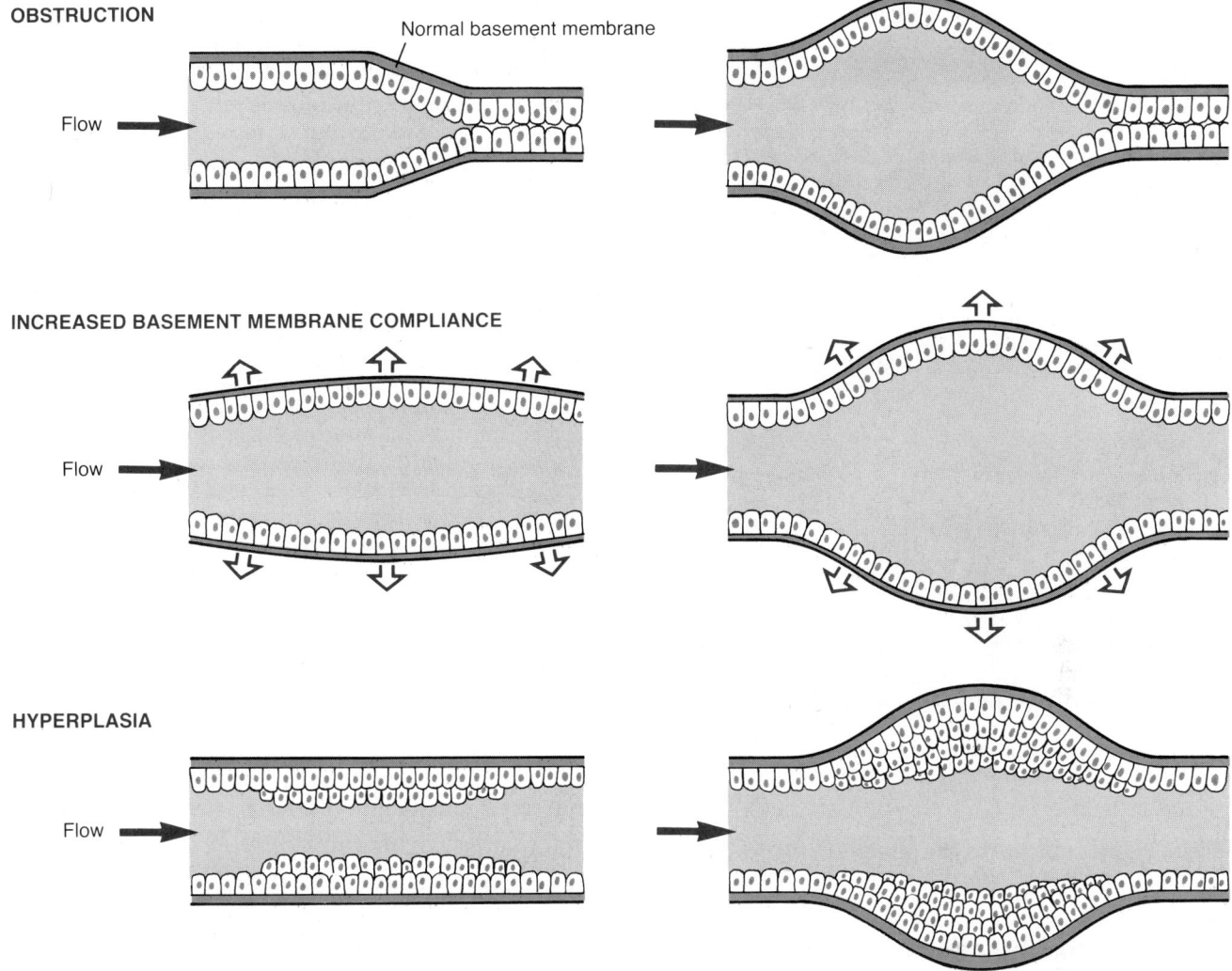

Figure 21–4. Mechanisms (not mutually exclusive) implicated in the pathogenesis of renal cystic disease: intratubular obstruction with cystic dilation proximal to the obstruction; increased basement membrane compliance secondary to a biochemical defect; and epithelial proliferation leading to epithelial hyperplastic lesions. (Adapted from Thompson, C.: Hosp. Pract. **23**:165, 1988.[20])

dilation proximal to obstructed sites; (2) a defect of the tubular basement membranes, causing loss of compliance of the tubular wall; and (3) a disorder in tubular epithelial cell growth, resulting in epithelial hyperplasia and cyst formation, possibly due to increased transepithelial secretion of solutes and water. These mechanisms are not mutually exclusive, and the three could indeed result from a primary defect in tubular cell metabolism, and tubular cell injury.

Cystic Renal Dysplasia

This disorder is due to an abnormality in metanephric differentiation *characterized histologically by the persistence in the kidney of abnormal structures — cartilage, undifferentiated mesenchyme, and immature collecting ductules — and by abnormal lobar organization.* Most cases are also associated with ureteral atresia. Renal dysplasia occurs as a sporadic disorder, without familial clustering.

Dysplasia can be unilateral or bilateral and is almost always cystic. Grossly, the kidney is usually enlarged, extremely irregular, and multicystic. The cysts vary in size from small microscopic structures to some that are several centimeters in diameter. They are lined by flattened epithelium. Histologically, although normal nephrons are present, many have immature ducts. **The characteristic feature is the presence of islands of undifferentiated mesenchyme often with cartilage** (Fig. 21–5).

Renal dysplasia is frequently associated with obstructive abnormalities of the ureter and lower urinary tract, and one concept holds that the dysplasia is caused by *intrauterine obstruction.* When unilateral, the dysplasia is discovered by the appearance of a flank mass that leads to surgical exploration and nephrectomy. Function in the opposite kidney is normal and such patients have an excellent prognosis

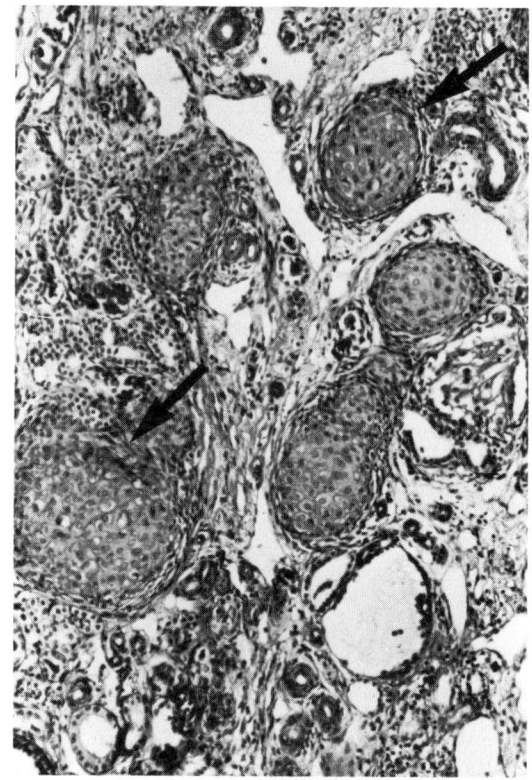

Figure 21–5. Renal dysplasia. Note disorganized architecture, dilated tubules, and islands of immature cartilage (arrow).

after surgical removal of the affected kidney. In bilateral renal dysplasia, renal failure may ultimately result.

Autosomal Dominant (Adult) Polycystic Kidney Disease

Adult polycystic kidney disease is a relatively common condition affecting roughly one of every 1000 persons and accounting for about 10% of cases requiring renal transplantation or chronic dialysis.[22] The pattern of inheritance is *autosomal dominant,* with very high penetrance, approaching 100% in those surviving through their 70s or 80s. The defective gene in most families is linked closely with markers (e.g., the α globin gene) on the short arm of chromosome 16,[23] but some pedigrees show no such linkage.[23a] The disease is universally bilateral; unilateral cases reported probably represent multicystic dysplasia. The cysts initially involve only portions of the nephrons, so that renal function is retained until about the fourth or fifth decade of life. In some patients, however, the first symptoms may appear in early childhood, in the teens, or as late as 70 or 80 years of age. In time, most patients develop hypertension or progress to chronic renal failure.

Grossly, the kidneys are usually bilaterally enlarged and may achieve enormous sizes, weights up to 4 kg for each kidney having been reported. The external surface appears to be composed solely of a mass of cysts, up to 3 to 4 cm in diameter, with no intervening parenchyma (Fig. 21–6). However, microscopic examination reveals functioning nephrons dispersed between the cysts. The cysts may be filled with a clear serous fluid or, more usually, with turbid, red-to-brown, sometimes hemorrhagic fluid. As these cysts enlarge, they may encroach upon the calyces and pelvis to produce pressure defects. The cysts arise from the tubules throughout the nephron and therefore have variable lining epithelia. The epithelial cells lining the cysts may be of proximal or distal tubule origin and the composition of cyst fluid within individual cysts reflects the type of epithelium lining these cysts—proximal or distal, indicating that the cyst epithelium has functional capacity. Occasionally, papillary epithelial formations and polyps project into the lumen. According to some,[21] these are reflections of disordered epithelial growth and may be the cause of intratubular obstruction. Occasionally, Bowman's capsules are involved in cyst formation, and glomerular tufts may be seen within the cystic space.

Clinically, many of these patients remain entirely asymptomatic until indications of renal insufficiency announce the presence of the underlying kidney disease. In others, hemorrhage or progressive dilation of cysts may produce pain. Excretion of blood clots causes renal colic. The larger masses usually apparent on abdominal palpation may induce a dragging sensation. Occasionally, the disease begins with the insidious onset of hematuria, followed by other features of progressive chronic renal disease such as proteinuria (rarely more than 2 gm per day), polyuria, and hypertension.

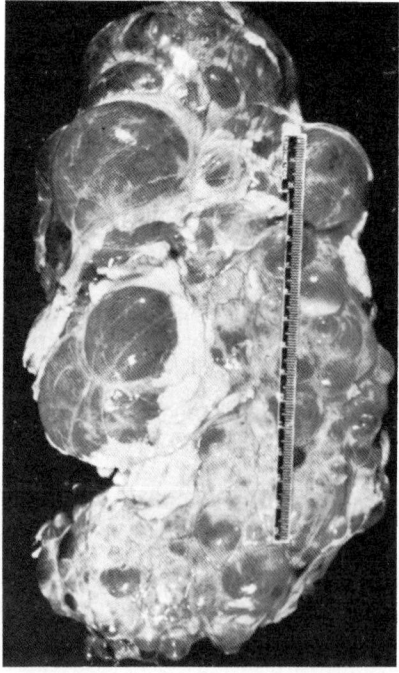

Figure 21–6. Adult polycystic kidney. Note its length of over 20 cm.

Patients with polycystic kidney disease also tend to have other congenital anomalies: *about 40% have one to several cysts in the liver (polycystic liver disease) that are usually asymptomatic.* Cysts occur much less frequently in the spleen, pancreas, and lungs. *Intracranial berry aneurysms in the circle of Willis are present in 10 to 30% of patients,* and subarachnoid hemorrhages from these account for death in about 10% of patients. Mitral valve prolapse also occurs,[24] consistent with a generalized defect in basement membranes in these patients.[25] The clinical diagnosis is made by radiologic imaging techniques; intravenous pyelography, which shows the elongated, stretched pelves and calyces; or CT scanning, which is highly sensitive and can detect cysts a few mm in diameter. Ultrasound is least invasive and can confirm the diagnosis. This form of chronic renal failure is quite remarkable in that patients may survive for many years with azotemia slowly progressing to uremia. Ultimately, about one third of adult patients die with renal failure; in another third, hypertension is responsible for death (cardiac disease, berry aneurysm); the remaining third die of unrelated causes.

Autosomal Recessive (Childhood) Polycystic Kidney Disease

This rare developmental anomaly is genetically distinct from adult polycystic kidney disease, having an *autosomal recessive* type of inheritance.[22] Perinatal, neonatal, infantile, and juvenile subcategories have been defined, dependent on time of presentation and presence of associated hepatic lesions. The first two are most common; serious manifestations are usually present at birth, and the young infant may succumb rapidly to renal failure.

> Kidneys are enlarged and have a smooth external appearance. On cut section, numerous small cysts in the cortex and medulla give the kidney a spongelike appearance. Dilated elongated channels are present at right angles to the cortical surface, completely replacing the medulla and cortex. Microscopically, there is saccular or, more commonly, cylindrical dilatation of all collecting tubules. The cysts have a uniform lining of cuboidal cells, reflecting their origin from the collecting tubules. The disease is invariably bilateral. **In almost all cases, there are multiple epithelium-lined cysts in the liver as well as proliferation of portal bile ducts.**

The patients with autosomal recessive kidney disease who survive infancy (infantile and juvenile form) may develop a peculiar type of hepatic fibrosis characterized by bland periportal fibrosis and proliferation of well-differentiated biliary ductules, a condition now termed *congenital hepatic fibrosis.* In older children, the hepatic picture in fact predominates. Such patients may develop portal hypertension with splenomegaly. Curiously, congenital hepatic fibrosis sometimes occurs in the absence of polycystic kidneys and has been reported occasionally in the presence of adult polycystic kidney disease.

Cystic Diseases of Renal Medulla

Although the names used for the two major types of medullary cystic disease are confusing, it is important to differentiate between the two types since one, *medullary sponge kidney,* is a relatively common and usually innocuous structural change, whereas the other, *nephronophthisis – uremic medullary cystic disease* complex, is almost always associated with renal dysfunction, and is a relatively common cause of chronic renal failure in children.[26]

MEDULLARY SPONGE KIDNEY. *The term medullary sponge kidney should be restricted to lesions consisting of multiple cystic dilatations of the collecting ducts in the medulla.* The condition occurs in adults and is usually discovered radiographically, either as an incidental finding or sometimes in relation to secondary complications. The latter include calcifications within the dilated ducts, infection, and urinary calculi. Renal function is usually normal. Grossly, the papillary ducts in the medulla are dilated and small cysts may be present. The cysts are lined by cuboidal epithelium or occasionally by transitional epithelium. Unless there is superimposed pyelonephritis, cortical scarring is absent. The pathogenesis is unknown.

NEPHRONOPHTHISIS – UREMIC MEDULLARY CYSTIC DISEASE (UMCD) COMPLEX. This is a group of progressive renal disorders that usually have their onset in childhood. The common characteristic is the presence of a variable number of *cysts in the medulla associated with significant cortical tubular atrophy and interstitial fibrosis.*[27] Although the presence of medullary cysts is important, the *cortical tubulointerstitial damage is the cause of the eventual renal insufficiency.* Four variants are recognized: (1) *sporadic, nonfamilial* (20%); (2) *familial juvenile nephronophthisis* (50%), inherited as a recessive disease; (3) *renal-retinal dysplasia* (15%), recessively inherited and associated with retinitis pigmentosa; and (4) *adult-onset medullary cystic disease,* dominantly inherited (15%). As a group this complex accounts for about 20% of cases of chronic renal failure in children and adolescents.

Affected children present first with polyuria and polydipsia, which reflect a marked tubular defect in concentrating ability. Sodium wasting and tubular acidosis are also prominent, findings consistent with initial injury to the distal tubules and collecting ducts. The expected course is progression to terminal renal failure over a period of five to ten years.

> Grossly, the kidneys are small, have contracted granular surfaces, and show cysts in the medulla, most prominently at the corticomedullary junction (Fig. 21 – 7). Small cysts are also seen in the cortices. The cysts are lined by flattened or cuboidal epithelium and are usually surrounded by either inflammatory cells or fibrous tissue. In the cortex

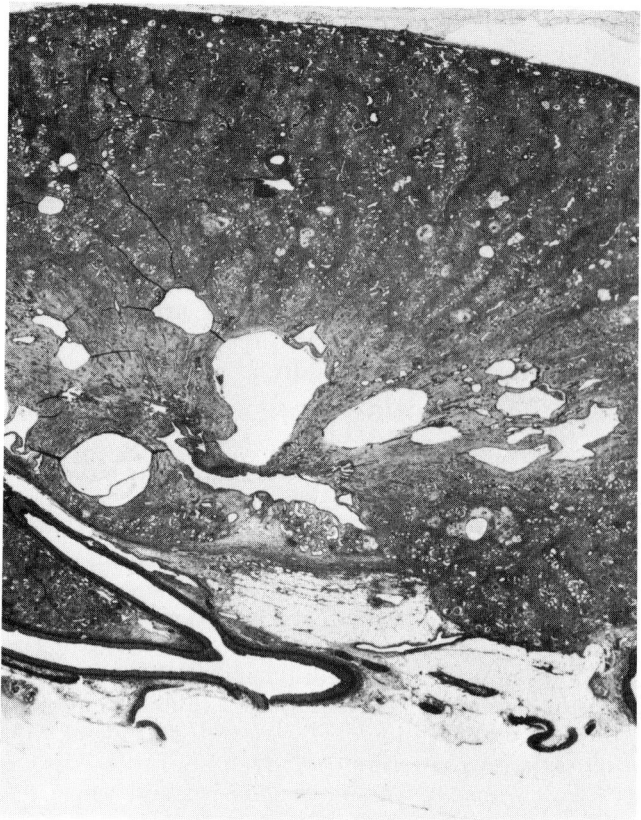

Figure 21–7. Uremic medullary cystic disease. Cut section of kidney showing cysts at corticomedullary junction and in medulla.

there is widespread atrophy and thickening of the basement membranes of proximal and distal tubules together with interstitial fibrosis. Some glomeruli may be hyalinized but, in general, glomerular structure is preserved.

There are few specific clues to diagnosis, because the medullary cysts may be too small to be visualized radiographically. The disease should be strongly considered in children or adolescents with otherwise unexplained chronic renal failure, a positive family history, and chronic tubulointerstitial nephritis on biopsy.

Acquired (Dialysis-Associated) Cystic Disease

The kidneys from patients with end-stage renal disease who have undergone prolonged dialysis sometimes exhibit numerous cortical and medullary cysts.[28] The cysts measure 0.5 to 2 cm in diameter, contain clear fluid, are lined by either hyperplastic or flattened tubular epithelium, and often contain calcium oxalate crystals. They probably form as a result of obstruction of tubules by interstitial fibrosis or by oxalate crystals. Tumors, usually of the renal adenoma type but occasionally adenocarcinomas, may be present in the walls of these cysts, and sometimes the

cysts bleed, causing hematuria. These complications are increasing in frequency with the growing population of patients with end-stage renal disease.

Simple Cysts

These occur as multiple or single cystic spaces that vary in diameter over wide limits. Commonly, they are 1 to 5 cm in size; translucent; lined by a gray, glistening, smooth membrane; and filled with clear fluid. Microscopically, these membranes are composed of a single layer of cuboidal or flattened cuboidal epithelium, which, in many instances, may be completely atrophic. These cysts are usually confined to the cortex, but may sometimes occur in the medullary portion of the kidney. Rarely, large massive cysts up to 10 cm in diameter are encountered.

Simple cysts are common post-mortem findings without clinical significance. On occasion, hemorrhage into them may cause sudden distention and pain, and calcification of the hemorrhage may give rise to bizarre radiographic shadows. The main importance of cysts lies in their differentiation from kidney tumors, when they are discovered either incidentally or because of hemorrhage and pain during life. Radiologic studies show that, in contrast to renal tumors (p. 1075), renal cysts have smooth contours, are almost always avascular, and give fluid rather than solid signals on ultrasound.

Table 21–1 summarizes the characteristic features of the principal cystic diseases.

GLOMERULAR DISEASES

Glomerular diseases constitute some of the major problems encountered in nephrology; indeed, chronic glomerulonephritis is the most common cause of chronic renal failure in man. Glomeruli may be injured by a variety of factors and in the course of a number of systemic diseases. Immunologic diseases such as systemic lupus erythematosus (SLE), vascular disorders such as hypertension and polyarteritis nodosa, metabolic diseases such as diabetes mellitus, and some purely hereditary conditions such as Fabry's disease often affect the glomerulus. These are termed *secondary glomerular diseases* to differentiate them from those in which the kidney is the only or predominant organ involved. The latter constitute the various types of *primary glomerulonephritis* (GN) or *glomerulopathy*. Here we shall discuss the various types of primary GN, and only briefly review the glomerular alterations in systemic diseases, which are covered in other parts of this book.

There are several types of glomerulonephritis, but no entirely satisfactory classification is available. Table 21–2 lists the most common forms that have reasonably well defined morphologic and clinical characteristics. In reviewing the specific types of GN, it is useful to consider each in terms of (1) clinical presentation, (2) the morphology of the glomerular

Table 21–1. Summary of Renal Cystic Diseases

	INHERITANCE	PATHOLOGIC FEATURES	CLINICAL FEATURES OR COMPLICATIONS	TYPICAL OUTCOME	DIAGRAMMATIC REPRESENTATION
Adult polycystic kidney disease	Autosomal dominant	Large multicystic kidneys, liver cysts, berry aneurysms	Hematuria, flank pain, urinary tract infection, renal stones, hypertension	Chronic renal failure beginning at age 40–60 years	
Childhood polycystic kidney disease	Autosomal recessive	Enlarged, cystic kidneys at birth	Hepatic fibrosis	Variable, death in infancy or childhood	
Medullary sponge kidney	None	Medullary cysts on excretory urography	Hematuria, urinary tract infection, recurrent renal stones	Benign	
Familial juvenile nephronophthisis	Autosomal recessive	Corticomedullary cysts, shrunken kidneys	Salt wasting, polyuria, growth retardation, anemia	Progressive renal failure beginning in childhood	
Adult-onset medullary cystic disease	Autosomal dominant	Corticomedullary cysts, shrunken kidneys	Salt wasting, polyuria	Chronic renal failure beginning in adulthood	
Simple cysts	None	Single or multiple cysts in normal-sized kidneys	Microscopic hematuria	Benign	
Acquired renal cystic disease	None	Cystic degeneration in end-stage kidney disease	Hemorrhage, erythrocytosis, neoplasia	Dependence on dialysis	

lesion, and (3) the cause and pathogenesis. The response of the glomerulus in all forms of injury is remarkably limited histologically and clinically, and only a small number of pathogenetic mechanisms are known. These will be summarized briefly before the specific types of GN are discussed.

Table 21–2. Glomerular Diseases

Primary Glomerulonephritis
   Acute diffuse proliferative glomerulonephritis (GN)
      Poststreptococcal
      Nonpoststreptococcal
   Crescentic (rapidly progressive) glomerulonephritis
   Membranous glomerulonephritis
   Lipoid nephrosis (minimal change disease)
   Focal segmental glomerulosclerosis
   Membranoproliferative glomerulonephritis
   IgA nephropathy
   Focal proliferative glomerulonephritis
   Chronic glomerulonephritis
Systemic Diseases
   Systemic lupus erythematosus
   Diabetes mellitus
   Amyloidosis
   Goodpasture's syndrome
   Polyarteritis nodosa
   Wegener's granulomatosis
   Henoch-Schönlein purpura
   Bacterial endocarditis
Hereditary Disorders
   Alport's syndrome
   Fabry's disease

CLINICAL MANIFESTATIONS

The clinical manifestations of glomerular disease are clustered into the five major glomerular syndromes described in Table 21–3 and on page 1016. Both the primary glomerulonephritides and systemic diseases affecting the glomerulus can result in these syndromes. Thus, a critical point in the clinical differential diagnosis is first to exclude the major systemic disorders, of which the major four are diabetes mellitus, SLE, vasculitis, and amyloidosis.

HISTOLOGIC ALTERATIONS

Various types of GN are characterized by one or more of four basic tissue reactions:

Table 21–3. The Glomerular Syndromes

Acute nephritis	Hematuria, azotemia, variable proteinuria, oliguria, edema, and hypertension
Rapidly progressive GN	Acute nephritis, proteinuria, and acute renal failure
Nephrotic syndrome	>3.5 gm proteinuria, hypoalbuminemia, hyperlipidemia, lipiduria
Chronic renal failure	Azotemia → uremia progressing over years
Asymptomatic hematuria or proteinuria	Glomerular hematuria; subnephrotic proteinuria

CELLULAR PROLIFERATION. Cellular proliferation is reflected by an increase in the number of cells in the glomerular tuft owing to proliferation of endothelial, mesangial, and epithelial cells. In certain diseases, there is also proliferation of the parietal epithelial cells that takes the form of a *crescent*, a histologic feature characteristic of diseases presenting clinically with rapidly progressive GN.

LEUKOCYTIC INFILTRATION. Neutrophils and monocytes infiltrate the glomerulus in some types of acute GN, and this is often accompanied by cellular proliferation.

GLOMERULAR BASEMENT MEMBRANE (GBM) THICKENING. By light microscopy, this change appears as thickening of the capillary walls best seen in sections stained with PAS. On electron microscopy such thickening can be resolved as either (1) thickening of the basement membrane proper, as occurs in diabetic glomerulosclerosis; or, more commonly, (2) deposition of amorphous electron-dense material representing precipitated proteins, on the endothelial or epithelial side of the basement membrane, or within the GBM itself. *By far the most common type of thickening is due to extensive subepithelial deposition, as occurs in membranous GN.* In most instances the deposits are thought to be immune complexes, although fibrin may also appear as an electron-dense material.

HYALINIZATION AND SCLEROSIS. Hyalinization or hyalinosis, as applied to the glomerulus, denotes the accumulation of material that is homogeneous and eosinophilic by light microscopy. By electron microscopy the material is extracellular and consists of amorphous substance (probably precipitated plasma protein) as well as increased amounts of basement membrane or mesangial matrix. This change results in obliteration of structural detail of the glomerular tuft (sclerosis) and usually denotes the end result of various forms of glomerular damage.

Additional alterations include fibrin deposition, intraglomerular thrombosis, or deposition of abnormal materials (amyloid, "dense deposits," lipid). Because many of the primary glomerulonephritides are of unknown cause, they are often classified by their histology, as can be seen in Table 21–2. The histologic changes can be further subdivided into *diffuse,* involving all glomeruli; *global,* involving the entire glomerulus; *focal,* involving only a certain proportion of the glomeruli; *segmental,* affecting a part of each glomerulus; and *mesangial,* affecting predominantly the mesangial region. These terms are sometimes appended to the histologic classifications.

PATHOGENESIS OF GLOMERULAR INJURY

Although much has yet to be learned, there has been considerable progress in our understanding of the pathogenesis of glomerular injury. It is best, for this discussion, to distinguish between (1) the primary mechanisms initiating glomerular injury and (2) the secondary, chemical mediators of glomerular damage. Regrettably, few of the *etiologic agents* triggering these events are known, and these will be noted in the discussion of the specific diseases.

Immune mechanisms clearly underlie the majority of primary glomerulonephritides and many of the secondary glomerular involvements[28–30] (Table 21–4). By far the most common mechanism is *antibody-mediated* injury, but cell-mediated mechanisms and activation of the alternate complement pathway also play a role.

Two basic forms of antibody-associated injury have been established: (1) injury by antibodies reacting *in situ* within the glomerulus, either with *insoluble fixed* (intrinsic) *glomerular antigens* or with circulating *antigens planted* within the glomerulus; and (2) injury resulting from deposition of *soluble circulating antigen-antibody complexes* in the glomerulus. These pathways are not mutually exclusive, and in man both seem to play a role.

In Situ Immune Complex Deposition

In this form of antibody-mediated injury, antibodies react directly with intrinsic tissue antigens. There are two well-established experimental models for anti–tissue-mediated glomerular injury, for which there are counterparts in human disease—antiglomerular basement membrane (anti-GBM) and Heymann's nephritis.

ANTI-GBM NEPHRITIS. *This term is now restricted to the type of injury in which antibodies are directed against intrinsic fixed antigens in the glomerular basement membrane, which induce a linear pattern of localization on immunofluorescence microscopy.* It has its experimental prototype in so-called Masugi or nephrotoxic nephritis, produced in rats by injections of anti–rat kidney antibodies prepared in rabbits by immunization with rat kidney tissue. The injected an-

Table 21–4. Immune Mechanisms of Glomerular Injury

Antibody-mediated Injury
  In situ immune complex deposition
  1. Fixed intrinsic tissue antigens (antitissue antibody–mediated GN)
    a. Anti-GBM nephritis
    b. Heymann nephritis
    c. ? Idiopathic human membranous GN
  2. Planted antigens
    a. Exogenous (drugs, lectins, infectious agents)
    b. Endogenous (DNA, immunoglobulins, immune complexes)
  Circulating immune complex deposition
  1. Endogenous antigens (e.g., thyroglobulin, DNA, tumor antigens)
  2. Exogenous antigens (e.g., infectious products)
  Cytotoxic antibodies
Cell-mediated Injury
Activation of Alternate Complement Pathway

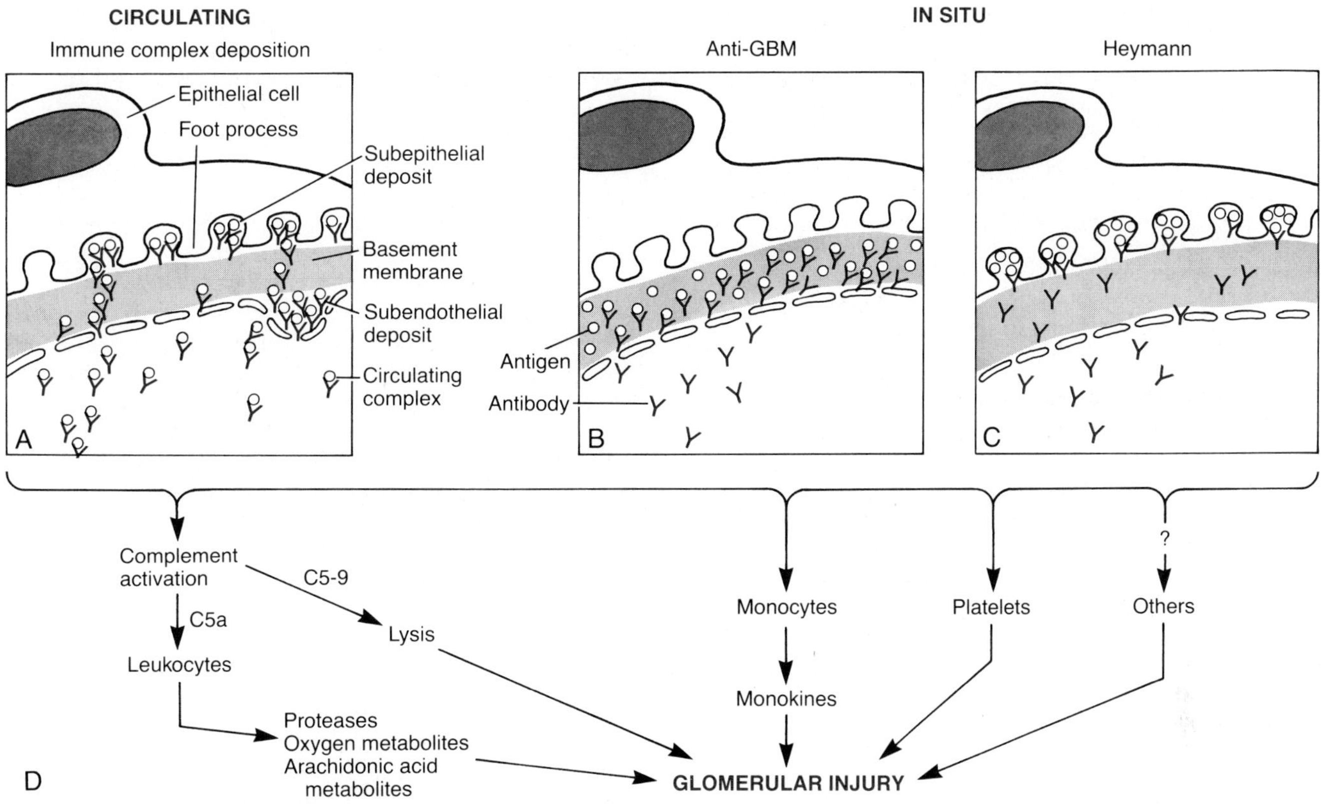

Figure 21–8. Antibody-mediated glomerular injury can result either from the deposition of circulating immune complexes *(A)* or from in situ formation of complexes *(B, C)*. Anti-GBM disease *(B)* is characterized by *linear* immunofluorescence patterns, whereas circulating and other lesions induced in situ develop *granular* patterns. The glomerular injury *(D)* results from mediators and toxic products derived from complement, neutrophils, monocytes, platelets, and other factors.

tibodies bind along the entire length of the GBM, *resulting in a homogeneous, diffuse linear immunofluorescent pattern* (Figs. 21–8B and 21–9B). This is contrasted with the granular lumpy pattern seen in other in situ models or after deposition of circulating immune complexes. To come back to Masugi's model, it should be noted that the deposited immunoglobulin of the rabbit is foreign to the host and thus acts as an antigen eliciting antibodies in the rat. This rat antibody then reacts with the rabbit immunoglobulin within the basement membrane, leading to further glomerular injury. This is referred to as the *autologous phase* of nephrotoxic nephritis, to distinguish it from the initial *heterologous phase* caused by the anti-GBM antibody. *The fluorescence in both instances is linear.* The nephritogenic "classic" GBM antigen appears to be a component of noncollagenous domain of collagen type IV.[31]

Anti-GBM nephritis accounts for less than 5% of human GN. It is well established as the cause of injury in Goodpasture's syndrome (p. 1031). Most instances of anti-GBM nephritis in humans are characterized by severe glomerular damage, with the development of rapidly progressive renal failure.

HEYMANN NEPHRITIS. Although classic anti-GBM nephritis is the one established form of immune injury

to intrinsic tissue antigen, other fixed antigens have been identified experimentally that initiate in situ immune deposition. One of these is the so-called *Heymann antigen.* The Heymann model of rat GN is induced by immunizing animals with preparations of proximal tubular brush border (Fig. 21–8C). The rats develop antibodies to brush border antigens, and a membranous GN, closely resembling human membranous GN, develops (p. 1034). The antigen is distributed along the visceral epithelial cell surface in an interrupted pattern; thus, the resultant pattern of immune deposition is *granular* and *interrupted,* rather than linear (Fig. 21–9A). On electron microscopy, the nephritis is characterized by the presence of numerous electron-dense deposits (presumably immune reactants) along the *subepithelial aspect* of the basement membrane. It is now clear that the GN results largely from the reaction of antibody with the Heymann antigen, a 330 kd glycoprotein (GP330) located in coated pits on the basal surface of visceral epithelial cells and expressed on the brush border also.[32] Antibody binding to the cell membrane is followed by complement activation and then by patching, capping, and subsequent shedding of the immune aggregates from the cell surface to form the characteristic subepithelial deposits (Fig. 21–10).[33] Unfortunately, despite the resemblance of the Heymann model to

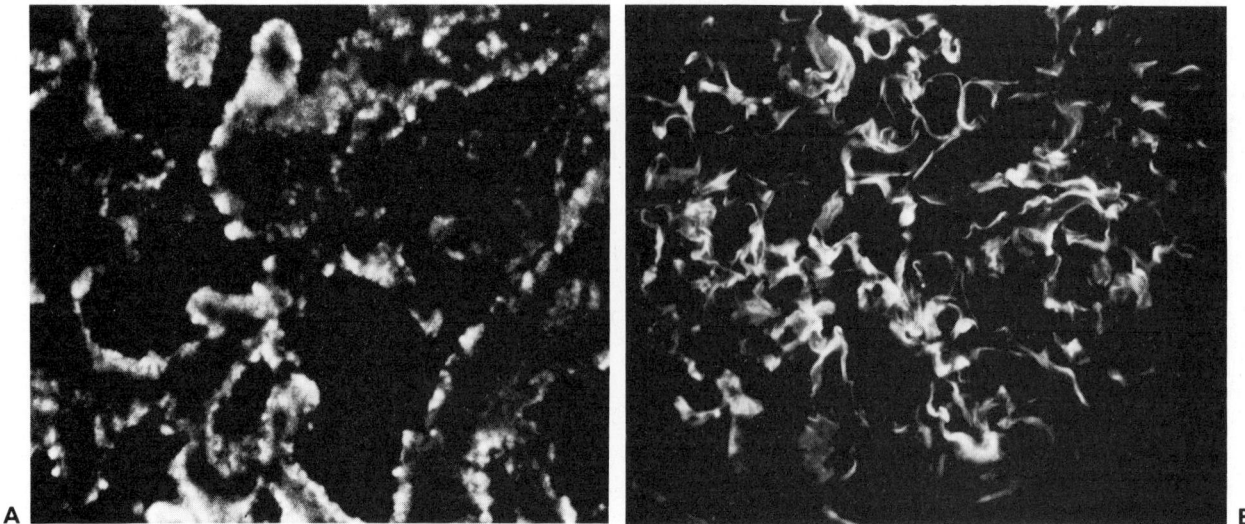

Figure 21–9. Two patterns of deposition of immune complexes as seen by immunofluorescence microscopy. *A, Granular,* characteristic of circulating and in situ immune complex nephritis; *B, linear,* characteristic of classic anti-GBM disease.

human membranous GN, the nature of the antigen in man is still unknown.

It must be apparent that, in humans, anti-GBM disease and the counterpart of Heymann nephritis are autoimmune diseases, caused by antibodies to endogenous tissue components. What triggers these autoantibodies is unclear, but any one of the several mechanisms responsible for autoimmunity, discussed earlier (p. 190), may be involved. Experimentally, several forms of autoimmune GN glomerulonephritis can

be induced by drugs (e.g., mercuric chloride), infectious products (endotoxin), and the graft-versus-host reaction.[34] In such models, there is an induced alteration of immune regulation associated with *polyclonal B-cell activation* (p. 191) and the induction of an array of autoantibodies which react with renal antigens.

ANTIBODIES AGAINST PLANTED ANTIGENS. Antibodies can react in situ with previously "planted" nonglomerular antigens. Such antigens may localize

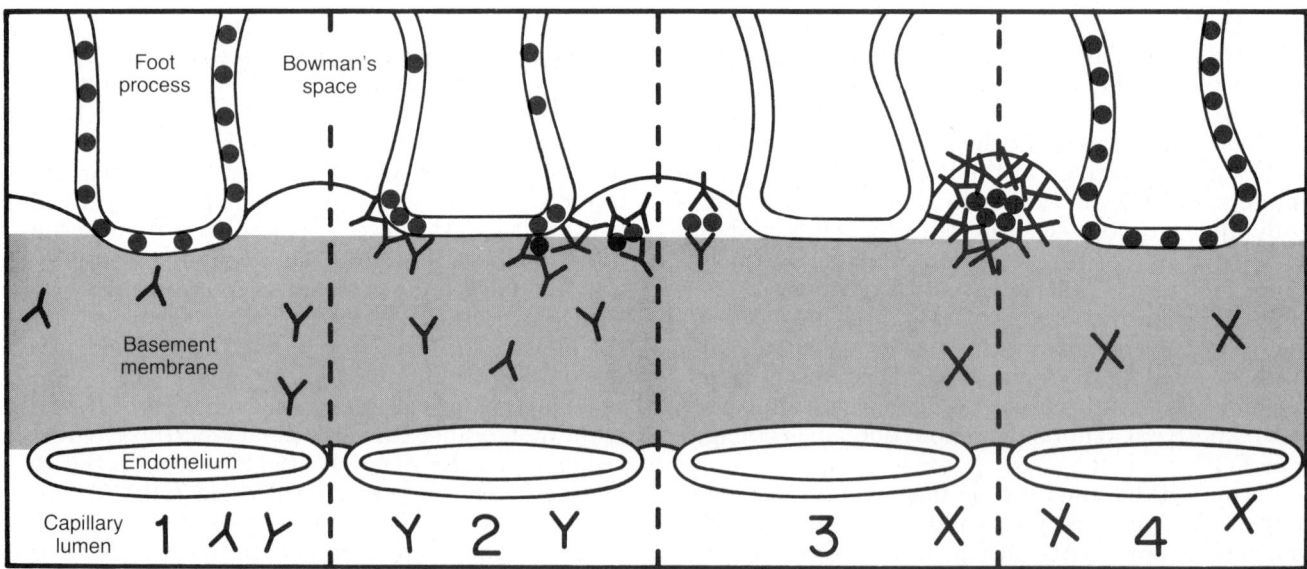

Figure 21–10. Heymann nephritis. Schematic drawing depicting the events occurring in rats injected with antibodies (Y) to rat tubular brush border antigen (gp 330), and reactive with gp 330 expressed on the plasma membrane of glomerular visceral epithelial cells *(dots, panel 1)*. Antibodies induce redistribution of Heymann immune complexes *(patching)* and subsequent *shedding* of complexes *(panel 2).* Owing to hydrodynamic forces of filtration the immune complexes initially aggregate and form detectable deposits in the filtration slits *(panels 3 and 4)*, where they increase in size when the autologous phase (X) occurs. When Heymann antibodies are no longer present in the circulation, gp 330 is re-expressed on the epithelial plasma membrane *(panel 4).* (From Andres, G.: Lab. Invest. *55:*513, 1986. Used by permission. © US & Canadian Academy of Pathology, Inc., 1986.)

in the kidney by interacting with various intrinsic components of the glomerulus. There is increasing experimental support for such a mechanism. Injections of *cationic* proteins, which bind to anionic sites in the GBM (p. 1012), followed by passively administered or actively induced antibody, result in immune complex GN, before or in the absence of circulating immune complexes.[35] Other planted antigens include lectins, which bind to capillary wall glycoprotein; DNA, which has an affinity for basement membrane components; bacterial products, such as endostreptosin, a protein of group A streptococci (p. 1029); and large aggregated proteins (e.g., aggregated IgG), which deposit in the mesangium because of their size. There is no dearth of other possible planted antigens, including viral, bacterial, and parasitic products and drugs. *Finally, immunoglobulins, complement components, and immune complexes themselves may potentially serve as planted antigens, because they continue to have reactive sites for further interactions with free antibody, free antigen, or complement.* Most of these planted antigens induce a granular or heterogeneous pattern of immunoglobulin deposition by fluorescence microscopy, the pattern found also in circulating immune complex nephritis, discussed next.

Circulating Immune Complex Nephritis

In this type of nephritis, glomerular injury is caused by the trapping of circulating antigen-antibody complexes within glomeruli. The antibodies have no immunologic specificity for glomerular constituents, and the complexes localize within the glomeruli because of their physicochemical properties and the hemodynamic factors peculiar to the glomerulus.

The pathogenesis of immune complex diseases (type III hypersensitivity reactions) was discussed in detail in an earlier chapter (p. 185). Here we shall briefly review the salient features that relate to glomerular injury.

The evocative antigens may be of endogenous origins, as in the case of the glomerulopathy associated with SLE (p. 193), or it may be exogenous, as is likely in the glomerulonephritis that follows certain streptococcal infections. Other antigens are implicated, including the surface antigen of the hepatitis B virus (HBsAg), various tumor antigens, *Treponema pallidum*, *Plasmodium falciparum*, and several viruses. Sometimes the inciting antigen is unknown. Whatever the antigen may be, antigen-antibody complexes are formed in the circulation and then trapped in the glomeruli, where they produce injury, in large part through the binding of complement. The glomerular lesions usually consist of leukocytic infiltration in glomeruli and proliferation of endothelial, mesangial, and epithelial cells. Electron microscopy reveals the immune complexes as electron-dense deposits or clumps that lie in the mesangium, or between the endothelial cells and the GBM *(subendothelial deposits)*, or between the outer surface of the GBM and the podocytes *(subepithelial deposits)* (Fig. 21-11). Deposits may be located at more than one site in a

given case. By immunofluorescence microscopy, *the immune complexes are seen as granular deposits either along the basement membrane or in the mesangium, or in both locations.* Once deposited in the kidney, immune complexes may eventually be degraded, mostly by phagocytic infiltrating monocytes and by mesangial cells, and the inflammatory changes may then subside. Such a course occurs when the exposure to the inciting antigen is short-lived and limited, as in most cases of poststreptococcal GN. However, if a continuous shower of antigens is provided, repeated cycles of immune complex formation, deposition, and injury may occur, leading to progressive GN. In some cases the source of chronic antigenic exposure is clear, such as in SLE, in which autoimmune injury to the tissues repeatedly releases nuclear and cytoplasmic antigens. In most cases, however, the antigen is unknown.

Several factors affect glomerular localization of antigen, antibody, or complexes. The molecular charge and size of these reactants are clearly important. Highly cationic immunogens tend to cross the GBM, and the resultant complexes eventually achieve a subepithelial location.[35] Highly anionic macromolecules are excluded from the GBM and either are trapped subendothelially or may, in fact, not be nephritogenic at all. Molecules with more neutral charge and their complexes tend to accumulate in the mesangium. Very large circulating complexes are not usually nephritogenic because they are cleared by the reticuloendothelial system and do not enter the GBM in sufficient quantities. The pattern of localization is also affected by changes in glomerular hemody-

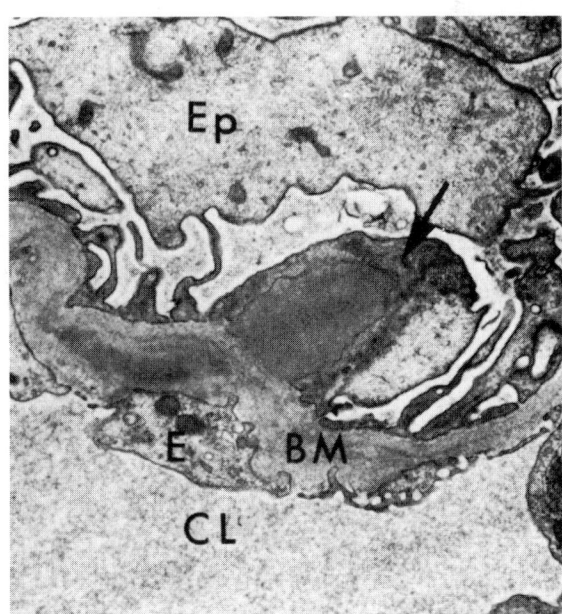

Figure 21-11. Electron-dense deposit in the subepithelial space *(arrow)*, characteristic of immune complex nephritis. BM = basement membrane; CL = lumen; E = endothelium; Ep = epithelium.

namics, mesangial function, and integrity of the charge-selective barrier in the glomerulus. These influences, as well as possible affinities of immune reactant to intrinsic glomerular components, underlie the variable pattern of immune reactant deposition and histologic change in the glomerulus.

Cytotoxic Antibodies

In addition to causing immune deposits, antibodies directed to glomerular cell antigens may cause direct cell injury—often without deposits. Antibodies to mesangial cell antigens, for example, cause mesangiolysis followed by mesangial cell proliferation[36]; antibodies to endothelial cell surface proteins cause endothelial injury[37]; and antibodies to certain visceral epithelial cell glycoproteins cause proteinuria in experimental animals.[38] This mechanism may well play a role in certain human immune disorders not associated with immune deposits.

To conclude the discussion of antibody-mediated injury, it must be stated that in the largest proportion of cases of human GN, the pattern of immune deposition is granular and along the basement membrane or in the mesangium. However, it is not clear in human GN whether the deposition has occurred in situ or via circulating complexes, or by both mechanisms—because, as discussed earlier, immune complex trapping can either initiate or be superimposed on in situ formation. It is best to consider that *antigen-antibody deposition in the glomerulus is a major pathway of glomerular injury; and that in situ immune reactions, trapping of circulating complexes, interactions between these two events, and local hemodynamic and structural determinants in the glomerulus all contribute to the morphologic and functional alterations in GN.*

Cell-Mediated Immunity in Glomerulonephritis

There is fragmentary and circumstantial evidence that sensitized T cells, as a reflection of cell-mediated immune reactions, can cause glomerular injury.[39] The idea is an attractive one, as it may account for the many instances of progressive GN in which either there are no immune deposits, or the deposits do not correlate with the severity of damage. Clues to its occurrence include the presence of macrophages and T lymphocytes in the glomerulus in some forms of human and experimental GN,[40] in vitro evidence of lymphocyte reactivity upon exposure to altered glomerular basement membrane antigen in progressive human GN, and a few successful attempts to transfer mild glomerular histologic alterations by lymphocytes in experimental GN.[39]

Activation of Alternate Complement Pathway

Alternate complement pathway activation occurs in the clinicopathologic entity called *membranoproliferative glomerulonephritis* (MPGN) (p. 1038), sometimes independently of immune complex deposition, and also in some forms of proliferative GN. This mechanism is discussed further on page 1039.

Mediators of Immunologic Glomerular Injury

Once immune reactants have localized in the glomerulus, glomerular damage ensues, mediated by several possible mechanisms (see Fig. 21–8D).

1. *Neutrophils.* These cells infiltrate the glomerulus in certain types of GN owing to activation of complement, resulting in generation of chemotactic agents (mainly C5a), and also via Fc-mediated immune adherence. Neutrophils release proteases, which cause GBM degradation; arachidonic acid metabolites; and oxygen-derived free radicals. The free radicals cause cell injury and also induce the release of latent metalloenzymes that can damage GBM components.[41,42] In some experimental models, depletion of neutrophils or complement inhibits both proteinuria and the histologic change. However, this mechanism applies only to some forms of GN, as many types show few neutrophils in the damaged glomeruli.

2. *C5b-9.* C5b-9, the terminal membrane attack complex of complement, can produce glomerular damage independently of the presence of neutrophils. In addition to causing cell lysis, it stimulates mesangial cells to produce various chemical mediators, including protease, oxygen-derived free radicals, interleukin-1, and prostaglandins.[43]

3. *Monocytes and macrophages.* Monocytes and macrophages infiltrate the glomerulus in many forms of human and experimental proliferative GN.[39] Depletion of monocytes prevents the proteinuria and histologic alterations in experimental nephritis. Activated macrophages release a vast number of biologically active molecules, and it is likely that some of these participate in the evolution of GN.

4. *Platelets.* Platelets aggregate in the glomerulus during immune-mediated injury. Their release of arachidonic acid metabolites and growth factors may play a role in some of the manifestations of GN. Antiplatelet agents have beneficial effects in both human and experimental GN.

5. *Glomerular cells.* Resident glomerular cells, particularly mesangial cells, can be stimulated to produce several inflammatory mediators, including oxygen free radicals, IL-1, arachidonic acid metabolites, and growth factors.[44] In the absence of leukocytic infiltration they may well initiate inflammatory responses in the glomerulus.

6. *Coagulation system.* The coagulation system may also be a mediator of glomerular damage. Fibrin is frequently present in the glomeruli in GN, and fibrinogen may leak into Bowman's space, serving as a stimulus to cell proliferation. Fibrin deposition is mediated largely by stimulation of macrophage procoagulant activity.[45] Pretreatment of animals with anticoagulants or defibrinating agents protects from the development of proliferative glomerular lesions

in some experimental models of GN, and this has led to the use of anticoagulant therapy in human GN.

Nonimmune Mechanisms of Glomerular Injury

There are other, largely nonimmune, mechanisms that may lead to glomerular damage in certain renal diseases, such as diabetic nephropathy and lipoid nephrosis, and these will be reviewed in the discussion of the specific diseases. However, nonimmune mechanisms in one important and common type of glomerular damage that leads to progressive glomerulosclerosis need to be addressed here.[46]

It has been amply documented that once any renal disease, glomerular or otherwise, destroys sufficient functioning nephrons to reduce the glomerular filtration rate (GFR) to about 30 to 50% of normal, progression to end-stage renal failure proceeds inexorably (although at variable rates), until renal failure ensues. Such patients develop proteinuria and their kidneys show widespread glomerular sclerosis. In some instances, such progression is the result of persistence or recurrence of the initial glomerular injury, as is the case in patients with chronic SLE. In others, it is due to glomerular damage induced by hypertension, which is a frequent complication of renal disease. Recent studies, however, suggest that progressive sclerosis may be initiated by the adaptive changes that occur in the relatively unaffected glomeruli of diseased kidneys.[47] Such a mechanism is suggested from experiments in rats subjected to ablation of renal mass by subtotal nephrectomy. Compensatory hypertrophy of the remaining glomeruli serves to maintain renal function in these animals, but proteinuria and focal glomerulosclerosis soon develop, leading eventually to total glomerular obsolescence, and if the renal ablation is severe, death of the animals in uremia ensues. The glomerular hypertrophy is associated with distinct hemodynamic changes, including increases in single nephron GFR, glomerular blood flow, and glomerular transcapillary pressure (capillary hypertension). Interventions that prevent the glomerular hypertrophy and blunt the hemodynamic changes (particularly the capillary hypertension) protect these animals from progressive glomerulosclerosis. The sequence of events (Fig. 21-12) leading to sclerosis entails endothelial and epithelial cell injury, increased glomerular permeability to proteins, accumulation of proteins in the mesangial matrix, and fibrin deposition. This is followed by proliferation of mesangial cells, increased deposition of mesangial matrix, and sclerosis of glomeruli.[47,48] This results in further reductions in nephron mass and a vicious circle of continuing glomerulosclerosis. As we shall see, this mechanism may play a role in the progressive renal failure in a number of chronic renal diseases. We now turn to a consideration of specific types of GN.

ACUTE GLOMERULONEPHRITIS

Certain types of glomerular disease are characterized anatomically by inflammatory alterations in the glomeruli and clinically by a complex of findings classically referred to as *the syndrome of acute nephritis.* The nephritic patient usually presents with hematuria, red cell casts in the urine, azotemia, oliguria, and mild-to-moderate hypertension. The patient also commonly has proteinuria and edema, but these are not as severe as those encountered in the nephrotic syndrome, discussed later. The acute nephritic syndrome may occur in such multisystem diseases as SLE and polyarteritis nodosa. Typically, however, it is characteristic of acute proliferative GN.

Acute Poststreptococcal (Proliferative) Glomerulonephritis

This is a fairly common glomerular disease that usually appears one to two weeks after a streptococcal infection of the throat or occasionally of the skin. It occurs most frequently in children 6 to 10 years of age, but adults of any age can be affected. The onset is generally abrupt and is heralded by the manifestations of acute nephritis.

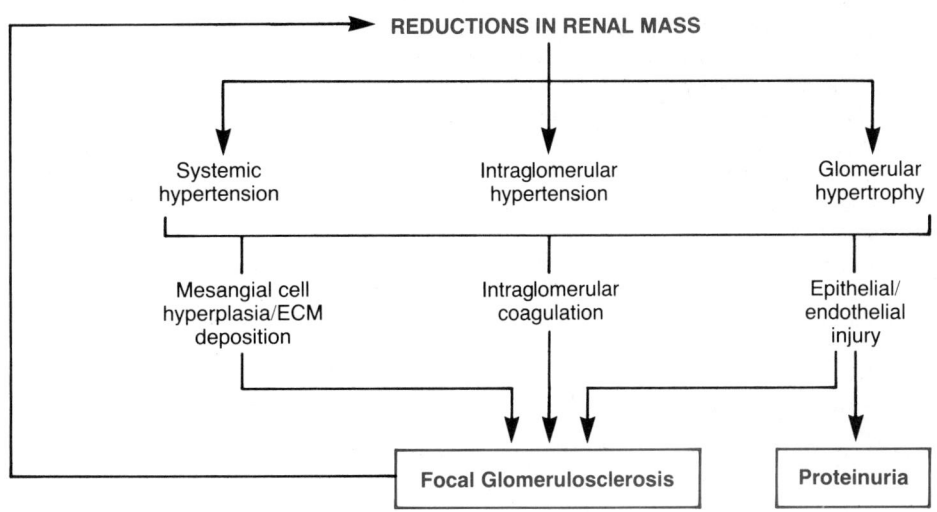

Figure 21–12. Nonimmune mechanisms in progressive glomerulosclerosis caused by reductions in renal mass. The adaptive changes in glomeruli (hypertrophy and glomerular capillary hypertension), as well as systemic hypertension, cause epithelial and endothelial injury and resultant proteinuria. The mesangial response, involving mesangial cell proliferation and extracellular matrix (ECM) production together with intraglomerular coagulation, causes the glomerulosclerosis. This results in further loss of functioning nephrons and a vicious circle of progressive glomerulosclerosis.

ETIOLOGY AND PATHOGENESIS. Only certain strains of group A beta-hemolytic streptococci are nephritogenic, over 90% of cases being traced to types 12, 4, and 1, which can be identified by typing of M protein of the cell wall. Skin infections are responsible for two thirds of cases in the southern United States and are commonly associated with overcrowding and poor hygiene.

Poststreptococcal GN is an immunologically mediated disease. The latent period between infection and onset of nephritis is compatible with the time required for the building up of antibodies. Elevated titers to one or more of the streptococcal exoenzymes, e.g., antistreptolysin-O (ASO), are present in a great majority of patients. Serum complement levels are low, compatible with involvement of the complement system as a mediator of the immune reaction. The presence of granular immune deposits of immunoglobulin and complement in the glomeruli suggests an immune complex–mediated mechanism, and so does the finding of electron-dense deposits seen under the electron microscope. The streptococcal antigenic component(s) responsible for the immune reaction has eluded identification for years. A cytoplasmic antigen called *endostreptosin* and several *cationic* streptococcal antigens are present in affected glomeruli,[49] but whether these represent "planted antigens," or part of circulating immune complexes, or both, is unknown. Additionally, cross-reacting cell-mediated reactions to GBM altered by streptococci have been implicated in cases of progressive poststreptococcal GN.[50]

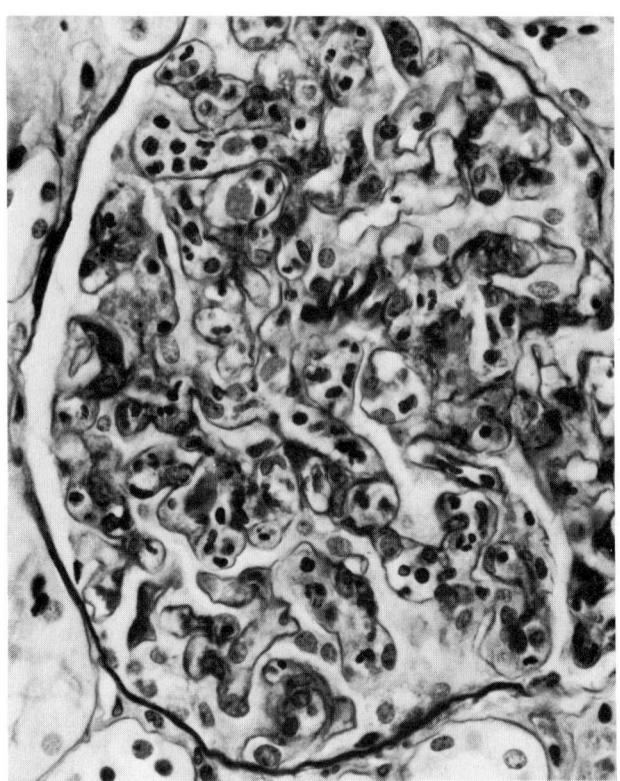

Figure 21–13. Poststreptococcal glomerulonephritis. Glomerular hypercellularity is due to intracapillary leukocytes and proliferation of intrinsic glomerular cells.

MORPHOLOGY. In fatal cases, the cortical surface appears red-brown and smooth, often dotted by fine, punctate petechiae produced by acute inflammatory rupture of glomerular capillaries.

The classic diagnostic picture is one of enlarged, hypercellular, relatively bloodless glomeruli (Fig. 21–13). The hypercellularity is caused by (1) proliferation of endothelial and mesangial cells and, in many cases, epithelial cells; and (2) infiltration by leukocytes, both neutrophils and monocytes. The proliferation and leukocyte infiltration are diffuse, i.e., involving all lobules of all glomeruli. There is also swelling of endothelial cells, and the combination of proliferation, swelling, and leukocyte infiltration obliterates the capillary lumina. Small deposits of fibrin within capillary lumina and mesangium can be demonstrated by special stains. There may be interstitial edema and inflammation, and the tubules often contain red cell casts and may show evidence of degeneration.

By **immunofluorescence microscopy** there are granular deposits of IgG and complement in the mesangium and along the basement membrane. Although present, they are often focal and sparse. The characteristic **electron microscopic findings** are the discrete, amorphous, electron-dense deposits on the epithelial side of the membrane, often having the appearance of "humps" (Fig. 21–11), presumably representing the antigen-antibody complexes trapped at the epithelial cell surface. Subendothelial and intramembranous deposits are sometimes seen, and there is often swelling of endothelial and mesangial cells. In the great majority of cases the glomerular changes begin to subside approximately four to six weeks after the onset of disease. In some cases they may persist for months, however, and are accompanied by persistent hypercellularity in the mesangial area with excessive deposition of mesangial matrix. Persistence of such abnormalities for prolonged periods may augur progression to chronic GN.

CLINICAL COURSE. In the classic case, a young child abruptly develops malaise, fever, nausea, oliguria, and hematuria (smoky or cocoa-colored urine) one to two weeks after recovery from a sore throat. Red cell casts in the urine are one of the most diagnostic findings. Proteinuria is generally mild (less than 1 gm), although it may reach 3 gm or even nephrotic levels. Edema may be limited to the periorbital areas but may subsequently progress, and hypertension is usually mild to moderate. In adults, the onset is more apt to be atypical, with the sudden appearance of hypertension or edema, frequently with elevation of BUN. During epidemics caused by nephritogenic streptococcal infections, GN may be entirely asymptomatic, discovered only when screening for microscopic hematuria. Important laboratory findings include elevations of ASO and other exoenzyme titers, a decline in the serum concentration of C3, and the presence of cryoglobulins in the serum.

Over 95% of children with poststreptococcal GN totally recover either spontaneously or with conservative therapy aimed at maintaining sodium and water balance. Microscopic hematuria, mild proteinuria, and histologic changes confined to the mesangium may persist in some patients for several weeks or months, but even then complete long-term recovery is the rule. A small minority of children (perhaps under 1%) do not improve, become severely oliguric, and develop a rapidly progressive form of GN (to be described later). Another 1 to 2% may undergo slow progression to chronic GN with or without recurrence of an active nephritic picture. Prolonged and persistent heavy proteinuria and abnormal GFR mark patients with an unfavorable prognosis.

In adults, the disease is probably less benign. Although the overall prognosis in epidemics is good, in only about 60% of *sporadic* cases do the patients recover promptly. Some patients develop rapidly progressive GN. In the remainder the glomerular lesions fail to resolve quickly, as manifested by persistent proteinuria, hematuria, and hypertension. In some of these patients the lesions eventually clear totally, but others develop chronic GN.

NONSTREPTOCOCCAL ACUTE GN. Although most patients with acute GN have poststreptococcal disease, a similar form has been reported sporadically in association with other bacterial agents (such as staphylococcal endocarditis, pneumococcal pneumonia, and meningococcemia), viral diseases (such as hepatitis B, mumps, varicella, and infectious mononucleosis) and parasitic infections (malaria, toxoplasmosis). In all of these, granular immunofluorescent deposits and subepithelial humps characteristic of immune complex nephritis are present.

CRESCENTIC (RAPIDLY PROGRESSIVE) GLOMERULONEPHRITIS (RPGN)

This form represents a *clinicopathologic syndrome* in which glomerular damage is accompanied by rapid and progressive decline in renal function, frequently with severe oliguria or anuria, usually resulting in irreversible renal failure in weeks or months.[51,52] *The syndrome is characterized histologically by the accumulation of cells in Bowman's space in the form of "crescents."* Thus, the terms *crescentic* and *extracapillary GN* are used synonymously. Hematuria is a common finding, but proteinuria is variable and hypertension and edema may or may not be present.

RPGN may occur in the course of three groups of diseases that can affect the glomerulus (Table 21–5): (1) poststreptococcal or postinfectious RPGN, (2) GN associated with systemic diseases, and (3) idiopathic RPGN. Here we shall describe postinfectious RPGN and Goodpasture's syndrome, as examples of a multisystem disorder, and idiopathic RPGN.

Table 21–5. Rapidly Progressive (Crescentic) Glomerulonephritis (RPGN)

Postinfectious RPGN
Systemic diseases
  Systemic lupus erythematosus
  Goodpasture's syndrome
  Vasculitis (e.g., polyarteritis nodosa)
  Wegener's granulomatosis
  Henoch-Schönlein purpura
  Essential cryoglobulinemia
Idiopathic RPGN

Postinfectious RPGN

Most patients with poststreptococcal or postinfectious GN recover, but in a small proportion intractable oliguria persists, anuria may ensue, and renal failure develops within weeks or months. This complication is rare in children but somewhat more common in adults. The initial clinical manifestations and pathogenetic mechanisms are similar to those of the diffuse proliferative GN: ASO serum titers are usually elevated, serum complement levels are reduced, and there is granular deposition of IgG and C3 in the glomeruli. Histologically, in addition to the diffuse proliferation and leukocyte infiltration, there is widespread crescent formation. Although all forms of RPGN have a dismal prognosis, the postinfectious type tends to fare better, and in some series up to 50% of patients may recover sufficient renal function to escape the necessity for long-term dialysis or transplantation.

Goodpasture's Syndrome

Goodpasture's syndrome is an acute, often fulminating disorder characterized by pulmonary hemorrhages and acute GN, commonly of the rapidly progressive type. Its peak incidence is in the third decade, with a 3:1 male female ratio. The pulmonary involvement usually precedes the onset of nephritis and is, the dominant cause of morbidity and mortality (p. 794). Here our interest is in the glomerular involvement.

ETIOLOGY AND PATHOGENESIS. Although pulmonary hemorrhage and GN may coexist in a variety of other conditions, such as SLE, Wegener's granulomatosis, scleroderma, and polyarteritis nodosa, the term *Goodpasture's syndrome is used here, in the strictest sense, to denote a disease that is the result of damage by anti–glomerular basement membrane antibodies that also cross react with alveolar basement membranes.* Immunofluorescent studies reveal the characteristic continuous linear staining for IgG seen in experimental anti-GBM nephritis. When immunoglobulins are eluted from glomeruli, they react in vitro with GBM, and when they are injected into monkeys, glomerular disease with typical linear staining is found in glomeruli. Circulating anti-GBM antibodies can be readily detected in the serum of most patients with Goodpasture's syndrome, and IgG may also be present in a linear fashion along the alveolar basement membranes. Experimentally, anti-GBM antibodies induce renal lesions as well as lung hemorrhage, provided the lung is previously injured (e.g., by oxygen toxicity[53] or by gasoline vapors).[54] Thus, the renal and lung injuries appear to be the result of antibodies against an antigen common to both basement membranes. The Goodpasture antigen resides in the noncollagenous portion of collagen type IV.[55] What triggers the formation of these antibodies is unclear. Exposure to viruses or hydrocarbon solvents (found in paints and dyes) has been implicated in some patients, as have been various drugs (e.g., rifampicin) and cancers. Cigarette smoking appears to play a permissive role, since most patients who develop pulmonary hemorrhage are smokers.[51] There is a high prevalence of DRW2 haplotype in Goodpasture's syndrome,[56] a finding consistent with the genetic predisposition to autoimmunity.

MORPHOLOGY. The lesions of Goodpasture's syndrome are similar to those of idiopathic RPGN and will be described together. In cases with mild renal involvement or early in the disease, there is focal and segmental proliferation of endothelial and mesangial cells with fibrinoid necrosis in glomerular tufts and focal infiltration by leukocytes. **This lesion may be present early, but more often as renal involvement progresses the picture is soon dominated by striking formation of extracapillary crescents** (Fig. 21–14).

Crescents are formed by proliferating parietal epithelial cells, accompanied by infiltrating macrophages, neutrophils, and occasionally lymphocytes. The macrophages are

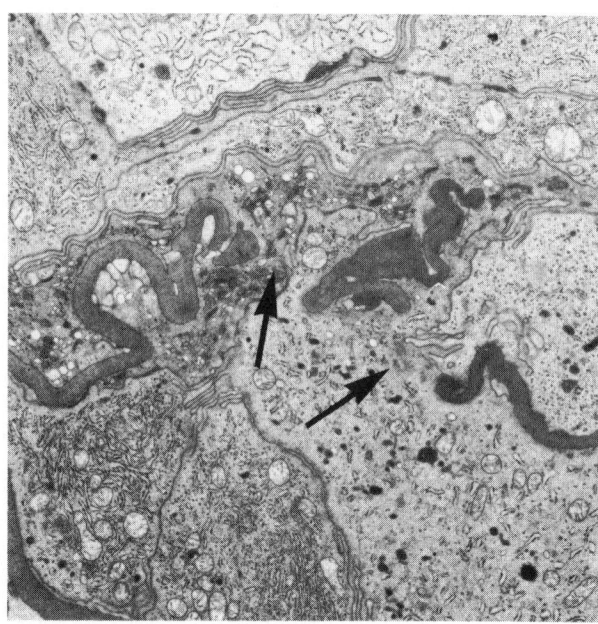

Figure 21–15. Rapidly progressive glomerulonephritis. Electron micrograph showing characteristic wrinkling of GBM with focal disruptions in its continuity *(arrows).*

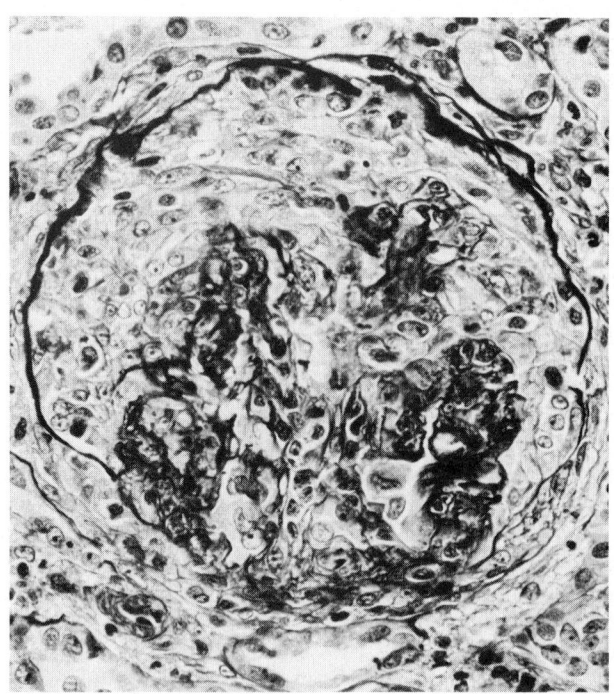

Figure 21–14. Crescentic glomerulonephritis. Glomerular tuft is collapsed. Note that the crescent is in Bowman's space (PAS stain).

activated and have abundant cytoplasm. Sequential renal biopsies have indicate that these crescents form quite rapidly and may be fully developed within a few days of onset of nephritis. Crescents compress and distort the capillary lumina, and many of them occlude the opening into the proximal renal tubule. **Fibrin is universally present in these lesions, often deposited among the interstices of the crescent.**

On electron microscopy the glomerulus discloses extensive fibrin deposition, epithelial and endothelial degeneration, and **characteristic focal disruptions of the GBM,** which may be filled with either fibrin or infiltrating leukocytes (Fig. 21–15). As mentioned earlier, immunofluorescent staining for immunoglobulins and complement reveals the uniform linear pattern characteristic of anti-GBM disease.

CLINICAL COURSE. The course may be dominated by recurrent hemoptysis or even life-threatening pulmonary hemorrhage (p. 794). Although milder forms of glomerular injury may subside, the renal involvement is usually progressive over a matter of weeks. When renal failure develops, dialysis support is necessary. Immunofluorescence or radioimmunoassays for circulating anti-GBM antibodies are helpful in the diagnosis, but severity of the disease does not correlate well with antibody titers. Dramatic remission may follow intensive plasmapheresis (plasma exchange) combined with steroids and cytotoxic agents. This therapy appears to reverse both pulmonary hemorrhage and renal failure. Plasma exchange presumably removes both the anti-GBM antibodies responsible for initiating the damage and the secondary circulating mediators. Despite therapy, patients may eventually require chronic dialysis or transplantation. Transplantation is usually delayed for several months to reduce the small but definite risk of recurrence of the disease in the transplanted kidney.

Idiopathic RPGN

In about half the patients presenting with RPGN, the conditions cited in Table 21–5 can be excluded; such cases are referred to as idiopathic RPGN. A flulike syndrome may precede the onset, but most often the signs of azotemia (weakness, nausea, vomiting), oliguria, hematuria, and proteinuria herald the disease.

Immunofluorescence microscopy of glomeruli in such patients shows linear fluorescence in about one fourth (anti-GBM disease), granular fluorescence in about one fourth, and scanty or no immune deposits in about one half of patients. This is thus not a distinctive entity but is best viewed as an ominous pathway that may follow many types of GN of differing causes and pathogeneses and having in common severe glomerular damage.[56]

The prognosis for most untreated forms of RPGN is bleak, the vast majority of these patients eventually requiring long-term dialysis or transplantation. Therapy with high-dose corticosteroids or plasma exchange may be helpful, particularly when instituted in less severely oliguric patients early in the course.

NEPHROTIC SYNDROME (NS)

Certain glomerular diseases (membranous GN, lipoid nephrosis, focal sclerosis) virtually always produce the nephrotic syndrome. In addition, many other forms of primary and secondary GN discussed in this chapter may evoke it. It is convenient, therefore, before presenting the major causes of NS, to discuss this clinical complex.[57] NS has the following features:

1. Massive proteinuria with the daily loss of 3.5 gm or more of protein (less in children).
2. Hypoalbuminemia with plasma albumin levels less than 3 gm per dl.
3. Generalized edema.
4. Hyperlipidemia.

The syndrome is fundamentally the *result of excessive glomerular permeability to plasma proteins, and thus heavy proteinuria is its prime characteristic.* The heavy proteinuria leads to depletion of serum albumin levels below the compensatory synthetic abilities of the liver, with consequent hypoalbuminemia and a reversed albumin-globulin ratio. Increased renal catabolism also contributes to the hypoalbuminemia. The generalized edema is, in turn, the consequence of the loss of colloid osmotic pressure of the blood and the accumulation of fluid in the interstitial tissues. There is also *sodium and water retention,* which aggravates the edema. This appears to be due to several factors, including compensatory secretion of aldosterone, mediated by the hypovolemia-en-

hanced antidiuretic hormone secretion; stimulation of the sympathetic system; and a reduction in the secretion of natriuretic factors, such as atrial peptides. Edema is characteristically soft and pitting, most marked in the periorbital regions and dependent portions of the body. It may be quite massive with pleural effusions and ascites.

The largest proportion of protein lost in the urine is albumin, but globulins are also excreted in some diseases. The ratio of low- to high-molecular-weight proteins in the urine in various cases of NS determines the so-called "selectivity" of proteinuria. A *highly selective proteinuria* consists mostly of low-molecular-weight proteins (albumin 66,000; transferrin 76,000), whereas a *poorly selective proteinuria* consists of higher-molecular-weight proteins in addition to albumin.

The genesis of the *hyperlipidemia* in the nephrotic syndrome is complex.[58] Most patients have increased VLDL and/or LDL and a decrease in HDL. In addition, the proportion of cholesterol to triglycerides in each lipoprotein fraction is increased. These defects seem to be due, in part, to *increased synthesis of lipoproteins in the liver, coupled with decreased catabolism.* HDL, but not the larger lipoproteins, is also lost in the urine when severe proteinuria occurs. *Lipiduria* follows the hyperlipidemia, because not only albumin molecules but also lipoproteins leak across the glomerular capillary wall. The lipid appears in the urine either as free fat or as "oval fat bodies" representing lipoprotein resorbed by tubular epithelial cells and then shed along with the degenerated cells. Whether associated hyperlipidemia increases the risk of atherosclerosis and coronary heart disease is controversial.

These patients are particularly vulnerable to *infection,* especially with staphylococci and pneumococci. The basis for this vulnerability could be related to loss of immunoglobulins or low-molecular-weight complement components (e.g., factor B) in the urine. *Thrombotic and thromboembolic complications* are also quite common in NS. The hypercoagulable state is due in part to loss of anticoagulant factors (e.g., antithrombin III) and antiplasmin activity through the leaky glomerulus. Thrombocytosis and marked increases in serum factors V, VII, and VIII and fibrinogen also occur. *Renal vein thrombosis,* once thought to be a cause of NS, is most often a consequence of this hypercoagulable state.

A compilation of the forms of renal involvement that give rise to NS is presented in Table 21–6. Several features are noteworthy in this table. Among children, the great preponderance of cases of NS is the consequence of primary renal disease. The outstanding cause is lipoid nephrosis (65%), and membranous GN accounts for only 5%. In adults, primary renal disease is less predominant. Most important is membranous glomerulonephritis (40%). Systemic diseases such as diabetic glomerulosclerosis, amyloidosis, and lupus nephritis make a substantial contribution to the spectrum of NS in adults.

Table 21–6. Causes of Nephrotic Syndrome

	PREVALENCE* (PER CENT)	
	Children	Adults
Primary Glomerular Disease		
Membranous GN	5	40
Lipoid nephrosis	65	15
Focal segmental glomerulosclerosis	10	15
Membranoproliferative GN	10	7
Other proliferative GN (focal, "pure mesangial," IgA nephropathy)	10	23
Systemic Diseases		
Diabetes mellitus		
Amyloidosis		
Systemic lupus erythematosus		
Drugs (gold, penicillamine, "street heroin")		
Infections (malaria, syphilis, hepatitis B, AIDS)		
Malignancy (carcinoma, melanoma)		
Miscellaneous (bee-sting allergy, hereditary nephritis)		

* Approximate prevalence of primary disease = 95% in children, 60% in adults.
Approximate prevalence of systemic disease = 5% in children, 40% in adults.

MEMBRANOUS GLOMERULONEPHRITIS (MGN)

Membranous glomerulonephritis, or membranous nephropathy, is a major cause of the nephrotic syndrome in adults. It is characterized by the presence of electron-dense, immunoglobulin-containing deposits along the epithelial (subepithelial) side of the basement membrane.[59] Early in the disease, the glomeruli may appear normal by light microscopy, but well-developed cases show *diffuse thickening of the capillary wall.*

MGN may occur in association with known disorders or etiologic agents,[59] which it would be well to bear in mind (secondary MGN). These include the following:

1. Malignant epithelial tumors, particularly carcinoma of the lung and colon and melanoma.[60]
2. Systemic lupus erythematosus.
3. Exposure to inorganic salts (gold, mercury).
4. Drugs (penicillamine, captopril).
5. Infections (chronic hepatitis B, syphilis, schistosomiasis, malaria).
6. Metabolic disorders (diabetes mellitus, thyroiditis).

In about 85% of patients, the condition is truly "idiopathic."

ETIOLOGY AND PATHOGENESIS. Because of the uniform presence of immunoglobulins and complement in the subepithelial deposits and of the similarity of the lesions with experimental immune complex diseases, it is believed that MGN is a form of chronic antigen-antibody–mediated disease.[61] In MGN associated with other disorders, specific antigens can sometimes be implicated. For example, MGN occurs in 10% of patients with SLE, presumably owing to DNA–anti-DNA complex deposition (p. 193). Exogenous (hepatitis B, Treponema antigens) or endogenous (thyroglobulin) antigens have been identified within deposits in some cases. In the vast majority of cases, however, including patients with idiopathic MGN, the antigens are still unknown.

Genetic susceptibility is suggested by the increased prevalence of HLA-DR/3 in European and HLA-DR/2 in Japanese patients with MGN. This suggests possible defects in immune regulation, and indeed an imbalance in T-helper and T-suppressor lymphocyte function has been reported in these patients.[61]

Circulating immune complexes are found in only 15 to 25% of cases, and thus an in situ immune reaction involving glomerular or planted antigen is postulated to account for the subepithelial immune deposits. The lesions bear a striking resemblance to those of experimental Heymann nephritis, which, as you recall, is induced by antibodies to an intrinsic tissue antigen present in the visceral epithelial cells (p. 1025). Susceptibility to Heymann nephritis in rats is also linked to the HLA locus, which influences the ability to elaborate antibodies to the nephritogenetic antigen. The possibility thus exists that idiopathic MGN, like Heymann nephritis, is an autoimmune disease, linked to susceptibility genes, and caused by antibodies to an as yet unidentified renal antigen.

Begging the question of the nature of the immune deposits, how does the glomerular capillary wall become leaky? In the absence of neutrophils, monocytes, or platelets, and the virtually uniform presence of complement, current work points to a direct action of C5b-9, the membrane-attack complex of complement, as described previously (p. 1028).

MORPHOLOGY. The kidneys are large, swollen, and pale. By light microscopy, the glomeruli appear either normal or exhibit (in the early stages of the disease) **uniform, diffuse thickening of the glomerular capillary wall** (Fig. 21–16A). By electron microscopy, irregular dense deposits can be seen between the basement membrane and the overlying epithelial cells, the latter appearing swollen and having lost their foot processes (Fig. 21–16B and D). Basement membrane material is laid down between these deposits, appearing as irregular spikes protruding from the GBM. These spikes are best seen by silver stains, which color the basement membrane black. In time, these spikes thicken to produce domelike protrusions; with progression of the disease, these eventually close over the immune deposits, burying them within a markedly thickened, irregular membrane. Immunofluorescence demonstrates that the granular deposits contain both immunoglobulins and complement (Fig. 21–16C). As the disease advances, the membrane thickening progressively encroaches upon the capillary lumina, and sclerosis of the mesangium may occur, and, in the course of time, glomeruli become totally hyalinized. The epithelial cells of the proximal tubules contain hyaline droplets, reflecting protein reabsorption. In the advanced stage of the disease, tubular atrophy and interstitial fibrosis occur, and indeed the kidneys may become contracted, finely granular, and scarred, closely resembling those in other forms of chronic GN.

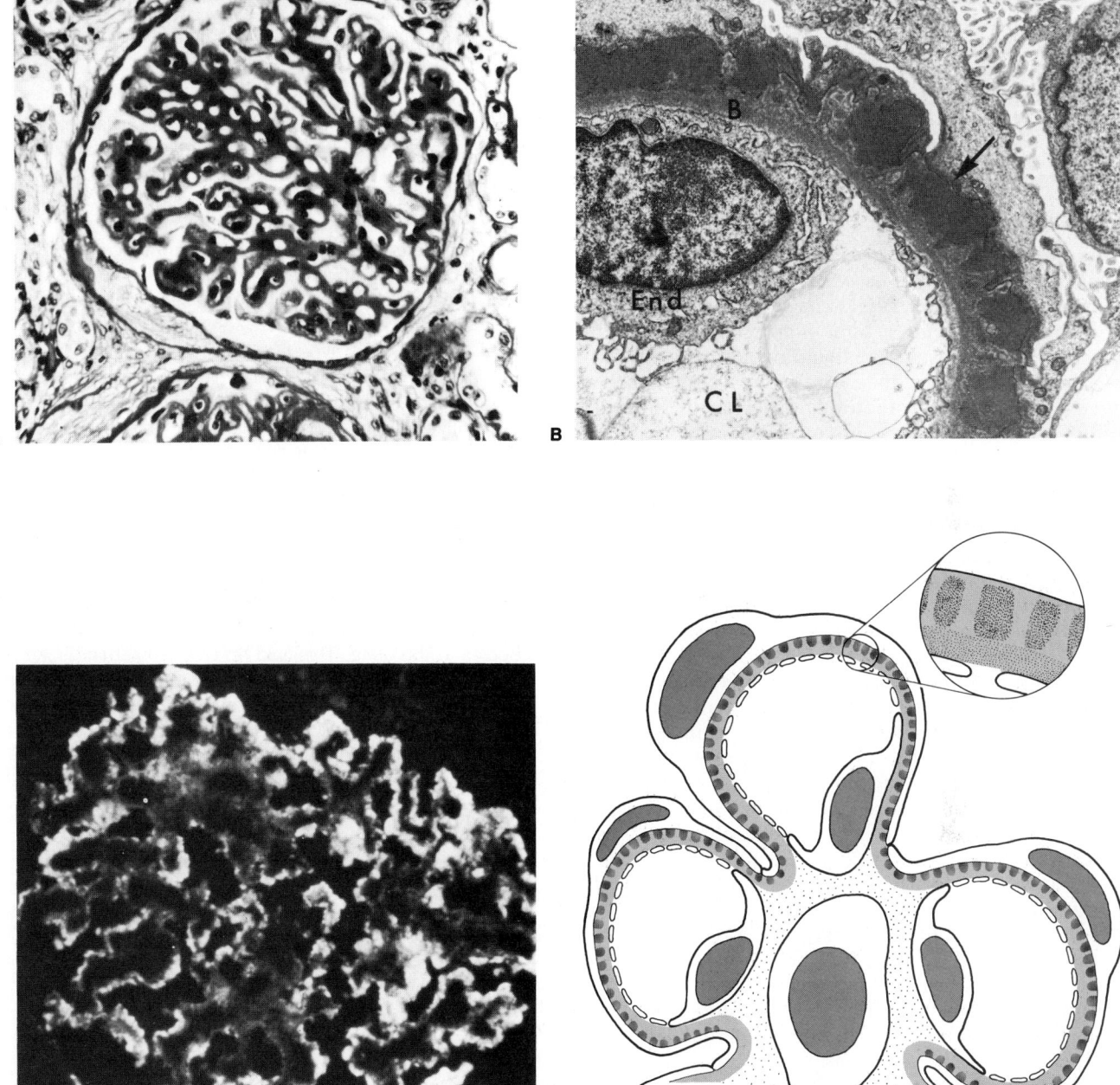

Figure 21–16. Membranous glomerulonephritis. *A*, PAS stain. Note diffuse thickening of capillary wall without increase in number of cells. *B*, Electron micrograph showing electron-dense deposits *(arrow)* along epithelial side of basement membrane (B). Note obliteration of foot process overlying deposits. CL = Capillary lumen; End = endothelium; Ep = epithelium. *C*, Characteristic granular immunofluorescent deposits of IgG along GBM. *D*, Diagrammatic representation of membranous GN.

CLINICAL COURSE. In a previously healthy individual this disorder usually begins with the insidious onset of the nephrotic syndrome or, in 15% of patients, with non-nephrotic proteinuria. Hematuria and mild hypertension are present in 15 to 35% of cases. It is necessary in any patient with MGN to first rule out the secondary causes described earlier.

The course is irregular,[62] but in 70 to 90% proteinuria is irreversible and in about 50% the disease progresses to renal insufficiency over an unpredictable span of two to 20 years. Progression is associated with increasing sclerosis of glomeruli, rising BUN, relative reduction in the severity of proteinuria, and development of hypertension. Perhaps 10 to 30% of patients have a more benign course, with partial or complete remissions. Renal vein thrombosis may occur as a reflection of the hypercoagulability. Because of the notoriously variable course of the disease, it has been difficult to evaluate the effectiveness of corticosteroids or immunosuppressive therapy in controlling the proteinuria or progression to chronic renal insufficiency.[63a]

MINIMAL CHANGE DISEASE (MCD) (LIPOID NEPHROSIS)

These terms are used to describe a disorder in which the nephrotic syndrome is associated with diffuse loss of foot processes of epithelial cells in glomeruli that appear virtually normal by light microscopy. MCD is the most common cause of NS in children (see Table 21–6), and the peak incidence is between 2 and 6 years of age.[63] The disease sometimes follows a respiratory infection (25% of cases) or routine prophylactic immunization (10%). Its most characteristic feature is its usually dramatic response to corticosteroid therapy.

ETIOLOGY AND PATHOGENESIS. These are essentially unknown. By fluorescence microscopy there is no deposition of immunoglobulins or complement in glomeruli, and by electron microscopy no deposits are seen, excluding classic immune complex mechanisms. Nevertheless, several features of the disease point to an immunologic basis,[64] including (1) the clinical association with respiratory infections and prophylactic immunizations; (2) the response to corticosteroid and immunosuppressive therapy; (3) the association with other atopic disorders (e.g., eczema, rhinitis); (4) the increased prevalence of HLA-B8 or HLA-DR7 in patients with minimal change disease associated with atopy (suggesting a possible genetic predisposition); (5) the increased incidence of MCD in patients with Hodgkin's disease, in whom defects in T cell–mediated immunity are well recognized; and (6) reports of the elaboration of lymphokine-like activity by lymphocytes of patients with MCD cultured with renal tissue. Such findings have led to *speculations* that lipoid nephrosis involves some dysfunction of T-cell immunity, eventually resulting in the elaboration of a lymphokine-like circulating substance that increases the permeability of the glomerular wall.

More has been learned about the molecular basis of protein leakage in this condition.[65] An early event in MCD and experimental aminonucleoside nephrosis (a model that mimics MCD) appears to involve *loss of glomerular polyanion* (p. 1012). This reduction in negative charge is associated with two defects: (1) enhanced filtration of circulating polyanions, mainly albumin, resulting in proteinuria, and (2) a change in epithelial cell shape leading to the familiar disappearance of foot processes. The first seems to involve loss of heparan sulfate proteoglycan, and the second a reduction of the sialoglycoprotein cell coat. How the glomerular polyanion loss is brought about, however, is mysterious. It could conceivably result from the action of some circulating factor or from a metabolic defect that affects the ability of visceral epithelial cells to elaborate basement membrane components, a notion consistent with the pronounced epithelial alterations in this disease.

MORPHOLOGY. The glomeruli are normal; there is no thickening of basement membranes and no cellular proliferation (Fig. 21–17). Occasionally, there is a mild increase in mesangial matrix. **By electron microscopy** the basement membrane appears morphologically normal, and no electron-dense material is deposited. **The principal lesion is in the visceral epithelial cells, which show a uniform and diffuse effacement of foot processes,** these being replaced by a rim of cytoplasm often showing vacuolization, swelling, and villous hyperplasia (Fig. 21–18). This change, often incorrectly termed "fusion" of foot processes, actually represents simplification of the epithelial cell architecture with flattening and swelling of foot processes rather than actual cell fusion. It should be noted that such foot process loss is also present in other proteinuric states (e.g., MGN, diabetes). It is only when fusion is associated with normal glomeruli that the diagnosis of minimal change disease can be made. The visceral epithelial changes are completely reversible after corticosteroid therapy and remission of the proteinuria. The term **lipoid nephrosis** was initially coined because of the presence of lipid in tubules and fat bodies in the urine. This lipid reflects glomerular leakage and reabsorption of lipoprotein. The protein reabsorption droplets appear as hyaline droplets or fatty vacuoles in the proximal convoluted tubules. Immunofluorescence studies show no immunoglobulin or complement deposits.

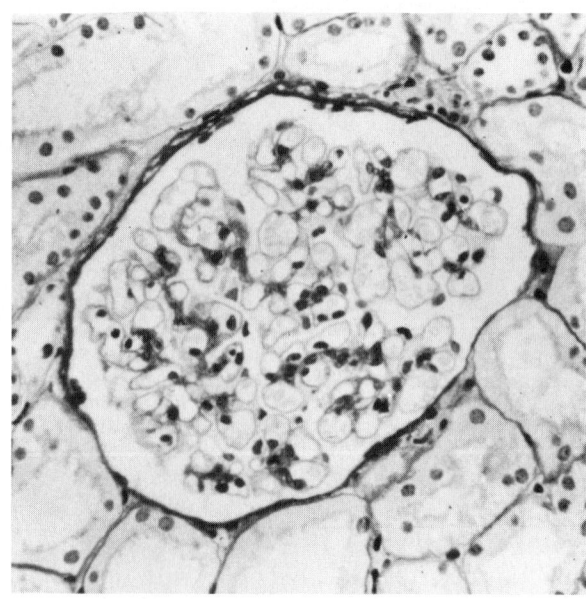

Figure 21–17. Minimal change disease. Thin section of glomerulus stained with PAS. Note thin basement membrane and absence of proliferation. Compare with membranous glomerulonephritis in Figure 21–16 A.

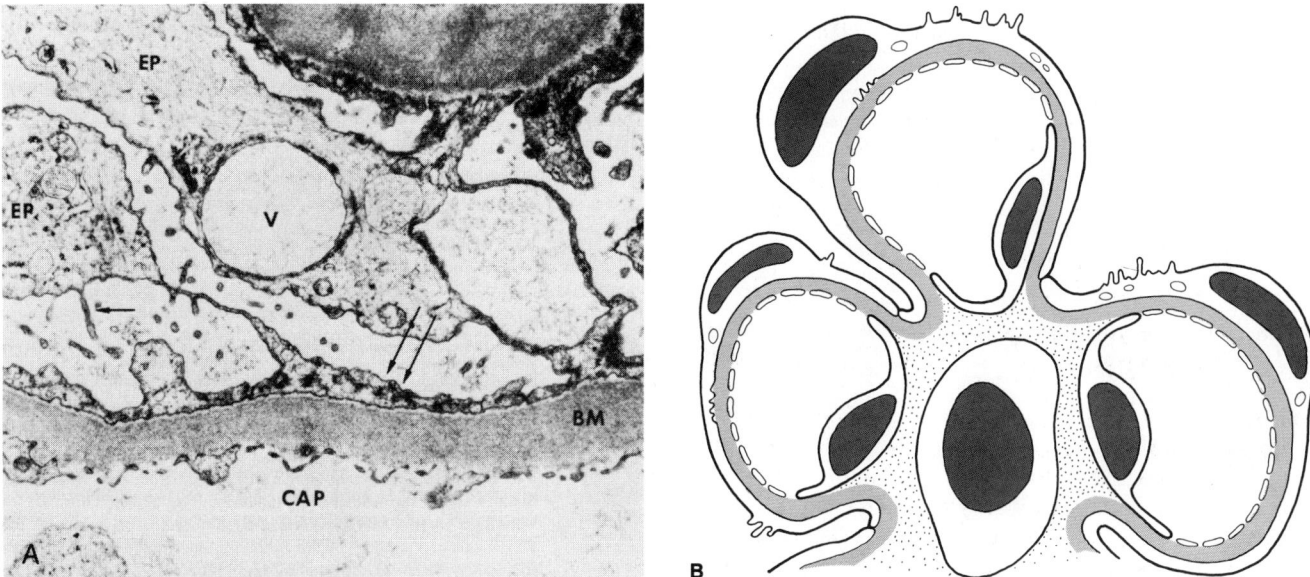

Figure 21–18. *A,* Ultrastructural characteristics of minimal change disease: loss of foot processes *(double arrows),* absence of deposits, vacuoles (v) and microvilli in visceral epithelial cells *(single arrow). B,* Schematic representation of minimal change disease, showing diffuse loss of foot processes.

CLINICAL COURSE. Despite massive proteinuria, renal function remains good and there is commonly no hypertension or hematuria. The proteinuria usually is highly selective. It may be impossible, however, short of renal biopsy, to differentiate MCD from MGN in the early stages of both diseases. The great majority (over 90%) of children with MCD exhibit a rapid response to corticosteroid therapy. However, the nephrotic phase may recur and some patients may become "steroid-dependent." Nevertheless, the long-term prognosis for patients is excellent, and even steroid-dependent disease resolves when children reach puberty.[63] Adults have a similarly good prognosis.[65a]

FOCAL SEGMENTAL GLOMERULOSCLEROSIS (FSG)

As the name implies, *this lesion is characterized by sclerosis of some, but not all, glomeruli (thus, it is focal), and in the affected glomeruli only a portion of the capillary tuft is involved (thus, it is segmental).* Focal segmental glomerulosclerosis is frequently accompanied clinically by the nephrotic syndrome or heavy proteinuria.[66]

FSG can be classified further into (1) *idiopathic FSG,* (2) *FSG superimposed on another primary glomerular lesion* (such as IgA nephropathy) (p. 1040), and (3) *secondary FSG,* associated with other known disorders or etiologic agents. Secondary FSG is a recognized manifestation of heroin abuse and of the acquired immunodeficiency syndrome (AIDS),[67] and it also occurs in advanced stages of other nonglomerular renal disorders, such as reflux nephropathy, analgesic abuse nephropathy, and unilateral renal agenesis.

Idiopathic FSG accounts for 10 and 15% of cases of nephrotic syndrome seen among children and adults, respectively. About 80% of patients with this lesion have a nephrotic syndrome but differ from the usual patients with MCD in the following respects: (1) they have higher incidence of hematuria, reduced GFR, and hypertension; (2) their proteinuria is more often nonselective; (3) they respond poorly or not at all to corticosteroid therapy; (4) many progress to chronic GN, and at least 50% develop end-stage renal disease within 10 years; and (5) immunofluorescence microscopy shows deposition of IgM and C3 in the sclerotic segment.

MORPHOLOGY. As seen by light microscopy, the segmental lesions may involve only a minority of the glomeruli and may be missed if insufficient glomeruli are present in the biopsy specimen. The lesions initially involve the juxtamedullary glomeruli, although they subsequently become more generalized. In the sclerotic segments there is collapse of basement membranes, increase in mesangial matrix, and deposition of hyaline masses **(hyalinosis),** often with lipoid droplets (Fig. 21–19). Glomeruli not exhibiting segmental lesions either appear normal on light microscopy or may show increased mesangial matrix and mesangial proliferation. On electron microscopy, nonsclerotic areas show the diffuse loss of foot processes characteristic of MCD, but in addition there is **pronounced, sometimes focal denudation of the epithelial cells.** Masses of electron-dense amorphous material and lipid granules are also present within the sclerotic areas. By immunofluorescence, IgM and C3 are present within the hyaline masses in the sclerotic areas. In addition to the focal sclerosis, there is often rather pronounced hyaline thickening of afferent arterioles, and occasionally there are glomeruli that are com-

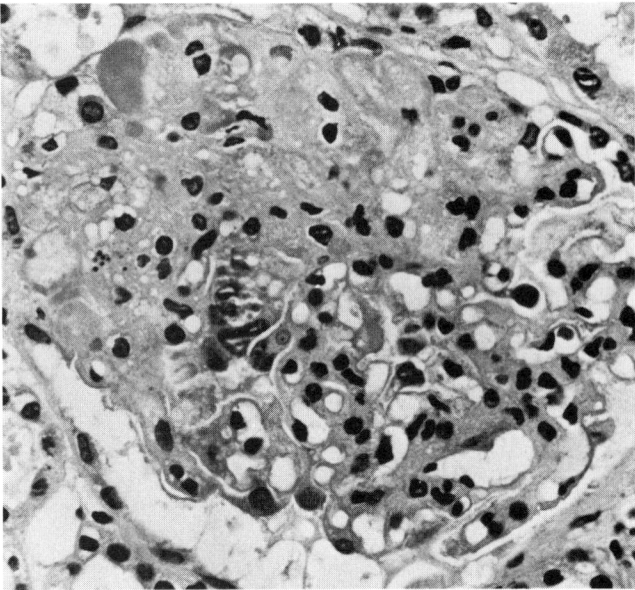

Figure 21–19. Segmental sclerosis. Note hyaline mass (11 o'clock) and lipid (small vacuoles) in sclerotic area.

pletely sclerosed (global sclerosis). With the progression of the disease, increased numbers of glomeruli become involved, sclerosis spreads within each glomerulus, and there is increase in mesangial matrix. In time this leads to total sclerosis of glomeruli with pronounced tubular atrophy and interstitial fibrosis. This advanced picture would be difficult to differentiate from other forms of chronic GN.

PATHOGENESIS. Whether idiopathic FSG represents a distinct disease or is simply a phase in the evolution of a subset of patients with MCD is a matter of debate.[68,69] The characteristic degeneration and focal disruption of visceral epithelial cells are thought to represent an accentuation of the diffuse epithelial cell change typical of MCD. *It is this epithelial damage that is the hallmark of FSG.* The hyalinosis and sclerosis represent entrapment of plasma proteins in extremely hyperpermeable foci and mesangial cell reaction to such proteins and to fibrin deposits. The recurrence of proteinuria in patients with focal sclerosis who receive renal allografts, sometimes within 24 hours of transplantation, suggests a systemic factor such as a circulating toxin as the cause of the epithelial damage.

As was noted, *secondary FSG* can occur as a complication of other nonglomerular renal diseases causing reduction in functioning renal tissue, particularly reflux nephropathy (p. 1055) and unilateral agenesis (p. 1018). These may lead to progressive glomerulosclerosis and renal failure. The pathogenesis of FSG in this setting may be related to the adaptive glomerular hypertrophy and capillary hypertention occurring in remnant functioning nephrons of these kidneys, as detailed earlier (p. 1029). In the FSG associated with AIDS, recent studies have identified HIV I protein in visceral epithelial cells, pointing again to possible epithelial cell injury in the development of the lesions.[70]

CLINICAL COURSE. As mentioned earlier, there is little tendency for spontaneous remission in idiopathic FSG, and responses to corticosteroid therapy are infrequent. In general, children have a better prognosis than adults. Progression of renal failure occurs at variable rates. About 20% of patients follow an unusually rapid course *(malignant focal sclerosis)*, with intractable massive proteinuria ending in renal failure within two years. FSG is particularly malignant in patients with AIDS.[67] Recurrences are seen in 25 to 50% of patients receiving allografts.

MEMBRANOPROLIFERATIVE GLOMERULONEPHRITIS (MPGN)

As the term implies, this group of disorders is characterized histologically by *alterations in the basement membrane and proliferation of glomerular cells.*[71] Because the proliferation is predominantly in the mesangium, a frequently used synonym is *mesangiocapillary GN.* MPGN accounts for 5 to 10% of cases of idiopathic NS in children and adults. Some patients present only with hematuria or proteinuria in the non-nephrotic range, and others have a combined nephrotic-nephritic picture. Although the histologic appearance of MPGN probably underlies a heterogeneous group of causes, two types are recognized on the basis of distinct ultrastructural, immunofluorescent, and probably pathogenic findings: type I and type II MPGN.[72]

MORPHOLOGY. By light microscopy, both types are similar. The glomeruli are large and hypercellular. The hypercellularity is produced largely by proliferation of mesangial cells, although infiltrating leukocytes and parietal epithelial crescents are present in many cases. The glomeruli have a "lobular" appearance, accentuated by the proliferating mesangial cells (Fig. 21–20). The GBM is clearly thickened, often focally, most evident in the peripheral capillary loops. The glomerular capillary wall often shows a "double-contour" or "tram-track" appearance, especially evident in silver or PAS stains (Fig. 21–21). This is caused by "splitting" of the basement membrane because of the inclusion within it of processes of mesangial cells extending into the peripheral capillary loops, so-called **mesangial interposition.**

Types I and II have altogether different ultrastructural and immunofluorescent features (Fig. 21–22 A–D).

Type I MPGN (two thirds of cases) is characterized by the presence of **subendothelial electron-dense deposits.** Mesangial and occasional subepithelial deposits may also be present (Fig. 21–22). By immunofluorescence, C3 is deposited in a granular pattern, and IgG and early complement components (C1q and C4) are often also present, suggesting an immune complex pathogenesis.

In type II lesions, the lamina densa of the GBM is trans-

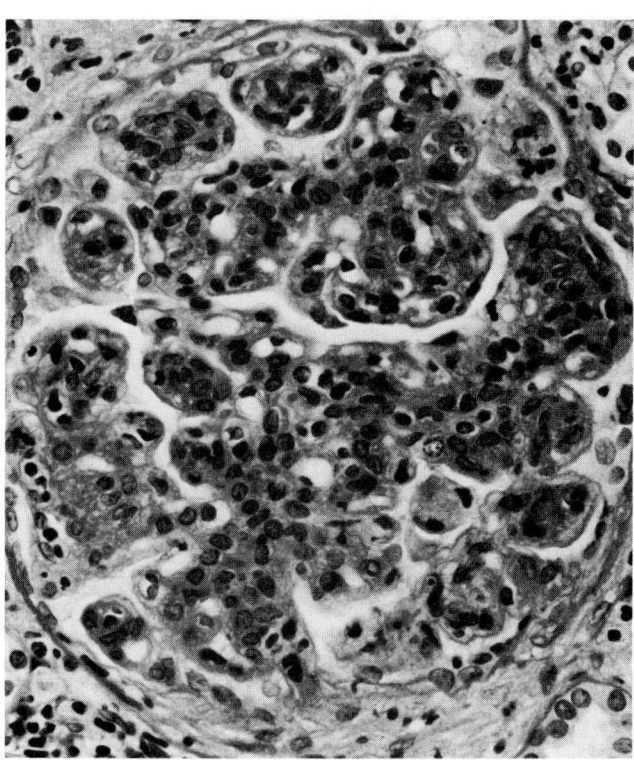

Figure 21-20. Membranoproliferative GN, showing mesangial cell proliferation, basement membrane thickening, leukocyte infiltration, and accentuation of lobular architecture.

formed into an irregular, ribbon-like, extremely electron-dense structure, due to the **deposition of dense material** of unknown composition in the GBM proper, giving rise to the term **dense-deposit disease.** In type II, C3 is present in irregular granular-linear foci in the basement membranes on either side, but not within the dense deposits. C3 is also present in the mesangium in characteristic circular aggregates (mesangial rings). **IgG is usually absent**, as are the early-acting complement components (C1q and C4).

A rare variant (type III) is segregated because it exhibits both subendothelial and subepithelial deposits, associated with GBM disruption and reduplication. **Its clinical features are similar to those of type I.**

PATHOGENESIS. *Although there are exceptions, most cases of type I MPGN present evidence of immune complexes in the glomerulus and activation of both classic and alternate complement pathways.*

Conversely, most patients with dense-deposit disease (type II) have abnormalities that suggest *activation of the alternate complement pathway.*[73] These patients have a *decreased serum C3*, but normal C1 and C4, the immune complex–activated early components of complement. They also have diminished serum levels of factor B and properdin, components of the alternate complement pathway. In the glomeruli C3 and properdin are deposited, but not IgG. Recall that, in the alternate complement pathway, C3 is directly cleaved to C3b (Fig. 21-23). The reaction depends on the initial interaction of C3 with such substances as bacterial polysaccharides, endotoxin, aggregates of IgA in the presence of factors B and D, and magnesium. This leads to the generation of C3bBb, the alternate pathway C3 convertase. The alternate C3 convertase is labile, being degraded by factors I and H, but it can be stabilized by properdin. Almost all patients with dense-deposit disease have in their serum a factor termed *C3 nephritic factor (C3NeF)*, which acts at the same step as properdin, helping to stabilize the alternate C3 convertase by binding to it (Fig. 21-23). *C3NeF is, in fact, an immunoglobulin of the IgG class, suggesting that it is an autoantibody to the alternate C3 convertase.* If this suggestion is correct, dense-deposit disease would be added to the category of *autoimmune diseases.* It is interesting that, in addition to increased consumption of C3, there is decreased C3 synthesis by the liver, further contributing to the profound hypocomplementemia. How these complement defects are translated into glomerular injury is unclear, but it has *not* been possible to induce glomerular damage in experimental animals by prolonged activation of the alternate complement pathway. However, the importance of the complement defects is underlined by the presence of C3NeF activity in some patients with a genetically determined disease, *partial lipodystrophy*, some of whom develop type II MPGN.

CLINICAL COURSE. Few remissions occur spontaneously in either type, and the disease follows a slowly progressive but unremitting course. Steroids may slow this progression considerably. Some patients develop numerous crescents and a clinical picture of rapidly progressive GN. About 50% develop chronic renal failure within ten years. There is a high inci-

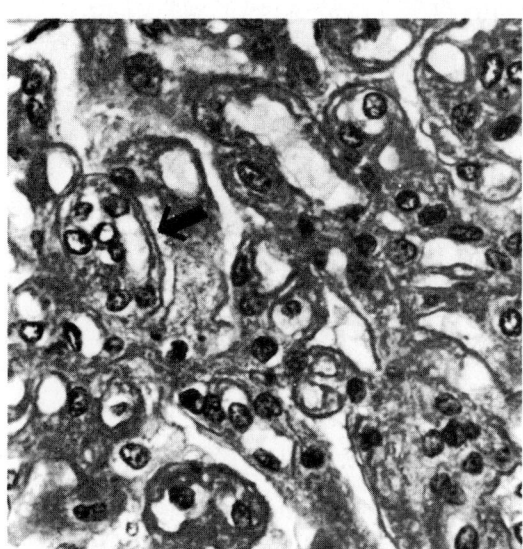

Figure 21-21. Detail of glomerular basement membrane (GBM) in membranoproliferative glomerulonephritis (PAS stained). Note splitting of GBM, giving characteristic "double-contour" or "tram-track" pattern (arrow).

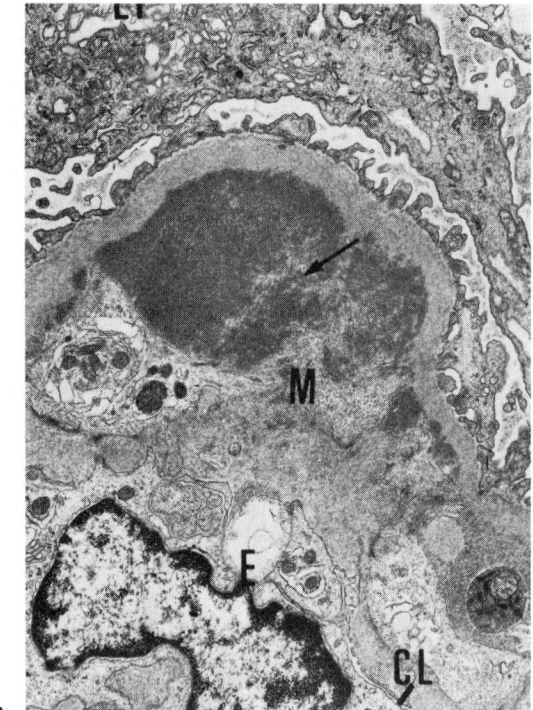
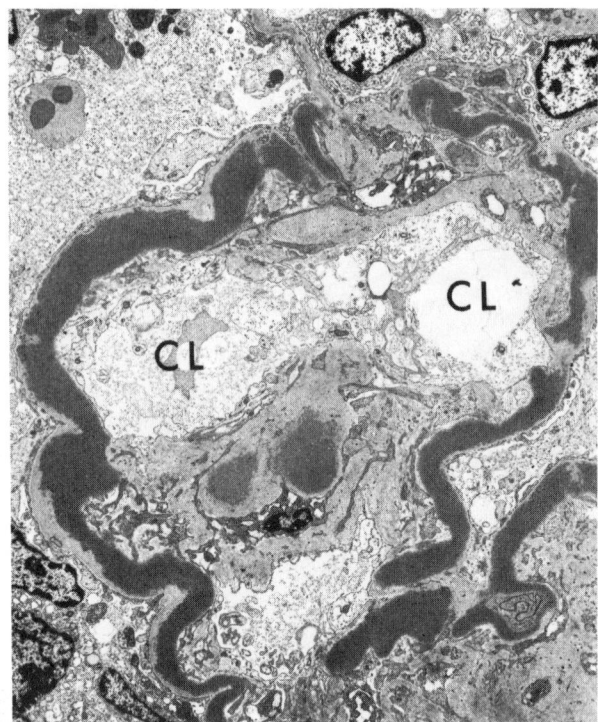

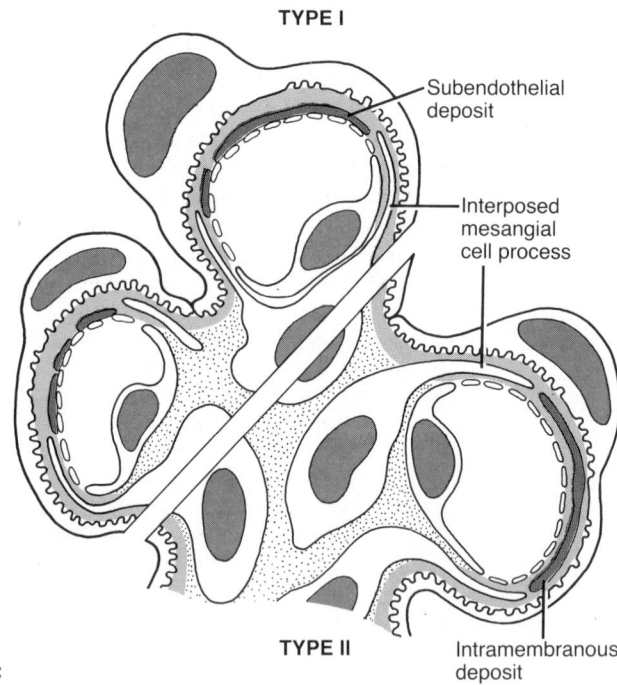

Figure 21–22. *A,* Membranoproliferative glomerulonephritis, type I. Note large subendothelial deposit
(arrow) incorporated into mesangial matrix (M)
through process of "mesangialization" (see text).
E = endothelium; EP = epithelium; CL = capillary
lumen. *B,* Type II MPGN, dense-deposit disease.
There are markedly dense homogeneous deposits
within basement membrane proper. CL = capillary
lumen. *C,* Schematic representation of patterns in the
two types of membranoproliferative glomerulonephritis, as seen by electron microscopy. In type I,
there are *subendothelial deposits;* type II is characterized by *intramembranous dense deposits* (dense
deposit disease). In both, mesangial interposition
gives the appearance of split basement membranes
when viewed with the light microscope.

dence of recurrence in transplant recipients, particularly in type II disease.

Histologic alterations very similar to MPGN
(mostly type I) occur in association with SLE,
hepatitis B antigenemia, infected ventriculoatrial
shunts, schistosomiasis, alpha₁-antitrypsin deficiency, chronic liver diseases, and certain malignancies.

IgA NEPHROPATHY (BERGER'S DISEASE)

*This form of glomerulonephritis is characterized by the
presence of prominent IgA deposits in the mesangial
regions detected by immunofluorescence microscopy.*[75] The disease can be suspected by light microscopic examination, but diagnosis is made only by im-

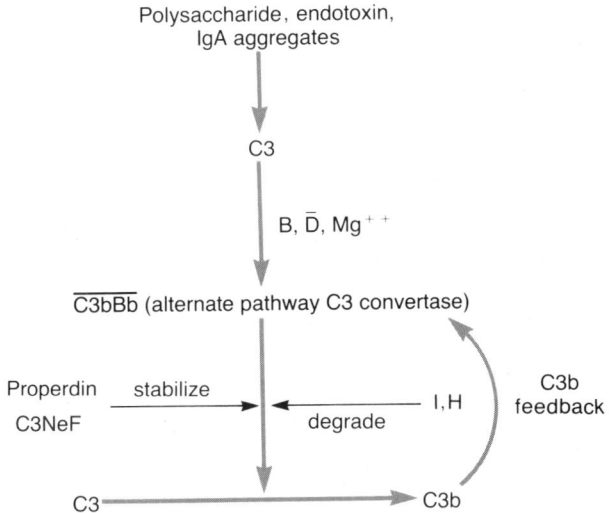

Polysaccharide, endotoxin,
IgA aggregates

$\downarrow$

C3

$\downarrow$ B, $\overline{\text{D}}$, Mg^{++}

$\overline{\text{C3bBb}}$ (alternate pathway C3 convertase)

Properdin
C3NeF — stabilize → ← degrade — I,H   C3b feedback

C3 ——————→ C3b

Figure 21–23. The alternate complement pathway. Note that C3NeF, present in the serum of patients with MPGN, acts at the same step as properdin, serving to stabilize the alternate pathway C3 convertase, thus enhancing C3 breakdown and causing hypocomplementemia.

munocytochemical techniques (Fig. 21–24). *IgA nephropathy is a very frequent cause of recurrent gross or microscopic hematuria,* and one of the most common types of glomerulonephritis. Mild proteinuria is usually present, and occasionally the nephrotic syndrome may develop.[75] Rarely a patient may present with rapidly progressive crescentic GN.

MORPHOLOGY. Histologically, the lesions vary considerably. The glomeruli may be normal or may show mesangial widening and segmental proliferation confined to some glomeruli (focal GN), diffuse mesangial proliferation (mesangioproliferative), or, rarely, overt crescentic GN. Focal segmental glomerulosclerosis can also be seen, particularly in patients with heavy proteinuria. The characteristic immunofluorescent picture is of **mesangial deposition**

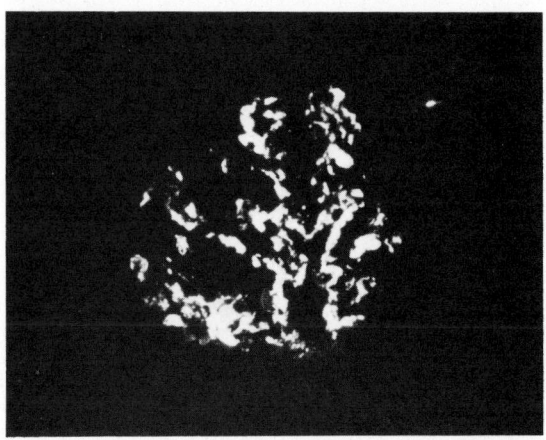

Figure 21–24. IgA nephropathy. Characteristic immunofluorescence deposition of IgA, principally in mesangial regions.

of IgA (Fig. 21–24), often with C3 and properdin and lesser amounts of IgG or IgM. Early complement components are usually absent. Electron microscopy confirms the presence of electron-dense deposits in the mesangium in the vast majority of cases. In some biopsies, prominent hyaline thickening of arterioles is present, a feature associated with a greater likelihood of progression to chronic renal failure.

PATHOGENESIS. The exclusive mesangial deposition of IgA suggests entrapment of large circulating aggregates or complexes in the mesangium, and the absence of C1q and C4 in glomeruli points to activation of the alternate complement pathway. You will recall that aggregated IgA is a known activator of the alternate pathway. Circulating IgA immune complexes are present in patients with IgA nephropathy and correlate with episodes of clinical activity. Up to 50% of patients have elevated IgA serum levels. A genetic influence is suggested by the occasional occurrence in families and in HLA identical brothers, and the increased frequency of certain HLA (e.g., HLA B35 and D4) and complement phenotypes in some populations.[75a] There is also evidence of defective phagocytic function of the mononuclear phagocyte system in such patients. Taken together, these clues suggest a genetic or acquired abnormality leading to increased mucosal IgA synthesis in response to respiratory or gastrointestinal exposure to environmental agents (such as viruses, bacteria, or food proteins). Circulating IgA aggregates or complexes are then entrapped in the mesangium, where they activate the alternate complement pathway.[75,76] In support of this scenario, IgA nephropathy occurs with increased frequency in patients with celiac disease (p. 876) and dermatitis herpetiformis (p. 1305), in whom intestinal mucosal defects are well defined.

CLINICAL COURSE. The disease affects children and young adults and may occur within a day or two of mucosal infections of the respiratory, gastrointestinal, or urinary tract. Typically the hematuria lasts for several days and then subsides, only to return every few months. IgA nephropathy is clinically a heterogeneous disease. Although most patients have an initially benign course, the disease appears to be slowly progressive: it is estimated that chronic renal failure develops in up to 50% of cases over a period of 20 years. Onset in old age, heavy proteinuria, hypertension, and the presence of vascular sclerosis or crescents on biopsy are clues to an increased risk of progression. Recurrence of IgA deposits in transplanted kidneys occurs in 50% of cases, but with seemingly limited clinical consequence in most of these.

FOCAL PROLIFERATIVE GLOMERULONEPHRITIS

Focal glomerulonephritis represents a histologic entity in which glomerular proliferation is restricted to seg-

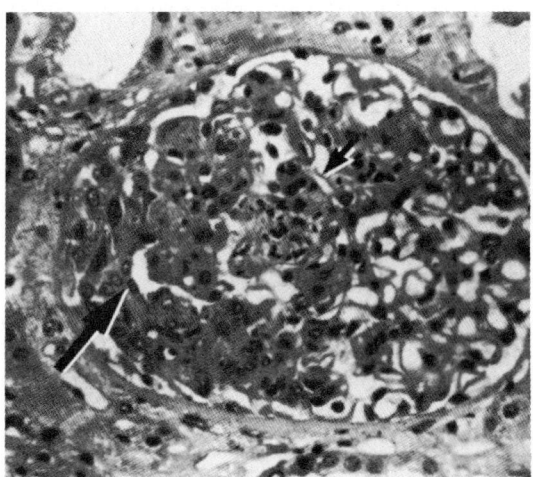

Figure 21–25. Focal glomerulonephritis in lupus erythematosus. There is segmental proliferation *(long arrow)* and necrosis *(small short arrow).* In the necrotic area there are neutrophils and fragmented nuclei (nuclear dust). The remainder of the glomerulus is not involved.

ments of individual glomeruli and commonly involves only a certain proportion of glomeruli. The lesions are predominantly proliferative and should be differentiated from those of focal sclerosis. Focal necrosis and fibrin deposition within the lesions may occur (Fig. 21–25).

Focal GN occurs under two circumstances:

1. It may be an early or mild manifestation of a systemic disease that sometimes involves entire glomeruli; among these are systemic lupus erythematosus, polyarteritis nodosa, Henoch-Schönlein purpura, Goodpasture's syndrome, subacute bacterial endocarditis, Wegener's granulomatosis, and **IgA** nephropathy.
2. It can occur unrelated to any systemic disease and constitutes a form of primary focal GN. The clinical manifestations may be subclinical, characterized by recurrent microscopic or gross hematuria or nonnephrotic proteinuria, but occasional cases present with a nephrotic syndrome.

CHRONIC GLOMERULONEPHRITIS

Chronic glomerulonephritis is best considered an end-stage pool of glomerular disease fed by a number of streams of glomerulonephritis, most of which have been described earlier in this chapter (Fig. 21–26). Poststreptococcal GN is a rare antecedent of chronic GN, except in adults. Patients with rapidly progressive GN, if they survive the acute episode, usually progress to chronic GN. Membranous glomerulonephritis, membranoproliferative glomerulonephritis, and IgA nephropathy progress more slowly to chronic renal failure, whereas focal sclerosis often advances rather rapidly into chronic GN. *Nevertheless, in any series of patients with chronic GN, about 20% of cases arise mysteriously with no antecedent history of any of the well-recognized forms of early GN.* These cases must represent the end result of relatively asymptomatic forms of GN, either known or still unrecognized, that progress to uremia.

MORPHOLOGY. The kidneys are symmetrically contracted and have diffusely granular, cortical surfaces. Each generally weighs in the range of 100 gm. On section, the cortex is thinned and there is increase in peripelvic fat. The glomerular histology depends on the stage of the disease. In early cases, the glomeruli may still show evidence of the primary disease (e.g., membranous or membranoproliferative GN). However, there eventually ensues hyaline obliteration of glomeruli, transforming them into acellular eosinophilic PAS-positive masses (Fig. 21–27). The hyaline represents a combination of trapped plasma proteins, increased mesangial matrix, basement membrane–like material, and collagen. Because hypertension is an accompaniment of chronic GN, arterial and arteriolar sclerosis may be conspicuous. Marked atrophy of associated tubules,

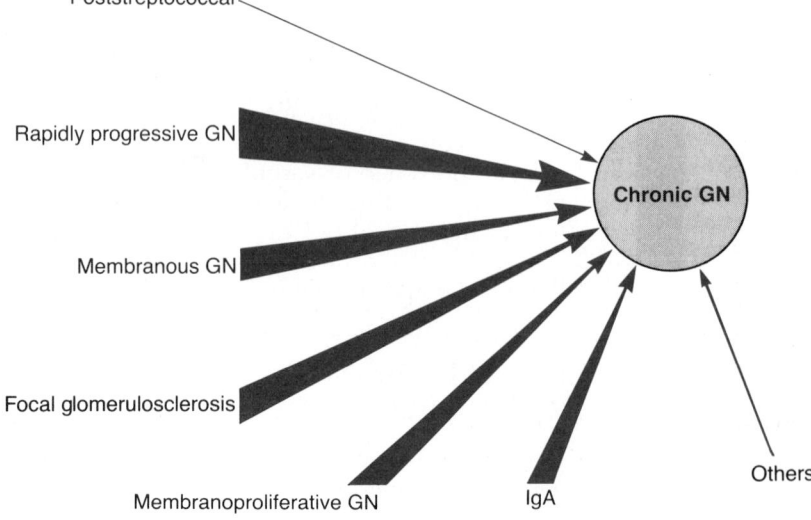

Figure 21–26. Primary glomerular diseases leading to chronic glomerulonephritis. The thickness of the arrows reflects the approximate proportion of patients in each group progressing to chronic GN. Poststreptococcal (1 to 2%); rapidly progressive (crescentic) (90%); membranous (50%); focal glomerulosclerosis (50 to 80%); MPGN (50%); IgA nephropathy (30 to 50%).

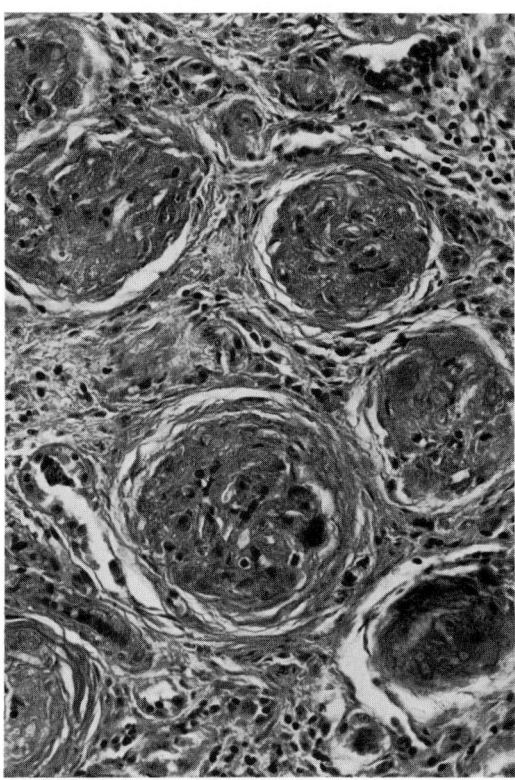

Figure 21–27. Chronic glomerulonephritis. Glomeruli are totally replaced by hyaline connective tissue.

irregular interstitial fibrosis, and lymphocytic infiltration also occur.

Kidneys from patients with end-stage disease on long-term dialysis exhibit a variety of so-called "dialysis changes" that are unrelated to the primary disease. These include arterial intimal thickening caused by accumulation of smooth muscle–like cells and a loose, proteoglycan-rich stroma; calcification, most obvious in glomerular tufts and tubular basement membranes; extensive deposition of calcium oxalate crystals in tubules and interstitium; acquired cystic disease (p. 1022); and increased numbers of renal adenomas and borderline adenocarcinomas.

Patients dying with GN also exhibit pathologic changes **outside** the kidney that are related to the uremic state and are also present in other forms of chronic renal failure (p. 1016). Often clinically important, these include **uremic pericarditis, uremic gastroenteritis, secondary hyperparathyroidism with nephrocalcinosis and renal osteodystrophy, left ventricular hypertrophy due to hypertension, and pulmonary changes of diffuse alveolar damage often ascribed to uremia (uremic pneumonitis).**

CLINICAL COURSE. In most patients, chronic GN develops insidiously and slowly progresses to death in uremia over a span of years or possibly decades (see discussion of chronic renal failure, p. 1016). Not infrequently, patients present with such nonspecific complaints as loss of appetite, anemia, vomiting, or weakness. In some, the renal disease is suspected with the discovery of proteinuria, hypertension, or azotemia on routine medical examination. In others, the underlying renal disorder is discovered in the course of investigation of edema. *Most patients are hypertensive, and sometimes the dominant clinical manifestations are cerebral or cardiovascular.* In all, the disease is relentlessly progressive, although at widely varying rates. In nephrotic patients, as glomeruli become obliterated, the protein loss in the urine diminishes. If patients with chronic GN are not maintained on continued dialysis or if they do not receive a renal transplant, the outcome is invariably death.

Table 21–7 summarizes the main clinical and histologic features of the major forms of primary GN.

GLOMERULAR LESIONS ASSOCIATED WITH SYSTEMIC DISEASE

Many immunologically mediated, metabolic, or hereditary systemic disorders are associated with glomerular injury, and in some (e.g., SLE and diabetes mellitus) the glomerular involvement is a major clinical manifestation. Most of these diseases have been discussed elsewhere in this book. Here we shall briefly recall some of the lesions and discuss only those not considered in other sections.

Systemic Lupus Erythematosus

The various types of lupus nephritis are described and illustrated in detail on page 198. As discussed, SLE gives rise to a heterogeneous group of lesions and clinical presentations.[77] The clinical manifestations include recurrent microscopic or gross hematuria, acute nephritis, the nephrotic syndrome, chronic renal failure, and hypertension. Histologically, glomerular changes are classified into mesangial lupus nephritis, focal GN, diffuse proliferative GN, and diffuse membranous GN.

Henoch-Schönlein Purpura

This syndrome consists of *purpuric skin lesions characteristically involving the extensor surfaces of arms and legs as well as buttocks; abdominal manifestations including pain, vomiting, and intestinal bleeding; non-migratory arthralgia; and renal abnormalities.* Not all components of the syndrome need be present and individual patients may have purpura, abdominal pain, or urinary abnormalities as the dominant feature. The disease is most common in children 3 to 8 years old, but it also occurs in adults, in whom the renal manifestations are usually more severe. There is a strong background of atopy in about one third of patients. The onset often follows an upper respiratory infection. Renal manifestations occur in one third of patients and include gross or microscopic hematuria, proteinuria, and nephrotic syndrome. A small number of patients, mostly adults, develop a rapidly progressive form of GN with many crescents.

Histologically, the renal lesions vary, according to the severity of the disease, from mild focal mesangial proliferation to diffuse mesangial proliferation to

Table 21–7. Summary of Major Primary Glomerulonephritides

DISEASE	MOST FREQUENT CLINICAL PRESENTATION	PATHOGENESIS	PATHOLOGY		
			Light Microscopy	*Fluorescence Microscopy*	*Electron Microscopy*
Poststreptococcal glomerulonephritis	Acute nephritis	Antibody-mediated; circulating or planted antigen	Diffuse proliferation; leukocytic infiltration	Granular IgG and C3 in GBM and mesangium	Subepithelial humps
Goodpasture's syndrome	Rapidly progressive GN	Anti-GBM	Proliferation; crescents	Linear IgG and C3; fibrin in crescents	No deposits; GBM disruptions; fibrin
Idiopathic RPGN	Rapidly progressive GN	Mixed (see text)	Proliferation; focal necrosis; crescents	25% linear IgG and C3 25–50% granular 25–50% negative or equivocal	No deposits Deposits may be present No deposits
Membranous glomerulonephritis	Nephrotic syndrome	Antibody-mediated; ?in situ	Diffuse capillary wall thickening	Granular IgG and C3; diffuse	Subepithelial deposits
Lipoid nephrosis	Nephrotic syndrome	Unknown, loss of glomerular polyanion	Normal; lipid in tubules	Negative	Loss of foot processes; no deposits
Focal segmental glomerulosclerosis	Nephrotic syndrome; non-nephrotic proteinuria	Unknown	Focal and segmental sclerosis and hyalinosis	Focal; IgM and C3	Loss of foot processes; epithelial denudation
Membrano-proliferative glomerulo-nephritis Type I Type II	Nephrotic syndrome Hematuria Chronic renal failure	(I) Immune complex (II)Autoantibody; alternate complement pathway activation	Mesangial proliferation; basement membrane thickening; splitting	(I) IgG + C3; C1 + C4 (II) C3 ± IgG; no C1 or C4	(I) Subendothelial deposits; (II) Dense-deposit disease
IgA nephropathy	Recurrent hematuria and/or proteinuria	Unknown; see text	Focal proliferative GN; mesangial widening	IgA + IgG, M, and C3 in mesangium	Mesangial and paramesangial dense deposits
Chronic glomerulonephritis	Chronic renal failure	Variable	Hyalinized glomeruli	Granular or negative	—

relatively typical crescentic GN. Whatever the histologic lesions, the prominent feature by fluorescence microscopy is the *deposition of IgA, sometimes with IgG and C3 in the mesangial region* in a distribution similar to that described for IgA nephropathy.[78] This has led to the belief that Berger's disease and Henoch-Schönlein purpura are perhaps spectra of the same disease. The skin lesions consist of subepidermal hemorrhages and a necrotizing vasculitis involving the small vessels of the dermis. IgA is also present in such vessels. Vasculitis can also occur in other organs such as the gastrointestinal tract, but is rare in the kidney.

The course of the disease is quite variable, but recurrences of hematuria may persist for many years after onset. Patients with the more diffuse lesions or with the nephrotic syndrome have a somewhat poorer prognosis, and renal failure occurs in those with the crescentic lesions.

Bacterial Endocarditis

Glomerular lesions occurring in the course of subacute bacterial endocarditis have long been known

and were termed "focal embolic GN." It is now clear, however, that these lesions are not embolic in nature and simply represent a type of immune complex nephritis initiated by bacterial antigen-antibody complex. Clinically, hematuria and proteinuria of various degrees characterize this entity, but an acute nephritic presentation is not uncommon, and even rapidly progressive GN may occur in rare instances. It must be apparent by now that the histologic lesions, when present, generally reflect these clinical manifestations. Milder forms have a focal and segmental necrotizing GN, whereas more severe ones exhibit a diffuse proliferative GN, and the rapidly progressive forms show large numbers of crescents. GN in acute endocarditis is rare, except in some patients with coagulase-positive *Staphylococcus aureus* endocarditis in whom a diffuse proliferative GN occurs (p. 1031).

Diabetic Glomerulosclerosis

Diabetes mellitus is a major cause of renal morbidity and mortality. End-stage kidney disease occurs in up to 30% of juvenile diabetics and accounts for 20% of deaths in patients under age 40. By far the most common lesions involve the glomeruli and are associated clinically with three glomerular syndromes, including non-nephrotic proteinuria, nephrotic syndrome, and chronic renal failure. However, diabetes also affects the arterioles, causing *arteriolar sclerosis;* increases susceptibility to the development of pyelonephritis, and particularly *papillary necrosis;* and causes a variety of tubular lesions. The term *diabetic nephropathy* is applied to the conglomerate of lesions that often occur concurrently in the diabetic kidney.

Proteinuria, sometimes in the nephrotic range, occurs in about 55% of juvenile- and 30% of adult-onset diabetics. It is usually discovered 12 to 22 years after the clinical appearance of diabetes, and (particularly in juvenile diabetics) often heralds the progressive development of chronic renal failure ending in death or end-stage disease within a period of four to five years. The morphologic changes in the glomeruli include (1) capillary basement membrane thickening, (2) diffuse diabetic glomerulosclerosis, and (3) nodular glomerulosclerosis.[79]

MORPHOLOGY

CAPILLARY BASEMENT MEMBRANE THICKENING. Widespread thickening of the glomerular capillary basement membrane (GBM) occurs in virtually all diabetics, irrespective of the presence of proteinuria, and is part and parcel of the diabetic microangiopathy described earlier (p. 1003). Pure capillary basement membrane thickening can be detected only by electron microscopy. Careful morphometric studies demonstrate that this thickening begins as early as two years after the onset of juvenile diabetes, and by five years amounts to about a 30% increase.[80] The thickening continues progressively, and usually concurrently with mesangial widening (Fig. 21–28). Simultaneously there is thickening of the tubular basement membranes.

DIFFUSE GLOMERULOSCLEROSIS. This consists of diffuse increase in mesangial matrix with mild proliferation of mesangial cells, and is always associated with the overall thickening of the GBM. The increase in mesangial volume appears to lag slightly behind basement membrane widening but becomes pronounced after ten to 20 years of diabetes. The matrix depositions are PAS positive. The changes almost always begin in the vascular stalk and sometimes seem continuous with the invariably present hyaline thickening of arterioles (Fig. 21–29). As the disease progresses, the mesangial areas expand further and obliterate the mesangial cells, gradually filling the entire glomerulus **(obliterative diabetic glomerulosclerosis).**

NODULAR GLOMERULOSCLEROSIS. This is also known as **intercapillary glomerulosclerosis or Kimmelstiel-Wilson disease.** The glomerular lesions take the form of ovoid or spherical, often laminated, hyaline masses situated in the periphery of the glomerulus. They lie within the mesangial core of the glomerular lobules and often are surrounded by peripheral patent capillary loops (Fig. 21–30). Usually, not all the lobules in the individual glomerulus are involved. **Uninvolved lobules and glomeruli all show striking diffuse glomerulosclerosis.** The nodules are PAS positive and contain lipids and fibrin. Often they contain trapped mesangial cells. As the disease advances, the individual nodules enlarge and eventually compress and engulf capillaries, obliterating the glomerular tuft (Fig. 21–28). As a consequence of the glomerular and arteriolar lesions, the kidney suffers from ischemia, develops tubular atrophy and interstitial fibrosis, and undergoes overall contraction in size.

Most workers believe that nodular glomerulosclerosis and the diffuse lesion are fundamentally similar lesions of the mesangium. The nodular lesion, however, is virtually pathognomonic of diabetes, so long as care is taken to exclude membranoproliferative (lobular) GN, the GN asso-

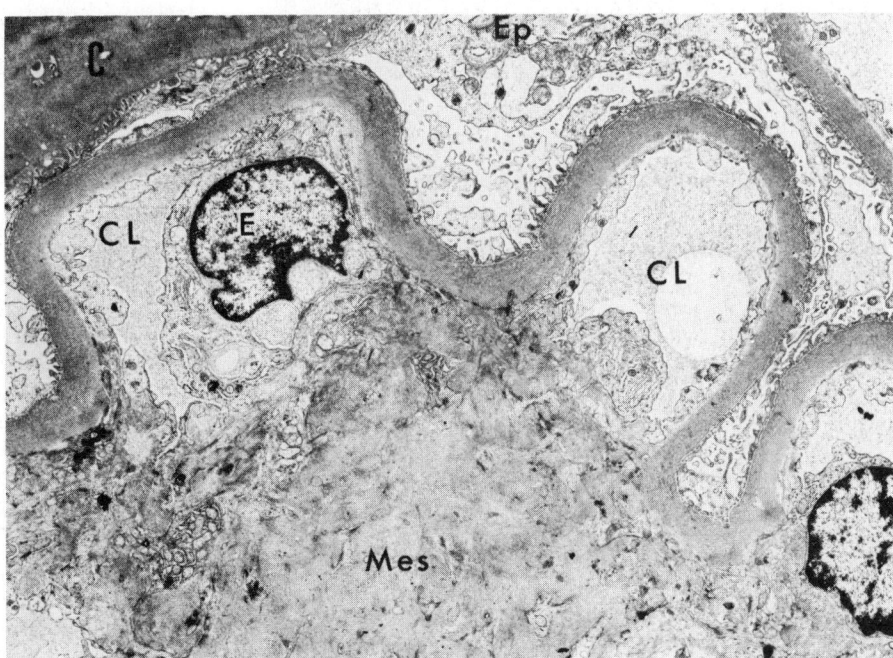

Figure 21–28. Electron micrograph of advanced diabetic glomerulosclerosis. Note massive increase in mesangial matrix (Mes) encroaching on glomerular capillary lumina (CL). GBM and Bowman's capsule (C) are markedly thickened. Ep = epithelium; E = endothelium.

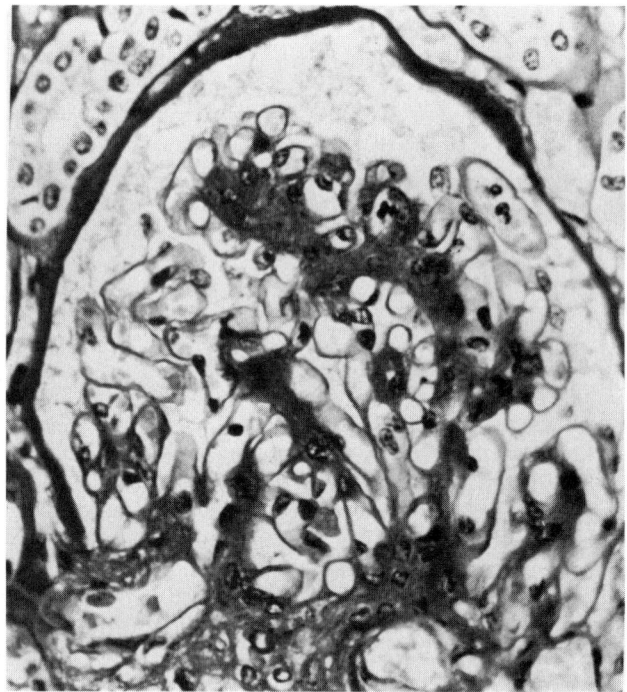

Figure 21–29. Diffuse diabetic glomerulosclerosis with diffuse mesangial thickening.

ciated with light-chain disease (p. 1047), and amyloidosis. Approximately 15 to 30% of long-term patients with diabetes develop nodular glomerulosclerosis, and in most instances it is associated with renal failure. It is rarely encountered in those who have had diabetes for less than ten years, except perhaps in a few juvenile diabetics with rapidly advancing disease.[79]

MINOR LESIONS. The **fibrin cap** appears as a homogeneous, brightly eosinophilic, crescentic subendothelial deposit in a peripheral capillary of a lobule and is also encountered in the nondiabetic person. The **capsular drop** is an eosinophilic, focal thickening of the parietal layer of Bowman's capsule, which apparently hangs into the uriniferous space. The capsular drop is PAS positive and contains plasma proteins. Both constitute plasma protein deposits that have escaped from the capillary lumen owing to capillary wall injury.

PATHOGENESIS. The pathogenesis of diabetic glomerulosclerosis is intimately linked with that of the generalized diabetic microangiopathy, discussed on page 1003. The principal points to remember are as follows:

1. The bulk of the evidence suggests that diabetic glomerulosclerosis is not a separate genetic defect in diabetics but *is caused by the metabolic defect*, i.e., the insulin deficiency, or the resultant hyperglycemia, or some other aspects of glucose intolerance.
2. Biochemical alterations in diabetic GBM have been described, including increased amount and synthesis of collagen type IV and fibronectin, and de-

creased synthesis of proteoglycan heparan sulfate.[81] Some of these alterations—for example, the increased collagen type IV and fibronectin—can be directly induced in cultured endothelial cells by high glucose concentrations.[82]

3. *Nonenzymatic glycosylation* of proteins, known to occur in diabetics and exemplified by hemoglobin A1c, may contribute to the glomerulopathy. For example, as detailed previously (p. 1000), advanced glycosylation end products in basement membrane collagen can interfere with its association with other extracellular components (i.e., proteoglycans) and thus with glomerular barrier function.

4. One recent hypothesis implicates *hemodynamic changes* in the initiation or modulation of diabetic glomerulosclerosis. It is well known that early-onset juvenile diabetics, particularly those with imperfectly controlled hyperglycemia, have an increased GFR, increased glomerular filtration area, and glomerular hypertrophy.[80] Hyperfiltration has been observed in experimental streptozotocin-induced diabetes in rats, where it is associated with proteinuria and can be reversed by diabetic control.[83] There is some experimental evidence that the contractile ability of mesangial cells is reduced by a hyperglycemic or insulin-deficient environment[84]; this could result in glomerular vasodilation, an increase in intraglomerular plasma flow and filtration pressure, and hyperfiltration. It has been speculated that the subsequent morphologic alterations in the mesangium are somehow influenced by the glomerular hypertrophy and hemodynamic changes, akin to the adaptive responses to reductions in renal mass (p. 1029).

CLINICAL COURSE. The clinical manifestations of diabetic glomerulosclerosis are linked to those of diabetes, as discussed on page 1005. Glomerular involvement is associated with proteinuria, which may be mild and asymptomatic initially but gradually increases to nephrotic levels in some patients. The increased GFR typical in early-onset diabetics is then

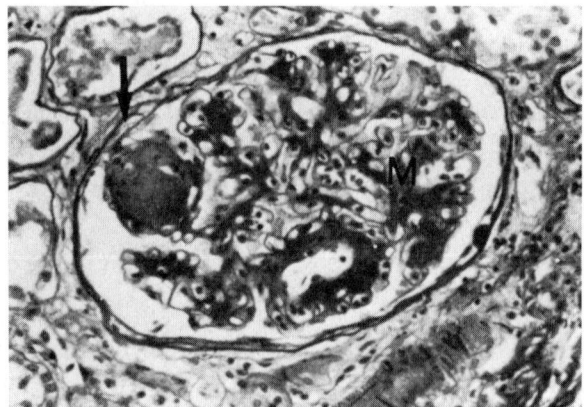

Figure 21–30. Diffuse and nodular diabetic glomerulosclerosis (PAS stain). Note diffuse increase in mesangial matrix (M) and characteristic acellular PAS-positive nodule *(arrow)*.

followed by progressive loss of GFR, leading to end-stage renal failure within a period of five years.

Diabetic glomerulosclerosis is more frequent, more severe, and more progressive in type I (insulin-dependent) diabetics. Systemic hypertension may precede the development of proteinuria and renal insufficiency. Indeed, recent evidence suggests that the risk of renal disease in type I diabetics is associated with a genetic predisposition to hypertension, and that hypertension increases the susceptibility to develop diabetic nephropathy in the presence of poor hyperglycemic control.[85] At present the vast majority of patients with end-stage diabetic nephropathy are maintained on long-term dialysis, and a few receive renal transplantation. Diabetic lesions may recur in the renal allografts, but whether these will eventually result in progressive loss of graft function is unknown. Whether precise control of the blood sugar in diabetes will prevent the glomerulopathy is still unsettled.

Amyloidosis

Disseminated amyloidosis, whether it conforms to the so-called primary or secondary pattern of distribution, may be associated with deposits of amyloid within the glomeruli (p. 210). The typical amyloid fibrils are present within the mesangium and subendothelium, and occasionally within the subepithelial space. Eventually, they obliterate the glomerulus completely. Recall that deposits of amyloid also appear in blood vessel walls and in the kidney interstitium. Amyloid can be detected on light microscopy by special stains, particularly by the characteristic birefringence after staining with Congo red. Patients with glomerular amyloid may present with heavy proteinuria or the nephrotic syndrome, and later, owing to destruction of glomeruli, die in uremia. Characteristically, kidney size tends to be either normal or slightly enlarged.

Other Systemic Disorders

Goodpasture's syndrome (p. 1031), *polyarteritis nodosa* (p. 571), and *Wegener's granulomatosis* (p. 574) are commonly associated with glomerular lesions and have been discussed earlier. Suffice it to say here that the glomerular lesions in these three conditions can be very similar. In the early or mild forms of involvement there is focal and segmental, sometimes necrotizing, GN and most of these patients will have hematuria with rather mild decline in GFR. In the more severe cases associated with rapidly progressive GN, there are also extensive necrosis, fibrin deposition, and the formation of epithelial crescents. It should be recalled, however, that these diseases have different pathogenetic mechanisms. Goodpasture's syndrome is mediated by anti-GBM antibodies and exhibits linear fluorescence of immunoglobulin and complement, whereas polyarteritis nodosa and Wegener's granulomatosis are of somewhat more obscure causation, although circulating immune complexes are frequently present in the former.

Essential mixed cryoglobulinemia is another rare systemic condition in which deposits of cryoglobulins composed principally of IgG-IgM complexes induce cutaneous vasculitis, synovitis, and focal or diffuse proliferative glomerulonephritis.

Plasma cell dyscrasias (p. 739) may also induce glomerular lesions. *Multiple myeloma* is associated with (1) amyloidosis, (2) deposition of monoclonal cryoglobulins in glomeruli, and (3) peculiar nodular lesions resembling those seen in nodular diabetic glomerulosclerosis and ascribed to the deposition of nonfibrillar light chains. This *light-chain nephropathy* also occurs in the absence of overt myeloma, usually associated with deposition of kappa chains in glomeruli.[86] The glomeruli show PAS-positive mesangial nodules, lobular accentuation, and mild mesangial hypercellularity and need to be differentiated from diabetic nodules and membranoproliferative GN. These patients usually present with proteinuria or the nephrotic syndrome, hypertension, and slowly progressive azotemia.

HEREDITARY NEPHRITIS

Hereditary nephritis refers to a group of hereditary-familial renal diseases associated primarily with glomerular injury.[87] The clinical, pathologic, and genetic features of the various types appear to be heterogeneous. The most well-studied entity is so-called *Alport's syndrome, the name usually given to the disease in which nephritis is accompanied by nerve deafness and various eye disorders, including lens dislocation, posterior cataracts, and corneal dystrophy.* Males tend to be affected more frequently and more severely than females and are more likely to progress to renal failure. Females, however, are not completely spared. The most common presenting sign is gross or microscopic hematuria, frequently accompanied by erythrocyte casts. Proteinuria may occur and, rarely, the nephrotic syndrome develops. Symptoms appear at ages 5 to 20 and the onset of overt renal failure is between ages 20 and 50 in males. The auditory defects may be subtle, requiring extensive testing. The mode of inheritance is heterogeneous, being either X-linked or autosomal dominant in most pedigrees.[87a] In the X-linked variety, the defective gene has been localized to the middle of the long arm of the X chromosome.[88]

Histologically, the glomeruli are always involved. The most common early lesion is segmental proliferation or sclerosis, or both. There is increase in mesangial matrix, and in some patients the persistence of fetal-like glomeruli. In some kidneys, glomerular or tubular epithelial cells acquire a foamy appearance due to accumulation of neutral fats and mucopolysaccharides (**foam cells**). As the disease progresses, there is increasing glomerulosclerosis, vascular narrowing, tubular atrophy, and interstitial fibrosis. With the electron microscope, characteristic basement membrane lesions are found in some (but not all) patients with

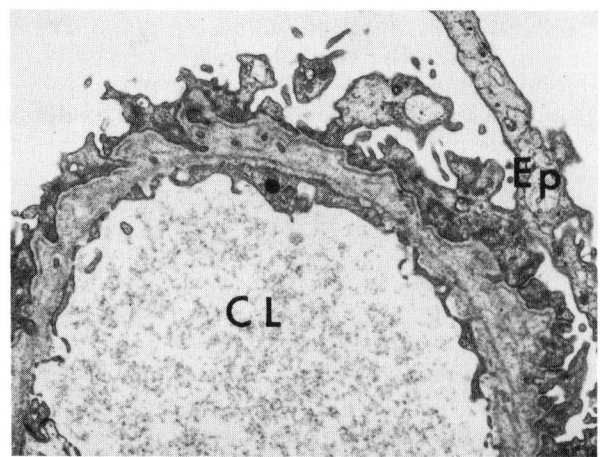

Figure 21–31. Hereditary nephritis. Electron micrograph of glomerulus with irregular thickening of basement membrane, lamination of lamina densa, and foci of rarefaction. Such changes may be present in other diseases but are most pronounced and widespread in hereditary nephritis. CL = capillary lumen; Ep = epithelium.

hereditary nephritis. The basement membrane shows irregular foci of thickening or attenuation, with pronounced splitting and lamination of the lamina densa (Fig. 21–31). Similar alterations are found in the tubular basement membranes. Although such basement membrane changes may be seen focally in diseases other than hereditary nephritis, they are most widespread and pronounced in patients with this disorder.

The nature of the basement membrane defect is not clear, but it is most likely the result of a disturbance in the synthesis of some GBM component. Indeed, glomeruli of some patients with familial nephritis lack the "Goodpasture's" antigen; i.e., they fail to react with anti-GBM antibodies derived from patients with Goodpasture's syndrome.[88a]

DISEASES OF TUBULES

Under this heading we will discuss *acute tubular necrosis* and a limited number of alterations that affect the proximal or distal tubular segments. In point of fact, most types of injury affecting the tubules also involve the interstitial tissue, and thus are discussed later under *tubulointerstitial diseases*.

ACUTE TUBULAR NECROSIS (ATN) AND ACUTE RENAL FAILURE

Acute tubular necrosis is a major cause of acute renal failure (ARF). The latter term refers to a syndrome associated with acute suppression of renal function, often accompanied by severe oliguria and, rarely, anuria. ARF can be caused by diverse clinical conditions that include the following:[89]

1. *Organic vascular obstruction.* ARF may be caused by diffuse involvement of the intrarenal vessels, such as in polyarteritis nodosa, malignant hypertension, and the hemolytic uremic syndrome. In rare instances, ARF may be due to bilateral occlusion of renal arteries by thromboemboli or by external compression.
2. *Severe glomerular disease,* such as rapidly progressive glomerulonephritis.
3. *Acute tubulointerstitial nephritis,* most commonly occurring as a hypersensitivity to drugs (p. 1057).
4. *Massive infection* (pyelonephritis), especially when accompanied by papillary necrosis (p. 1054).
5. *Disseminated intravascular renal coagulation* with cortical necrosis of the kidneys (p. 1070).
6. *Urinary obstruction* by tumors, prostatic hypertrophy, or blood clots (so-called postrenal acute renal failure).
7. *Acute tubular necrosis.*

Acute tubular necrosis (ATN) is the designation for all forms of acute renal failure associated with destruction of tubular epithelial cells. Two distinctive patterns were defined by Oliver and coworkers in their classic studies:[90] (1) *ischemic or tubulorrhectic ATN* occurs in cases that have in common a preceding hypotensive episode (shock), causing severe renal hypoperfusion and ischemia; (2) *nephrotoxic ATN* results from the ingestion, injection, or inhalation of some toxic agent that directly damages tubular cells. It must be emphasized at the outset that *morphologic evidence of tubular necrosis is present in both forms,*[91] but whereas it may be obvious in some types of nephrotoxic ATN, it is focal and often subtle in ischemic ATN. Clinical recognition of ATN is of particular importance because it represents a reversible disorder compatible with full recovery of normal renal function and morphology and of the patient.

Ischemic ATN appears most often after an episode of shock produced by severe bacterial infections; large cutaneous burns; massive crushing injuries; or any medical, surgical, or obstetric event complicated by peripheral circulatory collapse (thus the term "shock kidneys"). ATN is surprisingly uncommon when the shock is due to massive hemorrhage alone (e.g., following rupture of an aneurysm or laceration of a large artery).

A special form of ischemic ATN, so-called *pigment-induced ATN,* is associated with massive *hemoglobinuria* or *myoglobinuria.* The former occurs after conditions of massive hemolysis and the latter when there is severe skeletal muscle injury (rhabdomyolysis) and release of myoglobin into the circulation. Myoglobinuria is being recognized with increased frequency as a cause of acute renal failure not only after extensive traumatic injury, but also with nontraumatic rhabdomyolysis induced by strenuous exercise, heat stroke, drug coma (with resultant muscle compression), and alcohol abuse. Although these pigments may have some direct toxicity to tubules, the circumstances in which they induce ATN are almost always associated with dehydration and anoxia.

Ischemic ATN is characterized by focal tubular necrosis at multiple points along the nephron, with large skip areas in between, often accompanied by rupture of basement membranes (tubulorrhexis) and occlusion of tubular lumina by casts (Fig. 21–32). Nephron microdissection studies show that relatively small lengths of tubules are affected.[90] The straight portion of the proximal tubule and the ascending thick limb in the renal medulla are especially vulnerable, but focal necrotic lesions may also occur in the distal tubule, often in conjunction with casts. Although tubular necrosis may be difficult to see in regular histologic sections, careful light microscopic studies show focal necrosis of single cells or small clusters of cells in over 90% of cases.[91]

Eosinophilic hyaline casts, as well as pigmented granular casts, are extremely common, particularly in distal tubules and collecting ducts (Fig. 21–33). These casts consist principally of Tamm-Horsfall protein (a specific urinary glycoprotein normally secreted by the cells of ascending thick limb and distal tubules) in conjunction with hemoglobin, myoglobin, and other plasma proteins. Other common findings in ischemic ATN are interstitial edema and accumulations of leukocytes within dilated vasa recta. In the absence of overt tubular necrosis, these latter two findings should raise the suspicion of ischemic acute renal failure. In

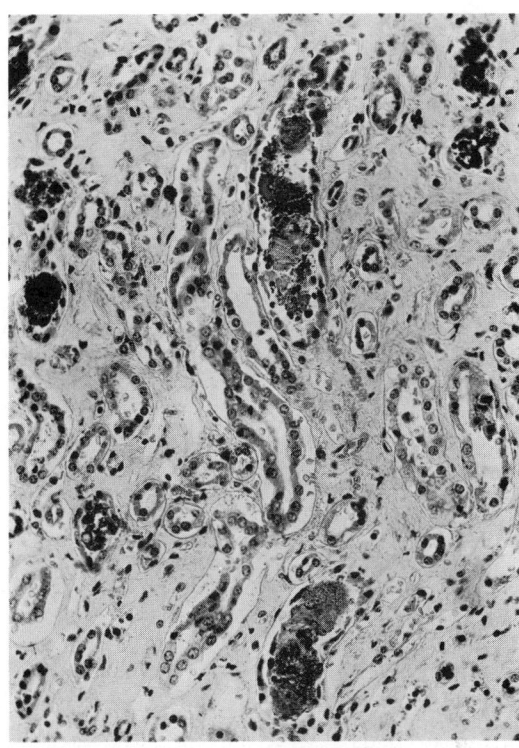

Figure 21–33. Ischemic ATN. Granular pigment casts are seen in collecting tubules. Some of the tubular epithelial cells in affected tubules are necrotic, whereas others are flattened, stretched out, and regenerating.

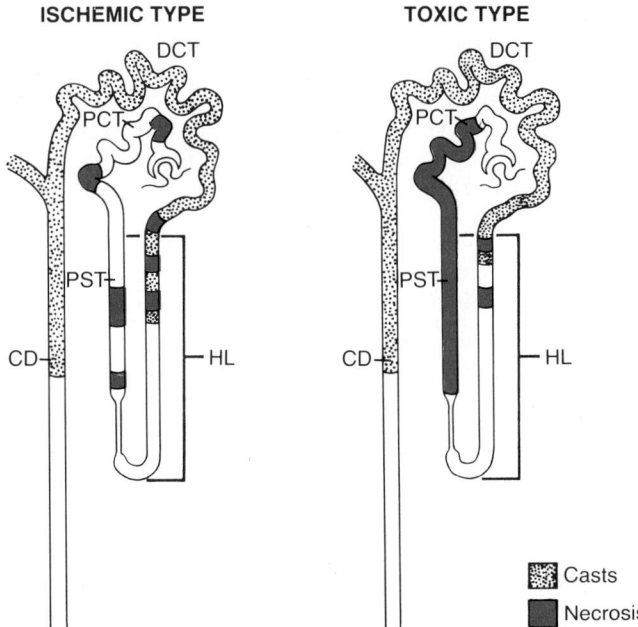

Figure 21–32. Patterns of tubular damage in ischemic and toxic ATN. In ischemic type, tubular necrosis is patchy, relatively short lengths of tubules are affected, and straight segments of proximal tubules (PST) and ascending limbs of Henle's loop (HL) are most vulnerable. In toxic ATN, extensive necrosis is present along proximal tubule segments (PCT) with many toxins (e.g., mercury), but necrosis of distal tubule, particularly ascending Henle's loop, also occurs. In both types, lumina of distal convoluted tubules (DCT) and collecting ducts (CD) contain casts.

patients who come to autopsy or who are biopsied after the first week of illness, there is often evidence of **epithelial regeneration:** flattened epithelial cells with hyperchromatic nuclei and mitotic figures are often present. In the course of time, this regeneration repopulates the tubules so that if survival occurs no residual evidence of damage can be seen. Glomeruli are remarkably normal, even by electron microscopy, although fibrin deposition and platelet thrombi have been reported in some cases.

Nephrotoxic ATN is caused by a wide variety of drugs and toxins, including antibiotics (gentamicin, cephalosporin), anesthetics (methoxyflurane), contrast media, chemotherapeutic agents (cyclosporine), heavy metals (mercury, lead, arsenic), organic solvents (carbon tetrachloride, methyl alcohol, ethylene glycol), and poisons (mushrooms, insecticides, herbicides).

Characteristic of toxic ATN is acute tubular injury, most obvious in the proximal convoluted tubules (Figs. 21–32 and 21–34). Histologically, the tubular necrosis may be entirely nonspecific but is somewhat distinctive in poisoning with certain agents. With mercuric chloride, for example, severely injured cells not yet dead may contain large acidophilic inclusions. Later, these cells become totally necrotic, are desquamated into the lumen, and may

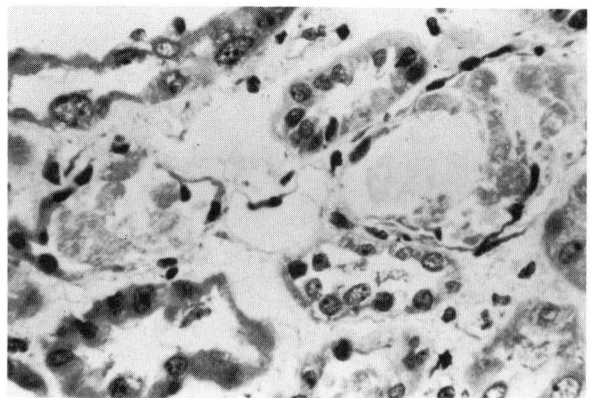

Figure 21–34. Toxic ATN. In center, two tubules show loss and desquamation of epithelial cells. (Courtesy of Dr. Kim Solez.)

undergo calcification. Carbon tetrachloride poisoning, in contrast, is characterized by the accumulation of neutral lipids in injured cells but, again, such fatty change is followed by necrosis. Ethylene glycol produces marked ballooning and hydropic or vacuolar degeneration of proximal convoluted tubules. Calcium oxalate crystals are often found in the tubular lumina in such poisoning. Because shock and ischemia are so frequently present in toxic ATN, focal necrosis of the distal nephron also occurs.

PATHOGENESIS. The sequence of events leading to acute renal failure and oliguria in ischemic or toxic renal failure has been the subject of extensive study and controversy.[89,91] Four principal mechanisms have been proposed: (1) failure of glomerular filtration due to decreased renal perfusion pressure or *persistent preglomerular vasoconstriction,* possibly related to the activity of the renin-angiotensin system; (2) destruction of the tubular integrity with leakage of tubular fluid into the interstitium *(tubular back leak or tubular back flow);* (3) *tubular obstruction* by either interstitial edema or intratubular casts; and (4) a *direct effect* on the permeability properties of the glomerular capillary wall.

Evidence has been marshaled from numerous experimental studies in favor of one or another of these hypotheses. A possible scheme incorporating some of these mechanisms is summarized in Figure 21–35. It is thought that both ischemia and nephrotoxins initially induce some type of tubular damage. Two segments of the tubules appear to be especially vulnerable to damage: *the proximal straight tubule and the medullary thick ascending limb,* the latter because of its high energy requirement and the relatively limited blood flow and oxygen supply to the renal medulla.[92] Tubular damage has at least three consequences, each of which contributes to the eventual development of oliguria.

1. Arteriolar vasoconstriction, which has been ascribed to various activation of vasoconstrictive agents (angiotensin II, thromboxane, catecholamines)

or loss of vasodilator effects (prostaglandin). How tubular damage triggers these events is unclear. Whatever the mechanism, vasoconstriction results in decreases in renal blood flow, glomerular filtration, tubular fluid flow, and oliguria.

2. The necrotic debris from tubular cells, together with proteinaceous material derived from either blood or tubular cells, results in cast formation. These casts increase proximal intratubular pressure and therefore further decrease GFR.

3. Back leak of tubular fluid into the interstitium, due to tubular damage, further decreases tubular fluid flow. The oliguria is thought to be the consequence of all these events.

4. Additionally, there is evidence that ischemia or toxins may directly affect glomerular ultrafiltration or vascular reactivity. For example, ischemia blunts the effects of several vasodilators, possibly by inhibiting the production of endothelium-derived relaxation factor (EDRF).[93] It could also stimulate release of endothelin, a potent vasoconstrictor.[93a]

Although some investigators argue for the primacy of one or the other of the cited mechanisms, it may be that a combination of all these effects in some individuals results in acute renal failure. One or the other may predominate according to the inciting cause of ATN.

CLINICAL COURSE. The nephrotoxic and ischemic forms of ATN are important causes of acute and reversible renal failure. Although the course may be variable, it can be divided into *initiating, maintenance,* and *recovery* stages.[94] *The initiating phase* is usually dominated by the inciting medical, surgical, or obstetric event or, in the case of toxins, by the extrarenal toxic manifestations of such chemicals. It represents the period of time between injury and the develop-

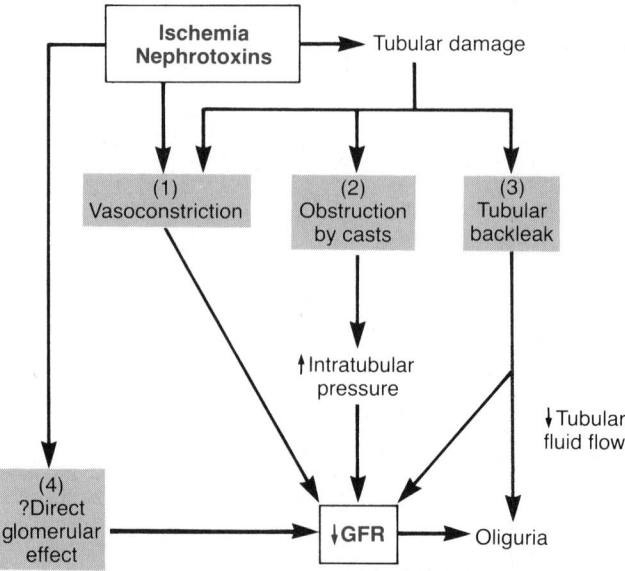

Figure 21–35. Possible pathogenetic mechanisms in acute renal failure. Sequence of events 1, 2, 3, and 4 are described in text.

ment of acute renal failure that cannot be reversed by treatment of the causes of injury or other extrarenal factors.

The maintenance stage is characterized by sustained decreases in urine output to between 40 and 400 ml per day (oliguria), with salt and water overload, rising blood urea nitrogens, hyperkalemia, metabolic acidosis, and other manifestations of uremia dominating this phase. With appropriate attention to balance of water and blood electrolytes, including dialysis, the patient can be carried over this oliguric crisis.

The recovery phase is heralded by a steady increase in urine volume that may reach up to 3 liters per day. The tubules are still damaged, so that large amounts of water, sodium, and potassium are lost in the urinary flood. *Hypokalemia, rather than hyperkalemia, becomes a clinical problem.* There is a peculiar increased vulnerability to infection at this stage. Eventually renal tubular function is restored, with improvement in concentrating ability. At the same time, BUN and creatinine levels begin to return to normal. Subtle tubular functional impairment may persist for months, but most patients who reach the recovery phase eventually recover completely.

The prognosis of ATN depends on the clinical setting surrounding its development. Ninety-five per cent recovery is expected with nephrotoxic ATN when the toxin has not caused serious damage to other organs, such as the liver or heart. Conversely, in shock related to overwhelming sepsis or extensive burns, the mortality rate may rise to 60 to 80%.

It should be noted that up to 50% of patients with ATN may not have oliguria, and may in fact have increased urine volumes. This so-called nonoliguric ATN occurs particularly often with nephrotoxins such as methoxyflurane, and generally it tends to follow a more benign clinical course.

TUBULOINTERSTITIAL DISEASES

This group of renal diseases is characterized by histologic and functional alterations that involve predominantly the tubules and interstitium.[95] Glomerular and vascular abnormalities may also be present but either are mild or occur only in advanced stages of these diseases. The point to emphasize is that *the tubulointerstitial diseases have diverse causes and different pathogenetic mechanisms* (Table 21–8). When the etiologic agent is evident, the disorder is identified by cause or by associated disease (e.g., analgesic nephritis, irradiation nephritis). However, in some cases, the etiologic agents are unknown and the term idiopathic tubulointerstitial nephritis (TIN) is used.

TIN can be acute or chronic. Acute TIN has an acute clinical onset and is characterized histologically by interstitial edema, often accompanied by leukocytic infiltration and focal tubular necrosis. In *chronic interstitial nephritis* (CIN) there is infiltration

Table 21–8. Tubulointerstitial Diseases

Infections
  Acute bacterial pyelonephritis
  Chronic pyelonephritis (including reflux nephropathy)
  Other infections (viruses, parasites, etc.)
Toxins
  Drugs
    Acute hypersensitivity interstitial nephritis
    Analgesic nephritis
  Heavy metals
    Lead, cadmium
Metabolic Diseases
  Urate nephropathy
  Nephrocalcinosis (hypercalcemic nephropathy)
  Hypokalemic nephropathy
  Oxalate nephropathy
Physical Factors
  Chronic urinary tract obstruction
  Radiation nephritis
Neoplasms
  Multiple myeloma
Immunologic Reactions
  Transplant rejection
  Tubulointerstitial disease associated with glomerulonephritis
  Sjögren's syndrome
Vascular Diseases
Miscellaneous
  Balkan nephropathy
  Nephronophthisis–medullary cystic disease complex
  Other rare causes (sarcoidosis)
  "Idiopathic" interstitial nephritis

with mononuclear cells, prominent interstitial fibrosis, and widespread tubular atrophy.

Clinically, these conditions are distinguished from the glomerular diseases by the absence, in early stages, of such hallmarks of glomerular injury as nephritic or nephrotic syndromes and by the presence of defects in tubular function. The latter may be quite subtle and include impaired ability to concentrate urine, evidenced clinically by polyuria or nocturia; salt wasting; diminished ability to excrete acids (metabolic acidosis); or isolated defects in tubular reabsorption or secretion. The advanced forms, however, may be difficult to distinguish clinically from other causes of renal insufficiency.

Some of the specific conditions listed in Table 21–8 are discussed elsewhere in this book. In this section we deal principally with pyelonephritis and interstitial diseases induced by drugs.

PYELONEPHRITIS (PN) AND URINARY TRACT INFECTION

Pyelonephritis is a renal disorder affecting tubules, interstitium, and renal pelvis and is one of the most common diseases of the kidney. It occurs in two forms. *Acute PN* is caused by bacterial infection and is the renal lesion associated with urinary tract infection. *Chronic PN* is a more complex disorder: bacterial infection plays a dominant role, but other factors (vesicoureteral reflux, obstruction) are critically involved in its pathogenesis.

The term *urinary tract infection* (UTI) implies involvement of either the bladder (cystitis) or the kidneys and their collecting systems (pyelonephritis), or both. UTIs are extremely common disorders. It is important to realize, however, that bacterial infection of the urinary tract may be completely asymptomatic (asymptomatic bacteriuria) or may remain localized to the bladder without the development of renal infection. However, UTI always carries the potential of spread to the kidney, and it is often difficult clinically to distinguish infection that is confined to the bladder from that which also affects renal tissue.

ETIOLOGY AND PATHOGENESIS. The dominant etiologic agents, accounting for over 85% of cases of UTI, are the gram-negative bacilli that are normal inhabitants of the intestinal tract.[95] By far the most common is *E. coli*, followed by Proteus, Klebsiella, and Enterobacter. *Streptococcus faecalis*, also of enteric origin, and staphylococci can also produce renal infection; virtually every other bacterial and fungal agent can also cause renal infection.

In most patients with UTI, the infecting organisms are derived from the patient's own fecal flora. This is thus a form of *endogenous infection*. There are two routes by which bacteria can reach the kidneys: (1) through the bloodstream (hematogenous infection), and (2) from the lower urinary tract (ascending infection) (Fig. 21–36). Although the hematogenous route is the less common of the two by far, acute pyelonephritis does result from seeding of the kidneys by bacteria from distant foci in the course of septicemia or infective endocarditis; hematogenous infection is more likely to occur in the presence of ureteral obstruction, in debilitated patients, in patients on immunosuppressive therapy, and with nonenteric organisms, such as staphylococci and certain fungi.

Ascending infection is clearly the most common pathway by which bacteria reach the kidney. Normal human bladder and bladder urine are sterile. The first step in the pathogenesis of ascending infection appears to be *colonization of the distal urethra and introitus* (in the female) by coliform bacteria. Current studies suggest that colonization is influenced by the ability of bacteria to adhere to vaginal or urethral mucosal cells.[96] Such bacterial adherence involves the P-fimbriae (pili) of bacteria that interact with receptors on the surface of uroepithelial cells that are identical to the glycosphingolipids of the P blood group system.[97]

From the urethra organisms may then gain entrance into the bladder during urethral catheterization or other instrumentation. Long-term catheterization, in particular, carries a high risk of infection. In the absence of instrumentation, *urinary infections are much more common in females and in the age group of 15 to 40 years, the ratio of females to males affected being 8:1.* This has been variously ascribed to the shorter urethra in females, the absence of antibacterial properties such as are found in prostatic fluid, hormonal changes affecting adherence of bacteria to the mucosa, and urethral trauma during sexual inter-

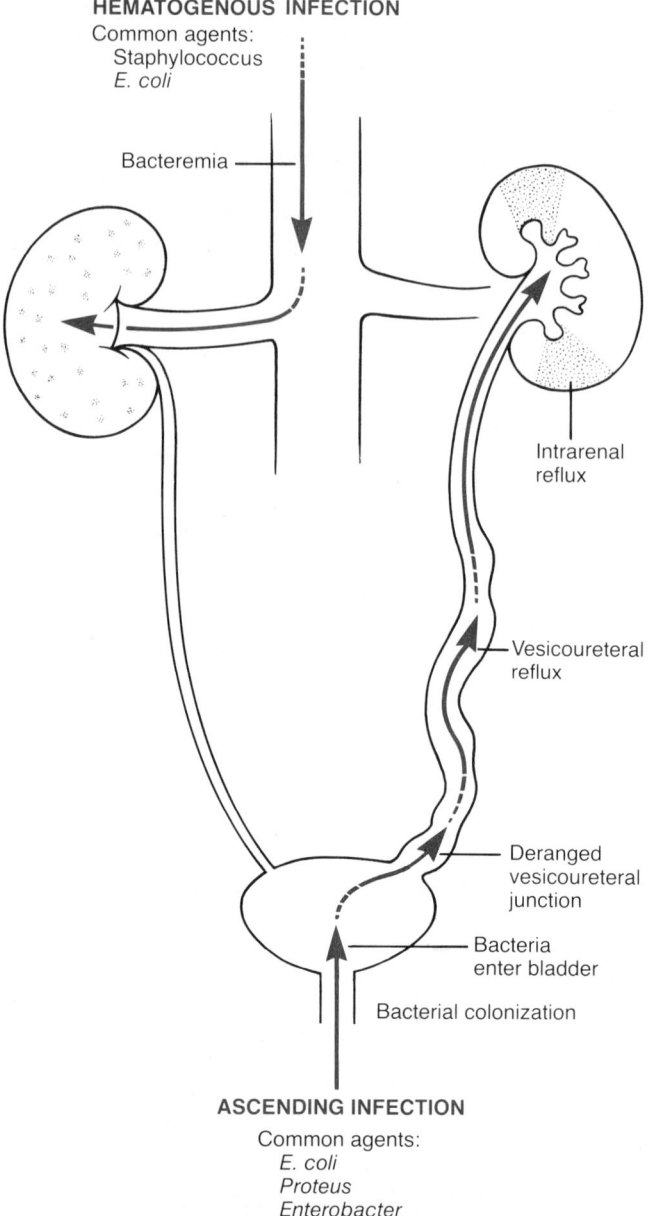

HEMATOGENOUS INFECTION
Common agents:
    Staphylococcus
    E. coli

Bacteremia

Intrarenal reflux

Vesicoureteral reflux

Deranged vesicoureteral junction

Bacteria enter bladder

Bacterial colonization

ASCENDING INFECTION
Common agents:
    E. coli
    Proteus
    Enterobacter

Figure 21–36. Schematic representation of pathways of renal infection. *Hematogenous* infection results from bacteremic spread. More common is *ascending infection,* which results from a combination of urinary bladder infection, vesicoureteral reflux, and intrarenal reflux.

course (the latter accounting for the well-recognized entity of "honeymoon cystitis"), or a combination of all these factors.[96]

Under normal conditions, organisms introduced into the bladder are cleared by the continual flushing of voiding and by other poorly understood antibacterial mechanisms. However, with outflow obstruction or bladder dysfunction, the natural defense mechanisms of the bladder are overwhelmed, setting the stage for UTI. Obstruction at the level of the urinary bladder results in incomplete emptying and increased residual volume of urine. In the presence of stasis, bacteria introduced into the bladder can multiply unhindered without being unceremoniously flushed out or destroyed by the bladder wall. Accordingly UTI is particularly frequent among patients with urinary tract obstruction, such as may occur with benign prostatic hypertrophy, tumors, calculi, or pregnancy.

Once cystitis has occurred, it may remain localized in the urinary bladder for years without ascension to the kidney. In some individuals, however, *incompetence of the vesicoureteral junction* allows urine (and bacteria) to be actively propelled up one or both ureters during micturition (*vesicoureteral reflux* [VUR]).[98] VUR can be documented radiologically by the *voiding cystourethrogram*, in which the bladder is filled with a radiopaque dye and the patient is instructed to void. In normal individuals the dye exits only through the urethra; VUR is prevented by virtue of the oblique insertion of the ureter in the bladder wall, so that the ureter is compressed during micturition. In the presence of reflux, dye is seen refluxing into the ureter, often all the way to the renal pelvis (Fig. 21–37). In *children*, reflux is due to a congenital, inherited[99] absence or shortening of the intravesical portion of the ureter (Fig. 21–38), such that the ureter is not compressed during micturition. In adults, VUR can also be caused by bladder diverticula and neurogenic factors, but its consequences are less serious than in children and infants. In addition, bladder infection itself, probably as a result of the action of bacterial or inflammatory products on ureteral contractility, can cause or accentuate VUR, particularly in children.[99a]

From the pelvis, bacteria can be propelled

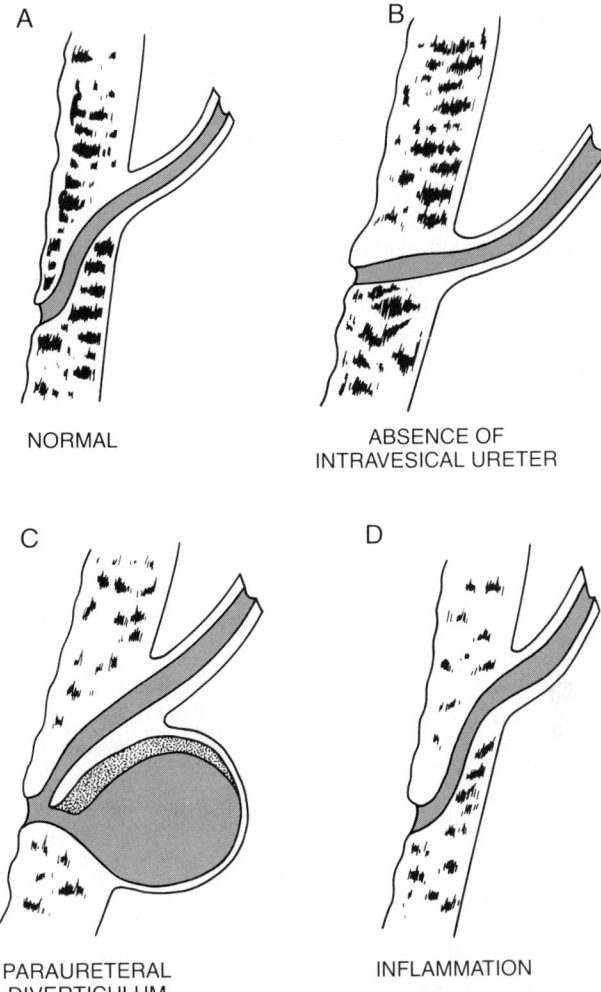

NORMAL

ABSENCE OF
INTRAVESICAL URETER

PARAURETERAL
DIVERTICULUM

INFLAMMATION

Figure 21–38. Causes of vesicoureteric reflux. In normal individuals (A), the intravesical portion of the ureter is oblique. The most common cause is congenital complete or partial absence of intravesical ureter (B). Paraureteral diverticula (C) and inflammation (D) also cause VUR.

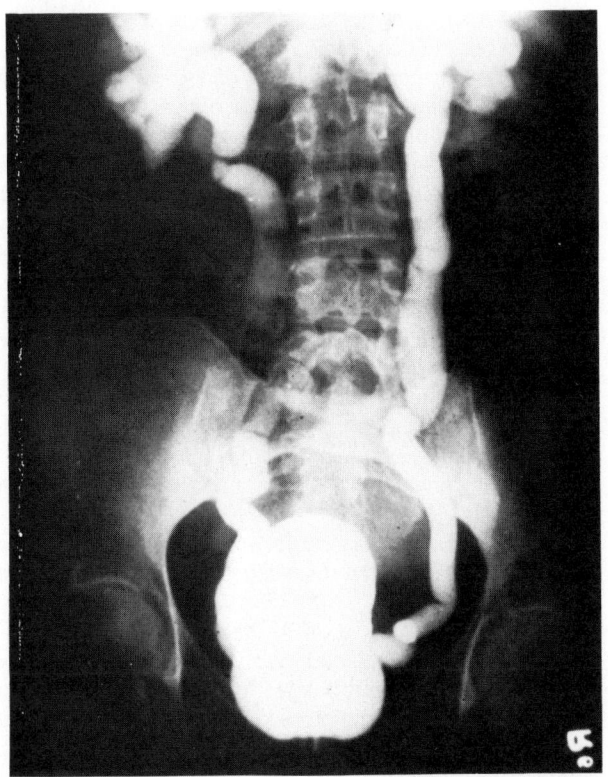

Figure 21–37. Vesicoureteral reflux demonstrated by a voiding cystourethrogram. Dye injected into bladder refluxes into both dilated ureters, filling pelvis and calyces.

through the collecting ducts of the pyramids into the cortex by a process called *intrarenal reflux* (Fig. 21–36). The dye also fills the collecting ducts of pyramids and fans out into the cortex in the shape of a V or U. This *intrarenal reflux* is the mechanism by which bacteria spread into the renal parenchyma. The basis for intrarenal reflux lies in the anatomic configuration of papillae.[98] Many "normal" papillae in human infants are not of the simple, convex, pointed type depicted in textbooks, but have concave or deeply indented tips with widened ducts of Bellini opening into the calyx. Such papillae are potentially refluxing, in that the orifices of their ducts cannot be occluded by a raised intrapelvic pressure. Two thirds of normal kidneys possess at least one potentially refluxing papilla; they are located most often in the upper and lower poles of the kidneys, the usual sites of intrarenal reflux and pyelonephritic scars. *High-grade obstruction, however, can cause infection of papillae throughout the kidney.* Figure 21–36 summarizes the various steps in hematogenous and ascending infection.

Acute Pyelonephritis

Acute PN is an acute suppurative inflammation of the kidney caused by bacterial infection — whether hematogenous and induced by septicemic spread, or ascending and associated with VUR.

MORPHOLOGY. The hallmarks of acute PN are **patchy interstitial suppurative inflammation and tubular necrosis.** The suppuration may occur as discrete focal abscesses involving one or both kidneys, or as large, wedge-shaped areas of coalescent suppuration (Fig. 21–39). The distribution of these lesions is unpredictable and haphazard, but in PN associated with reflux, damage occurs most commonly in the lower and upper poles.

In the very early stages, the neutrophilic infiltration is limited to the interstitial tissue. By the time most kidneys are examined, however, the reaction has ruptured into tubules and produced a characteristic abscess with the destruction of the engulfed tubules (Fig. 21–40). Since the tubular lumina present a ready pathway for the extension of the infection, large masses of neutrophils frequently extend along the involved nephron into the collecting tubules. Characteristically, the glomeruli appear to be resistant to the infection. Large areas of severe necrosis, however, eventually destroy the glomeruli, and fungal PN (e.g., Candida) often affects glomeruli.

Three complications of acute PN are encountered in special circumstances. **Necrotizing papillitis,** or **papillary necrosis,** is seen mainly in diabetics and in those with uri-

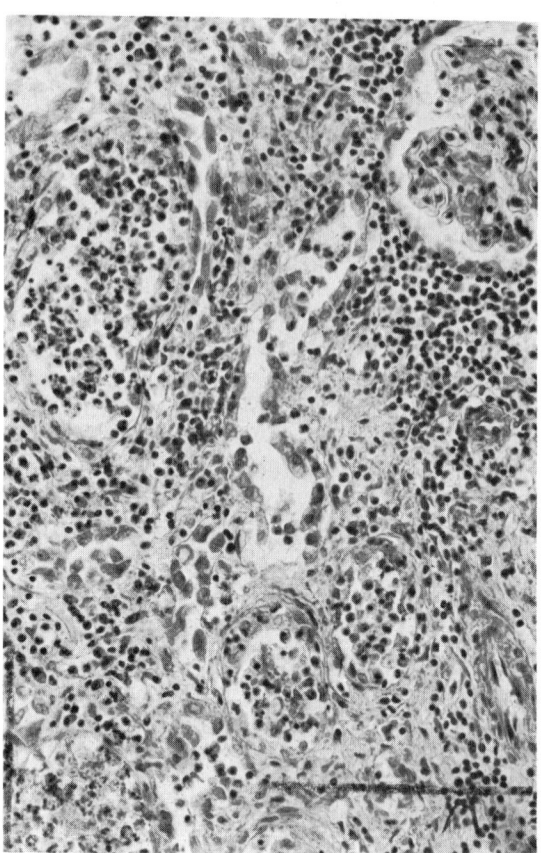

Figure 21–40. Acute pyelonephritis marked by an acute neutrophilic exudate within tubules and renal substance.

nary tract obstruction. Papillary necrosis is usually bilateral but may be unilateral. One or all of the pyramids of the affected kidney may be involved. On cut section, the tips or distal two thirds of the pyramids have gray-white to yellow necrosis that resembles infarction. The junction of the necrotic papillae with the preserved proximal portion of the pyramid is usually sharply defined and outlined by a narrow zone of hyperemia (Fig. 21–41). Microscopically, the necrotic tissue shows characteristic coagulative infarct necrosis, with preservation of outlines of tubules. The leukocytic response is limited to the junctions between preserved and destroyed tissue.

Pyonephrosis is seen when there is total or almost complete obstruction, particularly when it is high in the urinary tract. The suppurative exudate is unable to drain and thus fills the renal pelvis, calyces, and ureter, producing pyonephrosis.

Perinephric abscess implies extension of suppurative inflammation through the renal capsule into the perinephric tissue.

After the acute phase of PN, healing occurs. The neutrophilic infiltrate is replaced by one that is predominantly mononuclear with macrophages, plasma cells, and (later) lymphocytes. The inflammatory foci are eventually replaced by scars that can be seen on the cortical surface as fibrous depressions. Such scars are characterized microscopically by atrophy of tubules, interstitial fibrosis, and lymphocyte

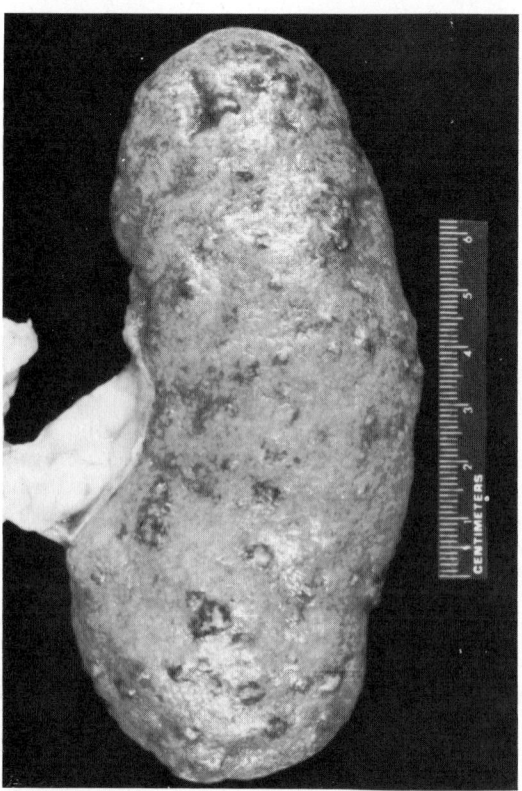

Figure 21–39. Acute pyelonephritis. Cortical surface is dotted with abscesses.

infiltrate and may resemble scars produced by ischemic or other types of injury to the kidney. **However, the pyelone-phritic scar is almost always associated with inflammation, fibrosis, and deformation of the underlying calyx and pelvis,** reflecting the role of ascending infection and VUR in the pathogenesis of the disease.

CLINICAL COURSE. Acute PN is often associated with specific predisposing conditions, some of which were covered in the discussion of pathogenetic mechanisms. These include

1. *Urinary obstruction,* either congenital or acquired.
2. *Instrumentation* of the urinary tract, most commonly catheterization.
3. *Vesicoureteric reflux.*
4. *Pregnancy.* Four to 6% of all pregnant women develop bacteriuria sometime during pregnancy, and 20 to 40% of these eventually develop symptomatic urinary infection if not treated.
5. *Patient's sex and age.* After the first year of life (when congenital anomalies in males commonly become evident) and up to around age 40, infections are much more frequent in females, and in the absence of obstruction and instrumentation, urinary infection in this age group is almost exclusively a disease of females. With increasing age, the incidence in males rises owing to the development of prostatic hypertrophy and frequent instrumentation.
6. *Preexisting renal lesions.* These cause intrarenal scarring and obstruction.
7. *Diabetes mellitus.* Acute PN is probably caused by more frequent instrumentation, the general suscepti-

bility to infection, and the neurogenic bladder dysfunction exhibited by patients.
8. *Immunosuppression and immunodeficiency.*

When acute PN is clinically apparent, the onset is usually sudden, with pain at the costovertebral angle and systemic evidence of infection, such as fever and malaise. There are usually indications of bladder and urethral irritation, such as dysuria, frequency, and urgency. The urine contains many leukocytes (pyuria) derived from the inflammatory infiltrate, but pyuria does not differentiate upper from lower urinary tract infection. The finding of leukocyte casts (pus casts) indicates renal involvement, because casts are formed only in tubules. The diagnosis of infection is established by quantitative urine culture. True infection can usually be differentiated from contamination by the presence of over 10^3 to 10^5 pathogenic organisms per milliliter in the urine. It is frequently difficult to differentiate cystitis alone from PN, as the symptoms referable to upper urinary tract infection may be absent. As mentioned earlier, pus casts, if present, always indicate kidney involvement.

Uncomplicated acute PN usually follows a benign course and the symptoms disappear within a few days after the institution of appropriate antibiotic therapy. Bacteria, however, may persist in the urine, the frequency of recurrence of infection with new serologic types of *E. coli* or other organisms being as high as 30% in some series. Such bacteriuria then either disappears or may persist sometimes for years. In the presence of unrelieved urinary obstruction, diabetes mellitus, and immunocompromise, acute PN may be more serious, leading to repeated septicemic episodes. The superimposition of papillary necrosis often leads to acute renal failure.

Chronic Pyelonephritis (CPN) and Reflux Nephropathy

CPN is a chronic tubulointerstitial renal disorder in which *chronic tubulointerstitial inflammation and renal scarring are associated with pathologic involvement of the calyces and pelvis* (Fig. 21–42). Pelvocalyceal damage is important in that virtually all the diseases listed in Table 21–8 produce chronic tubulointerstitial alterations, but except for CPN and analgesic nephropathy, none affects the calyces. CPN is an important cause of end-stage kidney disease. In various series, CPN is found in 11 to 20% of patients in renal transplant or dialysis units (30 to 50% being caused by chronic GN).

CPN can be divided into two forms: chronic obstructive and chronic reflux–associated.

CHRONIC OBSTRUCTIVE PN. We have seen that obstruction predisposes the kidney to infection. Recurrent infections superimposed on diffuse or localized obstructive lesions lead to recurrent bouts of renal inflammation and scarring, resulting in a picture of CPN. In this condition, the effects of obstruction obviously contribute to the parenchymal atrophy, and

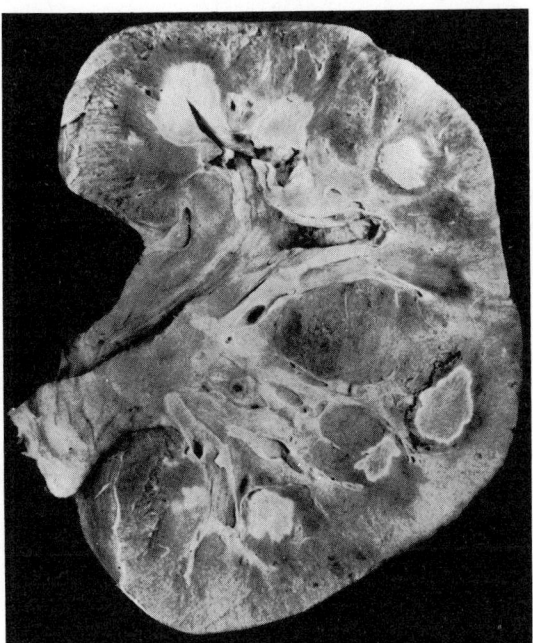

Figure 21–41. Papillary necrosis. Areas of pale gray necrosis are limited to papillae.

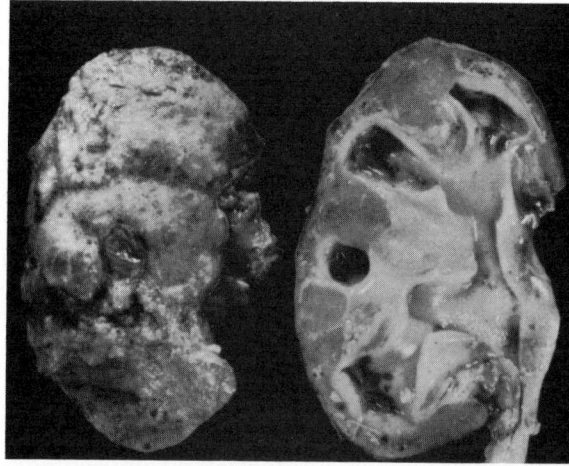

Figure 21–42. Chronic pyelonephritis. Surface *(left)* is irregularly scarred. Cut section *(right)* reveals characteristic dilatation and blunting of calyces. Ureter is dilated and thickened — a finding consistent with chronic vesicoureteral reflux.

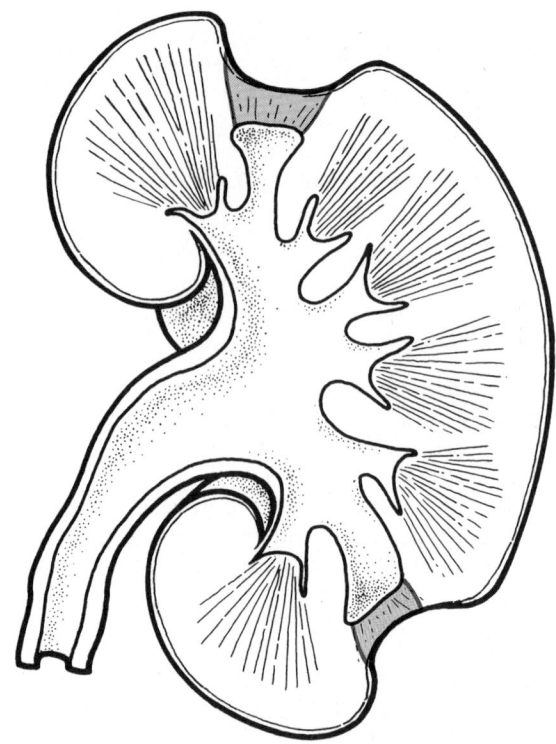

Figure 21–43. Coarse scars of chronic pyelonephritis associated with vesicoureteral reflux. The scars are usually polar and are associated with underlying blunted calyces.

indeed it is sometimes difficult to differentiate the effects of bacterial infection from those of obstruction alone. The disease can be bilateral, as with congenital anomalies of the urethra (posterior urethral valves), resulting in fatal renal insufficiency unless the anomaly is corrected; or unilateral, such as occurs with calculi and unilateral obstructive anomalies of the ureter.

REFLUX NEPHROPATHY (CHRONIC REFLUX–ASSOCIATED PN). This is by far the more common form of chronic pyelonephritic scarring. Renal involvement in reflux nephropathy occurs early in childhood, as a result of superimposition of a urinary infection on congenital VUR and intrarenal reflux, the latter conditioned by the number of potentially refluxing papillae. Reflux may be unilateral or bilateral; thus, the resultant renal damage either may cause scarring and atrophy of one kidney or may involve both and lead to chronic renal insufficiency. Whether VUR causes renal damage in the absence of infection (sterile reflux) is uncertain, as it is difficult clinically to rule out remote infection in a patient first seen with pyelonephritic scarring.

> **MORPHOLOGY.** The characteristic morphologic changes of CPN are seen on gross rather than on microscopic examination (Fig. 21–42). The kidneys usually are irregularly scarred; if bilateral, the involvement is asymmetric. This contrasts with chronic glomerulonephritis, in which the kidneys are diffusely and symmetrically scarred. The hallmark of CPN is the coarse, discrete, corticomedullary scar overlying a dilated, blunted, or deformed calyx (Figs. 21–43 and 21–44). The scars can vary from one to several in number and many affect one or both kidneys. Most are in upper and lower poles, consistent with the frequency of reflux in these sites.
>
> The microscopic changes involve predominantly tubules and interstitium (Fig. 21–45). The tubules show atro-

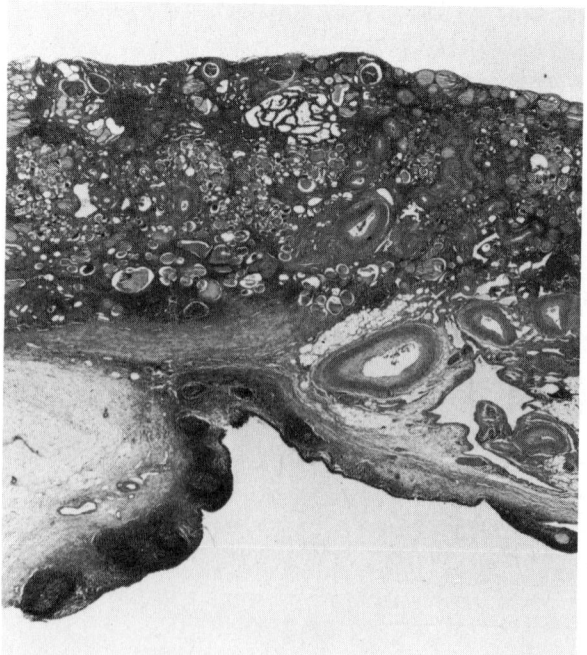

Figure 21–44. Chronic pyelonephritis. Low-power view to show corticomedullary renal scar with an underlying dilated deformed calyx. Note inflammatory infiltrate with lymphoid follicles around calyx.

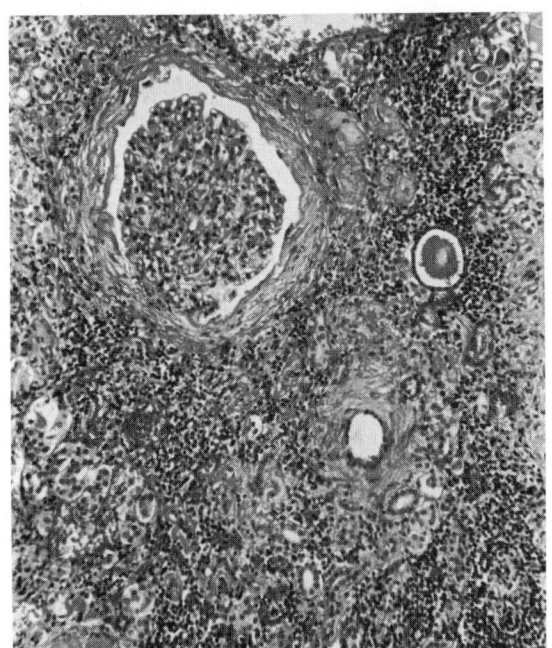

Figure 21–45. Cortex in CPN showing interstitial chronic inflammation, marked tubular atrophy, and occasional dilated tubules. Glomerulus is normal, but there is periglomerular fibrosis.

phy in some areas and hypertrophy in others, or dilatation. Dilated tubules may be filled with colloid casts, a pattern referred to as **thyroidization.** There are varying degrees of chronic interstitial inflammation and fibrosis in the cortex and medulla. In the presence of active infection, there may be neutrophils in the interstitium and pus casts in the tubules. Arcuate and interlobular vessels disclose obliterative endarteritis in the scarred areas, and in the presence of hypertension hyaline arteriolosclerosis is seen in the entire kidney. There is often fibrosis around the calyceal mucosa as well as marked chronic inflammatory infiltrate. Lymphoid follicles may appear in the calyceal wall (Fig. 21–44). Glomeruli may appear normal except for periglomerular fibrosis, but a variety of glomerular changes may be present, including ischemic fibrous obliteration as well as proliferation and necrosis ascribed to hypertension. Patients with CPN and reflux nephropathy who develop proteinuria in advanced stages exhibit secondary **focal segmental glomerulosclerosis,** as described later.

Xanthogranulomatous PN is an unusual and relatively rare form of CPN characterized by accumulation of foamy macrophages intermingled with plasma cells, lymphocytes, polymorphonuclear leukocytes, and occasional giant cells.[100] Often associated with Proteus infections and obstruction, the lesions sometimes produce large, yellowish-orange nodules that may be confused with renal cell carcinoma.

CLINICAL COURSE. Chronic obstructive PN may be insidious in onset or may present the clinical manifestations of acute recurrent PN with back pain, fever, frequent pyuria, and bacteriuria. CPN associated with reflux may have a silent insidious onset. These pa-

tients come to medical attention relatively late in the course of their disease because of the gradual onset of renal insufficiency and hypertension, or because of the discovery of pyuria or bacteriuria on routine examination. Reflux nephropathy is a common cause of hypertension in children. Loss of tubular function—in particular of concentrating ability—gives rise to polyuria and nocturia. Pyelography is required for the diagnosis. Pyelograms show the affected kidneys or kidney to be smaller than normal, often asymmetrically contracted, with characteristic coarse scars and blunting and deformity of the calyceal system. Significant bacteriuria may be present, but in the late stages it is often absent. Some of these patients develop severe and intractable hypertension, which contributes to the progressive renal failure.

Although proteinuria is usually mild, some patients with pyelonephritic scars develop significant proteinuria, even in the nephrotic range, usually many years after the scarring has occurred and often in the absence of continued infection, persistent VUR, or hypertension.[101] The appearance of proteinuria is a poor prognostic sign and many such patients proceed to chronic end-stage renal failure. Renal biopsies show focal segmental glomerulosclerosis superimposed on the tubulointerstitial damage caused by CPN. The glomerular lesions are probably attributable to the adaptive glomerular alterations secondary to loss of renal mass caused by pyelonephritic scarring (p. 1029).

TUBULOINTERSTITIAL NEPHRITIS INDUCED BY DRUGS AND TOXINS

Toxins and drugs can produce renal injury in at least three ways: (1) they may trigger an interstitial immunologic reaction, exemplified by the acute hypersensitivity nephritis induced by such drugs as methicillin; (2) they may cause acute renal failure (p. 1049) by direct tubular damage (such as in mercuric chloride poisoning) or by some other poorly understood mechanisms (e.g., the antibiotic aminoglycosides such as gentamicin); and (3) they may cause subtle but cumulative injury to tubules that takes years to become manifest, resulting in chronic renal insufficiency. The latter type of damage is especially treacherous, as it may be clinically unrecognized until significant renal damage has occurred. Such is the case with analgesic abuse nephropathy, which is usually detected only after the onset of chronic renal insufficiency.

Acute Drug-Induced (Hypersensitivity) Interstitial Nephritis

This is a well-recognized adverse reaction to a constantly increasing number of drugs. First reported after the use of sulfonamides, acute tubulointerstitial nephritis has occurred most frequently with synthetic penicillins (methicillin, ampicillin), but other synthetic antibiotics (rifampin), diuretics (furosemide, thiazides), nonsteroidal anti-inflammatory agents (phenylbutazone), and miscellaneous drugs (phenindione, cimetidine) have also been implicated.[94,102] The disease begins about 15 days (range, 2 to 40) after exposure to the drug and is characterized by fever, eosinophilia (which may be transient), hematuria, mild proteinuria, sterile pyuria, and a skin rash, the latter being present in about 25% of patients. A *rising serum creatinine level or acute renal failure with oliguria develops in about 50% of cases*, particularly in older patients. The azotemia typically resolves after withdrawal of the offending drug, although it may take several months for renal function to return to normal.

> Grossly, the kidneys are usually slightly enlarged. Histologically, the abnormalities are in the interstitium, which shows pronounced edema and infiltration by mononuclear cells, principally lymphocytes and macrophages (Fig. 21–46). Eosinophils and neutrophils may be present, often in large numbers, and plasma cells and basophils are sometimes found in small numbers. With some drugs (e.g., methicillin, thiazides), interstitial granulomas with giant cells may be seen. Variable degrees of tubular necrosis and regeneration are present.

Many features of the disease suggest an immunologic basis for its development.[102a]

1. Clinical evidence of hypersensitivity includes the latent period, the eosinophilia and skin rash, the fact that the onset of nephropathy is not dose related, and

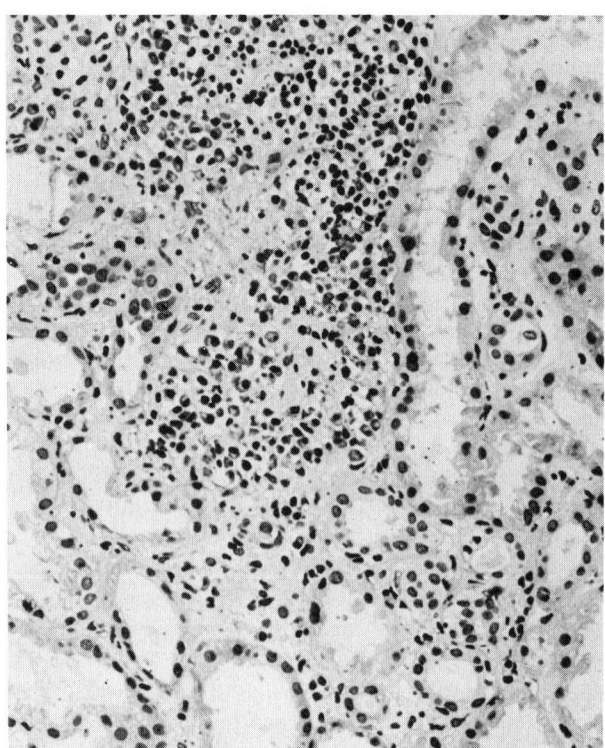

Figure 21–46. Acute drug-induced interstitial nephritis. Note interstitial inflammation and edema.

the recurrence of hypersensitivity following re-exposure to the same or a cross-reactive drug.

2. Immunofluorescence studies in rare cases have disclosed linear staining for IgG and complement along the tubular basement membranes (TBM), and circulating antibody to tubular basement membranes has been found in the circulation in some patients.

3. IgE serum levels are increased in some patients, and IgE-containing plasma cells and basophils are sometimes present in the lesions, suggesting that a type I IgE-mediated hypersensitivity may be involved in the pathogenesis.

4. Finally, the mononuclear or granulomatous infiltrate, together with positive skin tests to drug haptens, suggests a delayed-hypersensitivity type reaction (type IV).

The most likely sequence of pathogenetic events is that the drugs act as haptens, which, during secretion by tubules, covalently bind to some cytoplasmic or extracellular component of tubular cells and become immunogenic. The resultant injury is then due to antibody and cell-mediated immune reactions to tubular cells or their basement membranes.

It is important to recognize drug-induced renal failure because withdrawal of the drug is followed by recovery, although irreversible damage may occur occasionally in older subjects.

Analgesic Nephritis (Analgesic Abuse Nephropathy)

This is a form of chronic renal disease caused by excessive intake of analgesic mixtures and characterized morphologically by chronic tubulointerstitial nephritis with renal papillary necrosis.

First reported in Switzerland in 1953, analgesic nephropathy is of worldwide distribution, and in some parts of Australia and Western Europe it ranks as one of the most common causes of chronic renal insufficiency.[103] Its incidence in the United States is low, but in certain areas (e.g., the Southeast) it accounts for about 13% of cases of end-stage renal disease.[104] The renal damage was first ascribed to phenacetin, but the analgesic mixtures consumed often contain, in addition, aspirin, caffeine, acetaminophen (a metabolite of phenacetin), and codeine. Patients who develop this disease usually ingest large quantities of analgesic mixtures. The minimum requirements for the development of renal damage are 2 to 3 kg of phenacetin taken over a period of three years.

PATHOGENESIS. Experimentally, papillary necrosis is readily induced by a mixture of aspirin and phenacetin, usually combined with water depletion. Most patients consume phenacetin-containing mixtures, and cases ascribed to ingestion of aspirin, phenacetin, or acetaminophen alone are uncommon. It is now clear that in the sequence of events leading to renal damage, *papillary necrosis occurs first and cortical tubulointerstitial nephritis is a secondary phenomenon.* The phenacetin metabolite acetaminophen injures cells by both *covalent binding and oxidative damage*. The ability of aspirin to inhibit prostaglandin synthesis suggests that this drug may induce its potentiating effect by inhibiting the vasodilatory effects of prostaglandin, thus predisposing the papilla to ischemia. Thus, the papillary damage may be due to a combination of direct toxic effects of phenacetin metabolites as well as ischemic injury to both tubular cells and vessels, a notion consistent with the morphologic findings and with the synergistic effects of drug combinations.

MORPHOLOGY. Grossly, the kidneys are either normal or slightly reduced in size, and the cortex exhibits depressed and raised areas, the depressed areas representing cortical atrophy overlying necrotic papillae. On cut section, the papillae show various stages of necrosis, calcification, fragmentation, and sloughing. **This gross appearance contrasts with the papillary necrosis seen in diabetic patients, in which all papillae are at the same stage of acute necrosis.** Microscopically, the papillary changes may take one of several forms: in early cases there is patchy necrosis and widening of the interstitium, but in the advanced form the entire papilla is necrotic, often remaining in place as a structureless mass with ghosts of tubules and foci of dystrophic calcification (Fig. 21–47). If segments or entire portions of the papilla have been sloughed and excreted in the urine, the underlying calyx appears dilated, accounting for some of the diagnostic radiologic features of the disease.

The cortical changes consist of loss and atrophy of these tubules, and interstitial fibrosis and inflammation. These changes are mainly due to obstructive atrophy caused by the tubular damage in the papilla, but superimposed pyelonephritic changes may be present. **The cortical columns of Bertin are characteristically spared from**

this atrophy. The small vessels in the papilla and submucosa of the urinary tract exhibit characteristic PAS-positive basement membrane thickening (analgesic microangiopathy).

CLINICAL COURSE. Analgesic nephropathy is more common in women than in men and is particularly prevalent in individuals with recurrent headaches and muscular pain, in psychoneurotic patients, and in factory workers. The renal findings may be slight before the onset of chronic renal insufficiency. Inability to concentrate the urine occurs early, as would be expected with lesions in the papilla. Acquired distal renal tubular acidosis contributes to the development of renal stones. Headache, anemia, gastrointestinal symptoms, and hypertension are common accompaniments of analgesic nephropathy. The anemia in particular is out of proportion to the renal insufficiency, owing to damage to red cells by the phenacetin metabolites. Pyuria occurs in almost 100% of patients; although the urine is often sterile, urinary tract infection complicates about 50% of patients. Occasionally, entire tips of necrotic papillae are excreted, and these may cause gross hematuria or renal colic due to obstruction of the ureter by necrotic fragments. Intravenous pyelography (IVP) will often disclose the characteristic picture of absent papillae, but if the papillae remain in place the IVP may be entirely normal. Progressive impairment of renal function may lead to chronic renal failure, but *with proper therapy of any infection and drug withdrawal, renal function may either stabilize or actually improve.*

Unfortunately, a serious complication sometimes occurs in patients with analgesic nephropathy who have survived because of their discontinuance of the offending drugs—namely, the development of *transitional papillary carcinoma of the renal pelvis.*[105] Whether the carcinogenic effect is due to a metabolite of phenacetin or to some other component of the analgesic compounds is unsettled.

TUBULOINTERSTITIAL DISEASES CAUSED BY METABOLIC DISTURBANCES

Urate Nephropathy

Three types of nephropathy can occur in patients with hyperuricemic disorders (p. 1355). *Acute uric acid nephropathy* is caused by the precipitation of uric acid crystals in the renal tubules, principally in collecting ducts, leading to obstruction of nephrons and the development of acute renal failure. This type is particularly apt to occur in patients with leukemias and lymphomas who are undergoing chemotherapy; the drugs increase the destruction of neoplastic nuclei and the elaboration of uric acid. Precipitation of uric acid is favored by the acidic pH in collecting tubules.

Chronic urate nephropathy or gouty nephropathy occurs in patients with more protracted forms of hy-

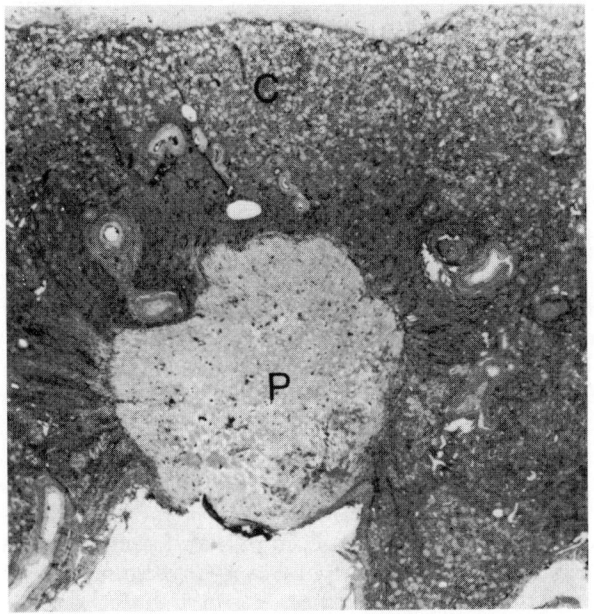

Figure 21–47. Analgesic nephropathy. Cortex (C) is scarred and papilla (P) is transformed to a necrotic, structureless mass.

peruricemia. The lesions are ascribed to the deposition of monosodium urate crystals in the acidic milieu of the distal tubules and collecting ducts, as well as in the interstitium. *These deposits have a distinct histologic appearance, in the form of birefringent, needle-like crystals present either in the tubular lumina or in the interstitium* (Fig. 21–48). The urates induce a *tophus* often surrounded by foreign body giant cells, other mononuclear cells, and a fibrotic reaction. Tubular obstruction by the urates causes cortical atrophy and scarring. Arterial and arteriolar thickening is also common in these kidneys, owing to the relatively high frequency of hypertension in patients with gout. Clinically, urate nephropathy is a subtle disease associated with tubular defects that may progress slowly, but the condition should be suspected in patients with prolonged hyperuricemia. Patients with gout who actually develop a chronic nephropathy commonly have evidence of increased exposure to lead (mostly by way of "moonshine" whiskey contaminated with lead).[106]

The third renal syndrome in hyperuricemia is *nephrolithiasis;* uric acid stones are present in 22% of patients with gout and 42% of those with secondary hyperuricemia (p. 1074).

Hypercalcemia and Nephrocalcinosis

Disorders characterized by hypercalcemia, such as hyperparathyroidism, multiple myeloma, vitamin D intoxication, metastatic bone disease, or excess calcium intake (milk-alkali syndrome), may induce the formation of calcium stones (p. 1074) and deposition of calcium in the kidney (nephrocalcinosis). Extensive degrees of calcinosis, under certain conditions, may lead to a form of chronic tubulointerstitial disease and renal insufficiency.[106] The first damage induced by the hypercalcemia is at the *intracellular level*, in the tubular epithelial cells, resulting in mitochondrial

Table 21–9. Renal Involvement by Nonrenal Neoplasms

1. Direct tumor invasion of renal parenchyma
   Ureters → obstruction
   Artery → renovascular hypertension
2. Hypercalcemia
3. Hyperuricemia
4. Amyloidosis
5. Excretion of abnormal proteins (multiple myeloma)
6. Radiotherapy
7. Chemotherapy
8. Infection
9. Glomerulopathy
   Immune complex GN (carcinomas)
   Lipoid nephrosis (Hodgkin's disease)

distortion and evidence of cell injury. Subsequently, calcium deposits can be demonstrated within the mitochondria, cytoplasm, and basement membrane. Calcified cellular debris then aids in obstruction of the tubular lumina and causes obstructive atrophy of nephrons with interstitial fibrosis and nonspecific chronic inflammation. Atrophy of entire cortical areas drained by calcified tubules may occur and this accounts for the alternating areas of normal and scarred parenchyma seen in such kidneys.

The earliest functional defect is an inability to elaborate a concentrated urine, which appears to be related to decreased transport of chloride in the ascending thick segment. Other tubular defects, such as tubular acidosis and salt-losing nephritis, may also occur. With further damage, a slowly progressive renal insufficiency develops. This is usually due to nephrocalcinosis, but many of these patients also have calcium stones and secondary PN. Renal calcification can be obvious radiologically and these patients often have calcifications in other organs and in blood vessels.

TUBULOINTERSTITIAL LESIONS CAUSED BY NEOPLASTIC DISEASES

Nonrenal malignant tumors, particularly those of hematopoietic origin, affect the kidneys in a number of ways (Table 21–9).[107] The most common involvements are tubulointerstitial, caused by complications of the tumor (hypercalcemia, hyperuricemia, obstruction of ureters) or therapy (irradiation, hyperuricemia, chemotherapy, infections in immunosuppressed patients). As the survival rate of patients with malignant neoplasms increases, so do these renal complications. Here we shall limit the discussion to the renal lesions in multiple myeloma that sometimes dominate the clinical picture in patients with this disease.

Multiple Myeloma (Myeloma Kidney)

Renal involvement is a common and sometimes ominous manifestation of multiple myeloma (p. 739), overt renal insufficiency occurring in half the patients with this disease.[107] The main cause of renal dysfunction is related to Bence Jones (light-chain) protein-

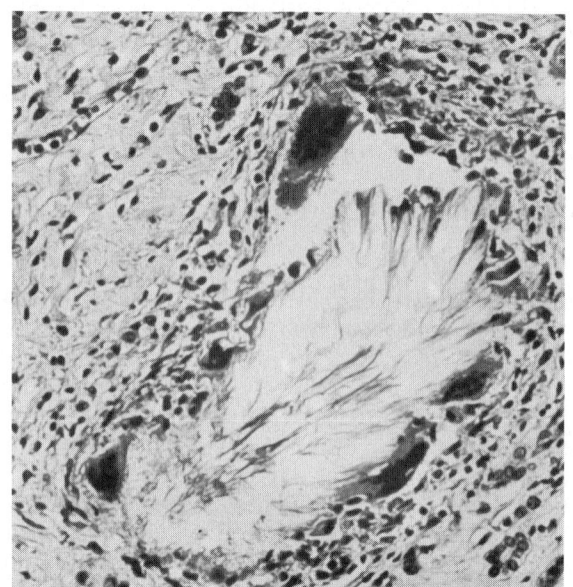

Figure 21–48. Urate crystals in renal medulla. Note inflammatory reaction with giant cells around needle-like crystals.

uria, because renal failure correlates well with the presence and amount of such proteinuria and is extremely rare in its absence.[108] Two mechanisms appear to account for the renal toxicity of Bence Jones proteins. First, some of these light chains appear to be directly toxic to epithelial cells; second, Bence Jones proteins combine with the urinary glycoprotein (Tamm-Horsfall protein) under acidic conditions to form large, histologically distinct tubular casts that obstruct the tubular lumina and also induce a peritubular inflammatory reaction. Other factors that may contribute to renal failure include (1) vascular disease in the usually elderly population affected with myeloma; (2) hypercalcemia and hyperuricemia, which are often present in these patients; (3) amyloidosis, which occurs in 6 to 24% of patients with myeloma; and (4) urinary tract obstruction with secondary pyelonephritis.

Grossly, the kidneys usually are normal but sometimes are shrunken and pale because of extensive interstitial scarring. The most prominent changes are histologic. The tubular casts appear as pink-to-blue amorphous masses, sometimes concentrically laminated, filling and distending the tubular lumina. Many of the casts are surrounded by multinucleate giant cells, derived from either reactive tubular epithelium or possibly mononuclear phagocytes (see Fig. 15–36, p. 742). The epithelium surrounding the cast is often necrotic, and the adjacent interstitial tissue usually shows a nonspecific inflammatory response. Occasionally, the casts erode their way from the tubules into the interstitium and here evoke a granulomatous inflammatory reaction.

Clinically, the renal manifestations are of several types. In the most common form, *chronic renal failure* develops insidiously and usually progresses slowly over a period of several months to years. Another form occurs suddenly, sometimes in the absence of obvious previous renal impairment, and is manifested by *acute renal failure* with oliguria. ARF commonly occurs in patients with other precipitating factors, such as dehydration, hypercalcemia, acute infection, and administration of nephrotoxic antibiotics. *Proteinuria* occurs in 70% of patients with myeloma; the presence of significant non–light-chain proteinuria (e.g., albumin) suggests secondary amyloidosis or light-chain glomerulopathy (p. 1047).

OTHER TUBULOINTERSTITIAL DISORDERS

Immunologically Mediated Tubulointerstitial Disease

Immunologic tubulointerstitial reactions are clearly involved in rejection of renal transplants, and we have seen earlier that a hypersensitivity reaction is the cause of acute interstitial nephritis induced by drugs. In addition, tubulointerstitial damage may be induced by immunologic mechanisms similar to those involved in glomerulonephritis (i.e., *tubular immune complex disease and antitubular basement membrane antibody disease*).[109]

Tubular immune complex disease is characterized by an immunofluorescent pattern of staining of granules containing immunoglobulin and complement along the tubular basement membrane and in the interstitium. (Fig. 21–49A): In humans, immune complex tubular deposits are seen in patients with accompanying glomerulonephritis: 50% of patients with lupus nephritis and occasional patients with membranoproliferative glomerulonephritis, mixed cryoglobulinemia, and Sjögren's syndrome. It is thought that the complexes contribute to the tubulointerstitial damage in these conditions.[110]

In antitubular basement membrane (anti-TBM) antibody disease, immunofluorescence discloses smooth, continuous linear accumulations of immunoglobulin and complement along the basement membrane of the proximal tubules (Fig. 21–49B). In man, anti-TBM antibodies frequently occur in conjunction with anti-GBM nephritis in Goodpasture's syndrome and rapidly progressive GN, suggesting that cross-reactive autoantibodies to both glomerular and tubular basement membrane are formed in these conditions. More unusually, they occur in other types of GN, drug-induced hypersensitivity, and idiopathic interstitial nephritis.

Radiation Nephritis

This condition, which follows therapeutic irradiation of tumors in the regions of the kidneys,[111] is now an uncommon complication, as damaging radiation levels can be predicted and the kidneys appropriately shielded. Doses of greater than 2300 rad in less than five weeks are sufficient to cause renal damage. The clinical presentation may be acute, beginning six to 12 months after radiation, and characterized by edema, hypertension (often malignant), anemia, proteinuria, and renal insufficiency (*acute radiation nephritis*). Other patients present more than 18 months after irradiation with hypertension (benign or malignant) or proteinuria. Histologically, all renal structures are affected; there is glomerular hyalinization, severe interstitial fibrosis and inflammation, tubular atrophy, and sometimes striking vascular thickening. In some instances, tubulointerstitial damage is out of proportion to the vascular or glomerular damage, but in the presence of severe hypertension, fibrinoid necrosis and hyperplastic changes in arterioles are common.

DISEASES OF BLOOD VESSELS

Renal vessels are affected secondarily by virtually all forms of renal disease. Here we are concerned with those disorders in which the vascular lesions are the primary cause of disease and in particular those associated with hypertension. Within this group, benign and malignant nephrosclerosis are of preeminent im-

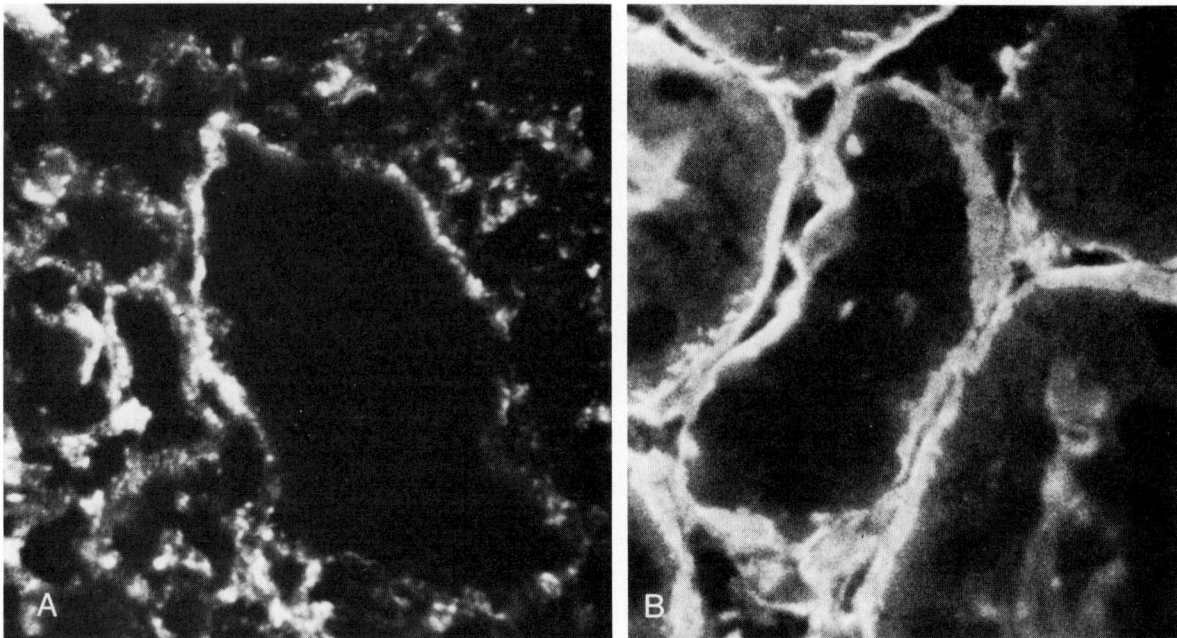

Figure 21–49. Immunofluorescent patterns of *(A)* immune complex (granular) and *(B)* antitubular basement membrane antibody-mediated tubulointerstitial nephritis. (Courtesy of Dr. Helmut Rennke.)

portance. Because the kidney and its diseases are intimately related to hypertension, it is first necessary to review briefly the subject of hypertension.

HYPERTENSION

Elevated blood pressure is a staggering health problem for three reasons: it is very common, its effects are sometimes devastating, and it remains asymptomatic until late in its course. Its effects are widespread, and no organ is spared. Hypertension has been identified as the single most important risk factor in both coronary heart disease and cerebrovascular accidents; it may also lead directly to congestive heart failure (hypertensive heart disease) and to chronic renal insufficiency. There is no magic threshold of blood pressure above which an individual is considered hypertensive and below which he or she is safe. Rather, the detrimental effects of blood pressure increase continuously as the pressure increases. Hypertension, then, must be defined somewhat arbitrarily. Most would agree that a sustained diastolic pressure above 90 mm Hg is an essential feature. A sustained systolic pressure above 140 mm Hg also constitutes hypertension, but its clinical consequences differ somewhat from diastolic hypertension. By means of these criteria, the prevalence of hypertension in large screening programs is about 25%. The prevalence increases with age, although when present in young adults it tends to be more severe. Blacks are affected about twice as often as whites and apparently are more vulnerable to complications. Although females are hypertensive more often than males, this sex preponderance is limited to the older age groups, in which the disease is

likely to be relatively benign. Under the age of 50 years, hypertension is more common in males.

Ninety to 95% of hypertension is idiopathic and apparently primary (essential hypertension). Of the remaining 5 to 10%, most are secondary to renal disease or, less often, to renal artery stenosis (renovascular hypertension). Less frequently, hypertension is the result of endocrine, vascular or psychogenic factors, as shown in Table 21–10. Both essential and secondary hypertension may be either benign or malignant, ac-

Table 21–10. Types of Hypertension

Primary or Essential Hypertension
Secondary Hypertension
  Renal
    Acute glomerulonephritis
    Chronic renal disease
    Renal artery stenosis
    Renal vasculitis
    Renin-producing tumors
  Endocrine
    Adrenocortical hyperfunction (Cushing's syndrome)
    Oral contraceptives
    Pheochromocytoma
    Acromegaly
    Myxedema
    Thyrotoxicosis (systolic)
  Vascular
    Coarctation of aorta
    Polyarteritis nodosa
    Aortic insufficiency (systolic)
  Neurogenic
    Psychogenic
    Increased intracranial pressure
    Polyneuritis, bulbar poliomyelitis, others

cording to the clinical course. In most cases hypertension remains fairly stable over years to decades and, unless a myocardial infarction or cerebrovascular accident supervenes, is compatible with a long life. This form of the disorder is termed *benign hypertension* and produces a renal lesion known as *benign nephrosclerosis.* About 5% of hypertensive persons show a rapidly rising blood pressure, which, untreated, leads to death within a year or two. Appropriately enough, this is called *accelerated* or *malignant hypertension,* and the corresponding renal lesion *malignant nephrosclerosis.* The morphology and clinical course of the two renal lesions, benign and malignant nephrosclerosis, will be considered separately later. First we discuss what is known of the cause and pathogenesis of hypertension in general.

Mechanisms of Hypertension

The search for the origins of essential hypertension[112-115] has been most frustrating. Much more has been learned about the pathogenesis of the secondary forms of hypertension, and so we will review first the more well-established mechanisms that cause secondary hypertension.

REGULATION OF NORMAL BLOOD PRESSURE.

As is well known, the magnitude of the arterial pressure is dependent on two fundamental hemodynamic variables: *cardiac output* and *total peripheral resistance* (Fig. 21–50). For the most part, the total peripheral resistance is accounted for by resistance of the arterioles. This in turn is determined by the thickness of the arteriolar wall in relation to lumen size *and* the effects of neural and hormonal influences that either constrict or dilate these vessels. Vasoconstricting agents are angiotensin II, catecholamines, thromboxane, leukotrienes and endothelin. Vasodilators are kinins and prostaglandins. These mediators act by

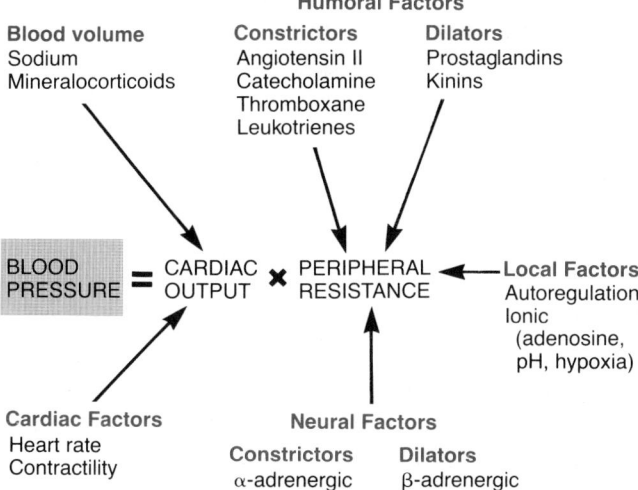

Figure 21–50. The influence of cardiac output and peripheral resistance in the regulation of blood pressure. (See text.) (Adapted from Kaplan, N.: Systemic hypertension. *In* Braunwald, E. (ed.): Heart Disease. 3rd ed. Philadelphia, W.B. Saunders, 1988, p. 828.)

binding specific receptors on the surface of smooth muscle cells. Certain metabolic products, such as lactic acid, hydrogen ions, and adenosine, as well as hypoxia, are also local vasodilators. An important property intrinsic to resistance vessels is *autoregulation,* a process by which increased blood flow to such vessels leads to vasoconstriction. This is an essentially adaptive mechanism, probably mediated by the local levels of adenosine, designed to protect from hyperperfusion; the resultant vasoconstriction leads to increased cardiac workload, reduction of cardiac output, and correction of hyperperfusion. *Arterial hypertension can best be considered a disease dependent on factors that may alter the relationship between blood volume and total arteriolar resistance* (Fig. 21–50).

MECHANISMS OF RENAL HYPERTENSION.

The kidney participates in the control of blood pressure by influencing both peripheral resistance and blood volume. It is no surprise, therefore, that hypertension is common in a variety of renal disorders.[114]

Three groups of factors that control blood pressure may be deranged in renal hypertension: (1) *vasoconstrictive factors, principally the renin-angiotension system,* (2) *factors that maintain salt and volume homeostasis,* and (3) *vasodepressor factors.* These three mechanisms are interrelated but will be discussed separately.

1. *Renin-angiotensin system.*[113] The kidney plays a major role in regulation of normal blood pressure through the elaboration of renin and the subsequent formation of angiotensin II (Fig. 21–51). *Angiotensin II is the major effector molecule of the renin-angiotensin axis.* It alters blood pressure by increasing both peripheral resistance and blood volume. The former effect is achieved largely by its ability to cause vasoconstriction through direct action on vascular smooth muscle; the latter effect is caused by stimulation of aldosterone secretion which increases distal tubular reabsorption.

Under normal conditions, the increased renin secretion is quickly corrected by negative feedback mechanisms that tend to suppress renin release and bring circulating renin levels back to normal. For example, increased blood pressure diminishes stretch receptor stimulation in the afferent arteriole and therefore diminishes renin secretion; similarly, the increased extracellular fluid volume consequent to aldosterone secretion increases GFR, thus decreasing proximal sodium reabsorption, and through the sensors in the macula densa diminishes renin secretion. Finally, angiotensin II itself appears to suppress juxtaglomerular cell secretion directly. Thus, in the presence of normal renal function, plasma renin values are restored to normal.

Increased renin secretion plays an important role in the following forms of renal hypertension: (a) unilateral renal artery stenosis (renovascular hypertension (p. 1068); (b) malignant hypertension, in which extremely high levels of renin and aldosterone have

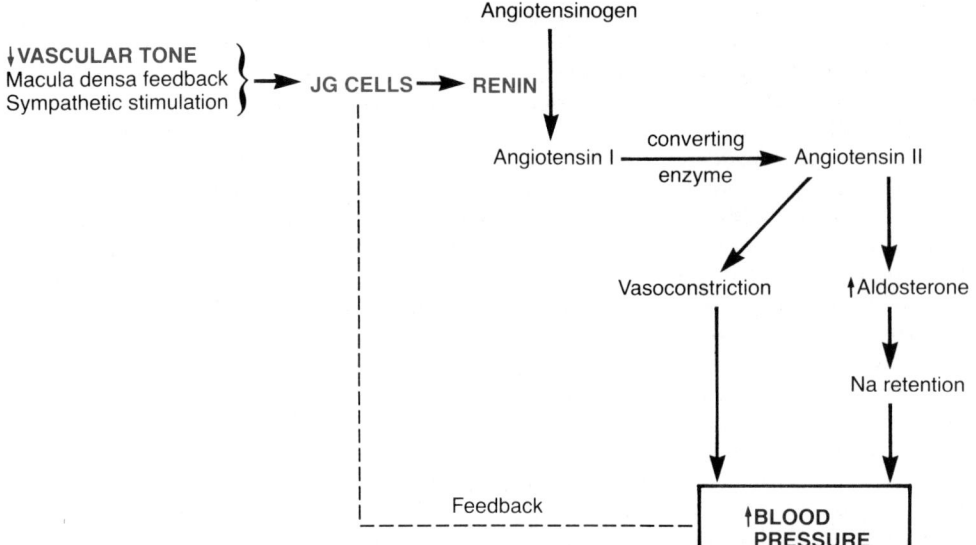

Figure 21–51. Renin-angiotensin system.

been measured; (c) vasculitides; (d) some cases of unilateral chronic PN or reflux nephropathy; (e) renin-secreting juxtaglomerular cell tumors, renal cell carcinoma, or Wilms' tumors; (f) some cases of chronic renal failure of diverse causation.

2. *Sodium homeostasis.*[114] You may recall that extracellular fluid volume (and therefore blood volume and cardiac output) is regulated mostly by total body sodium levels. The kidney is intimately involved in the complex process of sodium homeostasis. One mechanism already discussed is the renin-angiotensin system, which, as mentioned, affects distal tubular reabsorption of sodium through the mediation of aldosterone secretion. Two other renal factors have bearing on sodium homeostasis: *the glomerular filtration rate (GFR)* and *natriuretic factors.*[115] When blood volume is reduced, the GFR falls; this in turn leads to increased reabsorption of sodium by proximal tubules in an attempt to conserve sodium and expand blood flow. Natriuretic factors include *atrial natriuretic factor* (atriopeptin), a group of peptides secreted by heart atria in response to volume expansion.[116] These peptides cause natriuresis by increasing GFR and inhibiting sodium reabsorption at a distal site.

Sodium retention due to failure of these homeostatic mechanisms is probably the most important factor responsible for hypertension in patients with parenchymal renal diseases, including chronic renal failure. Increased total exchangeable sodium and ECF volume are found in such patients, and there is marked improvement of blood pressure when these excesses are removed.

3. *Renal vasodepressor substances.* The kidney produces a variety of vasodepressor or antihypertensive substances, which presumably counterbalance the vasopressor effects of angiotensin. The vasodepressor substances include the prostaglandins, a urinary kallikrein-kinin system, platelet-activating factor (**PAF**), and some neutral renomedullary lipids.[117] Although renal hypertension could theoretically result from

loss of such factors, clear evidence for such a mechanism is wanting.

To summarize, from the point of view of pathogenesis, two categories of renal hypertension can be recognized — those associated with excessive renin secretion (e.g., renovascular hypertension) and those associated with volume excess (e.g., acute glomerulonephritis). In some cases of chronic renal failure, a mixture of both patterns is seen.

The mechanism of other secondary forms of hypertension is heterogeneous. In *primary aldosteronism,* the major cause is aldosterone-induced sodium retention causing increased blood volume; in *pheochromocytoma,* the tumor in the renal medulla secretes epinephrine and norepinephrine, which cause vasoconstriction and increased cardiac contractility; *oral contraceptives,* a common cause of secondary hypertension, seem to activate the renin-angiotensin mechanism; and in *polyarteritis nodosa* there are marked increases in renin production.

MECHANISMS OF ESSENTIAL HYPERTENSION. By definition, essential hypertension is idiopathic, *but it is believed that a combination of genetic and environmental factors together is responsible for the condition.*[112] There is a rather high degree of concordance in levels of blood pressure among twins, siblings, and families. The increased prevalence of hypertension among blacks, the recognition in hypertensive families of hypertension in infants and children, and the development by inbreeding of various strains of spontaneously hypertensive rats all point to a genetic predisposition. The inheritance appears to be polygenic.

Environmental factors clearly influence the development of hypertension. This is illustrated by the lower prevalence of hypertension in Chinese people living in their native country than in the Chinese living in the United States. Behavior patterns, stress, obesity, and the intake of oral contraceptives all have important implications, but it is the relationship of *dietary sodium* to essential hypertension that has stimulated the most interest. Although the evidence is by no means unambiguous, most workers now agree that *in those with a genetic predisposition, high sodium intake predisposes to or may lead to hypertension.* People living in remote areas in Asia, South America, and Africa who have diets very low in sodium chloride show little evidence of essential hypertension. When some of these groups migrate to coastal towns where the salt intake is high, they begin to get their share of hypertension. The daily consumption of salt in such "civilized" areas as the United States, Europe, and Japan is 8 gm or more and correlates with an 8 to 25% incidence of hypertension. Experimentally susceptible strains of rats develop hypertension when fed high-sodium diets, but remain normotensive on low-salt diets.

Given that high salt intake and heredity play a role, what is it that is inherited? Many possibilities exist, but three are being currently pursued (Fig. 21–52).[112]

1. *A primary defect in renal sodium excretion.* This hypothesis contends that there is an initial *nonstructural* genetic defect in the kidney's ability to excrete salt and water in response to the inevitable periodic increases in pressure — so-called *arterial pressure natriuresis.*[117] The latter is an autoregulatory phenomenon that helps the normal kidney exposed to small increases in pressure to excrete excess quantities of water and salt, until the individual's blood pressure falls back to a level low enough to stop the pressure diuresis. Loss of this natriuretic response results in increased blood and ECF volumes, and eventually to increased peripheral vascular resistance and blood pressure. At the higher setting of blood pressure, enough additional sodium can be excreted by the kidneys to equal intake and prevent fluid retention. Thus, an altered but steady state of sodium excretion is achieved (resetting of pressure natriuresis).

2. *A defect in cell membrane sodium or calcium transport.* A defect in sodium transport has been shown in red blood cells of hypertensive subjects and is assumed to be generalized; a defect in sodium transport in *vascular smooth cells* would result in increased *intracellular calcium*, which, by stimulating myosin phosphorylation, heightens vascular reactivity to vasoconstrictive agents. The same effect would result from a primary defect in calcium transport, and indeed such a defect has been reported in fat cells and platelets from hypertensives.

3. *A primary heightened sympathetic response to stress or other neurogenic influences.* The resultant increases in vasoconstrictive agents raises blood pressure by increasing peripheral resistance and eventually extracellular fluid volume.

These three theories are not mutually exclusive, and high sodium intake clearly influences blood pressure in all three settings. In addition, once hypertension has been established from any cause, *structural changes occur in the small muscular arteries and arterioles* — the primary resistance vessels of the circulation. These changes include smooth muscle proliferation, hypertrophy, and fibrosis and result in thickening of the vessel wall and narrowing of the lumen. Such structurally abnormal vessels become even more narrowed under the influence of constrictive agents, and also are less responsive to vasodilatory agents — thus contributing to increased vascular resistance.

Figure 21–52 depicts a hypothetical sequence of

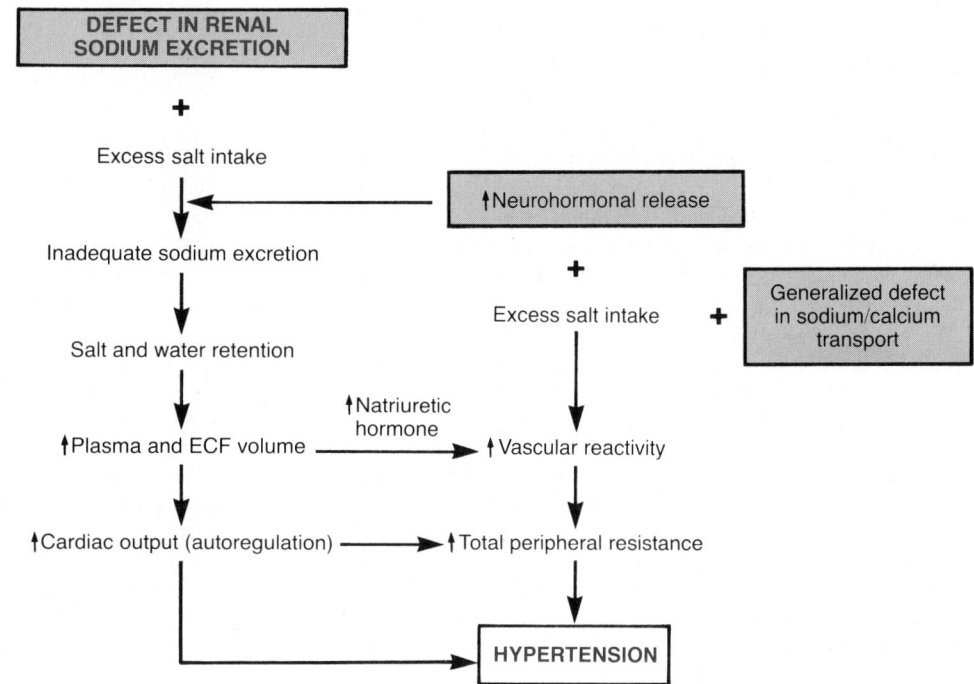

Figure 21–52. Hypothetical scheme for pathogenesis of essential hypertension implicating genetic defects in renal sodium excretion, or in sodium/calcium transport, or causing increased neurohormonal release — coupled with excess salt intake. Increased cardiac output and increased total peripheral resistance contribute to the hypertension.

events that is consistent with the mechanisms outlined. Essential hypertension is thus a complex disorder that may have more than one cause. It may be initiated by a disturbance in any of the factors that control normal blood pressure, many of which are environmental (stress, salt intake, estrogens) but act in the genetically predisposed individual. In established hypertension, both increased blood volume and increased peripheral resistance contribute to the increased pressure.

We shall now examine some of the renal vascular disorders associated with hypertension.

Benign Nephrosclerosis

Benign nephrosclerosis (BNS), the term used for the kidney of benign hypertension, is always associated with hyaline arteriolosclerosis. Some degree of BNS, albeit mild, is present at autopsy in many individuals over age 60. The frequency and severity of the lesions are increased in young age groups in association with hypertension and diabetes mellitus.

MORPHOLOGY. Grossly, the kidneys are either normal in size or moderately reduced to average weights between 110 and 130 gm. The cortical surfaces have a fine, even granularity that resembles grain leather (Fig. 21–53). On section, the loss of mass is due mainly to cortical narrowing.

The primary histologic characteristic of BNS is narrowing of the lumina of arterioles and small arteries, caused by thickening and hyalinization of the walls (Fig. 21–54*A*). Hyaline arteriolosclerosis occurs to some degree in normotensive individuals after the fifth decade, but it is more severe and frequent in patients with hypertension and diabetes mellitus. The hyaline material is composed of plasma proteins, lipids, and basement membrane material.

Consequent to the hyaline vascular narrowing, there is patchy ischemic atrophy, which consists of (1) foci of tubular atrophy and interstitial fibrosis and (2) a variety of glomerular alterations. The latter include collapse of glomerular basement membranes, deposition of collagen within Bowman's space, periglomerular fibrosis, and total sclerosis of glomeruli.

In addition to arteriolar hyalinization, the larger interlobular and arcuate arteries exhibit a characteristic lesion that consists of reduplication of the elastic lamina and increased fibrous tissue in the media, with consequent narrowing of the lumen. This change, called **fibroelastic hyperplasia,** often accompanies hyaline arteriolosclerosis and increases in severity with age and in the presence of hypertension.

It must be emphasized that renal biopsies of many patients with essential hypertension show no arteriolosclerosis. Thus, hyaline arteriolosclerosis cannot be the cause of hypertension. However, the possibility remains that the development of hyaline arteriolosclerosis may cause renal ischemia and may sustain or aggravate high blood pressure by activating the renin-angiotensin system.

Uncomplicated benign nephrosclerosis alone rarely causes renal insufficiency or uremia. There are usually moderate reductions in renal plasma flow, but the GFR is normal or slightly reduced. Occasionally, there is mild proteinuria. Patients with moderate degrees of benign nephrosclerosis appear to have lost an element of renal reserve and are thus more prone to develop azotemia in the face of volume depletion, surgical stress, or gastrointestinal hemorrhage. Renal failure may supervene in 1 to 5% of patients with severe, prolonged hypertension, but in most patients it results from the development of the malignant or accelerated phase of hypertension, discussed next.

Malignant Phase of Hypertension (Malignant Nephrosclerosis)

Malignant nephrosclerosis is the form of renal disease associated with malignant or accelerated phase of hypertension.[119] This dramatic pattern of hypertension may occasionally develop in previously normotensive individuals, but more often is superimposed on preexisting benign essential hypertension or on an underlying chronic renal disease, particularly glomerulonephritis or reflux nephropathy. It is also a frequent cause of death from uremia in patients with scleroderma (p. 204). Malignant hypertension is relatively uncommon, occurring in less than 5% of all patients with elevated blood pressure. In its pure form, it usually affects younger individuals, with a high preponderance in males and in blacks.

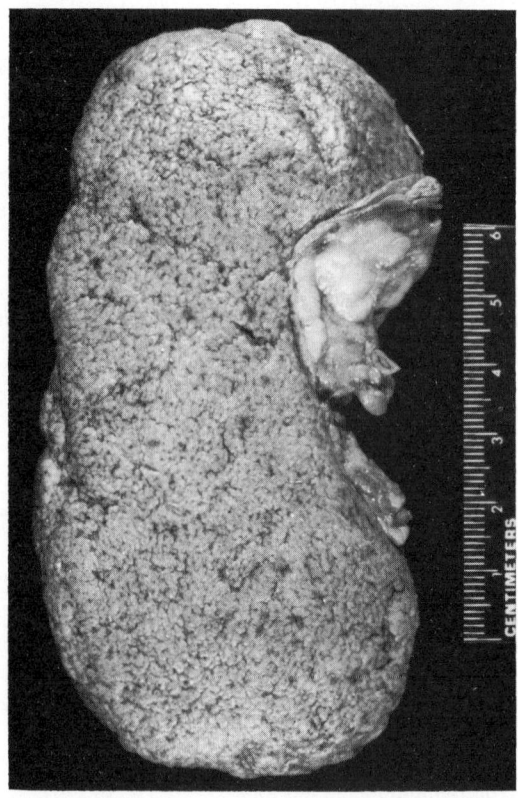

Figure 21–53. Benign nephrosclerosis illustrating fine granularity of surface.

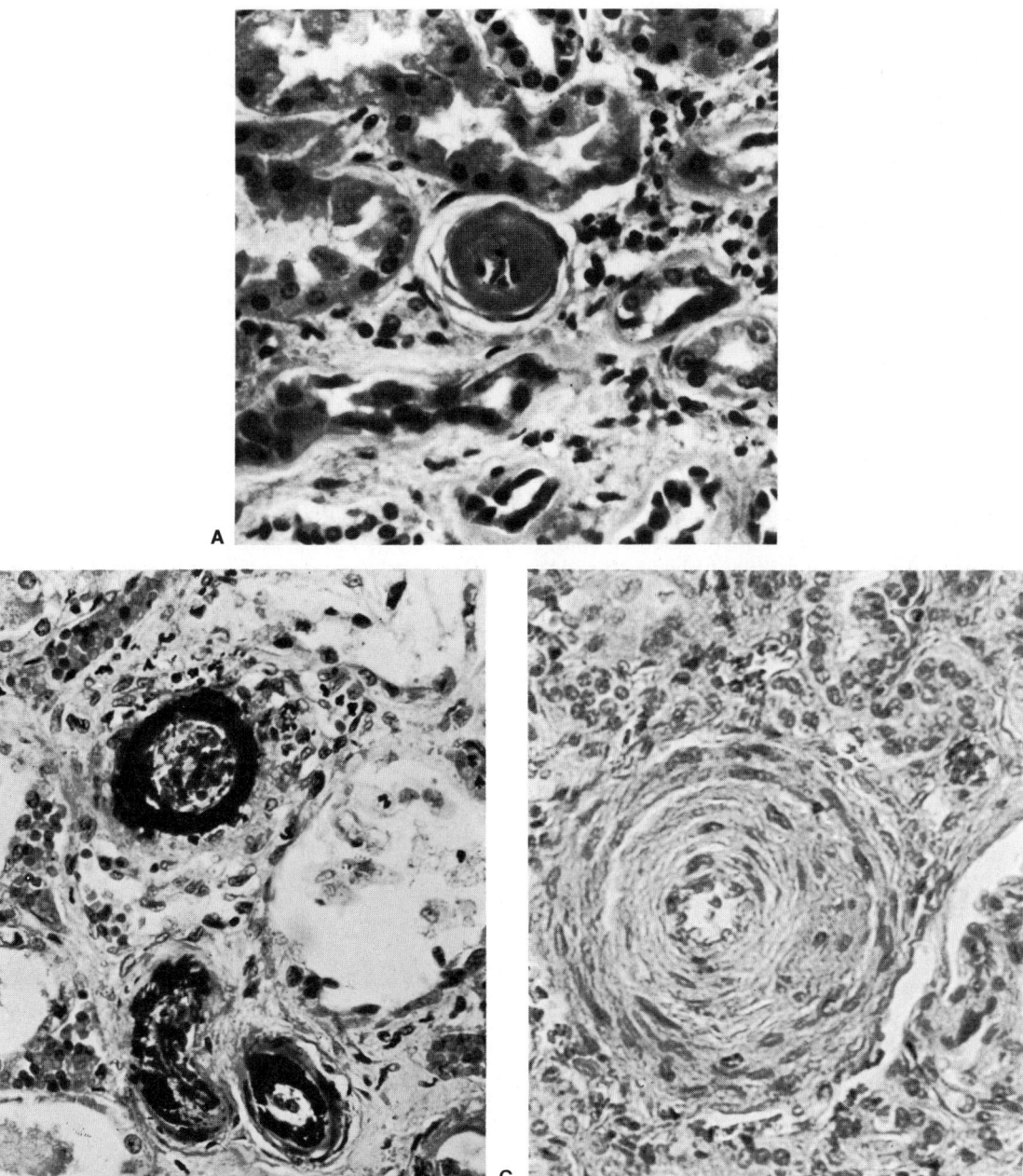

Figure 21–54. *A*, Hyaline arteriolosclerosis. Arteriolar wall is hyalinized and lumen is markedly narrowed. Note also interstitial fibrosis and tubular atrophy. *B*, Necrotizing arteriolitis of malignant nephrosclerosis with fibrinoid degeneration of walls of arterioles and small arteries. *C*, Hyperplastic arteriolitis of malignant hypertension (onionskinning).

MORPHOLOGY. Grossly, the kidney size is dependent on the duration and severity of the hypertensive disease. Small, pinpoint petechial hemorrhages may appear on the cortical surface from rupture of arterioles or glomerular capillaries, giving the kidney a peculiar "flea-bitten" appearance.

Two histologic alterations characterize malignant hypertension:

1. **Fibrinoid necrosis of arterioles.** This appears as an eosinophilic granular change in the blood vessel wall, which stains positively for fibrin by histochemical or immunofluo-

rescent techniques (Fig. 21–54*B*). In addition, there is often an inflammatory infiltrate within the wall, giving rise to the term **necrotizing arteriolitis.**

2. In the interlobular arteries and arterioles there is intimal thickening caused by a proliferation of elongated, concentrically arranged cells, smooth muscle cells, together with fine concentric layering of collagen. This alteration is known as **hyperplastic arteriolitis,** also referred to as "onionskinning" (Fig. 21–54*C*). The lesion correlates well with renal failure in malignant hypertension. Sometimes the glomeruli become necrotic and infiltrated with neutrophils, and

the glomerular capillaries may thrombose (**necrotizing glomerulitis**). The arteriolar and arterial lesions result in considerable narrowing of all vascular lumina, with ischemic atrophy and infarction distal to the abnormal vessels.

PATHOGENESIS. The rapidly mounting levels of arterial pressure often appear without any apparent cause. Malignant hypertension, however, is usually associated with remarkably high levels of renin, angiotensin, and aldosterone. Whatever the initial stimulus for the hyperreninemia, experimental studies suggest that vasoconstriction and the severe increases in blood pressure accentuate the vascular necrosis that occurs in arterioles of the kidney and other organs. Such an increase in blood pressure causes endothelial injury, platelet thrombosis, and intravascular coagulation; by producing ischemia, these perpetuate the vicious circle of hyperreninemia in malignant hypertension. Alternatively, the intravascular coagulation may well *initiate* the malignant phase; this view is suggested by the observation that intravascular coagulation in patients with microangiopathic hemolytic disorders *precedes* the appearance of increased blood pressure (p. 1070). Whatever the mechanism of malignant hypertension, the cause of the renal insufficiency is the profound ischemic change resulting from the arteriolar and arterial narrowing.

CLINICAL COURSE. The full-blown syndrome of malignant hypertension is characterized by diastolic pressures greater than 130 mm Hg, papilledema, encephalopathy, cardiovascular abnormalities, and renal failure. Most often, the early symptoms are related to increased intracranial pressure and include headaches, nausea, vomiting, and visual impairments, particularly the development of scotomas or spots before the eyes. "Hypertensive crises" are sometimes encountered, characterized by episodes of loss of consciousness or even convulsions. At the onset of rapidly mounting blood pressure, there is marked proteinuria and microscopic or sometimes macroscopic hematuria, but no significant alteration in renal function. Soon, however, renal failure makes its appearance. The syndrome is a true medical emergency requiring the institution of aggressive and prompt antihypertensive therapy before the development of irreversible renal lesions. Before introduction of the new antihypertensive drugs, malignant hypertension was associated with a 50% mortality rate within three months of onset, progressing to 90% within a year. At present, however, about 50% of patients will survive five years, and further progress is still being made. Ninety per cent of deaths are caused by uremia and others by cerebral hemorrhage or cardiac failure.

Renal Artery Stenosis

Unilateral renal artery stenosis is a relatively uncommon cause of hypertension, responsible for 2 to 4% of cases, but it is of importance because it is the most common curable form of hypertension, surgical treatment being successful in 70 to 80% of carefully selected cases in humans.[120] Furthermore, much of our knowledge of renal mechanisms in hypertension has come from studies of experimental and human renal artery stenosis.

The classical experiments of Goldblatt in 1934 showed that constriction of one renal artery in dogs results in hypertension, and that the magnitude of the effect is roughly proportional to the amount of constriction. Later experiments in rats confirmed these results, and in time it was shown that the hypertensive effect, at least initially, is due to stimulation of renin secretion by cells of the juxtaglomerular apparatus. A large proportion of patients with renovascular hypertension have elevated plasma or renal vein renin levels, and almost all show a reduction of blood pressure when given competitive antagonists of angiotensin II. Further unilateral renal renin hypersecretion can be normalized after renal revascularization, in association with a decrease in blood pressure. Other factors, however, play a role in the maintenance of renovascular hypertension, including sodium retention and, possibly, inhibition of medullary vasodepressor substances.[121]

The most common cause of renal artery stenosis (70% of cases) is occlusion by an atheromatous plaque at the origin of the renal artery. This lesion occurs more frequently in males, the incidence increasing with advancing age and diabetes mellitus. The plaque is usually concentrically placed, and superimposed thrombosis often occurs. The second type of lesion leading to stenosis is so-called **fibromuscular dysplasia** of the renal artery. This is a heterogeneous group of lesions characterized by fibrous or fibromuscular thickening and may involve the initima, the media, or the adventitia of the artery. These lesions are thus subclassified into intimal, medial, and adventitial hyperplasia—the medial type being by far the most common (Fig. 21–55). The stenoses, as a whole, are more common in females and tend to occur in younger age groups (i.e., in the third and fourth decades). The lesions may consist of a single well-defined constriction or a series of narrowings, usually in the middle or distal portion of the renal artery. They may also involve the segmental branches and may be bilateral. Fibromuscular dysplasia can often be differentiated from atherosclerotic stenosis by arteriography, as lesions tend to be segmental, with alternating segments of thickening and thinning of the vessels. The pathogenesis of the dysplasia is unknown.

The ischemic kidney is usually reduced in size and shows signs of diffuse ischemic atrophy, with crowded glomeruli, atrophic tubules, interstitial fibrosis, and focal inflammatory infiltrate. The juxtaglomerular apparatus may disclose hyperplasia and increased granularity. The arterioles in the ischemic kidney are usually protected from the effects of high pressure, thus showing only mild arteriolosclerosis, in contrast to the contralateral nonischemic kidney, which may exhibit hyaline arteriolosclerosis, depending on the severity of the preceding hypertension.

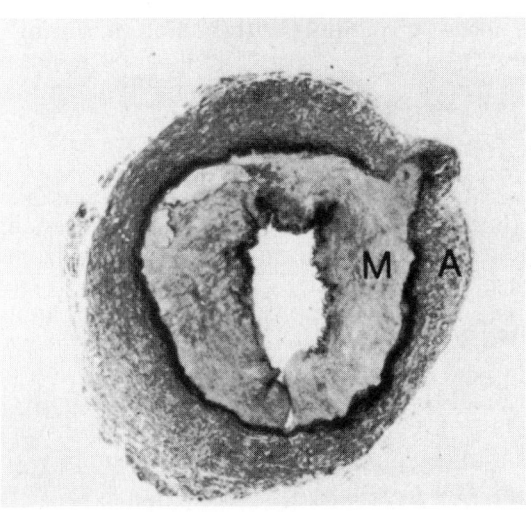

Figure 21–55. Fibromuscular dysplasia of renal artery, medial type (elastic tissue stain). Media shows marked fibrous thickening, and lumen is stenotic. M = media; A = adventitia. (Courtesy of Dr. Seymour Rosen, Beth Israel Hospital, Boston.)

CLINICAL COURSE. Few distinctive features suggest the presence of renal artery stenosis and, in general, these patients resemble those presenting with essential hypertension. Occasionally, a bruit can be heard on auscultation of the kidneys. *An intravenous pyelogram shows (1) a delay in the appearance of the contrast agent on the stenotic side,* owing to diminished blood flow and GFR; *(2) a small kidney,* owing to the ischemic atrophy and decreased blood volume; and *(3) delayed hyperconcentration of contrast material.* Arteriography is required to localize the stenotic lesion. Increased renin in the renal vein on the stenotic side and response to angiotensin antagonists favor a good outcome after surgical correction of the stenosis. In properly selected patients, the cure rate after surgery is about 90% in fibromuscular dysplasias and 60 to 75% in atherosclerotic stenosis.

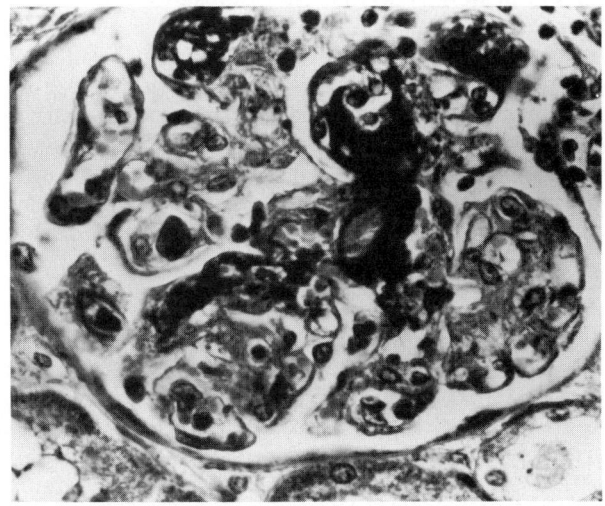

Figure 21–56. Thrombi *(center)* in glomerular capillaries characteristic of intravascular coagulation and microangiopathic disorders.

RENAL DISEASE ASSOCIATED WITH MICROANGIOPATHIC HEMOLYTIC ANEMIA

A group of diseases with overlapping clinical manifestations are characterized morphologically by thrombosis in the interlobular arteries, afferent arterioles, and glomeruli together with necrosis and thickening of the vessel walls (Fig. 21–56), and clinically by *microangiopathic hemolytic anemia, thrombocytopenia, renal failure, and manifestations of intravascular coagulation.* The morphologic changes are similar to those seen in malignant hypertension, but in these conditions they may precede development of hypertension or may be seen in its absence. The diseases include (1) childhood hemolytic uremic syndrome, (2) adult hemolytic uremic syndrome, (3) thrombotic thrombocytopenic purpura, and (4) scleroderma. Although these disorders may have diverse causes, *endothelial injury* and *intravascular coagulation* appear to be shared pathogenetic mechanisms.

Childhood Hemolytic Uremic Syndrome

Although relatively uncommon, this is one of the main causes of acute renal failure in children. It is characterized by the *sudden onset, usually after a gastrointestinal or flulike prodromal episode, of bleeding manifestations* (especially hematemesis and melena), *severe oliguria, hematuria, a microangiopathic hemolytic anemia, and (in some patients) prominent neurologic changes.* Hypertension is present in about half the patients. Up to 75% of patients are infected with *verocytotoxin-producing E. coli.*

The most important findings are in the kidney. Grossly, the kidneys may show patchy or widespread renal cortical necrosis. Microscopically, the glomeruli show thickening of capillary walls, due largely to endothelial and subendothelial swelling, and deposits of fibrin-related materials in the capillary lumina, subendothelially, and in the mesangium. Interlobular and afferent arterioles show fibrinoid necrosis and intimal hyperplasia and are often occluded by thrombi.

If the renal failure is managed properly with dialysis, mortality is limited to 10 to 15%, most patients experiencing complete recovery. In some patients, organization of the thrombi leads to chronic ischemia, and these individuals develop chronic renal insufficiency and hypertension. It is now thought that verocytotoxin plays a role in the pathogenesis of this disorder (p. 1070).

Adult Hemolytic Uremic Symdrome

A syndrome similar to that just described in children occurs in adults under a variety of settings:

1. In pregnant women with complications of pregnancy, such as placental hemorrhage or retained placental fragments.

2. In women in the postpartum period. This so-called *postpartum renal failure* usually occurs after an uneventful pregnancy, one day to several months following delivery, and is characterized by microangiopathic hemolytic anemia, oliguria, anuria, and initially mild hypertension. The condition has a grave prognosis, although in milder cases recovery may occur. The renal lesions are identical to those described in the childhood uremic syndrome.

3. In association with contraceptive agents. Women taking oral contraceptives have an increased risk of hypertension; in addition, both malignant nephrosclerosis and a typical hemolytic uremic syndrome develop with a greater frequency than in women not taking contraceptive agents.

4. In association with infection, such as typhoid fever, *E. coli* septicemia, viral infections, and shigellosis.

The clinical and morphologic features are more or less similar to those in children.

Thrombotic Thrombocytopenic Purpura

This entity, discussed earlier (p. 695), is manifested by fever, neurologic symptoms, hemolytic anemia, thrombocytopenic purpura, and the presence of thrombi in glomerular capillaries and afferent arterioles. The disease is more common in females, and most patients are under 40 years of age. The entity differs from hemolytic uremic syndrome in that central nervous system involvement is the dominant feature, whereas renal involvement occurs in only about 50% of patients. In addition, biochemical evidence of intravascular coagulation is uncommon. Histologically, eosinophilic granular thrombi are present predominantly in the terminal part of the interlobular arteries, afferent arterioles, and glomerular capillaries. The thrombi contain both platelets and fibrin and are found in arterioles of many organs throughout the body. Untreated, the disease was once highly fatal, but exchange transfusions and corticosteroid therapy have reduced mortality to less than 50%.

Pathogenesis of Microangiopathic Disorders

The fibrin deposition in small vessels, the presence of microangiopathic hemolytic anemia, and the biochemical abnormalities all point to the importance of disseminated intravascular coagulation (DIC). The lesions resemble those found in the generalized Shwartzman phenomenon, in which intravascular coagulation plays an important role. Current evidence points to endothelial injury as a major factor in initiating these pathologic events, particularly in HUS associated with gram-negative infections. Endotoxin activates endothelial cells to become thrombogenic, and the verocytotoxins of *E. coli* are cytotoxic to endothelial cells, both in vitro and in vivo. It is also possible that agents that predispose to the hemolytic uremic syndrome do so by inducing immunologic endothelial injury. Indeed, antibodies to endothelium are present in the serum of patients with hemolytic uremic syndrome.[123]

ATHEROEMBOLIC RENAL DISEASE

Embolization of fragments of atheromatous plaques from the aorta or renal artery into intraparenchymal renal vessels occurs in elderly patients with severe atherosclerosis, especially after surgery on the abdominal aorta, aortography, or intra-aortic cannulization.[124] These emboli can be recognized in the walls of arcuate and interlobular arteries by their content of cholesterol crystals, which appear as rhomboid clefts. The clinical consequences of atheroemboli vary according to the number of emboli and the preexisting state of renal function. Frequently, they have no functional significance. However, acute renal failure may result in elderly patients in whom renal function is already compromised, principally after abdominal surgery on atherosclerotic aneurysms. Chronic atheroembolization, with subsequent vascular fibrosis and narrowing, may cause foci of ischemic atrophy.

SICKLE CELL DISEASE NEPHROPATHY

Sickle cell disease in both the homozygous and heterozygous forms may lead to a variety of alterations in renal morphology and function, some of which, fortunately uncommonly, produce clinically significant abnormalities. The various manifestations are termed "sickle cell nephropathy."

The most common clinical and functional abnormalities are *hematuria* and a *diminished concentrating ability*. These are thought to be largely due to accelerated sickling in the hypertonic hypoxic milieu of the renal medulla, which increases the viscosity of the blood during its passage through the vasa recta, leading to plugging of vessels and decreased flow. Microangiographic studies of autopsied kidneys from patients with sickle cell disease disclose focal occlusions of the vasa recta, and functional studies show a diminished medullary blood flow. Patchy *papillary necrosis* may occur in both homozygotes and heterozygotes; this is sometimes associated with cortical scarring. *Proteinuria* is also common in sickle cell disease, occurring in about 30% of patients. It is usually mild to moderate, but on occasion the overt nephrotic syndrome arises, associated with a membranoproliferative glomerular lesion.

DIFFUSE CORTICAL NECROSIS

This is an uncommon condition that occurs most frequently following an obstetric emergency such as abruptio placentae (premature separation of the placenta), septic shock, or extensive surgery. When bilateral and symmetric, it is uniformly fatal, but patchy cortical necrosis may permit survival. The cortical destruction has all the earmarks of ischemic necrosis.

Glomerular and arteriolar microthrombi are found in some but by no means all cases; if present, they clearly contribute to the necrosis and renal damage. There are some authorities who believe that the primary lesion is a functional vasospasm of arteries and arterioles and that the intravascular coagulation is a secondary phenomenon. The two mechanisms, DIC and vasoconstriction, are not mutually exclusive and may act in concert or individually in specific cases.

> The gross alterations of the massive ischemic necrosis are sharply limited to the cortex (Fig. 21–57). The histologic appearance is that of acute ischemic infarction. The lesions may be patchy, with areas of apparently better preserved cortex. Intravascular and intraglomerular thromboses may be prominent but are usually focal, and occasionally acute necroses of small arterioles and capillaries may be present. Hemorrhages occur into the glomeruli, together with the precipitation of fibrin in the glomerular capillaries.

Massive acute cortical necrosis is of grave significance since it gives rise to sudden anuria, terminating rapidly in uremic death. Instances of unilateral or patchy involvement are compatible with survival.

RENAL INFARCTS

The kidneys are favored sites for the development of infarcts, as one fourth of the cardiac output passes through these organs. Although thrombosis in advanced atherosclerosis and the acute vasculitis of polyarteritis nodosa may occlude arteries, most infarcts are due to embolism. The major source of such emboli is mural thrombosis in the left atrium and ventricle as a result of myocardial infarction. Vegetative endocarditis, thrombosis in aortic aneurysms, and aortic atherosclerosis are less frequent sites for the origin of emboli.

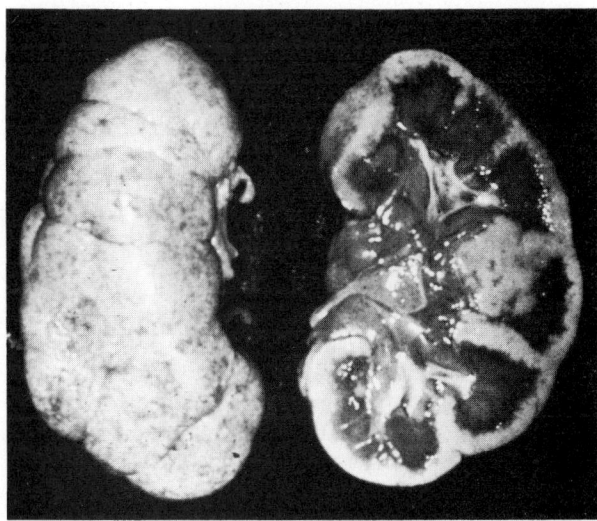

Figure 21–57. Diffuse cortical necrosis. Pale ischemic necrotic areas are confined to cortex and columns of Bertin.

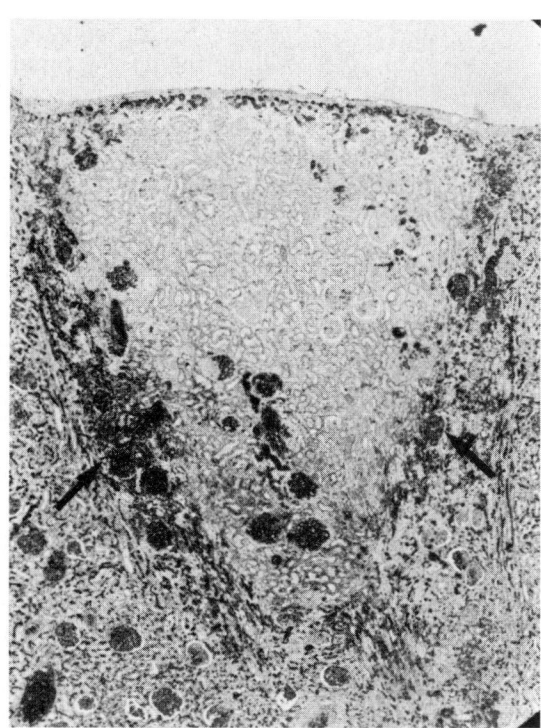

Figure 21–58. Renal infarction at low power, illustrating wedge shape, shadowy outlines of necrotic renal substances, and darker peripheral zone of leukocytic infiltration (arrows).

> Because the arterial supply to the kidney is of the "end-organ" type, most infarcts are of the "white" anemic type. They may occur as solitary lesions or be multiple and bilateral. Within 24 hours infarcts become sharply demarcated, pale, yellow-white areas that may contain small irregular foci of hemorrhagic discoloration. They are usually ringed by a zone of intense hyperemia.
>
> On section, they are wedge-shaped, with the base against the cortical surface and the apex pointing toward the medulla (Fig. 21–58). There may be a very narrow rim of preserved subcortical tissue that has been spared by the collateral capsular circulation. In time, these acute areas of ischemic necrosis undergo progressive fibrous scarring, giving rise to depressed, **pale, gray-white scars** that assume a V shape on section. The histologic changes in renal infarction have already been covered in Chapter 3.

Many renal infarcts are clinically silent. Sometimes, pain and tenderness localized to the costovertebral angle occurs, and this is associated with the showers of red cells in the urine. Large infarcts of one kidney are a well-known basis for hypertension.

URINARY TRACT OBSTRUCTION (OBSTRUCTIVE UROPATHY)

Recognition of urinary obstruction is important *because obstruction increases susceptibility to infection and to stone formation, and unrelieved obstruction al-*

most always leads to permanent renal atrophy, termed *hydronephrosis* or *obstructive uropathy.* Fortunately, many causes of obstruction are surgically correctable or medically treatable.

Obstruction may be sudden or insidious, partial or complete, unilateral or bilateral; it may occur at any level of the urinary tract from the urethra to the renal pelvis. It can be caused by lesions that are *intrinsic* to the urinary tract or *extrinsic* lesions that compress the ureter. The common causes are as follows[125] (Fig. 21–59):

1. *Congenital anomalies:* posterior urethral valves and urethral strictures, meatal stenosis, bladder neck obstruction; ureteropelvic junction narrowing or obstruction; severe vesicoureteral reflux.
2. *Urinary calculi.*
3. *Benign prostatic hypertrophy.*
4. *Tumors:* carcinoma of the prostate, bladder tumors, contiguous malignant disease (retroperitoneal lymphoma), carcinoma of the cervix or uterus.
5. *Inflammation:* prostatitis, ureteritis, urethritis, retroperitoneal fibrosis.
6. *Sloughed papillae or blood clots.*
7. *Normal pregnancy.*
8. *Functional disorders:* neurogenic (spinal cord damage with bladder paralysis) and other functional abnormalities of the ureter, bladder, and urethra (often termed *dysfunctional obstruction*).

Hydronephrosis is the *term used to describe dilatation of the renal pelvis and calyces associated with progressive atrophy of the kidney due to obstruction to the outflow of urine.* Even with complete obstruction, glomerular filtration persists for some time because the filtrate subsequently diffuses back into the renal interstitium and perirenal spaces, where it ultimately returns to the lymphatic and venous systems. Because of this continued filtration, the affected calyces and pelvis become dilated, often markedly so. The high pressure in the pelvis is transmitted back through the collecting ducts into the cortex, causing renal atrophy, but it also compresses the renal vasculature of the medulla, causing a diminution in inner medullary plasma flow. The medullary vascular defects are reversible, but if protracted, obstruction will lead to medullary functional disturbances. Accordingly, the initial functional alterations are largely tubular, manifested primarily by impaired concentrating ability. Only later does the GFR begin to diminish. Experimental studies indicate that serious irreversible damage occurs after about three weeks of complete obstruction and three months of incomplete obstruction.

MORPHOLOGY. When the obstruction is sudden and complete, the reduction of glomerular filtration usually leads to mild dilatation of the pelvis and calyces but sometimes to atrophy of the renal parenchyma. When the obstruction is subtotal or intermittent, glomerular filtration is not suppressed and progressive dilatation ensues. De-

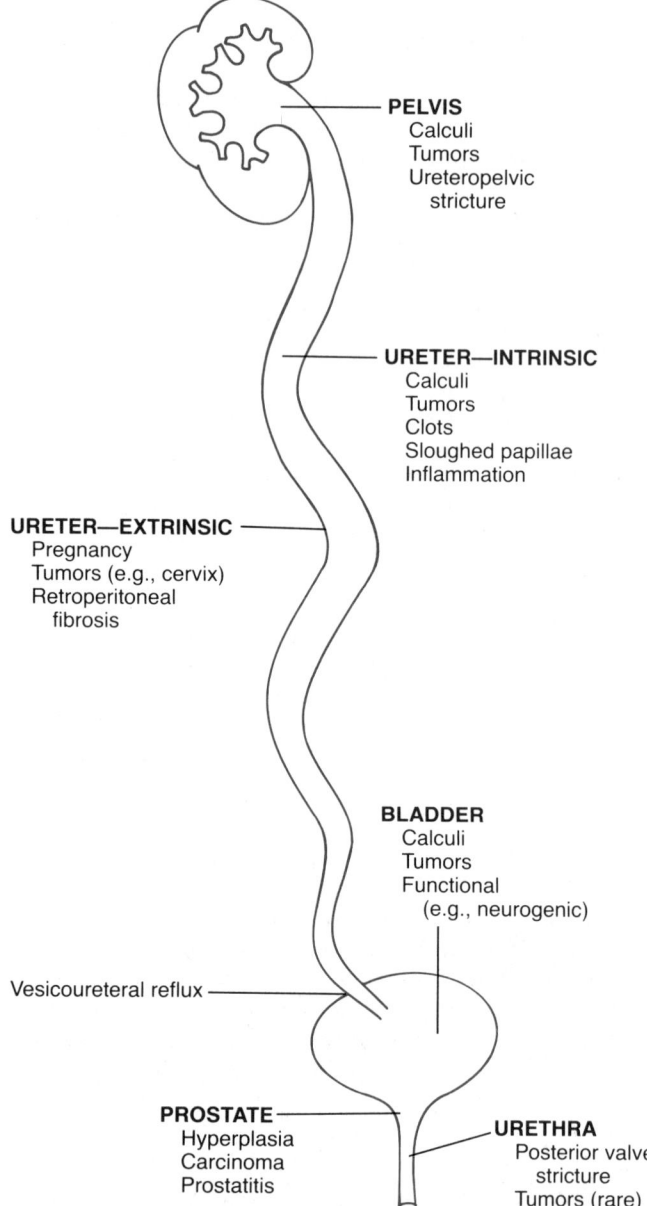

PELVIS
Calculi
Tumors
Ureteropelvic
stricture

URETER—INTRINSIC
Calculi
Tumors
Clots
Sloughed papillae
Inflammation

URETER—EXTRINSIC
Pregnancy
Tumors (e.g., cervix)
Retroperitoneal
fibrosis

BLADDER
Calculi
Tumors
Functional
(e.g., neurogenic)

Vesicoureteral reflux

PROSTATE
Hyperplasia
Carcinoma
Prostatitis

URETHRA
Posterior valve
stricture
Tumors (rare)

Figure 21–59. Obstructive lesions of the urinary tract.

pending on the level of urinary block, the dilation may affect first the bladder or ureter and then the kidney.

Grossly, the kidney may have slight-to-massive enlargement. The earlier features are those of simple dilatation of the pelvis and calyces. Histologically, the picture is one of cortical tubular atrophy with interstitial fibrosis. Progressive blunting of the apices of the pyramids occurs, and eventually these become cupped. In far-advanced cases, the kidney may become transformed into a thin-walled cystic structure having a diameter of up to 15 to 20 cm (Fig. 21–60) with striking parenchymal atrophy, total obliteration of the pyramids, and thinning of the cortex.

CLINICAL COURSE. *Acute obstruction* may provoke pain attributed to distention of the collecting system or renal capsule. Most of the early symptoms are produced by the basic cause of the hydronephrosis. Thus, calculi lodged in the ureters may give rise to renal colic, and prostatic enlargements to bladder symptoms.

Unilateral, complete, or partial hydronephrosis may remain silent for long periods of time, since the unaffected kidney can maintain adequate renal function. Sometimes its existence first becomes apparent in the course of intravenous pyelography. It is regrettable that this disease tends to remain asymptomatic, because it has been shown that in its very early stages, perhaps the first few weeks, relief of such obstruction is compatible with reversion to normal function. *Ultrasound* is a very useful noninvasive technique in the diagnosis of obstructive uropathy.

In *bilateral partial obstruction,* the earliest manifestations are those of inability to concentrate the urine, reflected by polyuria and nocturia. Some patients will have acquired distal tubular acidosis, renal salt wasting, and secondary renal calculi, *and a typical picture of tubulointerstitial nephritis* with scarring and atrophy of the papilla and medulla. Hypertension is common in such patients.

Complete bilateral obstruction results in oliguria or anuria and is incompatible with long survival unless the obstruction is relieved. Curiously, after relief of

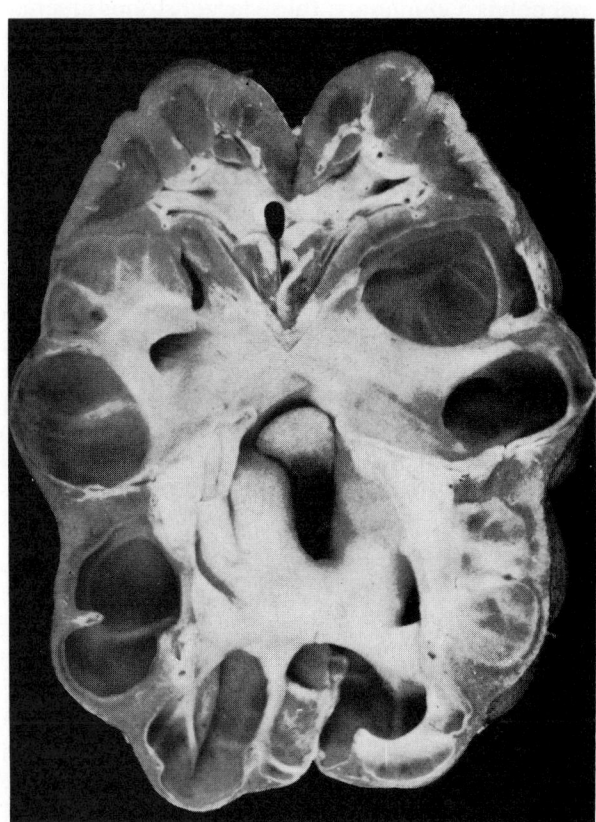

Figure 21–60. Hydronephrosis of kidney, with marked dilatation of pelvis and calyces and thinning of renal parenchyma.

Table 21–11. Types of Renal Stones

	PER CENT OF ALL STONES
Calcium oxalate (phosphate)	75
Idiopathic hypercalciuria (50%)	
Hypercalcemia and hypercalciuria (10%)	
Hyperoxaluria (5%)	
Enteric (4.5%)	
Primary (0.5%)	
Hyperuricosuria (20%)	
No known metabolic abnormality (25%)	
Struvite (Mg; NH$_3$; Ca; PO$_4$)	10–15
Renal infection	
Uric acid	6
Associated with hyperuricemia	
Associated with hyperuricosuria	
Idiopathic (50%)	
Cystine	1–2
Others or unknown	±10

complete urinary tract obstruction, postobstructive *diuresis* occurs. This can often be massive, with the kidney excreting large amounts of urine rich in sodium chloride. The diuresis is caused by (1) excretion of excess ECF retained during the period of obstruction ("unloading"), (2) effects of retained urea that act as a poorly reabsorbable solute, and possibly (3) an impaired response to antidiuretic hormone.[126]

UROLITHIASIS

Stones may form at any level in the urinary tract, but most arise in the kidney. Urolithiasis is a frequent clinical problem, with an annual incidence in the United States of 7 to 21 cases per 10,000 population.[127] From the clinical standpoint, it is said that seven to ten in every 1000 hospital admissions in the United States are for kidney stones. Males are affected more often than females, and the peak age of onset is between 20 and 30 years. Familial and hereditary predisposition to stone formation has long been known. Many of the inborn errors of metabolism, such as gout, cystinuria, and primary hyperoxaluria, provide good examples of hereditary disease characterized by excessive production and excretion of stone-forming substances.

CAUSE AND PATHOGENESIS. There are four types of calculi (Table 21–11): (1) *most stones (about 75%) are calcium-containing,* composed largely of calcium oxalate, or calcium oxalate mixed with calcium phosphate; (2) another 15% are so-called *"triple stones"* or *struvite stones,* composed of magnesium ammonium phosphate; (3) *6% are uric acid stones;* and (4) *1 to 2% are made up of cystine.* An organic matrix of mucoprotein, making up 1 to 5% of the stone by weight, is present in all calculi. Although there are many causes for the initiation and propagation of stones, *the most important determinant is an increased urinary concentration of the stones' constituents, such that it exceeds their solubility in urine (supersaturation).*[14,128] A *low* *urine volume* in some metabolically normal patients may also favor supersaturation.

Calcium oxalate stones (Table 21–11) are associated in about 10% of patients with both *hypercalcemia and hypercalciuria*, occasioned by hyperparathyroidism, diffuse bone disease, sarcoidosis, renal tubular acidosis, and other hypercalcemic states. About 50% have *hypercalciuria without hypercalcemia.* This so-called "idiopathic hypercalciuria" is thought to be caused by several factors, including hyperabsorption of calcium from the intestine (absorptive hypercalciuria) and an intrinsic impairment in renal tubular reabsorption of calcium (renal hypercalciuria). An inherited defect in calcium transport, related to an increase in calcium-magnesium ATPase activity, has recently been reported in these patients.[128a] Up to 20% of calcium-containing stones are associated with increased uric acid secretion (*hyperuricosuria*), with or without hypercalciuria. The mechanism of stone formation in this setting involves "nucleation" of calcium oxalate by uric acid crystals in the collecting ducts. Five per cent are associated with *hyperoxaluria*, either hereditary (primary oxaluria), or more commonly acquired by intestinal overabsorption in patients with enteric diseases. This so-called "enteric hyperoxaluria" also occurs in vegetarians, as much of their diet is rich in oxalates. *In 25% of patients with calcium stones, there is neither hypercalcemia nor hypercalciuria*, and stone formation remains unexplained (idiopathic calcium stone disease).

Magnesium ammonium phosphate stones are formed largely following infections by urea-splitting bacteria (such as Proteus and some staphylococci), which convert urea to ammonia. The resultant alkaline urine causes the precipitation of magnesium ammonium phosphate salts. These form some of the largest stones, as the amounts of urea excreted normally are huge (Fig. 21–61). Indeed, so-called *staghorn calculi* are almost always associated with infection.

Uric acid stones are common in patients with hyperuricemia, such as gout, and diseases involving rapid cell turnover, such as the leukemias. However, *more than half of all patients with urate calculi have neither hyperuricemia nor increased urinary excretion of uric acid.* In this group, it is thought that an unexplained tendency to excrete urine of pH below 5.5 may predispose to uric acid stones, as uric acid is insoluble in relatively acidic urine. In contrast to the radiopaque calcium stones, uric acid stones are radiolucent.

Cystine stones are associated with a genetically determined defect in the renal transport of certain amino acids, including cystine.

It can thus be appreciated that increased concentration of stone constituents, changes in urinary pH, decreased urine volume, and the presence of bacteria influence the formation of calculi. *However, many calculi occur in the absence of these factors, and conversely patients with hypercalciuria, hyperoxaluria, and hyperuricosuria often do not form stones.* It has, therefore, been postulated that changes in the urinary content of mucoproteins that form the organic matrix

of uroliths may be important or, alternatively, that there is a deficiency in inhibitors of crystal formation in urine. The list of such inhibitors is long, including pyrophosphate, diphosphonate, citrate, and a recently described glycoprotein called *nephrocalcin*, but no consistent deficiency of any of these substances has been demonstrated in stone formers.

> Stones are unilateral in about 80% of patients. The favored sites for their formation are within the renal calyces and pelves and in the bladder. If formed in the renal pelvis, they tend to remain small, having an average diameter of 2 to 3 mm. These may have smooth contours or may take the form of an irregular, jagged mass of spicules. Often, many stones are found within one kidney (Fig. 21–61A). Occasionally, progressive accretion of salts leads to the development of branching structures known as staghorn stones, which create a cast of the pelvic and calyceal system (Fig. 21–61B).

CLINICAL COURSE. Stones are of importance when they obstruct urinary flow or produce ulceration and bleeding. They may be present without producing any symptoms or significant renal damage. In general, smaller stones are most hazardous, as they may pass into the ureters, producing pain referred to as colic (one of the most intense forms of pain) as well as ureteral obstruction. Larger stones cannot enter the ureters and are more likely to remain silent within the renal pelvis. Commonly, these larger stones first manifest themselves by hematuria. Stones also predispose to superimposed infection, both by their obstructive nature and by the trauma they produce.

TUMORS OF THE KIDNEY

Both benign and malignant tumors occur in the kidney. In general, the benign tumors are incidental findings at autopsy and rarely have clinical significance. Malignant tumors, on the other hand, are of great importance clinically and deserve considerable emphasis.[129,130] By far the most common of these malignant tumors is renal cell carcinoma, followed by Wilms' tumor, which is found in children, and finally urothelial tumors of the calyces and pelves.

BENIGN

Cortical Adenoma

Small, discrete adenomas having origin in the renal tubules are found rather commonly (7 to 22%) at autopsy.

> These are usually under 2 cm in diameter. They are present invariably within the cortex and appear grossly as pale yellow-gray, discrete, seemingly encapsulated nodules. Microscopically, several variants are recognizable. Some tumors are composed of complex, branching, papil-

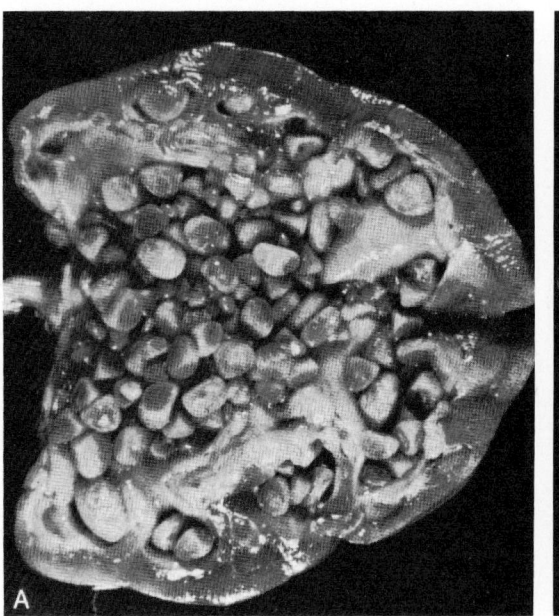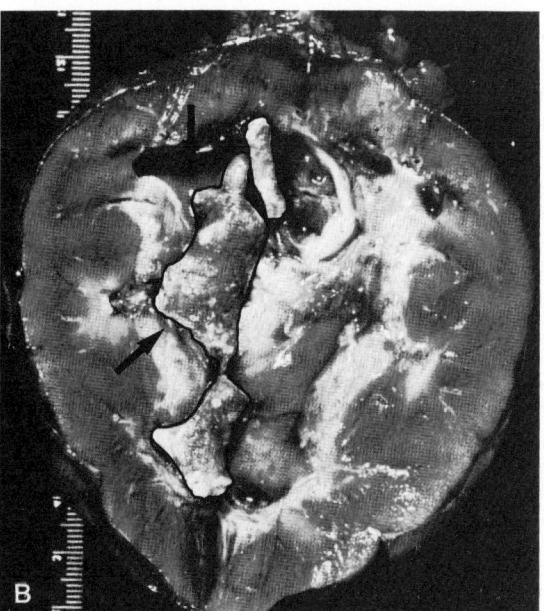

Figure 21–61. Nephrolithiasis, *A.* Multiple, somewhat rounded stones are present in expanded pelvis and calyces. Nephrolithiasis, *B.* A fractured stag-horn calculus *(arrows and outline)* is present in dilated pelvis.

lomatous structures with numerous complex fronds that project into a cystic space. In others, cells grow in tubules, glands, cords, and totally undifferentiated masses of cells.

The cell type for all these growth patterns is quite regular and free of atypia. The cells are cuboidal to polygonal in shape, have regular small, central nuclei, and have a cytoplasm that may be partially or totally filled with lipid vacuoles.

By histologic criteria, these tumors do not differ from renal cell adenocarcinoma. In this differential, the size of the tumor has been used as a diagnostic feature; tumors over 3 cm in diameter are likely to metastasize, whereas those under 3 cm rarely do. This is obviously useful as a rule of thumb only, because adenocarcinomas may arise from adenomas. In addition, although most renal adenomas are incidental findings at autopsy, some of borderline size (2 to 3 cm) may be detected clinically during angiography (usually to rule out renal artery stenosis) or surgery. It seems appropriate to consider and treat those of borderline size as early cancers.

Renomedullary Interstitial Cell Tumor (Renal Fibroma or Hamartoma)

Occasionally, at autopsy, small foci of gray-white firm tissue, usually under 1 cm in diameter, are found within the pyramids of the kidneys. Microscopic examination of these discloses fibroblast-like cells and collagenous tissue. Ultrastructurally, the cells have features of renal interstitial cells. The tumors have no malignant propensities and, contrary to previous views, are not associated with hypertension. Rarely, one finds small, gray, hamartomatous nodules within the renal substance, composed of abundant amounts of fibrous tissue, small cords of tubular cells, and prominent vessels.

Miscellaneous Benign Tumors

As might be anticipated, any other form of mesenchymal benign tumor may occur in the kidney, such as hemangioma and *angiomyolipoma.* The latter is thought to be a hamartomatous malformation consisting of vessels, smooth muscle, and fat. However, *angiomyolipomas are common in patients with tuberous sclerosis,* a disease characterized by lesions of the cerebral cortex that produce epilepsy and mental retardation, as well as a variety of skin abnormalities.

A rare but interesting tumor is the so-called *renin-producing juxtaglomerular cell tumor.* These tumors usually occur in younger individuals and are associated with hypertension. Histologically, they resemble *hemangiopericytomas* (p. 591), but granules similar to those in normal juxtaglomerular cells are seen with the electron microscope. Not all renin-secreting tumors are juxtaglomerular cell tumors, as *some renal cell carcinomas and Wilms' tumors have been shown to secrete renin.*

Oncocytoma is a benign epithelial tumor composed of large eosinophilic cells having small, rounded, benign-appearing nuclei. Ultrastructurally, the cells have numerous prominent mitochondria. The tumors are usually well encapsulated. However, they may achieve a large size (up to 12 cm in diameter) and thus should be differentiated from renal cell carcinomas.[131]

MALIGNANT

Renal Cell Carcinoma (Hypernephroma, Adenocarcinoma of Kidney)

Renal cell carcinomas represent about 1 to 3% of all visceral cancers and account for 85 to 90% of all renal cancers in adults. They occur most often in older individuals, usually in the sixth and seventh decades of life, showing a definite male preponderance in the ratio of 3 : 1. Because of their gross yellow color and the resemblance of the tumor cells to clear cells of the adrenal cortex, it was once thought that they arose from adrenal "rests," accounting for the term *hypernephroma*. It is now clear that these tumors arise from tubular epithelium and are therefore renal adenocarcinomas.

In laboratory animals, renal adenocarcinomas are readily induced by a variety of carcinogens, including chemical and viral agents, but few of these are potential carcinogens in humans. Epidemiologic studies show a greater frequency of adenocarcinoma of the kidney in cigarette, pipe, and cigar smokers. Genetic factors may play a role.[132] Nearly two thirds of patients with the von Hippel–Lindau syndrome develop bilateral, often multiple renal cell carcinomas.[133] Dominantly inherited aberrations in chromosomes 3 and 8 and in chromosomes 3 and 11 occur in some families with renal adenocarcinoma and similar translocations have been recently reported in sporadic cases.[134]

MORPHOLOGY. In its macroscopic appearance, the tumor is quite characteristic. It may arise in any portion of the kidney, but more commonly it affects the poles, particularly the upper one. Usually these neoplasms occur as solitary unilateral lesions. They are spherical masses, 3 to 15 cm in diameter, composed of bright yellow–gray-white tissue that distorts the renal outline. Commonly there are large areas of ischemic, opaque, gray-white necrosis, foci of hemorrhagic discoloration, and areas of softening. The margins are usually sharply defined and confined within the renal capsule (Fig. 21–62). However, small satellite nodules are often found in the surrounding substance, providing clear evidence of the aggressiveness of these lesions. As the tumor enlarges, it may bulge into the calyces and pelvis, and eventually may fungate through the walls of the collecting system to extend even into the ureter. One of the striking characteristics of this tumor is its tendency to invade the renal vein and grow as a solid column of cells within this vessel. Further extension produces a continuous cord of tumor in the inferior vena cava and even in the right side of the heart. Occasionally, the tumor grows through the capsule to invade the adrenal and perinephric fat.

Histologically the growth pattern varies from papillary to solid, trabecular (cordlike), or tubular (resembling tubules).[135] In any single tumor, all variations in patterns of growth may be present. The most common tumor cell type is the **clear cell,** having a rounded or polygonal shape and abundant clear cytoplasm (Fig. 21–63); the latter on special stains contains glycogen and lipids. Twelve per cent of carcinomas consist of **granular** cells, which have a moderately eosinophilic cytoplasm, and 14% grow as spindle-shaped cells resembling mesenchymal tumors. Nuclear atypia is highly variable and shows some correlation with prognosis. Most tumors are well differentiated (grades I and II), but some (grade IV) show marked nuclear atypia with formation of bizarre nuclei and giant cells (Fig. 21–64). The stroma is usually scanty but highly vascularized.

CLINICAL COURSE. The three classic diagnostic features of *costovertebral pain, palpable mass,* and *hematuria* unfortunately appear in only 10% of cases. The most reliable of the three is hematuria, which eventually appears in about 90% of cases. However, the hematuria is usually intermittent and may be microscopic; thus, the tumor may remain silent until it attains a large size. At this time, it gives rise to generalized constitutional symptoms such as fever, malaise, weakness, and weight loss. This pattern of asymptomatic growth occurs in many patients, so that the tumor may have reached a diameter of over 10 cm when it is discovered.

Renal cell carcinoma is classified as one of the great "mimics" in medicine, because it tends to produce a diversity of systemic symptoms not related to the kidney. In addition to the fever and constitutional symptoms mentioned earlier, renal cell carcinomas produce a number of paraneoplastic syndromes (p. 294), ascribed to abnormal hormone production, including *polycythemia, hypercalcemia, hypertension, feminization or masculinization, Cushing's syndrome, eosinophilia, leukemoid reactions,* and *amyloidosis.*

One of the common characteristics of this tumor is its *tendency to metastasize widely before giving rise to any local symptoms or signs.* In 25% of new patients with renal cell carcinoma, there is radiologic evidence of metastases at presentation. The most common loca-

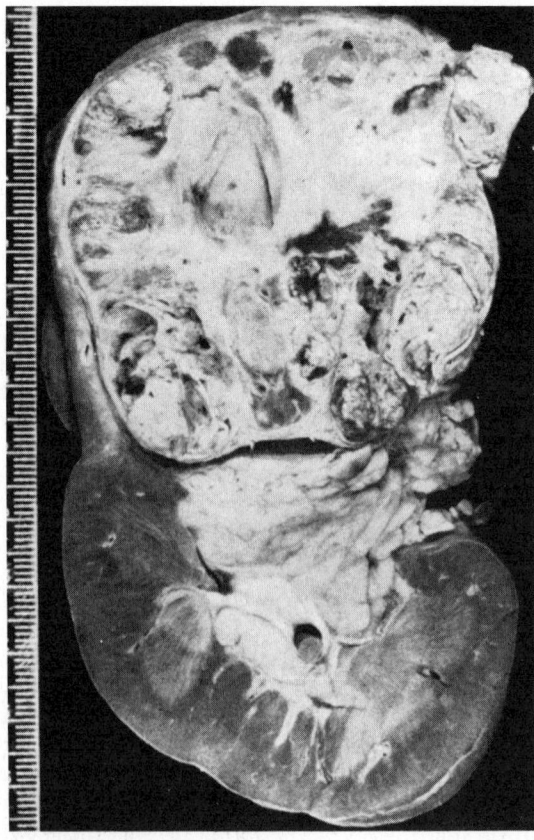

Figure 21–62. Renal cell carcinoma. Typical cross section of spherical neoplasm in one pole of kidney. Note necrosis and hemorrhages in tumor.

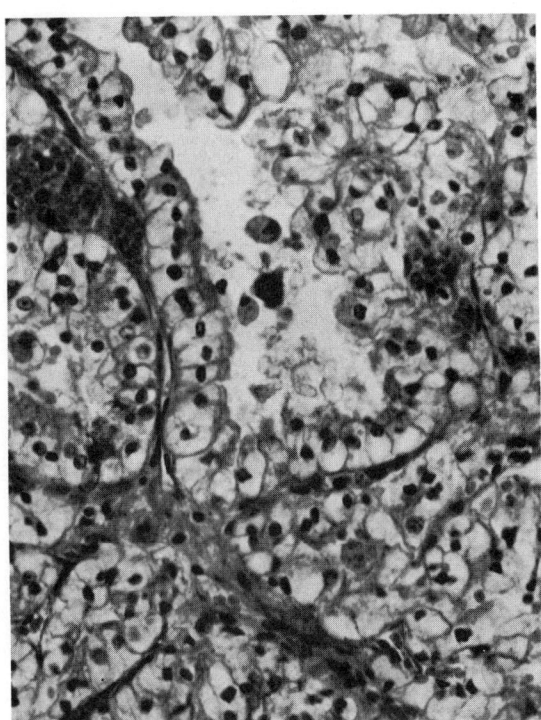

Figure 21–63. Renal cell carcinoma. Characteristic clear cell type.

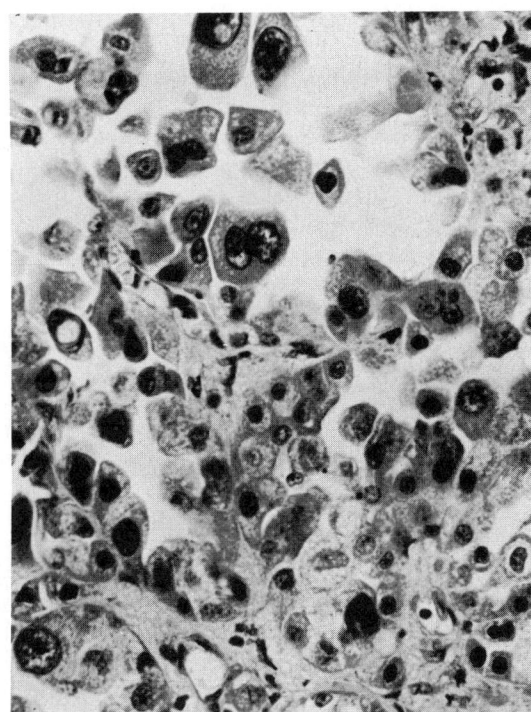

Figure 21–64. Renal cell carcinoma. Solid cell anaplastic variant.

tions of metastasis are the lungs (over 50%) and bones (33%), followed in order by the regional lymph nodes, liver and adrenals, and brain. In 10 to 15% of cases, the primary tumor metastasizes across the midline to the opposite kidney.

These tumors manifest some of the most bizarre growth behaviors in the realm of neoplasia. Sudden explosive growth with widespread metastasis is matched by slow, silent, asymptomatic growth for years. In a small number of cases, solitary metastases have occurred so that removal of the metastasis and the primary tumor has produced a cure. In still other instances, the metastases have mysteriously appeared in patients who have had nephrectomies 10 to 20 years before the discovery of the metastatic focus.

It is essential that renal cell carcinomas be diagnosed at the earliest possible stage, which is usually accomplished during the investigation of hematuria in a middle-aged or elderly patient. Renal ultrasonography, nephrotomography, CT scanning, and intravenous pyelography aid in the differential diagnosis of a simple cyst from a tumor. Urinary cytology may also be helpful in identifying tumor cells.

The average five-year survival of patients with renal cell carcinoma is about 45%, and up to 70% in the absence of distant metastases. With renal vein invasion or extension into the perinephric fat, the figure is reduced to approximately 15 to 20%. Nephrectomy is the treatment of choice.

Wilms' Tumor (Nephroblastoma)

This childhood tumor, derived from the renal blastema, consists of a mixture of primitive renal epithe-lial and stromal elements as well as heterologous tissues. Peak incidence is two to four years, but rare cases occur in adults. The tumor is characterized by a number of karyotypic defects, notably deletions in the short arm of chromosome 11, which may play a role in its pathogenesis.[136]

Grossly, these tumors are generally large, expansile, spherical masses that totally dwarf the kidney. In certain cases, they may grow so large as to produce distention of the abdomen and a readily observable mass on casual inspection. They are usually unilateral but, in 5 to 10% of cases, bilateral tumors are encountered. On section, these tumors have a very variegated surface dependent on the tissue types produced. Myxomatous, soft, fish-flesh areas; solid gray, hyaline cartilaginous tissue; and areas of hemorrhagic necrosis are the common components. They often invade the capsule and perirenal tissues.

Histologically, the tumor consists of nests and sheets of primitive blastema with intervening mesenchyme (Fig. 21–65). Abortive tubules are frequently seen with surrounding spindle cell stroma often having a sarcomatoid pattern. Abortive glomeruli may also be present. In addition, striated muscle, smooth muscle, collagenous fibrous tissue, cartilage, bone, fat cells, and areas of necrotic tissue containing cholesterol crystals and lipid macrophages may be seen. The degree of anaplasia in the stromal component generally correlates with prognosis.[137]

Most children with these neoplasms present with a large abdominal mass that may be unilateral or, when very large, may extend across the midline and down into the pelvis. Hematuria, pain in the abdomen following some hemorrhagic incident, intestinal obstruction, and the appearance of hypertension are other patterns of presentation. In a considerable number of these patients, pulmonary metastases are present at the time of primary diagnosis.

Up to the mid-1960s, the five-year survival of these patients was tragically low (10 to 40%), a tragedy rendered the more poignant because of the age of the patients. However, the combined use of chemotherapy, radiotherapy, and surgery has produced dramatic results in patients whose lesions were previously thought to be inoperable. Most large centers now report up to 90% long-term survivals if the tumors are available for primary treatment with the three modalities mentioned. Even recurrences can be successfully treated.

Urothelial Carcinomas of Renal Pelvis

Approximately 5 to 10% of primary renal tumors occur in the renal pelvis. These tumors span the range from apparently benign papillomas to frank papillary carcinomas but, as with bladder tumors, the benign papillomas are difficult to differentiate from the low-grade papillary cancers (p. 1092).

Renal pelvic tumors usually become clinically apparent within a relatively short time because they lie within the pelvis and, by fragmentation, produce noticeable hematuria. They are almost invariably small when discovered (Fig. 21–66). These tumors are almost never palpable clinically; however, they may block the urinary outflow and lead to palpable hydronephrosis and flank pain. Histologically, pelvic tumors are the exact counterpart of those found in the

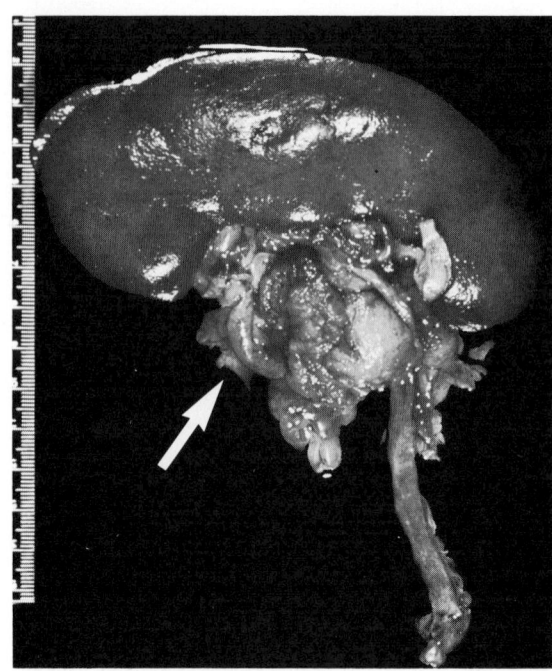

Figure 21–66. Urothelial carcinoma of renal pelvis. Pelvis has been opened to expose nodular irregular neoplasm *(arrow).*

urinary bladder; for further details, reference should be made to that section (p. 1092).

Occasionally, urothelial tumors may be multiple, involving the pelvis, ureters, and bladder. In 50% of renal pelvic tumors there is a preexisting or concomitant bladder urothelial tumor.[138] Histologically, there are also foci of atypia or carcinoma in situ in grossly normal urothelium remote from the pelvic tumor. All these facts point to a generalized "field" effect, caused by a carcinogenic influence on urothelium. There is a strikingly increased incidence of urothelial carcinomas of the renal pelvis and bladder in patients with analgesic nephropathy, but the precise carcinogen in these conditions is at present unknown.[139]

Infiltration of the wall of the pelvis and calyces is common, and renal vein involvement likewise occurs. For this reason, despite their apparent small, deceptively benign appearance, the prognosis for these tumors is not good. Five-year survivals vary from 50 to 70% for low-grade superficial lesions to 10% with high-grade infiltrating tumors.

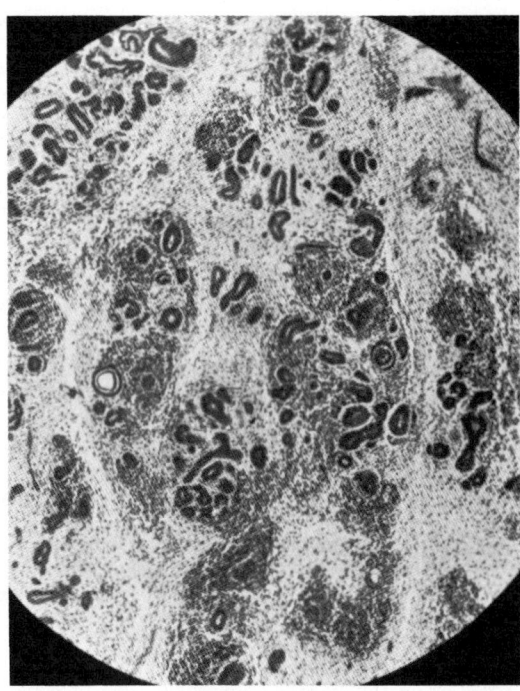

Figure 21–65. Wilms' tumor, illustrating sheets of primitive blastema with tubule formation surrounded by loose stroma.

1. Kriz, W., and Sakai, T.: Morphological aspects of glomerular function. *In* Davison, A. (ed.): Nephrology. Vol. 1. Philadelphia, W.B. Saunders Co., 1988, pp. 3–23.

2. Kanwar, Y.S., and Venkatachalam, M.A.: Morphology of the glomerulus and juxtaglomerular apparatus. *In* Handbook of Physiology, Section of Renal Physiology. 2nd ed. Washington, D.C., American Physiological Society (in press).

3. Price, R.G., and Hudson, B.G. (eds.): Renal Basement Membranes in Health and Disease. London, Academic Press, 1987.

4. Deen, W.M., et al.: Heterologous model of glomerular size selectivity: Application to normal and nephrotic humans. Am. J. Physiol. *249*:374, 1985.

5. Farquhar, M.G., et al.: Current knowledge of the functional architecture of the glomerular basement membrane. *In* Kuehn, R., et al. (eds.): New Trends in Basement Membrane Research. New York, Raven Press, 1982, pp. 57–71.

6. Rennke, H.G., et al.: Role of molecular charge in glomerular permeability. J. Cell Biol. *67*:638, 1975.

7. Cotran, R.S., and Rennke, H.G.: Anionic sites and the mechanisms of proteinuria. N. Engl. J. Med. *309*:1050, 1983.

8. Michael, A.F., et al.: The glomerular mesangium. Contrib. Nephrol. *40*:7, 1984.

9. Schlondorff, D.: The glomerular mesangial cell: An expanding role for a specialized pericyte. FASEB J. *1*:272, 1987.

10. Schreiner, G.F., and Cotran, R.S.: Localization of an Ia-bearing glomerular cell in the mesangium. J. Cell Biol. *94*:483, 1982.

11. Barajas, L., et al.: Pathology of the juxtaglomerular apparatus. *In* Tisher, C., and Brenner, B. (eds.): Renal Pathology with Clinical and Functional Correlations, Vol. I. Philadelphia, J.B. Lippincott, 1989, p. 877.

12. Bohman, S.-O.: The ultrastructure of the renal interstitium. *In* Cotran, R.S., et al. (eds.): Tubulo-interstitial Nephropathies. Contemporary Issues in Nephrology. Vol. 10. New York, Churchill Livingstone, 1983, pp. 1–34.

13. Krakauer, H.: The recent US experience in the treatment of end-stage renal disease by dialysis and transplantation. N. Engl. J. Med. *308*:1558, 1983.

14. Brenner, B.M., Coe, F., and Rector, F. (eds.): Clinical Nephrology. Philadelphia, W.B. Saunders Co., 1987.

15. Schrier, R.W., and Gottschalk, C.W. (eds.): Diseases of the Kidney. Boston, Little, Brown & Co., 1988.

16. Seldin, D., and Giebisch, G. (eds.): The Kidney. Physiology and Pathophysiology. New York, Raven Press, 1985.

17. Brenner, B.M., and Rector, F. (eds.): The Kidney. 4th ed. Philadelphia, W.B. Saunders Co., 1989.

18. Massry, S.G., and Glassock, R.J. (eds.): Textbook of Nephrology. 2nd ed. Baltimore, Williams & Wilkins, 1989.

19. Berstein, J.: A classification of renal cysts. *In* Gardner, K.D. (ed.): Cystic Diseases of the Kidney. New York, John Wiley & Sons, 1976, pp. 7–30.

20. Thompson, C.: The spectrum of renal cystic diseases. Hosp. Pract. *23*:165, 1988.

21. Gardner, K.D.: Pathogenesis of human cystic renal disease. Ann. Rev. Med. *39*:185, 1988.

22. Welling, L.W., and Grantham, J.J.: Cystic diseases of the kidney. *In* Tisher, C. and Brenner, B.M. (eds.): Renal Pathology with Clinical and Functional Correlations, Vol. II. Philadelphia, J.B. Lippincott, 1989, p. 1233.

23. Reeders, S.T., et al.: Two genetic markers closely linked to adult polycystic kidney disease on chromosome 16. Br. Med. J. *292*:851, 1986.

23a. Kimberling, W.J.: Linkage heterogeneity of autosomal dominant polycystic kidney disease. N. Engl. J. Med. *319*:914, 1988.

24. Hossack, K.F., et al.: Echocardiographic findings in autosomal dominant polycystic kidney disease. N. Engl. J. Med. *319*:907, 1988.

25. Carone, F.A., et al.: Basement membrane antigens in polycystic renal disease. Am. J. Pathol. *130*:466, 1988.

26. Bernstein, J., and Gardner, K.: Hereditary tubulo-interstitial nephropathies. Contemp. Issues Nephrol. *10*:335, 1983.

27. Cantini, A., et al.: Familial juvenile nephronophthisis: A review and differential diagnosis. Clin. Pediatr. Rev. *25*:90, 1986.

28. Grantham, J.J., and Levine, E.: Acquired cystic disease: Replacing one kidney disease with another. Kidney Int. *28*:99, 1985.

29. Hoedemaeker, Ph.J.: Experimental glomerulonephritis. *In* Davison, A.M. (ed.): Nephrology. Vol. 1. Philadelphia, W.B. Saunders Co., 1988, pp. 409–440.

30. Wilson, C., and Dixon, F.: The renal response to immunologic injury. *In* Brenner, B.M., and Rector, F. (eds.): The Kidney. 3rd ed. Philadelphia, W.B. Saunders Co., 1986, pp. 800–891.

31. Saus, J., et al.: Identification of the Goodpasture antigen as the alpha 3(IV) chain of collagen IV. J. Biol. Chem. *263*(26):13374, 1988.

32. Kerjaschki, D., and Farquhar, M.: The pathogenic antigen of Heymann nephritis is a membrane glycoprotein of the renal proximal tubule brush border. Proc. Natl. Acad. Sci. USA *79*:5557, 1982.

33. Andres, G., et al.: Formation of immune deposits and disease. Lab. Invest. *55*:550, 1986.

34. Goldman, M., et al.: Polyclonal activation and experimental nephropathies. Kidney Int. *34*:141, 1988.

35. Gallo, G.R., et al.: Nephrogenicity and differential distribution of glomerular immune complexes related to immunogen charge. Lab. Invest. *48*:353, 1983.

36. Wilson, C.B., et al.: Selective glomerular cell injury–antimesangial cell antibodies. *In* Davison, A.M. (ed.): Nephrology. Vol. 1. Philadelphia, W.B. Saunders Co., 1988, pp. 509–522.

37. Matsuo, S., et al.: Glomerulonephritis induced in the rabbit by antiendothelial antibodies. J. Clin. Invest. *79*(6):1798, 1987.

38. Mendrick, D.L., and Rennke, H.G.: Induction of proteinuria in the rat by a monoclonal antibody against SGP-115/107. Kidney Int. *33*:818, 1988.

39. Schreiner, G.F., et al.: Macrophages and cellular immunity in experimental glomerulonephritis. Semin. Immunopathol. *5*:251, 1982.

40. Nolasco, F.G., et al.: Intraglomerular T cells and monocytes in nephritis: Study with monoclonal antibodies. Kidney Int. *31*:1160, 1987.

41. Johnson, R.J., et al.: Participation of the myeloperoxidase-(H_2O_2)-halide system in immune complex nephritis. Kidney Int. *32*:342, 1987.

42. Shah, S.V., Baricos, W.H., and Basci, A.: Degradation of human glomerular basement membrane by stimulated neutrophils. J. Clin. Invest. *79*:25, 1987.

43. Lovett, D., et al.: Activation of glomerular mesangial cells by the terminal membrane attack complex of complement. J. Immunol. *138*:2473, 1987.

44. Lovett, D.F., and Sterzel, R.B.: Cell culture approaches to the analysis of glomerular inflammation. Kidney Int. *30*:246, 1986.

45. Tipping, P.G., Worthington, L.A., and Holdsworth, S.R.: Quantitation and characterization of glomerular procoagulant activity in experimental glomerulonephritis. Lab. Invest. *56*:155, 1987.

46. Olson, J.L., and Heptinstall, R.H.: Non-immunologic mechanisms of glomerular injury. Lab. Invest. *59*:564, 1988.

47. Rennke, H.G.: Structural alterations associated with glomerular hyperfiltration. *In* Mitch, W.E., et al. (eds.): The Progressive Nature of Renal Disease. New York, Churchill Livingstone, 1986, p. 111.

48. Klahr, S., et al.: The progression of renal disease. N. Engl. J. Med. *318*:1657, 1988.

49. Vogt, A., et al.: Cationic antigens in post-streptococcal glomerulonephritis. Clin. Nephrol. *20*:271, 1983.

50. Fillit, H., and Zabriskie, J.B.: Cell-mediated immunity in glomerulonephritis. Am. J. Pathol. *109*:225, 1982.

51. Couser, W.G.: Rapidly progressive glomerulonephritis. Classification, pathogenetic mechanisms, and therapy. Am. J. Kidney Dis. *11*:449, 1988.

52. Glassock, R.J., et al.: Primary glomerular disease. *In* Brenner, B.M., and Rector, F.C., Jr. (eds.): The Kidney. 3rd ed. Philadelphia, W.B. Saunders Co., 1986, pp. 929–1013.

53. Downie, G.H., et al.: Experimental anti-alveolar basement membrane mediated injury. J. Immunol. *129*:2647, 1982.

54. Yamamoto, T., and Wilson, C.D.: Binding of anti-basement membrane antibody to alveolar basement membrane after intratracheal instillation in rabbits. Am. J. Pathol. *126*:497, 1987.

55. Kefalides, N.A.: The Goodpasture antigen and basement membranes. Lab. Invest. *56*:1, 1987.

56. Lewis, E.J., and Schwartz, M.M.: Idiopathic crescentic GN. Sem. Nephrol. *2*:193, 1982.

57. Brenner, B.M., and Stein, J.H. (eds.): Nephrotic Syndrome. Contemporary Issues in Nephrology. Vol. 9. New York, Churchill Livingstone, 1982.

58. Kaysen, G.A.: Hyperlipidemia in the nephrotic syndrome. Am. J. Kidney Dis. *12*:548, 1988.

59. Arnaout, M.A., et al.: Membranous glomerulonephritis. Contemporary Issues in Nephrology. *9*:199, 1982.

60. Alpers, C., and Cotran, R.S.: Neoplasia and glomerular injury. Kidney Int. *30*:465, 1986.

61. Couser, W.G., and Abrass, C.K.: Pathogenesis of membranous nephropathy. Ann. Rev. Med. *39*:517, 1988.

62. Davison, A.M., et al.: The natural history of renal function in

untreated idiopathic membranous GN in adults. Clin. Nephrol. *22*:61, 1984.

63. Habib, R., and Kleinknecht, C.: The primary nephrotic syndrome of childhood: Classification and clinicopathologic study of 406 cases. Pathol. Annu. *6*:417, 1971.

63a. Relman, A.S.: What have we learned about the treatment of idiopathic membranous nephropathy with steroids? (Editorial). N. Engl. J. Med. *320*:248, 1989.

64. Grupe, W.E.: Minimal change disease. Semin. Nephrol. *2*:241, 1982.

65. Seiler, M.W., et al.: Pathogenesis of polycation-induced alterations of glomerular epithelium. Lab. Invest. *36*:48, 1977.

65a. Korbet, S.M., et al.: Minimal change glomerulopathy of adulthood. Am J. Nephrol. *8*:291, 1988.

66. Goldzer, R.H., et al.: Focal segmental glomerulosclerosis. Annu. Rev. Med. *35*:429, 1984.

67. Bourgoigne, E.T., et al.: The nephropathy related to acquired immune deficiency syndrome. Adv. Nephrol. *17*:113, 1988.

68. Rosen, S., et al.: Progress in human pathology: Glomerular disease. Hum. Pathol. *12*:964, 1981.

69. Border, W.A.: Distinguishing minimal-change disease from mesangial disorders. Kidney Int. *34*:419,1988.

70. Cohen, A., et al.: HIV-associated nephropathy: Direct viral infection of the kidneys? Lab. Invest. *58*:19A, 1988.

71. Donadio, J.V., and Holley, K.E.: Membranoproliferative glomerulonephritis. Semin. Nephrol. *2*:204, 1982.

72. Kim, Y., et al: Idiopathic membranoproliferative glomerulonephritis. Contemporary Issues in Nephrology. *29*:237, 1982.

73. Schreiber, R.D., and Muller-Eberhard, H.J.: Complement and renal disease. *In* Zabriskie, J.B., et al. (eds.): Clinical Immunology of the Kidney. New York, John Wiley & Sons, 1982, pp. 77–108.

74. Clarkson, A.R. (ed.): IgA Nephropathy. Boston, Martinus Nijhoff, 1987.

75. Julian, B.A. (ed.): IgA Nephropathy—a national symposium. Am. J. Kidney Dis. *12*:337, 1988.

75a. Julian, B.A., et al.: Familial clustering and immunogenetic aspects of IgA nephropathy. Am. J. Kidney Dis. *12*:366, 1988.

76. Emancipator, S.N., and Lamm, M.E..: IgA nephropathy: Pathogenesis of the most common form of glomerulonephritis. Lab. Invest. *60*(2):168, 1989.

77. Hill, G.S.: Systemic lupus erythematosus and mixed connective tissue disease. *In* Heptinstall, R.H. (ed.): Pathology of the Kidney. Boston, Little, Brown & Co., 1983, pp. 839–906.

78. Levy, M., et al.: Anaphylactoid purpura nephritis in childhood: Natural history and immunopathology. Adv. Nephrol. *6*:183, 1976.

79. Bloodworth, J.M.B., Jr., and Greider, M.H.: The endocrine pancreas and diabetes mellitus. *In* Bloodworth, J.M.B., Jr. (ed.): Endocrine Pathology. Baltimore, Williams & Wilkins Co., 1982, pp. 556–722.

80. Osterby, R., and Gundersen, H.G.: Glomerular size and structure in diabetes mellitus. Diabetologica *11*:225, 1975.

81. Kanwar, Y.S., et al.: Decreased *de novo* synthesis of glomerular proteoglycans in diabetes: Biochemical and autoradiographic evidence. Proc. Natl. Acad. Sci. U.S.A. *80*:2272, 1983.

82. Cagliero, E., et al.: Increased expression of basement membrane components in human endothelial cells cultured in high glucose. J. Clin. Invest. *82*:735, 1988.

83. Anderson, S., and Brenner, B.M.: Pathogenesis of diabetic glomerulopathy. Hemodynamic considerations. Diabetes Metab. Rev. *4*:163, 1988.

84. Kreisberg, J.I.: Insulin requirement for contraction of cultured rat glomerular mesangial cells in response to angiotensin II: A possible role for insulin in modulating glomerular hemodynamics. Proc. Natl. Acad. Sci. U.S.A. *79*:4190, 1982.

85. Krowleski, A.S., et al.: Predisposition to hypertension and susceptibility to renal disease in insulin-dependent diabetes mellitus. N. Engl. J. Med. *318*:141, 1988.

86. Venkataseshan, V.H., et al.: Morphologic variants of eight-chain deposit disease in the kidney. Am. J. Nephrol. *8*:273, 1988.

87. Grunfeld, J.P.: The clinical spectrum of hereditary nephritis. Kidney Int. *27*:83, 1985.

87a. Grunfeld, J.P., et al.: Advances in the understanding of inherited renal diseases. *In* Davison, A.M. (ed.): Nephrology. Vol. 1. Philadelphia, W.B. Saunders Co., 1988, pp. 409–440.

88. Brummer, H., et al.: Localization of the gene for X-linked Alport's syndrome. Kidney Int. *34*:507, 1988.

88a. Savage, C.O.S., et al.: The Goodpasture's antigen in Alport's syndrome: Studies with monoclonal antibodies. Kidney Int. *30*:107, 1986.

89. Brezis, M., et al.: Acute renal failure. *In* Brenner, B.M., and Rector, F. (eds.): The Kidney. 4th ed. Philadelphia, W.B. Saunders Co., 1986, pp. 735–799.

90. Oliver, J., et al.: The pathogenesis of acute renal failure associated with traumatic and toxic injury, renal ischemia, nephrotoxic damage, and the ischemic episode. J. Clin. Invest. *30*:1307, 1951.

91. Solez, K.: The pathogenesis of acute renal failure. Int. Rev. Exp. Pathol. *24*:278, 1983.

92. Heyman, S.N., et al.: Acute renal failure with selective medullary injury in the rat. J. Clin. Invest. *82*:401, 1988.

93. Couger, J.D., et al.: Smooth muscle calcium and endothelium-derived relaxation factor in the abnormal vascular responses of acute renal failure. J. Clin. Invest. *82*:532, 1988.

93a. Firth, J.D., et al.: Endothelin: an important factor in acute renal failure? Lancet *2*:1179, 1988.

94. Anderson, R.J., and Schier, R.W.: Clinical spectrum of oliguric and nonoliguric acute renal failure. *In* Brenner, B.M., and Stein, J.H. (eds.): Acute Renal Failure. Contemporary Issues in Nephrology. Vol. 6. New York, Churchill Livingstone, 1980, pp. 1–16.

95. Cotran, R.S., et al.: Tubulo-interstitial nephropathies. *In* Brenner, B.M., and Rector, F. (eds.): The Kidney. 3rd ed. Philadelphia, W.B. Saunders Co., 1986, pp. 1143–1173.

96. Rubin, R., et al.: Urinary tract infection, pyelonephritis and reflux nephropathy. *In* Brenner, B.M., and Rector, F. (eds.): Philadelphia, W.B. Saunders Co., The Kidney, 4th ed. 1989 (in press).

97. Kunin, C.M.: Detection, Prevention and Management of Urinary Tract Infections. 4th ed. Philadelphia, Lea & Febiger, 1987.

98. Hodson, C.J., and Cotran, R.S.: Vesicoureteral reflux, reflux nephropathy, and chronic pyelonephritis. *In* Cotran, R.S., et al. (eds.): Tubulo-interstitial Nephropathies. Contemporary Issues in Nephrology. Vol. 10. New York, Churchill Livingstone, 1983, pp. 83–120.

98a. Hodson, C.J., et al. (eds.): Reflux nephropathy update. Contrib. Nephrol. *39*:1, 1984.

99. Chapman, C.J., et al.: Vesicoureteral reflux. Segregation analysis. Am. J. Med. *20*:577, 1985.

99a. Jorgensen, T.M.: Pathogenetic factors in vesicoureteral reflux. Neurourol. Urodyn. *5*:153, 1986.

100. Goodman, M., et al.: Xanthogranulomatous pyelonephritis (XGP): A local disease with systemic manifestations: Report of 23 patients and review of the literature. Medicine *58*:171, 1979.

101. Cotran, R.S.: Glomerulosclerosis in reflux nephropathy. Kidney Int. *21*:528, 1982.

102. Appel, G.B., and Kunis, C.L.: Acute tubulo-interstitial nephritis. Contemp. Issues Nephrol. *10*:151, 1983.

102a. Adler, S., et al.: Hypersensitivity phenomena and the kidney. Role of drugs and environmental agents. Am. J. Kidney Dis. *5*:75, 1985.

103. Kincaid-Smith, P.: Analgesic abuse and the kidney. Kidney Int. *17*:250, 1980.

103a. Kincaid-Smith, P.: Analgesic nephropathy. Aust. N.Z. J. Med. *18*:251, 1988.

104. Gonwa, T.A., et al.: Chronic renal failure and end-stage renal disease in northwest North Carolina. Importance of analgesic-associated nephropathy. Arch. Intern. Med. *141*:462, 1981.

105. Bengtsson, U., et al.: Malignancies of the urinary tract and their relation to analgesic abuse. Kidney Int. *13*:107, 1978.

106. Wedeen, R.P., and Batuman, V.: Tubulointerstitial nephritis induced by heavy metals and metabolic disturbances. *In* Cotran, R.S., et al. (eds.): Tubulo-interstitial Nephropathies. Contemporary Issues in Nephrology. Vol. 10. New York, Churchill Livingstone, 1983, pp. 212–241.

107. Pirani, C.L., et al.: Tubulo-interstitial disease in multiple myeloma and other nonrenal neoplasias. Contemp. Issues Nephrol. *10*:287, 1983.

108. Hill, G.S., et al.: Renal lesions in multiple myeloma: Their relationship to associated protein abnormalities. Am. J. Kidney Dis. *2*:423, 1983.

109. Bannister, K.M.: Immunological mechanisms in experimental

models of TIN. *In* Davison, A.M. (ed.): Nephrology, Vol. 1. Philadelphia, W.B. Saunders Co., 1988, pp. 618–634.

110. McCluskey, R.T.: Immunologically mediated tubulo-interstitial nephritis. *In* Cotran, R.S., et al. (eds.): Tubulo-interstitial Nephropathies. Contemporary Issues in Nephrology. Vol. 10. New York, Churchill Livingstone, 1983, pp. 121–150.

111. Arruda, J.A.L.: Radiation nephritis. *In* Cotran, R.S., et al. (eds.): Tubulo-interstitial Nephropathies. Contemporary Issues in Nephrology. Vol. 10. New York, Churchill Livingstone, 1983, pp. 275–286.

112. Kaplan, N.M.: Systemic hypertension: Mechanisms and diagnosis. *In* Braunwald, E. (ed.): Heart Disease. 3rd ed. Philadelphia, W.B. Saunders Co., 1988, pp. 819–861.

113. Skeggs, L.T.: Current concepts and historical perspectives of renal pressor mechanisms. J. Hypertens. (Suppl.) *4*:53, 1986.

114. Gayton, A.C., et al.: Current concepts and perspectives of renal volume regulation in relationship to hypertension. J. Hypertens. (Suppl.) *4*:547, 1986.

115. Olmer, M., et al. (eds.): Electrolytes, hormones and blood pressure. Kidney Int. *34* (Suppl. 25):S1, 1988.

116. Genest, J., and Cantin, M.: Atrial natriuretic factor. Circulation *75*(Suppl. 1):118, 1987.

117. Muirhead, E.E., et al.: Renal medullary system of blood pressure control. J Hypertens. (Suppl.) *4*:527, 1986.

118. Guyton, A.C., et al.: A systems analysis approach to understanding long-range arterial blood pressure control and hypertension. Circ. Res. *35*:159, 1974.

119. Perez-Grovas, H., and Herrera-Acosta, J.: Mechanism and treatment of malignant hypertension. Semin. Nephrol. *11*(5):416, 1988.

120. Dzau, V.J., et al.: Renovascular hypertension: An update on pathophysiology, diagnosis and treatment. Am. J. Nephrol. *3*:172, 1983.

121. Swales, J.D., et al.: Renovascular hypertension. Role of the renal medulla in pathogenesis and reversal. *In* Davison, A. (ed.): Nephrology, Vol. II. Philadelphia, W.B. Saunders Co., 1988, p. 917.

122. Drummond, K.N.: Hemolytic uremic syndrome. Then and now. N. Engl. J. Med. *312*:116, 1985.

122a. Richardson, S.E.: Hemolytic uremic syndrome associated with verocytotoxin-producing E. coli infections. Hum. Pathol. *19*:1102, 1988.

123. Leung, D.Y., et al.: Lytic anti-endothelial cell antibodies in haemolytic-uraemic syndrome. Lancet *2*:183, 1988.

124. McGowan, J.A., and Greenberg, A.: Atheroembolic renal disease. Am. J. Nephrol. *6*:135, 1986.

125. Arruda, J.A.L.: Obstructive uropathy. Contemp. Issues Nephrol. *10*:248, 1983.

126. Klahr, S., et al.: Urinary tract obstruction. *In* Brenner, B.M., and Rector, F. (eds.): The Kidney. 3rd ed. Philadelphia, W.B. Saunders Co., 1986, pp. 1443–1490.

127. Consensus Conference: Prevention and treatment of kidney stones. JAMA *260*:977, 1988.

128. Coe, F.L., and Parks, J.H.: Pathophysiology of kidney stones and strategies for treatment. Hosp. Pract. *23*:185, 1988.

128a. Bianchi, G., et al.: Abnormal red-cell calcium pump in patients with idiopathic hypercalcemia. N. Engl. J. Med. *319*:897, 1988.

129. Mostofi, F.K.: Tumors of the kidney. *In* Churg, J., et al. (eds.): Renal Disease—Current Status. Baltimore, Williams & Wilkins Co., 1979, pp. 356–410.

130. Lohr, E., and Leder, L.D. (eds.): Renal and Adrenal Tumors. Heidelberg, Germany, Springer-Verlag, 1987.

131. Choi, H., et al.: Renal oncocytoma: A clinicopathologic study. Cancer *51*:1887, 1983.

132. Kantar, A.F.: The epidemiology of renal cell carcinoma in Connecticut. J. Natl. Cancer Inst. *57*:495, 1976.

133. Bollack, C. (ed.): Recent advances in renal cell carcinomas. *In* Progress in Surgery. Vol. 17. New York, S. Karger, 1983.

134. Kovacs, G., et al.: Consistent chromosome 3p deletion and loss of heterozygosity in renal cell carcinoma. Proc. Natl. Acad. Sci. U.S.A. *85*:1571, 1988.

135. Brodsky, G.L., and Garnick, M.B.: Neoplasms in the adult kidney. *In* Tisher, C.C., and Brenner, B.M. (eds.): Renal Pathology. Philadelphia, J.B. Lippincott Co., 1989.

136. Ganick, D.J.: Wilms' tumor. Hematol. Oncol. Clin. North Am. *1*(4):659, 1987.

137. Beckwith, J.B.: Wilms' tumor and other renal tumors of childhood. J. Urol. *136*:320, 1986.

138. McCarron, J.P., et al.: Tumors of the renal pelvis and ureter: Current concepts and management. Semin. Urol. *1*:75, 1983.

139. McCredie, M., et al.: Phenacetin and papillary necrosis: Independent risk factors for renal pelvic cancer. Kidney Int. *30*(1):81, 1986.

The Lower Urinary Tract

URETERS

NORMAL

The ureters arise as budlike outgrowths from the mesonephric or wolffian ducts. These buds elongate to produce the long, definitive tubular structures found in the adult. They grow into the metanephric anlage, which covers them in the form of a cap. Tubular projections from the blind end give rise to the collecting tubules. These eventually anastomose with the distal convoluted tubules of the renal nephron and thus provide drainage for the functioning nephron.

In the normal adult of average size, the ureters are approximately 30 cm in length and about 5 mm in diameter. They lie throughout their course in a retroperitoneal position. As they enter the pelvis, they pass anterior to either the common iliac or the external iliac artery. In the female pelvis, they lie close to the uterine arteries and are therefore vulnerable to injury in operations on the female genital tract. There are three points of slight narrowing: at the ureteropelvic junction, where they enter the bladder, and where they cross the iliac vessels, all providing loci where renal calculi may become impacted when they pass from the kidney to the bladder.

On histologic section, ureters are composed of three distinct coats: an outer fibrous investment; a thick muscular coat with the fibers traveling, for the most part, in a circular fashion but with, however, a less well-developed longitudinal layer of muscle; and a lining mucosa of transitional epithelium (urothelium) resembling that found in the renal pelvis and bladder. This epithelium rests on a well-developed basement membrane. Active peristaltic waves propel urine through the ureters into the bladder. As the ureters enter the bladder, they pursue an oblique course, terminating in a slitlike orifice. The obliquity of this intramural segment of the ureteral orifice permits the enclosing bladder musculature to act as a sphincteric valve, blocking the upward reflux of urine even in the presence of marked distention of the urinary bladder. As discussed earlier, a defect in the intravesical portion of the ureter leads to vesicoureteral reflux.

PATHOLOGY

As a generalization, the processes in which the ureters become involved are most commonly primary in either the kidney or the bladder. Ureteral involvement, then, is usually overshadowed clinically and anatomically by the accompanying underlying disorders. Here we shall briefly describe certain congenital anomalies and obstructive lesions.[1,2]

CONGENITAL ANOMALIES

Congenital anomalies of the ureters occur in about 2 or 3% of all autopsies. They are, for the most part, of only incidental interest and have little clinical significance. Rarely, certain anomalies may contribute to obstruction to the flow of urine and thus cause clinical disease. Anomalies of the ureterovesical junction, potentiating reflux, are discussed on page 1052.

Double and bifid ureters. Double ureters (derived from a double or split ureteral bud) are almost invariably associated either with totally distinct double renal pelves or with the anomalous development of a very large kidney, having a partially bifid pelvis terminating in separate ureters. Double ureters may pursue separate courses to the bladder, but commonly are joined within the bladder wall and drain through a single ureteral orifice.

Ureteropelvic junction obstruction (UPJ), a relatively uncommon congenital disorder, results in hydronephrosis (p. 1071). It is usually present in male infants, more commonly in the left ureter, but it can be bilateral in 20% of cases. It has been ascribed to abnormal organization of smooth muscle bundles at the UPJ, excess stromal deposition of collagen between smooth muscle bundles, or extrinsic compression by aberrant renal vessels.

Diverticula, saccular outpouchings of the ureteral wall, are uncommon lesions. They appear as congenital or acquired defects and are of importance as pockets of stasis and secondary infections. Dilatation, elongation, and tortuosity of the ureters *(hydroureter)* may occur as congenital anomalies or as acquired defects. Congenital hydroureter is thought to reflect some neurogenic defect in the innervation of the ureteral musculature. The acquired form is seen in Chagas' disease, in low ureteral obstruction, or in pregnancy. Massive enlargement of the ureter is known as *megaloureter* and is probably due to a functional defect of ureteral muscle. These anomalies are sometimes associated with some congenital defect of the kidney.

INFLAMMATION

Ureteritis may develop as one component of urinary tract infections. The morphologic changes are entirely nonspecific. Only infrequently does such ureteritis make a significant contribution to the clinical problem.

Persistence of infection or repeated acute exacerbations may give rise to chronic inflammatory changes within the ureters.

In certain cases of long-standing chronic ureteritis, specialized reaction patterns are sometimes observed. The accumulation or aggregation of lymphocytes in the subepithelial region may cause slight elevations of the mucosa and produce a fine granular mucosal surface **(ureteritis follicularis).** At other times, the mucosa may become sprinkled with fine cysts varying in diameter from 1 to 5 mm **(ureteritis cystica).** Chronic urinary tract infection is the most common antecedent of this interesting lesion, but it may also occur in the absence of any other disorder. The cysts are related to **Brunn's nests,** which are clusters of transitional epithelium beneath the urothelial surface. These sequestered epithelial nests give rise to small submucosal cysts. The cysts appear on the surface of the mucosa as small (0.1 to 0.5 cm), clear, thin-walled (hemispheric) vesicles (Fig. 22–1). They may aggregate to form small, grape-

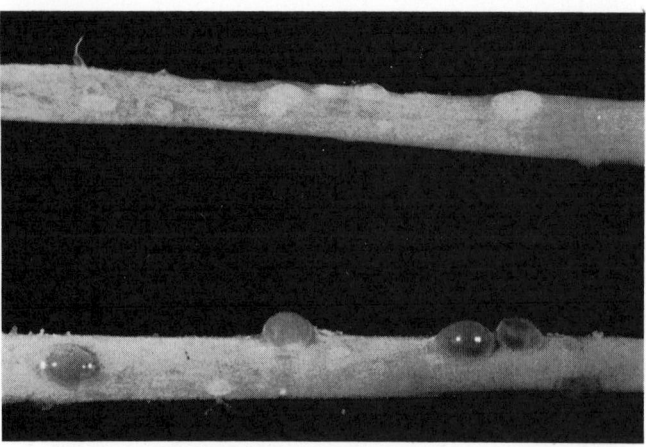

Figure 22–1. Ureteritis cystica.

like clusters. Histologic sections through such cysts demonstrate a lining of modified transitional epithelium with some flattening of the superficial layer of cells.

TUMORS

Primary neoplasia of the ureter is very rare, metastatic seeding from other primary lesions occurring much more often than primary growths.

Small *benign tumors* of the ureter are generally of mesenchymal origin. They include the usual variety of neoplasms derived from fibrous tissue, blood vessels, lymphatics, and smooth muscle. These appear as well-encapsulated, submucosal nodules less than 1 cm in diameter, which are rarely of sufficient size to cause obstruction of the ureteral lumen.

The primary *malignant tumors* of the ureter follow the identical patterns of those arising in the renal pelvis, calyces, and bladder, because all these structures are lined by the same transitional epithelium (urothelium).[3] They are found most frequently during the sixth and seventh decades of life, and are sometimes multiple and occasionally concurrent with similar neoplasms in the bladder or renal pelvis. Prognosis depends on the stage and extent of the lesion.

OBSTRUCTIVE LESIONS

A great variety of pathologic lesions may obstruct the ureters and give rise to hydroureter, hydronephrosis, and sometimes pyelonephritis. Obviously, it is not the ureteral dilatation that is of significance in these cases, but the consequent involvement of the kidneys. The latter has been detailed on page 1071. Here, some of the causes of ureteral obstruction will be discussed. These may be conveniently separated into intrinsic ureteral disease and extrinsic lesions that compress the ureters (see also Fig. 21–59).

INTRINSIC

These will be mentioned in order of clinical importance.

CALCULI. Calculous obstruction of the ureters not only is the most frequent cause of obstruction but also, at the same time, is the cause of one of the most intense forms of pain encountered in clinical practice — renal colic. Ureteral calculi almost invariably arise within the kidney and are more fully considered on page 1073. They vary from small, round-to-ovoid formations to irregular crystalline deposits, usually less than 0.5 cm in diameter. Stones larger than this do not enter the ureteropelvic junction, and therefore remain within the pelvis. The usual sites of impaction, as mentioned, are at loci of ureteral narrowing: the ureteropelvic junction; where the ureters enter the bladder; and where they cross the iliac vessels.

STRICTURES. Narrowing by strictures may occur from either congenital anomalous development or acquired deformities. Acquired strictures may be caused by operative trauma. Because of the close anatomic relationship of the ureter to the uterine arteries, ureteral damage occasionally occurs in pelvic surgery. Intrinsic inflammation or periureteral inflammatory reactions, occurring, for example, in chronic salpingitis, diverticulitis, sclerosing retroperitonitis, and adhesions following peritonitis, may also lead to narrowing or obstruction. Congenital ureteropelvic junction obstruction has been described in earlier sections.

TUMORS. Malignant tumors and, quite rarely, benign tumors may give rise to obstruction. The manner in which they produce impairment of urinary flow is twofold: first, by formation of an intraluminal mass, and second, by invasion and thickening of the underlying wall with consequent narrowing of the lumen.

BLOOD CLOT. Hematuria arising in the kidney or in a ureteral lesion may be sufficiently massive to permit the formation of clots, which may lodge and cause obstruction. This magnitude of bleeding is most often associated with calculi, tumors, or papillary necrosis.

EXTRINSIC

PREGNANCY. Ureteral dilatation is a frequent accompaniment of pregnancy. It is still not known whether the dilatation results from endocrine causes, physiologic relaxation of smooth muscle, or pressure upon the ureters at the pelvic brim.

ENDOMETRIOSIS. Endometriosis can affect the ureter proper, but more commonly, obstruction is associated with adjacent pelvic endometriosis that involves the serosa of the ureter.

TUMORS. Malignant tumors of the rectum, prostate, bladder, and female pelvic organis, particularly endometrial and cervical carcinoma, are major causes of narrowing of the ureters, either by external pressure or by direct invasion of the ureteral wall. This sequence of events constitutes one of the major complications of advanced carcinoma of the cervix. Retroperitoneal sarcomas, including lymphomas, and metastatic involvement of periureteral lymph nodes all behave in a similar fashion.

INFLAMMATION. It has already been indicated that periureteral inflammations may involve the ureters secondarily and, in the course of healing, cause scarring that may give rise to significant narrowing.

SCLEROSING RETROPERITONITIS (RETROPERITONEAL FIBROMATOSIS). This entity of obscure origin is an uncommon cause of ureteral narrowing or obstruction, and comes to medical attention by causing hydronephrosis.[5]

It is characterized by ill-defined fibrous masses that begin over the sacral promontory, encircle the lower abdominal aorta, and extend laterally through the retroperitoneum to enclose and encroach on the ureters. Microscopically, the inflammatory fibrosis is marked by a prominent inflammatory infiltrate of lymphocytes, often with germinal centers, plasma cells, and eosinophils. Sometimes, foci of fat necrosis and granulomatous inflammation are seen in and about the fibrosis.[5a]

The etiology of this condition is obscure. In some instances there is a history of intake of the drug methysergide, an ergot derivative used for migraine. However, most cases have no obvious cause. Several cases have been reported with similar fibrotic changes in other sites (referred to as mediastinal fibrosis, sclerosing cholangitis, and Riedel's (fibrosing) thyroiditis), suggesting that the disorder is systemic in distribution but preferentially involves the retroperitoneum. Thus, a systemic autoimmune reaction, sometimes triggered by drugs, has been proposed.

URINARY BLADDER

NORMAL

The bladder exists almost entirely as an extraperitoneal structure situated deep within the pelvis. It is in contact with the peritoneal cavity only in its most superior anterior aspect, where the peritoneum reflects from the anterior abdominal wall over the dome of the bladder. The close relationship of the female genital tract to the bladder is of considerable significance. It makes possible the spread of disease from one tract to the other. In middle-aged and elderly females, relaxation of pelvic support leads to prolapse (descent) of the uterus, pulling with it the floor of the bladder. In this fashion, the bladder is protruded into the vagina, creating a pouch — *cystocele* — that fails to empty readily with micturition. In the male, the seminal vesicles and prostate have similar close relationships, being situated just posterior and inferior to the neck of the bladder. Thus, enlargement of the prostate, so common in middle to later life, constitutes an important cause of urinary tract obstruction.

HISTOLOGY OF NORMAL UROTHELIUM. The normal bladder is lined by a uniform transitional epithelium, which rests on a thin basal lamina.[6] In humans the normal urinary mucosa is rarely more than seven to eight cells thick and consists of three zones (Fig. 22–2). The *superficial zone* consists of a single layer of large, flattened cells that cover relatively large areas, giving rise to the term "umbrella" cells. An *intermediate zone* contains four to five layers when the bladder is maximally stretched, and six to eight when it is fully contracted. The *basal zone* consists of a single layer of small cells that are cylindrical in contracted bladders and flattened in distended ones. Thickening (hyperplasia) of this mucosal layer and irregularity of the cell and nuclear size and shape are seen in inflammatory, preneoplastic, and neoplastic states. Indeed, cellular atypia is an almost invariable antecedent to the development of neoplasms. Ultrastructurally, bladder epithelium is characterized by unique scalloped, concave, rigid membrane plaques — the *asymmetric unit membrane* (AUM) plaque — present mostly on the luminal surface of such cells (Fig. 22–3). These plaques form one side of the *fusiform vesicles*, which are intracytoplasmic structures unique to urothelium. Bladder epithelium also contains numerous desmosomes, which increase in number from basal to superficial layers.

Several variants of this normal mucosal pattern may be encountered. Nests of urothelium or inbudding of the surface epithelium may be found occasionally in the mucosal lamina propria; these are sometimes referred to as *Brunn's nests*. Although in the past such changes have been thought to result from chronic inflammatory stimulation of the bladder mucosa, they may merely represent normal variations in morphology. Similarly, small cystic inclusions lined by cuboidal or columnar epithelium are sometimes found in the lamina propria.

PATHOLOGY

Diseases of the bladder, particularly inflammation (cystitis), constitute an important source of clinical

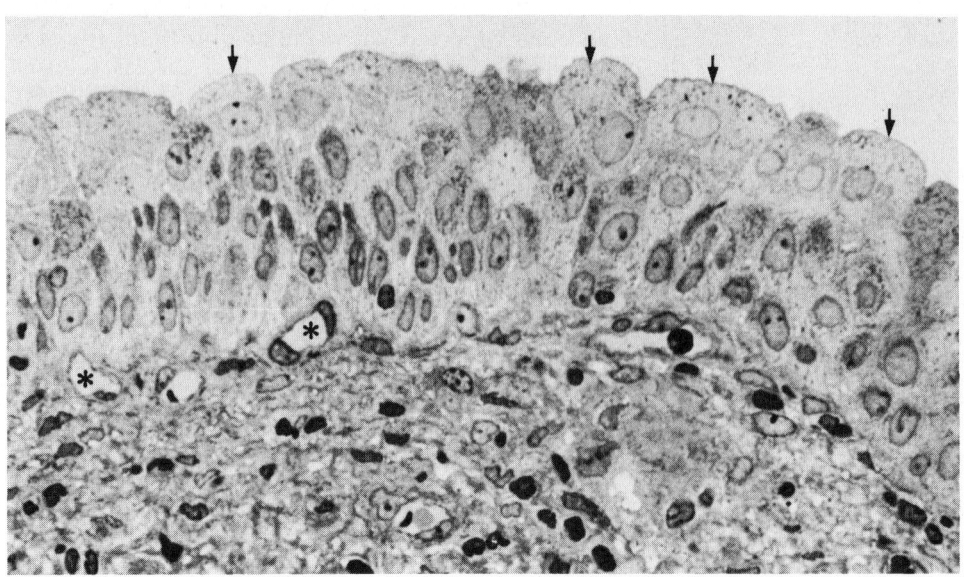

Figure 22–2. Human urinary bladder epithelium consists of superficial, intermediate, and basal zones. The superficial zone contains a single layer of large, so-called "umbrella" cells *(arrows)*. The intermediate zone is several cell layers thick. The basal zone is composed of a single layer of small, cylindrical cells. Submucosal capillaries in the contracted bladder characteristically invaginate into the subepithelial basement membrane *(asterisks)* (×530). (From Pauli, B.U., et al.: The ultrastructure and pathobiology of urinary bladder cancer. *In* Cohen, S., and Bryan, G.T. (eds.): The Pathology of Bladder Cancer. Boca Raton, CRC Press, 1984.)

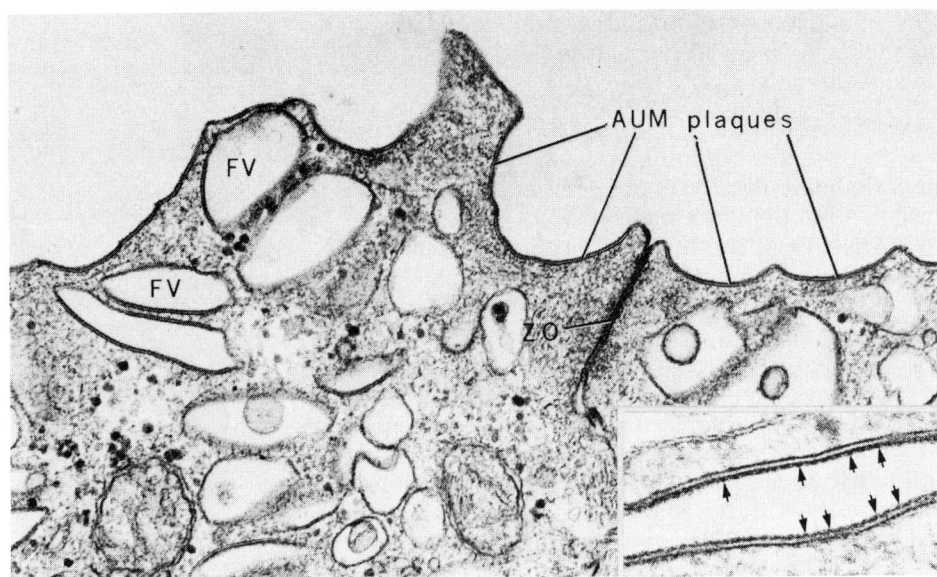

Figure 22–3. Luminal surface of two superficial cells of dog urinary bladder, joined by a zonula occludens intercellular junction (ZO). The luminal membrane has a scalloped appearance due to the presence of rigid, curved, AUM plaques alternating with short segments of symmetric unit membrane, which serve as "hinge" areas. Intracytoplasmic fusiform vesicles (FV) are lined by AUM plaques (×52,000). *Inset:* The thicker leaflets of the AUM plaque of fusiform vesicles face inward, lining the intravesicular space. This leaflet contains particulate membrane components (*arrows*) (×160,000). (From Alroy, J.: Ultrastructure of canine urinary bladder carcinoma. Vet. Pathol. *16:*693, 1979.)

signs and symptoms. Usually, however, these disorders are more disabling than lethal. Cystitis is particularly common in young women of reproductive age and in older age groups of both sexes. Tumors of the bladder are an important source of both morbidity and mortality.

CONGENITAL ANOMALIES

DIVERTICULA. A bladder or vesical diverticulum consists of a pouchlike eversion or evagination of the bladder wall. Diverticula may arise as congenital defects but more commonly are acquired lesions from persistent urethral obstruction. They are uncommon in persons under the age of 50 and are more prevalent in males, presumably because of the causal role of enlargement of the prostate.

The *congenital form* may be due to a focal failure of development of the normal musculature or to some urinary tract obstruction during fetal development. Alternatively, diverticula may develop from budlike outgrowths of the fetal bladder. In any event, *some musculature is retained within the wall* of such diverticula, although it may be thinner than normal.

In the *acquired variety* the diverticula have markedly thinned musculature and, in the more advanced lesions, may have virtually *no intrinsic musculature* but only a mucosa with tunica propria. Acquired diverticula are usually multiple (Fig. 22–4). In both forms, the diverticulum usually consists of a round-to-ovoid, saclike pouch that varies from less than 1 cm to 5 to 10 cm in diameter. The musosal lining may show inflammation as well as glandular or squamous metaplastic changes.

Diverticula are of clinical significance because they constitute sites of urinary stasis and predispose to infection and the formation of bladder calculi. They may also predispose to vesicoureteric reflux. Rarely, carcinomas may arise in bladder diverticuli.

EXSTROPHY. Exstrophy of the bladder implies the presence of a developmental failure in the anterior wall of the abdomen and the bladder, so that the bladder either communicates directly through a large defect with the surface of the body or lies as an opened sac.[7] The exposed bladder mucosa is subject to the development of infections that often spread to upper levels of the urinary system. In the course of persistent chronic infections, the mucosa often becomes converted into an ulcerated surface of granulation tissue, and the preserved marginal epithelium becomes transformed into a stratified squamous type. There is an increased tendency toward the development of

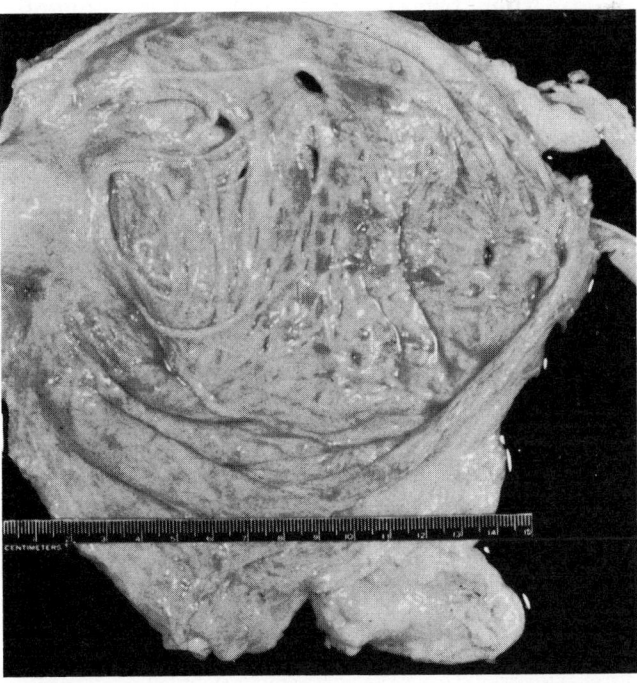

Figure 22–4. Acquired diverticula of bladder. Note bladder distention as indicated by 15 cm rule and trabeculation of wall.

carcinoma, mostly adenocarcinoma. These lesions are amenable to surgical correction, and long-term survival is possible.

MISCELLANEOUS ANOMALIES. *Vesicoureteral reflux* is the most common and serious anomaly. As a major contributor to renal infection and scarring it is discussed in detail on page 1053.

Absence of the bladder and hypoplasia are very uncommon congenital defects. Occasionally, an incomplete transverse septum may create a so-called hourglass deformity. Abnormal connections between the bladder and the vagina, rectum, or uterus may create congenital vesicouterine fistulas.

Rarely, the *urachus* may remain patent in part or in whole (persistent urachus). When it is totally patent, a fistulous urinary tract is created that connects the bladder with the umbilicus. At times, the umbilical end or the bladder end remains patent, while the central region is obliterated. A sequestered umbilical epithelial rest or bladder diverticulum is formed that may provide a site for the development of infection. At other times, only the central region of the urachus persists, giving rise to *urachal cysts,* lined by either transitional or metaplastic epithelium. Carcinomas, mostly adenocarcinomas, have been reported to arise in such cysts.

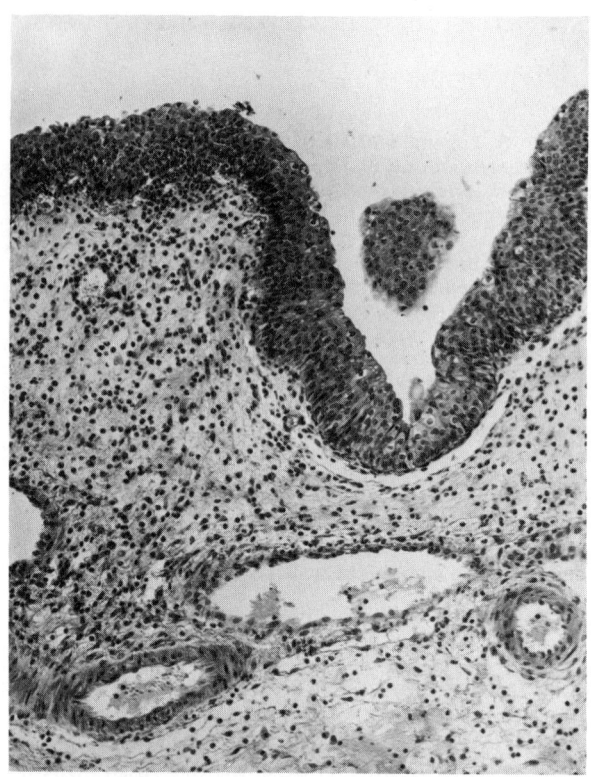

Figure 22–5. Chronic cystitis with a subepithelial mononuclear infiltrate and marked dilatation of blood vessels.

INFLAMMATIONS

ACUTE AND CHRONIC CYSTITIS

The pathogenesis of cystitis and the common bacterial and mycotic etiologic agents were discussed in the consideration of urinary tract infections. As emphasized earlier, bacterial pyelonephritis is frequently preceded by infection of the urinary bladder, with retrograde spread of microorganisms into the kidneys and their collecting systems. The common etiologic agents of cystitis are the coliforms—*E. coli,* followed by Proteus, Klebsiella, and Enterobacter.[8] *Tuberculous* cystitis is almost always a sequel to renal tuberculosis. *Candida albicans* (monilia) and, much less often, cryptococcal agents cause cystitis, particularly in immunosuppressed patients or those receiving long-term antibiotics. Schistosomiasis is rare in the United States but is extremely common in certain Middle Eastern countries, notably Egypt. Viruses (e.g., adenovirus), the chlamydia, and mycoplasma may also be causes of cystitis. Patients receiving *cytotoxic antitumor drugs,* such as cyclophosphamide and busulfan, sometimes develop hemorrhagic cystitis.[9] Finally, radiation of the bladder gives rise to *radiation cystitis.*

MORPHOLOGY. The great majority of cases of cystitis take the form of nonspecific acute or chronic inflammation of the bladder. Grossly, there is hyperemia of the mucosa, sometimes associated with exudate. When there is a hem-

orrhagic component, the cystitis is designated **hemorrhagic cystitis.** This form of cystitis sometimes follows radiation injury or antitumor chemotherapy and is often accompanied by epithelial atypia. Adenovirus infection also causes a hemorrhagic cystitis.

The accumulation of large amounts of suppurative exudate may merit the designation of **suppurative cystitis.** When there is ulceration of large areas of the mucosa, or sometimes the entire bladder mucosa, this is known as **ulcerative cystitis.** In cystitis associated with long-term indwelling catheters, the mucosa bulges into the lumen, forming polyps **(polypoid cystitis).**

Persistence of the infection leads to **chronic cystitis,** which differs from the acute form only in the character of the inflammatory infiltrate. There is more extreme heaping up of the epithelium with the formation of a red, friable, granular, sometimes ulcerated surface. Chronicity of the infection gives rise to fibrous thickening in the tunica propria and consequent thickening and inelasticity of the bladder wall.

The histologic findings of most of these variants of acute and chronic nonspecific cystitis are exactly those that can be anticipated in any such nonspecific inflammation (Fig. 22–5). Mention might be made of a special form of chronic inflammatory reaction, the aggregation of lymphocytes into lymph follicles within the bladder mucosa and underlying wall, creating a variant of chronic cystitis known as **cystitis follicularis.**

All forms of cystitis are characterized by a triad of symptoms: (1) frequency, which in acute cases may necessitate urination every 15 to 20 minutes; (2) lower abdominal pain localized over the bladder region or in the suprapubic region; and (3) dysuria—pain or burning on urination. Associated with these localized changes, there may be systemic signs of inflammation such as elevation of temperature, chills, and general malaise. In the usual case, the bladder infection does not give rise to such a constitutional reaction.

The local symptoms of cystitis may be disturbing, but these infections are more important as antecedents to pyelonephritis. Cystitis is sometimes a secondary complication of some underlying disorder such as prostatic enlargement, cystocele of the bladder, calculi, or tumors. These primary diseases must be corrected before the cystitis can be relieved.

SPECIAL FORMS OF CYSTITIS

There is a multiplicity of so-called special variants of cystitis that are distinctive by either their morphologic appearance or their causation.

ULCERATIVE INTERSTITIAL CYSTITIS (HUNNER'S ULCER).
This is a persistent chronic cystitis occurring most frequently in women and associated with inflammation and fibrosis of all layers of the bladder wall.[10] A localized ulcer is often present. The condition is of unknown etiology, but is often highly incapacitating and difficult to treat.

EMPHYSEMATOUS CYSTITIS.
This occurs most frequently in diabetics and is associated with gas bub-

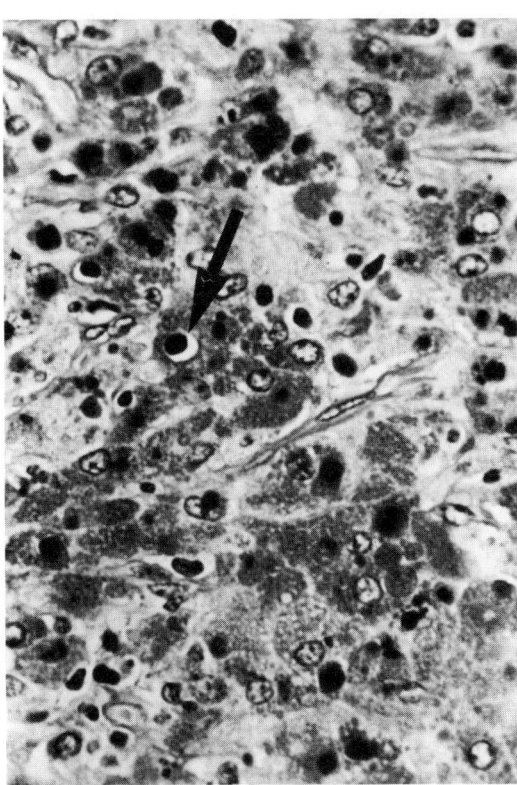

Figure 22–7. Malakoplakia, PAS stain. Note large macrophages with granular cytoplasm and round, dense Michaelis-Gutmann bodies *(arrow)*.

bles in the submucosal connective tissue. It is presumably caused by gas-forming bacteria. Giant cells often surround the gas bubbles.

MALAKOPLAKIA.
This designation refers to a *peculiar pattern of vesical inflammatory reaction characterized macroscopically by soft yellow, slightly raised, mucosal plaques 3 to 4 cm in diameter* (Fig. 22–6).[11] The surrounding mucosa is generally edematous, hyperemic, and inflammatory. Histologically, the plaques are made up of closely packed, large, foamy macrophages with occasional multinucleate giant cells and interspersed lymphocytes. The macrophages have an abundant granular cytoplasm. The granularity is PAS positive and due to phagosomes stuffed with particulate and membranous debris of bacterial origin. In addition, laminated mineralized concretions known as Michaelis-Gutmann (MG) bodies are typically present, both within the macrophages and between cells (Fig. 22–7). Similar lesions have been described in the colon, lungs, bones, kidneys, prostate, and epididymis. Malakoplakia occurs with increased frequency in immunosuppressed transplant recipients.[12]

The genesis of the malakoplakic lesion is still uncertain. Current opinion favors the hypothesis that the unusual-appearing macrophages and giant phagosomes result from defects in the phagocytic process. Thus, the phagosomes become overloaded with bacteria. The MG bodies are thought to result from the

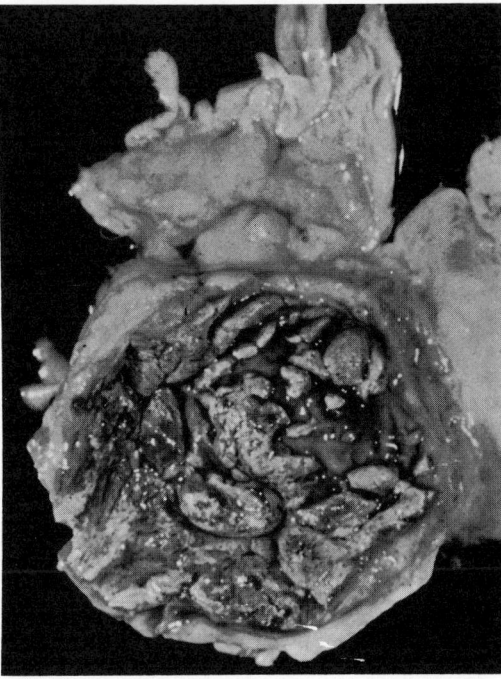

Figure 22–6. Malakoplakia of bladder, showing classic, broad, flat, inflammatory plaques.

deposition of calcium phosphate and other minerals on these overloaded, perhaps disintegrating phagosomes.

CYSTITIS CYSTICA. In long-standing chronic inflammation, nests of transitional bladder mucosa may become buried and give rise to small, cystic, mucosal inclusions. The accompanying gross and microscopic histologic features are identical with those already described in the renal pelvis and ureter. Occasionally, the epithelium is transformed by metaplasia to being mucus-secreting and columnar, producing *cystitis glandularis.*

EOSINOPHILIC CYSTITIS. This rare condition is characterized by a chronic cystitis with abundant eosinophils in the subepithelial connective tissue, together with fibrosis and, occasionally, giant cells. The etiology is unknown.[13]

In all these forms of cystitis, mucosal epithelial hyperplasia may occur, requiring differentiation from neoplastic lesions.[14]

NEOPLASMS
EPITHELIAL TUMORS

Approximately 95% of neoplasms of the bladder are of urothelial origin; the remainder are largely mesenchymal tumors of myoblastic, fibroblastic, or endothelial origin, similar to those arising elsewhere in the body. The epithelial tumors, most of which are malignant, are of interest for many reasons. First, these are rather common tumors: there are some 38,000 new cases of bladder cancer each year in the United States, and 10,000 deaths from the disease. Second, as we shall see, there is now substantial evidence that a long prodrome of widely dispersed mucosal epithelial hyperplasia and progressive atypia antedates the appearance of these neoplasms, rendering them at least theoretically subject to early detection; and third, although many of these tumors are initially of low histologic grade, they are often multiple and recurrent. With each recurrence, the tumors may show greater atypia and worse prognosis. It is therefore difficult to manage these tumors and to predict the outcome.

Table 22–1 presents a simplified classification of bladder tumors consistent with most current views;[15-17] Figure 22–8 illustrates the main features of each.

Table 22–1. Classification of Epithelial Bladder Tumors

Transitional cell papilloma
Transitional cell carcinoma
Grade I ⎫
Grade II ⎬ Invasive and noninvasive
Grade III ⎭
Carcinoma in situ
Squamous cell carcinoma
Adenocarcinoma
Mixed carcinoma
Undifferentiated carcinoma

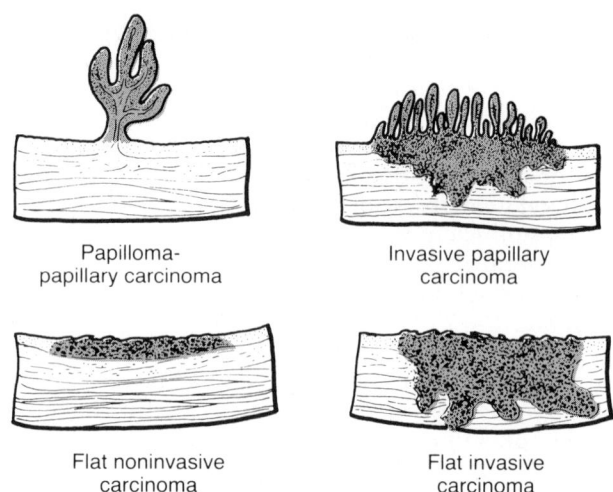

Papilloma-papillary carcinoma

Invasive papillary carcinoma

Flat noninvasive carcinoma

Flat invasive carcinoma

Figure 22–8. Four morphologic patterns of bladder tumors.

TRANSITIONAL CELL PAPILLOMA

These benign mucosal neoplasms, which may arise anywhere within the bladder, are difficult to distinguish from grade I papillary carcinomas and indeed some classification schemes consider them as grade I tumors. Pure papillomas are rare, representing about 2% of bladder tumors.

> Papillomas usually arise singly, but multiple and sequential lesions may occur at varied and random locations. The individual tumor is usually a small (0.5 to 2.0 cm), delicate, soft, branching structure, superficially attached to the mucosa by a slender stalk. The individual finger-like papillae have a central core of loose fibrovascular tissue covered by normal-appearing transitional cells (Fig. 22–9) **seven or fewer layers in thickness** (Table 22–2). The cells recapitulate the normal architecture of transitional urinary tract epithelium.

The usual papilloma is readily removed by transurethral resection, since it is attached only to the mucosa. The frequency of recurrence varies among series. However, there are numerous reported instances in which new growths reappear. The regrowth may again be benign, but sometimes it exhibits more marked irregularity of the epithelial cells sufficient to merit the diagnosis of transitional cell carcinoma. However, less than 10% ultimately develop invasive carcinoma.

CARCINOMA

Bladder cancers account for 3% of cancer deaths in the United States.[18] Although the incidence of these cancers has steadily increased over the past three decades in the United States, the death rate has remained relatively constant, probably as a result of improved methods of early diagnosis and treatment.

The three basic types are transitional cell carci-

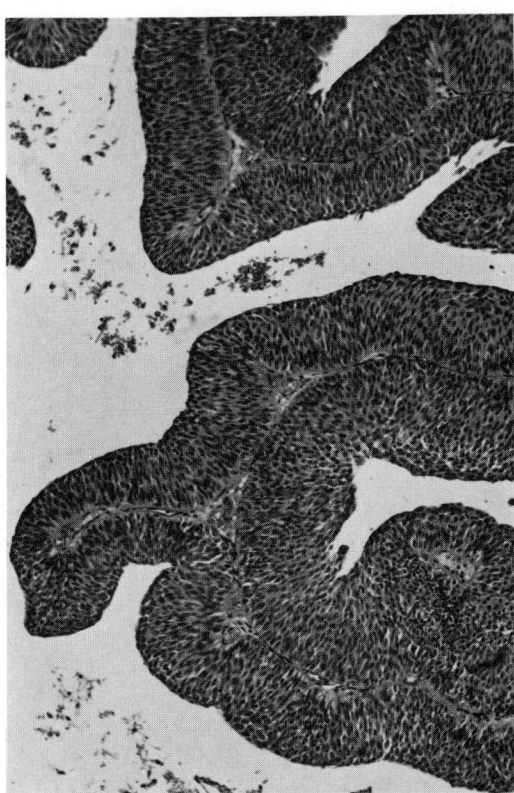

Figure 22–9. Low-power view of typical papillomatous growth of bladder. Note delicate axial stromal framework.

noma, squamous cell carcinoma, and adenocarcinoma. Approximately 90% are basically transitional cell carcinomas, 5% are squamous cell carcinomas, and 5% are mixed; adenocarcinomas are rare.

INCIDENCE. The incidence of carcinoma of the bladder resembles that of bronchogenic carcinoma, being more common in males than in females, in industrialized than in developing nations, and in urban than in rural dwellers. The male : female ratio for transitional cell tumors is approximately 3 : 1, whereas for squamous cell tumors it approaches 3 : 2. About 80% of patients are between the ages of 50 and 80. Squamous cell carcinomas occur frequently where bilharzial *(Schistosoma haematobium)* infections of the bladder are common. They represent 10 to 40% of all malignant tumors in Egypt.

EPIDEMIOLOGY AND PATHOGENESIS. A number of environmental factors increase the risk of bladder cancer.[18] *Occupational exposure to beta-naphthylamine, 4-aminobiphenyl, 4-nitrobiphenyl, and 4,4-diaminobiphenyl has been clearly demonstrated to be carcinogenic.*[19] These compounds are intermediaries in the synthesis of a wide range of azo dyes and pigments used in textile, printing, plastic, rubber, and cable industries. Bladder cancers occur among workers after a mean exposure of approximately 20 years, accounting for up to a 50-fold increased incidence in those exposed.

As mentioned, there is increased incidence of bladder cancer in patients harboring *Schistosoma haematobium* in their bladders. It is not certain whether the parasites elaborate a carcinogenic agent into the urine or instead cause local inflammation and subsequent hyperplastic and eventually neoplastic changes in the bladder mucosa. In either event, schistosomal cancers have a distribution within the bladder somewhat different from that seen in occupational exposure or spontaneous occurrence, arguing for a local effect.[20]

Certain *metabolites of tryptophan-kynurenine,* and some of its closely related compounds, are excreted in increased amounts in patients with bladder cancer. L-Tryptophan enhances chemically induced carcinogenesis.[21] Tryptophan metabolites induce tumors in mice when incorporated in cholesterol pellets inserted into the bladder.

Cyclophosphamide, an immunosuppressive agent used in immune diseases, causes hemorrhagic cystitis and atypia in the urothelium, and increases the risk of bladder cancer by close to ten times after 12 years of treatment.[22]

The risk of bladder cancer is two to four times greater among male cigarette *smokers* than among nonsmokers. Smoking pipes, cigars, and smokeless tobacco also increases risk.[22a] Transitional cell carcinomas of the pelvis, ureter, and bladder are also more common in patients with *analgesic abuse nephropathy* (p. 1058).

MORPHOLOGY. Before going into details of the major forms of bladder cancer, it is necessary to clarify the terminology used to describe the patterns of growth employed in the grading and staging of these neoplasms.[23]

Table 22–2. Morphology of Urothelial Transitional Cell Tumors

	HYPERPLASIA (>7 LAYERS)	SUPERFICIAL CELL LAYER	"CLEAR" CYTOPLASM	PLEOMORPHISM	NUCLEAR POLARIZATION	NUCLEAR CROWDING	CHROMATIN	MITOSES
Papilloma	None	Preserved	Present	None	Normal	None	Normal	Rare
TCC-I*	Variable	Variable	Often absent	Variable	Slightly abnormal	Slight	Fine—regular	Uncommon
TCC-II	Variable	Absent	Often absent	Variable	Abnormal	Moderate	Fine—regular	Common
TCC-III	Prominent	Absent	Absent; vacuoles common	Prominent	Absent	Moderate	Coarse—usually irregular	Prominent

* TCC = transitional cell carcinoma—grades I, II, III.

From Murphy, W.M.: Current topics in the pathology of bladder cancer. *Pathol. Annu. 18:*1, 1983.

The gross appearance of all vesical cancers may be described or categorized as:

1. Papillary—exophytic polypoid lesions attached by a stalk to the mucosa. Penetration of the basement membrane by the neoplastic cells may or may not be present.

2. Flat lesions—growing as plaque-like thickenings of the mucosa without the formation of well-defined papillary structures. The neoplasm may be in situ or invasive (more often the latter), and these neoplasms generally tend to be more anaplastic than the papillary lesions.

3. Noninvasive—thickening of the mucosa by proliferation of cells similar to those seen in carcinoma, but without penetration of the basement membrane.

4. Invasive—penetrating the mucosal basement membrane into the bladder wall, and possibly into contiguous structures.

Grading of the transitional cell neoplasms is based on the degree of atypia exhibited by the cancer cells as shown in Table 22–2.

GRADE I. The tumor cells display some atypia but are well differentiated and closely resemble normal transitional cells. Mitoses are rare. There is a significant increase in the number of layers of cells, i.e., more than seven layers, but only slight loss of polarity (Fig. 22–10).

GRADE II. The tumor cells are still recognizable as of transitional origin. The number of layers of cells is increased (often over ten), as is the number of mitoses, and there is greater loss of polarity. Greater variability in cell size, shape, and chromaticity is present.

GRADE III. The tumor cells are barely recognizable as of transitional origin, and all the changes mentioned under grade II are more aggravated. In particular, there is evident disarray of cells with loosening and fragmentation of the superficial layers of cells (Fig. 22–11).

There are several **staging** schemes for bladder cancer. The simplest is as follows:

STAGE 0. Carcinoma is limited to the mucosa.
STAGE A. Carcinoma invades the lamina propria but not the muscularis.
STAGE B$_1$. Carcinoma invades superficial muscle layer.
STAGE B$_2$. Carcinoma invades deep muscle.
STAGE C. Carcinoma invades perivesical region.
STAGE D$_1$. Carcinoma exhibits regional metastases.
STAGE D$_2$. Carcinoma exhibits distant metastases.

Against this background we can now turn to the individual types of tumors.

Transitional cell carcinomas range from noninvasive to invasive lesions, from flat to papillary, and from well-differentiated (grade I) to highly anaplastic, aggressive cancers (grade III). Almost 70% are papillary, noninvasive, and of low cytologic grade (I); 25 to 30% are invasive and of variable grades of cytologic atypia.

Papillary neoplasms have a complicated fernlike structure composed of a delicate connective tissue stalk, covered by transitional epithelium that ranges from grade I (Fig. 22–10) to grade III (Fig. 22–11). Most of these papillary

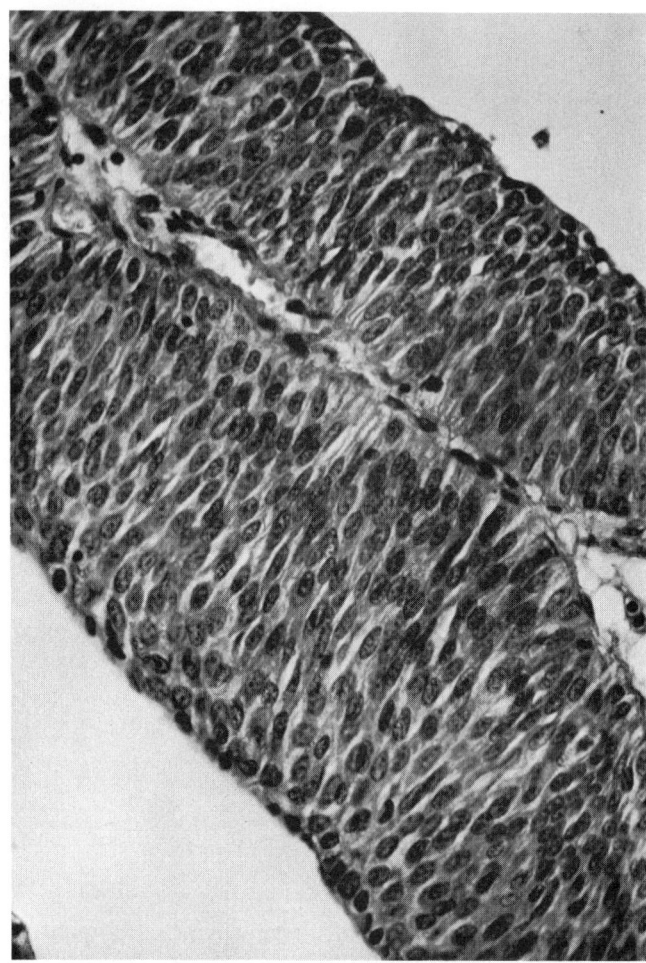

Figure 22–10. Papillary carcinoma of bladder, Grade I. Epithelium is hyperchromatic, slightly disorderly, and over seven cells thick. Compare well-differentiated transitional epithelium with lesion in Figure 22–11.

lesions appear as small, red, elevated excrescences varying in size from less than 1 cm in diameter to large masses up to 5 cm in diameter. Multicentric origins may produce separate tumors (Fig. 22–12). Some grade II and grade III papillary cancers spread over wide areas of the bladder wall (Fig. 22–13).

Grade I lesions are almost always papillary. Grade II neoplasms also are most often papillary but may be flat. Both the papillary and the flat patterns may be invasive or noninvasive. The grade III transitional cell carcinomas represent the other end of the spectrum of anaplasia. Some of these lesions retain a papillary configuration, but many are flat or fungating necrotic, sometimes ulcerative, tumors, which have unmistakably invaded deeply. In one series, 6% of grade I, but 82% of grade III tumors, were invasive.[24] However, **carcinoma in situ** (see later), a flat noninvasive transitional grade III lesion, is often present in areas adjacent to carcinomas.[16] Invasive tumors may extend only into the bladder wall, but the more advanced stages invade the adjacent prostate, seminal vesicles, ureters, and retroperitoneum, and some produce fistulous communications to

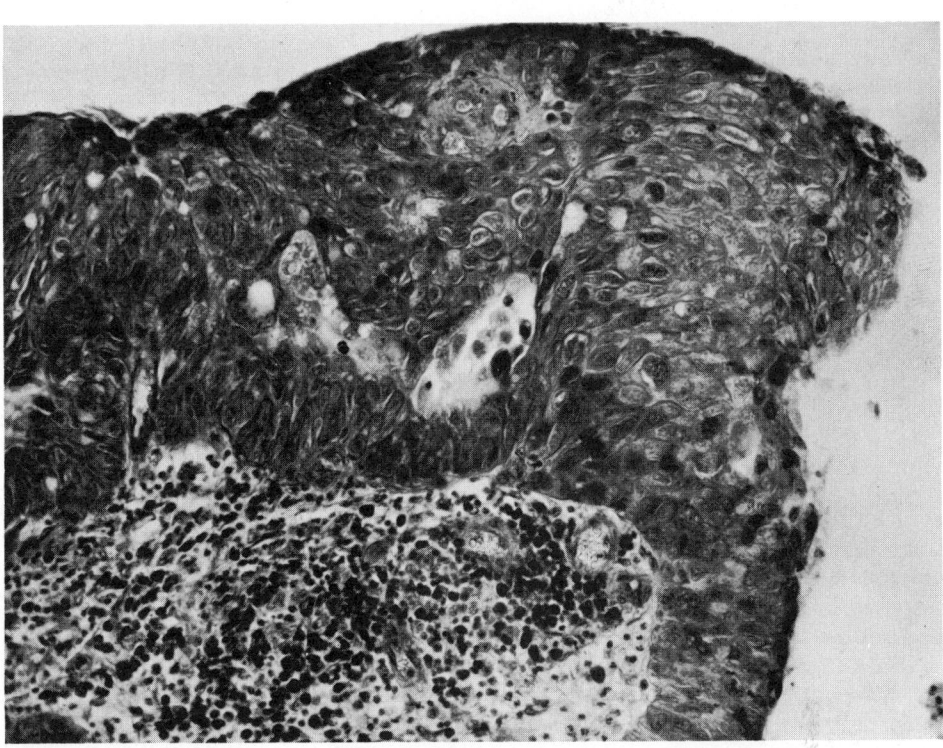

Figure 22–11. Papillary carcinoma of bladder, grade III, for comparison with Figure 22–10. Note loss of orderly normal transitional growth.

the vagina or rectum. About 40% of these deeply invasive tumors metastasize to regional lymph nodes. Hematogenous dissemination, principally to the liver, lung, and bone marrow, generally occurs late, and only with highly anaplastic tumors.

The **squamous cell carcinoma** in pure form accounts for about 5% of all bladder carcinomas. Transitional cell carcinomas with areas of squamous metaplasia are much more frequent. **Squamous cell carcinomas may be in situ but much more often are invasive, fungating tumors or infiltrative and ulcerative.** True papillary patterns are almost never seen. The level of cytologic differentiation varies widely, from the highly differentiated lesions producing abundant keratohyaline pearls to very anaplastic giant cell tumors showing no evidence of squamous differentiation.

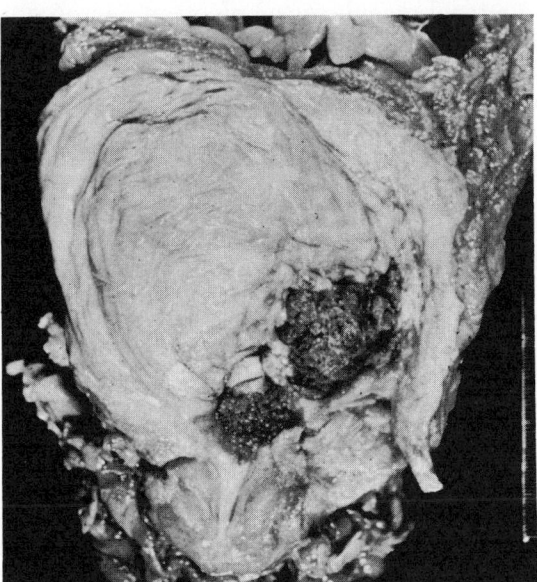

Figure 22–12. Papillary transitional cell carcinoma of bladder. Two discrete lesions in trigonal area.

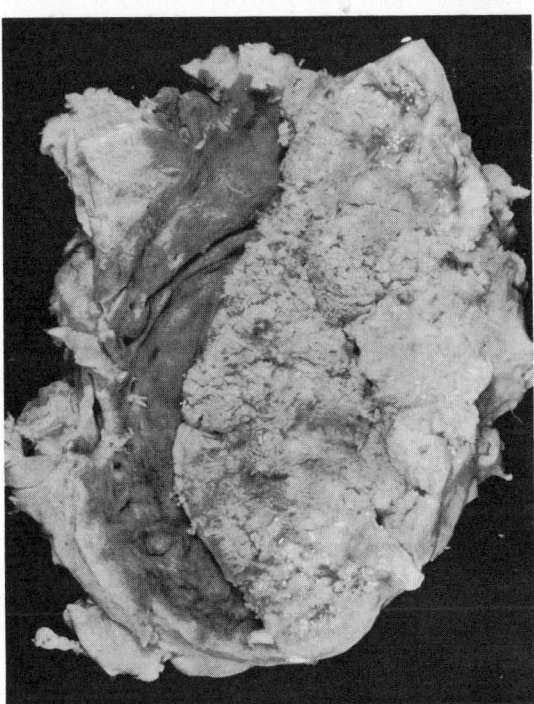

Figure 22–13. Transitional cell carcinoma. Entire right side of bladder is overgrown by spreading lesion.

Adenocarcinomas of the bladder are rare. These tumors may arise from urachal remnants, from periurethral and periprostatic glands, from cystitis cystica, or from metaplasia of transitional epithelium. Rare variants are the highly malignant **signet cell carcinoma** and the relatively nonaggressive **mesonephric or nephrogenic adenoma.**

CARCINOMA IN SITU. Studies of chemically induced bladder cancer in animals have shown that a series of progressive changes occur in bladder epithelium, culminating in the formation of bladder tumors.[16] These include *hyperplasia, dysplasia* (atypical hyperplasia), and *carcinoma in situ.* Similar changes occur in humans,[17,24–26] usually in association with fully developed tumors, and there is great current interest in detecting such lesions and determining their malignant potential before full-fledged cancer has developed.

Hyperplasia is characterized by a significantly increased number of epithelial cell layers, beyond the seven found in normal bladder. The cells show some de-differentiation, in that they usually resemble the basal cells of epithelium. The change can be focal or multifocal or can involve large areas of the mucosa.

Atypical hyperplasia and dysplasia are associated with significant nuclear atypicalities, which may be mild, moderate, or severe; increased mitotic activity; and evidence of de-differentiation.

Carcinoma in situ is the best studied of these lesions in humans. The lesions are flat and consist of highly anaplastic, overtly malignant cells with numerous mitoses, confined to the mucosa. They are most frequently detected in patients with previous or simultaneous papillary and invasive tumors, being present in from 5% to as many as 90% of such patients (the latter high figure being derived from cystectomy specimens in which the entire mucosa is histologically "mapped"[27]). It is reasonable to assume that all overt cancers must have passed through an in situ phase, but the natural history of in situ lesions is still uncertain. In the most thorough studies, about 55% of patients had developed invasive carcinoma within five years. Most workers now believe that these lesions are part and parcel of the generalized influence of a putative carcinogen on urothelium, and further, that these flat lesions are the precursors of *invasive* cancer in patients who also harbor noninvasive transitional cell carcinomas of various grades. Although carcinoma in situ is almost certainly precancerous, the malignant potential of hyperplasia and dysplasia is unknown.

CLINICAL COURSE OF BLADDER CANCER. All bladder tumors classically produce painless hematuria. This is their dominant and sometimes only clinical manifestation. Occasionally, frequency, urgency, and dysuria accompany the hematuria. When the ureteral orifice is involved, pyelonephritis or hydronephrosis may follow.

All transitional cell cancers, whatever their grade, have a tendency to recur following excision, and usually the recurrence exhibits greater anaplasia. Overall, 60 to 80% of grade I papillary carcinomas recur, whereas 80 to 90% of grade III lesions do so. In many instances, the recurrence is seen at a different site and the question of a new primary tumor must be entertained. Transitional cell tumors seem to be prime examples of neoplasms arising in a "restless epithelium."

The prognosis depends on the histologic pattern of the neoplasm, on the histologic grade, and principally on the clinical stage when first diagnosed. There is a strong correlation between the grade and the stage of the lesion. For the benign papilloma there is good agreement that the five-year survival is over 90%, with a simple local resection or fulguration. Failure to achieve 100% survival relates to either misdiagnosis or recurrence. For the malignant lesions, 30 to 80% five-year survival has been achieved for cancers that have not infiltrated more deeply than the superficial layers of the muscular wall of the bladder. With deeper invasion of the bladder wall, but no extension into surrounding structures, the five-year survival is only 10 to 30%. In general, the transitional cell cancers have a better prognosis than the squamous cell neoplasms. For the latter, approximately 70% of patients are dead within one year. In all forms of bladder cancer, death is usually caused by either progressive infiltration of the ureters leading to bacterial and obstructive renal disease, or dissemination of the cancer.

The difficulty of predicting aggressive clinical behavior in tumors of seemingly similar histologic grades has led to a search for modern cytologic flow cytometric, immunologic, and ultrastructural markers for aggressive tumors.[28–30] Tumors that are more likely to behave as malignant tumors (recur, invade, metastasize) have been shown to (1) lack blood group antigens on their cell surfaces, (2) exhibit alterations in junctional complexes on electron microscopic examination, (3) manifest abnormal karyotypes, (4) exhibit amplified or mutated oncogenes, and (5) show polyploidy and aneuploidy by flow cytometric analysis of cells.

MESENCHYMAL TUMORS

BENIGN. A great variety of benign mesodermal tumors may arise in the bladder. Collectively, they are rare. The most common is *leiomyoma.* They all tend to grow as isolated, intramural, encapsulated, oval-to-spherical masses, varying in diameter up to several centimeters. Occasionally, they assume submucosal pedunculated positions. They have the histologic features of their counterparts elsewhere.

SARCOMAS. Sarcomatous growths may also involve the bladder. As a group, they tend to produce large masses (varying up to 10 to 15 cm in diameter) that protrude into the vesical lumen. Their soft, fleshy, gray-white gross appearance suggests their sarcomatous nature.

One form, rhabdomyosarcoma, which deserves special mention, takes one of two forms. The "adult" form occurs mostly in adults over 40 years of age and shows a range of histology similar to rhabdomyosarcomas of striated muscle (p. 1375). The other variant is the embryonal rhabdomyosarcoma, encountered chiefly in infancy or childhood. This type of neoplasm tends to grow in large, polypoid projections into the bladder lumen, producing grapelike clusters of soft, fleshy tissue. These malignancies, also called *sarcoma botryoides*, are similar to those that occur in the female genital tract (p. 1138).

SECONDARY TUMORS

Secondary malignant involvement of the bladder is most often by direct extension from primary lesions in nearby organs, cervix, uterus, prostate, and rectum, in the order given. They may, on casual inspection of the bladder, appear as primary squamous cell carcinomas of this organ. Hemorrhage, ureteral obstruction, and vesicovaginal fistulas are the common sequelae.

OBSTRUCTION

Obstruction to the bladder neck is of major clinical importance, not only for the changes induced in the bladder, but also because of its eventual effect on the kidney. A great variety of intrinsic and extrinsic diseases of the bladder may narrow the urethral orifice and cause partial or complete vesical obstruction. In the male, the most important lesion is enlargement of the prostate gland due either to nodular hyperplasia or to carcinoma (Fig. 22–14). Vesical obstruction is somewhat less common in the female and is most often caused by cystocele of the bladder. The more infrequent causes can be listed as (1) congenital narrowings or strictures of the urethra; (2) inflammatory strictures of the urethra; (3) inflammatory fibrosis and contraction of the bladder following varying types of cystitis; (4) bladder tumors—either benign or malignant—when strategically located; (5) secondary invasion of the bladder neck by growths arising in perivesical structures, such as the cervix, vagina, prostate, and rectum; (6) mechanical obstructions caused by foreign bodies and calculi; and (7) injury to

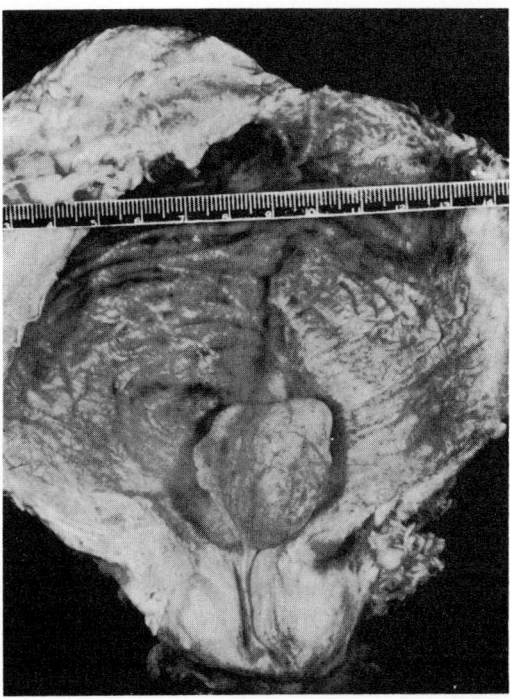

Figure 22–14. Hypertrophy and trabeculation of bladder wall secondary to polypoid hyperplasia of prostate.

the innervation of the bladder causing neurogenic or cord bladder.

In the early stages, there is only some thickening of the bladder wall, presumably due to hypertrophy of the smooth muscle. The mucosal surface at this time may be entirely normal. With progressive hypertrophy of the muscular coat, the individual muscle bundles greatly enlarge and produce trabeculation of the bladder wall. In the course of time, crypts form and may then become converted into true acquired diverticula.

In some cases of acute obstruction or in terminal disease when the patient's normal reflex mechanisms are depressed, the bladder may become extremely dilated. The enlarged bladder may reach the brim of the pelvis or even the level of the umbilicus. In these cases, the bladder wall is markedly thinned and the trabeculation becomes totally inapparent.

URETHRA

INFLAMMATIONS

Urethritis is classically divided into gonococcal and nongonococcal urethritis. As noted earlier, gonococcal urethritis is one of the earliest manifestations of this venereal infection. Nongonococcal urethritis is very common, and can be caused by a variety of bacteria, among which *E. coli* and other enteric organisms predominate. In females urethritis is often accompanied by cystitis and in males by prostatitis. In many instances bacteria cannot be isolated. Various strains of chlamydia (e.g., *C. trachomatis*) are the cause of 25

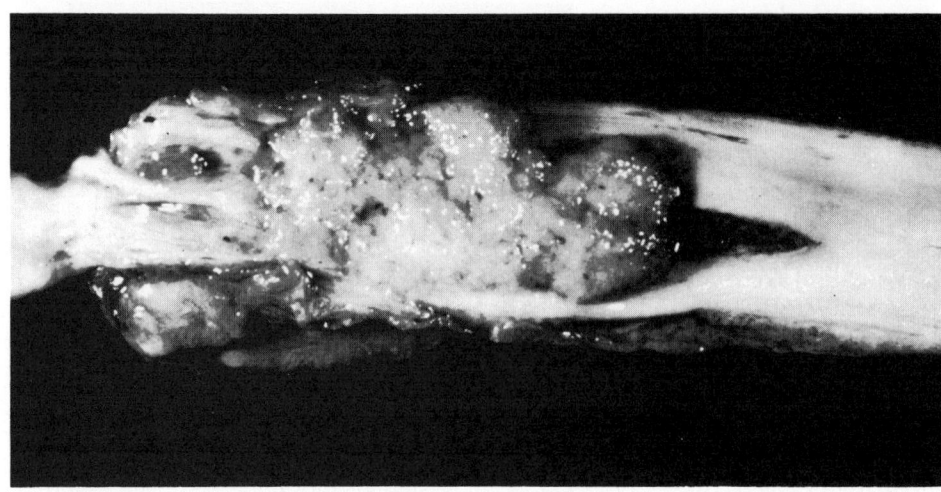

Figure 22–15. Carcinoma of urethra with typical fungating growth.

to 60% of nongonococcal urethritis in males and about 20% in females.[31,32] Mycoplasma *(Ureaplasma urealyticum)* also accounts for the symptoms of urethritis in many cases. Urethritis is also one component of *Reiter's syndrome*, which comprises the clinical triad of arthritis, conjunctivitis, and urethritis.

The morphologic changes are entirely typical of inflammation in other sites within the urinary tract. The urethral involvement is not itself a serious clinical problem, but may cause considerable local pain, itching, and frequency, and may represent a forerunner of more serious disease in higher levels of the urogenital tract.

TUMORS

CARUNCLE

Urethral caruncle is an inflammatory lesion presenting a small, red, painful mass about the external urethral meatus in the female. Caruncles may be found at any age but are more common in later life. The lesion consists of a hemispherical, friable, 1 to 2 cm nodule that occurs singly, either just outside or just within the external urethral meatus. It may be covered by an intact mucosa but is extremely friable, and the slightest trauma may cause ulceration of the surface and bleeding. Histologically, it is composed of a *highly vascularized, young, fibroblastic connective tissue, more or less heavily infiltrated with leukocytes.* The overlying epithelium, where present, is either transitional or squamous cell in type. Surgical excision affords prompt relief and cure.

BENIGN TUMORS

Papillomas of the urethra occur usually just within or on the external meatus. In this location, tumors in the spectrum of the veneral condylomas, discussed on page 1135, also arise.

CARCINOMA

Carcinoma of the urethra is an uncommon lesion. It tends to occur in advanced age and, in most instances, begins about the external meatus or on the immediately surrounding structures, such as the glans penis, or the introitus in the female. Some apparently begin just inside the external meatus or even at a higher level within the urethra. Those that occur at and protrude from the external meatus appear as warty, papillary growths that at first resemble the sessile papillary carcinomas described in the bladder. As they progress, they tend to become ulcerated on their surfaces and to assume the characteristics of a fungating, ulcerating lesion (Fig. 22–15).

Most of these malignancies are squamous cell carcinomas. The papillary lesions that protrude from the external meatus are apt to show a transitional cell growth that further heightens their similarity to bladder carcinoma. Uncommonly, an adenocarcinomatous growth pattern is found.

1. Petersen, R.O.: Urologic Pathology. Philadelphia, J.B. Lippincott Co., 1986.
2. Hill, G.S. (ed.): Uropathology. New York, Churchill-Livingstone, 1989.
3. McCarron, J.P., and Vaughn, E.D.: Tumors of the renal pelvis and ureter: current concepts and management. Semin. Urol. *1*:75, 1983.
4. Akaza, H., et al.: Clinical evaluation of urothelial tumors of the renal pelvis and ureter based on a new classification system. Cancer *59*:1369, 1987.
5. Mitchinson, M.J.: Retroperitoneal fibrosis revisited. Arch. Pathol. Lab. Med. *110*:784, 1986.
5a. Osborne, B.M., et al.: Idiopathic retroperitoneal fibrosis. Hum. Pathol. *18*:735, 1987.
6. Pauli, B.U.: The ultrastructure and pathobiology of urinary bladder cancer. *In* Chone, S., and Bryan, G.T. (eds.): The Pathology of Bladder Cancer. Boca Raton, CRC Press, 1984.
7. Engel, R.M., and Wilkinson, H.A.: Bladder extrophy. J. Urol. *104*:699, 1970.
8. Kunin, C.M.: Detection, Prevention, and Management of Urinary Tract Infections. 4th ed. Philadelphia, Lea & Febiger, 1987.

9. Poole, D.: Busulfan-induced hemorrhagic cystitis. J. Urol. *130:*347, 1983.

10. Messing, E.M., and Stamey, T.: Interstitial cystitis. Urology 2:381, 1978.

11. Smith, B.H.: Malakoplakia of the urinary bladder. A study of twenty-four cases. Am. J. Clin. Pathol. *43:*409, 1965.

12. Biggar, W., et al.: Malakoplakia and immunosuppressive therapy. Am. J. Pathol. *19:*5, 1985.

13. Littleton, R.H., et al.: Eosinophilic cystitis. J. Urol. *127:*132, 1982.

14. Young, R.H.: Pseudoneoplastic lesions of the urinary bladder. Pathol. Annu. 23(1):67, 1988.

15. Mostofi, F.K., et al.: Histological typing of urinary bladder tumors. Classification of Tumors *19.* Geneva, WHO, 1973.

16. Koss, L.G.: Tumors of the urinary bladder. Atlas of Tumor Pathology II, Series 2. Washington, D.C., Armed Forces Institute of Pathology, 1975.

17. Murphy, W.M.: Current topics in the pathology of bladder cancer. Pathol. Annu. *18:*1, 1983.

18. Matanoski, G.M., and Elliott, E.A.: Bladder cancer epidemiology. Epidemiol. Rev. *3:*203, 1981.

19. Schulte, P.A., et al.: Risk factors for bladder cancer in a cohort exposed to aromatic amines. Cancer *58:*2156, 1986.

20. EL-Bolkainy, M.N.: The impact of schistosomiasis on the pathology of bladder cancer. Cancer *48:*2043, 1981.

21. Fukushima, S., et al.: Effect of L-tryptophan and sodium saccharin on urinary tract carcainogenesis initiated by *N*-(4-5(nitro 2-furyl)-2-thiazolyl) formamide. Cancer Res. *41:*3100, 1981.

22. Bjergaard, J.P., et al.: Carcinoma of the urinary bladder after treatment with cyclophosphamide for non-Hodgkin's lymphomas. N. Engl. J. Med. *318:*1028, 1988.

22a. Hartge, P., et al.: Bladder cancer risk and pipes, cigars and smokeless tobacco. Cancer *55:*901, 1985.

23. Cummings, K.B.: Diagnosis, staging and classification of bladder tumors. Semin. Urol. *1:*7, 1983.

24. Koss, L.G.: Evaluation of patients with carcinoma *in situ* of the bladder. Pathol. Annu. *17:*353, 1982.

25. Fukui, I., et al.: Carcinoma in situ of the urinary bladder. Cancer *59:*164, 1987.

26. Hofstädter, F., et al.: Urothelial dysplasia and carcinoma in situ of the bladder. Cancer *57:*356, 1986.

27. Koss, L.G.: Mapping of the urinary bladder: Its impact on the concepts of bladder cancer. Hum. Pathol. *10:*553, 1979.

28. Coon, J.S., et al.: Markers in the analysis of human bladder carcinoma. Adv. Pathol. *1:*201, 1988.

29. Juhl, B.R., et al.: A,B,H antigen expression in transitional cell carcinomas of the urinary bladder. Cancer *57:*1768, 1986.

30. Weinstein, R.S., et al.: Blood group antigens and ploidy as prognostic factors in urinary bladder carcinoma. *In* Fenoglio-Preiser, C., and Weinstein, R.S. (eds.): New concepts in neoplasia as applied to diagnostic pathology. Baltimore, Williams & Wilkins, 1986.

31. Berger, R.E.: Urethritis and epididymitis. Semin. Urol. *1:*138, 1983.

32. Fihn, S.D., and Stamm, W.E.: The urethral syndrome. Semin. Urol. *1:*121, 1983.

Male Genital System

PENIS

The penis can be affected by congenital anomalies, inflammations, and tumors, the most important of which are inflammations and tumors. The venereal infections, e.g., syphilis and gonorrhea, usually begin with penile lesions. Carcinoma of the penis, although not one of the more common neoplasms in North America, still accounts for about 1% of cancers in males.

CONGENITAL ANOMALIES

The penis is the site of many varied forms of congenital anomalies, only some of which have clinical significance. These range from congenital absence and hypoplasia to hyperplasia, duplication, and other aberrations in size and form. For the most part, these deviations in size and form are extremely uncommon and readily apparent on inspection. Certain other anomalies are more frequent and, therefore, have greater clinical significance.

HYPOSPADIAS AND EPISPADIAS

Malformation of the urethral groove and urethral canal may create abnormal openings either on the *ventral surface of the penis (hypospadias) or on the dorsal surface (epispadias).* Such anomalies are commonly associated with failure of normal descent of the testes and with malformations of the urinary tract.[1] Even when isolated, these urethral defects may have clinical significance, because often the abnormal opening is constricted, producing partial urinary ob-

struction and an attendant hazard of spread of bacterial contamination from the obstructed penile urethra into the bladder and remainder of the urinary tract. Moreover, these anomalies may have more serious consequences. When the orifices are situated near the base of the penis, normal ejaculation and insemination are hampered or totally blocked. These lesions, therefore, are possible causes of sterility in the male.

PHIMOSIS

When the orifice of the prepuce is too small to permit its normal retraction, the condition is designated phimosis. Such an abnormally small orifice may result from anomalous development but may also be produced by inflammatory scarring of the prepuce. Phimosis is important because it interferes with cleanliness and permits the accumulation of secretions and detritus under the prepuce, favoring the development of secondary infections and possibly carcinoma. When a phimotic prepuce is forcibly retracted over the glans penis, marked constriction and subsequent swelling may block the replacement of the prepuce, creating what is known as *paraphimosis.* This condition not only is extremely painful, but it also may be a potential cause of urethral constriction and serious acute urinary retention.

INFLAMMATIONS

Inflammations of the penis almost invariably involve the glans and prepuce and include a wide variety of **1099** specific and nonspecific infections. The specific infections — syphilis, gonorrhea, chancroid, granuloma inguinale, lymphopathia venereum, genital herpes — are sexually transmitted and were discussed in Chapter 7. Only the nonspecific infections causing so-called balanoposthitis need description here.

BALANOPOSTHITIS

Balanoposthitis is a nonspecific infection of the glans and prepuce caused by a wide variety of organisms, e.g., staphylococci, streptococci, coliform bacilli, and (less often) the gonococci. It is usually encountered in patients having phimosis or a large, redundant prepuce that interferes with cleanliness and predisposes to bacterial growth within the accumulated secretions and smegma. Such inflammations, if neglected, may lead to frank ulcerations of the mucosal covering of the glans. If they persist and become chronic, they lead to further inflammatory scarring of the phimosis, with aggravation of the underlying condition. The inflammatory reaction is nonspecific, and correct identification of the specific agent requires bacterial smears and cultures.

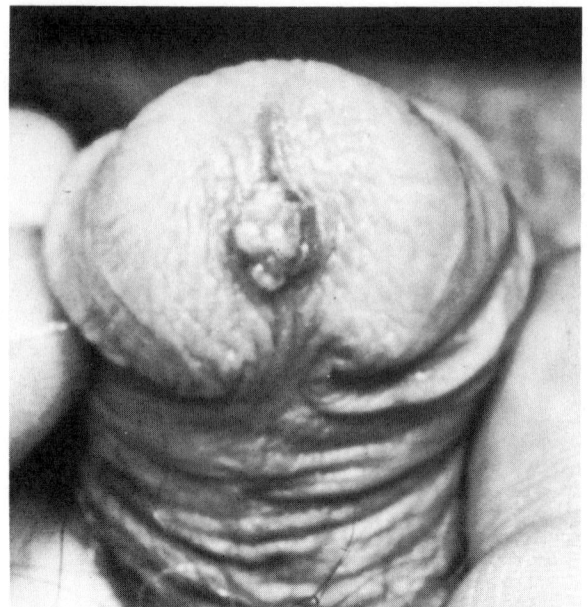

Figure 23 – 1. Condyloma acuminatum of penis.

TUMORS

Tumors of the penis are, on the whole, uncommon. The most frequent neoplasms are carcinomas and a benign epithelial tumor — condyloma acuminatum. However, in addition to the clearly defined benign and malignant categories there are some conditions that fall into an intermediate zone. These include the locally invasive giant condyloma (verrucous carcinoma) and Bowen's disease, which has the potential of developing into cancer.

BENIGN TUMORS

Condyloma Acuminatum

This benign tumor is caused by human papilloma virus (HPV). It is related to the common wart (verruca vulgaris) and may occur on any moist mucocutaneous surface of the external genitals in either sex. There is mounting evidence that HPV and associated diseases are sexually transmitted. In recent studies 64 to 69% of the male consorts of women with genital HPV infection were found to have condylomata acuminata or HPV-related penile intraepithelial neoplasia.[2,3] Of the various antigenically and genetically distinct types of HPV that have been identified, types 6 and 11 have been clearly associated with condylomata acuminata.[4] The antigens and genome of these HPV types can be demonstrated in most lesions by immunoperoxidase and DNA hybridization techniques, respectively.

As mentioned, condylomata acuminata may occur on the external genitalia or perineal areas. On the penis, these lesions occur most often about the coronal sulcus and inner

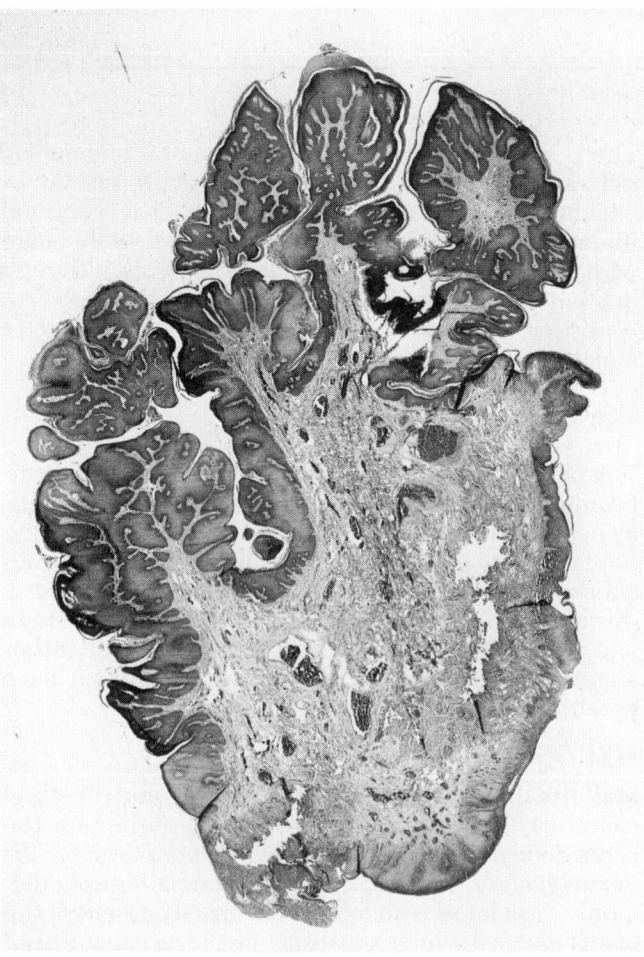

Figure 23 – 2. Condyloma acuminatum of penis. Low magnification reveals the papillary (villous) architecture. (Courtesy of Dr. Jag Bhawan, Boston University School of Medicine, Boston, MA.)

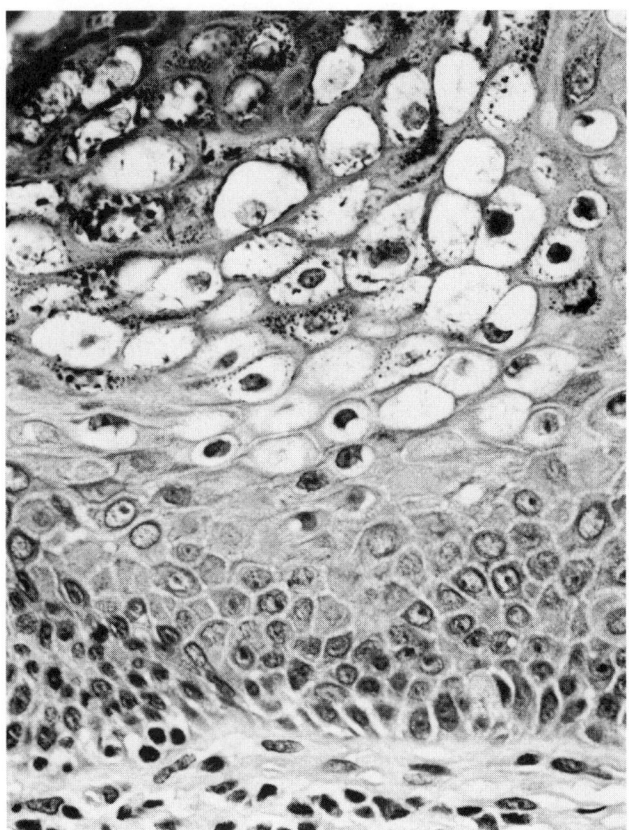

Figure 23–3. Condyloma acuminatum of penis. The epithelium shows vacuolization (koilocytosis) characteristic of human papilloma virus (HPV) infection. (Courtesy of Dr. Jag Bhawan, Boston University School of Medicine, Boston, MA.)

surface of the prepuce. They consist of single or multiple sessile or pedunculated, red papillary excrescences that vary from one to several millimeters in diameter (Fig. 23–1). Histologically, a branching, villous, papillary connective tissue stroma is covered by a thickened hyperplastic epithelium that may have considerable superficial hyperkeratosis and thickening of the underlying epidermis (acanthosis) (Fig. 23–2). The normal orderly maturation of the epithelial cells is preserved. Clear vacuolization of the prickle cells (koilocytosis), characteristic of HPV infection, is noted in these lesions (Fig. 23–3). The basement membrane is usually intact and there is no evidence of invasion of the underlying stroma. As far as we know, the vast majority of these lesions remain benign throughout their course.

Condylomata acuminata are uncommon before puberty. Their presence in small children should arouse the suspicion of sexual abuse.[5]

Giant Condyloma (Buschké-Lowenstein Tumor, Verrucous Carcinoma)

Giant condyloma, as implied by its name, is much larger than condyloma acuminatum. It presents usually as a solitary exophytic lesion which may cover and destroy much of the penis. Like condyloma acuminatum it is believed to be of viral origin, as HPV 6 and 11 can be demonstrated within the tumor cells by DNA hybridization.[6] Unlike condyloma acuminatum, it is locally invasive and has a tendency for recurrence. However, giant condylomata differ from the unambiguously malignant squamous cell carcinomas in that they rarely, if ever, metastasize. Thus with respect to biologic behavior giant condylomata occupy an intermediate position between the truly benign condyloma acuminatum and the squamous cell carcinoma.

Microscopically, the giant condyloma exhibits both upward and downward growth patterns. The exophytic part is almost indistinguishable from condyloma acuminatum, including the characteristic koilocytic change in the superficial layers. In its lower portion the hyperplastic epithelium penetrates the underlying tissues along a broad front in the form of bulbous downgrowths. Unlike squamous cell carcinoma the pegs of epithelium are composed of well-differentiated squamous epithelium with no cellular atypia.

Finally, a note about terminology. Giant condyloma is often referred to as Buschké-Lowenstein tumor, after the names of the authors who first recognized it as an entity distinct from condyloma acuminatum. Subsequently, histologically identical lesions in the oral cavity were labeled *verrucous carcinomas*, and hence many authors prefer to apply this term to the genital lesions as well.[7]

CARCINOMA IN SITU

From the discussion in Chapter 6 it will be recalled that carcinoma in situ is a histologic term used to describe epithelial lesions having the cytologic changes of malignancy confined to the epithelium with no evidence of local invasion or distant metastases. It is considered a precancerous condition because of its potential to evolve into invasive cancer. In the external male genitalia, three lesions that display histologic features of carcinoma in situ have been described: *Bowen's disease, erythroplasia of Queyrat*, and *bowenoid papulosis*. Whether these are distinct clinical entities or instead are variants of a single underlying disorder is controversial, as will be evident from the following brief descriptions.

Bowen's disease occurs in the genital region of both males and females, usually in those over the age of 35 years. In males it is prone to involve the shaft of the penis and the scrotum. Grossly it appears as a solitary thickened, gray-white, opaque plaque with shallow ulceration and crusting. Histologically the epidermis shows proliferation with numerous mitoses, some atypical. The cells are markedly dysplastic with large hyperchromatic nuclei, and there is total lack of orderly maturation (Fig. 23–4). Nevertheless *the dermal-epidermal border is sharply delineated by an intact basement membrane*. Over the span of years, Bowen's disease may become invasive and transform into typical squamous cell carcinoma. The frequency of such transition is not well established, but it is believed to be around 10%. Another curious feature said to be associated with Bowen's disease is

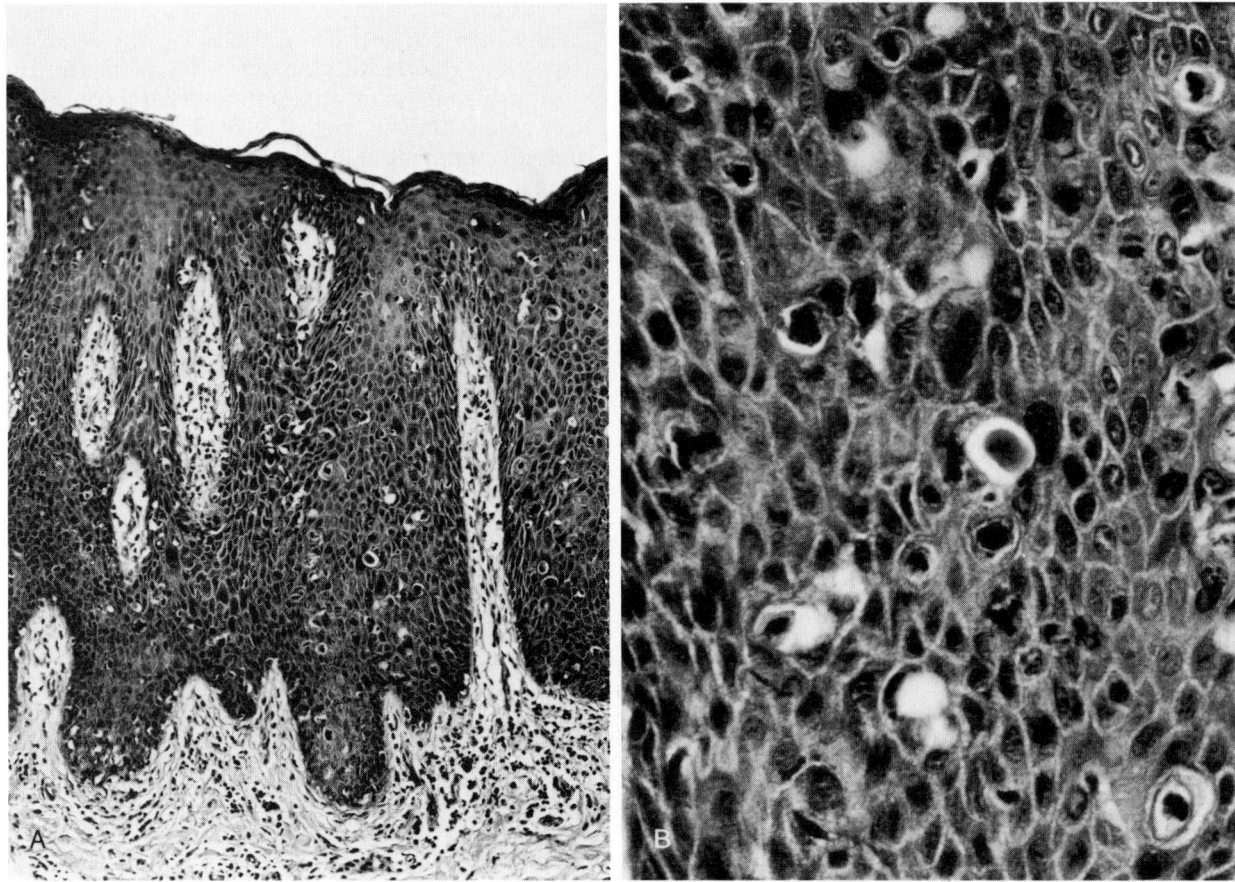

Figure 23–4. Bowen's disease (carcinoma in situ) of penis. *A,* Low magnification shows an intact basement membrane. *B,* Higher magnification reveals dysplastic epithelial cells with several mitoses. (Courtesy of Dr. Jag Bhawan, Boston University School of Medicine, Boston, MA.)

an association with visceral cancer. According to some authors, approximately one third of the patients develop carcinomas of the respiratory, gastrointestinal, or urinary tract. However, this view has been challenged and hence this issue remains unresolved.[8,9]

Erythroplasia of Queyrat generally appears on the glans and prepuce as a red, soft plaque. Histologically the dysplasia is of variable severity, ranging from mild disorientation of cells to a picture indistinguishable from that of Bowen's disease. Like Bowen's disease it has the potential to develop into invasive carcinoma. However, in contrast to Bowen's disease, there is no reported association with visceral malignancy. Because the relationship between Bowen's disease and internal malignancy remains unresolved, it should be apparent that the distinction between erythroplasia of Queyrat and Bowen's disease is at best tenuous.

Bowenoid papulosis, the third member of the carcinoma in situ "family" of lesions affecting the external genitalia, occurs in sexually active adults. Clinically it differs from Bowen's disease by the younger age of patients and the presence of multiple (rather than solitary), pigmented (reddish brown) papular lesions. In some cases the lesions may be verrucoid and readily mistaken for condyloma acuminatum. How-

ever, histologically bowenoid papulosis is indistinguishable from Bowen's disease.[10] It is of interest to note that although HPV type 16 DNA sequences can be detected in over 80% of cases by hybridization studies, viral antigens are detected infrequently. This suggests that despite integration of HPV DNA in the genome, the level of virus production is low. The association of HPV-16 with bowenoid papulosis, a precancerous lesion, is of interest in view of the possible role of this serotype HPV in the causation of cancers in the female genital tract [4] (p. 1136).

CARCINOMA

Squamous cell carcinoma of the penis represents about 1% of cancers in males in the United States. Because protection against this malignancy is apparently conferred by circumcision, the incidence among different population groups varies widely throughout the world. Carcinoma of the penis is virtually unknown among Jews, in whom ritual circumcision is performed in the first days of life. It is extremely rare among Moslems, in whom circumcision is performed before the tenth year of life. In regions of the world where circumcision is not routinely practiced, carcinoma of the penis is correspondingly more common;

for instance, it is reported to represent about 12% of all malignant tumors in the Orient.[11] The protection conferred by circumcision has traditionally been ascribed to its effectiveness in preventing accumulation of smegma, believed by some to be a source of as yet unidentified carcinogens. However, as with certain cancers of the female genital tract, there is some evidence suggesting a possible causal association with HPV types 16 and 18.[12] It is possible, therefore, that the protective effect of circumcision may be due to an associated improvement of penile hygiene, reducing the likelihood of exposure to potentially oncogenic viruses. Carcinomas are usually found in patients between the ages of 40 and 70.

> The lesion usually begins on the glans or inner surface of the prepuce near the coronal sulcus. The first observable changes are a small area of epithelial thickening accompanied by graying and fissuring of the mucosal surface. With progression, an elevated leukoplakic papule is produced that often ulcerates when a diameter of approximately 1 cm is reached. Despite the obviousness of such lesions, by the time most patients seek medical attention large characteristic malignant ulcers are present, having necrotic, secondarily infected bases with ragged, irregular, heaped-up margins (Fig. 23–5). In far-advanced lesions, the ulceroinvasive disease may have destroyed virtually the entire tip of the penis or large areas of the shaft. A second pattern of macroscopic tumor growth is the papillary tumor that simulates the condyloma and progressively enlarges to form a cauliflower-like, ulcerated, fungating mass. Histologically, both the papillary and ulceroinvasive lesions are squamous cell carcinomas exactly resembling those that occur elsewhere on the skin surface.

CLINICAL COURSE. Carcinoma of the penis is a slowly growing, locally metastasizing lesion,[13] which

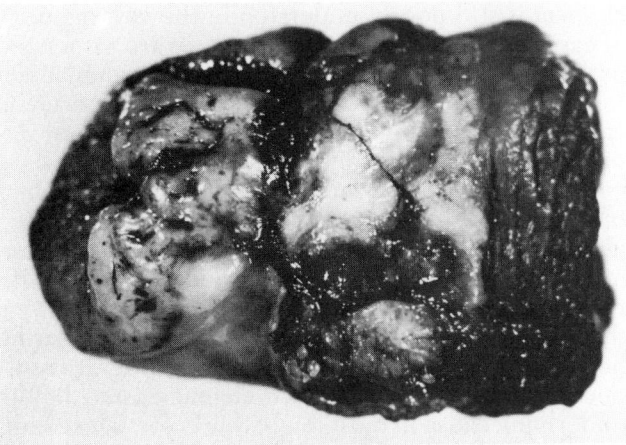

Figure 23–5. Squamous cell carcinoma of penis with typical shaggy fungating ulcerations. (Courtesy of Dr. Fred Silva, Department of Pathology, Southwestern Medical School, Dallas, TX.)

often has been present for a year or more before it is brought to medical attention. Such delay is occasioned sometimes by the existence of a phimosis that completely hides the developing lesion, but more often by unawareness of the significance of the developing papule. The lesions are nonpainful until they undergo secondary ulceration and infection. Frequently they bleed. Metastases to inguinal and iliac lymph nodes characterize the early stage, and widespread dissemination is extremely uncommon until the lesion is far advanced. The prognosis is related to the stage of advancement of the tumor. In persons with limited lesions without invasion of the penile shaft, there is a 95 to 100% three-year survival rate, whereas tumors that invade the shaft of the penis and the regional lymph nodes yield only a 30 to 50% three-year survival rate.

TESTIS AND EPIDIDYMIS

The major pathologic involvements of the testis and epididymis are quite distinct. In the case of the epididymis the most important and frequent involvements are inflammatory diseases, whereas in the testis the major lesions consist of tumors. However, their close anatomic relationship permits the extension of any of these processes from one organ to the other.

CONGENITAL ANOMALIES

With the exception of incomplete descent of the testes (cryptorchidism), congenital anomalies are extremely rare and include absence of one or both testes, fusion of the testes (so-called *synorchism*), and the formation of relatively insignificant cysts within the testis.

CRYPTORCHIDISM

Cryptorchidism is synonymous with undescended testes and is found in approximately 0.3 to 0.8% of the adult male population.[14] This anomaly represents a complete or incomplete failure of the intra-abdominal testes to descend into the scrotal sac.

It will be recalled that in the fetus the testis arises within the celomic cavity and then, by differential growth of the body as well as more rapid proliferation of the caudal end of the urogenital ridge, the testis comes to lie within the lower abdomen or brim of the pelvis, a process referred to as the internal descent. Following this, it descends through the inguinal canal into the scrotal sac—the external descent. On this basis, *malpositioned testes may be found at any point in this pathway of descent*. The precise cause of cryptorchidism is still poorly understood. The vast majority of cases are idiopathic, but some cases are associated with specific mechanical, genetic, and hormonal factors. Among mechanical factors, a short spermatic cord or a narrow inguinal canal may be of causal significance. Cryptorchidism may be one of several congenital defects in chromosomal disorders such as trisomy 13. Because a normally functioning hypothalamic-pituitary axis is essential for testicular development and descent, cryptorchidism is associated with rare hormonal disorders that are characterized by a deficient secretion of luteinizing hormone–releasing hormone. Although formal proof is lacking, it is suspected that subtle hormonal deficiencies may be the underlying cause in most idiopathic cases. The condition is completely asymptomatic, and it is found by the patient or the examining physician only when the scrotal sac is discovered not to contain the testis.

> Cryptorchidism is unilateral in the majority of cases, but it may be bilateral in 25% of patients. Contrary to previous beliefs, histologic changes in the malpositioned testis begin as early as two years of age. They are characterized by an arrest in the development of germ cells associated with marked hyalinization and thickening of the basement membrane of the spermatic tubules. Eventually the tubules appear as dense cords of hyaline connective tissue outlined by prominent basement membranes (Fig. 23–6). There may be concomitant increase in interstitial stroma and usually some hyperplasia of Leydig cells. As might be expected with progressive tubular atrophy, the cryptorchid testis is small in size and is firm in consistency owing to fibrotic changes. Surprisingly, histologic deterioration, leading to a paucity of germ cells, has also been noted in the contralateral (descended) testis in patients with unilateral cryptorchidism. This, as we shall discuss later, has important implications in the management of cryptorchidism.

Cryptorchidism is of more than academic interest for many reasons. When the testis lies in the inguinal canal, it is particularly exposed to trauma and crushing against the ligaments and bones. A concomitant inguinal hernia frequently accompanies such malposition of the testis. From the morphologic changes, it is apparent that bilateral cryptorchidism may result in sterility. However, infertility is also noted in a significant number of cases with uncorrected unilateral cryptorchidism because, as mentioned earlier, the contralateral descended testis may also be deficient in germ cells. In addition the undescended testis is at a 10- to 40-fold greater risk of developing testicular cancer (p. 1108) than is the descended testis. Hence the undescended testis requires surgical correction, preferably before histologic deterioration sets in at around 2 years of age.[15] Unfortunately, the placement of the testis within the scrotum does not preclude the possibility of a cancer developing at a later date, nor can fertility be taken for granted. Indeed, malignant change may occur in the contralateral, normally descended testis. These observations suggest that, at least in some cases, cryptorchidism is associated with an intrinsic defect in testicular development and cellular differentiation unrelated to anatomic position, and hence the associated changes cannot be corrected by orchiopexy (surgical repositioning).

REGRESSIVE CHANGES

ATROPHY

Atrophy is the only important regressive change that affects the scrotal testis, and it may have a number of causes. These can be listed as (1) progressive atherosclerotic narrowing of the blood supply in old age; (2) the end stage of an inflammatory orchitis, whatever the etiologic agent; (3) cryptorchidism; (4) hypopituitarism; (5) generalized malnutrition, or cachexia; (6) obstruction to the outflow of semen; and (7) irradiation. In addition, (8) prolonged administration of female sex hormones, such as is used in treatment of patients with carcinoma of the prostate, may lead to atrophy, and (9) exhaustion atrophy may follow the persistent stimulation produced by high levels of follicle-stimulating pituitary hormone. The gross and microscopic alterations follow the pattern already described for cryptorchidism. When the process is bilateral, as it frequently is, sterility results. Atrophy or sometimes improper development of the testes occasionally occurs as a primary failure of genetic origin. The resulting condition, called Klinefelter's syndrome, represents a sex chromosomal disorder that is discussed in detail on page 133 along with other cytogenetic diseases.

INFLAMMATIONS

Inflammations are distinctly more common in the epididymis than in the testis. It is classically taught that, of the three major specific inflammatory states, *gonorrhea and tuberculosis almost invariably arise in the epididymis, whereas syphilis affects first the testis.*

NONSPECIFIC EPIDIDYMITIS AND ORCHITIS

Epididymitis and possible subsequent orchitis are commonly related to infections in the urinary tract (cystitis, urethritis, genitoprostatitis), which presumably reach the epididymis and the testis through either the vas deferens or the lymphatics of the spermatic cord.

The cause of epididymitis varies with the age of the patient. Although uncommon in children, epididymitis in childhood is usually associated with a congenital genitourinary abnormality and infection with gram-negative rods. In sexually active men under the age of 35 years, the sexually transmitted pathogens *Chlamydia trachomatis* and *Neisseria gonorrhoeae* are the most frequent culprits. In men over the age of 35, the common urinary tract pathogens such as *E. coli*

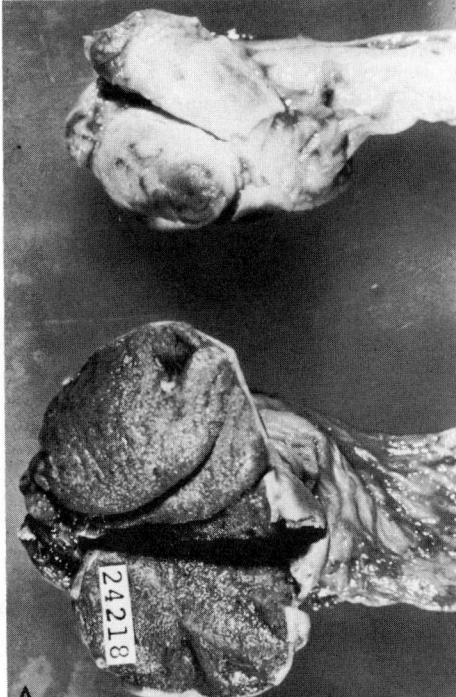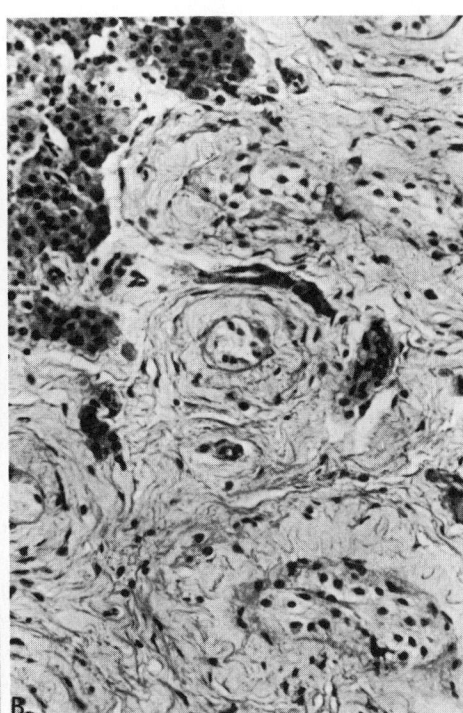

Figure 23–6. Testicular atrophy. *A,* The atrophic testis *(above)* is small and is replaced by white fibrous scars. Compare with cut surface of a normal testis *(below). B,* Microscopically, the tubules are visible as shadowy structures with markedly thickened basement membranes. Note the prominence of Leydig cells in upper left corner. (Courtesy of Dr. Fred Silva, Department of Pathology, University of Texas Health Science Center, Dallas.)

and *Pseudomonas* are responsible for most infections.[16]

The bacterial invasion sets up a nonspecific acute inflammation characterized by congestion, edema, and a white cell infiltration chiefly by neutrophils, macrophages, and lymphocytes. Although the infection, in the early stage, is more or less limited to the interstitial connective tissue, it rapidly extends to involve the tubules and may progress to frank abscess formation or complete suppurative necrosis of the entire epididymis. Usually, having involved the epididymis, the infection extends either by direct continuity or through tubular channels or lymphatics into the testis to evoke a similar inflammatory reaction within the testis. Such inflammatory involvement of the epididymis and testis is often followed by fibrous scarring, which, in many cases, leads to permanent sterility. Sterility may result from inflammatory obstruction of the excretory pathways or may be due to the intense pressure placed on the blood supply of the testis by the development of edema within a tight, fibrous, enclosing tunica albuginea. Thus, even when suppurative necrosis has not occurred, extensive inflammations may be followed by considerable atrophy of spermatic tubules and loss of spermatogenesis. Usually the interstitial cells of Leydig are not totally destroyed and are believed to be capable of regeneration when partially injured, so that sexual activity is not disturbed. Any such nonspecific infection may become chronic.

GRANULOMATOUS (AUTOIMMUNE) ORCHITIS

Among middle-aged men, a rare cause of unilateral testicular enlargement is nontuberculous, granulomatous orchitis. It usually presents as a moderately tender testicular mass of sudden onset sometimes associated with fever. However, it may appear insidiously as a painless testicular mass mimicking a testicular tumor, hence its importance.[17] Histologically, the orchitis is distinguished by granulomas seen both within spermatic tubules and in the intertubular connective tissue. The lesions closely resemble tubercles but differ somewhat in having plasma cells and occasional neutrophils interspersed within the enclosing rim of fibroblasts and lymphocytes. Although an autoimmune basis is suspected, the cause of these lesions remains unknown.

SPECIFIC INFLAMMATIONS

Gonorrhea

Extension of infection from the posterior urethra to the prostate, seminal vesicles, and thence to the epididymis is the usual course of a neglected gonococcal infection. Inflammatory changes similar to those described in the nonspecific infections occur, with the development of frank abscesses in the epididymis, resulting in extensive destruction of this organ. In the more neglected cases, the infection may thence spread to the testis and produce a suppurative orchitis (p. 344).

Mumps

About 25 to 30% of cases of mumps in males occur in persons 10 years of age or older. In this pubertal and postpubertal group, orchitis may develop and has been reported in approximately 20% of male patients who sought the care of a physician. Obviously, this sample is biased by the undoubted fact that many cases of mumps without orchitis do not come to medical attention, and only the more severe cases, particularly those with testicular involvement, are likely to be included in reported surveys. Most often, the acute interstitial orchitis develops about one week following onset of swelling of the parotid glands. Rarely, cases of orchitis precede the parotitis or may be unaccompanied by parotid gland involvement.

The testicular involvement is unilateral in approximately 70% of the cases. In the acute stage, the inflammatory reaction is characterized by intense interstitial edema and mononuclear infiltration, consisting chiefly of lymphocytes, plasma cells, and macrophages. Neutrophils are usually not prominent, but in the more intense inflammatory responses frank suppuration may develop and the tubular lumina may become filled with purulent exudate (Fig. 23–7). Because the process usually is unilateral, remains largely interstitial, and is characteristically patchy and haphazard, healing of the inflammatory reaction is usually not associated with infertility.

Tuberculosis

Tuberculosis almost invariably begins in the epididymis and may spread to the testis. On all but rare occasions, such lesions reflect a tuberculous infection elsewhere in the body, almost invariably in the lungs. Rarely, tuberculous epididymitis has followed apparently isolated renal tuberculosis. In many of these cases, there is associated tuberculous prostatitis and

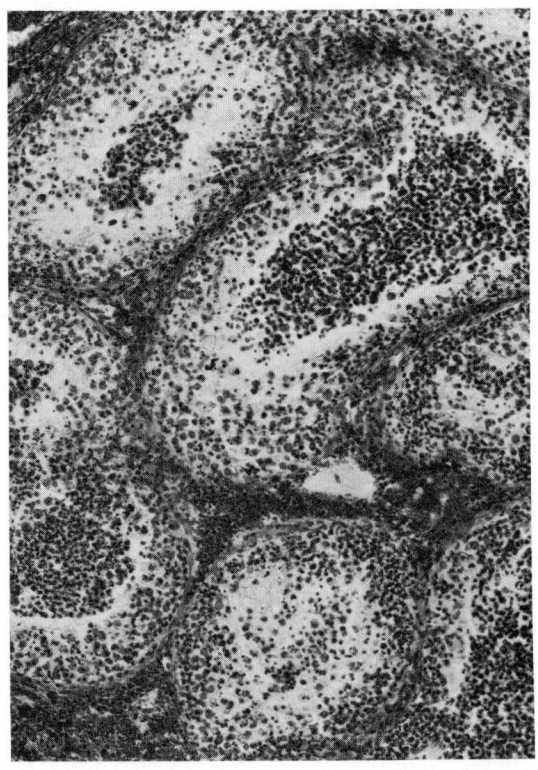

Figure 23–7. Acute severe mumps orchitis with extensive interstitial and intratubular exudation.

seminal vesiculitis, and it is believed by some that epididymitis usually represents a secondary spread from these other involvements of the genital tract. However, the epididymal involvement as a metastatic dissemination through the blood cannot be excluded, even in those cases with involvement of the organs in the urogenital system.

> The infection invokes the classic morphologic reactions of tuberculosis. Numerous tubercles become confluent to produce large caseous masses that, in the course of time, may obliterate the entire epididymal structure. By continuity or lymphogenous spread, such infections may extend into the adjacent regions of testis, but in most cases this organ is spared for long periods. The inflammatory involvement is followed, in the course of weeks or months, by progressive fibrous scarring and sometimes calcification.

Syphilis

The testis and epididymis are affected in both acquired and congenital syphilis, but *almost invariably the testis is involved first by the infection.* In many cases, the orchitis is not accompanied by epididymitis.

> The morphologic pattern of the reaction takes two forms: the production of gummas, or a diffuse interstitial inflammation characterized by edema and lymphocytic and plasma cell infiltration with the characteristic hallmark of all syphilitic infections, i.e., obliterative endarteritis with perivascular cuffing of lymphocytes and plasma cells. In the early case, the gummas cause a nodular enlargement and the characteristic yellow-white foci of necrosis. The diffuse reaction causes swelling and induration. In the course of time, whether or not the morphologic reaction is that of the already described gumma formation or diffuse inflammation, progressive fibrous scarring follows, which in turn leads to considerable tubular atrophy and, sometimes, sterility.

Miscellaneous Infections

The testis and epididymis are involved by hematogenous metastatic dissemination of organisms in a wide variety of infectious diseases, such as leprosy, typhoid fever, brucellosis, and meningococcal and rickettsial infections, and in some fungal diseases such as blastomycosis and actinomycosis. In all these instances, the testicular and epididymal involvement is only one small component of the systemic disorder, and the local inflammatory changes resemble those found in the systemic disease.

VASCULAR DISTURBANCES

TORSION

Twisting of the spermatic cord may cut off the venous drainage and the arterial supply to the testis. Usually,

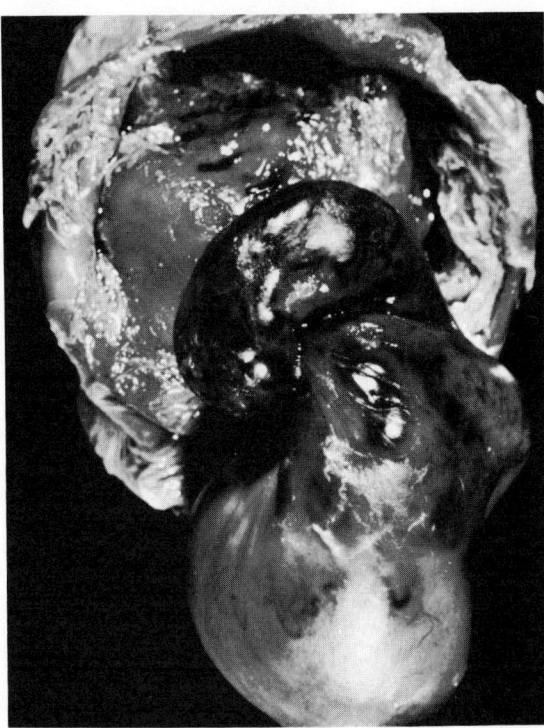

Figure 23–8. Torsion of testis.

however, the thick-walled arteries remain patent so that intense vascular engorgement and venous infarction follow. The usual precipitating cause of such torsion is some violent movement or physical trauma. In most instances, however, there are predisposing causes, such as incomplete descent, absence of the scrotal ligaments or the gubernaculum testis, atrophy of the testis so that it is abnormally mobile within the tunica vaginalis, abnormal attachment of the testis to the epididymis, or other abnormalities.

> Depending on the duration and severity of the process, the morphologic changes may range from those of merely intense congestion to widespread extravasation of blood into the interstitial tissue of the testis and epididymis. In more extreme instances, hemorrhagic or even anemic infarction of the entire testis may occur (Fig. 23–8). In these late stages, the testis is markedly enlarged and is converted virtually into a sac of soft, necrotic, hemorrhagic tissue. The leukocytic reaction is very variable and depends on the free access of blood via the arterial system. Usually the blood flow is so impaired that leukocytic infiltration is not a prominent feature and the process essentially resembles one of pure coagulative necrosis without considerable inflammatory reaction.

TESTICULAR TUMORS

Testicular neoplasms span an amazing gamut of anatomic types. Approximately 95% arise from germ cells. Most of these germinal tumors are highly aggressive cancers capable of rapid and wide dissemina-

tion, although with current therapy the outlook for these patients has improved considerably. Many when limited to the testis can be cured, and even with disseminated tumors complete remissions can sometimes be achieved. Nongerminal tumors, in contrast, are generally benign, but some elaborate steroids leading to interesting endocrinologic syndromes.

CLASSIFICATION AND HISTOGENESIS. Classifications of the testicular tumors abound and, regrettably, vary widely. The major problems are the differing concepts of the histogenesis of these lesions and the endless variability in morphology among the various forms of neoplasms as well as within a single tumor. As one might guess, totipotential germ cells that become cancerous are not inhibited in their lines of differentiation. The most authoritative and readily understood classification in the United States has been offered by Mostofi. More recently the WHO has presented a classification of testicular tumors (Table 23–1) that differs in only minor aspects from the Mostofi classification.[18]

The latter classification is based on the view that the vast majority of tumors in the testis arise from the testicular germ cells (Fig. 23–9).[19] The germ cells may give rise to seminoma, reflecting gonadal differentiation, or they may transform into totipotential tumor cells represented by embryonal carcinoma. According to this view, embryonal carcinomas contain stem cells for all nonseminomatous tumors. Depending on the degree and line of differentiation of embryonal carcinoma cells, tumors with different histologic patterns result. The most undifferentiated state is represented by pure embryonal cell carcinoma, whereas choriocarcinoma and yolk sac tumor represent commitment of the tumor stem cells to differentiate into specific extraembryonic cell types.

Table 23-1. WHO Pathologic Classification of Testicular Tumors

GERM CELL TUMORS
Tumors of one histologic pattern
    Seminoma
    Spermatocytic seminoma
    Embryonal carcinoma
    Yolk sac tumor (embryonal carcinoma infantile type)
    Polyembryoma
    Choriocarcinoma
    Teratomas
      Mature
      Immature
      With malignant transformation
Tumors showing more than one histologic pattern
    Embryonal carcinoma plus teratoma (teratocarcinoma)
    Choriocarcinoma and any other types (specify types)
    Other combinations (specify)
SEX CORD-STROMAL TUMORS
Well-differentiated forms
    Leydig cell tumor
    Sertoli cell tumor
    Granulosa cell tumor
Mixed forms (specify)
Incompletely differentiated forms

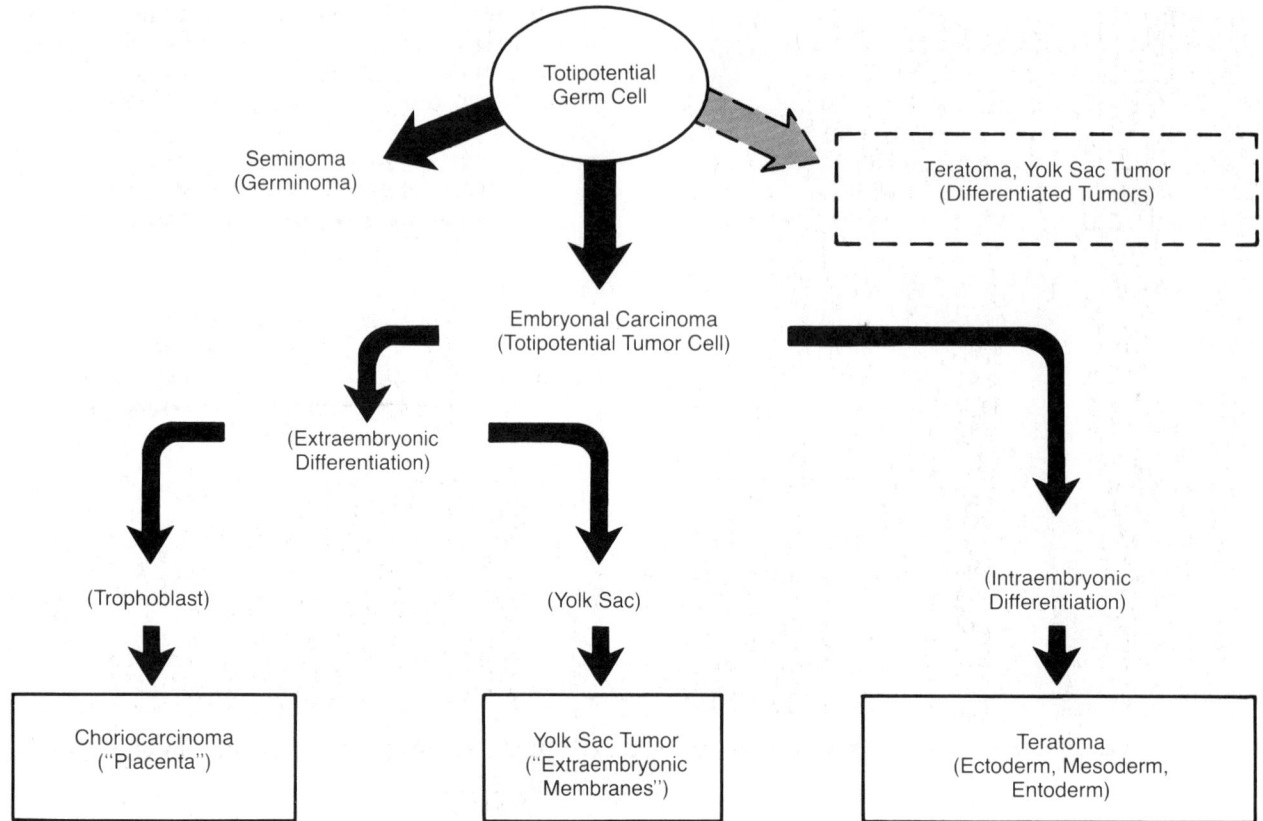

Figure 23-9. Histogenesis of testicular tumors.

Teratoma, on the other hand, results from differentiation of the embryonic carcinoma cells along the lines of all three germ cell layers, and therefore teratomas contain the greatest variety of neoplastic cells and tissues. In some cases (depicted by broken arrow, Fig. 23-9), differentiated tumors such as teratoma or yolk sac tumor seem to arise directly from the totipotential germ cell, and not through an intermediate stage of embryonal carcinoma.[20] This scheme provides a rational explanation for the apparently bewildering array of histologic patterns and is supported by the following observations: (1) the frequent, but not invariable, coexistence of embryonal carcinoma and teratoma in the testis; (2) the presence of teratoma or choriocarcinoma in the metastasis of a tumor, which in its primary site appears to be an embryonal carcinoma; and (3) the ultrastructural similarity between seminoma cells and normal primitive germ cells.[21]

Although this scheme is widely accepted in North America, it should be pointed out that an alternative hypothesis, which forms the basis of the British system of classification, differs significantly from this view. A comparative analysis of the British and WHO classifications is beyond the scope of this chapter and may be found in a review of this subject.[18] Although histogenetic classifications are of value in understanding the heterogeneity of testicular tumors, the student will be relieved to note that from a clinical standpoint there are only two important categories of germ cell tumors: seminomas and nonseminomatous tumors. As will be discussed later, this clinical distinction has important bearings on treatment and prognosis.

GERM CELL TUMORS

The incidence of testicular tumors in the United States is approximately two per 100,000 males. They cause about 0.15% of all male cancer deaths. In the 15- to 34-year age group, when these neoplasms have a peak incidence, they constitute the most common tumor of males and cause approximately 10% of all cancer deaths. Two smaller peaks of incidence are encountered in infancy and in later life.

PATHOGENESIS. As with all neoplasms, little is known about the ultimate cause of germinal tumors. However, several predisposing influences may be important: (1) cryptorchidism, (2) genetic factors, and (3) testicular dysgenesis, all of which may contribute to a common denominator—germ cell maldevelopment. Reference has already been made (p. 1104) to the increased incidence of neoplasms in *undescended testes*. In most large series of testicular tumors, approximately 10% are associated with cryptorchidism.[14] The higher the location of the undescended testicle (intra-abdominal vs. inguinal), the greater is the risk of developing cancer. The factors impinging on the cryptorchid testis that contribute to this increased risk of oncogenesis are not clear. It seems unlikely that the abnormal environment of the misplaced testis is related to the increased risk of carcinogenesis, as there is also an increased incidence of tumors in the contralateral, normally positioned testes. Furthermore there are virtually no data to prove that surgical repositioning (orchiopexy) eliminates or even reduces the risk of cancer development. Thus it seems that there are common predisposing factors, possibly hormonal, associated with both testicular cancer and cryptorchidism.[22] Nevertheless, it is recommended that ectopic testis should be repositioned surgically because it is easier to detect cancer in scrotal testis than in a testis in the groin or the abdomen.

Genetic predisposition also seems to be important, although no well-defined pattern of inheritance has been identified. In support, striking racial differences in the incidence of testicular tumors can be cited. Blacks in Africa have an extremely low incidence of these neoplasms, which is unaffected by migration to the United States. Testicular dysgenesis, a rare condition associated with endocrine abnormalities, also seems to predispose to tumor development, as malignant germ cell tumors develop in approximately 25% of dysgenetic testes.[23]

In summary, it appears that some abnormality in the development of germ cells may be the common denominator in predisposition to testicular cancer. Although such abnormalities are overt and severe only in some cases (e.g., cryptorchidism), more subtle aberrations may well underlie most cases. The changes may be genetically determined or perhaps may result from the interplay of genetic, environmental (e.g., carcinogens), and endocrine factors (Fig. 23–10).

With this background of pathogenesis, we can discuss the morphologic patterns of germ cell tumors followed by the clinical features common to most germinal tumors. The student can take comfort in the fact that some of the tumors listed in Table 23–1 are sufficiently rare to justify exclusion from the following discussion.

About 60% of germinal tumors are composed of a single cell type when examined by routine histologic

procedures. However, in one recent study in which tumor markers (discussed later) and histology were applied together, only 32% of the germ cell tumors appeared to belong to the group with a single histologic type.[18] These "pure" types will be described first, followed by some comments about the mixed patterns. Only then will the staging and clinical features common to most germ cell tumors be presented.

Seminoma

Seminomas are the most common type of germinal tumor (30%) and the type most likely to produce a uniform population of cells. They almost never occur in infants; they peak in the fourth decade, somewhat later than the collective peak.

Three histologic variants of seminoma are described: typical (85%), anaplastic (5 to 10%), and spermatocytic (4 to 6%). The last-mentioned has been segregated into a separate category in the WHO classification and will be discussed later. All produce bulky masses, sometimes ten times the size of the normal testis.

The typical seminoma has a homogeneous, gray-white, lobulated cut surface, usually devoid of hemorrhage or necrosis (Fig. 23–11). In over half the cases, the entire testis is replaced. The anaplastic variant has a similar macroscopic appearance. Generally, the tunica albuginea is not penetrated, but occasionally extension to the epididymis, spermatic cord, or scrotal sac occurs.

Microscopically, the typical seminoma, presumably derived from the proliferation of primary germ cells, presents sheets of uniform, so-called "seminoma cells" divided into poorly demarcated lobules by delicate septa of fibrous tissue. **The classic "seminoma cell" is large and round-to-polyhedral and has a distinct cell membrane, a cleared or watery-appearing cytoplasm, and a large, central hyperchromatic nucleus with one or two prominent nucleoli.** Mitoses are infrequent. The cytoplasm contains varying amounts of glycogen and, rarely, lipid vacuoles. Tumor giant cells may be present as well as syncytial giant cells; the latter resemble the syncytiotrophoblast of the placenta both morphologically and in that they contain human chorionic gonadotropins (HCG). In this subset of patients, serum HCG levels are also elevated (p. 1114). The amount of stroma in typical seminomas varies greatly. Sometimes it is scant and at other times abundant. Usually, well-defined fibrous strands are present, creating lobules of neoplastic cells. The septa are infiltrated with lymphocytes in 80% of cases (Fig. 23–12). In about 20% of tumors, the septa also bear prominent granulomatous reactions, i.e., aggregates of histiocytes enclosed within a rim of fibroblasts, lymphocytes, and occasional foreign body giant cells.

The anaplastic seminoma, as the name indicates, presents greater cellular and nuclear irregularity with more frequent tumor giant cells and many mitoses. Most critical to the identification of this pattern are the size of the cells and the presence of three or more mitoses per high-power field. Well-developed lymphocytic and granulomatous reactions are infrequent.

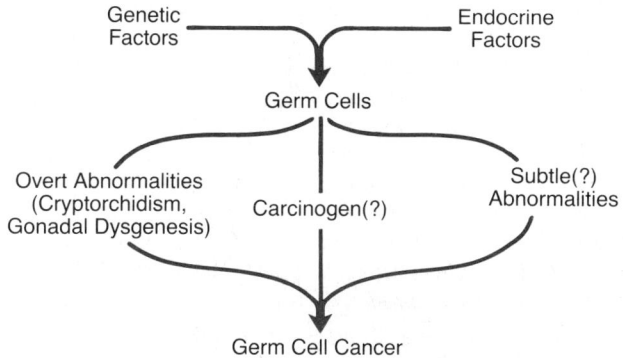

Figure 23–10. Pathogenetic pathways in the development of germ cell tumors of the testis.

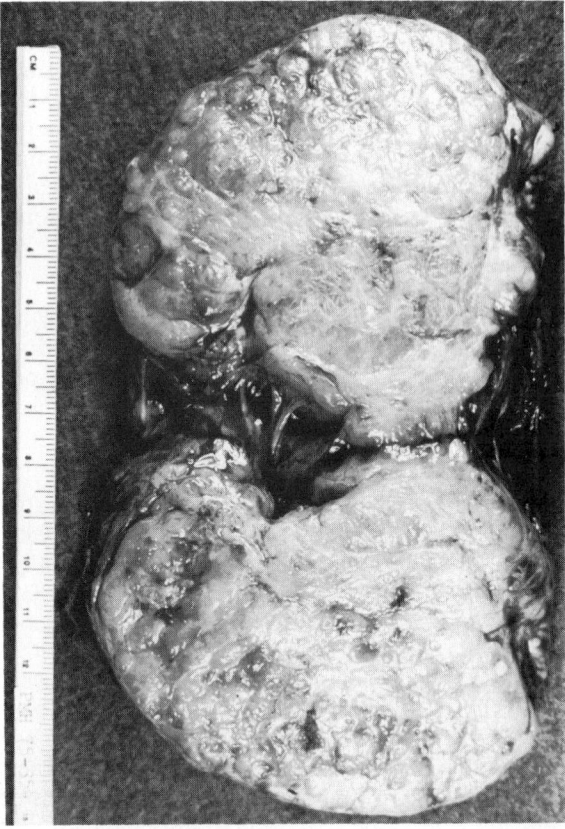

Figure 23-11. Seminoma. Testis is enlarged and virtually replaced by lobulated, homogeneous, gray-white tumor tissue. Hemorrhage and necrosis are not prominent. (Courtesy of Dr. Fred Silva, Department of Pathology, University of Texas Health Science Center, Dallas.)

Spermatocytic Seminoma

Although related by name, there is little in common between spermatocytic and classic seminomas. Both clinically and histologically, spermatocytic seminoma appears to be a distinctive tumor. It is an uncommon tumor, the reported incidence being approximately 4 to 6% of all seminomas. The age of involvement is much later than for most testicular tumors: affected individuals are mostly over the age of 65 years. Unlike classic seminoma, it is a slow-growing tumor that rarely if ever produces metastases, and hence the prognosis is excellent.

Grossly, spermatocytic seminoma tends to be larger than classic seminoma and presents with a pale gray, soft, and friable cut surface. Spermatocytic seminomas have three cell populations, all intermixed: (1) medium-sized cells (15 to 18 μm), the most numerous, which contain a round nucleus and eosinophilic cytoplasm; (2) smaller cells (6 to 8 μm), with a narrow rim of eosinophilic cytoplasm resembling secondary spermatocytes; and (3) scattered giant cells (50 to 100 μm), either uni- or multinucleate. Thus, marked variation in tumor cell size is an important microscopic feature. Unlike classic seminomas, there are no lymphocytes in the tumor, and mitoses are more common. With the electron microscope, tumor cells show nuclear and cytoplasmic features of spermatocytic maturation, thus justifying the term spermatocytic seminoma.

Embryonal Carcinoma

Embryonal carcinomas occur mostly in the 20- to 30-year age group. Although considerable progress has

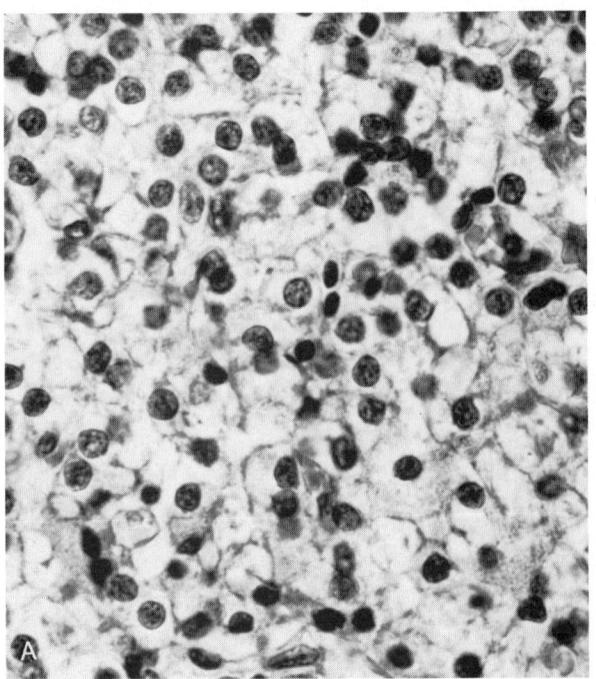

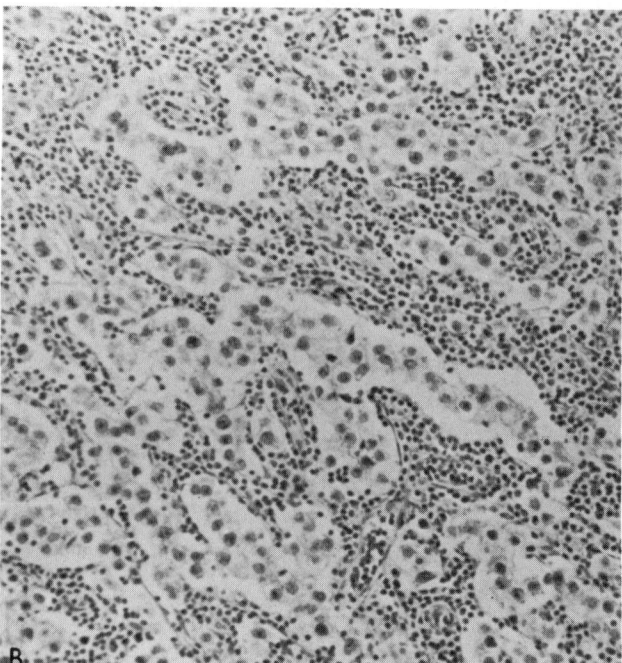

Figure 23-12. *A,* Microscopic detail of large, cleared seminoma cells. *B,* Seminoma with abundant lymphoid infiltrate (lower magnification than *A*).

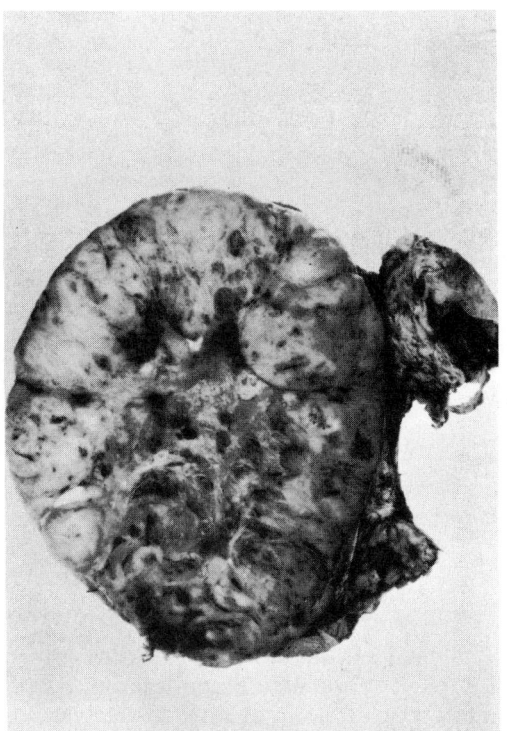 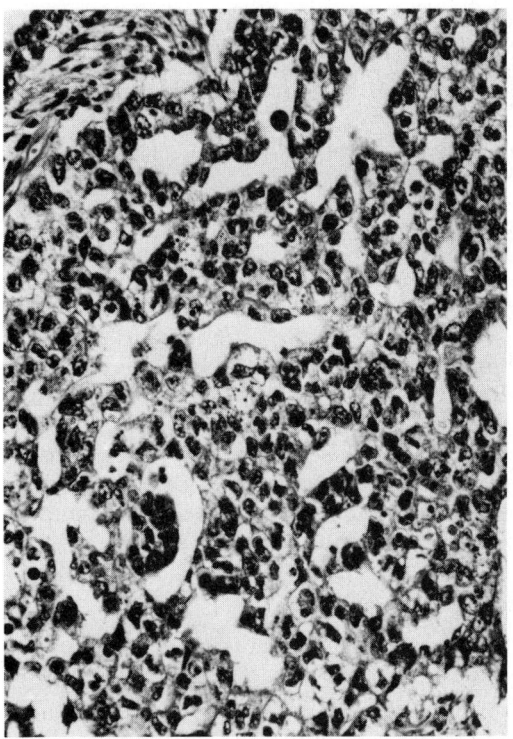

Figure 23–13   **Figure 23–14**

Figure 23–13. Embryonal carcinoma with extensive mottled necrosis and hemorrhage.

Figure 23–14. Embryonal carcinoma growing in a glandular and papillary pattern. (Courtesy of Dr. Fred Silva, Department of Pathology, University of Texas, Southwestern Medical School, Dallas, Texas.)

been made in treating these tumors with chemotherapy, they are more aggressive and lethal than seminomas.

Grossly, the tumor is often a small lesion that does not replace the entire testis. Larger, bulky tumors may be found but are the exception. On cut surfaces the mass is basically gray-white, but often variegated, poorly demarcated at the margins, and punctuated by foci of hemorrhage or necrosis (Fig. 23–13). Extension through the tunica albuginea into the epididymis or cord is not infrequent. **Histologically, the cells grow in glandular, alveolar, or tubular patterns, sometimes with papillary convolutions** (Fig. 23–14). **More undifferentiated lesions may present sheets of cells.** The neoplastic cells have an epithelial appearance and are large, anaplastic, and embryonic in aspect, with angry-looking hyperchromatic nuclei having prominent nucleoli. Unlike the case with seminoma, the cell borders are usually indistinct and there is considerable variation in cell and nuclear size and shape. Mitotic figures and tumor giant cells are frequent. **Within this background, syncytial cells containing HCG or cells containing alpha-fetoprotein (AFP), or both, may be detected by immunoperoxidase techniques. Because HCG and AFP are products of trophoblastic and yolk sac cells, respectively, their presence is indicative of a mixed tumor.**

If tumors containing HCG or AFP, or both, are excluded,

it is estimated that pure embryonal cell carcinomas constitute about 3% of testicular germ cell tumors. However, if one includes mixed tumors, embryonal carcinoma cells are present in about 45% of tumors.

Yolk Sac Tumor

Also known as infantile embryonal carcinoma or endodermal sinus tumor, the yolk sac tumor is the most common testicular tumor in infants and children. In adults, the pure form of this tumor is rare; instead yolk sac elements frequently occur in combination with embryonal carcinoma.

Grossly, the tumor is nonencapsulated, and on cross section it presents a homogeneous, yellow-white, mucinous appearance. Characteristic on microscopic examination are spaces of varying size lined by flattened-to-cuboidal epithelial cells. In addition, papillary structures or solid cords of cells may be found. In some tumors the so-called endodermal sinuses may be seen; these consist of a mesodermal core with a central capillary and a visceral and parietal layer of cells resembling primitive glomeruli. More typically the tumor cells have vacuolated cytoplasm, and in some cases the vacuoles coalesce to form large cleared spaces. Present within and outside the cytoplasm are eosinophilic, hyalin-like globules in which AFP and alpha-1-antitrypsin can be demonstrated by immunocytochemical staining. The presence of AFP in the tumor cells is highly characteristic and it underscores their differentiation into yolk sac cells.

Polyembryoma

This tumor in its pure form is extremely rare. Most often it forms a component of embryonal carcinoma or teratoma. It consists of so-called "embryoid bodies" that may appear in the form of a disc, a cavity, or a tubular structure. The disc resembles embryonic disc and is made up of undifferentiated, large epithelial cells; the cavity that represents the amniotic space is lined by flattened epithelial cells. These embryoid structures are surrounded by loose mesenchyme in which trophoblastic elements may be seen.

Choriocarcinoma

This highly malignant form of testicular tumor is composed of both cytotrophoblast and syncytiotrophoblast. Identical tumors may arise in the placental tissue (p. 1176), ovary, or sequestered rests of totipotential cells, e.g., in the mediastinum or abdomen. Fortunately, in its "pure" form it is a rare testicular tumor. As emphasized later, foci of choriocarcinoma are much more common in mixed patterns.

Despite their aggressive behavior, pure choriocarcinomas are usually small lesions. **Often they cause no testicular enlargement and are detected only as a small palpable nodule.** Because they are rapidly growing, they may outgrow their blood supply, and sometimes the primary testicular focus is replaced by a small fibrous scar, leaving only widespread metastases. On the other hand, the primary lesion may be a hemorrhagic, large bulky mass of clotted blood in which tiny bits of gray tumor, or indeed no tumor, can be identified. It is the necrotic hemorrhagic appearance that is most characteristic of these neoplasms. Histologically the tumors contain two cell types (Fig. 23–15). The syncytiotrophoblastic cell is large and has many irregular or lobular hyperchromatic nuclei and an abundant eosinophilic vacuolated cytoplasm. As might be expected, HCG can be readily demonstrated in the cytoplasm of syncytiotrophoblastic cells. The cytotrophoblastic cells are more regular and tend to be polygonal with distinct cell borders and clear cytoplasm; they grow in cords or masses and have a single, fairly uniform nucleus. Often the syncytial cells cap a cluster of cytotrophoblastic cells, but well-formed placental villi are never seen. Although most tumors contain both cellular elements, the presence of syncytiotrophoblast alone, documented by the presence of HCG in the cytoplasm, is considered adequate for diagnosis. These viable tumor cells are generally scattered within large areas of hemorrhage or necrotic tumor, or both. More anatomic details are available in the discussion of these neoplasms in the female genital tract (p. 1177).

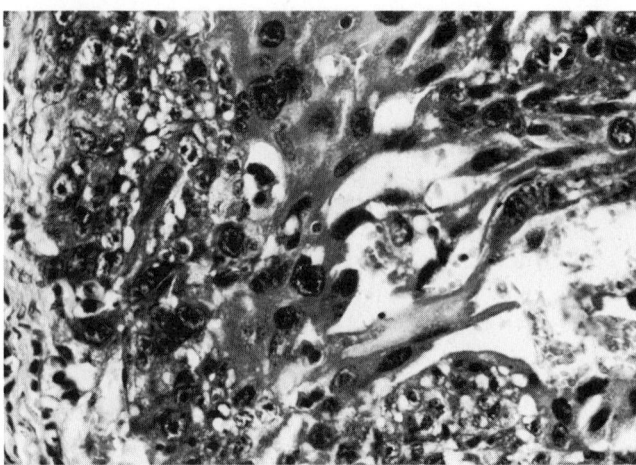

Figure 23–15. Choriocarcinoma of the testis showing an admixture of syncytiotrophoblast and cytotrophoblast.

Teratoma

The designation teratoma refers to a group of complex tumors having various cellular or organoid components reminiscent of normal derivatives from more than one germ layer. They may occur at any age from infancy to adult life. Indeed, teratomas are some of the more common tumors in infants and children; in the pure form teratomas constitute about 40% of testicular tumors in infants, but only 2 to 3% of germ cell tumors in adults. As with embryonal carcinomas, their frequency in combination with other histologic types is about 45%.[18]

Histologically, three variants are recognized based on the degree of differentiation.

Mature teratomas are composed of a heterogeneous, helter-skelter collection of differentiated cells or organoid structures such as neural tissue, muscle bundles, islands of cartilage, clusters of squamous epithelium, structures reminiscent of thyroid gland, bronchial or bronchiolar epithelium, and bits of intestinal wall or brain substance, all embedded in a fibrous or myxoid stroma (Fig. 23–16). All the elements are differentiated. This mature variant occurs with relatively greater frequency in infancy and childhood. Similar tumors may occur in adults, but there is a far greater risk of small hidden foci of immature or malignant components that may escape detection despite rigorous sampling of the lesion. Thus, although teratomas may appear entirely mature and benign, such a diagnosis in an adult must be made with circumspection. Dermoid cysts, common in the ovary (p. 1164), are rare in the testis. They represent a special form of mature teratoma.

Immature teratomas can be viewed as intermediate between mature teratoma and embryonal carcinoma. Unlike the mature teratoma, elements of the three germ cell layers are incompletely differentiated and not arranged in organoid fashion. Even though the differentiation is incomplete, the nature of the embryonic tissue can be clearly identified; thus, poorly formed cartilage, neuroblasts, loose

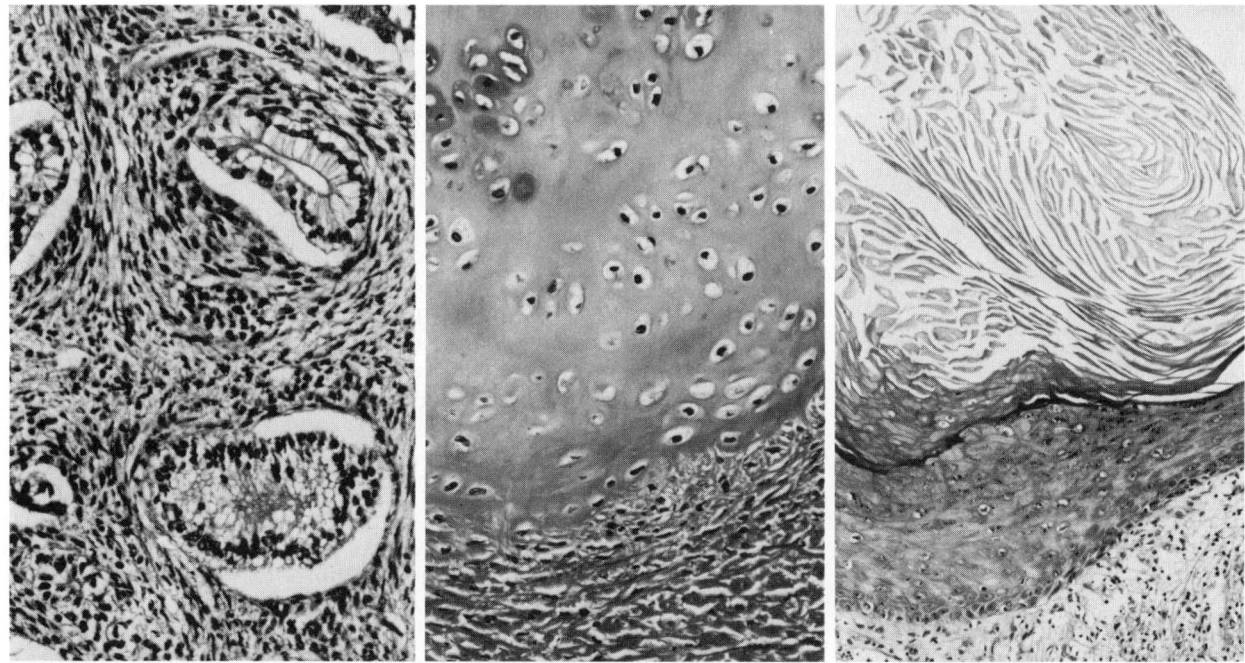

Figure 23–16. Mature teratoma. Three different fields from the same tumor with (1) well-differentiated mucus-secreting gland reminiscent of colonic (endodermal) mucosa on the left; (2) hyaline cartilage (mesodermal) in the middle; and (3) squamous stratified keratinizing epithelium (ectodermal) on the right. (Courtesy of Dr. Fred Silva, Department of Pathology, University of Texas, Southwestern Medical School, Dallas, Texas.)

mesenchyme, and clusters of glandular structures may be seen lying helter-skelter. In some areas, more mature forms of these tissues may also be seen. Although these tumors are clearly malignant, they may not display clear-cut cytologic features of malignancy.

In contrast, the third variant—**teratoma with malignant transformation**—shows clear evidence of malignancy in derivatives of one or more germ cell layers. Thus, there may be a focus of squamous cell carcinoma, mucin-secreting adenocarcinoma, or a sarcoma. Immature and frankly malignant teratomas occur more commonly in adults.

Owing to the wide variety of tissues present in teratomas, the gross appearance is understandably variable. Teratomas, whether mature or immature, reveal on gross inspection a variegated cut surface with minute cysts, islands of translucent cartilage, and possibly foci of bone, all embedded within a gray-white solid matrix (Fig. 23–17). They often cause testicular enlargement, sometimes producing bulky masses.

In the child, differentiated mature teratomas may be expected to behave as benign tumors, and almost all these patients have a good prognosis. In the adult, it is difficult to be certain because, as pointed out, even apparently differentiated mature teratomas may harbor minute foci of cancer. It would require meticulous serial sectioning of all these large neoplasms to uncover the small foci of cancer in some. Thus, some writers say that all teratomas in the adult should be considered malignant. Clinical experience has proved,

however, that some solid mature teratomas are indeed benign and can be cured by surgical removal of the affected testis.

Mixed Tumors

About 60% of testicular tumors are composed of more than one of the "pure" patterns. The most common mixture is that of teratoma, embryonal carcinoma, yolk sac tumor, and HCG-containing syncytiotrophoblast. Tumors with such a combination constitute 14% of testicular germ cell tumors. Other combinations include seminoma with embryonal carcinoma and embryonal carcinoma with teratoma. The latter has been called teratocarcinoma. In most instances the prognosis is worsened by the inclusion of more aggressive elements: e.g., the teratoma with a focus of choriocarcinoma has a poorer outlook than that of pure teratoma, but better than that of pure choriocarcinoma. It is noteworthy that metastases of these mixed tumors may be composed of one or more of the various neoplastic components, and indeed a new line of differentiation sometimes appears.

CLINICAL FEATURES. From a clinical standpoint tumors of the testis are segregated into two broad categories: *seminoma* and *nonseminomatous* germ cell tumors (NSGCT). The latter is an umbrella designation that includes tumors of one histologic type such as embryonal cell carcinoma as well as those with more than one histologic pattern. As will be evident from the later discussion, seminomas and NSGCT not only present with somewhat distinctive clinical features, but more importantly they also differ with re-

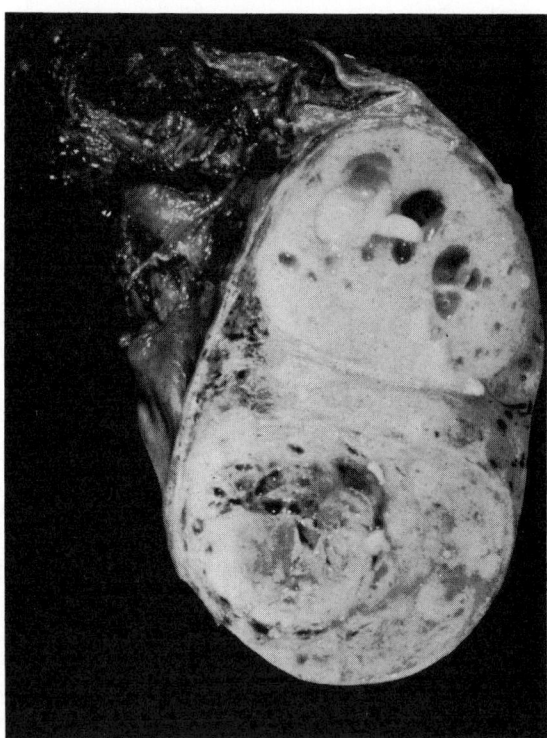

Figure 23–17. Teratoma of testis. The variegated cut surface reflects the multiplicity of tissue found histologically.

spect to therapy and prognosis. First we will offer some general comments on the clinical manifestations of testicular tumors as a group. *Painless enlargement of the testis* is the most common presenting feature of germ cell neoplasms. Indeed, any testicular mass should be considered neoplastic unless proved otherwise. Clinical differentiation between various types of germ cell tumors is at best imperfect as there are no distinctive clinical features to the testicular masses produced by these tumors.

Testicular tumors have a characteristic mode of spread, the knowledge of which is helpful in treatment. Lymphatic spread is common to all forms of testicular tumors, and in general retroperitoneal para-aortic nodes are the first to be involved. Subsequent spread may occur to mediastinal and supraclavicular nodes. Hematogenous spread is primarily to the lungs, but liver, brain, and bones may also be involved. Although most testicular tumors metastasize "true," the histology of metastases may sometimes be different from that of the testicular lesion. Thus an embryonal carcinoma may present a teratomatous picture in the secondary deposits. Conversely, a teratoma may show foci of choriocarcinoma in the lymph nodes. As discussed earlier (p. 1109), if one accepts the view that all these tumors are derived from totipotential germ cells, the apparent "forward" and "backward" differentiation seen in different locations is not entirely surprising.

With this background we can highlight the differences between seminoma and NSGCT. Seminomas tend to remain localized to the testis for a long period

of time and hence approximately 70% present in clinical stage I (see later). In contrast, approximately 60% of patients with NSGCT present with advanced clinical disease (Stages II and III). Metastases from seminomas typically involve lymph nodes. Hematogenous spread occurs later in the course of dissemination. NSGCT not only metastasize earlier but also utilize the hematogenous route more frequently. The rare choriocarcinoma is the most aggressive of NSGCT. It may not cause any testicular enlargement, but instead spreads predominantly and rapidly by the bloodstream. Therefore, lungs and liver are involved early in virtually every case. From a therapeutic viewpoint seminomas are extremely radiosensitive, whereas NSGCT are relatively radioresistant. To summarize, as compared to seminomas, NSGCT are biologically more aggressive and in general have a poorer prognosis.

Much progress has been achieved in the treatment of testicular tumors by utilizing sophisticated techniques for clinical staging and study of tumor associated markers. In addition to careful physical examination, staging involves abdominopelvic computed tomography (CT) for detection of nodal and visceral metastases, chest radiographs with lung tomography or CT scanning, and assessment of biologic markers. Three stages are defined:

- Stage I: tumor confined to the testis
- Stage II: distant spread confined to retroperitoneal nodes below the diaphragm
- Stage III: metastases outside the retroperitoneal nodes or above the diaphragm

Stages II and III are further subdivided ("early" or "advanced") on the basis of tumor burden in the secondary deposits.

Germ cell tumors of the testis often secrete polypeptide hormones and certain enzymes that can be detected in blood by very sensitive assays. Such "biologic markers" include HCG, AFP, placental alkaline phosphatase, placental lactogen, and lactic dehydrogenase. Of these, only the first two (i.e., HCG and AFP) are widely utilized and have proved to be of value in the diagnosis and management of testicular cancer.

AFP is the major serum protein of the early fetus and is synthesized by the fetal gut, liver cells, and yolk sac. One year after birth, the serum levels of AFP fall to less than 16 ng/ml, which is undetectable except by the most sensitive assays. HCG is a glycoprotein consisting of two dissimilar polypeptide units called alpha and beta. It is normally synthesized and secreted by the placental syncytiotrophoblast. The beta subunit of HCG has unique sequences not shared with other human glycoprotein hormones, and therefore the detection of HCG in the serum is based on a radioimmunoassay using antibodies to its beta chain. As might be expected from the histogenesis and morphology, elevated levels of these markers are most often associated with nonseminomatous tumors. In one large series, 9% of seminomas, 44% of teratomas, 88% of embryonal carcinomas, 86% of teratocarcinomas, 75% of yolk sac tumors, and all cases of choriocarcinoma demonstrated elevated levels of serum HCG or AFP, or both.[24] Yolk sac tumors produce AFP exclusively, and choriocarcinomas elaborate only HCG. However, most patients (but not all) with teratoma, embryonal carcinoma, and teratocarcinoma have elevations of both AFP and HCG simultaneously because they frequently contain yolk sac cells and syncytiotrophoblasts. In passing, it might be noted that elevated serum levels of AFP are also encountered with liver cell carcinomas. In the context of testicular tumors, the value of serum markers is threefold:

• In the diagnosis of testicular masses.
• In the staging of testicular germ cell tumors. For example, following orchiectomy persistent elevation of HCG or AFP indicates Stage II disease even if the lymph nodes appear of normal size by CT scanning.
• In monitoring the response to therapy. Following eradication of tumors, there is a rapid fall in serum levels of AFP and HCG. With serial measurements, it is often possible to predict recurrence before the patients become symptomatic or develop any other clinical signs of relapse.

The presence of elevated serum HCG levels in some patients with seminoma is not fully understood. Could all the serum HCG be produced by the syncytial giant cells known to occur in some seminomas, or should one suspect a mixed tumor with elements of choriocarcinoma? Should these patients be treated like others with NSGCT? Definite answers are not yet available, but some authorities believe that the presence of elevated serum HCG level in a patient with seminoma calls for a more aggressive therapeutic approach.

The therapy and prognosis of testicular tumors depend largely on clinical stage and on the histologic type. Seminoma, which is extremely radiosensitive and tends to remain localized for long periods, has the best prognosis. More than 90% of patients with Stage I and II disease can be cured. Among nonseminomatous tumors, the histologic subtype does not influence the prognosis significantly, and hence these are treated as a group. Although they do not share the good prognosis of seminoma, studies report considerable success in achieving significant remissions with excision followed by aggressive chemotherapy.[25] Currently, a 75 to 90% two-year survival rate for Stage I disease, and 50% two-year survival rate for Stage II disease, is being reported.

TUMORS OF SEX CORD–GONADAL STROMA

As indicated in Table 23–1, these tumors are subclassified on the basis of their presumed histogenesis and differentiation. The two most important members of this group—Leydig cell tumors (derived from the stroma) and Sertoli cell tumors (derived from the sex cord)—are described here.

Leydig (Interstitial) Cell Tumors

Tumors of Leydig cells are particularly interesting because they may elaborate androgens or androgens and estrogens and, indeed, some have also elaborated corticosteroids. Leydig cell tumors, however, are quite uncommon, accounting for approximately 2% of all testicular tumors in several large series.[26] They arise at any age, although the majority of the reported cases have been noted between 20 and 60 years of age. As with other testicular tumors, the most common presenting feature is testicular swelling, but in some patients gynecomastia may be the first symptom. In children hormonal effects, manifested primarily as sexual precocity, are the dominating features.

These neoplasms range from small nodules less than 1 cm in diameter to bulky masses 10 cm in diameter. On cut surface they can often be recognized by a distinctive, uniform, yellow-brown hue. Histologically, tumorous Leydig cells usually are remarkably similar to their normal forebears in that they are large and round or polygonal, and they have an abundant granular eosinophilic cytoplasm with a round central nucleus. Cell boundaries are often indistinct. The cytoplasm frequently contains lipid granules, vacuoles, or lipochrome pigment, but, most characteristically, rod-shaped crystalloids of Reinke occur in about one third of the tumors. As in the case of other endocrine tumors, they may display variability in cell and nuclear size and shape, often with binucleate or multinucleate cells. These do not necessarily indicate that the tumor is malignant: most are benign; only 10% are invasive and produce metastases.

Sertoli Cell Tumors (Androblastoma)

These tumors may be composed entirely of Sertoli cells or may have a component of granulosa cells. Some induce endocrinologic changes. Either estrogens or androgens may be elaborated but only infrequently in sufficient quantity to cause precocious masculinization or feminization. Occasionally, as with Leydig cell tumors, gynecomastia appears.

These neoplasms may appear as firm, small nodules or rarely as bulky masses causing considerable testicular enlargement. On cross section the surface is homogeneous gray-white to yellow. Histologically, in the classic form the cells are quite distinctive and are either tall, columnar, or polyhedral, having abundant, usually vacuolated cytoplasm. Quite distinctive is the tendency for these cells to grow in cords highly reminiscent of spermatic tubules. The great majority of Sertoli cell tumors are benign, but occasional tumors (approximately 10%) are more anaplastic and pursue a malignant course.

TESTICULAR LYMPHOMA

Although not primarily a tumor of the testis, testicular lymphoma is included here because affected patients present with only a testicular mass. *Lymphomas account for 5% of testicular neoplasms and constitute the most common form of testicular cancer in men over the age of 60.* In most cases, disseminated disease follows detection of the testicular mass, only rarely does it remain confined to the testis.[27] The histologic type in almost all cases is the diffuse large cell lymphoma (p. 714). The prognosis is extremely poor, unless the disease is found to be confined to the testis.

ADENOMATOID TUMORS

These are *benign,* slow-growing nodules that arise in the epididymis. They usually have an encapsulated, firm, gray-white macroscopic appearance and are rarely larger than a few centimeters in size. On microscopic examination, they contain variable amounts of stroma and an admixture of cells that seem to have an epithelial origin. These apparent epithelial cuboidal cells may line cystic spaces, form small apparent glandular patterns, or be disposed in cords and nests. Occasionally, these cells contain vacuoles that do not react with the usual fat or glycogen stains. The origin of these uncommon tumors is believed to be the mesothelium.

MISCELLANEOUS LESIONS OF TUNICA VAGINALIS

Brief mention should be made of the tunica vaginalis. As a serosa-lined sac immediately proximal to the testis and epididymis, it may become involved by any lesion arising in these two structures. Clear serous fluid may accumulate from neighboring infections or tumors *(hydrocele).* The tunica may fill up with fluids when there is systemic edema, as in cardiac failure or renal disease; at other times, when the processus vaginalis has failed to close completely, peritoneal fluid may seep in and accumulate. Considerable enlargement of the scrotal sac is produced, which can be readily mistaken for testicular enlargement. However, by transillumination it is usually possible to define the clear, translucent character of the contained substance, and many times the opaque testis can be outlined within this fluid-filled space. When infected, as in the course of a tap or by the extension of organisms directly from infections within the testis or epi-

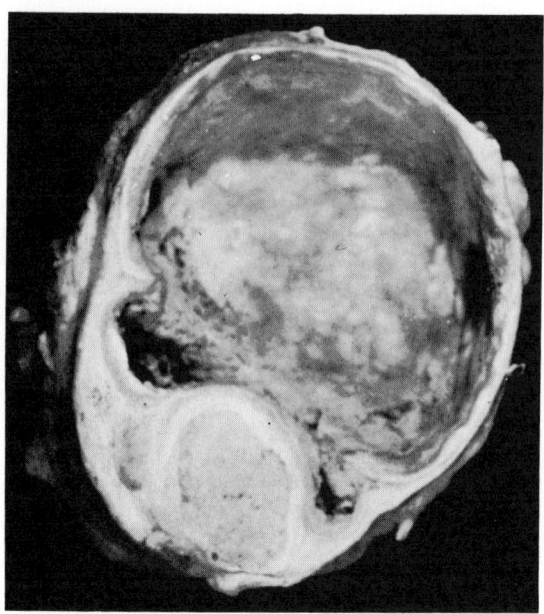

Figure 23–18. An infected hydrocele sac. The wall is thick and fibrous and has a shaggy lining.

didymis or through the lymphohematogenous route, the serosa-lined membrane may be converted to a shaggy, thickened, fibrous wall and the serous fluid may be transformed to frank pus (Fig. 23–18).

Hematocele indicates the presence of blood in the tunica vaginalis. It is an uncommon condition usually encountered only when there has been either direct trauma to the testis or torsion of the testis with hemorrhagic suffusion into the surrounding tunica vaginalis, or in hemorrhagic diseases associated with widespread bleeding diatheses. Tumorous invasion may evoke a hydrohematocele.

Chylocele refers to the accumulation of lymphatic fluid in the tunica and is almost always found in patients with elephantiasis who have widespread and severe lymphatic obstruction. For clarity's sake, mention should be made of the *spermatocele* and *varicocele,* which refer respectively to small cystic accumulations of either semen or blood in the spermatic cord. In the spermatocele, the cyst usually represents a dilatation of one of the ducts in the head of the epididymis; in the case of varicocele, it might be more properly described as a cystic varix of one of the veins of the spermatic cord.

PROSTATE

Consideration of prostatic diseases will be facilitated by a brief introduction to the normal anatomy of the prostate. In the normal adult, the prostate weighs approximately 20 gm. It is a retroperitoneal organ encircling the neck of the bladder and urethra and is devoid of a distinct capsule. Classically, the prostate has been divided into five lobes, to which are attrib-

uted distinctive significance in the development of tumors and benign enlargements. These five lobes include a posterior, middle, and anterior lobe and two lateral lobes. However, other investigators deny the clear definition of these five lobes and suggest that, in the course of development, the five become fused into only three distinct lobes—two major lateral lobes and a small median lobe, which presumably includes the classic posterior lobe. Cross section of the gland, however, fails to disclose well-defined lobes, and only two lateral masses can be found on either side of the urethra, as well as a much thinner median lobe, which forms the floor of the urethra.

Histologically, the prostate is a compound tubuloalveolar gland, which, in one plane of section, presents small to fairly large glandular spaces lined by epithelium. Characteristically, the glands are lined by two layers of cells: a basal layer of low cuboidal epithelium covered by a layer of columnar mucus-secreting cells. In many areas, there are small villous projections or papillary inbuddings of the epithelium. These glands all have a distinct basement membrane and are separated by an abundant fibromuscular stroma. The prostate is an endocrine-dependent organ. However, our knowledge of its endocrine relationships is still incomplete. Testicular androgens are clearly of prime importance in controlling prostatic growth since castration leads to atrophy of the prostate. There is some evidence that prolactin acts synergistically with androgens. In addition, normal prostate cells have cytoplasmic receptors for estrogens and progesterone, hinting at a possible influence of the female sex hormones. It is beyond the scope of this book to delve into the complexities of the hormonal effects and relationships in the normal prostate physiology; these may be found in a review by Coffey and Isaacs.[28]

The only three pathologic processes that affect the prostate gland with sufficient frequency to merit discussion are inflammation, benign nodular enlargement, and tumors. Of these three, the benign nodular enlargements are by far the most common and occur so often in advanced age that they can almost be construed as a "normal" aging process. Prostatic carcinoma is also an extremely common lesion in the male and one, therefore, that merits careful consideration. The inflammatory processes are, for the most part, of less clinical significance and can be treated briefly.

INFLAMMATIONS

Prostatitis may be divided into three categories: *acute* and *chronic bacterial prostatitis* and *chronic abacterial prostatitis.*[29] Differentiation among these entities is based on bacteriologic and microscopic examination of fractionated urine specimens and expressed prostatic secretions. The presence of prostatic inflammation is documented by the presence of more than 10 to 12 leukocytes per high power field in prostatic secretions obtained by transrectal prostatic massage. In bacterial prostatitis (acute or chronic), cultures of urine or expressed prostatic secretions are positive for bacterial growth. However, in chronic abacterial prostatitis the urine cultures and prostatic secretions are consistently negative for bacterial growth despite unambiguous evidence of prostatic inflammation (Fig. 23–19). Distinction between the three forms of prostatitis is important because treatment differs. In the ensuing discussion the three conditions will be characterized first, and then the morphologic features of all the forms will be described together.

Acute bacterial prostatitis consists of an acute focal or diffuse suppurative inflammation in the prostatic substance. The bacteria responsible are similar in type and in incidence to those that cause urinary tract infections (UTI). Thus, most cases are caused by various strains of *E. coli.* Most of the remaining infections are due to Klebsiella, Proteus, Pseudomonas, Enterobacter, and Serratia. Among gram-positive bacteria, only Enterococcus and *Staphylococcus aureus* are significant as causative agents. The organisms become implanted in the prostate usually by direct extension from the posterior urethra or from the urinary bladder, but occasionally they seed the prostate by the lymphohematogenous routes from distant foci of infection. Invasion from the rectum has also been proposed. One of the most common clinical sequences

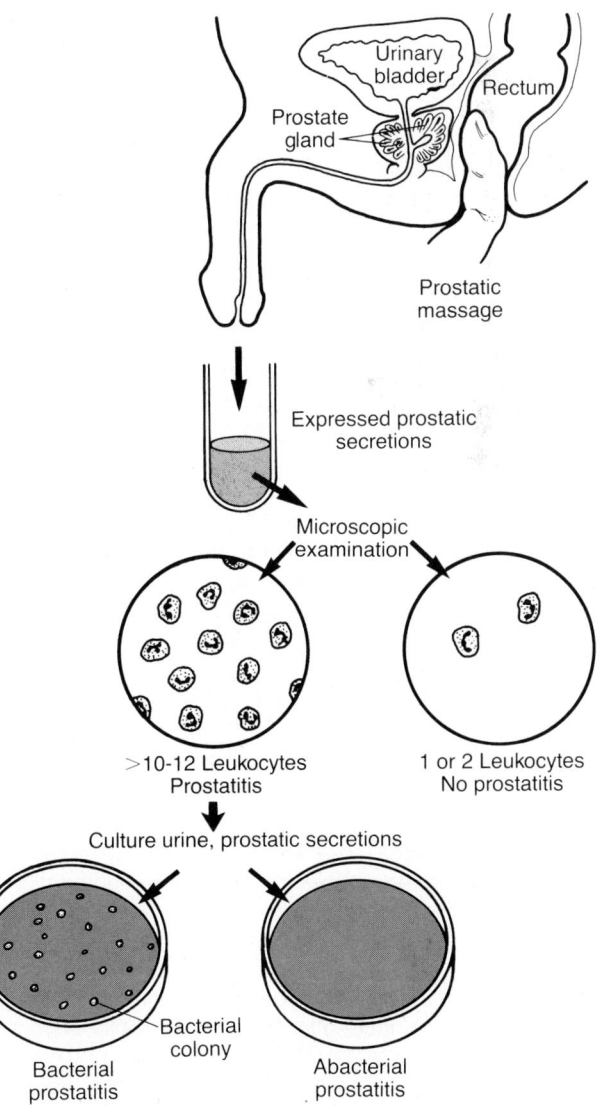

Figure 23–19. Prostatitis—bacterial and abacterial.

encountered is prostatitis following some surgical manipulation on the urethra or prostate gland itself, such as catheterization, cystoscopy, urethral dilatation, or resection procedures on the prostate. Clinically, acute bacterial prostatitis is easy to diagnose. It is associated with fever, chills, and dysuria. On rectal examination the prostate is exquisitely tender and boggy. Examination of expressed prostatic secretions by prostatic massage is usually avoided because it carries with it the risk of inducing bacteremia and because the diagnosis can be readily established by urine culture and clinical features.

Chronic bacterial prostatitis is difficult to diagnose and treat. It may present with low back pain, dysuria, and perineal and suprapubic discomfort. Alternatively, it may be virtually asymptomatic. *A very common historical characteristic is recurrent urinary tract infections (cystitis, urethritis) caused by the same organism.* Because most antibiotics penetrate the prostate poorly, bacteria find safe haven in the parenchyma and constantly seed the urinary tract. Except when there is an acute flare-up, the prostate is normal on rectal examination. Diagnosis of chronic bacterial prostatitis depends upon the documentation of leukocytosis in the expressed prostatic secretions along with positive bacterial cultures in the prostatic secretions and urine. The mode of development of chronic bacterial prostatitis is not well understood. In a minority of cases it represents a sequel to acute prostatitis. In some cases it follows urethral or prostatic manipulation, sometimes without a well-defined episode of acute inflammation. However, in the great majority of instances it appears insidiously and without obvious provocation. The implicated organisms are the same as those cited as causes of acute prostatitis.

Chronic abacterial prostatitis is the most common form of prostatitis seen today.[30] *Clinically it is indistinguishable from chronic bacterial prostatitis. However, there is no history of recurrent urinary tract infection.* Expressed prostatic secretions contain more than 10 to 12 leukocytes per high power field, but bacterial cultures are uniformly negative. Because the affected patients are usually sexually active males, several sexually transmitted pathogens have been implicated. The prime suspects are *Chlamydia trachomatis* and *Ureaplasma urealyticum,* two pathogens that have also been implicated in the causation of nongonococcal urethritis (p. 1095).

Acute prostatitis may appear as minute, disseminated abscesses; as large, coalescent focal areas of necrosis; or as a diffuse edema, congestion, and boggy suppuration of the entire gland. When these reactions are fairly diffuse, they cause an overall soft, spongy enlargement of the gland.

Histologically, depending on the duration and severity of the inflammation, there may be minimal stromal leukocytic infiltrate accompanied by increased elaboration of prostatic secretion or leukocytic infiltration within gland spaces (Fig. 23–20). When abscess formation has occurred, focal or

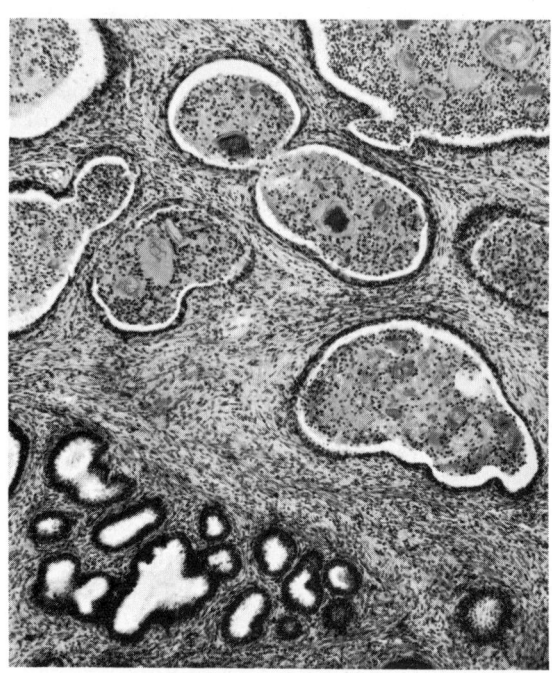

Figure 23–20. Acute prostatitis. Gland lumina are filled with neutrophils, and stroma contains a sprinkling of similar leukocytes.

large areas of the prostatic substance may become necrotic. Such inflammatory reactions may totally subside and leave behind only some fibrous scarring. Alternatively, they may become chronic, particularly when the excretory ducts are plugged and the infection continues to smolder within walled-off minute abscesses in the prostatic substance.

Chronic prostatitis, both bacterial and abacterial, when correctly diagnosed, should be restricted to those cases of inflammatory reaction in the prostate characterized by the aggregation of numerous lymphocytes, plasma cells, and macrophages, as well as neutrophils, within the prostatic substance. It should be pointed out that, in the normal aging process, aggregations of lymphocytes are prone to appear in the fibromuscular stroma of this gland. All too often, such nonspecific aggregates are diagnosed as chronic prostatitis, even though the pathognomonic inflammatory cells, i.e., the macrophages and neutrophils, are not present.

BENIGN ENLARGEMENT

NODULAR HYPERPLASIA (BENIGN PROSTATIC HYPERTROPHY OR HYPERPLASIA)

Nodular hyperplasia, still referred to by the redundant term benign prostatic hyperplasia (all hyperplasias are benign), is an extremely common disorder in men over age 50. It is characterized by the formation of large, fairly discrete nodules in the periurethral region of the prostate. When sufficiently large, the nodules compress and narrow the urethral canal to cause partial, or sometimes virtually complete, obstruction of the urethra.

INCIDENCE. Although reports vary slightly, a careful examination of the prostate in an unselected series of autopsies disclosed nodular hyperplasia in approximately 20% of the men 40 years of age, a figure that increases to 70% by age 60, and to 90% by the eighth decade of life.[31] With this prevalence, it has been argued that nodular hyperplasia is not truly a disease but rather a normal aging process; this is a dilemma we can leave to the semanticists. Clinically significant nodular hyperplasia is much less prevalent. Not more than 5 to 10% of men with this condition require surgical treatment for relief of urinary tract obstruction; in the remainder the condition is of little clinical significance. For obscure reasons the disease appears about a decade earlier in blacks than in whites, and it is somewhat more common in Protestants than in Jews and Catholics.

ETIOLOGY. Although the cause of nodular hyperplasia is still uncertain, the available evidence suggests that both androgens and estrogens are involved in its genesis.[32] Much evidence relating to the hormonal basis of nodular hyperplasia has been obtained in dogs, the only animal species that develops prostatic hyperplasia with aging. In both humans and dogs, hyperplasia of the prostate develops only in the presence of intact testes. In castrated young dogs it is possible to induce prostatic hyperplasia by administration of androgens, an effect markedly enhanced by simultaneous administration of 17-beta-estradiol, thus pointing to possible synergism between androgens and estrogens. Dihydrotestosterone, which is derived from plasma testosterone, is believed to be the ultimate mediator of prostatic growth.[33] Prostate epithelial cells contain cytoplasmic receptors for dihydrotestosterone; the expression of these receptors is enhanced by estrogens. There is no difference between levels of plasma testosterone in patients with prostatic hyperplasia and in age-matched controls; indeed, plasma testosterone levels decline after the age of 60 years. With aging, estradiol levels increase in men (absolute or relative to testosterone). Thus it is conceivable that despite the declining output of testosterone associated with aging, the increase of estrogens "sensitizes" the prostate to the growth promoting effects of dihydrotestosterone (Fig. 23–21). This hypothesis seems plausible and attempts to explain the role of androgens as well as the synergistic effects of estrogens, but formal proof is still lacking.

MORPHOLOGY. In the usual case of nodular enlargement, the prostatic nodules weigh between 60 and 100 gm. However, not uncommonly, aggregate weights of up to 200 gm are encountered, and even larger masses have been recorded. Careful studies by McNeal have demonstrated that nodular hyperplasia of the prostate originates almost exclusively in the preprostatic region.[34] This area, which lies proximal to the verumontanum, corresponds to the "inner" periurethral portion of the classically defined middle and lateral lobes. This distribution is in striking contrast to that of prostatic carcinoma, which usually involves the posterior lobe.

From their origin in this strategic location, the nodular

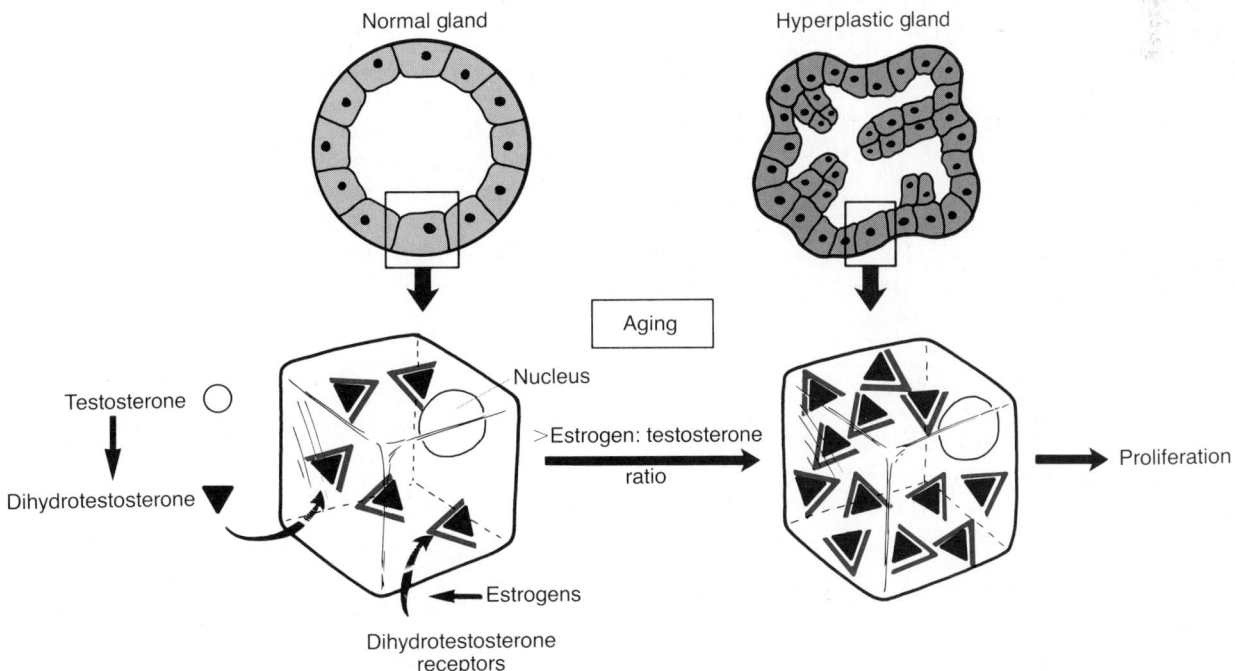

Figure 23–21. Diagrammatic representation of the possible roles of estrogen, testosterone, and the dihydrotestosterone receptors in the pathogenesis of nodular prostatic hyperplasia.

enlargements may encroach upon the lateral walls of the urethra to compress it to a slitlike orifice while, at the same time, nodular enlargement of the middle lobe may project up into the floor of the urethra as a hemispheric mass directly beneath the mucosa of the urethra (Fig. 23–22). At other times, the middle lobe enlargement may assume even a long, slender, delicate, polypoid appearance attached by a narrow neck; in many of these instances, it appears to act as a ball-valve obstruction to the mouth of the urethra.

On cross section of the affected prostate, the nodules usually are fairly readily identified because of the compression of the remainder of the prostatic tissue about the nodule (Fig. 23–23). As pointed out earlier, they usually arise from the inner prostatic mass, and only rarely do they extend to the outer perimeter of the gland. The nodule itself varies in color and consistency, depending, as will be shown, on whether it is primarily due to fibromuscular stromal hypertrophy and hyperplasia or to glandular proliferation. In those that are primarily glandular, the tissue has a yellow-pink soft consistency, which is fairly discretely demarcated from the more gray, glistening, firm, compressed prostatic capsule. Usually a milky-white prostatic fluid oozes out of these areas. In those primarily due to fibromuscular involvement, the nodule itself is also pale gray, tough, and fibrous; does not exude fluid; and is less clearly demarcated from the surrounding prostatic capsule.

Although the nodules do not have true capsules in the sense that benign neoplasms are encapsulated, the compressed surrounding prostatic tissue creates a plane of cleavage about them, utilized by the surgeon in the enu-

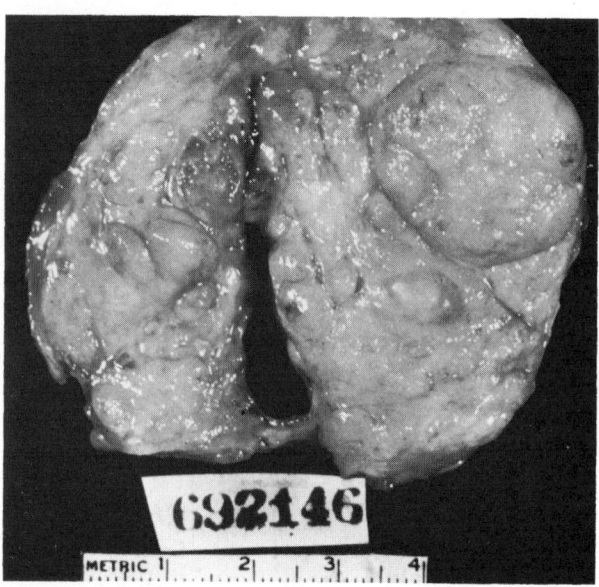

Figure 23–23. Nodular hyperplasia of prostate. Cut surface shows well-defined nodules of various sizes. (Courtesy of Dr. Fred Silva, Department of Pathology, University of Texas Health Science Center, Dallas.)

cleation of prostatic masses in so-called suprapubic prostatectomies. A considerable amount of prostatic tissue remains behind so that, at a later date, it is entirely possible for recurrent nodules to develop or for the patient to develop a carcinoma.

Microscopically, the nodularity may be due mainly to glandular proliferation or dilatation or to fibrous or muscular proliferation of the stroma. All three elements are involved in almost every case, although the epithelial element predominates in most cases. It takes the form of aggregations of small to large to cystically dilated glands, lined by two layers, an inner columnar and an outer cuboidal or flattened epithelium, based on an intact basement membrane (Fig. 23–24). The epithelium is characteristically thrown up into numerous papillary buds and infoldings, which are more prominent than in the normal prostate.

In certain cases, many small glands are formed that may simulate the pattern of adenocarcinoma. Usually the glandular size is sufficiently large to be visible on hand lens inspection of the tissue section. Frequently these glands contain inspissated secretion, granular desquamated epithelial cells, and numerous corpora amylacea. When the fibromuscular hypertrophy or hyperplasia predominates, it may produce aggregates of almost solid spindle cells free of glands. Not infrequently, aggregates of lymphocytes are found within the stroma, probably related to senile atrophic death of cells. Two other histologic changes are frequently found: (1) foci of squamous metaplasia and (2) small areas of infarction. The former tend to occur in the margins of the foci of infarction as nests of metaplastic, but orderly, squamous cells.

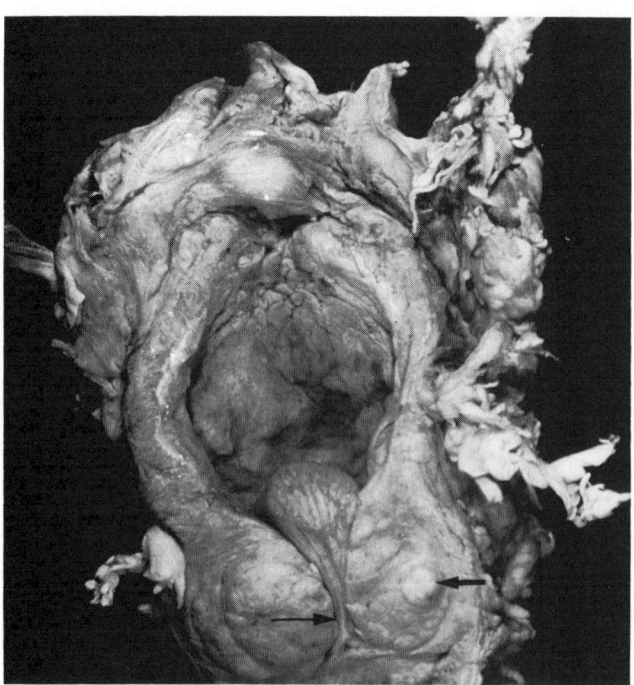

Figure 23–22. Nodular prostatic hyperplasia. Prostatic urethra and urinary bladder have been opened anteriorly to disclose enlarged prostatic gland that narrows urethral lumen to a slit *(small arrow)*. Note evident nodularity within prostatic gland *(large arrow)*. Urinary bladder is enlarged with hypertrophy of wall.

CLINICAL COURSE. Although nodular enlargement is an extremely common condition, it has been

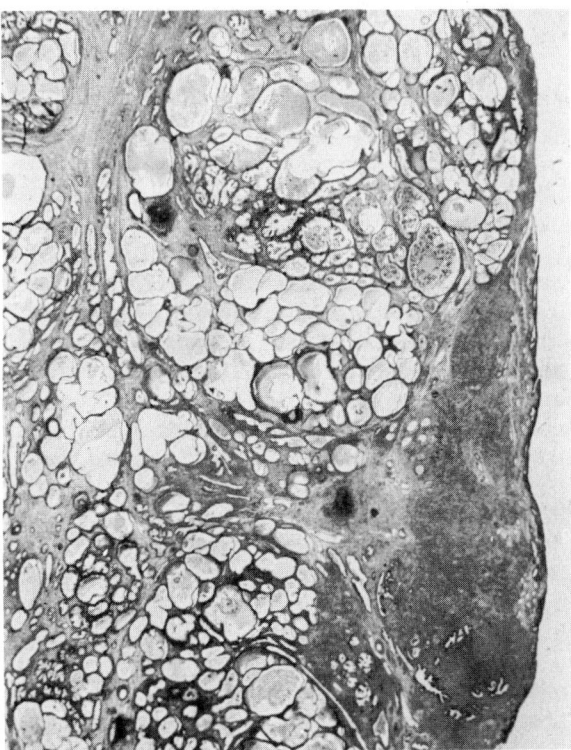
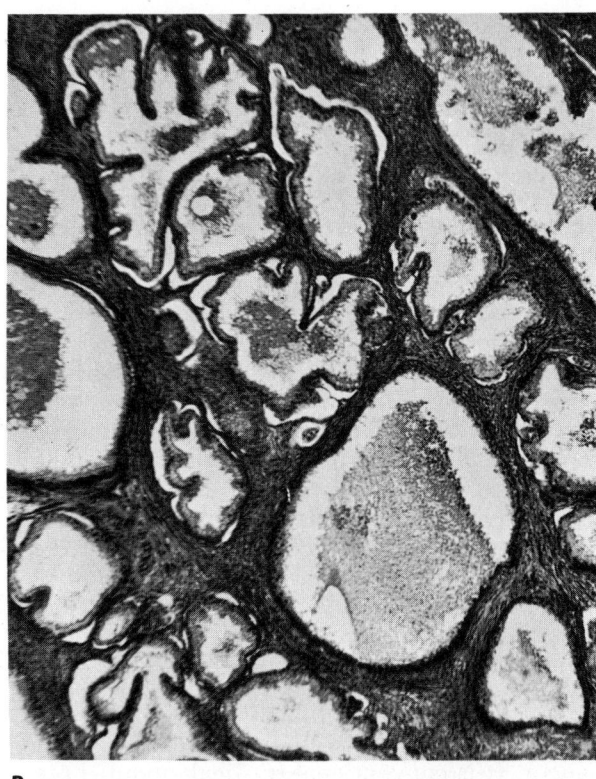

A **B**

Figure 23–24. Nodular hyperplasia of prostate. *A,* Low-power view shows proliferation of glands, some cystically dilated, with formation of nodules. (Courtesy of Dr. Fred Silva, Department of Pathology, University of Texas Health Science Center, Dallas.) *B,* High-power view shows hyperplastic glands with single epithelial layer, thrown into small papillary folds.

pointed out already that in only a small percentage of those affected does the lesion produce clinical symptoms. Symptoms, when produced, relate to two secondary effects: (1) compression of the urethra with difficulty in urination; and (2) retention of urine in the bladder with subsequent distention and hypertrophy of the bladder, infection of the urine, and the development of cystitis and renal infections.

These patients have frequency, nocturia, difficulty in starting and stopping the stream of urine, overflow dribbling, and dysuria (painful micturition). In many cases, sudden, acute urinary retention appears for unknown reasons and persists until the patient receives emergency catheterization. In addition to these difficulties in urination, prostatic enlargement results in the inability to empty the bladder completely. Presumably this is due to the raised level of the urethral floor so that, at the conclusion of micturition, a considerable amount of residual urine is left. This residual urine provides a static fluid that is vulnerable to infection. On this basis, catheterization or surgical manipulation provides a real danger of the introduction of organisms and development of pyelonephritis.

Many secondary changes occur in the bladder, such as hypertrophy, trabeculation, and diverticulum formation (p. 1095). Hydronephrosis or acute retention, with secondary UTI and even azotemia or uremia, may develop.

Finally, it should be noted that despite earlier claims that nodular hyperplasia predisposes to cancer of the prostate, most studies deny any association and hence nodular hyperplasia is not currently considered to be a premalignant lesion.

TUMORS

CARCINOMA

Carcinoma of the prostate is the most common form of cancer in males (followed closely by lung cancer) and the third leading cause of cancer death. It is currently estimated that slightly over 100,000 new cases are detected every year, of which approximately one third prove to be lethal.[35] In addition to these lethal neoplasms, there is an even more frequent anatomic form of prostatic cancer in which the cancer is discovered as an incidental finding, either at postmortem examination or in a surgical specimen removed for other reasons, e.g., nodular hyperplasia. In almost all these instances, the lesions are small and comprise only microscopic foci. The natural history of these occult carcinomas is not entirely clear, as is discussed later.

INCIDENCE. Cancer of the prostate is a disease of men over 50. The age-adjusted incidence in the United States is 69 per 100,000. Much more revealing, however, are the age-specific rates, which are 4.8 in the 45- to 49-year age group, but increase to a staggering 513 between the ages of 70 and 75.[36] The prevalence of latent prostatic cancer is even higher. In one series, approximately 30% of all the prostates removed at autopsy harbored a latent carcinoma.[37] There are some remarkable and puzzling national and racial differences in the prevalence of this disease. Prostatic cancer is extremely rare in Orientals. The prevalence rate among Japanese is in the range of three to four, and for the Chinese in Hong Kong only one, as compared with a rate of 50 to 60 among whites in the United States. The disease is even more prevalent among blacks, and indeed U.S. blacks not only have a markedly higher age-adjusted death rate from prostatic cancer than the white male population of the United States but also the highest rate among 24 countries having reasonably accurate mortality data.[38] Whites, in contrast, ranked fifteenth in the order. These differences are thought to be due to environmental influences, because in Japanese migrants to the United States the incidence of the disease seems to have risen, but not nearly to the level of that of native-born Americans.[39]

ETIOLOGY. Little is known about the causes of prostatic cancer. It is conventional to speak about three major factors—age, race, and the endocrine system.[40] To this triad a fourth might be added: environmental influences. The association of this form of cancer with advancing age, and the enigmatic differences among races, have already been mentioned. Could these be related to environmental influences? The tendency for the incidence of this disease to rise among those enjoying a low-incidence rate when they migrate to a high-incidence locale is consistent with a role for environmental influences, but if such influences exist, they remain unidentified.

The role of the endocrine system in the induction of prostatic cancer is also poorly understood, but one observation has been well established since the pioneer work of Huggins and Hodges.[41] The growth of metastatic prostatic cancer in men can usually be arrested or retarded for a time by castration or the administration of estrogens, or both. This has led to the assumption that androgens play a causal role. It has been impossible to document this hypothesis, however, and many studies have failed to establish a causal relationship between steroid hormone levels—estrogens, androgens, or adrenal steroids—in the blood or urine and the development of prostatic cancer.[42] *It seems more likely that the role of hormones in the evolution of this tumor is essentially permissive.* It appears that androgens are required for the maintenance of the prostatic epithelium, which is then transformed by as yet undefined carcinogens.

As mentioned previously, *nodular hyperplasia of the prostate has been suggested as a precursor, but most experts do not believe that this benign lesion has any relationship to the development of cancer.*[43] Any

concurrence of the two conditions could be a reflection of the prevalence of both diseases in aging men.

MORPHOLOGY. Carcinoma of the prostate arises in all but rare instances in the peripheral zone of the gland, classically in a posterior location, rendering it readily palpable on rectal examination. The origin may be multifocal, but by the time most lesions are discovered the multiple foci have coalesced into a poorly delimited cohesive area of cancer (Fig. 23–25). Characteristically, on cross section of the prostate, **the neoplastic tissue is gritty and firm, but when embedded within the prostatic substance it may be extremely difficult to visualize and be more readily apparent on palpation.** It should be noted, however, that uncommonly prostatic cancers are not hard, particularly those lesions that do not evoke a stromal proliferative reaction. The tumor tissue is usually somewhat yellower than the surrounding tissues and is therefore distinctive, but at other times it is gray-white and therefore blends imperceptibly into the background. Spread of prostate cancer occurs by direct local invasion and through the bloodstream and lymph. Local extension most commonly involves the seminal vesicles and the base of the urinary bladder, which may result in ureteral obstruction. Hematogenous spread occurs chiefly to the bones, particularly the axial skeleton,

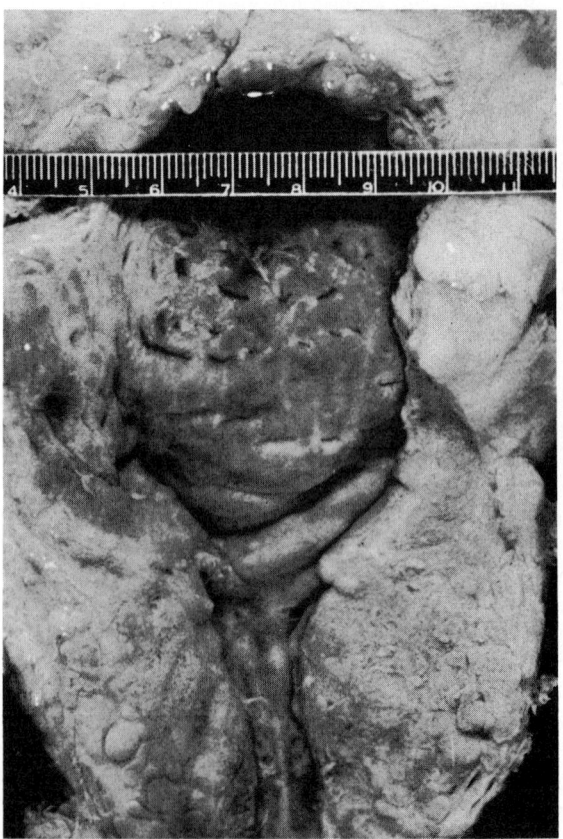

Figure 23–25. Carcinoma of prostate. Carcinomatous tissue cannot be distinguished within prostate itself but has invaded floor of urethra and infiltrated into vesicle neck.

but some lesions spread widely to viscera. Massive visceral dissemination is an exception rather than the rule. The bony metastases may be osteolytic, but osteoblastic lesions are frequent and in males point strongly to prostatic cancer. The bones commonly involved, in descending order of frequency, are lumbar spine, proximal femur, pelvis, thoracic spine, and ribs. Lymphatic spread occurs initially to the obturator nodes followed by perivesical, hypogastric, iliac, presacral, and para-aortic nodes. Only recently has it been appreciated that lymph node spread occurs frequently and often precedes spread to the bones. As we shall discuss later, metastases to the lymph nodes in apparently localized prostatic cancer have a significant impact on the prognosis.

Histologically most lesions are adenocarcinomas that produce well-defined, readily demonstrable gland patterns. In well-differentiated tumors the glands are either small or medium-sized with a single uniform layer of cuboidal or low columnar epithelium. Occasionally the glands are somewhat larger with a papillary or cribriform pattern. The cytoplasm of the tumor cells is pale and often granular, and the nuclei are round or oval and vesicular. Mitotic figures are extremely uncommon. When well-differentiated tumors occur in sharply delimited rounded masses, they have to be distinguished from nodular hyperplasia. In general, malignant acini are smaller and closely spaced, "back to back" with little intervening stroma, and are lined by a single layer of cells (Fig. 23–26). However, not all prostatic cancers are

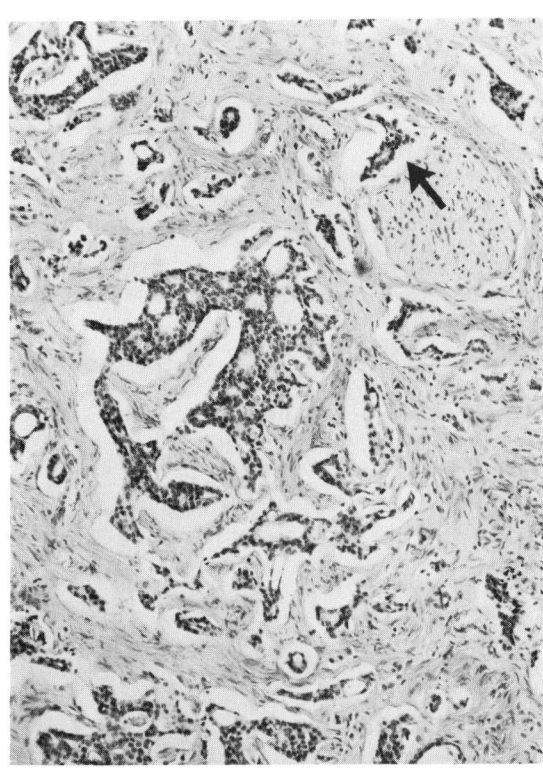

Figure 23–27. Carcinoma of prostate. Cords of tumor cells permeate stroma. Perineurial invasion is present *(arrow).*

well differentiated. In some poorly differentiated tumors the glandular pattern is apparent only on careful examination; the tumor cells in such cases tend to grow in cords, nests, or sheets. Concomitantly, the cells display obvious cytologic features of malignancy with prominent acidophilic nucleoli and increased mitotic activity. Stromal production may be scant or quite extensive in certain lesions, producing a scirrhous-like consistency to the neoplasm.

The frequent uniformity of cells and lack of anaplasia contribute to the histologic difficulties of diagnosing carcinomas of the prostate. The most reliable hallmarks of malignancy are clear evidence of invasion of the capsule with its lymphatic and vascular channels and/or perineurial invasion (Fig. 23–27). The perineurial spaces, which are involved in most cases, are not lined by endothelium and they do not represent lymphatics, as formerly believed.

Epidermoid carcinoma, adenoid cystic carcinoma, and transitional cell carcinoma are rare forms of prostatic cancer.

GRADING AND STAGING. Carcinomas of the prostate, like most other forms of cancer, are graded and staged. Regrettably, several grading systems have been described, but none is universally accepted. A detailed discussion of grading will not be presented here. Suffice it to say that all grading systems attempt to define histologic criteria (the arrangement and appearance of malignant glands, and the degree of anaplasia of cancer cells) by which tumors of differing

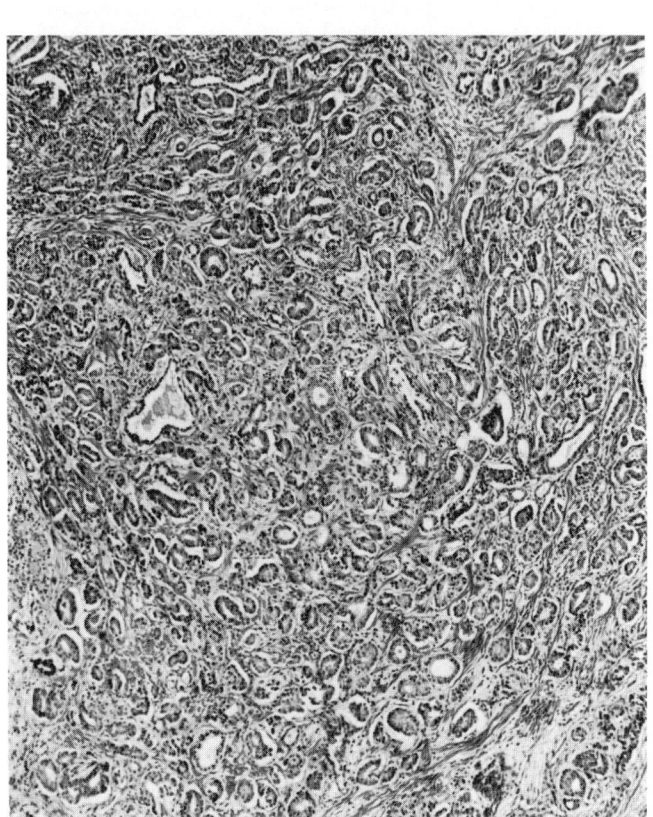

Figure 23–26. Well-differentiated adenocarcinoma of the prostate. Note numerous small acini lying "back to back."

Table 23–2. Staging of Prostate Cancer*

STAGE	PER CENT WITH POSITIVE LYMPH NODES
A. Incidental or clinically unsuspected cancer, detected in tissue removed for apparently benign disorders	
A1 Well differentiated lesions occupying less than 5% of resected specimen	2
A2 More than 5% of cancer in resected specimen or poorly differentiated lesion	23
B. Tumors palpable by rectal digital examination but confined to prostate	
B1 Tumor confined to one lobe	18
B2 Tumor extending to both lobes	35
C. Tumors that have extended locally beyond the prostate, but not produced clinically evident distant metastases	
C1 Tumor not involving seminal vesicles	50
C2 Extensive periprostatic spread with involvement of seminal vesicles	80
D. Tumors with distant metastases	
D1 Patients who are presumed to be Stage A, B, or C clinically but are found to have pelvic lymph node metastases at surgery or by aspiration cytology	100
D2 Clinical evidence of osseous or distant visceral spread	100

* Modified from Catalona, W.J.: Diagnosis, staging, and surgical treatment of prostatic carcinoma. Arch. Intern. Med. *147*:361:1987. Other authors use slightly different criteria for staging.

biologic behavior can be segregated. For example, the Gleason system is based on the degree of glandular differentiation and growth pattern of tumor in relation to the stroma. The Gaeta system, on the other hand, is based on the degree of glandular differentiation as well as nuclear cytology. *Grading is of particular importance in prostatic cancer because there is in general an excellent correlation between the prognosis and the degree of differentiation.* Not surprisingly, therefore, there is also a good correlation between histologic grading and clinical staging.[44]

Staging of prostatic cancer is also very important in the selection of the appropriate form of therapy and in establishing a prognosis. A staging system that is widely utilized in the United States is depicted in Table 23–2.

It will be noted that clinical staging is somewhat imperfect because many patients in stages A2, B, and C have unsuspected lymph node metastases that are discovered only during surgery or subsequent histologic examination. This is particularly relevant because most authorities believe that lymph node spread is indicative of systemic disease that is incurable by current surgical or radiotherapeutic modalities.[45] Because of the grave impact of lymph node spread on prognosis, several techniques, including lymphangiography, CT scanning, and fine needle aspiration biopsy of pelvic nodes under CT control, are employed to assess the status of draining lymph nodes. However, the utility of these procedures in detecting microscopic metastases is limited. Recent studies suggest that DNA ploidy of tumor cells is a useful adjunct to staging in the management of prostatic cancer.[45a]

CLINICAL COURSE. Approximately 35% of males over age 50 harbor Stage A cancer of the prostate.[37] This incidence increases with age and approaches 60% or more in men past the age of 80 years. These latent cancers are asymptomatic and are discovered incidentally at autopsy or in tissue removed for nodular hyperplasia of the prostate. The long-term signifi-

cance of these lesions is still not entirely clear. It is generally accepted that the majority of patients with stage A1 cancer do not show evidence of progressive disease when followed for 8 to 10 years. However, 5 to 10% of patients do develop local or distant spread. This is more likely in younger patients (<60 years) who have a longer life expectancy. For patients in this age group, some authorities recommend careful follow-up studies so that if progression occurs, the cancer may be detected early, at a stage amenable to surgical cure.[46] Stage A2 lesions are more ominous. Approximately 30 to 50% can be expected to progress over a period of 5 years with a mortality of 20% if left untreated.

About 5 to 10% of patients with overt prostatic cancer are discovered in Stage B. These patients do not have urinary symptoms, and the lesion is discovered by the finding of a suspicious nodule on rectal examination. You recall that most prostatic cancers arise in a subcapsular location removed from the urethra and, therefore, urinary symptoms occur late. Most of these lesions are destined to progress unless eradicated by surgery or radiation.

Over 75% of patients with prostatic cancer present with Stage C or D cancer. They come to clinical attention usually because of urinary symptoms such as difficulty in starting or stopping the stream, dysuria, frequency, or hematuria. Pain is a late finding reflecting involvement of capsular perineurial spaces. Some patients in Stage D come to attention because of back pain caused by vertebral metastases. *The finding of osteoblastic metastases in bone is virtually diagnostic of this form of cancer in males* (Fig. 23–28). The outlook for these patients is bleak.

Careful rectal digital examination is a very useful and direct method for detection of early prostatic carcinoma, because the posterior location of most tumors renders them easily palpable. A transperineal or transrectal biopsy can confirm the diagnosis. Several procedures are employed to determine the extent of disease. The involvement of lymph nodes may be de-

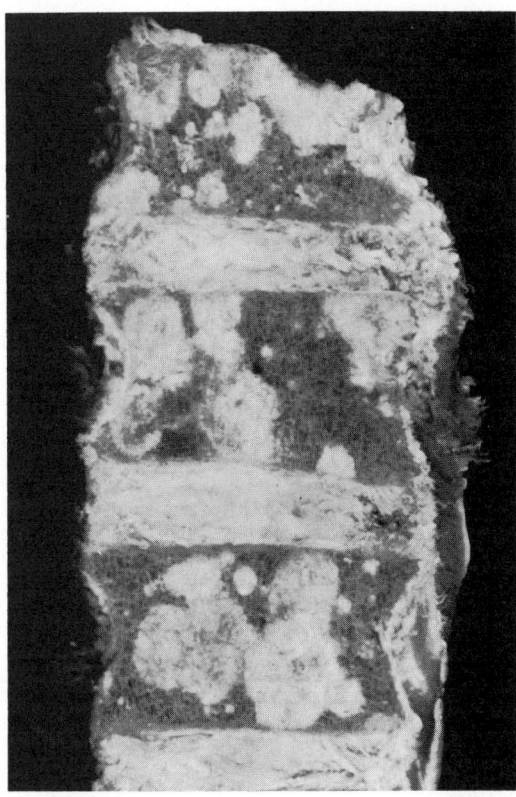

Figure 23–28. Metastatic osteoblastic prostatic carcinoma within vertebral bodies.

tected by CT scans or lymphangiography. Because microscopic metastases may be missed by either of these two procedures, some centers employ pelvic lymphadenectomy as a staging procedure in selected patients. Osseous metastases may be detected by skeletal surveys or the much more sensitive radionuclide bone scanning. It should be noted, however, that bone scans, although highly sensitive, have a low specificity. Any bony lesion (e.g., Paget's disease) that results in new bone formation and increase in blood flow will be seen as a "hot" spot in a bone scan.

Both normal and malignant prostatic epithelia produce acid phosphatase, which can be detected in serum. Other tissues (e.g., red cells) also contain acid phosphatase isoenzymes that can be distinguished from prostatic acid phosphatase by biochemical (enzymatic) or immunologic techniques. *Elevations of serum acid phosphatase levels are found only with cancer that has extended beyond the capsule or metastasized.* Although earlier studies claimed that a radioimmunoassay could be used to detect localized (Stage A) prostatic cancer, subsequent experience has not sustained this optimism. Currently, therefore, most investigators do not believe that radioimmunoassay is superior to the enzymatic assay as a routine laboratory procedure for the staging of prostatic cancer.[47] In addition to its value in staging, measurement of serum acid phosphatase is of value in monitoring of patients. There is a good correlation between response to treatment and a decrease in acid phosphatase. Conversely, cancer progression is usually associated with an increase in serum levels.

Prostate-specific antigen is another marker of some value in tissue diagnosis and the management of prostate cancer. It should be noted that this antigen is found in both normal and neoplastic epithelium, and it is therefore a differentiation antigen rather than a tumor-specific antigen. The immunohistochemical detection of prostate-specific antigen is very valuable in deciding whether a metastatic tumor originated in the prostate. As expected, such metastases are also positive for prostatic acid phosphatase. Recent studies suggest that assays of prostate-specific antigen in the serum may also be valuable in staging and in monitoring the therapeutic response of prostate cancer.[48,49]

Cancer of the prostate is treated by surgery, radiotherapy, and hormonal manipulations. As might be expected, surgery and radiotherapy are most suited for treatment of patients with localized (Stage A or B) disease. Fifty to 80% of patients in this group can expect to live for 10 years. Endocrine therapy is the mainstay for treatment of advanced, metastatic carcinoma. Because prostatic cancer cells are dependent on androgens for their sustenance, the aim of endocrine manipulations is to deprive the tumor cells of testosterone.[50] This can be achieved by orchiectomy, administration of estrogens or synthetic agonists of luteinizing hormone–releasing hormone (LHRH). Although estrogens can inhibit testicular androgen synthesis directly, their principal effect appears to be suppression of pituitary luteinizing hormone (LH) secretion, which in turn leads to reduced testicular output of testosterone. Synthetic analogs of LHRH act similarly. Long-term administration of LHRH agonists (after an initial transient increase in LH secretion) suppresses LH release, achieving in effect a pharmacologic orchiectomy. Despite all forms of treatment, patients with disseminated cancers have a 10 to 40% ten-year survival rate.

1. Opitz, J.M: Editorial comment: Hypospadias. Am. J. Med. Genet. *21:*57, 1985.

2. Sand, P.K., et al.: Evaluation of male consorts of women with genital human papilloma virus infection. Obstet. Gynecol. *68:*679, 1986.

3. Barrasso, R., et al.: High prevalence of papillomavirus-associated penile intraepithelial neoplasia in sexual partners of women with cervical intraepithelial neoplasia. N. Engl. J. Med. *317:*916, 1987.

4. Howley, P.: On human papilloma viruses. N. Engl. J. Med. *315:*1089, 1986.

5. Stringel, G., et al.: Condyloma acuminata in children. J. Petiatr. Surg. *20:*499, 1985.

6. Boshart, M., and zur Hausen, V.: Human papillomaviruses in Buschké-Lowenstein tumors: Physical state of the DNA and identification of a tandem duplication in the non-coding region of a human papilloma virus 6 subtype. J. Virol. *58:*963, 1986.

7. McKee, P.M., et al.: Penile verrucous carcinoma. Histopathology *7:*897, 1983.

8. Graham, J.H., and Helwig, E.G.: Bowen's disease and its relationship to systemic cancer. Arch. Dermatol. *83:*738, 1961.

9. Andersen, S.L.C., et al.: Relationship between Bowen disease and internal malignant tumors. Arch. Dermatol. *108:*367, 1973.

10. Obalek, S., et al.: Bowenoid papulosis of the male and female genitalia: Risk of cervical neoplasia. J. Am. Acad. Dermatol. *14*:433, 1986.

11. Persky, L., and de Kernion, J.: Carcinoma of the penis. CA *36*:258, 1986.

12. McCance, D.J., et al.: Human papillomavirus types 16 and 18 in carcinomas of the penis from Brazil. Int. J. Cancer *37*:55, 1986.

13. Merrin, C.E.: Cancer of the penis. Cancer *45*:1973, 1980.

14. Sheldon, C.C.: Undescended testis and testicular torsion. Surg. Clin. North Am. *65*:1303, 1985.

15. Colodny, A.H.: Undescended testis — is surgery necessary? N. Engl. J. Med. *314*:510, 1986.

16. Bardin, E., and Berger, R. E.: Sexually transmitted diseases in men. Primary Care *12*:761, 1985.

17. Klein, F.A., et al.: Bilateral granulomatous orchitis: Manifestation of idiopathic systemic granulomatosis. J. Urol. *134*:762, 1985.

18. Mostofi, F.K., and Sesterhenn, I.A.: Pathology of germ cell tumors of testes. Prog. Clin. Biol. Res. *203*:1, 1985.

19. Pierce, G.B., Jr., and Abell, M.A.: Embryonal carcinoma of the testis. *In* Sommers, S.C. (ed.): Pathology Annual. New York, Appleton-Century-Crofts, 1970, p. 27.

20. Damajanov, I.: Recent advances in the understanding of the pathology of testicular germ cell tumors. World J. Urol. *2*:17, 1984.

21. Jacobsen, G.K., et al.: Carcinoma in situ of testicular tissue adjacent to malignant germ cell tumors: A study of 105 cases. Cancer *47*:2660, 1981.

22. Henderson, B.E., et al.: Risk factors for cancer of testis in young men. Int. J. Cancer *23*:598, 1979.

23. Kaplan, J.H., et al.: Testicular tumors of germ cell origin. I. Epidemiology, pathogenesis, clinical presentation, and diagnosis. Postgrad. Med. *70*:114, 1981.

24. Javadpour, N.: Tumor markers in testicular cancer — an update. Prog. Clin. Biol. Res. *203*:141, 1985.

25. Drasga, R.E., et al.: The chemotherapy of testicular cancer. CA *32*:66, 1982.

26. Kim, I., et al.: Leydig cell tumors of the testis. Am. J. Surg. Pathol. *9*:177, 1985.

27. Doll, D.C., and Weiss, R.B.: Malignant lymphoma of testis. Am J. Med. *81*:515, 1986.

28. Coffey, D.S., and Isaacs, J.T.: Control of prostate growth. Urology *17*(Suppl. 3):17, 1981.

29. Orland, S.M., et al.: Prostatitis, prostatosis and prostatodynia. Urology *15*:439, 1985.

30. Shortliffe, L.M.D.: Prostatitis. Primary Care *12*:787, 1985.

31. Berry, S.J., et al.: The development of human benign prostatic hyperplasia with age. J. Urol. *132*:474, 1984.

32. Wilson, J.D.: The pathogenesis of benign prostatic hyperplasia. Am. J. Med. *68*:745, 1980.

33. Wilson, J.D.: The testes and the prostate. A continuing relationship. N. Engl. J. Med. *317*:628, 1987.

34. McNeal, J.: Normal and pathologic anatomy of prostate. Urology *17*(Suppl. 3):11, 1981.

35. Silverberg, E., and Lubera, J.: Cancer statistics, 1989. CA *39*:3, 1989.

36. Hutchinson, G.B.: Incidence and etiology of prostatic cancer. Urology *17*(Suppl. 3):4, 1981.

37. Guileyardo, J.M., et al.: Prevalence of latent prostate carcinoma in two U.S. populations J. Natl. Cancer Inst. *65*:311, 1980.

38. Jackson, M.S., et al.: Characterization of prostatic cancer among blacks. A continuation report. Cancer Treat. Rep. *61*:167, 1977.

39. Dunn, J.E.: Cancer epidemiology in populations of the United States — with emphasis on Hawaii and California — and Japan. Cancer Res. *35*:3240, 1975.

40. Catalona, W.J., and Scott, W.W.: Carcinoma of the prostate. *In* Walsh, P.C., et al. (eds.): Campbell's Urology. Fifth edition. Philadelphia, W.B. Saunders Co., 1986, p. 1463.

41. Huggins, C., and Hodges, C.V.: Studies of prostatic cancer. I. The effect of castration, of estrogen, and of androgen injections on serum phosphatase in metastatic carcinoma of the prostate. Cancer Res. *1*:203, 1941.

42. Zumoff, B., et al.: Abnormal levels of plasma hormones in men with prostate cancer: Evidence towards a two disease theory. Prostate *3*:579, 1982.

43. Greenwald, P., et al.: Cancer of the prostate among men with benign prostatic hyperplasia. J. Natl. Cancer Inst. *53*:335, 1974.

44. Gaeta, J.F.: Glandular profiles and cellular patterns in prostatic cancer grading. Urology *17*(Suppl.3):33, 1981.

45. Huben, R.P., and Murphy, G.P.: Prostate cancer: An update. CA *36*:274, 1986.

45a. Koss, L.G.: The puzzle of prostatic carcinoma. Mayo Clin. Proc. *63*:193, 1988.

46. Whitmore, W.: Stage A prostate cancer. J. Urol. *136*:883, 1986.

47. Heller, J.E.: Prostatic acid phosphatase: Its current clinical status. J. Urol. *137*:1091, 1987.

48. Chu, T.M., and Murphy, G.P.: What is new in tumor markers for prostate. Urol. *27*:487, 1986.

49. Stamey, T.A., et al.: Prostate specific antigen as a serum marker for adenocarcinoma of the prostate. N. Engl. J. Med. *317*:909, 1987.

50. Smith, J.A., Jr.: New methods of endocrine management of prostatic cancer. J. Urol. *137*:1, 1987.

Female Genital Tract

NORMAL

EMBRYOLOGY. Some knowledge of the embryology is important to understand the congenital anomalies of the female genital tract and the histogenesis of various tumors.[1] The *primordial germ* cells can be identified in the wall of the yolk sac by the fourth week of gestation; by the fifth or sixth week, they migrate into the *urogenital ridge* — the site of subsequent development of the urogenital system. The mesodermal epithelium of the urogenital ridge then begins to proliferate to produce the epithelium of the eventual gonad. In the presence of 46 XX chromosomes, the dividing germ cells are incorporated into proliferating epithelial cells to form what eventually becomes the organized ovary. Thus the ovary develops primarily from mesoderm (which gives rise to both surface epithelium and stroma), except for the germ cells, which are endodermal.[2] Failure of germ cells to develop in the urogenital ridge causes a spectrum of diseases from absence of ovaries to premature menopause. Arrest of normal migration in the midline

accounts for the extragonadal distribution of germ cell tumors in the midline structures — retroperitoneum, mediastinum, and even pineal gland.

Another important structure in female genital development is the *müllerian duct*. At about the sixth week, invagination of the coelomic lining epithelium creates a groove whose lips later fuse to form the lateral *müllerian* (or *paramesonephric*) *ducts*. Müllerian ducts first become apparent high on the dorsal wall of the coelomic cavity and then progressively grow caudally to enter the pelvis, where they swing medially *to fuse*. Further caudal growth brings these fused ducts into contact with the *urogenital sinus*, the area on the caudal surface of the embryo that eventually becomes the vestibule of the external genitalia. With relatively uncomplicated transformations, the unfused portions mature into the fallopian tubes, and the fused caudal portion into the uterus and the vagina. The upper portion of the vagina is generally held to be of müllerian origin, and the lower portion probably derived from the urogenital sinus. *It is apparent that the entire lining of the uterus and tubes is derived from coelomic epithelium.* The embryogenesis here serves to explain the various histologic patterns of those ovarian tumors derived from coelomic epithelium, as we shall see.

In males, *müllerian inhibiting substance*[3] produced by the developing testis causes regression of the müllerian ducts. Parallel to the müllerian ducts are the paired *wolffian* (or *mesonephric*) *ducts,* which in the male are destined to form the epididymis and the vas deferens. Normally, the mesonephric duct regresses in the female. Remnants, however, may persist into adult life as epithelial inclusions about the hilus of the ovary and mesosalpinx, designated respectively the epoophoron and paroophoron. If the caudal portions of this mesonephric anlage persist, they may appear as epithelial inclusions within the wall of the lower uterine segment and cervix, and as epithelial rests in the lateral walls of the vagina. Sometimes in the vagina these rests produce cysts that are known as *Gartner's duct cysts.*

ANATOMY. During active reproductive life, the *ovaries* measure about 4 cm in length, 2.5 to 3 cm in width, and 1 to 1.5 cm in thickness. The ovary is divided into a cortex and a medulla. Ordinarily, the cortex consists of a layer of closely packed spindle cells that resemble plump fibroblasts, separated by only a scant intercellular ground substance. The outermost portion directly beneath the surface epithelium is compacted into a thin layer of relatively acellular collagenous connective tissue. Thickening of this layer may accompany ovarian dysfunction. By puberty, follicles and ova in varying stages of maturation are found within the outer cortex. With each menstrual cycle, one follicle develops into a graafian follicle en route to ovulation. Corpora lutea of varying ages, as well as the corpora albicantia, are also present in the cortex of the adult.

The medulla of the ovary is made up of a more loosely arranged mesenchymal tissue. Occasionally, large, round to polygonal, epithelial-appearing cells are buried within the medulla in the hilar region. These "hilus" cells, presumed to be vestigial remains of the gonad from its primitive "ambisexual" phase, are steroid producing, and thus resemble the interstitial cells of the testis. Rarely, these cells give rise to masculinizing tumors.

In the *fallopian tube,* the mucosa is thrown up into numerous high, delicate folds that on cross section produce a papillary appearance. The lining epithelium of the tube is made up of three cell types: ciliated columnar cells; nonciliated, columnar, secretory cells; and so-called intercalated cells, which may simply represent inactive secretory cells.

The uterus varies in size, depending on the age and parity of the individual. During active reproductive life, it weighs about 50 gm and measures 8 cm in length, 5 to 6.5 cm in breadth in the fundic region, and 3 cm in thickness (1.5 cm of anterior and of posterior myometrium). Pregnancies may leave small residual increases in these dimensions (up to 70 gm in weight), because the uterus rarely involutes com-

pletely to its original size. Postmenopausally, the atrophic changes may cause diminution to 5 to 6 cm in length, 3 cm in width, and 1.5 to 2 cm in thickness.

The uterus has three distinctive anatomic and functional regions: the cervix, the lower uterine segment, and the corpus. The *cervix* is further divided into the vaginal portio and the endocervix. The anatomic portio is that portion of the cervix visible to the eye on vaginal examination. It is covered by a stratified nonkeratinizing squamous epithelium reflected off the vaginal vaults onto the cervix. This squamous epithelium covers the entire anatomic portio and extends more or less up to the central dimple that comprises the external os. In the normal cervix of nulliparous women, this os is virtually closed. The endocervix is normally not exposed and is lined by columnar, mucus-secreting epithelium that dips down into the underlying stroma to produce crypts sometimes designated as endocervical glands.

The *squamocolumnar junction* is of considerable importance, because most cervical carcinomas arise at this site. The position of the junction is variable. The original anatomic junction is at the cervical os (Fig. 24–1, *left*). However, in virtually all adult women who have borne children, the columnar endocervical epithelium migrates downward from the cervical os and thus is visible to the naked eye. This is referred to as an *ectropion* or *ectopic* endocervix (Fig. 24–1, *middle*). An ectropion appears red or pink on visual examination and is thus often called by clinicians an *erosion,* which is a misnomer because the mucosal layer is actually intact. Ectropions become gradually re-epithelialized by squamous epithelium (squamous metaplasia), producing the so-called *transformation zone* (Fig. 24–1, *right*); in postmenopausal women, this zone is high, above the external os, and thus this critical area is not visible to the naked eye. As we shall see, it is this transformation zone that must be biopsied to exclude carcinoma or precancerous lesions. The *lower uterine segment,* or *isthmus,* is the portion between the endocervix and the endometrial cavity.

ENDOMETRIAL HISTOLOGY AND MENSTRUAL CYCLE. The endometrial changes that occur during the menstrual cycle are keyed to the rise and fall in the levels of ovarian hormones, and the student should be familiar with the complex but fascinating interactions among hypothalamic, pituitary, and ovarian factors underlying maturation of ovarian follicles, ovulation, and the menstrual cycle. Suffice it to say that under the influence of the pituitary follicle-stimulating and luteotropic hormones (FSH and LH), development and ripening of a single ovum occurs, and estrogen production by the enlarging ovarian follicle progressively rises during the first two weeks of the classic 28-day menstrual cycle. It reaches a peak, presumably just before ovulation, and then falls. Following ovulation, the estrogen levels again begin to rise to a plateau at about the end of the third week, but these levels are never as high as the preovulatory peak. The

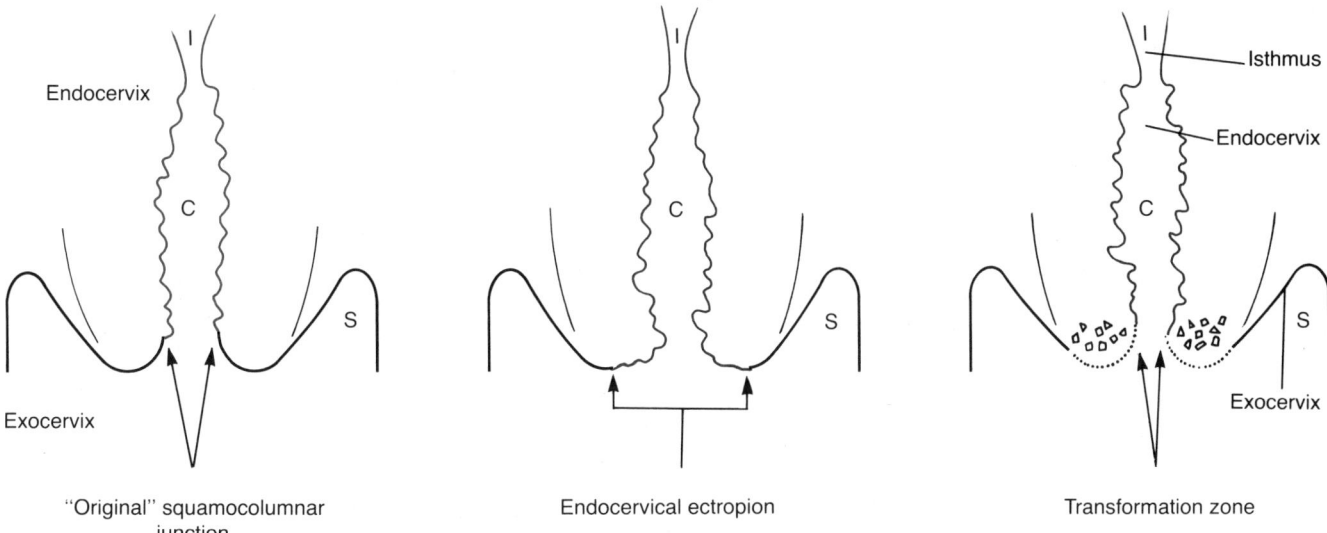

Endocervix

Exocervix

"Original" squamocolumnar
junction

Endocervical ectropion

Isthmus

Endocervix

Exocervix

Transformation zone

Figure 24–1. Schematic representation of normal cervix and transformation zone. *Left,* Diagram of a portio completely covered with native squamous epithelium. Squamocolumnar junction is at external os. *Middle,* Denotes an endocervical columnar ectropion with squamocolumnar junction located on exocervix below external os. *Right,* Indicates areas of ectropion now covered with squamous epithelium (stippled line). This area is the cervical transformation zone. (Modification from Ferenczy, A., and Winkler, B.: Anatomy and histology of the cervix. *In* Kurman, R. (ed.): Blaustein's Pathology of the Female Genital Tract. 3rd ed. New York, Springer-Verlag, 1987. Reproduced with permission.)

level of this hormone then progressively falls, beginning three to four days before the onset of menstruation. Progesterone, produced by the corpus luteum, rises throughout the last half of the menstrual cycle to fall to basal levels just before the onset of menstrual bleeding.

"Dating" the endometrium by its histologic appearance is helpful clinically to assess hormonal status, document ovulation, and determine causes of endometrial bleeding and infertility. We can begin with the shedding of the upper one-half to two-thirds of the endometrium during the menstrual period (Fig. 24–2). The basal third does not respond to the ovarian steroids and is retained at the conclusion of the menstrual flow. From the basal third of this preovulatory proliferative phase of the cycle, there is extremely rapid growth of both glands and stroma. The glands are straight, tubular structures lined by quite regular, tall, columnar cells. Mitotic figures are numerous, and there is no evidence of mucus secretion or vacuolation (Fig. 24–3). The endometrial stroma is composed of thickly compacted spindle cells that have scant cytoplasm but abundant mitotic activity.

At the time of ovulation, the endometrium slows in its growth, and it ceases apparent mitotic activity within days immediately following ovulation. The postovulatory endometrium is marked by basal secretory vacuoles beneath the nuclei in the glandular epithelium (Fig. 24–4). The secretory activity becomes more prominent during the third week of the menstrual cycle, and the basal vacuoles appear to push past the nuclei to appear above and below the nuclei, which are thus aligned at midpoint in the cell. When secretion is maximal, between 18 and 24 days, the

glands are dilated. Tortuosity of the glands, which is well developed by the fourth week, produces a serrate margin to the glands when cut in their long axis (Fig. 24–5). During the last week of the cycle, rupture of some of the columnar epithelial cells releases secretion into the gland lumina. The cells thus emptied, the glands begin to shrink, becoming narrower and "saw-toothed"—an appearance referred to as *secretory exhaustion.* The stroma between the glands becomes edematous, and the spiral arterioles become more prominent. At this time, 24 days, stromal mitoses reappear. There is now a considerable increase in ground substance and edema between the stromal cells. In the nonpregnant state, three to four days before the menstrual flow, the stromal cells become hypertrophied and accumulate a considerable amount of pink cytoplasm to produce so-called *predecidual changes.* The escape of blood into the stroma marks the beginning of menstrual shedding. In the premenstrual and menstrual phases, the endometrial stroma contains scattered neutrophils and occasional lymphocytes. The normal presence of such leukocytes is to be particularly noted because these white cells are ordinarily considered to be indicators of an inflammatory reaction.

The proliferative phase should therefore be readily differentiated from the secretory phase. *The hallmark of the proliferative phase is mitotic activity in glandular and stromal cells. Ovulation should be fairly well denoted by the basal vacuolation of the columnar epithelial cells of the glands.* When ovulation fails to occur, there is no secretory vacuolation in the endometrial glands, and the characteristic stromal edema and later decidual transformation are absent.

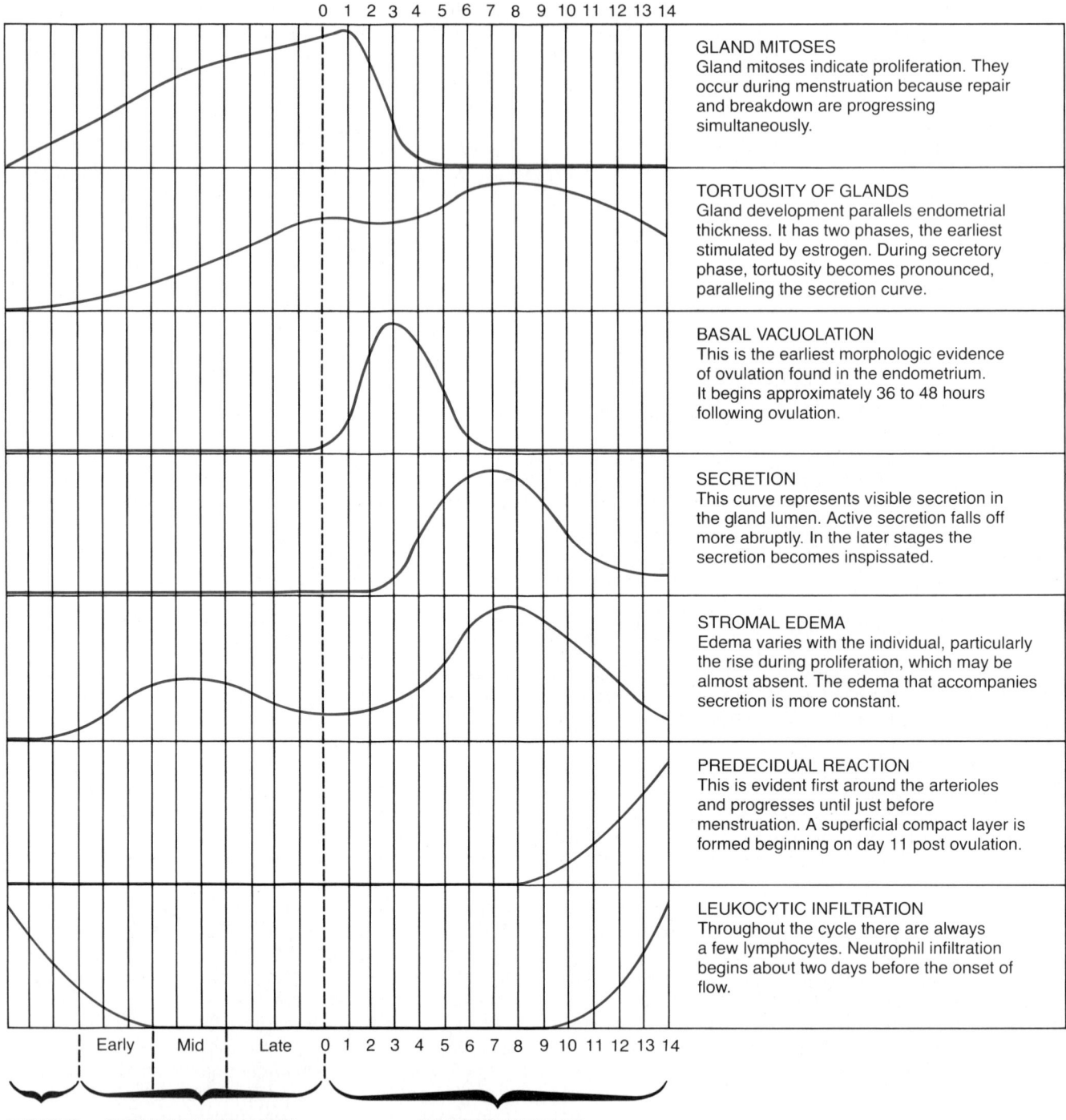

Figure 24–2. **Approximate quantitative changes in seven morphologic criteria found to be most useful in dating human endometrium.** **(Modified from Noyes, R.W.: Normal phases of the endometrium. *In* Norris, H.J., et al. (eds.): The Uterus. Baltimore, Williams & Wilkins Co., 1973.)**

PATHOLOGY

Diseases of the female genital tract are numerous and extremely common in clinical and pathologic practice. They include complications of pregnancy, in-

flammations, tumors, and hormonally induced defects. The following discussion presents the major entities that compose the majority of clinical problems.

Details can be found in current books of obstetric and gynecologic pathology and medicine.[4-10] The pathologic conditions peculiar to each segment of the female genital tract will be discussed separately, but first we shall briefly review pelvic inflammatory disease and other infections because they can affect many of the segments concomitantly.

FEMALE GENITAL INFECTIONS

A large variety of organisms can infect the female genital tract and in total account for a great deal of suffering and morbidity. Some, such as candidal infections and trichomoniasis, are extremely common and may cause significant discomfort but are not func-tionally significant. Others, such as gonorrhea, are major causes of female infertility, and others still, such as mycoplasma infections, are implicated in spontaneous abortions. And currently, viruses, prin-cipally the human papilloma viruses, appear to be in-volved in the pathogenesis of vulvar and cervical cancer.

Many of these infections are sexually transmitted, including gonorrhea, chancroid, granuloma ingui-nale, lymphogranuloma venereum, syphilis, myco-plasma, chlamydia, herpes, and human papilloma virus.[11] A few, such as moniliasis, tuberculosis, and trichomoniasis, are not. Most of these conditions have

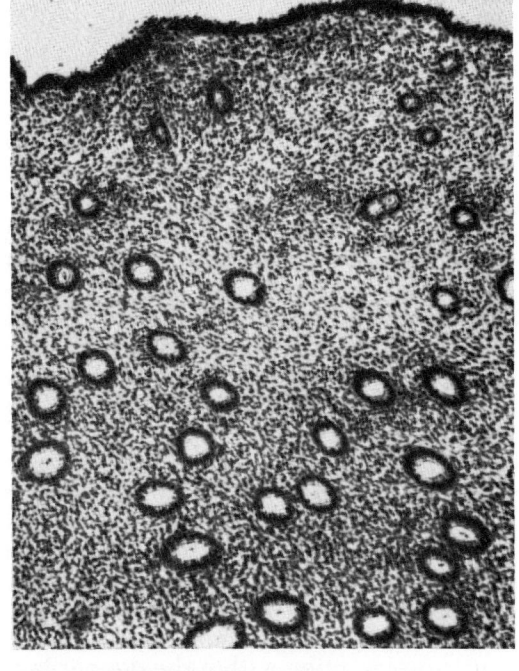

Fig. 24–3

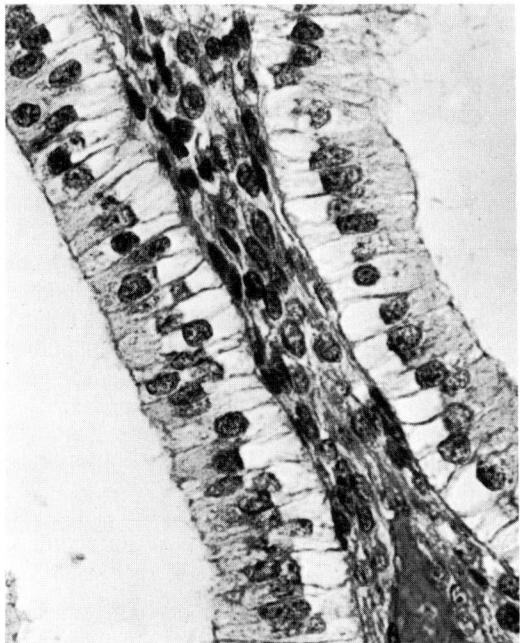

Fig. 24–4

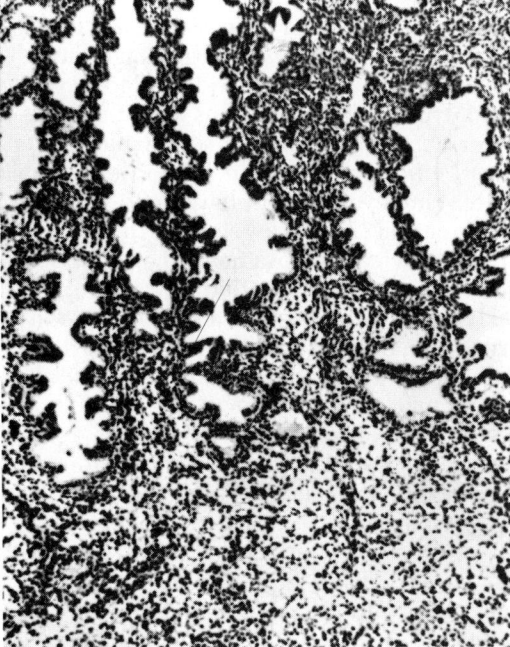

Fig. 24–5

Figure 24–3. Normal proliferative endometrium, il-lustrating tubelike pattern of glands.

Figure 24–4. Postovulatory endometrium with prom-inent subnuclear vacuoles and alignment of nuclei.

Figure 24–5. Late secretory endometrium with tortu-osity of glands, producing serrate margins.

(All three from Noyes, R.N., et al.: Fertil. Steril. *1*:3, 1950. Courtesy of Dr. A. Hertig.)

been adequately considered in Chapter 7. Here we shall only touch on selected aspects relevant to the female genital tract, but will discuss gonorrheal and polymicrobial pelvic inflammatory disease at some length.

Herpes simplex infection is common and usually involves the vulva, vagina, and cervix.[11] The frequency of genital herpes has increased dramatically in the past two decades, particularly in teenagers and young women, and herpes simplex virus type II (HSV II) infection is now one of the major sexually transmitted diseases. The lesions begin three to seven days after sexual relations and consist of painful red papules in the vulva that progress to vesicles and then coalescent ulcers. Cervical and vaginal involvement causes severe leukorrhea. There may be systemic symptoms such as fever, malaise, and tender inguinal lymph nodes. The vesicles and ulcers contain numerous virus particles, accounting for the high transmission rate during active infection. The lesions heal spontaneously in one to three weeks, but as with herpetic infections elsewhere, the latent infection persists, and about two-thirds of affected women suffer recurring relapses. Relapses are less painful and transmission is less likely from contact with asymptomatic carriers. In the pregnant mother, the risk of newborn, frequently fatal infection with herpes is particularly high when the virus particles are present at the time of delivery.

Mycotic and *yeast infections,* principally with *Candida albicans,* occur frequently. About 10% of women are thought to be carriers of vulvovaginal fungi. Diabetes mellitus, oral contraceptives, and pregnancy enhance the development of lesions, which consist of small white surface patches similar to monilial lesions elsewhere (p. 386). They are accompanied by leukorrhea and pruritus. The diagnosis is made by finding the organism in wet mounts of the lesions.

Acute or chronic vaginal infections are often caused by *Trichomonas vaginalis,* a large, flagellated, ovoid protozoan that can be readily identified in wet mounts of vaginal discharge. Infections with this organism may occur at any age but are somewhat more common in postmenopausal women. This infection is associated with a thick vaginal discharge and itching; when the inflammation is well developed, the underlying vaginal and cervical mucosa has a characteristic brilliant fiery red, sometimes called "strawberry," appearance. Histologically, there is a suppurative inflammatory reaction, but it is usually quite superficial and involves only the vaginal mucosa and immediately subjacent lamina propria.

Mycoplasma species account for some cases of vaginitis and cervicitis and have been implicated in spontaneous abortion and pelvic inflammatory disease.

Gardnerella is a gram-negative, small bacillus that is implicated in cases of vaginitis when other organisms (trichomonas, fungi) cannot be found.

Chlamydia trachomatis (p. 327) causes cervicitis in most instances. However, in some patients it ascends to the uterus and fallopian tubes, resulting in endometritis and salpingitis, and thus is one of the causes of pelvic inflammatory disease, discussed next.

PELVIC INFLAMMATORY DISEASE

Pelvic inflammatory disease (PID) is an ascending infection that begins in the vulva or vagina but usually spreads upward through the entire genital tract, involving more or less all the structures in the female genital system. The *gonococcus* continues to be a common cause of PID, which is the most serious complication of gonorrhea in women. The basic biology of gonococcal infections was discussed earlier (p. 343). Besides gonorrhea, infections following spontaneous or induced abortions and normal or abnormal deliveries are important in the production of PID. *Such postabortion and postpartum PIDs are polymicrobial and are caused by staphylococci, streptococci, coliform bacteria, and Clostridium perfringens. Chlamydia* infection is now another well-recognized cause of PID.

Gonococcal inflammation begins usually in Bartholin's glands and other vestibular glands, or in Skene's ducts and periurethral glands, or sometimes in the endocervical glands. From any of these loci, the organisms spread upward over the mucosal surfaces, eventually to involve the tubes and tubo-ovarian region. In such spread, the adult vagina is remarkably resistant. In the child, presumably because of a more delicate lining mucosa, vulvovaginitis may develop. The nongonococcal bacterial infections that follow induced abortion, dilatation and curettage of the uterus, and other surgical procedures on the female genital tract are thought to spread from the uterus upward through the lymphatics or venous channels rather than on the mucosal surfaces. These infections therefore tend to produce less mucosal involvement but more reaction within the deeper layers.

With the gonococcus, approximately two to seven days after inoculation of the organism, inflammatory changes appear in the affected glands. The mechanisms by which the gonococcus adheres to epithelial cells and then invades were reviewed previously (p. 343). Wherever it occurs, gonococcal disease is characterized by an acute suppurative reaction accompanied by the copious outpouring of pus. In gonococcal infections, the inflammatory changes are largely confined to the superficial mucosa and underlying submucosa. Smear of the exudate should disclose the intracellular gram-negative diplococcus, but absolute confirmation requires cultural identification. In most acute cases, with therapy, the infection promptly subsides and does not involve the upper levels of the genital tract. If spread occurs, a gonorrheal endometritis may develop, but more often the endometrium is remarkably spared, for obscure reasons. Once within the tubes, an **acute suppurative salpingitis** ensues. The tubal serosa becomes hyperemic and layered with fibrin, the tubal fimbriae are similarly involved, and the lumen fills with purulent exudate that may leak out of the fimbriated end. In the course of days or weeks, the tubal fimbriae may seal or become plastered against the ovary to create a **salpingo-oophoritis.** Pus may collect in these sealed tubes to cause **distention (pyosalpinx).** So enclosed, the infection tends to smolder and becomes chronic for months and even years. In the course of time the infecting organisms may disappear. The pus then undergoes slow proteolysis and the contents of the tubes are transformed to a thin, serous fluid **(hydrosalpinx). Tubo-ovarian abscesses** may result from collections of exudate in which the tube is sealed against the ovary.

PID caused by staphylococci, streptococci, and the other puerperal invaders tends to have less exudation within the lumina of the tube and less involvement of the mucosa, with a greater inflammatory response within the deeper layers. The infection tends to spread throughout the wall to involve the serosa, and may often track into the broad ligaments, pelvic structures, and peritoneum. Bacteremia is a more frequent complication of streptococcal or staphylococcal pelvic inflammatory disease than of gonococcal infections.

PID causes pelvic pain, dysmenorrhea, menstrual abnormalities, and sometimes manifestations of an acute abdomen. The complications of PID include (1) peritonitis; (2) intestinal obstruction due to adhesions between the small bowel and the pelvic organs; (3) bacteremia, which may potentially induce endocarditis, meningitis, and suppurative arthritis; and (4) infertility, one of the most feared consequences of long-standing chronic PID.

In the early stages, gonococcal infections are readily controlled with antibiotics, although regrettably, penicillin-resistant strains have emerged. When the infection becomes walled off in suppurative tubes or tubo-ovarian abscesses, it is difficult to achieve a sufficient level of antibiotic within the centers of such suppuration to control these infections effectively. Postabortion and postpartum PIDs are also amenable to antibiotics but are far more difficult to control than the gonococcal infections. Sometimes, it becomes necessary to remove the organs surgically.

VULVA

Diseases of the vulva in the aggregate constitute only a small fraction of gynecologic practice. Many are inflammatory dermatologic diseases that affect hair-bearing skin elsewhere on the body may also occur on the vulva, so that vulvitis may be encountered in psoriasis, eczema, and allergic dermatitis. The vulva is also prone to skin infections, because it is constantly exposed to secretions and moisture. Nonspecific vulvitis is particularly likely to occur in the blood dyscrasias, uremia, diabetes mellitus, malnutrition, and the avitaminoses. Most skin cysts (epidermal inclusion cysts) and tumors can also occur in the vulva. Here we shall discuss Bartholin's cyst, vulvar dystrophy, and tumors of the vulva.

BARTHOLIN'S CYST

Bartholin's vulvovaginal glands are frequently involved in gonorrheal infections, although at times other organisms may be responsible for the inflammatory reaction. Acute adenitis may result in abscess formation, which needs to be drained for relief. A chronic form, with asymptomatic intervals alternating with acute exacerbations, also occurs. If the main duct of the gland is blocked, a *Bartholin's cyst* results. This may become quite large, up to 3 to 5 cm in diameter. The lesion is fairly common and occurs at all ages. The cyst is lined by either the transitional epithelium of the normal duct or cells that are flattened by the increased intracystic pressure. The cysts produce pain and local discomfort but are otherwise of no systemic significance.

VULVAR DYSTROPHY

A heterogeneous group of lesions of the vulva present as opaque, white, plaquelike mucosal thickenings that are sometimes pruritic and scaly. In the past, clinicians have used the term "leukoplakia" to designate these lesions—an unfortunate choice of words, because white plaques may underlie a variety of histologic patterns, some of which are clearly benign but others premalignant or malignant.[12] Indeed, when biopsy is done on such "leukoplakic" lesions, they are found to represent any one of the following conditions: (1) vitiligo (loss of pigment); (2) an inflammatory dermatosis (e.g., psoriasis, chronic dermatitis [p. 1296]); (3) carcinoma in situ, Paget's disease, or even invasive carcinoma; and (4) a variety of alterations of unknown etiology that elude proper classification. Considerable confusion existed in the past because of imprecise words (e.g., kraurosis vulvae, leukoplakia, atrophic vulvitis), but a nomenclature developed by the International Society for the Study of Vulvar Disease now places the different lesions in this group under the single heading of *dystrophy.*

The 1986 version of the nomenclature recognizes two varieties of dystrophy:[13] (1) *lichen sclerosus,* a characteristic disorder manifested by epithelial thinning and subepithelial fibrosis, and (2) *squamous hyperplasia,* characterized by epithelial hyperplasia and hyperkeratosis. The two forms may coexist in different areas of the same vulva, and the lesions are often multiple, making their clinical management particularly difficult.

LICHEN SCLEROSUS. Lichen sclerosus is a disorder of the skin that can occur anywhere on the body and in all age groups. It consists of yellowish-blue papules or macules that eventually coalesce and evolve into thin, gray, parchment-like areas. The lesions become easily irritated, leading to fibrosis and scarring. For this reason the condition has been called "chronic atrophic vulvitis."

The skin becomes pale gray and parchment-like, the labia are atrophied, and the introitus is narrowed. The entire vulvar area becomes smooth, with loss of the usual skin folds, and the skin may assume a glazed red appearance as the subcutaneous vessels become more apparent. Histologically, there is apparent thinning of the epidermis, with disappearance of the rete pegs and replacement of the underlying dermis by dense collagenous fibrous tissue (Fig. 24-6). There is often marked hyperkeratosis, and a mononuclear cell infiltrate about blood vessels.

Clinically, this disease occurs in all age groups but is most common after menopause. Genetic as well as autoimmune and hormonal factors have been implicated in its pathogenesis.[14] At all ages, the disorder tends to be slowly developing, insidious, and progressive. It causes considerable discomfort and predisposes to acute infection, but is usually of little systemic significance. Lichen sclerosus is not considered a premalignant lesion.[15]

SQUAMOUS HYPERPLASIA. Previously called "hyperplastic dystrophy," this lesion denotes hyper-

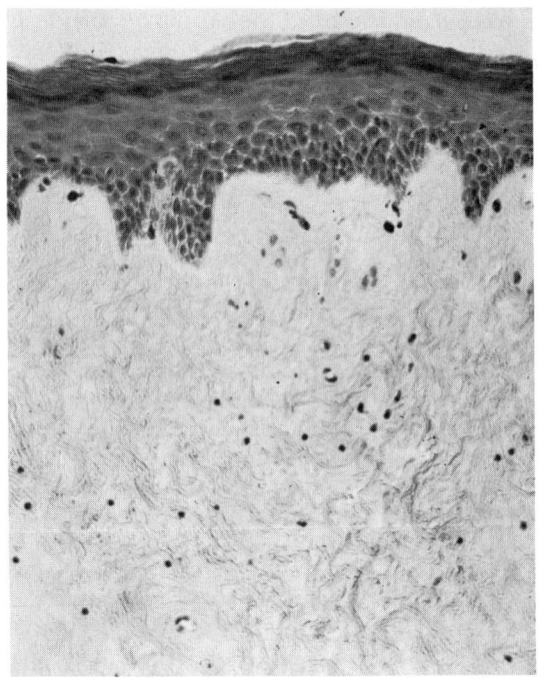

Figure 24-6. Lichen sclerosus illustrating atrophy of epidermis and dense sclerosis of dermis with total atrophy of dermal adnexal structures. (Courtesy of Dr. Arthur Hertig.)

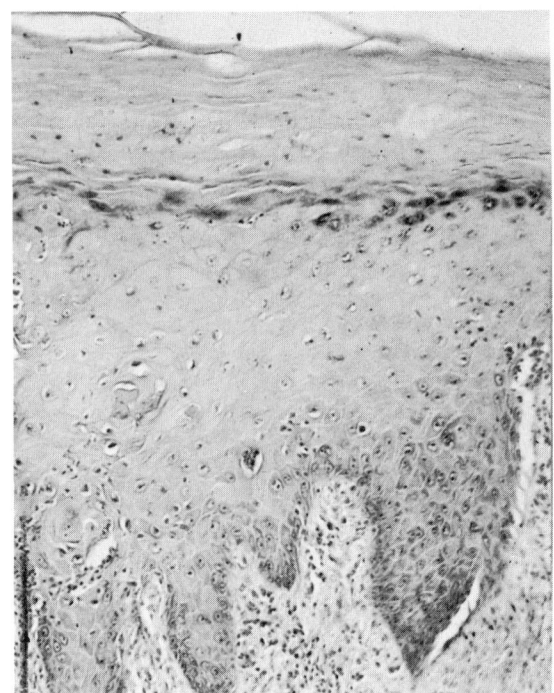

Figure 24-7. Squamous hyperplasia. Marked epithelial hyperplasia and hyperkeratosis present clinically as leukoplakia. (Courtesy of Dr. Arthur Hertig.)

plasia of the squamous epithelial lining, frequently with hyperkeratosis. The epithelium is thickened and may show increased mitotic activity in both the basal and prickle cell layers (Fig. 24-7). The hyperplastic epithelial changes show no atypia, but if they do, the current trend is to consider the lesions as *dysplasia* (p. 1136).[14]

Leukocytic infiltration of the dermis is sometimes pronounced. In the absence of atypia in the epithelium, squamous hyperplasia does not progress to carcinoma. Its pathogenesis is unknown, but this lesion may be a nonspecific reaction to vulvar irritants.

It is important to remember, however, that lesions that appear clinically as white plaques may be benign without the propensity to become cancerous (e.g., vitiligo, chronic dermatitis), hyperplastic, atypical, or malignant. Biopsy is therefore indicated in all lesions, even those that are remotely suspicious.

TUMORS

Tumors of the vulva are the most important lesions to affect this region. Many types have been recorded, both benign and malignant, including fibromas, neurofibromas, angiomas, sweat gland tumors, carcinomas, malignant melanomas, and various types of mesenchymal sarcoma. All these forms are uncommon and, moreover, are histologically analogous to similar tumors occurring elsewhere in the body. Therefore, attention is focused on the more common tumors and other proliferative lesions distinctive of the vulva.

CONDYLOMA ACUMINATUM

Benign verrucous protuberances of the vulva occur in three forms. (1) By far the most common is the *condyloma acuminatum,* a virus-induced squamous papilloma also called "venereal wart." (2) A much rarer form is the usually discrete *squamous papilloma,* which may be indistinguishable from condyloma acuminatum but is usually single, occurs in older age groups, and is not venereally transmitted; these squamous papillomas may be the forerunners of carcinoma in rare cases. (3) The *syphilitic condyloma latum* is described on page 370.

Condylomata acuminata are sexually transmitted, benign tumors that have a distinctly verrucous gross appearance (Fig. 24–8).[16] Although they may be solitary, they are more frequently multiple, involving perineal, vulvar, and perianal regions; the vagina; and, rarely, the cervix. The lesions are identical to those found on the penis and around the anus in males (p. 1100). Histologically, they consist of a tree-like proliferation of stratified squamous epithelium supported by a fibrous stroma (Fig. 24–9). Acanthosis, parakeratosis, hyperkeratosis, and a perinuclear vacuolization of epithelium (called *koilocytosis*) are present. There is usually a mild degree of atypicality which is increased when the lesions are painted with podophyllin, the chemical often used to treat these lesions.

The growth is induced by the human papilloma virus (HPV). HPV (mostly types 6 and 11)[17] has been recovered from the lesions, identified by molecular hybridization techniques, and localized in epithelial cells by electron microscopy and with the immuno-

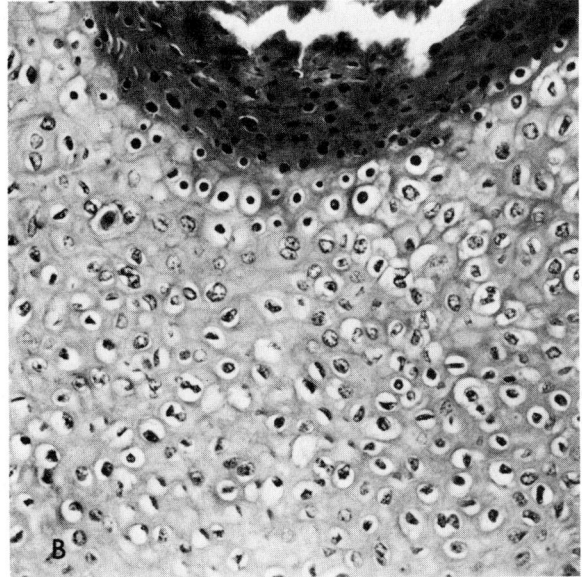

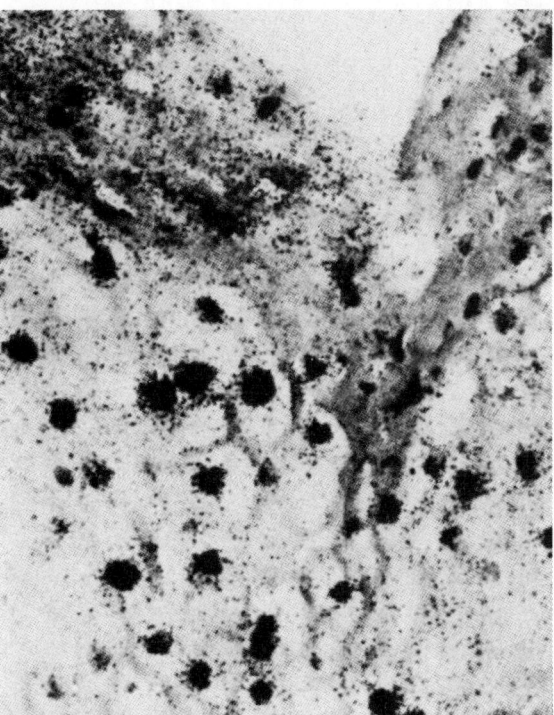

Figure 24–9. *Top,* High-power view of epithelial hyperplasia in condyloma acuminatum. Cytoplasmic vacuolization (koilocytosis) and oval nuclei in superficial layers are characteristic. *Bottom,* In situ hybridization autoradiogram of condyloma, using 35s labeled HPV 6/11 probe, showing positive nuclei of koilocytotic cells. (From Gupta, L., et al.: Am. J. Pathol. *127:*208, 1987. Used by permission.)

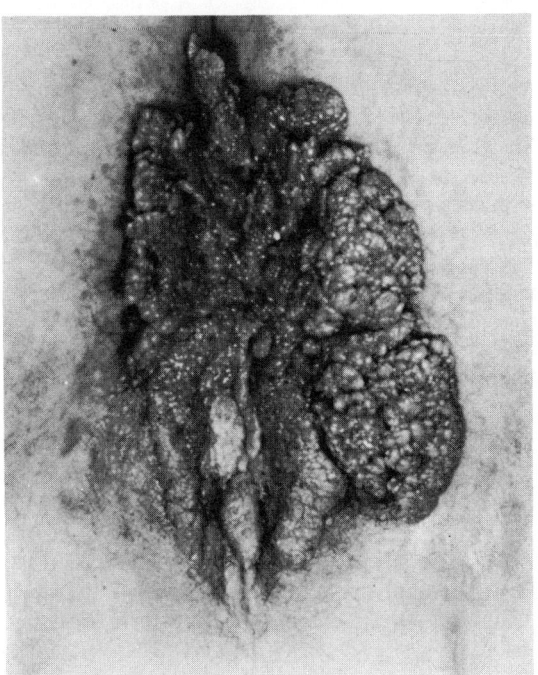

Figure 24–8. Numerous condylomas of vulva, almost obscuring labia minora. (Courtesy of Dr. Arthur Hertig.)

peroxidase technique. The condyloma acuminatum itself is not considered to be a precancerous lesion, having diploid or polyploid rather than the aneuploid DNA content of precancerous cells. However, patients with condylomas may also have HPV infection of other genital sites, and thus condylomas may sometimes *coexist* with areas of dysplasia, or carcinoma in situ,[18] a finding that may account for the reported carcinomas arising from them.

PAPILLARY HIDRADENOMA

This benign tumor arises from the modified apocrine sweat glands of the vulva. It presents as a sharply circumscribed nodule, most commonly on the labia majora or interlabial folds. This rare tumor can be mistaken for carcinoma by the clinician because of its tendency to ulcerate, and by the pathologist because of its complex histologic appearance, which consists of tubular ducts lined by a single or double layer of nonciliated columnar cells, with a layer of flattened "myoepithelial cells" underlying the epithelium. These myoepithelial elements are characteristic of sweat glands and sweat gland tumors. Hidradenoma is a benign lesion, and when completely excised it does not recur.

DYSPLASIA AND CARCINOMA

Carcinoma of the vulva is an uncommon malignancy that represents about 3% of all genital cancers in the female.[19] It is most common in those over the age of 60, but is increasing in frequency in younger age groups. Eighty-five per cent of these malignant tumors are squamous cell carcinomas, the remainder being basal cell carcinomas, melanomas, or adenocarcinomas.

In a considerable number of instances, the squamous cell carcinomas are preceded by vulvar dysplasia, also termed vulvar intraepithelial neoplasia (VIN). The latter is characterized by nuclear and epithelial atypia, increased mitoses, and lack of surface differentiation. The spectrum of dysplastic changes[13] ranges from mild dysplasia (VIN I), to moderate dysplasia (VIN II), to severe dysplasia and *carcinoma in situ* (VIN III). Carcinoma in situ, called Bowen's disease by dermatologists, is an intraepithelial squamous cell carcinoma that presents as either white (leukoplakia) or dark lesions. Identical lesions are encountered in the male (p. 1101).

Dysplasia is appearing with increasing frequency in women under the age of 40. The lesions are sometimes multicentric and may coexist with microinvasive or more deeply penetrating carcinomas. About 30% are also associated with in situ or invasive *cervical* or *vaginal carcinoma*, suggesting a common carcinogen. Indeed, human papilloma virus (types 16, 18 and others) is present in some 90% of cases of VIN.[20] However, actual progression of an in situ cancer to invasive carcinoma occurs in only about 5% of patients, and then principally in those who are elderly or immunosuppressed. Spontaneous regression of vulvar carcinoma in situ has also been observed, typically when these lesions occur in women in their late teens or twenties, or in pregnant women.[21]

Any regions of the vulva may be affected by cancer and, in fact, a small percentage arise from the perineal skin about the rectum. These tumors begin as small areas of epithelial thickening that resemble leukoplakia but, in the course of time, progress to create firm, indurated, **exophytic** tumors or ulcerated and endophytic lesions. Histologically, these tumors are almost invariably rather well-differentiated squamous cell carcinomas, with the formation of keratohyaline pearls and prickle cells (Fig. 24–10).

The tumors infiltrate locally for a period of weeks to months and tend to metastasize at a relatively early stage to the regional nodes. In about 65% of cases, vulvar carcinoma has metastasized to the regional nodes at the time of discovery. The nodes affected are the inguinal nodes and the nodes within the pelvis, about the rectum, and about the iliac vessels and bifurcation of the aorta. Such nodal metastasis is correlated more with the size and duration of the lesion than with the degree of differentiation of the squamous cell growth. Ultimately, lymphohematogenous dissemination involves the lungs, liver, and other internal organs.

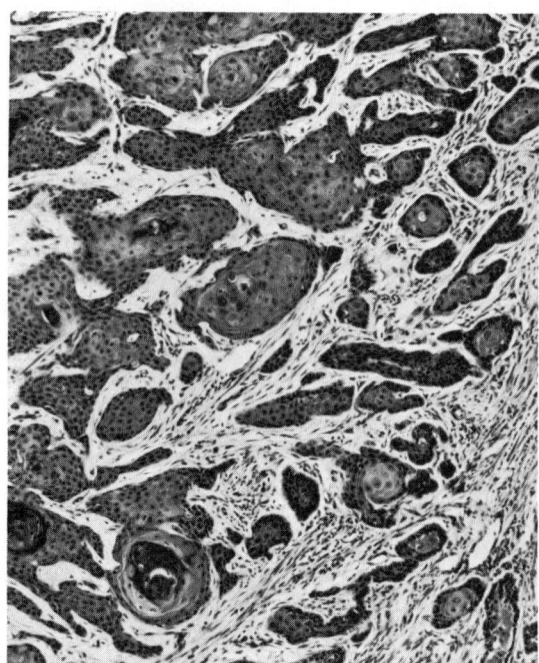

Figure 24–10. Carcinoma of vulva at medium power, illustrating typical invasive cords of squamous cell carcinoma.

Although vulvar carcinomas are external tumors that are obviously apparent to the patient and the clinician, many are misinterpreted as dermatitis, eczema, or leukoplakia for long periods.

The clinical manifestations evoked are chiefly those of pain, local discomfort, itching, and exudation, because superficial secondary infection is common. Lesions less than 2 cm in diameter have a 60 to 80% five-year survival rate after treatment with one-stage vulvectomy and lymphadenectomy; larger lesions with lymph node involvement yield a less than 10% five-year survival rate.

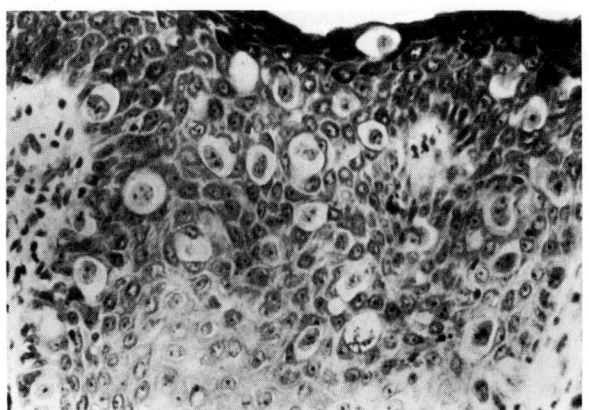

Figure 24–11. Paget's disease of vulva, with clusters of large clear tumor cells within squamous epithelium.

Verrucous carcinoma is a special type of highly differentiated squamous cell carcinoma that presents as a large fungating tumor. It may resemble condyloma acuminatum histologically. Local invasion confirms the malignant nature of the lesion, but it rarely metastasizes and can be cured by wide excision. It is particularly resistant to irradiation.

Basal cell carcinomas and adenocarcinomas, the latter arising in Bartholin's glands or sweat glands, also occur in the vulva but are uncommon.

EXTRAMAMMARY PAGET'S DISEASE

This curious and rare lesion of the vulva, and sometimes the perianal region, is similar in its skin manifestations to Paget's disease of the breast[22] (p. 1198). As a vulvar neoplasm it manifests as a red, crusted, sharply demarcated, maplike area, occurring usually on the labia majora. It may be accompanied by a palpable submucosal thickening or tumor. *The diagnostic microscopic feature of this lesion is the presence of large, anaplastic tumor cells lying singly or in small clusters within the epidermis and its appendages.* These cells are rendered distinctive by a clear halo that sets them off from the surrounding epithelial cells (Fig. 24–

11). The halo is due to a high content of cytoplasmic mucopolysaccharide, which can be visualized by such special stains as PAS, alcian blue, and mucicarmine. On electron microscopy, Paget's cells exhibit apocrine or eccrine differentiation, but some also have features of keratinocytes.[23]

In contrast to Paget's disease of the nipple, in which 100% of cases show an underlying ductal breast carcinoma, vulvar lesions are most frequently confined to the epidermis of the skin and adjacent hair follicles and sweat glands. An underlying or adjacent sweat gland adenocarcinoma is uncommon. It is thus assumed that the Paget's cells arise de novo from primitive intraepithelial precursors capable of differentiating along multiple lines. In some cases, however, for obscure reasons Paget's disease of the vulva is associated with carcinoma of the breast, bladder, or vulva. The prognosis of Paget's disease is poor in the cases with associated carcinoma, but intraepidermal Paget's disease may persist for many years, even decades, without the development of invasion. Paget's cells can be present beyond the confines of the gross lesions; thus there are recurrences if surgical excision is not adequate. Occasional untreated cases eventually become invasive.

MALIGNANT MELANOMA

Melanomas of the vulva are uncommon, representing 5 to 10% of all vulvar cancers and 2% of all melanomas in women. Their peak incidence is in the sixth or seventh decade; they tend to have the same biologic and histologic characteristics as melanomas occurring elsewhere and are capable of widespread metastatic dissemination. The overall survival rate is around 32%. Early in its evolution the melanoma is sometimes confined to the epithelium, where it may resemble Paget's disease both grossly and histologically. It can be differentiated by its uniform reactivity, using immunoperoxidase techniques, with antibodies to S100 protein, and by its lack of content of carcinoembryonic antigen (CEA) and mucopolysaccharides.

VAGINA

The vagina is a portion of the female genital tract that is remarkably free from primary disease. In the adult, inflammations often affect the vulva and perivulvar structures and spread through the vagina to the cervix without significant involvement of the vagina. The major serious primary lesion of this structure is the very uncommon primary carcinoma. The remaining entities can therefore be cited quite briefly.

CONGENITAL ANOMALIES

Atresia and total absence of the vagina are both extremely uncommon. The latter usually occurs only when there are severe malformations of the entire genital tract. Septate, or double, vagina is also a very uncommon anomaly that arises from failure of total fusion of the müllerian ducts.

Gartner's duct cysts are relatively common lesions, found along the lateral walls of the vagina and derived from wolffian duct rests. They are 1- to 2-cm, fluid-filled cysts that occur submucosally. Rarely, they may enlarge up to 5 to 6 cm. The lining epithelium is at times cuboidal and at times columnar, or may even be transitional in form. Mixtures of these epithelial types are common. The cysts should be differentiated from the more ominous tumor masses.

TUMORS

The malignant tumors of the vagina of clinical significance in terms of frequency and biologic behavior are *carcinomas* and *sarcoma botryoides*. However, benign neoplasms and non-neoplastic lesions that simulate tumors also arise in the vagina. Epithelial papillomas, fibromas, leiomyomas, and hemangiomas are uncommon and resemble their counterparts in other sites. Foci of endometriosis may arise in the vagina and masquerade as a neoplasm (p. 1147). Gartner's duct cysts and other epithelial inclusion cysts may also present as intravaginal masses.

CARCINOMA

Primary carcinoma of the vagina is an extremely uncommon cancer accounting for about 1% of malignant neoplasms in the female genital tract. Its peak incidence is in the sixth and seventh decades of life, but rarely, it occurs in younger women.

Squamous Cell Carcinoma

Over 95% of vaginal carcinomas are *squamous cell carcinomas*, usually of the well-differentiated type.[24] The peak age incidence is between 60 and 70 years, and most patients are over 50.

> Most often the tumor affects the upper posterior vagina, particularly along the posterior wall at the junction with the exocervix. It begins as a focus of epithelial thickening, progressing to a plaquelike mass that extends centrifugally and invades, by direct continuity, the cervix and perivaginal structures such as the urethra, urinary bladder, and rectum. The lesions in the lower two-thirds metastasize to the inguinal nodes, whereas upper lesions tend to involve the regional iliac nodes and, in late advanced stages, distant organs via the blood.

These lesions first come to the patient's attention by the appearance of irregular spotting or the development of a frank vaginal discharge (leukorrhea). At other times, they remain totally silent and become clinically manifest only with the onset of urinary or rectal fistulas.

Adenocarcinoma

Adenocarcinomas are rare but have received considerable attention because of the increased frequency of *clear cell adenocarcinomas* in young women whose mothers had been treated with diethylstilbestrol (DES) during pregnancy (for a threatened abortion).[25] Fortunately, less than 0.14% of such DES-exposed young women develop adenocarcinoma. These tumors are usually discovered between the ages of 15 and 20 and are often composed of vacuolated, glycogen-containing cells; hence, the term "clear cell" (Fig. 24–12).

> The tumors are most often located on the anterior wall of the vagina, usually in the upper third, and vary in size from 0.2 to 10 cm in greatest diameter. These cancers can also arise in the cervix.
>
> A probable precursor of the tumor is *vaginal adenosis*, a condition in which glandular columnar epithelium of müllerian type either appears beneath the squamous epithelium or replaces it.[26] Adenosis presents clinically as red, granular foci contrasting with the normal pale pink, opaque vaginal mucosa. Microscopically the glandular epithelium may be either mucus-secreting, resembling endocervical mucosa, or so-called tuboendometrial, often containing cilia. Adenosis has been reported in 35 to 90% of the offspring of estrogen-treated mothers, but as mentioned earlier, malignant transformation is extremely rare.

Because of its insidious, invasive growth, vaginal cancer (squamous and adenocarcinoma) is difficult to cure. Thus early detection by careful follow-up is mandatory in DES-exposed women. Surgery and irradiation have successfully eradicated DES-related tumors in up to 80% of cases.

Extension of cervical carcinoma to the vagina is much more common than primary malignancies of the vagina. Accordingly, before a diagnosis of primary vaginal carcinoma can be made, a pre-existing cervical lesion must be ruled out.

EMBRYONAL RHABDOMYOSARCOMA

Also called sarcoma botryoides, this is an interesting but very uncommon vaginal tumor most frequently found in infants and in children under the age of 5. The tumor consists predominantly of malignant em-

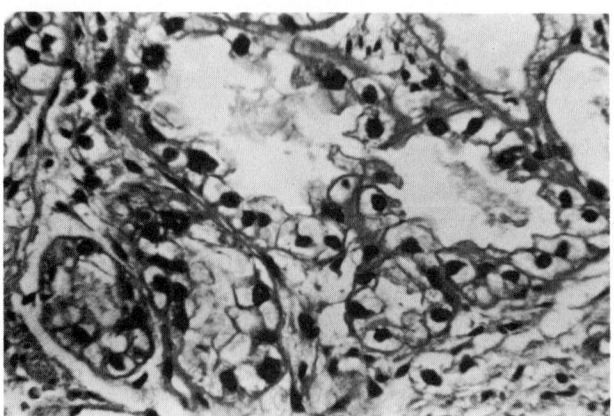

Figure 24–12. Clear cell adenocarcinoma of vagina, DES related, showing vacuolated tumor cells forming glands.

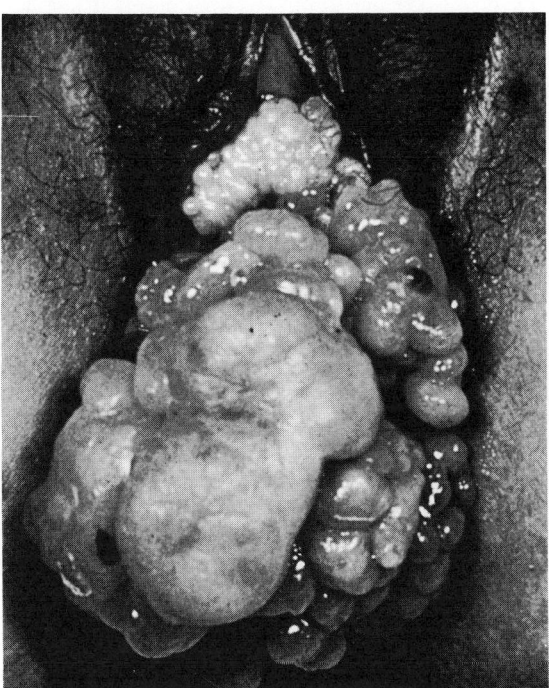

Figure 24-13. Sarcoma botryoides (embryonal rhabdomyosarcoma) of vagina appearing as a polypoid mass protruding from vagina. (Courtesy of Dr. Arthur Hertig.)

bryonal rhabdomyoblasts and is thus a type of rhabdomyosarcoma.[27]

Grossly, these tumors tend to grow as polypoid, rounded, bulky masses that sometimes fill and project out of the vagina; they have the appearance and consistency of grapelike clusters (hence the designation "botryoides," grapelike) (Fig. 24-13). Histologically, the tumor cells are small and have oval nuclei, with small protrusions of cytoplasm from one end, so that they resemble a tennis racket. Rarely, striations can be seen within the cytoplasm. Beneath the vaginal epithelium the tumor cells are crowded in a so-called cambium layer, but in the deep regions they lie within a loose fibromyxomatous stroma that is edematous and may contain many inflammatory cells. For this reason, the lesions can be mistaken for benign inflammatory polyps, leading to unfortunate delays in diagnosis and treatment.

These tumors tend to invade locally and cause death by penetration into the peritoneal cavity or by obstruction of the urinary tract. Radical surgery, unpleasant as it is for the young female, coupled with chemotherapy appears to offer the best results in cases diagnosed sufficiently early.

CERVIX

Lesions of the cervix are extremely common if one includes the great abundance of minor inflammatory changes designated as nonspecific cervicitis. In fact, excessive inflammatory vaginal discharge, referred to clinically as leukorrhea, constitutes one of the most common clinical complaints in gynecologic practice. However, the cervix is also extremely vulnerable to the development of cancer. As will be re-emphasized presently, cervical carcinoma alone is responsible for about 5% of all cancer deaths in women.

INFLAMMATIONS

Inflammations of the cervix are extremely frequent. They are caused by a variety of bacteria, many of which compose the normal flora of the vagina. This form of banal inflammation is referred to as nonspecific cervicitis. However, it should not be inferred that all nonspecific cervicitis is without serious significance, because as will be pointed out, it may predispose to serious complications in a small percentage of cases. In addition to this commonplace type of cervicitis, there are many types of specific cervical inflammations, i.e., gonorrhea, syphilis, chancroid, and tuberculosis, described in Chapter 7.

ACUTE AND CHRONIC CERVICITIS

Depending on the histologic criteria selected for the establishment of this diagnosis, some degree of cervical inflammation may be found in virtually all multiparous and in many nulliparous adult women. It is extremely doubtful whether the minor involvements are of any clinical consequence.

ETIOLOGY AND PATHOGENESIS. Specific infections by gonococci, *Trichomonas vaginalis, Candida albicans,* mycoplasma, Gardnerella, and herpes (mostly type II) are responsible for many cases of either acute or chronic cervicitis. *However, the most commonly identified organisms are endogenous vaginal aerobes and anaerobes*—streptococci, enterococci, *Escherichia coli,* and staphylococci. The vagina and the cervix normally contain a mixed flora that includes such organisms. Predisposing causes to infection must then be sought. Trauma of childbirth, instrumentation in the course of gynecologic treatment, hyperestrinism, hypoestrinism, intercourse, excessive secretion of the cervical glands, and high alkalinity of the cervical mucus have all been cited as predisposing influences.

MORPHOLOGY.   Cervicitis may be divided into an acute and a chronic phase.

Excluding gonococcal infections, **acute cervicitis** is most commonly encountered postpartally and is usually caused by either staphylococci or streptococci. Microscopically, there is stromal edema, infiltration by polymorphonuclear leukocytes, and, frequently, focal loss of the lining mucosa.

Chronic cervicitis is far more common than acute cervicitis. Grossly, chronic cervicitis appears as a reddening, swelling, and granularity around the margins of the external cervical os. Histologically, the infiltration is largely mononuclear (Fig. 24–14). Inflammatory stenosis of the cervical glands may yield cystic dilatations designated as **nabothian cysts.** The chronic inflammatory cells may accumulate into lymphoid follicles, **follicular cervicitis** (Fig. 24–15).

In addition to the inflammation, the cervical and endocervical mucosa exhibit other changes. The epithelium may show hyperplasia and **reactive atypia,** characterized by epithelial disorganization and nuclear alterations not to be confused with the changes of dysplasia (p. 1142). In the course of these changes, the epithelial cells are depleted of their normal content of glycogen. The loss of glycogen accounts for the failure of these areas to stain brown with Schiller's solution (an iodine preparation), as detailed on page 1144.

In certain cases, in the region of the external os, tongues of stratified squamous epithelium may extend down from the surface mucosa into the endocervical glands (Fig. 24–16). These changes are designated **squamous metaplasia of endocervical glands.** This form of epithelial alteration merits careful attention because it can be mistaken, on casual inspection, for the infiltrative growth of squamous cell carcinoma.

CLINICAL COURSE.   Infectious cervicitis is central to the propagation of sexually transmitted diseases by

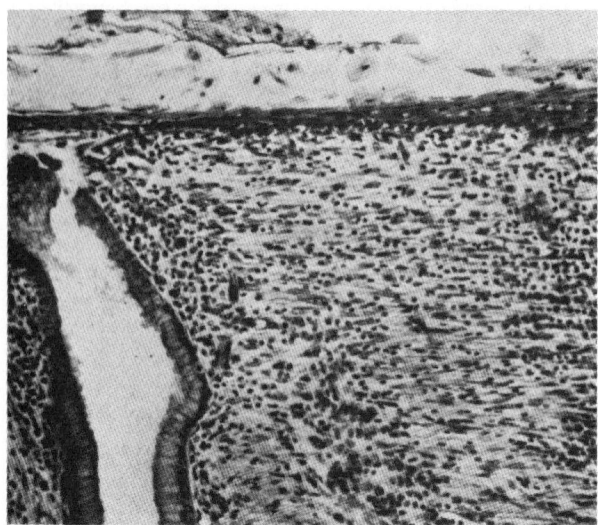

Figure 24–15. Chronic cervicitis. An inflammatory infiltrate is present in submucosal tissue.

ascension to the upper genital tract or by transmission through the placenta to the fetus and neonate (Fig. 24–17).[28] Nonspecific cervicitis, on the other hand, may be an asymptomatic lesion that is discovered in the course of routine gynecologic examination, or because of leukorrhea or when the cervix is removed for other causes. Diagnosis may be made by simple visual examination of the cervix when the changes are well defined, but at times infectious cervicitis may be difficult to differentiate from the much more serious conditions of dysplasia or cancer. Colposcopy, which allows a magnified view of vaginal and cervical mucosa, has greatly facilitated follow-up or direct biopsy of suspicious lesions. Ultimately, the differentiation rests on histologic examination of biopsy specimens.

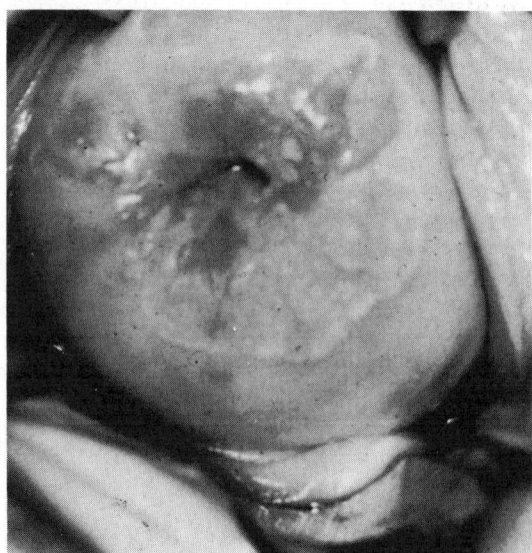

Figure 24–14. Chronic cervicitis as viewed through a speculum. The inflammatory area rims the external os. (Courtesy of Dr. Arthur Hertig.)

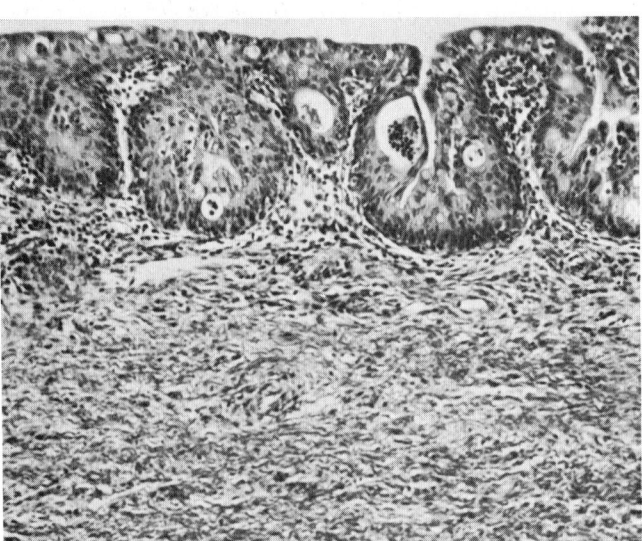

Figure 24–16. Chronic cervicitis with squamous metaplasia that has obliterated the endocervical glands. Note marked subepithelial inflammation. (Courtesy of Dr. Arthur Hertig.)

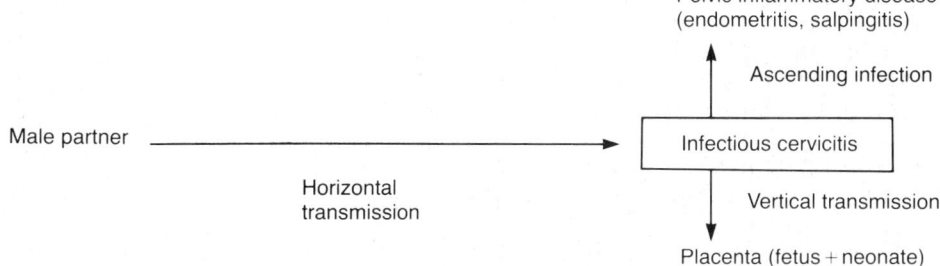

Figure 24–17. The central role of infectious cervicitis in the propagation of sexually transmitted disease. (Modified from Winkler, B., and Richart, R.M.: Cervical-uterine pathologic considerations in pelvic infection. *In* Zatuchni, G.I., et al. (eds.): Intrauterine Contraception. Advances and Future Prospects. New York, Harper & Row, 1985.)

TUMORS

BENIGN

Although the cervix may develop a wide variety of neoplasms, 95% of cervical tumors are represented by benign polyps and carcinoma.

Endocervical Polyps

Endocervical polyps are relatively innocuous, inflammatory, non-neoplastic tumors that occur in 2 to 5% of adult women. Perhaps the major significance of polyps lies in their production of irregular vaginal "spotting" or bleeding that arouses suspicion of some more ominous lesion.

Most polyps arise within the endocervical canal and vary from small and sessile to large, 5-cm masses that may protrude through the cervical os (Fig. 24–18). All are soft, almost mucoid, and are composed of a loose fibromyxomatous stroma harboring dilated, mucus-secreting endocervical glands, and often accompanied by inflammation. In almost all instances, simple curettage or surgical excision effects a cure.

Microglandular Endocervical Hyperplasia

This benign cervical lesion occurs in women receiving progestogen-containing oral contraceptive agents. Clinically the lesion resembles a cervical polyp, and histologically it is composed of a mass of tightly packed proliferating glands or tubules, with occasional focal squamous metaplasia. At times the epithelium may show atypical changes. Occasionally the lesions occur in the absence of contraceptive drug ingestion. The importance of the lesions lies in their possible confusion with endocervical adenocarcinoma.[29]

MALIGNANT

Dysplasia and Carcinoma

No form of cancer better documents the remarkable effects of early cancer diagnosis and curative therapy on the mortality rate than cancer of the cervix. Fifty years ago, carcinoma of the cervix was the leading cause of cancer deaths in women in the United States, but the death rate has dropped remarkably to its present rank as the eighth cause of cancer mortality, causing about 7000 deaths (behind lung, breast, colon, pancreas, ovary, lymph nodes, and blood). In sharp contrast to reduced mortality, the frequency is increasing. There are about two to three times as many newly diagnosed cases of invasive carcinoma of the cervix yearly, and seven to eight times as many new patients are discovered to have carcinoma in situ. In 1989 there are an estimated 13,000 cases of new invasive cancer and 50,000 of carcinoma in situ.[30] It is thus evident that *well over half of invasive cancers are cured by effective therapy, and even more important, most lesions are discovered while still in situ and amenable to eradication by timely and appropriate treatment.*

Credit for these dramatic gains is owed largely to the effectiveness of the Papanicolaou cytologic test in detecting cervical carcinoma during its incipiency and to the accessibility of the cervix to colposcopy and biopsy. The widespread application of the "Pap smear," followed by colposcopy and biopsy, has documented that carcinoma of the cervix arises in a series of stepwise epithelial changes ranging from progressively more severe dysplasia to invasive carcinoma. More is known about the life history of this form of cancer than of any other. Indeed, the entire concept

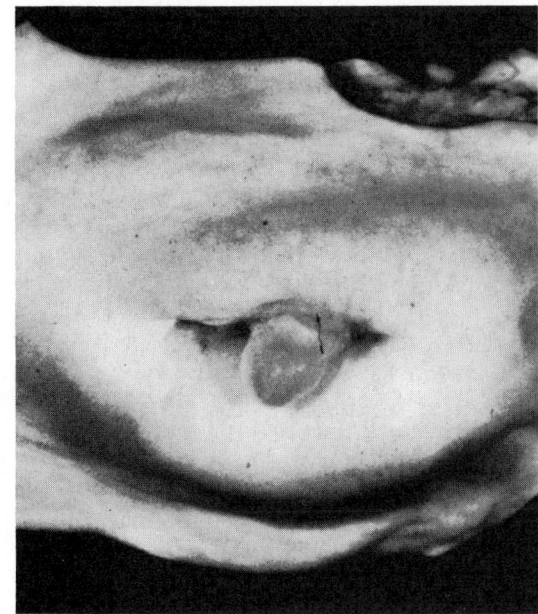

Figure 24–18. Endocervical polyp, protruding through external os.

of "in situ" cancer originated from studies of this neoplasm.

Carcinoma of the cervix may occur at any age from the second decade of life to senility. The peak incidence is occurring at an increasingly younger age: 40 to 45 years for invasive cancer and about 30 years for in situ lesions. Deaths begin in the fourth decade, and the mortality rate rises with age. Only a few decades ago, all of these unfortunate events were delayed at least ten years, strongly suggesting that oncogenic influences, possibly viruses (as will be noted later), are now at work earlier in life.

PATHOGENESIS. Many risk factors for cervical carcinoma have been identified. Among them, the following are most important:

1. Early age at first intercourse
2. Multiple sexual partners
3. "High-risk" male sexual partners — i.e., those who are promiscuous, who have a former wife with cervical cancer, or who have a history of penile condylomas.

All other risk factors can be related to these three influences, including the higher incidence of cervical carcinoma in lower socioeconomic groups, the higher incidence in married women (increasing with the number of marriages and children), the rarity of cervical carcinoma in virgins and nuns, and the high incidence in prostitutes. No longer considered significant risk factors are birth control pills, vague agents in semen, and lack of circumcision in the male sexual partner (implicating some putative carcinogen in smegma).

The epidemiology of cervical cancer strongly suggests sexual transmission of an oncogenic agent, most probably a virus, from male to female, at an early age. Although herpes simplex virus type II (HSV II) was once suspected, the finger currently points to *human papillomavirus as an important factor in cervical oncogenesis.*

Human Papillomavirus (HPV). As noted earlier, this virus is the known cause of the venereally transmitted vulvar condyloma acuminatum (p. 1135); it is also suspected to be an oncogenic agent in a variety of other squamous tumors or proliferative lesions of skin and mucous membranes, as detailed in the neoplasia chapter (p. 275).[33] There is mounting evidence for HPV involvement in cervical cancer.[34]

The strongest evidence is that HPV DNA is detected by hybridization techniques in 75 to 100% of patients with cervical condylomas, precancerous cervical dysplasia, and invasive carcinoma.

The cervical condylomas can be verrucous, like those of the vulva, but are much more often flat lesions (flat condylomas). Although there is overlap in the HPV types present in various lesions, HPVs 6 and 11 (low-risk HPVs) are found most frequently in condylomas, whereas HPVs 16, 18, and 31 (high-risk HPVs) are more often present in carcinoma.[35] Mixed low- and high-risk types are found in dysplasias. The condylomas are associated with the typical squamous vacuolization called koilocytosis, but this change is very uncommon in carcinoma and high-grade dysplasia.

The precise reasons for these associations between HPV types and lesions are unclear. One scenario is that low-risk HPVs (types 6 and 11) lead to productive infection associated with unintegrated episomal viral DNA. Full viral expression in infected cells is thus characterized by cell proliferation, cell maturation, koilocytosis, and other features distinctive of condylomas. High-risk HPVs (16 and 18), on the other hand, are associated with a greater proportion of viral DNA becoming integrated into the host genome. One current model for tumor progression with HPV is that the virus induces transformation by integration into the cellular sequence, possibly near a proto-oncogene.[33] Indeed, it has recently been shown that HPV types 16 and 18, *but not 6 and 11,* cooperate with the *ras* oncogene in causing transformed tumorigenic foci in cultured cells.[36] The putative transforming sequence of the HPV virus, the E6 to E7 open reading frame, is consistently transcribed in the squamous cancer cells, arguing for a similar role for HPV in vivo.

It has also been recently shown that male partners of women with lower genital tract cancer exhibit small penile or posterior urethral lesions harboring HPV.[37]

The evidence is, of course, incomplete, and all the associations cited might be independent consequences of promiscuity or may indeed follow the earliest precancerous lesion. But on balance, the current consensus is that the high-risk HPV types — 16, 18, and others — by integrating into host DNA, act as cancer *promoters,* which in concert with co-carcinogens (initiators) lead to cervical carcinoma. Co-carcinogens could be other viruses, such as herpes simplex type II (which are known to occur with high frequency in patients with cervical cancer), bacteria, and other environmental agents.[32,33] These co-carcinogens would explain the variable outcome of precursor lesions with the same histology and infections with similar types of viruses. Figure 24–19 presents one attempt to explain the role of HPV in cervical carcinogenesis.

DYSPLASIA AND CARCINOMA IN SITU (CERVICAL INTRAEPITHELIAL NEOPLASIA). One of the most significant advances in the therapy of neoplasia has been the realization that cervical carcinoma arises from *precursor lesions.*[38,39] *Most cervical cancer is the end stage of a continuum of progressively more atypical changes in which one stage merges imperceptibly with the next.* The first and apparently earliest change is the appearance of atypical cells in the basal layers of the squamous epithelium, but nonetheless with persistence of the normal differentiation toward the prickle and keratinizing cell layers. *The atypical cells show changes in nucleocytoplasmic ratio, loss of polar-*

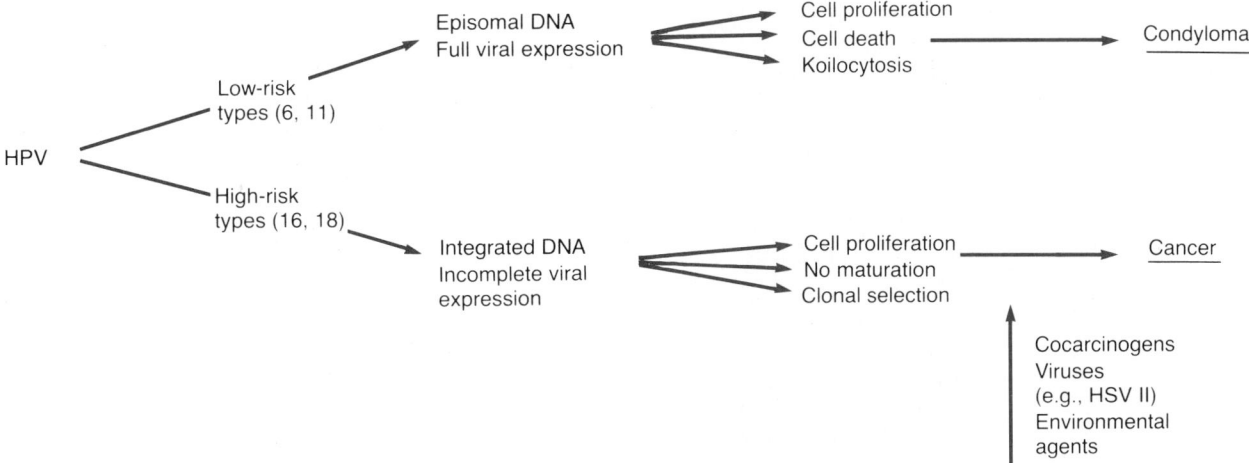

Figure 24–19. Hypothetical scheme for the role of human papillomavirus in cervical neoplasia. Cocarcinogens may act as different steps of this scheme.

ity, increased mitotic figures, and pleomorphism — in other words, all the hallmarks of malignant cells. As the lesion evolves, there is progressive involvement of more and more layers of the epithelium, until it is totally replaced by atypical cells, exhibiting no surface differentiation.

Precancerous lesions are classified by one or the other of two schemes, as shown in Figure 24–20.

1. The most widely used term is *dysplasia*, which literally means "bad molding" or, in more scientific terms, disordered development. Dysplasia is subdivided into mild, moderate, and severe, depending on the proportion of the thickness of squamous epithelium involved by atypical cells. Full-thickness involvement is *carcinoma in situ* (Figs. 24–20 and 24–21).

2. The second approach emphasizes that the dysplastic changes represent a spectrum of the same basic change, i.e., cervical intraepithelial neoplasia (CIN). Grade 1 CIN represents less than one-third involvement of the thickness of epithelium; grade 2, one-third to two-thirds; and grade 3 two-thirds to full thickness, thus *carcinoma in situ.*

Whatever terms are used, CIN almost always begins at the squamocolumnar junction, in the transformation zone; grade 1 may progress to the next higher grade during a ten-year follow-up period, grade 2 may progress to grade 3, and so on.[40] In one study, 50% of women with CIN 1 progressed to grade 3 (carcinoma in situ) and 28% either progressed to grade 2 or remained at grade 1 for nine years.[40] The more severe the grade of dysplasia, the shorter is the

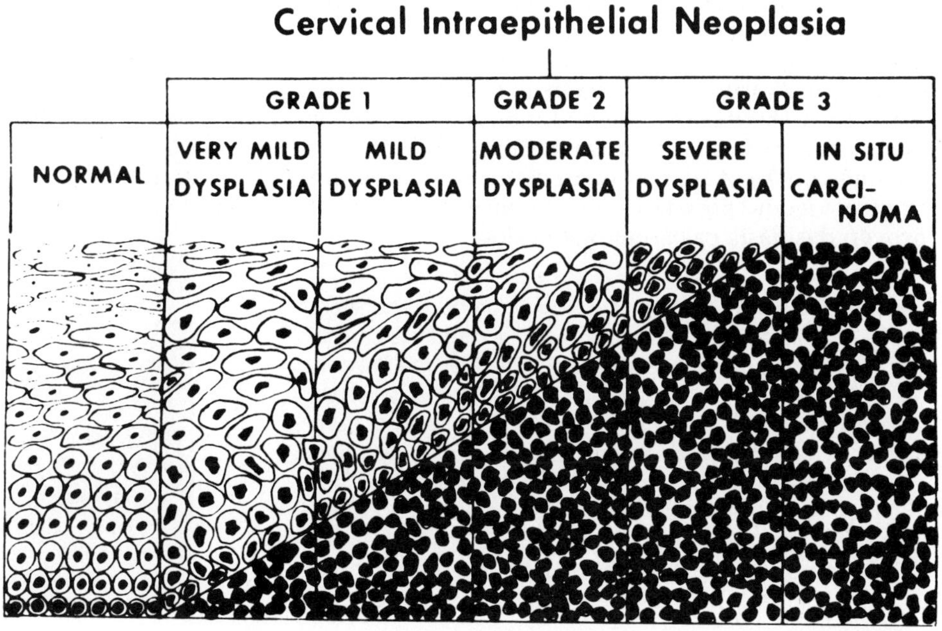

Cervical Intraepithelial Neoplasia

	GRADE 1		GRADE 2	GRADE 3	
NORMAL	VERY MILD DYSPLASIA	MILD DYSPLASIA	MODERATE DYSPLASIA	SEVERE DYSPLASIA	IN SITU CARCINOMA

Figure 24–20. Schematic representation of cervical cancer precursors. CIN grades 1, 2, and 3 correspond to traditional mild dysplasia, moderate dysplasia, and severe dysplasia-to-CIS, respectively. They are characterized by progressive increase in number of undifferentiated, malignant cells and decrease in superficial cell differentiation paralleling increasing severity of CIN. (Modified from A. Ferenczy and B. Winkler.[38] Cervical intraepithelial neoplasia and neoplasia. *In* Kurman, R. [ed.]: Blaustein's Pathology of the Female Genital Tract. 3rd ed. New York, Springer-Verlag, 1987. Reproduced with permission.)

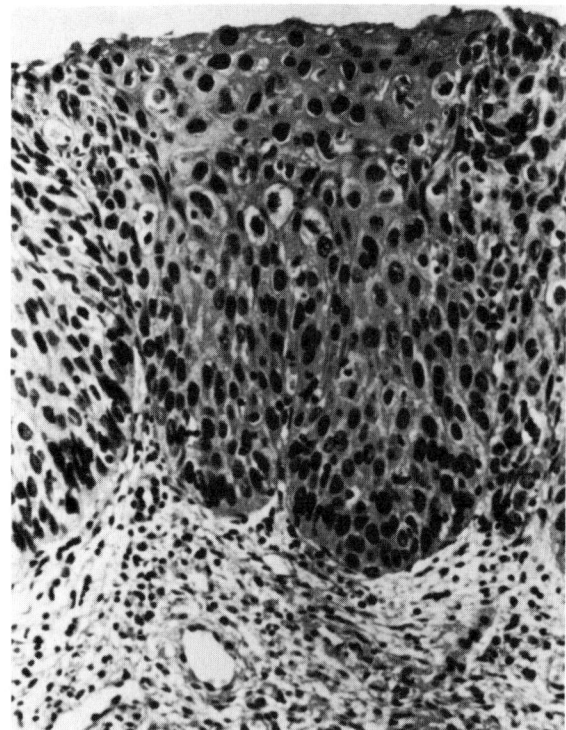

Figure 24–21. Focus of carcinoma in situ of cervix (CIN grade 3), showing markedly atypical cells occupying full thickness of epithelium. (Courtesy of Dr. D. Antonioli.)

time span for the development of carcinoma in situ. *The rates of progression, however, are by no means uniform, and in general, it is difficult, if not impossible, for a clinician using any technique to predict the outcome in an individual patient.* Careful follow-up is the only recourse. Regression does occur, but only in very mild lesions and flat condylomas.

Carcinoma in situ (CIN 3) is clearly a precursor of invasive carcinoma. This conclusion is based on three pieces of evidence: (1) the finding of foci of carcinoma in situ and invasive carcinoma simultaneously in the same cervix, usually in adjacent areas; (2) the development of invasive carcinoma in up to 71% of women followed without treatment for a minimum of 12 years after a diagnosis of carcinoma in situ; and (3) the fact that most (but not all) new cases of invasive carcinoma originate from a population of women with previously proven dysplasia or carcinoma in situ.

MORPHOLOGY. In situ carcinoma produces no alteration recognizable to the naked eye. The diagnosis can be suspected only on the basis of the Schiller test, the Papanicolaou smear, or colposcopy. The Schiller test involves painting the cervix with a solution of iodine and potassium iodide. The normal cervical epithelium is rich in glycogen and stains a mahogany brown. The cancerous focus, because it is depleted of glycogen, fails to stain. It should be cautioned that this method may yield false-positive results because areas of inflammation may also fail to stain with the Schiller solution. The changes seen on colposcopy are detailed later (p. 1145).

Histologically, dysplastic cells and mitotic figures can be seen in the entire thickness of epithelium. The individual cell can be small, or large and keratinizing, or large and nonkeratinizing. Sometimes the anaplastic changes extend along the surface into the underlying endocervical glands, but such superficial spread should not be construed as invasion, because the basement membranes of these glands are not penetrated.

Invasive cervical carcinoma manifests in three somewhat distinctive patterns: **fungating (or exophytic), ulcerating, and infiltrative cancer.** The most common variant is the fungating tumor, which produces an obviously neoplastic mass that projects above the surrounding mucosa (Fig. 24–22).

Advanced cervical carcinoma extends by direct continuity to involve every contiguous structure, including the peritoneum, urinary bladder, ureters, rectum, and vagina. Local and distant lymph nodes are also involved. Distant metastasis occurs to the liver, lungs, bone marrow, and other structures.

Histologically, 65% of tumors are **large cell, nonkeratinizing,** and moderately well-differentiated; some 25% are **large cell, keratinizing,** producing keratohyalin, epithelial pearls, and prickle cells; and the rest are composed of **small undifferentiated squamous cells.**

Cervical cancer is staged as follows:

Stage 0. Carcinoma in situ (CIN 3).

Stage I. Carcinoma confined to the cervix.

Ia. Preclinical carcinoma, i.e., diagnosed only by microscopy, but showing:

Ia1 Minimal microscopic invasion of stroma (minimally invasive carcinoma).

1a2 Microscopic invasion of stroma of less than 5 mm in depth (microinvasive carcinoma).

Ib. Histologically invasive carcinoma of the cervix that is greater than stage 1a2.

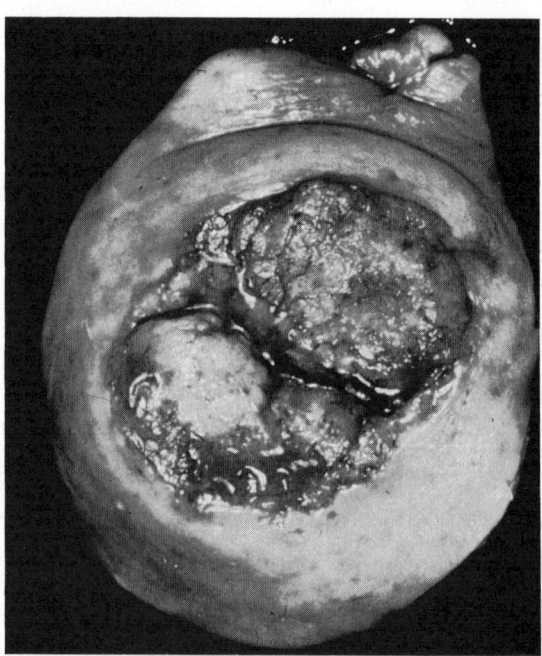

Figure 24–22. Carcinoma of cervix, well advanced.

Stage II. Carcinoma extends beyond the cervix but not onto the pelvic wall. Carcinoma involves the vagina, but not the lower third.

Stage III. Carcinoma has extended onto pelvic wall. On rectal examination, there is no cancer-free space between the tumor and the pelvic wall. The tumor involves the lower third of the vagina.

Stage IV. Carcinoma has extended beyond the true pelvis or has involved the mucosa of the bladder or rectum. This stage obviously includes those with metastatic dissemination.

Ten to 25% of cervical carcinomas comprise **adenocarcinomas, adenosquamous carcinomas, undifferentiated carcinomas,** or other rare histologic types. The **adenocarcinomas** presumably arise in the endocervical glands. They look grossly and behave like the squamous cell lesions, but arise in a slightly older age group. The **adenosquamous carcinomas** have mixed glandular and squamous patterns and are thought to arise from the reserve cells in the basal layers of the endocervical epithelium. They tend to have a less favorable prognosis than squamous cell carcinoma of similar stage. **Clear cell adenocarcinomas** of the cervix in DES-exposed women are similar to those occurring in the vagina (p. 1138).

CLINICAL COURSE. It is apparent from the preceding discussion that cancer of the cervix evolves slowly over the course of many years. The peak incidence of invasive carcinoma is in the fifth decade; that of in situ lesions is in the 30s, and dysplasias can arise in young women in their teens. During the long evolution, the cytologic abnormalities produce no clinical manifestations. Such nonspecific symptoms as increased vaginal discharge may be present. For these reasons, it is generally acknowledged that periodic Papanicolaou smears should be performed on all women after they become sexually active. Cytologic examination merely detects the possible presence of a cervical cancer; it does not make an absolute diagnosis, which requires histologic evaluation of appropriate biopsy specimens.

By *colposcopy,* the alterations that accompany dysplasia[41] include areas of white epithelium and abnormal patterns referred to as "mosaic or punctuation" patterns (Fig. 24–23). These are by no means diagnostic of cervical neoplasia, but their presence has been correlated with disease in many cases. Highly abnormal vascular patterns regularly accompany invasive cervical cancer. Ultimately, when these

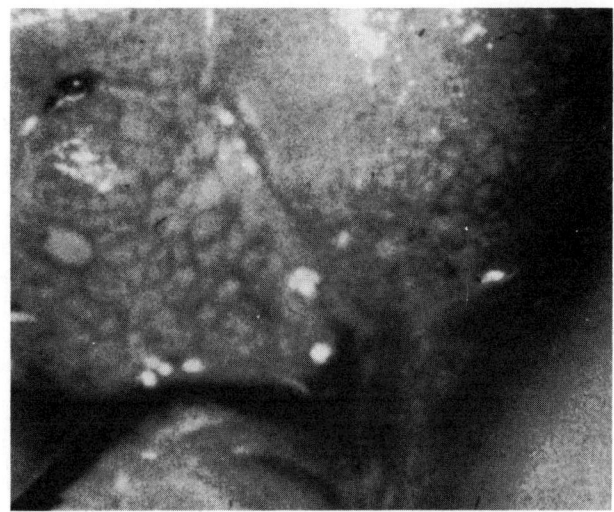

Figure 24–23. Colposcopic view of cervical mucosa showing characteristic mosaic pattern of cervical dysplasia. (Courtesy of Dr. D. Antonioli, Beth Israel Hospital, Boston.)

cancers become clinically overt, they usually produce irregular vaginal bleeding, leukorrhea, pain on coitus, and dysuria.

The treatment of carcinoma of the cervix depends on the stage of the neoplasm, and for invasive carcinomas includes surgical excision, radiation alone, or combined surgery and radiation. The prognosis and survival as well depend largely on the stage at which cancer is first discovered.[42] With stage 0, 100% cure should be effected. With current methods of treatment, there is a five-year survival rate of about 80 to 90% with stage I, 75% with stage II, 35% with stage III, and 10 to 15% with stage IV disease. Most patients with stage IV cancer die as a consequence of local extension of the tumor—e.g., into and about the urinary bladder and ureters, leading to ureteral obstruction, pyelonephritis, and uremia—rather than of metastatic disease.

As for the treatment of dysplasia and carcinoma in situ, there is no need for hasty radical surgery for these lesions. Many preinvasive lesions can be localized by colposcopy and eradicated by laser ablation, cryotherapy, electrocoagulation, or at the most, conization (removal of a cone of cervical mucosa and submucosa) for CIN 3. As long as the patient can be followed by means of periodic Papanicolaou smears of colposcopy, much can be gained from a conservative and individualized approach.[43]

BODY OF UTERUS AND ENDOMETRIUM

The uterus, stimulated continually by hormones, denuded monthly of its endometrial mucosa, and inhabited periodically by fetuses, is subject to a variety of disorders, the most common of which result from endocrine imbalances, complications of pregnancy, and neoplastic proliferation. Together with the lesions that affect the cervix, the lesions of the corpus of the uterus and the endometrium account for the great preponderance of gynecologic practice.

CONGENITAL ANOMALIES

Hypoplasia of the uterus is encountered in a variety of endocrine disorders. Such small uteri are referred to clinically as infantile. Most are due to ovarian or pituitary hypofunction. Strictly speaking, such failure of growth is not a congenital anomaly but an acquired defect.

Various anomalies may derive from the imperfect fusion of the primitive müllerian ducts. These consist of many patterns that vary from simple notching of the fundus to a partial septum that divides the fundus but not the cervix, to total division of the uterus by a septum into two endometrial cavities, a *septate uterus*. The most extreme anomaly is a completely *double uterus with double cervix*, each organ receiving only one tube. Such anomalies are perfectly compatible with normal fertility and normal menstrual cycles, but sometimes result in interesting and confusing clinical problems. Pregnancy in one half of a septate uterus may be accompanied by bleeding from the unaffected half or by a second conception. Pregnancy may occur in one half of the uterus after the other half has already developed a pregnancy, so-called superfetation.

INFLAMMATIONS

The endometrium and myometrium are relatively resistant to infections. Acute endometritis and myometritis are thus uncommon clinical problems. Acute reactions are virtually limited to bacterial infections that arise following delivery or miscarriage. Retained products of conception are the usual predisposing influence. The most common causative agents are the group A hemolytic streptococci, although the staphylococci and other bacteria are sometimes involved. The inflammatory response is chiefly limited to the interstitium and is entirely nonspecific. Removal of the retained gestational fragments by curettage is promptly followed by remission of the infection.

CHRONIC ENDOMETRITIS. Chronic inflammation of the endometrium occurs in the following settings:[44] (1) in patients suffering from chronic PID (p. 1132); (2) in tuberculosis, either from miliary spread or more commonly from drainage of tuberculous salpingitis (Fig. 24–24); (3) in postpartal or postabortal endometrial cavities, usually due to retained gestational tissue; and (4) in patients with intrauterine contraceptive devices (IUDs). The chronic endometritis in all these cases represents a secondary disease, and under these circumstances there is a plausible cause for the endometrial inflammation.

In about 15% of cases no such primary cause is obvious, yet plasma cells (which are not present in normal endometrium) are seen together with macrophages and lymphocytes. Some women with this so-called "nonspecific" chronic endometritis have such gynecologic complaints as abnormal bleeding, pain, discharge, and infertility. Chlamydia may be involved in the pathogenesis but may be difficult to culture. Importantly, such patients respond to antibiotic therapy, often preventing unnecessary hysterectomy for relief of chronic pain.

ADENOMYOSIS

Adenomyosis refers to the presence of nests of endometrium in the myometrium of the uterine wall. It is believed to represent an abnormal growth activity of the endometrium, reflecting a downgrowth of the basal zone of the endometrium into the myometrium. It is found at postmortem examination in 15 to 20% of uteri, depending on the criteria used for the diagnosis and the zeal with which it is sought.

> Adenomyosis may cause uterine enlargement and irregular thickening of the uterine wall, but the uterus appears unremarkable in many cases. In some cases the included endometrium is functional, menstruates, and therefore produces nests or cysts of red-brown blood pigmentation within the myometrium (Fig. 24–25).

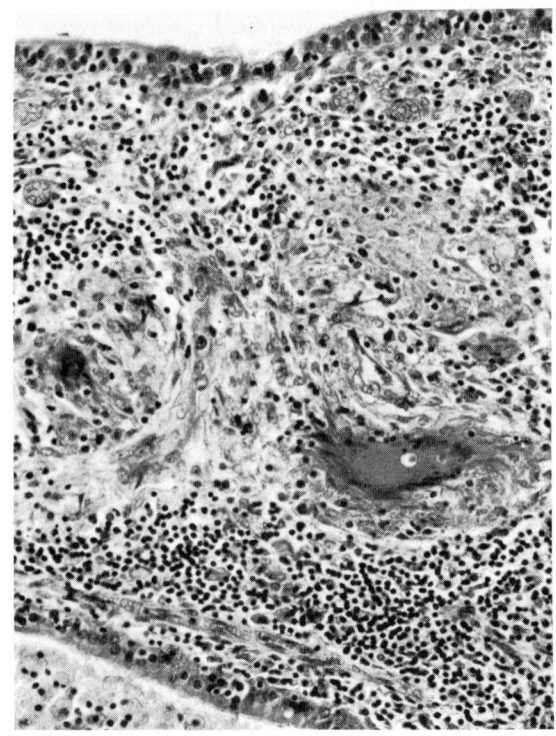

Figure 24–24. Tuberculous endometritis. Note granuloma with giant cells.

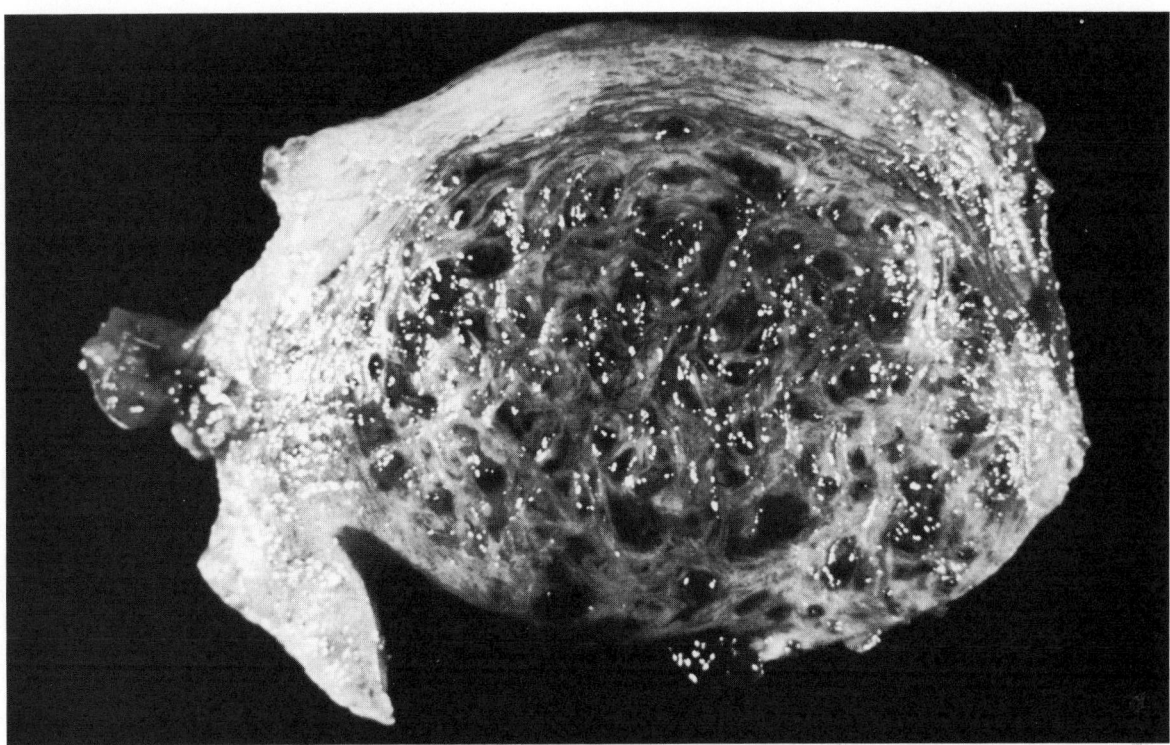

Figure 24–25. Adenomyosis. An unusual variant with functional endometrial nests producing foci of hemorrhagic cysts within uterine wall. (Courtesy of Dr. Arthur Hertig.)

The histologic diagnosis rests on the identification of buried endometrial stroma and glands between the muscle bundles of the myometrium. In most instances, the nests are composed of typical glands enclosed within a spindle cell stroma (Fig. 24-25). Occasionally, the nests are composed only of stroma, designated as **benign stromal nodules** (p. 1155). For a justifiable diagnosis of adenomyosis, the endometrial nests should be one low-power field or more (2 to 3 mm) below the endomyometrial junction.

Patients with adenomyosis frequently have menorrhagia, colicky dysmenorrhea, dyspareunia, and pelvic pain, particularly during the premenstrual period.

ENDOMETRIOSIS

Endometriosis is the term used to describe the presence of endometrial glands or stroma in abnormal locations *outside the uterus*. It occurs in the following sites, in descending order of frequency: (1) ovaries, (2) uterine ligaments, (3) rectovaginal septum, (4) pelvic peritoneum, (5) laparotomy scars, and (6) rarely in the umbilicus, vagina, vulva, or appendix. Endometriosis is an important clinical condition; it often causes infertility, dysmenorrhea, pelvic pain, and other problems. The disorder is principally a disease of women in active reproductive life, most often in the third and fourth decades.

Three possibilities (not mutually exclusive) have been invoked to explain the origin of these dispersed lesions (Fig. 24–26).[45]

1. The *regurgitation theory* proposes menstrual backflow through the fallopian tubes and subsequent implantation. Indeed, retrograde menstruation through the fallopian tubes occurs regularly even in normal women. However, this theory cannot explain lesions in the lymph nodes or lungs, for example.
2. The *metaplastic theory* proposes endometrial differentiation of coelomic epithelium, which in the last analysis is the origin of the endometrium itself. This theory, too, cannot explain endometriotic lesions in the lungs or lymph nodes.
3. The *vascular or lymphatic dissemination theory* has been invoked to explain extrapelvic or intranodal implants.

Genetic, hormonal, and immune factors have also been postulated to increase susceptibility of some women to endometriosis.

MORPHOLOGY. The foci of endometrium are almost invariably under the influence of the ovarian hormones and, therefore, undergo the cyclic menstrual changes with periodic bleeding. As a result, these foci appear as red-blue to yellow-brown nodules implanted on the serosal surfaces or

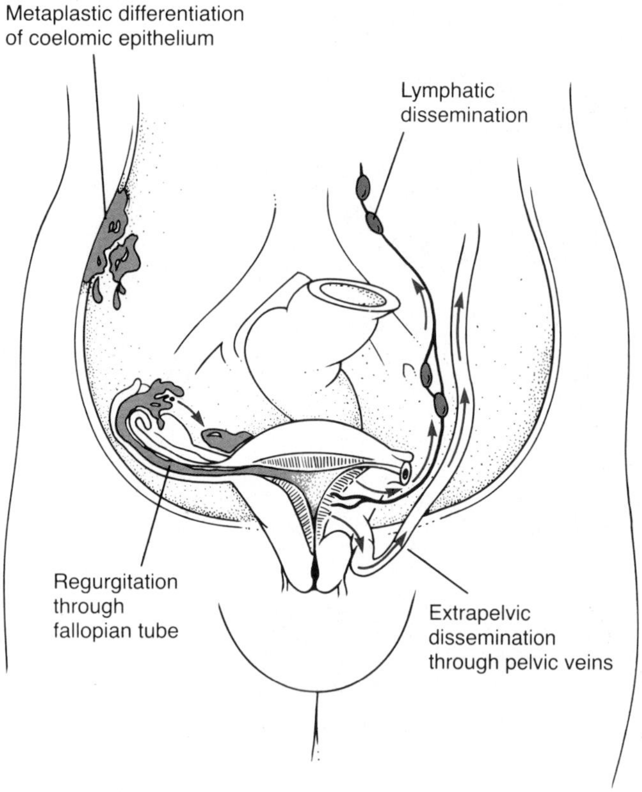

Metaplastic differentiation
of coelomic epithelium

Lymphatic
dissemination

Regurgitation
through
fallopian tube

Extrapelvic
dissemination
through pelvic veins

Figure 24–26. Depiction of the potential origins of endometrial implants.

apparently lying beneath the surface in the sites mentioned. When the accumulation of blood is extensive, its organization causes interadherence of structures, obliteration of the pouch of Douglas, and distortion and total fibrosis in and about the tubes and ovaries. The ovaries may become markedly distorted by large cystic spaces (3 to 5 cm in

Table 24–1. Causes of Abnormal Uterine Bleeding by Age Group

AGE GROUP	CAUSE(S)
Prepuberty	Precocious puberty (hypothalamic, pituitary, or ovarian origin)
Adolescence	Anovulatory cycle
Reproductive age	Complications of pregnancy (abortion, trophoblastic disease, ectopic pregnancy)
	Organic lesions (leiomyoma, adenomyosis, polyps, endometrial hyperplasia, carcinoma)
	Anovulatory cycle
	Ovulatory dysfunctional bleeding (e.g., inadequate luteal phase)
Perimenopause	Anovulatory cycle
	Irregular shedding
	Organic lesions (carcinoma, hyperplasia, polyps)
Postmenopause	Organic lesions (carcinoma, hyperplasia, polyps)
	Endometrial atrophy

diameter) filled with brown blood debris to form so-called chocolate cysts (Fig. 24–27A).

The histologic diagnosis of endometriosis is sometimes readily made (Fig. 24–27B) but may be obscure in advanced, florid, long-standing cases because, as the disease progresses, the fibroproliferative response obliterates recognizable features. A definite histologic diagnosis requires two of the three following features: glands, stroma, and hemosiderin pigment.

CLINICAL COURSE. Clinical signs and symptoms usually consist of severe dysmenorrhea and pelvic pain due to the intrapelvic bleeding and periuterine adhesions. Dyspareunia may be present for the same reason. Pain of defecation reflects rectal wall involvement, and dysuria reflects involvement of the serosa of the bladder. Intestinal disturbances may appear when the small intestine is affected. Menstrual irregularities are common. Infertility is the presenting complaint in 30 to 40% of women.

FUNCTIONAL MENSTRUAL DISORDERS (DYSFUNCTIONAL UTERINE BLEEDING)

During active reproductive life, the normal monthly cyclic shedding and regrowth of the endometrium is a finely balanced mechanism. It is controlled by the rise and ebb of pituitary and ovarian hormones, not only in regulated, absolute amounts, but also in carefully integrated, relative levels. This finely adjusted proliferation of a new endometrial mucosa each month is subject to many aberrations that cause either hyperplasia or atrophy of the endometrium.[46]

By far the most common problem is the occurrence of excessive bleeding during or between menstrual periods. The causes of abnormal bleeding from the uterus are many and vary among women of different age groups (Table 24–1). In some instances, bleeding is the result of a well-defined organic lesion such as leiomyoma, carcinoma, or polyp, but *the largest single group is so-called dysfunctional uterine bleeding.* This is defined as abnormal bleeding in the absence of an organic lesion of the endometrium or uterus.[47]

ANOVULATORY CYCLE. In most instances, dysfunctional bleeding is due to the occurrence of an *anovulatory cycle,* which results in excessive and prolonged estrogenic stimulation without the development of the progestational phase that regularly follows ovulation. In a small percentage of patients, lack of ovulation is the result of (1) an endocrine disorder, such as thyroid disease, adrenal disease, or pituitary tumors, (2) a primary lesion of the ovary such as a functioning ovarian tumor (granulosa-theca cell tumors, p. 1167) or polycystic ovaries (p. 1157), or (3) a generalized metabolic disturbance such as marked

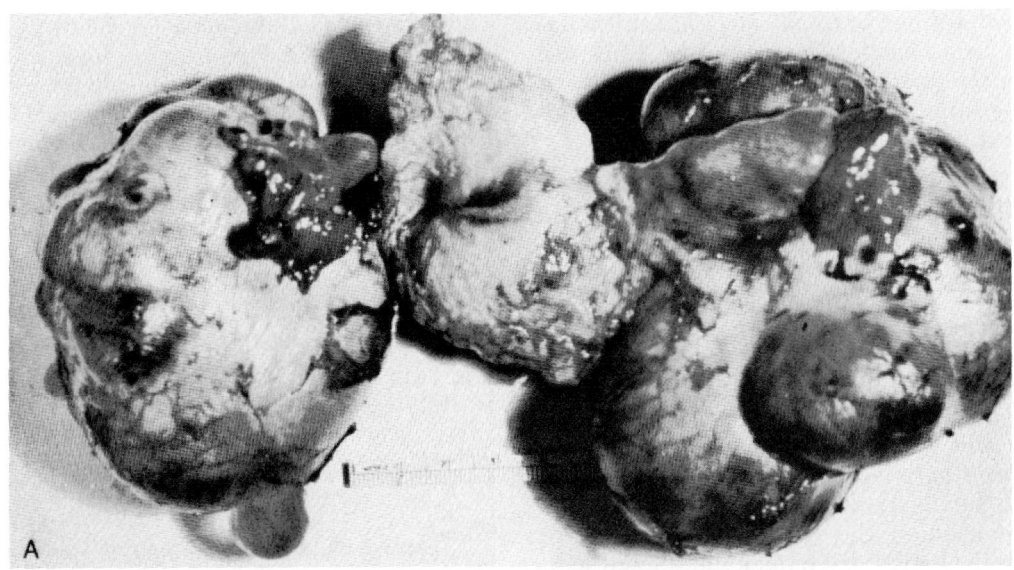

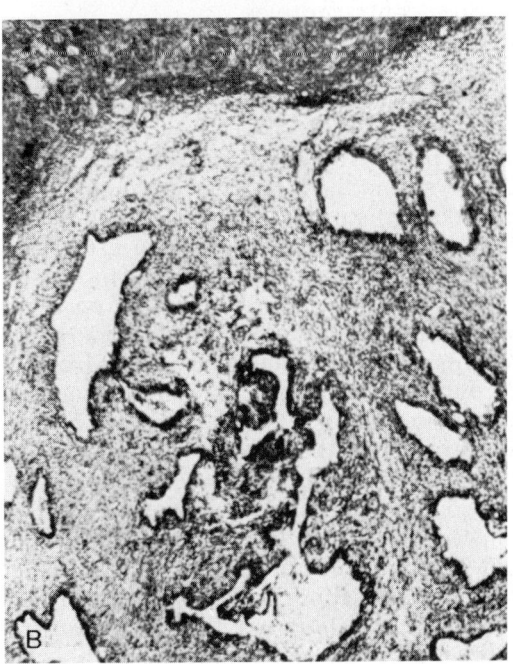

Figure 24–27. A, Endometriosis. Ovaries are converted into enlarged irregular masses by large "chocolate cysts." *B,* Classic diagnostic endometriosis of ovary with readily recognized, well-formed endometrium within ovarian stroma. (Courtesy of Dr. Arthur Hertig.)

obesity, severe malnutrition, or any chronic systemic disease. In most patients, however, anovulatory cycles are unexplainable, probably occurring because of subtle hormonal imbalances. Anovulatory cycles are most common at menarche and about the time of menopause.

Failure of ovulation results in *prolonged and excessive action of estrogens,* with no evidence of the endometrial secretory activity. The *proliferative endometrium* shows mild degrees of hyperplasia characterized histologically by mitotic activity and an increase in gland size. *Patients with endometrial carcinoma are more likely to have a history of repeated anovulatory cycles.*

INADEQUATE LUTEAL PHASE. This term refers to the occurrence of inadequate corpus luteum function and low progesterone output, with an irregular ovulatory cycle. Clinically, the condition often manifests as infertility and either increased bleeding or amenorrhea. Endometrial biopsy performed at an estimated postovulatory date shows secretory endometrium, which, however, lags in its secretory characteristics.

MISCELLANEOUS REACTIVE ENDOMETRIAL CHANGES

SENILE CYSTIC ENDOMETRIAL ATROPHY. In the postmenopausal woman, the endometrium normally atrophies and becomes a rudimentary layer composed only of the basal glands. For obscure reasons, in some women the glands, instead of shrinking, become *cysti-*

cally dilated by flattened or totally atrophic epithelial cells.[46] Such cystic changes should not be confused with cystic hyperplasia, in which the cystic glands are lined by proliferating as well as flattened cells and the stroma is hyperplastic.

ORAL CONTRACEPTIVES AND INDUCED ENDO-METRIAL CHANGES. As might be suspected, the use of oral contraceptive containing synthetic or derivative ovarian steroids induces a wide variety of endometrial changes, depending on the steroid use and the dose. A common reaction pattern is discordance between glandular and stromal activities.[48] Implied here is the presence of inactive, nonproliferative, nonsecretory glands surrounded by a lush stroma showing large cells with abundant cytoplasm and considerable mitotic activity. This stromal reaction is reminiscent of the decidua of pregnancy. When such therapy is discontinued, the endometrium reverts to normal. All these changes have been minimized with the newer low-dose contraceptives.

ENDOMETRIAL HYPERPLASIA

Endometrial hyperplasia is another cause of abnormal bleeding that differs from the functional endometrial disorders inasmuch as the origin of the bleeding is a variety of disordered glandular and stromal growth patterns. *Endometrial hyperplasia is important because of its special relationship to endometrial carcinoma.* Almost 40 years ago, Hertig and Sommers[49] proposed a progression of endometrial changes from hyperplasia through a spectrum of atypical changes leading eventually, in some cases, to endometrial carcinoma. Numerous studies have since largely confirmed the malignant potential of endometrial hyperplasia, and the concept of a continuum of atypical changes culminating in carcinoma.[50]

Although it is easy to recognize both ends of the spectrum of endometrial abnormality — benign hyperplasia on one end and frank adenocarcinoma on the other — there is little uniformity as to the terms or histologic criteria to be used for intermediate stages, or gray zones. Despite this confusion, most authors agree that *increased cancer risk correlates best with the degree of cytologic (cellular) atypia* accompanying hyperplasia.[50-53] Thus, 2% of untreated hyperplasias *without* cellular atypia progress to carcinoma, whereas 23% with atypical hyperplasia progress to

carcinoma.[54] Cellular atypia is usually, but not always, associated with a *complex glandular architecture.*

Endometrial hyperplasia occurs around the time of, or after, menopause and is associated clinically with abnormal or excessive uterine bleeding. The hyperplasia results from an abnormally high and prolonged level of estrogenic stimulation with diminution or absence of progestational activity. These conditions are encountered in the Stein-Leventhal syndrome (p. 1157), functioning granulosa and theca cell tumors of the ovary (p. 1167), excessive adrenocortical function, and prolonged administration of estrogenic substances. These are the same influences postulated to be of pathogenetic significance in endometrial carcinoma (p. 1153), a point that speaks to the precancerous potential of hyperplasia.

Simple hyperplasia, without atypia (also known as cystic or mild hyperplasia), is characterized by the presence of glands of various sizes, including many that are cystic (Figs. 24–28 and 24–29*A*). The epithelial lining may be cuboidal or tall columnar and occasionally multilayered. Mitoses are scant, but typical proliferative endometrium may be admixed with the dilated glands. The stroma between glands also is frequently increased. **These lesions rarely progress to adenocarcinoma.** Cystic hyperplasia should be differentiated from senile cystic atrophy; in the latter, the stroma is atrophic, and the dilated glands are lined by flattened epithelial cells.

Complex hyperplasia (also known as moderate or adenomatous hyperplasia **without** atypia) exhibits an increase in the number and size of endometrial glands, with a disparity in their size and irregularity in their shape. The glands are crowded. Papillary buddings into the glands are formed, as are finger-like outpouchings into the adjacent endometrial stroma. The lining epithelium is hyperplastic, and there is frequent stratification of the epithelium surrounding the lumina. (Figs. 24–28 and 24–29*B*). **In the absence of cytologic atypia,** less than 5% of these lesions develop carcinoma.

Atypical hyperplasia is also known as complex or adenomatous hyperplasia **with** atypia. In addition to glandular crowding and complexity, the distinguishing feature is **cellular atypia** of the hyperplastic epithelium, consisting of cytomegaly, loss of polarity, hyperchromatism, prominence of nucleoli, and altered nuclear cytoplasmic ratio (Fig. 24–30). This atypia could be mild, moderate, or severe. Mitotic figures are common. In the most severe forms, cytologic

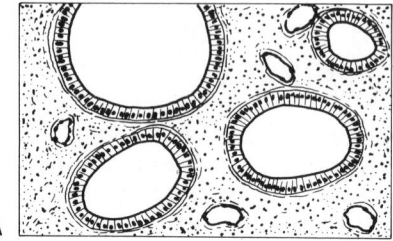
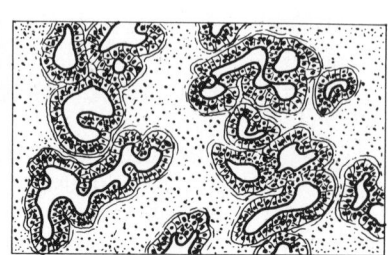

Figure 24–28. Diagram of simple *(A)* and complex *(B)* hyperplasia of endometrium. Complex hyperplasia (also called adenomatous hyperplasia) can occur *with* or *without* cellular atypia.

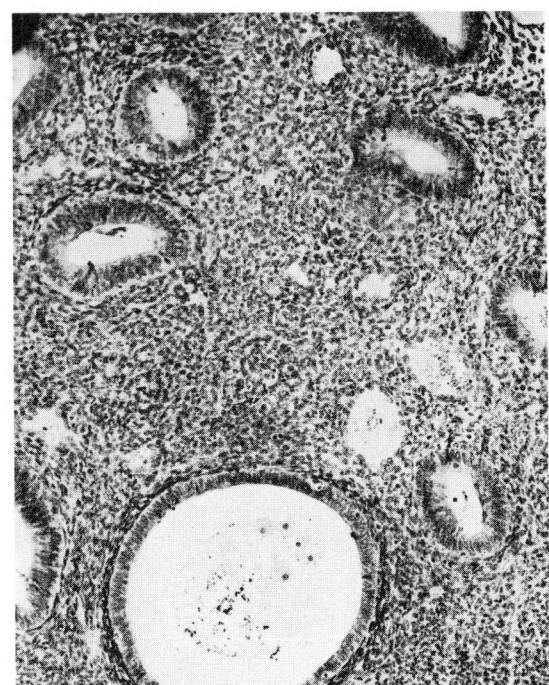

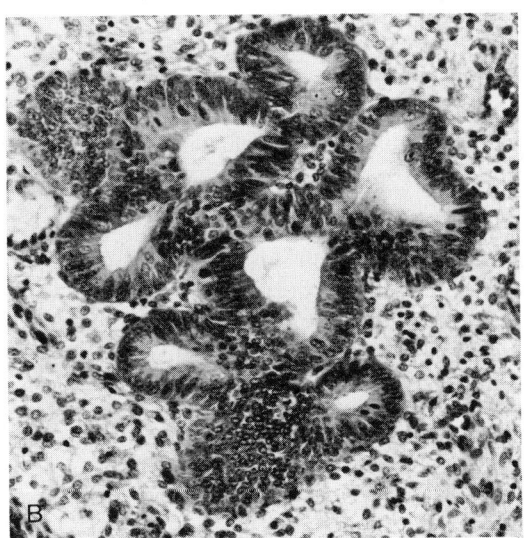

Figure 24–29. *A,* Simple (cystic, mild) hyperplasia with dilatation of glands. *B,* Complex hyperplasia of a nest of closely packed glands in right side of field. (Courtesy of Dr. Arthur Hertig.)

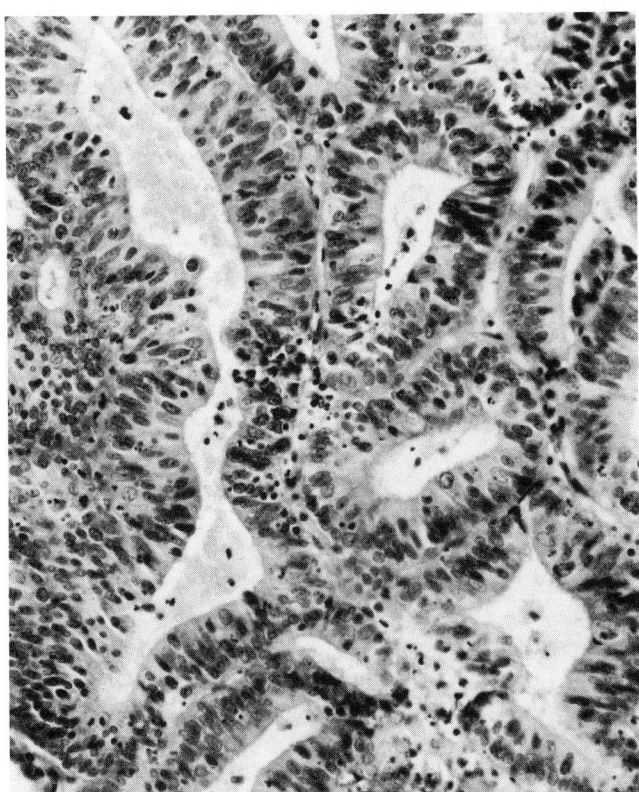

Figure 24–30. Severe atypical hyperplasia. Note both marked crowding of glands and cellular atypia.

and architectural atypia may resemble frank adenocarcinoma, but the term **carcinoma in situ,** suggested by some authors, is now out of favor.

All types of hyperplasia produce abnormal bleeding in the form of either spotting between periods or excessive menstrual flow. Distressing as these symptoms are, the role of hyperplasia in the genesis of endometrial cancer is far more important. As noted, *the increased risk from cystic hyperplasia is minimal but atypical hyperplasias are potentially precancerous lesions;* predictions cannot be made for the individual patient, but in general, the more severe the atypia, the greater the risk. *It is important, therefore, in any assessment of an endometrial hyperplastic lesion, for the pathologist to indicate the degree of atypia in a manner clearly understandable by the clinician.*

TUMORS

The uterine corpus, including its endometrium and myometrium, is affected by a great variety of neoplastic growths. These can be benign or malignant and arise from (1) the endometrial glands (endometrial polyp, endometrial carcinoma), (2) the endometrial stroma (stromal nodule and stromal sarcoma), (3) the müllerian mesoderm differentiating into both glandular and stromal elements (mixed mesodermal tumors), or (4) the smooth muscle of the myometrium (leiomyoma, leiomyosarcoma). The most common of these tumors are the endometrial polyps, leiomyomas, and endometrial carcinomas.

BENIGN

Benign Endometrial Polyps

Endometrial polyps are sessile masses that project into the endometrial cavity. They may be single or multiple, and are usually 0.5 to 3.0 cm in diameter but occasionally large and pedunculated (Fig. 24–31). They are somewhat more common at or near menopause. Smaller polyps are usually asymptomatic, incidental findings, whereas larger ones may ulcerate, degenerate, and cause clinical bleeding. Histologically, they are generally of two types, made up of (1) functional endometrium, paralleling the cycle of the surrounding nonpolypoid endometrium, or (2) more commonly, hyperplastic endometrium, mostly of the cystic variety. Such polyps may develop in association with generalized endometrial hyperplasia and are responsive to the growth effect of estrogen, but exhibit no progesterone response (Fig. 24–32). Malignant change in an initially benign endometrial polyp is rare.

Leiomyoma

Leiomyomas are the most common tumors in women. They are also referred to as myomas and, in colloquial usage, as "fibroids." The tumors are found in about one in four women in active reproductive life. They are more common in blacks.

It is known that leiomyomas regress and even calcify postmenopausally. Castration makes them atrophy. During pregnancy there is sometimes a rapid increase in their size, accompanied by cellular proliferation. On all these bases, the tumors are thought to be caused by excessive estrogenic stimulation. Experimental proof in animals is lacking, however, and it is perhaps more accurate, then, to regard uterine leiomyomas as endocrine-dependent lesions whose growth depends on estrogens.

Leiomyomas are sharply circumscribed, discrete, round, firm, gray-white tumors varying in size from small, barely visible nodules to massive tumors that fill the pelvis. Except in rare instances, they are found within the myometrium of the corpus. Only infrequently do they involve the uterine ligaments, lower uterine segment, or cervix. They can occur within the myometrium **(intramural),** beneath the serosa **(subserosal),** or in immediate proximity to the endometrium **(submucosal).** Frequently, the submucosal masses protrude into the endometrial cavity (Fig. 24–33), and the subserosal tumors become pedunculated and appear as bulbous polyps with firm, round heads (Fig. 24–34).

Whatever their size, the characteristic whorled pattern of smooth muscle bundles on cut section usually makes these lesions readily identifiable on gross inspection. Large tumors may develop areas of yellow-brown to red softening **(cystic degeneration).** In advanced ages, the masses atrophy, tending to become more collagenous, firm, and sometimes partially or completely calcified.

Histologically, the leiomyoma is composed of whorling bundles of smooth muscle cells that resemble the architecture of the uninvolved myometrium (Fig. 24–35). Usually, the individual muscle cells are uniform in size and shape, and have the characteristic oval nucleus and long, slender bipolar cytoplasmic processes. Mitotic figures are scarce, and giant cells and anaplasia are not present.

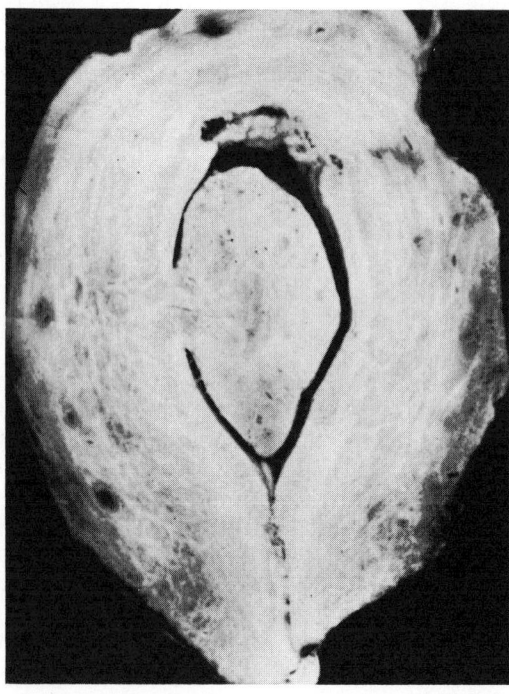

Figure 24–31. Large pedunculated polyp within endometrial cavity, viewed on cross section.

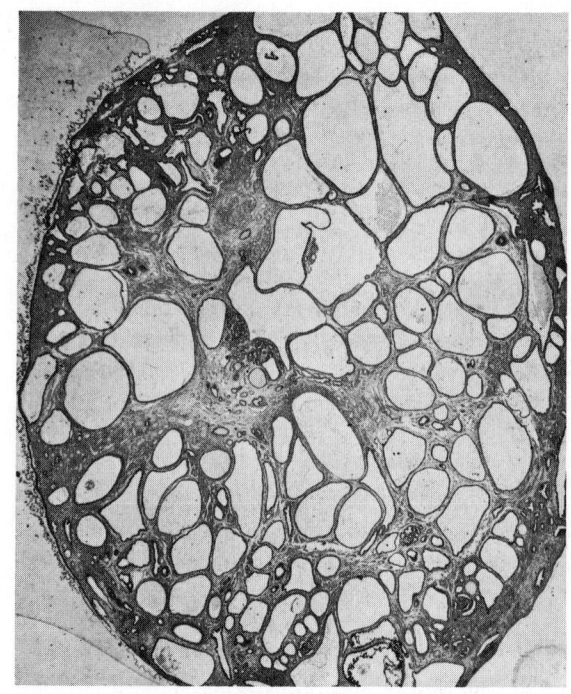

Figure 24–32. Cystic endometrial polyp at low power, illustrating cystic dilatation of glands. (Courtesy of Dr. Arthur Hertig.)

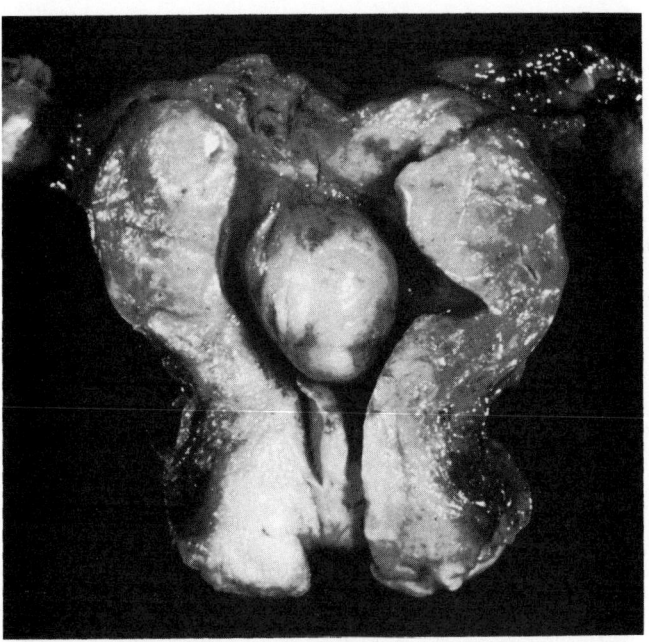

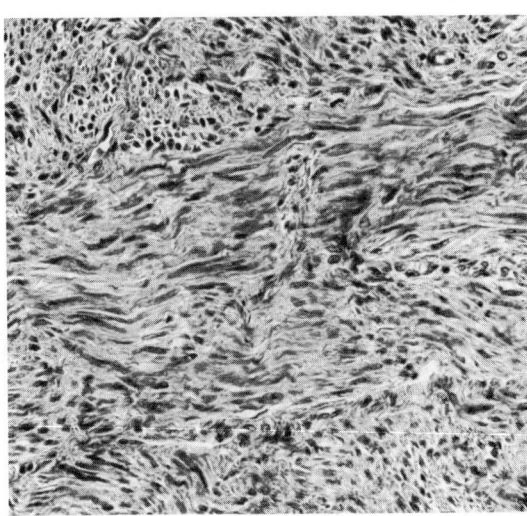

Figure 24–35. Leiomyoma showing bundles of well-differentiated, regular, spindle-shaped smooth muscle cells.

Figure 24–33. Submucosal leiomyoma appearing as a bulbous polyp, protruding into endometrial cavity.

Leiomyomas of the uterus may be asymptomatic or may cause a variety of symptoms, the most important of which is profuse bleeding at the time of the menstrual period. Pain, pressure on the urinary bladder causing urinary frequency, and impaired fertility are other clinical manifestations.

Leiomyomas frequently undergo rapid increase in size during pregnancy, and at this time, these tumors may have considerable hypertrophy of indi-

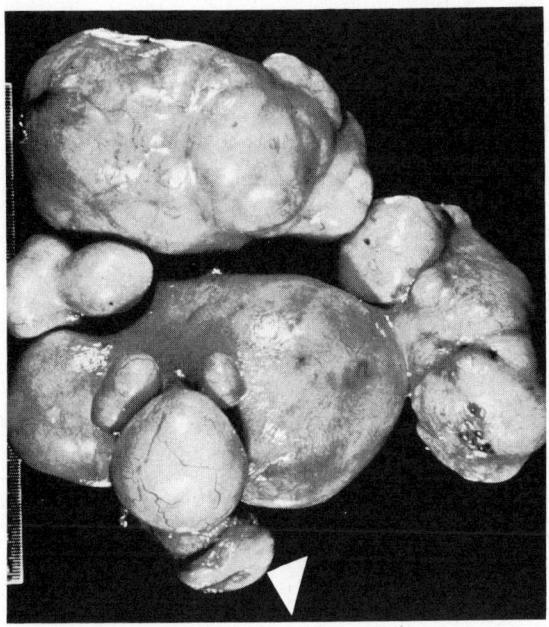

Figure 24–34. Multiple subserosal leiomyomas of uterus. Uterine body is "lost" in irregular mass, but cervix is visible as most dependent portion of specimen (*arrowhead*).

vidual cells with some variability in nuclear and cell size, as well as some mitotic figures. Myomas in pregnant women increase the frequency of spontaneous abortion, fetal malpresentation, uterine inertia, and postpartum hemorrhage. Malignant transformation is said to occur but is rare (p. 1155).

MALIGNANT

Carcinoma of the Endometrium

Endometrial carcinoma is the most common *invasive* cancer of the female genital tract and accounts for 7% of all invasive cancer in women (excluding skin cancer). At one time, it was far less common than cancer of the cervix, but earlier detection and eradication of in situ cervical cancer and an increase in endometrial carcinomas in younger age groups have reversed this ratio. There are now 34,000 new endometrial cancers per year, compared with 13,000 new invasive cervical cancers.[30] However, endometrial lesions tend to arise postmenopausally and cause irregular bleeding, permitting their diagnosis while they are still confined to the uterus and therefore curable by surgery or radiotherapy. Thus, endometrial carcinoma accounts for about 3000 deaths annually in the United States, less than half as many as caused by invasive cervical cancer.[30]

INCIDENCE. Carcinoma of the endometrium is uncommon in women under age 40. The peak incidence is in the 55- to 65-year-old woman. *A higher frequency of this form of neoplasia is seen with:* (1) *obesity*; (2) *diabetes* (abnormal glucose tolerance is found in over 60%); (3) *hypertension*; and (4) *infertility* — women who develop cancer of the endometrium tend to be single and nulliparous and to give a history of functional menstrual irregularities consistent with anovulatory cycles. Infrequently, both endometrial and breast carcinomas arise in the same patient.

PATHOGENESIS. There is quite compelling evidence that carcinoma of the endometrium is influenced by *prolonged estrogen stimulation:*[55]

1. Endometrial carcinoma is sometimes preceded by endometrial hyperplasia, which, as has been discussed (p. 1150), is related to hyperestrinism, and patients who develop endometrial carcinoma frequently have a history of anovulatory cycles.
2. Patients with ovarian estrogen-secreting tumors have higher risk of endometrial cancer (p. 1167).
3. Endometrial cancer is extremely rare in women with ovarian agenesis and in those castrated early in life.
4. Exogenous estrogens used to control menopausal symptoms are associated with increased risk.
5. Prolonged administration of large doses of diethylstilbestrol in laboratory animals has resulted in the production of endometrial polyps, hyperplasia, and carcinoma.
6. In postmenopausal women there is greater synthesis of estrogens in body fats from adrenal and ovarian androgen precursors. The amount of estrone thus produced is proportionate to total body weight, a finding that may partly explain why there is increased risk of endometrial cancer with age and obesity.

There is, however, a subset of patients with endometrial cancer who have no evidence of hyperestrinism. These non–estrogen-related cancers tend to occur in older women, are not preceded by hyperplasia, and are usually more aggressive.[56]

MORPHOLOGY. Grossly, endometrial carcinoma presents either as a localized polypoid tumor or as a diffuse tumor involving the entire endometrial surface (Fig. 24–36).[57] Myometrial extension produces subserosal and serosal nodules, and eventually the tumor spreads to the periuterine structures by direct continuity. Spread into the broad ligaments may create a clinically palpable mass. Eventually dissemination to the regional lymph nodes occurs, and in the late stages the tumor may be hematogenously borne to the lungs, liver, bones, and other organs.

Histologically, most endometrial carcinomas (about 85%) are **adenocarcinomas** characterized by more or less well-defined gland patterns lined by malignant stratified columnar epithelial cells (Fig. 24–37). They may be well differentiated (grade 1), having a prominent, easily recognizable glandular pattern; moderately differentiated (grade 2), showing well-formed glands mixed with solid sheets of malignant cells; or poorly differentiated (grade 3), characterized by solid sheets of cells with barely recognizable glands and a great degree of nuclear atypia and mitotic activity.

Ten to 20% of endometrial carcinomas contain foci of squamous differentiation. Squamous elements most commonly are histologically benign in appearance (called **adenocarcinoma with squamous metaplasia or adenoacanthoma**), but are sometimes frankly malignant (termed

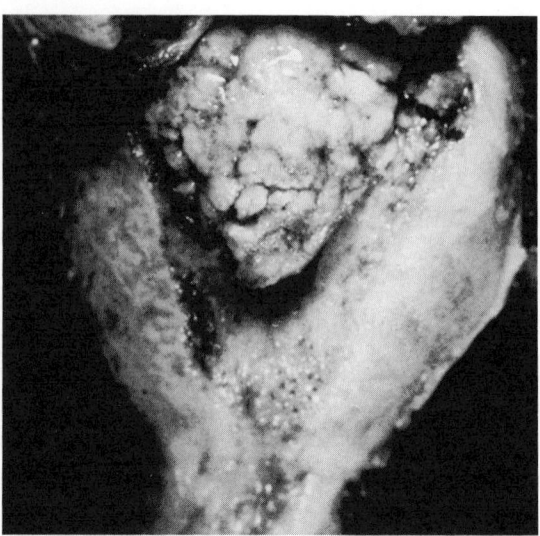

Figure 24–36. Endometrial carcinoma, presenting as a fungating mass in fundus of uterus.

adenosquamous carcinoma if over 10% of the tumor is squamous).[58]

Other rare histologic types of endometrial carcinoma are **clear cell carcinoma, mucinous adenocarcinoma, secretory carcinoma,** and **papillary serous carcinoma.** The last, in particular, is a highly malignant form of uterine cancer.

Staging of endometrial adenocarcinoma is as follows:[59]

Stage I. Carcinoma is confined to the corpus uteri itself.

Stage II. Carcinoma has involved the corpus and the cervix.

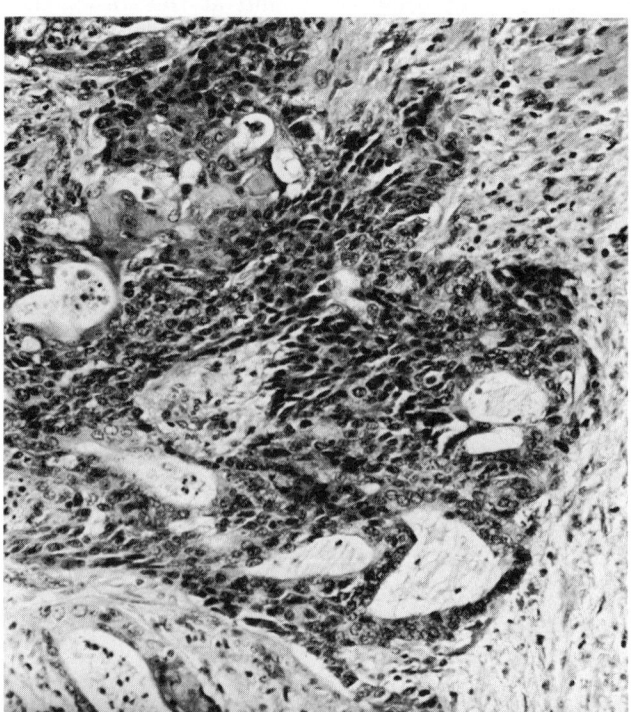

Figure 24–37. Endometrial adenocarcinoma, showing solid and gland components, focal squamous change *(upper left)*, and myometrial invasion. (Courtesy of Dr. William Welch.)

Stage III. Carcinoma has extended outside the uterus but not outside the true pelvis.

Stage IV. Carcinoma has extended outside the true pelvis or has obviously involved the mucosa of the bladder or the rectum.

Cases in various stages can also be subgrouped with reference to histologic type of adenocarcinoma as follows:

G1. Well-differentiated adenocarcinoma.

G2. Differentiated adenocarcinoma with partly solid areas.

G3. Predominantly solid or entirely undifferentiated carcinoma.

CLINICAL COURSE. Carcinoma of the endometrium may be asymptomatic for a long time. The most common manifestation is irregular vaginal bleeding accompanied by excessive leukorrhea. Uterine enlargement in the early stages may be deceptively absent. Cytologic examination of vaginal smears is helpful, but ultimately the diagnosis must be established by curettage and histologic examination of the tissue.

As would be anticipated, the prognosis is heavily dependent on the clinical stage of the disease when discovered, and to some degree also on the histologic grade.[60] Fortunately the great majority of women (about 80%) have stage I disease clinically, and histologically have well- or moderately well-differentiated lesions. Surgery, alone or in combination with irradiation, yields close to 90% five-year survival in stage I disease. This rate drops to 30 to 50% in stage II, and to less than 20% in any of the other, more advanced stages of the disease.

Mesenchymal Tumors

Collectively, sarcomas make up 5% or less of uterine tumors; mixed mesodermal tumors, leiomyosarcomas, and endometrial stromal sarcomas are the most common variants.[61,62]

MALIGNANT MIXED MESODERMAL TUMORS (MIXED MÜLLERIAN TUMORS).

These malignant and relatively rare tumors of the endometrium, are generally regarded as being derived from primitive stromal cells, originally derived from müllerian mesoderm.[63] They are called mixed tumors because they consist of malignant glandular and stromal sarcomatous elements, and the latter tend to differentiate into a variety of malignant mesodermal components, including muscle, cartilage, and even osteoid that exhibits a variety of mesenchymal differentiated antigens.[64] The tumor occurs in postmenopausal women and manifests like adenocarcinoma, with postmenopausal bleeding. Many affected patients give a history of previous radiation therapy.

Grossly, such tumors are bulky and polypoid, and may protrude into the vagina. On histology, much of the tumor may consist of endometrial adenocarcinoma, which tends to be poorly differentiated, but the glandular elements are intermixed with anaplastic, spindle-shaped stromal cells that have bizarre nuclei and numerous mitoses. As mentioned, the sarcomatous part may differentiate into recognizable smooth or striated muscle cells, cartilage, adipose tissue, and bone (**heterologous** mixed tumors). When these heterotopic structures are not present, the tumor consists simply of glands and malignant mesenchyme, and the terms **carcinosarcoma** and **homologous mixed tumors** are applied to such lesions. The tumors are highly malignant and have a five-year survival rate of 25 to 30%.

LEIOMYOSARCOMAS.

These uncommon malignancies almost always arise directly from the myometrium. Their origin from a pre-existing leiomyoma is a controversial issue, but the consensus holds that these cancers are extremely rare complications of the very common benign leiomyoma.

Leiomyosarcomas grow within the uterus in two somewhat distinctive patterns; bulky, fleshy masses that invade the uterine wall; or polypoid masses that project into the uterine lumen. Histologically, they show a wide range of atypia, from those that are extremely well differentiated to anaplastic lesions that have the cytologic abnormalities of wildly growing sarcomas (Fig. 24-38). Many of the borderline, well-differentiated sarcomas are difficult to delineate from cellular leiomyomas. Histologic features indicative of leiomyosarcoma include (1) more than ten mitoses per ten high-power fields (HPF), with or without cellular atypism; and (2) five to ten mitoses per ten HPF with cellular atypism. Leiomyosarcomas with **myxoid** or **epithelioid** features may have fewer than five mitoses per HPF and still behave aggressively.[65]

Leiomyosarcomas are equally common before and after menopause, with a peak incidence at 40 to 60 years of age. These tumors have a striking tendency to recur after removal, and in over half the

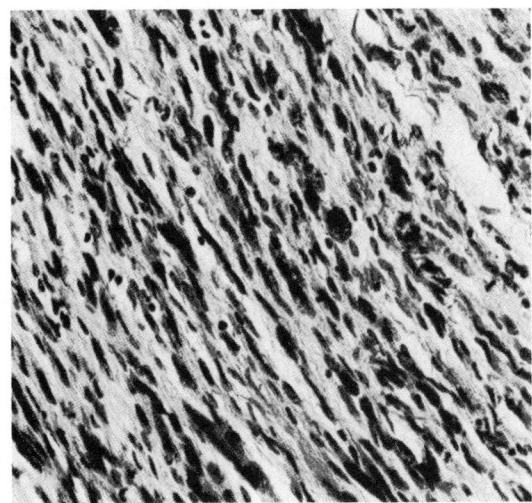

Figure 24-38. Leiomyosarcoma. Cells are large and irregular and have hyperchromatic nuclei.

cases eventually metastasize to distant organs such as lungs, bone, and brain. Dissemination throughout the abdominal cavity is also encountered. The five-year survival rate averages about 40%. The well-differentiated lesions have a better prognosis than the anaplastic lesions, which have a very low five-year survival rate of about 10 to 15%.

ENDOMETRIAL STROMAL TUMORS. Strands and nests of more or less well-differentiated endometrial stroma are sometimes encountered in the myometrium. The cytologic differentiation of the stromal cells ranges from patterns virtually indistinguishable from the normal endometrial stroma to obviously sarcomatous anaplasia. These involvements have been divided into three categories: (1) *benign stromal nodules* (p. 1147), (2) *low-grade stromal sarcoma, or endolymphatic stromal myosis,* and (3) *endometrial stromal sarcoma.*

Low-grade stromal sarcoma refers to the appearance of masses of well-differentiated endometrial stroma lying between muscle bundles of the myometrium, which can be differentiated from *benign stromal nodules* only by the tendency of the stromal nests to penetrate lymphatic channels (hence the term endolymphatic stromal myosis). About half of these tumors recur, sometimes after 10 to 15 years; distant metastases and death from tumor occur in about 15% of cases.

Endometrial stromal sarcoma is the overtly cancerous counterpart of endolymphatic stromal myosis. The cells display a wide range of atypia from fairly well-differentiated stromal cells, which nonetheless vary in size and shape and have frequent mitoses, to highly undifferentiated lesions with wild pleomorphic tumor giant cells. As with all sarcomas, these cancers invade vessels and are capable of widespread metastasis. Five-year survival rates average 50%.

FALLOPIAN TUBES

The most common disorders in these structures are inflammations, followed in frequency by ectopic (tubal) pregnancy (p. 1171) and endometriosis.

INFLAMMATIONS

SUPPURATIVE SALPINGITIS (PELVIC INFLAMMATORY DISEASE). Salpingitis may be caused by any of the pyogenic organisms, i.e., streptococci, staphylococci, coliforms, and gonococci. In spite of effective antibiotics, the gonococcus still accounts for over 60% of cases of suppurative salpingitis. In almost all instances, these tubular infections are a part of the pelvic inflammatory disease (PID) described on page 1132 (Fig. 24–39).

TUBERCULOUS SALPINGITIS. Another type of salpingitis encountered is almost invariably a secondary complication of a focus of tuberculosis elsewhere in the body. Presumably, the tubes are seeded hematogenously, and then the process spreads to other organs in the genital tract, such as the endometrium, and to the peritoneal cavity. Tuberculous salpingitis is extremely uncommon in the United States and accounts for probably not more than 1 to 2% of all forms of salpingitis. However, it is more common in parts of the world where tuberculosis is frequent and is an important cause of infertility in these areas.

TUMORS

Only rarely do tumors arise within the fallopian tubes. The most common forms of tumor, which hardly merit

such a designation, are minute, 0.1- to 2-cm, translucent cysts filled with clear serous fluid, found near the fimbriated end of the tube or in the broad ligaments, and referred to as *parovarian cysts* or *hydatids of Mor-*

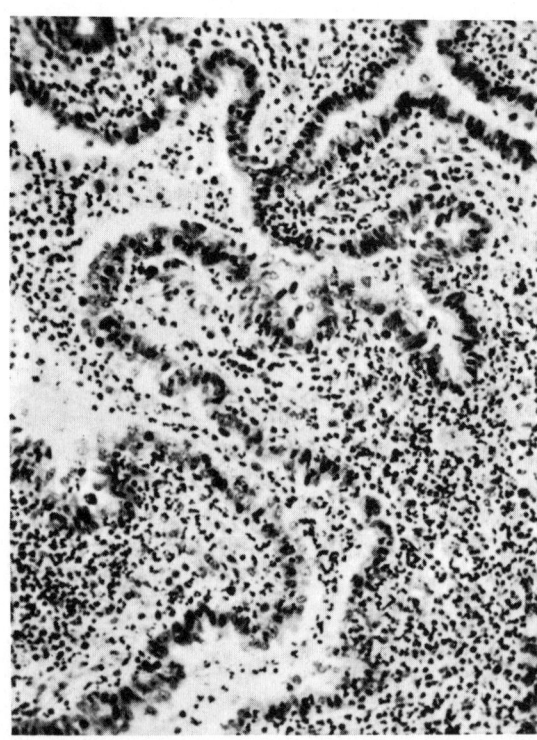

Figure 24–39. Acute salpingitis with a diffuse neutrophilic exudate within both the mucosal folds and the lumen.

gagni. Some of these cysts are presumed to arise in remnants of wolffian duct and are of little more than academic significance.

Carcinoma of the fallopian tubes is rare. The tumor arises from the mucosal lining of the tubes (usually near the distal ends), grows as an adenocarcinoma, spreads by continuity to adjacent structures, and may metastasize in the late stages to distant organs such as the lungs and bones.

Equally rarely, adenomatoid tumors (mesotheliomas) occur subserosally on the tube or sometimes in the mesosalpinx. These small nodules are the exact counterparts of those already described in relation to the testes or epididymides (p. 1116) and are benign.

OVARIES

Tumors and cysts are the most common types of lesions encountered in the ovary. Intrinsic inflammations of the ovary are uncommon, and periovarian inflammations are usually secondary to involvement of the adjacent tube. Endometriosis does affect the ovary but usually in conjunction with the pelvic endometriosis described earlier.

NON-NEOPLASTIC CYSTS

FOLLICULAR AND LUTEAL CYSTS

Follicular cysts in the ovary are so common as to be virtually physiologic. They originate in unruptured graafian follicles or in follicles that have ruptured and immediately sealed.

> These cysts are usually multiple. They range in size from 1 to 8 cm in diameter, are filled with a clear serous fluid, and are lined by a gray, glistening membrane. Histologically, granulosal lining cells can be identified when the intraluminal pressure has not been too great. As the cysts increase in size, however, the lining cells atrophy under pressure of the contained fluid (Fig. 24–40). Occasionally, large cysts may become palpable and cause pelvic pain. Rarely, the increased production of estrogen stimulates endometrial hyperplasia. Follicular cysts can be diagnosed on ultrasound.
>
> **Luteal cysts** may be formed in much the same way, usually by the immediate sealing of a corpus hemorrhagicum. These cysts are lined by a rim of bright yellow luteal tissue containing luteinized cells. Occasionally they rupture and cause a peritoneal reaction. With numerous luteal cysts, the aggregate production of hormone may induce endometrial hyperplasia.

POLYCYSTIC OVARIES

Polycystic ovaries (the Stein-Leventhal syndrome) are characterized by *persistent anovulation, fibrotic cystic ovaries,* associated with excessive production of androgens, increased conversion of androgen to estrogen, and inappropriate secretion of gonadotropins by the pituitary. The disorder is one of young women who present with oligomenorrhea, infertility, hirsutism, and sometimes obesity.[66]

> The ovaries are usually twice normal size, are gray-white with a smooth outer cortex, and are studded with subcortical cysts 0.5 to 1.5 cm in diameter. Histologically, there is a thickened fibrosed outer tunica, sometimes referred to as "cortical stromal fibrosis," beneath which are innumerable cysts lined by granulosal cells with a hypertrophic and hyperplastic luteinized theca interna. There is a conspicuous absence of corpora lutea.

The principal biochemical abnormalities that can be identified in most patients are excessive production of androgens, high levels of luteinizing hormone, and low levels of follicle-stimulating hormone. For years, these endocrine abnormalities were attributed to some primary ovarian dysfunction, because large wedge resections of the ovaries reverse the clinical and endocrinologic abnormalities and restore fertility

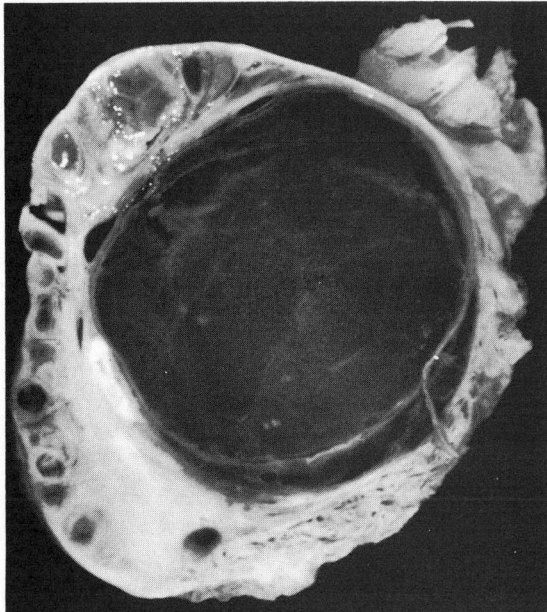

Figure 24–40. Follicular-luteal cysts of ovary, showing one large cyst and multiple subcortical smaller cavities.

in most patients. It is now believed, however, that the ovarian and hormonal changes are probably the result of unbalanced or asynchronous release of FSH and LH by the pituitary, which is in turn related to some disruption of hypothalamic control of pituitary secretion. Presumably, reduction in size of the ovarian mass by wedge resections corrects the condition because it reduces the volume of ovarian tissue that can respond to pituitary hormones.

TUMORS

Tumors of the ovary are common forms of neoplasia in women.[67,68] Among cancers of the female genital tract, the incidence of ovarian cancer ranks below only carcinoma of the cervix and the endometrium. Ovarian cancer accounts for 6% of all cancers in the female and is the fifth most common form of cancer in women in the U. S. (excluding skin cancer). In addition, because many of these ovarian neoplasms cannot be detected early in their development, they account for a disproportionate number of fatal cancers, being responsible for almost half of the deaths from cancer of the female genital tract. There are numerous types of ovarian tumors, both benign and malignant. About 80% are benign, and these occur mostly in young women between the ages of 20 and 45 years. The malignant tumors are more common in older women, between 40 and 65 years.

Risk factors for ovarian cancer are much less clear than for other genital tumors.[69] Most case control studies agree on two risk factors: nulliparity and family history. There is a higher frequency of carcinoma in unmarried women and in married women with low parity. Estrogen therapy seems to have no effect. Indeed, there is less risk of developing ovarian cancer in women 40 to 59 years of age who have taken oral contraceptives.[70] Gonadal dysgenesis in children is associated with a higher risk of ovarian cancer.

The classification of ovarian tumors given in Table 24–2 and Figure 24–41 is a simplified version of the WHO Histological Classification of Ovarian Tumors, which separates ovarian neoplasms according to the most probable tissue of origin. It is now believed that tumors of the ovary arise ultimately from one of three ovarian components: (1) *the surface coelomic epithelium*, which embryologically has the potential of differentiating into epithelium that resembles closely that of fallopian tubes (ciliated, serous, columnar cells), the endometrial lining (nonciliated, columnar cells), or the endocervical glands (tall, mucus-secreting, nonciliated cells); (2) *the germ cells*, which migrate to the ovary from the yolk sac and are totipotential; and (3) *the stroma of the ovary*, which includes the sex cords, forerunners of the endocrine apparatus of the postnatal ovary. There is, as usual, a group of tumors that defy classification, and finally there are secondary or metastatic tumors, the ovary being a common site of metastases from a variety of other cancers.

Table 24–2. Ovarian Neoplasms

Tumors of surface epithelium	Serous tumors
	Serous cystadenoma
	Borderline serous tumor
	Serous cystadenocarcinoma
	Adenofibroma and cystadenofibroma
	Mucinous tumors
	Mucinous cystadenoma
	Borderline mucinous tumor
	Mucinous cystadenocarcinoma
	Endometrioid carcinoma
	Clear cell adenocarcinoma
	Brenner tumor
	Undifferentiated carcinoma
Germ cell tumors	Teratoma
	Benign (mature, adult)
	Cystic teratoma (dermoid cyst)
	Solid teratoma
	Malignant (immature)
	Monodermal or specialized (e.g., carcinoid, struma ovarii)
	Dysgerminoma
	Endodermal sinus tumor
	Choriocarcinoma
	Others (embryonal carcinoma, polyembryoma, mixed germ cell tumors)
Sex cord–stromal tumors	Granulosa-theca cell tumors
	Granulosa cell tumor
	Thecoma
	Fibroma
	Sertoli-Leydig cell tumor (androblastoma)
	Gonadoblastoma
Unclassified tumors	
Metastatic tumors	

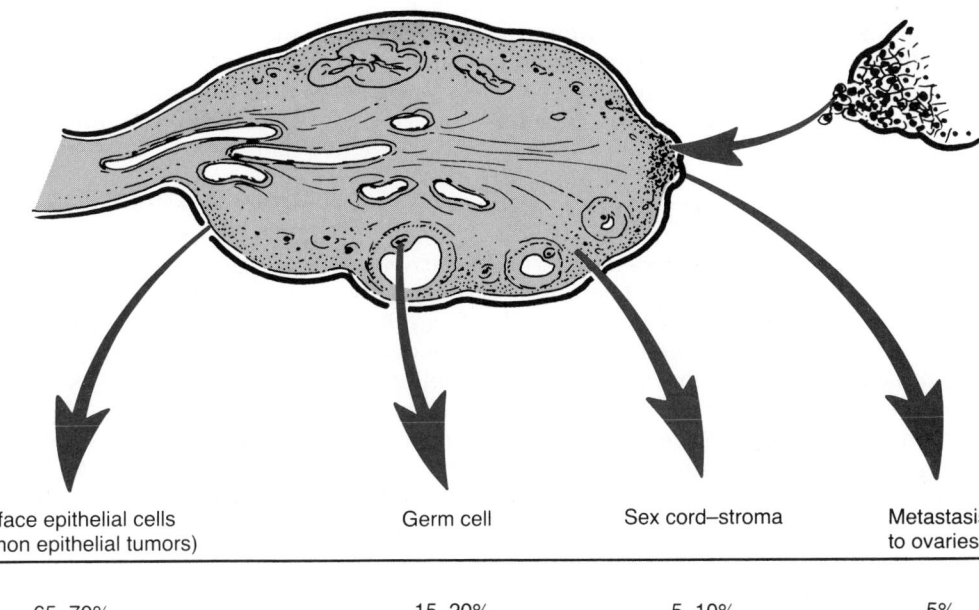

Origin	Surface epithelial cells (common epithelial tumors)	Germ cell	Sex cord–stroma	Metastasis to ovaries
Frequency	65–70%	15–20%	5–10%	5%
Age group affected	20 + years	0–25 + years	All ages	Variable
Types	• Serous tumor • Mucinous tumor • Endometrioid tumor • Clear cell tumor • Brenner tumor • Unclassifiable	• Teratoma • Dysgerminoma • Endodermal sinus tumor • Choriocarcinoma	• Fibroma • Granulosa–theca cell tumor • Sertoli-Leydig cell tumor	

Figure 24–41. Derivation of various ovarian neoplasms and some data on their frequency and age distribution.

Although some of the specific tumors have distinctive features and are hormonally active, the clinical characteristics of most ovarian tumors are similar, and the vast majority are nonfunctional. These tumors tend to produce relatively mild symptoms until they have reached a large size. Malignant tumors have usually spread outside the ovary by the time a definitive diagnosis is made. Some of these tumors tend to be bilateral. Table 24–3 lists these tumors and their subtypes and shows the frequency of bilateral occurrence. Abdominal pain and distention, urinary and gastrointestinal tract symptoms due to compression by tumor or cancer invasion, and abdominal and vaginal bleeding are the most common symptoms. The

Table 24–3. Certain Frequency Data for Major Ovarian Tumors

TYPE	PERCENTAGE OF MALIGNANT OVARIAN TUMORS	PERCENTAGE THAT ARE BILATERAL
Serous	40	
Benign (60%)		25
Borderline (15%)		30
Malignant (25%)		65
Mucinous	10	
Benign (80%)		5
Borderline (10%)		10
Malignant (10%)		20
Endometrioid carcinoma	20	40
Undifferentiated carcinoma	10	—
Clear cell carcinoma	6	40
Granuloma cell tumor	5	5
Teratoma		
Benign (96%)		15
Malignant (4%)	1	Rare
Metastatic	6	>50
Others	3	—

benign forms may be entirely asymptomatic and occasionally are unexpected findings on abdominal or pelvic examination or during surgery.

TUMORS OF SURFACE (COELOMIC) EPITHELIUM

The great majority of primary neoplasms in the ovary fall within this category.[71] There are three major types of such tumors, *serous, mucinous,* and *endometrioid.* Mixtures of these epithelia occasionally occur in the same tumor. In some tumors, the epithelium is so undifferentiated that it is unclassifiable. Neoplasms composed of these three cell types range from clearly benign to frankly cancer; however, between these two extremes fall a group of intermediate tumors that are best considered low-grade cancer and are called *carcinomas of low malignant potential* (or tumors of borderline malignancy).[72]

These neoplasms run the gamut from small to massive tumors that sometimes fill the pelvis and even the abdominal cavity. Many of the serous and mucinous varieties are cystic; thus the terms *cystadenoma* or *cystadenocarcinoma.* Solid areas are often interspersed. As one ascends the scale of aggressiveness, papillary projections into the cystic lumina become more prominent, multiloculation more complex, and solidification of cystic spaces more complete. In general, unilocular cysts with few papillary projections and no solid areas tend to be benign, whereas multiloculated cysts that are highly papillated with frequent solid areas are likely to be malignant.

Serous Tumors

These common *cystic neoplasms are lined by tall, columnar, ciliated epithelial cells and are filled with serous fluid,* the two distinctive features of these tumors. Together the benign, borderline, and malignant types account for about 30% of all ovarian tumors. In the overall spectrum of serous tumors, about 60% are benign, 15% borderline, and 25% malignant. The serous cystadenocarcinomas account for approximately 40% of all cancers of the ovary. As with all ovarian tumors, these serous lesions occur at any age, but are most common between the ages of 20 and 50, the malignant forms being seen later in life.

The benign, borderline, and malignant variants are usually large, spherical or ovoid cysts that average 10 to 15 cm in diameter but may be as large as 40 cm. The smaller masses usually have only a single cystic cavity, but as they enlarge they may become multilocular, and then they lose their symmetric external aspect (Fig. 24–42). In the cystadenoma, the serosal and inner linings are smooth and glistening. The **cystadenocarcinomas** often have small, solid

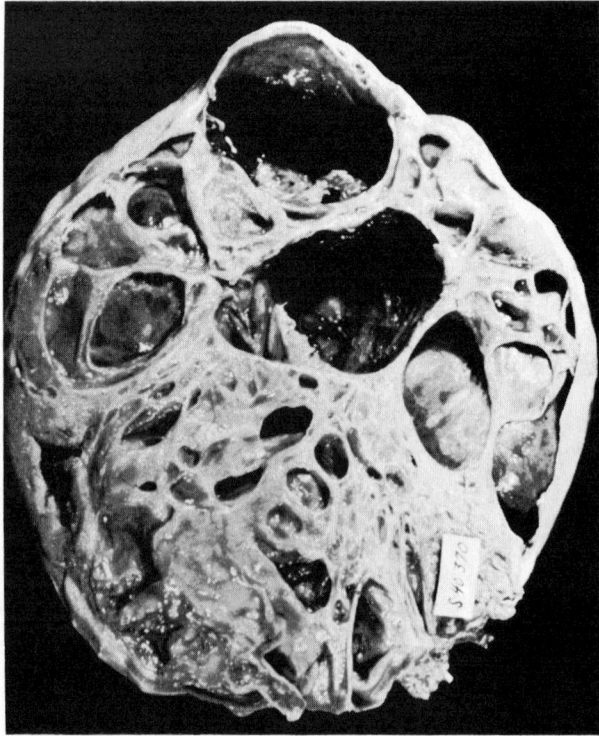

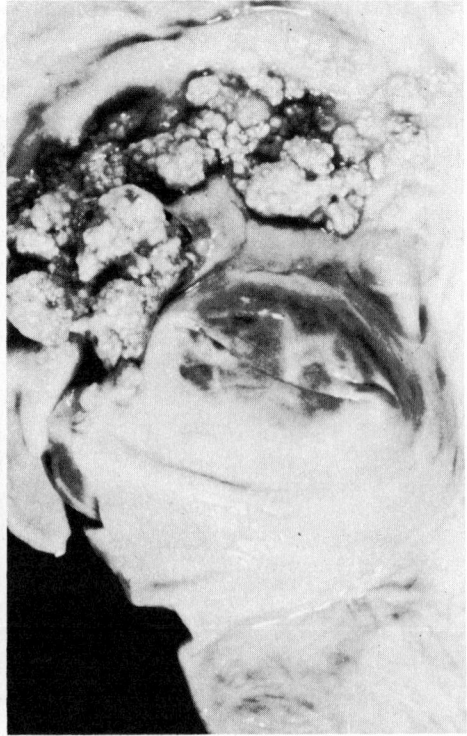

Fig. 24–42

Fig. 24–43

Figure 24–42. Multilocular serous cystadenoma of ovary on cross section.

Figure 24–43. Multilocular serous cystadenocarcinoma of ovary. Close-up of papillary excrescences that have penetrated covering serosa.

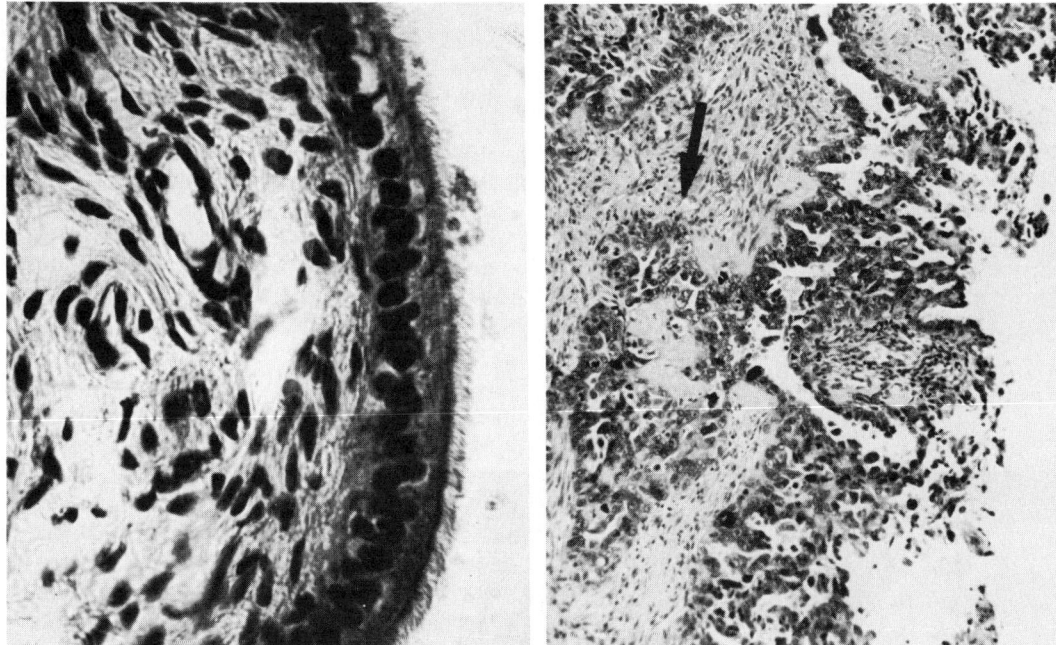

Fig. 24–44   **Fig. 24–45**

Figure 24–44. Histologic detail of classic ciliated columnar lining epithelial cells of a serous cystadenoma.

Figure 24–45. Papillary serous cystadenocarcinoma of ovary with loss of orientation and piling up of atypical epithelium.

nodularities or irregular thickenings either directly beneath the serosa or protruding through it. They tend to develop papillary projections or large masses or thickenings of the wall that jut into the cystic cavities. The papillary tendency, the solid projecting masses, the presence of totally solid locules, and penetration or nodularity of the capsule are all important indicators of probable malignancy (Fig. 24–43). Only 20% of benign tumors occur bilaterally, but 30% of borderline tumors and approximately two-thirds of malignant forms affect both ovaries.

Histologically, the lining epithelium in the smooth areas of the cysts is composed of a single layer of tall columnar epithelium. The cells are ciliated, dome shaped, and serous secreting (Fig. 24–44). Microscopic papillae may be found. The histologic features that denote malignancy consist of piling up of the epithelial lining into more than one layer; invasion of the underlying stroma or capsule of the cyst; the formation of large, solid, epithelial masses that usually represent the jutting areas cited in the gross description; and frank penetration or invasion of the cyst wall (Fig. 24–45). The individual tumor cells in the carcinomatous lesions display the usual features of all malignancy, and with the more extreme degrees of atypia, the cells may become quite undifferentiated.

The histologic criteria for borderline or low malignant potential tumors are obviously imprecise but include, in varying combinations, stratification of epithelial cells, apparent detachment of epithelial clusters from their site of origin, moderate mitotic activity, and nuclear atypia, **but lack of obvious invasion of the stroma.** The last is a sine qua non for outright cystadenocarcinoma.

All ovarian neoplasms derived from surface epithelium or ovarian stroma tend to produce similar clinical manifestations, which will be discussed later. Here it is important to cite some of the prognostic data for the borderline and cancerous lesions. The ten-year survival rate for the overt cancers is on the order of 10 to 20%, but for the borderline serous neoplasms it is approximately 75%.

Mucinous Tumors

These tumors closely resemble their serous counterparts. They are somewhat less common than the serous forms, accounting for about 25% of all ovarian neoplasms. They occur principally in middle adult life and are rare before puberty and after menopause. Eighty per cent are benign, 10 to 15% are borderline, and 5 to 10% are malignant. Indeed, mucinous cystadenocarcinomas are relatively uncommon and account for only 10% of all ovarian cancers.

Grossly, the mucinous tumors resemble the serous cystadenomas and cystadenocarcinomas. However, in contrast to serous tumors, the mucinous tumors are more apt to be unilateral. Approximately 5% of the benign forms and only 20% of the carcinomas are bilateral (contrasted with serous tumors, in which 20 to 30% of benign tumors and 65% of carcinomas are bilateral). Mucinous tumors tend to produce larger cystic masses, and some have been recorded with weights of over 25 kg! They tend to be more strikingly multiloculated and are filled with sticky, gelatinous fluid rich in glycoproteins (Fig. 24–46).

Two to 5% of ovarian mucinous tumors are complicated by a condition designated **pseudomyxoma peritonei.** The peritoneal cavity becomes filled with a glairy mucinous material resembling the cystic contents. Multiple tumor implants are found on all the serosal surfaces, and extensive interadherence and adhesion of the viscera produce a matting together of the abdominal contents (Fig. 24–47). This fortunately rare form of pseudomyxoma peritonei is similar to that encountered in rupture of a carcinomatous mucocele of the appendix.

Histologically, the tumors are identified by the apical mucinous vacuolation of the tall columnar lining epithelial cells and the absence of cilia (Fig. 24–48). The characteristics that applied to serous cystadenocarcinoma (i.e., piling up of epithelium, formation of papillae and complicated glandular structures, atypia of epithelial cells, invasion of the capsule, and formation of solid masses of tumor) also apply to the segregation of the mucinous variants into benign, borderline, and malignant tumors. In 5 to 10% of these mucinous tumors, nodules of a dermoid cyst or Brenner tumor are found in the wall of a cystic space.

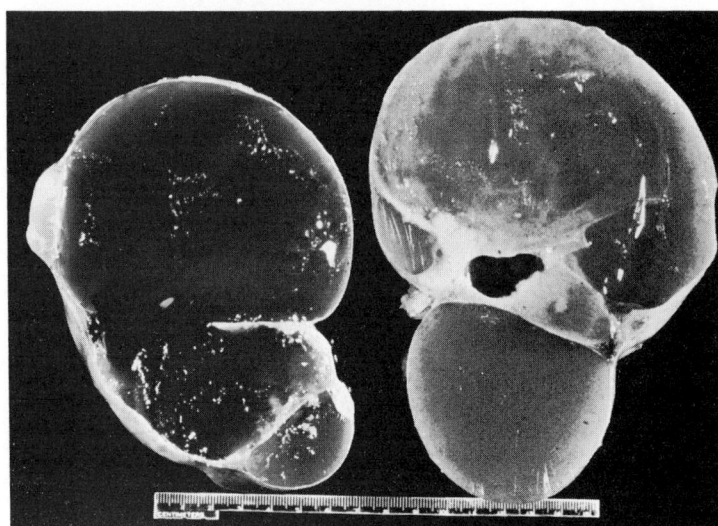

Figure 24–46. Bilateral mucinous cystadenomas of ovary. Tumors were fixed before sectioning to demonstrate gelatinous nature of cystic contents. Note 15-cm rule.

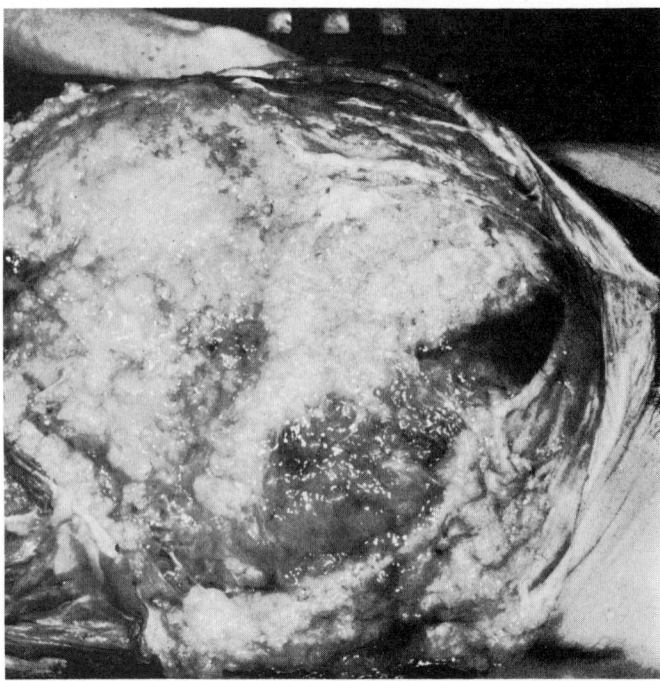

Figure 24–47. Pseudomyxoma peritonei (ovarian), viewed at autopsy with abdominal wall laid back to expose massive overgrowth of gelatinous metastatic tumor.

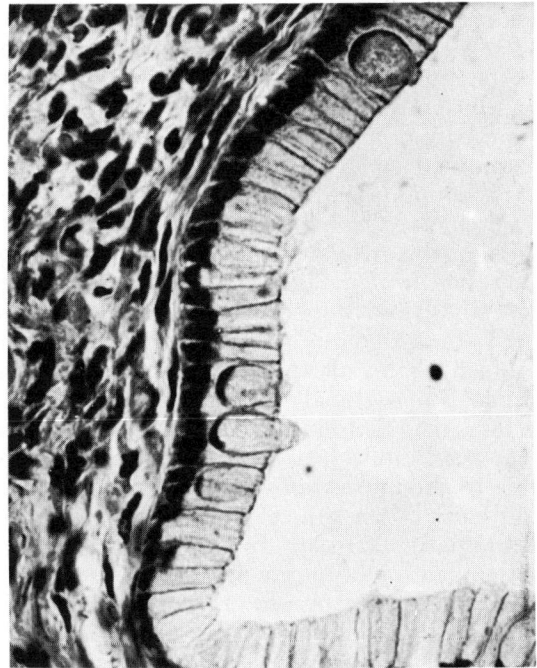

Figure 24–48. Histologic detail of classic nonciliated, mucin-secreting, columnar lining epithelium of a mucinous cystadenoma of ovary. (Courtesy of Dr. Arthur Hertig.)

The importance of differentiating between borderline and malignant mucinous tumors is made clear by the reported 70% ten-year survival rate in patients with borderline lesions, in contrast with a 35% rate for the overt carcinomas. With tumors localized to the ovary, the ten-year survival rate for borderline lesions is 95%, compared with 60% for carcinomas.

Endometrioid Tumors

These neoplasms account for approximately 20% of all ovarian cancers. Most are carcinomas, but benign forms exist, as do borderline tumors of low malignant potential.[73] They are distinguished from serous and mucinous tumors by the presence of tubular glands bearing a close resemblance to benign or malignant endometrium. For obscure reasons, 15 to 30% of endometrioid carcinomas are accompanied by a carcinoma of the endometrium. It is not thought that one represents metastatic spread from the other.

Although about 15% of cases with endometrioid carcinoma also harbor benign endometriosis, most endometrioid tumors are thought to arise de novo from ovarian coelomic epithelium.[74]

Grossly, endometrioid carcinomas present as a combination of solid and cystic areas. These tumors do not achieve the monstrous proportions of their mucinous cousins. The cysts are lined by a velvety surface from which may protrude polypoid masses or papillae.

Forty per cent of patients with endometrioid carcinoma have involvement of both ovaries. Such bilaterality usually, but not always, implies extension of the neoplasm beyond the female genital tract. Histologically, glandular patterns bearing a strong resemblance to those of endometrial origin are seen. In some cases, there are foci of squamous differentiation, recapitulating the pattern of adenoacanthomas of the endometrium. Similarly, some tumors have foci resembling serous or mucinous carcinomas. The overall five-year survival rate is 40 to 50%. The survival data are modified by the level of differentiation of the epithelial component.

Clear Cell Adenocarcinoma

This uncommon pattern of surface epithelial tumor of the ovary is characterized by large epithelial cells with abundant clear cytoplasm. Because these tumors sometimes occur in association with endometriosis or endometrioid carcinoma of the ovary, and resemble clear cell carcinoma of the endometrium, they are now thought to be of müllerian duct origin and, indeed, variants of endometrioid adenocarcinoma.[75]

The clear cell tumors of the ovary can be predominantly solid or cystic. In the solid neoplasm, the clear cells are arranged in sheets or tubules. In the cystic variety, the neoplastic cells line the spaces. The five-year survival rate is approximately 50% when the tumors are confined to the ovaries. Some patients with small, well-differentiated tumors may have no recurrence. With spread beyond the ovary, a survival of five years is exceptional.

Cystadenofibroma

The cystadenofibroma is essentially a variant of the serous cystadenoma in which there is more pronounced proliferation of the fibrous stroma that underlies the columnar lining epithelium. These benign tumors are usually small and multilocular and have rather simple papillary processes that do not become so complicated and branching as those found in the ordinary cystadenoma. The epithelial lining is usually quite regular. Carcinomatous transformation is rare. Borderline lesions with cellular atypia also occur, but their malignant potential is much less than that of borderline serous tumors.

Brenner Tumor

This usually solid ovarian neoplasm is characterized by a dense fibrous stroma punctuated by nests of transitional cells resembling those lining the urinary bladder. Less frequently, the nests contain microcysts or glandular spaces lined by columnar, mucin-secreting cells. Brenner tumors are uncommon and account for no more than 2% of ovarian neoplasms. As stated earlier, Brenner tumors are occasionally encountered in mucinous cystadenomas. This fact and other evidence suggest that these tumors arise from coelomic epithelial inclusion cysts through metaplasia of the cyst lining to transitional epithelium.[76]

These neoplasms are usually unilateral (approximately 90%) and vary in size from small lesions less than 1 cm in diameter to massive tumors up to 20 and 30 cm. Although generally solid, they occasionally are cystic. The fibrous stroma, resembling that of the normal ovary, is marked by sharply demarcated nests of epithelial cells (Fig. 24–49). The epithelial cells consist of solid nests resembling the epithelium of the urinary tract, often with mucinous glands in their center. Infrequently, the stroma is composed of somewhat plump fibroblasts resembling theca cells. Such neoplasms may have hormonal activity, and in support of such a notion are the reported instances of the concurrence of Brenner tumors and endometrial carcinoma. The vast majority of Brenner tumors are benign, but borderline and malignant counterparts have been reported.

Clinical Course of Surface Epithelial Tumors

All these tumors of the ovary tend to produce the same clinical manifestations. The two most prominent complaints are low abdominal pain and abdominal enlargement. Gastrointestinal complaints, urinary frequency, dysuria, pelvic pressure, and many other

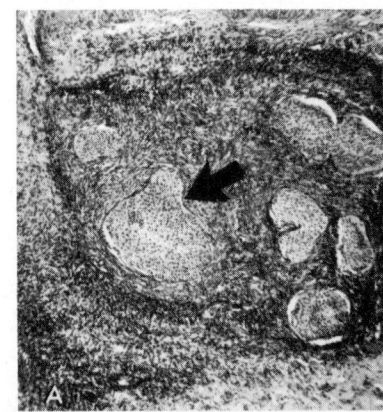
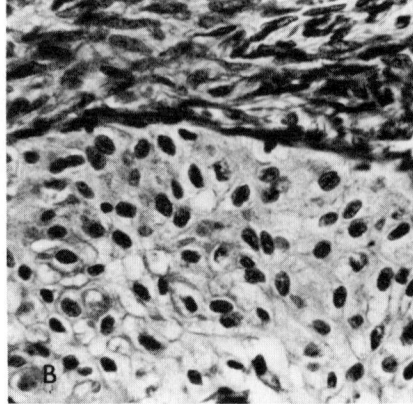

Figure 24–49. Brenner tumor. *A*, Low-power micrograph showing spindle cell component and nests of epithelial cells *(arrow)*. *B*, High-power detail of characteristic epithelial nests.

symptoms may appear. When benign, the lesions are easily resected with cure. However, the malignant forms tend to cause the progressive weakness, weight loss, and cachexia characteristic of all malignancies.

The carcinomas extend through the capsule of the tumor to seed the peritoneal cavity. Massive ascites is common with such dissemination to the abdominal cavity. Characteristically, this fluid is filled with diagnostic exfoliated tumor cells. The peritoneal seeding that these malignancies produce is quite distinctive: they tend to seed all serosal surfaces diffusely with 0.1- to 0.5-cm nodules of tumor. These surface implants rarely invade the underlying parenchyma of the organ. The regional nodes are often involved, and metastases may be found in the liver, lungs, gastrointestinal tract, and elsewhere. Metastasis across the midline to the opposite ovary is discovered in about half the cases by the time of laparotomy, and from this point the patients usually run a progressive downhill course to death within one to two years.

These tumors grow slowly and often remain undiagnosed until very large; thus, many patients with ovarian carcinoma are first seen with lesions that are no longer confined to the ovary. This is perhaps the primary reason for the relatively poor five- and ten-year survival rates for these patients, compared with rates in cervical and endometrial carcinoma. For these reasons, specific biochemical markers for tumor antigens or tumor products in the plasma of these patients are being sought vigorously. One such marker is a high molecular weight glycoprotein present in over 80% of serous and endometrioid carcinomas, known as CA-125, and detected by a monoclonal antibody (OC 125).[77]

GERM CELL TUMORS

Germ cell tumors represent 15 to 20% of all ovarian tumors.[78] The vast majority (95%) are benign cystic teratomas, but the remainder, *which are found principally in children and young adults*, have a higher incidence of malignant behavior and pose problems in histologic diagnosis and in therapy. They bear a remarkable homology to germ tumors in the male testis (p. 1108), and arise from germ cell differentiation in a similar manner (see Fig. 25–50).

Teratomas

Teratomas are divided into three categories: (1) mature (benign), (2) immature (malignant), and (3) monodermal or highly specialized.

MATURE (BENIGN) TERATOMAS. The vast majority of benign teratomas are cystic and are better known in clinical parlance as *dermoid cysts*. This designation alludes to the fact that they are lined by apparent skin with all of its associated adnexal structures and are typically filled with a sebaceous cheesy secretion in which is found matted hair. These neoplasms are invariably benign and are presumably derived from the ectodermal differentiation of totipotential

GERM CELL

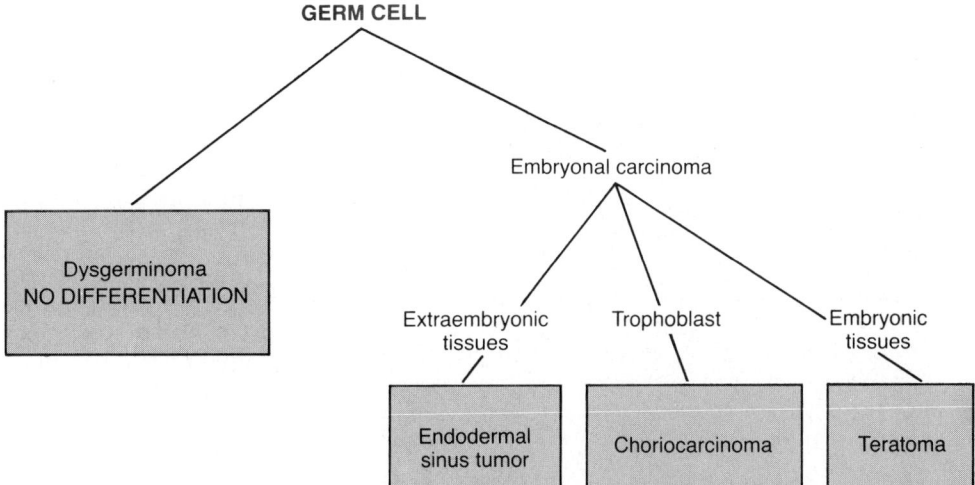

Dysgerminoma
NO DIFFERENTIATION

Embryonal carcinoma

Extraembryonic tissues

Trophoblast

Embryonic tissues

Endodermal sinus tumor

Choriocarcinoma

Teratoma

Figure 24–50. Histogenesis and interrelationships of tumors of germ cell origin.

cells. Cystic teratomas are usually found in young women during the active reproductive years.

The tumors are bilateral in 10 to 15% of cases. Characteristically, they are unilocular cysts that on section have a thin wall lined by an opaque, gray-white, wrinkled, apparent epidermis. From this epidermis, hair shafts frequently protrude. Within the wall, it is common to find tooth structures and areas of calcification. The lumen of the cyst is filled with a sebaceous secretion that is admixed with strands of hair (Fig. 24–51).

Histologically, the cyst wall is composed of stratified squamous epithelium with underlying sebaceous glands, hair shafts, and other skin adnexal structures (Fig. 24–52). In most cases, structures from other germ layers can be identified, such as cartilage, bone, thyroid tissue, and other organoid formations (Fig. 24–53). Dermoid cysts are sometimes incorporated within the wall of a mucinous cystadenoma. **About 1% of the dermoids undergo malignant transformation of any one of the component elements —e.g., thyroid carcinoma, melanoma—but most commonly squamous cell carcinoma.**

In rare instances, a teratoma is **solid** but is composed entirely of benign-looking heterogeneous collections of tissues and organized structures derived from all three germ layers. These tumors presumably have the same histogenetic origin as dermoid cysts but lack preponderant differentiation into ectodermal derivatives. These neoplasms behave in a benign fashion and can be adequately treated by simple surgical extirpation. **They should be differentiated from the malignant, immature teratomas, which almost always are largely solid.**

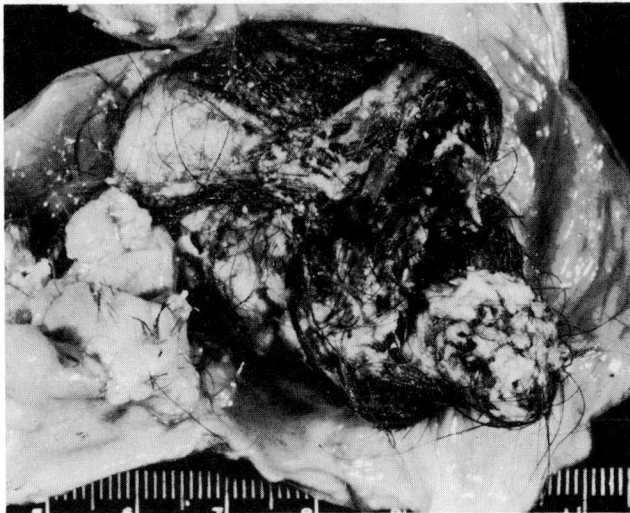

Figure 24–51. Opened dermoid cyst of ovary. Abundant hair and sebaceous material is evident.

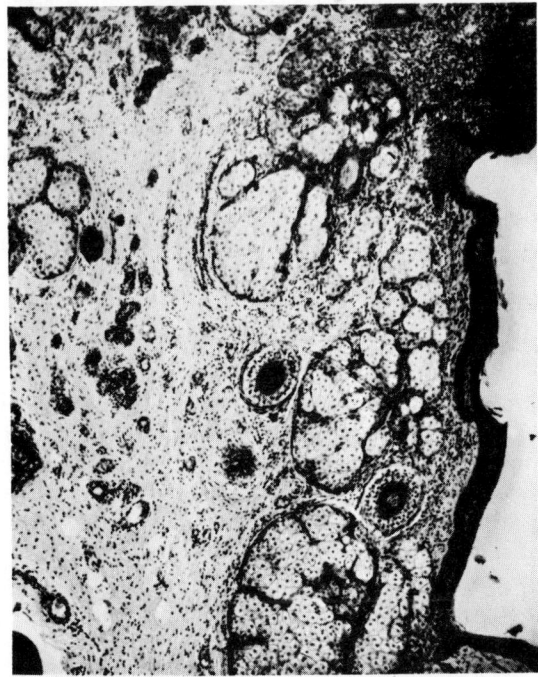

Figure 24–52. Dermoid cyst. Low-power view of lining epithelium, illustrating almost complete resemblance to skin. (Courtesy of Dr. Arthur Hertig.)

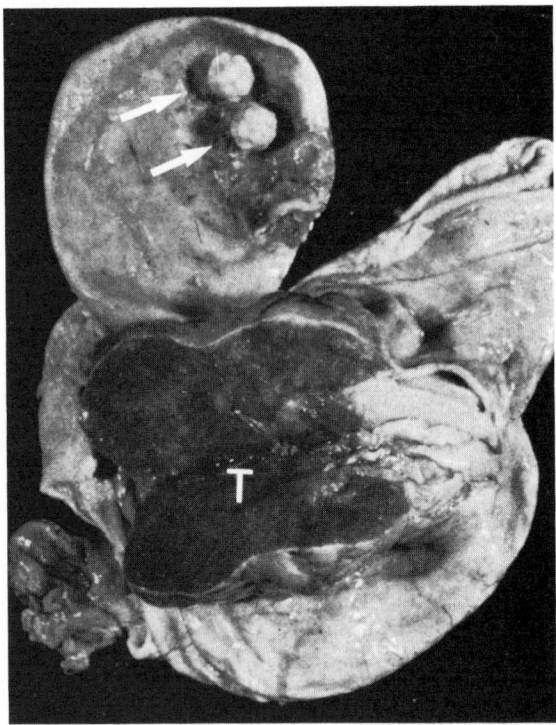

Figure 24–53. Dermoid cyst of ovary, opened to illustrate several abortive tooth structures *(arrows)* and a darker area of thyroid substance (T).

The clinical symptoms are those of all ovarian neoplasms, i.e., abdominal pain, mass, and occasionally, gastrointestinal complaints or disturbances in the menstrual cycle. There is a higher than usual rate of sterility. Torsion, rupture, infection, and an unexplained autoimmune anemia may complicate the picture. These tumors are resectable and curable.

The origin of teratomas has been a matter of fascination for centuries. Some common beliefs blamed witches, nightmares, or adultery with the devil. The current *parthenogenetic* theory suggests origin from a primordial germ cell. The karyotypes of all benign ovarian teratomas are 46,XX. From the results of chromosome-banding techniques and the distribution of electrophoretic variants of enzymes in the normal and teratoma cells, Linder and his group[80] suggested that tumors arise from an ovum after the first meiotic division. Other derivations have been proposed.[80a]

IMMATURE (MALIGNANT) TERATOMAS. These are rare tumors composed of a wide variety of tissue elements in varying stages of differentiation, but they differ from benign teratomas in that *embryonic* (rather than adult) *elements* derived from more than one of the three germ layers are usually present. The tumor is found chiefly in prepubertal adolescents and young women, the mean age being 18.[81]

The tumors are bulky and have a smooth external surface. On section they have a solid or predominantly solid structure. There are areas of necrosis and hemorrhage. Hair, grumous material, cartilage, bone, and calcification may be present. Microscopically, there are varying amounts of immature tissue differentiating toward cartilage, glands, bone, muscle, nerve, and others. The main determinant of extraovarian spread in immature teratomas is the histologic grade of tumor (I–III), which depends primarily on the degree of immaturity of various elements and the presence of neuroepithelium (Fig. 24–54).

Immature teratoma is a malignant tumor that usually grows rapidly and penetrates its capsule early. Spread and metastases are common. With grade I histology and tumors confined to the ovary, the survival rate is excellent, but most patients when seen have advanced tumor, and thus the overall five-year survival rate is poor.

In some cases there is coexistence of immature teratoma with other germ cell tumors (choriocarcinoma, endodermal sinus tumor, and embryonal carcinoma).

MONODERMAL OR SPECIALIZED TERATOMAS. The specialized teratomas are a remarkable group of tumors, the most common of which are *struma ovarii* and *carcinoid.* Struma ovarii is composed entirely of mature thyroid tissue. Interestingly, these thyroidal neoplasms may hyperfunction, producing hyperthyroidism. The ovarian carcinoid, which presumably arises from intestinal epithelium in a teratoma, might in fact be functioning, producing 5-hydroxytryptamine and the carcinoid syndrome. Primary ovarian

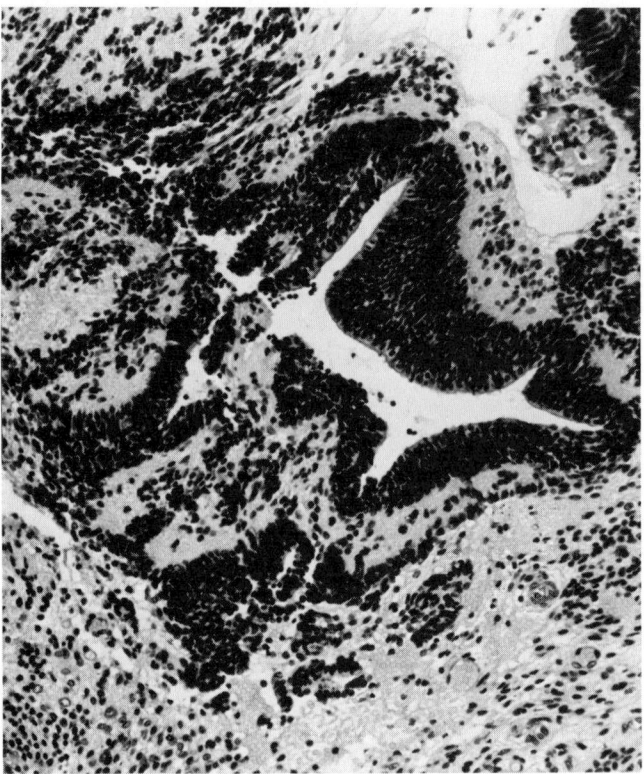

Figure 24–54. Immature teratoma of ovary, illustrating primitive neuroepithelium. (Courtesy of Dr. Janice Lage.)

carcinoid must be distinguished from ovarian metastasis of an intestinal carcinoid. Most fascinating is the *strumal carcinoid*, a combination of struma ovarii and carcinoid in the same ovary.

Dysgerminoma

The dysgerminoma[82] is best remembered as the ovarian counterpart of the seminoma of the testis. Like the latter, it is composed of large vesicular cells having a cleared cytoplasm, well-defined cell boundaries, and centrally placed regular nuclei. Relatively uncommon tumors, the dysgerminomas account for about 2% of all ovarian cancers, yet form about half of malignant germ cell tumors. They may occur in childhood, but 75% occur in the second and third decades. Some occur in patients with gonadal dysgenesis, including pseudohermaphroditism. Most of these tumors have no endocrine function. A few produce elevated levels of chorionic gonadotropin and may have syncytiotrophoblastic giant cells on histologic examination.

Usually unilateral (80 to 90%), they most frequently are solid tumors, ranging in size from barely visible nodules to masses that virtually fill the entire abdomen. On cut surface, they have a yellow-white to gray-pink appearance and are often soft and fleshy. Histologically, the dysgerminoma cells are dispersed in sheets or cords separated by scant fibrous stroma. As in the seminoma, the fibrous stroma is infiltrated with mature lymphocytes and occasional granulomas. Occasionally, small nodules of dysgerminoma are encountered in the wall of an otherwise benign cystic teratoma; conversely, predominantly dysgerminomatous tumor may contain a small cystic teratoma.

All dysgerminomas are malignant, but the degree of histologic atypia is variable and only about one-third are aggressive. Thus, a unilateral tumor that has not broken through the capsule and has not spread has an excellent prognosis (up to 96% cure rate) after simple salpingo-oophorectomy. These neoplasms are radiosensitive, and even those that have extended beyond the ovary can generally be controlled by radiotherapy.

Endodermal Sinus (Yolk Sac) Tumor

This tumor is rare but is the second most common malignant tumor of germ cell origin. It is thought to be derived from a multipotential embryonal carcinoma by selection and differentiation toward yolk sac structures[74] (see Fig. 24–50). Like the yolk sac, the tumor is rich in alpha-fetoprotein and alpha-1-antitrypsin. Its characteristic histologic feature, papillary projections composed of a central blood vessel enveloped by immature epithelium, is a recapitulation of the yolk sac endodermal sinus of Duval of the rat placenta. Conspicuous intracellular and extracellular hyaline droplets are present in all tumors, and some of these can be stained for alpha-fetoprotein by immunoperoxidase techniques.

Most patients are children or young women presenting with abdominal pain and a pelvic mass.

The tumors grow rapidly and aggressively, and once were almost uniformly fatal within two years of diagnosis, but recent combination chemotherapy has measurably improved the outcome.

Choriocarcinoma

More commonly of placental origin, the choriocarcinoma may arise in the ovary from the teratogenous development of germ cells. It is generally held that such an origin can be certified only in the prepubertal girl, because after this age the neoplasm may well have arisen in an ovarian ectopic pregnancy.

Most ovarian choriocarcinomas exist in combination with other germ cell tumors, and pure choriocarcinomas are extremely rare. Histologically, they are identical with the more common placental lesions (p. 1176). These ovarian primaries are ugly tumors that generally have metastasized widely through the blood stream to the lungs, liver, bone, and other viscera by the time of diagnosis.

As with all choriocarcinomas, they elaborate high levels of chorionic gonadotropins that are sometimes helpful in establishing the diagnosis or highlighting recurrences. In contrast to choriocarcinomas arising in placental tissue, those arising in the ovary are highly fatal cancers.

Other Germ Cell Tumors

These include (1) *embryonal carcinoma*, another highly malignant tumor of primitive embryonal elements, histologically similar to tumors arising in the testes (p. 1110); (2) *polyembryoma*, a malignant tumor containing so-called embryoid bodies (p. 1112); and (3) *mixed germ cell tumors* containing various combinations of dysgerminoma, teratoma, endodermal sinus tumor, and choriocarcinoma.

SEX CORD–STROMAL TUMORS

Included in this category are all ovarian neoplasms originating either from the sex cords of the embryonic gonad (which precede the differentiation of gonadal mesenchyme into male or female) or from the stroma of the ovary.[83] Thus, granulosa cell, theca cell, and luteal cell neoplasms having such histogenetic origins fall within this category. Moreover, because theca cells are the source of ovarian steroids, many of these neoplasms are functional and have feminizing effects. The embryonic sex cords may differentiate along masculine lines to give rise to Sertoli-Leydig cell tumors, also known as androblastomas or arrhenoblastomas. However, some of these Sertoli-Leydig cell tumors either have no function or have estrogenic effects.

Granulosa-Theca Cell Tumors

This designation embraces ovarian neoplasms composed of varying proportions of granulosa cells and theca cells, which may be luteinized. At one end of the spectrum are tumors composed almost entirely of granulosa cells, *granulosa cell tumors*, and at the other are pure *thecomas*. Collectively, these neoplasms account for about 5% of all ovarian tumors. Although they may be discovered at any age, approximately two thirds occur in postmenopausal women.

Granulosa cell tumors are usually unilateral and vary from microscopic foci to large, solid, and cystic encapsulated masses. Tumors that are endocrinologically active have a yellow coloration to their cut surfaces, produced by contained lipids. The pure thecomas are solid-firm tumors.

The granulosa cell component of these tumors takes one of many histologic patterns. The small, cuboidal-to-polygonal cells may grow in anastomosing cords, sheets, or strands. In occasional cases, small, distinctive, glandlike structures filled with an acidophilic material recall immature follicles (Call-Exner bodies) (Fig. 24–55). When these structures are evident, the diagnosis is rendered considerably more simple. In the thecoma component, the cells may be disposed in large sheets of cuboidal-to-polygonal cells that gradually change into plump spindle cells resembling the theca lutein cells.

Pure thecomas are composed of large sheets or poorly defined areas of plump spindle cells that closely resemble those of the fibroma (Fig. 24–56). The distinction between the theca cell and the fibrocyte cannot be made with certainty. Characteristically, theca cells contain lipid droplets, but only clinical or biochemical evidence of hormone production by the tumor distinguishes functional theca cells from fibroblasts.

These tumors have clinical importance for two reasons: (1) their potential elaboration of large amounts of estrogen and (2) the definite hazard of malignancy in the granulosa cell forms. Functionally active tumors (usually those having a large thecal component) may produce precocious sexual development in prepubertal girls. In adult women, they may be associated with endometrial hyperplasia, cystic disease of the breast, and endometrial carcinoma. About 10 to 15% of patients with steroid-producing tumors eventually develop an endometrial carci-

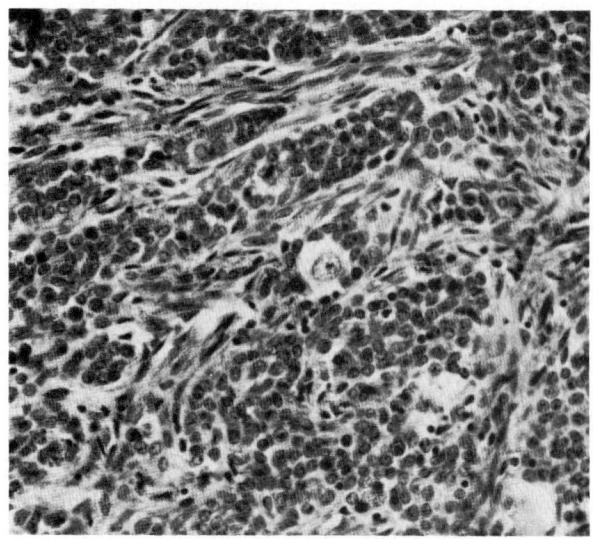

Figure 24–55. Granulosa cell tumor.

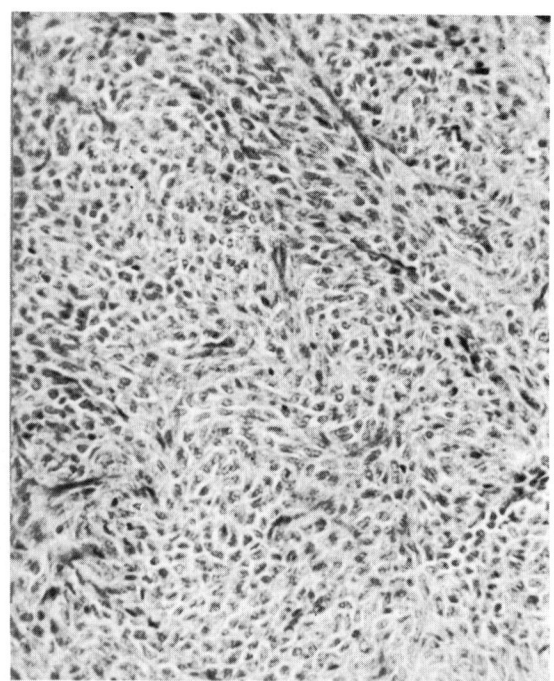

Figure 24–56. Theca luteoma composed of plump, differentiated stromal cells. Note resemblance to a fibroma. (Courtesy of Dr. Arthur Hertig and Armed Forces Institute of Pathology.)

noma. Occasional granulosa cell tumors produce androgens, masculinizing the patient.

The additional clinical significance of these tumors lies in the fact that all are potentially malignant. It is difficult, from the histologic evaluation of granulosa cell tumors, to predict their biologic behavior.[84] The estimates of clinical malignancy (recurrence, extension) range from 5 to 25%, but recurrences are amenable to surgical therapy. Recurrences are within the pelvis and abdomen and may appear many years (10 to 20) after removal of the original tumor. The ten-year survival rate is approximately 85%. *Tumors composed predominantly of theca cells are almost never malignant.*

Fibroma

Fibromas arising in the ovarian stroma are a relatively common form of ovarian neoplasm and account for about 4% of all types. Some are pure fibromas, but others contain theca elements and are termed fibrothecomas. Pure fibromas are nonfunctioning.

The fibromas of the ovary are unilateral in about 90% of cases and usually are solid, spherical, or slightly lobulated, encapsulated, hard, gray-white masses covered by glistening, intact ovarian serosa (Fig. 24–57). Histologically, they are composed of well-differentiated fibroblasts with a more or less scant collagenous connective tissue interspersed between the cells.

In addition to the relatively nonspecific findings of pain and pelvic mass, the tumors may be accompanied by two curious associations. The first is *ascites*, found in about 40% of cases, in which the tumors measure more than 6 cm in diameter. Uncommonly, there is also hydrothorax, usually only of the right side. This combination of findings, i.e., *ovarian tumor, hydrothorax, and ascites*, is designated *Meigs' syndrome.* The genesis is unknown. The second association is with the *basal cell nevus syndrome*, described on p. 1288. Rare fibrous tumors with few or no mitotic figures per ten high-power fields have a malignant course and are regarded as fibrosarcomas.[85]

Sertoli-Leydig Cell Tumors (Androblastoma)

These tumors recapitulate, to a certain extent, the cells of the testis at various stages of development.[86] They commonly produce masculinization or at least defeminization, but a few have estrogenic effects. They occur in women of all ages, although the peak incidence is in the second and third decades. The embryogenesis of such male-directed stromal cells remains a puzzle.

These tumors are unilateral and resemble granulosa-theca cell neoplasms. The cut surface is usually gray-white and solid.

Histologically, the well-differentiated tumors exhibit tubules composed of Sertoli cells or Leydig cells interspersed with stroma (Fig. 24–58). The intermediate forms show only outlines of immature tubules and large eosinophilic Leydig cells. The poorly differentiated tumors have a sarcomatous pattern with a disorderly disposition of epithelial cell cords. Leydig cells may be absent. Heterologous elements, such as mucinous glands, bone, and cartilage, may be present in some tumors.

The incidence of recurrence or metastasis by Sertoli-Leydig cell tumors is less than 5%. These neo-

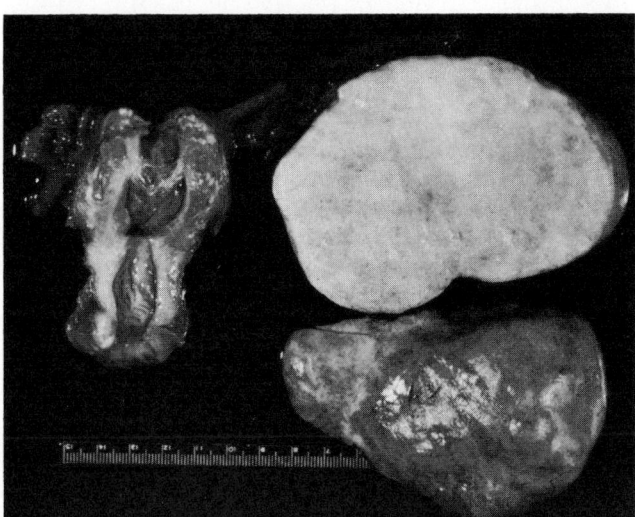

Figure 24–57. Large bisected fibroma of ovary apparent as a white, firm mass *(right).* **The uterus is to the left.**

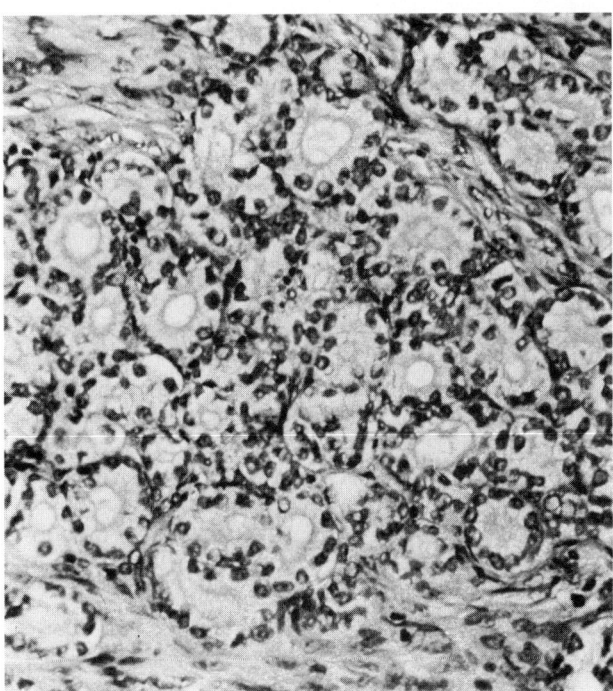

Figure 24–58. Sertoli cell tumor showing well-differentiated Sertoli cell tubules. (Courtesy of Dr. Noel Weidner.)

plasms may block normal female sexual development in children and may cause defeminization of adult females, manifested by atrophy of the breasts, amenorrhea, sterility, and loss of hair. The syndrome may progress to striking virilization, i.e., hirsutism, male distribution of hair, hypertrophy of the clitoris, and voice changes.

Other Sex Cord–Stromal Tumors

Hilus cell tumor (pure Leydig cell tumor) is rare and is characterized histologically by large, lipid-laden cells with distinct borders; ultrastructurally by the presence of Reinke crystals typical of Leydig cells, and a granular cytoplasm; and clinically by evidence of masculinization, with hirsutism, voice changes, and clitoral enlargement. The tumors are unilateral. The most consistent laboratory finding is an elevated 17-ketosteroid excretion level unresponsive to cortisone suppression. Treatment is surgical excision. True hilus cell tumors are almost always benign. Occasionally such pure Leydig cell tumors occur in the stroma, not in the hilus (nonhilar Leydig cell tumor).

Stromal luteoma is a small, benign tumor rarely over 3 cm in diameter composed of pure lutein cells. The tumor may produce the clinical effects of androgen, estrogen, or progestogen stimulation.

Pregnancy luteoma is a specific lesion, almost certainly not a neoplasm, occurring in women in the last trimester of pregnancy or immediately post partum. The cells resemble those of the corpus luteum of pregnancy, being large and eosinophilic but with little fat. They have been associated with virilization in the pregnant patients and in female infants born to some of the patients.

Lipid cell tumor is an imprecise term used for ovarian tumors with large, vacuolated cells that cannot be clearly categorized as Leydig cell tumors (hilar or stromal), stromal luteoma, or pregnancy luteoma. Malignancy is found in 25% of such tumors, but no histologic criteria have proved useful in predicting their metastatic potential. They are frequently virilizing.

Gonadoblastoma is an uncommon tumor thought to be composed of germ cells and sex cord–stroma derivatives. It occurs in individuals with abnormal sexual development and in gonads of indeterminate nature. Patients usually present with amenorrhea, virilization, and abnormal genitalia. Eighty per cent are phenotypic females and 20% are phenotypic males with undescended testicles and female internal secondary organs. This neoplasm has also been observed in hermaphrodites and among phenotypic females with normal menstrual cycles. Microscopically, the tumor consists of nests of a mixture of germ cells and sex cord derivatives resembling immature Sertoli and granulosa cells. A coexistent dysgerminoma occurs in 50% of the cases. The prognosis is excellent if the tumor is completely excised.

METASTATIC TUMORS

The ovary is more often involved by metastatic processes than any of the other pelvic genital organs. Three groups of malignancies contribute to high incidence: carcinomas arising within the other pelvic organs; carcinomas arising in the upper gastrointestinal tract, i.e., stomach, biliary tract, and pancreas; and carcinoma of the breast. The term Krukenberg tumor is sometimes applied to bilateral metastatic ovarian tumors composed of mucin-producing, signet-ring cancer cells, and the vast majority of such metastases are of gastric origin and cause massive enlargement of the ovaries.

GESTATIONAL AND PLACENTAL DISORDERS

Diseases of pregnancy and pathologic conditions of the placenta are important causes of intrauterine or perinatal death, congenital malformations, intrauterine growth retardation, maternal death, and a great deal of morbidity for both mother and child.[7,88] Here we shall discuss only a limited number of disorders in which knowledge of the morphologic lesions contributes to an understanding of the clinical problem.

PLACENTAL INFLAMMATIONS AND INFECTIONS

Infections may occur in the placenta *(placentitis, villitis)*,[89] in the fetal membranes *(chorioamnionitis)*, and in the umbilical cord *(funisitis)*.[90] They reach the placenta by two pathways: (1) ascending infection through the birth canal and (2) hematogenous (transplacental) infection. *Ascending infections* are by far the most common and are most often bacterial; in almost all such instances, premature rupture of the membranes provides the portal of entry for the organisms. Sexual intercourse has been implicated in enhancing ascending infections.[91] The amniotic fluid may be cloudy and contains purulent exudate. The chorioamnion is histologically the site of a leukocytic polymorphonuclear infiltration with accompanying edema and congestion of the vessels. When the infection extends beyond the membranes, it may involve the umbilical cord and placental villi with similar inflammatory changes. In the umbilical cord, in particular, there is often acute vasculitis.

Uncommonly, bacterial infections of the placenta and fetal membranes may arise by the *hematogenous spread* of bacteria, and under these circumstances the fetal membranes may be intact; histologically, the villi are most often affected (villitis).

Syphilis, tuberculosis, listeriosis, toxoplasmosis, candidiasis, and various viral (rubella, cytomegalovirus, herpes simplex) and mycoplasma infections can also affect the placenta. Villous inflammation may also occur without obvious cause, but infections or environmental factors are suspected.[92]

PLACENTAL ABNORMALITIES AND TWIN PLACENTAS

Abnormalities in placental shape, structure, and implantation are not uncommon. Accessory placental lobes, bipartite placenta (placenta made up of two equal segments), and *circumvallate* placenta (having an extrachorial part) are examples of abnormalities that have limited clinical significance.

Placenta accreta[93] denotes abnormal adherence of the placenta to the uterine wall, such that separation does not occur after delivery. *It is caused by partial or complete absence of the decidua.* It is important for two reasons: (1) postpartum bleeding, often life-threatening, occurs because of failure of placental separation; (2) in up to 60% of cases it is associated with *placenta previa*, a condition in which the placenta implants in the lower uterine segment or cervix. Placenta previa can cause serious antepartum bleeding and premature labor. Many cases of *placenta previa-associated accreta* occur in cesarean section scars.

TWIN PLACENTATION. As should be well known, twins arise from fertilization of two ova (dizygotic) or from division of one fertilized ovum (monozygotic). There are four basic types of twin placentas.[94] Dizygotic twins will have *dichorionic, diamniotic* placentas, which however, may occasionally be fused when the implantations are close together. *Monozygotic twins* have either dichorionic placentas, as described, or monochorionic placentas. *Monochorionic* placentas, depending on the time at which splitting occurs, result in two separate amnions *(monoorionic, diamniotic)* or one single amniotic sac *(monoorionic, monoamniotic)* (Fig. 24–59).

SPONTANEOUS ABORTION

Ten to 15% of *recognized* pregnancies terminate in spontaneous abortion. However, recent studies using highly sensitive immunoassay of chorionic gonadotropin to detect pregnancy identified an additional 22% loss of presumably fertilized and implanted ova in otherwise healthy women.[95] The causes for this early loss of pregnancy are still mysterious, but as one good writer said, "There's many a slip 'twixt implantation and the crib." [96]

The causes of *recognized* spontaneous abortion are both fetal and maternal. Defective implantation inadequate to support fetal development, and death of the ovum or fetus in utero because of some genetic or acquired abnormality constitute the major origins of spontaneous abortion. Numerous studies have indicated bizarre chromosomal abnormalities in over one-half of spontaneous abortuses.[97]

Maternal influences, which are less well understood, include inflammatory diseases, both localized

to the placenta and systemic, uterine abnormalities, and possibly trauma. The role of trauma is generally overemphasized and must be considered a rare-to-exceptional trigger of spontaneous abortion. Toxoplasma, mycoplasma, listeria, and viral infections have also been implicated as causes of abortion.

> The morphologic changes usually seen in endometrial curettage specimens depend, of course, on the interval between fetal death and passage of the products of conception.[98] Generally, there are focal areas of decidual necrosis with intense neutrophilic infiltrations, thromboses within decidual blood vessels, and considerable amounts of hemorrhage, both recent and old, within the necrotic decidua. Placental villi may be markedly edematous and devoid of blood vessels. The changes encountered in the ovum or fetus are highly variable. In many spontaneous abortions, no fetal products can be identified, but when they are present, they should be carefully examined for anomalies that would suggest specific genetic or karyotypic defects.

As indicated earlier, chromosomal studies often yield striking abnormalities in many of the defective fetuses. Such studies are recommended in three circumstances: (1) habitual or recurrent abortion; (2) after prenatal diagnosis of karyotypic abnormality; and (3) when there is a malformed fetus.

ECTOPIC PREGNANCY

Ectopic pregnancy is the term applied to implantation of the fetus in any site other than normal uterine location. The most common abnormal location is within the tubes (approximately 90%).[99] The other sites are the ovary, the abdominal cavity, and the intrauterine portion of the fallopian tube (interstitial pregnancy). Ectopic pregnancies occur about once in every 150 pregnancies. *The most important* predisposing condition in 35 to 50% of patients is pelvic inflammatory disease with chronic salpingitis. Other factors are peritubal adhesions due to appendicitis or endometriosis, leiomyomas, and previous surgery. Fifty per cent, however, occur in tubes that are apparently normal. Whether intrauterine contraceptive devices increase risk is controversial.

Ovarian pregnancy is presumed to result from the rare fertilization and trapping of the ovum within the follicle just at the time of its rupture. Abdominal pregnancies may develop when the fertilized ovum drops out of the fimbriated end of the tube. In all these abnormal locations, the fertilized ovum undergoes its usual development with the formation of placental tissue, amniotic sac, and fetus, and the host implantation site develops decidual changes.

In tubal pregnancy the placenta is poorly attached to the wall of the tube. *Intratubal hemorrhage* may thus occur from partial placental separation

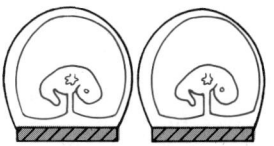

Dichorionic diamnionic   Dichorionic diamnionic (fused)

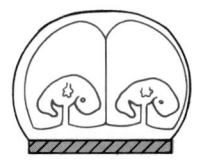

Monochorionic diamnionic   Monochorionic monoamnionic

—— Chorion —— Amnion ▨ Placenta

Figure 24–59. Diagrammatic representation of the various types of twin placentation and their membrane relationships. (Adapted from Gersell, D., et al.: *In* Kurman, R. (ed.): Blaustein's Pathology of the Female Genital Tract. New York, Springer-Verlag, 1987.)

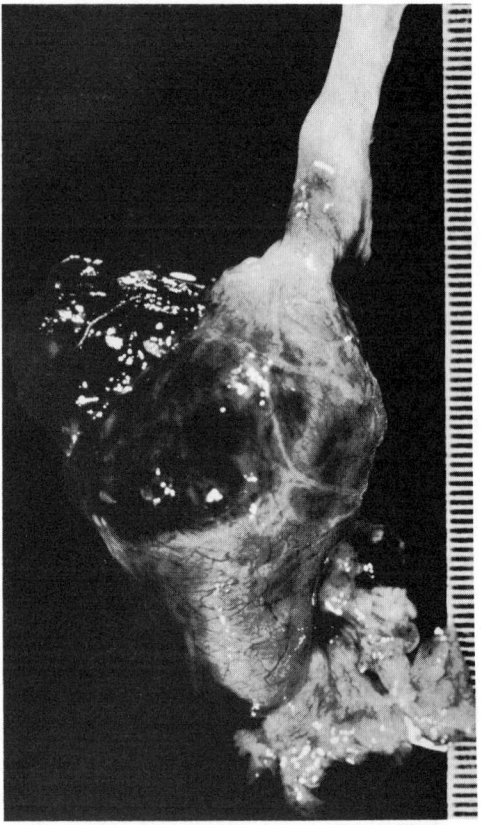

Figure 24–60. Tubal pregnancy with marked dilatation and rupture of distal end of tube by the contained pregnancy and subsequent hemorrhage.

without tubal rupture (Fig. 24–60). Tubal pregnancy is the most common cause of hematosalpinx, and when such intratubal hemorrhage is found, this underlying cause should always be suspected. More often the burrowing placental tissue invades the wall, weakens the tubal wall, and causes *tubal rupture and intraperitoneal hemorrhage*. This is the usual fate of tubal pregnancies, commonly occurring two to six weeks after onset of pregnancy. Less commonly, the tubal pregnancy may undergo *spontaneous regression* and resorption of the entire gestation. Still less commonly, the tubal pregnancy is extruded through the fimbriated end into the abdominal cavity *(tubal abortion)*.

The clinical course of ectopic pregnancy is punctuated by the onset of severe abdominal pain when rupture of the tube leads to a pelvic hemorrhage. Very often, with tubal rupture, the patient rapidly passes into a shocklike state accompanied by all the classic signs of an acute abdomen. Early diagnosis becomes critical. Chorionic gonadotropin assays, ultrasound studies, and laparoscopy with endometrial biopsy may be helpful, since, decidual changes develop here in less than half the cases and, in the absence of chorionic villi, are consistent with ectopic pregnancy. It must be remembered that rupture of a tubal pregnancy constitutes a medical emergency.

TOXEMIA OF PREGNANCY (PRE-ECLAMPSIA AND ECLAMPSIA)

Toxemia of pregnancy refers to a symptom complex characterized by hypertension, proteinuria, and edema (pre-eclampsia). It occurs in about 6% of pregnant women, usually in the last trimester, and more commonly in primiparas than in multiparas. Certain of these patients become more seriously ill, developing frank coma, and some have episodes of convulsions. To this more severe form, the term *eclampsia* is applied. Patients with eclampsia develop *disseminated intravascular coagulation* (DIC) with lesions in the liver, kidneys, heart, placenta, and sometimes the brain. This is not true of all cases. Moreover, there is no absolute correlation between the severity of eclampsia and the magnitude of the anatomic changes.

PATHOGENESIS. The many theories on the nature of toxemia of pregnancy[100] are beyond our scope, and only brief comments will be made on the three events that seem to be of prime importance in this disorder: *hypertension, placental ischemia,* and *DIC* (Fig. 24–61).

The mechanism of *toxemic hypertension* appears to involve the renin-angiotensin mechanism and prostaglandins. Normal pregnant women develop a resistance to the vasoconstrictive and hypertensive effects of angiotensin, but women with toxemia lose such resistance, developing a tendency to hypertension. *Prostaglandins* of the E series, produced in the uteroplacental vascular bed during pregnancy, are thought to mediate the normal resistance of pregnant women to angiotensin, and prostaglandin production is indeed decreased in the placenta of toxemic women. Thus, the increase in angiotensin hypersensitivity, characteristic of toxemia, may be due to *decreased synthesis of prostaglandin*. There is also evidence that renin production by the toxemic placenta is increased, another potentially vasoconstrictive event.

The initial cause of the hormonal disturbances (decreased prostaglandins, increased renin) by the placenta is unclear, but clinical and experimental data suggest that *reduced uteroplacental blood flow* and consequent *placental ischemia* are early events that mark the critical point for the development of symptoms and lesions of eclampsia.[101] A possible explanation for such reduced flow may lie in the vascular changes occurring in the uterine spiral arteries, consisting of fibrinoid necrosis and accumulation of foamy macrophages in the necrotic vessel wall, a condition called *acute atherosis* (Fig. 24–62). Because these vascular changes are similar to those that occur in immunologic reactions (such as allograft rejection), an immunologic basis for the initial vascular lesion in uteroplacental vessels has been suggested.

As to the pathogenesis of *DIC* in toxemia, endothelial damage, abnormalities in the levels and activi-

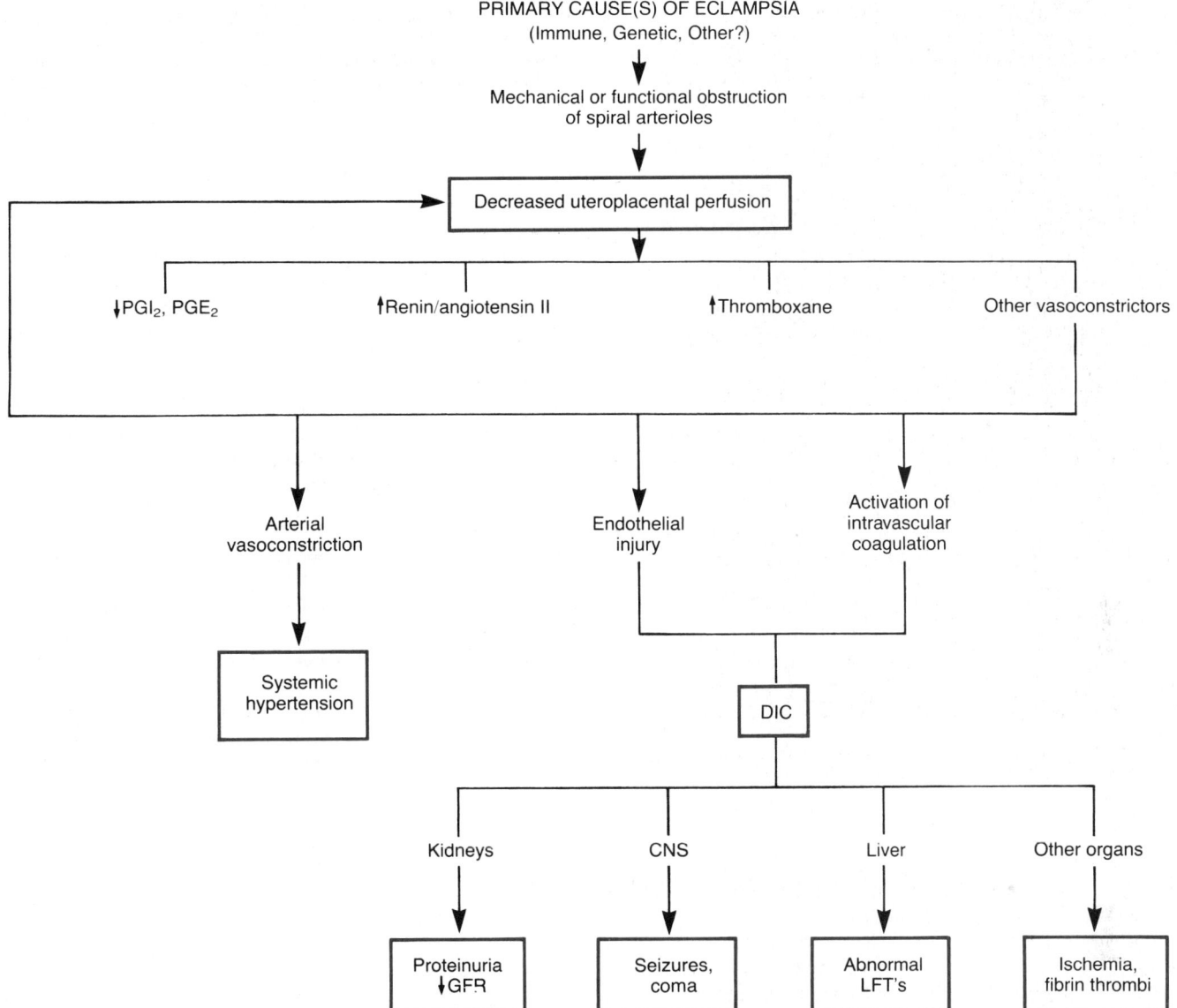

Figure 24–61. Proposed sequence of events in the pathogenesis of toxemia of pregnancy. The main features are: 1) decreased uteroplacental perfusion, 2) increased vasoconstrictors and decreased vasodilators, resulting in local and systemic vasoconstriction, and 3) disseminated intravascular coagulation (DIC). (Adapted from Friedman, S. A., Obstet. Gynecol., 71:122, 1988. Reprinted by permission of The American College of Obstetricians and Gynecologists.)

ties of coagulation factors, and primary platelet alterations may play a role.[102] For example, during toxemia the placental ischemia leads to a higher output of thromboplastic substances, and antithrombin III levels are reduced. Antiplatelet agents have beneficial effects. The characteristic lesions in eclampsia are in large part due to thrombosis of arterioles and capillaries throughout the body, particularly in the liver, kidneys, brain, pituitary, and placenta.

Figure 24–61 presents a hypothetical schema for the pathogenesis of eclampsia.

MORPHOLOGY. The **liver** lesions, when present, take the form of irregular, focal, subcapsular, and intraparenchymal hemorrhages. On histologic examination, there are fibrin thrombi in the portal capillaries with foci of characteristic peripheral hemorrhagic necrosis.

The **kidney** lesions are variable. Glomerular lesions are diffuse, at least when assessed by electron microscopy. They consist of striking swelling of endothelial cells, the deposition of fibrinogen-derived amorphous dense deposits on the endothelial side of the basement membrane, and mesangial cell hyperplasia. Immunofluorescent studies confirm the abundance of fibrin in glomeruli. In the more well-defined cases, fibrin thrombi are present in the glomeruli and capillaries of the cortex. These lead to microinfarcts throughout the cortex. When the lesion is far advanced, it may produce complete destruction of the cortex in the pattern referred to as bilateral renal cortical necrosis (p. 1070).

The **brain** may have gross or microscopic foci of hemor-

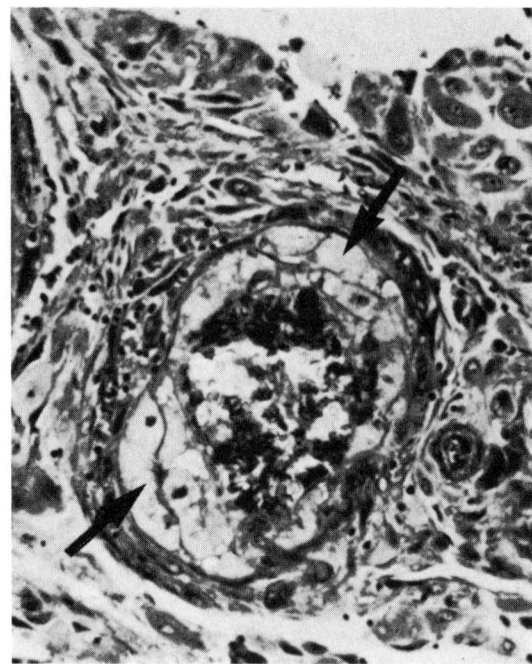

Figure 24–62. Acute atherosis of uterine vessels in eclampsia. Note foamy subendothelial macrophages *(arrows).*

rhage along with small-vessel thromboses. Similar changes are often found in the **heart** and the **anterior pituitary.**

The **placenta** is the site of variable changes. (1) Placental infarcts, which occur in normal full-term placentas, are larger and more numerous. (2) There is increased frequency of retroplacental hematomas. (3) There is increased evidence of villous ischemia: formation of prominent syncytial knots, thickening of trophoblastic basement membrane, and villous hypovascularity. (4) Alterations in the walls of **uterine** vessels, characterized by fibrinoid necrosis and intramural lipid deposition (acute atherosis) (see Fig. 24–62).

CLINICAL COURSE. *Pre-eclampsia* usually starts after the 32nd week of pregnancy, but begins earlier in patients with hydatidiform mole or pre-existing kidney disease or hypertension. The onset is usually insidious, characterized by hypertension and edema, with proteinuria following within several days. Headaches and visual disturbances are common. *Eclampsia* is heralded by central nervous system involvement, including convulsions and eventual coma. Mild and moderate forms of toxemia can be controlled by bed rest, a balanced diet, and antihypertensive agents, but induction of delivery is the only definitive treatment of established pre-eclampsia and eclampsia. Proteinuria and hypertension usually disappear within one or two weeks after delivery, except in patients in whom these findings predated the pregnancy.

GESTATIONAL TROPHOBLASTIC DISEASE

Gestational trophoblastic disease (GTD) constitutes a spectrum of tumors and tumor-like conditions characterized by proliferation of pregnancy-associated trophoblastic tissue of progressive malignant potential. The lesions include the *hydatidiform mole (complete and partial), the invasive mole,* and the frankly malignant *choriocarcinoma.*[103] GTD is important for the following reasons:

1. The hydatidiform mole is a common complication of gestation, occurring about once in every 1000 to 2000 pregnancies.
2. It has become possible, by monitoring the circulating levels of human chorionic gonadotropin (HCG), to determine the early development of persistent trophoblastic disease.
3. Choriocarcinoma, once a dreaded and uniformly fatal complication, is now highly responsive to chemotherapy in most cases.

HYDATIDIFORM MOLE (COMPLETE AND PARTIAL)

Hydatidiform mole is characterized by cystic swelling of the chorionic villi, accompanied by variable trophoblastic proliferation. The most important reason for the correct recognition of true moles is that they are the most common precursors of choriocarcinoma.[104] Most patients present in the fourth or fifth month of pregnancy with vaginal bleeding and with a uterus that is usually, but not always, larger than expected for the duration of pregnancy. These moles can occur at any age during active reproductive life, but the risk is higher in pregnant women in their teens or between the ages of 40 and 50 years. For poorly explained reasons, the incidence varies considerably in different regions of the world: 1 in 1000 pregnancies in the United States, but 10 in 1000 in Indonesia.[105]

Table 24–4. Features of Complete versus Partial Hydatidiform Mole

FEATURE	COMPLETE MOLE	PARTIAL MOLE
Karyotype	46,XX (46,XY)	Triploid
Villous edema	All villi	Some villi
Trophoblast proliferation	Diffuse; circumferential	Focal; slight
Atypia	Often present	Absent
Serum HCG	Elevated	Less elevated
HCG in tissue	++++	+
Behavior	2% choriocarcinoma	Rare choriocarcinoma

TYPES AND PATHOGENESIS. Two types of benign, noninvasive moles—complete and partial—can be differentiated by histologic, cytogenetic, and flow cytometric studies (Table 24–4).[106–108]

In *complete (or classic mole)*, all or most of the villi are edematous and there is diffuse trophoblast hyperplasia. Cytogenetic studies of these moles show that over 90% have a 46,XX diploid pattern, all derived from the sperm (a phenomenon called *androgenesis*). They are presumed to be derived from fertilization, by a single sperm of an egg that has lost its chromosomes (Fig. 24–63A). The remaining 10% are from the fertilization of such an empty egg by two sperms (46,XX and 46,XY). In both circumstances, the embryo dies early and thus *complete moles show no fetal parts*.

In *partial moles*, some of the villi are edematous and others show only minor changes; the *trophoblastic proliferation is focal*. In these moles, the karyotype is triploid (e.g., 69,XXY) or even occasionally tetraploid 92,XXXY. The moles result from fertilization of an egg with two sperms, one bearing 23,X and the other 23,Y (Fig. 24–63B). The embryo is viable for weeks, and thus *fetal parts may be present* when the resultant mole is aborted. In contrast to complete moles, partial moles are rarely followed by choriocarcinoma.

MORPHOLOGY. In most instances, moles develop within the uterus, but they may occur in any ectopic site of pregnancy. When discovered, usually in the fourth or fifth month of gestation, the uterus is usually larger (but may be normal-sized, or even smaller) than anticipated for the duration of the pregnancy. The uterine cavity is filled with a delicate friable mass of thin-walled, translucent, cystic, grapelike structures (Fig. 24–64). Careful dissection may disclose a small, usually collapsed amniotic sac. Fetal parts

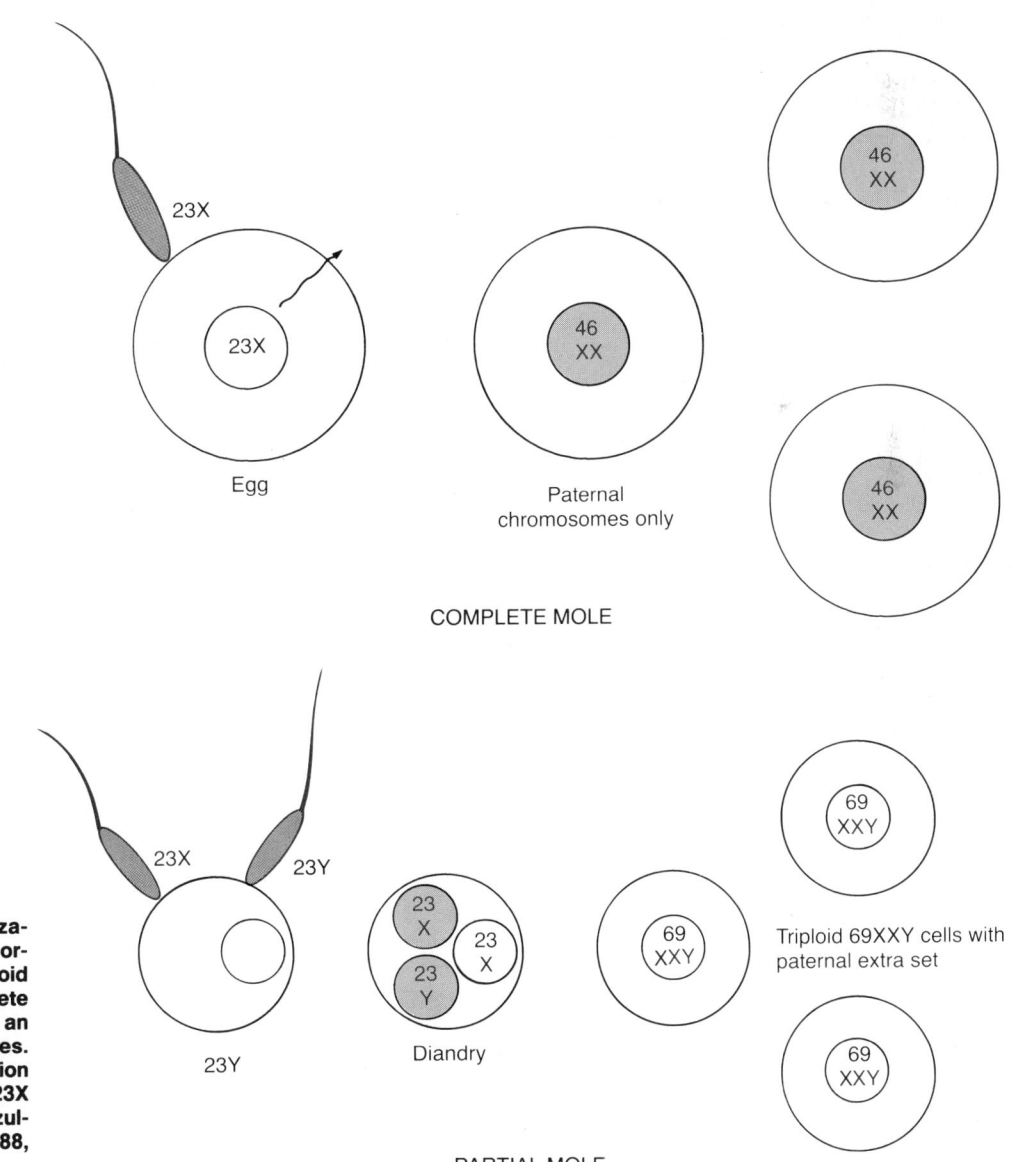

COMPLETE MOLE

PARTIAL MOLE

Figure 24–63. Patterns of fertilization to account for chromosomal origin of complete (46XX) and triploid partial moles (XXY). In a complete mole, a single sperm fertilizes an egg that has lost its chromosomes. Partial moles are due to fertilization of an egg by two sperms—one 23X and one 23Y. (Adapted from Szulman, A.E.: J. Reprod. Med. 29:288, 1984.)

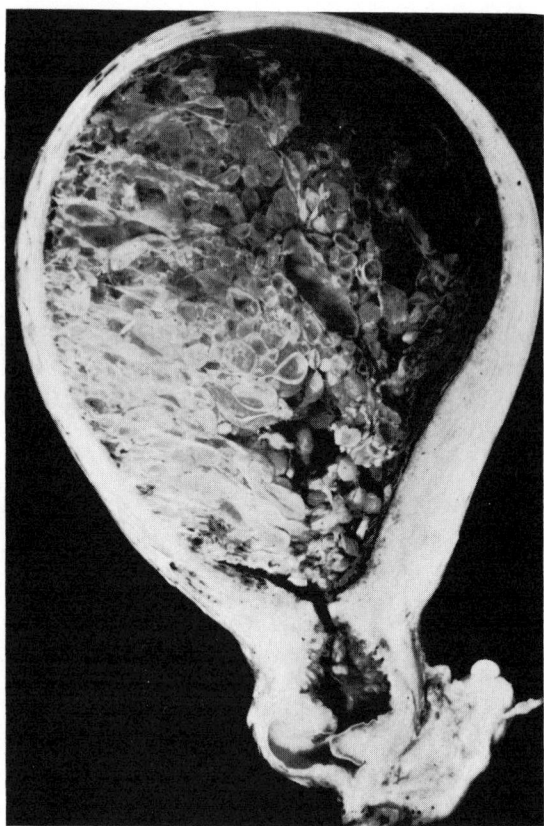

Figure 24–64. Hydatidiform mole. Uterus is filled with the classic mass of grapelike clusters. (Courtesy of Dr. Arthur Hertig. From Anderson, W.A.D.: Textbook of Pathology. St. Louis, C. V. Mosby Co., 1971.)

are rarely seen in complete moles but are more common in partial moles.

Microscopically, the **complete mole** shows hydropic swelling of chorionic villi and virtual absence or inadequate development of vascularization of villi. The central substance of the villi is a loose, myxomatous, edematous stroma, and they may be covered by a layer of chorionic epithelium, both cytotrophoblast and syncytial trophoblast (Fig. 24–65). At the opposite end of the spectrum are moles having similar cystic dilation of villi, accompanied, however, by circumferential and striking proliferation of the chorionic epithelium to produce sheets and masses of both cytotrophoblast and syncytial trophoblast. Histologic grading to predict the outcome of moles has been supplanted by careful following of the HCG levels.

In **partial moles** (Fig. 24–65*A*), the villous edema involves only a proportion of villi, and the trophoblastic proliferation is focal and slight.

CLINICAL COURSE. Most patients have abnormal uterine bleeding that usually begins early in the course of the pregnancy and is accompanied by the passage of a thin, watery fluid and bits of tissue seen as small, grapelike masses. The uterine enlargement is more rapid than anticipated. Ultrasound examination permits a definitive diagnosis in most cases.

In the classic case, quantitative analysis of HCG shows levels of hormone in both blood and urine greatly exceeding those produced by a normal pregnancy of similar age. Serial hormone determinations will indicate a rapidly mounting level that climbs faster than the usual normal single or even multiple pregnancy.

Once the diagnosis is made, the mole must be removed by thorough curettage. In patients over 35 years not desirous of further childbearing, hysterectomy is advocated by most gynecologists. The course following curettage alone depends on the malignant potential of the removed uterine contents. From many studies, it is clear that 80 to 90% of these moles remain benign and give no further difficulty. Ten per cent develop into invasive moles and 2.5% into choriocarcinoma.[109]

Proper follow-up with *periodic determination of HCG levels is essential* in these patients. A rise in such levels for the β subunit of the hormone heralds complications such as persistence of molar fragments or, more ominously, the development of invasive mole or choriocarcinoma.

INVASIVE MOLE

This is defined as a cellular mole that penetrates and may even perforate the uterine wall. There is invasion of the myometrium by well-developed embryonic villi, accompanied by proliferation of both cyto- and syncytiotrophoblast. The tumor is locally destructive and may invade parametrial tissues. Hydropic villi may embolize to distant sites such as lungs and brain but do not grow in these organs as true metastases, and even before the advent of chemotherapy they eventually regressed. Clinically, the tumor is manifested by vaginal bleeding and irregular uterine enlargement. It is *always* associated with a persistently elevated HCG level and varying degrees of luteinization of the ovaries. The tumor responds very well to chemotherapy. Although invasive mole is biologically benign, rupture of the uterus may lead to hemorrhage.

CHORIOCARCINOMA

Gestational choriocarcinoma is an epithelial malignancy of trophoblastic cells derived from any form of previous normal or abnormal pregnancy.[110] Although most cases arise in the uterus, ectopic pregnancies provide extrauterine sites of origin. Choriocarcinoma is a rapidly invasive, widely metastasizing malignancy, but once identified, it responds well to chemotherapy.

INCIDENCE. This is an uncommon condition that arises in 1 in 20,000 to 30,000 pregnancies in the U.S. It is much more common in some Asian and African

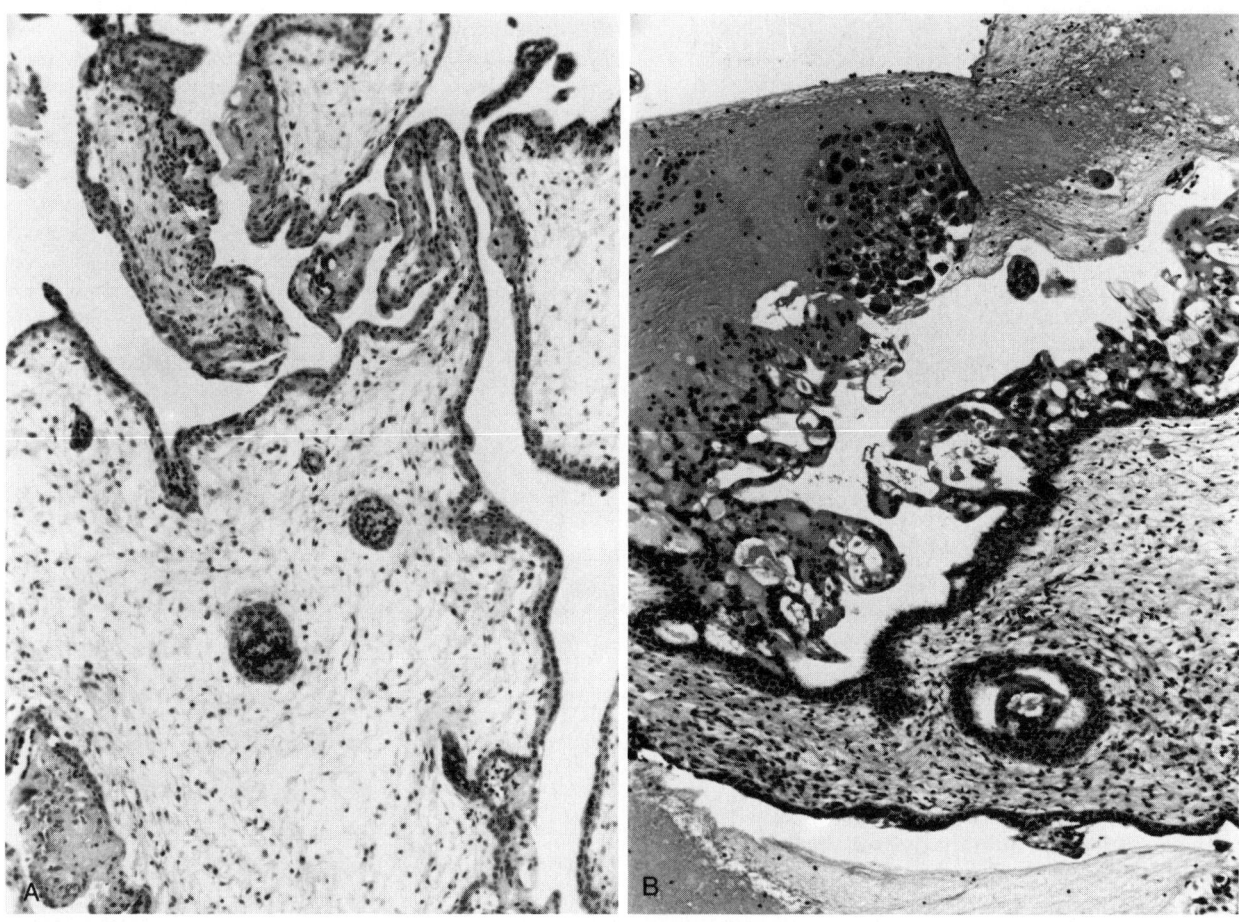

Figure 24–65. *A,* Partial mole showing villous edema and minimal focal epithelial hyperplasia. *B,* Complete mole with widespread trophoblast hyperplasia. (Courtesy of Dr. Janice Lage.)

countries, e.g., 1 in 2500 pregnancies in Ibadan. It is preceded by several conditions: 50% arise in hydatidiform moles, 25% in previous abortions, approximately 22% in normal pregnancies, and the rest in ectopic pregnancies and genital and extragenital teratomas. About 1 in 40 hydatidiform moles may be expected to give rise to a choriocarcinoma, in contrast to 1 in approximately 150,000 normal pregnancies.

MORPHOLOGY. Classically, the choriocarcinoma is a soft, fleshy, yellow-white tumor with a marked tendency to form large pale areas of ischemic necrosis, foci of cystic softening, and extensive hemorrhage. Histologically, it is a purely epithelial cellular malignancy that does not produce chorionic villi and that grows, as do other cancers, by the abnormal proliferation of both cyto- and syncytiotrophoblast (Figs. 24–66 and 24–67). It is sometimes possible to identify anaplasia within such abnormal proliferation replete with abnormal mitoses. The tumor invades the underlying myometrium, frequently penetrates blood vessels and lymphatics, and in some cases extends out onto the uterine serosa and adjacent structures. In its rapid growth, it is subject to hemorrhage, ischemic necrosis, and secondary inflammatory infiltration.

In fatal cases, metastases are found in the lungs, bone marrow, liver, and other organs. Occasionally, metastatic choriocarcinoma is discovered without a detectable primary in the uterus (or ovary), presumably because the primary has undergone total necrosis.

CLINICAL COURSE. Classically, the uterine choriocarcinoma does not produce a large, bulky mass. It becomes manifest only by irregular spotting of a bloody, brown, sometimes foul-smelling fluid. This discharge may appear in the course of an apparently normal pregnancy, after a miscarriage, or following a curettage. Sometimes the tumor does not appear until months later. Usually, by the time the tumor is discovered locally, radiographs of the chest and bones already disclose the presence of metastatic lesions. The HCG titers are elevated to levels above those encountered in hydatidiform moles. However, occasional tumors produce little hormone, and some tumors have become so necrotic as to become functionally inactive.

Widespread metastases are characteristic of these tumors. Favored sites of involvement are the lungs (50%) and vagina (30 to 40%), followed in de-

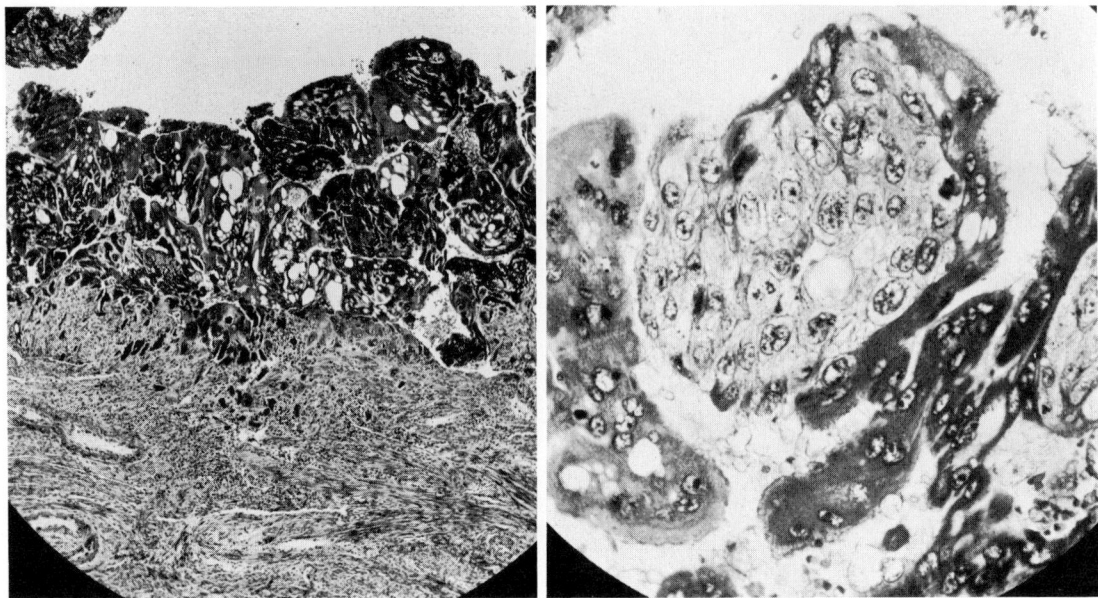

Fig. 24-66   **Fig. 24-67**

Figure 24-66. Low-power view of choriocarcinoma of uterine wall showing invasion of underlying myometrium.

Figure 24-67. High-power detail of choriocarcinoma illustrating the two types of epithelial cells—cytotrophoblast and syncytiotrophoblast.

scending order of frequency by the brain, liver, and kidney.

The *treatment* of trophoblastic neoplasms depends on the type and stage of tumor, and includes evacuation of the contents of the uterus, surgery, and chemotherapy. The results of chemotherapy for *gestational* choriocarcinoma are spectacular and have resulted in up to 100% cure or remission in all patients except some who had high-risk metastatic trophoblastic disease. Many of the cured patients have had normal subsequent pregnancies and deliveries. By contrast, nongestational choriocarcinomas are much more resistant to therapy.

PLACENTAL SITE TROPHOBLASTIC TUMOR

This rare tumor is characterized by the presence of proliferating trophoblastic tissue deeply invading the myometrium and is composed largely of *intermediate trophoblast.* These cells are usually mononuclear, rather than syncytial, but are larger and have more abundant cytoplasm than the regular cytotrophoblast. This lesion differs from choriocarcinoma in the absence of cytotrophoblastic elements and in the low level of HCG production. The tumors are locally invasive, but many are self-limited and subject to cure by curettage. However, malignant variants have been reported; they are distinguished by a high mitotic index, extreme cellularity, extensive necrosis, local spread, or even widespread metastases. About 10% result in disseminated metastases and death.[111]

1. McLean, J.M.: Embryology and anatomy of the female genital tract and ovary. *In* Fox, H. (ed.): Haines and Taylor's Obstetrical and Gynaecologic Pathology. 4th ed. Edinburgh, Churchill Livingstone, 1987, pp. 1-50.

2. Parmley, T.: Embryology of the female genital tract. *In* Kurman, R. (ed.): Blaustein's Pathology of the Female Genital Tract. New York, Springer Verlag, 1987, p. 1.

3. Donahoe, P.K.: The diagnosis and treatment of infants with intersex abnormalities. Pediatr. Clin. North Am. *34*(5):1333, 1987.

4. Kurman, R. (ed.): Blaustein's Pathology of the Female Genital Tract. 3rd ed. New York, Springer-Verlag, 1987.

5. Gompel, E., and Silverberg, S.: Pathology in Gynecology and Obstetrics. 3rd ed. Philadelphia, J.B. Lippincott Co., 1985.

6. Fox, H. (ed.): Haines and Taylor's Obstetrical and Gynaecologic Pathology. 4th ed. Edinburgh, Churchill Livingstone, 1987.

7. Lavery, J.P. (ed.): The Human Placenta. Rockville, MD, Aspen Publishers, Inc., 1987.

8. Danforth, D.N. (ed.): Obstetrics and Gynecology. 5th ed. Philadelphia, Harper & Row, 1988.

9. Buchsbaum, H. (ed.): Gynecology and Obstetrics. Hagerstown, Harper & Row, 1988.

10. Knapp, R.C., and Berkowitz, R.S.: Gynecologic Oncology. New York, Macmillan Publishing Co., 1986.

11. Holmes, K. (ed.): Sexually transmitted disease. New York, McGraw-Hill Book Co., 1984.

12. Sanchez, N.P., and Mihm, M.C., Jr.: Reactive and neoplastic epithelial alterations of the vulva. J. Am. Acad. Dermatol. *6*:378, 1982.

13. Report of the ISSVD Terminology Committee. Proceedings of the VIII World Congress (1986), Stockholm, Sweden. J. Reprod. Med. *31*:973, 1986.

14. Wilkinson, E.J., and Friedrich, E.G.: Diseases of the vulva. *In* Kurman, R. (ed.): Blaustein's Pathology of the Female Genital Tract. New York, Springer-Verlag, 1987, pp. 3-96.

15. Hart, W.R., et al.: Relation of lichen sclerosus et atrophicus of the vulva to the development of carcinoma. Obstet. Gynecol. *45*:369, 1975.

16. Lynch, P.J.: Condyloma acuminata. Clin. Obstet. Gynaecol. *28*:142, 1985.

17. Gissman, L., et al.: Human papilloma virus type 6 and 11 DNA

sequences in genital and laryngeal papillomas. Proc. Natl. Acad. Sci. (USA) *80:*560, 1983.

18. Crum, C.: Vulvar intraepithelial oncoplasia: The concept and its application. Hum. Pathol. *13:*127, 1982.

19. Zaino, R.J.: Carcinoma of the vulva, urethra, and Bartholin's glands. Contemp. Issues Surg. Pathol. *9:*119, 1987.

20. Gupta, J., et al.: Association of human papilloma virus type 16 with neoplastic lesions of the vulva by in-situ hybridization. Am. J. Pathol. *127:*206, 1987.

21. Powell, L.C., et al.: Carcinoma in situ of the vulva: a clinicopathologic study of 50 cases. J. Reprod. Med. *31:*808, 1986.

22. Michael, H., and Roth, L.M.: Paget's disease, skin appendage tumors, and cysts of the vulva. Contemp. Issues Surg. Pathol. *9:*25, 1987.

23. Stegner, H.E.: Ultrastructure of preneoplastic lesions of the vulva. J. Reprod. Med. *31:*815, 1986.

24. Pride, G.L., et al.: Primary invasive squamous carcinoma of the vagina. Obstet. Gynecol. *53:*218, 1979.

25. Herbst, A.L.: Clear cell adenocarcinoma and the current status of DES-exposed females. Cancer *48:*484, 1981.

26. Scully, R.E., and Welch, W.R.: Pathology of the female genital tract after prenatal exposure to diethylstilbestrol. *In* Herbst, A.L., and Bern, H.A. (eds.): Developmental Effects of Diethylstilbestrol in Pregnancy. New York, Thieme-Stratton, 1981, pp. 26–45.

27. Copeland, L.J., et al.: Sarcoma botryoides of the female genital tract. Obstet. Gynecol. *66:*262, 1985.

28. Winkler, B., and Richart, R.M.: Cervical-uterine pathologic considerations in pelvic infection. *In* Zatuchni, G.I., et al. (eds.): Intrauterine Contraception. New York, Harper & Row, 1985, pp. 438–449.

29. Wilkinson, E., and Dufour, D.R.: Pathogenesis of microglandular hyperplasia. Obstet. Gynecol. *47:*189, 1976.

30. Silverberg, E., and Lubera, J.: Cancer statistics. Cancer *39:*1, 1989.

31. Editorial: Papilloma virus and neoplasia. Lancet *1:*712, 1988.

32. zur Hausen, H., and Schneider, A.: The role of human papilloma viruses in human urogenital cancer. *In* Salzman, N., and Howley, P. (eds.): The Papovavirirididae. New York, Plenum Press, 1987, pp. 245–263.

33. zur Hausen, H.: Papilloma viruses in human cancer. Cancer *59:*1692, 1987.

34. Bonfiglio, T., and Stoler, M.: Papilloma virus and cervical cancer. Hum. Pathol. *19:*621, 1988.

35. Crum, C.P., et al.: Cervical papillomaviruses segregate within morphologically distinct precancerous lesions. J. Virol. *54:*675, 1985.

35a. Beckmann, A.M., et al.: Human papilloma virus type 16 in multifocal neoplasia of the female genital tract. Int. Gynecol. Pathol. *7:*39, 1988.

36. Storey, A., et al.: Comparison of the in-vitro transforming activities of HPV types. EMBO J. *6:*1850, 1988.

37. Campari, M.J., et al.: Increased risk of cervical neoplasia in women with pelvic condyloma. Lancet *1:*943, 1985.

38. Ferenczy, A., and Winkler, B.: Cervical intraepithelial neoplasia and condyloma. *In* Kurman, R. (ed.): Blaustein's Pathology of the Female Genital Tract. 2nd ed. New York, Springer-Verlag, 1987, pp. 177–218.

39. Richart, R.M.: Causes and management of cervical intraepithelial neoplasia. Cancer *60:*1951, 1987.

40. Richart, R.M., and Barron, B.B.: A follow-up study of patients with cervical dysplasia. Am. J. Obstet. Gynecol. *105:*386, 1969.

41. Creasman, W.T., et al.: The abnormal PAP smear—what to do next. Cancer *48:*515, 1981.

42. Rotman, M., et al.: Prognostic factors in cervical carcinoma: Implications in staging and management. Cancer *48:*560, 1981.

43. Richart, R.M., et al.: An analysis of long-term follow-up results in patients with cervical intraepithelial neoplasia treated by cryotherapy. Am. J. Obstet. Gynecol. *137:*823, 1980.

44. Rotterdam, H.: Chronic endometritis. A clinicopathologic study. Pathol. Annu. 13 (Part 2):209, 1978.

45. Fox, H., and Buckley, C.H.: Current concepts of endometriosis. Clin. Obstet. Gynecol. *11:*279, 1984.

46. Dahlenbach-Hellweg, G.: Histopathology of the Endometrium. 3rd ed. New York, Springer-Verlag, 1985.

47. Gurpids, E., et al.: Estrogen metabolism in normal and pathologic endometrium. Am. J. Obstet. Gynecol. *129:*809, 1977.

48. Ober, W.B.: Effects of oral and intrauterine administration of contraceptives on the uterus. Hum. Pathol. *8:*513, 1977.

49. Hertig, A.T., and Sommers, S.C.: Genesis of endometrial carcinoma. I. Study of prior biopsies. Cancer *2:*964, 1949.

50. Norris, H.J., et al.: Endometrial hyperplasia and carcinoma: Diagnostic considerations. Am. J. Surg. Pathol. *7:*839, 1983.

51. Kurman, R.J., and Norris, H.J.: Endometrial hyperplasia and metaplasia. *In* Kurman, R.J. (ed.): Blaustein's Pathology of the Female Genital Tract. 3rd ed. New York, Springer-Verlag, 1987.

52. Hendrickson, M.R., and Kempson, R.L.: Non-neoplastic endometrial metaplasias: Proliferations frequently misdiagnosed as adenocarcinoma. Lab. Invest. *40:*23, 1979.

53. Kraus, F.: High risk and premalignant lesions of the endometrium. Am. J. Surg. Pathol. *9:*31, 1985.

54. Kurman, R.J., et al.: The behavior of endometrial hyperplasia. A long-term study of untreated hyperplasia in 170 patients. Cancer *56:*403, 1985.

55. Henderson, B.E., et al.: The epidemiology of endometrial cancer in young women. Br. J. Cancer *47:*749, 1983.

56. Smith, M., and McCartney, A.J.: Occult high risk endometrial cancer. Gynecol. Oncol. *22:*254, 1985.

57. Gusberg, S.B.: Endometrial carcinoma. *In* Gusberg, S.B., et al. (eds.): Female Genital Cancer. New York, Churchill-Livingstone, 1988.

58. Connelly, P.J., et al.: Carcinoma of the endometrium III. Analysis of 865 cases of adenocarcinoma and adenocanthoma. Obstet. Gynecol. *59:*569, 1982.

59. Cowles, T.A., et al.: Comparison of clinical and surgical staging in patients with endometrial carcinoma. Obstet. Gynecol. *66:*413, 1985.

60. Hendrickson, M.R., et al.: Adenocarcinoma of the endometrium: analysis of 256 cases with disease limited to uterine corpus. Analysis of prognostic variables. Gynecol. Oncol. *12:*373, 1982.

61. Bard, D.S., and Zuna, R.E.: Sarcomas and related neoplasms of the uterine corpus. A brief review of the natural history, prognostic factors, and management. Obstet. Gynecol. Annu. *10:*237, 1981.

62. Christopherson, W.M., and Richardson, M.: Uterine mesenchymal tumors. Pathol. Annu. *16:*215, 1981.

63. Geisinger, K.R., et al.: Malignant mixed Mullerian tumors. Cancer *54:*1281, 1987.

64. Chung, M.T., et al.: Expression of various antigens by different components of uterine mixed Mullerian tumors. Acta Pathol. *38:*35, 1988.

65. Buscema, J., et al.: Epithelioid leiomyosarcoma. Cancer *47:*1192, 1986.

66. McKenna, T.J.: Pathogenesis and treatment of polycystic ovary syndrome. N. Engl. J. Med. *318:*558, 1988.

67. Scully, R.E.: Ovarian tumors. A review. Am. J. Pathol. *87:*686, 1977.

68. Langley, F.A., and Fox, H.: Ovarian tumors. Classification, histogenesis, etiology. *In* Fox, H. (ed.): Haines and Taylor's Obstetrical and Gynaecologic Pathology. 4th ed. Edinburgh, Churchill Livingstone, 1987, pp. 542–555.

69. McGowan, L., et al.: The woman at risk for developing ovarian cancer. Gynecol. Oncol. *73:*25, 1979.

70. Cramer, D.W., et al.: Factors affecting the association of oral contraceptives and ovarian cancer. N. Engl. J. Med. *307:*1047, 1982.

71. Blaustein, A.: Surface (germinal) epithelium and related ovarian neoplasms. Pathol. Annu. *16:*247, 1981.

72. Hart, W.R.: Ovarian epithelial tumors of borderline malignancy (carcinomas of low malignant potential). Hum. Pathol. *8:*541, 1977.

73. Snyder, R.R., et al.: Endometrial proliferative and low malignant potential tumors of the ovary. Am. J. Surg. Path. *12:*661, 1988.

74. Teilum, G.: Special Tumors of Ovary and Testis and Related Extragonadal Lesions. Philadelphia, W.B. Saunders Co., 1976.

75. Shevchuk, M.M., et al.: Clear cell carcinoma of the ovary: A clinicopathologic study and review of the literature. Cancer *47:*1344, 1981.

76. Shevchuk, M.M., et al.: Histogenesis of Brenner tumors. I. Histology and ultrastructure. II. Histochemistry and CEA. Cancer *46:*2607, 1980.

77. Altaras, M.M., et al.: The role of cancer antigen CA 125 in the management of various epithelial carcinomas. Gynecol. Oncol. *30:*26, 1988.

78. Kurman, R., and Norris, H.J.: Germ cell tumors of the ovary. Pathol. Annu. *13:*291, 1978.

79. Talerman, A.: Germ cell tumors of the ovary. *In* Kurman, R. (ed.): Blaustein's Pathology of the Female Genital Tract. New York, Springer-Verlag, 1987, pp. 657–715.

80. Linder, D., et al.: Pathogenetic origin of benign ovarian teratomas. N. Engl. J. Med. *292:*63, 1975.

80a. Mutter, G.L.: Teratoma genetics and stem cells: a review. Obstet. Gynecol. Surv. *42:*661, 1987.

81. Norris, H.J., et al.: Immature (malignant) teratoma of the ovary. A clinical and pathological study of 58 cases. Cancer *37:*2359, 1976.

82. Gordon, T., et al.: Dysgerminoma, a review of 158 cases from the Emil Novak ovarian tumor registry. Obstet. Gynecol. *58:*497, 1981.

83. Young, R.H., and Scully, R.: Ovarian sex cord-stromal tumors. Recent progress. Int. J. Gynecol. Pathol. *1:*101, 1982.

84. Bjorkholm, E., and Sifversward, C.: Prognostic factors in granuloma cell tumors. Gynecol. Oncol. *1:*261, 1981.

85. Prat, J., and Scully, R.E.: Cellular fibromas and fibrosarcomas of the ovary. Cancer *47:*2663, 1981.

86. Roth, L.M., et al.: Sertoli-Leydig cell tumors: A clinicopathologic study of 34 cases. Cancer *48:*187, 1981.

87. Scully, R.E.: The ovary. *In* Wolfe, H. (ed.): Endometrial Pathology. New York, Springer-Verlag, 1986.

88. Benirschke, K., and Driscoll, S.G.: The Pathology of the Human Placenta. New York, Springer Verlag, 1967.

89. Grossman, J.H.: Infections affecting the placenta. *In* Lavery, J.P. (ed.): The Placenta. Rockville, MD, Aspen Publishing, 1987, pp. 131–134.

90. Gersell, D.J., et al.: Diseases of the placenta. *In* Kurman, R. (ed.): Blaustein's Pathology of the Female Genital Tract. New York, Springer-Verlag, 1987, p. 769.

91. Naeye, R.L., and Peters, E.C.: Cancer and consequences of premature rupture of fetal membranes. Lancet *1:*192, 1980.

92. Kurlow, W.F., and Fox, H.: Villitis of unknown etiology. Placenta *5:*395, 1984.

93. Morison, J.E.: Placenta accreta: A clinicopathologic review of 67 cases. Obstet. Gynecol. Annu. *7:*107, 1978.

94. Lage, J.M., et al.: The twin placenta. *In* Lavery, J.P. (ed.): The Placenta. Rockville, MD, Aspen Publishing, 1987. p. 67.

95. Wilcox, A.J.: Incidence of early loss of pregnancy. N. Engl. J. Med. *319:*189, 1988.

96. Little, A.B.: There's many a slip 'twixt implantation and the crib. N. Engl. J. Med. *319:*241, 1988.

97. Baldwin, V.J., et al.: Diagnostic pathologic investigation of the malformed conceptus. *In* Rosenberg, H.S., and Bernstein, J. (eds.): Perspectives in Pediatric Pathology. New York, Masson Publishing, U.S.A., 1982, pp. 85–108.

98. Rushton, D.I.: Examination of products of conception from previable human pregnancies. J. Clin. Pathol. *34:*819, 1981.

99. Hockberger, R.S.: Ectopic pregnancy. Obstet. Gynecol. Emerg. *5:*481, 1987.

100. Weiner, C.P.: The clinical spectrum of preeclampsia. Am. J. Kidney Dis. *9:*312, 1987.

101. Friedman, S.A.: Preeclampsia: A review of the role of prostaglandins. Obstet. Gynecol. *71:*122, 1988.

102. Rubin, P.C., and Horn, L.: Preeclampsia, platelets and platelet therapy. Hosp. Pract. *23:*69, 1988.

103. Goldstein, D.P., and Berkowitz, R.S.: Gestational Trophoblastic Neoplasms: Clinical Principles of Diagnosis and Management. Vol. 14. Philadelphia, W.B. Saunders Co., 1982.

104. Elston, C.W.: Gestational tumors of trophoblast. *In* Anthony, P.P., and MacSween, R. (eds.): Recent Advances in Histopathology. New York, Churchill Livingstone, 1981, pp. 149–161.

105. Bracken, M.B., et al.: Epidemiology of hydatidiform mole and choriocarcinoma. Epidemiol. Rev. *6:*52, 1984.

106. Szulman, A.E.: Syndromes of hydatidiform mole. Partial vs. complete. J. Reprod. Med. *29:*288, 1984.

107. Surti, U., et al.: Tetraploid partial hydatidiform moles: Two cases with a triple paternal contribution and a 92XXXY karyotype. Hum. Genet. *72:*15, 1986.

108. Lage, J.M., et al.: Hydatidiform moles. Application of flow cytometry to diagnosis. Am. J. Clin. Pathol. *89:*596, 1988.

109. Lurain, J.R., et al.: Natural history of hydatidiform mole after primary evacuation. Am. J. Obstet. Gynecol. *145:*591, 1983.

110. Berkowitz, R.S., and Goldstein, D.P.: Gestational trophoblastic disease. *In* Moosa, A.R., et al. (eds.): Comprehensive Textbook of Oncology. Baltimore, Williams & Wilkins Co., 1989.

111. Finkler, N.J., et al.: Clinical experience with placental site trophoblastic tumors at the New England Trophoblastic Disease Center. Obstet. Gynecol., *71:*854, 1988.

NORMAL

EMBRYOLOGY. The breast is a modified skin sweat gland that develops into a complex functional structure in the female, but remains as a rudimentary organ in the male. It arises from an epidermal thickening on the ventral surface of the body at approximately the sixth week of fetal development. Bilateral ridges (the milk line) develop between the upper and lower limb buds. These ridges totally atrophy except for several persistent thickenings, which later give rise to the nipples. During the second trimester of fetal life, cords of cells grow downward from the basal layer of the epidermis and later give rise to the primary mammary ducts. At first solid, the cords eventually develop lumina so that, at the time of birth, rudimentary branching ducts are present, which fan out in a small area about the region of the nipple and the areola.

Development of the breast is by no means complete at the time of birth. Progressive growth and branching of the mammary ducts occur at a very slow pace during prepubertal life. Mammary development ceases at about this stage in the male. In the female, before the onset of menstruation, the growth rate increases with branching of ducts and proliferation of the interductal stroma. During adolescence, stromal growth is responsible for most of the increase in the mass of the breast, but at the same time the terminal small ducts give rise to many small, blind, saccular outpouchings. Under the influence of the ovarian hormones and the hormones of pregnancy, further changes occur, to be described.

ANATOMY AND HISTOLOGY. Only a few features of the gross anatomy, of special interest to pathology, bear repetition at this time. The resting mammary gland consists of about 20 lobes, each of which is subdivided into *lobules*, the functional units of the mammary parenchyma (Fig. 25–1). Each lobe drains through a separate main excretory or *lactiferous duct* into the nipple. Just beneath the nipple, the lactiferous ducts exhibit a small dilated segment, called the *lactiferous sinus*. Successive branchings of the lactiferous ducts distally eventually lead to the terminal ducts. Before puberty, this complex system of branching ducts ends blindly, but at the beginning of menarche, it proliferates distally, giving rise to some 30 epithelium-lined *ductules* or *acini*. Each terminal duct and its ductules compose the *terminal duct lobular units* (Fig. 25–1).

The areola, nipple, and mouths of the main lactiferous ducts are covered by stratified squamous epithelium. It soon becomes transformed into a pseudostratified columnar and then double-layered cuboidal epithelium that lines the major breast ducts. As the ducts branch and become smaller, the epithelium tends to become a single layer of cells, but in the smaller ducts and sometimes even in the ductules, a low flattened layer of cells (*myoepithelial cells*) can be identified beneath the more prominent lining epithelium. Myoepithelial cells contain myofilaments oriented parallel to the long axis of the duct. A basement membrane follows faithfully the contour of ducts and ductules.[1] These are enclosed in a loose, delicate, myxomatous stroma that contains a scattering of lymphocytes (*intralobular connective tissue*), and the individual lobules are enclosed within a denser, collagenous, fibrous *interlobular stroma*.

Just as the endometrium rises and ebbs with each menstrual cycle, so does the breast.[2] Following the menstrual period, with the progressive rise in estrogen, the ductal and ductular cells begin to proliferate and continue to develop throughout the menstrual cycle. During the secretory phase of the menstrual cycle, under the influence of progesterone, proliferation of the terminal duct structure increases, and there is vacuolization and increased mitotic activity of basal epithelial cells. The stromal cells proliferate and

1181

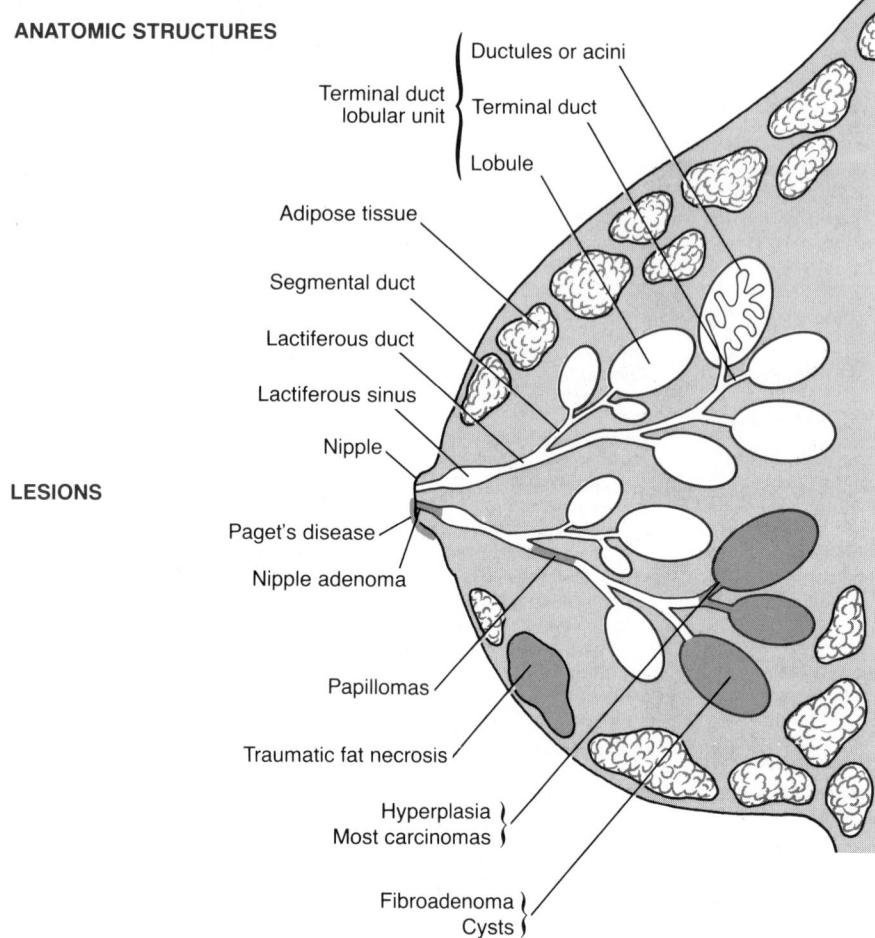

ANATOMIC STRUCTURES

Ductules or acini

Terminal duct lobular unit

Terminal duct

Lobule

Adipose tissue

Segmental duct

Lactiferous duct

Lactiferous sinus

Nipple

LESIONS

Paget's disease

Nipple adenoma

Papillomas

Traumatic fat necrosis

Hyperplasia
Most carcinomas

Fibroadenoma
Cysts

Figure 25–1. Anatomy of the breast and major lesions at each site within the various units.

there is, in addition, stromal edema. This combined stimulatory effect of estrogen and progesterone on the intralobular breast elements accounts for the sense of fullness commonly experienced by women during the premenstrual phase of the cycle. When menstruation occurs, the fall in estrogen and progesterone levels is followed by desquamation of epithelial cells, atrophy of the intralobular connective tissue, disappearance of stromal edema, and overall shrinkage in the size of the ducts and gland buds. Considerable numbers of lymphocytes accumulate in the periductal tissue.

It is only with the onset of pregnancy that the breast assumes its complete morphologic maturation and functional activity. From each gland bud, numerous true secretory glands pouch out to form grapelike clusters. As a consequence, there is a reversal of the usual stromal-glandular relationship so that, by the end of pregnancy, the breast is composed almost entirely of glands separated by a relatively scant amount of stroma. The secretory glands are lined by cuboidal

cells, and in the third trimester, secretory vacuoles of lipid material are found within the cells. Immediately following birth the secretion of milk begins (Fig. 25–2). Certain breast tumors arising during pregnancy exhibit similar secretory changes (lactating adenoma).

Following lactation, the glands once again regress and atrophy, the ducts shrink, and the total breast size diminishes remarkably. However, complete regression to the stage of the normal virginal breast usually does not occur, and some increases of glandular parenchyma remains as a permanent residual.

With the menopause, the ducts and gland buds further atrophy with more shrinkage of the intra- and interlobular stroma. The gland buds may almost totally disappear in the very aged, leaving only ducts to create a morphologic pattern that comes close to that of the male. However, in most women there is sufficient persistent estrogenic stimulation, possibly of adrenal origin, to maintain the vestigial remnants of gland buds that differentiate even the very aged female breast from the male breast.

FEMALE BREAST

PATHOLOGY

Lesions of the breast are preponderantly confined to the female. In the male, the breast is a rudimentary structure relatively insensitive to endocrine influences and apparently resistant to neoplastic growth. In the female, on the other hand, the more complex breast structure, the greater breast volume, and the extreme sensitivity to endocrine influences all predispose this organ to a number of pathologic conditions.

Most diseases of the breast take the form of palpable, sometimes painful, nodules or masses. Although fortunately most are benign, cancer of the breast is the second most common cause of cancer deaths and one of the most dreaded diseases of women. In this chapter, therefore, the conditions to be described should be considered in the terms of their possible confusion clinically with cancer.[3-5]

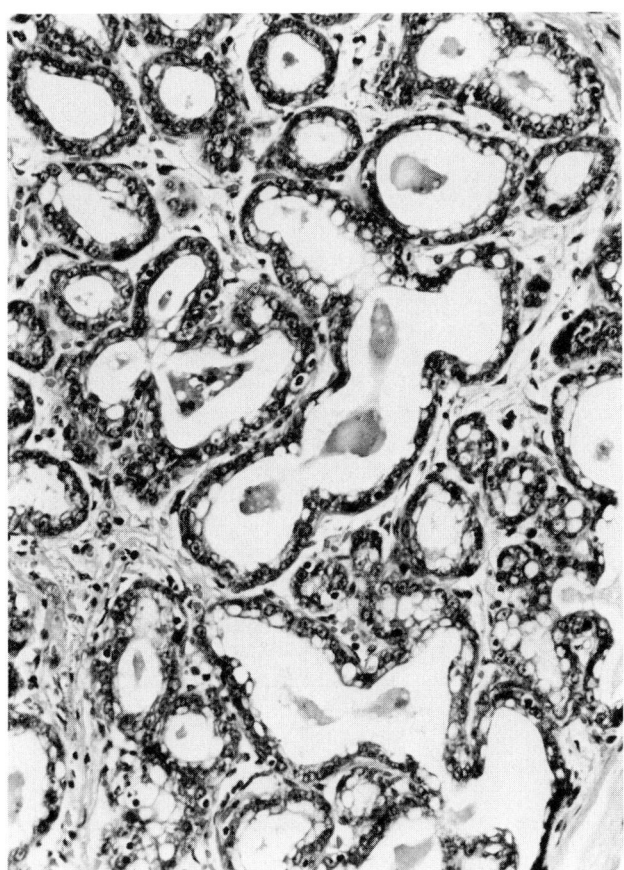

Figure 25–2. Lactating breast. Note the hyperplasia of glands, vacuolization of cells, and secretion in lumina.

An overall perspective of the frequency of various breast problems can be gained from an analysis of a large series of patients with breast complaints who were seen in a surgical outpatient department.[6] About 30% of the women were considered, after careful evaluation, to have no breast disease. Almost 40% were diagnosed as having fibrocystic changes. Slightly over 10% had biopsy-proven cancer, and about 7% had a benign tumor (fibroadenoma). The remainder were suffering from a miscellany of benign lesions (Fig. 25–3). Three features of this study deserve particular note: (1) *A significant proportion of women having no recognizable breast disease have sufficient irregularity of the "normal" breast tissue to cause concern and to necessitate clinical evaluation;* (2) *fibrocystic changes are the dominant breast problem;* and (3) *cancer, unhappily, is all too frequent.*

CONGENITAL ANOMALIES

These anomalies run the gamut from congenital absence to abnormal numbers of breasts, but as a group these entities are of limited clinical significance.

SUPERNUMERARY NIPPLES OR BREASTS. These result from the persistence of epidermal thickenings along the milk line, both below the adult breast and above it in the anterior axillary fold. Rarely, the disorders that affect the normally situated breast may arise in these heterotopic foci, and occasionally the cyclic changes of the menstrual cycle cause painful premenstrual enlargements.

ACCESSORY AXILLARY BREAST TISSUE. The chief importance of such tissue lies in the fact that it may give rise to tumors that appear to be outside the breast, and therefore are commonly misidentified as

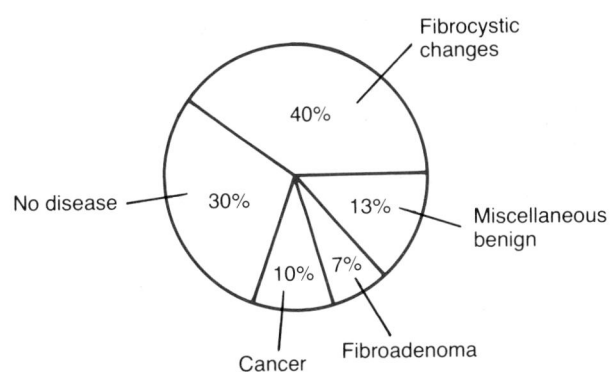

Figure 25–3. Representation of the findings in a series of women seeking evaluation of apparent breast "lumps."

lesions of the axillary lymph nodes or even as metastases from an occult breast cancer.

CONGENITAL INVERSION OF NIPPLES. This occurs in many women, particularly those who have large or pendulous breasts. Commonly, this inversion is corrected during the growth activity of pregnancy, or it may sometimes be corrected by simple traction upon the nipples. Nipple inversion is of clinical significance, since it may frustrate attempts at nursing and may also be confused with acquired retraction of the nipple, sometimes observed in mammary cancer and in inflammations of the breasts.

INFLAMMATIONS

Inflammations of the breast are, on the whole, uncommon and consist of only a relatively few forms of acute and chronic disease. Of these, the most important is nonspecific acute mastitis, virtually confined to the lactating period. Breast abscesses are included under the heading of acute mastitis. The other forms of mastitis consist of plasma cell mastitis or mammary duct ectasia (an entity of obscure etiology) and posttraumatic lesions.

ACUTE MASTITIS AND BREAST ABSCESS

During the early weeks of nursing, the breast is rendered vulnerable to bacterial infection by the development of cracks and fissures in the nipples. The disease is not confined to the postpartum state, however, and may be predisposed to by eczema and other dermatologic conditions of the nipples. From this portal of entry, *Staphylococcus aureus* usually, or streptococci less commonly, invade the breast substance.

Usually the disease is unilateral. The staphylococcus tends to produce a localized area of acute inflammation that may progress to the formation of single or multiple abscesses. The streptococcus tends to cause, as it does in all tissues, a diffuse spreading infection that eventually involves the entire organ. Surgical drainage and antibiotic therapy may limit the spread of the infection, but when extensive necrosis occurs, the destroyed breast substance is replaced by fibrous scar as a permanent residual of the inflammatory process. Such scarring may create a localized area of increased consistency sometimes accompanied by retraction of the skin or the nipple, changes that may later be mistaken for a neoplasm.

MAMMARY DUCT ECTASIA

This condition is characterized chiefly by dilatation of ducts, inspissation of breast secretions, and marked periductal and interstitial chronic granulomatous inflammatory reaction, sometimes associated with large numbers of plasma cells *(plasma cell mastitis).*[5] This disorder tends to occur in the fifth or sixth decade of life, usually in multiparous women, and is thought to result from obstruction of ducts due to inspissation of secretions. The etiology is unknown, but the association with pituitary adenomas or elevated prolactin levels suggests a role for prolactin secretion in the pathogenesis.[7]

The condition usually affects a single area of breast substance drained through one of the major excretory ducts. A poorly defined area of induration, thickening, or ropiness results. On section, thick, cheesy material can be extruded from the ducts by slight pressure.

The dilated ducts are filled by granular, necrotic, acidophilic debris that contains principally lipid-laden macrophages (Fig. 25–4). The lining epithelial cells of the ducts may persist in small foci, but for the most part are necrotic and atrophic. The periductal and interductal inflammation is manifested by heavy infiltrates of inflammatory cells, i.e., neutrophils, lymphocytes, and histiocytes, and in some cases with a striking predominance of plasma cells. Occasionally, there is a granulomatous inflammation around cholesterol deposits. Fibrosis may eventually produce skin retraction that can be confused with carcinoma.

This lesion is of clinical significance because it can be mistaken for a carcinoma clinically, grossly, and by mammography.

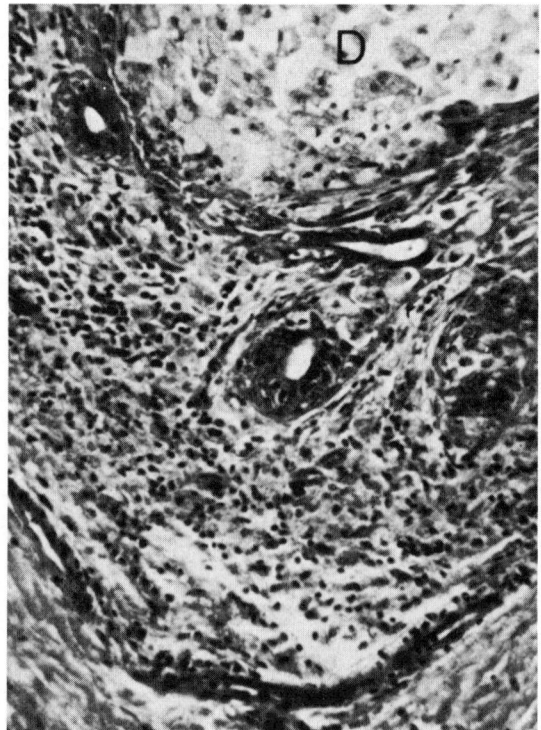

Figure 25–4. Duct ectasia. Duct at top (D) is partially filled with lipid-laden macrophages. Ductal epithelium is destroyed, and periductal tissues are infiltrated with leukocytes, mostly plasma cells.

FAT NECROSIS

Focal necrosis of fat tissues in the breast, followed by an inflammatory reaction, is an uncommon lesion that tends to occur as an isolated, sharply localized process in one breast. If strict criteria are used to differentiate this entity from mammary duct ectasia, almost all patients give a history of trauma.[5]

> In the early stages, the focus may consist of hemorrhage and, later, central liquefactive necrosis of fat. Still later, it may be an ill-defined nodule of gray-white, firm tissue, containing small foci of chalky white or hemorrhagic debris.
>
> Histologically, the central focus of necrotic fat cells is surrounded by lipid-filled macrophages and an intense neutrophilic infiltration. Then, over the next few days, progressive fibroblastic proliferation, increased vascularization, and lymphocytic and histiocytic infiltration wall off the focus. By this time, the central necrotic fat cells have disappeared and may be represented only by foamy, lipid-laden macrophages and spicules of crystalline lipids. Still later, foreign body giant cells, calcium salts, and blood pigments make their appearance, and eventually the focus is replaced by scar tissue or is encysted and walled off by collagenous tissue (Fig. 25–5).

The major clinical significance of the condition is its possible confusion with a tumor, when fibrosis has

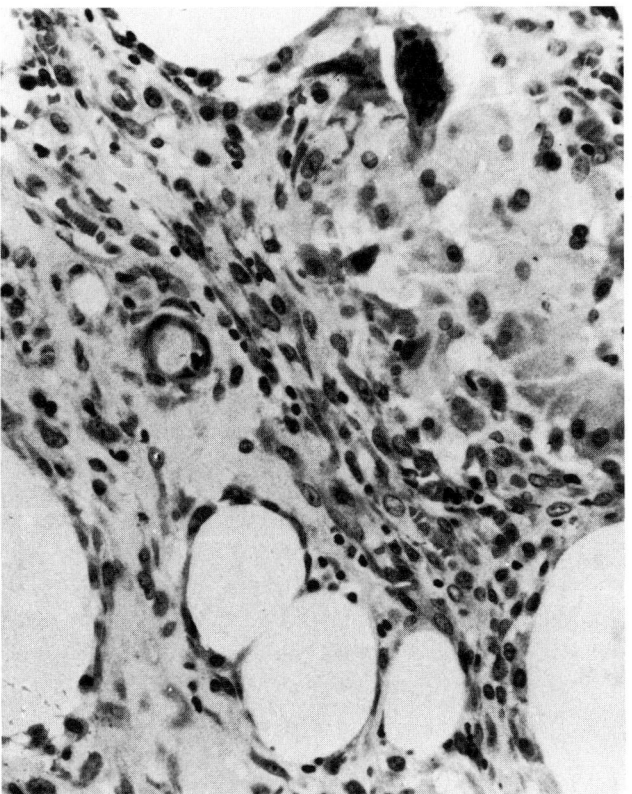

Figure 25–5. Fat necrosis. Note foamy macrophages and giant cell (*top right*), inflammation, and beginning fibrosis.

created a clinically palpable mass, and focal calcification is seen on mammography.

GALACTOCELE

A galactocele represents a cystic dilatation of a duct occurring during lactation. Occasionally, a single duct is affected to produce an isolated cyst, but more often multiple ducts are involved. During the acute phase, the palpable nodules are tender and, when exposed, contain a milky fluid enclosed within thin, dilated ductal walls. Secondary infection may convert these areas to foci of acute mastitis or abscess formation.

FIBROCYSTIC CHANGES (FIBROCYSTIC DISEASE)

These designations are applied to a miscellany of morphologic changes in the female breast ranging from those that are entirely innocuous to those that are associated with increased risk of carcinoma. One feature of all these changes is that they may produce palpable lumps—although some of the changes are so mild as to be clinically silent and so common as to be present in some 60 to 90% of breasts in routine autopsies.[8] The terminology of this condition and of the individual morphologic changes is, unfortunately, one of its most confusing aspects. Despite the many "good-byes to fibrocystic disease,"[9] however, the term seems to be ingrained in clinical usage. "Fibrocystic change" is probably more appropriate, since the alterations are often of no clinical significance.[10]

As noted, fibrocystic changes encompass a wide variety of morphologic features. These run the gamut from lesions that consist principally of cysts, to those characterized by an overgrowth of the fibrous stroma, to lesions in which both stromal and epithelial proliferation occurs, to other types in which epithelial proliferation predominates.[5] It is a notoriously pleomorphic disorder in which variable morphologic patterns are encountered in different patients, in different areas of the same lesion, or even in different microscopic fields of one slide. Despite this marked variability, it is possible to distinguish three dominant patterns of morphologic change: (1) *cystic formation and fibrosis* (simple fibrocystic change and gross cysts), (2) *epithelial hyperplasia* (ductal and lobular), and (3) *sclerosing adenosis.* Of these three, ductal and lobular hyperplasia—particularly when atypical—is the variant that is associated with increased risk for carcinoma.[11]

INCIDENCE AND PATHOGENESIS. Together these variants compose the single most common disorder of the breast and account for over one half of all surgical operations on the female breast. It is difficult to express an incidence of this condition in the general adult female population because of the variable criteria used for its diagnosis and because of the selective nature of the material studied. In a study of the so-called normal breast, i.e., in unselected post-mortem cases, significant disease was found in 29% and minimal disease was found in an additional 24%.[12] Haagensen estimates that at least 10% of women develop clinically apparent cystic disease.[13] The condition is unusual before adolescence, is diagnosed frequently between the ages of 20 and 40, peaks at or just before the menopause, and rarely develops after the menopause. However, premenopausal lesions may persist into more advanced years.

Hormonal imbalances are considered to be basic to the development of this multipatterned disorder. The excess of estrogens may represent an absolute increase, as in the rarely associated functioning ovarian tumors, or may be related to a deficiency of progesterone, as seen in anovulatory women. Experimentally, estrogen injections induce mammary cysts and hyperplastic lesions, particularly in mice.[14] There is also some evidence of abnormal end-organ metabolism of hormones in the pathogenesis of cystic disease.[15] Oral contraceptive use decreases the risk of fibrocystic disease,[16] presumably because it supplies a balanced source of progesterone and estrogen.

CYSTS AND FIBROSIS
(Simple Fibrocystic Change)

This is the most common type of alteration, characterized by an increase in fibrous stroma associated with dilatation of ducts and formation of cysts of various sizes. Haagensen pleads for differentiating *gross cysts*, over 3 mm in diameter, from *microcysts*.[13] He points out that microcysts are found so commonly in all women in the middle years of life that they cannot be construed as disease or as justification for surgery.

Grossly, a large cyst may be formed within one breast, but the disorder is usually multifocal and often bilateral (Fig. 25–6). As a result of the stromal overgrowth and cystic dilatation of the ducts, the involved areas have an ill-defined diffuse increase in consistency and discrete nod-

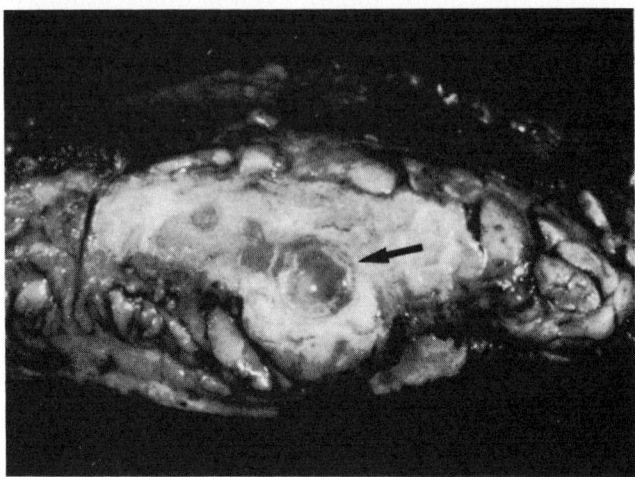

Figure 25–6. Cystic change of breast. Cross section reveals one large (*arrow*) and several smaller cysts.

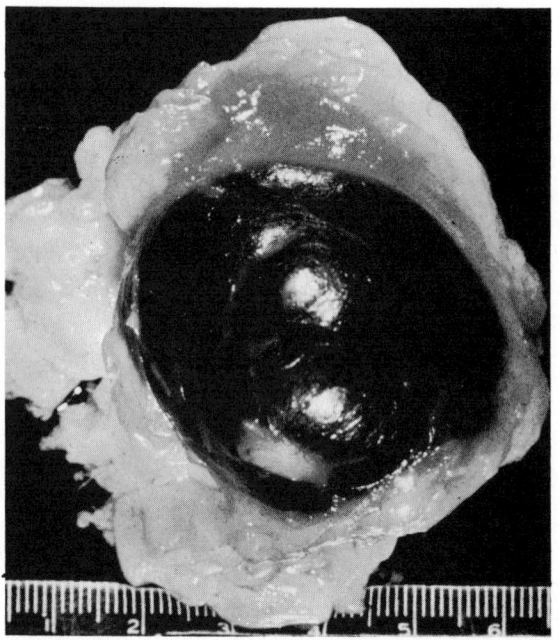

Figure 25–7. Cystic change of breast. A large, unopened, blue dome cyst.

ularities. Closely aggregated, small cysts produce a shotty texture. Larger, particularly solitary, cysts evoke the greatest alarm as isolated firm masses that are deceptively unyielding. On section, the cysts vary from less than 1 cm to up to 5 cm in diameter. Unopened, these cysts are brown to

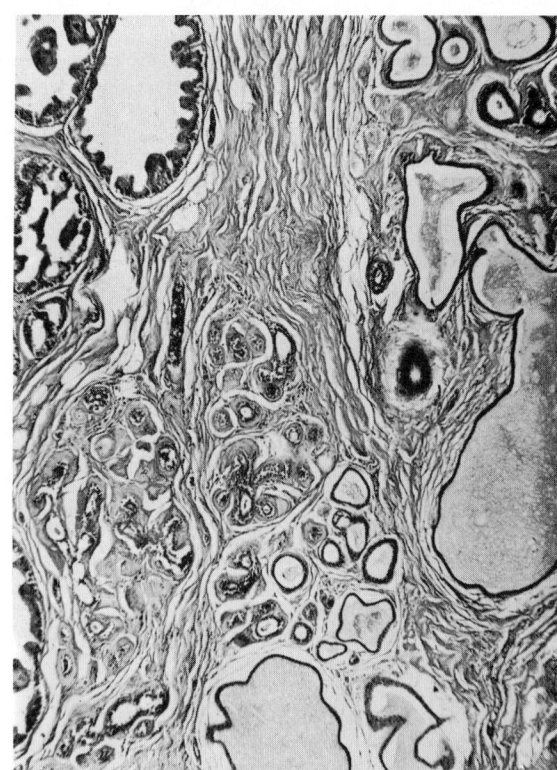

Figure 25–8. Cystic change of breast. Multiple cystic spaces, some filled with precipitated fluid with stromal fibrosis. Others (top left) exhibit apocrine metaplasia (see Fig. 25–9).

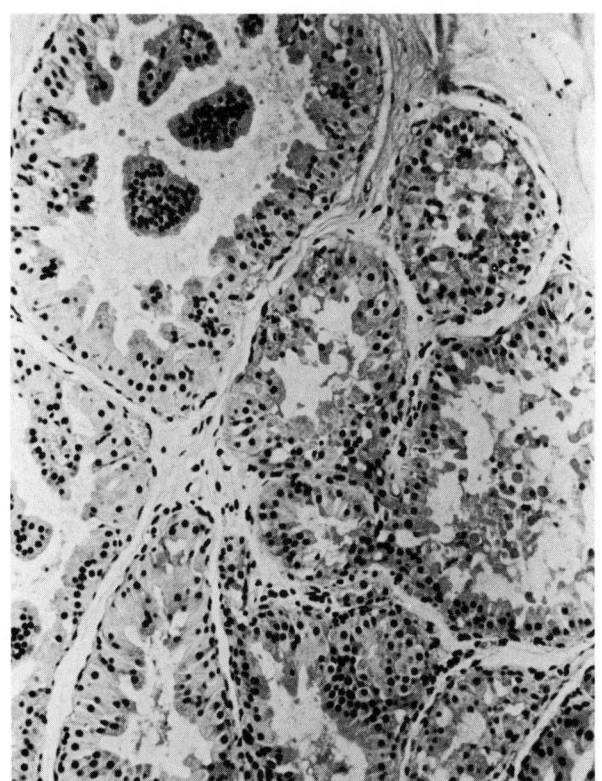

Figure 25–9. Apocrine metaplasia. Lining epithelium is high columnar and faintly staining (eosinophilic with H and E stain).

blue **(blue-dome cysts)** owing to the contained semitranslucent, turbid fluid (Fig. 25–7). Usually the cysts are filled with serous, turbid fluid, but intracystic hemorrhage, inspissation of secretions, or inflammation may modify the contents. Histologically, in smaller cysts, the epithelium is more

cuboidal to columnar and is sometimes multilayered in focal areas (Fig. 25–8). In larger cysts, it may be flattened or may even be totally atrophic. Occasionally, epithelial proliferation leads to piled-up masses or small papillary excrescences. Frequently, cysts are lined by large polygonal cells having an abundant granular, eosinophilic cytoplasm, with small, round, deeply chromatic nuclei, so-called **apocrine metaplasia;** such apocrine epithelium is found not uncommonly in the normal breast and is **virtually always benign.** Epithelial overgrowth and papillary projections are common in cysts lined by apocrine epithelium (Fig. 25–9).

The stroma about all forms of cysts is usually compressed fibrous tissue, having lost its normal, delicate, myxomatous appearance. Stromal lymphocytic infiltrate is common in this and all other variants of fibrocystic disease.

EPITHELIAL HYPERPLASIA

The fibrocystic changes can be accompanied by epithelial hyperplasia affecting the ducts and ductules, and as mentioned earlier, it is this histologic variant that increases the risk of the subsequent development of carcinoma.[3–5,10,17] This is not to say that all foci of epithelial hyperplasia (termed *epitheliosis* by British pathologists) are premalignant, leading inevitably to carcinoma; indeed, only a small proportion apparently are. But it is this pattern of alteration that should concern the pathologist, who is called to differentiate among benign hyperplasia, atypical but still noncancerous hyperplasia, and carcinoma. The more severe and atypical the hyperplasia, the greater the risk of developing cancer.[18] These hyperplasias may sometimes coexist with other fibrocystic changes, but on occasion they form the predominant pattern.

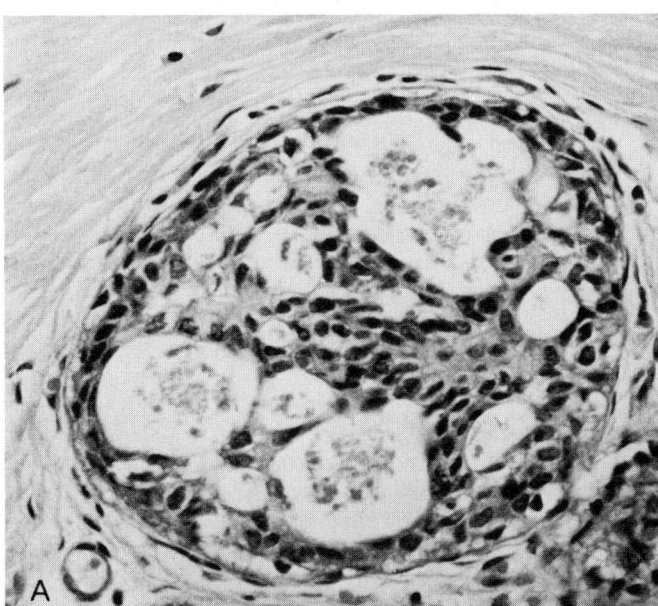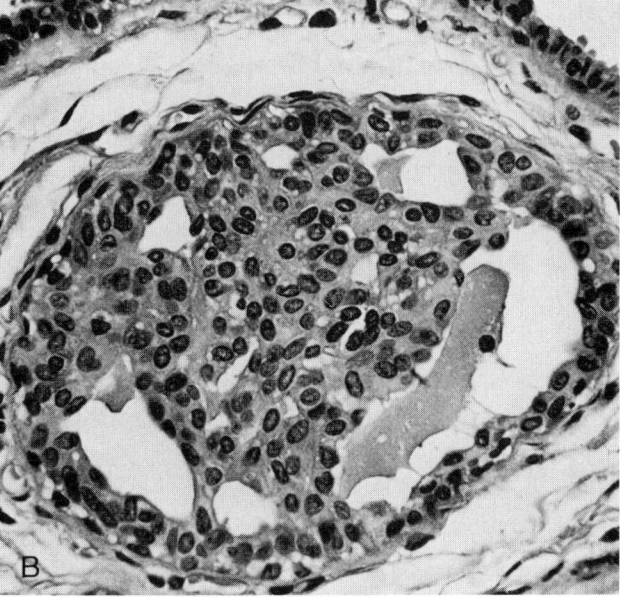

Figure 25–10. *A,* Moderate duct epithelial hyperplasia. Note cells fill part of the duct lumen. *B,* More florid duct epithelial hyperplasia, with irregular lumina at the periphery—so-called fenestrations. (Courtesy of Dr. Noel Weidner.)

The gross appearance is variable and may be overshadowed by the accompanying fibrosis, cysts, or adenosis. Microscopically, proliferation causes an increase in the layers of the duct-lining epithelium beyond the usual double layer. Sometimes the proliferating epithelium takes the form of solid masses extending and encroaching into the duct lumen, partially obliterating it, but usually irregular lumina **(so-called fenestrations)** can be discerned at the periphery of the cellular masses (Fig. 25–10). Alternatively, papillary epithelial projections may grow into the lumen **(ductal papillomatosis)** (Fig. 25–11). If extensive, this is termed **florid papillomatosis.** Both papillary and solid proliferations may sometimes show various degrees of cellular and architectural atypia **(atypical hyperplasia).** The differentiation from intraductal carcinoma (p. 1194) may be difficult in individual cases, especially if the tissue samples examined are inadequate. In general, greater cellular uniformity, more regular sharply defined gland lumina (so-called **cribriform pattern**), and nuclear hyperchromasia favor intraductal carcinoma.

Atypical lobular hyperplasia is the term used to describe hyperplasias of the terminal duct and ductules (acini) that have some — but not all — the features of lobular carcinoma in situ, described on page 1195. Cytologically, the atypical cells of atypical lobular hyperplasia resemble those of lobular carcinoma in situ but do not fill or distend more than 50% of the terminal duct units.[3] Atypical lobular hyperplasia, particularly when it affects ducts (rather than only acini), is associated with an increased risk of invasive carcinoma.[18a]

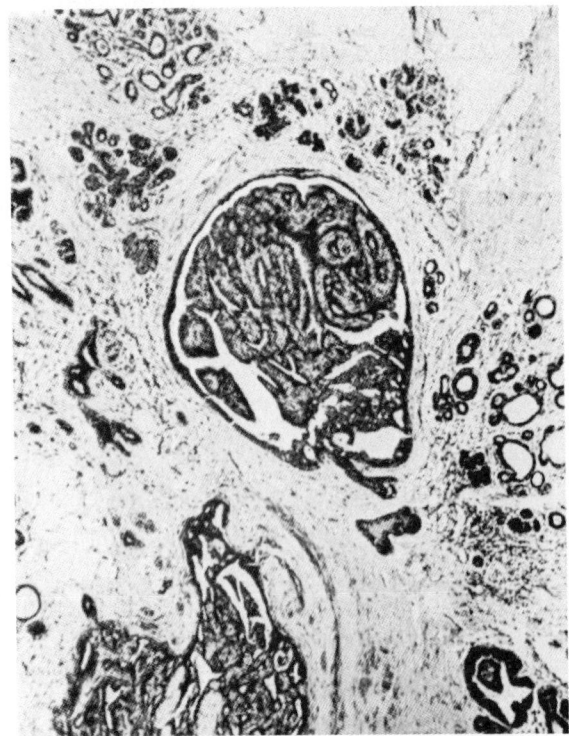

Figure 25–11. Papillary epithelial hyperplasia in fibrocystic disease. Two ducts show hyperplastic epithelium thrown into papillary projections. Note also fibrosis and small cysts. (Courtesy of Dr. Noel Weidner.)

SCLEROSING ADENOSIS

This variant is characterized histologically by *intralobular fibrosis and proliferation of small ductules or acini.* It is less common than cysts or epithelial hyperplasia.

Grossly, areas of sclerosing adenosis can be masked by the cystic changes but sometimes they have **hard cartilaginous consistency that begins to approximate that found in breast cancer.** On section, the involved area is not well localized and does not have the chalky yellow-white foci and streaks that identify breast carcinoma, an important gross differential feature.

Proliferation of small ducts, canaliculi, and gland buds may yield masses of small gland patterns, or nests and cords of cells within a fibrous stroma. The lobular arrangement is maintained. Usually, in such an area, many or at least some well-defined glands can be identified, but frequently they are closely aggregated so that glands lined by single or multiple layers of cells are backed up to each other **(adenosis).** At other times, the stromal overgrowth distorts and compresses the glands. Occasionally, the fibrous growth may totally compress the lumina to create the appearance of solid cords or strands of cells lying within the dense stroma, a histologic pattern that at times verges on the appearance of carcinoma (Fig. 25–12).

To the inexperienced, the histologic differentiation of a florid case of sclerosing adenosis from frank cancer may be difficult. When clearly defined cysts and apocrine elements are present, or when the epithelial structures preserve their glandular regularity, the distinction is made more readily.

OTHER LESIONS

Pure *fibrosis* is an infrequent variant in which a relatively well-delineated mass is associated with dense stromal fibrous tissue unaccompanied by cysts or epithelial hyperplasia.[19] It does not predispose to carcinoma.

Radial scar (benign sclerosing ductal proliferation) is characterized histologically by ductal proliferation with an abundant central fibrosis and elastosis, giving it the gross and microscopic appearance of a scar.[20] It is often associated with other features of cystic disease. It may be difficult to differentiate from a special type of cancer called tubular carcinoma.

CLINICAL SIGNIFICANCE OF FIBROCYSTIC CHANGES

The many patterns of breast pathology included under the designation fibrocystic change have clinical importance for two reasons: (1) They produce masses in the breast that require differentiation from carcinoma, and (2) *some* may predispose to the subsequent development of carcinoma.[21]

Certain clinical features of fibrocystic disease tend to differentiate it from cancer, but the only cer-

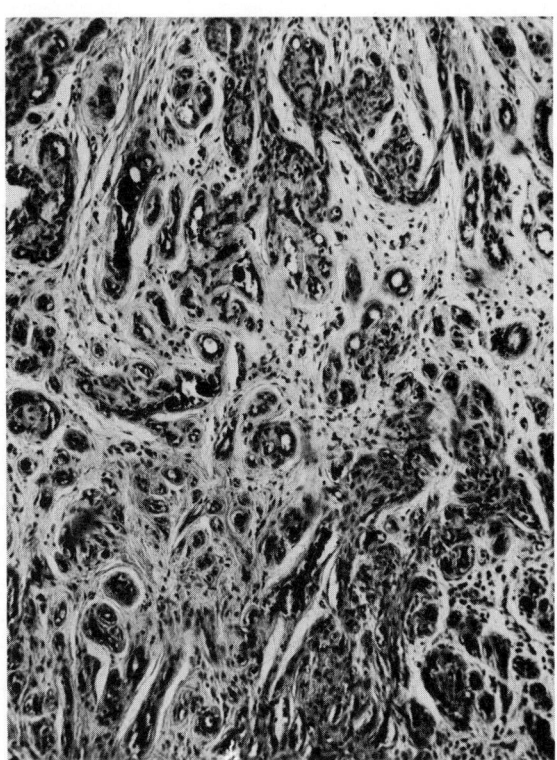

Figure 25–12. Sclerosing adenosis of the breast. The epithelial hyperplasia has produced the nests of cells, which appear quite disorderly. The overgrowth of fibrous tissue enmeshes and partially obliterates many of the epithelial nests, creating a pattern to be differentiated from the infiltrative growth of a cancer.

tain way of making this distinction is biopsy and pathologic examination. The following features favor the diagnosis of a benign lesion: bilateral involvement, multiple nodules, and pain prior to the menstrual period. These benign lesions occur in a somewhat younger age group, but unless the patient is in the first two decades of life (when carcinoma of the breast is rarely encountered), the age of the patient is a slender thread.

What is the relationship between the morphologic alterations of fibrocystic disease and carcinoma? Although there are many opinions, *the balance of evidence suggests that patients with some morphologic variants of fibrocystic disease, especially those with epithelial hyperplasia, have a higher than expected attack rate of cancer of the breast.* Current opinion places the increased risk of different lesions as follows:

• *No increased risk of breast carcinoma:* fibrosis, cystic changes (micro or macro), apocrine metaplasia, sclerosing adenosis, mild hyperplasia.
• *Slightly increased risk — 1.5 to 2 times:* hyperplasia moderate to florid, ductal papillomatosis (marked).
• *Significantly increased risk — 5 times:* atypical hyperplasia, ductal or lobular with duct involvement.
• *A family history of breast cancer increases the risk in all categories* — e.g., to about 10-fold with atypical hyperplasia.

Fortunately, only some 5% of biopsies reveal atypical epithelial hyperplasia. Thus the majority of women having "lumps" related to fibrocystic change can be reassured that there is little or no increased predisposition to cancer.

In summary, *the association between fibrocystic disease and cancer is proportional to the degree of epithelial hyperplasia and atypia seen.* In a study of 301 patients in whom a histologic diagnosis of *atypical hyperplasia* was made on biopsy but in whom the breast was not removed, the cumulative risk of breast cancer (both in situ and infiltrating) was 10% at 55 months.[22]

TUMORS

Neoplasms constitute the most important, albeit not the most common, lesions of the female breast. A great variety of tumors may occur in the female breast, made up as it is of a covering integument, adult fat, mesenchymal connective tissue, and epithelial structures. These tumors run the gamut of the neoplasms that may arise from stratified squamous epithelium, glandular structures, and mesenchymal connective tissue. Some may be listed as skin papillomas, squamous cell carcinomas of the skin, adenomas, papillomas of ducts, carcinomas of glandular or duct origin, and virtually every variety of benign and malignant mesenchymal tumor, such as fibroma and fibrosarcoma, granular cell myoblastoma, chondroma and chondrosarcoma, lipoma and liposarcoma, osteoma and osteogenic sarcoma, and angioma and angiosarcoma. Only the more common tumors specialized to the breast, however, will be discussed.

FIBROADENOMA

The most common benign tumor of the female breast is the fibroadenoma. As the name implies, it is *a new growth composed of both fibrous and glandular tissue.* Occurring at any age within the reproductive period of life, it is somewhat more common before age 30. Multiple small areas closely resembling a fibroadenoma are sometimes found in cases of cystic disease, termed *fibroadenomatosis.*

The fibroadenoma grows as a **spherical nodule that is usually sharply circumscribed and freely movable from the surrounding breast substance.** These tumors frequently occur in the upper outer quadrant of the breast. They vary in size from under 1 cm to giant forms 10 to 15 cm in diameter **(giant fibroadenoma),** but most are surgically removed when 2 to 4 cm in diameter (Fig. 25–13). On section they are firm, rubbery, and grayish white.

The histologic pattern is essentially one of delicate, cellular, fibroblastic stroma enclosing glandular and cystic spaces lined by epithelium. Intact, round-to-oval gland spaces may be present, lined by single or multiple layers of cells (pericanalicular fibroadenoma) (Fig. 25–14). In other

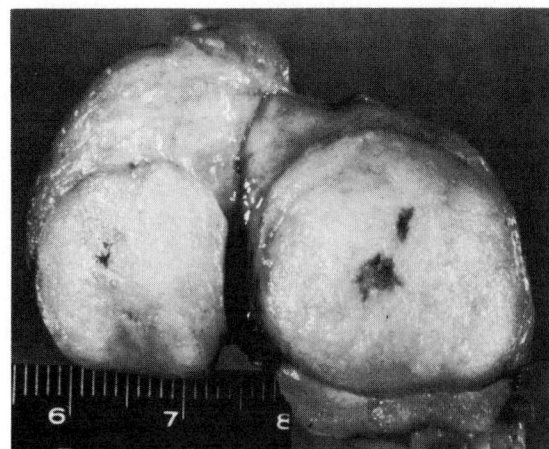

Figure 25–13. Fibroadenoma. Discrete mass bulges above level of surrounding breast tissue.

areas, the connective tissue stroma appears to have undergone more active proliferation with compression of the gland spaces. In consequence, glandular lumina are collapsed or compressed into slitlike, irregular clefts, and the epithelial elements then appear as narrow strands or cords of epithelium lying within the fibrous stroma (intracanalicu-

lar fibroadenoma) (Fig. 25–15). Both pericanalicular and intracanalicular patterns often coexist in the same tumor.

Quite rarely, the connective tissue element is scant, and the entire tumor may be composed of fairly densely packed glandular or acinar spaces lined by a single or double layer of cells **(tubular adenoma).** This pattern is most often seen in the lactating breast, and frequently the epithelium shows secretory activity similar to that in the surrounding breast substance **(lactating adenoma)** (see Fig. 25–2).

Fibroadenoma usually appears as a solitary, discrete, freely movable nodule within the breast. Slight increase in size may occur during the late phases of each menstrual cycle, and pregnancy may stimulate growth. Postmenopausally, regression or calcification may result. Although this lesion presents fairly distinctive clinical characteristics, it nonetheless requires surgical excision for absolute verification of its benign nature. Rarely in situ lobular or ductal carcinomas arise in or involve fibroadenomas.

PHYLLODES TUMOR

Infrequently, fibroadenomas may grow to very massive proportions, reaching diameters of 10 to 15 cm,

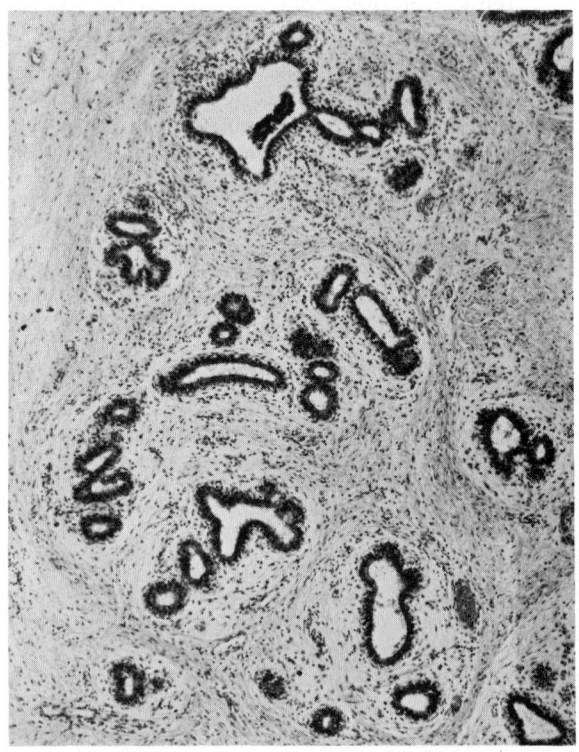

Fig. 25–14

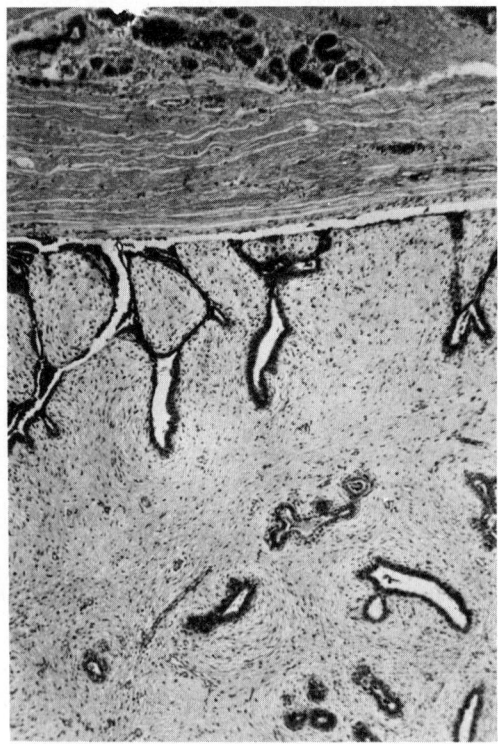

Fig. 25–15

Figure 25–14. Fibroadenoma showing morphology referred to as pericanalicular variant.

Figure 25–15. Fibroadenoma. Margin of nodule, with capsule and separation from compressed breast substance above. Growth is in part intracanalicular, particularly near capsule, with compression of gland spaces. Toward bottom, pattern is pericanalicular.

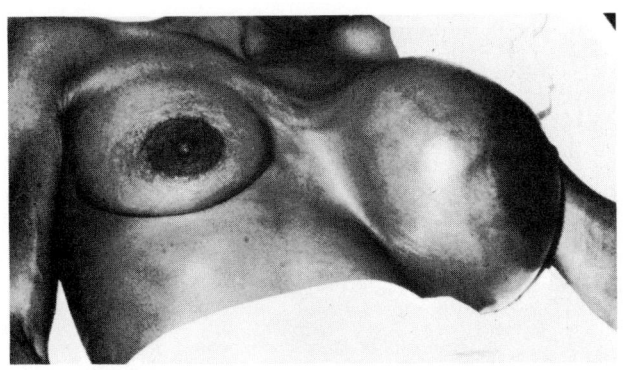

Figure 25–16. Malignant cystosarcoma phyllodes. Enlargement and distortion of breast.

the so-called *giant fibroadenomas*. Some of these large, bulky tumors become lobulated and cystic and on gross section exhibit leaflike clefts and slits (phyllodes). They have been designated *cystosarcoma phyllodes*, an unfortunate term since such lesions can be either benign or malignant. They may distort the breast, produce bulges in the skin surface, and even cause pressure necrosis of the overlying skin (Fig. 25–16). In these ulcerated lesions, the capsule of the tumor may rupture, and the growth may fungate through the skin to appear as an irregular mass. However, even this bizarre clinical behavior does not of necessity imply malignancy. Histologically, these lesions tend to have a more cellular myxoid stroma than do the usual fibroadenomas. The most ominous change is the appearance of *increased stromal cellularity, anaplasia, and high mitotic activity* (Fig. 25–17).[23] Malignant transformation is invariably accompanied by rapid increase in size, usually with invasion of adjacent breast tissue by malignant stroma. Malignant lesions may recur, but tend to remain as localized lesions for some time. However, in time, metastasis to

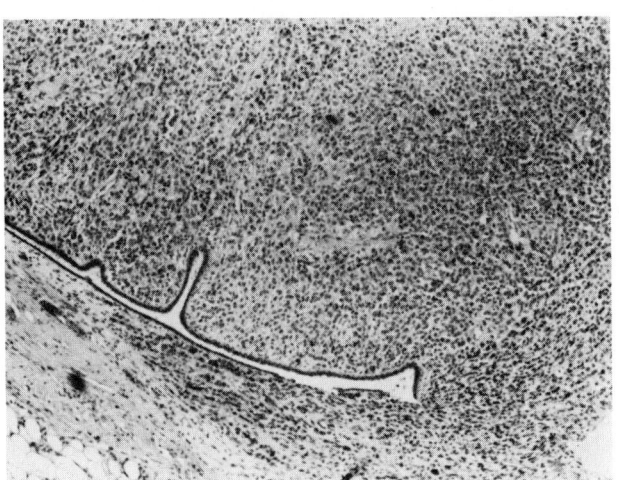

Figure 25–17. Malignant cystosarcoma phyllodes. Pleomorphic hypercellular stromal cells and a compressed ductal structure (left lower corner).

distant sites occurs in about 15% of cases. Most writers caution that, in many instances, anaplastic changes may be found in masses that nonetheless are innocent clinically, and therefore overdiagnosis and overtreatment must be guarded against.[24] Thus the term "phyllodes tumor" is preferable for these lesions.[24] The degree of histologic benignity or malignancy should be noted, dependent on the cytologic atypia and number of mitoses in stromal cells.

INTRADUCTAL PAPILLOMA

As the name implies, this is a neoplastic papillary growth within a duct. Most of these lesions are solitary and are found within the principal lactiferous ducts or sinuses. They present clinically as a result of (1) the appearance of serous or bloody nipple discharge; (2) the presence of a small subareolar tumor, a few millimeters in diameter; and (3) rarely, nipple retraction.

The tumors are usually very small, rarely more than 1 cm in diameter, and are therefore difficult to locate both clinically and anatomically. As mentioned, they are usually located in the major ducts, close to the nipple. They consist of friable, delicate, villous, branching growths within a dilated duct or cyst. Histologically, the tumor is composed of multiple papillae, each having a connective tissue axis covered by cuboidal or cylindrical epithelial cells (Fig. 25–18). In the truly benign papilloma, two cell types are seen in the centrally situated luminal mass—epithelial and myoepithelial.[5] The distinction between a benign but atypical intraductal papilloma and an intraductal papillary carcinoma may be difficult. In general, severe cytologic atypia, the absence of myoepithelial cells, abnormal mitotic figures, pseudostratification, the absence of a vascular connective tissue core, the presence of cell strands bridging the duct lumen (forming a so-called **cribriform pattern**), and the absence of hyalinization or apocrine metaplasia favor a malignant rather than benign papillary tumor.

Complete excision of the duct system should be performed in order to avoid local recurrences. The present consensus is that most solitary intraductal papillomas are benign and are *not* the precursors of papillary carcinoma. However, *multiple intraductal papillomas* should be distinguished from the group, since they are more likely to recur and are associated with an increased risk of development of carcinoma. They form poorly delineated, palpable tumors in which multiple papillary lesions in ducts occupy peripheral sectors of the breast,[25] and are best considered in the spectrum of epithelial hyperplasias associated with fibrocystic disease.

Nipple adenoma[26] and *florid papillomatosis of the nipple*[27] are terms used to describe tumors of the nipple exhibiting papillary hyperplasia of the duct epithelium, intermixed with fibrosis. They should be differentiated from carcinoma.

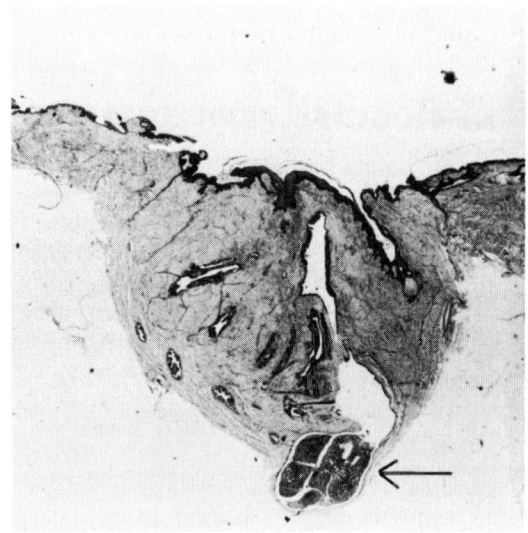

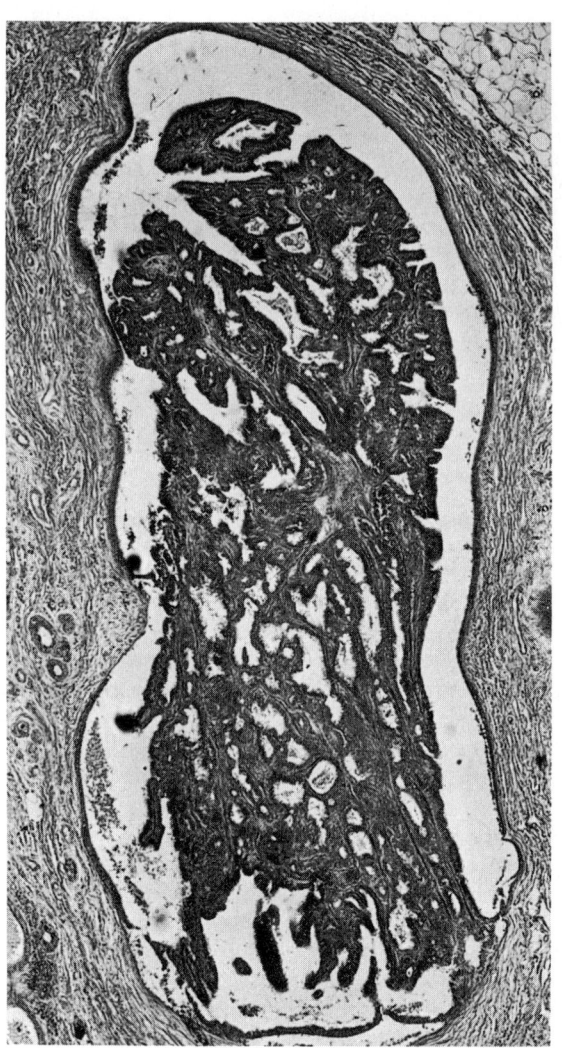

Figure 25–18. Intraductal papilloma. *A,* Low-power view of nipple showing tumor in lactiferous duct *(arrow). B,* High-power view showing well-differentiated papillary tumor.

CARCINOMA

The unqualified term "breast cancer" implies a carcinoma arising in the ductal and glandular structure of the breast. *Breast carcinoma causes some 20% of cancer deaths among females* and has been called "the foremost cancer" in women. Understandably, then, breast cancer has received a great deal of appropriate publicity and has been the focus of intensive study relative to its origins, diagnostic methods, and treatment.[28,29] Despite all the efforts, however, little ground has been gained, and the age-adjusted death rate from breast cancer in females in the United States has virtually remained stable over the past 30 years, now being about 27 per 100,000.[30] One of every 11 women in the United States will develop breast cancer and 43,000 die each year of the disease. It is both ironic and tragic that a neoplasm arising in an exposed organ, readily accessible to self-examination and clinical diagnosis, continues to exact such a heavy toll.

INCIDENCE AND EPIDEMIOLOGY. Cancer of the female breast is rarely found before the age of 25. It may occur at any age thereafter, with a peak incidence at or after the menopause.

Few cancers have been subjected to more intensive epidemiologic study. Observations bearing on the incidence of this disease can be summarized as follows:[31]

• *Geographic influences:* Five times more common in the United States than in Japan and Taiwan.
• *Genetic predisposition:* Well defined. The magnitude of risk is in proportion to number of close relatives with breast cancer and age when cancer occurred in relatives. The younger the relatives at time of developing cancer and the more bilateral cancers, the greater the genetic predisposition. There are uncommon high-risk families with apparent autosomal dominant transmission and familial association of breast and ovarian carcinomas.
• *Increasing age:* Uncommon before age 20, but then a steady rise to the time of menopause, followed by a slower rise throughout life.
• *Length of reproductive life:* Risk increases with early menarche and late menopause.

- *Parity:* More frequent in nulliparous than in multiparous women.
- *Age at first child:* Increased risk when over 30 at time of first child.
- *Obesity:* Increased risk attributed to synthesis of estrogens in fat depots.
- *Exogenous estrogens:* Still controversial, but some data show moderately increased risk with high-dosage therapy of menopausal symptoms.
- *Oral contraceptives:* No clear-cut increased risk; attributed to balanced content of estrogens and progestins in currently used oral contraceptives.[32-35]
- *Fibrocystic changes with atypical epithelial hyperplasia:* Increased risk, as noted in earlier discussion of this condition.
- *Carcinoma of the contralateral breast or endometrium:* Increased risk.
- *Diet and environmental agents:* High-lipid diets and moderate alcohol consumption[36] increase risk slightly.

ETIOLOGY AND PATHOGENESIS. Despite extensive studies, the ultimate origin or origins of breast carcinoma remains a mystery. However, the epidemiologic data cited above and extensive studies of mammary tumors in mice point to three sets of influences that may be important: (1) genetic factors, (2) hormonal imbalances, and (3) environmental factors. In animals, viruses can clearly interact with these influences to cause cancer, but no such viral etiology has yet been documented in humans.

Genetic predisposition undoubtedly exists, as evidenced by the markedly increased risk in first-degree relatives of cancer patients. In mice, high cancer strains can be achieved by genetic inbreeding. However, there is no understanding of how these factors operate in the induction of the neoplasm. Conceivably, they may influence the availability of hormone receptors in breast epithelial cells, as will be discussed.

Endogenous estrogen excess, or more accurately, hormonal imbalance, is thought to play a significant role. Many of the risk factors mentioned — long duration of reproductive life, nulliparity, and late age at first child — all imply increased exposure to estrogen peaks during the menstrual cycle. Functioning ovarian tumors that elaborate estrogens (p. 1167) are associated with breast cancer in postmenopausal women. Recent studies have confirmed associations among excess urinary estrogens, frequency of ovulation, age of menarche, and increased breast cancer risk.[37] There are also hints of how the estrogens might act. Normal breast epithelium possesses estrogen and progesterone receptors. These have been identified in some but not all breast cancers.[38] A variety of growth promoters (e.g., transforming growth factor α [TGF-α] and platelet-derived growth factor [PDGF]) and growth inhibitors (TGF-β) are secreted by human breast cancer cells, and many studies suggest that they are involved in tumor progression (see p. 287). Production of these growth factors is estrogen dependent, and it is possible that interactions between circulating hormones, hormone receptors on cancer cells, and autocrine growth factors induced by tumor cells play a role in breast cancer progression.[39]

Of the *environmental influences,* the effect of diet is controversial, but there are ardent advocates of the thesis that high dietary fat constitutes a significant predisposition.[40] Coffee addicts will be pleased to know that there is no substantial evidence that caffeine consumption increases the risk, but recent studies suggest that moderate alcohol consumption is associated with a 1.5 increased risk of breast cancer.[36]

The role of *viruses* in human breast cancer has been pursued since Bittner's brilliant discovery in 1936 that a filterable agent, transmitted through the mother's milk, causes breast cancer in suckling mice.[41] The virus, called mouse mammary tumor virus (MMTV), was later identified as a retrovirus. Subsequently there were many hints of the existence of an analogous virus in breast cancer of humans, but the findings have not been conclusive. Currently there is some interest in homologies between proviral DNA sequences of MMTV and the human genome, suggesting the presence of a yet unisolated latent retrovirus in certain human tissues.[42] There are also unconfirmed studies reporting the presence of reverse transcriptase or particles with properties of retroviruses in cancerous breast tissue.[43]

More has been learned recently of the possible contributions of *oncogenes* to breast cancer.[44] In particular, amplification of the HER-2/neu gene (which is similar to the gene for the receptor to epidermal growth factor) has been found in from 5% to as much as 30% of cancerous breast tissue,[45] associated with overexpression of the protein product of the gene in carcinoma cells (Fig. 25–19).[46] Insertion of an activated neu oncogene in transgenic mice results in the formation of breast adenocarcinomas. It has been suggested that this single-step induction of cancer may be one explanation of the high incidence of human breast cancer, since cancer can presumably result from the mutational activation of only one gene.[47] Amplification of the c-ras and c-myc genes, and insertional mutagenesis in the c-myc locus, have also been described in human breast cancer.[48] Finally, inactivation and structural rearrangements of the retinoblastoma gene (p. 291) in breast tumors suggest that mutations in cancer suppressor genes may play a role in breast cancer.[49]

CLASSIFICATION AND DISTRIBUTION. Curiously, carcinoma is more common in the left breast than in the right, in a ratio of 110:100. The cancers are bilateral or sequential in the same breast in 4% or more of cases.

Among breast carcinomas small enough for their general areas of origin to be identified, approximately 50% arise in the upper outer quadrant; 10% in each of the remaining quadrants; and about 20% in the central or subareolar region. As will be seen, the site of

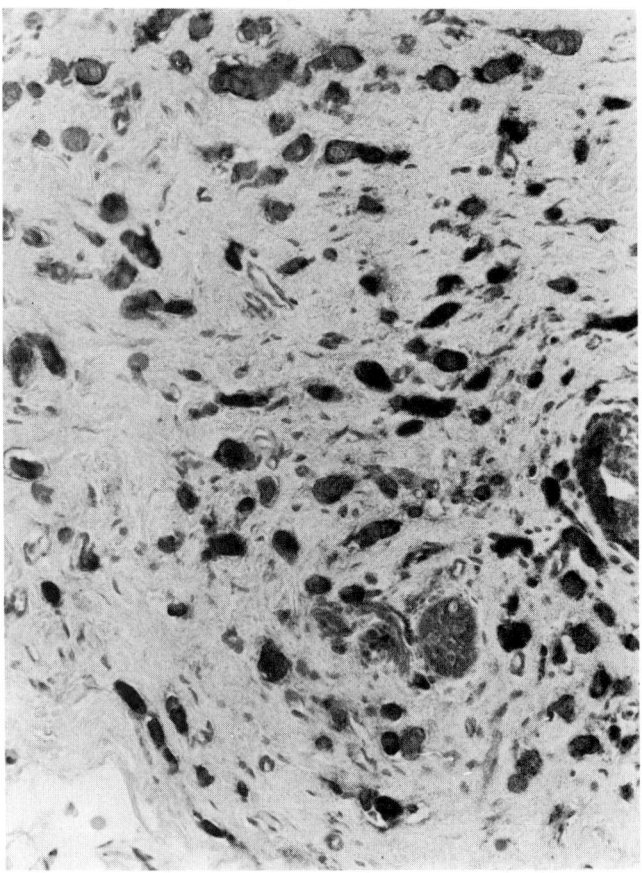

Figure 25–19. Immunoperoxidase stain of infiltrating breast carcinoma, stained with an antibody to the neu-oncogene product. Note darkly stained infiltrating cancer cells containing gene product. (Courtesy of Dr. Andrea Dawson.)

origin influences the pattern of nodal metastasis to a considerable degree.

An overview of the range in tumor types is provided by the following classification adopted from the World Health Organization.[50]

A. Noninvasive (noninfiltrating)
    1. Intraductal carcinoma
    2. Intraductal papillary carcinoma
    3. Lobular carcinoma in situ
B. Invasive
    1. Invasive ductal carcinoma—not otherwise specified (NOS)
    2. Invasive lobular carcinoma
    3. Medullary carcinoma
    4. Colloid carcinoma (mucinous carcinoma)
    5. Paget's disease
    6. Tubular carcinoma
    7. Adenoid cystic carcinoma
    8. Invasive comedocarcinoma
    9. Apocrine carcinoma
    10. Invasive papillary carcinoma

Only the more common types will be discussed. The incidence of the various types of infiltrating carcinomas collected from a national study is shown in Table 25–1.

Table 25–1. Incidence of Histologic Types of Invasive Breast Cancer

	%
Invasive duct carcinoma	
Pure	52.6
Combined with other types	22.0
Medullary carcinoma	6.2*
Colloid carcinoma	2.4
Paget's disease	2.3
Other pure types	2.0
Other combined types	1.6
Infiltrating lobular carcinoma	4.9
Combined lobular and ductal	6.0

Modified from Fisher, E., et al: The pathology of invasive breast cancer: A syllabus derived from the findings of the National Surgical Adjuvant Breast Project. Cancer *36*:1, 1975.
* With strict histologic criteria, medullary carcinoma incidence is 1%.[54]

Noninvasive (In Situ) Carcinoma

INTRADUCTAL CARCINOMA. Over 90% of breast carcinomas arise within the ducts. As long as the tumor remains within the confines of the ductal basement membranes, it constitutes a noninfiltrating intraductal carcinoma. It begins as an atypical proliferation of ductal epithelium that eventually completely fills and plugs the ducts with neoplastic cells. Grossly, the tumor is usually a poorly defined focus of slightly increased consistency caused by the marked dilatation and solidification of the ducts. When the breast is sectioned, cordlike ducts are found filled with necrotic and cheesy tumorous tissue. This substance can be readily extruded upon slight pressure, hence the designation **comedocarcinoma.** Histologically, the ducts are dilated and filled with neoplastic anaplastic epithelial cells that plug the lumina; sometimes there is central necrosis (Fig. 25–20). The growth pattern is sometimes **cribriform,** indicating the presence of ductlike structures within the primary dilated ducts (Fig. 25–21). Rarely, these intraductal carcinomas have a predominantly papillary pattern and are called **intraductal papillary carcinomas.** Invasive carcinoma develops in 28% of women treated with biopsy alone, over a period of 15 years, usually in the same region as the original tumor.[51]

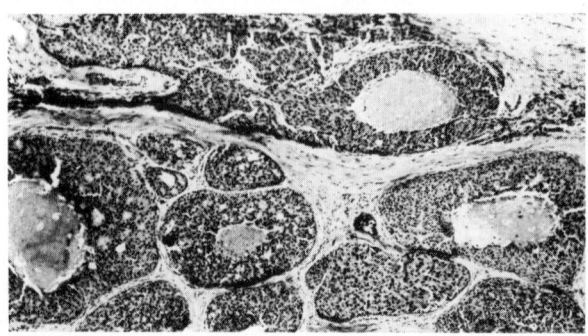

Figure 25–20. Comedocarcinoma. Intraductal proliferation of malignant cells. Note central necrosis.

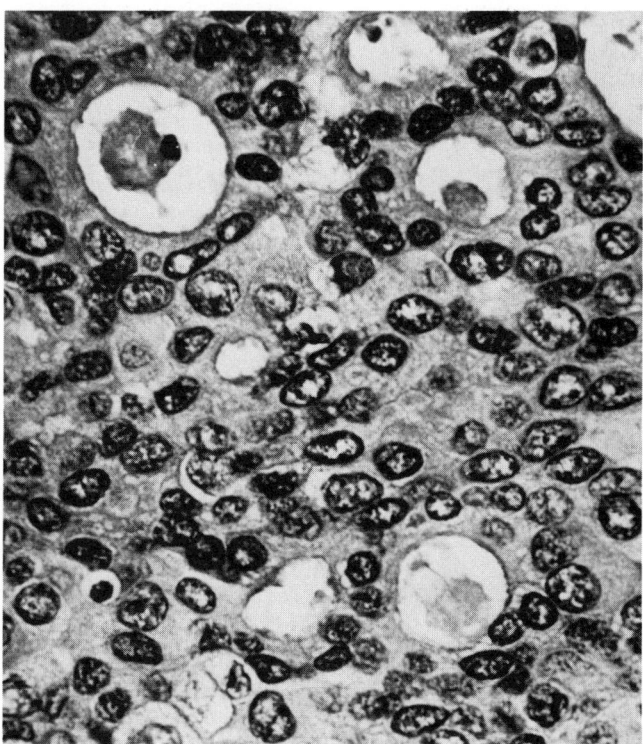

Figure 25–21. High magnification of intraductal carcinoma, showing cribriform pattern, and large cells with hyperchromatic nuclei: Compare with Figure 25–10, which shows hyperplastic lesions.

LOBULAR CARCINOMA IN SITU. This is a histologically unique lesion manifested by proliferation, in one or more terminal ducts and/or ductules (acini), of cells that are loosely cohesive, are somewhat larger than normal, and have rare mitoses and oval or round nuclei with small nucleoli (Fig. 25–22). These lesions can be seen in breasts removed for fibrocystic disease, in the vicinity of invasive carcinoma, or admixed with the foci of intraductal carcinoma. The frequency with which such change may develop into invasive carcinoma varies.[52] Both breasts are at equal risk. In a survey of 99 patients **not** treated with mastectomy and followed for 24 years,[53] the frequency of subsequent carcinoma developing in the same or **contralateral** breast was 30%, nine times greater than expected for the general population. **The infiltrating carcinomas that subsequently developed in both studies were either ductal or lobular.**

Infiltrating (Invasive) Duct Carcinoma

As mentioned, this is the most common type of breast cancer. Most exhibit marked increases in dense fibrous tissue stroma, giving the tumor a hard consistency **(scirrhous carcinoma).** These growths occur as fairly sharply delimited nodules of **stony-hard** consistency that average 2 cm in diameter and rarely exceed 4 to 5 cm. On palpation, they may have an infiltrative attachment to the surrounding structures with fixation to the underlying chest wall, dim-

pling of the skin, and retraction of the nipple (Fig. 25–23). The mass is quite characteristic on cut section. **It is retracted below the cut surface, has a hard cartilaginous consistency, and produces a grating sound when scraped.** Within the central focus, there are small pinpoint foci or streaks of chalky white, necrotic tumor (Fig. 25–24) and small foci of calcification.

Histologically, the **tumor consists of anaplastic duct lining cells disposed in cords, solid cell nests, tubes, glands, anastomosing masses, and mixtures of all these.** In some, clear-cut intraductal components can also be seen (Fig. 25–25). The cells are disseminated in a fibrous stroma. The cytologic detail of tumor cells varies from small cells with moderately hyperchromatic regular nuclei to huge cells with large irregular and hyperchromatic nuclei. Frequently invasion of perivascular and perineural spaces as well as blood and lymphatic vessels is readily evident (Fig. 25–26).

MEDULLARY CARCINOMA. This variant accounts for about 1% of all mammary carcinomas and tends to produce large fleshy tumor masses up to 5 to 10 cm in diameter.[54] These tumors do not have the striking desmoplasia (formation of fibrous tissue) of the usual carcinoma, and therefore are distinctly more yielding on external palpation and on cut section. On section, the tumor has a soft, fleshy consistency, and tends to be discrete (Fig. 25–27). Foci of necrosis and hemorrhage are large and numerous. Histologically, the carcinoma is characterized by (1) solid, syncytium-like sheets of large cells with vesicular, often

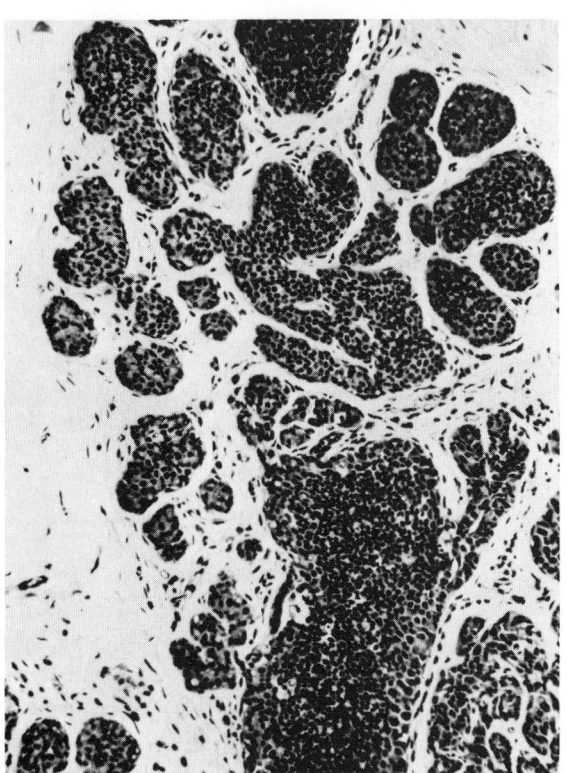

Figure 25–22. Lobular carcinoma in situ. Note proliferation of well-differentiated tumor cells in terminal ducts and ductules.

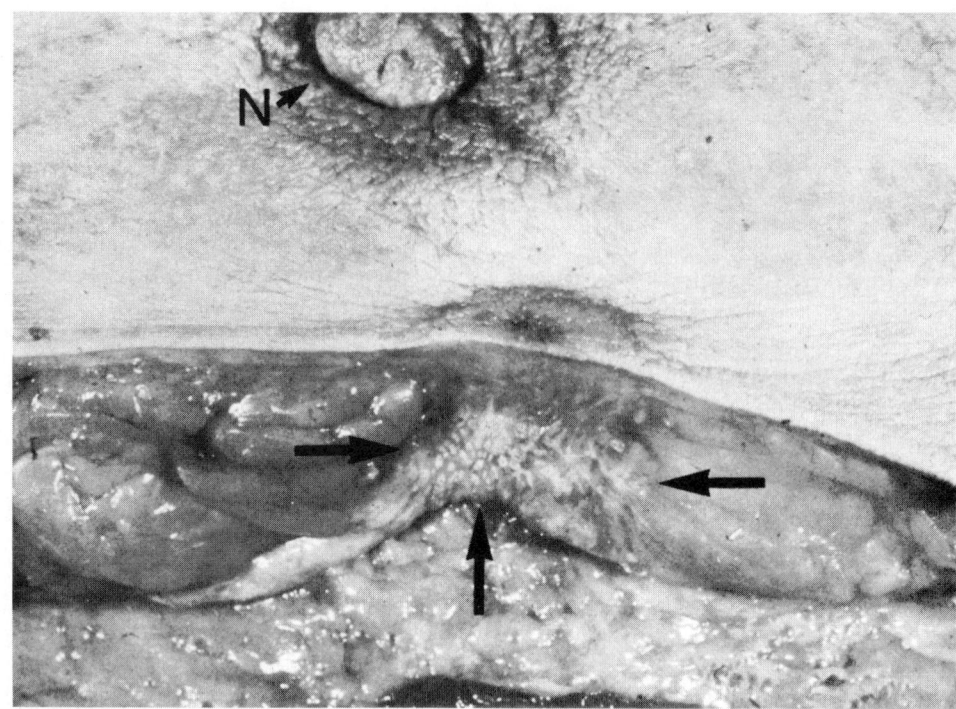

Figure 25–23. Carcinoma of breast, infiltrating *(arrows)*. Tumor is transected through middle, and breast is viewed obliquely to illustrate retracted mass and fixation to and dimpling of attached skin. (N = nipple.)

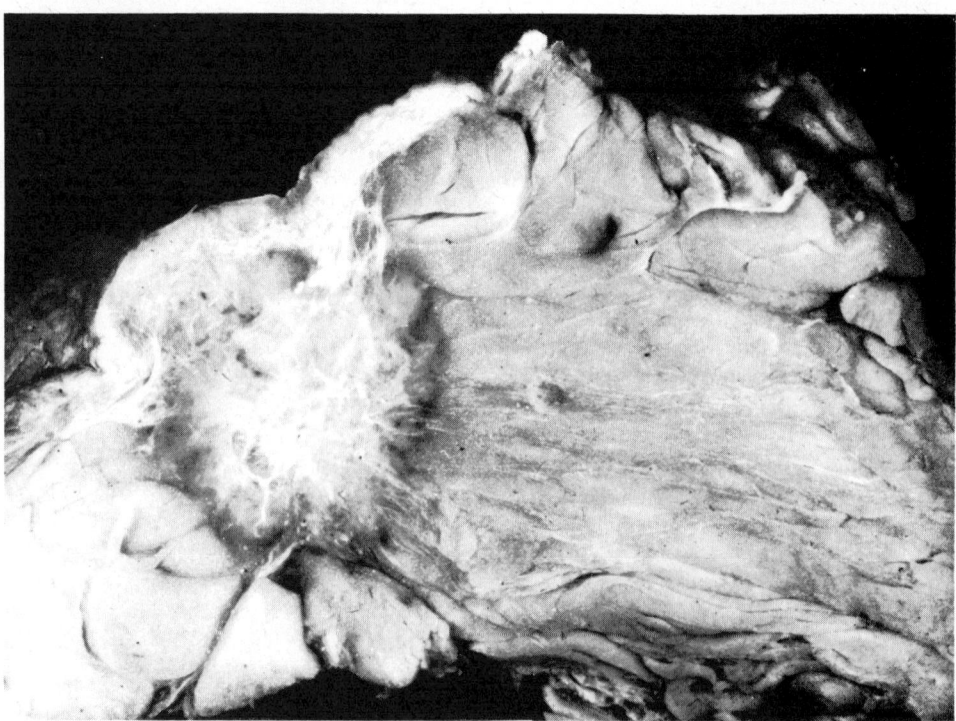

Figure 25–24. Carcinoma of breast, infiltrating. Cut surface illustrates lack of demarcation, fixation to skin, and chalky foci of necrosis within mass.

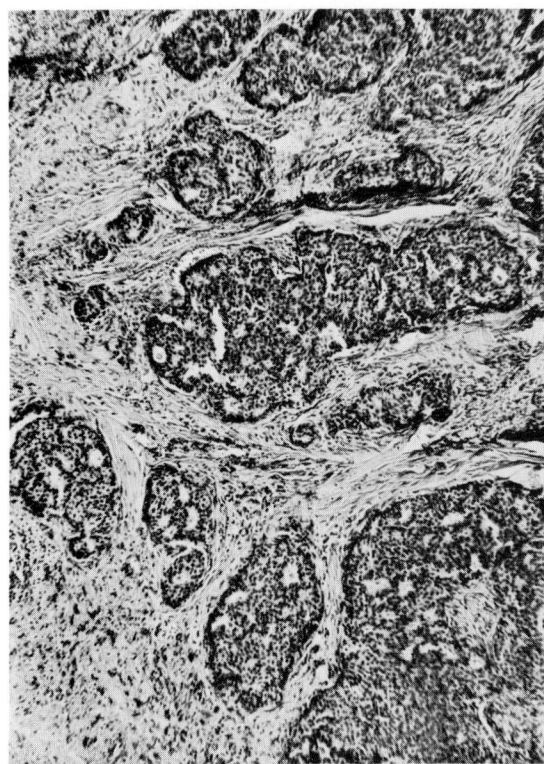

Figure 25–25. Ductal carcinoma. Tumor cells fill ducts and have invaded stroma.

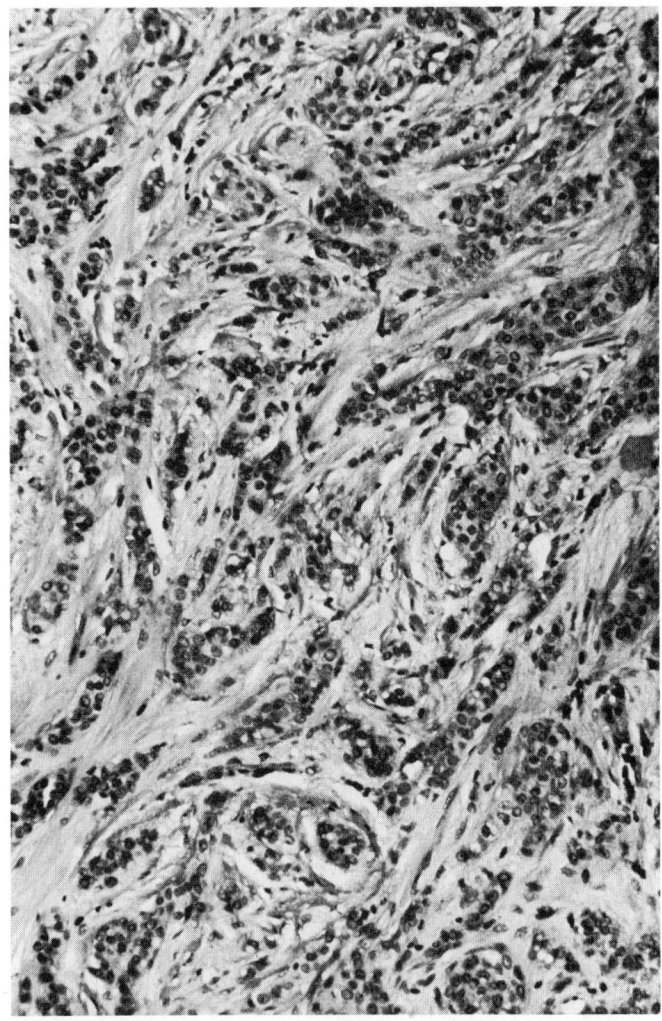

Figure 25–26. Infiltrating duct carcinoma. Note cords of cells infiltrating stroma.

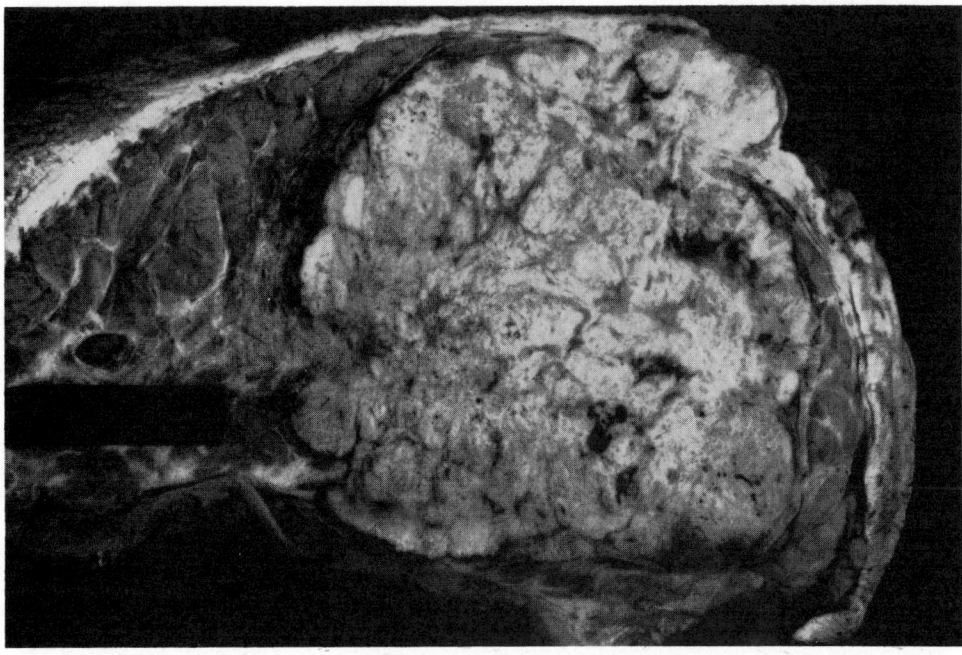

Figure 25–27. Carcinoma of breast, medullary type. The large bulky mass appears deceptively discrete.

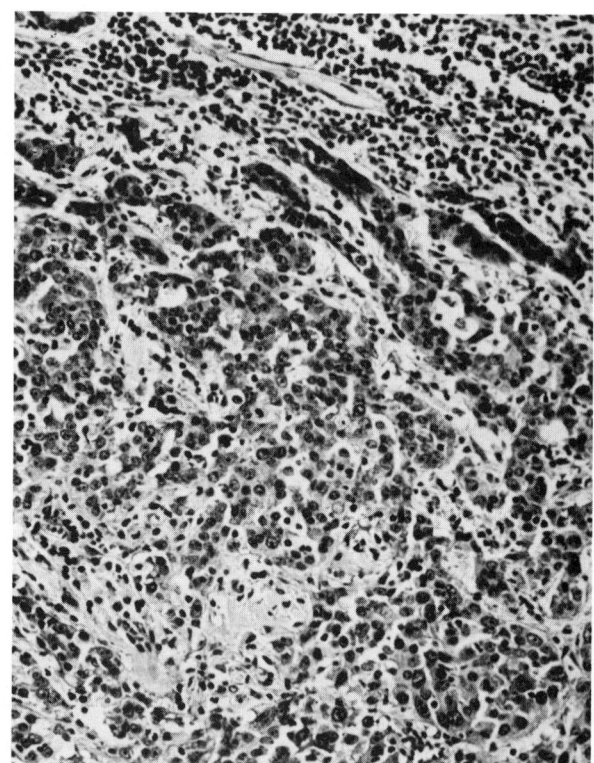

Figure 25-28. Medullary carcinoma with lymphoid infiltrate. Note lymphocytes infiltrating syncytial epithelial tumor.

pleomorphic nuclei, containing prominent nucleoli and frequent mitoses. The syncytial cells occupy over 75% of the tumor, and there is complete absence of microglandular structure and (2) a moderate-to-marked lymphocytic infiltrate between these sheets, with a scant fibrous component (Fig. 25-28). It is the lymphoid infiltrate that gives these tumors their special significance, since such tumors have a distinctly better prognosis than the usual infiltrating duct carcinomas, even in the presence of axillary lymph node metastases. The ten-year survival rate for these tumors is 70 to 90%.[54,55]

COLLOID OR MUCINOUS CARCINOMA.

This unusual variant tends to occur in older women and grows slowly over the course of many years, producing large, gelatinous masses. The tumor is extremely soft and has the consistency and appearance of pale gray-blue gelatin. It may occur in pure form or in association with other types.[56]

Histologically, this tumor usually takes on one of two patterns of growth, which may coexist in a single lesion. In the "pure" mucinous carcinomas there are large lakes of lightly staining, amorphous mucin that dissect and extend into contiguous tissue spaces and planes of cleavage. Floating within this mucin are small islands and isolated neoplastic cells, sometimes forming glands (Fig. 25-29). Vacuolation of at least some of the cells is characteristic. In "mixed" mucinous tumors the tumor exhibits large areas with mucin as well as areas of typical nonmucinous duct carcinoma.

The survival rate is appreciably greater in pure colloid carcinoma than in the usual infiltrating duct carcinoma, and lymph node metastases are infrequent.[57]

PAGET'S DISEASE.

Paget's disease of the nipple is a specialized form of ductal carcinoma that arises in the main excretory ducts of the breast and extends to involve the skin of the nipple and areola.[58] As a consequence of this malignant invasion of the skin, eczematoid changes occur in the nipple and areola. Careful morphologic study of these lesions has demonstrated beyond doubt that **ductal carcinoma, with or without invasion, invariably antedates the skin change.** Since Paget's disease of the nipple implies extension to the skin, the prognosis is somewhat less favorable than in the simple noninvasive ductal carcinoma. About 30 to 40% of these women have metastases at the time of surgery.

The most striking gross characteristics of this lesion involve the skin. The skin of the nipple and areola is frequently fissured, ulcerated, and oozing. There is surrounding inflammatory hyperemia and edema, and occasionally total nipple ulceration. An underlying lump or mass is only rarely present.

The histologic hallmark of this entity is the involvement of the epidermis by malignant cells, referred to as Paget cells. These cells are large, anaplastic, and hyperchromatic and are usually surrounded by a clear zone or halo (Fig. 25-30). The halo can be stained with such mucopolysaccharide stains as alcian blue. In addition to the Paget cells, the other histologic criteria of ductal carcinoma are present.

LOBULAR CARCINOMA.

Lobular carcinoma is a relatively distinct morphologic form of mammary cancer[59,60] that probably arises from the terminal ductules of the breast

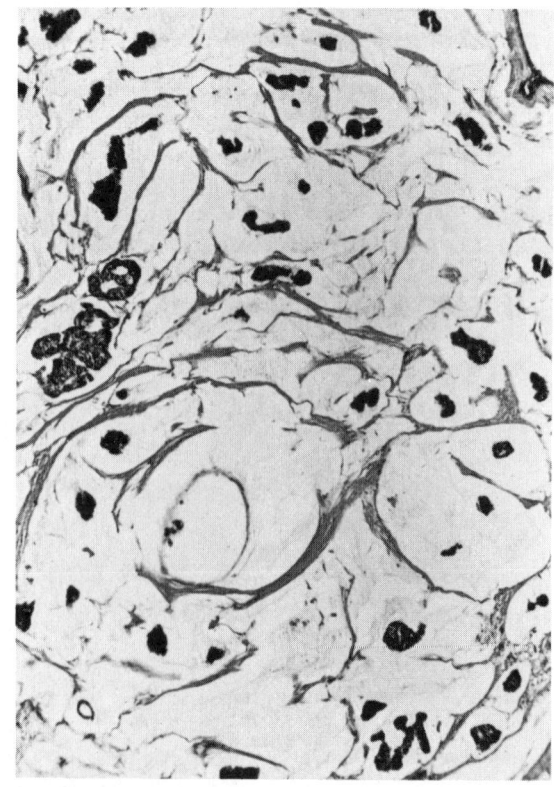

Figure 25-29. Colloid carcinoma. Note lakes of lightly staining mucin with small islands of tumor cells.

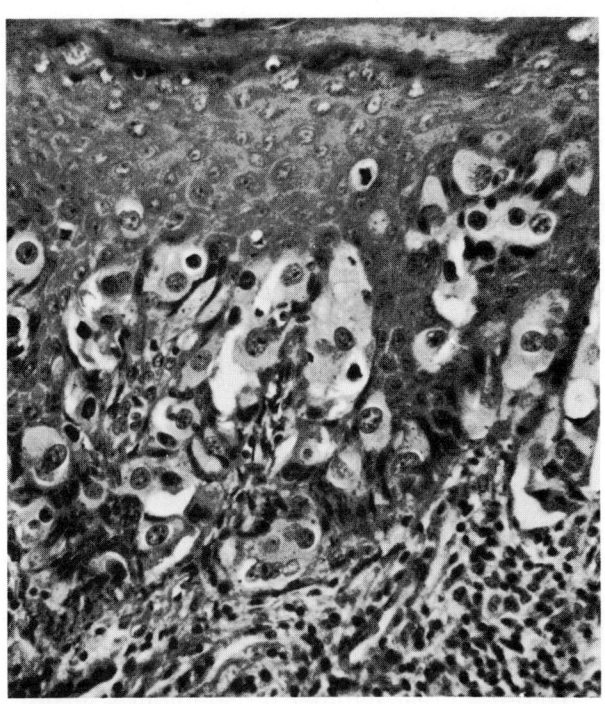

Figure 25–30. Paget's disease of breast. Classic Paget cells dot the epithelium.

to block the local area of skin drainage and cause lymphedema and thickening of the skin, a change that has for years been referred to as **peau d'orange** (orange peel). When the tumor involves the main excretory ducts, particularly in the intraduct variety, **retraction of the nipple** may develop. Certain carcinomas tend to infiltrate widely through the breast substance, involve the majority of the lymphatics, and produce acute swelling, redness, and tenderness of the breast, referred to clinically as **inflammatory carcinoma.** This is not a special morphologic pattern but merely implies widespread dissemination. It tends to develop with pregnancy.

The utilization of **mammography** has directed attention to the calcium content of mammary cancers, since the appearance of radiodense deposits has been regarded as an important radiologic feature of carcinoma. Foci of calcification are indeed present in 60% of cancers if special stains for calcium are done, although routine H and E sections may miss many of these. However, the incidence of calcific opacifications in benign lesions approaches that in malignant tumors, and furthermore over 40% of cancers are not substantially calcified.

Spread of the tumor eventually occurs through the lymphohematogenous routes. The pathways of lymphatic dissection are in all possible directions: **lateral** to the axilla, **superior** to the nodes above the clavicle and the neck, **medial** to the other breast, **inferior** to the abdominal viscera and lymph nodes, and **deep** to the nodes within the chest, particularly along the internal mammary arteries. The

lobule. Although making up only 5 to 10% of breast carcinomas, **invasive lobular carcinomas** are of particular interest for at least two reasons: (1) They tend to be bilateral far more frequently than those arising in ducts (the likelihood of cancer in the contralateral breast being on the order of 20%); (2) they tend to be multicentric within the same breast.

Grossly, the tumor is rubbery and poorly circumscribed, but sometimes appears as a typical scirrhous type. Histologically, it consists of strands of infiltrating tumor cells, often only one cell in width (in the form of an "Indian file"), loosely dispersed throughout the fibrous matrix (Fig. 25–31). The cells are small and uniform-staining with relatively little cytologic pleomorphism. Irregularly shaped solid nests and sheets may also occur in continuity with the single-file pattern. The tumor cells are frequently arranged in concentric rings about normal ducts, this pattern being virtually diagnostic of invasive lobular carcinoma. However, differentiation between ductal and lobular infiltrating carcinoma may very often be quite difficult, and in some tumors mixed ductal and lobular patterns, as well as intermediate cancers, exist (Table 25–1). Indeed, most duct carcinomas probably arise also from the terminal ductules.

FEATURES COMMON TO ALL INVASIVE CANCERS.
There are additional morphologic features common to all infiltrative breast carcinomas, whatever the histologic types. As focal lesions, they extend progressively in all directions. In the course of time, they may become adherent to the deep fascia of the chest wall and thus become **fixed in position.** Extension to the skin may cause not only fixation but also **retraction and dimpling of the skin,** an important characteristic of malignant growth. At the same time, the lymphatics may become so involved as

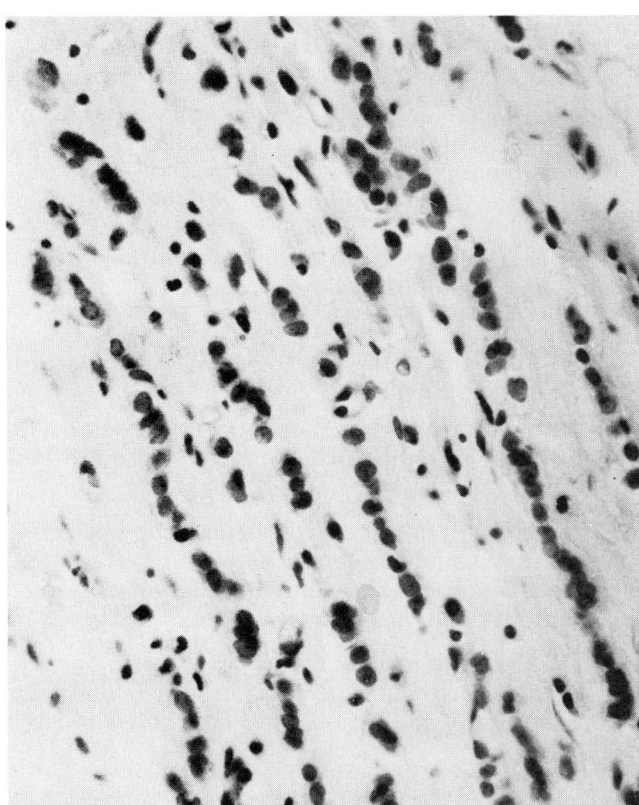

Figure 25–31. Carcinoma of breast, infiltrating lobular type. A single file of tumor cells are embedded within a dense fibrous stroma.

two most favored directions of drainage are the axillary nodes and the nodes along the internal mammary artery.

Overall, about two thirds of all patients have metastases to lymph nodes at the time of initial diagnosis of breast cancer. **The pattern of nodal spread is heavily influenced by the location of the cancer in the breast.** Tumors arising in the outer quadrants involve the axillary nodes alone in about 50% of cases, and have both internal mammary and axillary involvement in an additional 15% of cases. In contrast, cancers arising in the inner quadrants and center of the breast affect the axilla alone in about 25% of cases. In an additional 40%, internal mammary nodes are affected, often with axillary involvement.[5] The supraclavicular nodes are the third most favored site of nodal spread. As will be seen, nodal involvement seriously prejudices the prognosis. Distant metastases via the bloodstream may affect virtually any organ of the body. Favored sites for dissemination are the lungs, bones, liver, and adrenals. Some of the most bizarre metastatic involvements, such as spread to the pituitary gland, eyes, and skin, are seen in this form of cancer.

GRADING AND STAGING OF BREAST CANCER. The many histologic grades and stages of breast cancer have been subdivided into smaller homogeneous groups to standardize comparisons of results of various therapeutic modalities among clinics.[62] From the histologic classification described earlier, cancers may be roughly divided as follows:

Nonmetastasizing: intraductal or comedocarcinoma without stromal invasion; in situ lobular carcinoma.

Uncommonly metastasizing: pure extracellular mucinous or colloid cancer; medullary cancer; tubular adenocarcinoma; infiltrating papillary; adenoid cystic carcinoma.

Moderately to highly metastasizing: all other types.

The American Joint Committee on Cancer Staging divides the clinical stages as follows:

STAGE I. A tumor less than 5 cm in diameter without nodal involvement and no metastases.

STAGE II. A tumor less than 5 cm in diameter with involved but movable axillary nodes and no distant metastases.

STAGE III. All breast cancers of any size with possible skin involvement, pectoral and chest wall fixation, and nodal involvement including axillary nodes, fixed but without disseminated metastases.

STAGE IV. Any form of breast cancer with or without nodal involvement, pectoral fixation, skin ulceration, or chest wall fixation, but having disseminated metastases.

CLINICAL COURSE. Cancers of the breast are usually first discovered by the patient or physician as a solitary, painless mass in the breast. The older the patient with a single breast mass, the more likely is it to be cancer. When first discovered, these cancers are deceptively freely movable and delimited. Accordingly, the differential diagnosis extends to virtually every disorder in this chapter, including the variants of fibrocystic disease, fat necrosis, scarring of an abscess, and benign tumors. Many cancers are first detected by the patient during self-examination. On the average, these lesions are 4 cm in diameter when first found, and approximately two thirds have already spread to axillary or other nodes. Intraductal cancers, which rarely produce palpable masses, more often come to attention by the appearance of a discharge (sometimes hemorrhagic) from the nipple.

Because early treatment of localized disease is the best hope of total eradication, an enormous effort is being made to identify breast cancers at an early stage. Currently, emphasis is being placed on more frequent, regular medical examinations and mammography, xeroradiography, and thermography as screening techniques. Mammography in particular can detect small and early cancers and indeed has uncovered a great number of carcinomas in situ or cases of "minimal cancer." A recently completed massive screening study has shown unequivocal increases in survival for women with mammography-detected cancers—not only in women over 50, as previously thought, but also in women 40 to 49 years of age and even younger.[64] Thus, the present consensus is to recommend mammography at age 40 and every one or two years thereafter, except in high-risk groups, in whom screening could begin earlier.[65]

A number of factors influence the prognosis of breast cancer.

1. *The size of the primary tumor,* tumors of less than 2 cm being associated with favorable prognosis.
2. *Lymph node involvement and the number of lymph nodes exhibiting metastases.* For example, with no histologic involvement of axillary lymph nodes the five-year survival is close to 80%; those with one to three positive nodes have a 50% five-year survival. Disease-free survival falls off to 21% in the presence of four or more positive nodes.
3. *The histologic type and grade of tumor.* This has been discussed earlier, but can be appreciated from an older study of 30-year follow-up of 1458 consecutive operable infiltrating cancers treated by radical mastectomy. The survival for intraductal carcinoma was 74%; for papillary carcinoma, 65%; for medullary carcinoma, 58%; for colloid, 58%; for infiltrating lobular, 34%; and for infiltrating ductal, 29%.
4. *The presence or absence of estrogen and progesterone receptors.* As discussed earlier, estrogen is thought to be a promoter in breast carcinogenesis, possibly by its influence on autocrine growth factor production by cancer cells. The number of estrogen receptors in breast cancer cells can be high, intermediate, or absent and is proportional to the degree of cell differentiation and of the potential responsive-

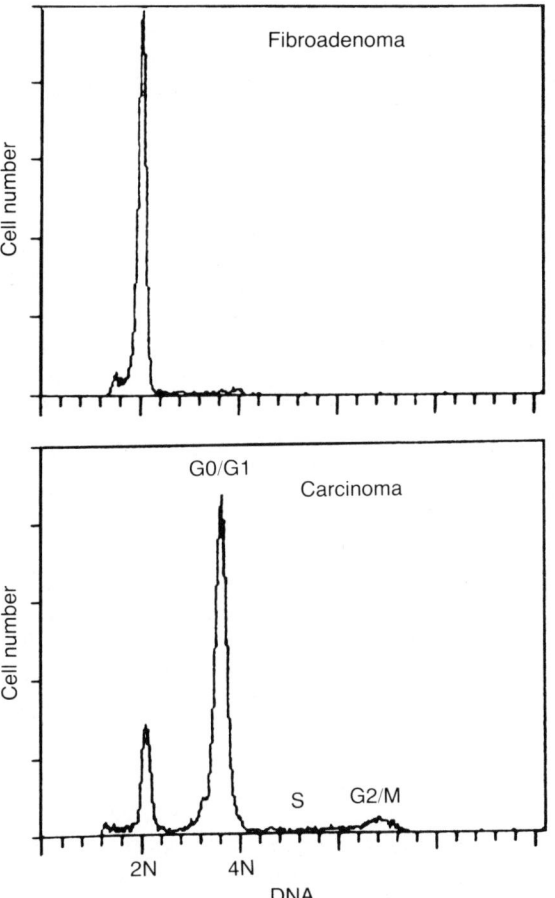

Figure 25–32. Flow cytometric histograms of a benign breast tumor *(top)* and ductal carcinoma *(bottom)*. The histogram of the benign lesion contains a single peak representing G0/G1 phase euploid nuclei having 2N DNA content. The histogram of the malignant lesion shows, in addition, an aneuploid population having near-tetraploid G0/G1 phase DNA content. (Courtesy of Dr. David Weinberg, Department of Pathology, Brigham and Women's Hospital.)

ness of the tumor to antiestrogen ablation by oophorectomy or tamoxifen. Seventy percent of tumors with estrogen receptors regress after hormonal manipulation, whereas only 5% of those that are negative respond to these procedures. The highest response rates to endocrine ablation are in patients with tumors containing both estrogen and progesterone receptors.[66] On the whole, cancers with high levels of estrogen receptors have a better prognosis than those with intermediate levels or no receptors.

5. *The proliferative rate, and the presence of aneuploidy* (increased and scattered DNA values) as measured by flow cytometry. The tumor's nuclear DNA content is a strong indicator of poor outcome—in particular, the fraction of cells scattered outside the modal peaks of DNA histograms (Fig. 25–32) correlates with poor behavior.[67,68]

6. *The presence of amplified or activated oncogenes.* The clinical utility of finding such oncogenes in tumor tissue is still unproved,[69] but some studies have corre-

lated certain oncogenes (e.g., the neu-oncogene[46]) with aggressive behavior.

Other obvious poor prognostic signs include extensive edema or multiple nodules in the skin of the breast, fixation to the chest wall, spread to internal mammary lymph nodes, supraclavicular metastases, inflammatory carcinoma, and of course, distant metastases.

Overall, *axillary node status* is the single most important prognostic factor for patients with early breast cancer. However, 20 to 30% of patients with histologically negative lymph nodes will suffer recurrences and die of their disease within ten years. For these reasons, there are continued searches for better biologic markers of prognosis[70] and more effective treatment modalities.[71] Current therapeutic approaches include combinations of simple mastectomy or segmental resection of the mass (lumpectomy) with or without lymph node dissection, postoperative irradiation, and chemotherapy—with ardent proponents for each of the many combinations.[72]

The overall five-year survival for stage I cancer is 80%; for stage II, 65%; for stage III, 40%; and for stage IV, 10%. It should be noted that recurrence may appear late, even after ten years, but with each passing year free of disease, the prognosis improves. In the overall view of breast cancers, the ten-year survival is still no more than 50%.

Thus, this discussion of breast cancer ends virtually where it began. The clinical problem is monumental despite great efforts to solve it, and there is much yet to be learned.

MISCELLANEOUS MALIGNANCIES. Malignant neoplasia may arise from the skin of the breast, sweat glands, sebaceous glands, and hair shafts, or from the connective tissues and fatty stroma. These tumors are identical to their counterparts found in other sites of the body. Those arising from skin grow as basal or squamous cell carcinoma. Cancers arising in the skin adnexa grow as carcinomas of sweat gland or sebaceous gland origin. Malignancies of the stroma are, of course, sarcomas and include fibrosarcomas, myxosarcomas, liposarcomas, angiosarcomas, chondrosarcomas, and osteogenic sarcomas, the last-named primarily derived from metaplastic differentiation of the fibroblasts. Of the same origin are the rare primary malignant lymphomas. As a general rule, sarcomas occur in the same age range as carcinomas and differ chiefly in their rate of growth. They tend to produce large, bulky, fleshy masses that cause rapid increase in breast size with considerable distortion of breast contour. Attachment to the skin surface and ulceration are, perhaps, more common with this rapid growth than with carcinomas. Sarcomas as a group spread via the lymphatics to the axillary nodes, but also frequently mestastasize via the blood to distant organs, particularly the lungs. The clinical outlook in these cases is poor. *Angiosarcomas,* in particular, are the most rapidly fatal of breast tumors.[72]

PATHOLOGY

The rudimentary male breast is relatively free from pathologic involvement. Only two processes occur with sufficient frequency to merit consideration.

GYNECOMASTIA

Gland lobules are not found in the normal male breast. As in the female, the male breast is subject to hormonal influences, but is considerably less sensitive than the female. Nonetheless, enlargement of the male breast (gynecomastia) may occur in response to excesses of estrogen. It is encountered under a variety of normal and abnormal circumstances.[73] It may be found at the time of puberty or in the very aged, in the latter presumably owing to a relative increase in adrenal estrogens as the androgenic function of the testis fails. It is one of the manifestations of Klinefelter's syndrome (p. 133) and may occur in those with functioning testicular neoplasms such as Leydig cell and, rarely, Sertoli cell tumors. It may occur at any time during adult life when there is cause for hyperestrinism. The most important cause of hyperestrinism in the male is cirrhosis of the liver, since the liver is responsible for metabolizing estrogen.

Grossly, the lesion may be unilateral or bilateral. A button-like, subareolar enlargement develops. In farther advanced cases, the swelling may simulate the adolescent female breast.

Microscopically, there is proliferation of a dense, periductal hyaline, collagenous connective tissue, but more striking are the changes in the epithelium of the ducts.[74] There is marked hyperplasia of the ductal linings with the piling up of multilayered epithelium (Fig. 25–33). The individual cells are fairly regular, columnar to cuboidal with regular nuclei. Occasionally there may be some variation in cell size and considerable disorientation of the heaped-up lining cells. Anaplasia is absent.

The lesion is readily apparent on clinical examination, and must be differentiated only from the seldom-occurring carcinoma of the male breast. Gynecomastia is chiefly of importance as an indicator of hyperestrinism, suggesting the possible existence of a functioning testicular tumor, or the possible presence of cirrhosis of the liver. Gynecomastia may also be seen in chronic marijuana smokers and heroin addicts, and may sometimes occur without apparent cause.

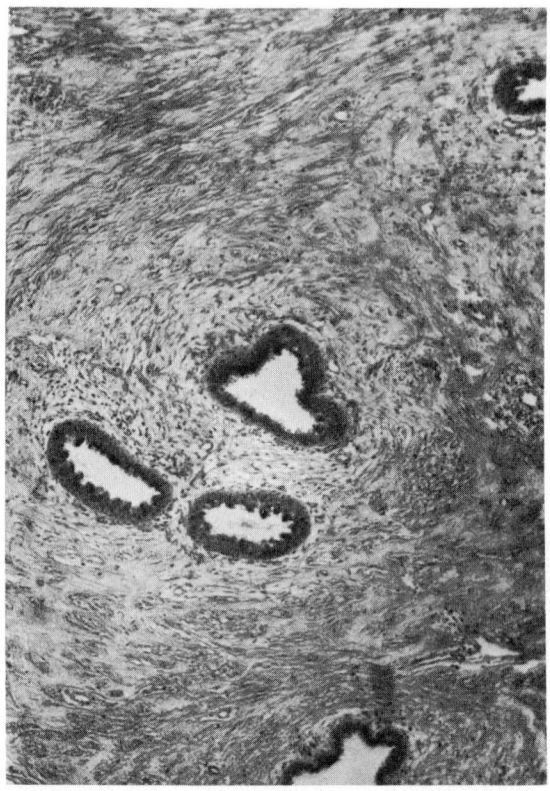

Figure 25–33. Gynecomastia. There is diffuse interductal fibrosis and hyperplasia of lining epithelium.

CARCINOMA

Carcinoma arising in the male breast is a very rare occurrence, with a frequency ratio to breast cancer in the female of 1:100. It occurs in advanced age. Because of the scant amount of breast substance in the male, the malignancy rapidly infiltrates to become attached to the overlying skin and underlying thoracic wall. Ulceration through the skin is perhaps more common than in the female. These tumors behave exactly as do the invasive ductal carcinomas in the female, but on the whole tend to have less striking desmoplasia and, hence, less of the hard, scirrhous quality.[73] Some resemble infiltrating lobular carcinoma. Dissemination follows the same pattern as in women, and axillary lymph node involvement is present in about one half of cases at the time of discovery of the lesion. Distant metastases to the lungs, brain, bone, and liver are common.

1. Stirling, J.W., and Chandler, J.A.: The fine structure of the normal, resting terminal ductal-lobular unit of the female breast. Virchows Arch. (A) 372:205, 1976.

2. Longacre, T.A., and Bartow, S.A.: A correlative morphologic study of human breast and endometrium in the menstrual cycle. Am. J. Surg. Pathol. *10*(6):382, 1986.

3. Page, D.L., and Anderson, T.J.: Diagnostic Histopathology of the Breast. New York, Churchill-Livingstone, 1988.

4. Carter, D.: Interpretation of Breast Biopsies. New York, Raven Press, 1988.

5. Azzopardi, J.G. (ed.): Problems in Breast Pathology. Philadelphia, W.B. Saunders Co., 1979.

6. Ellis, H., and Cox, P.J.: Breast problems in 1,000 consecutive referrals to surgical out-patients. Postgrad. Med. J. *60*:653, 1984.

7. Shousha, S., et al.: Mammary duct ectasia and pituitary adenoma. Am. J. Surg. Pathol. *12*:180, 1988.

8. Love, S.M., et al.: Fibrocystic "disease" of the breast—a non-disease? N. Engl. J. Med. *307*:1010, 1982.

9. Hutter, R.V.P.: Goodbye to "fibrocystic disease." N. Engl. J. Med. *312*:179, 1985.

10. Consensus Statement by the Cancer Committee of the College of American Pathologists: Is "fibrocystic disease" of the breast precancerous? Arch. Pathol. Lab. Med. *110*:171, 1986.

11. Dupont, W.D., and Page, D.L.: Risk factors for breast cancer in women with proliferative breast disease. N. Engl. J. Med. *312*:146, 1985.

12. Frantz, V.K., et al.: Incidence of chronic cystic disease in so-called "normal breast." A study based on 225 postmortem examinations. Cancer *4*:762, 1951.

13. Haagensen, C.D., et al. (eds.): Breast Carcinoma: Risk and Detection. Philadelphia, W.B. Saunders Co., 1981.

14. Wellings, S.R.: Development of human breast cancer. Adv. Cancer Res. *31*:287, 1980.

15. Bradlow, H.L., et al.: Steroid hormone accumulation in human breast cyst fluid. Cancer Res. *41*:105, 1981.

16. Parazzini F., et al.: Risk factors for pathologically confirmed benign breast disease. Am. J. Epidemiol. *120*:115, 1984.

17. Jensen, H.M., et al.: Preneoplastic lesions in human breast. Science *191*:295, 1976.

18. McDivitt, R.W.: Breast carcinoma. Hum. Pathol. *9*:3, 1978.

18a. Page, D.L., et al.: Ductal involvement by cells of atypical lobular hyperplasia in the breast. Hum. Pathol. *19*:201, 1988.

19. Rivera-Pomar, J.M., et al.: Focal fibrous disease of the breast. Virchows Arch. [A] *386*:59, 1980.

20. Andersen, J.A., et al.: A symposium on sclerosing duct lesions of the breast. Pathol. Annu. *21* (Part 11):145, 1986.

21. Harris, J.R., et al.: Breast Disease. Philadelphia, J.B. Lippincott Co., 1987.

22. Ashikari, R., et al.: A clinicopathologic study of atypical lesions of the breast. Cancer *33*:310, 1974.

23. Hart, W.R., et al.: Cystosarcoma phyllodes: A clinicopathologic study of 26 hypercellular periductal stromal tumors of the breast. Am. J. Clin. Pathol. *70*:211, 1978.

24. Ward, R.M., and Evans, H.L.: Cytosarcoma phyllodes. A clinicopathologic study of 26 cases. Cancer *58*:2282, 1986.

25. Rapotti, M., et al.: Association of breast carcinoma and intraductal papillomas. Histopathology *8*:963, 1984.

26. Perzin, K.H., and Lattes, R.: Papillary adenoma of the nipple: A clinical pathologic study. Cancer *29*:996, 1972.

27. Rosen, P.P., and Caicco, A.: Florid papillomatosis of the nipple. Am. J. Surg. Pathol. *87*:101, 1986.

28. Shingleton, W.W., and McCarty, K.S.: Breast carcinoma—an overview. Gynecol. Oncol. *26*:271, 1987.

29. Donegan, W.L., and Spratt, J.S. (eds.): Cancer of the Breast, 3rd ed. Philadelphia, W.B. Saunders Co., 1988.

30. Silverberg, E., and Lubera, J.: Cancer statistics. Cancer *39*:1, 1989.

31. Rico, M.: Breast cancer: Risk factors and etiology. Mt. Sinai J. Med. *51*:300, 1984.

32. The Cancer and Steroid Hormone Study of the Centers for Disease Control and the National Institute of Child Health and Human Development: Oral-contraceptive use and the risk of breast cancer. N. Engl. J. Med. *315*:405, 1986.

33. Miller, A.B., and Bulbrook, R.D.: VICC multidisciplinary project on breast cancer. Int. J. Cancer *37*:173, 1986.

34. Editorial: Oral contraceptives and breast cancer. Lancet *2*:665, 1986.

35. The Cancer and Steroid Hormone Study of the Centers for Dis-

ease Control and the National Institute of Child Health and Human Development: Oral contraceptive use and the risk of breast cancer. N. Engl. J. Med. *315*:405, 1986.

36. Schatzkin, A., Jones, D.Y., et al.: Alcohol consumption and breast cancer in the epidemiologic follow-up study of the first National Health and Nutrition Examination Survey. N. Engl. J. Med. *316*:1169, 1987.

37. McMahon, B., et al.: Urine estrogens, frequency of ovulation and breast cancer risk. Int. J. Cancer *40*(6):721, 1987.

38. Wittliff, J.L.: Steroid hormone receptors in breast cancer. Cancer *53*:630, 1984.

39. Lippman, M.E., et al.: Growth regulatory peptide production by human breast carcinoma cells. J. Steroid Biochem. *30*:53, 1988.

40. Wynder, E.L., and Rose, D.P.: Diet and breast cancer. Hosp. Pract. *19*:73, 1984.

41. Bittner, J.J.: Some possible effects of nursing on mammary gland tumor incidence in mice. Science *84*:162, 1936.

42. Ono, M., et al.: Nucleotide sequence of human endogenous retrovirus genome related to MMTV. J. Virol. *60*:589, 1986.

43. Al-Sumidaie, A.M., et al.: Particles with properties of retrovirus in patients with breast cancer. Lancet *1*:5, 1988.

44. Lippman, M.E.: Oncogenes in breast cancer. N. Engl. J. Med. *319*:1281, 1988.

45. Shamon, D.J., et al.: Human breast cancer: correlation of relapse and survival with the HER-2/NEU oncogene. Science *235*:177, 1987.

46. Ali, I.V., et al.: Amplification of c-erb-B2 and aggressive human breast tumors? Science *240:*1795, 1988.

47. Muller, W., et al.: Single step induction of mammary adenocarcinoma in transgenic mice bearing the activated c-neu oncogene. Cell *54*:105, 1988.

48. Marge, B., et al.: Insertional mutagenesis of the myc locus by a line sequence in a human breast carcinoma. Nature *333*:87, 1988.

49. T'Ang, A., et al.: Structural rearrangements of the retinoblastoma gene in human breast cancer. Science *242:*263, 1988.

50. The World Health Organization Histologic Typing of Breast Tumors (2nd ed.): Am. J. Clin. Pathol. *78*:806, 1982.

51. Page, D., et al.: Intraductal carcinoma of the breast: follow up after biopsy only. Cancer *49*:751, 1982.

52. Andersen, J.A.: Lobular carcinoma *in situ:* An approach to rational treatment. Cancer *39*:2597, 1977.

53. Rosen, P.P.: Lobular carcinoma *in situ* of the breast. Am. J. Surg. Pathol. *2*:225, 1978.

54. Rapier, V., et al: Medullary breast carcinoma. A reevaluation of 95 cases of breast cancer with inflammatory stroma. Cancer *61*:2503, 1988.

55. Ridolfi, R.L., et al.: Medullary carcinoma of the breast. A clinicopathologic study with a 10-year follow-up. Cancer *40*:1305, 1977.

56. Silverberg, S.G., et al.: Colloid carcinoma of the breast. Am. J. Clin. Pathol. *55*:355, 1971.

57. Rasmussen, B.B., et al.: Prognostic factors in primary mucinous breast carcinoma. Am. J. Clin. Pathol. *87*:155, 1987.

58. Ashikari, R., et al.: Paget's disease of the breast. Cancer *26*:680, 1970.

59. Wheeler, J.E., and Enterline, H.T.: Lobular carcinoma of the breast: *in situ* and infiltrating. Pathol. Annu. *11*:61, 1976.

60. Ashikari, R., et al.: Infiltrating lobular carcinoma of the breast. Cancer *31*:110, 1973.

61. Ensebi, V., et al.: Morphofunctional differentiation in lobular carcinoma of the breast. Histopathology *1*:301, 1977.

62. Bears, O.H.: Staging of cancer of the breast as a guide to therapy. Cancer *53*:592, 1984.

63. Harris, J.R., et al.: Cancer of the breast. *In* DeVita, V.T., et al. (eds.): Cancer Principles and Practice of Oncology. Philadelphia, J.B. Lippincott Co., 1985, pp. 1119–1177.

64. Seidman, H., et al.: Survival experience in the breast cancer detection demonstration project. Cancer *37*:258, 1987.

65. Adair, F.E., et al.: Long-term follow-up of breast cancer patients: The 30-year report. Cancer *33*:1145, 1974.

66. Mirecki, D.M., and Jordan, V.C.: Steroid hormone receptors and human breast cancer. Lab. Med. *16*:287, 1985.

67. Fallenius, A.G., et al.: Prognostic significance of DNA measurements in 409 consecutive breast cancer patients. Cancer *62*:331, 1988.

68. Clark, G.M., et al.: Prediction of relapse or survival in patients with node-negative breast cancer. N. Engl. J. Med. In press.

69. Thor, A.: Genetic alterations in breast carcinoma. Hum. Pathol. In press.

70. Hollingshead, A.C.: Biological markers of breast cancer: a review. Cancer Invest. *5*(6):581, 1987.

71. DeVita, D.T., Jr.: Breast cancer therapy: Exercising all our options. N. Engl. J. Med. *320*:527, 1989.

72. Suhrlane, L.G.: An overview of contemporary management of breast carcinoma. Obstet. Gynecol. Clin. North Am. *14*:783, 1987.

73. Hultborn, R., et al.: Male breast carcinoma. A study of the total material reported to the Swedish Cancer Registry 1958–1967 with respect to clinical and histological parameters. Acta Oncol. *26*:241, 1987.

The Endocrine System

Ronald A. DeLellis, M.D.

The endocrine system consists of a highly integrated set of glands and widely distributed neuroendocrine cells whose primary function is the control of homeostasis. In the following sections, each of the endocrine glands is discussed individually. It should not be forgotten, however, that the neuroendocrine cells (formerly referred to as APUD cells) may also be involved in a variety of pathologic processes, some of which have already been presented in chapters on the lung, pancreas, and gastrointestinal tract.[1,2]

INTRODUCTION

Diseases of the endocrine system may result from a vast array of pathogenetic mechanisms leading to abnormalities in the biosynthesis and secretion of hormones, or in the interactions of hormones with specific receptors in target cells, or in postreceptor responses.[3] The sequelae of such abnormalities include underproduction or overproduction of hormones and the clinical appearance of hypo- or hyperfunctional states. From the vantage point of the individual patient, the pathophysiologic hallmark of endocrine disease is the inability to maintain homeostasis.

Common to all endocrine systems is the control of target organ secretion by feedback mechanisms that operate at multiple levels. For example, when cortisol levels are insufficient to maintain homeostasis, the inhibitory effects of cortisol on the secretion of corticotropin releasing hormone (CRH) and on the secretion of adrenocorticotropin (ACTH) are reduced.[4] CRH then stimulates ACTH, which, in turn, activates the biosynthesis of cortisol in the adrenal cortex. When cortisol levels become adequate to meet metabolic demands, CRH and ACTH synthesis is suppressed. Hormonal feedback may be controlled by many factors, including hormones (as in the control of cortisol biosynthesis by CRH and ACTH), cations, metabolites, osmolarity, or extracellular fluid volume.

Diseases of the endocrine system may be understood in the context of the broad categories of "too much or too little" hormone.[5] Genetic disorders with enzymatic deficits in hormone synthesis and destructive lesions both may result in hypofunction. In genetic disorders with diminished hormone synthesis, affected endocrine glands undergo hyperplasia as a consequence of persistent stimulation of the gland by tropic hormones. In those cases in which the endocrine glands are affected by infection or an autoimmune process, they are unable, for the most part, to undergo hyperplasia because of the destructive nature of the basic disease process.

Hypofunction due to abnormalities of control mechanisms, with decreased production of tropic hormones, is associated with atrophy of the end-organ. For example, destructive lesions of the pituitary may result in secondary thyroid and adrenal failure. The administration of exogenous hormones will also result in atrophy of end-organs as a result of suppression of synthesis of tropic hormones.

Hyperfunction may result from end-organ autonomy or from abnormalities of control mechanisms, leading to increased levels of tropic hormones or other stimulating factors. In the setting of endocrine hyperfunction, autonomy refers to relative or absolute independence from the major control mechanism. Most functionally autonomous lesions prove to be benign or malignant neoplasms. When the levels of end-organ hormones are increased, the corresponding tropic hormone is decreased. As a result, those portions of the end-organ unaffected by tumor will undergo atrophy. Some forms of hyperplasia may occasionally function in an autonomous fashion. Hyperfunction may also result from abnormalities of control mechanisms, with increased levels of tropic hormones or other factors leading to hyperplasia of the end-organ.

NORMAL

No organ packs so much critical function into so little space as the pituitary. In the adult it weighs about 0.5 gm and measures 10 to 15 mm in greatest diameter. It is composed of two functionally separate components—the anterior lobe (adenohypophysis) made up of a mixture of secretory cells, and a posterior lobe (neurohypophysis) representing an extension of the brain. The anterior lobe is derived from an evagination of the roof of the primitive oral canal called Rathke's pouch, which extends superiorly toward the base of the brain to come to lie anterior to an outpouching of the floor of the third ventricle, constituting the anlage of the posterior lobe. Growth of the sphenoid bone creates the enclosing sella turcica, the floor of which detaches Rathke's pouch from its origins. Occasionally, rests of epithelial cells persist within or below the sphenoid as accessory, and sometimes functional, pharyngeal pituitary tissue. In contrast, the connection to the base of the brain persists as the pituitary stalk, which provides direct anatomic continuity between the neurohypophysis and hypothalamus. A thick extension of the dura called the diaphragma sellae roofs over the sella; it has a central orifice through which the stalk passes. If this aperture is too large for the stalk or there are other diaphragmatic defects, the arachnoid mater may herniate through when there is a prolonged increase in cerebrospinal fluid (CSF) pressure to compress the pituitary.

The blood supply to the pituitary has many similarities to that of the liver.[6] Some is derived from branches of the internal carotid arteries, but most is furnished by a portal system derived from capillaries in the floor of the third ventricle. By coalescence these capillaries form long parallel vessels that course along the surface of the pituitary stalk, eventually to connect with vascular sinusoids in the anterior lobe. There are also portal interconnections between the stalk and the anterior and posterior lobes. Thus, releasing and inhibiting factors synthesized in the hypothalamus are readily delivered to the anterior and posterior lobes via the processes of axonal transport and neuroendocrine secretion.

Histologically the posterior and anterior lobes are totally dissimilar. The posterior lobe is composed of tangled nerve fibers through which are scattered occasional glia-like pituicytes. Electron microscopy reveals that the unmyelinated nerve fibers contain numerous membrane-bound secretory granules of stored posterior pituitary hormones. There is no pars intermedia in the human, but its location is sometimes marked by small colloid-filled cysts or clefts. The anterior lobe is composed of round-to-polygonal epithelial cells arranged in cords and nests separated by a rich fibrovascular network. At one time the cells of the anterior lobe were classified as eosinophils, basophils, or chromophobes on the basis of their uptake of acidic and basic dyes, but the distinctions were at best unsatisfactory. Electron microscopy and immunocytochemical methods using specific hormonal antibodies now reliably distinguish the various cells responsible for secretion of each of the anterior pituitary hormones. Each tropic hormone is produced by one type of cell and stored in secretory granules of somewhat distinctive size and nature. The gonadotropins (FSH and LH), however, are both elaborated by one cell type.[7] By immunocytochemical methods, about 25% of the anterior pituitary cells do not apparently contain any of the known hormones and so conform to the "chromophobes" of the past. Electron microscopy of these cells, however, usually reveals a few secretory granules, and so they are thought to be sparsely granulated rather than nonfunctional.

The hypothalamus is a major regulator of both anterior and posterior pituitary secretory activity.[8] The neurohypophyseal hormones, vasopressin (antidiuretic hormone, ADH) and oxytocin, are produced in neurosecretory cells in the hypothalamus and are then transported within vesicles along the axons that end in the posterior lobe. In contrast, adenohypophyseal function is regulated by "releasing" and "inhibiting" factors synthesized in the hypothalamus and carried to the anterior pituitary through the portal system. Without delving into all the details, releasing factors have been well characterized for thyrotropin (TSH), luteinizing hormone (LH), follicle-stimulating hormone (FSH), corticotropin (ACTH), and growth hormone (GH). Prolactin (PRL) secretion is stimulated by a number of factors, the most important of which is thyrotropin releasing hormone (TRH). TRH stimulates prolactin release with much the same dose-response characteristics as stimulation of TSH release. Dopamine is the major prolactin inhibitory factor (PIF). This amine suppresses virtually all aspects of PRL secretion and also inhibits cell division and DNA synthesis of these cells. A second hypothalamic release inhibiting factor is somatostatin (SRIH).[9] This tetradecapeptide inhibits the secretion of growth hormone and TSH. Under certain conditions, SRIH also inhibits the secretion of PRL and ACTH. Somatostatin production is not limited to the hypothalamus, and its effects extend beyond the inhibition of GH and TSH release. Other influences also contribute to the regulation of anterior secretory function. Hormones elaborated by target endocrine glands in negative feedback loops inhibit anterior lobe cells. For example, thyroid hormones inhibit thyrotroph activity and glucocorticoids do the same with corticotrophs.

PATHOLOGY

Disorders of the pituitary may be divided into those involving primarily the anterior lobe and those involving the posterior lobe. However, certain lesions such as tumors, for example, may damage both.

Diseases affecting predominantly the adenohypophysis come to attention either as the consequence of increased or decreased production of tropic hormones or because of local space-occupying effects. Obviously, small lesions may remain entirely occult whatever their nature and may be discovered only at autopsy. The term hyperpituitarism is used to mean increased secretion of one or more of the tropic hormones of the anterior lobe, generally by a functioning tumor. Hyperpituitarism may also be hypothalamic in origin or related to loss of feedback inhibition by target organ hormones. Hypopituitarism has more varied origins and appears whenever there is destruction of at least 75% of the anterior lobe. Infrequently, it is hypothalamic in origin.

The local consequences of anterior pituitary disease can be divided into three patterns.[10] (1) Enlargement of the sella turcica, as demonstrated by x-ray, CT scan, or MRI, is a major marker of pituitary disease and is caused by any expansile lesion such as a neoplasm or chronic edematous enlargement of the gland. (2) Visual disorders may bring the pituitary pathology to the patient's attention. Classically it takes the form of bilateral homonymous hemianopsia, but other field defects are sometimes encountered. They result from encroachment of an expanding pituitary lesion on the immediately adjacent optic chiasm or optic nerves. (3) Infrequently, large pituitary tumors bulge upward into the floor of the brain and raise intracranial pressure sufficiently to produce headache, nausea, and vomiting reminiscent of a brain tumor (Fig. 26–1). Frequently the individual patient has more than one of these findings. On occasion the hyperpituitarism is suddenly converted to hypopituitarism when a neoplasm undergoes spontaneous infarction as it outgrows its blood supply. The major

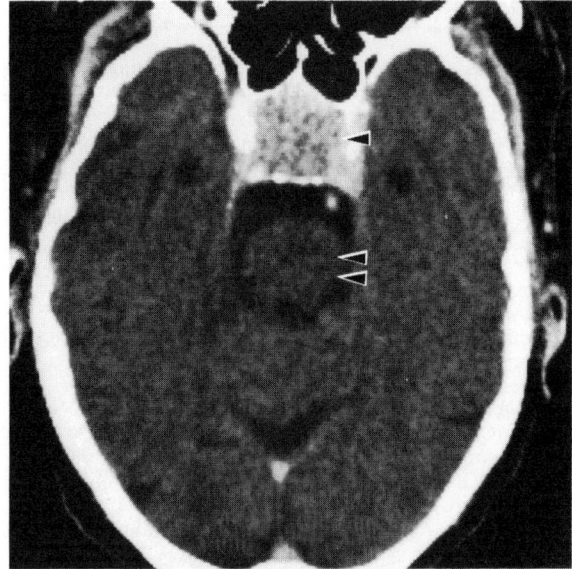

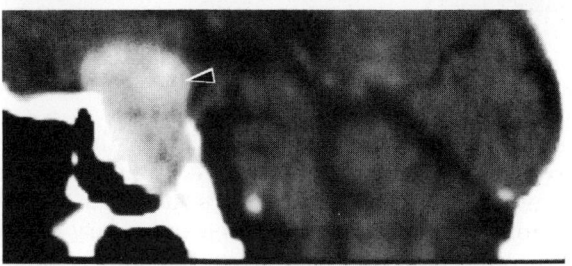

Figure 26–1. *Above,* CT scan of transverse plane of skull at level of pituitary fossa, revealing enlargement of sella caused by an expansile pituitary adenoma *(arrow).* Compare its size with transverse dimension of brain stem *(double arrow). Below,* Computer reconstruction of the same tumor in sagittal plane *(arrow).* It has bulged out of sella turcica, producing a moderately enlarged suprasellar mass. (Courtesy of Dr. Calvin Rumbaugh, Department of Radiology, Brigham and Women's Hospital, Harvard Medical School.)

anterior pituitary diseases can be encompassed within two categories: (1) hyperpituitarism — anterior lobe tumors, and (2) disorders associated with hypopituitarism.

HYPERPITUITARISM — ANTERIOR LOBE TUMORS

For all practical purposes, hyperfunction of the anterior pituitary means an adenoma; carcinomas of the anterior lobe are exceedingly rare. The great majority of adenomas elaborate a single tropic hormone. For unknown reasons, PRL-secreting, GH-secreting, and ACTH-secreting adenomas constitute about 70% of functional tumors, collectively (Table 26–1). Neoplasms producing TSH, LH, and FSH are very uncommon.[11]

On occasion an adenoma is associated with the production of two hormones, most often GH and PRL, and both these hormones can sometimes be identified

Table 26–1. Classification of Pituitary Adenomas

TUMOR TYPE	INCIDENCE (%)	CLINICAL FEATURES
Prolactinoma	**30.5**	Amenorrhea,
Sparsely granulated (C)*	(30)	galactorrhea,
Densely granulated (A)*	(<0.5)	infertility (females)
		Impotence, loss of
		libido (males)
Growth Hormone	**17**	Acromegaly,
Sparsely granulated (C)	(9)	gigantism
Densely granulated (A)	(8)	
Mixed Growth Hormone–	**9.5**	Acromegaly ± fea-
Prolactin (A, C)		tures of prolactin-
		oma
Adrenocorticotropin	**14**	
Functioning (B)*	(8)	Cushing's, Nelson's
Silent (C)	(6)	No specific syndrome
Gonadotropin (C)	**2.5**	Hormonally silent
Thyrotropin (C)	**<1**	Hyperthyroidism
Plurihormonal (C)	**2.5**	Variable
Nonfunctional (C,A)	**23**	Hormonally silent
Null cell	(17)	
Oncocytoma	(6)	

* A, acidophilic; B, basophilic; C, chromophobic.
Adapted from References 12 and 13.

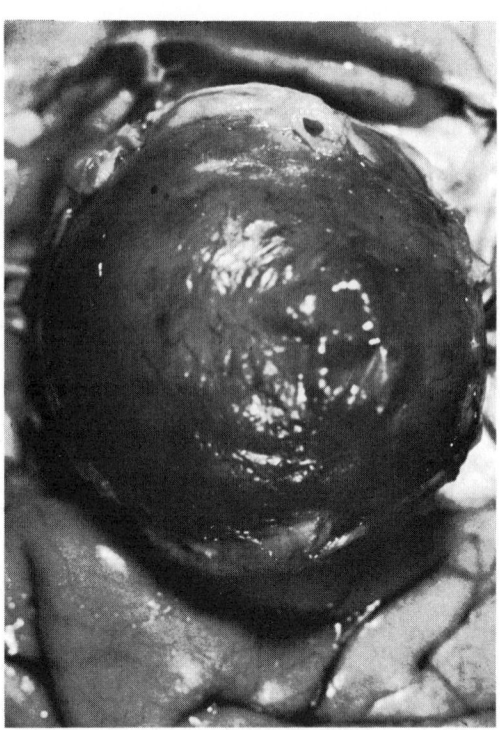

Figure 26–2. Close-up detail of a pituitary adenoma still attached to brain. Compressed vessels and nerves are apparent about periphery.

in one cell type. In some other instances the immunoperoxidase method reveals only a single hormone in the tumor cells, and the excess production of the other hormone must be attributed to a secondary effect of the neoplasm on the hypophyseothalamic regulatory apparatus. There are also rare instances of plurihormonal adenomas producing two or more hormones arising in distinct populations of cells. At the other extreme are the nonfunctional adenomas that, by virtue of their expansile growth, destroy the surrounding normal parenchyma and so lead to hypopituitarism (Table 26–1).[12]

It is impossible on gross examination and light microscopy with routine tissue stains to reliably differentiate one type of adenoma from another. Ultimate confirmation requires the use of immunocytochemical methods.[12-14] Adenomas, whatever the cell type, range from microscopic foci (referred to, when less than 10 mm in diameter, as microadenomas) to large masses sometimes approaching 10 cm in diameter. Among the functional adenomas, those producing GH generally tend to be the largest, possibly because the endocrinopathy they produce develops insidiously (Fig. 26–2). PRL- and ACTH-secreting lesions range widely in size from microadenomas to expansile masses. Microadenomas are surprisingly common and have been found in up to 27% of an unselected series of autopsies, of which half were PRL secreting.[15] Whether such lesions represent true neoplasms or foci of hyperplasia is unknown. Contributing to the dilemma is the fact that many of these small lesions are poorly encapsulated, an unusual feature for benign neoplasms. However, even large adenomas sometimes have only a delicate capsule that may well be incomplete.

Large pituitary adenomas expand the sella turcica, erode the clinoid processes, and sometimes, because of

the poor encapsulation, rupture through the diaphragma to injure the optic chiasm or optic nerves. **They may also penetrate into surrounding structures.** Thus, adenomas may give the deceptive appearance of invasion into the cavernous sinuses, the nasal sinuses, the base of the brain, or other contiguous structures. Such aggressive local behavior does not imply malignancy. On transection the neoplasms are usually soft, red-brown, and discrete, despite the lack of a capsule and despite extension along broad fronts into contiguous structures. Larger lesions may develop foci of ischemic necrosis, cystic softening, and hemorrhages (sometimes called **pituitary apoplexy**). Occasionally, very large adenomas undergo virtual total infarction as the expansile pressure compresses their blood supply. The non-neoplastic anterior lobe may be relatively preserved, may be markedly attenuated, or may have disappeared, depending on the size of the neoplasm. Microscopically, all adenomas have a fairly uniform appearance. The cells are arranged in sheets, cords, or nests having only a delicate, vascularized stroma. Sometimes, pseudoglandular or papillary formations are produced (Fig. 26–3). Small or large foci of coagulative necrosis may be present. Some neoplasms show considerable cellular and nuclear pleomorphism. When such cytologic changes are found in neoplasms that have extended beyond the sella, the question of malignancy arises. To avoid overdiagnosis, **most experts require evidence of metastatic dissemination for the diagnosis of carcinoma of the anterior pituitary.** As might be expected, the more differentiated the cells, the more abundant are the cytoplasmic granules, but lesions

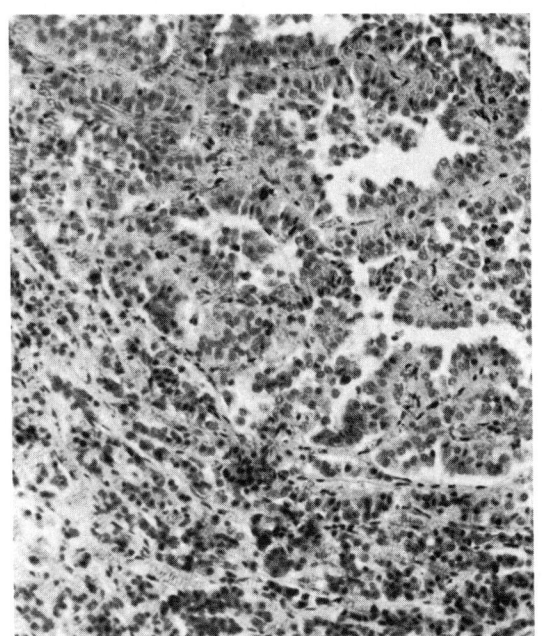

Figure 26–3. A pituitary adenoma illustrating a tendency to papillary growth and poor demarcation from surrounding pituitary substance. Tumor cells are uniform in size and compress adjacent normal gland *(below)*.

composed almost entirely of sparsely granulated cells may have marked secretory activity, accounting for the past dilemma of so-called functioning chromophobe adenomas (Fig. 26–4).

Adenomas associated with the production of GH (somatotroph adenomas) and/or PRL are usually composed of densely or sparsely granulated cells (Table 26–1; Fig. 26–4).[12] The former reveal brightly eosinophilic, orange-to-red cytoplasmic granules with conventional stains **(eosinophilic adenomas).** Sparsely granulated cells suggest **chromophobe adenomas.** In contrast, neoplasms associated with ACTH secretion (corticotroph adenomas) usually have abundant granules, stain darkly, and react strongly with the PAS stain and so are called **basophilic adenomas.** A distinctive alteration, referred to as Crooke's hyaline change and sometimes seen in the corticotrophs, will be discussed in the consideration of Cushing's syndrome (p. 1257).

Primary carcinomas of the anterior lobe should be mentioned. They are rare, are usually sufficiently undifferentiated so that the cell type of origin cannot be identified, and only rarely elaborate hormones. Metastatic lesions have been reported in lymph nodes, liver, bones, and heart but are exceptionally rare.[12]

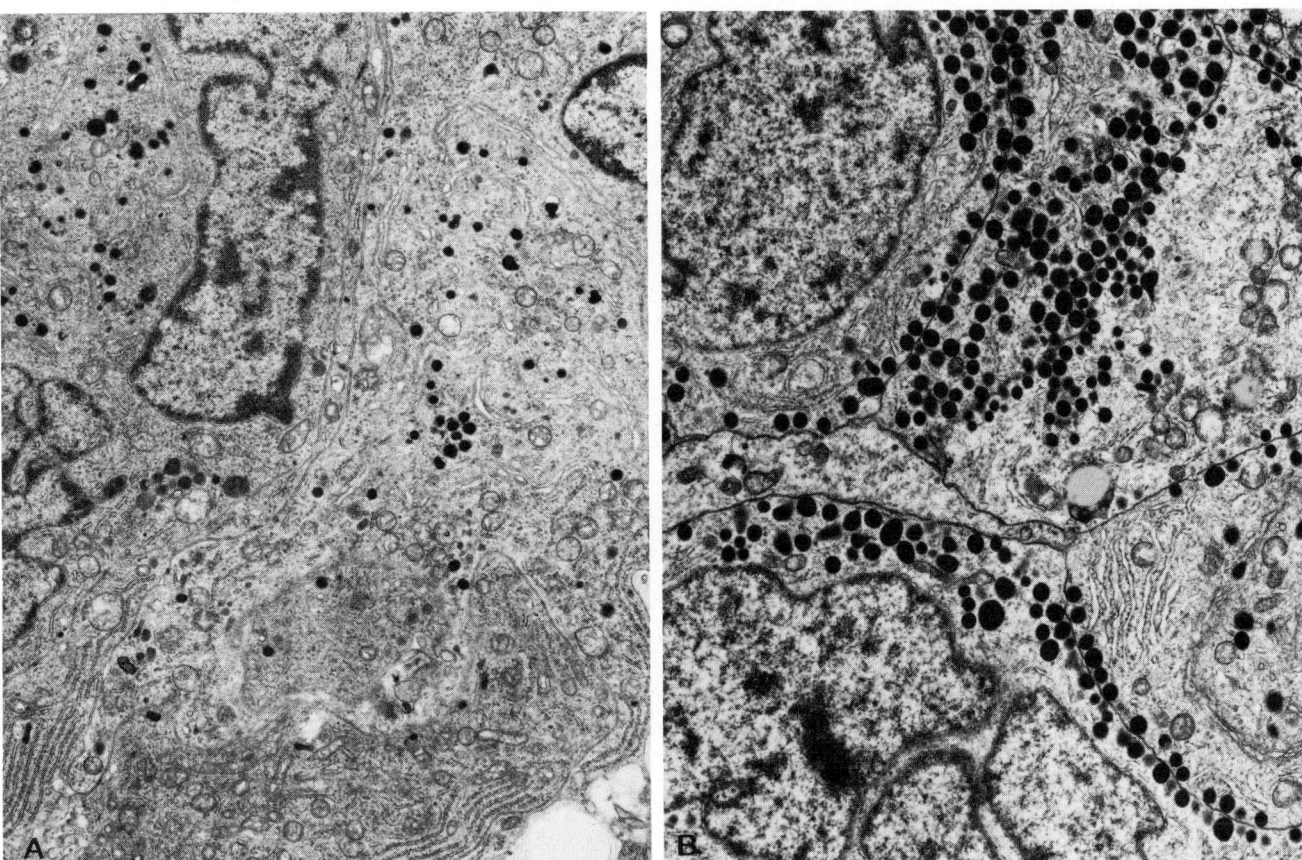

Figure 26–4. *A,* Electron micrograph of a sparsely granulated prolactinoma. The tumor cells contain abundant granular endoplasmic reticulum (indicative of active protein synthesis) and small numbers of secretory granules (6000 ×). *B,* Electron micrograph of densely granulated growth hormone–secreting adenoma. The tumor cells are filled with large membrane-bound secretory granules (6000 ×). (Courtesy of Dr. Eva Horvath, St. Michael's Hospital, Toronto, Ontario.)

CLINICAL COURSE. Pituitary adenomas occur in both sexes at any age but are somewhat more common in men, particularly between the ages of 20 and 50. Rarely, the pituitary tumor is accompanied by lesions in other endocrine glands in MEN I (p. 1007).[16]

Hyperprolactinemia is now recognized to be the most common endocrinopathy caused by pituitary tumors. Classically, it is marked by an amenorrhea-galactorrhea syndrome in women.[17] Since these manifestations are so overt, PRL-secreting adenomas are usually discovered while very small, i.e., microadenomas. The correlation between prolactin levels and galactorrhea is poor. For example, some patients with elevated prolactin levels do not lactate and lactation may continue without prolactinemia. There are, however, many other causes of hyperprolactinemia and/or amenorrhea and galactorrhea; for example, lesions in the hypothalamus, drugs that impair dopaminergic transmission (methyldopa, reserpine), and estrogen therapy. Thus, the clinical diagnosis of a prolactinoma requires not only elevated plasma levels of PRL but also evidence of an anterior lobe mass. When these neoplasms arise in males, they usually come to attention because of local effects, and so the adenomas generally are much larger. Rarely, they cause decreased libido or infertility. These features may be caused by inhibition of gonadotropin secretion or by interference with gonadotropin effects.

Excess secretion of GH by somatotroph adenomas induces gigantism in the prepubertal child and acromegaly in adults. Gigantism appears when the epiphyses have not fused and the high plasma levels of somatotropin, mediated by the hepatic production of growth factors including somatomedin C, stimulate extraordinary skeletal growth to produce the pathetic circus giants of the past, sometimes 8 to 9 feet tall. Despite the size of these individuals, myopathies, neuropathies, and arthropathies appear early in life, reducing these giants to tottering hulks. Fortunately, this condition has virtually disappeared because of early recognition and removal of the adenoma. Acromegaly, on the other hand, is the second most common hyperpituitary state. The essential hormonal feature of acromegaly is absence of the normal suppressibility of growth hormone by glucose. The disordered growth is far more insidious than gigantism, and although it may begin in early adult life, the physical changes are usually not recognized until years to decades later. Most striking is the enlargement and coarsening of the facial features, hands, and feet—namely, "megaly" of the acral parts. When fully expressed, the protruding jaw, thick lips, overly large tongue, and accentuated orbital and frontal ridges can be recognized at a distance (Fig. 26–5). A host of metabolic changes may also be present, among which are glucose intolerance (and sometimes overt diabetes mellitus), osteoporosis, and hypertension. Also, these patients frequently have visual field defects and enlargement of the sella because somatotropic adenomas often have become large by the time they are discovered. An identical clinical picture may occur by the ectopic secretion of growth hormone

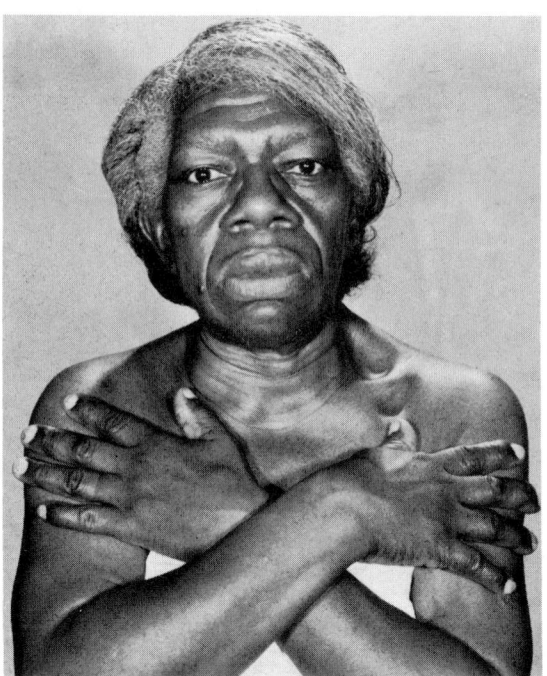

Figure 26–5. Acromegaly in a 60-year-old woman.

releasing factor by pancreatic endocrine tumors or carcinoids.

Corticotropin-secreting adenomas produce secondary adrenocortical hyperfunction, known as pituitary Cushing's syndrome or Cushing's disease. An analogous hyperadrenal state (described on p. 1254) may also be caused by adrenal functioning tumors, ectopic production of ACTH by nonendocrine cancers (such as those of the lung), and exogenous adrenal steroids. It is sufficient to note here that the pituitary adenomas giving rise to Cushing's syndrome are usually small, often conform to microadenomas, and rarely cause signs and symptoms related to tumorous enlargement of the pituitary.

Numerous other complexities are introduced by the possible effects of the secretory adenoma on the surrounding non-neoplastic pituitary gland. Thus, pressure on the posterior pituitary may impair ADH secretion and add an element of diabetes insipidus to the endocrinopathy. Analogously, an ACTH-secreting adenoma may sometimes lead to hypothyroidism by destruction of the non-neoplastic thyrotrophs. The variable clinical patterns produced by secretory adenomas are almost endless, but it should not be forgotten that they could have their origin in a nonendocrine cancer: for example, the ectopic production of hormones by a small cell bronchogenic carcinoma.

DISORDERS ASSOCIATED WITH HYPOPITUITARISM

Hypofunction of the adenohypophysis may result from lesions in the hypothalamus or in the anterior lobe of the pituitary. Hypothalamic lesions are on the whole extremely rare: Only the suprasellar craniopharyngioma, glioma, and germ cell tumor occur with sufficient frequency to merit description (see later). Such tumors may produce a variety of clinical syndromes including diabetes insipidus, growth acceleration, stunting of growth, and delayed puberty.[18] *More commonly, hypopituitarism arises from destructive processes directly involving the adenohypophysis, the three most common being nonsecretory adenomas, Sheehan's pituitary necrosis, and the empty sella syndrome.* Together they account for over 90% of instances of panhypopituitarism. The remaining causes of pituitary insufficiency include metastatic neoplasms, disruption of blood supply by systemic arteritis or thrombosis of cavernous venous sinuses, inflammatory destruction of the anterior lobe by sarcoidosis or infections, surgical or radiation ablation of the pituitary, and a variety of metabolic disorders. Whatever the underlying disorder, pituitary hypofunction is unlikely to be manifest until at least 75% of the anterior lobe is destroyed. With panlobar destruction, the impairment usually involves multiple tropic hormones and most often becomes evident in the following temporal sequence: gonadotropins, GH (particularly in children), TSH, ACTH, and lastly, PRL.

Rarely, the pituitary insufficiency manifests itself as an isolated or monotropic hormone deficiency, most often a lack of GH, less often a gonadotropic insufficiency, and still more infrequently a deficiency of ACTH or TSH. No satisfactory explanation has been offered to explain these unihormonal lacks, but without proof they are attributed to lesions primary in the hypothalamus.[19]

The clinical manifestations of destructive lesions of the adenohypophysis are extremely variable, and many will be mentioned along with the various causative conditions. Only a few comments are necessary here.

Lack of GH per se in the adult is virtually undetectable except by radioimmunoassay. In the prepubertal child it causes symmetric retardation of growth, so-called *pituitary dwarfism*. Frequently, sexual development is also retarded. This form of dwarfism must be differentiated from that of hypothyroidism (cretinism). The latter is typified by characteristic "mongoloid" facies and, most notably, striking mental retardation that contrasts with the normal facial features and mentality of pituitary dwarfs. In female adults the consequences of hypogonadotropism are amenorrhea, loss of axillary and pubic hair, sterility, and atrophy of the ovaries and external genitalia. In the male, hypogonadotropism is manifested by testicular atrophy, sterility, and loss of axillary and pubic hair. Often there is a notable absence of hair or recession of the hairline. All these manifestations are directly related to loss of gonadal function followed by atrophy. Other deficits may induce hypothyroidism related to a lack of TSH, or hypoadrenalism related to a deficiency of ACTH, followed in time by atrophy of the thyroid and adrenals. Thus, thyroid, adrenal, or gonadal insufficiency related to deficits of pituitary tropic hormones must be differentiated from

primary disorders of these organs. More is said about these difficult differential diagnoses in the consideration of the various endocrine glands, but it suffices here to note that most important are radioimmunoassays for serum levels of tropic hormones. The destructive process, whatever its nature, may also affect the posterior pituitary and add to the symptom complex. It should be noted that panhypopituitarism rarely, if ever, induces weight loss, and so the older designation of "Simmonds' cachexia" is clearly inappropriate.

Most of the destructive lesions that cause hypopituitarism have already been described elsewhere, and remarks will be confined to the four most common causes.

NONSECRETORY (CHROMOPHOBE) PITUITARY ADENOMAS

These tumors may present as space-occupying lesions (discussed on p. 1207) or as tropic hormone insufficiencies. With nonfunctional pituitary adenomas, the hormonal deficits develop slowly over the span of years, and so these tumors often achieve quite large size before they are discovered. On gross inspection they cannot be differentiated from secretory adenomas, but histologically they are apparently composed sometimes of sparsely granulated chromophobes. In other tumors the cells may be small and undifferentiated and have only a scant, cleared cytoplasm (null cell adenomas) or an abundant eosinophilic granular cytoplasm that is literally packed with mitochondria (oncocytic adenomas).[12] Immunoelectron microscopy often discloses, in both the null cell and the oncocytic patterns, small secretory granules about 100 nm in diameter, which fail to react with any of the antisera to known pituitary tropic hormones.[12] Chromogranin proteins, however, are frequently demonstrable in null cell adenomas.[20]

SHEEHAN'S SYNDROME

Also known as *post-partum pituitary necrosis*, this syndrome results from sudden infarction of the anterior lobe precipitated by obstetric hemorrhage or shock.[21] It has been hypothesized that during pregnancy the anterior pituitary gland enlarges to almost twice its normal size, compressing the vascular sinusoids supplied largely by the portal network at venous pressure. Thus, sudden systemic hypotension precipitates ischemic necrosis of much or all of the anterior lobe, sparing the posterior lobe, which is less vulnerable to anoxia (Fig. 26–6). However, other pathogenetic mechanisms may be involved, such as DIC or (more rarely) sickle cell anemia, cavernous sinus thrombosis, temporal arteritis, or traumatic injury of vessels. The incidence appears to be increased in individuals with long-standing diabetes mellitus. With these varied origins, Sheehan's syndrome may be encountered in nonpregnant females as well as in males. In most instances there is destruction of 95 to 99% of the anterior lobe, most evident as a gonadotropic deficiency having the features described but possibly ac-

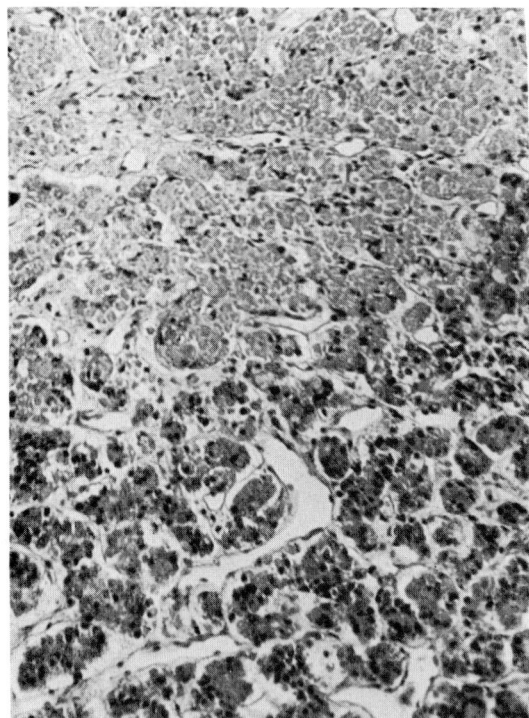

Figure 26-6. Sheehan's syndrome. A recent infarct of pituitary evident as pale-staining shadowy outlines of cells, which contrast with normal nucleated cells immediately below.

companied by failure of lactation in the puerperium. Concomitantly the deficiency of TSH and ACTH may induce hypothyroidism and adrenocortical insufficiency.[22] Less extensive destruction of the anterior lobe may be asymptomatic or may present as loss of only one of the tropic hormones. Strangely, the loss of pituitary function may not become evident for years after the initiating event, attributed to continued destruction of marginal viable cells as they become trapped in the postinfarction scarring. With substitution therapy or with incomplete destruction of the pituitary, long survival is possible, as indeed is childbearing.

Whatever the pathogenesis, the infarcted adenohypophysis at the outset appears soft, pale, and ischemic or hemorrhagic. Over time the ischemic area is resorbed and replaced by fibrous tissue. In some long-standing cases, the gland scars down to a fibrous nubbin weighing less than 0.1 gm, attached to the wall of an empty sella.

EMPTY SELLA SYNDROME

This uncommon condition has a number of origins. Most often it is related to herniation of the arachnoid through some deficit in the diaphragma sellae — either an abnormally large aperture through which the hypophyseal stalk passes or a defect elsewhere. The CSF pressure eventually causes atrophy of the pituitary, creating the appearance of an empty sella (Fig. 26-7). Other possible causes are Sheehan's syn-

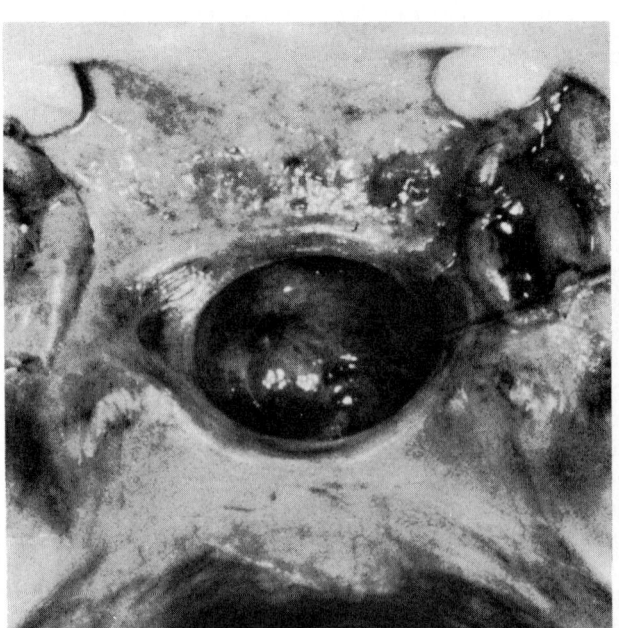
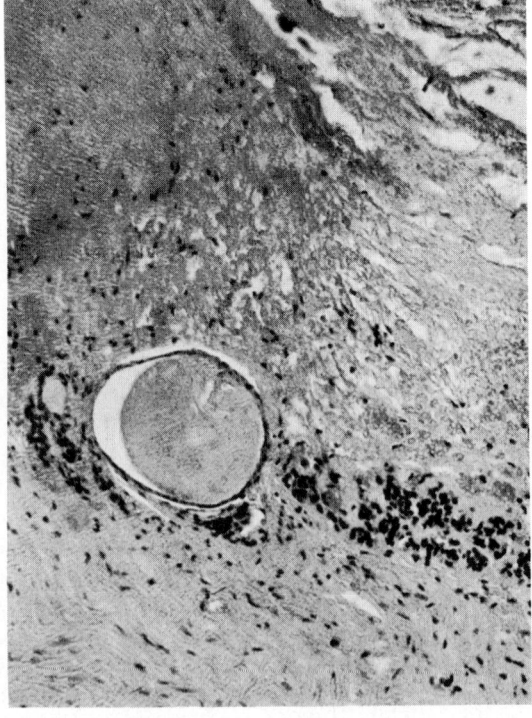

Figure 26-7. *A,* In situ view of sella turcica in a patient dying of far-advanced pituitary insufficiency. Residual gland substance remains in situ and can be seen as a minute nubbin of tissue protruding from midline of posterior wall of sella *(below). B,* Microscopic view of anterior lobe of pituitary illustrated in *A.* Complete fibrous atrophy of anterior lobe is evident above pars intermedia, indicated in photograph by cystic space. Posterior lobe is below and appears normal.

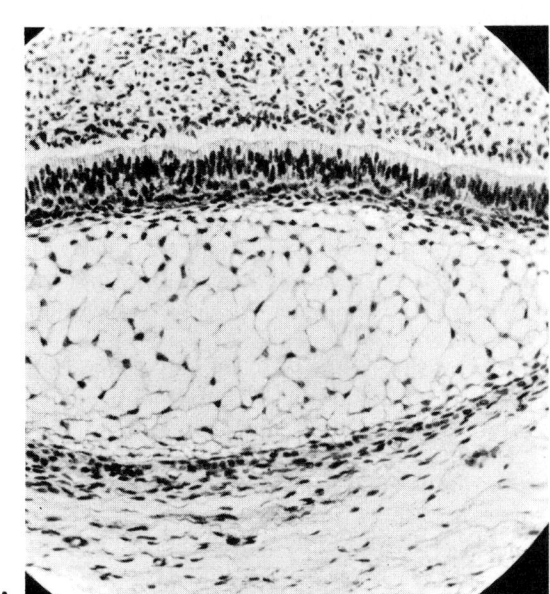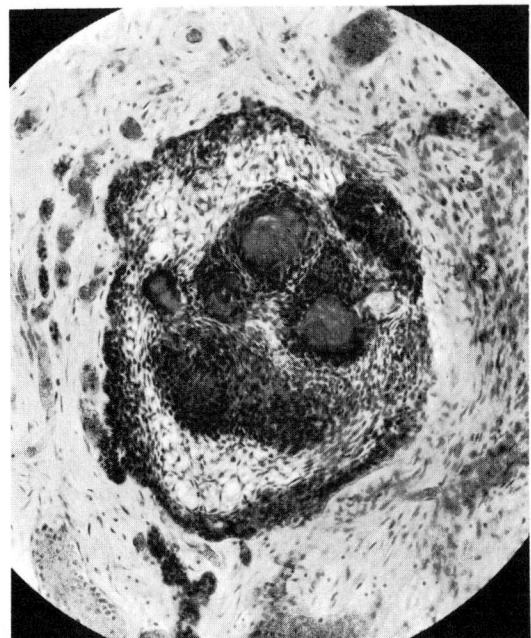

Figure 26–8. *A*, Embryonic tooth bud to illustrate similarity of cytology to cells of adamantinoma. *B*, Craniopharyngioma (adamantinoma). A nest of cells illustrating central squamous elements embedded in a loose cellular structure.

drome, total infarction of an adenoma followed by fibrous scarring, and ablation of the gland by either surgery or radiation.[23] In most individuals with this condition, sufficient parenchyma is preserved to prevent pituitary insufficiency, but occasionally there is either panhypopituitarism or inadequate secretion of one or more of the tropic hormones. In some cases the sella is not only empty but also enlarged, and so on radiography or CT scan is easily mistaken for an expansile pituitary neoplasm.

HYPOTHALAMIC SUPRASELLAR TUMORS

Neoplasms in this location are extremely uncommon but may induce hypofunction or hyperfunction of the anterior pituitary, diabetes insipidus, or combinations of these manifestations.[24] The most commonly implicated lesions are gliomas (sometimes arising in the chiasm) and craniopharyngiomas; germ cell tumors and lipomas may also appear as extreme rarities. Among these tumors only the craniopharyngioma is not considered elsewhere. Derived from vestigial remnants of Rathke's pouch, some arise within the sella but most are suprasellar. Most commonly seen in children and young adults, they are usually benign.

Craniopharyngiomas constitute up to 5% of all intracranial neoplasms. Averaging 3 to 4 cm in diameter, they may be encapsulated and solid but more commonly are cystic and sometimes multiloculated.[24] The cysts contain dark brown, oily fluid in which can be found granular debris as well as glittering cholesterol crystals. Over three fourths of these tumors contain sufficient calcification to be visualized radiographically, providing an important clinical diagnostic aid. In their strategic location, they often encroach on the optic chiasm or nerves and not infrequently bulge into the floor of the third ventricle and base of the brain.

The histologic pattern is quite variable and recapitulates the enamel organ of the tooth (Fig. 26–8). Thus, these tumors are also known as **adamantinomas** or **ameloblastomas.** Nests or cords of stratified squamous or columnar epithelium are embedded in a loose fibrous stroma. Often the nests of squamous cells gradually merge into a peripheral layer of columnar cells. In the cystic variants, the lining stratified squamous or columnar epithelium may be flat and regular, or thrown up into papillary projections. Calcification and metaplastic bone formation occur in the necrotic centers of the solid tumors as well as in the cystic variety. Infrequently, anaplastic changes are encountered in the epithelial cells, but cancerous behavior is rare. Craniopharyngiomas may stimulate considerable gliosis in the surrounding brain tissue.

POSTERIOR PITUITARY SYNDROMES

Disorders arising out of posterior pituitary dysfunction are exceedingly rare. Most relate to primary suprasellar hypothalamic lesions that will be detailed below. The consequences of dysfunction of the posterior pituitary take the forms of ADH deficiency or inappropriate release. The only known functions of oxytocin are potentiation of uterine contraction during labor, and stimulation of contraction of lactating glands in the breast to force milk into the excretory ducts during suckling. No well-defined syndrome associated with excessive or inappropriate release has been described.

ADH deficiency induces diabetes insipidus, characterized by polyuria and excessive thirst (polydipsia). The origins of this syndrome include (1) neoplastic or inflammatory involvement of the hypothalamo-hypophyseal axis (such as pituitary adenomas, metastatic cancer, abscesses, meningitis, tuberculosis, and sarcoidosis); (2) surgical or radiation injury to the hypothalamo-hypophyseal axis (such as surgical or irradiation hypophysectomy); (3) severe head injuries; and (4) idiopathic causes. Occasionally, patients with idiopathic diabetes insipidus have regressive alterations of obscure etiology of ganglion cells in the hypothalamus. Rarely, the idiopathic form of this syndrome is familial and apparently inherited as a mendelian dominant.

Inappropriate ADH secretion implies persistent release of ADH unrelated to the plasma osmolarity. Thus, there is excessive reabsorption of water from the glomerular filtrate, abnormal retention of water with expansion of the extracellular fluid volume, consequent hyponatremia and hemodilution, and the inability to excrete a dilute urine. The most common cause of inappropriate ADH secretion is paraneoplastic elaboration of ADH by nonendocrine tumors, particularly oat cell bronchogenic carcinoma, accounting for more than four fifths of all cases. Other neoplasms associated with ectopic production of ADH include thymoma, carcinoma of the pancreas, and lymphoma. Infrequently, disorders of the central nervous system underlie this syndrome, such as intracerebral hemorrhages or thromboses, subarachnoid hemorrhage, subdural hematoma, and infections in and about the CNS. Pulmonary disorders including pneumonia and tuberculosis have also been associated with the inappropriate secretion of ADH.

THYROID GLAND

CLINICAL SYNDROMES
  ASSOCIATED WITH THYROID
  DISEASE
Hyperthyroidism
Hypothyroidism
  Cretinism
  Myxedema
THYROIDITIS
Hashimoto's Thyroiditis

Subacute Granulomatous (de
  Quervain's) Thyroiditis
Subacute Lymphocytic
  (Painless) Thyroiditis
Riedel's Thyroiditis (Struma)
GRAVES' DISEASE
DIFFUSE NONTOXIC GOITER
  AND MULTINODULAR GOITER

Diffuse Nontoxic (Simple) Goiter
Multinodular Goiter
TUMORS
Adenomas
Other Benign Tumors
Malignant
  Papillary carcinoma
  Follicular carcinoma

Medullary carcinoma
Undifferentiated carcinoma
Other malignant tumors
MISCELLANEOUS LESIONS
Congenital Anomalies
Atrophy of Thyroid
Systemic Thyroidal Changes

NORMAL

The thyroid gland develops as a tubular evagination from the root of the tongue, called the foramen cecum. It grows downward in front of the trachea and thyroid cartilage to reach the position it will occupy in the adult. The distal end of this structure proliferates to form the adult gland, while the remainder degenerates and disappears, usually by the fifth to sixth week of development. Persistence of the vestigial tubular structure provides a source for the later development of thyroglossal cysts. Incomplete descent may lead to the formation of the thyroid at loci abnormally high in the neck, producing a lingual or aberrant subhyoid thyroid. Excessive descent leads to substernal thyroid glands. Rarely, lateral aberrant thyroid nodules develop, but these developmental anomalies are largely confined to the anterior triangle of the neck medial to the sternocleidomastoid muscle. Isolated follicles or groups of follicles have been identified outside the gland in perithyroid soft tissue in almost 90% of normal adults.[25] Malformations of branchial pouch differentiation may result in intrathyroidal sites for the thymus or parathyroid glands. The implication of these deviations from the norm may become all too evident in the patient who has a total thyroidectomy and subsequently develops hypoparathyroidism.

In the adult, the normal thyroid gland weighs 20 to 25 gm. Two large lateral lobes are connected in the midline by a broad isthmus from which, on occasion, a pyramidal lobe may protrude superiorly. Occasionally, in a very thin person, this normal pyramidal structure may be mistaken for a thyroid nodule. The close relationship of the recurrent laryngeal nerve and the parathyroid glands makes the latter extremely vulnerable to injury during thyroid surgery, and also to involvement by spreading malignancy or inflammation.

Histologically, the thyroid consists of variably sized follicles that, in three dimensions, compose spheres that are lined by regular cuboidal cells. In addition to the usual cellular organelles, numerous fine microvilli extend from the apical surface of the cells into the follicular colloid, within which is stored the thyroglobulin.[26] The microvilli participate in the mobilization of thyroid hormone from the thyroglobulin. In the normal gland, the follicles are separated by a delicate fibrous tissue stroma, which is compacted in some places into fibrous septa that traverse the gland. Small collections of lymphocytes are occasionally found in the stroma. Dispersed within the follicles are the calcitonin-secreting C-cells, which are derived from the neuroectoderm.[27] C-cells in the normal adult are concentrated at the junctions of the upper and middle thirds of the lateral lobes, along the central axes. These cells are extremely difficult to identify in normal glands without the use of immunocytochemical stains for the localization of calcitonin. However, they are more prominent in neonates and in adults with hypercalcemia or hypergastrinemia.

The active circulating hormones of the thyroid are triiodothyronine (T_3) and thyroxine (T_4).[28,29] The following steps are involved in the synthesis of these products: (1) Iodide trapping, an active process requiring energy. Normally the thyroid-serum, iodide ratio in humans is about $50 : 1$. (2) Oxidation of iodide within the thyroid cell to some form capable of iodinating tyrosine residues in the thyroglobulin. The oxidation is effected by an iodide peroxidase. (3) Iodination occurring at the microvillous interface between colloid and thyroid cell to form mono- and diiodotyrosine (MIT and DIT). (4) Coupling of MIT and DIT to form T_3 or coupling of two DITs to form T_4, again involving the peroxidase.

The release of T_3 and T_4 from the thyroglobulin involves the endocytosis of thyroglobulin and the proteolysis of the thyroglobulin within the follicular cells. The microvilli of the follicular cells reach out and enclose small fragments of the colloid to form membrane-bound vesicles that fuse with lysosomes to produce phagolysosomes.[30,31] The phagolysosome migrates to the basal portion of the epithelial cells, and during this passage, lysosomal proteases and peptidases split out T_3 and T_4, which are discharged at the base of the cell into the perifollicular capillaries. During this process some MITs and DITs are simultaneously released and deiodinated for salvage of the iodides.

Once released into the blood, T_4 is almost totally bound to an alpha globulin — thyroxine-binding globulin (TBG). Other plasma proteins, including prealbumin and albumin, participate to a lesser extent in this binding. T_3 is bound less firmly by TBG and very little by other plasma proteins. Because the metabolic state of cells is regulated by the unbound fraction, unbound or free T_3 is more available to the cells of the body than is the small fraction of free T_4. Alterations in the plasma levels of TBG may modify the metabolic state. Situations associated with increased TBG levels are pregnancy, ingestion of oral contraceptives and other forms of estrogen, diffuse liver disease, and possibly some genetic derangements. Decreased levels of TBG are seen with advanced liver disease, protein-losing nephropathies, adrenogenic steroid therapy, and possibly genetically conditioned syndromes.

The metabolic function of the thyroid hormones is a large and complex subject, well reviewed elsewhere.[32,33] It can be oversimplified by stating that at the cellular level thyroid hormone appears to interact with the nucleus, probably through nuclear hormone-binding receptors, and also with mitochondria to stimulate oxidative phosphorylation with the formation of ATP. Thyroidal hormones also enhance transmembrane transport and enzyme activity. With all these actions the hormones, more specifically the unbound or free fractions, stimulate virtually all metabolic processes, both synthetic and catabolic. In effect, then, the hormones provide the spark that keeps the metabolic machine running. As will be seen, a deficiency of the hormones significantly slows the machine, whereas an excess speeds it to the point at which it begins to consume itself.

From the physiologic standpoint, the thyroid gland is one of the most sensitive organs in the body. It responds to many stimuli and is in a constant state of adaptation. During puberty, pregnancy, and physiologic stress from any source, the gland increases in size and becomes more active. Changes in activity and size may even be noted during a normal menstrual period. This extreme functional lability is reflected in transient hyperplasia of the thyroidal epithelium. At this time, thyroglobulin is resorbed and the follicular cells become tall and columnar, sometimes forming small infolded buds or papillae. When the stress abates, involution occurs, i.e., the height of the epithelium falls, colloid accumulates, and the follicular cells resume their normal size and architecture. Failure of this normal balance between hyperplasia and involution may produce major or minor deviations from the usual histologic pattern.

The function of the thyroid gland can be inhibited by a variety of chemical agents, collectively referred to as goitrogens (Fig. 26-9). Because they suppress T_3 and T_4 synthesis, increased levels of TSH and subsequent hyperplastic enlargement of the gland (goiter) follow. Most important among these compounds are certain drugs used in the treatment of hyperthyroidism. The antithyroid agents thiourea and mercaptoimidazole inhibit the oxidation of iodide and block coupling of the iodotyrosines into T_3 and T_4. Thus, thyroid hormones cannot be produced; there is diminished negative feedback on the pituitary and hypothalamus, and the result is increased levels of TSH and TRH with stimulation of the gland, resulting in thyroid hyperplasia and enlargement. Iodide, when given to patients with thyroid hyperfunction, also blocks the release of thyroid hormones but through different mechanisms. Iodides in large doses inhibit proteolysis of thyroglobulin. Thus, thyroid hormone is synthesized and incorporated within increasing amounts of colloid, but it is not released into the blood. The gland following thiourea therapy lacks thyroglobulin-colloid and is extremely cellular, but with iodine treatment the follicles become distended with thyroglobulin and the stromal vascularization compressed, creating the appearance of an inactive gland.

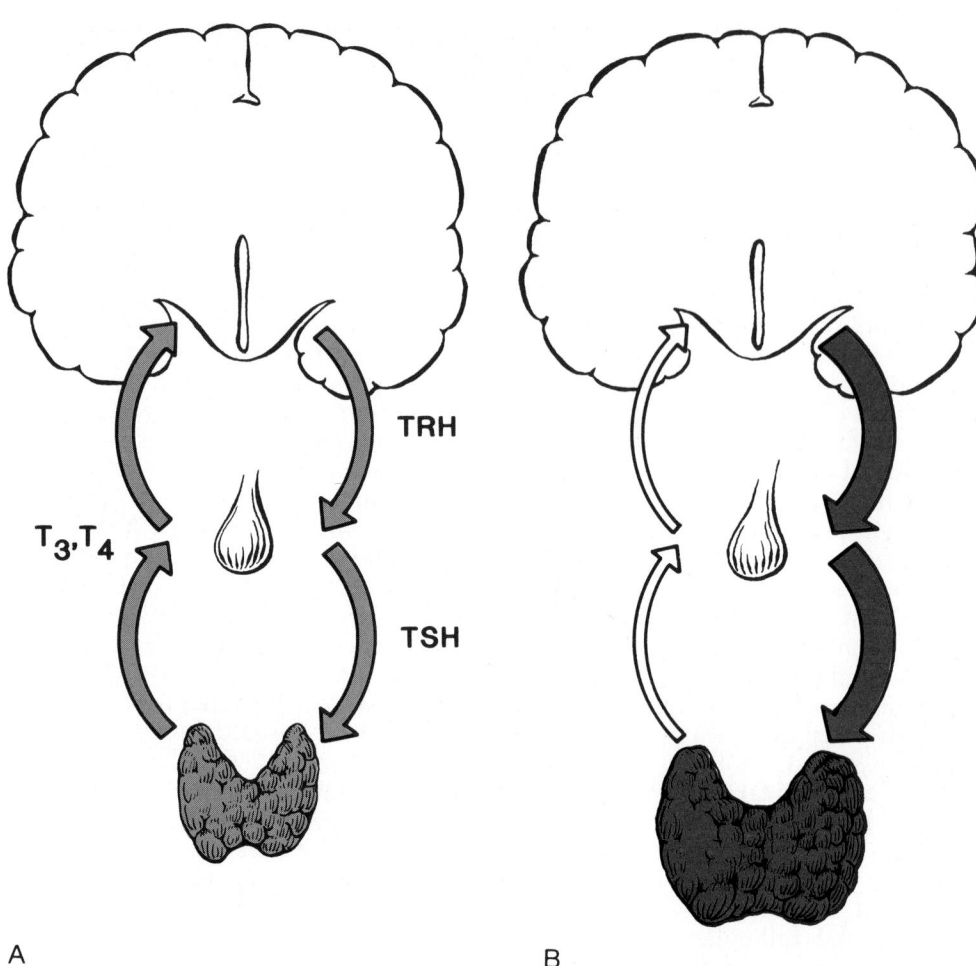

A

B

Figure 26-9. *A,* Thyroid hormone synthesis is controlled by both hypothalamic TRH and pituitary TSH secretion in a classic negative feedback loop. Low levels of T_3 and T_4 stimulate the release of TSH and TRH. TSH stimulates the thyroid to synthesize T_3 and T_4. When T_3 and T_4 levels rise sufficiently, the release of TRH and TSH is suppressed. *B,* In individuals with biosynthetic defects in T_3 and T_4 synthesis, TRH and TSH are increased. The persistent stimulation of the thyroid by TSH results in the development of thyroid enlargement (goiter).

Some of the numerous tests currently available to assay normal thyroid gland function include measurement of serum TSH and TRH by radioimmunoassay.[34] The serum levels of total T_3 and T_4 and the precise levels of free T_3 and T_4 can also be determined. Another measure of thyroid activity is the ability to take up an administered dose of radioactive iodine (RAI uptake). A functional evaluation of the gross anatomy of the thyroid is provided by a scintiscan, after administration of a radionuclide of iodide or technetium pertechnetate. The scan will disclose focal lesions such as tumors that are nonfunctioning ("cold nodules") or hyperactive masses ("hot nodules"), aberrant thyroid tissue, and functioning metastases of thyroid cancer, wherever they are located.

PATHOLOGY

Diseases of the thyroid are of great importance because most are amenable to medical or surgical management. *They present principally as hyperthyroidism, hypothyroidism, and diffuse or focal enlargement of the gland.* Some concept of the relative frequency of the more common forms of thyroid disease can be gained from a screening survey of individuals in a small northeastern town in the United States.[35] A total of 5.8% of the population was found to have thyroid abnormalities. In order of frequency, the following conditions were identified: simple (nonfunctional) symmetric enlargement, hyperthyroidism, multinodular goiter, thyroiditis, and a solitary nodular goiter (presumably an adenoma). No cases of cancer were identified. An essentially similar distribution of the various thyroid disorders was reported from a British community.[36] Thus, goitrous thyroid enlargement without manifestations of thyroid hyperfunction is the most common presentation in these two surveys, followed in frequency by hyperthyroidism.

There is no simple correlation between morphologic lesions of the thyroid and resultant clinical manifestations. For example, a multinodular goiter in one instance may be associated with normal thyroid function, in another with hyperfunction, and in yet another with hypofunction. It is best, therefore, at the outset to present the clinical syndromes of hyperthyroidism and hypothyroidism and then discuss the various thyroid lesions in some rational morphologic sequence, relating each to its possible clinical significance.

CLINICAL SYNDROMES ASSOCIATED WITH THYROID DISEASE

HYPERTHYROIDISM

Hyperthyroidism is a hypermetabolic state encountered much more often in females, caused by an increased output of T_4 and T_3. It is manifested by nervousness, palpitations, rapid pulse, fatigability, muscular weakness, weight loss with good appetite, diarrhea, heat intolerance, warm skin, excessive perspiration, emotional lability, menstrual changes, a fine tremor of the hand (particularly when outstretched), eye changes, and variable enlargement of the thyroid gland.

Typically, the skin is warm, moist, and flushed, related both to peripheral vasodilation to increase the heat loss and to the general hyperdynamic circulatory state. **Eye changes often call attention to the hyperthyroidism.** Typically, patients have a wide-eyed stare produced by retraction of the upper eyelid and upper lid lag as it falls behind the globe on slow downward gaze. In Graves' disease there is also protrusion of the globe (proptosis) secondary to immunoinflammatory changes in the retro-orbital tissues (Fig. 26–10). **Cardiac manifestations are among the earliest and most consistent features of hyperthyroidism.** Tachycardia, palpitations, and cardiomegaly are common. Cardiac arrhythmias occasionally appear and are often supraventricular. The basis for these arrhythmias is not clear. Myocardial changes, such as foci of lymphocytic and eosinophilic infiltration, mild fibrosis in the interstitium, fatty changes in myofibers, and an increase in size and number of mitochondria, have been described.[37] These changes are not frequent and other possible concomitant pathogeneses have not been rigorously ruled out, so that debate continues about so-called **thyrotoxic cardiomyopathy.** The cardiomegaly is equally obscure and is vaguely attributed to a cardiac hyperdynamic state induced by increased formation of or response to catecholamines. Other explanations have been offered, but it suffices to say that much is uncertain; only uncommonly does cardiac failure occur in these patients, usually in the elderly in whom other cardiac diseases are often present.

Other findings throughout the body include atrophy and fatty infiltration of skeletal muscle, sometimes with focal interstitial lymphocytic infiltrates; minimal fatty changes in the liver, sometimes accompanied by mild periportal fibrosis and a mild lymphocytic infiltrate; osteoporosis; and generalized lymphoid hyperplasia with lymphadenopathy.

Hyperthyroidism may be caused by a variety of disorders (Table 26–2). The three common causes collectively account for virtually 99% of cases. Among these, Graves' disease is the most frequent, particularly in patients under 40 years of age. This disease is also known as diffuse toxic goiter to differentiate it from the thyrotoxicosis related to toxic nod-

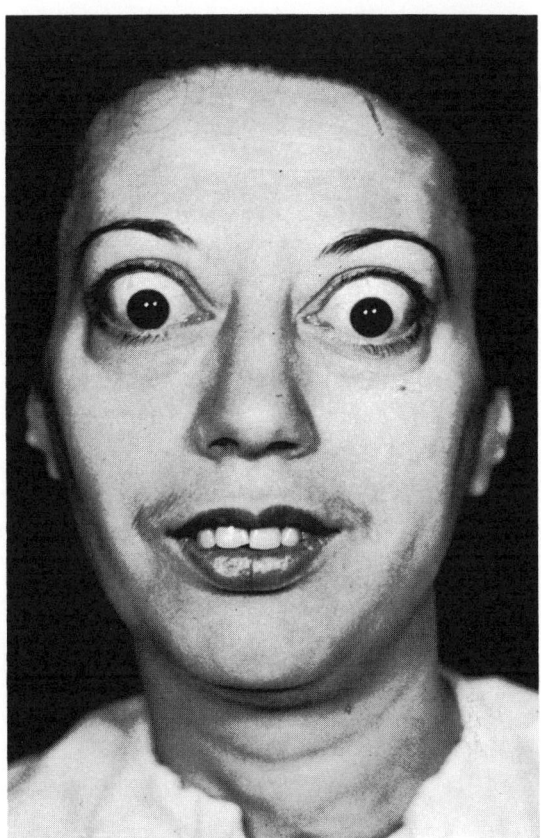

Figure 26–10. Hyperthyroidism in a 27-year-old woman.

ular goiter, whether it is a solitary nodule (presumably an adenoma) or multinodular (Fig. 26–11).[38] Only a few brief comments are merited on the rare causes of hyperthyroidism. Metastatic, well-differentiated thyroid carcinoma may sometimes elaborate sufficient thyroid hormones to cause hyperthyroidism. Similarly, acute or subacute thyroiditis during the stage of active cell injury may be associated with sufficient release of stored hormones to induce transient manifestations of hyperthyroidism. Choriocarcinomas and hydatidiform moles may produce not only chorionic gonadotropin but also sometimes a TSH-like material.[39] Increased levels of thyroid hormones are rarely caused by TSH-secreting pituitary tumors or pituitary stimulation by excessive hypothalamic

Table 26–2. Disorders Associated with Hyperthyroidism

COMMON
Diffuse toxic hyperplasia (Graves' disease)
Toxic multinodular goiter
Toxic adenoma
UNCOMMON
Acute or subacute thyroiditis
Hyperfunctioning thyroid carcinoma
Choriocarcinoma or hydatidiform mole
TSH-secreting pituitary adenoma
Neonatal thyrotoxicosis associated with maternal Graves' disease
Struma ovarii (ovarian teratomatous thyroid)
Iodide-induced hyperthyroidism
Iatrogenic (exogenous) hyperthyroidism

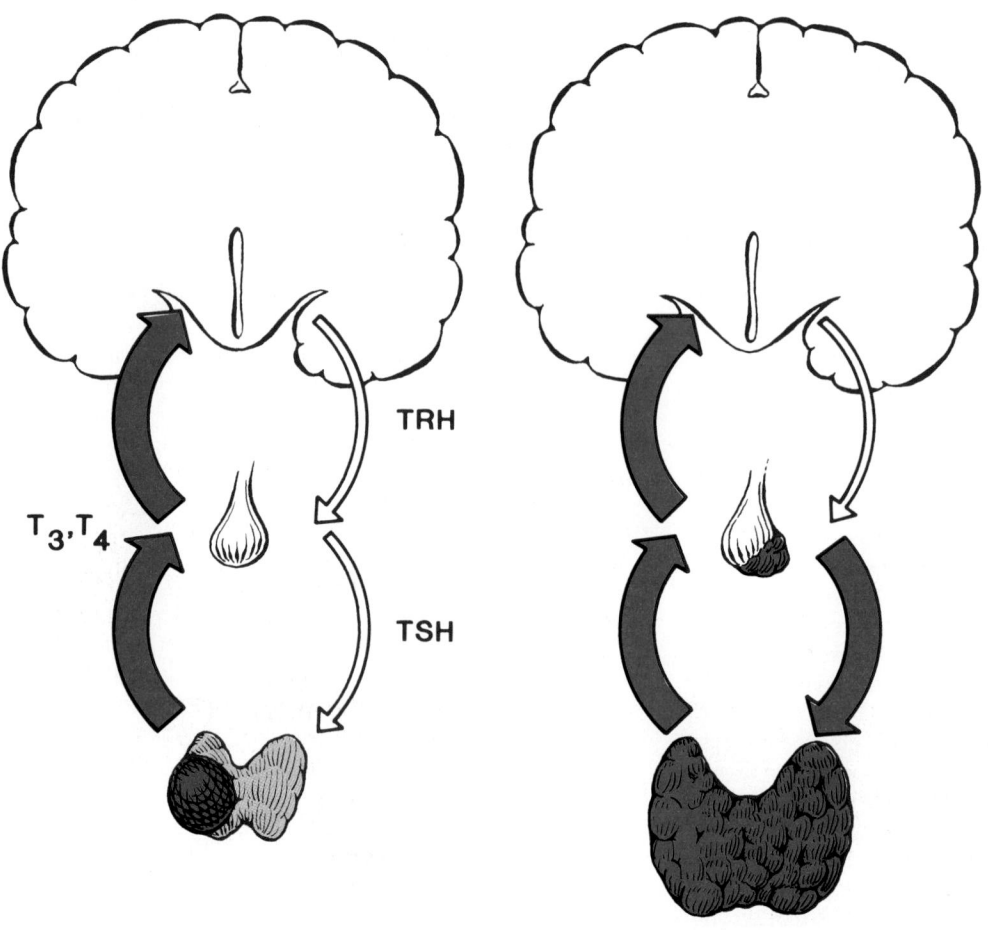

T₃,T₄ — TRH — TSH

A   B

Figure 26-11. Hyperthyroidism may be caused by a toxic adenoma that suppresses TSH production by the pituitary *(A)* or by a pituitary neoplasm producing excess TSH *(B)*.

release of TRH (Fig. 26-11).[40] Thyroid hyperfunction can be also induced by excess iodine ingestion in patients with various thyroid disorders. This pattern is sometimes referred to as jodbasedow disease. It is unclear at present how the iodine ingestion precipitates the thyrotoxicosis.[41] Equally rarely, patients receiving thyroid hormone medication for hypothyroidism or for other reasons (misguided attempts at weight control) may develop iatrogenic or factitious hyperthyroidism. In all the foregoing situations, the same hypermetabolic syndrome results.

The diagnosis of hyperthyroidism may be readily apparent from the clinical manifestations, or the signs and symptoms may be so subtle that resort must be made to laboratory evidence. Characteristically, there is an increase in the serum concentrations of T_4 and T_3, particularly the latter. Sometimes a decrease of thyroxine-binding globulin increases both the proportion and the amount of free T_4 and T_3. The radioactive iodine uptake is also increased. With Graves' disease, there are additional immunologic findings, and with thyrotoxicosis secondary to neoplastic or nodular goitrous involvement of the gland, there may be abnormalities in the scintiscan.

Finally, brief mention should be made of thyrotoxic crisis or storm. Although poorly understood, this clinical emergency usually occurs in patients with unrecognized or inadequately treated thyrotoxicosis. It is precipitated by subtotal thyroidectomy before adequate control of the thyrotoxic state has been established, but it may also arise with severe infection, trauma, or any other form of acute stress in the hyperthyroid patient. Severe hypermetabolism erupts, marked by fever, tachycardia, and often cardiac irregularities and failure, leading soon to progressive mental obtundation and coma. Emergency measures are necessary to control the desperate situation, but it is nonetheless fatal in 20 to 25% of patients.

HYPOTHYROIDISM

Any structural or functional derangement of the thyroid that significantly impairs its output of hormone will lead to the hypometabolic state of hypothyroidism. The clinical manifestations of the hormone lack depend on the age when it first appears. When present during development and infancy, it results in cretinism with its associated physical and mental retardation. The term "cretin" was derived from the French "chrétien," meaning Christian or Christ-like, and was applied to these unfortunates because they were considered to be so mentally retarded as to be incapable of sinning! When hypothyroidism first appears in older children or adults, it is termed myxedema. This designation calls attention to the accumulation of hydrophilic mucopolysaccharides in connective tissue throughout the body, leading to a distinctive, edematous, doughy thickening of the skin that is resistant to pitting.

The causes of hypothyroidism in both infants and adults can be divided into several categories, as in Table 26–3. Among these various disorders, the most frequent in the United States is ablation of the gland by either surgery or radiation. Sometimes an overly generous subtotal thyroidectomy for the treatment of hyperthyroidism is followed by insufficient thyroid function. On occasion it is necessary to remove the thyroid to adequately excise a primary neoplasm. The gland may also be ablated by radiation, whether in the form of radioiodine administered for the treatment of hyperthyroidism or in the form of exogenous irradiation employed in the treatment of some nearby neoplasm, e.g., lymphoma. The next most common cause of hypothyroidism is so-called primary idiopathic myxedema. There is now substantial evidence that this condition is autoimmune in origin.[42] It suffices for now to note that autoantibodies that block the TSH receptors have been identified and proposed as the cause of primary hypothyroidism.[43] Together, these two forms of thyroidal inadequacy account for 80 to 90% of all cases of hypothyroidism. Infrequently, hypothyroidism stems from a developmental failure, synthetic defect, or forms of thyroid disease that produce, among other things, a goiter. Even more infrequently, hypothyroidism arises because of a disorder in the hypothalamus or adenohypophysis that reduces serum TSH levels, or because of some peripheral resistance to thyroid hormone.

Cretinism

This usually preventable, and therefore all the more tragic, condition is marked by retardation of both physical and intellectual growth. It is seldom apparent at birth but, depending on the severity of hormone lack, becomes evident over ensuing weeks to months. By the time the changes become unmistak-

Table 26–3. Causes of Hypothyroidism

Deficiency of thyroid parenchyma
  Surgical or radiation ablation
  Primary idiopathic myxedema (?autoimmune)
  Agenesis, hypoplasia, or dysplasia of thyroid

Goitrous hypothyroidism
  Hashimoto's thyroiditis
  Endemic iodine deficiency
  Exogenous goitrogenic agents
  Iodide-induced

Suprathyroidal disorders
  Hypopituitarism
  Hypothalamic lesions

Peripheral resistance to thyroid hormones

ably evident they are largely irreversible, and so a strong case can be made for routine screening of neonates for possible thyroid hormone lack. The first and most sensitive laboratory abnormality to appear is an increase in serum TSH level related to loss of feedback inhibition. In time, serum T_4 and then T_3 concentrations fall. The initial clinical manifestations are feeding problems; constipation; a hoarse, husky cry; somnolence; and failure to thrive. With time, the abdomen becomes protuberant, the skin grows dry, and there is delay in the appearance of the deciduous teeth, accompanied by impaired skeletal growth leading to dwarfism. The fully developed syndrome is characterized by dry, rough skin; widely set eyes; periorbital puffiness, a flattened, broad nose; and an overly large protuberant tongue. There is delay in closure of the fontanelles and, late in life, delay in closure of the epiphyses along with other epiphyseal abnormalities. The radiographic findings are so distinctive as to be virtually diagnostic. When the thyroid deficit is present during early fetal development, as may occur with severe iodine lack, agenesis of the thyroid, or a congenital biosynthetic defect, there is retarded development of the brain and the child manifests deaf-mutism, spasticity, and severe mental deficiency, giving rise to the term "neurologic cretinism."[44] If the hormone lack is less severe or appears later in development, there is milder impairment but still some degree of mental deficiency, called hypothyroid cretinism.

The terms *endemic cretinism* and *sporadic cretinism* should be clarified here. Endemic cretinism occurs wherever endemic goiter is prevalent, generally related to a dietary lack of iodine. Often, both parents of the affected infant are goitrous. Sporadic cretinism, in contrast, is usually caused by some congenital developmental failure in thyroid gland formation (sporadic athyreotic cretinism) or by some biosynthetic defect in thyroid hormone formation.[45] In most instances, the hormonal lack in the neonate is not as severe as in endemic cretinism, and so the mental retardation is more subtle at birth and difficult to detect. However, it also provides a greater opportunity, if recognized relatively early, to institute appropriate therapy and prevent fully developed cretinism.

Myxedema

The term myxedema is applied to hypothyroidism in the older child or adult. The clinical manifestations vary with the age of onset of the deficiency. The older child shows signs and symptoms intermediate between those of the cretin and the adult with hypothyroidism. In the adult the condition appears very insidiously and may take years to reach the level of clinical suspicion. Basically it is characterized by slowing of physical and mental activity. The initial symptoms are fatigue, lethargy, cold intolerance, and general listlessness and apathy. Speech and intellectual functions become slowed. With the passage of time, periorbital edema develops along with a thickened, dry, coarse skin. Eventually the facial features become thickened and the tongue enlarged, and the distinctive peripheral edema described earlier worsens. At this time there is extreme physical and mental torpor. Other systems share in the general lethargy with decreased sweating, constipation, and slowness of motor function. The cardiac output is also decreased because of a reduction in both stroke volume and heart rate. An increase in peripheral vascular resistance and a decrease in blood volume result in narrowing of the pulse pressure, prolongation of the circulation time, and decreased flow to the peripheral tissues. It is the reduced circulation in the skin that accounts for the sensitivity to the cold. In well-advanced myxedema the heart is flabby and enlarged, with dilated chambers. Histologically, there is sometimes swelling of the myofibers with some loss of striations, accompanied by an increase of interstitial mucopolysaccharide-rich edema fluid. A similar fluid sometimes accumulates within the pericardial sac. To these changes the term *myxedema heart* or *hypothyroid cardiomyopathy* has been applied. There may also be some retardation in skeletal growth and in CNS development; however, the latter is more characteristic of cretinism.

Although the diagnosis of myxedema can often be made on the basis of the clinical findings, it usually requires laboratory confirmation. As in the infant and child with cretinism, the serum levels of T_4 and T_3 are subnormal. In primary hypothyroidism, such as occurs with thyroid disease, the TSH level is elevated owing to loss of feedback inhibition of the pituitary. However, in the uncommon instance in which the hypothyroidism is related to some hypothalamic/hypophyseal disorder and loss of tropic stimulation of the thyroid gland, the TSH levels are abnormally low. Recognition of this form of so-called trophoprivic hypothyroidism is of great importance because it is often accompanied by depressed ACTH levels and adrenocortical insufficiency. In such circumstances, treatment of the hypothyroid state with thyroid hormone and stimulation of the general metabolic activity of the body may precipitate a crisis of adrenal insufficiency. With this overview of the clinical consequences of disturbed thyroid function, we can turn to the disorders causing it.

THYROIDITIS

A variety of ill-defined forms of thyroiditis may be produced by microbial seeding of the thyroid. Almost always the infection is primary elsewhere and the agents blood-borne; rarely, there is direct traumatic seeding of the gland. Sometimes, immunologic incompetence potentiates these infective forms of thyroiditis. The most frequent causes are *Staphylococcus aureus*, streptococci, Salmonella, Enterobacter, tuberculosis, and fungi (Candida, aspergilli, Mucormycetes). Viral thyroiditis is a special case, discussed later (Fig. 26–12). The thyroid may also be involved in sarcoidosis. Whatever the cause, the inflammatory

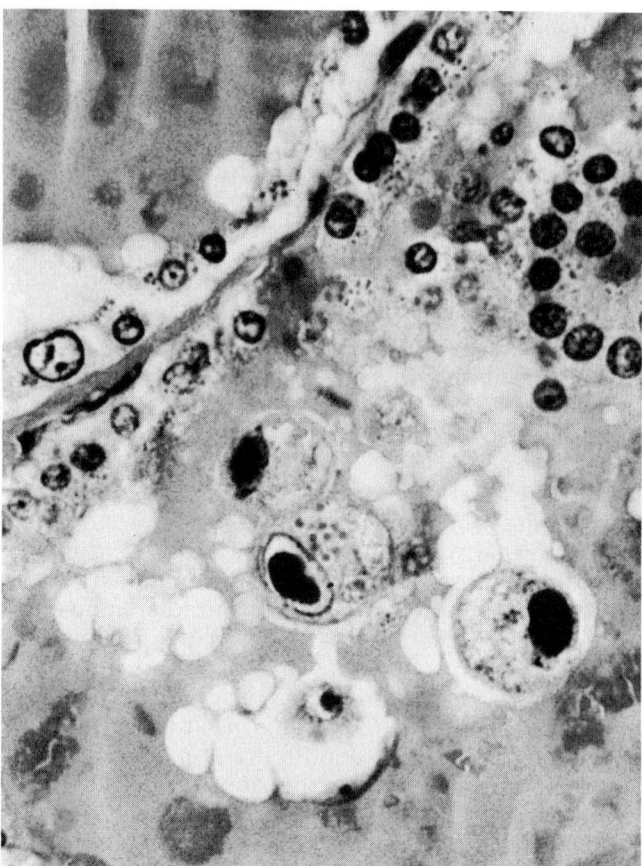

Figure 26–12. Cytomegalovirus producing large intranuclear inclusions may involve the thyroid in patients with AIDS or in individuals with other forms of immunosuppression.

involvement may cause painful enlargement of the gland, but almost always the condition is transient and self-limited or controllable with appropriate therapy. Thyroid function usually is not significantly affected, and there are few residual effects except for possible small foci of scarring. Much more common and clinically significant are the following more or less well-defined forms of thyroiditis: (1) Hashimoto's thyroiditis, (2) subacute granulomatous thyroiditis, (3) subacute lymphocytic thyroiditis, and (4) Riedel's thyroiditis (struma).[46,47]

HASHIMOTO'S THYROIDITIS

Marked by an intense infiltrate of lymphocytes admixed with plasma cells that virtually replaces the thyroid parenchyma (Fig. 26–13), this chronic form of thyroiditis is of importance on several scores: (1) It is the most common cause of goitrous hypothyroidism in regions having a sufficiency of iodine; (2) it is a major cause of nonendemic goiter in children; and (3) it is the first-described and the archetype of organ-specific autoimmune diseases.[48] The thyroid enlargement is generally painless; although diffuse, it may be asymmetric and may sometimes appear lobulated. Most patients with long-standing Hashimoto's disease become hypothyroid, but a few in midcourse develop hyperthyroidism, sometimes called *hashitoxicosis*. This concurrence is more than fortuitous, since there are many similarities in the autoimmune reactions in Hashimoto's thyroiditis and Graves' thyrotoxicosis. Because of all the immunologic abnormalities, Hashimoto's thyroiditis is also sometimes called *autoimmune thyroiditis*. Another synonym is *struma lymphomatosa*, denoting the striking replacement of the thyroid parenchyma by lymphoid cells.

Hashimoto's thyroiditis is predominantly a disease of women, with a female:male ratio of 10:1. Most cases occur between the ages of 30 to 50, but some are noted in children. The possibility of some genetic predisposition is suspected because of the familial occurrence of the disease and because of a well-defined association with HLA-DR5. There is also a greater-than-chance association with other diseases of presumed autoimmune origin, including systemic lupus erythematosus, Sjögren's syndrome, rheumatoid arthritis, pernicious anemia, adult-onset diabetes, and Graves' disease. However, it should be noted that the last-named condition tends to be associated with HLA-DR3 in whites.

ETIOLOGY AND PATHOGENESIS. Few doubt the autoimmune origin of this form of chronic thyroidi-

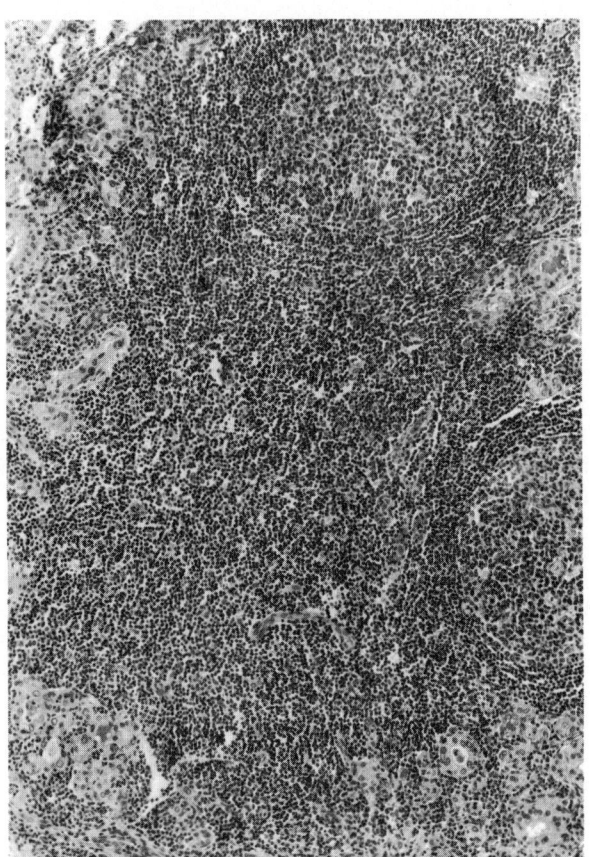

Figure 26-13. Hashimoto's thyroiditis. The thyroid parenchyma is largely replaced by a heavy lymphocytic infiltrate containing two evident lymphoid follicles. Only some marginal thyroid follicles are present in the field.

tis.[49] A variety of pathogenetic mechanisms, including antibody-dependent cell-mediated toxicity, antibody-dependent complement-mediated cytotoxicity, direct T-cell killing, and immune complex deposition with a localized Arthus type reaction, have been implicated. *The basic defect is thought to be a genetically conditioned deficiency in antigen-specific suppressor T cells.* As a consequence, there is uncontrolled attack on the follicular cells by cytotoxic T cells, and simultaneously unregulated T-helper cell participation in the B-cell formation of autoantibodies. The supporting evidence is as follows. A variety of autoantibodies against thyroid-cell antigens can be identified in virtually all patients with this condition, most consistently TSH-receptor antibodies and thyroid microsomal antibodies.[50] About half the patients also have antibodies to thyroglobulin and, less constantly, to follicular cell membranes, thyroid hormones themselves, and a colloid component other than thyroglobulin. The TSH-receptor autoantibodies are of particular interest; by binding to receptors, they mimic the action of TSH, but studies indicate that these receptor autoantibodies can be separated into those that stimulate hormone synthesis (thyroid-stimulating immunoglobulins—TSI) and those that initiate thyroid growth (thyroid-growth immunoglobulins—TGI).[51] To complicate matters further, "blocking" antibodies for each of these subsets can be identified.[43] Two scenarios can therefore be proposed in the pathogenesis of Hashimoto's disease: (1) The TSH-receptor autoantibodies may be largely TGI, i.e., those that stimulate growth with a relative paucity of TSI, which stimulate hormone synthesis; or (2) both TSI and TGI autoantibodies are present, but also TSI-blocking antibodies. These issues are now under investigation, but in either instance goitrous enlargement occurs without hyperfunction.[52] It is speculated, therefore, that HLA-DR5 individuals are in some way genetically predisposed to the production of the pathogenetic antibodies. Interestingly, patients with Graves' hyperthyroidism have virtually an identical complement of thyroidal autoantibodies but, with the HLA-DR3 genotype, express more of the TSI.

Hashimoto's thyroiditis is characterized by extensive loss of thyroid parenchyma, but despite all the immunologic alterations, the precise mechanisms of follicular cell destruction are uncertain. Recent studies have demonstrated that thyroid follicular cells in patients with Hashimoto's disease regularly express HLA-DR antigens, and have provided evidence that the thyroid cells are capable of activating T lymphocytes and presenting antigen directly to intrathyroidal T lymphocytes.[53] Since gamma interferon can induce HLA-DR expression by thyroid follicular cells and since viral infections may antedate endocrine autoimmunity, it has been suggested that gamma interferon locally produced by lymphocytes secondary to viral infection may result in HLA-DR expression by the follicular cells. This may be the initial inductive event in autoimmune thyroid disease.

MORPHOLOGY. There are two major morphologic variants of Hashimoto's thyroiditis. The **classic form** is characterized by rubbery, firm, usually symmetric, moderate enlargement of the gland. The capsule is intact and only rarely adherent to surrounding structures, while the parenchyma has a pale gray, fleshy cut surface with accentuation of normal lobulations. Although the macroscopic changes could be mistaken for neoplastic replacement, the symmetry of the involvement and the integrity of the capsule argue against a neoplasm. The differentiation can be more difficult when there is asymmetric enlargement.

Microscopically, **there is extensive replacement of the gland by lymphoid cells, including plasma cells, immunoblasts, transformed lymphocytes, and macrophages, with the formation of lymphoid germinal centers** (Fig.26–13).[47] Isolated follicles or clusters of follicles persist, but they are often atrophic and contain sparse, deeply staining colloid. The persistent follicular epithelium is transformed into so-called **Hürthle cells** or **oncocytes** having an abundant brightly eosinophilic granular cytoplasm packed with mitochondria and lysosomes. Hürthle cells produce little or no T_4, T_3, or thyroglobulin. They are thought to represent a degenerated state of the follicular epithelium, are not specific for Hashimoto's thyroiditis, and are found in many other forms of thyroid injury.[54] Such fibrosis as is present is usually delicate and largely confined to the interlobular septa.

The other, much less common morphologic pattern is called **fibrosing** Hashimoto's thyroiditis and is characterized by modest thyroid enlargement, a more intense fibrosis, and a less prominent lymphoid infiltrate.[55] The follicular atrophy is often more severe, with conversion of persistent follicular epithelium into either Hürthle cells or squamous cells. The fibrosing reaction does not extend beyond the capsule, differentiating this pattern of Hashimoto's disease from Riedel's struma.

CLINICAL COURSE. The cardinal clinical feature of Hashimoto's thyroiditis is goitrous enlargement of the thyroid gland associated with hypothyroidism in a middle-aged woman. At the outset only a goiter may be present, but in those with the fibrosing variant the enlargement may be subtle and the major feature is hypothyroidism. Only infrequently does the thyroid enlarge rapidly enough to cause pain and tenderness. In time, hypothyroidism becomes evident in most patients, but it worsens only very slowly over the course of years and is sometimes virtually static. Thus, early in the disease the patient is metabolically normal, but the serum **TSH** levels may be mildly elevated. At this time the **RAI** uptake and **PBI** may be mildly increased because of deranged thyroidal function, with the secretion of hormonally inactive iodoproteins. Notably, the serum T_4 and T_3 levels are normal. As the hypothyroidism becomes more established, the **RAI** uptake and T_4 and T_3 levels decline. Despite all the clinical evidence, needle biopsy is often required to confirm the diagnosis. There is no increased prevalence of thyroid carcinoma in these glands; however, the incidence of lymphoma appears to be increased.[56,57]

SUBACUTE GRANULOMATOUS (DE QUERVAIN'S) THYROIDITIS

The term *subacute thyroiditis* is restricted to a distinctive form of self-limited inflammation of the thyroid gland, which is also referred to as *giant cell* or *pseudogranulomatous thyroiditis*. The peak incidence is in the second to fifth decades of life, with a female : male ratio of $3:1$.[58,59]

Although the cause is still uncertain, considerable circumstantial evidence suggests a viral etiology.[60] For example, there is a more-than-chance association between onset of the thyroiditis and some form of viral infection (mumps, influenza, adenovirus, Coxsackie, ECHO viruses). Moreover, antibodies to the causative agents of these infections can be identified in about half the cases. Clinically, the condition is reminiscent of an infection with fever, painful tender enlargement of the thyroid gland, and a self-limited course measured in months.[61] A possible role for autoimmunity has been raised but has been largely excluded. Significant levels of thyroid autoantibodies are present in only a minority of patients, do not correlate with the course of the disease, and are transitory.[62]

MORPHOLOGY. The gland may be subtly or markedly enlarged. Sometimes, the enlargement appears asymmetric or focal on palpation of the neck, but more often the whole gland is irregularly involved. It may be slightly adherent to surrounding structures. On cut section the involved areas are firm and yellow-white and stand out from the more rubbery, normal brown thyroid substance. Histologically, the changes are patchy and depend on the stage of the disease. Early in the active inflammatory phase, scattered follicles may be entirely disrupted and replaced by neutrophils forming microabscesses. **Later, the more characteristic features appear in the form of aggregations of macrophages about damaged follicles, admixed with multinucleate giant cells enclosing naked pools or fragments of colloid** (Fig. 26–14).[47] The inflammatory foci more or less resemble granulomas, hence the designation "granulomatous thyroiditis." In later stages of the disease, a chronic inflammatory infiltrate and fibrosis may replace the foci of injury. Different histologic stages are sometimes found in the same gland, suggesting waves of destruction over a period of time. A morphologically similar pattern may result from vigorous palpation of the gland, which may lead to mechanical disruption of follicles (so-called palpation thyroiditis).[63]

CLINICAL COURSE. The presentation of this condition is extremely variable. Basically, three patterns can be identified: (1) an acute systemic febrile reaction with elevation of the sedimentation rate; (2) sudden painful enlargement of the gland, sometimes

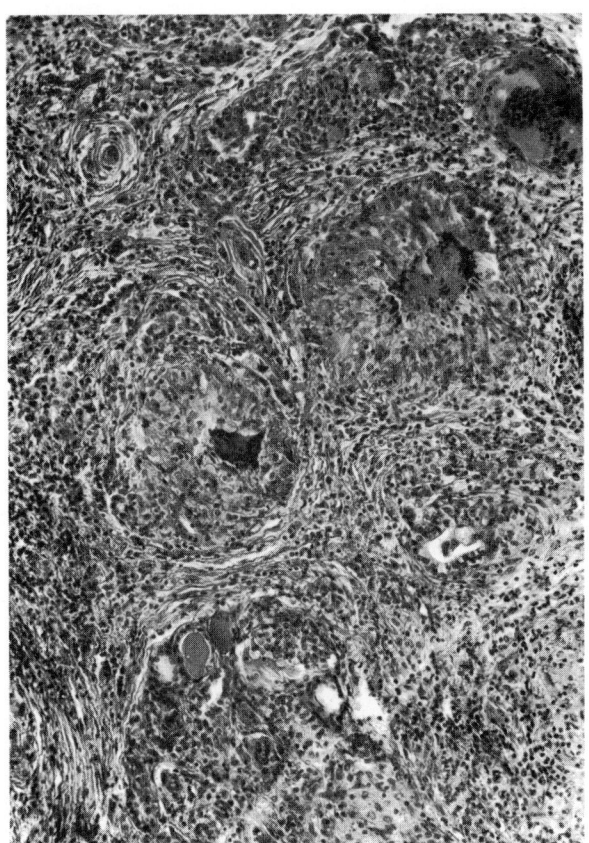

Figure 26–14. Subacute thyroiditis. Two granulomatous foci enclosing remnants of colloid are evident in midfield. Note large giant cell *(above right)*. (Courtesy of Dr. Merle Legg, New England Deaconess Hospital.)

mimicking "sore throat" or "earache"; or (3) less painful enlargement accompanied by transient manifestations of hyperthyroidism. Obviously, more than one may coexist in the same patient. Whatever form the disease takes at onset, the condition is self-limited, and over the span of weeks to months the tenderness usually abates along with the fever and manifestations of hyperthyroidism. Indeed, with extensive destruction of the gland, transient hypothyroidism may supervene. Laboratory tests of thyroid function can be anticipated to a considerable extent. Characteristically, the T_3 and T_4 levels are increased and the RAI uptake is low. Presumably, T_3 and T_4 are released as a result of damage to the follicles, while the low RAIU is caused by T_3- and T_4-induced suppression of TSH. The quantities of circulating T_3 and T_4 may be sufficient to induce transient hyperthyroidism. Extensive damage to the gland may induce a transient phase of hypothyroidism with a fall in plasma hormone levels. Following recovery, generally within five to six months, normal thyroid function resumes and the various laboratory test results return to normal. Scattered foci of fibrous scarring, rarely sufficient to cause asymmetry of the gland or to masquerade as tumorous involvement, may remain. In very rare instances, the disease may be characterized by repeated exacerbations and remissions over many months.

SUBACUTE LYMPHOCYTIC (PAINLESS) THYROIDITIS

This poorly understood condition constitutes, in essence, a painless variant of subacute granulomatous thyroiditis. It is also distinctive anatomically, inasmuch as the only changes in the gland are foci of lymphocytic infiltration, sometimes accompanied by an increase in interstitial fibrous tissue. There is no tendency to formation of lymphoid germinal centers and few, if any, plasma cells. Subacute painless thyroiditis usually comes to attention because of goitrous enlargement of the gland or hyperthyroidism, or both. One survey indicated that subacute lymphocytic thyroiditis was responsible for about 15% of all cases of hyperthyroidism in North America.[64] In the absence of hyperthyroidism and with only modest goitrous enlargement, the condition may well pass unrecognized, particularly since it is self-limited and without sequelae.

The origin of this form of thyroiditis and its place in the spectrum of thyroiditis are obscure. There is no association with previous viral infections, and the autoimmune reactions are inconstant and evanescent. Generally, the T_3 and T_4 levels are increased, while the RAIU is low. Antithyroid antibodies may be identified in relatively low titers. Although this form of thyroiditis may occur at any age, it is most common in the post-partum period. There is no evidence that it constitutes a precursor of Hashimoto's disease or that it leads to so-called primary idiopathic myxedema and permanent hypothyroidism.

RIEDEL'S THYROIDITIS (STRUMA)

This rare form of chronic thyroiditis is characterized pathologically by a fibrosing reaction that destroys more or less all the thyroid gland while simultaneously extending beyond the thyroid capsule into surrounding structures in the neck. Because of the woody hardness of the thyroid, it is sometimes called *ligneous thyroiditis.* The female : male ratio is approximately 3 : 1, and most affected individuals are in the fourth to seventh decades of life. The disease, although rare, assumes importance because it is easily confused with a thyroid malignancy. Patients may have manifestations of an obstructive, invasive process, including stridor, dysphagia, recurrent laryngeal nerve paralysis, dyspnea, or even suffocation. More often, however, the chief complaint is merely a painless lump in the neck.

The etiology of this condition is unknown.[65] It does not appear to be an end stage of any other form of thyroiditis, despite many morphologic overlaps with the fibrosing variant of Hashimoto's disease. Riedel's thyroiditis is not accompanied by significant titers of thyroid autoantibodies or the exuberant lymphoid infiltration seen in Hashimoto's disease. Similar fibrosing reactions sometimes are also present elsewhere, suggesting some systemic, possible familial, fibrosclerosing derangement.[66]

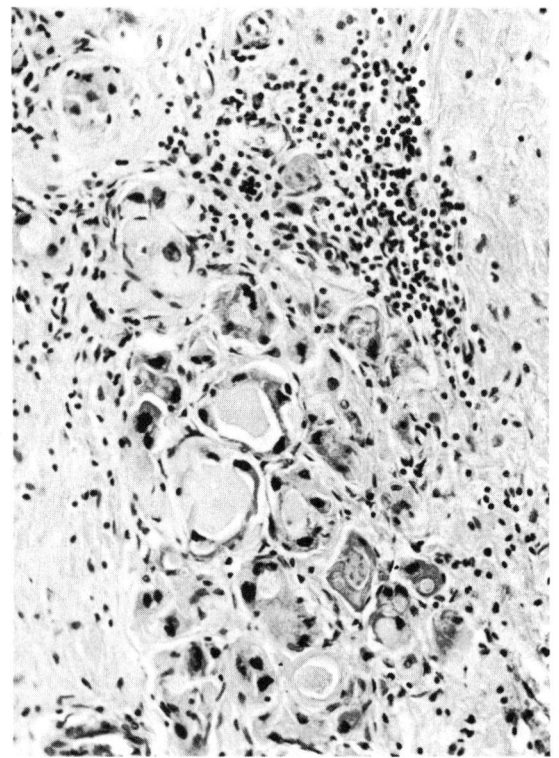

Figure 26–15. High-power view of a Riedel's thyroiditis illustrating extensive fibrosis, scant lymphocytic infiltration, and a few residual distorted thyroid follicles.

MORPHOLOGY. The entire thyroid may be normal in size or slightly enlarged but is usually markedly contracted. **It is stony hard, pale gray, and asymmetric, having apparent nodularity on clinical palpation.** Sometimes, only a lobe or a portion of a lobe is involved. The capsule is involved in the inflammatory process, producing dense adherence to surrounding structures such as the carotid sheath, trachea, and neck muscles—hence, the simulation of cancer.

Histologically there is no specific diagnostic feature of this disorder. In advanced cases, the parenchyma is markedly atrophic and is replaced by masses of dense collagenous fibrous tissue (Fig. 26–15). Scattered throughout this scarring, there is a focal lymphocytic infiltration. Such epithelial elements as remain show varying stages of pressure atrophy, nuclear enlargement, and oncocytic transformation.

CLINICAL COURSE. The prominent clinical features of this condition have already been cited. About 25 to 50% of patients are hypothyroid; the remainder are euthyroid. The major clinical significance of this condition is its differentiation from thyroid cancer. Because needle biopsy of the woody thyroid is difficult, surgical exploration may be necessary. Moreover, splitting the isthmus surgically may be required to relieve pressure on the trachea. Overall, the prognosis is good, and the fibrosing reaction rarely pro-

gresses to the extent that surgical excision is necessary.

GRAVES' DISEASE

The term *Graves' disease* is restricted to a syndrome marked by hyperthyroidism caused by a hyperfunctioning diffuse hyperplastic goiter, accompanied by infiltrative ophthalmopathy and sometimes infiltrative dermopathy. The most striking features of the ophthalmopathy, when present, are lid lag, upper lid retraction, stare, weakness of eye muscles, diplopia, periorbital edema, and notably proptosis to the point at which the lids cannot close. More consistent is an increase in intraocular pressure, evident only on special testing.[67] All these ocular abnormalities are believed to arise from immunologically mediated chronic edematous inflammation of the extraocular muscles and retro-orbital tissues. The dermopathy takes the form of localized areas of edematous skin over the dorsa of the legs or feet. The lesions are quite discrete and may have a plaquelike or nodular conformation. Despite the fact that the dermopathy is typical of Graves' disease, it is present in only 10 to 15% of cases. Perplexingly, it has been referred to as localized myxedema. *Thus, although Graves' disease is said to consist of a triad of major abnormalities, the dermopathy may be lacking and the ophthalmopathy may not be readily evident, so that diagnosis may rest largely on the documentation of thyrotoxicosis related to diffuse toxic goiter.*

Graves' disease is relatively common, occurring in about 0.4% of the United States population, and may arise at any age, with a peak incidence in the third and fourth decades. The female:male ratio is 5:1. There is a well-defined association with HLA-DR3, and familial predisposition has been frequently noted.[68] There is also a well-defined association between Graves' disease and other autoimmune thyroid disorders, notably Hashimoto's thyroiditis and, less strikingly, primary (?autoimmune) myxedema. You may recall that hyperthyroidism sometimes supervenes on pre-existing Hashimoto's thyroiditis, and conversely the morphologic changes in Graves' disease have some similarities to those of Hashimoto's thyroiditis. As might be expected, other autoimmune diseases such as pernicious anemia occur with greater-than-chance frequency in patients with Graves' disease.

ETIOLOGY AND PATHOGENESIS. The evidence is quite compelling that the thyroid gland changes are autoimmune in origin and initiated by IgG autoantibodies reactive with domains of the plasma membranes that include the receptor for TSH.[49] These antibodies thereupon activate adenyl cyclase and initiate a chain of reactions leading to thyroid growth, increased vascularity, and hypersecretion of T_3 and T_4 (Fig. 26–16). The essential nature of the autoimmune

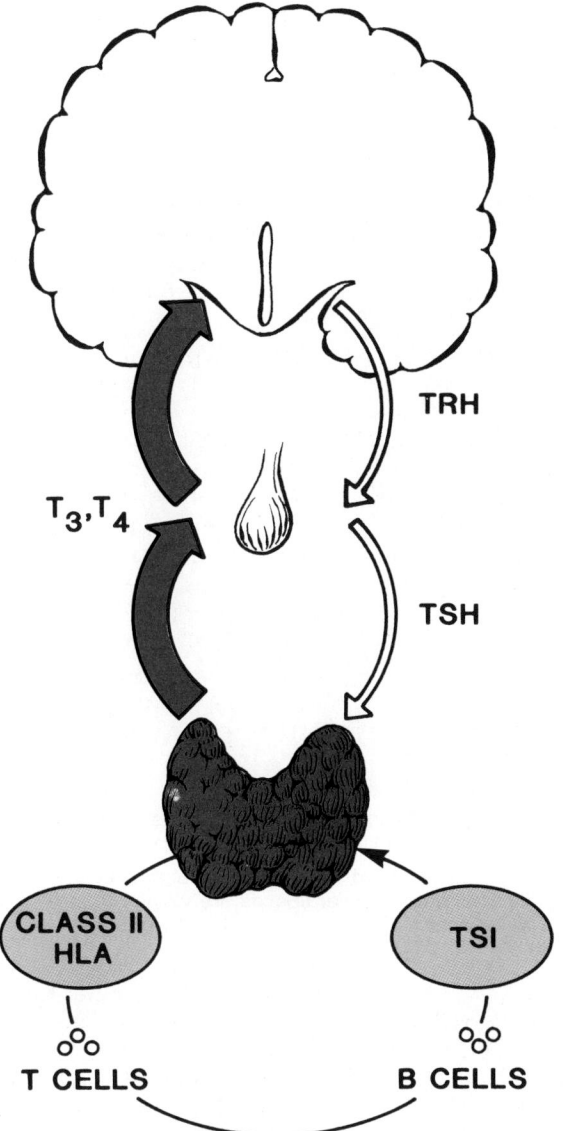

Figure 26–16. In individuals with Graves' disease, thyroid-stimulating immunoglobulins (TSI) stimulate the thyroid to produce excess T_3 and T_4, resulting in the suppression of TRH and TSH production. A genetic defect in T-suppressor cells potentiates the formation of the autoantibodies.

reaction is almost identical to that described in Hashimoto's thyroiditis (p. 1221), arising because of a defect in antigen-specific suppressor T cells. Moreover, hyperthyroidism itself may have an adverse effect on generalized suppressor T-lymphocyte function, and this may be a self-perpetuating factor in Graves' disease. Thus, the stage is set for an abnormal humoral reaction with the formation of autoantibodies to TSH-receptor antigens. It is theorized that immune response genes of the HLA-DR3 genotype account for the defect in antigen-specific suppressor T cells. TSH autoantibodies, which subsume the function of TSH by binding to the follicular cell receptors, can be identified in nearly all patients with Graves' disease.[69]

The TSH autoantibodies are of two categories: thyroid-stimulating immunoglobulins (TSI) that induce hyperfunction, and thyroid-growth immunoglobulins (TGI) that initiate growth.[51] As mentioned earlier, blocking antibodies for each of these immunoglobulins have been identified. Thus, in Graves' disease, both the TSI and the TGI fractions account for the increased output of thyroid hormones and the glandular hyperplasia. By contrast, in Hashimoto's thyroiditis there is expression mainly of TGI with either a failure in production of TSI or the elaboration of TSI-blocking antibody.[42]

The question must be raised: If genetic predisposition underlies the development of Graves' disease, why does it appear only in the third and fourth decades of life? One hypothesis invokes the concept that the disease appears only when chance mutation gives rise to autoreactive B cells that cannot be held in check because of the genetic defect in suppressor cell function. Alternatively, progressive decline in suppressor cell function may occur with the passing years, leading eventually to a critical threshold. Yet again, cumulative stress, either physical or emotional, may impair lymphocyte function in genetically predisposed individuals to potentiate the development of Graves' disease.[70] Thyrotoxicosis in animals depresses suppressor T-cell function, and in humans control of the hyperfunction with therapy tends to restore suppressor function to normal.[71]

Evidence is accumulating that the ophthalmopathy of Graves' disease is also autoimmune in origin.[72] A fairly intense lymphocytic infiltrate is present in the intra- and extraocular eye muscles as well as in the retro-orbital fibrofatty tissues, and a circulating autoantibody against a soluble eye muscle antigen can be identified in most patients.[73] The association of this ocular autoimmune reaction with past, present, or future thyroid dysfunction in 80 to 90% of cases may be explicable by more recent findings that monoclonal antibodies to eye muscle antigens cross react with thyroid microsomes.[74] So it is that the thyroid and orbital autoimmune reactions are separate but related.

MORPHOLOGY. In most cases of diffuse hyperplasia, the gland is usually uniformly but not markedly enlarged. It is **uncommon** to observe **more than threefold** increases in weight up to 80 to 90 gm. The capsule is intact and not adherent. On cut section, the parenchyma has a soft, yielding, red-brown, meaty appearance closely resembling the cross section of normal muscle. Preoperative iodine administration causes the accumulation of colloid and alters this gross appearance.

The dominant histologic feature is excessive cellularity of the parenchyma. This is imparted by an increase in height of the lining epithelium to form tall columnar cells, and an increase in the number of cells, causing them to pile up in papillary buds and encroach on the colloid (Fig. 26–17). For the most part, these papillae represent **simple, non-**

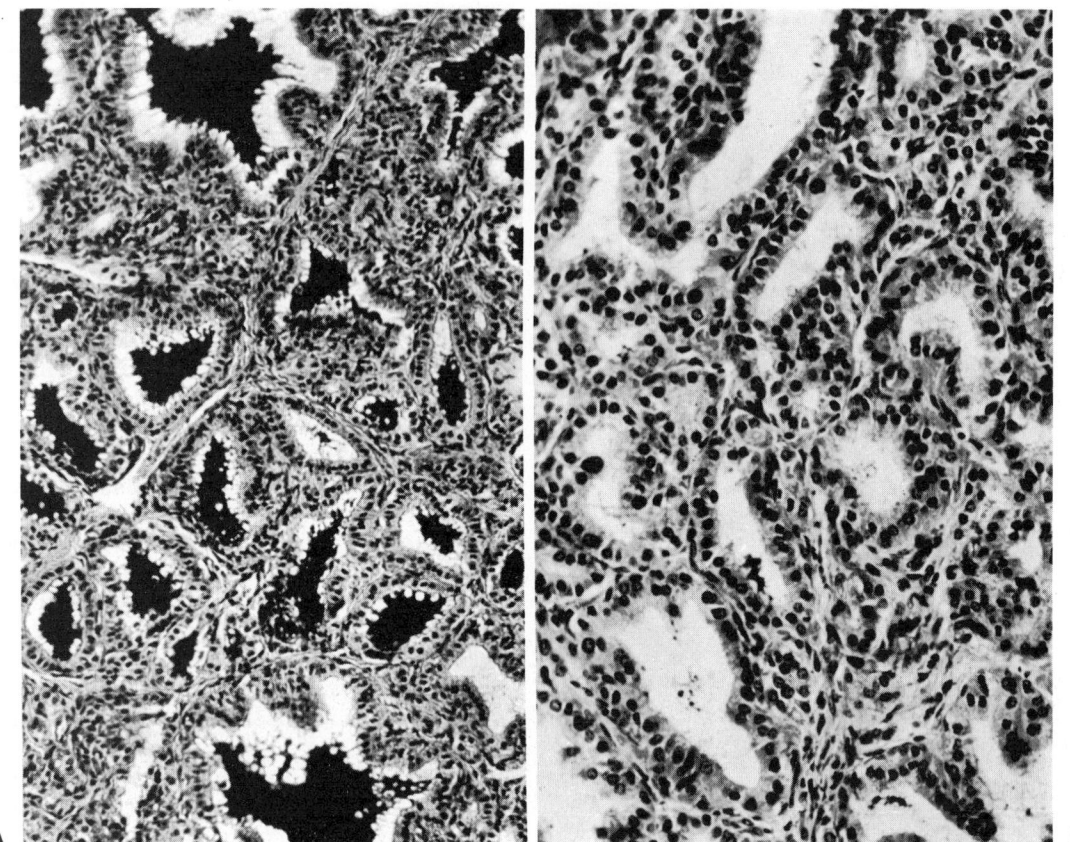

Figure 26–17. *A*, Microscopic view of diffuse thyroid hyperplasia. Cellularity of follicles and resorption of colloid are evident. High columnar epithelium and small projections into follicular spaces are visible. *B*, High-power view of diffuse thyroid hyperplasia, illustrating total absence of colloid, increase in height of epithelium, and buckling of lining cells into follicular spaces.

branching projections, which are usually slightly elevated above the level of the surrounding epithelium. Occasionally, the papillae are sufficiently large to mushroom out and virtually fill the follicles. The cells may show slight variation in size and shape, but no striking atypicality is present. The Golgi apparatus is hypertrophied, the mitochondria increased in number, and the microvilli more abundant. Colloid is markedly diminished and, when present, has a thin, pale pink, watery appearance. The interfollicular stroma shows a striking increase in the amount of lymphoid tissue, and in some areas, large lymphoid follicles are produced. The accumulation of lymphoid tissue in the thyroid is only one aspect of the generalized lymphoid hypertrophy found throughout the body, with enlargement of lymph nodes and thymus and hyperplasia of the lymphoid tissue of the spleen. There is inevitably a markedly increased vascularization of the thyroid gland.

This classic histologic pattern may be significantly altered by preoperative medication. Iodine promotes colloid storage, devascularization, and involution of the gland, whereas thiouracil tends to produce marked hyperplasia. Thus, it is impossible to evaluate correctly, from histologic examination, the amount of functional activity of pretreated surgical specimens.

When present, the exophthalmos is related to an increase in the volume of the extraocular muscles and orbital tissues secondary to edema, increased deposits of hydrophilic mucopolysaccharides, fibrosis, and lymphocytic infiltrates (infiltrative ophthalmopathy). The compressive forces account for the increased intraocular pressure. Later, fibrosis and contractures of the extraocular muscles occur and lead to the incoordination of eye movements, diplopia, and sometimes ophthalmoplegia.[75]

CLINICAL COURSE. Graves' disease presents, principally in young women, as thyrotoxicosis (p. 1217) associated with modest symmetric enlargement of the thyroid gland. When the ophthalmopathy and the dermopathy already described are also present, the diagnosis is almost certain. Confirmation usually requires one or more of the following findings: increased radioactive iodine uptake and above-normal serum levels of T_4 and T_3.

In most cases of Graves' disease the thyrotoxicosis is persistent, but it may wax and wane in severity over time. There are many ways of controlling it, but these forms of treatment are without effect on the ophthalmopathy. In most cases the eye changes run a benign course and spontaneously remit. The condition can, however, become progressively worse when the proptosis precludes closure of the lids, with corneal injuries and ulcerations and, ultimately, loss of the eye(s). On a happier note, there is little evidence to suggest an increased frequency of thyroidal cancer in patients with Graves' disease.

DIFFUSE NONTOXIC GOITER AND MULTINODULAR GOITER

Diffuse nontoxic goiter and multinodular goiter are the consequences of compensatory hypertrophy and hyperplasia of follicular epithelium secondary to some derangement that hampers thyroid hormone output. The degree of thyroid enlargement is proportional to the level and duration of thyroid hormone lack, but optimally, in most cases, the increased thyroid mass eventually achieves a euthyroid state, although hypo- or hyperthyroidism may result in some cases. At the outset the goitrous enlargement is diffuse, but for poorly understood reasons and in the course of time it is likely to become nodular, as described below. This progression is not inevitable, and indeed, during the diffuse stage, the gland may revert to normal if, for example, the impediment to thyroid hormone output abates.

DIFFUSE NONTOXIC (SIMPLE) GOITER

This designation specifies a form of goiter that (1) diffusely involves the entire gland without producing nodularity, and (2) is not associated with either hyper- or hypofunction. Because the enlarged follicles are filled with colloid, the term *colloid goiter* has been applied to this condition. It occurs in both an endemic and a sporadic distribution.

The term *endemic goiter* refers to the high incidence of simple goiter in particular geographic locales, namely, in over 10% of the population. It is extremely common throughout the world and is thought to affect over 200 million individuals. It is most prevalent in mountainous areas such as the Alps, Andes, and Himalayas but may also occur in non-mountainous regions remote from the sea. With this distribution a deficient intake of iodine is the dominant cause of the disease.[76] Simple goiter was at one time moderately prevalent in the Great Lakes region of North America, but the incidence has markedly decreased with the use of iodized salt. The lack of iodine leads to decreased synthesis of thyroid hormone and a compensatory increase in TSH, leading to follicular cell hypertrophy and hyperplasia with the generation of new follicles and goitrous enlargement. The enlarged mass of follicular cells increases hormone output until an euthyroid state is achieved.

Variations in the prevalence of endemic goiter in locales with similar levels of iodine deficiency point to the existence of other causative influences, particularly dietary substances referred to as goitrogens.[77] Calcium and fluorides in the water supply promote goiter formation. A number of foods, including cabbage, cassava, cauliflower, Brussels sprouts, turnips,

and others belonging to the Brassica and Cruciferae plants, have been documented to be goitrogenic in animals and may be associated with goiter in humans. To be clinically significant the food must be consumed in large quantity or represent the major portion of the diet, as noted in native populations subsisting largely on cassava root.[78] Cassava contains a thiocyanate that inhibits iodide transport within the thyroid, worsening any possible concurrent iodine deficiency. Pollution of water supplies may also in some way be goitrogenic. Depending on the severity of iodine lack and goitrogenic influences, the thyroid enlargement may appear in early childhood, but usually it peaks at about puberty or soon thereafter, affecting females more often than males. Severe iodine deficiency during fetal development may produce cretinism.

Nonendemic or sporadic simple goiter is much less common than the endemic variety. There is a striking female preponderance with a ratio of 8 : 1 and a peak incidence at puberty or in young adult life. The cause of this condition is rarely evident. Although it is natural to assume that increased levels of TSH stimulate the glandular enlargement, it has not been possible to document elevated levels of the pituitary hormone in all patients, perhaps because the elevations are slight or are transitory. Alternatively, an intrathyroidal mechanism has been invoked. Earlier (p. 1215) it was pointed out that a reduction in the intrathyroidal level of iodine, whatever the basis, enhances the adenyl cyclase response to TSH, initiating growth, but there is as yet no proof of this mechanism in sporadic goiter. Conceivably, a number of influences act in concert. For example, a minimal iodine lack, when coupled with increased demand for thyroid hormones, might lead to goiter formation. Sporadic goiters, especially in girls, are prone to appear first at puberty, a time of increased physiologic demand. During pregnancy, increased levels of the thyroid-binding globulins (TBG), perhaps estrogen-induced, and raised iodide clearance by the kidney may lower the levels of free T_3 and T_4 and reduce feedback inhibition of TSH. Dietary goitrogens may be superimposed on these causal influences. Other very uncommon causes of sporadic goiter are a hereditary defect in hormone transport and synthesis of excess amounts of TBG, reducing the proportion of free thyroid hormones.[79,80] Finally, there are the inborn biosynthetic errors in iodine metabolism.

The four major hereditary biosynthetic defects[81] in thyroid hormone synthesis, all transmitted as autosomal recessive conditions, can be characterized as follows: (1) iodide transport defect, (2) organification defect, (3) dehalogenase defect, and (4) iodotyrosine coupling defect.

In the transport defect, the thyroid and salivary glands and stomach are unable to trap or concentrate iodide or other anions such as perchlorate; the precise basis of the transport defect remains unclear. In the organification defect, an apparent lack of peroxidase limits the redox reaction, in which an electron is split off iodide before it combines with tyrosine. A subset of this group has concomitant deafness, referred to as Pendred's syndrome. The dehalogenase defect is characterized by an inability to recapture the iodide in MIT and DIT released from colloid along with T_4 and T_3. The fourth syndrome constitutes an inability to couple iodotyrosyl residues to form T_4 and T_3 and may actually embrace a number of defects all leading to impaired hormone synthesis. Depending on the severity of the biosynthetic defect, the development of a goiter may permit the output of sufficient thyroid hormone to maintain the euthyroid state. Obviously, with more severe biosynthetic defects, there is hypothyroidism along with the goitrous enlargement. Indeed, such errors in hormone synthesis may be responsible for cretinism.

MORPHOLOGY. Two stages can be identified in the evolution of the diffuse nontoxic goiter, the first being the hyperplastic stage and the second the colloid involution. In the stage of hyperplasia, the gland is modestly enlarged and rarely exceeds 100 to 150 gm. It is diffusely, symmetrically involved and markedly hyperemic. Histologically, the follicular epithelium is columnar and the newly generated follicles are small with only scanty colloid. The duration of the hyperplastic stage is extremely variable. With the increased mass of cells a euthyroid state is achieved, and follicular cell growth ceases and is followed by colloid accumulation.[82] At this stage, follicles enlarge as they become filled with colloid and the epithelium undergoes progressive flattening (Fig. 26–18). Indeed, it may be reduced to a thin layer of attenuated cells. For reasons that are unclear, **the accumulation of colloid is not uniform throughout the gland, and some follicles are hugely distended, while others remain small and may even retain small papillary infoldings of hyperplastic cells.** Now the thyroid becomes markedly enlarged, sometimes to 500 gm or more. The accumulated colloid produces a marked increase in consistency and a gelatinous, glistening cut surface. It is this phase of nontoxic diffuse enlargement that is referred to as **colloid goiter.** The pathogenetic mechanism underlying such colloid involution is obscure but presumably reflects the synthesis of thyroid hormone–poor glycoprotein.

CLINICAL COURSE. The clinical significance of nontoxic diffuse goiter depends largely on its ability to achieve a state of euthyroidism, which is generally the rule. Rare patients are hypothyroid and the TSH level is almost invariably elevated, as it may be to a lesser extent in marginally euthyroid individuals. The goitrous enlargement may be nonvisible, even with the head raised, or plainly evident to the casual observer on the street. During the early stages, administration of iodine brings about regression of the goiter, but later it is without effect. Perhaps the major significance of the diffuse goiter is that it is a forerunner of a nodular goiter.

MULTINODULAR GOITER

Nearly all long-standing simple goiters become transformed into multinodular goiters. They may be nontoxic or sometimes may induce thyrotoxicosis (toxic multinodular goiter), which differs from Graves' disease insofar as there is no associated ophthalmopathy or dermopathy and the hypermetabolism is usually less severe. Rarely, multinodular goiters are associated with hypothyroidism. Whatever their functional state, *multinodular goiters produce the most extreme thyroid enlargements and are more frequently mistaken for neoplastic involvement than any other form of thyroid disease.* Since they derive from simple goiter, they occur in both sporadic and endemic forms, having the same female-to-male distribution and presumably the same origins but affecting older individuals because they are late complications. However, there is no clear understanding of the basis for the transformation into the nodular pattern. Normal thyroid cells are heterogeneous with respect to iodinating capacity, peroxidase content, endocytic response to TSH, and ability to replicate.[83] The development of nodules may, therefore, reflect the generation of new metabolically heterogeneous follicles derived from genetically distinct cells and cell clusters existing in the normal gland. It is speculated that, with follicular hyperplasia, generation of new follicles, and uneven accumulation of colloid throughout the follicles, tensions and stresses are produced within the thyroid gland that lead to rupture of follicles and vessels followed by hemorrhages, scar-

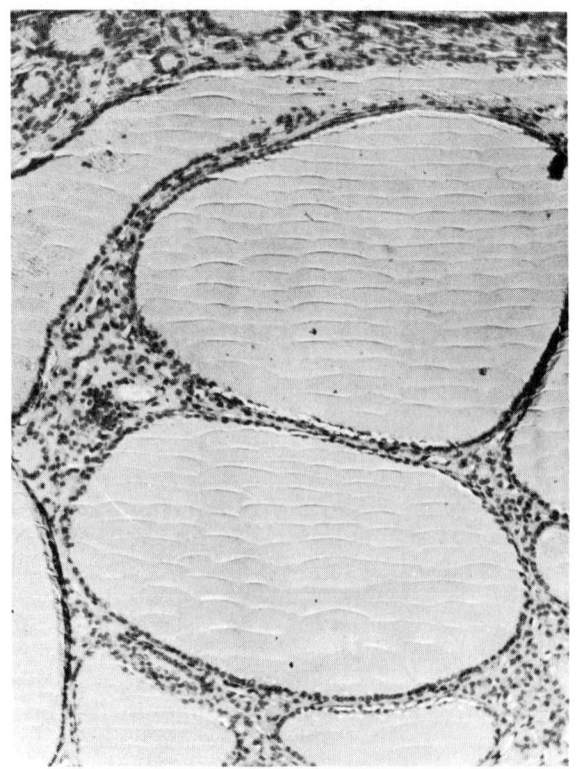

Figure 26–18. Diffuse, nontoxic goiter. Follicles are distended with colloid, and epithelial lining is flattened.

ring, and sometimes calcifications. The scarring adds to the tensions, and in this cyclical manner nodularity appears. Moreover, the pre-existent stromal framework of the gland may more or less enclose areas of expanded parenchyma, contributing to the nodularity.[84]

MORPHOLOGY. The multinodular goiter is marked by its heterogeneity. **Typical features include (1) nodularity created by islands of colloid-filled or hyperplastic follicles; (2) random irregular scarring; (3) focal hemorrhages and hemosiderin deposition; (4) focal calcifications in areas of scarring; and (5) microcyst formations.**

The goitrous enlargement may be monstrous and achieve a weight of over 2000 gm. The pattern of enlargement is quite unpredictable and may involve one lobe far more than the other, producing lateral pressure on midline structures such as the trachea and esophagus (Fig. 26–19). In other instances, the goiter grows behind the sternum and clavicles to produce the so-called **intrathoracic or plunging goiter.** Occasionally, most of it is hidden behind the trachea and esophagus, yet in other instances one nodule may so stand out as to impart the clinical appearance of a solitary nodule. On cut section there is an overall heterogeneous multinodularity; some of the nodules are poorly circumscribed, but others appear to accumulate scarring and condensation of the thyroid stroma about themselves to create the appearance of complete encapsulation similar to that found in the true adenoma. Thus have arisen the terms **adenomatous goiter** and **multiple colloid adenomatous goiter** as synonyms for this condition (Fig. 26–20).

CLINICAL COURSE. From the clinical standpoint, multinodular goiters are of importance because of (1) size and location of the goitrous mass; (2) possible

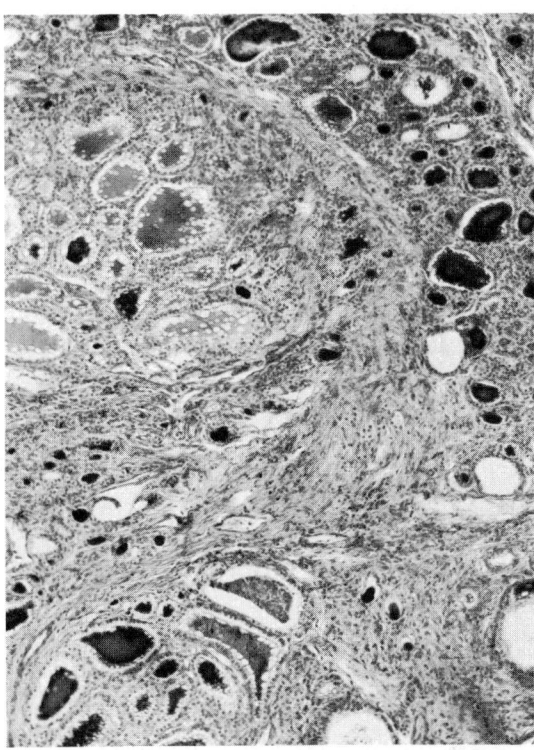

Figure 26–20. Multinodular goiter illustrating scarring and variation in size of follicles.

abnormal function, usually thyrotoxicosis; and (3) their differentiation from neoplasms. When sufficiently enlarged, the goiter may cause not only cosmetic disfigurement but also dysphagia, a choking sensation, and (with compression of the trachea) an inspiratory stridor. These manifestations are particularly prominent when the goiter enlarges into the thoracic inlet behind the sternum. Such symptoms may induce a superior vena caval syndrome, i.e., distention of the veins of the neck and upper extremities, edema of the eyelids and conjunctiva, and syncope on coughing. Hemorrhages into the goiter may induce sudden painful enlargement, worsening the obstructive symptoms.

In fewer than half the patients, hyperfunction appears—toxic multinodular goiter. Although it basically resembles the thyrotoxicosis of Graves' disease, there are several significant differences. Ophthalmopathy and dermopathy do not appear and, when present, probably represent the superimposition of Graves' disease; the thyrotoxicosis is, in general, nil to moderate; and cardiovascular manifestations tend to predominate, possibly because toxic multinodular goiter usually appears in older patients who are likely to have underlying heart disease. Thus, atrial fibrillation, tachycardia, and sometimes heart failure may be encountered. The radioactive iodine uptake and serum levels of T_3 and T_4 may be only slightly elevated. Scintiscans of the gland reveal one of two patterns: The radioiodine may accumulate in patchy foci throughout the gland or, less commonly, in only one or a few nodules. What accounts for this

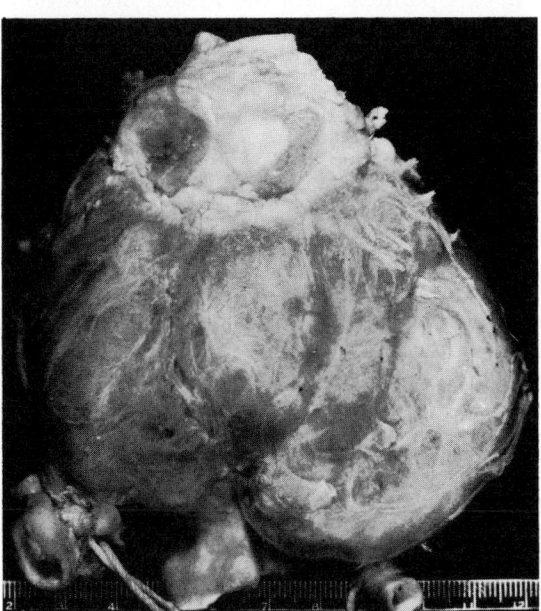

Figure 26–19. Multinodular goiter removed with trachea attached. Asymmetry and enlargement of gland are apparent.

variation is not known, but the latter pattern suggests suppression of much of the parenchymal function by hyperfunction of one or a few foci.

The differentiation of a multinodular goiter, toxic or nontoxic, from a neoplasm may be simple or difficult, both clinically and anatomically. When the multinodularity involves the entire gland, it is highly likely to represent a goiter rather than a neoplasm. Thyroid cancer sometimes spreads throughout the gland, but in such circumstances the nodular enlargement is usually of relatively short duration and not present for decades, as is generally the case with multinodular goiter. The major difficulty arises when the enlargement of a single focus outpaces the rest of the gland. Ultrasonography and CT scan may be helpful in ruling out neoplasia by revealing widespread diffuse multinodularity. Suppression of TSH by the administration of thyroid hormone is more likely to induce regression of a non-neoplastic nodule than of an autonomous tumor, but functioning adenomas also sometimes respond, and the converse is true about nodules within a goiter. A vast amount of literature has accumulated on the differential diagnosis, as discussed below.[85,86]

TUMORS

Nodules in the thyroid have always commanded a great deal of attention because they are sometimes visible, are often palpated by the patient, and always raise the question of cancer.[87] Most authorities say clinically palpable thyroid nodules are present in 4 to 7% of adults in the United States, but clinically evident cancers of the thyroid are rare, as you will see.[88] The prevalence of nodules in children has been reported to vary between 0.22 and 1.5%, depending on the series studied; it increases linearly at a rate of 0.08% per year, beginning at an early age and extending to the eighth decade.[89] The prevalence of thyroid nodules of all types is increased fivefold in individuals exposed to ionizing irradiation. The annual incidence of thyroid cancer in the United States is approximately 25 to 35 cases per million population, accounting for about 0.4% of cancer deaths.[90] It follows, therefore, that only a few clinically palpable nodules (of the order of 1 to 2 per 1000) are cancers. Reports from surgical clinics, however, point to a much higher incidence of cancer in nodular glands, with estimates ranging up to 20 to 30%. Such data can only reflect selection bias with surgical exploration of only the most ominous lesions. *It can reasonably be concluded that thyroid nodules are very common, but thyroid cancer is very uncommon.*

Despite all the epidemiologic data, the patient is not a statistic, and so every nodule demands careful appraisal. Short of anatomic study, there are no certain methods of differentiating nontumorous nodules from benign or malignant neoplasms. Approximately 50% of clinically apparent single nodules prove to be dominant nodules of multinodular goiters on pathologic examination.[89] Of the true solitary nodules, 70 to 80% prove to be adenomas, while 10 to 20% are carcinomas. A variety of other lesions, including foci of thyroiditis, cysts, and areas of fibrosis, account for most of the remainder of other "solitary" nodules. It is evident from these findings that many lesions of the thyroid may present as nodules, and indeed, in 10% of the cases no thyroid abnormality is present.

A discussion of current diagnostic approaches is far beyond our scope, but a few deserve mention because of their anatomic relevance. For years the cornerstone of clinical appraisal of a nodular thyroid has been the scintiscan, following the administration of radioiodine. Most thyroid cancers, and many adenomas, cannot accumulate significant quantities of radioiodine and so appear as nonfunctioning "cold" nodules. Although most adenomas and carcinomas are "cold" lesions, so are nonfunctioning nodules in multinodular goiter and focal enlargements in Hashimoto's thyroiditis. It is estimated that only about 20% of "cold" nodules prove to be malignant. Moreover, some adenomas and a rare cancer may be "hot," i.e., may take up radioiodine. Thus, although scintiscans suggest probabilities, they are not definitive.

Thyroglobulin can be detected in the serum of up to 90% of healthy adults and is, therefore, not a useful predictor of malignancy in individuals with nodular thyroid disease. However, measurements of thyroglobulin may be a useful predictor of tumor recurrence or metastasis in individuals who have had surgical ablation of all thyroid tissue or who have been treated with I-131.[91]

Fine needle aspiration biopsy represents a highly reliable approach for the diagnosis and classification of thyroid nodules and is of particular value in screening patients for subsequent surgery.[92] The procedure is relatively painless, and the results are often available while the patient is still in the office. In several series, about 60% of adequate aspirates proved to be benign, 5% were clearly malignant, and the remainder were indeterminate or cytologically suspicious for malignancy. The incidence of malignancy in the suspicious category, as determined by subsequent surgical removal of the lesion, has been reported to range from 15 to 40%. A clearly benign diagnosis in this situation has the potential to reduce the risk and cost of surgery. However, it should be noted that about 80% of aspirates are insufficient or otherwise unsuitable for definitive interpretation.

As reliable as any are the following simple observations. A solitary nodule is more suspect of being neoplastic than multiple nodules, for reasons that must now be obvious. The younger the patient (under the age of 40), the greater is the likelihood of neoplasia, because non-neoplastic nodularity, such as may be produced by Hashimoto's thyroiditis or multinodular goiter, tends to appear in older individuals. Both of these non-neoplastic disorders are significantly more common in women than in men, and thus a nodule in a male is more ominous than one in a female.

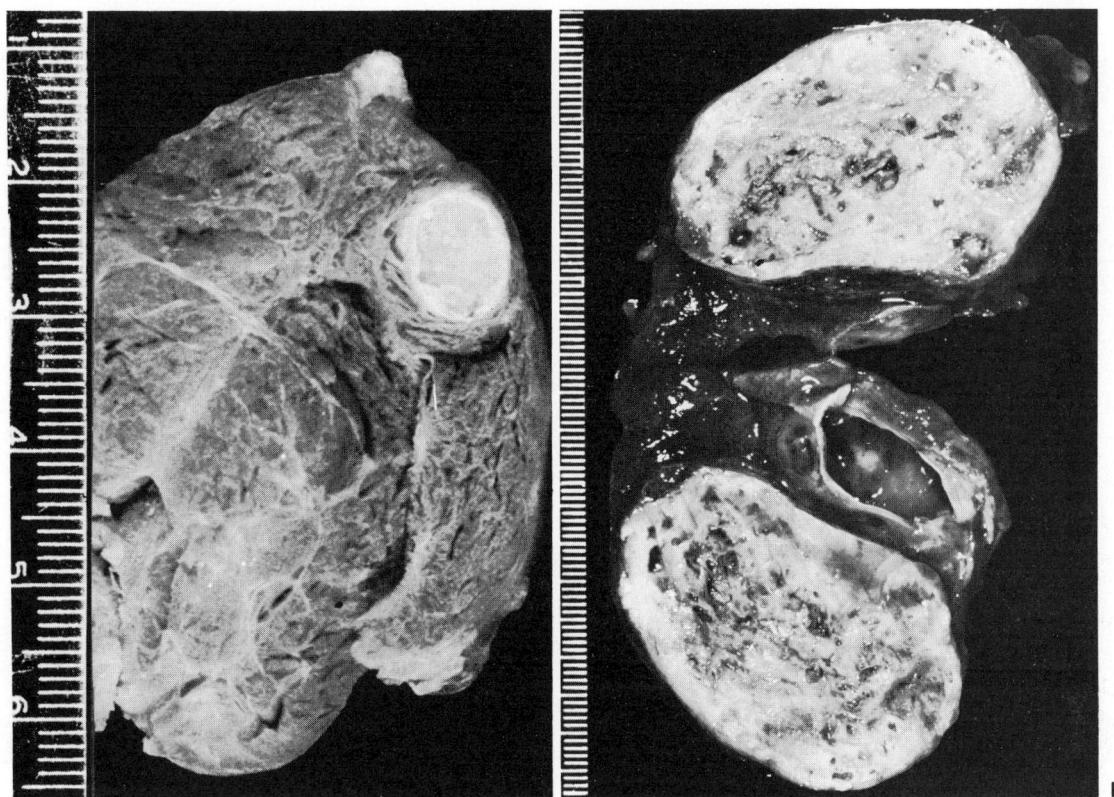

Figure 26–21. *A* and *B,* Adenomas of thyroid. View of cross section of nodules against background of darker normal thyroid tissue.

ADENOMAS

Virtually all adenomas of the thyroid gland present as solitary, discrete, small (under 4 cm) nodules (Fig. 26–21). The classification of adenomas continues to be unsettled. On histologic grounds, a variety of patterns can be identified that recapitulate stages in the embryogenesis of the normal thyroid, and hence are sometimes specified as *fetal, embryonal, simple,* and *colloid adenomas.* However, all adenomas contain follicles of varying size and in variable proportions. Hence, all might well be called *follicular adenomas.* A somewhat less common variant has branching papillary excrescences protruding into microcystic spaces; such lesions have been referred to as *papillary cystadenomas.* However, most pathologists now consider all papillary neoplasms of the thyroid to represent carcinomas, as discussed below. One additional rare lesion is the so-called *Hürthle cell adenoma.*

MORPHOLOGY. All adenomas will be described as a more or less cohesive group, indicating such distinctive patterns as can be discerned. As stated, they are generally solitary lesions rarely exceeding 3 cm in diameter, readily defined from the surrounding thyroid substance. Infrequently, two or even more adenomas are present. On cross section they range from pale tan to gray, are soft and fleshy, and sometimes have foci of softening, hemorrhage, or central fibrosis with calcification.

The histologic differentiation of a nodule within a multinodular goiter from an adenoma is difficult not only clinically but also anatomically. **The morphologic criteria used to identify an adenoma are (1) complete fibrous encapsulation, (2) a clear distinction between the architecture inside and outside the capsule, (3) compression of the thyroid parenchyma around the adenoma, and (4) lack of multinodularity in the remaining gland** (Fig. 26–22). None of these features alone is sufficient, but collectively they are quite reliable. All adenomas are characterized by some variation in the size and number of follicles as well as in the abundance of interfollicular stroma. At one extreme is the lesion composed of closely packed cells forming cords or trabeculae, with only here and there a small abortive follicle. This architecture is reminiscent of embryonic thyroid parenchyma before the development of well-formed follicles, accounting for the sometimes-used designation **embryonal** or **trabecular adenoma.** Another pattern is composed of small follicles containing little or no colloid, separated by an abundant, loose connective tissue. Here the architecture mimics the embryogenesis of the thyroid gland one step after the embryonal stage—hence the term **fetal adenoma.** The next identifiable variant is composed of closely packed follicles of normal size, sometimes termed a **simple adenoma.** Proceeding along this inexact and probably futile hair-splitting is the **colloid adenoma,** having large follicles filled with colloid and lined by flat epithelium (Fig. 26–23). A reasonable argument can be made to merely divide all these adenomas into **microfollicular**

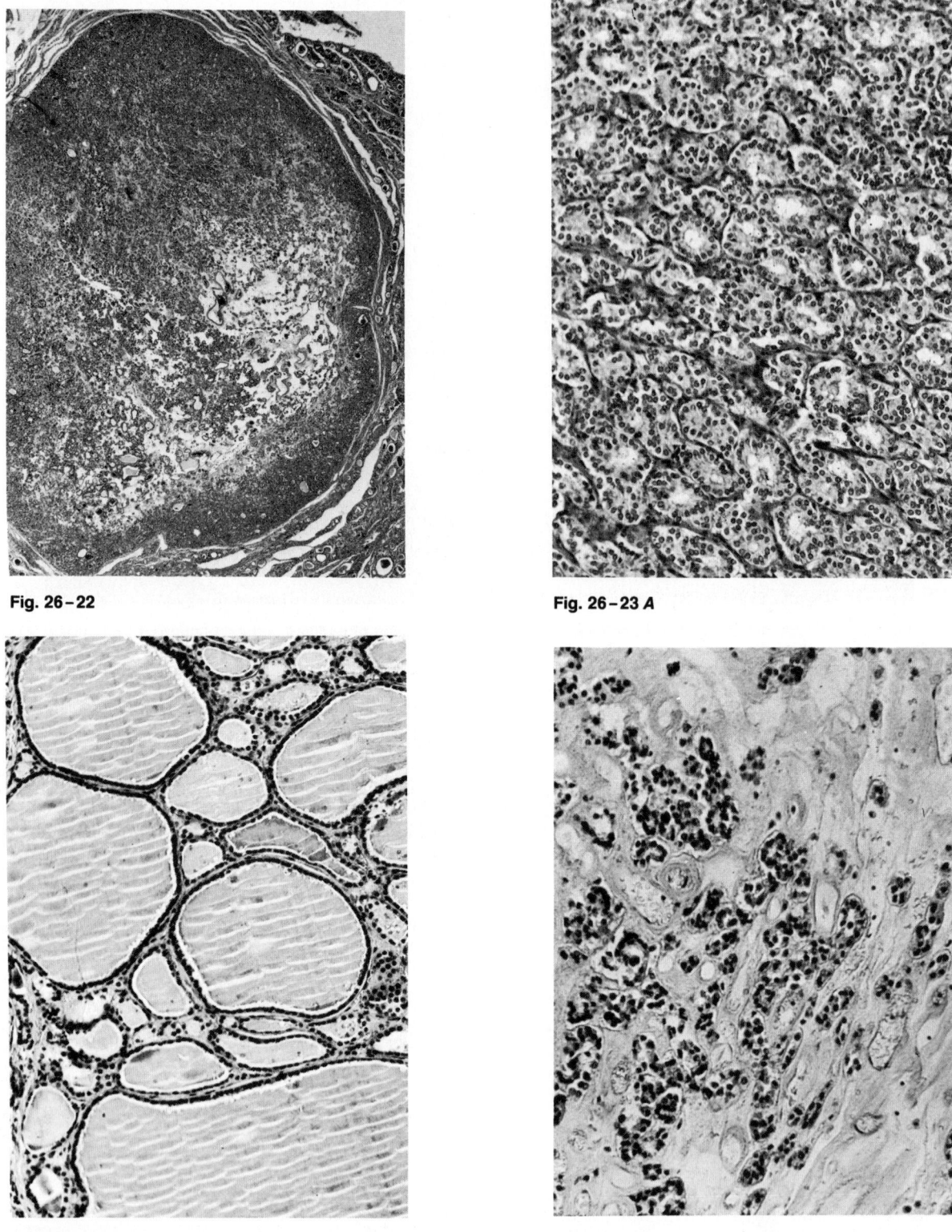

Fig. 26–22

Fig. 26–23 *A*

Fig. 26–23 *B*

Fig. 26–23 *C*

Figure 26–22. Low power view of follicular adenoma of thyroid, illustrating discrete encapsulation and demarcation from surrounding thyroid substance.

Figure 26–23. *A* to *C,* Three types of follicular adenoma, illustrating variability in acinar size, colloid content, and amount of interstitial connective tissue. *C* represents the type formerly referred to as a fetal adenoma.

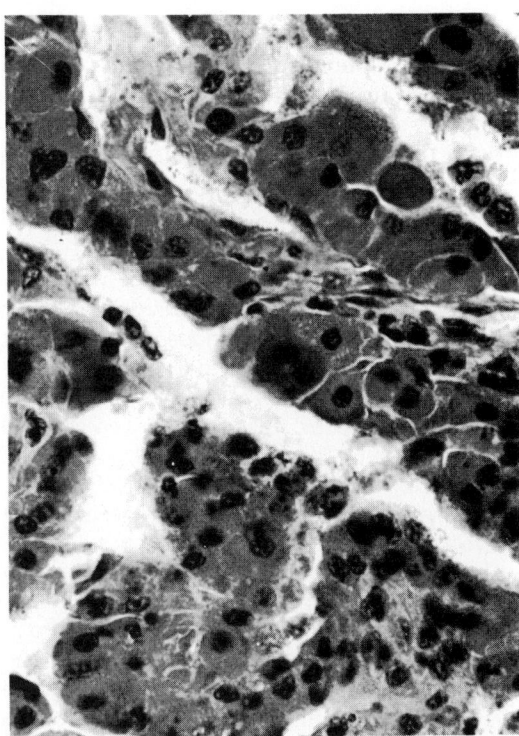

Figure 26-24. High-power detail of the cells that constitute a Hürthle cell adenoma. Considerable variability in size and shape of cells is evident. The abundant cytoplasm demonstrates a fine granularity.

and **macrofollicular** patterns, recognizing that all have the same clinical significance. Only the Hürthle cell adenoma is histologically distinctive, being composed of large granular cells identical to those encountered in various non-neoplastic thyroidal lesions (p. 1222), usually arranged in a trabecular pattern (Fig. 26-24). Infrequently, follicular adenomas exhibit some variability in cell morphology, including the presence of spindle-shaped cells. To express such changes, the term **atypical adenoma** has been applied, but it should not be construed as implying a drift toward cancer.

The principal importance of adenomas is their clinical differentiation from cancers, as has already been emphasized. In addition, they may (1) slowly increase in size to cause pressure symptoms in the neck; (2) achieve a certain size and then plateau, apparently as the expansile pressure restricts blood supply; (3) suddenly enlarge and become painful owing to intralesional hemorrhages; and (4) rarely, hyperfunction to cause hyperthyroidism that is usually mild and unassociated with ophthalmopathy. Most adenomas are "cold" nodules, but some, particularly those associated with hyperfunction, accumulate sufficient radioiodine to appear as "hot" nodules. Although theoretically autonomous, an adenoma occasionally has some dependence on TSH and so can be induced to regress by the administration of thyroid hormones, which suppress TSH secretion. Finally, there is the issue of malignant transformation of an adenoma. At one time these benign lesions were thought to be a serious risk, but there currently is doubt that even the "atypical adenomas" ever become cancerous. Past impressions probably reflect biopsy sampling errors of well-differentiated follicular carcinomas, at one time inappropriately labeled "angioinvasive adenomas" (p. 1237).

OTHER BENIGN TUMORS

Solitary nodules of the thyroid gland may also prove to be cysts.[93] The great preponderance of these lesions represent cystic degeneration of a follicular adenoma; the remainder probably arise in multinodular goiters. They are often filled with a brown, turbid fluid containing blood, hemosiderin pigment, and cell debris. Additional benign rarities include dermoid cysts, lipomas, hemangiomas, and teratomas (seen mainly in infants).

MALIGNANT

Thyroid cancers cause about 7000 deaths annually in the United States, with a $2-3:1$ female:male ratio. There are a number of anatomic subtypes of thyroid carcinoma, as indicated in Table 26-4.[94,95] Each of these anatomic patterns has its own distinctive biology and clinical significance. At one end of the spectrum are the often "benign" papillary carcinomas; at the other end are the undifferentiated carcinomas that must be rated among the most aggressive cancers of humans. Fortunately, the great preponderance of carcinomas fall into the so-called well-differentiated category, i.e., papillary and follicular lesions.

Since 1935 the overall incidence of thyroid carcinoma has tripled, but it is not certain whether this increase is real or artifactual. Favoring a real increase is the well-documented contribution of external radiation of the thyroid gland to the induction of cancer.[96] Irradiation during childhood has incurred the greatest risk.[97] From 4 to 9% of individuals irradiated during infancy for such trivial conditions as tonsillar or thymic enlargement, acne, and other skin disorders have developed thyroid carcinoma after a mean latent period of 20 years. Increased risk for thyroid carcinoma has been associated particularly with high doses

Table 26-4. Classification of Thyroid Malignancies

TYPE	FREQUENCY (%)
Papillary carcinoma (including mixed papillary and follicular types)	60-70
Follicular carcinoma (including clear cell, Hürthle cell, and insular types)	20-25
Medullary (C-cell) carcinoma	5-10
Undifferentiated carcinoma (including small cell, giant cell, and spindle cell types)	10
Epidermoid carcinoma	<1
Other tumors (lymphoma, sarcoma, metastatic carcinoma)	<1

of irradiation, young age at the time of exposure, and female sex.[98] From a different vantage point, 80% of children who develop thyroid carcinoma have received therapeutic radiation. Among the Japanese, 6.7% of individuals exposed to the atomic bomb have developed thyroid cancers.[99] Small wonder that there is present concern in the United States about the disposal of nuclear wastes. The nuclear accident at Three Mile Island in 1979 and the more recent accident at Chernobyl also give pause for thought despite reassurances that the risk is less than one case per 10 million exposed.[100] The only dubious comfort regarding the relationship of thyroid cancer to irradiation derives from the fact that the great preponderance of these thyroid cancers are either papillary or follicular, and only very rarely one of the anaplastic variants. There is no current evidence of an increased incidence of thyroid cancer in patients receiving either the relatively small doses of radiant energy involved in scintiscans or the larger doses inherent in the treatment of hyperthyroidism with radioiodine.[101]

Before turning to the various anatomic patterns, the clinical staging of thyroid cancers should be presented. The following is most widely used:

Stage I. Intrathyroidal lesions.
Stage II. Cancers lacking fixation to surrounding structures but with movable cervical metastases.
Stage III. Cancers with local fixation or fixed cervical nodes.
Stage IV. Cancers with distant metastases.

Although the staging of thyroid cancers is obviously of importance in estimating the prognosis, the histologic type is of much greater significance.

Papillary Carcinoma

Under this designation are included the benign-appearing lesions, formerly termed papillary adenoma, as well as the overt carcinomas, because experience has taught that all papillary neoplasms have the potential for spread and cancerous behavior. As Table 26–4 indicates, papillary carcinomas may be "pure," but over half contain an admixture of follicular elements. Even Solomon would have difficulty in appropriately subclassifying the infinite range of mixtures encountered. Long-term follow-up of patients with these mixed lesions, however, indicates that, *regardless of the precise proportions, all neoplasms containing some papillary areas have identical biologic behavior;* the great majority of all papillary lesions are indolent, with an excellent prognosis. About 10 to 20% first come to attention by spread to regional nodes with the production of cervical lymphadenopathy.

Whether pure or mixed, papillary carcinomas are the most common form of thyroid cancer in adults and children.[102] They tend to occur rather evenly through the third to seventh decades but account for at least 80% of thyroid cancers in individuals under 40 years

of age, largely because the less well differentiated neoplasms tend to occur in older persons. The tumors usually present as an incidental, painless lump in the neck, but occasionally they may be sufficiently large to produce obvious masses. *Not infrequently, the primary lesion remains occult and the first sign of the disease is metastatic enlargement of a cervical lymph node.*

Papillary carcinomas range from microscopic foci found incidentally in thyroids or lymph nodes removed for other reasons to nodules up to 10 cm in diameter (Fig. 26–25). Depending on the rigorousness of the search at autopsy, unsuspected microscopic foci of papillary carcinoma have been found in about 10% of cases! Indeed, about 20 to 75% of these cancers are multifocal in the gland.[102] Larger nodules are generally unencapsulated and invasive locally but may have apparent, poorly developed encapsulation. Penetration of the capsule of the thyroid gland occurs in about 20% of cases and is somewhat more common in the more anaplastic lesions. Such extension worsens the prognosis. Sometimes there are cystic spaces into which papillary fronds project, giving rise to the term papillary cystadenocarcinoma. The cut surfaces of these neoplasms may be furry, owing to the myriad of tiny papillae. Occasional tumors show dense fibrous sclerosis throughout the neoplasm, sometimes punctuated by focal calcification (so-called sclerosing carcinomas) (Fig. 26–26). **The pathognomonic histologic feature of all lesions is a complicated,**

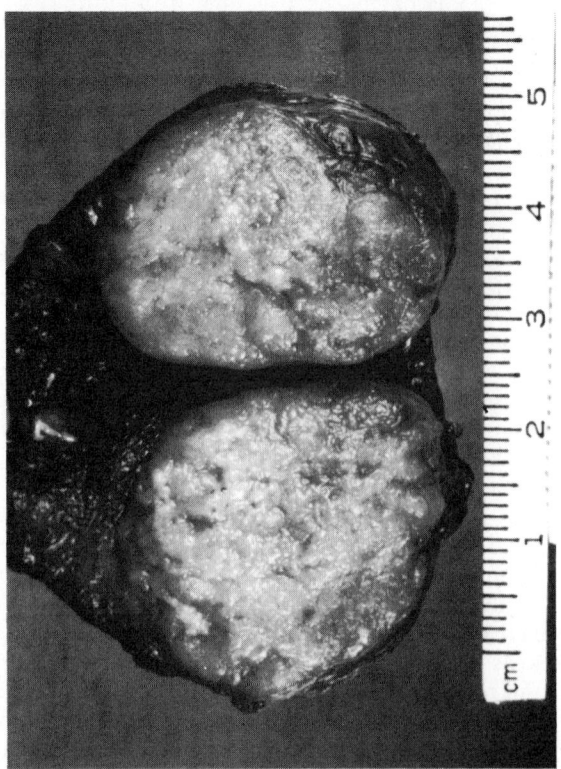

Figure 26–25. A papillary carcinoma showing deceptive apparent encapsulation. (Courtesy of Dr. Merle Legg, New England Deaconess Hospital.)

of the tip of a papilla. Psammoma bodies are rarely encountered in other forms of thyroid neoplasia and so, when present, point strongly to the diagnosis of a papillary adenocarcinoma. Thyroglobulin can be demonstrated immunocytochemically in the vast majority of primary and metastatic papillary carcinomas, and this feature may aid the pathologist in predicting the site of origin of a metastatic papillary neoplasm. Ultrastructural studies reveal numerous mitochondria, an abundant rough endoplasmic reticulum, and apical microvilli, similar to those seen in normal follicular cells.[26]

Papillary carcinomas are notorious for their extremely indolent growth and their propensity to metastasize to lymph nodes, particularly in the neck. The presence of isolated neoplastic thyroid follicles in cervical lymph nodes removed for other reasons may be the first clue to the presence of a papillary thyroid carcinoma. However, these tumors may also metastasize hematogenously to lungs and bone. Many appear as incidental asymptomatic nodules that have been present for months to years before being brought to

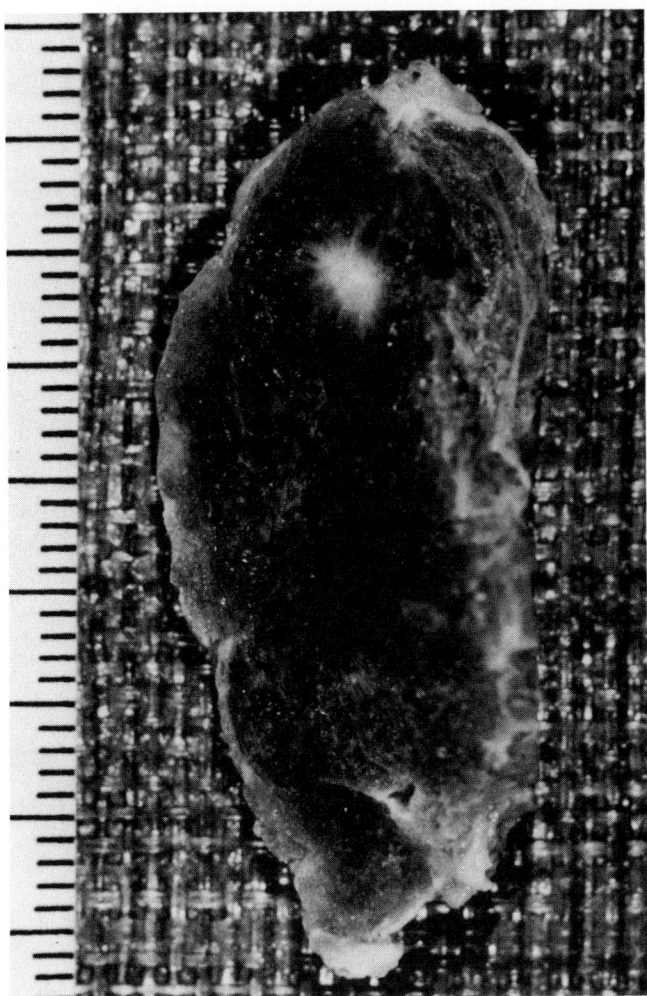

Figure 26–26. An occult sclerosing papillary carcinoma (small pale nodule) that was associated with lymph node metastases despite its small size. (Courtesy of Dr. Richard Sampson, Newton-Wellesley Hospital, Newton, Massachusetts.)

branching, treelike pattern most sharply outlined by the papilliform axial fibrovascular stroma. In the benign-appearing so-called adenomas, this framework is covered by a single layer of well-oriented regular cuboidal epithelium (Fig. 26–27). In areas the tumor cells may form colloid-containing follicles. All degrees of atypicality and disorientation of cells, piling-up of epithelium, invasion of the stalk and capsule, and formation of glands or sheets of cells may be encountered in the more obviously aggressive lesions (Fig. 26–28). Foci of squamous metaplasia are encountered frequently.

In more than half these neoplasms the nuclei assume a distinctive "ground-glass" appearance.[103] The nuclear membranes are distinct, but the nucleoli and nuclear chromatin are barely discernible. Ground-glass nuclei have been used as the sole criterion for classifying a tumor as papillary, even in the absence of papillae.[104] Almost half of all papillary lesions contain laminated calcific spherules known as **psammoma bodies** (Fig. 26–29). They range in size up to 0.1 μm and often are located in the fibrous axial stroma

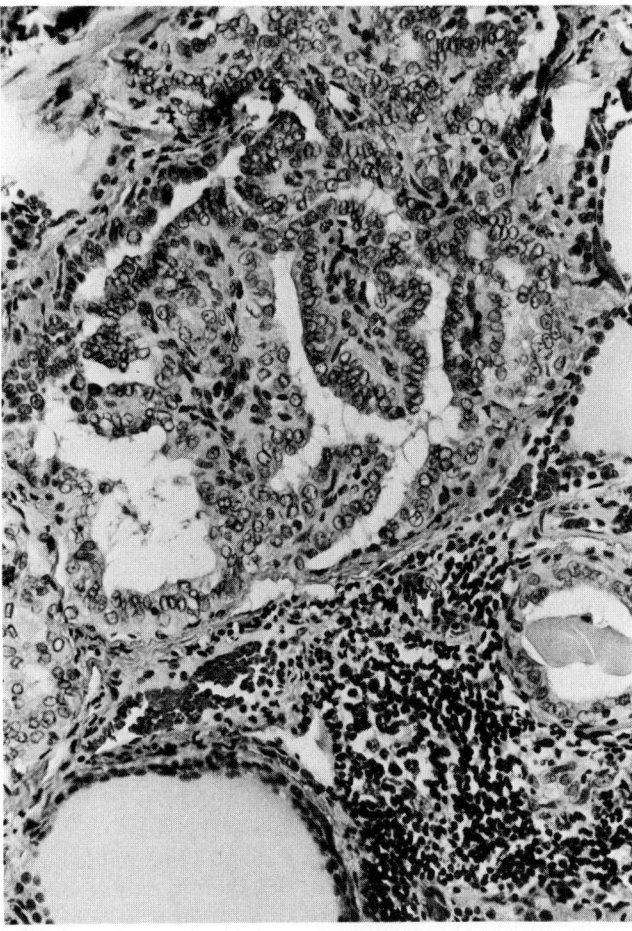

Figure 26–27. Intrathyroidal metastasis of a "benign-appearing" papillary carcinoma. Foci of intrathyroidal metastases are commonly seen in association with thyroid cancers of the papillary type.

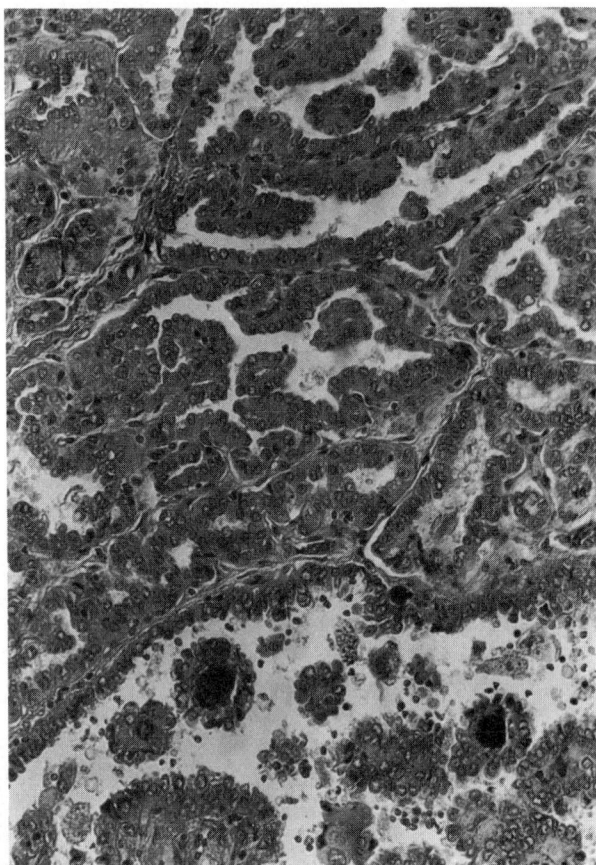

Figure 26–28. Papillary carcinoma of thyroid, showing obvious piling up and anaplasia of cells with some gland formations. Compare with better differentiated lesion of Fig 26–27. Note psammoma bodies within papillae in lower field. (Courtesy of Dr. Merle Legg, New England Deaconess Hospital.)

clinical attention. Others slowly but progressively enlarge and rarely induce disfiguring masses, dysphagia, dysphonia, or dyspnea. Whatever the presentation, all slowly increase in size and sometimes spread beyond the confines of the gland. In one analysis of a large series of cases, about 40% of the lesions had spread beyond the thyroid capsule at the time of initial diagnosis; a similar proportion had metastasized to regional lymph nodes; and 10% had metastasized more widely, e.g., to lungs, bones, and other areas.[105] It has been estimated that up to 20% of children may have evidence of lung metastasis at the time of initial diagnosis.[106] Asymptomatic pulmonary metastases may exist for many years. Overall, 70 to 80% of patients with this form of neoplasia survive at least ten years. Despite an innocuous facade, however, some of these lesions behave as usual cancers. Bearing on the outlook are the following factors: (1) The prognosis is significantly worse with extrathyroidal extension; (2) prognosis and cure are correlated with the degree of differentiation, although this factor is less important than local spread; (3) there is a tendency to more aggressive disease, particularly in males older than 45

years; and (4) the duration of the tumor is significant —there is a suggestion that highly malignant neoplasms emerge over time from pre-existing low-grade lesions.[105] Although papillary carcinoma has a very good prognosis in children, relapses may occur 20 to 35 years after the initial treatment.

Follicular Carcinoma

This pattern accounts for about one quarter of all thyroid cancers, and it is biologically more aggressive than papillary carcinoma. *Critical to the segregation of follicular from papillary carcinomas is the absence of (1) ground-glass nuclei, (2) well-formed papillae, and (3) psammoma bodies.* The presence of any of these morphologic features, even in neoplasms composed largely of follicular elements, seems to portend the biologic course of papillary carcinoma.[107] Follicular carcinoma occurs more often in females than males and has a peak incidence in the fifth and sixth decades. A diagnosis of follicular carcinoma implies up to a 70% mortality at five years.[108]

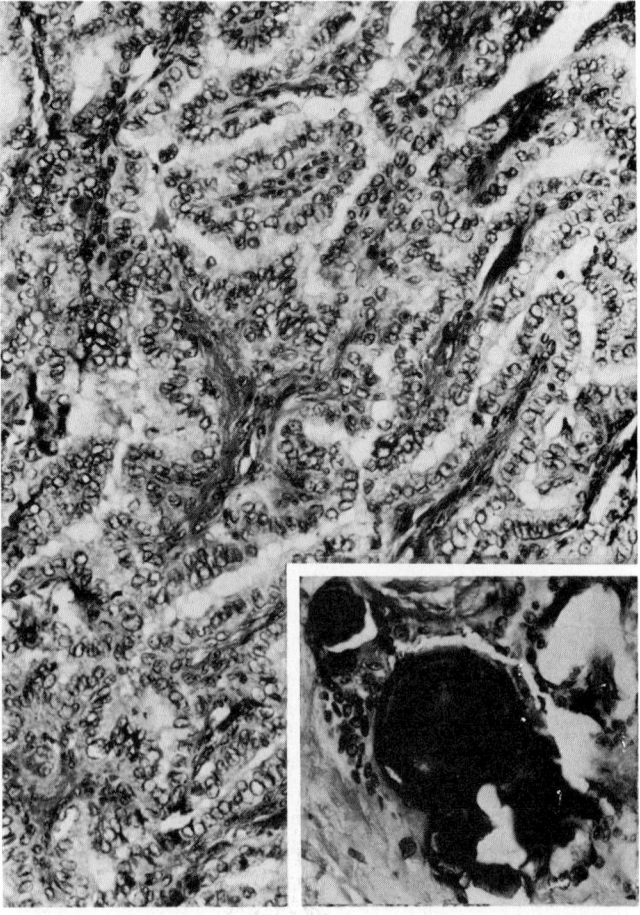

Figure 26–29. High-power view of a papillary carcinoma shows fibrovascular stalks covered by a single layer of epithelium with ground glass (Orphan-Annie eye) nuclei. The inset shows typical calcified psammoma bodies.

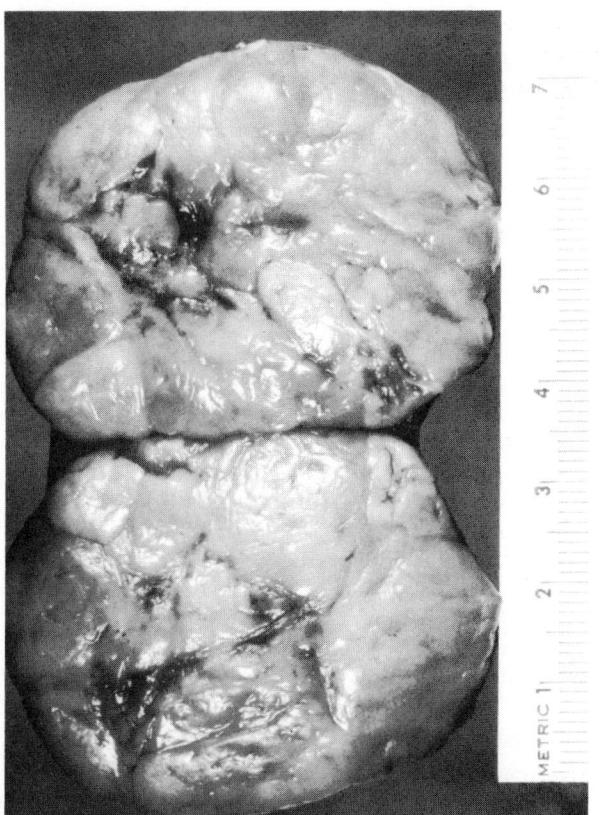

Figure 26–30. Cut surface of a follicular carcinoma with complete replacement of thyroid lobe. (Courtesy of Dr. Merle Legg, New England Deaconess Hospital.)

Anatomically, these tumors take one of two gross forms: (1) a small nodule, seemingly encapsulated, closely resembling a follicular adenoma; and (2) an obvious invasive mass, perhaps occupying an entire lobe.[109] The adenoma-like lesion has been called an **angioinvasive adenoma** but more properly is termed an **angioinvasive encapsulated carcinoma.** The second pattern is that of an obvious cancerous mass causing irregular enlargement of the gland. The tumorous gray-white tissue overgrows the thyroid, replaces large parts of it, and extends through the capsule to become adherent to or invade the trachea, muscles, skin, and great vessels of the neck (Figs. 26–30 and 26–31). In this infiltrative progression, the recurrent laryngeal nerves are often trapped. Both the localized and the invasive forms often have an abundant fibrous stroma. Hemorrhages, cyst formations, and areas of necrosis are frequently present.

Microscopically, the pattern is that of adenocarcinoma with considerable range in follicular size and differentiation. Thus, some carcinomas have a basically trabecular pattern with only small abortive follicle formations, resembling the embryonal pattern of follicular adenoma, whereas others produce well-defined follicles containing colloid (Fig. 26–32). In such lesions, the differentiation from normal thyroid architecture is difficult. These extremely well differentiated, colloid-producing adenocarcinomas, when found in metastatic sites, have in former years been referred to as **be-**

nign, metastasizing struma (Fig. 26–33). The invasiveness of these lesions is also quite variable. As pointed out, in the localized adenoma-like pattern there may be only penetration of the apparent capsule, and in the more overt aggressive lesions there is frequently extension beyond the gland capsule and vascular invasion, both features serving to differentiate these lesions from adenomas. In contrast to the papillary carcinoma, follicular carcinomas have a strong tendency to invade blood vessels and metastasize hematogenously. Lymphatic and lymph node dissemination is much less common. Thyroglobulin may be demonstrated immunohistochemically in the vast majority of follicular carcinomas.

There are several rare variant histologic patterns of the follicular carcinoma. In one, the cells have a very clear cytoplasm and closely resemble the clear cell renal carcinoma (hypernephroma) (p. 1075).[95] In the other variant the cells are large and have an abundant acidophilic cytoplasm with small pyknotic central nuclei, closely simulating Hürthle (oxyphil) cells. Neither of these histologic variations alters the biologic course of these neoplasms. The so-called insular type of thyroid carcinoma represents an aggressive form of follicular carcinoma, showing a predominantly solid growth

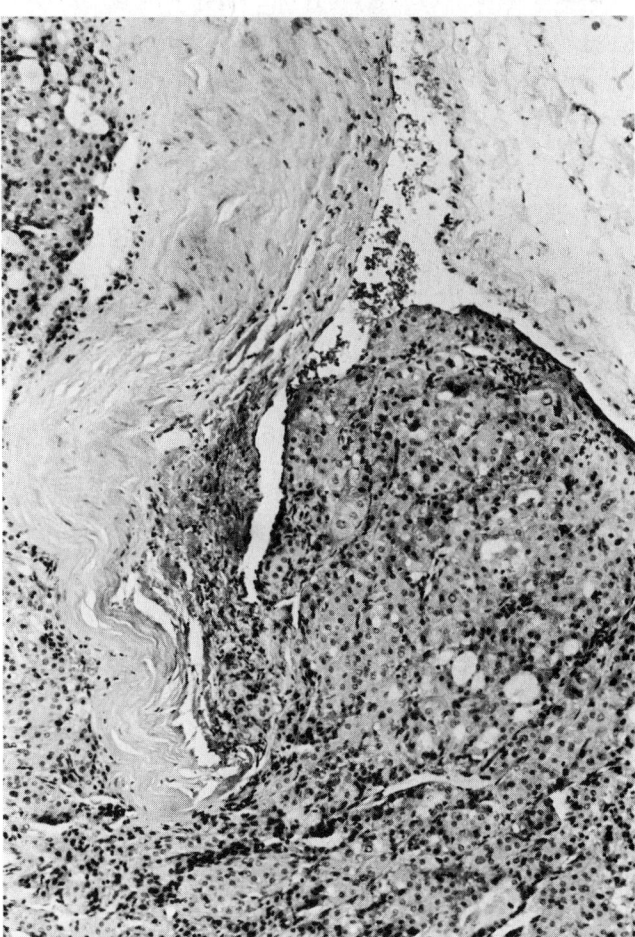

Figure 26–31. This oxyphilic follicular carcinoma has penetrated its connective tissue capsule.

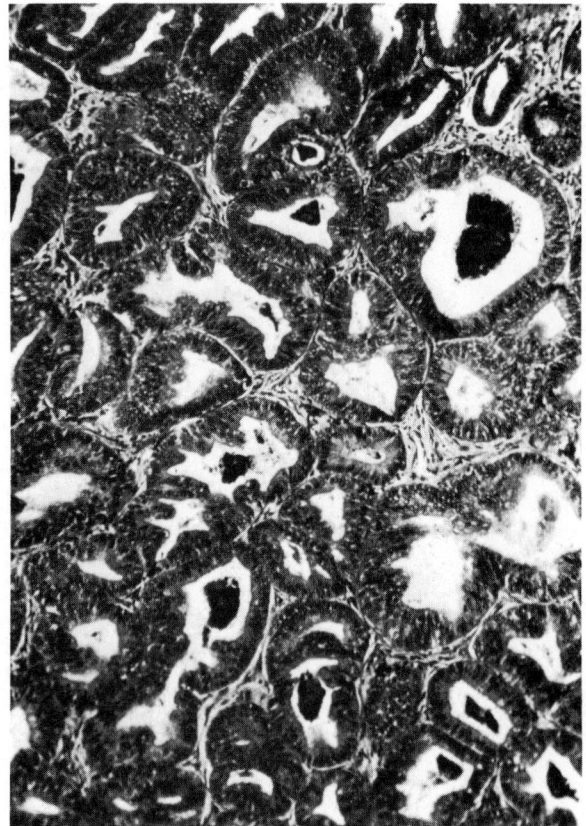

Figure 26–32. Follicular carcinoma of thyroid. A few of the glandular lumina contain recognizable colloid.

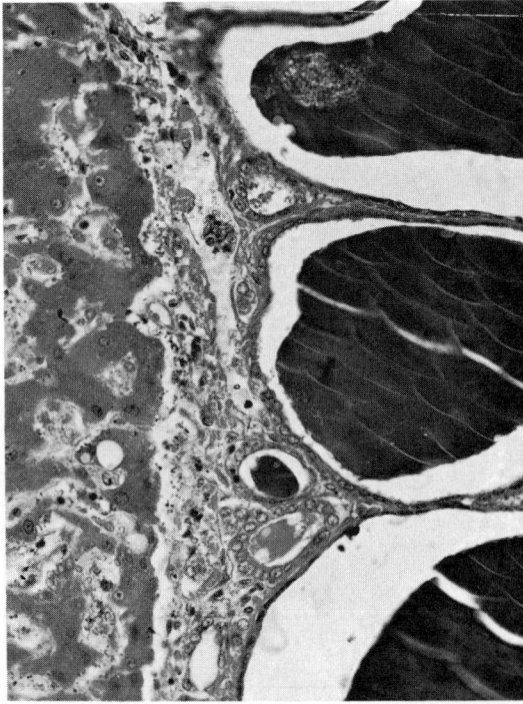

Figure 26–33. High-power detail of follicular cancer of thyroid that has metastasized to liver. Normal liver cells *(on left)* can be seen in approximation to extremely well-differentiated thyroid tissue, demonstrating abundant colloid and deceptively benign-appearing follicular epithelium.

pattern.[110] These tumors may bear a striking resemblance to medullary carcinomas but are thyroglobulin-positive and calcitonin-negative by immunohistochemistry.

The clinical presentation of follicular thyroid cancer is that of either a solitary enlarging nodule or (more often) an irregular, firm, nodular thyroid enlargement. In both presentations the mass slowly expands over the years but at a somewhat more rapid pace than that of the papillary carcinoma. Metastases may not become evident for some time, but eventually most lesions, when left untreated, disseminate through the bloodstream to the lungs, bones, and other distant sites.

The prognosis is heavily dependent on the stage of the neoplasm at the time diagnosed and on its response to therapy. Stages I and II cancers are generally curable by surgery. Because many of the well-differentiated lesions elaborate thyroglobulin and colloid, these neoplasms, even in stages III and IV, can sometimes be remarkably controlled by the administration of TSH, followed by radioiodine.

Medullary Carcinoma

This form of cancer, although one of the less frequent types (approximately 5 to 10%), is the most versatile of the thyroid carcinomas. Derived from parafollicular (C) cells within the thyroid, *medullary carcinoma is a prototypic neuroendocrine neoplasm. It has three distinctive features: (1) its amyloid stroma, (2) its genetic associations, and (3) its elaboration of calcitonin and other peptides.*[111–113] Amyloid deposits are present in the stroma of most, but not all, medullary carcinomas. The amyloid in these tumors is derived from the neoplastic C-cells and represents altered calcitonin molecules. With respect to genetic associations, perhaps 80 to 90% of these neoplasms occur sporadically, usually in adults, but 10 to 15% are encountered in children and teenagers in well-defined genetic syndromes, all transmitted by autosomal dominant patterns of inheritance.[114] Cytogenetic studies have linked the specific genetic defect to chromosome 10, and such analyses have the potential for prenatal and neonatal diagnosis of the disorder.[115]

Sipple's syndrome constitutes the association of pheochromocytoma with medullary carcinoma of the thyroid, sometimes coupled with either an adenoma or hyperplasia of the parathyroid glands. Thus, Sipple's syndrome is one of the multiple endocrine neoplasia (MEN) syndromes, classified as type IIa (p. 1007). In MEN IIb, medullary carcinoma of the thyroid and pheochromocytomas are associated with mucosal neuromas without parathyroid abnormalities. Patients with type IIb MEN also may exhibit a marfanoid habitus. Much less well characterized are the familial clusterings of medullary thyroid carcinoma unassociated with pheochromocytoma. Approximately 80 to 90% of medullary cancers secrete calcitonin, providing the opportunity to screen for this neoplasm by radioimmunoassay.[116] Somatostatin and gastrin-releasing peptide (bombesin) are also commonly elaborated by C-cell neoplasms.[113] They may produce histaminase, prostaglandins, and (more rarely) ACTH, vasoactive intestinal peptide (VIP), and serotonin. Calcitonin and/or prostaglandins induce diarrhea in about 30% of patients. The ACTH may be responsible for Cushing's syndrome, and the serotonin has in rare instances led to the carcinoid syndrome. It is evident that medullary carcinoma may be associated with a variety of clinical presentations.

Grossly, two patterns can be discerned—discrete tumors in one lobe, or numerous nodules that usually involve both lobes (Fig. 26–34). The sporadic neoplasms tend to originate within one lobe and with further growth may metastasize to the contralateral lobe. The familial tumors, on the other hand, are commonly bilateral and multicentric early in their course. In both, the tumor tissue may be soft and fleshy or firm and gritty and ranges from gray-white to yellow-brown. There may be foci of hemorrhage and necrosis in larger lesions, and some may have spread outside the thyroid capsule. About half the larger sporadic tumors have metastasized at the time of diagnosis. Histo-

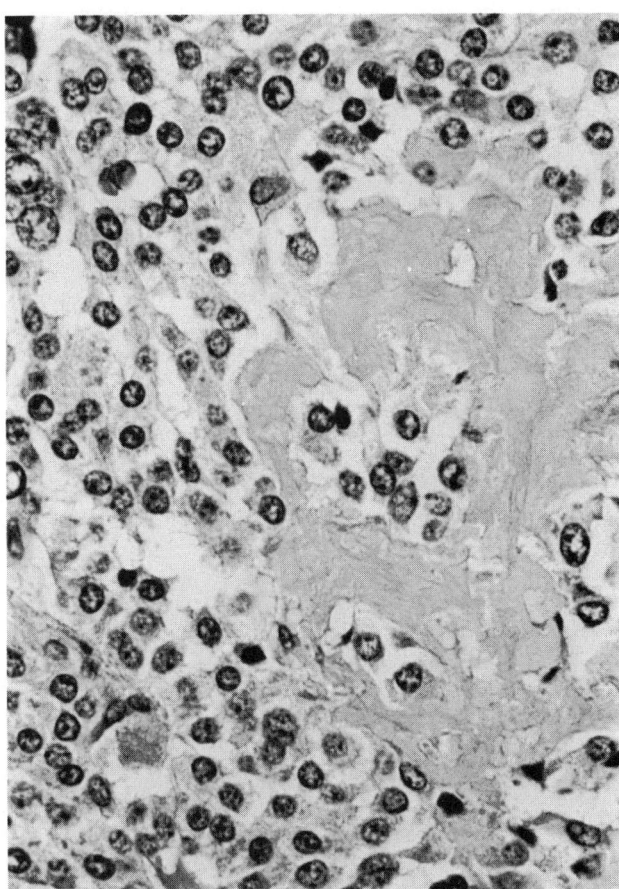

Figure 26–35. Medullary carcinoma with amyloid stroma. High-power detail revealing round-to-polygonal tumor cells with an abundant intercellular amyloidic stroma. (Courtesy of Drs. M. Warhol and L. Weiss, Department of Pathology, Brigham and Women's Hospital, Harvard Medical School.)

logically, these neoplasms have a range of cytologic patterns, from round-to-polygonal cells mimicking the histology of many other neuroendocrine cell tumors to spindle cells having a sarcomatoid appearance. Either cellular pattern may be disposed in organoid nests separated by a fibrovascular, amyloid-containing stroma; sometimes the nests acquire a pseudopapillary or follicular appearance (Fig. 26–35).[117] Alternatively, the cells, usually the spindle pattern, may be disposed in sheets. Occasional residual normal follicles may be entrapped within the substance of a medullary carcinoma; rare examples of mixed follicular and medullary carcinoma have also been reported.[117] Ultrastructural studies usually disclose in all cytologic patterns membrane-bound secretory granules that represent sites of storage of calcitonin and other peptides (Fig. 26–36).[112] Multiple foci of C-cell hyperplasia occasionally accompany the neoplasm in familial cases but are rarely, if ever, found in association with the sporadic tumors.[116]

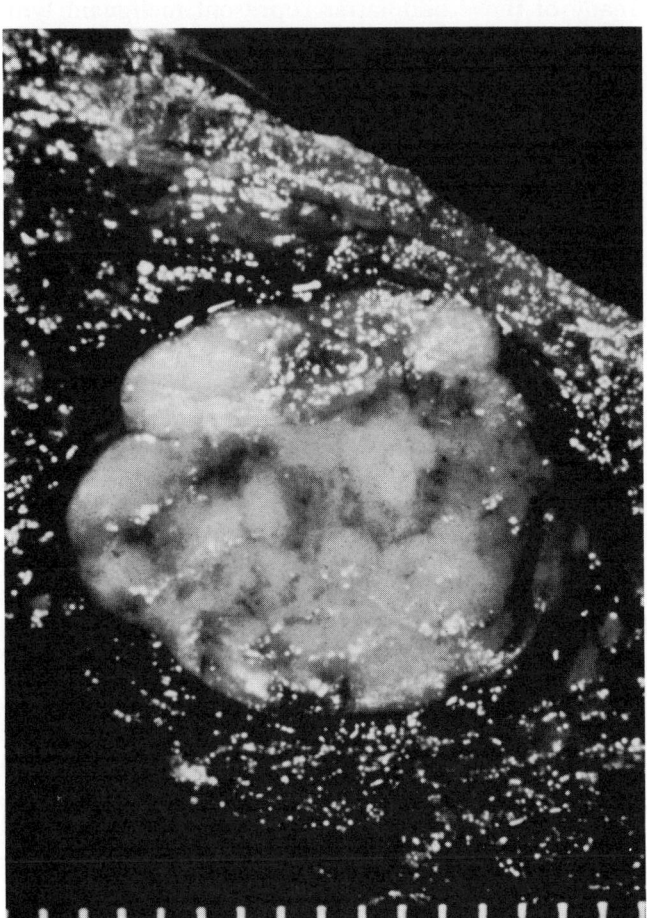

Figure 26–34. Medullary carcinoma of thyroid. These tumors typically show a solid pattern of growth and do not have connective tissue capsules.

Prospective studies of calcitonin secretory reserve have been of particular value in identifying family members at risk for the development of medullary carcinoma. In some instances, the precursor of medul-

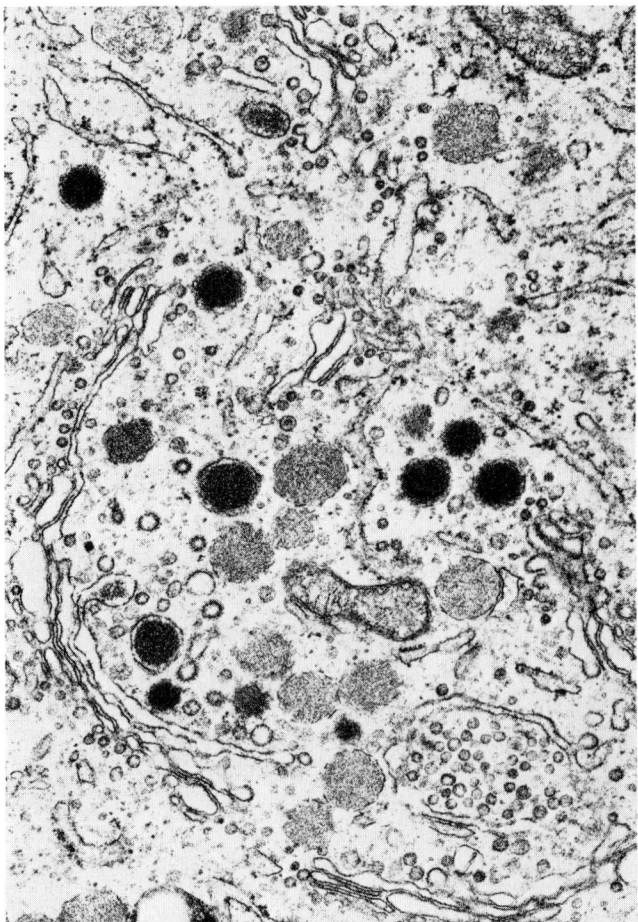

Figure 26–36. Electron micrograph of medullary thyroid carcinoma. These tumors contain membrane-bound secretory granules that are the sites of storage of calcitonin and other peptides (30,000 ×).

lary carcinoma (C-cell hyperplasia) has been identified on the basis of progressive abnormalities in calcium and/or pentagastrin-induced calcitonin secretion. Early thyroidectomy in these individuals has been effective in preventing the later development of carcinoma.

As mentioned earlier, there are significant differences in the clinical presentation of the sporadic and familial lesions. The mean age of diagnosis of the sporadic disease is the fifth to sixth decade, whereas that of the familial disease is the second to third decade. As a result of prospective screening studies in an extensively studied cohort, the mean age at diagnosis of very early C-cell disease, including C-cell hyperplasia and microscopic carcinoma, was 11.8 years.[118] The familial disease may also be masked by the clinical manifestations emanating from an associated pheochromocytoma (p. 1263) or parathyroid lesion (p. 1243). However, diarrhea related to calcitonin secretion or the production of other factors is a common manifestation in both forms. With early diagnosis often possible in the familial form, a recent study has demonstrated that 85% of patients were disease-free

11 years after thyroidectomy.[118] However, with the larger, more advanced sporadic neoplasms, the mean survival approaches five years. Death is usually related to recurrence, extension beyond the capsule, and metastasis, commonly to regional nodes, lung, liver, and bone.

Undifferentiated Carcinoma

About 10 to 15% of all thyroid carcinomas belong to this group. These tumors usually occur in the seventh and eighth decades of life and include some of the most malignant neoplasms encountered in humans.[95]

By the time these patients are seen clinically, most neoplasms have usually involved large areas of the thyroid gland and, indeed, have extended beyond its confines to produce bulky masses, readily apparent on clinical inspection. Several histologic variants can be identified. *Small cell carcinomas* are made up of compact, closely packed, cuboidal-to-polygonal cells, growing in cords or clusters, separated by a fibrous but non–amyloid-containing stroma. Numerous mitoses are present, but giant cells are infrequent. In another variant of small cell carcinoma, there are sheets of extremely small cells, having round, dark nuclei that indeed closely resemble atypical lymphocytes. Several studies have revealed, however, that many of these neoplasms represent malignant lymphomas rather than carcinomas.[119]

The *giant cell carcinoma* is one of the most wild human neoplasms and is composed of highly anaplastic cells, some of which are extremely large and pleomorphic, having multiple or multilobate nuclei; other cells may assume a spindle shape; still others may appear as elongated cytoplasmic ribbons. Numerous mitoses, bizarre mitoses, and giant nuclei are characteristic. Infrequently there are admixtures of papillary and follicle formations. These differentiated foci may represent residua of previously existing low-grade thyroid carcinomas. Invasion beyond the capsule, blood vessel involvement, and foci of infarct necrosis highlight the aggressive rapid growth of these forms of neoplasia (Fig. 26–37).

Other Malignant Tumors

Both Hodgkin's disease and non-Hodgkin's lymphoma may involve the thyroid in the course of their systemic dissemination, but both types of disease may also *arise* in the *thyroid* in the absence of systemic dissemination of a lymphoma primary elsewhere. Although most non-Hodgkin's lymphomas have been classified as large cell type, cell marker studies now suggest that they are transformed B cells and, in the terminology of Lukes and Collins, would be referred to as immunoblastic lymphomas (p. 714).[120] The mean age at the time of diagnosis is 60 to 70 years, and females are involved three or four times more commonly than males. Hashimoto's thyroiditis may precede the development of thyroid lymphomas in some cases.[121]

Sarcomas of the thyroid gland—fibrosarcoma, hemangiosarcoma, osteogenic sarcoma—are ex-

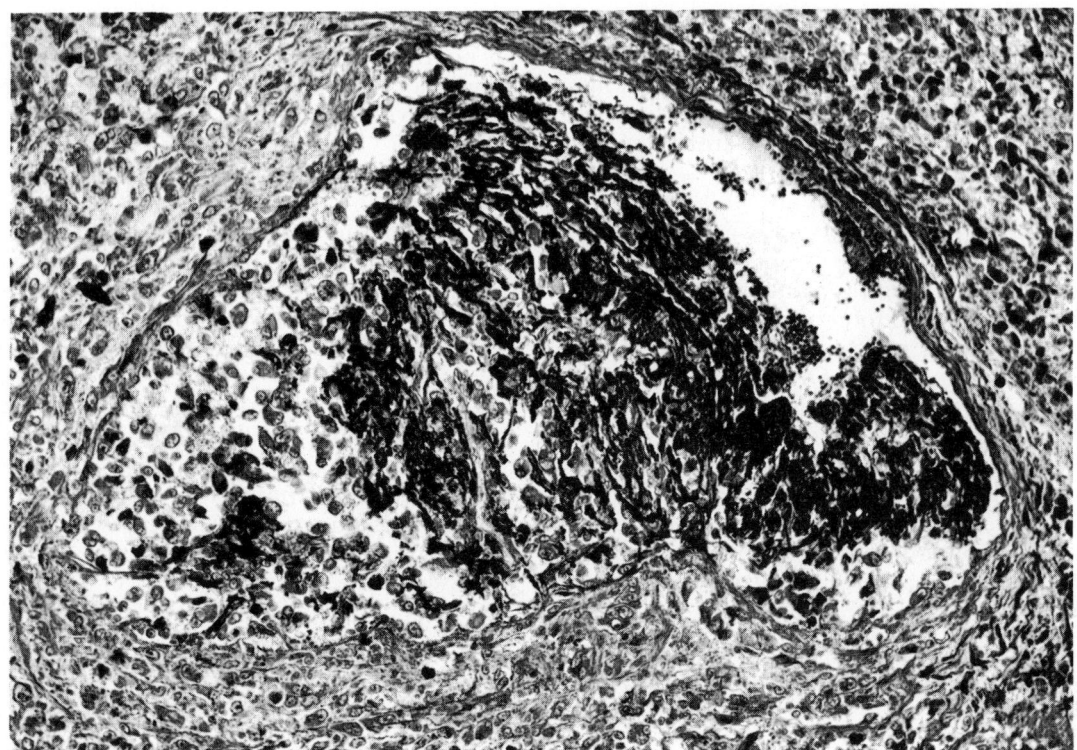

Figure 26–37. A highly undifferentiated anaplastic cancer of thyroid showing vascular invasion and thrombosis of the involved vessel.

tremely rare primary neoplasms. The diagnosis of such lesions must be made with due consideration for the fact that undifferentiated carcinomas may assume a sarcomatoid appearance. The demonstration of keratin type intermediate filaments, however, indicates that the tumor is of epithelial rather than mesenchymal origin.[122]

Squamous cell carcinomas may also arise within the thyroid gland but are exceptionally rare. More commonly, squamous cell carcinoma may invade the thyroid from an adjacent tracheal or esophageal primary tumor.

MISCELLANEOUS LESIONS

This noncommittal heading is adopted to cover some congenital anomalies of the thyroid gland and sundry other involvements, some encountered in systemic diseases.

CONGENITAL ANOMALIES

Thyroglossal duct or *cyst* is the most common clinically significant congenital anomaly. A persistent sinus tract may remain as a vestigial remnant of the tubular development of the thyroid gland. Parts of this tube may be obliterated, leaving small segments to form cysts. These occur at any age and may not become evident until adult life. Mucinous, clear secretion may collect within these cysts to form either spherical masses or fusiform swellings, rarely over 2 to 3 cm in diameter. These are present in the midline of the neck anterior to the trachea. Segments of the duct and cysts that occur high in the neck are lined by stratified squamous epithelium, which is essentially identical with that covering the posterior portion of the tongue in the region of the foramen cecum. Those anomalies that occur in the lower neck more proximal to the thyroid gland are lined by epithelium resembling the thyroidal acinar epithelium. Characteristically, subjacent to the lining epithelium there is an intense lymphocytic infiltrate. Superimposed infection may convert these lesions into abscess cavities.

The main significance of these lesions is that (1) they create masses in the neck requiring differentiation from more serious neoplasms; (2) they may communicate with the skin to produce persistent draining sinuses; (3) sometimes the persistent duct drains into the base of the tongue; and (4) these anomalous structures are rare sources for the development of malignancy.[123] *Agenesis and dysgenesis of the thyroid gland* are uncommon congenital anomalies. In many instances there appears to be total failure of development of the normally situated thyroid gland. Aberrant rests of *ectopic thyroid* are rare congenital anomalies. They are located most often at the base of the tongue but sometimes along the course of the thyroglossal duct. As mentioned at the outset, the ectopic rests are almost always located within the anterior triangle of the neck, and so may be mistaken for an enlarged lymph node or sometimes for a metastasis from a very well differentiated carcinoma of the thyroid. In most cases, these remnants are supernumerary to the definitive thyroid gland. Only infrequently do they represent the only thyroid tissue in the individual. When the definitive thyroid is lacking and there is little or no aberrant tissue to replace it, athyreotic cretinism may result.

ATROPHY OF THYROID

Atrophy of the thyroid gland is a nonclinical term applied by morphologists to total or near-total replacement of the thyroidal substance by fibrous tissue when the cause is uncertain. Often, only scattered rests of thyroid parenchyma persist along with foci of lymphocytic infiltration in the fibrous atrophy. Such follicular cells as persist may have undergone squamous metaplasia or transformation into Hürthle cells having abundant, finely granular eosinophilic cytoplasm. It is impossible from the morphologic examination to determine the cause of the atrophic process, but the possibilities include (1) panhypopituitarism; (2) acute or subacute thyroiditis (bacterial, viral); (3) irradiation; and (4) primary, idiopathic (autoimmune) hypothyroidism.

SYSTEMIC THYROIDAL CHANGES

Notable in this category are systemic amyloidosis, with deposits in the stromal connective tissue chiefly about vessels, and hemochromatosis, with the accumulation of hemosiderin pigment within thyroidal epithelium and within fibroblasts in the stroma. These involvements rarely produce functional abnormalities. The thyroid may be seeded by any blood-borne infection or disseminated disease, as pointed out in the consideration of thyroiditis (p. 1220). It is sometimes seeded by metastatic cancers, including lymphomas and leukemias. Necropsy studies have identified thyroid involvement in 4 to 24% of patients dying of disseminated cancer.[124]

PARATHYROID GLANDS

PRIMARY HYPERPARATHY-
   ROIDISM
Adenomas
Carcinoma
Primary Hyperplasia
SECONDARY HYPERPARATHY-
   ROIDISM
HYPOPARATHYROIDISM
Pseudo- and Pseudopseudohy-
   poparathyroidism

NORMAL

The parathyroid glands are derived from the pharyngeal pouches — the upper glands from the endoderm of the fourth pouch, and lower pair from the third pouch. About 90% of individuals have four parathyroid glands, but there may be as many as six or as few as two. There is, therefore, hazard in unnecessarily removing even a single gland in a patient who might have only one gland left. In the adult, the parathyroid is a yellow-brown, ovoid, encapsulated nodule weighing approximately 35 to 40 mg. It measures from 4 to 6 mm in length, 2 to 4 mm in width, and 0.5 to 2 mm in thickness. The superior glands are almost always located close to the upper posterior aspect of the thyroid, but the inferior glands are much more footloose and may be found anywhere from the lower pole of the thyroid down to the deepest recesses of the thymus.

In early infancy and childhood, the parathyroids are composed almost entirely of solid sheets of chief cells. With increasing age, the amount of stromal fat increases to reach a maximum of approximately 30% at about the age of 25 years. Thereafter the proportion of stromal fat to parenchyma remains relatively constant.[125,126] After the age of 25, the precise amount of fat is determined largely by constitutional factors; fat individuals have fat glands and vice versa! The poles of the glands often contain more fat than do the central regions.

Parathyroid chief cells compose the majority of the gland and vary from light to dark pink with H and E stains, depending on their glycogen content: the more glycogen, the lighter or clearer the cell. They are polygonal, 12 to 20 μ in diameter and have central, round, uniform nuclei. In addition to the usual cellular organelles, they have a large Golgi complex, a moderate number of mitochondria, lipofuscin pigment, and secretory granules.[127] *Oxyphil cells,* found throughout the normal parathyroid in adults, either singly or in small clusters, are slightly larger than chief cells, have a brightly acidophilic cytoplasm, and are tightly packed with mitochondria. Glycogen granules are also present in these cells, whereas secretory granules are sparse or absent. The chief cell is the progenitor of the other forms and is the major source of parathyroid hormone. Transitional oxyphils are indeed more numerous than oxyphils.

Parathyroid hormone (PTH) is a peptide containing 84 amino acids derived from a longer "pre-pro" form by sequential cleavage within chief cells. Following secretion, PTH is rapidly split (with a half-life of minutes) into an amino-terminal (N) fragment of 34 amino acids having an even shorter half-life, and a carboxy-terminal (C) fragment with a half-life of several hours. Most radioimmunoassays measure the serum level of the C fragments, which are more readily titered because of their longer half-life, but the biologic activity of PTH resides in the N fragments. The C fragment, so far as is known, has no biologic activity.[128]

As is well known, the function of PTH is the maintenance of normal levels of ionized calcium in the extracellular fluid. The hormone binds to membrane receptors of target cells to stimulate adenylate cyclase, leading to an increase in intracellular cAMP. At the same time it facilitates the flow of calcium out of blood into cells. It thus appears that cAMP and calcium cooperate in serving as the ultimate mediators of the physiologic actions of PTH, but the precise steps involved are unknown. Maintenance of normocalcemia is mediated by direct effects on kidney and bone and indirect effects on the intestine.[129] Absorption of calcium from the gut is enhanced largely by the vitamin D metabolite $1\alpha,25\text{-(OH)}_2D_3$, whose synthesis in the kidney is regulated by PTH. At the same time it directly reduces renal excretion of calcium by enhancing its reabsorption from the glomerular filtrate, increases phosphate excretion, and increases the rate of dissolution of bone mineral, involving two separable sequences. First, there is an immediate efflux of calcium from bone into blood. This is followed by a more prolonged release of bone calcium as a consequence of increased resorption of bone. Whether this action is related to increased osteoclastic activity or reduced osteoblastic activity, leading to a net catabolic effect, is not clear.[130] All actions of PTH serve to increase serum calcium. In turn, PTH secretion is regulated by the serum calcium level in a classic feedback loop. The complex relationships among phosphate, vitamin D, and PTH in the maintenance of normocalcemia were discussed earlier (p. 441).

PATHOLOGY

The anatomic disorders of the parathyroid gland are best considered in relation to their effects on func-

tion, i.e., hyperparathyroidism and hypoparathyroidism. The former can be further divided into primary hyperparathyroidism, which results from disorders intrinsic to the glands that produce hypersecretion of PTH with hypercalcemia and hypophosphatemia, and secondary hyperparathyroidism, also associated with excessive production of PTH but basically characterized by some apparent resistance in the target tissues to the action of the hormone. Thus, in secondary hyperparathyroidism the physiologic actions of PTH are more or less blocked, with resultant hypocalcemia and hyperphosphatemia. The low serum calcium levels stimulate parathyroid function and, in time, induce hyperplastic changes. The following discussion, therefore, covers primary hyperparathyroidism, secondary hyperparathyroidism, hypoparathyroidism, and the uncommon pseudohypoparathyroidism.

PRIMARY HYPERPARATHYROIDISM

Primary hyperparathyroidism is the cause of hypercalcemia in up to 30% of cases, and its incidence is about 1:800 in adults (Table 26–5). The major biochemical features of primary hyperparathyroidism include (1) elevated serum levels of PTH, (2) hypercalcemia, (3) hypophosphatemia, and (4) excessive urinary excretion of calcium. A number of clinical consequences follow, some early, others only after some long period of hyperfunction, and thus the clinical presentation depends on the duration of the metabolic derangement.[131] Neuromuscular weakness and fatigability appear early and insidiously in most patients. Neuropsychiatric disturbances may range from depression, anxiety, and psychoses to mental obtundation and even coma. More specific are renal stones or nephrocalcinosis (p. 1073) incident to the hypercalciuria. These were once found in 50 to 70% of patients, but with earlier diagnosis of the condition, they are now present in less than 25%. Increased mobilization of skeletal calcium followed by bone resorption and remodeling may in time give rise to so-called osteitis fibrosa cystica (p. 1326), diagnostic of hyperparathyroidism. These bony changes appear only after some long period (years) of parathyroid hyperfunction. They were once present in 80 to 90%

Table 26–5. Clinical Causes of Hypercalcemia

DIAGNOSIS	% OF CASES
Malignancy (nonparathyroid)	34.4
Hyperparathyroidism	34.2
Vitamin D excess	12.1
Hyperthyroidism	3.9
Milk alkali syndrome	3.9
Immobilization	2.3
Idiopathic	0.9
Sarcoidosis	0.9
Dysproteinemias	0.6
Addison's disease	0.6
Laboratory error	13.4

of cases but now are found in only 10 to 15%.[132] A number of other changes may also be present, but they are less constant. Hypertension is a common finding in over half the patients; however, the hypertension may not be alleviated by surgical removal of the parathyroid lesion. Persistence of the hypertension may be due to the development of renovascular changes incident to the prolonged hypertension. Pancreatitis is sometimes associated with hyperparathyroidism, as noted on page 984, but for reasons that are not entirely clear. Peptic ulcers are also more prevalent; this is attributed to increased secretion of gastrin secondary to elevated serum levels of calcium or PTH, but a direct causal association has been challenged. Cholelithiasis has been reported in 25 to 35% of patients, presumably due to increased calcium levels in the bile with the formation of insoluble calcium bilirubinates. Finally, the hypercalcemia may give rise to metastatic calcifications in soft tissues, vessels, and joints, as described on page 36. The deposition of calcium pyrophosphate in the joints causes disabling chondrocalcinosis in about 15 to 20% of cases (p. 1360).[133]

As indicated, the clinical picture of primary hyperparathyroidism has undergone change over the past years. At one time the condition passed unrecognized until "stone and bone" disease brought it to attention. Today, the diagnosis is often made fortuitously by a routine determination of serum calcium as one of the multiphasic laboratory tests routinely employed in clinical practice. Thus, most patients are asymptomatic or have vague complaints only in retrospect.[134] However, it must be cautioned that the mere identification of hypercalcemia by the laboratory cannot be equated with hyperparathyroidism. It may have many causes, as indicated in Table 26–5.

Nonparathyroid malignancy is the most common cause of hypercalcemia in the hospitalized patient. In some of these cases the elevated serum calcium is related to direct resorption of bone by the cancer (multiple myeloma) or by its osteolytic metastases (from cancers of the breast, lung [squamous cell], kidney, and other sites). Sometimes, however, the hypercalcemia occurs in the absence of skeletal metastases and is related to the elaboration of some calcium-mobilizing humoral agent such as prostaglandin E_2, osteoclast-activating factor, vitamin D–like substances, PTH, or PTH-like substances.[135] Transforming growth factor-alpha and other tumor-derived growth factors have the capacity to bind to parathyroid hormone receptors, and their combined actions lead to increased bone resorption and increased renal tubular calcium resorption.[136] There is a regrettable tendency to refer to these syndromes as "pseudohyperparathyroidism," when in reality they represent paraneoplastic syndromes.

Analyses of large series of cases of primary hyperparathyroidism reveal single adenomas in 80% of cases, while 2 to 3% of patients may harbor double adenomas. Carcinomas occur in 2 to 3% of individuals. About 15% of patients have evidence of primary parathyroid hyperplasia.[127,137] Included in this compilation are instances in which the parathyroid pathology is a component of familial polyendocrine syndromes such as multiple endocrine neoplasia (MEN) I, MEN IIa, and other more rare familial hypercalcemic hyperparathyroid constellations.[131] The MEN syndromes are discussed on page 1007; it suffices to note here that they may be associated with either adenomas or hyperplasia of the parathyroids.[16]

ADENOMAS

These benign tumors may be extremely small and difficult to locate even at surgical exploration.[127] They may occur in either sex at any age, with a peak incidence in the middle decades of life. Although the vast majority of adenomas occur singly, occasionally two adenomas are found dispersed among the four glands. The interpretation of double adenomas is uncertain. Are they merely coincidental neoplasms, or is the enlargement of two glands an incomplete form of hyperplasia that usually involves all four glands, but sometimes asymmetrically, giving the false impression of multiple adenomas? Although initial studies suggested that parathyroid adenomas were polyclonal, more recent studies employing powerful molecular biologic methods indicate that many are, in fact, monoclonal and represent true neoplasms.[138,139] In any case, it is evident that, in the surgical excision of an adenoma, all four glands must be visualized to discover possible double or polyglandular enlargements.

Adenomas average 0.5 to 5.0 gm in weight. Occasionally, however, they are as large as 10 to 20 gm, and extreme weights of over 100 gm have been reported. For obscure reasons, adenomas are most often located in the inferior parathyroid glands.[140] However, they may be found in such ectopic sites as the thymus, thyroid, or pericardium or behind the esophagus, sometimes creating the proverbial surgical problem of "the needle in the haystack." They are well encapsulated, soft, yielding, yellow-to-tan-to-red lesions. **Some are composed of pure cell types, but others display mixed cell populations** (Fig. 26–38). The most common variant is composed principally of chief cells, but many transitional and oxyphil cells are often present also. The cells of adenomas are arranged in large islands or broad bands. Occasional adenomas are composed of follicular structures that may bear a striking resemblance to thyroid follicles. Mitoses are generally absent. The chief cells are frequently slightly larger than normal, with variations in cell and nuclear size. Sometimes, hyperchromatic pleomorphic nuclei are present in these lesions, with occasional binucleate forms—features that are of some importance since they help to distinguish primary adenomas from hyperplasia. Infrequently, the adenoma is composed predominantly of water-clear cells; however, here again chief cells and oxyphils may be found. A functioning adenoma composed largely of oxyphil cells is extremely unusual. Whatever the type, cells are disposed in solid sheets or masses, but occasionally the tumor is separated into apparent lobules by traversing bands of fibrous tissue. At other times, a well-vascularized stroma produces cords of cells, and occasionally glandlike patterns are seen. **The presence of a rim of normal or atrophic (suppressed) parathyroid tissue with scattered fat cells can be seen external to the capsule, serving to differentiate the adenoma from diffuse hyperplasia.** The remaining glands in individuals with single adenomas are normal or atrophic (suppressed). While the parenchymal cells of adenomas are devoid of intracellular fat, the suppressed parathyroid chief cells adjacent to the adenoma or present in remaining glands contain intracellular fat deposits.[141]

Electron microscopy has not revealed many differences between these neoplastic cells and their normal counterparts.[142] Distinctive in many cells is a concentric laminated pattern of smooth-faced cisternae, termed annulate lamellae, in the region of the Golgi complex.[143] This structure has been identified in many experimental tumors, and there is the suggestion that it is involved in protein synthesis or some other synthetic activity.

CARCINOMA

Carcinoma of the parathyroid glands is a rare cause of primary hyperfunction. The manifestations are similar to those of "benign" hyperparathyroidism but tend to be exaggerated, with more marked and earlier bone changes and a greater tendency to renal stones — "bone and stone disease."[144] All agree that there are undoubted cases of nonfunctioning carcinomas of the parathyroid glands, but the close anatomic similarity between such lesions and carcinomas arising in the thyroid has led to the commonly accepted criterion that the diagnosis of a carcinoma arising in the parathyroid requires the demonstration of hyperfunction. There is great difficulty in distinguishing between the pleomorphism of adenomas and the mild anaplasia of some carcinomas. As a consequence, it has also been proposed that, for a diagnosis of malignancy, one of the three following features must be present: (1) metastases, either to regional nodes or to distant organs; (2) capsular invasion; or (3) local recurrence following resection. It should be remembered, however, that adenomas and even hyperplastic glands that have been excised incompletely may also recur.[145]

Most of the carcinomas described have been small, and in fact, some have been less than 1 gm in weight. They are often irregular in shape and show lobulation and pseudopod formation and sometimes adherence to surrounding structures. This feature often serves to alert the surgeon to the possibility of a carcinoma. They are usually considerably firmer than adenomas. The major histologic features that help to distinguish a carcinoma from an adenoma are (1) a trabecular growth pattern, (2) mitotic figures, (3) thick fibrous bands, (4) capsular invasion, and (5) blood vessel invasion.[146] When these lesions metastasize, they usually affect the regional nodes alone. Rarely, they may spread to distant sites, such as the lungs, as well as below the diaphragm. Survival for many years is the rule, and death results more often from the complications of hyperparathyroidism than from the spread of the lesion.

PRIMARY HYPERPLASIA

This designation is applied to diffuse hyperplastic enlargement, usually of all four parathyroid glands.[127] However, the hyperplasia may be asymmetric and leave one or two glands deceptively unenlarged, accounting for the controversy relative to multiple adenomas versus asymmetric hyperplasia. The dispute is heightened by a lack of understanding of the basis of the hyperplasia. Many hypotheses have been offered invoking excessive urinary excretion of calcium leading to a mild hypocalcemia, subtle end-organ resistance to PTH calling for increased parathyroid gland function, and previous neck irradiation stimulating cell replication. In the last analysis, however, the cause of the primary hyperplasia is unknown. Whatever its origins, primary hyperplasia accounts for 15% of cases of primary hyperparathyroidism, and is caused most often by chief cell hyperplasia (12%) and less commonly by clear cell hyperplasia (3%).

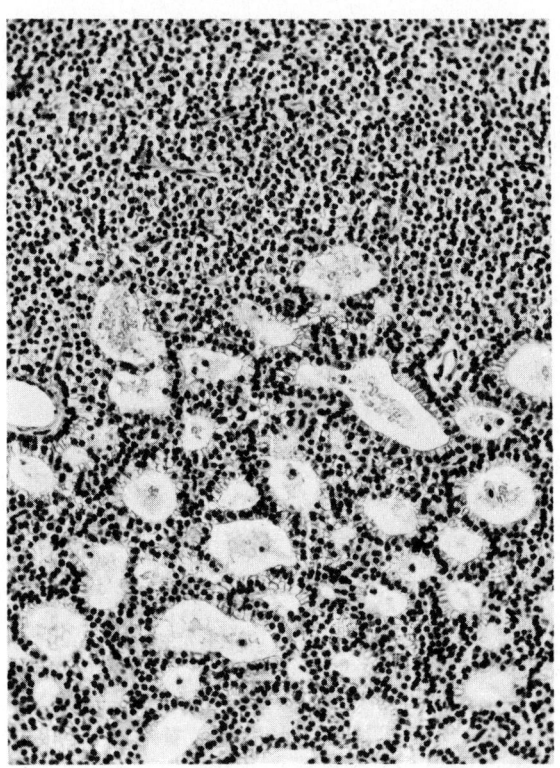

Figure 26–38. Parathyroid adenoma containing chief cells, oxyphils, and a few water-clear ("wasserhelle") cells growing in sheets and glandular patterns.

Chief cell hyperplasia must be described separately from clear cell hyperplasia, since there are both gross and microscopic differences. In **chief cell hyperplasia,** the total weight of all glands may be less than 1 gm, although an upper range in the order of 10 gm has been recorded. Often, one or two glands are significantly larger than the remainder.[147] The glands vary in color from yellow to tan to red-brown and often contain small cysts.

The histologic pattern of the hyperplastic glands is quite variable (Fig. 26–39). The chief cells are arranged in cords, sheets, and occasionally glandular patterns, sometimes with dispersed stromal fat cells. However, **usually there are areas of solid parathyroid cells devoid of stromal fat, a microscopic feature of great importance in distinguishing hyperplasia from normal glands.** Rarely, in chief cell hyperplasia, the glands are composed almost completely of oxyphil cells or a mixture of groups of chief cells, oxyphils, and transitional cells.[147] Primary chief cell hyperplasia may be either diffuse or nodular with respect to the overall growth pattern. The nodular forms of hyperplasia are often extremely difficult to distinguish histologically from adenomas. The parenchyma adjacent to foci of nodular hyperplasia appears diffusely hyperplastic, and biopsies of other glands will also reveal evidence of hyperplasia in contrast to the atrophy adjacent to true adenomas.

In contrast, **clear cell hyperplasias** are usually

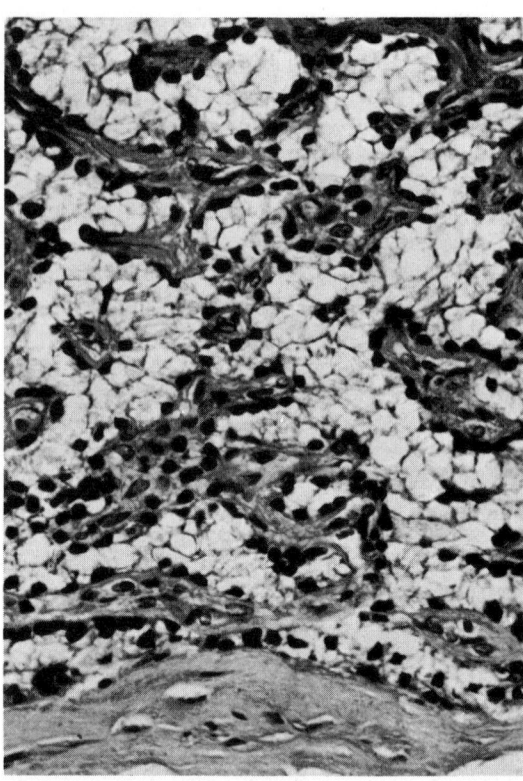

Figure 26–40. A detail of marked primary parathyroid hyperplasia showing a clear cell pattern.

marked by greater enlargement of the glands than in chief cell hyperplasia. Aggregate weights of over 10 gm are not uncommon. In clear cell hyperplasias the glands are most often characterized by a uniform distribution of variably enlarged cells (8 to 40 μm) with pale, vacuolated cytoplasm. Usually, all four parathyroid glands are completely replaced by the clear cells, and there are few residual fat cells or oxyphil cells (Fig. 26–40). The cytoplasm is not actually cleared but can be resolved under the electron microscope as being filled by small, seemingly empty vacuoles of uncertain origin—derived either from the Golgi apparatus or from the granular endoplasmic reticulum.[148]

SECONDARY HYPERPARATHYROIDISM

Secondary hyperparathyroidism is characterized by compensatory hypersecretion of PTH in response to end-organ resistance to PTH, resulting in depressed blood calcium levels.[149] *Primary hyperparathyroidism is usually marked by hypercalcemia, whereas secondary hyperparathyroidism is characterized by hypocalcemia,* albeit sometimes mild. The most important cause of secondary hyperparathyroidism is chronic renal insufficiency. Chronic hypocalcemia and secondary hyperparathyroidism also may be encountered in vitamin D deficiency, intestinal malabsorption syndromes with inadequate absorption of vi-

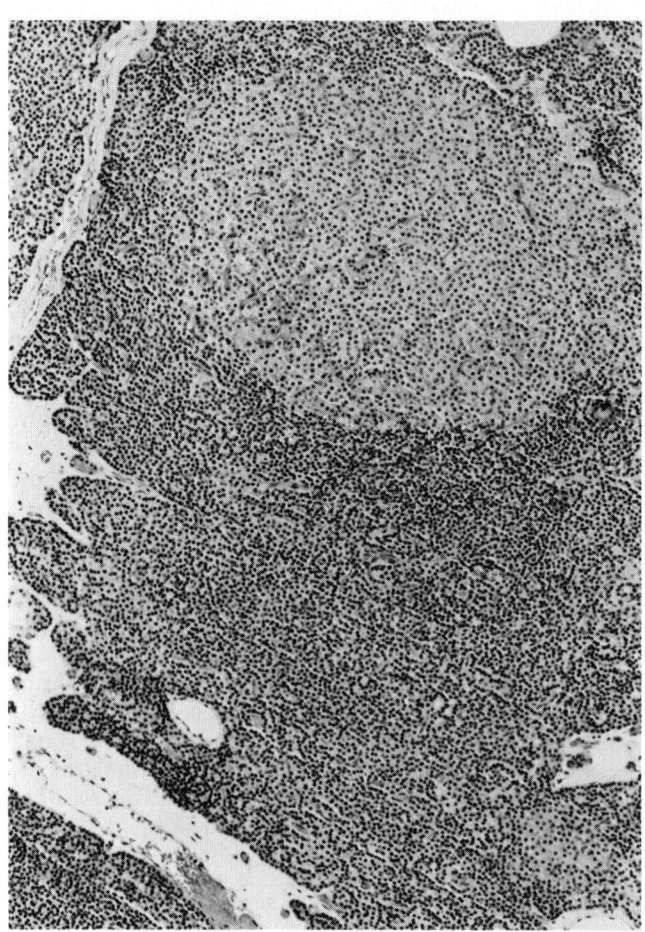

Figure 26–39. Primary chief cell hyperplasia of parathyroid glands. This parathyroid contains almost no stromal fat. The nodule in the top of the illustration is composed of transitional oxyphil type cells.

tamin D and calcium, and pseudohypoparathyroidism (p. 1248).

The sequence of events leading to the parathyroid compensatory hyperfunction in the various clinical circumstances mentioned is poorly understood. Although resistance to PTH and hypocalcemia are postulated, they are difficult to establish in many instances. Moreover, many more complexities are probably involved. For example, in chronic renal failure the initial stimulus is probably reduction of ionized calcium in the extracellular fluid secondary to renal retention of phosphate. The hyperphosphatemia and damaged renal parenchyma (underlying the renal failure) combine to reduce the renal production of $1\alpha,25\text{-}(OH)_2D_3$. Decreased intestinal absorption follows. There is also impaired mobilization of calcium from the skeleton, attributed to resistance to PTH. Compensatory hyperfunction of the parathyroids ensues. Generally, however, the manifestations of such hyperfunction are less prominent than those associated with primary hyperparathyroidism.

The anatomic changes in the parathyroid glands consist principally of hyperplasia of the chief cells. This usually affects all glands, but not infrequently, one, two, or even three may be spared. The basis for such asymmetric involvement is obscure. Islands of oxyphils are often present, and the fat is usually largely replaced by hyperplastic cells (Fig. 26–41).

In many instances the glands revert to normal if

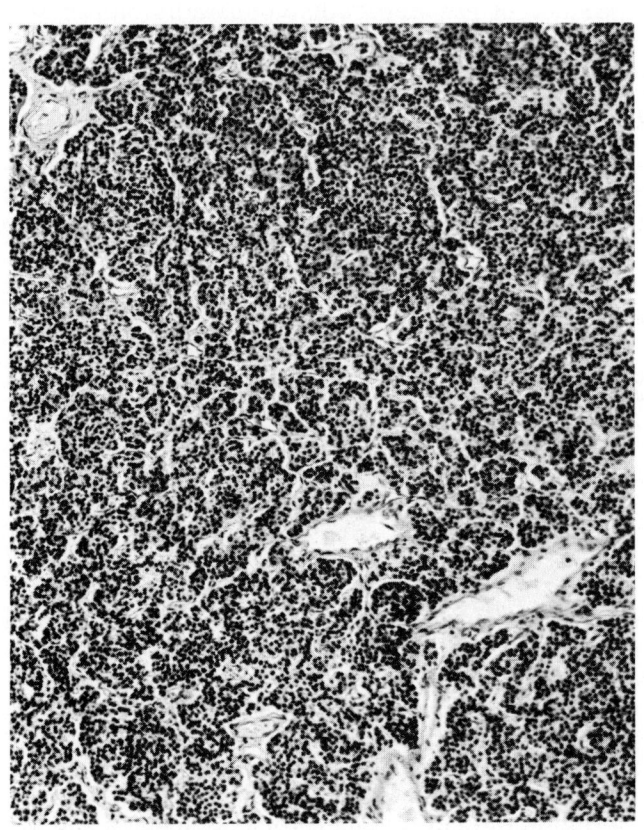

Figure 26–41. Diffuse secondary hyperplasia of parathyroid, illustrating extensive replacement of the normally contained fat.

the basic clinical derangement is brought under control by, for example, renal transplantation or vitamin D supplementation. With long-standing secondary hyperplasia and greater glandular enlargement, however, reversion to normal may not occur, contributing to the possibility that *secondary hyperplasia may in time convert into autonomous primary hyperplasia, which is sometimes referred to as tertiary hyperparathyroidism.*[150]

HYPOPARATHYROIDISM

Hypoparathyroidism may arise whenever there is inadequate secretion of PTH or the hormone is biologically ineffective.[151] Under these circumstances the diminished physiologic action of PTH on the kidney and bone leads to hypocalcemia and hyperphosphatemia. Reduced end-organ sensitivity to PTH may also induce hypoparathyroidism. A constellation of clinical changes is associated with hypoparathyroidism, but since the resultant syndrome is largely metabolic and clinical with scant anatomic changes, it will be discussed only briefly. With milder expressions of the syndrome, the clinical manifestations are exceedingly subtle and almost undecipherable without the documentation of hypocalcemia. At the other extreme are the more overt expressions marked by:

• *Increased neuromuscular excitability,* related to the decreased serum ionized calcium concentration. Classically, this is elicited by tapping along the course of the facial nerve, which induces contractions of the muscles of the eye, mouth, or nose (Chvostek's sign). More dramatic is the development of tetany with muscle cramps, carpopedal spasms, laryngeal stridor, and convulsions.
• *Mental changes* ranging from irritability to depression and frank psychosis.
• *Neurologic signs suggesting an intracranial tumor* with elevated CSF pressure and papilledema.
• *Intracranial calcifications* visualized by skull x-rays in approximately 20% of patients with chronic hypoparathyroidism, sometimes leading to a parkinsonian-like syndrome.
• *Calcification of the lens,* leading to cataract formation.
• *Abnormalities in cardiac conduction* (mainly prolongation of the Q-T interval and T-wave changes).
• *Abnormalities of dentition* with defective enamel, dental hypoplasia, and delayed eruption of teeth.

Many disorders may be associated with hypoparathyroidism. Postsurgical hypoparathyroidism has been reported following thyroidectomy, surgery for hyperparathyroidism, and radical neck dissections for cancer; its reported frequency ranges from 0.2 to 10%.[152] A familial syndrome of uncertain mode of transmission is thought to represent a form of autoimmune disease, but apparent autoimmune disease may also appear without an obvious hereditary background. In both instances the hypoparathyroidism is often accompanied by hypoadrenalism, autoimmune thyroid disease, insulin-dependent diabetes mellitus, and pernicious anemia, all suspected of also being autoimmune.[153,154] There is frequently associated mucocutaneous candidiasis, alopecia areata, and vitiligo; studies point to deranged T-suppressor cell function as the basis of the autoimmune reactions and vulnerability to fungal infections.[155] DiGeorge's syndrome, as discussed on page 222, is a form of congenital immunodeficiency state characterized by a T-cell deficiency secondary to thymic hypoplasia, but, for our interests, also accompanied by parathyroid hypoplasia. There are still other causes of hypoparathyroidism such as postradiation, metastases to the parathyroid glands, and suppression of PTH secretion by prolonged hypercalcemia, but all are exceedingly uncommon.

PSEUDO- AND PSEUDOPSEUDO-HYPOPARATHYROIDISM

Pseudohypoparathyroidism is a rare hereditary disorder, perhaps transmitted as an X-linked dominant trait, characterized by signs and symptoms of hypoparathyroidism, with hypocalcemia and hyperphosphatemia, associated, however, with normal or even elevated levels of circulating PTH.[156] End-organ unresponsiveness mainly in the kidney is postulated because the circulating hormone is biologically active. Rare reports suggest restoration of normal sensitivity to PTH following the administration of large doses of $1\alpha,25\text{-}(OH)_2D_3$. The distinctive features of pseudohypoparathyroidism are short stature, round face, short neck, abnormally short metacarpal and metatarsal bones, and particularly an abnormally short fourth and fifth metacarpal and metatarsal (Albright's hereditary osteodystrophy). Some patients have reduced intelligence. The hormone resistance in pseudohypoparathyroidism is presumably due to a defect in the interaction of PTH with the guanine nucleotide, binding protein (G-protein).[157] Deficient binding to G-unit limits the production of cAMP and impairs hormone responsiveness. These individuals fail to show an increase in urinary cAMP after intravenous infusion of PTH. Resistance to the actions of other hormones also may be apparent in individuals with G-unit deficiency. While almost all patients with G-unit deficiency show the phenotypic characteristics of Albright's hereditary osteodystrophy, those individuals with normal G-unit activity do not. Other patients with pseudohypoparathyroidism may have defects distal to cAMP formation. You may recall that end-organ resistance to PTH may lead to secondary hyperparathyroidism, and it is likely that some patients with pseudohypoparathyroidism develop some of the stigmata of secondary hyperparathyroidism.

Pseudopseudohypoparathyroidism is characterized by a clinical picture identical to that of pseudohypoparathyroidism except that these patients have no hypocalcemia or hyperphosphatemia and apparently have a relatively normal urinary cAMP response to PTH. Some workers, however, have questioned the existence of pseudopseudohypoparathyroidism as a defined entity.

ADRENAL CORTEX

NORMAL

The adrenal glands are highly complex endocrine organs consisting of the steroid-secreting cortical cells and the catecholamine-producing medullary (chromaffin) cells. Each of these compartments, although encased in a common connective tissue capsule, represents an anatomically and functionally discrete unit. The medulla is derived from the neural crest, while the cortex is mesodermal in origin, derived from the urogenital ridge. Before birth the adrenal cortex is composed largely of a wide fetal zone, but after birth the fetal zone begins to undergo a series of involutional changes. In a few months the three definitive cortical zones appear: the subcapsular zona glomerulosa, the intermediate zona fasciculata, and the inner zona reticularis.

The normal adrenal in the adult weighs 4 to

5 gm.[158] In individuals dying after prolonged illnesses, the adrenals may be considerably larger, presumably as a result of stress-induced ACTH stimulation of the glands. The normal adrenal cortex is yellow-brown owing largely to its content of lipochrome pigment and in some part to stored steroid precursors—free and esterified cholesterol, triglycerides, and phospholipids. The *zona glomerulosa* constitutes approximately 10 to 15% of the cortex. It consists of closely packed groups and clusters of cuboidal-to-columnar cells with darkly staining nuclei and scanty cytoplasm containing only a few lipid droplets. Ultrastructurally, the most prominent feature is an abundant anastomosing network of smooth endoplasmic reticulum. The mitochondria are filamentous and have lamellar cristae like those in most other organs.

The *zona fasciculata* constitutes 80% of the cortex. It is organized into long cords or columns of polyhedral cells somewhat larger than those of the glomerulosa that have a central darkly staining nucleus and a cytoplasm filled with fine vacuoles. The lipids within these vacuoles are mostly cholesterol and cholesterol esters, which are dissolved out in the usual paraffin sections. Such cells are variously referred to as "clear" or "light" cells. The fasciculata cells have an elaborate smooth endoplasmic reticulum, stacks of granular endoplasmic reticulum, and a prominent Golgi apparatus. However, mitochondria are less numerous and more variable in size and shape, and the cristae are tubulovesicular in configuration. The abundant storage of cholesterol is interpreted as reserve substrate for the biosynthesis of steroid hormones. In the unstressed individual, the fasciculata cells are lipid-rich, whereas stress is associated with lipid depletion.

In the *zona reticularis*, the parallel cords give way to irregularly arranged clusters that abut the medulla and in the aggregate make up about 5 to 10% of the total cortex. The cells basically resemble those of the fasciculata, but the cytoplasm is nonvacuolated, is deeply acidophilic, and contains large accumulations of lipochrome pigment. Thus, these cells are called "dark" or "compact" cells. They possess an abundant smooth endoplasmic reticulum and numerous mitochondria having cristae intermediate between those in the other two zones. The fasciculata and reticularis represent a single functional zone capable of synthesizing and secreting glucocorticoids and sex steroids.[159]

The *mineralocorticoids*, the most important of which is *aldosterone*, are synthesized primarily in the zona glomerulosa. The *glucocorticoids*, of which the most active is cortisol, are synthesized in the zonae reticularis and fasciculata. Analogously, testosterone, the major adrenal *androgen*, is also synthesized in the inner two zones. Although synthesis of the glucocorticoids and adrenal androgens is under hypothalamic–anterior pituitary ACTH control, aldosterone secretion is largely independent of ACTH and is regulated by the serum levels of potassium and renin-angiotensin. An additional factor controlling the secretion of aldosterone is a 26,000 dalton glycoprotein that has been found in extracts of pituitary, urine, and plasma.[160]

Increased levels of ACTH, whether of exogenous or endogenous origin, induce hyperplasia of the inner two zones, not affecting the zona glomerulosa (Fig. 26–42); conversely, loss of anterior pituitary function leaves the zona glomerulosa relatively unaffected while causing atrophy of the remainder of the cortex.

ACTH is a 39 amino acid peptide derived from a much longer peptide (proopiomelanocortin, POMC), which is cleaved first into a carboxy-terminal fragment containing not only ACTH but also beta lipotropin, beta endorphin, and beta melanotropin.[161] The amino-terminal fragment has no steroidogenic effect but contains a gamma melanotropin.[124] Thereafter, ACTH is cleaved from the carboxy-terminal fragment. Certain extrapituitary neoplasms such as bronchogenic carcinomas and others (p. 294) may also elaborate ACTH or ACTH-like substances. Release of ACTH in the anterior pituitary is effected by corticotropin-releasing factor (CRH) secreted into the pitui-

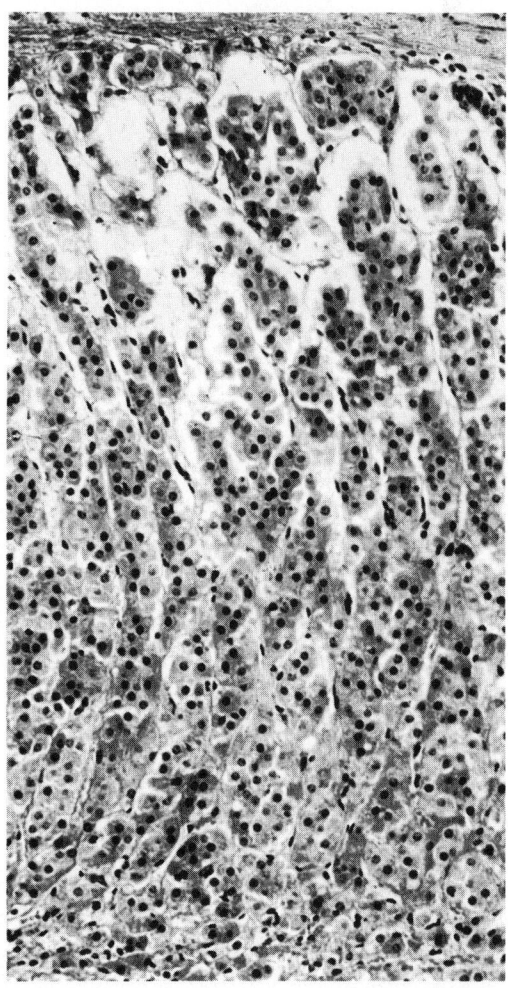

Figure 26–42. Human adrenal cortex in stress—complete lipid depletion. Cells of cortex are exclusively "dark" (compact) in type.

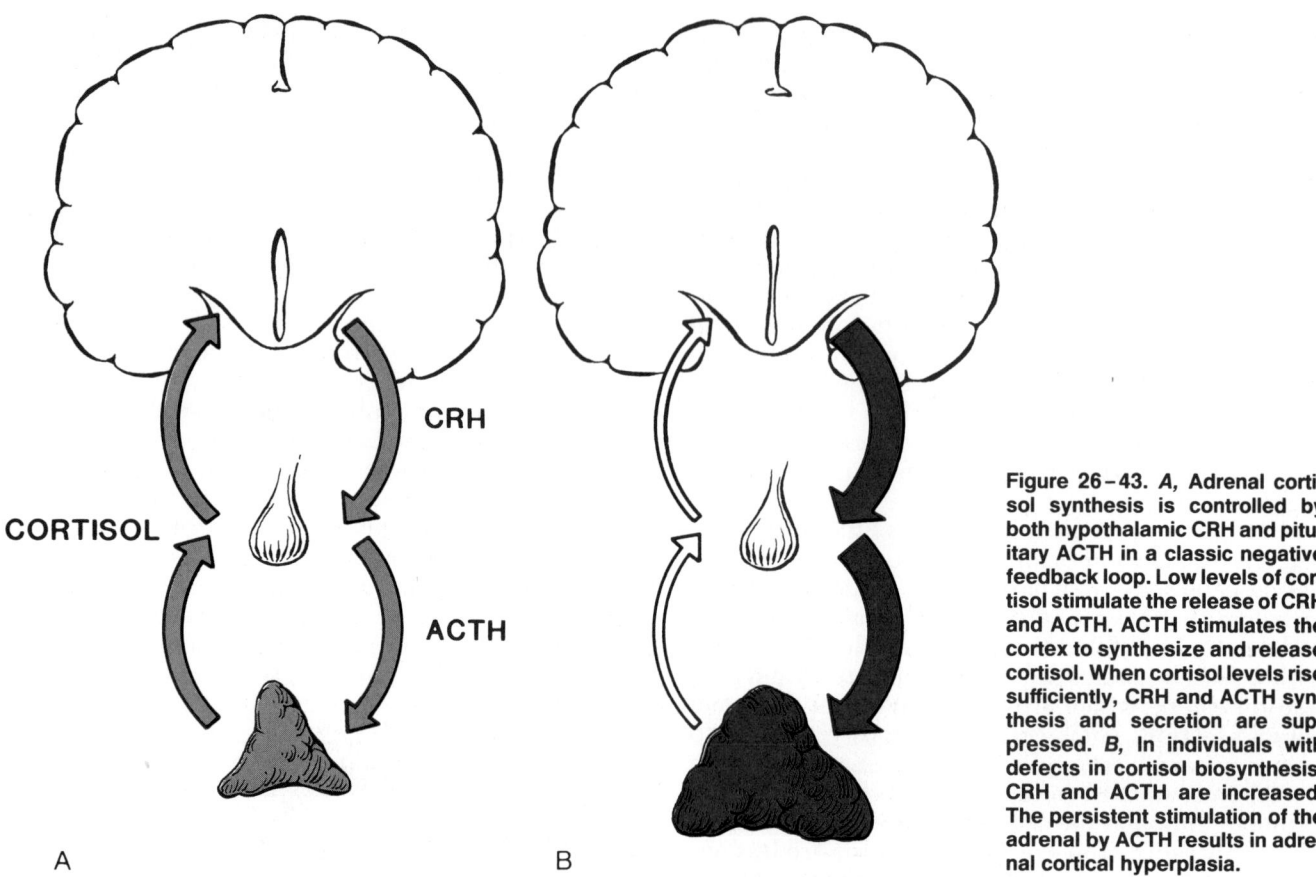

A   B

Figure 26-43. *A,* Adrenal cortisol synthesis is controlled by both hypothalamic CRH and pituitary ACTH in a classic negative feedback loop. Low levels of cortisol stimulate the release of CRH and ACTH. ACTH stimulates the cortex to synthesize and release cortisol. When cortisol levels rise sufficiently, CRH and ACTH synthesis and secretion are suppressed. *B,* In individuals with defects in cortisol biosynthesis, CRH and ACTH are increased. The persistent stimulation of the adrenal by ACTH results in adrenal cortical hyperplasia.

tary stalk–portal vascular system by the hypothalamus, as discussed earlier (Fig. 26–43).

The clinical manifestations of most adrenal disorders can be interpreted in terms of their impact on the production and hence the function of the adrenal steroids (Fig. 26–44).

Cortisol increases protein breakdown and nitrogen excretion. It increases the appetite and promotes the deposition of fat in the facial, cervical, and truncal regions. It increases hepatic gluconeogenesis by mobilization of glycogenic amino acids from bone, muscle, connective tissue, and elsewhere, and simultaneously retards the uptake of glucose by muscle cells. It impairs the antibacterial action of phagocytes and also stabilizes membranes of cells and lysosomes and impedes endothelial sticking of leukocytes and diapedesis. By unknown pathways it induces lysis of lymphoid tissues, particularly T cells. This steroid blocks inflammatory and immunologic responses and may predispose to serious infections. By its membrane actions, cortisol inhibits the migration of water into cells and tends to expand the extracellular fluid (ECF) volume. The consequences of these functions are readily observed in patients with disorders that increase or decrease the synthetic activity of the inner two zones of the adrenal cortex.

Aldosterone has two principal actions: (1) It is a major regulator of ECF volume, and (2) it is the major regulator of potassium metabolism. An excess of al-

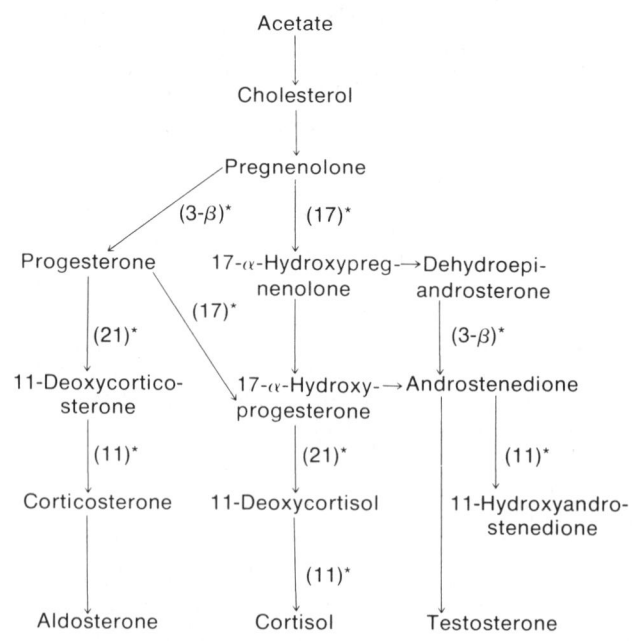

*Enzyme involved:

3-β = 3-β-hydroxysteroid dehydrogenase
11 = 11-hydroxylase
17 = 17-hydroxylase
21 = 21-hydroxylase

Figure 26-44. Pathways of steroid synthesis.

dosterone leads to sodium retention, loss of potassium, expansion of ECF volume, and hypertension. A deficiency induces the converse.[162]

Testosterone and the androgenic steroids accentuate male characteristics and inhibit female characteristics. Thus, excesses of androgens lead to virilization in the female, manifested principally by hirsutism, amenorrhea, clitoral enlargement, atrophy of the breasts and uterus, deepening of the voice, acne, and receding hairline. Masculinization is difficult to detect in the adult male but can lead to precocious puberty in male children.

PATHOLOGY

The pathology of the adrenal cortex can be divided essentially into three categories: (1) disorders that reduce the output of adrenal steroids, (2) disorders characterized by excess steroid production, and (3) lesions that have no functional effect. Inflammatory and regressive processes and, rarely, some tumors may destroy sufficient functioning cortical tissue to lead to adrenocortical hypofunction. Since the adrenal cortex has an enormous reserve of functional activity, the destructive processes, then, must wipe out most of the functioning cortical tissue before insufficiency develops. On the other hand, hyperplastic or neoplastic processes, by the production of increased amounts of steroids, lead to hyperfunction. To understand these syndromes, the biosynthesis of the steroids and the enzyme systems that play a role in this synthetic process must be known. In this area of pathology, as in so many others, function cannot be separated from structure.

DEVELOPMENTAL ANOMALIES

Adrenocortical hyperplasias are the most important of the congenital disorders. Because all cause striking alterations and increases in steroid synthesis resulting in adrenogenital syndromes, they will be discussed in the section on hyperadrenalism. Several rare anomalies remain to be considered here.

CONGENITAL ADRENAL HYPOPLASIA

Two distinct hypoplastic adrenal lesions occur in the newborn or young child.[163] In one, the small adrenals are seen in the anencephalic, usually stillborn fetus, and the term *anencephalic type* is applied. The gland consists only of a provisional or adult cortex and no fetal zone. In some cases of anencephaly and acardia, the adrenals may be absent. In the second, the *cytomegalic type,* an equally small adrenal (combined weight less than 1 gm) and a distinctive histologic pattern are found. The cortex consists of large, com-

pact eosinophilic cells several times the size of normal adrenal cells (cytomegaly). This cytomegalic type of adrenal hypoplasia should not be confused with cytomegalic inclusion disease, which is a very different condition. The cause of cytomegalic adrenal hypoplasia is still unknown, but is possibly familial with an X-linked or autosomal recessive pattern of inheritance. When it is recognized promptly and replacement steroid therapy is instituted, long survival is possible.[164]

ECTOPIC ADRENALS

Accessory adrenal tissue may be found retroperitoneally anywhere from the diaphragm to the pelvis. Although most ectopic adrenals consist entirely of cortex, some, particularly in the region of the celiac ganglion, may also contain medulla. Rests of adrenal cortex are also found in the subcapsular regions of the kidney, testis, and ovarian cortex. Occasionally, ectopic arenal cortical tissues may be found in the wall of an inguinal hernia sac, where they are sometimes called Marchand's rests. Ectopic adrenals may undergo hyperplasia in individuals with Cushing's disease and may rarely serve as the sites of origin of neoplasms.[165]

HYPOFUNCTION OF ADRENAL CORTEX (HYPOADRENALISM)

Adrenocortical hypofunction may be caused by any anatomic or metabolic lesion of the cortex that impairs the output of cortical steroids, or it may be secondary to a deficiency of ACTH (Table 26–6). The distinctive clinicoanatomic patterns of adrenocortical insufficiency are (1) primary chronic adrenocortical insufficiency (Addison's disease), (2) primary acute adrenocortical insufficiency (adrenal crisis), and (3) secondary adrenocortical insufficiency.

Table 26–6. Adrenocortical Insufficiency

PRIMARY INSUFFICIENCY	SECONDARY INSUFFICIENCY
Loss of Cortex	***Hypothalamic Pituitary Disease***
Idiopathic (autoimmune)	Neoplasm, infection
Infection (mycobacteria, fungi)	***Hypothalamic Pituitary Suppression***
Acute hemorrhagic necrosis	Long-term steroid administration
Amyloidosis	Steroid-producing neoplasms
Sarcoidosis, hemochromatosis	
Metastatic carcinoma	
Bilateral adrenalectomy	
Metabolic Failure in Hormone Production	
Congenital adrenal hyperplasia	
Drug-induced inhibition of cortical cell function	

PRIMARY CHRONIC ADRENOCORTICAL INSUFFICIENCY (ADDISON'S DISEASE)

Addison's disease is a rare condition caused by any chronic destructive process in the adrenal cortex. Clinical manifestations appear insidiously at any age, but usually not until at least 90% of the functioning cells have been destroyed.

ETIOLOGY AND PATHOGENESIS. Among the many possible origins of primary chronic adrenal insufficiency, only two—idiopathic adrenalitis/atrophy and tuberculosis—account for most cases. All the remaining potential causes, such as amyloidosis, metastatic cancer, sarcoidosis, and hemochromatosis, are extremely rare, and moreover, when present, may not destroy the functional reserve. Tuberculosis, usually secondary to pulmonary disease, was once the dominant cause of Addison's disease, but it now accounts for less than 25% of cases, having been supplanted by so-called idiopathic adrenalitis/atrophy. In some cases of Addison's disease, small atrophic adrenal glands are found. There may be a cortical infiltrate of lymphocytes, or merely marked cortical atrophy. Presumably the noninflammatory glands represent the end stage of a previously more active destructive process. There are many hints that this condition is autoimmune in origin.[166] Adrenal autoantibodies can be identified in 60 to 75% of patients, and their absence in tuberculous involvement suggests that they are not merely secondary phenomena but instead play a causal role.[126]

So-called *autoimmune Addison's disease* has occurred along with pernicious anemia, insulin-dependent diabetes mellitus, chronic mucocutaneous candidiasis, hypoparathyroidism, hypogonadism, and autoimmune thyroid disorders. This polyglandular autoimmune syndrome has been divided into two distinctive subsets, both of which occur as sporadic and familial diseases.[154] Type I is characterized by at least two of the triad of Addison's disease, hypoparathyroidism and mucocutaneous candidiasis. Other autoimmune disorders may or may not be present. The other, type II, also known as *Schmidt's syndrome*, is characterized by Addison's disease with autoimmune thyroid disease and/or insulin-dependent diabetes mellitus, but hypoparathyroidism or candidiasis is not present. This subset is clearly associated with HLA-A1 and B8 haplotypes, which is not true of the other subgroup. The autoimmune reactions in type I have been related to a defect in T-suppressor cell function.[155] In any event, although adrenocortical insufficiency may be the sole disorder in a patient, it is more often accompanied by some other form of endocrinopathy or systemic disease.[167]

MORPHOLOGY. A variety of anatomic changes may be present in the cortex, depending on the cause of the cortical destruction. When associated with a systemic disease (e.g., tuberculosis, histoplasmosis) or primary cancer elsewhere, specific histologic changes are present. With so-called idiopathic atrophy, the anatomic changes are less specific. The glands are small and irregularly contracted and may have a combined weight of as little as 2 to 3 gm. Indeed, it may be difficult to identify such glands in the periadrenal fat. The medulla is unaltered, but the cortex appears to have collapsed about it. There is focal or general absence of cortical cells, and such intervening cells as are present are usually large with an abundant eosinophilic cytoplasm and large irregular nuclei. A loose fibrous tissue, heavily infiltrated with lymphocytes, may occupy the areas between and about the islands of residual epithelial cells, or the cortical cells may be merely atrophic with little or no lymphocytic infiltrate (Fig. 26–45).

CLINICAL COURSE. Nearly all patients with primary chronic adrenocortical insufficiency insidiously and progressively develop weakness, fatigability, anorexia, nausea and vomiting, weight loss, hypotension, and hyperpigmentation of the skin and some-

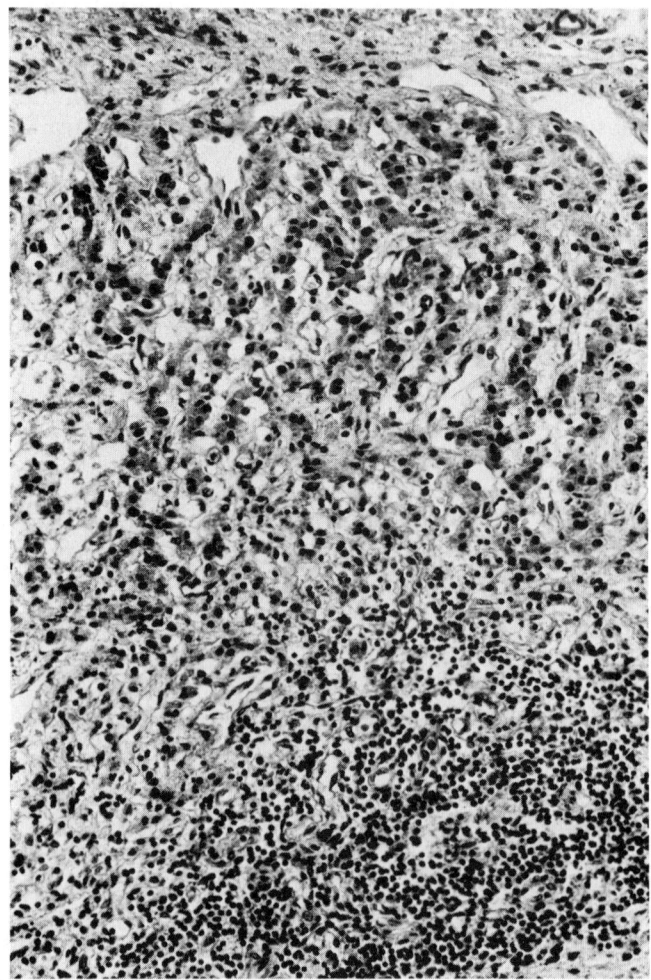

Figure 26–45. Autoimmune adrenalitis. In addition to loss of all but a subcapsular rim of cortical cells, there is an extensive mononuclear cell infiltrate.

times of the mucous membranes. Less consistently present are diarrhea, constipation, salt craving, and ill-defined abdominal pain that sometimes becomes sufficiently severe to mimic an "acute abdomen." The weakness may become so profound as to confine the individual to bed and even impair speech. Blood pressure may fall below 80/50 and induce syncope on sudden standing. The pigmentation appears as an accentuated sun tan on both exposed and unexposed skin, apparently as a consequence of loss of feedback inhibition of pituitary function and increased synthesis of both ACTH and POMC related peptides. Sometimes the mucous membranes develop brown-black patches. All the laboratory values may be within the normal range in mild expressions of Addison's disease. However, as the adrenocortical insufficiency becomes more marked, the serum levels of sodium, chloride, bicarbonate, and glucose fall, as well as the plasma cortisol and urinary steroid excretory products such as 17-ketosteroids and 17-hydroxycorticoids. The serum potassium is elevated largely because of aldosterone deficiency, contributing to the salt wasting, lowered circulating blood volume, and hypotension.

When the diagnosis of adrenocortical insufficiency has been established, it is necessary to determine whether it is primary (related to adrenal dysfunction), or secondary (having its origins in the anterior pituitary or hypothalamus). The skin pigmentation may be of value in the differential diagnosis, since it is not seen in secondary adrenocortical insufficiency. More direct and definitive is measurement of the plasma ACTH level or testing of the adrenocortical functional reserve by ACTH or CRH administration. Although Addison's disease is readily managed by steroids, death may occur when the disease is unrecognized because of acute adrenal insufficiency superimposed on the chronic condition, hyperkalemic cardiac arrhythmias, or a hypoglycemic cerebral crisis (addisonian crisis). Any of these complications may be precipitated by stress, including intercurrent illness in an already fragile metabolic state.

PRIMARY ACUTE ADRENOCORTICAL INSUFFICIENCY

Acute adrenocortical insufficiency may appear in three settings: It can occur (1) as a "crisis" in patients with chronic Addison's disease, precipitated by any form of stress that requires an immediate increase in steroid output from glands incapable of responding; (2) from too rapid withdrawal of steroids from patients whose adrenal glands have been suppressed by chronic steroid administration, or from failure to increase the level of administered steroids during stress in a bilaterally adrenalectomized patient; (3) in otherwise healthy individuals as the result of massive hemorrhagic destruction of the adrenals (adrenal apoplexy). In neonates, extensive adrenal hemorrhages may follow prolonged and difficult delivery associated with considerable trauma and hypoxia. The neonatal adrenal is particularly predisposed, since it is

large for the body size, it has little periadrenal fat, and its large medullary venous sinuses are fragile and have poorly developed muscular walls. Moreover, newborn infants are often deficient in prothrombin for at least several days after birth. In adults, the hemorrhagic destruction of the adrenals is most often related to a bacteremic infection, and in this setting it is called the Waterhouse-Friderichsen syndrome.

Waterhouse-Friderichsen Syndrome

This catastrophic cause of acute adrenocortical insufficiency is most often caused by meningococcemia.[168] Sometimes these patients have a preceding overt meningitis, but in other instances the first manifestations of the meningococcal infection relate to the meningococcemia. Less commonly, the Waterhouse-Friderichsen syndrome is seen with bacteremic infections due to pneumococci, staphylococci, or *Haemophilus influenzae*. Whatever the cause, the disease may be literally explosive. Soon after the onset of the infectious febrile reaction, systemic hemorrhagic manifestations appear. Showers of cutaneous petechiae and purpura can be seen in the skin. Presumably at the same time there are hemorrhages into the adrenals and other internal organs and surfaces. The patient may go into circulatory collapse and die within 24 hours. Blood cultures invariably disclose the causative organism. The organism can sometimes be cultured from hemorrhagic skin lesions that may become focally necrotic if the patient survives long enough. However, more often the skin lesions are related to the development of disseminated intravascular coagulation (DIC).

Anatomically, widespread petechiae, purpura, and hemorrhages are found throughout the body, particularly in the skin, mucous membranes, and serosal surfaces. The adrenals are likewise hemorrhagic and partially necrotic. In some children, the adrenals appear as virtual sacs of clotted blood (Fig. 26–46). The bleeding begins in the zona reticularis or the medulla and may be confined to these regions. More often, it extends throughout the medulla and cortex, at first penetrating between the cords of cortical cells toward the capsule and eventually engulfing these cells. Classically, even in those cases in which the entire adrenal appears to be replaced by blood clot, microscopic examination discloses nests and strands of preserved cortical cells. In essence, the morphologic changes are those of a bleeding diathesis, probably related to the development of DIC. Sometimes the endotoxemia causes an acute interstitial myocarditis.

The cause of the circulatory collapse appears to be predominantly the overwhelming bacteremia and toxemia; however, cardiac failure, arrhythmias, and the acute adrenocortical insufficiency may play significant contributory roles. When this condition is recognized promptly (within hours) and appropriately treated with massive doses of antibiotics and steroids, survival and complete recovery are possible. Uncommonly, the meningococcemia pursues a

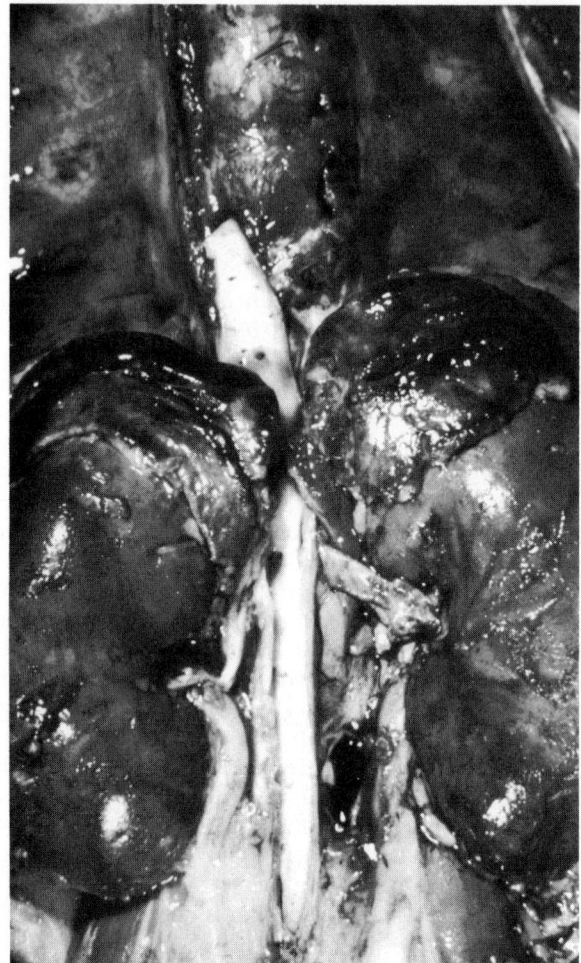

Figure 26–46. Waterhouse-Friderichsen syndrome in a child. The dark, hemorrhagic adrenal glands are distended with blood.

chronic or recurrent course and produces a vasculitis indistinguishable from hypersensitivity leukocytoclastic vasculitis (p. 573).

SECONDARY ADRENOCORTICAL INSUFFICIENCY

Any disorder of the hypothalamus and pituitary, such as metastatic cancer, infection, infarction, or irradiation, that reduces the output of ACTH will lead to a syndrome of hypoadrenalism having many similarities to Addison's disease. Analogously, prolonged administration of exogenous glucocorticoids will suppress the output of ACTH to induce a similar syndrome. *With secondary disease the hyperpigmentation of primary Addison's disease is lacking, since tropic hormones are low.* The manifestations also differ inasmuch as secondary hypoadrenalism is characterized by deficient cortisol and androgen output but normal or near-normal aldosterone synthesis. Thus, in adrenal insufficiency secondary to pituitary malfunction there is no marked hyponatremia and hyperkalemia, although a liberal intake of water may induce dilutional lowering of the serum sodium level.

ACTH deficiency may be selective, but in some instances it is only one part of panhypopituitarism, associated with multiple primary tropic hormone deficiencies. The differentiation of secondary disease from Addison's disease can be confirmed with demonstration of low levels of plasma ACTH in the former. In patients with primary disease, the destruction of the adrenal cortex does not permit a response to exogenously administered ACTH in the form of increased plasma levels of cortisol, whereas in those with secondary hypofunction, there is a prompt rise in plasma cortisol levels.

Depending on the extent of ACTH lack, the adrenals may be moderately to markedly reduced in size.[169] They may come to have a leaflike appearance and, indeed, be extremely difficult to find in the periadrenal fat. The cortex may be reduced to a thin ribbon having an unusually heavy fibrous capsule and scattered subcapsular cortical cells composed largely of zona glomerulosa. The medulla is unaffected (Fig. 26–47).

HYPERFUNCTION OF ADRENAL CORTEX (HYPERADRENALISM)

Just as there are three basic types of corticosteroids elaborated by the adrenal cortex-glucocorticoids, mineralocorticoids, and sex steroids—so there are three distinctive hyperadrenal clinical syndromes: (1) Cushing's syndrome, characterized by an excess of cortisol; (2) aldosteronism, with excess production of aldosterone; and (3) adrenogenital syndromes with an excess of sex steroids (Table 26–7). Mixed syndromes may also occur.[165]

CUSHING'S SYNDROME

Cushing's syndrome represents a distinctive constellation of clinical features associated with prolonged overproduction of cortisol. Clinical and laboratory findings include impaired glucose tolerance, overt diabetes (in approximately 20%), "moon facies," "buffalo hump," abdominal striae, and (in men) loss of libido, impotence, and oligospermia.[170] Some of these abnormalities, such as the obesity, deranged glucose

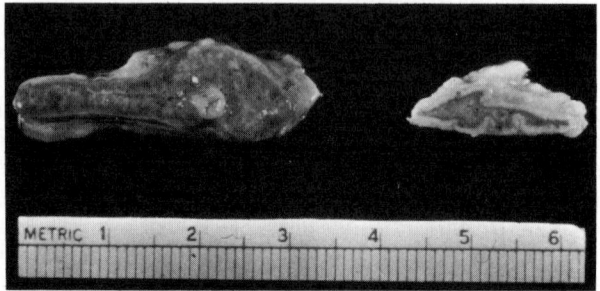

Figure 26–47. Cross section of an atrophic adrenal *(right)*. Compare with normal adrenal cross section *(left)*.

Table 26–7. Syndromes of Adrenocortical Hyperfunction

CLINICAL SYNDROME	ADRENAL PATHOLOGY
Cushing's Syndrome (Hyper-cortisolism)	
Pituitary-based (Cushing's disease)	Diffuse cortical hyperplasia with or without small areas of nodularity
Adrenal neoplasm	Adenoma and carcinoma equally common in adults; carcinoma more common in children
Ectopic production of ACTH or CRH	Diffuse cortical hyperplasia with or without small areas of nodularity
Multinodular adrenal disease	
Multinodular hyperplasia	Diffuse hyperplasia with nodules up to 3 cm
Microadenomatous dysplasia	Small pigmented nodules with atrophy of intervening cortex
Conn's Syndrome (Hyperal-dosteronism)	
Adrenal neoplasm	Adenoma (very common), carcinoma (rare)
Cortical hyperplasia	Hyperplasia of zona glomerulosa
Virilization (Adrenogenital Syndrome)	
Adrenal neoplasm	Adenoma (rare), carcinoma (common)
Enzymatic defects in cortisol biosynthesis (CAH)	Diffuse and nodular cortical hyperplasia
Feminization	
Adrenal neoplasm	Adenoma (rare), carcinoma (common)
Mixed Syndromes	Adenoma (rare), carcinoma (common)

metabolism, and mental disorders, are directly attributable to the increased glucocorticoids, but many have more complex origins. Excess production of testosterone probably contributes to the appearance of hirsutism and acne in women. The testosterone and the cortisol inhibition of pituitary release of gonadotropins accounts for menstrual irregularities. The bruisability and osteoporosis are poorly understood, but it is speculated that steroid suppression of collagen synthesis deprives subcutaneous vessels of their connective tissue support, and similar suppression of osteoid matrix formation underlies the osteoporosis. It suffices to note that, although Cushing's syndrome is characterized by overproduction of cortisol, other secondary derangements contribute to its full expression.

PATHOGENESIS. The term "Cushing's syndrome" encompasses four distinct pathogenetic syndromes, all marked by hypercortisolism (Figs. 26–48 and 26–49).[171]

1. *About 60 to 70% of cases can best be identified as "pituitary Cushing's syndrome,"* which was the first type to be described by Harvey Cushing.[172] Perhaps because he was a neurosurgeon, most of his patients had well-defined pituitary basophilic adenomas, presumably composed of corticotropin-secreting cells. On this account, Cushing's *syndrome* related to an adenoma (some would include all forms of the pituitary subgroup) is sometimes referred to as Cushing's *disease.* More recently, it has become evident that many patients with pituitary Cushing's syndrome do not have a discrete solitary adenoma, but instead have multiple corticotroph microadenomas. Moreover, a significant minority have no apparent pituitary lesion, giving rise to the concept of "hypothalamic Cushing's syndrome."[173] Not rigorously ruled out in some of the cases attributed to hypothalamic origins are undetected pituitary microadenomas. In any event, *pituitary Cushing's syndrome is characterized by bilateral adrenal hyperplasia and, in most cases, readily measurable elevated plasma levels of ACTH.* Sometimes, however, the elevations are very modest or indeed undetectable. No satisfactory explanation has been offered for the failure to find elevated levels of ACTH, but the possibilities have been raised of abnormal sensitivity of adrenocortical cells to even normal levels of ACTH, or loss of the normal circadian rhythm of ACTH secretion inducing unremitting stimulation of the adrenals by low levels of ACTH (Table 26–8).[174] *Whatever the nature of the pituitary dysfunction, the hypercortisolism can be suppressed by high doses of administered glucocorticoids such as dexamethasone, inducing a fall in levels of serum cortisol and its urinary excretory products (e.g., 17-hydroxycorticosteroids). This response serves as a clinical diagnostic test of the pituitary variant of Cushing's syndrome* (Table 26–8).

2. *About 20 to 25% of cases are best termed adrenal Cushing's syndrome.* The source of the excess cortisol is a functioning neoplasm of the adrenal cortex, more often an adenoma than a carcinoma in adults. Rarely, there is no well-defined neoplasm but only apparently autonomous nodular hyperplasia. Adrenocortical carcinomas tend to produce the most marked hypercortisolism. In those instances due to a unilateral neoplasm, the uninvolved adrenal cortex and that in the opposite gland undergo atrophy because of suppression of ACTH secretion. *Adrenal Cushing's syndrome is marked by low serum levels of ACTH and failure of administered high doses of glucocorticoid to suppress the levels of serum cortisol and its urinary excretory products* (Table 26–8).[5]

3. *About 10 to 15% of cases are "ectopic Cushing's syndrome,"* in which nonendocrine cancers elaborate ACTH or some biologically active fragment of the hormone.[175] Most commonly implicated are bronchogenic carcinoma (60%), malignant thymoma (15%), and pancreatic neoplasms, usually islet cell (10%), but a variety of other tumors have also been implicated. An elevated plasma level of ACTH is almost uniformly present. In passing, sensitive radioimmunoassays have documented that the great majority of bronchogenic carcinomas contain ACTH-like material, but in most instances it represents a nonbiologically active fragment of the large precursor peptide from which ACTH is cleaved.[176] Very rarely, a visceral cancer produces corticotropin-releasing factor or a closely related product as the basis for the ectopic Cushing's syndrome.[177] *As in the pituitary variant, the adrenal*

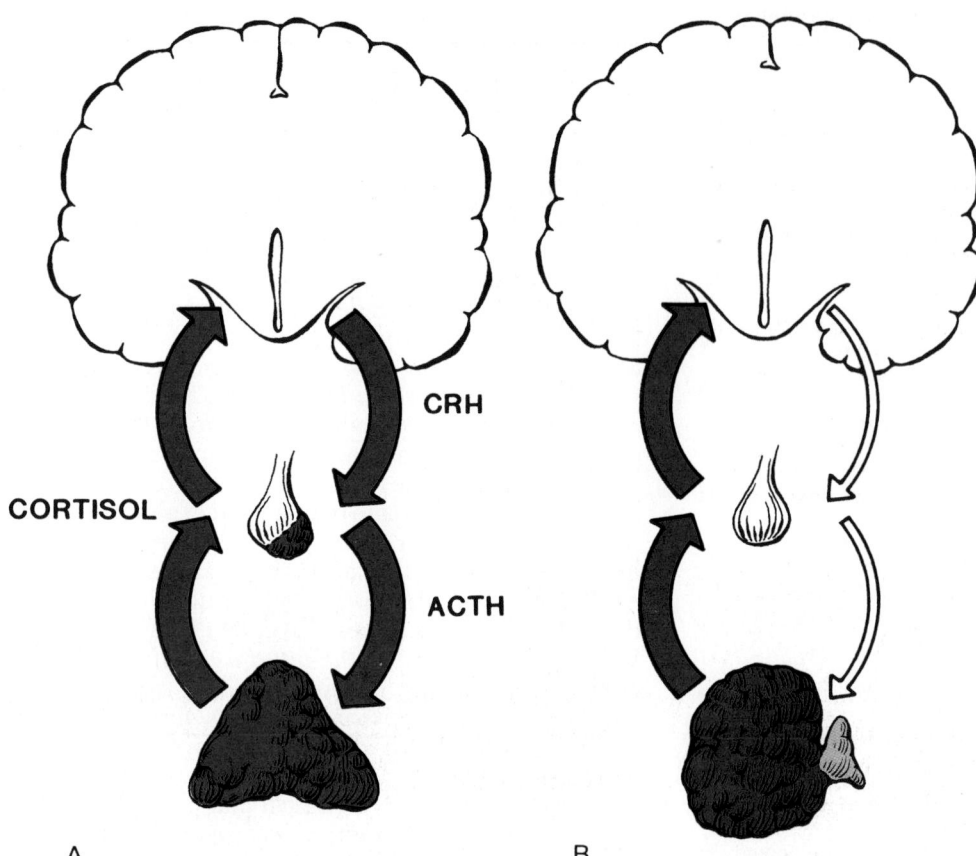

Figure 26–48. Cushing's syndrome *(A)* may be caused by a pituitary lesion producing excess ACTH or by a hypothalamic lesion producing excess CRH. In both instances both cortisol and ACTH levels are increased. *(B)* In individuals with Cushing's syndrome associated with a cortical adenoma, the ACTH levels are suppressed and the adjacent adrenal cortex is atrophic.

glands undergo bilateral cortical hyperplasia, but with ectopic disease the ACTH secretion cannot be suppressed by high doses of glucocorticoid, and so there is no fall in levels of serum cortisol or its excretory products.

Iatrogenic Cushing's syndrome may arise from the long-term use of glucocorticoids, for example, as an immunosuppressant in transplant recipients or in those having an autoimmune disorder. Should a patient receiving long-term steroids die, bilateral cortical atrophy related to suppression of ACTH secretion may be present.

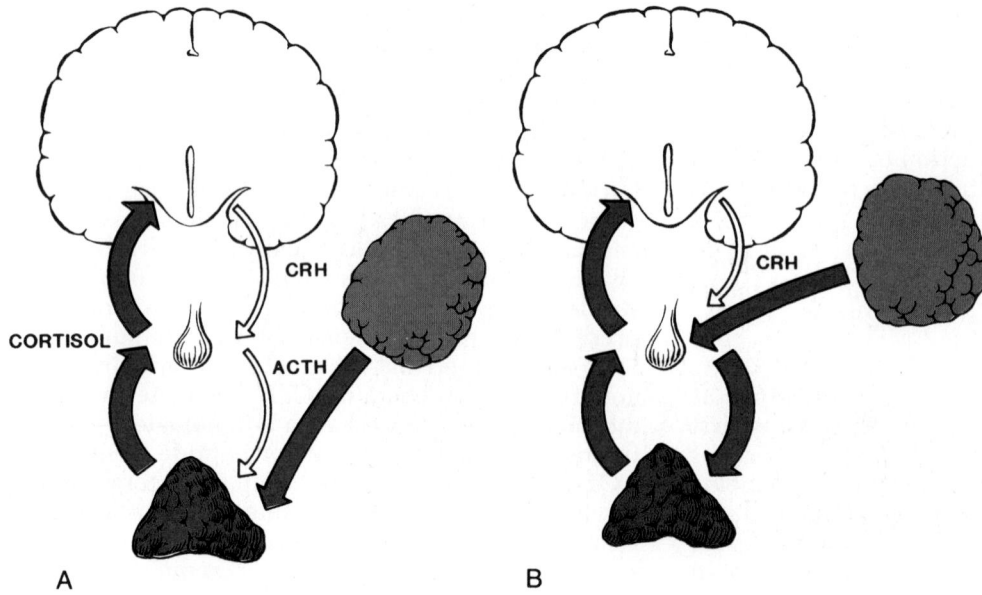

Figure 26–49. Cushing's syndrome may result from the direct stimulation of the adrenal cortex by an extra pituitary neoplasm producing ACTH ectopically *(A)*. Alternatively, Cushing's syndrome may result from ectopic production of CRH *(B)*.

Table 26-8. Differential Diagnosis of Cushing's Syndrome

	PLASMA CORTISOL	PLASMA ACTH	GLUCOCORTICOID RESPONSE TO DEXAMETHASONE	GLUCOCORTICOID RESPONSE TO ACTH
Diagnosis				
Normal	Normal rhythm	Normal rhythm	Decrease with low dose	Increase
Adrenal neoplasm	Normal or high No rhythm	Low	No decrease	No change
Pituitary-based hyperplasia	Normal or high No rhythm	High	Partial decrease with low dose Decrease with high dose	Increase
Ectopic ACTH syndrome	Normal or high No rhythm	High	No decrease	No change
Multinodular hyperplasia	Normal or high No rhythm	Variable	Variable	Variable, some increase
Microadenomatous dysplasia	Normal or high No rhythm	Low	No decrease	No change

Adapted from Page, D. L., et al.: Tumors of the Adrenal. A.F.I.P. (Fascicle 23). Washington, D.C., 1986.

MORPHOLOGY. The basic lesions of Cushing's syndrome are found in the pituitary and adrenal glands.

In the **pituitary,** irrespective of the cause of Cushing's syndrome, the increased levels of cortisol produce feedback effects on the nontumorous corticotrophs, referred to as **Crooke's hyaline degeneration of the basophils.** Infrequently, the corticotrophs in adenomas display the same changes.[178] The perinuclear or patchy foci of cytoplasm take on a basophilic hyalinization that obscures underlying details. Electron microscopy indicates that the hyalin is made up of aggregates of intermediate filaments.[179] The basis for this change is not known. In most cases of the pituitary variant of Cushing's syndrome, adenomas or microadenomas composed of densely granulated or sparsely granulated corticotrophs also are present, as discussed on page 1208. There are no adequate data on how often the anterior pituitary lacks any evidence of neoplasia (suggesting only a hypothalamic dysfunction) in cases that otherwise satisfy the criteria of the "pituitary" syndrome.[180]

The changes in the adrenals may take the form of (1) bilateral cortical hyperplasia, which is sometimes nodular, in response to ACTH of either pituitary or ectopic origin (Fig. 26-50); (2) adrenal cortical neoplasm, benign or malignant; (3) nodular hyperplasia; or (4) adrenocortical atrophy, associated with exogenous steroid administration.

Hyperplasia induced by ACTH is usually diffuse and bilateral but sometimes nodular. The extent of the hyperplasia is obviously a function of the duration and level of the ACTH excess.[169] It may be so subtle that the adrenals may be of normal weight. However, the term "normal" only depicts the subtlety of the hyperplasia compatible with excess elaboration of cortisol. With more marked ACTH production, as is encountered in some nonendocrine cancers, the adrenals are markedly enlarged, sometimes to a collective weight of 25 gm or more. Histologically, the cortex is widened and is composed predominantly of lipid-poor reticularis type cells.

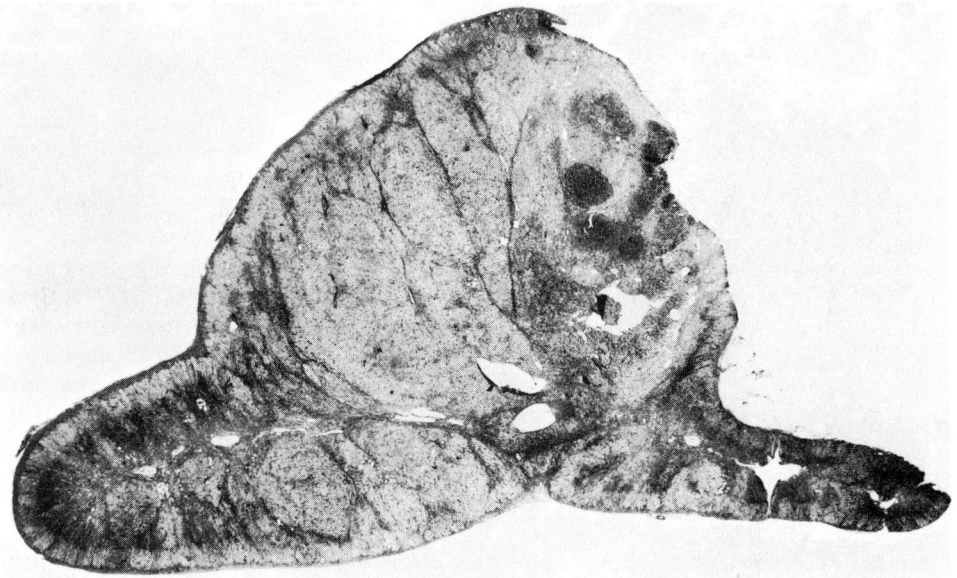

Figure 26-50. Irregular, nodular adenomatous hyperplasia of adrenal from a patient with Cushing's syndrome.

The term "multinodular" or "pseudoadenomatous hyperplasia" has been used to describe adrenals in which there is bilateral diffuse and nodular hyperplasia. Individual nodules may measure up to 3 cm in diameter and each adrenal may weigh up to 30 to 50 gm![181] This entity is unusual and appears to be related more to pituitary-dependent hyperplasia than to an autonomously functioning cortical neoplasm. Adrenal nodular dysplasia (microadenomatous adrenal) is a rare entity occurring predominantly in infancy and childhood.[182] The adrenals have a near-normal weight, but the cortex is studded with heavily pigmented nodules measuring 0.1 to 0.5 cm in diameter. The cortex between the nodules is typically atrophic, in contrast to the diffuse cortical hyperplasia that is present in multinodular hyperplasia. In these cases, ACTH is low or undetectable, indicating autonomous adrenal hyperfunction.

Adenomas or carcinomas of the adrenal cortex, as the source of the cortisol secretion, are not macroscopically distinctive from nonfunctioning adrenal neoplasms (Fig. 26–51). Histologically, the adenomas present varying admixtures of "clear" and "compact" cells similar to those of the normal zona fasciculata, but compact cells may predominate (Fig. 26–52). Similarly, the adrenal cancers in Cushing's syndrome display the same range in cellular pleomorphism encountered in nonfunctioning cancers (p. 1261).[165] The cortex adjacent to functional cortical neoplasms is atrophic, as is the contralateral cortex.

The distinction between a cortical adenoma and a cortical carcinoma associated with Cushing's disease may, at

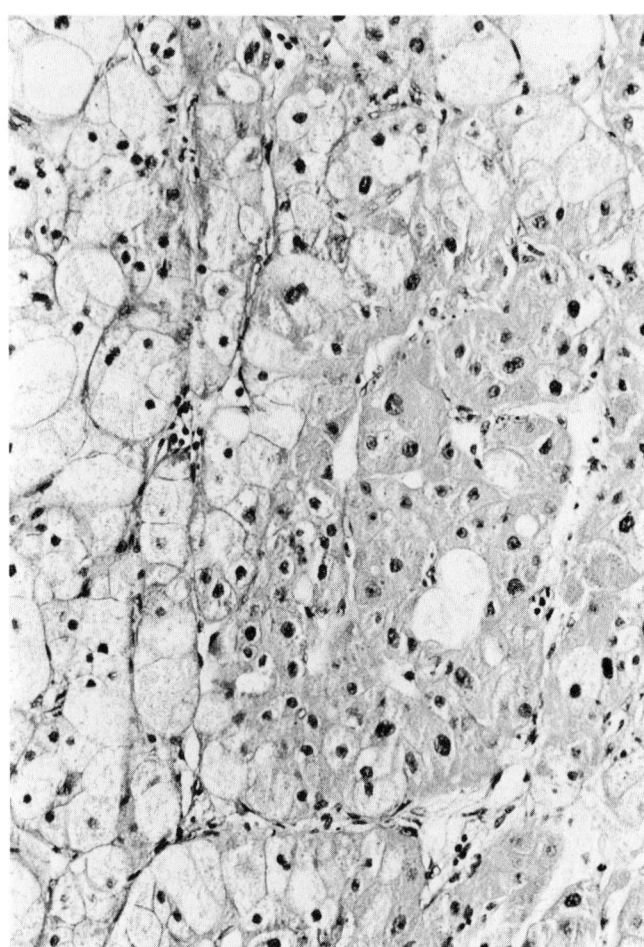

Figure 26–52. Cortical adenoma associated with Cushing's syndrome. Some of the cells are clear (lipid rich), while others contain little or no lipid (compact cells).

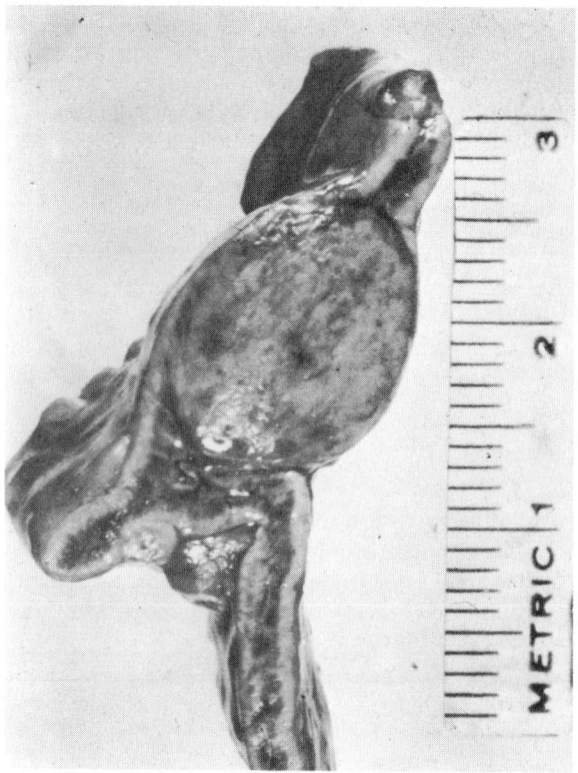

Figure 26–51. A small adrenal adenoma productive of Cushing's syndrome.

times, be extremely difficult. Most adenomas weigh 40 to 60 gm, whereas most carcinomas are more than 100 gm.[165] Carcinomas are more likely to show areas of necrosis, broad fibrous bands, nuclear anaplasia, and high mitotic activity.

The atrophic adrenal associated with exogenous steroid administration is a small, shrunken organ having a barely visible rim of cortex surrounding the medulla. The glands may be reduced to a collective weight of 3 to 6 gm. Histologically, it is evident that the atrophy affects primarily the inner two zones of the cortex, sparing to an extent the aldosterone-secreting zona glomerulosa, which is not dependent on ACTH. The severity of these atrophic changes is, of course, a function of the level of suppression of ACTH secretion and its duration.

CLINICAL COURSE. Cushing's syndrome generally appears in middle adult life, and is three times more common in women than in men. When it occurs in childhood, it is most often related to an adrenal neoplasm. The presenting features mentioned at the outset are more or less the same, irrespective of the underlying cause of the hypercortisolism. However, when related to ectopic production of ACTH by a nonadrenal cancer, the shortened clinical course may truncate the development of the complete syndrome. Most commonly observed under these circumstances are weakness, muscle wasting, hypokalemia, hyperglycemia, and (sometimes) hyperpigmentation. Truncal obesity, hirsutism, bruisability, and osteoporosis may not have time to develop.

It is beyond our scope to go into the diagnosis of Cushing's syndrome and the differential diagnosis of the various patterns. It is enough to note that the diagnosis rests mainly on the documentation of hypercortisolism, and the differential diagnosis on the cortisol-secretory response to an administered large dose of corticosteroid (dexamethasone) and on other testing procedures that are described in standard endocrinology texts (Table 26–8).

Brief mention should be made of *Nelson's syndrome*, encountered in patients with pituitary corticotroph adenomas who are bilaterally adrenalectomized because the primary pituitary tumor cannot be eradicated. Under these circumstances, progressive enlargement of the pituitary adenoma may follow as the feedback inhibition of cortisol is removed, often accompanied by intense pigmentation, presumably related to excess production of ACTH and POMC-derived peptides.

PRIMARY (LOW-RENIN) HYPERALDOSTERONISM — CONN'S SYNDROME

In 1955, Conn first described a patient with *hypertension, neuromuscular symptoms, renal potassium wasting, and elevated levels of aldosterone, all associated with an adrenocortical adenoma.*[183] These features were all attributable to the "autonomous" hypersecretion of aldosterone, which promotes sodium retention and potassium loss. The sodium retention leads to expansion of extracellular fluid volume and elevation of blood pressure, with concomitant suppression of renin production. In the absence of circulatory insufficiency, physiologic adjustments prevent progressive expansion of ECF volume and overt edema. The renal potassium wasting induces hypokalemia, hypokalemic alkalosis, and muscular weakness as well as other neuromuscular abnormalities and electrocardiographic changes.

Primary or autonomous hyperaldosteronism must be differentiated from secondary hyperaldosteronism. The latter refers to the secretion of aldosterone in response to increased levels of renin-angiotensin. Overproduction of renin by the kidneys occurs mainly with (1) any cause of renal ischemia, (2) any edematous state, and (3) a renin-producing neoplasm. Decreased renal blood flow and perfusion pressure occur, for example, in renal artery stenosis and malignant nephrosclerosis with its hyperplastic arteriolosclerosis. Secondary aldosteronism is also encoun-

tered in situations with developing edema as sodium is retained, e.g., in the nephrotic syndrome. Rarely, a renin-producing tumor or oral contraceptives induce elevated levels of aldosterone. A special form of secondary disease is known as *Bartter's syndrome*, characterized by renal juxtaglomerular cell hyperplasia, hyperreninemia, hyperaldosteronism, and hypokalemia. Inappropriately, blood pressure is often low, raising the issue of blood pressure refractoriness to the actions of renin-angiotensin.[184] Whatever its origins, *secondary aldosteronism is associated with sodium retention and potassium wasting, but notably with high renin output, in contrast to the low renin levels of primary aldosteronism.*

PATHOGENESIS. *There are three distinct clinicoanatomic forms of primary aldosteronism (Table 26–7; p. 1255).*[185] *The common form in adults is caused by an aldosterone-producing adenoma, accounting for 50 to 90% of cases.* Very rarely, an adrenal carcinoma induces this pattern of the condition. Second, particularly common in children but sometimes encountered in adults, is *idiopathic hyperaldosteronism*, sometimes called *congenital hyperaldosteronism* when the onset is in childhood owing to bilateral adrenal hyperplasia. This pattern has also been called pseudoprimary aldosteronism. Third and much more rare is a subset called *glucocorticoid-suppressible hyperaldosteronism.*[186] Little is known about the adrenal histologic findings in this third pattern, but adrenal hyperplasia has been observed in several surgical patients.

MORPHOLOGY. Aldosterone-secreting adenomas are usually less than 2 cm in diameter. For unknown reasons, the left adrenal gland is involved in slightly more than 60% of cases. Macroscopically, they are bright yellow and nonencapsulated.[187] Cytologically, these tumors show a mixture of cell types, including lipid-laden "clear" cells, compact cells, and hybrid forms. Electron microscopic studies indicate that cells of the adenoma sometimes possess lamellar mitochondrial cristae identical to those in glomerulosa cells, whereas others interestingly possess tubulovesicular cristae identical to those in the cells of the zona fasciculata. When cells of such adenomas are cultured in vitro, they produce, as would be expected of such a mixture of cell types, aldosterone and cortisol.[188]

In cases in which there is no adrenal neoplasm, most patients have bilateral hyperplasia of the zona glomerulosa, sometimes nodular. Very rarely, the hyperplasia is unilateral, as judged by measurement of the aldosterone levels in the venous efflux of each gland. Supporting this surprising finding is the fact that unilateral adrenalectomy is curative in these cases. The cells making up the diffuse and nodular hyperplasia are largely lipid-laden, with occasional masses of compact cells. The hyperplastic foci may extend into the inner cortex in tongue-like fashion. It is of interest that functional studies in vitro indicate that the hyperplastic cortical cells, as exemplified by those in the macronodules, synthesize not only aldosterone but also cortisol. Thus, the micronodular and the diffuse adrenal hyperplasia may reflect some unknown proliferative stimulus that induces simultaneously hyperfunction and hyperplasia of zona glomerulosa cells and glucocorticoid-secreting cells.

The adrenal carcinomas associated with hyperaldosteronism are not morphologically different from nonfunctioning neoplasms.[165]

CLINICAL COURSE. Primary aldosteronism is generally an insidious disease that can be diagnosed only by having a high index of suspicion. *Moderate hypertension (diastolic pressure 100 to 125 mmHg) is the predominant manifestation,* sometimes associated with mild frontal headaches, chronic fatigue, and weakness, but obviously these are quite nonspecific. It must be appreciated, however, that less than 1% of hypertensive individuals have primary aldosteronism. Rarely, there are more distinctive neuromuscular findings in the form of paralyses or tetany secondary to hypokalemia. *Only the laboratory evidence is diagnostic—hypernatremia, hypokalemia, alkalosis, excessive potassium excretion, low plasma renin activity, and (with adenomas) elevated nonsuppressible aldosterone levels.*[189]

Even more difficult than establishing the diagnosis of primary aldosteronism is determining its cause. The identification of an adenoma is both difficult and critical: difficult because the lesions are frequently small, and critical because the decision must be made about which side to operate on. Radioscans and CT scans may suffice, but in most instances adrenal vein catheterization (a difficult procedure with many limitations) is necessary to measure the levels of aldosterone in the venous efflux from each gland. When it is equally elevated in the effluent of both adrenal veins, bilateral hyperplasia is most likely. A number of other clinical approaches can be used and have been briefly characterized by Ganguly and colleagues.[190] It need only be emphasized in closing that recognition of an aldosterone-producing adenoma offers the satisfying opportunity of curing a form of hypertension.

ADRENAL VIRILISM AND CONGENITAL ADRENAL HYPERPLASIA (CAH)

Adrenal virilism, most readily recognized in females, can appear at any age with an androgen-secreting adenoma or carcinoma. These tumors are similar histologically to those associated with Cushing's syndrome; however, the virilizing adenomas tend to be considerably larger than adenomas associated with Cushing's syndrome and are more often highly pigmented.[165] Rarely, cortical neoplasms may also be associated with feminization.

A similar syndrome may arise as a metabolic disorder related to enzymatic defects in the biosynthesis of cortical steroids, leading to cortisol deficiency. The resultant increased levels of ACTH stimulate unaffected pathways of steroidogenesis, notably those involved in the production of adrenal androgens. Depending on the specific enzymatic defect and its effects on steroid biosynthesis, these inborn errors of metabolism may present as "pure" virilization, salt wasting, or "mixed" syndromes. As might be anticipated, the elevated levels of ACTH induce adrenocortical hyperplasia (Fig. 26–53).

At least eight distinctive clinical syndromes are encompassed under the term "congenital adrenal hyperplasia."[191] All are characterized by a congenital deficiency of a specific biosynthetic enzyme. All variants are autosomal recessive, and within a particular family all members inherit the same enzyme deficiency. *The clinical manifestations of each syndrome are determined largely by the functional properties of the steroid intermediates that build up because of the enzyme lack, and by the completeness of the enzyme block and resultant cortisol deficiency.* The understanding of the various syndromes is greatly facilitated by referral to the pathways of steroid synthesis shown in Figure 26–44, page 1250.

The most common deficiency involves 21-hydroxylase. Neonatal screening studies reveal an incidence of 1 in 5000 to 1 in 15,000 in white populations but a considerably higher incidence in certain Alaskan Eskimo tribes. Females with classic 21-hydroxylase deficiency are born with clitoral enlargement, fused labioscrotal folds, and a urogenital sinus that may be manifested as a phallic urethra. The internal reproductive organs, on the other hand, are normal. Males may show bilateral cryptorchidism and hypospadias. In approximately two thirds of individuals with this deficiency, aldosterone synthesis is also affected. These patients have the salt-wasting form of the disease with hyponatremia and hyperkalemia. Without treatment, this form of 21-hydroxylase deficiency may result in death in the first two weeks of life. A nonclassic form of 21-hydroxylase deficiency syndrome occurs in about 0.3% of the white population and in 3% of European Jews. Affected individuals develop signs of virilization during late childhood or at

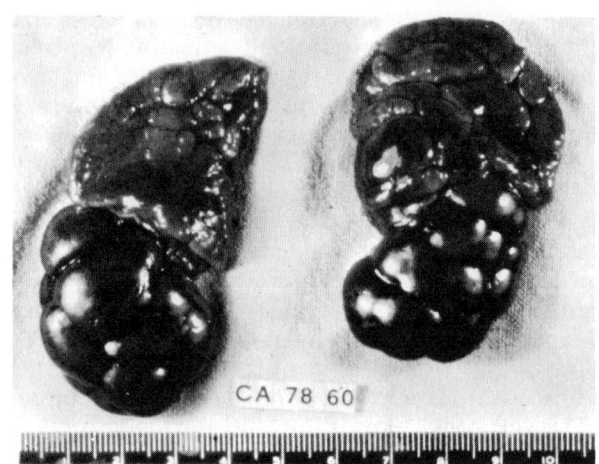

Figure 26–53. Adrenogenital syndrome in an infant with massive nodular enlargement of adrenals to the point at which they approximate the size of kidneys.

puberty, and this particular form of the syndrome may be an important cause of infertility. Occasional patients with the biochemical abnormality may remain asymptomatic.

21-Hydroxylase deficiency is a monogenic autosomal trait, closely linked to the HLA major histocompatibility complex on the short arm of chromosome 6. Salt wasting is associated with HLA-Bw 60, simple virilization with HLA-Bw 51, and nonclassic disease with HLA-B14;DR1.[192]

The second most common deficiency involves 11-hydroxylase and has an incidence of 1 in 100,000. A higher incidence has been noted in Israel, particularly among Moroccan Jews. In this disorder, 11-deoxycortisol is not converted to cortisol, and accumulated precursors are shunted into the androgen pathway. Additionally, deoxycorticosterone is not converted to corticosterone, and the increased levels lead to hypertension and hypokalemia. There is considerable heterogeneity in the 11-hydroxylase deficiency syndrome, and the disorder is not HLA linked.

The remaining forms of CAH are uncommon.[191] For example, a lack of 17-hydroxylase results in diminished secretion of glucocorticoids and sex steroids, and shunts steroidogenesis into the mineralocorticoid pathway. As a consequence, hypertension and hypokalemia develop, analogous to that in primary aldosteronism. The deficiency of androgens in males suppresses male differentiation and results in pseudohermaphroditism. Untreated females have sexual infantilism.

The adrenals in CAH are strikingly enlarged and may be 10 to 20 times normal weight (Fig. 26–53). The glands have a typical cerebriform configuration and are tan to brown on cross section. Microscopically, there is diffuse and nodular cortical hyperplasia. A deficiency of desmolase, an enzyme involved in the synthesis of testosterone, is characterized by extensively vacuolated cells with cholesterol clefts and giant cells, while other types of CAH are morphologically indistinguishable. Biochemical analysis of the adrenal glands revealing a specific enzyme deficiency is the only laboratory method to differentiate the other forms of CAH. On clinical grounds, differentiation depends on the specific manifestations, serum levels of the various steroids, and the urinary levels of their excretory products. When one of the virilizing syndromes is diagnosed early in life, the daily administration of glucocorticoids to suppress pituitary ACTH will stop the virilization, but reconstructive surgery may be necessary to correct abnormalities in the genitals.[193]

NONFUNCTIONAL CORTICAL NEOPLASMS

It is evident from preceding sections that the proliferative lesions of the adrenal cortex range from diffuse hyperplasia to nodular hyperplasia to benign and malignant tumors, and that all these proliferative proc-

esses may be associated with steroidogenesis. In addition, there are nonfunctional benign and malignant tumors of the adrenal cortex.[165]

Adrenal adenomas or *nodules* are found in about 2% of adult autopsies; very few produce excess steroids. For years, however, the controversy has persisted as to whether some apparently nonfunctional adenomas may produce hypertension in the nature of a "forme fruste" of Conn's syndrome.[194] Some workers have suggested that these adenoma-like lesions are a consequence rather than a cause of hypertension. In hypertensive individuals, adrenal capsular arteries and arterioles often undergo sclerosis, which may lead to areas of cortical atrophy. Nodules may develop as a form of compensatory hyperplasia in such a setting.[195] It is apparent that such nodules increase in frequency with age and that they are commonly multicentric and bilateral. Usually, nonfunctional adenomas are poorly encapsulated masses of yellow-orange adrenocortical tissue ranging up to 2.5 cm in diameter. Some nestle within the adrenal cortex, others appear to be within the medulla, and still others protrude under the capsule (see Fig. 26–51). Some may achieve a larger size and exhibit areas of hemorrhage, cystic degeneration, and calcification. The encapsulation may be poorly defined and may appear at places to be deficient. In contrast to functional adenomas, which are associated with atrophy of the adjacent cortex, the cortex adjacent to nonfunctional adenomas is of normal thickness.

Some *cortical carcinomas* may not be associated with the biosynthesis of steroid hormones. These tumors are highly malignant and usually large when discovered, many exceeding 20 cm in diameter.[165,196] On cut section they are predominantly yellow but frequently have hemorrhagic, cystic, and necrotic areas (Fig. 26–54). Many appear to be more or less encapsulated. Histologically, they range from lesions showing mild degrees of atypia to wildly anaplastic neoplasms composed of monstrous giant cells (Fig. 26–55). Between these extremes are found cancers with moderate degrees of anaplasia, some predominantly composed of spindle cells. Carcinomas, particularly those of bronchogenic origin, may metastasize to the adrenals, and they may be extremely difficult to differentiate from primary cortical carcinomas.

Adrenal cancers have a strong tendency to invade the adrenal vein, vena cava, and lymphatics. Metastases to regional and periaortic nodes are common, as well as distant hematogenous spread to the lungs and other viscera. Bone metastases are unusual.[196]

OTHER MASS LESIONS OF THE ADRENAL

Adrenal cysts are relatively uncommon lesions; however, with the use of sophisticated abdominal imaging techniques, the frequency of these lesions appears to be increasing.[165] The larger cysts may produce an abdominal mass and flank pain. It should be remem-

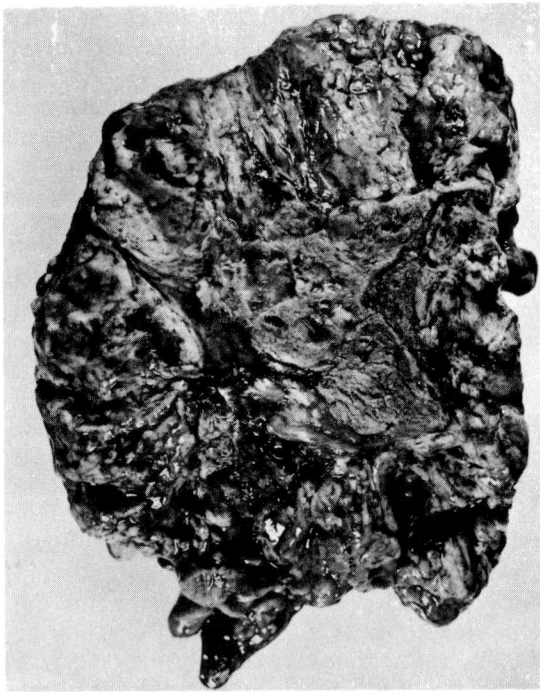

Figure 26–54. Adrenal carcinoma. Tumor is large, hemorrhagic, and necrotic. Very little viable tissue is present.

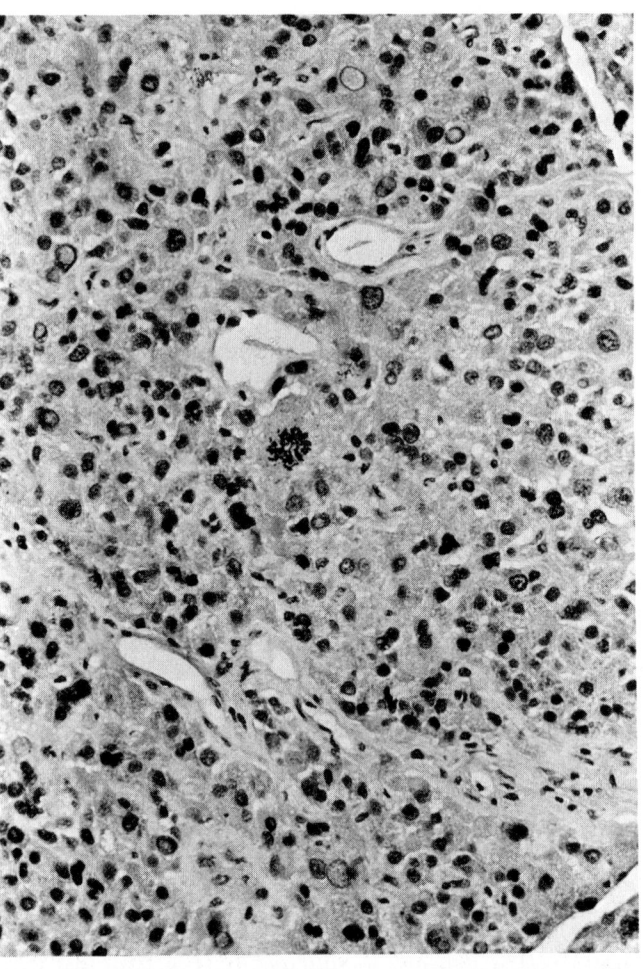

Figure 26–55. Adrenal carcinoma. In contrast to the cytologic uniformity of adenomas, adrenal carcinomas frequently show nuclear atypia and numerous mitoses.

bered that both cortical and medullary neoplasms may undergo necrosis and cystic degeneration and may present as "nonfunctional" cysts. Other types of adrenal cysts may be of parasitic origin (predominantly echinococcal). So-called pseudocysts of the adrenal most probably develop initially as lymphangioendothelial type cysts.

The adrenal myelolipoma is an unusual lesio composed of mature fat and hematopoietic cells.[1] Although most of these lesions represent incident findings, occasional myelolipomas may reach massive proportions. Foci of myelolipomatous change may be seen in cortical tumors and in adrenals with cortical hyperplasia.

ADRENAL MEDULLA

PHEOCHROMOCYTOMA
NEUROBLASTOMA AND GAN-
  GLIONEUROMA
TUMORS OF EXTRA-ADRENAL
  PARAGANGLIA

NORMAL

A unified concept of the paraganglionic system encompassing the adrenal medulla (intra-adrenal para-

ganglia) and the widely distributed paraganglia associated with branchiomeric, intravagal, paravertebral, and visceral autonomic ganglia was first proposed almost a century ago.[197] The branchiomeric and intravagal paraganglia are associated with the parasympathetic nervous system, while the paravertebral and visceral paraganglia are associated with the sympathetic nervous system.[198] With the exceptions of the adrenal medulla and the organ of Zuckerkandl, the locations of sympathetic paraganglia are variable and they are not known by individual names. Paraganglionic cells are typical neuroendocrine cells that synthesize and secrete both catecholamines and a variety of regulatory peptides. The adrenal medulla is the body's major source of epinephrine. Embryologically, it is derived from cells of the primitive neuroectoderm (neural crest) that differentiate to form adrenal medullary chromaffin cells (pheochromocytes), autonomic ganglion cells, and extra-adrenal paraganglionic cells.

The chromaffin cell is characterized by intracytoplasmic granules that appear brown after fixation in dichromate fixatives (e.g., Zenker's) as the result of oxidation and polymerization of the catecholamines stored in the granules. The granules are sharply delineated and electron dense. Epinephrine is the major catecholamine, but also present is norepinephrine, the ratio of these two in the normal state being 5–6 : 1. During the biosynthesis of catecholamines, tyrosine is converted to DOPA and dopamine in the cytosol of the chromaffin cell.[199] Dopamine then enters the secretory granules for conversion into norepinephrine. The latter exits the granule and is converted into epinephrine in the cytosol; epinephrine then re-enters the granule for storage prior to its release into the peripheral circulation. The principal metabolites of the catecholamines are metanephrine, normetanephrine, vanillylmandelic acid (VMA), and homovanillic acid (HVA). Catecholamines are the most abundant constituent of the chromaffin granule on a molar basis but account for only 20% of the dry weight. Other components of the granule include ATP and other nucleotides, chromogranin proteins, neuropeptides, ascorbate, glycosaminoglycans, and enzymes that function in the production and processing of granule constituents.[199]

PATHOLOGY

The most significant disorders arising in the medulla are neoplasms. Rarely, hyperplasia of chromaffin cells may also occur. As can be surmised from the cell types indigenous to the medulla, the tumors include pheochromocytomas, neuroblastomas, and ganglioneuromas.

PHEOCHROMOCYTOMA

This neoplasm is uncommon but of great interest because it usually induces hypertension related to the production of catecholamines. Most of these neoplasms secrete a combination of norepinephrine and epinephrine, predominantly the former. Occasionally a tumor elaborates only one or the other, and a rare tumor produces only dopamine and is not associated with hypertension.[200] Occasionally, pheochromocytomas may also produce ACTH and may be associated with Cushing's syndrome. *Although only about 0.1 to 0.2% of hypertensive persons have an underlying pheochromocytoma,* resection of the neoplasm produces a dramatic cure of what is otherwise a potentially lethal disease. The tumors occur at any age, with a peak incidence in the fourth and fifth decades.[201]

These neoplasms may arise wherever chromaffin cells are found. By convention, those arising in the medulla are called pheochromocytomas (intra-adrenal paragangliomas), whereas neoplasms arising elsewhere are referred to collectively as extra-adrenal paragangliomas.[198] About 97% of all these tumors are situated within the abdomen, and 70 to 90% within the adrenals, more often on the right than the left. In about 10 to 20% of cases there are bilateral neoplasms. The remainder of intra-abdominal tumors, sometimes several tumors, are located along the aorta, often at the bifurcation in the region of the organ of Zuckerkandl.[202] Infrequently, a solitary neoplasm or multiple neoplasms arise in thoracic paravertebral ganglia, in the wall of the urinary bladder, or in other sites harboring paraganglionic cells. Although only about 5% of adrenal tumors are malignant, extra-adrenal paragangliomas arising in the retroperitoneum are more likely to pursue a malignant course.[203]

Approximately 80 to 90% of pheochromocytomas occur sporadically, and most often these are solitary neoplasms.[165] The remaining 10 to 20% are associated with four, possibly more, familial syndromes, some of which are characterized by multiple endocrine neoplasms (MEN) and other lesions (p. 1007). The concurrence of multiple endocrine tumors raises the possibility of some widespread stimulus to neoplasia in the family of neuroendocrine cells. In some of the familial syndromes, the tumors may arise outside the adrenals.

One hereditary pattern is simply familial predisposition to pheochromocytomas, transmitted as an autosomal dominant trait. The tumors tend to arise in childhood and are multiple or bilateral in more than half the cases. *A second familial syndrome is MEN type IIa, also known as Sipple's syndrome.*[16] Briefly, it comprises the concurrence of pheochromocytoma, medullary carcinoma of the thyroid, and parathyroid hyperplasia or adenoma. This condition is thought to be transmitted as an autosomal dominant trait. It is distinguished from the simple familial syndrome by a later onset (fourth decade of life), a greater tendency to intermittent or paroxysmal hypertension, fewer pheochromocytomas outside the adrenals, and a strong tendency (60 to 100%) to bilaterality. *A third familial subgroup, designated MEN type IIb* (or sometimes MEN III) is characterized by pheochromocytoma, medullary carcinoma of the thyroid, and mucosal neuromas, but rarely parathyroid lesions; there may be an associated marfanoid habitus. This subset is also transmitted as an autosomal dominant trait, but the two MEN syndromes are distinct. *A fourth familial syndrome is the association of pheochromocytoma with von Recklinghausen's neurofibromatosis and other neurocutaneous phakomatosis syndromes.* A less well defined subset is marked by the association of pheochromocytoma with von Hippel–Lindau disease. It is evident that the pheochromocytoma is a "social animal" that may live a solitary life, but often consorts with a number of interesting conditions.

MORPHOLOGY. It should be noted at the outset that, in the MEN syndromes, the adrenal medullary involvement may take the form of diffuse or nodular hyperplasia, sometimes accompanied by one or more discrete neoplasms.[203] There is the suggestion, then, that the pheochromocytomas may arise through a sequence of diffuse hyperplasia, nodular hyperplasia, and, finally, an overt neoplasm in this setting. Significantly, occasional intramedullary tumors are associated with diffuse hyperplasia in the opposite medulla. Rarely, diffuse hyperplasia of the medulla may occur in a sporadic fashion and may be associated with signs and symptoms of catecholamine hypersecretion.[204]

The average weight of a pheochromocytoma is 100 gm, but variations from just over 1 gm to almost 4000 gm have been recorded.[165] The larger tumors are well demarcated by either connective tissue or compressed cortical or medullary tissue. Fibrous trabeculae, richly vascularized, pass

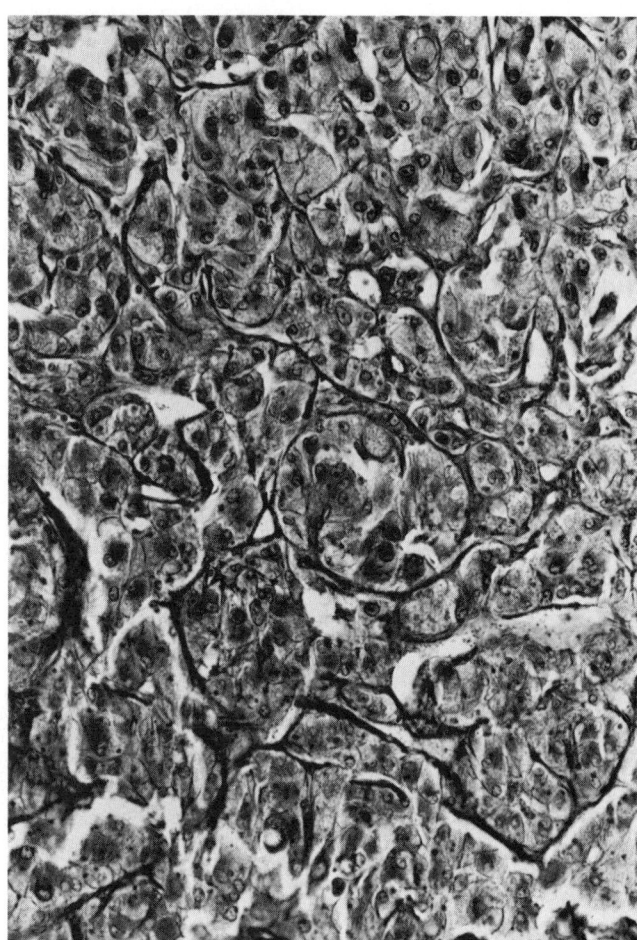

Figure 26–57. Pheochromocytoma. The cells are typically arranged in nests resembling those normally found in the medulla.

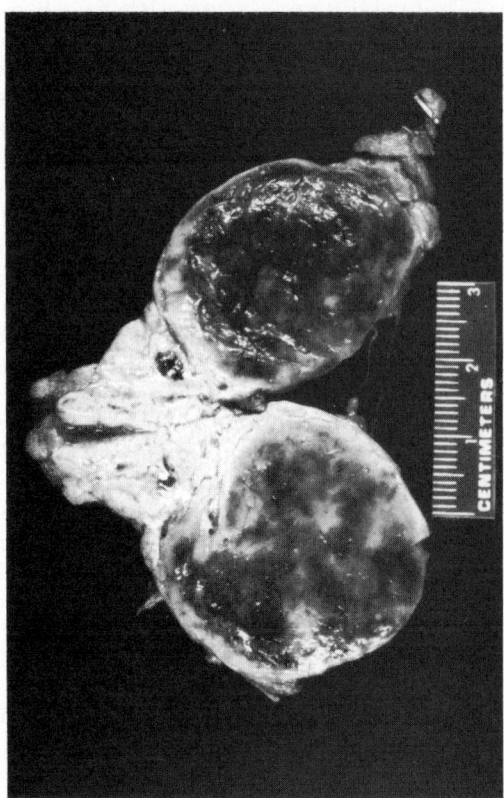

Figure 26–56. Pheochromocytoma of adrenal. Tumor is well encapsulated and exhibits hemorrhagic dark mottling.

into the tumor and produce a lobular pattern. In many tumors, remnants of the adrenal gland can be seen, stretched over the surface or attached at one pole. On section, the cut surface has a pale gray or light brown color, and areas of hemorrhage, necrosis, or cyst formation can be observed, particularly in the larger lesions (Fig. 26–56). When a suitable dichromate fixative (Zenker's or Helly's solution) is used, the tumor turns brown-black owing to oxidation of stored catecholamines—hence, the term chromaffin.

The cytologic patterns in pheochromocytomas are quite variable.[205] The tumors are composed of mature-appearing chromaffin cells, which possess an abundant basophilic cytoplasm in which secretory granules can be seen in dichromate-fixed tissue or with the electron microscope (Figs. 26–57 and 26–58).[206] The functional activity of a neoplasm cannot be judged by the abundance of granules, since actively secreting neoplasms may contain few granules. The cells are arranged either in large trabeculae, punctuated by thin-walled sinusoids often lined by the tumor cells themselves, or in small alveoli, each surrounded by fibrovascular stroma derived from the tumor capsule (Fig. 26–57). Various patterns may be found in any one tumor. Cellular and

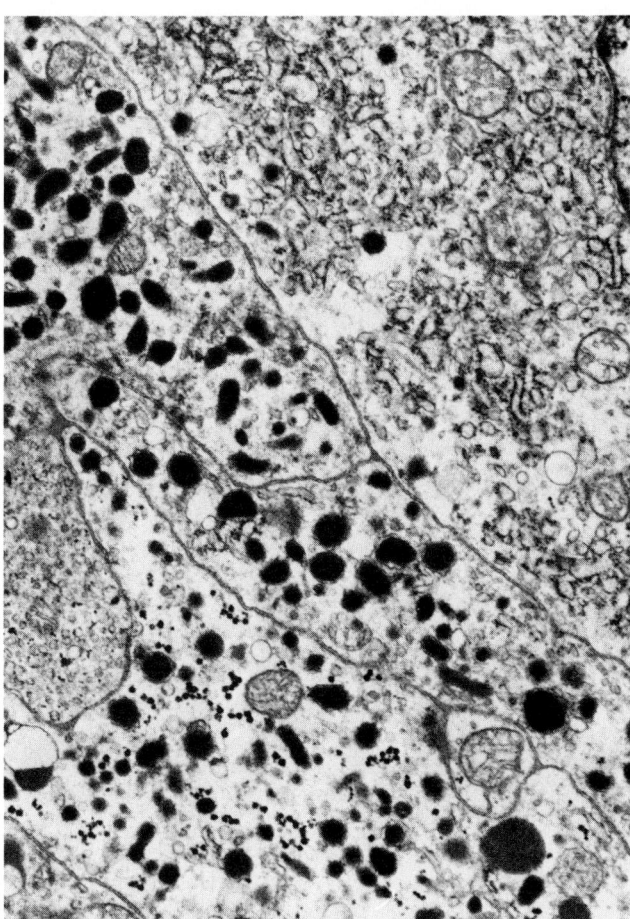

Figure 26–58. Electron micrograph of pheochromocytoma. This tumor contains membrane-bound secretory granules in which catecholamines are stored (30,000 ×).

nuclear pleomorphism is often noted, especially in the alveolar group of lesions, and giant and bizarre cells are commonly seen. Mitotic figures are rare; moreover, they do not imply malignancy. Occasionally, tumor cells can be found lying in the capillaries or sinusoids. This is not indicative of malignancy, since it has been observed in tumors that are benign in their behavior.

Since malignant and benign pheochromocytomas may have an identical histologic appearance, the diagnosis of malignancy cannot be made by histologic examination of the tumor alone.[165] The general histologic criteria of malignancy, when applied to pheochromocytomas, lead only to misdiagnosis. The only absolute criterion upon which a diagnosis of malignancy can be made is the presence of distant metastases. Overall, about 5 to 10% of pheochromocytomas are malignant, with higher frequencies in some of the familial syndromes. Metastases occur most frequently in the related lymph nodes, liver, lungs, and bones, and survival after diagnosis rarely exceeds three years.

An important part of the evaluation of these neoplasms is the demonstration of increased levels of catecholamines in fresh tissue samples of the neoplasms by either biochemical or histochemical techniques.

CLINICAL COURSE. *The dominant clinical feature in patients with pheochromocytoma is hypertension.*[207] About one third of patients have sustained hypertension rendered distinctive by paroxysmal attacks. In another third, the hypertension is intermittent; in the remaining third, it is sustained without paroxysms. The paroxysms may be precipitated by emotional stress, exercise, changes in posture, and palpation in the region of the tumor. The elevations of pressure are induced by the sudden release of catecholamines that may acutely precipitate congestive heart failure, pulmonary edema, myocardial infarction, ventricular fibrillation, cerebral hemorrhage, and even death. The cardiac complications are attributable, at least in some instances, to what has been called *catecholamine cardiomyopathy* or *catecholamine heart muscle disease.* The myocardial changes have been attributed to ischemic damage secondary to the catecholamine-induced vasomotor constriction of the myocardial circulation. Histologically, there are focal areas of myocytolysis and occasionally myofiber necrosis and interstitial fibrosis, sometimes with mononuclear inflammatory infiltrates.[208] These cardiac lesions are often superimposed upon hypertensive changes or alterations incident to coronary artery disease, and so, not surprisingly, patients may have anginal chest pain.

The sudden release of catecholamines may provoke a number of other symptoms during or following the paroxysm, including headache, sweating, anxiety or fear of impending death, tremor, fatigue, nausea and vomiting, abdominal pain, and visual disturbances. These findings in combination with the hypertension, particularly if paroxysmal, point strongly to the appropriate diagnosis.[201] Measurement of urinary catecholamines and their metabolites, principally metanephrine and VMA, is necessary to confirm it.[209] Other diagnostic approaches are also available, such as a hypertensive response to provocative agents, a hypotensive response to adrenergic blockade, plasma assays of catecholamines, and others. The clonidine suppression test has been found to be particularly valuable in confirming the diagnosis in atypical cases. This agent suppresses plasma catecholamines in normal individuals but has little or no effect in patients with pheochromocytomas.[210] Even when excess production of catecholamines has been established, the questions arise: Is it caused by a neoplasm and where is it located? You recall that multiple neoplasms may be present or, uncommonly, there may be no neoplasm, only hyperplastic lesions in chromaffin tissues. Most tumors are larger than 2 cm and can be detected reliably by CT or MRI scan. In some instances, however, resort must be made to intra-abdominal exploration.

NEUROBLASTOMA AND GANGLIONEUROMA

Neuroblastoma is one of the common solid tumors of childhood and ranks along with Wilms' tumor, glioma, and leukemia as a principal form of cancer in the young. Approximately 80% of these neoplasms are found in children under the age of five years, 35% are found in those under two years, and only infrequently are they encountered in those over the age of 15 years. Small neoplasms found in infancy have been reported as in situ neuroblastomas, and these lesions have a high frequency of apparent spontaneous regression.[165]

Although neuroblastomas may occur sporadically, there is evidence that at least some cases have a heredofamilial basis. In such cases the neoplasms may involve both adrenals or have multiple primary extra-adrenal sites of origin. Transmission by an autosomal dominant gene has been proposed, with reports of several pairs of twins being affected and of another family in which each of four siblings had a neuroblastoma.

MORPHOLOGY. Arising from neural crest cells, neuroblastomas are found in a variety of locations. The adrenal medulla or cells in the adjacent retroperitoneal tissues account for 50 to 80% of neoplasms in most reported series. The second most common location is within the posterior mediastinum, usually in paravertebral sites. The remaining neoplasms occur in the pelvis, in the cervical region, in the lower abdominal sympathetic chain, rarely within the posterior cranial fossa, or in other locations.

Macroscopically, the growths are lobular and soft. The cut surface is red-gray, and areas of hemorrhage, necrosis, and cyst formation may be obvious as the tumor increases in size. Calcification is common, and this can help in radiologic localization.

Histologically, the cells are small with hyperchromatic nuclei and are arranged in solid sheets in the most undifferentiated forms of the tumor. On occasion, these tumors may be difficult to distinguish from lymphomas and other small cell tumors of infancy and childhood.[211] In characteristic lesions, rosettes (Homer-Wright pseudorosettes) are formed in which the tumor cells occupy the periphery and young nerve fibrils grow into the center of each rosette (Fig. 26–59). Careful search of the tumor will often reveal this type of structure.

Metastases develop rapidly and widely. In addition to local infiltration and lymph node metastases, there is a pronounced tendency to spread by the blood to liver, lungs, and bones. Extensive bony metastases, particularly to the skull and orbit, with exophthalmos is referred to clinically as **Hutchinson-type neuroblastoma.** Widespread dissemination throughout the bone marrow is another distinctive pattern of spread. Many putative cases of Ewing's tumor of bone represent metastases from an occult primary neuroblastoma. Massive metastasis to the liver is designated the **Pepper-type syndrome.**

Differentiation to varying levels may be found in neuroblastomas. The tumor may completely differentiate to a **ganglioneuroma** composed of a fibrous and Schwann cell–rich stromal background through which ganglion cells are scattered (Fig 26–60). All intermediate levels of differ-

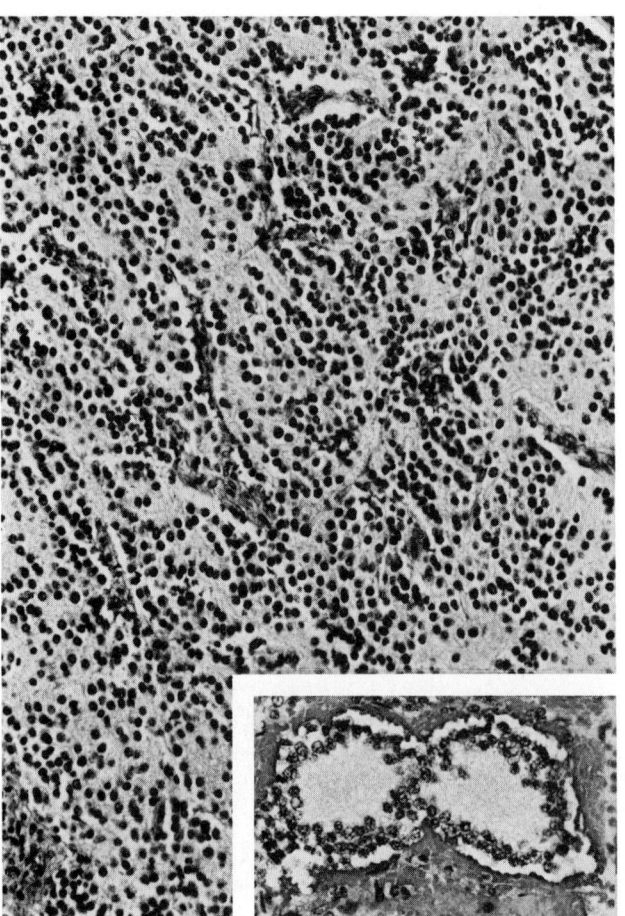

Figure 26–59. Adrenal neuroblastoma. This tumor is composed of small cells embedded in a finely fibrillar matrix. Homer-Wright pseudorosettes are illustrated in the inset.

entiation between the pure neuroblastoma and the pure ganglioneuroma may be encountered, and such lesions are referred to as **ganglioneuroblastomas.** Prognosis is dependent in part on the extent of differentiation within the tumors.[212] This has permitted the grouping of patients into those with favorable (94% two-year survival) and unfavorable (39% two-year survival) prognosis.[213]

CLINICAL COURSE. The manifestations of neuroblastomas are extremely varied but usually relate to the rapid growth of the neoplasm. Loss of energy and weight, pallor, abdominal protrusion, irregular fever, and generalized malaise are all probably related to rapid tumor growth and resorption of necrotic tumor products. Also, more than 90% of neuroblastomas elaborate catecholamines, principally norepinephrine.[161] Thus, assays of catecholamine metabolites provide diagnostic screening techniques as well as supportive diagnostic evidence. In contrast to patients with pheochromocytomas, however, hypertension is rare. Metastases may be located in bizarre locations, such as in the orbit or scalp, subcutaneously, and elsewhere. Sometimes the appearance of these

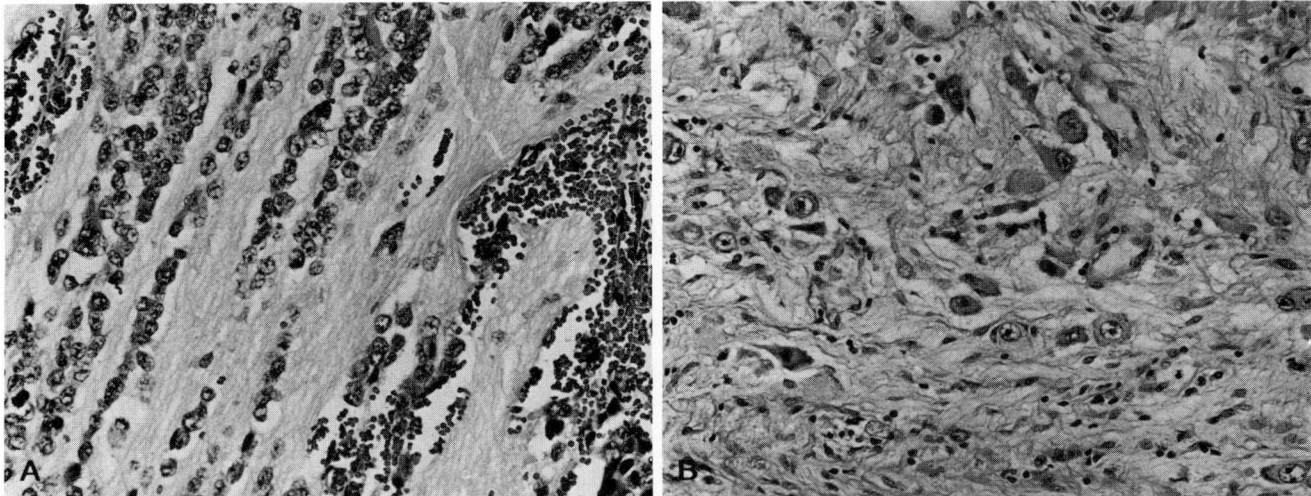

Figure 26–60. *A,* Differentiating neuroblastoma (ganglioneuroblastoma). Differentiating neuroblastoma cells show nuclear enlargement and enlargement of nucleoli. *B,* Ganglioneuroma. The tumor cells are almost identical to normal ganglion cells. The stroma consists of spindle-shaped Schwann cells.

metastases precedes the identification of the primary neoplasm. Indeed, except for patients in whom the neoplasm is present at or before birth, metastatic dissemination is already present in approximately three fourths of patients by the time diagnosis is made.[214]

Prognosis in patients with neuroblastomas is dependent upon a number of variables, the most important of which are the age at diagnosis and the stage of the disease. Stage I disease refers to tumors that are confined to the structure or organ of origin, while stage II refers to tumors that extend beyond the site of origin but do not cross the midline. Stage III tumors have crossed the midline and may or may not have associated lymph node involvement. In stage IV disease, there is evidence of metastatic disease involving the skeleton, viscera, or distant nodal sites. A special prognostic category is referred to as *IVs.*[214] These individuals have evidence of microscopic metastatic disease involving skin, liver, or bone marrow. Most patients with *IVs* disease are less than one year old and have an excellent prognosis, in contrast to patients with stage IV disease. High levels of ferritin and neuron-specific enolase have an adverse effect on prognosis, while high ratios of urinary vanillylmandelic acid to homovanillic acid are associated with a more favorable prognosis.[214] Inhibition of sheep erythrocyte rosettes after incubation of the patient's T cells in autologous plasma, on the other hand, is associated with a poor prognosis.

Cytogenetic studies have revealed a characteristic 1P deletion in tumor cells, homogeneously staining regions and double minute chromosomes.[215] There also appears to be a direct relationship between the number of N-myc oncogene copy numbers and biologic aggressiveness.[216] In contrast to the high N-myc copies in patients with stage IV disease, those individuals with stage IVs have normal levels of N-myc.

TUMORS OF EXTRA-ADRENAL PARAGANGLIA

The branchiomeric and intravagal paraganglionic system (parasympathetic paraganglia) is represented principally by the carotid, vagal, and jugulotympanic bodies, although similar collections of cells have been demonstrated in other sites such as the paranasal or laryngeal regions.[198] Some of these paraganglia respond to variations in the blood oxygen and carbon dioxide tensions and may be concerned with the regulation of respiration. Because of this property of chemoreception, some authors have referred to tumors arising from the parasympathetic paraganglia as chemodectomas. The currently preferred terminology for these lesions, however, is paraganglioma, with an indication of the anatomic site of origin (e.g., carotid body paraganglioma).

Neoplasms arising from the aorticosympathetic paraganglia have been referred to as extra-adrenal pheochromocytomas because of their histologic, biochemical, and clinical similarities to adrenal pheochromocytomas. However, the preferred terminology is simply paraganglioma, with an indication of the anatomic site of origin (e.g., paraganglioma of the organ of Zuckerkandl). In contrast, branchiomeric and intravagal paragangliomas are rarely associated with signs and symptoms of catecholamine hypersecretion.

Paragangliomas are rare, occur in both males and females, and are found mostly in persons between the ages of 30 and 60 years. They usually occur singly and sporadically, but may be familial and, in some cases, multiple.[217] They can be of great clinical importance, because depending on their site of origin, 10 to 50% of these tumors may recur following resection, and overall about 10% metastasize widely to cause death.[218]

Typically, these tumors range from 1 to 6 cm in diameter and are firm and tan-red. Despite encapsulation, well-developed or scant, they are often densely adherent to adjacent vessels and difficult to excise. Histologically, most are composed of well-differentiated neuroendocrine cells disposed in small clusters (zellballen) or cords separated by prominent fibrovascular stroma. Distinctive within the cells in most tumors are dark neurosecretory granules that contain catecholamines. Sometimes the cells are spindle-shaped. Mitoses are usually infrequent, but occasional tumors are overtly anaplastic and pleomorphic and contain numerous mitoses. Although most paragangliomas are benign, about 10% of those in the carotid body and as many as 50 to 60% of those arising elsewhere recur following resection. The more obviously anaplastic lesions may disseminate widely and cause death.[219]

THYMUS

THYMIC AGENESIS AND
   HYPOPLASIA
THYMIC HYPERPLASIA
TUMORS
Thymomas

NORMAL

Once an organ buried in obscurity within the mediastinum, the thymus has risen to a star role in cell-mediated immunity, as detailed in Chapter 5. Here our interest centers on the disorders of the gland itself.

The thymus is embryologically derived from the third and, inconstantly, the fourth pair of pharyngeal pouches along with the lower pair of parathyroid glands. Not surprisingly, one or two parathyroids occasionally become enclosed within the thymic capsule, an aberrance that may plague the parathyroid surgeon. At birth, the thymus weighs 10 to 35 gm and continues to grow in size until puberty, when it achieves a maximum weight of 20 to 50 gm. Thereafter it undergoes progressive atrophy to little more than 5 to 15 gm in the elderly. This age-related involution is accompanied by replacement of the thymic parenchyma by fibrofatty tissue. The rate of thymic growth in the child and involution in the adult is extremely variable, and so it is difficult to determine weight appropriate for age.[220]

The fully developed thymus is pyramid-shaped, encapsulated, and composed of two fused lobes. Fibrous extensions of the capsule divide each lobe into numerous lobules. The thymus is divided into cortical and medullary regions that consist of epithelial cells and lymphocytes. The lymphocytes include immature (cortical) and mature (medullary) T cells, small numbers of B lymphocytes, and occasional macrophages. The cortical lymphocytes contain terminal deoxynucleotidyl transferase (TdT) and express reactivities with the monoclonal antibodies OKT6 and OKT10.[221] Medullary thymocytes, on the other hand, exhibit the phenotypic characteristics of peripheral blood T lymphocytes.[222]

Scattered so-called myoid cells having many ultrastructural and antigenic similarities to skeletal muscle are also present, which may bear on the pathogenesis of myasthenia gravis. In addition, other cell types are present in scant numbers, as pointed out in the discussion of tumors. The epithelial cells, which often have long extended reticular processes (not readily seen in usual sections), form a loose meshwork within the lobule. Ultrastructural studies of these cells reveal unmistakable evidence of their epithelial nature, such as desmosomes, cytoplasmic tonofilaments, and the many other organelles found in epithelial cells. The large spaces between the epithelial cells are filled with lymphocytes. The division of each lobule into a dark cortex and a lighter medulla is the consequence of a greater concentration of lymphocytes in the cortex as compared with the medulla.[223]

The epithelial cells within the medulla are aggregated into concentric onionskin layers of keratinized cells, creating Hassall's corpuscles (Fig. 26–61). Two special histologic features should be emphasized. Well-developed B-cell lymphoid follicles with germinal centers are, on the whole, rare in the normal thymus. When numerous and prominent, they must be construed as pathologic and, as will be seen, are associated with a number of extrathymic disorders, notably myasthenia gravis.[223] Similarly, plasma cells are usually absent in the normal thymus and, when present, imply some inflammatory change.

There is no longer doubt that the thymus in its role as a central lymphoid organ in cell-mediated immunity is a secretory organ. Several factors have been described, each by an independent group of investigators, and variously named thymic humoral factor,

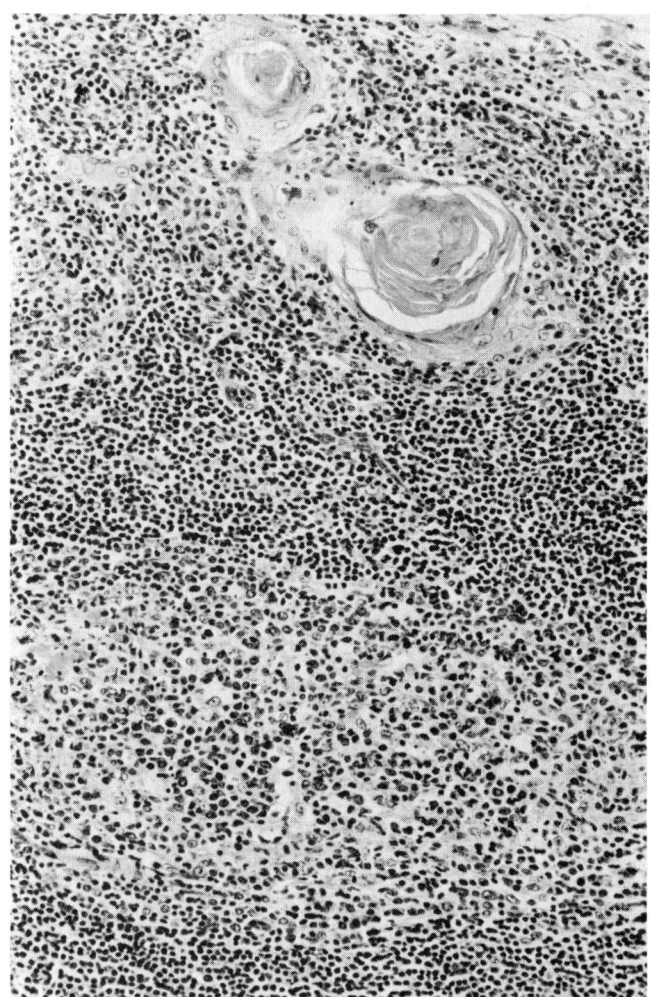

Figure 26–61. Thymic lymphoid hyperplasia in a patient with myasthenia gravis. A Hassall's corpuscle is seen in the upper portion of the illustration. A lymphoid follicle is present in the lower portion.

thymosin, thymin, and thymopoietin.[224] These factors, when added to cultures of thymic cells, can induce the appearance of T-cell differentiation markers, activate cyclic GMP or AMP, and induce mature T-cell functions. Whether all factors are truly distinctive is unclear at present, but without doubt one or more is necessary to maintain immunologic competence of peripheral T cells. Also, the thymus plays a role in the maintenance of tolerance and immune surveillance.

PATHOLOGY

Morphologic lesions in the thymus are associated with a diversity of conditions ranging from immunologic to hematologic to neoplastic.[223] Fortunately, thymic lesions are limited in type and can be adequately encompassed within the following categories: (1) thymic agenesis and hypoplasia, (2) thymic hyperplasia, and (3) thymic neoplasia. The thymic changes associated with myasthenia gravis are referred to on page 1367.

THYMIC AGENESIS AND HYPOPLASIA

Despite the difficulty in estimating thymic size normal for age, there can be no doubt that under certain clinical circumstances the thymus is abnormally small, either as a congenital defect or as an acquired disorder. Congenital thymic agenesis or hypoplasia is encountered in neonates and infants having one of the following immunodeficiency states: reticular dysgenesis, combined immunodeficiency disease, ataxia-telangiectasia, or the DiGeorge or Nezelof syndrome.[225] In the DiGeorge syndrome there is concomitant agenesis of the parathyroid glands. The thymus in these conditions may be completely absent and represented by a fibrous pad; or sometimes it is composed of scattered lymphocytes embedded within fibrous tissue. All these immunodeficiencies are marked by severe T-cell and variable B-cell defects.

Acquired hypoplasia is a normal consequence of aging, but it may appear suddenly in the young as a result of severe stress, malnutrition, irradiation, or following the use of cytotoxic drugs or glucocorticoids. The histologic changes depend on the time elapsed since the insult. Early there are focal areas of cytolysis that may later be replaced by fibrosis. Undoubtedly, previous episodes of cytolysis are masked by subsequent regeneration, but some foci of fibrosis may persist.

THYMIC HYPERPLASIA

Thymic hyperplasia is exceedingly difficult to evaluate by the weight of the gland, because of the wide range of normal variation at every age level. *The most reliable criterion of hyperplasia is the appearance of lymphoid follicles within the thymus*, creating what is referred to as *thymic follicular hyperplasia*. Although true hyperplasia has been said to develop in the absence of follicle formation, the burden of proof is on those who make such a diagnosis.[223]

In follicular hyperplasia, the gland may be normal in weight but more often is slightly enlarged. Germinal centers are located principally in the medulla, resulting in compression and atrophy of the cortex. The lymphoid follicles are not different from those encountered in lymph nodes and contain both dendritic reticular cells and B lymphocytes (Fig. 26–61).[220] Although follicular hyperplasia may occur in chronic inflammatory and immunologic states, it is most frequently encountered in myasthenia gravis. In this condition, autoantibodies to acetylcholine receptors at neuromuscular junctions impair transmission of motor impulses; it is thought that in some cases thymic hyperplasia with the formation of activated lymphoid follicles of B cells participates in the formation of the autoantibodies. Thymic lymphoid hyperplasia is seen in up to 85% of all patients with myasthenia gravis, but the frequency of this change decreases in individuals greater than 60 years of age. Follicular thymic hyperplasia is not exclusive to myasthenia gravis; it is also found in Graves' disease, Addison's disease, systemic lupus erythematosus, scleroderma, and rheumatoid arthritis (all having autoimmune origins) and in a variety of liver diseases that are less clearly immunologic in origin. The relationship between the thymic changes and these disorders is unclear. Rarely, germinal centers are found in the thymic glands of patients who have died of apparently unrelated disease.

TUMORS

In the past, there has been a practice of referring to all tumors primary in the thymus as thymomas. As pointed out, the basic cell type in the thymus is the epithelial cell; the rich component of lymphocytes is viewed as a migratory population that comes and goes. Thus, *the term thymoma is restricted to neoplasms of thymic epithelial cells, regardless of the abundance or scarcity of the lymphoid component.* Both non-Hodgkin's lymphomas and Hodgkin's disease may also arise in the thymus and may stimulate the proliferation of epithelial cells. The latter was once called a granulomatous thymoma but now is recognized as Hodgkin's disease arising in the thymus. Similarly, there are many other cell types scattered through the thymus, e.g., neuroendocrine cells, fibroblasts, myoid cells, vascular elements, and sometimes sequestered rests of germ cells. A tumor composed of neuroendocrine cells is thus termed a thymic carcinoid or neuroendocrine tumor. Germ cell tumors may also arise within the thymus.[223]

THYMOMAS

True thymomas are rare but nonetheless are one of the most common mediastinal neoplasms, particularly those in the anterosuperior mediastinum.[223] They are intriguing tumors because of their associations with a number of systemic disorders, notably myasthenia gravis, hematologic cytopenias, hypogammaglobulinemia, various collagen-vascular diseases, and nonthymic cancers, to mention only the more frequent. Most thymomas (about 90%) are benign and are composed of epithelial cells having a rich or scant lymphocytic infiltration. The lymphocytes are not neoplastic and possess markers of normal cortical thymocytes (TdT,OKT6,OKT10 positive), medullary (mature) thymocytes, or admixtures of cortical and medullary lymphocytes. About 10% of thymomas are malignant. Most of these cancers have little or no cytologic

atypia, and so the determination of malignancy rests entirely on demonstration of invasion beyond the capsule or, more certainly, on the presence of lymphatic or hematogenous spread.[220] *Rarities are cytologically malignant tumors segregated from malignant thymomas by being called thymic carcinomas.*[170] Thymic carcinomas, like all cancers, have the potential of aggressive local spread and metastasis. They have been well reviewed and because of their great rarity will not be discussed further.[226]

MORPHOLOGY. Whatever their histology, all thymomas are lobulated, apparently encapsulated gray, yellow, or tan masses ranging in size from 1 to 20 cm in greatest diameter. They vary from soft to firm and frequently have focal areas of hemorrhage. Cysts are often present in the larger lesions, sometimes many centimeters in diameter.

The epithelial component of benign thymomas displays a range of patterns (Fig. 26–62). In most neoplasms the epithelial cells resemble those of the normal cortex, having poorly defined cytoplasmic outlines and being visible mostly as large, pale, vesicular nuclei. Their epithelial nature can be documented by the ultrastructural identification of desmosomes and tonofilaments and by the demonstration of keratin proteins by immunohistochemistry.[227] The next most frequent variant has oval to spindle-shaped epithelial cells. Uncommonly, the cells assume a sarcomatoid appearance, readily mistaken for some form of mesenchymal neoplasm. The term "spindle-cell thymoma" is sometimes applied to this morphologic pattern; it tends to be associated with hypogammaglobulinemia and red cell aplasia but not with myasthenia gravis.[228] Other epithelial patterns include reticular and squamoid differentiation. In the latter, there may be formation of Hassall's corpuscles, but they are not frequent.

All epithelial variants have a rich or scant lymphocytic infiltrate of T cells (Fig 26–62). Some of the lymphocytes appear to be activated and are therefore larger than T cells in the peripheral circulation. The abundance of mitotic figures in these cells suggests some form of mitogenic stimulus. Neoplasms having a great many lymphocytes are readily mistaken histologically for non-Hodgkin's lymphoma. Careful scrutiny, however, will disclose epithelial cells or, in a few cases, Hassall's corpuscles indicative of a thymic epithelial origin.

As noted, malignant thymomas, as distinct from benign thymomas and thymic carcinomas, can be differentiated only by penetration and extension beyond the fibrous capsule or more distant spread.

In contrast to epithelial thymomas, thymic neuroendocrine tumors are characterized by the presence of cells with varying numbers of peptide hormone–containing secretory granules. Most of these tumors resemble carcinoid tumors, but some may appear identical to oat cell carcinomas of the lung. Indeed, it may be impossible to differentiate a primary thymic oat cell carcinoma from a mediastinal metastasis of a bronchogenic oat cell carcinoma. Thymic endocrine tumors may produce a variety of ectopic hormones, including ACTH.

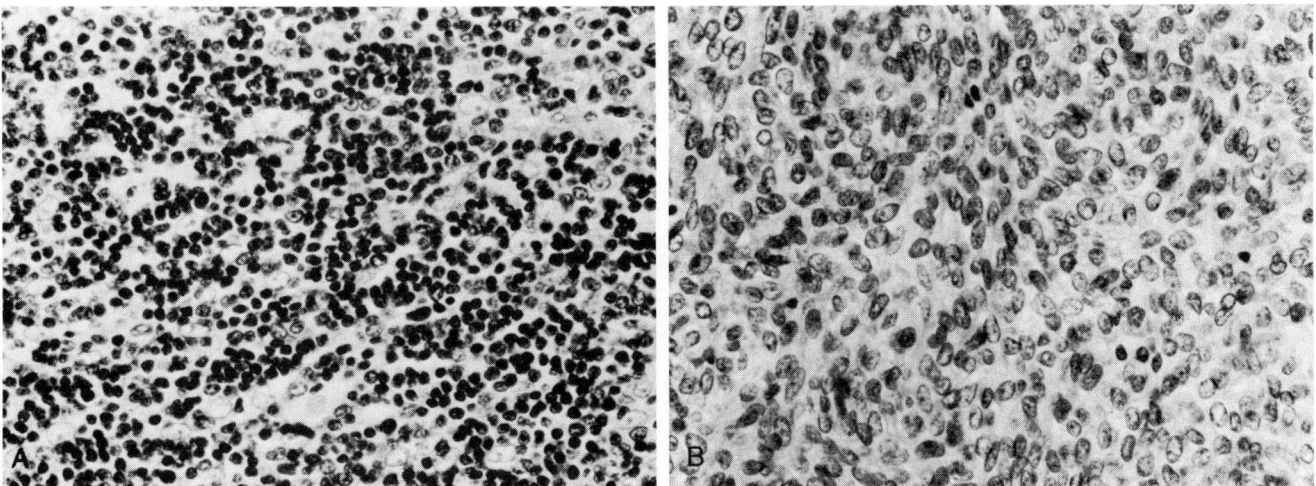

Figure 26–62. *A,* Predominantly lymphocytic thymoma. The pale cells represent epithelial cells, which are difficult to see among the lymphoid cells. *B,* Spindle cell thymoma. The tumor cells have a spindle shape, and there are few lymphocytes within the lesion.

CLINICAL COURSE. The mean age of patients with thymomas is 50 years; in children they are rare but have a poor prognosis. Males and females are affected equally often, as are whites and blacks.[229] The clinical presentation is extremely varied but can be categorized into three basic patterns: (1) neoplasms that are entirely asymptomatic and are discovered incidentally on chest radiography, during cardiac surgery, or at autopsy; (2) neoplasms that cause local pressure effects such as cough, dyspnea, difficulty in swallowing, or signs of vena caval compression; and (3) neoplasms associated with systemic disorders. There is no consensus in the literature on the frequency of each of these three presentations, but the following ranges can be offered. About 10 to 50% of patients are asymptomatic, 10 to 30% have local signs and symptoms, and 30 to 40% have an associated disease. The broad range of associated systemic diseases reported raises the questions of how many are coincidental and how many are causally related to the thymic lesion (Table 26–9). Most of these associated systemic diseases are probably of autoimmune origin, although the precise mechanisms of these associations are unknown.

The prognosis in patients with thymic neoplasms is directly related to the aggressiveness of the lesion and to the presence and nature of an associated systemic disease. The following generalizations can be made. Benign thymomas are slow-growing neoplasms. When well encapsulated and noninvasive, they can be completely excised and cured, but recurrence (still benign) rarely follows. In the small minority of malignant thymomas or thymic carcinomas with spread to the pleura or elsewhere, despite surgical resection and postoperative irradiation, over half may be expected to result in death within five to ten years. A concomitant systemic disease has a strong adverse effect; about two thirds of such individuals followed for three to five years died, most often of an uncontrolled infection and sometimes of another complication related to the associated disease.[230]

Table 26–9. Thymomas and Associated Diseases

DISEASE	PATIENTS WITH THYMOMA (%)
Myasthenia gravis	15–44
Cytopenias (red cell aplasia, thrombocytopenia, neutropenia, pancytopenia)	21
Carcinoma	17
Hypogammaglobulinemia	6
Polymyositis	5
Systemic lupus erythematosus	2
Other diseases: Hashimoto's disease, rheumatoid arthritis, pernicious anemia, scleroderma	Rare

NORMAL

The rarity of clinically significant lesions justifies considerable brevity in the consideration of the pineal gland. It is a minute, pine cone–shaped organ (hence its name), weighing 100 to 180 mg, and lying between the superior colliculi at the base of the brain. It is composed of a loose, neuroglial stroma enclosing nests of large, epithelial-appearing pineocytes. Silver impregnations reveal that these cells have long, slender processes reminiscent of primitive neuronal precursors. Although a large number of neurotransmitter substances such as dopamine, octopamine, serotonin, and others can be extracted from the pineal, the only abundant biologically active substance secreted by it is melatonin. The functions of melatonin in humans are poorly understood, but it can be found in the blood, cerebrospinal fluid, and urine. The levels of this hormone have a diurnal rhythm significantly higher during the night than in the day. Administration of melatonin to humans induces sleepiness, and so this secretory product may play some role in maintaining the awake-sleep rhythm. Despite anecdotal observations to the contrary, large pathology texts do not stimulate melatonin secretion! In addition, melatonin is believed to suppress, at least in animals, the release of gonadotropic hormones, and so it may be more than coincidental that pineal tumors that destroy the gland cause precocious puberty almost exclusively in males. However, injury to the immediately adjacent hypothalamus may simultaneously destroy structures normally involved in pubertal development.

Calcification of the pineal occurs with age. It often first becomes visible at the time of puberty, but calcification has also been seen in infants. There appears to be no correlation between the level of calcification and pineal function.[231]

PATHOLOGY

Pineal tumors account for less than 1% of brain neoplasms. Most (50 to 70%) arise from embryonic germ cells sequestered in the midline pineal. As with testicular tumors arising in germ cells, they most commonly take the form of so-called *germinomas* replicating the testicular seminoma or ovarian dysgerminoma (p. 1109). Other lines of germ-cell differentiation include embryonal carcinomas; choriocarcinomas; mixtures of germinoma, embryonal carcinoma, and choriocarcinoma; and, uncommonly, typical teratomas (usually benign).[232] Whether to characterize these germ-cell neoplasms as pinealomas is still a subject of debate. Thought today favors the restriction of the term to neoplasms arising from the parenchymal and stromal elements of the pineal gland itself.

PINEALOMAS

These neoplasms are divided into two categories, pineoblastomas and pineocytomas, based on their level of differentiation, which in turn correlates with their neoplastic aggressiveness.

Pineoblastomas are encountered mostly in young people and appear as soft, friable, gray masses punctuated with areas of hemorrhage and necrosis. They typically invade surrounding structures, i.e., hypothalamus, midbrain, and lumen of the third ventricle. Histologically, they are composed of masses of pleomorphic cells two to four times the diameter of an erythrocyte. Large hyperchromatic nuclei appear to occupy almost the entire cell, and mitoses are frequent. The cytology is that of the medulloblastoma-neuroblastoma of the brain (p. 1419). Large, poorly formed rosettes are sometimes present in the pineoblastoma, reminiscent of these "first cousins" in the brain. A further similarity is the tendency of pineoblastomas to spread via the cerebrospinal fluid. As might be expected, the enlarging mass may compress the aqueduct of Sylvius, giving rise to internal hydrocephalus and all its consequences. Survival beyond one to two years is rare.

In contrast, *pineocytomas* occur mostly in adults and are much slower growing than the pineoblastomas. They tend to be well-circumscribed, gray, or hemorrhagic masses that compress but do not infiltrate surrounding structures. *Histologically, they exhibit divergent glial and neuronal differentiation.* On the one hand, the neoplasm may be largely astrocytomatous (p. 1414). On the other hand, it may be composed largely of neuronal precursor cells, which are uniform round cells having darkly staining, round-to-oval, fairly regular nuclei. Particularly distinctive of the pineocytoma is the creation of large rosettes rimmed by rows of pineocytes. The centers of these rosettes are filled with eosinophilic cytoplasmic material representing tumor-cell processes. These cells are set against a background of thin, fibrovascular, anastomosing septa that divide the tumor into lobular masses. Occasional mitotic figures and giant cells are present.[233]

In addition to the monomorphic pineocytomas composed largely of one line of differentiation, there are many instances in which mixed patterns are encountered, in part astrocytic, in part pineocytomatous, sometimes having neuronal type cells. Such neoplasms are highly reminiscent of the ganglioglioma (p. 1418).

The clinical course of patients with pineocytomas is prolonged, averaging seven years. The manifestations are the consequence of its pressure effects and consist of visual disturbances, headache, mental deterioration, and sometimes dementia-like behavior. The lesions being located where they are, it is understandable that successful excision is at best very difficult.

1. Pearse, A.G.E.: The cytochemistry and ultrastructure of polypeptide hormone–producing cells of the APUD series and the embryologic, physiologic and pathologic implications of the concept. J. Histochem. Cytochem. 17:303, 1969.

2. Le Douarin, N.: On the origin of pancreatic endocrine cells. Cell 53:169, 1988.

3. Wilson, J.D., and Foster, D.F.: Williams Textbook of Endocrinology. Philadelphia, W.B. Saunders, 1985.

4. Taylor, A.L., and Fishman, L.M.: Corticotropin releasing hormone. N. Engl. J. Med. 319:213, 1988.

5. Hershman, J.M.: Endocrine Pathophysiology. A Patient Oriented Approach. Philadelphia, Lea & Febiger, 1988.

6. Besser G.M.: The hypothalamus and pituitary. Clin. Endocrinol. 6:1, 1977.

7. Pelletier , G., et al.: Identification of human anterior pituitary cells by immunoelectron microscopy. J. Clin. Endocrinol. Metab. 46:534, 1978.

8a. Federman, D.D.: Endocrinology. In Rubenstein, E., and Federman, D.D. (eds.): Scientific American Medicine (Section 3). New York, Scientific American, Inc., 1988.

8. Daughaday, W.H.: The anterior pituitary. In Wilson, J.D., and Foster, D.F. (eds.): Williams Textbook of Endocrinology. Philadelphia, W.B. Saunders, 1985, p. 568.

9. Reichlin, S.: Somatostatin (Parts 1 and 2). N. Engl. J. Med. 309:1495; 1556, 1983.

10. Cook, D.M.: Pituitary tumors—current concepts of diagnosis and therapy. West. J. Med. 133:189, 1980.

11. Saeger, W., and Ludecke, D.K.: Pituitary adenomas with hyperfunction of TSH. Virchows Arch. (Pathol. Anat.) 394:255, 1982.

12. Kovacs, K., and Horvath, K.: Tumors of the Pituitary Gland (Fascicle 21). Washington, D.C., Armed Forces Institute of Pathology, 1983.

13. Horvath, E., and Kovacs, K.: Pathology of prolactin cell adenomas. Semin. Diagn. Pathol. 3:4, 1986.

14. Adelman, L.S.: The pathology of pituitary adenomas. In Post, K.D., et al. (eds.): The Pituitary Adenoma. New York, Plenum Medical Book Co., 1980, p. 47.

15. Burrow, G.N., et al.: Microadenomas of the pituitary and abnormal sellar tomograms in an unselected autopsy series. N. Engl. J. Med. 304:156, 1981.

16. DeLellis, R.A., et al.: Multiple endocrine neoplasia syndromes: Cellular origins and inter-relationships. Int. Rev. Exp. Pathol. 28:163, 1986.

17. McCarty, K.S., Jr., et al.: Pituitary pathology associated with abnormalities of prolactin secretion. Clin. Obstet. Gynecol. 23:367, 1980.

18. Sung, D.I.: Suprasellar tumors in children. A review of clinical manifestations and managements. Cancer 50:1420, 1982.

19. Jialal, I., et al.: Hypopituitarism. A 3-year study. S. Afr. Med. J. 59:590, 1981.

20. Lloyd, R.V., et al.: Immunohistochemical localization of chromogranin in human hypophyses and pituitary adenomas. Arch. Pathol. Lab. Med. 109:517, 1985.

21. Sheehan, H.L.: Post partum necrosis of the anterior pituitary. J. Pathol. Bacteriol. 45:189, 1937.

22. Grimes, H.G., and Brooks, M.H.: Pregnancy in Sheehan's syndrome. Report of a case and review. Obstet. Gynecol. Surv. 35:481, 1980.

23. Spaziante, R.: The empty sella. Surg. Neurol. 16:418, 1981.

24. Rubinstein, L.: Tumors of the Central Nervous System (Fascicle G). Washington, D.C., Armed Forces Institute of Pathology, 1972.

25. Komorowski, R.A., and Hanson, G.A.: Occult thyroid pathology in the young adult. An autopsy study of 138 patients without clinical thyroid disease. Hum. Pathol. 19:689, 1988.

26. Johannesen, J.V., et al.: The fine structure of human thyroid cancer. Hum. Pathol. 9:385, 1978.

27. Delellis, R. A., et al.: C-cell hyperplasia: An ultrastructural analysis. Lab Invest. 36:237, 1977.

28. Rapoport, B., and DeGroot, L.J.: Current concepts of thyroid physiology. Semin. Nucl. Med. 1:265, 1971.

29. Davies, A.G.: Thyroid physiology. Br. Med. J. 2:206, 1972.

30. Stein, O., and Gross, J.: Metabolism of 125-I in the thyroid gland studied with electron microscopic radioautography. Endocrinology 75:787, 1964.

31. Seljelid, R.: Endocytosis of thyroglobulin and the release of thyroid hormone. Scand. J. Clin. Lab. Invest. (Suppl.) 22:106, 1968.

32. Sterling, K.: Thyroid hormone's action at the cell. N. Engl. J. Med. 300:117; 173, 1979.

33. Oppenheimer, J.H.: Thyroid hormone action at the cellular level. Science 203:971, 1979.

34. Caldwell, G., et al: A new strategy for thyroid function testing. Lancet 1:1117, 1985.

35. Baldwin, D.B., and Rowett, D.: Incidence of thyroid disorders in Connecticut. J.A.M.A. 239:742, 1978.

36. Tunbridge, W. M. G., et al.: The spectrum of thyroid disease in a community: the Whickham survey. Clin. Endocrinol. 7:481, 1977.

37. Skelton, C.L.: The heart and hyperthyroidism. N. Engl. J. Med. 307:1206, 1982.

38. Werner, S.C.: Toxic goiter. In Werner, S.C., and Ingbar, S.H. (eds.): The Thyroid. 4th ed. Hagerstown, Harper & Row, 1978, p. 591.

39. Amir, S.M., et al.: In vitro responses to crude and purified hCG in human thyroid membranes. J. Clin. Endocrinol. Metab. 51:51, 1980.

40. Emerson, C.H., and Utiger, R.D.: Hyperthyroidism and excessive thyrotropin secretion, N. Engl. J. Med. 287:328, 1972.

41. Dorfman, S.G.: Hyperthyroidism, usual and unusual causes. Arch. Intern. Med. 137:995, 1977.

42. Doniach, D.: Hashimoto's thyroiditis and primary myxoedema viewed as separate entities. Eur. J. Clin. Invest. 11:245, 1981.

43. Drexhage, H.A., et al.: Thyroid growth-blocking antibodies in primary myxedema. Nature 289:594, 1981.

44. Hamilton, W.: Endemic cretinism. Dev. Med. Child. Neurol. 18:386, 1976.

45. Hamilton, W.: Sporadic cretinism. Dev. Med. Child. Neurol. 18:384, 1976.

46. Hurley, J.R.: Thyroiditis. DM 24:3, 1977.

47. Volpe, R.: The pathology of thyroiditis. Hum. Pathol. 9:429, 1978.

48. Volpe, R.: Immunoregulation in autoimmune thyroid disease. N. Engl. J. Med. 316:44, 1987.

49. Strakosch, C.R., et al.: Immunology of autoimmune thyroid disease. N. Engl. J. Med. 307:1499, 1982.

50. Volpe, R.: Autoimmunity in the endocrine system. Monogr. Endocrinol. 20:19, 1981.

51. Drexhage, H.A., et al.: Evidence for thyroid-growth-stimulating immunoglobulins in some goitrous thyroid diseases. Lancet 2:287, 1980.

52. Rose, N.R., et al.: T-cell regulation in autoimmune thyroiditis. Immunol. Rev. 55:299, 1981.

53. Botazzo, G.F., et al.: Role of aberrant HLA-DR expression and antigen presentation in induction of endocrine autoimmunity. Lancet 2:1115, 1983.

54. Friedman, N.B.: Cellular involution in the thyroid gland: Significance of the Hürthle cells in myxedema, exhaustion atrophy, Hashimoto's disease and the reactions to irradiation, thiouracil therapy and subtotal resection. J. Clin. Endocrinol. Metab. 9:874, 1949.

55. Katz, S.M., and Vickery, A.L.: The fibrosing variant of Hashimoto's thyroiditis. Hum. Pathol. 5:161, 1974.

56. Compagno, J., and Oertel, J.E.: Malignant lymphoma and other lymphoproliferative disorders of the thyroid gland. Am. J. Clin. Pathol. 74:1, 1980.

57. Crile, G., Jr.: Struma lymphomatosa and carcinoma of the thyroid. Surg. Gynecol. Obstet. 147:350, 1978.

58. De Pauw, B.E., and De Rooy, H.A.M.: De Quervain's subacute thyroiditis. Neth. J. Med. 18:70, 1975.

59. Greene, J.N.: Subacute thyroiditis. Am. J. Med. 51:97, 1971.

60. Volpe, R.: Subacute thyroiditis. In Soto, R.J., et al. (eds.): Progress in Clinical and Biological Research. New York, Alan R. Liss, 1981, p. 115.

61. Volpe, R.: Subacute (de Quervain's) thyroiditis. Clin. Endocrinol. Metab. 8:81, 1979.

62. Strakosch, C.R., et al.: Thyroid-stimulating antibodies in patients with subacute thyroiditis. J. Clin. Endocrinol. Metab. 46:345, 1978.

63. Carney, A.J., et al.: Palpation thyroiditis (multifocal granulomatous folliculitis). Am. J. Clin. Pathol. 64:639, 1975.

64. Dorfman, S.G., et al.: Painless thyroiditis and transient hyperthyroidism without goiter. Ann. Intern. Med. 86:24, 1977.

65. Katsikas, D., et al.: Riedel's thyroiditis. Br. J. Surg. 63:929, 1976.

66. Meyer, S., and Hausman, R.: Occlusive phlebitis in multifocal fibrosclerosis. Am. J. Clin. Pathol. 65:274, 1976.

67. Gamblin, G.T., et al.: Prevalence of increased intraocular pressure in Graves' disease—evidence of frequent subclinical ophthalmopathy. N. Engl. J. Med. 308:420, 1983.

68. Farid, N.R., and Bear, J.C.: The human major histocompatibility complex and endocrine disease. Endocr. Rev. 2:50, 1981.

69. Smyth, P.P.A., et al.: The prevalence of thyroid-stimulating antibodies in goitrous disease assessed by cytochemical section bioassay. J. Clin. Endocrinol. Metab. 54:357, 1982.

70. Monjan, A.A., and Collector, M.I.: Stress-induced modulation of the immune response. Science 196:307, 1977.

71. Aoki, N., et al.: Studies on suppressor cell function in thyroid diseases. J. Clin. Endocrinol. Metab. 48:803, 1979.

72. Burman, K.D., and Baker, J.R., Jr.: Immune mechanisms in Graves' disease. Endocr. Rev. 6:183, 1985.

73. Kodama, K., et al.: Demonstration of a circulating autoantibody against a soluble L-muscle antigen in Graves' ophthalmopathy. Lancet 2:1353, 1982.

74. Editoral: Autoimmune endocrine exophthalmos. Lancet 2:1378, 1982.

75. Gorman, C.: Ophthalmopathy of Graves' disease. N. Engl. J. Med. 308:453, 1983.

76. Clements, F.W.: Endemic goitre. W.H.O. Mongr. Ser. 62:83, 1976.

77. Editorial: Dietary goitrogens. Lancet 1:394, 1982.

78. Delange, F., et al.: Nutritional factors involved in the goitrogenic action of cassava. Ottawa Int. Develop. Res. Ctr., 1982.

79. Refetoff, S., and Selenkow, H.A.: Familial thyroxine-binding globulin deficiency in a patient with Turner's syndrome (XO). N. Engl. J. Med. 278:1081, 1968.

80. Beienwaltes, W.H., et al.: Hereditary increase in the thyroxin-binding sites in the serum alpha globulin. Trans. Assoc. Am. Physicians 74:170, 1961.

81. Zonana, J., and Rimoin, D.L.: Genetic disorders of the thyroid gland. Med. Clin. North Am. 59:1263, 1975.

82. Studer, H., and Ramelli, F.: Simple goiter and its variants: Euthyroid and hyperthyroid multinodular goiters. Endocr. Rev. 3:40, 1982.

83. Peter, H.J., et al.: The pathogenesis of "hot" and "cold" follicles in multinodular goiters. J.C.E.M. 55:941, 1982.

84. Ramelli, F., et al.: Pathogenesis of thyroid nodules in multinodular goiter. Am. J. Pathol. 109:215, 1982.

85. Taylor, S.: Sporadic nontoxic goiter. In Werner, S.C., and Ingbar, S.H. (eds.): The Thyroid. A Fundamental and Clinical Text. 4th ed. Hagerstown, Harper & Row, 1978, p. 505.

86. Van Herle, A.J., and Uller, R.P.: Thyroid cancer classification. Clinical features, diagnosis and therapy. Pharmacol. Ther. 2:215, 1977.

87. Klonoff, D.C., and Greenspan, F.S.: The thyroid nodule. Adv. Intern. Med. 27:101, 1982.

88. Vander, J.B., et al.: The significance of nontoxic thyroid nodules. Final report of a 15-year study of the incidence of thyroid malignancy. Ann. Intern. Med. 69:537, 1968.

89. Rojiski, M.T., and Gharib, H.: Nodular thyroid disease. Evaluation and Management. N. Engl. J. Med. 313:428, 1985.

90. DeGroot, L.J.: Thyroid carcinoma. Med. Clin. North Am. 59:1233, 1975.

91. Van Herle, A.J.: Serum thyroglobulin measurement in the diagnosis and management of thyroid disease. Thyroid Today 4:1, 1981.

92. Colacchio, T.A., et al.: Fine needle cytological diagnosis of thyroid nodules: Review and report of 300 cases. Am. J. Surg. 140:568, 1980.

93. Wang, C.A., et al.: The role of needle biopsy in evaluating solitary cold thyroid nodules. Proc. 7th Int. Thyroid Conf. Thyroid Research. Excerpta Med. Int. Serv. 378:568, 1975.

94. Meissner, W.A.: Diseases of the thyroid. In Werner, S.C., and Ingbar, S.H. (eds.): The Thyroid. A Fundamental and Clinical Text. 4th ed. Hagerstown, Harper & Row, 1978, p. 444.

95. Rosai, J., et al.: Undifferentiated and poorly differentiated thyroid carcinoma. Semin. Diagn. Pathol. 2:137, 1985.

96. Roudebush, C.P., et al.: Natural history of radiation-associated thyroid cancer. Arch. Intern. Med. 138:1631, 1978.

97. Refetoff, S., et al.: Continuing occurrence of thyroid carcinoma after irradiation to the neck in infancy and childhood. N. Engl. J. Med. 292:171, 1975.

98. Editorial: Radiation-induced thyroid cancer. Lancet 2:21, 1985.

99. Sampson, R.J., et al.: Thyroid carcinoma in Hiroshima and Nagasaki. J.A.M.A. 209:65, 1969.

100. Devall, L., et al.: Initial observations of fallout from the reactor accident of Chernobyl. Nature 231:91, 1986.

101. Rall, J.E.: The effects of radiation on the thyroid gland. A quantitative analysis. In Soto, R.J., et al. (eds.): Physiopathology of Endocrine Diseases and Mechanisms of Hormone Action. New York, Allen R. Liss, 1981, p. 29.

102. Frauenhofer, C.M., et al.: Thyroid carcinoma. A clinical and pathological study of 125 cases. Cancer 43:2414, 1979.

103. Hapke, M.R., and Dehner, L.P.: The optically clear nucleus: A reliable sign of papillary carcinoma of the thyroid. Am. J. Surg. Pathol. 3:31, 1971.

104. Chen, K.T.K., and Rosal, J.: Follicular variant of thyroid papillary carcinoma. A clinicopathologic study of six cases. Am. J. Surg. Pathol. 1:123, 1977.

105. Tscholl-Ducommun, J., and Hedinger, C.E.: Papillary thyroid carcinomas: Morphology and prognosis. Virchows Arch. (Pathol. Anat.) 396:19, 1982.

106. Tubiana, M., et al.: Long-term results and prognostic factors in patients with differentiated thyroid carcinoma. Cancer 55:794, 1985.

107. Rosai, J., et al.: Papillary carcinoma of the thyroid. A discussion of its several morphological expressions with particular emphasis on the follicular variant. Am. J. Surg. Pathol. 1:809, 1983.

108. Franssila, K.: Is the differentiation between papillary and follicular carcinoma valid? Cancer 32:853, 1973.

109. Meissner, W.A.: Follicular carcinoma of the thyroid. Am. J. Surg. Pathol. 1:171, 1977.

110. Carcangiu, M.L., et al.: Poorly differentiated ("insular") thyroid carcinoma. A reinterpretation of Langhans' "Wuchernde Struma." Am. J. Surg. Pathol. 8:655, 1984.

111. Hazard, J.B.: The C cells (parafollicular cells) of the thyroid gland and medullary thyroid carcinoma. Am. J. Pathol. 88:213, 1977.

112. DeLellis, R.A., and Wolfe, H.J.: The pathobiology of the C-cell. Pathol. Annu. 16:25, 1981.

113. Uribe, M., et al.: Medullary carcinoma of the thyroid gland: clinical, pathological and immunohistochemical features with review of the literature. Am. J. Surg. Pathol. 9:577, 1985.

114. Schimke, R.N., and Hartman, W.H.: Familiar amyloid-producing medullary thyroid carcinoma and pheochromocytoma: A distinct genetic entity. Ann. Intern. Med. 63:1027, 1965.

115. Matthew, C.G.P., et al.: A linked genetic marker for multiple

endocrine neoplasia type 2A on chromosome 10. Nature *328*:527, 1987.

116. Wolfe, H.J., et al.: C-cell hyperplasia preceding medullary thyroid carcinoma. N. Engl. J. Med. *289*:437, 1973.

117. Albores-Saavedra, J., et al.: Medullary carcinoma. Semin. Diagn. Pathol. *2*:137, 1985.

118. Gagel, R.F., et al.: The clinical outcome of prospective screening for multiple endocrine neoplasia, type 2A. N. Engl. J. Med. *318*:478, 1988.

119. Devine, R.M., et al.: Primary lymphoma of the thyroid: A review of the Mayo Clinic experience through 1978. World J. Surg. *5*:33, 1981.

120. Burke, J.S., et al.: Malignant lymphomas of the thyroid, a clinico-pathologic study of 35 patients including ultrastructural observations. Cancer *39*:1587, 1977.

121. Kapadia, S.B., et al.: Malignant lymphoma of the thyroid gland: A clinicopathologic study. Head Neck Surg. *4*:270, 1982.

122. Stanta, G., et al.: The biochemical and immunohistochemical profile of thyroid neoplasia. Pathol. Annu. *23*:129, 1988.

123. Saharia, P.C.: Carcinoma arising in thyroglossal duct remnant: Case reports and review of the literature. Br. J. Cancer *62*:689, 1975.

124. Woolner, L.B., et al.: Classification and prognosis of thyroid carcinoma. Am. J. Surg. *102*:354, 1961.

125. Dufour, D.R., et al.: The normal parathyroid revisited. Hum. Pathol. *13*:717, 1982.

126. Grimelius, L., et al.: Anatomy and histopathology of human parathyroid glands. Pathol. Annu. *16*:1, 1981.

127. Castleman, B., and Roth, S.I.: Tumors of the Parathyroid Gland. Washington, D.C., Armed Forces Institute of Pathology, 1978.

128. Rosenblatt, M.: Pre-proparathyroid hormone: intracellular transport and processing. Min. Electrolyte Metab. *8*:118, 1982.

129. Martin, K.J.: The peripheral metabolism of parathyroid hormone. N. Engl. J. Med. *301*:1092, 1979.

130. Raisz, L.G., and Kream, B.E.: Regulation of bone formation. N. Engl. J. Med. *309*:29; 83, 1983.

131. Wells, S.A., Jr., et al.: Primary hyperparathyroidism. Curr. Probl. Surg. *17*:398, 1980.

132. Mallette, L.E., et al.: Primary hyperparathyroidism: Clinical and biochemical features. Medicine *53*:127, 1974.

133. Health, H., III, et al.: Primary hyperparathyroidism: Incidence, morbidity, and potential economic impact in a community. N. Engl. J. Med. *302*:189, 1980.

134. Coffey, R.J., et al.: The surgical treatment of primary hyperparathyroidism. A 20-year experience. Ann. Surg. *185*:518, 1977.

135. Sharp, C.F., Jr., et al.: Abnormal bone and parathyroid histology in carcinoma patients with pseudohyperparathyroidism. Cancer *49*:1449, 1982.

136. Mundy, G.R.: Ectopic hormonal syndromes in neoplastic disease. Hosp. Pract. *22*:113, 1987.

137. Thompson, N.W., et al.: The anatomy of primary hyperparathyroidism. Surgery *92*:814, 1982.

138. Fialkow, P.J., et al.: Multicellular origin of parathyroid "adenomas." N. Engl. J. Med. *297*:696, 1977.

139. Arnold, A., et al.: Monoclonality and abnormal parathyroid hormone genes in parathyroid adenomas. N. Engl. J. Med. *318*:658, 1988.

140. Kay, S.: The abnormal parathyroid. Hum. Pathol. *7*:127, 1976.

141. Roth, S.I., and Gallagher, M.D.: The rapid identification of normal parathyroid glands by the presence of intracellular fat. Am. J. Pathol. *84*:521, 1976.

142. Nisson, O.: Studies on the ultrastructure of the human parathyroid glands in various pathological conditions. Acta Pathol. Microbiol. Scand. (A) *263*(Suppl):5, 1977.

143. Elliott, R.L., and Arhelger, R.B.: Fine structure of parathyroid adenomas. Arch. Pathol. *81*:200, 1966.

144. Shane, E., and Bilezikian, J.P.: Parathyroid carcinoma: A review of 62 patients. Endocr. Rev. *3*:218, 1982.

145. Davies, D.R.: The surgery of primary hyperparathyroidism. Clin. Endocrinol. Metab. *3*:253, 1974.

146. Schantz, A., and Castleman, B.: Parathyroid cancer: a study of 70 cases. Cancer *31*:600, 1973.

147. Castleman, B., et al.: Parathyroid hyperplasia in primary hyperparathyroidism. A review of 85 cases. Cancer *38*:1668, 1976.

148. Roth, S.I.: The ultrastructure of primary water cell hyperplasia of the parathyroid gland. Am. J. Pathol. *61*:233, 1970.

149. Massry, S.G., and Ritz, E.: The pathogenesis of secondary hy-perparathyroidism of renal failure: Is there a controversy? Arch. Intern. Med. *138*:853, 1978.

150. David, D.S., et al.: Hypercalcemia after renal transplantation: Long term follow-up data. N. Engl. J. Med. *289*:398, 1973.

151. Nusynowitz, M.L., et al.: The spectrum of the hypoparathyroid states: A classification based on physiologic principles. Medicine *55*:105, 1976.

152. Schneider, A.B., and Sherwood, L.M.: Pathogenesis and management of hypoparathyroidism and other hypocalcemic disorders. Metabolism *24*:871, 1975.

153. Daneman, D., et al.: Hypoparathyroidism and pseudohypoparathyroidism in childhood. Clin. Endocrinol. Metab. *11*:211, 1982.

154. Neufeld, M., et al.: Two types of autoimmune Addison's disease associated with polyglandular autoimmune (PGA) syndromes. Medicine *60*:335, 1981.

155. Arulanantham, K., et al.: Evidence for defective immunoregulation in the syndrome of familial candidiasis endocrinopathy. N. Engl. J. Med. *300*:164, 1979.

156. Spiegel, A.M., et al.: Pseudohypoparathyroidism: The molecular basis for hormone resistance—a retrospective. N. Engl. J. Med. *307*:679, 1982.

157. Farfel, Z., et al.: Defect of receptor cyclase coupling protein in pseudohypoparathyroidism. N. Engl. J. Med. *303*:237, 1980.

158. Tannenbaum, M.: Ultrastructural pathology of the adrenal cortex. In Sommers, S.C. (ed.): Endocrine Pathology Decennial. New York, Appleton-Century-Crofts, 1975, p. 423.

159. Neelon, F.A.: Adrenal physiology and pharmacology. Urol. Clin. North Am. *4*:179, 1977.

160. Carey, R.M., et al.: Idiopathic aldosteronism: A possible role for aldosterone stimulating factor. N. Engl. J. Med. *311*:94, 1984.

161. Elpper, B.A., and Mains, R.E.: Structure and biosynthesis of proadenocorticotropin/endorphin and related peptides. Endocr. Rev. *1*:1, 1980.

162. Vaughan, N.J.A., et al.: The diagnosis of primary hyperaldosteronism. Lancet *1*:120, 1981.

163. Dehner, L.P.: Pediatric Surgical Pathology. Baltimore, Williams & Wilkins, 1987, p. 550.

164. Lindgren, S.: Congenital primary adrenal hypoplasia. Acta Pathol. Microbiol. Scand. *70*:541, 1967.

165. Page, D.L.: Tumors of the Adrenal (Fascicle 23). Washington, D.C., Armed Forces Institute of Pathology, 1986.

166. Maisey M.N., and Lessof, M.H.: Addison's disease: A clinical study. Guys Hosp. Rep. *118*:363, 1969.

167. Williams, G.H.: The adrenal manifestations of systemic diseases. Clin. Endocrinol. Metab. *8*:527, 1979.

168. Bohm, N.: Adrenal cutaneous and myocardial lesions in fulminating endotoxinemia. Pathol. Res. Pract. *174*:92, 1982.

169. O'Hare, M.J., et al.: The pathology of adrenal cortical neoplasia: A correlated structural and functional approach to the diagnosis of malignant disease. Hum. Pathol. *10*:137, 1979.

170. Ross, E.J., et al.: Cushing's syndrome: Diagnostic criteria. Q.J. Med. *35*:149, 1966.

171. Gold, E.M.: The Cushing's syndromes: Changing view of diagnosis and treatment. Ann. Intern. Med. *90*:829, 1979.

172. Cushing, H.: The basophil adenomas of the pituitary body and their clinical manifestations (pituitary basophilism). Bull. Johns Hopkins Hosp. *50*:137, 1932.

173. Krieger, D.T.: The central nervous system and Cushing's disease. Med. Clin. North Am. *62*:261, 1978.

174. Fehm, H.L., and Voigt, K.H.: Pathophysiology of Cushing's disease. Pathobiol. Annu. *9*:225, 1979.

175. Imura, H., et al.: Studies on ectopic ACTH-producing tumors. II. Clinical and biochemical features of 30 cases. Cancer *35*:1430, 1975.

176. Gewirtz, G., and Yalow, R.S.: Ectopic ACTH production in carcinoma of the lung. J. Clin. Invest. *53*:1022, 1974.

177. Belsky, J.L., et al.: Cushing's syndrome due to ectopic production of corticotropin releasing factor. J.C.E.M. *60*:496, 1985.

178. Felix, I.A., et al.: Massive Crooke's hyalinization in corticotroph cell adenomas of the human pituitary. A histological, immunocytological, and electron microscopic study of three cases. Acta Neurochirurg. *58*:235, 1981.

179. DeCicco, F.A., et al.: Fine structure of Crooke's hyaline change in the human pituitary gland. Arch. Pathol. *94*:65, 1972.

180. Tyrrell, J.B., et al.: Cushing's disease. Selective trans-sphenoidal resection of pituitary microadenomas. N. Engl. J. Med. *298*:753, 1978.

181. Symington, T.: The adrenal cortex. *In* Bloodworth, J.M.B. (ed.): Endocrine Pathology. General and Surgical. Baltimore, Williams & Wilkins, 1982.

182. Shenoy, B.V., et al.: Bilateral primary pigmented nodular adrenal cortical disease. Rare cause of the Cushing syndrome. Am. J. Surg. Pathol. *8*:835, 1984.

183. Weinberger, M.H., et al.: Primary aldosteronism: Diagnosis, localization and treatment. Ann Intern. Med. *90*:386, 1979.

184. Editorial: Bartter's syndrome. Lancet *2*:721, 1976.

185. Ferriss, J.B., et al.: Primary hyperaldosteronism. Clin. Endocrinol. Metab. *10*:419, 1981.

186. Ganguly, A., et al.: Anomalous postural aldosterone response in glucocorticoid-suppressible hyperaldosteronism. N. Engl. J. Med. *305*:991, 1981.

187. Neville, A.M., and Symington, T.: Pathology of primary aldosteronism. Cancer *19*:1854, 1966.

188. Hornsby, P.J., et al.: Functional and morphological observations on rat adrenal zone glomerulosa cells in monolayer culture. Endocrinology *95*:1240, 1974.

189. McGuffin, W.L., Jr., and Gunnelis, J.C., Jr.: Primary aldosteronism. Urol. Clin. North Am. *4*:227, 1977

190. Ganguly, A., et al.: Primary aldosteronism. The etiologic spectrum of disorders and their clinical differentiation. Arch. Intern. Med. *142*:813, 1982.

191. White, P.C., et al.: Congenital adrenal hyperplasia. N. Engl. J. Med. *316*:159, 1987.

192. Speiser, P.W., et al.: Molecular genetic analysis of non-classic steroid 21-hydroxylase deficiency associated with HLA-B14, Drl. N. Engl. J. Med. *319*:19, 1988.

193. Ross, G., Jr., et al.: Our experience with the adrenogenital syndrome. A review of 16 cases. J. Urol. *115*:462, 1976.

194. Russell, R.P., et al.: Adrenal cortical adenomas and hypertension. A clinical pathologic analysis of 690 cases with matched controls and a review of the literature. Medicine *51*:211, 1972.

195. Dobbie, J.W.: Adrenal cortical nodular hyperplasia. The aging adrenal. J. Pathol. *99*:1, 1969.

196. Hutter, A.M., and Kayhoe, D.E.: Adrenal cortical carcinoma. Am. J. Med. *41*:572, 1966.

197. Kohn, A.: Die Paraganglien. Arch. Mikr. Anat. *52*:262, 1903.

198. Glenner, G.G., and Grimley, P.M.: Tumors of the Extra-Adrenal Paraganglionic System (Including Chemoreceptors) (Fascicle 9). Washington, D.C., Armed Forces Institute of Pathology, 1974.

199. Kirshner, N.: Biosynthesis of catecholamines. *In*: Handbook of Physiology, Endocrinology. Section 7, Volume 6. Washington, D.C., American Physiological Society, 1975, pp. 341–355.

200. Falterman, C.J., and Kreisberg, R.: Pheochromocytoma: Clinical diagnosis and management. South. Med. J. *75*:321, 1982.

201. Manger, W.M., and Gifford, R.W., Jr.: Pheochromocytoma. New York, Springer-Verlag, 1977.

202. Atuk, N.O.: Pheochromocytoma: Diagnosis, localization and treatment. Hosp. Pract. *18*:187, 1983.

203. Melicow, M.M.: One hundred cases of pheochromocytoma (107 tumors) at the Columbia Presbyterian Medical Center 1926–1976. Cancer *40*:1987, 1977.

204. Rudy, F.R., et al.: Adrenal medullary hyperplasia: A clinicopathologic study of four cases. Hum. Pathol. *11*:650, 1980.

205. Symington, T., and Goodall, A.L.: Studies in phaeochromocytoma. Pathological aspects. Glasgow Med. J. *34*:75, 1953.

206. Wilson, R.A., and Ibanez, M.L.: A comparative study of 14 cases of familial and nonfamilial pheochromocytomas. Hum. Pathol. *9*:181, 1978.

207. Goldfien, A.: Phaeochromocytoma. Clin. Endocrinol. Metab. *10*:607, 1981.

208. Garcia, R., and Jennings, J.: Pheochromocytoma masquerading as a cardiomyopathy. Am. J. Cardiol. *29*:568, 1972.

209. Bravo, E.L., and Gifford, R.W.: Pheochromocytoma: Diagnosis, localization and management. N. Engl. J. Med. *311*:1298, 1984.

210. Bravo, E.L., et al.: Clonidine suppression test: A useful aid in the diagnosis of pheochromocytoma. N. Engl. J. Med. *305*:623, 1981.

211. Triche, T.J., and Askin, F.B.: Neuroblastoma and the differential diagnosis of small-, round-, blue- cell tumors. Hum. Pathol. *14*:568, 1983.

212. Beckwith, J.B., and Perrin, E.V.: In situ neuroblastomas: A contribution to the natural history of neural crest tumors. Am. J. Pathol. *43*:1089, 1963.

213. Shimada, H., et al.: Histopathologic prognostic factors in neuroblastic tumors: Definition of subtypes of ganglioneuro-blastoma and an age-linked classification of neuroblastomas. J. Natl. Cancer Inst. *73*:405, 1984.

214. Evans, A.E., et al.: Prognostic factors in neuroblastoma. Cancer *59*:1853, 1987.

215. Brodeur, G.M., et al.: Cytogenetic features of human neuroblastomas and cell lines. Cancer Res. *41*:4678, 1981.

216. Brodeur, G.M., et al.: Clinical implications of oncogene activation in human neuroblastomas. Cancer *58*:541, 1986.

217. Grimley, P.M., and DeLellis, R.A.: Multisystem neuroendocrine neoplasia. *In* Henson, D.E., and Albores-Saavedra, J. (eds.): The Pathology of Incipient Neoplasia. Philadelphia, W.B. Saunders, 1986, p. 425.

218. Lack, E.E., et al.: Paragangliomas of the head and neck region. A pathobiologic study of tumors from 71 patients. Hum. Pathol. *10*:191, 1979.

219. Someren, A., and Karcoiglu, Z.: Malignant vagal paraganglioma. Report of a case and review of the literature. Am. J. Clin. Pathol. *68*:400, 1977.

220. Levine, G.D., and Rosal, J.: Thymic hyperplasia and neoplasia. A review of current concepts. Hum. Pathol. *9*:495, 1978.

221. Masaoka, A., et al.: Study of the ratio of lymphocytes to epithelial cells in thymoma. Cancer *40*:1222, 1977.

222. Mokhtar, N., et al.: Thymoma: Lymphoid and epithelial components mirror the phenotype of the normal thymus. Hum. Pathol. *15*:378, 1984.

223. Rosai, J., and Levine, G.D.: Tumors of the Thymus (Fascicle 13). Washington, D.C., Armed Forces Institute of Pathology, 1976.

224. Schulof, R.S., et al.: Thymic physiology and biochemistry. Adv. Clin. Chem. *26*:203, 1987.

225. Rosen, F.S., et al.: Primary immunodeficiency diseases. WHO Meeting Report. Clin. Immun. Immunopathol. *28*:450, 1983.

226. Snover, D.G., et al.: Thymic carcinoma. Five distinctive histological variants. Am. J. Surg. Pathol. *6*:451, 1982.

227. Battifora, H.: Recent progress in the immunohistochemistry of solid tumors. Semin. Diagn. Pathol. *1*:251, 1984.

228. Robins-Browne, R.M., et al.: Thymoma, pure red cell aplasia, pernicious anaemia and candidiasis: A defect in immunohomeostasis. Br. J. Haematol. *36*:5, 1977.

229. Salyer, W.R., and Eggleston, J.C.: Thymoma, a clinical and pathological study of 65 cases. Cancer *37*:229, 1976.

230. LeGolvan, D.P., and Abell, M.R.: Thymomas. Cancer *39*:2142, 1977.

231. De Martino, C., et al.: Electron microscopic study of impuberal and adult rats pineal body. Experientia *20*:556, 1964.

232. Rubinstein, L.J.: Cytogenesis and differentiation of pineal neoplasms. Hum. Pathol. *12*:441, 1981.

233. Borit, A., et al.: The separation of pineocytoma from pineoblastoma. Cancer *45*:140B, 1980.

George F. Murphy, M.D.   *Martin C. Mihm, Jr., M.D.*

THE SKIN AS A PROTECTIVE ORGAN

More than 100 years ago, the noted pathologist Rudolph Virchow portrayed the skin as a protective covering for more delicate and functionally sophisticated internal viscera.[1] At that time, the skin was appreciated primarily as a passive barrier to fluid loss and mechanical injury. By routine light microscopy, early investigators could visualize only the tough epidermal layer composed of stratified squamous epithelial cells, the leathery underlying dermis, and the cushion of subcutaneous fat that lay beneath. Amazingly, this level of understanding changed little over the century that followed. During the past three decades, however, enormously productive avenues of scientific inquiry have demonstrated skin to be a complex organ in which precisely regulated cellular and molecular interactions govern many crucial responses to our environment.

We now know that skin is composed of a number of interdependent cell types (Fig. 27–1). *Melanocytes* within the epidermis are cells responsible for the production of a brown pigment (melanin) that represents an important endogenous screen against harmful ultraviolet rays in sunlight. *Langerhans* cells[2,3] are dendritic histiocytic cells that take up and process antigenic signals and communicate this information to lymphoid cells. *Squamous epithelial cells (keratinocytes)* are no longer conceived of as "an inert mass," as Virchow wrote,[1] or as simply factories for the synthesis of keratin protein, but rather are viewed as major sites for the biosynthesis of soluble molecules (cytokines) important in the functional regulation of adjacent epidermal cells and cells forming the nearby dermal microenvironment.[4,5]

Factors affecting the delicate homeostasis that exists among skin cells may result in conditions as diverse as wrinkles and hair loss, blisters and rashes, and even life-threatening cancers and disorders of immune regulation. For example, chronic exposure to sunlight fosters premature cutaneous aging, blunting of immunologic responses to environmental antigens, and the development of a variety of premalignant and malignant cutaneous neoplasms. Ingested agents, such as therapeutic drugs, may result in an enormous number of skin rashes, or exanthems. And internal disorders, such as diabetes mellitus, amyloidosis, and lupus erythematosus, also may have important manifestations in the skin.

As our only external organ, the skin is the first to be evaluated by physical examination. It represents a window to internal well-being or disease. The pages that follow describe examples of important and commonly encountered diseases of the skin that have not been detailed in other chapters (scleroderma, vascular neoplasms, malformations, vasculitis, and lichen sclerosis are described in other sections of this text) and that have characteristic and instructive diagnostic features. Particular attention will be given to gross and microscopic correlations and to pathogenesis.

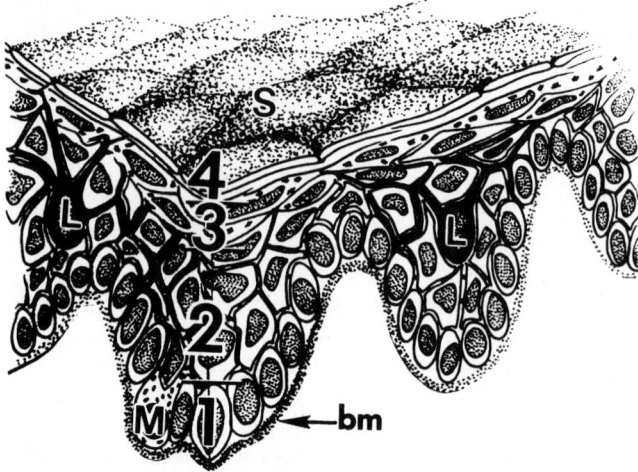

Figure 27–1. Cells composing normal epidermis. The majority are keratinocytes that undergo progressive upward maturation from ovoid cells of the basal layer cell (1) that rest on the basement membrane (bm), to more polyhedral stratum spinosum cells (2), then to flattened stratum granulosum (granular) cells (3), and finally to anucleate cells of the epidermal surface(s), the stratum corneum (4). Dendritic melanocytes (M) and Langerhans cells (L) are interspersed in relatively low numbers within the epidermal layer.

Awareness of the myriad manifestations of cutaneous pathology both clinically and microscopically should enhance general medical acumen as well as an understanding of the pathologic basis of diseases of the skin.

DISORDERS OF PIGMENTATION AND MELANOCYTES

Skin pigmentation historically has had major societal implications. Cosmetic desire for increased pigmentation (tanning) has resulted in many deleterious alterations that will be described in the pages that follow. Focal or widespread loss of pigmentation not only renders individuals extraordinarily vulnerable to the harmful effects of sunlight (as in albinism) but also has resulted in severe emotional stresses, and in some cultures, profound social and economic discrimination (as in vitiligo). Change in pre-existing pigmentation may signify important primary events in the skin (e.g., malignant transformation of a mole) or disorders of internal viscera (e.g., in Addison's disease).

VITILIGO

Vitiligo is a common disorder characterized by partial or complete loss of pigment-producing melanocytes within the epidermis. All races are affected, but lesions are most noticeable in darkly pigmented individuals. Lesions may be entirely unapparent in lightly pigmented skin until tanning occurs in the surrounding normal skin, or until the skin is exposed to Wood's ultraviolet long-wave light ("black light"), which enhances visually covert differences in pigmentation.

Clinically, lesions are asymptomatic, flat, well-demarcated zones (macules) of pigment loss (Fig. 27–2). Their size varies from few to many centimeters, and their distribution often involves the wrists, axillae, and perioral, periorbital, and anogenital skin. Rarely, total body involvement may occur. Sometimes extensor surfaces are involved preferentially, raising the possibility of a role for repeated trauma in the induction of lesions (a characteristic also seen in other skin conditions and known as the Koebner phenomenon).

Histologically, vitiligo is characterized by loss of melanocytes, as defined by electron microscopy. This is in contrast to some forms of *albinism,* in which melanocytes are present but no melanin pigment is produced because of a lack of or defect in the tyrosinase enzyme. Both conditions may be differentiated from other forms of hypopigmentation (unrelated to the absence of melanocytes or tyrosinase enzyme) by demonstrating diminished or absent activity of melanocyte tyrosinase on the melanin pigment precursor dopa (dihydroxyphenylalanine). This histochemical stain is useful because melanocytes or their melanogenic potential cannot be reliably quantified in routine H and E sections.

Why are melanocytes progressively lost or destroyed in vitiligo? Theories of pathogenesis include (1) autoimmunity, (2) neurohumoral factors, and (3) self-destruction of melanocytes by toxic intermediates of melanin synthesis. Most evidence supports autoimmune causation, focusing on the presence of circulating antibodies against melanocytes[6] and the association of vitiligo with disorders possibly involving autoimmune mechanisms, such as pernicious anemia, Addison's disease, and autoimmune thyroiditis. Recently, abnormalities in Langerhans cells[7] and T lymphocytes in the peripheral blood[8] have also been described, suggesting that aberrations in cell-mediated immunity may also be operative in the patho-

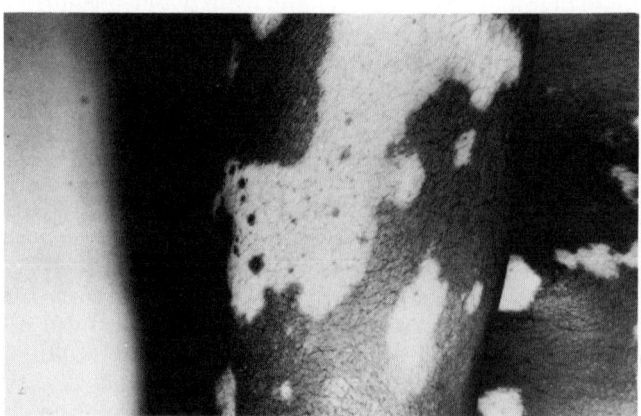

Figure 27–2. Vitiligo. Well-demarcated zones of pigment loss result from loss of melanocytes that produce small melanin granules.

genesis of vitiligo. Interestingly, repigmentation may be induced therapeutically by the selective use of ultraviolet (UV) light of the A wavelength in individuals made more sensitive to its effect(s) by the photosensitizing drug psoralen (a treatment known as PUVA[9]). Such an approach may result in photostimulation of residual melanocytes, possibly residing in low numbers in or about hair follicles.

FRECKLE (EPHELIS)

Freckles are the most common pigmented lesions of childhood in light-skinned Caucasians. Their ubiquitous and inconsequential nature accounts for their more common depiction in Norman Rockwell portraits than in standard dermatologic texts.

Freckles are small (1 to 10 mm), tan-red or light brown macules that first appear in early childhood after sun exposure. Once present, they will fade and reappear in a cyclic fashion with winter and summer, respectively.

> The observed hyperpigmentation of the freckle is the result of increased amounts of melanin pigment within basal keratinocytes; melanocytes are relatively normal in number, although they may be slightly enlarged. It is unclear as to whether the freckle represents a focal abnormality in pigment production by a discrete field of melanocytes, enhanced pigment donation to adjacent basal keratinocytes, or both.

MELASMA

Melasma is a masklike zone of facial hyperpigmentation commonly seen in pregnancy; hence its designation as "the mask of pregnancy." It presents as poorly defined, blotchy macules involving the cheeks, temples, and forehead bilaterally. Sunlight may accentuate this pigmentation, which often resolves spontaneously, particularly after the end of pregnancy.

> Histologically, two patterns have been recognized:[10] an **epidermal type,** in which there is increased melanin deposition in the basal layers, and a **dermal type,** characterized by macrophages in the superficial (papillary) dermis that have phagocytized melanin from the adjacent epidermal layer (a process referred to as **melanin pigment incontinence**). These two types may be distinguished by the use of a Wood's light (see p. 1278). This is important because melasma of the epidermal type may respond to the topical bleaching agent hydroquinone.

The pathogenesis of melasma appears to relate to functional alterations in melanocytes resulting in enhanced pigment transfer to basal keratinocytes or to dermal macrophages. Apart from its association with pregnancy, melasma may occur during the administration of oral contraceptives or hydantoins, or it may be idiopathic. One study indicates that subclinical ab-

normalities in ovarian hormone production may underlie the pathogenesis of some cases of idiopathic melasma.[11]

LENTIGO

Until now, we have been addressing disorders of pigmentation that do not involve proliferation of melanocytes. The term lentigo (plural, lentigenes) refers to a common benign hyperplasia of melanocytes occurring at all ages, but often in infancy and childhood. There is no sex or racial predilection, and the cause and pathogenesis are unknown. These lesions may involve mucous membranes as well as the skin, and they appear as small (5 to 10 mm), oval, tan-brown macules. Unlike freckles, lentigenes do not darken when exposed to sunlight.

The essential histologic feature of the lentigo is melanocytic hyperplasia that produces a hyperpigmented basal cell layer in the epidermis in a linear fashion. So characteristic is this linear hyperplasia that the term lentiginous is often used to describe similar patterns of growth in unrelated melanocytic tumors. Elongation and thinning of the rete ridges are also commonly seen in a lentigo.

NEVOCELLULAR NEVUS (PIGMENTED NEVUS, MOLE)

Most of us have at least a few moles and probably regard them as mundane and uninteresting. It may be surprising to learn, then, that moles or nevi represent one of the most diverse, dynamic, and biologically instructive tumors of the skin! Strictly speaking, the term nevus denotes any congenital lesion of the skin. Nevocellular nevus, however, refers to any congenital or acquired neoplasm of melanocytes.

Clinically, common acquired nevocellular nevi are tan-to-brown, uniformly pigmented, small (usually less than 1 cm), solid regions of elevated skin (papules) with well-defined, rounded borders (Fig. 27–3A). There are numerous clinical and histologic types of nevocellular nevi, and the clinical appearance may be quite variable. The *common acquired nevus* is usually dark brown and raised centrally, surrounded by a tan, flat (macular) area. On the other hand, *congenital nevocellular nevi* may be large and contain numerous hairs; so-called *blue nevi* have a deep blue-gray color that may be confused with malignancy of melanocytes. The *compound nevus of Spitz* (spindle cell and epithelioid cell nevus) is a lesion that occurs predominantly in childhood. It usually grows rapidly and has a pink-to-tan color. *Halo nevi* are surrounded by a vitiligo-like zone of hypopigmentation, often associated with inflammation of the nevocellular nevus. Most acquired (noncongenital) nevocellular nevi develop during childhood and early adulthood. True congenital lesions are present at birth, although they may become clinically prominent only with time, and they often involve large segments of

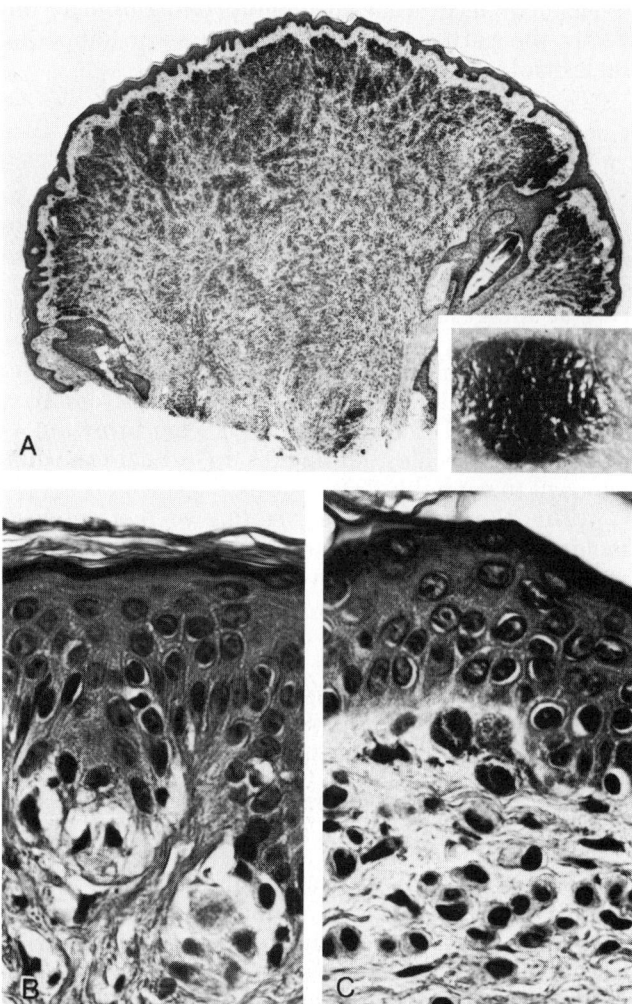

Figure 27–3. Nevocellular nevus. Lesions are symmetric and uniform in clinical (A, inset) and histologic (A) appearance. Junctional nevi (B), characterized by rounded nests of nevus cells at the dermoepidermal junction, may progress with time to become compound and pure dermal nevi (C), exhibiting migration of nevus cells into the underlying dermis.

ble to predict these histologic variations clinically, although compound and dermal nevi tend to be more elevated than junctional nevi. With progressive downgrowth into the dermis, nevus cells undergo an intriguing cytologic and histochemical change termed maturation. Whereas early nests at the dermoepidermal junction tend to be pigmented (type A cells), nevus cells within the superficial dermis tend to be nonpigmented and arranged in cords or fascicles (type B cells). In the lower papillary and upper reticular dermis, individual nevus cells frequently become spindle-shaped and cluster to resemble neural tissue (type C cells).[12,13] This amazing metamorphosis appears to correlate with progressive aging of lesions and with enzymatic changes in these cells (e.g., loss of tyrosinase activity in nonpigmented type B and C cells and acquisition of cholinesterase activity in nerve cell–like type C cells). **This sequence of maturation of individual nevus cells is of diagnostic importance in distinguishing some benign nevi from malignant melanoma** (see later).

In addition to nevocellular nevi with classic histologic features, there are a number of variants. Many true **congenital nevi** exhibit infiltration of the lower dermis and subcutaneous fat, with small clusters of nevus cells intimately associated with neurovascular bundles and skin appendages. **Blue nevi** are characterized by highly dendritic nevus cells (as opposed to the rounded cell typical of most melanocytic nevi) that are very heavily pigmented. When these cells are located within the middle to deep dermis, a blue to gray-blue color is appreciated clinically. **Compound nevi of Spitz** are formed by spindle-shaped and plump "epithelioid" (epithelium-like) nevus cells that frequently show striking nuclear irregularities, resulting in confusion with malignant melanoma. **Halo nevi** are associated with a brisk lymphocytic response that may indicate the attempt of immune mechanisms to eradicate nevus cells. Conceivably, they have acquired some early characteristics of malignancy, although most are believed to be benign biologically at the time of their removal.

the body surface ("garment" or "bathing trunk" nevi). Such large congenital lesions may undergo malignant degeneration.

All nevocellular nevi are composed of melanocytes that have been transformed into cells that little resemble the dendritic forms from which they arose. Nevus cells are round to oval in shape and contain uniform nuclei without prominent nucleoli. These cells form well-defined, rounded aggregates of cells (nests) that initially grow along the dermoepidermal junction (Fig. 27–3B). Such lesions are called **junctional nevi,** and when they are accompanied by lentiginous proliferation of melanocytes, they are referred to as lentiginous junctional nevi. With time, nevus cells begin to grow downward into the dermis to become **compound nevi,** in which epidermal nests and dermal nests coexist. Finally, older lesions may lose their epidermal components to become **dermal nevi** (Fig. 27–3C). It is not always possi-

Although nevocellular nevi are common, their clinical and histologic diversity necessitates thorough knowledge of their appearance and natural evolution lest they be confused with other skin conditions, notably malignant melanoma. The biologic importance of some nevi, however, resides in their recent recognition as an important model of tumor progression (dysplastic nevi and the heritable melanoma syndrome).

DYSPLASTIC NEVI

The association of nevocellular nevi with malignant melanoma was made over 160 years ago,[14] although it was not until 1978 that a true precursor of malignant melanoma was described in detail. In 1978, Clark and colleagues detailed the characteristics of lesions they termed "BK" moles[15] (a name derived from the first letters of the last names of the initial two families studied). These investigators not only described a cutaneous lesion of marked practical significance in the identification and prophylactic monitoring of individuals at high risk to develop melanoma, but also identified a process that could be easily seen and studied on the skin and that served as a model for the progression of many tumors from dysplasia to malignancy.

Clinically, BK moles — or dysplastic nevi, as they are frequently called — are larger than most acquired nevi (often greater than 6 mm) and may occur as hundreds of lesions on the body surface (Fig. 27–4A). They are flat macules to slightly raised plaques and usually show variability in pigmentation (variegation) and borders that are irregular in contour. Unlike ordinary moles, dysplastic nevi have a tendency to occur on non–sun-exposed, as well as on sun-exposed, body surfaces. Dysplastic nevi have been documented in multiple members of families with the heritable melanoma syndrome.[16] In these cases, genetic analyses have demonstrated the trait to be inherited as an autosomal dominant, possibly involving a susceptibility gene located on the short arm of chromosome 1, near the Rh locus.[17] Dysplastic nevi imply an increased risk that the patient will develop malignant melanoma in clinically unaffected skin as well as in pre-existing nevi. Dysplastic nevi undergo malignant transforma-

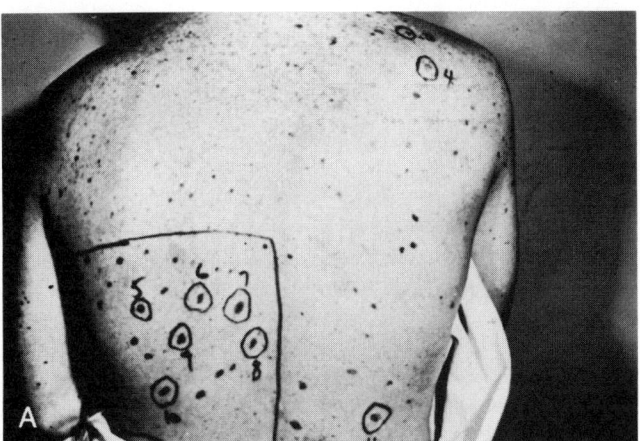
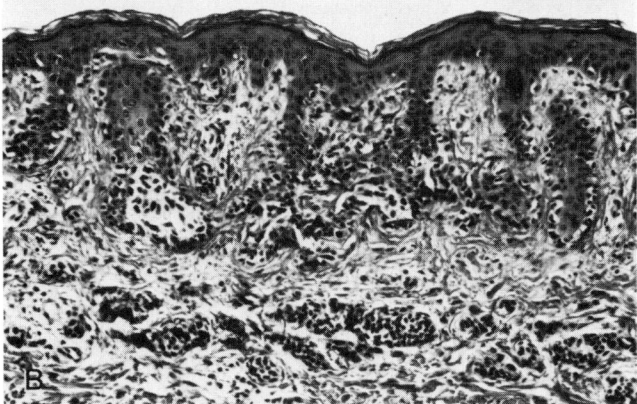

Figure 27–4. Dysplastic nevi. *A,* Multiple irregular, darkly pigmented lesions on the back of a young patient. *B,* Histologically, poorly formed and coalescent nests of nevus cells as well as lentiginous hyperplasia are present along the dermoepidermal junction. These nevi often have an asymmetric architecture and are accompanied by fibrosis within the superficial dermis.

tion at a much higher frequency than ordinary moles, and transitions from these lesions to early melanoma have actually been documented clinically and histologically within a period as short as several weeks. However, most dysplastic nevi are clinically stable lesions.

Histologically (Fig. 27–4B), dysplastic nevi have characteristic features. They generally consist of compound nevi with both architectural and cytologic evidence of abnormal growth (atypia). **Nevus cell nests within the epidermis may be enlarged and exhibit abnormal fusion or coalescence of adjacent nests. As part of this process, single nevus cells begin to replace the normal basal cell layer along the dermoepidermal junction, producing so-called lentiginous hyperplasia** (recall the definition of this term earlier). Individual nevus cells may deviate from their round shapes to become more fusiform, and cytologic atypia consisting of irregular, often angulated, nuclear contours and hyperchromasia are frequently observed. Associated alterations also occur in the superficial dermis. These consist of a usually sparse lymphocytic infiltrate, loss of melanin pigment from presumably destroyed nevus cells, phagocytosis of this pigment by dermal macrophages (melanin pigment incontinence), and a peculiar linear fibrosis surrounding the epidermal rete ridges that are involved by the nevus. All of these features assist in the histologic recognition of a dysplastic nevus.

Several lines of evidence support the concept that *the dysplastic nevus is a precursor of malignant melanoma.* In one study[18] it was shown that in a large number of families prone to the development of melanoma, over 5% of family members developed melanoma over an eight-year follow-up period, and new melanomas occurred only in individuals with dysplastic nevi. From this database, it was concluded that the actuarial probability of persons with the dysplastic nevus syndrome developing melanoma is 56% at age 59! Dysplastic nevi also demonstrate expression of some cell surface antigens that are intermediate between those present on benign nevocellular nevi and malignant melanoma.[19] Karyotypic abnormalities have been documented in members of melanoma-prone families with dysplastic nevi,[20] suggesting that chromosome instability may contribute to the pathogenesis of hereditary melanoma. In addition, cells cultured from such individuals show abnormal vulnerability to the deleterious effects of ultraviolet irradiation.[21] Clinical documentation of progression of dysplastic nevi to melanoma exists,[22] and these two entities are frequently encountered together in tissue sections.[23] Because dysplastic nevi occur in the skin, an organ readily accessible to study, their biologic course and progression have provided an important model for the evolution of malignancy in general. Accordingly, Clark and associates[24] have proposed six steps whereby benign nevi may undergo aberrant differentiation to become dysplastic, and eventually, metastasizing malignant tumors (Fig. 27–5). Parallels

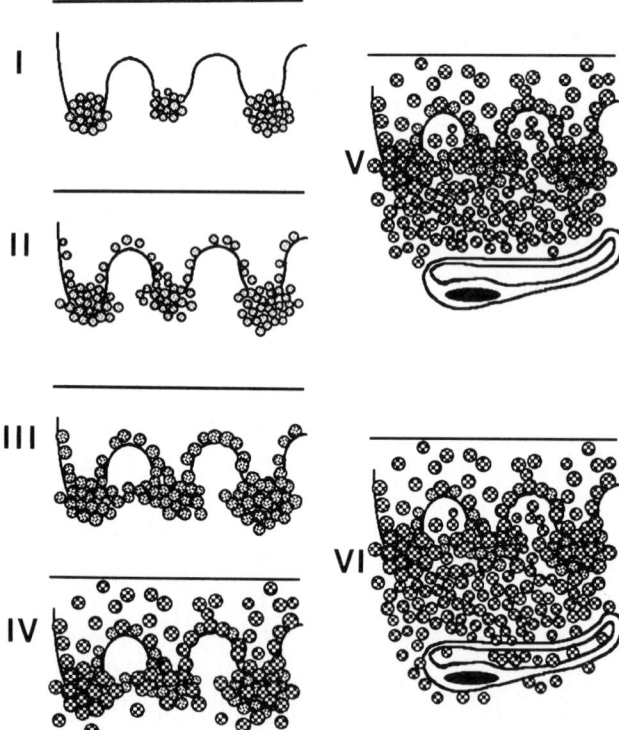

Figure 27–5. Steps of tumor progression in nevocellular nevi. Ordinary junctional nevus (I) develops lentiginous component (II), cells become enlarged and atypical (III), and they begin to coalesce and invade more superficial layers of the epidermis (IV; in situ melanoma). Finally they invade the dermis as an expansive nodule (V), a stage that correlates with acquisition of potential for vessel invasion and metastasis (VI).

may be found in neoplasia involving other organ systems.

MALIGNANT MELANOMA

Malignant melanoma is a relatively common neoplasm that not long ago was considered deadly. Today, as a result of increased public awareness of the earliest manifestations of this neoplasm, most melanomas are cured surgically.[25] Nonetheless, the incidence of melanoma is on the rise, necessitating vigorous surveillance for its development and ongoing study to determine its pathogenesis.

As with epithelial malignancies of the skin (see later), sunlight appears to play an important role in the development of malignant melanoma. For example, men commonly develop this tumor on the upper back, whereas women have a relatively high incidence on both the back and the legs. Lightly pigmented individuals are at higher risk for the development of melanoma than darkly pigmented individuals. Sunlight, however, does not seem to be the only predisposing factor, and the presence of a pre-existing nevus (e.g., a dysplastic nevus), hereditary factors, or even exposure to certain carcinogens (as in the case of experimental melanomas in rodent models) may play a role in lesion development and evolution.[26]

Clinically, malignant melanoma is usually asymptomatic, although itching may be an early manifestation. The most important clinical sign of the disease is change in color in a pigmented lesion. Unlike benign (nondysplastic) nevi, melanomas are variegated in pigmentation, appearing in shades of black, brown, red, dark blue, and gray (Fig. 27–6A). Occasionally, zones of white or flesh-colored hypopigmentation are also present. The borders of melanomas are not smooth, round, and uniform, as in nevocellular nevi, but irregular and often "notched." Melanomas occur at a variety of sites in addition to the skin including the scalp, oral and anogenital mucosal surfaces, nail beds, conjunctivae, orbit, and even the esophagus and leptomeninges. Because of this, careful clinical examination is necessary for definite exclusion of this diagnosis in a given individual.

Central to understanding the complicated histology of malignant melanoma is the concept of radial and vertical growth.[27] *Simply stated, radial growth indicates the tendency of a melanoma to grow horizontally within the epidermal and superficial dermal layers, often for a prolonged period of time. During this stage*

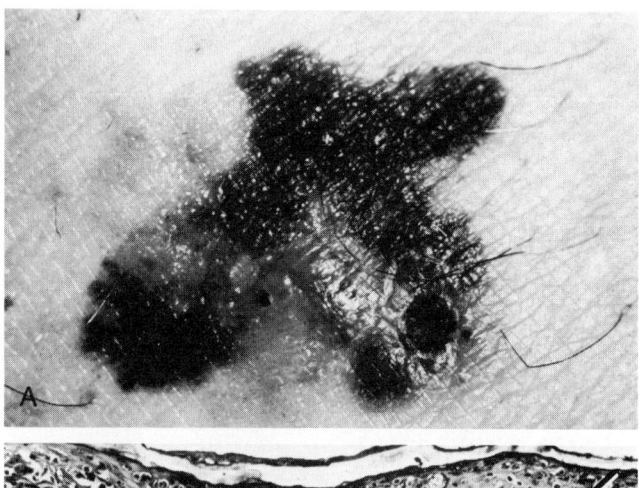

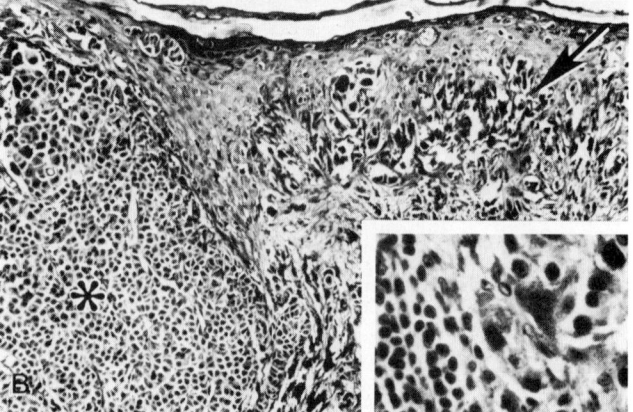

Figure 27–6. Malignant melanoma. *A,* Clinically, lesions are irregular in contour and pigmentation. *B,* Flat macular areas correlate with the radial growth phase *(arrow),* raised areas usually correspond to nodular aggregates of malignant cells (*) in the vertical phase of growth. Note in the inset the difference between melanoma cells (upper right half of inset) and a small focus of benign, presumably pre-existing nevus cells (lower left half of inset).

of growth (analogous to stage IV of Clark's model of tumor progression, Fig. 27–5), melanoma cells do not have the capacity to metastasize. With time, the pattern of growth assumes a vertical component, and the melanoma now grows downward into the deeper dermal layers as an expansile mass lacking cellular maturation (stage V, Fig. 27–5). This event is heralded clinically by the development of a nodule in the relatively flat radial growth phase, and correlates with the emergence of a clone of cells with true metastatic potential.[28] Interestingly, the probability of metastasis in such a lesion may be predicted by simply measuring in millimeters the depth of invasion of this vertical growth phase nodule below the granular cell layer of the overlying epidermis (Fig. 27–7).[29]

Individual melanoma cells usually are considerably larger than nevus cells. They contain large nuclei with irregular contours having chromatin characteristically clumped at the periphery of the nuclear membrane and prominent red (eosinophilic) nucleoli. These cells grow as poorly formed nests or as individual cells at all levels of the epidermis and, in the dermis, as expansile, balloon-like nodules (Fig. 27–6B). Different morphologic variants of radial growth phases have been recognized and termed superficial spreading, lentigo maligna, and acral-lentiginous types.[30] **The nature and extent of the vertical growth phase, however, determines the biologic behavior of malignant melanoma,** and thus it is important to observe and record vertical growth phase parameters in a pathology report (Fig. 27–7).[31]

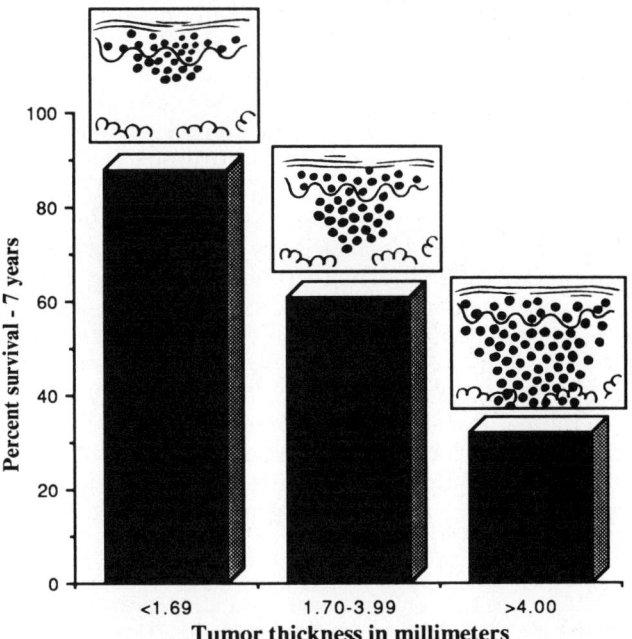

Figure 27–7. Graph of seven-year survival versus thickness of the vertical growth phase nodule in malignant melanoma. Note the dramatic and consistent decline in survival with increasing tumor thickness. (Adapted from Clark, W.C., Jr., et al.: The biologic forms of malignant melanoma. Hum. Pathol. *17*:443, 1986.)

Revolutionary advances have occurred during the past decade concerning our understanding of the fundamental biology and practical therapy of malignant melanoma. It is becoming apparent that melanoma cells in the vertical phase of growth possess distinctive antigenic, cytogenetic, and biosynthetic abnormalities that may assist in overall understanding of the metastatic process.[32,33] There is a growing appreciation of the role of the immune response in preventing the emergence and progression of melanoma, particularly with respect to local imbalances in immune regulation that may result from ultraviolet light exposure, creating a permissive environment for tumorigenesis.[34] Of enormous practical importance is that accurate recognition of early stages of melanoma development has led to conservative strategies for surgical removal that have resulted in dramatic increases in survival. In the United States, the five-year survival of persons with melanoma in 1945 was about 40%; in 1983 it was 83%.[34a] Many modalities of exquisitely specific tumor destruction are now being tested. One such method utilizes laser energy of a predetermined wavelength, energy level, and pulse duration to selectively destroy pigmented melanosomes within melanocytes, or potentially within tumor cells.[35]

BENIGN EPITHELIAL TUMORS

Benign epidermal neoplasms are common and usually biologically inconsequential, although they may represent significant sources of psychologic discomfort for the patient. These tumors, derived from the keratinizing stratified squamous epithelium of the epidermis and hair follicles (keratinocytes) and the ductular epithelium of cutaneous glands, may recapitulate the cell layers from which they arise. Clinically, they are often confused with malignancy, particularly when they are pigmented or inflamed, and histologic examination of a biopsy specimen is frequently required to establish a definitive diagnosis. Appearance of these neoplasms in certain clinical settings (such as in the case of the explosive development of multiple seborrheic keratoses, described below) provides important insights into basic mechanisms responsible for the genesis of some of these lesions.

SEBORRHEIC KERATOSES

These common epidermal tumors occur most frequently in middle-aged or older individuals. They arise spontaneously and may become particularly numerous on the trunk, although the extremities, head, and neck may also be involved. In blacks, multiple small lesions on the face are termed *dermatosis papulosa nigra.*

Clinically, seborrheic keratoses (also called senile keratoses) have characteristic features. They appear as round, flat, coinlike plaques that vary in diameter from millimeters to several centimeters (Fig.

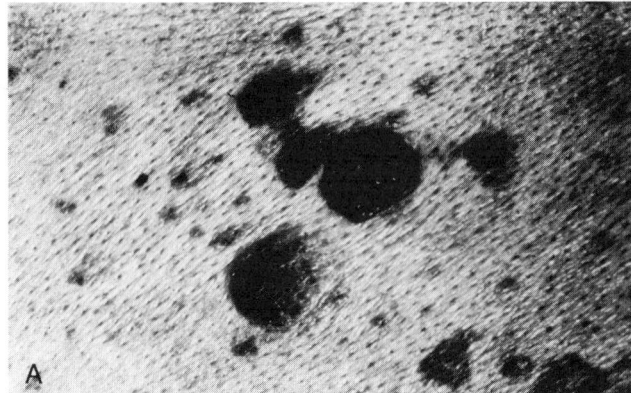

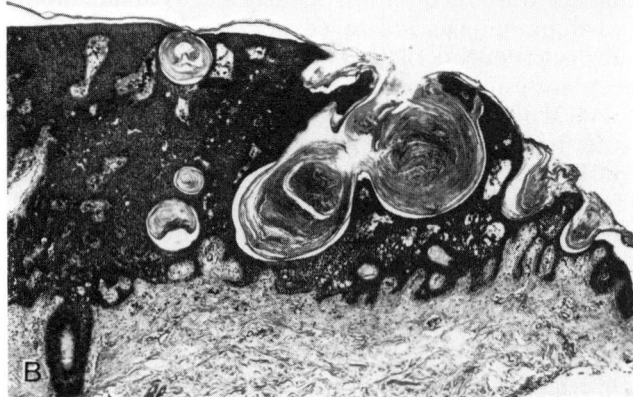

Figure 27–8. Seborrheic keratoses. Multiple coinlike pigmented lesions on the back (*A*) are composed of well-demarcated, orderly proliferations of basaloid cells forming small, keratin-filled cysts (*B*).

27–8*A*). They are uniformly tan to dark brown in color and usually show a velvety to granular surface. Lesions may give the impression that they are "stuck on" and that they may be easily peeled off. Inspection with a hand lens will usually reveal small, round, porelike ostia impacted with keratin (a feature helpful in differentiating these pigmented lesions from melanomas).

Histologically, these neoplasms are exophytic and demarcated sharply from the adjacent epidermis (Fig. 27–8*B*). They are composed of sheets of small cells that most resemble basal cells of the normal epidermis. Variable melanin pigmentation is present within these basaloid cells, accounting for the brown coloration clinically. Exuberant keratin production (hyperkeratosis) occurs at the surface of seborrheic keratoses, and small keratin-filled cysts (horn cysts) and downgrowths of keratin into the main tumor mass (pseudo–horn cysts) are characteristic features. The pseudo–horn cysts correlate with the keratin-filled ostia that are seen on the surface of the lesion. Interestingly, when seborrheic keratoses become irritated and inflamed, they undergo squamous differentiation[36] and are characterized by foci of "whirling" squamous cells resembling eddy currents in a stream. A biologic explanation for this intriguing phenomenon awaits discovery. When seborrheic kera-

toses involve the epithelium of hair follicles, they may grow in an endophytic fashion, and they generally also show the effects of inflammation; such lesions are termed **inverted follicular keratoses**.

It is tempting to dismiss the seborrheic keratosis as a mundane lesion. It is easily removed by curettage or freezing, and it poses no significant risk of malignancy. However, when this tumor occurs explosively in large numbers, as part of a paraneoplastic syndrome *(sign of Leser-Trelat)*, important pathogenetic issues arise. In a recent report, for example, a patient was noted to have developed the sign of Leser-Trelat in association with the occurrence of a malignant melanoma.[37] The melanoma was shown to produce an alpha-transforming growth factor (a growth factor closely related to epidermal growth factor). Because this factor exerts its effects by interaction with receptors on basal keratinocytes, it was hypothesized that the seborrheic keratoses were related to its abnormal production by the melanoma. Interestingly, when the melanoma was excised surgically, the number of seborrheic keratoses decreased.

ACANTHOSIS NIGRICANS

This term is used to describe thickened (acanthosis = hyperplasia of the stratum spinosum of the epidermis), hyperpigmented zones of skin involving most commonly the flexural areas (axillae, skin folds of the neck, groin, and anogenital regions). It is an important cutaneous marker for associated benign and malignant conditions, and, accordingly, is divided into two types.[38] The *benign type* constitutes about 80% of all cases. It develops gradually and usually occurs in childhood or during puberty. It may occur (1) as an autosomal dominant trait with variable penetrance; (2) in association with obesity or endocrine abnormalities (particularly with pituitary and pineal tumors and with diabetes); and (3) as part of a number of rare congenital syndromes. As with seborrheic keratoses, acanthosis nigricans may result from abnormal production of epidermal growth-promoting factors by a variety of tumors.[37] This latter occurrence may account for many instances of the *malignant type,* in which lesions arise in middle-aged and older individuals, often in association with an underlying adenocarcinoma. Because the occurrence of acanthosis nigricans may precede the overt clinical symptoms and signs of the underlying process, knowledge and recognition of this entity is of great diagnostic importance.

All forms of acanthosis nigricans have similar histologic features. The epidermis is not flat, but undulates sharply to form numerous repeating peaks and valleys. Variable hyperplasia (as judged by total epidermal cells per body surface area) may be seen, although the overall epidermal thickness may appear normal. There is also hyperkeratosis and slight basal cell layer hyperpigmentation (but no melanocytic hyperplasia). Most of the clinically appreciated hyperpigmentation is the result of the epidermal changes, and not excess or abnormally distributed melanin pigment.

FIBROEPITHELIAL POLYP

The fibroepithelial polyp has many names (acrochordon, squamous papilloma, skin tag) and is probably one of the most common cutaneous lesions. It is generally detected as an incidental finding in middle-aged and older individuals and is seen on the neck, trunk, face, and intertriginous areas as a soft, flesh-colored, baglike tumor attached to the skin surface by a small, often slender stalk.

Histologically, these tumors are merely fibrovascular cores covered by benign squamous epithelium. It is not uncommon to discover ischemic necrosis in histologic sections (the result of torsion that produced the pain and swelling that precipitated their removal).

Fibroepithelial polyps are usually biologically inconsequential, although they have been associated with diabetes and intestinal polyposis. It is of interest that along with nevocellular nevi (discussed earlier) and hemangiomas (see later), they often become more numerous or prominent during pregnancy.

EPITHELIAL CYST (WEN)

Epithelial cysts are common lesions formed by the downgrowth and cystic expansion of the epidermis or of the epithelium forming the hair follicle. These cysts are filled with keratin and variable amounts of admixed, lipid-containing debris derived from sebaceous secretions. Clinically, they are subcutaneous, well-circumscribed, firm, and often moveable nodules. When large, they may be dome-shaped and flesh-colored and often become painful upon traumatic rupture.

Histologically, epithelial cysts are divided into several types according to the structural components of their walls. The **epidermal inclusion cyst** has a wall nearly identical to the epidermis and is filled with laminated strands of keratin. The **pilar** or **trichilemmal cyst** has a wall that resembles follicular epithelium, without a granular cell layer and filled by a more homogeneous mixture of keratin and lipid. The **dermoid cyst** is similar to the epidermal inclusion cyst, but it also shows multiple appendages (such as small hair follicles) budding outward from its wall. Finally, **steatocystoma multiplex** constitutes a curious cyst with a wall resembling the sebaceous gland duct from which numerous compressed sebaceous lobules originate. The importance of recognition of this cyst derives from the often dominantly heritable nature of the lesion.

KERATOACANTHOMA

Keratoacanthoma is a remarkable, rapidly developing neoplasm that clinically and histologically may mimic well-differentiated squamous cell carcinoma (p. 1287), but it heals spontaneously, without treatment! Men are more often affected than women, and lesions most frequently affect sun-exposed skin of Caucasians over 50 years of age.[39]

Clinically, keratoacanthomas appear as flesh-colored, dome-shaped nodules with a central, keratin-filled plug, imparting a crater-like topography. Lesions range in size from 1 cm to several centimeters and have a predilection for the cheeks, nose, ears, and dorsa of the hands.

Histologically, keratoacanthomas are characterized by a central, keratin-filled crater, surrounded by proliferating epithelial cells that extend upward in a liplike fashion over the sides of the crater and downward into the dermis as irregular tongues (Fig. 27–9A). This epithelium is composed of enlarged, often cytologically atypical, cells that have a characteristically "glassy" eosinophilic cytoplasm (Fig. 27–9B) and produce keratin abruptly (without the development of an intervening granular cell layer). This mode of keratinization is analogous to that of the normal hair follicle and similar to that seen in the pilar cyst described earlier, giving rise to speculation that the keratoacanthoma is a neoplasm of follicular epithelium. The early tumor infiltrates into the collagen and elastic fibers and entraps them. Little, if any, host inflammatory response is present during this rapidly proliferative phase, but as the lesion evolves, there is some stromal response that is fibrotic and contains numerous inflammatory cells.

Because certain well-differentiated squamous cell carcinomas may closely resemble keratoacanthomas histologically, more sensitive methods are currently being sought to assist in this differential diagnosis. Markers for the degree and uniformity of keratinocyte differentiation may indicate subtle differences between these two neoplasms. For example, antibodies to the protein involucrin, a marker for terminal keratinocyte differentiation, appear to separate some keratoacanthomas from squamous cell carcinomas by indicating more complete terminal differentiation of the former.[40,41] The role of host immunity in the determination of the biologic behavior of keratoacanthomas is only now being examined. The intriguing possibility exists that the clinical course of keratoacanthoma (regression) and squamous cell carcinoma (progression) may be more the result of differences in host immune responsiveness than of differences inherent in the biologic aggressiveness of these two morphologically similar neoplasms.

ADNEXAL (APPENDAGE) TUMORS

There are literally hundreds of benign neoplasms arising from cutaneous appendages.[42] Although some

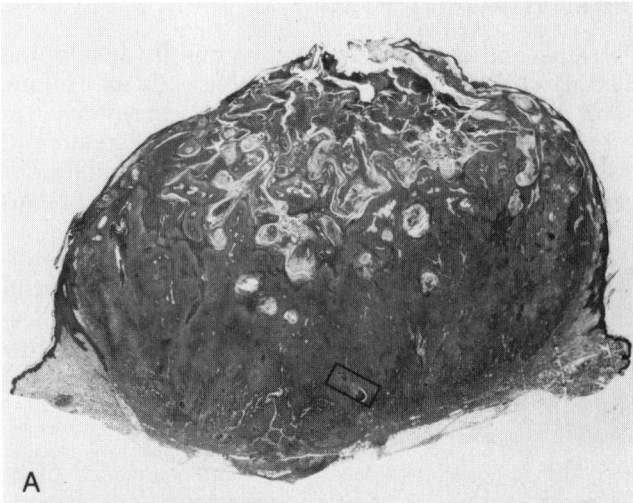

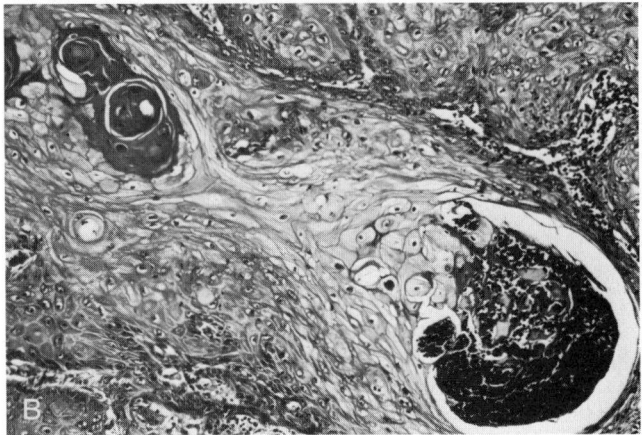

Figure 27–9. Keratoacanthoma. *A,* At low power, the crater-like architecture may be appreciated. *B,* Higher power of the small rectangle in *A.* These tumors are composed of large, glassy squamous cells that form islands of keratin (upper left). The dark mass in the lower right corner is a characteristic aggregate of neutrophils within the tumor.

show no aggressive behavior and remain localized, they may be confused with certain types of cutaneous cancers (e.g., basal cell carcinoma, p. 1282). Certain appendage tumors are associated with mendelian patterns of inheritance and occur as multiple disfiguring lesions. In some instances, these lesions serve as markers for internal malignancy, as in the case of multiple trichilemmomas and breast carcinoma of Cowden's syndrome.[43] Selected examples are provided here to illustrate neoplasms of hair follicles, eccrine glands, and apocrine glands.

Clinically, appendage tumors are often nondescript, solitary or multiple papules and nodules. Some have a predisposition for occurrence on specific body surfaces. For example, the *eccrine poroma* occurs predominantly on the palms and soles. The *cylindroma,* an appendage tumor with apocrine differentiation, usually occurs on the forehead and scalp (Fig. 27–10*A*), where coalescence of nodules with time may

produce a hatlike growth, hence the name *"turban tumor."* These lesions may be dominantly inherited and first appear early in life. *Syringomas,* lesions of eccrine differentiation, on the other hand, usually occur as multiple, small, tan papules in the vicinity of the lower eyelids. *Trichoepitheliomas,* showing follicular differentiation, are dominantly inherited when they are seen as multiple, semitransparent, dome-shaped papules that involve the face, scalp, neck, and upper trunk.

> Histologically, appendage tumors do not always resemble their normal adnexal counterparts, and differentiation pathways are revealed only by electron microscopy and enzyme histochemistry.[41] The **cylindroma,** for example, is composed of islands of basaloid cells that seem to fit together like pieces of a jigsaw puzzle within a fibrous dermal matrix (Fig. 27–10*B*). The **syringoma** does show some eccrine ductular differentiation within small, tadpole-like islands and strands of basaloid epithelium (Fig. 27–10*C*). The **trichoepithelioma** is a proliferation of basaloid cells that forms hair follicle–like structures (Fig. 27–10*D*). The **trichilemmoma** is a localized proliferation of pale pink, glassy cells that resembles the uppermost portion of the hair follicle (infundibulum).

Although most appendage tumors are benign, malignant variants do exist. *Sebaceous carcinoma,* for example, arises from the meibomian glands of the eyelid and may show an aggressive biologic course with systemic metastases. *Eccrine* and *apocrine carcinomas* are often confused with metastatic adenocarcinomas to the skin because of their tendency for abortive gland formation.

PREMALIGNANT AND MALIGNANT EPIDERMAL TUMORS

ACTINIC KERATOSIS

Prior to the development of overt malignancy of the epidermis, a series of progressively dysplastic changes occurs, a phenomenon analogous to the atypia that precedes carcinoma of the squamous mucosa of the uterine cervix (p. 1141). Because this dysplasia is usually the result of chronic exposure to sunlight and is associated with build-up of excess keratin, these lesions are called actinic keratoses. As would be expected, they occur in a particularly high incidence in lightly pigmented individuals. Exposure to ionizing radiation, hydrocarbons, and arsenicals may induce similar lesions.

> Lesions are usually less than 1 cm in diameter; are tan-brown, red, or skin-colored; and have a rough, sandpaper-like consistency. Some lesions may produce so much keratin that a "cutaneous horn" develops (Fig. 27–11*A*). Skin

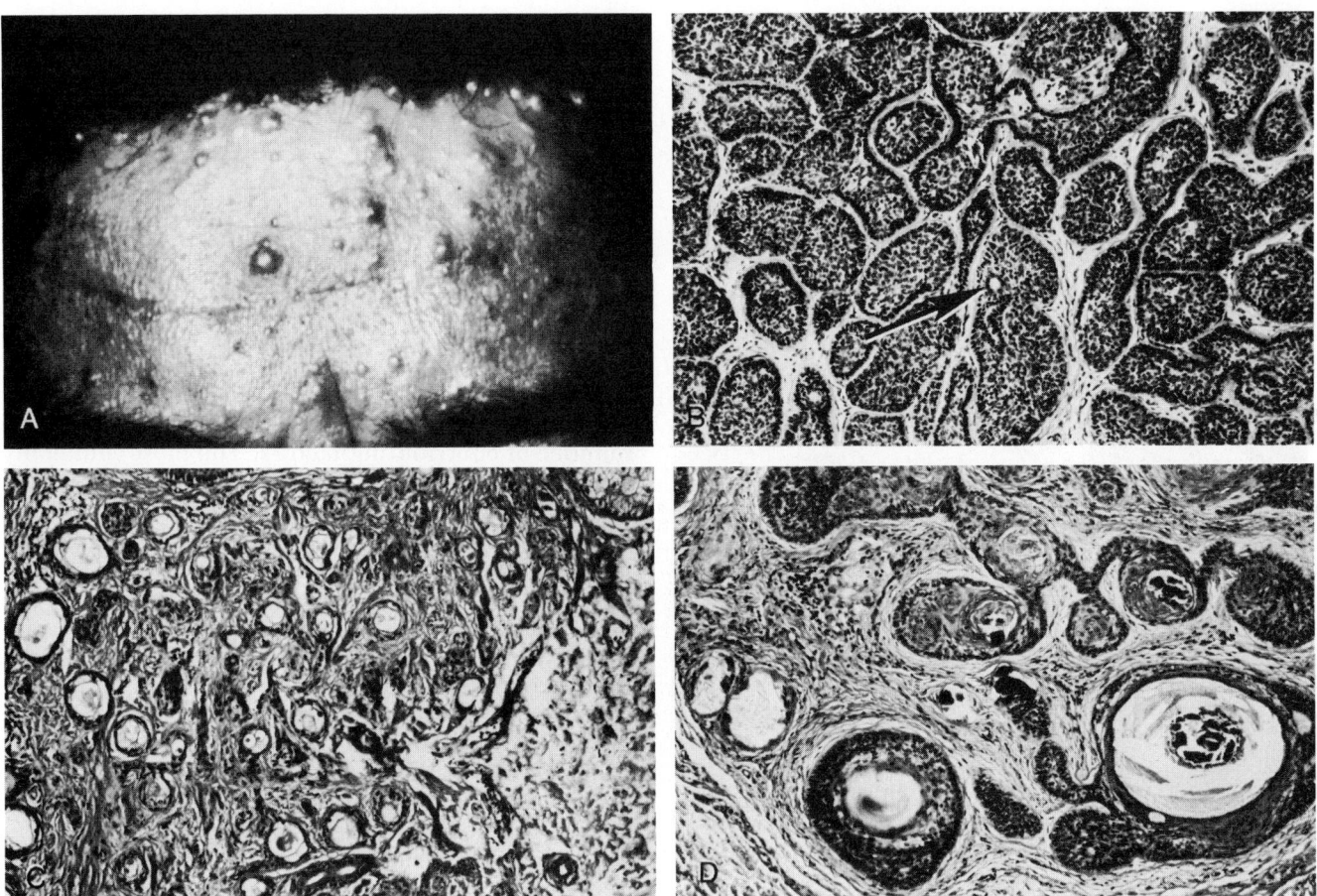

Figure 27–10. Adnexal tumors. Although the clinical appearance is often nondescript (*A* shows multiple cylindromas), the histologic features of each are characteristic. *B,* Cylindroma; *C,* syringoma; *D,* trichoepithelioma. Note the rare ducts in the cylindroma *(arrow),* and the numerous ducts in the syringoma. The trichoepithelioma resembles primitive hair follicle differentiation.

sites commonly involved by sun exposure (face, arms, dorsum of hands) are most frequently affected. The lips may also develop similar lesions (actinic cheilitis).

Cytologic atypia is first seen in the lowermost layers of the epidermis and may be associated with hyperplasia of basal cells (Fig. 27–11A), or, alternatively, with early atrophy that results in diffuse thinning of the epidermal surface of the lesion. The atypical basal cells in the lesions usually have evidence of dyskeratosis with pink or reddish cytoplasm. Also, intercellular bridges are present, in contrast to basal cell carcinoma cells (p. 1288), in which the cytoplasm is usually basophilic and the cells lack intercellular bridges that are identifiable by light microscopy. The dermis contains thickened, blue-gray elastic fibers (elastosis), a probable result of abnormal dermal elastic fiber synthesis by sun-damaged fibroblasts[44] within the superficial dermis. The stratum corneum is thickened and, unlike normal skin, nuclei in the cells in this layer are often retained (a pattern termed parakeratosis). These chronic alterations contrast sharply with the acute changes that occur as a result of sunburn—namely, dermal edema, degranulation of mast cells, and individual cell necrosis within the basal cell layer of the epidermis.[45]

Whether all actinic keratoses would eventuate in skin cancer (usually squamous cell carcinoma), if given enough time, is conjectural. However, enough do become malignant to warrant local eradication of these precursor lesions. This can usually be accomplished by gentle curettage, freezing, or topical application of chemotherapeutic agents.

SQUAMOUS CELL CARCINOMA

Squamous cell carcinoma is the most common tumor arising on sun-exposed sites of older people. Except for lesions on the lower legs, males have a higher incidence of these tumors than women. Implicated as predisposing factors, in addition to sunlight, are industrial carcinogens (tars and oils), chronic ulcers and draining osteomyelitis, old burn scars, ingestion of arsenicals, ionizing radiation, and in the oral cavity tobacco and betel nut chewing. Patients with xeroderma pigmentosum (p. 274) and immunosuppressed individuals also have a high incidence of this neoplasm. *Although these tumors may remain locally confined, they possess a low, but significant, potential for metastasis.*

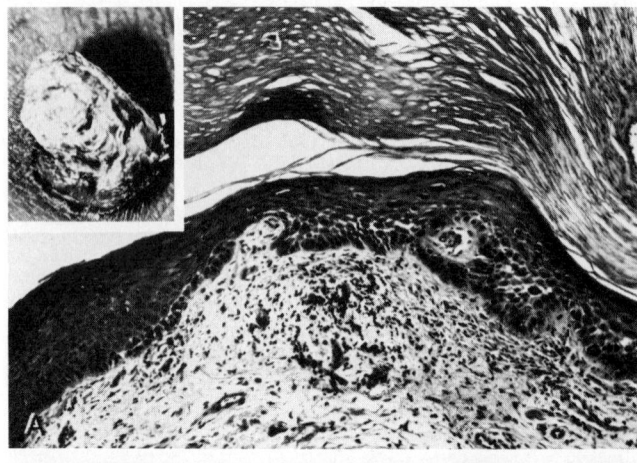

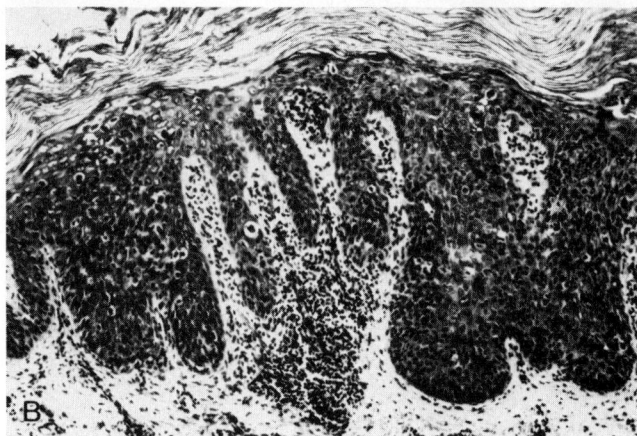

Figure 27–11. *A,* Actinic keratosis. Basal cell layer atypia (normal epidermis on left) is associated with marked hyper- and parakeratosis that may result in the clinical appearance of a horn *(inset). B,* Progression to full-thickness atypia heralds the development of squamous cell carcinoma in situ.

Squamous cell carcinomas that have not invaded through the basement membrane of the dermatoepidermal junction **(in situ carcinoma)** appear as sharply defined, red scaling plaques. More advanced, invasive lesions are nodular, show variable keratin production appreciated clinically as hyperkeratosis, and may ulcerate (Fig. 27–12). Well-differentiated lesions may be indistinguishable from keratoacanthoma (p. 1285). When the mucosa is involved, a zone of white thickening is seen, an appearance caused by a variety of disorders and referred to clinically as **leukoplakia.**

Unlike actinic keratoses, squamous cell carcinoma in situ is characterized by highly atypical cells at all levels of the epidermis (Fig. 27–11*B*). When these cells break through the basement membrane, the process has become invasive. Invasive squamous cell carcinoma (Fig. 27–12) exhibits variable differentiation, ranging from tumors formed by polygonal squamous cells arranged in orderly lobules and exhibiting numerous large zones of keratinization to neoplasms formed by highly anaplastic, rounded cells with foci of necrosis and only abortive, single-cell kera-

tinization (dyskeratosis). These tumors may be so poorly differentiated that electron microscopy for the detection of keratinocyte intercellular attachment sites (desmosomes) or reaction of tissue with antibodies to keratin or epithelial membrane-associated antigens may be necessary to definitively establish cell lineage.

These skin tumors are usually discovered while small and resectable; fewer than 5% have metastases to regional nodes.

The pathogenesis of squamous cell carcinoma of the skin is complex, because it is likely that there are a number of contributing factors. The most commonly accepted exogenous cause is exposure to ultraviolet light with subsequent DNA damage and associated mutagenicity. Individuals who are immunosuppressed, as a result of chemotherapy or organ transplantation or who have xeroderma pigmentosum are at increased risk of developing neoplasms.[46] A considerable proportion of these are squamous cell carcinomas, implicating aberrations in local immune networks in the skin in the production of an atmosphere permissive to neoplasia. Sunlight, in addition to its effect on DNA, also seems to have a direct and at least a transient immunosuppressive effect on skin by affecting the normal surveillance function of antigen-presenting Langerhans cells in the epidermis.[47] In experimental animals, it now appears that although Langerhans cells responsible for T-lymphocyte activation are injured by ultraviolet light, similar cells responsible for the selective induction of suppressor lymphocyte pathways are resistant to UV damage.[48,49] Such a phenomenon could result in local imbalances in T-cell function that would favor tumorigenesis and progression. DNA sequences of certain viruses (e.g., human papillomavirus HPV36) have been detected recently in DNA extracted from potential precursors of squamous cell carcinoma,[50] suggesting a role for these agents in the evolution of certain cutaneous epithelial neoplasms. Finally, certain chemical agents appear to have direct mutagenic effects by producing DNA adducts with subsequent oncogene activation.[51]

BASAL CELL CARCINOMA

Basal cell carcinomas are common, slow-growing tumors that rarely metastasize. They have a tendency to occur at sites subject to chronic sun exposure and in lightly pigmented people. As with squamous cell carcinoma, the incidence of basal cell carcinoma rises sharply with immunosuppression and in patients with inherited defects in DNA replication or repair (xeroderma pigmentosum, p. 274). The rare, dominantly inherited basal cell nevus syndrome[52] is associated with the development of numerous basal cell carcinomas in early life and with abnormalities of bone, nervous system, eyes, and reproductive organs.

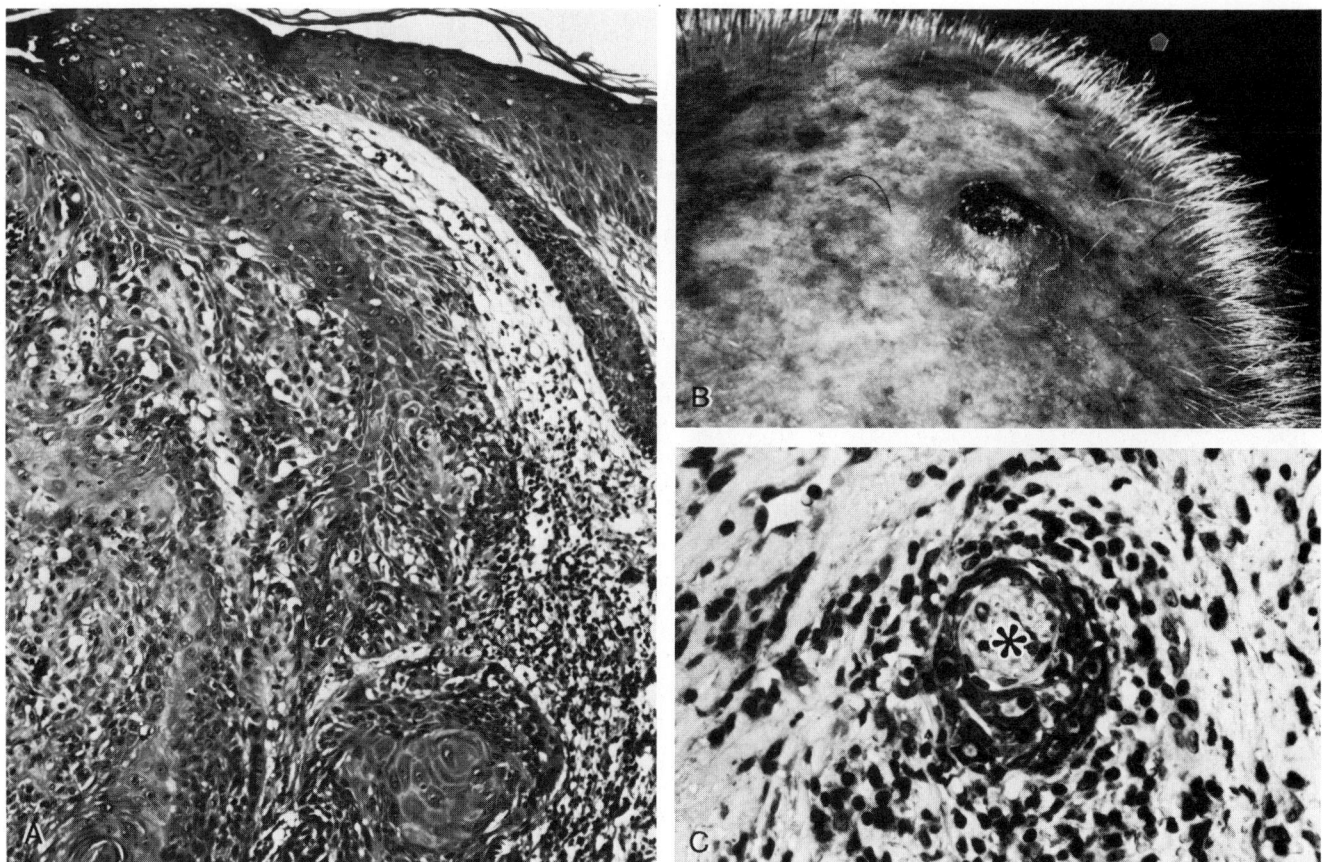

Figure 27–12. Invasive squamous cell carcinoma. *A,* Tongues of atypical squamous epithelium have transgressed the basement membrane, invading deeply into the dermis. *B,* Such lesions are often nodular and ulcerated clinically. *C,* Tumor cells highlighted by staining with labeled antibodies to keratin are surrounding a dermal nerve twig (*), indicative of the locally aggressive nature of this neoplasm.

Macroscopically, these tumors present as pearly papules often containing prominent, dilated subepidermal blood vessels (telangiectasias) (Fig. 27–13*A*). Some tumors contain melanin pigment and, thus, appear similar to nevocellular nevi or melanomas. Advanced lesions may ulcerate, and extensive local invasion of bone or facial sinuses may occur after many years of neglect or in unusually aggressive tumors, justifying the past designation "rodent ulcers."

Histologically, tumor cells resemble those in the normal basal cell layer of the epidermis. They arise from the epidermis or follicular epithelium and do not occur on mucosal surfaces. Two patterns are seen, either **multifocal growths** originating from the epidermis and extending over several square centimeters or more of skin surface (multifocal superficial type), or **nodular lesions** growing downward deeply into the dermis as cords and islands of variably basophilic cells with hyperchromatic nuclei, embedded in a mucinous matrix, and often surrounded by many fibroblasts and lymphocytes (Fig. 27–13*B*). The cells forming the periphery of the tumor cell islands tend to be arranged radially with their long axes in approximate parallel alignment (palisading). The stroma shrinks away from the epithelial tumor nests, creating clefts or separation artifacts that assist in differentiating basal cell carcinomas from certain appendage tumors also characterized by proliferation of basaloid cells.

The indolent clinical behavior of basal cell carcinoma may relate in part to the marked inflammatory infiltrate of T lymphocytes that usually accompanies these tumors. Hyperplasia of Langerhans cells, apposition of T cells to necrotic tumor cells, and markers of functional activation on these T cells have all been documented, supporting the notion that local immunity is important in limiting the growth of these commonly encountered and usually curable tumors.[53,54]

MERKEL CELL CARCINOMA

This rare neoplasm is derived from the infrequent and functionally obscure *Merkel cell* of the epidermis, a neural crest–derived cell putatively important for tactile sensation in lower animals.

Clinically,[55] these tumors occur as flesh-colored, usually solitary nodules on the head, neck, and extremities of elderly individuals. Metastases occur to regional lymph nodes

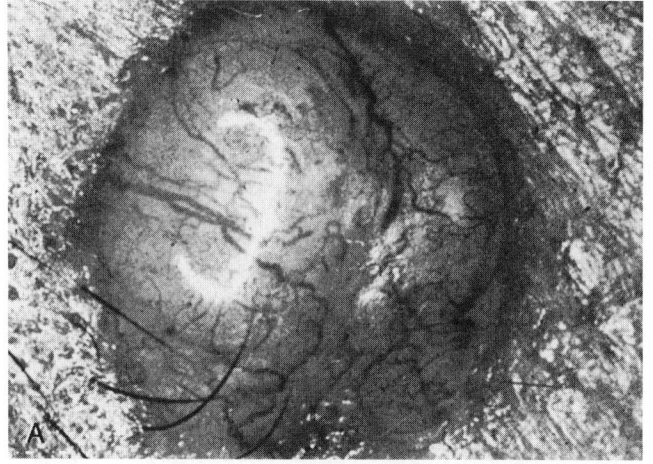

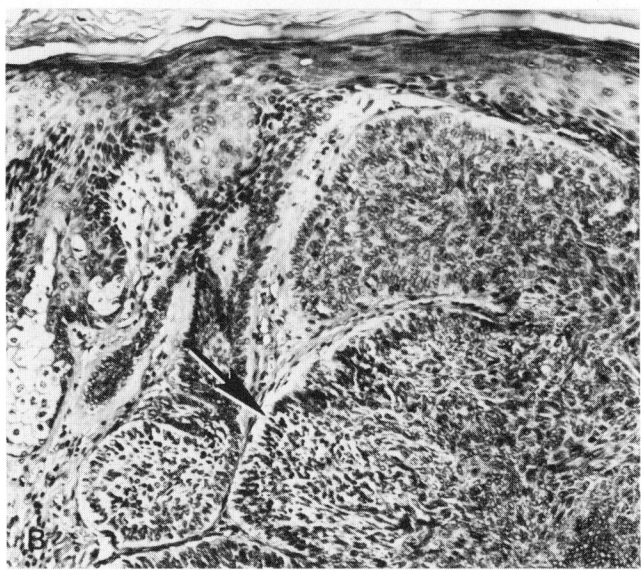

Figure 27–13. Basal cell carcinoma. Pearly telangiectatic nodules (*A*) are composed of nests of basaloid cells within the dermis (*B*) that are often separated from the adjacent stroma by thin clefts (*arrow*).

in more than half the patients, and widespread metastases resulting in death occur in almost one fifth of affected individuals.

Histologically, this tumor closely mimics metastatic small cell carcinoma to the skin (e.g., oat cell carcinoma from the lung; p. 800). Anastomosing cords and sheets of small round cells with pale nuclei, scant cytoplasm, and numerous mitotic figures are present in the dermis and give a trabecular or network-like appearance to the tumor. By electron microscopy, these cells resemble normal Merkel cells in that they contain scattered, membrane-bound, 120- to 210-μm, dense-core granules[56] similar to those seen in other tumors of neuroendocrine origin. They express antigenic markers common to both neuroendocrine and epithelial cells,[57] suggesting that they probably represent true epithelial cells that have undergone neuroendocrine differentiation.

TUMORS OF THE DERMIS

The dermis is composed of a variety of different elements, including smooth muscle, pericytes, fibroblasts, neural tissue, and endothelium. All of these components can give rise to neoplasia within the skin, but many of these tumors also arise in soft tissue and viscera unrelated to skin (e.g., leiomyosarcoma) or occur as part of a syndrome primarily affecting another organ system (e.g., as with cutaneous neurofibromas in neurofibromatosis). In this section, therefore, only representative dermal neoplasms that arise primarily in the skin, that have unique characteristics in the skin, or that have not been detailed in other chapters are considered.

BENIGN FIBROUS HISTIOCYTOMA

Benign fibrous histiocytoma refers to a heterogeneous family of morphologically and histogenetically related benign dermal neoplasms of fibroblasts and histiocytes. They are also discussed on page 1373. These tumors are usually seen in adults, and often occur on the legs of young to middle-aged women.

On gross inspection, these neoplasms are tan to brown, firm papules (Fig. 27–14*A*). Lesions are asymptomatic to slightly tender, and their size may increase and decrease slightly over time. Actively growing lesions may reach several centimeters in diameter, and, with time, they often become flattened. The tendency for fibrous histiocytomas to dimple inward upon lateral compression is helpful in distinguishing them from nodular melanomas, which protrude outward when similarly manipulated.

The most common form of fibrous histiocytoma is referred to as a **dermatofibroma.** These tumors are formed by benign, spindle-shaped fibroblasts arranged in a well-defined, nonencapsulated mass within the mid-dermis (Fig. 27–14*B*). Extension of these cells into the subcutaneous fat is frequently observed. The majority of cases demonstrate a peculiar form of overlying epidermal hyperplasia, characterized by lateral thinning and downward elongation of hyperpigmented rete ridges (''dirty fingers'' pattern). Although foamy histiocytes may be seen in dermatofibromas, they are generally not conspicuous. Other tumors are composed predominantly of these foamy histiocytes admixed with a paucity of fibroblasts. Finally, variants containing numerous blood vessels and deposits of hemosiderin may be encountered (**sclerosing hemangiomas**).

The histogenesis of fibrous histiocytomas remains a mystery. Many cases have a history of antecedent trauma, suggesting an abnormal response to injury, perhaps analogous to the deposition of increased amounts of altered collagen in a hypertrophic scar or keloid.

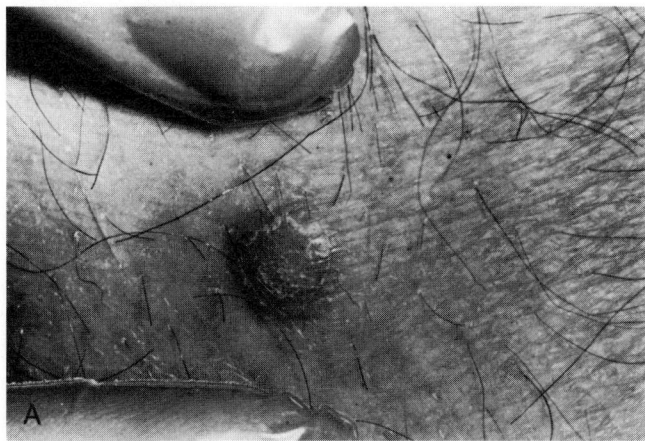

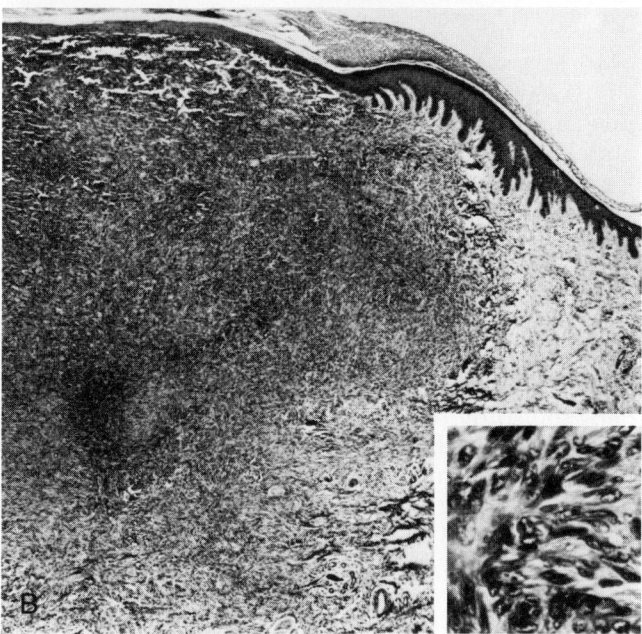

Figure 27–14. Benign fibrous histiocytoma (dermatofibroma). Upon excision, this firm, tan papule on the leg (*A*) shows a localized nodular proliferation of benign-appearing fibroblasts within the dermis (*B; inset*). Note the characteristic overlying epidermal hyperplasia near the edge of the lesion.

DERMATOFIBROSARCOMA PROTUBERANS

Like dermatofibroma, dermatofibrosarcoma protuberans is primarily a proliferation of fibroblasts. It is best regarded as a well-differentiated, primary fibrosarcoma of the skin. These tumors are slow-growing, and, although they are locally aggressive, they rarely metastasize.

Clinically, they are firm, solid nodules that arise most frequently on the trunk. They often develop as aggregated "protuberant" tumors within a firm (indurated) plaque and may ulcerate.

Microscopically, these neoplasms are very cellular, composed of fibroblasts arranged radially, reminiscent of blades of a pinwheel, a pattern referred to

as storiform. Mitoses are usually present but are not as numerous as in a fibrosarcoma (see p. 1377). In contrast to the dermatofibroma, the overlying epidermis is generally thinned and extension from the dermis into subcutaneous fat is frequently present, hindering attempts at complete surgical removal.

XANTHOMAS

Xanthomas are tumorous collections of foamy histiocytes within the dermis. They are best regarded as tumor-like enlargement and accumulation of these cells, as opposed to true neoplasms. They may be associated with familial (p. 561) or acquired disorders resulting in hyperlipidemia, with lymphoproliferative malignancies, or without any underlying disorder.

On the basis of clinical appearance, xanthomas are divided into five types. Because identification of these types may provide important clinical markers of the underlying hyperlipoproteinemia, the classes of lipid abnormality (types I to V) are specified for each kind of clinical lesion.[58] *Eruptive xanthomas* (types I, IIB, III, IV, V) occur as sudden showers of yellow papules that wax and wane according to variations in plasma triglyceride and lipid content. They occur on the buttocks, posterior thighs, knees, and elbows. *Tuberous* (types IIA, III; rarely IIB, IV) and *tendinous* (types IIA, III; rarely IIIB) *xanthomas* occur as yellow nodules; the latter frequently are found on the Achilles tendon and the extensor tendons of the fingers. *Plane xanthomas* (type III; IIA associated with primary biliary cirrhosis) are linear yellow lesions in the skin folds, especially the palmar creases. *Xanthelasma* (types IIA, III; also without lipid abnormality) refers to soft yellow plaques on the eyelids.

Histologically, all types are characterized by dermal accumulation of benign-appearing histiocytes with abundant, finely vacuolated (foamy) cytoplasm. Multinucleate giant cells often are present. They may exhibit a central or peripheral cluster of nuclei surrounded by lipid-laden cytoplasm, so-called Touton giant cells. Cholesterol (free and esterified), phospholipids, and triglycerides are present within cells. The cellularity of the infiltrate is variable, and with the exception of xanthelasma, lesions may also be surrounded by inflammatory cells and fibrosis about the central zone of lipid-laden cells.

DERMAL VASCULAR TUMORS; KAPOSI'S SARCOMA

Benign vascular neoplasms (capillary and cavernous hemangiomas), malformations (nevus flammeus or "port-wine stain"), and malignant vascular tumors (angiosarcomas) are not infrequently encountered in the skin, and are discussed in depth in Chapter 12 (p. 587); Kaposi's sarcoma, on the other hand, is a distinctive vascular proliferative process that most often arises primarily in the skin, where its features are most distinctive. Prior to the epidemic of AIDS, this disease characteristically presented in the United States as a slowly progressive but malignant mesenchymal neoplasm that most commonly occurred on the lower extremities of middle-aged and older men (male-female ratio of 10:1) of Mediterranean origin.[59] In Africa and in individuals with AIDS, more aggressive forms of Kaposi's sarcoma are characteristic (p. 591).

> Kaposi's sarcoma presents a spectrum of lesions consisting of red-purple coalescent macules, papules, and plaques (Fig. 27–15A). The earliest lesions may at first resemble a petechia or may be a red papulonodule. As the lesions enlarge, spongy nodular tumors arise measuring 7 cm or more in diameter. In disseminated disease (aggressive forms), mucosal surfaces, lymph nodes, salivary glands, and viscera may be involved. Bleeding from intestinal involvement is a common and serious complication.
>
> Early lesions of Kaposi's sarcoma may be extremely difficult to diagnose histologically.[60] However, the formation of irregular and angulated spaces lined by flattened and elongated endothelial cells in close proximity to normal vessels of the superficial dermis and periadnexal connective tissue is an important diagnostic finding. In more fully developed lesions, there are numerous bland-appearing spindle cells insidiously infiltrating collagen bundles (Fig. 27–15B). In some areas, these cells form slitlike spaces that may contain rows of red blood cells characteristically arranged in a "boxcar" pattern. At the margins, abnormal vascular proliferations infiltrate and separate the surrounding collagen bundles. Mitoses are common. Hemosiderin is focally deposited throughout the tumor, presumably the result of rupture of the poorly formed vascular channels. Individual endothelial cells may contain minute, round, pink cytoplasmic droplets. Occasional plasma cells are characteristically identified at the periphery of the tumor. Kaposi's sarcoma associated with AIDS cannot be reliably differentiated by histologic features alone from the form not associated with immune deficiency.

Growing public awareness of what once was a rare and relatively indolent neoplasm in the United States has evolved as a result of the more aggressive form of Kaposi's sarcoma that develops in many individuals afflicted with AIDS (p. 224). A direct pathogenic link between human immunodeficiency virus and the vascular proliferation typical of Kaposi's sarcoma, however, has not been established. Controversy exists concerning the cell of origin of this tumor, with some favoring blood vessel endothelium and others supporting lymphatic endothelium.[61,62] Perhaps the study providing evidence that minute lymphatic-venous channels occur as the earliest stage of lesion formation[63] assists in reconciling these seemingly conflicting notions. Another intriguing discovery is the recent recognition that subtly atypical vessels are present even in *uninvolved* skin of patients with AIDS-related Kaposi's sarcoma,[64–66] suggesting that widespread endothelial growth disturbances may characterize this disorder.

TUMORS OF CELLULAR IMMIGRANTS TO THE SKIN

Aside from tumors that arise directly from epidermal and dermal cells, several proliferative disorders of the skin involve primarily cells whose progenitors have arisen elsewhere, but which exhibit a peculiar homing to the cutaneous microenvironment. Examples of such cells are epidermal Langerhans cells, which arise from precursors in the bone marrow and which, in their mature form, traffic freely from skin to regional lymph nodes by way of dermal lymphatics (p. 1298; see Fig. 27–20); T lymphocytes that are normally in residence in low numbers in the dermis and epidermis; and dermal mast cells derived from marrow precursors. The proliferative lesions to be discussed in this section—namely, histiocytosis X, cutaneous T-cell lymphoma, and mastocytosis—are primary cutaneous disorders that arise from these three cell types, respectively.

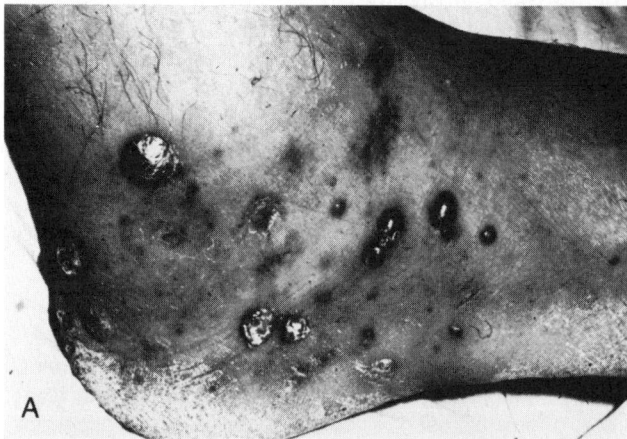
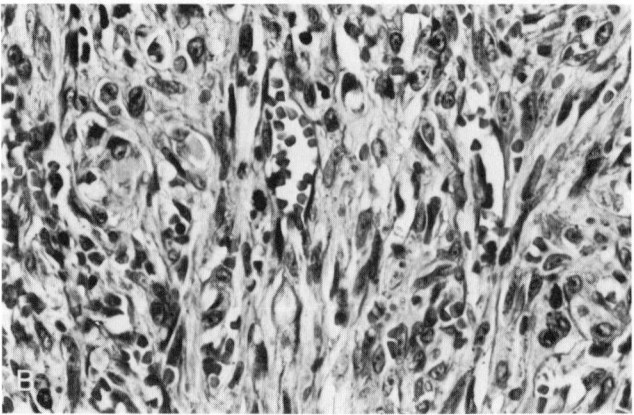

Figure 27–15. Kaposi's sarcoma. A, Multiple hemorrhagic plaques and nodules on the extremity. **B,** Even aggressive lesions may show a remarkably bland histologic appearance, consisting of a cellular proliferation of spindle cells forming slitlike spaces often filled with red blood cells.

HISTIOCYTOSIS X

Histiocytosis X has been described in detail in a previous chapter (p. 745). In the skin, this condition presents in multiple forms, including solitary or multiple lesions ranging from papules to nodules to scaling erythematous plaques that, in infants, may resemble seborrheic dermatitis (p. 1283).

Histologically, histiocytosis X involving the skin has several patterns, all of which may show marked infiltration of the skin. The first is that of a diffuse dermal infiltrate of large, round-to-ovoid cells with pale pink cytoplasm containing indented, often bland nuclei (Fig. 27–16A). A second pattern is composed of similar cells that are clustered into small aggregates that resemble granulomas. The third is characterized by a dermal infiltrate of cells with foamy, xanthoma-like cytoplasm. Variable numbers of eosinophils may also be observed, particularly with the first pattern. Because these patterns are not specific, ultrastructural identification of specific organelles (Birbeck granules), characteristic of the Langerhans cells from which histiocytosis X cells are believed to originate, is helpful. Likewise,

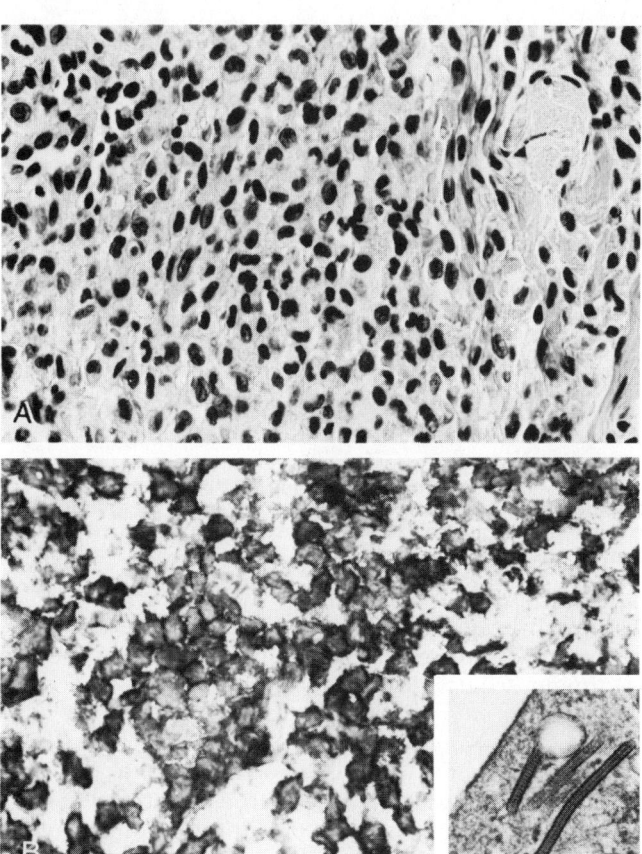

Figure 27–16. Histiocytosis X. *A*, Dermal infiltration by bland mononuclear cells with infolded nuclei presents a nonspecific histologic pattern. *B*, However, immunohistochemical demonstration of the Langerhans cell CD1 antigen by the use of anti-T6 antibody or ultrastructural detection of Birbeck granules *(inset)* permitted accurate diagnosis in this case.

special immunohistochemical methods to identify cell surface markers common to Langerhans cells and histiocytosis X cells (CD1 antigen)[67] may be necessary to establish a definitive histologic diagnosis (Fig. 27–16B).

MYCOSIS FUNGOIDES (CUTANEOUS T-CELL LYMPHOMA)

Cutaneous T-cell lymphoma (CTCL) represents a spectrum of lymphoproliferative disorders affecting the skin. Two types of malignant T-cell disorders were originally recognized: mycosis fungoides (MF), a chronic proliferative process, and a nodular eruptive variant, *mycosis fungoides d'emblée*. It is now known that a variety of presentations of T-cell lymphoma occur, including MF, the eruptive nodular type, and an adult T-cell leukemia or lymphoma type.[67a] The latter disorder may have a rapid progressive downhill course.

Mycosis fungoides is the T-cell lymphoproliferative disorder that arises primarily in the skin and that may evolve into generalized lymphoma.[68] Most affected individuals have disease that remains localized to the skin for many years; a minority have rapid systemic dissemination. This condition may occur at any age, but most commonly it afflicts persons over 40 years of age.

Clinically, lesions of the MF type of CTCL include scaly, red-brown patches; raised, scaling plaques that may even be confused with psoriasis; and fungating nodules. Eczema-like lesions typify early stages of disease when obvious visceral or nodal spread has not occurred. However, even at these stages, karyotypic abnormalities of lymphocytes in blood and lymph nodes may be observed. Raised, indurated, irregularly outlined, erythematous plaques may then supervene (Fig. 27–17A). Development of multiple, large (up to 10 cm or more in diameter), red-brown nodules correlates with systemic spreading. Lesions may affect numerous body surfaces, including the trunk, extremities, face, and scalp. In some individuals, seeding of the blood by malignant T cells is accompanied by diffuse erythema and scaling of the entire body surface (erythroderma), a condition known as *Sézary syndrome* (p. 716).

The hallmark of CTCL of the mycosis fungoides type histologically is the identification of the **Sézary-Lutzner** cells. These are T-helper cells (CD4 antigen-positive) that characteristically form bandlike aggregates with the superficial dermis (Fig. 27–17B) and invade the epidermis as single cells and small clusters (**Pautrier's microabscesses**). These cells have markedly infolded nuclear membranes, imparting a "hyperconvoluted" or "cerebriform" contour (Fig. 27–17C). Although patches and plaques show pronounced epidermal infiltration by Sézary-Lutzner cells (epidermotropism), in nodular lesions the ma-

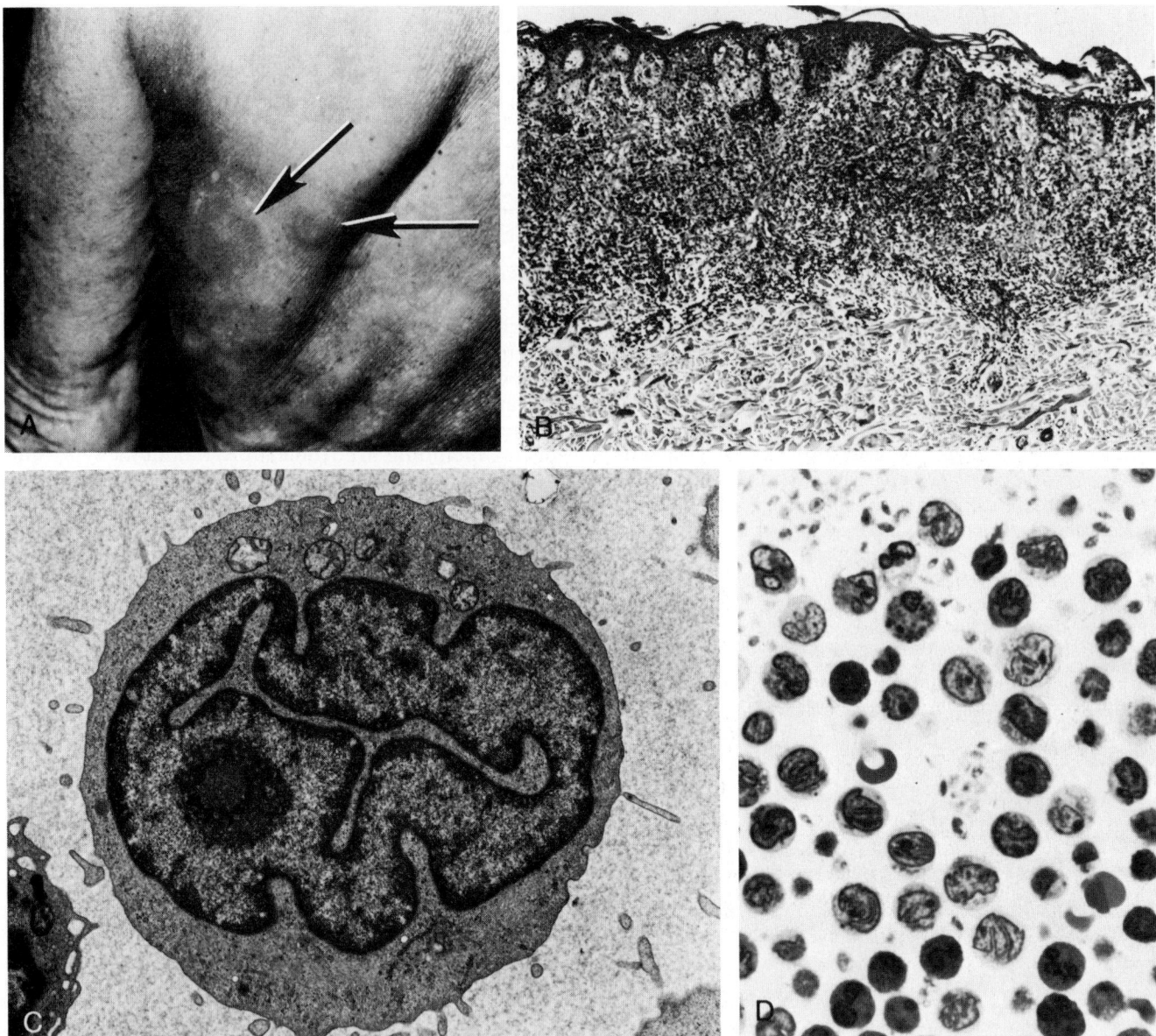

Figure 27–17. Cutaneous T-cell lymphoma. The histologic correlate of ill-defined erythematous, often scaling plaques (*A*) is an infiltrate of atypical lymphocytes that show a tendency to accumulate beneath the epidermal layer (*B*) and to invade the epidermis as small Pautrier microabscesses. *C,* Unlike most benign lymphocytes, these cells have markedly irregular nuclear contours. *D,* With advanced disease, they may be detected in white cell fractions (buffy coat) of the peripheral blood.

lignant T cells often lose this epidermotropic tendency, grow deeply into the dermis, and, eventually, seed lymphatics and the peripheral circulation (Fig. 27–17D).

The cause of CTCL is under active investigation. The recent discovery that a highly aggressive form of T-cell lymphoma or leukemia in adults is caused by infection of helper T cells by a specific retrovirus (human T-cell leukemia virus or HTLV-I)[68] (p. 734) raises the possibility that conventional CTCL may also have an infectious causation. In at least one case of mycosis fungoides, a new retrovirus (HTLV-V) has been described.[69] Therapy for CTCL is conservative for early lesions (topical corticosteroids and chemo-therapeutic agents and ultraviolet light therapy), but for advanced disease, aggressive chemotherapeutic regimens are employed.

MASTOCYTOSIS

The term *mastocytosis* refers to a spectrum of rare disorders characterized by proliferation of mast cells in the skin and, in some instances, in other organs. A localized cutaneous form of the disease that affects predominantly children and accounts for more than 50% of all cases is termed *urticaria pigmentosa*. These lesions are multiple, although solitary mastocytomas may also occur, usually shortly after birth. About 10% of patients with mast cell disease have overt systemic mastocytosis, with mast cell infiltration of many organs. These individuals are often adults, and unlike the case with localized cutaneous disease, the prognosis may be poor.

The clinical picture of mastocytosis is highly variable. In urticaria pigmentosa, lesions are multiple and widely distributed, consisting of round-to-oval, red-brown, nonscaling papules and small plaques. Solitary mastocytomas present as one or several tan-brown nodules that may be pruritic or exhibit blister formation. In systemic mastocytosis, skin lesions similar to those of urticaria pigmentosa are accompanied by

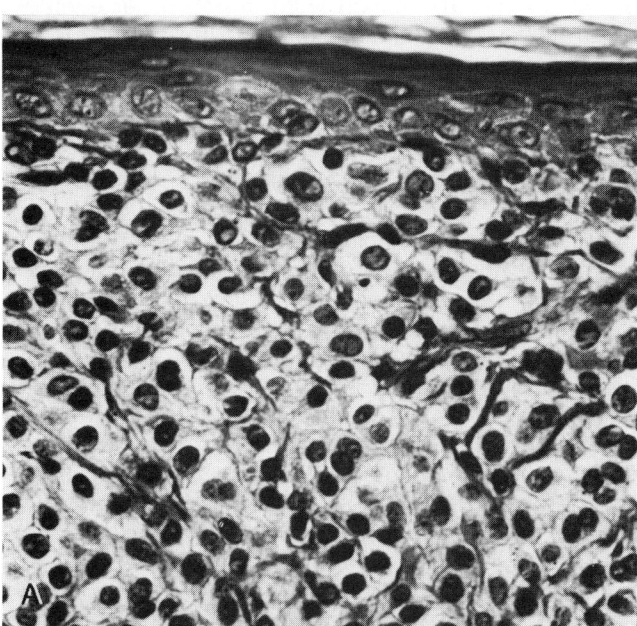

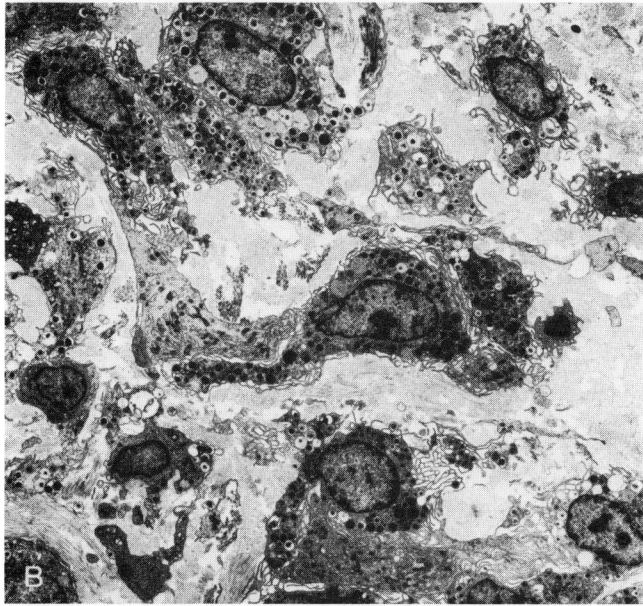

Figure 27–18. Mastocytosis. *A,* Numerous ovoid cells with uniform, centrally located nuclei are observed in the dermis. *B,* By electron microscopy, most of these cells are found to contain cytoplasmic granules typical of mast cells.

mast cell infiltration of bone marrow, liver, spleen, and lymph nodes. Many of the signs and symptoms of mastocytosis are due to the effects of histamine, heparin, and other substances released as a result of degranulation. *Darier's sign* refers to a localized area of dermal edema and erythema (wheal) that occurs when lesional skin is rubbed. *Dermatographism* refers to an area of dermal edema, resembling a hive that occurs in normal skin as a result of localized stroking with a pointed instrument. Pruritus and flushing triggered by certain foods, temperature changes, alcohol, and certain drugs (morphine, codeine, aspirin); watery nasal discharge (rhinorrhea); rarely gastrointestinal or nasal bleeding, possibly due to the anticoagulant effects of heparin; and bone pain as a result of osteoblastic and osteoclastic involvement may all be seen in systemic disease.

> The histologic picture varies, from a subtle increase in the numbers of spindle-shaped and stellate mast cells about superficial dermal blood vessels to large numbers of tightly packed, round-to-oval mast cells in the upper to mid-dermis (Fig. 27–18A) in urticaria pigmentosa or solitary mastocytoma. Variable fibrosis, edema, and small numbers of eosinophils may also be present. Mast cells may be difficult to differentiate from lymphocytes in routine, H and E–stained sections, and special "metachromatic" stains (toluidine blue or Giemsa) must be used to visualize their granules. Even with these stains, extensive degranulation may result in failure to detect these cells by light microscopy, and ultrastructural analysis must then be performed (Fig. 27–18B).

Whether mastocytosis is a true neoplasm or instead represents altered maturation or proliferation of these cells as a result of abnormalities in their local microenvironment is at present unsettled. In this regard, the mastocytosis syndromes may share biologic features in common with histiocytosis X (discussed earlier). The recent discovery of new markers for mast cell biosynthetic products (e.g., proteases within mast cell granules[70]) should assist in future characterization of normal and proliferating mast cells in the skin.

ACUTE INFLAMMATORY DERMATOSES

Inflammatory dermatoses are usually mediated by local or systemic immunologic factors, although the causes for most remain a mystery. Literally thousands of specific inflammatory dermatoses exist. Although some have both acute and chronic stages, others are most characteristic either in their early or their late stages. Many lesions resolve before chronic changes can occur. In general, acute lesions last from days to weeks and are characterized by inflammation (often marked by mononuclear cells, not neutrophils), edema, and, in some, epidermal, vascular, or subcutaneous injury. Chronic lesions, on the other hand, persist for months to years and often show significant components of altered epidermal growth (atrophy or hyperplasia) or dermal fibrosis. The lesions discussed here are selected as examples of the more commonly encountered dermatoses within the acute category.

URTICARIA

Urticaria (hives) refers to a common disorder of the skin characterized by localized mast cell degranulation and resultant dermal microvascular hyperpermeability, culminating in pruritic wheals. More than 20% of people experience urticaria at some time during their lives. Angioedema is closely related to urticaria and is characterized by edema of both the dermis and the subcutaneous fat. In the very uncommon hereditary angioneurotic edema there are recurrent attacks of angioedema involving the skin, gastrointestinal tract, and larynx.

Clinically, urticaria most often occurs between the ages of 20 and 40, although all age groups are susceptible. Individual lesions develop and fade within hours (usually less than 24 hours), and episodes may last for days or persist for months. Persistent urticaria may simply be the result of inability to eliminate the causative antigen, or may herald underlying disease (e.g., collagen-vascular disorders, Hodgkin's disease). When individual lesions themselves last for more than 24 hours (regardless of whether the overall episode is short or persistent), underlying vasculitis should be considered (see later). Lesions vary from small, pruritic papules to large edematous plaques. In Caucasian skin they appear pale pink. Individual lesions may coalesce to form annular, linear, or arciform configurations. Sites of predilection for urticarial eruptions include any area exposed to pressure, such as trunk, distal extremities, and ears.

> The histologic features of urticaria may be so subtle that many biopsy specimens, at first, resemble normal skin. Usually there is a very sparse superficial perivenular infiltrate consisting of mononuclear cells and rare neutrophils. Unlike mastocytosis (which may have an urticarial component if degranulation has occurred), urticaria does not demonstrate an increase in dermal mast cells. Collagen bundles are more widely spaced than in normal skin, a result of superficial dermal edema fluid that does not stain in routinely prepared tissue. Superficial lymphatic channels are dilated in an attempt to accommodate this transudated edema fluid.

Most urticaria results from antigen-induced release of vasoactive mediators from mast cell granules via sensitization with specific IgE antibodies.[71] This *IgE-dependent* degranulation can follow exposure to a number of antigens (pollens, foods, drugs, insect venom) and specifically results from bridging of cell-bound IgE molecules by multivalent ligand, as discussed on page 173. *IgE-independent* urticaria may result from substances that, in certain individuals, incite directly the degranulation of mast cells, such as opiates, certain antibiotics, curare, and radiographic contrast media. Another cause of IgE-independent urticaria is exposure to chemicals, such as aspirin, that suppress prostaglandin synthesis from arachidonic acid. Hereditary angioneurotic edema is the result of an inherited deficiency of Cl activator (Cl esterase inhibitor) that results in uncontrolled activation of the early components of the complement system (so-called complement-mediated urticaria).[72] Urticaria associated with necrotizing vasculitis and serum sickness may be caused by a similar mechanism. In some individuals, urticaria and even anaphylaxis may result from exposure to the sun, cold, pressure, or even exercise.[73] The mechanisms of these forms of this disorder are not entirely understood, although some appear to show distinctive morphologic features on ultrastructural analyses of degranulated mast cells.[74]

ACUTE ECZEMATOUS DERMATITIS

Eczema is a clinical term that embraces a number of pathogenetically different conditions. All are characterized by red, papulovesicular, oozing, and crusted lesions early on that with persistence eventuate into raised, scaling plaques. Eczema is an example of a disorder that has an acute phase which, if untreated, goes to a chronic eruption. Although the histopathologic features of most of these conditions are similar, clinical differences permit classification into the following categories: (1) allergic contact dermatitis; (2) atopic dermatitis; (3) drug-related eczematous dermatitis; (4) photoeczematous dermatitis; and (5) primary irritant dermatitis (Table 27-1).

The Greek word "eczema," meaning "to boil over,"[75] vividly describes the clinical appearance of acute eczematous dermatitis. The most obvious example is an acute contact reaction to poison ivy, characterized by pruritic, edematous, oozing plaques, often containing small and large blisters (vesicles and bullae) (Fig. 27-19A). Such lesions are prone to bacterial superinfection, which produces a yellow crust (impetigenization). Most acute eczematous dermatitis is pruritic, and scratching only serves to worsen this process by superimposing primary irritant dermatitis on the underlying process. With time, persistent lesions become less "wet" (fail to ooze or form vesicles) and become progressively scaly (hyperkeratotic) as the epidermis thickens (acanthosis). These more chronic lesions may produce psoriasis-like plaques clinically and histologically, and their perpetuation is often more the result of persistent rubbing or scratching than of immunologic hypersensitivity (see below).

> **Spongiosis — the accumulation of edema fluid within the epidermis —** characterizes acute eczematous dermatitis, hence the synonym "spongiotic dermatitis." Whereas in urticaria, edema is localized to the perivascular spaces of

Table 27–1. Classification of Eczematous Dermatitis

TYPE	CAUSE OR PATHOGENESIS	HISTOLOGY*	CLINICAL FEATURES
Contact dermatitis	Topically applied chemicals Pathogenesis: delayed hypersensitivity	Spongiotic dermatitis	Marked itching or burning or both; requires antecedent exposure
Atopic dermatitis	Unknown, may be heritable	Spongiotic dermatitis	Erythematous plaques in flexural areas; family history of eczema, hay fever, or asthma
Drug-related eczematous dermatitis	Systemically administered (e.g., penicillin)	Spongiotic dermatitis; eosinophils often present in infiltrate; deeper infiltrate	Eruption occurs with administration of drug; remits when drug is discontinued
Photoeczematous eruption	Ultraviolet light	Spongiotic dermatitis; deeper infiltrate	Occurs on sun-exposed skin; phototesting may help in diagnosis
Primary irritant dermatitis	Repeated trauma (rubbing)	Spongiotic dermatitis in early stages	Localized to site of trauma

* All types, with time, may develop chronic changes.

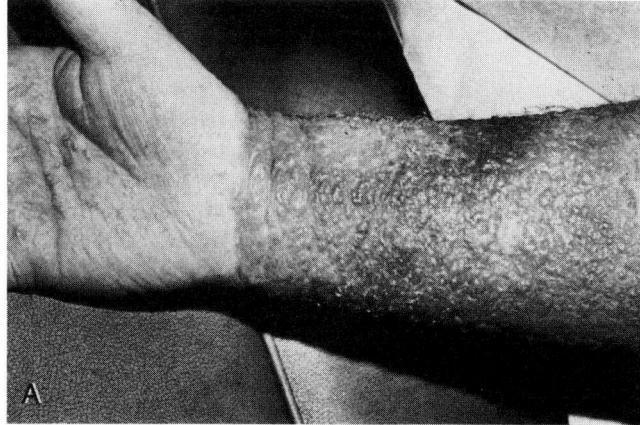

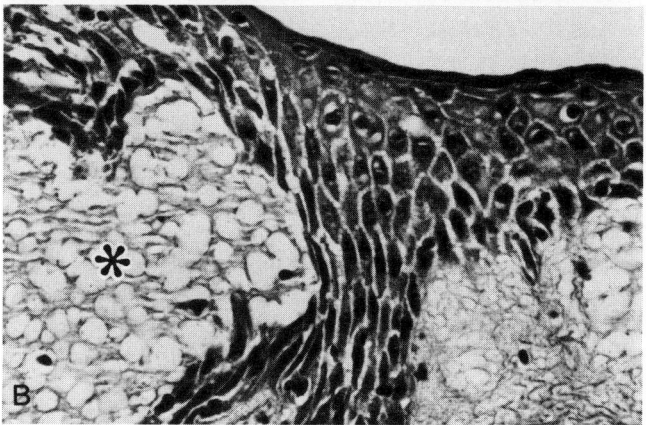

Figure 27–19. Eczematous dermatitis. *A,* In an acute allergic contact dermatitis, numerous vesicles appear at the site of antigen exposure (in this case, laundry detergent). *B,* Histologically, intercellular edema produces widened intercellular spaces within the epidermis, eventually resulting in small, fluid-filled intraepidermal vesicles (*).

the superficial dermis, in spongiotic dermatitis edema seeps into the intercellular spaces of the epidermis, splaying apart keratinocytes located primarily in the stratum spinosum. Intercellular bridges become prominent, giving a "spongy" appearance to the epidermis (Fig. 27–19*B*). Mechanical shearing of intercellular attachment sites (desmosomes) and cell membranes by progressive accumulation of intercellular fluid may result in the formation of intraepidermal vesicles.

During the earliest stages of the evolution of spongiotic dermatitis, there is a superficial, perivascular, lymphocytic infiltrate associated with papillary dermal edema and mast cell degranulation. The pattern and composition of this infiltrate may provide clues to the underlying cause[76]. For example, spongiotic dermatitis resulting from certain drugs will show a lymphocytic infiltrate, **often containing eosinophils,** and extending around deep as well as superficial dermal vessels. With time (days to weeks), the acute vesicular phase of spongiotic dermatitis may subside, giving rise to progressive epidermal hyperplasia with hyper- and parakeratosis.

The immunopathology of many examples of spongiotic dermatitis—the cutaneous delayed hypersensitivity response—has been the subject of active and productive investigation during the past decade. We now know that epidermal Langerhans cells serve as reticuloendothelial traps for a number of environmental (and potentially endogenous) antigens. Subsequent to antigen uptake, these specialized monocyte- or macrophage-like cells present this antigen to T-helper lymphocytes locally or, after migration, to draining lymph nodes.[77] These sensitized T cells, upon subsequent antigen challenge, may then produce an antigen-directed, local tissue reaction[78] (Fig. 27–20). The selective homing of these sensitized T cells to specific anatomic regions of skin accounts for the characteristic clinical localization of lesions and appears to be in part the result of expression of adhesion molecules for leukocytes on the membranes of

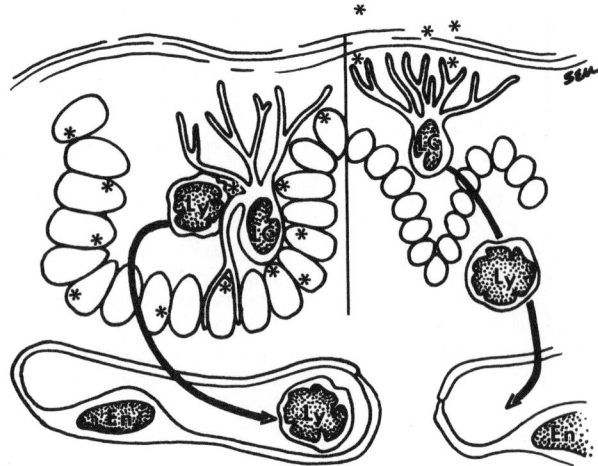

Figure 27–20. Immunopathology of cutaneous delayed hypersensitivity reaction. Antigen (*), either endogenous *(left)* or environmental *(right),* is taken up and presented by Langerhans cells (LC) to T-helper lymphocytes (Ly). Both cell types traffic freely by way of endothelium-lined (En) dermal lymphatics to regional lymph nodes, where antigen presentation may be amplified. Upon antigen challenge, these specifically sensitized T cells proliferate and infiltrate the skin, where they orchestrate the immune response.

postcapillary and venular endothelial cells lining superficial dermal vessels.[79,80] Cytokines such as interleukin-1[81] are actively synthesized by epidermal cells and are important initiators of the expression of these adhesion molecules.[82] These immunologic events, coupled with mast cell degranulation, result in vascular alterations, favoring the accumulation of edema fluid in the dermal and epidermal layers.

ERYTHEMA MULTIFORME

Erythema multiforme is an uncommon, self-limited disorder that appears to be a hypersensitivity response to certain infections and drugs. Unlike contact allergy (a form of spongiotic dermatitis), erythema multiforme is a prototype of a cytotoxic reaction pattern (one typified by extensive epithelial cell degeneration and death). This disorder affects individuals of any age and is associated with the following conditions: (1) infections such as herpes simplex, mycoplasma infections, histoplasmosis, coccidioidomycosis, typhoid, and leprosy, among others; (2) administration of certain drugs (sulfonamides, penicillin, barbiturates, salicylates, hydantoins, and antimalarials); (3) malignancy (carcinomas and lymphomas); and (4) collagen-vascular diseases (lupus erythematosus, dermatomyositis, and periarteritis nodosa). Clinically, patients present with an array of "multiform" lesions including macules, papules, vesicles, and bullae, as well as the characteristic target lesion consisting of a red macule or papule with a pale, vesicular or eroded center (Fig. 27–21A). Although lesions may be widely distributed, symmetric involvement of the extremities frequently occurs. An extensive and symptomatic febrile form of the disease,

which is more common in children, is called the Stevens-Johnson syndrome. Typically, erosions and hemorrhagic crusts involve the lips and oral mucosa, although the conjunctiva, urethra, and genital and perianal areas may also be affected. Infection of involved areas may result in life-threatening sepsis. Still another probable variant, termed *toxic epidermal necrolysis,* results in diffuse necrosis and sloughing of cutaneous and mucosal epithelial surfaces, producing a clinical situation analogous to an extensive third-degree burn.

Histologically, early lesions show a superficial perivascular, lymphocytic infiltrate associated with dermal edema and margination of lymphocytes along the dermoepidermal junction, where they are intimately associated with degenerating and necrotic keratinocytes. Prominent endothelial cell swelling may be noted. With time, there is upward migration of lymphocytes. Discrete and confluent zones of epidermal necrosis occur with concomitant blister formation (Fig. 27–21B). Epidermal sloughing leads to shallow erosions. Histologically the **"target lesion"** exhibits central necrosis surrounded by a rim of perivenular inflammation.

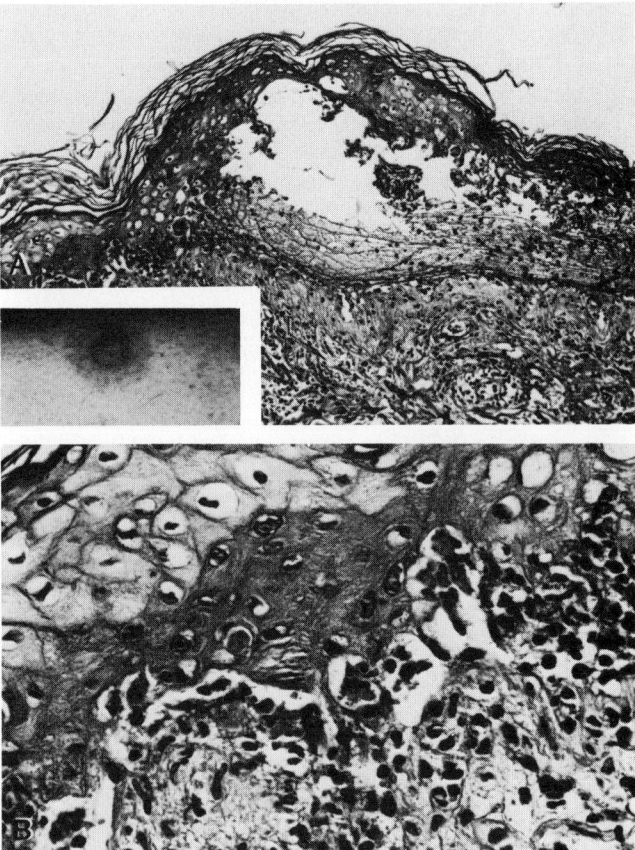

Figure 27–21. Erythema multiforme. A, The target-like clinical lesion *(inset)* is the result of a central blister or zone of epidermal necrosis surrounded by macular erythema. **B,** Higher magnification of a biopsy specimen from the erythematous edge shows numerous lymphocytes in intimate contact with degenerating basal epidermal cells.

Erythema multiforme has potential immunologic similarities to other conditions characterized by cytotoxic epidermal cell injury (e.g., acute graft-versus-host disease,[83] skin allograft rejection,[84] and fixed drug eruptions[85]). Unlike spongiotic dermatitis, many of the lymphocytes responsible for the cytotoxic response are of the suppressor-cytotoxic phenotype, expressing CD8 molecules on their surfaces. Moreover, marked vascular injury may also be seen in erythema multiforme, and some observers actually characterize this disorder as a form of lymphocyte-mediated vasculitis. The usual neutrophil-associated hypersensitivity vasculitis (*leukocytoclastic vasculitis*) is discussed on p. 573. Thus, the epithelial injury that characterizes erythema multiforme may be the combined result of direct cytotoxicity by infiltrating lymphoid cells, as well as a consequence of microvascular injury to the underlying nutrient vessels.

ERYTHEMA NODOSUM AND ERYTHEMA INDURATUM

Erythema nodosum is a type of *panniculitis.* The term panniculitis describes an inflammatory reaction in the subcutaneous fat that may affect (1) principally the connective tissue septa separating lobules of fat, or (2) predominantly the lobules of fat themselves. Acute and chronic variants are known. *Erythema nodosum* is the most common form of panniculitis and usually has an acute presentation. Its occurrence is often associated with infections (beta-hemolytic streptococcal infection, tuberculosis, and, less commonly, coccidioidomycosis, histoplasmosis, and leprosy), drug administration (sulfonamides, oral contraceptives), sarcoidosis, inflammatory bowel disease, and certain malignancies, but many times a cause cannot be elicited. Many types of panniculitis have a subacute to chronic course.

Panniculitis often involves the lower legs. Erythema nodosum presents acutely as poorly defined, exquisitely tender, erythematous nodules that may be felt better than seen. Fever and malaise may accompany the cutaneous signs. Over the course of weeks, lesions usually flatten and become bruiselike, leaving no residual clinical scars, while new lesions develop. Biopsy of a deep wedge of tissue is usually required to establish a definitive diagnosis.

Erythema induratum is an uncommon type of panniculitis that affects primarily adolescents and menopausal women. Although the cause is not known, most observers today regard this disorder as the result of a primary vasculitis affecting deep vessels supplying lobules of the subcutis, with subsequent necrosis and inflammation within the fat. Erythema induratum presents as an erythematous, slightly tender nodule that usually goes on to ulcerate. Originally considered a hypersensitivity response to tuberculosis, erythema induratum today most commonly occurs without an associated underlying disease.

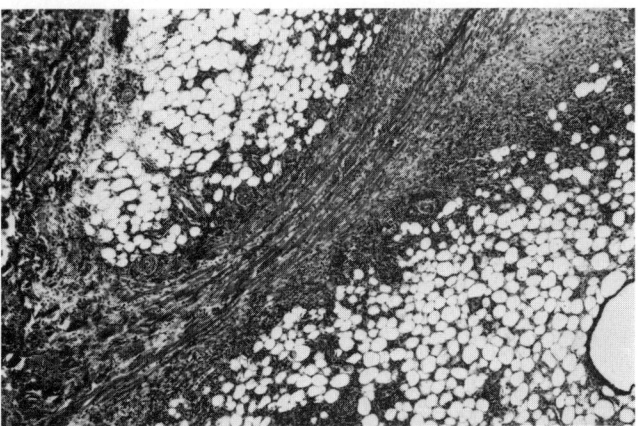

Figure 27–22. Erythema nodosum. A septum of the subcutaneous fat is preferentially infiltrated and widened by inflammatory cells.

The histopathology of erythema nodosum is distinctive. In early lesions, there is widening of the connective tissue septa owing to edema, fibrin exudation, and neutrophilic infiltration (Fig. 27–22). Later, infiltration by lymphocytes, histiocytes, multinucleated giant cells, and occasional eosinophils is associated with septal fibrosis. Vasculitis is not present. In the more chronic panniculitis—erythema induratum—on the other hand, the fat lobule is involved by granulomatous inflammation and zones of caseous necrosis. Early lesions show necrotizing vasculitis affecting small to medium-sized arteries and veins in the deep dermis and subcutis.

Erythema nodosum and erythema induratum are but two examples of many types of primary and secondary panniculitis. *Weber-Christian disease (relapsing febrile nodular panniculitis)* is a rare form of lobular, nonvasculitic panniculitis seen in children and adults. It is marked by crops of erythematous plaques or nodes, predominantly on the lower extremities, created by deep-seated foci of inflammation with aggregates of foamy histiocytes admixed with lymphocytes, neutrophils, and giant cells. Factitial panniculitis, as a result of self-inflicted trauma or injection of foreign or toxic substances, may result in profound problems in definitive clinical and pathologic diagnosis, and it may present a distinct set of therapeutic challenges. Deep mycotic infections in immunocompromised individuals may produce histologic changes that mimic primary panniculitis. Finally, disorders such as lupus erythematosus (see later) may occasionally have deep inflammatory components with associated panniculitis.

CHRONIC INFLAMMATORY DERMATOSES

This category focuses on those persistent inflammatory dermatoses that exhibit their most characteristic clinical and histologic features over many months to

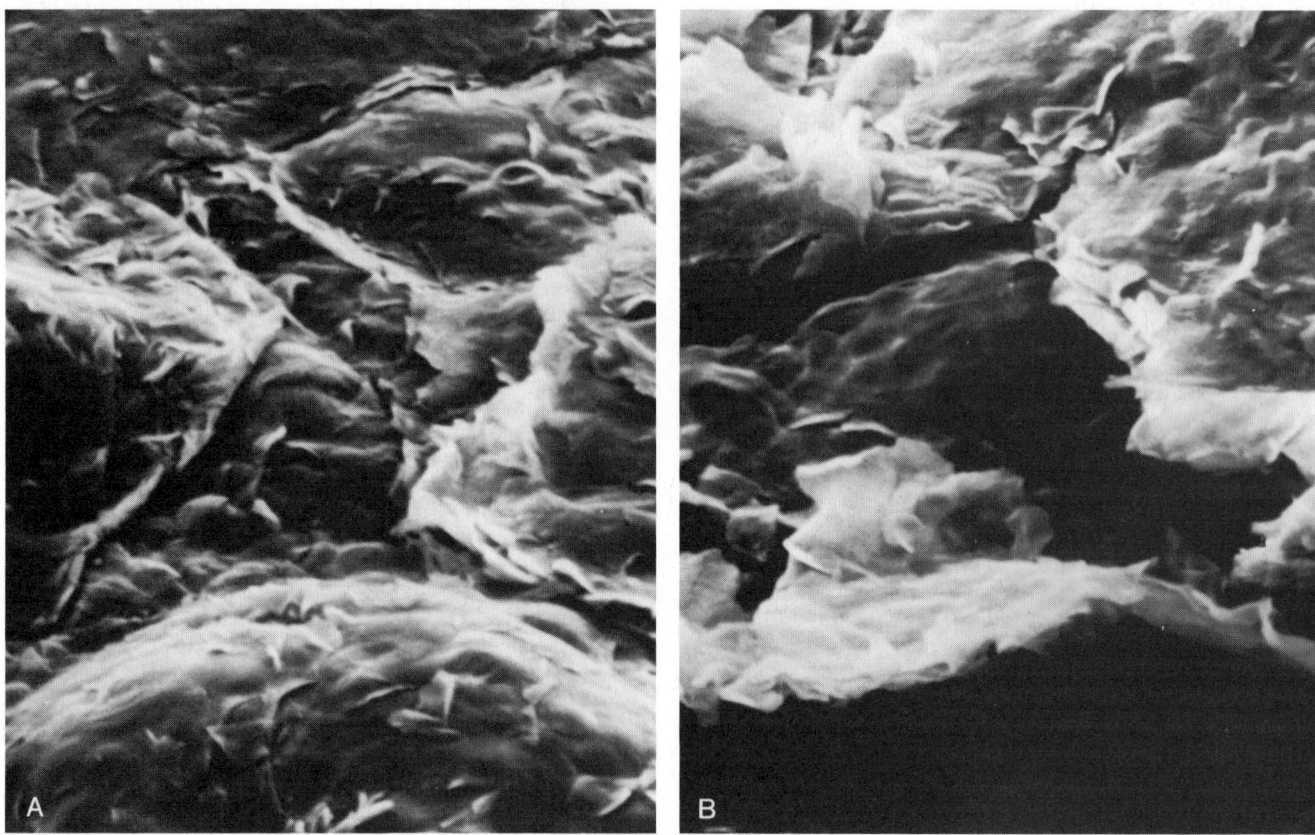

Figure 27–23. The surface morphology of hyperkeratosis assessed by scanning electron microscopy. Unlike the normal cutaneous surface (A) that is covered by relatively smooth and contiguous squamous cells of the stratum corneum, chronic dermatoses often exhibit excessive stratum corneum production (B), producing an irregular and roughened surface. (Courtesy of Dr. Robert Lavker, University of Pennsylvania.)

years. Unlike the normal cutaneous surface, the skin surface in some chronic inflammatory dermatoses is roughened as a result of excessive or abnormal scale formation and shedding (desquamation) (Fig. 27–23). However, not all scaling lesions are inflammatory. Witness the hereditary ichthyoses with fish-like scales as the result of some defect in the adhesive properties of cells in the stratum corneum.

PSORIASIS

Psoriasis is a common chronic inflammatory dermatosis affecting as many as 1 to 2% of people in the United States. The mean age of onset is 27, although persons of all ages may develop the disease. Psoriasis is sometimes associated with arthritis, myopathy, enteropathy, spondylitic heart disease, and AIDS. Psoriatic arthritis may be mild or produce deformities resembling the joint changes seen in rheumatoid arthritis.

Macroscopically, psoriasis most frequently affects elbows, knees, scalp, lumbosacral areas, intergluteal cleft, and glans penis. The most typical lesion is a well-demarcated, pink and salmon-colored plaque covered by loosely adherent scales that are characteristically silver-white in color (Fig. 27–24A). Variations exist, with some lesions occurring in annular, linear, gyrate, or serpiginous configurations. Psoriasis can be the cause of total body erythema and scaling known as **erythroderma.** Nail changes[86] occur in 30% of cases of psoriasis and consist of yellow-brown discoloration (often likened to an oil slick), pitting, dimpling, separation of the nail plate from the underlying bed (onycholysis), thickening, and crumbling. In the rare variant called **pustular psoriasis,** multiple small pustules form on erythematous plaques. This type of psoriasis is either benign and localized (hands and feet) or generalized and life-threatening, with associated fever, leukocytosis, arthralgias, diffuse cutaneous and mucosal pustules, secondary infection, and electrolyte disturbances.

Established lesions of psoriasis have a characteristic histologic picture. Increased epidermal cell turnover results in marked epidermal thickening (acanthosis), with regular downward elongation of the rete ridges and mitotic figures easily identified well above the basal cell layer, where, in normal skin, mitotic activity is confined (Fig. 27–24B). **The stratum granulosum is thinned or absent, and extensive overlying parakeratotic scale is seen.** This is in contrast to chronically irritated and traumatized lesions of eczematous dermatitis (termed **lichen simplex chronicus**), which may demonstrate psoriasis-like acanthosis, but which show increased thickness of the granular cell layer and

Determination of the pathogenesis of psoriasis is one of the most important challenges in dermatopathologic research. An increased incidence of disease in association with certain HLA types suggests that genetic factors participate in the predisposition for disease development. The genesis of new lesions at sites of trauma (termed the *Koebner phenomenon*) is undoubtedly providing some basic yet elusive pathogenetic clue. Evidence has recently been accumulated that psoriasis may be a type of complement-mediated reaction localized to the stratum corneum.[87] According to this hypothesis, exogenous or endogenous damage to the stratum corneum of certain individuals results in the unmasking of stratum corneum antigens. These antigens elicit the formation of specific autoantibodies that bind to the stratum corneum, fix complement, and activate the complement cascade. Release locally of C3a, C5a, and C567 then leads to neutrophil activation and accumulation, a phenomenon likely aided by arachidonic acid metabolites, including leukotrienes. Neutrophils within the stratum corneum then release neutral serine proteases, which unmask more antigen and perpetuate the process. Proliferative factors for underlying keratinocytes are released as a consequence of these events and result in increased epidermal turnover and the hyperplasia and scale formation so characteristic of psoriasis.

LICHEN PLANUS

"Pruritic, purple, polygonal papules" are the presenting signs of this disorder of skin and mucous membranes. Lichen planus is self-limiting and generally resolves spontaneously one to two years after onset, often leaving zones of postinflammatory hyperpigmentation (see later). Oral lesions may persist for years. Malignant degeneration has been noted to occur in chronic mucosal and paramucosal lesions of lichen planus, although the direct pathogenetic relationship has not been shown.[88]

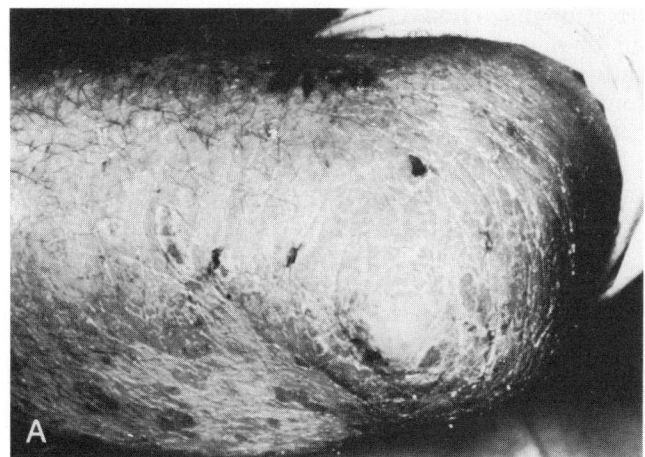

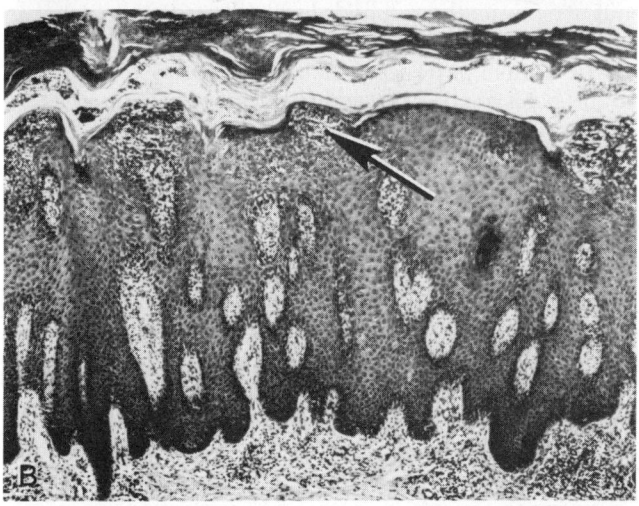

Figure 27–24. Psoriasis. A characteristic scaling plaque on the elbow (*A*) histologically demonstrates marked epidermal hyperplasia (*B*), parakeratotic scale, and importantly, minute microabscesses of neutrophils (*arrow*) within the superficial epidermal layers.

hyperkeratosis. Typical of psoriatic plaques is thinning of the portion of the epidermal cell layer that overlies the tips of dermal papillae (suprapapillary plates) and dilated, tortuous blood vessels within these papillae. This constellation of changes results in abnormal proximity of dermal vessels within the dermal papillae to the overlying parakeratotic scale, and it accounts for the characteristic clinical phenomenon of multiple, minute, bleeding points when the scale is lifted from the plaque **(Auspitz sign).** Although there is usually a superficial, perivascular, lymphocytic infiltrate in psoriasis, the most diagnostically helpful inflammatory cells are neutrophils that form small aggregates within slightly spongiotic foci of the superficial epidermis **(spongiform pustules)** and within the parakeratotic stratum corneum **(Munro's microabscesses).** In pustular psoriasis, larger abscess-like accumulations of neutrophils are present within the epidermis or directly beneath the stratum corneum; the degree of dermatitis may show occasional clinical and histologic similarities to psoriasis, and certain individuals are prone to develop both dermatoses.

Cutaneous lesions consist of itchy, violaceous, flat-topped papules that may coalesce focally to form plaques. These papules are often highlighted by white dots or lines called **Wickham's striae** (Fig. 27–25A). Multiple lesions are characteristic and are symmetrically distributed, particularly on the extremities, often about the wrists and elbows, and on the glans penis. In 70% of cases, oral lesions are present as white, reticulated, or netlike areas involving the mucosa. As in psoriasis, the Koebner phenomenon (see above) also may be seen in lichen planus.

Lichen planus is characterized histologically by a dense, continuous infiltrate of lymphocytes along the dermoepidermal junction that fills the papillary dermis (Fig. 27–25B). This zonation of inflammatory cells in the upper dermis has been called "lichenoid" or bandlike. The lymphocytes are intimately associated with basal keratinocytes, which show degeneration, necrosis, and a resemblance in size and contour to more mature cells of the stratum spinosum (squamatization). A consequence of this destructive infiltration of

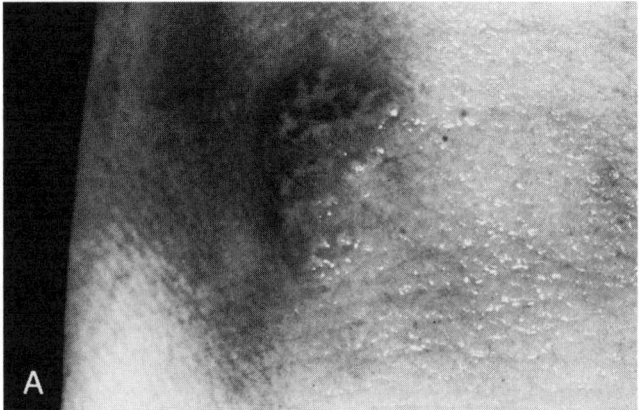

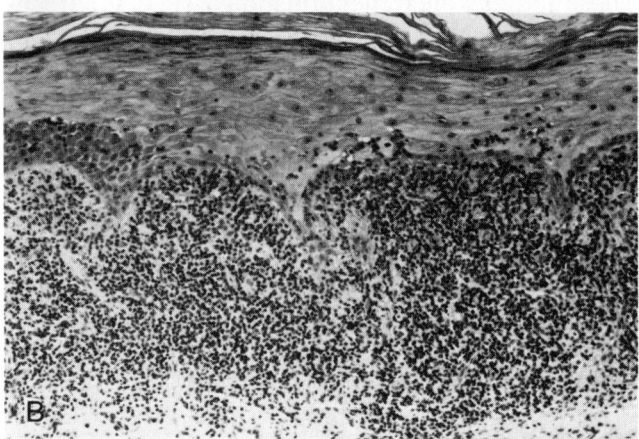

Figure 27–25. Lichen planus. *A,* **A small erythematous plaque covered with oil to render the stratum corneum translucent shows characteristic Wickham's striae.** *B,* **Biopsy of this lesion demonstrates the bandlike infiltrate of lymphocytes at the dermoepidermal junction and pointed rete ridges ("saw-toothing"; compare with Fig. 27–1).**

lymphocytes is a redefinition of the normal, smoothly undulating configuration of the dermoepidermal interface (refer to Fig. 27–1) to a more angulated zig-zag contour ("saw-toothing"). At times, basal cell destruction may become so pronounced that cleftlike spaces develop, resulting in clinical erosions. Anucleate, necrotic basal cells may become incorporated into the inflamed papillary dermis, where they are referred to as **colloid** or **Civatte bodies.** These keratin-filled, ghostlike remnants of epidermal cells may nonspecifically take up immunoglobulins to produce a characteristic pattern on direct immunofluorescence examination. Although this destructive relationship between lymphocytes and epidermal cells bears some similarities to erythema multiforme (discussed previously), lichen planus shows changes of chronicity—namely, epidermal hyperplasia (or rarely atrophy) and thickening of the granular cell layer and stratum corneum (hypergranulosis and hyperkeratosis, respectively). Lichen planus preferentially affecting the epithelium of hair follicles is referred to as **lichen planopilaris.**

The precise pathogenesis of lichen planus is not known. It is plausible that release of antigens at the levels of the basal cell layer and the dermoepidermal junction may elicit a cell-mediated immune response in lichen planus. Supporting this notion are data indicating that infiltrates of primarily T lymphocytes associated with hyperplasia of Langerhans cells are fundamental to lesion formation and evolution.[89]

LUPUS ERYTHEMATOSUS (LE)

The manifestations of systemic lupus erythematosus (SLE) have been described in detail on page 193. However, a localized, cutaneous form of LE, with no associated systemic manifestations, occurs and is called *discoid lupus erythematosus (DLE).* Patients who present with DLE usually do not go on to develop systemic disease. However, over one third of patients with SLE may exhibit, during their course, lesions that are clinically and histologically indistinguishable from those of discoid type. Thus, it is often impossible to distinguish patients with SLE from those with DLE on the basis of clinical and histologic inspection of skin lesions alone.

Cutaneous lesions usually consist of either poorly defined malar erythema (usually seen in systemic disease) or large, sharply demarcated erythematous scaling plaques (Fig. 27–26A). These "discoid" plaques may occur either in pure cutaneous LE or SLE. Cutaneous manifestations of LE may occur or worsen with sun exposure. The epidermal surface of lesions is shiny or scaly, and lateral compression often produces wrinkling, a sign of epidermal atrophy. Through this thinned epidermis, dilated and tortuous blood vessels (telangiectasia) and small zones of hypo- and hyperpigmentation may be seen. Small, keratotic plugs in follicular ostia may be appreciated with a hand lens and assist in differentiating LE from certain other inflammatory dermatoses.

Histologically, lesions of DLE are characterized by an infiltrate of lymphocytes along the dermoepidermal or the dermal-follicular epithelial junction, or both (Fig. 27–26B). Deep perivascular and periappendageal (e.g., around sweat glands) infiltrates are also observed. The basal cell layer generally shows diffuse vacuolization. Unlike classic lichen planus, however, the epidermal layer is markedly thinned or atrophied, with loss of the normal rete ridge pattern. Variable hyperkeratosis is present on the epidermal surface. Involved hair follicles also may show epithelial atrophy and their infundibula are frequently dilated and plugged with keratin. Periodic acid-Schiff (PAS) stain of established lesions reveals marked thickening of the epidermal basement membrane zone (Fig. 27–26C), and **direct immunofluorescence shows a characteristic granular band of immunoglobulin and complement along the dermoepidermal and dermal-follicular junctions (so-called lupus band test[90])** (Fig. 27–26D). This granular band may also be present in clinically normal skin in patients with systemic disease and is a helpful criterion in establishing the diagnosis. Infiltration of the subcuticular fat by lymphocytes, histiocytes, and plasma cells, often without significant epidermal changes, is seen in a rare cutaneous manifestation of lupus erythematosus called **lupus profundus.**

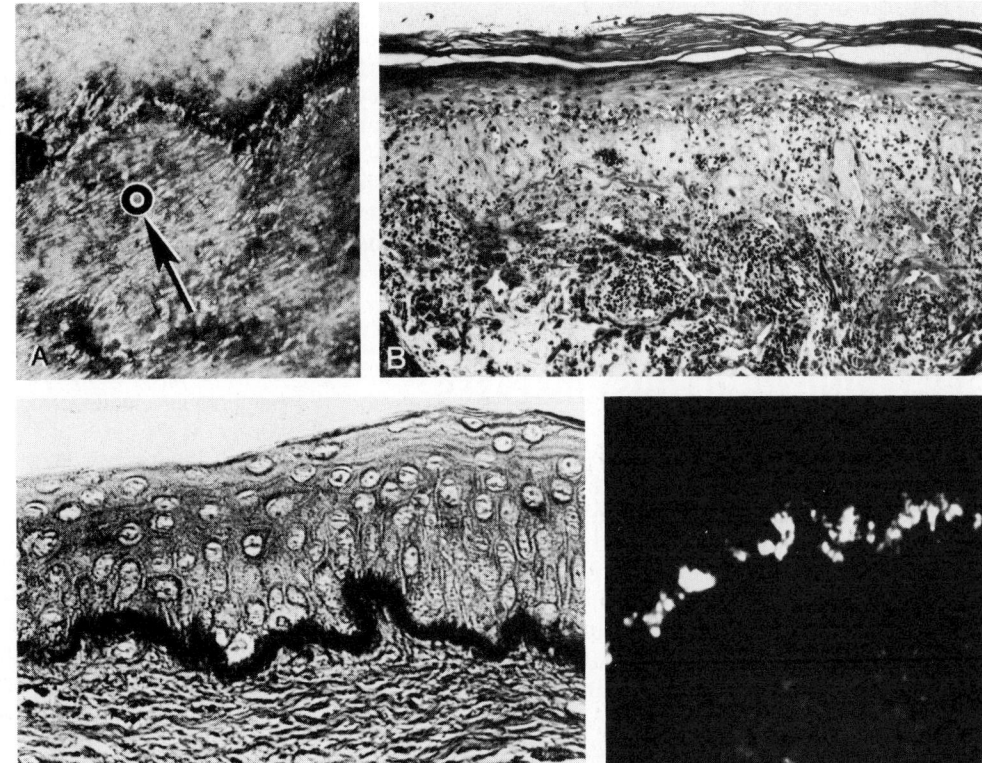

Figure 27–26. Lupus erythematosus. *A,* Discoid plaque shows erythema and excessive scale. The histology of a biopsy taken from the center of this plaque *(arrow)* is depicted in *B. B,* There is an infiltrate of lymphocytes within the superficial (and often deep) dermis, marked thinning of the epidermis, and hyperkeratosis. *C,D,* Chronic damage to the basal cell layer is characteristically associated with thickening of the basement membrane zone *(C)* and granular deposits of immunoglobulin and complement at the dermoepidermal junction *(D).*

The immunopathogenesis of lupus erythematosus is discussed extensively elsewhere in this text (p. 196). In the skin, it is believed that both humoral and cell-mediated mechanisms collaborate to result in destruction of pigment-containing basal cells.[91] Humoral mechanisms of injury may involve both formation and deposition of immune complexes and components C5b to C9 ("membrane attack complex"[92]; p. 53) in dermoepithelial basement membranes.

ACNE VULGARIS

Acne vulgaris is a chronic inflammatory dermatosis affecting the hair follicle. It is virtually universal in the mid-to-late teenage years, affecting both males and females, although males tend to have more severe disease. Acne is seen in all races, but it is said to be milder in Orientals. Acne vulgaris in adolescents is believed to occur as a result of physiologic hormonal variations and alterations in hair follicle maturation. The clinical features of acne may be induced or exacerbated by drugs (corticosteroids, ACTH, testosterone, gonadotropins, contraceptives, trimethadone, iodides, and bromides), occupational contactants (cutting oils, chlorinated hydrocarbons, and coal tars), and occlusive conditions such as heavy clothing and tropical climates. Some families seem to be particularly affected by acne, suggesting a heritable factor. The role of diet in acne has been greatly exaggerated.

Acne is divided into noninflammatory and inflammatory types, although both may coexist. The former consists of open and closed comedones (singular, comedo). **Open comedones** consist of small follicular papules containing a central black keratin plug. This color is the result of oxidation of melanin pigment (not dirt). **Closed comedones** are follicular papules without a visible central plug. Because the keratin plug is trapped beneath the epidermal surface, these lesions are potential sources of follicular rupture and inflammation. Inflammatory acne is characterized by erythematous papules, nodules, and pustules. Severe variants (e.g., acne conglobata) result in profound scarring and sinus tract formation.

Histologically, comedones form as an expanding mass of lipid and keratin within the midportion of the hair follicle. With gradual expansion, the follicle becomes dilated and the follicular epithelium and sebaceous glands atrophy. Resultant open comedones have large, patulous orifices, whereas those of closed comedones are identifiable only microscopically. Variable lymphohistiocytic infiltrates are present in and around affected follicles, and extensive acute and chronic inflammation accompanies follicular rupture. Dermal abscesses may form in association with rupture, and gradual resolution, often with scarring, ensues.

The pathogenesis of acne is incompletely understood. Endocrine factors have been implicated (especially androgens) because castrated persons never develop the condition, although these do not appear to be the sole or primary cause.[93] It has been postulated that bacterial lipases of the *Propionibacterium acnes* break down sebaceous oils, liberating highly irritating fatty acids and resulting in the earliest inflammatory phases of acne.[94] Inhibition of lipase production is a rationale for administration of antibiotics to patients with inflammatory acne.[95] More recently, a synthetic vitamin A derivative, 13-*cis*-retinoic acid, has resulted in remarkable clinical improvement in some cases of severe acne.[96]

BLISTERING (BULLOUS) DISEASES

Although vesicles and bullae (blisters) occur as a secondary phenomenon in a number of unrelated conditions (e.g., herpesvirus infection, spongiotic dermatitis, erythema multiforme, and thermal burns), there exists a group of disorders in which blisters are the primary and most distinctive features. These bullous diseases, as they are called, produce visually dramatic clinical lesions, and in some instances (e.g., pemphigus vulgaris) are uniformly fatal if untreated.

PEMPHIGUS

Pemphigus is a rare autoimmune blistering disorder resulting from loss of the integrity of normal intercellular attachments within the epidermis and mucosal epithelium.[97] The majority of individuals who develop pemphigus are in the fourth to sixth decades, and men and women are affected equally. There are four clinical and pathologic variants: (1) pemphigus vulgaris; (2) pemphigus vegetans; (3) pemphigus foliaceus; and (4) pemphigus erythematosus.

Pemphigus vulgaris, by far the most common type (accounting for over 80% of cases worldwide), involves mucosa and skin, especially the scalp, face, axilla, groin, trunk, and points of pressure. It may present as oral ulcers that persist sometimes for months before skin involvement appears. Primary lesions are very superficial vesicles and bullae that rupture easily, leaving shallow erosions covered with dried serum and crust. *Pemphigus vegetans* is a rare form that usually presents not with blisters but with large, moist, verrucous (wartlike), vegetating plaques studded with pustules on the groin, axilla, and flexural surfaces. *Pemphigus foliaceus* is a more benign form of pemphigus that occurs in an epidemic form in South America, as well as in isolated cases in other countries. Sites of predilection are the scalp, face, chest, and back, and the mucous membranes are only rarely affected. Bullae are so superficial that only zones of erythema and crusting, sites of previous blister rupture, are usually present on physical examination. *Pemphigus erythematosus* is considered to be a localized, less severe form of pemphigus foliaceus that may selectively involve the malar area of the face in a lupus erythematosus–like fashion.

The common denominator, histologically, in all forms of pemphigus is **acantholysis**. This term implies dissolution, or lysis, of the intercellular adhesion sites within a squamous epithelial surface. Acantholytic cells that are no longer attached to other epithelial cells lose their polyhedral shape and characteristically become rounded. In pemphigus vulgaris and pemphigus vegetans, acantholysis selectively involves the layer of cells immediately above the basal cell layer. (The vegetans variant has considerable overlying epidermal hyperplasia.) The **suprabasal acantholytic blister** that forms is characteristic of pemphigus vulgaris (Fig. 27–27). In pemphigus foliaceus, a blister forms by similar mechanisms, but, unlike the case with pemphigus vulgaris, selectively involves the superficial epidermis at the level of the stratum granulosum. Variable superficial dermal infiltration by lymphocytes, histiocytes, and eosinophils accompanies all forms of pemphigus.

Sera from patients with pemphigus contain antibodies (IgG) to intercellular cement substance of skin and mucous membranes.[98] This phenomenon is the basis for direct and indirect diagnostic immunofluorescence testing of skin and serum, respectively. Lesional sites show a characteristic netlike pattern of intercellular IgG deposits localized to sites of developed or incipient acantholysis. Although cultured skin exposed to pemphigus antiserum develops acantholysis, it now appears that at least some of the acantholytic process is not the direct result of antibody-induced damage, but rather is the consequence of synthesis and liberation of a serine protease, plasminogen activator, by epidermal cells, an event that is triggered by the pemphigus antibody.[99,100]

BULLOUS PEMPHIGOID

Originally considered to be a form of pemphigus, bullous pemphigoid has been recognized for almost the last four decades as a distinct and relatively common

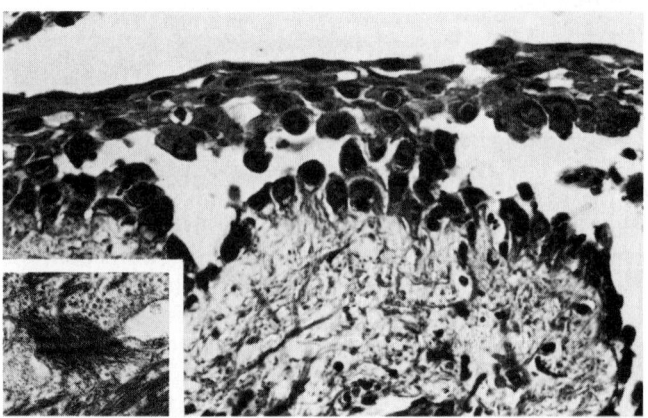

Figure 27–27. Pemphigus vulgaris. Suprabasal acantholysis results in an intraepidermal blister in which rounded (acantholytic) epidermal cells are identified. Dissolution of intercellular cement substance of keratinocyte attachment plaques (desmosomes [*inset*]) results in acantholysis in this disorder.

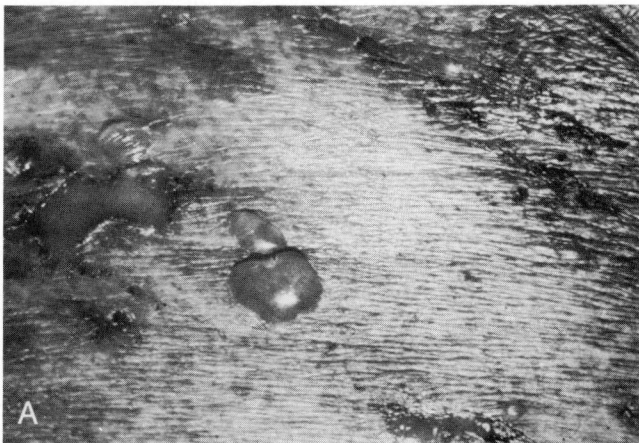

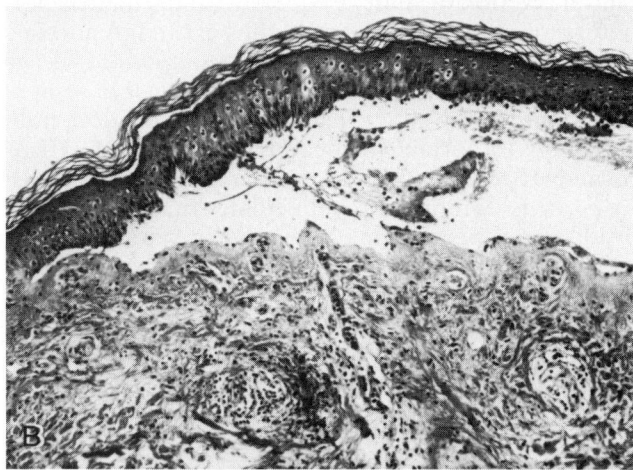

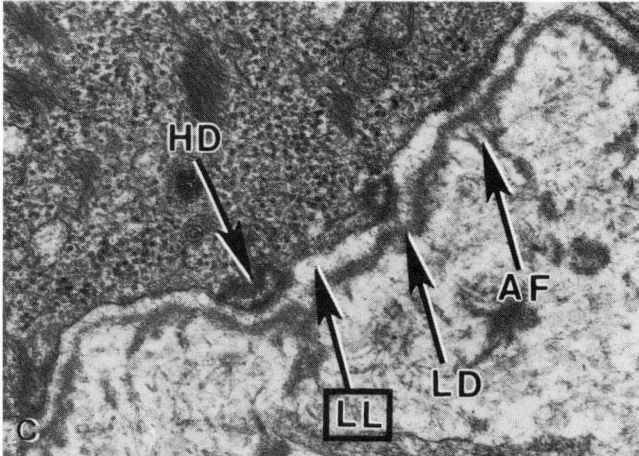

Figure 27–28. Bullous pemphigoid. Clinical bullae (*A*) result from basal cell layer vacuolization, producing a subepidermal blister (*B*). *C,* Bullous pemphigoid antigen is located in the lamina lucida (LL) of the basement membrane zone and in the lowermost portion of the basal cell cytoplasm. HD = hemidesmosome; LD = lamina densa; AF = anchoring fibrils.

autoimmune, vesiculobullous disease. Generally affecting elderly individuals, bullous pemphigoid shows a wide range of clinical presentations, with localized to generalized cutaneous lesions and involvement of mucosal surfaces.

Clinically, lesions are tense bullae, filled with clear fluid, on normal or erythematous skin (Fig. 27–28A). The size may reach 4 to 8 cm in diameter. The bullae do not rupture as easily as the blisters seen in pemphigus, and, if uncomplicated by infection, heal without scarring. Sites of occurrence include the inner aspects of the thighs, flexor surfaces of the forearms, axilla, groin, and lower abdomen. Oral involvement is present in up to one third of patients, usually following the development of cutaneous lesions. Some patients may present with urticarial plaques, with extreme associated pruritus. The immunopathologic features of these lesions, however, are identical to those of bullous lesions.

The separation of bullous pemphigoid from pemphigus, establishing the former as a distinctive entity, was based on the seminal observation of Lever that pemphigoid resulted from a **subepidermal, nonacantholytic** blister.[101] Early lesions show a superficial and sometimes deep perivascular infiltrate of lymphocytes and variable numbers of eosinophils, occasional neutrophils, superficial dermal edema, and associated basal cell layer vacuolization. The vacuolated basal cell layer eventually gives rise to a fluid-filled blister (Fig. 27–28B).

The immunopathology of bullous pemphigoid[102] features *linear* basement membrane zone deposition of immunoglobulin and complement (recall that the pattern for lupus erythematosus was similar, but granular in character). Ultrastructural studies have shown that circulating antibody reacts with antigen present in the narrow clear zone (lamina lucida) of the epidermal basement membrane that separates the underlying lamina densa from the plasma membrane of the basal cells (Fig. 27–28C). Some reactivity also occurs in the basal cell–basement membrane attachment plaques (hemidesmosomes). The antigen present at these sites has been named "bullous pemphigoid antigen" and is now recognized as a normal constituent of the dermoepidermal junction. In bullous pemphigoid, it is likely that the generation of autoantibodies to this basement membrane component results in the fixation of complement and subsequent tissue injury at this site via locally recruited neutrophils and eosinophils.

DERMATITIS HERPETIFORMIS

Dermatitis herpetiformis, first described by Duhring[103] in 1884, is a rare and fascinating entity characterized by urticaria and vesicles. Males tend to be affected more frequently than females, and the age of onset is often in the third and fourth decades, although disease has been known to develop at any age after weaning. A major association is with celiac disease (p. 876); both the vesicular dermatosis and the enteropathy respond to a diet free of gluten (see later).

The urticarial plaques and vesicles of dermatitis

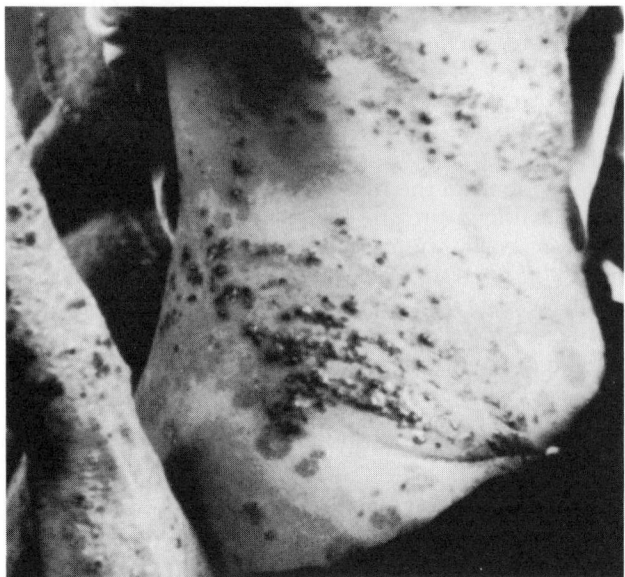

Figure 27–29. One of the original cases of dermatitis herpetiformis described by Duhring. (From the Duhring Collection of the Department of Dermatology of the University of Pennsylvania.)

herpetiformis are extremely pruritic. They characteristically occur bilaterally and symmetrically, involving preferentially the extensor surfaces, elbows, knees, upper back, and buttocks. Figure 27–29 illustrates one of the original Duhring cases. Vesicles are frequently grouped, as are those of true herpesvirus, and hence the name "herpetiform."

Histologically, the early lesions of dermatitis herpetiformis are characteristic. Fibrin and neutrophils accumulate selectively at the **tips of dermal papillae,** forming small "microabscesses" (Fig. 27–30*A*). The basal cells overlying these microabscesses show vacuolization, and minute zones of dermoepidermal separation (microscopic blisters) may occur at the tips of involved papillae. In time, these zones coalesce to form a true subepidermal blister. Eosinophils may occur in the infiltrates of older lesions, creating confusion with the histologic picture of bullous pemphigoid. Attention to the early alterations at the blister edge, however, usually allows for separation of these two disorders. By direct immunofluorescence, dermatitis herpetiformis shows granular deposits of **IgA** selectively localized in the tips of dermal papillae where they are deposited on anchoring fibrils (Fig. 27–30*B*; also refer to Fig. 27–28*C*).

Gluten is the protein moiety that persists subsequent to the removal of water and starch from defatted flour. Gliadin is a class of protein found in the gluten fraction of flour. Patients with dermatitis herpetiformis may develop antibodies of the IgA and IgG classes to gliadin and reticulin, a component of the anchoring fibrils that tether the epidermal basement membrane to the superficial dermis. In addition, individuals with certain histocompatibility types (HLA-B8 and HLA-DRw3) are particularly prone to this disease. It is tempting to speculate that genetically predisposed persons may develop IgA antibodies in the gut to components of dietary gluten, and that these antibodies (or immune complexes) then cross react or are deposited in the skin, resulting in clinical disease. Although it is clear that some individuals with dermatitis herpetiformis and enteropathy respond to a gluten-free diet (as with celiac disease, p. 876), the immunopathogenesis of the disease remains to be fully clarified.[104]

NONINFLAMMATORY BLISTERING DISEASES—PORPHYRIA, EPIDERMOLYSIS BULLOSA

To this point, we have discussed inflammatory blistering diseases. However, some primary disorders char-

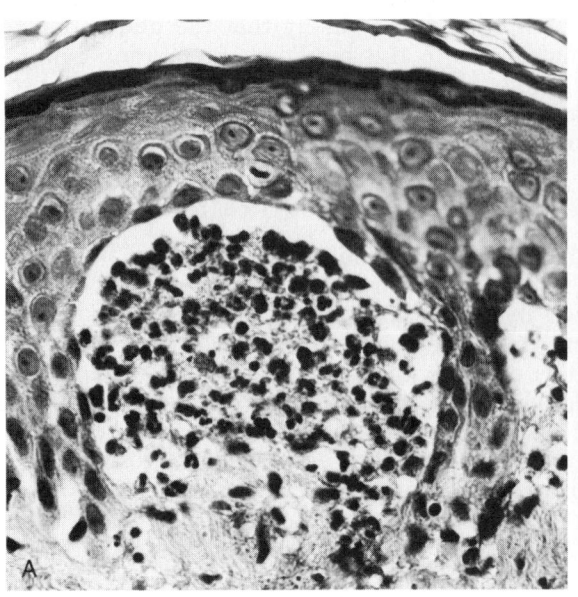
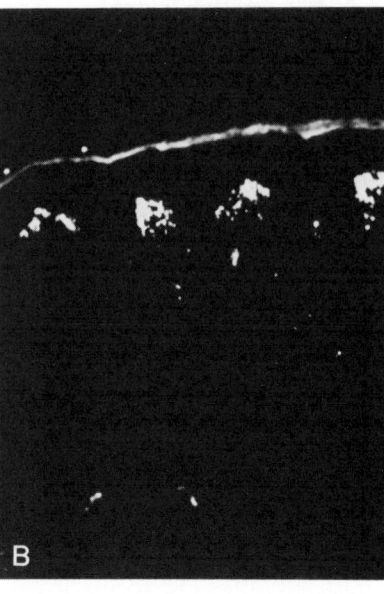

Figure 27–30. Dermatitis herpetiformis. *A,* Neutrophilic microabscess selectively involving the dermal papilla. *B,* Direct immunofluorescence demonstrates granular IgA deposits within four adjacent dermal papillae. These deposits are specifically localized to the anchoring fibrils (refer to Fig. 27–28*C*).

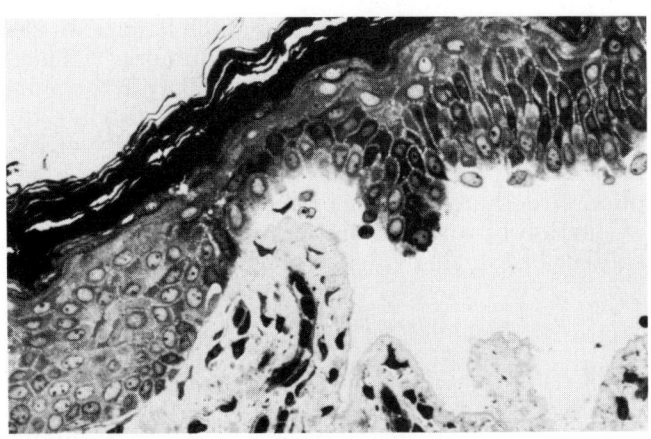

Figure 27–31. Epidermolysis bullosa. A noninflammatory subepidermal blister in this case has formed at the level of the lamina lucida.

acterized by vesicles and bullae are not mediated by inflammatory mechanisms. Two such diseases are *porphyria* and *epidermolysis bullosa.*

Porphyria refers to a group of uncommon inborn or acquired disturbances of porphyrin metabolism. Porphyrins are pigments normally present in hemoglobin, myoglobin, and cytochromes. The classification of porphyrias is based on both clinical and biochemical features. The five major types are (1) congenital erythropoietic porphyria; (2) erythrohepatic protoporphyria; (3) acute intermittent porphyria; (4) porphyria cutanea tarda; and (5) mixed porphyria. Cutaneous manifestations consist of urticaria and vesicles that heal with scarring and that are exacerbated by exposure to sunlight. The primary alterations by light microscopy are a *subepidermal vesicle with associated marked thickening of superficial dermal vessels.* The pathogenesis of these alterations is not well understood.

Epidermolysis bullosa is a group of disorders unified by the common link of blisters that develop at sites of pressure, rubbing, or trauma at or soon after birth. The different types of epidermolysis bullosa, however, are likely to be unrelated with regard to pathogenesis. In the *junctional type,* for example, blisters occur in otherwise histologically normal skin at precisely the level of the lamina lucida (Fig. 27–31). In the scarring *dystrophic types,* blisters develop beneath the lamina densa, presumably in association with rudimentary or defective anchoring fibrils. In the *simplex type,* degeneration of the basal cell layer of the epidermis results in clinical bullae. The histologic changes are so subtle that electron microscopy may be required to differentiate among these types in clinically ambiguous settings!

INFECTION AND INFESTATION

Although the skin is a protective organ, it frequently succumbs to the attack of microorganisms, parasites, and insects. We have already discussed the possible role of bacteria in the pathogenesis of common acne, and the dermatoses resulting from viruses are too numerous to list. In the setting of the immunocompromised patient, ordinarily trivial cutaneous infections may be life-threatening.

Many disorders, such as herpes simplex and herpes zoster, the viral exanthems, and deep fungal infections, are discussed in Chapter 7. Here we address a representative sampling of common infections and infestations whose primary clinical manifestations are in the skin.

VERRUCAE (WARTS)

Verrucae are common lesions of children and adolescents, although they may be encountered at any age. They are caused by papillomaviruses that belong to the DNA-containing papovavirus group. Transmission of disease usually involves direct contact between individuals, or autoinoculation. Verrucae are generally self-limiting, regressing spontaneously within six months to two years.

The classification of verrucae is based largely on clinical morphology and location. *Verruca vulgaris* is the most common type of wart. These lesions occur anywhere, but most frequently on the hands, particularly on the dorsal surfaces and periungual areas, where they appear as gray-white to tan, flat to convex, 0.1- to 1-cm papules with a rough, pebble-like surface (Fig. 27–32A). *Verruca plana,* or *flat wart,* is common on the face or the dorsal surfaces of the hands. These warts are slightly elevated, flat, smooth, tan papules that are generally smaller than verruca vulgaris. *Verruca plantaris* and *verruca palmaris* occur on the soles or palms, respectively. Rough, scaly lesions may reach 1 to 2 cm in diameter, coalesce, and be confused with ordinary calluses. *Condyloma acuminatum (venereal wart)* occurs on the penis, female genitalia, urethra, perianal areas, and rectum. These lesions appear as soft, tan, cauliflower-like masses that in occasional cases reach many centimeters in diameter.

Histologic features common to verrucae include epidermal hyperplasia that is often undulant in character (so-called verrucous or papillomatous epidermal hyperplasia— Fig. 27–32B) and cytoplasmic vacuolization (koilocytosis) that preferentially involves the more superficial epidermal layers producing zones of pallor surrounding infected nuclei. Electron microscopy of these zones reveals numerous viral particles within nuclei. Infected cells may also demonstrate prominent and apparently condensed keratohyaline granules and jagged eosinophilic intracytoplasmic keratin aggregates as a result of viral cytopathic effects. These cellular alterations are not as prominent in condylomas, hence their diagnosis is based primarily on hyperplastic papillary architecture containing wedge-shaped zones of koilocytosis.

It is now recognized that the clinically different types of warts just described result not solely because

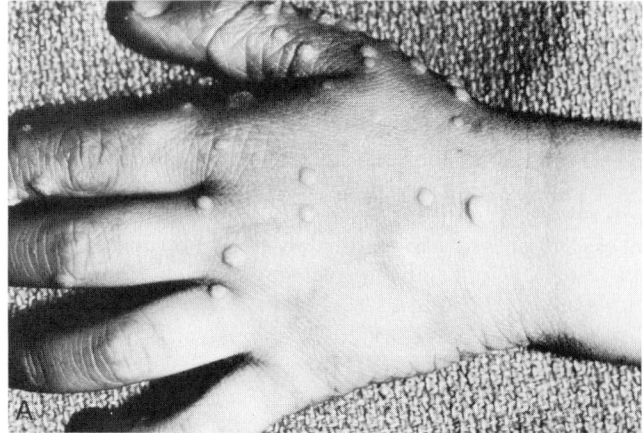

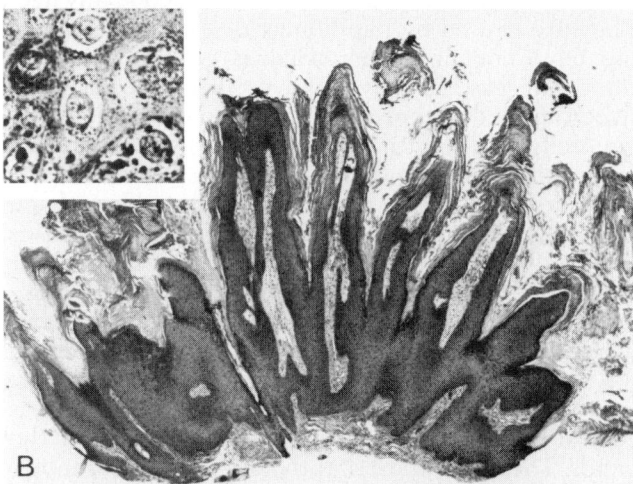

Figure 27–32. Verrucae. *A,* Multiple papules with rough, pebble-like surfaces are present. *B,* Histologically, such lesions show papillomatous epidermal hyperplasia and cytopathic alterations that include nuclear pallor and prominent keratohyaline granules *(inset).*

of the anatomically different sites in which they arise but also as a consequence of distinct types of human papillomavirus. Over 40 types of papillomavirus that can produce warts in humans have been identified in studies utilizing molecular hybridization and restriction enzyme analyses. For example, anogenital warts are caused predominantly by papillomavirus types 6, 11, 16, and 18. Interestingly, there is a tendency for lesions induced by type 16 to show some degree of associated dysplasia.[105] Moreover, type 16 has also been associated with in situ squamous cell carcinoma of the genitalia and with *bowenoid papulosis* (genital lesions of young adults with the histology of in situ carcinoma but with a biologic course of spontaneous regression).[106] These findings are relevant to previous observations of the association of types 16 and 18 with carcinomas of the uterine cervix.[107] The potential relationship of papillomavirus to carcinoma is reinforced by the rare heritable condition termed *epidermodysplasia verruciformis.* In this disorder, patients develop multiple flat warts, some of which evolve to become invasive squamous cell carcinoma. The ge-

nomes of papillomavirus types 5 and 8 have been detected in some of these cutaneous tumors.[108] Thus, the types of papillomavirus differ not only in the morphology of the lesions they produce but also in their oncogenic potential. The current availability of hybridization probes for viral DNA, which can be applied directly to histologic sections, will assist in the evaluation of warts exhibiting unusual growth clinically or histologic evidence of dysplasia.

MOLLUSCUM CONTAGIOSUM

Molluscum contagiosum is a common, self-limiting, viral disease of the skin caused by a poxvirus. The virus is characteristically brick-shaped, has a dumbbell-shaped DNA core, and measures 300 nm in maximum dimension. Infection is usually spread by direct contact, particularly among children and young adults.

Clinically, multiple lesions may occur on the skin and mucous membranes, with a predilection for the trunk and anogenital areas. Individual lesions are firm, often pruritic, pink to skin-colored umbilicated papules generally ranging in diameter from 0.2 to 0.4 cm. Rarely, "giant" forms occur measuring up to 2.0 cm in diameter. A curdlike material can be expressed from the central umbilication. Smearing this material onto a glass slide and staining with Giemsa reagent often shows diagnostic "molluscum bodies."

Microscopically, lesions show cuplike verrucous epidermal hyperplasia (Fig. 27–33A). The pathognomonic structure is the **molluscum body,** which occurs as a large (up to 35 μm), ellipsoid, homogeneous, cytoplasmic inclusion in cells of the stratum granulosum and the stratum corneum (Fig. 27–33B). These inclusions are eosinophilic in the blue-purple (on H and E stain) stratum granulosum and acquire a red to pale blue hue in the red stratum corneum. Numerous virions are present within molluscum bodies.

IMPETIGO

This common superficial infection of the skin usually caused by staphylococci or streptococci is discussed on page 338. Impetigo is frequently seen in normal children as well as in adults in poor health. Cultures most frequently grow coagulase-positive staphylococci or group A beta-hemolytic streptococci, or both. Nephritogenic strains of streptococcus cause impetigo, particularly in tropical areas and in the southern United States.[109]

The condition usually involves exposed skin, particularly that of the face and hands. Initially it is an erythematous macule, but multiple small pustules rapidly supervene. As pustules break, shallow erosions form, covered with drying serum, giving the characteristic clinical appearance of **honey-colored crust.** If the crust is not removed, new lesions form about the periphery and extensive epidermal

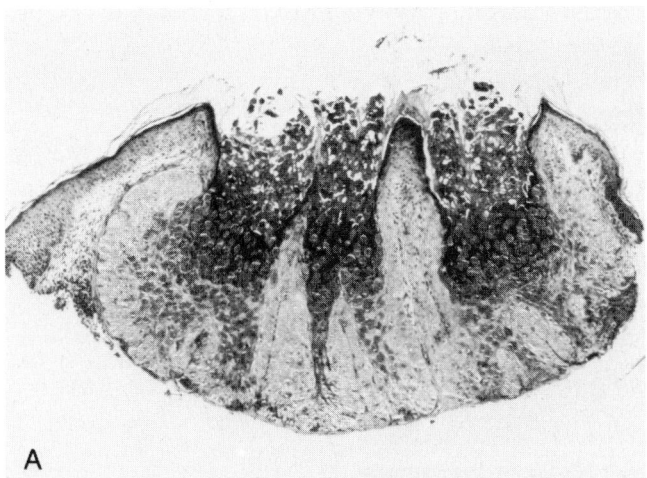

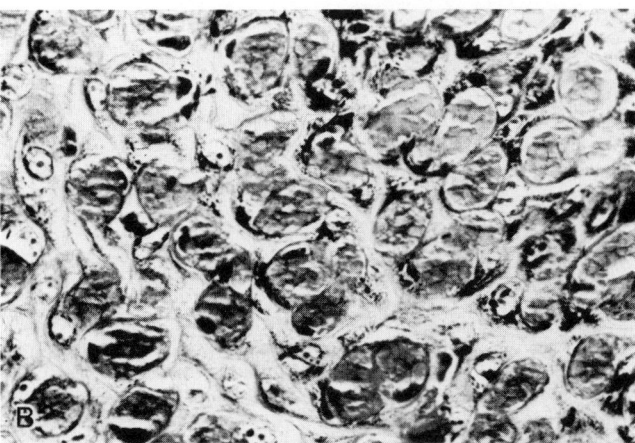

Figure 27–33. Molluscum contagiosum. A focus of cuplike verrucous epidermal hyperplasia (*A*) contains numerous cells with ellipsoid cytoplasmic inclusions (molluscum bodies) (*B*).

damage may ensue. A bullous form of impetigo occurs in children.

The characteristic microscopic feature of impetigo is accumulation of neutrophils beneath the stratum corneum, often with the formation of a subcorneal pustule. Special stains reveal the presence of bacteria in these foci. Nonspecific, reactive epidermal alterations and superficial dermal inflammation accompany these findings. Rupture of pustules results in superficial layering of serum, neutrophils, and cellular debris to form the characteristic clinical crust.

SUPERFICIAL FUNGAL INFECTIONS

As opposed to deep fungal infections, superficial fungal infections of the skin are confined to the stratum corneum, where they are caused primarily by dermatophytes. These organisms grow in the soil and on animals and produce a number of diverse and characterisitc clinical lesions.

Tinea capitis usually occurs in children and is only rarely seen in infants and adults. It is a dermatophy-

tosis of the scalp characterized by asymptomatic, often hairless patches of skin associated with mild erythema, crust formation, and scale. *Tinea barbae* is a dermatophyte infection of the beard area that affects adult men; it is a relatively uncommon disorder. *Tinea corporis*, on the other hand, is a common superficial fungal infection of the body surface that affects all ages, but particularly children. Predisposing factors include excessive heat and humidity, exposure to infected animals, and chronic dermatophytosis of the feet or nails. The most common type of tinea corporis is an expanding, round, slightly erythematous plaque with an elevated scaling border (Fig. 27–34A). *Tinea cruris* occurs most frequently in the inguinal areas of obese men during warm weather. Heat, friction, and maceration all predispose to its development. The infection usually first appears on the upper inner thighs, with gradual extension of moist, red patches that have raised, scaling borders. *Tinea pedis (athlete's foot)* affects 30 to 40% of the population at some time in their lives. There is diffuse erythema and scaling, often initially localized to the web spaces. Most of the inflammatory tissue reaction, however, has recently been shown to be the result of bacterial superinfection and not directly related to the primary dermatophytosis.[110] Spread to, or primary infection of, the nails is referred to as *onychomycosis*. This produces discoloration, thickening, and deformity of the nail plate. *Tinea versicolor* usually occurs on the upper trunk and is highly distinctive in appearance. Caused by *Malassezia furfur*, the lesions consist of groups of macules of all sizes, lighter or darker than surrounding skin, with a fine peripheral scale.

The histologic features of all dermatophytoses are variable, depending on the antigenic properties of the organism, the corresponding host response, and the degree of bacterial superinfection that occurs.[110] Fungal cell walls, rich in mucopolysaccharides, stain bright pink to red with PAS stain. They are present in the anucleate cornified layer of lesional skin, hair, or nails (Fig. 27–34B,C), and scraping of these areas and subsequent culture of organisms will usually produce colonial growth that permits definitive classification of the offending species (Fig. 27–34D). Reactive epidermal changes may produce a pattern that mimics a mild eczematous dermatitis.

ARTHROPOD BITES, STINGS, AND INFESTATIONS

Arthropods are ubiquitous, and we all are prone to the bites, stings, and other discomforts they cause. The arthropods include Arachnida (spiders, scorpions, ticks, and mites); Insecta (lice, bedbugs, bees, wasps, fleas, flies, and mosquitos); and Chilopoda (centipedes). All can cause skin lesions, but there is a wide variability in clinical patterns of reaction. Some persons suffer minimal symptoms, others considerable discomfort, and some may die as a consequence of a

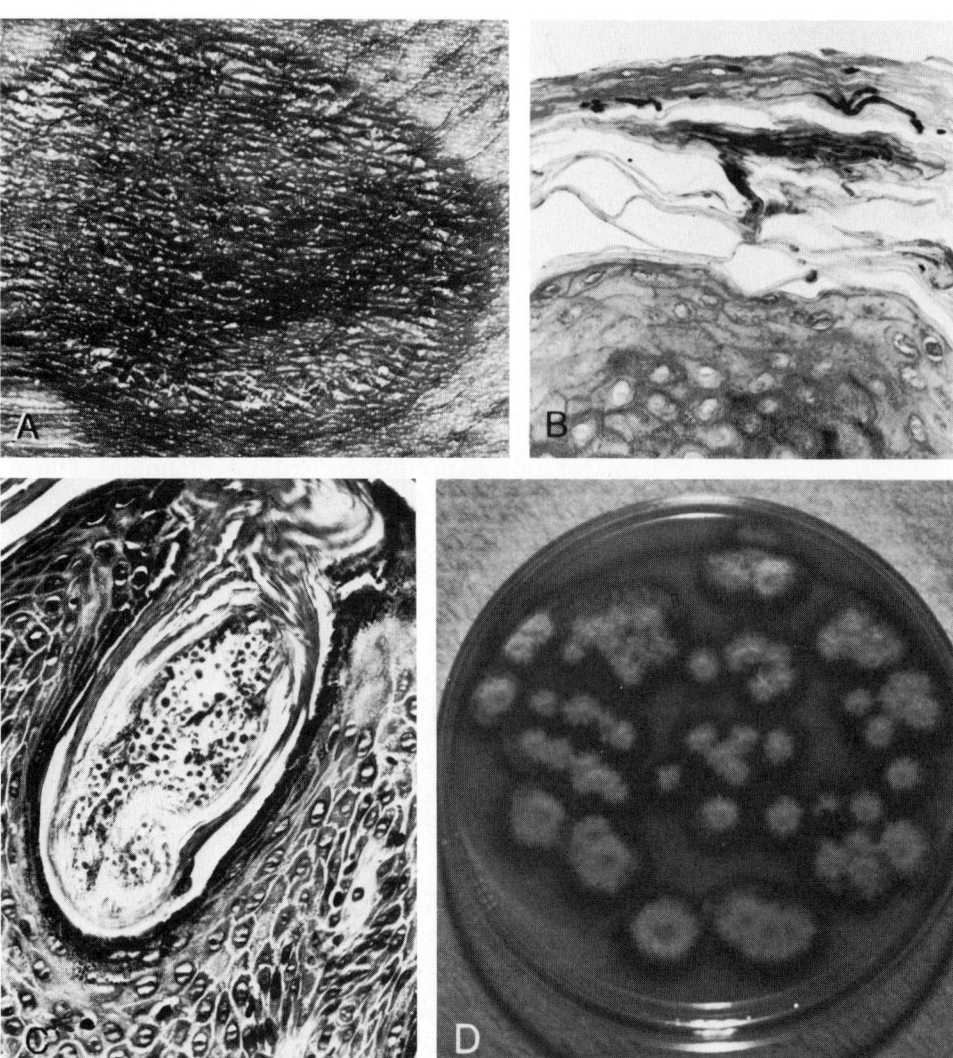

Figure 27–34. Tinea. *A,* A characteristic plaque of tinea corporis. PAS stain reveals hyphae (*B*) and yeast forms (*C*) within the stratum corneum and hair shaft in tinea corporis and tinea capitis, respectively. *D,* Scraping and culture of infected sites will often permit growth of offending organisms, facilitating their definitive classification.

bite or sting. Arthropods can produce lesions in several ways: (1) by direct irritant effects of insect parts or secretions; (2) by immediate or delayed hypersensitivity responses (including an anaphylactic reaction) to retained or injected body parts or secretions; (3) by specific effects of venoms (e.g., the black widow spider venom produces severe cramps and excruciating pain; the brown recluse spider venom contains potent enzymes that produce tissue necrosis); and (4) by serving as vectors for secondary invaders, such as bacteria, rickettsiae, and parasites.

Macroscopically, arthropod bites may be urticarial or inflamed papules and nodules, sometimes with ulceration, that may last for several weeks. In the case of the tick bite caused by the mite *Ixodes dammini,* the vector for the spirochete that causes Lyme disease (p. 366), a characteristic expanding, erythematous plaque (erythema migrans) develops. Such extensive necrosis may result from the bite of the brown recluse spider that radical, surgical excision of the involved area is often necessary. **Scabies** is a conta-

gious, pruritic dermatosis caused by the mite *Sarcoptes scabiei.* The female mite burrows under the stratum corneum, producing furrows (linear, poorly defined streaks, 0.2 to 0.6 cm in length) on the interdigital skin, palms, wrists, periareolar skin of women, and genital skin of men. **Pediculosis** is caused by the head louse, crab louse, and body louse. The disease is pruritic, and the louse, or its eggs, attached to hair shafts can usually be seen with the unaided eye (Fig. 27–35). In pediculosis of the scalp, impetigo and enlarged cervical lymph nodes may be frequent complications, especially in children. The pubic louse may be transmitted through sexual contact. Infection with the body louse ("vagabond's disease") is usually characterized by areas of hyperpigmentation and scratch marks (excoriations).

The histologic picture of arthropod bites is highly varied. The classic lesion shows a wedge-shaped perivascular infiltrate of lymphocytes, histiocytes, and eosinophils within the dermis. There may be a central zone of exceedingly focal epidermal necrosis, directly under which birefringent insect mouthparts may be found (the site of the bite is called the

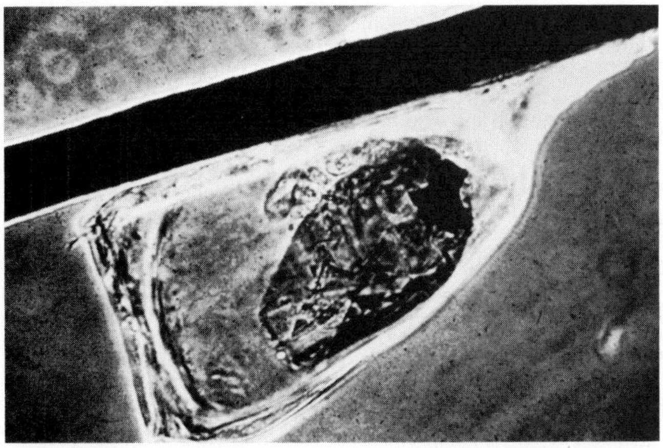

Figure 27–35. Pediculosis. Egg case (nit) of head louse attached to hair shaft.

punctum). In some bites, a primarily urticarial reaction is seen histologically, whereas in others the inflammatory infiltrate is so florid and dense that it may superficially resemble a cutaneous lymphoma. Spongiosis, resulting in intraepidermal blisters, is present in some biopsy specimens, and, in certain settings, insect bites even resemble bullous pemphigoid.

Careful correlation with a clinical history of exposure to insects and the gross finding of clustered or linear lesions facilitate the clinicopathologic diagnosis.

Acknowledgments

Dr. Gerald Lazarus graciously provided the clinical photographs. Clinical panels of Figures 27–3, 27–6, 27–15, 27–19, 27–28, and 27–34 were reproduced with permission from F.A. Davis Co., Philadelphia. Sharon E. Murphy provided the excellent medical illustrations. Ms. Diana Whitaker gave expert technical assistance in the preparation of illustrations. Finally, I thank the histotechnologists of the Dermatopathology Laboratory of the Hospital of the University of Pennsylvania for the superb slides, upon which the photomicrography was performed.

1. Virchow, R.: Cellular Pathology. London, John Churchill, 1860, p. 33.

2. Shelley, W.G., and Juhlin, L.: Langerhans cells form a reticuloendothelial trap for external contact antigens. Nature 261:46, 1976.

3. Murphy, G.F.: Cell membrane glycoproteins and Langerhans cells. Hum. Pathol. 16:103, 1985.

4. Kupper, T.: Epidermal cytokines. In Shevach, E., and Oppenheim, J. (eds.): The Immunophysiology of Cells and Cytokines. Oxford, Oxford University Press, 1988.

5. Sporn, M.D., and Roberts, A.B.: Peptide growth factors are multifunctional. Nature 332:217, 1988.

6. Hertz, K.C., et al.: Autoimmune vitiligo, detection of antibodies to melanin-producing cells. N. Engl. J. Med. 297:634, 1977.

7. Palkowski, M.R., et al.: Langerhans cells in hair follicles of the depigmenting C57B1/Ler-vit.vit mouse. A model for human vitiligo. Arch. Dermatol. 123:1022, 1987.

8. Grimes, P.E., et al.: T cell profiles in vitiligo. J. Am. Acad. Dermatol. 14:196, 1986.

9. Parrish, J.A.: Phototherapy of psoriasis and other skin diseases. In Regan, J.D., and Parrish, J.A. (eds.): The Science of Photomedicine. New York, Plenum Press, 1982.

10. Sanchez, N.P., et al.: A clinical, light microscopic, ultrastructural, and immunofluorescence study. J. Am. Acad. Dermatol. 4:698, 1981.

11. Perez, M., et al.: Endocrinologic profile of patients with idiopathic melasma. J. Invest. Dermatol. 81:543, 1983.

12. Reed, R.: Minimal deviation melanoma. In Mihm, M.C., Jr., and Murphy, G.F. (eds.): Pathobiology and Recognition of Malignant Melanoma. Baltimore, Williams & Wilkins, 1988, p. 111.

13. Murphy, G.F., and Mihm, M.C., Jr.: Origin and fate of pigmented nevi. In Williams, H.B. (ed.): Symposium on Vascular Malformations and Melanocytic Lesions. St. Louis, C.V. Mosby Co., 1983, p. 268.

14. Norris, W.: A case of fungoid disease. Edinburgh Med. Surg. J. 16:562, 1820.

15. Clark, W.H., Jr., et al.: Origin of familial malignant melanomas from heritable melanotic lesions: The BK mole syndrome. Arch. Dermatol. 114:732, 1978.

16. Reimer, R.R., et al.: Precursor lesions in familial melanoma: A new genetic preneoplastic syndrome. J.A.M.A. 239:744, 1978.

17. Greene, M.H., et al.: Familial cutaneous malignant melanoma: Autosomal dominant trait possibly linked to the Rh locus. Proc. Natl. Acad. Sci. U.S.A. 80:6071, 1983.

18. Greene, M.H., et al.: The high risk of melanoma in melanoma prone families with dysplastic nevi. Ann. Intern. Med. 102:458, 1985.

19. Ruiter, D.J., et al.: Major histocompatibility antigens and mononuclear inflammatory infiltrate in benign nevomelanocytic proliferations and malignant melanoma. J. Immunol. 129:2808, 1982.

20. Caporaso, N., et al.: Cytogenetics in hereditary malignant melanoma and dysplastic nevus syndrome: Is dysplastic nevus syndrome a chromosome instability disorder? Cancer Genet. Cytogenet. 24:299, 1987.

21. Smith, P.J., et al.: Abnormal sensitivity to UV-radiation in cultured skin fibroblasts from patients with hereditary cutaneous malignant melanoma and dysplastic nevus syndrome. Int. J. Cancer 30:39, 1987.

22. Tong, A.K.F., et al.: Dysplastic nevus: A formal histogenetic precursor of malignant melanoma. In Mihm, M.C., and Murphy, G.F. (eds.): Pathobiology and Recognition of Malignant Melanoma. Baltimore, Williams & Wilkins, 1988, p.10.

23. Rhodes, A.R., et al.: Dysplastic melanocytic nevi in histologic association with 234 primary cutaneous melanomas. J. Am. Acad. Dermatol. 9:563, 1983.

24. Clark, W.H., et al.: A study of tumor progression: The precursor lesions of superficial spreading and nodular melanoma. Hum. Pathol. 15:1147, 1985.

25. Mihm, M.C.: The clinical diagnosis, classification and histogenetic concepts of the early stages of cutaneous malignant melanomas. N. Engl. J. Med. 284:1078, 1971.

26. Mihm, M.C.: Malignant melanoma. In Demis, D.J. (ed.): Clinical Dermatology. Baltimore, Harper & Row, 1984, p. 104.

27. Murphy, G.F., et al.: Clinicopathologic types of malignant melanoma: Relevance to biologic behavior and diagnostic surgical approach. J. Dermatol. Surg. Oncol. 11:673, 1985.

28. Imber, M.J., and Mihm, M.C.: Biological and prognostic significance of vertical growth phase characteristics in malignant melanoma. In Mihm, M.C., and Murphy, G.F. (eds.): Pathobiology and Recognition of Malignant Melanoma. Baltimore, Williams & Wilkins, 1988, p. 19.

29. Breslow, A.: Thickness, cross-sectional areas and depth of invasion in the prognosis of cutaneous melanoma. Ann. Surg. 182:572, 1970.

30. Clark, W.H., et al: The developmental biology of primary cutaneous malignant melanoma. Semin. Oncol. 2:83, 1975.

31. Murphy, G.F., and Mihm, M.C.: Histologic reporting of malignant melanoma. In Mihm, M.C., and Murphy, G.F. (eds.): Pathobiology and Recognition of Malignant Melanoma. Baltimore, Williams & Wilkins, 1988, p. 79.

32. Thurin, J., et al.: GD2 ganglioside biosynthesis is a distinct biochemical event in melanoma tumor progression. FEBS Lett. 208:17, 1986.

33. Balaban, G.B., et al.: Karyotypic evolution of human malignant melanoma. Cancer Genet. Cytogenet. 19:113, 1986.

34. Granstein, R.D., et al.: Epidermal antigen-presenting cells in acti-

vation of suppression: Identification of a new functional type of ultraviolet radiation-resistant epidermal cells. J. Immunol. *132*:563, 1984.

34a. Rigall, D.S., and Friedman, R.J.: The rate of malignant melanoma in the United States: Are we making an impact? J. Am. Acad. Dermatol. *17*:1050, 1987.

35. Murphy, G.F., et al.: Organelle-specific injury to melanin-containing cells in human skin by pulsed laser irradiation. Lab. Invest. *49*:680, 1983.

36. Mevorah, B., and Mishima, Y.: Cellular response of seborrheic keratosis following croton oil irritation and surgical trauma. Dermatologica *131*:452, 1965.

37. Ellis, D.L., et al.: Melanoma, growth factors, acanthosis nigricans, the sign of Leser-Trelat, and multiple acrochordons. A possible role for alpha-transforming growth factor in cutaneous paraneoplastic syndromes. N. Engl. J. Med. *317*:1582, 1987.

38. Curth, H.O.: Classification of acanthosis nigricans. Int. J. Dermatol. *15*:592, 1976.

39. Fitzpatrick, T.B., et al.: Color Atlas and Synopsis of Clinical Dermatology. New York, McGraw-Hill Book Company, 1983, p. 284.

40. Murphy, G.F., et al.: Involucrin expression in normal and neoplastic human skin: A marker for keratinocyte differentiation. J. Invest. Dermatol. *82*:453, 1984.

41. Smoller, B.R., et al.: Keratoacanthoma and squamous cell carcinoma of the skin: Immunohistochemical localization of involucrin and keratin protein. J. Am. Acad. Dermatol. *14*:226, 1986.

42. Hashimoto, K., et al.: Tumors of Skin Appendages. Boston, Butterworths, 1987.

43. Starink, T.M., et al.: The cutaneous pathology of cutaneous lesions of Cowden's disease: New findings. J. Cutan. Pathol. *11*:331, 1984.

44. Thielmann, H.W., et al.: DNA repair synthesis in fibroblast strains from patients with actinic keratosis, squamous cell carcinoma, basal cell carcinoma, or malignant melanoma after treatment with ultraviolet light, N-acetoxy-2-acetyl-aminofluorene methyl methanesulfonate, and N-methyl-N-nitrosourea. J. Cancer Res. Clin. Oncol., *113*:171, 1987.

45. Parrish, J.A.: Responses of skin to visible and ultraviolet radiation. *In* Goldsmith, L.A. (ed.): Biochemistry and Physiology of the Skin. Oxford, Oxford University Press, 1983, p. 722.

46. Penn, I.: Neoplastic consequences of transplantation and chemotherapy. Cancer Detect. Prev., *1*(Suppl):149, 1987.

47. Cooper, K.D., et al.: Effects of ultraviolet radiation on human epidermal cell alloantigen presentation: Initial depression of Langerhans cell–dependent function is followed by the appearance of T6⁻Dr⁺ cells that enhance epidermal alloantigen presentation. J. Immunol. *134*:129, 1985.

48. Granstein, R.D.: Epidermal I-J-bearing cells are responsible for transferable suppressor cell generation after immunization of mice with ultraviolet radiation–treated epidermal cells. J. Invest. Dermatol. *84*:206, 1985.

49. Granstein, R.D., et al.: Epidermal cells in activation of suppressor lymphocytes: Further characterization. J. Immunol. *138*:4055, 1987.

50. Kawashima, M., et al.: Characterization of a new type of human papillomavirus (HPV) related to HPV5 from a case of actinic keratosis. Virology *154*:389, 1986.

51. Hochwalt, A.E., et al.: Mechanism of H-ras oncogene activation in mouse squamous carcinoma induced by an alkylating agent. Cancer Res. *48*:556, 1988.

52. Gorlin, R.J., et al.: The multiple basal cell nevi syndrome. Cancer *18*:89, 1965.

53. Murphy, G.F., et al.: Local immune response in basal cell carcinoma: Characterization by transmission electron microscopy and monoclonal anti-T6 antibody. J. Am. Acad. Dermatol. *8*:477, 1983.

54. Guillen, F.J., et al.: Expression of activation antigens by T cells infiltrating basal cell carcinomas. J. Invest. Dermatol. *85*:203, 1985.

55. Wick, M.R., et al.: Primary neuroendocrine carcinomas of the skin (Merkel cell tumors). A clinical, histologic, and ultrastructural study of thirteen cases. Am. J. Clin. Pathol. *79*:6, 1983.

56. Yoshida, Y., et al.: Merkel cell tumor of the skin: Ultrastructural and immunohistochemical studies. Acta Pathol. Japon. *34*:1433, 1984.

57. Drijkoningen, M., et al.: Merkel cell tumor of the skin: An immunohistochemical study. Hum. Pathol. *17*:301, 1986.

58. Lever, W.F., and Schaumburg-Lever, G.: Histopathology of the Skin. Philadelphia, J.B. Lippincott, 1983, p. 385.

59. Templeton, A.C.: Studies in Kaposi's sarcoma. Cancer *34*:634, 1972.

60. Gottlieb, G., and Ackerman, A.B.: Kaposi's Sarcoma: A Text and Atlas. Philadelphia, Lea & Febiger, 1988.

61. Jones, R.R., et al.: Histogenesis of Kaposi's sarcoma in patients with and without acquired immune deficiency syndrome (AIDS). J. Clin. Pathol. *39*:742, 1986.

62. Beckstead, J.H., et al.: Evidence for the origin of Kaposi's sarcoma from lymphatic endothelium. Am. J. Pathol. *119*:294, 1985.

63. Dictor, M.: Kaposi's sarcoma. Origin and significance of lymphaticovenous connections. Virchows Arch. (A) *409*:23, 1986.

64. Ruszczak, Z., et al.: Angioproliferative changes in clinically noninvolved, perilesional skin in AIDS-associated Kaposi's sarcoma. Dermatologica *175*:270, 1987.

65. Ruszczak, Z., et al.: Kaposi's sarcoma in AIDS. Multicentric angioplasia in early skin lesions. Am. J. Dermatopathol. *9*:388, 1987.

66. DeDobbler, G., et al.: Clinically uninvolved skin in AIDS: Evidence of atypical dermal vessels similar to early lesions observed in Kaposi's sarcoma. J. Cutan. Pathol. *14*:154, 1987.

67. Murphy, G.F., et al.: Distribution of T cell antigens in histiocytosis X cells. Quantitative immunoelectron microscopy using monoclonal antibodies. Lab. Invest. *48*:90, 1983.

67a. Knobler, R.M., and Edelson, R.L.: Lymphoma cutis: T cell type. *In* Murphy, G.F., and Mihm, M.C., Jr. (eds.): Lymphoproliferative Disorders of the Skin. Boston, Butterworths, 1980, p. 176.

68. Murphy, G.F.: Cutaneous T cell lymphoma. *In* Fenoglio-Preiser, C.M. (ed): Advances in Pathology. Chicago, Year Book Medical Publishers, 1988.

69. Manzari, V., et al.: HTLV-V: A new human retrovirus isolated in a Tac-negative T cell lymphoma/leukemia. Science *238*:1581, 1987.

70. Sayama, S., et al.: Human skin chymotrypsin-like proteinase chymase. Subcellular localization to mast cell granules and interaction with heparin and other glycosaminoglycans. J. Biol. Chem. *262*:6808, 1987.

71. Roitt, I.M., et al.: Immunology. St. Louis, C.V. Mosby Company, 1985, p. 199.

72. Frank, M., et al.: Hereditary angioedema. The clinical syndrome and its management. Ann. Intern. Med. *84*:580, 1976.

73. Sheffer, A.L., et al.: Exercise-induced anaphylaxis; a common, serious form of physical allergy associated with mast cell degranulation. J. Allergy Clin. Immunol. *75*:479, 1985.

74. Murphy, G.F., et al.: Morphologically distinctive forms of cutaneous mast cell degranulation induced by cold and mechanical stimuli; an ultrastructural study. J. Allergy Clin. Immunol. *80*:603, 1987.

75. Leider, M., and Rosenblum, M.: A Dictionary of Dermatologic Words, Terms, and Phrases. West Haven, CT, Dome Laboratories, 1976.

76. Murphy, G.F., et al.: Reaction patterns in the skin and special dermatologic techniques. *In* Moschella, S. (ed.): Dermatology. Philadelphia, W.B. Saunders Company, 1984, p. 104.

77. Toews, G.B., et al.: Langerhans cells: Sentinels of skin-associated lymphoid tissue. J. Invest. Dermatol. *75*:78, 1980.

78. Dvorak, A.M., et al.: Morphology of delayed-type hypersensitivity reactions in man. Lab. Invest. *34*:179, 1976.

79. Cotran, R.S., et al.: Induction and detection of human endothelial activation antigen in vivo. J. Exp. Med. *164*:661, 1986.

80. Messadi, D.V., et al.: Induction of an activation antigen on postcapillary venular endothelium in human skin organ culture. J. Immunol. *139*:1557, 1987.

81. Hanser, C.H., et al.: Interleukin I is present in normal human epidermis. J. Immunol. *136*:3317, 1986.

82. Bevilacqua, M.P., et al.: Interleukin I acts on cultured human vascular endothelium to increase the adhesion of polymorphonuclear leukocytes, monocytes, and related leukocyte cell lines. J. Clin. Invest. *76*:2003, 1985.

83. Guillen, F.J., et al.: Acute cutaneous graft-versus-host disease to minor histocompatibility antigens in a murine model: Evidence that large granular lymphocytes are the effector cells in the immune response. Lab. Invest. *137*:1874, 1986.

84. Guillen, F.J., et al.: Inhibition of rat skin allograft rejection by cyclosporin. In situ characterization of the impaired local immune response. Transplantation *41*:734, 1986.

85. Murphy, G.F., et al.: Cytotoxic T lymphocytes and phenotypically abnormal epidermal dendritic cells in fixed cutaneous eruptions. Hum. Pathol. *16*:1264, 1985.

86. Zaias, N.: Psoriasis of the nail. A clinical-pathologic study. Arch. Dermatol. *99*:567, 1969.

87. Beutner, E.H., et al.: Autoimmunity in psoriasis. *In* Beutner, E.H., et al. (eds.): Immunopathology of the Skin. New York, John Wiley and Sons, 1987, p. 703.

88. Kronenberg, K., et al.: Malignant degeneration of lichen planus. Arch. Dermatol. *104*:304, 1971.

89. Bhan, A.K., et al.: T cell subset populations in lichen planus: In situ characterization using monoclonal anti–T cell antibodies. Br. J. Dermatol. *105*:617, 1981.

90. Harrist, T.J., and Mihm, M.C.: The specificity and usefulness of the lupus band test. Arthritis Rheum. *23*:479, 1980.

91. Rubenstein, M.H., et al.: Lichen planus and lupus erythematosus: Two disorders with pigment incontinence of possible immunologically mediated origin. *In* Fitzpatrick, T.B., et al. (eds.): Biology of Diseases of Dermal Pigmentation. Tokyo, University of Tokyo Press, 1981, p. 151.

92. Biesecker, G., et al.: Cutaneous localization of membrane attack complex in discoid and systemic lupus erythematosus. N. Engl. J. Med. *306*:264, 1982.

93. Strauss, J.S., and Pochi, P.E.: Recent advances in androgen metabolism and their relation to the skin. Arch. Dermatol. *100:*621, 1969.

94. Voss, J.G.: Acne vulgaris and free fatty acids. Arch. Dermatol. *109*:849, 1974.

95. Webster, G.F., et al.: Inhibition of lipase production in *Propionibacterium acnes* by sub-minimal-inhibitory concentrations of tetracycline and erythromycin. Br. J. Dermatol. *104*:453, 1981.

96. Mills, O.H., and Kligman, A.M.: Treatment of acne by vitamin A (retinol). Semin. Dermatol. *1*:245, 1985.

97. Ahmed, A.R.: Clinical features of pemphigus. *In* Ahmed, A.R. (ed.): Clinics in Dermatology—Pemphigus. Philadelphia, J.B. Lippincott Company, 1983, p. 13.

98. Beutner, E.H., and Jordan, R.E.: Demonstration of skin antibodies in sera of pemphigus vulgaris in patients by indirect immunofluorescent staining. Proc. Soc. Exp. Biol. Med. *117*:505, 1964.

99. Hashimoto, K., et al.: Anti-cell surface pemphigus autoantibody stimulates plasminogen activator activity of human epidermal cells. J. Exp. Med. *157*:259, 1983.

100. Morioka, S., et al.: Involvement of urokinase-type plasminogen activator in acanthosis induced by pemphigus. J. Invest. Dermatol. *189*:474, 1987.

101. Lever, W.F.: Pemphigus. Medicine *32*:1, 1953.

102. Imber, M.J., et al.: The immunopathology of bullous pemphigoid. *In* Ahmed, A.R.: Clinics in Dermatology—Bullous Pemphigoid. Philadelphia, J.B. Lippincott Company, 1987, p. 81.

103. Duhring, L.: Dermatitis herpetiformis. J.A.M.A. *3*:225, 1984.

104. Hall, R.P.: The pathogenesis of dermatitis herpetiformis: Recent advances. J. Am. Acad. Dermatol. *16*:1129, 1987.

105. von Krogh, et al.: Advantage of human papillomavirus typing in the clinical evaluation of genitoanal warts. J. Am. Acad. Dermatol. *18*:495, 1988.

106. Ikenberg, H., et al.: Human papillomavirus type-16–related DNA in genital Bowen's disease and bowenoid papulosis. Int. J. Cancer *32*:563, 1983.

107. Zachow, K.R., et al.: Detection of human papillomavirus DNA in anogenital neoplasia. Nature *300*:771, 1982.

108. Ostrow, R., et al.: Human papillomavirus DNA in cutaneous primary and metastasized squamous cell carcinoma from patients with epidermodysplasia verruciformis. Proc. Natl. Acad. Sci. U.S.A. *79*:1634, 1982.

109. Dillion, H.C.: Streptococcal skin infection and glomerulonephritis. *In* Hoeprick, P.D. (ed.): Infectious Diseases. 2nd ed. New York, Harper & Row, 1977.

110. Leyden, J.J., and Kligman, A.M.: Interdigital athlete's foot. The interaction of dermatophytes and resident bacteria. Arch. Dermatol. *114*:1466, 1978.

The Musculoskeletal System

SKELETAL SYSTEM

NORMAL

Despite its seemingly static appearance, bone is a remarkably labile tissue throughout life. Remodeling, with the daily turnover of up to 1 gm of calcium, continues even after the skeleton has been fully formed. Involved in this process are the cells of bone—osteocytes, osteoblasts, and osteoclasts (Fig. 28–1). The osteocytes and osteoblasts are both uninucleate cells of mesenchymal origin. *Osteoblasts,* found most abundantly along bone-forming surfaces in adult life, have receptors for parathyroid hormone, have an abundance of ribosomes involved in the synthesis of mainly collagen propeptides, and are rich in collagenases, plasminogen activator, and *alkaline* phosphatase. The serum level of bone alkaline phosphatase reflects the level of neo-osteogenesis whatever the stimulus. *Osteocytes,* found within the lacunae, are merely osteoblasts that become incorporated within the bone matrix. *Osteoclasts,* of monocyte-macrophage origin, are multinucleated cells found along the cortical endosteal surface and the trabeculae in scalloped bays (Howship's lacunae) where mineralized bone is being actively resorbed. The contact surface of the osteoclast appears ruffled, which can be resolved as membranous or villous-like projections that close over crystals or microfragments of bone to form intracytoplasmic vesicles in which osteolysis is completed. These cells contain *acid* phosphatase, collagenases, dehydrogenases, proteases, and carbonic anhydrase, which undoubtedly play roles in the resorption of bone. Signals from osteoblasts appear to be involved in activation of osteoclastic bone resorption.[1] For example, parathormone-induced osteoclastic bone resorption will not occur in the absence of osteoblasts.

The osteoid matrix of bone is 90 to 95% type I collagen (embedded in ground substance of glycosaminoglycans) linked to some noncollagenous proteins, principally osteocalcin and osteonectin, both of which are vitamin K dependent, calcium-binding carboxyproteins (see below). Disorders in the synthesis of collagen, as in osteogenesis imperfecta (p. 1318), result in skeletal abnormalities. Particularly important in collagen is proline; after hydroxylation (requiring vitamin C), it provides the intra- and intermolecular links and bonding, conferring stability on the collagen fibers.

When active neo-osteogenesis is occurring, as for example in repair of fractures or in diseases with increased bone turnover, the collagen is first laid down in feltlike sheets along the endosteal and periosteal surfaces, as well as about trabeculae. At the outset the collagen fibers are haphazardly arranged, and when this osteoid is mineralized it is referred to as *woven bone.* Soon thereafter, the collagen fibers are remodeled and laid down in parallel array along lines of stress, providing much of the structural strength of bone. Mineralization of this mature osteoid produces *lamellar bone* (the lamellae being about 10 μm thick) (Fig. 28–2). There is a 12- to 15-day delay between the formation of osteoid and its mineralization, leav-

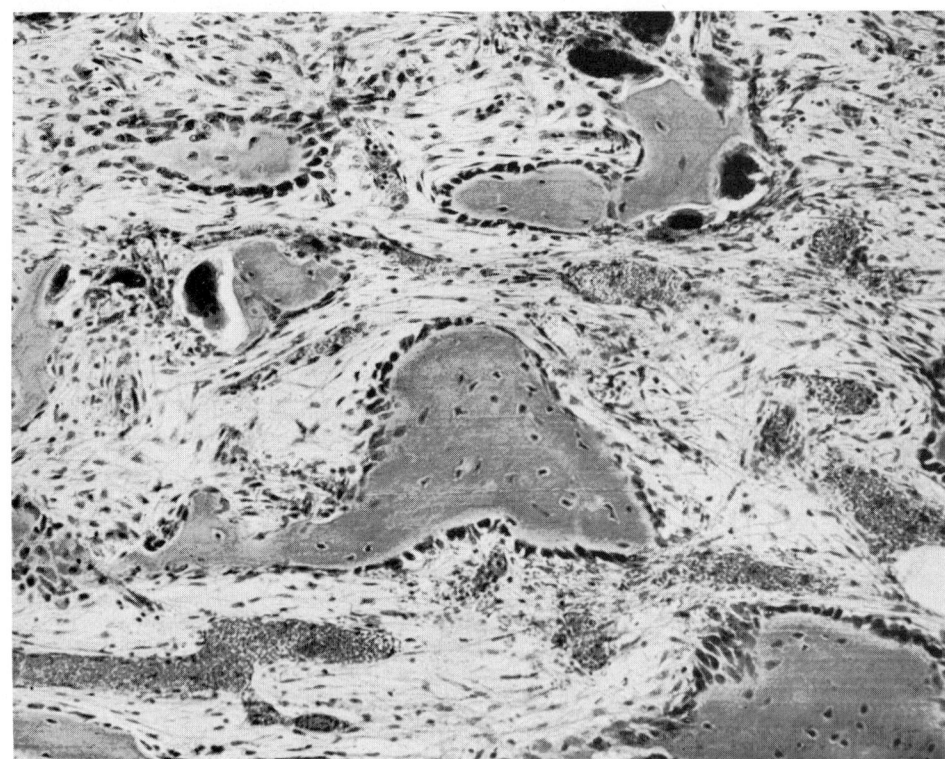

Figure 28-1. Normal bone with active osteoblastic and osteoclastic activity. There is slight fibrosis of marrow spaces.

Normal bone

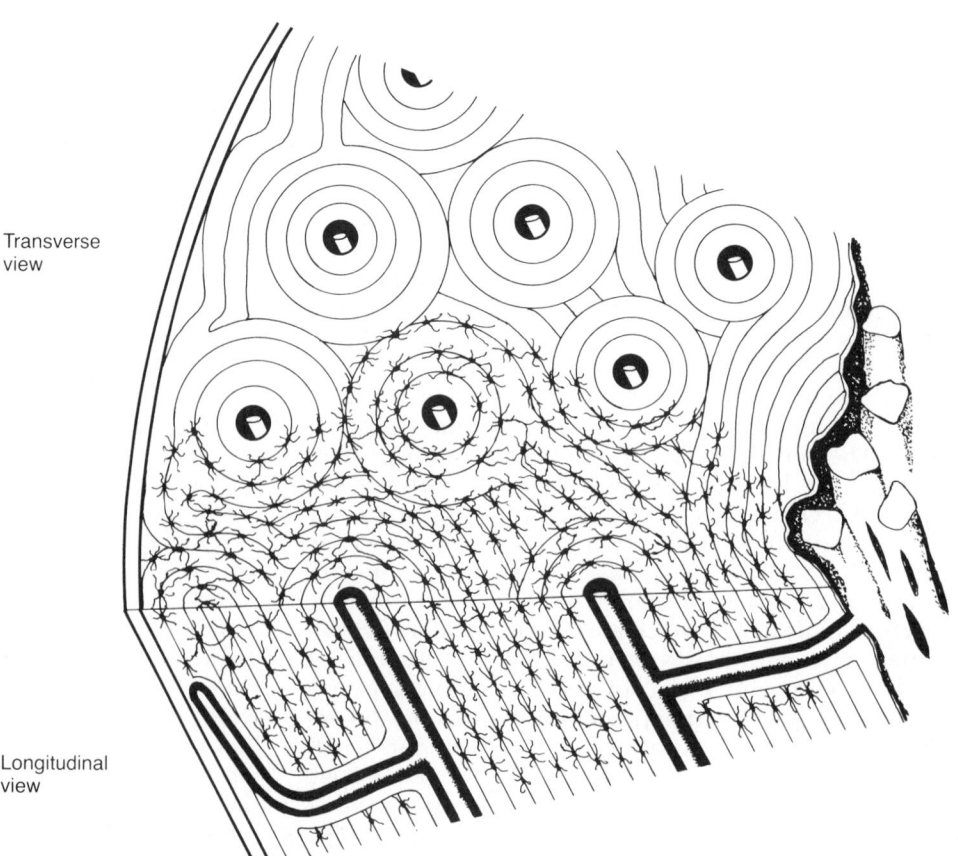

Transverse view

Longitudinal view

Figure 28-2. The schematic of normal bone structure reveals the concentric lamellae about vascular cores creating haversian systems in cortical bone. The individual lamellae are punctuated by osteocytic lacunae with their finely ramifying and interconnecting canals.

ing unmineralized osteoid seams up to 15 μm in thickness at bone-forming fronts. *A deficiency in the width and extent of the osteoid seams implies impaired osteoblastic function and reduced bone formation and, conversely, an increase in their width signifies unusually active bone formation or a delay in mineralization* (p. 445). Osteoid is recognized histologically by its eosinophilic appearance in H and E stains, in contrast to the basophilia of mineralized osteoid, namely bone. Special stains can highlight this distinction.

The *mineral phase of bone* is largely calcium hydroxyapatite—empiric formula $Ca_{10}(PO_4)_6(OH)_2$—admixed with trace amounts of other elements such as fluorides that favor crystallization and thus harden bones (and teeth). Initially, amorphous calcium phosphate is deposited, but with maturation it is converted into crystalline hydroxyapatite. There is still no agreement on the precise details of bone mineralization. The two favored theories are supersaturation of calcium and phosphate in the interstitial fluid bathing bone or selective binding to proteins such as osteocalcin and osteonectin that have an avidity for bone minerals. The important roles of vitamin D and parathyroid hormone in maintenance of the blood calcium levels were discussed on page 441. The rate of mineralization can be assessed by double tetracycline labeling. When administered to a subject, the antibiotic localizes at sites of active bone mineralization and in tissue section fluoresces under ultraviolet light. If given again 10 to 14 days later, the distance between the two fluorescent bands represents the amount of bone growth.[2]

BONE REMODELING

A large number of factors modify and regulate bone resorption and formation (Table 28–1). Up to age 30 to 40 years, resorption and replacement are nicely balanced. Thereafter osteoclastic resorption exceeds replacement with progressive slow loss of bone mass over the years.[3] Osteoporosis in adults represents in essence a disturbance in the balance of formation and resorption.

PATHOLOGY

The skeletal system is as subject to vascular, inflammatory, neoplastic, and endocrine diseases as the soft tissues of the body. Indeed, the constant turnover of bone makes it unusually vulnerable to adverse influences. Areas of bone necrosis sometimes appear following steroid therapy, trauma, and sometimes mysteriously—an example is Legg-Calvé-Perthes disease, called avascular necrosis of the femoral head, but in truth the cause is unknown. The bones also become secondarily involved by a number of dis-

Table 28–1. Some Factors Influencing Bone Metabolism*

	PREDOMINANT EFFECTS	
	On Resorption	*On Formation*
Calcium-regulating hormones		
Parathyroid hormone	+	+
1,25-Dihydroxyvitamin D	+	− (+)
Calcitonin	−	0
Systemic hormones		
Growth hormone	0	(+)
Glucocorticoids	(+)	−
Thyroid hormones	+	+
Insulin	0	+
Estrogens	(−)	(−)
Local factors		
Prostaglandin E$_2$	+	+
Interleukin-1	+	− (+)
Interferon-γ	−	−
Insulin-like growth factor 1	0	+
Transforming growth factor-β	− (+)	+

* Assignment of a predominant effect for each factor is based on current data (from in vivo studies if available). A plus sign denotes an increase; a minus sign a decrease; and a zero no effect. The symbols in parentheses indicate indirect mechanisms. For example, 1,25-dihydroxyvitamin D can increase bone formation by increasing the calcium and phosphorus supply, whereas growth hormone probably acts largely through insulin-like growth factor 1. Glucocorticoids can increase bone resorption indirectly by producing secondary hyperparathyroidism. The remaining symbols in parentheses represent indirect mechanisms that are probably mediated by changes in local prostaglandin E$_2$ production. Several other growth factors, not listed here, can increase bone resorption by increasing prostaglandin E$_2$ production.

From Raisz, L.G.: Local and systemic factors in the pathogenesis of osteoporosis. N. Engl. J. Med. *318:* 818, 1988.

orders primary elsewhere, for example, cancers. Not surprisingly, then, primary and secondary diseases of bone are varied and numerous.

HEREDITARY DISORDERS

Hereditary disorders of bone include a variety of relatively innocuous abnormalities and a number of systemic diseases that result in striking skeletal changes and sometimes great morbidity and mortality. Some of the more simple anomalies consist of failure of development of a bone (e.g., congenital absence of a phalanx, rib, or clavicle); the formation of extra bones (supernumerary ribs); the fusion of two adjacent digits (syndactylism); or the development of long spider-like digits (arachnodactylism). The association of the last anomaly with Marfan's syndrome was discussed on page 138. Other anomalies affect the skull and vertebral column and are frequently of great clinical importance, such as craniorachischisis (failure of closure of the spinal column and skull). This anomaly produces a persistent defect through which the meninges and central nervous system may herniate to produce a meningomyelocele or meningoencephalocele. In addition to these localized developmental defects, there are more important systemic disorders.

OSTEOGENESIS IMPERFECTA (OI)

Osteogenesis imperfecta, also known as "brittle bones," refers to a group of closely related, genetic, mostly hereditary disorders of collagen synthesis leading to changes mainly in the skeleton, but also in the sclerae, joints, ligaments, eyes, ears, teeth, and skin.[4] You recall that there are other hereditary disorders, such as Marfan's syndrome and Ehlers-Danlos syndrome, that have their origins in disordered synthesis of collagen or elastin, or both.[5]

The basic defect in all variants of OI is some abnormality in the synthesis of type I collagen (which constitutes about 90% of the matrix of bone). More specifically, each variant is characterized by mutations in a gene encoding the synthesis of pro-$\alpha1(1)$ or the pro-$\alpha2(1)$ chain, resulting in insufficient synthesis of normal collagen molecules, the formation of abnormal molecules that are unstable, or the formation of collagen molecules that cannot form helices.[6] Of recent date a model of this disease has been produced in transgenic mice by the introduction of a mutant gene for pro-alpha 1(1) collagen.[6a] On the basis of the specific biosynthetic abnormality, four major subsets of OI have been segregated, some having well-defined modes of inheritance and phenotypic changes (Table 28–2). There are still other, less well characterized variants.

Only a few general comments will be offered. The differing syndromes, it is evident, range from a variant (type II) that is uniformly fatal in the perinatal period, characterized by extraordinary bone fragility and multiple fractures in utero or immediately following birth, to variants marked by an increased predisposition to fracture but compatible with survival. Often present are blue sclerae, owing to their thin translucence with partial visualization of the underlying choroid; hearing loss related to bony abnormalities in the middle and inner ear; and dental imperfections (e.g., blue-yellow, small, misshapen teeth). *Morphologically, the basic change in all is "too little bone," thus constituting a type of osteopenia with marked thinning of the cortices and rarefication of the trabeculae.* Recognition of particular variants and their modes of inheritance is of importance in genetic counseling.

OSTEOPETROSIS

This hereditary metabolic disorder is also known as Albers-Schönberg disease or more graphically as "marble bones" to denote *the principal characteristics of overgrowth and sclerosis of bone with marked thickening of the cortex and narrowing or even filling of the medullary cavity.* Despite the "too much bone," the skeleton is abnormally brittle and fractures readily (like a piece of chalk).

Although classically two hereditary subsets have been described, it is now evident that each subset embraces a number of variants ranging from those compatible with survival into adult life to those causing death in infancy. One of the major subsets constitutes a so-called *malignant autosomal recessive pattern that becomes evident in utero or in infancy* because of the extreme density of the bones accompanied by progressive obliteration of the marrow cavity.

Table 28–2. Osteogenesis Imperfecta

	SUBTYPE	INHERITANCE	COLLAGEN DEFECT	MAJOR CLINICAL FEATURES
OI I	Postnatal fractures, blue sclerae	• Autosomal dominant	• Decreased synthesis pro-$\alpha1(1)$ • Abnormal pro-$\alpha1(1)$ or pro-$\alpha2(1)$ chains	• Compatible with survival • Normal stature • Skeletal fragility • Dentinogenesis imperfecta • Hearing impairment • Joint laxity • Blue sclerae
OI II	Perinatal lethal	• Most autosomal recessive • Some autosomal dominant ?New mutations	• Abnormally short pro-$\alpha1(1)$ chain • Unstable triple helix • Abnormal or insufficient pro-$\alpha2(1)$	• Death in utero or within days of birth • Skeletal deformity with excessive fragility and multiple fractures • Blue sclerae
OI III	Progressive deforming	• Heterogeneous	• Altered structure of propeptides of pro-$\alpha2(1)$ • Impaired formation triple helix	• Compatible with survival • Growth retardation • Multiple fractures • Progressive kyphoscoliosis • Blue sclerae at birth that become white • Hearing impairment • Dentinogenesis imperfecta
OI IV	Postnatal fractures, normal sclerae	• Autosomal dominant	• Short pro-$\alpha2(1)$ chain • Unstable triple helix	• Compatible with survival • Moderate skeletal fragility • Short stature • Sometimes dentinogenesis imperfecta

Others with features of Ehlers-Danlos syndrome

The consequent anemia and neutropenia usually result in early death from infections. Also seen are hepatosplenomegaly due to extramedullary hematopoiesis, hydrocephalus, and cranial nerve involvements (e.g., optic atrophy, deafness, and facial paralysis [narrowing of foramina]). *The adult pattern is relatively benign and is transmitted as an autosomal dominant.*[7] The anemia is not as severe, neurologic abnormalities are infrequent, and the main clinical feature is predisposition to fractures. *The common denominator among all variants is a hereditary defect in osteoclast function resulting in reduced bone resorption and hence net bone overgrowth, and indeed in some cases, there is also increased bone formation.* The precise nature of the osteoclast defect remains unknown,[8] but these cells are usually increased in number and often bizarre and exceptionally large. In animal models, bone marrow transplantation is sometimes curative, adding a new impetus to early diagnosis.

ACHONDROPLASIA

This autosomal dominant condition is characterized by a derangement in epiphyseal cartilaginous growth resulting in dwarfism. *The major defect occurs at the epiphyseal osteochondral junction with loss of the usual palisade of growing cartilaginous spicules that are normally destined to undergo provisional calcification and subsequent ossification. Premature ossification creates a transverse bony barrier at the osteochondral junction.*

> Anatomically, the skeletal changes reflect retarded endochondral bone formation; thus, the long bones are abnormally short, and—because appositional growth is not affected—unusually wide. The length of the spine is almost always normal, but the overall changes in body conformation lead to kyphoscoliosis or other vertebral deformities. The skull, not dependent on endochondral bone formation, appears unusually large.

Heterozygous individuals with this form of dwarfism have a normal longevity. They are usually recognizable on sight, often at birth, because of the head and body too large for the markedly shortened extremities. Mental and sexual development are normal and there is no reproductive deficit. Homozygosity results in severe disease that is usually fatal soon after birth.

HEREDITARY MULTIPLE AND SPORADIC SOLITARY EXOSTOSES

An *exostosis* is also known as an osteochondroma. *Despite the neoplastic designation, these lesions are developmental aberrations rather than neoplasms. They result from misdirected epiphyseal bone growth producing cartilage-capped bony projections from the lateral contours of endochondral bones. Exostoses may occur as sporadic solitary lesions, or in profusion in the hereditary disorder termed osteochondromatosis transmitted by autosomal dominant inheritance.* For reasons that are not clear, males are afflicted three times more often than females.

Exostoses most frequently appear on the long bones of the extremities in the metaphyses close to the epiphyseal region. Occasionally the pelvis, scapula, and ribs are involved, but only rarely are the small bones of the hands and feet. Although they arise from the epiphyseal cartilage, when the long bones grow they are left behind, progressively extending the distance from their points of origin (Fig. 28–3). Sometimes there is concomitant derangement in epiphyseal growth of the long bones of the extremities, causing bowing and shortening.

> **The lesions are usually mushroom-shaped and project 3 to 5 cm from the normal contour of the bone (Fig. 28–4). A layer of mature cartilage resembling an articular surface covers the head while the body of the head and pedicle are composed of well-formed bone having an outer cortex enclosing trabecular bone and a medullary cavity in continuity with that of the bone of origin.** Microscopically, the cartilage is usually mature and resembles that in the normal epiphysis, but foci of cartilage may persist within the cancellous centers of these lesions. The histologic details of the bone structure are otherwise normal.

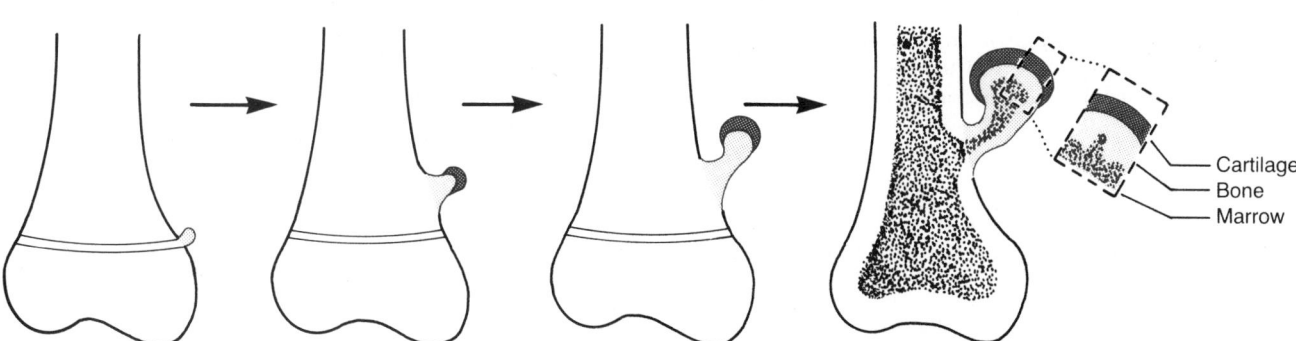

Cartilage
Bone
Marrow

Figure 28-3. A schematic of the development over time of an osteochondroma beginning with an outgrowth from the epiphyseal cartilage.

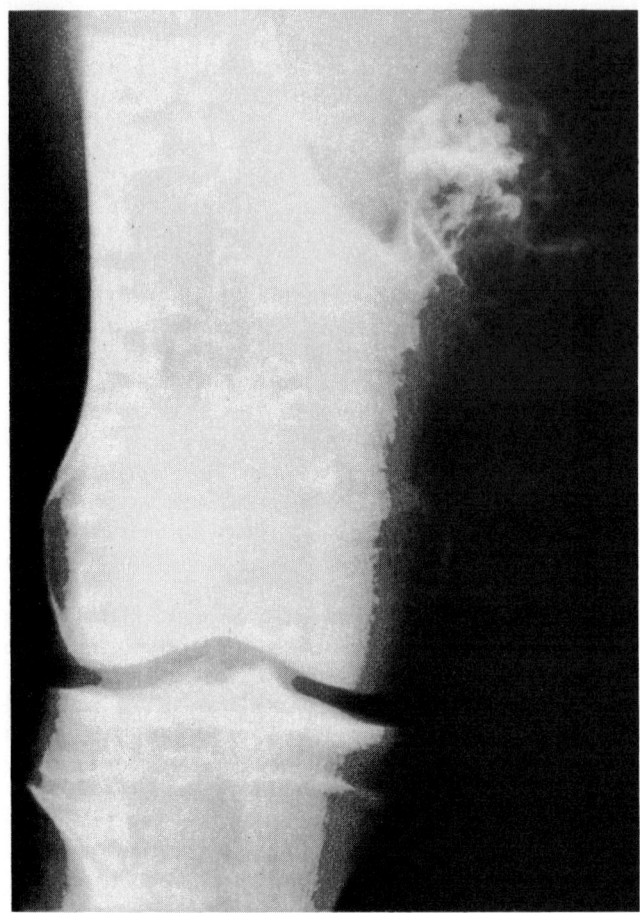

Figure 28-4. Mushroom-shaped osteochondroma (exostosis) of lower end of femur with its long axis pointing away from region of adjacent epiphysis. (Courtesy of Dr. Ashley Davidoff, Department of Radiology, Brigham and Women's Hospital, Boston.)

Whether solitary or multiple, they are rarely discovered before late childhood or adolescence, perhaps reflecting the time required for their development. Growth of the lesion usually stops at the time of epiphyseal closure but occasionally continues into adult life. Usually symptomless, exostoses come to attention as a chance radiographic finding. However, they can produce obvious external deformities or uncommonly impinge on a blood vessel or nerve. More important, chondrosarcomas may arise in one of the lesions, whether solitary or multiple. The risk is substantially greater with multiple lesions. Rarely, osteochondromatosis appears in the hereditary Gardner's syndrome (p. 897), characterized also by desmoid tumors, sebaceous cysts, and, most significantly, polyps of the colon that sometimes become carcinomatous.

INFECTIONS

In any blood-borne systemic disease, such as brucellosis, typhoid fever, the mycoses, tuberculosis, and bacterial endocarditis, the bone marrow may be seeded with organisms to produce small foci of infection. Usually these inflammatory lesions are of microscopic size, do not contribute materially to the clinical disease, and are of significance only as anatomic findings that aid in establishing the nature of the primary systemic disease. However, in addition to these insignificant lesions, more serious infections termed *osteomyelitis* may occur. The three most important are (1) pyogenic osteomyelitis, (2) tuberculosis, and (3) syphilis.

PYOGENIC OSTEOMYELITIS

Pyogenic osteomyelitis almost always is caused by bacteria, rarely by fungi. The organisms may reach the bone (1) through the bloodstream, (2) by extension of a contiguous infection, or (3) by direct traumatic (including surgical) introduction. The last two pathways account for most cases in developed countries—commonly involved are the jaws and skull bones from dental or sinus infections, the toes and feet in diabetics with chronic penetrating skin ulcers, and random other sites that were exposed to bone surgery. In the developing world, hematogenous osteomyelitis is more frequent. It tends to occur in long bones in children or in the vertebrae of adults.[9] Many infections resolve spontaneously and others are aborted by appropriate antibacterial treatment, accounting for the current decrease in the incidence of this disease. If unrecognized or inadequately treated, the infection may persist to become chronic, as still occurs in 20% of cases.[10]

ETIOLOGY AND PATHOGENESIS. Although hematogenous osteomyelitis may complicate an overt extraosseous infection, more often it appears as an apparent primary infection in previously healthy individuals. Bacteremias may occur from such trivial sources as insignificant injury to the intestinal mucosa; the mere vigorous chewing of hard foods, with or without apparent dental infection; and commonplace cuts and bruises of the skin. Local trauma may influence the location of the bone infection, but often it appears to be purely chance. Not unexpectedly, these infections are common and more severe in persons suffering from debilitation or some immunodeficiency.

Almost any pathogen may be responsible, but most often implicated is *Staphylococcus aureus* (80 to 90%) which is often penicillin-resistant, and less frequently *Escherichia coli*, Pseudomonas, Klebsiella, or various other pyogens. Mixed infections and anaerobes are common with osteomyelitis resulting from direct spread or introduction of organisms, as in postsurgical or postfracture osteomyelitis. In the neonatal period, *Hemophilus influenzae* and group B streptococci are frequent offenders. Osteomyelitis is a particular hazard in patients with sickle cell disease, and for unknown reasons, it is often caused by salmonellae. In drug addicts, Pseudomonas is the most common offender.[11] In a significant minority of cases, no organisms are recovered. They may have been eradicated by prior antibacterial therapy or the methods of isolation were inadequate.

MORPHOLOGY. In hematogenous osteomyelitis, the ends of the long bones are the most common sites involved. The reaction usually begins in the metaphyseal marrow where capillary flow is slowest, favoring lodgement of organisms. Eventually the build-up of exudative pressure leads to extension in both directions within the marrow cavity and sometimes to compromise of the vascular supply, favoring tissue damage. The inflammation may then **penetrate the endosteum** and enter the haversian and lacunar systems of the cortex to reach the periosteum **(periostitis).** During the growing years, the loose attachment of the periosteum may permit a sizeable **subperiosteal abscess** to form, which treks along the shaft of the long bone but is halted by the tight attachment at the epiphysis. In some cases, the suppuration ruptures through the periosteum to reach the surrounding soft tissues. Penetration of the cortex may produce single or multiple **sinus tracts** through the cortical bone. Lifting of the periosteum further impairs the blood supply in the affected region, and the combination of suppurative and ischemic injury may then cause necrosis of a small or large fragment of bone known as a **sequestrum.** This devitalized sequestrum, in the course of time, may be resorbed or is sometimes sloughed to form a free foreign body that on occasion dissects through to the skin. In this fashion, or by the direct penetration of the spreading infection, inflammatory **skin sinuses** may develop.

In infants in the first year of life, the epiphyseal plate is vascularized and infection may spread directly into the joint space to produce septic arthritis. In adults the cartilaginous plate resists bacterial invasion, and therefore the osteomyelitis rarely extends into the head of the bone, the epiphysis, or the joint cavity. However, when the infection is sufficiently severe, spread into the soft tissue provides a pathway to the head of the bone and the joint cavity. Such a complicating **suppurative arthritis** may result in extensive destruction of the joint and permanent disability (p. 1354). A basically similar pattern of reaction is seen with spinal osteomyelitis save that the contiguous intervertebral discs frequently become secondarily involved and then possibly adjacent vertebrae as well.

Not all instances of acute osteomyelitis follow such a spreading destructive course. The initial infection may be localized to a small area and become walled off to create a localized abscess that may undergo spontaneous sterilization or become a chronic nidus of infection **(Brodie's abscess).** In other instances, the infection, after having spread through a localized region of the bone, is contained by the natural resistive forces of the host or is controlled by therapy.

In some cases, the smoldering infection stimulates osteoblastic activity, particularly from the periosteum, forming new bone subperiosteally **(involucrum)** that encloses and envelops the inflammatory focus. New bone is also laid down about the focus of infection within the marrow cavity to further localize the infection. This neo-osteogenesis, if continued long enough, gives rise to a densely sclerotic

pattern of osteomyelitis referred to as **Garré's sclerosing osteomyelitis** (Fig. 28–5).

The histologic changes depend entirely on the stage of the osteomyelitis and its duration. **Basically, two elements can be identified: suppurative and ischemic destructive necrosis and fibrous and bony repair.**

CLINICAL COURSE. Hematogenous osteomyelitis usually manifests itself as an acute, febrile, systemic illness accompanied by symptoms referable to the local lesion. These children have malaise, fever, chills, and leukocytosis as well as marked-to-intense local pain that is frequently described as throbbing. Often there is redness, swelling, and tenderness in the overlying soft tissues. However, the presentation may be much more subtle with only unexplained fever, particularly in infants, or conversely only localized pain in the absence of fever in an adult. The diagnosis is confirmed by radiologic evidence of bone destruction. However, in the early stages of osteomyelitis (during the first ten days) the necrosis of bone may not be sufficiently advanced to produce radiographic changes. Radionuclide scans are helpful in such cases, showing accumulation of the tracer at sites of increased cellularity and vascularity. In about 60% of instances, blood cultures are positive, particularly during the stage of development of bone infection.

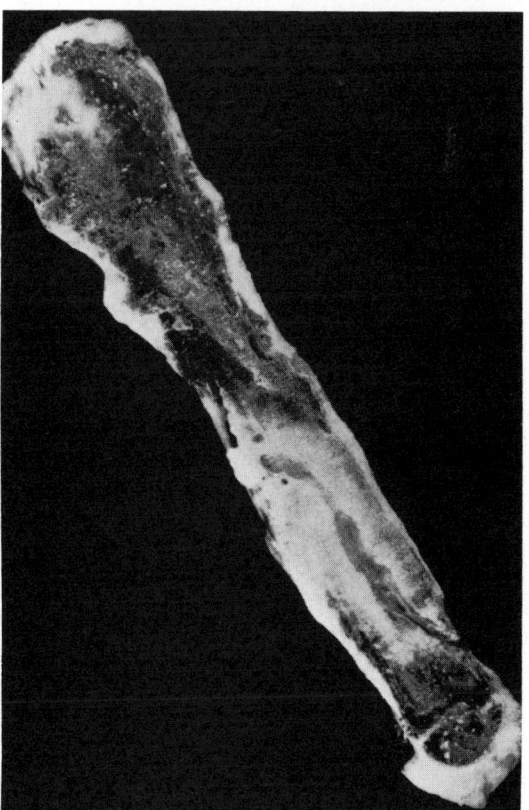

Figure 28-5. Sclerosing osteomyelitis as evidenced by dense, sclerotic, pale-appearing area in shaft.

Sometimes the course is complicated by spontaneous fracture of the weakened bone or by the extension of infection into adjacent joints. In addition to the local destruction, osteomyelitis is an important source for the hematogenous dissemination of infection, with the production of pyemic abscesses and focal soft tissue lesions elsewhere in the body, sometimes on the heart valves. The development of osteomyelitis is a feared complication of compound fractures that seriously delays and prejudices the quality of eventual repair. Amyloidosis is a potential complication of persistent chronic infections.

TUBERCULOSIS

Tuberculous osteomyelitis, analogous to pyogenic osteomyelitis, is now a rarity in industrialized nations. When seen, it occurs most often in elderly, debilitated, diabetic, or otherwise compromised hosts. Much more often the tuberculous infection of bone takes the form of miliary seeding of the marrow in the course of hematogenous dissemination of organisms from a primary source elsewhere, usually the lungs. The widely scattered granulomas are mainly of importance in providing a biopsy opportunity to diagnose the cause of a fever of unknown origin.

In developing countries, pulmonary and gastrointestinal tuberculosis are still common, as is commensurately destructive tuberculous osteomyelitis. Most victims are young adults or adolescents. Whatever the setting, the organisms are usually bloodborne, but in a few instances spread may occur by direct extension (e.g., from a pulmonary focus into a rib, or from tracheobronchial nodes into adjacent vertebrae).

Unlike pyogenic osteomyelitis, *tuberculous osteomyelitis tends to arise as an insidious chronic infection that is characteristically much more destructive and resistant to control.* The long bones of the extremities and the spine are favored sites of localization. Commonly, the infection extends through large areas of the medullary cavity and causes extensive necrosis of cortical bone, with the production of large and multiple sinuses into the soft tissues and through the skin. Extension through the epiphyseal cartilage into joint spaces and destruction of intervertebral discs make this a most disabling disease. When it occurs in the spine *(Pott's disease)*, compression fractures are prone to develop that result in serious deformities (kyphosis and scoliosis) and often lead to permanent damage as new bone formation fixes the spine in malalignment. The tuberculous exudation may extend from the vertebral bodies into the paravertebral muscles and, in one characteristic pattern, it extends along the sheath of the psoas muscle to produce a *psoas abscess.* Sometimes these infections present as cold fluctuating abscesses in the inguinal regions and inguinal nodes. Systemic amyloidosis may develop in protracted cases.

SYPHILIS

Today, in the United States, syphilitic involvement of bone is uncommon. It may occur in both congenital and acquired syphilis. In the *congenital form,* the junction of the metaphysis and the epiphysis is principally involved and is designated *osteochondritis.* When the periosteum, principally of the long bones, is involved alone, it is referred to as *periostitis.* The osteochondritis causes considerable disarray and destruction of the epiphyseal cartilage by the characteristic fibroproliferative inflammatory reaction of syphilis. The principal hallmarks are obliterative endarteritis and striking perivascular mononuclear cell infiltrations, principally of plasma cells. Reactive bone formation occurs from the surrounding vital periosteum. The periostitis produces a similar syphilitic granulation tissue between the cortical bone and the periosteum and is accompanied by the laying down of new bone to produce a characteristic "crew haircut" appearance or sclerosis of the cortex roentgenographically. When this thickening occurs on the tibia, it gives rise to the deformity recognized as *saber shin.*

Acquired syphilis may result in osteochondritis and periostitis, but it may also be manifested by the development of a frank syphilitic osteomyelitis, usually by the production of characteristic gummas within the marrow cavity of the bone. In the acquired forms, in addition to the long bones, the skull and vertebral column are affected.

FRACTURES

The speed of healing and perfection of repair of a fracture depend on whether the break has occurred in a previously normal bone or at some site of preexistent disease *(pathologic fracture).* Healing also depends on the extent and nature of the fracture. Fractures may be *complete* or *incomplete (greenstick), closed (simple)* with intact overlying tissue, *comminuted* when the bone has been splintered, and *compound* when the fracture site communicates with the skin surface. Incomplete closed fractures heal most rapidly with potentially complete reconstruction of the preexisting architecture. On the other hand, comminuted and compound fractures heal much more slowly with less satisfactory results. In the former, the devitalized bone splinters constitute impediments to repair; in the latter, possible infection contributes to bone destruction and impairment of blood supply and stimulates fibrosis, which interferes with bony healing. On this basis, the morphologic changes that are encountered in the healing of a fracture depend, to a considerable extent, on the nature of the fracture and the collateral problems involved. The basic sequence of events in the repair of a simple closed fracture are presented here.

Healing of a fracture represents a continuous process, but it can be divided for convenience into three distinct stages: (1) **organization** of hematoma at the fracture site, leading to a soft, weak **procallus;** (2) conversion of the weak procallus to fibrocartilaginous callus, which more effectively immobilizes the bone fragments; and (3) replacement of the fibrocartilaginous callus by osseous callus, which eventually will be remodeled along lines of weight-bearing to complete the repair.

Immediately after a fracture, hematoma fills the fracture cleft and surrounds the area of bone injury. The coagulation of this blood gives rise to a **loose fibrin mesh** that more or less seals off the fracture site and, at the same time, serves as a framework for the ingrowth of fibroblasts and new capillary buds. As occurs with a soft tissue injury, the clot undergoes organization to produce eventually a soft tissue callus that provides some anchorage for the bone fragments, but no structural rigidity.

However, the healing of a bone injury differs from the healing of a soft tissue injury from this point on. After the first few days, **newly formed cartilage and bone matrix** are evident in the fibrovascular response. By the end of the

first week, well-developed new bone and cartilage are dispersed through the soft tissue callus. In the course of succeeding days, new bone formation creates a large, fusiform, temporary bony **provisional callus** or **procallus** (Fig. 28–6).

This provisional callus creates a spindle-shaped, fairly effective splint. In an uncomplicated fracture, the provisional callus usually attains its maximal size at about the end of the second or third week. Over the subsequent course of time, this provisional callus is increasingly strengthened by the widening of the newly formed delicate bone spicules and is at the same time remodeled by osteoblastic and osteoclastic activity.

The remodeling process is directed by the muscle and weight-bearing stresses imposed on the bone. If the fracture has been well aligned and the original weight-bearing strains are restored, nearly perfect reconstruction of the bone is accomplished. In such reconstruction, the internal callus that fills the marrow space is also resorbed and, at some later date, roentgenograms may completely fail to demonstrate the site of previous injury.

Perfect repair may be not only impeded but also blocked

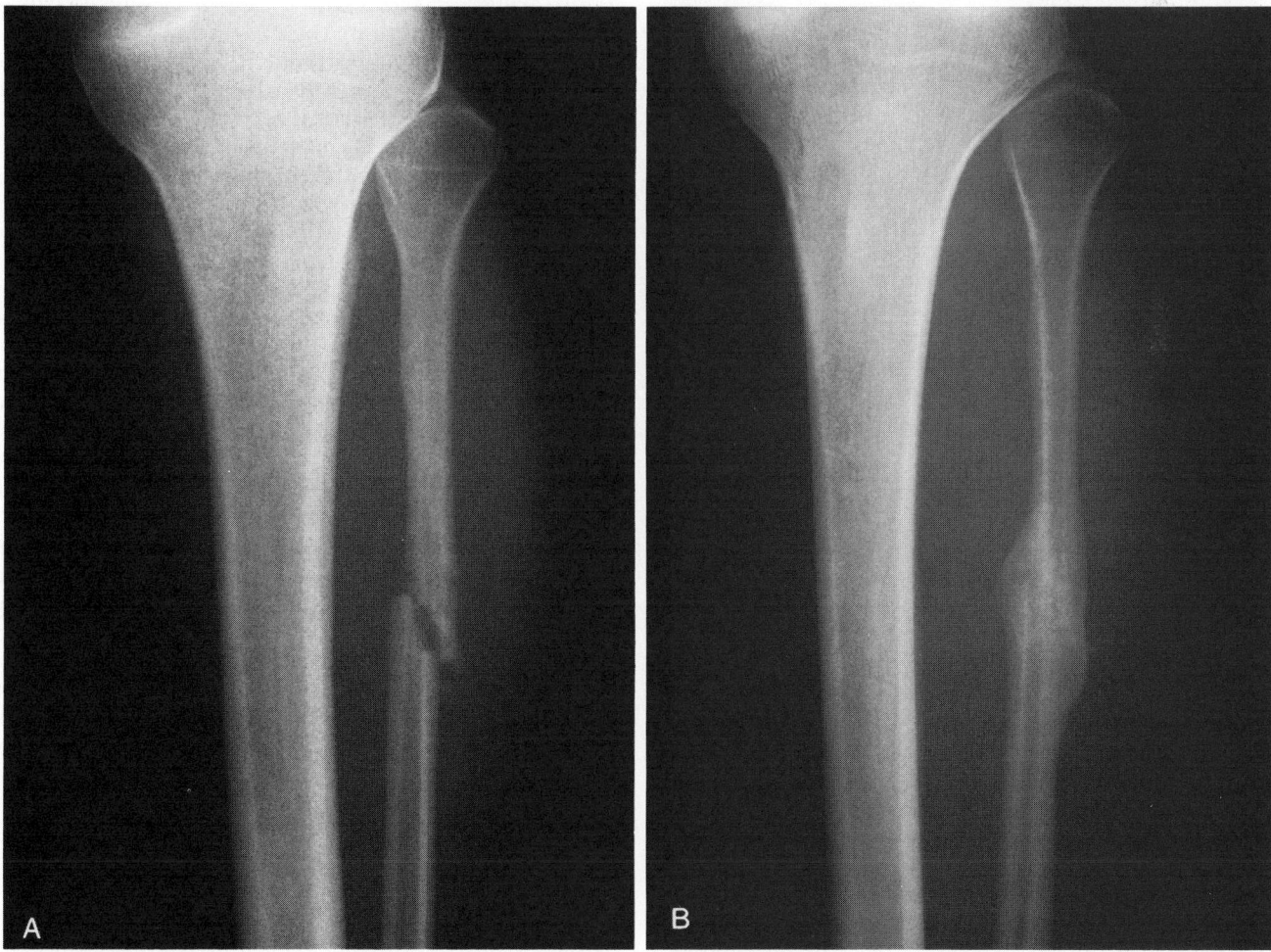

Figure 28-6. *A*, A recent fracture of the fibula. *B*, The marked callus formation six weeks later. (Courtesy of Dr. Barbara Weissman, Brigham and Women's Hospital.)

by many complications. Malalignment and comminution of the bone are almost inevitably followed by some permanent deformity. Moreover, the devitalized spicules of comminuted bone must be demineralized and the osteoid material resorbed. These processes delay healing, enlarge the provisional callus, and favor the formation of an overly large, deforming, permanent callus. Permanent obliteration of the marrow cavity may occur. Inadequate immobilization of the bone permits the continuance of twisting, shearing, and bending stresses. Under these circumstances, the laying down of a chondroid and osteoid matrix is slow and, in fact, may be blocked, so that the callus may be composed of only fibrous tissue and cartilage that perpetuate the abnormal mobility. An osseous callus may not form under these circumstances and a dense fibrous tissue remains as the end stage of the repair process, producing a **false joint (pseudoarthrosis).** Interposition of soft tissues tends to give rise to such fibrous, inadequate bony union. However, in any of these complications, if the interposed soft parts can be removed at a later date, or adequate immobilization eventually effected, ultimate adequate repair can be anticipated except perhaps in persons of advanced age suffering from arterial and venous inadequacies. Perhaps the most serious impediment to healing is infection of the fracture site, as feared in comminuted fractures. In this circumstance, the infection must be brought under control before bony union can be effected.

Systemic derangements may further unfavorably affect the end results. Inadequate levels of calcium and phosphorus, avitaminoses, systemic infections, generalized atherosclerosis that renders the area ischemic, and preexistent osteomalacia or osteoporosis are some of these unfavorable influences. Generally, with children and young adults, in whom most uncomplicated fractures are found, practically perfect reconstruction may be anticipated. In older age groups in whom fractures tend to occur on a background of some previous disease (e.g., osteoporosis, osteomalacia), repair is less perfect and often requires mechanical methods of immobilization to facilitate healing.

OSTEOPOROSIS

Osteoporosis is a very common disorder, particularly among the elderly, characterized by reduction in bone mass sufficient to render the skeleton fragile and vulnerable to fracture, but the "too little" bone that remains is otherwise normal. As you recall, remodeling of bone occurs throughout life. Peak bone mass occurs at about age 30; thereafter resorption outpaces formation with progressive loss of skeleton. Both sexes are affected, but the loss is greater in women than in men because the rate of loss significantly increases following the menopause; it is also more marked in whites than in blacks. *There is no clear line separating normal age-related bone loss from abnormal loss, but osteoporosis is said to exist when the reduction in bone mass produces pain and increased vulnerability to fractures.* About 15 million individuals in the United States suffer from primary osteoporosis.[12] When it

occurs in the later decades in men, it is referred to as *"senile osteoporosis"*; in women it often becomes manifest after the menopause, or *"postmenopausal osteoporosis"*; both terms are euphemisms for "idiopathic."[13] Infrequently, osteoporosis is encountered in young adults and sometimes in juveniles — also "idiopathic osteoporosis." In addition, excessive bone loss and osteoporosis also occur as a secondary phenomenon in hyperadrenocorticism (including prolonged exposure to exogenous glucocorticoids), hypogonadism in young males, thyrotoxicosis, hypopituitarism, pregnancy, malnutrition and malabsorption, chronic heparin administration, prolonged weightlessness in space, and other conditions. The combined frequency of these secondary variants is dwarfed by that of the idiopathic patterns.

PATHOGENESIS. The law of perversity states that the more common a condition, the less known about its cause — witness baldness, atherosclerosis, and cancer. Not surprisingly, the origins of primary osteoporosis are unknown, but the available evidence suggests strongly that *it is the result mostly of increased osteoclastic resorption coupled with some slowing of bone formation*[14] (Fig. 28 – 7). Every proposed causal mechanism has in some measure been refuted.

Genetic or constitutional factors determine the peak bone mass of an individual in early life, and hence the person's vulnerability to osteoporosis later. Differences in skeletal mass in males versus females and in blacks versus whites may explain in part the epidemiology of this disorder.

Reduced physical activity increases the rate of bone loss in experimental animals and humans. The mediator of this bone loss may be PGE_2 produced by osteoblasts. The bone loss (bone atrophy) seen in an immobilized or paralyzed extremity, the reduction of skeletal mass observed in astronauts subjected to a gravity-free environment for prolonged periods, and the higher bone density in athletes as compared with nonathletes all support a role for physical activity in preventing bone loss. Indeed, herein may lie a partial explanation for senile osteoporosis.

Estrogen deficiency in women and *androgen deficiency* in men have long been known to be important, but the mechanism of action of these hormones is obscure. There is some evidence that sex hormones stimulate osteoblasts and that postmenopausal osteoporosis can be prevented by supplemental estrogens. However, once osteoporosis has developed, steroids do not reverse the bone loss. Recourse has been made, therefore, to a secondary role for estrogens, as is discussed later.

Increased parathyroid hormone levels or function, or marginal to insufficient intake of vitamin D $(1,25[OH]_2D)$, despite wishful thinking, cannot be ascribed significant roles in the causation of osteoporosis.[15] Controlled studies of groups of postmenopausal women with osteoporosis have failed to document significant benefit from vitamin D supplementation of the diet.[16] The role of calcium intake is more contro-

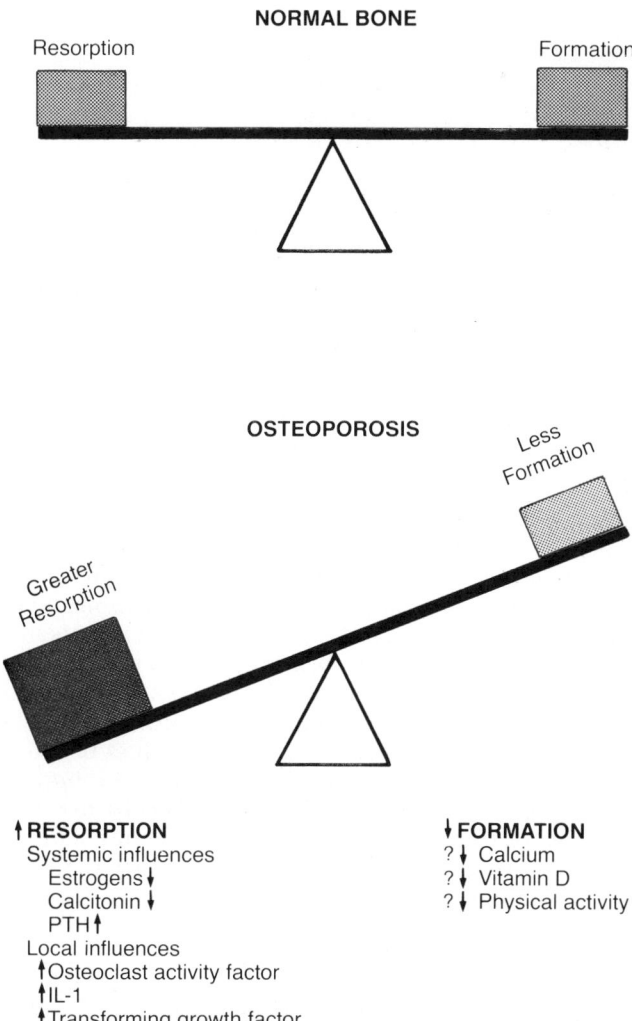

NORMAL BONE

Resorption   Formation

OSTEOPOROSIS

Less Formation

Greater Resorption

↑ RESORPTION
Systemic influences
   Estrogens ↓
   Calcitonin ↓
   PTH ↑
Local influences
  ↑Osteoclast activity factor
  ↑IL-1
  ↑Transforming growth factor

↓ FORMATION
? ↓ Calcium
? ↓ Vitamin D
? ↓ Physical activity

Figure 28-7. A schematic of the potential factors in osteoporosis leading to increased resorption and decreased formation of bone.

versial. Up to the recent past, calcium supplementation did not appear to be beneficial, but a recent survey of a cohort of men and women aged 50 to 79 years revealed an inverse correlation between their dietary intake of calcium in the preceding years and the risk of hip fracture.[16a]

Combined deficiencies of calcitonin and estrogen have been accorded pathogenetic significance. Circulating levels of calcitonin tend to be lower in women than in men, particularly in postmenopausal women. This hormone directly inhibits osteoclast activity and therefore bone resorption. It is theorized that a deficiency of estrogen and calcitonin, perhaps coupled with some parathyroid activity, may underlie osteoporosis, but regrettably the evidence is tenuous.

Local factors have also been invoked to explain the unequal involvement of regions of the skeleton.[14] Theoretical local mediators include PGE_2 formed by osteoblasts, which, depending on the level produced, can increase either bone resorption or bone formation. Several osteoclast-activating factors, such as in-

terleukin-1 (IL-1) (alpha and beta) and transforming growth factor (beta) produced locally by macrophages and lymphocytes, may contribute to regional bone resorption.

Much is speculative and so it would be premature to attempt any synthesis of the many possible mediators of this disease.

Although disuse or immobilization may lead to osteoporosis localized to an extremity, in the great preponderance of instances it is a systemic skeletal disease, although certain regions tend to be affected more than others. The bone loss is almost always greater in the vertebral bodies, femoral necks, and metacarpals than it is in the skull and midshafts of the long bones. Additional target sites are the distal radius, proximal humerus, proximal tibia, and pelvis. **The resorption usually begins at the corticoendosteal surface, resulting in enlargement of the medullary cavity and thinning of the cortex. Cancellous bone is also affected; trabecular plates may be converted to slender strands, sometimes with complete resorption or transection.** Because the vertebrae have a thin cortex normally and depend for their structural integrity on trabeculae, they are particularly vulnerable to microfractures and collapse, often referred to as **"vertebral crush-fracture syndrome"** (Fig. 28–8). Histologically, such bone as remains has a normal matrix and mineral content, and there is no accentuation of the osteoid seams. The increased bone resorption is often reflected in an increased number of somewhat bizarre osteoclasts, particularly at the corticoendosteal surface. Osteoblasts are normal in number or possibly increased.

CLINICAL COURSE. *Osteoporosis is a difficult condition to diagnose for three reasons: (1) it remains asymptomatic until the skeletal fragility is well advanced; (2) there is no easy way to determine the severity of the bone loss; and (3) it is only one of a group of skeletal disorders characterized by "too little" bone (the osteopenias), which are difficult to differentiate from each other.* Postmenopausal and age-related bone loss progresses unnoted until the skeletal fragility leads to (1) pain in the back, usually thoracic or lumbar, owing to compression-microfractures of the vertebrae, (2) significant loss of height or deformity of the spine such as lumbar lordosis or kyphoscoliosis related to vertebral collapse or crush, or (3) overt fractures most often of the distal radius (wrist), femoral neck, and vertebral bodies. Fractures in these three sites have a combined prevalence of 40% in women over the age of 65 years. About 30% of all nonagenarians sustain femoral neck fractures and 50% have vertebral crush fractures. These fractures result in 40,000 to 50,000 deaths annually, more than the combined mortality from carcinomas of breast and endometrium combined.

Determining the extent of bone loss is difficult because standard radiographs do not reliably disclose increased radiolucency until more than 30% of the

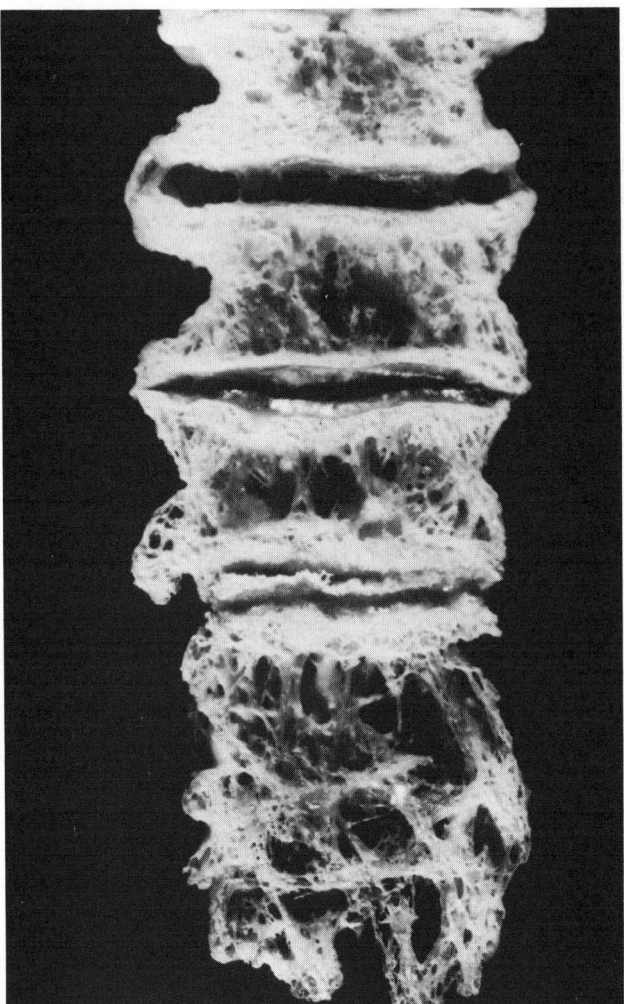

Figure 28-8. Vertebral osteoporosis in a specimen cleared of soft tissue, leaving only the residual bone structure. There is striking cortical thinning and loss of trabeculae with compression fracture of the upper three bodies. (Compare vertical dimensions with the lowest vertebra shown.)

bone mass has been lost. Moreover, the concentrations of calcium and inorganic phosphorus in the blood are usually normal in uncomplicated cases, as is the alkaline phosphatase level. The only procedures that provide accurate estimates of the extent of bone resorption are the highly specialized dual-photon absorptiometry, quantitative computed tomography, and neutron activation analysis of total-body calcium.

Even when significant reduction in the bone mass has been established, there arises the difficulty of differentiating osteoporosis from the other osteopenias, such as osteomalacia, osteogenesis imperfecta, osteitis fibrosa associated with hyperparathyroidism (in its early stages), renal osteodystrophy, and the bone loss encountered with various types of malignancy, particularly multiple myeloma. Because of the many difficulties, unless there is clear evidence of another form of osteopenia, osteoporosis is suspected whenever the skeletal mass is insufficient for the normal

stresses and strains of life in postmenopausal women and elderly men.

RICKETS AND OSTEOMALACIA

Rickets in the growing child and osteomalacia in the adult, skeletal disorders caused by vitamin D deficiency, were discussed on page 441. Although a dietary lack may underlie this deficiency, as was pointed out earlier it may have other origins: (1) inadequate exposure to sunlight with reduced endogenous synthesis of vitamin D precursors; (2) malabsorption of lipids, including vitamin D; (3) derangements in metabolism of vitamin D (as in chronic renal failure) (p. 1017); (4) end-organ resistance to vitamin D; and (5) other uncommon hereditary and acquired disorders of vitamin D metabolism. Whatever the cause of the functional inadequacy, *the fundamental skeletal defect is failure in bone mineralization resulting in excess unmineralized matrix and abnormally wide osteoid seams.* In the growing child, rickets may induce overt skeletal deformities, but in the adult osteomalacia presents only as a form of osteopenia with radiolucency of the skeleton and predisposition to fracture. In time, the mineralization defect in osteomalacia leads to decreased production of organic bone matrix and bone and thus a hybrid state of osteomalacia-osteoporosis evolves. The two forms of osteopenia are then difficult to differentiate both clinically and radiologically.

SKELETAL CHANGES IN HYPERPARATHYROIDISM — OSTEITIS FIBROSA (CYSTICA)

Chronic hyperparathyroidism, whether primary or secondary, depending on severity and duration, leads to a sequence of skeletal changes beginning with (1) demineralization, followed in time by (2) increased osteoclastic activity with resorption of bone and peritrabecular fibrosis (*osteitis fibrosa*), evolving ultimately into (3) more marked bone resorption and marrow fibrosis with the formation of micro- to macrocysts within the enlarged fibrotic marrow spaces (*osteitis fibrosa cystica*, also known as *von Recklinghausen's disease of bone*). The origins and pathophysiology of primary and secondary hyperparathyroidism are discussed on page 1243. Here we are concerned with the impact of excess parathormone on the skeleton, but first two points should be noted: (1) fully evolved osteitis fibrosa cystica is now uncommon because hyperparathyroidism is now discovered and treated at a much earlier stage than previously, thus aborting the development of advanced bony changes; and (2) the skeletal changes induced by the secondary hyperparathyroidism associated with chronic renal failure are rarely as marked as those seen with primary hyperparathyroidism. They are referred to as *renal osteodystrophy* and are frequently complicated by the effects of long-term dialysis and potential aluminum toxicity and so require separate consideration later.

As pointed out earlier, there is a sequence of bony changes over time in hyperparathyroidism. The earliest alteration is demineralization, leaving an excess of osteoid and producing a remarkable similarity to vitamin D–related osteomalacia. Soon, however, osteoclasts are activated with increased bone resorption first at the subperiosteal and endosteal surfaces and later generalized to the trabeculae. This resorption is accompanied by fibrosis beginning about the trabeculae. An increased number of somewhat bizarre-shaped osteoclasts are found lying within scalloped resorption cavities. In this manner the cortex and trabeculae are thinned and sometimes the latter are hollowed out or completely transected or resorbed. The bone loss is particularly evident as subperiosteal resorption of the phalanges and distal clavicle, creating "moth-eaten" surfaces and loss of the lamina dura (a dense, opaque radiographic line normally surrounding the tooth socket). As the bone resorption becomes more marked, microfractures and microhemorrhages occur, yielding hemosiderin-laden macrophages dispersed throughout a delicate fibrous tissue that fills the marrow spaces (osteitis fibrosa). With progression, the bone resorption, microhemorrhages, and fibrosis become more marked and often accompanied by the formation of macroscopically visible cysts within the fibrous tissue—osteitis fibrosa cystica (Fig. 28–9). Scattered within this background there may be so-called **brown tumors,** a particularly inappropriate designation since the lesions are not neoplastic. They represent foci of hemorrhage, perhaps related to microfractures that undergo organization with the release of hemosiderin and the accumulation of macrophages, fibroblasts, and multinucleate giant cells. These lesions have more than a passing similarity to true giant cell tumors (described on p. 1343), but are better referred to as **reparative giant cell granulomas** having none of the neoplastic potential of true giant cell tumors. Soft tissue metastatic calcifications sometimes appear in individuals with osteitis fibrosa cystica.

Only 10 to 15% of patients with primary hyperparathyroidism now have skeletal changes, for reasons given earlier. Secondary hyperparathyroidism is rarely sufficiently severe or prolonged to induce well-defined osteitis fibrosa cystica.

The clinical manifestations relating to the disease of bone are almost invariably overshadowed by the other manifestations of hyperparathyroidism. However, as indicated, there is sometimes a predisposition to fracture, to skeletal deformities under the stress of weight-bearing, and to joint pains and dysfunctions as the lines of normal weight-bearing are disturbed. The bony changes may regress or completely disappear following removal of the hyperplastic glands or functioning tumor in primary hyperparathyroidism. The skeletal radiologic rarefaction in advanced disease

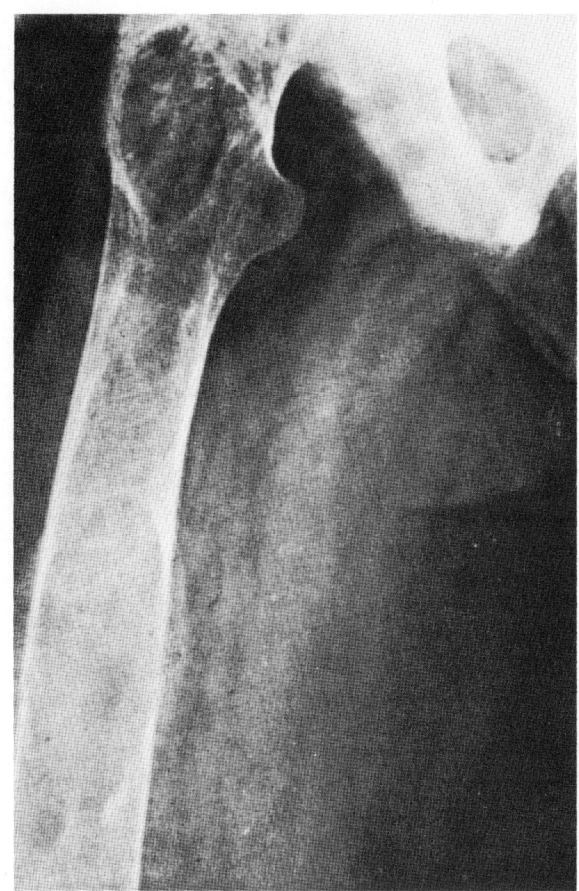

Figure 28-9. Advanced osteitis fibrosa cystica of femur in primary hyperparathyroidism due to a functioning adenoma. Cystic rarefaction is evident throughout shaft.

must be differentiated from the other forms of osteopenia (Fig. 28–10).

RENAL OSTEODYSTROPHY

This term is applied to a complex of bone changes that appear in the majority of patients with chronic renal failure. *Included are features of osteitis fibrosa cystica admixed with osteomalacia and sometimes, less prominently, areas of osteosclerosis.* These skeletal alterations tend to be more severe in the young and may be accentuated by long-term hemodialysis for reasons discussed later.[17] With protracted skeletal disease, metastatic calcifications may develop in the skin, eyes, arterial walls, and about the joints.

The pathogenesis of the melange of skeletal lesions is complex and will be simplified here.

• Chronic renal failure is characterized by phosphate retention and hyperphosphatemia.
• Hyperphosphatemia produces secondary hyperparathyroidism (p. 1246), possibly by direct action of the phosphate on the parathyroid glands, more likely indirectly by leading to hypocalcemia.
• Contributing to the hypocalcemia are (1) decreased

MAJOR FORMS OF OSTEOPENIA

Normal bone

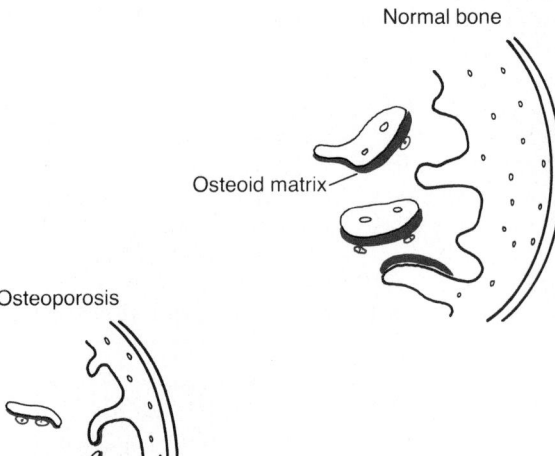

Osteoid matrix

Osteoporosis

Osteomalacia

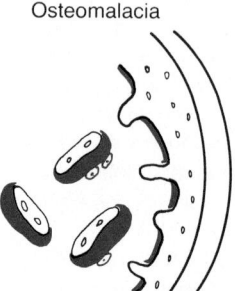

Osteitis fibrosa cystica

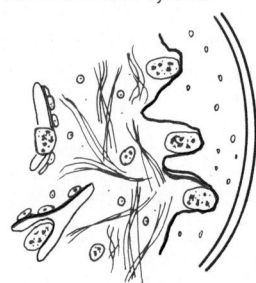

Figure 28-10. The major forms of osteopenia. In osteoporosis, the cortex and trabeculae are more slender than normal and there is no accentuation of osteoid matrix. In osteomalacia, there is an excess of unmineralized osteoid and hence a deficiency of mineralized bone. In osteitis fibrosa cystica, the "too little bone" is caused by marked osteoclastic resorption of cortex and trabeculae.

conversion of the vitamin D metabolite 25(OH)D to 1,25(OH)$_2$D by damaged, shrunken kidneys; (2) inhibition by phosphorus of the renal hydroxylase involved in the conversion of 25(OH)D to the active metabolite 1,25(OH)$_2$D; (3) reduced intestinal absorption of calcium because of the low levels of 1,25(OH)$_2$D; and (4) the opposite and reciprocal relationship that exists between serum ionized calcium and serum phosphorus.[18]

• Renal failure and low levels of 1,25(OH)$_2$D render bone more unresponsive to parathormone level and thus the parathyroids are stimulated to increased activity to maintain the serum calcium levels, an abnormality referred to as a "shift in the set point for calcium."

• The secondary hyperparathyroidism (p. 1246) accounts for the skeletal changes of osteitis fibrosa cystica.

• The lowered levels of 1,25(OH)$_2$D and serum calcium account for the changes of osteomalacia (p. 441).

Aluminum toxicity in patients with renal failure maintained for some period of time on hemodialysis may contribute to the skeletal changes in renal osteodystrophy.[19] The sources of aluminum are the dialysate solutions prepared from water with a high aluminum content and the use of oral aluminum phosphate binders. The aluminum localizes within newly laid down osteoid and interferes with normal mineralization, thus inducing changes of osteomalacia. It can be demonstrated within the osteoid by histochemical methods and by atomic absorption spectroscopy.[20] In passing, we might note, aluminum has also been implicated as the cause of "dialysis encephalopathy" and microcytic anemia in patients with chronic renal failure.

PAGET'S DISEASE (OSTEITIS DEFORMANS)

This idiopathic skeletal disease can be characterized as "matrix metabolic madness." At the outset it is marked by regions of furious osteoclastic bone resorption triggering reactive, disordered bone formation. The net effect at first is mobilization of bone, but with the passage of time, bone resorption slows and is more or less balanced by bone formation, which, however, is disordered and structurally inadequate. Eventually over the span of years a quiescent or inactive sclerotic stage ensues. *Thus Paget's disease is divided into (1) an initial osteolytic stage, followed by (2) a mixed osteolytic-osteoblastic stage, evolving ultimately into (3) a burnt-out quiescent osteosclerotic stage.*

This disorder usually begins after age 40 and becomes progressively more prevalent thereafter.[21] It is common in Caucasians in Europe, North America, Australia, and New Zealand and reaches a frequency in these countries of about 10% of males and 15% of females in the ninth decade of life. For unknown reasons the condition is rare in the native populations of Asia and Africa. *The involvement is monostotic in about 15% of cases and is polyostotic in the remainder, with notable variation in the stage of the process from one site to another.* Although it may be discovered as an incidental radiographic finding, it can produce a variety of skeletal, neuromuscular, and cardiovascular problems, the most serious of which is the development of a sarcoma in pagetic bone.

PATHOGENESIS. When Sir James Paget first described this condition over 100 years ago, he attributed the skeletal changes to an inflammatory process (hence the designation "osteitis deformans"). It is ironic that after numerous alternative causations have been proposed, currently in vogue is the following concept: *Paget's disease is a slow-virus infection by a paramyxovirus, likening this skeletal disorder to such slow-virus diseases as subacute sclerosing leukoencephalitis and kuru, also produced by the same family of viruses.*[22] Ultrastructurally, microcylindric inclu-

sions can be seen in the nuclei and cytoplasm of osteoclasts in affected areas of bone, and immunocytologic techniques using monoclonal antibodies disclose paramyxovirus antigens identical to those of the respiratory syncytial virus (RSV) and measles virus.[23] Furthermore, in situ hybridization has detected measles virus nucleotide sequences in pagetic osteoclasts. The presence of two closely related agents raises questions but has been explained by mutation of a single virus or by invoking the concept of synergistic action of two "incomplete slow viruses." Welcome as an established causation might be, prudence is indicated because no virus has been isolated from affected tissue.

MORPHOLOGY. Monostotic Paget's disease most often involves, in descending order of frequency, the tibia, iliac bone, femur, skull, vertebra, and humerus. Curiously, the rank order differs in the polyostotic disease in which the spine is most often involved (70%), followed closely by the pelvis (65%) and then in decending order the femur, skull, sacrum, tibia, humerus, and virtually any other bone in the skeleton.[24] In all sites of involvement the disease progresses through the three distinct phases mentioned (Fig. 28–11). In the skull, it tends to begin in the frontal and occipital regions, whereas in the long bones it begins in the

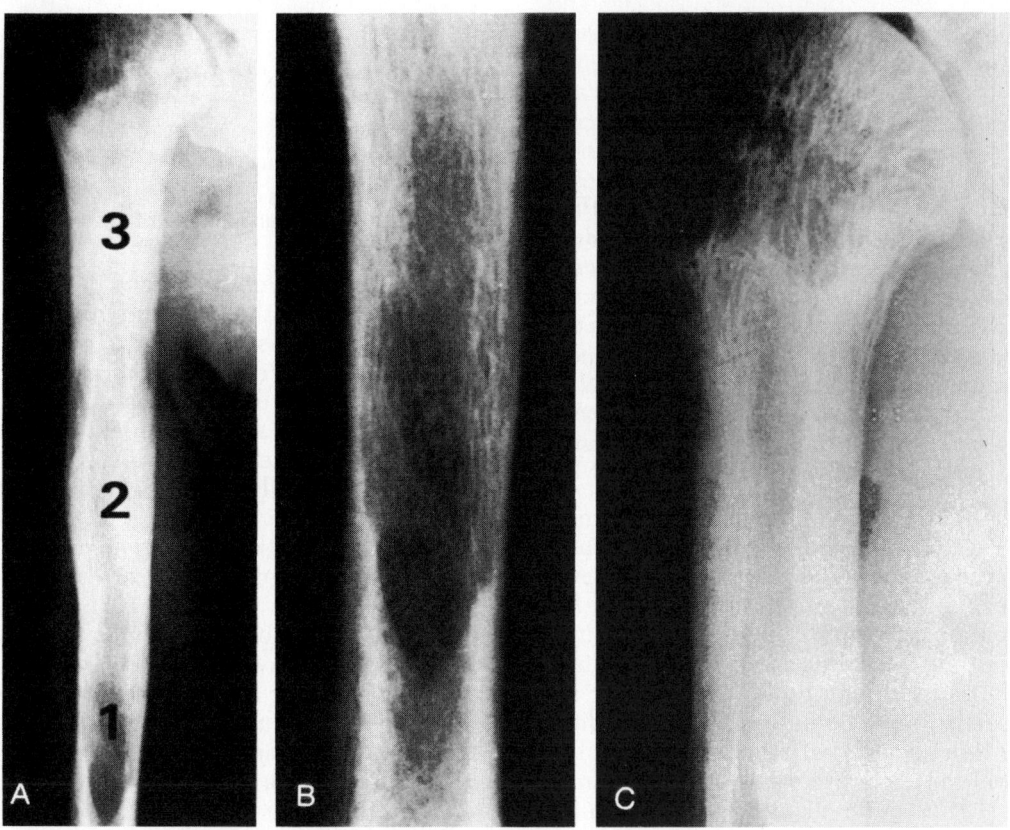

Figure 28-11. Paget's disease of the humerus. The three sequential stages, (1) lytic, (2) mixed, and (3) sclerotic, are shown in *A*. Area 1, the lytic stage, is seen in close-up in *B*. Area 2, the mixed stage (upper portion of *B*) reveals central and endosteal cortical resorption and replacement by less compact new bone. Area 3, the sclerotic stage, with irregular thickening of both cortical and trabecular bone, is seen in *C*. (From Maldague, B., and Malghem, J.: Dynamic radiologic pattern of Paget's disease of bone. Clin. Orthop. 217:127, 1987.)

subchondral ends. The initial osteolytic phase is marked by a disordered patchwork of areas of resorption produced by an increased number of overly large osteoclasts, some containing as many as 100 nuclei. With the electron microscope, the microcylindric inclusions mentioned earlier can be seen in the nuclei and cytoplasm of these osteoclasts. In the second mixed phase, the resorption is closely followed by new bone formation effected by an abundance of osteoblasts. However, the new matrix is haphazardly laid down, mostly in the form of woven bone, some of which may be converted into lamellar bone. **Because resorption and formation are uncoupled, mineralization of the matrix lags and osteoid seams persist to demarcate the margins of the newly laid down bone. In this manner, a tilelike or mosaic pattern of bone is created that is pathognomonic of Paget's disease** (Fig. 28–12). Concomitantly the adjacent marrow spaces fill with a loose, highly vascularized connective tissue. In the course of this active breakdown and build-up, the conformation of the bone as well as its internal structure is significantly altered, as will be pointed out later. Eventually, after many years, the condition is marked predominantly by bone formation and osteosclerosis as the disease appears to burn out. Because the new bone formation is disordered and poorly mineralized, it is soft and porous, lacks structural stability, and is vulnerable to fracture or deformation under stress.

As a consequence of the changes described, involved bones thicken and enlarge owing to both subperiosteal and endosteal bone formation. Concomitantly, the medullary spaces are diminished and demarcation between cortex and medullary cavity is obscured. During the osteolytic and mixed stages, the bone is soft and rubbery or has the consistency of dried bread. It can be cut readily with a knife. Anterior bowing of the femur and tibia characteristically develops as a consequence of weight-bearing, and the neck of the femur sags to a right angle. The skull is enlarged and irregularly thickened three- to fourfold with loss of differentiation between the tables and diploë. Coarsening of the facial bones may induce leontiasis ossea (lion-like facies). The cortex of the vertebrae becomes thickened, with poorly formed bone and coarsening of the trabeculae. Because of loss of structural strength, the vertebrae tend to collapse, often anteriorly, to produce a marked kyphosis.

CLINICAL COURSE. When symptomatic, the manifestations of Paget's disease are extremely variable, depending on the extent of the disease, the particular bones involved, and the development of superimposed complications. The usual initial manifestation is pain as a result of microfractures, compression of nerves as they pass through bony foramens, or secondary osteoarthritis.[25] Sometimes the condition comes to attention because with the thickening of the skull the patient notices a progressive increase in hat size (Fig. 28–13). Pagetic changes may lead to flattening of the base of the skull (platybasia) with narrowing of the foramen magnum, creating the danger of compression of the medulla. Foraminal narrowing with impingement on the eighth cranial nerve may cause hearing loss, but sometimes the hearing loss is

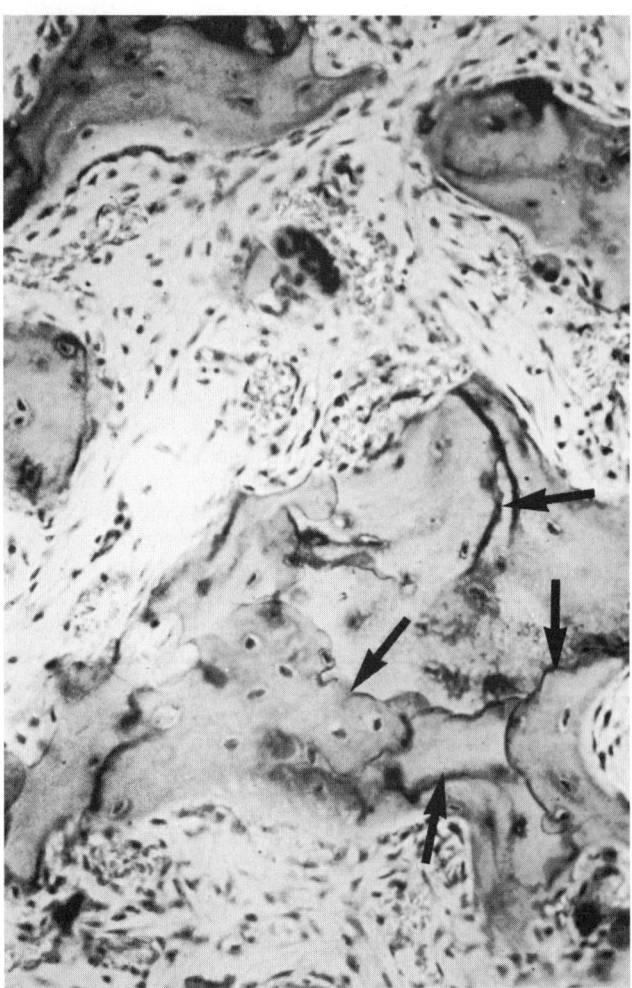

Figure 28-12. Paget's disease of the vertebrae, revealing the tile-like mosaic *(arrows)* and fibrosis of the intertrabecular spaces.

due to direct pagetic changes in the ossicles of the inner ear. Pain in the back and lower extremities may be caused by pressure on nerve roots or by vertebral microfractures. Vertebral fracture and compression of the spinal cord may cause paraplegia. Anterior bowing of the tibias and femurs is a common finding. Sclerotic bone, despite its density, is prone to fracture. Radiologically, affected bones are enlarged, and at first have patchy increased radiolucency during the stages of osteolytic and active disease. Later, they may become irregularly sclerotic with increased bone density. Typically there is marked elevation of the serum alkaline phosphatase and increased urinary excretion of hydroxyproline. The serum calcium level may be normal or high during the osteolytic stage.

Two additional features may be encountered: (1) hemodynamic changes, and (2) the development of a sarcoma in an area of involvement. Bony hypervascularity leads to warmth of the skin overlying affected areas of the skeleton. When the involvement is polyostotic and widespread, the vascularity acts as an arteriovenous shunt that sometimes leads to high output failure or exacerbation of an underlying cardiac disease.[26]

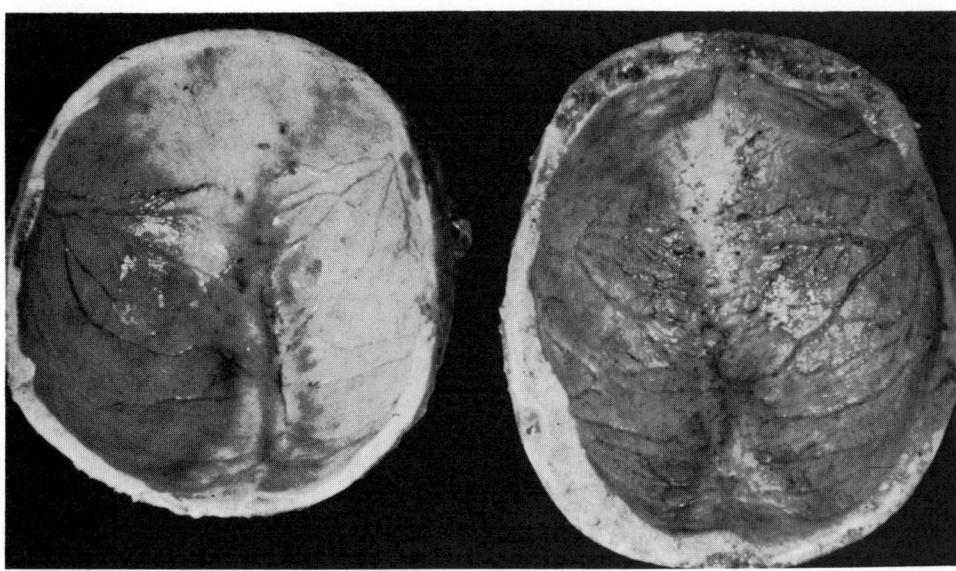

Figure 28-13. Paget's disease of skull. Irregular thickening of right calvarium is well brought out by comparison with normal control on left.

The most ominous complication, occurring in about 1% of patients, is the development of a sarcoma in an involved bone, *generally an osteogenic sarcoma, but sometimes fibrosarcoma or another form.*[27] Indeed, when a patient over 40 develops an osteosarcoma, there is a strong likelihood of underlying Paget's disease. The tumors tend to arise in the jaw, pelvis, or femur and are more aggressive than de novo neoplasms.

FIBROUS DYSPLASIA

This benign disorder of bone is best characterized as slow, progressive replacement of a localized area of bone by an abnormal proliferation of isomorphic fibrous tissue intermixed with poorly formed, haphazardly arranged trabeculae of woven bone. The changes seem to represent a focus of disordered maturation of bone with arrest at an immature stage of woven bone. The lesions appear in three distinctive but sometimes overlapping clinical patterns: (1) involvement of a single bone (monostotic); (2) involvement of several or many, but never all, bones (polyostotic); and (3) a special category of polyostotic fibrous dysplasia (*Albright's syndrome, McCune-Albright syndrome*) associated with café-au-lait skin pigmentations and endocrine dysfunctions, especially precocious sexual development.[28]

Monostotic fibrous dysplasia accounts for about 70% of all cases. It may arise in either sex, usually in childhood, and often comes to an arrest at puberty. The following sites are involved in descending order of frequency—ribs, femur, tibia, maxilla, mandible, calvarium, humerus, and other bones. The condition is often asymptomatic and discovered incidentally in a radiograph taken for other reasons. However, the lesions may cause tumorous distortion of the bony contours, disfigurement of the face or skull, or sometimes pain related to the expanding bone mass or to pressure on nerves. The monostotic pattern does not appear to be a precursor to the polyostotic form.

Polyostotic fibrous dysplasia without endocrine dysfunctions accounts for about 25% of all cases. It tends to appear at a slightly earlier age than the monostotic pattern and may progress into middle adult life. Both sexes are affected equally. The bony sites affected, in descending order of frequency, are the femur, skull, tibia, humerus, ribs, fibula, radius and ulna, mandible, vertebrae, and others. The lesions may be limited to a single limb or one side of the skeleton, but there is sometimes a bilateral distribution. In the polyostotic disease the craniofacial bones are affected in about 50% of persons with moderate dissemination of lesions, but the frequency reaches 100% in those with extensive disease. Also distinctive is a tendency to involve the shoulder and pelvic girdles; the development of severe, sometimes crippling deformities (e.g., shepherd-crook deformity of the proximal femur); and a marked predisposition to the development of spontaneous and often recurrent fractures.[29]

Polyostotic fibrous dysplasia in association with endocrinopathies accounts for about 3 to 5% of all cases. When accompanied by skin pigmentations and precocious sexual development, the multisystem disorder is referred to as Albright's syndrome or sometimes McCune-Albright syndrome. However, many other endocrine associations have been identified, including hyperthyroidism, Cushing's syndrome, acromegaly, hyperparathyroidism, vitamin D resistant rickets, and adenomas of various endocrine glands.[30] In the most common clinical presentation with precocious sexual development, females are affected much more often than males. There is a tendency for the bone lesions to be unilateral and for the skin pigmentations to be confined to the same side of the body. The areas of pigmentation are classically large, dark to "café-au-lait" macules having irregular serpiginous borders (coastline of Maine) found primarily on the neck, chest, back, shoulder, and pelvic region. There is no understanding of the association of the skeletal, skin, and endocrine derangements.[31]

MORPHOLOGY. Grossly in all clinical patterns, the bone lesions take the form of localized defects a few to many centimeters in diameter arising **within cancellous bone** that by enlargement erode into, but rarely through, the cortex. The involved bone may be expanded and distorted but a thin shell of subperiosteal cortical bone persists. Rarely, the cortex is eroded. The gray-red fibrous tissue of the lesions may be gritty or sandy to touch. Occasionally, cystic spaces, small hemorrhages, or foci of chondroid or myxomatous tissue are present. Histologically, **the lesions are composed of a mature, whorled, connective tissue (sometimes sufficiently cellular to resemble a fibroma) in which is laid down irregular trabeculae of woven bone** (Fig. 28–14). The osseous component is of variable prominence and sometimes is virtually absent. The haphazardly arrayed trabeculae are thin, lack osteoblasts, and appear to be formed through osseous metaplasia of the background fibrous tissue. Occasionally, there are calcified spherules or islands of cartilage within the connective tissue, sometimes with ossification of the cartilaginous inclusions. Osteoclastic giant cells are generally sparse and the vascularization varies from scant to abundant.

CLINICAL COURSE. Fibrous dysplasia pursues an unpredictable course. As mentioned, patients with monostotic lesions remain asymptomatic throughout life. In some instances, however, sufficient destruction of cortical bone leads to fracture. In other instances, particularly in persons with disseminated disease, there is a tendency to skeletal deformity and fracture, and when the facial bones are involved there may be severe distortions of the orbit, nose, and jaw. Generally, the earlier the age of onset, the more progressive is the condition. Areas of involvement have a distinctive ground-glass, well-demarcated lucent appearance on radiographs. Rarely, a sarcoma develops, most often an osteogenic sarcoma, or sometimes fibrosarcoma or chondrosarcoma.[32] In some of these instances there has been previous radiation therapy, but malignant transformation has been noted in the absence of such intervention.

FIBROUS CORTICAL DEFECT (NONOSSIFYING FIBROMA)

Fibrous cortical defects are extremely common *nonneoplastic developmental aberrations* seen chiefly in children, almost always in the femur, tibia, and fibula. They create irregular, sharply demarcated, lobular, radiolucent defects in the metaphyseal cortex that usually leave intact a thin, subperiosteal layer of cortical bone. The margins of these lesions are sometimes slightly sclerotic. Multiple and bilateral lesions are found in about half the cases. Often they consist of minute lesions only a few millimeters in diameter, but occasionally larger defects up to 4 to 5 cm are seen.

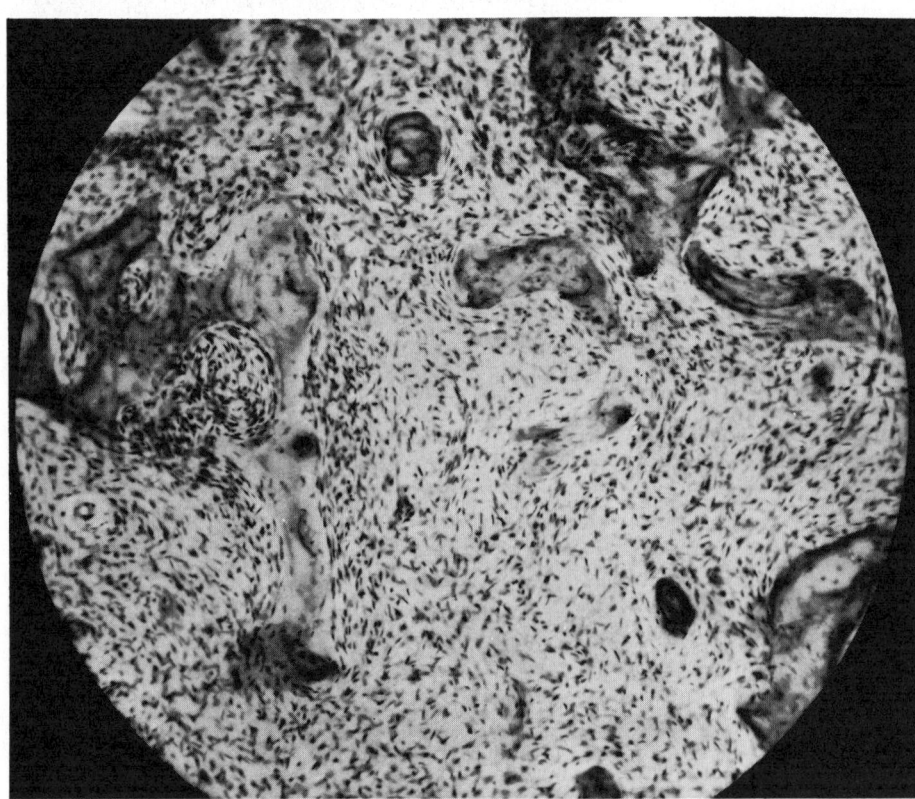

Figure 28-14. Fibrous dysplasia of bone, illustrating characteristic overgrowth of fibrous tissue and haphazardly scattered trabeculae of woven bone.

HYPERTROPHIC OSTEOARTHROPATHY

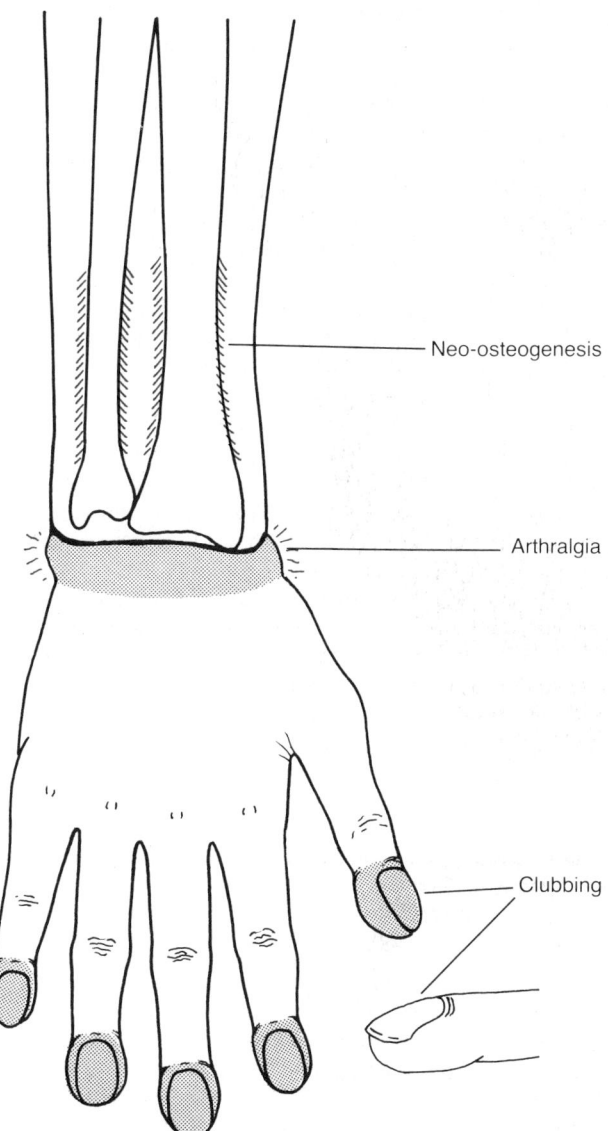

Figure 28-15. Hypertrophic osteoarthropathy depicting the three major components: (1) periosteal new bone formation at the ends of distal bones, (2) ill-defined arthralgia, and (3) clubbing of the fingertips.

The well-demarcated lesions are composed of soft gray tissue lying within the cortex with an intact shell of overlying bone. They are composed of cellular, whorled fibroblasts sometimes forming palisades. There may also be scattered lipid-laden macrophages and multinucleate benign cells, but no bone formation or anaplasia.

The major clinical significance of these osseous lesions derives from the following facts: *(1) being non-neoplastic, they do not become transformed into sarcomas; (2) they are generally asymptomatic, but* *larger lesions may cause pain and predispose to fracture; (3) they are extremely common and have been reported in almost one third of apparently normal children, both boys and girls; and (4) they often disappear spontaneously within a few years.*

HYPERTROPHIC OSTEOARTHROPATHY

This enigmatic disorder is characterized by *(1) periosteal new bone formation primarily at the distal ends of long bones, metatarsals, metacarpals, and proximal phalanges, (2) arthritis of the adjacent joints, and (3) clubbing of the digits* (Fig. 28–15). These three components usually appear in individuals having an underlying disease, most often bronchogenic carcinoma but sometimes other forms of intrathoracic cancer (pleural tumors, pulmonary metastases, mediastinal Hodgkin's disease), chronic lung infections, and chronic liver disease. Rarely hypertrophic osteoarthropathy occurs as an apparent primary idiopathic, sometimes familial, disorder.[33] *Clubbing alone* without the other two components may occur secondary to the same conditions but also with cyanotic heart disease, infective endocarditis or aortitis, ulcerative colitis, Crohn's disease, and cancer of the esophagus and colon. It too occurs rarely as a primary idiopathic reaction.

> The **periosteal bone changes** take the form of new bone formation beneath the periosteum accompanied by endosteal bone resorption, producing only barely visible roughening of the surface (visible radiologically as tufting along the bony contour). They may also comprise a complete enclosing shell visualized radiographically as bulbous enlargement of the phalanges. Identification of these changes on x-ray films sometimes provides the first clue to an occult cacinoma of the lung.
>
> The **arthritis** is nonspecific and comprises edematous thickening of the synovium associated with a mild infiltrate of lymphocytes and plasma cells.
>
> **Clubbing** results from an edematous fibrovascular overgrowth in the tips of the digits. As a consequence they become dusky and cyanotic, and the nails undergo rounding to develop a "watchglass" deformity. Here again clubbing may provide a valuable diagnostic clue to any one of the conditions mentioned earlier, but first and foremost to the possibility of a lurking bronchogenic carcinoma.

The cause of these changes is unknown, but increased blood flow produced by some neurogenic mechanism is suspected because vagotomy is sometimes beneficial. How one of the underlying conditions, say bronchogenic carcinoma, leads to such neurovascular alterations remains mysterious, but the relationship cannot be doubted as resection of the cancer reverses the changes.

TUMORS

Although tumors of bones are encountered infrequently in clinical practice, they are nonetheless of great clinical significance because many are highly malignant.

Primary bone tumors may arise from any of the elements indigenous to bone, including the diverse marrow cells as well as the vascular and neural components. Some concept of the variety of primary bone tumors and their frequency as encountered at the Mayo Clinic is provided in Table 28–3. Lest this array produce "neurogenic shock," it should be mentioned that many of these neoplasms (e.g., those derived from marrow, vascular, and neural cells) have been described elsewhere in this book. Moreover, the chordoma, which looms particularly large in the compilation presented (probably because of referrals), is in most clinics quite rare and so will also be omitted.

Certain useful generalizations can be made about the clinical presentation and distribution of bone tumors. The frequency of particular neoplasms is of importance in the differential diagnosis. In adults, *malignant tumors of bone are twice as common as benign.* By contrast, in the first decade of life, only a minority (15 to 20%) are malignant. Excluding malignant neoplasms of marrow origin (myeloma and leukemia), if all ages are included, *osteosarcoma is the most common cancer of bone,* followed by chondrosarcoma and Ewing's tumor. Among the benign tumors the exostoses (osteochondromas) predominate, followed by benign giant cell tumors.

There are significant contrasts in the age distributions of individual types of tumors.[34] The peak incidence of osteosarcoma is in the second decade, but chondrosarcomas are uncommon in the young; most occur after middle life. Ewing's sarcoma tends to occur in those under the age of 30 years, but giant cell tumors are rare under age 20. However, it should be cautioned—these age differentials merely express peak incidences, and osteosarcoma, for example, may arise in infancy or in the elderly, and chondrosarcoma may arise in the young.

The favored *skeletal locations for various tumors differ.* About half of all osteosarcomas occur about the knee, more often in the distal femoral metaphysis than in the proximal tibial metaphysis. Interestingly, these are sites of greatest skeletal growth activity. By contrast, chondrosarcomas tend to arise in the trunk, limb girdles, and proximal long bones, rarely in the hands and feet. Chondroblastomas and giant cell tumors are almost always located in the epiphyseal ends of long bones; in contrast, Ewing's sarcoma more often arises in the diaphysis. The location of a tumor is then of some differential value.

The *radiographic appearance of some lesions may be distinctive.* Certain neoplasms tend to be osteoblastic (e.g., the osteosarcoma), yielding radiodensities within the central region of the tumor and often in the extraskeletal extension of the invasive cancer. On the other hand, layered subperiosteal new bone

Table 28–3. Classification of 8542 Primary Tumors of Bone in Mayo Clinic Patients

HISTOLOGIC TYPE	TOTAL CASES	BENIGN	CASES	MALIGNANT	CASES
Hematopoietic	3401 (39.8%)			Myeloma	2932
				Malignant lymphoma	469
Chondrogenic	1822 (21.3%)	Osteochondroma	727	Primary chondrosarcoma	545
		Chondroma	245	Secondary chondrosarcoma	89
		Chondroblastoma	79	Dedifferentiated chondrosarcoma	79
		Chondromyxoid fibroma	39	Mesenchymal chondrosarcoma	19
Osteogenic	1638 (19.2%)	Osteoid osteoma	245	Osteosarcoma	1274
		Osteoblastoma	63	Parosteal osteosarcoma	56
Unknown origin	878 (10.3%)	Giant cell tumor	425	Ewing's tumor	402
				Malignant giant cell tumor	28
				Adamantinoma	23
Histiocytic origin	62 (0.7%)	Fibrous histiocytoma	10	Malignant (fibrous) histiocytoma	52
Fibrogenic	315 (3.7%)	Metaphyseal fibrous defect (fibroma)	99	Desmoplastic fibroma	9
				Fibrosarcoma	207
Notochordal	262 (3.1%)			Chordoma	262
Vascular	147 (1.7%)	Hemangioma	80	Hemangioendothelioma	60
				Hemangiopericytoma	7
Lipogenic	7 (0.1%)	Lipoma	6	Liposarcoma	1
Neurogenic	10 (0.1%)	Neurilemmoma	10		
Total	8542 (100%)		2028		6514

From Dahlin, D.C., and Unni, K.K.: Bone Tumors, 4th ed. Springfield, Illinois, Charles C Thomas, 1986, p. 8, by permission of Mayo Foundation.

formation—"onion-skinning"—is strong presumptive evidence of Ewing's tumor. Thus, in the morphologic evaluation of a neoplasm of bone, the frequency of various neoplasms, the age of the patient, the location of the lesion, and its radiographic appearance all are helpful in the differential diagnosis.

BONE-FORMING (OSTEOBLASTIC) TUMORS

Tumors in this category were at one time referred to as osteogenic neoplasms, and the malignant variant was referred to as osteogenic sarcoma. The term "osteogenic" is avoided here because it has been used confusingly to apply to tumors arising in bone as well as to those arising in extraosseous sites producing bone. Here we restrict the term "osteoblastic" to neoplasms of bone characterized by *the synthesis of osteoid matrix that may become mineralized.*

Osteoma

Osteomas are usually bossellated sessile tumors composed of densely sclerotic well-formed bone projecting out from the cortical surface, most often of the skull and facial bones. They often protrude into one of the air sinuses (frontal, ethmoid, and others) and sometimes from the mandible, maxilla, and inner and outer skull tables. Reactive bone growth from infection, trauma, or vascular malformations may produce lesions simulating an osteoma. These neoplasms may arise at any age, slightly more frequently in men than in women. They are composed of mature, irregularly laid down, broad bony trabeculae. The intertrabecular spaces are filled with fibrous tissue that is sometimes highly vascularized and may even contain foci of hematopoiesis. Osteomas are generally of little clinical significance and need not even be excised, unless they cause obstruction to a sinus cavity, impinge on the brain, or are disturbing cosmetically. They do not transform into other lesions but occasionally are associated with Gardner's syndrome.

Osteoid Osteoma and Osteoblastoma

The osteoid osteoma is a small benign neoplasm having no malignant potential. In contrast, the osteoblastoma is best viewed as a larger, more aggressive osteoid osteoma. Most of the following remarks are directed toward the more common osteoid osteoma.[35] Almost 90% of these lesions are encountered in persons between 5 and 25 years of age, and they occur twice as often in males as in females. *They evoke a surprising amount of pain for their size and are distinctive radiographically, appearing as a small radiolucent focus (the nidus) surrounded by densely sclerotic bone* (Fig. 28–16). With lesions located close to the periosteum there may be sufficient subperiosteal bone formation to produce fusiform thickening of the overlying cortex.[36] Controversy continues as to whether these lesions are true neoplasms or inflammatory reactions.

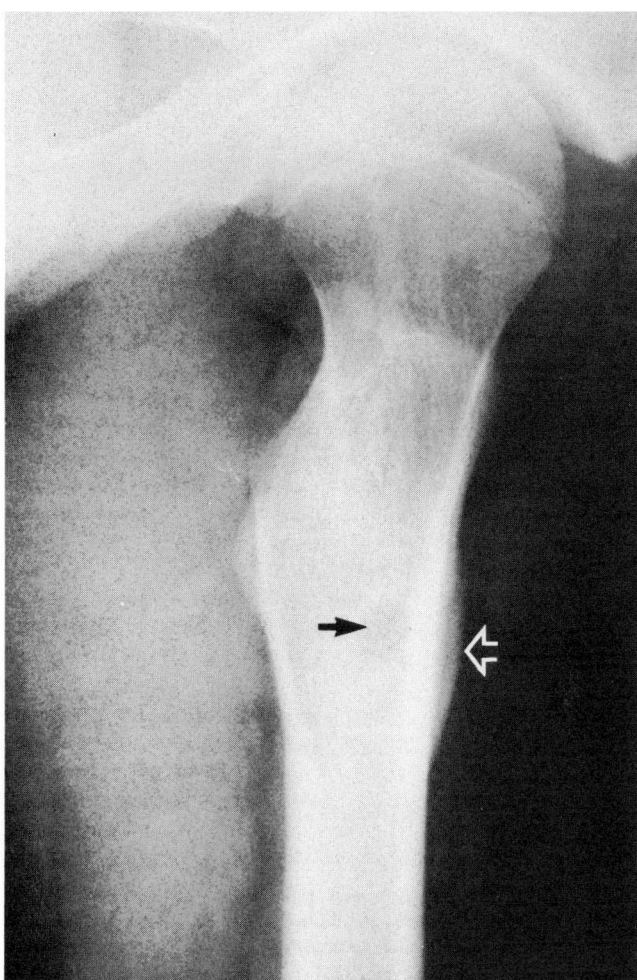

Figure 28-16. Osteoid osteoma of the femur illustrating the radiolucent nidus *(arrow)* and the adjacent thickening of the cortex *(open arrow).* (Courtesy of Dr. Barbara Weissman, Brigham and Women's Hospital.)

Osteoid osteomas are usually about 1 cm in diameter and most are located near the ends of the tibia and femur, but nearly every other bone in the body has been involved at one time or another. Most lesions are intracortical, but some may arise close to the endosteum or within cancellous bone. The nidus itself is composed of firm, red-gray tissue that is sometimes gritty because of the contained mineralized osteoid trabeculae. The surrounding bone is densely sclerotic. Microscopically, the nidus is initially composed of delicate trabeculae of osteoid rimmed by numerous osteoblasts and enclosed by a vascularized spindle cell stroma. At a later stage, tangled islands and trabeculae of partially mineralized osteoid become more prominent within the fibrous stroma, and still later densely packed irregular bone trabeculae are seen (Fig. 28–17).

These benign lesions are readily managed by local excision; even with recurrence malignant transformation does not occur.

The closely related *osteoblastoma,* sometimes called a *giant osteoid osteoma,* is a purely lytic tumor

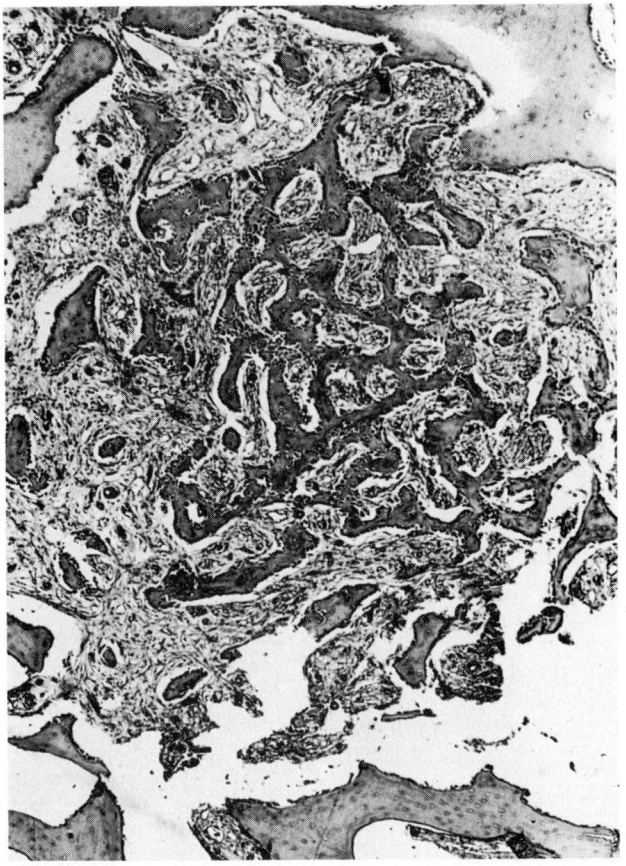

Figure 28-17. Osteoid osteoma. Low-power view of an entire lesion enclosed within sclerotic wide bone spicules. Lesion is composed of fibrous tissue and numerous anastomosing spicules of osteoid.

having a similar histologic appearance save that it does not evoke surrounding bone formation. It tends to be larger than the osteoid osteoma, is frequently located in the vertebrae or long bones, and does not cause pain. Although usually benign, about 10% recur following removal and some convert into osteosarcomas.[37]

Osteosarcoma ("Osteogenic" Sarcoma)

The osteosarcoma is best defined as a malignant tumor of mesenchymal cells, characterized by the direct formation of osteoid or bone by the tumor cells. Some are composed largely of fibroblastic cells, others have abundant bone formation, some show chondroid differentiation, and still others are highly vascular (telangiectatic), but all have tumor-produced osteoid marked by trapping of anaplastic tumor cells within the lacunae of the osteoid matrix. Excluding plasma cell myelomas, osteosarcomas are the most common form of primary cancer in bones.

On the basis of clinical setting, these neoplasms can be divided into two large categories, primary and secondary. *Primary osteosarcomas* arise de novo in the apparent absence of underlying bone disease or recognized carcinogenic influences. Most of these cancers appear in young persons under 20 years of age in the long bones before the epiphyses have closed, with a definite male preponderance. Those of the jaws usually arise in older individuals. *Secondary osteosarcomas* develop against a background of preexisting bone pathology or previous exposure to some potentially carcinogenic influence.[38] Most important is underlying disease (e.g., Paget's disease of bone, multiple enchondromas, multiple osteochondromas, chronic osteomyelitis, fibrous dysplasia, infarcts, and fractures of bone).[39] Bone irradiation also is a well-recognized predisposing influence. Secondary osteosarcomas usually occur in considerably older individuals; they account for about 6 to 10% of all osteosarcomas.

On the basis of site of origin within the bone, osteosarcomas have been divided into many subsets (e.g., medullary, intracortical) that need not concern us save to point out the parosteal (juxtacortical) variant. It is applied to the periosteum and usually is well differentiated, with a much better prognosis than the other variants (80% five-year survival). Most of the following remarks relate to the most common pattern of osteosarcoma, sometimes referred to as "conventional."

PATHOGENESIS. The origins of osteosarcomas are as mysterious as those of all other forms of cancer. However, a number of interesting observations have been made that can be considered under the categories of (1) genetic, (2) constitutional, and (3) environmental.

The evidence implicating *genetic factors* in the origin of some (possibly many) osteosarcomas mounts with each passing year. It is well established that about 40% of patients with retinoblastomas have a hereditary mutation in chromosome 13 within the q14 band.[40] Patients who survive their genetic retinoblastoma have about a 500-fold greater risk of developing an osteosarcoma. Subsequently, it was discovered that some osteosarcomas are associated with homozygous mutations at the "retinoblastoma locus" on chromosome 13 even in the absence of retinoblastomas.[41] It is hypothesized that the 13q14 locus constitutes a suppressor gene. Individuals who inherit a single mutation on one of the alleles are at risk of acquiring a somatic mutation in the other allele and, with homozygosity, of developing a retinoblastoma or osteosarcoma, or both.[42]

The *constitutional influences* in the genesis of osteosarcomas point mostly to a possible contributory role for unusually active bone growth. The well-known association between these neoplasms and Paget's disease could relate to active bone growth. The male preponderance and the peak frequency in youth are additional "straws in the wind." Of interest, large dogs, such as the Saint Bernard and Great Dane, have 13 times the frequency of bone sarcoma of smaller breeds (data are not available on the frequency in professional basketball players).

The best documented *environmental influence* is the effect of radiation, a well-recognized mutagen. In addition, there has been some tenuous evidence pointing to a virus; a cell-free agent derived from human osteosarcomas, when injected into hamsters, has been reported to produce an increased incidence of a variety of mesenchymal sarcomas, the most common being osteosarcoma.[43] Such an exogenous agent might fit with the fragmentary evidence of immunologic reactions to apparent tumor antigens, not only among patients harboring these neoplasms, but also among family members.[44] Although the pathogenetic puzzle has not been solved, progress has been made.

DISTRIBUTION OF OSTEOSARCOMA

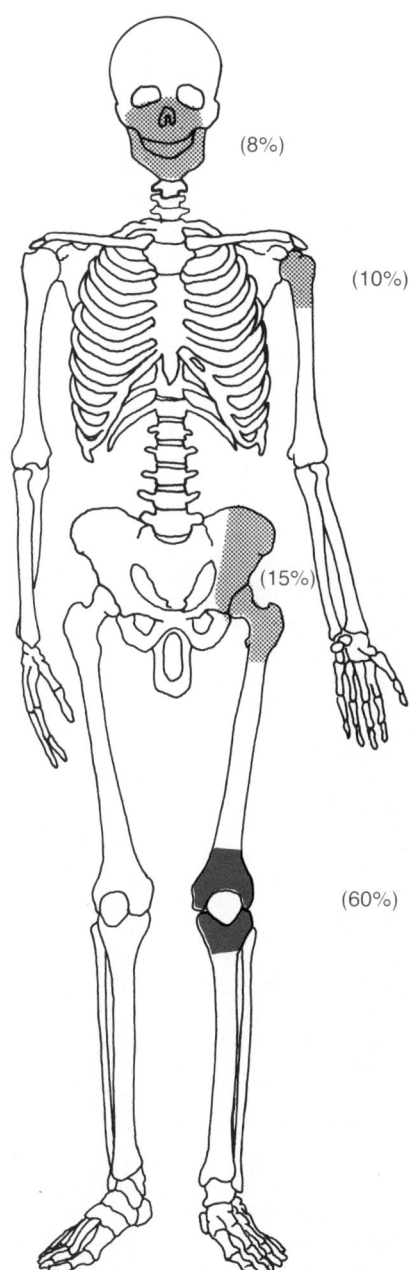

(8%)

(10%)

(15%)

(60%)

Figure 28-18. The major sites of origin of osteosarcomas. Numbers in parentheses are approximate percentages.

MORPHOLOGY. Most conventional osteosarcomas arise in the medullary cavity of the metaphyseal end of the long bones of the extremities: in decreasing order of frequency, in the lower end of the femur, upper end of the tibia, upper end of the humerus, and upper end of the femur. About 60 to 70% of all tumors arise close to the knee. However, any bone may be involved, and in persons over the age of 25 the incidence in flat bones (e.g., jaws, pelvis) and long bones is almost equal (Fig. 28–18). By the time of diagnosis, most osteosarcomas have broken through the cortex and periosteum and are bulky masses that often cause obvious swelling of the extremity. The neoplasms appear as gray-white, aggressive masses that often contain areas of hemorrhage and cystic softening (Fig. 28–19). They vary in consistency; some are largely fibroblastic and soft, whereas others have components of osteoid or chondroid and are firmer. As the neoplasm penetrates the cortex, it lifts the periosteum and a characteristic "Codman's triangle" is produced — the angle between the plane of the outer surface of the cortex and the elevated periosteum. This anatomic feature can often be visualized in radiographs, and although it is characteristic of osteogenic sarcoma, it is not pathognomonic. The tumor may

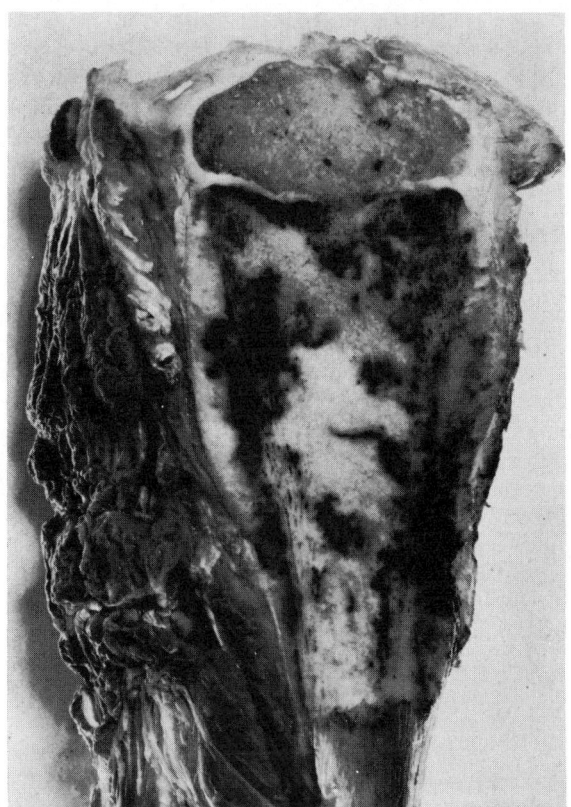

Figure 28-19. Osteosarcoma of upper end of tibia. White tumor with areas of necrosis and hemorrhage fills marrow cavity but has not penetrated epiphyseal plate. It has infiltrated through cortex and lifted periosteum on both lateral aspects.

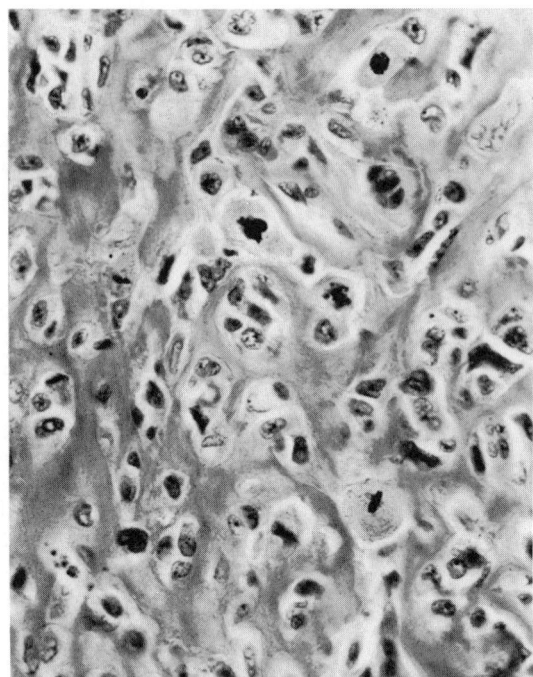

Figure 28-20. Osteoid produced by an osteogenic sarcoma. Note anaplasia and mitotic figures within trapped tumor cells.

spread widely in the narrow cavity, but it rarely penetrates the epiphyseal plate to involve the joint space; this may, however, occur after epiphyseal closure.

Histologically, these tumors vary in the richness of the osteoid or cartilaginous or vascular components, but **common to all is a basically anaplastic mesenchymal parenchyma that in places is punctuated by the formation of osteoid matrix by tumor cells.** Thus, frankly anaplastic cells are found lying within the lacelike patterns of osteoid matrix (Fig. 28-20). Islands of cartilage may also be formed by tumor cells. The mesenchymal cells between the osteoid or cartilaginous matrix are often wildly anaplastic, with numerous tumor giant cells, atypical mitoses, and striking hyperchromasia. The vascularization may be subtle or take the form of large, cavernous telangiectatic channels, distributed throughout the tumor — **telangiectatic osteosarcomas.**

Extraskeletal osteogenic sarcomas are rare. The most common sites of origin are the retroperitoneum, mediastinum, and breast, but sometimes they arise in internal organs such as the uterus or lungs.

Whatever the morphologic variant and site of origin, all osteosarcomas are aggressive lesions that metastasize widely through the bloodstream, usually first to the lungs, but also to other parenchymal organs and other osseous sites. In contrast, lymph node involvement, even in the local region, is unusual. Approximately 30 to 40% of patients have demonstrable pulmonary metastases when first seen, and more than 90% of those who die of the neoplasm have metastases to the lungs, bones, brain, and elsewhere.

CLINICAL COURSE. As with most malignant tumors of bone, the presenting clinical complaints are those of pain, tenderness, and swelling of the affected parts. Rapid growth is characteristic of many, sometimes producing expansion and enlargement of the limb or sudden fracture of the bone as the first symptom. The serum alkaline phosphatase level may be elevated but is usually of no diagnostic significance. Radiographs, CT scans, or MRI scans are distinctive in many instances. The radiodensity or radiolucency of the tumor varies according to the extent of bone formation. Lifting of the periosteum at Codman's triangle can sometimes be visualized but may be absent. Subperiosteal and soft tissue penetration of the tumor with its bony osteoid content may produce extraosseous radiodensities (Fig. 28-21). However, in almost all cases, biopsy of these neoplasms is necessary to confirm the diagnosis before radical surgical procedures are performed.

Advances in treatment have substantially improved the prognosis. In the past, the five-year survival with surgery alone was about 20%. Currently, combined surgery, radiation, and chemotherapy yield about a 60% five-year disease-free survival with a remarkably small incremental loss over the next five years.[45] In general, osteoblastic lesions respond the least favorably to therapy and fibroblastic lesions respond best.

Variant Osteosarcoma

As noted at the outset, conventional osteosarcoma generally arises de novo in the young and in the appendicular skeleton. *Secondary osteosarcomas* may

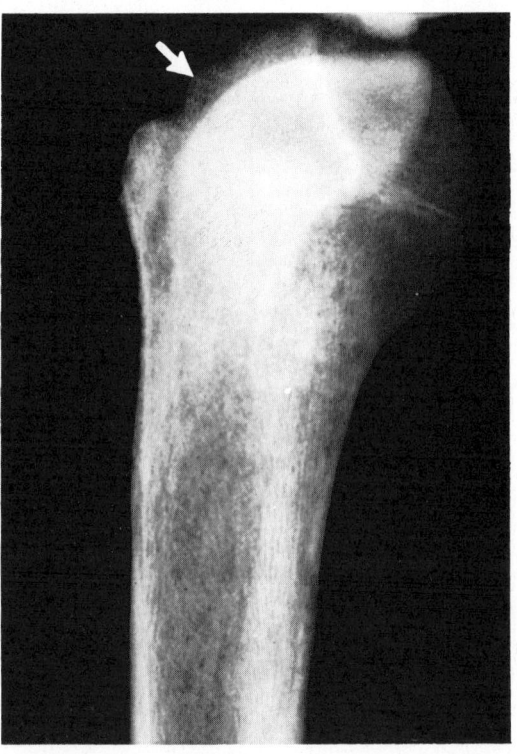

Figure 28-21. Osteosarcoma of humerus. Note bone formation visible external to cortex (arrow).

appear at any age, and frequently in the advanced years of life in those with Paget's disease. In this setting the bones most often involved are the pelvis, femur, humerus, tibia, skull, facial bones, and scapula, in descending order of frequency. Although the tumor is morphologically similar to the conventional lesions, it is usually more aggressive, and few patients survive more than two years despite therapy.

Another variant is *osteosarcoma of the jawbones*, arising generally in middle to later life. These neoplasms tend to have marked chondroid differentiation, and distant metastases are less frequent. Radical resection yields a significantly higher cure rate than is achieved with conventional neoplasms.

CHONDROMATOUS TUMORS

Exostosis, Osteochondroma

These benign cartilage-capped bony outgrowths from the surfaces of bones may occur as solitary sporadic lesions or less commonly as multiple lesions in the familial disorder osteochondromatosis. They were described earlier on page 1319 because they probably are disorders of bone development rather than true neoplasms. However, rarely they undergo sarcomatous transformation.

Chondroma, Enchondroma

The chondroma is a benign tumor composed of mature hyaline cartilage. Because such tumors most often arise centrally within the interior of a bone, they are frequently called *enchondromas*. It is believed that, like exostoses, chondromas arise from remnants of epiphyseal cartilage that are left behind.[46] Most often they occur singly, at any age and in either sex. Much less frequently, chondromas or enchondromas occur in multiple sites, often in childhood, in the nonhereditary disorder known as *enchondromatosis or Ollier's disease*. When the skeletal lesions are familial and accompanied by hemangiomas of the skin they have been called *Maffucci's syndrome*. The cartilaginous tumors in these systemic syndromes tend to be more cellular and have greater variability in cell morphology than the sporadic isolated lesions. *Whereas sarcomatous transformation of solitary sporadic chondromas is rare, with the multiple tumors in the systemic syndromes, the frequency of such transformation (usually into a chondrosarcoma) is about 30 to 50%.*[47]

> Most solitary lesions occur in the small bones of the hands and less often the feet. However, they also arise in other bones but are infrequent in the skull. In situ, they are firm, slightly lobulated, gray-blue, translucent masses rarely over 2 cm in diameter. Although they arise centrally, in their growth they may erode the adjacent cortex and cause expansion of the bone. Through and through penetration is rare and should raise the suspicion of malignancy.
>
> Histologically the tumor is composed of **masses or islands of hyaline cartilage enclosed within a vascular-**

ized fibrous stroma. Cartilage cells are irregularly dispersed throughout the matrix and are contained within clearly defined lacunar spaces. Multinucleated chondrocytes or marked cellular dysplasia is unusual and raises the possibility of cancer. Often there are **foci of calcification and even ossification, but the cells trapped within the osteoid matrix are not anaplastic, as is typical of osteosarcomas.**

Many chondromas are asymptomatic or are called to attention by the bony deformation they produce. Some cause pain, most often attributed to pathologic fracture. Radiologically, this tumor creates a lobulated area of rarefaction, often stippled or even opacified by calcifications. Lesions in the small bones of the hands and feet are almost always innocuous, but those in long bones raise the differential diagnosis of chondrosarcoma and so require complete excision. Occasionally, the recurrence of an apparently benign tumor reveals notable cellularity and anaplasia. Whether this implies true sarcomatous transformation of a benign lesion or instead misinterpretation of the original tumor continues to be disputed.

Chondromyxoid Fibroma

This uncommon benign tumor of bone, composed of chondroid, fibrous, and myxoid tissues in varying proportions, is of importance because it can be mistaken for a sarcoma. It tends to occur in the lower metaphysis of the femur and upper metaphysis of the tibia (about the knee joint) and less commonly in the upper metaphysis of the femur and virtually any other bone in the body, including the jaws.[48] The majority are found in the second and third decades of life, but sometimes much later, with a definite male preponderance.

> Most neoplasms are small (less than 5 cm in diameter), discrete, gray-white, lobulated masses, sharply delineated from the surrounding bone, which may be somewhat sclerotic. They are often located close to the epiphyseal region. Although they may encroach on the cortex or produce fusiform expansion of the bone, only rarely do they penetrate the periosteum.
>
> As the name indicates, histologically there are chondroid areas interspersed with myxomatous zones and fibrous zones. Foci of calcification may be present but are not usually prominent. Within the chondroid lobules, the matrix is well-developed and mature with single cells lying within lacunae, but toward the periphery of the lobules increased cellularity and gradual transition into the more cellular fibrous tissue or loose myxoid tissue are seen. Multinucleate giant cells with benign nuclei are sometimes dispersed in the fibromyxoid zones. **Significantly, in some areas there may be dysplastic cells having large irregular and sometimes multiple nuclei. In the context of the overall pattern of chondromyxoid fibroma, the cellular atypism does not denote cancerous transformation.**

Although small tumors may be asymptomatic, the larger ones come to attention because of pain, local swelling, or distortion of the contour of the bone. On radiographs, they appear as very sharply circumscribed areas of radiolucency with scattered foci of calcification and occasionally some marginal increased radiodensity. As noted earlier, correct identification of these neoplasms is most important because they rarely if ever become malignant, can be adequately treated by curettage, and even though possibly recurrent, pose no threat.

Chondroblastoma

This uncommon benign tumor is composed basically of a background of immature small chondrocytes having single, round to polygonal nuclei scattered among which are multinucleated giant cells with benign-appearing nuclei and islands of chondroid matrix.[49] Recognition of this lesion is of importance because some of its morphologic and radiographic features can be misinterpreted as a more ominous neoplasm, such as a giant cell tumor. *Chondroblastomas usually arise within the epiphyseal region of long tubular bones in individuals between 10 and 20 years of age with a male-to-female ratio of 2:1.* Most occur about the knee, but sometimes they are located in the pelvis, skull, ribs, vertebrae, and small bones of the feet. Although they often abut on the articular cartilage of a joint, they rarely break into the joint space, but may erode through the cortex to produce an extraosseous mass. This apparent destructiveness can be mistaken for a malignant neoplasm. Radiologically, they appear as a sharply delimited area of radiolucency traversed by trabeculation and mottled with calcific radiodensities.

MORPHOLOGY. These neoplasms rarely exceed 5 cm in diameter. On gross inspection, the tumor is soft, gray to pink, and often punctuated by gritty foci of calcification and areas of hemorrhage or necrosis. Occasionally, there is an abundant chondroid component imparting the consistency of a chondroma or chondrosarcoma. Extensive necrosis may produce grossly visible cystic spaces.

There is great variability microscopically. The dominant theme consists of sheets of round-to-oval cells (chondrocytes or chondroblasts) having rounded or polygonal nuclei often with a longitudinal groove.[50] Scattered mitotic figures are sometimes present. Dispersed within this background are benign multinucleate giant cells having a variable number of nuclei, but in general these cells are smaller than those in the giant cell tumor of bone. Lobules of chondroid material may be abundant or rare, and foci of calcification may be scattered or sufficiently numerous to fuse into lace-like patterns. Blood-filled spaces representing hemorrhage within foci of necrosis may be widely scattered or create the impression of an aneurysmal bone cyst.

Although these tumors may be asymptomatic and discovered only during radiographic studies, most come to attention because of local pain, tenderness, or complaints relative to the adjacent joint. Recognition of these lesions becomes of great importance because almost all are benign and the great danger is overdiagnosis and too radical treatment. There are, however, rare reports of chondroblastomas that have metastasized to the lungs—in the great majority of cases, following attempts at surgical removal, but rarely before any operative manipulation.[51] Despite these exceptional instances, chondroblastomas must be viewed as benign neoplasms, more often sinned against than sinner.

Chondrosarcoma

Among the primary bone cancers, excluding those of hematopoietic origin, chondrosarcoma is second only to osteosarcoma in frequency, occurring about half as often. Chondrosarcomas vary widely in their clinical behavior depending on the level of anaplasia, but most have a slow clinical evolution and metastasize late, providing a much better prognosis than the more aggressive osteosarcomas.

Most chondrosarcomas (approximately 75%) arise de novo and are referred to as "primary." The remaining "secondary" chondrosarcomas arise in preexisting, benign, cartilaginous tumors, such as in multiple enchondromatosis (Ollier's disease and Maffucci's syndrome), exostoses whether solitary or multiple, and rarely chondroblastoma. In addition, several variant types of chondrosarcomas have been segregated, least rare among them being the clear cell pattern, about which a few comments will be offered later. Primary chondrosarcoma occurs primarily in middle to later life, slightly more often in males.

MORPHOLOGY. The majority of primary chondrosarcomas arise in the central skeleton (i.e., ribs, shoulder, and pelvic girdles) and about the knee (Fig. 28–22). Although distal bones may be involved, there is a notable rarity of these neoplasms beyond the ankles and wrists. You will recall that, by contrast, the hands and feet are favored locations for chondromas. Most arise centrally within bone, but a few occur subperiosteally. They range in size from a few centimeters in diameter to large bulky masses. Whether peripheral or central, transection characteristically reveals lobules of gray-white translucent tissue (Fig. 28–23). Central necrosis may create cystic spaces. Spotty calcifications are typically present. The adjacent cortex may be thickened or eroded with extension of the tumor along broad fronts into the surrounding soft tissues.

The histologic distinction between well-differentiated chondrosarcomas and chondromas may be difficult.[52] The essential feature is the identification of anaplasia within the lacunar cells (i.e., hyperchromatic nuclei, two or more cells within a single lacuna, multinucleate cells, and bizarre tumor giant cells) (Fig. 28–24). On the basis of level of anaplasia, these neoplasms are graded 1 to 3, or sometimes 1 to 4, from least to most anaplastic. Of additional aid is evidence of permeation of the abutting cancellous bone with engulfment of normal trabeculae. Equally difficult is the differentiation of chondrosarcomas with foci of ossification from

DISTRIBUTION OF CHONDROSARCOMA

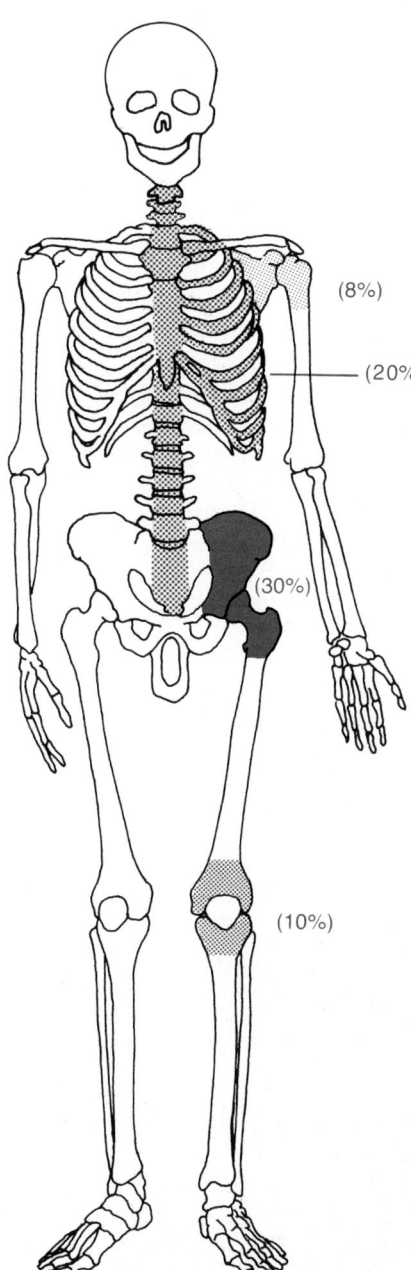

Figure 28-22. The major sites of origin of chondrosarcomas. Numbers in parentheses are approximate percentages. The remaining tumors are scattered throughout the skeleton, including the skull.

osteosarcomas with chondroid differentiation. In general, in the chondrosarcomas the bone formation occurs within cartilage, whereas in osteosarcomas it arises out of a background of anaplastic, osteoblastic-fibroblastic cells.[53]

One particular variant, the clear cell chondrosarcoma, has a distinctly better prognosis than conventional tumors or the other variant patterns. Such chondrosarcomas tend to arise in the epiphysis of the long bones, especially of the

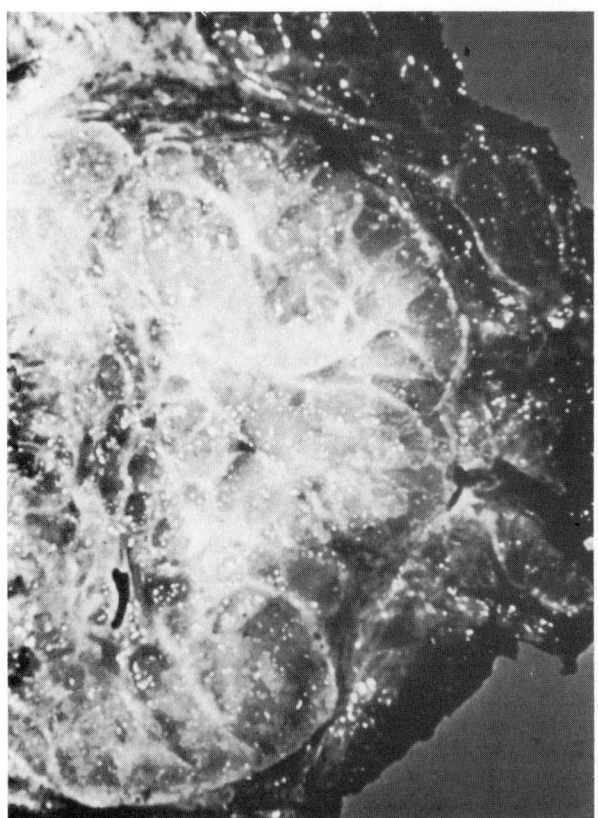

Figure 28-23. Lobulated translucent appearance of transected chondrosarcoma.

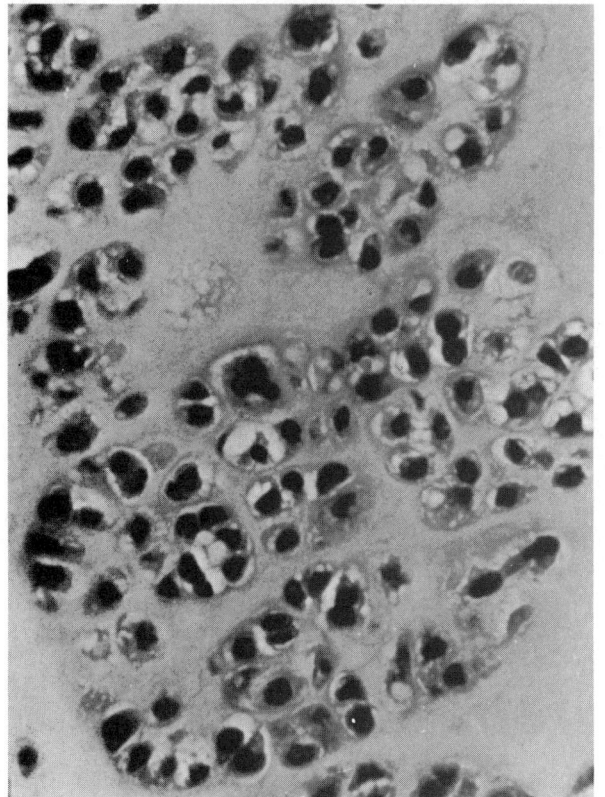

Figure 28-24. Anaplastic chondrocytes within a chondrosarcoma.

proximal femur and humerus, and are rendered distinctive by the cleared cytoplasm of the chondrocytes within the chondroid matrix.[54]

Because most of these neoplasms are remarkably indolent, they come to attention either as a mass that gradually enlarges for years and even decades or because of pain, presumably due to their expansile growth within the bone. Radiographs may be nearly diagnostic. Classically, there is a localized area of bone destruction punctuated by mottled densities from calcification or ossification. They may expand the contour of the bone with either thickening of the cortex or, in some instances, destruction of the cortex with extraosseus extension. It is the "snowstorm" of radiodensities within the lesion that is most pathognomonic.

In most series, about 80 to 90% of chondrosarcomas, whether primary or secondary, fall into grades 1 or 2. Whatever the grade, all require total removal or they stubbornly recur sometimes after five- to ten-year intervals. The higher the grade the more likely a recurrence and the shorter the interval to recurrence. Metastatic dissemination may eventually occur particularly with the higher grade tumors, most commonly to the lungs, liver, kidney, and brain. In one analysis, the five-year survival rates of patients with grades 1, 2, and 3 were 90%, 81%, and 43%, respectively.[55] None of the grades 0 or 1 lesions metastasized, whereas 70% of the grade 3 tumors disseminated. Thus, with chondrosarcomas, more than with most primary bone tumors, histologic analysis is of great prognostic significance.

TUMORS OF UNKNOWN ORIGIN

Two neoplasms—Ewing's sarcoma and giant cell tumors—are of uncertain histogenesis.

Ewing's Sarcoma

Ewing's sarcoma, composed of nondistinctive, small, round cells, has long posed a difficult morphologic and diagnostic problem because the cells lack distinctive features and so resemble those of malignant lymphomas, metastatic neuroblastomas, and other undifferentiated cancers. Some newer findings cited later may be helpful in this respect. When all misidentifications are excluded, Ewing's sarcoma is rare past the third decade of life and has a peak incidence in the second decade. The male preponderance is 2 to 1.[56]

Over the years, the cell of origin of Ewing's sarcomas has been held to be endothelial, pericytic, myeloid, osteoblastic, mesenchymal, or neuroectodermal. It is fruitless to present all of the conflicting evidence relevant to this controversy.[57] It will suffice to say here that the front-runner a few years ago was a mesenchymal cell, but it has been overtaken recently by the neuroectodermal cell for the following reasons. A unique and characteristic reciprocal translocation of a portion of the long arms of chromosomes 11 and 22 has been identified in these tumors.[58] This same chromosomal abnormality has been identified in peripheral neuroepitheliomas and in other neuroectodermal neoplasms. When Ewing's sarcoma cells in culture are exposed to agents known to induce cell differentiation, the nondescript tumor cells undergo neural differentiation.[59] There are, in addition, certain histologic similarities (mentioned later) between Ewing's sarcoma and other neoplasms of presumed neuroectodermal origin, but until there is documentation that the 11/22 chromosomal translocation is not found in non-neural tumors, the cell of origin of Ewing's sarcoma must still be considered uncertain.

MORPHOLOGY. Ewing's sarcoma may occur in any bone of the skeleton with some predilection for long tubular bones and the pelvis. It usually arises in the medullary cavity; origin in an epiphysis would be unusual. Characteristically, it involves large areas or even the entire medullary cavity. The lesional tissue is typically gray-white, is soft, and may be almost puriform. The bone may be expanded. Elevation of the periosteum and subperiosteal new bone for-

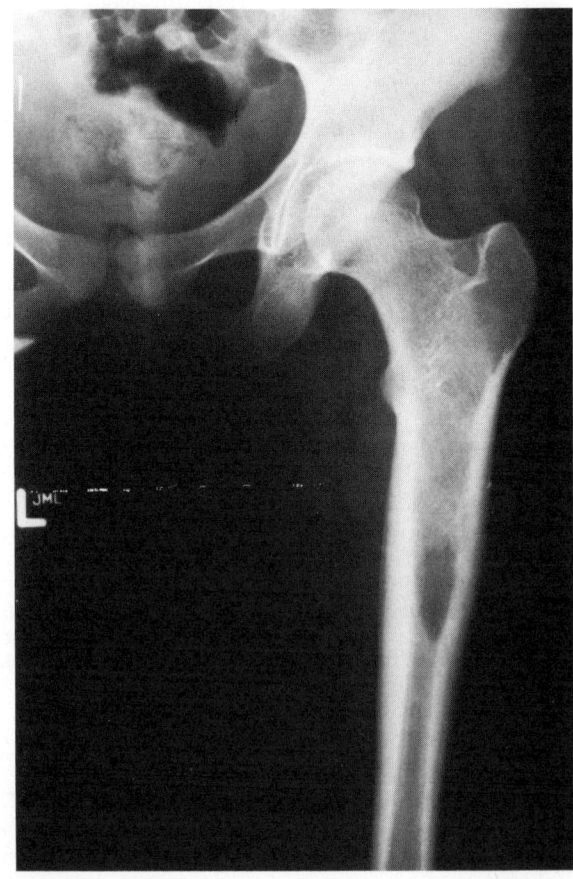

Figure 28-25. Ewing's sarcoma of the femur. The tumor has induced a lytic lesion in the metaphyseal region accompanied by subperiosteal new bone formation with widening of the shaft. (Courtesy of Dr. Herbert Gramm, New England Deaconess Hospital.)

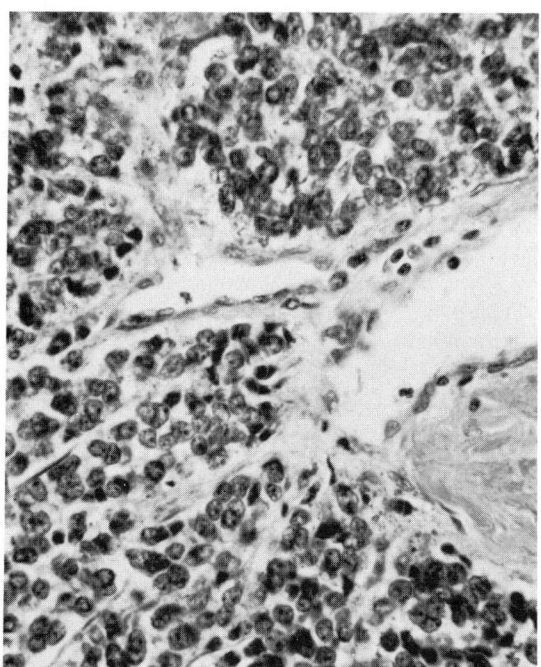

Figure 28-26. Ewing's sarcoma at high power, illustrating characteristic cytology.

mation is characteristic, producing a distinctive radiographic "onion-skin layering" about the cortex and widening the contour of the shaft (Fig. 28–25). Often the tumor ruptures through the cortex to extend into the surrounding soft tissues, sometimes producing a clinically palpable mass.

Histologically, the tumor is composed of sheets of quite uniform, small cells resembling lymphocytes, but they are considerably larger (Fig. 28–26). The cells in occasional tumors are more pleomorphic and have less regular nuclei, features that point to a poorer prognosis, but generally mitotic figures are scant. There is remarkably little intercellular stroma, and much of the tumor may be necrotic; often the best preserved areas rim blood vessels. The tumor cells sometimes ring a central clearing, creating **"pseudorosettes."** Significantly, this feature is typical of neuroblastomas. Intracytoplasmic glycogen (in appropriately preserved tissue) is a distinctive but not pathognomonic feature, as it is present in other primitive tumor cells, including those in osteosarcomas, rhabdomyosarcomas, and neuroblastomas. Equally suggestive of neural origin is the presence of neuron-specific enolase in the cells of some tumors, but most helpful is the identification of the 11/22 chromosomal translocation.

Tumors having identical morphologic features and composed of nondistinctive small round cells have appeared outside of the skeleton and are referred to as **extraosseous Ewing's sarcoma.**

Early in the course, Ewing's sarcoma may masquerade as osteomyelitis. Pain, swelling, tenderness of the affected part, dilated veins, elevated temperature, and increased sedimentation rate are all seen with this form of neoplasia, all suggestive of osteomyelitis. Moreover, at the outset there may be no radiographic changes or only a small focus of ill-defined radiolucency. However, in time, these tumors cause large areas of bone lysis as they erode the cancellous trabeculae and then the cortex from within outward. The continuity of the cortex may be interrupted, but usually the cortex is only mottled owing to spotty bone resorption. Elevation of the periosteum is present in about half of the cases, but it is also seen with osteogenic sarcoma. More typical, but not diagnostic of Ewing's sarcoma, is the radiographic subperiosteal new bone formation creating what has been referred to as "onion-skin layering."

Up to the recent past, the five-year survival rate was 10%. Currently, with combined surgery, chemotherapy, and (in selected cases) radiation, the five-year survival has been measurably improved to between 40 and 75%. Associated with poorer prognosis are pelvic origin and a markedly elevated sedimentation rate. Widespread hematogenous dissemination is the usual cause of death.

Giant Cell Tumors

Giant cell tumors are distinctive neoplasms because they are characterized by a profusion of multinucleate giant cells scattered throughout a stroma of mononuclear cells. The neoplastic elements are the stromal cells, not the giant cells. Because the giant cells have some similarity to osteoclasts, these neoplasms have also been inappropriately called *osteoclastomas.* As will become evident, however, the giant cells are not osteoclasts. Relatively uncommon neoplasms, the great majority occur between the ages of 20 and 40 years, with a slight female preponderance. They are distinctly rare in skeletally immature subjects and infrequent in the advanced years of life.[60] Three aspects of these neoplasms are of particular interest: (1) their cell of origin, (2) their differentiation from other giant cell–bearing lesions, and (3) their biologic behavior.

Speculation about *the histogenesis of these neoplasms* has filled many a "busy" hour for "osseo-oncologists" and fortunately (for them) no conclusion has been reached. The major issues are as follows: (1) Are the stromal mononuclear cells of monocyte-macrophage lineage or are they instead connective tissue cells, and (2) are the multinucleate giant cells derived from osteoclasts or fusion of mononuclear stromal cells?[61] Although still disputed, *the weight of evidence favors a mesenchymal origin for the mononuclear cells and that they are the progenitors of the giant cells.*[62]

The differentiation of these neoplasms from other giant cell-bearing lesions is as important as it is difficult. Multinucleate giant cells are a feature of many non-neoplastic as well as neoplastic lesions of bone. They are particularly prominent in so-called "brown tumors" seen in osteitis fibrosa cystica related to hyperparathyroidism, and in the giant cell granuloma (also called epulis) of the gingiva and jaw bones. These lesions are better referred to as *reparative giant cell granulomas* and are not true neoplasms. Multinu-

DISTRIBUTION OF GIANT CELL TUMORS

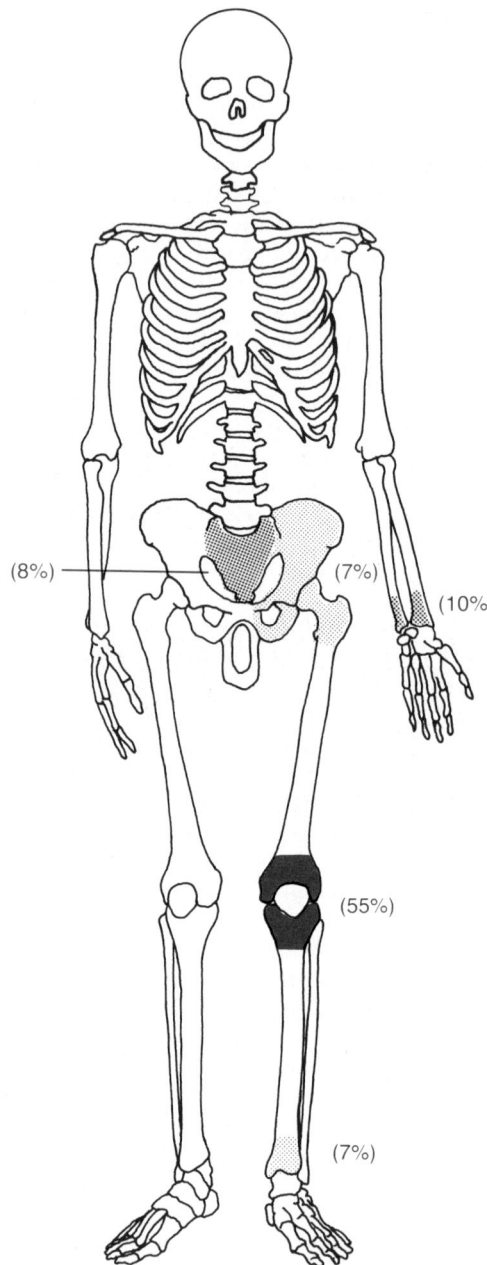

Figure 28-27. The major sites of origin of giant cell tumors. Numbers in parentheses are approximate percentages.

MORPHOLOGY.   Giant cell tumors nearly always arise within the epiphyses, but may then spread into the metaphyses or even through the articular cartilage into the joint space. **Over half of these lesions occur about the knee (in the distal femur, proximal tibia), or proximal fibula,** but virtually any other bone may be involved, including sacrum, pelvis, long bones of the forearm, and the small bones of the hands and feet (Fig. 28–27). Although most are solitary lesions, multiple or multicentric tumors are encountered rarely.[63]

Characteristically, they are multilobular and red-brown on cut surface, with prominent areas of hemorrhage, cyst formation, and foci of pale, yellow-white necrosis. Most are large and have undergone fairly rapid increase in size with clublike expansion of the end of the bone (Fig. 28–28). In this expansion the cortex may be thinned or even eroded. Rarely, the tumors penetrate into the surrounding soft tissue, but despite this invasive behavior, they tend to grow as cohesive masses along broad lobulated fronts.

Histologically, giant cell tumors are composed mainly of nondistinctive mononuclear cells having round to oval to spindle-shaped nuclei remarkably uniform in size. Mitotic figures are often numerous, even in lesions that later prove to be entirely curable by local resection. Scattered within this background are numerous giant cells having as many as 100 benign-appearing nuclei resembling those in the mononuclear cells (Figs. 28–29 and 28–30). There may be foci of necrosis, hemorrhage, hemosiderin deposition, and osteoid formation. Chondroid foci are unusual and when prominent strongly suggest the diagnosis of chondroblastoma. In the unusual giant cell tumors that are malignant from the outset, the stromal mononuclear cells are anaplastic.

cleate giant cells are also encountered in many benign and malignant bone tumors. Chondroblastomas in particular pose a challenging diagnostic problem because they have many multinucleate giant cells and moreover they often arise in the epiphyseal ends of bones, where giant cell tumors arise. Because the chondroblastoma is rarely malignant, but 3 to 10% of giant cell tumors prove to be malignant, the importance of the differential is evident.

The *biologic behavior of giant cell tumors* is an equally challenging feature of these neoplasms, as will become evident.

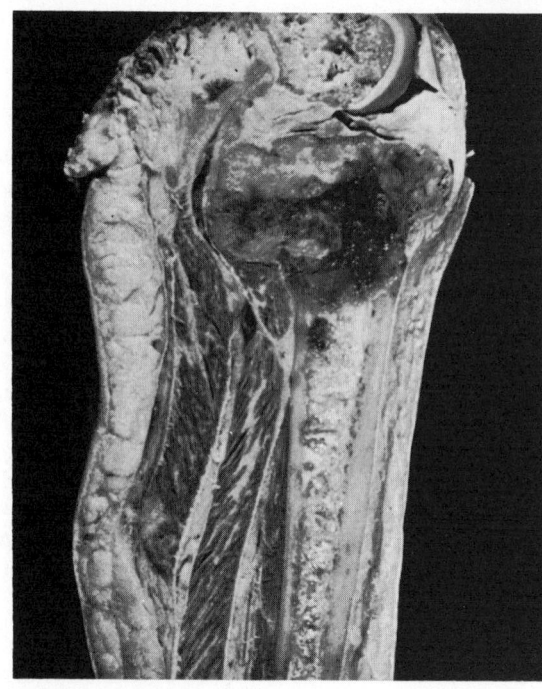

Figure 28-28. Benign giant cell tumor of upper end of tibia. Tumor has produced an ovoid enlargement, expanding epiphysis.

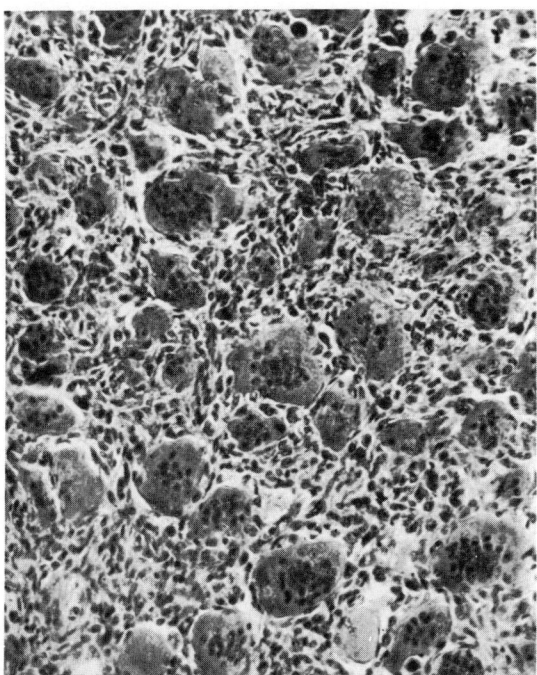

Figure 28-29. Benign giant cell tumor, illustrating abundance of multinucleate giant cells.

Patients with these neoplasms usually present with nonspecific complaints of local pain, tenderness, functional disability, and occasionally pathologic fracture. However, in many instances the tumors grow insidiously to massive size to produce externally palpable masses before discovery. Radiographs are

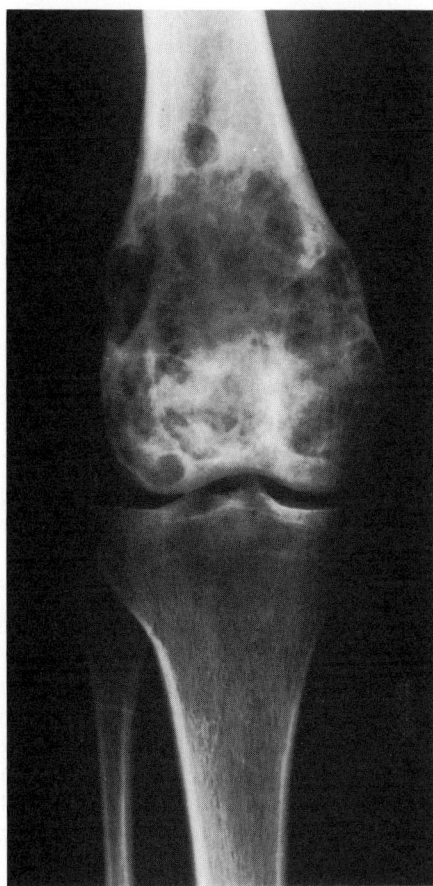

Figure 28-31. Giant cell tumor. The lytic lesion has expanded the lower end of the femur and abuts on the articular cartilage.

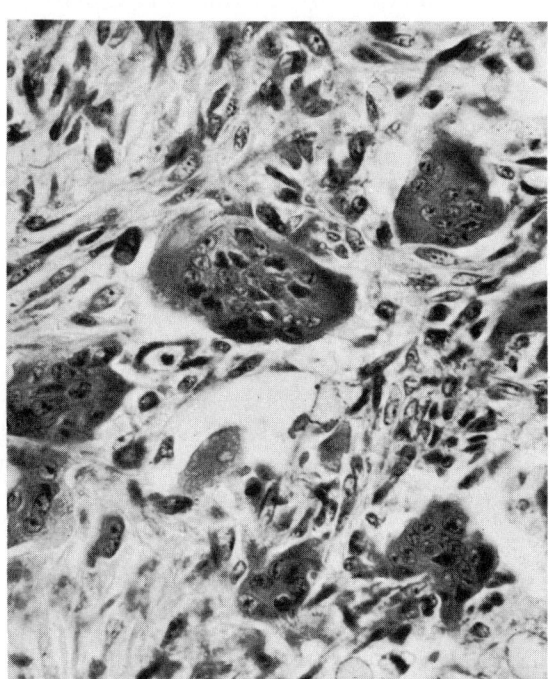

Figure 28-30. High-power detail of giant cells and well-differentiated stroma in benign giant cell tumor.

distinctive, but not pathognomonic, and reveal large, lytic, "soap-bubble" lesions within the epiphysis usually abutting on the articular cartilage (Fig. 28–31). Notably absent are stippling and calcifications. A thinned-out but usually preserved cortex surrounds the lesion, although, as was pointed out, aggressive neoplasms may break out or erode into the joint space.

The biologic unpredictability of these neoplasms complicates their clinical management. The great majority of giant cell tumors are benign histologically and can be eradicated by curettage or conservative resections to preserve function. However, *recurrences are very frequent (25 to 50%) and occur possibly as late as 20 to 30 years after the initial resection.* Most of the recurrences appear benign despite the fact that sometimes there are histologically "benign" metastases in the lungs. It is evident that prognostication based on histology is of little value with these lesions. In about 10% of recurrences, there are overt sarcomatous changes, frequently (but not always) in irradiated cases. In addition, a small number of giant cell tumors are overtly anaplastic and malignant from the outset. With these de novo and recurrent cancers, the five-year mortality rate is approximately 80%.

JOINS AND RELATED STRUCTURES

NORMAL

The joints of the skeleton vary widely in structure and function, and also in predisposition to disease. Those which are nearly rigid (e.g., the calvarial sutures, symphysis pubis) almost never are involved in disease. Joints having limited mobility (e.g., the vertebrae with their intervertebral discs) are frequent sources of symptoms, as every sufferer from a "bad back" knows. But remarkably little is known about the disorders causing such back pain save for such nebulous entities as muscular or ligamentous strains or "degeneration," rupture, or prolapse of intervertebral discs. Perhaps humans were not designed to walk on their "hind legs."

Much more is known about disorders of articulating diarthrodial joints. The ends of the bones in such joints are capped by articular cartilage and the joint space is lined by synovial membrane, save in the cartilaginous, weight-bearing areas. The surface of this membrane is thrown up into innumerable microvilli covered by a layer one to several cells deep, consisting of synoviocytes of two types. The more common, type A, is closely related to macrophages and is phagocytic and synthesizes degradative enzymes, principally collagenases. Type B synoviocytes synthesize mucinous hyaluronic acid. Underlying these surface cells is a thin layer of loose connective tissue containing variable numbers of mononuclear cells, interdigitating dendritic cells, blood vessels, lymphatics, and nerve filaments. The synovial fluid that lubricates diarthrodial joints is composed of a vascular transudate admixed with mucin. Normally the fluid is clear and viscid (owing to its contained glycoproteins), is colorless, contains fewer than 200 white cells/mm³ (mostly mononuclear leukocytes), and forms a mucinous clot on addition of acetic acid.

The articular cartilage is a unique connective tissue ideally suited to serve as an elastic shock absorber and wear-resistant surface. Although the ends of apposing bones within a joint are remarkably contoured to fit each other, there is not perfect congruence and, therefore, uneven load distribution. However, the maximum load per unit of area is limited in health by protective mechanisms such as increasing congruence with increasing load, marginal elasticity of the subchondral bone, and muscular adaptations to joint loading. Despite its lack of nerves, lymphatics, and blood vessels, articular cartilage is a metabolically active tissue. The contained chondrocytes synthesize the cartilaginous matrix. These cells also have the capacity to synthesize collagenases and other proteinases, and may thus contribute to degradation of the articular cartilage in disease. The bland-appearing cartilaginous matrix is in active turnover and highly specialized. It is composed mainly of collagen type II and proteoglycans, with smaller components of other glycoproteins and several proteinase inhibitors. The collagen fibers provide the structural integrity and the hydrophilic proteoglycans the resiliency because of the "bottle-brush" spatial configuration of these molecules and the large amounts of water bound between the "bristles." It is evident that diarthrodial joints are complicated hinges.

PATHOLOGY

Joint disease is commonplace in clinical medicine. Various surveys indicate that about 1 to 5% of the American population under 45, and 15 to 85% (depending on criteria) of older individuals suffer from some form of arthritis—mainly osteoarthritis and rheumatoid arthritis. Primary attention here is devoted to these two disorders, but other disorders such as gout and less common arthropathies also require consideration.

OSTEOARTHRITIS (OA) (DEGENERATIVE JOINT DISEASE, DJD)

Despite being the most common form of arthritis, little is known about the cause of OA. *Basically, this condition is characterized by progressive deterioration and loss of articular cartilage over the years, mainly in weight-bearing joints, leading to subchondral bony thickening and bony outgrowths — osteophytes ("spurs") — about the joint margins.* Mobility may be impaired, but destruction of the joint space and ankylosis do not occur. Sometimes one of the first manifestations of OA is the presence of knobby, bony protrusions at the margins of the distal interphalangeal joints creating nontender, harmless, subcutaneous *Heberden's nodes.*

OA occurs in two clinical patterns — primary and secondary. *Primary OA* is one of the dubious rewards of reaching the "golden years"; it appears de novo in a small number of individuals, mostly males in midlife, but the frequency increases steadily, particularly in women, to reach 80 to 85% of the population over the age of 70.[64] Fortunately, in many individuals, it is largely asymptomatic. *Secondary OA* may appear at any age in any previously damaged or congenitally abnormal joint. The relationship to age and previous injury account for the view that this form of arthritis is essentially a "wear and tear" phenomenon. Hence some have preferred the designation *"degenerative joint disease,"* but like an old soldier, historically sanctified "osteoarthritis" refuses to fade away.

The morphology will be presented before the consideration of pathogenesis.

MORPHOLOGY. The weight-bearing joints — vertebrae, hips, knees — bear the brunt of the disease, but in addition, the distal and proximal interphalangeal joints of the fingers and the first carpometacarpal and metatarsophalangeal joints may also be involved. The wrists, elbows, and shoulders are seldom involved. Usually the disease is limited to a few joints, but it can be widespread. The pattern of involvement is influenced by the cumulative stresses of life (e.g., the metatarsophalangeal joints in ballet dancers, the knees and hips in letter carriers). In experimental models of OA, the earliest changes are loss of proteoglycans and decreased metachromasia in the articular cartilage. There is concomitant focal loss of chondrocytes and in other areas reactive proliferation of cartilage cells marked by crowding of cells and increased basophilia of the matrix. These changes are followed by fissuring, pitting, and flaking of the articular cartilage and the development of vertical clefts, which may extend down to the subchondral bone. The regressive alterations are most marked in areas subjected to overloading (discussed later). With progression, the fissures deepen and pieces of cartilage break off, exposing subchondral bone, which becomes vascularized, thickened, and ivory-like (eburnation) as continued joint motion polishes the surface. In other areas, death of osteocytes or increased osteoclastic activity leads to bony rarefaction, microcyst formation, and sometimes microfractures.[65] The collective changes malform the contours of the ends of the bones, sometimes causing flattening or mushroom-like deformation of the articular ends of the bone.

Controversy continues as to whether inflammatory changes in the synovial membrane precede the cartilaginous changes or follow them. In any event, such synovitis as is present is nonspecific, is not severe, and does not form a pannus, as occurs in rheumatoid arthritis. Osseous metaplasia of synovial connective tissue or cartilaginous outgrowths from the margins of the joint that later become ossified create the osteophytes ("spurs") mentioned earlier. In the vertebrae, when closely apposed, they may cause some limitation of motion, but only rarely do they fuse to produce bony ankylosis (Fig. 28–32). The osteophytes produce the Heberden's nodes mentioned earlier. Fragments of spurs or cartilage may form free "joint mice."

PATHOGENESIS. Any theory of pathogenesis should satisfactorily incorporate the following observations.[66]

• Affected joints suffer from uneven overloading leading to altered lines of weight-bearing, deranged chondrocyte function and focal death, and reactive proliferation of chondrocytes.
• In developed OA, there are increased intra-articular levels of collagenase, neutral proteases, and degradative products of proteoglycans.
• Nonspecific synovitis is usually present in involved joints.

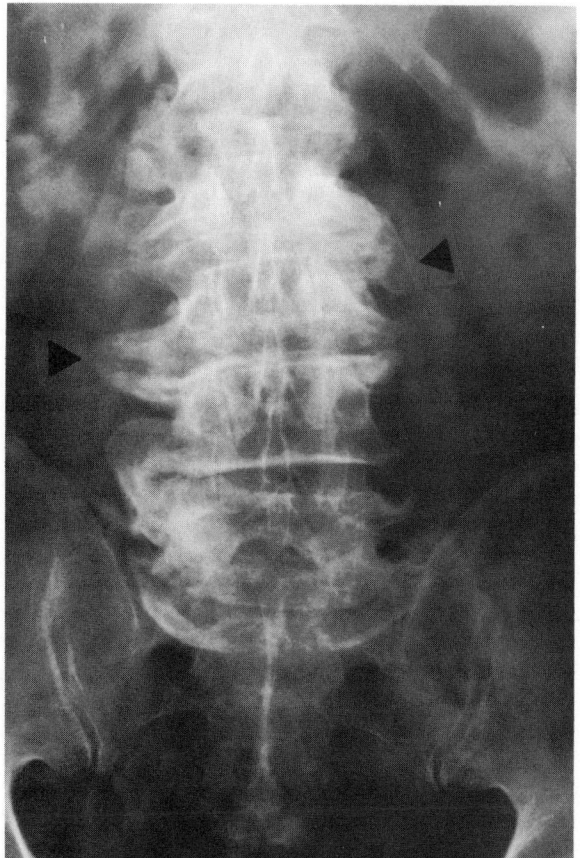

Figure 28-32. Extensive osteoarthritis with marked spur formations *(arrows)* **along lateral margins of intervertebral disc spaces. (Courtesy of Dr. John O'Connor, Boston University Medical Center.)**

• Remodeling of subchondral bone with the changes described is prominent in evolved OA, altering the support for the articular cartilage.

Two somewhat similar proposals have been made to accommodate these observations. They can be categorized as (1) the biomechanical theory and (2) the biochemical theory.

The *biomechanical theory* proposes that excessive joint loading produces altered stresses that derange normal chondrocyte function, leading to an imbalance between matrix mobilization and synthesis. Thus, some areas of cartilage become softened and vulnerable to flaking and fissuring. Chondrocyte injury might further predispose to release of collagenases and other proteases, contributing to the matrix and cartilage breakdown. The articular alterations might then produce a secondary synovitis with mononuclear cell infiltration, leading to release from monocytes or macrophages of inflammatory mediators such as IL-1 (mostly beta). This cytokine has the capacity to stimulate release of lytic enzymes from chondrocytes and synoviocytes and to inhibit proteoglycan synthesis. The changes in the subchondral bone may also be the consequence of altered weight-bearing, and by

weakening the underlying support, predispose to further cartilage injury. However, whether the bony changes antedate or follow the cartilage injury is uncertain.

The *biochemical theory* places more emphasis on early impairment of the integrity of cartilage by collagenases and other lytic enzymes.[67] This theory proposes that aging or abnormal stresses initiate the injury by inducing a synovitis with the release of enzymes and cytokines, damaging the metabolic integrity of the cartilage, which is then followed by the changes described.[68] The two theories differ only in the events that initiate the changes (Fig. 28–33). It is highly likely that both are correct in particular instances.

CLINICAL COURSE. Osteoarthritis is an insidious disease that may remain asymptomatic. When overt it is usually first noticed as transient slight stiffness or decreased mobility, most prominent in the morning on arising. Usually, after resuming motion for a short time, the stiffness, and sometimes the pain, subsides but recurs late in the day with prolonged use or undue activity. These manifestations are most prominent in the hips, knees, and back. Often even before definite

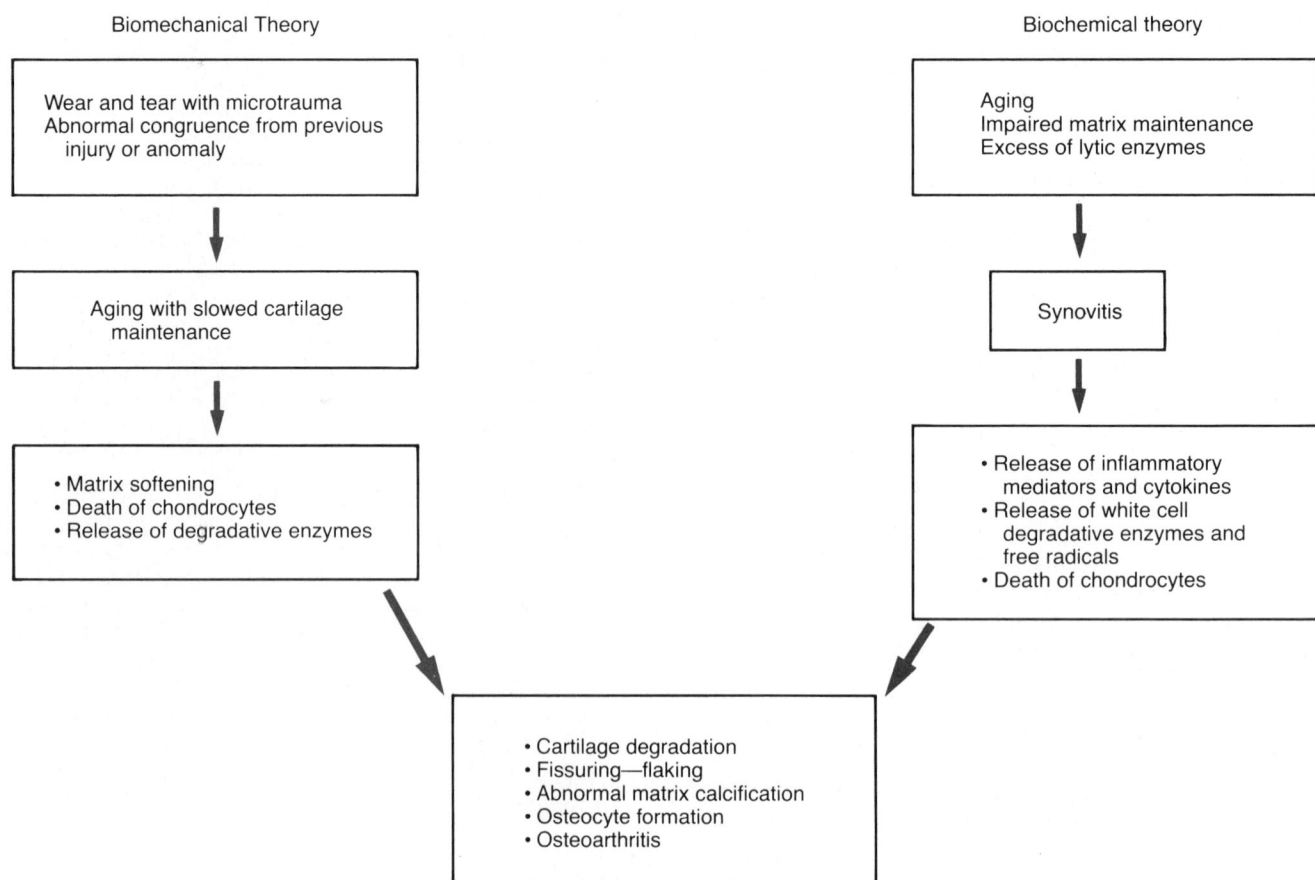

OSTEOARTHRITIS

Figure 28-33. Theories of the development of osteoarthritis.

joint discomfort comes to attention, Heberden's nodes may appear. They are more common in women than in men, have a familial distribution, and may be an autosomal dominant trait. With more advanced joint disease the pain and disability are more protracted. There is usually no evidence of local heat or tenderness, but the joints may have a restricted range of motion, small effusions, and crepitus. Osteophytes may impinge on spinal foramina and cause cervical and lumbar nerve root compression, with radicular pain, muscle spasms, muscle atrophy, and neurologic abnormalities. Involvement of the distal interphalangeal joints may cause stiffness and decreased mobility of the fingers.

There is no satisfactory means of preventing this condition nor any method known for its arrest. The disorder may stabilize for years at any stage but more often is slowly progressive over the remaining years of life, and joins atherosclerosis and cancer as a dividend of the "golden years."

RHEUMATOID ARTHRITIS (RA)

Rheumatoid arthritis is a multisystem, chronic, relapsing, inflammatory disease of unknown cause. Although the skin, eyes, heart, lungs, and other organs may be affected, *RA is basically a severe form of chronic synovitis that sometimes leads to destruction and ankylosis of affected joints.* On the other hand, in the fortunate individual the disease may be mild and of brief duration with little impairment of joint function. The course is highly unpredictable. It is estimated that about 1% of the world's population suffers from RA. Females are affected three times more often than males, with a peak prevalence in the third to fourth decades of life. There is an increased frequency of RA among first degree relatives and an approximately 30% concordance rate in monozygous twins. A complex association exists between RA and HLA genes. The major association is with HLA-DR4, present in about 70% of whites or Japanese with the disease as compared with 28% of controls. Relatively fewer black Americans and Israeli Jews have the DR4 haplotype.[69] Individuals who lack DR4 specificities have an increased frequency of DR1, but the linkage is less strong. The well-known association between HLA class II antigens and immune response genes raises the possibility of particular immunologic susceptibility to this disease.

Before the possible origins of this condition are considered, the morphology will be reviewed.

MORPHOLOGY

MUSCULOSKELETAL SYSTEM. The major anatomic changes are found in the joints. **RA generally first affects the small joints of the hands and feet, but then may involve, usually symmetrically, the wrists, elbows, ankles, and knees.** Typically, the proximal interphalangeal

and metacarpophalangeal joints are affected, but the distal interphalangeal joints are spared. Uncommonly, the upper cervical spine is involved, but for obscure reasons rarely the lumbosacral spine. Analogously, the hips are usually spared. The arthritis begins with a nondistinctive, inflammatory, edematous thickening of the synovia. With progression, **the characteristic changes appear in the form of a diffuse, proliferative synovitis with (1) marked thickening of the synovial membrane, forming edematous, villous projections that extend into the joint space, (2) multilayering of the synoviocytes over the thickened villous membrane, (3) an intense infiltration of the synovia with macrophages, lymphocytes, and plasma cells, sometimes with the formation of lymphoid follicles, and (4) in some instances, foci of fibrin deposition and necrosis within the synovia (Fig. 28–34). The exuberant inflammatory synovium that covers the articular surfaces is known as a pannus.** As the synovitis progresses, periarticular soft tissue edema may appear, which classically produces fusiform redness and swelling of the proximal interphalangeal joints. Eventually, the pannus fills the joint space, covering the articular surfaces. Release of enzymes and mediators from the highly vascularized, inflammatory

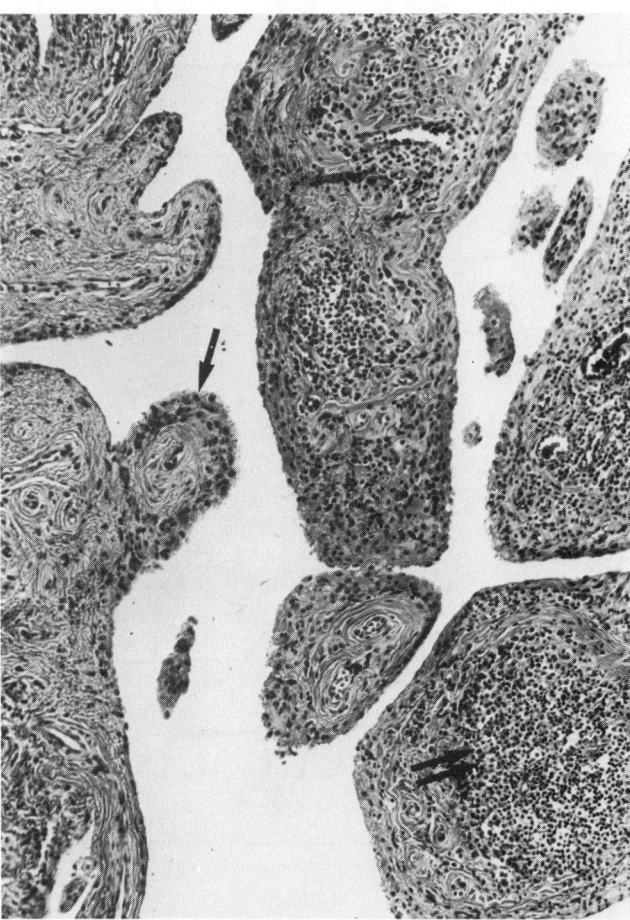

Figure 28-34. Rheumatoid arthritis. The villous hypertrophy of the synovium is shown with proliferation of the synoviocytes *(arrow)* and aggregates of inflammatory cells *(double arrows)* within the villi.

PROGRESSION OF RHEUMATOID ARTHRITIS

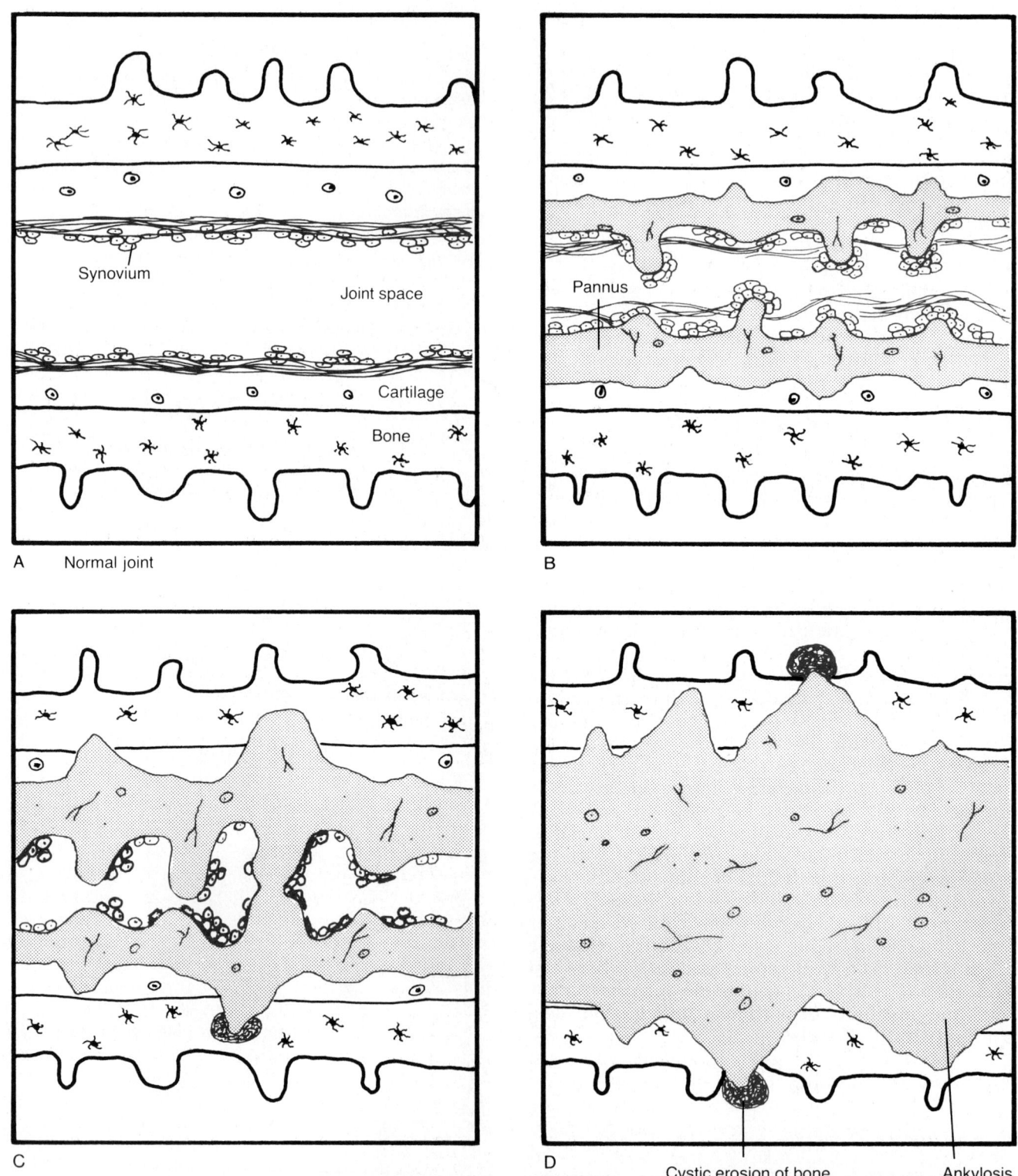

Figure 28-35. Rheumatoid arthritis — its progressive development. *A,* The normal joint with thin synovium. *B,* Polypoid fibrovascular thickening of the synovium with synoviocyte hyperplasia, producing a pannus that is eroding into articular cartilage. *C,* Continued growth of the pannus and erosion of cartilage with penetration into the subchondral bone and cyst formation. *D,* Complete filling of joint space with pannus producing ankylosis of the joint.

pannus progressively damages the cartilage. There follows invasion of the cartilage by the pannus, producing irregular erosions and sometimes fragmentation. The subchondral bone may also undergo demineralization and cystic resorption owing to released enzymes and pannus invasion. In time, the pannus undergoes organization, leading at first to bridging fibrous bands (fibrous ankylosis) and ultimately to bony ankylosis. In this manner, function is totally destroyed with the production of fairly typical joint deformities described later (Fig. 28–35).

While the early chronic inflammatory changes are developing in the synovial membrane, an acute inflammatory reaction takes place within the synovial fluid. Early in the disease, the volume increases, the fluid becomes turbid because of an accumulation of neutrophils, mononuclear leukocytes, and possibly red cells, and the mucin content is diluted (thus forming a poor mucin clot when exposed to dilute acetic acid). Some of the neutrophils, called **RA cells,** reveal granular intracytoplasmic inclusions of phagocytized immune complexes.

Tendinomuscular involvement frequently accompanies the arthritis. Focal areas of inflammation in tendons, muscles, and periarticular connective tissue may appear about inflamed joints; in addition, in more remote muscles, such inflammation is manifested by collections of lymphocytes, plasma cells, and macrophages.

SKIN. Subcutaneous **rheumatoid nodules** appear in about one quarter of the patients, particularly those with rapidly progressive disease. Favored sites are pressure points, such as elbows, backs of the forearms, and back of the skull. **They are firm, nontender, round to oval, palpable subcutaneous masses, rarely exceeding 2 cm in diameter. Histologically, they have a central focus of fibrinoid necrosis surrounded by an intense inflammatory infiltrate of palisaded epithelioid cells, external to which are numerous lymphocytes, macrophages, and plasma cells** (Fig. 28–36). Less commonly, rheumatoid nodules are found in the lungs, spleen, pericardium, myocardium, heart valves, aorta, and other internal organs.

BLOOD VESSELS. A nonspecific, **acute vasculitis** may appear in patients with severe RA and high titers of circulating immune complexes. The histologic changes range from a venulitis, most often in the skin, to random, sometimes systemic, necrotizing arteritis resembling polyarteritis nodosa. However, the kidneys are usually spared in rheumatoid arteritis. The cutaneous venulitis may produce palpable purpura, whereas cutaneous arteritis may cause large ischemic ulcers.

OTHER ORGANS. Nonspecific inflammatory changes or rheumatoid nodules may be found in the lungs, pleura, pericardium, myocardium, and peripheral nerves. Inflammatory changes in the **eyes** sometimes appear in the form of nonspecific conjunctivitis, keratoconjunctivitis, or uveitis.

ETIOLOGY AND PATHOGENESIS.

Most widely held, although not proved, is the view that RA is an autoimmune disease.[70] About 80% of patients with RA have a circulating autoantibody called rheumatoid

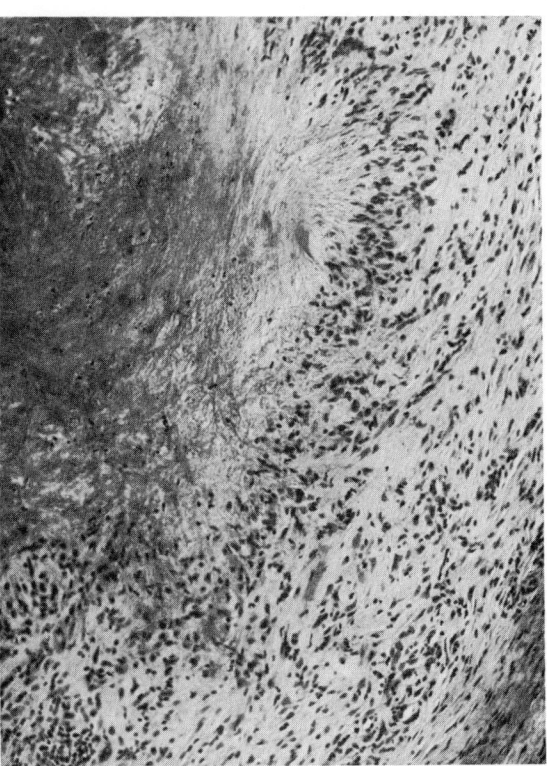

Figure 28-36. Subcutaneous rheumatoid nodule with an area of necrosis *(upper left)* **surrounded by a palisade of fibroblasts and white cells.**

factor (RF) against the Fc portion of autologous IgG. Most of the RF is IgM, but some is IgG, IgA, or IgE. All types of RF form immune complexes with autologous (?altered) IgG. The IgG-RF, in particular, is of interest because it is a rare instance in which the same molecule functions as the antigen and antibody. It appears to be also synthesized locally within joints and by self-association forms immune complexes within the articular spaces that activate complement with the formation of the strongly chemotactic fractions $C3_a$ and $C5_a$. The resultant accumulation of neutrophils contributes, as will be seen, to the pathogenesis of the joint disease. Other autoantibodies are also present in some patients with RA, including antinuclear antibodies, antibodies to collagen, and antibodies to cytoskeletal filamentous proteins. Circulating immune complexes are thought to underlie the wide-ranging extra-articular manifestations of RA.

Cell-mediated immunity is also activated in RA. The interface between the pannus with its numerous inflammatory cells and the cartilage is the site of most active cartilaginous destruction.[71] In the inflamed synovium, dendritic cells and macrophages (antigen-presenting) are scattered among a profusion of lymphocytes, predominantly T4 "helper-inducer" cells and fewer T8 "suppressor" cells. The proximity of T cells and antigen-presenting cells speaks in favor of a cell-mediated immune reaction.

What initiates the autoimmune reaction, and what mechanisms mediate the articular destruction?

The answers are unknown, but many possibilities have been raised, which fall into two general categories. The first proposes the existence of an extrinsic antigen, such as Epstein-Barr virus (EBV), which induces a synovitis, releasing articular antigens. Alternatively, virus-specific T cells might localize in the joints, either because of local accumulation of antigen or because of cross-reactive antigens within the joints. However, there is no substantial evidence linking the EBV or any other infectious agent with RA. The second general line of speculation invokes the possibility of an aberrant clone of DR4 or DR1 positive lymphocytes reactive against synovial antigens. Conceivably, nonspecific polyclonal activation by the EBV might augment the reactivity. These cells might then produce the joint injury. Both theoretical pathways could lead to T cell–B cell interactions with the production of the numerous autoantibodies described.

There is no shortage of potential mediators of the destruction of the cartilage and subjacent bone. These can be summarized briefly as follows.

- *Neutrophils* in the synovial fluid release reactive free radicals and lysosomal enzymes, initiating the inflammation, while released proteinases and proteoglycanases degrade the cartilage.[72] Simultaneously, the neutrophils generate prostaglandins (particularly PGE_2, which in vitro damages cartilage and bone) and leukotrienes, such as LTB_4, which augments the accumulation of neutrophils.
- *Synovial lining cells*, when activated by inflammation or phagocytosis of immune complexes, elaborate collagenase and large amounts of PGE_2 and IL-1 (mostly beta). The prostaglandins must also play an important role in causing the pain of the rheumatoid joint, because inhibition of cyclooxygenase by nonsteroidal anti-inflammatory drugs (e.g., aspirin) is very effective for symptomatic relief.[73] The contribution of IL-1 is discussed below.[73a]
- *Lymphocytes* are thought to play an important role. The predominant infiltrating cell, as noted earlier, is the T4 cell. In response to both the initiating antigen, whatever it may be, and appropriate class II molecules on antigen-presenting cells, the activated T cells produce a variety of lymphokines, such as interleukin 2, gamma-interferon, macrophage migration inhibition factor, and macrophage activating factor. Furthermore, as already noted, the T cells cooperate with the B cells in the production of the numerous autoantibodies characteristic of RA.
- *Macrophages* are considered the major players. Once "turned on" by T4 lymphocytes, macrophages elaborate—in addition to lytic enzymes and prostaglandins—a variety of monokines, including IL-1 and tumor necrosis factor (TNF). Currently, IL-1 is accorded a central role, because it is capable of (1) stimulating synthesis and release of collagenase by stellate or dendritic cells and synovial fibroblasts, (2) activating and stimulating chondrocytes with release of PGE_2, collagenase, and other lytic enzymes, (3)

inhibiting synthesis of proteoglycans by chondrocytes, (4) serving as an osteoclast-activating factor, and (5) acting as a chemoattractant for neutrophils and lymphocytes. *In short, IL-1 could well be a major mediator of rheumatoid arthritis.* We know less about TNF, but its functions more or less parallel those of IL-1.[74]

In summary, a large number of potential immunologic pathways have been identified leading to the release of cytokines and enzymes, which serve as the ultimate mediators of the chronic, proliferative, erosive synovitis characteristic of RA. However, what triggers these reactions remains unknown.

CLINICAL COURSE. As stated, the clinical course of RA is extremely variable. In most patients, the disease begins insidiously with malaise, fatigue, nonlocalized musculoskeletal pain, and sometimes low grade fever. Only later do joints become involved, sometimes monarticular, at other times oligoarticular, and in some instances, polyarticular (usually symmetrically). *Typically, there is local swelling, redness, and pain about the joints and particularly stiffness on arising or following inactivity.* In a minority of cases, the onset is acute, with polyarticular involvement almost from the outset and rapidly progressive deterioration of joint function. In the usual instance, the joint involvement slowly becomes more evident, with at first minimal limitation of motion that in time becomes marked. At this stage, radiographs may reveal juxta-articular osteopenia, narrowing of the joint space with loss of articular cartilage, and ultimately erosion of bone. *Characteristic deformities may develop, such as radial deviation of the wrist with ulnar deviation of the fingers* (Fig. 28–37).

Laboratory studies can support the diagnosis but are not definitive. Usually there is a mild anemia, an increased erythrocyte sedimentation rate, and RF seropositivity (in 80% of patients). However, it should be cautioned that a significant minority of patients, possibly a distinctive subset, lack RF and moreover RF is also present in up to 5% of normal individuals; it is also significantly increased in titer in other disease states, such as cirrhosis, sarcoidosis, leprosy, and viral hepatitis. However, there is some correlation between the severity and progression of the disease and the RF titer. Synovial fluid analysis, as pointed out, can support but not establish the diagnosis. The plasma IL-1 level is raised in active disease.

Extra-articular manifestations, although relatively infrequent, complicate the clinical diagnosis. Rarely they are the presenting features of the disease. They tend to develop in individuals with high titers of RF. Prominent among them are subcutaneous rheumatoid nodules, but pleuropulmonary, vascular, and arterial involvements make RA a multisystem disease that must be differentiated from other collagen-vascular diseases and other forms of arthritis. Because of the diagnostic difficulties, criteria have been established for the classification of RA into classic, definite, probable, and possible categories.[75]

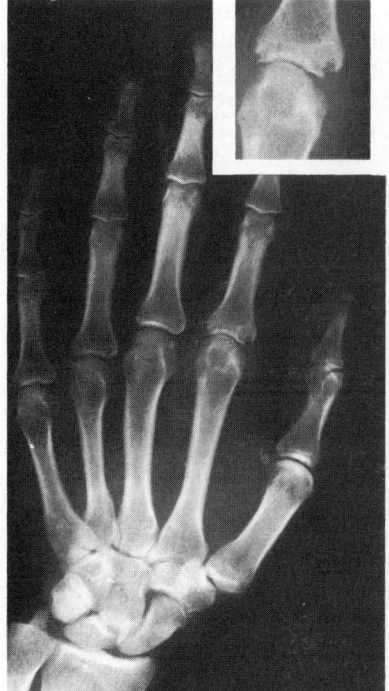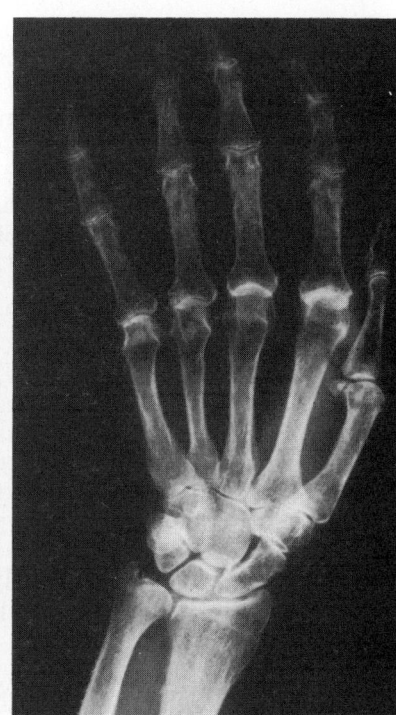

Figure 28-37. Rheumatoid arthritis. *A*, Early disease, most marked in second metacarpophalangeal joint where there is narrowing of joint space and marginal erosions on both radial and ulnar aspects of proximal phalanx *(see inset)*. *B*, More advanced disease with loss of articular cartilage, narrowing of joint spaces of virtually all the small joints, and ulnar deviation of fingers. There is dislocation of second, third, and fourth proximal phalanges produced by advanced articular disease. (Courtesy of Dr. John O'Connor, Boston University Medical Center.)

A **B**

It is difficult to prognosticate the course of RA. The fortunate patient with mild onset may have transient disease with no sequelae. In most patients, there is fluctuating activity over a period of years, with the greatest progression occurring during the initial four to five years. Sometimes, after a period of progressive damage, the disease becomes quiescent and stabilizes. At the other end of the scale are those unfortunate persons who go from acute onset to crippling deformity within a few years. Overall, life expectancy is shortened, with a roughly twofold increase in mortality over that expected for comparable cohorts. Some part of the increased mortality is caused by gastrointestinal bleeding related to long-term use of aspirin, by infections potentiated through chronic use of steroids, and by the development of reactive amyloidosis, particularly in those with protracted severe disease.

VARIANT JOINT INVOLVEMENTS

Variants of RA include juvenile RA, Felty's syndrome, and some cases of arthritis associated with Sjögren's syndrome. Some disorders, e.g., those associated with inflammatory bowel disease and ankylosing spondylitis, tend to attack joint ligamentous structures. Only a few are described here; several of the others are discussed elsewhere.

Juvenile rheumatoid arthritis is sometimes referred to as *Still's disease*. Approximately 5% of patients with RA are under 16 years of age and have the juvenile form of the disease. The disease differs from the usual form of RA in several respects. It is more often marked by an acute febrile onset, weeks to months before joint manifestations appear. About one third of patients have involvement of only one or a few joints, most often the knees or ankles. Generalized lymphadenopathy and hepatosplenomegaly are more prominent in this juvenile variant than in the classic disease. RF is present only infrequently. Despite these differences, the joint changes are identical to those in classic RA.[76] In passing we might note that occasionally the acute, febrile, systemic form of arthropathy may have its onset in adult life, when it is termed *Still's disease.*

Felty's syndrome is another variant of RA that comprises the constellation of splenomegaly, manifestations of hypersplenism such as leukopenia, and leg ulcers associated with the characteristic polyarticular RA. In these patients the hematologic derangements (p. 749) may dominate the clinical course.[77]

Ankylosing spondylitis, also known as *rheumatoid spondylitis* and *Marie-Strümpell disease*, is a distinctive form of inflammatory arthritis, mainly localized to the spine. The sacroiliac joints are always affected, but the hip and shoulder joints are involved only sometimes. The peripheral joints are rarely involved, as in classic RA. This is a disease predominantly of young men and is of unknown cause. There is, however, a strong association between this condition and HLA-B27, found in approximately 90 to 95% of patients. Hereditary influences appear to play a role, because about one quarter of close relatives also have symptomatic or asymptomatic spondylitis. There is also a small group of inflammatory diseases associated with HLA-B27 and ankylosing spondylitis, including inflammatory bowel disease, Reiter's syndrome, Yersinia arthritis, and acute anterior uveitis. In these settings, there is no male preponderance. The anatomic changes encountered in the spine and sacroiliac joints comprise inflammation of ligamentous insertions, e.g., on the vertebral bodies, followed eventually by fibrous and bony ankylosis. As a result, vertebral mobility is impaired, and in severe cases there is fusion of the vertebral bodies and immobilization of affected regions of the spine.

ARTHRITIS ASSOCIATED WITH RHEUMATIC FEVER

It will be remembered that acute rheumatic fever is classically associated with a *migratory polyarthritis* (p. 629). Although such joint involvement is a principal clinical manifestation of this disease, the arthritic involvement, usually spontaneously or with appropriate therapy, subsides to leave no permanent residual.

SUPPURATIVE ARTHRITIS

Suppurative arthritis, almost always acute, refers merely to a suppurative inflammation within a joint space. This type of inflammatory involvement is almost invariably initiated by bacterial invasion. Physical trauma, bleeding into a joint, or a metabolic disorder such as gout may evoke a leukocytic infiltrate that resembles, but is not, a valid suppurative arthritis. Bacteria usually seed the joint space in the hematogenous dissemination of an infection localized in some other organ of the body. Much less frequently, bacteria may invade the joint either by the direct spread of a neighboring infection, through a perforating injury, or during surgery.

The most common causes of suppurative arthritis are gonococci, staphylococci, streptococci, *Hemophilus influenzae,* and gram-negative bacilli (*Escherichia coli,* Salmonella, Pseudomonas, and others). Most instances of suppurative arthritis occur in adult life, more often in drug addicts and persons with reduced immunocompetence or debilitation (predominantly caused by staphylococci and gram-negative organisms). Gonococcal arthritis is mainly seen in sexually active young adults, more often in females with neglected infections. Acute arthritis may also develop in childhood, when *H. influenzae* is the most common etiologic agent. Suppurative arthritis associated with osteomyelitis is also frequently a childhood disorder. For reasons that are unclear, individuals with sickle cell anemia are particularly prone to Salmonella infections.

> Any joint may be involved, but those most frequently affected are the large joints such as the knee, hip, ankle, elbow, wrist, and shoulder. For obscure reasons, the sternoclavicular joint is an additional favored site. In most instances, the infection is limited to a **monarticular involvement.** The anatomic changes consist of a **nonspecific, acute suppurative infection virtually identical with similar infections in other regions of the body. Depending on the virulence of the causative agent and the chronicity of the infection, the inflammatory synovitis may ulcerate and involve the underlying articular cartilage.** It is therefore possible for suppurative arthritis to result in extensive destruction of joint surfaces and in fibrous bridging scars that seriously hamper joint function. Calcifications may further limit the mobility, but only infrequently produce permanent ankylosis.

The clinical manifestations are those of any local infection (i.e., redness, swelling, tenderness, and pain). Frequently, a systemic constitutional reaction is also present. Because of the destructive tendencies of chronic, suppurative infections, prompt recognition and effective therapy are necessary for the preservation of normal joint function. Overall, suppurative arthritis is an uncommon cause of permanent joint damage.

TUBERCULOUS ARTHRITIS

Tuberculous arthritis is almost invariably an insidious chronic disease. It may be encountered in adults but is more common in children, and arises either as a complication of tuberculous osteomyelitis or following hematogenous dissemination of organisms from a pulmonary or other focus of infection. It is usually monarticular in type. The most common site of localization is the spine (*Pott's disease* or *tuberculous spondylitis*) followed in frequency by the hip joint, knee, elbow, wrist, ankle, and sacroiliac joints.

The initial recognizable joint change is seeding of the synovium with small foci of inflammatory granulation tissue harboring solitary and confluent tubercles. Because these infections tend to take a chronic course, the inflammatory tissue creates a thick, felt-like covering over the articular surfaces (i.e., a *pannus*). The caseous necrotizing inflammation may extend from the pannus into the underlying articular surface, thus causing considerable ulceration and destruction, and erosion into the head of the bone. Sometimes the tuberculous infection erodes into the bone from the margin of the articular cartilage and, thus undermining it, causes it to fragment and slough. Conversely, tuberculous osteomyelitis may trek into the joint space to cause arthritis.

Tuberculous arthritis tends to be a much more destructive process than suppurative arthritis and frequently results in extensive fibrous bridging and obliteration of the joint space. Late calcification of the inflammatory tissue may lead to ankylosis of the joint. In other instances, the tuberculous infection may erode through the joint capsule to create draining skin sinuses. The precise diagnosis requires the identification of the characteristic morphologic tissue reaction or, more positively, the acid-fast bacilli. When a suppurative arthritis fails to yield a common pyogen by means of usual bacterial cultural methods, tuberculosis should be suspected!

LYME DISEASE

Initially called Lyme arthritis, this spirochetal infection involves multiple systems, principally the skin, heart, joints, and nervous system, hence the preferred designation "Lyme disease." The causative organism is *Borrelia burgdorferi*, which is transmitted to humans by the bite of several species of infected ixodid ticks, according to the locale. In the northeastern United States, where Lyme disease is most prevalent, the principal vector is *I. dammini*, whose reservoirs are field mice and the white-tailed deer. More details on transmission clinical features are offered in the previous discussion (p. 366); here our focus is on the arthritis.

Like most spirochetal infections, Lyme disease can be divided into three stages, the first stage being the rather characteristic skin lesion, the second stage being marked by involvements of the cardiac and nervous systems, and the third and late stage being dominated by arthritis resembling rheumatoid disease.[78] A transient, remitting, migratory polyarthritis may appear in the second stage weeks to months following the skin lesion. The knees are most commonly affected, followed, in decreasing frequency, by the shoulder, elbow, temporomandibular joint, ankle, and other joints. This transitory polyarthritis eventually passes without permanent joint damage. Much later, months to years, a chronic, symmetric polyarthritis appears in about 10% of cases, involving most often one or both knees, but sometimes small joints.

> The anatomic changes are highly reminiscent of rheumatoid arthritis and constitute chronic proliferative synovitis with pannus formation (p. 1349) and cartilage erosion. Two distinctive features of Lyme arthritis are hyperplastic "onion-skin" thickening of the walls of small arterioles (reminiscent of syphilis) and, in 25% of cases, visualization of the infectious agent by silver stains.[79] As with rheumatoid arthritis, some patients are left with permanent, disabling limitation of joint motion and joint deformities.

It is still not known whether the joint changes are a response to direct bacterial invasion or instead are immune-mediated. The effectiveness of antibiotics in controlling the activity of the joint involvement favors direct bacterial involvement.

GOUT AND GOUTY ARTHRITIS

Gout is the generic designation of a group of disparate conditions having in common (1) hyperuricemia, (2) recurrent attacks of acute arthritis triggered by crystallization of urates within joints, (3) intercritical periods (asymptomatic intervals) of varying length, and (4) eventually the development of chronic tophaceous gout marked by aggregates of urates mainly in and about joints, producing chronic and sometimes crippling gouty arthritis. Most, but not all, patients with chronic arthritis also develop urate nephropathy and uric acid nephrolithiasis. Although hyperuricemia is a sine qua non for the development of gout, it is not the sole determinant. A plasma urate level above 7 mg/dl is considered elevated because it exceeds the saturation value for urate at normal body temperature and blood pH. By this standard, 2 to 18% of the population of the Western world are hyperuricemic, but the overall prevalence of gout is in the range of 0.13 to 0.37%. Clearly, only a small fraction of hyperuricemic people develop gout, and equally clearly asymptomatic hyperuricemia may persist for life, and most experts would say it requires no treatment.

Both age and sex influence serum urate levels. They generally are quite low before puberty in both sexes; in males they reach adult levels in the third decade of life, but in females they do not reach such levels until after the menopause. Thus, the great majority of cases of gout occur in males, usually after the third decade. Females are almost never affected before the menopause. Genetic factors also play a role, as will soon be seen.

CLASSIFICATION. The various conditions associated with hyperuricemia and gout have been segregated into primary and secondary categories. *Primary gout* denotes those disorders in which the underlying biochemical defect causing the hyperuricemia is unknown or those cases in which, when the cause is known, the main manifestation of the defect is gout (Table 28–4).

PATHOPHYSIOLOGY. The pathogenesis of gout is the pathogenesis of hyperuricemia. Subsets of primary idiopathic gout have (1) overproduction of uric acid with normal excretion, (2) overproduction of uric acid with increased excretion, or (3) normal uric acid production with underexcretion.[80] From the clinical standpoint, patients with overproduction of urates and increased urinary excretion are at particular risk of urate nephrolithiasis, whereas the others with primary gout are not.

The precise metabolic or renal defect leading to overproduction or underexcretion of uric acid has not been defined. Genetic factors, however, may play a role because family studies suggest polygenic or multifactorial inheritance. In addition, environmental influences such as obesity or chronic alcoholism may be necessary to evoke the hyperuricemia in those persons with the inherited traits. To understand the potential biochemical basis for excess production of urates, it is necessary to review purine metabolism briefly[81] (Fig. 28–38). Several features are worthy of emphasis. Inosinic acid—inosine monophosphate, IMP—is central to the derivation of uric acid. It can be formed from ribose-5-phosphate in the so-called

Table 28–4. Classification of Hyperuricemia and Gout

TYPE	METABOLIC DISTURBANCE	INHERITANCE
Primary (90% of all cases)		
Enzyme defects undefined (idiopathic) (95–98% of primary gout)	Overproduction of uric acid with normal excretion	Multifactorial (polygenic)
	Overproduction of uric acid with increased excretion	Multifactorial (polygenic)
	Normal production of uric acid with underexcretion	
Associated with specific enzyme defects		
Hypoxanthine-guanine phosphoribosyltransferase deficiency (partial)	Overproduction of uric acid; increased purine biosynthesis de novo, driven by surplus PRPP	X-linked
PRPP synthetase variants; increased activity	Overproduction of PRPP and of uric acid	X-linked
Secondary (10% of all cases)		
Associated with increased nucleic acid turnover	Overproduction of uric acid (chronic hemolysis, polycythemia, leukemia, lymphoma)	
Associated with specific enzyme defects		
Glucose-6-phosphatase deficiency or absence	Overproduction plus reduced renal clearance of uric acid; glycogen storage disease, type I (von Gierke's disease)	Autosomal recessive
Hypoxanthine-guanine phosphoribosyltransferase deficiency "virtually complete"	Overproduction of uric acid; Lesch-Nyhan syndrome	X-linked
Associated with decreased excretion of uric acid	Reduced renal functional mass; inhibited tubular secretion of uric acid or enhanced tubular reabsorption of uric acid, or both	
Associated with certain drugs or intoxications	Overproduction of uric acid or underexcretion	

Adapted from Wyngaarden, J.B., and Keller, W.N.: Gout. *In* Stanbury, J.B., et al. (eds.): Metabolic Basis of Inherited Disease. 5th ed. New York, McGraw-Hill Book Co., 1983, p. 1043.

PRPP, 5-phosphoribosyl-1-pyrophosphate.

de novo pathway or in so-called salvage pathways from guanylic acid—GMP—hypoxanthine, or adenylic acid—AMP—(dotted pathways in Fig. 28–38). The rate-limiting step in the de novo pathway is the conversion of 5-phosphoribosyl-1-pyrophosphate (PRPP) into 5-phosphoribosylamine by amidophosphoribosyltransferase. GMP and AMP derived from endogenous or exogenous nucleic acids in the salvage pathways exert feedback inhibition of the amidotransferase involved in this conversion. Of significance to our later consideration of the Lesch-Nyhan syndrome is the generation of GMP from guanine and IMP from hypoxanthine in the salvage pathways, in both instances involving PRPP and the enzyme hypoxanthine-guanine phosphoribosyltransferase (HGPRT).

There are three important control points in purine metabolism: (1) *the activity of HGPRT* in the salvage pathways, (2) *the activity of the amidotransferase* in the de novo pathway, which is subject to feedback inhibition by GMP and AMP, and (3) *the availability of the substrate PRPP*, which is required in both the de novo and salvage pathways. The rare inborn error of metabolism involving HGPRT has helped to unravel these pathways.

HGPRT deficiency in the pathogenesis of hyperuricemia was recognized with the identification of the Lesch-Nyhan syndrome. It is characterized by an al-

most complete deficiency of this enzyme.[82] An X-linked disorder seen only in males, it is associated with *severe neurologic disease* marked by choreoathetosis, spasticity, self-mutilation, mental and growth retardation, hyperuricemia, and hyperuricosuria with uric acid calculi. Typical gouty arthritis is neither common nor a prominent clinical feature, and therefore the Lesch-Nyhan syndrome is usually considered an example of secondary gout. Since the original discovery of the Lesch-Nyhan syndrome, some cases of *partial deficiency of HGPRT* have been identified. Affected males usually have severe gouty arthritis, with onset at a young age (15 to 30 years), hyperuricaciduria, and a high incidence of renal stones. Neurologic manifestations that dominate the Lesch-Nyhan syndrome are either absent or relatively mild, hence the gout is categorized as "primary." Two mechanisms may be involved in the overproduction of uric acid in patients with a partial or complete deficiency of HGPRT and consequent impairment of the salvage pathways: (1) underutilization and accumulation of PRPP, and (2) lessened feedback inhibition of the "amidotransferase" involved in the de novo pathway. However, in the great majority of cases of primary gout, no specific enzyme or renal defect has been identified and so in these circumstances the condition remains "idiopathic."

In contrast with primary gout, most cases of secondary gout are caused by overproduction of uric acid. Many are associated with excessive breakdown of cells and increased turnover of nucleic acids (e.g., myeloproliferative disorders, leukemias, chronic hemolytic anemias, and multiple myeloma) and a consequent increase in the breakdown of purines to uric acid. *In all these cases there is an increased excretion of urates in the urine.* In a few patients with secondary gout, overproduction of uric acid results from inborn errors of metabolism in which, as mentioned earlier, gout is not the major clinical feature. One such condition is the Lesch-Nyhan syndrome. Another is type I glycogen storage disease (von Gierke's disease, p. 151), in which the inability to convert glucose-6-phosphate to glucose leads secondarily to excessive production of lactate. Hyperlactic acidemia stimulates purine biosynthesis and impairs the renal clearance of urate by poorly understood mechanisms. As a result, hyperuricemia in these patients is often marked.

Reduced excretion of uric acid by the kidney may cause secondary gout, but the serum elevation of urates is usually not sufficiently marked to produce the full-blown syndrome of gout. Any type of chronic renal disease reducing the glomerular filtration rate and tubular function—e.g., polycystic kidney disease and lead nephropathy (saturnine gout)—may lead to hyperuricemia. A large number of drugs decrease urate excretion, most notably various diuretics such as thiazides.[83] Other agents may induce hyperuricemia by undefined renal mechanisms, including low-dose aspirin, pyrazinamide, nicotinic acid, and ethanol. Other causes of secondary gout are sufficiently uncommon to not merit comment.

MORPHOLOGY. The distinctive morphologic features of gout are (1) acute arthritis, (2) chronic tophaceous arthritis, and (3) tophi in soft tissues.

Acute arthritis represents an acute inflammatory synovitis accompanied by a rich outpouring of polymorphonuclear leukocytes and macrophages, secondary to the formation of microcrystals of urates in the joint effusion. In order of frequency, joints of the great toe (90% of patients), instep, ankle, heel, knee, and wrist are involved, but ultimately any joint in the body may be affected. In most patients, however, involvement is limited to the lower extremities. Typically, one or two joints are affected at one time, but

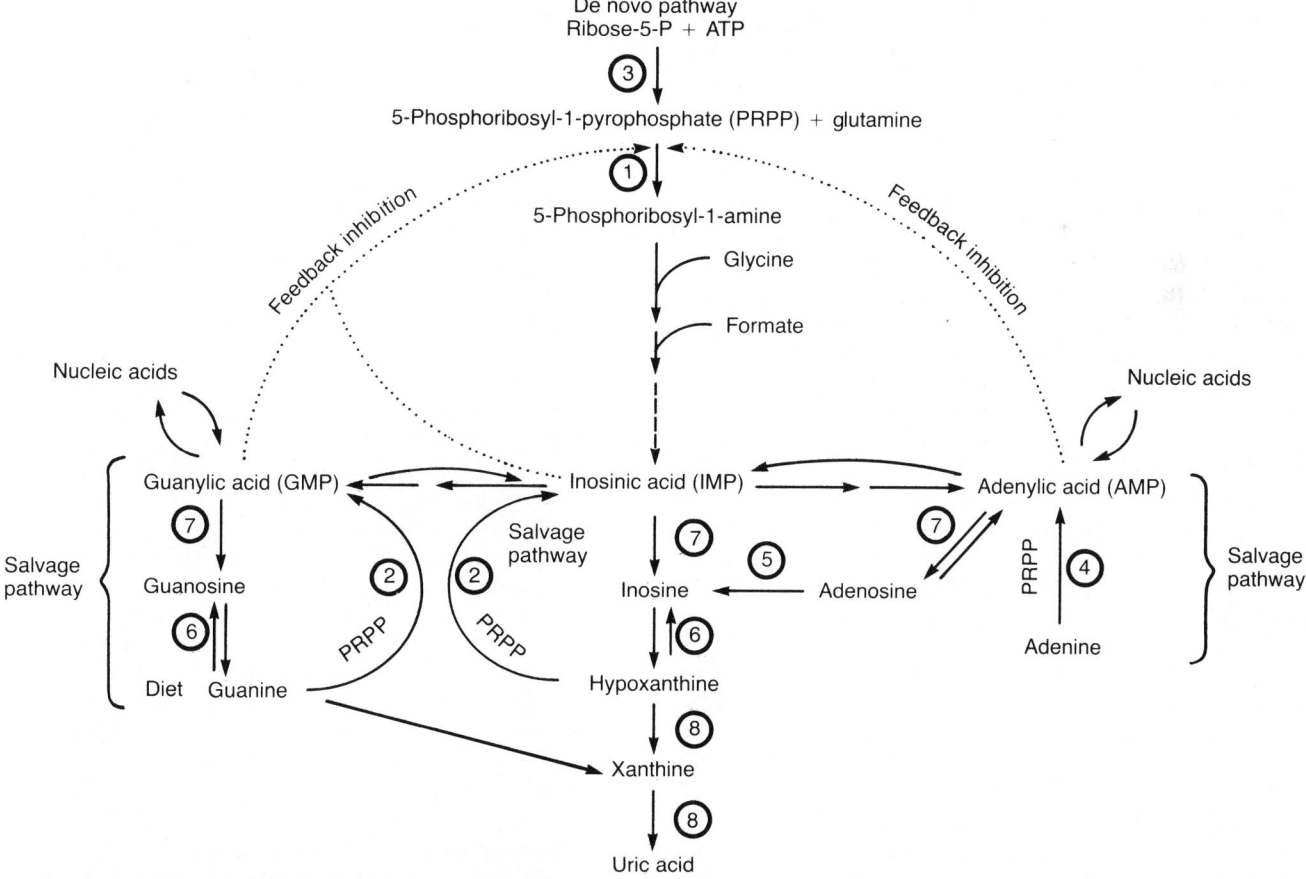

Figure 28-38. Outline of purine metabolism. (1) Amidophosphoribosyltransferase; (2) hypoxanthineguanine phosphoribosyltransferase; (3) PP-ribose-P synthetase; (4) adenine phosphoribosyltransferase; (5) adenosine deaminase; (6) purine nucleoside phosphorylase; (7) 5'-nucleotidase; (8) xanthine oxidase. (Modified from Kelley, W.N., and Wyngaarden, J.B.: Clinical syndromes associated with hypoxanthine-guanine phosphoribosyl transferase deficiency. *In* Stanbury, J.B., et al. [eds.]: Metabolic Basis of Inherited Disease. New York, McGraw-Hill Book Co., 1982, p. 1115. Copyright © 1982 by McGraw-Hill, Inc. Used by permission.)

rarely the disease is polyarticular. There is little doubt that the acute attack of arthritis is triggered by the formation of monosodium urate (MSU) crystals within the joint fluid and the synovial membrane.[84] The crystals are quite distinctive —long, needle-shaped, and birefringent. However, there is much uncertainty about the precise mechanisms that evoke the acute arthritis. Potential contributors are as follows:

• Hageman factor is activated by MSU crystals, leading to production of inflammatory mediators, including the kinins and complement fractions.
• Phagocytosis of the MSU crystals by neutrophils results in release of lysosomal products, toxic free radicals, and possibly prostaglandins and leukotrienes (LTB$_4$), augmenting the accumulation of neutrophils and the inflammatory reaction.
• Phagocytosis of MSU crystals by monocytes or macrophages may lead to the release of the potent inflammatory mediator IL-1 (and possibly tumor necrosis factor), known to have secondary actions such as stimulation and activation of collagenases derived from synoviocytes, chondrocytes, and other cells, as well as the other effects presented in the consideration of rheumatoid arthritis (p. 1349).[85]

Although the relative roles of the various chemical mediators and cytokines in the pathogenesis of acute gouty arthritis are still not clear, the significance of the leukocyte-crystal interaction is well established. Indeed, the therapeutic effect of colchicine in terminating an acute attack of gout is best explained by its ability to block several leukocyte functions (adhesiveness, migration, and movement of lysosomal granules), which depend on the integrity of the cytoskeleton.

Although the mechanisms outlined provide a reasonable explanation for joint inflammation, unresolved questions persist. What favors the microcrystallization of urates in joint fluids? Why are some joints affected while others are spared? Why are the acute attacks of gout self-limited? Relative to the events favoring crystallization, it is hypothesized that minimal trauma may cause shedding of surface cartilage laden with urates acting as seed crystals, or the cartilage trauma may mobilize urates absorbed into the matrix, increasing the synovial fluid concentration. It is interesting to note that MSU crystals have also been found in the synovial fluid of asymptomatic hyperuricemic subjects, but in gout, surface-coating immunoglobulins, albumin, or complement may favor their phagocytosis with activation of white cells. To explain the self-limited nature of acute gouty arthritis, it has been suggested that elevation of the local temperature brought about by inflammation enhances the solubilization of urate crystals, and the increased blood flow tends to wash the dissolved urates out of the joint.

Chronic arthritis evolves from the progressive precipitation of urates into the synovial linings of joints following recurrent attacks of acute arthritis. The urates may heavily encrust the articular surfaces (Fig. 28–39). Synovial proliferation and pannus formation follow and destroy the underlying articular cartilage. With progression, the subarticular bone becomes involved. In time, destruction of subchon-

dral bone, proliferation of marginal bone, and sometimes fibrous or bony ankylosis ensue, ultimately to cause chronic disabling arthritis. Deposits of urates (tophi) may appear in the periarticular tissues.

The tophus is the pathognomonic lesion of gout—a mass of urates, crystalline or amorphous, surrounded by an intense inflammatory reaction, composed of macrophages, lymphocytes, fibroblasts, and extraordinary foreign body giant cells (Fig. 28–40). The giant cells are distinctive and often appear as extended cytoplasmic masses, partially encircling the central aggregation of urates. Tophi commonly occur in the helix or antihelix of the ear, the olecranon and patellar bursae, and periarticular ligaments and connective tissues. In the kidney, tophi tend to be deposited in the medulla or pyramids and evoke a surrounding typical inflammatory reaction in the tubular interstitium. Less frequently, tophi are found in the skin of the fingertips, palms, or soles; nasal cartilages; aorta; myocardium; and aortic or mitral valves. Very rarely, tophi form in the eyes, tongue, larynx, penis, testis, or marrow cavities of bone, such as in the marrow spaces adjacent to intervertebral discs of the spine.[86] Tophi do not develop in the central nervous system, because of the relative impermeability of the blood-brain barrier to uric acid. The urate crystals are water soluble, and nonaqueous fixatives such as absolute alcohol are necessary to preserve them in histologic sec-

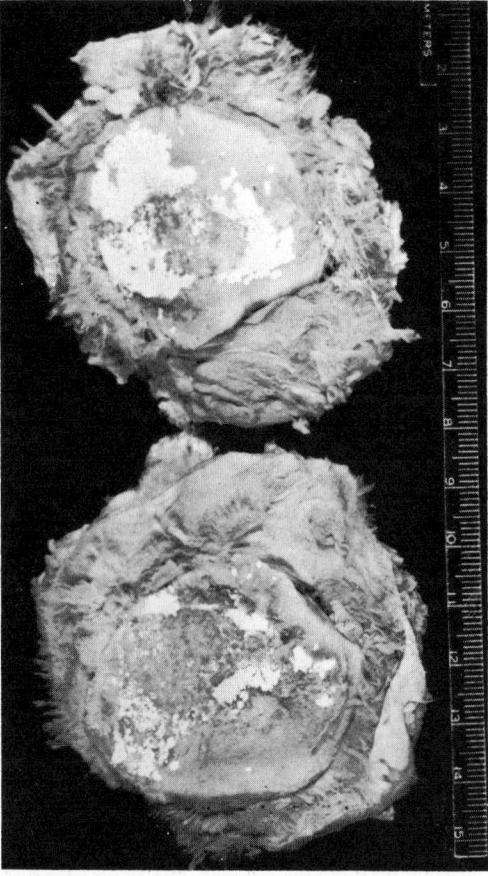

Figure 28-39. Gouty deposits of patella. Articular surfaces of patellas are encrusted with white deposits of urates.

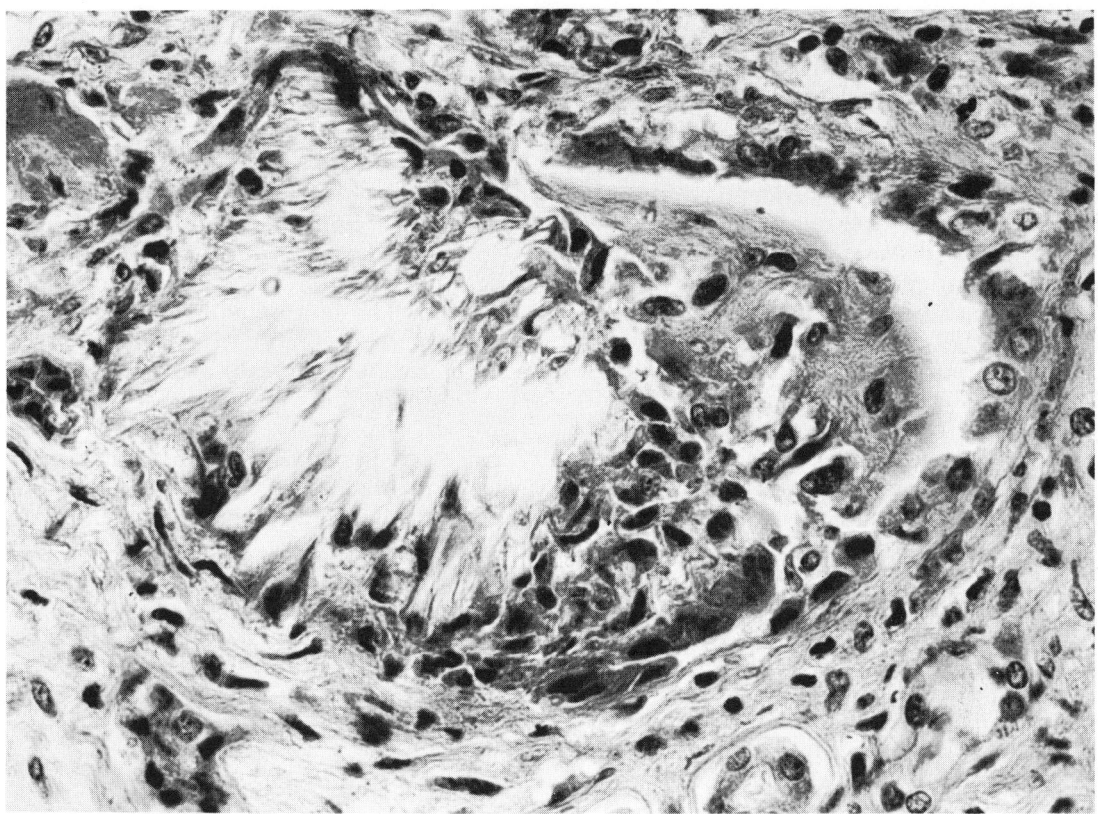

Figure 28-40. A tophus of gout. The group of slender urate crystals is surrounded by a reaction of fibroblasts, occasional lymphocytes, and giant cells.

tion. When preserved, they are brilliantly anisotropic when viewed with polarized light, or are demonstrable as crystalline or amorphous masses with silver staining techniques.

The **kidneys** are involved in the great majority of patients with chronic gouty arthritis. **Three types of renal diseases may develop: (1) acute uric acid nephropathy, (2) nephrolithiasis, and (3) chronic urate nephropathy.**[87] **Acute uric acid nephropathy** refers to the intratubular deposition of free uric acid crystals in the acid milieu of the collecting ducts, resulting in acute obstructive renal disease. This complication is seen most often in the secondary form of gout induced by the treatment of various myeloproliferative disorders with the acute destruction of myriad cells. **Uric acid nephrolithiasis** is related to hyperuricosuria and the formation of stones in the collecting system, favored by volume depletion and oliguria. **Chronic urate nephropathy** refers to the deposition of urates within the interstitial tissue of the medulla, sometimes with the formation of microtophi. However, because similar deposits sometimes develop in nongouty subjects, the changes are not specific. In addition, hypertensive nephrosclerosis may be present in chronic urate nephropathy, but it is not clear whether the hypertensive changes are merely coincidental in an aging population or are associated with the gouty diathesis.

CLINICAL CORRELATION. As mentioned, the natural history of gout evolves through three well-defined clinical phases: (1) asymptomatic hyperuricemia, (2) recurrent attacks of acute gouty arthritis interspersed with asymptomatic (intercritical) intervals, and (3) chronic gouty arthritis.

A long period of asymptomatic hyperuricemia almost always precedes the first acute attack of arthritis. As mentioned earlier, most hyperuricemic patients never develop symptomatic gout. The likelihood of developing the disease is correlated with both the duration and level of the hyperuricemia.

Acute gouty arthritis is characterized by the sudden onset of excruciating pain, almost always in a peripheral joint, usually in a lower extremity. At least 50% of the initial attacks involve the great toe, or less frequently the instep, ankle, or heel. Affected joints are red, hot, swollen, and tender; when accompanied by fever, these changes are readily mistaken for acute suppurative arthritis. In some patients a history can be obtained of some unusual form of stress immediately preceding the acute attack (e.g., physical or emotional fatigue, an alcoholic spree, or dietary overindulgence). The initial attack usually subsides with therapy or spontaneously in a few days to a few weeks, and is followed by an asymptomatic phase that may last from a few months to many years (so-called intercritical gout) or, in the particularly fortunate patient, for a lifetime. More often, however, a recurrence of the arthritis is experienced within several months to a few years, with increased likelihood of other joint involvement, longer duration of the acute phase, and more severe signs and symptoms.

Chronic gouty arthritis is the most disabling phase of the disease. It generally follows multiple recurrences of acute arthritis, over a span of years, of increasing severity with a tendency to involve more and more joints. Treatment for hyperuricemia and acute arthritis significantly reduces the risk of development of this chronic phase of disease, which appears now in only 10 to 15% of patients. Chronic involvement is insidious and may not become apparent until tophi can be palpated in the soft tissues about the joint, or until it is documented by radiographic evidence of joint damage. Limitation of motion ranges from mild to severe. Surprisingly, the soft tissue tophi are remarkably painless and nontender. For unknown reasons, with the development of the chronic phase of the disease, the attacks of acute arthritis tend to subside. About 90% of patients with chronic arthritis develop some degree of renal functional impairment. In some instances the functional deficit is marked, but the question always arises—does the renal insufficiency have unrelated origins and indeed is it the cause of the hyperuricemia? With hemodialysis, fewer patients (5 to 10%) are dying of gouty nephropathy. Nephrolithiasis is seen in a minority of patients, most under treatment for a myeloproliferative disorder.

The diagnosis of gout should not be missed by clinicians, because it affords them the uncommon and splendid opportunity of "doing good." An extensive armamentarium of drugs is available to inhibit uric acid synthesis, lower serum uric acid levels, abort or prevent acute attacks of arthritis, and mobilize tophaceous deposits. Generally, gout does not materially shorten the span of life, but it certainly may impair its quality.

CALCIUM CRYSTAL DEPOSITION ARTHRITIS

This cumbersome designation refers to acute and chronic inflammatory joint disease caused by the deposition of either crystals of calcium pyrophosphate (formerly called pseudogout and chondrocalcinosis) or basic calcium phosphates (hydroxyapatite) in the joint spaces. Inasmuch as the inflammatory changes in these arthropathies are related to crystal formation, they have many clinical and pathogenetic similarities to gout (p. 1355). Calcium crystal deposition usually occurs in those over the age of 50. Because of the aging population these arthropathies are being encountered increasingly frequently.[88] The pseudogout form can be classified into distinctive subsets: a hereditary type, a variant associated with metabolic disease, a sporadic idiopathic form, and one associated with trauma or surgery. The familial type is characterized by autosomal dominant transmission with complete penetrance after age 40. The associated metabolic diseases are principally primary hyperparathyroidism and hemochromatosis and, less commonly, hypothyroidism, gout, ochronosis, and Wilson's disease, as well as others.[88]

The pathogenesis of the pyrophosphate crystal deposition within joints is unclear. It does not appear to result solely from elevated levels in the blood or in the synovial fluid. There is some evidence that it begins with the formation of crystals within the articular cartilage followed by shedding into the joint space and fluid. The consequent inflammatory changes in the joints are attributed to the same theoretical mechanisms involved in urate arthropathy (i.e., aggregation of neutrophils, phagocytosis of crystals with release of lysosomal enzymes, and generation and release of collagenases and inflammatory mediators, such as prostaglandins, leukotrienes, and IL-1 by native and immigrant cells within the joints).

> The morphologic changes in **pseudogout** are somewhat distinctive. The involvement may be monarticular, oligoarticular, or polyarticular, but whatever the distribution the knees are most often affected, followed by ankles, wrists, elbows, hips, spine, and metatarsophalangeal joints. Affected joints reveal deposits of short, rhomboid, water-soluble crystals that produce chalky deposits on the articular cartilage, in the joint capsule and other intra-articular structures. In contrast, and for obscure reasons, in **hydroxyapatite arthropathy,** the joints affected are mainly the knees and shoulders (hence the designation "Milwaukee shoulder syndrome").

Whatever their chemical nature, the crystals at first induce an acute synovitis accompanied by an increased amount of turbid synovial fluid. In about half of the cases, the acute arthritis progresses to chronic disease with destruction of the articular cartilage and changes reminiscent of osteoarthritis. The radiographic appearance of these joints is somewhat distinctive, revealing calcification in the soft tissues as well as linear densities in the articular cartilage parallel to but separated from the underlying subchondral bone surface.

OTHER FORMS OF ARTHRITIS

Arthritis is a secondary feature of a number of extra-articular disorders. Some of these arthropathies are sufficiently significant clinically to merit mention here.

Reiter's syndrome is characterized by the triad of arthritis, conjunctivitis, and urethritis following either nongonococcal urethritis (p. 1095) or bacillary dysentery (p. 355). Mucocutaneous lesions sometimes also appear typically on the palms, soles, glans penis, and oral mucosa. The primary infections are sufficiently common to make this form of joint involvement the most common cause of arthritis in young men. Up to 90% of individuals are HLA-B27 –

positive. The histopathologic changes in the acute stages are nonspecific and comprise edematous thickening of the synovial membrane with an infiltrate primarily of neutrophils. If the disease persists to the stage of chronic arthritis, the changes come to resemble those seen in rheumatoid arthritis. However, rheumatoid factor and antinuclear antibodies are negative and the intra-articular complement level is not reduced.

Arthritis appears in 10 to 20% of cases of *inflammatory bowel disease.* It may involve peripheral joints or the vertebral column (spondylitis). The arthropathy of the large joints takes the form of a nonspecific, acute inflammatory synovitis analogous to that seen in acute rheumatoid disease, except that it is not progressive, is not accompanied by pannus formation, and usually subsides without residuals within weeks to months. The involvement of the vertebral column takes the form of ankylosing spondylitis indistinguishable from that already described (p. 1353).

Psoriatic arthritis appears in approximately 5% of patients with this common skin disease (p. 1300). Whatever the clinical pattern and particular joint involved, the changes closely resemble those described in rheumatoid disease, and indeed may lead to joint destruction and limitation of motion. As with the ankylosing spondylitis described earlier, psoriatic spondylitis has a strong association with HLA-B27. Although it is tempting to consider psoriatic arthritis as rheumatoid disease in patients with the skin condition, rheumatoid factor is almost never present.

MISCELLANEOUS LESIONS

PIGMENTED VILLONODULAR SYNOVITIS, NODULAR TENOSYNOVITIS (GIANT CELL TUMOR OF TENDON SHEATH)

These designations refer to several closely related conditions marked by proliferation of synovial membranes within joints and tendon sheaths accompanied by mononuclear cell infiltrations. Some are rendered distinctive by prominent hemosiderin deposition and others by numerous benign multinucleate giant cells. The synovial proliferative reaction tends to produce villous overgrowths that sometimes become bulbous and apparently neoplastic. *When the process is sharply localized and within a tendon sheath, it is referred to as nodular tenosynovitis, or, when giant cells are numerous, as giant cell tumor of tendon sheaths.*[89] *When it involves the intra-articular synovial membrane and there is accumulation of hemosiderin, the condition is referred to as pigmented villonodular synovitis.*

The nature of these conditions is unknown, and indeed whether they are basically inflammatory or neoplastic. Some of the relevant considerations are listed here.

Proinflammatory
  Frequent history of antecedent trauma
  Prominence of inflammatory infiltrate
  Analogous (not identical) experimental lesions induced by intra-articular injection of blood
  Similar changes observed in hemophiliacs with repeated intra-articular bleeding
  Villous hypertrophy of synovia seen in rheumatoid arthritis

Proneoplastic
  Failure to identify an etiologic agent
  Occasional cases of villonodular synovitis involve only a portion of synovial membrane
  Nodular accumulations within intra-articular synovia and in tendon sheaths are "tumorous"
  Occasional local recurrence of pigmented villonodular synovitis after excision of lesion

Although the morphology of nodular tenosynovitis (giant cell tumor) and pigmented villonodular synovitis have many features in common, they are best considered separately.

Nodular tenosynovitis occurs predominantly in the tendons of the fingers and much less frequently in those of the knees, hips, or elsewhere. It usually takes the form of a solitary, circumscribed, lobulated, small nodule (0.5 to 1.5 cm) closely applied to a tendon, and is sometimes lightly called a "fingeroma." Characteristically it is gray-pink to yellow-brown depending on the hemosiderin and lipid content. Microscopically, there are sheets of rounded or polygonal cells scattered through which are multinucleate, benign-appearing giant cells, lipid-laden macrophages, and many hemosiderin-laden, rounded or spindled cells. The lesion is usually enclosed within a well-defined capsule and is readily excised.

The changes in **pigmented villonodular synovitis comprise an exuberant villous, heavily pigmented synovial overgrowth covering all or at least most of the synovial surface of a joint.** Rarely is more than one joint affected. The knee is the most frequent target, followed by the hip. The villous projections may be several centimeters in length and frequently have bulbous tips. Some may disclose evidence of traumatic crushing or fragmentation. The overall appearance is that of a brown-to-rusty, tangled mat; however, the lesion may seemingly invade the articular cartilage and the joint capsule. Histologically, the changes are variable and undoubtedly modified by injury to the exuberant overgrowth. Basically, there are two components: (1) villous projections of the synovial membrane due to proliferation of surface synoviocytes and chronic inflammatory thickening of the synovial membrane, and (2) many pigment-laden and scattered lipid-laden histiocytes, occasional multinucleate giant cells sometimes also bearing hemosiderin pigment, and a nonspecific chronic inflammatory

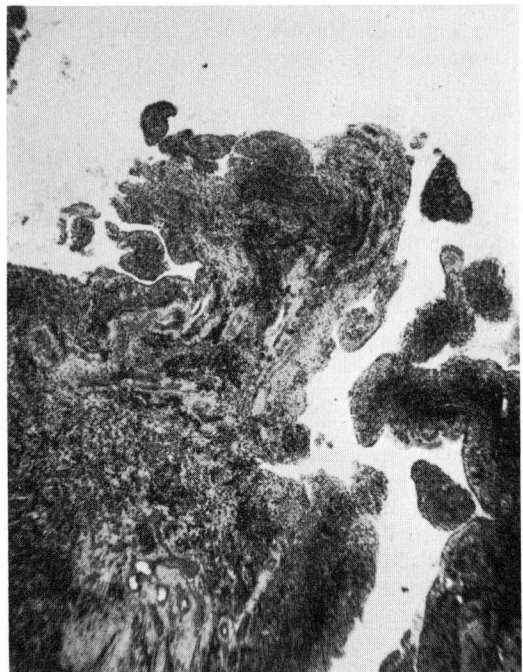

Figure 28-41. Villonodular synovitis, illustrating filamentous strands of inflammatory synovia.

infiltrate (Fig. 28-41). In some areas, the subsynovial cells are closely packed and recapitulate the appearance of the giant cell tumor of tendon sheaths.

Pigmented villonodular synovitis usually presents with pain, swelling, and limitation of motion, easily mistaken for rheumatoid or infective arthritis. Occasionally there is a history of joint "locking." It is cured by adequate excision, but recurrences have been reported, presumably following incomplete removal.

OTHER FORMS OF TENOSYNOVITIS

There are several forms of inflammation of the tendon sheaths produced by specific causes. For the most part these conditions are more uncomfortable than serious, rarely require surgical intervention, and hence only infrequently come to morphologic study.

So-called *traumatic tenosynovitis* is most often encountered in the wrists and hands of stenographers and in the upper extremities of laborers and artisans. Without proof, the nonspecific painful inflammation is attributed to excessive stress on particular tendons and their investing sheaths.

Suppurative tenosynovitis develops when a penetrating injury introduces usually common pyogens. Medical personnel are at particular risk because of accidental needle punctures. Almost always, the process responds to antibiotic therapy, but in rare instances the infection requires drainage.

Tuberculous tenosynovitis was at one time a complication of a primary tuberculous infection elsewhere, usually in the lungs, with hematogenous seeding of tendon sheaths. As in all other sites of localization, characteristic tuberculous granulomas develop within the synovial lining and may be followed by fibrosing adhesions. This form of tenosynovitis is now rare in the Western world.

BURSITIS

Bursitis (inflammation of the bursa) tends to be more common in males than in females, perhaps because of greater physical activity. These lesions are most often encountered in the subdeltoid bursa of the shoulder, the olecranon bursa of the elbow, the prepatellar bursa, and the radiohumeral bursa of the lateral radial head.

The cause is unknown. Trauma is believed to play an important role, but whether this acts as an initiating influence or a precipitating factor is still unclear. Bacterial invasion may be responsible for occasional flareups, but in most instances the aspirated fluid is sterile. Generally, no precise initiating influence can be identified except possibly a history of excessive exercise (e.g., tennis elbow).

In the early acute stages of the inflammatory condition, the bursa is distended with a watery or mucoid fluid. As the chronic stage is reached—the stage at which the lesion is usually excised—the bursal space is filled with a granular, brown, inspissated changed blood heavily admixed with gritty calcific precipitations. The wall is thick, tough, and fibrous and is often pigmented by the contained hemorrhage and hardened by calcification. The inner surface is usually shaggy and trabeculated, and often thick, fibrous bridging cords traverse the inner space.

Histologically, the walls are composed of dense fibrous tissue focally infiltrated by lymphocytes, plasma cells, and macrophages. The lining of the bursa is usually composed of granulation tissue or precipitated fibrin. Characteristically, there is marked focal vascularization of the wall of the cyst that often produces small, hemangiomatoid collections of capillary channels. Basophilic calcium deposits may be found trapped within the fibrinous lining material and within the wall.

The conditions are more painful than serious and presently are treated by supportive measures, the local instillation of cortisone or similar steroids, and, in the calcific stages, surgical excision.

GANGLION AND BAKER'S CYSTS

A *ganglion* is a small (1 to 1.5 cm) cystic lesion, almost always found in the collagenous connective tissue of a joint capsule or tendon sheath. A favored location is the small joints of the wrist, where it is usually palpable as a firm but yielding, pea-sized subcutaneous nodule. Ganglions are thought to arise from a focus of myxoid degeneration and cystic softening of connecting tissue. The central myxoid tissue, perhaps because of motion of the joint, becomes cystic, and condensation of the periphery yields an enclosing collagenous capsule. The lesion may be multilocular and may enlarge through coalescence of adjacent areas of myxoid cystic changes. The older concept that these cysts communicate with the joint space has proved erroneous.

Herniations of a joint space may occur, particularly into the popliteal space from the knee joint when there is a marked increase of intra-articular fluid or exudate, as in rheumatoid or suppurative arthritis. These herniations of the knee joint are known as *Baker's cysts.* The anatomic changes are those of the underlying predisposing articular disease.

DISEASES OF MUSCLE

BASIC PATHOLOGIC REACTIONS
NEUROGENIC DISEASE
Myasthenic Syndromes
    Myasthenia gravis
    Denervation atrophy

Myopathic Disease
    Inflammatory myopathies
    Muscular dystrophies
    Duchenne and Becker muscular dystrophies
    Myotonic dystrophy

INHERITED METABOLIC AND CONGENITAL MYOPATHIES
Inherited Metabolic Disorders
Congenital Myopathies
ACQUIRED METABOLIC AND TOXIC MYOPATHIES
NEOPLASMS

NORMAL

Skeletal (striated) muscle is an elegant example of adaptation of structure to function, in this case the production of movement and the stabilization of posture. A number of aspects of normal muscle fiber morphology and physiology are important to the understanding of muscle pathology.

By usual standards muscle fibers are very large, with a diameter as great as 100 μm and a length that ranges between 1 and 35 cm. Each cell is a syncytium that may contain up to several hundred nuclei that are small and spindle-shaped with dense chromatin and no visible nucleolus. Usually the nuclei are located just under the sarcolemma. Almost the entire cytoplasm of the muscle fiber is filled with *myofilaments,* which form the contractile apparatus. Each myofilament consists of overlapping thick and thin filaments, the main components of which are *myosin* and *actin,* respectively. These are interleaved in a repeating pattern called a *sarcomere* (Fig. 28–42). The major features of the sarcomere are the A band (anisotropic, mostly myosin), the I band (isotropic, mostly actin), and the Z line (band) (actin and associated molecules), which marks the boundary between adjacent sarcomeres[90] (Fig. 28–42). Shortening of the muscle fiber occurs by an increase in the overlap of the actin and myosin filaments with a corresponding reduction in sarcomere length. Tension is developed by the formation of cross-bridges between the two types of filament, a process controlled by a calcium activated ATPase that is part of the cross-bridge structure. This is called the sliding filament theory of muscle contraction.[91]

The cross-striations that are characteristic of skeletal muscle are easily visible with the light microscope. They occur because all the myofilaments in a fiber are maintained in register within sarcomeres by a network of intermediate filaments (desmin and vimentin) that form an internal cytoskeleton to which the contractile apparatus is anchored at the Z line.[92] The cytoskeleton is also attached to the sarcolemma through membrane skeleton proteins such as spectrin and vinculin.[93] This system enables the contractile force produced by the interaction of actin and myosin to be transmitted first to the sarcomere and then to the muscle tendon.

Muscle fibers are caused to contract by nerve action potentials at the motor end plate (myoneural or neuromuscular junction). After chemical transmission of the impulse across the synaptic gap by acetylcholine, the subsequent propagation of an action potential over the muscle cell membrane is followed by muscle fiber contraction, a phenomenon called excitation-contraction coupling. This is achieved through the T tubule system, which is a network of fine tubular extensions of the cell membrane into the muscle cell that transmit the action potential throughout the cell.

There are two functional types of muscle fiber. *"Slow-twitch" (type I) fibers* are high in myoglobin and oxidative enzymes, have many mitochondria, and are dark-staining with ATPase at pH 4.2. They are involved mainly in tonic contraction and the maintenance of posture. *"Fast-twitch" type II fibers* are

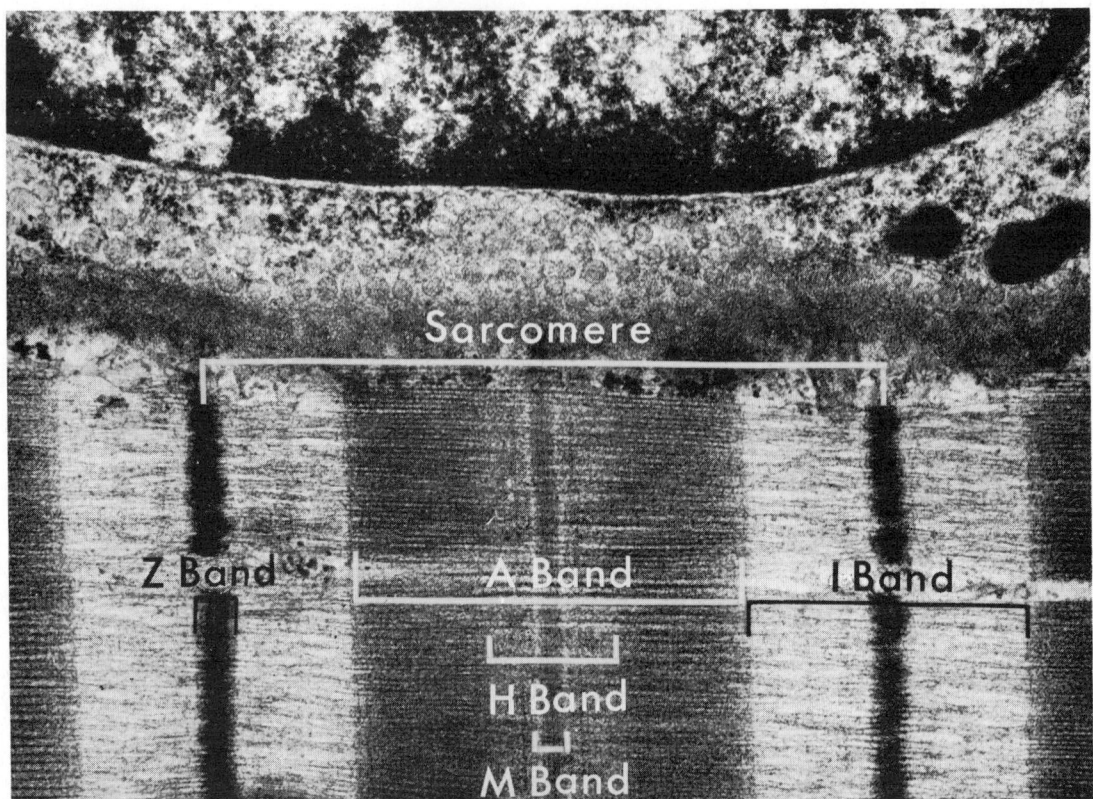

Figure 28-42. Electron micrograph of parts of two muscle fibers with the nucleus of one *(above)* and the most superficial myofibrils of the other *(below)*. Principal features of pattern of cross striations are identified on figure. (×34,000.) (Courtesy of Bloom, W., and Fawcett, D.W.: A Textbook of Histology. 9th ed. Philadelphia, W.B. Saunders Co., 1968, p. 277.)

richer in glycolytic enzymes, stain dark with ATPase at pH 9.4, and are more involved in rapid phasic contractions. Although in animals such as birds the fiber types are segregated into different muscles, human muscles contain both types of fibers in random array.

Muscle fiber type is determined by innervation. Each motor neuron innervates a group of muscle fibers called a *motor unit* that is dispersed among fibers from other motor units rather than being segregated from each other. ATPase stains that distinguish between type I and type II fibers produce a "checkerboard"-like pattern of dark and light staining fibers. If a muscle fiber is denervated and then reinnervated by another nerve, the muscle fiber will change its biochemical characteristics to match those of the fibers innervated by that particular neuron.

Muscle fibers are embedded in a delicate fibrous stroma called *endomysium* that also contains the blood vessels and nerves supplying it, and groups of muscle fibers are surrounded by slightly more prominent fibrous tissue called *perimysium.*

The easy accessibility of muscle means that it is frequently used in biopsy in the investigation of neuromuscular disease. In addition to routine histologic stains, electron microscopy is often necessary, particularly in the inherited metabolic diseases. However,

in many cases, histochemical stains and immunocytochemical markers are necessary.

PATHOLOGY

Muscle is affected secondarily in a number of systemic diseases such as sarcoidosis and various forms of arteritis. The latter may cause local ischemic necrosis directly, or, indirectly, produce denervation of the muscle fibers. A more specific process is the rhabdomyolysis associated with snake venoms, alcohol, and some drugs and viral infections. Muscle can be incidentally infected by bacterial infections spreading from adjacent tissues such as occurs, for example, with *Clostridium perfringens* in gas gangrene. Conversely, muscle is a specific target of infection, as for example in trichinosis (p. 416), in which the larval form of *Trichinella spiralis* encysts in muscle. These and other systemic involvements of skeletal muscle have already been mentioned in other portions of this text. Here we are concerned with the more specific

Table 28–5. Major Categories of Neurogenic and Myopathic Disease of Muscle

Neurogenic Disease
Myasthenic syndromes
Myasthenia gravis
Lambert-Eaton syndrome
Congenital myasthenia
Denervation atrophy
Myopathic Disease
Inflammatory myopathies
Polymyositis-dermatomyositis (p. 207)
Myositis associated with collagen
vascular disease
Muscular dystrophies
Duchenne or Becker
Limb girdle
Facioscapulohumeral
Myotonic dystrophy
Inherited metabolic and congenital
McArdle's syndrome (p. 153)
Mitochondrial myopathies
Nemaline myopathy
Hyper- or hypokalemic periodic paralysis
Central core disease
Centronuclear or myotubular myopathy
Congenital fiber–type disproportion
Acquired metabolic and toxic
Steroid-induced
Hypothyroid and thyrotoxic
Alcohol
Chloroquine
Epsilon-aminocaproic acid
D-Penicillamine
Procainamide

diseases of muscle that fall into two general categories, *neurogenic* and *myopathic* (Table 28–5), but first a consideration of some basic pathologic reactions of skeletal muscle cells.

BASIC PATHOLOGIC REACTIONS

The basic pathologic reactions of skeletal muscle fibers are atrophy, degeneration, regeneration, and various other myopathic changes.

Atrophy occurs when muscle fibers are denervated, unused, or deprived of their blood supply. The most marked atrophy follows denervation. The fibers become progressively smaller in volume, and, on cross section, often have an angulated appearance that is mostly a function of the pressure of adjacent normal-sized fibers. The reduction in volume that occurs is not accompanied by loss of nuclei so that the nuclear density rises and in very atrophic muscle there are characteristic clumps of overlapping nuclei with very little visible cytoplasm. If fibers are reinnervated, they are able to regenerate to their normal size.

Degeneration of muscle fibers occurs in a number of different diseases. It usually affects only a segment of the fiber, and the fiber is able to reconstitute itself from the remaining undamaged segments. Initially, the segment loses its distinctive striations and becomes more eosinophilic, appearing pink rather than red on H and E stains. Subsequently, inflammatory cells, notably macrophages, invade and digest the necrotic region.

Regeneration takes place by the activation and multiplication of myoblasts that are present in normal muscle as small spindle-shaped satellite cells.[93] In regeneration the initial proliferation occurs around the edges of the old muscle fiber, where the proliferating myoblasts form myotubes analogous to the myotubes found in muscle development. The growth and subsequent fusion of these myotubes reconstitutes the muscle fiber.[94] While this process is occurring, and also when muscle is regrowing after reinnervation, *the muscle fiber nuclei are found centrally in the cytoplasm, are markedly enlarged, and often have a prominent nucleolus*. The developing cytoplasm has a distinct basophilic tint on H and E stain, a reflection of the large number of ribosomes required to perform the protein synthesis necessary to reconstitute the cell. Subsequently, the cytoplasm loses its basophilic tint, and the nuclei return to their normal, small, spindle shape and subsarcolemmal location.

Other so-called *myopathic changes* are typically seen in primary muscle disease but are not specific to any particular type of disease, and indeed may be seen in neurogenic disease of muscle, particularly if it is of long duration. *Increased variation in fiber diameter*, with fibers both larger and smaller than normal, is seen in many circumstances and may occur in both neurogenic and myopathic disease. Similarly, an *increased number of central nuclei* is a very nonspecific indicator of disturbance in muscle fiber function. In normal muscle, central nuclei are found in only about 5% of fibers. *Hypercontraction (contraction bands similar to those seen in the heart)* of localized segments of muscle fibers where the sarcomeres are abnormally and excessively shortened are often seen around the edges of biopsy specimens, and are particularly frequent in Duchenne muscular dystrophy (p. 1368). *Ring fibers* are muscle fibers in which the peripheral myofilaments have become reoriented to run circumferentially and, on transverse sections, form a "ring" around the central, longitudinally oriented myofilaments. Ring fibers can be seen in a number of conditions but are particularly characteristic of myotonic dystrophy. *Fiber splitting* is the presence of what appear to be clefts in a single large fiber, splitting it up into a number of smaller daughter fibers. Notwithstanding its name, it is thought that this appearance may reflect defective regeneration, with failure of the regenerating myoblasts to completely fuse. *Endomysial and perimysial fibrosis and fatty infiltration* usually follow atrophy or inflammation, or both, in muscle. Their distribution and character are not usually helpful diagnostically, except for the characteristic perifascicular atrophy and fibrosis that occur in some cases of myositis.

NEUROGENIC DISEASE

MYASTHENIC SYNDROMES

Myasthenic syndromes are characterized by the combination of muscular weakness and fatigability. Myasthenia gravis is the most frequently encountered example, but there are also several forms of congenital myasthenia, an acquired Lambert-Eaton syndrome, and denervation atrophy.

Myasthenia Gravis (MG)

Myasthenia gravis is an autoimmune disease in which *the antigenic target is the acetylcholine receptor (AChR) of the postsynaptic membrane of the neuromuscular junction.* The resultant abnormalities of receptor number and function hamper or block transmission of the nerve impulse across the neuromuscular junction, transmission being most severely compromised when there is repetitive or tetanic stimulation. Clinically, this is reflected in the characteristic combination of weakness and fatigue that increases with activity in muscle groups.

> **MORPHOLOGY.** The principal nonimmunologic morphologic finding is a simplification of the neuromuscular junction (NMJ), in reality only an elaborate synapse. In the normal NMJ the postsynaptic membrane has elaborate infoldings, called junctional folds. Combined immunocytochemistry and bungarotoxin binding studies have shown that normally there is a high density of AChR on the postsynaptic membrane, concentrated mostly on the terminal expansions of the junctional folds.[95] In patients with MG, the junctional folds are greatly reduced or abolished, and the number of AChR is dramatically reduced.[96] Because neuromuscular transmission is a function of the number of membrane ionic channels that can open, a reduction in the number of channels will reduce signal transmission. By electron microscopic immunocytochemistry, both IgG and the "attack complex" of complement can be demonstrated at the neuromuscular junctions in the appropriate sites to affect AChR transmission.[97]

ETIOLOGY AND PATHOGENESIS. *Antibodies to the AChR receptor are present in the serum of about 85 to 90% of patients with MG, being found most frequently in patients with severe or generalized disease.*[98] The disease can be transmitted to mice by passive transfer of serum from patients with MG. There is, however, a poor correlation between the antibody titer and the severity of the disease. The antibody response in MG is polyclonal and directed against various components of the AChR. These antibodies accelerate degradation of the AChR, possibly by complement-mediated destruction of the junctional folds of the neuromuscu-

Figure 28-43. A schematic representation of the neuromuscular junction in myasthenia gravis showing degradation of acetylcholine receptors by specific antibodies and complement.

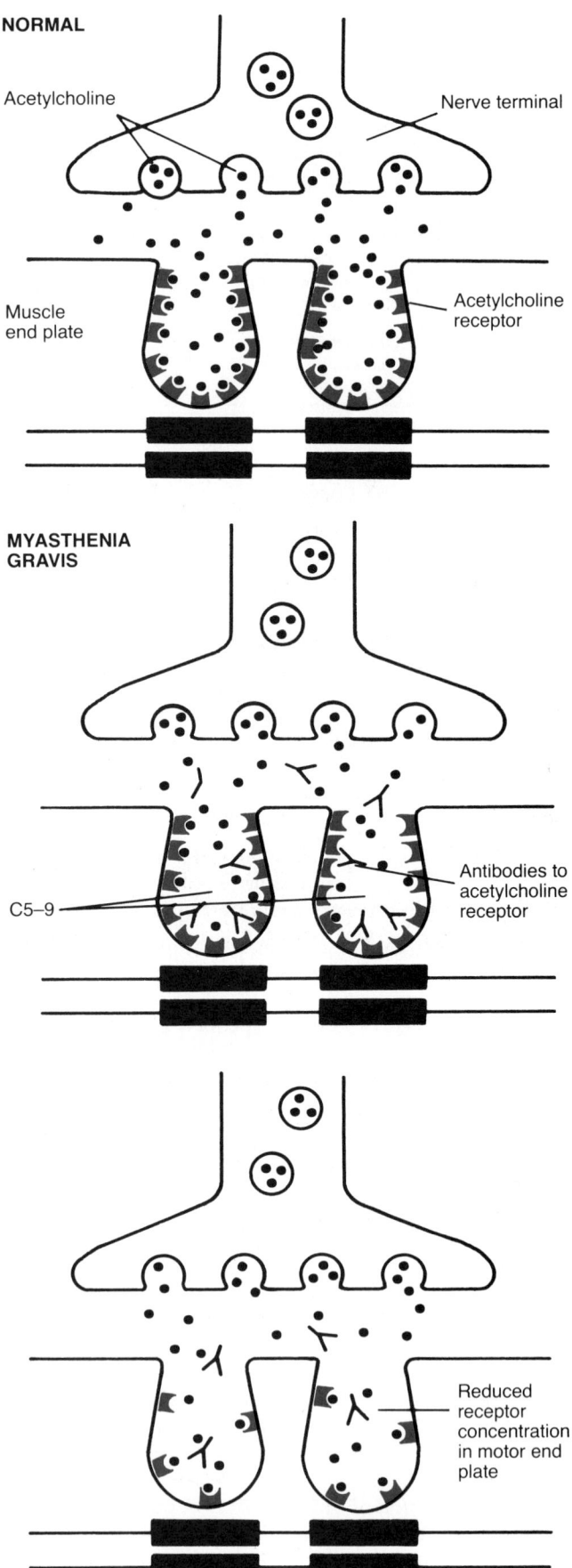

lar junction and by inhibition of acetylcholine binding (Fig. 28–43).[99]

Although only about 15 to 40% of the patients with MG have a thymoma, thymic hyperplasia is present in the majority of patients without thymoma (p. 1270), and thymectomy is an important modality of treatment. Cells that express AChR on their surfaces are present in both thymic tumors and tumor-free thymus.[100] So it is thought that, in susceptible individuals, antigen-presenting cells in the thymus sensitize B cells that produce the antibodies.[101] The thymus, then, appears to have a central role in the development of the autoimmunity in MG, although many of the details of its involvement remain to be clarified.

CLINICAL COURSE. Myasthenia gravis often presents as weakness and fatigability in the ocular musculature, usually in the form of ptosis or diplopia.[94] The symptoms may remain predominantly ocular but in the majority of patients the weakness and fatigability spread to other muscle groups, often involving other bulbar muscles and producing episodic dysphagia and dysarthria. Trunk and limb muscles are also frequently involved. There is a wide variation in the clinical course, and a frequently used clinical classification is based on a combination of distribution, severity, and rate of progression of the disease.[102] Another classification, based on the pattern of immunologic abnormalities, divides patients with MG into three groups (Table 28–6).[103]

Overall, there is about a 10% mortality that occurs mostly in patients with severe generalized disease and respiratory compromise. This is most frequent in patients with thymomas who also usually respond relatively poorly to anticholinesterase drugs. In recent years, there has been a substantial fall in mortality that is chiefly the result of improvements in respiratory care of acutely ill patients during myasthenic crises.

About 15% of patients with MG have other autoimmune diseases, a reflection of the generalized nature of the disturbance in immune function that occurs in MG. A wide variety have been described, including autoimmune thyroid disease, rheumatoid arthritis, pernicious anemia, SLE, and other collagen-vascular diseases.[104]

Other myasthenic syndromes include the Lambert-Eaton syndrome,[105] which in about two thirds of the cases is associated with a malignancy (usually a small cell carcinoma of the lung). There are also several congenital and familial myasthenic syndromes that relate to a variety of defects in acetylcholine biosynthesis and metabolism or in AChR function.[105]

Denervation Atrophy

Impairment in muscular function occurs in any form of peripheral neuropathy in which there is axonal degeneration that results in denervation of muscle fibers leading to secondary muscle atrophy. By contrast, in *demyelination* there is a conduction block that prevents nerve impulses from being transmitted to the muscle, but because the axon remains intact there is no denervation of the muscle and atrophy does not occur. *Amyotrophic lateral sclerosis* is an example of a muscle denervation disorder.

MORPHOLOGY. The major consequence of denervation is atrophy of the denervated muscle fiber with the production of small angulated fibers. Subsequently, the muscle fiber may be reinnervated by **collateral sprouting** from an adjacent nerve fiber and may regenerate up to its previous size. As was described, muscle fiber type is determined by innervation and, therefore, after reinnervation, its fiber type will be the same as that of the adjacent muscle fiber. Repeated episodes of denervation and reinnervation by collateral sprouting will therefore eventually produce clusters of muscle fibers of a single type, a phenomenon called **type grouping**.[106] Type grouping can be easily recognized on ATPase stains that differentiate between type I and type II fibers and is quite different from the random checkerboard pattern of intermingled type I and type II fibers seen in normal muscle. The corollary of type grouping is that, with further denervation, the muscle fibers that atrophy will also be in groups, called—not surprisingly—**group atrophy. Type grouping and group atrophy are therefore the pathologic hallmarks of denervation.** In long-standing neurogenic atrophy some myopathic changes may be superimposed on these basic neurogenic changes.

CLINICAL COURSE. Denervation is manifested by a combination of weakness and loss of muscle bulk. In conditions such as amyotrophic lateral sclerosis (ALS) (p. 1342), in which the process of denervation is relatively rapid, progressive *fasciculations* may also be present. These are fine, repetitive, multifocal contractions of small segments of the muscle belly that are a manifestation of denervation hypersensitivity. This hypersensitivity results from an increase in the number of acetylcholine receptors on the denervated muscle, which are found over the whole surface of the

Table 28–6. Classification of Myasthenia Gravis by Pattern of Immunologic Abnormalities

CLASSIFICATION	AGE	THYMOMA	SEX BIAS	HLA	AChR ANTIBODIES	STRIATED MUSCLE ANTIBODIES	OTHER ORGAN ANTIBODIES
1	—	+	—	—	+++	+++	—
2	>40	—	F	A1,B8,DRw3	++	+	+++
3	>40	—	M	A3,B7,DRw2	+	++	+++

muscle fiber rather than being concentrated in the region of the neuromuscular junction, as with innervated muscle. In this situation, small amounts of acetylcholine may cause propagated action potentials to occur and produce the local contractions in the denervated muscle. In ALS, fasciculations are often seen in the muscles of the shoulder girdle and are virtually pathognomonic if present in the tongue.

MYOPATHIC DISEASE

The myopathies have been subdivided into four groups, which are listed in Table 28–5, with a few examples of the specific diseases in each category. It should be emphasized that this is by no means a comprehensive list, but it is included to give a general idea of the range of disease that can affect muscle. Space permits discussion of only a few examples from even this abbreviated list.

Inflammatory Myopathies

The major inflammatory myopathies of microbiologic origin have been considered in Chapter 7 and will not be further considered here.

Muscular Dystrophies

This is a heterogeneous group of well-recognized muscle diseases that are probably best thought of as *progressive, primary, genetically determined myop-*athies. They therefore constitute a subgroup of inherited metabolic diseases of muscle, but convention currently dictates that they be considered separately. The major dystrophies are cited in Table 28–7.

Duchenne and Becker Muscular Dystrophies

Duchenne dystrophy is both the most common and the most devastating of the dystrophies. It occurs in about 1 in 3500 live-born males,[107] about two thirds of whom are the children of female carriers, the remaining third having suffered new mutations.

MORPHOLOGY. Pathologically, there is necrosis and attempted regeneration of individual muscle fibers (Fig. 28–44). The necrotic fibers are ingested by macrophages, and as the muscle fibers are destroyed, they are replaced by fibrofatty tissue that can occupy as much, or even a greater, volume than the muscle fibers it replaces. In the early stages of the disease, the diameters of the nondegenerating fibers range more widely than those of normal muscle with both hypertrophic and smaller than normal fibers. Other findings are central nuclei, hypercontracted segments of muscle fibers (contraction bands), and fiber splitting. In an end-stage biopsy, almost the entire muscle belly is replaced by fibrofatty tissue with only a few scattered surviving muscle fibers. This appearance is similar to the end stage of inflammatory muscle disease.

Table 28–7. Muscular Dystrophies

	INHERITANCE	AGE AT ONSET	MAJOR CLINICAL FEATURES	COURSE
Duchenne type	X-linked recessive	Early childhood	Symmetric weakness, initially pelvifemoral; later weakness in leg, shoulder girdle, and then trunk muscles; ''pseudohypertrophy'' of calves, reduced intelligence, cardiac involvement	Progressive; inability to walk by puberty; death by age 20
Becker type	X-linked recessive	Second decade	Milder variant of Duchenne type	''Benign''; ability to walk into adult life
Facioscapulohumeral	Autosomal dominant	Childhood to late adult life	Usually facial weakness first; scapular weakness; humeral weakness	''Benign'' course not progressive
Limb-girdle	Autosomal recessive	Variable onset first to sixth decade	Two variants: (1) pelvifemoral weakness; (2) shoulder girdle weakness	Variable progression; disability within 20 years
Myotonic dystrophy	Autosomal dominant	Infancy to middle adult life	Weakness and myotonia (difficulty in relaxation) of distal muscles (e.g., hands and feet); frontal baldness; cataracts; testicular atrophy; cardiac involvement	''Benign''; does not shorten life
Ocular myopathy	?Autosomal dominant	Variable	Group of syndromes all having weakness in extraocular muscles initially; sometimes involvement of face, neck, limbs	Rarely progressive

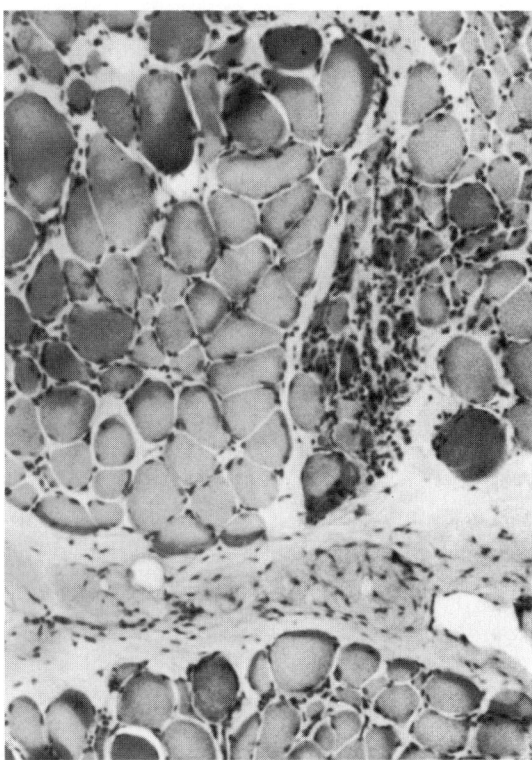

Figure 28-44. Duchenne's muscular dystrophy. Biopsy specimen of calf muscle. There is an obvious focus of active necrosis containing occasional mononuclear cells, reduplicated sarcolemmal nuclei, and some necrotic and necrotizing muscle fibers with internalization of sarcolemmal nuclei. The surrounding, better-preserved fibers reveal marked inequality of cross-sectional diameter with a slight interstitial fibrosis. (Courtesy of Dr. William Schoene, Department of Pathology, Brigham and Women's Hospital, Boston, and Harvard Medical School.)

ETIOLOGY AND PATHOGENESIS. The understanding of Duchenne dystrophy has been transformed by recent advances in cytogenetics and molecular biology that have identified the defective gene on the short arm of the X chromosome.[108,109] The defective gene is very large, and most of the defects are deletions of varying lengths. The product of the normal gene found within the muscle fiber proves to be a 400-kilodalton protein called dystrophin, which is present in only very small quantities (0.002% of total protein) in normal muscle but is deficient in the patients with Duchenne dystrophy that have been studied.[110] The protein has similarities to actinin (at its actin binding site) and also to spectrin (p. 1363), which is part of the "membrane skeleton." It is localized to the T-tubule system, which triggers the release of calcium after depolarization of the T tubule.[111] The function of dystrophin has not yet been elucidated, although it is currently hypothesized that its absence may disrupt the normal mechanism of controlled calcium release that is required for muscle fiber contraction, or that its absence weakens myocyte membranes, making these cells vulnerable to the stresses of contraction-relaxation. In this respect, it is significant that hypercontraction of sarcomeres and

contraction band formation are so frequent in Duchenne dystrophy. It is also speculated that a defect in dystrophin might also allow excess calcium entry and the inappropriate activation of proteases and phospholipases that could damage the muscle fiber.

The gene deletions in different affected families tend to be of different lengths and in Duchenne dystrophy the deletion also disrupts the reading frame of the DNA, so that the undeleted part of the gene cannot be normally transcribed. In the Becker variant, there is no disruption of the reading frame so that variable-length fragments of dystrophin are produced, which have a degree of normal function. This is thought to account for the relative mildness of this variant, with the less severe forms having, in general, larger residual protein fragments.

Because one third of the cases are thought to be sporadic new mutations, genetic analysis of families would not be able to detect more than two thirds of the cases. The isolation of the product of the defective gene raises the possibility of antenatal screening for all cases of this devastating disease.

CLINICAL COURSE. The disease becomes apparent in early childhood with progressive weakness that paradoxically produces hypertrophy of affected muscles, particularly in the calf, owing in part to fibrofatty replacement. This relative preservation of muscle bulk is maintained even in the face of increasingly severe weakness and incapacitation that, in the Duchenne variant, usually results in death before the age of 20 years. The milder (Becker) type, with a genetic defect at the same locus, has about one tenth the frequency of Duchenne dystrophy. There are, however, phenotypic variations of both conditions with relatively mild versions of Duchenne dystrophy and quite severe Becker variants.

Myotonic Dystrophy

This autosomal dominant disease resulting from a mutation in chromosome 19 is characterized by alterations in many systems of the body as well as muscle. The other major features in addition to the muscle disease are cataracts, frontal baldness in males, testicular atrophy, heart disease, and dementia.

MORPHOLOGY. Although there is no single pathognomonic feature, the overall appearance of muscle biopsy specimens in myotonic dystrophy is rather characteristic. The major features are an increased number of central nuclei, prominent ring fibers, and the presence of sarcoplasmic masses, which are regions of disorganized sarcoplasm devoid of normal striations. Other features are chains of nuclei and a type I fiber atrophy.

ETIOLOGY AND PATHOGENESIS. Myotonic dystrophy occurs in all racial groups that have been studied and has a frequency of about 5 per 100,000 population, with heterozygote frequency estimated to be approximately 13.5 per 100,000. Despite heterogeneity of both clinical expression and severity, the genetic defect appears to be homogeneous. The myotonic dystrophy gene is on chromosome 19 and closely linked to the genes for the C3 component of complement and peptidase D.[112,113] Given the power of current gene mapping and molecular biologic techniques, it is likely that more detailed information about the gene and its product will soon become available.

INHERITED METABOLIC AND CONGENITAL MYOPATHIES

INHERITED METABOLIC DISORDERS

Inherited metabolic disorders of muscle encompass a spectrum of enzyme deficiencies, most of which are in the pathways of energy metabolism. In myophosphorylase deficiency (McArdle's syndrome) (p. 152), acid maltase deficiency, and phosphofructokinase deficiency, the lesions are in the pathways of glycolysis. Enzyme deficiencies are also found in different aspects of carnitine metabolism (carnitine deficiency and carnitine palmitoyltransferase deficiency) and in the mitochondrial myopathies.

The *mitochondrial myopathies* are a group of disorders with defects in mitochondrial metabolism. The types of defect so far discovered are in *substrate transport* (carnitine metabolism and the pyruvate dehydrogenase complex), *energy conservation* (ATPase deficiency), and the respiratory chain (cytochrome deficiencies). With defects in structures as basic as the mitochondria, it is not surprising that the effects are widespread and this group merges into the mitochondrial encephalomyopathies (p. 1446). Neither the clinical expression nor the pathologic findings are particularly specific, and more than one biochemical defect may be found associated with a particular clinical syndrome. One of these conditions is the Kearns-Sayre syndrome, the most constant features of which are ophthalmoplegia, pigmentary degeneration of the retina, and heart block. Other findings include short stature, cerebellar ataxia, and hypogonadism. The major pathologic finding in these conditions is "ragged red fibers," which are reflections of the accumulation of excessive numbers of mitochondria that are often unusually large, have abnormal patterns of cristae, and may contain crystalloids. Unfortunately, the specific features of mitochondrial morphology seen in these diseases do not indicate the nature of the biochemical defect.

CONGENITAL MYOPATHIES

A heterogeneous group of diseases, some examples of congenital myopathies are listed in Table 28–8. Most of these conditions present as a "floppy infant" with symmetric weakness that is usually most severe proximally. Some diseases are associated with somatic features such as scoliosis, high arched palate, or elongated facies that probably in part reflect the effects of muscle weakness during development. It is not established that all are primary muscle conditions. For example, the congenital fiber type disproportion syndrome may well prove to be a form of spinal muscular atrophy in which the major pathology will be in the spinal cord.

Nemaline (rod body) myopathy is a congenital disorder, most cases having autosomal dominant transmission with reduced penetrance. It presents as hypotonia and weakness in infancy that delays motor development, which persists to some extent into adult life. Microscopically, muscle fibers contain nemaline rods, which, ultrastructurally, are made up of large masses of otherwise normal appearing Z band material.

ACQUIRED METABOLIC AND TOXIC MYOPATHIES

The major acquired metabolic myopathies are encountered in hypo- and hyperthyroidism and steroid-induced (usually iatrogenic) myopathy. Clinically they present with diffuse weakness and sometimes a degree of wasting.

The morphologic changes in muscle seen in these conditions are inconspicuous and there are no pathognomonic pathologic features. Their diagnosis is mostly a matter of exclusion of other causes combined with treatment of the hormone abnormality.

Among the toxins, alcohol, as usual, occupies a

Table 28–8. Congenital Myopathies

DISEASE	INHERITANCE	HISTOLOGIC FEATURES
Central core disease	Autosomal dominant	Amorphous central core in fibers (principally type I) with partial or complete lack of myofilaments and oxidative and glycolytic enzymes
Nemaline (rod body) myopathy	Sporadic Autosomal dominant Autosomal recessive	Dark-staining ovoid or elongated rods within types I and II fibers composed of filamentous structures with periodic lines perpendicular and parallel to long axis
Centronuclear (myotubular) myopathy	Variable	Nuclei occupy center of fiber, often absence of myofibrils about nuclei, numerous mitochondria and glycogen vacuoles
Congenital fiber–type disproportion	?Autosomal recessive ?Autosomal dominant	Type I fiber predominance, abnormally small type I fibers, normal or enlarged Type II, various ultrastructural alterations

prominent position and can produce acute rhabdomyolysis with the accompanying complications of myoglobinuria and possibly renal failure. Epsilonaminocaproic acid, which is used as an antifibrinolytic agent after subarachnoid hemorrhage, can also cause acute necrosis of muscle fibers. Chloroquine can produce a myopathy that pathologically has a vacuolar degeneration of the muscle fibers, and D-penicilla-

mine and procainamide can both produce a vasculitis that can affect muscle tissues.

NEOPLASMS

Neoplasms primary in muscle are uncommon and are considered along with other soft tissue tumors.

SOFT TISSUE TUMORS AND TUMOR-LIKE CONDITIONS

GRANULAR CELL TUMOR
BENIGN AND MALIGNANT FIBROUS HISTIOCYTOMA (MFH)
LIPOMA, LIPOSARCOMA
RHABDOMYOMA, RHABDOMYOSARCOMA (RMS)

LEIOMYOMA, LEIOMYOSARCOMA
FIBROMA, FIBROSARCOMA
SYNOVIAL SARCOMA
TUMOR-LIKE CONDITIONS
Palmar, Plantar, and Penile Fibromatosis

Desmoid (Aggressive Fibromatosis)
Nodular (Pseudosarcomatous) Fasciitis
Traumatic Myositis Ossificans

It is appropriate that our discussion of the disorders that make muscles "soft" be followed by a consideration of tumors and tumor-like conditions of the soft tissues. Conventionally, the term "soft tissue" applies to the skeletal muscles, fat, and fibrous tissue along with the vessels and nerves supplying these components of the body. The neoplasms of vessels and nerves are considered elsewhere. Here we are concerned only with a small group of tumorous lesions showing fat, fibrous, and muscle differentiation, which often constitute challenging clinical and morphologic differential diagnoses.[114]

Before discussing the individual entities, some clinicopathologic generalizations are in order that influence the prognosis of a patient with a soft tissue sarcoma.

• Accurate histologic classification contributes significantly to establishing the prognosis of a sarcoma. Unfortunately, distinguishing one from another is often difficult, particularly with poorly differentiated aggressive tumors. Great reliance must be placed on the immunohistochemistry of the intermediate filaments elaborated by the various cell types from which the soft tissue sarcomas arise.[115]
• Whatever the type, the grade of a soft tissue sarcoma is of great importance. Grading, usually I to IV, is based largely on the average number of mitoses per high power field, cellularity, pleomorphism, and an estimate of the extent of necrosis (presumably a reflection of rate of growth).[116]
• No agreement has been reached on the relative importance ascribed to each of these variables, but tumor size and extent of necrosis are each particularly significant.

• Staging determines the chances of successful excision of a tumor. Several staging systems have been proposed for these sarcomas; the one most widely used is presented in Table 28–9.
• As an independent variable, male sex is associated with a significantly poorer prognosis.

The significance of these considerations is borne out by a recent study based largely on histologic grade.[117] Adequate excision of low grade sarcomas (I-II) yielded a 96% six- (up to ten-) year survival, whereas grade III tumors yielded about an 85% survival, and grade IV about a 60% survival. When three to four of the risk factors — male sex, grade IV malignancy, large tumor size (>10 cm^2), and extensive necrosis — applied, the ten-year survival was about 15%, compared with about 70% when not more than one risk factor was present. It is apparent that many considerations are involved in the outlook of a patient with a soft tissue sarcoma.

GRANULAR CELL TUMOR

These histologically distinctive, almost always benign neoplasms have many points of interest. Debate about their histogenesis has persisted for years.[118] Early observations attributed these tumors to myoblastic cells, and so they were called *granular cell myoblastomas*. Succeeding reports have variously suggested mesenchymal, fibroblastic, or histiocytic derivations. Favored today is derivation from precursors of Schwann cells, supported by the presence of S-100 protein in many of these neoplasms.[119] They may occur at any age, most often in young to middle-aged adults with

Table 28–9. AJC Staging of Soft Tissue Sarcomas

DEFINITIONS OF TNMG

T: Primary tumor
T_1 Tumor less than 5 cm
T_2 Tumor 5 cm or greater

N: Regional lymph nodes
N_0 No histologically verified metastasis to regional lymph nodes
N_1 Histologically verified regional lymph node metastasis

M: Distant metastasis
M_0 No distant metastasis
M_1 Distant metastasis

G: Histologic grade of malignancy
G_1 Low (well differentiated)
G_2 Moderate (moderately well differentiated)
G_3 High (poorly differentiated)

DEFINITIONS OF STAGES

Stage I

| Stage Ia ($G_1T_1N_0M_0$): | Grade 1 tumor less than 5 cm in diameter with no regional lymph node or distant metastasis |
| Stage Ib ($G_1T_2N_0M_0$): | Grade 1 tumor 5 cm or greater in diameter with no regional lymph node or distant metastasis |

Stage II

| Stage IIa ($G_2T_1N_0M_0$): | Grade 2 tumor less than 5 cm in diameter with no regional lymph node or distant metastasis |
| Stage IIb ($G_2T_2N_0M_0$): | Grade 2 tumor 5 cm or greater in diameter with no regional lymph node or distant metastasis |

Stage III

Stage IIIa ($G_3T_1N_0M_0$):	Grade 3 tumor less than 5 cm in diameter with no regional lymph node or distant metastasis
Stage IIIb ($G_3T_2N_0M_0$):	Grade 3 tumor 5 cm or greater in diameter with no regional lymph node or distant metastasis
Stage IIIc ($G_{1-3}T_{1-2}N_1M_0$):	Tumor of any grade or size with regional lymph node but no distant metastasis

Stage IV

| Stage IVa ($G_{1-3}T_{1-2}N_{0-1}M_0$): | Tumor of any grade and any size that grossly invades bone, a major vessel, or a major nerve with or without regional lymph node metastasis but without distant metastasis |
| Stage IVb ($G_{1-3}T_{1-2}N_{0-1}M_1$): | Tumor with distant metastasis |

From Russell, W.O., et al.: A clinical and pathological staging system for soft tissue sarcomas. Cancer *40*:1562, 1977. As modified by The International Union Against Cancer, Hermanek P., et al.: TNM Classification of Malignant Tumours, 4th ed. Berlin, Springer-Verlag, 1987.

no sex preponderance. The two most common locations are the tongue and the subepidermal (and subcutaneous) tissues, particularly in the trunk and upper extremities. However, they have occurred in almost every other site in the body. Although rarely malignant they are often poorly encapsulated, with tongue-like projections simulating local invasiveness. *When located close to squamous epithelium, they induce pseudoepitheliomatous hyperplasia of the overlying epithelium that can easily be mistaken for a squamous cell carcinoma.*[120]

Granular cell tumors are generally small (less than 3 cm), firm, gray-white–to–yellow-tan, poorly circumscribed nodules on cross section. Almost invariably they are composed of nests and sheets of round-to-polygonal cells with distinct borders enclosing an abundant eosinophilic granular cytoplasm evenly distributed about small, usually centrally located, uniform nuclei (Fig. 28–45). Multinucleation, nuclear pleomorphism, and mitotic activity may be present, but only rarely. The histologic hallmark of these lesions is the prominent, variably sized cytoplasmic granules that are PAS positive and diastase resistant. With the electron microscope the granules are found to be mem-

brane-limited, autophagic vacuoles or phagolysosomes containing electron-dense amorphous material that can sometimes be resolved as disintegrating cellular organelles. Smaller vesicular bodies may also be present, contributing to the granularity.

Malignant granular cell tumors are rarities. Generally they are of larger size (over 8 to 10 cm), grow more rapidly, and are more obviously infiltrative at their margins. Nuclear hyperchromasia, pleomorphism, and mitoses are more prominent than in benign lesions, but the line of differentiation is at best tenuous. Incomplete excision may be followed by local recurrence or lymphatic or hematogenous dissemination, or both.

There are no distinguishing clinical features of granular cell tumors apart from their propensity for unusual locations, such as the tongue. Excision with a comfortable margin is curative. However, infiltrative projections left behind lead to a recurrence rate of 5 to 10% even with benign lesions. Secondary and tertiary reexcisions may still be curative. Perplexingly, in some instances, the benign granular cell tumor has failed to recur despite apparently incomplete removal. The associated pseudoepitheliomatous hyper-

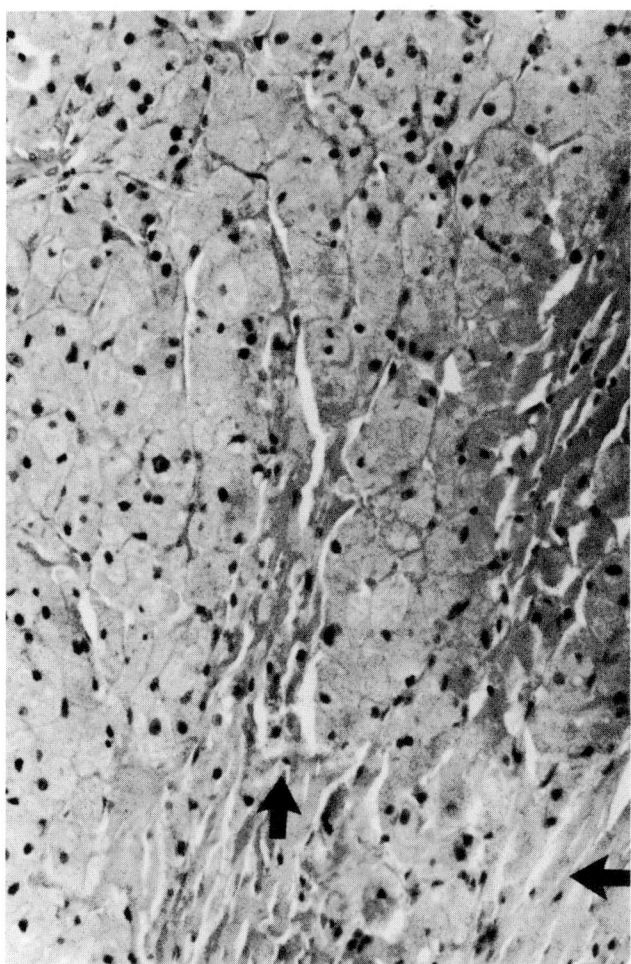

Figure 28-45. Granular cell tumor, illustrating a poorly demarcated border penetrating into subcutaneous collagenous fibrous tissue *(arrows)*. The rounded tumor cells have abundant granular cytoplasm, extremely small dark nuclei, and, for the most part, distinct cell borders.

plasia of the squamous mucosa can be mistaken for a primary squamous cell carcinoma.

BENIGN AND MALIGNANT FIBROUS HISTIOCYTOMA (MFH)

Fibrous histiocytomas, whether benign or malignant, are distinctive neoplasms because they are composed of a mixture of cells resembling fibroblasts, myofibroblasts, histiocytes, primitive mesenchymal cells, and cells having intermediate or mixed features (i.e., fibrohistiocytoid cells). Additional features include rich vascularization and varying numbers of giant cells (benign and malignant) and lipid-laden xanthomatous cells. The benign tumors occur preponderantly in the skin (p. 1290). Depending on the predominant pattern and location, these neoplasms have been called *dermatofibromas, fibroxanthomas, histiocytomas, xanthogranulomas, sclerosing hemangiomas,*

and giant cell tumors of tendon sheath. Here our attention is directed to the malignant fibrous histiocytoma (MFH) that occurs preponderantly in soft tissues, but also occasionally in bone.[121] These cancers represent 20 to 30% of soft tissue sarcomas. They may appear at any age with a peak incidence of the more common variants in the seventh decade, somewhat more commonly in males.

The histogenetic origins of the varied cell types in MFH, despite several decades of investigation, remain elusive. Favored today is the view that they arise from primitive mesenchymal cells capable of multidirectional differentiation.[122,123] In keeping with this histogenetic origin, many if not most cells in these neoplasms give positive immunoreactions for lysozyme, alpha-1-antitrypsin, alpha-1-antichymotrypsin, and Factor XIIIa, all classic markers of histiocytoid differentiation.

The sites of origin of soft tissue MFH are lower extremities (approximately 50%), upper extremities (approximately 20%), abdominal cavity including retroperitoneum (approximately 20%), and other sites uncommonly. Most arise in relation to skeletal muscle but some involve the deep fascia or less often subcutaneous tissue. The osseous tumors tend to occur about the knee, but sometimes elsewhere in the lower extremities, pelvis, or upper extremities. Rarely, MFH of bone appears to arise in two or more bones simultaneously, usually in the metaphysis. Being osteolytic, these neoplasms may erode through the cortex to invade surrounding soft tissues.

Soft tissue lesions are multilobulated, gray-white, fleshy, infiltrative, unencapsulated but deceptively circumscribed masses. Sometimes they are softer and translucent owing to an abundant myxoid stroma. Hemorrhages and areas of necrosis are common.

Five histologic variants of MFH have been described.[124] The most common is called storiform-pleomorphic and next most common myxoid MFH. The three less common variants — giant cell, inflammatory, and angiomatoid — will not be described because their designations are somewhat self-explanatory.

The **storiform-pleomorphic** variant is composed mainly of (1) polygonal histiocytoid cells with prominent oval nuclei and filopodial cytoplasmic extensions by EM; (2) spindle-shaped fibroblasts and myofibroblasts; and (3) smaller-sized nonspecialized polygonal to oval mesenchymal cells with small nuclei. **Characteristic is the tendency for the spindle cells to be disposed in a cartwheel (storiform) pattern often about slit-like vessels** (Fig. 28 – 46). In other areas, the cells are haphazardly oriented. Pleomorphism, mitotic activity, and hyperchromatic tumor giant cells as well as numerous slit-like vessels and scattered lymphocytes or plasma cells are present, in addition to variable benign multinucleate giant cells and xanthoma cells. There may also be bands or areas of collagenous fibrosis.

The **myxoid variant** of MFH is marked by areas of loose myxoid stroma interspersed with areas of cellularity. The transition zones may be gradual or abrupt. The myxoid areas are rich in acid mucopolysaccharides and contain dispersed spindled or sometimes stellate mesenchymal cells, some having coarse cytoplasmic vacuoles of mucopolysaccharides. The cellular areas more or less resemble those in the storiform variant. An abundant plexiform vascular network is present, as are scattered tumor giant cells and foreign body type giant cells. Recognition of the myxoid variant of MFH is of importance on two scores: (1) it can be confused histologically with benign lesions of nodular fasciitis and myxoma and myxoid liposarcoma (low grade) (p. 1380), and (2) as will be seen, it tends to have a better prognosis than other variants. The greater the amount of myxoid stroma, the better the prognosis. However, as with other soft tissue sarcomas, the location and stage of the lesion are the most important prognostic criteria. Tumors located near the surface come to attention earlier and thus tend to be smaller and more resectable than deep-seated masses. Metastases are present in almost 50% of storiform-pleomorphic lesions at the time of diagnosis, but in only 25% of myxoid tumors. Overall, the five-year survival is approximately 50%.

LIPOMA, LIPOSARCOMA

Tumorous collections of fatty tissue are extremely common lesions but not all are true neoplasms. For our purposes the benign lesions can be divided simply into (1) lipomas and (2) non-neoplastic lipomatous masses. The latter often appear within and between muscles, in the spermatic cord, and sometimes in association with tendon sheaths or nerve trunks. Infrequently, lipomatous masses involve an entire extremity or a large area of the trunk (lipomatosis). These non-neoplastic fatty collections are developmental in origin, but they can be difficult to differentiate from benign fatty neoplasms.

Lipomas are the most frequent soft tissue tumors. The peak incidence is in the fifth and sixth decades of life; they are rare under the age of 20 years. They arise most often in the subcutaneous regions of the back, shoulder, and neck, but no subcutaneous location is immune. Infrequently they occur in the anterior mediastinum, in the retroperitoneum, within the gastrointestinal wall, and in the deep tissues of the extremities. They tend to occur singly or in limited numbers, but about 5% of patients have multiple tumors, and in some instances a well-defined family history of similar tumors is found.

In subcutaneous locations, lipomas are generally small (1 to 4 cm in diameter) and have a delicate encapsulation that poorly delimits them from the surrounding adipose tissue. Hemorrhage and necrosis are uncommon. On microscopic section, most of these lesions are indistinguishable from adult fat, although occasional subcutaneous examples show cytologic atypia. However, admixtures of fibrous tissue (**fibrolipoma**) or proliferating blood vessels (**angiolipoma**) may be present, or, curiously, bone marrow elements (**myelolipoma**), which are most often encountered in the adrenal or retroperitoneal region.

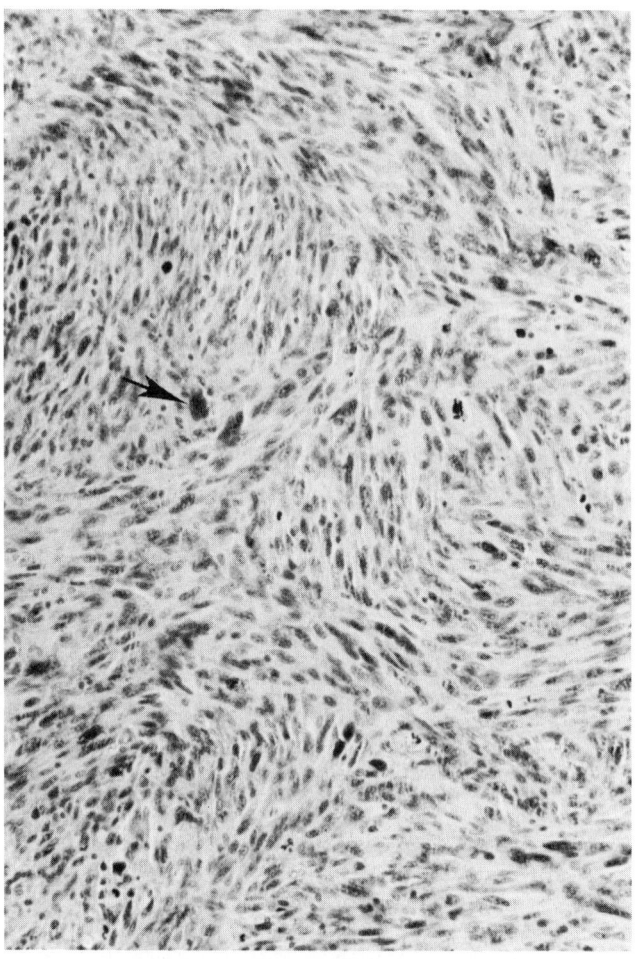

Figure 28-46. Malignant fibrous histiocytoma revealing fascicles of plump spindled cells of varying size arranged in a swirling (storiform) pattern. Giant cells *(arrow)* are present.

Subcutaneous lipomas are of little clinical significance save for their cosmetic effects and the necessity to differentiate them from more serious lesions. It is doubtful that liposarcomas ever arise in preexisting lipomas.

Liposarcomas are uncommon; they occur much less frequently than lipomas. They arise from primitive mesenchymal cells rather than adult fat cells, and so they may appear virtually anywhere in the body without regard to adipose tissue. The peak incidence of these neoplasms is in the fifth to seventh decade, but uncommonly they appear in children or in the very elderly.

In contrast to lipomas, most liposarcomas arise in deep structures such as the retroperitoneum and deep tissues of the thigh, and less frequently in the mediastinum, omentum, breast, and axilla. On gross inspection, these neoplasms tend to have a somewhat more opaque, gray-white–to–yellow appearance than lipomas. Sometimes there is an almost myxoid or gelatinous quality. They tend to be deceptively well-circumscribed and seemingly encapsulated, but they are frequently multilobular with projections insinuating between adjacent structures. They range from 5 to 10 cm in diameter and some become massive (40 kg). Areas of cystic softening, hemorrhage, and necrosis are frequent. Histologically, individual tumors tend to be fairly monomorphic, but four variants have been characterized: (1) well-differentiated, (2) myxoid, (3) round cell, and (4) pleomorphic.

The **well-differentiated liposarcoma** is easily misinterpreted as a lipoma. It is composed largely of adult-appearing fat cells, which, however, generally retain a rim of discernible cytoplasm about the large central fatty vacuole and in addition have subtle nuclear and nucleolar anaplasia. The nuclei may be scalloped because of the pressure of the intracytoplasmic fat vacuole(s). Interspersed among these cells are more immature lipoblasts with one or more small lipid droplets in an abundant cytoplasm. Mitoses and tumor giant cells are infrequent. Variable amounts of myxomatous tissue may be present. Occasional well-differentiated lesions have areas of dense, hyaline sclerosis or aggregated spindle cells closely simulating the malignant fibrous histiocytoma.

The **myxoid liposarcoma** is the most common variant. It contains primitive mesenchymal cells dispersed throughout a prominent mucopolysaccharide-rich ground substance (Fig. 28–47). The neoplastic cells range from adult-appearing fat cells to more pleomorphic stellate cells with minute vacuoles and cytoplasmic processes. Some cells crowded with vacuoles have scalloped nuclei. Tumor giant cells may be present, but are not common, and mitoses are few in number. Typically, the vascularization is prominent in the form of branching capillary channels that produce a "chicken-wire" pattern.

The **round cell liposarcoma** is composed of masses of small round cells having distinct acidophilic cytoplasm and dark, round-to-oval nuclei. These cells greatly resemble those in malignant lymphomas and Ewing's sarcoma. Important to the diagnosis are occasional cells containing fatty vacuoles (i.e., lipoblasts). Mitoses are more common in this pattern, and sometimes the cells are segregated into

small clusters or pseudoglandular arrangements by traversing strands of connective tissue. In some tumors, there is considerable anaplasia with large epithelium-like tumor cells, and in yet others, the lipoblasts tend to align in files reminiscent of carcinomas.

The **pleomorphic liposarcoma** is a highly undifferentiated, wildly anaplastic lesion extremely difficult to differentiate from other anaplastic soft tissue sarcomas. Ultimately, however, scattered lipoblasts can be found sometimes in the form of giant tumor cells with multivacuolated cytoplasm.

Because liposarcomas tend to arise within the abdominal cavity or deeply within the thigh, they are often large, bulky tumors when first brought to medical attention. They are difficult to excise and so recurrence is common (about 50%), irrespective of histologic type. Well-differentiated liposarcomas and myxoid tumors metastasize late or perhaps not at all, but in contrast, 85 to 90% of the round cell and pleomorphic variants give rise to metastases, most often to the lungs, visceral organs, and—curiously—serosal surfaces. Because the better differentiated variants predominate, the overall five-year survival rate is in the range of 60 to 70%.[125]

RHABDOMYOMA, RHABDOMYOSARCOMA (RMS)

So-called *rhabdomyomas* occur in two forms—cardiac and extracardiac—which surprisingly have little relationship to each other. *Cardiac rhabdomyomas (p. 653) are probably hamartomas* and are often associated with the hamartomatous condition tuberous sclerosis. Extracardiac rhabdomyomas are exceedingly rare and are more likely to be true neoplasms. Their rarity justifies considerable brevity and so it suffices to state merely that they are divided into adult and fetal types on the basis of the level of differentiation and maturation of the tumor parenchymal cells (i.e., the degree to which they resemble normal muscle cells).[126]

Rhabdomyosarcomas (RMS) occur much more frequently than rhabdomyomas and are one of the more common soft tissue sarcomas, especially in children, of the head and neck and urogenital regions. *They vary in histology and so have been divided into four subtypes—embryonal, botryoid, alveolar, and pleomorphic—but the botryoid pattern is basically a variant of the embryonal.* The embryonal subtype constitutes more than half of all cases of RMS. Aside from histologic differences among these variants, there are striking biologic contrasts. For example, pleomorphic RMS (a rare tumor) tends to occur in individuals over 45 years of age. In contrast, the other three variants are rare in adults; 90% occur before the age of 20.[127] Males are involved somewhat more often than females, and whites more often than blacks.

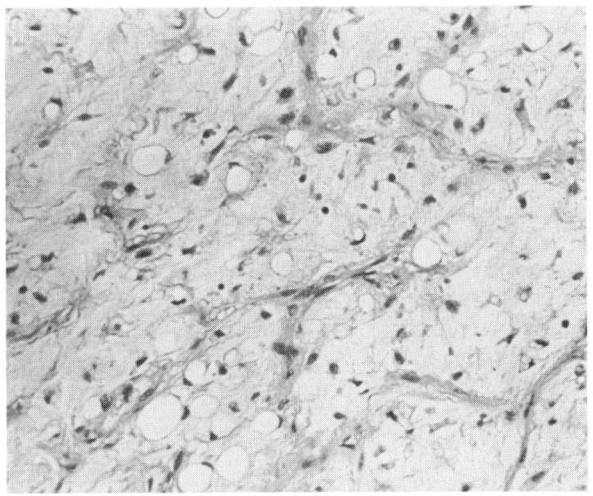

Figure 28-47. Myxoid liposarcoma with abundant ground substance in which are scattered adult-appearing fat cells and more primitive cells, some containing small lipid vacuoles.

RMS may arise anywhere in the body (e.g., brain, heart, orbit), and surprisingly less than one quarter arise in muscles. About 40% arise in the head and neck (orbit, nasal cavity, and nasopharynx), 30% in the genitourinary tract (paratesticular, urinary bladder, prostate, retroperitoneum, vagina, vulva), and 20 to 25% in the upper or lower extremities, mostly within muscles.[128]

Macroscopically, botryoid RMS differs from the other variants. It usually presents as a soft, multilobular, polypoid mass (having some remote resemblance to a cluster of grapes—hence "botryoid") projecting into the vagina, urinary bladder, or other space. The remaining patterns are nondistinctive, soft, gray-white, sarcomatous masses that vary widely in size. Those arising close to the surface of the body are discovered earlier and so are often small, whereas those in the retroperitoneum may be enormous.

Histologically, **embryonal RMS** is characterized by considerable cytologic variability, recapitulating the various stages in the morphogenesis of skeletal muscle cells. The least differentiated cell type is a primitive round-to-oval cell with a fairly uniform, dark, hyperchromatic nucleus. A better differentiated cell has more abundant cytoplasm and one or two larger hyperchromatic nuclei. Cross-striations can be seen within the cytoplasm in some of these cells. **Further differentiation yields more characteristic, elongated strap-shaped cells, with one or several nuclei, and long, extended cytoplasmic processes in which cross-striations are likely to be evident** (Fig. 28–48). In addition, usually scattered within these neoplasms are racquet-shaped cells with a single nucleus in the expanded end and tumor giant cells sometimes with peripherally arranged vacuoles separated by thin strands of cytoplasm ("spider cells"). The vacuoles are PAS-positive and contain glycogen. The better differentiated cells in these tumors will yield positive immunoperoxidase reactions to one or more of the following—desmin, actin, myosin, myoglobin.[129,130] Most valuable for certain identification of RMS are cross-striations, desmin, and myoglobin. Although an individual neoplasm may fail to have cross-striations, the majority should show immunoreactivity to desmin or myoglobin, or both, when proper technique is applied. To be noted, leiomyosarcomas and some presumed nonmuscle tumors may also yield positive reactions to desmin and myoglobin. Ultrastructural studies should help resolve diagnostic difficulties in doubtful cases (discussed later).

Botryoid RMS is basically a macroscopic variant of the embryonal pattern. The only distinctive histologic features are a recognizable normal epithelial covering derived from the structure into which the tumor protrudes, and deep to this a layer of somewhat closely packed tumor cells, the so-called cambium layer.

Alveolar RMS is characterized by interlacing strands of fibrovascular stroma creating a honeycomb pattern of spaces more or less filled with solid or loose clusters of small, round, undifferentiated tumor cells. Characteristically, the centers of these clusters of cells are less cohesive and sometimes necrotic, leaving only cells attached to the stromal framework and creating a remarkable likeness to pulmonary alveoli (Fig. 28–49). Mitoses may be numerous and sometimes are atypical. Some of the alveolar spaces

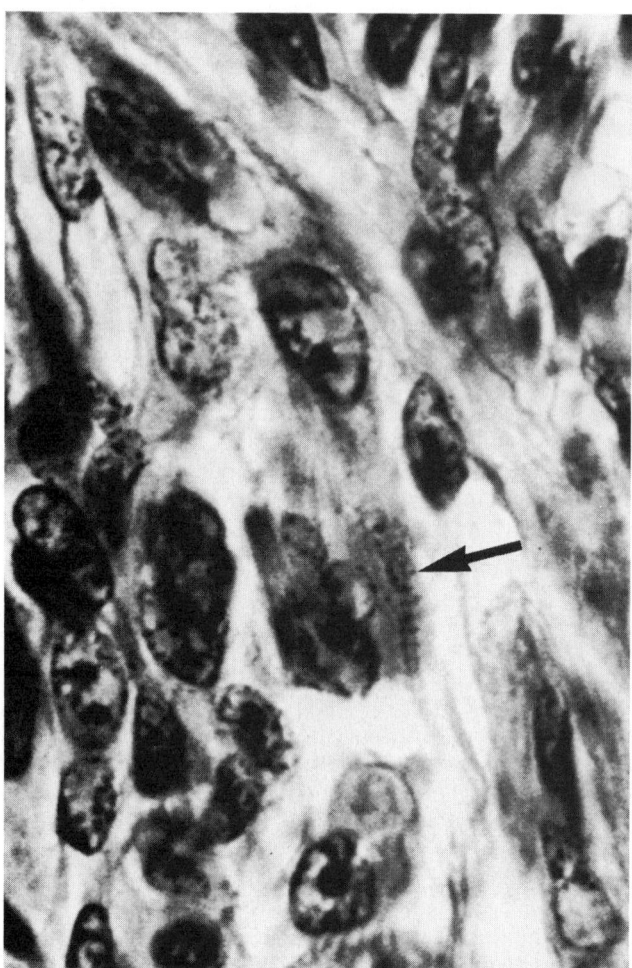

Figure 28-48. Embryonal rhabdomyosarcoma revealing the dark hyperchromatic nuclei and one better differentiated cell with ribbon-like cytoplasm containing pathognomonic cross striations *(arrow)*.

may contain spindle cells or multinucleated giant cells similar to those seen in the embryonal variants. The results of the various immunoperoxidase techniques are as given previously.

Pleomorphic RMS is characterized by large, atypical tumor cells (some having abundant eosinophilic cytoplasm), racquet cells, vacuolated "spider" cells, and more primitive rhabdomyoblasts loosely arranged and haphazardly oriented. Classic, elongated strap cells are infrequent and cross-striations are virtually nonexistent. Thus, identification of this variant is largely dependent on the immunoperoxidase or ultrastructural results discussed previously and later.[131] Many tumors diagnosed earlier as pleomorphic rhabdomyosarcomas are now called malignant fibrous histiocytomas.

Electron microscopy may be very helpful in identification of RMS. The most distinctive features, when present, are thick and thin myofilaments and ribosomal-myosin complexes.

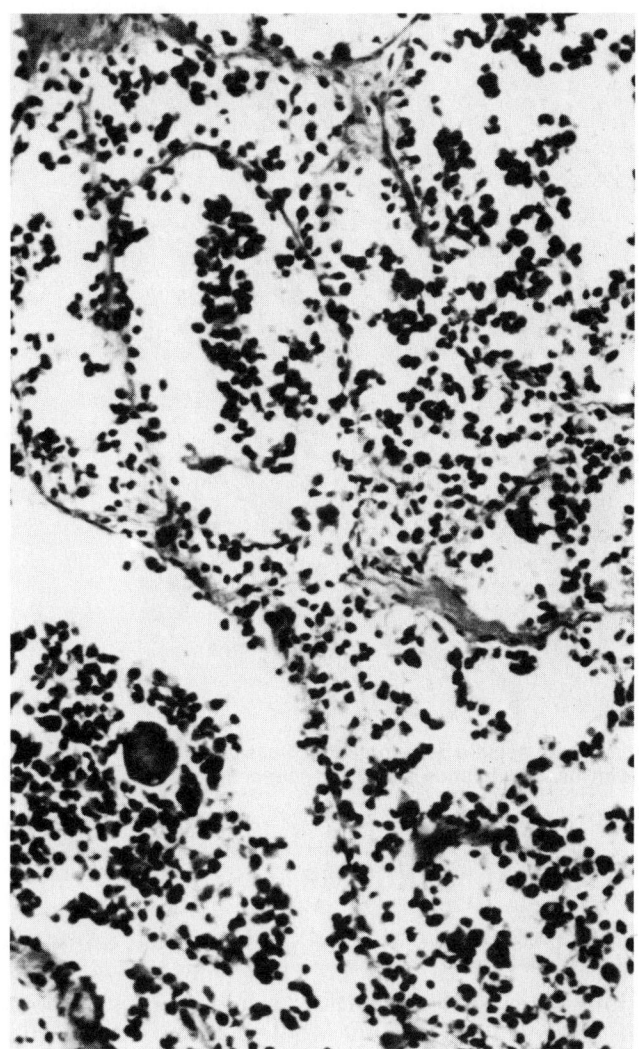

Figure 28-49. Embryonal rhabdomyosarcoma, in which small, dark, undifferentiated tumor cells have fallen away from the stromal framework, creating some resemblance to an alveolar pattern.

RMS usually presents as slowly or rapidly enlarging masses when located near the surface of the body. The more deeply situated neoplasms (e.g., retroperitoneal) have usually attained considerable size by the time of discovery. In general, neoplasms located on the extremities permit more complete surgical removal, whereas those arising in the head and neck tend to invade the bony walls of the orbit and sinuses or the vertebral foramina, precluding total excision. Incomplete removal and recurrence increase the risk of metastatic spread. Overall, about 20 to 40% of patients have lymph node or visceral (lung, lymph nodes, bone marrow, heart, brain, meninges, etc.) metastases at the time of diagnosis.[132]

Most studies confirm that, other factors being equal, the alveolar RMS tends to have a poorer prognosis and to occur in a slightly older age group, but all rhabdomyosarcomas are highly malignant.[133] Some of these tumors have proved to be responsive to combinations of surgery, radiation, and chemotherapy.

With such treatment, the median survival is now three to five years, some patients with smaller, localized lesions apparently being cured, and others with advanced disease at the time of diagnosis dying within months.

LEIOMYOMA, LEIOMYOSARCOMA

These benign and malignant smooth muscle neoplasms may present as soft tissue tumors, but about 95% of leiomyomas — and a substantial fraction of the malignant counterparts as well — occur within the female genital tract and are described on pages 1152 and 1155. However, several points might be made here: (1) additional favored sites of origin of leiomyosarcoma are retroperitoneum, wall of the gastrointestinal tract, and subcutaneous tissue; (2) highly cellular leiomyomas may be difficult to differentiate from well-differentiated leiomyosarcomas; (3) the latter must come into the consideration of all spindle cell soft tissue sarcomas.

FIBROMA, FIBROSARCOMA

Despite the widespread distribution of connective tissue throughout the body, fibromas are surprisingly limited in their sites of origin, and fibrosarcomas are one of the less common soft tissue tumors. Many lesions heretofore called fibromas have been reclassified as "fibromatosis" (p. 1380), and analogously many lesions diagnosed as "fibrosarcoma" have been reclassified as malignant fibrous histiocytomas or aggressive fibromatoses (desmoids) (p. 1373).

Fibromas most often arise in ovaries or along nerve trunks (neurofibroma). Circumscribed nodules referred to as "fibromas" occur about the teeth, but these may be reactive. Wherever they arise, the benign neoplasms are composed of typical spindled fibroblasts either closely packed with scant intervening collagen or separated by abundant collagen. They are usually firm, encapsulated, and pearly-gray on cross-section, and rarely they have areas of hemorrhagic cystic softening or necrosis. The cells may be laid down in random array or sometimes are aligned in broad ribbons. In most, mitoses are rare, but in so-called "cellular fibromas" scattered mitoses may be present; thus, the differentiation between these cellular lesions and fibrosarcomas may be difficult. Differentiation of fibromas from the leiomyomas also composed of spindle cells may be equally challenging. Fibroblastic nuclei tend to be spindle- or boat-shaped, whereas those within smooth muscle cells characteristically have blunt ends. Silver impregnation stains of fibromas typically reveal a delicate intercellular reticulin network.

Fibrosarcomas may occur anywhere in the body but are most common in the retroperitoneum, in the thigh,

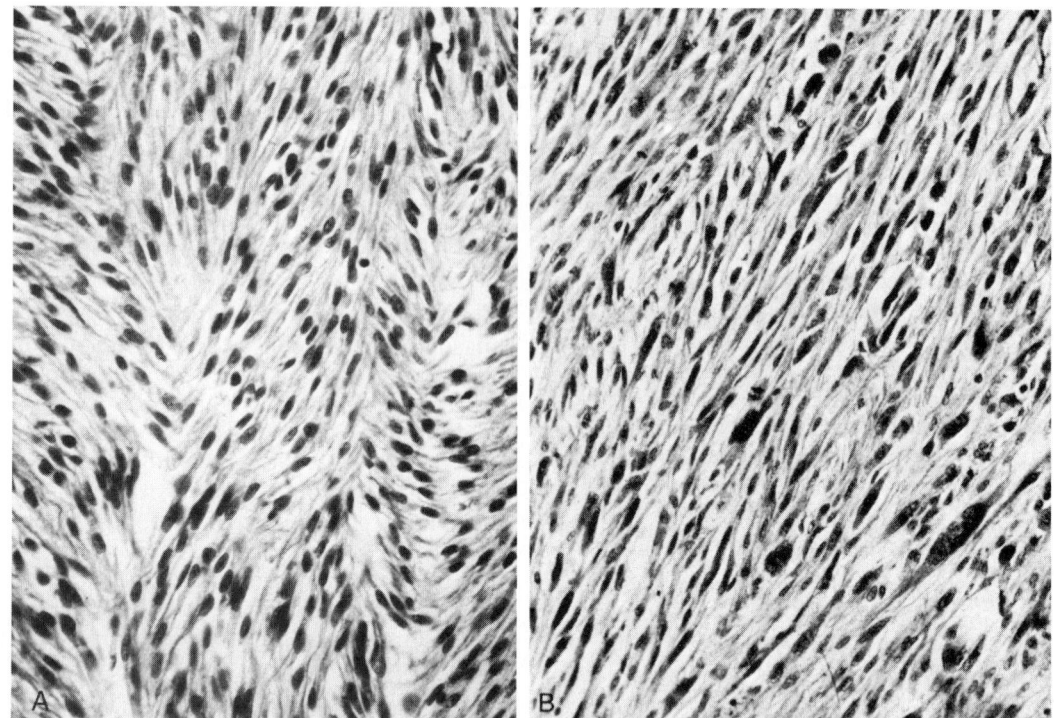

Figure 28-50. Fibrosarcoma. *A,* A better differentiated tumor with spindle cells forming a classic herringbone pattern. *B,* There is considerable anaplasia of cells with marked variation in size and shape. Scattered giant cells are readily evident.

about the knee, and in the distal extremities. Typically, these neoplasms are unencapsulated, infiltrative, soft, "fish-flesh" masses often having areas of hemorrhage and necrosis. Better differentiated lesions may appear deceptively encapsulated. Histologic examination discloses all degrees of differentiation, from slowly growing tumors that closely resemble "cellular fibromas" sometimes having spindled cells growing in a "herringbone" fashion to highly cellular neoplasms dominated by pleomorphism and frequent mitoses (Fig. 28–50). Distinguishing fibrosarcomas from leiomyosarcomas can be difficult. In addition to the special features cited in fibromas, electron microscopy of fibrosarcomas classically reveals fibroblastic or myofibroblastic differentiation, or both. Immunoperoxidase methods for desmin and muscle actin are usually negative or weak in the fibrosarcomas but positive in leiomyosarcomas.

The prognosis for patients with fibrosarcomas depends on the level of cytologic atypia, tumor size, and location. The prime modality of therapy for these neoplasms is surgical resection; radiation and chemotherapy have been added but have not been proved to be beneficial. Recurrence occurs in over half of the cases, and in about 25%, metastases are present at the time of diagnosis. Intervals as long as ten years have been recorded between excision of the neoplasm and the appearance of metastasis, even in the absence of local recurrence. Overall, 60 to 80% of patients survive five years with present methods of treatment.

SYNOVIAL SARCOMA

Synovial sarcomas are uncommon forms of soft tissue tumors. They range in behavior from aggressive lesions causing death within a few months, despite treatment, to extremely indolent tumors permitting cure or long survival. The latter group gave rise to the concept of "benign synovioma," but all of these neoplasms, even the most indolent, are sarcomas and potentially lethal. Most occur in the region of joints in close relationship to tendon sheaths, bursae, and joint capsules, but almost never within joint cavities. Very uncommonly, identical neoplasms appear remote from joints in the parapharyngeal region or the abdominal wall. Although the cell of origin of synovial sarcoma is still unclear, most of the evidence suggests that they arise not from synoviocytes but rather from multipotential mesenchymal cells.

The great majority occur in patients between the ages of 15 and 35 years, but older and younger persons may be affected. The male-to-female ratio is approximately 1.5:1. *The highly distinctive feature of these lesions (shared only by mesotheliomas) that helps to differentiate most of these neoplasms from other soft tissue sarcomas is their biphasic patterns of cell growth—distinct epithelial and well-defined spindle cell components.* However, a minority are predominantly monophasic, with either the epithelial or the spindle cells predominating. Many experts refuse to call such neoplasms "synovial sarcoma."[134]

Synovial sarcomas arise most often in the lower extremities (60%), more specifically about the knees, ankles, and feet, whereas about 25% arise in the upper arms between the shoulders and elbows. The remainder are widely scattered, such as in the parapharyngeal region and abdominal wall. Surprisingly few arise in the fingers and toes. They range in size from a few centimeters in greatest diameter to masses exceeding 15 cm. Smaller lesions tend to be slowly growing, sharply circumscribed, seemingly encapsulated, gray-white, round or multilobular, firm masses. Cystic spaces may be present. Larger lesions are more classically sarcomatous (i.e., soft, gray, fish-flesh in appearance with areas of cyst formation, hemorrhage, and necrosis). Sand-like calcifications may be palpable.

In the classic, biphasic lesion, cuboidal to columnar epithelial cells form cords, glands, microcystic spaces, or compact nests of cells. The nuclei are large, generally without marked variability in size, and the cytoplasm is abundant with distinct cell borders. Interspersed among these "epithelial" elements is the spindle cell, fibroblast-like component (Fig. 28–51). These cells tend to be laid down in interlacing bands with some greater variability in cell and nuclear size, but giant cells and mitotic figures are on the whole infrequent. In places, there are transitional zones where "epithelial cell"–fibroblast hybrids gradually blend into spindle cell elements. In other places the interface is quite abrupt. Uncommonly, as noted earlier, some synovial sarcomas are predominantly monophasic, but almost always traces of the classic biphasic pattern can be found (or the diagnosis should be reconsidered).

Helpful histologic features, when present, are focal calcifications usually in the spindled areas; PAS-positive, diastase-resistant secretions within the "epithelial cells"; and pseudoglandular cystic spaces. In addition, electron microscopy reveals irregular microvilli on the luminal surfaces of the "epithelial cells" abutting on the pseudoglandular or cystic spaces.[135] Analogous to the mesothelioma, both the spindle and "epithelial" components of synovial sarcomas have been found to contain cytokeratins with the immunoperoxidase method.[136]

In more than half of the cases, these neoplasms present as tender or painful deep-seated masses in close proximity to, but not involving, bone or the adjacent joint. Radiographs sometimes reveal spotty calcifications, and in about 15% of cases, the growth of the tumor extends to the bone, producing a periosteal reaction, erosion, or even invasion. Although most tumors grow slowly and have been present for years, some are rapidly enlarging and have already metastasized (20 to 25% of cases) to the lungs and elsewhere at the time of diagnosis. Local recurrence, which may be early or late following combined surgery and adjuvant therapy, is frequent, leading even-

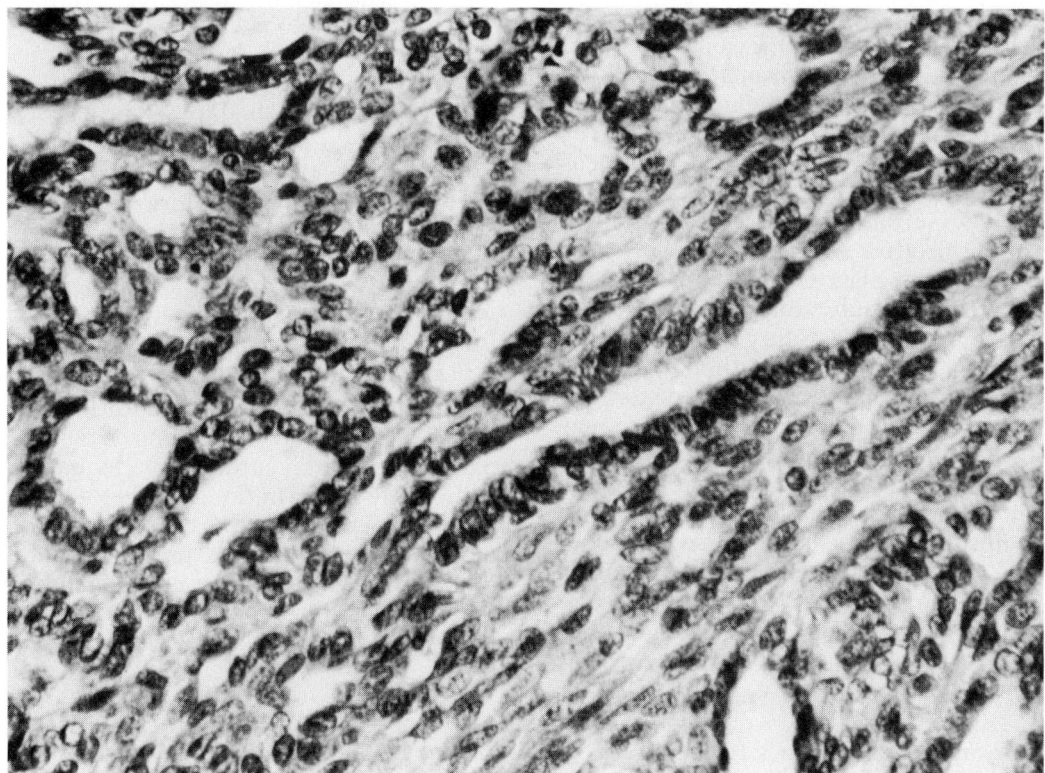

Figure 28-51. Synovial sarcoma revealing the classic biphasic spindle cell and epithelium-like histology.

tually to widespread metastases. The median five-year survival is about 45 to 50%.[137]

TUMOR-LIKE CONDITIONS

A few non-neoplastic entities require consideration here because they often mimic soft tissue tumors morphologically and clinically. Some of these lesions — the fibromatoses — fall in the gray area between reactive proliferations and neoplasms and range from those composed largely of dense collagen with sparse spindle cells to densely cellular tumor-appearing masses.

PALMAR, PLANTAR, AND PENILE FIBROMATOSIS

These more bothersome than serious lesions constitute a small group of superficial, largely collagenous fibromatoses. They are characterized by nodular or poorly defined aggregates of mature to somewhat immature fibroblasts dispersed throughout dense collagen. Ultrastructural studies indicate that many of these cells are myofibroblasts and therefore presumably contractile.[138] In the *palmar pattern (Dupuytren's contracture)*, the condition constitutes irregular or nodular subcutaneous thickening of the palmar fascia either unilaterally or bilaterally (50%). Over a span of years, attachment to the overlying skin causes puckering and dimpling, eventually resulting in a slowly progressive flexion contracture, mainly of the fourth and fifth fingers of the hand. Essentially similar changes are seen with *plantar fibromatosis* save that flexion contractures are uncommon and bilateral involvement is infrequent. In *penile fibromatosis (Peyronie's disease)*, a palpable induration or mass appears usually on the dorsolateral aspect of the penis. It may cause eventually abnormal curvature of the shaft or constriction of the urethra, or both.

It is significant that planter and palmar involvements appear in the same individual with greater than chance frequency, suggesting some genetic predisposition, but nothing is known about their cause. Although, not surprisingly, males are affected more frequently than females in Peyronie's disease, male predominance is true of the other patterns as well. In about 20 to 25% of cases, the palmar and plantar fibromatoses, after a period of time, stabilize and do not progress, and in some instances they resolve spontaneously. On the other hand, some recur after excision, particularly plantar lesions.

DESMOID (AGGRESSIVE FIBROMATOSIS)

Biologically, desmoids lie in the interface between exuberant fibroproliferations and low-grade fibrosarcomas. On the one hand, they present frequently as large, infiltrative masses that may recur after incomplete excision, whereas on the other hand, histologically they are composed of banal "tame-looking" fibroblasts that do not metastasize. They may occur at any age but are most frequent in the second to fourth decades.[139] They are sometimes divided into extra-abdominal, abdominal, and intra-abdominal, but all have essentially similar gross and microscopic features. *Extra-abdominal desmoids* occur in men and women with equal frequency and arise principally in the musculature of the shoulder, chest wall, back, and thigh.[140] *Abdominal desmoids* generally arise in the musculoaponeurotic structures of the anterior abdominal wall in women during or following pregnancy. *Intra-abdominal desmoids* tend to occur in the mesentery or pelvic walls, often in patients having Gardner's syndrome (p. 897).

Morphologically, these lesions occur as unicentric, gray-white, firm, unencapsulated, poorly demarcated masses varying from 1 to 15 cm in greatest diameter. They are rubbery and tough and infiltrate surrounding structures in an insidious manner such as between muscles, muscle bundles, and individual muscle cells. Histologically, the more central regions, presumably the oldest part of the growth, are largely densely collagenous, whereas the periphery is made up of plump, typical fibroblasts having moderate variation in cell and nuclear size, resembling a "low-grade" fibrosarcoma.[141] Mitoses are infrequent and, when present, are regular. Muscle cells or groups trapped within the growth are destroyed or atrophic. Sometimes, regenerative activity creates muscle giant cells having many sarcolemmal nuclei and abundant sarcoplasm.

The nature and origin of these masses remains obscure. The histologic appearance, their relationship to pregnancy, and the occasional history of antecedent trauma all suggest reaction to injury. The association with Gardner's syndrome raises the possibility of genetic influences. Estrogen receptor proteins have been identified in the fibroblasts in some, and similar desmoid-like masses have been produced in guinea pigs by the injection of estrogens, both observations pointing to endocrine influences.[142]

Of obvious importance is the differentiation of desmoids from sarcomas. In addition to their possibly being disfiguring or disabling they are occasionally painful. Although curable by adequate excision, they stubbornly recur in the local site when incompletely removed. The rare reports of metastasis of a desmoid must be interpreted as misidentification of a low-grade fibrosarcoma. We can conclude by recalling that "all that glitters is not gold" and analogously, all that "masses" is not neoplastic.

NODULAR (PSEUDOSARCOMATOUS) FASCIITIS

This reactive fibroproliferative lesion is probably more commonly mistaken for a neoplasm than any other non-neoplastic condition. Typically, these lesions present as palpable nodules or small masses most often in the extremities (but possibly elsewhere) in young and middle-aged adults of either sex.[143]

> Three somewhat distinctive macroscopic patterns are found. The most common by far is the **subcutaneous form** that extends from the superficial fascia outward into the subcutis as a discrete, rounded, gray-white lesion, usually less than 2 cm in diameter. The other, less common patterns are the **fascial form** that tends to spread along the fascia, and the **intramuscular variation** that extends deeply from the superficial fascia into the adjacent skeletal muscle. Although the classic subcutaneous form is well circumscribed, it is not encapsulated. The periphery often exhibits streaming extensions into the surrounding fat.[144]
>
> The histologic appearance varies with the age of the lesion and progresses through three phases—myxoid, cellular, and fibrosing. Common to all are plump, immature-appearing fibroblasts closely resembling those found in granulation tissue or tissue culture. Nuclei are large and "juicy," and nucleoli are often prominent giving some cells an ominous appearance and justifying the term "pseudosarcomatous." Although mitotic figures are frequent, they are almost never atypical. The early lesions are characterized by a myxoid pattern. They reveal short, irregular bundles or aggregates of fibroblasts scattered throughout a vascularized, mucopolysaccharide-rich matrix. As the lesion matures, it becomes cellular. Often the center is myxoid, while the more peripheral zones are cellular. The cellular phase is characterized by more closely packed, haphazardly arrayed, plump fibroblasts. In some instances, the fibroblasts are arrayed in bundles having a vague storiform (spoke-wheel) pattern. Intermixed with the fibroblasts are scattered lymphoid cells and red blood cells. Occasionally there are dispersed lipid-laden histiocytes and benign-appearing multinucleate giant cells (Fig. 28–52). The late fibrosing phase presumably represents a fully evolved lesion. Thick bundles of collagen are found between residual fibroblasts. The margins of these lesions permeate surrounding structures, and often there is entrapment of muscle cells and muscle giant cells within the margins. Foci of cartilage or osteoid or large atypical ganglion-like cells may be present in a special variant.[145]

It is evident that nodular fasciitis may produce a palpable tumorous mass readily mistaken for a sarcoma because of its apparent invasiveness and attachment to underlying fascia, and because of a rapid increase in size exceeding that of most cancers. However, after a period of rapid growth, the tumors tend to plateau in size, indicating progressive maturation. Recurrence following excision, even incomplete, is exceedingly rare and should lead to a reappraisal of the original diagnosis.

TRAUMATIC MYOSITIS OSSIFICANS

The final tumor-like lesion to be considered— myositis ossificans—has clearly been misnamed. It is

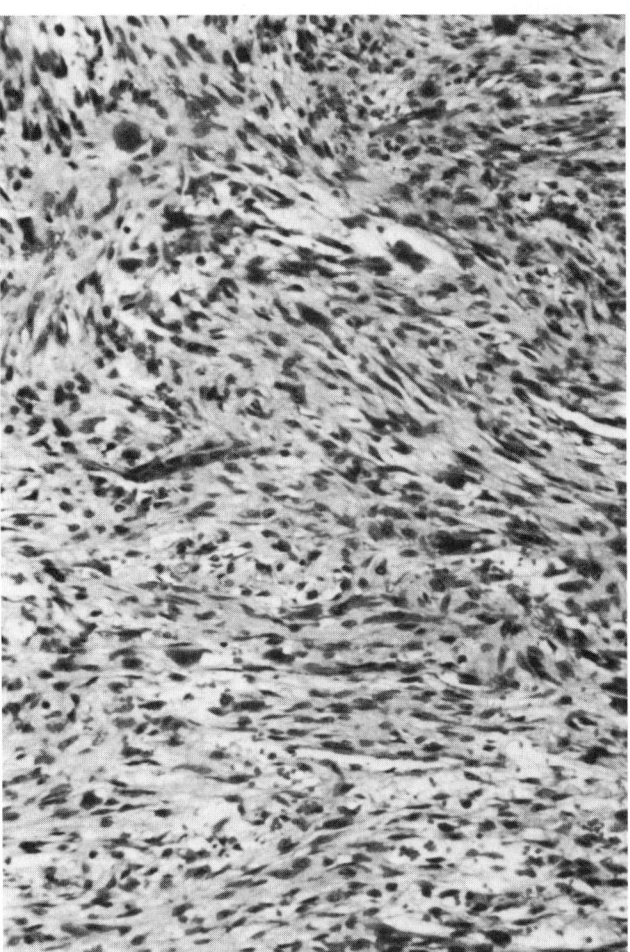

Figure 28-52. Nodular fasciitis. Cellular active margin of a lesion. There is considerable variation in nuclear size of plump fibroblasts with occasional cells approaching giant cells. Basis for term "pseudosarcomatous fibromatosis" is evident.

not restricted to skeletal muscles, it is not an inflammatory reaction, and it is not always "ossified." It is, however, a tumor-like lesion sometimes preceded by injury that develops most often in skeletal muscle, but sometimes in the subcutaneous fat. Favored locations are the extremities, particularly the quadriceps muscle in the leg and brachialis muscle in the arm. Most patients are young, athletically active males.

> Myositis ossificans begins with an area of pain, tenderness, and swelling presumably as a consequence of hemorrhage into a focus of injury in soft tissues. There follows a progressive sequence of ingrowth of a richly vascular, ossifying, fibroblastic tissue that ultimately produces a well-circumscribed, gray-white, unencapsulated, seemingly infiltrative mass, sometimes gritty, ranging to 5 to 8 cm in diameter. Histologically, the periphery of the mass has spicules of woven, often mineralized, bone surrounded by immature fibroblasts. This zone encloses an area of less well formed, less calcified osteoid dispersed in a looser cellular

fibrous tissue with plump, sometimes mitotically active fibroblasts. This organization suggests fibrous replacement and ossification of a hematoma from the periphery inward. Trapped within the margins are skeletal muscle fibers and regenerating muscle giant cells.

Clinically, in addition to the local symptoms of pain and tenderness, myositis ossificans produces a tumorous lesion that must be differentiated from a true neoplasm. The hard, localized bony mass often attached to the skeleton, the roentgenographic demonstration of bone density outside the normal bone, and the rich cellularity associated with bone formation may all be confused with an extraskeletal osteogenic sarcoma. Rare and controversial instances of malignant transformation have been reported.

1. Chambers, J.T.: The pathophysiology of the osteoclast. J. Clin. Pathol. *38*:241, 1985.

2. Fallon, M.D., and Teitelbaum, S.L.: The interpretation of fluorescent tetracycline markers in the diagnosis of metabolic bone diseases. Hum. Pathol. *13*:416, 1982.

3. Marcus, R.: Normal and abnormal bone remodeling in man. Annu. Rev. Med. *38*:129, 1987.

4. Tsipouras, P., and Ramirez, F.: Genetic disorders of collagen. J. Med. Genet. *24*:2, 1987.

5. Prockop, D.J., and Kivirikko, K.I.: Heritable diseases of collagen. N. Engl. J. Med. *311*:376, 1984.

6. Prockop, D.J.: Mutations in collagen genes. Consequences for rare and common diseases. J. Clin. Invest. *75*:783, 1985.

6a. Stacey, A., et al.: Perinatal lethal osteogenesis imperfecta in transgenic mice bearing an engineered mutant pro-alpha 1(1) collagen gene. Nature *131*:1, 1988.

7. Marks, S.C.: Osteopetrosis—multiple pathways for the interception of osteoclast function. Appl. Pathol. *5*:172, 1987.

8. Shapiro, F., et al.: Human osteopetrosis. Histologic, ultrastructural, and biochemical study. J. Bone Joint Surg. *62A*:384, 1980.

9. Ray, M.J., and Bassett, R.L.: Pyogenic vertebral osteomyelitis. Orthopedics *8*:506, 1985.

10. McHenry, M.C., et al.: Hematogenous osteomyelitis. Cleveland Clin. Q. *42*:125, 1975.

11. Waldfogel, F.A., and Vasey, H.: Osteomyelitis: The past decade. N. Engl. J. Med. *303*:360, 1980.

12. Martin, A.D., and Houston, C.S.: Osteoporosis, calcium, and physical activity. Can. Med. Assoc. J. *136*:587, 1987.

13. Silverberg, S.J., and Lindsay, R.: Postmenopausal osteoporosis. Med. Clin. North Am. *71*:41, 1987.

14. Raisz, L.G.: Local and systemic factors in the pathogenesis of osteoporosis. N. Engl. J. Med. *318*:818, 1988.

15. Kleerekoper, M., et al.: Nutritional, endocrine, and demographic aspects of osteoporosis. Orthop. Clin. North Am. *12*:547, 1981.

16. Nordin, B.E.C., et al.: Treatment of spinal osteoporosis in postmenopausal women. Br. Med. J. *280*:451, 1980.

16a. Holbrook, T.L., et al.: Dietary calcium and risk of hip fracture: 14 year prospective population study. Lancet *2*:1046, 1988.

17. Cushner, H.M., and Adams, N.D.: Review: Renal osteodystrophy—pathogenesis and treatment. Am. J. Med. Sci. *291*:264, 1986.

18. Slatopolsky, E.: The interaction of parathyroid hormone and aluminum in renal osteodystrophy. Kidney Int. *31*:842, 1987.

19. Nebeker, H.G., and Coburn, J.W.: Aluminum and renal osteodystrophy. Annu. Rev. Med. *37*:79, 1986.

20. Maloney, N.A., et al.: Histologic quantitation of aluminum in iliac bone from patients with renal failure. J. Lab. Clin. Med. *99*:206, 1982.

21. Barker, D.J.P.: The epidemiology of Paget's disease of bone. Br. Med. Bull. *40*:396, 1984.

22. Mirra, J.M.: Pathogenesis of Paget's disease based on viral etiology. Clin. Orthop. *217*:162, 1987.

23. Basle, M.F., et al.: On the trail of paramyxoviruses in Paget's disease of bone. Clin. Orthop. *217*:9, 1987.

24. Meunier, P.J., et al: Skeletal distribution of biochemical parameters of Paget's disease. Clin. Orthop. *217*:37, 1987.

25. Ouslander, J.G., and Beck J.C.: Paget's disease of bone. J. Am. Geriatr. Soc. *30*:410, 1982.

26. Henley, J.W., et al.: The cardiovascular system in Paget's disease of bone and the response to therapy with calcitonin and diphosphonate. Aust. N.Z. J. Med. *9*:390, 1979.

27. Seret, P., et al.: Sarcomatous degeneration in Paget's bone disease. J. Cancer Res. Clin. Oncol. *113*:392, 1987.

28. Lee, P.A., et al.: McCune-Albright syndrome. Long-term follow-up. J.A.M.A. *256*:2980, 1986.

29. Harris, W., et al.: The natural history of fibrous dysplasia. J. Bone Joint Surg. *44A*:207, 1962.

30. Harris, R.I.: Polyostotic fibrous dysplasia with acromegaly. Am. J. Med. *78*:539, 1985.

31. Mauras, N., and Blizzard, R.M.: The McCune-Albright syndrome. Acta Endocrinol. (Suppl.) *279*:207, 1986.

32. Nager, G.T., et al.: Fibrous dysplasia: A review of the disease and its manifestations in the temporal bone. Ann. Otol. Rhinol. Laryngol. (Suppl.) *92*:5, 1982.

33. Hausen-Flasche, J., and Nordberg, J.: Clubbing and hypertrophic osteoarthropathy. Clin. Chest Med. *8*:287, 1987.

34. Senac, M.O., et al.: Primary lesions of bone in the first decade of life: Retrospective survey of biopsy results. Radiology *160*:491, 1986.

35. Healey, J.H., and Ghelman, B.: Osteoid osteoma and osteoblastoma. Clin. Orthop. *204*:76, 1986.

36. Byers, P.D.: Solitary benign osteoblastic lesions of bone: Osteoid, osteoma, and osteoblastoma. Cancer *22*:43, 1968.

37. Kenan, S., et al.: Aggressive osteoblastoma. Clin. Orthop. *195*:294, 1985.

38. Dahlin, D.C., and Unni, K.K.: Bone tumors, 4th ed. Springfield, Illinois, Charles C Thomas, 1986, p. 269.

39. Dorfman, H.D.: Malignant transformation of benign bone lesions. Proc. Natl. Cancer Conf. 7:901, 1973.

40. Dryja, T.P., et al.: Molecular detection of deletions involving band q14 of chromosome 13 in retinoblastomas. Proc. Natl. Acad. Sci. U.S.A. *83*:7391, 1986.

41. Dryja, T.P., et al.: Chromosome 13 homozygosity in osteosarcoma without retinoblastoma. Am. J. Hum. Genet. *38*:59, 1986.

42. Wiggs, J., et al.: Prediction of the risk of hereditary retinoblastoma using DNA polymorphisms within the retinoblastoma gene. N. Engl. J. Med. *318*:151, 1988.

43. Finkel, M.P.: Pathogenesis of radiation and virus-induced bone tumors. Rec. Adv. Cancer Res. *54*:92, 1976.

44. Sinkovizs, J.G.: Bone sarcomas: Etiology and immunology. Can. J. Surg. *20*:494, 1977.

45. Sim, F.H., et al.: Osteosarcoma: State of the art. Minnesota Med. *69*:442, 1986.

46. Milgram, J.W.: The origins of osteochondromas and enchondromas, a histopathologic study. Clin. Orthop. *174*:264, 1983.

47. Liu, J., et al.: Bone sarcomas associated with Ollier's disease. Cancer *59*:1376, 1987.

48. Beggs, I.G., and Stoker, D.J.: Chondromyxoid fibroma of bone. Clin. Radiol. *33*:671, 1982.

49. Springfield, D.S., et al.: Chondroblastoma: A review of 70 cases. J. Bone Joint Surg. *67A*:748, 1985.

50. Levine, G.D., and Bensch, K.G.: Chondroblastoma—the nature of the basic cell. A study by means of histochemistry, tissue culture, electron microscopy, and autoradiography. Cancer *29*:1546, 1972.

51. Kyriakos, M., et al.: Metastatic chondroblastoma. Report of a fatal case with a review of the literature on atypical, aggressive, and malignant chondroblastoma. Cancer *55*:1770, 1985.

52. Mirra, J.M., et al.: A new histologic approach to the differentiation of enchondroma and chondrosarcoma of the bones. Clin. Orthop. *201*:214, 1985.

53. Kristensen, I.B., et al.: Chondrosarcoma. Increasing grade of malignancy and local recurrence. Acta Pathol. Microbiol. Immunol. Scand. *94*:73, 1986.

54. Taconis, W.K.: Clear cell chondrosarcoma: Report of three

cases and review of the literature. Diagn. Imaging Clin. Med. *55*:219, 1986.

55. Evans, H.L., et al.: Prognostic factors in chondrosarcoma of bone. A clinicopathologic analysis with emphasis on histologic grading. Cancer *40*:818, 1977.

56. Wilkins, R.M., et al.: Ewing's sarcoma of bone. Experience with 140 patients. Cancer *58*:2551, 1986.

57. Yunis, E.J.: Ewing's sarcoma and related small round cell neoplasms in children. Am. J. Surg. Pathol. (Suppl. 1) *10*:54, 1986.

58. Whang-Peng, J., et al.: Cytogenetic characterization of selected small round cell tumor of childhood. Cancer Genet. Cytogenet. *21*:185, 1986.

59. Cavazzana, A.O., et al.: Experimental evidence for a neural origin of Ewing's sarcoma of bone. Am. J. Pathol. *127*:507, 1987.

60. Eckardt, J.J., and Grogan, T.J.: Giant cell tumor of bone. Clin. Orthop. *204*:45, 1986.

61. Burmester, G.R., et al.: Delineation of four cell types comprising the giant cell tumor of bone. J. Clin. Invest. *71*:1633, 1983.

62. Goldring, S.R., et al.: Human giant cell tumors of bone. Identification and characterization of cell types. J. Clin. Invest. *79*:483, 1987.

63. Sim, F.H., et al.: Multicentric giant cell tumor of bone. J. Bone Joint Surg. *59A*:1052, 1977.

64. Moskowitz, R.W.: Primary osteoarthritis: Epidemiology, clinical aspects, and general management. Am. J. Med. *83(Suppl. 5A)*:5, 1987.

65. Wong, S.Y.P., et al.: The pathogenesis of osteoarthritis of the hip. Evidence for primary osteocyte death. Clin. Orthop. *214*:305, 1987.

66. Howell, D.S.: Pathogenesis of osteoarthritis. Am. J. Med. *80(Suppl. 4B)*:24, 1986.

67. Heinegard, D., et al.: Cartilage proteoglycans in degenerative joint disease. J. Rheumatol. *14(Suppl. 14)*:110, 1987.

68. Ehrlich, M.G., et al.: The role of proteases in the pathogenesis of osteoarthritis. J. Rheumatol. *14(Suppl. 14)*:30, 1987.

69. Gregersen, P.K., et al.: The shared epitope hypothesis. An approach to understanding the molecular genetics of susceptibility to rheumatoid arthritis. Arthritis Rheum. *30*:1205, 1987.

70. Maini, R.N., et al.: Autoimmunity in rheumatoid arthritis. An approach via a study of B lymphocytes. Rheum. Dis. Clin. North Am. *13*:319, 1987.

71. Bromley, M., and Woolley, D.E.: Histopathology of the rheumatoid lesion. Identification of cell types at sites of cartilage erosion. Arthritis Rheum. *27*:857, 1984.

72. Mainardi, C.L.: Biochemical mechanisms of articular destruction. Rheum. Dis. Clin. North Am. *13*:215, 1987.

73. Henderson, B., et al.: Mediators of rheumatoid arthritis. Br. Med. Bull. *43*:415, 1987.

73a. Eastgate, J.A., et al.: Correlation of plasma interleukin 1 levels with disease activity in rheumatoid arthritis. Lancet *2*:706, 1988.

74. Beutler, B., and Cerami, A.: Cachetin and tumor necrosis factors as two sides of the same biological coin. Nature *320*:584, 1986.

75. Clegg, D.O., and Ward, J.R.: Diagnostic criteria in rheumatoid arthritis. Scand. J. Rheumatol. *(Suppl.)65*:3, 1987.

76. Schaller, J.: Juvenile rheumatoid arthritis. Postgrad. Med. *61*:177, 1977.

77. Editorial: Felty's syndrome. Lancet *1*:540, 1978.

78. Goldings, E.A., and Jericho, J.: Lyme disease. Clin. Rheum. Dis. *12*:343, 1986.

79. Johnston, Y.E., et al.: Lyme arthritis spirochetes found in synovial microangiopathic lesions. Am. J. Pathol. *118*:26, 1985.

80. Wyngaarden, J.B., and Kelley, W.N.: Gout. *In* Stanbury, J.B., et al. (eds.): Metabolic Basis of Inherited Disease, 5th ed. New York, McGraw-Hill Book Co., 1982, p. 1043.

81. German, D.C., and Holmes, E.W.: Hyperuricemia and gout. Med. Clin. North Am. *70*:419, 1986.

82. Boss, G.R., and Seegmiller, J.E.: Hyperuricemia and gout. Classification, complications, and management. N. Engl. J. Med. *300*:1459, 1979.

83. German, D.C., and Holmes, E.W.: Gout and hyperuricemia. Diagnosis and management. Hosp. Pract. *21*:119, 1986.

84. Dreppe, P.A.: Crystal deposition and inflammation. Q. J. Med. *3*:309, 1984.

85. Di Giovine, F.S., et al.: Interleukin 1 (IL-1) as a mediator of crystal arthritis. Stimulation of T cell and synovial fibroblast mitogenesis by urate crystal–induced IL-1. J. Immunol. *138*:3213, 1987.

86. Chung, E.B.: Histologic changes in gout. Georgetown Med. Bull. *15*:269, 1962.

87. Dykman, D., et al.: Hyperuricemia and uric acid nephropathy. Arch. Intern. Med. *147*:1341, 1987.

88. McCarty, D.J.: Arthritis associated with crystals containing calcium. Med. Clin. North Am. *70*:437, 1986.

89. Myers, B.W., et al.: Pigmented villonodular synovitis: Light and electron microscopic studies. Semin. Arthritis Rheum. *12*:32, 1982.

90. Craig, R.: The structure of the contractile elements. *In* Engle, A., and Banker, B. (eds.): Myology. Vol. 1. New York, McGraw-Hill Book Co., 1976, p. 73.

91. Huxley, A.F.: The activation of striated muscle and its mechanical response. Proc. R. Soc. Biol. *178*:1, 1971.

92. Lazarides, E.: Intermediate filaments as mechanical integrators of cellular space. Nature *283*:249, 1980.

93. Pardo, J.V., et al.: A vinculin containing cortical lattice in skeletal muscle: Transverse lattice elements ("costameres") mark sites of attachment between myofibrils and sarcolemma. Proc. Natl. Acad. Sci. U.S.A. *80*:1008, 1983.

94. Grob, D., et al.: The natural course of myasthenia gravis and the effect of therapeutic measures. Ann. N.Y. Acad. Sci. *377*:652, 1981.

95. Engel, A.G., et al.: Ultrastructural localization of the acetylcholine receptor in myasthenia gravis and in its experimental autoimmune model. Neurology *27*:307, 1977.

96. Engel, A.G., et al.: The motor end plate in myasthenia gravis and in experimental autoimmune myasthenia gravis. A quantitative ultrastructural study. Ann. N.Y. Acad. Sci. *274*:60, 1976.

97. Engel, A.G.K., et al.: The ultrastructural localization of the acetylcholine receptor, immunoglobulin G, and the third and ninth complement components at the motor endplate and their implications for the pathogenesis of myasthenia gravis. *In* Aguayo, A.J., and Karpati, G. (eds.): Current Topics in Nerve and Muscle Research. Amsterdam, Excerpta Medica, 1978, p. 111.

98. Drachman, D.B., et al.: Humoral pathogenesis of myasthenia gravis. Ann. N.Y. Acad. Sci. *505*:90, 1987.

99. Lennon, V.: Immunologic mechanisms in myasthenia gravis—a model of a receptor disease. *In* Franklin, E.E. (ed.): Clinical Immunology Update: Reviews for Physicians. New York, Elsevier, 1979, p. 259.

100. Kirchner, T., et al.: Pathogenesis of myasthenia gravis. Acetylcholine receptor–related antigenic determinants in tumor-free thymuses and thymic epithelial tumors. Am. J. Pathol. *130*:268, 1988.

101. Scadding, G.K., et al.: Acetylcholine receptor antibody synthesis by thymic lymphocytes: Correlation with thymic histology. Neurology *31*:395, 1981.

102. Osserman, K.E., and Genkins, G.: Studies in myasthenia gravis: Review of a twenty-year experience in over 1200 patients. Mt. Sinai J. Med. (N.Y.) *38*:497, 1971.

103. Compston, D.A.S., et al.: Clinical, pathological, HLA antigen, and immunological evidence for disease heterogeneity in myasthenia gravis. Brain *103*:579, 1980.

104. Osserman, K.E.: Myasthenia gravis and thyroid disease: Clinical and immunological correlation. J. Mt. Sinai Hosp. *34*:469, 1967.

105. Engel, A.G.: Myasthenic syndromes. *In* Engel, A.G., and Banker, B. (eds.): Myology. Vol. 2. New York, McGraw-Hill Book Co., 1986, p. 1955.

106. Karpati, G., and Engel, W.K.: "Type grouping" in skeletal muscles after experimental reinnervation. Neurology *18*:447, 1968.

107. Moser, H.: Duchenne muscular dystrophy: Pathogenetic aspects and genetic prevention. Hum. Genet. *66*:17, 1984.

108. Hoffman, E.P., et al.: Conservation of the Duchenne muscular dystrophy in mice and humans. Science *238*:347, 1987.

109. Hoffman, E.P., et al.: Dystrophin: The protein product of the Duchenne muscular dystrophy locus. Cell *51*:919, 1987.

110. Hoffman, E.P., et al.: Characterization of dystrophin in muscle–biopsy specimens from patients with Duchenne's or Becker's muscular dystrophy. N. Engl. J. Med. *318*:1363, 1988.

111. Hoffman, E.P., et al.: Subcellular fractionation of dystrophin to the triads of skeletal muscle. Nature *330*:754, 1987.

112. Harper, P.S.: Myotonic disorders. *In* Engel, A., and Banker, B.

(eds.): Myology. Vol. 2. New York, McGraw-Hill Book Co., 1986, p. 1267.

113. Eiberg, H., et al.: Linkage relationship between the locus of C3 and 50 polymorphic systems. Assignment of C3 to the DM-SE-LU linkage group: Confirmation of C3-LES linkage; support of LES-DM synteny. *In* Proceedings of the Sixth International Congress on Human Genetics. New York, Alan Liss, 1983.

114. Enzinger, F.M., and Weiss, S.W.: Soft Tissue Tumors. St. Louis, C.V. Mosby Co., 1983.

115. Roholl, P.J.M., et al.: Application of markers in the diagnosis of soft tissue tumors. Histopathology *9*:1019, 1985.

116. Costa, J., et al.: The grading of soft tissue sarcomas. Results of a clinicohistopathologic correlation in a series of 163 cases. Cancer *53*:530, 1984.

117. Rooser, B., et al.: Prognostication in soft tissue sarcoma. A model with four risk factors. Cancer *61*:817, 1988.

118. Morrison, J.G., et al.: Granular cell tumors. Am. Surg. *53*:156, 1987.

119. Stephansson, K., and Wollman, R.L.: S100 protein in granular cell tumors (granular cell myoblastomas). Cancer *49*:1834, 1982.

120. Lack, E.E., et al.: Granular cell tumor: A clinicopathologic study of 110 patients. J. Surg. Oncol. *13*:301, 1980.

121. McCarthy, E.F., et al.: Malignant fibrous histiocytoma of bone. A study of 35 cases. Hum. Pathol. *10*:57, 1979.

122. Iwasaki, H., et al.: Malignant fibrous histiocytoma. Evidence of perivascular mesenchymal cell origin. Immunocytochemical studies with monoclonal anti-MFH antibodies. Am. J. Pathol. *128*:528, 1987.

123. Nemes, Z., and Thomazy, V.: Factor XIIIa and the classic histiocytic markers in malignant fibrous histiocytoma. Hum. Pathol. *19*:822, 1988.

124. Lagace, R.: The ultrastructural spectrum of malignant fibrous histiocytoma. Ultrastruct. Pathol. *11*:153, 1987.

125. Spittle, M.F., et al.: Liposarcoma — a review of 60 cases. Br. J. Cancer *24*:696, 1971.

126. Di Sant'Agnese, P.A., and Knowles, D.M., II: Extracardiac rhabdomyoma: A clinicopathologic study and review of the literature. Cancer *46*:780, 1980.

127. Molenaar, W.M., et al.: The rarity of rhabdomyosarcomas in the adult. A morphologic and immunohistochemical study. Pathol. Res. Pract. *180*:400, 1985.

128. Agamanolis, D.P., et al.: Tumors of skeletal muscle. Hum. Pathol. *17*:778, 1986.

129. Scupham, R., et al.: Immunohistochemical studies of rhabdomyosarcoma. Arch. Pathol. Lab. Med. *110*:818, 1986.

130. Miettinen, M.: Antibody specific to muscle actins in the diagnosis and classification of soft tissue tumors. Am. J. Pathol. *130*:205, 1988.

131. DeJong, A.S.H., et al.: Pleomorphic rhabdomyosarcoma in adults: Immunohistochemistry as a tool for its diagnosis. Hum. Pathol. *18*:298, 1987.

132. Gaiger, A.M., et al.: Pathology of rhabdomyosarcoma: Experience of the intergroup rhabdomyosarcoma study 1972–1978. National Cancer Institute Monograph 56, p. 19, 1981.

133. Hawkins, H.K., and Camacho-Velasquez, J.D.: Rhabdomyosarcoma in children. Correlation of form and prognosis in one institution's experience. Am. J. Surg. Pathol. *11*:531, 1987.

134. Soule, E.H.: Synovial sarcoma. Am. J. Surg. Pathol. *10(Suppl. 1)*:78, 1986.

135. Krall, R.A., et al.: Synovial sarcoma. A clinical, pathological, and ultrastructural study of 26 cases supporting the recognition of a monophasic variant. Am. J. Surg. Pathol. *5*:137, 1981.

136. Corson, J.M., et al.: Keratin proteins and carcinoembryonic antigen in synovial sarcomas: An immunohistochemical study of 24 cases. Hum. Pathol. *15*:615, 1984.

137. Rajpal, S., et al.: Synovial sarcoma. A review of treatment and survival in 52 patients. N.Y. State J. Med. *84*:17, 1984.

138. Gabbiani, G., and Majno, G.: Dupuytren's contracture: Fibroblast contraction? Am. J. Pathol. *66*:131, 1972.

139. Reitamo, J.J., et al.: The desmoid tumor. 1. Incidence, sex-, age-, and anatomical distribution in the Finnish population. Am. J. Clin. Pathol. *77*:665, 1982.

140. Markhede, G., et al.: Extra-abdominal desmoid tumors. Acta Orthopaed. Scand. *57*:1, 1986.

141. MacKenzie, D.H.: The fibromatoses. A clinicopathological concept. Br. Med. J. *4*:277, 1972.

142. Weiss, S.W., et al.: Estrogen receptor protein in bone and soft tissue tumors. Lab. Invest. *54*:689, 1986.

143. Shimizu, S., et al.: Nodular fasciitis: An analysis of 250 patients. Pathology *16*:161, 1984.

144. Weiss, S.W.: Proliferative fibroblastic lesions from hypoplasia to neoplasia. Am. J. Surg. Pathol. *10(Suppl. 1)*:14, 1986.

145. Bernstein, K.E., and Lattes, R.: Nodular (pseudosarcomatous) fasciitis. A nonrecurrent lesion: Clinicopathologic study of 134 cases. Cancer *49*:1668, 1982.

The Nervous System

James H. Morris, M.A., D.Phil., B.M., B.Ch.

To even the least introspective, the brain is an organ of enormous structural and physiologic complexity and unparalleled subtlety of operation. To an extent, both the complexity and the subtlety are manifested in the pathology of the brain, and this can make neuropathology seem very intimidating and obscure to the uninitiated. However, much of the apparent obscurity is only a reflection of the differences be-

tween the brain and other organs, and once these are appreciated many of the difficulties disappear. The major differences that have pathologic significance are:

1. The high degree of *localization of function* in the nervous system. This is perhaps the most important difference between the brain and the rest of the body,

and it has four major pathologically important consequences.

a. *Localization of function makes the brain inherently vulnerable to focal lesions that in other organs might go unnoticed or produce only trivial symptoms.* For example, the destruction of quite small areas of brain can severely impair specific functions such as speech and the ability to move one side of the body; by contrast, two-thirds of the renal mass can be destroyed without fatally compromising renal function. This vulnerability of the brain to small lesions is compounded by its very limited capacity to reconstitute damaged tissue. There has clearly been a serious error by the celestial committee in its design of an organ that is vital for biologic survival and yet is both the most vulnerable to, and the least tolerant of, focal damage.

b. The *localization of function in the brain causes the same pathologic process to manifest clinically in a completely different way when it affects a different part of the system.* For example, a meningioma (p. 1420) in the olfactory groove might manifest insidiously with unilateral anosmia (loss of sense of smell), but the same tumor impinging on the foramen magnum would produce a progressive and ultimately life-threatening quadriplegia from spinal cord compression.

c. *Localization of physiologic function has its pathologic counterpart in the selective vulnerability of types of neurons or specific regions of the brain to particular pathologic processes or etiologic agents.* For example, Purkinje cells of the cerebellum and hippocampal neurons are particularly susceptible to ischemia; herpes simplex virus type I initially attacks the temporal lobes; amyotrophic lateral sclerosis (ALS) affects only motor neurons.

d. In a rather different way, localization is important in pathologic diagnosis. Like other organs, the brain has only a limited repertoire of pathologic responses, so that the same type of pathologic change, e.g., neurofibrillary tangle formation, can occur in more than one disease. Hence, *pathologic diagnosis sometimes rests as much on the localization (distribution) of the pathologic change in the nervous system as on its character.*

2. *The nervous system has a number of anatomic and physiologic features that are peculiar to it and very much affect the way disease is expressed.* Some act as double-edged swords, conferring protection against one form of attack while increasing the vulnerability to a different kind of pathologic assault. The most important are the *skull,* which protects against trauma but makes possible raised intracranial pressure and herniation; the *cerebrospinal fluid,* which also protects against trauma but is the agent for the development of hydrocephalus and the dissemination of microorganisms and tumor cells in infective and carcinomatous meningitis; the *blood-brain barrier,* which stabilizes the intraparenchymal "milieu intérieur"; and the *absence of lymphatic drainage,* which in combination with the blood-brain barrier makes the

brain an immunologically privileged site but also renders it particularly susceptible to the accumulation of edema.

3. *Nervous system diseases fall into two general groups:*

a. Processes such as infections, trauma, and neoplasms, which occur both in the nervous system and in other organs.

b. Conditions unique to the nervous system, a category that includes the diseases of myelin and system degenerations of neurons. They are much rarer than diseases with systemic counterparts.

Because the nervous system is so large and complex it is nearly impossible pathologically to examine all its parts in detail. It is therefore important to determine which parts are involved clinically before undertaking a pathologic examination; in many cases a diagnosis is made only by correlating the clinical and pathologic findings.

NORMAL CELLS AND THEIR BASIC REACTIONS TO INJURY

The brain parenchyma is composed of neurons, neuroglia, and microglia. The neuroglia form a specialized supporting matrix in which the neurons are embedded, and the microglia are the nervous system counterpart of the monocyte-phagocyte system.

NEURONS

Neurons, with their network of axons, dendrites, and synaptic contacts, are the basic communicating units of the nervous system. They come in a large variety of shapes and sizes, ranging from the small granular cells of the cerebellum to the large Betz cells of the motor cortex. The archetypal neuron is the cortical pyramidal neuron that is triangular in outline and has a large watery nucleus with a prominent nucleolus. The cytoplasm contains clumps of rough-surfaced endoplasmic reticulum and free ribosomal rosettes (called Nissl substance) that stain strongly with basic dyes such as hematoxylin and cresyl violet (Nissl stain). Other special features of neuronal cytoplasm are microtubules, various types of synaptic vesicles,[1] and neurofilaments. Neurofilaments are the intermediate filament specific to neurons and are composed of three polypeptide chains with molecular weights of 68K, 150K, and 200K.[2]

In disease a variety of changes occur in neurons that are, to varying degrees, associated with specific etiologic agents or pathologic processes. Most of these will be discussed with the appropriate disease, but some more ubiquitous processes are better described here.

1. *Atrophy and degeneration.* In many of the system degenerations of neurons (p. 1426), the affected neurons atrophy and die without undergoing any specific morphologic change or inciting much glial reaction.

In some neuron systems, damage to one neuron may also provoke degeneration of the neuron with which it synapses, as happens, for example, in the visual system, where removal of the eye results in *trans-synaptic degeneration* of the neurons of the lateral geniculate body on which the retinal ganglion cells synapse.

2. *Intraneuronal body formation.* A number of the degenerative diseases are associated with intracytoplasmic neuronal bodies, notably neurofibrillary tangles (p. 1427), Lewy bodies (p. 1430), Pick bodies (p. 1429), and Hirano bodies (p. 1429).

3. *Intraneuronal storage.* Neurons may be the depository of stored substances in inborn errors of metabolism (e.g., Niemann-Pick disease, p. 146). Microscopically they are enlarged with an eccentrically placed nucleus. The distended cytoplasm usually appears granular regardless of the composition of the stored material. The ultrastructure of the material is sometimes diagnostic, but biochemical analysis of brain or some other tissue is usually the definitive diagnostic procedure.[3]

4. *Chromatolysis (axonal reaction).* If its axon is cut or damaged the cell body of the neuron may swell up, becoming round and pale staining (chromatolysis). There is loss, particularly centrally, of stainable Nissl substance and displacement of the nucleus to the periphery of the cell.

5. *Axonal degeneration.* Neuronal dysfunction may be manifested by inability to maintain its axon, which *dies back* from its distal terminal. This is most frequently seen in the peripheral nervous system (p. 1441), but also occurs in the CNS, notably at the upper end of the dorsal columns and the lower end of the corticospinal tract. *Spheroids* are circular or elongated granular bodies containing cell organelles. They are local dilatations of axons and are seen around the edges of infarcts, in axonal dystrophies, and in other situations of axonal damage.

NEUROGLIA

The neuroglial cells are the proletarians of CNS society, providing shelter and maintenance for the aristocratic neurons. They comprise astrocytes, oligodendrocytes, and ependymal cells.

Astrocytes

Hematoxylin and eosin stains of normal brain demonstrate only astrocyte nuclei that are round or oval and have fine granular chromatin. With special stains (such as Cajal gold sublimate) that reveal their cytoplasm, they emerge as stellate cells with processes that ramify to form a framework for the other brain cells (Fig. 29–1). Processes that end on blood vessels have expanded terminals called *foot processes* or *end feet*. Astrocytes are divided into *protoplasmic* and *fibrous* forms on the basis of the geometry of their processes; the protoplasmic form occurs mostly in gray matter and has frequently branched processes, whereas the fibrous astrocytes have long thin processes and are found mostly in white matter.

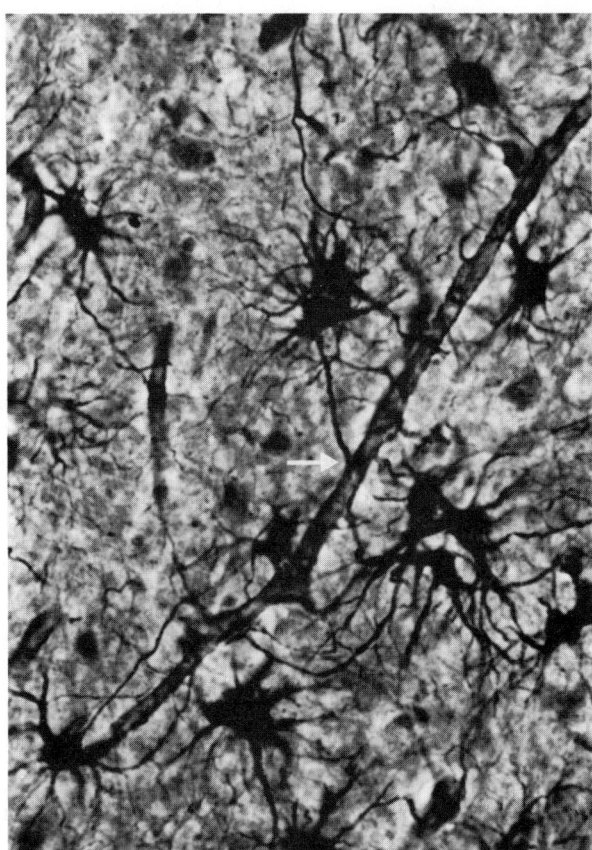

Figure 29–1. Astrocytes and their processes. Some processes are attached to blood vessels *(arrow)* (Cajal gold sublimate).

The functions of astrocytes are incompletely understood but probably include the provision of physical and biochemical support, insulation of the receptive surface of neurons, and interactions with capillary endothelial cells in the establishment and maintenance of the blood-brain barrier (p. 1389).[4] In damaged brain they act rather like fibroblasts in the rest of the body and form glial "scars," a process called *gliosis*. There is proliferation of fibrillary astrocytes and the formation of a feltwork of cellular processes. However, unlike the fibrosis that occurs in other organs, no collagen or equivalent extracellular fibrous protein is produced, so that a glial "scar" is composed entirely of cellular processes. The glial fibers contain abundant intermediate filaments, some of which are the specific glial fibrillary acidic protein (GFAP), although most are vimentin. GFAP is well demonstrated immunocytochemically, but astrocyte processes can also be stained by phosphotungstic acid–hematoxylin (PTAH) and Holzer stains. Early reactive astrocytes develop a conspicuous pink hyaline cytoplasm and are called *gemistocytic (stuffed) astrocytes*. The nucleus, which in this activated state may have a nucleolus, is often displaced to one side. As the reaction resolves, the astrocytes lose their cytoplasm but retain the processes and are then called *fibrillary astrocytes*. If a specific tract is damaged the gliosis tends to conform to the pattern of the tract and is called *isomorphic gliosis*, whereas in gross tissue destruction the gliosis is random and called *anisomorphic gliosis*.

Rosenthal fibers are eosinophilic, opaque, elongated, tapering or globular bodies that form in astrocyte processes.[5] They are strongly PTAH positive but GFAP negative. Ultrastructurally they are irregular, amorphous, electron dense, and surrounded by a feltwork of intermediate filaments. They are found in long-standing progressive gliosis, but are also typically present in juvenile pilocytic astrocytomas (p. 1414), which are very slow-growing tumors, and in Alexander's disease, an extremely rare form of leukodystrophy.

Corpora amylacea (polyglucosan bodies) accumulate with age in astrocyte processes, principally in the subpial and subependymal regions and around blood vessels. They are spherical, basophilic, PAS-positive, sometimes concentrically laminated structures with a diameter between 1 and 150 μm. Ultrastructurally they are composed of branched filaments approximately 8 nm in diameter, and their main biochemical component is glucose polymers with a small and variable content of phosphate and sulfate groups and less than 5% protein. The *Lafora bodies* seen in the perikarya of neurons in myoclonus epilepsy (Lafora's disease) are biochemically similar, as are the polyglucosan bodies that accumulate in astrocytes in *type IV glycogenosis* (amylopectinosis) and in a few other rare conditions.[6]

Oligodendrocytes

These cells are so called because, when visualized by special stains such as the Hortega carbonate, they have fewer and shorter processes than astrocytes. Hematoxylin and eosin stains only the small, dark, lymphocyte-sized nucleus, around which there is often a clear halo that although regularly present is an artifact of fixation. Ultrastructurally, the nucleus is eccentrically located in a cytoplasm containing many microtubules that makes it difficult to distinguish between oligodendrocyte processes and dendrites. Oligodendrocytes are found throughout the brain; in white matter they are frequently lined up along the myelinated fibers, but in gray matter they tend to cluster around the neurons, where they are called *satellite cells. The principal function of oligodendrocytes is the production and maintenance of the CNS myelin.* They are the counterpart of the Schwann cells of the peripheral nervous system (p. 1442), but unlike Schwann cells, oligodendrocytes contribute segments of myelin sheath to multiple axons. Because they produce myelin, diseases affecting oligodendrocytes manifest as disorders of myelin and myelination. The two major groups are the *leukodystrophies* (p. 1437), which are generalized, usually inherited disorders of myelin metabolism, and the acquired *demyelinating diseases* (p. 1422), such as multiple sclerosis, in which there is focal myelin loss.

Ependymal Cells

Ependymal cells form a single layer of cuboidal-to-columnar cells that line the cerebral ventricles and form the central canal of the spinal cord. They react to injury mainly by cell loss, the ensuing gaps being filled with glial fibers produced by the underlying astrocytes (ependymal granulations). Ependymal cells are also occasionally the target for infection, notably by cytomegalovirus (p. 1398).

Microglia

Microglial cells are found in all areas of the brain. Routine stains show only the small elongated nuclei, but special stains (Hortega carbonate) and electron microscopy reveal a few long angular cytoplasmic processes with few organelles but scattered dense bodies. In response to tissue damage, microglia proliferate and develop elongated nuclei (*rod cells*), and can form microscopic clusters (*microglial nodules*) around tiny foci of necrosis or dead neurons (*neuronophagia*). Some authorities consider that, after gross tissue destruction, microglial cells are capable of assuming the shape and function of macrophages (*gitter cells, compound granular corpuscles*), although it is clear that a large majority of the macrophages seen in the brain in necrotizing processes are derived from the blood.

Historically there have been two schools of thought about the origin of microglia, one that they are ectodermal and the other that they are mesodermal like the rest of the mononuclear-phagocyte (reticuloendothelial) system (MPS). Recent work suggests that, when activated, they have histochemical reactions similar to those of macrophages and quite different from the reactions of other glial cells.[7] It now seems that microglia are the representatives of the MPS in the nervous system.[8] As such, the name microglia, which tends to link them with the true glial cells, is misleading but probably unchangeable.

COMMON PATHOPHYSIOLOGIC COMPLICATIONS

The fixed and restricted volume of the cranial vault is one of the most important of the special anatomic features of the brain. It renders the brain susceptible to three interrelated pathophysiologic complications that occur in a number of different pathologic processes. *Increased intracranial pressure* is produced by any space-occupying lesion that sufficiently increases the volume of the intracranial contents. Frequently encountered examples of such space-occupying lesions are hemorrhage, neoplasm, abscess, cerebral edema, and hydrocephalus. However, both *cerebral edema* and *hydrocephalus* can themselves be a result of hemorrhage, neoplasm, or abscess, and the presence of either or both of these complications will exacerbate increased intracranial pressure from one of the other causes. This interaction among the three processes is one of the most frequently encountered and potentially dangerous complications of CNS disease.

INCREASED INTRACRANIAL PRESSURE AND HERNIATIONS OF THE BRAIN

Increased intracranial pressure is defined as an increase in the mean cerebrospinal fluid (CSF) pressure above 200 mm water (15 mm mercury) with the patient in the lateral decubitus position. It occurs whenever the volume of the intracranial contents increases beyond the slight leeway permitted by the compression of veins and displacement of CSF. Most cases of increased intracranial pressure are associated with a mass effect that can be either diffuse, as in the generalized brain edema of lead encephalopathy, or focal, such as that seen with tumors, abscesses, and hemorrhages.

Clinically, raised intracranial pressure causes symptoms such as headache that is typically worst in the mornings, mental slowness, and confusion, in addition to any focal signs that might result from the causative lesion. Papilledema may also be present.

On gross examination, when the increased intracranial pressure is due to an expansile process within the brain, there is either focal or diffuse flattening of the cortical gyri, sometimes associated with compressed or distorted ventricles. Because the cranial vault is partitioned by relatively rigid dural folds that form the falx cerebri and the tentorium cerebelli, a local expansion of the brain causes it to be displaced in relation to these partitions. If the expansion is sufficiently severe, a **herniation** of the brain will be produced.

Herniations are classified by the part that is herniated or the structure under which it has been pushed (Fig. 29–2). Expansion of one cerebral hemisphere may produce **subfalcine herniation** of the cingulate gyrus under the falx or may cause the medial temporal lobe to be forced into the gap between the cerebral peduncles and the tentorium, producing **uncinate (uncal) or transtentorial herniation**. Uncinate herniation may stretch and damage the oculomotor (III) nerve, thereby producing the well-known fixed, dilated pupil. If severe, the herniation may displace the midbrain enough to compress the contralateral cerebral peduncle against the free edge of the tentorium and cause a paralysis ipsilateral to the lesion, a famous false localizing sign. Downward movement of the posterior fossa contents results in **herniation of the cerebellar tonsils into the foramen magnum with compression of the medulla**, a process often called **coning. It is the compression of the medulla, with its vital respiratory center, that is the cause of death in patients with tonsillar herniation.** Upward as well as downward herniation of the posterior fossa contents can occur when a mass is located in the posterior fossa. Grossly swollen brain may also herniate through skull defects.

Severe herniations may also produce two other effects on the brain. First, they compress surface arteries against the unyielding edge of dural folds, possibly occluding the arteries and causing brain infarction. This can be seen when the posterior cerebral artery is compressed against the free edge of the tentorium in uncinate herniation, and when the callosal marginal branches of the anterior cerebral artery pass under the falx in subfalcine herniation. Second, with rapidly expanding supratentorial masses, there is both compression and downward displacement of the midbrain through the tentorium. Probably by rupture of penetrating arteries, this displacement produces linear hemorrhages, called **Duret hemorrhages**, in the mesencephalon and upper pons. Brain swelling severe enough to produce this complication is almost invariably fatal.

CEREBRAL EDEMA

The brain is particularly sensitive to edema not only because it has little room to expand, but also because *the brain has no lymphatic system to carry away excess fluid that accumulates.* Fluid and electrolyte movements into and out of the brain therefore need to be closely regulated, a function that is performed at the *blood-brain barrier.* The existence of this barrier is demonstrated by the exclusion from almost all regions of the brain of albumin-bound intravital dyes such as trypan blue.[9] The barrier is located at the capillary endothelial cells, which ultrastructurally have tight junctions and very few pinocytotic vesicles.[10,11] Recent studies suggest that the development of the barrier function in the cerebral capillaries is the result of an interaction between the astrocytes and the capillary endothelial cells.

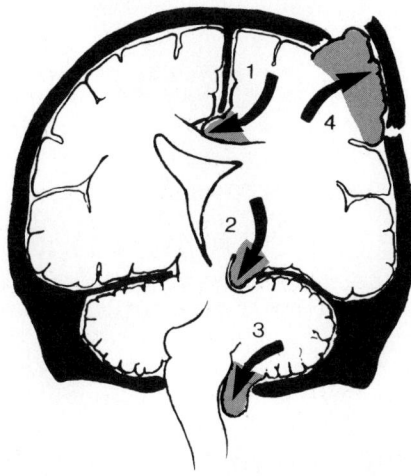

Figure 29–2. Herniations of the brain: (1) cingulate, (2) uncal (hippocampal), (3) cerebellar, and (4) transcalvarial. (From Fishman, R.A.: Brain edema. N. Engl. J. Med. 293:706, 1975. Reprinted, by permission, from The New England Journal of Medicine.)

Three types of cerebral edema are described.[12]

1. **Vasogenic edema is the accumulation of edema fluid in the extracellular space,** either through damaged capillaries that have lost their barrier function or through newly formed capillaries that have not yet established a barrier. **Vasogenic edema is the most common form of cerebral edema and occurs particularly in association with primary and metastatic tumors, abscesses, infarctions, contusions, and lead encephalopathy.** Neovascularization is particularly pronounced in tumors, especially metastatic tumors, and in abscess capsules. In vasogenic edema, white matter is conspicuously more affected than gray, and the edema may be focal or diffuse. If focal, the edema is more pronounced adjacent to its source.

Grossly, the edematous white matter is swollen and soft, and there may be gyral flattening over the affected region. Microscopically, there is microvacuolation and separation of myelin sheaths with generally poor staining, and lucent halos are seen around nuclei. Ultrastructural studies of experimental models of vasogenic edema show distention of astrocytic foot processes adjacent to cerebral capillaries.[13] If the edema is long-standing there may be demyelination (p. 1422) and axonal degeneration.

2. **Cytotoxic edema is the accumulation of excess intracellular water.** It predominantly affects gray matter and occurs in processes such as ischemia and water intoxication. The former results in damage to the metabolic machinery and membrane function of the cell with failure of electrolyte and water homeostasis, whereas the latter produces a hypo-osmolar state in the plasma that requires water to enter the cerebral cells to maintain osmotic equilibrium. Microscopically, the cells appear swollen and vacuolated.

3. **Interstitial edema** is seen in noncommunicating hydrocephalus when excess fluid crosses the ependymal lining of the ventricles and accumulates in the periventricular white matter.

So many conditions are associated with the development of cerebral edema that it is a very common clinical problem and often a major contributor to raised intracranial pressure, cerebral herniation, and even death. In many cases there is both vasogenic and cytotoxic edema, as for example in arterial occlusion or purulent meningitis in which both cells and blood vessels are damaged.

HYDROCEPHALUS

Hydrocephalus is the term for a marked increase in the volume of CSF with expansion of the cerebral ventricles (Figs. 29–3 and 29–4). CSF is produced by the choroid plexus in the lateral, third, and fourth ventricles and flows through the ventricular system to reach the subarachnoid space through the foramina of Luschka and Magendie. It is resorbed by the arachnoid villi along the dural venous sinuses.

Almost all cases of hydrocephalus result from a blockage somewhere along this pathway of CSF flow, although very occasionally, excess production of CSF by choroid plexus papillomas can produce hydrocephalus. When the blockage is in the CSF pathway

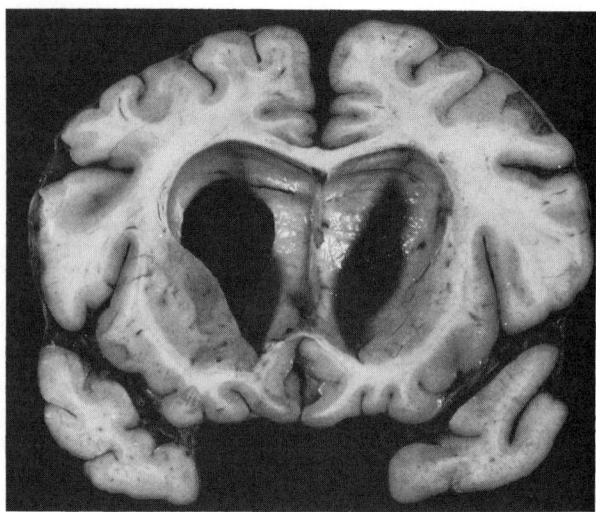

Figure 29–3. Hydrocephalus. Dilated lateral ventricles seen in a coronal section through frontal lobes.

within the brain, the hydrocephalus is called *noncommunicating*. If the obstruction to CSF flow is in the subarachnoid space or is caused by damage to or malfunction of the arachnoid villi, the result is a *communicating* hydrocephalus.

In infants and children, before fusion of the cranial sutures, hydrocephalus produces enlargement of the head. The incidence ranges from 0.2 to 5 per 1000 births, and there are many causes, including congeni-

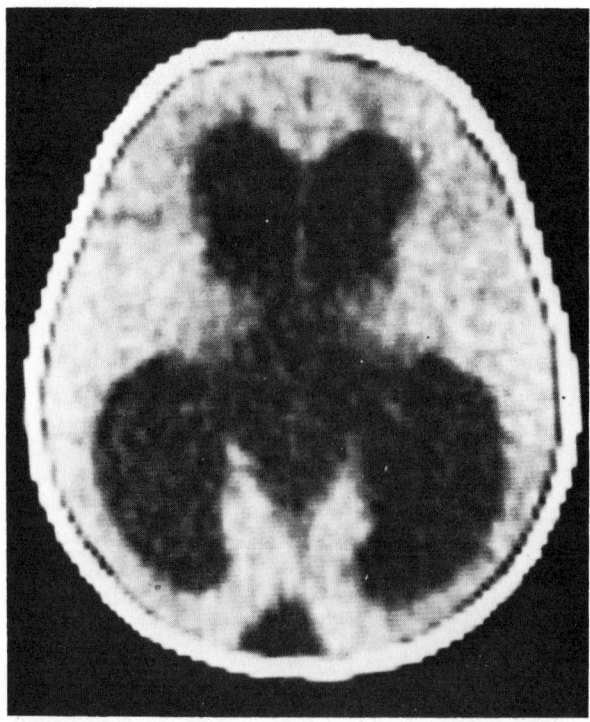

Figure 29–4. CT scan showing massively dilated ventricular system characteristic of hydrocephalus.

Table 29–1. Causes of Hydrocephalus

Noncommunicating hydrocephalus	
Congenital malformations	Stenosis of the aqueduct of Sylvius (a few cases are familial)
	Forking or atresia of the aqueduct of Sylvius
	Gliosis of the aqueduct of Sylvius
	Dandy-Walker syndrome (p. 1441)
	Arnold-Chiari malformation (p. 1439)
	Vascular malformations (e.g., aneurysm of the great vein of Galen)
Neoplasms	Ependymoma of the fourth ventricle (p. 1417)
	Choroid plexus papilloma of the fourth ventricle (p. 1418)
	Medulloblastoma (p. 1419)
	Colloid cyst of III ventricle (p. 1422)
	Other neoplasms adjacent to the ventricular system
Inflammatory processes	Meningitis and postmeningitic states
	Cerebellar abcess (compression of fourth ventricle)
	Other infections (e.g., cytomegalovirus)
Hemorrhage	Intraparenchymal hemorrhage (compression of ventricle)
	Intraventricular hemorrhage
	Epidural and subdural hematomas (usually unilateral; occur when there is a large midline shift and occlusion of a foramen of Monro)
Communicating hydrocephalus	
Overproduction of CSF	Choroid plexus papillomas (some only) (p. 1418)
	Other causes?
Deficient reabsorption of CSF	Postmeningitic states (e.g., pneumococcal and tuberculous meningitis)
	Subarachnoid hemorrhage
	Dural sinus thrombosis
	Deficiency of arachnoid villi (?)

Modified from Paine, R.S.: Hydrocephalus. Pediatr. Clin. North Am. *14*: 781, 1967.

tal malformations, infections, trauma, subarachnoid hemorrhage, and tumors (Table 29–1).[14] Genetic abnormalities, viruses, irradiation, and vitamin deficiencies have all been linked experimentally to congenital anomalies associated with hydrocephalus.

In adults, the onset of hydrocephalus may be acute and rapidly symptomatic or slow and insidious, depending upon the cause. Acute hydrocephalus is usually associated with processes such as trauma, infections, subarachnoid hemorrhage, or tumors (see Table 29–1) and is manifested as raised intracranial pressure. More slowly developing hydrocephalus produces symptoms such as dementia, gait disturbance, and incontinence, sometimes combined in a clinical syndrome called normal pressure hydrocephalus, a syndrome of unclear etiology that can be treated by ventricular shunting.[15]

Grossly, all forms of hydrocephalus produce dilated ventricles (see Figs. 29–3 and 29–4). With severe ventricular dilatation the ependymal lining of the ventricle is often damaged, and CSF may permeate into the periventricular white matter (interstitial edema). Unless the hydrocephalus is very severe and long-standing, the overlying cortex will usually be spared.

Hydrocephalus ex vacuo is really just another term for brain atrophy. It refers to the compensatory enlargement of the ventricles and increase in CSF volume that occur when the brain volume is reduced. It is seen in, for example, Alzheimer's (p. 1427) and Pick's disease (p. 1429). In hydrocephalus ex vacuo, CSF production, pressures, and flow patterns are normal.

INFECTIONS

The nervous system is susceptible to a large number of infectious agents of all types. Because the clinical pattern of disease and the types of infectious agent differ, it is appropriate to divide CNS infections into (1) infections of the meninges and CSF (meningitis) and (2) infections of brain parenchyma (encephalitis). Although these two categories are generally separable, a *meningoencephalitis* can occur if a meningitis extends into the parenchyma, or if, as commonly happens in encephalitis, some of the inflammatory reaction in the brain spills over into the CSF and adds symptoms of meningeal irritation to those of the encephalitis.

Because the nervous system is so well insulated from outside influences, organisms infecting it usually come from other organs and may evoke prodromal syndromes related to those organs.

There are four routes of infection of the nervous system.

1. The *bloodstream* is the most common portal of entry. Usually infection enters through the arterial circulation, but retrograde venous spread can occur through the veins of the face that have anastomotic connections through the orbit to the cerebral circulation. In acute bacterial endocarditis, septic emboli combine infection with infarction.

2. *Direct implantation* is almost invariably traumatic, and also sometimes iatrogenic—for example, from lumbar puncture, infected foreign bodies such as ventricular shunts and, in special circumstances (p. 1401) corneal transplants, and EEG needles.

3. *Local extension* of established infection in an air sinus (most often the mastoid or frontal) may erode through the bone to the meninges or brain. Local extension may also occur in patients, particularly neonates, with midline fusion defects such as meningomyelocele, in which there is a connection between an external surface and the nervous system.

4. The *peripheral nervous system* is the conduit for some viruses, specifically rabies and herpes simplex,

which first invade the peripheral nerve terminals and then ascend to the CNS.

Although not strictly infections, some bacteria that produce exotoxins, notably tetanus (p. 358), and diphtheria (p. 351) can seriously affect the nervous system without having actually to invade it.

MENINGITIS

The most important special anatomic feature of the nervous system that affects the pathophysiology of infections is that the brain is surrounded by meninges and bathed in CSF. The CSF provides both a culture medium for the infecting organisms and a rapid means of disseminating infection throughout the system once the outer defenses have been breached. *A meningitis is an inflammatory state of the leptomeninges (meninges) and subarachnoid space.* It is usually the result of an infection, but *chemical meningitis* may also occur, and infiltration of the subarachnoid space by tumor cells is conventionally referred to as *carcinomatous meningitis* (p. 1413) in spite of the fact that there is usually no inflammatory response.

Infectious meningitis can be broadly classified as *acute pyogenic* (usually bacterial), *acute lymphocytic* (usually viral), and *chronic* (bacterial or fungal).

Acute Pyogenic Meningitis

The most commonly encountered causal organisms are *Escherichia coli* in the neonate, particularly one with a neural tube defect; *Haemophilus influenzae* in infants and children; *Neisseria meningitidis* in adolescents and young adults (also the most common cause of epidemic meningitis because it is an oral commensal and can be transmitted through the air)[16]; and the *Pneumococcus*, particularly in the very young or the old, and following trauma.[17]

MORPHOLOGY. Grossly, the normally clear CSF is cloudy and sometimes frankly purulent (Fig. 29–5). The location of the exudate varies; in *H. influenzae* meningitis, for example, it is usually basal, whereas in pneumococcal meningitis it is more frequently densest over the cerebral convexities near the sagittal sinus.[18] From the areas of greatest accumulation, tracts of pus can be followed along blood vessels. When the meningitis is fulminant, the inflammation may extend into the ventricles, producing a ventriculitis.

Microscopically, polymorphonuclear leukocytes fill the entire subarachnoid space in severely affected areas and are found predominantly around the leptomeningeal blood vessels in less severe cases. In untreated meningitis, Gram stain reveals varying numbers of the causative organism, although they are frequently not present in treated cases. In fulminant meningitis, the inflammatory cells infiltrate the walls of the leptomeningeal veins and produce a venulitis that can lead to venous occlusion and a characteristic hemorrhagic infarction of the underlying brain (p. 1405). Arteritis is not common unless the meningitis is prolonged.

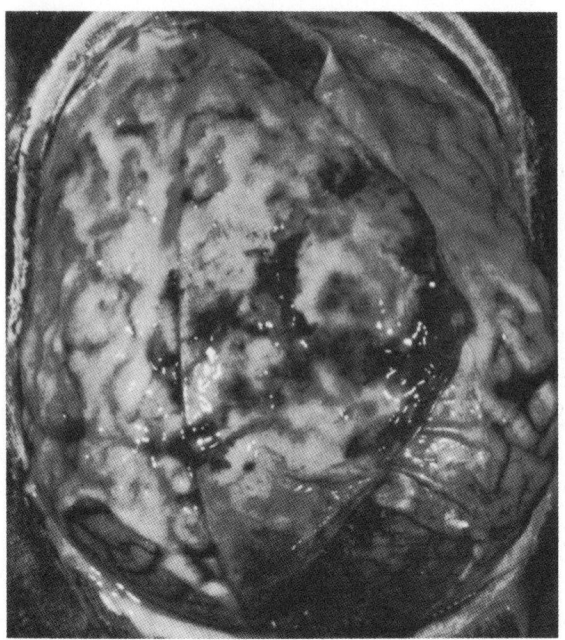

Figure 29–5. Pyogenic meningitis. A thick layer of suppurative exudate is disclosed beneath the folded-back dura.

CLINICAL COURSE. The typical patient with acute pyogenic meningitis has the general signs of infection with the added symptoms and signs of meningeal irritation: headache, photophobia, irritability, clouding of consciousness, and neck stiffness. *A spinal tap yields cloudy or frankly purulent CSF, under increased pressure, with up to 90,000 polymorphonuclear leukocytes per mm³, a raised protein level, and a markedly reduced sugar content.*[19] Bacteria may be seen on a smear or cultured, sometimes a few hours before the polymorphs appear.

In the pre-antibiotic era, pyogenic meningitis was frequently fatal. Recovery, when it occurred, was often accompanied by fibroblastic proliferation in the meninges that produced an adhesive arachnoiditis that in turn obliterated the subarachnoid space. If the obliteration sufficiently impeded CSF flow, hydrocephalus (p. 1390) would result and could also be fatal. Even with antibiotic treatment, hydrocephalus may still follow meningitis, particularly in pneumococcal meningitis, in which large quantities of the capsular polysaccharide of the organism produce a particularly glutinous exudate that encourages arachnoid fibrosis. A particular current problem is meningitis in the immunosuppressed patient. It may be caused by an unusual agent (such as Klebsiella or an anaerobic organism), and may have an atypical course and uncharacteristic CSF findings, all of which make the diagnosis more urgent and more difficult.[19]

An acute *chemical meningitis* can be caused by the release or insertion of an irritative substance, such as procaine or methotrexate, into the CSF. In these cases there is an increased number (pleocytosis) of polymorphonuclear leukocytes in the CSF, with a raised protein, but usually a normal sugar content, and of course organisms can be neither seen nor cultured.

Acute Lymphocytic Meningitis

Viral meningitis manifests in much the same way as bacterial meningitis with the clinical picture of meningeal irritation, but the course is generally less fulminant and the CSF findings are markedly different. *There is a lymphocytic rather than neutrophil pleocytosis; protein elevation is only moderate; and the sugar content is nearly always normal, in contrast to the reduced CSF sugar content in bacterial meningitis.* The viral meningitides are self-limiting, only symptomatic treatment being necessary, and there are none of the life-threatening complications seen in pyogenic meningitis. Many different viruses have been isolated from the CSF, including mumps, ECHO viruses, coxsackie virus, Epstein-Barr virus, and herpes simplex II, but at best, specific agents are identified in only two-thirds of the cases of presumed viral meningitis.

Chronic Meningitis

The archetype of chronic meningitis is that produced by *Mycobacterium tuberculosis*, but all the indolent meningeal infections (cited later) produce rather similar changes.

MORPHOLOGY. Grossly, the subarachnoid space contains a gelatinous or fibrinous exudate that is usually most obvious around the base of the brain and extending into the lateral sulci. Small focal densities may be visible, usually along the course of the cerebral vessels. Microscopically, the exudate is composed of chronic inflammatory cells with varying mixtures of lymphocytes, plasma cells, macrophages, and fibroblasts. The focal densities are tubercles, sometimes with caseous necrosis and giant cells. Arteries running through the subarachnoid space may show **obliterative endarteritis** with inflammatory infiltrates in their walls and marked intimal thickening. In late cases, there may be a dense fibrous adhesive arachnoiditis, most conspicuous around the base of the brain.

CLINICAL COURSE. Tuberculous meningitis usually manifests as generalized complaints of headache, malaise, mental confusion, and vomiting.[20] There is only a moderate CSF pleocytosis of up to 1000 cells per mm³ (the usual value is about 100), which are either entirely mononuclear cells, or a mixture of polymorphonuclear and mononuclear cells. The protein level is elevated, often strikingly so, and the sugar content typically is moderately reduced, although it may be normal. The worst complications of chronic meningitis are consequences of the continuing inflammatory reaction in the subarachnoid space. The arachnoid fibrosis may produce hydrocephalus, and the obliterative endarteritis can cause arterial occlusion and infarction of underlying brain, with consequences that depend on which artery is occluded. They may be catastrophic, as for example in the case of occlusion of the anterior spinal artery. The cranial nerves, which

necessarily pass through the subarachnoid space, may also be affected, either directly by the infection or indirectly by the continuing inflammatory reaction.

Other organisms that produce meningitis with similar chronic inflammatory and granulomatous features include bacteria such as *Treponema pallidum* (syphilis) and Brucella spp., and many of the fungi such as Coccidioides and Candida. Arachnoid fibrosis, obliterative endarteritis, and cranial nerve damage may also occur in conditions, such as sarcoidosis[21] and granulomatous arteritis,[22] that are granulomatous in character but not known to be infective.

Cryptococcal meningitis is especially frequent in debilitated or immunocompromised hosts. This organism sometimes elicits only a trivial inflammatory response even in the presence of large numbers of organisms. They can then be found widely in the subarachnoid space and also focally distending the Virchow-Robin spaces, producing characteristic "soap bubbles." In other cases, there is a marked chronic inflammatory and granulomatous reaction similar to that previously described, with all the usual complications. Clinically, the course may be fulminant and fatal in as little as two weeks, or indolent over months or even years. The CSF, particularly in indolent cases, may have few cells but a very high protein (over 500 mg per dl) and may contain the pathognomonic cryptococcal antigen. The mucoid encapsulated yeasts can also be visualized in the CSF by India ink preparations.[18]

SUBDURAL EMPYEMA

Bacterial or, occasionally, fungal infection of the skull bones or air sinuses can spread to the subdural space and produce a subdural empyema. The underlying arachnoid mater and subarachnoid space are usually unaffected, but the subdural pus may form a layer thick enough to compress the brain and produce a mass effect. Further, a thrombophlebitis may develop in the cerebral veins that cross the subdural space to reach the dural venous sinuses, and the resulting venous occlusion may produce infarction of the brain (p. 1405). With treatment, resolution of the empyema occurs from the dural side, and if it is complete, a thickened dura may be the only residual.

Clinically, most patients have a sinusitis with fever and then develop lethargy, coma, and focal neurologic signs, usually with neck stiffness. The CSF resembles that seen in brain abscesses, because both are parameningeal infective processes. If diagnosis and treatment are prompt, complete recovery is usual.

ENCEPHALITIS

Parenchymal infections of the brain have a very wide spectrum of clinical and pathologic expressions, all of which can be subsumed under the rubric *encephalitis*, because the term means only an inflammatory state of the brain. Pathologically, they range from focal necrotizing processes, exemplified by bacterial cerebritis with abscess formation, to diffuse infections causing only individual cell death, such as occurs in the arboviral encephalitides. Most are the result of bacterial, viral, or fungal infection.

Bacterial Encephalitides

The majority of bacterial CNS infections manifest as meningitides, although a meningoencephalitis may develop if bacteria invade the brain from a pre-existing meningitis. Primary parenchymal bacterial infection does occur but, because it usually causes focal tissue necrosis, produces in most cases a focal cerebritis that progresses to form a cerebral abscess. However, the parenchymal involvements of *Mycobacterium tuberculosis* and *Treponema pallidum* encephalitis are somewhat different.

Tuberculosis

As well as a chronic meningitis (p. 1393), tuberculosis may occur as a tuberculoma, which is a well-circumscribed intraparenchymal mass that may be up to several centimeters in diameter causing significant mass effect. Microscopically, there is usually a central core of caseous necrosis surrounded by a typically tuberculous granulomatous reaction. Organisms can often be seen with acid-fast stains, and calcification may occur in inactive lesions.

Although now rare in the United States and Europe, tuberculomas still constitute up to 25% of intracranial masses in India and South America. In about 25% of cases they are multiple, and in only about 50% of patients is there a previous history of tuberculosis.[23] Curiously, in children they are usually found in the posterior fossa, whereas in adults they are predominantly supratentorial.

Neurosyphilis

In modern Western practice, new cases of neurosyphilis are relatively rare, and what follows is a highly abbreviated description; fuller discussions can be found elsewhere.[24] Recent reports of atypical progression of neurosyphilis in AIDS,[25] however, suggest that we should not be lulled into the belief that the spirochete is necessarily an entirely spent force.

Neurosyphilis is a tertiary stage of syphilis, and occurs in only about 10% of the at risk population. Its major forms of expression are meningitic neurosyphilis, paretic neurosyphilis, and tabes dorsalis.

Meningitic neurosyphilis is a chronic meningitis (p. 1393) with all the complications thereof. Somewhat distinctive is an obliterative endarteritis (p. 1393) accompanied by a perivascular inflammatory reaction rich in plasma cells.

Paretic neurosyphilis is the outcome of *diffuse parenchymal invasion by the treponema, which results in widespread individual cell death and, consequently, brain atrophy.* Microscopically, there is loss of cortical neurons with proliferation of microglia (rod cells) and gliosis, which produces a "windswept" appearance of the cortex. Appropriate stains demonstrate the spiro-

chetes. As might be surmised from the pathology, paretic neurosyphilis manifests as an insidious but progressive loss of mental and physical functions with mood alterations (including the well-known delusions of grandeur), terminating in a dementia of the most extreme and bizarre variety (general paresis of the insane). Once the disease becomes symptomatic, treatment can arrest but not reverse the decline in neurologic function.

Tabes dorsalis (locomotor ataxia) is the result of damage by the spirochete to the sensory nerves in the dorsal roots, which produces, among other features, impaired joint position sense and resultant ataxia (locomotor ataxia); loss of pain sensation leading to skin and joint damage (Charcot joints); other sensory disturbances, particularly the characteristic "lightning pains"; and absence of deep tendon reflexes. Less well explained, but usually present, are Argyll Robertson pupils, which react to accommodation but not to light. Microscopically there is loss of both axons and myelin in the dorsal roots, with pallor and atrophy in the dorsal columns of the spinal cord.

Although these three forms of expression of neurosyphilis have been described separately, patients often show incomplete or mixed pictures, notably the combination of tabes dorsalis and general paresis (taboparesis).

Brain Abscess

Brain abscesses may arise by direct implantation of organisms (usually traumatic), local extension from adjacent foci (especially mastoiditis), or hematogenous spread (usually from a primary site in the heart, lung, or distal bones). Conditions particularly associated with the development of cerebral abscesses include *acute bacterial endocarditis*, which tends to produce multiple abscesses; *cyanotic congenital heart disease*, in which there is a right-to-left shunt and loss of pulmonary filtration of organisms; and *chronic pulmonary sepsis (bronchiectasis)*. The microflora of cerebral abscesses is very varied, but anaerobic organisms (of which streptococci and *Bacteroides fragilis* are the most common), aerobic streptococci, and staphylococci are the principal offenders.[26]

MORPHOLOGY. Abscess formation is the same in the brain as in any other organ, with the formation of a fibrous capsule around a focus of necrotizing cerebritis (Fig. 29–6). Though seemingly banal, this is in fact a rather unusual occurrence, being one of the few instances in which there is fibrosis with collagen production in the brain. As previously mentioned (p. 1387), astrocytes do not produce collagen, and the fibroblasts that produce this collagen are derived from the blood vessels that proliferate around the margin of the necrotic brain. It is probably this exuberant neovascularization that is responsible for the marked vasogenic edema (p. 1390) so characteristic around brain abscesses. Outside the fibrous capsule is a zone of gliosis. The inflammatory reaction, both acute and chronic, associated with the infection is reflected in the CSF by increased pressure,

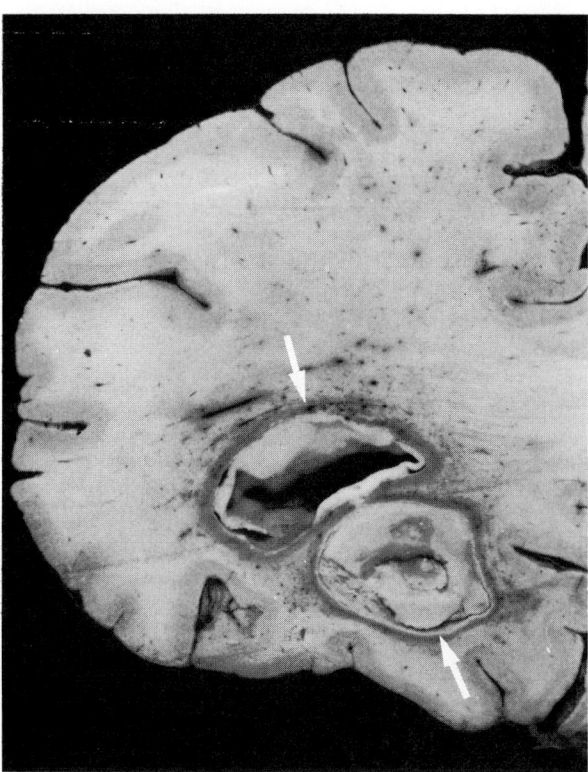

Figure 29–6. Frontal abscesses *(arrows).*

or even unknown, as in progressive multifocal leuko-encephalopathy (PML), in which there is only serologic evidence of previous infection. Rabies and herpes simplex are exceptions in which the virus enters the CNS through inoculation into, and ascent along, the peripheral nerves.

> The most characteristic histologic features of viral diseases are a perivascular and parenchymal mononuclear cell infiltrate (lymphocytes, plasma cells and macrophages) (Fig. 29–7), glial nodules (p. 1388), and neuronophagia (p. 1388). However, too much reliance should not be placed on these histologic features alone, because both mononuclear infiltrates and glial nodules can be seen in conditions in which viruses are not thought to be involved. A more direct expression of viral involvement is the usually intranuclear **inclusion body** seen in some viral infections. The only really specific inclusion is the cytoplasmic Negri body of rabies (p. 1397).
>
> The degree of **tropism** exhibited by some viruses is particularly striking in the nervous system.[28] Herpes zoster and poliomyelitis virus, for example, affect only specific subpopulations of neurons—the dorsal root ganglion cells and the anterior horn motor neurons, respectively. Other viruses affect whole classes of cells; the papovavirus of PML infects primarily oligodendroglia, and rabies virus attacks only neurons. Herpes simplex, although it infects all

> raised white cell count and protein level, but normal sugar content.[18] No organisms will be present unless the abscess has ruptured into a ventricle or the subarachnoid space.

CLINICAL COURSE. Cerebral abscesses are so destructive of tissue that patients almost invariably present with progressive focal deficits in addition to the general signs of raised intracranial pressure caused by the volume effect of the abscess.[27] A systemic or local source of infection is usually apparent, but a small systemic focus may have ceased to be symptomatic by the time the patient presents with evidence of cerebral infection. The increased intracranial pressure and progressive herniation can be fatal, and abscess rupture can lead to ventriculitis, meningitis, and sinus thrombosis. With surgery and antibiotics, the otherwise almost 100% mortality rate can be reduced to less than 20%.

Viral Encephalitis

Viral diseases in general have been discussed already (p. 312). Here, reference will be made only to those aspects that are germane to disease of the nervous system.

The CNS can be infected by many viruses, an event that has almost always been preceded by a primary infection, or at least colonization, elsewhere. Sometimes, as with varicella-zoster, the primary infection is another recognized disease, but it is often nonspecific, as in the gastroenteritis of poliomyelitis,

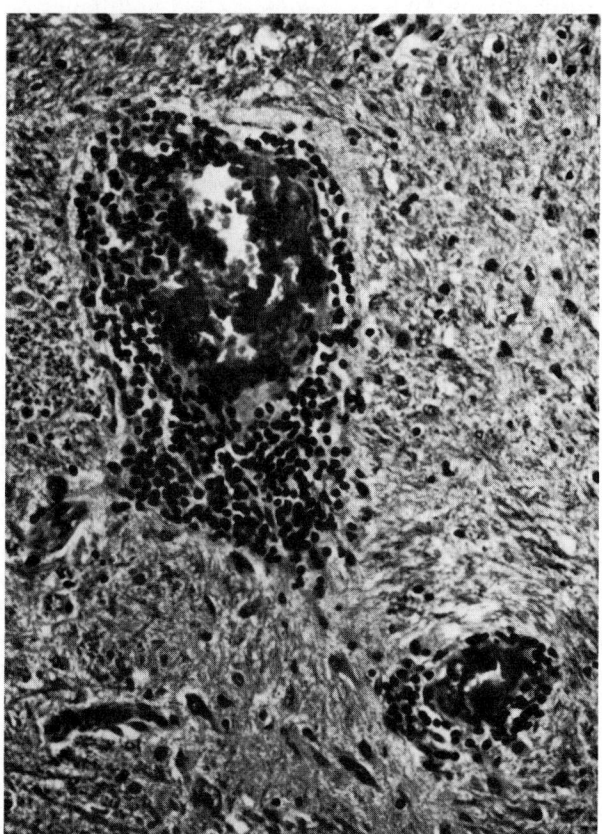

Figure 29–7. Perivascular mononuclear cell infiltrate typical of a viral infection (H and E stain).

types of neural cells, is at least initially geographically restricted, affecting principally the inferior frontal and temporal lobes. The origins of these different specificities are not entirely clear but they probably reflect receptor interactions between the host cells and the virus.

The capacity of some viruses for *latency* is also particularly important in the nervous system. Herpes simplex and varicella-zoster can remain latent in their host cells in the nervous system, to be reactivated months or years after the initial infection.

The *slow virus diseases* (p. 1399) have both a long latent period and an illness that, when it finally becomes apparent, pursues a prolonged clinical course that is quite unlike the usual pattern of an infectious disease.

It should not be thought that infections, overt or covert, compose the full gamut of viral effects on the CNS. Systemic viral infections are occasionally followed by an immune-mediated *perivenous encephalitis* (p. 1425) with no viral penetration of the nervous system. *Reye's syndrome* (p. 963),[29] a condition of unknown but possibly toxic etiology, occurs most frequently after viral infections, usually influenza or chicken pox, and is associated with severe and sometimes fatal brain edema. *Congenital malformations* can result from intrauterine viral infection, as occurs with rubella, and *postencephalitic Parkinsonism* (p. 1430) followed the presumed viral influenza epidemic during and after the First World War.

Brain biopsy, with direct identification and localization of the virus by labelling with specific antibodies attached to fluorescent markers, offers the most rapid means of diagnosis. In suitable cases the virus can be identified in minutes.[30] This is important principally in the diagnosis of herpes simplex encephalitis, for which there is a reasonably effective treatment. In other parts of the diagnostic jungle, however, and particularly with the latent and slow viruses, detection and identification are sometimes possible only with more arcane methods, such as co-cultivation and nucleic acid hybridization. Despite this array of diagnostic sophistication, a virus is identified in only 30 to 40% even of fatal cases of presumed "viral encephalitis."

Acute Viral Encephalitis

Excluding AIDS and related conditions (p. 1398), *about 1500 cases of presumed acute viral encephalitis are reported each year in the United States.*[31] In only about 500 of these is a virus actually identified. About a decade ago, almost all the diagnosed cases fell into one of five groups (number of cases for the year 1978 in parentheses): arboviral (143); enteroviral (40); associated with childhood infections (measles, mumps, chickenpox, rubella) (80); respiratory (70); other known agents (cytomegalovirus, herpes simplex, herpes zoster, Epstein-Barr virus) (99). Because so many types of virus can cause encephalitis, it is im-

practical to describe them separately. Only the most common and those with specific or illustrative features will be considered here.

ARTHROPOD-BORNE (ARBOVIRUS) ENCEPHALITIDES. These are the typical viral panencephalitides without conspicuous localizing features. They are responsible for most outbreaks of epidemic encephalitis. In the Western hemisphere the most important types are eastern and western equine, Venezuelan, St. Louis, and California. Types found elsewhere include Japanese B (Far East), Murray Valley (Australia and New Guinea), and tickborne (U.S.S.R. and Eastern Europe). All have vertebrate hosts and mosquito vectors, except for the tickborne. These viruses have many common properties, and some investigators wish to group them collectively as *encephaloviruses*. Clinically, there are global deficits, such as seizures, confusion, delirium, and stupor or coma, and often some focal features as well, such as reflex asymmetry and ocular palsies. *The CSF is usually colorless but with a slightly elevated pressure and, initially, a polymorph pleocytosis that rapidly converts to lymphocytes; the protein level is usually raised but sugar content is normal.*

Eastern equine encephalitis (EEE) can serve as the example for all the arboviruses. It was initially described in horses in 1933, and the first human cases were reported in 1939, when an outbreak in children followed an epidemic in horses. Serologic studies indicate that only about 5% of the exposed population develop encephalitis, but the mortality rate is about 80%. Some survivors recover completely, but others, especially young children, are left with serious disability.

Pathologically, EEE is a meningoencephalitis with perivascular inflammatory cells, many focal areas of necrosis, and selective neuronal necrosis with neuronophagia. In severe cases there may be a necrotizing vasculitis. Some cases have predominantly cortical involvement, whereas in others the basal ganglia bear the brunt of the disease. In both eastern and western equine encephalitis, large numbers of polymorphonuclear leukocytes appear in the brain and CSF early in the disease. CSF sugar content, however, is not decreased even when the cell count is exclusively polymorphonuclear.

The other arbovirus encephalitides differ in epidemiology and prognosis, but pathologically their appearance is very similar, except for variations in severity and a tendency for there to be fewer polymorphs.

The brain is the principal site of infection in the arboviral encephalitides, but there are other viral infections, such as measles, rubella, and chickenpox, in which encephalitis is only an occasional, though sometimes severe, complication. Most of these cases are probably examples of allergic perivenous encephalomyelitis (p. 1425), but with some viruses, such as

Epstein-Barr and mumps, the fact that the virus can be recovered from CSF is suggestive of true neurotropic infection.

HERPES SIMPLEX TYPE I (HSV-I). HSV-I (labialis) (p. 319) produces an encephalitis that occurs in any age group but is most common in children and young adults. Only about 10% of the patients have a history of prior labial herpes. Acyclovir has emerged as the most effective treatment, with which there is a mortality rate of about 30% (compared with 70% in controls), and about 30% make a complete recovery, but outcome is significantly influenced by the clinical state of the patient at the start of treatment.[32]

> In adults the encephalitis starts in, and most severely involves, the inferior and medial regions of the temporal lobes and the orbital gyri of the frontal lobes. The infection is grossly necrotizing and often hemorrhagic in the most severely affected regions. Perivascular inflammatory infiltrates are usually present, and intranuclear viral inclusion bodies may be found in both neurons and glial cells.

HSV-I encephalitis in neonates produces a panencephalitis similar to that seen with HSV-II. The basis of this difference is not known, but it is speculated that there are differences in surface receptors in neonatal and adult brains.

HERPES SIMPLEX TYPE II (HSV-II). HSV-II (genitalis) also affects the nervous system and is responsible for most cases of *herpetic viral meningitis*. More ominously, it causes a generalized, and usually severe, *encephalitis* in neonates that has been shown to occur in up to 50% of neonates born by vaginal delivery to women with *primary* HSV infection. The risk to the infant whose mother has *recurrent* genital herpes at the time of delivery has been shown to be very much lower.[33]

HERPES ZOSTER – VARICELLA. This infection in adults (commonly called "shingles") usually manifests as a vesicular skin eruption in the distribution of a dermatome (p. 320). Overt CNS involvement with herpes zoster is much rarer, but compensates by being correspondingly more severe. Two types of pathophysiologic processes have been described. First, herpes zoster has been associated with a *predominantly unilateral vasculopathy* that frequently manifests clinically as a delayed contralateral hemiparesis following unilateral zoster (shingles) in the distribution of the ophthalmic division (V1) of the fifth cranial (trigeminal) nerve.[34] Direct immunocytochemical and electron microscopic evidence of viral involvement has been obtained in a few of these cases. In some but not all cases, the vasculopathy is a granulomatous arteritis.[35] Second, in immunosuppressed patients, including those with AIDS, herpes zoster may cause a *multifocal encephalitis* with numerous sharply circumscribed lesions characterized by early demyelination and subsequent necrosis.[36,37] Inclusion bodies can easily be found in astrocytes, oligodendrocytes, and neurons.

POLIOMYELITIS. Poliovirus infections of the nervous system have largely been eliminated by immunization, a signal triumph for preventive medicine, because poliomyelitis is a disease with serious acute symptoms and major long-term morbidity. Poliovirus is an enterovirus that causes a nonspecific gastroenteritis. In a small fraction of the exposed population, however, it secondarily invades the nervous system, where it specifically attacks only lower motor neurons.

> **MORPHOLOGY.** Acute cases show typical viral disease features with mononuclear cell perivascular cuffs and neuronophagia of the anterior horn motor neurons of the spinal cord. The inflammatory reaction is usually confined to the anterior horns, and the damage is occasionally severe enough to produce cavitation. Although the motor cranial nuclei may sometimes be involved, there is rarely much neuron loss. Currently, the most commonly encountered examples of this disease are long-term survivors of symptomatic polio. These patients show loss of neurons and long-standing gliosis in the affected anterior horns of the spinal cord, atrophy of the anterior (motor) spinal roots, and neurogenic atrophy of the denervated muscle.

CLINICAL COURSE. Infection of the nervous system by poliomyelitis virus manifests initially with meningeal irritation (p. 1392), which may be its only effect. However, if the motor system is affected, *loss of motor neurons produces a flaccid paralysis with muscle wasting and hyporeflexia in the affected spinal segments that is the permanent neurologic residual of poliomyelitis.* In the acute disease, death can occur from paralysis of the respiratory muscles, and a myocarditis sometimes complicates, or terminates, the clinical course. Permanent cranial nerve (bulbar) weakness is rare, as is any evidence of encephalitis. In survivors, some recovery of muscle power is usual, but severe respiratory compromise is an important cause of long-term morbidity. Coxsackie viruses can cause a somewhat similar paralysis that, although occasionally severe, is usually transitory.

RABIES. This disease is transmitted by the bite of a rabid animal, usually a dog. It causes a severe encephalitis that is almost always fatal.

> **MORPHOLOGY.** Grossly, the brain shows intense edema and vascular congestion. Microscopically there is widespread neuronal degeneration and an inflammatory reaction that is most severe in the basal nuclei, midbrain, and floor of the fourth ventricle, particularly in the medulla. The spinal cord and dorsal root ganglia may also be involved. **Negri bodies** are the pathognomonic microscopic finding. They are **cytoplasmic, round to oval or bullet-shaped,**

sometimes multiple, eosinophilic inclusions that are aggregates of virus particles. They are found only in neurons, most frequently in the pyramidal neurons of the hippocampus and the Purkinje cells.[38,39]

The virus enters the CNS by ascent along the peripheral nerves from the wound site. The incubation period depends on the distance of the wound from the brain and varies between one and three months. Clinically, the onset is nonspecific, with malaise, headache, and fever, but the conjunction of these symptoms with local paresthesias around the wound is diagnostic. In advanced cases, the patient exhibits extraordinary CNS excitability; the slightest touch is painful, and minute movements provoke violent motor responses progressing to convulsions. There is meningismus and, as the disease progresses, flaccid paralysis. Periods of alternating mania and stupor progress to coma and death from respiratory center failure.

CYTOMEGALOVIRUS (CMV). This infection of the nervous system occurs in two patient populations, fetuses and the immunosuppressed. The outcome of in utero infection is a necrotizing periventricular infection that produces severe brain destruction followed later by microcephaly with a characteristic pattern of periventricular calcifications that reflects the ependymal location of the initial infection.[40] This susceptibility of the ependyma to infection is maintained in the immunosuppressed where infection often starts as an ependymitis that subsequently extends into the subependymal brain.[41] Outlying focal necrotizing lesions may also be found, with the characteristic large CMV-infected cells containing both intranuclear and cytoplasmic inclusion bodies. Particularly in AIDS, cytomegalovirus infection may also produce multiple microglial nodules, in some of which the typical CMV cells can be seen.[42]

HUMAN IMMUNODEFICIENCY VIRUS 1 (HIV-1, HTLV III, LAV) (p. 224). The nervous system is a major target for the human immunodeficiency virus, which ravages the system in a variety of guises. Viral antigen in the brain has been detected not only in cells of monocyte-macrophage origin but also, though in much smaller quantities, in neuroglial cells and perhaps in neurons. How HIV-1 gets into the nervous system has not been established, but current opinion favors macrophages as the vector and perhaps the principal reservoir of infection.[43] *At least four syndromes have been ascribed to the direct effects of the virus: (1) an acute aseptic meningitis or, more rarely, encephalitis, (2) a subacute encephalitis, (3) a vacuolar myelopathy, and (4) a peripheral neuropathy.*[44]

The **aseptic meningitis** resembles viral meningitis (p. 1393). In retrospective studies, it has occurred in about 10% of patients with HIV infection, usually around the time

of seroconversion. HIV has been isolated from the CSF in some of these patients.[44,45]

Subacute encephalitis is characterized pathologically by microscopic foci of multinucleated giant cells, macrophages, and lymphocytes (Fig. 29–8), together with adjacent microglial cells, reactive astrocytes, and some vacuolation and pallor of the surrounding myelin. This appearance is pathognomonic for HIV infection. The lesions are found mostly in the cerebral and cerebellar white matter, but in more severely affected cases may also be present in the diencephalon, brainstem, and spinal cord. Virus particles and viral proteins have been demonstrated to be present in at least some of the multinucleated giant cells by electron microscopy and immunocytochemistry, respectively.[46] In a recent autopsy study these foci were present in 28% of all patients with AIDS, and their presence correlated well with the presence of the AIDS dementia complex, although there was a poor correlation between the number of focal lesions in the brain and the clinical severity of the dementia.[47] Other less definitive findings are microglial nodules without the characteristic giant cells, areas of white matter pallor, and vacuolation. Although these findings are correlated with the clinical presence of AIDS dementia, the lesions themselves do not seem to produce either the type or the degree of damage to the brain that might be expected to produce a dementia. It is possible, if not probable, that the

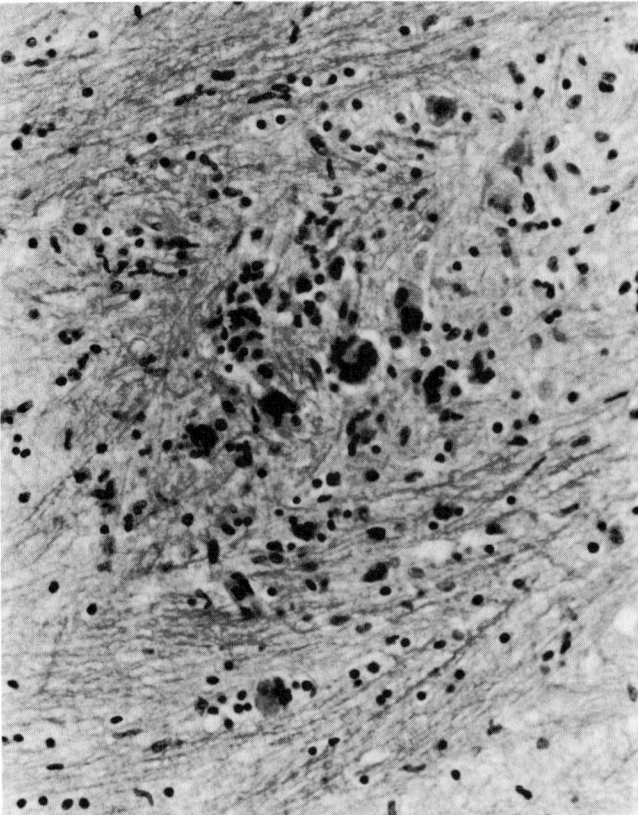

Figure 29–8. AIDS subacute encephalitis with several of the characteristic multinucleate giant cells that have been shown to contain HIV-1.

lesions seen pathologically represent only the tip of the iceberg as far as involvement of the brain with HIV-1 is concerned. Clinically, **some degree of AIDS dementia may be present in as many as two thirds of all patients with AIDS and can be the presenting syndrome.**[48,49]

Vacuolar myelopathy is found in 20 to 30% of patients at autopsy,[50] about half of whom have clinical signs and symptoms of spinal cord dysfunction. Pathologically, there is vacuolation and an accumulation of lipid-laden macrophages in the white matter of the cord that is very similar to that seen in subacute combined degeneration due to vitamin B$_{12}$ deficiency. The vacuolation is usually most severe in the lateral columns, less in the dorsal columns, and least in the anterior white columns. In the mild and moderately affected cases, most of the axons in the vacuolated areas are preserved, but in severe examples there is also disruption of axons. Although found throughout the length of the cord, the myelopathy is usually most severe at the middle and lower thoracic levels. A large fraction of the patients with vacuolar myelopathy also exhibit the AIDS dementia syndrome, but there is no apparent correlation between the severity of the dementia and the severity of the myelopathy.

The **peripheral neuropathy** (p. 1443) associated with HIV-1 comes in a variety of clinical guises. One version is a demyelinating neuropathy with focal inflammatory demyelination, from which HIV-1 can be cultured. A more acute syndrome rather like Guillain-Barré syndrome (p. 1444) has been described, and there is also a distal, predominantly sensory neuropathy. Although there is a large demyelinating component in all these peripheral nerve syndromes, a variable degree of axonal loss is also found. In patients with AIDS or AIDS-related complex, pathologic examination of peripheral nerves shows evidence of active disease in up to 95%, although only about 50% have clinical evidence of a peripheral neuropathy.[51]

Infection with HIV-1 is also associated with a significantly higher risk of opportunistic infections of the nervous system, notably *cytomegalovirus, varicella-zoster, and herpes simplex encephalitis, progressive multifocal encephalopathy (p. 1400), cryptococcosis (p. 1393), and toxoplasmosis (p. 1402)*. There is also a greatly increased risk of developing a *primary CNS lymphoma* (p. 1421) that is unusually aggressive and relatively resistant to treatment.[42,47,49,52–54]

Although HIV-1 is the best-characterized retrovirus infection of the nervous system, high levels of antibodies to another retrovirus, HTLV-1 (the cause of acute T-cell leukemia/lymphoma), are found in a condition called tropical spastic paraparesis. Although the precise etiologic connection is not clear, it seems likely that this disease also will prove to be retrovirus associated.

Slow Virus Diseases

Thus far we have been discussing viruses that, although they may remain latent for some time, cause acute illnesses that are recognizably infective in character.[55] The agents that cause slow virus diseases not only have a long latent period but also cause a disease that evolves very slowly and does not clinically resemble an acute infection at all. Since 1958, when this concept was formulated,[56] advances in our understanding have made it appropriate to divide them into two groups.[57]

1. Slow virus infections that have a known viral cause, specifically subacute sclerosing panencephalitis (SSPE), progressive multifocal leukoencephalopathy (PML), and progressive rubella panencephalopathy.[58]
2. Unconventional agent (spongiform) encephalopathies (kuru and Creutzfeldt-Jakob disease in humans) that have a distinct histologic appearance and are caused by agents that are not yet characterized but that do not appear to be conventional viruses.

SUBACUTE SCLEROSING PANENCEPHALITIS (SSPE).

SSPE (Dawson's encephalitis) is caused by measles virus and generally occurs in children but can be seen in adolescents and young adults. It has always been preceded by an attack of measles in the distant past, often unusually early in life, or, very occasionally, by previous immunization against measles. Clinically, SSPE usually starts with personality changes, followed by the development of involuntary movements and a slow but relentless neurologic deterioration over two to three years.

Grossly, the brain may be normal or unusually firm and may have regions of granularity or focal destruction. Microscopically, there is a perivascular and parenchymal lymphoplasmacytic infiltrate. Inclusion bodies are frequently present in oligodendroglia but are also found in neurons and astrocytes. Neuronophagia and extensive neuronal loss are seen in severely involved areas, and there is a dense fibrillary gliosis. Electron microscopy shows paramyxovirus nucleocapsid tubules characteristic of measles virus in the inclusion bodies.[59]

ETIOLOGY AND PATHOGENESIS. Although many inclusion bodies and viral particles can be seen in the brain, measles virus can be grown only if brain tissue is co-cultivated with other cells. The reason for this emerged from studies of the CSF, which in SSPE contains oligoclonal immunoglobulins directed against components of the virus.[60] However, no antibody is present to the M protein. This protein is associated with the inner surface of the viral coat and is important in the assembly and budding of the virus particle. For reasons currently undetermined, it appears that brain cells do not produce the M protein and therefore manufacture defective virus particles that are incapable of extracellular spread. The presence of this defect is the reason for the necessity to co-cultivate to obtain the virus, but in the patient it is also likely greatly to inhibit the rate of progression of the infection and so be at least part of the explanation for the fact that SSPE is a slow virus disease.[61,62]

PROGRESSIVE MULTIFOCAL LEUKOENCEPHALOPATHY (PML).

PML is a viral infection of oligodendrocytes that, because it kills the oligodendrocytes that produce myelin, causes demyelination as its principal pathologic effect. First described in 1958,[63] PML occurs in association with advanced hematologic malignancies and other immunosuppressed states (including AIDS).[64] Usually, the associated conditions have been present for months or years before PML occurs, and most cases are seen in adults, although it has been described in children.

ETIOLOGY. Two closely related papovaviruses have been implicated in PML, one called JC (the initials of a patient and unrelated to Creutzfeldt-Jakob disease), which accounts for almost all the cases, and SV40, which has been reported in only a very few cases.[65] Although no systemic syndrome has been described, about 65% of normal people have serologic evidence of exposure to JC virus by the age of 14 years.[66] It is not known whether PML results from a primary infection in a susceptible host or from the rekindling of an old infection.

Grossly, the affected white matter has irregular margins, a sunken gray translucent appearance, and a soft texture. Microscopically, there are numerous areas of demyelination ranging in size from microscopic foci to huge confluent regions affecting whole lobes. The cerebrum, brainstem, cerebellum, and, occasionally, the spinal cord can all be involved. The appearance of the oligodendrocytes is diagnostic; their nuclei are still spherical but grossly enlarged and contain inclusion bodies that range from violet smudges to discrete homogeneous eosinophilic masses. They are most frequent at the margins of the lesions. Within the lesions there are characteristic bizarre giant astrocytes with irregular, hyperchromatic, sometimes multiple nuclei. Reactive fibrillary astrocytes are scattered among the bizarre forms, and there are many foamy macrophages containing myelin debris, but strikingly little inflammatory reaction. Axons traversing the lesions are conspicuously preserved. Electron microscopy shows numerous papovavirus particles, often in paracrystalline arrays in the oligodendrocyte nuclei, and, sometimes, isolated virus particles in astrocyte nuclei.

Clinically, patients develop protean but focal and relentlessly progressive neurologic symptoms and signs, and both CT and MRI scans show extensive, often multifocal lesions in the hemispheric or cerebellar white matter with sparing of gray matter. No effective treatment is currently known.

Unconventional Agent (Spongiform) Encephalopathies

These are a group of diseases caused by transmissible agents that are not yet fully characterized but that seem to lack many of the features of ordinary viruses.[67] They comprise Creutzfeldt-Jakob disease and kuru in humans, scrapie in sheep and goats, and transmissible encephalopathy in mink. Microscopically they all have a characteristic *spongiform change* in the gray matter (Fig. 29–9), and their similarity is emphasized by the fact that scrapie and Creutzfeldt-Jakob tissue cause the same disease when injected into monkeys. Both kuru and Creutzfeldt-Jakob disease have been transmitted to other primates by a variety of parenteral routes, but most easily by intracerebral injection of infected tissue.[68] After a long latent period (usually about 18 months), the inoculated animals develop CNS changes similar to those seen in humans. Before describing the two conditions, a few words about their causation are in order.

ETIOLOGY AND PATHOGENESIS. The precise nature of the transmissible agent in these diseases remains elusive. Like a virus it is filterable, titrates cleanly, and has distinctive host specificities. Conversely, it is very resistant to formalin, ultraviolet and ionizing radiation, and other physicochemical agents that usually inactivate viruses. It also does not evoke any immune or inflammatory reaction in the host. Much recent work has focused on a heavily glycosylated protein of about 27K daltons that is closely associated with infectivity and is called prion protein (as a putative *pro*teinaceous *in*fective particle) by one major research group.[69] Surprisingly, this protein has proved to be a modification of a protein of about 30K

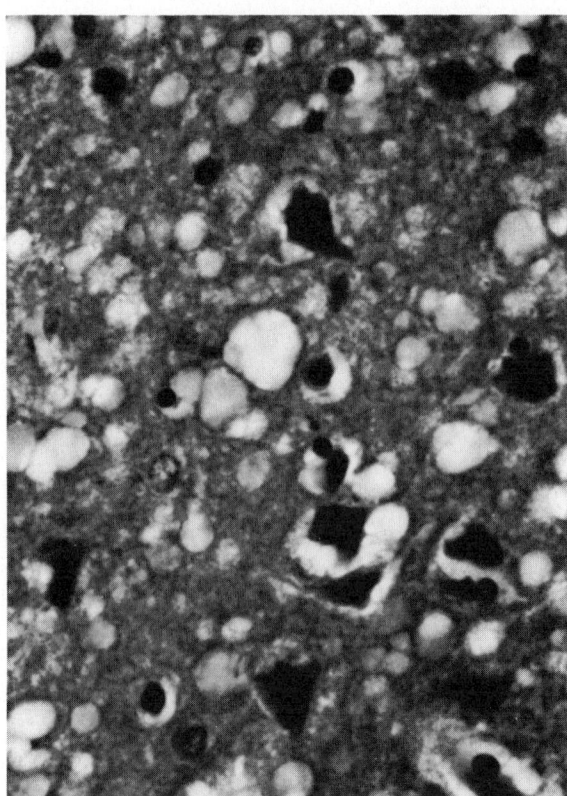

Figure 29–9. Status spongiosus—characteristic of unconventional agent infections. Vacuoles are located in the neuropil (the feltwork of cytoplasmic processes). Note absence of an inflammatory infiltrate. (H and E stain.)

daltons that is present in normal tissue and coded for in the normal genome.[70] Currently there is intense interest (and, not surprisingly, controversy) about whether there is any nucleic acid associated with this protein.[71] So far none has been found, and if this continues to be the case, the agent will prove unconventional indeed. However, much remains to be discovered, and radical changes may occur in our ideas about these agents.

SUBACUTE SPONGIFORM ENCEPHALOPATHY (CREUTZFELDT-JAKOB DISEASE, TRANSMISSIBLE AGENT DEMENTIA).

These are synonyms for a rare but well-characterized disease that manifests clinically as a rapidly progressive dementia. Despite the demonstrated transmissibility of its causative agent, it is sporadic in its occurrence, with a worldwide incidence of about one per million with no discernible pattern of exposure in the patient population. The natural mode of transmission in humans is wholly obscure,[72] but there are a few cases of iatrogenic transmission, notably via corneal transplantation, deep implantation electrodes,[73] and, most recently, contaminated preparations of human growth hormone.[74,75]

The progress of the dementia in Creutzfeldt-Jakob disease is so rapid that despite the degree of neuronal loss there is little if any gross atrophy of the brain (unlike Alzheimer's and Pick's diseases, in which there is often pronounced atrophy). Microscopically, the pathognomonic spongiform change (see Fig. 29–9) is seen in the cortex and sometimes other regions of gray matter, and consists of a variable vacuolation in the background neuropil.[76] In more advanced cases there is severe neuronal loss and marked reactive astrocytosis. No inflammatory infiltrate is present. Electron microscopy shows the vacuoles to be intracytoplasmic, membrane bound, and present in neuronal and glial processes (Fig. 29–10).[77] Kuru plaques (see later) occur in the cerebellar cortex in about 10% of cases.

CLINICAL COURSE. The clinical picture is usually quite typical, with the initial subtle changes being followed by a rapidly progressive dementia, often with pronounced startle myoclonus. The disease is uniformly fatal, with an average duration of only seven months, although a few patients survive for several years. All treatments have so far been unavailing.

KURU. This disease is confined to the Fore tribe of the eastern highlands of Papua–New Guinea, among whom the disease was transmitted by cannibalism. Recognition of this mode of spread led to the discovery of the transmissibility of the causative agent.[67] At one time kuru was the cause of death in 90% of the women of the Fore tribe, because it was mainly they who came into contact with or ate the brains of the deceased. With the cessation of cannibalism, new cases have stopped appearing. The morphologic changes are similar to those of Creutzfeldt-Jakob disease but are most prominent in the cerebellum and striatum. Kuru plaques, which are amyloid deposits

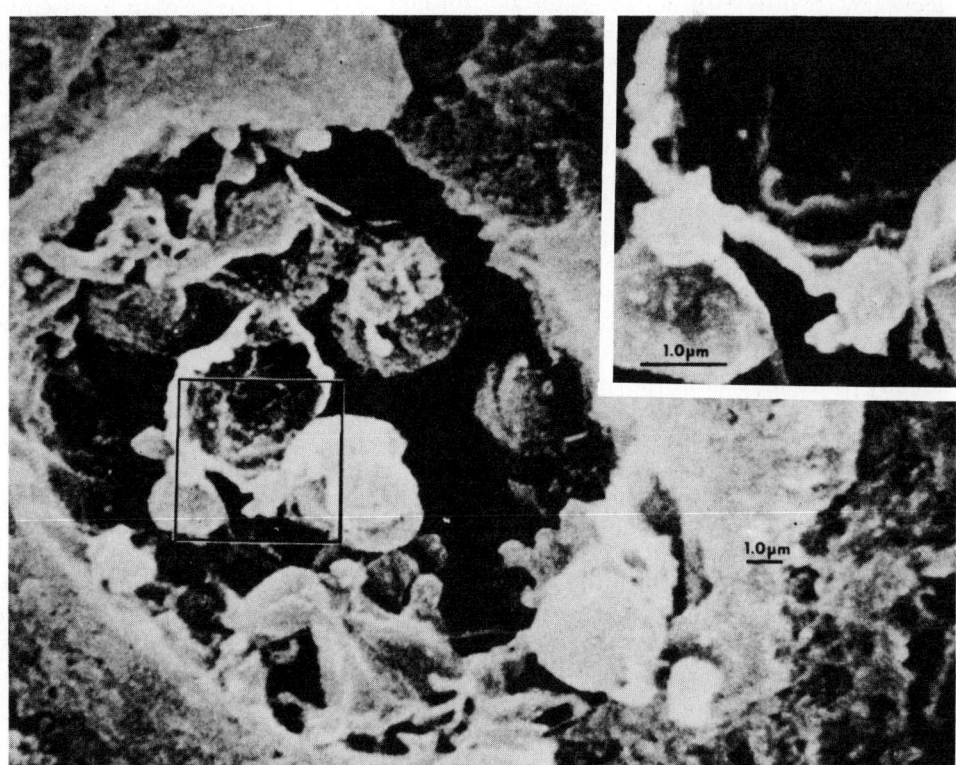

Figure 29–10. Scanning electron micrograph of a large vacuole in a monkey with transmitted Creutzfeldt-Jakob disease. Inset shows an enlargement of the area inside the small square. (From Chou, S.M., et al.: Transmission and scanning electron microscopy of spongiform change in Creutzfeldt-Jakob disease. Brain *103*:885, 1980.)

made up of the 27K dalton prion protein,[78] appear in the cerebellum in about 60% of cases. Clinically, there is cerebellar ataxia and a "shivering tremor" that progresses to complete motor incapacity and death from intercurrent infection or malnutrition in less than a year. Dementia is not prominent but may occur terminally.

FUNGAL INFECTIONS

As with the systemic deep mycoses (p. 386), fungal disease of the CNS, in the developed world, is most frequently encountered in patients who have cancer, notably lymphomas,[79,80] or who are otherwise immunocompromised (e.g., with AIDS).[81] The brain is usually involved only late in the disease, when there is widespread hematogenous dissemination of the fungus, most often *Candida albicans*, Mucor, *Aspergillus fumigatus*, and *Cryptococcus neoformans (Torula histolytica)*. Less frequently seen, and then usually in the endemic areas, are the more traditional agents, such as *Histoplasma capsulatum*, *Coccidioides immitis*, and *Blastomyces dermatitidis*. A broad range of other agents have also been encountered on rare occasions.

There are three basic patterns of fungal infection in the CNS: chronic meningitis, vasculitis, and parenchymal invasion.

Chronic meningitis has already been discussed (p. 1393) and will not be further considered here.

Vasculitis is most frequently seen with Mucor and Aspergillus, both of which have a marked predilection for invasion of blood vessel walls, but occasionally occurs with other organisms such as Candida. The resultant thrombosis of the affected vessel produces a cerebral infarction that is often strikingly hemorrhagic and that subsequently becomes septic from ingrowth of the causative fungus. Clinically, brain involvement is typically signalled by the development of cerebral infarction(s) in a patient with a systemic fungemia.

Parenchymal invasion, usually in the form of granulomas or abscesses, can occur with most of the fungi that affect the nervous system and often coexists with a meningitis. The most commonly encountered are Candida and Cryptococcus (p. 1393). Candida usually produces multiple microabscesses, with or without giant cell or granuloma formation that are not usually large enough to cause focal symptoms.

Although most fungi arrive in the brain by hematogenous dissemination, direct extension may also occur, particularly with Mucor, which has a predilection for growth in air sinuses, and Actinomyces, which in its craniofacial form may occasionally invade the brain.

OTHER INFECTIONS

Protozoal diseases such as malaria, toxoplasmosis, amebiasis, and trypanosomiasis; rickettsial infections such as typhus, Rocky Mountain spotted fever; and metazoal diseases such as cysticercosis and echinococcosis may also involve the CNS and are discussed in Chapter 7.

Cerebral toxoplasmosis merits special mention. Like cytomegalovirus encephalitis, it occurs in the fetus and in immunosuppressed adults. Primary maternal infection with toxoplasmosis, particularly if it occurs early in pregnancy, may be followed by a cerebritis in the fetus, with the production of multifocal cerebral necrotizing lesions similar to those seen in immunosuppressed adults, with correspondingly severe damage to the developing brain. In its acquired adult form, toxoplasmosis occurs only in the immunosuppressed population, is particularly common in AIDS,[82] and is treatable. Pathologically it is a progressive, multifocal, necrotizing, and often hemorrhagic encephalitis. The organisms are present in the characteristic pseudocysts and also free in the tissue. They are usually most easily found at the margins of the necrotic areas.

In this section, there has been a considerable bias towards infections encountered in the developed world. Outside these privileged areas, however, malaria, cysticercosis, and tuberculosis are probably the most common infections of the nervous system.

VASCULAR DISEASE

The importance of vascular disease of the brain can hardly be overstated, because notwithstanding a recent and gratifying decrease in its incidence,[83] cerebrovascular disease has been estimated to account for 50% of all neurologic problems encountered in general hospitals. The major categories of vascular disease are (1) hypoxia, ischemia, and infarction, (2) intracranial hemorrhage, and (3) hypertensive cerebrovascular disease.

HYPOXIA, ISCHEMIA, AND INFARCTION

Although the brain constitutes only 2% of the body weight it receives 15% of the resting cardiac output and accounts for 20% of the oxygen consumption, a reflection of the importance of aerobic metabolism to the brain. The brain may be deprived of oxygen in a variety of ways: *anoxic anoxia*, in which there is a low inspired pO_2; *anemic anoxia*, in which the oxygen carrier, hemoglobin, is reduced; *histotoxic anoxia*, which occurs in, for example, cyanide poisoning; and *stagnant (ischemic) anoxia*, when there is cessation of blood flow. *All these different forms of anoxia produce rather similar patterns of brain damage*, as indeed does *hypoglycemia*, which reduces aerobic metabolism by removing the substrate.[84]

The major reason for the similarity of all these lesions is that exposure to any form of severe hypoxia is rapidly followed by severe hypotension and subsequently, cardiac arrest, so that *"ischemia is the last common path of all forms of hypoxia."*[85] In animal experiments in which the circulation is artificially maintained, the brain is actually quite tolerant of hypoxia, but ischemia can be tolerated for only a very short time.[86] The principal difference between all the other forms of hypoxia and ischemic (stagnant) anoxia is that the cessation of blood flow that occurs in ischemia allows the local accumulation of metabolic products and pH changes, events that do not happen in the other types of anoxia. Of the cells of the nervous system, neurons are the most vulnerable to ischemia, being able to tolerate it for only three to four minutes without permanent damage. Lesser degrees of ischemia produce individual cell death of neurons, but if the ischemia is sufficiently severe or prolonged, the glial cells also die, producing complete necrosis of the tissue.

In clinical practice, two general types of acute ischemic injury are recognized:

1. *Ischemic (hypoxic) encephalopathy* occurs when there has been a generalized reduction of cerebral perfusion with widespread bilateral ischemic damage.
2. *Cerebral infarction* is the focal ischemic necrosis that follows very severe reduction or cessation of blood flow to a localized area of the brain.

Ischemic (Hypoxic) Encephalopathy

The brain has an almost constant level of metabolic activity, and autoregulation of the cerebral circulation maintains cerebral perfusion pressure, and hence blood flow, over a wide range of systemic blood pressures and intracranial pressures. This homeostasis is achieved principally by control of the cerebrovascular resistance. In normal persons adequate blood flow to the brain is maintained down to a systolic blood pressure of about 50 mm mercury, but cerebral atherosclerosis makes the brain vulnerable to smaller fluctuations of blood pressure. If perfusion pressure falls below the critical value, there is increasing tissue ischemia secondary to progressive reductions in cerebral blood flow, manifested clinically as ischemic encephalopathy.

As already mentioned the cells most vulnerable to ischemia are neurons, which suffer first reversible and then irreversible damage. Some types of neurons, notably the Purkinje cells of the cerebellum and the pyramidal cells in Sommer's sector of the hippocampus, are particularly susceptible to ischemia and are often the first to be damaged. The reasons for this *selective vulnerability* are not entirely clear, but attention is currently focused on the role of what are called *excitotoxins.* These are acidic excitatory neurotransmitters, notably glutamate and aspartate, that can cause cell death if their action is prolonged. The mechanism of their cytotoxicity is not certain, but one hypothesis is that prolonged action of one of these transmitters causes persistent opening of membrane channels. This results in an uncontrolled rise in intra-

cellular Ca^{++} and the inappropriate activation of calcium-dependent proteases and lipo-oxygenases.[87,88]

The changes seen in the brain depend upon the duration and severity of the ischemia and the length of survival. When the insult has been slight and transient, the nerve cells recover completely, and in patients who survive only a few hours no changes are seen regardless of the severity of the ischemic episode. In ordinary histologic preparations the first visible change occurs after survival for 12 to 24 hours. The affected neurons develop a strikingly eosinophilic cytoplasm and a small pyknotic nucleus, an appearance called **ischemic cell change** (red neurons). In the cortex, the process is widespread but not completely uniform, clusters of damaged cells being found next to unaffected cells even in the same cortical lamina. Subsequently the nerve cells die and disappear, being replaced by fibrillary gliosis. The pyramidal cell layers of the cortex are more severely affected than the granular layers, and in areas of greater destruction, the loss of the pyramidal cell layer produces the appearance of **laminar necrosis.**

The most severe ischemia is suffered by tissue supplied by the most distal branches of the cerebral arteries, and this may be sufficient to produce wedge-shaped areas of coagulation necrosis called **border zone or watershed infarcts** in the junctional zones between the major arterial territories. In the cerebral hemispheres, the border zone between the anterior and middle cerebral arteries seems to be most at risk. Damage to this region produces a linear parasagittal infarction, usually with some expansion over the lateral occipital gyri, the precise geometry of the infarct being governed by the degree of ischemia and the extent of local vessel narrowing. Border zone infarcts are almost invariably seen in the context of severe ischemic encephalopathy. In long-term survivors of ischemic encephalopathy, the degree of cortical atrophy reflects the amount of cortical destruction.

Ischemic encephalopathy occurs after episodes of profound systemic hypotension, such as, for example, after cardiac arrest when resuscitation has not been sufficiently expeditious. Its clinical expression reflects its pathologic severity. In mild cases, there may be only a transient post-ischemic confusional state with complete recovery, whereas the most severely affected patients lose almost all cortical functions and remain comatose or in a persistent vegetative state.

Cerebral Infarction

Almost all cerebral infarctions are caused by local vascular occlusions, including instances when cerebral arteries are compressed against dural folds during herniations (p. 1389) and can even occur without obstruction, as in border zone infarctions or when there is a reduction in perfusion pressure combined with a severe atherosclerotic stenosis.

Clinically, the symptoms and signs produced by cerebral infarctions are called strokes. *Stroke* is one of those old-fashioned terms that is clinically very useful but pathologically imprecise. It implies the acute onset of a focal neurologic syndrome, such as a hemiparesis, secondary to a vascular event. This may be either a vascular occlusion, producing an infarct, or a hemorrhage, (p. 1405) which also causes local destruction of tissue. Other types of focal lesions that cause local tissue destruction, such as a tumor or abscess, may also occasionally manifest with a focal syndrome of rapid onset mimicking a "stroke."

When there is an occlusion, whether an infarct occurs, and the size and shape of the infarct are determined by which vessel is occluded and by the pattern and extent of its anastomotic connections with adjacent vessels. In the case of the large internal carotid and vertebral arteries, the circle of Willis often provides complete collateral flow. The major cerebral arteries, such as the middle and anterior cerebral, have a partial anastomosis of their distal branches. Although a quite severe stenosis of such an artery can be tolerated, complete occlusion always causes an infarct that is, however, smaller than the whole territory supplied by the artery. Surprisingly, there is little or no anastomosis among the small cerebral arteries, so that occlusion of any of these vessels always causes an infarct. This inevitability of infarction with small vessel occlusions combines with the vulnerability of the brain to focal lesions in an ominous synergy. Together, they ensure that small or medium-sized arterial occlusions that would be almost unnoticed in other organs may be dramatically symptomatic in the brain, an arrangement that seems perverse even to the rational (and deliberate to the paranoid!).

Most vascular occlusions are either thrombotic or embolic. The vast majority of *thrombotic occlusions* are caused by atherosclerosis and occur either at the bifurcations of the carotid arteries in the neck, or in the vertebrobasilar system. If the circle of Willis is functioning, a carotid artery can be occluded without causing any symptoms at all, and there are many patients with asymptomatic carotid occlusions. However, if the anastomotic capacity of the circle of Willis is reduced by atherosclerosis or there is an abnormal pattern of cerebral circulation, an infarction may occur that can range in size from a small distal lesion in the territory of the middle cerebral artery to a catastrophic infarct of a whole hemisphere. The posterior circulation is not afforded the same degree of anastomotic protection, and atherosclerotic occlusion of the basilar artery usually is seriously incapacitating and often is fatal. Before total occlusion occurs, ephemeral focal neurologic symptoms and signs, called *transient ischemic attacks*, often point to significant atherosclerotic cerebrovascular disease.

Although atherosclerosis is by far the most common cause of thrombotic occlusion of a cerebral artery, other much rarer causes exist, notably the arteritides, including cranial arteritis and granulomatous arteritis of the nervous system.[89] They usually cause obstruction of smaller arteries than those occluded by atherosclerosis.

Emboli (p. 105) have a wide range of origins, and

usually cause occlusions of intracerebral arteries, often producing an infarct in only part of the territory of a major cerebral artery. Probably for hemodynamic reasons, cardiac and carotid emboli have a marked tendency to impact in the middle cerebral artery territory. As might be expected, very small emboli tend to affect the most distal branches of the artery in the border zone between the territories of the middle and anterior cerebral arteries. If numerous, such emboli may radiologically and pathologically simulate the border zone infarcts seen in severe ischemic encephalopathy.

Hemorrhagic infarcts result from the breakup of emboli. The bleeding is petechial in character and restricted to the infarcted cerebral cortex; the infarcted white matter does not become hemorrhagic, a difference that probably reflects the different caliber and density of vessels supplying the white matter. In anticoagulated patients, however, hemorrhage may be diffuse and massive. In this situation it may be difficult to distinguish pathologically between a hemorrhagic infarct and a lobar hemorrhage.

Grossly, **anemic infarctions** are not detectable until 6 to 12 hours after their occurrence. The earliest visible change is a slight discoloration and softening of the affected area, so that the gray matter architecture becomes blurred and the white matter loses its normal fine-grained

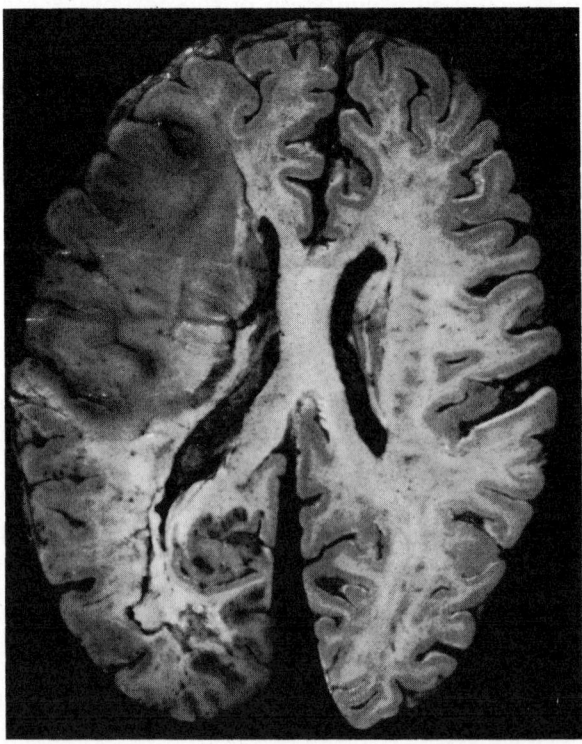

Figure 29–11. Section of brain showing both anemic and hemorrhagic infarcts. The anemic infarct is the large oval discolored region in the middle of the hemisphere *(upper left)*. The hemorrhagic infarct involves the cortex over the posteromedial region of the same hemisphere.

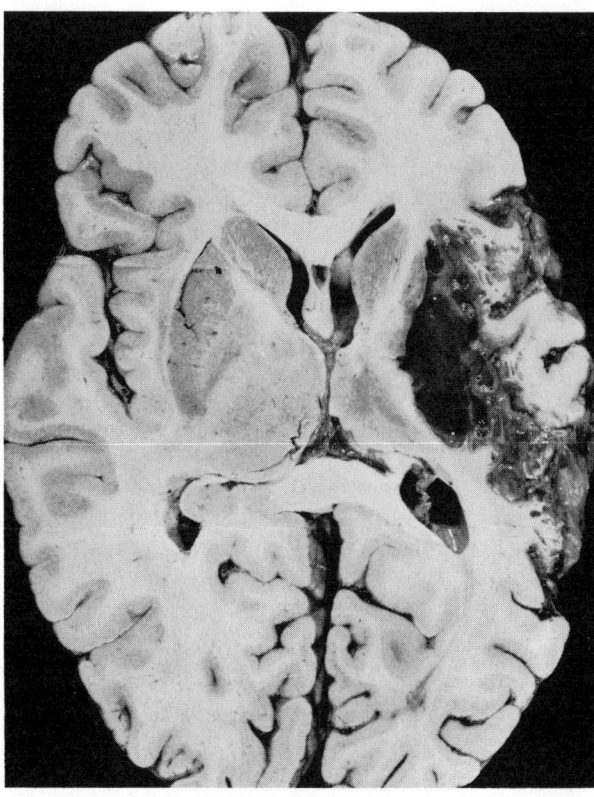

Figure 29-12. Old cystic infarct.

appearance (Fig. 29-11). After 48 to 72 hours, there is softening and disintegration of the infarcted area with pronounced edema of both the infarct and the adjacent tissue that may, in large infarcts, be sufficient to produce herniation. Resolution is associated with progressive tissue liquefaction and cyst formation; the latter may be traversed by fine trabeculations and surrounded by firm glial reaction (Fig. 29-12). The leptomeninges, when involved, become thickened and may form the outer wall of the cyst.

Histologically the process of resolution is very similar to that in any other necrotic tissue, there being an initial influx of polymorphonuclear leukocytes followed by a prolonged macrophage invasion with progressive digestion of the necrotic tissue. The major, and very important, difference is that no collagen scar tissue is formed because astrocytes do not produce collagen. Because fibroblasts, which in the brain are found only around blood vessels, do not have a role in the resolution of cerebral infarcts, the end result of cerebral infarct resolution is a cyst rather than a scar. This is fortunate, given what the formation of a contractile fibrous scar might do to the function of the adjacent intact brain! The astrocytosis that occurs in infarcts becomes prominent about the second week of resolution and in the final state produces a fibrillary gliosis that replaces and/or surrounds the necrotic region. Macrophages take a very long time to disappear entirely and may be found in the interstices of old infarcts even years later. The time required for an infarct to resolve ranges from weeks to many months, depending on its size.

The signs and symptoms associated with cerebral infarctions depend entirely on which region of the brain is infarcted, and textbooks of neurology should be consulted for a description of stroke syndromes.

Before we leave the subject of infarctions, *venous infarctions* must be mentioned. Because of the great collateralization of the cerebral venous drainage, infarction follows only either occlusion of a large sinus or widespread obstruction of smaller veins. It most commonly occurs with occlusion of the superior sagittal sinus, which itself is most often a consequence of the predisposition to thrombosis associated with cancer.[90] The infarctions are typically bilateral, multiple, parasagittal, and hemorrhagic, with hemorrhage into both gray and white matter. Clinically, they are often distinguished by the occurrence of particularly intractable seizures.

INTRACRANIAL HEMORRHAGE

Spontaneous (nontraumatic) intracranial hemorrhage falls into three general categories: (1) intracerebral (hypertensive), (2) subarachnoid (aneurysmal), and (3) mixed intraparenchymal and subarachnoid (arteriovenous malformation–associated).

Intracerebral Hemorrhage

Most spontaneous intracerebral hemorrhages are associated with a prior history of hypertension, but blood dyscrasias, bleeding into tumors, amyloid angiopathy, and silent angiomas are rarer causes of intracerebral hemorrhage.

ETIOLOGY AND PATHOGENESIS. The hypertensive hemorrhages result, it is thought, from rupture of microaneurysms called Charcot-Bouchard aneurysms that form at the bifurcations of small intraparenchymal arteries. Bursting destroys the aneurysm responsible for the hemorrhage and the adjacent brain tissue, but studies have shown an increasing number of these aneurysms in the arteries of the brain with age and length of history of hypertension.[91] In recent years the treatment of hypertension has resulted in a substantial reduction in the incidence of hypertensive cerebral hemorrhages.

The major sites of hypertensive hemorrhages are the putamen (55%), lobar white matter (15%), thalamus (10%), pons (10%), and cerebellar cortex (10%).

MORPHOLOGY. Gross inspection of a brain with, for example, a basal ganglia hemorrhage often shows obvious expansion of the affected hemisphere with flattening of the gyri. Uncinate herniation may be present as well as displacement of the midbrain to the opposite side from the hemorrhage. If the hemorrhage has ruptured into the ventricles, blood clot may be present around the foramina of Luschka and Magendie, where CSF enters the subarachnoid space from the ventricles. The cut surface of the brain shows blood clot separating the structures of the basal ganglia with relatively little gross tissue destruction (see Fig.

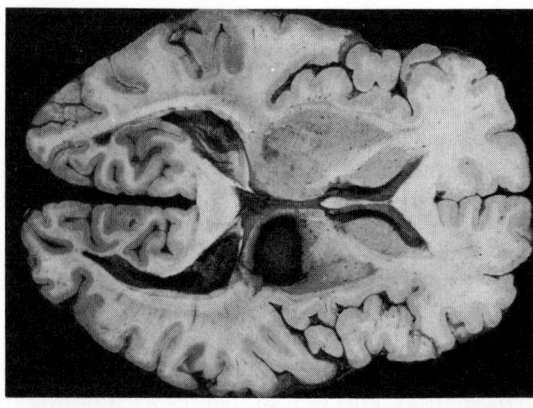

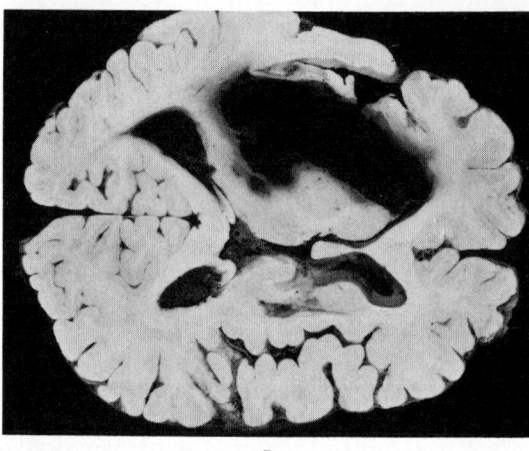

Figure 29-13. *A,* Hypertensive hemorrhage, thalamus. *B,* Massive hypertensive hemorrhage, rupturing into lateral ventricle.

29-13*B*). The parenchyma adjacent to the clot is usually somewhat edematous and often discolored by the degradation products of hemoglobin, especially if the hemorrhage is some days old. Small ring hemorrhages in the Virchow-Robin spaces of neighboring blood vessels are frequently seen. The mass effect of the blood clot causes distortion of the cerebral ventricles, the ipsilateral one being compressed, but there also may be hydrocephalus if the aqueduct of Sylvius or either of the foramina of Monro is occluded by the ventricular distortion. Rupture into a ventricle will be indicated by ventricular casts of blood clot (Fig. 29-13*A*). Resolution of a hemorrhage begins with the appearance of macrophages that, over a period of months, digest the clot, leaving a slit-like cavity surrounded by a zone of fibrillary astrocytosis containing scattered hemosiderin-laden macrophages.

CLINICAL COURSE. The advent of CT and MRI scans has led to some revision of our ideas about the natural history of intracerebral hemorrhages. They were thought to be usually large and frequently fatal, but scans have revealed that a number of smaller hemorrhages manifest clinically just like occlusive infarcts. Cerebral hemorrhage has been revealed to be not as invariably catastrophic as was previously

thought. This is not to say that it is benign! There is still an initial mortality rate of about 40%, and in the majority of such cases the hemorrhage has ruptured into the ventricles.[92] However, there is a relatively good prognosis for most survivors of the initial hemorrhage, probably because hemorrhages tend to separate tissue along planes of cleavage rather than destroy it. Thus, resolution of the mass of the hematoma may be accompanied by considerable restitution of function. Recurrent intracerebral hemorrhage is rare, in marked contrast to the situation with subarachnoid hemorrhages.

Supratentorial hemorrhages tend to present as progressive hemiplegias, whereas cerebellar hematomas in the posterior fossa produce symptoms such as ataxia, eye movement abnormalities, and intractable vomiting. Wherever its location, if there is substantial hemorrhage and mass effect, raised intracranial pressure, coma, and the syndromes of herniation rapidly come to dominate the clinical picture.

Subarachnoid Hemorrhage

Bleeding into the subarachnoid space is usually the result of rupture of an aneurysm or, more rarely, an arteriovenous malformation (p. 1408). Aneurysms can be developmental (berry, "congenital"), arteriosclerotic (fusiform), inflammatory (mycotic), or traumatic.

Berry aneurysms are the most common variety, accounting for 95% of aneurysms that rupture. They occur at bifurcations of the major cerebral arteries, the most common sites being (1) the junction of the carotid and posterior communicating arteries, (2) the anterior communicating artery, and (3) the major bifurcation of the middle cerebral artery in the Sylvian fissure (Fig. 29-14). Together these three sites ac-

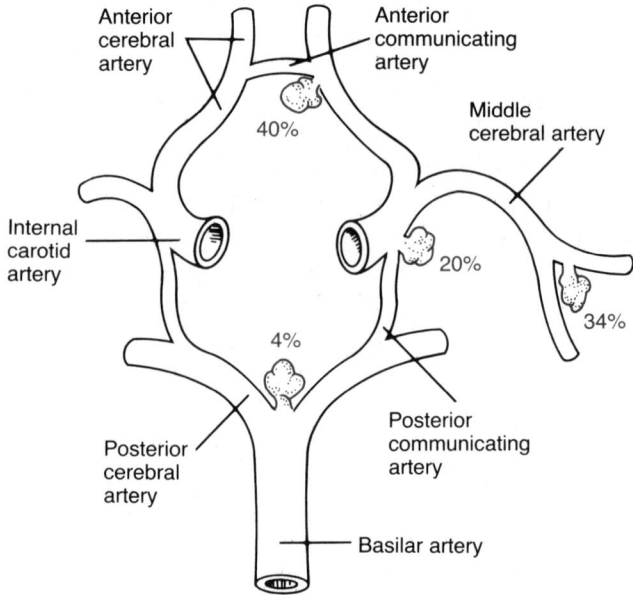

Figure 29-14. Common sites of berry aneurysms in the circle of Willis.

count for at least 85% of all ruptured berry aneurysms. Almost all the remainder are in the posterior circulation. In 20 to 30% of cases, berry aneurysms are multiple.

PATHOGENESIS. Although often called congenital aneurysms, *berry aneurysms are not present at birth; they develop because there is a discontinuity in the smooth muscle of the media at the carina of arterial bifurcations.* The arterial wall bulges out through the muscular defect to form a thin-walled saccular fundus, composed only of fibrous tissue in which there may be additional local degeneration and calcification (Figs. 29–15 and 29–16). Laminated blood clot and fibrin may be deposited on this attenuated wall. This insubstantial structure is a little like an inflated balloon, and it is not surprising that the activities that cause acute rises in intravascular pressure, such as straining at stool, lifting heavy weights and, discouragingly, sexual intercourse, are associated with their rupture. There is, however, no association between chronic hypertension and either the development or the rupture of berry aneurysms.

Most berry aneurysms are sporadic in occurrence, but some conditions are particularly associated with their presence, notably polycystic kidney disease and the prior existence of a cerebral arteriovenous malformation. There is angiographic evidence that aneurysms enlarge with time; the likelihood of rupture is increased when the diameter rises above 10

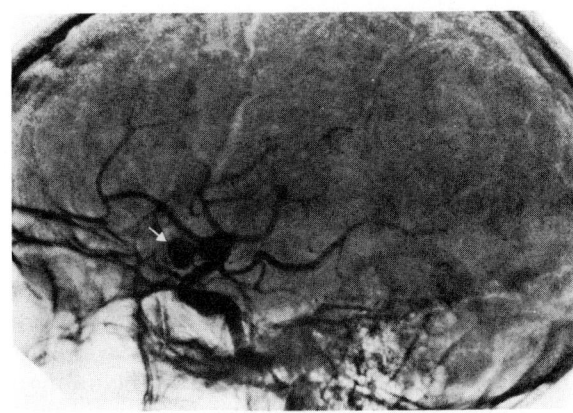

Figure 29–16. Cerebral arteriogram showing berry aneurysm arising from anterior communicating artery *(arrow).*

mm. However, not every aneurysm bursts, and small ones are not infrequent incidental findings on carotid angiography and at autopsy.

MORPHOLOGY. The common site of aneurysm rupture is in the thin-walled fundus, with consequences that depend on its orientation. If the fundus is pointing toward or applied to the surface of the brain, the escaping blood, at arterial pressure, may tunnel into the brain, sometimes reaching a ventricle and producing as much intraparenchymal as subarachnoid bleeding. This occurs in 15 to 40% of patients and is particularly common in those who succumb in the first week after rupture. Alternatively, the blood may lead directly into the subarachnoid space and produce the more typical clinical and pathologic presentation of a subarachnoid hemorrhage (Fig. 29–17).

CLINICAL COURSE. Patients usually complain of a sudden severe headache, typically "the worst headache I've ever had," and may rapidly lose consciousness. Between 25 and 50% of patients die with the

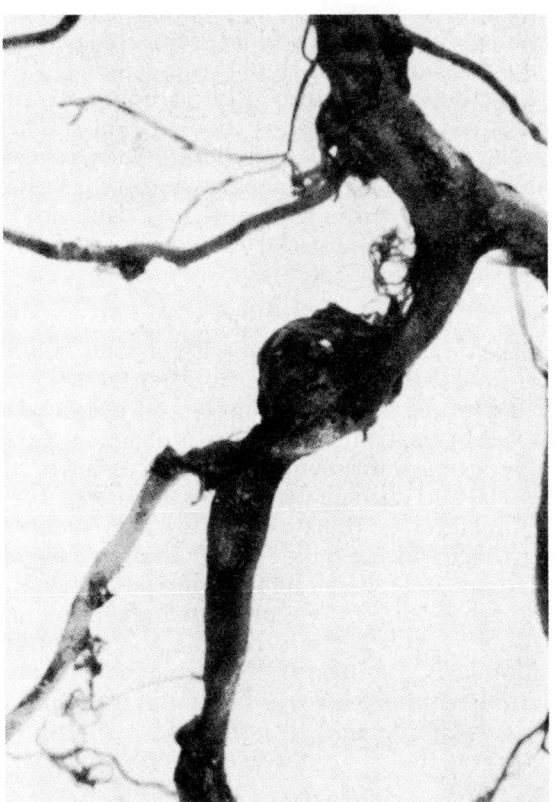

Figure 29–15. Berry aneurysm of middle cerebral artery. The vessels have been dissected away from the brain.

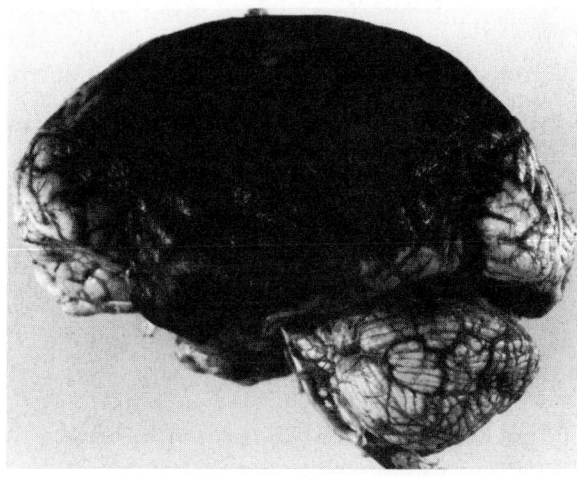

Figure 29–17. Subarachnoid hemorrhage covering the left cerebral hemisphere.

first rupture, but most patients who survive improve and recover consciousness in minutes. Rebleeding is common in the survivors, and it is currently not possible to predict in which patients rebleeding will occur. When it does, the prognosis is significantly more grave.

Four to nine days after rupture, regional arterial vasospasm can be demonstrated angiographically in about 40% of patients, but not all are symptomatic.[93] Postmortem examination of patients dying with vasospasm frequently reveals infarcts in the territories supplied by the affected vessels.[94] Experimentally, platelet products and red cell lysates, including oxyhemoglobin, cause vasoconstriction, but whether they play a role clinically is unknown.

Mixed CNS and Subarachnoid Hemorrhage (Vascular Malformations)

The principal source of these mixed hemorrhages are vascular malformations, which are conventionally divided into *arteriovenous malformations* (AVMs), *cavernous angiomas,* and *capillary telangiectases.*[5]

Arteriovenous malformations consist of tangles of abnormal vessels of various diameters, most of which have characteristics intermediate between those of arteries and veins. Ninety per cent are in the cerebral hemispheres, with half being predominantly superficial and the other half deeply situated. Within the brain, the abnormal vessels are separated by gliotic tissue, in which there is usually evidence of repeated episodes of bleeding. Irregular, often grossly enlarged arteries supply the AVM, and large draining veins can also usually be found.

Bleeding from AVMs is most frequent between the ages of 10 and 30 years and is rare after 60, with males being affected twice as often as females. In about two-thirds of cases the bleeding occurs into both the parenchyma and the subarachnoid space; in about 25% it is confined to the subarachnoid space; and in the remainder, it occurs only into the parenchyma. Bleeding and the development of seizures are the most common clinical presentations.

Cavernous hemangiomas (p. 588) are occasionally found in the brain. They may be multiple, and are sometimes the source of a usually small hemorrhage that will be symptomatic if located in a sensitive region such as the internal capsule or basis pontis. When a cavernous hemangioma is found incidentally, there is almost always some evidence of old hemorrhage and a surrounding fibrillary gliosis.

Capillary hemangiomas (p. 588) are also found in the brain but almost never bleed. Microscopically, they consist of thin-walled, capillary-sized vessels separated by normal neuropil. Almost invariably they remain undetected during life.

HYPERTENSIVE VASCULAR DISEASE

Hypertension has a number of adverse effects on the brain. We have already seen its association with hypertensive intracerebral hemorrhage, and, given its relationship to the development of atherosclerosis (p. 561), with occlusive atherosclerotic vascular disease and atheroembolic infarcts. Three other pathophysiologic processes are associated with hypertension: lacunae, subcortical leukoencephalopathy (Binswanger's disease), and hypertensive encephalopathy.

Lacunae

Lacunae (little lakes) are small necrotic foci ranging from 2 or 3 mm to 15 mm in diameter, most commonly found in the deep portions of the brain, especially the basal ganglia, thalamus, internal capsule, hemispheric white matter, and the pons. Most of them probably result from the occlusion of deep arterioles,[95] either by emboli or as a result of hypertensive arteriolosclerosis.[96] Pigmented macrophages are present in some lacunae, suggesting that they may have a hemorrhagic component or may have been minute hemorrhages. Because of their small size lacunae are often asymptomatic, but if in a vulnerable spot, such as the internal capsule or the basis pontis, they may produce symptoms, for example, a monoplegia.

Subcortical Leukoencephalopathy (Binswanger's Disease)

This name is given to a diffuse loss of predominantly deep hemispheric white matter seen in some hypertensive patients with a progressive dementia.[97] The affected white matter shows diffuse but irregular loss of both axons and myelin, and sometimes areas of relative demyelination, with widespread gliosis. There is marked arteriolar sclerosis of the long penetrating arteries of the white matter. The pathogenesis of this lesion is not clear, but it is thought that the severe arteriolar sclerosis may result in reduced perfusion of the deep white matter during periods of relative hypotension. This lesion frequently coexists with other lesions, notably atherosclerotic cerebrovascular disease.

Hypertensive Encephalopathy

This disease is associated not with chronic stable hypertension, but with malignant hypertension, and with the acute hypertension seen in eclampsia and acute nephritis. Clinically, there is headache, drowsiness, vomiting, and convulsions, progressing to stupor and coma, and if the diastolic pressure is greater than 130 mm mercury, there may be retinal exudates and hemorrhages with papilledema. Pathologically, cerebral edema, petechial hemorrhages, and fibrinoid necrosis of the walls of some small arteries and arterioles are usually seen.[98] There may be accumulations of fibrinous exudate around the damaged vessels and sometimes, in longer-surviving patients, a mild perivascular lymphocytic infiltrate. Experimentally, it has been shown that hypertensive encephalopathy is associated with a failure of autoregulation, a high cerebral blood flow, and a breakdown of the blood-brain barrier with the development of cerebral edema.[99]

VASCULAR DISEASE OF THE SPINAL CORD

The spinal cord has a unique pattern of blood supply, with one anterior and two posterior spinal arteries that are reinforced at several vertebral levels by tributaries of varying sizes from the intercostal and lumbar arteries. The most common vascular injury to the spinal cord is a low flow state that results from the interruption of many of these feeding tributaries. This is particularly associated with dissecting aortic aneurysms. The damage is usually concentrated in the gray matter of the anterior horns of the mid and lower thoracic cord. Occlusion of the anterior spinal artery is rarer, but may occur through compression of a herniated disc, thrombosed endarteritis (p. 1393), or embolism. Spinal cord hemorrhage is most commonly associated with trauma (p. 1412), although vascular malformations and tumors can also bleed.

TRAUMA

Cerebral trauma, a major cause of persisting neurologic handicap, most often affects relatively young people in general, and young males in particular, who may survive with varying degrees of incapacity for many years. Thus, brain trauma is an area of neuropathology with high costs to both the individual and society.

The most important anatomic feature that influences the effect of trauma on the brain is the skull. Although it acts as a shield against moderate forces, in more severe trauma the skull can turn into a weapon and cause brain damage.

The effects of trauma on the skull and brain depend on the shape of the object causing the trauma, the force of impact, and whether the head is in motion at the time of impact. A blow to the head may be penetrating or blunt, and may cause either an open or a closed injury. It is important to appreciate that *severe brain damage can occur in the absence of external injury, and conversely, severe external lacerations, and even skull fractures, do not necessarily indicate injury to the underlying brain.* The major structures affected by cranial trauma are the skull, dura, leptomeninges, and brain. Figure 29–18 is a diagrammatic summary of the ways that injuries to these structures may interact to produce brain damage.

Injuries affecting the brain fall into four groups: (1) skull fractures, (2) epidural hematomas, (3) subdural hematomas, and (4) parenchymal injuries.

SKULL FRACTURES

Fractures of the skull are common complications of cranial trauma. They may be closed or open, linear or comminuted, and they may be depressed. They may be either occult, or evident from the presence of blood or CSF draining from the nose or ears. Skull

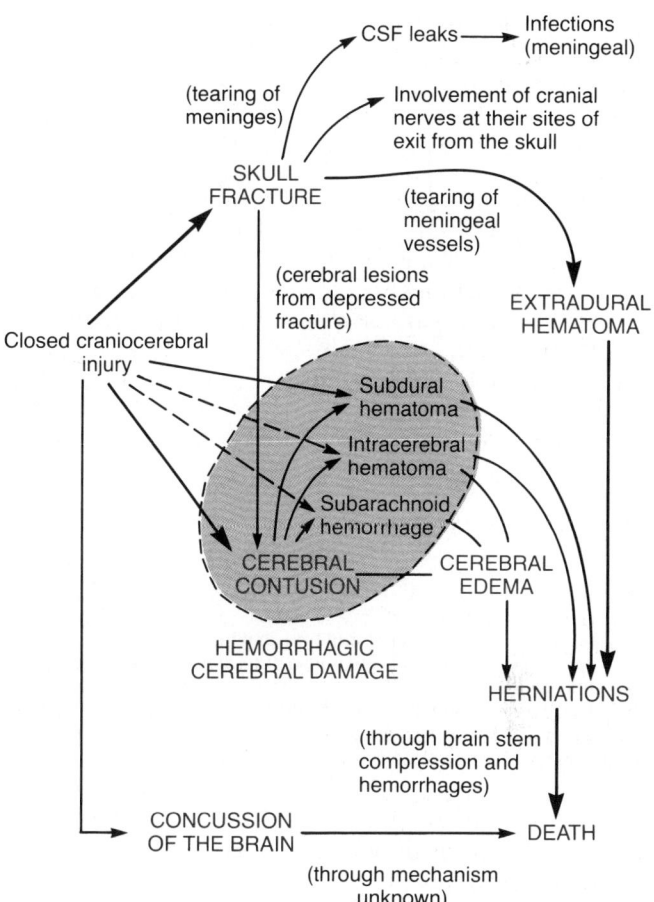

Figure 29–18. Major complications of closed craniocerebral injury. (From Escourolle, R., and Poirier, J.: Manual of Basic Neuropathology. 2nd ed. Philadelphia. W.B. Saunders Co., 1978, p. 65.)

fractures may be followed by the development of an epidural hematoma, or if they are comminuted or depressed, the brain may be injured directly by bone fragments.

EPIDURAL HEMATOMA

Epidural hematomas are localized collections of blood between the skull and the dura mater. They occur following rupture of one of the meningeal arteries, usually the middle meningeal, that run between the dura and the skull (Fig. 29–19). Because the dura is, in part, also the periostium of the skull and is firmly attached to it, a skull fracture is usually necessary to produce arterial rupture (Fig.29–20).[100] Because they are a result of *arterial* bleeding, epidural hematomas cause a rapid and progressive rise in intracranial pressure, usually within minutes to a few hours after the trauma. *Typically, patients recover consciousness from the initial trauma only to slip back into a progressively deepening coma.* Epidural hematomas are surgical emergencies that, if not drained, will produce, in rapid succession, uncinate herniation, tonsil-

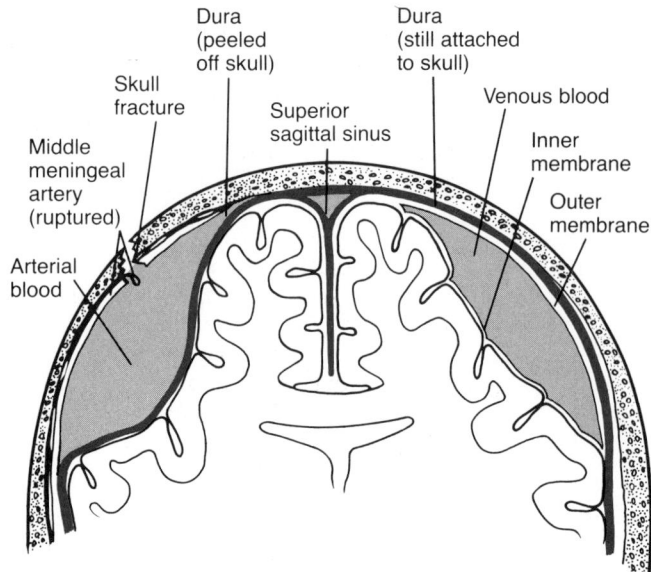

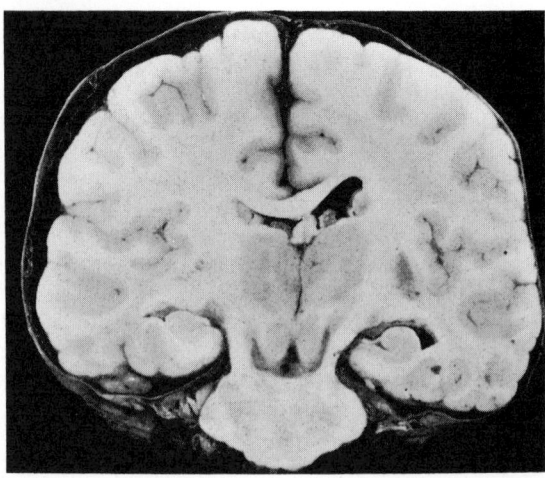

Figure 29–21. Subdural hematoma. The thin inner membrane can be seen between the clot and the leptomeninges (coronal section).

Figure 29–19. *A*, Epidural hematoma, in which rupture of a meningeal artery, usually associated with a skull fracture, leads to accumulation of arterial blood between the dura and the skull. *B*, In a subdural hematoma, damage to bridging veins between the brain and the superior sagittal sinus leads to the accumulation of blood between the dura and the brain.

noid (Figs. 29–19, 29–21, and 29–22). Because subdural hematomas depend for their origin on movement of the brain rather than the direct application of force, they are a reflection of inertial rather than impact forces. Consequently, they occur most commonly where the freedom of movement is greatest, i.e., over the convexities of the hemispheres, and are relatively uncommon where little relative movement is possible, such as the posterior fossa. Subdural he-

lar herniation, medullary compression, respiratory arrest, and death.

SUBDURAL HEMATOMA

Subdural hematomas result from rupture of bridging veins that connect the venous system of the brain to the large intradural venous sinuses. Because the brain, in its bath of CSF, can move within the skull but the venous sinuses are fixed, the displacement of the brain that occurs in trauma can tear some of these delicate veins at the point where they penetrate the dura. The resultant bleeding is into the subdural space between the inner surface of the dura and the arach-

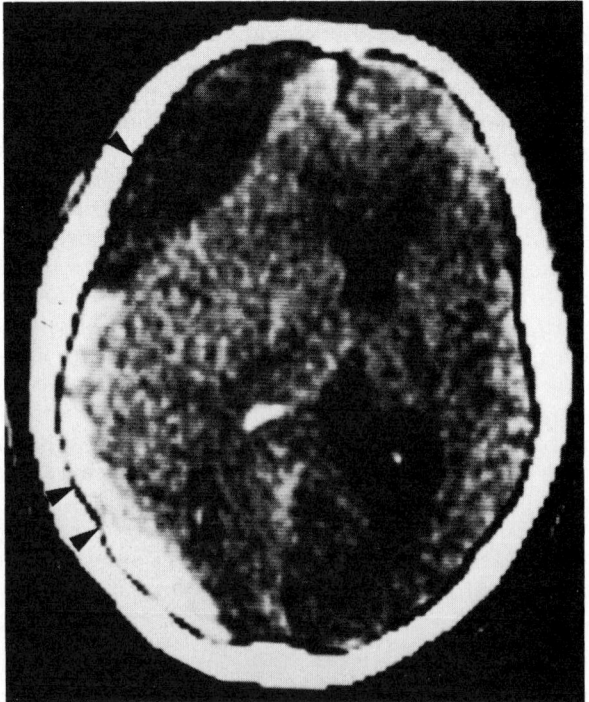

Figure 29–22. CT scan of subdural hematoma overlying and compressing left cerebral hemisphere and distorting ventricular system. Note that less dense blood elements remain in upper zone *(single arrow)* and heavier elements remain in lower dependent zone *(double arrow)*.

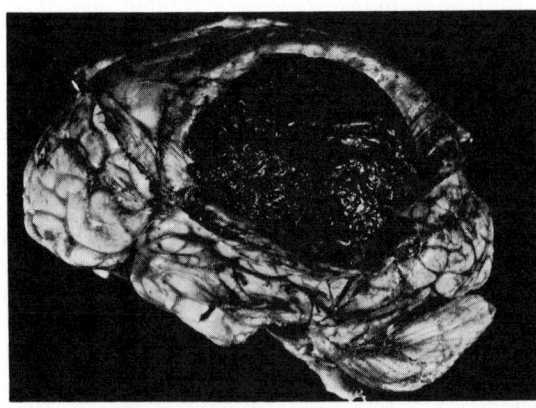

Figure 29–20. Epidural hematoma, the result of laceration of middle meningeal artery caused by fracture of skull.

matomas are classified as being either acute or chronic.

Acute subdural hematomas are usually associated with obvious trauma, and often with other brain injuries as well. *Unlike the case with epidural hematoma, because the bleeding in acute subdural hematoma is venous in origin and at a lower pressure, the onset of symptoms is generally delayed, and the lesion is manifested by a gradual decline in the level of consciousness and sometimes focal signs.* The outcome depends as much on the degree to which the brain is damaged as on the effectiveness of surgical drainage.

Chronic subdural hematomas are much less obviously symptomatic. Older people and alcoholics are common victims. In these patients, there is usually some atrophy of the brain and consequently an increased range of movement of the brain within the skull. This translates into a higher risk of rupturing the bridging veins, and in these patients subdural hematomas, which are often bilateral, may develop slowly following insignificant or even unnoticed trauma. Because they develop relatively slowly, the brain is able to accommodate to their mass effect. Chronic subdural hematomas can therefore produce a much greater degree of cerebral distortion and herniation than acute subdural hematomas before symptoms and signs develop (Fig. 29–23). The symptoms that do occur, such as confusion, inattention, and obtundation, are often vague in nature and insidious in onset. More rarely, seizures or a progressive hemiparesis may occur. A source of clinical confusion is that these symptoms may either mimic or be masked by concomitant disease, such as cerebrovascular disease or dementia. CT and MRI scans have greatly simplified the investigation of these cases.

Chronic subdural hematomas consist of accumulations of blood encased by an outer membrane underlying the dura and by an inner membrane that separates the blood from the arachnoid. Both membranes are composed of fi-

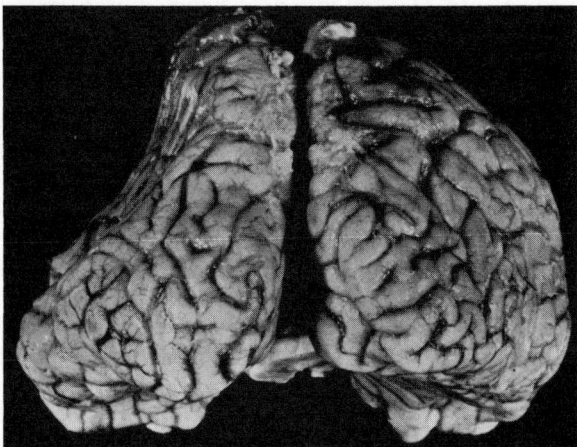

Figure 29–23. Deformed left cerebral hemisphere secondary to massive subdural hematoma.

brous tissue derived from the dura, from which clot resolution proceeds as it does elsewhere in the body. Electron microscopy shows that the vascular channels within the membranes have very thin, incompletely endothelialized walls, making them very susceptible to rebleeding with minimal trauma.

Treatment usually consists of surgical drainage, but rebleeding from the membranes sometimes requires a craniotomy for their removal.

A closely related lesion is the *subdural hygroma*, which is a subdural collection of sometimes blood-tinged CSF. It is thought usually to result from a tear in the arachnoid.[89]

PARENCHYMAL INJURIES

Trauma to the brain itself can be divided for the purposes of discussion into four categories: (1) concussion, (2) contusions and lacerations, (3) traumatic intracerebral hemorrhage, and (4) diffuse axonal injury. The separate category of birth injury is discussed on p. 518.

Concussion

Concussion is a transient loss of consciousness following head trauma. Its duration is usually short, though it may last for some hours, and there is almost always complete recovery. Animal experiments have shown that angular (rotational) acceleration of the head is more potent than translational (anteroposterior) movement in producing concussion (a scientific confirmation of the efficacy of the left hook!).[101] There is no established explanation for its occurrence, but an attractive hypothesis is that torsion of the midbrain may temporarily disrupt the function of the reticular activating system in the periaqueductal gray matter.

Contusions and Lacerations

These traumatic lesions of the brain are analogous to those found in other soft tissues. *Contusions* occur when blunt trauma crushes or bruises brain tissue without rupturing the pia. The most common sites of contusions are either directly related to trauma, in which case they may be at the site of impact (coup lesions) or at a point opposite (contrecoup lesions),[102] or indirectly related, occurring at points where the brain, as it moves, can strike against irregularities on the inner surface of the skull (e.g., the lesser wing of the sphenoid and the orbital ridges, which produce contusions at the frontal and temporal poles and on the orbitofrontal gyri) (Fig. 29–24). The occipital poles are rarely damaged by this mechanism.

Contusions usually affect only the crowns of the gyri, leaving the depths of the gyri intact, but there is often substantial attenuation of the underlying white matter that extends under adjacent intact cortex. Parenthetically, this is the opposite of what happens in ischemic lesions, in which the cortical lesion is usually

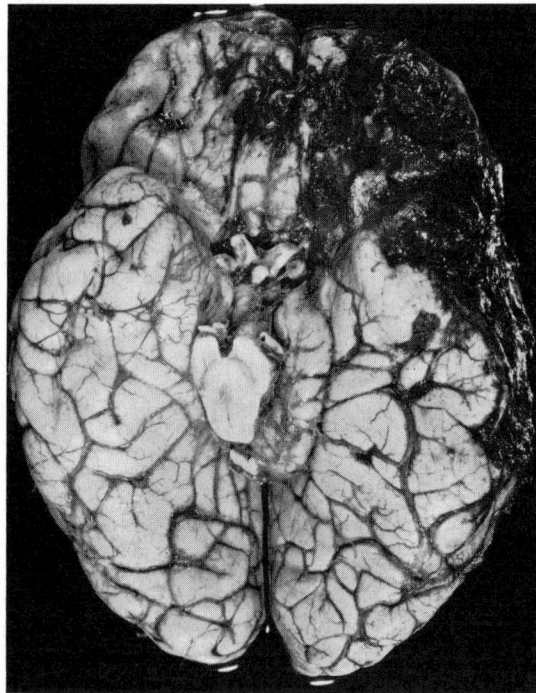

Figure 29–24. Severe contusions of left frontal and temporal lobes. There is also massive left uncal (hippocampal) herniation and compression of right cerebral peduncle.

more extensive than the damage to white matter. Histologically, acute contusions show foci of hemorrhagic gray matter that is subsequently removed by macrophages, leaving an irregular yellow-brown crater with a floor of reactive glial tissue, and often some leptomeningeal fibrosis. Because of their color, these old contusions are often called "plaques jaunes."

Lacerations are tears in the brain tissue produced by more severe blunt trauma that is often accompanied by other damage, such as fractures and local hemorrhage and necrosis. Resolution of lacerations is similar to that of contusions, except that it results in an irregular, yellow-brown gliotic scar that involves not only cortex and meninges but also deeper structures.

Traumatic Intracerebral Hemorrhages

Hemorrhages of this nature are entirely within the brain and do not extend to the surface. They are often multiple, involving the frontal and temporal lobes as well as the deep structures, and may be accompanied by contusions, lacerations, or diffuse axonal injury.[103] Their origin is not fully understood, but they probably result from direct rupture of intracerebral vessels at the time of trauma.

Diffuse Axonal Injury

This obscure type of injury is seen in patients who have severe neurologic impairment after trauma but do not have massive, grossly visible brain damage. Clinically, these patients are deeply comatose from the moment of injury and recover only to the point of

a persistent vegetative state. Microscopic examination of the brain shows widespread white matter damage in the form of *ruptured axons and spheroids (p. 1387).*[104,105] Older cases show microglial reaction, myelin degeneration, and, sometimes, microcavitation. There is some dispute over the pathogenesis of this lesion, but the most likely explanation is that shearing forces that occur during acceleration and deceleration of the brain cause rupture of the axons.

Complications of Trauma

Various complications may develop in patients who survive the initial insult (see Fig. 29–18). *Post-traumatic brain edema* may occur, especially in children, and herniation, brainstem compression, and Duret hemorrhage may follow. Skull fractures may provide a conduit for *infection*, especially from the ear or nose, and *hydrocephalus* may develop secondary to blood or infection in the ventricular system, aqueduct, or subarachnoid space.

In a few patients, for unknown reasons, death may occur shortly after trauma even though there is no apparent physical disruption of tissue.

Delayed sequelae of trauma include *post-traumatic epilepsy*, which usually occurs in patients who have sustained a cortical contusion or laceration, and very occasionally a *delayed intracerebral hemorrhage*, the so-called spät apoplexy, for totally obscure reasons.

Spinal Cord Trauma

Mechanical injury to the spinal cord occurs by penetration or compression. Penetrating wounds, usually stabbing or shooting, produce lacerations, sometimes combined with hemorrhage into the cord (hematomyelia). Compression injuries cause contusions, and are most commonly caused by subluxation, dislocation, or fracture of the vertebrae. They occur most commonly in the cervical and lumbar regions. Vertebral dislocation without permanent bone displacement sometimes causes only momentary cord compression, and the resulting "concussion" induces a transient loss of cord function from which there is usually complete recovery. Displacements and fractures of the vertebrae may produce contusions, lacerations, or even transection of the cord, from which there is usually severe permanent disability, if not complete paralysis. If, as for example in cervical spondylosis, the spinal canal is already narrowed, even small vertebral displacements may severely damage the cord.

In the spinal cord, associated vascular damage is often an important contributing factor, adding local ischemia, infarction, edema, and hemorrhage to the direct physical disruption. Epidural bleeding may also exacerbate damage from other causes. Further, because of the arrangement of the spinal vascular supply, ischemia may occur at some distance from the point of vascular injury, as occurs for example in severe thoracic and abdominal trauma, in which rupture of the intercostal arteries may produce severe cord ischemia and infarction (p. 1409).

TUMORS

Tumors of the nervous system can be divided into *primary intracranial tumors*, a term that covers all primary tumors developing in the cranial cavity, *primary brain tumors*, which arise from the constituent cells of the brain and do not include tumors such as meningiomas that occur in non-brain intracranial tissues, and *metastatic tumors*.

CLASSIFICATION. A modified version of the WHO classification of tumors of the nervous system is shown in Table 29–2. Each type of cell (with the exception of the microglial cell) is represented by at least one type of tumor. Tumors arising from nervous system parenchyma may have mixed cellularity, e.g., ganglioglioma, and tumors from primitive neuroectodermal cells may differentiate along both neuronal and glial lines within the same tumor, e.g., medulloblastoma. A major diagnostic difficulty arises from the wide range of histologic appearances among tumors of the nervous system. This can result in close morphologic similarities between tumors of quite different origin and prognosis, such as a fibrous meningioma and a fibrillary astrocytoma. Immunocytochemistry and special stains are particularly helpful in resolving this type of problem.

Table 29–2. Classification of Nervous System Tumors

Tumors of neuroglia	
Astrocytes	Astrocytoma
	Anaplastic astrocytoma
	Glioblastoma multiforme
	Pilocytic astrocytoma
Oligodendrocytes	Oligodendroglioma
Ependyma and its homologues	Ependymoma
	Myxopapillary ependymoma
	Subependymoma
	Choroid plexus papilloma
Tumors of neurons	Neuroblastoma
	Ganglioneuroblastoma
	Ganglioneuroma
Tumor of neurons and neuroglia	Ganglioglioma
Tumor of primitive undifferentiated cells	Medulloblastoma
Tumors of pineal cells	Pineoblastoma/Pineocytoma
Tumors of meninges	Meningioma
	Meningeal hemangiopericytoma
	Meningeal sarcoma
Tumors of nerve sheath cells	Schwannoma (neurilemmoma)
	Neurofibroma
Lymphomas	Primary
	Secondary
Malformative tumors	Craniopharyngioma
	Epidermoid cyst
	Dermoid cyst
	Colloid cyst
Metastatic tumors	

Modified from WHO.

BIOLOGIC PROPERTIES. In a manner similar to that seen with other types of brain disease, the unique anatomic and physiologic characteristics of the brain interact with the pathophysiology of the different tumor types to affect their growth, spread, treatment, and prognosis.

The essential bodily functions performed by the brain mean that *biologic malignancy has to be distinguished from histologic malignancy.* Some primary intracranial tumors are histologically benign but cannot be removed, and so shorten the life of the patient, thereby demonstrating "biologic malignancy." This usually occurs because *the tumor is located in a part of the brain that makes it impossible to remove even a well-circumscribed or trivially invasive neoplasm,* as for example in an ependymoma of the floor of the fourth ventricle or a meningioma surrounding the carotid artery.

The other major reason that most intracerebral tumors cannot be resected is that *many primary brain tumors have a marked propensity for infiltrative growth, so that individual tumor cells extend well beyond the margin of grossly visible tumor.* Even making allowance for the daunting prognosis of these neoplasms, an attempt at curative resection requires the sacrifice of too much functioning brain tissue to justify the procedure.

Intraneural seeding is a form of tumor dissemination made possible by the fact that the brain is surrounded by the CSF. In tumors that extend to the meninges or cerebral ventricles, tumor cells may be disseminated throughout the neuraxis via the CSF to form deposits on brain, spinal cord, and nerve roots that present clinically as a carcinomatous meningitis (p. 1392). Of the primary brain tumors, medulloblastomas frequently spread in this fashion, and sometimes astrocytomas also; among the metastatic tumors, breast cancer and adenocarcinoma and oat cell carcinoma of the lung are the principal offenders. *Extraneural metastases* from primary intracranial tumors are uncommon but are most likely to arise from a glioblastoma or medulloblastoma. Metastatic spread is encouraged by operative procedures that disrupt the integrity of the dura and subarachnoid space and by any form of ventricular shunting.

CLINICAL EFFECTS. As with other space-occupying lesions of the cranial cavity, tumors produce both local and general effects. The *local effects* of a tumor are determined more by its size and location than by its nature and are not clinically distinguishable from those caused by other types of space-occupying lesions. CT and MRI scans usually show a focal mass lesion of either increased or reduced density, often a midline shift, and other effects, such as edema (Fig. 29–25). The *general effects* of mass lesions have already been described (p. 1389), but a primary intracranial tumor, particularly if located in a so-called silent area such as the frontal lobe, may reach a large size before either local or general symptoms bring the patient to medical attention. This insidious onset is

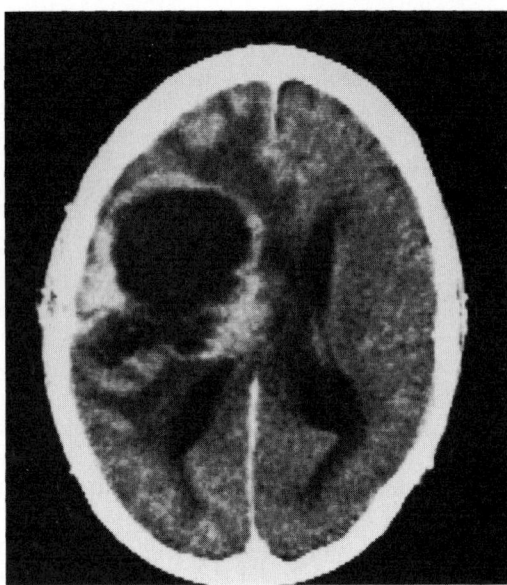

Figure 29–25. CT scan of large tumor in cerebral hemisphere showing ring enhancement with contrast material and pronounced peritumor edema.

somewhat more likely to occur with primary intracranial than with metastatic tumors, because the latter are more often surrounded by a zone of edema that makes even small masses rapidly symptomatic.

INCIDENCE AND DISTRIBUTION. In unselected series, primary intracranial tumors are present in about 1.2% of post-mortems and constitute approximately 9.2% of all primary neoplasms. They are one of the most common types of neoplasms in infants and children, become rarer in young adults and then increase again in frequency with age, but are unusual over the age of 70 years. Some tumors have a predisposition for specific sites, notably medulloblastomas, which are confined to the cerebellum, and pilocytic astrocytomas, which are found predominantly in the cerebellum and hypothalamus. In children approximately 70% of primary intracranial tumors are infratentorial, whereas in adults the converse is true, about 70% being supratentorial. There are also age prefer-

Table 29–3. Incidence of Intracranial Tumors

NEOPLASM	INCIDENCE (%)
Secondary metastases	25–30
Primary neoplasms	70–75
Gliomas	40–50
Glioblastoma	25–30
Astrocytoma	8–12
Ependymoma	2–3
Oligodendroglioma	2–3
Medulloblastoma	2–3
Meningioma	12–15
Acoustic nerve tumor	5–10

Modified from WHO.

ences, medulloblastomas, for example, being most common in the first two decades of life. The approximate relative incidences of the more common intracranial tumors in adults are shown in Table 29–3.

Only the most important or illustrative tumors are described here.

NEUROGLIAL TUMORS

Generically called gliomas, these tumors are derived from neuroectodermal glial cells. The most important clinical variants are astrocytomas and glioblastoma multiforme, pilocytic astrocytomas, oligodendrogliomas, ependymomas, and choroid plexus papillomas.

Astrocytoma and Glioblastoma Multiforme

Astrocytoma and glioblastoma multiforme account for about 80% of adult primary brain tumors. Pathologically they are divisible into three grades of progressively increasing anaplasia and rapidity of clinical progression: astrocytoma, anaplastic astrocytoma, and glioblastoma multiforme. The term glioblastoma requires a little clarification. In principle this term should apply to the most anaplastic form of any glial tumor, but in practice it has come to be used for the most anaplastic form of astrocytoma.

Astrocytomas in general are most common in late middle age, with the peak incidence of anaplastic astrocytomas occurring in the sixth decade and that of glioblastomas about ten years later. *An important property of astrocytic tumors is their marked tendency to become more anaplastic with time, so that a tumor initially diagnosed as an astrocytoma may, and frequently does, prove on later biopsy to be a glioblastoma multiforme.*[5] However, because of their infiltrative character, different areas of the same neoplasm may have quite different histologic appearances. Thus, a small biopsy taken from a less anaplastic area of a glioblastoma may give a misleadingly benign impression of the likely biologic behavior of the tumor.

Astrocytomas are poorly defined, gray-white, infiltrative tumors that expand and distort the underlying brain (Fig. 29–26). They are solid and, depending on their fibrillary content, may be firm or soft and gelatinous. They range from a few centimeters in diameter to enormous lesions that replace the major part of a cerebral hemisphere and extend through the commissures into the opposite hemisphere.

Histologically, astrocytomas may be composed of rather uniform populations of cells described as **protoplasmic, fibrillary, or gemistocytic** (p. 1387), but usually they contain a variety of astrocyte conformations, many of which cannot be classified as one of the classic cell types. Between the neoplastic cells there is usually a highly characteristic fibrillary background of astrocytic processes of varying density and caliber.

Anaplastic astrocytomas are not grossly distinguishable from astrocytomas. Microscopically, however, they

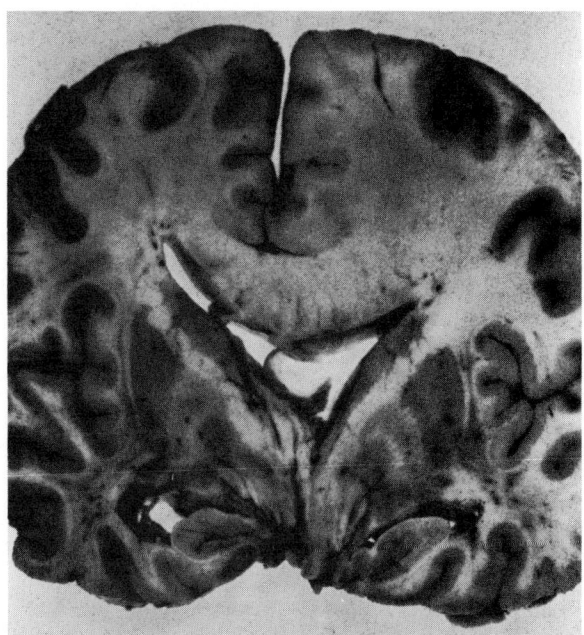

Figure 29-26. Diffuse astrocytoma. Expanded white matter of right cerebral hemisphere and thickened corpus callosum (coronal section).

have anaplastic features such as increased hypercellularity, nuclear and cytoplasmic pleomorphism and irregularity, and nuclear hyperchromatism (Fig. 29-27). Many, but not all, of these tumors have very characteristic proliferation and hyperplasia of the capillary endothelial cells that is not seen in less anaplastic tumors. **The presence of either vascular endothelial proliferation or a mitotic rate greater than 1 per 10 HPF is pathognomonic of anaplastic change,**[106] but neither feature is necessary for the diagnosis. Both anaplastic astrocytoma and glioblastoma are occasionally disseminated throughout the neuraxis via the CSF.

Glioblastoma multiforme is distinguished from the other types of astrocytoma by its variegated appearance; hence the term multiforme. Some regions may be white and firm, others yellow and soft, and foci of necrosis, cysts, and hemorrhages are common (Fig. 29-28A). Microscopically, **necrosis**, which may or may not have pseudopallisading around it (Fig. 29-28B),[107] distinguishes them from anaplastic astrocytomas, the other cellular features of anaplasia being the same. The endothelial proliferation is often very prominent and may form little clusters of capillaries

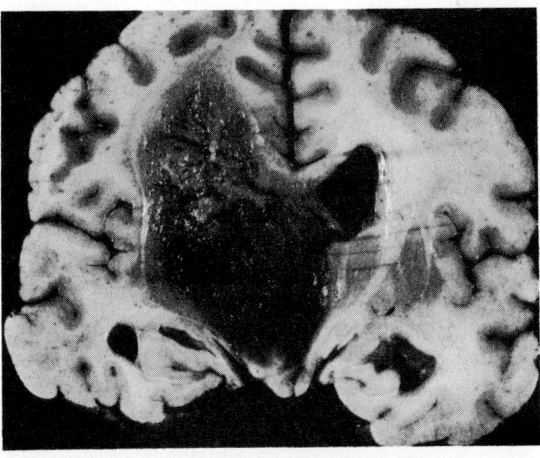

A

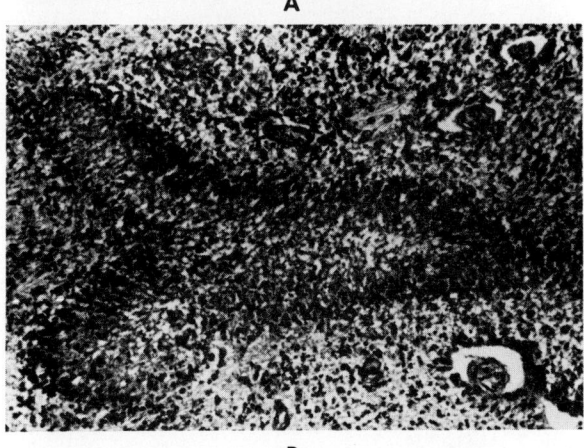

B

Figure 29-28. *A,* Glioblastoma multiforme appearing as a necrotic hemorrhagic infiltrating mass. *B,* Pseudopalisading (neoplastic cells aligned around a region of necrosis), hypercellularity, and pleomorphism in glioblastoma multiforme. (H and E stain.)

Figure 29-27. Anaplastic astrocytoma. There is hypercellularity and pleomorphism of the tumor cells and marked hyperplasia of the capillary endothelial cells *(arrows).*

called "glomeruli." Notwithstanding these anaplastic features, areas of more benign-appearing astrocytoma will usually be present as well. The presence of numerous large, bizarre-looking giant cells confers a slightly more favorable prognosis to this otherwise rapidly fatal tumor, and the term giant cell glioblastoma is sometimes applied to this variant.

The location and size of the tumor determines the clinical presentation. Almost all astrocytomas in adults occur in the cerebral hemispheres, although they are occasionally found in the spinal cord. Curiously, glioblastomas almost never arise in the cerebellum. With astrocytomas, the symptoms may remain static or progress only slowly for a number of years. Eventually, however, patients usually enter a period of more rapid clinical deterioration that is generally correlated with the appearance of anaplastic features and more rapid growth of the tumor. The prognosis for patients with glioblastoma is very poor. With current treatment, comprising palliative resection when feasible together with radiotherapy and steroids, the mean length of survival after diagnosis is only eight to ten months, with fewer than 10% of patients alive after two years. Survival is substantially shorter in older patients.[108] With anaplastic astrocytomas, the length of survival is more variable, but a high mitotic rate or the presence of endothelial hyperplasia tends to be associated with a poor prognosis.

Brainstem gliomas are a clinical subgroup of astrocytomas. They occur mostly in the first two decades of life and compose about 20% of the primary brain tumors in this age group. At autopsy about 50% of them are glioblastomas. With current radiother-apy, the five-year survival rate for the composite group, which includes all grades of astrocytoma, is between 25 and 40%.

Pilocytic Astrocytoma

These tumors are distinguished from other astrocytomas by their distinctive pathologic appearance and almost invariably benign behavior. They typically occur in children and young adults and usually are located in the cerebellum, but may also appear in the floor and walls of the third ventricle, the optic nerves, and, very occasionally, the cerebral hemispheres.

Grossly, pilocytic astrocytoma is often cystic, with the tumor confined to a mural nodule in the wall of the cyst (Fig. 29–29), but if solid, it may be well circumscribed or apparently infiltrative. Microscopically, the tumor is only moderately hypercellular and is composed of **pilocytic astrocytes**, which are bipolar cells with long, thin "hair-like" processes. **Rosenthal fibers** (p. 1388) and microcysts are often present. Vascular endothelial proliferation is also common, but in this tumor, unlike in the other astrocytomas, it does not imply an unfavorable prognosis, and other features of anaplasia are almost never seen.

These tumors grow very slowly, and in some ways act more like hamartomas than true neoplasms, patients having survived for more than 40 years after incomplete resection.

Oligodendroglioma

These tumors constitute about 5% of gliomas, are most common in middle life, affect both sexes about equally, and are found mostly in the cerebral hemispheres.

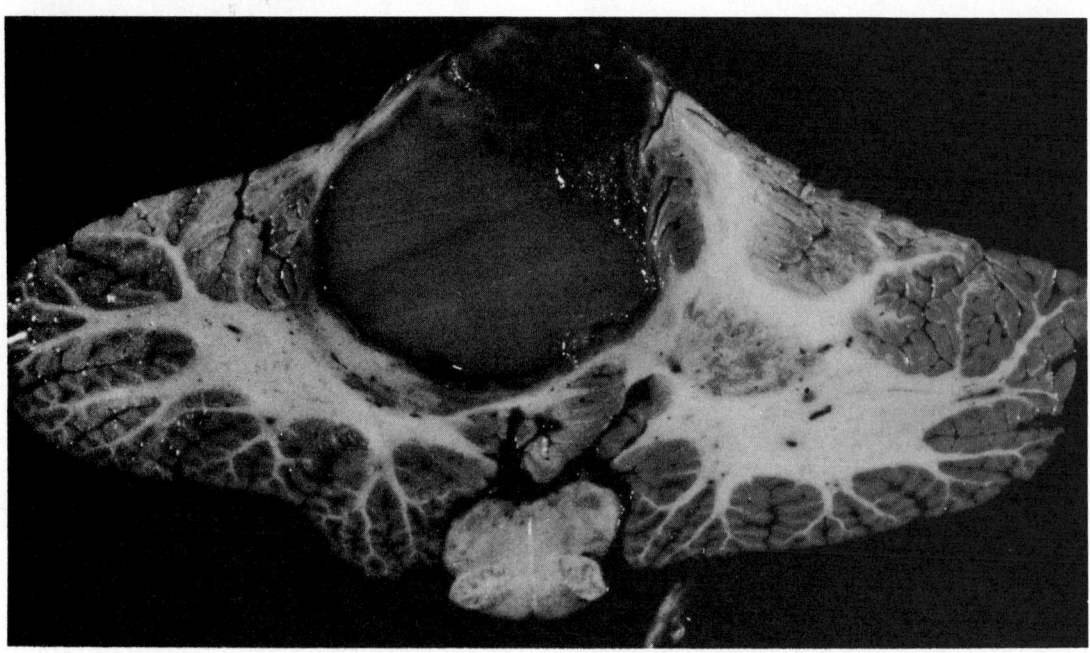

Figure 29–29. Juvenile pilocytic astrocytoma in cerebellum with nodule of tumor in cyst.

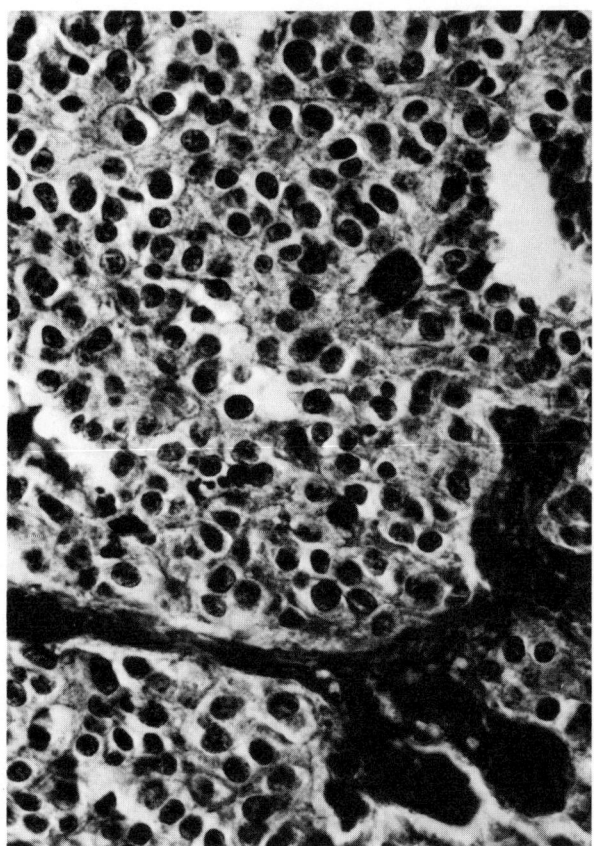

Figure 29–30. Oligodendroglioma. Cells are round and small and have perinuclear halos. (H and E stain.)

Grossly, oligodendrogliomas are well-circumscribed, gelatinous, gray masses, often with cysts, focal hemorrhage, and calcification (which is often a useful radiologic diagnostic feature). As with other gliomas, there is occasionally extension of the tumor into the subarachnoid space. Microscopically, the tumor is composed of sheets of regular cells with spherical nuclei containing finely granular chromatin surrounded by a clear halo of cytoplasm that, although regularly present and a valuable diagnostic feature, is an artifact of fixation (Fig. 29–30). Typically, a delicate network of anastomosing capillaries separates the tumor cells into clusters. The calcification, which is present in up to 90% of these tumors, ranges from microscopic foci to massive depositions. Anaplastic variants of these tumors show progressive, particularly nuclear pleomorphism that, in the most anaplastic examples, makes them difficult to recognize as oligodendrogliomas. Up to 50% of these tumors contain areas of astrocytoma that, if anaplastic, will determine the prognosis.

In these tumors there is a poor correlation between the microscopic features and prognosis, some having an indolent pattern of growth but other, similar-looking tumors behaving more like glioblastomas.[109,110] Undoubtedly part of the reason for this imprecision is the variable content of astrocytoma, which might not be present in a small biopsy specimen. Surgery and radiotherapy yield an average survival of about five years.

Ependymoma

Ependymomas are derived from the single layer of epithelium that lines the ventricles and extends down the center of the spinal cord as a remnant of the central canal. Although they may develop anywhere in this territory, in the first two decades of life, ependymomas typically occur in the fourth ventricle, where they constitute between 5 and 10% of the primary brain tumors in this age group. In middle life, the spinal cord is the most common location, where ependymomas constitute a large fraction of primary intraspinal neoplasms.[111,112]

In the fourth ventricle ependymomas are typically solid or papillary masses erupting from the floor of the ventricle. Although often well demarcated from adjacent brain, their proximity to the vital pontine and medullary nuclei usually makes complete extirpation impossible. In the intraspinal tumors, this sharp demarcation sometimes makes total removal, and therefore cure, possible. Microscopically, ependymomas are composed of cells with rather regular, round to oval or "carrot-shaped" nuclei with abundant granular chromatin. Between the nuclei there is a fine fibrillary background that may be very dense. Helpful diagnostic features include **ependymal canals** and **rosettes**, in which the tumor cells create arrays that resemble ependymal canals, and perivascular **ependymal pseudorosettes**, in which there is a dense array of long, delicate ependymal processes inserted into the wall of a blood vessel, producing a prominent nucleus-free halo around the vessel (Fig. 29–31). **Blepharoplasts**, which are the basal bodies of cilia, are stained by PTAH and are pathognomonic if present. Immunocytochemically, about 50% of ependymomas can be shown to contain the neuroglial intermediate filament glial fibrillary acidic protein (GFAP). Most tumors are well differentiated, but anaplastic tumors occur, the most anaplastic of which resemble glioblastomas.

Clinically, posterior fossa ependymomas often manifest with hydrocephalus secondary to progressive obstruction of the fourth ventricle rather than evidence of invasion of the pons or medulla. Some are disseminated through the CSF. However, their origin from the floor of the fourth ventricle usually means that even the least invasive tumors cannot be completely excised. Hence, even though they are usually slow growing and histologically benign, their prognosis is poor. An average survival of about four years following surgery and radiotherapy has been recorded. In ependymoma of the spinal cord, slowly progressive long tract signs and expansion of the cord by MRI and CT scans are common findings.

Myxopapillary ependymomas occur in the filum terminale of the spinal cord and, as implied by their name, may contain myxoid or papillary elements admixed with more typical ependymal cells. In the papillary component, cuboidal cells, sometimes with

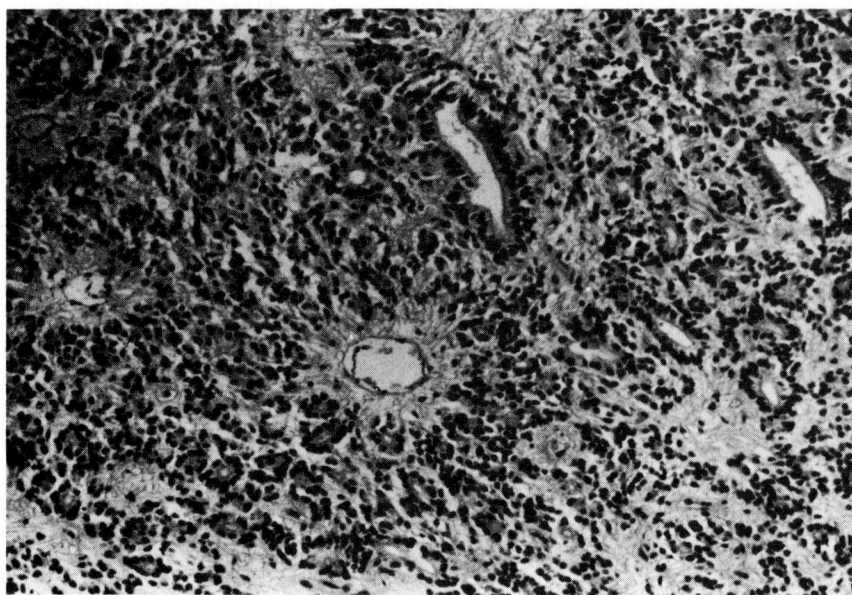

Figure 29–31. Ependymoma. Note tumor cells align themselves around tubular spaces resembling the ependymal cavity and also around blood vessels. (H and E stain.)

clear cytoplasm, are arranged around papillary cores containing connective tissue and blood vessels. Mucin-positive material may be present in the connective tissue elements of this tumor. As with other ependymomas, myxopapillary ependymomas are usually histologically benign. Their prognosis depends mostly upon whether they have erupted into the subarachnoid space and surrounded the roots of the cauda equina; if they have, complete surgical removal is very difficult and recurrence is likely.

Subependymomas are solid, sometimes calcified, very slow-growing nodules attached to the ventricular lining and protruding into the ventricle. They are usually asymptomatic findings at autopsy, but if they are sufficiently large or appropriately located, they may cause hydrocephalus or other focal findings. They are most often found in the lateral and fourth ventricles, and in the latter location, as with other fourth ventricular tumors, may be impossible to remove, although they are histologically benign. Microscopically, they have a very characteristic appearance, with clumps of ependymal-appearing nuclei scattered in a very dense, finely fibrillar background.

Choroid Plexus Papilloma

Choroid plexus papillomas can occur anywhere in the distribution of the choroid plexus and are most common in children, in whom they are most often found in lateral ventricles. In adults they are more often present in the fourth ventricle.

These tumors almost exactly recapitulate the structure of the normal choroid plexus and are markedly papillary growths. The papillae have connective tissue stalks covered with a cuboidal, or sometimes almost columnar, ciliated epithelium. There are very rare malignant examples, which so closely resemble metastatic adenocarcinomas that this diagnosis should be rigorously excluded before accepting the diagnosis of malignant choroid plexus papilloma.

Clinically, choroid plexus papillomas usually present with some variant of hydrocephalus due either to obstruction of the ventricular system by tumor or to overproduction of CSF.

TUMORS OF NEURONAL ORIGIN

In the central nervous system the major tumors of neuronal origin are neuroblastoma, ganglioneuroma (gangliocytoma), and ganglioglioma. There are many similarities between these tumors and their counterparts found in the adrenal medulla and other locations (p. 1265). All are rare and are usually found in children or young adults.

Neuroblastomas

These tumors occur mostly in the cerebral hemispheres in children. Microscopically they resemble peripheral neuroblastomas (p. 1266), being composed of small undifferentiated cells with characteristic rosettes. There is a desmoplastic variant that is characterized by the presence of a connective tissue stroma.[113]

Ganglioneuromas (Gangliocytomas) and Gangliogliomas

Tumors containing more differentiated neuronal elements that are sometimes so mature that they may resemble normal neurons are called ganglioneuromas. Ganglioneuromas (gangliocytomas) are the

CNS equivalent of the peripheral tumor of the same name, except that the reactive stroma in these tumors is glial. In gangliogliomas, the glial stroma itself is judged to be neoplastic, although the distinction between reactive changes and low-grade tumor can sometimes be very difficult.

Grossly, ganglioneuromas are well-circumscribed masses with focal calcification and small cysts usually found in the floor of the third ventricle, the hypothalamus, or the temporal lobe. Microscopically the ganglion cell component often comprises clumps of cells separated by a not very cellular stroma.

Most of these tumors are slow growing, but occasionally the glial component becomes frankly anaplastic and the tumor then runs a much more rapid course.

TUMORS OF PRIMITIVE OR UNDIFFERENTIATED CELLS

The most important member of this group is the medulloblastoma.

Medulloblastoma

This neoplasm of undifferentiated cells occurs in the cerebellum. It is overwhelmingly a tumor of the first two decades of life. In this age group medulloblastomas account for 25% of all primary brain tumors, although they occasionally occur in older persons.

Grossly, medulloblastomas are gray-white masses that sometimes appear to be well demarcated. In young children they are typically located in the vermis of the cerebellum (Fig. 29–32A), but in older patients they are more often found laterally in the hemispheres. Dissemination through the CSF with extensive ependymal and subarachnoid growth of tumor is almost the rule in medulloblastomas. Microscopically, they are very densely cellular tumors composed of sheets of small but moderately pleomorphic nuclei with varying chromatin density and very little if any visible cytoplasm (Fig. 29–32B). Some tumors show no detectable differentiation, but in others there is spongioblastic (glial) differentiation into spindle cells with delicate processes containing GFAP that resemble the primitive spongioblasts of early brain development. In a smaller fraction of these tumors, neuronal differentiation in the form of Homer-Wright rosettes (p. 1266) is present, and in a few of these tumors the primitive nature of the precursor cell is reflected in the presence of both neuronal and glial differentiation. **This capacity for both glial and neuronal differentiation is the major feature that distinguishes the medulloblastoma from almost all other primary brain tumors.** In these rapidly growing neoplasms, mitoses are often, but not always, easily found. The cell of origin of these tumors, the putative "medulloblast," has not been identified with cer-

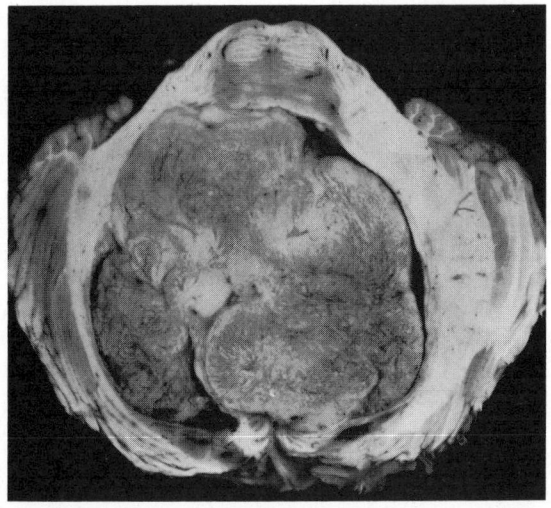

A

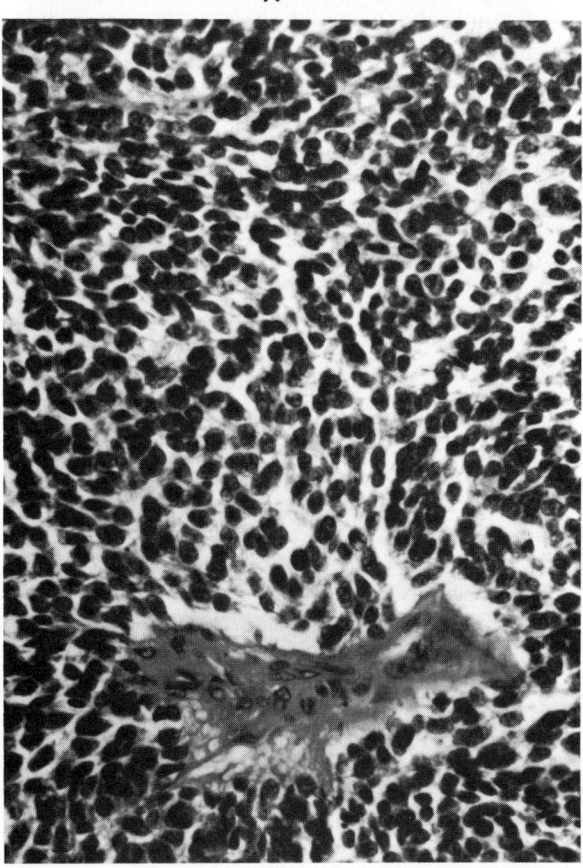

B

Figure 29–32. *A,* Medulloblastoma growing into fourth ventricle, distorting, compressing, and infiltrating surrounding structures. *B,* Medulloblastoma (H and E stain).

tainty, but a multipotential cell in the external granular layer of the cerebellum is a favored candidate.

Medulloblastomas that abut or extend into the meninges may develop a mesodermal fibrous stroma. These tumors are called desmoplastic medulloblastomas.

Clinically, patients present with signs of progressive cerebellar dysfunction or hydrocephalus. The high frequency of CSF dissemination of the tumor occasionally results in a spinal cord syndrome when the primary cerebellar lesion has not yet become symptomatic. This pattern of dissemination also necessitates treatment of the entire neuraxis; otherwise spinal recurrence is very common. A ten-year 50% survival rate is currently obtained with a combination of surgery and craniospinal radiotherapy.

TUMORS OF MENINGES

Meningioma

The term meningioma is used for tumors arising from the specialized arachnoid cap cells, although very occasionally other types of primary tumor also develop in the meninges. Meningiomas constitute about 20% of all primary intracranial tumors. Their most common sites of occurrence are in the front half of the head and include the hemispheric convexity, the falx cerebri, the lesser wing of the sphenoid bone, and the olfactory groove. Other rarer but clinically important locations are inside the cerebral ventricles, the cerebellopontine angle, the foramen magnum, and the spinal cord. Although meningiomas are usually solitary, multiple meningiomas do occur, and are particularly likely in von Recklinghausen's neurofibromatosis. Meningiomas are generally tumors of middle and later life and are more common in women (3:2 ratio). Some meningiomas have sex hormone receptors, and rapid growth during pregnancy is an occasional but well-described finding.

Grossly, meningiomas are usually irregular, bosselated masses firmly adherent to the dura that indent the surface of the brain but rarely invade it (Fig. 29–33A). Occasionally growth occurs in a plate-like form called meningioma-en-plaque. Meningiomas are usually firm solid tumors, often with a gritty texture. A whorl-like pattern may be detectable on their cut surfaces. Hyperostosis of the bone overlying a meningioma is common.

Histologically, there are three major patterns, **syncytial**, **fibroblastic**, and **transitional**, which constitute a spectrum of lesions rather than three distinct entities. **Syncytial meningiomas** recapitulate the normal appearances of arachnoid cap cells and form prominent cellular whorls and nodules. The nuclei are regular and oval, with finely granular chromatin and, not infrequently, cytoplasmic intrusions that give the nuclei a hollow appearance. The cell borders are indistinct, and electron microscopy shows a complex interdigitation of cell membranes with desmosomes and gap junctions. **Fibroblastic meningiomas** have spindle-shaped bipolar cells that resemble fibroblasts arranged in bands and swaths, and **transitional meningiomas** have intermediate characteristics and often contain psammoma bodies (p. 35) (Fig. 29–33B), which are also occasionally seen in the other variants. Various forms of degeneration can be seen, including xanthomatous and myxomatous degenera-

tion and bone and, rarely, cartilage formation. These configurations are largely of academic interest because they have no prognostic significance. However, **malignant meningiomas** do occasionally occur, either as unexceptional-looking tumors with a high mitotic rate, or as more frankly sarcomatous lesions that resemble fibrosarcomas. These tumors, unlike benign meningiomas, may invade the brain and even, very rarely, metastasize.

A tumor that requires special mention is the **hemangiopericytoma** (p. 591) of the meninges. Grossly, it is indistinguishable from a conventional meningioma. This entity is the subject of an arcane (one is tempted to say acrimonious) taxonomic debate, but its practical significance is that it can be mistaken for a somewhat atypical meningioma.[114] As with systemic hemangiopericytomas, however, and unlike ordinary meningiomas, it has a high likelihood of recurring even after apparently complete resection and tends to become more anaplastic with time.

Clinically, the symptoms caused by meningiomas depend upon their location, although their slow growth means that the onset of symptoms is often insidious and such a tumor may reach a large size before the patient seeks medical attention. The outcome similarly depends on location. Most can be entirely removed, and with little risk of recurrence, but if unfavorably placed, e.g., around the carotid artery, they may not be completely resectable and may cause severe morbidity or even mortality.

LYMPHOMAS (PRIMARY AND SECONDARY), LEUKEMIA

Systemic lymphomas may invade the nervous system and cause either a lymphomatous meningitis or, less frequently, parenchymal infiltration. The brain may also be the site of a primary lymphoma. In the past these tumors were called microgliomas, on the assumption that they were derived from microglial cells (p. 1388), but marker studies have shown that many of them are of B-lymphocyte origin.[115] Current practice is to use the same terminology as for extracranial lymphomas (p. 708), and such terms as "microglioma" and "reticulum cell sarcoma" should be discarded.

The emergence of AIDS has resulted in a marked increase in the incidence of primary CNS lymphomas, which are found in about 5% of cases. In these patients the spectrum of CNS lymphomas follows the same pattern as that seen in the rest of the body, the tumors being non-Hodgkin's lymphomas with a higher than usual incidence of intermediate- and high-grade neoplasms (p. 714).[53,54] Outside the AIDS population they are rare, constituting only about 0.02% of all lymphomas and 0.4% of primary brain tumors, and are most commonly seen in immunosuppressed patients, notably those with renal transplants,[116] and also in association with mycosis fungoides and dysproteinemias. Interestingly, no unequivocal case of primary CNS Hodgkin's disease has yet been described.

On CT scans primary CNS lymphomas often have a characteristic, but not pathognomonic, periventricular distribution and may be multifocal. Grossly, they may be nodular or may infiltrate the brain so diffusely that it can be very difficult to distinguish tumor from normal tissue. In this way lymphoma is one of the few tumors that mimics the infiltrative behavior of the glial neoplasms. The features of lym-

phomas have been described on p. 711, but in the brain, one of their most characteristic microscopic features is a tendency to infiltrate and expand the walls of blood vessels. This is well demonstrated by reticulin stains, which show a laminated network of reticulin around the affected vessel; a network that sometimes extends into the adjacent parenchyma when it is infiltrated by tumor.

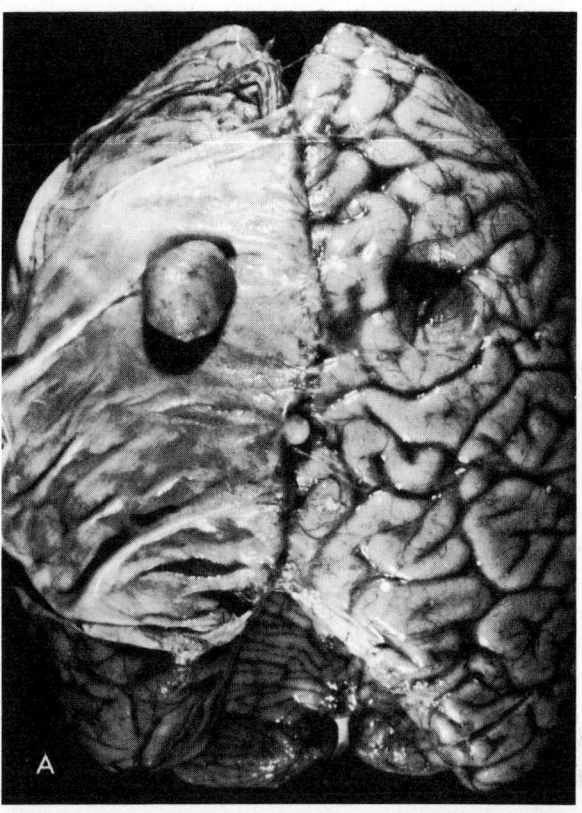

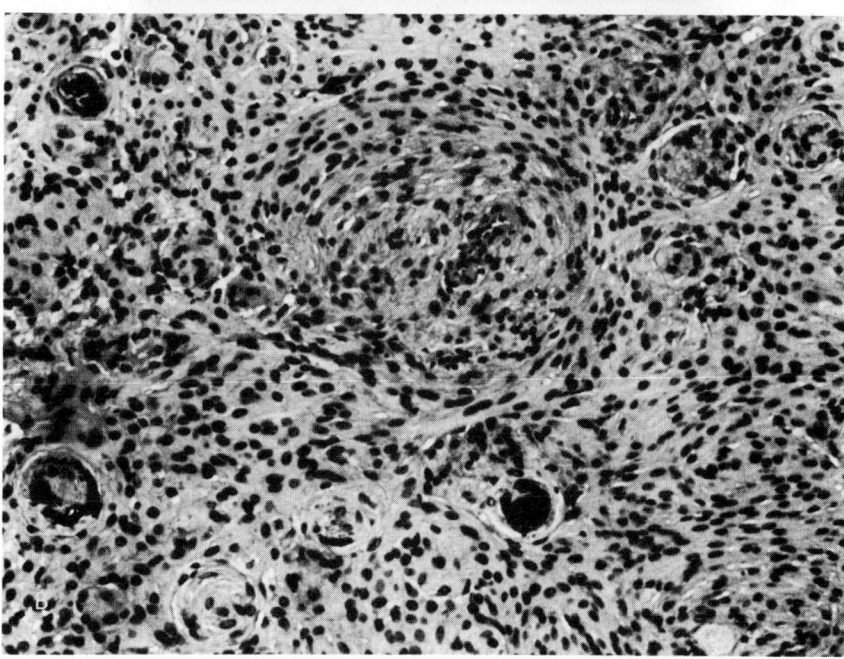

Figure 29–33. *A*, Reflected dura *(on left)* showing one large and one small *(in middle of illustration)* meningioma. Note prominent indentation of right cerebral hemisphere by the larger tumor. *B*, Transitional meningioma with hypercellularity, whorled pattern of cells, and psammoma bodies (H and E stain).

Clinically, although there is often a good initial response to steroids and radiation, CNS lymphomas do not have a good prognosis, mean survival being only about 18 months in patients treated with a combination of surgery, radiation, and chemotherapy.

Leukemias, like secondary lymphomas, may involve the dura and leptomeninges, but rarely invade the parenchyma. Focal intracranial hemorrhage may occur as a consequence of the bleeding diathesis that is frequently seen in these disorders. The hemorrhages are often multiple and may be life threatening or fatal.

OTHER INTRACRANIAL TUMORS

Colloid Cyst of Third Ventricle

Colloid cysts usually occur in young adults and account for about 2% of primary intracranial tumors. Their precise origin is uncertain but it is probably ependymal or paraphyseal (choroid plexus).

> A colloid cyst is 1 to 4 cm in diameter located in the anterior third ventricle, attached by its walls or by a short pedicle to the ventricular wall. It consists of a fibrous capsule lined by a cuboidal or low columnar, sometimes ciliated epithelium, often with interspersed mucous goblet cells. The cyst contents are of varying consistency, but are usually jelly-like and often PAS positive.

The significance of these lesions, like so much else in the nervous system, is a consequence of their location. The presence of a colloid cyst in the anterior third ventricle means that it can obstruct the foramina of Monro, block drainage of CSF from the lateral ventricles, and cause intermittent hydrocephalus that can be rapidly fatal. Surgical excision is curative but can be technically demanding.

Metastatic Tumors

About 25 to 30% of intracranial tumors are metastases. The vast majority are carcinomas, the five most common sites of origin, in order of frequency, being lung, breast, skin (melanoma), kidney, and gastrointestinal tract. These sites account for about 80% of all metastases. Some tumors, for example choriocarcinomas, although quite rare, have a high likelihood of metastasizing to the brain, whereas others, notably prostate tumors and squamous cell carcinoma of the head and neck, almost never do even when disseminated to adjacent bone.

> Grossly, metastatic intracranial tumors form sharply demarcated masses, often at the cortico–white matter junction, usually surrounded by a zone of edema. Carcinomatous meningitis, with tumor nodules studding the surface of the brain, spinal cord, and intradural nerve roots, is an occasional complication particularly associated with small cell carcinoma and adenocarcinoma of the lung and carcinoma of the breast. Microscopically, most metastases recapitulate their primaries, but in morphologically ambiguous cases, the sharp demarcation between metastatic tumor and the surrounding reactive brain contrasts markedly with the infiltrative behavior of many primary brain tumors, a helpful diagnostic feature.

Metastatic tumors present as mass lesions and may even occasionally be the presenting symptoms of a carcinoma. In general, treatment is symptomatic and palliative, although the greater precision possible with modern imaging techniques and stereotactic neurosurgical procedures more frequently allows removal of single, or even multiple, metastases, with benefit to the patient.

DEMYELINATING DISEASES

The major pathologic process in the demyelinating diseases is loss of the myelin sheaths that surround the axons, the axons themselves being relatively preserved. Demyelination results either from damage to the oligodendrocytes that produce the myelin or from a direct, usually immunologic or toxic assault on the myelin itself. The demyelinating diseases are therefore a group of conditions bound together not by a common etiology but by a type of pathologic process. Advances in our understanding have resulted in the transfer of many of the diseases previously included in the demyelinating disease category to more explicit etiologic categories. The *leukodystrophies* (inborn errors of metabolism), *progressive multifocal leukoencephalopathy* (slow virus diseases), and *central pontine myelinolysis* (toxic metabolic) are all examples of diseases in which the principal pathologic process is demyelination but which are described in their specific etiologic categories. The most important diseases still included in this category are *multiple sclerosis* and the *perivenous encephalomyelitides*.

MULTIPLE SCLEROSIS

Since its first description by Charcot in 1868, multiple sclerosis (MS) has been the subject of exhaustive study, and there is a great deal of interesting but currently inconclusive evidence about its pathogenesis. Most ongoing research relates to putative viral or autoimmune etiologies, but as yet there is no coherent theory of pathogenesis, and it should not be assumed that these etiologies must necessarily be the only candidates or that they are mutually exclusive.

ETIOLOGY AND PATHOGENESIS. Epidemiologically, there is a slight excess of females in the patient population, a higher incidence of disease in first-degree relatives, and an excess of HLA-A3, B7, and DR2 antigens in north European and Caucasian American patients.[117] The existence of a significant genetic susceptibility to MS is underlined by twin studies, one of which has shown a 25% concordance for the disease in monozygotic twins.[118] Multiple sclerosis is much more prevalent in the temperate higher latitudes in both the northern and southern hemispheres, but this effect is most apparent in patients of European origin, there being a notably low incidence of multiple sclerosis in Orientals, Africans, and American Indians. Migration studies have indicated that persons who emigrate from regions of high incidence to more tropical climes (and conversely) tend to retain the risk of their birthplace if they move after about the age of 15 years, but to adopt the risk of their new home if they move as children.[119]

The suggestion that an infectious agent may be involved has been reinforced by the occurrence of outbreaks of the disease in isolated communities, notably in the Faroe Islands. The outbreak there began when British troops were present during the Second World War, and new cases occurred long after their withdrawal, although it now seems to have died out. The pattern of incidence seems to suggest exposure to an agent that can predispose to the later development of MS.[120] Because the occupation introduced canine distemper to the islands, canine distemper virus, an agent antigenicially related to measles virus, was a favored candidate. However, intensive investigations have failed to substantiate its involvement, or indeed that of any other virus, in the etiology of MS. In light of this failure, it is provoking that the neighboring Orkney Islands, which have one of the highest incidences of multiple sclerosis in the world, have registered an apparent decline in the incidence of the disease following a reduction in canine distemper subsequent to a program of immunization.[121]

The demyelination in MS is accompanied by a prominent lymphocyte invasion into the plaques. Both T4 (helper/inducer) and T8 (suppressor/cytotoxic) cells are present, and although both types are most common at the edge of the plaques, they are present in different ratios in different areas.[122] This differential accumulation suggests that the balance of T-cell subsets in and around a plaque may influence its evolution, an inference that is supported by reports of a selective loss of the suppressor-inducer T-cell subset in the blood of some patients with progressive MS.[123] *Although these findings are presumptive evidence of a role for cell-mediated immunity in demyelination, the precise contribution remains elusive.* In relation to humoral immunity, the oligoclonal bands of immunoglobulins that are found in the CSF of patients with MS are probably epiphenomena that result from the trapping of activated B lymphocytes in the CNS. Unlike the oligoclonal immunoglobulins in SSPE (p. 1399), they are not directed against any known antigen; in the context of multiple sclerosis it is significant that the immunoglobulins are not anti-myelin antibodies.[124] Although helpful diagnostically, they do not seem to be etiologically significant.[125]

Present evidence concerning the pathogenesis of MS is thus both confusing and incomplete, but suggests that the disease is the result of an interaction involving genetic, environmental, and immune mechanisms, perhaps operating at different times in the patient's life.[126]

MORPHOLOGY. The external appearance of the brain and spinal cord is usually normal, or there is mild generalized atrophy. On sectioning, multiple, irregularly shaped, sharp-edged areas of demyelination called **plaques** are seen (Fig. 29–34). Occasionally, plaques have a diffuse rather than a sharp border or may be only faintly visible (shadow plaques). The appearance of plaques varies with their age, being initially slightly pink and swollen, but later becoming gray, sunken, and opalescent. They occur in gray and white matter, range from the just visible to many centimeters in diameter, and may be sparsely scattered or involve a large fraction of the brain and spinal cord. Although plaques have a predilection for the angles of the cerebral ventricles, they may occur anywhere in the CNS and are often distributed in a relatively symmetrical fashion on the two sides of the brain.

Microscopically, the earliest loss of myelin is seen around small veins and venules (perivenous demyelination).

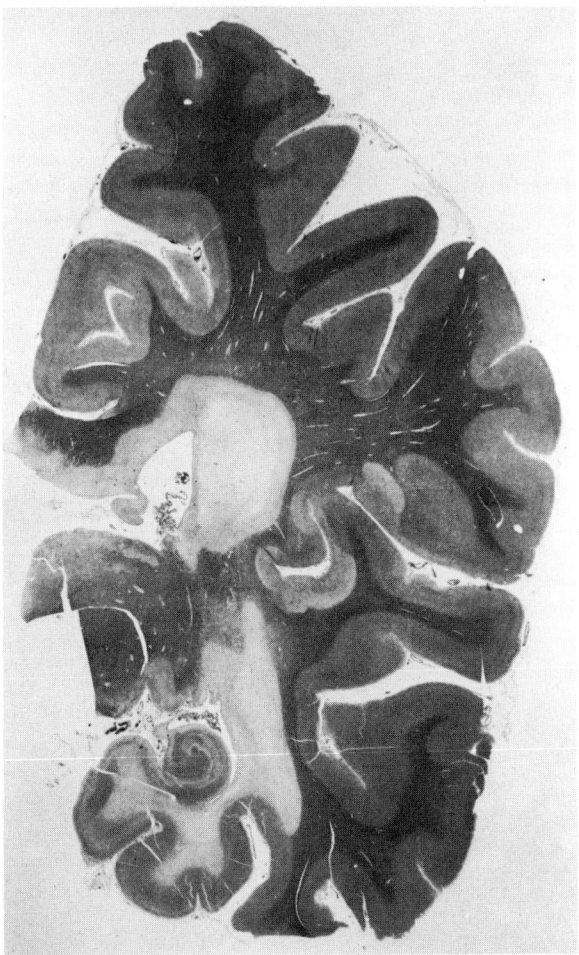

Figure 29–34. Multiple sclerosis. Unstained regions of demyelination (MS plaques) around lateral ventricle and in temporal lobe. (Luxol-fast-blue PAS stain for myelin.)

Mononuclear cells and lymphocytes are often present around these vessels. As the demyelination progresses, the perivenular foci expand to form the macroscopically visible plaques. In actively enlarging plaques, there is an inflammatory phalanx composed mostly of lymphocytes at the border between the demyelinated and normal areas. Within the plaque there is loss of oligodendroglia, and a pronounced reactive astrocytosis with many lipid-laden macrophages containing the debris of the degenerated myelin. The axons traversing the plaque are largely intact (Fig. 29–35). Old inactive plaques have profound myelin loss, an almost total absence of oligodendroglia, and scattered fibrillary astrocytes (Fig. 29–35). Although axons are relatively preserved, some loss is often detectable. In shadow plaques, the demyelinated area shades gradually into the white matter without a sharply defined border, and there may be only partial loss of myelin throughout the plaque.

CLINICAL COURSE. The onset of multiple sclerosis occurs between 20 and 40 years of age in about two thirds of the cases, and is rare before puberty and in patients more than 55 years old. Its natural history is very varied; a relapsing and remitting course over many years is the most common pattern, but some patients have only a few brief episodes of disability, whereas others have a relentless downhill course over months or even weeks. Common early manifestations are paresthesias, retrobulbar neuritis, mild sensory or motor symptoms in a limb, and cerebellar incoordination. Intellectual deterioration is not usually an early feature. As the disease progresses, remissions become less complete, and although not all patients become totally disabled, the end stage is too often ataxia, incontinence, paraplegia, and mental dysfunction due to widespread cerebral and spinal cord demyelination. There is no effective treatment, although ACTH and sometimes other immunosuppressive agents are administered during relapses, with some benefit.[127]

The variable clinical presentation of MS poses frequent diagnostic problems and, combined with differences in the pathologic appearance of the lesions at different stages of the disease, has led to the

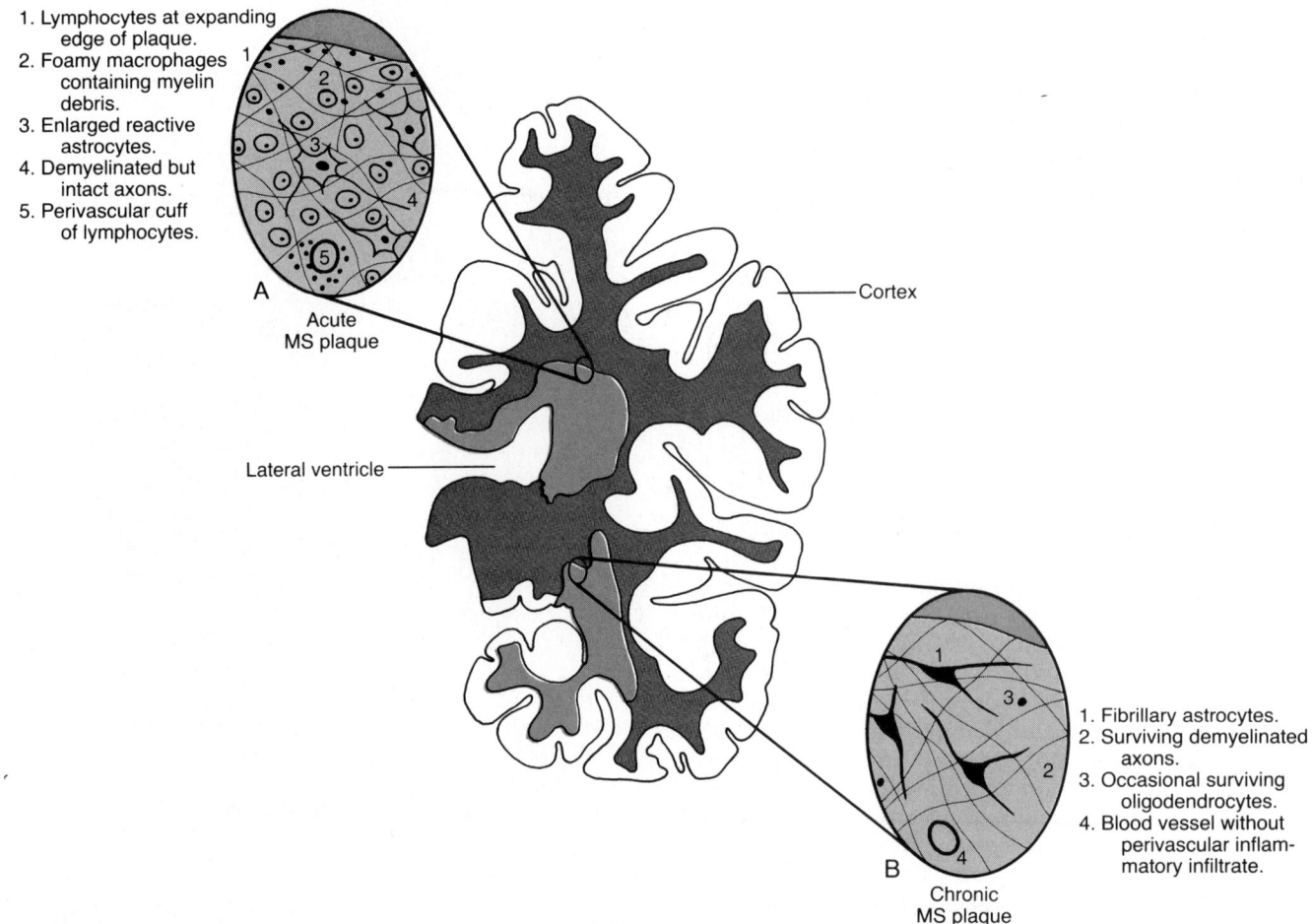

1. Lymphocytes at expanding edge of plaque.
2. Foamy macrophages containing myelin debris.
3. Enlarged reactive astrocytes.
4. Demyelinated but intact axons.
5. Perivascular cuff of lymphocytes.

A
Acute MS plaque

Cortex

Lateral ventricle

1. Fibrillary astrocytes.
2. Surviving demyelinated axons.
3. Occasional surviving oligodendrocytes.
4. Blood vessel without perivascular inflammatory infiltrate.

B
Chronic MS plaque

Figure 29–35. A diagrammatic representation of the cerebral hemisphere seen in Figure 29–34 with acute and chronic MS plaques.

emergence of a number of eponyms for what are probably only variants of the basic disease. In addition to the classical Charcot type described previously, they include the *Marburg* (acute progressive) variant and *Devic's disease* (neuromyelitis optica), in which typical MS plaques coexist with necrotic lesions in the spinal cord and demyelination in the optic nerves. Nowhere, however, has the terminology of multiple sclerosis been more confusing than in the vexing question of *Schilder's disease* (diffuse sclerosis). The difficulty has been resolved by the recognition that Schilder described at least two morphologically rather similar but quite different diseases, both of which were called Schilder's disease. One is what is now called adrenoleukodystrophy (p. 1438), and the other is probably a variant of MS characterized by giant plaques symmetrically affecting major portions of the cerebral hemispheres. Both of these conditions occur most frequently in children and are usually progressive rather than relapsing and remitting.

PERIVENOUS ENCEPHALOMYELITIS

The two diseases in this category are *acute disseminated encephalomyelitis* and *acute necrotizing hemorrhagic leukoencephalitis*. Both are monophasic, rapidly progressive illnesses that usually follow a viral infection, vaccination, or vague respiratory illness.

Acute disseminated encephalomyelitis (postinfectious and postvaccinial encephalomyelitis) is a rare condition that may occur during or shortly after a virus infection (measles, mumps, chickenpox, rubella), whooping cough, or vaccination. Spontaneous cases occur, and there are other, less well characterized antecedents. Clinically, there is headache, men-

ingismus, and lethargy progressing to coma, sometimes with the intercurrent development of focal neurologic signs. These symptoms develop between 5 and 14 days after the onset of the initiating event. Imaging studies usually show marked brain swelling. Although the disease is fatal in 15 to 20% of patients, the prognosis for recovery in the survivors is generally good; some patients, however, are left with relatively mild permanent residual effects.

> Grossly the brain looks normal or diffusely congested. Microscopically there are many foci of perivenous and perivenular demyelination (Fig. 29–36). Very early cases may show a polymorphonuclear leukocyte accumulation, but usually there is a variable mononuclear cell and lymphocytic cuff around veins in the affected regions. Similar cells and macrophages containing myelin debris are seen in the demyelinated regions, but axons are preserved.

Acute necrotizing hemorrhagic leukoencephalitis, a rare entity, is usually preceded by a nonspecific respiratory infection. Headache and fever rapidly progress to coma and, usually, death.

> Gross examination shows severe brain swelling and, on sectioning, multiple purpuric hemorrhages that are particularly prominent in the white matter and sometimes focally concentrated in one lobe. Histologically, as in acute disseminated encephalomyelitis, there is perivenular demyelination, but also acute necrosis of small blood vessels with fibrinoid degeneration, focal perivascular necrosis, and small ring hemorrhages. The inflammatory infiltrate is more pronounced, with an initial neutrophil invasion that is later

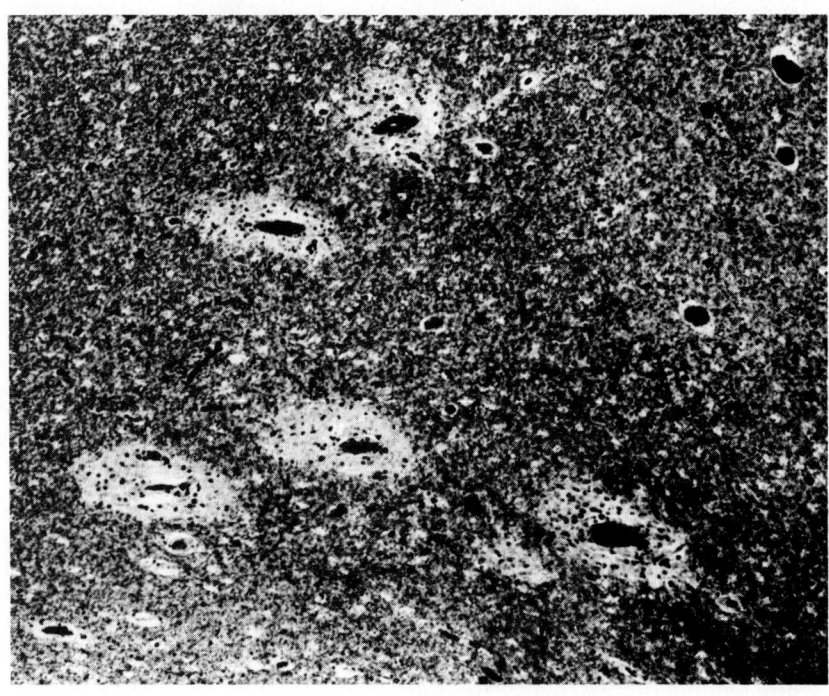

Figure 29–36. Postvaccinal encephalomyelitis. Note demyelination (lack of stain) around venules (stained black) (Woelcke stain).

replaced by lymphocytes and plasma cells. These inflammatory cells infiltrate the vessel walls and Virchow-Robin spaces and extend into the damaged parenchyma.

Both perivenous encephalomyelitides are considered to be allergic reactions against the nervous system. Acute disseminated encephalomyelitis is histologically very similar to *experimental allergic encephalomyelitis (EAE)*, which can be produced in animals by injections of myelin basic protein and myelin lipids. It is thought that the human disease is also a manifestation of an allergic reaction against myelin antigens.[128] In acute necrotizing hemorrhagic leukoencephalitis, there is a major vascular component in addition to any anti-myelin activity. It has been speculated that this vascular component possibly reflects immune complex deposition. There is some debate as to whether these two conditions are entirely distinct, because some cases are difficult to fit into either category and because experimentally, hyperimmune EAE resembles acute necrotizing hemorrhagic encephalomyelitis.[129] Notwithstanding these reservations, the two conditions generally tend to have different antecedent events and very different clinical courses and prognoses.

DEGENERATIVE DISEASES

The application of the label *degenerative* to the diseases discussed in this section should not be allowed to disguise the fact that it is a confession of ignorance. Like the demyelinating diseases, the degenerative diseases are a group of conditions unified only by some general clinicopathologic similarities, and thus they differ from most other categories of disease such as infections or vascular disease, which are bound by a common etiologic thread. There is no compelling reason to suppose that the so-called degenerative diseases have the same or even similar etiologies, and in almost all of these diseases, there is currently no coherent theory of etiology or pathogenesis. As with the demyelinating diseases, progress in understanding the degenerative diseases is reflected by their reassignment to more specific etiologic categories. This occurred with, for example, Creutzfeldt-Jakob disease (p. 1401), which was comfortably ensconced with the degenerative diseases until the demonstration of its transmissibility precipitated its removal to that of the unconventional agent (spongiform) encephalopathies. Although Huntington's disease is included in this section, recent advances mean that probably it will soon be more appropriately discussed as an inherited metabolic disease.

Two major common clinicopathologic features unite these seemingly disparate conditions and led to their being grouped together as the degenerative diseases. First, *they are diseases of neurons and tend to be selective, affecting one or more functional systems while leaving others relatively intact.* For example, in

Table 29–4. Degenerative Diseases

REGION(S) OF BRAIN AFFECTED	DISEASES
Cerebral cortex	Alzheimer's disease*
	Pick's disease*
Basal ganglia and brainstem	Huntington's disease*
	Idiopathic Parkinson's disease*
	Postencephalitic Parkinson's disease*
	Striatonigral degeneration*
	Shy-Drager syndrome*
	Hallervorden-Spatz syndrome
	Progressive supranuclear palsy*
Spinal cord and cerebellum	Olivopontocerebellar atrophy*
	Friedreich's ataxia*
	Ataxia-telangiectasia
Motor neurons	Motor neuron disease (amyotrophic lateral sclerosis [ALS])*
	ALS/parkinsonism/dementia of Guam
	Werdnig-Hoffmann disease*
	Kugelberg-Welander syndrome

* Discussed in text.

Parkinson's disease the nigrostriatal dopaminergic system is selectively, though not exclusively, damaged. Second, *they are generally symmetric and progressive.*

In other ways degenerative diseases differ among themselves quite sharply; some have a clear pattern of heritability, others are sporadic; some exhibit intracellular abnormalities of a greater or lesser specificity (e.g., Lewy bodies, neurofibrillary tangles), whereas in others the pathologic process is atrophy and degeneration of the affected neurons without specific features.

Degenerative diseases that affect similar regions of the brain tend to produce clinical syndromes with many similarities. For example, cortical and basal ganglia diseases tend to manifest as dementias and extrapyramidal movement disorders, respectively, and for ease of description it is empirically convenient to group them according to the part or parts of the brain that are principally affected. There is, in general, no reason to infer the existence of any etiologic association among the diseases in each group.

A list of the major degenerative diseases is given in Table 29–4, the most important of which are discussed in the text.

DEGENERATIVE DISEASES AFFECTING CEREBRAL CORTEX

The major cortical degenerative diseases are *Alzheimer's disease* and *Pick's disease*, and their principal clinical manifestation is dementia. They are, of course, not the only causes of dementia; there are many others, including cerebrovascular disease, encephalitis, hydrocephalus, and Creutzfeldt-Jakob disease. In the past, a distinction was made between presenile and senile dementia, with onset before and after the age of 65, respectively, but age as the criterion is no longer believed to be either pathologically valid or clinically useful.[130]

Alzheimer's Disease

Alzheimer's disease usually becomes clinically apparent as an initially subtle impairment of higher intellectual function or a disturbance of affect. Later, progressive disorientation, memory loss, and aphasia bespeak a more severe cortical dysfunction that eventually develops into a profound, mute, immobile dementia over five to ten years. Death is usually the result of an intercurrent infection, exacerbated by inanition and dehydration. Symptoms rarely begin before the age of 50 years, but in each succeeding decade there is a progressive increase in the incidence of Alzheimer's disease that is producing major medical, social, and economic problems in an aging society.[131] Most cases are sporadic in incidence, although at least 5 to 10% of cases (and perhaps more) are familial.[132] Identical pathologic changes occur in almost all patients with trisomy 21 (Down's syndrome) who survive beyond the age of about 45 years.[133]

MORPHOLOGY. Gross examination of the brain shows a variable degree of cortical atrophy with widening of the cerebral sulci that is most pronounced in the frontal, temporal, and parietal lobes. With significant atrophy there is compensatory ventricular enlargement secondary to loss of parenchyma (hydrocephalus ex vacuo, p. 1391) (Figs. 29–37 and 29–38). The major microscopic features of Alzheimer's disease are **neurofibrillary tangles, senile (neuritic) plaques, amyloid angiopathy, granulovacuolar degeneration, and Hirano bodies.** It is important to recognize that all these features may be present to a lesser degree in the brains of old people who are not demented[134]

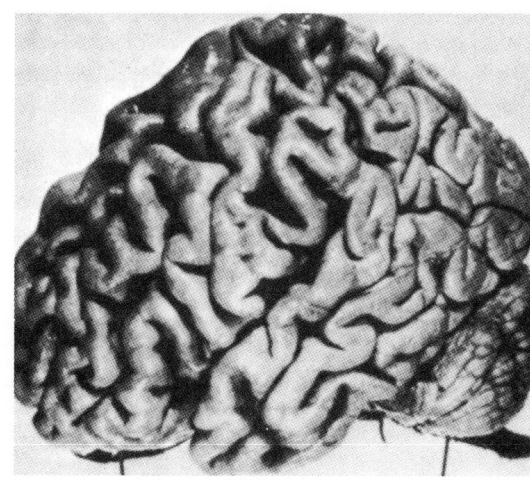

Figure 29–38. Alzheimer's disease. The brain shows diffuse cortical atrophy, particularly marked in frontal, parietal, and temporal lobes, with narrowing of gyri and widening of sulci. (Courtesy of Dr. Robert D. Terry.)

and that the pathologic diagnosis of Alzheimer's disease is based on the relative prominence of these features rather than their mere presence.[135]

Neurofibrillary tangles are bundles of filaments in the cytoplasm of the neuron that displace or encircle the nucleus. They are mildly basophilic with H and E stains, but strongly stained by silver (Bielschowsky) methods (Figs. 29–39 and 29–40). Ultrastructurally, they are composed of (mostly) paired helical filaments (PHF) with a diameter of 7 to 9 nm and a period of about 80 nm. Neurofibrillary tangles are very insoluble and remain visible and stainable in tissue sections as "ghost" tangles long after the death of the parent neuron. Immunocytochemical studies suggest that, when the neuron is still intact, a major surface antigen of the tangles is phosphorylated tau protein, which is a variety of microtubule-associated protein. The protein structure of the filaments of the "ghost" tangles (which interestingly are straight tubules, not PHF) has not yet been elucidated. Although they are characteristic of Alzheimer's disease, neurofibrillary tangles are not specific to this condition, being also found, in other regions of the brain, in progressive supranuclear palsy, dementia pugilistica, post-

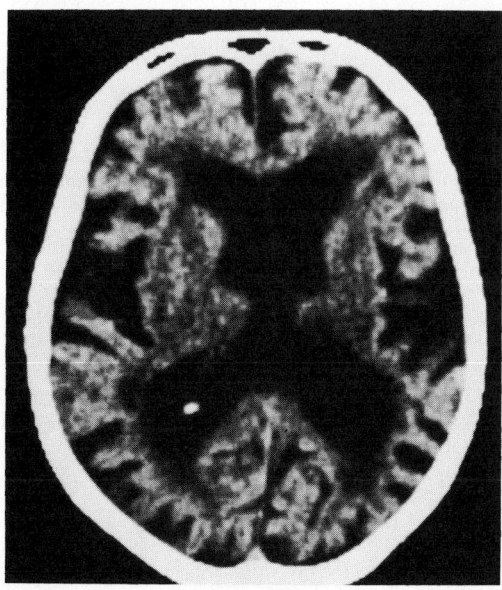

Figure 29–37. CT scan showing severe atrophy with gross dilatation of lateral ventricles and widening of cortical sulci.

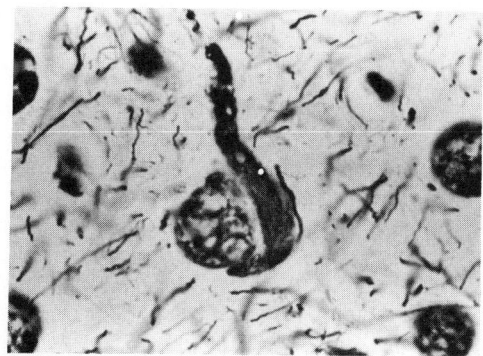

Figure 29–39. Neurofibrillary tangle consisting of a skein of silver-positive material with a neuron (Bodian stain).

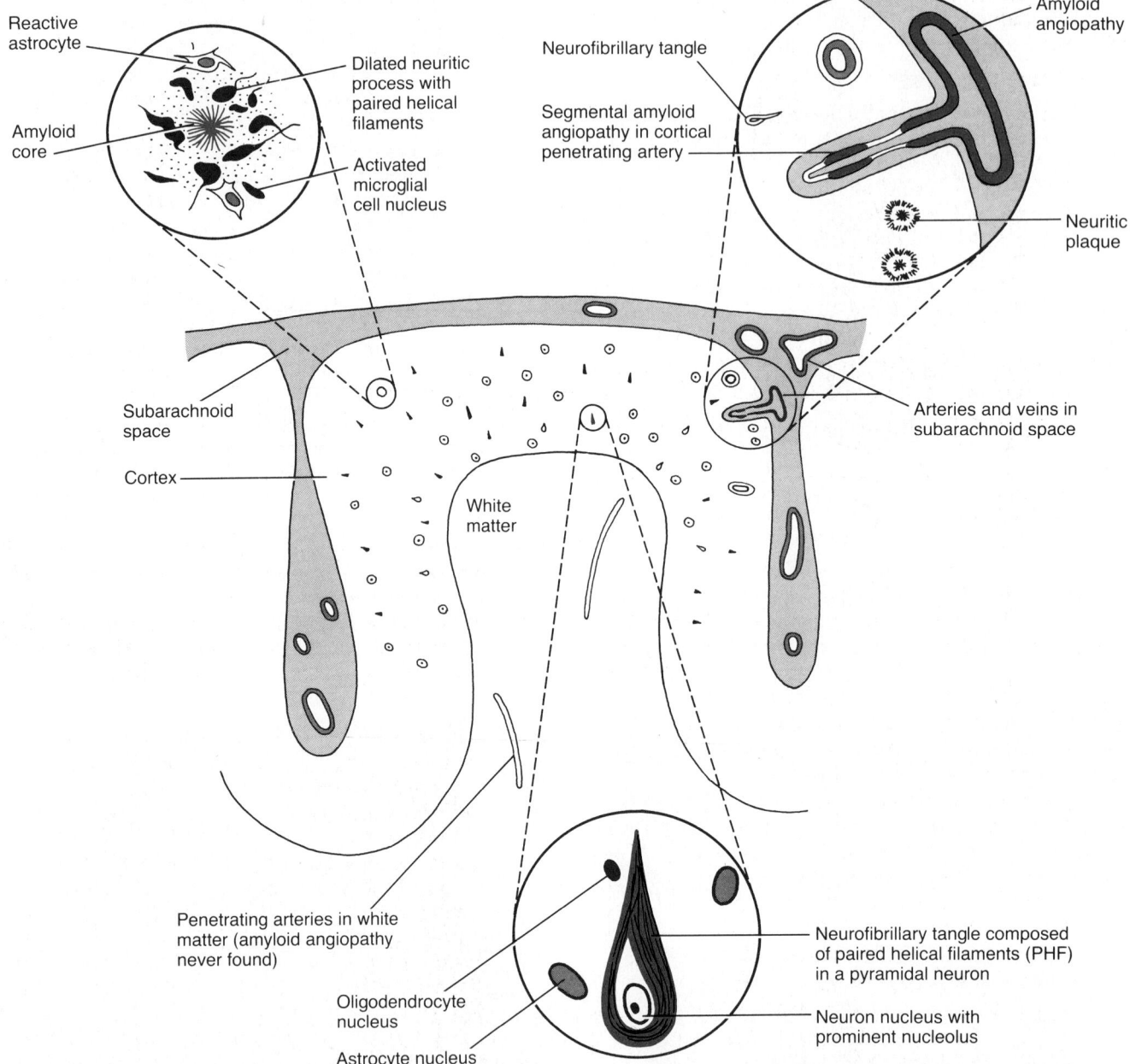

Figure 29–40. Diagrammatic representation of the major microscopic changes in the cortex in Alzheimer's disease. The cortex contains both neuritic plaques and neurofibrillary tangles, and amyloid angiopathy is present in subarachnoid and intracortical arteries and arterioles.

encephalitic Parkinson's disease, and the ALS Parkinsonism/dementia complex of Guam. They probably represent the end point of a number of different cellular pathophysiologic processes.[136]

Senile (neuritic) plaques are focal collections of dilated, tortuous, silver-staining neuritic processes found almost exclusively in the cerebral cortex. They range from 20 to 150 μm in diameter. Microglial cells and reactive astrocytes can be seen around the periphery. Early plaques have only neuritic processes, but later in their evolution they develop a central amyloid core around which a clear halo tends to form (Fig. 29–41). Electron microscopy and im-

munocytochemistry reveal that the silver-stained neuritic processes contain paired helical filaments similar to those found in neurofibrillary tangles.

In Alzheimer's disease, plaques and tangles are found extensively in the hippocampus and amygdala and in the whole of the cerebral cortex, although there is usually significant relative sparing of the primary motor and sensory cortices. In patients over 75 years of age, only neuritic plaques may be present in the cortex. Neurofibrillary tangles are also found in the basal forebrain nuclei (basal nucleus of Meynert), scattered in the raphe nuclei, and in the locus ceruleus.

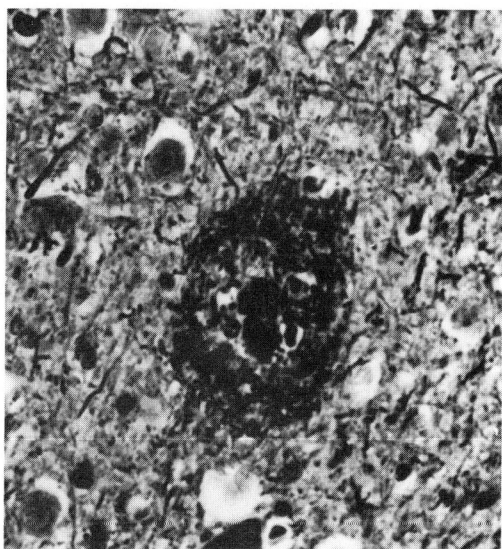

Figure 29–41. A senile (neuritic) plaque composed of a central, silver-positive amyloid core surrounded by a ring of cellular processes (Bielschowsky stain).

amyloid protein of the plaque core and cerebral vessels.[140] Genetic studies have shown that in familial Alzheimer's disease, the gene defect is located on chromosome 21,[141] a very provocative finding in the context of the almost invariable development of Alzheimer's disease in patients with trisomy 21! Even more intriguing is that the gene coding for the amyloid protein also turns out to be on chromosome 21, although not quite in the same location as the defect in familial Alzheimer's disease.[142] Further, the gene coding for cerebral amyloid has been shown to be expressed in neurons, but many are not apparently affected in Alzheimer's disease, such as the Purkinje cells of the cerebellum.[143] Current work is directed toward definition of the nature, function, and processing of the precursor protein that gives rise to the cerebral amyloid.[144] These findings are perhaps a long way from a practical treatment for this important disease, but they represent striking progress, particularly in comparison with some of the other degenerative diseases.

Pick's Disease

Pick's disease occurs far less frequently than Alzheimer's disease and produces a similarly profound dementia over about the same time course. Clinically it cannot reliably be distinguished from Alzheimer's disease, and there are also occasional familial cases.

Amyloid angiopathy is an almost invariable accompaniment of Alzheimer's disease. It is found in the intracortical and smaller subarachnoid arteries but never in the white matter vessels, and only very rarely in the arteries supplying the deep gray nuclei. The amyloid is similar to that of the plaque core and contains the beta peptide that is specific to Alzheimer's disease and the ageing brain and is quite different from other forms of amyloid (p. 210).

Granulovacuolar degeneration is the formation of small (5 μm diameter), clear intraneuronal cytoplasmic vacuoles, each of which contains an argyrophilic granule. The constituents of the granule are unknown, as is the pathophysiologic significance of this form of degeneration. The latter stricture also applies to the **Hirano bodies** seen in proximal dendrites as glassy eosinophilic inclusions. Ultrastructurally, they are composed of regular arrays of beaded filaments, which biochemical analysis shows to be mostly actin.[137] Although occasionally present in older normal persons, both these features can be found in up to 10% of the pyramidal cells of the hippocampus in Alzheimer's disease.

The brain in Pick's disease invariably exhibits a pronounced, although sometimes asymmetrical, atrophy of the frontal and temporal lobes with conspicuous sparing of the posterior two-thirds of the superior temporal gyrus and only very rare involvement of either the parietal or occipital lobe. The atrophy can be very severe, reducing the gyri to a thin wafer, the so-called knife blade atrophy or "walnut brain." This pattern of atrophy is usually sufficient to distinguish Pick's disease, sometimes called lobar atrophy, from Alzheimer's disease. Microscopically, neuronal loss is most severe in the outer three layers of the cortex, and may be severe enough superficially to resemble laminar necrosis (p. 1403). Some of the surviving neurons may exhibit a characteristic ballooning degeneration (Pick's cells) or contain **Pick bodies**, which are cytoplasmic, round to oval, filamentous inclusions that are only weakly eosinophilic but stain strongly with silver methods.[145] Ultrastructurally they are composed of neurofilaments, vesiculated endoplasmic reticulum, and paired helical filaments that are immunocytochemically similar to those found in Alzheimer's disease.[146] In severe cases there is marked attenuation of the subcortical white matter, which probably reflects the degree of loss of cortical neurons.

ETIOLOGY AND PATHOGENESIS. The basic defect in Alzheimer's disease is unknown. The number of neurofibrillary tangles and senile plaques is roughly correlated with the degree and duration of the dementia.[138] The most consistent biochemical abnormality is a deficiency of acetylcholine and its associated enzymes choline acetyl transferase and acetyl cholinesterase in the cerebral cortex, amygdala and hippocampus.[131] This is correlated with severe loss of the acetylcholine-containing neurons of the basal nucleus of Meynert in Alzheimer's disease, this nucleus being the major source of cholinergic input to the depleted areas.[139]

Most recent advances have come from genetic analysis and studies of the molecular biology of the

DEGENERATIVE DISEASES OF BASAL GANGLIA AND BRAINSTEM

Diseases affecting these regions of the brain frequently involve the extrapyramidal motor system and are associated with various types of movement disorder, such as rigidity, abnormal posturing, and chorea. The most important are Huntington's disease and the syndrome of Parkinsonism.

Huntington's Disease

This disease usually appears in persons between 20 and 50 years of age and is characterized by the combination of extrapyramidal or choreiform movements and a progressive dementia. It is inherited as an autosomal dominant, and by linkage analysis of what are called restriction fragment length polymorphisms, the genetic defect has been localized to a small segment on chromosome 4.[147] Those who inherit the disease from their fathers tend to become symptomatic much earlier in life than those who inherit it from their mothers, an effect that might occur through modulation of chromosomal gene expression by extrachromosomal, maternally inherited cytoplasmic components such as mitochondria. This combination of autosomal dominant inheritance with onset of symptoms often delayed until middle life turns Huntington's disease into a medical sword of Damocles hanging over the heads of the children of affected persons. For them, an already difficult personal situation is exacerbated by the dilemma as to whether they themselves should have children and perhaps pass on the disease. The localization of the gene marker to a fragment of chromosome 4 offers the hope of eventual antenatal diagnosis, and perhaps intervention.

ETIOLOGY AND PATHOGENESIS. The neurochemistry of this disease is complex, with some transmitter substances, such as GABA, acetylcholine, and substance P, being decreased and others either unchanged or even, as with somatostatin, increased.[148] Recent research has focused attention on the *N*-methyl-*D*-aspartic (NMDA) receptor, and the role of excitotoxins (p. 1403), notably quinolinic acid, a substance that is present in the brain and that may be increased in Huntington's disease. On injection, quinolinic acid can mimic some of the highly selective neurochemical changes that occur in Huntington's disease.[149] Excitotoxins are thought to cause cell damage and even death by producing prolonged opening of membrane ion channels, which allows the uncontrolled entry of, particularly, Ca^{++} into the cell. If this proves to be an important mechanism of cell death in Huntington's or any other disease, it raises the possibility of selectively blocking the receptor and perhaps preventing or at least ameliorating the damage. Initial experiments with a selective blocking agent, called MK-801, are being conducted in animals.

> **MORPHOLOGY.** On gross examination the brain is small (less than 1000 gm) and shows striking atrophy of the caudate nucleus and, less dramatically, the putamen.[151] The globus pallidus may be secondarily atrophied, and the lateral and third ventricles are dilated. Atrophy is frequently seen in the frontal lobe, less often in the parietal lobe, and only occasionally affects the entire cortex. Microscopically,

> there is severe loss of neurons, particularly in the dorsomedial part of the striatum, with striking preservation of the nucleus accumbens in the inferior striatum. Both the large and small neurons are affected, but loss of the small neurons generally seems to precede that of the larger. There is also a pronounced fibrillary gliosis that seems much greater than that usually seen in reaction to neuronal loss.[150]

CLINICAL COURSE. Affected patients develop a chorea characterized by jerky, hyperkinetic, sometimes dystonic movements affecting all parts of the body, and they may later develop parkinsonian features with bradykinesia and rigidity. Early signs of the dementia often are forgetfulness, disorganization, and affective disorders. The disease is relentlessly progressive, with an average course of about 15 years to death.

Parkinsonism

Parkinsonism is the name given to a disturbance of motor function characterized by expressionless facies, a stooped posture, slowness of voluntary movement, festinating gait (progressively shortened, accelerated steps), rigidity, and sometimes a characteristic "pill-rolling" tremor. It is named after James Parkinson, who described what is now called idiopathic Parkinson's disease in 1817, but *this type of motor disturbance is seen in a number of different conditions that have in common damage to the nigrostriatal dopaminergic system*. Parkinsonism may also be produced by drugs, particularly dopamine antagonists and toxins (notably 1-methyl-4-phenyl-1,2,3,6-tetrahydropyridine [MPTP]), that affect this system. The principal diseases that involve the nigrostriatal system are *idiopathic Parkinson's disease (paralysis agitans), postencephalitic parkinsonism, striatonigral degeneration, Shy-Drager syndrome*, and *progressive supranuclear palsy*.

Idiopathic Parkinson's Disease (Paralysis Agitans)

This is a progressive syndrome occurring from about age 50 onwards. As with Alzheimer's disease, it is seen with increasing frequency in older age cohorts. There is no evidence for a hereditary component. As well as the motor disorder, there are often less well-characterized changes in mental function, and a few patients with the pathologic findings of idiopathic Parkinson's disease present with a dementia clinically similar to that of Alzheimer's disease.[151]

> **MORPHOLOGY.** Pathologically, the only gross findings are pallor of the substantia nigra (Fig. 29–42) and locus ceruleus. Microscopically, there is loss of the pigmented neurons in these regions, and **Lewy bodies** may be found in some of the remaining neurons. These are intracytoplasmic, eosinophilic, round to elongated inclusions that often have a dense core surrounded by a paler rim.[152] Ultrastructurally Lewy bodies are composed of fine filaments,

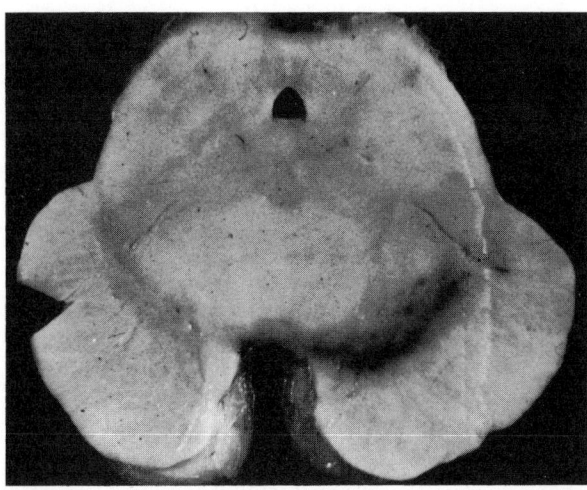

Figure 29–42. Idiopathic Parkinson's disease (paralysis agitans). Unilateral loss of pigment *(left)* in substantia nigra. This is a rare occurrence; most cases show bilateral depigmentation.

densely packed in the core but quite loose at the rim, and antibody studies have shown the presence of neurofilament antigens.[153] Lewy bodies may also be found in the cholinergic cells of the basal nucleus of Meynert, which particularly in patients with abnormal mental function is depleted of neurons. Rather similar inclusions are also occasionally found in large numbers in the cerebral cortex.

ETIOLOGY AND PATHOGENESIS. The dopaminergic neurons of the substantia nigra project to the striatum, and their degeneration in Parkinson's disease is associated with a reduction in the striatal dopamine content. The severity of the motor syndrome is proportional to the dopamine deficiency,[154] which can, at least in part, be corrected by replacement therapy with levodopa (the immediate precursor of dopamine); unlike dopamine, levodopa is able to cross the blood-brain barrier. Treatment does not, however, reverse the morphologic changes or arrest the progress of the disease, and with progression, drug therapy tends to become more difficult to manage and less effective.

An experimental model for this disease has emerged from the study of some young patients who developed an acute parkinsonian syndrome. On investigation most of these patients were found to have been exposed to MPTP as a contaminant in the illicit synthesis of meperidine analogs. Administration of MPTP to animals has produced selective damage to the neurons of the substantia nigra and a parkinsonian syndrome.[155] It is hoped that the elucidation of the mechanism of action of this toxin will throw some light on the etiology of idiopathic Parkinson's disease and possibly lead to new therapeutic approaches.[156]

Postencephalitic Parkinsonism

This form of Parkinson's disease is now very rare but was a relatively common sequela of the encephalitis that occurred during the great "influenza" epidemic of 1914–1918. Brain examinations of patients who died during the acute illness showed findings suggestive of a viral encephalitis (p. 1395), although a virus was neither isolated nor identified at the time. After months, or more commonly years, some patients who recovered from the encephalitis developed parkinsonism, but usually at an earlier age than in idiopathic Parkinson's disease, and the disease was not so progressive. Pathologically, these patients have depletion of the substantia nigra, but with the formation of neurofibrillary tangles rather than Lewy bodies.

Striatonigral Degeneration and Shy-Drager Syndrome

There is great variation in the pathologic findings in these diseases, and sometimes a relatively poor correlation between the clinical findings and the distribution of the pathologic changes.

Striatonigral degeneration is clinically similar to idiopathic Parkinson's disease but is resistant to levodopa treatment and pathologically different. There is grossly visible atrophy of the caudate and putamen, and microscopically, both nuclei show severe neuronal loss, particularly of the small neurons, and a marked gliosis. Loss of pigmented neurons also occurs, particularly in the zona compacta of the substantia nigra, but neither Lewy bodies nor neurofibrillary tangles are seen.

In the *Shy-Drager* syndrome, autonomic system failure is present in addition to the parkinsonism. The findings in the brain are variable; some cases are similar to idiopathic Parkinson's disease with Lewy bodies, whereas others resemble striatonigral degeneration with widespread neuronal loss. In the spinal cord there is loss of neurons from the intermediolateral column, these being the neurons of origin of the sympathetic system.

Progressive Supranuclear Palsy

Patients with this disorder usually present with loss of vertical gaze progressing to difficulty with all eye movements, associated with back rigidity, paroxysmal dysequilibrium, expressionless facies, and (often) increasing dementia. Onset is usually between the fifth and seventh decades, and death often occurs within five to seven years.[157]

There is widespread neuronal loss in the globus pallidus, subthalamic nucleus, substantia nigra, tectum, periaqueductal gray matter, and dentate nucleus of the cerebellum. The cerebral and cerebellar cortices are usually not involved. Neurofibrillary tangles (p. 1427) are found in most of the affected regions. Although generally (but not invariably) composed of straight filaments rather than paired helical filaments, they are immunocytochemically similar to the tangles found in Alzheimer's disease.[158]

SPINOCEREBELLAR DEGENERATIONS

This group of diseases affects, to varying degrees, the basal ganglia, brainstem, cerebellum, spinal cord, and peripheral nerves. Pathologically, there is simple atrophy and degeneration of the neurons in the affected areas with varying, usually mild, gliosis. Clinically, patients present with combinations of parkinsonism, cerebellar and sensory ataxia, spasticity, and peripheral motor and sensory defects that reflect the areas of the nervous system involved.

There is no satisfactory classification of the spinocerebellar ataxias, and historically many different, usually eponymous syndromes have been described. Genetically they may be dominant or recessive, or sporadic. In the inherited degenerations, even within a single pedigree there is great variation in clinical presentation. To compound the nosological problem, the disease may evolve over time in an affected individual from a predominantly spinal to a cerebellar symptomatology. Consequently, there are often many similarities among patients suffering from what are nominally different syndromes. Pathologically, patients are often found to have more widespread disease than their symptoms and signs would suggest, and syndromes that are clinically different may have similar or overlapping pathologic findings. The *olivopontocerebellar atrophy* complex is a good example of the taxonomic difficulties encountered in this group of diseases. An alternative approach, which has substantial practical merit, is to classify these patients as having dominant, recessive, or sporadic ataxia, and allow each affected individual or pedigree to define the course of the disease.[159] Taxonomic nihilism should not, however, be carried too far. Some spinocerebellar ataxias are relatively consistent enough or have sufficiently characteristic systemic associations to allow them to be reliably defined. *Friedreich's ataxia*, for example, has a distinctive neurologic presentation combined with a typical and prognostically significant cardiac lesion.

Olivopontocerebellar Atrophy

Olivopontocerebellar atrophy has such an inconstant and varied clinical expression that the term "heterogeneous system degeneration" is sometimes used. Even in the same family no two cases are exactly alike, and the heredity is no less varied: most cases are autosomal dominant (Menzel type), but others are autosomal recessive, and still others clearly nonfamilial. Neuronal loss is usually concentrated in the olive, pons, and cerebellum, but the basal ganglia and spinal cord can also be involved. Clinically, symptoms and signs include, in varying degrees and combinations, ataxia, eye and somatic movement abnormalities, dysarthria, and rigidity.

Friedreich's Ataxia

An autosomal recessive condition with a male preponderance, Friedreich's ataxia has an average age of onset of about 11 years, although a less common dominantly inherited variant manifests at about 20 years. An initial gait ataxia is followed by the development of hand clumsiness and dysarthria. Deep tendon reflexes

are absent, but the Babinski reflex is typically present. Joint position and vibratory sense are impaired, and there is sometimes loss of pain, temperature, and light touch senses. Most patients eventually become paralyzed over a course of about 20 years. Some patients have pes cavus and kyphoscoliosis, and there is a high incidence of concomitant diabetes and cardiac disease, the latter being manifested as cardiac arrthymias and congestive heart failure.[160]

> The spinal cord is small with loss of nerve fibers and gliosis in the posterior columns, distal corticospinal tract, and spinocerebellar tracts. Neuronal loss occurs in Clark's column; the VIII, X, and XII cranial nerve nuclei; the dentate nucleus, and in the Purkinje cells of the superior vermis. Loss of dorsal root ganglion cells is the cause of the visible degeneration of the dorsal columns. Systemically, the heart is enlarged and may have pericardial adhesions. There may be an interstitial myocarditis with focal or diffuse inflammatory infiltrates, and myofiber hypertrophy or, more rarely, necrosis.

The pathogenesis of Friedreich's ataxia is unknown, and although abnormalities have been reported in the activities of some mitochondrial enzymes, notably pyruvate and oxoglutarate dehydrogenases and malic enzymes, they have not been confirmed.

DEGENERATIVE DISEASES AFFECTING MOTOR NEURONS

Motor Neuron Disease (Amyotrophic Lateral Sclerosis [ALS] Complex)

Nowhere is the term *system degeneration* more appropriately applied than to this complex. All variants are characterized by degeneration in the pyramidal motor system. This system is composed of the *upper motor neurons* in the motor cortex, the axons of which traverse the internal capsule, brainstem and corticospinal tract, to synapse on the *lower motor neurons* in the cranial nerve motor nuclei and the anterior horns of the spinal cord.

CLINICAL COURSE. Four variants are recognized at presentation. The most common is *amyotrophic lateral sclerosis*, in which patients have loss of both lower motor neurons (muscular atrophy, fasciculations, and weakness) and upper motor neurons (hyper-reflexia, spasticity, and a Babinski reflex). In *progressive bulbar palsy* there is a predominance of cranial nerve and brainstem involvement. *Progressive muscular atrophy* exhibits only lower motor neuron signs, whereas in *primary lateral sclerosis* the patients have only upper motor neuron signs and symptoms. Most cases are sporadic, although a few familial cases have been reported, and males are more often affected than females. The onset is typically in late middle age, with a progressive and inevitably fatal course in two to six years. Bulbar palsy tends to run a shorter course, probably because of the earlier involvement of the respiratory and pharyngeal muscles.[161]

MORPHOLOGY. Grossly, lower motor neuron loss is manifested as muscular atrophy and a gray discoloration and atrophy of the anterior (motor) roots of the spinal cord that reflects the loss of myelinated axons. Degeneration of the upper motor neurons results in atrophy and pallor of the corticospinal tracts, which develop a dense, bone-white appearance, and occasionally in severe or long-standing cases, atrophy of the precentral gyrus.[162] The pathologic findings usually very much reflect the clinical picture, with simple atrophy and degeneration of neurons in the appropriate areas, and subsequent degeneration in the corticospinal tract (Fig. 29–43) or motor roots, depending on the clinical picture. Occasional active neuronophagia can be seen in the affected populations, and the remaining neurons may have a shrunken or ghost-like appearance.

ETIOLOGY AND PATHOGENESIS. The pathogenesis of motor neuron disease is unknown. A high prevalence of HLA-A3 and B12 haplotypes has been reported. Needless to say, many possible etiologies have been investigated, including viral, immunologic, and metabolic, but as yet no serious etiologic candidate has emerged.[163] However, a form of motor neuron disease occurs in the Chamorro people on the island of Guam that is also associated with a high incidence of concomitant parkinsonism and dementia. All cases are characterized by the presence of neurofibrillary tangles, and recent work has strongly suggested that this form of motor neuron disease is a toxic effect of the seed of the false sago palm *Cycas circinalis*, which is used by the Chamorro to make flour.[164] There is an interesting parallel with Huntington's disease, in that the toxic substance *B-N*-methylamino-*L*-alanine (L-BMAA) seems to be acting as an excitotoxin, the effect of which is attenuated by the NMDA (p. 1430) receptor blocker MK801. Although there is no suggestion that L-BMAA is the cause of motor neuron disease outside of Guam, its discovery has revived interest in the possibility that a long-term exposure to toxic substances may be etiologically significant.

Werdnig-Hoffmann Disease (Infantile Progressive Spinal Muscular Atrophy)

This infantile autosomal recessive condition manifests either at birth as a "floppy infant" or in the first months of life with rapidly progressive muscular weakness. Death usually ensues within a few months from respiratory failure or aspiration pneumonia. Pathologically, there is severe loss of lower motor neurons, degeneration of the motor axons of the anterior roots, and profound neurogenic atrophy of muscle.

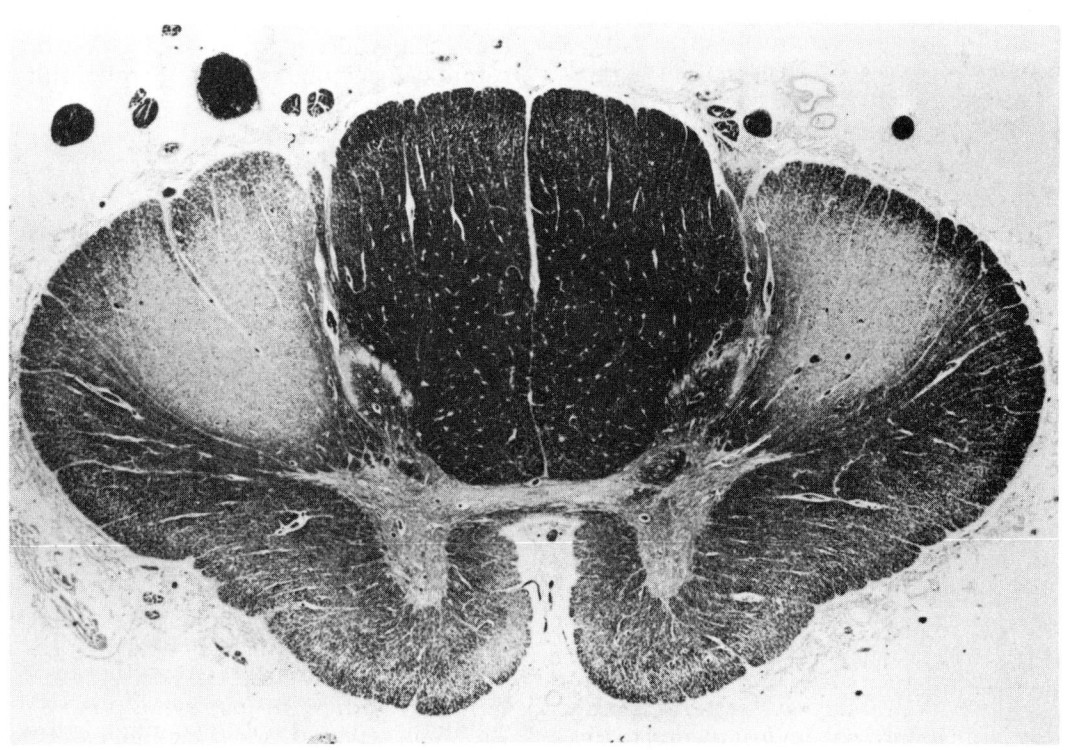

Figure 29–43. Amyotrophic lateral sclerosis. Cross section of spinal cord showing loss of myelinated fibers (lack of stain) in corticospinal tracts. At higher magnification, loss of anterior horn neurons can also be seen (Woelcke stain).

NUTRITIONAL, ENVIRONMENTAL, AND METABOLIC DISORDERS

NUTRITIONAL DISORDERS

The major vitamin deficiencies that affect the nervous system are those of thiamine (p. 450), nicotinamide (p. 453), and cobalamin (p. 455), all of which have been described in Chapter 8. Reference will be made here only to the neurologic manifestations of cobalamin deficiency.

Vitamin B₁₂ (Cobalamin) Deficiency (Subacute Combined Degeneration of the Spinal Cord [SACD])

The precise cause of the neurologic damage in cobalamin deficiency has not been elucidated, but some studies suggest a link to defective synthesis of methionine by the B_{12}-dependent enzyme methionine synthetase. Methionine acts as a donor of methyl groups required in the synthesis of choline, which is an important component of myelin.

MORPHOLOGY. Pathologically, there is degeneration of spinal cord white matter that is usually concentrated in the posterior and lateral white columns and most marked in the midthoracic region. The earliest lesions are in the body of the affected white column and extend outwards from these initial foci. In severe cases, the affected regions are atrophic and gray. Microscopically, the myelin sheaths initially are swollen but later disintegrate and are degraded by macrophages. There is axonal degeneration and a variable gliosis. This pattern of degeneration gives the tissue a characteristic loose and vacuolated appearance on light microscopy, which is also seen in the vacuolar degeneration of the spinal cord in AIDS (p. 1399). Gray matter is usually unaffected.

CLINICAL COURSE. Patients present with a subacute progressive spastic paraparesis, sensory ataxia, and marked paresthesias of the legs. Untreated, they may progress to total paralysis with trunk and lower limb anesthesia. Treatment with cobalamin can completely reverse early symptoms and signs but may only arrest progression if structural damage has occurred.

Cobalamin deficiency is also associated with an optic atrophy, an axonal peripheral neuropathy, and (rarely) a perivascular demyelination in the hemispheric white matter that is histologically similar to the spinal cord lesions.

ENVIRONMENTAL DISORDERS

The central and peripheral nervous systems are the target of a very large number of environmental toxins, some of the most important of which are listed in Table 29–5 together with an indication of their major effects. Among the major categories of neurotoxic substances are *metals*, *industrial chemicals*, and a range of *naturally occurring toxins*. Perhaps the most rapidly expanding category of neurotoxins, however, are those prescribed by doctors and otherwise known as *therapeutic agents*. Appearances to the contrary, this is not a recent phenomenon. Sir Anthony Carlisle (1768–1840) caustically remarked of the therapeutic agents available to him, "Calomel is poison and Digitalis kills people"!

Although the externally imposed hazards of the environment must not be minimized, the all too human propensity for self-administration of neurotoxins cannot be ignored. Ethyl alcohol, for example, is widely used and abused. There are also the so-called recreational substances that, in addition to their own addictive properties and neurotoxic side effects, may contain contaminants, such as MPTP (p. 1431), that are specific neurotoxins.

Alcohol-Related Conditions

Few medical students need to be told of the intoxicating properties of *ethyl alcohol*. Acutely, notwithstanding its socially disinhibiting effects, it produces a generalized cerebral depression that can be fatal. The Wernicke-Korsakoff syndrome,[165,166] a cerebellar degeneration, and a peripheral neuropathy are all seen in chronic alcohol abusers but are at least in part the consequences of thiamine deficiency (p. 450) rather than toxic effects of the alcohol itself. Likewise, although central pontine myelinolysis was first described in alcoholics, it appears to be an effect of therapeutic manipulation of the serum sodium level.

Methyl alcohol, by contrast, through its metabolite formic acid, has a direct toxic effect on the retina,[167] and there may also be a widely distributed cerebral damage that is probably the result of histotoxic anoxia.[168]

Radiation/Chemotherapy Leukoencephalopathy

The effects of radiation have been described in Chapter 9. However, the combination of cranial irradiation with some forms of chemotherapy, particularly intrathecal or high-dose intravenous methotrexate, sometimes produces a leukoencephalopathy with a well-characterized morphology but unknown pathogenesis.[169] Most lesions are in the periventricular or deep white matter and are composed of foci of coagulative necrosis containing many dilated axons that are often mineralized. There is little or no inflammatory reaction, and although radiation vascular changes (p. 507) have been described, they are not consistently present.

Morphologically similar but much smaller lesions have also been described in the pons. They have been seen in association with chemotherapy[170] but also in other conditions, such as AIDS (p. 1398), in which chemotherapy has not been administered.[171]

Central Pontine Myelinolysis

This lesion, as indicated by its name, consists of a region of demyelination in the central pons. The de-

Table 29-5. Neurotoxic Substances

AGENT	MAJOR EFFECT	PATHOLOGY
Metals		
Aluminum	Dialysis encephalopathy	No specific features
Arsenic	Encephalopathy	Pericapillary hemorrhage
	Peripheral neuropathy	Axonal degeneration
Lead		
Inorganic	Encephalopathy	Vascular damage
	Peripheral neuropathy	Axonal degeneration
Organic	Psychosis	Cortical and cerebellar neuron loss
Manganese	Parkinsonism	Neuron loss and gliosis
Mercury (organic)	Perioral paresthesias	Cerebellar and calcarine cortex atrophy
	Ataxia	
	Constriction of visual fields	
Industrial chemicals		
Acrylamide	Peripheral neuropathy	Axonal degeneration
	Ataxia	?
	Encephalopathy	?
Hexacarbon solvents	Peripheral neuropathy	Axonal degeneration
Ethyl alcohol	See discussion of thiamine deficiency (p. 450)	
Methyl alcohol	Visual loss	Neuronal loss
	Encephalopathy	Putamenal necrosis
Organophosphorus compounds	Autonomic symptoms	Axonal degeneration
	Peripheral neuropathy	
Naturally occurring toxins		
Buckthorn toxin	Muscular weakness	Demyelination
	Respiratory paralysis	
Lathyrus sativus (chickpeas)	Spastic paraplegia	Motor neuron degeneration
Drugs		
Clioquinol	Subacute myelo-optic neuropathy	Axonal degeneration
Hexachlorophene	Encephalopathy	Segmental demyelination
	Convulsions	
Isoniazid	Peripheral neuropathy	Axonal degeneration
Methotrexate	Encephalopathy	Necrotizing leukoencephalopathy
Vincristine	Peripheral neuropathy	Axonal degeneration
Hypertonic saline	Quadriparesis	Central pontine myelinolysis

myelination is symmetrically distributed about the midline and in severe cases may involve almost all the basis pontis. Microscopically, there is preservation of axons with loss of myelin and oligodendrocytes and, depending on the stage of evolution, a reactive astrocytosis and an accumulation of lipid-laden macrophages.

Clinically, smaller lesions may be asymptomatic, but a flaccid quadriplegia may occur with the large foci. The precise pathogenesis of the demyelination is not clear, but it appears to be associated with the correction of severe hyponatremia to normal or hypernatremic levels at a rate greater than 12 to 15 mmol per liter per day.[172-174] Rises of this rapidity usually require intravenous administration of sodium-containing solutions, particularly the use of hypertonic saline solutions, so the lesion is arguably iatrogenic in most cases.

METABOLIC ENCEPHALOPATHY

The blood-brain barrier ensures that the CNS neurons are insulated from the normal vagaries of the systemic biochemical milieu, but these defenses can be breached by large or prolonged changes. Effects can be seen with changes in both electrolytes and nonelectrolytes, and the resulting disturbance in cerebral function is referred to as a *metabolic encephalopathy.* Despite a sometimes profound disturbance in cerebral function, there may be only very minor morphologic changes in the brain, an appearance that reflects the predominantly biochemical nature of the cerebral disorder. Some causes of a metabolic encephalopathy may produce visible changes: *In hepatic encephalopathy,* there are often markedly dilated astrocytic nuclei, some of which may contain a glycogen dot and which are called Alzheimer II astrocytes. In diabetics, *hypoglycemic coma,* if not rapidly reversed, will cause neuronal loss in a pattern similar to that seen in ischemia (p. 1403). *Hyperglycemic coma* is more complicated, with changes in pH, electrolytes, and osmotic pressure all contributing to a cerebral dysequilibrium that can persist for several days after the serum parameters are returned to normal, presumably reflecting the time required to re-establish intracellular normality.

Table 29–6. Major Types of Metabolic Encephalopathy

Hepatic failure
Uremia
Diabetes (hypoglycemia and hyperglycemia)
Addison's disease (hyponatremia)
Hypercalcemia and hypocalcemia
Hyperthyroidism and hypothyroidism
Hypermagnesemia and hypomagnesemia
Acidosis and alkalosis (metabolic and respiratory)
CO_2 narcosis
Hypoxia

Some of the types of organ failure and biochemical derangement that are associated with a metabolic encephalopathy are listed in Table 29–6.

INBORN ERRORS OF METABOLISM

The variety and range of effects of inborn errors of metabolism on the nervous system are very wide, and many have effects both inside and outside the nervous system. In some cases, it is the balance of these effects that determines whether they manifest clinically as nervous system or systemic diseases. For example, in Wilson's disease, some patients present with hepatic failure and little or no nervous system involvement, whereas others present with choreoathetosis and dementia without hepatic failure. In phenylketonuria, although the inborn error is common to all tissues, the clinical manifestations are overwhelmingly in the nervous system.

To universal regret, there is no easily assimilable classification of these diseases, mostly because different biochemical lesions in a single metabolic pathway can produce quite different clinical manifestations, and abnormalities in different biochemical systems can result in a rather similar clinical picture. Thus for example, the sphingolipidoses, which are a subgroup of the lysosomal storage diseases, include systemic storage diseases, e.g., Gaucher's disease; neuronal storage diseases (Fig. 29–44), exemplified by Tay-Sachs disease and Niemann-Pick disease; and leukodystrophies in the form of metachromatic and globoid cell (Krabbe's) leukodystrophies.

Other general categories of inborn error of metabolism that produce effects on the nervous system include the mucopolysaccharidoses and glycogen storage diseases, and disorders of amino acid (phenylketonuria), copper (Wilson's disease) (p. 956), and purine and pyrimidine (Lesch-Nyhan syndrome) metabolism. This whole general topic is considered in Chapter 4, and here we will discuss only the mitochondrial encephalomyopathies and the leukodystrophies.

MITOCHONDRIAL ENCEPHALOMYOPATHIES

Over the past decade there has been a progressive, though incomplete, recognition of a rather diverse group of conditions that have in common a distur-

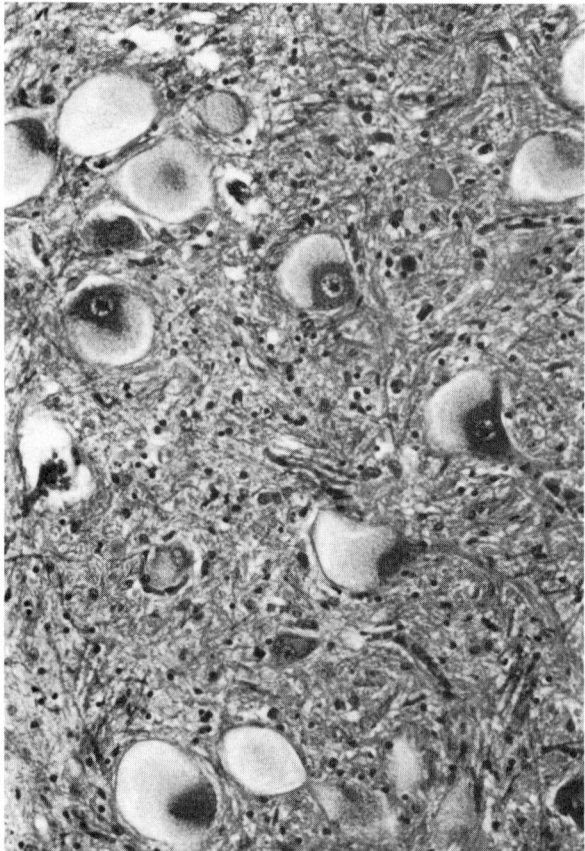

Figure 29–44. Neuronal storage disease. Anterior horn neurons are distended with stored lipid. (H and E stain.)

bance of mitochondrial energy metabolism (including the electron transport chain).[175] Clinically, these defects often produce combinations of muscle pathology with cerebral disease, in which sometimes the muscular pathology and sometimes the cerebral pathology dominates the clinical picture. The group includes conditions such as the very rare carnitine deficiency Kearns-Sayre syndrome[176] and Leigh's syndrome.

Subacute Necrotizing Encephalomyelopathy (Leigh's Syndrome)

Leigh's syndrome is an autosomal recessive disorder characterized by bilateral symmetric regions of necrosis in the thalamus, midbrain, pons, medulla, and spinal cord. In the necrotic region there is a prominent vascular proliferation, cribriform change, and gliosis.

Clinically, patients exhibit ataxia, weakness, hypotonia, seizures, and intellectual deterioration, and death usually occurs within a few years.

A number of patients with Leigh's syndrome have shown a reduction in cytochrome C oxidase activity in some organs, notably muscle and brain.[177] However, it appears likely that more than one type of mitochondrial defect is capable of producing this pathologic picture, because other patients have been described with a deficiency of the pyruvate dehydrogenase complex.

LEUKODYSTROPHIES

These are diseases of white matter in which the inborn error is known, or presumed to be, in the pathways of myelin metabolism. In those leukodystrophies in which the defect has been identified, it is a deficiency of a lysosomal degradative enzyme. Although the principal pathologic process is demyelination (there may also be some neuronal storage), it might, in view of the type of biochemical defect, be more helpful to think of them as *dysmyelinating* rather than *demyelinating* diseases. From their etiology, leukodystrophies might be expected to become manifest in early childhood as symmetrical disorders of myelination. In many cases, such as the childhood form of metachromatic leukodystrophy, they conform to this archetype, but as exemplified by adrenoleukodystrophy, there can be great phenotypic variation in spite of the apparently stereotypic nature of the biochemical defect.

Metachromatic leukodystrophy, Krabbe's disease, and adrenoleukodystrophy/adrenomyeloleukodystrophy will be discussed here. There are other, rarer leukodystrophies, ranging from simple sudanophilic to the eponymous leukodystrophy of Messrs. Pelizaeus and Merzbacher.

Metachromatic Leukodystrophy

An autosomal recessive disorder of sphingolipid metabolism, metachromatic leukodystrophy is marked by a deficiency of aryl-sulfatase A (cerebroside sulfatase) leading to the accumulation of galactosyl sulfatide and other lipids containing a galactosyl-3-sulfatide moiety.[178]

> The accumulated sulfatide appears as intra- and extracellular spherical granular masses 15 to 25 μm in diameter that stain positively with PAS and metachromatically with acid cresyl violet on frozen sections. In the CNS there is demyelination, and metachromatic material may be seen free in tissue spaces or within macrophages in the perivascular spaces. Although there is widespread demyelination in the cerebral hemispheres, the immediately subcortical axons and myelin are conspicuously spared (Fig. 29–45). In the peripheral nervous system there is also demyelination, and metachromatic material may be found in Schwann cells and macrophages.

The first symptoms of progressive motor impairment with mental deterioration and, sometimes, a peripheral neuropathy usually occur between one and four years of age, although there are rare adult forms. The diagnosis can be made prenatally by amniocentesis and enzyme analysis and in adults by measuring the urinary aryl-sulfatase A level, which is decreased or absent. Peripheral nerve biopsy may show myelin breakdown and sulfatide accumulation.

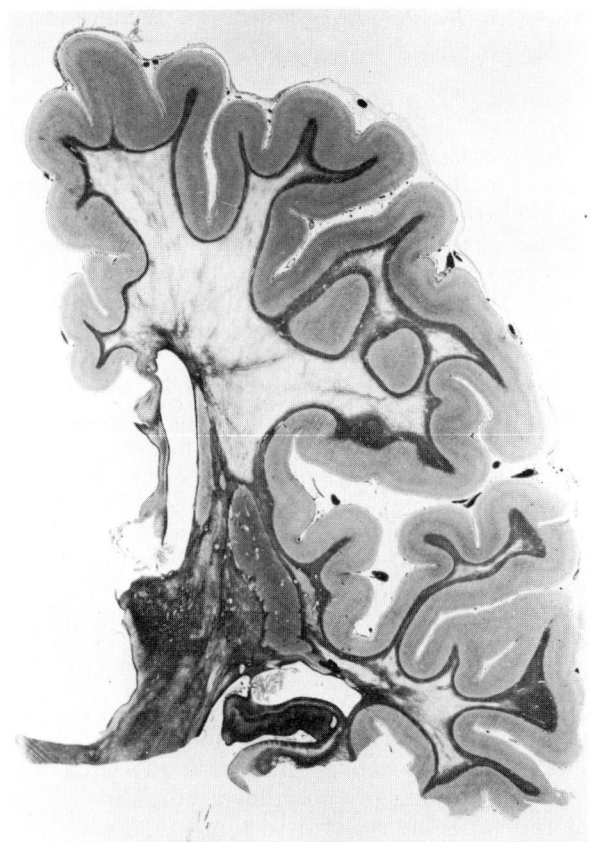

Figure 29–45. Metachromatic leukodystrophy. Demyelination is extensive. Subcortical fibers in cerebral hemisphere are spared. (Luxol-fast-blue PAS stain.)

Krabbe's Disease (Globoid Cell Leukodystrophy)

This condition is also an autosomal recessive disease, with a deficiency of galactocerebroside B galactosidase and the accumulation of galactocerebroside.[179]

> Histologically, in addition to the demyelination, there are characteristic large, sometimes multinucleate histiocytes (globoid cells), usually seen around blood vessels. On electron microscopy, the globoid cells have cytoplasmic inclusions composed of straight or curved, hollow tubular profiles, often with longitudinal striations of variable density and approximately 6 nm wide. Similar cytoplasmic inclusions have been found in Schwann cells, although demyelination in the peripheral nervous system is less common than in metachromatic leukodystrophy.

The onset of Krabbe's disease is usually in early infancy, generally in the first six months of life, and is marked by rigidity, instability, and decreased alertness. The disease is fatal, usually within 6 to 12 months of onset, with terminal blindness and deafness.

Adrenoleukodystrophy/ Adrenomyeloneuropathy

This imposing designation refers to an X-linked recessive disease leading to the accumulation of long-chain (C24-30) fatty acid esters of cholesterol. Although the precise biochemical defect is not known, it is considered likely that the condition is the result of a defect in peroxisome (microbody) function, because this is the organelle responsible for long-chain fatty acid oxidation.[180] All patients have adrenal insufficiency, but the disease has two quite different manifestations in the nervous system.

The *juvenile form* occurs in boys, usually with onset under the age of ten years, and has a relentless downhill course to death in three to four years. Pathologically, there are large plaques of demyelination in the cerebral hemispheres (adrenoleukodystrophy) resembling those seen in multiple sclerosis, and for this reason this variant was originally included in the Schilder's disease (p. 1425) complex.[181,182] In *adult males* there is a slowly developing spastic paraparesis and peripheral neuropathy (adrenomyeloneuropathy),[183] with cerebellar ataxia, varying degrees of intellectual deterioration, and hypogonadism. Both neurologic variants may occur in the same family, and transitional cases occur.[184] It is not known what determines this striking phenotypic variation in a disease that appears to be genetically homogeneous.

Ultrastructurally, pathognomonic inclusions, composed of long thin leaflets enclosing an electron lucent space, can be found in cerebral macrophages, adrenal cortical cells, and Schwann cells (Fig. 29–46).[185] Biochemically, the diagnosis is made by measuring the C26 : C20 fatty acid ratio in either serum or fibroblast culture.[3] Most of the female carriers, some of whom have minor symptoms, can also be identified permitting genetic counselling if desired.

MALFORMATIONS AND DEVELOPMENTAL DISEASES

To a large extent the embryologic development of the nervous system mirrors the complexity of the system itself. Hence, it is not surprising that there are a large number of different developmental anomalies. There is also considerable variation in the lesions, so that they do not always fit comfortably into one of the described categories.

One of the most important factors determining the nature of a developmental lesion is the timing of the insult. Different types of insult occurring at the same time during development are likely to produce rather similar types of malformation.[186]

In most malformations, the relative contributions of inherited and acquired factors are uncertain, although in conditions associated with chromosome anomalies, inherited factors are clearly predominant. Environmental agents known to cause malformations include (1) maternal and fetal infections (e.g., rubella), (2) drugs (e.g., thalidomide), (3) fetal anoxia and circulatory insufficiency, (4) physical agents, notably ionizing radiation, and (5) mechanical forces, such as amniotic bands.[187]

In this section it is not possible to do more than introduce the terms used for the most commonly encountered types of malformation, and to give some idea of the basic type of structural defect implied by the use of a given term. What follows has no pretense to be other than a basic lexicon, and no attempt has been made either to be comprehensive or to discuss what is known of the etiology or pathogenesis of the malformations described.[188,189]

NEURAL TUBE DEFECTS

Anencephaly

Anencephaly is the most common congenital malformation of the brain in humans, with a notably high incidence in Ireland and Wales (1 to 6 per 1000 live births, compared with 0.5 to 2 per 1000 in the U.S.),[190] and an excess of females in the patient population. It is associated with spina bifida (see later) in about 15% of cases. There is hypoplasia or absence of the calvaria, and the basal bones of the skull are thick and flattened, with shallow orbits and protuberant eyes. The only central nervous system elements that can be found are usually glial nodules in the area cerebrovasculosa at the base of the brain and a disorganized brainstem in the posterior fossa.

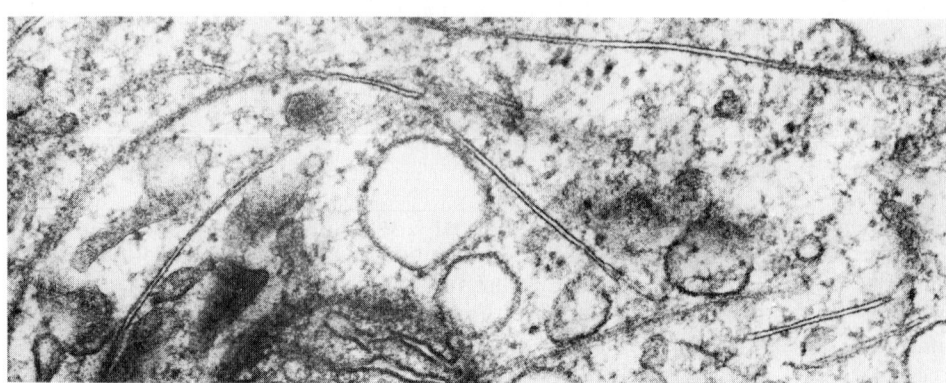

Figure 29–46. Electron micrograph of the characteristic curvilinear profiles seen in adrenoleukodystrophy. (From Schaumberg, H.H., et al.: Adreno-leukodystrophy (sex linked Schilder's disease): ultrastructural demonstration of specific cytoplasmic inclusions in the central nervous system. *Arch. Neurol. 31:*210, 1974.)

Cranial Meningocele and Encephalocele

These disorders result from defects in skull bones. They are most common in the occipital bone but may also be seen anteriorly at the fronto-ethmoidal junction and parietally. In an encephalocele, a portion of the brain, which may be very large, herniates through the defect. The herniated brain is grossly distorted and may have cortical anomalies. It is covered only by skin, which is liable to frequent ulceration and secondary infection.

Spinal Meningocele, Meningomyelocele, and Myelocele (Spina Bifida)

These are all associated with varying degrees of vertebral defects (spina bifida). The smallest degree of spina bifida is *spina bifida occulta*, in which there is only a defect in the vertebrae and no abnormality of the nervous system. Externally, its presence may be indicated by a skin dimple or hairy patch. In a *meningocele*, only dura and arachnoid herniate through the

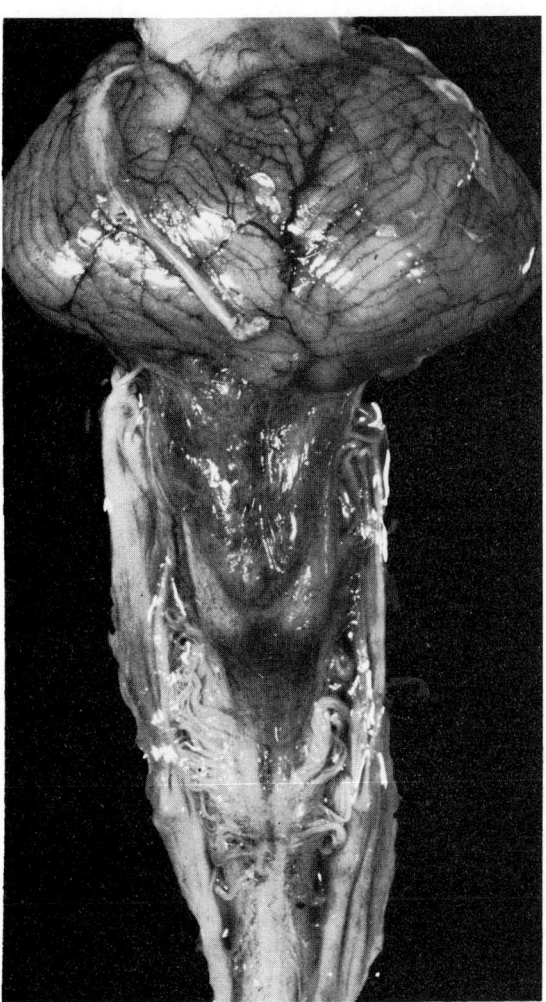

Figure 29–47. Arnold-Chiari malformation. Cerebellar tonsils are displaced into cervical canal.

bone defect, the spinal cord being in the normal position, normally formed, and functional. The term *meningomyelocele* is used when the spinal cord or spinal roots are also herniated, although, at least initially, they are still relatively normally formed. In a *myelocele* there has been defective closure of the cord, and it is present as an open discoid plate of neural tissue without any skin covering that leaks CSF and often has a superficial granulation reaction. All these spinal dysraphic states may be associated with hydrocephalus, which, if the cause is identifiable, is usually due to an Arnold-Chiari malformation (Chiari type II) (see later). Clinically, meningomyelocele and myelocele produce bladder and bowel dysfunction with motor and sensory defects in the legs, the severity of which reflects the degree of spinal cord abnormality. The neurologic defects often are exacerbated by the trauma and infection (meningitis and meningomyelitis) that are major and frequent complications of these malformations.

Chiari Malformation

This umbrella term encompasses a complex of abnormalities of the brainstem and cerebellum. Four types are described, of which type II (the *Arnold-Chiari malformation*) is the most common and is almost always associated with both hydrocephalus and a spinal dysraphism. The major components of the Chiari type II deformity are: (1) lengthening and downward displacement through the foramen magnum of the vermis and tonsils of the cerebellum, which form a compacted mass at the foramen magnum and over the upper cervical cord (Fig. 29–47); (2) distortion of the medulla with a characteristic Z kink at the cervicomedullary junction; and (3) a small, shallow posterior fossa with an enlarged foramen magnum.

Diastematomyelia and Diplomyelia

These terms describe partial and complete duplication of the spinal cord. If the region of duplication is contained within a single dural sac, it may be asymptomatic. However, when there are separate dural sacs, there is often a cartilaginous or bony spur between them. This form almost invariably becomes symptomatic because of the differential expansion of the vertebral bodies and spinal cord during growth, when the bony spur prevents the normal ascent of the conus medullaris to the vertebral L2 level and produces a syndrome called tethering of the cord.

WHOLE-BRAIN ABNORMALITIES
Microcephaly

Microcephaly is conventionally defined as an adult brain weighing less than 900 gm that has a relatively simplified gyral pattern but no gross structural defects. This term covers a whole variety of pathologic processes that can result in a microcephaly and is not at all etiologically specific. In some cases it is the result of an autosomal or sex-linked defect.

Megalencephaly

This term is applied to fully developed brains weighing more than 1800 gm. Although normal brains may weigh this much, such weight may be associated with extraordinary intelligence or mental retardation. A few conditions, notably tuberous sclerosis, cerebral lipidoses, and the leukodystrophy Alexander's disease, may be associated with an enlarged, heavy brain.

ABNORMALITIES OF HEMISPHERE FORMATION

Holoprosencephaly (Arhinencephaly)

These terms cover a spectrum of malformations in which there is incomplete formation of the hemispheres. The malformation ranges in severity from a relatively inconspicuous failure of formation of the olfactory bulbs (arhinencephaly) to cyclopia. In the more severe varieties there is no anterior separation of the hemispheres and a single common ventricle, often with fusion of the deep gray nuclei of the hemispheres. There are also associated abnormalities in facial structure, seen most dramatically in cyclopia.

Agenesis of the Corpus Callosum

This may occur as part of a larger complex malformation such as Aicardi's syndrome or as an isolated phenomenon, in which case it may be asymptomatic. Hypoplasia and partial absence of the corpus callosum also occur. In complete agenesis, the remnant of the corpus callosum is a longitudinally running band of fibers called the bundle of Probst, and the cingulate gyrus fails to form on the medial surface of the hemisphere. There is also gross dilatation of the occipital poles of the lateral ventricles.

ABNORMALITIES OF CELL MIGRATION AND GYRAL DEVELOPMENT OR FORMATION

Ectopias and Heterotopias

These abnormalities result from curtailment or arrest of neuronal migration from the germinal matrix in the periventricular region. They occur in both the cerebrum and cerebellum. The ectopic cells form irregular nodules or radial columns in the white matter at varying distances from their destinations. They are often seen in association with other malformations such as microcephaly and gyral abnormalities.

Agyria (Lissencephaly) and Pachygyria

These are both anomalies of the gyral formation with either none (agyria/lissencephaly) or a few broad malformed gyri (pachygyria). The cortex shows simplification, with only four layers, and there are often associated heterotopias.

Polymicrogyria

Polymicrogyria is the formation of an increased number of gyri, most of which have very shallow sulci, producing, paradoxically, the appearance of a pachygyria with broad, finely wrinkled gyri. The lesion may be focal or widespread. Microscopically, the cortex is simplified, with only four layers, often with an irregularly thickened second layer.

SCHIZENCEPHALY AND ENCEPHALOCLASTIC PORENCEPHALY

Schizencephaly and *encephaloclastic porencephaly* describe clefts in the brain. It is not absolutely clear that the defects they refer to are really distinct conditions, but conventionally, the term *schizencephaly* is used for a cleft with continuous, though abnormal, cortex across the base of the cleft. There is also white matter between the base of the cleft and the ependymal lining of the underlying ventricle. In *encephaloclastic porencephaly*, there is a defect in all the structures of the hemisphere, producing a cleft or "pore" in the brain that extends to the ependymal lining of the ventricle with often a communication between the ventricle and the subarachnoid space.

DEVELOPMENTAL AND PERINATAL HYPOXIC OR ISCHEMIC INSULTS

Ulegyria, état marbre, and periventricular leukomalacia are all examples of hypoxic or ischemic insults occurring relatively late in development, after the formation of all the major components of the brain, and they may occur together in the same brain.

Hydranencephaly

In hydranencephaly, large fractions of the cerebral hemispheres are reduced to diaphanous tissue composed only of leptomeninges and a gliotic molecular layer. In the archetypal examples, the posterior fossa contents, thalamus, and posterior cerebral artery territories are preserved, suggesting that the basic lesion is ischemia in the territory of the carotid arteries.

Ulegyria

The cortical gyri in ulegyria have a grossly attenuated cortex with marked loss of neurons and gliosis. The damage is concentrated in the depths of the sulci, often leaving the crowns of the gyri relatively intact. Ulegyria may be focal and unilateral or widespread and bilateral, depending upon the severity and distribution of the insult.

État Marbré (Status Marmoratus, Marbled State)

État marbré refers to a usually bilateral pattern of white streaks and spots in the lateral part of the corpus striatum that is thought to result from perinatal ischemic injury to the basal ganglia. The pattern is produced by the arrangement of bundles of myelinated fibers, together with focal loss of neurons and glial scarring in the affected regions.

Periventricular Leukomalacia

This lesion consists of poorly defined areas of coagulation necrosis in the deep hemispheric white matter at the angles of the ventricles. In long-standing cases there may be cavitation of the affected areas. The deep white matter is relatively poorly vascularized. In neonates, white matter is more vulnerable to hypoxia than gray matter; hence it is vulnerable to damage during the episodes of apnea and hypotension that occur in many of the patients in whom this lesion is seen.

CEREBELLUM/BRAINSTEM/SPINAL CORD ANOMALIES

Agenesis/Hypoplasia of the Cerebellum

This occurs in a variety of conditions and may be associated with defects elsewhere in the nervous system. It may be partial in topography, as occurs in asymmetrical hypoplasias, or in cell type, as when there is a selective absence of granule cells. In even quite severe hypoplasias there may be no clinical evidence of cerebellar dysfunction.

Dandy-Walker Malformation

Dandy-Walker malformation is characterized by absence or severe hypoplasia of the vermis of the cerebellum with gross cystic distention of the roof of the fourth ventricle, which bulges out posteriorly. There is also hydrocephalus with distended ventricles, and a variety of other malformations may be present, notably agenesis of the corpus callosum and anomalies of cell migration.

Syringomyelia and Syringobulbia

These anomalies tend to become manifest only later in life and, in some ways, are hard to think of as malformations, particularly as they may occur secondary to acquired lesions such as trauma, tumor, and hemorrhage. The defect that develops in the tissue is a syrinx (from the Greek for "tube") or tubular cavity. In idiopathic cases the cavity is usually largest in the cervical cord, extends for several spinal segments, and usually terminates in the lower thoracic cord. Involvement of the medulla (syringobulbia) is manifested by slit-like cavities or clefts.

Pathologically, the cord is distended and fluctuant, with the syrinx containing fluid that resembles CSF but has a much more variable protein content. The syrinx, which is asymmetrical and may or may not involve the central canal, is lined by dense gliotic tissue. It may involve both gray and white matter but almost always affects the anterior commissural fibers of the lateral spinothalamic tract.

Clinically, early findings usually include a loss of pain and temperature sensation in a cape-like distribution involving the shoulder girdle and chest. This reflects the fact that only the crossing fibers of the spinothalamic tract are damaged. Later, there may be local involvement of the anterior horns and of the long tracts in the spinal cord.

PHACOMATOSES

These are familial, slowly progressive neurocutaneous disorders that inhabit the borderland between malformations and neoplasia. They include neurofibromatosis (p. 139), von Hippel–Lindau disease (p. 588), Sturge-Weber disease (encephalotrigeminal angiomatosis), and tuberous sclerosis.

TUBEROUS SCLEROSIS (EPILOIA, BOURNEVILLE'S DISEASE)

This is an autosomal dominant condition of variable expression characterized clinically by mental retardation and seizures, both of which usually manifest in infancy or childhood. Other manifestations are adenoma sebaceum of the skin and visceral anomalies, notably renal angiomyolipomata, cardiac rhabdomyomata, and pancreatic cysts.

The characteristic lesions in the brain are **tubers**, firm whitish nodules ranging in size from barely visible to 1 or 2 cm in diameter. They are found in the cortex and the subependyma adjacent to the ventricles. Microscopically, the cortical tubers show loss or distortion of the cortical cytoarchitecture with maloriented, deformed, bizarre, and often enlarged neurons with a marked gliosis. The subependymal lesions form nodules protruding into the ventricles, an appearance that is sometimes referred to as "candle dripping." Microscopically, they are composed of large, sometimes multinucleate, bizarre astrocytes with a prominent fibrillary background. These lesions tend to enlarge slowly and to calcify, although they may also undergo neoplastic transformation to infiltrating astrocytomas.

THE PERIPHERAL NERVOUS SYSTEM

The peripheral nervous system (PNS) consists of the motor and sensory components of the cranial and spinal nerves, the autonomic nervous system with its sympathetic and parasympathetic divisions, and the peripheral ganglia. It is the conduit for sensory information to the CNS and for effector signals to the peripheral end organs such as muscle. Peripheral nerves are composed of groups of intermingling fascicles. Each fascicle consists of a bundle of individual nerve fibers embedded in loose connective tissue containing fibroblasts and collagen (*endoneurium*) that is encased by a multilayered membrane of flattened cells (*perineurium*). The nerve trunk is composed of a variable number of fascicles (up to 50 in a major nerve such as the sciatic) bound together by fibrous tissue (*epineurium*). The major arteries supplying the nerve

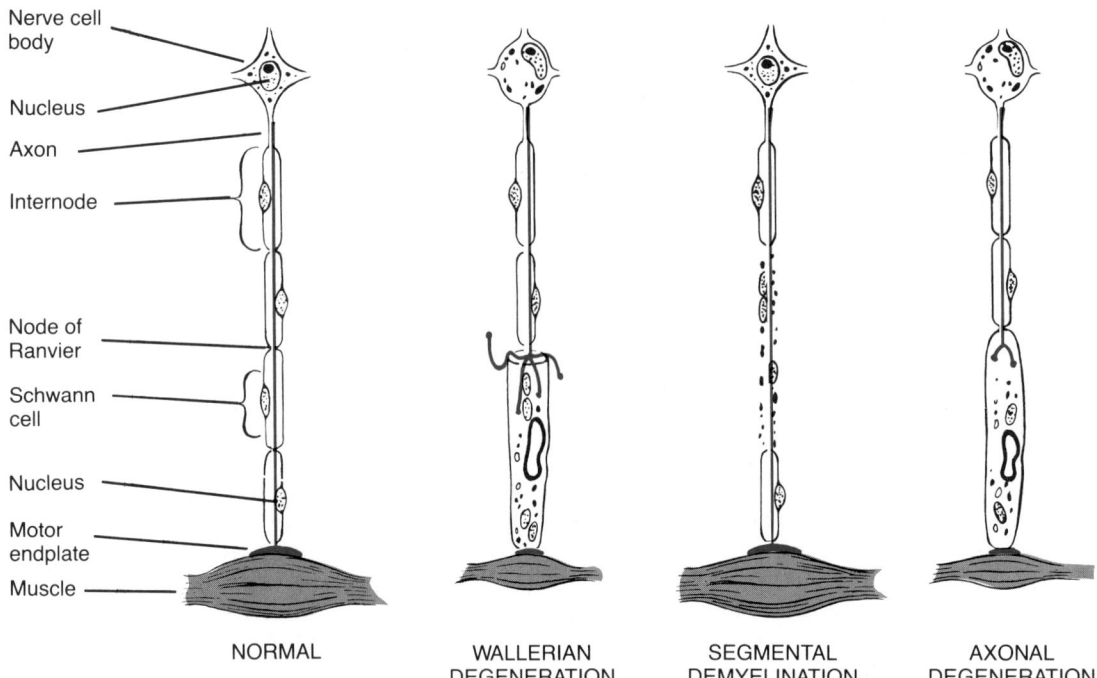

Figure 29–48. Pathologic reactions affecting peripheral nerve. (From Asbury, A.K., and Johnson, P.C.: Pathology of Peripheral Nerve. Philadelphia, W.B. Saunders Co., 1978, p. 51.)

run in the epineurium, and only terminal arterioles and capillaries are present within the fascicles. Nerve axons vary between 0.5 and 15 μm in diameter; and if greater than 2 μm, they have myelin sheaths produced by the *Schwann cells*, with larger-diameter axons having thicker myelin sheaths. The myelin is arranged in segments separated by *nodes of Ranvier*. Each peripheral myelin internode is produced by a single Schwann cell, unlike the multiple internodes produced by CNS oligodendrocytes (p. 1388).

PATHOLOGIC REACTIONS

Peripheral nerve has a very restricted range of pathologic reactions, and most commonly becomes symptomatic through either (1) the occurrence of one of the types of *degeneration* and the development of a *peripheral neuropathy* or (2) the formation of a tumor.

There are three basic degenerative processes, wallerian degeneration, axonal degeneration, and segmental demyelination (Fig. 29–48). Unlike in the brain, however, regeneration can also occur in the PNS.

Wallerian degeneration occurs after transection of the axon. Proximal to the transection, the axon degenerates back to the next node of Ranvier, and if the transection is sufficiently proximal, there will be chromatolysis (p. 1387) in the neuronal cell body. Distal to the transection, both the axon and its myelin sheath disintegrate and are digested by the Schwann cells, which proliferate and are able to function as facultative phagocytes.

Axonal degeneration occurs when dysfunction of

the neuron renders it unable to maintain its axon. The degeneration begins at the peripheral terminal of the axon and proceeds back toward the cell body, a process called "dying back."[191] There is often chromatolysis of the cell body. Schwann cell proliferation occurs in the region of active axonal degeneration, though it is usually less pronounced than that seen in wallerian degeneration. If the neuronal dysfunction can be halted or reversed, regeneration and some recovery of nerve function can occur.

Segmental demyelination, analogous to demyelination in the brain, is the selective loss of individual myelin internodes with preservation of the axon (Fig. 29–48). After an episode of demyelination, the remaining Schwann cells can proliferate and remyelinate the axons. However, the reconstituted myelin sheaths both are thinner than normal and have shorter internodal lengths. Both of these characteristics can be measured and are useful in the analysis of demyelinating peripheral neuropathies. Repeated episodes of demyelination and remyelination can occur and generate concentric arrangements of Schwann cell processes around the axon called "onion bulbs," which are found in the hypertrophic neuropathies (Fig. 29–49).

Regeneration occurs by the outgrowth of multiple sprouts from the distal end of the surviving segment of the axon. If there is no obstruction to their growth, the regenerating axons grow back down the nerve trunk at a rate of about 1 mm per day in association with the surviving Schwann cells that remain after digesting the degenerated axon and its myelin. If, as is frequently the case in wallerian degeneration, there is traumatic injury to the nerve with disruption of its fascicular architecture, interposed hematoma or fibrous scar may prevent the regenerating sprouts from entering the distal stump of the nerve. The obstructed regenerating axons then form a tangled, often painful mass of intertwined nerve fibers called an *amputation or traumatic neuroma.*

PERIPHERAL NEUROPATHY

Both diffuse demyelination and axonal degeneration tend to affect the longest axons first and produce a *peripheral polyneuropathy.* Polyneuropathies are typically symmetrical and present with distal signs and symptoms in the limbs, such as muscle weakness and loss of tendon reflexes, peripheral paresthesias, and a "glove and stocking" sensory loss. If the autonomic system is affected, there may be postural hypotension, constipation, or impotence. With axonal degeneration, muscle weakness will be accompanied by muscle fasciculation and wasting, but neither of these is present in demyelination, in which there is conduc-

tion failure but no denervation. To an extent, different etiologic agents tend preferentially to affect axons of different diameters, or sensory, motor, and autonomic axons to varying degrees. Clinically, the balance of symptoms and signs reflects the axons principally involved.

Although many etiologic agents produce diffuse damage, some pathologic processes that are focal (e.g., vasculitis, amyloid deposition) may affect only individual nerves. The result is a *mononeuropathy* or, if several nerves are affected, *mononeuritis multiplex.* However, even pathologically focal processes may present as a usually asymmetric *polyneuropathy* if they are widely distributed.

Pathologically, neuropathies are usually classified as being either *axonopathies,* in which there is "dying back" of the axon and degeneration of the nerve fiber, or *demyelinating,* with relative preservation of the axons. The types of etiology associated with peripheral neuropathies are: (1) nutritional deficiencies, e.g., thiamine; (2) toxins such as acrylamide and hexacarbons; (3) therapeutic agents, notably vincris-

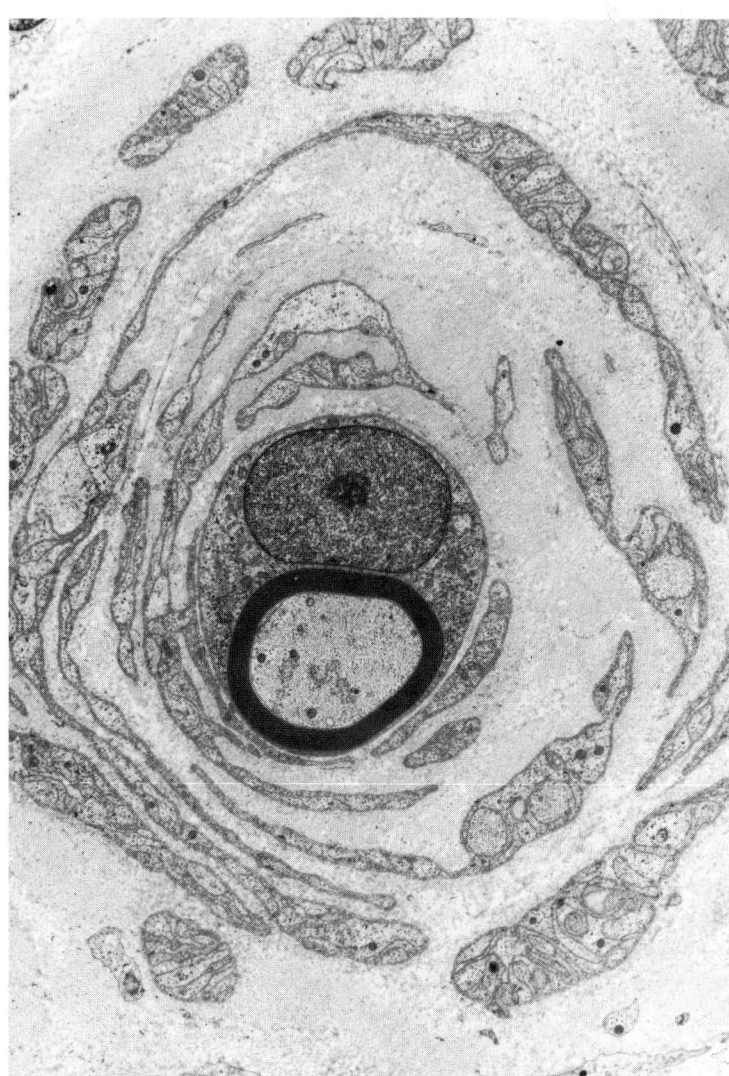

Figure 29–49. Electron micrograph showing onion-bulb formation (hypertrophic neuropathy). Myelinated fiber in center is surrounded by concentrically arranged Schwann cell cytoplasmic processes. Collagen is longitudinally oriented between these processes. (From Asbury, A.K., and Johnson, P.C.: Pathology of Peripheral Nerve. Philadelphia, W.B. Saunders Co., 1978, p. 142.)

tine and isoniazid; (4) systemic diseases, examples of which are arteritis, diabetes, and amyloid deposition; (5) inflammatory or demyelinating (autoimmune) disorders, as exemplified by the Guillain-Barré syndrome; and (6) a large number of hereditary neuropathies. These last may, as in the neuropathy of metachromatic leukodystrophy, have other organ involvements and a known cause, or may be idiopathic, as is the case in Charcot-Marie-Tooth disease (see below). There is no particular pathologic consistency within these etiologic groups, which may each contain examples of demyelinating or axonal neuropathies. In some neuropathies more than one process may be occurring; for example, in diabetic neuropathy, there is frequently both acute and chronic demyelination as well as axonal degeneration.

Most clinical classifications are based on the type of syndrome that develops, and a simplified version of a widely used classification is given in Table 29–7, with an indication for each clinical category of the predominant pathologic process encountered. Although this table seems to offer an impressive range of possible causes, between 30 and 70% of peripheral neuropathies clinically encountered remain undiagnosed as to etiology. Intensive evaluation of a series of such cases showed that whereas about 40% were probably hereditary and 20% were inflammatory or demyelinating, 25% still remained undiagnosed at the end of the evaluation.[192] In this chapter there is space for only one or two specific examples of neuropathies.

Of the peripheral neuropathies, perhaps the most commonly encountered and most clinically significant are those associated with *diabetes* (p. 1005) and *alcoholism*. It is unfortunate that both are predominantly axonal neuropathies without specific morphologic features. Pathologically, they show only axonal degeneration, usually with some evidence of attempted, though abortive, regeneration that is morphologically indistinguishable from the changes seen with many other causes of axonal degeneration.

Acute Idiopathic Polyneuritis (Landry-Guillain-Barré Syndrome)

This acute demyelinating neuropathy has been associated with a bewildering number of antecedents. About 40% of cases are associated with a "viral prodrome," with cytomegalovirus being implicated in about 15% of all cases, Epstein-Barr virus in about 5%, and Mycoplasma in 5%; 10% have had sundry allergic phenomena; 25% have a wide variety of other associations, including surgery; and the residual 25% have no known antecedent.[193]

ETIOLOGY AND PATHOGENESIS. An immunologic component to this disease is widely accepted.[194] In terms of cell-mediated immunity, lymphocytes accumulate in the endoneurium, but no B- or T-cell preference is apparent, and there is no evidence of cytotoxic T-cell activity directed against either Schwann cells or myelin.[195] Passive transfer with lymphocytes to experimental animals has not been accomplished. However, recent studies have demonstrated the presence of anti–peripheral nerve myelin antibodies during the acute phase of the disease[196] that, in a few cases, may be directed against gangliosides rather than the more conventional myelin antigens.[197] The presence of activated complement components in the CSF of patients during the acute phase of the illness may indicate a role for complement-fixing antibodies in the pathogenesis of the immune-mediated demyelination.[198] These findings reinforce the validity of recent studies that show that plasmapheresis, if carried out early in the course of the disease, can significantly shorten the clinical course of Guillain-Barré syndrome.[199,200]

MORPHOLOGY. Pathologically, focal collections of lymphocytes are found scattered throughout the endoneurium of peripheral nerves, although there is some predilection for the proximal nerve trunks.[194] Widespread focal demyelination is spatially associated with the areas of lymphocyte infiltration, and an accumulation of macrophages phagocytose the damaged myelin. Ultrastructurally, the earliest change is splitting of myelin lamellae, which are subsequently stripped off the axons and ingested by the macrophages, leaving the Schwann cells intact. The demyelination apparently occurs without the direct participation of the lymphocytes.

CLINICAL COURSE. Acute idiopathic polyneuritis manifests as a rapidly progressive, predominantly motor neuropathy with variable sensory features. In some cases, the muscular weakness may proceed so far proximally and be so profound that it produces facial diplegia and a potentially fatal respiratory paralysis. The CSF often but not always shows the classic "dissociation albuminocytologique," with a strikingly raised protein level but a normal or only slightly raised cell count.

Peroneal Muscular Atrophy (Charcot-Marie-Tooth Disease, Hypertrophic Type; Hereditary Sensory Motor Neuropathy [HSMN] Type I)

This is a dominantly inherited, slowly progressive sensorimotor neuropathy. Its major peripheral manifestations are wasting and weakness in the lower leg and foot giving the characteristic "inverted champagne bottle limb." Pathologically, the nerves are thickened, and there are prominent hypertrophic changes with "onion bulb" formation (see Fig. 29–49) indicative of repeated episodes of demyelination.[201]

Two other types of hypertrophic neuropathy are described: *Dejerine-Sottas disease*, which is a severe neuropathy occurring in young children, and Ref-

Table 29–7. Principal Neuropathic Syndromes

TYPE	PATHOLOGIC PROCESS	SYNDROME(S)
Acute ascending motor paralysis with variable sensory disturbance	Acute demyelinating neuropathy	Acute idiopathic polyneuritis (Landry-Guillain-Barré syndrome Infectious mononucleosis with polyneuritis Hepatitis and polyneuritis Diphtheritic polyneuropathy Toxic polyneuropathies, e.g., triorthocresyl phosphate
Subacute sensorimotor polyneuropathy Symmetric	Mostly axonal neuropathy	Alcoholic polyneuropathy and beriberi Arsenic polyneuropathy Lead polyneuropathy Vinca alkaloids and other intoxications
Asymmetric	Axonal neuropathy with focal and/or diffuse pathology	Diabetic neuropathy Polyarteritis nodosa and other arteritides Sarcoidosis
Chronic sensorimotor polyneuropathy Acquired	Axonal neuropathy with focal and/or diffuse pathology	Carcinomatous Paraproteinemias (demyelinating) Uremia Diabetes Connective tissue diseases Amyloidosis Leprosy
Inherited	Mostly chronic demyelination with hypertrophic changes	Peroneal muscular atrophy (Charcot-Marie-Tooth disease) Hypertrophic polyneuropathy (Dejerine-Sottas disease) Refsum's disease
Chronic relapsing polyneuropathy	Mixed pathology	Idiopathic polyneuritis Porphyria Beriberi and intoxications
Mononeuropathy or multiple neuropathy	Focal axonal or demyelinating pathology	Pressure palsies Traumatic palsies Serum neuritis Zoster Tumor invasion with neuropathy Leprosy

Adapted from Adams, R.D., and Asbury, A.K.: Diseases of the peripheral nervous system. *In* Petersdorf, R.G., et al. (eds.): Harrison's Principles of Internal Medicine. 10th ed. New York, McGraw-Hill Book Co., 1983, p. 2158.

sum's disease, which merits mention because of its association with raised levels of phytanic acid.[202]

PERIPHERAL NERVE TUMORS

Schwannomas (Neurilemmomas) and Neurofibromas

Despite their usually distinct clinical presentations and histologic features, both these tumors are derived from Schwann cells.

Grossly, both types of tumor have a white to gray color and a firm texture. **Schwannomas** are typically solitary, circumscribed, and encapsulated tumors eccentrically located on proximal nerves or spinal nerve roots (Fig. 29–50). Microscopically, they have regions of high and low cellularity called **Antoni A and B areas**, respectively. In the Antoni A tissue there may be foci of palisaded nuclei called **Verocay bodies**, and the blood vessels in schwannomas often have **hyaline thickening** around which there may be pseudopalisading of tumor nuclei.

Neurofibromas, by contrast, are not infrequently multi-ple, are usually but not always unencapsulated, and are often subcutaneous or produce fusiform enlargement of distal nerves. Microscopically, they usually consist of a loose pattern of interlacing bands of delicate spindle cells with elongated, slender, and sometimes wavy nuclei.

Immunocytochemically, both types of tumor contain S100 protein, a property that can be very useful in distinguishing them from tumors of fibrous tissue in morphologically ambiguous cases.[203] Similarly, both types of tumor may show quite marked nuclear pleomorphism and irregularity, and even occasionally giant cells, but these are not necessarily ominous findings. Myxoid or xanthomatous degeneration may also be seen. In schwannomas, no nerve fibers are present in the body of the tumor, although the residual nerve of origin of the tumor may be seen compressed to one side. Conversely, nerve fibers are found scattered throughout the tumor mass in neurofibromas, as if it had arisen by polyclonal growth of the Schwann cells with expansion of the entire nerve fascicle. This latter suggestion has obtained some support from studies in G6PD heterozygotes that show polyclonality of the neurofibroma tumor cells.[204] The distribution of nerve fibers within these

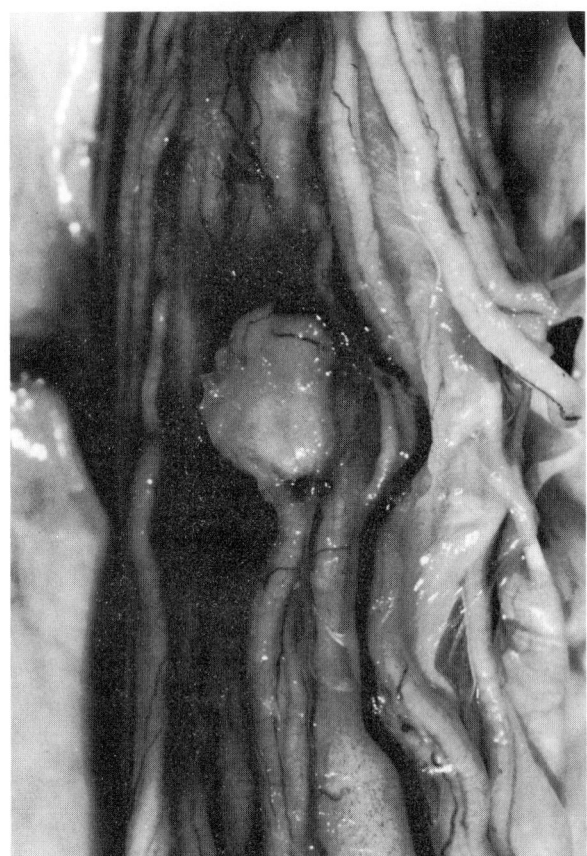

Figure 29–50. Schwannoma in cauda equina region.

tumors has some practical significance, as the compression to one side of the nerve of origin of a schwannoma admits the possibility of its removal without requiring transection of the nerve, an option not available for neurofibromas in which the entire nerve is involved in the tumor. The nerve fiber distribution is clinically important with acoustic (VIII cranial nerve) schwannomas: if the tumor is not too large, a skilled neurosurgeon may be able to remove the tumor and still preserve auditory function.

Malignant transformation may occur in both types of tumor, but is much rarer in schwannomas.[205] When it occurs, the tumor tends to lose its specific histologic characteristics and resemble a fibrosarcoma; perhaps consequentially, S100 protein also becomes a less reliable discriminant. Most cases of malignant neurofibroma are encountered in patients with von Recklinghausen's neurofibromatosis (p. 139).

Except in von Recklinghausen's disease, schwannomas are very much tumors of adults, manifesting most commonly in the fifth and sixth decades. The most serious symptoms are those produced by schwannomas on the cranial and spinal nerve roots. Acoustic schwannomas typically manifest with complaints of deafness and tinnitus, and, if the tumor is large enough, pressure palsies of the adjacent fifth and seventh cranial nerves or evidence of brainstem

compression and hydrocephalus. Spinal root neurilemmomas may present as slowly progressive cord compression or a cauda equina syndrome. With more distal tumors on nerve trunks, there may be local complaints in the territory of the affected nerve. Finally, there are the ubiquitous subcutaneous "lumps and bumps" that, if of neural origin, usually prove to be neurofibromas.

Epilogue

It is evident at the conclusion of this broad overview of the diseases of the nervous system that in number and diversity they rival the wondrous complexities of the nervous system itself.

1. Peters A., et al.: The Fine Structure of the Nervous System: The Neurons and Supporting Cells. Philadelphia, W.B. Saunders Co., 1976.
2. Lazarides, E.: Intermediate filaments as mechanical integrators of cellular space. Nature 283:249, 1980.
3. Kolodney, E.H., and Cable, W.J.L.: Inborn errors of metabolism. Ann. Neurol. 11:221, 1982.
4. Janzer, R.C., and Raff, M.C.: Astrocytes induce blood-brain barrier properties in endothelial cells. Nature 325:253, 1987.
5. Russell, D.S., and Rubenstein, L.J.: Pathology of Tumors of the Nervous System. 4th ed. Baltimore, Williams & Wilkins Co., 1977.
6. Robitaille, Y., et al.: A distinct form of adult polyglucosan body disease with massive involvement of central and peripheral neuronal processes and astrocytes. Brain 103:315, 1980.
7. Oehneichen, M.: Enzyme-histochemical differentiation of neuroglia and microglia: A contribution to the cytogenesis of microglia and globoid cells. Pathol. Res. Pract. 168:344, 1980.
8. Hickey, W.F., and Kimura, H.: Perivascular microglial cells of the CNS are bone-marrow derived and present antigen in vivo. Science 239:290, 1988.
9. Brightman, M.W., et al.: The blood-brain barrier to proteins under normal and pathological conditions. J. Neurol. Sci. 10:215, 1970.
10. Reese, T.S., and Karnovsky, M.S.: Fine structural localisation of a blood-brain barrier to exogenous peroxidase. J. Cell Biol. 34:207, 1967.
11. Bradbury, M.W.B.: The structure and function of the blood-brain barrier. Fed. Proc. 43:186, 1984.
12. Fishman, R.A.: Brain edema. N. Engl. J. Med. 293:706, 1975.
13. Manz, H.J.: The pathology of cerebral edema. Hum. Pathol. 5:291, 1974.
14. Katzman, R., and Pappius, H.M.: Brain Electrolytes and Fluid Metabolism. Baltimore, Williams & Wilkins Co., 1973.
15. Adams, R.S., and Victor, M.: Principles of Neurology. New York, McGraw-Hill Book Co., 1977.
16. Feigin, R.D., et al.: Epidemic meningococcal disease in an elementary school classroom. N. Engl. J. Med. 307:1255, 1982.
17. Carpenter, R.R., and Petersdorf, R.G.: The clinical spectrum of bacterial meningitis. Am. J. Med. 33:262, 1962.
18. Fishman, R. A.: Cerebrospinal fluid. In Asbury, A.K., et al. (eds.): Diseases of the Nervous System. Philadelphia, W.B. Saunders Co., 1980.
19. Lukes, S. A., et al.: Bacterial infections of the CNS in neutropenic patients. Neurology 34:269, 1984.
20. Case Records of the Massachusetts General Hospital (Case 2–1982): N. Engl. J. Med. 306:91, 1982.
21. Delaney, P.: Neurologic manifestations in sarcoidosis: Review of the literature, with a report of 23 cases. Ann. Intern. Med. 8:336, 1977.
22. Sabharwal, U.K., et al.: Granulomatous angiitis of the nervous system: Case report and review of the literature. Arthritis Rheum. 25:342, 1982.
23. DeAngelis, L.M.: Intracranial tuberculoma: Case report and review of the literature. Neurology 31:1133, 1982.
24. Harriman, D.G.F.: Bacterial infections of the central nervous system. In Adams, J.H., Corsellis, J.A.N., and Duchen, L.W. (eds.): Green-

field's Neuropathology. 4th ed. London, Arnold, Ltd., 1984, pp. 236–259.

25. Johns, D.R., et al.: Alteration in the natural history of neurosyphilis by concurrent infection with the human immunodeficiency virus. N. Engl. J. Med. *316*:1569, 1987.

26. Brewer, N.S., et al.: Brain abscesses: A review of recent experience. Ann. Intern. Med. *82*:571, 1975.

27. Shaw, M.D.M., and Russell, J.A.: Cerebellar abscesses: A review of 47 cases. J. Neurol. Neurosurg. Psychiatry *38*:429, 1975.

28. Johnson, R.T.: Selective vulnerability of neural cells to viral infection. Brain *103*:447, 1980.

29. Ede, R.J., and Williams, R.: Reye's syndrome in adults. Br. Med. J. *296*:517, 1988.

30. Tomlinson, A.H., et al.: Immunofluorescence staining for the diagnosis of herpes encephalitis. J. Clin. Pathol. *27*:495, 1974.

31. Centers for Disease Control: Encephalitis surveillance. Annual Summary, 1987. Issued 1988.

32. Whitley, R.J., et al.: Vidarabine versus acyclovir therapy in herpes simplex encephalitis. N. Engl. J. Med. *314*:144, 1986.

33. Brown, Z.A., et al.: Effects on infants of a first episode of genital herpes during pregnancy. N. Engl. J. Med. *317*:1246, 1987.

34. Hilt, D.C., et al.: Herpes zoster ophthalmicus and delayed contralateral hemiparesis caused by cerebral angiitis: Diagnosis and management approaches. Ann. Neurol. *14*:543, 1983.

35. Eidelberg, D., et al.: Thrombotic cerebral vasculopathy associated with herpes zoster. Ann. Neurol. *19*:7, 1986.

36. Horten, B., et al.: Multifocal varicella-zoster virus leukoencephalitis temporally remote from herpes zoster. Ann. Neurol. *9*:251, 1981.

37. Morgello, S., et al.: Varicella-zoster virus leukoencephalitis and cerebral vasculopathy. Arch. Pathol. Lab. Med. *112*:173, 1988.

38. Dupont, J.R., and Earle, J.M.: Human rabies encephalitis: A study of 49 fatal cases with a review of the literature. Neurology *15*:1023, 1975.

39. Sandhyamari, S., et al.: Pathology of rabies: A light and electron microscopic study with particular reference to the changes with prolonged survival. Acta Neuropathol. (Berlin) *54*:247, 1981.

40. Wolf, A., and Cowan, D.: Perinatal infections of the central nervous system. In Minkler, J. (ed.): Pathology of the Nervous System. New York, McGraw Hill, 1972, pp. 2565–2611.

41. Morgello, S., et al.: Cytomegalovirus encephalitis in patients with acquired immunodeficiency syndrome. Hum. Pathol. *18*:289, 1987.

42. Snider, W.D., et al.: Neurological complications of acquired immune deficiency syndrome: Analysis of 50 patients. Ann. Neurol. *14*:403, 1983.

43. Fauci, A.: The human immunodeficiency virus: Infectivity and mechanisms of pathogenesis. Science *239*:617, 1988.

44. Gabuzda, D.H., and Hirsch, M.S.: Neurologic manifestations of infection with human immunodeficiency virus. Ann. Intern. Med. *107*:383, 1987.

45. Carne, C.A., et al.: Acute encephalopathy coincident with seroconversion for anti-HTLV-III. Lancet *2*:1206, 1985.

46. Koenig, S., et al.: Detection of AIDS virus in macrophages in brain tissue from AIDS patients with encephalopathy. Science *233*:1089, 1986.

47. Petito, C.K., et al.: Neuropathology of acquired immunodeficiency syndrome (AIDS): An autopsy review. J. Neuropathol. Exp. Neurol. *45*:635, 1986.

48. Price, R.W., et al.: The brain in AIDS: Central nervous system HIV-1 infection and AIDS dementia complex. Science *239*:586, 1988.

49. Anders, K.H., et al.: The neuropathology of AIDS: UCLA experience and review. Am. J. Pathol. *124*:537, 1986.

50. Petito, C.K., et al.: Vacuolar myelopathy pathologically resembling subacute combined degeneration in patients with the acquired immunodeficiency syndrome. N. Engl. J. Med. *312*:874, 1985.

51. De la Monte, S.M., et al.: Peripheral neuropathy in the acquired immunodeficiency syndrome. Ann. Neurol. *23*:485, 1988.

52. Rosenberg, S., et al.: Neuropathology of acquired immunodeficiency syndrome (AIDS): Analysis of 22 Brazilian cases. J. Neurol. Sci. *76*:187, 1986.

53. Di Carlo, E.F., et al.: Malignant lymphomas and the acquired immunodeficiency syndrome. Arch. Pathol. Lab. Med. *110*:1012, 1986.

54. Yuen, T.S., et al.: Primary central nervous system lymphoma in acquired immune deficiency syndrome: A clinical and pathological study. Ann. Neurol. *20*:566, 1986.

55. Satyakam, B., et al.: Detection of human T-cell lymphoma/leukemia virus type 1 DNA and antigen in spinal fluid and blood of patients with chronic progressive myelopathy. N. Engl. J. Med. *318*:1141, 1988.

56. Sigurdsson, B.: Observations on the slow infections of sheep. Br. Vet. J. *110*:255, 307, 341, 1954.

57. Manz, H.J.: Pathology and pathogenesis of viral infections of the central nervous system. Hum. Pathol. *8*:3, 1977.

58. Townsend, J.J., et al.: Neuropathology of progressive rubella panencephalitis after childhood rubella. Neurology *32*:185, 1982.

59. Oyanagi, S., et al.: Histopathology and electron microscopy of three cases of subacute sclerosing panencephalitis (SSPE). Acta Neuropathol. (Berlin) *18*:58, 1971.

60. Tourtellotte, W.W., et al.: Quantification of de novo central nervous system IgG measles antibody synthesis in SSPE. Ann. Neurol. *9*:551, 1981.

61. Hall, W.W., et al.: Measles and SSPE virus proteins: Lack of antibodies to the M protein in patients with subacute sclerosing panencephalitis. Proc. Natl. Acad. Sci. USA. *76*:2047, 1979.

62. Choppin, P.W.: Measles virus and chronic neurological diseases. Ann. Neurol. *9*:17, 1981.

63. Astrom, K.E., et al.: Progressive multifocal leukoencephalopathy: A hitherto unrecognised complication of chronic lymphatic leukemia and Hodgkin's disease. Brain *81*:93, 1958.

64. Berger, J.R.: Progressive multifocal leukoencephalopathy associated with human immunodeficiency virus infection. Ann. Intern. Med. *107*:78, 1987.

65. Walker, D.L.: Progressive multifocal leukoencephalopathy and opportunistic viral infection of the central nervous system. In Vinken, P.J., and Bruyn, G.W. (eds.): Handbook of Clinical Neurology, Vol. 34. Infection of the Nervous System, Part II. Amsterdam, North-Holland Publishing Co., 1978, pp. 307–329.

66. Podgett, B.L., and Walker, D.L.: Prevalence of antibodies in human sera against JC virus, and isolate from a case of progressive multifocal leukoencephalopathy. J. Infect. Dis. *127*:467, 1973.

67. Gajdusek, D.C.: Unconventional viruses and the origin and disappearance of Kuru. Science *197*:943, 1977.

68. Gibbs, C.J., Jr., et al.: Creutzfeldt-Jakob disease (spongiform encephalopathy): Transmission to the chimpanzee. Science *161*:388, 1968.

69. Prusiner, S.B.: Prions and neurodegenerative diseases. N. Engl. J. Med. *317*:1571, 1987.

70. Oesch, B., et al.: A cellular gene encodes scrapie PrP 37-30 protein. Cell *40*:735, 1985.

71. Kretzschmar, H.A., et al.: Scrapie prion proteins are synthesised in neurons. Am. J. Pathol. *122*:1, 1986.

72. Masters, C.L., et al.: Creutzfeldt-Jakob disease: Patterns of worldwide occurrence and the significance of familial and sporadic clustering. Ann. Neurol. *5*:177, 1979.

73. Duffy, P., et al.: Possible person-to-person transmission of Creutzfeldt-Jakob disease. N. Engl. J. Med. *291*:692, 1974.

74. Brown, P.: Human growth hormone therapy and Creutzfeldt-Jakob disease: A drama in three acts. Pediatrics *81*:85, 1988.

75. Rappaport, E.B.: Iatrogenic Creutzfeldt-Jakob disease. Neurology *37*:1520, 1987.

76. Masters, C.L., and Richardson, E.P., Jr.: Subacute spongiform encephalopathy (Creutzfeldt-Jakob disease). Brain *101*:333, 1978.

77. Chou, S.M., et al.: Transmission and scanning electron microscopy of spongiform change in Creutzfeldt-Jakob disease. Brain *103*:885, 1980.

78. Kitamoto, T., et al.: Amyloid plaques in Creutzfeldt-Jakob disease stain with prion protein antibodies. Ann. Neurol. *20*:204, 1986.

79. Chernik, N.L., et al.: Central nervous system infections in patients with cancer. Cancer *40*:268, 1977.

80. Parker, J.C., et al.: The emergence of candidosis: The dominant post mortem cerebral mycosis. Am. J. Clin. Pathol. *70*:31, 1978.

81. Hooper, D.C., et al.: Central nervous system infection in the chronically immunosuppressed. Medicine *61*:166, 1982.

82. Navia, B.A., et al.: Cerebral toxoplasmosis complicating the acquired immune deficiency syndrome: Clinical and neuropathological findings in 27 patients. Ann. Neurol. *19*:224, 1986.

83. Whisnant, J.P.: The decline of stroke. Stroke *15*:160, 1984.

84. Brierly, J.B., and Graham, D.I.: Hypoxia and vascular disorders of the central nervous system. In Adams, J.H., Corsellis, J.A.N., and

Duchen, L.W. (eds.): Greenfield's Neuropathology. 4th ed. London, Arnold Ltd., 1984, pp. 125–207.

85. Schneider, M.: Survival and revival of the brain in anoxia and ischaemia. *In* Gastaut, H., and Meyer, J.S. (eds.): Cerebral Anoxia and the Electroencephalogram. Springfield, Ill., Charles C Thomas Pub., 1961, pp. 134–143.

86. Garcia, J.H., and Conger, K.A.: Ischemic brain injuries: Structural and biochemical effects. *In* Grenvile, A.K., and Safar, P. (eds.): Brain Failure and Resuscitation. London, Churchill Livingstone, 1981.

87. Rothman, S.M., and Olney, J.W.: Glutamate and the pathophysiology of hypoxic-ischemic brain damage. Ann. Neurol. *19*:105, 1986.

88. Coyle, J.T.: Kainic acid: Insights into excitatory mechanisms causing selective neuronal degeneration. Ciba Found. Symp. *126*:186, 1987.

89. Moore, P.M., and Cupps, T.R.: Neurological complications of vasculitis. Ann. Neurol. *14*:155, 1983.

90. Sigsbee, B., et al.: Non-metastatic superior sagittal sinus thrombosis complicating systemic cancer. Neurology *29*:139, 1979.

91. Cole, F.M., and Yates, P.O.: The occurrence and significance of intracerebral microaneurysms. J. Pathol. Bacteriol. *93*:393, 1967.

92. Douglas, M.A., and Haerer, A.F.: Long-term prognosis of hypertensive intracerebral hemorrhage. Stroke *13*:488, 1982.

93. Heros, R.C., et al.: Cerebral vasospasm after subarachnoid hemorrhage: An update. Ann. Neurol. *14*:599, 1983.

94. Hughes, J.T., and Schianchi, P.M.: Cerebral artery spasm. A histological study at necropsy of the blood vessels in cases of subarachnoid hemorrhage. J. Neurosurg. *48*:515, 1978.

95. Fisher, C.M.: Lacunar strokes and infarcts: A review. Neurology *32*:871, 1982.

96. Fisher, C.M.: The arterial lesions underlying lacunes. Acta Neuropathol. (Berlin) *12*:1, 1969.

97. Babikian, V., and Ropper, A.H.: Binswanger's disease: A review. Stroke *18*:2, 1987.

98. Chester, E.M., et al.: Hypertensive encephalopathy: A clinicopathologic study of 20 cases. Neurology *28*:928, 1978.

99. Dinsdale, H.B.: Hypertensive encephalopathy. Stroke *13*:717, 1982.

100. Adams, J.H.: Head injury. *In* Adams, J.H., Corsellis, J.A.N., and Duchen, L.W. (eds.): Greenfield's Neuropathology. 4th ed. London, Arnold, Ltd., 1984, pp. 85–124.

101. Genarelli, T.A., et al.: Diffuse axonal injury and traumatic coma in the primate. Ann. Neurol. *12*:564, 1982.

102. Dawson, S.L., et al.: The contrecoup phenomenon. Hum. Pathol. *11*:155, 1980.

103. Adams, J.H., et al.: Deep intracerebral (basal ganglia) haematomas in fatal non-missile head injury in man. J. Neurol. Neurosurg. Psychiatry *49*:1039, 1986.

104. Adams, J.H., et al.: Diffuse brain damage of immediate impact type. Brain *100*:489, 1977.

105. Adams, J.H., et al.: Diffuse axonal injury due to non-missile head injury in humans: An analysis of 45 cases. Ann. Neurol. *12*:557, 1982.

106. Fulling, K.H., and Garcia, D.M.: Anaplastic astrocytoma of the adult cerebrum. Prognostic value of histologic features. Cancer *55*:928, 1985.

107. Nelson, J.S., et al.: Necrosis as a prognostic criterion in malignant supratentorial, astrocytic tumors. Cancer *52*:550, 1983.

108. Burger, P.C., and Green, S.B.: Patient age, histologic features, and length of survival in patients with glioblastoma multiforme. Cancer *59*:1617, 1987.

109. Mork, S.J., et al.: Oligodendroglioma. Histologic evaluation and prognosis. J. Neuropath. Exp. Neurol. *45*:65, 1986.

110. Burger, P.C., et al.: Clinicopathologic correlation in the oligodendroglioma. Cancer *59*:1345, 1987.

111. Slooff, J.L., et al.: Primary Intramedullary Tumors of the Spinal Cord and Filum Terminale. Philadelphia, W.B. Saunders Co., 1964.

112. Ilgren, E.B., et al.: Ependymomas: A clinical and pathological study. Part 1 – Biologic features. Clin. Neuropathol. *3*:113, 1984.

113. Bennett, J.P., Jr., and Rubenstein, L.J.: The biologic behaviour of primary cerebral neuroblastoma: A reappraisal of the clinical course in a series of 70 cases. Ann. Neurol. *16*:21, 1984.

114. Kepes, J.J.: Meningiomas: Biology, Pathology and Differential Diagnosis. New York, Masson, 1982.

115. Taylor, C.R., et al.: An immunohistological study of immunoglobulin content of primary central nervous system lymphomas. Cancer *41*:2197, 1978.

116. Penn, I.: Development of cancer as a complication of renal transplantation. Transplant Proc. *9*:1121, 1977.

117. Compston, A.: Genetic factors in the etiology of multiple sclerosis. *In* McDonald, W.I., and Silberberg, D.H. (eds.): Multiple Sclerosis. London, Butterworths, 1986, pp. 56–73.

118. Ebers, G.C., et al.: A population based study of multiple sclerosis in twins. N. Engl. J. Med. *315*:1638, 1986.

119. Kurtzke, J.F.: Epidemiologic contributions to multiple sclerosis: An overview. Neurology *30*:61, 1980.

120. Kurtzke, J.F., and Hyllested, K.: Multiple sclerosis in the Faroe Islands. II. Clinical update, transmission, and the nature of MS. Neurology *36*:307, 1986.

121. Cook, S.D., et al.: Declining incidence of multiple sclerosis in the Orkney Islands. Neurology *35*:545, 1985.

122. McCullam, K., et al.: T cell subsets in multiple sclerosis. Gradients at plaque borders and differences in nonplaque regions. Brain *110*:1297, 1987.

123. Morimoto, C., et al.: Selective loss of the suppressor-inducer T-cell subset in progressive multiple sclerosis. N. Engl. J. Med. *316*:67, 1987.

124. Chou, C-H.J., et al.: Failure to detect antibodies to myelin basic protein or peptic fragments of myelin basic protein in CSF of patients with MS. Neurology *33*:24, 1983.

125. Ebers, G.C.: Oligoclonal banding in MS. Ann. N. Y. Acad. Sci. *436*:206, 1984.

126. Ellison, G.W., et al.: Multiple sclerosis. Ann. Intern. Med. *101*:514, 1984.

127. Weiner, H.L., and Hafler, D.A.: Immunotherapy of multiple sclerosis. Ann. Neurol. *23*:211, 1988.

128. Allen, I.V.: Demyelinating diseases. *In* Adams, J.H., Corsellis, J.A.N., and Duchen, L.W. (eds.): Greenfield's Neuropathology. London, Arnold, 1984, pp. 338–384.

129. Chou, S.M.: Acute hemorrhagic leucoencephalitis as a disseminated vasculomyelinopathy: Immunoperoxidase study. J. Neuropathol. Exp. Neurol. *41*:357, 1982.

130. Amaducci, L.A., et al.: Origin of the distinction between Alzheimer's disease and senile dementia: How history can clarify nosology. Neurology *36*:1497, 1986.

131. Katzman, R.: Alzheimer's disease. N. Engl. J. Med. *314*:964, 1986.

132. Heyman, A., et al.: Alzheimer's disease: Genetic aspects and associated clinical disorders. Ann. Neurol. *14*:507, 1983.

133. Wisniewski, K.E., et al.: Occurrence of neuropathological changes and dementia of Alzheimer's disease in Down's syndrome. Ann. Neurol. *17*:278, 1985.

134. Ulrich, J.: Alzheimer changes in nondemented patients younger than sixty-five: Possible early stages of Alzheimer's disease and senile dementia of Alzheimer type. Ann. Neurol. *17*:273, 1985.

135. Khachaturian, Z.S.: Diagnosis of Alzheimer's disease. Arch. Neurol. *42*:1097, 1985.

136. Selkoe, D.J.: Altered structural proteins in plaques and tangles: What do they tell us about the biology of Alzheimer's disease? Neurobiol. Aging *7*:425, 1986.

137. Goldman, J.E.: The association of actin with Hirano bodies. J. Neuropathol. Exp. Neurol. *42*:146, 1983.

138. Blessed, G., et al.: The association between quantitative measures of dementia and of senile changes in the cerebral gray matter of elderly subjects. Br. J. Psychiatry *114*:797, 1968.

139. Whitehouse, P.J., et al.: Alzheimer's disease and senile dementia: Loss of neurones in the basal forebrain. Science *215*:1237, 1982.

140. Selkoe, D.J., et al.: Conservation of brain amyloid protein in aged mammals and humans with Alzheimer's disease. Science *235*:872, 1987.

141. St. George-Hyslop, P.H., et al.: The genetic defect causing familial Alzheimer's disease. Maps on chromosome 21. Science *235*:885, 1987.

142. Tanzi, R.E., et al.: The genetic defect in familial Alzheimer's disease is not tightly linked to the amyloid B-protein gene. Nature *329*:156, 1987.

143. Bahmanyar, S., et al.: Localization of amyloid B protein messenger RNA in brains from patients with Alzheimer's disease. Science *237*:77, 1987.

144. Kang, J., et al.: The precursor of Alzheimer's disease amyloid A4 protein resembles a cell surface receptor. Nature *325*:733, 1987.

145. Munoz-Garcia, D., and Ludwin, S.: Classic and generalized var-

iants of Pick's disease: A clinicopathological, ultrastructural, and immunocytochemical comparative study. Ann. Neurol. *16*:467, 1984.

146. Perry, G., et al.: Filaments of Pick's bodies contain altered cytoskeletal elements. Am. J. Pathol. *127*:559, 1987.

147. Gusella, J.F., et al.: A polymorphic DNA marker genetically linked to Huntington's disease. Nature *306*:234, 1983.

148. Martin, J.B., and Gusella, J.F.: Huntington's disease: Pathogenesis and management. N. Engl. J. Med. *315*:1267, 1986.

149. Beal, M.F., et al.: Replication of the neurochemical characteristics of Huntington's disease by quinolinic acid. Nature *321*:168, 1986.

150. Vonsattel, J-P., et al.: Neuropathological classification of Huntington's disease. J. Neuropathol. Exp. Neurol. *44*:559, 1985.

151. Joachim, C.L., et al.: Clinically diagnosed Alzheimer's disease: Autopsy results in 150 cases. Ann. Neurol. *24*:50, 1988.

152. Bethlem, J., and Den Hartog Jager, W.A.: The incidence and characteristics of Lewy bodies in idiopathic paralysis agitans (Parkinson's disease). J. Neurol. Neurosurg. Psychiatry *23*:74, 1960.

153. Pappola, M.A.: Lewy bodies of Parkinson's disease. Arch. Pathol. Lab. Med. *110*:1160, 1986.

154. Hornykiewicz, O.: Brain neurotransmitter changes in Parkinson's disease. *In* Marsden, C.D., and Fahn, S. (eds.): Movement Disorders. London, Butterworth Scientific, 1982, pp. 41–58.

155. Forno, L.S., et al.: Locus ceruleus lesions and eosinophilic inclusions in MPTP-treated monkeys. Ann. Neurol. *20*:449, 1986.

156. Snyder, S.H., and D'Amato, R.J.: MPTP: A neurotoxin relevant to the pathophysiology of Parkinson's disease. Ann. Neurol. *36*:250, 1986.

157. Steele, J.: Progressive supranuclear palsy. Brain *95*:693, 1972.

158. Joachim, C.L., et al.: Tau antisera recognise neurofibrillary tangles in a range of neurodegenerative disorders. Ann. Neurol. *22*:514, 1987.

159. Haines, J.L.: Spinocerebellar ataxia in a large kindred: Age at onset, reproduction, and genetic linkage studies. Neurology *34*:1542, 1984.

160. Stumph, D.A.: Friedreich's ataxia and other hereditary ataxias. *In* Tyler, H.R., and Dawson, D.M. (eds.): Current Neurology. Vol. 1. Boston, Houghton-Mifflin Medical Division, 1978, pp. 86–118.

161. Tandon, R., and Bradley, W.G.: Amyotrophic lateral sclerosis. Part 1. Clinical features, pathology and ethical issues in management. Ann. Neurol. *18*:271, 1985.

162. Brownell, B., et al.: The central nervous system in motor neurone disease. J. Neurol. Neurosurg. Psychiatry *33*:338, 1970.

163. Tandon, R., and Bradley, W.G.: Amyotrophic lateral sclerosis. Part 2. Etiopathogenesis. Ann. Neurol. *18*:419, 1985.

164. Spencer, P.S., et al.: Guam amyotrophic lateral sclerosis–Parkinsonism–dementia linked to a plant excitant neurotoxin. Science *237*:517, 1987.

165. Victor, M., et al.: The Wernicke-Korsakoff syndrome. Philadelphia, F.A. Davis, 1971.

166. Reuler, J.B., et al.: Wernicke's encephalopathy. N. Engl. J. Med. *312*:1035, 1985.

167. Sharpe, J.A., et al.: Methanol optic neuropathy: A histopathological study. Neurology *32*:1093, 1982.

168. McLean, D.R., et al.: Methanol poisoning: A clinical and pathological study. Ann. Neurol. *8*:161, 1980.

169. Glass, J.P., et al.: Treatment-related leukoencephalopathy. Medicine *65*:154, 1986.

170. Breuer, A.C., et al.: Multifocal pontine lesions in cancer patients treated with chemotherapy and CNS radiotherapy. Cancer *41*:2112, 1978.

171. Vinters, H.V., et al.: Focal pontine leukoencephalopathy in immunosuppressed patients. Arch. Pathol. Lab. Med. *111*:192, 1987.

172. Laureno, R.: Central pontine myelinolysis following rapid correction of hyponatremia. Ann. Neurol. *13*:232, 1983.

173. Sterns, R.H., et al.: Osmotic demyelination syndrome following correction of hyponatremia. N. Engl. J. Med. *314*:1535, 1986.

174. Ayus, J.C., et al.: Treatment of symptomatic hyponatremia and its relation to brain damage. N. Engl. J. Med. *317*:1190, 1987.

175. DiMauro, S., et al.: Mitochondrial myopathies. Ann. Neurol. *17*:521, 1985.

176. Bresolin, N., et al.: Progressive cytochrome c oxidase deficiency in a case of Kearns-Sayre syndrome: Morphological, immunochemical and biochemical studies in muscle biopsies and autopsy tissues. Ann. Neurol. *21*:564, 1987.

177. DiMauro, S., et al: Cytochrome c oxidase deficiency in Leigh

syndrome. Ann. Neurol. *22*:498, 1987.

178. Kolodny, E.H., and Moser, H.W.: Sulfatide lipidosis: Metachromatic leukodystrophy. *In* Stanbury, J.B., et al. (eds.): The Metabolic Basis of Inherited Disease. 5th ed. New York, McGraw-Hill Book Co., 1983, pp. 881–905.

179. Suzuki, K., and Suzuki, Y.: Galactosylceramide lipidosis: Globoid cell leukodystrophy (Krabbe's disease). *In* Stanbury, J.B., et al. (eds.): The Metabolic Basis of Inherited Disease. 5th ed. New York, McGraw-Hill Book Co., 1983, pp. 857–880.

180. Rizzo, W.B., et al.: Adrenoleukodystrophy: Dietary oleic acid lowers hexacosanoate levels. Ann. Neurol. *21*:232, 1987.

181. Schaumberg, H.H., et al.: Adrenoleukodystrophy: A clinical and pathological study of 17 cases. Arch. Neurol. *32*:577, 1975.

182. Moser, H.W., et al.: Adrenoleukodystrophy: Survey of 303 cases: Biochemistry, diagnosis and therapy. Ann. Neurol. *16*:628, 1984.

183. Schaumberg, H.H., et al.: Adrenomyeloneuropathy: A probable variant of adrenoleukodystrophy. II. General pathologic, neuropathologic and biochemical aspects. Neurology *27*:1114, 1977.

184. O'Neill, B.P., et al.: The adrenomyeloneuropathy complex: Expression in four generations. Neurology *31*:151, 1981.

185. Schaumberg, H.H., et al.: Adrenoleukodystrophy (sex-linked Schilder disease): Ultrastructural demonstration of specific cytoplasmic inclusions in the central nervous system. Arch. Neurol. *31*:210, 1974.

186. Hicks, S.P.: Developmental malformations produced by radiation. A timetable of their development. Am. J. Roentgenol. *69*:279, 1953.

187. Kalter, H., and Warkany, J.: Congenital malformations: Etiologic factors and their role in prevention. N. Engl. J. Med. *308*:424, 491, 1983.

188. Larroche, J-C.: Malformations of the nervous system. *In* Adams, J.H., Corsellis, J.A.N., and Duchen, L.W. (eds.): Greenfield's Neuropathology. Arnold, London, 1984, pp. 385–450.

189. Friede, R.L.: Developmental Neuropathology. New York, Springer-Verlag, 1975.

190. Nevin, N.C., et al.: Influence of social class on the risk of recurrence of anencephalus and spina bifida. Dev. Med. Child Neurol. *23*:155, 1981.

191. Cavanagh, J.B.: The "dying back" process: A common denominator in many naturally occurring and toxic neuropathies. Arch. Pathol. Lab. Med. *103*:659, 1979.

192. Dyck, P.J., et al.: Intensive evaluation of referred unclassified neuropathies yields improved diagnosis. Ann. Neurol. *10*:222, 1981.

193. Dowling, P.C., and Cook, S.D.: Role of infection in Guillain-Barré: Laboratory confirmation of herpes viruses in 41 cases. Ann. Neurol. *9* (Suppl.):44, 1981.

194. Prineas, J.W.: Pathology of the Guillain-Barré syndrome. Ann. Neurol. *9* (Suppl.):6, 1981.

195. Iqbal, A., et al.: Cell mediated immunity in idiopathic polyneuritis. Ann. Neurol. *9* (Suppl.):65, 1981.

196. Koski, C.L., et al.: Clinical correlation with anti–peripheral-nerve myelin antibodies in Guillain-Barré syndrome. Ann. Neurol. *19*:573, 1986.

197. Ilyas, A.A., et al.: Serum antibodies to gangliosides in Guillain-Barré syndrome. Ann. Neurol. *23*:440, 1988.

198. Hartung, H-P., et al.: Guillain-Barré syndrome: Activated complement components C3a and C5a in CSF. Neurology *37*:1006, 1987.

199. French Cooperative Group on Plasma Exchange in Guillain-Barré Syndrome. Role of replacement fluids. Ann. Neurol. *22*:753, 1987.

200. Guillain-Barré Study Group. Plasmapheresis and acute Guillain-Barré syndrome. Neurology *35*:1096, 1985.

201. Smith, T.W., et al.: Charcot-Marie-Tooth disease associated with hypertrophic neuropathy. J. Neuropathol. Exp. Neurol. *40*:420, 1980.

202. Fardeau, M.: Pathology of Refsum Disease. *In* Dyck, P.J., et al. (eds.): Peripheral Neuropathy. Vol. 2. Philadelphia, W.B. Saunders Co., 1984, pp. 1693–1703.

203. Stefansson, K., et al.: S-100 protein in soft-tissue tumors derived from Schwann cells and melanocytes. Am. J. Pathol. *106*:261, 1982.

204. Fialkow, P.J., et al.: Multiple cell origin of hereditary neurofibromas. N. Engl. J. Med. *284*:298, 1971.

205. Burger, P.C., and Vogel, F.S.: Surgical Pathology of the Nervous System and its Coverings. 2nd ed. New York, Wiley Medical, 1982.

Daniel M. Albert, M.D.   *Thaddeus P. Dryja, M.D.*

CONGENITAL ANOMALIES

Chromosomal mutations and aneuploidies are often associated with ocular abnormalities. Among the most common are trisomy 13 and trisomy 21.

TRISOMY 13

Trisomy 13, called D-trisomy or Patau's syndrome in earlier classifications, results from accidental failure of disjunction of one pair of chromosomes during meiosis.[1] The condition is estimated to be present in 1 in 14,000 live births and usually proves lethal by six months of age. There is no sex predilection. This aberrant karyotype is associated with numerous systemic findings, which include mental retardation, low-set and malformed ears, cleft lip and/or palate, sloping forehead, polydactyly of hands and feet, and absence or hypoplasia of the olfactory lobes (arhinencephaly).

OCULAR ABNORMALITIES. Severe ocular anomalies occur in almost all cases. Abnormally small eyes (microphthalmos) are common. In rare instances the eyes may be fused, resulting in a cyclopia-like condition known as cyclopean synophthalmus. The most characteristic findings are areas of defective formation of the iris and ciliary body (colobomas), cataract, and a persistence of the embryonic vasculature of the vitreous known as persistent hyperplastic primary vitreous. These features are present in about 80% of eyes with this abnormality. A striking finding seen in about 65% of these eyes is cartilage present within the coloboma (Fig. 30–1). In about 75% of eyes with this condition the retina contains tubular and rosette-like structures known as dysplastic retina (Fig. 30–2).[2] Retinal folds

and microcystoid changes are also common. In about 60% of eyes there is evidence of defective development of cornea, iris, and anterior chamber angle (dysgenesis of the cornea and iris), with congenital glaucoma being seen in some instances.

TRISOMY 21

Trisomy 21, also known as Down's syndrome or mongolism, is discussed in some detail on page 129. It is characterized by a number of findings including severe mental retardation; a flat nasal bridge; an open mouth with a furrowed, protruding tongue and small, malformed teeth; prominent malformed ears with absent lobes; a flattened occiput; a broad neck, with loose skin at the back of the neck and over the shoulders; short, broad hands, with the little fingers being shortened and curved with dysplastic middle phalanges; abnormalities of the dermal ridge, including a transverse palmar crease; and cardiovascular and hematologic defects.

The **ocular findings,**[3] while far less severe than in trisomy 13, are distinctive. The eyes are usually set far apart (hypertelorism) and are associated with abnormalities of the lids, including oblique or arched palpebral fissures, epicanthus, and ectropion and eversion of the upper eyelids. The irides have a speckled appearance owing to the presence of ringlike foci of iris hypoplasia surrounding relatively normal iris stroma (Brushfield spots). In addition, the irides may show focal stromal hyperplasia. Cataracts are often present and are unusual in having abnormal anterior lens capsular excrescences.[4] A progressively cone-shaped cornea with ectasia of the central part (keratoconus) and retinal dysplasia may also be present. Additional ocular abnormali-

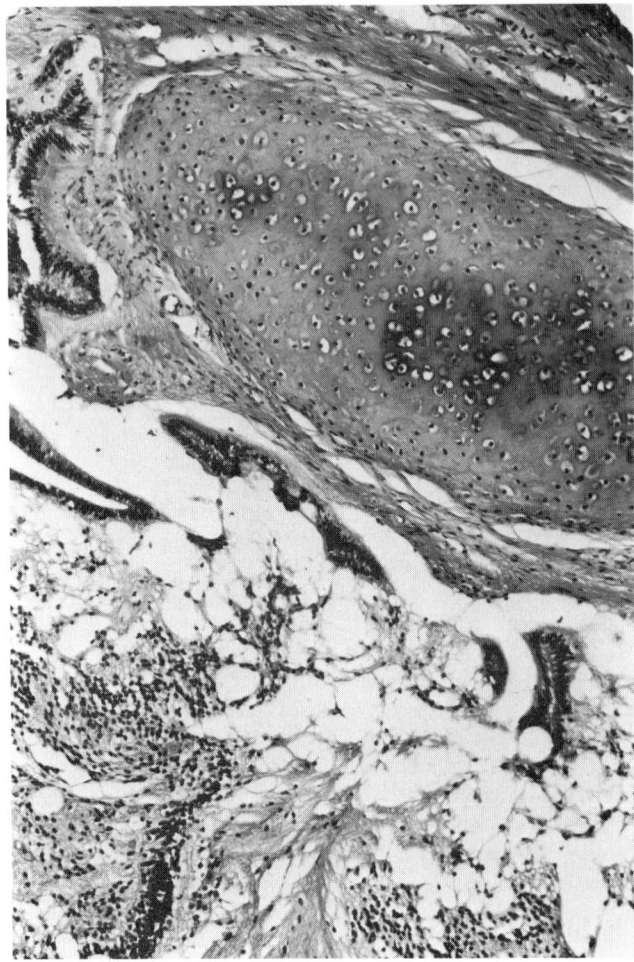

Figure 30–1. High-power view of eye with trisomy 13 showing a cartilaginous mass characteristic of this disorder.

ties include esotropia, high myopia, a hyperemic optic disc with an increased number of retinal vessels crossing its margin, retinal pigment epithelial atrophy seen both surrounding the disc and in a patchy distribution at the periphery of the retina, prominent whitened choroidal vessels, and chronic blepharoconjunctivitis.

INFECTIOUS EMBRYOPATHIES

A number of maternal infections during pregnancy may result in ocular abnormalities. Among the most toxic and severe are toxoplasmosis, cytomegalic inclusion disease, congenital rubella, and congenital syphilis. The latter two conditions are now considered.

Congenital Rubella Syndrome

The congenital rubella syndrome, also known as Gregg's syndrome, consists of cataracts, cardiovascular defects, mental retardation, and deafness. The syndrome is the result of maternal rubella infection during pregnancy. The rubella virus is able to pass through the placenta and infect the fetus, thus causing abnormal embryogenesis. If a woman contracts ru-

bella during the first month of pregnancy, her child has a 50% chance of being affected. Twenty falling to 7 percent of fetuses are affected if infection occurs during the second and third months.

The associated systemic findings include low birth weight, deafness, patent ductus arteriosus and other congenital heart defects, central nervous system abnormalities, pneumonitis, hepatomegaly, genitourinary anomalies, and other defects.

Ocular abnormalities found in the rubella syndrome[5] are primarily cataract, congenital glaucoma, iris abnormalities, and a pigmentary disturbance of the retina known as rubella retinopathy. The rubella cataract is quite distinctive on histologic examination because of the retention of cell nuclei in the centrally located embryonic nucleus of the lens, an area in which the cell nuclei normally disappear. It has also been shown that the rubella virus can survive within the lens for a number of years after birth. Consequently, surgery on rubella cataracts may lead to the release of virus into the interior of the eye and cause an endophthalmitis.

The iris has a poorly developed dilator muscle, and a

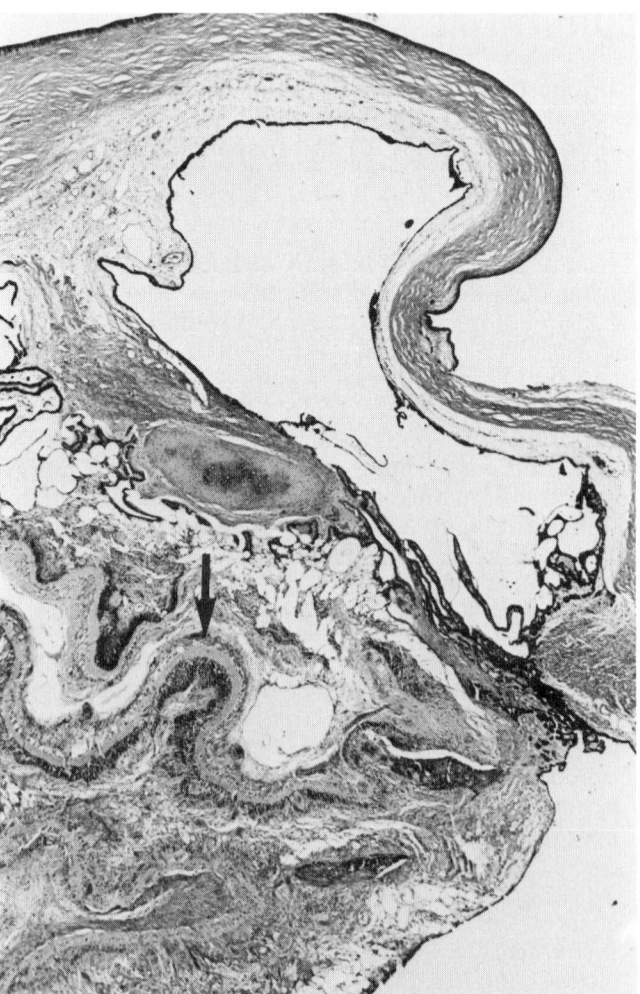

Figure 30–2. The anterior half of an eye with trisomy 13. The retina is dysplastic (arrow).

necrotic-appearing epithelium. In addition, chronic, non-granulomatous inflammation of the iris stroma is often present. These factors contribute to the inability of the iris to dilate normally, and result in the clinical appearance of a "leathery" iris. The ciliary body also shows pigment epithelium necrosis and nongranulomatous inflammation.

In instances in which congenital glaucoma is present, the anterior chamber angle shows the same abnormalities seen in other eyes with congenital glaucoma (p. 1466).

Rubella retinopathy is probably the most characteristic finding in this disorder. The principal defect is in the retinal pigment epithelium, which shows alternating areas of atrophy and hypertrophy; this gives rise to the clinically striking "salt-and-pepper" ophthalmoscopic appearance. In some cases, this retinal abnormality is progressive. Subretinal neovascularization may occur in some patients, usually between the ages of 10 and 18 years.

Congenital Syphilis

Although infrequently seen today, congenital syphilis results in marked ocular abnormalities.[6] The most common and characteristic finding is an inflammation of the stroma of the cornea (interstitial keratitis). This has a typical onset between 5 and 20 years of age. These changes are frequently associated with abnormalities in the teeth and deafness (Hutchinson's triad). Initially the cornea becomes edematous and is infiltrated by lymphocytes and plasma cells, accounting for the clinical appearance of clouding of the cornea. The involvement is often unilateral and may even occupy only a sector of the cornea. Blood vessels develop in the deep cornea just anterior to the basement membrane of the endothelium (Descemet's membrane). The inflammation often lasts for two to three months and is followed by regression, during which time the edema and inflammatory cells disappear but the blood vessels persist. Often, however, they are not filled with blood, and may be seen on slit-lamp biomicroscopy as delicate white "ghost vessels" corresponding to the empty vessels seen histopathologically. Subsequently the damaged corneal endothelium may produce excess basement membrane that may have a variety of clinical appearances.

CONJUNCTIVA

VITAMIN A DEFICIENCY AND BITOT'S SPOT

Bitot's spot is a thickened, bubbly-appearing lesion located at the limbus of the cornea seen in vitamin A deficiency (p. 439). It occurs most commonly in young male children and is a localized form of keratomalacia (see below). Histologically, one sees thickened keratinized epithelium. The conjunctival mucous cells are lost, and in severe cases the conjunctival epithelium may assume the appearance of skin epithelium with rete pegs (epidermidalization). *Corynebacterium xe-*

rosis bacteria are typically found in profusion within the lesion.

A more severe form of vitamin A deficiency is *keratomalacia*,[7] characterized by diffuse, severe keratinization of all mucous membrane epithelia. In the eye the corneal and conjunctival epithelia are involved (xerophthalmia). Hypovitaminosis A is also accompanied by *night blindness* due to degenerative changes in the retina. The condition occurs principally in children. Secondary bacterial infection and corneal ulceration may occur with subsequent *hypopyon, corneal necrosis and perforation, and panophthalmitis* (Fig. 30–3). Keratomalacia constitutes a leading cause of blindness in underdeveloped countries.

PINGUECULA AND PTERYGIUM

Pingueculae are raised yellowish lesions that characteristically occur in the conjunctiva near the nasal limbus of the cornea, are bilateral, and are seen in middle-aged and elderly patients. On histologic examination, there is breakdown of the collagen in the subepithelial tissue[8] (basophilic degeneration), resulting in gray-staining material with H and E that stains positively for elastin but is insensitive to elastase.

A *pterygium* is histologically identical to pinguecula but constitutes a winglike projection of vascularized tissue that extends onto the nasal cornea. Pterygia are usually bilateral but asymmetric. They cause dissolution of the anterior layers of the corneal stroma (Bowman's membrane). The epithelium overlying pterygia or pinguecula may show a variety of secondary changes including ancanthosis, hyperkeratosis, and dyskeratosis.

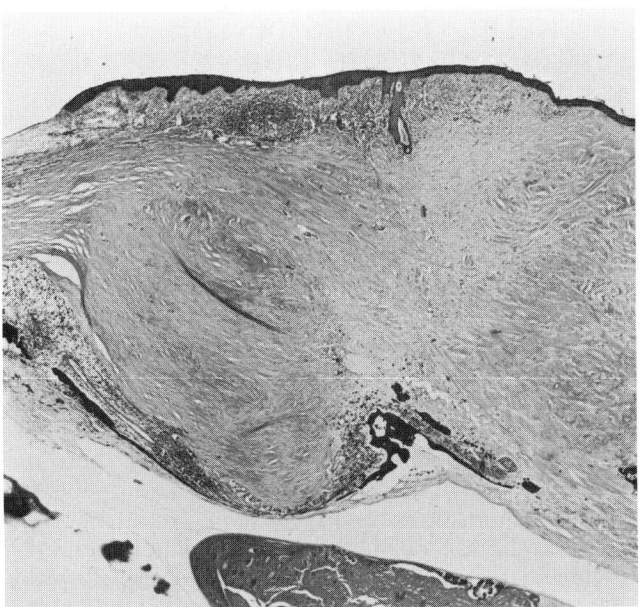

Figure 30–3. Area of corneal scarring in keratomalacia caused by vitamin A deficiency.

TRACHOMA

Trachoma, one of the world's major causes of blindness, is caused by *Chlamydia trachomatis* (p. 327). It affects primarily the conjunctival and corneal epithelium, ultimately causing cicatrization of this tissue. Its course can be divided into four stages (the MacCallan classification).[9]

> **Stage I** is characterized clinically by the formation of conjunctival follicles (subepithelial conjunctival inflammatory infiltrates) and diffuse punctate inflammation of the cornea. Subsequently there is growth of fibrovascular tissue in the substantia propria of the conjunctiva and onto the cornea (early **pannus**). Microscopically, the corneal epithelium contains cytoplasmic inclusion bodies composed of microcolonies of elementary bodies and larger basophilic initial bodies. Lymphocytes and plasma cells infiltrate the subepithelial tissue; polymorphonuclear leukocytes infiltrate the corneal and conjunctival epithelium.
>
> In **Stage II,** the inflammation becomes more florid, with the further formation of follicles and epithelial thickening. The corneal pannus becomes more severe. Histologically, large macrophages with phagocytized debris (Leber cells) are seen in the conjunctiva, accompanying the epithelial hyperplasia with round cell infiltration and subepithelial edema. In **Stage III,** the follicles disappear and cicatrization occurs, leaving in its wake inversion of the upper lid (cicatricial entropion) and misdirected lashes (trichiasis). On histologic examination, scattered lymphocytes and plasma cells can still be seen along with subepithelial scar tissue.
>
> In **Stage IV,** there is spontaneous arrest of the disease. However, the residual entropion and trichiasis lead to corneal damage, denuding the epithelium and leaving the cornea vulnerable to infection and further opacification due to scarring.

EPITHELIAL TUMORS OF THE CONJUNCTIVA AND LIDS

Carcinoma in situ of these structures appears clinically either as an opaque, white, shiny lesion (leukoplakia) or as a fleshy mass.[10] Histologically, the polarity of the epithelium is lost, and atypical pleomorphic cells are found throughout the entire thickness of the epithelium. Mitotic figures are commonly seen. The basal membrane of the epithelium is intact, and there is no invasion of the subepithelial tissue.

Squamous cell carcinoma shows the changes of carcinoma in situ, but there is also invasion by the tumor cells through the epithelial basement membrane into the superficial epithelial tissues.[11] Most commonly, squamous cell carcinoma of the conjunctiva shows only superficial invasion, and deep invasion and metastases are rarely seen.

Carcinoma derived from the mucus-secreting cells and squamous cells of the conjunctival epithelium *(mucoepidermoid carcinoma)* and *melanomas* of the conjunctiva also occur. Carcinoma derived from the basal cells of the conjunctival epithelium is almost never encountered.

CORNEA

ULCERATIVE INFLAMMATIONS

The cornea (proceeding inward) is composed of five layers: (1) the epithelium, (2) Bowman's membrane, (3) stroma, (4) Descemet's membrane, and (5) endothelium. Because of the cornea's lack of cellularity and absence of vascularity, numerous bacterial, viral, and fungal agents, including types usually considered noninfectious, can cause severe corneal infection. Corneal ulcers are a major cause of visual loss. Although they frequently respond to topical medication, they may necessitate corneal transplantation, and they sometimes lead to loss of the eye. Corneal ulcers are characterized by inflammation, necrosis, and loss of tissue. The ulcers can progress slowly over many weeks.

Herpetic Infections

The most common cause of central corneal ulcers is herpes simplex virus.[12] The characteristic clinical presentation is a dendritic ulcer.

> Initially the infection of the epithelium is characterized histologically by intranuclear inclusion bodies in corneal epithelial cells. There may be widespread epithelial edema, leading to bullae within the epithelium or between the epithelium and Bowman's layer of stroma. In chronic cases, inflammation of the corneal stroma may take the form of a localized discoid opacity **(disciform keratitis).** On histologic examination of a cornea with chronic herpetic keratitis, the stromal opacity is found to contain lymphocytes and plasma cells, with occasional multinucleated giant cells near the basement membrane of the endothelium. Intranuclear viral inclusion bodies are seen in corneal epithelial cells by light microscopy, and viral particles can be identified in the epithelial nucleus and cytoplasm by electron microscopy. With resolution of the infection, the cornea may be left scarred and vascularized.

DYSTROPHIES

Corneal dystrophies are primary corneal disorders, usually inherited, that show bilateral and usually symmetric involvement. These constitute an important group of corneal diseases. Three corneal dystrophies[13] involve the stroma and can lead to severely compromised visual acuity necessitating corneal transplant.

Granular dystrophy is an autosomal dominant disease that usually appears in the first or second decade of life and shows a slow and continuous progression. It is characterized by sharply defined, variably sized, white opacities or granules in the anterior portion of the stroma. Histologically these correspond to hyalin-like eosinophilic deposits, which by electron microscopy consist of dense granules.

Lattice dystrophy is also an autosomal dominant disease that usually begins in the first or second decade of life. It appears clinically as linear opacities forming a lattice configuration concentrated in the central portion of the anterior stroma. Histologically these opacities (composed of amyloid) are eosinophilic, metachromatic, periodic acid–Schiff positive and Congo red positive.

The most severe of the stromal dystrophies is *macular dystrophy,* which has an autosomal recessive mode of inheritance. This disease causes diffuse cloudiness of the anterior stroma with aggregates of gray-white opacities in the axial region. Macular dystrophy usually results in severe impairment of vision by 30 years of age. This disorder is a localized corneal mucopolysaccharidosis, which appears to result from a defect in the catabolism of corneal keratan sulfate. Histologically, one observes basophilic deposits that stain positive for acid mucopolysaccharides.

UVEA

The uvea is a vascular coat that includes the choroid, ciliary body, and iris. Uveitis comprises a large, heterogeneous group of disorders that have in common inflammation of one or more portions of the uveal tract.[14] Uveitis is classified in several different ways. Clinically it is often convenient to separate cases of uveitis according to the portions of the uveal tract involved (i.e., *iritis, cyclitis,* and *choroiditis*). Commonly, involvement of more than one part of the uvea and frequently the entire uvea *(panuveitis)* is seen. Another method of classification is based on etiology. Uveitis may result from trauma, systemic disease, or infection. In the vast majority of cases, however, a definitive clinical cause cannot be found.

From a histologic standpoint, the two broad categories of uveitis are *granulomatous uveitis,* characterized by the presence of giant cells and/or epithelioid cells, and *nongranulomatous uveitis,* in which only lymphocytes and plasma cells are the inflammatory components. Usually, histopathologic examination fails to reveal the cause of nongranulomatous uveitis. On the other hand, the etiologic agent can sometimes be identified in cases of granulomatous uveitis.

GRANULOMATOUS UVEITIS

Granulomatous uveitis is frequently caused by infectious agents. Among the bacterial causes are tuberculosis, leprosy, syphilis, and tularemia. Viral causes of granulomatous uveitis include cytomegalic inclusion disease and herpes zoster. The principal fungal causes of granulomatous uveitis are blastomycosis, cryptococcosis, coccidioidomycosis, aspergillosis, phycomycosis, candidiasis, and histoplasmosis. The most important parasitic causes are onchocerciasis and toxoplasmosis. In all these disorders, the inflammation is not limited to the uvea but involves the retina and often the vitreous and sclera as well. In some cases, as in cytomegalic inclusion disease or toxoplasmosis, the infection is primarily in the retina and secondarily involves the choroid.

Sarcoidosis

Granulomatous uveitis is a common complication of sarcoidosis. In about one third of patients with sarcoidosis, a granulomatous anterior uveitis occurs, characterized by "mutton fat" deposits of chronic inflammatory cells on the cornea *(keratic precipitates)*. Less commonly, granulomatous inflammation can be found involving the choroid (Fig. 30–4). The retina can be involved by sarcoidosis, characterized by retinal periphlebitis with "candle wax drippings" on or near retinal vessels, retinal hemorrhages, and whitish masses in the adjacent vitreous. Retinal sarcoidosis is frequently associated with central nervous system sarcoidosis and carries a grave prognosis. Commonly, sarcoid patients have granulomatous infiltrates in the conjunctiva. As a result, a conjunctival biopsy can be a relatively simple method for diagnosing sarcoidosis in a significant percentage of suspected cases. Histologically, discrete, noncaseating, granulomatous infiltrates are seen in the involved parts of the eye, similar to lesions found elsewhere in sarcoidosis (p. 427).

Sympathetic Ophthalmia

Sympathetic uveitis is a rare but noteworthy disease that is an important consideration in the treatment of ocular trauma.[15] This is a *bilateral* diffuse granulomatous uveitis that is generally associated with penetrating injuries to *one* eye, particularly those in which uveal prolapse or incarceration occurs. The cause is thought to be an autosensitivity against a putative antigen shared by the uveal melanocytes, retinal pigment epithelium, and neural retinal cells. Removal of the injured eye before the onset of sympathetic uveitis is the only method of preventing this disease. Sympathetic uveitis rarely occurs earlier than two weeks following an ocular injury. Consequently, the

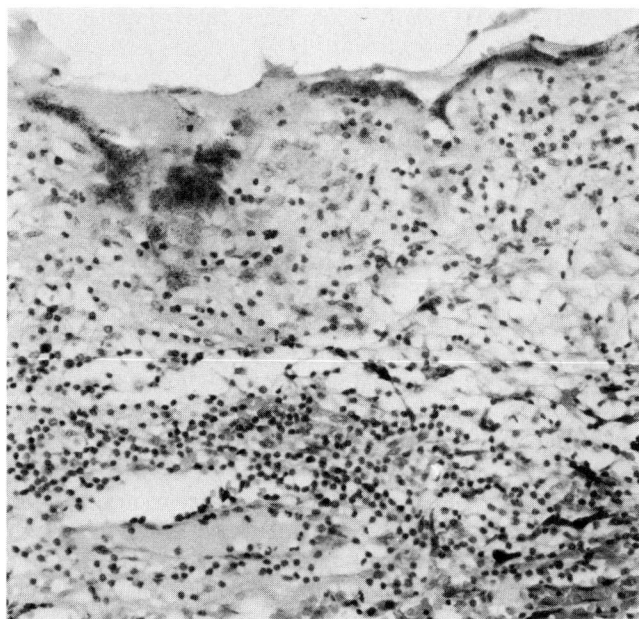

Figure 30–4. Granulomatous uveitis occurring in patient with sarcoid. Infiltrate is a mixture of lymphocytes and plasma cells.

clinician must weigh the likelihood of maintaining useful vision in the injured eye against the risk of developing this bilateral disease. Following the onset of inflammation, removal of the injured eye appears to result in milder inflammation in the noninjured or "sympathizing" eye. Occasionally, however, the injured eye ends up as the eye with better vision; so again, judicious evaluation of the prognosis for vision in the injured eye is called for. The initial symptoms are loss of accommodation, blurred vision, and photophobia in the sympathizing eye. The earliest clinical signs are the appearance of keratic precipitates seen with the slit lamp and of choroidal infiltrates seen on fundus examination and fluorescein angiography.

Sympathetic uveitis is a clinicopathologic diagnosis; hence, one must know the history and clinical findings as well as the histopathologic findings before making a precise diagnosis. The characteristic histopathologic signs are similar in both the injured (exciting) eye and the sympathizing eye: There is diffuse granulomatous uveal inflammation composed primarily of lymphocytes with clusters of epithelioid cells. Plasma cells typically are scant. Early in the course, eosinophils may be seen. The inflammation affects primarily the choroid with only mild involvement of the retina, usually appearing as a perivasculitis. Within the choroid the choriocapillaris usually shows less severe inflammation. Clusters of epithelioid cells are seen between Bruch's membrane and the retinal pigment epithelium forming **Dalen-Fuchs nodules.** Inflammation is usually present wherever melanocytes reside; consequently the emissary canals passing through the sclera and meninges of the optic nerve may show inflammation. Although necrosis is not characteristic, pigment granules can be found in the macrophages, suggesting that disordered melanocytes play a role in the pathogenesis of the disease. In eyes in which the lens is injured, a form of granulomatous inflammation called **phacoanaphylactic endophthalmitis** occurs in and about the lens in about 25% of patients with sympathetic uveitis.

The course of the disease is usually protracted with flare-ups and remissions. Inflammation can usually be controlled with long-term immunosuppressive treatment.

UVEAL MELANOMAS

Intraocular melanomas constitute the most common primary ocular malignancy in Caucasians. Although we describe here melanomas of the uveal tract (i.e., the iris, ciliary body, and choroid), melanomas also occur on the skin of the lid, on the conjunctiva, and even within the orbit. Moreover, in addition to the uveal melanocytes (the cells giving rise to uveal melanomas), a second population of pigmented cells exists within the eye: the pigment epithelium of the iris, ciliary body, and retina. The pigment epithelium is embryologically derived from the neural tube and can undergo non-neoplastic proliferation or reactive hy-

perplasia in response to a variety of stimuli, but only in rare instances will it undergo malignant transformation. The uveal melanocytes originate from the neural crest and possess long dendrite-like processes emanating from the center of the cell body, similar to dermal melanocytes. They never undergo reactive hyperplasia, but they are the origin of malignant melanomas of the eye.

The annual age-adjusted incidence of non-skin melanomas as reported in a major study was 0.7 per 100,000 population in the United States. Ocular tumors constitute 79% of all the noncutaneous melanomas reported. The annual age-adjusted incidence of ocular melanomas is about one-eighth that of melanoma of the skin in the United States. The risk of ocular melanoma for whites is eightfold higher than for blacks.

MORPHOLOGY. Most melanomas arise in the posterior choroid. They may spread laterally between the sclera and retina or may produce bulbous masses projecting into the vitreous cavity and pushing the retina ahead of them (Fig. 30–5). Callender[16] in 1931 devised the initial histologic classification relating the histologic appearance to prognosis for metastases. The Callender classification, in somewhat modified form, remains in general use today as follows:

Spindle A melanomas have cohesive tumor cells with small, spindle-shaped nuclei containing a central dark strip that is seen by electron microscopy to be a nuclear fold. Nucleoli are not distinct, cytoplasm is scant, and cell borders are difficult to identify. These constitute approximately 5% of ciliary body and choroidal melanomas. They have a very good prognosis, with only 8% of patients dead from metastases 15 years after enucleation.

Spindle B melanomas are composed of cohesive cells having distinct spindle-shaped nuclei with prominent nucleoli. The cells contain more cytoplasm than those in the spindle A lesion, and cell borders are difficult to discern by light microscopy. This cell type constitutes approximately 40% of ciliary body and choroidal melanomas. The **fascicu-**

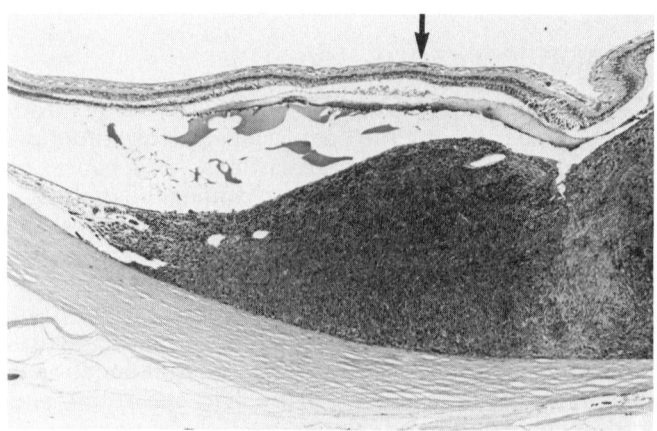

Figure 30–5. Choroidal melanoma with overlying retinal detachment *(arrow)* produced by a serous transudate.

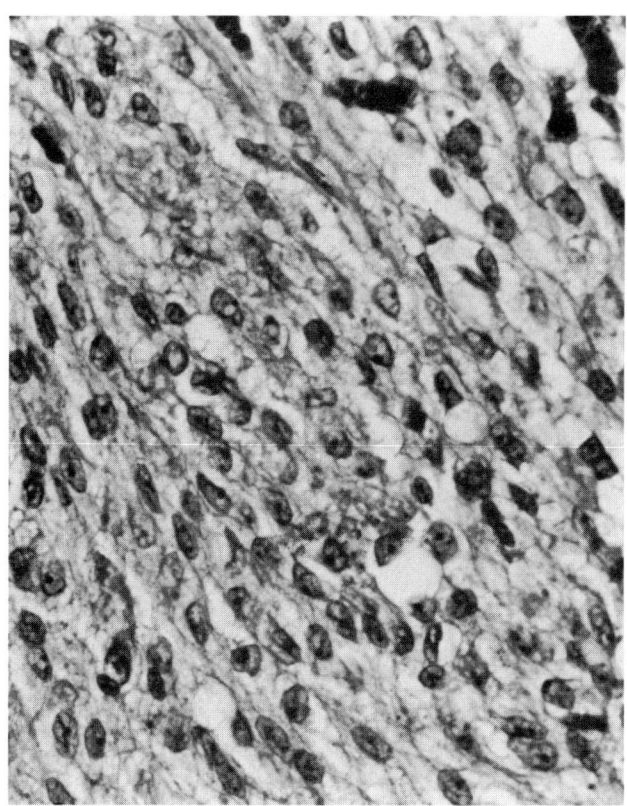

Figure 30–6. High-power view of cells composing choroidal melanoma. Majority are of epithelioid type, which carries a poor prognosis.

lar type of uveal melanoma is a subgroup of spindle B melanomas characterized by a palisading arrangement of the spindle-shaped cells, termed a fascicular pattern. These compose approximately 6% of choroidal melanomas. Spindle A and spindle B melanomas are the cell types seen in almost all iris melanomas. Approximately 15% of patients are dead from metastases 15 years after enucleation.

Epithelioid melanomas are composed of poorly cohesive, large cells with round nuclei and prominent nucleoli. Abundant eosinophilic cytoplasm and well-demarcated cell borders are seen (Fig. 30–6). This is the rarest type of the ciliary body and choroidal melanomas, occurring in only 3% of all cases. It has a poor prognosis, with 72% of patients dead after 15 years.

Mixed cell type melanomas are neoplasms having spindle cells (usually spindle B) together with a significant epithelioid population. This is the most common type of ciliary body and choroidal melanoma, accounting for about 40% of these lesions. Approximately 60% of patients are dead after 15 years.

Necrotic melanoma refers to a tumor so necrotic that the cell type cannot be identified. It occurs in only 7% of all ciliary body and choroidal tumors. The prognosis is similar to that for the mixed type.

For the sake of convenience, uveal melanomas are often considered in two primary categories: the spindle cell variety (combining spindle A and spindle B types) and the epithelioid, mixed, and necrotic types, or nonspindle cell variety. Slightly less than 50% of ciliary body and choroidal malignant melanomas are of the spindle cell variety; these have a good prognosis, with about 73% survival at 15 years. A little more than 50% are of the non–spindle cell variety, with a prognosis of about 35% survival at 15 years (because of the frequency of late metastases, "five-year cure rates" are less useful with this tumor than with most others). A number of other parameters have been correlated with survival. Features considered the most significant are cell type, largest dimension, scleral extension, and mitotic activity. Morphometry is also useful, with a high degree of pleomorphism of nucleoli indicating a poor prognosis.

CLINICAL PRESENTATION. An iris melanoma most commonly presents as a pigmented mass. It may also be somewhat light in color. Distortion of the pupil is frequently seen. A ciliary body melanoma may elicit episcleral vascular injection over it, may interfere with accommodation, and may cause a localized cataract. Both iris and ciliary body melanomas are causes of glaucoma. Choroidal melanoma may appear as a mass on routine ophthalmoscopic examination, and may cause retinal detachment, macular edema or detachment, or choroidal hemorrhage (Fig. 30–7). A melanoma in any position may extend through an emissary canal to the surface of the globe or may cause ocular inflammation.

For many years, enucleation was the primary treatment for ocular melanomas. Because it became evident that iris melanomas are usually of the spindle cell type and of low malignancy, the usual treatment is now to observe these and resect the tumor only when intraocular spread threatens the eye. Enucleation is still widely employed as treatment for large melanomas as well as for many medium-sized tumors. Radiation delivered by proton beam or by a radioactive scleral plaque is being used increasingly in the treat-

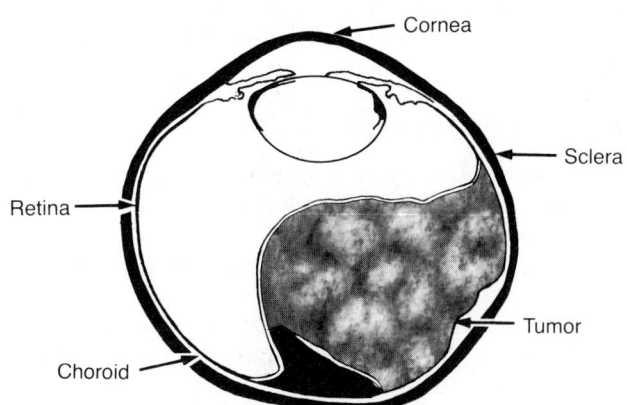

Figure 30–7. A representation of a choroidal melanoma seen on transection of the globe, appearing as a large, pigmented mass elevating and detaching the retina.

ment of melanomas. To be noted, sometimes an intraocular hemorrhage or the development of a cataract or glaucoma brings the melanoma to attention.

The pattern of metastatic disease in ocular melanoma differs from that of cutaneous melanoma because of the absence of lymphatic drainage from the uveal tract. Hepatic metastases predominate.

SECONDARY INTRAOCULAR NEOPLASMS

Secondary intraocular neoplasms may occur by direct extension of tumors of the ocular adnexae or by metastatic spread. Metastatic neoplasms, in fact, constitute the most common intraocular neoplasm.[17,18] Lung carcinoma is the most common metastatic lesion in men, usually occurring early in the course of the disease. Breast carcinoma is the most common metastatic tumor in women and usually occurs late in the course of the disease (Fig. 30–8). The relative frequency of metastases from other primary sites usually reflects the incidence and malignancy of the tumor. Metastatic intraocular tumors are bilateral in about 20 to 25% of cases.

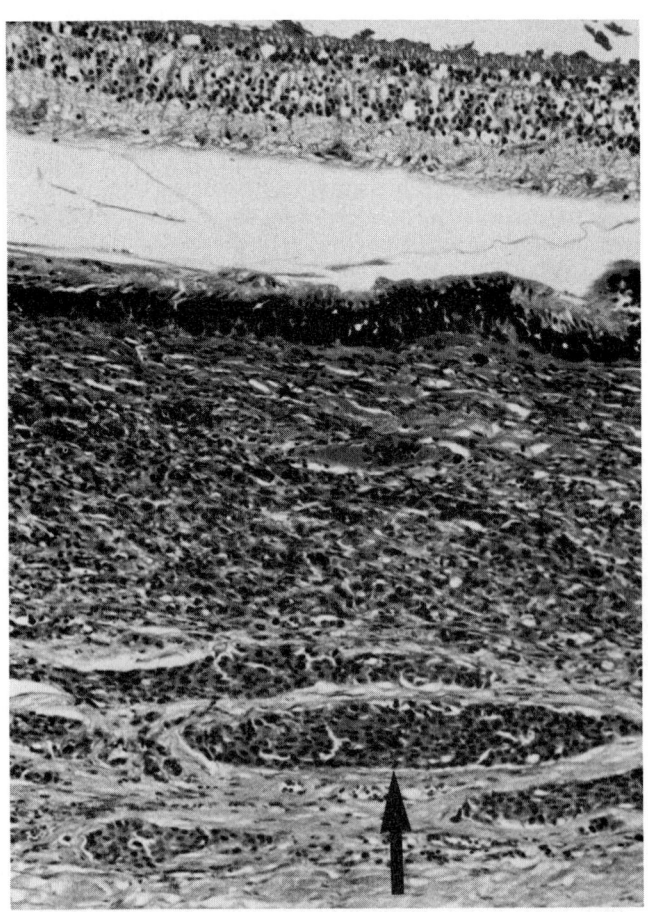

Figure 30–8. Breast carcinoma metastatic to the choroid (arrow). This is the most common form of choroidal metastases in women.

LENS

Cataracts, by definition, are opacities in the crystalline lens. They are a major cause of visual loss and blindness throughout the world. Among the many causes of cataracts are metabolic diseases, physical agents, ocular diseases, viruses, skin diseases, and aging. The most common type is idiopathic and develops in older individuals (so-called *senile cataracts*).

SENILE CATARACTS

A wide spectrum of cataracts develop as individuals become older.[19] Cataracts are examined by ophthalmologists using a slit lamp biomicroscope. This permits observation of many of the same changes in vivo that the pathologist sees under the microscope after the lens is removed. Consequently, we will first describe the changes that can be noted both on biomicroscopic examination of the patient and on light microscopic examination of the sectioned lens. Following this we will discuss changes seen on histologic examination only.

The most common change in the aging lens is *nuclear sclerosis* or compression of the lens fibers in the central portion of the lens. On examination the borders of the individual nuclear fibers are indistinct, and the nucleus as a whole stands out from the cortex more distinctly than normal. As the process progresses the nucleus may become brown ("brunescent cataract"). The earliest changes in the cortex are the appearance of wedge- or spokelike opacities that occur first at the lens equator and then progress into the anterior and posterior cortex (*cortical cataract*). Vacuoles often appear in the cortex of the lens, and the clefts show an accumulation of opaque debris of degenerated lens material (Morgagni's globules).

Another common type of senile cataract is marked by the development of granular opacities in the zone immediately anterior to the posterior capsule. These spread toward the periphery (*posterior subcapsular cataract*). A lens with an early or *immature cataract* frequently has an increased osmotic pressure as a result of the degenerated lens material and may imbibe water and swell (*intumescent cataract*). Eventually the entire lens may become involved in the degenerative process (*mature cataract*). The sclerotic nucleus may sink in the cortex when the latter becomes entirely liquefied (*Morgagnian cataract*). Occasionally, cataractous lenses may shrink after the lens capsule and epithelium degenerate, and lenticular debris passes into the aqueous humor (*hypermature cataract*). As the lens capsule becomes more permeable, allowing lens material to escape, the lenticular debris is engulfed by macrophages that may obstruct the aqueous outflow, resulting in *phacolytic glaucoma*. Cataractous lenses may eventually calcify; less commonly, lens material is partially or completely reabsorbed, leaving the residual lens capsule.

If cataract surgery is performed and some lens epithelium is left behind within the capsule, these cells may produce abortive opaque lens fibers that appear as large globules. In some instances of extracapsular extraction the anterior and posterior capsules of the lens may become apposed while the epithelium at the periphery forms abortive lens fibers having a doughnut shape *(Soemmering's ring cataract)*.

On examination of histologic sections, abnormalities of the epithelium may be seen. The most common finding is the migration of epithelium over the posterior lens capsule. The epithelial cells may enlarge and appear vacuolated (bladder cells); they may undergo necrosis and be partially or totally absent, or they may undergo fibrous metaplasia.

RETINA

The retina has a very complex structure, but can be summarized as having a basic three-neuron organization (Fig. 30–9). An electrical impulse generated by light impinging on the process of a photoreceptor cell (rod or cone) is transmitted through a bipolar neuron and then carried by the axon of a neuron to the lateral geniculate body, providing ultimately a visual image.

RETROLENTAL FIBROPLASIA (RETINOPATHY OF PREMATURITY)

Retrolental fibroplasia was a leading cause of blindness in infants in the United States and other countries between 1940 and the early 1950s and continues to occur with disturbing frequency. Terry in Boston was the first to define the clinical aspects of the condition, but it took a decade for its true nature to be recognized.[20] It occurs almost entirely in premature infants who have a history of oxygen therapy. The major risk factors in this disease are the level and duration of oxygen exposure and consequent formation of oxygen species of free radicals and the immaturity of the retinal circulation. The peripheral retinal vasculature, particularly on the temporal side, does not become fully formed until the end of fetal life. The least mature vessels are the most vulnerable to injury on exposure to oxygen. In babies of very low birth weight, the retinal vessels can apparently be injured by levels of arterial oxygen tension that are physiologic at term (i.e., approximately 90 mm Hg).

The present ability to maintain babies weighing as little as 600 gm at birth appears to be the reason for the rise in incidence of retrolental fibroplasia in recent years. The previously defined "safe" dose of oxygen (an ambient concentration of not more than 40%, which corresponds to a partial pressure in the arterial blood of 160 mm Hg) now is considered unsafe for extremely small infants. In addition, occasional examples of oxygen-induced retrolental fibroplasia at full term have been reported and are considered to be the result of a barely mature retinal vasculature in the extreme temporal periphery of these infants.

The initial stage in *the pathogenesis of retrolental fibroplasia*[21] is a vaso-obliterative phase in which there is a functional constriction of the immature retinal blood vessels followed by a structural obliteration. The peripheral retina consequently fails to vascularize. On cessation of exposure to oxygen the vasopro-

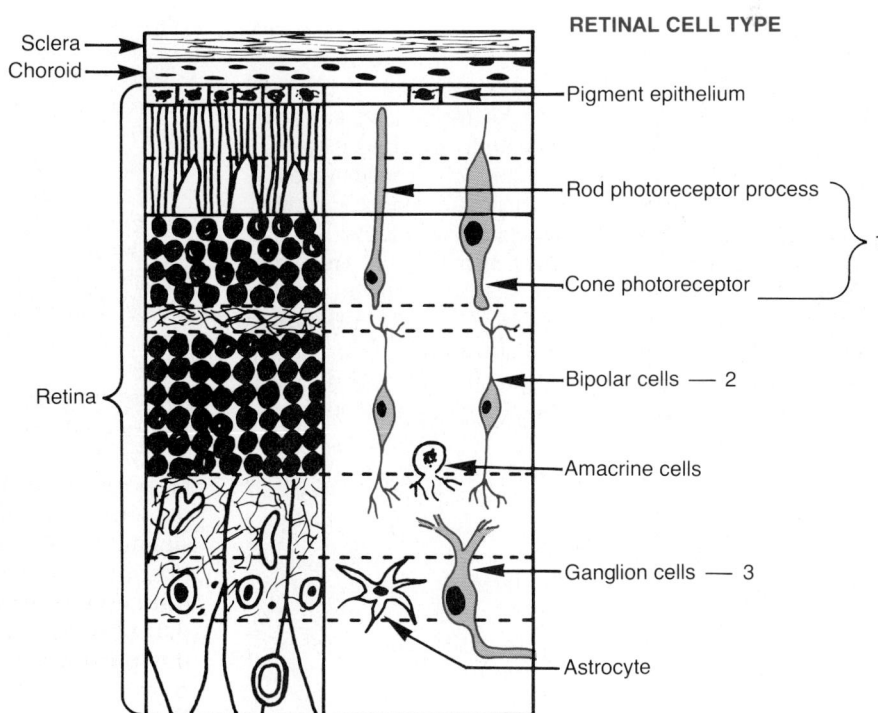

RETINAL CELL TYPE

Sclera
Choroid
Pigment epithelium
Rod photoreceptor process
Cone photoreceptor
Retina
Bipolar cells — 2
Amacrine cells
Ganglion cells — 3
Astrocyte

Figure 30–9. A schematic representation of the basic three-neuron organization of the retina. The three neurons comprise (1) photoreceptors (rods or cones), and (2) bipolar cells that interconnect the photoreceptors with (3) the ganglion cells, whose axon processes transmit the signal to the brain.

liferative phase ensues, in which there is an intense proliferation of vascular epithelium and fibroblasts occurring as a secondary response to retinal ischemia. This neovascularization begins at the junction of the avascular and vascularized portions of the retina, and the new vessels break through the internal limiting membrane of the retina and grow into the vitreous. These changes become apparent by about five to ten weeks after cessation of exposure to oxygen.

In about 25% of cases a cicatricial phase ensues, in which the fibrovascular component shrinks or contracts. The retrolental mass becomes increasingly pale, and retinal detachment occurs. The macula and posterior retinal vessels are displaced temporally, and areas of hemorrhage may be seen. Neovascularization on the iris may develop in later years, resulting in closed-angle glaucoma.

DIABETES MELLITUS

The incidence of diabetic retinopathy rises with the duration of the metabolic defect. With advances in therapy, the life span of diabetic patients has improved, and the prevalence of secondary retinal disease has greatly increased (p. 1004). Approximately 60% of diabetic patients develop retinopathy 15 to 20 years after the original diagnosis. Diabetic retinopathy ranks with glaucoma, macular degeneration, and cataract as a major cause of blindness in the United States and Europe. Further, about 2% of the diabetic population have visual impairment severe enough to be considered legally blind that is attributable to retinopathy.

Diabetic retinopathy is classified into two subgroups: (1) background or nonproliferative retinopathy, and (2) proliferative retinopathy.[22] Sometimes a "preproliferative" group is added.

BACKGROUND RETINOPATHY. Five types of structural capillary change can be recognized in background retinopathy. **Basement membrane** changes occur that are identical to those described for diabetic microangiopathy in general (p. 1003). These are characterized by varying degrees of thickening and are probably the result of increased synthesis of basement membrane components and the insudation of blood-borne constituents through an abnormally permeable endothelium.[23] **Pericyte degeneration,** as described by Cogan and coworkers,[24] is an almost invariable feature of diabetic retinopathy. It has been postulated that the pericytes exercise a contractile function and that their loss plays a role in the formation of microaneurysms and arteriovenous shunts. **Capillary microaneurysms** are also a dramatic feature of diabetic retinopathy and often its presenting clinical sign. These are rare in capillaries elsewhere in the body of the diabetic patient but do occur in several other retinal disorders. The presence of microaneurysms is associated with excessive permeability and frequent rupture resulting in focal serous exudates and hemorrhages. Microaneurysms may develop thromboses and become occluded, and subsequent examination of the retina by fluorescein angiography may give a misleading

impression of regression of the retinopathy. **Microvascular obstructions and nonperfusion of capillaries** occur in vessels in the posterior fundus that are lacking both pericytes and endothelium. Histologically these vessels are seen as tubes of basement membrane. **Cotton-wool spots** are often seen in these areas, and **scotomata** occur owing to degeneration of nerve fibers and ganglion cells. The nonperfusion provides a basis for the hypoxia that can later lead to proliferative retinopathy. Intraretinal vascular shunts occur in areas of ischemic retina and may show slow leakage. It seems probable that these arteriolar-venular shunts are the surviving vessels in areas of capillary closure.

Arteriolar hyalinization of the retinal arterioles occurs. This is thought to be due to increased permeability of the retinal circulation and insudation of plasma. Gradual narrowing of the arteriolar lumen follows, particularly around the mouths of branch vessels. Occlusion of precapillary arterioles accounts for the cytoid bodies (see below) seen in approximately one third of diabetic retinas.

In diabetic retinas there is a gradual increase in retinal vein caliber. Additional venous abnormalities occurring as a response to local ischemia include the formation of venous loops as well as "beading" of the blood column within veins. Obstruction of the central retinal vein or of a retinal branch vein may occur in the preproliferative stage of diabetic retinopathy.

PROLIFERATIVE RETINOPATHY. This occurs in response to severe ischemia and hypoxia of the retina. The presence of a retinally derived angiogenic factor that induces neovascularization has been postulated but not proved. The new vessels usually extend from the larger veins surrounded by areas of capillary closure, or they may arise from the region near the optic disc. Rarely they may arise from arterial vessels at the retinal periphery. The new capillaries contain both endothelial cells and pericytes but are incompletely formed and poorly supported. Initially they proliferate within the potential space between the inner limiting membrane of the retina and the posterior face of the vitreous, where they have a flat appearance. Subsequently they extend into the vitreous cavity. At this stage, bleeding is common as the vessels are stretched by the vitreous. After a variable period, the neovascularization is followed by the development of a fibrous component. At this stage the neovascular membrane is referred to as **retinitis proliferans.** The fibrous component increases the traction on the underlying retina, often culminating in retinal detachment.

HYPERTENSIVE AND ARTERIOSCLEROTIC RETINOPATHY

Hypertensive and arteriosclerotic changes in the retinal vessels provide useful prognostic clues to the physician. The Scheie[25] and Keith-Wagener[26] classifications, which assign stages to these diseases, will be followed in our consideration of the underlying histopathology, because the divisions are useful for teaching purposes. It should be remembered, however, that arteriosclerotic changes occur in close association with hypertensive retinopathy.

Hypertensive changes in the retinal arterioles

primarily involve diminution in their diameter. In acute severe hypertension, as in toxemia of pregnancy or at the onset of malignant hypertension, these initially appear as focal spasms. Usually in chronic hypertension, however, they narrow in a more diffuse, slowly progressive pattern. Sclerotic changes of the retinal arterioles involve a hyaline or "onionskin" thickening of the arteriolar walls with a narrowing of the lumen diameter (p. 570).

HYPERTENSIVE RETINOPATHY. Grade I hypertensive retinopathy involves a generalized narrowing of the arterioles, and **grade II** has, in addition, focal arteriolar spasms. **Grade III** includes, in addition to the narrowing and spasms, flame-shaped hemorrhages, dot-and-blot hemorrhages, cotton-wool spots, and hard waxy exudates. Histologically, flame-shaped hemorrhages are extravasated erythrocytes deposited in the retinal nerve fiber layer. The typical shape results from the confinement of the red blood cells within spaces between the nerve fibers, which run in a parallel fashion. Dot-and-blot hemorrhages, in contrast, are seen in the inner nuclear layer with spreading to the outer plexiform layer. Cotton-wool spots are microinfarctions of the nerve fiber layer. The interruption of axonal flow produces clusters of ganglion cell axons that have undergone bulbous dilatation at the site of ischemic damage or infarction. Each swollen axon assumes a shape resembling a cell — hence the term **cytoid (cell-like) bodies.** The hard or waxy exudates are composed of extravasated lipophilic material located in the outer plexiform layer. **Grade IV** hypertensive retinopathy encompasses all the changes of grade III plus optic disc edema.

GRADATION OF ARTERIOSCLEROTIC RETINOPATHY. Grade I arteriosclerotic retinopathy consists of an increase in the arteriolar light reflex. Histologically this corresponds to a subintimal hyaline deposition and a thickened arteriolar media and adventitia that causes the normally transparent arteriolar wall to become semiopaque. **Grade II** arteriosclerotic retinopathy has, in addition, arteriolar-venular crossing defects. At the site of crossing, the arteriole and venule share a common adventitia. The semiopaque wall of the arteriole obscures the venous blood column of the underlying venule. The various arteriovenous crossing changes are often collectively termed "arteriovenous nicking." **Grade III** arteriosclerotic retinopathy adds the presence of "copper-wire" arterioles. Here, as a result of subintimal hyaline deposition and thickening of the media and adventitia, the arteriolar wall is sufficiently opaque to reflect only a portion of the red color of the intravascular blood. **Grade IV** includes the presence of "silver-wire" arterioles. The opacity resulting from the sclerotic changes in the arteriolar wall is now sufficient to obscure entirely the intravascular blood, giving a white or silver pattern.

RETINITIS PIGMENTOSA

A variety of systemic and ocular diseases result in the degeneration of the retina, characterized by a loss of visual receptors. This is usually accompanied by focal proliferations of the adjacent retinal pigment epithelium, with migration of retinal pigment epithelial cells into the sensory retina *(pigmentary retinopathy)* (Fig. 30–10). *The term "retinitis pigmentosa" refers to several types of bilateral, progressive, pigmentary retinopathy, classified primarily according to the mode of inheritance.* Retinitis pigmentosa can occur as an autosomal dominant trait, as a recessive trait, or as a sex-linked recessive trait. Night blindness, as a result of the loss of rods, is usually an early symptom. The disease progresses to blindness in advanced stages. Ophthalmoscopically, the principal findings are retinal pigmentation distributed in a branching reticulated pattern along the course of retinal vessels creating a lattice-like appearance, a pale, waxy-appearing optic disc, attenuation of retinal blood vessels, and a posterior subcapsular cataract. Histologically, the photoreceptors gradually disappear, and the retinal pigment epithelium undergoes degeneration in some areas and migration and proliferation in others.[27] A glial membrane grows on the inner surface of the optic disc and spreads over the peripapillary retina.

MACULAR DEGENERATION

The macular region of the retina is the target for a variety of disorders. Factors that may predispose to degenerative lesions in this location include an absence of retinal vessels in the foveola and the exclusive dependence of the foveola on the underlying choroidal circulation, a majority of cones rather than rods, and a large population of ganglion cells.[28] Age-related macular degeneration (formerly called "senile" macular degeneration) is the most serious of the

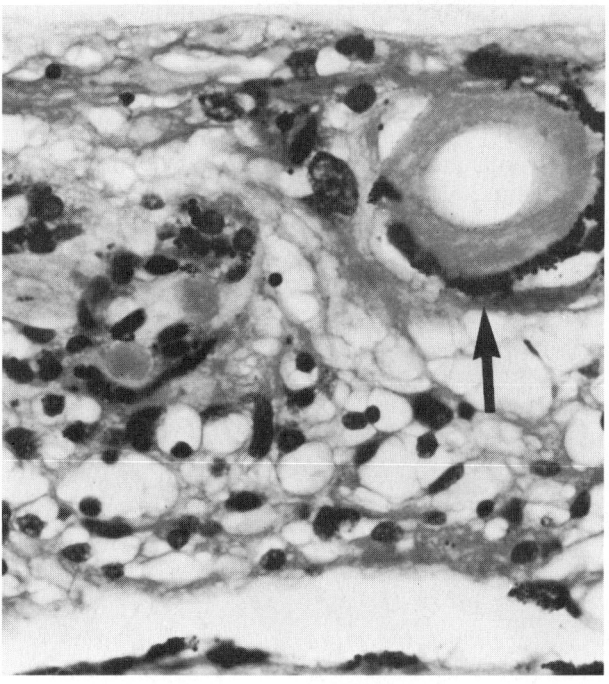

Figure 30–10. Atrophic retina seen in long-standing retinitis pigmentosa. Pigment-containing macrophages surrounding a vessel *(arrow)* give the clinical appearance of bone corpuscle pigmentation on ophthalmoscopic examination.

macular disorders and is a common cause of decreased central vision in the elderly.

Macular degeneration occurs either as an atrophic form or as an exudative (disciform) degeneration. In the atrophic form, Bruch's membrane, the membrane between the retinal pigment epithelium and the choroid, is thickened generally and focally. The discrete thickenings are called **drusen**. The choriocapillaris is often focally obliterated, and the pigment epithelium is focally atrophic and depigmented. The photoreceptors degenerate in the regions of atrophy of the retinal pigment epithelium. One complication of atrophic macular degeneration is the development of defects in Bruch's membrane. New vessels grow from the choroid through these defects. If untreated by laser photocoagulation the new vessels leak and produce exudates and hemorrhage under the retina. Organization of the hemorrhage and exudate is accompanied by retinal pigment epithelial proliferation and fibrous overgrowth. The end result is a fibrous scar in the macular region with degeneration of the neuroretina and permanent loss of central vision.

RETINAL DETACHMENT

A retinal "detachment" is a separation between the neurosensory retina and the retinal pigment epithelium (Fig. 30–11). This is an opening of the potential space that is a vestige of the original cavity of the embryonic optic vesicle. There are three major causes for retinal detachment[1]:

1. The accumulation of vitreous fluid beneath a retina containing a hole or tear. The break or tear in the retina often results from vitreous traction (i.e., a *rhegmatogenous retinal detachment*) (Fig. 30–12).
2. Exudative detachments in which fluid accumulates beneath an intact sensory retina, as in choroidal malignant melanoma, malignant hypertension, and types of severe choroiditis *(serous retinal detachment)*.
3. Traction detachments in which membranes form in the vitreous and lead to detachment of the retina in the absence of a retinal break. This may occur from many causes, including diabetes mellitus, or following

accidental trauma or complicated intraocular surgery.

The earliest histopathologic change following retinal detachment is degeneration of the outer retinal layers, because they are removed from their source of nourishment, the choriocapillaris.[29] Cystoid degeneration follows in the outer plexiform layer. The cystoid spaces may coalesce to form increasingly larger cysts. Glial proliferation frequently occurs in detached retinas. The subretinal space is filled with liquefied vitreous or serous fluid and may also contain inflammatory cells, blood, or tumor cells, depending on the nature of the detachment. The retinal pigment epithelium beneath the detached neural retina frequently shows proliferation and may contribute to the membranes on the retina.

RETINOBLASTOMA

Retinoblastoma is the most common malignant eye tumor of childhood and is responsible for approximately 1% of all deaths from cancer in the age group of newborns to 15 years. From a pathologic as well as from a clinical standpoint, retinoblastoma is unusual in several aspects when compared with most other solid tumors.[30] Retinoblastoma can be multifocal and often bilateral; it undergoes spontaneous regression more frequently than other tumors; retinoblastoma patients have a high incidence of second primary tumors, and retinoblastoma frequently occurs as a congenital tumor. The condition is hereditary in a significant number of cases.

Retinoblastoma is worldwide in distribution and affects all racial groups. Its frequency has been calculated to range from 1 in 34,000 to 1 in 15,000 live births. The incidence of retinoblastoma decreases with age, with the great majority of cases being diagnosed before the age of four years. It affects both sexes with equal frequency.

STUDIES OF THE RETINOBLASTOMA GENE. Retinoblastoma has long been recognized to occur in both *familial* and *sporadic* patterns. Familial cases typi-

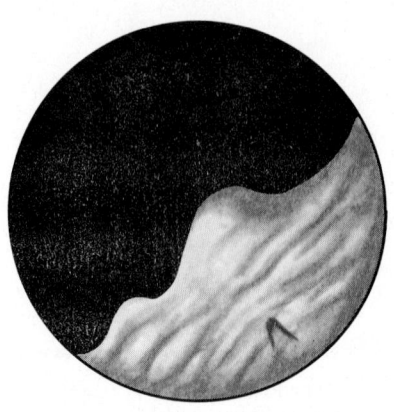
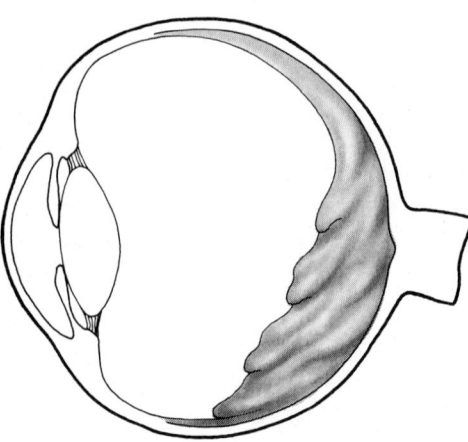

Figure 30–11. Retinal detachment. A common pattern with extensive lifting of the retina secondary to a tear and the accumulation of subretinal vitreous fluid as seen funduscopically (on the left) and diagrammatically (on the right).

hits correspond to mutations of the two homologous alleles at the retinoblastoma locus. In other words, one copy of the normal retinoblastoma gene in a retinal cell is sufficient to prevent the retinal cell from becoming malignant.

Retinoblastoma serves as a prototype of a diverse group of human cancers apparently caused by recessive loss-of-function mutations at distinct genetic loci, i.e., suppressor cancer genes (p. 289). These include osteosarcoma, Wilms' tumor, hepatoblastoma, rhabdomyosarcoma, uveal melanoma, bladder cell carcinoma, acoustic neuroma, and meningioma. As in retinoblastoma, in these tumors the normal "cancer suppressor gene" appears to be lost as a key step in malignant transformation. In some cases, it is known that different tumor types, such as retinoblastoma and osteosarcoma, arise after the loss of the same genetic locus.

Retinoblastoma is believed to arise from a cell of neuroepithelial origin, usually in the posterior retina. The tumors tend to be nodular masses, often with satellite seedings. On light microscopic examination, undifferentiated areas of these tumors are composed of small round cells with large hyperchromatic nuclei and scanty cytoplasm. The resemblance of these cells to undifferentiated retinoblasts, which are precursors of the differentiated retinal cells, led to the use of the term "retinoblastoma."

Differentiated structures are found within many retinoblastomas, the most characteristic of these being the rosettes described by Flexner and Wintersteiner (**Flexner-Wintersteiner rosettes;** Figs. 30–13 and 30–14). These structures consist of clusters of cuboidal or short columnar cells arranged around a central lumen. The nuclei are displaced away from the lumen, which by light microscopy appears to have a limiting membrane resembling the external limiting membrane of the retina. Photoreceptor-like elements protrude through the membrane, and some taper into fine filaments. Less common are the rosettes described by Wright: radial arrangements of cells around a central tangle of fibrils (**Homer Wright rosettes**). An additional differentiated structure is the **fleurette,** which represents an attempt at photoreceptor differentiation by tumor cells.

Tumor cells may disseminate through the choroidal vasculature or may spread beyond the eye through the optic nerve or subarachnoid space. Bone marrow aspiration, peripheral blood smears, and cerebral spinal fluid examinations are employed to assess the extent of spread in patients with metastatic retinoblastoma. In advanced cases, the tumor may penetrate through the sclera and grow in the orbit. Metastases to the preauricular and cervical lymph nodes commonly follow overt extraocular extension. The most common sites of distant metastases are the central nervous system, skull, distal bones, and lymph nodes.

Spontaneous necrosis or regression of a retinoblastoma is marked by calcification and severe inflammation. The mechanism responsible for spontaneous necrosis is unknown. Rarely, tumors composed of uniformly benign appearing cells exhibiting photoreceptor differentiation and

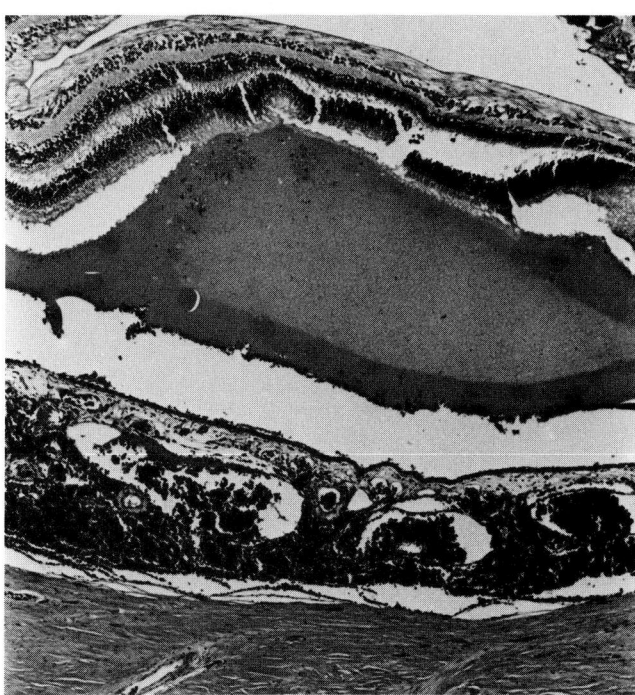

Figure 30–12. Retinal detachment with proteinaceous fluid separating retina above from underlying pigment epithelium and choroid.

cally develop multiple tumors that are bilateral, although they may be unifocal and unilateral. Of the sporadic *nonheritable* tumors, all are unilateral and unifocal.

Because of the sporadic and familial patterns, the genetic factors causing retinoblastoma were initially thought to be complex. In 1971, Knudson proposed that, minimally, two genetic events are required to trigger the development of retinoblastoma (p. 289). In hereditary retinoblastoma, the first of these retinal events occurs either through the inheritance of a mutant allele from a carrier parent or as a new germinal mutation. The second mutation in the retina is somatic. In contrast, Knudson argued, in sporadic cases, both the mutations are somatic and occur in retinal cells. Since the retinal cell that gives rise to a nonhereditary retinoblastoma must acquire two somatic mutations, and since the somatic mutation rate is low, all patients with nonhereditary retinoblastoma have only a single focus of tumor formation.

A major clue to the location of the retinoblastoma gene came with the observation in 1962 that patients with a deletion of one chromosome 13 homolog ("13 deletion syndrome") often develop retinoblastoma. Investigators observed that the deletions found in different patients with retinoblastoma all involve the q14 band. Subsequently, a DNA sequence was isolated corresponding to the messenger RNA transcript produced by the normal retinoblastoma gene.[31] This was the first isolation of a human gene governing cancer predisposition. This work led to confirmation of Knudson's earlier "two-hit hypothesis": the two

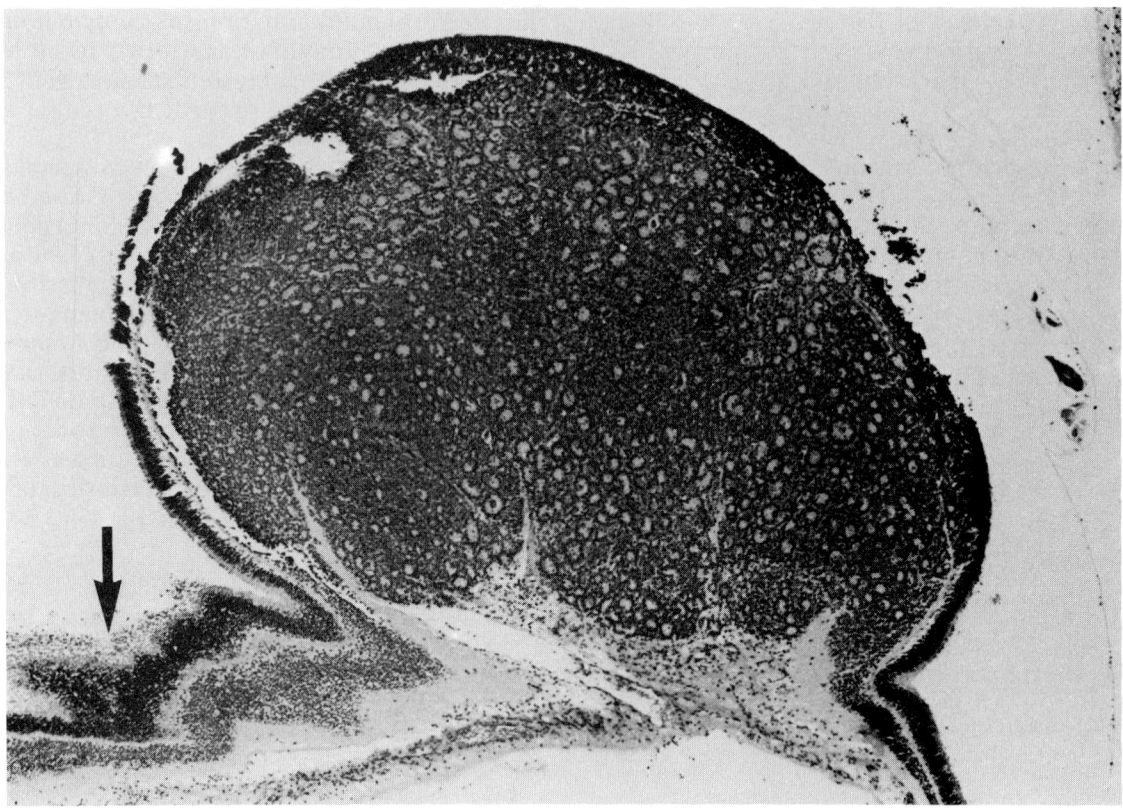

Figure 30–13. Focus of retinoblastoma arising from retina *(arrow)*.

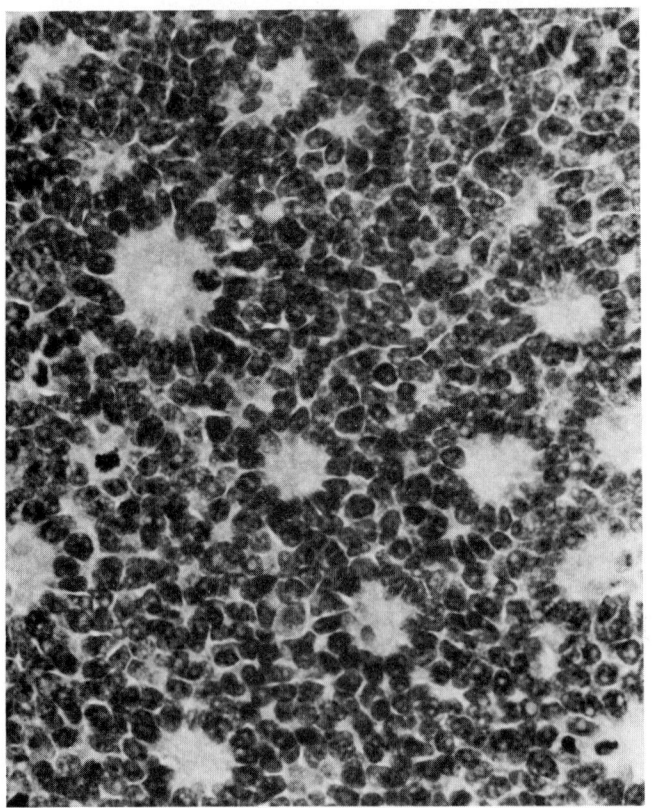

Figure 30–14. Higher power view of retinoblastoma showing differentiated rosettes (Flexner-Wintersteiner rosettes).

the formation of fleurettes have been reported. These have been referred to as **retinomas** or **retinocytomas** and are believed to be a benign variant of retinoblastoma.

VITREOUS

The vitreous has three components. The *primary vitreous* forms during the first month of fetal life in the space between the lens and the retina. It consists of two parts: (1) mesodermally derived tissue including the hyaloid vessel and its branches, and (2) a fibrillar meshwork of uncertain origin. The *secondary vitreous* or definitive adult vitreous forms during the second month of embryonic development. This portion is composed of 99% water bound with collagen and hyaluronic acid forming a hydrogel of high viscosity. The *tertiary vitreous* forms the suspensory ligament of the lens (zonules of Zinn) during the fourth month of gestation.

In primary familial amyloidosis, amyloid appears in the vitreous in sheetlike form.[32] The amyloid is thought to gain access to the vitreous through retinal blood vessels.

OPTIC NERVE

PAPILLEDEMA

Papilledema, or edema of the optic disc, results from increased intracranial pressure. There are several structural characteristics of the optic nerve that are believed to play a crucial role in the pathogenesis of papilledema.[33] The subarachnoid space surrounding the optic nerve is a direct extension of the subarachnoid space around the brain, with which it is normally in direct communication. Any increase in intracranial pressure is thus transmitted to the optic nerve. In addition, the central retinal vein draining the retina runs in the axial portion within the optic nerve for about 8 to 15 mm and then exits from the nerve and crosses the meninges. At this point it is vulnerable to occlusion from increased pressure in the subarachnoid space. The optic disc possesses a rich arterial blood supply from the central retinal artery and the choroidal arteries, supplied by the arterial circle of Zinn-Haller. The relevant differences between the arterial and venous pressure seem to be significant in the development of papilledema. Axonal swelling, however, appears to be the most important factor in the increase in tissue volume of the optic nerve head.

> Acutely, there is edema and vascular congestion of the nerve head. The physiologic cup is obliterated, and hemorrhages may be seen in the optic nerve or adjacent retinal nerve fiber layer. The sensory retina is displaced away from the edges of the optic disc by the edema, and folding of the retina and choroid are seen. With chronic papilledema, degeneration of nerve fibers, gliosis, and optic atrophy may occur.

OPTIC NEURITIS

Although optic neuritis, through common usage, implies an *inflammation* of the optic nerve, the term has come to also include certain vascular diseases and degenerative diseases that hinder optic nerve function.[34] True inflammatory causes of optic neuritis include direct spread of inflammation from the orbit, from the sinuses, or from within the eye itself. Optic neuritis may also occur as a result of the spread of infections within the central nervous system. Rarely, inflammation of the optic nerve occurs secondary to the spread of a distant infection. Vascular diseases causing optic neuritis include temporal arteritis, periarteritis nodosa, pulseless disease, and atherosclerosis.[35] Degenerative optic neuritis encompasses the demyelinating diseases, toxic conditions such as methyl alcohol poisoning or lead poisoning, and systemic diseases, including sarcoidosis, collagen diseases, hyperthyroidism, diabetes mellitus, and blood disorders. Optic neuritis is classified according to the topographic location in the coats of the optic nerve. *Perineuritis* signifies involvement of the leptomeninges around the optic nerve and is usually the result of direct spread from orbital inflammation or intraocular inflammations. *Periaxial neuritis* indicates involvement of the peripheral portions of the nerve as the result of extension from the leptomeninges. *Axial neuritis* implies involvement of the inner or central portion of the optic nerve as is seen in multiple sclerosis, vascular diseases, and toxic entities.

Transverse neuritis denotes complete cross-sectional destruction of a variable length of optic nerve, the classic example being the neuromyelitis optica of Devic.

The histopathologic findings in optic neuritis depend on whether the cause is inflammatory, ischemic, or degenerative. If chronic and severe, the common end stage is optic atrophy.

OPTIC ATROPHY

The ultimate result of progressive optic nerve diseases is optic nerve atrophy. Variations in the findings depend on the pathogenetic factors involved.[36] Common to all cases, however, are loss of both myelin and axis cylinders, glial proliferation (gliosis), thickening of the pial septa, and widening of the space separating the optic nerve and the meninges as a result of the loss of nerve parenchyma. In addition, the physiologic cup may appear wider or deeper than normal (Fig. 30–15).

TUMORS

Meningioma

Meningiomas arise from the meningothelial cells of the arachnoid. Most cases of meningioma of the optic nerve are extensions of tumors having their primary site within the cranium.[37] Less commonly, meningiomas may arise directly from the intraorbital or intracanalicular meninges of the optic nerve.

Orbital meningiomas are more common in females (5:1) and account for 3 to 10% of the orbital lesions that cause unilateral exophthalmos. The average age at onset is 38 years, with about 40% of the tumors occurring in patients under 20 years of age at the time of surgery. Associated neurofibromatosis is found in approximately 16% of patients. The menin-

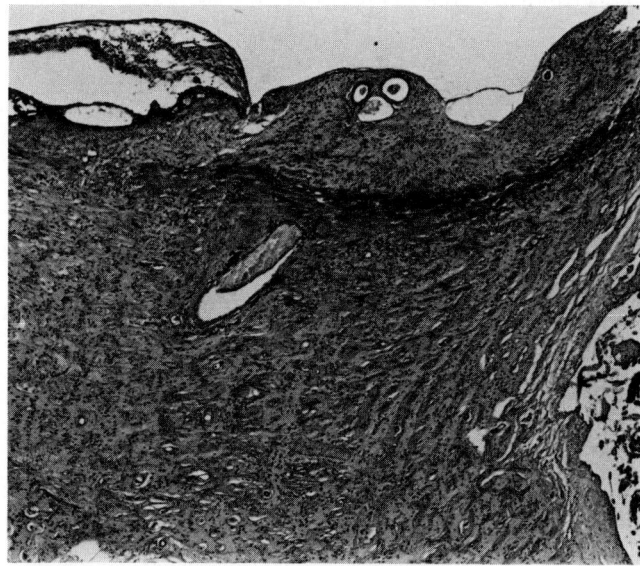

Figure 30–15. Optic atrophy showing loss of myelin and axis cylinders with marked proliferation of glial cells.

gioma may appear as an eccentric mass on one side of the optic nerve, and it may spread forward or backward along the nerve.[38] The tumor may also surround and compress the nerve.

Histopathologically, the neoplasms are indentical to those arising in the skull (p. 1420). Most primary intraorbital meningiomas are either of the *meningotheliomatous* (Fig. 30–16) or the *mixed* type. The *fibroblastic* and *angioblastic* types of meningiomas rarely, if ever, occur as primary tumors in the orbit.

Glioma

Optic nerve gliomas occur slightly more frequently in females than in males. The median age of onset is about five years, with over 80% of patients under 15 years of age. Gliomas occasionally develop in adults. Neurofibromatosis is present in about 10% of reported cases. The tumors are typically derived entirely from astrocytes, although oligodendrogliomas may occur.

Histologically three patterns are seen, all of which may occur in the same tumor. In **transitional** areas, the tumor merges with the normal optic nerve, but an increased number of glial cells are seen and are arranged in a less orderly fashion than in the normal nerve. The nerve bundles are enlarged by the increased number and size of glial cells, and the area has a finely reticulated appearance. The second pattern consists of coarsely **reticulated** and **myxomatous**

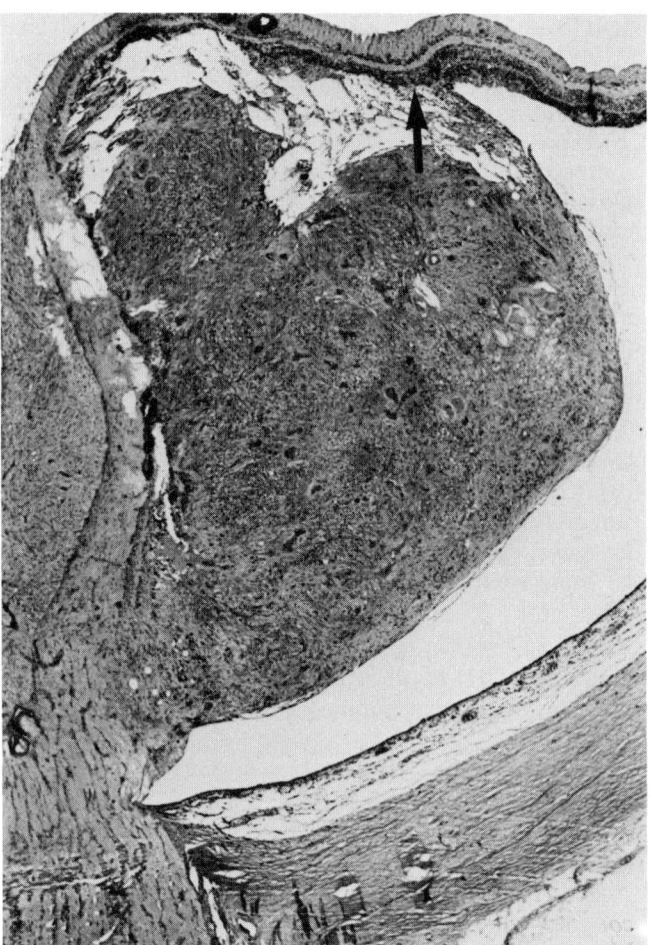

Figure 30–17. Glioma of optic nerve growing into globe and displacing retina *(arrow)*.

areas. The third pattern is that of **astrocytic areas,** in which spindle cell formation and cytoplasmic eosinophilic structures within astrocytes (Rosenthal fibers) (p. 1388) are often prominent. Gliomas may arise from the optic disc and grow intraocularly (Fig. 30–17). Optic nerve gliomas commonly result in visual loss. Intracranial extension and death are infrequent when a glioma is limited to the orbital portion of the optic nerve at the time of diagnosis and treatment.[39]

GLAUCOMA

Glaucoma is often mistakenly considered by non-ophthalmologists to be a discrete disease entity. It is, in fact, several different diseases, all of which are characterized by an intraocular pressure sufficiently elevated to produce ocular tissue damage.[40] Glaucoma is one of the leading causes of blindness among the 500,000 legally blind individuals in the United States. The three major categories of glaucoma are (1) *angle-closure glaucoma* (Fig. 30–18), (2) *open-angle glaucoma,* and (3) *congenital glaucoma.* The term "angle" refers to the angle of the anterior chamber formed by the junction of the uveal tract with the

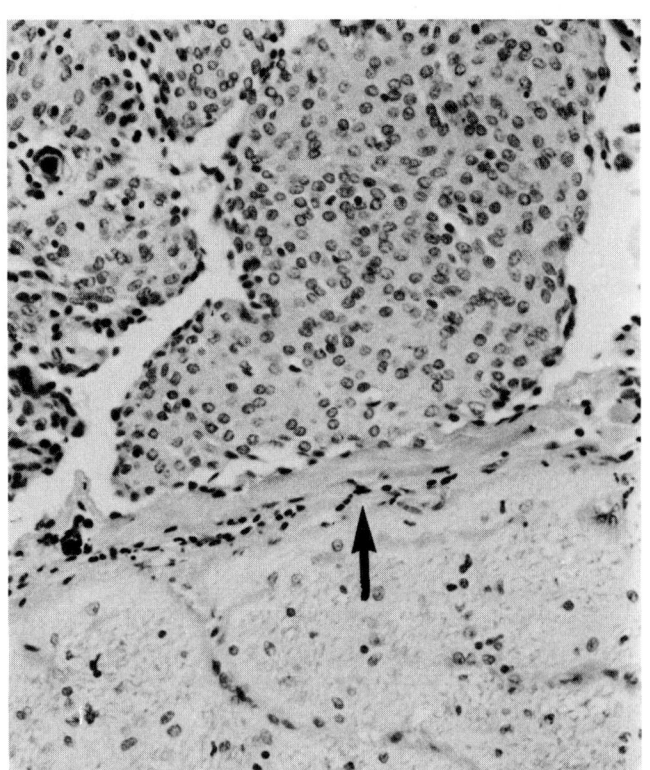

Figure 30–16. Meningotheliomatous meningioma surrounding optic nerve below, the edge of which is indicated by the arrow.

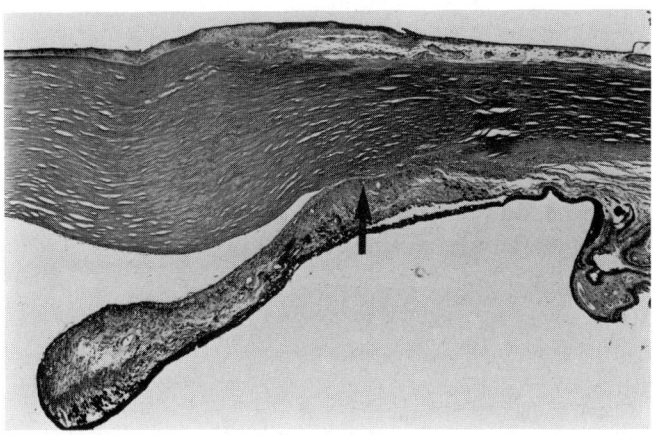

Figure 30–18. Long-standing chronic narrow-angle glaucoma with iris adhering to anterior cornea and angle sealed closed *(arrow)*.

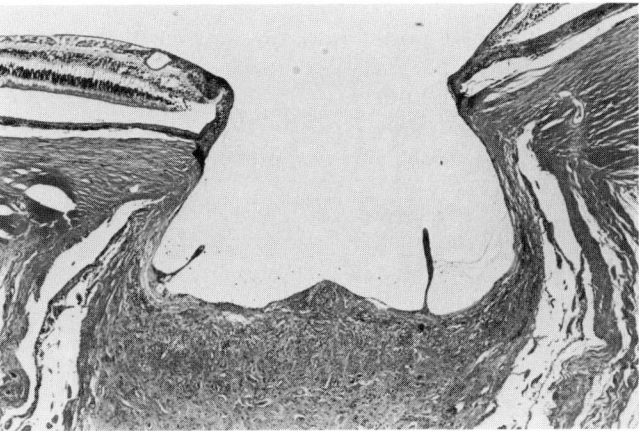

Figure 30–19. Glaucomatous cupping occurring in end-stage, open-angle glaucoma. Optic nerve is atrophic.

corneoscleral coat. This is the most important region for aqueous drainage.

Primary open-angle glaucoma accounts for about two thirds of all glaucoma seen in whites and has an incidence of between 0.5 and 1%. The incidence of primary open-angle glaucoma in blacks is about 1.5%. In open-angle glaucoma, the angle appears open but does not function properly in transporting aqueous humor out of the eye. The exact nature of the obstruction has not yet been recognized.

Eyes that develop *primary angle-closure glaucoma* are anatomically predisposed to the condition. Most commonly, the surface of the peripheral iris is close to the inner surface of the trabecular meshwork, resulting in a narrow or shallow anterior chamber angle.

Congenital glaucoma is usually an inherited autosomal recessive abnormality, although it can have an infectious etiology (e.g., rubella). The incidence of congenital glaucoma is about 1:5000 to 1:10,000 live births. Its cause (or causes) is controversial, with many theories having been proposed but none proven. A more detailed discussion of the types, causes, and mechanisms of glaucoma goes beyond the scope of this chapter but can be found elsewhere.[40]

Elevated intraocular pressure results in secondary effects on the ocular tissues, and many of these are common to the various types of glaucoma. From a visual standpoint, the most serious changes are those in the retina and optic nerve. It is thought that the mechanical force of the intraocular pressure on the nerve fibers as they course around the margin of the cup of the optic nerve may interfere with axoplasmic flow and produce axonal necrosis. In addition, impairment of the vascular supply to the optic nerve occurring in glaucoma may lead to ischemic necrosis of nerve fibers. The loss of nerve fibers leads to a characteristic cupped excavation of the optic disc (Fig. 30–19). The end result is gliosis, demyelination, and decrease in diameter of the nerve. The innermost portion of the retina consequently

undergoes atrophic changes, with thinning of the nerve fiber layer and degeneration and disappearance of the ganglion cells. Additional changes in long-standing glaucoma include intracellular and intercellular epithelial edema of the cornea, corneal stromal edema, degenerative pannus, and corneal scarring; cataracts; necrosis of the iris and the ciliary body stroma; neovascular membranes covering the iris; atrophy, hyalinization, and shortening of the ciliary processes; diffuse thickening of the ciliary body basement membrane; and venous stasis, sometimes with occlusion of the central retinal vein. In infants, the corneoscleral coat may become stretched and thinned as a result of chronically elevated intraocular pressure, producing an enlargement of the entire eye (buphthalmos). In adult eyes, sustained elevation of pressure may lead to bulging of the cornea or sclera. These areas are often lined by atrophic uveal tissue and are black clinically **(staphylomata.)**

PHTHISIS BULBI AND THE END STAGE OF DIFFUSE OCULAR DISEASE

With the exception of eyes enucleated because of intraocular tumors, the vast majority of the eyes sent to the pathology laboratory were removed because of blindness, pain, and disfigurement. The causes of the ocular changes are usually trauma, glaucoma, or intraocular inflammation. "End-stage" blind eyes are generally classified into one of three categories[41]: *Atrophy without shrinkage* refers to an eye of otherwise normal or enlarged size that has atrophy of the intraocular structures. An eye with long-standing glaucoma is an example of an eye in this category. If there is also atrophy of the globe, so that it is smaller than normal, the eye shows *atrophy with shrinkage.* *Atrophy with shrinkage and disorganization (phthisis bulbi)* describes an eye with a markedly thickened sclera and generalized disorganization of intraocular contents sufficiently severe to make them unrecognizable. The globe is small. The cornea is flattened,

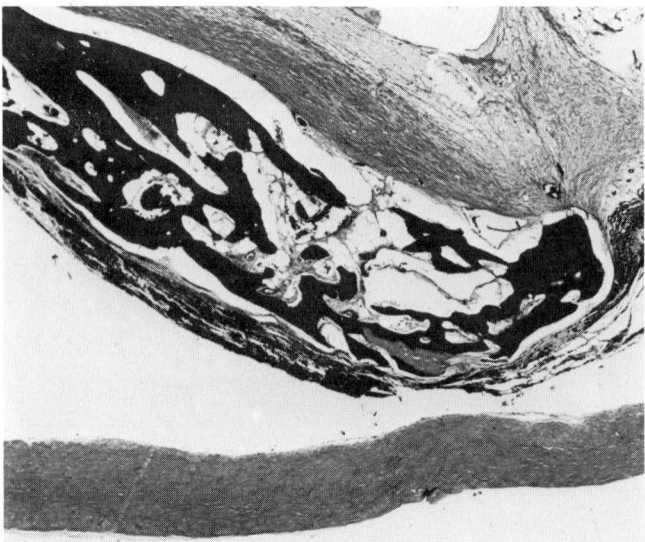

Figure 30–20. Bone deposition at the level of the retinal pigment epithelium occurring in phthisis bulbi.

shrunken, and scarred. The lens, if not previously removed or extruded, may be displaced and shows cataractous changes, often with calcium deposition. Most phthisical eyes contain a dense fibrous membrane running across the ciliary body (cyclitic membrane). Intraocular bone formation is a characteristic finding in phthisis bulbi (Fig. 30–20). This is a result of osseous metaplasia of the retinal pigment epithelium, and it forms without cartilage. A fatty marrow can be present within the bone, and in younger individuals, the marrow may possess hematopoietic elements. The retina is usually detached and reduced to a gliotic scar, and the optic nerve is markedly atrophic.

1. Green, W.R.: Retina. *In* Spencer, W.H. (ed.): Ophthalmic Pathology. An Atlas and Textbook, Vol. 2. 3rd ed. Philadelphia, W.B. Saunders Co., pp. 589–1921, 1985.

2. Lahav, M., Albert, D.M., and Wyand, S.: Clinical and histopathological classification of retinal dysplasia. Am. J. Ophthalmol. *75*:648, 1973.

3. Jaeger, E.A.: Ocular findings in Down's syndrome. Trans. Am. Ophthalmol. Soc. *78*:808, 1980.

4. Robb, R.M., and Marchevsky, A.: A pathology of the lens in Down's syndrome. Arch. Ophthalmol. *96*:1039, 1978.

5. Boniuk, M., and Zimmerman, L.E.: Ocular pathology in the rubella syndrome. Arch. Ophthalmol. *77*:455, 1967.

6. Contreras, F., and Pereda, J.: Congenital syphilis of the eye with lens involvement. Arch. Ophthalmol. *96*:1052, 1978.

7. Smith, R.S., Farrell, T., and Bailey, T.: Keratomalacia. Surv. Ophthalmol. *20*:213, 1975.

8. Austin, P., Jakobiec, E.A., and Iwamoto, T.: Elastoplasia and elastodystrophy as the pathologic basis of ocular pterygia and pingueculae. Ophthalmology *90*:96, 1983.

9. McCallan, A.F.: The epidemiology of trachoma. Br. J. Ophthalmol. *15*:369, 1931.

10. Spencer, W.H., and Zimmerman, L.E.: Conjunctiva. *In* Spencer, W.H. (ed.): Ophthalmic Pathology. An Atlas and Textbook, Vol. 1. 3rd ed. Philadelphia, W.B. Saunders Co., 1985, pp. 109–228.

11. Blodi, F.C.: Squamous cell carcinoma of the conjunctiva. Doc. Ophthalmol. *34*:93, 1973.

12. Dawson, C.R., Togni, B., and Moore, T.E. Jr.: Structural changes in chronic herpetic keratitis studied by light and electron microscopy. Arch. Ophthalmol. *79*:740, 1968.

13. Rodrigues, M.M., and Waring, G.O. III: Anterior and posterior corneal dystrophies. *In* Garner, A.C., and Klintworth, G.K. (eds.): Pathology of Ocular Disease. New York, Marcel Dekker, 1982, pp. 1153–1166.

14. Schlaegel, T.F. Jr.: Essentials of Uveitis. Boston, Little, Brown, & Co., 1969.

15. Lubin, J.R., Albert, D.M., and Weinstein, M.: Sixty-five years of sympathetic ophthalmia. A clinicopathologic review of 105 cases (1913–1978). Ophthalmology *87*:109, 1980.

16. Callender, G.R.: Malignant melanotic tumors of the eye: A study of histologic types in 111 cases. Trans. Am. Acad. Ophthalmol. Otolaryngol. *36*:131, 1931.

17. Ferry, A.P., and Font, R.L.: Carcinoma metastatic to the eye and orbit. I. A clinicopathologic study of 227 cases. Arch. Ophthalmol. *92*:276, 1974.

18. Ferry, A.P., and Font, R.L.: Carcinoma metastatic to the eye and orbit. II. A clinicopathologic study of 26 patients with carcinoma metastatic to the anterior segment of the eye. Arch. Ophthalmol. *93*:472, 1975.

19. Apple, D.J., and Rabb, M.F.: Ocular Pathology. Clinical Applications and Self-Assessment. 3rd ed. St. Louis, C.V. Mosby, 1985.

20. Ashton, N., Ward, B., and Serpell, G.: Effects of oxygen on developing retinal vessels with particular reference to the problem of retrolental fibroplasia. Br. J. Ophthalmol. *38*:397, 1954.

21. Garner, A.: Vascular disorders. *In* Garner, A.C., and Klintworth, G.K. (eds.): Pathobiology of Ocular Disease. New York, Marcel Dekker, 1982, pp. 1479–1575.

22. Yanoff, M., and Fine, B.: Ocular Pathology: A Text and Atlas. 2nd ed. New York, Harper & Row, 1982.

23. Ashton, N.: Vascular basement membrane changes in diabetic retinopathy. Br. J. Ophthalmol. *58*:344, 1974.

24. Cogan, D.G., Toussaint, D., and Kuwabara, T.: Retinal vascular patterns. IV. Diabetic retinopathy. Arch. Ophthalmol. *66*:366, 1961.

25. Scheie, H.G.: Evaluation of ophthalmoscopic changes of hypertension and arteriolar sclerosis. Arch. Ophthalmol. *49*:117, 1953.

26. Wagener, H., and Keith, N.: Diffuse arteriolar disease with hypertension and associated retinal lesions. Medicine *18*:317, 1939.

27. Gartner, S., and Henkind, P.: Pathology of retinitis pigmentosa. Ophthalmology *89*:1425, 1982.

28. Gass, J.D.M.: Stereoscopic Atlas of Macular Diseases. 3rd ed. St. Louis, C.V. Mosby Co., 1987.

29. Machemer, R., and Kroll, A.J.: Experimental retinal detachment in the owl monkey. VII. Photoreceptor protein renewal in normal and detached retina. Am. J. Ophthalmol. *71*:690, 1971.

30. Zimmerman, L.E.: Retinoblastoma and retinocytoma. *In* Spencer, W.H. (ed.): Ophthalmic Pathology. An Atlas and Textbook, Vol. 2. 3rd ed. Philadelphia, W.B. Saunders Co., 1985, pp. 1292–1351.

31. Friend, S.H., Bernards, R., Rogelj, S., et al.: A human DNA segment with properties of the gene that predisposes to retinoblastoma and osteosarcoma. Nature *323*:643, 1986.

32. Kaufman, H.E., and Thomas, L.B.: Vitreous opacities diagnostic of familial primary amyloidosis. N. Engl. J. Med. *261*:1267, 1959.

33. Heyreh, M.S., and Heyreh, S.S.: Optic disc edema in raised intracranial pressure. I. Evolution and resolution. Arch. Ophthalmol. *95*:1237, 1977.

34. Spencer, W.H.: Optic nerve. *In* Spencer, W.H. (ed.): Ophthalmic Pathology. An Atlas and Textbook, Vol. 3. 3rd ed. Philadelphia, W.B. Saunders Co., 1985, pp. 2337–2458.

35. Henkind, P., Charles, N.C., and Pearson, J.: Histopathology of ischemic optic neuropathy. Am. J. Ophthalmol. *69*:78, 1970.

36. Anderson, D.R.: Ascending and descending optic atrophy produced experimentally in squirrel monkeys. Am. J. Ophthalmol. *76*:693, 1973.

37. Karp, L.A., Zimmerman, L.E., Borit, A., and Spencer, W.H.: Primary intraorbital meningiomas. Arch Ophthalmol. *91*:24, 1974.

38. Cogan, D.G.: Tumors of the optic nerve. *In* Vinken, P.J., and Bruyn, B.W. (eds.): Handbook of Clinical Neurology, Vol. 17, Part II. New York, Elsevier Publishing Co., 1974.

39. Hoyt, W.F., and Baghdassarian, S.A.: Optic glioma of childhood: natural history and rationale for conservative management. Br. J. Ophthalmol. *53*:793, 1969.

40. Spencer, W.H.: Glaucoma. *In* Spencer, W.H. (ed.): Ophthalmic Pathology. An Atlas and Textbook, Vol. 1. 3rd ed. Philadelphia, W.B. Saunders Co., 1985, pp. 480–547.

41. Hogan, M.J., and Zimmerman, L.E.: Ophthalmic Pathology: An Atlas and Textbook. 2nd ed. Philadelphia, W.B. Saunders Co., 1962.

Index